THE MERCK MANUAL

FIFTEENTH EDITION

★

1st Edition – 1899
2nd Edition – 1901
3rd Edition – 1905
4th Edition – 1911
5th Edition – 1923
6th Edition – 1934
7th Edition – 1940
8th Edition – 1950
9th Edition – 1956
10th Edition – 1961
11th Edition – 1966
12th Edition – 1972
13th Edition – 1977
14th Edition – 1982
15th Edition – 1987

FIFTEENTH EDITION

THE MERCK MANUAL

OF

DIAGNOSIS AND THERAPY

Robert Berkow, M.D., *Editor-in-Chief*

Andrew J. Fletcher, M.B., B.Chir., *Assistant Editor*

Published by

MERCK SHARP & DOHME RESEARCH LABORATORIES

Division of

MERCK & CO., INC.

Rahway, N.J.

1987

MERCK & CO., INC.
Rahway, N.J.
U.S.A.

MERCK SHARP & DOHME
West Point, Pa.

MERCK SHARP & DOHME INTERNATIONAL
Rahway, N.J.

MERCK SHARP & DOHME RESEARCH LABORATORIES
Rahway, N.J. *West Point, Pa.*

MSD AGVET DIVISION
Woodbridge, N.J.

HUBBARD FARMS, INC.
Walpole, N.H.

MERCK CHEMICAL MANUFACTURING DIVISION
Rahway, N.J.

CALGON CORPORATION
Water Management Division
Pittsburgh, Pa.
Commercial Division
St. Louis, Mo.

KELCO DIVISION
San Diego, Calif.

Library of Congress Catalog Card Number 1-31760
ISBN Number 0911910-06-09
ISSN Number 0076-6526

First Printing—August 1987

Printed in the U. S. A.

FOREWORD

THE MERCK MANUAL first appeared in 1899 as a slender 262-page text titled MERCK'S MANUAL OF THE MATERIA MEDICA. It was expressly designed to meet the needs of general practitioners in selecting medications, noting that "memory is treacherous" and even the most thoroughly informed physician needs a reminder "to make him at once master of the situation and enable him to prescribe exactly what his judgment tells him is needed for the occasion." It was well received and, by the 6th Edition (1934), THE MERCK MANUAL had become highly valued by medical students and house staff also; by the end of World War II the pocket-sized manual was an established favorite ready-reference. Today THE MANUAL is the most widely used medical text in the world. While the book has grown to about 2500 pages, its primary purpose remains the same—to provide useful information to practicing physicians, medical students, interns, residents, and other health professionals.

Fewer physicians now attempt to manage the whole range of medical disorders that can occur in infants, children, and adults, but those who do must have available a broad spectrum of current and accurate information. The specialist requires precise information about subjects outside his area of expertise. All physicians need more and more information for study and examination purposes as well as for patient care. THE MERCK MANUAL continues to try to meet these needs, excluding only details of surgical procedures.

Precisely how do we attempt to meet these needs? First, from a disease orientation, THE MANUAL covers all but the most obscure disorders of mankind, not only those that a general internist might expect to encounter, but also problems of pregnancy and delivery, the more common and serious disorders of neonates, infants, and children, and many special situations. Disorders are mainly organized according to the organ systems primarily affected, on the basis of their etiology (as with most of the infectious diseases and disorders due to physical agents), or on the basis of disciplines (eg, gynecology, obstetrics, pediatrics, genetics, psychiatry). In addition, THE MANUAL contains information for special circumstances, such as radiation reactions and injuries, problems encountered in deep-sea diving, or dental emergencies. The entire book is updated for each new edition, and new subjects continue to be added, such as discussions of diagnostic and therapeutic procedures in gastroenterology, acquired immunodeficiency syndrome (AIDS), reproductive endocrinology, oncology, the management of severe and chronic pain, the value of hyperbaric O_2 therapy, and special considerations in drug treatment of infants and children. This edition has 114 pages (approximately 5%) more text than the preceding edition. We therefore urge you to check the Index whenever you require information, even on unusual subjects or those not commonly found in other texts.

A completely disease-oriented compendium, however, would have serious limitations. Since patients usually present with complaints or concerns that must be meticulously described, sorted, and deciphered, many chapters are devoted to discussions of symptoms and signs and how to elicit the historical and physical data required for diagnosis. Common clinical procedures and laboratory tests used as diagnostic and management aids are described with emphasis on their indications, contraindications, and possible complications. New and sophisticated laboratory and technologic procedures are also described, with comments on their uses, interpretations, and limitations.

Current therapy is presented for each disorder and supplemented with a separate section on clinical pharmacology that describes general principles, new ad-

vances (eg, the role of drug receptors, plasma concentration monitoring), details of pharmacologic groups and specific agents, and even a discussion on the use of placebos. The use of complex equipment (eg, respirators) is also described. Prophylaxis is emphasized wherever possible. Finally, reference guides are provided for checking normal values, calculating dosages, and converting weights, measures, and volumes to metric equivalents.

Can so many subjects be covered adequately in a single book? You, the reader, must make the ultimate judgment, but we believe the answer is in the affirmative. This edition required a concerted effort by many people, beginning with an internal analysis and critique of the previous edition, even though it enjoyed highly favorable reviews and outstanding reader acceptance. Sections of that book were then sent to outside experts, who had had nothing to do with its preparation, to solicit their most candid criticism. Published reviews and letters received from readers were analyzed. Next, the Editorial Board met to compare reviews and critiques and to plan this 15th Edition. Distinguished special consultants were enlisted to provide additional expertise. Then, 269 authors with outstanding qualifications, experience, and knowledge were engaged. Their manuscripts were edited repeatedly in-house to retain every valuable morsel of knowledge while eliminating sometimes elegant, but unneeded, words. Each manuscript was then reviewed by a member of the Editorial Board or a consultant. In many cases, additional special reviewers were invited to comment. Every mention of a drug and its dosage was reviewed by a separate outside consultant. The objectives of all these reviews were to ensure adequate and relevant coverage of each subject, accuracy, and simple and clean exposition. The authors then reworked, modified, and polished their manuscripts. Almost all of the manuscripts were revised at least 6 times; 15 to 20 revisions were not uncommon. We believe that no other medical text undergoes as many reviews and revisions as THE MERCK MANUAL.

Owing to the extensive subject matter covered and a successful tradition, the style and organization of THE MANUAL have some unique characteristics. Readers are urged to spend a few minutes reviewing the Guide for Readers (p. viii), the Table of Contents *at the beginning of each section,* and the Index (p. 2577). Scrutiny of the arrangement of subject headings within each section, of internal headings within a subject discussion, and of boldfaced terms in the text will reveal a pattern of outlining intended to aid study of the text.

The foregoing is a simplified review of the complex, arduous, and rewarding 5-year enterprise that culminates in the presentation of this 15th Edition of THE MERCK MANUAL. The members of the Editorial Board, special consultants, contributing authors, and in-house editorial staff and their affiliations are listed on the pages that follow. They deserve a degree of gratitude that cannot be adequately expressed here, but we know they will feel sufficiently rewarded if their efforts serve your needs.

We hope this edition of THE MERCK MANUAL will be a welcome aid to you, our readers—compatible with your needs and worthy of frequent use. Suggestions for improvements will be warmly welcomed and carefully considered.

Robert Berkow, M.D., *Editor-in-Chief*
MERCK SHARP & DOHME RESEARCH LABORATORIES
West Point, Pa. 19486

CONTENTS

GUIDE FOR READERS

- The **Contents** (p. vii) shows the pages where readers will find lists of Editorial Board members, consultants, and contributors, as well as abbreviations and symbols, titles of sections (groupings of related chapters), and the index. **Thumb-tabs** with appropriate abbreviations and section numbers mark each section and the index.
- Each **Section**, designated by the symbol §, begins with its own table of contents, listing chapters and subchapters in that section.
- **Chapters** are numbered serially from the beginning to the end of the book.
- The **Index** contains many cross-entries; page numbers in bold type signify major discussions of the topics. In addition, the text in THE MANUAL gives numerous cross-references to other sections and chapters.
- Each **Page Head** carries (1) the page number (page numbers and chapter numbers run serially from the beginning to the end of the book); (2) left-hand pages contain the section title, and (3) right-hand pages contain the chapter number and title.
- **Abbreviations and Symbols**, used liberally as essential space savers, are listed on pp. ix and x.
- The **Tables** and **Figures** found throughout the text are referenced appropriately in the index but are not listed in a table of contents.
- Section 22, **Special Subjects**, contains discussions such as **Geriatric Medicine, Aids for the Disabled Patient, Nuclear Medicine**, and **Hyperbaric Oxygen Therapy**, as well as **Laboratory Medicine** and **Ready Reference Guides.**
- **Drugs** are designated in the text by generic (nonproprietary) names. In the last chapter of the Clinical Pharmacology section, many of the drugs mentioned in the book are listed alphabetically, with each generic term followed by one or more trademarks.
- The authors, reviewers, editors, and publisher of this book have made extensive efforts to ensure that treatments, drugs, and dosage regimens are accurate and conform to the standards accepted at the time of publication. However, constant changes in information resulting from continuing research and clinical experience, reasonable differences in opinions among authorities, unique aspects of individual clinical situations, and the possibility of human error in preparing such an extensive text require that the reader exercise individual judgment when making a clinical decision and, if necessary, consult and compare information from other sources. In particular, the reader is advised to check the product information provided by the manufacturer of a drug product before prescribing or administering it, especially if the drug is unfamiliar or is used infrequently.

ABBREVIATIONS AND SYMBOLS

ACTH adrenocorticotropic hormone
ADH antidiuretic hormone
ADP adenosine diphosphate
AIDS acquired immunodeficiency syndrome
ALT alanine aminotransferase (formerly SGPT)
AST aspartate aminotransferase (formerly SGOT)
ATP adenosine triphosphate
bid 2 times a day
BMR basal metabolic rate
BP blood pressure
BSA body surface area
BUN blood urea nitrogen
C Celsius; centigrade; complement
Ca Calcium
CBC complete blood count
CF complement fixation, fixating
Ch. chapter
Ci curie
CK creatine kinase
Cl chloride; chlorine
cm centimeter
CNS central nervous system
CO carbon monoxide; cardiac output
CO_2 carbon dioxide
CPR cardiopulmonary resuscitation
CSF cerebrospinal fluid
CT computed tomography
cu cubic
D & C dilation and curettage
dL deciliter (= 100 mL)
DNA deoxyribonucleic acid
DTP diphtheria-tetanus-pertussis (toxoids/vaccine)
D/W dextrose in water
ECF extracellular fluid
ECG electrocardiogram
EEG electroencephalogram
ENT ear, nose, and throat
ESR erythrocyte sedimentation rate
F Fahrenheit
FDA U.S. Food and Drug Administration
ft foot; feet (measure)
FUO fever of unknown origin
GFR glomerular filtration rate
GI gastrointestinal
gm gram
G6PD glucose-6-phosphate dehydrogenase
GU genitourinary
h hour
Hb hemoglobin
HCl hydrochloric acid; hydrochloride
HCO_3 bicarbonate
Hct hematocrit
Hg mercury
HI hemagglutination-inhibition, inhibiting
HLA human leukocyte group A
Hz hertz (cycles/second)
ICF intracellular fluid
IgA, etc immunoglobulin A, etc
IM intramuscular(ly)
IPPB inspiratory positive pressure breathing
IU international unit
IV intravenous(ly)
IVU intravenous urography
K potassium
kcal kilocalorie (food calorie)
kg kilogram
17-KGS 17-ketogenic steroids
17-KS 17-ketosteroids
L liter
lb pound
LDH lactic dehydrogenase
LE lupus erythematosus
lt left
m meter
M molar
MCH mean corpuscular hemoglobin
MCHC mean corpuscular hemoglobin concentration
mCi millicurie
MCV mean corpuscular volume
mEq milliequivalent
mg milligram
Mg magnesium

MIC	minimum inhibitory concentration
min	minute
mIU	milli-international unit
mL	milliliter
mm	millimeter
mM	millimole
mo	month
mol wt	molecular weight
mOsm	milliosmole
MRC	Medical Research Council (units)
MRI	magnetic resonance imaging
N	nitrogen; normal (strength of solution)
Na	sodium
NaCl	sodium chloride
ng	nanogram (=millimicrogram)
nm	nanometer (=millimicron)
17-OHCS	17-hydroxycorticosteroids
OTC	over-the-counter (pharmaceuticals)
oz	ounce
P	phosphorus; pressure
P_{CO_2}	carbon dioxide pressure (or tension)
P_{O_2}	oxygen pressure (or tension)
Pa_{CO_2}	arterial carbon dioxide pressure
Pa_{O_2}	arterial oxygen pressure
PA_{O_2}	alveolar oxygen pressure
pg	picogram (=micromicrogram)
pH	hydrogen-ion concentration
po	orally
PPD	Purified Protein Derivative (tuberculin)
ppm	parts per million
prn	as needed
psi	pounds per square inch
q	every
q 4 h, etc	every 4 hours, etc
qid	4 times a day
R, r	roentgen
RA	rheumatoid arthritis
RBC	red blood cell
RF	rheumatic fever; rheumatoid factor
RNA	ribonucleic acid
rt	right
Sa_{O_2}	arterial oxygen saturation
SBE	subacute bacterial endocarditis
s.c.	subcutaneous(ly)
sec	second
SI	International System of Units
SLE	systemic lupus erythematosus
soln	solution
sp gr	specific gravity
sq	square
sq m	square meter
STS	serologic test(s) for syphilis
TB	tuberculosis
tbsp	tablespoon
tid	3 times a day
tsp	teaspoon
u.	unit
URI	upper respiratory infection
UTI	urinary tract infection
USPHS	United States Public Health Service
WBC	white blood cell
WHO	World Health Organization
wk	week
wt	weight
yr	year
μ	micro-
μL	microliter
μm	micrometer; micron
mμ	millimicron (=nanometer)
μCi	microcurie
μg	microgram
μmol	micromole
μOsm	micro-osmole
/	per
$<$	less than
$>$	more than
$\leq$	equal to or less than
$\geq$	equal to or more than
$\cong$	approximately equal to
$\pm$	plus or minus
§	section

EDITOR-IN-CHIEF

Robert Berkow, M.D.
Senior Director of Medical Literature
Merck Sharp & Dohme Research Laboratories
and
Clinical Professor of Medicine and of Psychiatry
Hahnemann University

ASSISTANT EDITOR

Andrew J. Fletcher, M.B., B.Chir.
Merck Sharp & Dohme Research Laboratories

EDITORIAL BOARD

CONSULTANTS

John J. Calabro, M.D.
Director of Rheumatology, St. Vincent Hospital; Professor of Medicine and Pediatrics, University of Massachusetts

Musculoskeletal Disorders

Ralph E. Cutler, M.D.
Professor of Medicine, Loma Linda University; Chief, Nephrology Section, Jerry L. Pettis Memorial VA Hospital, Loma Linda

Renal and Urologic Disorders

George E. Downs, Pharm.D.
Professor of Clinical Pharmacy, Philadelphia College of Pharmacy and Science

Pharmaceutical Preparations and Dosages

Charles S. Houston, M.D.
Professor of Environmental Health and Professor of Medicine (Emeritus), University of Vermont

Disorders Due to Physical Agents

Edward B. Lewin, M.D.
Head, Division of Pediatric Infectious Disease, Henry Ford Hospital; Associate Clinical Professor of Pediatrics and Communicable Diseases, University of Michigan

Pediatric Infectious Disease

José J. Llinas, M.D.
Clinical Professor of Psychiatry, University of Florida

Psychiatric Disorders

Hal B. Richerson, M.D.
Professor of Internal Medicine and Director of Allergy/Immunology Division, University of Iowa

Immunology; Allergic Disorders

Ruth W. Schwartz, M.D.
Clinical Professor of Obstetrics and Gynecology, University of Rochester

Gynecology and Obstetrics

Howard M. Spiro, M.D.
Gastroenterology Unit, Yale University

Gastrointestinal and Hepatobiliary Disorders

EDITORIAL STAFF

Ruth M. Heckler, Executive Editor
Arlene Elisabeth Dahlbeck, Senior Staff Editor
Frank E. Manson, Senior Staff Editor
Doris C. Smith, Senior Staff Editor
Catherine J. Humber, Medical Textbook Coordinator

CONTRIBUTORS

Meena Adhar, M.D.
University of Rochester
Diabetes Mellitus in Children

Hagop S. Akiskal, M.D.
Professor of Psychiatry, Associate Professor of Pharmacology, and Director of Affective Disorders Program, University of Tennessee, Memphis; Associate Director, Baptist Memorial Hospital Sleep Disorder Center
Mood Disorders

Philip O. Alderson, M.D.
Professor of Radiology and Director, Division of Nuclear Medicine, Columbia-Presbyterian Medical Center
Radionuclide Imaging of the Heart

James K. Alexander, M.D.
Professor of Medicine, Baylor College of Medicine; Chief of Cardiology, VA Medical Center, Houston
Pulmonary Embolism

Chloe G. Alexson, M.D.
Associate Professor of Pediatrics, University of Rochester
Congenital Heart Disease; Heart Failure

James R. Allen, M.D.
Assistant Director for Medical Science. AIDS Program, Center for Infectious Diseases, Centers for Disease Control, USPHS
Nosocomial Infection in the Newborn

Terry D. Allen, M.D.
Professor of Urology, University of Texas, Dallas
Intersex States

Roy D. Altman, M.D.
Professor of Medicine, University of Miami; Chief, Arthritis Division, VA Medical Center, Miami
Paget's Disease of Bone

Jacob V. Aranda, M.D., Ph.D
Professor of Pediatrics, Pharmacology, and Therapeutics, McGill University; Director, Apnea Treatment and Research Centre and Developmental Pharmacology and Perinatal Research Unit, Montreal Children's Hospital
Special Considerations of Drug Treatment in Neonates, Infants, and Children

Hugh Auchincloss, M.D.
Associate Clinical Professor of Surgery (Emeritus), Columbia University
Breast Disorders

Hervy E. Averette, M.D.
Professor and Director, Division of Gynecologic Oncology, University of Miami
Gynecologic Neoplasms

Richard F. Bakemeier, M.D.
Professor of Medicine and Director of Cancer Education, University of Colorado
Tumor Immunology

H. Scott Baldwin, M.D.
Chief Resident and Clinical Instructor, Department of Pediatrics, University of Rochester
Hemorrhagic Shock and Encephalopathy

Mark Ballow, M.D.
Professor of Pediatrics and Head, Division of Clinical Immunology, University of Connecticut
Immunologic Status of the Fetus and Newborn

Peter A. Banks, M.D.
Associate Professor of Medicine, Tufts University; Lecturer of Medicine, Harvard University
Pancreatitis

C. Redington Barrett, Jr., M.D.
Associate Professor of Clinical Medicine, Columbia University
Pulmonary Insufficiency; Acute Respiratory Failure

John G. Bartlett, M.D.
Chief, Division of Infectious Diseases, Johns Hopkins University
Pneumonia; Lung Abscess

Gerald L. Baum, M.D.
Professor of Medicine, Tel-Aviv University; Director, Pulmonary Division, Chaim Sheba Medical Center, Tel-Hashomer, Israel
Special Procedures—Pulmonary

Laurence H. Beck, M.D.
Professor of Medicine, University of Pennsylvania
Diuretics

Peter Beighton, M.D., Ph.D.
Professor, Department of Human Genetics, University of Cape Town, South Africa

Arthrogryposis Multiplex Congenita; Inherited Disorders of Connective Tissue; The Osteochondrodysplasias; The Osteopetroses; The Osteochondroses

Robert Berkow, M.D.
Editor-in-Chief, THE MERCK MANUAL; Clinical Professor of Medicine and of Psychiatry, Hahnemann University

Psychiatry in Medicine; Management of Chronic Disability; Anorexia Nervosa and Bulimia

Richard W. Besdine, M.D.
Travelers Professor of Geriatrics and Gerontology; Director, Travelers Center on Aging; and Associate Professor of Community Medicine and Health Care and of Internal Medicine, University of Connecticut

Geriatric Medicine

Don C. Bienfang, M.D.
Assistant Professor of Ophthalmology, Harvard University

Optic Nerve; Visual Pathways

Jacob D. Bitran, M.D.
Associate Professor of Medicine and Director of Clinical Research Development, University of Chicago

Oncology

F. William Blaisdell, M.D.
Professor and Chairman, Department of Surgery, University of California, Davis

Adult Respiratory Distress Syndrome

John H. Bland, M.D.
Professor of Medicine and Rheumatology, University of Vermont

Osteoarthritis

Harvey Blank, M.D.
Professor Emeritus, Department of Dermatology and Cutaneous Surgery, University of Miami

Herpes Gestationis; Impetigo, Ecthyma; Dermatologic Disorders; Reactions to Sunlight

M. Donald Blaufox, M.D., Ph.D.
Professor and Chairman, Department of Nuclear Medicine and Professor of Medicine and Radiology, Albert Einstein College of Medicine

Radiation Reactions and Injuries; Nuclear Medicine

Rodney Bluestone, M.B., F.R.C.P.
Clinical Professor of Medicine, University of California, Los Angeles

Vasculitis; Polyarteritis Nodosa

Philip K. Bondy, M.D.
Professor of Medicine, Yale University; Chief of Staff, VA Medical Center, West Haven

Adrenal Functional Disorders; Nonfunctional Adrenal Masses; Polyglandular Deficiency Syndromes; Congenital Adrenal Hyperplasia; Corticotropin and Corticosteroids

William K. Bottomley, D.D.S., M.S.
Professor and Chairman, Department of Oral Diagnosis, Georgetown University

Disorders of the Lips, Mouth, and Tongue; Dental Caries and Its Complications; Periodontal Disease; Preneoplastic and Neoplastic Lesions

Bernard B. Brody, M.D.
Clinical Professor of Medicine, Pathology, and Laboratory Medicine, University of Rochester; Senior Vice President of Medical Affairs, The Genesee Hospital

Laboratory Medicine

John G. Brooks, M.D.
Associate Professor of Pediatrics and Director of Pediatric Pulmonary Medicine, University of Rochester

Sudden Infant Death Syndrome

Marilyn R. Brown, M.D.
Associate Professor of Pediatrics, Chief of Pediatric GI/Nutrition Unit, and Director of Nutritional Support Service and Weight Control Clinic for Children and Adolescents, University of Rochester

Obesity (in Adolescence)

Felix E. Bruckner, M.B., F.R.C.P.
Head, Department of Rheumatology, St. George's Hospital; Honorary Senior Lecturer and Teacher, University of London, London, England

Neurogenic Arthropathy

Michael F. Bryson, M.D.
Clinical Associate Professor of Pediatrics, University of Rochester

Growth and Development from Birth Through Childhood; Failure to Thrive

Roger J. Bulger, M.D.
President, University of Texas Health Science Center, Houston; Professor of Medicine and Professor of Public Health, University of Texas, Houston

Rat-Bite Fever

John F. Burke, M.D.
Helen Andrus Benedict Professor of Surgery, Harvard University; Chief, Trauma Services, Massachusetts General Hospital
Burns

Benjamin Burrows, M.D.
Professor of Internal Medicine and Director, Division of Respiratory Sciences, University of Arizona

Acute Bronchitis; Chronic Obstructive Pulmonary Disease

John J. Calabro, M.D.
Director of Rheumatology, St. Vincent Hospital; Professor of Medicine and Pediatrics, University of Massachusetts

Ankylosing Spondylitis

Kathryn Lynn Cates, M.D.
Associate Professor of Pediatrics, University of Connecticut, Farmington

Immunologic Status of the Fetus and Newborn

Jesse M. Cedarbaum, M.D.
Assistant Professor of Neurology, Cornell University; Burke Rehabilitation Center

Disorders of Movement: Extrapyramidal and Cerebellar Disorders

Fredric L. Coe, M.D.
Director, Nephrology Program and Professor of Medicine and Physiology, University of Chicago

Urinary Calculi

Alan S. Cohen, M.D.
Chief of Medicine and Director, Thorndike Memorial Laboratory and Boston City Hospital; Conrad Wesselhoeft Professor of Medicine, Boston University
Amyloidosis

Sidney Cohen, M.D.
Richard Laylord Evans Professor of Medicine and Chairman, Department of Internal Medicine, Temple University

Disorders of the Esophagus

Bentley P. Colcock, M.D.
Senior Surgeon (Emeritus), Lahey Clinic; Associate Professor of Clinical Surgery, Boston University

Diverticular Disease

John J. Condemi, M.D.
Clinical Professor of Medicine, University of Rochester

Immunology and Allergic Disorders—Introduction; Biology of the Immune System; Hypersensitivity Reactions

Alastair M. Connell, M.D.
Vice President for Health Sciences, Virginia Commonwealth University

Bowel Obstruction; Appendicitis; Peritonitis; Meckel's Diverticulum

Jules Constant, M.D.
Clinical Associate Professor of Medicine, State University of New York, Buffalo

An Approach to the Cardiac Patient; Valvular Heart Disease

Mary Ann Cooper, M.D.
Associate Professor and Director of Research, Division of Emergency Medicine, Department of Surgery, University of Illinois

Electric Shock

Ralph E. Cutler, M.D.
Professor of Medicine, Loma Linda University; Chief, Nephrology Section, Jerry L. Pettis Memorial VA Hospital, Loma Linda

Clinical Evaluation of Genitourinary Disorders; Renal Failure; The Glomerular Diseases; Tubulointerstitial Disease; Infections of the Kidney, Urinary Tract, and Male Genital Tract; Vascular Disease; Inherited and Congenital Disorders; Childhood Polycystic Disease

David C. Dale, M.D.
Professor of Medicine, University of Washington

Infections in the Compromised Host; Leukopenia; Neutropenia

Ronald G. Davidson, M.D.
Professor of Pediatrics and Director, Program in Human Genetics, McMaster University, Hamilton, Ontario, Canada

General Principles of Medical Genetics

Anne L. Davis, M.D.
Associate Professor of Clinical Medicine, New York University; Assistant Director, Chest Service, Bellevue Hospital Center

Bronchiectasis; Atelectasis

W. Howard Davis, D.D.S.
Clinical Professor of Oral Surgery, University of Southern California; Associate Professor, Loma Linda University

Dental Emergencies

Norman L. Dean, M.D.
Associate Clinical Professor of Medicine, Yale University

Near-Drowning

Ronald Dee, M.D.
Assistant Clinical Professor of Surgery, Albert Einstein College of Medicine; Visiting Surgeon, Bronx Municipal Hospital Center; Consultant in Venous Diseases. United Hospital

Varicose Veins

Roger M. Des Prez, M.D.
Chief, Medical Services, VA Medical Center, Nashville; Professor of Medicine, Vanderbilt University

Tuberculosis; Other Mycobacterial Infections Resembling Tuberculosis

Victor G. deWolfe, M.D.
Resident Emeritus, Department of Peripheral Vascular Disease; Cleveland Clinic Foundation

Peripheral Vascular Disorders

Preston V. Dilts, Jr., M.D.
Bates Professor and Chairman, Department of Obstetrics and Gynecology, University of Michigan

Conception, Implantation, Placentation, and Embryology; Normal Pregnancy, Labor, and Delivery; Abnormalities and Complications of Pregnancy; Pregnancy Complicated by Disease; Abnormalities and Complications of Labor and Delivery; Postpartum Care

Eugene P. DiMagno, M.D.
Professor of Medicine, Mayo Medical School; Consultant in Gastroenterology and Internal Medicine, Mayo Clinic

Cancer of the Pancreas

Leonard S. Dreifus, M.D.
Professor of Medicine, Thomas Jefferson University; Chief, Cardiovascular Division, Lankenau Hospital

Cardiac Arrhythmias

Douglas A. Drossman, M.D.
Associate Professor of Medicine and Psychiatry, University of North Carolina, Chapel Hill; Co-Director, Medical-Psychiatric Liaison Group, North Carolina Memorial Hospital

Diagnostic and Therapeutic Gastrointestinal Procedures; Functional Dyspepsia and Other Nonspecific Gastrointestinal Complaints

David J. Drutz, M.D.
Director, Center for Cell Regulation and Professor of Medicine and Microbiology, University of Texas, San Antonio

Leprosy

Felton J. Earls, M.D.
Blanche F. Ittleson Professor of Child Psychiatry and Director, William Greenleaf Eliot Division of Child Psychiatry, Washington University

Childhood Psychosis

Elliot F. Ellis, M.D.
Professor of Pediatrics, State University of New York, Buffalo

Bronchial Asthma

Kent Ellis, M.D.
Professor of Radiology, Columbia University; Attending Radiologist, Columbia-Presbyterian Medical Center

Radiology

Harvey Feigenbaum, M.D.
Distinguished Professor of Medicine, Indiana University

Echocardiography

Robert Fekety, M.D.
Professor of Internal Medicine and Head, Division of Infectious Diseases, Department of Internal Medicine, University of Michigan

Bacterial Diseases Caused by Gram-Positive Cocci; Rheumatic Fever; Sydenham's Chorea

Murray M. Fisher, M.D., Ph.D.
Vice President, Research, Sunnybrook Medical Centre, University of Toronto, Ontario, Canada

Laboratory Evaluation of the Liver and Biliary System; Fatty Liver; Fibrosis and Cirrhosis; Liver Disease Due to Alcohol; Vascular Lesions of the Liver

Lawrence Fleckenstein, Pharm.D.
Department of Pharmacology, Division of Experimental Therapeutics, Walter Reed Army Institute of Research

Drug Absorption and Bioavailability; Drug Distribution; Antiemetics

Kathleen M. Foley, M.D.
Chief, Pain Service, Memorial Sloan Kettering Cancer Center; Associate Professor of Neurology and Pharmacology, Cornell University

Pain

Noble O. Fowler, M.D.
Professor of Medicine (Emeritus), Director of Cardiology, and Professor of Pharmacology and Cell Biophysics (Emeritus), University of Cincinnati

Pericardial Disease

Howard R. Foye, Jr., M.D.
Associate Professor of Pediatrics, University of Rochester

Behavioral Problems

Irwin N. Frank, M.D.
Professor of Urology, University of Rochester

Obstructive Uropathies; Myoneurogenic Disorders; Urinary Incontinence; Male Genital Lesions; Genitourinary Trauma; Neoplasms; Congenital Abnormalities—Kidney; Congenital Abnormalities—Ureter; Wilms' Tumor; Neuroblastoma

Emil Frei III, M.D.
Richard and Susan Smith Professor of Medicine, Harvard University; Director and Physician-in-Chief, Dana-Farber Cancer Institute

Lymphomas

Eugene P. Frenkel, M.D.
Professor of Internal Medicine and Radiology; Emma Freeman Professor for Research in Radiation Therapy; Chief, Division of Hematology-Oncology, University of Texas Health Science Center, Dallas

Anemias

Gerald Friedman, M.D., Ph.D.
Associate Clinical Professor of Medicine, Mount Sinai School of Medicine

Irritable Bowel Syndromes

Peter L. Frommer, M.D.
Deputy Director, National Heart, Lung, and Blood Institute

Sudden Cardiac Death

William A. Frosch, M.D.
Professor and Vice Chairman, Department of Psychiatry, Cornell University; Medical Director, Payne Whitney Clinic of The New York Hospital

Psychiatric Emergencies

Steven M. Fruchtman, M.D.
Assistant Professor of Medicine, Mount Sinai School of Medicine; Director, Bone Marrow Transplantation, Mount Sinai Hospital

Myeloproliferative Diseases

Michael C. Gelfand, M.D.
Clinical Associate Professor of Medicine and Pediatrics, Georgetown University

Immunologically Mediated Renal Diseases

Michael A. Gerber, M.D.
Associate Professor of Pediatrics, University of Connecticut

Neonatal Hepatitis B Virus Infection

Ray W. Gifford, Jr., M.D.
Senior Physician, Department of Hypertension and Nephrology and Vice Chairman, Division of Medicine, Cleveland Clinic Foundation

Hypertension

Martin Goldberg, M.D.
Dean and Vice President, and Professor of Medicine, Temple University

Diuretics

Harvey M. Golomb, M.D.
Professor of Medicine, University of Chicago; Director, Joint Section of Hematology/Oncology, Michael Reese Medical Center

Oncology

M. Jay Goodkind, M.D.
Clinical Associate Professor of Medicine, University of Pennsylvania; Attending in Medicine, Mercer Medical Center

Cardiac Tumors

Stephen Gryzan, M.D.
Senior Research Associate in Medicine, University of Pittsburgh

Cardiac Arrest and Cardiopulmonary Resuscitation

G. Peter Halberg, M.D.
Professor of Clinical Ophthalmology, New York Medical College; Chief, Glaucoma Service, St. Vincent's Hospital and Medical Center of New York

Congenital Glaucoma; Glaucoma; Contact Lenses

Caroline Breese Hall, M.D.
George Washington Goler Professor of Pediatrics and Medicine, University of Rochester

Acute Epiglottitis; Croup; Bronchiolitis

Robert W. Hamilton, M.D.
Associate Professor of Medicine/Nephrology, Wake Forest University
Dialysis and Filtration Procedures

Margaret R. Hammerschlag, M.D.
Associate Professor of Pediatrics, State University of New York, Health Science Center, Brooklyn
Neonatal Conjunctivitis

Paul G. St. J. Hammond, M.B., D.Phil., F.R.C.P.(C)
Associate Professor of Medicine, Loma Linda University; Assistant Chief of Nephrology, Jerry L. Pettis Memorial VA Hospital, Loma Linda
The Glomerular Diseases

James P. Harnisch, M.D.
Chief of Dermatology, Pacific Medical Center, Seattle; Clinical Associate Professor of Medicine, University of Washington
Diphtheria

Donald H. Harter, M.D.
Benjamin and Virginia T. Boshes Professor of Neurology and Chairman, Department of Neurology, Northwestern University; Chairman, Department of Neurology, Northwestern Memorial Hospital
Slow Virus Infections; Subacute Sclerosing Panencephalitis; Progressive Rubella Panencephalitis

Jack Hartstein, M.D.
Associate Professor of Clinical Ophthalmology, Washington University
Dyslexia

Herbert B. Hechtman, M.D.
Professor of Surgery, Harvard University; Surgeon, Brigham and Women's Hospital
Invasive Cardiovascular Procedures

Paul Henkind, M.D., Ph.D. (Deceased)
Dejur Professor and Chairman, Department of Ophthalmology, Albert Einstein College of Medicine; Director, Department of Ophthalmology, Montefiore Hospital and Medical Center
Retinopathy of Prematurity; Retinoblastoma; Retina

Werner Henle, M.D.
Professor of Virology (Emeritus), University of Pennsylvania; The Joseph Stokes, Jr. Research Institute, The Children's Hospital of Philadelphia
Infectious Mononucleosis

Jan V. Hirschmann, M.D.
Assistant Professor of Medicine, University of Washington; Assistant Chief of Medicine, VA Medical Center, Seattle
Prevention of Infection—Antimicrobial Chemoprophylaxis: Superficial Infections; Abscesses; Osteomyelitis

Basil I. Hirschowitz, M.D.
Professor of Medicine and Physiology, and Director, Division of Gastroenterology, University of Alabama, Birmingham
Disorders of the Stomach and Duodenum; Childhood Peptic Ulcer

Christopher H. Hodgman, M.D.
Director, Division of Child and Adolescent Psychiatry, and Associate Professor of Psychiatry and Pediatrics, University of Rochester
Adolescent Psychiatric Conditions; Suicide in Children and Adolescents

Robert A. Hoekelman, M.D.
Professor and Chairman, Department of Pediatrics, University of Rochester
Pediatrics and Genetics—Introduction; Health Management in Normal Neonates, Infants, and Children—Introduction; Health Supervision of the Well Child; Acute Infectious Gastroenteritis: Pinworm Infestation

Paul D. Hoeprich, M.D.
Professor of Medicine and Chief, Division of Medical Mycology, University of California, Davis
Erysipeloid; Listeriosis

James W. Holcroft, M.D.
Professor of Surgery, University of California, Davis
Adult Respiratory Distress Syndrome

Dorothy Reycroft Hollingsworth, M.D.
Professor of Reproductive Medicine and Medicine, University of California, San Diego
Pregnancy Complicated by Disease—Diabetes Mellitus; Pregnancy Complicated by Disease—Thyroid Disease

Richard B. Hornick, M.D.
Associate Dean for Affiliated Hospitals and External Relations and Professor, Department of Medicine, University of Rochester
Salmonella Infections; Shigellosis; Tularemia; Leptospirosis

Dorothy M. Horstmann, M.D.
John Rodman Paul Professor of Epidemiology and Professor of Pediatrics (Emeritus), Yale University

Poliomyelitis

Charles S. Houston, M.D.
Professor of Environmental Health and Professor of Medicine (Emeritus), University of Vermont

Heat Disorders; Cold Injury; High-Altitude Illness

Douglas W. Huestis, M.D.
Professor of Pathology and Chief of Immunohematology, University of Arizona

Blood Transfusion

Graham R. V. Hughes, M.D., F.R.C.P.
Consultant Physician, Rheumatology Department, and Head of Lupus-Arthritis Research Laboratories (Rayne Institute), St. Thomas' Hospital, London, England

Discoid Lupus Erythematosus: Systemic Lupus Erythematosus

Daniel A. Hussar, Ph.D.
Remington Professor of Pharmacy, Philadelphia College of Pharmacy and Science

Modification of Drug Response

Harold L. Israel, M.D.
Professor of Medicine (Emeritus), Thomas Jefferson University

Sarcoidosis

Michael Jacewicz, M.D.
Cornell University

Neurologic Disorders—Approach to the Patient; Disorders of Smell and Taste; Nutritional Neurologic Disorders; CNS Infections

George Gee Jackson, M.D.
Robert Wood Keeton Professor of Medicine and Chief, Section of Infectious Diseases, University of Illinois, Chicago

Respiratory Viral Diseases: Respiratory Syncytial Virus

Harry S. Jacob, M.D.
Professor of Medicine and Head, Division of Hematology, University of Minnesota

The Spleen

Ralph F. Jacox, M.D.
Professor of Medicine (Emeritus), University of Rochester

Wegener's Granulomatosis

Dennis M. Jensen, M.D.
Associate Professor of Medicine, University of California, Los Angeles

Gastrointestinal Bleeding

Karl D. Kappus, Ph.D.
Epidemiologist, Division of Viral Disease, Centers for Disease Control, USPHS

Rabies

Fred E. Karch, M.D.
Clinical Assistant Professor of Medicine, University of Rochester

Topical Antiseptics; Antiviral Drugs; Antihistamines

Dennis L. Kasper, M.D.
Director, Division of Infectious Disease, Beth Israel Hospital; Professor of Medicine, Harvard University

Bacteroides and Mixed Anaerobic Infections

Stephen I. Katz, M.D., Ph.D.
Chief, Dermatology Branch, National Cancer Institute

Herpes Gestationis; Impetigo, Ecthyma; Dermatologic Disorders; Reactions to Sunlight

Donald Kaye, M.D.
Professor and Chairman, Department of Medicine, Medical College of Pennsylvania

Antimicrobial Chemotherapy

Thomas Killip, M.D.
Professor of Medicine, Mount Sinai School of Medicine; Executive Vice President, Beth Israel Medical Center

Heart Failure; Myocardial Ischemic Disorders

Eric P. Kindwall, M.D.
Chief, Department of Hyperbaric Medicine, St. Luke's Hospital; Assistant Adjunct Clinical Professor of Pharmacology, Medical College of Wisconsin

Hyperbaric Oxygen Therapy

James R. Klinenberg, M.D.
Vice President for Professional Services, Cedars-Sinai Medical Center; Professor of Medicine, University of California, Los Angeles

Progressive Systemic Sclerosis; Polymyositis/Dermatomyositis

Arthur E. Kopelman, M.D.
Professor of Neonatology, East Carolina University

Perinatal Physiology; Parent-Infant Bonding: The Sick Neonate; Gestational Age and Birth Weight; Postmature Infant; Asphyxia and Resuscitation; Respiratory Disorders; Hematologic Problems; Metabolic Problems in the Newborn; Neonatal Pneumonia; Gastrointestinal Defects

Saul Krugman, M.D.
Professor of Pediatrics, New York University

Prevention of Infection—Immunization Procedures for Adults; Immunization Procedures Throughout Childhood

Gary L. Lage, Ph.D
Chairman, Department of Pharmacology and Toxicology and Professor of Toxicology, Philadelphia College of Pharmacy and Science

Drug Toxicity

Lewis Landsberg, M.D.
Professor of Medicine, Harvard University; Chief, Division of Endocrinology and Metabolism, Beth Israel Hospital

Multiple Endocrine Neoplasia Syndromes

Edward H. Lanphier, M.D.
Senior Scientist, Department of Preventive Medicine and Assistant Director for Research, The Biotron, University of Wisconsin

Medical Aspects of Diving and Work in Compressed Air

Louis Lasagna, M.D.
Professor of Pharmacology and Psychiatry, Dean of Sackler School of Graduate Biomedical Sciences, and Dean for Academic Affairs of the School of Medicine, Tufts University

Placebos

Daniel M. Laskin, D.D.S.
Professor and Chairman, Department of Oral and Maxillofacial Surgery and Director, Temporomandibular Joint and Facial Pain Research Center, Virginia Commonwealth University

Temporomandibular Joint Disorders

Ruth A. Lawrence, M.D.
Professor of Pediatrics and of Obstetrics and Gynecology and Director, Poison Center, University of Rochester

Management of the Normal Newborn—Initial Care; Complete Physical Examination; The First Few Days; Feeding; Hospital Accommodations; Infant Nutrition; Accidents and Poisonings

Chinh Trung Lê, M.D.
Chief, Pediatric Infectious Diseases, Kaiser Permanente Medical Center, Sacramento; Associate Clinical Professor, University of California, Davis

Antimicrobial Therapy for Newborns; Neonatal Listeriosis; Perinatal Tuberculosis

James B. Lee, M.D.
Professor of Medicine, State University of New York, Buffalo; Director, Division of Hypertension and Medical Director, Erie County Medical Center Skilled Nursing Facility

Prostaglandins, Thromboxanes, and Leukotrienes

Harvey Lemont, D.P.M.
Chairman, Department of Medicine, Pennsylvania College of Podiatric Medicine; Clinical Associate Professor of Medicine, Department of Dermatology, Hahnemann University

Common Foot Disorders

Roland A. Levandowski, M.D.
Assistant Professor of Medicine, University of Illinois, Chicago

Respiratory Viral Diseases

Gerald S. Levey, M.D.
Professor and Chairman, Department of Medicine, University of Pittsburgh; Chief of Medicine, Presbyterian-University Hospital

Thyroid; Congenital Goiters; Hypothyroidism; Hyperthyroidism

Daniel Levinson, M.D.
Associate Professor, Department of Family and Community Medicine, University of Arizona

Medical Aspects of Air Travel

Robert I. Levy, M.D.
Professor of Medicine, Columbia University

Anomalies in Lipid Metabolism

Edward B. Lewin, M.D.
Head, Division of Pediatric Infectious Disease, Henry Ford Hospital; Associate Clinical Professor of Pediatrics and Communicable Diseases, University of Michigan

Neonatal Sepsis; Neonatal Meningitis; Fever of Unknown Origin in Children

Harold I. Lief, M.D.
Professor of Psychiatry, University of Pennsylvania; Psychiatrist to the Pennsylvania Hospital

Psychosexual Disorders; Disorders of Sexual Function; The Medical Examination of the Rape Victim; Gender Identity Disorder of Childhood

Mortimer B. Lipsett, M.D. *(Deceased)*
Director, Clinical Center, National Institutes of Health; Professor of Medicine, Uniformed Services University of the Health Sciences

The Testes; Precocious Puberty

Larry I. Lipshultz, M.D.
Professor of Urology, Baylor College of Medicine

Infertility

Elliot M. Livstone, M.D.
Sarasota, Florida

Neoplasms of the Bowel

Henry S. Loeb, M.D.
Professor of Medicine, Loyola University; Program Director in Cardiology, VA Hospital, Hines

Shock

Mortimer Lorber, D.M.D., M.D.
Associate Professor of Physiology and Biophysics, Georgetown University

Dentistry in Medicine; Examination of the Oral Region

Robert G. Loudon, M.B., Ch.B.
Professor of Medicine and Director, Pulmonary Disease Division, University of Cincinnati

Approach to the Pulmonary Patient

Robert F. Mahler, M.D.
Consultant in Diabetes; Clinical Research Centre, Northwick Park Hospital, Harrow, Middlesex, England

Genetic Abnormalities of Carbohydrate Metabolism

Lois A. Maiman, Ph.D.
Assistant Professor of Pediatrics, University of Rochester

Special Considerations of Drug Treatment in Neonates, Infants, and Children—Compliance

Stephen E. Malawista, M.D.
Professor of Medicine and Chief, Section of Rheumatology, Yale University

Lyme Disease

S. Michael Marcy, M.D.
Clinical Professor of Pediatrics, University of Southern California; Consultant, Los Angeles Children's Hospital; Staff Pediatrician, Kaiser Foundation Hospital

Acute Infectious Neonatal Diarrhea

Alfonse T. Masi, M.D.
Professor of Medicine and Epidemiology, University of Illinois, Peoria; University of Illinois School of Public Health

Nonarticular Rheumatism; Regional Musculoskeletal Pain

Richard G. Masson, M.D.
Chief, Pulmonary Medicine, Framingham Union Hospital; Associate Professor of Medicine, Boston University

Pulmonary Function Tests

Alvin M. Mauer, M.D.
Professor of Medicine and Chief, Medical Oncology and Hematology, University of Tennessee, Memphis

The Leukemias

Elizabeth McAnarney, M.D.
Professor of Pediatrics and Chief, Division of General Pediatrics/Adolescent Medicine, University of Rochester

Physical Conditions in Adolescence—Developmental Conditions; Teenage Pregnancy and Conception

Daniel J. McCarty, M.D.
Will and Cava Ross Professor and Chairman, Department of Medicine, Medical College of Wisconsin

Chondrocalcinosis

Kenneth L. McCormick, M.D.
Associate Professor, Pediatric Endocrinology, University of Rochester

Diabetes Mellitus in Children

J. Allen McCutchan, M.D.
Associate Professor of Medicine, University of California, San Diego

Sexually Transmitted Diseases; Congenital Syphilis

Donald S. McLaren, M.D., Ph.D., F.R.C.P.
Reader in Clinical Nutrition, Department of Medicine, The Royal Infirmary, Edinburgh, Scotland

Nutrition—General Considerations; Undernutrition; Vitamin Deficiency, Toxicity, and Dependency; Element Deficiency and Toxicity; Nutritional Disorders

Daniel R. Mishell, Jr., M.D.
Professor and Chairman, Department of Obstetrics and Gynecology, University of Southern California

Family Planning

John P. Morgan, M.D.
Medical Professor and Director of Pharmacology Program, City University of New York; Associate Professor of Pharmacology and Medicine, Mount Sinai School of Medicine

Drug Dependence; General Central Nervous System Stimulants and Anorexiants

W. K. C. Morgan, M.D.
Professor of Medicine, University of Western Ontario; Director, Chest Diseases Service, University Hospital, London, Ontario, Canada

Occupational Lung Disease

José L. Muñoz, M.D.
Assistant Professor of Pediatrics, University of Rochester

Urinary Tract Infection in Children

Gary J. Myers, M.D.
Professor of Pediatrics and Neurology, University of Alabama, Birmingham

Birth Trauma; Seizure Disorders in the Newborn; Congenital Abnormalities—General Considerations; Musculoskeletal Defects; Neurologic Defects; Common Foot and Leg Problems in Children and Adolescents

Nancy M. Nealon, M.D.
Assistant Attending Neurologist, New York Hospital; Assistant Professor, Cornell University

Craniocervical Junction Abnormalities; Spinal Cord Disorders; Disorders of the Peripheral Nervous System; Muscular Dystrophies and Other Myopathies

John C. Nemiah, M.D.
Professor of Psychiatry, Dartmouth Medical School; Professor of Psychiatry (Emeritus), Harvard University

The Neuroses

Heber H. Newsome, M.D.
Professor and Vice-Chairman, Department of Surgery, Virginia Commonwealth University

Chronic Peritonitis

Robert A. Nozik, M.D.
Clinical Professor of Ophthalmology, University of California, San Francisco

Uveal Tract

Stephen E. Oshrin, Ph.D.
Director and Associate Professor of Audiology, University of Southern Mississippi

Clinical Measurement of Hearing in Children; Congenital Sensorineural Hearing Loss

William R. Panje, M.D.
Professor and Chairman, Otolaryngology—Head and Neck Surgery, University of Chicago

Neoplasms of the Head and Neck

William J. Parsons, M.D.
Associate Resident in Medicine, University of Rochester

Salmonella Infections

Robert F. Pass, M.D.
Associate Professor of Pediatrics, University of Alabama, Birmingham

Congenital Rubella; Congenital and Perinatal Cytomegalovirus Infection; Congenital Toxoplasmosis

Lawrence L. Pelletier, Jr., M.D.
Chief, Medical Service, Wichita VA Medical Center; Professor and Vice Chairman of Internal Medicine, University of Kansas, Wichita

Endocarditis

Peter L. Perine, M.D.
Professor and Director, Tropical Public Health, and Adjunct Professor of Medicine, Uniformed Services University of the Health Sciences

Endemic Treponematoses; Relapsing Fever

Robert G. Petersdorf, M.D.
President, Association of American Medical Colleges; formerly Dean, School of Medicine, and Vice-Chancellor for Health Sciences, University of California, San Diego

Manifestations of Infection; Bacteremia and Septic Shock; Enterobacteriaceae Infections; Familial Mediterranean Fever

Hart deC. Peterson, M.D.
Clinical Professor of Neurology in Pediatrics and Clinical Professor of Neurology, Cornell University

Cerebral Palsy Syndromes

Marjorie C. Pfaudler, R.N., B.S., M.A., Nursing Ed.
Associate Professor (Emeritus) of Nursing and Preventive, Family, and Rehabilitation Medicine, University of Rochester

Aids for the Disabled Patient

Sidney F. Phillips, M.D.
Professor of Medicine, Mayo Medical School; Director, Gastroenterology Unit and Consultant in Gastroenterology, Mayo Clinic
Diarrhea and Constipation; Gastroenteritis: Infective and Toxic

Nathaniel F. Pierce, M.D.
Professor of Medicine, Johns Hopkins University
Cholera

James J. Plorde, M.D.
Professor of Medicine and Laboratory Medicine, University of Washington; Chief, Microbiology Section, VA Hospital, Seattle
Bartonellosis; Parasitic Infections

Fred Plum, M.D.
Anne Parrish Titzell Professor of Neurology, Cornell University; Neurologist-in-Chief, New York Hospital
Disorders of the Cerebral Hemispheres and Higher Brain Functions; Headache; Seizure Disorders; Sleep Disorders; Cerebrovascular Disease; Trauma of the Head and Spine

Russell K. Portenoy, M.D.
Co-Director, Unified Pain Service and Assistant Professor of Neurology, Albert Einstein College of Medicine
Pain

Keith R. Powell, M.D.
Associate Professor of Pediatrics and Chief, Division of Pediatric Infectious Disease/Immunology, University of Rochester
Occult Bacteremia; Periorbital and Orbital Cellulitis

Douglas J. Pritchard, M.D.
Professor of Orthopedic Surgery, Mayo Clinic
Neoplasms of Bones and Joints

Samuel I. Rapaport, M.D.
Professor of Medicine and Pathology, University of California, San Diego
Hemorrhagic Disorders

C. George Ray, M.D.
Professor of Pathology and Pediatrics, University of Arizona
Viral Diseases—Introduction; Exanthematous Viral Diseases; Herpes Simplex; Pertussis; Measles; Rubella; Roseola Infantum; Erythema Infectiosum; Chickenpox; Enteroviral Diseases; Mumps; Reye's Syndrome; Kawasaki Syndrome

Robert W. Rebar, M.D.
Head, Division of Reproductive Endocrinology and Infertility and Professor, Department of Obstetrics and Gynecology, Northwestern University
Hypothalamic-Pituitary Relationships; Pituitary; Reproductive Endocrinology; Amenorrhea and Abnormal Genital Bleeding; Pituitary Dwarfism

John D. Reid, M.D.
Professor of Pathology, Northeastern Ohio Universities; Pathology Department, Robinson Memorial Hospital
Carcinoid Syndrome

James C. Reynolds, M.D.
Assistant Professor of Medicine, University of Pennsylvania
Disorders of the Esophagus

Hal B. Richerson, M.D.
Professor of Internal Medicine and Director of Allergy/Immunology Division, University of Iowa
Hypersensitivity Diseases of the Lungs

B. Lawrence Riggs, M.D.
Professor of Medicine, Mayo Medical School; Consultant, Division of Endocrinology and Metabolism, Mayo Clinic
Osteoporosis

Jean E. Rinaldo, M.D.
Associate Professor of Medicine, University of Pittsburgh; Director, Medical Intensive Care Unit, Presbyterian-University Hospital
Adult Respiratory Distress Syndrome

Leonor Rivera-Calimlim, M.D.
Associate Chairman and Associate Professor, Department of Pharmacology and Assistant Professor, Department of Medicine, University of Rochester
Drugs in Pregnancy; Drugs in Lactating Mothers; Antianxiety Drugs; Antipsychotic Drugs

Kenneth B. Roberts, M.D.
Assistant Professor of Pediatrics, Johns Hopkins University; Associate Pediatrician-in-Chief, Sinai Hospital of Baltimore
Fluid and Electrolyte Disorders in Infants and Children

William O. Robertson, M.D.
Professor of Pediatrics, University of Washington; Director, Washington Poison Network
Poisoning

Robert M. Rogers, M.D.
Professor of Medicine and Anesthesiology and Chief, Pulmonary Medicine, University of Pittsburgh

Cardiac Arrest and Cardiopulmonary Resuscitation; Pulmonary Alveolar Proteinosis

John Romano, M.D.
Distinguished University Professor of Psychiatry (Emeritus), University of Rochester

Psychiatric Disorders—Introduction; Schizophrenic Disorders; Paranoid Disorders

Beryl J. Rosenstein, M.D.
Associate Professor of Pediatrics, Johns Hopkins University; Director, Cystic Fibrosis Clinic, Johns Hopkins Hospital

Cystic Fibrosis

Findlay E. Russell, M.D., Ph.D.
Professor of Pharmacology and Toxicology, University of Arizona; Adjunct Professor of Neurology, University of Southern California

Venomous Bites and Stings

Paul S. Russell, M.D.
John Homans Professor of Surgery, Harvard University; Visiting Surgeon and Chief, Transplantation Unit, Massachusetts General Hospital

Transplantation

Edwin A. Rutsky, M.D.
Professor of Medicine and Director of Medical Dialysis Facilities, University of Alabama, Birmingham

Water, Electrolyte, Mineral, and Acid-Base Metabolism

David B. Sachar, M.D.
Director, Division of Gastroenterology, Mount Sinai Hospital; Professor of Clinical Medicine, Mount Sinai School of Medicine

Chronic Inflammatory Diseases of the Bowel; Antibiotic-Associated Colitis

Olle Jane Z. Sahler, M.D.
Associate Professor of Pediatrics and Psychiatry, University of Rochester

Recurrent Abdominal Pain

Jay P. Sanford, M.D.
Professor of Medicine and Dean, Uniformed Services University of the Health Sciences

Plague; Melioidosis; Cat-Scratch Disease; Chlamydial Diseases; Arbovirus and Arenavirus Diseases

James W. Sayre, M.D.
Associate Clinical Professor of Pediatrics, University of Rochester

Screening Procedures for Infants and Children; Common Feeding and Gastrointestinal Problems; Child Abuse and Neglect

Dennis R. Schaberg, M.D.
Associate Professor of Internal Medicine, University of Michigan

Pseudomonas Infections; Campylobacter fetus *and Vibrio Infections*

Kurt Schapira, M.D., F.R.C.P., F.R.C. Psych.
Department of Psychological Medicine, The Royal Victoria Infirmary, Newcastle upon Tyne, England

Suicidal Behavior

Albert P. Scheiner, M.D.
Professor of Pediatrics and Co-Director, Child Development Service, University of Massachusetts

Mental Retardation

George E. Schreiner, M.D.
Professor of Medicine and Director, Nephrology Division, Georgetown University

Nephrotoxic Disorders

H. Ralph Schumacher, Jr., M.D.
Professor of Medicine, University of Pennsylvania; Director, Rheumatology-Immunology Center, VA Medical Center, Philadelphia

Approach to the Patient with Joint Disease; Rheumatoid Arthritis; Juvenile Rheumatoid Arthritis

Arthur D. Schwabe, M.D.
Professor of Medicine and Chief, Division of Gastroenterology, University of California, Los Angeles

Abdominal Pain

Ruth W. Schwartz, M.D.
Clinical Professor of Obstetrics and Gynecology, University of Rochester

Gynecologic Practice and Approach to the Patient; Common Gynecologic Problems

Ronald Schworm, Ph.D.
Associate Professor of Clinical Pediatrics and Education and Education Discipline Coordinator, University of Rochester

Learning Disorders; Attention Deficit Disorder

William R. Shapiro, M.D.
Professor of Neurology, Cornell University; Head, Laboratory of Neurological Oncology, Memorial Sloan-Kettering Cancer Center

CNS Neoplasms; Demyelinating Diseases

Gordon C. Sharp, M.D.
Professor of Medicine and Pathology, and Director, Division of Immunology and Rheumatology and the Multipurpose Arthritis Center, University of Missouri, Columbia

Mixed Connective Tissue Disease

Martin A. Shearn, M.D.
Clinical Professor of Medicine, University of California, San Francisco

Sjögren's Syndrome

Roger C. Sider, M.D.
Associate Professor of Psychiatry, University of Rochester

The Psychiatric Interview

Fiorindo A. Simeone, M.D.
Professor of Medical Science (Emeritus), Brown University; Surgeon-in-Chief (Emeritus), Miriam Hospital

Arteriosclerosis, Atherosclerosis; Diseases of the Aorta and Its Branches

Jerome B. Simon, M.D., F.R.C.P. (C)
Associate Professor of Medicine, Queen's University; Head, Division of Gastroenterology, Kingston General Hospital, Kingston, Ontario, Canada

Hepatic and Biliary Disorders—Introduction; Clinical Features of Liver Disease; Hepatitis; Drugs and the Liver; Postoperative Liver Disorders; Hepatic Granulomas; Neoplasms of the Liver; Pregnancy Complicated by Disease—Hepatic Disorders

David P. Simpson, M.D.
Professor of Medicine and Head, Nephrology Section, University of Wisconsin

Renal Disease Associated with Systemic and Metabolic Syndromes; Anomalies in Kidney Transport

Margaret T. Singer, Ph.D.
Professor, Department of Psychology, University of California, Berkeley; Professor, Department of Psychiatry, University of California, San Francisco

Group Psychodynamics

Arthur T. Skarin, M.D.
Associate Professor of Medicine, Harvard University; Associate Physician, Dana-Farber Cancer Institute

Lymphomas

Charles B. Smith, M.D.
Chief, Medical Service, VA Hospital, Salt Lake City; Associate Chairman and Professor, Department of Medicine, University of Utah

Infectious Arthritis; Reiter's Syndrome; Behçet's Syndrome; Relapsing Polychondritis

Celia A. Snavely, M.S.W., A.C.S.W.
Senior Nephrology Social Worker, Piedmont Dialysis Center, Inc.

Psychosocial Aspects of Chronic Dialysis

James D. Snell, Jr., M.D.
Professor of Medicine and Director of Ambulatory Care Programs, Vanderbilt University

Tuberculosis; Other Mycobacterial Infections Resembling Tuberculosis

Gordon L. Snider, M.D.
Professor of Medicine, Boston University; Chief, Pulmonary Medicine Section, VA Hospital, Boston

Pleural Disorders; Pneumothorax

James B. Snow, Jr., M.D.
Professor and Chairman, Department of Otorhinolaryngology and Human Communication, University of Pennsylvania

Adenoid Hypertrophy; Retropharyngeal Abscess; Nose and Throat Disorders; Clinical Evaluation of Complaints Referable to the Ears; External Ear; Tympanic Membrane and Middle Ear; Inner Ear; Nose and Paranasal Sinuses; Nasopharynx; Oropharynx; Larynx; Motion Sickness

Selma E. Snyderman, M.D.
Professor of Pediatrics, New York University; Director, Metabolic Disease Center, New York University Medical Center

Anomalies in Amino Acid Metabolism

Norman Sohn, M.D.
Clinical Assistant Professor of Surgery, New York University; Associate Attending Surgeon, Lenox Hill Hospital

Anorectal Disorders

Gabriel Spergel, M.D.
Clinical Associate Professor of Medicine, State University of New York, Downstate Medical Center; Chief of Endocrinology, Lutheran Medical Center; Senior Staff Endocrinologist, Brookdale Hospital Medical Center

Pheochromocytoma

Wesley W. Spink, M.D.
Regents' Professor of Medicine and Comparative Medicine (Emeritus), University of Minnesota

Brucellosis

Howard M. Spiro, M.D.
Gastroenterology Unit, Yale University

Bezoars and Foreign Bodies

Sergio Stagno, M.D.
Professor of Pediatrics and Microbiology, University of Alabama, Birmingham

Congenital Rubella; Congenital and Perinatal Cytomegalovirus Infection; Congenital Toxoplasmosis

Walter E. Stamm, M.D.
Professor of Medicine, University of Washington; Head, Division of Infectious Diseases, Harborview Medical Center

Prevention of Infection—Barriers; Neisseria; Hemophilus Infections

Allen C. Steere, M.D.
Associate Professor of Medicine, Yale University

Lyme Disease

E. Richard Stiehm, M.D.
Head, Division of Immunology, Department of Pediatrics and Associate Director, Center for Interdisciplinary Research in Immunology Division, University of California, Los Angeles

Immunodeficiency Diseases; Acquired Immunodeficiency Syndrome; Immunologic Status of the Fetus and Newborn

Marvin J. Stone, M.D.
Chief of Oncology, Baylor University Medical Center; Clinical Professor of Internal Medicine, University of Texas, Dallas

Plasma Cell Dyscrasias

Albert J. Stunkard, M.D.
Professor of Psychiatry, University of Pennsylvania

Obesity; Anorexia Nervosa and Bulimia

Michael Sue, M.D.
Director of Gastroenterology, White Memorial Medical Center

Gastrointestinal Bleeding

Pavur R. Sundaresan, M.D., Ph.D.
Assistant Professor of Pharmacology, University of Rochester

Respiratory Drugs

J. Peter Szidon, M.D.
Professor of Medicine, Rush University

Cor Pulmonale; Goodpasture's Syndrome; Idiopathic Infiltrative Diseases of the Lung

John H. Talbott, M.D.
Clinical Professor of Medicine, University of Miami

Musculoskeletal and Connective Tissue Disorders—Introduction; Gout; Eosinophilic Fasciitis, Polymyalgia Rheumatica

Paul H. Tanser, M.D., F.R.C.P. (C)
Professor of Medicine, McMaster University; Chief of Medicine and Head of Cardiology, St. Joseph's Hospital, Hamilton, Ontario, Canada

Myocardial Disease

J. Richard Thistlethwaite, Jr., M.D., PhD.
Assistant Professor of Surgery, University of Chicago

Transplantation

Richard A. Thoft, M.D.
Professor and Chairman of Ophthalmology, University of Pittsburgh; Chief of Ophthalmology, Eye and Ear Hospital of Pittsburgh

Congenital Cataract; Ophthalmologic Disorders—Strabismus; Clinical Examination; Ocular Symptoms and Signs; Injuries; Orbit; Lacrimal Apparatus; Eyelids; Conjunctiva; Cornea; Cataract

Ronald G. Tompkins, M.D., Sc.D.
Instructor in Surgery, Harvard University; Research Associate, Massachusetts Institute of Technology

Burns

Thomas N. Tozer, Pharm.D., Ph.D.
Professor of Pharmacy and Pharmaceutical Chemistry, University of California, San Francisco

Pharmacokinetics and Drug Administration; Drug Elimination; Plasma Concentration Monitoring

Donald P. Tschudy, M.D.
Senior Investigator, Metabolism Branch, National Cancer Institute

Anomalies in Pigment Metabolism

Gerard M. Turino, M.D.
John H. Keating Senior Professor of Medicine, Columbia University; Director, Department of Medicine, St. Luke's-Roosevelt Hospital Center

Pulmonary Insufficiency: Respiratory Failure

John E. Ultmann, M.D.
Professor of Medicine; Director, Director of Cancer Research Center and Dean for Research and Development, University of Chicago

Oncology; Neoplasms of the Head and Neck

John P. Utz, M.D.
Professor of Medicine, Georgetown University

Nocardiosis; Actinomycosis; Systemic Fungal Diseases

George E. Vaillant, M.D.
Raymond Sobel Professor of Psychiatry, Dartmouth Medical School

Personality Disorders

Paul P. VanArsdel, Jr., M.D.
Professor of Medicine and Head, Allergy Section, University of Washington

Disorders Due to Hypersensitivity

Jack A. Vennes, M.D.
Professor of Medicine, University of Minnesota; VA Medical Center, Minneapolis

Extrahepatic Biliary Disorders

Wolfgang H. Vogel, Ph.D.
Professor of Pharmacology and Psychiatry and Human Behavior, Thomas Jefferson University

Neurotransmission

Jacob S. Walfish, M.D.
Clinical Assistant Professor, Mount Sinai School of Medicine

Antibiotic-Associated Colitis; Gas

Louis R. Wasserman, M.D.
Distinguished Service Professor (Emeritus) and Albert A. and Vera G. List Professor (Emeritus) of Medicine (Hematology), Mount Sinai School of Medicine

Myeloproliferative Disorders

William C. Watson, M.D., Ph.D.
Professor of Medicine, University of Western Ontario; Director of Gastroenterology, Victoria Hospital, London, Ontario, Canada

Malabsorption Syndromes

Michael Weintraub, M.D.
Associate Professor of Preventive, Family, and Rehabilitation Medicine, Pharmacology and Medicine, University of Rochester

Mechanism of Drug Action; Patient Compliance; Opioid Analgesics and Antagonists; Nonnarcotic Analgesics, Antipyretics, Nonsteroidal Anti-inflammatory Drugs

William Weiss, M.D.
Professor of Medicine (Emeritus), Hahnemann University

Tumors of the Lung

Thomas H. Weller, M.D.
Richard Pearson Strong Professor of Tropical Public Health (Emeritus), Harvard University

Cytomegalovirus Infections

Nanette K. Wenger, M.D.
Professor of Medicine (Cardiology), Emory University; Director, Cardiac Clinics, Grady Memorial Hospital

Syncope; Orthostatic Hypotension; Exercise and the Heart

Richard J. Whitley, M.D.
Professor of Pediatrics and of Microbiology and Director, General Clinical Research Center, University of Alabama, Birmingham

Neonatal Herpes Simplex Virus Infection

Francis C. Wood, Jr., M.D.
Associate Professor of Medicine, University of Washington; Director of Physician Education, Providence Medical Center

Disorders of Carbohydrate Metabolism

Walter S. Wood, M.D.
Professor and Chairman, Department of Community and Family Medicine, Loyola University

Anthrax; Clostridial Infections

Theodore E. Woodward, M.D.
Professor of Medicine (Emeritus), University of Maryland; Distinguished Physician, VA

Rickettsial Diseases

Verna Wright, M.D., F.R.C.P.
Professor of Rheumatology, University of Leeds, England

Psoriatic Arthritis

§1. INFECTIOUS AND PARASITIC DISEASES

1. MANIFESTATIONS OF INFECTION

A healthy individual lives in harmony with his normal body flora, but this balance may be disturbed by disease. **Host defenses** are an important factor in determining whether or not infection will occur. These include anatomic barriers, such as intact skin and the ciliated respiratory mucosa; physiologic barriers, such as gastric acid; immune factors, such as specific antibodies; and phagocytic cells, such as polymorphonuclear neutrophils and macrophages of the reticuloendothelial system. Unknown factors presumably are also involved.

The **microbes that cause disease** are sometimes members of the normal flora. For example, *Streptococcus pneumoniae* and the β-hemolytic *S. pyogenes*, which cause pneumococcal pneumonia and streptococcal pharyngitis, respectively, can exist as part of the normal throat flora. Disease can also be caused by microorganisms that are usually harmless or even beneficial members of the normal flora. An example of this is *Streptococcus viridans*, an organism that is usually a commensal in the mouth but that can cause endocarditis in a patient whose heart valve has been damaged by acute rheumatic fever.

Disease may be caused by a microorganism with a particular virulence for man. Most highly virulent pathogens (eg, *Yersinia [Pasteurella] pestis*, the causative organism of plague, and *Rickettsia rickettsii*, the causative organism of Rocky Mountain spotted fever) are not part of the normal body flora and predictably will cause disease in man.

Some of the more likely causative pathogens of some common bacterial infections are shown in TABLE 1–1.

Many **manifestations of infections** are not due to a direct action of the infecting organism and its products but reflect the response of the infected host, and may not

TABLE 1–1. CAUSATIVE PATHOGENS IN SOME COMMON BACTERIAL INFECTIONS

	Bronchitis, Acute	*Cellulitis*	*Cystitis*	*Endocarditis*	*Furuncles & Carbuncles*	*Impetigo*	*Meningitis*	*Osteomyelitis*	*Otitis Media*	*Pneumonia*	*Prostatitis*	*Pyelonephritis*	*Septicemia*	*Sinusitis*	*Tonsillitis & Pharyngitis*
Enterobacter spp.			X								✓	X	X		
Enterococcus.			✓	✓			✓				✓	✓			
Escherichia coli			X				✓			✓	X	X	X		
Hemophilus influenzae	X						X		X	✓				✓	✓
Klebsiella spp.			X							✓	✓	X	X		
Meningococcus							X						X		
Pneumococcus	X						X		X	X			X	X	
Proteus spp.			X						✓		X	X	X		
Pseudomonas aeruginosa			✓									✓	✓		
Staphylococcus aureus		X		X	X	X	✓	X	✓	✓	✓		X	X	
Staph. epidermidis (albus)		✓		✓	✓	✓						✓	✓	✓	
α-Hemolytic streptococcus.				X											
β-Hemolytic streptococcus.		X		✓		X	✓	✓	✓	✓			✓	✓	X

X = Commonly encountered pathogens; ✓ = Less commonly encountered pathogens.

appear in patients with impaired host defense mechanisms. They include inflammation at the site of the infection (absent in patients who lack polymorphonuclear leukocytes) and systemic manifestations such as malaise, fever, and chills. Breakdown of local defense barriers around a local inflammatory process may permit dissemination of infection or absorption of toxic material sufficient to cause constitutional symptoms. Bacteremia occurs when infection spreads from a local focus, either (1) along the lymphatics to the lymph nodes and then to the thoracic duct into the bloodstream, or (2) from entry into the bloodstream directly from an extravascular focus. Bacteria, viruses, rickettsias, parasites, and fungi can cause disseminated infection. Individuals with disseminated or generalized infections nearly always present with systemic symptoms if host responses are intact.

Manifestations of infectious diseases are protean because infectious agents differ widely and may involve any organ system of the body. Furthermore, many manifestations result from nonspecific host responses rather than from direct actions of infecting organisms.

Infectious illnesses often begin with generalized symptoms: malaise, listlessness,

inability to concentrate, and weakness. Myalgias, arthralgias, headache, and anorexia are common nonspecific complaints. Fever is the hallmark of most infections, but some patients may develop more serious symptoms, eg, hypotension, confusion, and dehydration. A catabolic response occurs at the onset of clinical illness, and weight loss may become prominent in protracted infections.

FEVER

Body temperature > 37.8 C (100 F) orally or 38.2 C (100.8 F) rectally is the cardinal finding in infectious diseases. Fever, exaggerating the normal diurnal variation in body temperature, usually is highest in the late afternoon and early evening. The febrile response is most pronounced in childhood and diminishes with age. **Hyperthermia,** *a temperature > 41.2 C (106 F)* rectally or orally, is rarely caused by infection and is usually a consequence of CNS disease or heat stroke.

The thermoregulatory centers in the hypothalamus control the temperature by altering skin circulation, sweating, and involuntary muscle activity (shivering). Fever associated with bacterial infection is due to direct action on that thermoregulatory center by endogenous pyrogen (interleukin-1—**IL-1/EP**), a protein with a molecular weight of about 15,000 kilodaltons that is a product of monocytes and microphages. IL-1/EP is synthesized in response to exogenous pyrogens such as bacteria, their endotoxins, viruses, parasites, other infectious agents, and immune complexes.

Chills raise the temperature to a new level set by the hypothalamus. A single chill typically precedes fever in pneumococcal pneumonia, streptococcal infection, osteomyelitis, tularemia, plague, leptospirosis, typhus, and influenza. However, a chill is not diagnostic of infection and may occur with use of antipyretics or with fever due to allergic reactions or malignancies. Repeated chills are common with aspirin administration and with bacteremias associated with acute pyelonephritis, biliary tract obstruction, endocarditis, and abscesses. **Sweats** usually connote defervescence and commonly occur when the temperature drops to its low diurnal point in the early morning **(night sweats).**

Fever occurs in many noninfectious diseases, including thyrotoxicosis, dehydration in infants and the elderly, ichthyosis and other generalized skin disorders, congenital absence of sweat glands, trauma, myocardial infarction, cerebral thrombosis or hemorrhage, peripheral arterial occlusion, malignant neoplasms, conditions causing intravascular hemolysis, serum sickness, periarteritis nodosa, rheumatic fever, rheumatoid arthritis, and erythema nodosum. When fever is the sole adverse reaction to drugs, the elevated temperature characteristically remains at a relatively constant level. Several fever patterns occur and, although some are associated with particular etiologic agents, the fever curve is usually of little diagnostic aid in the individual patient.

Diagnosis of fever of unknown origin (FUO): Usually fever is readily diagnosed because the agent causing the associated infection is identified or the fever subsides spontaneously or responds to treatment; but in some instances the fever continues and its cause escapes ready detection. *A fever documented to be at least 38.3 C (101 F) rectally for at least 3 wk without discovery of the cause despite extensive investigation for at least 1 wk is designated an FUO.* Differential diagnosis of FUO presents special problems because characteristic localizing symptoms or signs of a number of febrile diseases may be minimal or absent. Causes of fever in **infants and children** are discussed in Ch. 191. In **adults,** many conditions cause FUO, but infections, connective tissue disorders, occult neoplasms (particularly leukemia or lymphoma) are the most common causes. The history often gives important clues (eg, a history of drinking contaminated water suggests typhoid; of employment in meat-packing plants, brucellosis; of proximity to rats, typhus or leptospirosis; of being bitten by a rat, rat-bite fever). Usually the diagnosis requires frequent physical examinations, appropriate imaging

studies (including x-rays), ultrasonograms and CT scans, blood cultures, and serology. In about half the cases of FUO, the diagnosis requires biopsy of involved lymph nodes, subcutaneous nodules, chronic skin lesions, tender muscles, liver, or bone marrow. Blood cultures should be taken 1 to 3 times daily for several days, but a total of > 6 blood cultures is rarely indicated. Serologic tests should be repeated if typhoid, brucellosis, certain virus diseases, or a rickettsial disease is suspected, since a rise in titer as the disease progresses is more significant than a single titer. Malarial parasites must be sought. Liver-spleen scan should be performed in most patients; ultrasonography, arteriography, lymphography, and CT scans are of value in selected patients. Gallium scans are seldom helpful. With a thoughtful, individualized approach to FUO, the cause can be identified in 90% of patients.

Treatment of fever must be directed to its cause. In serious infections, antibiotic therapy may need to be instituted before results of cultures and sensitivity studies are known. In general, antipyretic therapy is only appropriate when the diagnosis is clear, but it should be considered when fever is debilitating, causes major symptoms, or affects CNS function. The average oral adult doses of antipyretics are aspirin 0.3 to 1.0 gm q 2 to 3 h or acetaminophen 0.3 to 0.6 gm q 4 h. Antipyretics should be given around-the-clock to mitigate acute swings in temperature; however, in some patients with high fever, antipyretics may cause a sudden fall in temperature associated with circulatory collapse. Safer ways to decrease temperature include cold compresses or sponging and use of cooling blankets. The oral temperature should not be reduced to < 38.3 C (101 F). Antipyretic drugs are ineffective in **neurogenic hyperpyrexia** caused by damage to the hypothalamus (eg, following a CVA or head trauma), and fever should be reduced by physical means. **Heatstroke** is discussed in Ch. 255. Maintaining fluid and electrolyte balance is important, and supplementary sodium chloride may be required. Nutrition should be provided by high-vitamin, high-protein diets in small, frequent feedings; a few patients with prolonged, debilitating fever may require parenteral hyperalimentation.

OTHER MANIFESTATIONS OF INFECTION

Hematologic Manifestations of Infection

Leukocytosis, *an increase in the number of leukocytes in the blood,* characterizes many infectious diseases. Not every kind of WBC is increased with every kind of infection; with most bacterial infections, leukocytosis is reflected primarily as neutrophilia. The demand for neutrophils in the tissues is first supplied by increased margination of mature, segmented polymorphonuclear leukocytes **(PMNs)** on the walls of capillaries. As the bone marrow storage pool of mature, segmented neutrophils is exhausted, the proportion of less mature band forms in the peripheral blood increases, and as band forms become depleted, metamyelocytes become the predominant form of neutrophil. Severe infections are sometimes accompanied by a **"leukemoid blood picture"** in which immature, mitotically active leukocytes, including myelocytes, promyelocytes, and myeloblasts, are released into the circulation; careful study may be required to differentiate leukemoid reactions from true leukemias.

In severe infections, the neutrophil stores and productive capacity of bone marrow may be incapable of keeping up with cellular utilization, and **neutropenia** (< 3000 PMN/μL) ensues. This is often an ominous prognostic finding. Diminished ability to mobilize white cells may contribute to the leukopenia found in chronic alcoholics (in whom folate deficiency may also be contributory) and in patients with diabetes mellitus or terminal shock. Neutropenia is frequent in salmonellosis, brucellosis, pertussis, and some rickettsial and viral infections. Abnormalities in neutrophils (eg, toxic granu-

lations, vacuolization of the cytoplasm, and Döhle bodies) may be signs of severe inflammation.

Antigen-antibody complexes appear to attract eosinophils. Therefore, **eosinophilia** (> 700 eosinophils/μL) is common in allergic diseases and helminthic infections, and may be found during the recovery phase in many bacterial infections. **Basophilia** generally is not a response to infectious processes. **Monocytosis** may be present in TB, brucellosis, syphilis, some rickettsial and protozoal infections, and SBE or during recovery from acute infections. **Lymphocytosis** (> 4,000 lymphocytes/μL) is typical in pertussis and is also seen in various chronic illnesses and during convalescence from acute infections.

Anemia that develops acutely in the course of an infectious disease results from bleeding or from direct destruction of RBCs. The alpha-lecithinase of *Clostridium perfringens* has been associated with hemolysis in vivo; and intraerythrocytic parasitization destroys red cells in malaria and bartonellosis. Cold agglutinins associated with *Mycoplasma pneumoniae*, infectious mononucleosis, or chlamydia infections may cause hemolysis. Chronic infections cause an anemia characterized by an inflammatory block in which there are normal or increased stores of iron in the reticuloendothelial system and decreases in plasma iron and total iron-binding capacity. Saturation of transferrin may be decreased. Cure of the infection is essential to correction of the anemia.

The **erythrocyte sedimentation rate (ESR)** is increased in almost all infectious diseases. Although the test has great sensitivity in indicating active disease, it lacks specificity; any disease that engenders an inflammatory response may be associated with an increased ESR.

Disseminated intravascular coagulation (DIC) (see Ch. 99) is most common in gram-negative infections, but may occur as part of severe gram-positive or viral infections as well.

Cardiovascular Manifestations of Infection

When there is fever, the pulse is usually increased about 10 beats/min/degree F. With some infections the rate is characteristically slower than would be predicted (eg, with salmonelloses including typhoid fever, tularemia, brucellosis, bacterial meningitides complicated by increased intracranial pressure, *Mycoplasma pneumoniae*, rickettsialpox, ornithoses, mumps, infectious hepatitis, Colorado tick fever, dengue, and factitious fever). Hypotension with or without shock can occur with severe infections, especially in patients with serious underlying diseases or with administration of antipyretics. **Septic shock** is discussed separately in Ch. 6.

Renal Manifestations of Infection

Febrile proteinuria—mild, transient proteinuria occurring with fever of any cause—most likely results from nonspecific increased permeability that lets more protein pass through the glomerular membrane. Some infections, such as poststreptococcal glomerulonephritis and the nephritis of SBE or parasitic infections, cause structural and functional changes in the kidney, probably as a consequence of immune complex deposition (see Ch. 149). Characteristic changes of immune-complex nephritis involve hematuria or proteinuria, which may be reversible, but in some instances causes permanent abnormalities in the urinary sediment as well as chronic renal failure. In many acute infections, prerenal azotemia occurs, with an increase in the BUN and with normal creatinine. Hypotension may lead to oliguria and, if progressive, to acute renal failure (see Ch. 6).

Hepatic Manifestations of Infection

Some hepatic dysfunction occurs in many infectious diseases, even without localization of the infectious agent in the liver. Jaundice associated with bacteremia generally indicates a poor prognosis. Intrahepatic cholestasis secondary to hepatocellular dys-

function is the usual finding. Jaundice may also accompany infections that cause massive hemolysis (malaria, bartonellosis, and gas gangrene). Other infectious agents damage hepatic cells (infectious hepatitis, serum hepatitis, infectious mononucleosis, cytomegalovirus, and yellow fever) or create space-occupying lesions (granulomas of TB, brucellosis, schistosomiasis, syphilitic gummas, amebic abscesses, and echinococcal cysts) that produce the laboratory findings of intrahepatic obstruction (mild elevation of direct bilirubin, elevated alkaline phosphatase and 5′-nucleotidase).

Central Nervous System Manifestations of Infection

Nonspecific manifestations of infection (eg, anxiety, confusion, delirium, stupor, convulsions, or coma) may occur without the presence of the infectious agent in brain tissue. These manifestations of cerebral malfunction usually are proportional to the severity of the infection. More focal findings will usually accompany actual invasion of the brain by infectious agents (see Ch. 125).

2. PREVENTION OF INFECTION

BARRIERS

To prevent transmission of infectious diseases within hospitals, special isolation procedures are used for patients who have or are suspected of having certain infections. (For infants, see also NOSOCOMIAL INFECTION IN THE NEWBORN under NEONATAL INFECTIONS in Ch. 186.) In deciding which diseases to isolate and choosing specific isolation procedures, the epidemiology of each infectious disease in the hospital setting must be considered. The usual source of the microorganism in question, its common mode of transmission, and the susceptibility of adjacent patients must all be considered. Not all infections spread readily from patient to patient, and hence not all infections require isolation. In the hospital, most microorganisms spread by direct or indirect contact (including droplet-spread); airborne transmission or contaminated vehicles such as food, water, or drugs rarely spread infection. Based on epidemiology, diseases can be sorted into categories of isolation.

Strict isolation prevents the spread of highly communicable or virulent diseases that can be readily transmitted by contact or airborne routes. It requires a private room with the door kept closed and with an independent air supply; gowns, masks, and gloves worn by all persons entering the room; handwashing in disinfectant material by all persons entering and leaving the room; and special handling of all articles leaving the room to insure their disinfection. **Contact isolation** prevents transmission of highly transmissible or epidemiologically important infections that do not warrant strict isolation. Diseases in this category are spread by close or direct contact. Masks, gowns, and gloves are indicated for close direct patient contact. A private room is indicated. **Respiratory isolation** prevents transmission of microorganisms through direct contact or droplets that are spread into the immediate environment by coughing, sneezing, or breathing. It requires a private room with the door kept closed; gowns and gloves are not necessary for visitors unless they plan to touch the patient, but they must wear masks; hands must be washed on entering and leaving the room; and articles directly contaminated with secretions must be disinfected upon leaving the room. **Tuberculosis isolation**, used for patients with known or suspected TB, differs from respiratory isolation only in that it requires a room with ventilation that does not empty into the general ventilation system. **Enteric precautions** prevent spread of diseases that occur through direct or indirect contact with infected feces or heavily contaminated articles. A private room is not required, although it may be desirable in some cases, particularly for children or adults who are uncooperative or have poor hygiene. Persons directly

contacting the patient must wear gowns, but masks are not necessary. Gloves are necessary only for persons having direct contact with the patient or with articles contaminated with fecal material; hands must be vigorously washed upon entering and leaving the room; and all articles contaminated with urine or feces must be disinfected or discarded. **Drainage/secretion precautions** prevent infection from spreading through direct or indirect contact with heavily contaminated dressings, or with purulent material or secretions from wounds or other body sites. Private rooms are not necessary; gowns must be worn by all persons directly contacting the patients, but masks are unnecessary. Gloves are required for persons touching infected areas or changing dressings; hands must be washed upon entering and leaving the room; and articles such as instruments, dressings, and linen must be disinfected or discarded. **Blood/body fluid precautions** prevent direct or indirect contact with potentially infected blood, secretions, or items contaminated with infected blood or secretions, and are particularly important in patients who have diseases associated with circulation of the etiologic agent in the blood; a private room is needed only for patients with poor hygiene. Masks are not needed; gloves should be worn for touching blood or body fluids, and gowns if soiling with blood or body fluids is likely. Hands should be washed immediately if contaminated with blood or body fluids, and needle-stick injuries should be carefully avoided. Contaminated articles should be discarded or bagged and decontaminated before reuse. Blood spills should be cleaned up immediately with 5.25% sodium hypochlorite (bleach) diluted 1:10 with water.

Rooms or areas used for isolation should have handwashing facilities and special containers for soiled linens and for waste disposal. Visiting should be restricted, and *all* visitors (professional or social) must wash their hands upon entering and leaving the isolation area. Handwashing remains the most important procedure for preventing microorganism transmission in the hospital. Vigorously washing for 10 to 20 sec with soap and water removes nearly all transiently acquired bacteria. Using antiseptic handwashing agents is probably unnecessary in routine patient care, but may be advisable before invasive procedures or in other special circumstances. If required, a mask should be worn over the nose and mouth and should be discarded and replaced as soon as it becomes moist. Masks and gowns are discarded into appropriate receptacles when the visitor leaves the isolation area. Whenever possible, disposable needles, syringes, eating utensils, dishes, and other items are used. Nondisposable items such as thermometers, stethoscopes, sphygmomanometers, and other instruments should be left in the patient's room for the duration of the isolation. Disposal of contaminated materials is important. Used gowns and soiled linens should be bagged immediately and labeled for sterilization by the hospital laundry. Disposable items should be placed in plastic bags and incinerated. Nondisposable items such as instruments or glassware should be rinsed in cold water, double-bagged, and labeled for decontamination. As indicated for each specific disease, items such as body discharges, blood, sputum, vomitus, excreta, soiled dressings, and uneaten food should be flushed down toilets or removed in labeled bags and incinerated. The room and furnishings should be disinfected when the isolation period is over. Details pertaining to each type of isolation are listed in TABLE 2–1.

Protective isolation (or **reverse isolation**) attempts to protect the infection-prone patient from contact with potentially harmful microorganisms. It is used for leukopenic or immunosuppressed patients, cancer patients, and others at high risk of infection but, when assessed critically in terms of preventing infection in the immunosuppressed host, it has little preventive value. In most hospitals protective isolation consists of a private room with closed door; gowns, masks, and gloves worn by all persons entering the patient's room; handwashing with a disinfectant upon entering and leaving the patient's room; and special disinfection of all items placed in the patient's room. More elaborate forms of protective isolation, used in centers treating many immunosup-

pressed patients, include special laminar air-flow rooms, serving sterilized food, and giving prophylactic, nonabsorbable oral antibiotics to reduce the patient's intestinal microorganisms. These measures, though effective, are expensive, time-consuming, and not available in most hospitals.

In all forms of isolation, patients experience loneliness, guilt, and anxiety. The necessity for isolation, the procedures to be used, and the anticipated period of isolation should be carefully explained to the patient, with reassurance that the illness, not the person, is being temporarily isolated.

ANTIMICROBIAL CHEMOPROPHYLAXIS

Antimicrobial chemoprophylaxis is used in 3 general situations: (1) to prevent acquisition of exogenous pathogens; (2) to prevent resident flora in one area of the body from entering normally sterile sites; (3) to prevent a dormant pathogen already in the body from causing disease. For successful prophylaxis, antimicrobial administration must be brief or the target organisms must have a stable antimicrobial susceptibility. Otherwise, drug resistance emerges and renders the regimen ineffective.

Prophylaxis Against Exogenous Pathogens

Accepted indications for prophylaxis include prevention of infections from *Streptococcus pyogenes* in patients with recent rheumatic fever or rheumatic heart disease (see Ch. 197) and those with recurrent cellulitis (see Ch. 4). Persons traveling to endemic areas should take antimalarial prophylaxis (see Ch. 13), and certain unvaccinated people should receive amantadine during influenza A epidemics (see Ch. 12).

Household contacts or those exposed to oral secretions of patients with meningococcal meningitis are at increased risk for developing meningococcal disease. They should receive rifampin 600 mg bid orally for 2 days if > 12 yr of age. Pediatric doses are 5 mg/kg bid for 2 days if < 1 yr old, 10 mg/kg bid orally for 2 days if ages 1 to 12.

For those traveling to high-risk areas for travelers' diarrhea, antimicrobial prophylaxis reduces the incidence. Doxycycline 100 mg/day orally or sulfamethoxazole-trimethoprim **(SMX/TMP)** one 400 mg/80 mg tablet bid orally is effective. Some physicians prefer to use bismuth subsalicylate (Pepto-Bismol®) tablets for prophylaxis and reserve SMX/TMP for treatment should diarrhea develop.

SMX/TMP, 25/5 mg/kg/day in 2 divided doses until completion of chemotherapy, may prevent *Pneumocystis carinii* pneumonia in certain high-risk patients undergoing cancer chemotherapy.

Prophylaxis Against Resident Flora Infecting Sterile Sites

Patients with severe neutropenia from cancer chemotherapy have a high risk of developing bacterial infections from resident flora of the alimentary canal. In many studies prophylactic SMX/TMP, 800/160 mg bid given until the neutrophil count exceeds $1000/mm^3$, reduces the incidence of infections, but results vary and in some centers this regimen is ineffective.

Children with recurrent otitis media may profit from prophylaxis with sulfisoxazole 500 mg bid or ampicillin 125 mg/day for age < $2^1/_2$ yr, 250 mg/day for age > $2^1/_2$ yr. Similarly, women with > 3 urinary tract infections per year may benefit from prophylaxis with SMX/TMP, 200/40 mg 3 times/wk.

Although its efficacy is unproven, most physicians recommend antimicrobial prophylaxis for certain patients with valvular or congenital heart disease when undergoing various dental and surgical procedures (see ENDOCARDITIS in Ch. 27).

Surgical Prophylaxis

Antimicrobial prophylaxis in surgery is warranted only when postoperative infections are common or unusually severe. These conditions occur primarily in 2 situ-

TABLE 2–1. HOSPITAL ISOLATION RECOMMENDATIONS*

NOTE: Careful handwashing before and after every patient contact is *mandatory*.

Disease	*Type of Isolation*	*Private Room*	*Mask*	*Gown*	*Gloves*	*Maximum Room Cleaning*	*Tray Precautions*	*Excreta & Excreta-Soiled Articles*	*Blood*	*Secreta & Secreta-Soiled Articles*	*Duration of Communicability*	*Comments*
Actinomycosis												
1. Draining lesions	DrS			(X)	(X)					X	Duration of drainage	
2. Other	N											
Agranulocytosis, leukopenia, other compromised hosts	PI	X	X	X	X						Duration of susceptibility	Isolate from patients with any suspected communicable disease
AIDS	B/BF	(X)		(X)	(X)			X	X	X	Duration of hospitalization	AIDS patients may generally share rooms
Burns												
1. Extensive	Con	D	X	(X)	(X)	X				X	Duration of skin lesions	Use careful dressing technic
2. Minor	DrS			(X)	(X)					X		
Chickenpox (varicella)	SI	X	X	X	X	X	X	X	X	X	For 7 days after first vesicles appear; for duration of illness in compromised host	Isolate from highly susceptible patients (eg, with eczema, burns, leukemia); pregnant women (late 3rd trimester) should not care for the patient; children should be admitted to a nonpediatric unit
Conjunctivitis												
1. Acute infectious of newborn	DrS			(X)	(X)					X	Until discharges from infectious mucous membranes have ceased	
2. Neonatal inclusion blenorrhea	DrS			(X)	(X)					X		

Cryptococcosis with draining wounds	DrS				(X)	(X)				X	Until drainage ceases	No isolation for other forms of cryptococcus
Diarrheal diseases												
1. Amebiasis	EnP			(X)	(X)			X				
2. Unknown etiology	EnP			(X)	(X)			X				Culture stools of obstetric patients with diarrhea; isolate patient until diagnosis is definite
3. Enterobiasis	EnP			(X)	(X)			X				
4. Gastroenteritis (in patients < 2 yr);	EnP	X		(X)	(X)	X	X	X			48 h after patient is asymptomatic or 1 negative stool culture	Babies should be isolated in suspect nursery
(in patients > 2 yr)	EnP			(X)	(X)			X				Same as for diarrheal diseases of unknown etiology
5. Nonbacterial gastroenteritis	EnP			(X)	(X)			X			48 h after patient is asymptomatic	
6. Salmonellosis & shigellosis (bacillary dysentery)	EnP			(X)	(X)	X	X	X			Until 3 stool cultures, taken 24 h apart & beginning 72 h after cessation of antibiotic therapy, are negative	Clean floors, soiled walls, & equipment, using a phenolic compound
7. Trichuriasis	EnP			(X)	(X)			X				
8. *Yersinia enterocolitica*	EnP			(X)	(X)			X				

(*Continued*)

* Abbreviations: AFB, TB isolation; B/BF, blood and body fluid precautions; Con, contact isolation; D, desirable but optional; DrS, drainage/secretion precautions; EnP, enteric precautions; N, no isolation or precautions; PI, protective isolation; RI, respiratory isolation; SI, strict isolation; X, all circumstances; (X), with direct contact. (Isolation criteria published by The Centers for Disease Control.)

TABLE 2–1. HOSPITAL ISOLATION RECOMMENDATIONS* *(Cont'd)*

NOTE: Careful handwashing before and after every patient contact is *mandatory*.

Disease	*Type of Isolation*	*Private Room*	*Mask*	*Gown*	*Gloves*	*Maximum Room Cleaning*	*Tray Precautions*	*Excreta & Excreta-Soiled Articles*	*Blood*	*Secreta & Secreta-Soiled Articles*	*Duration of Communicability*	*Comments*
Diphtheria	SI	X	X	X	X	X	X			X	Until 2 cultures, taken from nose & throat at least 24 h after cessation of antibiotic therapy, are negative	Carrier state usually lasts 2–4 wk, may last 6 mo
Encephalitis 1. Suspect arboviral	N											Isolation unnecessary
2. Mumps	RI	X	X							X	12–21 days after exposure & until swelling or other signs have cleared	Masks not required for personnel who have had mumps; personnel who have *not* had mumps should *not* care for patient Susceptible personnel should be vaccinated
3. Herpes simplex	N											Isolation unnecessary in absence of skin lesions
Gas gangrene	DrS			(X)	(X)					X	Duration of illness	Wear gloves during wound contact; greatest danger is transmission to pre- and postoperative patients
Gastroenteritis												See Diarrheal diseases
Head lice	Con	D		(X)	(X)						Until head lice and nits are gone	Caps to be worn by hospital personnel

Hemophilus influenzae pneumonia or epiglottitis	RI	X	X	(X)	(X)					X	Until 48 h of antibiotics	
Hepatitis 1. Asymptomatic HBsAg positive	B/BF			(X)	(X)		X	X	X	X	Until patient is negative for HBsAg	Transmitted through blood & fecal/oral route; discard needles with extra care to avoid accidental pricking; label all specimens *Bio-hazard*; γ-globulin for hospital personnel only if percutaneous prick occurs
2. Viral, all types	B/BF			(X)	(X)		X	X	X	X	Duration of illness	
Herpes simplex	Con	D	(X)	(X)	(X)					X	Duration of vesicle, pustule, or scab	
Herpes zoster 1. Disseminated	SI	X	X	X	X	X		X	X	X	Until all lesions are crusted & *dry*	Avoid contact with highly susceptible patients (those on steroids & immunosuppressive therapy, hemodialysis, etc); see Chickenpox
2. Local	Con	D		(X)	(X)					X		
Infections or colonization with multiple antibiotic-resistant gram-negative organisms	Con	D	(X)	(X)	(X)	X				X	Until resistant organisms are no longer recovered	Gram-negative bacilli resistant to gentamicin; clean floors, soiled walls, & equipment, using a phenolic compound
Malaria	B/BF			(X)	(X)				X		Duration of hospital stay	
Measles (rubeola)	RI	X	X	(X)	(X)					X	Isolation for 8–21 days after exposure & for 7 days after rash appears	Susceptible personnel should not care for patient
Meningococcemia	RI	X	X	(X)	(X)					X	Until 24 h after start of effective therapy	Chemotherapy for hospital personnel after intimate contact (eg, mouth-to-mouth resuscitation)

(*Continued*)

TABLE 2–1. HOSPITAL ISOLATION RECOMMENDATIONS* *(Cont'd)*

NOTE: Careful handwashing before and after every patient contact is *mandatory*.

Disease	*Type of Isolation*	*Private Room*	*Mask*	*Gown*	*Gloves*	*Maximum Room Cleaning*	*Tray Precautions*	*Excreta & Excreta-Soiled Articles*	*Blood*	*Secreta & Secreta-Soiled Articles*	*Duration of Communicability*	*Comments*
Meningitis 1. Meningococcal, *H. Influenzae*, bacterial of unknown etiology	RI	X	X	(X)	(X)					X	Until 24 h after start of effective therapy	Chemotherapy for hospital personnel after intimate contact (eg, mouth-to-mouth resuscitation)
2. Fungal	N											RI if associated with pulmonary disease; ExP for urinary tract infection
3. Tuberculosis	AFB	X	X	(X)	(X)					X	Until pulmonary disease has been ruled out	
4. Viral	Con		(X)	(X)	(X)			X		X	Duration of hospital stay	
Mumps	RI	X	X	(X)	(X)					X		Susceptible personnel should be vaccinated; masks required for young children
Pertussis (whooping cough)	RI	X	X	(X)	(X)					X	Duration of hospital stay	
Pneumocystis carinii	N											Isolate from immunosuppressed patients
Pneumonia (bacterial, viral, influenza)	Con	D	(X)	(X)	(X)					X	Duration of illness	See also Streptococcal & Staphylococcal infections & Infections with antibiotic-resistant organisms
Psittacosis (ornithosis)	DrS			(X)	(X)					X	Duration of illness	Patient should wear mask when anyone else is in room

Rabies	Con	X	(X)	(X)	(X)	X	X	X		X	Duration of illness	
Respiratory disease in children Croup, bronchiolitis	Con	X	(X)	(X)	(X)					X	Duration of illness	
Febrile undifferentiated exanthem or disease	Con	X	(X)	(X)	(X)			X		X	Duration of illness	
Roseola	N											No contact with patients < 4 yr of age
Rubella, congenital syndrome	Con	X	(X)	(X)	(X)			X	X	X	Duration of hospital stay	Infants with congenital rubella may excrete virus for 2 yr after birth
Rubella (German measles)	Con	X	(X)	(X)	(X)					X	12–21 days after exposure & for 5 days after onset of rash	Pregnant women (at risk during first 5 mo if antibody-negative or unknown) should *not* take care of patient; label all specimens *Bio-hazard*
Salmonellosis & shigellosis												See Diarrheal diseases
Staphylococcal diseases (coagulase-positive) 1. Abscesses, draining wounds, skin lesions a. Minor	DrS			(X)	(X)					X	Until drainage ceases	Mere colonization does not necessarily require isolation
b. Extensive	Con	X	(X)	(X)	(X)	X				X		
2. Pneumonia; draining abscess; tracheobronchitis	Con	X	(X)	(X)	(X)	X				X	Until organism is no longer recovered	Clean floors, soiled walls, & equipment, using a phenolic compound
Streptococcal diseases, Group A 1. Pneumonia	Con	X	(X)	(X)	(X)					X	Until 24 h after adequate antibiotic treatment	
2. Skin lesions a. Minor	DrS			(X)	(X)					X		
b. Extensive	Con	X	(X)	(X)	(X)	X				X		

(*Continued*)

TABLE 2–1. HOSPITAL ISOLATION RECOMMENDATIONS* *(Cont'd)*

NOTE: Careful handwashing before and after every patient contact is *mandatory.*

Disease	*Type of Isolation*	*Private Room*	*Mask*	*Gown*	*Gloves*	*Maximum Room Cleaning*	*Tray Precautions*	*Excreta & Excreta-Soiled Articles*	*Blood*	*Secreta & Secreta-Soiled Articles*	*Duration of Communicability*	*Comments*
Syphilis, mucocutaneous	DrS			(X)	(X)					X	Until 24 h after start of effective therapy	
Tuberculosis 1. Pulmonary (sputum-proven or suspected)	AFB	X	X	(X)	(X)	X	X			X	Until 2 wk after start of therapy; in minimal disease a shorter duration of isolation may be acceptable	Patient must wear mask when in contact with others; during transport in hospital, patient must wear mask & carry tissue & wax-paper bag; label all specimens *Bio-hazard;* use sputum bottles if possible
2. Extrapulmonary (open)	DrS			(X)	(X)					X		
Typhoid fever	EnP	D		(X)	(X)	X	X	X		X	Until 3 consecutive negative stool cultures, taken at least 24 h apart with patient off antibiotics for 72 h, are obtained	
Vaccinia 1. Local vaccination site	DrS			(X)	(X)							Isolate from highly susceptible patients (eg, with eczema, burns, leukemia)
2. Eczema vaccination & other generalized complications	Con	X	(X)	(X)	(X)	X	X			X	Duration of skin lesions	

ations: (1) transection of a mucosal surface that harbors a teeming population of resident bacteria, making wound contamination virtually unavoidable; (2) insertion of an orthopedic or cardiovascular prosthesis, where skin organisms in small numbers and ordinarily of low pathogenicity can cause infections with deep contamination of the wound.

Certain principles govern the timing and duration of prophylaxis. (1) To be effective, the antimicrobial must be present in the tissue during or only shortly after contamination. Prophylaxis started after surgery is ineffective. It should be given just before the operation. (2) The agent must sustain antibacterial levels throughout surgery. Once the wound is closed, however, contamination ceases, and no further drug administration is necessary. (3) The agent should be active against the major pathogens likely to be present. It need not be effective against *all* possible contaminating organisms, for the goal is not to eliminate all bacteria, but to reduce them to a level that the body's defense mechanisms can handle without developing purulence. For nearly all surgery, a single preoperative dose of an agent is satisfactory. Intraoperative doses are necessary only for prolonged surgery (> 4 h); postoperative doses are never necessary unless established infection is detected during the operation.

TABLE 2–2 lists the agent and dose recommended for the surgical procedures where prophylaxis is appropriate. Situations where prophylactic antibiotics are not indicated include hand lacerations, prostatectomy in patients with sterile preoperative urine, neurosurgical procedures (including insertion of ventricular shunts), and other clean surgery not included in the table. In patients with established infections, antibiotics are obviously indicated but function as *therapeutic* rather than *prophylactic* agents.

Prophylaxis Against Dormant Pathogens

This situation rarely arises. Patients with a positive tuberculin test presumably harbor live tubercle bacilli in their bodies, and under certain circumstances prophylaxis with isoniazid is recommended (see TUBERCULOSIS in Ch. 8).

IMMUNIZATION PROCEDURES FOR ADULTS

Vaccinations in the infant and child are discussed under IMMUNIZATION PROCEDURES THROUGHOUT CHILDHOOD in Ch. 182. Vaccinations to be considered in adults are diphtheria and tetanus toxoids, polio, measles, mumps, rubella, influenza, hepatitis B viral vaccines and pneumococcal polysaccharide vaccines. The indications for these immunizations are discussed under specific disorders.

---

3. ANTI-INFECTIVE DRUGS

TOPICAL ANTISEPTICS

Agents that kill or inhibit the growth of microorganisms when applied to living tissues without significant harm to the tissues.

Antiseptics are widely used but their efficacy and hazards are poorly understood. An ideal antiseptic should (1) possess high germicidal activity, a broad spectrum of effectiveness, and a wide margin of safety; (2) act promptly, even in the presence of exudate or necrotic tissue; (3) have prolonged therapeutic effectiveness; (4) have low surface tension for easy and effective topical application; and (5) be painless, stable, odorless, and nonstaining. Since no such product exists, therapeutic selection must be based on the most important characteristic required for each case. Several typical antiseptics are discussed here under broad chemical categories.

TABLE 2–2. ANTIMICROBIAL PROPHYLAXIS IN SURGERY

Procedure	Indications	Adult Dosage*
Abdominal surgery		
Gastroduodenal surgery	Gastric ulcer; gastric malignancy; hemorrhage; obstruction; long-term H_2-blocker therapy	Cefazolin 1 gm IM or IV
Appendectomy	All patients	Cefoxitin 1 gm IV
Colorectal surgery	All patients	Neomycin 1 gm and erythromycin 1 gm p o at 1 PM, 2 PM, and 11 PM the day before surgery *plus* cefoxitin 1 gm IV at anesthesia induction; delete oral antibiotics for bowel obstruction or emergency surgery
Biliary tract surgery	Age > 70; previous biliary tract surgery; obstructive jaundice; common duct obstruction; acute cholecystitis	Cefazolin 1 gm IM or IV
Cardiovascular surgery		
Cardiac surgery	Prosthetic valve insertion; coronary artery bypass	Cefazolin 1 gm IV q 4 h for duration of surgery
Peripheral vascular surgery	Abdominal aortic graft; lower extremity graft through groin incision	Cefazolin 1 gm IM or IV
Cardiac pacemaker insertion	All patients	Cefazolin 1 gm IM or IV
Pulmonary surgery		
Pulmonary resection	All patients	Cefazolin 1 gm IM or IV
Obstetric-gynecologic surgery		
Vaginal or abdominal hysterectomy	All patients	Cefazolin 1 gm IM or IV
Cesarean section	Ruptured membranes; labor	Cefazolin 1 gm IV after cord clamping
Otolaryngolic surgery		
Head and neck surgery	Incision through oral or pharyngeal mucosa	Cefazolin 1 gm IM or IV
Orthopedic surgery		
Artificial joint insertion	All patients	Cefazolin 1 gm IM or IV
Internal fixation of proximal femoral fracture	All patients	Cefazolin 1 gm IM or IV

* Unless otherwise stated, all IM doses should be given 1/2 to 1 h before surgery; IV doses should be given at anesthesia induction.

(Modified from "Rational Antibiotic Prophylaxis" by J. V. Hirschmann in *Hospital Practice*, November 1981. Copyright HP Publishing Company, 1981. Used with permission of HP Publishing Company and the author.)

Phenols: A 1 to 2% solution of phenol (carbolic acid) is effective against nonsporulating bacteria and fungi, but clinical usefulness is limited due to systemic toxicity manifested by CNS stimulation with muscle tremors and seizures, possibly followed by CNS depression, respiratory failure, and death. Several phenol derivatives are more effective and less toxic than phenol. **Hexylresorcinol** is a useful agent when applied in a 1:1000 dilution; its low surface tension allows effective penetration and spreading, but it may produce skin irritation.

Hexachlorophene, a chlorinated bis-phenol, is a highly effective bacteriostatic agent in concentrations of 2 to 5% against gram-positive organisms but is less active against gram-negative organisms. Although often used in combination with soaps, maximum effectiveness is only achieved with regular use when a deposit of hexachlorophene forms on the skin. This deposit exerts a prolonged bacteriostatic effect but is readily removed by soap. *Hexachlorophene should not be applied to denuded skin*, since excessive absorption results in systemic toxicity manifested by vomiting, abdominal cramps, diarrhea, disorientation, and seizures. Routine bathing of newborn infants with hexachlorophene soaps or solutions greatly reduces the incidence of staphylococcal infections, but CNS toxicity with cerebral degeneration has been reported, especially in premature and low-birth-weight infants. For this reason, *routine infant bathing with hexachlorophene preparations should be restricted* to nurseries having a serious risk of staphylococcal infections. It is wise to avoid bathing low-birth-weight and premature infants with such products.

Chlorhexidine is an effective antiseptic against gram-positive and to a lesser extent gram-negative bacteria when used as a 4% sudsing scrub or 1.0% aqueous solution. It is most effective as a 0.5% solution in 70% isopropyl alcohol. Antibacterial activity is cumulative with regular use and persists for > 6 h on gloved hands. Local skin reactions are unusual, but *contact with the eyes and ears should be avoided.* Chlorhexidine may cause hearing loss if it reaches the middle ear and should *not* be used as a skin antiseptic before ear surgery. It is effective in combination with silver sulfadiazine to control infection in burn wounds.

Alcohols: Ethyl alcohol (50 to 70% solution) and isopropyl alcohol (70 to 90% solution) are both effective antiseptics. Isopropyl alcohol is less volatile and has slightly greater antiseptic activity. Neither alcohol is suitable for sterilization, since they are not sporocidal. Alcohols are not used to disinfect wounds, since they form a coagulum with protein under which bacteria can thrive.

Iodine, an old and potent antiseptic, is highly effective, low in cost, and has low tissue toxicity. In a 1:20,000 solution, it is bactericidal after 1 min and sporocidal after 15 min. Iodine solutions are also fungicidal, amebicidal, and weakly virucidal. Iodine preparations are available as tincture of iodine, containing 2% iodine and 2.4% sodium iodide in 50% alcohol, and as iodine solution, containing 2% iodine and 2.4% sodium iodide in water. Despite the efficacy of iodine preparations, clinical applications have been limited by the disadvantages of skin staining, tissue irritation, pain, and occasional hypersensitivity reactions manifested by fever and generalized skin eruptions.

Iodophors are complexes of iodine, usually with a surface active agent. Following application, free iodine is slowly released for germicidal activity. Iodophors are somewhat less effective than the aqueous and alcoholic iodine solutions, but may be less irritating and less toxic. Iodophor compounds such as povidone-iodine are available in aerosol spray, ointment, shampoo, skin cleanser, solution, and vaginal douche preparations containing 0.5% to 1% available iodine.

Boric acid is weakly bacteriostatic and nonirritating to devitalized tissues and delicate eye structures. However, it is readily absorbed if applied to large or denuded skin areas and can cause severe systemic toxicity with GI disturbances, hypothermia, rash,

renal impairment, vascular collapse, shock, and death, particularly in infants and children. *Clinical use of boric acid should be limited to the ophthalmic preparations.*

Hydrogen peroxide as a 3% solution is a weak and very unstable antiseptic, but is useful for cleansing wounds. The brief antibacterial activity is due to the release of O_2, which also aids in the mechanical removal of tissue debris from wounds.

Mercury compounds exert antibacterial action by reversible binding to sulfhydryl enzymes in microorganisms. However, mercury compounds are highly toxic to tissues, they penetrate poorly, and their activity can be blocked by extraneous proteins. Therefore, these preparations are not recommended.

Silver nitrate solution in a 1:1000 dilution rapidly destroys most microorganisms. Silver nitrate as a 0.5% solution has been used extensively in the treatment of burns for reducing the incidence of infections and promoting eschar formation. Prolonged use may result in argyria, and bacterial reduction of silver nitrate to nitrite in the burn may cause methemoglobinemia. One to 2 drops of 1% silver nitrate ophthalmic solution is commonly used as prophylaxis for gonorrheal ophthalmia neonatorum, but may cause a chemical conjunctivitis, especially following repeated applications (see NEONATAL CONJUNCTIVITIS under NEONATAL INFECTIONS in Ch. 186).

Surface-active agents: Many anionic and cationic surfactants possess antiseptic properties. Most anionics are effective against gram-positive bacteria, while the cationics are effective against gram-positive and gram-negative bacteria as well as some fungi and viruses. Anionic and cationic surfactants inactivate each other, so cationic surface active agents cannot be used with ordinary soaps, which are anionic detergents. The mechanism of antimicrobial activity is not known but may be related to alterations in bacterial cell membrane permeability. The clinically useful cationic surfactants are the quaternary ammonium compounds such as **benzalkonium chloride, cetylpyridinium chloride,** and **benzethonium chloride**. They possess rapid onset of antiseptic action, good tissue penetration, and low systemic toxicity; the disadvantages are inactivation by soaps and formation of a film on the skin with a weakly antiseptic inner surface under which some bacteria may survive and grow, despite a highly bactericidal outer surface. Aqueous solutions of these antiseptics may become contaminated with resistant gram-negative bacteria and serve as a source of nosocomial infections.

Nitrofurazone is bactericidal against many gram-positive and gram-negative organisms in dilutions up to 1:75,000. It is clinically useful as a topical antiseptic on surgical wounds and superficial skin lesions, including burns, ulcers, and abrasions, but systemic toxicity may result from absorption from large wound areas. It is available as a 0.2% solution, cream, and ointment. Rash, pruritus, and, rarely, exfoliative dermatitis have been reported with this agent.

Miscellaneous agents: Mafenide acetate is a useful topical sulfonamide, available as an 8.5% cream, for applying to burns to prevent bacterial infection. It provides effective *prophylaxis* against both gram-positive and gram-negative organisms, especially *Pseudomonas aeruginosa*, but should not be used to treat established *Pseudomonas* infections. Unlike other sulfonamides, it is effective in the presence of pus and has a low incidence of hypersensitization. A disadvantage is severe pain on application or removal. Systemic absorption inhibits carbonic anhydrase activity in the renal tubule and may cause hyperchloremic acidosis. Mafenide hydrochloride is also available as a 5% solution.

Silver sulfadiazine is a topical antiseptic effective against most pathogenic bacteria and fungi, but some gram-negative organisms are resistant. It is clinically useful for burn treatment, where it both prevents and eradicates *Pseudomonas* infections. It rapidly penetrates the eschar and is painless on application and removal. However, sys-

temic absorption may result in the same toxicity as seen with any systemic sulfonamide.

ANTIMICROBIAL CHEMOTHERAPY

Antibacterial, antirickettsial, and antifungal agents are derived either from bacteria or molds (the *antibiotics*) or from total chemical synthesis. Antibiotics that are sufficiently nontoxic to the host are used as chemotherapeutic agents. They act on organisms by (1) inhibiting cell wall synthesis and activating enzymes that destroy the cell wall, (2) increasing cell membrane permeability, (3) interfering with protein synthesis, and (4) interfering with nucleic acid metabolism.

SELECTION OF A CHEMOTHERAPEUTIC AGENT

An ever-increasing number of antimicrobial drugs is available for treating infections. A working knowledge of the common pathogenic microorganisms is essential for best results. Although etiology can often be inferred from the onset and clinical features of a disease, cultures and antibiotic sensitivities are frequently desirable and are essential for the proper treatment of most serious infections. Experienced laboratory help must be available. It may be necessary to begin treatment in critically ill patients before culture and sensitivity studies are completed. In such cases, it is advisable to give maximum doses of the agent most likely to be effective from the outset, but culture specimens should always be taken before therapy is begun.

In vitro sensitivity of organisms is difficult to interpret unless test methods are standardized. In vitro sensitivity of an organism to an antimicrobial may *not* be a true index of the drug's clinical effectiveness, since efficacy depends in part on the pharmacology of the drug (absorption, distribution, concentration in fluids and tissues, protein binding sites, and rate of excretion or metabolism), the presence of drug interactions or of inhibiting substances, and the effectiveness of host defense mechanisms. Generally, however, agents active in vitro are therapeutically effective.

The choice of drug is not automatic even when the etiology of infection and the sensitivity of the causative organism are known. The nature and gravity of the illness, the toxicity of the drug, the patient's history of hypersensitivity or other serious reaction, and the cost of the drug must also be considered.

Penicillins, cephalosporins, vancomycin, aminoglycosides, and polymyxins are generally considered bactericidal, whereas erythromycin, tetracyclines, chloramphenicol, clindamycin, lincomycin, and sulfonamides are generally bacteriostatic. However, bactericidal agents may be bacteriostatic against certain microorganisms and vice versa. For example, chloramphenicol is bactericidal against pneumococci, and penicillin has poor bactericidal activity against enterococci.

In most infections, including pneumococcal pneumonia and UTI, there seems to be no advantage of bactericidal over bacteriostatic agents. However, bactericidal activity seems to be necessary in infections where host defense mechanisms are at least partially lacking either at the local site or systemically. Some examples are endocarditis, meningitis, and serious gram-negative bacillary infection in the leukopenic patient. In such infections better results are obtained with bactericidal agents than with bacteriostatic agents.

Combinations of antimicrobial agents are often necessary in serious infections before the infecting organism's antimicrobial susceptibility pattern is known in order to guarantee antimicrobial activity against the organism. Combinations are also frequently required in mixed infections and are superior to single agents in treating certain infections, such as TB, where resistance of the microorganism tends to develop when one agent is used. Antibiotic combinations are required to treat enterococcal endocarditis, where an aminoglycoside must be added to penicillin to produce adequate bactericidal

activity; otherwise, the relapse rate is very high. Combinations also seem to be important in leukopenic patients with serious *Pseudomonas aeruginosa* infection; an aminoglycoside (eg, tobramycin) plus an antipseudomonal penicillin (eg, ticarcillin) may give better results than either agent alone.

Administration: Parenteral administration, preferably IV, is usually mandatory in severe infection; oral preparations are often used for maintenance once the infection is under control. Therapy should be continued until there is objective evidence that active systemic infection has been absent for several days (eg, absence of fever, leukocytosis, and abnormal laboratory findings).

Administration of antimicrobials to patients with impaired kidney function must be carefully supervised, since many antimicrobials are excreted mainly in the urine. Such patients run the risk of having drug concentrations in blood and tissue rise to toxic levels because of renal insufficiency. They may tolerate the usual doses for the first 24 h, but subsequent doses must be reduced or the intervals between doses prolonged. Dosages must be carefully supervised in infants (see NEONATAL INFECTIONS in Ch. 186) and the elderly for the same reason.

COMPLICATIONS OF CHEMOTHERAPY

Undesirable effects may follow the use of any chemotherapeutic agent and can involve most organ systems. These adverse effects may be due to direct toxicity or to hypersensitivity. Reactions do not always require cessation of treatment, especially if the offending drug is the only effective one available. The severity and type of reactions, their expected course, the possibility of influencing them by proper management, and the gravity of the infection must all be considered when deciding whether or not to continue the agent.

Cutaneous reactions are mostly due to hypersensitivity and may occur with any drug. Morbilliform and other eruptions, purpura, erythema multiforme, erythema nodosum, and exfoliative dermatitis may occur. Contact dermatitis may develop in persons handling antibiotics. **Other manifestations of hypersensitivity** include fever; angioedema; serum sickness, possibly with subsequent polyarteritis or SLE; and, rarely, anaphylactic shock (mainly with penicillin). **Oral reactions** occur most commonly with the broad-spectrum antibiotics and include dryness, burning, soreness, and itching of the mouth and tongue; stomatitis; acute glossitis; cheilosis; and black or brown coating of the tongue. **GI reactions** include nausea, vomiting, diarrhea, pseudomembranous colitis (caused by *Clostridium difficile*), *Candida* infections (oral, pharyngeal, rectal, and perianal), liver damage, jaundice, hepatitis, and steatorrhea. **Urinary tract complications** include hematuria (penicillins and sulfonamides); crystalluria, acute tubular necrosis, and obstruction to urine flow (sulfonamides); and nephrotoxicity (polymyxin, neomycin, gentamicin, tobramycin, amikacin, netilmicin, kanamycin, and vancomycin). **Neurologic reactions** include peripheral neuritis (nitrofurantoin), paresthesias (streptomycin, polymyxin), 8th nerve damage (streptomycin, neomycin, vancomycin, kanamycin, gentamicin, tobramycin, netilmicin, and amikacin), psychosis or convulsions (cycloserine), and respiratory paralysis (polymyxin, kanamycin and other aminoglycosides, colistin). **Hematologic complications** include hemolytic anemia (sulfonamides, the nitrofurans, nalidixic acid), eosinophilia (sensitization to any of the antibiotics), aplastic anemia (chloramphenicol), thrombocytopenia, and leukopenia. **Electrolyte disturbances** include potassium loading (potassium penicillin G), sodium loading, and hypokalemic alkalosis (carbenicillin, ticarcillin).

Organisms may develop **resistance** to any antimicrobial agent. The resistance may appear rapidly or after long or repeated courses of therapy. Therefore, infections must be promptly controlled by (1) identifying the causative organism, (2) determining its in vitro sensitivity, and (3) providing effective in vivo concentrations of the drug. Initially

inadequate doses promote the development of resistance, and thereafter even greatly increased doses may fail to control the infection.

For a discussion of superimposed infections by resistant organisms, see Ch. 7.

MISUSES OF CHEMOTHERAPY

Antibacterial agents are often used in the absence of a valid indication (such as for viral illness) or used improperly with poor clinical results. The most frequent misuse is probably in the treatment of fever per se. Fever is not necessarily due to bacterial infection. Without strong evidence of microbial invasion, chemotherapy should be delayed, if possible, until clinical and laboratory studies confirm the presence of an infection and guide the choice of an appropriate agent.

Common misuses and errors include (1) choice of an ineffective antibiotic, (2) inadequate or excessive doses, (3) use in infections such as uncomplicated viral disease, (4) improper route of administration, (5) continued use after bacterial resistance has developed, (6) continued use in the presence of a serious toxic or allergic reaction, (7) stopping effective therapy prematurely, (8) failure to alter chemotherapy when superimposed infections with resistant organisms occur, (9) use of improper combinations of chemotherapeutic agents, and (10) reliance on chemotherapy or prophylaxis to the exclusion of surgical intervention (eg, drainage of localized infection and removal of a foreign body).

PENICILLINS

Penicillin G-like agents	Ampicillin-like agents	Penicillinase-resistant penicillins	Broad-spectrum (antipseudomonal) penicillins
Penicillin G*†	Ampicillin*†	Cloxacillin*	Azlocillin†
Penicillin V*	Amoxicillin*	Dicloxacillin*	Carbenicillin*†
Procaine penicillin G†	Amoxicillin and clavulanate*	Methicillin†	Mezlocillin†
Benzathine penicillin G†	Cyclacillin*	Nafcillin*†	Piperacillin†
	Bacampicillin*	Oxacillin*†	Ticarcillin†
	Hetacillin*		Ticarcillin and clavulanate†

Other: Amdinocillin†

* Orally absorbed; † parenteral

The penicillins are a large group of bactericidal antibiotics having the **6-aminopenicillanic acid (6-APA)** nucleus in common. Penicillins affect only actively multiplying bacteria. Their antibacterial action seems to reside in their ability to inhibit metabolic functions vital to bacterial cell wall synthesis, and to activate enzymes that destroy the cell wall.

Pharmacology

Penicillins are distributed rapidly to most body fluids and tissues after IV or IM injection, more slowly after oral administration. Concentrations are low in normal joint, ocular, pericardial, and pleural fluids. However, with active inflammation the penicillins penetrate well into most body fluids and spaces. Penetration into the CSF also varies, but the levels are often therapeutic when the meninges are inflamed. High concentrations are found in the liver, bile, lungs, intestine, and skin.

Penicillins are reversibly bound to plasma protein. Only the free agent is active, and activity occurs when the complex dissociates. A highly bound penicillin may be thera-

peutically comparable to one less strongly bound if it is inherently more potent (has a lower minimum inhibitory concentration) against a specific organism.

Penicillin is largely excreted unchanged but some is metabolized. Penicilloic acid, a metabolite of benzylpenicillin, appears to be an important intermediate in the formation of certain antigenic determinants in vivo and may be an important factor in allergic reactions. Benzylpenicilloyl-polylysine is available as a skin test for determining sensitivity to penicillin. (See also in Ch. 21.)

Excretion of penicillins occurs, with varying rapidity, mainly by a renal tubular mechanism and to a lesser degree via the bile. However, nafcillin is excreted mainly by the liver. Parenteral penicillin G is so rapidly absorbed and excreted that repository preparations have been formulated; these slowly release the antibiotic from the injection site, thereby producing a lower, but more prolonged, blood concentration. The penicillinase-resistant penicillins differ significantly in their degree of oral absorption and serum binding, and in their rate of urinary excretion.

Indications

Penicillin G is the antibiotic of choice for infections caused by pneumococci, meningococci, aerobic and anaerobic streptococci, gonococci, non-penicillinase-producing staphylococci, syphilis, actinomycosis, anthrax, and yaws. It is useful in ratbite fever and infections caused by *Listeria*, *Corynebacterium*, and *Clostridium*. The other penicillin G-like penicillins can be substituted for penicillin G in some of these conditions as indicated.

Ampicillin and the ampicillin-like agents (eg, amoxicillin) have a spectrum of activity very similar to penicillin G. The only difference is greater activity against certain gram-negative bacilli such as nonpenicillinase-producing *Hemophilus influenzae*, some *E. coli*, *Proteus mirabilis*, *Salmonella*, and *Shigella*.

The addition of clavulanate, a beta-lactamase inhibitor, to amoxicillin adds activity against beta lactamase producing staphylococci, *H. influenzae* and *N. gonorrhoeae*.

Amdinocillin has activity against *E. coli*, *Klebsiella*, *Enterobacter*, *Citrobacter*, *Shigella*, and *Salmonella*. It acts synergistically with other beta-lactam antibiotics against many strains of gram-negative bacilli. Amdinocillin has poor activity against gram-positive bacteria.

The **penicillinase-resistant penicillins** are active only against staphylococci and streptococci (including pneumococci but not enterococci). Their primary use is for infections caused by penicillinase-producing staphylococci.

The **broad-spectrum (antipseudomonal) penicillins** have activity similar to ampicillin but in addition are active against *Enterobacter* and *Pseudomonas aeruginosa*. Mezlocillin, azlocillin, and piperacillin are also active against many strains of *Klebsiella*. The addition of clavulanate to ticarcillin adds activity against *Klebsiella*, *Serratia*, and *Bacteroides*, and against beta-lactamase producing strains of staphylococci, *H. influenzae*, and *N. gonorrhoeae*.

Adverse Reactions

True toxic reactions seldom occur, but the penicillins are potent sensitizers and 2 types of allergic reactions are not uncommon: (1) immediate, including anaphylaxis (with the possibility of sudden death), urticaria, and angioneurotic edema, and (2) delayed, including serum sickness, various rashes such as macular, papular, and morbilliform, and exfoliative dermatitis that usually appear after 7 to 10 days of therapy. Previous hypersensitivity to any penicillin is generally a *contraindication* to their use, although untoward effects are not always repeated on future exposures. Patients with mild reactions are sometimes given penicillin at a later date, after appropriate skin tests (see DRUG HYPERSENSITIVITY in Ch. 21, and TYPE I REACTIONS in Ch. 20). A patient who suffers a serious reaction *should not be given penicillin again*, except with special precautions in unusual circumstances when no substitute can be found.

Mild allergic responses may disappear even if penicillin is continued, subside quickly if it is stopped, or may be managed with an oral antihistamine. More severe reactions may require epinephrine and corticosteroids. Specific treatment for urticaria is given in Ch. 21; for exfoliative dermatitis, in Ch. 230; for serum sickness, in DRUG HYPERSENSITIVITY in Ch. 21; and for anaphylactic shock, in ATOPIC DISEASES also in Ch. 21.

CNS toxicity may occur with high penicillin doses, especially if renal function is reduced. All penicillins can cause nephritis (most common with methicillin), Coombs-positive hemolytic anemia, leukopenia, or thrombocytopenia. Leukopenia seems to occur most often with nafcillin. While any penicillin used in very high IV doses can interfere with platelet function and cause bleeding, this is most prone to occur with carbenicillin and ticarcillin, especially in patients with renal insufficiency. Pseudomembranous colitis (caused by *C. difficile*) can follow use of any penicillin, but is probably more likely to occur with oral than parenteral administration.

Other reactions include pain at the site of IM injection, thrombophlebitis when the same site is used repeatedly for IV injection, and GI disturbances with oral preparations. Black tongue may occur, more often with oral preparations, and is due to irritation of the glossal surface and keratinization of the superficial layers. Superinfection by nonsusceptible bacteria or fungi may occur as with other antibiotics.

ADMINISTRATION AND DOSAGE

Penicillin G and Its Congeners

The antibacterial spectrums of penicillins G and V are similar. Penicillin G is highly effective in vitro against many, but not all, species of gram-positive and -negative cocci. Some gram-negative bacilli are susceptible to very large parenteral doses of penicillin G, but most, except *Hemophilus influenzae*, gonococci, and meningococci, are beyond the range of clinically practicable doses. Clinical use of penicillin V is primarily for infections due to susceptible gram-positive organisms; it should *not* be used to treat infections caused by *Neisseria* or *Hemophilus* species. These compounds are inactivated by penicillinase and are contraindicated for infections caused by organisms elaborating that enzyme.

Penicillin G is highly effective in gonorrhea; infections due to meningococci, pneumococci, and β-hemolytic and anaerobic streptococci; most cases of SBE; fusospirochetal diseases; anthrax; streptobacillosis; actinomycosis; and all stages of syphilis. Most community as well as hospital-acquired staphylococcal infections are penicillin G-resistant. Penicillin G may be used to prevent streptococcal pharyngitis, recurrent rheumatic fever, acute gonococcal urethritis, and SBE (after surgical procedures such as dental extractions). Penicillin G is marketed in many forms, the most important of which are discussed here.

Penicillin G may be given IM or IV, but is usually given IV because IM injection is painful. When high serum concentrations are required, as in meningitis or enterococcal endocarditis, IV dosage must be used. The usual IV dosage in adults is 5 to 30 million u./day by continuous IV drip or in divided doses q 2 to 4 h. Severe infections in children are treated with 75,000 to 100,000 u./kg in divided doses. Injection intrathecally, intracisternally, or into pleural or joint spaces is rarely necessary.

Repository forms of penicillin G are given IM, the slow absorption from IM depots providing prolonged therapeutic blood levels. The **aqueous suspension of procaine penicillin G** is used most extensively; blood levels may be detectable for as long as 12 to 48 h. Doses of 600,000 u. bid suffice for most penicillin-susceptible infections. For uncomplicated gonorrhea the dose is 4.8 million u. IM plus 1 gm probenecid orally. A

single IM injection of 600,000 u. of **benzathine penicillin G** produces detectable blood levels for 1 wk or longer. A dose of 1,200,000 u. IM once/mo is used in preventing recurrent rheumatic fever. Syphilis of < 1 yr duration is treated with 2.4 million u. IM. Syphilis of longer duration is treated with 3 weekly injections of 2.4 million u.

Oral penicillin G is used in mild to moderate infections such as scarlet fever and streptococcal pharyngitis and is *not* recommended for severe infections because it is incompletely absorbed. The usual oral dose is 400,000 to 800,000 u. q 6 h for 10 days. Children receive 25,000 to 90,000 u./kg/day in divided doses. For maximum absorption it should be given 1 h before a meal.

Penicillin V is given orally only. It is acid-resistant and better absorbed than oral penicillin G and is usually preferred when penicillin is to be given orally. Like penicillin G, it is indicated in mild to moderate infections due to streptococci, pneumococci, and susceptible staphylococci. It is *not* effective in gonorrhea. For most infections, the usual oral dose is 400,000 to 800,000 u. (250 to 500 mg) q 6 h. Children receive 25 to 50 mg/kg/day in divided doses.

Ampicillin and Its Congeners

Ampicillin is primarily indicated for infections with certain gram-negative organisms and for enterococcal infections, but is ineffective against *Klebsiella*, *Enterobacter*, and *Pseudomonas* species. It is effective in UTI due to susceptible *Escherichia coli* and *Proteus mirabilis*, and in meningitis due to susceptible *H. influenzae*, pneumococci, and meningococci. Ampicillin compares favorably with the tetracyclines in treating the exacerbations of bronchitis caused by *H. influenzae*. Cholangitis and cholecystitis due to susceptible organisms may respond, since biliary levels of the drug are high. Ampicillin is effective in typhoid fever caused by sensitive organisms. Combined with probenecid it has been effective in some chronic typhoid carriers. Ampicillin appears to be effective in shigellosis and salmonellosis, although antimicrobials are usually not needed in uncomplicated *Salmonella* gastroenteritis.

Ampicillin may be given orally, IM, or IV; oral absorption is variable, and may be decreased when the drug is given with food. Peak blood levels are attained about 2 h after oral or 1 h after IM administration; significant activity lasts for several hours. Orally, the dose in adults and children weighing > 20 kg is usually 250 to 500 mg q 6 h; in children < 20 kg it is 50 to 100 mg/kg/day in divided doses. Parenterally the dose is 1 to 2 gm q 4 to 6 h in adults and 25 to 50 mg/kg/day in divided doses in children. For meningitis and bacteremia the dose is 150 to 200 mg/kg/day IV in adults and children. The dose for uncomplicated gonorrhea is 3.5 gm plus 1 gm probenecid orally.

Skin rashes, particularly delayed responses, occur more often with ampicillin than with other penicillins, but the reported incidence varies greatly. It is high in conditions often associated with a rash. Patients with infectious mononucleosis are especially prone to react to ampicillin with a characteristic skin eruption. Most ampicillin rashes are probably not allergic in origin.

Hetacillin and **bacampicillin** are orally administered esters of ampicillin that are hydrolyzed to ampicillin following absorption. The antimicrobial spectrum and clinical indications are the same as for oral ampicillin. Hetacillin is used in the same doses as ampicillin. Bacampicillin results in higher blood levels and is used in doses of 400 to 800 mg bid in adults and 25 to 50 mg/kg/day in 2 divided doses in children.

Amoxicillin is similar to ampicillin except that it is absorbed better in the GI tract and is less active against *Shigella*. Amoxicillin causes fewer GI effects and is given q 8 h instead of q 6 h for ampicillin. It is available only for oral use. The dose is 0.75 to 1.5 gm/day in 3 divided doses for adults and 20 to 40 mg/kg/day in 3 divided doses for children. The dose for uncomplicated gonorrhea is 3 gm plus 1 gm probenecid orally. **Cyclacillin** has activity and indications similar to ampicillin but results in higher blood

levels. The adult dose is 250 to 500 mg qid. The dose in children is 50 to 100 mg/kg/day in divided doses.

Amoxicillin plus clavulanate is equivalent in activity to amoxicillin but is also active against beta-lactamase producing strains of staphylococci, *H. influenzae* and *N. gonorrhoeae*. It is used in the same doses as amoxicillin based on its content of amoxicillin.

Amdinocillin is indicated only for treatment of urinary tract infection caused by *E. coli*, *Klebsiella* species, and *Enterobacter* species. Amdinocillin is given IM or IV to adults and children in a dose of 10 mg/kg q 4 h in serious infections.

Penicillinase-Resistant Penicillins

Methicillin, oxacillin, nafcillin, cloxacillin, and **dicloxacillin** are primarily indicated for infections due to penicillinase-producing coagulase-positive staphylococci. Methicillin-resistant strains are almost always resistant to the other 4 agents. These agents also constitute adequate treatment for pneumococcal, group A streptococcal, and susceptible *S. epidermidis* infections. They are ineffective against enterococci, gonococci, and gram-negative bacilli.

Methicillin is not absorbed orally and must be injected parenterally. The usual dose for adults is 6 to 12 gm/day IV, 50 to 150 mg/kg/day IV in newborns, and 200 to 300 mg/kg/day IV for children in 6 divided doses. **Nafcillin** and **oxacillin** are used in the same parenteral dosage as methicillin. The 3 agents are therapeutically equivalent. Of the 3 agents, methicillin is the most likely to produce nephritis, nafcillin to produce leukopenia, and oxacillin to produce elevation of liver enzymes.

Nafcillin, oxacillin, cloxacillin, and dicloxacillin are available for oral use in treating *non-serious* staphylococcal infections. However, the absorption of nafcillin is poor and that of oxacillin is variable. Dicloxacillin and cloxacillin are absorbed well. Dicloxacillin results in twice the blood levels as equivalent doses of cloxacillin, but the protein binding of dicloxacillin is higher. The oral dosage for nafcillin or oxacillin is 500 mg to 1 gm q 4 to 6 h in adults, and 50 to 100 mg/kg/day in divided doses in children; for cloxacillin 250 to 500 mg q 6 h in adults, and 50 to 100 mg/kg/day in divided doses in children; and for dicloxacillin 250 mg q 6 h in adults, and 25 mg/kg/day in divided doses in children.

Broad-Spectrum (Antipseudomonal) Penicillins

Carbenicillin and **ticarcillin** are carboxypenicillins with activity similar to ampicillin (most gram-positive cocci, except penicillin G-resistant staphylococci, and most *E. coli* and *Proteus mirabilis*). In addition they are active against most *Pseudomonas aeruginosa* (these antibiotics are usually used in combination with an aminoglycoside for Pseudomonas infections), *Enterobacter* species, and indole-positive *Proteus*; infections caused by these organisms are their major indications. Enterococci are relatively resistant and activity is lacking against *Klebsiella* and *Serratia*. The only difference between carbenicillin and ticarcillin is that the latter is about twice as active as carbenicillin against *Pseudomonas aeruginosa*. Both drugs are used parenterally and should be reserved for serious infections; the dose is 500 mg/kg/day IV of carbenicillin and 250 mg/kg/day IV of ticarcillin in divided doses q 4 h in adults and children. As these agents contain about 5 mEq of sodium/gm, sodium loading is a potential problem with IV use. Hypokalemic alkalosis may result from loss of cation with the nonreabsorbable anion in the urine. Interference with platelet function and bleeding has been noted with very high blood levels and has been seen particularly in patients with renal insufficiency.

Ticarcillin plus clavulanate has a broader spectrum of activity than ticarcillin, including activity against beta-lactamase producing *N. gonorrhoeae*, staphylococci, and *H. influenzae*, as well as *Klebsiella*, *Serratia*, and Bacteroides. The IV dose is the same as for ticarcillin based on its ticarcillin content.

Carbenicillin indanyl sodium is an oral preparation that is used only for treatment of

UTIs and chronic bacterial prostatitis. The dosage is 1 to 2 tablets (each containing 382 mg of carbenicillin) qid.

Mezlocillin, azlocillin, and **piperacillin** are ureidopenicillins available only for parenteral use. Mezlocillin has a spectrum like ticarcillin but also has activity against many *Klebsiella* and *Serratia*. Azlocillin and piperacillin have spectrums similar to mezlocillin but are 4 to 8 times more active against *Pseudomonas*. The ureidopenicillins are more active against enterococci than the carboxypenicillins. As with carbenicillin and ticarcillin, the ureidopenicillins should be reserved mainly for serious infections; the dose is 250 mg/kg/day IV in divided doses q 4 h. These agents contain about 2 mEq of sodium/gm and are therefore less likely than carboxypenicillins to cause sodium loading. They are also less likely to interfere with platelet function.

CEPHALOSPORINS

First Generation	Second Generation	Third Generation
Cefadroxil*	Cefaclor*	Cefoperazone†
Cefazolin†	Cefamandole†	Cefotaxime†
Cephalexin*	Cefonicid†	Ceftizoxime†
Cephalothin†	Cefoxitin†	Ceftriaxone†
Cephapirin†	Cefuroxime†	Moxalactam†
Cephradine*†	Ceforanide†	Ceftazidime†

* Orally absorbed
† Parenteral

The cephalosporins are bactericidal agents with both gram-positive and gram-negative activity. They work by inhibiting bacterial cell wall synthesis in a manner similar to the penicillins and are widely distributed to most body fluids and tissues after administration. Concentrations in most body fluids are sufficient to treat infection, especially in the presence of inflammation (which enhances diffusion). However, penetration into the vitreous humor of the eye and into the CSF is relatively poor. Some of the cephalosporins (especially some of the 3rd generation cephalosporins) do achieve high enough CSF levels to treat meningitis.

Cephalosporins are reversibly bound to plasma protein and only the free agent is active. Cephalothin, cephapirin, and cefotaxime are metabolized to the desacetyl forms that in general have less antibacterial activity than the parent forms. Cefoperazone is excreted primarily in the bile. Ceftriaxone, although not excreted in the bile to the same extent as cefoperazone, is eliminated to a significant extent (33 to 67%) via this route. All of the other cephalosporins and their desacetyl metabolites (if any) are excreted mainly in the urine. Most of the cephalosporins are excreted by tubular secretion as well as glomerular filtration.

Indications

Although it is often stated that the cephalosporins are the drugs of choice for few infections, they have become the most widely used and recommended agents for many situations. Because of their relative safety and broad spectrum of activity, they are frequently recommended for prophylaxis for orthopedic, abdominal, and pelvic surgery and are often used in infections caused by gram-negative bacilli and gram-positive cocci. The cephalosporins have no advantages over the penicillins against gram-positive cocci, but do have definite advantages against gram-negative bacilli.

It is useful to classify the cephalosporins as first, second, and third generation. The **first-generation cephalosporins** are active against gram-positive cocci, with the exception of enterococci and both coagulase-positive and -negative staphylococci that are resistant to methicillin; they are also active against most strains of *E. coli*, *P. mirabilis*,

and *Klebsiella pneumoniae*. The **second-generation cephalosporins** have a somewhat expanded spectrum against gram-negative bacilli as detailed below.

The available **third-generation cephalosporins** have much greater activity against *E. coli*, *Klebsiella*, *Enterobacter*, *P. mirabilis*, indole-positive *Proteus*, and *Serratia*. Their in vitro activity against *P. aeruginosa* is comparable to that of ticarcillin, but their gram-positive activity is less than that of the first-generation cephalosporins. Their activity against anaerobic organisms is inferior to that of cefoxitin. Ceftazidime exhibits activity against Pseudomonas comparable to piperacillin. Ceftazidime, cefotaxime, ceftizoxime, ceftriaxone, and moxalactam penetrate sufficiently into the CSF for use in meningitis caused by highly susceptible *E. coli*, *Klebsiella*, *Enterobacter*, and *Proteus* and other gram-negative bacilli and are now considered the drugs of choice. Ceftazidime can also be used in Pseudomonas meningitis; however, cefotaxime, ceftizoxime, ceftriaxone, and moxalactam are not sufficiently effective. Ceftriaxone has a very long plasma half-life (8 h), and can be used in once-a-day dosage. It penetrates into the spinal fluid in high concentrations and has been used in therapy of meningitis (caused by *H. influenzae*, *N. meningitidis*, *S. pneumoniae*, and gram-negative enteric bacilli) in twice-a-day dosing.

Adverse Reactions

Pain at the site of IM injection and thrombophlebitis following IV use can occur with all cephalosporins. Hypersensitivity reactions such as rash, urticaria, and anaphylaxis seem to be less common with cephalosporins than with penicillins. Cross-sensitivity between cephalosporins and penicillins is probably uncommon, and cephalosporins can be given cautiously to patients with a history of delayed hypersensitivity to a penicillin. However, if there was an immediate reaction to a penicillin, cephalosporins should not be used.

Cephalothin in combination with gentamicin results in more nephrotoxicity than when gentamicin is used alone. All cephalosporins can produce pseudomembranous colitis (caused by *C. difficile*). Leukopenia, thrombocytopenia, and a positive Coombs' test can occur with cephalosporin therapy.

Cefamandole, moxalactam, and cefoperazone have a disulfiram-like effect and cause nausea and vomiting with ethanol ingestion; they can also cause elevations in the prothrombin time and partial thromboplastin time that is reversible with vitamin K. Moxalactam can also interfere, dose dependently, with platelet function.

Administration and Dosage

First-Generation Cephalosporins

These cephalosporins all have the same spectrum with the major differences being pharmacologic. All have good activity against all gram-positive cocci (except for enterococci and methicillin-resistant, coagulase-positive and negative-staphylococci), and most *E. coli*, *P. mirabilis*, and *K. pneumoniae*. Cephalexin, cephradine, and cefadroxil are well absorbed following oral administration. Because cefadroxil is excreted more slowly than the other two, it results in more sustained serum and urine levels. Of those used parenterally, cephalothin and cephapirin are equivalent pharmacologically. Cefazolin results in serum concentrations that are 3 times higher and more sustained than those of cephalothin or cephapirin, but it is more protein bound. Cephradine by IM injection results in serum concentrations equivalent to those achieved with the oral preparation. None of the first-generation cephalosporins can reach sufficient CSF concentrations to treat meningitis.

Cefadroxil is used orally in adults in a dose of 500 mg to 1 gm q 12 h. The dose in children is 30 mg/kg/day in 2 divided doses.

Cephalexin and **cephradine** are used orally in a dose of 250 mg to 1 gm q 6 h in adults and 25 to 100 mg/kg/day in 4 divided doses in children. Cephradine is used IM or IV

in doses of 2 to 8 gm/day in adults and 50 to 100 mg/kg/day in children in divided doses q 4 to 6 h.

Cephalothin and **cephapirin** are used IM or IV in doses of 0.5 to 2 gm q 4 to 6 h in adults. In children the dosage for cephalothin is 100 mg/kg/day and for cephapirin 40 to 80 mg/kg/day IM or IV in divided doses.

Cefazolin is used IM or IV in doses of 0.5 to 2 gm q 6 to 8 h in adults and 25 to 100 mg/kg/day in divided doses in children.

Second-Generation Cephalosporins

These cephalosporins differ in their antibacterial spectrum. Cefaclor, which is only available orally, has increased activity over first-generation cephalosporins against *H. influenzae*. Cefamandole, cefonicid, ceforanide, and cefuroxime, which are only available for parenteral use, have increased activity against *H. influenzae*, *E. coli*, and *Enterobacter* spp. Cefoxitin (which is actually a cephamycin) is more active than first-generation cephalosporins against indole-positive *Proteus*, *Serratia*, anaerobic gram-negative bacilli (including *B. fragilis*), and some *E. coli*, *Klebsiella*, and *P. mirabilis*. Cefuroxime is the only available second-generation cephalosporin that penetrates into the CSF sufficiently to be effective in meningitis (pneumococcal, meningococcal, *H. influenzae*, and *S. aureus*).

Cefaclor is used orally in doses of 0.25 to 0.5 gm q 8 h in adults and 20 to 40 mg/kg/day in divided doses in children.

Cefamandole is used IM or IV in doses of 500 mg to 2 gm q 4 to 8 h in adults and 50 to 150 mg/kg/day in divided doses in children. Cefamandole may elevate the prothrombin and partial thromboplastin time (reversible with vitamin K) and has an antabuse-like effect.

Cefonicid has a very long plasma half-life (4 h) and can be given once a day at a dosage of 0.5 to 2 gm IM or IV in adults.

Cefoxitin has more in vitro activity against anaerobic bacteria than any other cephalosporin available. It is active against most strains of *B. fragilis* and other *Bacteroides* spp. The adult dosage is 1 to 2 gm IM or IV q 4 to 8 h. In children the dose is 80 to 160 mg/kg/day in divided doses.

Cefuroxime is used IM or IV in doses of 750 mg to 1.5 gm q 6 to 8 h in adults and 50 to 100 mg/kg/day in divided doses in children. In bacterial meningitis, higher doses such as 3 gm IV q 8 h in adults and 200 to 240 mg/kg/day IV in children in divided doses are recommended.

Ceforanide has a long plasma half-life (2.9 h). The adult dose is 0.5 to 1 gm q 12 h IM or IV. In children the dose is 20 to 40 mg/kg/day in divided doses q 12 h.

Third-Generation Cephalosporins

These drugs have excellent activity against *Enterobacteriaceae*. Cefotaxime, ceftizoxime, and ceftriaxone have very similar in vitro activity and have good activity against many gram-positive cocci, but not as good as the first-generation cephalosporins, and moxalactam and cefoperazone are even less active against gram-positive cocci. Moxalactam has good activity against *B. fragilis*, but not as good as cefoxitin. Cefoperazone is less active than moxalactam, cefotaxime, ceftizoxime, or ceftriaxone against *Enterobacteriaceae* but is more active against *Pseudomonas aeruginosa*. Spinal fluid levels of cefotaxime, ceftizoxime, ceftriaxone, ceftazidime, and moxalactam (but not cefoperazone) are sufficient to treat meningitis caused by highly susceptible organisms. In general, meningitis caused by *H. influenzae*, meningococci, and *Enterobacteriaceae* can be treated with cefotaxime, ceftriaxone, ceftazidime, ceftizoxime, and moxalactam. Pneumococcal meningitis can be treated with cefotaxime, ceftizoxime, and ceftriaxone but not moxalactam because of greater resistance of pneumococci to moxalactam.

Cefoperazone differs from the other available cephalosporins in being excreted pri-

AMINOGLYCOSIDES

Streptomycin	Gentamicin	Amikacin
Neomycin	Tobramycin	Netilmicin
Kanamycin		

The aminoglycosides are bactericidal antibiotics that bind to the 30S ribosome and inhibit bacterial protein synthesis. They are active only against aerobic gram-negative bacilli and staphylococci. Activity against streptococci and anaerobes is poor. Aminoglycosides have been used in combination with a penicillin in enterococcal endocarditis. Neomycin and kanamycin have a limited antibacterial spectrum and are more toxic than the other aminoglycosides. Neomycin should not be used parenterally. Kanamycin is used to a limited extent parenterally.

Pharmacology

All of the aminoglycosides have similar pharmacokinetic properties. They are poorly absorbed orally and must be used parenterally for systemic infection.

As the aminoglycosides are toxic and are absorbed from areas of denuded skin, such as burns, it is important to be cautious even in their topical use. They are absorbed well from the peritoneum, pleural cavity, and joints and *should never be instilled in these cavities.*

After injection, the aminoglycosides are distributed mainly in the ECF. Protein binding is low. Even in the presence of inflammation, concentrations in tissues and secretions are much less than plasma levels. The major exceptions are urine, the otic perilymph, and renal cortical tissue, which selectively binds aminoglycosides resulting in concentrations higher than in plasma. In the presence of inflammation, levels > 50% of serum concentrations can be achieved in synovial, pleural, pericardial, and peritoneal fluids. Levels in bile are 25 to 75% of those in serum. With biliary obstruction, levels are much lower. Penetration of aminoglycosides into the eye, CSF, and respiratory secretions is poor even with inflammation. When aminoglycosides are used to treat meningitis, in addition to IV administration, it is necessary to give intrathecal injections to achieve adequate therapeutic spinal fluid levels.

Aminoglycosides are excreted unchanged into the urine by glomerular filtration. They all have the same half-life in plasma of 2 to 3 h. With renal insufficiency the half-life rises markedly. In order to avoid toxic blood levels, it is essential to modify the maintenance dosages of aminoglycosides in patients with renal insufficiency—either by decreasing the dose or increasing the interval between doses, or both.

Because of the distribution properties of aminoglycosides, dosing in obese patients should be based on a weight equal to lean body wt plus 50% of the adipose mass. In patients with excessive ECF as in edema, the dose should be calculated based on total body wt. Patients with burns and cystic fibrosis have decreased plasma levels and may require higher doses. Anemia tends to increase plasma levels.

Aminoglycosides are inactivated in vitro by antipseudomonal penicillins (eg, carbenicillin) and the 2 agents should not be mixed together in vitro. In vivo inactivation of the aminoglycoside can occur in patients with renal failure receiving both a penicillin and aminoglycoside with long intervals between doses of aminoglycoside.

Indications

With the exception of streptomycin, which has a more limited antimicrobial spectrum, all aminoglycosides have good activity against gram-negative aerobic bacilli but lack activity against anaerobes. Neomycin and kanamycin lack activity against *P. aeruginosa*, whereas gentamicin, tobramycin, amikacin, and netilmicin have good activity against this organism. The aminoglycosides are active against staphylococci but not against streptococci, including pneumococci.

Streptomycin has limited uses because of the resistance of many bacteria. It is used

marily in the bile. It is associated with an antabuse-like reaction and with elevated prothrombin and partial thromboplastin times reversible with vitamin K. The adult dose is 2 to 6 gm/day IM or IV in divided doses q 6 to 12 h. However, doses up to 12 gm/day have been used.

Cefotaxime is given IM or IV in doses of 1 to 2 gm q 4 to 6 h to adults and 50 to 180 mg/kg/day in divided doses in children.

Ceftizoxime is given IM or IV to adults in doses of 1 to 2 gm q 6 to 8 h and to children in doses of 50 to 200 mg/kg/day in divided doses.

Ceftriaxone is given IM or IV in a dose of 1 to 2 gm once or twice a day to adults. In children 50 to 75 mg/kg/day (not to exceed 2.0 gm) is given in 2 equally divided doses. In children with meningitis, 100 mg/kg/day (not to exceed 4.0 gm) is given in divided doses q 12 h. For uncomplicated gonorrhea a single IM dose of 250 mg is used.

Moxalactam has been associated with an antabuse-like reaction and also with elevated prothrombin and partial thromboplastin times. It can also interfere with platelet function. It is recommended that patients who receive moxalactam be given vitamin K 10 mg/wk prophylactically. As the platelet dysfunction is dose-related, bleeding times should be monitored in patients with normal renal function who receive > 4 gm of moxalactam/day for > 3 days or in any patient with impaired renal function. Moxalactam is given IM or IV in doses of 500 mg to 2 gm q 6 to 12 h to adults, but as much as 12 gm/day has been used. In children doses are 50 mg/kg q 6 to 8 h; up to 200 mg/kg/day in divided doses has been used.

Ceftazidime is given IM or IV in doses of 1 to 2 gm q 8 to 12 h in adults and 30 to 50 mg/kg q 8 h (not to exceed 6 gm each day) in children.

Other Beta-Lactam Antibiotics

Imipenem is an extremely active parenteral antibiotic with a spectrum against almost all gram-positive and -negative organisms, both aerobic and anaerobic. Enterococci, *Bacteroides fragilis*, and *Pseudomonas aeruginosa* are susceptible. However, most strains of methicillin-resistant staphylococci are resistant.

Imipenem is formulated with cilastatin sodium, a substance that was developed in order to inhibit the renal metabolism of imipenem and maintain adequate antibacterial levels. Imipenem-cilastatin is given IV in a dose of 0.5 to 1.0 gm q 6 h in adults and children 12 yr or older.

Aztreonam is a parenteral antibiotic with excellent activity against gram-negative aerobic bacilli including *P. aeruginosa*. Gram-positive organisms and anaerobes are resistant to aztreonam.

Clavulanic acid has poor antibiotic activity but inhibits the beta-lactamases produced by many bacteria. It is absorbed orally and can be given parenterally also. When used in combination with amoxicillin orally or ticarcillin parenterally these agents become effective against certain organisms that otherwise are resistant; eg, amoxicillin plus clavulanic acid is effective against beta-lactamase producing staphylococci and *H. influenzae* (see above under PENICILLINS).

Cefotetan, a cephamycin antibiotic, has in vitro activity against gram-negative bacteria similar to that of cefotaxime and moxalactam, but it is less active against *Enterobacter aerogenes*, and has no useful activity against *Pseudomonas*. Cefotetan has activity against gram-positive organisms similar to that of moxalactam, but is significantly less active against pneumococci. Activity against anaerobes is similar to that of cefotaxime.

The proper dosage of cefotetan and route of administration should be determined by the condition of the patient, severity of the infection, and susceptibility of the causative organism. The usual adult dosage is 1 or 2 gm IV or IM q 12 h for 5 to 10 days.

for brucellosis, tularemia, and plague. It is also a companion drug with isoniazid and rifampin in the treatment of TB and with penicillin or vancomycin in the treatment or prophylaxis of streptococcal endocarditis.

Neomycin and **kanamycin** should be limited to oral or topical (eye, ear) use because of toxicity. They are used orally for bowel preparation before surgery or in the treatment of hepatic coma to reduce GI bacterial populations and ammonia production. Topical use should be limited to small amounts in small areas, since absorption and toxicity can occur.

Gentamicin, tobramycin, amikacin, and **netilmicin** should be used only in the treatment of serious gram-negative bacillary infection. Gentamicin is also used as a companion drug with a penicillin or vancomycin in the treatment of enterococcal or *S. aureus* endocarditis or in prophylaxis of enterococcal endocarditis. Gentamicin and tobramycin are very similar in antimicrobial activity against gram-negative bacilli with only two differences: Tobramycin is more active against *P. aeruginosa*, and gentamicin is more active against *S. marcescens*.

Resistance of gram-negative bacilli to gentamicin and tobramycin has occurred in some hospitals, and such infections in these institutions cannot be treated with these agents. The resistance is most commonly due to a plasmid-mediated enzymatic alteration of the aminoglycoside.

Amikacin has the same spectrum of activity as gentamicin and tobramycin but is less susceptible to enzymatic inactivation. Therefore, amikacin has great value in the management of infections caused by gram-negative bacilli resistant to gentamicin and tobramycin. Amikacin should probably be reserved for use in these resistant infections. Resistance to amikacin usually means resistance to all currently available aminoglycosides.

Netilmicin has the same spectrum of activity as gentamicin and tobramycin. It is less susceptible to enzymatic alteration than gentamicin or tobramycin but more susceptible than amikacin. It seems to have no advantages over the other agents.

Adverse Reactions

All aminoglycosides are **nephrotoxic** and **ototoxic**. Aminoglycosides can cause **paresthesias** and **peripheral neuropathy. Hypersensitivity reactions** may occasionally occur.

Neomycin and kanamycin are more toxic than the other aminoglycosides and should no longer be used parenterally. Furthermore, large oral doses of neomycin or kanamycin (eg, 12 gm/day) can produce a **malabsorption syndrome**. In addition, although oral absorption is poor, enough can be absorbed to produce renal or ototoxicity with prolonged use, especially in patients with renal insufficiency. Streptomycin has very little nephrotoxicity. Gentamicin may be more nephrotoxic than tobramycin, amikacin, and netilmicin. Nephrotoxicity is reversible and is more likely to occur with large doses, high blood levels, or long duration of therapy, and in elderly patients, those with preexisting renal disease, those who are dehydrated, and those receiving furosemide or cephalothin.

Streptomycin and gentamicin are more likely to produce vestibular damage than hearing loss, whereas amikacin, netilmicin, and kanamycin are more likely to produce hearing loss than vestibular damage. Vestibular damage from streptomycin is common with prolonged use and in patients with impaired renal function. The symptoms and signs are vertigo, nausea, vomiting, nystagmus, and loss of equilibrium. Tobramycin affects vestibular and auditory function equally. The 8th nerve toxicity is often *irreversible* and is more likely to occur with larger doses, higher blood levels, or longer duration of therapy and in elderly patients, those with renal insufficiency, those with preexisting auditory impairment, and those receiving ethacrynic acid, furosemide, or bumetanide. Patients receiving aminoglycosides for longer than 2 wk or those with known potentiating factors for ototoxicity should be monitored with serial audiograms.

Administration and Dosage

Streptomycin is given IM in doses of 0.5 to 1 gm q 12 h to adults and 10 to 20 mg/kg q 12 h to children in therapy of infections other than TB. For TB in adults, 1 gm is usually given once/day for several months and thereafter 2 to 3 times/wk.

Neomycin is available for topical, oral, and rectal use and as a bladder irrigant. The oral or rectal dose is 1 to 2 gm q 6 h.

Kanamycin, no longer recommended for parenteral use, is used orally in a dose of 8 to 12 gm/day in divided doses.

Gentamicin and **tobramycin** are given IM or IV in a dose of 1 to 1.7 mg/kg q 8 h in adults and 2 to 2.5 mg/kg q 8 h in children. For treatment of meningitis, gentamicin is given intrathecally 10 mg once a day in adults and 1 to 2 mg once a day in small children. Gentamicin is also available for topical use.

Amikacin 15 mg/kg/day in divided doses is given IM or IV bid in adults and children.

Netilmicin 3 to 6.5 mg/kg/day is given IM or IV in 2 or 3 equally divided doses in adults or children.

To minimize the possibility of ototoxic and nephrotoxic reactions, dosage should be decreased in patients with impaired renal function. Following a normal loading dose (1.0 to 1.7 mg/kg for gentamicin or tobramycin or 7.5 mg/kg for amikacin), smaller doses can be given at the customary intervals or normal doses can be given at increased intervals. It is probably best to give decreased doses at normal or somewhat increased intervals to avoid long time periods with subtherapeutic blood levels. Nomograms are available to calculate dosages based on serum creatinine or creatinine clearance values, but they are inaccurate. With changing renal function no nomogram will give useful information. The simplest method is to give the loading dose and then, as maintenance doses, to give the loading dose divided by the serum creatinine value (assuming a stable creatinine) at the usual intervals.

The best approach is to give the usual loading dose and then a 2nd dose estimated on the basis of a nomogram. Serum concentrations should be measured just before (trough) and 60 min after the 2nd and periodic subsequent IM doses or 30 min after the 2nd and periodic subsequent 30-min infusions of the drug. The peak concentration is the level 60 min after an IM injection and is equivalent to the level 30 min after the end of a 30-min infusion. Doses should be adjusted to give serum peak levels of 4 to 8 μg/mL for gentamicin and tobramycin, 16 to 25 μg/mL for amikacin, and 5 to 10 μg/mL for netilmicin. Troughs > 2 μg/mL for gentamicin, tobramycin, and netilmicin, and > 5 μg/mL for amikacin indicate retention of drug and a greater chance of toxicity. Therapy must be aimed at achieving adequate peak levels q 8 h for gentamicin, tobramycin, and netilmicin, and q 12 h for amikacin. When doses are adjusted and serum levels are stable, levels can be measured every other day or twice/wk.

IV injections of aminoglycosides should always be given slowly and these agents should *never be injected into a body cavity*, since neuromuscular blockade with respiratory arrest can occur. This complication is especially likely in patients with myasthenia gravis or in those receiving curare-like drugs and is reversible with neostigmine or IV administration of calcium.

ERYTHROMYCIN, LINCOMYCIN, AND CLINDAMYCIN

Lincomycin and clindamycin are similar in structure and activity. Erythromycin, lincomycin, and clindamycin are absorbed when taken orally and can also be given parenterally. All are primarily bacteriostatic agents that work by binding to the 50S subunit of the ribosome thus inhibiting bacterial protein synthesis.

These agents are active against aerobic and anaerobic gram-positive cocci, with the exception of enterococci, and also have activity against gram-negative anaerobes.

Pharmacology

Following oral or parenteral administration these agents diffuse well into body fluids, with the exception of CSF. Excretion is mainly in the bile and dosage adjustments are not required in the presence of renal failure.

Indications

Erythromycin is active against gram-positive cocci (including anaerobes), with the exception of enterococci; but many *S. aureus* strains are now resistant and it should not be used in serious *S. aureus* infection. Erythromycin is also active against *Mycoplasma pneumoniae, Chlamydia trachomatis, Legionella pneumophila* and other *Legionella, Corynebacterium diphtheriae, Campylobacter,* and *Treponema pallidum.* Erythromycin is the substitute of choice in group A streptococcal and pneumococcal infections when penicillin cannot be used. It should not be used to treat meningitis. It is the drug of choice in *M. pneumoniae* and *Legionella* infection, in *C. diphtheriae* carriers, and in *Campylobacter* gastroenteritis. Although it has activity against anaerobic gram-negative bacilli, its activity is much less than that of clindamycin. Erythromycin has been used orally in combination with an oral aminoglycoside as a bowel preparation before GI tract surgery.

Clindamycin has a similar spectrum to that of erythromycin, except that it has poor activity against *Mycoplasma.* It is *not* a reliable drug in serious *S. aureus* infection. The major advantage of clindamycin over erythromycin is its much greater activity against anaerobic bacteria, especially *Bacteroides* sp (including *B. fragilis*). The principal use of clindamycin is in serious infections caused by anaerobic microorganisms, especially when *B. fragilis* is likely to be present. Clindamycin cannot be used in CNS infection because penetration into the brain and spinal fluid is poor.

Lincomycin has a spectrum similar to that of clindamycin but it is less active and is not as well absorbed after oral intake. Therefore, clindamycin is the preferable agent.

Adverse Reactions

Erythromycin commonly causes GI tract disturbances, including nausea, vomiting, and diarrhea. Cholestatic jaundice occurs with erythromycin estolate and less often with erythromycin ethylsuccinate. The jaundice usually appears after 10 days of administration but can occur earlier if the agent has been given previously. Erythromycin is not given IM because of severe pain and it may cause phlebitis when used IV. Hypersensitivity reactions are rare. Transient auditory impairment has rarely been noted with IV use of erythromycin or large oral doses of the estolate.

Clindamycin and lincomycin can cause diarrhea, which is sometimes severe. Pseudomembranous colitis due to *C. difficile,* may result. Hypersensitivity reactions may occur with lincomycin and clindamycin.

Administration and Dosage

Erythromycin base, estolate, ethylsuccinate, and **stearate** can all be given orally in adult doses of 250 mg to 1 gm q 6 h. The dose in children is 30 to 100 mg/kg/day in divided doses. IV therapy is rarely required, but when necessary (as in severe Legionnaires' disease), continuous infusion is preferred; however, intermittent infusion (over 20 to 60 min) at intervals not more than q 6 h is also effective. **Erythromycin lactobionate** and **gluceptate** are used IV in doses of 15 to 20 mg/kg/day in 4 divided doses. Up to 4 gm/day have been used in very severe infections in adults.

Clindamycin is used orally in doses of 150 to 450 mg q 6 h in adults and 8 to 20 mg/kg/day in 4 divided doses in children. The IM or IV dosage is 600 mg to 2700 mg/day in adults and 15 mg to 40 mg/kg/day in children in 3 or 4 equal doses.

Lincomycin has been superseded by clindamycin, which has better activity and absorption. The oral dose of lincomycin is 500 mg q 6 to 8 h in adults and 30 to 60 mg/kg/day in children in 3 or 4 divided doses. The usual IM dose is 600 mg q 12 to 24

h in adults and 10 mg/kg q 12 to 24 h in children. The usual IV dose is 600 mg q 8 to 12 h in adults and 10 to 20 mg/kg/day in divided doses in children.

TETRACYCLINES

Oxytetracycline	Demeclocycline	Doxycycline
Tetracycline	Methacycline	Minocycline

These drugs are closely related bacteriostatic antibiotics, similar in antibacterial spectrum and toxicity. They work by binding to the 30S subunit of the ribosome and inhibiting bacterial protein synthesis. They are effective against many α-hemolytic streptococci, nonhemolytic streptococci, gram-negative rods, rickettsias, spirochetes, *E. histolytica*, *Mycoplasma*, and *Chlamydia*. Tetracycline-resistant strains of pneumococci account for about 5% of isolates from pneumococcal pneumonia patients. Infections due to Group A β-hemolytic streptococci should not be treated with a tetracycline, since as many as 25% of the organisms may be resistant when tested in vitro. Serious staphylococcal disease is also not a primary indication for tetracyclines. Bacterial resistance to one tetracycline is generally accompanied by cross resistance to the others.

Pharmacology

The tetracyclines are variably absorbed after oral administration. About 60 to 80% of oxytetracycline, demeclocycline, and tetracycline and 95% or more of doxycycline and minocycline are absorbed. Food interferes with absorption of tetracyclines with the exception of doxycycline and minocycline. Absorption of tetracyclines is decreased in the presence of antacids containing Al, Ca, and Mg, and preparations containing Fe. The half-lives in plasma are about 8 h for oxytetracycline and tetracycline; 16 h for demeclocycline and methacycline; and 17 to 20 h for doxycycline and minocycline.

Tetracyclines penetrate into most tissues and body fluids. However, CSF levels are not reliably therapeutic. Minocycline, because of its high lipid solubility, is the only tetracycline that penetrates into tears and saliva in levels high enough to eradicate the meningococcal carrier state. All tetracyclines, except doxycycline, are excreted primarily in the urine by glomerular filtration, and their blood levels increase in the presence of renal insufficiency. Doxycycline is excreted mainly in the feces. All tetracyclines are partially excreted in bile resulting in high biliary levels. They are then partially reabsorbed.

Indications

Tetracyclines are primarily used in treating UTI, rickettsial infections, chlamydial infections, *Mycoplasma* infections, acute exacerbations of chronic bronchitis, shigellosis, brucellosis, granuloma inguinale, and chancroid, and as alternative therapy to penicillin in gonorrhea and syphilis. Penicillinase-producing gonococci are relatively resistant to tetracycline.

Adverse Reactions

All orally administered tetracyclines produce varying degrees of GI side effects such as nausea, vomiting, and diarrhea, and can cause pseudomembranous (*C. difficile*) colitis. With IV use thrombophlebitis is common. Tetracyclines can cause staining of teeth, hypoplasia of dental enamel, and abnormal bone growth in children < 8 yr and in the fetuses of pregnant women. *Therefore, tetracyclines should be avoided after the 1st trimester of pregnancy and in children < 8 yr of age.* In infants, pseudotumor cerebri with increased intracranial pressure and bulging fontanelles may occur.

All tetracyclines have an antianabolic effect and increase protein breakdown. In patients with renal insufficiency this can result in worsening of uremia by increasing

the urea and acid load to the kidney. Outdated tetracyclines can degenerate and cause a Fanconi syndrome. With excessive blood levels resulting from large doses, IV use, or renal insufficiency, fatal acute fatty degeneration of the liver may occur, especially during pregnancy. Tetracyclines (especially demeclocycline) can cause photosensitivity. Demeclocycline also can cause nephrogenic diabetes insipidus. Minocycline commonly causes vertigo.

Administration and Dosage

Oxytetracycline and **tetracycline** are therapeutically equivalent, but tetracycline is by far the most commonly used. Both are usually given orally in doses of 250 to 500 mg q 6 h to adults and 25 to 50 mg/kg/day in 4 divided doses to children. IM injection is very painful and the IV route is preferred for parenteral therapy. Tetracycline can be given IV in doses of 250 to 500 mg (rarely 1 gm) q 12 h to adults and 10 to 20 mg/kg/day in 2 equal doses to children. These agents are available as ointments for ophthalmic and other topical use.

Demeclocycline and **methacycline** are used orally 600 mg/day in adults and 6 to 12 mg/kg/day in children in 2 to 4 divided doses.

Doxycycline is used orally or IV in adults in a dose of 200 mg in 2 divided doses on the first day and thereafter, 100 mg/day in a single daily dose or 2 divided doses; 100 mg q 12 h for the entire course of therapy has also been used. In children 5 mg/kg/day divided in 2 doses is given orally or IV on the first day and thereafter 2.5 mg/kg/day as a single daily dose or divided in 2 doses; 5 mg/kg/day divided in 2 doses has also been used for the whole course of therapy. Doxycycline is the only tetracycline that is excreted normally in renal failure.

Minocycline is given orally or IV in a dose of 200 mg followed by 100 mg q 12 h in adults. In children, the dose is 4 mg/kg followed by 2 mg/kg q 12 h orally or IV. For the meningococcal carrier state 100 mg orally q 12 h for 5 days has been successful in adults, but vestibular dysfunction is common especially in women.

MISCELLANEOUS ANTIMICROBIALS

CHLORAMPHENICOL

Chloramphenicol is primarily bacteriostatic. It binds to the 50S subunit of the ribosome and inhibits bacterial protein synthesis. It has a wide spectrum of activity against gram-positive and -negative cocci and bacilli (including anaerobes), *Rickettsia*, *Mycoplasma*, and *Chlamydia*. Chloramphenicol therapy should be restricted to serious infections when other agents are not as effective or are more toxic. The major reason for restricting its use is the rare but potentially lethal complication of aplastic anemia.

Pharmacology: Chloramphenicol is well absorbed orally but not IM. Parenteral therapy should be IV. The drug is distributed widely in body fluids and therapeutic concentrations are achieved in CSF. It is metabolized in the liver to the inactive glucuronide. Both chloramphenicol and the glucuronide metabolite are excreted in the urine. Because of hepatic metabolism, active chloramphenicol does not accumulate in the plasma of patients with renal insufficiency.

Indications: Chloramphenicol is one of the drugs of choice in the following infections: (1) typhoid fever and other serious *Salmonella* infections; (2) meningitis caused by *H. influenzae* resistant to ampicillin or when ampicillin or a third-generation cephalosporin cannot be used; (3) meningococcal or pneumococcal meningitis in a penicillin allergic patient; (4) serious infection caused by *B. fragilis* (including CNS infection); and (5) rickettsial infection not responding to tetracycline or in which tetracycline cannot be used. Chloramphenicol is effective (bactericidal) in *H. influen-*

zae, meningococcal, and pneumococcal meningitis. It is only bacteriostatic and relatively ineffective in meningitis caused by *E. coli* and other *Enterobacteriaceae*.

Adverse reactions: Two types of bone marrow depression may be caused by chloramphenicol, a reversible dose-related interference with Fe metabolism, and an irreversible idiosyncratic form of aplastic anemia. The **reversible form**, which is particularly likely to occur with high doses, a prolonged course, and in patients with liver disease, is manifested by increased serum Fe, increased saturation of iron-binding capacity, decreased reticulocytes, vacuolization of RBC precursors, anemia, leukopenia, and thrombocytopenia.

Irreversible idiosyncratic aplastic anemia occurs in < 1:25,000 patients given chloramphenicol. The onset may be delayed until after therapy has been discontinued. There may be a genetic predisposition.

Optic neuritis and peripheral neuropathy may be seen with prolonged use of chloramphenicol. Nausea, vomiting, and diarrhea may occur. Hypersensitivity reactions are uncommon.

The **gray baby syndrome** (see in ANTIMICROBIAL THERAPY FOR NEWBORNS in NEONATAL INFECTIONS in Ch. 186), which is often fatal, occurs in neonates given standard doses of chloramphenicol. It is related to high blood levels resulting from an inability of the immature liver to metabolize chloramphenicol.

Administration and dosage: The dose of chloramphenicol in adults and children is 50 mg/kg/day orally or IV in divided doses q 6 h. In meningitis and occasionally other serious infections, 100 mg/kg/day in divided doses are used. Children 1 mo of age or less should not be given > 25 mg/kg/day to avoid the gray baby syndrome. Chloramphenicol should not be given to women in labor.

Chloramphenicol should not be used topically because small amounts may be absorbed and possibly cause aplastic anemia.

VANCOMYCIN

Vancomycin is a bactericidal antibiotic that inhibits cell wall synthesis. It is active against all gram-positive cocci and bacilli, including *S. aureus* and *S. epidermidis* strains that are resistant to penicillins and cephalosporins. Vancomycin also has bacteriostatic activity against enterococci. All gram-negative bacilli are resistant to vancomycin.

Pharmacology: Vancomycin is not absorbed orally and must be given IV for treatment of systemic illness. It penetrates into body fluids including pleural, pericardial, synovial, ascitic, and CSF. Therapeutic levels are found in bile. It is excreted unchanged by glomerular filtration; therefore, it is retained in the presence of renal insufficiency. Serum concentrations must be measured and doses decreased in patients with decreased renal function.

Indications: Vancomycin is the agent of choice in treating serious infections caused by gram-positive organisms resistant to penicillins and cephalosporins (eg, *S. aureus* and *S. epidermidis* resistant to methicillin). Vancomycin is also the drug of choice for serious staphylococcal infection and endocarditis caused by viridans streptococci or enterococci when penicillins or cephalosporins cannot be used because of drug allergy. For treating enterococcal endocarditis, an aminoglycoside must be used concurrently with vancomycin.

Vancomycin orally is an agent of choice in *Clostridium difficile* colitis (antibiotic-associated colitis) and *S. aureus* enterocolitis.

Adverse reactions: Common side effects are phlebitis and chills and fever during IV infusion. Rash may be seen. Nephrotoxicity occurs occasionally, and deafness may be associated with very high blood levels, usually in patients with renal insufficiency.

When used in patients with impaired renal function, blood levels should be monitored to keep peak plasma concentrations below 30 μg/mL.

Infusion should be slow to avoid the "red-neck syndrome," in which there is a flushing of the skin on the neck and shoulder area, malaise, and a shock-like state.

Administration and dosage: The dose in adults is 500 mg IV q 6 h or 1 gm q 12 h. In children the dose is 44 mg/kg/day IV in divided doses. Infusions should be given over at least 30 min and preferably 60 min. The oral dose for *C. difficile* colitis is 125 to 500 mg q 6 h in adults and 44 mg/kg/day in 4 equally divided doses in children.

In patients with renal failure requiring dialysis, 0.5 to 1 gm of vancomycin given IV **once/week** will provide therapeutic levels.

Metronidazole

Metronidazole is a microbicidal agent that is active only against protozoa, such as *Giardia lamblia*, *Entamoeba histolytica*, and *Trichomonas vaginalis* (see Protozoal Diseases in Ch. 13; also Trichomoniasis in Ch. 14) and strictly anaerobic bacteria. It is not active against aerobic or microaerophilic bacteria.

Pharmacology: Metronidazole is absorbed well when given orally. It is distributed widely in body fluids and penetrates into the CSF in high concentrations. Metronidazole and its metabolites are excreted mainly in the urine.

Indications: Metronidazole is used mainly in the treatment of protozoal infections and in serious infections caused by anaerobes, particularly *B. fragilis*, that are resistant to other antimicrobial agents. Metronidazole has also been used successfully in treating *Gardnerella* vaginitis and Crohn's disease. The major use in infections caused by anaerobes is in intra-abdominal and pelvic infections. Metronidazole has poor activity against microaerophilic gram-positive cocci, and therefore, it is not very effective in lung abscess. It is effective in the treatment of meningitis or brain abscess caused by susceptible anaerobes. It has also been used for prophylaxis of infections associated with bowel surgery and in treatment of *C. difficile* colitis.

Adverse reactions: These include nausea, vomiting, headache, seizures, syncope, other CNS reactions, and peripheral neuropathy. Rash, fever, and reversible neutropenia have been reported. Metronidazole has caused cancer in mice and rats, but the risk to humans is unknown. A disulfiram-like reaction may occur if alcohol is ingested.

Administration and dosage: The oral dose in adults for anaerobic bacterial infection is 7.5 mg/kg q 6 h. The IV dose in adults with anaerobic bacterial infection is 15 mg/kg followed by 7.5 mg/kg q 6 h. An oral dose of 250 mg qid for 10 days has been used in adults with *C. difficile* colitis. For *Gardnerella* vaginitis 500 mg orally bid for 7 days is usual. An oral daily dose of 800 mg in divided doses has been used in adults with Crohn's disease.

Rifampin (RMP)

RMP is an antibiotic that inhibits DNA-dependent RNA polymerase leading to suppression of RNA synthesis. It has a very broad spectrum of activity against most gram-positive and -negative organisms (including *Pseudomonas aeruginosa*) and *Mycobacterium* sp. Because of rapid emergence of resistant bacteria, use of RMP is restricted to treatment of mycobacterial infections (see Tuberculosis in Ch. 8) and relatively few other indications as listed below.

Pharmacology: RMP is well absorbed when taken orally and distributed widely in body tissues and fluids including the CSF. It is metabolized in the liver and eliminated in the bile, and to a much lesser extent, in the urine, but dose adjustments are not necessary in the presence of renal insufficiency.

Indications: RMP and isoniazid are major drugs in TB therapy. RMP is also an important agent in therapy of atypical mycobacterial infection and leprosy.

In nonmycobacterial infection the indications are limited. RMP is the drug of choice for eradication of the meningococcal and *H. influenzae* (Type B) carrier state in prevention of meningitis caused by these organisms. It may also be useful in combination with a penicillin, cephalosporin, or vancomycin in therapy of staphylococcal endocarditis and staphylococcal osteomyelitis. RMP has been effective when used along with a penicillin or cephalosporin in eradicating the nasal carrier state in patients with recurrent staphylococcal furunculosis.

Adverse reactions: Heartburn, nausea, vomiting, and diarrhea may occur. CNS effects such as headache, drowsiness, ataxia, and confusion have been reported. Rash, fever, thrombocytopenia, leukopenia, and hemolytic anemia all occur and are thought to be related to hypersensitivity. The most serious side effect is hepatitis, which occurs much more often when isoniazid and RMP are used together than when either is used alone. Renal insufficiency thought to be due to hypersensitivity has occurred. RMP stains the urine, saliva, sweat, and tears an orange color.

RMP has many drug interactions (see under TUBERCULOSIS in Ch. 8).

Administration and dosage: The dose to eliminate the meningococcal carrier state is 600 mg orally bid for 2 days in adults and 10 mg/kg bid for 2 days in children. To liminate the *H. influenzae* (Type B) carrier state, 600 mg/day orally is continued for 4 days in adults. In children 20 mg/kg/day is given orally in one dose each day for 4 days. For staphylococcal infections 300 mg orally bid has been used in combination with a penicillin, a cephalosporin, or vancomycin.

ISONIAZID AND ETHAMBUTOL

Isoniazid and ethambutol are discussed under TUBERCULOSIS in Ch. 8.

SPECTINOMYCIN

Spectinomycin is a bactericidal antibiotic that binds to the 30S subunit of the ribosome thus inhibiting bacterial protein synthesis. It is used only in the treatment of gonococcal infections and should be reserved for patients allergic to penicillin, for the treatment of infections caused by *N. gonorrhoeae* that produce penicillinase, and for patients who fail to respond to therapy with penicillin, ampicillin, amoxicillin, or tetracycline. Spectinomycin is not effective in gonococcal pharyngitis.

A single IM dose of 2 gm is given for gonococcal urethritis, cervicitis, and proctitis. Side effects other than hypersensitivity reactions and fever are rare with the dose used. Spectinomycin is excreted by glomerular filtration.

POLYPEPTIDES

Polymyxin B   Colistin   Bacitracin

Polymyxin B and **colistin (polymyxin E)** are toxic and *their use should be restricted to topical application*, particularly since there are safer and more effective agents available (eg, aminoglycosides and antipseudomonal penicillins). They are bactericidal antibiotics with activity against gram-negative aerobic bacilli including *Pseudomonas aeruginosa*. Polymyxin B and colistin are not active against *Proteus* spp and have no activity against gram-positive organisms. Both act by disrupting the bacterial cell membrane.

Polymyxin B and colistin are not absorbed when given orally. They are used topically (eg, ear, eye, urinary bladder).

Bacitracin is a bactericidal antibiotic active only against gram-positive organisms,

and a few gram-negative organisms such as gonococci and meningococci. It inhibits cell wall synthesis and is nephrotoxic and should not be used parenterally. It is commonly used topically and is effective orally in treatment of *C. difficile* colitis.

SULFONAMIDES

The sulfonamides are synthetic bacteriostatic antimicrobial agents with a wide antibacterial spectrum encompassing most gram-positive and many gram-negative organisms. Especially among the latter, however, many strains of an individual species may be resistant. Sulfonamides inhibit multiplication of bacteria by acting as competitive inhibitors of para-aminobenzoic acid in the folic acid metabolism cycle. Bacterial sensitivity is the same for the various sulfonamides, and cross-resistance is absolute.

Most sulfonamides are absorbed rapidly and well by mouth, the small intestine being the major site of absorption. Parenteral administration is difficult, since the soluble sulfonamide salts are highly alkaline and irritating to the tissues.

Pharmacology

The sulfonamides are widely distributed throughout all tissues. High levels are achieved in pleural, peritoneal, synovial, and ocular fluids. CSF levels are effective in meningeal infections. When given in pregnancy, high levels are achieved in the fetus. Sulfonamides are loosely and reversibly bound in varying degrees to serum albumin. Since the bound sulfonamide is inactive and nondiffusible, the degree of binding can affect antibacterial effectiveness, distribution, and excretion. The antibacterial action of sulfonamides is inhibited by pus.

The sulfonamides are metabolized mainly by the liver to acetylated forms and glucuronides, both therapeutically inactive. Excretion is primarily renal by glomerular filtration with minimal tubular secretion or reabsorption.

The relative insolubility of most sulfonamides, especially their acetylated metabolites, may cause them to precipitate in the renal tubules. The more soluble analogs, such as sulfisoxazole and sulfamethoxazole, should be chosen for systemic therapy, and the patient must be well hydrated. To avoid crystalluria and renal damage, fluid intake should be sufficient to produce a urinary output of 1200 to 1500 mL/day. Sulfonamides should not be used in the presence of renal insufficiency.

Indications

Sulfonamides are currently used in only specific circumstances. These are (1) UTI; (2) nocardiosis; (3) in combination with pyrimethamine in the treatment of toxoplasmosis; (4) as a substitute for penicillin in prophylaxis of rheumatic fever; (5) as prophylaxis against susceptible meningococcal strains; (6) as sulfasalazine in ulcerative colitis; (7) as silver sulfadiazine or mafenide in burns; (8) in chloroquine-resistant *Plasmodium falciparum* infection; (9) for dermatitis herpetiformis; and (10) in combination with trimethoprim (see below).

Sulfisoxazole and sulfamethoxazole are the major agents used for UTI. Sulfadiazine is rarely used because of the danger of crystalluria.

Adverse Reactions

These include (1) GI reactions, such as nausea, vomiting, and diarrhea; (2) hypersensitivity reactions, such as rashes, the Stevens-Johnson syndrome (see ERYTHEMA MULTIFORME in Ch. 237), vasculitis, serum sickness, anaphylaxis, and angioedema; (3) crystalluria, oliguria, and anuria; (4) hematologic reactions, such as methemoglobinemia, agranulocytosis, thrombocytopenia, kernicterus in the newborn, and hemolytic anemia in patients with G6PD deficiency; (5) photosensitivity; and (6) neurologic effects, such as peripheral neuritis, insomnia, and headache. The Stevens-Johnson syndrome seems more likely to occur with long-acting sulfonamides than short-acting sulfonamides. Kernicterus can result from administration of sulfonamides to the

mother at term or to the newborn, because sulfonamides displace bilirubin from albumin in the newborn. Therefore, pregnant women near term and newborns should not be given sulfonamides. Other side effects include hypothyroidism, hepatitis, potentiation of sulfonylureas with consequent hypoglycemia, and potentiation of coumarin anticoagulants. Activation of quiescent lupus erythematosus has been reported. The incidence of side effects is different for the various sulfonamides, but cross-sensitivity is common.

Administration and Dosage

Many sulfonamides are available, but doses will be given only for some of the more commonly used ones.

Systemic sulfonamides: An initial loading dose is commonly recommended, but it is unnecessary and should not be used in treating UTI (the major use for sulfonamides) and is rarely needed for most other indications.

Sulfisoxazole is used in a dose of 1 gm q 4 to 6 h in adults. (If used, the loading dose is 2 to 4 gm.) In children 150 mg/kg/day is given orally in 6 divided doses; the loading dose if used is 75 mg/kg. The IV dose in adults and children is 100 mg/kg/day divided into doses q 6 h; the loading dose if used is 50 mg/kg.

Sulfamethoxazole is used orally in a dose of 1 gm bid to tid in adults and 25 to 30 mg/kg bid in children; loading doses are 2 gm in adults and 50 to 60 mg/kg in children.

Sulfadiazine is used in the same dosage as sulfisoxazole. **Sulfamethizole** is used in a dose of 500 to 1000 mg tid to qid in adults and 30 to 45 mg/kg/day in 4 divided doses in children.

Topical sulfonamides: Silver sulfadiazine and mafenide are used topically to prevent infection in burns (see Ch. 254; also TOPICAL ANTISEPTICS in Ch. 3). **Sufacetamide** is useful in the treatment of ocular infections.

TRIMETHOPRIM/SULFAMETHOXAZOLE

Trimethoprim/sulfamethoxazole **(TMP/SMX)** is a fixed combination (1:5) of the 2 drugs and is usually bacteriostatic. Both agents block the folic acid metabolism cycle of bacteria and are much more active together than either agent alone. Sulfonamides are competitive inhibitors of the incorporation of *p*-aminobenzoic acid. TMP prevents reduction of dihydrofolate to tetrahydrofolate. TMP/SMX is active against most gram-positive and -negative organisms. However, *P. aeruginosa* and *B. fragilis* are usually resistant.

Pharmacology: Both TMP and SMX are well absorbed orally and are excreted into the urine. They have similar half-lives of about 9 h in plasma and penetrate well into tissues and body fluids including the CSF. The dosage ratios are fixed so as to result in a 20:1 ratio of SMX to TMP in blood and tissues, which is optimal for maximal antibacterial activity.

Indications: TMP/SMX is effective in UTI. It is one of the few agents effective in chronic bacterial prostatitis, but cures only a minority of patients even when given for 12 wk. It is effective in the prophylaxis of UTI in women who have multiple reinfections. TMP/SMX is the drug of choice for treatment of *Pneumocystis carinii* pneumonia. It is also effective in prophylaxis of this infection in children with malignancies. It is useful in treatment of typhoid fever, especially when ampicillin and chloramphenicol cannot be used. TMP/SMX is effective in shigellosis, otitis media, gonorrhea, and acute exacerbations of chronic bronchitis.

Adverse reactions: The side effects are the same as those already listed for sulfonamides. Although both TMP and SMX can cause identical side effects, TMP is less

likely to do so. When it does, nausea, vomiting, rash, and folate deficiency (resulting in macrocytic anemia) are those most likely to occur.

Administration and dosage: The usual oral dose in adults is 2 regular strength tablets (each tablet contains 80 mg TMP and 400 mg SMX) or one double strength tablet (160 mg TMP and 800 mg SMX) bid. The usual oral dose in children is 8 mg/kg TMP and 40 mg/kg SMX daily in 2 divided doses. The IV dose in adults and children is 8 mg/kg TMP and 40 mg/kg SMX daily in 2 divided doses.

Much higher doses (20 mg/kg/day TMP and 100 mg/kg/day SMX in 4 divided doses) are used in the treatment of *P. carinii* pneumonia. Much lower doses (40 mg TMP and 200 mg SMX each night) are used for prophylaxis of UTI.

Trimethoprim

For patients allergic to sulfonamides, trimethoprim alone has been used mainly in the treatment of chronic bacterial prostatitis and in the prophylaxis and treatment of UTI. The pharmacology and side effects are listed under TMP/SMX, above. The dose in adults for UTI is 100 mg orally q 12 h.

AGENTS USED ONLY FOR URINARY TRACT INFECTION

Nitrofurantoin	Nalidixic acid	Methenamine mandelate
	Cinoxacin	Methenamine hippurate

Nitrofurantoin

Nitrofurantoin is used orally for the treatment or prophylaxis of UTI. It is active against *E. coli* and *Klebsiella-Enterobacter* spp, but *Pseudomonas* and many strains of *Proteus* are resistant. It is absorbed well when given orally but does not give antibacterial blood levels. However, urinary levels are high. Nitrofurantoin is *contraindicated* in patients with renal insufficiency, since serious toxicity is possible. Although an IV preparation is available, it should not be used as there are less toxic and equally or more effective parenteral agents available for treatment of UTI.

The side effects are nausea and vomiting, which are less likely to occur with use of the macrocrystalline form. Fever, rash, and hypersensitivity pneumonitis as well as progressive pulmonary interstitial fibrosis may occur. Paresthesias, followed by a severe polyneuropathy can result if the drug is not discontinued, especially in patients with renal failure. Hemolytic anemia can occur in patients with G6PD deficiency. Leukopenia and hepatotoxicity have also been reported.

The oral dose is 50 to 100 mg qid in adults and 5 to 7 mg/kg/day in 4 divided doses in children. A single nightly dose of 50 to 100 mg may decrease the number of episodes in women with frequent reinfections of the urinary tract.

Quinolones

Nalidixic acid and **cinoxacin** are oral antimicrobial quinolones used only in the treatment of UTI. They are active against *E. coli*, *Klebsiella-Enterobacter*, and *Proteus* but not *Pseudomonas*. However, bacteria tend to become rapidly resistant. These drugs are well absorbed when given orally and result in very low blood levels. They are excreted in the urine, giving antibacterial urinary concentrations. *They should not be used in the presence of renal insufficiency.*

The side effects are nausea, vomiting, rash, fever, headache, psychosis, and seizures. Papilledema with the headache may occur in children. Photosensitivity reactions have been reported. Thrombocytopenia, leukopenia, or hemolytic anemia (sometimes associated with G6PD deficiency) may occur.

Nalidixic acid is given in a dose of 1 gm qid in adults. The dose in children is 55 mg/kg/day in 4 divided doses.

Cinoxacin is given in a dose of 1 gm/day in adults in 2 or 4 divided doses.

Methenamine Mandelate and Methenamine Hippurate

These are oral agents used only for the suppression or prophylaxis of UTI. They are absorbed well and are excreted into the urine in high concentrations. These agents have no intrinsic antibacterial activity, but at a pH of 5.5 or less, mandelic and hippuric acids are antibacterial and methenamine is converted to formaldehyde, which is antibacterial. These agents are active against *E. coli* and to a lesser extent against other bacilli.

It is often necessary to add an oral acidifying agent such as methionine or ascorbic acid to reduce the urinary pH to 5.5 or less. When *Proteus* infections occur, the methenamines are usually not active because *Proteus* produce urease and alkalinize the urine.

The side effects are nausea, vomiting, rash, dysuria (especially with high doses), and metabolic acidosis, especially with the addition of acidifying agents and in the presence of renal insufficiency. *The methenamines should not be used in patients with renal insufficiency.*

Methenamine mandelate is used in adults in a dose of 1 gm qid. Children > 6 yr receive half the adult dose.

Methenamine hippurate is used in adults and children > 12 yr in a dose of 1 gm bid. The dose in children 6 to 12 yr is 0.5 to 1.0 gm bid.

ANTIVIRAL DRUGS

Difficulties with antiviral chemotherapy arise because of the obligatory dependence of viruses on host cell metabolism for replication and because few virus-specific enzyme systems are presently vulnerable to chemotherapeutic intervention. Agents that block viral replication also block normal host cell processes, and the limits between effective and toxic doses are very narrow. Some of the clinically useful antiviral agents have a wide variety of side effects and a relatively low therapeutic index. Patients receiving these agents must be monitored carefully. Further, some resistant virus strains have developed in patients receiving initially effective therapy.

Chemotherapeutic intervention can occur (1) at the time of viral particle attachment to host cell membranes, (2) during uncoating of viral nucleic acids, (3) by blocking transcription in some deoxyriboviruses and riboviruses that require a virus-specific DNA-dependent RNA polymerase, (4) by blocking translation at the level of viral messenger RNA (which must be different from mammalian host cell messenger RNA, since the interferon-induced translation inhibitory protein can recognize the difference), and (5) by blocking specific virus-coded enzymes produced in the host cells that are essential for viral replication but not for normal host cell metabolism.

Amantadine is primarily used for influenza *prophylaxis* and appears to act at the early stage of virus-host interaction, blocking either virus penetration into the host cells or uncoating. Given orally, 90% of the drug may be recovered unchanged in the urine; about 50% of a single dose is recovered in 20 h. Amantadine is partially protective against influenza A infection and is recommended for prophylactic treatment of high-risk patients during influenza A epidemics. Prophylaxis is immediate. Antibody formation following influenza infection apparently is not blocked. In addition, when the drug is given as *treatment* early in the clinical course symptoms are reduced and the illness is shortened by 1 to 2 days. Side effects include CNS reactions (eg, nervousness, insomnia, dizziness, lightheadedness, slurred speech, ataxia, inability to concentrate, hallucinations, and depression); skin rashes; and anorexia, nausea, and constipation. Side effects usually develop within 48 h after starting amantadine and often resolve during continued use. Amantadine has anticholinergic activity and may intensify peripheral and central adverse effects of other anticholinergic drugs administered concomitantly. The usual prophylactic dose is 100 mg orally bid for the duration of the epidemic. For children aged 1 to 9 yr, the daily dose is 4.4 to 8.8 mg/kg in 2 divided

doses, not to exceed 150 mg/day. When used for treatment of influenza A virus infections, the usual adult dose is 100 mg orally bid for 5 days. Since amantadine is eliminated by the kidney, the dose should be reduced for the elderly and for patients with renal impairment.

Ribavirin, a purine nucleoside analog, has activity against several RNA and DNA viruses. Its mechanism of action is uncertain. When administered as a small particle aerosol, ribavirin has been effective in treating young adults with **influenza A or B infections**. The aerosol has also been effective in infants with **respiratory syncytial virus (RSV) infections**.

In a recent clinical trial, ribavirin therapy significantly reduced mortality from **Lassa fever**. IV administration of ribavirin, 2 gm loading dose then 1 gm q 6 h for 4 days followed by 0.5 gm q 8 h for 6 days, was more effective than oral therapy, and the best results occurred when treatment was started within 6 days after the onset of fever. The most common side effect was hemolysis, with the Hct of some patients dropping 20%.

Idoxuridine (IDU) apparently acts by being phosphorylated and incorporated into newly synthesized DNA, irreversibly replacing thymidine and producing an abnormal and essentially nonfunctional DNA molecule. The drug acts on both viral and host cell DNA and is *highly toxic to host cells*. Clinical use of IDU has been limited to topical therapy because of its high systemic toxicity. An ophthalmic preparation has been used to treat **herpes simplex keratoconjunctivitis**, but is less effective for recurrent herpes keratitis, probably because of the development of drug-resistant virus strains. Two topical ophthalmic preparations are available: a 0.1% aqueous solution and a 0.5% ointment. One drop of the solution is instilled conjunctivally q 1 h during waking hours and q 2 h at night. The ointment is given 5 times/day (q 4 h), with the last dose at bedtime. Treatment should be continued for 3 to 5 days after healing is complete to lessen the chance of recurrence. Ophthalmic IDU may cause irritation, pain, pruritus, and inflammation or edema of the eyelids; rare allergic reactions and photophobia have also been reported.

Vidarabine (adenine arabinoside, Ara-A) interferes with viral DNA synthesis and is effective in the treatment of **herpes simplex virus infections**. Ophthalmic preparations of vidarabine are effective for acute keratoconjunctivitis and recurrent superficial keratitis caused by herpes simplex virus types 1 and 2. Vidarabine appears less susceptible to the development of drug resistant viral strains than idoxuridine, and IDU resistant infections often respond to vidarabine therapy. A 3% ophthalmic ointment is available and is given 5 times/day (q 3 h). Treatment should be continued for several days after complete healing to prevent recurrent infection. Possible side effects include tearing, irritation, pain, photophobia, and superficial punctate keratitis.

Systemic vidarabine for herpes simplex encephalitis has reduced mortality from 70% to 28%. It is most effective when therapy is initiated early; little benefit ensues when therapy is started after the patient is comatose. Systemic vidarabine is given as an IV infusion of 15 mg/kg/day over 12 h for 10 days. Side effects include nausea, vomiting, tremor, and phlebitis at the infusion site. Bone marrow toxicity and hepatotoxicity may occur with high doses. Recent clinical trials indicate that acyclovir is more effective than vidarabine in biopsy proven herpes simplex encephalitis.

Vidarabine is also useful in **varicella-zoster infections** in immunosuppressed patients. Given as an IV infusion of 10 mg/kg/day for 5 to 7 days, it reduces cutaneous and visceral dissemination, shortens the period of viral shedding, and lessens the morbidity from postherpetic neuralgia. Again, recent studies have shown that acyclovir is more effective than vidarabine.

Neonatal herpes infections have also been treated with IV vidarabine. In one report mortality was reduced from 74 to 38%, but 1 yr later only 29% of the vidarabine treated infants with CNS or disseminated disease were considered normal.

Trifluridine (trifluorothymidine), a thymidine analog, interferes with DNA synthesis and is effective in treating acute **herpes keratitis** caused by herpes simplex virus types 1 and 2. Trifluridine is as effective as vidarabine and may be effective in patients who have not responded to idoxuridine or vidarabine. The marrow-suppressive effect of trifluridine precludes systemic use. A 1% ophthalmic solution is available, and 1 drop should be instilled into the affected eye q 2 h while the patient is awake. The maximum recommended dose is 9 drops/day until the corneal ulcer is re-epithelialized, then 5 drops/day (1 drop q 4 h) for 7 days. If there is no improvement in 7 days, another agent should be considered. Side effects include burning or stinging in the eye and palpebral edema; less frequently, punctate keratopathy and hypersensitivity reactions may develop.

Acyclovir is phosphorylated by herpes specific viral enzyme (thymidine kinase), forming the active triphosphate compound that inhibits the viral DNA polymerase. Some strains of herpes simplex and varicella-zoster do not produce thymidine kinase and are acyclovir resistant. In clinical use a 5% topical ointment reduces viral shedding and improves the rate of healing in primary genital herpes infections; however, it does not prevent or delay recurrent episodes and it is relatively ineffective in treating *recurrent* infections. The ointment is applied q 3 h (6 times/day) for 7 days. Transient burning and stinging have been reported. Topical acyclovir has also been useful in limited mucocutaneous infections in immunocompromised patients.

Oral acyclovir is effective for both primary and recurrent **genital herpes infections.** It is poorly absorbed after oral administration with a bioavailability of only 15 to 30%. Treatment with acyclovir, 200 mg orally 5 times/day, shortens the clinical course, reduces pain, and decreases viral shedding. The drug should be given for 10 days in primary infection and for 5 days in recurrent episodes. In recurrent episodes, oral acyclovir is most effective when it is started at the first sign of recurrence. Side effects are infrequent with oral administration, but nausea, vomiting, diarrhea, headache, and rashes have been reported. As with topical therapy, oral acyclovir does not eliminate the latent infection. In patients with frequent recurrences, therapy with acyclovir, 200 mg orally tid for up to 6 mo, suppresses recurrent episodes; but they recur again when treatment is stopped.

Oral acyclovir has also been effective in treating **mucocutaneous herpes simplex infections** and in suppressing recurring **herpes infections** in immunocompromised patients.

Acyclovir given by IV infusion reduces viral shedding, promotes scabbing and healing of lesions, and lessens pain in immunocompromised patients with mucocutaneous herpes simplex infection. The usual adult dosage is 5 mg/kg IV q 8 h for 7 days, and children < 12 yr can be given 250 mg/m² q 8 h. Infusions should be given slowly over at least 1 h to prevent deposition of acyclovir crystals in renal tubules. Patients receiving acyclovir IV should be well hydrated, and dosage should be reduced in patients with renal impairment. Reported side effects include phlebitis at the infusion site, rash, and possible neurotoxicity resulting in lethargy, confusion, seizures, or coma.

IV acyclovir is also effective for **varicella-zoster infections** in immunosuppressed patients. Given as 500 mg/m² IV q 8 h, acyclovir reduced viral shedding, promoted healing of lesions, and decreased pain; it was more effective than IV vidarabine.

In clinical trials acyclovir 10 mg/kg IV q 8 h was also more effective than vidarabine for treating **herpes simplex encephalitis.** It reduced mortality and also improved functional capacity of the survivors. As with vidarabine, the best response was in younger patients who began therapy before onset of coma.

Levamisole is an experimental immunotropic drug whose exact mechanism of action in viral illness is not understood. In clinical trials, pain was dramatically relieved with levamisole therapy in **acute genital herpes**, but recurrent genital herpes responded only when both partners were treated simultaneously. The dosage for acute infection is 50 mg levamisole orally tid for 4 days with a 2nd course of treatment after 10 to 14 days.

Recurrent genital herpes requires 50 mg levamisole orally tid for 2 consecutive days each week for 4 to 8 wk.

Investigational prophylactic use of levamisole in children with a history of frequent wintertime **viral respiratory infections** decreased the number of viral URIs and the duration and severity of the illnesses. The levamisole dosage was 1.25 mg/kg orally bid for 2 consecutive days each week during the winter months. Side effects with levamisole are uncommon and may include nervousness, nausea, vomiting, diarrhea, dysosmia, metallic taste, and skin rash.

Interferon is a natural cellular product released from infected host cells in response to viral or other foreign nucleic acids. It is detectable as early as 2 h after infection. Its complex mechanism of action has not been fully established, but it selectively blocks translation and/or transcription of viral RNA, stopping viral replication without disturbing normal host cell function. Interferon is not virus-specific and may be active against many viruses; however, it is species specific and can be used only in the same species as initially produced it. Recombinant DNA technics now allow production of human interferon from bacterial cells.

Interferon use remains investigational. Recent clinical studies have shown that α_2-interferon nasal spray can prevent URIs from rhinoviruses. Interferon also proved beneficial in immunocompromised patients with varicella-zoster infections. Combined antiviral therapy with either acyclovir or vidarabine plus interferon was useful in patients with chronic active hepatitis B infections. Recombinant DNA technology has made interferons available in adequate quantities and many clinical trials are now underway.

ANTIFUNGAL DRUGS

(See Ch. 9)

4. SUPERFICIAL INFECTIONS

CELLULITIS

(See also ORBITAL CELLULITIS in Ch. 216)

A diffuse, spreading, acute inflammation within solid (nonhollow) tissues, characterized by hyperemia, leukocytic infiltration, and edema without cellular necrosis or suppuration. It is most commonly evident in the skin and subcutaneous structures but may involve deeper areas.

Etiology

Streptococcus pyogenes (Group A β-hemolytic streptococcus) is the commonest cause of superficial cellulitis; diffuse spread of infection occurs because streptokinase, DNAse, and hyaluronidase—enzymes produced by the organism—break down cellular components that otherwise would contain and localize the inflammatory process. β-Hemolytic streptococci of other serologic groups (eg, B, C, and G) are less frequent causes of cellulitis. *Staphylococcus aureus* occasionally produces a superficial cellulitis typically less extensive than that of streptococcal origin and usually only in association with an open wound or cutaneous abscess. Superficial cellulitis caused by other organisms occurs rarely and generally only when impaired host defenses, such as granulocytopenia or tissue ischemia, prevent localization of infection or when certain forms of trauma, such as animal bites or immersion injuries, introduce unusual pathogens into the skin.

Symptoms and Signs

The lower extremities are the most common sites of infection. A cutaneous abnormality (eg, skin trauma, ulceration, tinea pedis, or dermatitis) often precedes the infection; areas of lymphedema or other edema seem especially susceptible. Scars from saphenous vein removal for cardiac or vascular surgery are common sites for recurrent cellulitis, especially if tinea pedis is present. Frequently, however, no predisposing condition or site of entry is evident. The major findings are local erythema and tenderness, frequently with lymphangitis and regional lymphadenopathy. The skin is hot, red, and edematous, often with an infiltrated surface resembling the skin of an orange (*peau d'orange*). The borders are usually indistinct, but in **erysipelas** (see also in Ch. 231), a type of cellulitis, the raised margins are sharply demarcated. Petechiae are common; large areas of ecchymosis, rare. Vesicles and bullae may develop and rupture, occasionally with necrosis of the involved skin. Systemic manifestations (fever, chills, tachycardia, headache, hypotension, and delirium) sometimes occur and may precede the cutaneous findings by several hours, but many patients do not appear ill. Leukocytosis is common, but not constant.

Diagnosis

The diagnosis usually depends on the clinical findings. The responsible organism is difficult to isolate, even with aspiration or skin biopsy of the infected area, unless pus has formed or there is an open wound. Blood cultures are only occasionally positive. Serologic tests, especially measurement of anti-DNAse B, will confirm a streptococcal etiology, but are usually unnecessary.

Although cellulitis and deep vein thrombosis are easily differentiated clinically, many physicians confuse the two entities when edema occurs in the lower extremities. The major differences are (1) skin temperature: hot in cellulitis, normal or cool with deep venous thrombosis; (2) skin color: red in cellulitis, normal or cyanotic with deep venous thrombosis; and (3) skin surface: a *peau d'orange* appearance in cellulitis, smooth in deep venous thrombosis. Lymphangitis and regional lymphadenopathy, frequent in cellulitis, do not occur with deep venous thrombosis.

Course and Prognosis

Local abscesses form occasionally and require incision and drainage. Serious but rare complications include development of severe necrotizing subcutaneous infection (streptococcal gangrene or necrotizing fasciitis) and bacteremia with metastatic foci of infection. Even in the preantibiotic era, however, most cases of superficial cellulitis resolved spontaneously. Recurrences in the same area were common, sometimes causing serious damage to the lymphatics, chronic lymphatic obstruction, marked edema, and, rarely, elephantiasis. With antibiotic therapy, such complications are uncommon. Symptoms and signs of superficial cellulitis usually resolve after a few days of antibiotics, but often the clinical manifestations worsen initially, presumably from the abrupt death of organisms and release of their enzymes.

Treatment

Penicillin is the drug of choice. For mild, outpatient cases, penicillin V 250 mg qid, or a single dose of benzathine penicillin 1.2 million u. IM is adequate. For severe infections requiring hospitalization, aqueous penicillin G 400,000 u. IV q 6 h is indicated. For penicillin-allergic patients, erythromycin 250 mg orally qid is an effective alternative for mild infections, and parenteral clindamycin 150 mg IV q 6 h can be used for severe cases. When pus or an open wound is present, results of a Gram stain should dictate antibiotic choice. Cellulitis in a neutropenic patient requires antibiotics effective against enteric gram-negative bacilli (eg, gentamicin 1.5 mg/kg q 8 h and carbenicillin 5 gm q 4 h) until culture results are available. In patients with recurrent leg cellulitis, treatment of concomitant tinea pedis often eliminates the sources of

streptococci that may reside in the inflamed, macerated tissue. If such therapy is unsuccessful or not indicated, recurrent cellulitis can be prevented by benzathine penicillin 1.2 million u. IM monthly, or either penicillin V or erythromycin 250 mg qid orally for 1 wk each month. Immobilizing and elevating the affected area help reduce edema; cool, wet dressings may help relieve local discomfort.

LYMPHADENITIS

Inflammation of lymph nodes.

Etiology

Any pathogen—bacterial, viral, protozoal, rickettsial, or fungal—can cause lymphadenitis. The lymph node involvement may be generalized, with systemic infections, or confined to regional lymph nodes draining a local area of infection. **Infections with prominent regional lymphadenopathy** include streptococcal disease, TB or nontuberculous mycobacterial disease, tularemia, plague, cat-scratch disease, primary syphilis, lymphogranuloma venereum, chancroid, and genital herpes simplex. **Generalized lymph node enlargement** is frequent in infectious mononucleosis, cytomegalovirus infection, toxoplasmosis, brucellosis, secondary syphilis, and disseminated histoplasmosis.

Symptoms, Signs, and Diagnosis

Lymph node enlargement from edema and leukocytic cellular infiltration, the major sign of lymphadenitis, may be asymptomatic or may cause pain and tenderness. With some infections the overlying skin is inflamed, occasionally with cellulitis; abscess formation may occur, and penetration to the skin will produce draining sinuses.

Lymphadenitis and its cause are usually apparent. Occasionally, however, lymph node aspiration and culture or excisional biopsy may be necessary.

Treatment and Course

Treatment depends on the underlying cause. With resolution of the primary process, lymph node enlargement usually resolves, but firm, nontender lymphadenopathy sometimes persists. Hot, wet applications may help relieve symptoms of acutely painful lymph nodes. Abscesses require surgical drainage (see Ch. 5).

ACUTE LYMPHANGITIS

Acute inflammation of the subcutaneous lymphatic channels, usually caused by Streptococcus pyogenes.

Symptoms, Signs, and Diagnosis

Streptococci most commonly enter the lymphatic channels from an abrasion, wound, or infection (usually cellulitis) on an extremity. Red, irregular, warm, and tender streaks develop on an extremity and extend proximally from a peripheral lesion toward regional lymph nodes, which are typically enlarged and tender. Systemic manifestations such as fever, shaking chills, tachycardia, and headache are common, often are more severe than the cutaneous findings would suggest, and occasionally precede any evidence of significant local infection. Leukocytosis, sometimes marked, is usual.

Diagnosis is based on the symptoms and signs. As in cellulitis, culture of the responsible organism is uncommon unless there is pus, an open wound, or bacteremia.

Course and Treatment

Bacteremia with metastatic foci of infection may occur, often with startling rapidity. Rarely, cellulitis with suppuration, necrosis, and ulceration may develop along the course of the involved lymph channels. Most cases respond rapidly to antibiotic therapy, as discussed under CELLULITIS, above.

CUTANEOUS ABSCESSES

Localized collections of pus causing fluctuant soft-tissue swelling surrounded by erythema. (See also FOLLICULITIS; FURUNCLES; CARBUNCLES in Ch. 231.) Local cellulitis, lymphangitis, regional lymphadenopathy, fever, and leukocytosis are variable accompanying features. These abscesses usually follow minor skin trauma.

Organisms isolated from cutaneous abscesses are typically the bacteria indigenous to the skin of the involved area. Abscesses in the perineal region (inguinal, vaginal, buttock, and perirectal) contain organisms found in the stool, commonly anaerobes alone or a combination of aerobes and anaerobes. *Peptococcus, Peptostreptococcus, Lactobacillus, Bacteroides,* and *Fusobacterium* species are the predominant anaerobic isolates; α- and nonhemolytic streptococci are the most frequent aerobes. For abscesses on the trunk, extremities, axillae, or head and neck, aerobes alone or a mixture of aerobic and anaerobic flora is usual. The most frequent anaerobic species are *Peptococcus* and *Proprionibacterium*; the most common aerobic organisms are *Staphylococcus aureus* and *epidermidis. S. aureus,* found in less than half of cutaneous abscesses in any location, typically occurs in pure culture.

Treatment of cutaneous abscesses is incision of the fluctuant area, thorough evacuation of pus from the abscess cavity with careful probing to remove loculations, irrigation with normal saline, and loose packing with a gauze wick that is removed 24 to 48 h later. Local heat and elevation of the affected area, if possible, may hasten resolution of the tissue inflammation. Gram stain, culture, and antibiotic therapy are unnecessary, unless the patient has signs of systemic infection, compromised host defenses, or facial abscesses in the area drained by the cavernous sinus.

NECROTIZING SUBCUTANEOUS INFECTIONS

(Necrotizing Fasciitis; Synergistic Necrotizing Cellulitis)

Severe infections, typically due to a mixture of aerobic and anaerobic organisms, that cause necrosis of subcutaneous tissue, usually including the fascia. When the male genitalia are involved, this infection is called **Fournier's disease.**

Etiology, Pathogenesis, and Pathology

While *Streptococcus pyogenes* (Group A streptococcus) alone may occasionally cause these infections, usually they are caused by a mixture of aerobic and anaerobic bacteria, the most common isolates being aerobic streptococci other than Group A, aerobic gram-negative bacilli, anaerobic gram-positive cocci, and *Bacteroides* species.

These organisms reach the subcutaneous tissue by extension from a contiguous infection or trauma to the area. The trauma, often minor, may be thermal, chemical, or mechanical, including surgical procedures. Involvement of the extremities, the most common site, may occur from infected cutaneous ulcers or infectious complications of previous trauma. Involvement of the perineum, the second most common site, is usually a complication of preceding surgery, perirectal abscesses, periurethral gland infection, or retroperitoneal infections from perforated abdominal viscera.

The major gross pathologic findings are edema and necrosis of the subcutaneous tissues, including adjacent fascia; widespread undermining of surrounding tissue; occlusion of small subcutaneous vessels, leading to dermal gangrene, and absent or minimal muscle involvement. Microscopic abnormalities include intense leukocytic infiltration, microabscess formation, and necrosis in the subcutaneous tissue and adjacent fascia. The subcutaneous arterioles and venules are often completely occluded.

The combination of ischemia, edema, and inflammation in the subcutaneous tissue decreases PO_2 and permits growth of obligate anaerobes like *Bacteroides,* and promotes anaerobic metabolism by facultative organisms like *E. coli.* This anaerobic metabolism often produces hydrogen and nitrogen, relatively insoluble gases, that may accumulate in subcutaneous tissues and cause crepitus or roentgenographically detectable gas.

Patients with diabetes mellitus seem predisposed to these infections. Possible explanations include (1) small vessel disease, causing tissue hypoxia and therefore promoting anaerobic bacterial metabolism; (2) defective leukocyte function; and (3) elevated tissue glucose, providing abundant nutrients for bacterial growth.

Symptoms and Signs

The skin overlying the infection is tender, red, hot, and swollen; with progression, violaceous discoloration, bullae, crepitus, and dermal gangrene may develop. Fever, nearly always present, typically is accompanied by systemic toxicity, including tachycardia and altered mental status ranging from confusion to obtundation. Evidence of intravascular volume depletion, including hypotension, is frequent.

Laboratory Findings

Polymorphonuclear leukocytosis is usual. With diabetics, the blood glucose is elevated and ketoacidosis may occur. Decreased intravascular volume causes concentrated urine and increased serum creatinine and BUN. Radiographs of the affected area often demonstrate soft-tissue gas.

Diagnosis

Red, hot, tender, and markedly edematous skin suggests an underlying necrotizing subcutaneous infection. Rapid progression or the development of bullae, ecchymoses, dermal gangrene, fluctuance, crepitus, or roentgenographically visible soft-tissue gas confirms the necessity for surgical exploration. Blood cultures should be obtained. Pus aspirated into a syringe percutaneously or during surgery provides the best material for Gram stain and aerobic and anaerobic cultures.

Prognosis

The mortality rate is about 30%. Factors associated with a poor prognosis include old age, the presence of other medical problems, delayed diagnosis and therapy, and insufficiently extensive surgery.

Treatment

Gram stain of pus should determine antibiotic choice. Since both aerobes and anaerobes are usually present, gentamicin combined with clindamycin, or chloramphenicol alone, will usually be appropriate pending culture results. Large quantities of IV fluids are needed to replace losses into the tissues.

The major element of therapy is extensive incision and debridement. The area involved is typically greater than anticipated by the overlying skin abnormalities, and the incision should be extended until an instrument or finger can no longer separate the skin and subcutaneous tissue from the deep fascia. The most common error is insufficient surgical exposure, and repeating the operation 1 to 2 days later is usually prudent to insure adequate incision and debridement of all affected areas. Amputation of an extremity may be necessary.

---

5. ABSCESSES

Collections of pus, usually caused by bacterial infection, in tissues, organs, or confined spaces.

This chapter covers the basic elements of abscess formation; the clinical characteristics of common and important abscesses, based on their location in the body; and the principles of treatment. Specific organisms involved vary greatly and are also discussed elsewhere in the text under appropriate headings (see especially, "Abscesses" in the index). In particular, the frequency, importance, and complexities of mixed anaerobic

infections are receiving increasing attention; they are discussed in Ch. 8. Cutaneous abscesses are discussed in Ch. 4.

Pathogenesis

Organisms causing an abscess may enter the tissue by (1) direct implantation (eg, penetrating trauma with an unsterile object); (2) spread from an established, contiguous infection; (3) dissemination via lymphatic or hematogenous routes from a distant site; or (4) migration from a location where they are resident flora into an adjacent, normally sterile area because of disruption of natural barriers (eg, perforation of an abdominal viscus causing an intra-abdominal abscess).

Predisposing factors to abscess formation include impaired host defense mechanisms (eg, abnormal leukocyte function); the presence of foreign bodies; obstruction to normal drainage of the urinary, biliary, or respiratory tracts; tissue ischemia or necrosis; hematoma or excessive fluid accumulation in tissue; and trauma.

Abscesses begin as **cellulitis** (see Ch. 4). Separation of cellular elements by fluid or by space created by cellular necrosis from another cause provides an area where leukocytes can accumulate and form the abscess. Progressive dissection by pus or the necrosis of surrounding cells expands the abscess. Highly vascularized connective tissue may then invade and surround the necrotic tissue, leukocytes, and debris to limit further spread.

Symptoms, Signs, and Complications

The symptoms and signs of cutaneous or subcutaneous abscesses are heat; swelling; tenderness; redness over the affected site; and, possibly, fever, especially when surrounding cellulitis is present. For deep-seated abscesses the major findings are local pain and tenderness and systemic symptoms, especially fever, but also such nonspecific complaints as anorexia, weight loss, and fatigue. In some locations the predominant manifestation is abnormal organ function, eg, hemiplegia with a brain abscess.

Complications of abscesses include bacteremia, with spread of infection to distant sites; rupture into adjacent tissue; bleeding from vessels eroded by inflammation; impaired function of a vital organ; and inanition from the systemic effects of anorexia and tissue catabolism.

Treatment

Healing usually requires removing the contents of the abscess, since they can provoke further inflammation. Rupture of the abscess may result in spontaneous drainage, sometimes with formation of chronic draining sinuses, into adjacent tissue or to the outside surface of the body. Without spontaneous or surgical drainage, an abscess occasionally resolves slowly after proteolytic digestion of the pus produces a thin, sterile fluid that is resorbed into the bloodstream. Incomplete resorption leaves a cystic loculation within a fibrous wall, where calcium salts sometimes accumulate to form a calcified mass.

The major elements of adequate drainage are thorough removal of pus, necrotic tissue, and debris (often necessitating blunt dissection to disrupt the fibrous walls surrounding loculated suppuration), and elimination of dead space that provides a locus for further accumulation of organisms, leukocytes, and debris (often accomplished by packing with gauze—capillary action draws up liquified contents and keeps the wound clean and dry—or by using various types of drains). Predisposing conditions, eg, obstruction or the presence of a foreign body, require correction if possible.

Systemic antimicrobial agents active against the responsible organisms are indicated for deep-seated infections, but are rarely effective without concurrent surgical drainage. Gram stains, cultures, and sensitivity studies of purulent material removed by aspiration or drainage of the abscess provide an indispensable guide to antibiotic choice by identifying the infecting organisms and their antimicrobial susceptibility.

INTRA-ABDOMINAL ABSCESSES

The 3 types of intra-abdominal abscesses are (1) **intraperitoneal,** (2) **retroperitoneal,** and (3) **visceral.** Though the clinical features vary, most of these abscesses cause fever, leukocytosis, and an increased ESR. Pain, if present, usually occurs near the abscess. Paralytic ileus, either generalized or localized near the infection, may develop, and nonspecific GI symptoms, such as anorexia, nausea, vomiting, and diarrhea or constipation, are common.

Many intra-abdominal abscesses develop when perforation or inflammation disrupts the GI tract; the infecting organisms, a complex mixture of anaerobic and aerobic bacteria, are part of the normal bowel flora. The most important isolates from these abscesses are aerobic gram-negative rods, eg, *E. coli* and *Klebsiella,* and anaerobes, especially *Bacteroides fragilis*; effective antimicrobial therapy requires agents active against these organisms. For patients with normal renal function, giving a combination of an aminoglycoside, such as gentamicin 1.5 mg/kg q 8 h, and clindamycin 600 mg q 6 h is effective. Cefoxitin alone, 2 gm q 6 h, is a reasonable alternative, except with previous antibiotic administration or hospital-acquired infections, when an aminoglycoside like gentamicin should be added.

Nearly all intra-abdominal abscesses require drainage, either by surgery or by percutaneous catheters. Drainage through indwelling catheters placed by CT or ultrasonic guidance may be appropriate when (1) no more than 2 abscess cavities are present; (2) the drainage route does not traverse bowel or uncontaminated organs, pleura, or peritoneum; (3) there is no source of continued contamination, such as a perforated viscus; or (4) the pus is thin enough to pass through the catheter.

INTRAPERITONEAL ABSCESSES

The 3 types of abscesses in this group, **subphrenic, midabdominal,** and **pelvic,** develop from generalized peritonitis due to causes such as trauma, perforated abdominal viscera, or localized peritonitis resulting from infection in a contiguous site. With generalized peritonitis, the effects of gravity and intra-abdominal pressure favor localization to the subphrenic spaces, pelvis, and paracolic gutters lateral to the ascending and descending colon.

SUBPHRENIC ABSCESSES

The subphrenic space, arbitrarily defined as lying below the diaphragm and above the transverse colon, consists of 4 subdivisions. On the right side are the suprahepatic and subhepatic spaces. On the left side, the subhepatic and suprahepatic spaces freely communicate and constitute a single combined subphrenic space. The other left-sided space, behind the stomach and anterior to the pancreas, is the lesser sac. About 55% of subphrenic abscesses are right-sided, 25% left-sided, and 20% multiple.

Etiology and Pathogenesis

Most subphrenic abscesses arise from direct contamination of the area following local disease, injury, or, most frequently, surgery. They develop from peritonitis secondary to another cause, such as perforated viscus; extension from an abscess in an adjacent organ; or, most commonly, as a postoperative complication of abdominal surgery, especially on the biliary tract, duodenum, or stomach. The peritoneum may be contaminated during or after surgery, from such events as anastomotic leaks. Some abscesses follow spread of infection through the peritoneal cavity from a distant site of contamination (eg, appendicitis). Factors favoring movement of fluid into subphrenic spaces include the negative pressure in the area generated during the diaphragmatic movement of respiration, and greater intra-abdominal pressure in the lower abdomen,

promoting fluid movement superiorly. In a few patients, no predisposing cause is evident (primary subphrenic abscess); presumably, a subclinical peritonitis occurred.

Symptoms and Signs

Clinical manifestations of subphrenic abscesses usually begin subtly within 3 to 6 wk following surgery, but occasionally do not appear for several months. Fever, nearly always present, may be the only evidence of the abscess. Nonspecific constitutional symptoms such as anorexia and weight loss are common. The most frequent findings relate to the thorax and abdomen. Nonproductive cough, chest pain, dyspnea, and shoulder pain may occur from the effects of the infection on the adjacent diaphragm. Rales, rhonchi, or a friction rub may be audible. Dullness to percussion and decreased breath sounds are present when basilar atelectasis, pneumonia, or pleural effusion occurs.

The most common abdominal complaint, pain, is often accompanied by localized tenderness. A mass, wound drainage, or sinus tracts at the previous abdominal incision site are sometimes present. Abdominal distention and hypoactive bowel sounds from paralytic ileus are common.

Diagnosis

Leukocytosis occurs in most patients, and anemia is frequent. Blood cultures are occasionally positive.

Chest x-rays are usually abnormal. The common findings are ipsilateral pleural effusion, elevated or immobile hemidiaphragm, pneumonitis, and atelectasis. Plain abdominal films may reveal extraintestinal gas in the abscess, displacement of adjacent organs, or a soft-tissue density representing the abscess.

Ultrasonic examination is especially helpful in right-sided subphrenic abscesses. The left-sided subphrenic area is more difficult to examine because of the gas-filled stomach, splenic flexure, aerated lung, and ribs. Moreover, because the spleen varies in shape and size and may contain few echoes, it can resemble an abscess.

CT detects most intra-abdominal abscesses, but the subdiaphragmatic area may be difficult to assess, to ascertain whether an abnormality lies just above or below the diaphragm. CT is especially helpful when the left upper quadrant is the likely site of infection or during the postoperative period, when wounds, dressings, and drains make ultrasonic examination difficult.

Complications, Prognosis, and Treatment

Subdiaphragmatic abscesses may extend into the thoracic cavity and cause an empyema, a lung abscess, or pneumonia. Intra-abdominal complications include incisional breakdown and fistula formation. Occasionally, the abscess may compress the inferior vena cava and cause lower extremity edema.

The mortality of subphrenic abscesses is 25 to 40%; deaths occur from uncontrolled infection, malnutrition, and complications of prolonged hospitalization such as pulmonary emboli and nosocomial infections.

The **treatment** is surgical or percutaneous catheter drainage. Antibiotics are adjuncts but not satisfactory substitutes. Adequate nutrition is critical during the often prolonged hospital course.

MIDABDOMINAL ABSCESSES

Midabdominal abscesses, lying between the transverse colon and the pelvis, include **right and left lower-quadrant** and **interloop abscesses.**

Right lower-quadrant abscesses develop most commonly as complications of acute appendicitis and less frequently from colonic diverticulitis, regional enteritis, or a perforated duodenal ulcer with drainage down the right paracolic gutter. Typically, fever, right lower-quadrant tenderness, and a mass develop following symptoms sug-

gesting acute appendicitis. The mass may cause partial or complete small-bowel obstruction. Leukocytosis is usual. **Treatment** includes antibiotics plus surgical drainage. Appendiceal abscesses, however, usually resolve on antibiotic therapy alone.

Left lower-quadrant abscesses usually occur from perforation of a diverticulum in the descending or sigmoid colon, less commonly from a perforated colonic carcinoma. The symptoms are those of acute diverticulitis: left lower-quadrant pain, anorexia, and mild nausea followed by fever, leukocytosis, and development of a palpable mass. **Treatment** usually consists of antibiotic therapy plus surgery, although some diverticular abscesses resolve with antimicrobial therapy alone. Some surgeons drain the abscess and perform a diverting colostomy, resect the diseased bowel in a 2nd operation, and close the colostomy in a 3rd. Others resect the diseased bowel and bring out the proximal colon as an end colostomy and the distal bowel as a mucous fistula; 2 to 3 mo later, they perform an end-to-end anastomosis.

Interloop abscesses, loculations of pus between the folded surfaces of the small and large intestines and their mesenteries, are complications of bowel perforation, anastomotic disruption, or Crohn's disease. The manifestations may be very subtle. Fever and leukocytosis are often the only features; abdominal tenderness, signs of paralytic ileus, or a palpable mass sometimes occur. Plain abdominal films occasionally suggest the diagnosis by the presence of bowel-wall edema, separation of bowel loops, localized ileus, and air-fluid levels on upright films. **Treatment** is surgical drainage and appropriate antibiotics.

Pelvic Abscesses

Pelvic abscesses usually are complications of acute appendicitis, pelvic inflammatory disease, or colonic diverticulitis. The major symptoms are fever and lower abdominal pain. Abscesses in the Douglas' cul-de-sac, adjacent to the colon, may cause diarrhea; contiguity to the bladder may result in urinary urgency and frequency. Abdominal tenderness is common, and the abscess is usually palpable on vaginal or rectal examination. Leukocytosis is typically present.

Treatment is surgical drainage (through the vagina or rectum) and antibiotics—clindamycin and an aminoglycoside (tobramycin or gentamicin) being a good initial choice pending culture results. Large abscesses may be drained via percutaneous catheters. With abscesses due to pelvic inflammatory disease, some gynecologists treat the patient with fluids, bed rest, and antibiotics and reserve surgery for failure to respond after several days, presence or suspicion of a ruptured abscess, an abscess amenable to drainage via culdotomy or another extraperitoneal route, or uncertain diagnosis.

RETROPERITONEAL ABSCESSES

Anterior Retroperitoneal Abscesses

These abscesses are complications of acute appendicitis, colonic perforation from diverticulitis or tumor, gastric or duodenal perforation, regional enteritis, or pancreatitis. The major symptoms are fever, abdominal or flank pain, nausea and vomiting, weight loss, and pain in the hip, leg, or knee from psoas muscle involvement. The major findings on examination are fever, abdominal or flank tenderness, and a palpable mass. Pain on extension of the hip is frequent. Leukocytosis is usual. Abnormalities on plain film examination include extraintestinal gas in the abscess, displacement of adjacent organs (such as kidney or colon), and loss of the psoas muscle shadow. Chest films may show ipsilateral diaphragmatic elevation, with or without pleural effusion. Abnormalities shown by excretory urogram include renal or ureteral displacement or hydronephrosis from ureteral obstruction. Barium studies of the intestinal tract may show displacement of adjacent viscera. CT often defines retroperitoneal

abscesses when other studies are negative or equivocal. **Treatment** is usually surgical or percutaneous catheter drainage and antibiotics, although some abscesses resolve with antimicrobial therapy alone. Complications of untreated infection include extension along fascial planes to involve the anterior abdominal wall, thigh, hip, psoas muscle, subphrenic spaces, mediastinum, and pleural cavities. Sometimes intraperitoneal rupture occurs, causing acute bacterial peritonitis.

PERINEPHRIC ABSCESSES

Perinephric abscess nearly always occurs from rupture of a renal parenchymal abscess into the perinephric space between the kidney and its surrounding fascia (Gerota's capsule). Some of these abscesses are staphylococcal and follow hematogenous spread of infection to the kidney from another site, usually cutaneous, with symptoms classically developing 1 to 3 wk after the skin lesions. More commonly, however, perinephric abscesses arise from pyelonephritis, often associated with renal calculous disease, the usual infecting organisms being *E. coli*, *Proteus*, or other aerobic gram-negative rods. Patients are often diabetic.

Symptoms and Signs

The major symptoms are fever, chills, and unilateral flank or abdominal pain, frequently with dysuria. Most patients are febrile and have unilateral flank or abdominal tenderness, often with a palpable mass. Nausea, vomiting, and hematuria occur occasionally. In some patients fever is the only manifestation.

Diagnosis

Leukocytosis and pyuria are common, but not universal. A majority of patients have positive urine cultures; blood cultures are positive in 20 to 40%. Perinephric abscess usually differs clinically from acute pyelonephritis by longer duration of symptoms before hospitalization and by fever following the start of antibiotic therapy; both usually last > 5 days with perinephric abscess and < 5 days with acute pyelonephritis.

Chest x-rays are abnormal in about half the patients, revealing ipsilateral pneumonia, atelectasis, pleural effusion, or an elevated hemidiaphragm. In about half the patients, plain abdominal films are also abnormal, showing a mass, calculi, loss of the psoas shadow, or extraintestinal gas in the perinephric area from infection with gas-forming organisms. Findings on excretory urogram, abnormal in about 80% of cases, may include nonvisualizing or poorly visualizing kidney, distorted calyces, anterior renal displacement, and unilateral renal fixation, best demonstrated by fluoroscopy or inspiration-expiration films. Ultrasound and CT are alternative diagnostic technics that are positive in nearly all perinephric abscesses.

Prognosis and Treatment

The overall mortality rate is about 40%, but prompt diagnosis and therapy usually portend an excellent outcome, especially if the patient has no serious underlying disease. Treatment is surgical drainage and sometimes nephrectomy (if the kidney is extensively involved by infection or stones), and systemic antimicrobial therapy. A reasonable initial choice, pending results of blood, urine, and abscess cultures, is gentamicin.

VISCERAL ABSCESSES

SPLENIC ABSCESSES

Etiology

Most splenic abscesses occur from uncontrolled infection elsewhere and are small, multiple, and clinically silent abnormalities found incidentally at autopsy. Clinically

evident splenic abscesses usually are solitary and arise from (1) systemic bacteremia (eg, endocarditis or salmonellosis) that originated in another site and is now causing infection in a previously normal spleen; (2) infection, presumably of hematogenous origin, in a spleen damaged by blunt or penetrating trauma (with superinfection of a hematoma), bland infarction (such as occurs in hemoglobinopathies, especially sickle trait or hemoglobin SC disease), or other diseases (malaria, hydatid cysts); or (3) extension from a contiguous infection, such as a subphrenic abscess. The most common infecting organisms are staphylococci, streptococci, anaerobes, and aerobic gram-negative rods, including salmonella.

Symptoms, Signs, and Diagnosis

The major symptoms are subacute onset of fever and left-sided pain, often pleuritic, in the flank, upper abdomen, or lower chest that may radiate to the left shoulder. The left upper-quadrant is commonly tender to palpation, and splenomegaly is typical. Rarely, a splenic friction rub is audible. Leukocytosis is usual, and blood cultures sometimes grow the infecting organisms.

Radiographic findings may include a left upper-quadrant mass; extraintestinal gas in the abscess from gas-forming organisms; displacement of other organs, including kidney, colon, and stomach; elevated left hemidiaphragm; and left pleural effusion.

A liver-spleen radionuclide scan, a CT scan, and ultrasonic scanning should demonstrate intrasplenic defects with abscesses larger than 2 to 3 cm.

Complications and Treatment

Complications of untreated abscesses include hemorrhage into the abscess cavity or rupture into the peritoneum, bowel, bronchus, or pleural space. Splenic abscess is a rare cause of sustained bacteremia in endocarditis despite appropriate chemotherapy. Treatment consists of systemic antibiotics and splenectomy.

PANCREATIC ABSCESSES

Etiology

Pancreatic abscesses typically develop in a site of pancreatic necrosis, including pseudocysts, following an attack of acute pancreatitis. The usual organisms are bowel flora—aerobic gram-negative rods and anaerobes, but how they reach the pancreas is uncertain. Staphylococcus and candida are surprisingly frequent isolates, as well.

Symptoms and Signs

In most cases the patient improves after an attack of pancreatitis, but one to several weeks later fever, abdominal pain and tenderness, nausea, vomiting, and, sometimes, paralytic ileus occur. Less commonly, the abscess develops shortly after the attack begins. In these cases the fever, leukocytosis, and abdominal findings so common in acute pancreatitis fail to resolve as quickly as usual; persistence of these features for longer than about 7 days should suggest an abscess. An abdominal mass is palpable in about half the cases.

Diagnosis

The serum amylase may be elevated, but often is normal. Leukocytosis, however, is usually present. The serum alkaline phosphatase may be increased and the albumin decreased. Blood cultures occasionally grow the responsible organism, and sometimes ascitic fluid is positive when cultured.

Chest x-rays often demonstrate left-sided abnormalities, such as a pleural effusion, basilar atelectasis, pneumonia, or an elevated hemidiaphragm. Plain abdominal films or barium studies of the GI tract may reveal extraintestinal gas in the pancreatic area or displacement of adjacent structures. Ultrasound may show a fluid-filled pancreatic mass, whose contents may have multiple echoes from debris or loculations within the

abscess. CT may show within the pancreas a low-density mass that may contain gas and that fails to enhance following intravenously administered contrast material.

Complications, Prognosis, and Treatment

Complications of undrained abscesses include perforation into contiguous structures; erosion into adjacent vessels, such as the left gastric, splenic, and gastroduodenal arteries, with exsanguination; and further abscess formation, a frequent occurrence that necessitates reoperation. Even with appropriate surgical and antimicrobial therapy, the mortality rate is about 40%.

Treatment includes surgical drainage or percutaneous catheter drainage (which, however, is much less successful in pancreatic diseases than in other intra-abdominal abscesses) and systemic antibiotic therapy. A reasonable choice until culture results are available is chloramphenicol alone or a combination of clindamycin and an aminoglycoside like tobramycin or gentamicin.

HEPATIC ABSCESSES

Etiology and Pathogenesis

Hepatic abscesses are usually amebic or bacterial (pyogenic). Bacterial abscesses occur from (1) ascending cholangitis in a biliary tract partially or completely obstructed by stone, tumor, or stricture; (2) portal bacteremia from an intra-abdominal site, such as diverticulitis or appendicitis; (3) systemic bacteremia originating from a distant location, with organisms reaching the liver via the hepatic artery; (4) direct extension from an adjacent infection outside the biliary tract; and (5) trauma, either penetrating, with direct implantation of bacteria into the liver, or blunt, causing a hematoma that becomes secondarily infected. A cause is typically obvious, but sometimes the abscess is unexplained. Most abscesses are single, but multiple (usually microscopic) abscesses are common with systemic bacteremia or complete biliary tract obstruction.

Streptococci or staphylococci are the most common bacteria when the infection results from systemic bacteremia. Abscesses originating from a biliary tract infection usually contain aerobic gram-negative rods—eg, *E. coli* and *Klebsiella*, while those secondary to portal bacteremia from an intra-abdominal infection typically contain both aerobic gram-negative bacilli and anaerobic bacteria.

Symptoms and Signs

With multiple abscesses from systemic bacteremia or biliary tract infection, the onset is usually acute and the principal clinical features of the predisposing disease predominate. With single abscesses, a subacute onset of symptoms occurs over several weeks. Fever is a major, and sometimes the sole, complaint, but most patients also have such symptoms as anorexia, nausea, weight loss, and weakness. Right upper-quadrant pain or tenderness and hepatomegaly occur in about half the cases; right pleuritic chest pain is seen occasionally. Jaundice is usually apparent only with biliary tract obstruction.

Diagnosis

Common blood test abnormalities include anemia, leukocytosis, elevated ESR, increased alkaline phosphatase, decreased albumin, and mildly elevated bilirubin. Blood cultures are positive in a substantial minority of patients. About half the patients have chest x-rays demonstrating right-sided basilar atelectasis, pleural effusion, pneumonia, or an elevated hemidiaphragm.

An abscess larger than 2 cm can usually be detected on radionuclide liver scan or ultrasound examination, which can usually differentiate fluid-filled masses from solid ones and help to distinguish liver abscesses from neoplasms. CT scan may demonstrate the abscess when the other studies are negative.

In the patient with symptoms of liver abscess and a defect on radionuclide, ultrasound, or CT scans, the most important clinical distinction is between a pyogenic and an amebic abscess. Amebic abscesses respond well to chemotherapy alone—metronidazole, chloroquine, or emetine—and usually do not require surgical drainage. Features suggesting an amebic etiology are age < 50; single, rather than multiple, defects; a history of diarrhea, especially if bloody; *Entamoeba histolytica* in the stool; and absence of a condition predisposing to bacterial abscesses. Most importantly, nearly all patients with amebic liver abscesses have a positive serology for *E. histolytica.*

Complications, Prognosis, and Treatment

Complications of hepatic abscesses include subphrenic abscess formation, bleeding into the abscess cavity, and rupture into the lung, pleural cavity, or peritoneum. With correct diagnosis and appropriate therapy, the mortality rate is 10 to 30%; those with multiple abscesses have a higher mortality rate than those with a single abscess.

Treatment includes antimicrobial agents and removal of pus, preferably with percutaneous drainage by needle aspiration or an indwelling catheter. Surgery is indicated for patients with a coexisting process requiring laparotomy and those failing to respond to nonoperative management. When the bacteriology is unknown, chloramphenicol alone or a combination of clindamycin and an aminoglycoside like tobramycin or gentamicin should provide adequate coverage until the infecting organisms are identified. To help prevent relapses, antibiotic therapy is usually continued for several weeks following drainage. Some abscesses will resolve with antibiotic therapy alone.

URINARY TRACT ABSCESSES

PROSTATIC ABSCESSES

Prostatic abscesses develop as complications of urinary tract infections, especially acute prostatitis, urethritis, and epididymitis. The usual patient is 40 to 60 yr and has frequency, dysuria, or urinary retention. Perineal pain, evidence of acute epididymitis, hematuria, and a purulent urethral discharge are less common signs. Fever is present in some patients. Rectal examination may show prostatic tenderness and fluctuance, but often prostatic enlargement is the only abnormality, and sometimes the gland feels normal.

Leukocytosis is common. Although pyuria and bacteriuria are frequent, the urine may be completely normal. Blood cultures are positive in a small minority of patients.

Prostatic fluctuance, a purulent urethral discharge, continued or recurrent urinary infections despite antimicrobial therapy, and persistent perineal pain should suggest a prostatic abscess. Many of these abscesses, however, are discovered unexpectedly during prostatic surgery or endoscopy; bulging of a lateral lobe into the prostatic urethra or rupture during instrumentation reveals the abscess.

Treatment is drainage by transurethral evacuation or perineal incision plus appropriate antibiotics. The usual infecting organisms are aerobic gram-negative bacilli or, less frequently, *Staphylococcus aureus.*

HEAD AND NECK ABSCESSES

(See also RETROPHARYNGEAL ABSCESS under BACTERIAL INFECTIONS in Ch. 191 and PERITONSILLAR CELLULITIS AND ABSCESS in Ch. 210)

SUBMANDIBULAR SPACE INFECTION

(Ludwig's Angina)

A rapidly spreading, bilateral, indurated cellulitis occurring in both the sublingual and submaxillary spaces without abscess formation or lymphatic involvement. Ludwig's an-

gina usually develops from dental or peridontal infection, especially of the 2nd and 3rd mandibular molars. It may occur in association with problems caused by poor dental hygiene (eg, gingivitis and dental sepsis), tooth extractions, or trauma (eg, fractures of the mandible, lacerations of the floor of the mouth, peritonsillar abscess). Although not a true abscess, Ludwig's angina resembles one clinically and is treated similarly. Untreated, it may be fatal.

The major manifestations are pain in the area of the involved tooth; severe, tender induration of the submandibular region; trismus; dysphonia; drooling and inability to swallow; and dyspnea and stridor from laryngeal edema and tongue elevation. Fever, chills, and tachycardia are usually present. X-rays of the head and neck are useful to assess the degree of soft-tissue swelling and airway obstruction. **Complications** can include asphyxiation, aspiration pneumonia, lung abscess, and metastatic sepsis.

Treatment includes establishment of an adequate airway, which may require tracheostomy (NOTE: *Obstruction of the airway can progress within hours, and the patency of the airway must be assessed frequently*); penicillin in high doses to treat the oral anaerobes that cause the infection; and incision to drain whatever fluid is present and to relieve the pressure of the swollen, infected tissues. If the patient is allergic to penicillin, chloramphenicol, clindamycin, or a cephalosporin may be used.

PHARYNGOMAXILLARY ABSCESSES

The pharyngomaxillary (lateral pharyngeal, parapharyngeal, or pterygomaxillary) space is a cone-shaped compartment lateral to the pharynx, extending from the sphenoid bone at the base of the skull to the hyoid bone. The styloid bone divides this space into an anterior compartment, closely related to the tonsillar fossa medially and the internal pterygoid muscle laterally, and a posterior compartment containing the carotid sheath and the cranial nerves emerging from their foramina in the base of the skull.

Pharyngomaxillary abscesses usually arise from infections in the pharynx, including the nasopharynx, adenoids, and tonsils. Less common sources are dental infections, parotitis, and mastoiditis. Fever, sore throat, and malaise are usually present. With infections limited to the anterior compartment, trismus, induration along the angle of the jaw, and medial bulging of the tonsil and lateral pharyngeal wall occur. With posterior compartment infection, swelling of the posterior pharyngeal wall and parotid space develops. Trismus is minimal or absent. Involvement of the internal jugular vein within the carotid sheath causes shaking chills, high fever, and bacteremia. Erosion of the internal, external, or common carotid arteries causes profuse hemorrhage. Inferior spread of infection results in neck swelling that obliterates the space beneath the angle of the mandible. **Treatment** is surgical drainage and high-dose penicillin, which is effective against *Streptococcus pyogenes* and the oral anaerobes usually responsible for the infection.

SUPPURATIVE PAROTITIS

Suppurative parotitis, an infection ascending from the mouth, is usually due to *Staphylococcus aureus*, which normally colonizes the opening to Stensen's duct. This infection typically occurs in the elderly or chronically ill patient with a dry mouth from decreased oral intake, from medications with atropine-like effects such as antihistamines or phenothiazines, or following general anesthesia. Fever, chills, and unilateral pain and swelling mark the sudden onset. The gland is firm and tender, with erythema and edema of the overlying skin. Frank pus, expressed from Stensen's duct on compressing the gland, typically shows gram-positive cocci in clumps.

Treatment is a penicillinase-resistant penicillin when *Staphylococcus aureus* is re-

sponsible; the antibiotic choice is determined by Gram stain and culture if another organism causes the infection. Improved hydration and oral hygiene are important. Sialagogues (eg, lemon drops) and massage of the gland help promote drainage through the duct. Surgery is rarely necessary, unless the patient fails to improve after several days of medical management.

MUSCULOSKELETAL ABSCESSES

PYOMYOSITIS

Abscess formation deep within large striated muscles. Muscle abscesses are uncommon. They may develop by spread from a contiguous bone or soft-tissue infection or from a hematogenous route. The latter is thought to be the mechanism of pyomyositis. Presumably, asymptomatic bacteremia occurs with localization of organisms in a muscle damaged by previous, often unrecognized, trauma. Pyomyositis is rare in the USA, but may occur in compromised hosts. It is common in many tropical areas and affects both children and adults, especially the malnourished. The most frequent sites are the quadriceps, gluteus, shoulder, and upper arm muscles, with multiple areas of involvement in about 40% of patients. The initial symptoms are cramping pain followed by edema, worsening discomfort, and mild fever. The muscle may feel indurated at this time. Later, edema and tenderness increase, with obvious fluctuance developing in about half the patients. Leukocytosis is common. In the early indurated stage, needle aspiration may be negative; later it yields thick, yellow pus, nearly always growing *Staphylococcus aureus.* Occasional cases are due to *Streptococcus pyogenes* or *E. coli.* **Treatment** is antibiotic therapy with a penicillinase-resistant penicillin. In the nonsuppurative phase, antibiotics alone suffice; with pus, incision and drainage are mandatory. The extent of involvement at surgery is frequently much greater than anticipated on clinical evaluation.

HAND ABSCESSES

(See also Paronychial Infections in Ch. 231)

Felon

A felon, an infection of the pulp space of the finger pad, nearly always follows minor finger injury (eg, a splinter or needle prick). Severe local pain, heat, and redness occur, often with lymphangitis and lymphadenopathy. Leukocytosis is common. The abscess rapidly enlarges to involve multiple septae in the distal pulp compartment. Osteitis is a frequent, and osteomyelitis an occasional, complication. **Treatment** is prompt incision, with division of the fibrous septae, to insure adequate drainage.

Purulent Tenosynovitis

Purulent tenosynovitis occurs from penetrating injury to the flexion creases of the fingers, most commonly the index, middle, and ring fingers. Infection within the tendon sheaths causes rapid tissue destruction and impairment of the gliding mechanisms, leading to loss of finger motion. The major signs are generalized swelling and inflammation of the finger, tenderness over the flexor tendon sheaths, careful maintenance of a flexed finger position, and exquisite pain on active or passive finger extension. Fever, lymphangitis, lymphadenitis, and leukocytosis are usual. **Treatment** is surgical drainage plus antibiotics. Gram stain of the pus should dictate antibiotic choice; streptococci and staphylococci are the usual pathogens.

6. BACTEREMIA AND SEPTIC SHOCK

Bacteremia connotes *invasion of the circulation by bacteria.* The term **septicemia** is reserved for *situations in which bacteremia is associated with clinical manifestations of infection.* Bacteremia commonly, and usually transiently, accompanies various surgical manipulations (eg, incision of an abscess); or it may result from colonization of indwelling intravenous devices and urethral catheters. (For infants, see also NEONATAL SEPSIS AND NEONATAL MENINGITIS under NEONATAL INFECTIONS in Ch. 186.) Bacteremia may be intermittent or sustained, and may cause severe consequences. In patients who abuse IV narcotics, gram-positive bacteremia is common and may lead to right-sided bacterial endocarditis even in the absence of cardiac murmurs. The bacteremia of left-sided bacterial endocarditis is usually sustained and may be prolonged. Gram-negative bacteremia is usually intermittent and generally follows primary infection in the GU tract, biliary tree, GI tract, lungs, or, less commonly, skin, bones, or joints. In many patients with chronic diseases no primary focus of infection is apparent.

Symptoms and Signs

Few clinical manifestations are unique to bacteremia. Although variable, fever is almost always present and may be intermittent, with wide diurnal variations (septic, or "spiking"). Chills are common at the onset. Skin eruptions are also common, and may be petechial, purpuric, papular, pustular, or vesicular. Usually gram-negative bacteremia begins abruptly with chills, fever, nausea, vomiting, diarrhea, and prostration.

Diagnosis

The presence of bacteremia is established by blood cultures, which should be performed for both aerobic and anaerobic organisms. A single negative culture does not exclude bacteremia; moreover, in some patients, especially those with prior antibiotic therapy, blood cultures never do become positive. If the patient is not very ill, no more than 6 blood cultures should be performed. In severely ill patients, 2 blood cultures taken 30 min apart before treatment is instituted should suffice. In most cases, treatment is required before results of blood cultures become available.

Complications

Metastatic infection of the meninges or of serous cavities, such as the pericardium or larger joints, may occur. Endocarditis (see also ENDOCARDITIS in Ch. 27) may be the sequel of bacteremia if the pathogen is a streptococcus or staphylococcus, but rarely occurs as a result of gram-negative bacteremias. **Metastatic abscesses** may occur almost anywhere and, when extensive, produce symptoms and signs characteristic of infection in the organ affected. Multiple abscess formation is particularly common with staphylococcal bacteremia. Bacteremia may result in **septic shock,** which is discussed separately, below.

Prognosis

Transient bacteremias associated with surgical procedures, indwelling IV catheters, or urinary catheters are often undetected and probably do not require therapy. However, persistent bacteremia is dangerous; the prognosis depends on the ability to eliminate the source of infection with surgery or antibiotics, and on the status of the underlying disease. When multiple organisms are recovered consistently (polymicrobial bacteremia), a poor outcome can be expected. Bacteremia unresponsive to treatment because of inadequate antibiotic therapy, poor host resistance, or delay in diagnosis is often fatal.

Treatment of bacteremia is discussed below with septic shock.

SEPTIC SHOCK

When bacteremia is associated with inadequate tissue perfusion, especially with gram-negative organisms or meningococci, **septic shock** with hypotension, vascular collapse, renal failure, and death may ensue. Septic shock usually occurs when bacteremia is due to gram-negative organisms and generally in hospitalized patients with underlying diseases. Predisposing factors include diabetes mellitus; cirrhosis; leukemia; lymphoma; disseminated carcinoma; surgical procedures; antecedent infection in the urinary, biliary, or GI tracts; indwelling IV catheters; treatment with antibiotics, steroids, cytotoxic agents, or inhalation equipment. Septic shock occurs more often in the elderly and in the newborn.

The pathogenesis of septic shock depends upon vasoconstriction of the small arteries and veins, which leads to increased peripheral vascular resistance, pooling of blood in the microcirculation, and decreased cardiac output. With poor perfusion there is tissue anoxia and the decreased blood volume results in hypotension and oliguria. These vasoactive phenomena are related largely to release of endotoxin, the lipopolysaccharide moiety of gram-negative bacillary cell walls, into the circulation.

Symptoms and Signs

Manifestations of bacteremia (see above) usually appear first. When septic shock develops, there are, in addition, tachycardia; tachypnea; hypotension; cool, pale extremities (often with peripheral cyanosis); mental obtundation; and oliguria. Occasionally the findings are subtle, especially in elderly, debilitated patients or infants. Unexplained hypotension, increasing confusion and disorientation, hyperpnea, or oliguria due to decreased renal blood flow may be the only early clues to gram-negative shock. As shock progresses, inadequate renal perfusion may lead to acute renal failure. Congestive heart failure, respiratory insufficiency, and coma may progress to death.

Different hemodynamic patterns are characteristic of endotoxin-related shock. Some patients have normal blood volume, venous pressure, circulation time, and cardiac output, but have decreased peripheral resistance. These patients have warm, dry skin; often they also have cirrhosis. The prognosis in this type of **"warm shock"** is good unless local acidosis, a consequence of ineffective tissue perfusion and impaired oxygen utilization, eventuates in decreased blood volume, central venous pressure, and cardiac output, with hypotension and oliguria. This hemodynamic pattern may be present initially or may follow a period of warm shock.

Most patients with septic shock have deficiencies in several clotting factors, probably due to their consumption in the process of disseminated intravascular coagulation (see Ch. 99). Respiratory failure characterized by decreased pulmonary compliance and irreversible hypoxia, called **"shock lung"** (see Ch. 35), may ensue even after hemodynamic abnormalities have been corrected.

Laboratory Findings

Laboratory data in bacteremia and septic shock vary greatly and depend in many instances on the cause and stage of hemodynamic decompensation. Usually, leukocytosis of between 15,000 and 30,000 WBC/μL with a left shift is present. However, relative or absolute leukopenia may be present in severe cases, particularly early in the course. The platelet count is usually decreased. Urinalysis reveals no specific abnormality. Initially the urine sp gr is increased. However, if oliguria persists, isosthenuria may develop. The BUN and creatinine are increased, and creatinine clearance declines. Electrolytes vary considerably, with a trend toward hyponatremia and hypochloremia. Potassium may be low or high, depending upon the ability of the kidney to excrete this ion.

Respiratory alkalosis, with a low P_{CO_2} and increased arterial pH, is present early and

compensates for lactic acidemia. Serum bicarbonate is usually low, while blood lactate is increased. As shock progresses, metabolic acidosis supervenes. Hypoxemia with P_{O_2} < 70 mm Hg is common. Hemodynamic measurements vary as described above. The ECG shows depressed ST segments with T wave inversions and various arrhythmias.

Treatment

Overall mortality in septic shock ranges from 50 to 90%. If mild to moderate lactic acidemia is present, the prognosis is good, but if lactic acidosis is severe, the outcome is likely to be fatal. Poor results often follow failure to institute therapy soon enough. Once severe lactic acidemia and decompensated metabolic acidosis become established, shock is often irreversible despite therapy. Because most patients likely to develop septic shock are in the hospital before the symptoms and signs of shock appear, this grave complication of infection is often avoidable by vigilant care.

Patients with septic shock should be treated in intensive care units. Pulmonary artery and systemic pressures, arterial and venous pH, arterial blood gases, blood lactate, renal function, and electrolytes should be monitored frequently. Cutaneous vasoconstriction provides a clue to peripheral vascular resistance, but does not accurately reflect blood flow to kidney, brain, or gut. Therefore, hourly urine output should be used to monitor splanchnic blood flow and visceral perfusion. Indwelling urinary catheters are usually required.

Fluid therapy: The central venous pressure **(CVP)** or pulmonary artery pressure should be measured in every patient, and fluid replacement given until the CVP reaches 10 to 12 cm of water or until the pulmonary wedge pressure reaches 12 to 15 mm Hg. Blood volume should be replaced with blood if anemia is present; otherwise, plasma, dextran, human serum albumin, or appropriate electrolyte solutions (usually dextrose-saline with bicarbonate, which is preferable to lactate) are used. Oliguria in the presence of hypotension is not a contraindication to continuing vigorous fluid therapy. The quantity of fluid required often far exceeds the normal blood volume and may amount to 8 to 12 L in a few hours.

Respiration should be supported with nasal oxygen, tracheal intubation, or tracheostomy as necessary. The pulmonary artery pressure may be the best guide for anticipating incipient pulmonary edema. Treatment of shock lung is described in Ch. 35.

Parenteral, bactericidal antibiotics should be administered after cultures of blood and appropriate sites have been taken. Usually at the onset of bacteremia or septic shock, while awaiting cultures and sensitivities, an etiologic diagnosis entails an educated guess based on previous cultures from a primary focus or on the setting in which infection occurs. Pus must be drained and foreign bodies and necrotic tissue must be removed. Failure to do so often results in a poor outcome despite antibiotic therapy. Specific therapy is the same as for the primary infection, but more intense. Since *early* administration of antibiotics may be critical to save the patient's life, an effective regimen for bacteremia of unknown etiology before antimicrobial sensitivities are known is gentamicin or tobramycin 3 to 5 mg/kg/day IM or IV plus either nafcillin 4 to 8 gm/day IV or a parenteral cephalosporin. Carbenicillin or ticarcillin 30 gm/day IV may be added if *Pseudomonas* is suspected. As soon as cultures have revealed the putative pathogen, unnecessary agents are stopped. Antibiotics should be continued for several days after shock has resolved and the primary focus of infection has healed adequately.

Vasoactive drugs, particularly alpha-receptor blocking agents (eg, phenoxybenzamine) or beta-receptor stimulators (eg, isoproterenol) have been of value in septic shock. Dopamine is now the preferred agent because it enhances renal perfusion. The response to therapy is determined clinically, and return of perfusion to normal is the best guide to stopping vasopressors.

Adrenal corticosteroids in large doses support peripheral resistance and mitigate the

cellular injury evoked by endotoxin. While some consider their use controversial, most clinicians will give 30 mg/kg methylprednisolone as a bolus and repeat it at 6- to 12-h intervals for 24 to 48 h.

Control of hemorrhage, with fresh frozen plasma when it is a consequence of clotting factor deficiency or with platelets when due to thrombocytopenia, is important.

Surgical intervention to drain abscesses or excise infected tissues—eg, infarcted bowel, inflamed gallbladder, infected uterus, or pyonephrosis—should be performed. The patient's condition, although grave, may continue to deteriorate unless the septic focus is removed or drained.

Other therapeutic modalities are indicated, depending on the patient's clinical status, and include mannitol or furosemide to induce diuresis in patients with oliguria, a rapidly acting digitalis preparation in patients with heart failure, and, occasionally, heparin in patients with disseminated intravascular coagulation.

---

7. INFECTIONS IN THE COMPROMISED HOST

Infections ranging from minor to fatal, caused by normally nonpathogenic organisms in patients whose host defense mechanisms have been compromised. Mainly, the problems presented take place in the hospital setting and are the price of medical advances that have enabled us to deal more effectively with previously unmanageable disorders. Nosocomial infection in the newborn is discussed under NEONATAL INFECTIONS in Ch. 186.

Etiology

Host defense mechanisms—physiologic, anatomic, or immunologic—may be altered or breached by disease or trauma, or by procedures or agents used for diagnosis or therapy. Infections occurring in this setting, also called **opportunistic infections**, are seen if antimicrobial therapy alters the normal relationship between host and microbe, or if host defense mechanisms have been altered by burns, anemia, other infections, neoplasms, metabolic disorders, irradiation, foreign bodies, immunosuppressive or cytotoxic drugs, corticosteroids, or diagnostic or therapeutic instrumentation.

The underlying alteration predisposes the patient to infections from his usually nonpathogenic endogenous microflora or from ordinarily harmless, saprophytic organisms acquired by contact with other patients, hospital personnel, or equipment. Management is complicated by the fact that the organisms that opportunistically take advantage of the compromised host usually are resistant to antibiotics. These organisms may be bacteria, fungi, viruses, or other parasites, and the precise character of the host's altered defenses determines which organisms are most likely to be involved.

1. Antibiotic resistance and impaired anatomic host defense mechanisms: Antimicrobial treatment alters the normal microflora of the skin, mucous membranes, and GI tract and may result in colonization of these organs. Colonization per se is harmless unless followed by **superinfection** (invasion by endogenous or environmental organisms resistant to the antibiotic being given), which is demonstrable microbiologically or clinically. Factors predisposing to superinfection include extremes of age, chronic infection or other debilitating disease, excessive doses of one or several antimicrobials, and use of broad-spectrum antibiotics either singly or in combination. The wider the antimicrobial spectrum, the greater the danger of superinfection. Superinfections usually appear on the 4th or 5th day of chemotherapy and may convert a benign, self-limited disease into a serious, prolonged, or even fatal one. They are most often caused by endogenous gram-negative enteric bacilli, fungi, and resistant staphylococci. The

diagnosis of superinfection by a normally commensal organism is certain only when the organism is recovered from blood, CSF, or body cavity fluid.

Nosocomial (hospital-acquired) infections are usually acquired from the hospital environment or personnel, the patient's own microflora, or inadequately sterilized equipment, and are commonly due to *Enterobacter*, *Klebsiella*, *Serratia*, *Pseudomonas*, *Proteus*, or *Candida*. They may replace strains of *Escherichia coli* and many gram-positive organisms, especially when a susceptible patient is given a broad-spectrum antibiotic or massive doses of any antibiotic.

Patients with extensive **burns** or those undergoing diagnostic or therapeutic **procedures that breach normal anatomic barriers** to infection (eg, tracheostomy, inhalation therapy, urinary tract instrumentation, indwelling urethral or IV catheters, surgery, and surgical prostheses) are vulnerable to infection by endogenous or exogenous (acquired from the environment) antibiotic-resistant organisms. Gram-negative bacteria, particularly *Pseudomonas* and *Serratia*, and other multiple-antibiotic–resistant organisms, alone or in combination with staphylococci, cause soft-tissue infections and bacteremia in severely burned patients. Significant bacteriuria develops in patients with indwelling urethral catheters and increases the risk of cystitis, pyelonephritis, and gram-negative rod bacteremia. Polyethylene IV catheters may cause sepsis, especially when thrombophlebitis from irritating IV solutions is present. Sepsis due to gram-negative organisms alone or in combination with staphylococci and *Candida* may arise in current or prior IV infusion sites and range from local suppuration to severe and sometimes fatal systemic infection. Patients with endotracheal tubes or tracheostomies and others who require repeated tracheal suctioning or inhalation therapy with equipment containing a reservoir of nebulization fluid may develop bronchopulmonary infection, usually with nosocomial gram-negative organisms.

2. Impaired cellular or humoral host defense mechanisms: Such **neoplastic** and **immunodeficiency diseases** as leukemia, aplastic anemia, Hodgkin's disease, and myeloma are characterized by selective defects in host resistance. Patients with hypogammaglobulinemia, myeloma, macroglobulinemia, or chronic lymphatic leukemia tend to have deficient humoral immune mechanisms and to develop pneumococcal and *Hemophilus* pneumonia (see also PNEUMONIA IN THE COMPROMISED HOST in Ch. 40) and bacteremia. Patients with Hodgkin's disease or acute leukemia, and those receiving intensive **immunosuppressive** or **irradiation therapy** frequently develop gram-negative bacteremia secondary to pneumonia. Since these patients also tend to have depressed cellular immune mechanisms, serious infection with *Aspergillus*, *Candida*, *Cryptococcus*, *Histoplasma*, *Mucor*, *Nocardia*, or *Staphylococcus* is frequent; herpes zoster, cytomegalovirus, *Pneumocystis*, and *Toxoplasma* infections also occur. **AIDS** is accompanied by yet another group of infections, including those caused by *Pneumocystis*, atypical mycobacteria, herpes simplex and zoster, giardia, cryptosporidia, isospora, and many others. (AIDS is discussed in Ch. 19.)

Cytotoxic drugs enhance the susceptibility of tissues to infection by direct cytotoxic action, resulting in severe leukopenia and thrombocytopenia; depression of the immune response, particularly cell-mediated immunity; and an altered inflammatory response. Most opportunistic infections in these patients result from the severe leukopenia.

Corticosteroids alter many aspects of host defenses; one of the most important is inhibition of the movement of leukocytes into the inflammatory exudate. Corticosteroids may reactivate healed pulmonary TB, histoplasmosis, coccidioidomycosis, and blastomycosis. Patients receiving corticosteroid treatment (especially in high dose) for RA, ulcerative colitis, asthma, sarcoidosis, SLE, and pemphigus, and patients with **Cushing's syndrome** have increased susceptibility to infection from usual and unusual

bacteria; they also tend to develop infections with *Aspergillus*, *Candida*, *Cryptococcus*, *Mucor*, and *Nocardia*.

Prophylaxis

Awareness of the patterns of infections that occur in the compromised host helps greatly in early recognition of infections and initiation of appropriate therapy. It is important to be aware of the specific site of breached defense, the type of defense system that has been weakened or lost, and the characteristics of organisms prevalent in a particular institution, based on continuous epidemiologic hospital surveillance.

Antibiotic prophylaxis (see also ANTIMICROBIAL CHEMOPROPHYLAXIS in Ch. 2) is indicated for various conditions, including rheumatic fever and bacterial endocarditis, TB contacts, recurrent urinary tract infections, recurrent otitis media, bacterial infections in granulocytopenic patients, and some types of *Neisseria* infections. Prophylaxis with antibiotics is also indicated following vaginal and abdominal hysterectomies; colonic, rectal, cardiac, joint, and vascular surgery; and prostatectomies in patients with previous urinary tract infections. On the other hand, use of broad-spectrum antibiotics, massive doses of any antibiotic, or prophylactic use of systemic antibiotics may ultimately result in infection with resistant bacteria. Patients receiving antimicrobial therapy should be watched for signs of superinfection.

Active or passive immunization helps prevent some types of infections. Active immunizations can prevent influenza and pneumococcal infections in individuals with heart and lung diseases. Pneumococcal vaccination is effective for splenectomized and sickle cell disease patients. Hepatitis B vaccine should be given to patients receiving blood products repeatedly. Passive immunizations can prevent or ameliorate herpes zoster, hepatitis A and B, measles, and rubella in immunosuppressed subjects. Severe hypogammaglobulinemia may require maintenance with immune serum globulin.

The use of **barriers to control and prevent infection** is discussed in detail in Ch. 2. Strict **asepsis** should be maintained in diagnostic and therapeutic manipulative procedures. **Urethral catheters** must be connected to closed sterile drainage bags and the system kept closed. Attendants should wear sterile gloves during **endotracheal** or **tracheostomy suctioning,** and suction catheters should be sterile, disposable, and used only once. Masks, tubing, nebulizer jars, and other components of respiratory therapy equipment that connect directly to a patient's airway should be sterilized by steam or gas prior to use and should be changed daily. When steam or gas sterilization is not possible, the equipment should be disinfected with a 2% glutaraldehyde or 2% acetic acid wash followed by thorough rinsing and drying. Alternatively, nebulization of 0.25% acetic acid through the equipment, followed by careful rinsing, is usually satisfactory for daily cleaning of a respirator after it has been assigned to a patient. Special care should be taken to be sure the gas jets have been completely cleaned.

When possible, **IV therapy** should be given through metal or scalp vein needles. IV catheters should be inserted securely, covered with a sterile protective dressing, and removed after 48 h or at the first sign of phlebitis. An ointment of neomycin, polymyxin B, and bacitracin or an iodine ointment (eg, povidone-iodine), applied daily to the cannulation site and the emerging catheter, may help in preventing infection. Thrombophlebitis usually responds to catheter withdrawal and local application of hot compresses.

Treatment

The organisms of opportunistic infection tend to be resistant to most commonly used antibiotics and are difficult to treat once established. Treatment periods often must be longer than usual. Short-term therapy may be merely suppressive unless the underlying condition can be corrected (eg, removal of urethral or IV catheters, or tracheostomy closure). Cultures, and possibly tissue biopsy (eg, for *Pneumocystis* infections—see in Ch. 40), should be obtained before starting or altering antibacterial

treatment, but at times, while awaiting laboratory results, therapy on the basis of clinical-bacteriologic diagnosis and presumptive sensitivity may need to be instituted. When possible, corticosteroid dosage and immunosuppressive chemotherapy should be reduced while treating opportunistic infections. Severely granulocytic patients with documented infection may benefit from granulocyte transfusions.

Further details of treatment are given elsewhere in the book, in discussions of specific underlying disorders or procedures and specific organisms.

---

8. BACTERIAL DISEASES

CAUSED BY GRAM-POSITIVE COCCI

STAPHYLOCOCCAL INFECTIONS

Epidemiology

Pathogenic staphylococci are ubiquitous. They are *normally* carried in the anterior nares of about 30%, and on the skin of about 20%, of healthy adults; hospital patients or personnel have slightly higher rates of carriage. Penicillin-resistant strains are common, especially in hospitals. Certain patients are predisposed to staphylococcal infections: newborns, nursing mothers, and patients with influenza, chronic bronchopulmonary disorders (eg, cystic fibrosis, pulmonary emphysema), leukemia, neoplasms, renal transplants, tracheostomies, burns, chronic skin disorders, surgical incisions, diabetes mellitus, and indwelling intravascular plastic catheters. Patients receiving adrenal steroids, irradiation, immunosuppressives, or antitumor chemotherapy are also at an increased risk. Predisposed patients may acquire antibiotic-resistant staphylococci from other colonized areas of their own bodies or from infected hospital personnel who may be asymptomatic carriers. Patient-to-patient transmission via the hands of personnel is the most important means of spread.

Unlike other staphylococcal diseases, **staphylococcal food poisoning** (see STAPHYLOCOCCAL FOOD POISONING in Ch. 57) is caused by ingestion of a preformed enterotoxin produced by staphylococci in contaminated food, not by infection with the organism itself. Victims of staphylococcal food poisoning usually are healthy otherwise.

Symptoms, Signs, and Diagnosis

The site of the staphylococcal infection determines its clinical picture. Common presentations include furuncles, carbuncles, abscesses, pneumonia, bacteremia, endocarditis, osteomyelitis, enterocolitis, and gastroenteritis. These are discussed in further detail in other appropriate sections of THE MANUAL, as listed in the Index.

Staphylococcal abscesses, toxic epidermal necrolysis (see Ch. 237), and the "scalded skin syndrome" (see Ch. 231): **Neonatal infections** usually appear within 6 wk after birth. Most commonly seen are pustular or bullous skin lesions, generally located in the axillary, inguinal, or neck skin folds; but multiple subcutaneous abscesses, exfoliation, bacteremia, meningitis, or pneumonia may also occur. Microscopic examination of the pus discloses polymorphonuclear neutrophils and staphylococci, often within the leukocytes.

Nursing mothers who develop breast abscesses or mastitis 1 to 4 wk postpartum should be considered as having penicillin-resistant staphylococcal infections, most probably derived from the nursery via the infant.

Postoperative infections ranging from "stitch abscesses" to extensive wound involvement commonly are due to staphylococci. Such infections may appear within a few days or not until several weeks after an operation; they are particularly likely to be delayed in onset if the patient received antibiotics at the time of surgery. The toxic

shock syndrome (see below) may occur as a complication of a postoperative staphylococcal infection.

Furuncles and **carbuncles** are discussed in Ch. 231.

Staphylococcal pneumonia (see in Ch. 40) should be suspected in patients with influenza who develop dyspnea, cyanosis, or persistent or recurrent fever, and in patients hospitalized with chronic bronchopulmonary disease or other high-risk diseases who develop fever, tachypnea, cough, cyanosis, and leukocytosis. In neonates, staphylococcal pneumonia is characterized by abscess formation, rapid development of pneumatoceles, and, often, complicating empyema. Microscopic examination of patients' sputum discloses numerous large gram-positive cocci, occasionally within neutrophils.

Staphylococcal bacteremia may occur with any localized staphylococcal abscess and in severely burned patients is a common cause of death, generally 2 to 4 wk after injury. Symptoms and signs are discussed in Ch. 6. Persistent fever is usual and may be associated with shock. Bacterial endocarditis (see in INFECTIVE ENDOCARDITIS in Ch. 27) may develop. Diagnosis is established by positive blood cultures.

Staphylococcal osteomyelitis (see also Ch. 114): Acute hematogenous osteomyelitis occurs predominantly in children, causing chills, fever, and pain over the involved bone. Redness and swelling subsequently appear. Periarticular infection frequently results in effusion, suggesting septic arthritis rather than osteomyelitis. The WBC count is usually > 15,000 and blood cultures are often positive. X-ray changes are not apparent for 10 to 14 days; it may be longer before bone rarefaction and periosteal reaction are detected. Radionuclide bone scans often become abnormal earlier. The differential diagnosis is usually not difficult if the delayed development of abnormalities on x-ray and bone scan is appreciated.

Staphylococcal enterocolitis is suggested when hospitalized patients develop fever, ileus, abdominal distention, hypotension, or diarrhea—especially if they have had recent abdominal surgery, broad-spectrum antibiotics, or antibiotics for preoperative bowel preparation. If microscopic examination of the stools discloses leukocytes and clumps of staphylococci, the diagnosis is likely. It is important to rule out infection with toxigenic *Clostridium difficile,* which is the most common cause of antibiotic-associated colitis (see Ch. 60).

Prophylaxis

Aseptic precautions (eg, thorough hand washing between patient examinations, sterilization of equipment) are important. Infected patients and their bedding should be isolated from other vulnerable patients. Hospital personnel with active staphylococcal infections, even of a local nature (eg, boils), should not be allowed in contact with patients or equipment until their infections have been cured. Asymptomatic nasal carriers need not be excluded from patient contact unless the strains are particularly dangerous and the individual is the suspected source of an outbreak.

Treatment

Management includes abscess drainage, antibacterial therapy (parenterally, in a seriously ill patient), and general supportive measures. Cultures should be obtained before instituting or altering antibacterial regimens. Hospital-acquired staphylococci and most community-acquired strains usually are resistant to penicillin G, ampicillin, carbenicillin, streptomycin, and the tetracyclines. These antibiotics should not be used unless the organisms have been proved to be susceptible.

Most strains are susceptible to penicillinase-resistant penicillins (methicillin, oxacillin, nafcillin, cloxacillin, dicloxacillin), cephalosporins (cephalothin, cefazolin, cephalexin, cephradine, cefamandole, cefoxitin, and the newer third-generation cephalosporins), gentamicin, vancomycin, lincomycin, and clindamycin. One of the penicillins is usually the agent of choice, although the cephalosporins and vancomycin

are equally effective. Many staphylococcal strains are also sensitive to erythromycin, kanamycin, bacitracin, and chloramphenicol. Chloramphenicol and bacitracin, however, are seldom indicated because they are potentially toxic and alternative agents are available.

The choice and dosage of an antibiotic agent depend on the site of the infection, the severity of the illness, and the sensitivity of the organism. Infections caused by methicillin-resistant *Staphylococcus aureus* **(MRSA)** isolates are being encountered with increasing frequency in the USA, especially in tertiary-care and large city hospitals. Intravenous drug abusers with endocarditis and burned patients with skin infections are the 2 most important groups infected with these organisms, which can spread within hospitals and into the community to compromised and debilitated patients. Isolates are usually resistant to nafcillin, oxacillin, cloxacillin and *all* the cephalosporins. Frequently, because of technical factors, laboratory reports falsely indicate that these organisms are susceptible to cephalosporins; thus, cephalosporins are not reliable for treating these infections. Resistance to aminoglycosides and macrolides (erythromycin, lincomycin and clindamycin) is also common. Vancomycin given intravenously is the drug of choice for treating these infections. The usual dose for adults with normal renal function is 500 mg IV q 6 h or 1000 mg IV q 12 h infused over at least an hour. Dosages must be adjusted when renal function is compromised. Duration of therapy is based upon the infection site and the patient's response, but usually is 2 to 4 wk. Sulfamethoxazole-trimethoprim in a range of 50 SMX/10 TMP to 75 SMX/15 TMP/mg/kg/day, in divided doses taken at 8- or 12-h intervals for 2 to 4 wk, for adults is a useful alternative to vancomycin for treating MRSA infections. In staphylococcal enterocolitis, a nonabsorbed antistaphylococcal agent such as vancomycin 250 to 500 mg q 6 h is given orally, in combination with systemic therapy.

TOXIC SHOCK SYNDROME (TSS)

A syndrome characterized by high fever, vomiting, diarrhea, confusion, and skin rash that may rapidly progress to severe and intractable shock. This syndrome was first described in children (8 to 17 yr old) in 1978. In 1980, a large number of cases began to be recognized, predominantly in young women (age 13 to 52 yr), almost always associated with menstruation and the use of vaginal tampons. The incidence is not known, but estimates made from small series suggest about 3 cases/100,000 menstruating women. Overall, about 700 cases were reported in the USA in 1980. By 1981, after widespread publicity, as well as withdrawal of some vaginal tampons from the market, the incidence in women dropped precipitously. About 15% of cases occur in men, usually postoperatively. Less severe instances of the syndrome that may lack some of the manifestations are fairly common.

Etiology and Pathogenesis

The exact cause of TSS is unknown, but almost all cases have been found to have an infection with exotoxin-producing strains of phage-group I *Staphylococcus aureus*. These cases appear to be caused by the same toxin, now called the toxic shock toxin. The organism has been found in mucosal (nasopharynx, vagina, trachea) or sequestered (empyema, abscess) sites. In menstruating women it has been found in the vagina in almost every case and the affected women used vaginal tampons for their menses. During the past few years, tampon manufacturers have been modifying the absorbent material to increase absorbency and more completely obstruct outflow from the vagina. Presumably, women most at risk are those with preexisting *S. aureus* colonization of the vagina who also use tampons on a continuous basis for their menses. Conceivably, mechanical factors related to tampon use result in the bacterial exotoxin being able to enter the bloodstream through a mucosal break or via the uterus to the peritoneal cavity. The syndrome may occur as a complication of a postoperative staphylococcal wound infection that is often minor, deep, and difficult to detect.

Symptoms and Signs

The onset is sudden, with fever of 102 to 105 F (39 to 40.5 C) that remains elevated and that is associated with headache, sore throat, nonpurulent conjunctivitis, profound lethargy, intermittent confusion without focal neurologic signs, vomiting, profuse watery diarrhea, and a diffuse, sunburnlike erythroderma. The syndrome may progress rapidly (within 48 h) to hypotension, orthostatic syncope, and shock. Between the 3rd and 7th days after onset, desquamation of the skin occurs and may lead to epidermal sloughing, particularly of the skin of the palms and soles.

Other organ systems are usually involved, resulting in mild nonhemolytic anemia, moderate leukocytosis with a predominance of immature granulocytes, and early thrombocytopenia followed by thrombocytosis. Although clinically important bleeding phenomena rarely occur, the prothrombin time and partial thromboplastin time tend to be elevated. Particularly in children, impaired perfusion of the extremities may be associated with profound hypotension. Renal dysfunction, characterized by diminished urine output and increases in BUN and creatinine, is almost universal. Laboratory evidence of hepatocellular dysfunction (hepatitis) and skeletal myolysis are common during the 1st wk of illness. Cardiopulmonary involvement occurs, manifested by peripheral and pulmonary edema (despite abnormally low central venous pressures, suggesting adult respiratory distress syndrome).

Mortality rates range between 8 and 15%, but may not reflect the true incidence, since these figures are probably based on recognition of only more severe cases. Recurrence is common in women who continue to use tampons during the first 4 mo following an episode of TSS, although there is evidence that women treated with antibiotics to eradicate *S. aureus* do not fit this pattern.

Diagnosis

TSS resembles Kawasaki syndrome (mucocutaneous lymph node syndrome—see also in Ch. 191), but can usually be differentiated on clinical grounds. Shock usually is not seen in Kawasaki syndrome; the skin rash is maculopapular in Kawasaki syndrome, but a diffuse erythema in TSS; azotemia and thrombocytopenia are rarely seen in Kawasaki syndrome and are common in TSS. Kawasaki syndrome generally occurs in children < 5 yr of age and the staphylococcal exotoxin is different from that in TSS. Other disorders to be considered in differential diagnosis are scarlet fever, Reye's syndrome, the staphylococcal scalded-skin syndrome, meningococcemia, Rocky Mountain spotted fever, leptospirosis, and viral exanthematous diseases. These are ruled out by specific differences in the clinical picture and appropriate cultures and serologic studies.

Treatment

Patients suspected of having TSS should be hospitalized immediately and treated intensively. Tampons should be removed at once when the diagnosis is suspected. Immediate consideration must be given to supportive care, particularly adequate fluid and electrolyte replacement to prevent or treat hypovolemia, hypotension, or shock. Since shock may be profound and resistant, large quantities of fluid and electrolyte are sometimes required. Specimens for Gram stain and culture should be obtained from mucosal surfaces and blood. After these specimens have been obtained, it is appropriate to treat with a β-lactamase-resistant penicillin or a cephalosporin. Whether antibiotics modify the acute course of the illness is unclear, but eradicating staphylococcal foci does appear to protect against recurrences.

In addition to eradicating *S. aureus*, precise recommendations for prevention (primary or secondary) cannot be made with certainty. However, it seems prudent to advise women to avoid constant use of tampons throughout the menstrual period, intermittently using napkins or other hygienic measures. Additionally, it may be advisable to avoid newer designs of tampons promoted for maximum absorbency.

STREPTOCOCCAL INFECTIONS

Classification

Streptococcal infections can be classified **microbially** according to characteristics of the streptococcus and **clinically** according to the type of infection.

When grown on sheep-blood agar, β-hemolytic streptococci produce zones of clear hemolysis around each colony; α-streptococci (commonly called *Streptococcus viridans*) are surrounded by green discoloration due to incomplete hemolysis; and γ-streptococci are nonhemolytic. An additional classification, based on carbohydrates present in the cell wall, divides streptococci into the Lancefield Groups A through H and K through T. The members of Group D include enterococcal (*Streptococcus faecalis, S. durans, S. faecium*) and nonenterococcal (*S. bovis, S. equinus*) species. Group G streptococci may also cause infections, particularly endocarditis and septic arthritis. Extracellular Group A streptococcal antigens evoking antibody responses play important roles in the diagnostic tests to be described later.

Clinically, streptococcal infections can be divided into 3 broad groups: (1) the **carrier state,** in which the patient harbors streptococci without apparent infection; (2) **acute illnesses,** often suppurative, caused by streptococcal invasion of tissues; and (3) **delayed, nonsuppurative complications.** The nonsuppurative complications are the inflammatory states of acute rheumatic fever, chorea (discussed in Chs. 197 and 198), and glomerulonephritis (in Ch. 150). They occur most commonly about 2 wk after a clinically overt streptococcal infection, but the infection may be asymptomatic and the interval may be under or over 2 wk.

Clinical Manifestations

The symptoms and signs of acute invasive streptococcal infections depend on the affected tissue, the organism, the state of the host, and the host's response.

A **carrier state** exists when streptococci can be identified in material taken from a site that shows no evidence of inflammation. Group D streptococci are normally found in the gut, γ-streptococci in the throat and respiratory tract. β-Hemolytic streptococci of Groups A, B, C, and G—the groups generally regarded as pathogenic for man—can be cultured regularly from normal-looking throats of asymptomatic patients, and the term "carrier state" is usually reserved for such pharyngeal discoveries. The carrier state has importance as a cause of misdiagnosis in many pharyngeal or respiratory illnesses, since bacteriologic demonstration does not prove that a streptococcus is responsible for the associated clinical manifestations. Throat cultures from carriers usually yield only small numbers of organisms, while those from persons with significant infections are strongly positive.

Acute streptococcal infections can be *primary*, invading normal tissue, or *secondary*, invading tissue compromised by trauma or other disease. The organism in primary invasions is usually the Group A β-hemolytic streptococcus and the site is usually the pharynx. Secondary invasions can be caused by γ-hemolytic streptococci, by Group D streptococci, or by Group A organisms. Group A erysipelas can occur in previously normal or in edematous skin, or a streptococcal cellulitis can be imposed on traumatized skin or in subcutaneous tissue predisposed by venous insufficiency. A viral pneumonia or degenerative lung disease may be followed by a streptococcal pneumonia; *S. viridans* or Group D streptococci may cause bacterial endocarditis; Group D streptococci are frequently found in urinary tract infections; and the endometritis of a postpartum uterus is often due to enterococci or Group A organisms. Group D streptococci have been recognized as common causes of nosocomial wound infections. The eyes, ears, joints, bone, and gut are other sites of secondary streptococcal invasion. Infections with Group B β-hemolytic streptococci *(Streptococcus agalactiae)* are important causes of neonatal sepsis (see in NEONATAL SEPSIS in Ch. 186). In adults, sporadic

cases of bacteremia, endocarditis, urinary tract infections, pneumonia, and meningitis have been observed. In addition, Group B β-hemolytic streptococci have been recovered frequently from elderly diabetic patients with cellulitis complicating severe peripheral vascular disease.

Primary or secondary infections can spread through the affected tissues and along lymphatic channels to regional lymph nodes, and can also produce bacteremia. The development of suppuration depends on the severity of infection and the susceptibility of tissue.

The most common type of streptococcal disease is **primary pharyngeal infection with the Group A β-hemolytic organism**. In its typical form, the infection is manifested by sore throat, fever, a beefy red pharynx, and tonsillar exudate. This form occurs in about 20% of patients with Group A infections; the remainder are asymptomatic, have fever or mild sore throat alone and resemble viral pharyngitis, or have nonspecific symptoms such as headache, malaise, nausea, vomiting, or tachycardia. Convulsions may occur in children. The cervical and submaxillary nodes may enlarge and become tender. In children < 4 yr, rhinorrhea is frequent and sometimes the sole manifestation. None of these symptoms (including sore throat) and none of the signs (including pharyngeal exudate or occasional palatal petechiae) are specific for streptococcal infection, and any or all of these clinical features can occur in viral infections, particularly with the adenoviruses and in infectious mononucleosis. The only sign or symptom statistically associated with serologically confirmed streptococcal disease is cervical adenitis. Cough, laryngitis, and stuffy nose are uncharacteristic of streptococcal infection, and their presence suggests that other etiologic agents or complications coexist or have exclusive responsibility for the clinical ailment. Definitive diagnosis rests on the laboratory technics described later.

Though formerly a common ailment, **scarlet fever** (scarlatina) is uncommon today, probably because antibiotic therapy prevents the streptococcus from progressing in individual patients or causing massive epidemics. Scarlet fever is associated with Group A streptococcal strains that produce an erythrogenic toxin, leading to a diffuse pink-red cutaneous flush that blanches on pressure. The rash, an additional feature of an illness that otherwise resembles streptococcal pharyngitis, is seen best on the abdomen, on the lateral chest, and in cutaneous folds. Among the characteristic manifestations of the rash are **circumoral pallor** surrounded by a flushed face, a **"strawberry tongue"** (inflamed papillae protruding through a bright red coating), and **Pastia's lines** (dark red lines in the creases of skin folds). A similar tongue can be seen in the toxic shock (see above) and Kawasaki (see in Ch. 191) syndromes. The upper layer of the previously reddened skin often desquamates after the fever subsides. The course and management of scarlet fever are the same as for other clinically evident Group A infections.

Streptococcal pyoderma (impetigo) is covered in BACTERIAL INFECTIONS in Ch. 191.

Laboratory Diagnostic Tests

Acute streptococcal inflammation is regularly associated with an elevation both in ESR (usually > 50 in the Westergren test or uncorrected Wintrobe value) and in WBC count (about 12,000 to 20,000), with 75 to 90% neutrophils, many of which are young forms. The urine commonly shows no specific changes except those attributable to fever (eg, proteinuria).

The presence of streptococci can be established directly and promptly in material taken from the inflammatory site and examined by bacteriologic technics: overnight incubation on a sheep-blood agar plate or, for Group A organisms, immediate staining with fluorescent antibodies. The fluorescent method obviates the need, when organisms are grown in culture, for serologic testing to differentiate Group A organisms from other β-hemolytic streptococci, but the fluorescence may often produce false-

positive reactions with hemolytic staphylococci. There are also a number of diagnostic kits for rapid identification of Group A streptococcus. These are subject to false-positive and some false-negative results, but are nonetheless useful.

These direct tests can show that streptococci are *present* but *proof of infection* is obtained indirectly from streptococcal antibodies in the serum. The ASO titer rises in only 75 to 80% of infections, and, for completeness, streptococcal antihyaluronidase, antideoxyribonuclease B, antidiphosphopyridine nucleotidase, and antistreptokinase can also be used. Penicillin given early (within the first 5 days) for symptomatic streptococcal pharyngitis may delay the appearance and decrease the magnitude of the antibody response to streptolysin O. Patients with streptococcal pyoderma usually do not have a significant ASO response.

A single value of one antibody titer is only a crude index of recent streptococcal infection. Confirmation requires comparing sequential specimens for recent *changes* in titer, since a single value may be high as a result of slow "decay" of antibodies from a long antecedent infection. Conversely, a single value lower than the laboratory's upper limit of normal may represent an elevation for an individual patient. Sera need not be taken more often than every 2 wk and may be as far apart as 2 mo. A significant rise (or fall) in titer should span at least 2 tube dilutions, since a 1-tube increment may be due to laboratory variation. For greatest accuracy, the sera under comparison should be saved and tested on the same day, with the same reagents, by the same technician.

Streptozyme, an inexpensive, easily performed test for antibodies to streptolysin O, hyaluronidase, deoxyribonuclease B, and other streptococcal antigens, correlates best with an elevated ASO titer. False-positive results are seen in 3 to 5% of cases. However, 25 to 50% of patients with borderline serologic responses to specific streptococcal extracellular antigens will have false-negative agglutination with the streptozyme test.

Because of the time interval between serial specimens, serologic testing is not useful in managing acute invasive streptococcal infections, where diagnosis depends on clinical manifestations and results of bacteriologic tests. Serial antibody tests are particularly useful, however, in diagnosing poststreptococcal inflammatory states. Evidence of a recent Group A streptococcal infection is critical for diagnosing rheumatic fever, which can generally be ruled out if no change in titer is demonstrated in a properly performed "serial run" with measurement of other appropriate antibodies besides ASO.

Course and Treatment

The secondarily invasive streptococcal infections can be life-threatening, particularly for a debilitated patient. Septicemias, puerperal sepsis, endocarditis, and pneumonias due to streptococci were frequent causes of death in the preantibiotic era, and remain serious, especially if the infecting organism is an enterococcus. Though Group A streptococci and *S. viridans* are almost always sensitive to penicillin, enterococci are relatively resistant and require treatment with an aminoglycoside in addition to penicillin or ampicillin.

The primary pharyngeal infections, including scarlet fever, ordinarily have a finite course; the fever will drop after several days and recovery is complete within 2 wk. Antibiotics shorten the clinical illness in young children, especially those with scarlet fever, but they have little effect on the symptoms of streptococcal pharyngitis in adolescents or adults. Their value is primarily to prevent local suppurative events such as peritonsillar abscess (quinsy), otitis media, sinusitis, and mastoiditis. Most important, they are used to thwart the nonsuppurative complications that may follow untreated Group A infections.

Penicillin is the best therapeutic agent for an established Group A streptococcal infection. A single injection of benzathine penicillin G, at a dose of 600,000 to 900,000 u. IM for small children and 1.2 million u. IM for adolescents or adults, will usually

suffice. Since the injection is often painful, oral therapy may be preferred if the patient can be trusted to maintain the regimen. The minor differences of absorption among the diverse oral preparations of penicillin do not seem as important as an adequately high dosage and duration of the regimen. At least 200,000 u. (and preferably 400,000 u.) of penicillin G taken on an empty stomach or 125 mg (to 250 mg) of penicillin V should be taken qid for at least 10 days to achieve the effect of a single injection of benzathine penicillin G. The 10-day course *must be completed* even though the patient has become asymptomatic. An alternative plan for patients considered unreliable or unable to take oral medication is to give 3 injections of procaine penicillin (each usually less painful than the one large benzathine dose): 600,000 u. IM is given on the 1st, 4th, and 7th days.

When penicillin is contraindicated, erythromycin 0.5 gm or clindamycin 0.3 gm may be given orally twice daily for 10 days. Clindamycin is preferred when children have relapses of chronic tonsillitis. Sulfadiazine, which is bacteriostatic, should not be used to treat an established infection, though it is useful in preventing streptococcal infections. Tetracycline is undesirable because a significant number of Group A streptococci are resistant to it; moreover, in the young it may discolor growing teeth.

Antistreptococcal therapy can often be withheld for 1 or 2 days, until bacteriologic verification has been obtained, without significantly increasing the risk of suppurative or nonsuppurative complications of streptococcal pharyngitis. An effective plan is to begin oral penicillin when infection is suspected and specimens for laboratory tests have been obtained. The treatment can be stopped if laboratory tests fail to confirm the presence of streptococci. Otherwise, oral treatment is continued or replaced by an injectable agent.

Other symptoms of streptococcal infection can be treated with agents such as analgesics or antipyretics for sore throat, headache, or fever. Bed rest is unnecessary unless the patient wants it. Isolation technics are no longer warranted. Among the infected patient's close associates in family or friends, those who are symptomatic or have a history of poststreptococcal complications should be examined for streptococci, then appropriately treated with antibiotics.

RHEUMATIC FEVER

(See Ch. 197)

PNEUMOCOCCAL INFECTIONS

Bacteriology

The pneumococcus (formerly called *Diplococcus pneumoniae* and now designated *Streptococcus pneumoniae*) is a gram-positive encapsulated diplococcus, the adjacent surfaces of the cocci being rounded and the ends pointed to give a lancet shape. It sometimes appears as short chains; in old cultures or in purulent exudates, some of the organisms may appear pink. The capsule, visible in ordinary smears stained with methylene blue, consists of a complex polysaccharide that determines serologic specificity and contributes to the virulence and pathogenicity. Some of the 85 or more specific types show cross-reactivity. In the **Neufeld quellung reaction,** the best method for determining type specificity, the capsule swells in the presence of type-specific rabbit antiserum; since this swelling does not occur with other bacteria and does not occur clearly with pneumococci of other types, this method establishes both the species and type of organism. For clinical diagnosis, polyvalent antiserum against some groups of specific types is available commercially or from the Centers for Disease Control of the USPHS, and a serum against all types is available from the Danish

Serum Institute in Copenhagen. Typing may also be carried out by specific agglutination or by immunoelectrophoresis against specific antisera. The specific type of pneumococcal antibody in serum or other body fluids may be determined by counterimmunoelectrophoresis against type-specific polysaccharides.

Distribution of specific serotypes of pneumococci varies among isolates from different clinical types of infections, in carriers, at different times, and in different locations; the most common types in recent serious infections have been types 1, 3, 4, 7, 8, and 12 in adults and types 6, 14, 19, and 23 in infants and children. The capsular polysaccharides are antigenic in humans and produce type-specific serologic and protective antibody against the whole organism; a polyvalent vaccine containing polysaccharides of 23 types that account for about 87% of pneumococcal infections is available (see Prophylaxis below).

Recovery from pneumococcal infection is usually associated with development of circulating type-specific antibodies.

Epidemiology

Pneumococci commonly inhabit the human respiratory tract, particularly in winter and early spring, when they may be cultured from up to half of the population at any given time. The organisms spread from person to person in droplets, but true epidemics of pneumococcal pneumonia or other infections are rare. Isolation of patients for pneumococcal infections is therefore not generally required.

The patients most susceptible to serious and invasive pneumococcal infections are those with lymphoma, Hodgkin's disease, multiple myeloma, splenectomy, other serious debilitating diseases or immunologic deficiencies, and sickle cell disease. Damage to the respiratory epithelium by chronic bronchitis or common respiratory viruses, notably influenza virus, may predispose to pneumococcal invasion of the pulmonary parenchyma and pneumonia. Pneumococcal pneumonias are highly prevalent among gold and diamond miners in South Africa and New Guinea.

Diseases Caused by Pneumococcus

Pneumonia: Pneumonia, the most frequent serious infection caused by the pneumococcus, is usually lobar, but may present as bronchopneumonia or as tracheobronchitis without clearly defined parenchymal involvement (see PNEUMOCOCCAL PNEUMONIA in Ch. 40).

Acute purulent empyema of the pleura: Pneumococcus, the most common cause, accounts for about 15% of all empyemas, but < 3% of cases of pneumococcal pneumonia are complicated by empyema (in contrast to sterile pleural effusions, which are more common). The exudate may resolve spontaneously or during therapy of the pneumonia; or it may become thick and fibrinopurulent, sometimes loculated, and require surgical drainage. (See Treatment below and also in Chs. 40 and 47.)

Acute otitis media: The pneumococcus causes about ½ of all cases of acute otitis media in infants (after the newborn period) and children. About ⅓ of all children in most populations have an attack of acute pneumococcal otitis media in the first 2 yr of life, and recurrent otitis due to pneumococcus is common. Mastoiditis, meningitis, and lateral sinus thrombosis, fairly common complications of otitis media in the preantibiotic days, are rare. (See TABLE 1–1 in Ch. 1 and also ACUTE OTITIS MEDIA in Ch. 206.)

Acute sinusitis: The pneumococcus may cause infections of the paranasal sinuses. Infection of the ethmoidal or sphenoidal sinus may extend into the meninges and produce bacterial meningitis. Sinusitis may become chronic and mixed with other bacteria. (See TABLE 1–1 in Ch. 1 and also SINUSITIS in Ch. 208.)

Acute bacterial meningitis: Except for *H. influenzae* meningitis in children and epi-

demic meningococcal meningitis, the pneumococcus is one of the most frequent etiologic agents of acute bacterial (purulent) meningitis in all age groups. Pneumococcal meningitis may be secondary to (1) bacteremia from other foci (notably pneumonia), (2) an infection of the ear, mastoid process, or paranasal sinuses (notably the ethmoidal or sphenoidal sinuses), or (3) basilar fracture of the skull involving one of these sites or the cribriform plate. (For the clinical aspects, see ACUTE BACTERIAL MENINGITIS in Ch. 125.)

Pneumococcal bacteremia: Bacteremia may accompany the acute phase of pneumococcal pneumonia or meningitis and, of course, is a major manifestation of pneumococcal endocarditis. Pneumococcal bacteremia may also be an apparently primary infection (ie, without another focus) in susceptible patients (see Epidemiology above) or may occur in an otherwise normal patient during the course of a simple, febrile, viral URI (common cold). In some such cases the pneumococcus is first discovered at autopsy in an infected paranasal sinus, internal ear, or mastoid.

Pneumococcal endocarditis: Pneumococcal endocarditis may complicate the bacteremia accompanying pneumonia or meningitis, or it may occur in patients who have no clinically apparent focus that accounts for the bacteremia. It may occur in patients with or without prior history or evidence of valvular heart disease and rarely may even be fatal without changing murmurs, petechiae, or embolic phenomena. Pneumococcal endocarditis may produce a corrosive valvular lesion, with sudden rupture or fenestration leading to rapidly progressive congestive heart failure; prompt removal and replacement of the diseased valve may be life-saving. It may be possible to visualize the valvular lesion and vegetations by echocardiography or nuclear scanning methods. (See also INFECTIVE ENDOCARDITIS in Ch. 27.)

Pneumococcal peritonitis: Peritonitis caused by pneumococcus, once a common complication of lipoid nephrosis but now seen only rarely, occurs most often in young girls, presumably as an ascending infection from the vagina through the fallopian tubes. The symptoms are similar to those of other causes of acute bacterial peritonitis; the infection responds rapidly to treatment with penicillin. (See also PERITONITIS in Ch. 55.)

Pneumococcal arthritis: The pneumococcus, an uncommon cause of acute purulent (septic) arthritis, can usually be demonstrated by direct smear and by culture of the aspirated purulent synovial fluid. It is usually a complication of pneumococcemia from another focus, especially meningitis or endocarditis. The clinical picture and therapy are similar to those of septic arthritis caused by other gram-positive cocci. (See INFECTIOUS ARTHRITIS in Ch. 108.)

Prophylaxis

A polyvalent pneumococcal polysaccharide vaccine, commercially available, is directed against the 23 types that account for > 80% of serious pneumococcal infections. It produces specific antibodies against nearly all of these types in most children > 2 yr of age and most adults, reducing pneumonia and other bacteremic infections by about 80% and mortality from such infections by 40%. Its antigenicity and protective effects in infants and young children have not been clearly demonstrated. In the recommended dose of 50 μg of each type in physiologic saline, it is relatively free of side reactions. Protection may last for several years, but in the highly susceptible, especially children, revaccination after 3 yr or more is desirable.

The vaccine is indicated for persons with chronic cardiac disease, chronic bronchitis and bronchiectasis, diabetes, and metabolic disorders, and for elderly and debilitated persons in chronic care facilities. Preliminary data suggest that the vaccine may prevent pneumonia and bacteremia in most but not all patients with sickle cell anemia and in splenectomized patients > 2 yr. The vaccine may not be effective in preventing

pneumococcal meningitis complicating basilar fracture of the skull, and is currently not recommended for pregnant females, children < 2 yr, splenectomized patients with Hodgkin's disease, or anyone hypersensitive to the components of the vaccine. Penicillin V 250 mg bid to qid for 5 days at the onset of a common cold may prevent recurrences of pneumococcal pneumonia in patients with chronic bronchitis; however, tetracycline or ampicillin (or one of its derivatives) is preferred in patients whose sputum may also contain *Hemophilus influenzae*.

Treatment

The preferred therapy for all pneumococcal infections is penicillin G, to which pneumococci of all serotypes have been highly susceptible. (For treatment of pneumococcal pneumonia and of pleural empyema, see PNEUMOCOCCAL PNEUMONIA in Ch. 40.) Generally, doses of procaine penicillin G 600,000 u. IM q 6 to 12 h or penicillin V 250 to 500 mg orally q 3 or 4 h are given for 5 to 7 days for acute pneumococcal otitis media, sinusitis, or arthritis; in arthritis, however, parenteral treatment is preferred and should be kept up for an additional week. Pneumococcal meningitis or endocarditis require much larger doses of penicillin G potassium for injection—24 million u./day given by intermittent (q 2 h) or continuous IV infusion and maintained for 10 days to 2 wk after the patient is afebrile and cultures of blood and CSF are sterile.

Antibiotic resistance: Where strains of pneumococci with marked resistance to penicillin and other antibiotics have been reported (eg, Great Britain, South Africa, New Guinea), it is necessary to test for susceptibility to antibiotics. These strains are rarely encountered in the USA, so routine susceptibility testing is not necessary.

For patients with pneumococcal pneumonia, meningitis, or endocarditis who are allergic to penicillin, see PNEUMOCOCCAL PNEUMONIA in Ch. 40 and INFECTIVE ENDOCARDITIS in Ch. 27. Patients with endocarditis should be followed closely for evidence of changing murmurs or sudden or progressive heart failure; the latter requires prompt surgical intervention.

CAUSED BY GRAM-NEGATIVE, AEROBIC COCCI

NEISSERIA

Organisms of the genus *Neisseria* include *N. meningitidis*, an important cause of meningitis, bacteremia, and other serious infections in both children and adults; *N. gonorrhoeae*, a major cause of sexually transmitted diseases, including urethritis, cervicitis, proctitis, pharyngitis, salpingitis, and epididymitis; and numerous saprophytic *Neisseria* species that commonly inhabit the oropharynx, vagina, or colon but rarely cause human disease. Morphologically, organisms of the genus *Neisseria* can be recognized by their characteristic colonial morphology (small, translucent colonies with umbilicated centers and crenated margins), by Gram stain (small gram-negative cocci, often in chains or pairs), and by their positive oxidase reactions. *N. meningitidis* and *N. gonorrhoeae* can be distinguished from one another and from saprophytic strains on the basis of sugar fermentation reactions or by immunofluorescence. *Neisseria* grow well on solid media containing blood or serum and thrive in a reduced O_2 atmosphere with 5 to 10% CO_2 at 35 to 37 C. Chocolate agar incubated in a candle jar provides a suitable environment.

Since each of the medically important *Neisseria* species is principally responsible for infections of a particular site, gonorrhea infections are discussed in Chs. 14, 153, 171, and 219. Meningococcal infections are discussed under ACUTE BACTERIAL MENINGITIS in Ch. 125.

CAUSED BY GRAM-POSITIVE BACILLI

ERYSIPELOID

An acute, but slowly evolving, skin infection caused by Erysipelothrix rhusiopathiae.

Etiology

Erysipelothrix rhusiopathiae (insidiosa), a gram-positive, noncapsulated, nonsporulating, nonmotile, microaerophilic bacillus with worldwide distribution, is primarily an animal pathogen, especially for swine. Infection in man is chiefly occupational and typically follows a penetrating hand wound in persons who handle fish or animal tissues (eg, butchers).

Symptoms, Signs, and Diagnosis

Within a week of injury a characteristic raised, purplish-red, nonvesiculated, indurated maculopapule appears, accompanied by itching and burning. Local swelling, though sharply demarcated, may inhibit use of the hand. The border of the lesion may slowly extend outward. Regional lymphatic involvement is absent. The disease is usually self-limiting; discomfort and disability may persist for 2 to 3 wk. Bacteremia is rare but may result in septic arthritis or infective endocarditis (without known valvular heart disease in half the patients).

The characteristic lesion and its course are diagnostic. Culture of a needle aspirate or biopsy specimen taken from the advancing edge of a lesion may yield *Erysipelothrix rhusiopathiae*.

Treatment

Benzathine penicillin G 1.2 million u. IM (600,000 u. in each buttock), or erythromycin 0.5 gm qid orally for 7 days, is curative.

ANTHRAX

(Malignant Pustule; Woolsorter's Disease)

A highly infectious disease of animals, especially ruminants, that is transmitted to man by contact with the animals or their products.

Etiology and Epidemiology

The causative organism, *Bacillus anthracis*, is a large, gram-positive, facultatively anaerobic, encapsulated rod. The spores resist destruction and remain viable in soil and animal products for decades. Human infection is usually through the skin but has followed ingestion of contaminated meat. Inhaling spores under adverse conditions (eg, the presence of an acute respiratory infection) may result in pulmonary anthrax **(woolsorter's disease)**, which is often fatal.

Anthrax is an important animal disease. Disease in man is rare, mainly occurring in countries without public health regulations that prevent industrial exposure to infected goats, cattle, sheep, and horses, or to their products.

Symptoms, Signs, and Diagnosis

The occupational history is most important. The organism may be demonstrated in cultures or in gram-stained smears from cutaneous lesions and, in the pulmonary form, from throat swabs and sputum. Mouse inoculation may permit isolation of the organism when primary cultures are unsuccessful.

The incubation period varies from 12 h to 5 days (generally, 3 to 5 days). The **cutaneous form** begins as a red-brown papule that enlarges with considerable peripheral erythema, vesiculation, and induration. Central ulceration follows, with serosanguineous exudation and formation of a black eschar. Local lymphadenopathy may be present, occasionally with malaise, myalgia, headache, fever, nausea, and vomiting.

Pulmonary anthrax follows rapid multiplication of spores in the mediastinal lymph nodes. Severe hemorrhagic necrotizing lymphadenitis develops and spreads to the adjacent mediastinal structures. Serosanguineous transudation, pulmonary edema, and pleural effusion occur. Initial symptoms are insidious and resemble influenza. Fever increases; within a few days, severe respiratory distress develops, followed by cyanosis, shock, and coma. Hemorrhagic meningoencephalitis may develop. Lung x-ray may show diffuse patchy infiltration; the mediastinum is widened because of enlarged hemorrhagic lymph nodes. Without early specific and generalized supportive treatment, a fatal outcome may ensue.

Prevention and Treatment

A vaccine, composed of a culture filtrate, is available for those at high risk (veterinarians, laboratory technicians, employees of textile mills processing imported goat hair).

Treatment of the cutaneous form with procaine penicillin G 600,000 u. IM bid prevents systemic spread and induces gradual resolution of the pustule. Tetracycline 2 gm/day in 4 divided doses orally is also effective.

For pulmonary anthrax, early and continuous IV therapy with penicillin G 10 million u./day may be lifesaving. Corticosteroids may be of value, but have not been adequately evaluated. If treatment is delayed (usually because the diagnosis is missed), death is likely.

NOCARDIOSIS

An acute or chronic, often disseminated, granulomatous-suppurative infectious disease caused by the aerobic gram-positive microorganism Nocardia asteroides, *a soil saprophyte.*

Etiology and Epidemiology

The organism usually enters the body via the lung; rarely, via the GI tract or skin. This uncommon disease occurs worldwide at all ages, but incidence is greatest in older adults and more frequent in men than in women. Those who are debilitated or receiving immunosuppressive therapy are most susceptible, but approximately half the patients have no preexisting disease.

Symptoms and Signs

Most cases of disseminated nocardiosis begin as pulmonary infections. Pulmonary nocardiosis may resemble actinomycosis, but *N. asteroides* is more likely to disseminate hematogenously with abscess formation in the brain or, less frequently, in the kidney or in multiple organs. **Skin or subcutaneous abscesses** occur in ⅓ of cases. With **lung lesions**, the most frequent symptoms—including cough, fever, chills, chest pain, weakness, anorexia, and weight loss—resemble those of TB or suppurative pneumonia. In the **metastatic brain abscesses** that occur in ⅓ of cases, the symptoms are severe headache and focal and motor disturbances.

Diagnosis, Prognosis, and Treatment

Diagnosis is by identification of the microorganism in tissue or culture. Though closely related to *Actinomyces israelii*, *N. asteroides* is not clubbed and becomes arranged in loose clusters of interlacing, slender, branching filaments rather than in the true "sulfur granule" form.

Without treatment, the disease is usually fatal. In those receiving appropriate therapy, the prognosis is poorest in the presence of immunosuppressive therapy, better in CNS infection, and best (> 50% survival) in instances where the lesions occur only in the lungs. *Nocardia* organisms are usually resistant to penicillin in vivo. Sulfonamide **treatment** in a dose that maintains a blood concentration of 12 to 15 mg/dL (eg, with

sulfadiazine 4 to 6 gm/day orally) must be continued for several months, since most cases respond slowly. Some patients have responded only to amikacin.

ACTINOMYCOSIS

A chronic infectious disease characterized by multiple draining sinuses and caused by the anaerobic gram-positive microorganism Actinomyces israelii, *often present as a commensal on the gums, tonsils, and teeth.*

Incidence and Pathology

The disease is seen most often in adult males. In the cervicofacial form, the most common portal of entry is decayed teeth; pulmonary disease results from aspiration of oral secretions; abdominal disease, from a break in the mucosa of a diverticulum or the appendix.

The characteristic lesion is an indurated area of multiple, small, communicating abscesses surrounded by granulation tissue. Disease spreads to contiguous tissue and, rarely, hematogenously. Other anaerobic bacteria are usually also present.

Symptoms and Signs

There are 4 clinical forms. (1) The **abdominal form** affects the intestines (usually the cecum and appendix) and the peritoneum. Pain, fever, vomiting, diarrhea or constipation, and emaciation are characteristically present. An abdominal mass with signs of partial intestinal obstruction appears, and draining sinuses and fistulas may develop in the abdominal wall. (2) The **cervicofacial form (lumpy jaw)** usually begins as a small, flat, hard swelling, with or without pain, under the oral mucosa or the skin on the neck, or as a subperiosteal swelling of the jaw. Subsequently, areas of softening appear and develop into sinuses and fistulas with a discharge that contains the characteristic "sulfur granules" (rounded or spherical, usually yellowish, granules up to 1 mm in diameter). The cheek, tongue, pharynx, salivary glands, cranial bones, meninges, or brain may be affected, usually by direct extension. (3) In the **thoracic form**, involvement of the lungs resembles TB. Extensive invasion may occur before chest pain, fever, and productive cough appear. Perforation of the chest wall, with chronic draining sinuses, may result. (4) In the **generalized form**, hematogenous spread occurs to the skin, vertebral bodies, brain, liver, kidney, ureter, and (in women) the pelvic organs. More recently, this disease has been a local complication of the contraceptive intrauterine device (IUD).

Diagnosis

This is based on clinical symptoms, x-ray findings, and demonstration of *A. israelii* in sputum, pus, or biopsy specimen. In pus or tissue, the microorganism appears as tangled masses of branched and unbranched wavy filaments, or as the distinctive "sulfur granules." These consist of a central mass of tangled filaments, pus cells, and debris, with a midzone of interlacing filaments surrounded by an outer zone of radiating, club-shaped, hyaline and refractive filaments that take the eosin stain in tissue but are positive on Gram stain.

Lung lesions must be distinguished from those of TB and neoplasms. Lesions in the abdomen occur most frequently in the ileocecal region and are difficult to diagnose, except at laparotomy or when draining sinuses appear in the abdominal wall. Aspiration liver biopsy should be avoided because of the danger of inducing a persistent sinus. A tender, palpable mass suggests appendiceal abscess or regional enteritis. Nodules in any location may simulate malignant growths.

Prognosis and Treatment (see also in Ch. 267)

The disease is slowly progressive. Prognosis relates directly to early diagnosis, is

most favorable in the cervicofacial form, and is progressively worse in the pulmonary, abdominal, and generalized forms.

Most cases respond to medical treatment but, owing to the extensive induration and relatively avascular fibrosis, response is slow and treatment must be continued for at least 8 wk and occasionally for > 1 yr. Extensive and repeated surgical procedures may be required. Aspiration is indicated for small abscesses and drainage for large ones. (See TABLE 2–1 under BARRIERS in Ch. 2.) Penicillin G, at least 12 million u./day IV, should be given initially; penicillin V 1 gm orally qid may be substituted after about 2 wk. Tetracycline 500 mg orally q 6 h may be given instead of penicillin. Treatment must be continued for several weeks after apparent clinical cure.

CAUSED BY GRAM-NEGATIVE, FACULTATIVELY ANAEROBIC BACILLI

ENTEROBACTERIACEAE INFECTIONS

The Enterobacteriaceae comprise *Salmonella, Shigella, Escherichia, Klebsiella, Enterobacter, Serratia, Proteus, Morganella, Providencia, Yersinia,* and other less common genera. These organisms are readily cultured on ordinary media; they ferment glucose, reduce nitrates to nitrites, and are oxidase-negative and catalase-positive. Only the clinically important organisms that are not discussed in other chapters are covered here.

Escherichia coli normally inhabits the GI tract. If normal anatomic barriers are disrupted, the organism may spread to adjacent structures or invade the bloodstream. The site most often infected by *E. coli* is the urinary tract, which is colonized from without; but hepatobiliary, peritoneal, cutaneous, and pulmonary infections are not uncommon. *E. coli* is an important cause of bacteremia, which often occurs without an overt portal of entry. This organism is also an "opportunistic invader," causing disease in patients who have defects in host resistance due to other disease (eg, cancer, diabetes, cirrhosis) or who have received treatment with steroids, radiation, antineoplastic drugs, or antibiotics.

E. coli bacteremia is common in neonates, particularly premature infants (see ACUTE INFECTIOUS NEONATAL DIARRHEA under NEONATAL INFECTIONS in Ch. 186), and certain strains (enteropathogenic *E. coli*) cause diarrhea in infants and traveler's diarrhea in adults.

When *E. coli* infection is suspected on clinical grounds, the **diagnosis** must be confirmed by culture and appropriate biochemical tests; Gram stain does not differentiate *E. coli* from other gram-negative bacteria.

Treatment may be started empirically, and then should be modified on the basis of antibiotic sensitivity studies. Most strains are sensitive to the tetracyclines, chloramphenicol, ampicillin, carbenicillin, the cephalosporins, the aminoglycosides, and trimethoprim-sulfamethoxazole. In many instances, therapy also requires surgery to drain pus, excise necrotic lesions, or remove foreign bodies.

***Klebsiella-Enterobacter-Serratia* infections** are usually acquired in the hospital, mainly by patients with diminished host resistance. In general, these organisms are more resistant to antimicrobials than *E. coli*. As a rule, *Klebsiella, Enterobacter,* and *Serratia* cause infections in the same sites as does *E. coli* and they are also an important cause of bacteremia. They tend to respond to extended spectrum penicillin (ticarcillin, carbenicillin, piperacillin) and the aminoglycosides; however, many isolates are resistant to multiple antibiotics and sensitivity studies are essential. The sensitivity of *Klebsiella* to the cephalosporins differentiates them from *Enterobacter*, which are generally resistant to these drugs.

Klebsiella pneumonia (see in Ch. 40), a rare pulmonary infection characterized by

severe pneumonia (sometimes with expectoration of dark brown or red-currant-jelly sputum), lung abscess formation, and empyema, is most common in diabetics and in patients with alcoholism. If treated early enough, it responds to cephalosporins and aminoglycosides.

Proteus species encompass gram-negative organisms that do not ferment lactose and are characterized by their spreading trait. There are 4 species, *P. mirabilis*, *P. vulgaris*, *P. morganii*, and *P. rettgeri*. *P. mirabilis* causes most human infections and is distinguished from the others by its failure to form indole. These organisms are normally found in soil, water, and the flora of normal feces. They are often cultured from superficial wounds, draining ears, and sputum, particularly in patients whose normal flora has been eradicated by antibiotic therapy. They may also cause deep-seated infections (particularly in the ears and mastoid sinuses, peritoneal cavities, and urinary tracts of patients with chronic urinary tract infections or with renal or bladder stones) and bacteremia.

P. mirabilis is sensitive to ampicillin, carbenicillin, ticarcillin, piperacillin, the cephalosporins, and the aminoglycosides. The other 3 species tend to be more resistant, but, generally, are sensitive to the 3 penicillins mentioned; they are not sensitive to ampicillin. They are also sensitive to gentamicin, tobramycin, and amikacin.

SALMONELLA INFECTIONS

The 2200 known serotypes of *Salmonella* may be grouped into those (1) highly adapted to humans, (2) adapted to nonhuman hosts, or (3) unadapted to specific hosts. The first group includes *S. typhi*, *S. paratyphi A, B*, and *C*, and *S. sendai*, which are pathogenic only in humans and commonly cause enteric fever. The 2nd group causes disease almost exclusively in animals, but 2 strains within this group, *S. dublin* and *S. choleraesuis*, are also pathogenic in humans. The 3rd group includes > 2000 serotypes that are ubiquitous in nature. Most strains within this group cause gastroenteritis and account for 85% of all *Salmonella* infections in the USA. *Salmonella* is a major cause of bacterial diarrheal illness worldwide.

TYPHOID FEVER

A systemic infectious disease caused by S. typhi *and characterized by fever, prostration, abdominal pain, and a rose-colored rash.* It is the prototype of the *Salmonella* infections causing enteric fever.

Epidemiology and Pathology

About 400 cases of typhoid fever have been reported annually in the USA over the last decade. Typhoid bacilli are shed in the feces of asymptomatic carriers or the stool or urine of patients with active disease. Inadequate handwashing and failure to use toilet paper after defecation may spread *S. typhi* to communal food or water supplies. In endemic areas where adequate sanitary measures are generally lacking, *S. typhi* is transmitted more frequently by water than by food. In developed countries, transmission is chiefly by food that has been contaminated by healthy carriers during its preparation. Flies may spread the organism from feces to food. Occasional transmission by direct contact (anal-oral route) has been documented as occurring in children during play and in homosexuals. Rarely, hospital personnel who have not taken adequate enteric precautions (see TABLE 2-1 in Ch. 2) have acquired the disease when changing soiled bedclothes of infected patients.

The organism enters the body via the GI tract and gains access to the bloodstream via the lymphatic channels. Monocytic inflammation occurs in the ileum and colon, within the lamina propria and Peyer's patches. Local tissue necrosis is common at these sites. Ulceration, hemorrhage, and intestinal perforation may result in severe cases.

Carriers: About 3% of untreated patients shed organisms in their stool for > 1 yr and are referred to as "chronic enteric carriers." Some carriers have no history of clinical illness and apparently were asymptomatically infected. Obstructive uropathy related to schistosomiasis infection may predispose certain typhoid patients to develop a urinary carrier state. Most of the estimated 2000 carriers in the USA have chronic biliary disease and are female and elderly. Epidemiologic data indicate that typhoid carriers are more likely than the general population to acquire hepatobiliary cancer.

Symptoms and Signs

The incubation period (generally 8 to 14 days) is inversely related to the number of organisms ingested. Onset is usually gradual, with fever, headache, arthralgias, pharyngitis, constipation, anorexia, and abdominal pain and tenderness. Less common symptoms include dysuria, nonproductive cough, and epistaxis.

Without therapy, the temperature rises in steps over 2 to 3 days and remains elevated (usually to 39.4 to 40 C [103 to 104 F]), for another 10 to 14 days, begins to fall gradually at the end of the 3rd wk, and reaches normal levels during the 4th wk. Sustained fever is often accompanied by relative bradycardia and prostration. CNS symptoms such as delirium, stupor, or coma occur in severe cases. In about 10% of patients discrete, pink, blanching lesions (**"rose spots"**) appear in crops on the chest and abdomen during the 2nd wk of illness and resolve in 2 to 5 days. Splenomegaly, leukopenia, anemia, liver function test abnormalities, proteinuria, and a mild consumptive coagulopathy are common. Late in the disease, when intestinal lesions are most prominent, florid diarrhea occurs. The stool may contain blood. Atypical presentations such as pneumonitis, fever only, or symptoms consistent with UTI may delay diagnosis.

Convalescence may last several months. Antibiotic treatment markedly reduces the severity and duration of the disease.

Complications

Complications occur mainly in untreated patients or when treatment is delayed. **Intestinal bleeding** is occult in about 20% of patients; in 10% the stool contains gross blood. In about 2% severe bleeding occurs during the 3rd wk of illness, with a mortality rate of about 25%. **Intestinal perforation,** usually involving the distal ileum, occurs in 1 to 2% of cases. An acute abdomen and leukocytosis during the 3rd wk of illness may suggest perforation. **Pneumonia** may develop during the 2nd or 3rd wk and is usually due to pneumococcal infection, though *S. typhi* can also cause an infiltrative process. **Acute cholecystitis** and **hepatitis** may occur. **Bacteremia** occasionally leads to focal infections such as osteomyelitis, endocarditis, meningitis, soft tissue abscesses, glomerulitis, or GU tract involvement.

Relapses: In 8 to 10% of untreated patients, signs and symptoms similar to the initial clinical syndrome may be seen about 2 wk after defervescence. For unclear reasons, antibiotic therapy during the initial illness increases the incidence of febrile relapse to 15 to 20%. If antibiotic therapy is reinstituted at the time of relapse, the fever abates rapidly, unlike the slow defervescence seen during the primary illness. Occasionally a 2nd relapse occurs.

Diagnosis

Diagnosis is ultimately based on isolation of typhoid bacilli from culture sites, though the clinical setting and hematologic abnormalities may suggest typhoid fever. Typhoid bacilli are usually cultured from the blood during only the first 2 wk of illness, while stool cultures are usually positive from the 3rd to 5th wk. Urine cultures are often positive. Cultures of bone marrow aspirates, liver biopsies, and rose spots may also yield the organism.

Typhoid bacilli contain antigens (O and H) that stimulate the host to form corresponding antibodies. A four-fold rise in O and H antibody titers in paired specimens

acquired 2 wk apart indicates *S. typhi* infection. However, this test, the Widal agglutination reaction, is only moderately sensitive (30% of culture-proven cases have negative tests) and lacks specificity (many nontyphoidal *Salmonella* strains have cross-reacting O and H antigens; cirrhosis is associated with nonspecific antibody production causing a falsely positive Widal test). Tests are being sought that will detect *S. typhi* antigens in the serum or urine early in the course of the illness.

The differential diagnosis includes other *Salmonella* infections causing enteric fever, the major rickettsioses, leptospirosis, disseminated TB, malaria, brucellosis, tularemia, infectious hepatitis, *Yersinia enterocolitca* infection, or lymphoma. Early in its clinical course typhoid fever may resemble viral upper respiratory or urinary tract infections.

Prognosis

Prior to the introduction of antibiotics, the mortality rate among typhoid fever patients was about 12%. Death usually resulted from intestinal hemorrhage or perforation. With prompt antibiotic therapy, the mortality is < 1%. Most deaths occur in the malnourished, infants, and the elderly. Stupor, coma, or shock reflects severe disease and a poor prognosis.

Prophylaxis

Primary preventive measures include purified drinking water, effective sewerage systems, pasteurization of milk, prevention of chronic carriers from handling food, and adequate patient isolation precautions (see TABLE 2–1 in Ch. 2). Compulsory surveillance and case finding are essential in controlling epidemics.

The acetone-treated, heat-killed vaccine currently available provides only partial protection; therefore, vaccine is administered only to individuals with known exposure to *S. typhi* (eg, during epidemics) and to those at high risk of exposure. The latter group includes laboratory personnel working with *S. typhi* and travelers (including military personnel) who anticipate significant exposure in endemic areas. The vaccine is given in two 0.5-mL doses s.c. 1 mo apart. Children > 6 mo and < 10 yr of age should receive two 0.25-mL doses s.c. 1 mo apart. Care should be taken to avoid intradermal administration, since this may cause a severe local reaction.

Travelers in endemic areas should avoid ingesting raw leafy vegetables and other foods stored or served at room temperature. Recently prepared foods (served hot or chilled), bottled carbonated beverages, and raw foods peeled by the consumer are generally safe. Unless water is known to be safe, it should be boiled or chlorinated prior to drinking.

Treatment

Antibiotics markedly decrease the severity and duration of clinical illness and also reduce complications and mortality. Chloramphenicol, the drug of choice, is given orally or IV starting with one dose of 15 to 20 mg/kg, then 50 mg/kg/day in divided doses q 8 h for 14 days. When chloramphenicol-resistant strains are suspected, ampicillin may be given IV, IM, or orally (or amoxicillin given orally) 100 mg/kg/day in divided doses q 6 h for 14 days. Penicillin-allergic patients can be given trimethoprim 8 mg/kg/day plus sulfamethoxazole 40 mg/kg/day in 2 or 3 divided doses for 14 days.

Severely toxic patients may be given **glucocorticoids** in addition to antibiotics. Defervescence and clinical improvement usually follow. Prednisone 20 to 40 mg/day orally (or equivalent) for the first 3 days of treatment usually suffices. Higher doses of glucocorticoids (dexamethasone 3 mg/kg IV initially, followed by 1 mg/kg q 6 h for 48 h total) are used only in patients with marked delirium, coma, or shock.

As **supportive measures,** adequate nursing care and special attention to enteric precautions are critically important. Compulsory handwashing and proper stool disposal are mandatory. Nutrition should be maintained with frequent feedings. Patients are generally kept at bed rest while febrile. Salicylates (which may cause hypothermia and hypotension) as well as laxatives and enemas should be *avoided.* Diarrhea may be

minimized with a clear liquid diet and, if necessary, parenteral nutrition. Fluid and electrolyte therapy and blood replacement may be needed.

In the event of **intestinal perforation** and associated peritonitis, broader gram-negative and anaerobic antibiotic coverage is recommended. Surgical intervention plus antibiotics is preferred in treating perforation, though medical therapy alone has been moderately successful.

Relapses are treated the same as the initial illness, though duration of antibiotic therapy seldom needs to be > 5 days.

Convalescence: Three negative stool cultures at weekly intervals must be acquired during convalescence to exclude a carrier state. Typhoid bacilli may be isolated for as long as 3 mo after the acute illness in individuals who do not become carriers.

Carriers must be reported to the local health department and prohibited from handling food. If gallbladder pathology is present, cholecystectomy with 1 to 2 days of preoperative and 2 to 3 wk of postoperative antibiotics (ampicillin 6 gm/day IV in 4 divided doses) usually cures the carrier state. In carriers with normal biliary tracts, the cure rate is about 60% with antibiotics such as ampicillin 1.5 gm qid orally or IV for 6 wk or amoxicillin 2 gm tid orally for 4 wk.

OTHER SALMONELLA INFECTIONS

The epidemiology of the other Salmonelloses is similar to but more complicated than that of *S. typhi*, since disease may also occur in humans by direct and indirect contact with numerous species of infected animals, their derived foodstuffs, and their excreta. Infected meat-producing animals, poultry, raw milk, eggs, and egg products are common sources of *Salmonellae*. Other reported sources include infected pet turtles, carmine red dye, and contaminated marijuana.

Each *Salmonella* serotype can produce any or all of the clinical syndromes described below, though a given serotype is often associated with a specific syndrome. Subtotal gastrectomy, achlorhydria (or ingestion of antacids), sickle cell anemia, splenectomy, louse-borne relapsing fever, malaria, bartonellosis, cirrhosis, leukemia, and lymphoma predispose to *Salmonella* infection. Except for typhoid fever, *Salmonella* infections remain a significant public health problem in the USA, where the most common *Salmonella* serotypes (listed in descending order by frequency of isolates) include *S. typhimurium* (causing 35% of reported *Salmonella* infections), *S. enteritidis*, *S. heidelberg*, *S. newport*, *S. infantis*, *S. agona*, *S. montevideo* and *S. saint-paul*.

Symptoms and Signs

Salmonella infection may present clinically as a gastroenteritis, enteric fever, a bacteremic syndrome, or focal disease. An asymptomatic carrier state may also occur.

Gastroenteritis, which usually appears 12 to 48 h after ingestion of organisms, starts with nausea and crampy abdominal pain followed by diarrhea, fever, and sometimes vomiting. Usually the stool is watery, but a few patients have paste-like semisolid stools. Rarely, mucus or blood is present. The disease is usually mild, lasting 1 to 4 days. Occasionally a more severe and protracted illness reminiscent of cholera may occur. In stool specimens stained with methylene-blue, white cells are often seen and indicate colitis. Diagnosis is confirmed by culturing *Salmonella* from stool specimens or rectal swabs.

Enteric fever is a systemic syndrome characterized by fever, prostration, and septicemia. The prototype of this syndrome, typhoid fever, is described above. An identical presentation, though often less severe, is caused by *S. paratyphi A, B,* and *C,* and *S. sendai*.

Bacteremia is rare in patients with gastroenteritis. *S. choleraesuis* (which almost never produces gastroenteritis), *S. typhimurium*, and *S. heidelberg*, among others, can cause a sustained bacteremic syndrome lasting 1 wk or more. Though blood cultures are positive, stool cultures are generally negative.

Focal manifestations of *Salmonella* infection may occur with or without sustained bacteremia. In patients with bacteremia, localized infection may occur, involving the GI tract (liver, gallbladder, appendix, etc), endothelial surfaces (atherosclerotic plaques, ileofemoral or aortic aneurysms, heart valves), pericardium, meninges, lungs, joints, bones, GU tract, and soft tissues. Preexisting solid tumors will occasionally be seeded and develop abscesses that may, in turn, become a source of *Salmonella* bacteremia. *S. choleraesuis* and *S. typhimurium* are the pathogens most commonly causing focal infection.

Carriers: Persistent shedding of organisms in the stool for 1 yr or longer occurs in 0.2 to 0.6% of patients with nontyphoidal *Salmonella* infections. These carriers do not appear to play a major role in large outbreaks of gastroenteritis.

Prophylaxis

Case reporting is essential. Preventing contamination of foodstuffs by infected animals and humans is of primary importance. Proper cooking, handling, storage, and refrigeration of poultry, meat, eggs, etc is imperative. Infected animals (eg, pet turtles) and potentially contaminated substances (eg, carmine red dye) must be identified and controlled. Freshly passed stool specimens are preferable to rectal swabs in detecting *Salmonella* carriers. The preventive measures for travelers discussed under TYPHOID FEVER, above, apply to most other enteric infections as well.

Treatment

Gastroenteritis is treated symptomatically with fluids and bland diet (see SHIGELLOSIS below and General Principles of Treatment in Ch. 57). Antibiotics prolong excretion of the organism and are, therefore, unwarranted in uncomplicated cases. Elderly nursing home patients and infants, because of increased mortality risk, should be treated with antibiotics (ampicillin or amoxicillin 50 to 100 mg/kg/day orally in divided doses for 3 to 5 days). **Systemic** or **focal disease** should be treated with antibiotic doses as outlined above for typhoid fever. Sustained bacteremia is generally treated for 4 to 6 wk. Abscesses should be drained surgically; at least 4 wk of antibiotic therapy should follow the surgery. Infected aneurysms, heart valves, etc usually require surgical intervention and prolonged courses of antibiotics. **Carriers** are treated as described above for typhoid enteric carriers.

SHIGELLOSIS

(Bacillary Dysentery)

An acute infection of the bowel, caused by Shigella *organisms.*

Etiology and Epidemiology

The genus *Shigella* is divided into 4 major subgroups (A, B, C, and D), which are subdivided into serologically determined types. The genus is worldwide in distribution, but *Shigella flexneri* (B) and *S. sonnei* (D) are found more widely than *S. boydii* (C) and the particularly virulent *S. dysenteriae* (A). *S. sonnei* is the most common isolate found in the USA.

The source of infection is the excreta of infected individuals or convalescent carriers. Direct spread is by the fecal-oral route; indirect spread, by contaminated food and inanimate objects. Waterborne disease is unusual. Flies serve as mechanical vectors. Epidemics occur most frequently in overcrowded populations with inadequate sanitation. Bacillary dysentery is particularly common in younger children living in endemic areas; adults are relatively resistant to infection and usually have less severe disease.

Convalescents and subclinical carriers are significant infection hazards, but true long-term carriers are rare. Infection imparts little or no immunity, since reinfection with the same strain is possible.

Pathology and Pathophysiology

Shigella organisms penetrate the mucosa of the lower intestine and cause mucus secretion, hyperemia, leukocytic infiltration, edema, and often superficial mucosal ulcerations. The entire colon and often the lower ileum are involved in severe cases. The subacute form, seen almost exclusively in adults, is limited to the lower half of the colon. This pathological picture describes *Shigella* dysentery, a syndrome frequently preceded by a nonspecific, watery diarrhea. In many patients, dysentery does not occur after the diarrheal phase. The watery diarrhea associated with infection caused by *Shigella* organisms is probably mediated by an enterotoxin that causes increased secretory activity of the intestinal epithelial cells.

Symptoms, Signs, and Course

The incubation period is 1 to 4 days. In young **children,** onset is sudden, with fever, irritability or drowsiness, anorexia, nausea or vomiting, diarrhea, abdominal pain and distention, and tenesmus. Within 3 days, blood, pus, and mucus appear in the stools. The number of stools generally increases rapidly to 20 or more/day, and weight loss and dehydration become severe. The untreated child may die in the first 12 days; if not, acute symptoms subside by the 2nd wk.

Most **adults** are afebrile, with nonbloody and nonmucous diarrhea and little or no tenesmus. However, onset may be characterized by episodes of griping abdominal pain, urgency to defecate, and passage of formed feces, initially, which temporarily relieves the pain. These episodes recur with increasing severity and frequency. Diarrhea becomes marked, with soft or liquid stools containing mucus, pus, and often blood. Rectal prolapse and consequent fecal incontinence may result from severe tenesmus. The disease usually resolves spontaneously in adults: mild cases in 4 to 8 days, severe cases in 3 to 6 wk. Significant dehydration and electrolyte loss with circulatory collapse and death is largely limited to infants under age 2 yr and to debilitated adults.

In the rare **choleriform type** of bacillary dysentery, onset is sudden, with rice-water or serous (occasionally bloody) stools. The patient may vomit and become rapidly dehydrated.

S. dysenteriae causes a rare form with delirium, convulsions, and coma, but little or no diarrhea; it may be fatal in 12 to 24 h.

Secondary bacterial infections may occur, especially in debilitated and dehydrated patients. Severe mucosal ulcerations may cause significant acute blood loss. Other complications are uncommon, but include toxic neuritis, arthritis, myocarditis, and, rarely, intestinal perforation. Bacillary dysentery does not become chronic and is not an etiologic factor in ulcerative colitis. However, patients with the HLA-B27 genotype probably have a significant association of Reiter's syndrome following shigella infection.

Laboratory Findings

The bacillus is found in the stools, but bacillemia and bacilluria are rare. Though the WBC count is often reduced at onset, it averages 13,000. Hemoconcentration is common. Plasma CO_2 is usually low, reflecting the diarrhea-induced metabolic acidosis.

Diagnosis

This is facilitated by a high index of suspicion during outbreaks and in endemic areas. The commonest form, watery diarrhea, is indistinguishable from other bacterial, viral, and protozoan infections that induce secretory activity of intestinal epithelial cells. In patients who develop the acute form of bacillary dysentery, ie, small-volume stools containing blood and mucus, the differential diagnosis should include invasive *Escherichia coli*, *Salmonella*, *Yersinia*, *Campylobacter*, amebiasis, and viral diarrheas. The mucosal surface, as seen through a proctoscope, will be diffusely erythematous, with numerous small ulcers. Swabs of material taken from the ulcers should be smeared and cultured. These swabs, as well as fresh stool specimens, need to be cul-

tured immediately. Smears stained with methylene blue or Wright's stain will reveal sheets of leukocytes. The bacteria on these smears have no characteristic silhouette to allow for a specific diagnosis. Only a positive culture assures the diagnosis.

Prophylaxis

To prevent spread by contaminated food, water, and flies requires good sanitation, with the following precautions: thorough handwashing before handling food; immersion of soiled garments and bedding of dysentery patients in covered buckets of soap and water until they can be boiled; use of screens on houses; use of mosquito netting. Patients and carriers should be managed by proper isolation technics (especially stool isolation). A live oral vaccine is being developed, and field trials in endemic areas seem successful.

Treatment

Fluid therapy: See Ch. 84. Diarrhea usually causes isotonic dehydration (equal salt and water loss), with metabolic acidosis and significant potassium loss. Thirst from dehydration can lead to a proportionately excessive water intake, causing hypotonicity. Dysentery without diarrhea will not produce significant fluid loss.

In infants, especially in hot climates, the fluid lost through sweat and respiration, added to the severe diarrhea, may cause hypertonic serum (see Ch. 185). Premature administration of high-solute fluids (milk, tube feedings, "homemade" electrolyte mixtures) may cause damaging hypertonicity, including convulsions.

Infant feedings: See treatment of ACUTE INFECTIOUS GASTROENTERITIS under BACTERIAL INFECTIONS in Ch. 191.

Antibiotics: The decision to use antibiotics requires consideration of several factors, including the severity of the disease, age of the patient (for children, see treatment in ACUTE INFECTIOUS GASTROENTERITIS under BACTERIAL INFECTIONS in Ch. 191), adequacy of sanitation, the likelihood of further transmission, and the possibility of engendering antibiotic-resistant organisms. With proper fluid replacement, antibiotics are often unnecessary, and resistance to them is now widespread, varying with the species. *S. sonnei* isolates are likely to be resistant to ampicillin and tetracycline, but despite resistance to tetracycline, successful therapy has been achieved by administering the drug 3 gm (in adults) over a 1-h period, eg, 1 gm given at the beginning, middle, and end of the hour. Trimethoprim with sulfamethoxazole (as for typhoid fever—see under SALMONELLA INFECTIONS, above) will eradicate organisms quickly from the intestine. Ampicillin 3 gm/day for 5 days will cure most *S. flexneri* infections.

Other treatment: A hot-water bottle helps relieve abdominal discomfort. Absorbent and demulcent methylcellulose preparations do little to alleviate diarrhea and tenesmus. Anticholinergics and paregoric should be avoided in patients with shigellosis. Opiates will induce intestinal stasis, prolong the febrile state, and permit continued organism excretion in the stool. However, individualized use of opiates may be necessary if pain, discomfort, and anxiety are pronounced. Continuous use of opiates should be avoided.

The patient's progress should be followed until the stools are consistently free of *Shigella*.

CHOLERA

(Asiatic or Epidemic Cholera)

An acute infection involving the entire small bowel, characterized by profuse watery diarrhea, vomiting, muscular cramps, dehydration, oliguria, and collapse.

Etiology, Epidemiology, and Pathophysiology

The causative organism is *Vibrio cholerae*, serogroup 01, a short, curved, motile, aerobic rod. Susceptibility varies among individuals. Since the vibrio is sensitive to

gastric acid, hypo-and achlorhydria are predisposing factors. Persons living in endemic areas gradually acquire a natural immunity.

Cholera is spread by ingestion of water, seafoods, and other foods contaminated by the excrement of persons with symptomatic or asymptomatic infection. Outbreaks of the disease may be explosive and brief or may be protracted. Cholera is endemic in portions of Asia, the Middle East, Africa, and the Gulf Coast of the USA. Cases imported into Europe, Japan, and Australia have caused localized outbreaks. In endemic areas, outbreaks usually occur during warm months and the incidence is highest in children; in newly infected areas, epidemics may occur during any season and all ages are equally susceptible. Both the El Tor and classic biotypes of *V. cholerae* can cause severe disease; however, mild or asymptomatic infection is much more common with the El Tor biotype. A similar mild form of gastroenteritis caused by non-cholera vibrios is discussed in this chapter under *Campylobacter* and Noncholera Vibrio Infections.

The manifestations of cholera result from the loss of isotonic, watery stools rich in sodium, chloride, bicarbonate, and potassium. *V. cholerae* produces a protein enterotoxin, the enzymes mucinase and neuraminidase, several hemagglutinins, and other less clearly defined substances. The enterotoxin induces hypersecretion of an isotonic electrolyte solution by an intact small-bowel mucosa. The roles of mucinase and neuraminidase in pathogenesis are unclear. Mucinase may be important in reducing a protective effect of intestinal mucin, while neuraminidase may alter the structure of gangliosides in mucosal cell membranes, increasing the content of the specific ganglioside (GM_1) that binds the enterotoxin. A cell-associated hemagglutinin may aid the process of mucosal colonization.

Clinical Course and Prognosis

The incubation period is 1 to 3 days. Cholera can be subclinical; a mild, uncomplicated episode of diarrhea; or a fulminant, potentially lethal disease. Abrupt, painless, watery diarrhea with vomiting is usually the initial finding; stool loss may exceed 1 L/h but is usually much less. The resultant severe water and electrolyte depletion leads to intense thirst, oliguria, muscle cramps, weakness, and marked loss of tissue turgor, with sunken eyes and wrinkled skin. Hypovolemia, hemoconcentration, oliguria and anuria, and serious metabolic acidosis with potassium depletion (but with normal serum sodium concentration) occur and, if untreated, circulatory collapse with cyanosis and stupor may follow. Prolonged hypovolemia can cause renal tubular necrosis.

Uncomplicated cholera is self-limited; recovery occurs within 3 to 6 days. The fatality rate exceeds 50% in untreated severe cases, but is reduced to $< 1\%$ with prompt and adequate fluid and electrolyte therapy. Most patients are free of *V. cholerae* within 2 wk, but a few become chronic biliary carriers.

Diagnosis

The diagnosis is confirmed by isolation of *V. cholerae,* serogroup 01, in cultures from direct rectal swabs or fresh stools and its subsequent identification through agglutination by specific antiserum. Cholera must be distinguished from clinically similar disease caused by enterotoxin-producing strains of *Escherichia coli* and from the watery diarrhea with dehydration produced occasionally by salmonella and shigella infections.

Prophylaxis

Proper disposal of human excrement and purification of water supplies are essential in controlling cholera. Precautions also include using boiled water and avoiding uncooked vegetables. Cholera vaccine gives partial protection in endemic areas, but booster injections are required every 6 mo. Prompt prophylaxis with tetracycline 500 mg orally q 6 h in adults (12 mg/kg q 6 h in children $<$ 8 yr of age) for 8 doses is useful in preventing secondary cases among household contacts of cholera patients.

Treatment

Rapid correction of hypovolemia and metabolic acidosis, and prevention of hypokalemia are the objectives. For seriously dehydrated patients or those unable to drink, IV infusion should be started promptly with either (a) Ringer's lactate solution; (b) a solution of 8 gm glucose, 4 gm sodium chloride, 6.5 gm sodium acetate, and 1.0 gm potassium chloride per liter; or (c) a 2:1 mixture of normal saline and 0.17 M (1/6 M) sodium lactate. Patients in shock require 100 mL/kg; milder cases require only 50 to 80 mL/kg. The infusion should be given very rapidly until BP is normal and pulse is strong. The remainder is then given over a period of 2 h in adults; over 4 to 6 h in children. Water should also be given freely by mouth. Children given either normal saline-sodium lactate or Ringer's lactate solution require additional potassium, which can be supplied by adding potassium chloride 10 to 15 mEq/L to the IV solution or by giving potassium bicarbonate (1 mL/kg of a 100 gm/L solution) orally qid.

Amounts for replacement of continuing losses should equal measured stool volume. Adequacy of hydration is confirmed by frequent clinical evaluation (pulse rate and strength, skin turgor, and urine output).

Plasma, plasma volume expanders, and vasopressors do not correct the water and electrolyte loss and *should not be used.*

Initial IV rehydration followed by oral or nasogastric administration of a glucose- or sucrose-electrolyte solution is effective in replacing stool losses and is particularly useful in epidemic areas where supplies of parenteral fluids may be limited. Patients with mild disease who are able to drink may be given the oral solution immediately, to eliminate the need for IV infusion. A solution of 20 gm glucose or 40 gm sucrose, 3.5 gm sodium chloride, 2.9 gm trisodium citrate, dihydrate (or 2.5 gm sodium bicarbonate), and 1.5 gm potassium chloride per liter of drinking water should be warmed to 25 to 37 C (77 to 99 F) and given ad libitum in amounts at least equal to stool and vomitus losses. Solid food should be withheld until vomiting stops and appetite returns.

Early treatment with tetracycline (adults: 500 mg orally q 6 h for 48 h; children < 8 yr: 50 mg/kg/day in 4 divided doses, for 48 h) eradicates vibrios, reduces stool volume by 50%, and terminates diarrhea within 48 h. Furazolidone (adults: 100 mg orally q 6 h for 48 to 72 h; children: 5 mg/kg/day in 4 divided doses, for 48 to 72 h) can be used for tetracycline-resistant strains.

TULAREMIA

(Rabbit or Deer-fly Fever)

An acute infectious disease, usually characterized by a primary local ulcerative lesion, profound systemic symptoms, a typhoidlike state, bacteremia, and, not infrequently, atypical pneumonia.

Etiology and Epidemiology

The causative organism, *Francisella tularensis*, is a small, pleomorphic, nonmotile, nonsporulating, aerobic bacillus that enters the body by ingestion, inoculation, or contamination. It can penetrate unbroken skin. Of the 2 major species of *F. tularensis,* Types A and B, Type A is more virulent for man. It is found in rabbits. Type B, usually a mild ulceroglandular infection, comes from rodents. Transmission among animals is by blood-sucking arthropods and by cannibalism.

Hunters, butchers, farmers, fur-handlers, and laboratory workers are most commonly infected. Most cases result from contact with (especially in skinning) infected wild rabbits; others follow handling of other infected animals or birds, contact with infected ticks or other arthropods, and, rarely, eating undercooked infected meat or drinking contaminated water. Man-to-man transmission has not been reported.

Pathology

In disseminated cases, characteristic focal necrotic lesions in various stages of evolution are scattered throughout the body. They are minute (1 mm) to large (8 cm), whitish-yellow, and commonly found in lymph nodes, spleen, liver, kidney, and lung. In most cases, however, necrotic foci are seen externally as the primary lesions found on the finger, eye, or mouth; in pneumonia, foci of necrosis occur in the lung. Microscopically, the focal necrosis is surrounded by monocytes and young fibroblasts, in turn surrounded by large collections of lymphocytes. There may be severe systemic toxicity, but no toxins have been demonstrated.

Symptoms and Signs

The 4 clinical types of tularemia are **ulceroglandular,** 87% of cases, with primary lesions on the hands or fingers; **oculoglandular,** 3%, with inflammation of ipsilateral lymph nodes, probably caused by inoculation of the eye from an infected finger or hand; **glandular,** 2%, with regional lymphadenitis but no primary lesion, is usually cervical and suggests oral ingestion of the bacteria; and **typhoidal,** 8%, a systemic illness with abdominal pain and fever. Tularemic pneumonia may be primary or may be associated with the ulceroglandular manifestations of tularemia.

Onset occurs suddenly, 1 to 10 (usually 2 to 4) days after contact, with headache, chills, nausea, vomiting, fever of 39.5 or 40 C (103 or 104 F), and severe prostration. Extreme weakness, recurring chills, and drenching sweats develop. Within 24 to 48 h an inflamed papule appears at the infection site (finger, arm, eye, or roof of the mouth), except in glandular or typhoidal tularemia. The papule rapidly becomes pustular and ulcerates, producing a clean ulcer crater with a scanty, thin, colorless exudate. The ulcers are usually single on the extremities, but multiple in the mouth or eye. Usually, only one eye is affected. Regional lymph nodes enlarge and may suppurate and drain profusely. A typhoidlike state frequently develops by the 5th day, and the patient may show signs of an atypical pneumonia, in which symptoms are those of other pneumonias (see Ch. 40). Delirium may accompany tularemic pneumonia and lead to an initial neurologic diagnosis. Signs of consolidation are frequently present, but suppression of breath sounds and occasional rales may be the only signs in lobular tularemic pneumonia. A dry, nonproductive cough is present, and is associated with a retrosternal burning sensation. A nonspecific roseola-like rash may appear at any stage of the disease. The spleen is often enlarged and perisplenitis may occur. Leukocytosis is common, but the WBC count may be normal with only an increased proportion of polymorphonuclears. In untreated cases, temperature remains elevated for 3 to 4 wk and falls by lysis. Mediastinitis, lung abscess, and meningitis are rare complications.

One attack confers immunity. Mortality is almost nil in treated cases and about 6% in untreated cases. Death is usually from overwhelming infection, pneumonia, meningitis, or peritonitis. Relapses are uncommon, but occur in inadequately treated cases.

Diagnosis

A history of even slight contact with a wild rodent or of exposure to arthropod vectors, the sudden onset of symptoms, and the characteristic primary lesion are usually diagnostic. Laboratory infections are frequently typhoidal or pneumonic, with no demonstrable primary lesion, and are difficult to diagnose. Recovery of the organism from the lesion, lymph nodes, or sputum is diagnostic. Agglutination tests usually become positive after the 10th day and almost never before the 8th day. A rising titer supports the diagnosis. The serum of brucellosis patients may also react positively to tularemic antigens, but usually in much lower titers.

Prophylaxis

Wild rabbits and other rodents should be handled with great caution, especially in endemic areas. The organisms may be present in the animal and in tick feces on the animal's fur. Protective clothing should be worn and all ticks removed at once. Wild

birds and game must be thoroughly cooked before eating; any water that may be contaminated must be disinfected before use.

This organism is so highly infectious that the diagnostic laboratory must have appropriate protective hoods before attempting isolation. Extreme caution is required in handling infected tissues or culture media.

Treatment

The agent of choice is streptomycin, 0.5 gm IM q 12 h until the temperature is normal; thereafter, 0.5 gm/day for 5 days. Gentamicin 3 to 5 mg/kg/day in 3 divided doses is also effective. Chloramphenicol or tetracycline 500 mg orally q 6 h may be given until the temperature is normal, and then 250 mg qid for 5 to 7 days; however, relapses occasionally occur with these 2 drugs, and they may not prevent node suppuration. Supportive therapy for pneumonia is the same as for pneumococcal pneumonia (see Ch. 40).

Continuous wet saline dressings are beneficial for primary skin lesions and may diminish the severity of the lymphangitis and lymphadenitis. Large abscesses may be drained, but this is rarely necessary unless therapy is delayed. In ocular tularemia, application of warm saline compresses and use of dark glasses give some relief; 1% homatropine 4 drops q 4 h may be instilled in severe cases. Intense headache usually responds to codeine 15 to 60 mg orally or s.c. q 3 to 4 h.

PLAGUE

(Bubonic Plague; Pestis; Black Death)

An acute, severe infection appearing in a bubonic or pneumonic form, caused by the bacillus Yersinia pestis.

Etiology, Epidemiology, and Transmission

The causative organism, *Y. pestis* (*Pasteurella pestis*), is a short bacillus that often shows bipolar staining, especially with Giemsa stain, and may resemble "safety pins."

Plague occurs primarily in wild rodents (eg, rats, mice, squirrels, prairie dogs), in whom it may be acute, subacute, or chronic, and murine or sylvatic, depending on whether urban or rural rodents are infected. Massive human epidemics have occurred (eg, the "Black Death" of the Middle Ages); more recently, infection has occurred sporadically or in limited outbreaks.

Plague is transmitted from rodent to man by the bite of an infected flea vector. Man-to-man transmission occurs from inhalation of droplet nuclei spread by coughing patients with bubonic or septicemic plague who have developed pulmonary lesions; primary pneumonic plague is the result. Recently in endemic areas in the USA, a number of cases have been associated with household pets, especially cats. Transmission from cats can be by bite or, if the cat has pneumonic plague, by inhalation of infected droplets.

Symptoms and Signs

Bubonic plague is the most common form. The incubation period varies from a few hours to 12 days, but is usually 2 to 5 days. Onset is abrupt and often associated with chills; the temperature rises to 39.5 to 41 C (103 to 106 F). The pulse may be rapid and thready; hypotension may occur. Enlarged lymph nodes **(buboes)** appear with or shortly before the fever. The femoral or inguinal lymph nodes are most commonly involved (50%), followed by axillary (22%), cervical (10%), or multiple (14%) node involvement. The nodes are typically extremely tender and firm, with considerable edema around them. The overlying skin is smooth and reddened, but often is not warm. A primary cutaneous lesion, varying from a small vesicle with slight local lymphangitis to an eschar, occasionally appears at the bite. The patient may be restless, delirious, confused, and incoordinated. The liver and spleen may be palpable. The

WBC count is usually 10,000 to 20,000 with a predominance of immature and mature neutrophils. The nodes may suppurate in the 2nd wk. The mortality in untreated patients is about 60%, most deaths occurring from sepsis in 3 to 5 days.

Primary pneumonic plague has a 2- to 3-day incubation period, followed by abrupt onset of high fever, chills, tachycardia, and headache, often severe. Cough, not prominent initially, develops within 20 to 24 h; sputum is mucoid at first, rapidly shows blood specks, and then becomes uniformly pink or bright red (resembling raspberry syrup) and foamy. Tachypnea and dyspnea are present, but not pleurisy. Signs of consolidation are rare and rales may be absent. Chest x-rays show a rapidly progressing pneumonia. Most untreated patients die within 48 h after onset of symptoms.

Other forms of plague: Septicemic plague usually occurs with the bubonic form as an acute, fulminant illness. It may be fatal before bubonic or pulmonary manifestations predominate. **Pharyngeal plague** and **plague meningitis** are less common forms. **Pestis minor,** a benign form of bubonic plague, usually occurs only in endemic areas. Lymphadenitis, fever, headache, and prostration subside within a week.

Diagnosis

This is based on recovery of the organism, which may be cultured from blood, sputum, or lymph node aspirate. Needle aspiration of a bubo is preferable, since surgical drainage may disseminate the organisms. *Y. pestis* can be grown on ordinary culture media or isolated by animal (especially guinea pig) inoculation. Serologic tests include CF, passive hemagglutination, and immunofluorescent staining of a node, secretions, or tissues. A vaccination history does not exclude plague in the differential diagnosis, since clinical illness may occur in vaccinated persons.

Prophylaxis and Treatment

Prevention is based on rodent control and the use of repellents to minimize bites by fleas. Immunization with standard killed plague vaccine gives protection and is recommended for travelers to Southeast Asia.

Treatment should be immediate upon suspicion of plague; prompt treatment reduces mortality to below 5%. In septicemic or pneumonic plague, treatment must begin within 24 h. Streptomycin 30 mg/kg/day IM in 4 equal doses at 6-h intervals for 7 to 10 days is the regimen of choice. Many authorities give higher initial dosages, up to 0.5 gm IM q 3 h for 48 h. Alternative agents include tetracycline 30 mg/kg IV or orally in divided doses. For persons with plague meningitis, chloramphenicol is the drug of choice: a loading dose of 25 mg/kg IV, followed by 50 mg/kg/day in divided doses IV or orally.

Routine aseptic precautions are adequate for patients with bubonic plague. Primary or secondary pneumonic plague requires strict isolation of the patient. All pneumonic plague contacts should be kept under medical surveillance; their temperatures should be taken q 4 h for 6 days. If this is not possible, chemoprophylaxis with tetracycline 1 gm/day orally for 6 days is an alternative, but is not ideal, because of the potential danger of producing drug-resistant strains.

PSEUDOMONAS INFECTIONS

Pseudomonas aeruginosa, a gram-negative, oxidase-positive, motile rod, frequently grows on agar in yellow-green iridescent colonies because two pigments, pyocyanin and fluorescin, are diffused into the medium.

Epidemiology

Pseudomonas can be found occasionally in the axilla and anogenital areas of normal skin, but rarely in stools of adults unless antibiotics are being given. The organism is commonly a contaminant of lesions populated with more virulent organisms, but occasionally it causes infection in tissues that are exposed to the external environment. The

most serious infections occur in debilitated patients with diminished resistance due to other disease and/or therapy. *Pseudomonas* infections occur most often in hospitals, where the organism is frequently found in moist areas such as sinks, antiseptic solutions, and urine receptacles. Cross-infection from patient to patient on hands of personnel may occur in outbreaks of urinary tract infection, on burn wards, and in premature-infant nurseries.

Pseudomonas infections can develop in many anatomic locations, including skin, subcutaneous tissue, bone, ears, eyes, urinary tract, and heart valves. The site varies with the portal of entry and the patient's particular vulnerability. In burns, the region below the eschar can become heavily infiltrated with organisms serving as a focus for subsequent bacteremia—an often lethal complication of burns. Bacteremia without a detectable urinary focus, especially if due to *Pseudomonas* species other than *aeruginosa,* should raise the possibility of contaminated IV fluids, medication, or antiseptics used in placing the IV.

Symptoms and Signs

Clinical presentation depends upon the site involved. Otitis externa with purulent drainage, commonly seen in tropical climates, is the commonest form of *Pseudomonas* infection involving the ear. Ocular involvement with *Pseudomonas* generally presents as corneal ulceration, most often following trauma, but contamination of contact lenses or lens fluid has been implicated as causing infection in some cases. *Pseudomonas* osteomyelitis is unusual, although the organism may be found in draining sinuses, especially following trauma or deep puncture wounds.

Pseudomonas is a common cause of urinary infection and usually is seen in patients who have had urologic manipulation or have obstructive uropathy. After *Pseudomonas* has joined with other gram-negative rods in colonizing the oropharynx in hospitalized patients, pulmonary infection can occur in association with endotracheal intubation, tracheostomy, or IPPB treatment. *Pseudomonas* bronchiolitis is common late in the course of cystic fibrosis; isolates have a characteristic mucoid colonial morphology.

Blood isolates of *Pseudomonas* are common in burns and patients with underlying malignancy. The clinical presentation is that of gram-negative sepsis, sometimes with **ecthyma gangrenosum,** which is a helpful clinical clue. This characteristic skin lesion consists of purple-black areas about 1 cm in diameter with an ulcerated center and surrounding erythema; it is found most often in the axillary or anogenital areas. Rarely, *Pseudomonas* causes endocarditis, usually after open-heart surgery on prosthetic valves or in IV drug abusers. Right-sided endocarditis can be treated medically, but usually the infected valve must be removed to cure an infection involving mitral, aortic, or prosthetic valves.

Treatment

When infection is localized and external, treatment with 1% acetic acid irrigations or topical agents such as polymyxin B or colistin is effective. Necrotic tissue must be debrided and abscesses must be drained. When parenteral therapy is required, 5 mg/kg/day in divided doses of the aminoglycoside antibiotic tobramycin or gentamicin inhibits most *Pseudomonas.* With clinical response, dosage can be reduced to 3 mg/kg/day to minimize adverse side effects. Dosage must be reduced in renal insufficiency. Amikacin should be used in treating *Pseudomonas* that has enzyme-mediated resistance to tobramycin and gentamicin. Several penicillins, including carbenicillin, ticarcillin, piperacillin, mezlocillin, and azlocillin, are active against *Pseudomonas.* Ticarcillin is most often used at doses from 16 to 20 gm/day. Piperacillin and azlocillin are active in vitro against some strains resistant to ticarcillin. In systemic infections or in granulocytopenic patients, an aminoglycoside active against *Pseudomonas* should be combined with an antipseudomonal penicillin. Infections confined to the urinary tract can often be treated with indanyl carbenicillin, an oral preparation useful for urinary infections.

CAUSED BY ANAEROBIC BACILLI

Increased clinical awareness and therapeutic efficacy have followed improved technics for isolating and delineating anaerobic bacteria. The anaerobes can be divided into spore formers (ie, the clostridia) and an extending taxonomy of other strict and facultative saprophytic gram-negative and gram-positive anaerobes that in the appropriate environment can destroy tissue.

CLOSTRIDIAL INFECTIONS

Clostridia are anaerobic, spore-forming, gram-positive bacilli that exist widely in nature, being found in dust, soil, vegetation, and the GI tracts of humans and animals. Though nearly 100 *Clostridium* species have been identified, relatively few cause disease in humans or animals (see TABLE 8–1). The pathogenic species, in the vegetative form, produce various tissue-destructive and neural exotoxins that have been biochemically and serologically delineated.

TABLE 8–1. CLOSTRIDIAL DISEASES

Disease	*Agent*	*Major Types in Man*	*Exotoxin*
Tetanus	*C. tetani*		Tetanospasmin
Botulism	*C. botulinum*	A, B, E	Neurotoxin (acetylcholine blocks)
Food poisoning	*C. perfringens*	A (variants?)	Enterotoxin
Antibiotic-associated colitis	*C. difficile*		Cytotoxin, enterotoxin
Necrotizing enteritis	*C. perfringens*	C (?)	
Histotoxic infections: local, uterine, wound infections (myositis, myonecrosis, anaerobic cellulitis)	*C. perfringens,* *C. novyi,* *C. septicum*	A–E A–D A	Lecithinase, protease, collagenase, fibrinolysin, hyaluronidase, deoxyribonuclease, leukocidin

The most frequent manifestations of colonization by clostridia in humans are benign, self-limited food poisoning (see *Clostridium perfringens* FOOD POISONING in Ch. 57) and incidental wound contamination. Lethal clostridial diseases, including gas gangrene (myonecrosis), tetanus, and botulism, are relatively rare but can follow trauma, injection of "street" drugs by addicts, and contamination in home food canning.

NEUROTOXIC CLOSTRIDIAL DISEASE

Botulism

(See in Ch. 57)

Tetanus

(Lockjaw)

An acute infectious disease characterized by intermittent tonic spasms of voluntary muscles. Spasm of the masseters accounts for the name "lockjaw."

Etiology and Pathogenesis

Tetanus is caused by an exotoxin (tetanospasmin) elaborated by *Clostridium tetani*, a slender, motile, gram-positive, anaerobic, sporulating bacillus. Spores remain viable for years and can be found in soil and in animal feces. Tetanus may follow trivial as well as overtly contaminated wounds, depending on a suitably reduced oxidation-reduction potential in the injured tissues. In the USA, drug addicts in particular are prone to develop tetanus, as are patients with burns or surgical wounds. Infection may also develop in the postpartum uterus and a newborn's umbilicus **(tetanus neonatorum)**. Clinical disease does not confer immunity.

The toxin enters the CNS along the peripheral motor nerves, or it may be bloodborne to the nervous tissue. The tetanospasmin binds to the ganglioside membranes of nerve synapses and blocks release of the inhibitory transmitter from the nerve terminals, thereby causing a generalized tonic spasticity upon which intermittent tonic convulsions are usually superimposed. Once fixed, the toxin cannot be neutralized.

Symptoms and Signs

The incubation period ranges from 2 to 50 (usually 5 to 10) days. The most frequent symptom is **stiffness of the jaw.** Other symptoms include difficulty in swallowing; restlessness; irritability; stiff neck, arms, or legs; headache; fever; sore throat; chilliness; and tonic spasms. Later, the patient has difficulty opening his jaws **(trismus)**; spasm of the facial muscles produces a characteristic expression with a fixed smile and elevated eyebrows **(risus sardonicus)**. Rigidity or spasm of abdominal, neck, and back muscles—even opisthotonos—may be present. Sphincteral spasm causes urinary retention or constipation. Dysphagia may interfere with nutrition. Painful generalized tonic spasms with profuse sweating are characteristic and are precipitated by minor disturbances such as a draft or noise, or by jarring the bed. The patient's sensorium usually is clear, but coma may follow repeated spasms. During generalized spasms, chest wall rigidity or glottal spasm interferes with respiration, causing cyanosis or fatal asphyxia; since the patient is unable to speak, the immediate cause of death may not be apparent.

The patient's temperature is only moderately elevated except when a complicating infection, such as pneumonia, is present. Respiratory and pulse rates are increased. Reflexes are often exaggerated. Moderate leukocytosis is usual.

Localized tetanus can occur, with spasticity of a group of muscles near the wound but without trismus. The spasticity may persist for weeks.

Diagnosis

A history of a wound in a patient with muscle stiffness or spasm is suggestive. A slight wound may have been overlooked. Tetanus can be confused with meningoencephalitis of other bacterial or viral origin, but the combination of an intact sensorium, normal CSF, and muscle spasms suggests tetanus. Trismus must be distinguished from local causes such as a peritonsillar or retropharyngeal abscess or another local infection. The phenothiazines can induce a tetanus-like rigidity, but other signs of basal ganglia dysfunction are usually evident.

C. tetani sometimes can be cultured from the wound, but its absence does not negate the diagnosis.

Prognosis

The prognosis is poorer if the incubation period is short and symptoms progress rapidly, or if treatment is delayed. Mortality is highest in young and old patients and in drug abusers. The course tends to be milder when there is no demonstrable focus of infection.

Prophylaxis

Immunization: Primary immunization against tetanus with either the fluid or adsorbed toxoid is superior to giving antitoxin at the time of injury. When a pregnant woman is immunized, both active and passive immunity will occur in the fetus; the former occurs at a gestational age of 5 to 6 mo with a booster at 8 mo. Passive immunity develops with maternal toxoid given before a gestational age of 6 mo. For routine DTP immunization and booster recommendations, see TABLE 182–4 in IMMUNIZATION PROCEDURES THROUGHOUT CHILDHOOD in Ch. 182.

At the **time of injury** (see also TABLE 8–2), 0.5 mL of toxoid elicits a protective antibody level in a *previously immunized patient*; this booster dose is not necessary if it is known beyond doubt that the patient has received a booster within the past 5 yr. An *inadequately immunized patient* should be given tetanus immune globulin (human) 250 to 500 u. IM, depending on the wound potential and not on age or body wt. At the same time, the first of three 0.5-mL doses of adsorbed tetanus toxoid should be given s.c. or IM at another injection site. The 2nd and 3rd doses of toxoid are given at monthly intervals. Tetanus antitoxin 3000 to 5000 u. IM (Caution: *Made from horse or bovine serum; see Serum Sickness in Ch. 21*) should be used *only* if tetanus immune globulin (human) is not available.

TABLE 8–2. GUIDELINES FOR IMMUNIZING PATIENTS WHO HAVE OPEN WOUNDS

History	*Susceptibility to Tetanus/ Immunization Recommended*		
	None	*Moderate*	*High*
Fully immunized and < 5 yr since booster	0	0	0
Fully immunized and 5–10 yr since booster	0	Td	Td
Fully immunized and > 10 yr since booster	Td	Td	Td
Incompletely immunized or uncertain	Td	Td and TIG-H* (250 u.)	Td and TIG-H** (500 u.)

* Tetanus immune globulin not to be given if patient is known to have had 2 primary doses of toxoid.
** To be given at different sites with different syringes.

Wound care: Prompt, careful wound debridement, especially of deep puncture wounds, is essential, since dirt and dead tissue promote multiplication of *C. tetani*. Penicillin and the tetracyclines are effective against *C. tetani* but are not substitutes for adequate debridement.

Treatment

Therapy involves maintaining an adequate airway; early and adequate use of human immune serum globulin; neutralizing nonfixed toxin; preventing further toxin production; sedation; controlling muscle spasm, hypertonicity, fluid balance, and intercurrent infection; and continuous nursing care.

General principles: The patient should be kept in a quiet room. The patient should be intubated and an adequate airway should be maintained in moderate or severe cases. Tracheostomy should be done when intubation is expected to be prolonged—ie, 7 to 10 days. Mechanical ventilation may be necessary and is essential when controlled respirations have been instigated by neuromuscular blockade (see Management of Muscle Spasms, below). O_2 should be humidified. Gastric intubation facilitates feeding; however, IV hyperalimentation avoids the hazard of aspiration secondary to feed-

ing by gastric tube. Since constipation is usual, stools should be kept soft; a rectal tube may help to control distention. Bladder catheterization is required if urinary retention occurs. Respiratory toilet, frequent turning, and forced coughing are essential to prevent pneumonia. Codeine is useful for pain. Patients with protracted tetanus may manifest a very labile and overactive sympathetic nervous system, including periods of hypertension, tachycardia, and myocardial irritability. Ongoing monitoring is indicated, and use of adrenergic blockers, α- or β-blockers, may be indicated, including using propranolol, bethanidine, or labetalol.

Antitoxin: The benefit of antiserum depends primarily on how much tetanospasmin is already bound to the synaptic membranes. A single IM injection of 3000 u. of tetanus immune globulin (human) should be given. Antitoxin of animal origin is far less preferable, since the patient's serum antitoxin level is not as well maintained and there is considerable risk of serum sickness. If horse serum must be used, however, the usual dose is 50,000 u. IM or IV (CAUTION: *see SERUM SICKNESS in Ch. 21 for necessary precautions*). Human immune globulin or animal antitoxin can be injected directly into the wound, but this is not as important as proper wound excision and debridement.

Management of muscle spasms: Diazepam is the drug of choice to counter muscle rigidity and induce sedation. The most severe cases may require 10 to 20 mg q 3 h by IV push. Less severe cases can be controlled with 5 to 10 mg q 2 to 4 h orally. A total daily dose of 10 to 15 mg/kg is used in children and 50 mg/kg in neonates. Diazepam may not preclude reflex spasms, and effective respiration may require neuromuscular blockade with pancuronium bromide (*d*-tubocurarine, in contrast to pancuronium bromide, may manifest histamine release with unwanted hypotension).

Antibiotics: Although the role of antibiotic therapy is minor in contrast to wound debridement, either penicillin G 2 million u. IV q 6 h or tetracycline 500 mg IV q 6 h should be given. Neither is likely to prevent secondary infections (eg, pneumonia). If pneumonia develops, cultures of the sputum or trachea should be taken, sensitivity tests performed, and an appropriate antibiotic given if necessary. If the patient has an indwelling urethral catheter, the urine should be cultured frequently and antimicrobial therapy given if indicated (see also in Ch. 153).

Immunization: Since immunity does not follow clinical tetanus, the patient should receive a full immunizing course of toxoid after he leaves the hospital.

HISTOTOXIC CLOSTRIDIAL DISEASE

Etiology and Pathogenesis

The ubiquitous, saprophytic, and usually endogenous clostridia become pathogenic when the tissues show a reduced oxidation-reduction potential, a high lactate concentration, and a low pH. Such an abnormal anaerobic environment may develop with primary arterial insufficiency or after severe penetrating or crushing injuries. The deeper and more severe the wound, the more prone the patient is to anaerobic infection, especially if there has been even minimal foreign-particle contamination. Clostridial lesions tend to be self-perpetuating once the clostridia have assumed the vegetative form and are producing toxins.

Severe clostridial sepsis may complicate intestinal perforation and obstruction. *C. perfringens* infection may, rarely, complicate simple appendicitis. Clostridia (usually *C. perfringens* Type A) have been implicated in cholecystitis, peritonitis, ruptured appendix, meningitis, otitis media, lung abscess, brain abscess, endocarditis, pyelonephritis, and osteomyelitis. A clostridial origin should always be suspected in omphalitis of the newborn. Clostridial infections may complicate initially aerobic local tissue or organ infections that have become anaerobic by extensive necrosis. Tumors, tissues devitalized by radiation, and even parenteral injection sites can also be susceptible to clos-

tridial infection. Debilitated patients with burns, neoplastic disease, or leukemia and patients with diabetes mellitus (because of associated occlusive vascular disease) are at a high risk of developing clostridial infections. The anaerobic environment of intestinal lymphoma and carcinoma permits endogenous *C. perfringens* invasion and replication, resulting in severe local or, rarely, septicemic clostridial disease.

Clinical Types

Uterine Clostridial Infection

This may be a fatal complication of septic abortion; rarely, it also can follow relatively uncomplicated pelvic surgery or childbirth. The patient is toxic and febrile, the lochia is foul-smelling, and the uterus is tender. Gas sometimes escapes through the cervix. Hemolytic anemia may develop as a result of clostridial septicemia and the effect of the toxin lecithinase on the RBC membrane. With severe hemolysis and coexistent toxicity, acute renal failure is to be expected. The mortality rate is then about 50%.

Early **diagnosis** requires a high index of suspicion. Early and repeated Gram stains and cultures of the lochia and blood are indicated, though *C. perfringens* occasionally can be isolated from the healthy vagina and lochia. X-rays may show local gas production.

Treatment consists of debridement by curettage, and administration of penicillin G 10 million u./day for at least 1 wk. Hysterectomy may be necessary and lifesaving if debridement by curettage is insufficient. Early renal dialysis is needed if acute tubular necrosis develops.

Clostridial Wound Infections

These may occur as local cellulitis, local or spreading myositis, or, most seriously, progressive myonecrosis **(gas gangrene)**. Infection develops hours or days after injury occurs, usually in an extremity after severe crushing or penetrating trauma that results in much devitalized tissue. Similar spreading myositis or myonecrosis may occur in operative wounds, particularly in patients with underlying occlusive vascular disease.

Clostridial cellulitis (anaerobic cellulitis) occurs as a localized infection in a superficial wound, usually 3 or more days after initial injury. Infection may spread extensively along fascial planes, but toxicity is much less severe than in patients with extensive myonecrosis. The exudate is foul-smelling, serous, and brown, with evident crepitation and abundant bubbling of gas. Discoloration and gross edema of the extremity are rare. In clostridial infections associated with primary vascular occlusion of an extremity, extension beyond the line of demarcation and progression to severe toxic myonecrosis are rare.

An initially localized deep **clostridial myositis** rapidly spreads by toxin production in an anaerobic environment, causing edema, gas production, and subsequent myonecrosis. In **myonecrosis**, the exudate is serous and brown, but not necessarily foul-smelling. Pain, tenderness, and edema are usually severe, with dramatic progression over a period of hours. Late in the course, gas crepitation can be felt in about 80% of cases. The wound site may be pale initially, but it becomes red or bronze and finally turns blackish-green. The affected muscle is a lusterless pink, then deep red, and finally gray-green or mottled purple. The patient becomes progressively toxic, though often alert until the terminal stage. In contrast to uterine clostridial infection, septicemia and overt hemolysis are rare with gas gangrene of the extremities, even in terminally ill patients.

Though localized cellulitis, myositis, and spreading myonecrosis may be sufficiently distinctive to permit clinical differentiation and appropriate treatment, precise **diagnosis** often requires thorough surgical wound exploration and visual evaluation of tissue involvement. X-rays may show local gas production. Appropriate anaerobic and aero-

bic cultures of wound exudate should be taken, to identify the organism. Smears show gram-positive clostridial rods. Typically, there are few polymorphonuclear leukocytes in the exudate. Free fat globules may be demonstrated using Sudan stain. Many wounds, particularly if open, are contaminated with both pathogenic and nonpathogenic clostridia without evident invasive disease. The significance of this must be determined clinically.

Other anaerobic and aerobic bacteria, including members of the family Enterobacteriaceae and *Bacteroides, Streptococcus*, and *Staphylococcus* species, alone or mixed, frequently cause clostridia-like severe cellulitis, extensive fasciitis, or gas gangrene in traumatic and postoperative wounds. If polymorphonuclear leukocytes are abundant and the smear shows many chains of cocci, an anaerobic streptococcal or staphylococcal infection should be suspected. An abundance of gram-negative rods may indicate infection with one of the Enterobacteriaceae or a *Bacteroides* species. (See also BACTEROIDES AND MIXED ANAEROBIC INFECTIONS, below.)

Anaerobic wound infections, particularly those due to Clostridium *species, can progress from initial injury through the stages of cellulitis to myositis to myonecrosis with shock, toxic delirium, and finally death within one to several days.* Early suspicion and intervention are essential. Anaerobic cellulitis uniformly responds to treatment; however, established and progressive myositis with an associated systemic toxemia has a mortality rate of 20% or more.

Treatment requires thorough wound debridement, including removal of foreign material and all devitalized tissue. Amputation of an extremity may even be necessary. Penicillin G 10 to 20 million u./day IV should be given as soon as clostridial disease is suspected clinically. Cephalothin 6 to 8 gm/day IV or tetracycline 2 gm/day IV may be substituted in penicillin-allergic patients.

Detection of specific antigenic toxins in the wound or blood is useful only in the rare instance of botulism acquired through a wound portal. For **wound botulism**, early administration of specific or polyvalent antitoxin (see BOTULISM in Ch. 57) is valuable. Polyvalent heterologous antiserum is available for gas gangrene, but its value is questionable compared to that of thorough wound debridement and use of penicillin. Hyperbaric O_2 is helpful in extensive myonecrosis, particularly in extremities, as a supplement to antibiotics and surgery. However, few chambers large enough for surgical and nursing care are available.

Necrotizing Enteritis

In addition to *C. perfringens* food poisoning, clostridia occasionally cause acute inflammatory, sometimes necrotizing, disease in the small and large bowels. A similar process may occur in patients being treated for leukemia. Such clostridial enterotoxemias can occur as isolated cases or as outbreaks and some appear due, at least in part, to contaminated meat. Pig-bel, for example, which occurs in New Guinea, presumably results from eating pork contaminated by *C. perfringens* Type C; it varies from mild diarrhea to fulminant toxemia with dehydration, causing shock and sometimes death. Newborn infants and young children seem to be at greater risk than adults.

Diarrhea Associated with Clostridium difficile

C. difficile, the proximate cause of antibiotic-associated colitis (see also Ch. 60), is frequently exogenous and has not only been incriminated in nosocomial diarrhea but also as an infrequent cause of diarrhea of children in the community. *C. difficile*-induced diarrhea occurs both alone and in limited outbreaks, transferred from person to person. Antibiotic-induced changes in the GI flora are the dominant predisposing host factor. Both a cytotoxin (A) and an enterotoxin (B) are demonstrable. The natural history varies from an asymptomatic carrier state, particularly in infants, to a severe necrotizing colitis. Rarely, limited tissue dissemination occurs.

BACTEROIDES AND MIXED ANAEROBIC INFECTIONS

Hundreds of species of nonsporulating anaerobes, in concentrations up to 10^{11}/gm, are part of the normal flora of the skin and of the mouth, intestinal tract, vagina, and other mucous membranes of the body. If this harmonious commensal relationship is disrupted (eg, by surgical or other trauma, poor blood supply, tissue necrosis), a few of these species can cause severe infections that are associated with high morbidity and mortality. Because aerobic and anaerobic bacteria frequently are found in the same infected site, the anaerobes may be overlooked unless appropriate procedures for isolation and culture are used. Recent improvements in these procedures and in taxonomy are revealing the pathogenic mechanisms, synergistic interactions, and spectrums of the infections they cause. Anaerobes can be the major cause of infection in the pleural spaces and the lungs; in bones and joints; in intra-abdominal, gynecologic, CNS, upper respiratory tract, and cutaneous infections; and in bacteremia and endocarditis (see TABLE 8–3).

Etiology and Pathogenesis

A useful classification is based on gram-stain characteristics. The principal anaerobic gram-positive cocci that produce disease are the peptococci and the peptostreptococci. The principal anaerobic gram-negative bacilli belong to the Bacteroides family, which includes the *Bacteroides fragilis* and *Bacteroides melaninogenicus* groups as well as the genus *Fusobacterium*. The *B. fragilis* group is part of the normal **bowel flora** and includes the anaerobic pathogens most frequently isolated from infections. The distinct species that comprise this group (*B. fragilis, B. thetaiotaomicron, B. distasonis, B. vulgatus*, and *B. ovatus*) are classified together because they were formerly designated as subspecies of *B. fragilis*. The organisms in the *B. melaninogenicus* group and *Fusobacterium* spp are part of the indigenous **oral flora**. The *B. melaninogenicus* group are primarily pigment-producing Bacteroides and include *B. gingivalis, B. asaccharolyticus*, and *B. melaninogenicus*. Recently the terminology of this group was changed so that some distinct species are listed.

TABLE 8–3. RECOVERY OF ANAEROBIC BACTERIA IN VARIOUS DISEASES

Disease Category	Percentage of Cases with Anaerobes Isolated	Disease Category	Percentage of Cases with Anaerobes Isolated
Head and Neck		**Female Genital Tract**	
Nontraumatic brain abscess	89	Pelvic abscess	88
Chronic sinusitis	53	Pelvic inflammatory disease	25
Perimandibular space infection	96	**Soft Tissue**	
Chest		Wound infection following elective colonic surgery	85
Aspiration pneumonia	75	Cutaneous abscess	60
Lung abscess	90	Diabetic foot ulcer	63
Empyema	72	Nonclostridial crepitant cellulitis	75
Intra-abdominal Sepsis		Pilonidal sinus	73
Abscess of peritonitis	89	**Bacteremia**	
Appendiceal	96	All blood cultures	9
Liver abscess	52	Intra-abdominal sepsis	73
		Septic abortion	63
		Decubitus ulcers	63

Anaerobic infections are distinct from those caused by other bacteria because (1) they tend to occur as localized collections of pus or abscesses, (2) the reduced P_{O_2} tension and low oxidation-reduction potential that prevail in avascular and necrotic tissues are critical for the survival of anaerobes, and (3) when bacteremia occurs, it is only rarely associated with disseminated intravascular coagulation and purpura.

Anaerobic infections are most often secondary to mechanical disruption of anatomical barriers contiguous to mucosal surfaces, where they exist as normal flora (eg, anaerobic pulmonary infections occur most often by aspiration of normal mouth flora). After entry by this route, organisms can spread hematogenously to distant sites.

Some anaerobic bacteria possess distinct virulence factors; those of *B. fragilis* probably account for its frequent isolation from clinical specimens despite its relative rarity in normal flora. This organism has a polysaccharide capsule that apparently stimulates abscess formation. An experimental model of intra-abdominal sepsis has shown that *B. fragilis* alone can cause abscesses, whereas other Bacteroides species require the synergistic effect of a facultative organism.

Symptoms and Signs

Since symptoms and signs of infection vary according to the site involved and the predisposing conditions, individual infections caused by mixed-anaerobic organisms are covered elsewhere in this book. Clinical syndromes caused by mixed-anaerobic bacteria include dental abscesses, mandibular osteomyelitis, periodontitis, necrotizing gingivitis, necrotizing ulcerative mucositis (cancrum oris), gangrenous pharyngitis (Vincent's angina), chronic sinusitis and otitis media, Ludwig's angina, brain abscess, aspiration pneumonia, lung abscess, empyema, peritonitis, intra-abdominal abscess, liver abscess, endometritis, parametrial abscess, pelvic peritonitis, nongonococcal tubo-ovarian abscess, anaerobic cellulitis, human bite infections, decubitus ulcer and ischemic ulcer infections, and septic thrombophlebitis. Although anaerobes are relatively rare in osteomyelitis and in infective endocarditis, they should be considered.

Clinical clues that anaerobic organisms are present are based on awareness of the etiologic and pathogenetic mechanisms described above and include infection adjacent to mucosal surfaces bearing anaerobic flora; ischemia, neoplasm, penetrating trauma, foreign body, or perforated viscus; spreading gangrene involving skin, subcutaneous tissue, fascia, and muscle; feculent odor in pus or infected tissues; abscess formation; gas in tissues; septic thrombophlebitis; and failure to respond to routine antibiotics.

Bacteremia complicating mixed-anaerobic infections may result in fever, rigors, and a critically ill patient. Shock and disseminated intravascular coagulation may occur, although the latter is extremely rare in pure Bacteroides sepsis.

When a Gram stain of pus from an infected site shows mixed pleomorphic bacterial flora, anaerobic infection should be considered. When the culture from an obviously necrotic, infected site showing mixed flora by Gram stain is reported as showing no growth, only α-hemolytic streptococci, or a single aerobic species such as *Escherichia coli*, the implication is that anaerobic microorganisms failed to grow because of inadequate transportation or bacteriologic technics.

Diagnosis

Special technics of specimen collection, transport, and culture are necessary to isolate and identify pathogenic anaerobes. **Cultures free of contamination by normal flora must be obtained**, since contaminants easily may be mistaken for pathogens. Blood, pleural fluid, transtracheal aspirates, pus obtained by direct aspiration, culdocentesis and suprapubic aspirates, and biopsies of normally sterile sites are free of contamination and may be cultured for anaerobes. When liquid specimens are obtained by needle and syringe, air should be expelled from the syringe and the needle should be inserted into a sterile rubber stopper.

Brief **exposure to air** may kill some of the more fastidious anaerobes, such as those found in pulmonary infections, but the most virulent of the anaerobic species are somewhat O_2 tolerant. *B. fragilis* will not grow aerobically but will survive for a few hours in the presence of O_2. **Transit time to the laboratory should be rapid**; delays can lead to overgrowth of aerobic bacteria and result in failure to identify anaerobes.

Gram stains and aerobic cultures should be performed on all specimens. Some anaerobes have characteristic morphology that may be identified on Gram stain. In the laboratory, anaerobic cultures should be plated on special media and incubated anaerobically for 48 to 72 h before examination. Anaerobic culture results may not be available for 3 to 5 days, and often the clinician must start therapy before the results are available. Susceptibility data may not be available for 1 wk or more after initial culture and may not be reliable in many laboratories. However, if the species of bacteria is known, in most instances susceptibility patterns can be predicted; therefore, many laboratories do not perform anaerobic susceptibility tests routinely.

Prevention

Preventive measures include early treatment of localized infection to prevent bacteremia and metastatic disease: cleansing, removal of foreign bodies, reestablishment of circulation, and early antimicrobial treatment of traumatic wounds. Early surgical exploration, drainage, closure of bowel perforation, and antimicrobial treatment of penetrating abdominal wounds are all essential for optimal results. Bowel preparation, eg, with neomycin and erythromycin, should be used when patients are undergoing elective colonic surgery. Parenteral antibiotics have also been used prophylactically in the immediate postoperative period. Several potentially useful regimens ae available, including cefoxitin or a combination of either metronidazole or clindamycin with gentamicin or tobramycin.

Prognosis

Morbidity and mortality from anaerobic and mixed bacterial sepsis tend to be as great as from sepsis caused by a single aerobic organism. Additionally, anaerobic infections often are complicated by deep-seated tissue necrosis. The overall mortality rate for severe intra-abdominal sepsis and mixed anaerobic pneumonias tends to be high, and *B. fragilis* bacteremia is an important cause of mortality.

Treatment

Treatment involves administration of antibiotics and appropriate surgical procedures. Many studies of therapy in *B. fragilis* infections have shown cures in $> 80\%$ of cases.

Antimicrobial therapy of anaerobic infections usually must be started before definitive laboratory results are available (see above) and sometimes is successful even when *some* of the bacterial species in a mixed infection are resistant to the antimicrobial agent, especially if adequate drainage is used. Treating anaerobes as important pathogens in mixed infection reduces the number of organisms found in wounds and the number of abscesses formed. Abscesses and inciting sites of infection, such as organ perforations, must be closed or drained. Devitalized tissue, foreign bodies, and necrotic tissue must be removed. Any closed-space infections, such as empyemas, must be drained and, whenever possible, the blood supply should be reestablished. Septic thrombophlebitis may require vein ligation as well as antimicrobial agents.

Penicillin G is the antibiotic of choice for treating anaerobic infections arising from oral-pharyngeal sources. The recommended dose varies with the site and severity of the infection; for example, in treating lung abscesses, a dose of 6 to 12 million u./day IV for 4 wk is recommended. Infrequently, infections arising from oral bacteria fail to respond to penicillin and should be treated with one of the drugs effective against

penicillin-resistant anaerobes (see below). In patients allergic to penicillin, clindamycin or metronidazole are useful.

Infections arising from a colonic source, which are likely to contain *B. fragilis*, present a different problem because *B. fragilis* is known to be resistant to the penicillins. There are several commonly accepted alternative forms of therapy. Comparative studies have not shown any advantage to any single regimen. One regimen for intra-abdominal sepsis or any infection arising from a colonic source is clindamycin 600 mg q 6 or 8 h IV, or metronidazole 500 mg q 8 h IV. Either of these is given with an aminoglycoside to cover aerobic enteric gram-negative flora; eg, gentamicin 5 mg/kg/day in 3 divided doses. Serum levels of gentamicin should be monitored because of known nephrotoxicity and ototoxicity. Cefoxitin, a second-generation cephalosporin, or third-generation cephalosporins such as cefotaxime or moxalactam are also effective against the anaerobic bacteria in peritonitis. Therefore, any of these agents can be used as alternative therapies for intra-abdominal sepsis. Another effective drug is chloramphenicol (succinate derivative) given in initial doses of 30 to 60 mg/kg/day IV, depending on the severity of the illness. However, because of rare cases of idiosyncratic aplastic anemia, this drug should be used only when other options are not satisfactory. Chloramphenicol and the cephalosporins listed above are active against anaerobes, including *B. fragilis*, and against the aerobic enteric gram-negative bacterial flora, and can be used alone (rather than in combination with an aminoglycoside). Failure of a known *B. fragilis* infection to respond to chloramphenicol, clindamycin, or cefoxitin suggests relative drug resistance and may warrant changing to another agent, provided that foci of infection have been drained adequately.

Campylobacter AND NONCHOLERIC VIBRIO INFECTIONS

Campylobacter INFECTIONS

Campylobacter species are motile, curved, microaerophilic, gram-negative rods associated with septic thrombophlebitis, bacteremia, endocarditis, and diarrhea.

Epidemiology

Three species are believed to be human pathogens. *Campylobacter fetus fetus* is primarily associated with bacteremia in adults, often with underlying predisposing disease such as diabetes or malignancy. *C. jejuni* is implicated as a cause of meningitis in infants and it, as well as *C. coli*, causes diarrheal disease. The latter is being recognized with increasing frequency. Although contact with infected animals and ingestion of contaminated food or water have been implicated, the source of the infecting organisms frequently is obscure.

Symptoms and Signs

Bacteremia without localized infection and diarrhea are the most common presentations. Fever of 38 to 40 C (100 to 104 F) that follows a relapsing or intermittent course is the only constant feature of systemic campylobacter infection, although abdominal pain and hepatosplenomegaly are frequent. This infection can also present as SBE, septic arthritis, meningitis, or an indolent FUO. Enteritis resembling salmonellosis or shigellosis affects all ages, but peak incidence appears to be in the 1- to 5-yr age group. The diarrhea is watery and sometimes becomes bloody; WBCs are seen in stained smears of stool.

Diagnosis

Diagnosis, particularly to differentiate from ulcerative colitis (see Ch. 59), requires microbiologic evaluation. *Campylobacter* can be recovered from blood and various body fluids by using standard culture media, but isolation from stool requires selective

media. Skirrow's medium using 7% lysed horse-blood agar with added vancomycin, polymyxin B, and trimethoprim has been used successfully.

Treatment

Various antibiotics alone and in combination have been used. Tetracycline or chloramphenicol in a divided dosage of 2 gm/day orally for 10 to 14 days should eradicate the organisms in most instances. Erythromycin 1 to 2 gm/day in 4 divided doses has been effective in treating campylobacterial diarrhea.

NONCHOLERIC VIBRIO INFECTIONS

These vibrios are biochemically or serologically distinct from *V. cholerae* and produce wound infections, enteric sepsis, or diarrhea, depending on the species involved.

Etiology and Epidemiology

The vibrios of importance (other than cholera, which is discussed above under BACTERIAL DISEASES CAUSED BY GRAM-NEGATIVE, FACULTATIVELY ANAEROBIC BACILLI) are *V. parahemolyticus*, *V. mimicus*, *V. alginolyticus*, *V. vulnificus*, and the so-called "nonagglutinable" **(NAG)** vibrios. *V. parahemolyticus* is a halophilic organism incriminated in food-borne (in inadequately cooked seafood, usually shrimp) outbreaks of diarrhea in Japan and in coastal areas of the USA.

Symptoms, Signs, and Diagnosis

After a 15- to 24-h incubation period, the illness, which usually begins acutely with cramping abdominal pain, watery diarrhea (stools may be bloody and contain polymorphonuclear leukocytes), tenesmus, weakness, and sometimes low-grade fever, subsides spontaneously in 24 to 48 h. The organism neither produces enterotoxin nor invades the bloodstream, but it does damage the gut mucosa. NAG vibrios may cause a cholera-like illness, and they have been isolated from wounds and blood. Neither *V. alginolyticus* nor *V. vulnificus* causes enteritis, but both can cause marine wound infection. *V. vulnificus*, when ingested by a compromised host (often an individual with chronic liver disease), crosses the gut mucosa *without* enteritis and produces septicemia with a high mortality rate.

Wound and bloodstream infections are readily diagnosed with routine cultures. When enteric infection is suspected, vibrio organisms can be cultured from stool on thiosulfate-citrate-bile-sucrose (TCBS) medium; contaminated seafood also yields positive cultures.

Treatment

Noncholeric vibrio infections have been treated with a wide range of antibiotics. Limited experience suggests that 2 gm/day orally of tetracycline or chloramphenicol in divided doses should be effective. Close attention to repleting volume and electrolyte losses in diarrheal disease is needed.

CAUSED BY AEROBIC BACILLI

HEMOPHILUS INFECTIONS

The nonmotile, small gram-negative rods or coccobacilli comprising the genus *Hemophilus* require specific factors (X and/or V) for growth. Most *Hemophilus* species grow well on chocolate agar incubated at 37 C in air. Many *Hemophilus* species are normally found in the upper respiratory passages of both children and adults and rarely cause disease.

H. influenzae, the species most important in causing human disease, is a leading cause of meningitis, bacteremia, septic arthritis, pneumonia, tracheobronchitis, otitis

media, conjunctivitis, sinusitis, and acute epiglottitis in young children. These infections, as well as endocarditis, may occur in adults, but do so far less commonly. They are discussed in Ch. 40 and under ACUTE EPIGLOTTITIS in Ch. 191, MENINGITIS in Ch. 125, and INFECTIOUS ARTHRITIS in Ch. 108. Most *H. influenzae* strains that cause serious infections in children or adults are encapsulated, type b strains. Other *Hemophilus* strains may cause respiratory infections or, less commonly, endocarditis. *H. ducreyi* causes the venereal disease chancroid (see Ch. 14).

BRUCELLOSIS

(Undulant, Malta, Mediterranean, or Gibraltar Fever)

An infectious disease characterized by an acute febrile stage with few or no localizing signs and a chronic stage with relapses of fever, weakness, sweats, and vague aches and pains.

Etiology and Epidemiology

The causative microorganisms of human brucellosis are *Brucella abortus* (cattle), *B. suis* (hogs), *B. melitensis* (sheep and goats), and *B. rangiferi* (*B. suis* biotype 4; Alaskan and Siberian caribou); *B. canis* (dogs) has caused sporadic infections. Brucella infections of deer, horses, moose, hares, chickens, and desert rats have also been reported. Brucellosis is acquired by direct contact with secretions and excretions of infected animals, and by ingesting cow, sheep, or goat milk or milk products (eg, butter and cheese) containing viable *Brucella* organisms. It is rarely transmitted from person to person. Most prevalent in rural areas, brucellosis is an occupational disease of meatpackers, veterinarians, farmers, and livestock producers; children are less susceptible. Distribution is worldwide.

Clinical Course

The incubation period varies from 5 days to several months (average, 2 wk). Symptoms vary, especially in the early stages. Onset may be sudden and acute, with chills and fever, severe headache, pains, malaise, and occasionally diarrhea; or insidious, with mild prodromal malaise, muscular pain, headache, and pain in the back of the neck, followed by a rise in evening temperature. The total WBC count usually is normal or reduced, with a relative or absolute lymphocytosis. As the disease progresses, the temperature increases to 40 or 41 C (104 or 105 F), then subsides gradually to normal or near-normal in the morning, when profuse sweating occurs.

Typically, the intermittent fever persists for 1 to 5 wk, followed by a 2- to 14-day remission with symptoms greatly diminished or absent; the febrile phase then recurs. Sometimes this pattern occurs only once; occasionally, however, subacute or chronic brucellosis ensues, with repeated febrile waves (undulations) and remissions recurring over months or years. In some patients, fever may be only transient.

After the initial phase, constipation usually is pronounced; anorexia, weight loss, abdominal pain, joint pain, headache, backache, weakness, irritability, insomnia, mental depression, and emotional instability occur. Splenomegaly appears, and lymph nodes may be slightly or moderately enlarged; hepatomegaly may be present in up to 50% of patients.

Patients with acute, uncomplicated brucellosis usually recover in 2 to 3 wk. **Complications** are rare but include SBE, meningitis, encephalitis, neuritis, orchitis, cholecystitis, hepatic suppuration, and bone lesions. It is usual for chronic disease to result in prolonged ill health. The disease is rarely fatal.

Diagnosis

A definitive diagnosis is usually based upon recovery of the organism from the blood, and less often from CSF, urine, or tissues. However, serological results are of major importance also, and agglutination tests are particularly valuable when a titer is 1:100 or higher. Brucella agglutination tests should include the simple procedure of identifying site of IgG and IgM immunoglobulins. IgG globulins indicate active disease, even with titers below 1:100. Therefore, when the agglutination test is positive in the absence of bacteriologic evidence, diagnosis is based on a history of exposure to infected animals or animal products (eg, ingestion of unpasteurized milk), epidemiologic data, and the characteristic clinical findings and course. Intradermal tests with *Brucella* antigens are of little value in diagnosing active brucellosis.

Prophylaxis

Pasteurization of milk and eating only aged cheese are the most important prophylactic measures. Persons handling animals or carcasses that are likely to be infected should wear goggles (or glasses) and rubber gloves and should protect skin breaks from bacterial invasion. Every effort should be made to detect the infection in animals and control it at its source.

Treatment

Tetracycline 0.5 gm is given orally qid for 21 days and should be repeated if relapses occur. Seriously ill patients are also given streptomycin 1 gm IM q 12 h for 1 wk, then 0.5 gm IM q 12 h or 1 gm IM daily for an additional 7 to 14 days. Prednisone 20 mg orally tid for 5 or 7 days can be given simultaneously with the antibiotics if toxemia is present. Severe musculoskeletal pains, especially over the spine, may require codeine 15 to 60 mg orally or s.c. q 4 to 6 h.

Activity should be restricted in acute cases, with bed rest recommended during febrile periods.

MELIOIDOSIS

A glanderslike infection of man and animals, caused by Pseudomonas pseudomallei *and endemic in Southeast Asia, in North Queensland, Australia, and (recently recognized) in Central, West, and East Africa.* This bacillus can be isolated from soil and water. Man may contract melioidosis by contamination of skin abrasions or burns, by ingestion, or by inhalation, but not directly from infected animals or patients.

Symptoms and Signs

Illness may be asymptomatic or occur in various forms. Clinically inapparent infection may be latent for years. Mortality is < 10%, except in acute septicemic melioidosis. In endemic areas, melioidosis is likely to be one of the infections seen in patients with AIDS.

Acute pulmonary infection, the most common form, varies from mild to an overwhelming necrotizing pneumonia. Onset may be abrupt or gradual, with headache, anorexia, pleuritic or dull aching chest pain, and generalized myalgia. Fever is usually over 39 C (102 F). Cough, tachypnea, and rales are characteristic; sputum may be blood-tinged. Chest x-rays usually show upper-lobe consolidation, frequently cavitating and resembling TB. Nodular lesions, thin-walled cysts, and pleural effusion may also be present. The WBC count ranges from normal to 20,000.

Acute septicemic infection: Onset may be abrupt, with disorientation, extreme dyspnea, severe headache, pharyngitis, upper abdominal colic, diarrhea, and pustular skin lesions. High fever, tachypnea, a bright erythematous flush, and cyanosis are present.

Muscle tenderness may be striking. There may be signs of arthritis or meningitis. Pulmonary signs may be absent, or rales, rhonchi, and pleural rubs may be present. Chest x-rays usually show irregular nodular (4 to 10 mm) densities. The liver and spleen may be palpable. Liver function tests, AST (SGOT), and bilirubin often are abnormal. The WBC count is normal or slightly increased.

Chronic suppurative infection: Secondary abscesses may develop in the skin, lymph nodes, or any organ. Osteomyelitis is a relatively common presentation. Patients may be afebrile. An acute suppurative form is uncommon.

Diagnosis

Culture of *P. pseudomallei* (which grows on most laboratory media in 48 to 72 h) and HA, agglutination, and CF tests on paired sera aid in diagnosis.

Treatment

Inapparent infection needs no treatment. **Mildly ill patients** are given trimethoprim/sulfamethoxazole **(TMP/SMX)**, TMP 20 mg/SMX 100 mg/kg/day (eg, 4 tablets, each containing 80 mg of TMP and 400 mg of SMX, orally qid in 70-kg adult), for a minimum of 30 days, or tetracycline or chloramphenicol 40 mg/kg/day orally. **Moderately ill patients** are given 2 antimicrobials (eg, TMP/SMX plus tetracycline or ceftazidime or ceftriaxone) for 30 days, then tetracycline alone or TMP/SMX alone for 30 to 120 days. **Severe acute melioidosis** is treated with TMP/SMX (5.0 mg of TMP/kg q 6 h) IV plus ceftazidime (30 mg/kg q 8 h) IV or ceftriaxone (loading dose of 75 mg/kg followed by 50 mg/kg q 12 h) IV. The dosage should be tapered as clinical improvement occurs. TMP/SMX should be used as for mildly ill patients, for 30 to 120 days.

BARTONELLOSIS

(Bartonella bacilliformis Infection; Carrion's Disease)

A bacterial infection, caused by Bartonella bacilliformis *and seen only in South America, that can be characterized by an acute febrile anemia (Oroya fever) or a chronic cutaneous eruption (Verruga peruana).*

Etiology, Epidemiology, and Pathogenesis

The organism, a small, motile, aerobic, gram-negative bacillus that can be cultured on enriched media, is passed from human to human by the phlebotomine sandfly. Sporadic cases and epidemics occur only at certain altitudes of the Andes in Colombia, Ecuador, and Peru where the vector is found. In nonimmune individuals, the bartonella invade the bloodstream, attach to the surface of erythrocytes, and initiate anemia. They also invade capillary endothelial cells and produce vascular occlusion. This stage of disease is frequently complicated by superimposed bacteremia caused by salmonella or other coliform organisms. As immunity develops, the numbers of bacteria in the blood and in endothelial cells sharply decrease. After a latent period they reappear in the skin and subcutaneous tissue, where they apparently cause hemangioid lesions.

Symptoms and Signs

Oroya fever is characterized by sudden fever, weakness, pallor, muscle and joint pain, severe headache, and, in many cases, delirium and coma. Mortality rates may exceed 50% in untreated patients. **Verruga peruana** may occur in patients with or without previous symptoms of Oroya fever. The skin lesions, ranging from 0.2 to 4 cm in diameter, may be nodular or eroding in nature. They occur in series of crops, usually on the limbs and face, that may persist for from months to years and may be accompanied by pain and fever.

Diagnosis

During the acute phase, the organisms may involve 90% of the erythrocytes and can be easily seen on a stained smear of peripheral blood. During the cutaneous stage, the organisms can be demonstrated in the lesions. Although the peripheral blood smear is usually negative at this stage, bartonella may be recovered from the blood by culture. Salmonellosis, malaria, and amebiasis are important intercurrent infections.

Prophylaxis and Treatment

The sandfly vector can be controlled with insect repellents and residual insecticides. Antimicrobial therapy rapidly terminates the acute febrile illness and hastens involution of cutaneous lesions. Bartonellosis responds to tetracycline and chloramphenicol, but because often it is complicated by salmonella bacteremia, chloramphenicol 2 to 4 gm/day in divided doses for 7 days is the treatment of choice.

LISTERIOSIS

(See also Neonatal Listeriosis under Neonatal Infections in Ch. 186)

Infection caused by Listeria monocytogenes *and having manifestations that vary according to pathogenesis, site, and age of the patient.*

Etiology, Incidence, and Epidemiology

L. monocytogenes, a gram-positive, non-acid-fast, noncapsulated, nonsporulating, motile, microaerophilic bacillus that is β-hemolytic, is found worldwide and afflicts mammals, birds, arachnids, and crustaceans. Of the 7 major serotypes, Types 4b, 1b, and 1a account for most human listerioses in the USA. Incidence, highest in neonates and in persons > 40, peaks in July and August. It may be significant that 25% of listeriosis patients have a preexisting disease (eg, cirrhosis, lymphomas, solid tumors). Also, immunodeficiencies, acquired naturally (as with AIDS) or artificially (eg, as part of cancer therapy), are associated with an increased frequency of listeriosis. Infection with *L. monocytogenes* has been proved to occur via ingestion (contaminated cows' milk, cheese products) and direct contact (antepartum and intrapartum from mother to child; exposure of veterinarians to listerial abortions in livestock and of butchers in slaughtering infected animals). Epizootic disease appears to be related to epidemic listeriosis.

Clinical Forms and Diagnosis

In adults, **meningitis** is the most common form of listeriosis and, unlike in other bacterial meningitides, cerebritis (ranging from diffuse encephalitis to abscesses) occurs in up to 20% of cases. **Endocarditis** is a rare form, as is **typhoidal listeriosis** with bacteremia and high fever and without localizing symptoms and signs. **Oculoglandular** infection, with ophthalmitis and regional lymph node involvement, follows conjunctival inoculation and, if untreated, may progress to bacteremia and meningitis.

Listerial infections may be suspected but not definitely diagnosed clinically; isolation of *L. monocytogenes* is necessary for diagnosis. *The laboratory must be informed of the possibility of listeriosis when specimens are sent for culture* because the organism is easily confused with diphtheroids. In all listerial infections, IgG agglutinin titers peak 2 to 4 wk after onset.

Treatment

For meningitis in adults, penicillin G 75,000 to 100,000 u./kg should be given IV q 4 h and continued for 10 to 14 days after defervescence. For endocarditis and typhoidal listeriosis, both penicillin G (75,000 to 100,000 u./kg IV q 4 h) and tobramycin (1.7 mg/kg IV q 8 h) should be given until 4 wk after defervescence. Oculoglandular

listeriosis should respond to erythromycin 30 mg/kg/day orally as 4 equal doses q 6 h, continued until 1 wk following defervescence.

CAUSED BY MYCOBACTERIA

TUBERCULOSIS

(See also PERINATAL TUBERCULOSIS under NEONATAL INFECTIONS in Ch. 186)

An acute or chronic infection caused by Mycobacterium tuberculosis *and, rarely in the USA, by* M. bovis. TB is characterized clinically by a lifelong balance between the host and the infection, in which pulmonary or extrapulmonary foci may reactivate at any time, often after long periods of latency. TB is characterized pathologically by the formation of tubercles made up of giant cells and epithelioid cells, by a tendency for fibrosis to occur, and by caseation, a unique form of nonliquefying necrosis.

Etiology

M. tuberculosis is an acid-fast, nonmotile rod that is characteristically sensitive to isoniazid **(INH)** and produces niacin and the enzyme catalase. INH-resistant mutants generally lose their ability to produce catalase, but remain niacin-positive. *M. bovis* is also sensitive to INH, but does not produce niacin. Other pathogenic mycobacteria (except *M. leprae*) are highly INH-resistant and catalase-positive, and almost all are niacin-negative.

Epidemiology

Infection occurs primarily by inhalation. Infectious droplets, which are aerosolized by coughing and dry while suspended in air, may contaminate the air in closed spaces for long periods. Fomites such as dishes and bedclothes are not important vectors. In areas where bovine TB has not been eliminated, transmission may occur by ingestion of contaminated milk. Direct inoculation occasionally occurs in laboratory workers.

Case rates vary markedly with such factors as age, race, socioeconomic status, and geography. In the USA, 20,000 new cases and 1800 deaths are being reported annually; almost 15% of the cases involve extrapulmonary sites. In the USA, most active disease occurs in older individuals (particularly nonwhite males); in contacts of active cases; in persons known to have had clinical TB in the past who were never adequately treated with drugs; and in immigrants from Southeast Asia, Africa, and Central and South America (many of whom show resistance to one or more antituberculous drugs).

Pathogenesis

A nonsensitized host has no specific immunologic defense against TB. Infection usually begins in the lower or middle lung fields. With little host reaction and no symptoms, the bacilli spread readily to the draining lymph nodes and, via the bloodstream, can reach any other organ. With the development of tuberculin hypersensitivity 4 to 10 wk later, a small area of pneumonitis develops, multiplication of intracellular bacilli is inhibited at both the initial and metastatic foci, and the infection is usually quickly *arrested*.

The frequency with which infection develops into disease depends on the person's age and the intensity of exposure. Smear-negative, culture-positive cases have little infectiousness, and extrapulmonary cases have almost none. A large percentage of infants and ≥ 10% of adolescents and young adults in household contact with smear-positive cases will develop active disease. The postinfancy prepubertal child and the middle-aged adult are much more resistant; in old age susceptibility rises again. Ex-

cept in infants, the risk of tuberculin conversion due to a very small inoculum developing into disease is probably quite low. If active disease develops, it usually does so within 1 to 2 yr of infection. In the remainder, foci of infection in the lung and elsewhere may remain dormant but viable and at risk of reactivation for many years. Factors favoring reactivation include waning immunity (due to immunosuppressive or prolonged corticosteroid therapy, old age, malnutrition, alcoholism, or intercurrent illness—eg, uncontrolled diabetes or malignancy of the lymphatic or hematologic systems), local injury (destructive pulmonary processes such as lung abscess, cancer, surgery, or local joint or back injury), and some poorly understood intercurrent processes (silicosis, gastric resection).

Prophylaxis

Vaccination with BCG (an attenuated strain of *M. tuberculosis*), still useful in certain parts of the world and in certain groups where TB is prevalent (> 20% of secondary school children positive to tuberculin), is now rarely used in the USA.

Chemoprophylaxis usually consists of **INH** alone, 300 mg daily in adults, 6 to 10 mg/kg in children, for 12 to 18 mo, given as a single dose in the morning. In Southeast Asians and other groups with a high incidence of INH resistance, multiple drug therapy should be given as for treatment of established, drug-resistant disease. Treating **tuberculin-negative** individuals is sometimes appropriate; eg, when brief exposure of an infant to a known infectious risk (eg, the mother) cannot be avoided, or when an exposed person has a reduced immune response for any reason. Chemoprophylaxis is indicated in certain **tuberculin-positive** individuals without overt disease: children under age 20; individuals with pulmonary infiltrates of unknown etiology; persons receiving prolonged corticosteroid therapy; the postgastrectomy patient with x-ray evidence of a quiescent or inactive focus of pulmonary TB; and all patients with silicosis. Chemoprophylaxis of recent tuberculin converters is appropriate in those of any age when epidemiologic factors suggest that recent infection is likely and in the relatively young. However, in some—particularly middle-aged and older adults—an apparent tuberculin conversion may actually represent the so-called **booster effect**. This occurs when injection of tuberculin, which itself produces a negative reaction, stimulates residual tuberculin hypersensitivity from a remote infection so that a subsequent test will be positive. The booster effect develops in < 1 wk and persists for > 1 yr. The confusion can be avoided by repeating an initially negative 5 TU tuberculin test in 1 wk and assuming that in that brief interval a 2nd positive test will represent boosting rather than a new infection.

Hospitalizing or isolating a patient under treatment is not necessary to prevent spread. The major risk of contagion is before diagnosis; in 10 to 14 days, patients on adequate treatment become noninfectious, despite continued positive sputum by laboratory tests.

PULMONARY TUBERCULOSIS

Childhood Type

Hilar lymphadenopathy is the hallmark of childhood pulmonary TB. Mediastinal nodes draining the initial area of pneumonitis become massively enlarged, usually unilaterally, causing bronchial compression resulting in a brassy, nonproductive cough or, particularly in very young children with flaccid small bronchi, atelectasis distal to bronchial compression. **Serofibrinous pleurisy** with effusion (see PLEURAL TUBERCULOSIS, below) occasionally occurs soon after infection. **Progressive primary TB** is uncommon, but caseation and, very rarely, cavity formation may result. **Hypersensitivity**

syndromes include phlyctenular keratoconjunctivitis (a brisk ocular inflammatory reaction to locally deposited tubercle bacilli) and erythema nodosum. Both are rare, probably occur in association with development of tuberculin hypersensitivity, usually are self-limited, and respond to corticosteroids.

Treatment is the same as for adults (see Treatment, in ADULT TYPE, below), except that the dose of INH (10 mg/kg, up to 300 mg) is larger, since children are more resistant to INH induction of pyridoxine deficiency and resulting peripheral neuritis. Corticosteroids may be helpful when bronchial compression by enlarged nodes produces symptoms.

Adult Type

Most pulmonary TB in adults is seen initially in the apical areas of the lung, which have been seeded by bloodstream-spread from an often undetectable primary focus in the lower lung. Progression of the metastatic apical focus takes place while the initial focus is healing. It may occur after a long period of latency, but usually occurs within 2 yr of initial infection. Chronic apical TB can also result from new (exogenous) infection in persons previously infected. Caseous necrosis, liquefaction, and cavity formation in the apical areas permit spread of infection via the bronchi; new cavities typically form in the apical and subapical areas on that side and later in the opposite lung. Prior to drug therapy, 50% of cases with cavitary TB were fatal; healing of cavities is now the rule with appropriate drug treatment.

TB in the aged differs in some important ways from the usual form of adult apical TB. At least in the USA, most persons over age 65 are now tuberculin-negative because they have never been infected or because tuberculin hypersensitivity and specific cellular immunity have disappeared when ancient infections have died out (5 to 10% of tuberculin reactions revert to negative each year). Infection in these individuals frequently causes an indolent, nondescript, unresolving lower-lobe bronchopneumonia, difficult to diagnose because of relatively sparse bacillary content as compared to upper-lobe disease. Also, calcified hilar nodes from remote infections can erode into a bronchus, spilling infectious caseous material and causing distal spread of infection into the middle or lower lobe. Other late consequences of calcified hilar nodes include midesophageal traction diverticula and, rarely, bronchoesophageal fistulas.

Symptoms and Signs

Pulmonary TB is asymptomatic at first; signs usually become apparent when the lesion is large enough to be visible on x-ray. Systemic symptoms of fever, malaise, and weight loss are often so gradual as to be unnoticed.

Cough is due to irritative secretions draining into the bronchi from sloughing areas of lung tissue. It is most frequently associated with cavitation and at first occurs only in the morning, as a result of material accumulated in the bronchi overnight. **Sputum**, scanty at first, increases with progressive pulmonary excavation. In a caseous liquefying lesion, it is green and purulent. In chronic disease, with less excavation, the sputum becomes yellowish and mucoid. **Hemoptysis**, occasionally the first symptom, may be due to endobronchial involvement with granulation tissue or to erosion of an artery by an enlarging cavity. It may vary from slight bloody streaking of the sputum to massive, though seldom fatal, hemorrhage. **Pleural** or **chest wall pain** occurs with pleural involvement. **Dyspnea** is common during acute febrile periods. Acute dyspnea may result from a spontaneous pneumothorax or rapidly developing pleural effusion. Rarely, endobronchial spread of infectious secretions causes oral ulcers, painful laryngeal involvement with hoarseness, or gastrointestinal TB that may first call attention to the pulmonary disease.

The pace of the illness varies widely. Particularly in Eskimos, American Indians, and

some blacks, the entire upper lobe may be involved together with systemic symptoms, suggesting lobar pneumonia. In others, symptoms may be minimal or absent despite extensive cavity formation and marked fibrosis. Undiagnosed and highly infectious patients may remain in relatively good health for prolonged periods.

Extensive pulmonary TB compromises pulmonary function, and some patients may succumb to respiratory failure or to pulmonary hypertension and cor pulmonale. **Extrapulmonary TB** is discussed below.

Diagnosis

Pulmonary TB is often first suspected on the basis of chest x-ray findings. An apical lesion is most common; a small mottled density is characteristic of early reinfection. However, an unexplained infiltrate in any area of the lung may be due to TB. Rarefaction may indicate beginning liquefaction and cavitation. Laminagrams help to visualize cavities.

Microscopic identification of acid-fast rods on direct examination of sputum is good presumptive evidence, but it does not exclude other mycobacterial diseases. Histologic evidence of tubercle formation in pulmonary or other tissue is strong but also presumptive evidence for the same reason. Fiberoptic transbronchial lung biopsy often facilitates provisional diagnosis when sputum is negative; however, negative biopsy results do not exclude the diagnosis.

Definitive diagnosis requires cultural identification of *M. tuberculosis* or *M. bovis.* Since *M. tuberculosis* grows slowly, culture is time-consuming and results may not be available for 3 to 6 wk. An early morning sputum collection is the best source. Alternatively, sputum swallowed during the night may be obtained by aspirating gastric contents immediately after the patient awakens and prior to his leaving the bed. The specimen should also be plated on media containing various concentrations of INH, streptomycin, and, if possible, other antituberculous drugs for initial drug sensitivity studies. A high degree of INH resistance, with the ability to form catalase, is often the first evidence that the infection is due to another mycobacterial species.

The **tuberculin test** is an important adjunct to diagnosis. The standard test material, purified protein derivative **(PPD)**, is stabilized by including a polysorbate detergent in the diluent. First strength tuberculin (1 tuberculin unit or **TU**) is useful in individuals in whom a high degree of hypersensitivity might be anticipated, such as young children. Most epidemiologic data are based on 5 TU (intermediate strength). Second strength PPD is 250 TU. Antigen can be applied by the scratch (Pirquet's) test and by multiple-puncture tine and Heaf tests, but the most satisfactory method is careful intradermal administration (Mantoux test). Palpable induration (not erythema) of over 10 mm 48 h after administration of 5 TU by the Mantoux technic is diagnostic of tuberculous infection, though not necessarily of *active* TB. A smaller reaction (5 to 9 mm of induration) is labeled doubtful and may be due to infection with other mycobacteria. Many patients with active TB do not react to 5 TU and some patients seriously ill with proven TB do not initially react to 250 TU; they usually become positive with clinical improvement. *Accordingly, a negative tuberculin test does not exclude a diagnosis of TB.*

Treatment

Principles of drug therapy: (1) At least 2 drugs are required for treating pulmonary TB; in extensive disease, 3 drugs are desirable. In populations with a large percentage of drug-resistant infections, 4 drugs are advisable. (2) Response to drug therapy and prognosis as to potential relapse can be predicted by the rapidity of sputum conversion from positive to negative. When this occurs within 3 mo, successful outcome without adding a third or fourth drug is usual. When sputum conversion is delayed past 4 or 5 mo, the probability of an emerging drug-resistant population is greater and 2 new drugs to which the infection is known to be sensitive should be added. (3) Since most

treatment failures are based on lack of patient compliance, the least inconvenient and disagreeable drug regimen is preferred. (4) INH should be part of all treatment regimens except in the unusual circumstance of unacceptable drug toxicity, and probably when rifampin **(RMP)** is being given for retreatment of INH-resistant TB. (5) Therapy with drug regimens other than those containing both INH and RMP should be continued at least 18 to 24 mo after sputum has become negative for tubercule bacilli. Regimens containing both INH and RMP can be as short as 9 mo. (6) INH + RMP has been widely accepted as initial therapy for all patients, administered for 9 mo, with streptomycin **(SM)** or ethambutol **(EMB)** added during the first 2 to 3 mo in advanced cases or where there is suspicion of drug resistance. This regimen carries some risk of increased hepatotoxicity and no better final outcome than INH + EMB in moderate disease or INH + EMB + SM (2 mo) in advanced disease, given for 18 to 24 mo. There is concern that noncompliant patients who take drugs irregularly may develop resistance to both major agents in regimens containing both INH and RMP. (7) Ultrashort regimens using 4 drugs (INH, RMP, pyrazinamide **[PZA]**, and either SM or EMB) are particularly valuable in patients in whom supervision is mandatory. (8) In end-stage renal diseases INH and RMP can be used in regular doses, administered after dialysis when the latter is used. The dose of EMB should be reduced to 8 to 10 mg/kg and PZA to 12 to 20 mg/kg. Aminoglycosides should not be used ordinarily. *Pyridoxine supplementation is mandatory in uremia.*

Initial treatment regimens: (See TABLE 8–4.) In generally well individuals with moderately advanced disease, the INH + EMB regimen is simple, nontoxic, and effective. In extensive disease and in patients with markedly compromised general health, INH + EMB + SM (SM for 2 mo) and INH + RMP or INH + RMP + EMB (EMB for 2 mo) are equally effective, differing only in that the last 2 regimens can be discontinued after 9 mo. In the 1st and 3rd regimens, when bacteriologic response is favorable and the infection is known to be drug sensitive, SM or EMB is usually given only during the initial 2 or 3 mo. Patients such as alcoholics in whom compliance problems make continued supervision highly desirable are often best treated with short-course (6 mo) 4-drug regimens with hospitalization for the 2- or 3-mo period of intensive therapy.

Retreatment regimens: (See TABLE 8–4.) Principles of the therapy of treatment failures are complex. In general, if rifampin **(RMP)** has not been given previously, it is the keystone of retreatment, in combination with at least 1 and preferably 2 other drugs also not previously given.

Specific antimicrobial drugs: Isoniazid (INH) is bactericidal and the least toxic (see also in Ch. 72), least expensive, and most easily administered antituberculous agent (see TABLE 8–4 for dosages). Concentrations in the CSF are approximately 20% of those in the serum; with meningeal inflammation, the concentration approaches that in the serum. Penetration into other tissues is also excellent.

Toxic reactions: Transient minor **elevations of serum transaminase** occur in as many as 10% of patients; **jaundice** is seen in about 1%; fatalities due to severe liver injury, histologically resembling chronic active hepatitis, occur in about 0.1% of some treatment groups. *The risk increases progressively with age, and is further increased in daily users of alcohol.* Minor transaminase elevations (< 5 × normal) usually subside without stopping the drug but must be closely followed. Jaundice is usually associated with symptoms of hepatitis; *to avoid fatality, the drug must be stopped and not given again.*

INH-induced **pyridoxine deficiency**, which may cause peripheral neuritis, is dose-related and occurs in about 2% of patients taking the usual 300-mg daily dose but in > 10% of those taking INH in increased dosages. Routine administration of pyridoxine, 50 to 100 mg/day, is necessary in those receiving increased INH dosage and in patients in whom baseline pyridoxine deficiency might be expected, such as alcoholic, uremic, or cancer patients; those who are pregnant; and those with malnutrition of any

sort. Many administer pyridoxine in the same dosage in all cases, although the need for this has not been established. If pyridoxine-deficiency peripheral neuritis does develop, INH should be discontinued temporarily and pyridoxine 300 mg/day administered until symptoms disappear. INH can then be resumed together with a reduced pyridoxine dosage. **INH hypersensitivity** may be manifested by fever, skin rash, and, rarely, agranulocytosis. **Drug interactions**: INH interferes with phenytoin metabolism; phenytoin blood levels should be monitored to avoid toxicity.

Rifampin (RMP) is at least as potent as INH against rapidly metabolizing organisms and more potent than INH against slowly metabolizing persisting organisms. Once begun it should be continued throughout the course of treatment. Administering INH + RMP results in slightly more hepatotoxicity than INH alone. Other untoward effects include serum-sickness-like syndromes, thrombocytopenia, and, rarely, acute renal failure. These are uncommon when dosage is given daily, but occur more frequently with dosage intervals > 72 h and especially with doses > 600 mg given on a less-than-daily basis. The drug should be given orally on an empty stomach (see TABLE 8–4 for dosages). It is always administered with at least one other drug to which the infecting microbial population is sensitive, since resistance can develop promptly and when it does all drug effect is lost. **Drug interactions** occur with many drugs; RMP has been reported to accelerate the metabolism of coumarin anticoagulants, oral contraceptives, corticosteroids, digitoxin, oral hypoglycemic agents, and methadone, and occasionally to cause osteomalacia due to enhanced metabolism of vitamin D.

Streptomycin (SM), the 3rd major antituberculous agent, is given IM in a dosage of 1 gm/day for adults; after the initial response to treatment has been established, the dosage may be reduced to 1 gm 3 times/wk. (See also TABLE 8–4 for dosages.) Compromised renal function is a relative contraindication to its use; when SM is required

TABLE 8–4. SUGGESTED SCHEME OF TREATMENT FOR TUBERCULOSIS

	*Recommended Regimen**
Initial Treatment, Pulmonary	
Chemoprophylaxis†	INH for 12–18 mo
Minimal disease	INH + EMB for 18 mo
Moderately advanced or far advanced disease	INH + EMB for 18–24 mo INH + EMB + SM (SM for 2 mo; INH + EMB for 18–24 mo) INH + RMP for 9 mo INH + RMP + EMB (EMB for 2 mo, INH + RMP for total of 9 mo)
Short-course therapy	INH + RMP + PZA + SM or EMB daily for 2 or 3 mo followed by INH + RMP (standard doses) daily for total of 6 mo
Re-treatment, Pulmonary	
Drug-sensitive	As above
INH-resistant‡	RMP + 2 other effective§ drugs
INH- + EMB- + SM- + RMP-resistant	3 effective§ drugs; preference, in order: capreomycin, pyrazinamide, ethionamide, cycloserine, kanamycin, amikacin. (No more than one aminoglycoside should be given at the same time)

(*Continued*)

TABLE 8–4. SUGGESTED SCHEME OF TREATMENT FOR TUBERCULOSIS (*Cont'd*)

	*Recommended Regimen**
Intermittent Supervised Initial Treatment	INH + EMB + SM daily for 2 mo followed by twice weekly INH 15 mg/kg + either EMB 50 mg/kg or SM 25–28 mg/kg INH + RMP (with or without SM for 2 mo) daily followed by twice weekly INH 15 mg/kg + RMP 600 mg or 10 mg/kg (usual dose) INH + RMP + PZA + SM or EMB daily for 2 or 3 mo followed by INH 15 mg/kg + RMP (usual dose) twice weekly for total of 6 mo
Extrapulmonary (life-threatening)	
Miliary, meningeal, renal, spinal, pericardial	INH + SM or INH + RMP (with or without SM)
Extrapulmonary (other)	
Lymphatic, bone & joint, excluding spinal; pleural; peritoneal; GU, excluding renal; upper airways (laryngeal, oral, middle ear) in the absence of concomitant pulmonary disease (rare); GI in the absence of pulmonary disease (uncommon)	INH + EMB or INH + RMP
Pregnancy	INH + RMP for 9 mo (SM + PZA is contraindicated)

* INH = isoniazid 300 mg/day (single dose in the morning) in adolescents and adults, 10 to 30 mg/kg (single dose) in infants and small children. For chemoprophylaxis in children, 6 to 10 mg/kg (single dose in the morning).

EMB = ethambutol 25 mg/kg/day for 2 mo or until sputum becomes negative or while under close observation; reduced to 15 mg/kg/day for prolonged or relatively unsupervised use (single dose in adults; divided dose in older children; not used in younger children).

SM = streptomycin 1 gm/day (single dose) in adults; 20 mg/kg (single dose) in children. Usually discontinued after 8 to 16 wk when sputum conversion has occurred promptly in regimens initially containing 3 drugs.

RMP = rifampin 600 mg/day (single dose) in adults; 15 to 20 mg/kg (single dose) in children.

PZA = pyrazinamide 30 to 35 mg/kg in divided doses; usually 1.5 gm in small adults and 2.5 gm in large adults.

† Instances in which progressive infection has not been established (see chemoprophylaxis above).

‡ With exception of RMP-containing regimens, INH included in spite of in vitro resistance.

§ Effective here means that the infecting microbial population is sensitive to that drug.

despite the presence of azotemia, the dosage must be reduced and serum drug concentrations should be monitored. The minimal inhibitory serum concentration for sensitive strains of *M. tuberculosis* is 0.2 μg/mL, 20 to 50 times less than the peak serum concentration after a 1-gm dose. CSF penetration is poor. Intrathecal SM is **not recommended.**

SM causes selective toxicity for the 8th cranial nerve, particularly the vestibular apparatus, and the vestibular injury tends to be permanent. Since patients over age 50 may become permanently ataxic, they should not be given SM if possible. Caloric testing of vestibular function and audiologic examination are recommended before and during treatment. SM may also cause allergic reactions, including drug fever,

agranulocytosis, and a serum-sickness-like illness. Flushing, itching, and fullness of the head immediately after injection are bothersome histamine-like reactions not necessarily associated with the more serious allergic and toxic signs.

Ethambutol (EMB) is a most desirable companion drug to INH (especially when RMP cannot be used with INH when RMP is the drug of choice). EMB is well absorbed by mouth. The recommended dosages are given in TABLE 8–4. Some authorities do not give EMB to children, especially young children; other authorities prescribe it for older children if clinical testing for optic neuritis is carried out. Optic neuritis with visual field constriction and loss of ability to distinguish the color green, a dose-related side effect, is completely reversible when detected early. EMB should be avoided in uremia; when this is impossible it should be administered at a decreased dosage, 8 to 10 mg/kg.

Pyrazinamide (PZA) is very important to the success of ultrashort (6 mo) multiple-drug regimens. It is thought to be particularly effective against organisms in caseous material or inside of cells existing at an acid pH. At the dosage (1.5 to 2.5 gm/day) and duration (2 or 3 mo) used, hepatotoxicity has not been a problem; the major side effect is arthralgia or frank arthritis, probably due to induction of hyperuricemia.

Capreomycin, ethionamide, cycloserine, kanamycin, and **amikacin** are effective and useful in special situations (see TABLE 8–4), but their use is limited by toxicity.

Other modes of therapy: Bed rest and **hospitalization** are indicated by the patient's general condition. Since patients receiving chemotherapy become noninfectious rapidly, most can quickly return to work and other normal activity. **Surgical resection** has limited usefulness. If sputum conversion is delayed, drug resistance emerges, or thick-walled cavities or dense confluent disease persists after 5 to 9 mo of effective chemotherapy, resection may be performed provided that the remaining pulmonary function will be adequate. When resection is performed because of drug resistance, 2 drugs not previously given are administered together with the drugs previously given.

Adjunctive corticosteroid therapy may be advantageous in patients with extensive disease and profound hypoxemia and toxicity (as in extensive miliary TB or extensive bronchogenic spread); those who remain toxic, anemic, catabolic, and febrile for many weeks despite effective chemotherapy; and those with tuberculous meningitis. For patients who remain toxic and catabolic, prednisone 30 to 40 mg/day is sufficient. In patients in whom the inflammatory response is life-threatening, an initial larger dose (60 mg/day) is advisable. Guided by whether or not the symptoms reappear, the dosage is progressively decreased after 2 or 3 wk and then discontinued. Using corticosteroids in tuberculous pleurisy and pericarditis is controversial. Corticosteroids are also used for replacement (rather than pharmacologic) therapy in patients with coexistent Addison's disease.

EXTRAPULMONARY TUBERCULOSIS

Extrapulmonary TB represents an increasing proportion of cases. It may result from lymphohematogenous spread; dissemination of contaminated pulmonary secretions via the bronchi to the upper air passages, mouth, and GI tract (intracanalicular spread); or direct extension to contiguous tissue. Sites seeded by lymphohematogenous spread prior to the development of tuberculin hypersensitivity may be undetectable for some time and then appear as an isolated clinical syndrome or syndromes without evidence of recent or remote pulmonary TB. Extrapulmonary lesions produced by intracanalicular spread respond promptly to drug therapy for the pulmonary disease and rarely achieve clinical prominence.

Treatment differs from that of cavitary pulmonary TB (see TABLE 8–4 and the preceding discussions of specific drugs for dosages and other details of drug regimens). The drug regimen is determined by urgency rather than by the possibility of emerging

resistance. Prompt treatment with a multiple-drug regimen may be required when the anatomic location carries special risk, as in tuberculous meningitis, pericarditis, or spondylitis (Pott's disease). Initial treatment with INH + EMB is adequate when there is no immediate threat of loss of vital function, as in tuberculous lymphadenitis, peritonitis, or peripheral arthritis.

Miliary Tuberculosis

(Generalized Hematogenous or Lymphohematogenous Tuberculosis)

When metastatic foci are located near blood vessel lumina, development of hypersensitivity and its attendant necrosis may result in secondary reseeding of the bloodstream, causing **early postprimary tuberculous septicemia (hyperacute miliary TB).** High fever and general toxicity are usually present. Tuberculous meningitis is a common complication, particularly in young children. Early in the course, the chest x-ray may be negative because the inflammatory foci are small; the tuberculin test may also be negative. Choroidal tubercles are usually present and are important in diagnosis. Cultures of sputum or gastric contents are often positive; urine cultures are occasionally positive even without demonstrable GU involvement. Examination and culture of the bone marrow or liver may provide the only evidence of tuberculous infection; fiberoptic transbronchial lung biopsy is more often productive than either bone marrow or liver biopsy. **Maximally effective drug therapy** is indicated, usually with INH + SM or INH + RMP.

Late hematogenous dissemination or chronic hematogenous TB: That intermittent nonprogressive episodes of bloodstream-spread from chronic organ foci of TB are the rule is evidenced by the frequency with which choroidal tubercles and hepatic granulomas may be seen in chronic pulmonary TB. However, particularly in the elderly and in patients with compromised immunity, multiple, widely spread episodes of bloodstream seeding, usually from extrapulmonary and previously undetected foci in lymph nodes or bones, may accelerate into progressive hematogenous disease. This may produce a serious febrile illness much like that occurring soon after initial infection, or may produce a less acute process with low grade or absent fever, anemia, and wasting. In some, the usual cellular components of the inflammatory process may be lacking, a process termed **nonreactive TB**, in which myriads of tubercle bacilli exist in the tissues with only a sparse nonspecific cellular response. The clinical manifestations may be extremely subtle, consisting simply of loss of appetite and weight, and failure to thrive. Fever may be absent. Marrow involvement occasionally produces syndromes resembling primary hematologic diseases such as refractory anemia, thrombocytopenia, and leukemoid reaction. Often no pulmonary disease is evident, and the tuberculin test often is negative.

Diagnosis may be established by culture of any body fluid or tissue. Bone marrow and liver biopsies are important, and fiberoptic transbronchial lung biopsy more important. *The key to diagnosis is keeping the syndrome in mind*, and, in the absence of contraindications, it may be appropriate to assess results of a therapeutic trial of INH + EMB. Response is prompt; abrupt improvement in health, nutrition, and vigor generally supports the diagnosis. When the diagnosis is established on histologic or cultural grounds rather than by response to therapeutic trial, double drug **therapy** with INH + SM or INH + RMP is usually recommended.

Central Nervous System Tuberculosis

Tuberculous meningitis develops following rupture of a metastatic subependymal focus of TB into the subarachnoid space (not via bloodstream contamination of the CSF). With complicating miliary disease, it usually develops several weeks after the initial manifestations of the miliary process, but it often is seen in the absence of other

evidence of active TB. Incidence is highest in children aged 1 to 5 yr, but the disease may occur at any age. Symptoms may be acute and resemble bacterial meningitis, or may be chronic with emphasis on headache and perhaps behavioral changes. Usually, however, there are alterations in consciousness, ranging from drowsiness to stupor or coma; various cranial nerve or long-tract signs may be present. Permanent sequelae include convulsive disorders, communicating hydrocephalus, subarachnoid block, mental retardation, and focal neurologic abnormalities.

Diagnosis is suspected in the presence of active TB or a history of TB or of exposure to it. The tuberculin test is usually positive, but confirmation is by CSF examination. When 4 serial spun sediment specimens are examined, the result is positive in > 75%. In most cases, the cell count is between 100 and 600/μL and is principally mononuclear. However, polymorphonuclear cells may predominate, especially early in the course of the illness. CSF protein concentration is usually elevated, and the CSF glucose content is typically less than half that in a simultaneously obtained blood sample. A low CSF glucose content and mononuclear pleocytosis are characteristic, but may also accompany fungal meningitis, meningeal involvement with carcinoma or lymphoma, and, rarely, partially treated bacterial meningitis. CSF culture is usually positive (even when cells are scant), but therapy must begin before these long-delayed results are available.

Treatment consists of maximum chemotherapy, usually with INH + SM or INH + RMP. Adjunctive therapy with corticosteroids (eg, prednisone 60 mg/day orally in 4 divided doses) is recommended for inflammatory complications. The symptoms of meningeal inflammation are an excellent guide to duration of corticosteroid therapy and rapidity of dosage tapering. Usually, initial dosage is given for about 2 wk and discontinued by 4 to 6 wk. Cranial CT scans often are abnormal, revealing round parenchymal lesions, basilar arachnoiditis, hydrocephalus, and vascular infarction when present.

Tuberculomas produce symptoms of mass brain lesions, usually without signs of infection, and are most often discovered at craniotomy for intracranial mass. Removal carries a risk of spread of infection and, accordingly, **chemotherapy** (INH + RMP for 18 mo) is always administered after resection. When a tuberculoma or (as is often the case) tuberculomas are discovered on CT scan and diagnosis seems secure because of the presence of associated active TB, medical therapy without excision often is superior to surgical treatment and chemotherapy. In areas in which tuberculomas are common, craniotomy and biopsy for diagnosis followed by medical therapy without excision has produced superior results.

Spinal cord TB may occur with or without clinical meningitis and may produce symptoms of a mass lesion, peripheral nerve involvement, or some combination.

Pleural Tuberculosis

Pleural TB occurs in at least 2 forms differing in pathogenesis and clinical import. **Primary serofibrinous pleurisy with effusion** may occur without discernible pulmonary parenchymal disease. It most often occurs soon after initial infection but may be seen any time during the course of pulmonary TB. The necrotizing effect of hypersensitivity causes a subpleural focus to rupture suddenly into the pleural space and produce an allergic effusion of mononuclear cells, protein, and pleural fluid enzyme (LDH) concentrations characteristic of exudates. Systemic symptoms may be marked or entirely lacking. A high degree of reactivity to tuberculin is commonly present. Pleural effusions with a mononuclear pleocytosis in a tuberculin-positive individual should be considered tuberculous unless proved otherwise. Tubercle bacilli are rarely seen on direct examination of the fluid; culture is positive in about ⅓ of the cases. Thoracoscopy or thoracotomy reveals many small tubercles studding the pleural surfaces. Pleu-

ral needle biopsy should be performed; histologic evidence of granuloma formation is present in most patients, stainable organisms will be seen in many, and culture of the biopsy specimen is often positive. **Treatment** is usually with INH alone. Although the pleural involvement is usually self-limited and resolves with no visible residua or, rarely, with some pleural fibrosis, most untreated patients develop progressive TB in the lung or elsewhere within 5 yr.

Tuberculous empyema is usually a chronic and generally progressive complication of an established focus of chronic pulmonary TB. The pleural fluid is frankly purulent and loculation is common. Bronchopleural fistula may be the initial cause or a complication of the empyema, and surgical drainage is usually required for resolution. When spontaneous pneumothorax is followed by a tuberculous empyema or bronchopleural fistula, surgical drainage is usually required in addition to chemotherapy as for established pulmonary TB.

Tuberculous Pericarditis

Tuberculous pericarditis is usually due to direct extension from involved mediastinal nodes, or, rarely, to hematogenous dissemination. It may begin acutely, with systemic symptoms and rapid development of compromised cardiac function, or it may be indolent, sometimes becoming apparent only as constrictive pericarditis. There may be no evidence of coexistent TB in the lungs or elsewhere, but the tuberculin test is usually positive.

The presence of a pericardial effusion or constrictive pericarditis can be readily established, but it is often difficult to establish etiology. The risk of morbidity is considerable, and some mortality is associated with pericardiocentesis; the fluid obtained rarely provides prompt evidence of TB, since culture reports not only are delayed but also are positive in less than half the cases. Pericardial biopsy by a subxiphoid approach is a safe, small operation that will provide tissue for histologic study and culture, but even then the reports may be false-negative.

Therapy requires a maximal chemotherapeutic regimen, usually INH + SM or INH + RMP. There is uncertainty concerning the proper use of corticosteroids and surgery in treatment; corticosteroid treatment combined with antimycobacterials may prevent chronic scarring and constriction in some cases, although this is not certain and is risky when etiologic diagnosis is in doubt. Pericardiocentesis may be necessary to relieve or prevent cardiac tamponade but is not without risk and should be performed in controlled situations, preferably a cardiac catheterization laboratory. Pericardiectomy is indicated for chronic constrictive or restrictive pericarditis. When pericardial effusion is associated with considerable hemodynamic compromise, excisional pericardial biopsy and drainage through a subxiphoid approach is usually sufficient.

Genitourinary Tuberculosis

Tuberculous pyelonephritis begins as a small cortical focus, seeded hematogenously, and progresses after the infection reaches the medulla. Local symptoms may be subtle or absent (though fever and weight loss may be present) and the patient often appears to be in surprisingly good health. Renal cavities may be seen on IVP as calyceal deformities with areas of reflux of the dye from the pelvis to the interstitial area. When the process is longstanding, renal calcification and pyelographic evidence of pyelonephritis may be the only signs. Symptoms of lower urinary tract involvement due to intracanalicular spread from the kidneys to the ureters, bladder, seminal vesicles, and even prostate are variable. Cystitis with pyuria but no culturable bacterial pathogens suggests tuberculous infection. Once the infection reaches the pelvis, inflammation of other genitourinary organs develops. Indolent, draining, perineal fistulas or an unexplained epididymal mass may be the first evidence of genitourinary TB.

Treatment consists of multiple-drug therapy, usually INH + SM, or possibly, in older or uremic individuals, INH + EMB. Frequent pyelograms are indicated during treatment to detect possible ureteral constriction. Nephrectomy is seldom indicated.

Tuberculous salpingo-oophoritis is probably acquired hematogenously. It may remain clinically silent or may present as acute or chronic pelvic inflammatory disease and may cause sterility. Laparotomy may be required for diagnosis. Culture of uterine scrapings or culture and biopsy of cervical lesions is occasionally diagnostic. Response to **chemotherapy** (INH + EMB) is usually prompt; surgery is unnecessary in most cases.

Tuberculosis of the Gastrointestinal Tract

TB may occur anywhere in the GI tract as superficial mucosal ulcerations caused by continuous surface contamination, or as hyperplastic involvement of a viscus wall presenting as an obstructing lesion. The latter may occur without obvious active pulmonary TB and is almost always discovered during surgery for a suspected carcinoma. Where bovine TB is common, contaminated milk may produce primary lesions in the GI tract, most frequently in the oropharynx. Superficial mucosal involvement of the **small and large intestine** may result in profound malabsorption, and TB of the **cecum**, probably the most frequent form of intestinal TB, may cause obstruction or bleeding with diarrhea. Unexplained perirectal ulcers or fistulas should be investigated by biopsy to see if they are tuberculous.

Treatment of gastrointestinal TB is with INH + EMB.

Tuberculous Peritonitis

Tuberculous peritonitis may be due to spread from adjacent lymph nodes, a GI focus, or tuberculous salpingo-oophoritis. Clinically, it ranges from an indolent illness with a doughy-feeling abdomen, local tenderness, and systemic signs of infection, to a process resembling acute bacterial peritonitis. The peritoneal exudate is usually mononuclear.

The main consideration in differential diagnosis is peritoneal carcinomatosis. Peritoneoscopy with biopsy under direct vision or a limited laparotomy are the best ways to make a diagnosis. Prompt response to antituberculous **chemotherapy** (INH + EMB) is expected.

Tuberculosis of the Adrenals

TB of the adrenals occurs occasionally as a result of hematogenous dissemination. The glands may be totally destroyed, causing adrenal cortical insufficiency (Addison's disease). **Treatment** is with INH + EMB and corticosteroid replacement therapy.

Tuberculosis of the Liver

TB of the liver is frequent in patients with both pulmonary and extrapulmonary TB, but it is seldom of clinical importance. Granulomas usually heal without scarring, but occasionally symptoms resembling obstructive or infiltrative liver disease (jaundice, hepatomegaly) may be seen. **Diagnosis** is made by liver biopsy, and a portion of the tissue obtained should be cultured. The serum alkaline phosphatase and 5′-nucleotidase tend to be elevated. **Treatment** is that of hematogenous TB; no specific treatment of the liver is indicated. Tuberculoma, tuberculous cholangitis, and tuberculous pylephlebitis are all extremely rare.

Tuberculosis of Bones and Joints

TB of a peripheral joint is usually a chronic, monarticular, purulent arthritis involving the hip, knee, elbow, or wrist. Diagnosis usually requires biopsy. Rarely, cystic areas of osteomyelitis due to TB are found in the long bones or digits. Response to **chemotherapy** (INH alone) is usually prompt. Immobilization and avoidance of weight bearing may be required to relieve pain.

Tuberculous spondylitis (Pott's disease) is a serious form of TB; neurologic damage frequently occurs. Symptoms are variable. Nagging local back pain may be present and may be referred to the anterior abdominal wall and mistaken for appendicitis or another abdominal disorder. A tender, prominent spinal process may develop because of anterior wedging of 2 vertebral bodies. A paraspinal abscess may extend and present as a mass in the groin or the supraclavicular space; symptoms may develop because tissue is dissected by the abscess. A paraspinal abscess that compresses the spinal cord or granulation tissue that intrudes on the anterior aspects of the cord may cause symptoms ranging from minor loss of bowel and urinary sphincter control to abrupt and irreversible paraplegia.

X-rays reveal anterior destruction of 2 or more adjacent vertebral bodies, loss of the intervertebral disk, anterior wedging of the vertebrae, and presence of a paraspinal abscess in some combination. Spondylitis due to staphylococci, gram-negative enterobacteria, and, less commonly, fungus infections such as blastomycosis may produce similar clinical and x-ray evidence. If active TB is present elsewhere in the body, a strong presumptive **diagnosis** of tuberculous spondylitis can be made. However, needle biopsy or surgical exploration of the lateral aspects of the vertebral column is often necessary to provide tissue for culture and histologic study.

Treatment with chemotherapy, usually INH + SM, and limited bed rest is usually satisfactory in neurologically uncomplicated disease. Posterior spinal fusion is safe and probably contributes to the firmness of healing (if instability of the spine is likely), but morbidity following prolonged immobilization is substantial. A major conflict surrounds the usual orthopedic recommendation that the spinal column be explored and debrided extensively along its anterior aspect. Serious worsening of the neurologic status of the patient has occurred and the procedure should be *avoided* if possible, except when mandated by progressive paralysis of legs or sphincters.

Tuberculous Lymphadenitis

Before the control of bovine TB, most tuberculous lymphadenitis occurred as **scrofula**, cervical lymphadenitis due to primary infection in the oropharyngeal lymphatic tissue. Scrofula, now rare in this context, is common in other mycobacterial infections. Currently, TB of the lymph nodes represents lymphohematogenous spread from a primary pulmonary focus. The process may be disseminated or localized. Diagnosis is usually made by excisional biopsy. Response to INH plus EMB is usually prompt and complete.

Tuberculosis of the Mouth, Middle Ear, Larynx, and Bronchial Tree

TB of the mouth is almost always associated with a pulmonary cavity, but an oral ulcer or a tooth socket that does not heal after dental extraction may suggest an otherwise silent pulmonary cavitary lesion. **Tuberculous otitis media**, presumably seeded via the eustachian tube, is characterized by persistent drainage and multiple perforations of the tympanic membrane. Profound conductive hearing loss and intracranial complications may occur. **Tuberculous involvement of the larynx** is rare and

usually due to infectious bronchial secretions, or, occasionally, to hematogenous spread. Severe pain may occur on swallowing and hoarseness is common. Laryngeal carcinoma must be excluded. **Bronchial TB** invariably accompanies cavitary pulmonary TB. The draining bronchi are superficially infected, granulation tissue forms, and, rarely, cicatrization and obstruction occur. Hemoptysis in pulmonary TB often originates from inflamed bronchial mucosa. Considerable bronchial distortion is almost always present following extensive pulmonary TB. Response of these types of TB to any INH-containing drug regimen is prompt and excellent.

OTHER MYCOBACTERIAL INFECTIONS RESEMBLING TUBERCULOSIS

Mycobacteria other than the tubercle and lepra bacillus cause disease in man pathologically and clinically similar to TB. The most important species include *M. intracellulare*, *M. kansasii*, *M. xenopi*, *M. scrofulaceum*, *M. marinum*, *M. fortuitum*, *M. chelonei*, and *M. ulcerans*. The organisms are INH-resistant, catalase-positive, and niacin-negative. They may cause chronic pulmonary disease and, rarely, (usually in immunologically compromised patients) disseminated disease in adults, cutaneous abscesses and granulomas, and, particularly in children, bone and joint involvement, lymphadenitis, and disseminated disease including meningitis. The frequency of fatal disseminated *M. intracellulare* infection in AIDS has recently been emphasized. Person-to-person transmission does not occur; the organisms presumably exist in the environment.

Pulmonary disease: *M. intracellulare*, *M. kansasii*, and *M. xenopi* are most frequently involved, but any of the nontuberculous mycobacteria can cause chronic pulmonary disease. The typical patient is male, white, and middle-aged and has underlying chronic pulmonary disease, most frequently with persisting cavitation. Systemic symptoms are uncommon. Usually such cases are stabile or slowly progressive, but progressive pulmonary insufficiency may develop. *M kansasii* and *M. xenopi* are fairly responsive to antituberculous chemotherapy. The other nontuberculous mycobacteria are much more drug-resistant and the efficacy of chemotherapy is far from clear. Pulmonary resection of infected cavities is rarely possible because of coexisting lung disease and has not been shown to be beneficial.

Cutaneous disease: "Swimming pool" granuloma is a protracted but self-limited superficial granulomatous ulcerating infection caused by *M. marinum* contracted from contaminated swimming pools and occasionally from home aquariums. The infection is pathologically similar to TB. Healing occurs spontaneously, though RMP may hasten healing. *M. ulcerans* causes an indolent, progressive, cutaneous and subcutaneous ulcerative process seen only in Africa and Australia. *M. chelonei abscessus* and *M. fortuitum* have caused injection abscesses that require drainage and sometimes excision.

Bone and joint involvement: Widespread lytic bone disease may rarely occur in children. Joint involvement, and, more rarely, cutaneous fistula formation may occur as complications. The infections are usually drug-resistant, but RMP, EMB, and SM may be tried.

Lymphadenitis: In the USA, these organisms probably cause infectious granulomatous lymphadenitis more frequently than does the tubercle bacillus. The portal of entry is probably the eye, pharynx, GI tract, or abraded skin. Many cases are due to local spread from the site of primary infection. Response to drug therapy varies; surgical excision is recommended when the process persists.

Disseminated disease is rare, occurring particularly in children and in immunologically compromised older individuals. It may resemble malignant reticuloendotheliosis,

except that the causative organisms are readily recovered. Meningitis may also occur, and, rarely, extensive miliary-like pulmonary involvement. Treatment with maximum chemotherapy (INH, SM, RMP, or another combination based on sensitivity testing) is usually tried, almost always with disappointing results.

Other processes: *M. chelonei* has been associated with microepidemics of sternal and mediastinal infection following cardiac surgery. *M. chelonei* and *M. fortuitum* have caused infection of the prosthetic devices used for augmentation mammoplasty.

LEPROSY

(Hansen's Disease)

A chronic infectious disease caused by Mycobacterium leprae, *an organism with suspected high infectivity but low pathogenicity and with a predilection for cooler regions—skin, mucous membranes, and peripheral nerves.*

Etiology and Distribution

M. leprae, an acid-fast bacillus, is the etiologic agent. Leprosy has a prolonged incubation period (from 1 to 30 yr) and progresses slowly. Transmission, most probably via infected nasal discharges, possibly occurs also by fomites and arthropods. Only about 5% of contacts acquire the disease; others appear to be immune. Leprosy is found mainly within a broad equatorial band that includes Southeast Asia, Africa, and South America. Of the estimated 12 to 20 million cases, about 2000 are in the continental USA. Endemic foci exist in Texas, Louisiana, and Hawaii. The disease is also seen in California, Florida, New York City, and other areas where immigrants from endemic areas have settled.

Types and Clinical Course

In all types, lesions of the skin and peripheral nerves dominate early clinical findings. Leprosy is classified on a spectrum reflecting degrees of host immunity (Ridley-Jopling classification).

Indeterminate leprosy is difficult to diagnose. The earliest skin lesion, usually a poorly defined, hypopigmented or erythematous macule 1 or 2 cm in diameter, generally shows nonspecific inflammation involving blood vessels, sweat and sebaceous glands, hair follicles, and cutaneous nerves. Organisms are few and may not be detected, but a presumptive diagnosis can be made if the cutaneous nerves are inflamed. The lesions tend to heal spontaneously, but may progress to any of the 3 more distinct types.

Tuberculoid leprosy (TT) is characterized by skin lesions that are localized initially to the skin or peripheral nerves. Lesions of the skin tend to be large, well-defined, single or few in number, anesthetic, and asymmetric. The inflammatory response is intense, with epithelioid and Langhans' cells resembling a tubercle surrounded by many lymphocytes. Bacilli are few and difficult to find. Caseation necrosis may destroy nerve bundles, with resulting focal paralysis. Resistance to the infection is high, and spontaneous recovery may occur; however, peripheral nerves can be destroyed.

Lepromatous leprosy (LL) is a generalized infection involving skin, oral, nasal, and upper respiratory mucous membrane, the anterior aspect of the eye, cutaneous and peripheral nerve trunks, the reticuloendothelial system, adrenal glands, and testes. The entire body surface may be involved so diffusely that no distinct lesion is identifiable and there is a continuous, high-grade leprosy bacillemia. When individually discernible, the numerous small skin lesions have poorly defined margins. Macules are most common; papules, nodules, or plaques also occur. Numerous bacilli are easily found in tissue specimens. Patient resistance to *M. leprae* is low, and untreated disease is progressive.

Borderline (dimorphous) leprosy has clinical and pathologic features of both TT and LL "polar" types in various combinations, and subclassification, from borderline-tuberculoid **(BT)** to mid-borderline **(BB)**, to borderline-lepromatous **(BL)**, depends on the relative numbers of bacilli, lymphocytes, epithelioid cells, and macrophages. *M. leprae* usually are numerous. Borderline forms of leprosy are unstable and may regress ("reversal reaction") toward the TT form or progress ("downgrading reaction") toward the LL form, depending on the effects of treatment and shifts in the patient's immunologic status.

Nerve lesions: In all stages of all forms of leprosy, *M. leprae* invades peripheral nerves, particularly the terminal cutaneous branches (producing anesthesia of a skin lesion) or the nerve trunk (producing anesthesia along its cutaneous innervation). Advanced disease results in "glove and stocking" anesthesia, or a pattern consistent with "mononeuritis multiplex." Paralysis and deformity follow sensory loss. Facial paralysis usually is limited to lagophthalmos, which may end in blindness from trauma and infection involving the insensitive cornea. Claw-hand, foot-drop, and claw-toe deformities are common and may be accompanied by ulcers and secondary infection. Insensitivity leads to neglected injuries (eg, destruction of the fingers, resulting in a "mitten hand"); about 25% of patients have some disfigurement and disabling deformity.

In LL, peripheral nerves may be enlarged, yet the patient may show little clinical change or deformity. Sensory loss may be widespread, but motor impairment develops insidiously over several years. Reflexes are not affected. Impairment of touch and temperature sensation occurs early, whereas deep-pain perception and proprioception are lost later. In TT, caseation necrosis may destroy segments or entire fascicles of the nerve and produce more sudden paralysis. Painful neuritides usually are associated with "acute reaction" episodes.

Acute reactions: Reversal reactions, seen in all but pure LL, apparently result from spontaneous increases in patients' cell-mediated immunity to *M. leprae*. In a reversal, eg, from borderline toward TT, the lesions become erythematous and edematous and may progress to necrosis and ulceration. **Erythema nodosum leprosum (ENL) reactions,** by contrast, probably are mediated by humoral factors and resemble the Arthus phenomenon (see TYPE III HYPERSENSITIVITY REACTIONS in Ch. 20). ENL occurs in LL patients and in some BL cases with dominant LL features. Multiple painful erythematous nodules develop that may form pustules or progress to ulceration and necrosis. ENL often is accompanied by fever and sometimes by neuritis, lymphadenopathy, arthritis, iridocyclitis, orchitis, glomerulonephritis, and leukocytosis.

Other manifestations (mainly in progressive BL and LL types): Nasal stuffiness and epistaxis occur early; later, ulceration and necrosis destroy supporting cartilages, causing nasal deformity and collapse. Earlobe enlargement and loss of eyebrows are common. Isolated lesions of the lip, tongue, and palate must be differentiated from malignancy.

Leprosy affects the eyes in several ways: by direct infection, acute reaction, or damage of the zygomatic branch of the facial nerve, which leads to paralysis of the orbicularis oculi muscle. Conjunctivitis, keratitis, corneal ulceration, iridocyclitis, anterior choroiditis, and glaucoma may occur and, if untreated, may lead to blindness.

Orchitis, often leading to atrophy, and gynecomastia occur in advanced LL. Peripheral lymph nodes enlarge and may develop abscesses. In advanced LL, the spleen, bone marrow, liver, and kidney are involved and amyloidosis occasionally develops; death may then be due to renal failure.

Diagnosis

Leprosy may mimic other diseases involving the skin and peripheral nerves. The

diagnosis is established by biopsy. Skin smears indicate the extent and progress of the disease. The **lepromin test** (intradermal injection of autoclaved bacilli from human lepromas) usually is positive in TT and negative in LL polar types. An early positive lepromin reaction in tuberculin-negative *children* (it is positive in nearly all normal adults) is considered diagnostic. (Lepromin is not available commercially.) Recent studies based on detection of *M. leprae*-specific phenolic glycolipid I give rise to the possibility of a serodiagnostic test for leprosy in the forseeable future.

Prophylaxis and Treatment

Control requires active case-finding and early treatment. A patient controlled by therapy poses no public health problem. Results of prophylaxis with BCG vaccine or dapsone in highly endemic areas have been inconclusive. In the USA, contacts without disease should be examined every 6 to 12 mo. Careful, long-term follow-up of exposed children is essential. Cure by immediate active therapy can be expected if a lesion is found early.

The 4 principal drugs for treating leprosy are dapsone (4,4′-diaminodiphenyl sulfone, DDS), rifampin, clofazimine, and ethionamide.

Dapsone inhibits microbial folate synthesis and is weakly bactericidal. Side effects from doses of 100 mg/day or less are infrequent. Mild anemia is common. Since patients with G6PD deficiency may experience more severe hemolysis, they should be given antileprosy drugs not related to the sulfones. Agranulocytosis is a potentially serious, but rare, complication. (Peripheral neuropathy, reported in other diseases, is attributed to doses of dapsone considerably larger than those used in leprosy.) **Clofazimine,** a weakly bactericidal phenazine dye derivative, also can suppress leprosy reactions. The drug produces relatively few side effects in most patients, but does cause skin pigmentation that light-complexioned patients may find objectionable. Especially with doses > 100 mg/day, GI distress is a major problem in some patients. **Rifampin** is strongly bactericidal for *M. leprae*. It sometimes causes chills, fever, headache, myalgias, thrombocytopenia, or renal failure; its principal drawback, especially in underdeveloped countries, is cost. Rifampin also may produce reddish discoloration of body secretions. **Ethionamide** is weakly bactericidal; its principal toxicities are GI and hepatic. Hepatotoxicity may be augmented by concomitant rifampin therapy.

Leprosy therapy is complicated by the increasing prevalence of sulfone-resistant *M. leprae*. Hence, dapsone monotherapy is a calculated risk and is no longer considered ideal for any form of the disease. Using drug combinations may reduce the incidence of secondary resistance to dapsone and other drugs. It is hoped that shorter courses of therapy may prove efficacious, as they have in multidrug TB regimens.

In vitro methods do not measure the susceptibility of *M. leprae* to antimicrobial agents. Footpads of mice are inoculated with biopsy-derived bacilli, then bacillary survival is measured to determine the effectiveness of the dosage of antimicrobials added to the diet. Footpad-testing facilities are available in the USA (eg, National Hansen's Disease Center; Carville, Louisiana). In countries where they are not available and accurate susceptibility information cannot be obtained, multidrug regimens reduce the possibility that a resistant organism will go untreated. When animal-testing facilities are available, biopsy material should be submitted for analysis, and therapy altered appropriately when test results become available 6 to 9 mo later.

TABLE 8–5 summarizes alternative regimens for treating leprosy. WHO recommendations are appropriate where resources are limited and costs of drugs and patient follow-up are major problems. The other listed regimens should be used in developed countries.

Most patients will be treated as though infected with dapsone-sensitive *M. leprae*. Drug resistance should be suspected if the disease progresses or relapses, if bacilli are

TABLE 8–5. LEPROSY TREATMENT REGIMENS

Leprosy Type	*Patients with Dapsone-Sensitive* M. leprae	*Patients with Dapsone-Resistant* M. Leprae	*WHO Study Group Recommendation*
	Regimen	Regimen	Regimen
Indeterminate and TT	Dapsone 100 mg/day* and rifampin 600 mg/day‡	Clofazimine 50–100 mg/day*† and rifampin 600 mg/day‡	Dapsone 100 mg/day‡ and rifampin 600 mg/mo‡§
BT	Dapsone 100 mg/day** and rifampin 600 mg/day‡	Clofazimine 50–100 mg/day** and rifampin 600 mg/day‡	Dapsone 100 mg/day‡ and rifampin 600 mg/mo‡§
BB	Dapsone 100 mg/day†† and rifampin 600 mg/day‡‡ ± clofazimine 50–100 mg/day† ± ethionamide 250–500 mg/day	Clofazimine 50–100 mg/day†† and rifampin 600 mg/day‡‡ ± ethionamide 250–500 mg/day *or* rifampin + ethionamide††	Dapsone 100 mg/day‡‡ and rifampin 600 mg/mo§‡‡ and clofazimine* 50 mg/day‡‡ and clofazimine 300 mg/mo§‡‡
BL or LL	Dapsone 100 mg/day§§ and rifampin 600 mg/day‡‡, ± clofazimine 50–100 mg/day ± ethionamide 250–500 mg/day	Clofazimine 50–100 mg/day§§ and rifampin 600 mg/day‡‡ ± ethionamide 250–500 mg/day *or* rifampin + ethionamide§§	Dapsone 100 mg/day‡‡ and rifampin 600 mg/mo§‡‡ and clofazimine 50 mg/day‡‡ and clofazimine 300 mg/mo§‡‡

Abbreviations: TT, tuberculoid type; BT, borderline tuberculoid; BB, mid-borderline; BL, borderline lepromatus; LL, lepromatous.

* Until 3 yr beyond negativity
† Clofazimine is available from the National Hansen's Disease Center, Carville, LA.
‡ For at least 6 mo
§ Supervised
** Until 5 yr beyond negativity
†† Until 10 yr beyond negativity
‡‡ For at least 2 yr
§§ For life

(Modified from WHO Study Group, Chemotherapy of Leprosy for Control Programmes, 1982, *Technical Report Series* No. 675, Geneva. Used with permission.)

found in new lesions, or if there is no response to treatment in 3 to 6 mo. Concern about drug resistance should be confirmed with mouse-footpad drug sensitivity studies before therapy is changed.

Although paucibacillary cases (eg, indeterminate, TT, and perhaps BT) may heal spontaneously, every active case should be treated so that cure can be expected. In most cases of multibacillary disease (BB, BL, or LL), the disease may be cured or arrested. Medication must be taken regularly, and in adequate dosages, since small doses or interrupted therapy may produce drug-resistant *M. leprae*, with exacerbation or relapse of the disease, even after several years of inactivity. Therapy should *not* be interrupted during reactional states.

Mild **reactional states** are treated with bed rest, analgesics, and sedatives. More severe reactions may be managed with bed rest and corticosteroids, thalidomide, or clofazimine.

Prednisone 30 to 60 mg/day is given when a serious complication, such as rapid onset of paralysis, necessitates immediate treatment. After the desired response, the dosage is cut gradually. If therapy is required for more than several months, prednisone should be replaced by thalidomide or clofazimine.

Thalidomide, an experimental drug in the USA but available through the National Hansen's Disease Center, Carville, Louisiana, is the treatment of choice for ENL reactions. The initial dose of 300 mg/day may be continued for several months. Because of teratogenicity, it is **contraindicated** in women of childbearing age. The drug does not affect the underlying disease.

Clofazimine is slow-acting and seldom given initially to control acute reaction. Usually it supplements antileprosy drugs prescribed for patients with chronic recurring ENL. The initial dosage, 300 mg/day, may be decreased to a minimum of 100 mg 3 times/wk in case of severe GI complaints. Treatment becomes less effective when doses are given at intervals of a week or more. Clofazamine may be the only alternative to prolonged high-dose corticosteroid therapy for severe reactions.

Moderate reactions are sometimes treated with other drugs, including potassium antimony tartrate (tartar emetic), stibophen, and chloroquine.

DDS or other specific therapy for the disease must be continued during episodes of acute reaction, or the disease deteriorates and becomes chronic; therapy is discontinued only if thalidomide or clofazimine fails to control the acute reaction or the patient experiences serious steroid side effects.

Immediate recognition and treatment of eye **problems** are essential. ENL iridocyclitis is an emergency. The pupil is dilated, using atropine eyedrops or ointment 1% q 6 h for 3 days and then once daily until the reaction subsides. Hydrocortisone drops or ointment 1.5% is also applied q 4 h for the first 3 days, then bid until the inflammation subsides. These drugs are given in addition to the treatment for the ENL reaction. Lagophthalmos is another serious complication, especially when associated with corneal anesthesia. Corneal dryness is treated with commercial artificial teardrops or ophthalmic mucin substitutes. Physiotherapeutic measures are instituted to strengthen weakened eyelid muscles; if no improvement follows, surgery is indicated. Glaucoma and cataracts may follow iridocyclitis. In general, the patient should be referred to an ophthalmologist for management of these problems.

Supportive care is important to protect insensitive eyes, hands, and feet from repeated infections and injuries that lead to blindness and mutilation. Deformities may be corrected surgically to improve function. Shoes can be built to conform to residual deformity and bear weight evenly. The patient must understand his problems and their potential dangers and observe early changes. Physicians at the National Hansen's Disease Center in Carville, Louisiana, are always available to the medical profession for consultation on leprosy-related matters.

CAUSED BY SPIROCHETES

SYPHILIS

(See Ch. 14)

ENDEMIC TREPONEMATOSES

(Endemic Syphilis, Yaws, and Pinta)

Chronic nonvenereal spirochetal infections, spread by body contact. Treponema pallidum II **(endemic syphilis),** *T. pertenue* **(yaws),** and *T. carateum* **(pinta)** are morphologically and serologically indistinguishable from *T. pallidum* **(syphilis).**

Endemic syphilis is mainly found in arid countries of the eastern Mediterranean and West (Sahel) Africa; yaws, in humid equatorial countries; and pinta, among the Indians of Mexico, Central America, and northern South America.

Clinical Course

Endemic syphilis (nonvenereal syphilis, bejel) begins in childhood as a mucous patch, usually on the buccal mucosa, followed by papulosquamous and erosive papular lesions of the trunk and extremities. Periostitis of the bones of the legs is common. Gummatous lesions of the nose and soft palate develop in later stages.

Yaws (frambesia) begins as a granulomatous or macular lesion at the inoculation site, usually on the legs, after an incubation period of several weeks. The lesion heals but is followed by a generalized eruption of soft granulomas of the face, extremities, and buttocks, often at mucocutaneous junctions. These granulomas heal slowly and may relapse. Keratotic lesions may develop on the soles and cause painful ulcerations ("crab" yaws). Destructive lesions may develop later, including periostitis (particularly of the tibia), proliferative exostoses of the nasal portion of the maxillary bone **(goundou),** juxta-articular nodules, gummatous skin lesions, and, ultimately, mutilating facial ulcers, particularly around the nose **(gangosa).**

Pinta begins at the inoculation site as small papules that progress to erythematous plaques in several months. Erythematous, squamous patches develop later, mainly on the extremities, face, and neck. After several years, slate-blue patches develop, usually symmetrically and generally on the face and extremities and over bony prominences; these later become depigmented, resembling vitiligo. Hyperkeratosis may occur on the soles and palms.

Diagnosis and Treatment

Diagnosis is made from the typical appearance of lesions in persons from endemic areas. The Venereal Disease Research Laboratory **(VDRL)** and fluorescent treponemal antibody absorption **(FTA-ABS)** tests are positive but do not distinguish these diseases from venereal syphilis. Early lesions are often darkfield-positive for spirochetes indistinguishable from *T. pallidum.*

In each disease, one IM injection of 1.2 million u. of benzathine penicillin G produces healing, with rapid disappearance of the spirochetes. Children < 100 lb should receive 600,000 u. Destructive lesions leave a scar. Public health control of each disease is based on active case finding and the prophylactic treatment of family and childhood contacts with benzathine penicillin.

RELAPSING FEVER

(Tick, Recurrent, or Famine Fever)

An acute infectious disease caused by several species of spirochetes, transmitted by lice or ticks, and characterized by recurrent febrile paroxysms lasting 3 to 5 days, separated by intervals of apparent recovery.

Etiology and Epidemiology

Relapsing fever is the term applied to recurrent fevers, clinically similar but etiologically distinct, caused by different *Borrelia* spirochetes. The insect vector may be the soft ticks of the genus *Ornithodoros* or the body louse, depending on geographic location. The louse-borne relapsing fevers are endemic only in parts of Africa and South America; the tick-borne, in the Americas, Africa, Asia, and Europe. In the USA, the disease is generally confined to the western states, where occurrence is highest between May and September.

The various species of *Borrelia* are morphologically similar. They are delicate, threadlike organisms 8 to 30 μ long, with pointed ends and 4 to 10 large, irregular coils. They appear in the blood during a paroxysm, and can be found in internal organs, especially the spleen and brain.

The louse is infected by feeding on a patient during the febrile stage. The spirochetes are not transmitted directly to man, but are released and enter abraded skin or bites when the louse is crushed. Ticks acquire the spirochetes from rodents acting as reservoirs, and infect man when spirochetes in the tick's saliva or coxal fluid (excreta) enter the skin as the tick bites. Congenital borreliosis has also been reported.

Symptoms, Signs, and Prognosis

Patients who have been exposed to *Borrelia* while visiting in an endemic area may become symptomatic after leaving the area, since the incubation period ranges from 3 to 11 days (median, 6 days). Sudden chills usher in the disease, followed by high fever, tachycardia, severe headache, vomiting, muscle and joint pain, and often delirium. An erythematous macular or purpuric rash may appear early over the trunk and extremities; conjunctival, subcutaneous or submucous hemorrhages may be present. Mild polymorphonuclear leukocytosis may occur. Late in the course of the fever, jaundice, hepatomegaly, splenomegaly, myocarditis, and cardiac failure may appear, especially in cases of louse-borne disease. Fever remains high for 3 to 5 days, then clears abruptly by crisis. The duration of illness ranges from 1 to 54 days (median, 18 days).

The patient is usually asymptomatic for several days to a week or more; relapse, related to the cyclic development of the parasites, occurs with a sudden return of fever and, often, arthralgia and all the former symptoms and signs. Jaundice is more common during relapse. The illness clears as before, but from 2 to 10 similar paroxysms may follow at intervals of 1 to 2 wk. The paroxysms become progressively less severe, and recovery eventually occurs as the patient develops immunity.

The mortality rate is generally low (0 to 5%) but may be considerably higher in very young, old, malnourished, or debilitated persons, or during epidemics of louse-borne fever.

Complications can include abortion, ophthalmitis, exacerbation of asthma, and erythema multiforme. Iritis or iridocyclitis and CNS involvement can occur.

Diagnosis

Relapsing fevers may be confused with Lyme arthritis, malaria, dengue, yellow fever, leptospirosis, typhus, influenza, and the enteric fevers. The diagnosis is suggested by the recurrent fever and confirmed by the appearance of spirochetes in the blood during a paroxysm. Darkfield examination or thick and thin Wright- or Giemsa-stained blood smears will disclose the spirochetes (acridine orange stain for examination of blood or tissue is more sensitive than Wright-Giemsa peripheral blood smears). Because the tick feeds transiently and painlessly at night, most patients do not give a history of tick bite. In tick-borne infection, intraperitoneal injection of the patient's blood into a mouse or rat produces large numbers of spirochetes in the animal's tail blood within 3 to 5 days.

Prophylaxis

Dusting undergarments and inner surfaces of clothing with DDT, malathion, or lindane powders will protect against relapsing fever resulting from infestations of body lice. Tick-borne infections are more difficult to prevent because of the inadequacy of insect control measures (see ROCKY MOUNTAIN SPOTTED FEVER in Ch. 10).

Treatment

Therapy should be started early in the paroxysm or during the afebrile stage, but should be avoided near the end of a paroxysm because of the danger of a **Herxheimer reaction** (rigors, fever, and a rise in BP, followed by a fall in BP to near shock levels), which is regularly seen and occasionally fatal in louse-borne infection. Personnel and equipment should be available in the event of the reaction. The severity of the Herxheimer reaction may be lessened in tick-borne relapsing fever by giving acetaminophen 0.65 gm orally 2 h before and 2 h after the first dose of tetracycline or erythromycin. In tick-borne fever, tetracycline or erythromycin 0.5 gm orally q 6 h is given for 5 to 10 days; a single 0.5-gm oral dose of either drug cures louse-borne fever. Erythromycin estolate should be given in proportionately reduced doses in children < 8 yr of age. When vomiting or severe disease precludes oral administration, tetracycline 500 mg in 100 or 500 mL of saline may be given IV once or twice/day.

Dehydration and electrolyte imbalance should be corrected with parenteral fluids. Codeine 30 to 60 mg orally q 4 to 6 h may be used to relieve severe headache. Nausea and vomiting should be treated with dimenhydrinate 50 to 100 mg orally or rectally (or 50 mg IM) q 4 h, or with prochlorperazine 5 to 10 mg orally or IM 1 to 4 times/day. If heart failure occurs, specific therapy is indicated (see Ch. 27).

LEPTOSPIROSIS

(Weil's Disease or Syndrome; Infectious [Spirochetal] Jaundice; Canicola Fever)

An inclusive term for all infections due to an organism of the genus Leptospira, *regardless of serotype.* About 170 serotypes have been identified. A single serotype may cause various clinical features, or a single syndrome (eg, aseptic meningitis) may be caused by multiple serotypes.

Epidemiology

Leptospirosis, a zoonosis, occurs in several domestic and wild animal hosts and varies from inapparent illness to fatal disease. A carrier state exists in which animals shed leptospires in their urine for months. Human infections occur by direct contact with an infected animal's urine or tissue, or indirectly by contact with contaminated water or soil. Abraded skin and exposed mucous membranes (conjunctival, nasal, oral) are the usual portals of entry in man. Infection occurs at any age. At least 75% of those infected are males. Leptospirosis can be an occupational disease (eg, of farmers or sewer and abattoir workers), but most patients are exposed incidentally during recreational activities. Dogs, immersion (eg, swimming) in contaminated water, and rats are the most common probable sources. The 40 to 100 cases reported annually in the USA occur mainly in late summer and early autumn. Because of lack of distinctive clinical features, probably many cases are not diagnosed and reported.

Clinical Features

The incubation period ranges from 2 to 20 (usually 7 to 13) days. The disease is characteristically biphasic. The **leptospiremic phase** is abrupt in onset, with headache, severe muscular aches, chills, and fever. Conjunctival suffusion is characteristic, usually appearing on the 3rd or 4th day. Spleno-and hepatomegaly are uncommon. This phase lasts 4 to 9 days, with recurrent chills and fever that often spikes to > 39 C (102 F). Defervescence follows; then, on the 6th to 12th day of illness, the **second** or

"immune" phase occurs, correlating with appearance of antibodies in the serum. Fever and earlier symptoms recur and meningismus may develop. CSF examination after the 7th day discloses pleocytosis in at least 50% of the patients. Iridocyclitis, optic neuritis, and peripheral neuropathy occur infrequently. If acquired during pregnancy, leptospirosis may cause abortion even during the convalescent period.

Weil's syndrome is a form of severe leptospirosis with jaundice and, usually, azotemia, hemorrhages, anemia, disturbances in consciousness, and continued fever. Onset is similar to that of less severe forms; the signs of hepatocellular and renal dysfunction appear from the 3rd to 6th day. Renal abnormalities include proteinuria, pyuria, hematuria, and azotemia. Hemorrhagic manifestations are due to capillary injury. Thrombocytopenia may occur. Hepatic damage is minimal, and complete healing occurs.

Aseptic meningitis may occur with any serotype. The CSF cell count is between 10 and 1000/μL (usually < 500), with predominantly mononuclear cells. CSF sugar is normal; protein is < 100 mg/dL. Most patients with aseptic meningitis do not manifest significant disease of liver and kidney.

Mortality is nil in anicteric patients. With occurrence of jaundice, the mortality rate is about 15%; in patients over 60, the rate is doubled.

Laboratory Findings

The WBC count is normal or slightly elevated in most cases but may reach 50,000 in severely ill, icteric patients. Leukocytosis > 15,000 suggests liver involvement. There are usually > 70% neutrophils, a finding that may help to differentiate leptospirosis from viral illnesses. In jaundiced patients, intravascular hemolysis may cause marked anemia. Serum bilirubin, usually < 20 mg/dL, may reach 40 mg/dL in severe infection; BUN is usually < 100 mg/dL. These findings indicate liver and renal involvement.

Investigations include the search, toward the end of the 1st wk, for spirochetes in the blood and assay for antibodies in serum. Blood is drawn for staining, darkfield examination for spirochetes, culture, guinea pig inoculation, and acute-phase serologic antibodies. Leptospires may be isolated from the blood, urine, or CSF during the first phase by inoculation onto Fletcher's medium. After the 1st wk, *Leptospira* may be found in the urine and guinea pig inoculation may be positive. Serologic technics, including slide and microscopic agglutination tests and an indirect fluorescent antibody method, may be used during this second phase.

Diagnosis

Meningitis or meningoencephalitis, influenza, hepatitis, acute cholecystitis, and renal failure must be included in the differential diagnosis. With the enteroviruses, which commonly cause aseptic meningitis, there is usually no history suggesting biphasic illness. Such a history favors leptospirosis or perhaps cytomegalovirus infections. Diagnosis is established by laboratory identification of the organism (see above).

Prophylaxis and Treatment

In chemoprophylactic trials conducted during recent outbreaks in military personnel who were training in Panama, doxycycline 100 mg/day, if continued during the period of exposure, prevented disease. Antibiotics such as penicillin, streptomycin, the tetracyclines, chloramphenicol, and erythromycin are effective in experimental infections, but their value in man is uncertain. They are not beneficial if given later than 4 days after onset of the disease. In severe illness, penicillin G 6 to 12 million u./day IM or IV or tetracycline 2 gm/day orally or IV is often recommended. Fluid and electro-

lyte therapy are necessary for azotemia or jaundice. Isolation is not required, but care is needed in disposing of urine.

RAT-BITE FEVER

Rat-bite fever represents 2 clinically similar but etiologically distinct diseases that may follow a rodent bite. **Streptobacillary rat-bite fever,** caused by the pleomorphic gram-negative bacillus *Streptobacillus moniliformis*, is more common in the USA than **spirillary rat-bite fever,** caused by *Spirillum minus*. Rat-bite fever follows up to 10% of rat bites. It is mainly a disease of ghetto dwellers and the socially deprived, and it is also a hazard to biomedical laboratory personnel.

Streptobacillary Rat-Bite Fever

S. moniliformis is present in the oropharynx of healthy rats. Epidemics have been associated with ingestion of unpasteurized, contaminated milk **(Haverhill fever),** but infection is usually a consequence of a bite by a wild rat or mouse; weasels and other rodents have also been implicated. Patients may be bitten in their sleep. There have been < 20 cases reported in the USA over the past decade, but in England in 1983 an epidemic associated with ingestion of raw milk at a boarding school involved 208 school children.

The primary wound usually heals promptly, but after an incubation period of 1 to 22 (usually < 10) days, the patient abruptly develops a viral-like syndrome with chills, fever, vomiting, headache, and back and joint pains. The WBC count ranges between 6,000 and 30,000. A morbilliform, petechial rash appears in about 3 days on the hands and feet of most patients. Polyarthralgia or arthritis, usually affecting the large joints asymmetrically, develops in many patients within a week and may persist for several days or for months if untreated. Bacterial endocarditis and abscesses in the brain or other tissues are rare but serious complications. Patients have presented with infected pericardial effusion and infected amniotic fluid.

Streptobacillary rat-bite fever usually can be differentiated on clinical grounds from spirillary rat-bite fever, but can be confused with Rocky Mountain spotted fever, infection with Coxsackie B virus, and meningococcemia. **Diagnosis** is confirmed by culturing the organism from blood or joint fluid. Agglutinins develop during the 2nd or 3rd wk and are diagnostically important if the titer increases.

Treatment consists of either procaine penicillin G 1.2 million u./day IM or penicillin V 2 gm/day orally for 7 to 10 days. Erythromycin 2 gm/day orally may be an alternative in cases of penicillin hypersensitivity.

Spirillary Rat-Bite Fever (Sodoku)

Spirillum minus infection is acquired through a rat or, occasionally, a mouse bite. The wound usually heals promptly, but inflammation recurs at the site after an incubation period of 4 to 28 (usually > 10) days, accompanied by a relapsing fever and regional lymphadenitis. The WBC count ranges between 5,000 and 30,000. VDRL tests are false-positive in half the patients. A roseolar-urticarial rash sometimes develops, but is less prominent than the streptobacillary rash. Systemic symptoms commonly accompany the fever. Arthritis is rare. In untreated patients, 2-to 4-day cycles of fever usually recur for 4 to 8 wk but, rarely, febrile episodes recur for > 1 yr.

Diagnosis is made by demonstration of the spirillum in blood smears or tissue from the lesions or lymph nodes, or by Giemsa stain or darkfield examination of blood from inoculated mice. If the physician is unaware of previous rat bite in cases with long incubation periods, he may easily confuse the disease with malaria, meningococcemia, or *Borrelia recurrentis* infection, all of which are characterized by relapsing fever.

Treatment: Procaine penicillin G 1.2 million u./day IM or, for patients allergic to penicillin, tetracycline 2 gm/day orally is given for 7 days.

PRESUMPTIVE BACTERIAL DISEASES

CAT-SCRATCH DISEASE

A zoonotic infection characterized by regional lymphadenitis that follows a skin papule at the site of a cat scratch.

Etiology

Although an etiologic agent has not been cultured, small gram-negative pleomorphic bacilli have been demonstrated in sections of lymph nodes and the primary papules in 3/4 of a group of patients meeting the clinical criteria for cat-scratch disease. The organisms can be demonstrated with Warthin-Starry silver impregnation stain or with Brown-Hopp's tissue Gram stain. Several animals are thought to be carriers, particularly cats, because > 90% of cases follow cat scratches.

Symptoms and Signs

A few days after a minor scratch, a papule or pustule develops at the site in 50 to 90% of patients. The typical primary lesion is an erythematous, crusted papule (rarely, a pustule), 2 to 6 mm in diameter. Regional lymphadenopathy develops within 2 wk, usually unilaterally and in relation to the scratch site (ie, axillary, epitrochlear, submandibular, cervical, or inguinal). The nodes are initially firm and tender, but later become fluctuant and may drain with fistula formation. Pathologic examination of involved nodes shows hyperplasia, a granulomatous response, and then suppurative necrosis and microabscess formation. The bacilli are in the walls of capillaries and in macrophages. Fever, malaise, headache, and anorexia accompany the lymphadenopathy. Erythema nodosum, thrombocytopenic purpura, Parinaud's syndrome (conjunctivitis associated with palpable preauricular lymph nodes), and osteolytic lesions occur but are uncommon. Encephalitis is a rare but severe complication, usually occurring one or more weeks after onset. The skin lesion and lymphadenopathy will subside spontaneously within 2 to 5 mo. Complete recovery is usual.

Diagnosis, Treatment, and Prognosis

Diagnostic criteria include persistent (> 3 wk) regional lymphadenopathy, a history of cat contact, characteristic histopathology, negative studies for other common causes of lymphadenitis, and a positive intradermal skin test with cat-scratch antigen (not commercially available).

Therapy with tetracycline may shorten the course. Surgical excision may be necessary, especially if fistulas drain. **Prognosis** is excellent.

---

9. SYSTEMIC FUNGAL DISEASES

(Systemic Mycoses)

The major systemic mycoses are discussed in this chapter. Dermatophytoses and other skin infections can be found in Ch. 232; pulmonary disorders caused by hypersensitivity to fungi are discussed in Ch. 43; fungal diseases affecting the GU system can be found in Ch. 153.

General Diagnostic Principles

Several considerations are important in the diagnosis of the systemic mycoses.

1. Many of the causative fungi are "opportunists," and are not usually pathogenic unless they enter a compromised host. (See also Ch. 7.) Opportunistic fungal infections are particularly apt to occur and should be anticipated in patients after ionizing (x-)

irradiation and during therapy with corticosteroids, immunosuppressives, or antimetabolites; they also tend to occur in patients with azotemia, diabetes mellitus, bronchiectasis, emphysema, TB, Hodgkin's disease or other lymphoma, leukemia, AIDS, or burns. Candidiasis, aspergillosis, phycomycosis, nocardiosis, and cryptococcosis are typical opportunistic infections.

2. Fungal diseases occurring as primary infections may have a typical geographic distribution. For example, in the USA, coccidioidomycosis is virtually confined to the Southwest, while histoplasmosis occurs in the East and Midwest, especially in the Ohio and Mississippi River valleys. Blastomycosis is restricted to North America and Africa; paracoccidioidomycosis, often called South American blastomycosis, is confined to that continent. However, travelers can develop a symptomatic infection some time after returning from such endemic areas.

3. The major clinical characteristic of virtually every systemic mycosis is its chronic course. Septicemia or acute pneumonia is rare. Lung lesions develop slowly. Months or years may elapse before medical attention is sought or a diagnosis is made.

4. Symptoms are rarely intense, but fever, chills, night sweats, anorexia, weight loss, malaise, and depression may all be present.

5. When a fungus disseminates from a primary focus in the lung, the manifestations may be characteristic. For example, cryptococcosis usually appears as meningitis, progressive disseminated histoplasmosis as hepatic disease, and blastomycosis as a skin lesion.

6. Delayed cutaneous hypersensitivity and serologic tests are available for only 3 or 4 of the infections discussed in this chapter. Even in these, the tests may become positive either so late (eg, coccidioidomycosis) or so infrequently (eg, blastomycosis) that they are of no diagnostic value in the acutely ill patient.

7. The diagnosis is usually confirmed by isolating the causative fungus from sputum, bone marrow, urine, blood, or CSF, or from lymph node, liver, or lung biopsy. When the fungus is a commensal of humans or is prevalent in their environment (eg, *Candida*, *Aspergillus*), it is difficult to interpret its isolation from such specimens as sputum, and confirmation of tissue invasion is necessary to attribute an etiologic role to it.

8. In contrast to viral and bacterial diseases, fungal infections can be diagnosed histopathologically with a high degree of reliability. It is the distinctive fungal morphology, not the tissue reaction, that permits specific etiologic identification.

9. Even when the microorganism has been demonstrated histopathologically in tissues, the activity of the disease must be established before treatment is begun. Culture of the causative microorganism or such clinical and laboratory findings as fever, leukocytosis, elevated ESR, abnormal liver function, worsening of chest film findings, or elevated serum globulins are helpful as indications for therapy.

General Therapeutic Principles

General medical care, surgery, and chemotherapy constitute modes of treatment for systemic fungus infections. **Ketoconazole,** a new antifungal imidazole derivative, appears to have major advantages: oral dosage and broad antifungal activity with minimal adverse effects; but testosterone and adrenalcorticoid synthesis may be blocked, usually transiently, and serious hepatotoxicity may occur. From 200 to 400 mg orally once a day with a meal may be given for prolonged periods to establish and maintain clinical remission or to prevent reinfection.

Amphotericin B, a fungicidal and fungistatic antibiotic, is covered in detail here because it is used in many systemic mycoses. Indications and directions for other therapeutic measures are given below in the discussions of specific mycoses. Amphotericin B has reversed the prognosis of many fungal infections. An initial IV dose of 0.1 mg/kg/day is increased by 0.05 to 0.10 mg/kg every day until 1.0 mg/kg (but not exceeding 50 mg/dose) is given daily or every other day. The antibiotic is dissolved in

5% D/W (optimal concentration, 0.1 mg/mL). (CAUTION: *Saline solution precipitates the drug and should not be used. Follow the manufacturer's instructions in preparing and storing solutions.*)

The drug should be given over a 2- to 6-h period. Reactions are usually mild, but some patients may experience chills, fever, headache, anorexia, nausea, and, occasionally, vomiting, particularly with the initial infusions. The severity of reactions may be reduced by giving aspirin or an antihistamine (eg, diphenhydramine 50 mg) before, after 3 h, and at the end of treatment. If this therapy is ineffective, hydrocortisone 25 to 50 mg IV may be given at the beginning of each amphotericin B infusion.

Chemical thrombophlebitis may occur; adding heparin (300 u.) to the infusion (or into the tubing just prior to starting the injection) may lessen the incidence.

The BUN or serum creatinine should be determined before and periodically during treatment. A slight increase can be ignored. A moderate rise, up to 50 mg/dL in the BUN or 3.5 mg/dL in the serum creatinine, may be reversed by giving the drug on alternate days; if the rise is not reversed, treatment should be discontinued until the levels approach normal. If this requires only a few days, treatment can be resumed with the previous dose, but if a longer period is necessary, therapy should be restarted with a smaller dose. Serum potassium should be determined regularly, since hypokalemia is common and occasionally is dramatic and dangerous. Oral liquid supplements are usually sufficient; rarely, potassium IV (not added to the amphotericin B infusion) may be necessary (see DISTURBANCES IN POTASSIUM METABOLISM, in Ch. 84).

Intrathecal injection may be indicated in meningitis, but great care must be taken to ensure proper dose and volume: 50 mg of amphotericin B should be painstakingly dissolved in 10 mL of sterile water. The total volume should then be diluted in a 250-mL bottle of 5% D/W from which 10 mL has been removed. From 0.5 mL (0.1 mg) to 5.0 mL (1.0 mg) should then be drawn into a 10-mL syringe, further diluted to 10 mL with CSF, and injected *slowly* (over at least 2 min). A lumbar, cisternal, or ventricular (by an Ommaya reservoir) site may be used.

HISTOPLASMOSIS

An infectious disease caused by Histoplasma capsulatum, *characterized by a primary pulmonary lesion and occasional hematogenous dissemination, with ulcerations of the oropharynx and GI tract, hepatomegaly, splenomegaly, lymphadenopathy, and adrenal necrosis.*

Etiology and Incidence

H. capsulatum in tissue is an oval budding cell 1 to 5 μ in diameter. Infection follows inhalation of dust that contains the spores. Severe disease is more frequent in men.

Chest x-ray surveys in certain geographic areas have demonstrated many residents with symptomless, nontuberculous, occasionally calcified pulmonary lesions; delayed cutaneous hypersensitivity reactions to histoplasmin suggest widespread but subclinical infection. The highest incidence of such hypersensitivity is in the Ohio and Mississippi River valleys. The largest single outbreak, affecting over 100,000, occurred in Indianapolis.

Symptoms and Signs

There are 3 recognized forms of the disease. The **primary acute form** causes symptoms (fever, cough, malaise) indistinguishable in endemic areas (except by culture) from otherwise undifferentiated URI or grippe-like disease. The **progressive disseminated form** follows hematogenous spread from the lungs and is characterized by hepatomegaly, lymphadenopathy, splenomegaly, and, less frequently, oral or GI ulceration. Addison's disease is an uncommon but serious manifestation. The lesions in the liver are granulomatous, show the intracellular fungus, and may lead to hepatic calcification. Addison's disease of other etiology, lymphoma, Hodgkin's disease, leukemia, and

sarcoidosis must be differentiated. The **chronic cavitary form** produces pulmonary lesions indistinguishable, except by culture, from cavitary TB. The principal manifestations are cough, increasing dyspnea, and eventually disabling respiratory embarrassment. That histoplasmosis is a cause of uveitis has been postulated but not proved.

Diagnosis

Culture of *H. capsulatum* is diagnostic. Specimens for culture may be sputum, lymph nodes, bone marrow, liver biopsy, blood, urine, or oral ulcerations. Tissues may be examined microscopically after staining (Gomori's methenamine silver, periodic acid-Schiff, or Gridley). Delayed cutaneous hypersensitivity and serologic tests are of no diagnostic value, since they are usually negative early in the disease.

Prognosis and Treatment

The acute primary form is usually benign; it is fatal only in those rare cases with massive infection. The progressive disseminated form has a 90% fatality rate. In the chronic cavitary form, death results from severe respiratory insufficiency.

Primary acute disease rarely requires chemotherapy (see amphotericin B and also ketoconazole in General Therapeutic Principles, above). The disseminated form responds to amphotericin B; in the chronic cavitary form, the fungi disappear with therapy, but fibrotic lesions show little change.

COCCIDIOIDOMYCOSIS

(San Joaquin or Valley Fever)

An infectious disease, caused by the fungus Coccidioides immitis, *occurring in a* **primary form** *as an acute, benign, self-limiting respiratory disease, or in a* **progressive form** *as a chronic, often fatal, infection of the skin, lymph nodes, spleen, liver, bones, kidneys, meninges, and brain.*

Etiology, Incidence, and Pathology

The disease is endemic in the southwestern USA and occurs most frequently in men aged 25 to 55. Infection is acquired by inhalation of spore-laden dust. Individuals contracting the disease while traveling through endemic areas may not develop manifestations until later, after leaving the area.

The basic pathologic change is an acute, subacute, or chronic granulomatous process with varying degrees of fibrosis. Lesions may show central necrosis; the organisms are surrounded by lymphoctyes and by plasma, epithelioid, and giant cells. Cavitation or granuloma ("coin lesion") formation may occur in chronic lung infection.

Symptoms and Signs

Primary pulmonary coccidioidomycosis, the more common form, may occur asymptomatically, as a mild URI, as acute bronchitis, occasionally with pleural effusion, or as pneumonia. Symptoms, in descending order of frequency, include fever, cough, chest pain, chills, sputum production, sore throat, and hemoptysis. Physical signs may be absent, or occasional scattered rales and areas of dullness to percussion may be present. Leukocytosis is present and the eosinophil count may be high. Some patients develop **"desert rheumatism,"** a more recognizable form with conjunctivitis, arthritis, and erythema nodosum.

Progressive coccidioidomycosis develops from the primary form; evidence of dissemination may appear a few weeks, months, or, occasionally, years after primary infection or long residence in an endemic area. Symptoms include continuous low-grade fever, severe anorexia, and loss of weight and strength. Progressive cyanosis, dyspnea, and mucopurulent or bloody sputum are present in the pulmonary type. The

bones, joints, skin, viscera, brain, and meninges may be involved as the disease spreads.

Diagnosis

Coccidioidomycosis should be suspected in a patient with an obscure illness who has been or is in an endemic area. Diagnosis is established by finding the characteristic spherules of *C. immitis* in sputum, gastric washings, pleural fluid, CSF, pus from abscesses, biopsy specimens, or exudate from skin lesions by direct examination or by culture of the fungus. In the tissues, the fungus appears as thick-walled, nonbudding spherules, 20 to 80 μ in diameter.

A delayed cutaneous hypersensitivity reaction to coccidioidin or spherulin usually appears 10 to 21 days after infection, but is characteristically absent in progressive disease. Precipitating and CF antibodies are present regularly and persistently in the progressive form but only transiently in acute primary cases.

Prognosis and Treatment

For primary pulmonary coccidioidomycosis, treatment is not needed and the outlook is excellent. The progressive type, however, is fatal in 55 to 60% of cases. Either amphotericin B or ketoconazole (see amphotericin B and also ketoconazole in General Therapeutic Principles, above) is indicated in all patients with the progressive form. Results are less satisfactory than in blastomycosis or histoplasmosis. Meningitis may require intrathecal amphotericin B administration, usually prolonged for years. Untreated meningitis is fatal.

CRYPTOCOCCOSIS

(Torulosis)

An infectious disease due to the fungus Filobasidiella neoformans *(formerly known as* Cryptococcus neoformans *or* Torula histolytica), *with a primary focus in the lung and characteristic spread to the meninges and occasionally to the kidneys, bone, and skin.*

Incidence and Pathology

Distribution is worldwide. In the USA, more cases occur in the Southeast and in men aged 40 to 60. Individuals with Hodgkin's disease or AIDS are particularly susceptible.

CNS lesions include diffuse meningitis, meningeal granulomas, infarcts, areas of softening, increase in neuroglia, or extensive tissue destruction. Cutaneous lesions appear as acneiform pustules or granulating ulcers. Subcutaneous and visceral lesions are deep nodules or tumorlike masses filled with gelatinous material. Acute inflammation is minimal or absent, but infiltration with lymphocytes and fibroblasts, and with plasma, "foam," and giant cells, is seen occasionally.

Symptoms and Signs

Meningitis with headache is the most common form. The patient seeks medical care because of blurred vision or is brought to the physician because of such mental disturbances as confusion, depression, agitation, or inappropriate speech or dress. CSF examination shows elevated protein and cell count (mostly lymphocytes) in about 90% of patients, and decreased glucose in 50%; *F. neoformans* can be seen on India ink examination in 60%, but antigen can be detected by latex agglutination test in > 90%.

Though the infection is acquired via the respiratory route with a primary focus in the lung, it has only recently been recognized that a benign, rarely progressive, pulmonary form occurs, often as a complication of other lung disease. Cough or other symptoms of the underlying pathologic changes in the lung are usually present.

The kidney is the next most common organ involved. *F. neoformans* can be cultured from the urine in about 30% of patients with cryptococcal meningitis. Although renal

infection is usually asymptomatic, pyelonephritis with renal papillary necrosis has been reported.

Skin lesions (pustules or ulcers) and bone lesions (osteomyelitis) are seen less frequently.

Diagnosis

This is strongly suggested by finding, with an India ink preparation, the budding yeast surrounded by a clear capsular area in sputum, pus, other exudates, or CSF. Similar encapsulated yeast forms, seen on proper staining of fixed tissues, are also almost diagnostic. The latex particle agglutination test for antigen is useful with CSF, blood, and urine. Culture and identification of the causative fungus confirm the diagnosis.

Prognosis and Treatment

For the meningitic form, combined amphotericin B/flucytosine therapy is best: amphotericin B 20 mg/day IV and flucytosine 150 mg/day orally for 6 wk. Patients with nonprogressive pulmonary disease may need no treatment. Skin, bone, and renal infections require therapy, though these forms are intermediate in severity.

Alternatively, once sensitivity has been demonstrated, flucytosine 150 mg/kg/day orally at 6-h intervals may be given for nonmeningitic forms. Flucytosine is not metabolized significantly when taken orally; it is excreted primarily by the kidney. Renal and hematologic status should be determined before therapy, and the drug must be given with caution to patients with impaired renal function or bone marrow depression. Frequent (ie, twice weekly) monitoring of renal, hematologic, and hepatic function is essential throughout therapy, in order to vary appropriately the interval between doses.

Adverse reactions include GI disturbances; rash; anemia; leukopenia; thrombocytopenia; occasionally, elevation of hepatic enzymes, BUN, and creatinine; and, infrequently, confusion, hallucination, or headache. Leukopenia, thrombocytopenia, and, occasionally, elevated SGOT have occurred, which can be due to the drug, to underlying disease, to the infection, or to a combination of all three.

BLASTOMYCOSIS

(North American Blastomycosis; Gilchrist's Disease)

An infectious disease caused by the fungus Blastomyces dermatitidis, *primarily involving the lungs and occasionally spreading hematogenously, characteristically to the skin.*

Etiology and Incidence

The site in nature of the causative fungus is not established, but association with beavers has been suggested in a recent outbreak. Most reported cases are from the USA, chiefly in the southeastern states and the Mississippi River valley, and in men aged 20 to 40. A sufficient number of cases from widely scattered sites in Africa now precludes geographic limitation of the disease name. Disease occurs prominently in dogs and may be a harbinger of that in man.

Symptoms and Signs

Pulmonary form: Primary pulmonary blastomycosis frequently forms patches of bronchopneumonia that appear, on chest film, to fan out from the hilum like a neoplastic growth. Onset is usually insidious. A dry hacking or productive cough, chest pain, fever, chills, drenching sweats, and dyspnea are initial symptoms.

Systemic form: Sites of hematogenous spread include skin, prostate, epididymis, testis, bone, subcutaneous tissue, and, rarely, oral or nasal mucosa. The vertebrae, tibia, and femur are more commonly involved than other bones; swelling, heat, and tenderness are present over the lesion. Genital tract lesions are characterized by painful swelling.

Skin lesions begin as papules or papulopustules on exposed surfaces and spread slowly. Painless miliary abscesses, varying from pinpoint to 1 mm in diameter, develop on the advancing borders. Irregular, wartlike papillae form on the surfaces. As the lesions enlarge, the center heals with a typical atrophic scar. A fully developed individual lesion appears as an elevated verrucous patch measuring 2 cm or larger with an abruptly sloping, purplish-red, abscess-studded border. Ulceration may occur if bacteria are present.

Diagnosis

Diagnosis is by culture and identification of *B. dermatitidis*. Diagnosis is almost as certain if thick-walled budding yeasts, about 15 μ in diameter and without a capsule, are seen on direct examination of pus, sputum, or exudate, or after appropriate tissue fixation and staining. Skin and serologic tests are of no value.

Pulmonary disease must be distinguished from TB, other fungus infections, and bronchogenic carcinoma. Skin lesions resemble sporotrichosis, TB, iodism, or, especially, basal cell carcinoma. Genital involvement mimics TB.

Prognosis and Treatment

In most untreated patients, the disease is slowly and fatally progressive. Amphotericin B (see General Therapeutic Principles, above) is highly effective. Improvement begins within a week, with rapid disappearance of organisms.

Hydroxystilbamidine isethionate is occasionally useful (eg, in patients with a renal disorder or with nonprogressive blastomycosis limited to the skin). However, storage and administration are difficult, and the manufacturer's instructions for use must be carefully followed. Dosage is begun with 25 mg/day IV and increased by increments of 25 mg/day until 225 mg/day is reached; this dose is continued until a total of 8 gm has been given. Alleviation of symptoms usually begins after 14 days, but little improvement in the lesions is noted before 30 days. Improvement usually continues for 3 to 6 mo after the last dose. Occasionally, the course of treatment must be repeated. Rarely, facial numbness in the sensory distribution of the 5th cranial nerve occurs. Fever occurring near the end of the first week of therapy suggests a Herxheimer-like reaction.

Ketoconazole is effective in about 75% of patients.

PARACOCCIDIOIDOMYCOSIS

(South American Blastomycosis)

An infectious disease of the skin, mucous membranes, lymph nodes, and internal organs, caused by the fungus Paracoccidioides brasiliensis (*formerly* Blastomyces brasiliensis). The disease occurs only in South and Central America, most frequently in men aged 20 to 50, and especially in the coffee-growers of Brazil and Colombia.

Symptoms and Signs

Disease is now believed to be acquired by the respiratory route with a primary focus of infection in the lung, although there are 4 clinical forms. (1) The **cutaneous form** occurs most often on the face, frequently at the nasal and oral mucocutaneous borders. The typical lesion is a slowly expanding ulcer with a granular base and numerous pinpoint yellowish-white areas in which the fungus is abundant. Regional lymph nodes enlarge, become necrotic, and discharge necrotic material through the skin. (2) In the **lymphatic form**, there is massive painless enlargement of the cervical, supraclavicular, or axillary lymph nodes. (3) In the **visceral form**, the liver, spleen, and abdominal lymph nodes enlarge. Abdominal pain may be the first symptom. (4) In the **mixed type**, cutaneous, lymphatic, and visceral lesions are present simultaneously.

Diagnosis and Treatment

Identification of *P. brasiliensis* in pus, biopsy, or culture is diagnostic. Treatment with amphotericin B (see General Therapeutic Principles, above) is effective; sulfona-

mides are suppressive but not curative. Ketoconazole (see General Therapeutic Principles, above) currently appears to be the preferable drug on the basis of its efficacy, oral route of administration, and potential for prolonged duration of treatment.

SYSTEMIC CANDIDIASIS

(Candidosis; Moniliasis)

Invasive disease caused by Candida *spp, especially* C. albicans, *and manifested by septicemia, endocarditis, meningitis, or, rarely, osteomyelitis.* Topical *Candidal* spp infections are discussed in other appropriate sections of THE MANUAL.

Etiology and Incidence

The infections are usually caused by *C. albicans* or by *C. tropicalis* in immunosuppressed patients. Superficial candidiasis is universal, but patients with leukemia, or with organ transplants, or receiving immunosuppressive or antibacterial therapy are especially prone to *C.* spp septicemia. *C.* spp (frequently *C. parapsilosis*) endocarditis is related to intravascular trauma such as cardiac catheterization, surgery, or indwelling venous catheters. An endogenous alcohol syndrome has been attributed to fermentation by the fungus in the gut.

Symptoms and Signs

C. spp **endocarditis** resembles bacterial disease, with fever, heart murmur, splenomegaly, and anemia; large vegetations and emboli to major vessels are frequently differential features. Renal involvement is usually found on laboratory and autopsy examination. *C.* spp **septicemia** often resembles gram-negative bacterial sepsis in frequency of fever, shock, azotemia, oliguria, renal shutdown, and fulminant course. *C.* spp **meningitis** is chronic, like cryptococcal meningitis, but lacks the latter's usually fatal outcome when untreated. *C.* spp **pyelonephritis** and pulmonary disease are less well characterized. **Osteomyelitis** and a related disease, spondylodiscitis (infection of the intervertebral disk) have been encountered, notably in intravenous drug addicts.

Diagnosis

Because *C.* spp are commensals of man, their culture from sputum, mouth, vagina, urine, stool, or skin must be interpreted cautiously. To confirm the diagnosis, the culture must be complemented by a characteristic clinical lesion, exclusion of other etiology, and histologic evidence of tissue invasion. Culture from blood or CSF, however, establishes infection and supports the appropriate clinical impression: septicemia, endocarditis, or meningitis.

Treatment

Such predisposing conditions as diabetic acidosis must first be controlled. In systemic candidiasis, amphotericin B IV is preferable therapy (see General Therapeutic Principles, above). As an alternative, flucytosine may be given as for cryptococcosis (see above) if the isolate is sensitive to it. Ketoconazole (see General Therapeutic Principles, above) appears promising, notably for chronic mucocutaneous candidiasis (see CHRONIC MUCOCUTANEOUS CANDIDIASIS in Ch. 18).

ASPERGILLOSIS

An infectious disease of the lung, with occasional hematogenous spread, caused by various Aspergillus *spp, especially* A. fumigatus. A noninvasive pulmonary disorder may also occur as an allergic reaction to *A. fumigatus* (see ALLERGIC BRONCHOPULMONARY ASPERGILLOSIS in Ch. 43) or other species.

Etiology, Symptoms, and Signs

The fungus, an "opportunist," appears after antibacterial or antifungal therapy (to which it is usually resistant) in bronchi damaged by bronchitis, bronchiectasis, or TB.

The "fungus ball" (aspergilloma), a characteristic form of the disease, appears on the chest film as a dense round ball, capped by a slim meniscus of air, in a cavity; it is composed of a tangled mass of hyphae, fibrin, exudate, and a few inflammatory cells. Aspergillomas usually occur in old cavitary disease (eg, TB). Symptoms (cough, productive sputum, dyspnea) and findings on physical examination or chest film are usually those of the underlying disease. However, hemoptysis has been a disturbing and even occasionally fatal complication. In the presence of leukemia, organ transplantation, or corticosteroid or immunosuppressive therapy, dissemination to the brain and kidneys may occur. The clinical picture in this form is a typical septicemia: fever, chills, hypotension, prostration, and delirium. Another form, termed chronic necrotizing pulmonary aspergillosis, is akin to chronic suppurative lung disease.

Diagnosis and Treatment

Because the *A.* spp are commensals of man, their culture from sputum, mouth, or bowel must not be considered diagnostic unless a clinically compatible illness is present, other causes have been eliminated, and tissue invasion has been demonstrated. In disseminated and pulmonary disease, amphotericin B should be given IV (see General Therapeutic Principles, above), although tolerated doses are usually ineffective, since most strains are resistant. Ketoconazole, so far, has not been any more effective.

PHYCOMYCOSIS

(Mucormycosis, Zygomycosis)

A term that includes numerous clinical conditions associated with the presence of broad, nonseptate hyphae. In most cases, the fungus has been visualized in tissues only microscopically. When cultured, it has been either a *Rhizopus, Absidia, Mucor,* or *Basidiobolus* spp. One form of the disease, subcutaneous phycomycosis, occurs in southeast Asia and Africa as a self-limited, multiple, grotesque, subcutaneous swelling of the neck and chest. **Rhinocerebral phycomycosis**, more familiar in the USA, is a fulminant and usually fatal primary infection of the nose, sinus, or orbit seen in patients with diabetic acidosis or immunosuppressive disorders or drugs. Severe pain, fever, orbital cellulitis, proptosis, purulent nasal drainage, and gangrenous and necrotic destruction of the nasal septum, palate, or orbital or sinus bones are usually present. Early invasion of vessels and spread to the brain causes convulsions, aphasia, and hemiplegia. The clinical appearance is diagnostic, but bacterial abscesses, histoplasmosis or TB of the oral cavity, or lethal midline granuloma occasionally mimics rhinocerebral phycomycosis. It has been difficult to culture the fungi clearly present in tissues at biopsy or autopsy. **Treatment** includes control of the underlying acidosis and amphotericin B, given empirically, since the causative fungus has not usually been available for sensitivity studies. Surgery, principally incisional and excisional, is important initially and has increased survival rates in patients with underlying diabetes mellitus.

MADUROMYCOSIS

(Madura Foot; Mycetoma)

A infectious disease of the feet (and occasionally the upper extremity), characterized by chronicity, tumefaction, and multiple sinus formation, and progressing unless excised or amputated; death occurs occasionally in neglected cases.

About half the cases are caused by *Nocardia* spp, the remainder by some 20 different fungi and bacteria. The disease is most prevalent in the tropics and southern USA and is usually contracted between ages 21 and 40.

Symptoms, Signs, and Diagnosis

The first lesion may be a small papule, a deep-seated fixed nodule, a vesicle with an indurated base, or an abscess that ruptures and produces a fistula. Early lesions are

granulomatous but are later surrounded by a dense fibrous capsule and intersected by fibrous trabeculae. Lesions are usually nontender unless secondary infection is present. The disease progresses slowly; 6 to 8 papules or abscesses may form in succession and then disappear. Months or years may pass before muscles, tendons, fascia, and bone are destroyed.

In advanced cases, the foot characteristically appears as a grotesque, swollen, club-shaped mass of cystlike areas with multiple draining and intercommunicating sinuses and fistulas that discharge an "oily" or serosanguineous fluid. Characteristic fungus granules in the discharge measure 0.5 to 2 mm, are irregularly shaped, and vary in color. The patient is able to walk until deformity or muscle wasting intervenes. Systemic symptoms are rare. The course may be prolonged for ≥ 10 yr; the patient eventually may die from sepsis or intercurrent disease, unless the infecting organism is sensitive to an antimicrobial agent. Diagnosis is made from the clinical course, appearance, and demonstration of the characteristic colored granules in the exudate.

Treatment

Cases caused by *Actinomyces* spp should be treated with penicillin or a tetracycline (see ACTINOMYCOSIS in Ch. 8); those caused by *Nocardia* spp, with a sulfonamide (see NOCARDIOSIS in Ch. 8). If the fungus is sensitive, amphotericin B or ketoconazole may be helpful. Amputation of the limb may be required to prevent fatal spread of secondary bacterial infection.

SPOROTRICHOSIS

An infectious disease caused by the plant saprophyte Sporothrix schenckii, *and characterized by the formation of nodules, ulcers, and abscesses, usually confined to the skin and superficial lymph channels but occasionally affecting the lung or other tissues (eg, synovial membranes).* Farm laborers and horticulturists, especially those handling barberry bushes or sphagnum moss, are most often infected.

Symptoms and Signs

The most common form, cutaneous-lymphatic, occurs characteristically on the arm and hand. The primary lesion, usually on the finger, begins as a small, movable, nontender, subcutaneous nodule that slowly enlarges, adheres to the skin, becomes pink and later necrotic, and finally ulcerates. In a few days or weeks, similar discolored subcutaneous nodules appear along the course of the lymphatics draining the area. Local pain, heat, and general symptoms (fever, chills, malaise, or anorexia) are notably absent.

Inhalation of the fungus may cause pneumonia, localized infiltrates, or cavities (sometimes bilateral). Symptoms are relatively mild, and the course is chronic.

Though *S. schenckii* has only rarely been cultured from the blood, it seems reasonable to explain other extracutaneous disease as hematogenous dissemination either from a subclinical cutaneous lesion or, perhaps more likely, from a pulmonary focus. Bone, periosteum, or synovium is involved in 80% of such cases; muscle and eye, in others. Involvement of the spleen, liver, kidney, genitalia, or CNS is rare.

Diagnosis

Diagnosis is by culture and identification of *S. schenckii*. Unlike other pathogenic fungi, *S. schenckii* is rarely seen in fixed tissue, even with special stains.

Prognosis and Treatment

The cutaneous-lymphatic form is chronic, indolent, and rarely fatal. It responds readily to potassium iodide saturated solution, initially 1 mL orally tid, increased by 1 mL/day to an optimal dose of 3 to 4 mL tid. The solution may be diluted in water or other beverage and should be taken after meals. Therapy must be continued and may be well tolerated for prolonged periods. However, iodism may appear at any time as an

irritative phenomenon of the skin and mucous membranes (eg, rashes, coryza, conjunctivitis, stomatitis, laryngitis, bronchitis). When symptoms develop, the dose should be decreased or the drug temporarily discontinued. After a 1- to 2-wk interruption, the drug may be cautiously resumed at a lower dosage. It may be considered essential to continue iodide medication despite iodism; in such cases, iodide sensitivity may lessen or disappear despite continued therapy.

In disseminated disease, IV amphotericin B (see General Therapeutic Principles, above) may be helpful, since about 30% of patients have died, in some instances despite extensive treatment with iodides.

CHROMOMYCOSIS

(Chromoblastomycosis; Verrucous Dermatitis)

An infectious disease caused by Hormodendrum pedrosoi, H. compactum, *or* Phialophora verrucosa, *and characterized by warty cutaneous nodules which slowly develop into large papillomatous vegetations that tend to ulcerate.* Incidence is worldwide, but highest in the tropics. The disease is prevalent from age 30 to 50, principally in men.

Symptoms, Signs, and Diagnosis

The infection, usually unilateral, begins on the foot and leg, or sometimes on other exposed parts, especially where the skin is broken. The early lesion is a small, itching, enlarging papule resembling ringworm. The patch is dull red or violaceous in color, is sharply demarcated, and has an indurated base. New crops projecting 1 or 2 mm above the skin may appear several weeks or months later along the paths of lymphatic drainage. Hard, dull red or grayish cauliflower-like nodules may develop in the center of the patch and gradually cover the infected extremities. Lymphatics may be blocked, itching may be present, and secondary infection may lead to ulceration. From 4 to 15 yr may elapse before the entire extremity is involved.

In late cases, the diagnosis is made from the clinical appearance. Early lesions may be mistaken for dermatophytoses and must be differentiated by finding the characteristic dark brown septate bodies in pus or biopsy specimens.

Prognosis and Treatment

The disease is rarely fatal, but complete surgical excision is the treatment of choice. A few reports suggest that amphotericin B, instilled into the lesion, may be effective even in advanced cases. Recently, flucytosine has been the recommended chemotherapy (see dosage for nonmeningitic forms in CRYPTOCOCCOSIS, above).

RHINOSPORIDIOSIS

A probably infectious disease caused by Rhinosporidium seeberi, *characterized by large, friable, sessile or pedunculated polyps on the mucous membranes of the nose, eyes, larynx, and vagina, and occasionally on the skin of the ears or penis.* The disease, apparently contracted by swimming in stagnant water, occurs most often in boys and young men in India and Ceylon. The diagnosis is established by identifying the ovoid spores (measuring 7 to 9 μ) in smears, or by demonstrating the characteristic spore-filled sporangia (200 to 300 μ) in biopsy material.

Prognosis and Treatment

The disease is rarely fatal, but the patient may die of secondary infection. Complete excision of the early lesions is curative.

GEOTRICHOSIS

A term used to include a variety of conditions, none yet characterized or studied, in a patient from whom Geotrichum candidum *has been cultured.* Since the microorganism is

a commensal of man, culture from the mouth and bowel is etiologically meaningless. There have been rare reported cases of fungemia.

PENICILLIOSIS

A term used to include the rarely encountered, disparate instances when a species of apparently multiplying Penicillium *has been recovered from deep tissues* (eg, the brain, orbit, or kidney). Like *Candida* and *Geotrichum*, *Penicillium* is a commensal in the bowel and is found in stool.

---

10. RICKETTSIAL DISEASES

A variety of illnesses manifested by sudden onset, a course of fever of one to several weeks, headache, malaise, prostration, peripheral vasculitis, and, in most cases, a characteristic rash. Most rickettsias are maintained in nature by a cycle involving an animal reservoir and an insect vector (usually an arthropod) that infects humans.

Most of the members of the order Rickettsiales are obligate intracellular organisms that resemble viruses and bacteria. Like bacteria, they possess metabolic enzymes, have cell walls, utilize O_2, and are susceptible to antibiotics; like viruses, they require living cells for growth. Most are pleomorphic coccobacilli that stain purple with Giemsa, pink to red with Castaneda, and bright red with Giménez stains. During convalescence they usually induce serum agglutinins against specific *Proteus* strains **(Weil-Felix reaction)** and various types of antibodies to specific rickettsial antigens. Since many of the rickettsias are localized to geographic areas, knowing where the patient lives or has recently traveled often helps in diagnosis.

In some rickettsioses, rickettsias multiply at the site of an arthropod attachment and produce a local lesion (eschar). They penetrate the skin or mucous membranes and multiply in the endothelial cells of small blood vessels, causing a vasculitis consisting of endothelial proliferation, perivascular infiltration, and thrombosis. The endovasculitis is responsible for the rash, encephalitic signs, and gangrene of skin and tissues.

Rickettsioses comprise 4 groups: (1) **typhus**—epidemic typhus, Brill-Zinsser disease, murine (endemic) typhus, and scrub typhus; (2) **spotted fever**—Rocky Mountain spotted fever, Eastern tick-borne rickettsioses, and rickettsialpox; (3) **Q fever**; and (4) **trench fever**.

EPIDEMIC TYPHUS

(European, Classic, or Louse-Borne Typhus; Jail Fever)

An acute, severe, febrile disease characterized by prolonged high fever, intractable headache, and a maculopapular rash. The agent, Rickettsia prowazekii, *is transmitted by lice.*

Etiology and Epidemiology

Rickettsia prowazekii is prevalent worldwide and transmitted to man in feces of the human body louse, *Pediculus humanus*, when a puncture wound is contaminated by scratching. Dried louse feces may also infect the mucous membranes of the eyes or oral cavity. Lice become infected on febrile patients and transmit illness to susceptible humans. Man is the natural reservoir of infection. A human form of epidemic typhus fever has been identified in the USA that is occasionally contracted after contact with flying squirrels or their ectoparasites; the illness is generally milder than classic typhus and is identified by serologic methods.

Symptoms and Signs

Following the 7- to 14-day incubation, fever, headache, and prostration begin suddenly. Temperature reaches 40 C (104 F) in several days and remains at a high level,

with slight morning remission, for about 2 wk. Headache is generalized and intense. Small pink macules appear on the 4th to 6th day, usually in the axillae and on the upper trunk; they rapidly cover the body, usually sparing the face, soles, and palms. Later the lesions become dark and maculopapular; in severe cases, the rash becomes petechial and hemorrhagic. Splenomegaly occurs in some cases. Hypotension occurs in most seriously ill patients, and vascular collapse, renal insufficiency, encephalitic signs, ecchymosis with gangrene, and pneumonia are poor prognostic signs. Fatalities are rare in children < 10 yr, but mortality increases with age and may reach 60% in those > 50.

Prophylaxis

Immunization and louse control are highly effective. Live and killed vaccines are available. Lice may be eliminated by dusting infested persons with DDT, malathion, or lindane.

For **diagnosis** and **treatment**, see DIFFERENTIAL DIAGNOSIS OF RICKETTSIAL DISEASES and THERAPY OF RICKETTSIAL DISEASES, below.

BRILL-ZINSSER DISEASE

Recrudescence of epidemic typhus, occurring years after an initial attack.

Etiology and Epidemiology

Patients who develop Brill-Zinsser disease either acquired epidemic typhus earlier in life or lived in an endemic area. *R. prowazekii* persist as viable organisms long after recovery. Apparently when host defenses falter, rickettsia are activated, causing recurrent typhus. Lice that feed on patients may acquire infection and transmit the agent. Also, *R. prowazekii* may be isolated from the blood of such patients by animal inoculation.

The disease is sporadic, occurring at any season and in the absence of infected lice. A history of epidemic typhus or residence in an endemic area is helpful.

Symptoms and Signs

The illness, almost always mild, resembles epidemic typhus in the character of the rash, circulatory disturbances, and hepatic, renal, and nervous system changes. The remittent febrile course lasts about 7 to 10 days; the rash is often evanescent or absent. Mortality is nil.

For **diagnosis** and **treatment**, see DIFFERENTIAL DIAGNOSIS OF RICKETTSIAL DISEASES and THERAPY OF RICKETTSIAL DISEASES, below.

MURINE (ENDEMIC) TYPHUS

(Rat-Flea Typhus; Urban Typhus of Malaya)

An acute febrile disease clinically similar to, but milder than, epidemic typhus, caused by Rickettsia typhi (mooseri) *and transmitted to humans by rat fleas.*

Etiology and Epidemiology

The causative agent, *R. typhi (mooseri)*, resembles other rickettsias morphologically, in staining characteristics, and in intracellular parasitism. The animal reservoir is wild rats, mice, and other rodents; the agent is transmitted to man by rat fleas (*Xenopsylla cheopis*). This illness, sporadic and worldwide in distribution, is more prevalent in congested areas where rats abound, but the incidence is low.

Symptoms and Signs

Following an incubation of 6 to 18 days (mean 10), a shaking chill develops, associated with headache and fever. The fever lasts about 12 days and terminates by lysis. The rash and other manifestations are similar to those of epidemic typhus but are

much less severe. The early exanthem is sparse and discrete. Although mortality is low, fatalities may occur in elderly patients.

Prophylaxis

Incidence of murine typhus has been decreased by reducing rat and rat-flea populations through securing foundations of food depots and granaries and by dusting rat runs, burrows, and harborages with DDT or another residual insecticide. There is no effective vaccine.

For **diagnosis** and **treatment**, see DIFFERENTIAL DIAGNOSIS OF RICKETTSIAL DISEASES and THERAPY OF RICKETTSIAL DISEASES, below.

SCRUB TYPHUS

(Tsutsugamushi Disease; Mite-Borne Typhus; Tropical Typhus)

A mite-borne infectious disease caused by Rickettsia tsutsugamushi *and characterized by fever, a primary lesion, a macular rash, and lymphadenopathy.*

Etiology and Epidemiology

This disease occurs in the Asiatic-Pacific area bounded by Japan, India, and Australia; *R. tsutsugamushi* is transmitted in nature by trombiculid mites (usually *Leptotrombidium akamushi* and *L. deliensis*) transovarially and by feeding on forest and rural rodents, including rats, voles, and field mice. Human infection follows a chigger (mite larva) bite.

Symptoms and Signs

After an incubation period of 6 to 21 days (average 10 to 12 days), onset is sudden, with fever, chilliness, headache, and generalized lymphadenopathy. At onset of fever, a local lesion (eschar) often develops at the site of the chigger bite. The lesion is more common in Caucasians than in Asians, in whom it is rare. It begins as a red, indurated lesion about 1 cm in diameter and eventually vesiculates, ruptures, and becomes covered with a black scab; regional lymph node enlargement occurs. Fever rises during the 1st wk, often to 40 to 40.5 C (104 to 105 F). Headache is severe and commonly present, as is conjunctival injection. A macular rash develops on the trunk during the 5th to 8th day of fever and often extends to the arms and legs. It may disappear rapidly or become maculopapular and intensely colored. Cough is present during the 1st wk of fever, and pneumonitis may develop during the 2nd wk. In severe cases, pulse rate increases, blood pressure decreases, and delirium, stupor, and muscular twitching develop. Splenomegaly may be present, and interstitial myocarditis is more common than in other rickettsioses. In untreated patients, high fever may persist for 2 wk or more, then fall by lysis over several days. With specific therapy, defervescence usually begins within 36 h and recovery is prompt and uneventful.

Prophylaxis

Clearing brush and spraying infested areas with residual insecticides eliminate or decrease mite populations. Mite repellents, eg, dimethyl phthalate or benzyl benzoate, should be used by individuals likely to be exposed.

For **diagnosis** and **treatment**, see DIFFERENTIAL DIAGNOSIS OF RICKETTSIAL DISEASES and THERAPY OF RICKETTSIAL DISEASES, below.

ROCKY MOUNTAIN SPOTTED FEVER (RMSF)

(Spotted Fever; Tick Fever; Tick Typhus)

An acute febrile disease caused by Rickettsia rickettsii *and transmitted by ixodid ticks.*

Etiology, Epidemiology, and Pathology

R. rickettsii is limited to the Western Hemisphere. Initially recognized in the Rocky Mountain states, it occurs in practically all states (except Maine, Hawaii, and Alaska)

in the USA, especially on the Atlantic seaboard. Hard-shelled ticks (family Ixodidae) harbor *R. rickettsii*, and infected females transmit the agent transovarially to their progeny. Ticks are the natural reservoir, and animals provide blood nourishment. *Dermacentor andersoni* (the wood-tick) is the principal vector in the western USA; *D. variabilis* (dog tick) and *Ambloyomma americanum* (lone-star tick) are common vectors in the eastern and southern USA. The organism is also maintained in rabbits and other small mammals. RMSF occurs mainly from May to September, when adult ticks are active and persons are most apt to be in areas infested by ticks. In southern states, cases occur throughout the year. The incidence is high in children under age 15 and in others who frequent tick-infested areas for work or recreation. It is unlikely that RMSF is transmitted directly from person to person via infectious aerosol produced by the cough of a patient with respiratory-tract involvement.

Small blood vessels are the sites of the characteristic pathologic lesion. Rickettsia propagate within damaged endothelial cells, and vessels may be blocked by thrombi. The major sites of vasculitis are the skin, subcutaneous tissues, CNS, lungs, heart, kidneys, liver, and spleen.

Symptoms and Signs

A history of tick bite is elicited in about 70% of patients. The incubation period averages 7 days but varies from 3 to 12 days; the shorter the incubation period, the more severe the infection. Onset is abrupt, with severe headache, chills, prostration, and muscular pains. Fever reaches 39.5 or 40 C (103 or 104 F) within several days and remains high (for 15 to 20 days in severe cases), though morning remissions may occur. An unproductive, harassing cough develops. On about the 4th day of fever, a rash appears on the wrists, ankles, palms, soles, and forearms; it rapidly extends to the neck, face, axilla, buttocks, and trunk. Often a warm water or alcohol compress will bring out the rash. Initially macular and pink, it becomes maculopapular and darker. In about 4 days, the lesions become petechial and may coalesce to form large, hemorrhagic areas that later ulcerate. The rash can be noted as early as the first day of illness or as late as day 6, with rapid development of petecheae. Uncommonly there is no rash. Neurologic symptoms include headache, restlessness, insomnia, delirium, and coma, all indicative of an encephalitis. Hypotension develops in severe cases. Hepatomegaly may be present, but jaundice is infrequent. Localized pneumonitis may occur. Untreated patients may develop such complications as pneumonia, tissue necrosis, and circulatory failure, with such sequelae as brain and heart damage. Cardiac arrest with sudden death occasionally occurs in fulminant cases.

Prognosis

Starting antibiotic therapy early has significantly reduced mortality, which was formerly about 20%. The current 7% mortality rate is largely due to delay in initiating specific treatment. No serious sequelae result if therapy is instituted early.

Prophylaxis

A tissue-culture–derived, inactivated vaccine is under development for use in persons who frequently encounter ticks during work or recreation. Tick repellents such as dimethyl phthalate should be used by all who live or work in tick-infested areas. Good personal hygiene should be practiced, with frequent searches for ticks, particularly in children. Engorged ticks should be removed with care and not crushed between the fingers because of danger of transmission. Gradual traction of the head part with a small forceps will dislodge the tick. The point of attachment should be swabbed with alcohol. Although no practical means exist to rid entire areas of ticks, tick populations may be reduced in endemic areas by controlling small-animal populations; spraying the area with DDT, dieldrin, or chlordane is also helpful.

In the event of tick bite in a known endemic area of RMSF it is best not to give antibiotics immediately, but caution the patient or parent about early clinical signs. If

sustained fever, headache, and malaise occur with or without a rash, antibiotics effective for rickettsial disease should be initiated promptly.

For **diagnosis** and **treatment**, see DIFFERENTIAL DIAGNOSIS OF RICKETTSIAL DISEASES and THERAPY OF RICKETTSIAL DISEASES, below.

TICK-BORNE RICKETTSIOSES OF THE EASTERN HEMISPHERE

(North Asian Tick-Borne Rickettsiosis; Queensland Tick Typhus; African Tick Typhus [Fièvre Boutonneuse])

Mild to moderately severe febrile diseases, transmitted by ixodid ticks and characterized by an initial lesion, satellite adenopathy, and an erythematous maculopapular rash.

Etiology and Epidemiology

The etiologic agents of the 3 diseases in this category (listed above) belong to the spotted fever group of rickettsia and, with *R. rickettsii* and *R. akari*, possess common group antigens that are demonstrated by agglutination, complement fixation, rickettsiae microagglutination, and indirect fluorescent antibody reactions. North Asian tick-borne rickettsiosis, caused by *R. sibirica*, is found in Armenia, Central Asia, Siberia, and Mongolia; Queensland tick typhus, caused by *R. australis*, in Australia. Fièvre boutonneuse, the prototype of the 3, caused by *R. conorii*, occurs throughout the African continent, in India, and in areas of Europe and the Mideast adjacent to the Mediterranean, Black, and Caspian Seas. It often is known by the area in which it occurs (eg, Indian tick typhus, Marseilles fever).

The epidemiology of these tick-borne rickettsioses resembles that of spotted fever in the Western Hemisphere. Ixodid ticks and wild animals maintain the rickettsias in nature; if humans intrude accidentally into the cycle, they break the transmission chain. In certain areas, the cycle of fièvre boutonneuse involves domiciliary environments, with the brown dog tick, *Rhipcephalus sanguineus*, as the dominant vector. Transovarial transmission of rickettsias occurs in various ticks.

Symptoms, Signs, and Prognosis

The 3 tick-borne rickettsioses of the Eastern Hemisphere resemble one another closely; they are milder than spotted fever. After a 5- to 7-day incubation period, fever, malaise, headache, and conjunctival injection develop. With the onset of fever a local lesion appears (termed **eschar**, or, in fièvre boutonneuse, **tache noire**), a small button-like ulcer 2 to 5 mm in diameter with a black center. Usually the regional or satellite lymph nodes are enlarged. About the 4th day of fever, a red maculopapular rash appears on the forearms and extends to most of the body, including the palms and soles. Fever lasts into the 2nd wk of illness. Complications are rare. Death is rare except among aged or debilitated patients.

For **diagnosis** and **treatment**, see DIFFERENTIAL DIAGNOSIS OF RICKETTSIAL DISEASES and THERAPY OF RICKETTSIAL DISEASES, below.

RICKETTSIALPOX

(Vesicular Rickettsiosis)

A mild, self-limited, febrile disease with an initial local lesion and a generalized papulovesicular rash, caused by Rickettsia akari *and transmitted from its murine host by mites.*

First observed in New York City, rickettsialpox has also occurred in other US areas and in Russia, Korea, and Africa. The vector, a small, colorless mite, *Allodermanyssus sanguineus*, is widely distributed. It infects the house mouse (*Mus musculus*) and some species of wild mice, and can transmit *R. akari* transovarially. Humans may be infected by either chigger or adult mite bites.

Symptoms and Signs

An eschar resembling the tache noire of fièvre boutonneuse appears about 1 wk before onset of fever. Initially a small papule 1 to 1.5 cm in diameter, it develops into a small ulcer with a dark crust that heals leaving a scar; regional lymphadenopathy is present. The fever is intermittent and lasts about a week, with chills, profuse sweating, headache, photophobia, and muscle pains. Early in the febrile course, a generalized maculopapular rash with intraepidermal vesicles appears, sparing palms and soles. The disease is mild; no deaths have been reported.

Prophylaxis

Mouse harborages must be destroyed and the vector controlled by residual insecticides.

For **diagnosis** and **treatment**, see DIFFERENTIAL DIAGNOSIS OF RICKETTSIAL DISEASES and THERAPY OF RICKETTSIAL DISEASES, below. Treatment is usually not indicated because the disease is so mild.

Q FEVER

An acute disease characterized by sudden onset of fever, headache, malaise, and interstitial pneumonitis, caused by Coxiella burnetii (Rickettsia burnetii). In contrast to other rickettsial diseases, the illness is not associated with a cutaneous exanthem or agglutinins for *Proteus* strains (Weil-Felix reaction).

Etiology and Epidemiology

The route of infection is usually inhalation of infected aerosols. Worldwide in its distribution, Q fever is maintained as an inapparent infection in domestic animals; sheep, cattle, and goats are the principal reservoirs for human infections. *C. burnetii* persists in feces, urine, milk, and tissues (especially the placenta), so that fomites and infective aerosols form easily. Cases occur among workers whose occupations bring them in close contact with domestic animals or their products. The disease can also be contracted by ingesting infective raw milk.

C. burnetii is also maintained in nature through an animal-tick cycle. In the USA, Q fever was first recognized in persons bitten by *Dermacentor andersoni*. Various arthropods, rodents, other mammals, and birds are naturally infected and may play a role in human infection.

Symptoms and Signs

The incubation period varies from 9 to 28 days (average 18 to 21 days). Onset is abrupt, with fever, severe headache, chilliness, severe malaise, myalgia, and, often, chest pains. Fever may rise to 40 C (104 F) and persist for 1 to > 3 wk. Rash is absent. A nonproductive cough with x-ray evidence of pneumonitis often develops during the 2nd wk of illness. Mortality is < 1% in untreated patients, and even lower with antibiotic therapy.

In fatal Q fever, lobar consolidation usually occurs and the gross appearance of the lungs may resemble that of bacterial pneumonia. However, histologic changes in Q fever pneumonia are similar to those of psittacosis and some viral pneumonias. An intense interstitial infiltrate about the bronchioles and blood vessels extends into the adjacent alveolar walls. Plasma cells are numerous. The bronchiolar lumina may contain polymorphonuclear leukocytes. The alveolar lining cells are swollen, and the alveoli contain desquamated lining cells and large mononuclear cells.

There is an acute form of Q-fever hepatitis, and in about 1/3 of patients with the protracted type, hepatitis is present. In this type there is fever, malaise, hepatomegaly with right upper abdominal pain, and possibly jaundice. Headache or respiratory signs are frequently absent. Liver biopsy specimens show diffuse granulomatous changes,

and *C. burnetii* may be identified by immunofluorescence. Lobar pneumonia may be particularly severe in aged or debilitated patients. There are several forms of chronic Q fever, such as chronic hepatitis and endocarditis. Chronic Q fever hepatitis must be differentiated from other liver granulomas, eg, TB, sarcoidosis, histoplasmosis, brucellosis, tularemia, and syphilis. Endocarditis caused by *C. burnetii* is serious but uncommon. Clinically, it simulates SBE, with aortic valve involvement more common. Routine blood cultures are persistently negative.

Diagnosis

Diagnosis is made by clinical suspicion and by demonstrating phase I type antibodies in the patient's serum. Clinically during early stages, Q fever simulates many infectious diseases (eg, influenza, other viral infections, salmonellosis, malaria, hepatitis, brucellosis) and later on, many forms of bacterial, viral, and mycoplasmal pneumonias. Contact with animals, animal products, or ticks is an important clue.

C. burnetii may be isolated from the blood. The Weil-Felix reaction is negative. Specific CF and agglutinating antibodies appear during convalescence. Agglutination tests are more sensitive than CF tests; fluorescent antibody tests are helpful. *C. burnetii* exists in 2 phases, I and II; antibodies against Phase I organisms are rarely produced in infected human serum, but when present indicate chronic Q fever.

Prophylaxis

Animal-to-man transmission must be prevented: milk should be pasteurized; dust control in pertinent industries is essential; and animal placentas, feces, and urine should be incinerated. The sputum and urine of Q fever patients should be autoclaved and the patient isolated. Vaccines made from Phase I rickettsias are effective and should be used to protect slaughterhouse and dairy workers, rendering plant workers, herders, woolsorters, farmers, and others at risk. These vaccines are not available commercially, but may be obtained from special laboratory groups—eg, the US Army Medical Research Institute of Infectious Diseases in Frederick, Maryland.

Treatment (See also Therapy of Rickettsial Diseases, below)

Tetracycline and chloramphenicol are effective. In acute disease, treatment should be continued until the patient has been afebrile for about 5 days. The course of illness may be shortened by giving tetracycline 250 mg orally q 4 or 6 h. Chloramphenicol may be used in young children.

In endocarditis, treatment needs to be prolonged and tetracycline is preferred. Some cures without surgical intervention have been reported, but when antibiotic treatment is only partially effective, it is necessary to replace damaged valves. Clear-cut regimens for chronic hepatitis have not been determined.

TRENCH FEVER

(Wolhynian Fever; Skin-Bone Fever; Quintan Fever)

A rare louse-borne febrile disease observed mainly in military populations during World Wars I and II.

Etiology and Epidemiology

The causative organism, *Rochalimaea (Rickettsia) quintana*, grows extracellularly, unlike other rickettsias, and multiplies in the gut lumen of the body louse. One strain has been cultivated in blood agar. *R. quintana* is transmitted to man by the rubbing of infected louse feces into abraded skin or into the conjunctiva. Humans are the reservoir, since *R. quintana* persists in the blood for months after clinical recovery. The disease is endemic in Mexico, Tunisia, Eritrea, Poland, and the USSR.

Symptoms and Signs

Following a 14- to 30-day incubation period, onset is sudden, with fever, weakness, dizziness, headache, and severe back and leg pains. Fever may reach 40.5 C (105 F)

and persist for 5 to 6 days. In about half the cases, fever recurs 1 to 8 times at 5- to 6-day intervals. A transient macular or papular rash and, occasionally, hepatomegaly and splenomegaly are present. Although recovery is usually complete in 1 to 2 mo and mortality is negligible, the illness may be prolonged and debilitating.

The disease is marked by persistent rickettsiemia present during the initial attack, during relapses (which are common), and throughout the symptomatic periods between relapses. Rickettsiemia may persist for long periods, and clinical relapse has been reported 10 yr after the original attack.

Diagnosis

The disease may be suspected in persons living where louse infestation is heavy. Leptospirosis, typhus fever, relapsing fever, and malaria must be ruled out. The organism may be identified by xenodiagnosis: normal body lice excrete *R. quintana* about 1 wk after ingesting the patient's blood. Antibodies can be demonstrated by fluorescence or CF tests during convalescence.

Prophylaxis and Treatment

Body lice must be controlled (see EPIDEMIC TYPHUS, above). *R. quintana* is highly sensitive to in vitro chloramphenicol and the tetracyclines, but there are no reliable data regarding clinical efficacy. Aspirin and codeine are indicated for control of discomfort.

DIFFERENTIAL DIAGNOSIS OF RICKETTSIAL DISEASES

Differentiating the rickettsioses from other acute infectious diseases is difficult during the first several days before the rash. A history of lousiness, flea infestation, or tick bite in known endemic areas of typhus, or of Rocky Mountain spotted fever **(RMSF)** or other tick-borne rickettsial disease is a helpful clue.

The rash of **meningococcemia**, which may be pink, macular, maculopapular, or petechial in the subacute form, and petechial confluent or ecchymotic in the fulminant type, resembles RMSF or epidemic typhus. The meningococcal rash develops rapidly in the acute type and when ecchymotic is usually tender to palpation; the rickettsial rash usually appears on about the 4th febrile day and gradually, over several days, becomes petechial.

RMSF is often confused with measles. In **rubeola**, the rash begins on the face, spreads to the trunk and arms, and soon becomes confluent; the rash of **rubella** usually remains discrete. Postauricular lymph nodes and lack of toxicity favor rubella.

In murine typhus, the illness is milder than in RMSF or epidemic typhus, the rash is nonpurpuric, nonconfluent, and less extensive; renal and vascular complications are uncommon. Differentiating RMSF from murine typhus may be difficult and require the results of specific serologic reactions. (Treatment cannot be delayed until this distinction is made.) Epidemic louse-borne typhus fever causes all of the profound physiologic and pathologic abnormalities of RMSF, including peripheral vascular collapse, shock, cyanosis, ecchymotic skin necrosis, gangrene of digits, azotemia, renal failure, delirium, and coma. The rash of epidemic typhus usually appears first over the axillary folds and trunk; later it spreads peripherally, rarely involving the palms, soles, and face. Local eschars occur in patients with scrub typhus, rickettsialpox, and, occasionally, spotted fever. The epidemiologic history often helps in differentiation. The rash in rickettsialpox is vesicular, whereas in tick-borne typhus it is often obviously maculopapular. In ulceroglandular **tularemia** (associated with an eschar) and other forms of tularemia, there is no exanthem.

Rickettsialpox, a member of the spotted fever group, is mild; there is usually an initial eschar at the point of the mite attachment, and the rash, in the form of vesicles

with surrounding erythema, is sparse. **Varicella** must be ruled out, since similar oral lesions occur in both diseases.

A rash in Q fever is unusual and in trench fever is sparse.

Patients with scrub typhus have all of the clinical and pathologic manifestations of RMSF and epidemic typhus. Scrub typhus occurs in different geographic areas; there is frequently an eschar with satellite adenopathy.

Several types of confirmatory **laboratory tests** aid diagnosis: serologic tests, isolation and identification of *R. rickettsii* from blood or tissues, or identification of the agent in skin or other tissues by immunofluorescence technics.

Serologic tests, to be useful, require 3 serum samples during the 1st, 2nd, and 4th to 6th wk of illness.

Weil-Felix reaction: Strains of *Proteus* OX-19 are agglutinated by sera of patients with epidemic or murine typhus fever or RMSF; however, they provide no specificity for these diseases. In RMSF and other tick-borne rickettsioses, agglutinins for *Proteus* OX-19 and OX-2 appear; *Proteus* OX-K agglutinins occur in scrub typhus. The Weil-Felix reaction is not significantly reactive in patients with rickettsialpox, Brill-Zinsser disease, Q fever, or trench fever.

A single convalescent serum titer of 1/160 to 1/320 is usually diagnostic, but a demonstrated rise in titer is of greater value. *Proteus* agglutinins may appear as early as the 5th day and are generally present by the 12th febrile day. A maximum titer is generally reached in early convalescence and declines rapidly to nondiagnostic levels in several months. In approximately 10% of cases, *Proteus* agglutinins fail to appear. When antibiotics are given during the first few days of illness, the titer may be delayed, but it usually reaches the same level.

Complement-fixation reaction: The various rickettsial diseases can be differentiated by using group-specific, soluble rickettsial antigens. Using specific rickettsial antigens, the serologic patterns of RMSF and typhus are distinctive. In the USA, epidemic typhus occurs as Brill-Zinsser disease (recurrent epidemic typhus fever) and human-related flying squirrel epidemic typhus. Spotted fever and typhus group rickettsiae possess 2 types of CF antigens; the soluble fraction is common to all members of the group, while purified fractions are more specific for individual rickettsiae. Various member-diseases of the spotted fever group, such as RMSF, rickettsialpox, fièvre boutonneuse, north Asian tick-borne rickettsiosis and Queensland tick typhus, may be distinguished by use of type-specific washed rickettsial-body antigen. Antibodies during response to a primary infection of RMSF and typhus are usually 19S globulins. CF antibodies appear during the 2nd and 3rd wk of these illnesses and later in those treated with antibiotics within the first 3 to 5 days of illness. Under these circumstances, a later convalescent specimen should be taken at 4 to 6 wk. In Brill-Zinsser disease, antibodies appear rapidly after several days of illness and are 7S type. Q fever antigens are specifically diagnostic. In acute infections, antibodies to phase II antigens appear; phase I antibodies indicate chronic infection such as hepatitis or endocarditis.

Other serologic tests: Using purer antigens, other serologic procedures for rickettsioses not only distinguish between specific rickettsial infections but also help determine the type of immunoglobulin in acute (IgM) and late or recurrent (IgG) illnesses such as Brill-Zinsser disease (recurrent typhus fever). The Weil-Felix and CF tests are useful for routine diagnosis; microscopic agglutination (MA), immune fluorescence antibody (IFA), and hemaglutination (HA) reactions are valuable for identification and are becoming standard procedures. IFA and CF tests help confirm trench fever. *R. akari* shares a common antigen with other members of the spotted fever group but can be differentiated from them by demonstrating a rising titer of specific CF antibodies. *R. conori*, *R. sibirica*, and *R. australis* share a common antigen with *R. rickettsii* and *R.*

akari, but are differentiated by CF and mouse toxin neutralization tests and by cross-immunity tests in guinea pigs.

Isolating and identifying rickettsia: If isolation is attempted, blood should be obtained, prior to antibiotic treatment, from febrile patients with spotted or typhus fever. Male guinea pigs are inoculated intraperitoneally with 2 to 4 mL of defibrinated blood or emulsified clot. Details of how to establish infection may be found in standard laboratory texts.

Identification of *R. rickettsii* in tissues: Immunofluorescence technics have been used to detect *R. rickettsii* and *R. prowazekii* in tissues of chick embryos, guinea pigs, and vector ticks. Identifiable rickettsiae have been visualized in skin lesions of patients with RMSF as early as the 4th day of illness or as late as the 10th day. Rickettsia may be stained by IFA technic in formalized tissues.

THERAPY OF RICKETTSIAL DISEASES

Those principles necessary for treating all rickettsioses are (1) specific chemotherapy and (2) supportive care. Measures advisable for all rickettsioses are described here; variations are described in specific subsections, above.

Prompt alleviation of signs and symptoms occurs if therapy begins early, when the rash first appears. *Since untreated patients with RMSF may become moribund or die before definitive serologic data are available, treatment should begin as soon as a presumptive diagnosis is made.*

Chloramphenicol and the tetracyclines are specifically effective; they are rickettsiostatic, not rickettsiocidal. Optimal antibiotic regimens are (1) chloramphenicol, an initial oral dose of 50 mg/kg or (2) tetracycline, 25 mg/kg. The same dosage is given subsequently in daily doses divided equally and given at 6-to 8-h intervals until the patient improves and has been afebrile for about 24 h. IV preparations are used for the loading dose and subsequent doses in patients too ill to take oral medication. In critically ill patients who are first observed late in the course of severe illness, large doses of corticosteroids, given for about 3 days in combination with specific antibiotics, are recommended. All patients with rickettsioses respond promptly to antibiotic treatment when it is initiated early in illness, before serious tissue changes have occurred. Obvious clinical improvement is usually noted within 36 to 48 h, with defervescence in 2 to 3 days. In scrub typhus the response is even more dramatic. In those patients first treated during the later stages, clinical improvement is slower and fever extends over longer periods. Patients seriously ill with the typhus spotted fever group often have circulatory collapse, oliguria, anuria, azotemia, anemia, hyponatremia, hypochloremia, edema, and coma that must be managed. In mildly and moderately ill patients these alterations are absent, making management less complicated.

Proper mouth care, swabbing the oral cavity and using mouthwashes, may help prevent gingivitis and parotitis. Turning the patient frequently will help avert pressure sores over bony prominences and prevent aspiration pneumonia. Negative nitrogen balance can be avoided by generous protein supplements with frequent feedings. Protein intake of 2 to 3 gm protein/kg of normal body weight, with adequate carbohydrate and fat to make the diet palatable, is usually well tolerated. In uncooperative patients when there is no abdominal distention, IV alimentation or hourly liquid protein feedings by gastric tube are helpful.

In critically ill patients, attention is given to parenteral alimentation with glucose and amino acid supplements. Small whole blood transfusions are indicated when anemia is present. Judicious use of serum albumin may improve the circulation. With oliguria, anuria, and azotemia, the circulation should not be overloaded; results of

laboratory tests and clinical judgment guide therapy. In the rare instances of clear-cut evidence of acute renal failure, dialysis is indicated.

---

11. CHLAMYDIAL DISEASES

The organisms responsible for psittacosis, lymphogranuloma venereum **(LGV)**, trachoma, and and inclusion conjunctivitis, are now classified in the genus *Chlamydia* (*Bedsonia*, *Miyagawanella*), which is divided into 2 species: *C. psittaci*, which causes psittacosis, and *C. trachomatis*, which consists of several strains that cause LGV, trachoma, and inclusion conjunctivitis. *C. trachomatis* has also been shown to cause a number of sexually transmitted diseases, including nongonococcal urethritis and epididymitis in the male, cervicitis, urethritis, and pelvic inflammatory disease in women, Reiter's syndrome in HLA-B27 haplotype individuals, and neonatal conjunctivitis and pneumonia transmitted from an infected mother to her newborn. In some studies, *C. trachomatis* has been implicated in 20% of adults with pharyngitis.

The chlamydias are nonmotile, obligate intracellular parasites. Although originally considered viruses because they multiply in the cytoplasm of host cells, the chlamydias are more closely related to bacteria, since they contain both DNA and RNA, have a cell wall chemically similar to that of gram-negative bacteria, possess ribosomes, grow well in the yolk-sacs of embryonated eggs, and are susceptible to the tetracyclines and erythromycin. Chlamydia can be isolated from infected secretions or tissues in appropriate tissue cultures.

PSITTACOSIS is discussed in Ch. 40; the sexually transmitted diseases LGV and urethritis are in Ch. 14; epididymitis is in LOWER URINARY TRACT AND MALE GENITAL TRACT INFECTIONS in Ch. 153, and REITER'S SYNDROME is in Ch. 108; NEONATAL CONJUNCTIVITIS and NEONATAL PNEUMONIA are in NEONATAL INFECTIONS in Ch. 186; and the ophthalmic disorders TRACHOMA and INCLUSION CONJUNCTIVITIS are in Ch. 219.

---

12. VIRAL DISEASES

INTRODUCTION

Viruses: *The smallest of parasites; intracellular molecular particles, in some instances crystallizable, with a central core of nucleic acid and an outer cover of protein; wholly dependent on cells (bacterial, plant, or animal) for reproduction*. The nucleic acid core (RNA or DNA) represents the basic infectious material that in many cases can penetrate susceptible cells and initiate infection alone.

Though most viruses are invisible in the light microscope (size variation, about 0.02 to 0.3 μ), they can be seen by electron microscopy and measured by various biophysical and biochemical methods. Like most other parasites, viruses stimulate host antibody production.

Several hundred different viruses may infect man. Many have been recognized only recently, so their clinical effects or even relationships are not fully delineated. Many viruses usually produce inapparent infections and only occasionally overt disease; nevertheless, because of their wide (sometimes universal) prevalence and their numerous distinct serotypes, they create important medical and public health problems.

The viruses occurring primarily in man are spread chiefly by man himself, mainly via respiratory and enteric excretions. Such viruses (see TABLE 12-1) are found in all parts of the world, their spread being limited by inborn resistance, prior immunizing

infections or vaccines, sanitary and other public health control measures, and, in a few instances, by chemoprophylactic agents.

Many viruses pursue their biologic cycles chiefly in animals, man being only a secondary or accidental host. The zoonotic viruses (see TABLE 12–2), in contrast to the specifically human agents, are limited to those geographic areas and environments able to support their extrahuman natural cycles of infection (vertebrates or arthropods, or both).

Two properties of certain viruses are noteworthy because of their implications: (1) oncogenicity and (2) prolonged incubation. **Oncogenic properties** of some animal viruses are well known (eg, Rous sarcoma of chickens, Shope rabbit papilloma, murine leukemia viruses). Three human retroviruses called human T-lymphotrophic viruses **(HTLV)** have now been described. HTLV types I and II appear to cause some human T cell leukemias and lymphomas, and HTLV type III is the cause of AIDS. Epstein-Barr virus has also been found in association with malignancies, such as African Burkitt's lymphoma and lymphomas in immunosuppressed organ transplant recipients. The **prolonged incubation** periods of some viruses have led to the term, **"slow" viruses**. Kuru, a rare disease confined to natives of New Guinea and characterized by chronic degeneration of the CNS, has been transmitted and passed in primates. Symptoms appear after an incubation period of about 18 mo. The implications are clear: some of the chronic degenerative diseases, previously with no known etiology, now appear to be due to slow virus infections. Besides kuru, these include subacute sclerosing panencephalitis, progressive multifocal leukoencephalopathy, Creutzfeldt-Jakob disease, and progressive rubella encephalitis. (See SLOW VIRUS INFECTIONS below and SUBACUTE SCLEROSING PANENCEPHALITIS and PROGRESSIVE RUBELLA ENCEPHALITIS in Ch. 191.)

Diagnosis of Viral Infections

In theory, most viral infections can, by some means, be recognized; in practice, diagnosis often remains difficult. A few viral diseases can be diagnosed accurately on clinical and epidemiologic grounds (eg, several well-known exanthems), but many diagnoses depend on retrospective tests (eg, serologic examination of acute and convalescent sera), unless an adequately equipped diagnostic virology laboratory is available in the community for more rapid diagnosis by such procedures as culture or immunofluorescence microscopy. During large epidemics (eg, of influenza), laboratory diagnosis of early cases may aid in recognizing and managing subsequent cases. Many state health laboratories and the National Centers for Disease Control also offer diagnostic assistance.

Viruses of man and animals are isolated from secretions, excretions, and tissues by inoculating susceptible animals, chick embryos, and cultures of living cells. Presence of the virus usually is indicated by disease and antibody responses in the animals or by cytopathogenic effects and antigen production in tissue cultures. Specific diagnostic details are discussed in THE MANUAL in relation to the discussion of each disease.

Prophylaxis and Treatment

Viral diseases are not susceptible to antibiotics, but particularly in those liable to superinfection with bacterial pathogens, antibiotics are used to prevent complications. The efficacy of such treatment is debatable, and indiscriminate use of antibiotics in viral infections (eg, measles) may be harmful.

The barriers—chiefly intracellular multiplication—to effective use of chemotherapeutic or chemoprophylactic drugs against viruses and viral diseases are being breached, if not broken. Examples are trifluorothymidine or acyclovir for herpes simplex keratitis, amantadine or rimantadine for influenza A, vidarabine or acyclovir for severe herpes simplex or varicella-zoster infections, and possibly ribavirin aerosol for influenza, parainfluenza, and respiratory syncytial viruses. There is also a potential for the use of interferon, a protein of low molecular weight that is produced by certain cells when they have been stimulated (eg, by bacteria, some viruses, or nucleic acids)

TABLE 12–1. HUMAN VIRAL DISEASES: NATURAL CYCLE CHIEFLY IN MAN; PERSON-TO-PERSON SPREAD*

Virus Groups & Categories	*No. Known Serotypes*	*Most Important*		*Prevalence, Distribution*	*Diagnostic Leads*	*Specific*	
		Syndromes	Serotypes			Therapy	Prophylaxis
Respiratory							
Influenza A, B, & C	3	Influenza; AFRD; acute bronchitis & pneumonia; croup	A (with many possible subtypes), B, C	Epidemic, occasionally pandemic (A, B); endemic (C)	Clinical & epidemiologic features; serologic; virus isolation	Amantadine (A)	Vaccine (moderately effective) Amantadine (A)
Parainfluenza 1–4	4	AFRI (children); acute bronchitis & pneumonia; croup	1, 2, 3	1: Local epidemic; 1 & 3: widely in children	Clinical not defined; serologic; virus isolation	None	Vaccines under study
Mumps	1	Parotitis, orchitis, meningoencephalitis	1	Global; most children; some adults	Clinical features; serologic; virus isolation	None	Vaccine
Adenoviruses	41	AFRD (children); ARD (adults); APCF; EKC; viral pneumonia; acute follicular conjunctivitis; diarrhea	1–10, 14, 21, 40, 41	1–3, 5–7: Children 4, 7, 14, 21: Adults 8: Local EKC 40, 41: Diarrhea in childhood	APCF, EKC: Clinical features Most: Serologic & virus isolation	None	Vaccine (4,7) for military epidemic situations
Reoviruses	3	Mild RI	(?)	Widely in children; may be same as in animals	Serologic; virus isolation	None	None
Respiratory syncytial	1	U & L RI (infants); mild URI (adults)	1 (?)	Pediatric clinics & hospital wards	Serologic & isolation & identification of viruses	None	None
Infectious mononucleosis	1	Infectious mononucleosis	Epstein-Barr virus	Widespread; apparent chiefly in young adults	Heterophil agglut.; diff. WBC count; specific serology	None	None

Rhinoviruses	(?)	Common cold; acute coryza with or without fever	>95; probably 100's	Universal; especially in cold months	Clinical features	None	None
Enteric							
Polioviruses	3	Poliomyelitis (paralytic); aseptic meningitis; AFRD (children)	1, 2, 3	Almost universal; + in warm months; + at younger ages	Paralysis typical; serologic; virus isolation	None	Vaccines: Live (oral) Killed (injected)
Coxsackieviruses	30 (A's: 24; B's: 6)	Herpangina; epidemic pleurodynia; aseptic meningitis; myocarditis; pericarditis; AFRD (children); paralytic disease; fever & exanthem	A's: 2, 4–10, 16, 21, 23 B's: 1–6	Varies with types; most persons infected; + in warm months; + in children	Virus isolation; serologic difficult, due to so many serotypes	None	None
Echoviruses and "high-numbered" enteroviruses	36**	Aseptic meningitis; fever & exanthem; meningoencephalitis with rash; diarrhea neonatorum; paralytic disease; myocarditis; pericarditis; ARD	4, 6, 8, 11, 14, 16, 18, 20, 30	As for coxsackieviruses	As for coxsackieviruses	None	None

(Continued)

* Developments are so rapid that no summary can be fully up to date. Main abbreviations: **AFRD,** acute febrile respiratory disease; **AFRI,** acute febrile respiratory illness; **APCF,** acute pharyngoconjunctival fever; **ARD,** acute respiratory disease; **EKC,** epidemic keratoconjunctivitis; **LRI,** lower respiratory illness; **RI,** respiratory illness; **URI,** upper respiratory illness.

** Echovirus types 9, 10, and 28 have been reclassified; these numbers are no longer used; more recently described enteroviruses have been designated as types 68 to 72.

TABLE 12–1. HUMAN VIRAL DISEASES: NATURAL CYCLE CHIEFLY IN MAN; PERSON-TO-PERSON SPREAD *(Cont'd)*

Virus Groups & Categories	*No. Known Sero-types*	*Most Important*		*Prevalence, Distribution*	*Diagnostic Leads*	*Specific*	
		Syndromes	Serotypes			Therapy	Prophylaxis
Enteric *(Cont'd)* Epidemic gastroenteritis	(?)	Epidemic nausea & vomiting	Rotaviruses; "Norwalk" agents; astro-viruses, adenovirus types 40 & 41; caliciviruses; "coronavirus-like" agents	Local epidemics (children); + in colder months	Clinical & epidemiologic features, electron microscopy of diarrheal stools; serologic	None	Rotavirus vaccines under study
Exanthems Rubeola	1	Measles; encephalomyelitis	1 known	Almost universal; monkeys also infected; CNS involvement rare	Clinical features; serologic; virus isolation	None	Vaccines
Rubella	1	German measles	1 (?)	Universal; birth defects from infection during 1st trimester of pregnancy	Clinical & epidemiologic features; serologic	None	Vaccines
Varicella-zoster	1	Chickenpox	1 known	Almost universal (children); occasionally in adults	Clinical features; serologic; virus isolation	Acyclovir	Immune globulins
	Same	Herpes zoster	Same	Common in adults; reactivation or reinfection	Same	Acyclovir	None

Herpes simplex	2	Herpes labialis; herpetic gingivostomatitis; dermatitis; keratoconjunctivitis; encephalitis; vulvovaginitis; neonatal disseminated disease	2 established	Recurrent labial, almost universal; gingivostomatitis frequent in infants & children; others rare	Clinical features; serologic; virus isolation	Acyclovir or vidarabine	None
Roseola infantum	1 (?)	Rose rash, infants (Exanthem subitum)	Not isolated	Widespread; early childhood	Clinical features	None	None
Erythema infectiosum	1 (?)	"Fifth" disease; rash, malaise	1 known	Sporadic outbreaks	Atypical exanthems	None	None
Persistent (Latent)							
Cytomegaloviruses (salivary gland)	1	Congenital defects (cytomegalic inclusion disease); hepatitis (CMV mononucleosis) Disseminated disease (compromised host)	1 established	Virus widespread; recognized disease uncommon	Clinical features; serologic; virus isolation	None	None

(Continued)

TABLE 12–1. HUMAN VIRAL DISEASES: NATURAL CYCLE CHIEFLY IN MAN; PERSON-TO-PERSON SPREAD *(Cont'd)*

Virus Groups & Categories	*No. Known Sero-types*	*Most Important*		*Prevalence, Distribution*	*Diagnostic Leads*	*Specific*	
		Syndromes	Serotypes			Therapy	Prophylaxis
Persistent (Latent) *(Cont'd)* Hepatitis							
1. Type A	1	Hepatitis A	1 established	Widespread; often epidemic	Clinical & epidemiologic features	None	γ-Globulin;
2. Type B	1	Hepatitis B	1 established	Widespread	Clinical features; serologic	None	Strict aseptic precautions; screening for hepatitis B surface antigen; vaccine; γ-globulin
3. Non-A, Non-B	?	? Hepatitis C	?	Similar to Types A and B	Clinical features; serologic exclusion of Types A & B	None	None
4. Type D	1	"Delta" hepatitis	1 established	Associated with IV drug abuse and use of whole blood and derivatives; can only infect in the presence of hepatitis B infection	Serologic	None	None
Papovavirus	1	Warts (Verrucae)	Not definitely established	Universal; common; often recurrent	Clinical examination & biopsy	Interferon (?)	None
Molluscum contagiosum	1	Molluscum contagiosum tumors	1 established	Infrequent	Clinical examination & biopsy	None	None

Table 12–2. VIRUSES TRANSMITTED FROM NATURE TO MAN (ZOONOSES)

Virus Groups & Categories	No. Known Sero-types	Most Important: Syndromes	Most Important: Serotypes	Prevalence, Distribution	Diagnostic Leads	Specific: Therapy	Specific: Prophylaxis
Arboviruses* Group A	>250	1. Western equine encephalitis (WEE)	Same designations as clinical syndromes	1. N. & S. America	Serologic; patho-logic; virus isolation	None	Effective vac-cines can be made; except for yellow fever, none in general use
		2. Eastern equine encephalitis (EEE)		2. N. & S. America			
		3. Venezuelan equine encephalitis (VEE)		3. Gulf states to S. America			
		4. Chikungunya encephalitis		4. Africa, S.E. Asia, India			
		5. Mayaro disease		5. S. America, Trinidad			
Group B		1. Yellow fever		1. Africa, Cen. & S. America			
		2. Dengue 1–4		2. Tropics & subtropics worldwide			
		3. Japanese encephalitis		3. Asia, Australia, New Zealand			
		4. Murray Valley encephalitis		4. Australia, New Guinea			
		5. St. Louis encephalitis		5. N. & S. America			
		6. Russian spring-summer encephalitis		6. USSR, E. Central Europe, Malaya			
		7. Omsk hemorrhagic fever		7. USSR			
		8. Kyasanur Forest disease		8. India			
		9. Powassan		9. N. America			

(Continued)

*See also Table 12–5 in Arbovirus and Arenavirus Diseases, below. Arthropod vectors of most arboviruses are one or more genera and species of mosquitoes, ticks (Russian spring-summer encephalitis, Crimean hemorrhagic fever), and sandflies (Phlebotomus fever). Arbovirus Groups A and B are now reclassified as Togaviruses.

TABLE 12–2. VIRUSES TRANSMITTED FROM NATURE TO MAN (ZOONOSES) *(Cont'd)*

Virus Groups & Categories	*No. Known Sero-types*	*Most Important*		*Prevalence, Distribution*	*Diagnostic Leads*	*Specific*	
		Syndromes	Serotypes			Therapy	Prophylaxis
Arboviruses *(Cont'd)*							
Group C (Bunyamwera supergroup)		1. Bunyamwera and 13 others 2. Marituba and 12 others 3. California encephalitis and 8 related types 4. Hantaan and related types	Same designations as clinical syndromes	1. Africa, S. America, Finland, USA 2. S. America, Central America 3. Probably worldwide; common in midwest USA 4. Northern Asia, Europe, USA (?); chief reservoir: rodents	Serologic; patho-logic; virus isolation	None	Effective vac-cines can be made; none in general use
Phlebotomus fever group		1. Naples, Sicilian fevers 2. Punta Toro, Chagres fevers 3. Candiru fever		1. Italy, India, Egypt 2. Panama 3. Brazil			
Ungrouped		1. Rift Valley fever 2. Crimean-Congo hemorrhagic fever		1. E. Africa, Egypt 2. USSR, Central Africa, W. Pakistan			
Orbivirus	1	Colorado tick fever	1 known	Western USA	Serologic; virus isolation	None	None
Rabies	1	Rabies (Hydrophobia)	1 known	Worldwide; domestic & wild animals; infrequent in man	Hist'y, clin. & path. findings; virus isolation	None	Effective vaccines available

Herpesvirus simiae (B virus)	1	Encephalomyelitis	1 known	Chiefly lab. workers exposed to monkeys, simian tissue cultures	Virus isolation	None	None
Arenaviruses*	≥11	1. Lassa fever 2. Machupo (Bolivian hemorrhagic fever) 3. Junin (Argentinian hemorrhagic fever) 4. Lymphocytic choriomeningitis	Same designations as clinical syndromes	1. Africa 2. S. America 3. S. America 4. Worldwide; chief reservoir: rodents	Virus isolation, serology	None	None
Unclassified viruses	2	1. Marburg virus (hemorrhagic fever) 2. Ebola virus (hemorrhagic fever)		1. Africa 2. Africa	Virus isolation, serology	None	None

and that nonspecifically inhibits replication of a wide range of viruses in the cells of the host producing it. (See also ANTIVIRAL DRUGS in Ch. 3.)

In many common, undifferentiated illnesses—the most frequent manifestations of prevalent viruses—decisions concerning the use of chemotherapeutic agents or antibiotics are often complicated by the difficulties of making definitive diagnoses. In such instances, the best guides are the severity and course of the illness, blood and x-ray findings, and clinical judgment. Because antibiotics cannot influence most viral illnesses favorably, lack of response should suggest stopping the antibiotics.

Effective virus vaccines in general use for active immunity include those for influenza, measles, mumps, poliomyelitis, rabies, rubella (German measles), hepatitis B, and yellow fever. An effective adenovirus vaccine is available, but should be used only in groups subject to high risk, such as military recruits. Specific immune globulins are also available for passive immune prophylaxis. (See also IMMUNIZATION PROCEDURES FOR ADULTS in Ch. 2, and IMMUNIZATION PROCEDURES THROUGHOUT CHILDHOOD in Ch. 182.)

EXANTHEMATOUS VIRAL DISEASES

(See also MEASLES, RUBELLA, ROSEOLA INFANTUM, ERYTHEMA INFECTIOSUM, and CHICKENPOX under VIRAL INFECTIONS in Ch. 191)

HERPES ZOSTER

(Shingles; Zona; Acute Posterior Ganglionitis)

An acute CNS infection involving primarily the dorsal root ganglia and characterized by vesicular eruption and neuralgic pain in the cutaneous areas supplied by peripheral sensory nerves arising in the affected root ganglia.

Etiology, Incidence, and Pathology

Herpes zoster is caused by the varicella-zoster virus, the same virus that causes chickenpox. It may be activated by local lesions involving the posterior root ganglia, by systemic disease, particularly Hodgkin's disease, or by immunosuppressive therapy. It may occur at any age but is most common after age 50. Inflammatory changes occur in the sensory root ganglia and in the skin of the associated dermatome. In some instances, the inflammation may involve the posterior and anterior horns of the gray matter, the meninges, and the dorsal and ventral roots.

Symptoms and Signs

Prodromal symptoms of chills and fever, malaise, and GI disturbances may be present for 3 or 4 days before distinctive features of the disease develop, with or without pain along the site of the future eruption. On about the 4th or 5th day, characteristic crops of vesicles on an erythematous base appear, following the cutaneous distribution of one or more posterior root ganglia. The involved zone is usually hyperesthetic, and the associated pain may be severe. The eruptions occur most often in the thoracic region and spread unilaterally. They begin to dry and scab about the 5th day after their appearance. Zoster may become generalized. If dissemination occurs or the lesions persist > 2 wk, an underlying malignancy or immunologic defect becomes more suspect.

One attack of herpes zoster usually confers immunity (recurrence is estimated to be 2% or less). Most patients recover without residua, except for occasional scarring of the skin. However, postherpetic neuralgia may persist for months or years, most frequently in the elderly.

Geniculate zoster (Ramsay Hunt syndrome) results from involvement of the geniculate ganglion. Pain in the ear and facial paralysis (rarely permanent) occur on the involved side. Vesicular eruptions are present in the external auditory canal and on the auricle, the soft palate, and the anterior pillar of the fauces. (See also HERPES ZOSTER OTICUS in Ch. 207.)

Ophthalmic herpes zoster (see also in Ch. 220) follows involvement of the gasserian ganglion, with pain and a vesicular eruption in the distribution of the ophthalmic division of the 5th nerve. A 3rd nerve palsy may be present. Vesicles on the tip of the nose indicate the nasociliary branch of the 5th nerve and the cornea are involved, and corneal ulcerations and opacities may develop.

Diagnosis

Though difficult in the preeruption stage, diagnosis is made readily after the vesicles appear in characteristic distribution. Pleurisy, trigeminal neuralgia, Bell's palsy, and, in children, chickenpox must be differentiated. The pain may resemble that of appendicitis, renal colic, cholelithiasis, or colitis, depending on the location of the involved nerve. Herpes simplex virus may produce nearly identical zosteriform lesions. Herpes simplex tends to recur, but herpes zoster rarely does. The viruses can be differentiated serologically and by culture.

Treatment

There is no specific therapy. However, a corticosteroid, if given early, may relieve pain and prevent or reduce later post-zoster pain in severe cases, particularly in the elderly. The initial dose should be relatively large (eg, prednisone 50 mg/day orally for an adult), and duration should not exceed 3 wk; all the precautions associated with prescribing corticosteroids should be observed. Locally applied wet compresses are soothing. Aspirin 600 mg, alone or with codeine 15 to 60 mg, orally q 4 to 6 h, may relieve pain. Tricyclic antidepressants (eg, amitriptyline) have been reported to be helpful when analgesics alone do not relieve the pain. Recent trials suggest that immunosuppressed patients with herpes zoster may benefit from treatment with vidarabine or acyclovir IV, if begun before dissemination develops.

For treatment of ophthalmic herpes zoster, see Ch. 220. (CAUTION: *Before using corticosteroids one must be certain that the disease is not acute ocular herpes simplex, in which corticosteroids are* ***contraindicated;*** *close supervision and follow-up of the patient are required*)

RESPIRATORY VIRAL DISEASES

Viral infections of the respiratory tract are acute illnesses with local and systemic manifestations. Coryza (common cold), pharyngitis, laryngitis (including croup), and tracheobronchitis are common respiratory syndromes. Infectious asthma can resemble an allergic reaction. Viral pneumonia is often unrecognized. Febrile syndromes without respiratory symptoms mimic systemic bacterial infections. In infants, such illnesses probably are caused more often by viruses than by bacterial sepsis. In adults, acute febrile "flu" can be produced by many viruses. In individuals, the syndrome is not distinguishable clinically from the specific infection described below under influenza.

THE COMMON COLD

(Upper Respiratory Infection, URI; Acute Coryza)

An acute, usually afebrile, viral infection of the respiratory tract, with inflammation in any or all airways, including the nose, paranasal sinuses, throat, larynx, and often the trachea and bronchi.

Etiology

Many viruses cause the common cold, including rhino-, influenza, parainfluenza, respiratory syncytial, corona, adeno-, certain echo-, and coxsackieviruses. More than 100 sero-specific rhinovirus types have been established and many viruses are still untyped. Pinpointing the specific etiology of each illness by virus isolation or serologic tests is impractical. However, only a few of the viruses are important at any one time

and the causes of the common cold have a striking seasonal relation. Spring, summer, and fall colds are more often picornavirus (rhino-, echo-, and coxsackie-) infections; late fall and winter colds are most frequently paramyxo- or myxovirus (influenza, parainfluenza, and respiratory syncytial) infections.

Predisposing factors have not been clearly identified. Chilling of the body surface will not by itself induce colds, and susceptibility is not affected by either the person's health and nutrition or upper respiratory tract abnormalities (eg, enlarged tonsils or adenoids). Upon exposure, infection may be facilitated by excessive fatigue, emotional distress, or allergic nasopharyngeal disorders and during the midphase of the menstrual cycle.

Pathogenic bacteria inhabiting the nasopharynx infrequently cause purulent complications such as otitis media and sinusitis. Bronchitis of viral etiology also can become secondarily infected by bacteria.

Symptoms and Signs

Onset is abrupt after a short (1 to 3 days) incubation period. Illness generally begins with nasal or throat discomfort, followed by sneezing, rhinorrhea, and malaise. Characteristically, it is an afebrile illness, but fever of 38 to 39 C (100 to 102 F) can occur, especially in infants and children. Pharyngitis is regularly present early; laryngitis and tracheitis with substernal tightness and burning discomfort vary with the individual and with the etiologic agent. Nasal secretions, watery and profuse during the first day or two of symptoms, become more mucoid and purulent; mucopurulent nasal discharge does not necessarily indicate a bacterial suprainfection. Hacking cough with scanty sputum often lasts into the 2nd wk. An exacerbation of persistent bronchitis after a cold is common in people with chronic respiratory tract disease. Severe tracheobronchial involvement with purulent sputum suggests primary or secondary bacterial infection. Exacerbation of bronchoconstriction in asthmatics and bronchitic patients is frequently initiated by a common cold. Purulent sinusitis or otitis media are bacterial complications. In the absence of complications, symptoms normally resolve in 4 to 10 days.

Diagnosis

Clinical symptoms and signs are nonspecific. Bacterial infections, allergic rhinorrhea, and other disorders also cause upper respiratory tract symptoms and at their onset may be confused with primary coryza. Differentiation depends on the course of the symptoms. Transient pharyngitis without exudate or adenopathy (except adenovirus infections) signifies a viral rather than a bacterial cause. The presence of fever and more severe symptoms usually differentiates influenza. A substantial leukocytosis indicates a disorder other than an uncomplicated common cold.

If exudate is present, a smear for microscopic examination is recommended, with attention given to the number of polymorphonuclear cells and the character of the bacteria. Eosinophilia in secretions suggests an allergic etiology. In the early phase of an epidemic of viral respiratory infections, nasopharyngeal washings or garglings should be sent to local public health or academic laboratories for specific virus identification and serum specimens should be collected for serologic confirmation.

Prophylaxis

Immunity is type-specific. Effective experimental vaccines have been prepared for single types of rhinoviruses or paramyxoviruses, but the large number of types and strains of causative viruses has precluded production of a useful vaccine.

Many measures to prevent acquisition and spread of common colds have been tried, including polyvalent bacterial vaccines, alkalis, citrus fruits, vitamins, ultraviolet light, and glycol aerosols, but none has been effective. In controlled trials, large (as much as 2 gm/day) prophylactic oral doses of vitamin C have not altered the frequency of acquisition of common rhinovirus colds or the amount of virus shedding, but some

studies have shown a reduced duration of disability among persons who took as much as 8 gm/day on the first day of disease; virus shedding is not reduced. Intranasal application of alpha interferon, 1 to 2 million u. q 8 to 12 h, limits acquisition of rhinovirus infection and virus shedding under controlled conditions. It might promise clinical benefit in patients at risk for greater morbidity from colds, such as people with asthma or bronchitis. Prophylactic administration of an interferon inducer has shown protective and beneficial effects; however, biologic and logistic limitations prevent practical use.

Conscientious handwashing may be beneficial for family units, where most viral respiratory infections are spread, since many viruses, particularly rhinoviruses, are spread by person-to-person contact via contaminated secretions on fingers. The use of nasal wipes that have been treated to inactivate the virus has been suggested, but they have not been proven to decrease spread and they are more expensive than regular tissues.

Treatment

A warm, comfortable environment and measures to avoid direct spread of infection are recommended for all persons. Rest at home is indicated for children, preadolescents, and all febrile patients. Though antipyretics and analgesics are commonly used, their benefit, except on fever, is doubtful. Under some conditions, aspirin can increase virus shedding while producing only slight symptomatic improvement and therefore its regular use is not recommended unless symptoms are severe enough to keep the patient at home in relative isolation. If influenza is the etiology of the cold, aspirin may increase the risk of Reye's syndrome in children.

Oral phenylpropanolamine 15 to 50 mg, 0.5% phenylephrine or ephedrine nose drops or spray, or a nasal inhaler (not more often than q 3 or 4 h) can provide temporary nasal decongestion. Steam inhalations help relieve chest tightness. Cough is infrequently severe in the common cold. If present, follow the recommendations for treatment of bronchitis or influenza. In persons with nasal allergy, antihistamines reduce rhinorrhea, but they are of no use in other people. Ascorbic acid or high doses of citrus juices are popular, mostly on lay recommendation; no adequate scientific data confirm any benefit. Antibiotics do not affect viruses and are *not recommended* unless a specific bacterial complication develops.

RESPIRATORY SYNCYTIAL VIRUS (RSV)

(See under VIRAL INFECTIONS in Ch. 191)

INFLUENZA

(Grippe; Grip; "Flu")

A specific acute viral respiratory disease characterized by fever, coryza, cough, headache, malaise, and inflamed respiratory mucous membranes. It usually occurs as an epidemic in the winter. Prostration, hemorrhagic bronchitis, pneumonia, and sometimes death occur in severe cases.

Etiology

Influenza is caused by one of the myxoviruses. These are RNA viruses 80 to 120 nm in size with a core of helical nucleic acid and a soluble nucleoprotein (NP or S) antigen. On the basis of the reaction of this antigen with specific antibody in a CF test, influenza viruses are classified into Types A, B, and C. The virion has a limiting membrane and is enveloped in a coat composed principally of 2 glycoproteins, one having hemagglutinating activity **(HA)** and one having enzymatic activity as a neuraminidase **(NA)**. Both are strain-specific antigens. Myxoviruses attach to a specific glycoprotein receptor for the hemagglutinin on the cell surface. The virus is engulfed, its envelope fuses with the vacuolar membrane, and the viral genetic material enters the cell. After intracellular replication of the viral components, the virus is assembled

at the cell surface and is released from the cell by a budding process in which the viral NA participates.

Different serotypes of influenza A viruses are numbered H_0N_1, H_1N_1, H_2N_2, and H_3N_2 according to the major surface antigens of strains that have caused epidemics of disease in humans since the virus was first isolated in 1933. Currently both H_3N_2 and H_1N_1 types are causing prevalent disease. Usually only the most recent serotype causes epidemics, but strains of similar antigenic composition can recycle after several years of absence, probably by genetic reconstruction of infectious viruses, rather than re-emergence from a reservoir. Influenza B viruses show strain-specific variations, but the cross-relationship among strains is much greater than with influenza A. Specific numbers are not assigned to the Type B surface antigens. Influenza C is not a prevalent virus, and serotypes, if they occur, are not defined.

Epidemiology

Influenza A virus is the most frequent single cause of clinical influenza, which is also caused by influenza B, paramyxo-, and rarely by rhino- or echoviruses. Spread is by person-to-person contact and airborne droplet spray contaminates articles with viruses that can transmit infection. Influenza produces widespread sporadic respiratory illness every year. Acute epidemics occur about every 3 yr, generally nationwide during late fall or early winter. A major shift in the prevalent antigenic type of influenza A virus has occurred about once in a decade and has resulted in an acute pandemic. Persons of all ages are afflicted, but prevalence is highest in school children, and severity is greatest in the very young, aged, or infirm. **Persons at high risk** of developing severe disease are those with chronic pulmonary diseases; those with valvular heart disease with or without congestive heart failure, or other heart disease with pulmonary edema; pregnant women in the 3rd trimester; and persons who are aged, very young, or confined to bed. Influenza B, but not influenza C, has caused equally severe disease.

Epidemics often occur in 2 waves—the first in students and active family members, the second mostly in shut-ins and persons in semi-closed institutions. Influenza B causes epidemics about every 5 yr and is much less often associated with pandemics. Influenza C is an endemic virus that sporadically causes mild respiratory disease.

Symptoms and Signs

During the 48-h incubation period, transient asymptomatic viremia is quite likely before symptoms of infection, and virus replication localizes in the respiratory tract. Influenza A or B is sudden in onset, with chilliness and fever up to 39 to 39.5 C (102 to 103 F) developing over 24 h. Prostration and generalized aches and pains (most pronounced in the back and legs) appear early. Headache is prominent, often with photophobia and retrobulbar aching. Respiratory tract symptoms may be mild at first, with sore throat, substernal burning, nonproductive cough, and sometimes coryza; later the respiratory disease becomes dominant. Cough can be severe and productive. The skin, especially on the face, is warm and flushed. The soft palate, posterior hard palate, tonsillar pillars, and posterior pharyngeal wall may be reddened, but there is no exudate. The eyes water easily and the conjunctiva may be mildly inflamed. Usually, after 2 to 3 days, acute symptoms subside rapidly and fever ends, though fever lasting up to 5 days may occur without complications. Abnormal bronchociliary clearance and altered bronchiolar air flow are regularly present. Weakness, sweating, and fatigue may persist for several days or occasionally for weeks.

In severe cases, hemorrhagic bronchitis and pneumonia are frequent and can develop within hours. Fulminant fatal viral pneumonia occasionally occurs; dyspnea, cyanosis, hemoptysis, pulmonary edema, and death may proceed as soon as 48 h after onset of the influenza. Such severe disease is most likely to occur during a pandemic caused by a new influenza A serotype and in persons at high risk.

Complications

Secondary bacterial infection of the bronchi and sometimes pneumonia are suggested by persistence of fever, cough, and other respiratory symptoms for more than 5 days. Pneumonia should be suspected if dyspnea, cyanosis, hemoptysis, rales, a secondary rise in temperature, or a relapse develops. With pneumonia, cough increases and purulent or bloody sputum is produced. Crepitant or subcrepitant rales can be detected over the involved pulmonary segments. The bacterial etiology of this secondary pneumonia is related to age and environment. Pneumococci, streptococci, and *Hemophilus influenzae* are common causes, especially in ambulatory nonhospitalized or young patients. Pneumococci, staphylococci, and *Klebsiella pneumoniae* are the most common causes in older, infirm, or hospitalized patients. (See also Ch. 40.)

Encephalitis, myocarditis, and myoglobinuria may also occur as complications of influenza, usually during convalescence. The virus is rarely recovered from affected organs and the specific relationship and pathogenesis of these diseases cannot be positively established. However, an increase in such diseases regularly follows influenza A pandemics. Reye's syndrome (see under MISCELLANEOUS INFECTIONS in Ch. 191), characterized by encephalopathy, fatty liver, hypoglycemia, and lipidemia, has been prominently associated with epidemics of influenza B.

Diagnosis

Clinical influenza is a common experience and a frequently made lay diagnosis. The specific viral disease cannot be diagnosed clinically except during epidemics. In the early stages of infection or in uncomplicated cases, chest examination is usually normal. In mild cases, the symptoms are those of a febrile or afebrile common cold. Pulmonary symptoms may be those of bronchitis or atypical pneumonia, especially during epidemics. In distinguishing influenza from other respiratory tract infections, one should consider the season and whether an influenza epidemic is in progress; the mode of onset and severity of symptoms; and the presence or absence of a tonsillar or pharyngeal exudate, other signs of localized infection, or evidence of suppurative disease. The leukocyte count is normal in uncomplicated cases; sometimes a leukopenia with a relative lymphocytosis may be present. Fever and severe constitutional symptoms differentiate influenza from the common cold. No exudate is present over the tonsils and pharyngeal wall as it is in hemolytic streptococcal tonsillitis and sometimes with adenoviral infection. Petechiae or ulcers on the palate might signify infectious mononucleosis or a herpes or coxsackie viral infection.

A **specific diagnosis** of influenza can be made by virus isolation, demonstration of viral NA activity in secretions, or serologic tests. During the first several days, the virus can be recovered from respiratory secretions. The specimen can be collected as sputum, but more often throat washings are obtained by gargling a buffered saline solution, usually with a small amount of protein such as albumin or gelatin; if necessary, diluted skim milk can be used. A rapid diagnosis can be made if the specimen cleaves a fluoroscent product, 4-methyl umbelliferyl alpha ketoside of N-acetyl neuraminic acid from a labeled substrate by specific NA activity. The recently prevalent strains of influenza virus have not been difficult to isolate in either tissue cultures or embryonated eggs. During epidemics, it is important to isolate and identify influenza viruses early. For this purpose, State Health Laboratories and, through them, the National Centers for Disease Control and International Influenza Reference Centers assist in strain identification.

Leukocytosis, with juvenile granulocytes in the blood smear, is a valuable diagnostic sign of complicating bacterial pneumonia. Purulent sputum should be smeared, gram-stained, and examined for leukocytes and bacteria. Sputum and blood cultures and other examinations should be made to identify the specific bacterial species and to determine the extent of secondary infection.

Serologic tests used are predominantly CF and HI tests. Serial serum specimens are

best, the first collected at the onset of illness and another a week or more later. The 2 specimens are tested simultaneously to demonstrate a rise in the specific antibody titer. If only a single serum specimen is available after the disease is already well developed, a high CF antibody titer may indicate recent infection; the HI titer may reflect previous infection or vaccination.

Prognosis

Recovery is the rule in uncomplicated influenza. However, viral pneumonia and other virus-related complications may cause death in some patients, especially those identified above as being at high risk. Chemotherapy decreases the fatality rate of severe secondary bacterial pneumonia.

Prophylaxis

Vaccines that include the prevalent strains of influenza viruses effectively reduce the incidence of infection among vaccinees for 1 or 2 yr after vaccination. The immunity is less when appreciable antigenic drift occurs in the virus; when a major antigenic mutation occurs, no significant protection is afforded unless the new strain is incorporated into the vaccine. Vaccine is prepared as inactivated whole virus or as subunits of the virus, either semi-purified viral hemagglutinin or disrupted virion components. Both types of vaccine are equally protective. Under development are attenuated live virus vaccines given intranasally. They have the advantage of eliciting specific secretory antibody at the portal of virus entry.

Vaccination is especially important for the aged and for patients with cardiac, pulmonary, or other chronic diseases. Pregnant women whose 3rd trimester occurs during the winter months should be vaccinated also. Immunization, preferably in the fall, usually consists of 1 dose of vaccine, but when new strains arise primary immunization should consist of 2 injections, given 1 mo apart, of vaccine containing the new strains. After vaccination, about 2 wk is required to develop immunity. Because immunity from vaccination lasts only 1 or 2 yr, an annual booster dose early in the fall is required for optimal protection. Primary or booster doses are 0.5 to 1 mL s.c. or IM. With the presently available purified vaccines, local or constitutional reactions are uncommon or minor, except sometimes in children. Children < 13 yr should receive split virus vaccine, since the side effects are fewer. Also, because children have had reduced exposure to multiple wild strains of influenza virus, both a primary and a booster dose (0.5 mL each for children 3 to 12 yr, 0.25 mL each for children 6 to 35 mo) 1 mo apart are recommended unless vaccination has been administered in prior years.

Amantadine 100 mg orally bid (for adults) can be used prophylactically against influenza A. It is ineffective against influenza B. During influenza A epidemics, it should be given to family members and other close contacts of patients and to persons at high risk of increased morbidity from influenza. During administration of amantadine, persons at high risk of infection who have not been vaccinated previously should receive vaccine; then amantadine may be discontinued in 3 wk. If vaccine cannot be given, amantadine must be continued for the duration of the epidemic, usually 6 or 8 wk. Amantidine causes nervousness, insomnia, or other side effects in 7% of people. Rimantadine (presently an investigational new drug in the USA) is an analog of amantadine and has different pharmacokinetics and causes fewer adverse effects at a comparable dose. It can be used as an alternative to amantadine with approximately equal efficacy.

Influenza renders the patient temporarily immune to reinfection with the same virus serotype and incompletely immune to variants from antigenic drift.

Treatment

Amantadine has a beneficial effect on fever and respiratory symptoms if given early in uncomplicated influenza A. It has no clinical benefit when used for pneumonia, but might improve the recovery of pulmonary function. Ribavirin (see in RESPIRATORY

SYNCYTIAL VIRUS under VIRAL INFECTIONS in Ch. 191) administered by small-particle aerosol can shorten the duration of fever and reduce virus shedding in severe cases of influenza A or B infection, and may favorably reverse the course of primary influenzal pneumonia.

The basic treatment for most patients is symptomatic. The patient should remain in bed or rest adequately and avoid exertion during the acute stage and for 24 to 48 h after the temperature becomes normal. If constitutional symptoms of acute uncomplicated influenza are severe, antipyretics and analgesics (eg, for adults, aspirin 600 mg, or acetaminophen 650 mg, orally q 4 h) are helpful. To relieve nasal obstruction, 1 or 2 drops of 0.25% phenylephrine may be instilled into the nose periodically. Steam inhalation may alleviate respiratory symptoms somewhat and also prevent drying of secretions. Treatment of respiratory symptoms may be unnecessary in less severe cases. Complicating bacterial infections require appropriate antibiotics.

PARAINFLUENZA VIRUSES

Three principal, closely related viruses causing a number of respiratory illnesses varying from the common cold to influenza-like pneumonia, with febrile croup as their most common severe manifestation.

Etiology

The parainfluenza viruses are RNA paramyxoviruses and consist of 4 serologically distinct agents categorized as Types 1, 2, 3, and 4. Early human isolates of parainfluenza Types 1 and 3 were called "hemadsorption **(HA)** viruses." The initial Type 2 isolates were designated "croup-associated **(CA)** viruses." Though the 4 types tend to cause diseases of different severity, they share common antigens, as evidenced by cross-reactive antibody responses, and are similar structurally and biologically. Type 4 has antigenic cross-reactivity with mumps. Though each type of parainfluenza virus has a corresponding serotype that causes specific diseases in animals, cross-infection of animals to man or vice versa either does not occur or the transfer is very inefficient. The corresponding strains of animal origin for Types 1, 2, and 3 are Sendai virus (mice), Simian virus 5 (SV-5), and shipping fever virus of cattle (SF-4).

Epidemiology

Infections with Types 1 and 3 are common in early childhood; sharp localized outbreaks occur in nurseries, schools, pediatric wards, and orphanages. Widespread community epidemics are prevented by almost universal immunity in adults and reinfection usually causes a mild URI. Infection with each type produces different epidemiologic patterns. Parainfluenza infections occur in all seasons, but epidemic disease in the fall is more likely to be due to Type 1, which comprises ½ of the isolates. The epidemic types, 1 and 2, tend to recur reciprocally every other year. Type 3 disease is endemic, highly contagious, occurs in all seasons, and causes ⅓ of the infections. The incubation period is usually 24 to 48 h with Type 3, and 4 to 5 days with Type 1. Type 2 is more sporadic and causes modest epidemics of infantile croup (acute laryngotracheobronchitis). The parainfluenza viruses are a chief cause of this condition. Type 4 causes mild respiratory illness, but only rarely.

Second and even third infections with the same strains of virus, particularly with Types 1 and 3, are not uncommon, though the partial immunity developed during previous episodes may reduce the spread and severity of subsequent infections.

Symptoms and Signs

The most common illness produced in children is an acute febrile respiratory infection that is clinically indistinguishable from influenza or other respiratory virus infection occurring in the same age group. Onset is marked by fever and moderate coryza. The degree of malaise is directly related to the height of the fever. In many cases, the

temperature does not exceed 38 or 39 C (101 or 102 F); in others, it may peak several times to 40 C (104 F). Moderate sore throat and a dry cough usually develop early in the disease. Hoarseness and croup are prominent symptoms in many cases; this **acute laryngotracheobronchitis** (see CROUP under VIRAL INFECTIONS in Ch. 191) is the most severe and dangerous manifestation of parainfluenza virus infections in children.

Fever may subside promptly or continue for 2 or 3 days. In some patients, particularly those who develop lower respiratory tract involvement, fever lasting a week or more may recur one or more times.

Bronchitis and "walking" pneumonia often develop during or after the initial acute episode in children and sometimes adults infected with Type 3. Pneumonia is detected by auscultation that reveals moist rales in one or more lung areas and by chest x-ray. Bacterial complications are not common.

Diagnosis

A specific diagnosis of parainfluenza infection cannot be made clinically. Virus isolation and identification require tissue culture inoculation. CF, HI, and hemadsorption-neutralization tests with acute and convalescent sera will confirm a parainfluenza infection but serologic cross-reactions can make it difficult to identify the specific parainfluenza virus without a virus isolate.

Prognosis

Except for infantile croup, illnesses due to the parainfluenza viruses, although frequent, are usually mild, self-limited, and of brief duration. The bronchitis and pneumonia associated with Type 3 infections seldom cause serious disability and are rarely, if ever, fatal.

Prophylaxis and Treatment

No effective vaccine is available and there is no specific therapy. Rest and a comfortable environment are the best remedies. Aspirin is not recommended unless the fever is high or the symptoms prevent sleep. If necessary, antitussives (eg, dextromethorphan 1 to 1.5 mg/kg/day orally in 6 divided doses) will suppress cough. For treatment of croup, see that discussion under VIRAL INFECTIONS in Ch. 191.

ADENOVIRUSES

A group of many viruses, some of which cause acute febrile disorders characterized by inflammation of the respiratory and ocular mucous membranes and hyperplasia of submucous and regional lymphoid tissue.

Etiology

Adenoviruses are DNA viruses 60 to 90 nm in size. The virion is shaped like an icosahedron. Three major antigens can be directly related to the capsid structures. Most important is the hexon, a 6-sided capsomere comprising 240 of the 252 capsomeres. It reacts with specific antisera in a non–type-specific CF reaction and thus serves as a group antigen to identify all types of adenoviruses. Virus-neutralizing antibody, however, is type-specific. The 2nd major antigen is associated with a penton, a 5-sided capsomere located at the 12 common vertices of the 20 triangles that form the icosahedron. It is a type-specific antigen that can be differentiated in neutralization or HI tests. The 3rd antigen is a fiber antigen related to the threadlike structure extending from the apices of the virion. Not infrequently, adenoviruses have another smaller DNA virus associated with them, called **adenoassociated virus (AAV)**. It is a defective virus that requires complementation by adenovirus in order to replicate. The importance of AAV in adenovirus infections is not known.

Epidemiology

About 4 to 5% of clinically recognized respiratory illnesses in civilian populations are caused by adenoviruses. Of the 41 known serotypes, only a few have been adequately observed in relation to human disease to determine their prevalence and ability to produce illness (see TABLE 12–3). **Different serotypes have quite different epidemiologies**: Types 1, 2, and 5 cause sharp, limited outbreaks of respiratory or enteric illness during the first few months or years of life. Type 2 has been relatively more common in some of these episodes. In older children and adults, Type 3 causes a characteristic syndrome of acute pharyngoconjunctival fever **(APC)**, especially among patrons of summer camps and swimming pools. Acute respiratory disease **(ARD)** occurs in military camps and is caused by Types 4, 7, 14, and 21. In some countries, ARD epidemics have also been apparent among civilian populations, but not in the USA. Epidemic keratoconjunctivitis **(EKC)** is caused by one of several types and is seen largely among persons in industrial plants and eye clinics.

Adenoviruses also often primarily infect the intestinal tract, usually without causing symptoms, although enteritis, mesenteric adenitis, and intussusception can occur. Fol-

TABLE 12–3. SYNDROMES CAUSED BY ADENOVIRUSES

Disease	*Serotypes Implicated* Common	Less Common	Comments
Respiratory only:			
Acute febrile respiratory disease of children	1, 2, 3, 5, 6	Other types	Probably the most frequent manifestation of adenoviruses; Types 1, 2, & 5 endemic; Type 3 occasionally epidemic; more prevalent during cold months
Acute respiratory disease (ARD)	4, 7	14, 21	Epidemic in military recruits; sporadic in adult civilians; Types 4 & 7 infections rare in children
Viral pneumonia:			
Infants	7	1, 3	Rare; occurs in hospital nurseries; may be fatal; similar to Goodpasture's inclusion body pneumonitis
Adults	4, 7	3	Predominantly associated with acute respiratory disease; cold agglutinins not developed
Ocular only:			
Acute follicular conjunctivitis	3, 7	2, 4, 6, 9, 10, 21	Sporadic; adults chiefly affected; in children, usually associated with respiratory & systemic effects
Epidemic keratoconjunctivitis (EKC)	8 (classic)	3, 7 (mild)	Epidemic; adults mainly affected; widespread in Japan, rare in USA
Combined respiratory & ocular:			
Acute pharyngoconjunctival fever (APC)	3, 7	1, 2, 5, 6, 14, 21	Epidemic in children; sporadic in adults; summer epidemics frequently associated with swimming in pools or lakes

lowing infection with Types 1, 2, and 5, the virus may remain latent in the tonsils and adenoids; about 80% of excised tonsils yield such virus.

The ratio of manifest disease to infection rates varies with the different syndromes and serotypes and according to the season when infected. In winter, infection of military recruits with adenovirus Types 4 or 7 causes recognizable illness in most cases and about 25% require hospitalization for fever and lower respiratory tract disease. APC occurs in a high proportion of Type 3 infections in the summer. The ratio of illness to infection is lower with Types 1, 2, 5, and some of the less studied, higher-numbered adenoviruses.

Pathology

Adenoviral infections are rarely fatal and have few, if any, recognizable long-term pathologic effects. Some deaths have occurred with giant-cell pneumonia associated with adenovirus Types 3, 4, or 7. Autopsies have disclosed microscopically an extensive and unique inclusion body pneumonia, the intranuclear inclusions appearing to be similar to those considered characteristic of adenoviral cellular invasions in tissue cultures. Biopsies of superficial lesions produced by adenoviruses in conjunctival and pharyngeal mucosa show capillary dilation, occasional submucous hemorrhage, and mononuclear leukocyte infiltration, but no intranuclear inclusions. The conjunctivitis caused by the common respiratory types of adenoviruses is usually benign, but sometimes they cause keratoconjunctivitis, as does Type 8, with production of corneal opacities and impaired vision.

Symptoms and Signs

Acute febrile respiratory disease is the usual manifestation of known adenoviral infection in children. Adenoviruses Types 1, 2, 3, 5, and 6 have been isolated most commonly, though infection with these types is often not directly associated with any specific illness. Infection is airborne or waterborne (by swimming), or acquired by direct contact. The incubation period is 2 to 5 days. In a typical outbreak confined to a household or nursery, some affected children have fever only, without localizing signs; others have fever and pharyngitis; others have fever with pharyngitis, tracheitis, and bronchitis, a moderately persistent nonproductive cough, and, rarely, pneumonia. Cough with adenoviral pneumonia has been confused with pertussis in children. Pharyngeal lymphoid hypertrophy sometimes persists and leads to eustachian tube obstruction and possibly otitis media. Regional lymph nodes are frequently enlarged and sometimes tender, but they never suppurate. Laboratory findings are generally within normal limits, though some children may show a lymphocytosis.

A disease syndrome designated **ARD (acute respiratory disease)** has been observed in military recruits during 2 periods of troop mobilization. Adenovirus Types 4 and 7 have been reported in most outbreaks in the USA, but Types 14 and 21 have also been incriminated. ARD is marked by malaise, fever, chills, and headache. Respiratory manifestations include nasopharyngitis, hoarseness, and dry cough. The disease may resemble streptococcal pharyngitis with exudate on the faucial pillars and posterior pharyngeal wall. Cervical adenopathy is present, but the nodes are not as tender as in streptococcal pharyngitis. Viremia and viruria have been demonstrated and there may be a fine erythematous macular rash on the body, but the viruria occurring with these respiratory strains of adenoviruses does not produce symptoms like those of the epidemic hemorrhagic cystitis that occurs as a primary disease with Type 11. Physical signs are minimal except in about 10% of patients, who develop rales and x-ray evidence of pneumonia. Fever usually subsides within 2 to 4 days; convalescence, while uneventful, may require another 10 to 14 days.

Viral pneumonia of infants, due chiefly to Type 7, is a rare but specific clinicopathologic entity. Small outbreaks have occurred in France, South Africa, the USA, China,

and Japan, with fatalities due to extensive pneumonia. Onset is sudden, affecting infants in the first few days or weeks of life up to 2 to 3 yr, with high fever and rapid upper and lower respiratory tract involvement. The pneumonia is lobular but may be so extensive as to suggest lobar pneumonia. Several fatal cases developed a maculopapular rash and encephalitis, with focal necrosis apparent in the brain, skin, and lungs.

Acute pharyngoconjunctival fever (APC) produces the clinical triad of fever, pharyngitis, and conjunctivitis. Infection is sometimes waterborne. The incubation period is 5 to 8 days. Adenovirus Types 3 and 7 have been reported in nearly all outbreaks. In a typical outbreak, 50% or more of the patients have all 3 components, while others may have only 1 or 2. The conjunctivitis is initially unilateral and sometimes painful. Involvement of the lower respiratory tract may occur in addition to pharyngitis. The illness usually subsides within a week, but follicular conjunctivitis may persist for another week.

Conjunctivitis without constitutional symptoms appears to be a rather common manifestation of infection with several different adenovirus serotypes. It occurs most often in young adults, chiefly parents of children with APC, and is self-limited and benign. Onset is sudden and usually unilateral. Symptoms and signs include a foreign-body sensation in the eye, lacrimation, and focal erythema of the palpebral and bulbar conjunctiva. The discharge is mucoid but not purulent. The other eye is subsequently involved in about half the patients, usually less severely. Persistent follicular enlargement of submucous lymphoid tissue under the palpebral conjunctiva, even resembling early trachoma, may be seen about 2 to 4 days after onset. Preauricular and posterior cervical lymphadenopathy, more prominent on the same side as the more involved eye, is usual. A mild sore throat occasionally develops, often on the same side as the affected eye. The course is usually mild, though focal conjunctival hemorrhages and extensive periorbital edema occasionally occur.

Epidemic keratoconjunctivitis (EKC) is a specific, sometimes severe, epidemic disease caused by adenovirus, especially Type 8. Observed for many years in Japan, it became epidemic in the USA during World War II, chiefly among shipyard workers on both coasts. It has occurred only sporadically in this country since then, but widespread epidemics have occurred in Europe and Asia. Onset is sudden, one eye showing redness and chemosis followed by periorbital swelling, preauricular lymphadenopathy, and superficial corneal opacities. Unlike herpetic keratitis, it does not result in corneal ulceration; local pain like that from foreign-body irritation is usual, however. The other eye may become involved within a week. Systemic symptoms and signs are mild or absent. The illness usually lasts 3 or 4 wk, though opacities may persist much longer and vision has sometimes been permanently impaired.

Mild, transient corneal involvement has been observed in eye infections (eg, APC) with other adenoviruses (Types 3, 4, and 7), but the opacities are seldom noticeable except to an ophthalmologist.

Diagnosis

Clinical identification of adenoviral infection is only presumptive, except in typical APC, EKC, and ARD in military recruits; in these conditions the clinical or epidemiologic characteristics, or both, are unique. During the acute stages of adenoviral illnesses, the virus can be isolated for 7 to 10 days from respiratory and ocular secretions, and frequently from feces and urine. Several serologic procedures (CF, HI, and neutralization tests) can be performed on acute and convalescent sera. A fourfold rise in the serum antibody titer indicates recent adenoviral infection. The CF test is group-specific for any adenovirus serotype. HI and neutralization tests are type-specific. Commercial antigen is available for the CF test but not for the latter 2 tests.

Prognosis

Adenoviral infections are generally benign and of relatively short duration. Except for rare cases of fulminating primary pnuemonia in young infants and military recruits, even severe adenoviral pneumonia is not fatal.

Prophylaxis

Live Type 4 and 7 adenovirus vaccine, given orally in an enteric-coated capsule, has markedly reduced ARD in military populations. Spread of the vaccine virus among family members with intimate contact can occur, but it is of no apparent importance. The live oral vaccine is neither recommended nor available for civilian use. Vaccines for other serotypes have not been developed. Among civilians, adenoviruses causing outbreaks of adenovirus conjunctivitis are spread by contact with contaminated objects (towels, instruments, etc), by secretions, or by finger transmission. Proper sterilization, gloving and hand washing before and after examination of infected patients, and avoidance of multiple patient exposures to ophthalmologic instruments are recommended to prevent transfer of virus.

Treatment

Treatment is symptomatic and supportive. Bed rest at home or infirmary care may be required during the acute febrile period. Aspirin is not recommended unless headache and malaise are distressing; analgesics such as codeine are rarely necessary. Severe pneumonia in infants and EKC require early hospitalization and close supervision to prevent death in the former and permanently impaired vision in the latter. Topical corticosteroids relieve symptoms and shorten the course of EKC and adenoviral conjunctivitis. Such therapy is dangerous in ulcerative corneal conditions, however, and should always be supervised by an ophthalmologist.

HERPES VIRUSES

HERPES SIMPLEX

A recurrent viral infection characterized by the appearance on the skin or mucous membranes of single or multiple clusters of small vesicles, filled with clear fluid, on slightly raised inflammatory bases.

Etiology

The infecting agent is the relatively large herpes simplex virus **(HSV)**, also known as herpesvirus hominis. There are 2 HSV strains, HSV-1 and HSV-2. HSV-1 commonly causes herpes labialis and keratitis; HSV-2 is usually genital and is transmitted primarily by direct contact with lesions, most often venereally. The time of initial HSV infection is often obscure, except in the primary systemic infection that is occasionally seen in infants (see NEONATAL HERPES SIMPLEX VIRUS INFECTION under NEONATAL INFECTIONS in Ch. 186) and is characterized by generalized or localized cutaneous and mucosal lesions accompanied by severe constitutional symptoms. Localized infections ordinarily occur more frequently in childhood, but may be delayed until adult life. Presumably, the virus remains dormant in the skin or nerve ganglia, and recurrent herpetic eruptions can be precipitated by overexposure to sunlight, febrile illnesses, physical or emotional stress, or certain foods and drugs. The trigger mechanism is often unknown.

Symptoms and Signs

The lesions may appear anywhere on the skin or mucosa, but are most frequent about the mouth, on the lips, on the conjunctiva and cornea, and on the genitalia. Following a short prodromal period of tingling discomfort or itching, small tense

vesicles appear on an erythematous base. Single clusters vary in size from 0.5 to 1.5 cm, but several groups may coalesce. Herpes simplex on skin tensely attached to underlying structures (eg, the nose, ears, or fingers) may be painful. The vesicles persist for a few days, then begin to dry, forming a thin yellowish crust. Healing usually begins 7 to 10 days after onset and is complete by 21 days. Healing may be slower, with secondary inflammation, in moist body areas. Individual herpetic lesions usually heal completely, but recurrent lesions at the same site may cause atrophy and scarring.

Variations and Complications

Genital herpes is discussed in Ch. 14, herpes simplex keratitis in Ch. 220, and primary and recurrent herpetic stomatitis and herpes labialis in ORAL HERPETIC MANIFESTATIONS in STOMATITIS in Ch. 247. Gingivostomatitis and vulvovaginitis may occur as a result of herpes infection in infants or young children. Symptoms include irritability, anorexia, fever, gingival inflammation, and painful ulcers of the mouth and occasionally of the vulva and vagina. In infants and sometimes in older children, primary infections may cause extensive organ involvement and fatal viremia. Women with HSV-2 infection late in pregnancy may transmit the infection to the fetus, with the development of severe viremia (see in NEONATAL HERPES SIMPLEX VIRUS INFECTION under NEONATAL INFECTIONS in Ch. 186). Herpes simplex occasionally causes severe encephalitis (see ACUTE VIRAL ENCEPHALITIS AND MENINGITIS in Ch. 125). HSV-2 has also been associated with usually self-limited aseptic meningitis or lumbosacral myeloradiculitis syndromes. **Kaposi's varicelliform eruption (eczema herpeticum)** is a potentially fatal complication of infantile or adult atopic eczema; patients with extensive atopic dermatitis should **avoid** exposure to persons with active herpes simplex. Herpes simplex may be followed by typical erythema multiforme, but the relationship is sometimes uncertain because a variety of other infectious agents and drugs can induce an identical syndrome.

Diagnosis

Herpes simplex may be confused with herpes zoster, but the latter rarely recurs and usually causes more severe pain and larger groups of lesions that are distributed along the course of a sensory nerve. Differential diagnosis also includes varicella, genital ulcers or gingivostomatitis due to other causes, and vesicular dermatoses, particularly dermatitis herpetiformis and drug eruptions. When herpes simplex is suspected, cultures for the virus, a progressive increase in serum antibodies (in primary infections), and biopsy findings confirm the diagnosis.

Treatment

In superficial infections, topical agents such as idoxuridine **(IDU)**, trifluorothymidine, or acyclovir are sometimes effective (see discussions of specific herpetic disorders). Smallpox vaccinations have been used prophylactically but may be dangerous and should *not* be used.

Gentle cleansing with soap and water is recommended, but keeping lesions moist may aggravate the inflammation and delay healing.

In secondary infections, topical antibiotics (eg, neomycin-bacitracin ointment) or, if severe, systemic antibiotics are indicated.

In herpes simplex with systemic manifestations, vigorous supportive therapy (control of electrolyte balance, parenteral fluid, blood transfusions, and systemic antibiotics) may be necessary. Systemic treatment with acyclovir or vidarabine has been used in serious herpes infections, such as disseminated neonatal disease, and acyclovir therapy has been of particular benefit in some cases of herpes simplex encephalitis. Acyclovir is now available in an oral preparation for suppressing recurrent eruptions of genital herpes.

CYTOMEGALOVIRUS (CMV) INFECTION

(Cytomegalic Inclusion Disease)

(See also CONGENITAL AND PERINATAL CYTOMEGALOVIRUS INFECTION under NEONATAL INFECTIONS in Ch. 186)

A virus infection occurring congenitally, postnatally, or at any age, and ranging in severity from a silent infection without consequences, through disease manifested by fever, hepatitis, pneumonitis, and (in neonates) severe brain damage, to stillbirth or perinatal death. The restrictive appellation "cytomegalic inclusion disease" refers to the intranuclear inclusions found in enlarged infected cells.

Etiology and Epidemiology

The human cytomegaloviruses ("salivary gland viruses") are a subgroup of agents within the herpes group of viruses, all of which have the propensity for remaining latent in man. Molecular analysis of the DNA of CMV isolates reveals minor strain-specific differences that are useful markers in epidemiological investigation. Cytomegaloviruses are highly host-specific and cannot be propagated in laboratory animals or in most nonhuman cell cultures.

The cytomegaloviruses are ubiquitous. Infected individuals may excrete virus in the urine or saliva for months; virus may be demonstrable in human cervical secretions, semen, feces, and milk; fresh blood or organs (eg, kidneys) from asymptomatic infected donors may produce disease in susceptible recipients. Infection may be acquired transplacentally, during birth, or by contact with infected secretions or excretions at any time thereafter. High infection rates may occur at early ages in closed populations such as orphanages and infant day care centers, and are the rule in active male homosexual groups. Prevalence in the general population increases gradually with age; 60 to 90% of adults have experienced infection.

Symptoms and Signs

Congenital infection: The extent of the pathologic process is highly variable. Infection may be manifested only by cytomegaloviruria in an otherwise apparently normal infant. At the other extreme, CMV infection may cause abortion, stillbirth, or postnatal death from hemorrhage, anemia, or extensive hepatic or CNS damage. (See CONGENITAL AND PERINATAL CYTOMEGALOVIRUS INFECTION under NEONATAL INFECTIONS in Ch. 186.)

Acquired infection: Infections acquired postnatally or later in life are often asymptomatic. An acute febrile illness, termed **cytomegalovirus mononucleosis** or **cytomegalovirus hepatitis,** may result from iatrogenic or spontaneous contact with CMV. **Postperfusion syndrome** develops 2 to 4 wk after transfusion with fresh blood containing CMV and is characterized by fever lasting 2 to 3 wk, hepatitis of variable degree with or without jaundice, a characteristic atypical lymphocytosis resembling that of infectious mononucleosis, and occasionally a rash. In patients receiving immunosuppressive therapy, CMV infections, acquired or due to reactivation of a latent process, may cause pulmonary, GI, or renal involvement. This complication is of major import, with a 50% attack rate and high associated mortality in some reported transplantation series. Disseminated CMV infection is common in the terminal phase of AIDS.

Diagnosis

CMV may be isolated from urine, other body fluids, or tissues by inoculation of human fibroblastic cell cultures. However, CMV may be excreted for months or years after infection and cytomegaloviruria must be interpreted accordingly. The appearance of specific CF antibodies during illness provides supportive evidence. New, more rapid approaches based on demonstrating CMV in secretions or tissues by immunofluorescence with commercially available monoclonal antibodies, or by in situ hybridization, are promising.

Congenital infection must be differentiated from bacterial, viral (eg, rubella), and protozoan (eg, toxoplasmosis) infections. Acquired infection must be differentiated from viral hepatitis and infectious mononucleosis. The absence of pharyngitis or lymphadenopathy, and a negative heterophil antibody test, help to rule out infectious mononucleosis.

Treatment

No specific therapy is available. CMV, compared to other herpes-related viruses, is resistant to acyclovir. Pre- and postoperative use of interferon-alpha in renal transplant recipients reduces the consequences of the CMV reactivation syndrome.

CENTRAL NERVOUS SYSTEM VIRAL DISEASES

RABIES
(Hydrophobia)

An acute infectious disease of mammals, especially carnivores, characterized by CNS irritation followed by paralysis and death.

Etiology and Epidemiology

The etiologic agent is a neurotropic virus often present in the saliva of rabid animals. The use of monoclonal antibodies has revealed that rabies virus, previously thought to be stable, is as unstable in tissue culture as is the influenza virus. Several serotypes have been defined in the laboratory and from street isolates collected from different parts of the world. Identification of distinct virus serotypes is providing new information of value in epidemiology and vaccine production.

Rabid animals transmit the infection by biting animals or humans. Rabies may also be acquired by exposure of a mucous membrane or fresh skin abrasion to infected saliva. Four cases of apparent respiratory infection have been reported, 2 following laboratory exposure and 2 from the atmosphere of a cave infested by millions of guano bats. Worldwide, rabid dogs still present the highest risk to man. In the USA, where vaccination has largely controlled canine rabies, bites of infected wild animals have caused most cases of human rabies since 1960.

Infected dogs may have either **furious rabies,** characterized by agitation and viciousness, followed by paralysis and death; or **dumb rabies,** in which paralytic symptoms predominate. Rabid wild animals may show "furious" behavior, but less obvious changes (diurnal activity of normally nocturnal bats, skunks, and foxes; lack of normal fear of humans) are more likely.

Pathology

The virus has an affinity for nervous tissue. It travels from the site of entry via peripheral nerves to the spinal cord and the brain, where it multiplies; subsequently it continues through efferent nerves to the salivary glands and into the saliva. Postmortem examination shows vessel engorgement and associated punctate hemorrhages in the meninges and brain; microscopic examination shows perivascular collections of lymphocytes but little destruction of nerve cells. The presence of intracytoplasmic inclusion bodies **(Negri bodies),** usually in the cornu Ammonis, is pathognomonic of rabies, but these are not always found.

Symptoms and Signs

In man, the incubation period varies from 10 days to > 1 yr (average, 30 to 50 days). It is usually shortest in patients with extensive bites or bites about the head or trunk. The disease commonly begins with a short period of mental depression, restlessness, malaise, and fever. Restlessness increases to uncontrollable excitement, with excessive salivation and excruciatingly painful spasms of the laryngeal and pharyngeal muscles.

The spasms, which result from reflex irritability of the deglutition and respiration centers, are easily precipitated—eg, by a slight breeze or an attempt to drink water. As a result, the patient cannot drink, though his thirst is great (hence, "**hydrophobia**"). Death from asphyxia, exhaustion, or general paralysis formerly occurred within 3 to 10 days, but with modern supportive care patients may survive much longer.

Diagnosis

The fluorescent antibody test and virus isolation have replaced examination of the animal's brain for Negri bodies as the preferred method of diagnosis. An asymptomatic dog or cat that bites a human should, when practicable, be confined and observed by a veterinarian for 10 days. If the animal remains healthy, it can be safely concluded that it was not infectious at the time of the bite. When the biting animal was apparently rabid or was a wild animal (ie, whenever a biting animal must be proved uninfected to avoid human treatment), it should be killed immediately and the brain submitted to a diagnostic laboratory for fluorescent antibody testing.

In patients, diagnosis is suggested by a history of a compatible animal bite (infrequently absent) and confirmed by viral testing once the characteristic clinical symptoms appear. The diagnosis should be considered in cases with severe, progressive encephalitis or ascending paralysis with encephalitis. The latter presentation occurs in 20% of human rabies cases, and appears more often after exposure to rabid bats and possibly after postexposure therapy with nerve-tissue vaccines available in some countries outside the USA. Hysteria due to fright may follow a bite and give the impression of rabies, but the symptoms should subside promptly once the patient is assured that he is in no immediate danger and can be protected from rabies.

Control

Prevention and control require restraint of dogs by their owners and impoundment of stray dogs. Immunizing 70% or more of the canine population has effectively restricted transmission of the disease, even in areas where rabies is endemic among wildlife.

Controlling rabies in wildlife reservoirs is more difficult, especially when the wildlife host population is dense. Locally, rabies becomes self-limiting because it decimates susceptible hosts until epidemic disease can no longer be propagated. Adequate systematic reductions of host species yield the same result and prevent spread; however, these expensive control efforts are best limited to locales where human contact with wildlife is high (eg, campgrounds).

Prophylaxis

Postexposure: Rabies rarely occurs in man if proper local and systemic prophylaxis is carried out immediately after exposure. **Local wound treatment** may be the most valuable preventive measure. The contaminated area should be cleansed immediately and thoroughly with a 20% solution of medicinal soft soap. Deep puncture wounds should be flushed, using a catheter and soapy water. Cauterizing or suturing the wound is not advised.

Systemic postexposure prophylaxis (see TABLE 12–4) should be started immediately (1) if the animal is rabid or develops rabies during confinement or (2) if a domestic animal that is not available for observation or examination was behaving in an atypical manner or its biting was unprovoked *and* there is rabies in the area. Among wild animals, skunks, raccoons, foxes, and bats are particularly suspect and, unless proved uninfected by examination, their bites generally necessitate rabies treatment. Rabbits and rodents (including squirrels, chipmunks, rats, and mice) are rarely infected and their bites seldom justify rabies treatment. State or local health departments may be consulted on these decisions.

TABLE 12–4. POSTEXPOSURE ANTIRABIES GUIDE

The following guide should be used in conjunction with knowledge of the animal species involved, circumstances of the bite or other exposure, vaccination status of the animal, and presence of rabies in the region. Advice from local or state public health officials may be sought to help determine the need for prophylaxis.

Animal and Its Condition		*Treatment of Exposed Human**
Species	Condition at Time of Attack	
Wild		
Skunk, Fox, Coyote, Raccoon, Bat, other wild carnivore	Regard as rabid unless proven negative by laboratory test	RIG† + HDCV‡
Domestic		
Dog, Cat	Healthy (and available for observation)	None§
	Escaped (unknown)	Consult public health officials. If treatment is indicated, give RIG† + HDCV
	Rabid or suspected rabid	RIG† + HDCV
Others		
Including Livestock, Rodents, Rabbits	Consider individually: Bites of rodents almost never require prophylaxis	

RIG = Human rabies immune globulin; HDCV = Human diploid cell vaccine; ARS = Antirabies serum, equine.

* Clean bites with soap and water. For rabies prophylaxis, give both RIG† and HDCV immediately.

† If RIG is unavailable, use ARS.

‡ Discontinue vaccine if fluorescent antibody tests of animal killed at time of attack are negative.

§ Begin RIG + HDCV at first sign of rabies in biting dog or cat during holding period (10 days).

(Adapted from USPHS Advisory Committee on Immunization Practices [ACIP] Recommendations, *Morbidity and Mortality Weekly Report* Vol. 33, No. 28, 1984.)

Administration of rabies immune globulin or antirabies serum for **passive immunization** followed by vaccine for **active immunization** gives the best specific postexposure prophylaxis. Both passive and active immunizing products should be used concurrently but never administered in the same anatomic site. The preferred products are human rabies immune globulin **(RIG)** for passive immunization with human diploid cell rabies vaccine **(HDCV)** for active immunization. HDCV produces a superior immune response and fewer adverse reactions than older vaccines. If RIG is unavailable, antirabies serum **(ARS)** of equine origin may be substituted for RIG. RIG is preferred over ARS because ARS has a much higher risk of adverse reactions. For **passive immunization,** RIG is given only once—at the beginning of antirabies prophylaxis. The recommended dose is 20 IU/kg. If possible, up to ½ of the total dose is infiltrated around the wound; the remainder is given IM. If ARS is used, 40 u./kg is given in the same manner.

Active immunization with HDCV should also begin immediately. HDCV is given in a series of five 1-mL IM injections (the deltoid area is preferred) beginning on the day of exposure, followed by injections on days 3, 7, 14, and 28. Because antibody response has been uniformly satisfactory following this regimen, routine serologic testing is not

recommended unless the patient is thought to be immunodeficient. The World Health Organization also recommends that a 6th injection be given 90 days after the 1st injection. Local reactions at the injection site are usually minor, and systemic reactions are rarely associated with primary immunization. Prophylaxis should not be interrupted because of minor adverse reactions that can be managed with antihistamines, anti-inflammatory, and antipyretic agents; for serious systemic or neuroparalytic reactions, consideration should be given to evaluating the patient's risk of developing rabies before discontinuing vaccination. Testing the patient's serum for rabies antibody titer may provide essential information in such cases. Individual assistance in each situation may be sought from the state health department or the Centers for Disease Control, Atlanta, GA, 30333.

Preexposure: Because of the relative safety of HDCV, prophylactic vaccination of persons with a high risk of exposure to rabid animals is justified. Such persons include those in frequent contact with potentially rabid animals (eg, veterinarians, animal handlers, spelunkers), laboratory workers handling tissues infected with rabies virus, and individuals who reside or stay for an extended period in foreign countries where rabies in dogs is prevalent. HDCV is given in the deltoid area in a series of three 1-mL IM injections, with the 2nd injection 7 days after the 1st, and the 3rd one 2 or 3 wk later. Routine confirmation of antibody titer following this regimen is not required. However, persons with a continued high risk of exposure should have their sera tested for antibody at 2-yr intervals and have a booster dose of HDCV if the titer is inadequate. Hypersensitivity reactions, presumed to be Type III, have occurred in about 5% of those given these booster doses. If a previously immunized person (postexposure or HDCV preexposure regimen) is bitten by a rabid animal, he should receive two 1-mL injections of HDCV, one dose immediately and another 3 days later. Passive immunization is not given. Preexposure immunization gives greater protection and reduces the postexposure regimen; it does *not* eliminate the need for prompt postexposure prophylaxis.

Treatment

If rabies develops, treatment is symptomatic. Vigorous supportive treatment is **recommended** and expert consultation should be sought to assist in clinical management. Although death from rabies was once considered inevitable if symptoms developed, recovery has occurred following aggressive, vigorous, supportive treatment to control respiratory, circulatory, and CNS symptoms.

SLOW VIRUS INFECTIONS

(See also SUBACUTE SCLEROSING PANENCEPHALITIES and PROGRESSIVE RUBELLA PANENCEPHALITIES in Ch. 191)

In these slowly developing, progressive diseases, responses to viral infections appear many years after the initial infections. The etiology may be conventional viruses or infectious agents lacking some properties of conventional viruses.

PROGRESSIVE MULTIFOCAL LEUKOENCEPHALOPATHY

A rare, rapidly progressive, demyelinating CNS disorder that occurs mainly in patients with underlying depression of cell-mediated immunity.

Etiology and Epidemiology

The disease is caused by the JC virus, a human papovavirus that replicates in human fetal glial cell tissue cultures. It is commonly associated with disorders of the reticuloendothelial system, such as leukemia and lymphoma, but may occur in any disease with concomitant depression of cell-mediated immunity (eg, AIDS). A few cases have

occurred in patients without a detectable immune disorder. The disease affects adults of all ages, men more frequently than women.

Symptoms, Signs, and Diagnosis

Onset may be gradual or insidious, but the course is relentlessly progressive. The duration from onset of symptoms to death is usually 1 to 4 mo. The neurologic findings reflect diffuse asymmetrical involvement of the cerebral hemispheres. Pyramidal tract involvement manifested by hemiparesis is the most commonly encountered finding. Progressive intellectual impairment of varying severity occurs in $2/3$ of patients. Aphasia, dysarthria, and hemianopsia are other frequent findings. Sensory changes and cerebellar and brainstem signs may be present. Occasionally an incomplete or complete transverse myelitis appears. Headaches and convulsive seizures are rare.

CSF studies, skull x-rays, and cerebral angiograms are normal. Abnormalities in radioactive and CT brain scan have been noted. The EEG commonly shows diffuse and focal abnormalities corresponding to the underlying asymmetric pathology, but these findings are not pathognomonic. Serologic studies do not confirm the diagnosis because $2/3$ of a normal population have antibodies against JC virus and underlying immunologic abnormalities in most patients with progressive multifocal leukoencephalopathy make serologic tests unreliable. Brain tissue confirms the diagnosis by identifying the JC virus, using IFA staining or electron microscopic agglutination.

Treatment

There have been isolated reports of favorable therapeutic responses to cytosine or adenine arabinoside, but no treatment has been proven effective.

CREUTZFELDT-JAKOB DISEASE
(Subacute Spongiform Encephalopathy)

A progressive, inevitably fatal, slow virus disease of the CNS, characterized by progressive dementia and myoclonic seizures and affecting adults in mid-life.

Etiology and Epidemiology

The disease occurs throughout the world, but little is known about its mode of transmission. Human-to-human transmission has occurred inadvertently during organ transplantation and by the use of contaminated brain electrodes, and the incidence of neurosurgical procedures is more common in Creutzfeld-Jakob patients than would be expected by chance. The disease has developed in several patients who were treated with human growth hormone when they were children. The agent has been recovered from the CSF. It occurs primarily in adults, men and women alike, with peak incidence in the late 50s. A familial form of the disease as well as the more common sporadic form has been described.

The disease can be transmitted to primates and small rodents; it causes scrapie-like tissue damage. The infectious agent (called a "prion" by some) appears similar to the agent that causes scrapie of sheep. It is unusually resistant to inactivation by heat, formalin, or exposure to ultraviolet light or x-rays. Abnormal fibrils, similar to those observed in preparations of scrapie-infected brain, have been recovered from Creutzfeldt-Jakob brains. A nucleic acid has not been demonstrated in preparations that cause the disease but PrP, a protein of a single molecular species, has been associated with infective fractions.

Symptoms and Signs

Dementia, invariably present and often the first manifestation of illness, is commonly evidenced by self-neglect, apathy, or irritability. Some patients complain of easy fatigability, somnolence, or insomnia or other sleep disorders. Disorientation may be

noted and may progress to profound and global intellectual defects. Other abnormalities of higher cortical function—eg, aphasia, apraxia, dyslexia, dysgraphia, agnosia, left-right disorientation, and unilateral neglect—may occur. Palmomental and snout reflexes are frequently present.

Myoclonus, often provoked by sensory stimuli, usually appears within the first 6 mo of the illness. Cerebellar disturbances also occur. Corticospinal tract involvement is common, as manifested by extensor plantar reflexes, clonus, and hyperreflexia. In certain cases, anterior horn cell involvement is prominent, with muscular atrophy and fasciculations. Signs of basal ganglia involvement, such as hypokinesia, dystonic posturing, cogwheel rigidity, tremor, and choreathetoid movements may develop. Cranial nerve palsies may be noted occasionally. Ocular disturbances are frequent and include visual field defects, diplopia, dimness or blurring of vision, and vision agnosia. In a variant of the disorder, the Gerstmann-Sträussler-Scheinker's disease, patients have a chronic cerebellar ataxia and amyloid plaque deposition in brain.

The disease ends in death after a 3- to 12-mo illness, commonly with a complicating pneumonia; 5 to 10% may have clinical courses of 2 yr or more.

Diagnosis

The CSF is normal, but may harbor the infectious agent. A CT brain scan may show cerebral and cerebellar atrophy. The EEG often shows a local or generalized disorganization, which progresses to a characteristic pattern of paroxysms of sharp waves and spikes against the slow background or, in some cases, a "burst suppression" pattern of low voltage activity. Creutzfelt-Jakob disease should be considered in a patient with a rapidly progressive dementia appearing in mid-adult life, especially if accompanied by myoclonic seizures. There are no specific tests, but the diagnosis can be confirmed by finding the typical spongiform vacuolar changes and astrocytic proliferation in brain tissue. Plaques of amyloid proteins have been observed in diseased brain.

Treatment

To prevent transmission of the disease, *caution must be exercised in handling fluids and other materials from patients suspected to have Creutzfeld-Jakob disease.* The infective agent can be destroyed by autoclaving and other treatments, but many standard methods of sterilization, such as exposure to formalin, may be ineffective in destroying the agent. Steam autoclaving at 132 C for 1 h or immersion in sodium hydroxide for 1 h is recommended for sterilization.

Treatment is nonspecific and symptomatic.

KURU

A progressive neurologic disorder transmitted during cannibalistic rites and occurring only in natives of the New Guinea highlands. The scrapie-like infectious agent appears to enter the body during cannibalistic practices (ritual feasts at which the brains of dead relatives are eaten). The infectious origin of the illness has been confirmed by inoculating brain material into higher primates and other animals. The cannibalistic practices have now been abandoned, and kuru has been virtually eliminated.

Symptoms and Signs

Patients exhibit various movement disorders; ie, cerebellar abnormalities, rigidity of the limbs, and clonus. Occasionally, coarse athetosis and choreiform movements are present and the patient shows an exaggerated startle response. Emotional lability is present, with pathologic bursts of laughter. Dementia may be present in advanced stages. In a terminal state, the patient is generally totally placid, mute, and unresponsive. Death is caused by severe decubitus or hypostatic pneumonia and usually occurs from 3 to 12 mo after onset of the disease.

Diagnosis and Treatment

Laboratory tests are unrevealing. The diagnosis is made by noting characteristic spongiform changes, amyloid plaques, and astrocytic proliferation in brain tissue. There is no treatment for the disorder.

ARBOVIRUS AND ARENAVIRUS DISEASES

Arboviruses: *Viruses maintained in nature through transmission between vertebrate and hematophagous arthropod hosts; they multiply in both.* **Arenaviruses**: *Lymphocytic choriomeningitis and morphologically related viruses usually transmitted by rodents but that can also show man-to-man transmission.* Current taxonomy, based on viral morphology, structure, and function, has eliminated the term *arbovirus*. "Arboviruses" are now distributed among 5 families. Terms for virus families end in *-viridae*; terms designating genera end in *-virus*. Genera and families without genera are tabulated in TABLE 12–5.

ARBOVIRUS ENCEPHALITIDES

The arboviruses (**ar**thropod-**bo**rne viruses) number > 250; at least 80 immunologically distinct arboviruses cause disease in humans. Arboviruses are transmitted among vertebrates by biting insects, chiefly mosquitoes and ticks. Birds are often important sources of infection for mosquitoes, which then transmit the infection to horses, other domestic animals, and humans. Man is a "dead-end" host (ie, incidental to the natural cycle and ineffective in virus perpetuation) for most of the agents, but is a definitive host (ie, part of the natural cycle and necessary for transmitting the infection) in urban yellow fever, phlebotomus fever, chikungunya, and dengue. The agents are widely distributed throughout the world, depending on the availability of lower vertebrate hosts and appropriate vectors.

In the USA, Western equine encephalitis (**WEE**) occurs throughout the country in all age groups, but a disproportionate number of cases occur in children < 1 yr old. Eastern equine encephalitis (**EEE**) occurs in the eastern USA, mainly in young children and persons > 55 yr, and has a higher mortality rate than WEE. In children < 1 yr old, WEE and EEE tend to be severe, with permanent neurologic sequelae. Epidemics of both WEE and EEE are associated with epizootics in horses. Urban and rural outbreaks of St. Louis encephalitis have occurred throughout the USA; morbidity and mortality are greatest in older age groups. The California encephalitis virus group is distributed primarily in the North Central States and New York, and mainly affects children in rural or suburban areas.

Symptoms, Signs, and Treatment

Arboviruses may cause CNS syndromes (including aseptic meningitis and encephalitis), minor nonspecific febrile illnesses, and, most commonly, inapparent infection. Except in epidemics, the clinical findings in meningitis and encephalitis rarely permit specific identification. Headache, drowsiness, fever, vomiting, and stiff neck are the usual presenting symptoms. Tremors, mental confusion, convulsions, and coma may develop rapidly. Paralysis of the extremities occasionally occurs. Treatment is supportive, as in other viral encephalitides (see in Ch. 125).

YELLOW FEVER

An acute arbovirus infection of variable severity, characterized by sudden onset, fever, a relatively slow pulse, and headache. Intense albuminuria, jaundice, and hemorrhage, especially hematemesis, are characteristic but occur only in the proportionately few severe cases.

TABLE 12–5. IMPORTANT "ARBOVIRUS" AND ARENAVIRUS DISEASES IN MAN: CLINICAL AND EPIDEMIOLOGIC FEATURES

Major Clinical Syndrome	*Viral Agent/ Disease*	*Genus*	*Vector*	*Major Distribution*
Fever, malaise, headaches, myalgia	Colorado tick fever	Arbovirus	Tick	Western USA, western Canada
	Phlebotomus fever	Phlebovirus	Sandfly	Mediterranean Basin, Balkans, Middle East, Pakistan, India, China, eastern Africa, Panama, Brazil
	Venezuelan equine encephalitis	Alphavirus	Mosquito	Argentina, Brazil, northern S. America, Panama, Mexico, Florida
	Rift Valley fever	Phlebovirus	Mosquito	S. Africa, E. Africa, Egypt
Fever, malaise, headaches, myalgia, lymphadenopathy, rash	Dengue fever	Flavivirus	Mosquito	Southeast Asia, Africa, Oceania, Australia, S. America, Mexico, Caribbean
	West Nile fever	Flavivirus	Mosquito	Africa, Middle East, southern France, USSR, India, Indonesia
Fever, malaise, headaches, myalgia, arthralgia, rash	Chikungunya	Alphavirus	Mosquito	Africa, India, Guam, Southeast Asia, New Guinea
	Mayaro virus disease	Alphavirus	Mosquito	Brazil, Bolivia
	Ross River virus disease	Alphavirus	Mosquito	Australia, New Guinea, Solomon Islands, Samoa, Cook Islands
	Sindbis virus disease	Alphavirus	Mosquito	Africa, Australia, USSR, Finland, Sweden
Fever with CNS involvement	Eastern equine encephalitis	Alphavirus	Mosquito	Atlantic & Gulf Coasts, USA; Caribbean; upper New York; western Michigan
	Western equine encephalitis	Alphavirus	Mosquito	USA, Canada, Central & S. America
	St. Louis encephalitis	Flavivirus	Mosquito	USA, Caribbean
	Venezuelan equine encephalitis	Alphavirus	Mosquito	Argentina, Brazil, northern S. America, Panama, Mexico, Florida

(Continued)

TABLE 12–5. IMPORTANT "ARBOVIRUS" AND ARENAVIRUS DISEASES IN MAN: CLINICAL AND EPIDEMIOLOGIC FEATURES *(Cont'd)*

Major Clinical Syndrome	*Viral Agent/ Disease*	*Genus*	*Vector*	*Major Distribution*
Fever with CNS involvement *(Cont'd)*	California group virus	Bunyavirus	Mosquito	North Central States, New York, USA
	Japanese encephalitis	Flavivirus	Mosquito	Japan, Korea, China, India, Philippines, Southeast Asia, eastern USSR
	Powassan virus	**Flavivirus**	**Tick**	**Eastern Canada, New York**
	Murray Valley encephalitis	**Flavivirus**	**Mosquito**	**Australia, New Guinea**
	Kyasanur Forest disease	**Flavivirus**	**Tick**	**India**
	Tick borne encephalitis virus	**Flavivirus**	**Tick**	**Europe, USSR**
	Lymphocytic choriomeningitis	**Arenavirus**	**Rodent**	**USA, Argentina, Germany, Balkans**
Fever, malaise, headaches, myalgia, hemorrhagic signs	Yellow fever	Flavivirus	Mosquito	Central & S. America, Africa
	Dengue hemorrhagic fever	Flavivirus	Mosquito	Southeast Asia, Oceania, Caribbean
	Kyasanur Forest disease	Flavivirus	Mosquito	India
	Omsk hemorrhagic fever	Flavivirus	Tick	USSR
	Crimean-Congo hemorrhagic fever	Nairovirus	Tick	Africa, eastern Europe, Middle East, USSR
	Hantaan virus	Bunyaviridae, genus not established	Rodent	Korea, Japan, USSR, Balkans, Scandinavia
	Machupo virus	Arenavirus	Rodent	Bolivia
	Junin virus	Arenavirus	Rodent	Argentina
	Lassa fever	Arenavirus	Rodent, man to man	W. Africa
	Marburg virus	Filoviridae	Unknown, man to man	Zimbabwe, Kenya, Uganda
	Ebola virus	Filoviridae	Unknown, man to man	Zaire, Sudan

(Modified from "Arbovirus Injections" by J. P. Sanford in *Harrison's Principles of Internal Medicine*, edited by R. G. Petersdorf et al, ed. 10, 1983. Copyright 1983 by McGraw-Hill, Inc. Used with permission of the McGraw-Hill Book Company.)

Etiology and Epidemiology

The virus of **urban yellow fever** is transmitted by the bite of an *Aedes aegypti* mosquito infected 2 wk previously by feeding on a viremic patient. **Jungle (sylvatic) yellow fever** is transmitted by *Haemogogus* and other forest canopy mosquitoes that acquire the virus from wild primates. Yellow fever is endemic in central Africa and areas of South and Central America.

Symptoms and Signs

(1) Period of incubation: *3 to 6 days.* Prodromal symptoms are usually absent. **(2) Period of invasion**: *2 to 5 days.* Onset is sudden, with fever of 39 to 40 C (102 to 104 F). The pulse, usually rapid initially, by the 2nd day becomes slow for the degree of fever present **(Faget's sign)**. The face is flushed and the eyes are injected; the tongue margins are red and the center is "furred." Nausea, vomiting, constipation, epigastric distress, headache, muscle pains (especially in the neck, back, and legs), severe prostration, restlessness, and irritability are common symptoms. If mild, the illness ends at this stage after 1 to 3 days. **(3) Period of remission**: In moderate or severe illness, the fever falls by crisis 2 to 5 days after onset and a remission of several hours or days ensues. **(4) Period of intoxication**: *3 to 9 days.* The fever recurs but the pulse remains slow. Jaundice, extreme albuminuria, and hematemesis ("black vomit"), the three characteristic clinical features, appear. Oliguria or anuria may occur, and petechiae and mucosal hemorrhages are common. The patient is dull, confused, and apathetic. Delirium, convulsions, and coma occur terminally. **(5) Period of convalescence**: Usually short, except in the most severe cases. There are no known sequelae.

Diagnosis and Laboratory Findings

Albuminuria occurs in 90% of patients, usually on the 3rd day, and may reach 20 gm/L in severe cases. The WBC count is usually low and drops to 1500 to 2500 by the 5th day; leukocytosis may occur terminally. Experimental evidence suggests that disseminated intravascular coagulation may occur. Serum bilirubin is mildly elevated.

The clinical features are nonspecific during the period of invasion, but the diagnosis is suggested by Faget's sign. During the period of intoxication, the characteristic triad of intense albuminuria, jaundice, and hematemesis should suggest the diagnosis. Diagnosis is confirmed by isolation of the virus from the blood, by a rising antibody titer, or at autopsy by the characteristic midzonal liver cell necrosis. Needle biopsy of the liver during illness is **contraindicated** by the risk of hemorrhage.

Prognosis

Up to 10% of clinically diagnosed cases end fatally but overall mortality is actually lower, since many mild or inapparent infections are undiagnosed.

Prophylaxis

Active immunization with the 17D strain of live attenuated yellow fever virus vaccine (0.5 mL s.c. every 10 yr) effectively prevents outbreaks and sporadic cases. In the USA, the vaccine is given only at USPHS-authorized Yellow Fever Vaccination Centers. Countries vary in vaccination requirements; current information and addresses of vaccination centers can be obtained from state and local health departments.

To prevent further mosquito transmission, patients should be isolated in well-screened rooms sprayed with residual insecticides. Since infection can be transmitted through laboratory accidents, hospital and laboratory personnel should be careful to avoid self-inoculation with patients' blood.

Eradication of urban yellow fever requires widespread mosquito control and mass immunization. During sylvatic outbreaks, work in the area should be discontinued pending immunization and mosquito control.

Treatment

Management is supportive and directed toward alleviating major symptoms. Complete bed rest and nursing care are important. Correction of fluid and electrolyte imbalance is imperative (see Ch. 84).

Hemorrhagic tendencies should be combated with calcium gluconate 1 gm IV once or twice/day, or with phytonadione (see VITAMIN K DEFICIENCY, in Ch. 81). Transfusion may be necessary. Therapy with heparin should be considered if there is evidence of disseminated intravascular coagulation (low fibrinogen levels, prolonged thrombin time, thrombocytopenia, and elevation of fibrin split products in full-blown cases; in less acute forms some of these laboratory findings may not occur and heparin may not be necessary). Typical heparin dosage is 50 to 100 u./kg initially, then 10 to 15 u./kg/h, given by IV infusion.

Nausea and vomiting may be alleviated with dimenhydrinate 50 to 100 mg orally or rectally, or 50 mg IM, q 4 to 6 h; or with prochlorperazine 5 to 10 mg orally, parenterally, or rectally q 4 to 6 h. Fever may be reduced with tepid-water sponge baths. Headaches may require codeine 15 to 60 mg orally or s.c. q 4 to 6 h, or meperidine 50 to 100 mg orally or IM q 4 to 6 h.

DENGUE

(Breakbone or Dandy Fever)

An acute febrile disease characterized by sudden onset, with headache, fever, prostration, joint and muscle pain, lymphadenopathy, and a rash that appears simultaneously with a second temperature rise following an afebrile period. A hemorrhagic fever syndrome associated with dengue occurs primarily in children (see below).

Dengue is endemic throughout the tropics and subtropics; outbreaks have occurred in the Caribbean, including Puerto Rico and the US Virgin Islands, since 1969. Cases have also been imported in tourists returning from Tahiti. The causative agent, a flavivirus with 4 distinct serogroups, is transmitted by the bite of *Aëdes* mosquitoes.

Symptoms and Signs

Following an incubation period of 3 to 15 (usually 5 to 8) days, onset is abrupt, with chills or chilly sensations, headache, postorbital pain on moving the eyes, lumbar backache, and severe prostration. Extreme aching in the legs and joints occurs during the first hours of illness. The temperature rises rapidly to as high as 40 C (104 F), with relative bradycardia and hypotension. The bulbar and palpebral conjunctivas are injected, and a transient flushing or pale pink macular rash (particularly of the face) usually appears. The spleen may be soft and slightly enlarged. Cervical, epitrochlear, and inguinal lymph nodes are usually enlarged.

Fever and other symptoms persist for 48 to 96 h, followed by rapid defervescence with profuse sweating. This ushers in an afebrile period, with a sense of well-being, that lasts about 24 h. A second rapid temperature rise follows, usually with a lower peak than the first, producing a "saddle-back" temperature curve. A characteristic maculopapular eruption appears simultaneously, usually spreading from the extremities to cover the entire body except the face, or distributed patchily over the trunk and extremities. The palms and soles may be bright red and edematous. The fever, rash, and headache and other pains constitute the **"dengue triad."** Cases have occurred without the second febrile period.

Mortality is nil in typical dengue. Convalescence is often prolonged, lasting several weeks, and is accompanied by asthenia. An attack produces immunity for a year or more.

Laboratory Findings and Diagnosis

Leukopenia is present by the 2nd day of fever; by the 4th or 5th day, the WBC count has dropped to 2000 to 4000 with only 20 to 40% granulocytes. Moderate albuminuria and a few casts may be found.

Dengue may be confused with Colorado tick fever, typhus, yellow fever, or other hemorrhagic fevers. Serologic diagnosis may be made by HI and CF tests using paired sera, but is complicated by cross-reactions with other flavivirus antibodies.

Prophylaxis and Treatment

Prevention requires control or eradication of the mosquito vector. To prevent transmission to mosquitoes, patients in endemic areas should be kept under mosquito netting until the second bout of fever has abated. **Treatment** is symptomatic. Complete bed rest is important. Aspirin 600 mg and codeine 15 to 60 mg orally q 4 h may be given for severe headache and myalgia.

DENGUE HEMORRHAGIC FEVER

(DHF; Philippine, Thai, or Southeast Asian Hemorrhagic Fever)

An acute disease occurring primarily in children living where dengue is endemic, and characterized by an abrupt febrile onset followed by hemorrhagic manifestations and circulatory collapse. It is prevalent in Southeast Asia, China, and Cuba. Most patients are under age 10.

Symptoms and Signs

Onset is abrupt, with fever, headache, nausea, vomiting, abdominal pain, cough, pharyngitis, and dyspnea. Shock occurs 2 to 6 days after onset, with sudden collapse or prostration, cool clammy extremities (the trunk is often warm), weak thready pulse, and circumoral cyanosis. Bleeding tendencies occur, usually as purpura, petechiae, or ecchymoses at injection sites; sometimes as hematemesis, melena, or epistaxis; and occasionally as subarachnoid hemorrhage.

Hepatomegaly is common, as is bronchopneumonia with or without bilateral pleural effusions. Myocarditis may be present. Mortality ranges from 6 to 30%; most deaths occur in infants < 1 yr old.

Laboratory Findings and Diagnosis

Hemoconcentration (Hct $> 50\%$) is present during shock; the WBC count is elevated in 1/3 of the patients. Thrombocytopenia ($< 100{,}000/\mu L$), a positive tourniquet test, and a prolonged prothrombin time are characteristic and indicative of the coagulation abnormalities. Minimal proteinuria may be present. AST (SGOT) levels may be moderately increased. Serologic tests usually show high CF antibody titers against flaviviruses, suggestive of a secondary immune response.

One of the criteria established by the WHO for diagnosing DHF is acute onset of fever that is high and continuous, lasting for 2 to 7 days. Another criterion is hemorrhagic manifestations, including at least a positive tourniquet test and any of the following: petechiae, purpura, ecchymoses, bleeding gums, hematemesis, or melena; enlargement of the liver; thrombocytopenia ($\leq 100{,}000/\mu L$); hemoconcentration (Hct increased by $\geq 20\%$). Criteria for dengue shock syndrome are a rapid weak pulse with narrowing of the pulse pressure (≤ 20 mm Hg) or hypotension with cold, clammy skin and restlessness.

Treatment

The degree of hemoconcentration, dehydration, and electrolyte imbalance must be evaluated immediately and monitored closely for the first few days, since shock may occur or recur precipitously. Cyanotic patients should be given O_2. Vascular collapse

and hemoconcentration require immediate and vigorous fluid replacement, preferably with a crystalloid solution such as Ringer's lactate (overhydration must be avoided). Plasma or human serum albumin should also be given if there is no response in the first hour. Fresh blood or platelet transfusions may control bleeding. Agitated patients may be given paraldehyde, chloral hydrate, or diazepam. Hydrocortisone, pressor amines, α-adrenergic blocking agents, and vitamins C and K are of doubtful value.

LYMPHOCYTIC CHORIOMENINGITIS (LCM)

An acute viral infection caused by an RNA virus now classified as an arenavirus, usually appearing as an influenza-like illness or aseptic meningitis, which may be associated with rash, arthritis, orchitis, or parotitis.

LCM infection is endemic in rodents. Human infection results most commonly from exposure to dust or food contaminated by the gray house mouse or hamsters, which harbor the virus for life and excrete it in urine, feces, semen, and nasal secretions. When transmitted by mice the disease occurs primarily in adults, in the winter.

Symptoms and Signs

An influenza-like illness develops 5 to 10 days after exposure. Fever, usually 38.5 to 40 C (101 to 104 F), with rigors is uniform. Other symptoms in over half the patients include malaise, weakness, myalgia (especially in the lumbar area), retro-orbital headache, photophobia, anorexia, nausea, and light-headedness. Less common symptoms include sore throat and dysesthesia. In the first week of illness, physical findings are few; there may be relative bradycardia and pharyngeal injection without exudate. After 5 days to 3 wk, patients may improve for 1 or 2 days. Many then relapse with recurrent fever, headache, skin rashes, swelling of metacarpophalangeal and proximal interphalangeal joints, meningeal signs, orchitis, parotitis, and alopecia of the scalp. Patients with aseptic meningitis almost always recover without sequelae. With encephalitis, up to 33% of patients have neurologic residua.

Laboratory Findings, Diagnosis, and Treatment

Leukopenia (WBC, 2000 to 3000) and thrombocytopenia (platelets, 50,000 to 100,000) are almost uniform during the first week of illness. Chest radiographs may reveal basilar pneumonitis. In patients with meningeal signs, the CSF usually contains several hundred cells/μL, but occasionally > 1000. Lymphocytes predominate (> 80%), even early. Decreased CSF glucose, with concentrations as low as 15 mg/dL, has been reported in up to 25% of patients, but in most instances the CSF is normal.

Clinical manifestations cannot be differentiated from those of many other viral meningitides.

Diagnosis can be made by isolating the virus from the CSF or by a rise in complement fixing neutralizing antibody.

Therapy is supportive.

LASSA FEVER

A serious systemic arenavirus infection that involves most visceral organs but spares the CNS.

Etiology and Epidemiology

After Lassa fever was first recognized in Lassa, Nigeria in 1969, outbreaks occurred in Nigeria, Liberia, and Sierra Leone. Cases have been imported into the USA and the United Kingdom. *Mastomys natalensis*, a small rat that commonly inhabits houses and is widespread in Africa, is a reservoir of the virus. Most human cases probably result from contamination of food with rodent urine, but human-to-human transmission can

occur through contact with urine, feces, saliva, vomitus, or blood. The outbreaks in Nigeria and Liberia were primarily hospital-associated, spreading from an index case to hospital workers or other patients. In Sierra Leone, where most cases were acquired outside of hospitals, 6% of the residents in the endemic area had antibody against Lassa virus, while only 0.2% were recognized as having had clinical disease. About 2/3 of the cases have been women, a predilection that may relate to exposure rather than to differences in susceptibility.

Symptoms and Signs

The incubation period is 1 to 24 days, 10 days being usual. The onset of severe symptoms is gradual; most patients have symptoms for 4 to 5 days before hospitalization. The initial symptoms—sore throat, fever, chilliness, headache, myalgia, and malaise—are followed by anorexia, vomiting, and pains in the chest and epigastrium. The sore throat becomes more severe during the 1st wk; patches of white or yellow exudate may appear on the tonsils and may coalesce into a pseudomembrane. Early in the course, relative bradycardia is common. Generalized nontender lymphadenopathy occurs in some patients. During the 2nd wk, severe lower abdominal pain and intractable vomiting are common. Facial and neck swelling and conjunctival edema are seen in 10 to 30%. Occasionally, patients have tinnitus, epistaxis, bleeding from the gums and venipuncture sites, maculopapular rashes, cough, and dizziness. During the acute stage, systolic BPs of < 90 mm Hg with pulse pressures of < 20 mm Hg occur in 60 to 80% of patients. During the 2nd wk, patients who will recover defervesce, while fatally ill patients often develop shock, clouded mental status, agitation, rales, pleural effusion, and, occasionally, grand mal seizures. The illness lasts from 7 to 31 days (average, 15 days) in those who survive and 7 to 26 days (average, 12 days) in fatal cases.

Laboratory Findings and Diagnosis

Hct values are normal. Early, in 1/3 of the patients the WBC count drops to < 4000, with relative neutrophilia. Platelet counts remain normal. Urinalyses reveal proteinuria, which is often massive. Chest radiographs may show basilar pneumonitis and pleural effusions. AST (SGOT) and ALT (SGPT) values become elevated (10 × normal), as do levels of creatine phosphokinase (CPK) and lactic dehydrogenase (LDH). The diagnosis may be made by demonstrating a four-fold rise in antibody titer with an indirect fluorescent antibody technic or by Lassa IgM antibodies.

Prognosis

The severity of infection correlates with the level of viremia, elevations in transaminase values, and fever. Mortality rates have varied between 16 and 45%; however, in women who were pregnant or delivered within 1 mo, mortality was 50%. Among survivors, late sequelae include deafness in about 5% and occasional instances of alopecia, iridocyclitis, and transient blindness.

Prophylaxis and Treatment

In Sierra Leone, barrier nursing (surgical masks, gowns, and gloves) has been effective. In the USA, maximum isolation, including use of goggles, high efficiency masks, and a negative pressure room with no air circulation, is recommended. Surveillance of contacts also is recommended.

Management is supportive and directed toward alleviating major symptoms. *Correction of fluid and electrolyte imbalance is imperative.* In a study of the antiviral agent ribavirin, 19 of 20 patients treated within 6 days of onset with a 2-gm IV loading dose followed by 1 gm q 6 h for 4 days then 0.5 gm q 8 h for another 6 days survived, while 11 of 18 who received no therapy and 10 of 16 who received convalescent plasma died.

13. PARASITIC INFECTIONS

(NOTE: Several of the drugs mentioned in this chapter are not available commercially in the USA but may be obtainable as investigational drugs from the Parasitic Diseases Branch of the Centers for Disease Control in Atlanta, Georgia.)

LABORATORY DIAGNOSIS OF PARASITIC INFECTIONS

(See TABLE 13–1)

Detecting an intestinal parasite is contingent on many factors, among which are quality and number of specimens; for instance, many protozoa, unlike helminths, are shed in sporadic numbers, and repeated examinations may almost double the yield.

For intestinal ova or parasites, 3 stool specimens should, preferably, be collected consecutively every other day. Alternatively, the series may be shortened to 3 consecutive days. Duodenal aspirates or string test specimens may be required. Posttreatment follow-up examinations should be started 2 wk after completion of therapy for helminthic, 4 wk for protozoan, and 6 wk for *Taenia* infections.

Except for a few specific tests, usually no special preparations are required before collecting a stool other than to ensure against contamination with urine, water, dirt, or disinfectants. However, antibiotics, contrast material purgatives, and antacids will adversely affect detection of parasites or decrease to below detectable levels the number of parasites passed; it may be several weeks before such stools become suitable for examination, depending on how soon the interfering compounds are cleared from the GI tract.

Freshly passed stools should be sent to the examining laboratory within 15 min, particularly if they are unformed or diarrheal (ie, likely to contain motile trophozoites). Do not attempt to keep specimens warm while they are in transit to the laboratory. Formed stools may be refrigerated (*not* frozen) if the examination cannot be effected immediately. If facilities exist, portions of fresh specimen should be emulsified (1 part feces to 3 parts fixative) in polyvinyl alcohol **(PVA)** and 5 to 10% aqueous formalin. Thin fecal smears fixed in Schaudinn's fixative are also useful. Such preserved specimens are suitable for mailing.

Anal swabs are useful for detecting pinworms and tapeworms but are unsatisfactory specimens for parasitologic examination.

Specimens collected by sigmoidoscopy should be considered, particularly from patients with a history of amebiasis but a negative series of routine stool examinations. The sigmoidoscopic material should be examined immediately. The specimen is collected with a curette or Volkman's spoon; cotton swabs are unsatisfactory. Sigmoidoscopic specimens and rectal and bladder biopsies should be examined immediately.

For patients with a negative series of stools, one may elect to do the string test for *Giardia* and *Strongyloides*. Instructions should be obtained from the laboratory.

PROTOZOAL DISEASES

AMEBIASIS

(Entamebiasis)

An infection of the colon caused by Entamoeba histolytica. *It is most commonly asymptomatic, but symptoms ranging from mild diarrhea to dysentery may occur.*

TABLE 13–1. COLLECTING AND HANDLING SPECIMENS FOR LABORATORY DIAGNOSIS OF PARASITIC INFECTIONS

Affected Organ System	*Parasite*	*Optimal Specimen*	*Collection Details*	*Comments*
Blood	*Plasmodium* spp.	Thick & thin smears from capillary blood (ie, finger or earlobe, using disposable lancet) or 5–10 mL fresh anticoagulated blood Thin smears are made same as hematology differential slides; for thick smears, place drop of blood on meticulously clean glass slide & mix into area about 5/8″ in diameter Place slide on flat surface; allow blood to dry gently & dust-free before sending slide to laboratory	Collect every 6 h for 3 days Be certain all alcohol disinfectant has evaporated before collecting blood specimen Smears may be made from the tube or anticoagulated blood up to 1 h after collected Slowly dry in covered dish	Wright's or Giemsa stain Glass slides must be very clean If there is any doubt about ability to prepare good slides, collect anticoagulated blood in a tube & send to laboratory for preparation of slides & staining
	Trypanosoma spp.	Place & coverslip drop of capillary blood from a fingerstick onto clean glass slide Alternatively, send 5–6 mL of anticoagulated blood to laboratory		Wright's or Giemsa stain
	Microfilariae	Send 5–10 mL of anticoagulated blood If first specimen is negative, collect one or more to be concentrated For African onchocerciasis, "skin snips" from thigh, buttocks, iliac crest For American onchocerciasis, "skin snips" from scalp, buttocks, face	*Wuchereria bancrofti* & *Brugia malayi:* collect between 10 PM & 2 AM *Loa loa, Acanthocheilonema perstans,* & *Mansonella ozzardi:* collect between 10 AM & 6 PM For "skin snips," see below under Skin	Wright's or Giemsa stain

Bone Marrow	*Leishmania* spp	Bone marrow aspirates or thin air-dried smears	Centrifuge 5–10 mL of anticoagulated blood & make buffy coat smears	Wright's or Giemsa stain
Central Nervous System	*Naegleria* *Hartmannella* *Acanthameba* group	Fresh spinal fluid	Asceptic collection Keep specimen temperature	If immediate examination by light of phase microscopy is not possible, fix slides in PVA, Schaudinn's fixative, or 5–10% formalin
Intestinal System Biopsies Jejunal Duodenal	*Giardia lamblia* *Strongyloides*	Collected & placed in sterile jar or tube with a little saline, or placed on coverslipped glass microscope slide	Examine immediately	
Rectal	*Entamoeba histolytica* *Schistosoma mansoni* *Schistosoma japonicum*	For schistosomes: biopsy from level of dorsal fold (Houston valve), about 9 cm from anus		
Feces	*Entamoeba histolytica* Other amebas	3 freshly passed stools collected in AM every other day	If unformed or diarrheal, specimen should be examined within 15 min Formed stools may be refrigerated until examined (see also accompanying text)	Schaudinn's fixative, PVA, or 5–10% formalin
	Giardia lamblia	3 freshly passed stools collected in AM every other day	If initial series of 3 specimens is negative, examine 3 more, 1/wk Duodenal aspirates (string test) may be necessary (see accompanying text)	
	Cryptosporidia	3 freshly passed stools collected daily	Jejunal biopsy may yield organism in stool-negative patients.	If immediate examination is not possible, preserve in 2.5% potassium dichromate or 10% buffered formalin. Fresh and dichromate-preserved stool is infectious.

(Continued)

TABLE 13–1. COLLECTING AND HANDLING SPECIMENS FOR LABORATORY DIAGNOSIS OF PARASITIC INFECTIONS *(Cont'd)*

Affected Organ System	*Parasite*	*Optimal Specimen*	*Collection Details*	*Comments*
Intestinal System *(Cont'd)* Feces *(Cont'd)*	*Trichuris trichiura* *Ascaris lumbricoides* Hookworm *Strongyloides* Tapeworms Flukes	Up to 3 stools collected daily	Not critical to examine immediately May be refrigerated	
	Enterobius vermicularis	Cellophane tape or anal swab	Collect from area around anus; patient should be resting & quiet for several hours before collecting specimen—usually in AM before bowel movement or bath	
Sigmoidoscopy (Proctoscopy)	*Entamoeba histolytica*	Fresh scrapings collected with a curette or Volkmann's spoon; or with a surgical instrument snip off a piece of mucosa; or aspirate lesion with a 1-mL serologic pipette with a rubber bulb Cotton-tipped swabs are not satisfactory	If patient has not had a bowel movement shortly before sigmoidoscopy is begun, he should be purged and the procedure not started for 2–3 h Specimen must be examined immediately or fixed for later examination	
Respiratory Tract Sputum	*Paragonimus westermani*	Fresh sputum	Instruct patient carefully	
Aspirates (tracheal, broncheal)	*Entamoeba histolytica* *Strongyloides* *Echinococcus granulosus* Hookworm *Ascaris*	Any aspirated material; also drainage material	If amebiasis is suspected, specimen should be examined as soon as possible or preserved for later examination	

Lung biopsy	All listed above under Respiratory Tract + *Pneumocystis carinii*	Open lung biopsy Percutaneous biopsy under fluoroscopy	Collect into sterile container If needle biopsy, add sterile saline	For *Pneumocystis carinii*, lung biopsy is best
Skin	*Onchocerca volvulus*	For African cases, "skin snips" from thigh, buttocks, iliac crest For American cases, "skin snips" from face, scapula, buttocks	For "skin snips," disinfect skin with alcohol, insert 25-gauge needle just under epidermis, raise it, & slice off small piece of tissue with a scalpel or razor blade; bleeding should not occur	
	Leishmania spp. *Entamoeba histolytica*	Ulcer bed	In amebiasis or leishmaniasis, parasites typically are found in the lesion/ulcer wall rather than in the pus	
	Taenia solium *Echinococcus granulosus*	Regular biopsy technic		
Urogenital System Vagina Urethra Prostatic secretions	*Trichomonas* spp	1 sterile swab in a tube with small amount of sterile saline	Females should not douche for 3–4 days before collecting specimen Send to laboratory as soon as possible, before trichomonads stop moving	
Bladder	*Schistosoma haematobium*	Biopsy from area around the trigone		

Etiology, Epidemiology, and Incidence

There are 2 forms of *E. histolytica*: the motile trophozoite and the cyst. The trophozoite, the parasitic form, dwells in the bowel lumen, where it feeds on bacteria or tissue. With diarrhea, the fragile trophozoites pass unchanged in the liquid stool and rapidly die. If diarrhea is not present, the organisms usually encyst before leaving the gut. The cyst, the infective form of the organism, resists environmental changes and may be spread either directly from person to person or indirectly via food or water. **Direct spread** appears to be more common in the USA, where it occurs in situations of compromised personal hygiene (eg, among sexual partners, particularly male homosexuals and institutionalized, mentally retarded individuals). **Indirect spread** is more frequent in areas of the world where sanitation is poor, including migrant labor camps and Indian reservations in the USA. Fruits and vegetables may be contaminated when they are fertilized by human feces, washed in polluted water, or prepared by an asymptomatic cysts-passer. Faulty hotel and factory plumbing has resulted in 2 water-borne epidemics; more commonly, amebiasis is sporadic. The infection rate in the USA is about 1%. The carrier rate may exceed 50% in areas of the world where sanitation is poor.

Controlling the spread of *E. histolytica* requires preventing access of human feces to the mouth. The high incidence of asymptomatic carriers complicates the problem.

Pathogenesis

Excystation of ingested cysts occurs in the small intestine. The released trophozoites are carried to the colon, where they grow and multiply in the bowel lumen as commensals. Pathogenicity appears to be limited to a small number of *E. histolytica* zymodemes that regularly invade tissue. Changes in the virulence of these organisms or the host's resistance may lead to extensive tissue damage and disease.

The trophozoites penetrate the mucous membrane mainly in regions of fecal stasis—the cecum, appendix, ascending colon, sigmoid colon, and rectum. The earliest lesion is a small abscess, usually in the submucosa; later, ulcers form that tend to be ragged and undermined. The lesions are focal and discrete in mild cases, but may spread and become confluent, with hemorrhage, edema, and sloughing of large areas of mucosa. Although penetration by the ameba is limited by the muscular coat, it is occasionally destroyed and perforation results; amebas enter the radicles of the portal vein and are carried to the liver. Most of the amebas are probably destroyed, but one or more large hepatic abscesses develop if the survivors are numerous and multiply. Further spread of the disease is usually by direct extension from the liver into the pleura, right lung, and pericardium.

Symptoms and Signs

Because of the infrequency of virulent strains, most patients, particularly those living in temperate climates, are asymptomatic. Symptoms occur with tissue invasion and may be so vague as to be recalled only after successful therapy, but more often intermittent diarrhea and constipation, flatulence, and cramping abdominal pain occur. There may be tenderness over the liver and ascending colon, and the stools may contain mucus and blood.

Amebic dysentery, common in the tropics but uncommon in temperate climates, is characterized by episodes of frequent semifluid or fluid stools that often contain blood, flecks of mucus, and hordes of active trophozoites. Slight fever may be present. Between relapses, symptoms diminish to recurrent cramps and loose or very soft stools due to colitis, yet emaciation and anemia increase.

Complications and Sequelae

Hepatic amebiasis: Tender hepatomegaly frequently accompanies amebic colitis. This syndrome, formerly termed "diffuse amebic hepatitis," probably reflects a nonspecific periportal inflammation and not amebic liver infection. **Liver abscess** may

develop during or 1 to 3 mo after an attack of dysentery, or may be unassociated with dysentery. Abscesses occur most frequently in male adults. The abscesses are usually single and develop insidiously, but symptoms may begin abruptly in non-immune patients. Symptoms include pain or discomfort over the liver, aggravated by movement and occasionally referred to the right shoulder; intermittent fever; sweats; chills; nausea; vomiting; weakness; and weight loss. Jaundice is unusual and, when present, is low-grade. The abscess may perforate into the subphrenic space, right pleural cavity, right lung, and other adjacent organs.

Symptoms of **subacute appendicitis** may occur during clinical or subclinical amebic infection as a result of diffuse amebic invasion of the appendix and cecum. Surgery in such cases often results in peritonitis and death. If there is reasonable suspicion that the symptoms are of amebic origin, it is advisable to delay surgery for 48 to 72 h in order to observe the effects of chemotherapy (see Treatment, below).

Penetration of the muscle layers of the colon occasionally results in a vigorous granulomatous reaction, producing tissue masses or ameboma that may obstruct the bowel and be mistaken for carcinoma.

The lungs, brain, and other organs are occasionally infected by **hematogenous spread** from the intestines. Skin lesions, especially around the perineum and buttocks, and, particularly, traumatic and operative wounds are occasionally infected with amebas.

Diagnosis

Intestinal amebiasis, suggested by the clinical picture and epidemiologic setting, is confirmed by demonstration of *E. histolytica* in the stool or tissues. Wet mounts of liquid and semiformed stools should be examined immediately for motile trophozoites. Bloodstained flecks of mucus in the stool are more likely to contain amebas. Formed stool should be examined, by direct and concentration methods, for cysts. If examination is delayed, a portion of the stool should be placed in a preservative for cysts (5% formalin) and trophozoites (polyvinyl alcohol). Diagnosis may require examination of 3 to 6 stool specimens. Since antibiotics, antacids, antidiarrheal agents, enemas, and intestinal radiocontrast agents may interfere with recovery of the parasite, their administration should be postponed until the stool has been examined.

Proctoscopy often demonstrates mucosal lesions in symptomatic patients. The lesions should be aspirated and the material examined for trophozoites. Biopsy specimens from the lesions may also show trophozoites.

Extraintestinal amebiasis is more difficult to diagnose. Stool examination is usually negative, and recovery of the trophozoite from pus is uncommon. In patients suspected of having an amebic liver abscess, a therapeutic trial of amebicides may be the single most helpful diagnostic tool.

Serologic tests are positive in almost all patients with amebic liver abscess and in > 80% of those with acute amebic dysentery. However, since antibody titers may persist for months or years, serologic tests are less helpful in endemic areas. The tests are positive in only about 10% of asymptomatic carriers, suggesting that tissue invasion is a prerequisite for antibody formation. The indirect HA and enzyme-linked immunosorbent assays are the most sensitive tests available.

Differential Diagnosis

Nondysenteric amebiasis is often misdiagnosed as irritable bowel syndrome, regional enteritis, or diverticulitis. **Amebic dysentery** may be confused with bacillary dysentery, salmonellosis, schistosomiasis, or ulcerative colitis. In contrast to bacillary dysentery, the stools in amebic dysentery are more fecal and less frequent and watery. They characteristically contain tenacious mucus and flecks of both fresh and altered blood. Unlike shigellosis, salmonellosis, and ulcerative colitis, they do not contain large numbers of leukocytes.

Hepatic amebiasis and amebic abscess must be differentiated from other hepatic in-

fections, including abscesses due to bacterial infection and infected echinococcus cysts. Fever, local pain and tenderness, and hepatomegaly are significant findings. Serologic tests are usually positive in hepatic amebiasis; amebas are found in the stools in about 1/3 of cases.

When an abscess is present, the liver is usually enlarged and tender, but it may not be palpable. X-rays may show elevation and fixation, or impaired excursion of the right leaf of the diaphragm. Radioisotopic liver scanning CT may show the extent of the abscess, while ultrasonic scanning may demonstrate it to be fluid-filled. The alkaline phosphatase may be elevated. The abscesses contain thick, semifluid material ranging from yellow to chocolate brown and composed of cytolyzed remains of tissue. A needle biopsy may show necrotic tissue, but motile amebas are difficult to find in the abscess material and cysts are not present.

Treatment

General: This is directed at relieving symptoms, replacing blood, and correcting fluid and electrolyte losses.

Chemotherapy:

Course A (asymptomatic intestinal amebiasis): Metronidazole, iodoquinol, or diloxanide furoate may be given orally. For adults, metronidazole 750 mg orally tid for 10 days is recommended; for children, 35 to 50 mg/kg/day orally in 3 divided doses, also for 10 days. The comparable dose of iodoquinol is 650 mg tid, or 30 to 40 mg/kg/day in 3 divided doses for children. For both, the drug is given for 20 days. Diloxanide furoate is given for 10 days, 500 mg tid in adults and 20 mg/kg/day in 3 doses for children.

Course B (symptomatic intestinal amebiasis): Metronidazole should be given *in combination* with iodoquinol. In severe dysentery, emetine 1 mg/kg/day (maximum 65 mg) or dehydroemetine 1 to 1.5 mg/kg/day (maximum 90 mg) given by deep s.c. or IM injection may be added to the above regimen until symptoms are controlled (maximum 5 days). (CAUTION: *Emetine and dehydroemetine are toxic; patients receiving them should be confined to bed and placed on cardiac monitors. Therapy should be stopped promptly if such signs of toxicity as tachycardia, hypotension, muscular weakness, marked GI effects, or dermatoses appear.*) Pregnancy and cardiac disease are **contraindications.**

Course C (extraintestinal amebiasis): Metronidazole, given in the dosage mentioned above, is the drug of choice. Alternatively, emetine or dehydroemetine can be given for 5 days in the manner described for severe amebic dysentery. If one of the latter 2 drugs is used, it should be combined with oral chloroquine phosphate to diminish the risk of relapse. The dosage is 1 gm/day orally for 2 days, then 500 mg/day for 3 wk. The dose for children is 10 mg/kg/day (maximum 600 mg/day) for the same duration.

Emetine, dehydroemetine, or chloroquine can be used in a therapeutic trial. A favorable response is so characteristic that it constitutes an important diagnostic aid. A therapeutic trial of metronidazole, however, may lead to an erroneous diagnosis, since it is also effective against many anaerobic bacteria that commonly cause pyogenic liver abscess.

Criteria of cure: Since amebiasis tends to relapse, stools should be reexamined with reasonable frequency—if feasible, 1, 3, and 6 mo after treatment. Recurrence of GI symptoms does not require amebicidal drug therapy unless parasitic relapse has been proved by demonstration of *E. histolytica.*

GIARDIASIS

An infection of the small intestine caused by Giardia lamblia. It is commonly asymptomatic, but clinical manifestations ranging from flatulence to malabsorption may occur.

Etiology and Epidemiology

The *G. lamblia* trophozoite attaches itself to the mucosa of the duodenum and jejunum by means of a central sucker and multiplies by binary fission. The organisms are passed in normal stool as cysts. In this resistant form, they spread the disease from host to host by fecal-oral routes, either directly, as between children or sexual partners, or indirectly via food or water. Water-borne epidemics involving remote mountain streams, well water, and chlorinated community systems have all been implicated. Both humans and wild animals may serve as reservoirs.

The infection is found worldwide, especially in areas of poor sanitation and in children; rates > 50% have been noted in day care centers. Infection rates are also high among travelers, male homosexuals, and patients with gastrectomies, decreased gastric acidity, chronic pancreatitis, and immunoglobulin deficiencies. In the USA, about 4% of stools submitted for parasitologic examination contain *G. lamblia* cysts.

Pathogenesis and Symptoms and Signs

Symptoms are commonly absent or mild, but intermittent nausea, eructation, flatulence, epigastric pain, abdominal cramps, and diarrhea may occur. In severe cases, malabsorption can lead to significant weight loss and bulky, malodorous stools. The severity of the malabsorption is related to the degree of infection, but the pathogenesis of these manifestations is unknown. Mechanical blockade of the microvilli, damage to their brush border, altered mobility, and mucosal invasion resulting in T cell mediated mucosal damage have all been suggested as possible mechanisms.

Diagnosis

Finding the organism in the stool or duodenal secretions is diagnostic. In acute infections the parasite can be readily found in the stool; in chronic cases excretion is irregular, requiring repeated stool examinations. Alternatively, duodenal contents—obtained with a nylon string (Enterotest®) or by aspirations through a gastric tube—can be examined for trophozoites.

Treatment

Of the 3 drugs available in the USA for treatment of giardiasis, the most frequently recommended is quinacrine 100 mg tid for 5 days. Although it is highly effective (70 to 95% cure rate), it may produce GI disturbances and, rarely, toxic psychosis. Metronidazole 250 to 750 mg tid for 7 days is equally effective and better tolerated, but it is not currently licensed for use in giardiasis and there is concern over its potential teratogenicity and/or carcinogenicity. Furazolidone is less effective than either of these agents but is available as a suspension, making it useful in children. Although the FDA has approved it, it has induced neoplasia in experimental animals.

Household and sexual contacts should be examined and, if infected, treated. Pregnant women should be treated only if they show significant symptoms.

MALARIA

A protozoan infection characterized by paroxysms of chills, fever, and sweating, and by anemia, splenomegaly, and a chronic relapsing course.

Etiology and Epidemiology

Malarial parasites of 4 types, each with a different biologic pattern, may affect man: *Plasmodium vivax*, *P. falciparum*, *P. malariae*, and *P. ovale*. Infection occurs through the bite of an infected anopheles mosquito, transfusion of blood from an infected donor, or use of a common syringe by drug addicts.

Most hyperendemic malarious areas are in the tropics. Chemotherapeutic agents and insecticides have made autochthonous malaria rare in the USA and many other parts of the world, but visitors from malarious areas and returning tourists may introduce the infection; returning armed forces personnel have caused small sporadic epidemics.

Pathogenesis

The life cycle of the malarial parasite begins when a female anopheles mosquito, feeding on a patient with malaria, ingests blood containing gametocytes. These undergo sexual development (sporogony) within the mosquito, to end as sporozoites located in the insect's salivary glands. The mosquito injects the sporozoites into man, and the parasite multiplies asexually in the liver parenchymal cells. Little is known of the pathologic changes accompanying this asymptomatic fixed-tissue **(exoerythrocytic)** phase. After a period of maturation ranging from days to months (average, 2 to 4 wk), merozoites are released and invade the RBCs, initiating the clinical or **erythrocytic** phase. *P. vivax* and *P. ovale* exoerythrocytic parasites persist in the liver cells, periodically "seeding" the bloodstream with new merozoites to cause a relapse. *P. falciparum* and *P. malariae* do not persist in the liver cells; however, in untreated infections erythrocytic parasites may persist from months (*P. falciparum*) to years (*P. malariae*) and produce recrudescent clinical disease.

All 4 parasites multiply asexually within the RBCs (schizogony) to produce a new generation of merozoites. The RBCs rupture and these merozoites are released into the circulating plasma to enter intact RBCs and repeat the erythrocytic cycle. Except in falciparum infections, it is unusual for > 1% of the RBCs to become infected. Gametocytes rather than merozoites are formed in some RBCs. These gametocytes cannot self-replicate, and they die unless ingested by the anopheles mosquito for completion of the sexual cycle.

Pathology

After prolonged untreated malarial infection or repeated relapses, persistent hepatosplenomegaly develops. The spleen is usually soft and full of malarial pigment. The sinusoids are filled with numerous parasitized RBCs and the macrophages contain ingested malarial pigment. The Kupffer cells may be distended with parasites and pigment. There are no characteristic changes in other organs except the presence of scattered malarial pigment in macrophages. In fatal falciparum malaria, however, the brain is slate gray and punctate hemorrhages are often scattered throughout the brain substance as the result of capillary occlusion with parasite-infected RBCs.

Symptoms and Signs

The incubation period is usually 10 to 35 days, often followed by a short (2 to 3 days) prodrome of irregular low-grade fever, malaise, headache, myalgia, and chilly sensations that is frequently misidentified and treated as influenza.

In **vivax** and **ovale malaria,** the primary attack begins abruptly with a shaking chill, followed by fever and sweats with irregularly remittent fever. Within a week the typical paroxysmal pattern of the disease is established. The initial chill may be preceded by a short period of malaise or headache. The fever lasts from 1 to 8 h; after it subsides, the patient feels well until the next rigor. A rigor occurs q 48 h in uncomplicated vivax malaria.

In **falciparum malaria,** there may be a chilly sensation rather than a shaking chill; the temperature rises gradually and falls by lysis. The paroxysm may last 20 to 36 h, there is more prostration than in vivax malaria, and headache is prominent. During intervals between paroxysms, which are exceedingly variable (36 to 72 h), the patient usually feels miserable and has a low-grade fever.

In **malariae malaria,** the disease more frequently begins abruptly with a paroxysm, which then recurs at 72-h intervals.

In falciparum malaria, fever of 40 C (104 F) or severe headache, drowsiness, delirium, confusion, or parasitemia in excess of 100,000 organisms/cu mm may indicate impending **cerebral malaria,** usually a fatal complication and most commonly seen in infants, pregnant women, and nonimmune travelers to endemic areas. Delirium may accompany high fever in vivax malaria, but cerebral manifestations are uncommon.

In both falciparum and vivax malaria, the periodicity of the chills and fever is influenced by numerous factors, including dual infection (by more than 1 plasmodium species), strain differences, and immunity. The WBC count is usually normal, with an increased percentage of lymphocytes and monocytes. Mild jaundice usually develops if the disease persists untreated, and the spleen and liver become enlarged. Hypoglycemia is common and severe in patients with intense parisitemia and may be exaggerated with quinine therapy.

Chronic malaria with low-grade parasitemia occurs in partially immune subjects in hyperendemic areas and may be accompanied by malaise, listlessness, periodic headache, anorexia, fatigue, and mild fever. These symptoms may culminate in acute attacks of chills and fever, considerably milder and of shorter duration than in the primary attack.

Blackwater fever, a rare complication, is characterized by intravascular hemolysis and hemoglobinuria. It occurs, perhaps exclusively, in chronic falciparum malaria, especially in patients treated with quinine. Primaquine may cause hemolysis in individuals with G6PD deficiency (see Curative Therapy, below).

Diagnosis

Periodic attacks of chills and fever without apparent cause should always suggest malaria, particularly if the individual has been in a malarious area within the year and if the spleen is enlarged. Demonstration of the parasite in the stained blood smear is diagnostic; more than one smear may be required, since the intensity of parasitemia varies. It is important to identify the type of plasmodium, as this will influence therapy and prognosis.

If fever persists after adequate antimalarial therapy in patients with suspected malaria, the original diagnosis was probably wrong.

Prognosis

Untreated vivax malaria subsides spontaneously in 10 to 30 days, but may recur at variable intervals. The prognosis becomes less favorable if intercurrent infection supervenes or if the individual was in poor general health when the attack began. Antimalarial therapy produces excellent results in vivax and falciparum malaria. Untreated falciparum malaria has a high mortality rate.

Prophylaxis and Suppression Therapy

Attempts to induce immunity with vaccines are still experimental. Patients with malaria, however, gradually develop immunity that considerably modifies the clinical course. This immunity has a degree of strain specificity.

Preventive measures include control of mosquito breeding places and use of residual insecticide sprays in homes and outbuildings, screens (or mosquito netting where screens are not feasible) on doors and windows, and mosquito repellents and sufficient clothing (particularly after sundown, to protect as much of the skin surface as possible against mosquito bites). Contact between malaria patients and mosquitos must be prevented to avoid further spread of infection.

Chloroquine phosphate 500 mg (300-mg base) (children, 5-mg base/kg) orally once/wk protects travelers to malarious areas by suppressing the erythrocytic infection and the clinical manifestations of malaria. Although not effective in suppressing chloroquine-resistant *P. falciparum*, chloroquine prophylaxis should, nevertheless, be taken by travelers to East Africa, Asia, and Latin America, where such strains are found, to suppress coexisting chloroquine-sensitive plasmodium species. The addition of 25 mg of pyrimethamine and 500 mg of sulfadoxine (available in a combination tablet in endemic areas) to the weekly chloroquine regimen is usually effective in suppressing chloroquine-resistant falciparum malaria. However, as this drug combination has been associated with several cases of severe cutaneous reactions, its use should be limited to

those planning prolonged stays in areas of intense malaria transmission. These drugs should be started 2 wk before arrival in the area and continued for 6 wk after leaving, since this continued use eradicates *P. falciparum* and *P. malariae*. In other types of malaria, primaquine must be given in addition to chloroquine (see Curative Therapy, below).

Treatment

1. Treatment of the acute attack: The drug of choice in all types of malaria except drug-resistant falciparum malaria is chloroquine. The dose is 1 gm of chloroquine phosphate (600-mg base) (children, 10-mg base/kg) orally, followed by 500 mg (300-mg base) (children, 5-mg base/kg) in 6 h, and then 500 mg (300-mg base)/day for 2 days. The total dose for adults is 2.5 gm (1.5-gm base). Patients who are comatose or vomiting may be given chloroquine hydrochloride 250 to 375 mg (200- to 300-mg base) IM q 6 h (children, 5-mg base/kg q 12 h). Oral therapy with chloroquine phosphate should be resumed as soon as possible.

Chloroquine-resistant strains of *P. falciparum* (any case contracted in East Africa, Central or South America, or the Far East may be resistant) should be treated with quinine, pyrimethamine, and a sulfonamide, all given concurrently. Quinine sulfate 600 mg tid (children, 25 mg/kg/day in 3 doses) is given orally for 3 days. If oral therapy is precluded, 600 mg of quinine dihydrochloride (children, 25 mg/kg/day in 3 doses) may be diluted in 300 mL saline or glucose and given IV over 30 min. The dose may be repeated q 8 h, but oral therapy should be restarted as soon as possible. In cases with renal failure, the dose is limited to 600 mg once/day. Quinine may cause tinnitus and, occasionally, drug fever or allergic purpura. If quinine dihydrochloride is not immediately available, the antiarrhythmic agent quinidine gluconate can serve as a satisfactory substitute. The dose is 800 mg, administered as described for quinine dihydrochloride. Careful electrocardiographic monitoring should be employed. Pyrimethamine 25 mg bid (children $<$ 10 kg, 6.25 mg/day; 10 to 20 kg, 12.5 mg/day) is given orally for 3 days. It is a folate antagonist and may cause or accentuate anemia. Sulfadiazine 500 mg orally qid (children, 100 to 200 mg/kg/day in 4 doses, to a maximum of 2 gm/day) is given for 5 days.

2. Curative therapy: Because *P. falciparum* and *P. malariae* parasites do not have a persistent hepatic (exoerythrocytic) phase, the disease is cured once the acute attack is adequately treated as outlined above.

In other types of malaria, the exoerythrocytic and erythrocytic parasites must be eradicated to prevent relapse. Primaquine phosphate 26.3 mg (15-mg base)/day (children, 0.3-mg base/kg/day) orally for 14 days accomplishes this in 80 to 90% of primary infections. It may be given at the same time as chloroquine or afterward. A second course of primaquine may be given if relapse occurs. Primaquine may cause intravascular hemolysis in patients with G6PD deficiency, and patients should be screened for this deficiency prior to treatment. Abdominal cramps and methemoglobinuria may also occur with primaquine. Primaquine should not be given to pregnant women.

3. Gametocidal therapy: Gametocytes usually appear 2 to 3 days after onset of the erythrocytic phase and may persist for long periods, particularly in falciparum malaria. They do not produce symptoms, but indicate preexisting infection and serve as a source of infection for the anopheles mosquito.

P. vivax and *P. malariae* gametocyte development can be prevented by suppression with chloroquine (see Prophylaxis and Suppression Therapy, above), or by adequate and prompt treatment of the acute attack. *P. falciparum* gametocytes, once developed, are resistant to suppressive drugs, but are susceptible to primaquine; 15 mg (base)/day for 3 days or a single 45-mg dose will sterilize the gametocytes.

LEISHMANIASIS

A group of conditions caused by a species of Leishmania *and transmitted by several phlebotomine sandflies.* Manifestations may be visceral, mucocutaneous, or cutaneous, and the strain of the infecting organism and the host's immunologic status apparently can greatly modify the clinical manifestations. The incubation period is weeks to months.

KALA-AZAR

(Visceral Leishmaniasis; Dumdum Fever)

Epidemiology, Pathogenesis, and Findings

Kala-azar occurs in India, China, Russia, Africa, the Mediterranean basin, and several South and Central American countries. Children and young adults are particularly susceptible. The protozoa (*L. donovani*) invade the bloodstream and localize in the reticuloendothelial system, causing fever, pronounced splenomegaly, emaciation, and pancytopenia. The fever is seldom sustained and recurs irregularly. The liver and lymph nodes may become enlarged. Hypergammaglobulinemia is present. The parasite may be demonstrated in needle biopsy of the liver, spleen, bone marrow, skin lesions, or lymph nodes, or in cultures from these tissues or from blood. Sensitive serologic tests have been developed but are not generally available. The leishmanin skin test is negative during active disease. The fatality rate is 90% in untreated cases but generally below 10% in treated cases.

Treatment

General: Bed rest, oral hygiene, and good nutrition are important. Transfusions are useful for anemia; antibacterial chemotherapy is indicated for bacterial complications.

Specific: Pentavalent antimony compounds and aromatic diamidines are the drugs of choice. Sodium antimony gluconate (sodium stibogluconate) is given once daily, slowly IV or IM in distilled water. The generally accepted dosage is 0.1 mL (10 mg antimony)/kg/injection (maximum, 600 mg antimony/day; minimum, 200 mg/day) for 6 to 10 days. If toxic effects (nausea, vomiting) appear, the drug should be given on alternate days, its dosage reduced, or its administration stopped. Three 10-day courses as above, separated by 10-day intervals, may be given in resistant (African) cases. Kala-azar encountered in the Sudan is resistant to antimony; pentamidine 4 mg/kg/day IM for up to 15 days must be used instead.

ORIENTAL SORE

(Cutaneous Leishmaniasis; Tropical Sore; Delhi or Aleppo Boil)

Epidemiology and Findings

Oriental sore occurs in China, India, the Near East, the Mediterranean basin, and Africa as far south as Nigeria and Angola. It is characterized by single or multiple sharply demarcated, ulcerating, granulomatous, autoinoculable skin lesions. Secondary infection is usual. The only systemic symptoms are those due to secondary infection. *Leishmania tropica* or *L. major* may be demonstrated in smears or cultures of curettings from the sides or base of the ulcer. The leishmanin skin test is positive. Healing occurs spontaneously in 2 to 18 mo, leaving a depressed scar.

Treatment

Excellent results are obtained by infiltrating the indurated edge and base of the ulcer with 6 mL of sodium antimony gluconate 3 or 4 times every other day. CO_2 snow, infrared therapy, and radiotherapy may also be effective. When lesions are numerous,

sodium antimony gluconate should be given parenterally as for kala-azar, above. Antibiotics are indicated for secondary infections.

American Leishmaniasis
(Espundia; Forest Yaws; Uta; Chiclero Ulcer)

This disease may manifest itself as localized cutaneous ulcers resembling oriental sore or as metastatic mucocutaneous lesions known as *Espundia*. The localized lesions, caused by *L. mexicana*, usually occur on the face; they are known as chiclero ulcers, since they primarily affect persons who enter forests to gather chicle. Uta, a similar disease found in Peru, is caused by *L. braziliensis peruviana*. *Espundia*, which causes ulcerative lesions of the nose and pharynx, occurs in southern Mexico and Central and South America. It is caused by *L. braziliensis braziliensis*. Untreated, the disease may persist for years, with death resulting from secondary infection. **Diagnosis** is by demonstrating the parasites in biopsy material or by culture of material from the ulcer edge.

Treatment of the early cutaneous lesions is as recommended above for oriental sore. The extensive lesions of later stages require sodium antimony gluconate or pentamidine as for kala-azar (see above).

Diffuse Cutaneous Leishmaniasis

This form of the disease, characterized by widespread skin lesions resembling those of lepromatous leprosy, presumably results from a specific defect of cell-mediated immunity to the leishmanial organism. In South America, it is caused by *L. mexicana amazonensis*; in Ethiopia, by *L. tropica aethiopica*. The diagnosis is made by demonstrating the organisms in the skin lesions. The disease is resistant to treatment.

TRYPANOSOMIASIS
(African Sleeping Sickness; Chagas' Disease)

A chronic disease caused by protozoa of the genus Trypanosoma. *T. brucei* var. *gambiense* and *rhodesiense* produce African sleeping sickness (Gambian and Rhodesian trypanosomiasis); *T. cruzi* causes Chagas' disease (South American trypanosomiasis), seen in South and Central America. The African forms of trypanosomiasis are spread by the bite of the tsetse fly (genus *Glossina*). Chagas' disease is transmitted by contamination of the bite wound of the "assassin" or "kissing" reduviid bugs (*Triatoma* and related Reduviidae) with the infected feces of the insect.

Symptoms, Signs, and Course

African trypanosomiasis is characterized by irregular fever, generalized lymphadenopathy (particularly of the posterior cervical chain), cutaneous eruptions, and areas of painful localized edema. CNS symptoms, such as tremors, headache, apathy, and convulsions, later predominate and progress to coma and death. Rhodesian trypanosomiasis is more severe and more often fatal than Gambian trypanosomiasis.

Acute **Chagas' disease** occurs predominantly in young children and is characterized in the early stages by fever, lymphadenopathy, hepatosplenomegaly, and facial edema. Rarely, meningoencephalitis or convulsive seizures may occur, sometimes causing permanent mental or physical defects or death. Acute myocarditis is common and may be fatal. Chronic Chagas' disease may be mild or even asymptomatic, or may be accompanied by myocardiopathy, megaesophagus, and megacolon, with fatal outcome. These late manifestations probably result from lymphocyte-mediated destruction of muscle tissue and nerve ganglions during the acute stage of the disease. In Brazil and Argentina the disease is often severe; in Chile, usually mild.

Diagnosis

Recognition of African trypanosomiasis depends on demonstration of the trypanosomes. Early in the disease, they may be found in smears of peripheral blood or in fluid aspirated from an enlarged lymph node. In advanced stages, they may be found only in the CSF. A number of serologic tests, including a card agglutination test, have been employed as screening tests.

Chagas' disease is identified by demonstration of trypanosomes in the peripheral blood or leishmanial forms in a lymph node biopsy, or by animal inoculation or culture, xenodiagnosis, or serologic tests.

Prophylaxis

Prophylaxis against African trypanosomiasis includes protection against the vector flies, avoidance of endemic areas, or chemoprophylaxis. Pentamidine 4 mg/kg IM every 3 to 6 mo confers a high degree of protection against the Gambian form of disease, but its use in the Rhodesian variety is controversial. Pentamidine may mask infection and cause renal failure and, on occasion, diabetes; therefore it should be used only in persons in great danger of being infected.

Reduviid bugs, the vectors of Chagas' disease, inhabit poorly constructed houses and outbuildings. Residual spraying with 5% γ-benzene hexachloride is most effective in controlling the vector. Patching wall cracks and cementing over dirt floors also help to eliminate the vectors.

Treatment

There is no satisfactory treatment for Chagas' disease. Prolonged administration of nifurtimox, a nitrofurazone derivative, may effect parasitologic cure. Chronic organ damage, however, appears irreversible.

Suramin is the drug of choice for both early Rhodesian and Gambian trypanosomiasis. It is given IV as a 10% solution in distilled water; an initial test dose of 100 mg (to exclude hypersensitivity) is followed by 1 gm on the next day and on days 3, 7, 14, and 21, for a total of 5 gm. (CAUTION: *Renal impairment*)

Melarsoprol, a trivalent arsenical, is more toxic than the above drugs, but is effective in all stages of Gambian and Rhodesian trypanosomiasis. It should be used when the CNS is involved. Patients with minimal to moderate neurologic involvement are given three 3-day courses of 3.6 mg/kg/day IV, each course 2 wk apart. Melarsoprol causes the usual arsenical toxicity: GI, neurologic, and renal.

Patients with severe neurologic involvement may develop a reactive encephalopathy when given melarsoprol. Prior treatment with suramin may help to avert this complication, which is apparently due to release of trypanosomal antigen. Suramin is given in 2 to 4 alternate-day doses of 250 to 500 mg IV. Melarsoprol is then given in 3 daily or alternate-day doses of 1.5, 2.0, and 2.2 mg/kg IV. After a 7-day interval, 3 doses of melarsoprol, 2.5, 3.0, and 3.6 mg/kg/day, are given; after another 7-day interval, a third course of 3.6 mg/kg/day is given for 3 days. A new experimental drug, α-difluoromethylornithine **(DFMO)** appears to be more effective and less toxic than melarsoprol in treating CNS disease.

TOXOPLASMOSIS

A generalized or CNS granulomatous disease caused by Toxoplasma gondii. Asymptomatic infections are common; serologic surveys show that 7 to 94% of various populations are infected. The disease occurs worldwide.

Etiology and Pathogenesis

T. gondii is a small intracellular protozoan parasite that can infect any warm-blooded animal. It invades and multiplies asexually within the cytoplasm of nucleated

host cells. With the development of host immunity, multiplication slows and tissue cysts are formed. Sexual multiplication occurs in the intestinal cells of cats (and apparently only cats); oocysts form and are shed in the stool. Transmission may occur transplacentally, by ingestion of raw or undercooked meat containing tissue cysts, or, perhaps most importantly, by exposure to oocysts in soil contaminated with cat feces.

Symptoms and Signs

Neonatal congenital toxoplasmosis (see also CONGENITAL TOXOPLASMOSIS under NEONATAL INFECTIONS in Ch. 186) is acquired transplacentally, the mother presumably having acquired a primary infection at conception or later during pregnancy. Abortion may ensue if infection occurs early in pregnancy. Infection later in pregnancy may result in miscarriage or stillbirth, or in the birth of a living child with clinical disease. The disease may be severe, fulminating, and rapidly fatal, or there may be no symptoms at all. Symptoms of subacute infection may begin shortly after birth, but more often appear months or several years later. Chronic chorioretinitis; severe jaundice; hepatosplenomegaly; maculopapular rash; thrombocytopenic purpura; intracerebral calcification; convulsions, opisthotonos, psychomotor disturbances, or other CNS symptoms; and hydrocephalus or microcephaly are common. Blindness and severe mental retardation may result. Chronic disease, with relapses, occurs in patients who survive the subacute phase. Visceral lesions, aside from those in the liver, are unusual and heal more readily than CNS lesions.

Acquired toxoplasmosis is seldom symptomatic and is usually recognized serologically. However, symptomatic infection may present in any of 3 ways:

1. The more common **mild lymphatic form** may resemble infectious mononucleosis. It is characterized by cervical and axillary lymphadenopathy, malaise, muscle pain, and irregular low fever. Mild anemia, hypotension, leukopenia, lymphocytosis, and slightly altered liver function may be present. More commonly, it presents as asymptomatic cervical lymphadenopathy.
2. An acute, **fulminating, disseminated infection** occurs primarily in immunologically incompetent patients, often with a rash, high fever, chills, and prostration. Some patients may develop meningoencephalitis, hepatitis, pneumonitis, or myocarditis.
3. **Chronic toxoplasmosis** causes severe retinochoroiditis (posterior uveitis); muscular weakness, weight loss, headache, and diarrhea may be present. Symptoms are vague and indefinite, and diagnosis is difficult. In the USA, uveitis is seldom due to *Toxoplasma* infection.

Diagnosis

The diagnosis is usually established serologically. IgM antibodies, which are detected by the indirect fluorescent antibody procedure (IgM-IFA), appear during the 1st wk of illness, peak within 1 to 2 wk, and revert to normal within 3 wk to several months. IgG antibodies arise more slowly, peak in 1 or 2 mo, and then may remain high and stable for months to years. They are also detected with the indirect fluorescent-antibody **(IgG-IFA)** technic, but may also be measured with the Sabin-Feldman dye, indirect hemagglutination, and the CF tests. A positive IgM-IFA test (> 1:20) or a 2-tube rise in one of the IgG tests usually indicates the presence of acute disease. Acute disease should also be assumed present if the IgG-IFA or dye test titers exceed 1:1000 in the presence of lymphadenopathy in a pregnant woman or encephalitis in an immunocompromised host.

The parasite has been isolated during the acute phase of the disease by injecting mice with biopsy material from lymph nodes, muscle, or other tissues.

Prognosis

The prognosis is poor in congenital toxoplasmosis acquired during the 1st trimester. Affected children die in infancy or suffer chronic destructive CNS lesions. Infections

acquired during the 3rd trimester are usually asymptomatic. The prognosis in acquired postnatal toxoplasmosis is good. The general mildness of postnatally acquired infection is indicated by the large number of persons with latent or cured toxoplasmosis, and by the fact that the disease is rarely fatal in adults. Reactivation of toxoplasmosis in immunosuppressed patients usually ends in death.

Treatment

Acute toxoplasmosis of newborns, pregnant women, and immunosuppressed patients should be treated with standard oral doses of trisulfapyrimidines or sulfadiazine plus pyrimethamine 25 mg (1 mg/kg for children) daily for 3 to 4 wk. The hematologic toxicity of pyrimethamine can be minimized by daily administration of folinic acid (10 mg). Since pyrimethamine is teratogenic in animals, sulfonamides alone should be used in the first trimester of pregnancy. Other patients with active disease do not require specific therapy unless a vital organ (eye, brain, heart) is involved or constitutional symptoms are severe and persistent. Corticosteroids are often useful in these situations to control the inflammatory reaction. Periodic blood counts need to be obtained during therapy to monitor pyrimethamine hemotoxicity.

BABESIOSIS

A cosmopolitan infection of animals caused by intraerythrocytic parasites of the genus Babesia. Human disease is rare. The organisms are transmitted by hard-bodied ticks and produce a febrile hemolytic anemia. In splenectomized patients the infection has a high mortality rate and closely resembles falciparum malaria, with high fever, hemolytic anemia, hemoglobinuria, jaundice, and renal failure. A patient with an intact spleen has a milder illness that usually resolves spontaneously in weeks or months. Most cases in the USA have been of this milder type and have been acquired on offshore islands of New York and Massachusetts. **Diagnosis** requires demonstration of the parasites, which resemble those of malaria, in Giemsa-stained smears of peripheral blood. In contrast to *Plasmodium* spp., however, neither gametocytes nor malaria pigment can be seen. The presence of tetrads and basket-shaped parasites is also helpful.

Treatment is usually not required in patients with intact spleens. In infections that are life-threatening, clindamycin 300 to 750 mg IV q 6 h and quinine 650 mg orally q 6 h appear to be effective.

CRYPTOSPORIDIOSIS

A diarrheal disease of vertebrates produced by protozoa of the genus Cryptosporidia. The illness is acute and self-limited, except in the immunocompromised, where it is chronic, severe and life-threatening.

Etiology, Epidemiology, and Pathogenesis

Cryptosporidia are small (2 to 6 μm) basophilic spherules that inhabit the microvillous border of the intestinal epithelium, arranged in rows along the brush border of the jejunum. There they multiply asexually until the host mounts an immunologic response. Infective **oocysts** are shed into the intestinal lumen and passed in the feces. Following its ingestion by another vertebrate, the oocyst releases **sporozoites** that attach themselves to the epithelial surface and initiate a new cycle of infection. Cryptosporidiosis involves most vertebrate groups. All parasite strains appear morphologically identical and are currently considered a single species. Human infections may result from zoonotic spread or direct person-to-person contact and perhaps via food and water. Children, travelers to foreign countries, male homosexuals, and medical personnel caring for patients with cryptosporidiosis are at particular risk. In western countries, 1 to 4% of children with gastroenteritis harbor cryptosporidia; in developing countries, 4 to 11% of such children have cryptosporidiosis.

The nature of the diarrhea suggests that it is caused by an enterotoxin. Bowel changes are limited to mild villous atrophy, crypt enlargement, and a minimal mononuclear infiltrate of the lamina propria.

Symptoms, Signs, and Diagnosis

In the normal host, onset is explosive, with profuse, watery diarrhea and abdominal cramping 4 to 14 days after exposure. Symptoms generally persist for 5 to 11 days, then rapidly abate. In the immunocopromised host (eg, marasmic and malnourished children, individuals with congenital hypogammaglobulinemia, those receiving immunosuppressive drugs for cancer therapy or organ transplantation, and patients with AIDS), onset is more gradual and the diarrhea more severe, with daily fluid losses of up to 15 to 20 L. Unless the underlying immunologic defect is corrected, the diarrhea may continue persistently or remittently for life.

Recovering acid-fast oocysts from the stool confirms the diagnosis. Their excretion is most intense during the first 4 days of illness but persists for the duration of the diarrhea. Using the formalin-diethyl acetate sedimentation or Sheather's sugar flotation stool concentration procedure enhances yield in specimens with few oocysts.

Prophylaxis and Treatment

Stools of patients with cryptosporidiosis are highly infectious; stool precautions should be instituted, particularly in cancer chemotherapy and transplantation units, where spread of the disease can be catastrophic.

No uniformly effective, specific anticryptosporidial therapy is available, although some patients have responded at least temporarily to spiramycin, furazolidone or α-difluoromethylornithine **(DFMO)**. Reversal of malnutrition, withdrawal of immunosuppressive agents, and bone marrow transplantation have resulted in cure. Oral and parenteral rehydration should be employed as necessary.

DISEASES CAUSED BY WORMS

INTESTINAL NEMATODES

ENTEROBIASIS

(See TABLE 13–2 in this chapter and PINWORM INFESTATION in MISCELLANEOUS INFECTIONS in Ch. 191)

TRICHURIASIS

(Whipworm Infection; Trichocephaliasis)

An infection caused by Trichuris trichiura *and characterized by abdominal pain and diarrhea.*

Etiology, Pathogenesis, and Epidemiology

Infection results from ingestion of eggs that have incubated in soil for 2 or 3 wk. The larva hatches in the small intestine, migrates to the colon, and embeds its anterior head in the mucosa. Mature females produce about 5000 eggs/day, which are passed in the stool.

This parasite is found principally in the subtropics and tropics, where poor sanitation and a warm, moist climate provide the conditions necessary for incubating the eggs in soil. Clinically significant infections are uncommon in the USA.

Symptoms, Signs, and Diagnosis

Only heavy infection causes symptoms—abdominal pain and diarrhea. Very heavy infections may cause intestinal blood loss, anemia, weight loss, appendicitis, and, in children and parturient women, rectal prolapse.

The characteristic barrel-shaped eggs are usually readily found in the stool.

Prophylaxis and Treatment

Prevention depends upon adequate toilet facilities and good personal hygiene.

Mebendazole 100 mg orally bid for 3 days has been highly effective and is the drug of choice. The drug should not be used in pregnancy because it is teratogenic in animals. Light infections (those that require stool concentration procedure for their detection) do not require treatment.

ASCARIASIS

An infection caused by Ascaris lumbricoides *and characterized by early pulmonary and later intestinal symptoms.*

Etiology, Epidemiology, and Pathogenesis

The life cycle of the ascarids resembles that of *Trichuris* except for a phase of larval migration through the lungs. Once the larva hatches, it migrates through the wall of the small intestine and is carried by the lymphatics and bloodstream to the lungs. Here it passes into an alveolus, ascends the respiratory tract, and is swallowed. It matures in the jejunum, where it remains as an adult worm. Disease may be caused by both the larval migration through the lung and the presence of the adult worm in the intestine. Malabsorption may result with heavy worm loads; the pathogenesis is not clearly understood.

The disease occurs worldwide but is concentrated in warm, poorly sanitated areas where it is maintained largely by the indiscriminate defecation and ingestion habits of children.

Symptoms, Signs, and Diagnosis

Fever, cough, wheezing, eosinophilic leukocytosis, and migratory pulmonary infiltrates may be present during the phase of larval migration through the lungs. Heavy intestinal infection may cause abdominal cramping and, occasionally, intestinal obstruction. Adult worms may rarely obstruct the appendix, or the biliary or pancreatic ducts.

Infection with the adult worm is usually diagnosed by finding eggs in the stool. Occasionally, adult worms are passed in the stool or vomited. Larvae are occasionally found in the sputum during the pulmonary phase.

Prophylaxis

Prevention requires adequate sanitation. Drug prophylaxis has been successful in endemic areas.

Treatment

Pyrantel pamoate 11 mg/kg (maximum, 1 gm) in a single oral dose, or mebendazole 100 mg bid for 3 days is also effective. Mebendazole should not be used in pregnancy (see TRICHURIASIS, above).

HOOKWORM DISEASE

A symptomatic infection caused by Ancylostoma duodenale *or* Necator americanus *and characterized by abdominal pain and iron-deficiency anemia.* Asymptomatic hookworm infection is more common than symptomatic disease.

Etiology, Pathogenesis, and Epidemiology

The life cycles of the 2 worms are similar. Eggs are discharged in the stool, hatch in the soil after a 1- to 2-day incubation period, and release a free-living larva that molts a few days later and becomes infective to humans. The larvae penetrate human skin, reach the lung via the lymphatics and blood, ascend the respiratory tract, are swal-

TABLE 13–2. COMMONLY ENCOUNTERED

Condition	Causative Organism (Synonyms or Varieties)	Geographic Distribution	Source of Infection	Portal of Entry (& Stage)
Roundworms				
Ascariasis	*Ascaris lumbricoides* (Giant intestinal roundworm)	Cosmopolitan, more common in warm, moist climates	Fecal contamination of soil (eggs) Contaminated vegetables	Mouth (embryonated eggs)
Hookworm infection	a) *Ancylostoma duodenale* (Old World type) b) *Necator americanus* (Tropical type)	a) Temperate & warm, moist climates b) Warm, moist climates	Fecal contamination of soil (larvae)	Skin, usually feet, possibly mouth (filariform larvae)
Strongyloidiasis	*Strongyloides stercoralis* (Threadworm)	Southern USA, moist tropics	Fecal contamination of soil (larvae)	Skin, usually feet (filariform larvae)
Trichuriasis	*Trichuris trichiura* (Whipworm)	Warm, moist climates Uncommon in USA	Fecal contamination of soil (eggs)	Mouth (embryonated eggs)
Enterobiasis	*Enterobius vermicularis* (*Oxyuris vermicularis;* pinworm, seatworm)	Cosmopolitan, esp. in children	Eggs from contaminated fomites Anus-finger-mouth	Mouth (embryonated eggs)
Tapeworms				
Dwarf Tapeworm infection	*Hymenolepis nana*	Southern USA, in children Cosmopolitan	Eggs contaminating environment	Mouth (eggs)
Beef Tapeworm infection	*Taenia saginata*	Cosmopolitan	Inadequately cooked or raw infected beef	Mouth (cysticercus larvae in infected beef)
Pork Tapeworm infection	*Taenia solium*	Rare in USA; common in Latin America, Asia, USSR, E. Europe	Inadequately cooked or raw infected pork	Mouth (cysticercus larvae in infected pork)
Fish Tapeworm infection	*Diphyllobothrium latum*	Northern Minn. & Mich.; Canada Cosmopolitan	Infected fresh-water fish	Mouth (larvae in infected fresh-water fish flesh)

INTESTINAL PARASITIC INFECTIONS

Most Common Symptoms	*Diagnostic Findings*	*Therapeutic Agents*	*Remarks*
Bronchial symptoms, eosinophilia* (larval stage) Colicky pains, "acute abdomen"	Immature eggs in stool Worms evacuated in stool, occasionally vomited	Pyrantel pamoate Mebendazole	May block intestine, biliary or pancreatic duct
Abdominal pain, anemia, cardiac insufficiency, retarded growth	Immature eggs in stool	Pyrantel pamoate Mebendazole	Prophylaxis: Use sanitary latrines, wear shoes, treat infected persons
Radiating pain in pit of stomach, diarrhea, linear urticaria	Larvae in stool Larvae in duodenum	Thiabendazole	Prophylaxis: As for hookworm May persist for decades
Diarrhea, abdominal pain, anemia, weight loss	Immature eggs in stool	Mebendazole	May produce dysenteric syndrome or acute appendicitis; rectal prolapse in children
Perianal & perineal pruritus	Eggs in perianal swabs; adult worms per anum	Pyrantel pamoate Mebendazole	Often involves entire family
Diarrhea, abdominal discomfort, in massive infections in children	Eggs in stool	Niclosamide Praziquantel	May be symptomless
Usually asymptomatic, anal passage of proglottids, abdominal distress, "acute appendix"	Proglottids of adult worms in stool; eggs near anus	Niclosamide Praziquantel	May be symptomless Prophylaxis: Thoroughly cook all suspected beef
Similar to *T. saginata*	Eggs and proglottids of adult worms in stool; eggs near anus	Niclosamide Praziquantel	May be symptomless Ingested eggs may produce human cysticercosis Prophylaxis: Thoroughly cook all pork in infected areas
Mild GI symptoms; may cause pernicious anemia	Immature eggs in stool	Niclosamide Praziquantel	May be symptomless Prophylaxis: Thoroughly cook or freeze fresh-water fish

(Continued)

* Note: Eosinophilia often accompanies intestinal helminthiasis.

TABLE 13–2. COMMONLY ENCOUNTERED

Condition	Causative Organism (Synonyms or Varieties)	Geographic Distribution	Source of Infection	Portal of Entry (& Stage)
Tapeworms *(Cont'd)*				
Sparganosis	*Diphyllobothrium mansoni*	Several areas, incl. southern USA Cosmopolitan	a) Drinking water containing infected Cyclops (primary host) b) Direct contact with flesh of intermediate host	a) Usually mouth (larval stages) b) Skin
Echinococcus	*Echinococcus granulosus*	Sheep-raising areas of the world, Alaska, Utah, Arizona, Nevada	Canine feces	Mouth (eggs)
Protozoa				
Amebiasis	*Entamoeba histolytica*	Cosmopolitan; common in warm, moist climates	Feces-contaminated water, food, fomites	Mouth (cyst)
Giardiasis	*Giardia lamblia*	Cosmopolitan	Human feces, water, mammal feces	Mouth (cyst)
Flukes				
Intestinal	a) *Fasciolopsis buski* b) *Heterophyes, Metagonimus*	In USA only as rare infections imported from Orient or tropics	a) Vegetation b) Fresh-water fish	Mouth (encysted metacercarial larva)
Hepatic	a) *Fasciola hepatica* (sheep liver fluke) b) *Clonorchis sinensis*	a) Cosmopolitan in sheep-raising countries b) Orient	a) Watercress containing metacercarial cysts b) Fresh-water fish	a) Mouth (encysted metacercarial larva) b) Mouth (encysted larva)

INTESTINAL PARASITIC INFECTIONS *(Cont'd)*

Most Common Symptoms	*Diagnostic Findings*	*Therapeutic Agents*	*Remarks*
Inflamed subcut. tissue containing sparganum larva	Sparganum larva in subcut. tissues	Surgical excision	Adult worm in intestine of various nonhuman mammals
Abdominal mass, pain, pulmonary "coin lesion," cough, hemoptysis	Compatible history, liver or lung cyst, positive serology	Surgical excision Mebendazole	Patients with small, calcified hepatic cysts & Alaskan variety pulmonary cyst require surgery only if symptomatic
a) Intestinal 1. Mild 2. Dysentery b) Amebic abscess	Trophozoite stage or cyst in stool	a) 1. Metronidazole, Iodoquinol, or Diloxanide furoate† 2. Metronidazole & Iodoquinal + Emetine† or Dehydroemetine† b) Metronidazole *or* Emetine† & Chloroquine phosphate	Amebiasis may be asyndromic in individuals or populations
Mucous diarrhea, abdominal pain, weight loss	Vegetative stage or cyst in stool	Metronidazole Quinacrine	Prevalent in children in day-care centers and patients with immunoglobulin deficiencies. A cause of "travelers' diarrhea"
Usually asymptomatic abdominal pain, diarrhea, at times intestinal obstruction	Eggs in stool	a) Praziquantel b) Praziquantel	Primary intermediate hosts are fresh-water snails
Hepatic colic, cholecystitis	a) Immature eggs in stool or biliary drainage b) Eggs in stool & duodenal contents	a) Praziquantel b) Praziquantel	a) Sheep infected in USA, but few confirmed human infection b) Infections in USA from imported dried or pickled fish

(Continued)

† Available in USA from Center for Disease Control.

TABLE 13–2. COMMONLY ENCOUNTERED

Condition	Causative Organism (Synonyms or Varieties)	Geographic Distribution	Source of Infection	Portal of Entry (& Stage)
Flukes *(Cont'd)*				
Pulmonary	*Paragonimus westermani* (Orient) *Paragonimus* spp.	a) Africa b) Orient, extensive foci c) Latin America d) Rarely, USA and Canada	Crabs or crayfishes containing metacercarial cysts	Mouth (encysted metacercarial larva)
Blood (Schistosomiasis)	a) *Schistosoma japonicum* b) *S. mansoni* c) *S. haematobium*	a) Orient b) Africa, Latin America c) Africa, Near East	Infested water containing fork-tailed larvae from snail hosts	Skin (active fork-tailed cercariae)

lowed, and, about a week after skin penetration, reach the intestine. They attach by their mouths to the mucosa of the upper small intestine and suck blood.

About 25% of the world's population is infected with hookworms. Infection is most common in warm, moist areas with poor sanitation. *A. duodenale* is found in the Mediterranean basin, India, China, and Japan. *N. americanus* is found primarily in tropical areas of Africa, Asia, and the Americas; it is the species found in the USA.

Symptoms and Signs

A pruritic maculopapular rash ("ground itch") may develop at the site of larval penetration. Larval pulmonary migration occasionally causes pulmonary symptoms (see ASCARIASIS, above). Adult worms often cause epigastric pain. Whether iron-deficiency anemia and hypoalbuminemia result from intestinal blood loss depends upon whether the gut losses are replaced in the diet; this, in turn, is related to the worm load and to dietary adequacy. Growth retardation, cardiac failure, and anasarca may accompany chronic severe blood loss. In most infections, however, anemia does not develop.

Diagnosis

In symptomatic infections, the typical eggs are usually readily detected in the stool. If the stool is not examined for several hours, the eggs may hatch and release larvae that may be confused with those of *Strongyloides*.

Prophylaxis

Preventing soil pollution and avoiding direct skin contact with the soil are effective but impractical measures in most endemic areas. Periodic mass treatment and dietary iron supplements may be effective.

Treatment

General supportive treatment and correction of anemia take first priority. Anemia usually responds to oral iron therapy, but parenteral iron or blood transfusions may be required in severe cases. Anthelmintic therapy may be given as soon as the patient's condition is stable. Several effective agents are available. Pyrantel pamoate 11 mg/kg

INTESTINAL PARASITIC INFECTIONS *(Cont'd)*

Most Common Symptoms	*Diagnostic Findings*	*Therapeutic Agents*	*Remarks*
Peribronchiolar distress, with hemoptysis	Immature eggs in stool or sputum Serology	Praziquantel	Related species in wild mammals and hogs in USA
Dysentery, fibrosis of intestinal or bladder walls, hepatic fibrosis (a,b), hematuria (c)	Embryonated eggs in stool (a,b), or urine (c)	a) Praziquantel b) Praziquantel or Oxamniquine c) Praziquantel or Metrifonate‡	Related flukes cause "swimmer's itch" in bathers in USA and elsewhere

‡ Not available in USA.

(maximum, 1 gm) orally is given in a single dose. Mebendazole 100 mg orally bid for 3 days is equally effective but should not be used in pregnant women (see TRICHURIASIS, above).

STRONGYLOIDIASIS
(Threadworm Infection)

An infection caused by Strongyloides stercoralis *and characterized by eosinophilia and epigastric pain.*

Etiology, Pathogenesis, and Epidemiology

The life cycle closely resembles that of the hookworm, except that the eggs hatch while still in the intestine, and larvae rather than ova are passed in the stool. The larvae generally molt in the soil and develop into the infective filariform stage. Occasionally, the larvae molt in the intestine or on the perianal skin, and the filariform larvae then invade the host directly ("autoinfection" or "hyperinfection") without going through a soil phase. This can result in an extremely heavy worm load.

The disease is endemic in the tropics, is generally found in the same climatic and sanitary conditions favorable to the spread of hookworm, and may also occur in temperate areas in unsanitary, crowded institutions.

Symptoms, Signs, and Diagnosis

Transient bouts of linear urticaria and erythema may accompany autoinfection. Pulmonary manifestations similar to those seen in ascariasis (see above) may occur as a result of larval migration through the lungs. Heavy intestinal infection may cause epigastric pain and tenderness, vomiting, and diarrhea. Potentially fatal massive autoinfection and widespread larval migration, often accompanied by severe enterocolitis and gram-negative bacteremia, may occur in immunodepressed patients.

Larvae are found in the stool; several specimens should be examined, since only a few larvae may be present. Examination of duodenal aspirates or jejunal biopsies may also demonstrate the larvae.

Prophylaxis and Treatment

Prevention is generally as above, for hookworm. Thiabendazole 25 mg/kg bid orally for 2 or 3 days is effective treatment. In disseminated disease, treatment should be continued for 5 days.

TISSUE NEMATODES

TRICHINOSIS
(Trichiniasis)

A parasitic disease caused by Trichinella spiralis, *characterized initially by GI symptoms, and later by periorbital edema, muscle pains, fever, and eosinophilia.*

Etiology, Pathogenesis, and Epidemiology

Infection with the roundworm *T. spiralis* results from eating raw or inadequately cooked or processed pork or pork products (rarely, meat of bears and some marine mammals) containing encysted larvae (trichinae). The cyst wall is digested in the stomach or duodenum and the liberated larvae penetrate the duodenal and jejunal mucosa. Within 2 days, the larvae mature sexually and mate, after which the males play no further role in disease causation. The females burrow into the intestinal wall and begin to discharge living larvae by the 7th day. Each female may produce over 1000 larvae. Larviposition continues for about 4 to 6 wk, after which the female worm dies and is digested. The minute (0.1 mm) larvae are carried by the lymphatic and portal circulation to the bloodstream, and from there to various tissues and organs. Only those larvae reaching skeletal muscle survive; they penetrate individual fibers, causing myositis. They grow to 1 mm in length, coil up, encyst, and eventually calcify. Encystment is complete by the end of the 3rd mo. The larvae may remain viable for several years. The diaphragm and tongue, and the pectoral, eye, and intercostal muscles are especially involved. Larvae reaching the myocardium and other nonskeletal muscles are surrounded by a focus of inflammatory reaction and die. In animals, the encysted larvae are the source of infection for the next host.

Trichinosis occurs worldwide but is rare or absent in native populations of the tropics and where swine are fed root vegetables, as in France. In the USA, it has become sporadic and less frequent; outbreaks are usually caused by consumption of ready-to-eat pork sausages.

Symptoms and Signs

The clinical course is variable and the severity depends upon the number of invading larvae, the tissues invaded, and the physiologic condition of the patient. Many patients remain asymptomatic. GI symptoms and slight fever may appear within 1 or 2 days after ingestion of infected meat, but manifestations of systemic larval invasion usually do not appear for 7 to 15 days. Edema of the upper eyelids appears suddenly about the 11th day of infection and is one of the earliest and most characteristic signs. This may be followed by subconjunctival and retinal hemorrhages, pain, and photophobia. Muscle soreness and pain, urticaria, subungual hemorrhage, thirst, profuse sweating, fever, chills, weakness, prostration, and rapidly rising eosinophilia may develop shortly after the ocular signs. Soreness is especially pronounced in the muscles of respiration, speech, mastication, and swallowing. Severe dyspnea, sometimes causing death, may occur. Fever is generally remittent, rising to 39 C (102 F) or higher, remaining elevated for several days, and then falling gradually. Eosinophilia usually begins in the 2nd wk, reaches its height (20 to 40% or more) in the 3rd or 4th wk, then gradually declines. It may be obscured by concomitant bacterial infection. Lymphadenitis, encephalitis, meningitis, visual or auditory disorders, pneumonitis, pleurisy, and myocar-

ditis may develop in the 3rd to 6th wk, as the widely disseminated larvae outside the skeletal muscles are destroyed by inflammatory reaction; if myocardial failure develops, it occurs between the 4th and 8th wk. Most symptoms disappear by about the 3rd mo, although vague muscular pains and fatigue may persist for months.

Diagnosis

During the intestinal stage of infection, symptoms are nonspecific and no diagnostic laboratory procedures are available. Diarrhea, nausea, vomiting, and other GI disturbances may be recalled later by the patient. A history of ingesting ready-to-eat pork sausage or insufficiently cooked pork, bear, or walrus meat, followed by acute gastroenteritis or acute facial edema (particularly of the upper eyelids) is helpful in diagnosis. Eosinophilic leukocytosis usually appears within 2 wk of infection. Muscle biopsy performed during the 4th wk of infection may demonstrate larvae or cysts. Even when trichinae cannot be demonstrated in the biopsy specimen, a diffuse myositis may indicate active trichinosis. The parasite is rarely found in the infected meat, or in the patient's stool, blood, or CSF.

Commercially available skin test antigens are unreliable and their use is discouraged. Available serologic tests include CF, indirect fluorescent antibody, and (the most widely used) bentonite flocculation. False negative results can occur occasionally with each; therefore, 2 or more tests should be employed routinely. (Recently, a highly sensitive enzyme-linked immunosorbent assay has been introduced. This test becomes positive 10 to 14 days prior to the other serologic tests and may eventually supplant them.) Since these tests may also remain positive for years, they are of most value if they are initially negative and then turn positive.

Skeletal manifestations of trichinosis must be differentiated from acute rheumatic fever, acute arthritis, angioedema, and myositis; **febrile states** from TB, typhoid fever, sepsis, undulant fever; **pulmonary manifestations** from pneumonitis; **neurologic manifestations** from meningitis, encephalitis, and poliomyelitis; and **eosinophilia** from Hodgkin's disease, eosinophilic leukemia, and polyarteritis nodosa.

Prognosis

This is good in most cases. Unfavorable prognostic signs are the absence of an eosinophilic response, or a sudden fall in the eosinophil level to 1% or zero during the acute phase.

Prophylaxis

Trichinosis can be prevented by thoroughly cooking all pork and pork products. Larvae can generally be rendered nonviable by freezing the meat at –15 C for 3 wk or –18 C for 1 day; however, larvae from arctic mammals appear to survive even colder temperatures. Hogs should not be fed raw garbage, since it may contain infected pork wastes.

Treatment

Symptomatic and supportive therapy is aimed at assisting the patient to survive the acute toxemia, which terminates when the larvae become encysted. Muscular pains are usually relieved by bed rest, but may require analgesics such as aspirin or codeine. Corticosteroids are indicated for patients with severe allergic manifestations or myocardial or CNS involvement. Prednisone 20 to 60 mg/day orally in divided doses is given for 3 or 4 days; dosage is then gradually reduced and the drug is discontinued in 10 days.

Thiabendazole, 25 mg/kg bid orally for 5 to 10 days, is highly effective against the parasite, but the clinical response is variable.

TOXOCARIASIS
(Visceral Larva Migrans)

A widely distributed clinical syndrome resulting from invasion of human viscera by nematode larvae (eg, Toxocara canis *and* cati, *normally intestinal parasites of dogs and cats), with subsequent prolonged migration of the larvae through the body.* It usually occurs as a relatively benign disease in children aged 2 to 4, but may afflict older patients.

Etiology and Pathogenesis

The source of infection is the fully embryonated egg of the parasite found in soil contaminated by feces of infected dogs and cats. Children's sandboxes are attractive defecating sites for cats and are a potential hazard. The eggs may be transferred either directly to the mouth as the child plays in or eats (geophagia) the contaminated soil or indirectly through contaminated food or other objects. The incubation period varies from weeks to several months, depending on the intensity and number of exposures and on the sensitivity of the patient.

The eggs hatch in the intestine after ingestion. Liberated larvae penetrate the intestinal wall and are widely disseminated in the body by the systemic circulation. Almost any tissue may be involved, particularly the CNS, eye, liver, lung, and heart. The larvae may remain alive for many months, causing damage by their wanderings and by tissue sensitization. They produce a focal granulomatous reaction, though the larvae themselves may be difficult to demonstrate in tissue sections. The parasites do not complete their development in the human body.

Symptoms, Signs, and Diagnosis

Clinically, patients present with fever, cough or wheezing, and hepatomegaly. Skin rash, splenomegaly, and recurrent pneumonia occur in some patients. Eye lesions (chorioretinitis), which may be mistaken for retinoblastoma, may be seen in older children and adults, usually in the absence of other clinical manifestations of disease.

High eosinophilia (> 60%), hepatomegaly, pneumonitis, fever, and hyperglobulinemia are suggestive. Liver biopsy and demonstration of a larva or its fragments in the typical granulomatous lesion may be helpful in the diagnosis. Reliable serologic tests have been developed recently. The prognosis is good; the disease is self-limited (6 to 18 mo in the absence of reinfection).

Prophylaxis and Treatment

Infected pet dogs and cats, particularly those under 6 mo of age, should be dewormed regularly (under veterinary direction), and children's sandboxes should be covered when not in use.

No proven treatment is available. Thiabendazole 25 to 50 mg/kg for 7 to 10 days is probably the treatment of choice; or diethylcarbamazine 2 mg/kg tid orally after meals for 2 to 4 wk may be helpful, although it has no demonstrable activity against ascarids. Prednisone 20 to 40 mg/day orally, with reduced dosage after 3 to 5 days, helps to control symptoms.

FILARIASIS

A group of diseases occurring in tropical and subtropical countries and caused by Filarioidea.

Etiology and Pathogenesis

Wuchereria bancrofti is found only in humans; *Brugia malayi* is often spread to man from animal hosts. The adult filarioidea live in the human lymphatic system. Microfilariae released by gravid females are found in the peripheral blood, usually at night. Infection is spread by many species of mosquitoes; vectors of *W. bancrofti* are *Aedes*,

Culex, and *Anopheles*; of *B. malayi*, *Anopheles* and *Mansonia*. The microfilariae are ingested by the mosquito, undergo development in the insect's thoracic muscles, and, when mature, migrate to its mouthparts. When the infected mosquito bites a new host, the microfilariae penetrate the bite puncture and eventually reach the lymphatics, where they develop to the adult stage.

Pathology

Inflammation and fibrosis occurring in the vicinity of the juvenile and adult worms produce progressive lymphatic obstruction. The microfilariae probably do not contribute directly to the host reaction.

Symptoms and Signs

The incubation period may be as short as 2 mo. The "prepatent" period (from time of infection to appearance of microfilariae in the blood) is at least 8 mo. Clinical manifestations depend on the severity of the infection; they may include lymphangitis, lymphadenitis, orchitis, funiculitis, epididymitis, lymph varices, and chyluria. Chills, fever, headache, and malaise may also be present. Elephantiasis and other late severe sequelae occur with long-time residence in endemic areas and repeated reinfection. An aberrant form of filariasis (tropical eosinophilia) is characterized by hypereosinophilia, presence of microfilariae in the tissues but not the blood, and high titers of antifilarial antibodies (tropical eosinophlia). Clinically, the patient may present with lymphadenosplenomegaly or with cough, bronchospasm, and chest infiltrates.

Diagnosis

Microfilariae may be found in blood or lymph fluid. A number of serologic tests are available, but are not completely reliable. Antigen detection procedures are being investigated.

Prophylaxis and Treatment

Promising results have been obtained in controlling filariasis by combining mass treatment and mosquito control.

Diethylcarbamazine 2 mg/kg orally tid after meals for 3 to 4 wk eliminates microfilariae from the bloodstream and, in many patients, also kills adult worms or impairs their reproductive capacity. The result is permanent clearing of the microfilariae. Severe allergic reactions and abscess formation may follow use of diethylcarbamazine, but may be controlled by antihistamines or corticosteroids.

Surgical intervention is indicated only to alleviate certain types of elephantiasis, especially of the scrotum. Elephantiasis of the legs is treated by elevation and elastic bandages.

ONCHOCERCIASIS
(River Blindness)

A disease resulting from infection by Onchocerca volvulus *and characterized by fibrous nodules in the skin and subcutaneous tissues.* Ocular findings are common; blindness may result. The disease, spread by the bite of black flies (*Simuliidae*), occurs in southern Mexico, Guatemala, Venezuela, Colombia, Yemen, and central Africa. **Diagnosis** depends on demonstration of microfilariae in skin snips or nodules.

Treatment

Microfilariae, but not adult worms, are destroyed by diethylcarbamazine, which is given orally after meals. Since an allergic reaction to the dead microfilariae can result in ocular damage if the eye is involved in the infection, initial dosage is limited to 0.1 to 0.2 mg/kg/day. Dosage is gradually increased to 2 to 3 mg/kg tid and then maintained at this level for 1 wk. An antihistamine and prednisone 20 to 40 mg/day orally may be necessary to prevent the acute allergic inflammation in and around the eye that

follows the rapid destruction of numerous microfilariae. A new agent, ivermectin, destroys microfilaria more slowly than diethylcarbamazine and its use is less frequently accompanied by serious allergic reactions. Its final role in the treatment of this disease remains to be determined.

Adult worms are eliminated by surgically removing the nodules; suramin (CAUTION: *Toxicity*) in a test dose of 100 mg IV, followed by 5 weekly injections of 1 gm IV, is also effective.

LOIASIS
(Calabar Swellings)

A form of filariasis found in west and central Africa, caused by Loa loa, *and transmitted by the bite of flies of the genus* Chrysops. The disease is characterized by localized transient swellings (calabar swellings) caused by migration of adult worms in the subcutaneous tissues. The worms may also migrate across the eye beneath the conjunctiva. Microfilariae are found in the calabar swellings and peripheral blood; eosinophilia is common.

Treatment

Diethylcarbamazine 2 mg/kg orally tid after meals for 14 days kills both the microfilariae and adult worms. Since allergic reactions are common during the first part of treatment, an antihistamine and prednisone 10 to 30 mg/day orally should be given concurrently during the first 4 days of treatment.

DRACUNCULIASIS
(Dracontiasis; "Fiery Serpent"; Guinea Worm)

A disease caused by the presence of the guinea worm (Dracunculus medinensis) *in subcutaneous tissues.* It is endemic in India, Pakistan, the Near East, tropical Africa, certain West Indies islands, and the Guianas. Infection follows ingestion of water containing infected crustacea (*Cyclops*). The larvae penetrate the intestinal wall, mature in the retroperitoneal space, migrate to the subcutaneous tissue, and produce skin ulcers through which the female discharges larvae. Intense local itching and burning may result. **Diagnosis** is possible only after the adult worm reaches its destination under the skin, at which time its head may be seen in the base of the ulcer, or larvae may be demonstrated in the discharge.

Treatment consists of slow extraction of the adult worm by gradual traction on its head over a period of 10 days. Administering thiabendazole 25 mg/kg bid for 2 days or niridazole 25 mg/kg in 3 divided doses for 3 days leads to rapid symptomatic improvement; it is uncertain whether the worms are killed or just expelled. Surgical removal is not recommended. Septic and foreign-body reactions should be treated with antibiotics and removal as indicated.

DIROFILARIASIS
(Heartworm)

Dirofilaria immitis, a large filaria, lives in the right heart of dogs. Microfilariae are released into the peripheral blood, where they are taken up by several species of mosquitoes. If they are subsequently transmitted to man by an infected mosquito (an exceedingly rare event), they find their way to the lung to produce well-defined pulmonary nodules. The patient may experience chest pain, cough, and, occasionally, hemoptysis. **Diagnosis** is made by histologic examination of pulmonary nodules. A reliable serologic test has been described. No treatment is indicated.

TREMATODES

SCHISTOSOMIASIS
(Bilharziasis)

A visceral parasitic disease caused by blood flukes of the genus Schistosoma.

Etiology, Pathogenesis, and Epidemiology

The schistosomes that affect man are digenetic trematodes. Fresh-water snails are the intermediate hosts. Human infection follows contact (by bathing, wading, etc) with the free-swimming cercariae of the parasite that penetrate the skin and are carried to the intrahepatic portal circulation, where they mature in 1 to 3 mo. The adult worms then migrate to the venules of the bladder or intestines. Three species produce most clinical disease: *S. haematobium* causes symptoms in the GU system or the lower colon and rectum; *S. mansoni* and *S. japonicum* cause disturbances in the small intestine, colon, and rectum. *S. mekongi* is found in the Mekong River area of Indochina. In its epidemiology, disease manifestations, and response to therapy, it closely resembles *S. japonicum*.

The disease is endemic in Africa, the Middle East, and Cyprus (*S. haematobium*); Egypt, areas of northern and southern Africa, certain West Indies islands, and the northern 2/3 of South America (*S. mansoni*); and Japan, central and south China, the Philippines, the Celebes, Thailand, and Laos (*S. japonicum*). *S. mansoni* is frequently encountered in Puerto Ricans residing in the USA.

Several schistosome species do not dwell in man, but are capable of causing dermatitis **("swimmer's itch")** and are seen in the USA as well as elsewhere. The definitive hosts are usually migratory birds; both fresh and salt water mollusks serve as intermediate hosts.

Symptoms and Signs

Initially, a pruritic papular dermatitis appears where the cercariae entered the skin. In "swimmer's itch" the disease never progresses beyond this point. In other forms, the adult worm develops in the liver, causing fever, eosinophilia, and often urticaria, hepatosplenomegaly, and lymphadenopathy. When the adults migrate to the viscera, the damage caused by the reaction to their eggs produces symptoms referable to the affected visceral structures (cystitis, chronic diarrhea). Hepatic cirrhosis, portal hypertension and resulting splenomegaly, ascites, and esophageal varices may occur from inflammation and fibrosis around eggs that have been carried back to the liver by the portal blood flow, especially in *S. mansoni* and *S. japonicum* infections. With the establishment of venous collaterals, eggs may be transported to other organs of the body as well. Eggs of *S. haematobium* and *S. mansoni* may cause pulmonary damage; those of *S. japonicum* and *S. mansoni* may cause CNS damage.

Diagnosis

Eggs are found in the stool (*S. japonicum* and *mansoni*) or urine (*S. haematobium*), or in rectal or bladder biopsies. Repeated stool examinations using concentration technics may be necessary. Positive serologic tests are not sufficient basis for therapy, but should lead to a vigorous search for eggs. Only the demonstration of living eggs in a patient warrants initiation of treatment.

Prophylaxis

Control of the disease is difficult and depends upon proper disposal of urine and feces, use of molluscacides, provision of a pure water supply, and treatment with anthelmintics.

Treatment

Since the severity of schistosomiasis depends on the intensity of infection, the aim of therapy is to reduce the worm load. Prolonged or repeated courses of antischistosomal agents in an attempt to effect a cure are unwarranted. Praziquantel, a recently introduced antihelminthic, is the preferred treatment for all 3 types of schistosomiasis. For *S. haematobium* and *S. mansoni* it is given as a single 40 mg/kg dose. For *S. japonicum* and *S. mekongi*, the recommended dose is 60 mg/kg in 3 divided doses over a single day.

Patients should be examined for the presence of living eggs 3 and 6 mo after treatment. Retreatment is indicated if egg excretion has not decreased markedly.

CLONORCHIASIS

An inflammation of the liver resulting from ingesting cysts of the fluke Clonorchis sinensis.

Etiology and Epidemiology

Clonorchis sinensis is an important liver fluke of humans (see SCHISTOSOMIASIS above and TABLE 13–2 for other flukes infesting humans): it lives for 20 to 50 yr in the biliary tree and passes operculated eggs into the feces. The egg, on reaching fresh water, hatches into a free-swimming miracidium that is ingested by the intermediate snail host. After multiplication and further development within the snail, thousands of free-living cercariae are released and must enter 2nd intermediate hosts—eg, freshwater fish, such as the carp and salmon, where they encyst to form metacercariae. Infections follow ingestion of raw, dried, salted, or pickled fish containing these metacercariae. The larvae are released in the duodenum, enter the common bile duct, and migrate to the 2nd-order bile ducts (or, occasionally, the gallbladder and pancreatic ducts), where they mature in about 1 mo into adult, flat flukes varying from a few mm to several cm in length. Endemic in the Far East (where dogs, cats, pigs, and other animals also serve as reservoirs), the infection is found elsewhere most frequently among immigrants from that area and in fish imported from there.

Symptoms, Signs, and Complications

Light infections are usually asymptomatic. Apparent cases occur mainly in adults, when the worm load accumulates to > 500. Initially the patient may have fever, chills, tender hepatomegaly, mild jaundice, and eosinophilia. The mature worms, feeding on secretions from the biliary duct mucosa and possibly on cellular elements, cause chronic cholangitis with inflammation of the biliary tree, proliferation of the biliary epithelium, and progressive portal fibrosis. In heavy infections (10,000 to 20,000 flukes), portal fibrosis may be associated with portal hypertension and may extend into the liver parenchyma, with resulting liver cell death and fatty change. Jaundice is usually caused by biliary obstruction due to a mass of flukes or stone formation. Other complications of severe clonorchiasis include cholangiocarcinoma (a metaplastic change in the irritated biliary epithelium), suppurative cholangitis, and chronic pancreatitis.

Diagnosis

Clinical and epidemiologic findings often suggest the diagnosis, which can be confirmed only by finding the eggs in the feces or duodenal contents. The light brown, ovoid eggs measure 29 × 16 μm, have a conspicuous opercular rim and a posterior knob, and are difficult to distinguish from the eggs of the trematodes *Metagonimus*, *Heterophyes*, and *Opisthorchis*. Alkaline phosphatase and bilirubin may be elevated. Eosinophilia is variable. A plain film of the abdomen occasionally demonstrates intrahepatic calcification. In acute symptomatic disease, liver scan is usually negative but may show multiple areas of diminished uptake, and percutaneous transhepatic cholan-

giography often shows dilatation of peripheral intrahepatic bile ducts. The adult worms (5 × 15 mm in diameter) look like round filling defects.

Prophylaxis and Treatment

Thorough cooking of freshwater fish prevents infection. Praziquantel, 75 mg/kg in 3 divided doses over a single day, is highly effective. Biliary obstruction may require surgery.

CESTODES

BEEF TAPEWORM INFECTION

(*Taenia saginata* Infection; Taeniasis Saginata)

A usually asymptomatic infection of the intestinal tract caused by the cestode Taenia saginata.

Etiology, Pathogenesis, and Epidemiology

The adult worm inhabits the human intestinal tract and is composed of a small head (scolex), 1 to 2 mm in diameter, and up to 1000 hermaphroditic proglottids that give the worm its characteristic ribbonlike shape. The worm measures 4.5 to 9 m (15 to 30 ft). Egg-bearing proglottids are passed in the stool and ingested by cattle. The eggs hatch in the cattle, invade the intestinal wall, and are carried by the bloodstream to striated muscle, where they encyst (cysticercus stage). Humans are infected by ingesting the cysticercus in raw or undercooked beef.

The infection is particularly common in Africa, the Middle East, Eastern Europe, Mexico, and South America. Infection in the USA is uncommon, but still occurs in California and New England.

Symptoms, Signs, and Diagnosis

The infection is usually asymptomatic, although epigastric pain, diarrhea, and weight loss may occur. Occasionally, the patient may feel an active proglottid crawling through the anus.

The diagnosis is usually made by finding the characteristic proglottids or, more rarely, the scolex in the stool. The perianal area may also be examined by pressing the sticky side of cellophane tape against the area, placing the tape on a glass slide, and microscopically examining it for eggs deposited by ruptured proglottids.

Prophylaxis

Infection may be prevented by thoroughly cooking beef at a minimum of 56 C (133 F) for 5 min. Meat inspection and adequate toilet facilities also help to control infection.

Treatment

A single dose of 2 gm niclosamide is given as 4 tablets (500 mg each) that are chewed one at a time and swallowed with a small amount of water. The worm is then usually digested by the time it is passed. The stool should be rechecked in 3 mo and 6 mo to make certain a cure has been obtained.

Alternatively, praziquantel can be used in a single 10 mg/kg dose.

PORK TAPEWORM INFECTION

(*Taenia solium* Infection; Cysticercosis)

An intestinal infection caused by the adult cestode Taenia solium. Infection with the larvae (cysticerci) causes **cysticercosis**, an occasional occurrence in man.

Etiology, Pathogenesis, and Epidemiology

The adult *T. solium* measures 2.5 to 3 m (8 to 10 ft) in length, and is composed of a scolex armed with several hooklets and a body composed of 1000 proglottids. The gravid proglottids have fewer uterine branches than gravid *T. saginata* proglottids have. The life cycle resembles that of *T. saginata* except that hogs rather than cattle serve as the normal intermediate hosts. Humans may also act as intermediate hosts either by ingesting the eggs directly, or by regurgitating gravid proglottids from the intestine to the stomach where the embryos are released, penetrate the intestinal wall, and are carried to the subcutaneous tissue, muscle, viscera, and CNS. Viable cysticerci cause only a mild tissue reaction; dead larvae, however, provoke a vigorous reaction.

T. solium infections are frequent in Asia, Russia, Eastern Europe, and Latin America; infection in the USA is rare.

Symptoms and Signs

Infection with the adult worm is usually asymptomatic. Heavy larval infection (cysticercosis) may cause muscle pains, weakness, fever, or, if the CNS is involved, meningoencephalitis or epilepsy.

Diagnosis

In adult worm infections, eggs may be found in the perianal area or stool. The proglottids or scolex must be recovered from the stool and examined in order to differentiate *T. solium* from *T. saginata*. Cysticercosis should be suspected in any patient who lives in an endemic area and develops neurologic findings. Calcified cysticerci may be seen on x-ray. Encysted larvae may occasionally be recovered in biopsied subcutaneous nodules. Reliable serologic tests have been developed recently; cross-reactivity has been shown with echinococciasis.

Prophylaxis and Treatment

Infection may be prevented by thoroughly cooking pork.

The intestinal infection is treated as described above for *T. saginata*. However, since these agents result in proglottid disintegration, with release of eggs, their use could theoretically cause cysticercosis.

FISH TAPEWORM INFECTION
(Diphyllobothriasis)

An intestinal infection caused by the adult cestode Diphyllobothrium latum.

Etiology, Pathogenesis, and Epidemiology

The adult worm possesses several thousand proglottids, and measures 4.5 to 9 m (15 to 30 ft) in length. Operculated ova (*D. latum* are the only eggs of the tapeworm group that are operculated) are released from the proglottid in the intestinal lumen and are passed in the stool. The egg, as it hatches in fresh water, releases the embryo, which is eaten by small crustaceans. They may, in turn, be ingested by a fish. Humans are infected by eating raw or undercooked infected fish.

The infection occurs in Europe (particularly Scandinavia), Japan, Africa, South America, Canada, and, in the USA, in Florida and the North Central States. Uncooked "lutefisk" or "gefilte fish" often harbor infection.

Symptoms, Signs, and Diagnosis

Infection is usually asymptomatic, although mild GI symptoms may be noted. Rarely, an anemia that resembles pernicious anemia may develop, presumably because of host-tapeworm competition for vitamin B_{12}.

Operculated eggs are easily found in the stool.

Prophylaxis and Treatment

All fresh-water fish should be thoroughly cooked, or frozen at -10 C (14 F) for 48 h. Treatment requires niclosamide or praziquantel (see BEEF TAPEWORM INFECTION, above).

ECHINOCOCCIASIS

(*Echinococcus granulosus* Infection)

A tissue infection of humans caused by the larval stage of Echinococcus granulosus.

Etiology, Epidemiology, and Pathogenesis

The adult worm is found in the small intestines of dogs, wolves, and other canines. It measures 5 mm in length and consists of a scolex and 3 proglottids. The terminal or gravid proglottid splits, releasing into the stool eggs that are morphologically identical to those of *T. saginata*. These eggs pass to the external environment and are ingested by an intermediate host, eg, sheep, moose, or human; the embryos penetrate the intestinal wall and the portal circulation carries them to the liver, or beyond to the lung, brain, kidney, bones, and other tissues. Surviving larvae develop into hydatid cysts that slowly enlarge to produce pressure symptoms. The cyst is fluid-filled and contains scolices, brood capsules, and 2nd-generation (daughter) cysts containing infectious scolices. When the intermediate is eaten by a carnivore the scolices are released into the GI tract, where they develop into adult worms.

The dog is the principal definitive host and the sheep the most common intermediate. (In Alaska and western Canada, wolves act as the definitive host and moose as the intermediate.) Human infection, often acquired in childhood during play with infected dogs, is most common in the sheep-raising areas of the world, including South Africa, Australia, New Zealand, the Middle East, central Europe, and South America. In the USA, autochthonous cases have been reported among southwestern Indian, California Basque, and Utah shepherds.

Symptoms and Signs

The majority of cysts are found in the liver, where, after remaining asymptomatic for decades, they finally produce abdominal pain or a palpable mass. Jaundice may occur if the bile duct is obstructed. Rupture into the bile duct, abdominal cavity, peritoneal cavity, or lung may produce fever, urticaria, or a serious anaphylactoid reaction. The released scolices may produce metastatic infection. Pulmonary cysts are usually discovered on routine chest x-ray. Some rupture, and cough, chest pain, and hemoptysis result.

Diagnosis

Radioisotopic and ultrasonic scanning will reveal the fluid-filled liver cysts. Chest x-ray may demonstrate a round, often irregular, pulmonary mass of uniform density. The skin test is usually positive but lacks both sensitivity and specificity. Serologic tests are positive in approximately 60% of pulmonary and 90% of hepatic lesions.

Prophylaxis and Treatment

Dogs in sheep-raising areas should be wormed repeatedly. The carcasses and offals of sheep should be destroyed to prevent access of dogs to material containing hydatid cysts.

Surgical excision offers the only hope of cure. Patients with small hepatic cysts or pulmonary lesions acquired in Alaska need surgery only if they are symptomatic or the cysts enlarge with time; all others require surgery. Mebendazole may be helpful in ameliorating symptoms of patients with inoperable disease.

14. SEXUALLY TRANSMITTED DISEASE (STD)

The incidence of STDs, among the most common communicable diseases in the world, steadily increased from the 1950s to the 1970s, but stabilized in the past decade. Diseases such as nonspecific urethritis, trichomoniasis, chlamydial infections, genital candidiasis, genital and anorectal herpes and warts (all discussed in this chapter), scabies, pediculosis pubis, and molluscum contagiosum (see Chs. 233 and 234) probably are more prevalent than the 5 historically defined venereal diseases—syphilis, gonorrhea, chancroid, lymphogranuloma venereum, and granuloma inguinale. However, because the former group is not consistently reported, incidence figures are not available. For gonorrhea, it is estimated that > 250 million persons worldwide, and close to 3 million in the USA, are infected annually. For syphilis, annual worldwide incidence is estimated at 50 million persons, with 400,000 in the USA annually needing treatment. Other infections, including salmonellosis, giardiasis, amebiasis, shigellosis, campylobacter, hepatitis A and B, and cytomegalovirus infection, sometimes are sexually transmitted. Strong associations between cervical cancer (see also Chs. 105 and 173) and herpesviruses and papillomaviruses have been discovered. Since 1978, an epidemic, sometimes-fatal, retroviral infection—acquired immunodeficiency syndrome **(AIDS)**—has spread rapidly in certain groups of homosexual men in western countries and among heterosexuals in Africa (see Ch. 19).

STD incidence has risen despite advances in diagnosis and treatment that rapidly render patients noninfectious and cure the majority. Factors responsible for this paradox include changes in sexual behavior, eg, widespread use of contraceptive pills and devices; more varied sexual practices, including orogenital and anorectal contact; emergence of strains of organisms less sensitive to antibiotics; symptomless carriers of infecting agents; a highly mobile population; a high level of sexual activity in some homosexual men; ignorance of the facts by physicians and the public; and reticence of patients in seeking treatment.

STD control depends on having good facilities for diagnosis and treatment; tracing and treating all sexual contacts of the patients; continuing to observe those who received treatment to ensure that they have been cured; educating doctors, nurses, and the public; counseling patients about responsible sexual behavior; and developing methods for producing artificial immunity against infection.

GONORRHEA

An acute infectious disease of the epithelium of the urethra, cervix, rectum, pharynx, or eyes, that may give rise to bacteremia and result in metastatic complications.

Etiology and Epidemiology

The causative organism, *Neisseria gonorrhoeae*, can be identified in discharges (by direct smear or after culture) as pairs or clumps of gram-negative, kidney-shaped diplococci, often intracellular and with their adjacent surfaces slightly concave.

The disease usually spreads by sexual contact. Women are frequently symptomless carriers of the organisms for weeks or months and often are identified by tracing sexual contacts. Symptomless infection is also common in the oropharynx and rectum in homosexual men, and has been found occasionally in the urethras of heterosexual men in some geographic regions.

Gonorrhea occurs in the vagina of prepubertal girls, most of whom are infected by adults, through either sexual abuse or, rarely, fomites.

Symptoms and Signs

In men, the incubation period is from 2 to 14 days. The onset usually begins with mild discomfort in the urethra, followed a few hours later by dysuria and a purulent

discharge. Frequency and urgency of micturition develop as the disease spreads to the posterior urethra. Examination shows a purulent, yellowish-green urethral discharge: the lips of the meatus may be red and swollen.

In women, symptoms usually begin within 7 to 21 days after infection. Symptoms generally are mild, but in a few women the onset may be severe, with dysuria, frequency, and vaginal discharge. The cervix and deeper reproductive organs are the sites most frequently infected, followed by the urethra, rectum, Skene's ducts, and Bartholin's glands. The cervix may be reddened and friable, with a mucopurulent or purulent discharge. Pus may be expressed from the urethra on pressure against the symphysis pubis or from Skene's ducts or Bartholin's glands. Salpingitis is a common complication (see Ch. 171).

In women or homosexual men, rectal gonorrhea is common. It usually is symptomless in women, but perianal discomfort and a rectal discharge may occur. Severe rectal infection is more common in homosexual men. Patients may note mucopus coating their stools, perianal excoriation may be present, and proctoscopy may show mucopus on the rectal wall. **Gonococcal pharyngitis** from orogenital contact is being recognized more frequently. Although often there are no symptoms or signs, some patients may complain of a sore throat and discomfort on swallowing, and the pharynx and tonsillar area may be red, sometimes with a mucopurulent exudate and occasionally with edema of the uvula and faucial pillars.

In female infants and prepubertal girls, irritation, erythema, and edema of the vulva with a purulent vaginal discharge may be accompanied by proctitis. The child may complain of soreness or dysuria and the parents may notice staining of the underclothes.

Diagnosis

A gram-stained smear of urethral discharge allows rapid identification of the gonococcus in most men. However, the cervical Gram stain is only about 60% sensitive in women. Identification of the gonococcus by culture of genital exudate should always be done for women and for men with negative or equivocal urethral Gram stains. Cultures should be performed in both sexes when symptoms of rectal or pharyngeal infection are present, as Gram stains are *unreliable* (insensitive and nonspecific). Exudates from the urethra, cervix, rectum, and other infected sites are inoculated onto a suitable medium (eg, Modified Thayer-Martin medium) and incubated at 35 to 36 C for 48 h in an atmosphere containing 3 to 10% carbon dioxide (a candle jar may be used). Some colonies become visible after 24 h, but most appear after 48 h. The colonies are small, circular, transparent, and usually 1 to 4 mm in diameter. Complete identification depends on characteristic appearance on Gram stain; on the oxidase test, in which positive colonies turn purple and later black on exposure to 1% di- or tetramethyl-*p*-phenylenediamine HCl; and on fermentation reactions. All *Neisseria* are oxidase-positive. *N. gonorrhoeae* ferments dextrose (glucose), but not maltose or sucrose. The meningococcus (*N. meningitidis*) ferments dextrose and maltose, but not sucrose. Nonpathogenic *Neisseria* spp ferment either 3 or more carbohydrates, or none, and are usually inhibited by antibiotics (eg, colistin, vancomycin, nystatin) in selective media.

If adequate laboratory facilities are not immediately available, the specimen may be inoculated onto a transport medium for transfer to a laboratory. Containers with suitable media and self-contained carbon dioxide supply are commercially available. For successful growth of gonococci, the specimens must be subcultured within 48 h, preferably within 24 h. Reliable serologic tests for gonococci are not yet available for routine clinical use.

Complications

In men treated early, postgonococcal urethritis is the most common sequel. It is often due to the presence of other organisms (eg, *Chlamydia trachomatis*) that were acquired simultaneously with gonorrhea but have longer incubation periods and do not respond to penicillin. Less dramatic discharge or dysuria recurs 7 to 14 days following penicillin treatment for gonorrhea. **Epididymitis** (see Ch. 153), another important complication, is usually unilateral; if bilateral, sterility may result. Infection descends from the posterior urethra along the vas deferens to the lower pole of the epididymis. The testicle is painful, and the epididymis and spermatic cord become hot, tender, and swollen. A secondary hydrocele may follow. Abscesses of Tyson's and Littré's glands, periurethral abscesses, infection of Cowper's glands and the prostate, urethral stricture, and infection of the seminal vesicles are less common complications.

In women, salpingitis is the most important clinical problem (see Ch. 171).

In either sex, disseminated gonococcal infection (DGI) with bacteremia may occur, but it is more common in women. Nearly all strains of gonococci from DGI are serum resistant, but only a small portion of persons infected with serum-resistant gonococci acquire systemic disease. The patient presents with a mild febrile illness, malaise, migratory polyarthralgias or polyarthritis, or a few pustular skin lesions, often on the periphery of the limbs (each symptom is present in about ⅔ of the patients). The genital infection is often symptomless, but bacteriologic tests of the genital secretions may demonstrate gonococci. In about ½ of cases, the organism can be grown from the bloodstream (blood cultures are most often positive in the first week) or joint fluid. By using immunofluorescent technics, sometimes the gonococcus can be demonstrated in the pus from skin lesions. Any potential source of bacteremia should be cultured. Patients with DGI almost never have simultaneously positive blood and synovial fluid cultures. Bacteremia has serious potential sequelae; pericarditis, endocarditis, meningitis, and perihepatitis occasionally occur and rarely can be fatal.

Gonococcal arthritis, possibly a different type of DGI, also is more frequent in women than in men and genital manifestations may be minimal or absent. The onset is acute, with fever, severe pain, and limitation of movement (usually in a single joint or a few joints, as opposed to DGI, which involves multiple joints). The joint is swollen and tender, and the overlying skin is hot and red. Synovial fluid is increased, and aspiration produces pus from which gonococci can be isolated, stained, and cultured. Analysis should be done and treatment started immediately because early destruction of the articular surfaces of the joint occurs. Any purulent joint effusion should be considered septic and treated until proved otherwise.

Ocular infections may occur in the newborn (see under NEONATAL INFECTIONS in Ch. 186) or in adults (see Ch. 219).

Treatment

Blood for serologic tests for syphilis **(STS)** should always be obtained before treatment is started, and the patient should be carefully examined to exclude other STDs. STS should be repeated 3 mo later.

The infectious nature of gonorrhea should be explained to the patient, who should abstain from sexual activity until cure is confirmed. Men should also be advised not to squeeze the penis in a search for urethral discharges. All sexual contacts of the patient should be traced, examined, and given treatment.

The Centers for Disease Control now consider 3 treatment regimens to be coequal: (1) aqueous procaine penicillin G 4.8 million u. IM (divided, at 2 sites) plus probenecid 1 gm orally given simultaneously; (2) ampicillin 3.5 gm or amoxicillin 3.0 gm orally given simultaneously with probenecid 1 gm; and (3) tetracycline 500 mg orally qid for 5 days. Patients with uncertain reliability should be given one of the single-dose regimens. For suspected rectal infection, the penicillin regimen is preferred. For suspected

pharyngeal infection, ampicillin should be *avoided.* Patients who fail therapy or who have possible penicillin-resistant gonorrhea can be given spectinomycin 2 gm IM or cefoxitin 2 gm mixed with 4 mL of 0.5% lidocaine. Penicillin-allergic patients (unless pregnant) should be given spectinomycin or tetracycline. Gonococci that cause **DGI** are usually very sensitive to penicillin. In **gonococcal arthritis,** in which sterile joint effusions may persist for 7 to 14 days, adding an anti-inflammatory medication seems beneficial. Repeated drainage is usually unnecessary, but initially the joint is kept immobilized in an optimal functional position. Passive range of motion should be started as soon as possible, as well as quadriceps-setting exercises, if the knee is involved. As soon as the pain subsides, more active exercises, with stretching, active range of motion, and muscle strengthening, should be done at least twice daily. Over 95% of patients treated for gonococcal arthritis recover complete joint function.

One week after treatment, to confirm that the patient is cured and no longer infectious, specimens from accessible infected sites (except joints) should be cultured. Ideally, a second test for cure should be performed 2 wk later and STS carried out 3 mo after treatment, but most incubating syphilis is cured by the treatment for gonorrhea. Many recurrent infections are reinfections. However, penicillin-resistant gonococci are occurring in the USA and have become endemic in many parts of the world. In patients who fail therapy and deny reexposure or have acquired gonorrhea in areas with endemic penicillin-resistant strains, culture and tests for penicillin resistance are indicated.

For treatment of specific complications, see appropriate chapters elsewhere in THE MANUAL.

SEXUALLY TRANSMITTED CHLAMYDIAL AND UREAPLASMAL INFECTIONS

(Nongonococcal Urethritis [NGU]; Nonspecific Urethritis [NSU]; Mucopurulent Cervicitis; Nonspecific Genital Infections)

Etiology and Incidence

The sexually transmitted causes of most cases of cervicitis and urethritis in women, urethritis in men, and proctitis and pharyngitis in both sexes have been identified. Terms previously used to describe the nongonococcal forms of these infections, nonspecific urethritis **(NSU)** or nongonococcal urethritis **(NGU)**, are inexact. This group of sexually transmitted infections, although not reportable, may be the most common STDs in the USA. The causal agents include *Chlamydia trachomatis* (responsible for about 50% of cases of NGU and most cases of nongonococcal mucopurulent cervicitis) and *Ureaplasma urealyticum*, but some cases remain unexplained.

Symptoms and Signs

In men, symptoms of urethritis generally appear between 7 and 28 days after intercourse, usually with mild dysuria and discomfort in the urethra and a clear to mucopurulent discharge. Although the discharge may be slight and the symptoms mild, they are frequently more marked early in the morning when the lips of the meatus often are stuck together with dried secretions. On examination the meatus may be red, with evidence of the dried secretions on underclothes. Occasionally the onset is more acute, with dysuria, frequency, and a copious purulent discharge.

Proctitis and pharyngitis may develop following rectal and orogenital contact.

Most **women** are asymptomatic, although vaginal discharge, dysuria, frequency, pelvic pain, and dyspareunia, as well as symptoms of proctitis and pharyngitis, may occur. Cervicitis with characteristic yellow, mucopurulent secretion may be seen.

Diagnosis

Diagnosis is based on bacteriologic examination to exclude gonorrhea in men and other causes of discharge in women, including herpes, trichomoniasis, and candidiasis. **In men,** gram-stained slides of the urethral discharge will show many polymorphonuclear leukocytes and some epithelial cells, but no pathogenic organisms. In mild cases, evidence of urethritis may require examination of urine, which shows ≥ 5 PMN/× 1000 (oil) field. If the diagnosis is in doubt, examination is made on first-voided, morning urine. If infection is present, usually urethral swabbing produces enough material for laboratory examination to confirm the diagnosis. *C. trachomatis* can be grown on culture in nearly half the cases, but requires inoculation of tissue cultures. The introduction of specific monoclonal antibodies and fluorescent staining to identify chlamydia in genital secretions allows most laboratories to diagnose *C. trachomatis*. **In women,** Gram stain of a purulent cervical discharge often shows many leukocytes, but no gonococci.

See also PROCTITIS, below.

Complications

In men, local complications include epididymitis (especially chlamydial infections in men < 35 yr) and urethral stricture; in women, bartholinitis, cysts of Bartholin's glands, salpingitis, and Fitz-Hugh–Curtis syndrome (perihepatitis). Chlamydial salpingitis is increasingly recognized as an important source of morbidity and has focused attention on the diagnosis and treatment of chlamydial infections in women. A serious systemic complication is Reiter's syndrome, consisting of nonspecific urethritis, polyarthritis, and conjunctivitis or uveitis (see Ch. 108).

Chlamydial ophthalmia neonatorum is increasingly recognized in infants born to women with chlamydial cervicitis (see under NEONATAL INFECTIONS in Ch. 186).

Treatment

Uncomplicated infections are treated with tetracycline 500 mg orally q 6 h or doxycycline 100 mg/day for 7 days. Patients who relapse or develop complications require longer courses (tetracycline 500 mg or doxycycline 100 mg/day orally q 6 h for 21 to 28 days). **In pregnant women**, erythromycin (500 mg orally q 6 h for at least 7 days) should be substituted for tetracycline; if this schedule cannot be tolerated, a lower dosage can be used for a longer interval. Infected Bartholin's glands may require aspiration, drainage, or surgical removal. About 20% of the patients have one or more relapses on follow-up and require retreatment. They may become anxious, and should be assured that they will eventually be cured.

If appropriate treatment is not given, the signs and symptoms usually subside within 4 wk in about 60 to 70% of patients, but may persist in women and result in chronic pelvic infection and its sequelae—pain, infertility, or ectopic pregnancy.

Patients should be advised to abstain from sexual intercourse until treatment is completed and symptoms subside. Sexual partners should be examined and treated. Treated persons should be followed for 3 mo with regular clinical examinations. STS should be done before treatment and after 3 mo.

SYPHILIS

(Lues)

A contagious systemic disease caused by the spirochete Treponema pallidum, *characterized by sequential clinical stages and by years of symptomless latency*. It can affect any tissue or vascular organ of the body and be passed from mother to fetus (congenital syphilis).

Classification (see TABLE 14–1)

TABLE 14–1. CLASSIFICATION OF SYPHILIS

Acquired	*Congenital*
Early infectious syphilis **Primary** stage Chancre; regional lymphadenopathy **Secondary** stage Immediately follows primary stage Characterized by varied dermatologic lesions that mimic several disorders (eg, skin rashes, erosions of mucous membranes, alopecia) **Latent** stage (asymptomatic; may persist indefinitely or be followed by late stage, below) **Early latent syphilis** (infection < 2 yr* duration; infectious lesions may recur) **Late latent syphilis** (infection > 2 yr* duration) **Late** or **tertiary** stage (symptomatic; not contagious) **Benign tertiary (late benign) syphilis** **Cardiovascular syphilis** **Neurosyphilis**	**Early congenital syphilis** (symptomatic) The overt disease seen in infants up to age 2 **Late congenital syphilis** (symptomatic) The stigmas seen in later life (eg, Hutchinson's teeth, scars of interstitial keratitis, bony abnormalities) (Congenital syphilis can also exist in a permanently latent, or asymptomatic, state.)

* For reporting purposes, the division is sometimes made on a 4-yr rather than a 2-yr basis.

ACQUIRED SYPHILIS

Etiology and Pathology

T. pallidum is a delicate spiral organism about 0.25 μm wide and from 5 to 20 μm long. It can be identified by morphology and motility, using a darkfield microscope or fluorescent technics (see under Diagnosis, below). It does not grow on artifical media and cannot survive for long outside the human body, but remains viable for several days in tissue culture.

In acquired syphilis, *T. pallidum* enters the body through the mucous membranes or skin. Within hours the organisms reach the regional lymph nodes and rapidly disseminate throughout the body. The host reacts by perivascular infiltration of lymphocytes, plasma cells, and, later, fibroblasts. The resulting swelling and proliferation of the endothelium of the smaller blood vessels leads to **endarteritis obliterans**. Healing occurs with scar tissue formation. In late syphilis, hypersensitivity to *T. pallidum* leads to gummatous ulcerations and necrosis. Inflammatory changes are replaced by degenerative processes, especially in the cardiovascular and central nervous systems.

The CNS is invaded early in the infection, and during the secondary stage of the disease > 30% of patients have an abnormal CSF (see TABLE 117–1 in Ch. 117). During the first 5 to 10 yr after infection, the disease principally involves the meninges and blood vessels and results in **meningovascular neurosyphilis**; later the parenchyma of the brain and spinal cord are damaged, which leads to **parenchymatous neurosyphilis**. Involvement of the cerebral cortex and overlying meninges results in **general paresis**. Degeneration of the posterior columns and root ganglia of the spinal cord results in **tabes dorsalis**.

Epidemiology

Infection is usually transmitted by sexual contact, including orogenital and anorectal, and occasionally by kissing or close bodily contact. Recently, promiscuous homosexual men have been at the greatest risk in the USA. Untreated patients with primary

or secondary syphilis who have skin lesions are the most infectious. Early latent syphilis is potentially infectious during mucocutaneous relapses, but late latent syphilis is not. Tertiary syphilis is not contagious. Infection with syphilis does not confer lasting immunity against subsequent reinfection, particularly if treatment is given early in the course of the disease.

Symptoms, Signs, and Course

The incubation period of primary syphilis can vary from 1 to 13 wk, but is usually from 3 to 4 wk. The disease can appear in any stage without a history of prior stages and remote from the time of initial infection. Because the disease has diverse clinical manifestations and is now relatively rare in the USA, clinicians there may find it difficult to recognize.

Primary syphilis: The primary lesion or **chancre** generally appears within 4 wk of infection and heals within 4 to 8 wk in untreated patients. At the inoculation site, a red papule develops and soon erodes to form a painless ulcer. It is usually single, occasionally multiple, with an indurated, hard base. It does not bleed, but when abraded exudes a clear serum containing numerous *T. pallida*. A red areola may surround it. The regional lymphatic nodes usually enlarge painlessly and are rubbery, discrete, and nontender. Primary chancres occur on the penis, anus, and rectum in men; the vulva, cervix, and perineum in women. Chancres may also be found on the lips, tongue, buccal mucosa, tonsils, or fingers, and rarely on other parts of the body, and often produce such minimal symptoms that they are ignored.

Secondary syphilis: Cutaneous rashes usually appear within 6 to 12 wk after infection and are most florid after 3 to 4 mo. (About 25% of patients have a healing primary chancre.) The lesions may be transitory or may persist for months. In untreated patients they frequently heal but fresh ones may appear within weeks or months. Over 80% of patients have mucocutaneous lesions, 50% have generalized enlargement of the lymph nodes, and about 10% have lesions of the eyes (uveitis), bones (periostitis) and joints, meninges, kidney (glomerulitis), liver, and spleen. Mild constitutional symptoms of malaise, headache, anorexia, nausea, aching pains in the bones, and fatigability are often present, as well as fever, anemia, jaundice, albuminuria, and neck stiffness. At this stage a small number of patients develop acute syphilitic meningitis, with headache, neck stiffness, cranial nerve lesions, deafness, and occasional papilledema.

Syphilitic skin rashes may simulate a variety of dermatologic conditions (see Diagnosis, below). Usually they are symmetric and more marked on the flexor and volar surfaces of the body, especially the palms and soles. The rashes generally occur in crops, and may be macules, papules, pustules, or squamous lesions. The individual spots are pigmented in black persons and pinkish or pale red in whites, are round and tend to become confluent and indurated, and generally do not itch. They eventually heal, usually without leaving a scar, but in some patients there may be areas of residual hyper- or depigmentation.

The surface of the mucous membranes frequently becomes eroded, forming mucous patches that are circular and often grayish-white with a red areola. These patches occur mostly in the mouth; on the palate, pharynx, larynx, glans penis, or vulva; or in the anal canal and rectum. Papules developing at the mucocutaneous junctions and in moist areas of the skin become hypertrophic, flattened, and dull pink or gray; are called **condylomata lata;** and are extremely infectious. The hair often falls out in patches, leaving a "moth-eaten" appearance.

Frequently, there is a generalized, nontender, rubbery, discrete enlargement of the lymph nodes affecting the cervical, suboccipital, epitrochlear, axillary, and inguinal groups. The liver and spleen may be palpable in some patients.

Latent syphilis: In the early latent period (> 1 yr after infection), infectious mucocutaneous relapses may occur during the first year, but after 2 yr the development of further contagious lesions is rare and the patient appears normal. The latent stage may last for a few years or for the rest of the patient's life. In untreated cases, about 1/3 of those infected develop late or tertiary syphilis. This may not occur for many years after the initial infection.

Late or **tertiary syphilis:** Clinical description of the lesions of late syphilis may be divided into (1) benign tertiary syphilis of the skin, bone, and viscera, (2) cardiovascular syphilis, and (3) neurosyphilis.

Lesions of **benign tertiary syphilis** usually develop within 3 to 10 yr of infection and have almost vanished in the antibiotic era. The typical lesion is a **gumma,** a chronic granulomatous reaction that leads to necrosis and fibrosis. It is frequently localized, but may diffusely infiltrate an organ or tissue. With localized lesions, an area of central necrosis is surrounded by granulation tissue. Gummas are indolent, increase slowly in size, heal gradually, and leave scars. Gummatous lesions may develop in the skin, where they result in nodular, ulcerative, or squamous skin eruptions. If they are subcutaneous, they result in punched-out ulcers with sloughing, washed-leather–appearing bases that heal leaving typical tissue-paper scars. Often they occur in submucous tissue, especially of the palate, nasal septum, pharynx, and larynx, and lead to tissue destruction with perforation of the palate or septum. They are most common on the leg just below the knee, the upper trunk, the face, and the scalp, but may occur almost anywhere in the body, including the stomach, lung, liver, testicle, and choroid of the eye.

Diffuse gummatous infiltration affects the tongue and leads to chronic interstitial glossitis with leukoplakia and deep fissure formation. Carcinoma is a common sequel.

Benign tertiary syphilis of the bones results in either periostitis with bone formation or osteitis with destructive lesions. The patient complains of a deep, boring pain, characteristically worse at night. A lump or swelling may be noticed if the area involved is superficial.

Cardiovascular syphilis produces thoracic aneurysm, narrowing of the coronary ostia, or aortic valvular insufficiency that usually appears 10 to 25 yr after the initial infection. (See in AORTITIS in Ch. 29.)

Symptomatic neurosyphilis produces various clinical syndromes that develop in about 5% of untreated syphilitics. **Asymptomatic neurosyphilis** generally precedes symptomatic neurosyphilis and is found in about 15% of those originally diagnosed as having latent syphilis, in 12% of those with cardiovascular syphilis, and in 5% of those with benign tertiary syphilis. In asymptomatic neurosyphilis, abnormalities may be present in the CSF (see Diagnosis, below).

Meningovascular neurosyphilis: When the cerebral cortex is principally involved, headache, dizziness, poor concentration, lassitude, insomnia, neck stiffness, and blurred vision occur. Mental confusion, epileptiform attacks, papilledema, aphasia, and mono- or hemiplegia may also be present. Cranial nerve palsies and pupillary abnormalities occur with basal meningitis. The **Argyll Robertson pupil,** which occurs almost exclusively in neurosyphilis, is a small irregular pupil that reacts normally to accommodation but not to light.

When the spinal cord is involved there may be bulbar symptoms, weakness and wasting of the muscles of the shoulder girdle and arms, a slowly progressive spastic paraplegia with bladder symptoms, and in rare cases, a transverse myelitis with sudden flaccid paraplegia and loss of sphincter control.

Parenchymatous neurosyphilis: General paresis or **dementia paralytica** generally affects patients in their 40s or 50s. The onset usually is insidious and manifested by behavior

changes. There may be convulsions, aphasia, or transient hemiparesis, but more commonly irritability, difficulty in concentrating, memory deterioration, defective judgment, headaches, insomnia, or fatigue and lethargy occur. The patient's hygiene and grooming deteriorate; emotional instability leads to frequent weeping and temper tantrums; asthenia, depression, and delusions of grandeur with lack of insight may be present.

Physical signs include tremors of the mouth, tongue, outstretched hands, and whole body; pupillary abnormalities; dysarthria; brisk tendon reflexes; and, in some cases, extensor plantar responses. The handwriting usually is shaky and illegible. Signs of posterior column involvement accompany taboparesis. The lesions of **tabes dorsalis (locomotor ataxia)** result in pain, ataxia, sensory changes, and loss of tendon reflexes. Onset is slow and insidious. The first and most characteristic symptom usually is an intense, stabbing pain (lightning pain) in the legs that occurs in crops and recurs at irregular intervals. Later, unsteadiness of gait develops that is worse in the dark. The patient may walk on a broad base with the feet wide apart. There may be a feeling of walking on foam rubber, with hyperesthesia and paresthesia. Loss of bladder sensation leads to urine retention, incontinence, and recurrent infections. Impotence is common.

The majority of patients with tabes dorsalis are thin and have a characteristic sad-looking, tabetic facies. Argyll Robertson pupils usually are present and there may be primary optic atrophy. Examination of the lower limbs discloses hypotonia, diminished or absent tendon reflexes, impaired vibration and joint position sense, ataxia in the heel-shin test, and absence of deep pain sensation. **Romberg's sign** is positive and there is ataxia on walking. The bladder is frequently palpably enlarged.

Visceral crises appear as paroxysms of pain in various organs, the most common being gastric crises with vomiting. Rectal, bladder, and laryngeal crises also occur. **Trophic lesions**, secondary to hypoesthesia of the skin or periarticular tissues, may develop in the later stages of the disease. Trophic ulcers may develop on the soles of the feet, penetrate deeply and involve the underlying bone. **Charcot's arthropathy,** a painless disorganization of a joint, with bony swelling and an abnormal range of movement, is a common manifestation.

Diagnosis

Diagnostic studies for syphilis should include a clinical history, a thorough physical examination, serologic tests, darkfield examination of fluids from lesions, CSF tests, radiologic examination, and investigations of all personal contacts where relevant.

Darkfield examination: In darkfield microscopy, light is directed obliquely through the slide so that rays striking any organisms on the slide cause them to appear as bright objects against a dark background. The external morphology and motility of spirochetes present in exudates and tissue fluids from primary and secondary lesions may thus be observed and identified. Experience and skill are needed in taking the specimens and identifying the organism by its regular coils, corkscrew rotation, watchspring movements, and angulation. The organism must be distinguished from nonpathogenic spirochetes, which may be part of the normal flora.

Serologic tests for syphilis (STS): Two principal classes of STS aid in diagnosing syphilis and other treponemal diseases: (1) screening, nontreponemal tests using lipoid antigens detect syphilitic reagin, and (2) specific treponemal tests detect antitreponemal antibodies.

The screening tests most frequently used are the **Venereal Disease Research Laboratory (VDRL)** and the **rapid plasma reagin (RPR)** tests. Specific treponemal tests include the **fluorescent treponemal antibody-absorption (FTA-ABS)** test, the ***Treponema pallidum* hemagglutination assay (TPHA),** and the ***T. pallidum* immobilization (TPI)** test.

The **VDRL test** is a flocculation test for syphilis in which reagin antibody (not to be confused with the reaginic antibodies that mediate allergy) in the patient's serum

reacts visibly with cardiolipin, the antigen. A number of conditions (eg, acute infectious hepatitis) can increase serum reagin and produce a reactive VDRL test. Results are reported as reactive, weakly reactive, borderline, or nonreactive. Reactive and weakly reactive sera are considered positive for syphilitic antibodies. All reactive and weakly reactive VDRL tests should be confirmed by one of the more specific **FTA-ABS tests.**

The screening tests are easy to perform and inexpensive, but they lack the specificity of the treponemal tests and sometimes give biologic false-positive **(BFP)** results. A BFP reaction (defined as a reactive reaginic test, but a nonreactive treponemal test) may be a clue to the presence of autoimmune or collagen vascular disorders, viral infection, or various conditions with alterations in immunoglobulins. Quantitative reaginic tests give declining titers following treatment and become negative by 1 yr in primary and 2 yr in secondary cases. Reaginic tests do not become positive until 3 to 6 wk after the initial infection. Since the chancre usually develops before this, an early negative STS cannot rule out syphilis. If the screening tests are positive, the more specific treponemal tests are performed. In patients with undiagnosed genital lesions, the reaginic tests should be repeated at 2-wk intervals for the first 6 wk before the diagnosis of syphilis can be excluded. The treponemal tests usually become positive after infection has been established 3 to 4 wk and remains so for many years despite effective treatment.

CSF examination: Before treatment is given in all but the early (< 1 yr) infectious cases, examination of the CSF is recommended to exclude neurosyphilis. The cell count and differential, total protein, and VDRL or other nonspecific (reaginic) serologic tests are usually performed. The value of treponemal tests of CSF is unclear.

Immediate **diagnosis of primary syphilis** depends on demonstrating *T. pallidum* in exudates taken from the chancre by darkfield microscopy. If initial results are negative, the examinations should be repeated and serologic tests ordered. Aspirates from lymph node punctures may demonstrate *T. pallidum* in some cases, especially where topical antiseptics or antibiotics have reduced organisms in the chancre below detectable levels.

Differential diagnosis of genital ulceration includes herpes genitalis, chancroid, lymphogranuloma venereum, scabies, mucous patches of secondary syphilis, erosive balanitis, Behçet's disease, gummatous ulceration, epithelioma, granuloma inguinale, tuberculous ulceration, and trauma; dual infections with 2 pathogens (eg, herpes simplex and treponemá) are not rare. **All genital ulcers should be considered syphilitic until proved otherwise.** Because physicians frequently overlook the possibility of syphilis, extragenital chancres are often misdiagnosed.

Diagnosis of secondary syphilis: Because syphilis can mimic most skin diseases, any undiagnosed cutaneous eruption or mucosal lesion should be considered syphilitic, especially if it is associated with generalized lymphadenopathy or occurs in patients at risk of syphilis. The diagnosis is established by demonstrating *T. pallidum* on darkfield examination or by positive STS. These are reactive in virtually all cases, often with a high titer of reaginic antibody. Common errors are misdiagnosing secondary syphilis as a drug eruption, pityriasis rosea, rubella, infectious mononucleosis, erythema multiforme, pityriasis rubra pilaris, or fungal infection. Condylomata lata may be mistaken for warts, hemorrhoids, or pemphigus vegetans; scalp lesions for ringworm or alopecia areata; and mucous patches for various other conditions.

Diagnosis of latent syphilis is made by excluding the other forms of syphilis in patients with persistently positive reaginic and treponemal STS, but without clinical evidence of active syphilitic lesions. The CSF is normal and the heart and aorta are normal on clinical and radiologic examination. Latent acquired syphilis must be differentiated from latent congenital syphilis (see in NEONATAL INFECTIONS in Ch. 186), latent yaws and other treponemal diseases found in patients from tropical areas, and

BFP reactions. Many patients give no history of primary or secondary manifestations, and it must be presumed that they were asymptomatic during the early stages, the manifestations were trivial or ignored, or the diagnosis was missed.

Diagnosis of tertiary syphilis: In **benign tertiary syphilis,** STS will be positive in most cases, but differentiation from coincidental granulomatous conditions may be difficult without biopsy. In **cardiovascular syphilis,** symptoms and signs are sometimes so typical that a clinical diagnosis can easily be made. However, it may be confirmed by echocardiographic and radiologic examination, ECG, and STS. The CSF should be examined, as neurosyphilis and cardiovascular syphilis often occur concurrently. In **asymptomatic neurosyphilis,** the CSF usually shows an elevated cell count, increased protein, and positive reaginic test. In **paresis,** treponemal test in serum is positive and the CSF is always abnormal, usually with an elevated cell count of 7 to 100 lymphocytes, increased protein, and positive reaginic test. In **tabes dorsalis** the treponemal tests are usually positive, but the reaginic screening tests may be negative. The CSF usually shows an increased cell count, a raised protein, and weakly positive STS. In many advanced cases the CSF may be normal.

Treatment

In **primary and secondary syphilis,** all the implications should be explained to the patient. All sexual contacts of the past 3 mo (in cases of primary syphilis) and those up to 1 yr (in cases of secondary syphilis) should be examined, treated, and informed that they may be contagious. They should not have any form of sexual relations until they and their sexual partners have been examined and have completed treatment.

Penicillin is the antibiotic of choice for all stages of syphilis. A serum level of 0.03 IU/mL for 6 to 8 days is required to cure early infectious syphilis. Benzathine penicillin G 2.4 million u. IM will produce a satisfactory blood level for 2 wk (1.2 million u. is usually given in each buttock). Two additional injections of 2.4 million u. q 7 days should be given for secondary syphilis of > 1 yr in duration. Alternatively, aqueous procaine penicillin G 600,000 u./day IM for 10 days may be given, but offers no advantage. For penicillin-allergic patients, erythromycin 500 mg orally q 6 h for 15 days or tetracycline (at the same dosage) may be used. Because these latter regimens require the patient's compliance, they should be monitored closely.

Patients with **early and late latent syphilis** should be treated with penicillin to prevent subsequent development of tertiary manifestations. Benzathine penicillin G at a total dosage of 7.2 million u. may be given as single injections of 2.4 million u. IM once/wk for 3 wk. Alternatively, aqueous procaine penicillin G 600,000 u./day IM for 14 days may be given. Those sensitive to penicillin may be treated with erythromycin 500 mg q 6 h for 15 days. **Benign tertiary syphilis** is treated in the same way as latent syphilis, above; however, for those who cannot tolerate penicillin and are treated with erythromycin, a second course of erythromycin at the same dosage 3 mo later is advisable.

Cardiovascular syphilis: Treatment is the same as for latent syphilis, above, but procaine penicillin G usually is given for a total of 21 days.

Neurosyphilis: Penicillin is given as in latent syphilis, above, but, if used, procaine penicillin G should be given for a total of 21 days. Treatment of asymptomatic neurosyphilis prevents development of symptomatic neurosyphilis but usually does not reverse established symptoms. Chlorpromazine 25 or 50 mg orally or IM is effective in controlling restless patients with paresis; analgesics should be used freely for tabetic patients with lightning pains. Carbamazepine 200 mg orally tid or qid is sometimes effective in controlling the pains.

Over 50% of the patients with early infectious syphilis, especially those with secondary syphilis, will have a **Jarisch-Herxheimer reaction** within 6 to 12 h after the initial

treatment. The reaction—manifested by general malaise, fever, headache, sweating, rigors, and a temporary exacerbation of the syphilitic lesions—usually subsides within 24 h and is not dangerous to the patient apart from the anxiety it may produce. However, patients with general paresis or those with a high CSF cell count are likely to develop a Herxheimer reaction that occasionally causes serious disorders, such as seizures, a hemiplegia, or a monoplegia. The Herxheimer reaction should be explained to the patient before treatment is started. Herxheimer reactions may be confused with penicillin allergy and may provide a clue to coexistent syphilis in persons treated with penicillin for other conditions, such as gonorrhea.

Posttreatment Surveillance

The importance of repeated tests to confirm a permanent cure should be explained to the patient before treatment. Examinations and quantitative reaginic tests should be made (at 1, 3, 6, and 12 mo or until no reaction is found, whichever period is longer). Following successful treatment, lesions heal rapidly, serologic titers fall, and the reagin tests usually become negative within 9 to 12 mo. The treponemal tests, such as the FTA-ABS and the TPHA, usually remain positive for years or even for the rest of the patient's life. The CSF should be examined after 1 yr of surveillance. If the VDRL remains positive for > 1 yr or if the titer starts to rise, more intensive re-treatment should be considered. Serologic or clinical relapse is uncommon, but occasionally occurs about the 6th to 9th mo and most commonly in the nervous system. Relapse requires re-treatment with a more intensive regime of antibiotics, but the possibility of reinfection should also be considered and investigated. If all the clinical and serologic examinations remain satisfactory for 2 yr after treatment, the patient can be reassured that cure is complete and permanent and he need not return.

Patients with **latent syphilis** should be kept under surveillance at intervals of 3, 6, 12, 18, and 24 mo, and those with persistently positive serologic tests should be seen annually indefinitely. The prognosis is excellent. Patients with **benign tertiary syphilis** should be examined at regular intervals after treatment, and those with **cardiovascular syphilis** should be followed throughout their lives.

In **asymptomatic neurosyphilis,** the CSF should be examined q 6 mo until it has been normal for 2 yr; if the CSF is abnormal, it should be examined q 3 mo until it is normal, and then annually for 2 yr more. Tabes dorsalis tends to progress despite treatment, and a careful watch should be kept for urinary tract infections.

CONGENITAL SYPHILIS

(See in NEONATAL INFECTIONS in Ch. 186)

TRICHOMONIASIS

Etiology

Trichomonas vaginalis, a flagellate protozoan found in the GU tract of either sex is a common cause of vaginitis. The organism is usually pear-shaped, with average dimensions of 7 × 10 μm, but occasionally as long as 25 μm. It has 4 flagella anteriorly and a fifth flagella embedded in an undulating membrane. The organism, found more commonly in females, affects about 20% of them during their reproductive years and causes vaginitis, urethritis, and possibly cystitis. *T. vaginalis* is more difficult to detect in males, probably causes urethritis, prostatitis, and cystitis, and may account for as much as 5 to 10% of all cases of male urethritis in some areas. Most infected males are asymptomatic carriers, but are infectious to their sexual partners.

Symptoms and Signs

In females, onset typically is accompanied by a copious, greenish-yellow, frothy vaginal discharge associated with irritation and soreness of the vulva, perineum, and

thighs, and with dyspareunia and dysuria. Some females have only a slight discharge, and many are symptom-free carriers for long periods, although symptoms may develop at any time. The infection frequently coexists with gonorrhea. In severe cases, the vulva and perineum may be inflamed, with edema of the labia. The vaginal walls and surface of the cervix may show punctate, red "strawberry" spots, but frequently are normal or have a small amount of discharge in the vaginal fornices. Complications, including bartholinitis, skenitis, and cystitis, are rare.

Males generally are asymptomatic. Some may have a transient, frothy, or purulent urethral discharge with dysuria and frequency, usually early in the morning; mild urethral irritation and, occasionally, moisture at the urethral meatus; and discomfort in the perineum or deeper in the pelvis. A subpreputial discharge may appear in uncircumcised men. Epididymitis and prostatitis are the only known complications.

Diagnosis

In females the diagnosis can usually be made immediately by examining a sample of vaginal secretion taken from the posterior fornix under either a darkfield, phase contrast, or ordinary light microscope. The lashing movements of the flagella and striking motility of the oval-shaped organisms are readily observed. The organism can be cultured on a suitable medium. Trichomoniasis is also commonly diagnosed on a Papanicolaou smear. Tests should be done to exclude gonorrhea and other STDs.

If the **male patient** is examined early in the morning before urinating, a slight mucoid discharge may be present and there may be some fine threads in the 2-glass urine test. A wet film of the urethral secretions in males should be examined microscopically for trichomonads and cultures inoculated. Examining the centrifuged deposit of urine and prostatic secretions may also be helpful.

Treatment

Metronidazole, 2 gm orally once, will cure up to 95% of women submitting to initial treatment if sexual partners are treated simultaneously. Because the effectiveness of single-dose regimens in men is unclear, men should be treated with 250 mg tid for 7 days. Metronidazole may cause leukopenia, disulfiram-like adverse interactions with alcohol, or candidal superinfections. Metronidazole is relatively contraindicated in pregnancy, although no human data suggest it is dangerous to the fetus after the first trimester. Povidone-iodine should also be avoided. All sexual partners should be examined and treated and patients should abstain from intercourse until a cure is established.

GENITAL CANDIDIASIS

Etiology

Yeast infections of the genital tract caused by *Candida albicans* are increasing in frequency, especially in women. Uncommonly transmitted sexually, the infection usually spreads from the patient's normal skin or intestinal flora. The increased incidence is primarily due to widespread use of broad-spectrum antibiotics and the large number of women taking oral contraceptives, although better diagnostic methods may also contribute. Other predisposing factors include pregnancy, menstruation, diabetes mellitus, constrictive undergarments, and use of immunosuppressive drugs and corticosteroids. *Systemic* candidiasis is evidence of severe underlying disease or immunologic abnormality and is rarely a complication of genital infection.

Symptoms and Signs

Women usually develop vulval irritation and vaginal discharge. Frequently the irritation is severe and the discharge scanty. The vulva may be reddish and swollen, with excoriation and fissuring. The vaginal wall may be covered with a white, cheesy mate-

rial or may appear normal. **Men** often are symptomless, but may complain of irritation and soreness of the glans penis and prepuce, especially after intercourse. Occasionally they may notice a slight urethral discharge. The glans penis and prepuce are reddish on examination, and there may be vesicles or erosions. White, cheesy material may adhere to the surface. In severe cases the prepuce may be edematous, causing phimosis (constriction of the foreskin).

Diagnosis

An immediate diagnosis can be made by taking smears from the vagina, glans penis, prepuce, or urethra and looking for *C. albicans* under the microscope by the potassium hydroxide method of Gram stain (gram-positive, oval, budding, yeastlike cells having typical elongated, filamentous pseudohyphae). Culture media, such as Sabouraud's, should also be inoculated; this procedure increases the number of positive findings by 25% and confirms the presence of *C. albicans*. Since candidiasis is rarely transmitted sexually, tests should be done for coexisting STDs only if clinically or epidemiologically indicated.

Treatment

Once the diagnosis and the underlying cause have been identified, predisposing conditions such as antibiotic therapy should be controlled to avoid recurrences.

Vaginal candidiasis can be treated locally with (1) nystatin, 2 tablets of 100,000 u. each being inserted high into the vagina for 14 nights before retiring; (2) clotrimazole, one 100-mg vaginal tablet/day for 6 days or 200 mg/day for 3 days; or (3) miconazole 100 mg/day intravaginally for 7 days. An oral regimen of ketoconazole 200 mg bid for 6 days has produced satisfactory results.

Candidal balanoposthitis is treated by carefully washing the genitalia with soap and water, drying with a clean towel, and applying nystatin cream bid for 7 to 10 days. Urethritis may be treated with daily irrigations of a 100,000-u./mL nystatin suspension, but usually it is secondary to balanitis and does not require additional treatment.

Relapse is common in either sex and may be due to reinfection by the sexual partner or, more commonly, from the normal flora in combination with a provoking condition. Occasionally contraceptive pills must be discontinued for several months during treatment. Women who require antibiotics recurrently or for prolonged periods or have other unavoidable predispositions may require prophylaxis with any of the treatment regimens.

BALANOPOSTHITIS; BALANITIS

Inflammation of the glans penis and the prepuce.

Etiology

Balanoposthitis (balanitis when in the circumcised) may be caused by complications of gonorrhea, trichomoniasis, candidiasis, Reiter's syndrome, and primary or secondary syphilis. Other causes include fixed drug eruptions, contact dermatitis, psoriasis, lichen planus, seborrheic dermatitis, lichen sclerosus et atrophicus, and erythroplasia of Queyrat. In many cases no cause can be found. Balanoposthitis is often associated with a tight prepuce. The subpreputial secretions become infected with anaerobic bacteria, with resulting inflammation and tissue destruction. Diabetes mellitus predisposes to balanoposthitis.

Symptoms and Signs

Soreness, irritation, and a subpreputial discharge often occur 2 or 3 days after sexual intercourse. Phimosis (constriction of the foreskin) due to edema of the surface of the glans penis and prepuce may be present. Both may be eroded with superficial ulcerations. The inguinal lymphatic nodes may be tender and enlarged.

Diagnosis

Common STDs should be excluded by smears and cultures of material from the inflamed surface, STS performed, and the urine tested for glucose.

Treatment

The appropriate treatment should be given if a specific cause is found. Saline washes should be carried out several times daily if no cause can be found. Subpreputial irrigations should be given if there is true phimosis. Oral sulfonamides, which will not mask incubating syphilis, should be given if there is significant secondary infection. Circumcision should be considered in patients with persistent phimosis once the inflammation has resolved.

VULVITIS

(See in Ch. 171)

CHANCROID

An acute, localized, contagious disease characterized by painful genital ulcers and suppuration of the inguinal lymphatic nodes.

Etiology

The causative agent is *Hemophilus ducreyi*, a short, slender, gram-negative bacillus with rounded ends that is usually found in chains or groups. It generally will grow on nutritionally enriched culture media containing hemin and albumin.

Symptoms and Signs

The incubation period is 3 to 7 days. Small, painful papules rapidly break down to become shallow ulcers with ragged, undermined edges. Each ulcer is shallow, nonindurated, painful, and surrounded by a reddish border. Ulcers vary in size and often coalesce. Phagedenic erosion occasionally leads to marked tissue destruction. The inguinal lymphatic nodes become tender, enlarged, and matted together, and form a fluctuant abscess (bubo) in the groin. The skin over the abscess may become red and shiny and may break down to form a sinus. Autoinoculation may result in new lesions. Complications include phimosis, urethral stricture, urethral fistula, and severe tissue destruction. Chancroid may coexist with other causes of genital ulcers and may occur in epidemic form.

Diagnosis

Diagnosis usually has been based on clinical findings, since culture of the organism is difficult and the polymicrobial flora of ulcers makes microscopic identification uncertain. However, attempts should be made to identify *H. ducreyi* in material taken from the edge of the ulcers or pus from a bubo. Cultures should also be attempted on media containing fresh defibrinated rabbit blood or the patient's own serum. Biopsy from an ulcer edge may be helpful, but the changes are often nonspecific. Tests to exclude other STDs should be performed—especially STS and culture for herpes, if available.

Treatment

Trimethoprim/sulfamethoxazole (160 and 800 mg), 1 tablet q 12 h, or erythromycin 500 mg q 6 h for at least 10 days are the drugs of choice. Increasing resistance to sulfonamides alone and tetracycline have rendered these drugs less effective. Buboes should be aspirated, not incised. All sexual contacts should be examined and the patient kept under surveillance for 3 mo, with regular STS.

LYMPHOGRANULOMA VENEREUM

(LGV; Lymphopathia Venereum; Lymphogranuloma Inguinale)

A sexually transmitted chlamydial disease having a transitory primary lesion followed by suppurative lymphangitis and serious local complications.

Etiology

LGV is caused by a limited number of immunotypes of *Chlamydia trachomatis* distinct from the agents causing trachoma, inclusion conjunctivitis, urethritis, and cervicitis. The disease is found mostly in tropical and subtropical areas.

Symptoms and Signs

After an incubation period of from 3 to 12 or more days, a small, transient, nonindurated vesicular lesion is formed that ulcerates rapidly, heals quickly, and may pass unnoticed. Usually, the first symptom is unilateral tender enlargement of the inguinal lymphatic nodes, which progresses to form a large, tender, fluctuant mass that adheres to the deep tissues and inflames the overlying skin. Multiple sinuses may develop and discharge purulent or bloodstained material. Healing eventually occurs with scar formation, but the sinuses can persist or recur.

The patient may complain of fever, malaise, headaches, joint pains, anorexia, and vomiting. Backache is common in women, in whom the initial lesions may be on the cervix or upper vagina and result in enlargement and suppuration of perirectal and pelvic lymphatics. If the rectal wall is involved in women or homosexual men, an ulcerative proctitis with bloodstained purulent rectal discharges may ensue.

Chronic inflammation obstructs the lymphatic vessels and leads to edema, ulcerations, and fistula formation. Large polypoid masses develop, and gross swellings may eventually result in genital elephantiasis. Rectal strictures may be found in females and male homosexuals.

Diagnosis

Clinical diagnosis can be confirmed by a CF test in which a rising titer of antibody may be demonstrated. A microimmunofluorescence test **(microIF)** measures type-specific antibody and distinguishes various serotypes of antibody. Cross-reactions, however, are common. Isolation on cell culture is sometimes possible, but is limited to a relatively few centers. Commercially available immunofluorescence kits using monoclonal antibodies should increase the availability of specific tests. In the absence of microIF and cell culture, diagnosis can be made by a careful history, clinical examination, and the presence of high or rising titers of complement-fixing antibodies.

Treatment

Tetracycline 500 mg orally q 6 h for 10 to 14 days is the treatment of choice, producing rapid healing of early lesions. Erythromycin, chloramphenicol, and rifampin are also effective. Fluctuant buboes should be aspirated, not incised. Abscesses and fistulas usually require surgery, but rectal strictures can usually be dilated. Elephantiasis is treated by plastic surgery. All sexual contacts should be examined, and the patient should be kept under observation for 6 mo after apparently successful treatment.

GRANULOMA INGUINALE

A chronic granulomatous condition usually involving the genitalia and probably spread by sexual contact.

Etiology

Granuloma inguinale is rare in temperate climates but is common in some tropical and subtropical areas. It is believed to be caused by a gram-negative, intracellular

bacillus found in mononuclear cells and known as *Donovania granulomatis* and recently renamed *Calymmatobacterium granulomatis*.

Symptoms and Signs

The incubation period varies from about 1 to 12 wk. The initial lesion is a painless, beefy-red nodule that slowly develops into a rounded, elevated, velvety, granulomatous mass. Sites of infection are the penis, scrotum, groin, and thighs in males; the vulva, vagina, and perineum in females; the anus and buttocks in homosexual males; and the face in both sexes. There is no lymphadenopathy, and the disease spreads by continuity and autoinoculation. Progress is slow, but eventually the lesions may cover the genitalia. Healing also is slow and scar tissue forms. Secondary infection is common and can cause gross tissue destruction. Anemia, cachexia, and death may follow in neglected cases, and hematogenous dissemination to bones, joints, or liver occurs occasionally.

Diagnosis

Bright, beefy-red, granulomatous lesions are characteristic. Confirmation of the diagnosis is made microscopically by demonstrating Donovan bodies (intracytoplasmic bacilli in macrophages stained by Giemsa or Wright's stain) in smears taken from edge scrapings of the lesions. Biopsy specimens from such scrapings contain many plasma cells, but few mononuclear cells.

Treatment

Streptomycin, tetracycline, erythromycin, chloramphenicol, and trimethoprim/sulfamethoxazole produce satisfactory healing of the lesions. Streptomycin will not mask incubating syphilis, is given 1 gm IM q 12 h for 21 days, and remains effective in some areas. Tetracycline is given 500 mg orally q 6 h for 10 to 14 days. Treatment should result in a response in 7 days, but should be continued for 3 wk or until lesions have been healed to minimize relapses. The patient's sexual contacts should be located and thoroughly examined. Surveillance after apparently successful treatment should be for 6 mo and should include STS.

GENITAL HERPES

Infection of the skin of the genital area or perirectal area by herpes simplex.

Etiology

Infection of the genital and anorectal skin and mucosa, usually with herpes simplex virus **(HSV)** type 2 but also (in $\cong$ 5%) type 1, is the most common cause of genital ulceration in developed countries. It is moderately contagious and usually spreads by sexual contact. Lesions frequently develop 4 to 7 days after contact, and the condition tends to recur because the virus establishes latent infection of the sacral sensory nerve ganglia, from which it reactivates and reinfects the skin.

Symptoms and Signs

Primary lesions are more painful, prolonged, and widespread than those of recurrent outbreaks. Itching and soreness usually precede a small patch of erythema on the skin or mucous membranes. A small group of painful vesicles develops; they erode and form several superficial, circular ulcers with a red areola. If secondary infection occurs, the ulcers may coalesce to form a larger ulcer. The ulcers become crusted after a few days and usually heal in about 10 days, with scarring. The inguinal lymphatic nodes are usually slightly enlarged and tender. The ulcers are usually painful.

Lesions may occur on the prepuce, glans penis, and shaft of the penis in males, and on the labia, clitoris, perineum, vagina, and cervix in women. They may occur around the anus and in the rectum in homosexual males or rectally exposed females. In addi-

tion to pain in primary infections, the patient may experience generalized malaise, fever, and difficulty with micturation (because of bladder paresis or dysuria) or with walking.

Diagnosis

Clinical diagnosis is confirmed by taking material from the base of ulcerated lesions on a cotton wool swab (or by aspiration from a vesicle), placing it in a suitable virus transport medium, and inoculating tissue cultures. A characteristic cytopathic effect is produced within 24 to 48 h. Paired sera, taken at 10- to 14-day intervals, may show a rise in antibody titer in primary infections. Immediate diagnosis can be made by finding characteristic multinucleate giant cells in Wright-Giemsa stained smears of cells from lesions (Tzanck preparation).

Complications

Genital herpes may be complicated by aseptic meningitis, transverse myelitis, or autonomic nervous system dysfunction involving the sacral regions. Aseptic meningitis presents with fever, headache, vomiting, photophobia, and nuchal rigidity 3 to 12 days after onset of primary or recurrent genital lesions. WBCs range from 10 to > 1000 cells, preodminantly lymphocytes, and the CSF protein may be slightly elevated. The disease almost always resolves spontaneously in a few days without sequelae. Symptoms of autonomic dysfunction, including inability to urinate, constipation, and impotence in men, frequently complicate primary infection. Less commonly, the syndrome of transverse myelitis affecting the legs complicates primary infections.

Hematogenous dissemination of virus to the skin, joints, liver, or lung occasionally occurs in apparently immunologically normal patients, but is more common in immunosuppessed or pregnant patients.

Extragenital lesions, usually involving the buttock, groin, or thigh area, may occur in either primary or recurrent disease by either neuronal spread or direct inoculation. The latter mechanism accounts for occasional infections of the fingers or eye. Extension into the genitals or urinary system is extremely rare. Bacterial superinfection of herpes ulcers is uncommon, although herpes may coexist with *Treponema pallidum*, *Hemophilus ducreyi*, or *Candida albicans*.

By far the most common complication of genital herpes is recurrent disease, usually confined to one side of the body, milder than the initial attack, and associated with prodromal symptoms that may be severe. The likelihood and rate of recurrences are greater with HSV type 2 (80%) than type 1 (50%). Recurrences vary greatly in their courses, but may be quite frequent and may be prolonged over many years. Reinfection with different strains of type 2 virus can also occur.

Treatment

Acyclovir, available in IV, topical, and oral forms, effectively treats primary herpetic infections of the mouth, genitalia, and rectum. It (1) reduces viral shedding and symptoms in severe primary infections, (2) marginally reduces shedding and symptoms in recurrent disease, (3) cures chronic infections in immunocompromised patients, and (4) when used prophylactically, reduces rates of recurrence. However, even early treatment of primary infections does not abort latent infections or prevent recurrences. Oral acyclovir seems likely to become standard outpatient therapy for most of the indications listed above. Patients with severe primary disease or immunocompromised patients with chronic progressive lesions (eg, acquired immunodeficiency syndrome [**AIDS**]) should receive oral acyclovir 200 mg q 4 h 5 times/day for 5 days or, if necessary, acyclovir 5 mg/kg IV q 8 h. Prophylaxis for severe recurrent disease with acyclovir 200 mg orally tid dramatically reduces the rate and severity of recurrences.

GENITAL WARTS

(Condylomata Acuminata; Moist or Venereal Warts)

Etiology and Incidence

Genital warts are caused by papilloma viruses (human papilloma virus **[HPV]** types 1, 2, 6, 11, 16, and 18) and usually are transmitted sexually. They have an incubation period of from 1 to 6 mo, and occur most commonly on warm, moist surfaces in the subpreputial area, the coronal sulcus, within the urethral meatus, and on the shaft of the penis in males; and on the vulva, the vaginal wall, the cervix, and the perineum in females. They are particularly common in the perianal region and rectum in homosexual males.

Genital wart infections in the USA have increased in the past 10 yr at twice the rate of genital herpes and are medically important, especially for future cancers.

Symptoms and Signs

Genital warts usually appear as soft, moist, minute, pink or red swellings that grow rapidly and become pedunculated. Usually several of them are found in the same area and look like cauliflower. Occasionally they are solitary. During pregnancy and in the presence of chronic discharge they may grow more rapidly and disseminate.

Diagnosis

Genital warts usually can be identified by their appearance, but must be differentiated from the flat-topped condylomata lata of secondary syphilis. Atypical or persistent warts should be biopsied to exclude carcinoma. Women with cervical warts should not be treated until the result of a Pap smear is available to guide therapy.

Treatment

No treatment is completely satisfactory.

Genital warts may be removed by electrocauterization under local or general anesthesia, or by freezing with a cryoprobe. Extensive lesions may require surgical excision. Topical applications of podophyllin or trichloroacetic acids are widely used, often require repeated applications, and frequently fail. For **urethral lesions,** thiotepa has been effective. Topical 5-fluorouracil applied 2 to 3 times a day by the patient is highly effective in the urethra in men, but the patient should be watched for acute, but rare, urethral obstruction. Removal with a resectoscope under general anesthesia may be the most satisfactory treatment. Circumcision may prevent recurrence.

Sexual contacts should be examined and STS performed initially and after 3 mo. Relapse is frequent and requires re-treatment.

Need for follow-up of patients and their sexual partners with genital warts (types 6, 11, 16, and 18) has radically changed with the knowledge that many women with external warts may develop dysplastic changes of the uterine cervix or invasive carcinoma that must be found early and treated. Finding HPV type 16 or 18 in Bowenoid papulosis and in bladder cancers is also cause for regular follow-up examinations. The fact that type 16 integrates with the host's cell DNA rather than remaining as an episome, as with other types of wart virus, may account for its greater invasiveness and its possibly lesser susceptibility to interferon treatment. All physicians who treat genital warts must insist on careful cervical cytological or colposcopic examination of women at yearly or shorter intervals to detect early cancer.

Interferon, especially alpha, intralesionally or IM, has also cleared intractable lesions of skin and genitals. Its optimal administration and long-term results are under study in several countries. Caution is suggested by reports of patients with Bowenoid papulosis of the genitals (type 16) wherein, after initial disappearance of the lesions with interferon-beta, the lesions reappeared as invasive cancers.

PROCTITIS

Inflammation of the anorectal mucosa.

Etiology

Proctitis is caused by gonococci, herpes simplex virus, primary and secondary syphilis, both LGV and non-LGV immunotypes of *Chlamydia trachomatis*, and human papilloma viruses. It is usually a disease of women and homosexual men who practice anal-receptive intercourse.

Proctitis, usually acquired by direct implantation of pathogens on the rectal mucosa, is also associated with sexually transmitted enteric infections that are probably acquired by fecal-oral contamination. A search for bacterial and parasitic agents associated with these syndromes (see below) is important because the same sexual practices (anogenital and ano-oral contact) may transmit both syndromes, signs and symptoms overlap, and several pathogens may coexist.

Symptoms and Signs

Patients may complain of rectal pain or soreness, tenesmus, blood or pus coating their stools, or rectal discharge. Proctoscopy may show focal or diffuse inflammation or ulceration of the mucosa with mucopurulent secretions.

Diagnosis

Proctitis is diagnosed by clinical appearance and finding abundant neutrophils in smears of material swabbed from the mucosa. Specific diagnosis can be made by Gram stain (gonorrhea), Tszank preparation for multinucleate giant cells and tissue culture (herpes), serology (syphilis or chlamydia), or clinical appearance (rectal warts).

Treatment

Therapy depends on the specific etiologic agent. **Gonococcal proctitis** responds to the standard IM regimens of procaine penicillin or spectinomycin, but less consistently to oral regimens of penicillins or tetracyclines. **Primary herpetic proctitis** in immunocompetent persons and chronic progressive disease in the immunocompromised respond to acyclovir 200 mg orally q 4 h or 5 mg/kg IV q 8 h for 5 days. **Chlamydial proctitis** with both LGV and non-LGV strains responds to tetracycline 500 mg orally qid for 14 days. Treatment of **anorectal syphilis** is similar to that for other forms of primary and secondary syphilis. **Perirectal or intrarectal warts** (condylomata acuminata) may be treated with cytotoxic agents (podophyllin or 5-fluorouracil), trichloroacetic acid, laser, cryosurgery, electrocautery, or simple excision.

SEXUALLY-TRANSMITTED ENTERIC INFECTIONS

Various bacterial (shigella, campylobacter, or salmonella), viral (hepatitis A), or parasitic (giardia or amoeba) pathogens are transmitted efficiently by sexual practices that promote fecal-oral contamination. Although the bacterial pathogens may coexist with or cause proctitis, they usually produce symptoms (diarrhea, fever, bloating, nausea, and abdominal pain) suggesting disease more proximal in the GI tract. Multiple infections are frequent, especially in homosexual men with many sexual partners. Asymptomatic infections also occur with all these pathogens, and are the rule with *Entamoeba histolytica*, which is usually of a nonpathogenic type in homosexual men in western countries. Diagnosis and treatment of these conditions are discussed in Ch. 57.

ACQUIRED IMMUNODEFICIENCY SYNDROME (AIDS)

(See Ch. 19)

15. DISEASES OF UNCERTAIN ETIOLOGY

SARCOIDOSIS

A multisystem granulomatous disorder of unknown etiology, characterized histologically by epithelioid tubercles involving various organs or tissues, with symptoms dependent on the site and degree of involvement.

Etiology and Incidence

The cause is unknown. A single provoking agent or disordered defense reactions triggered by a variety of insults may be responsible; genetic factors may be important. Sarcoidosis occurs predominantly between ages 20 and 40 and is most common among northern Europeans and American blacks; the lifetime risk of developing sarcoidosis is 1.15% in Swedish men and 1.6% in Swedish women. The incidence in advanced countries exceeds that of TB.

Pathology

The characteristic histopathologic findings are multiple noncaseating epithelioid granulomas, with little or no necrosis, that may resolve completely or proceed to fibrosis. They occur commonly in mediastinal and peripheral lymph nodes, lungs, liver, eyes, and skin, and less often in the spleen, bones, joints, skeletal muscle, heart, and CNS.

Symptoms and Signs

Symptoms depend on the site of involvement and may be absent, slight, or severe. Function may be impaired by the active granulomatous disease or by secondary fibrosis. Fever, weight loss, and arthralgias may be initial manifestations. Persistent fever is especially common with hepatic involvement. Peripheral lymphadenopathy is common and usually asymptomatic. Even insignificant nodes may contain granulomas.

Mediastinal adenopathy often is discovered by routine chest x-ray. X-ray findings of bilateral hilar and right paratracheal adenopathy are virtually pathognomonic; adenopathy occasionally is unilateral. **Diffuse pulmonary infiltration** may accompany or follow the adenopathy; this infiltration may have a diffuse fine ground-glass appearance on x-ray, may occur as reticular or miliary lesions, or may be present as confluent infiltrations or large nodules that resemble metastatic tumors. Pulmonary involvement, which may also occur without visible adenopathy, is usually accompanied by cough and dyspnea, but these symptoms may be minimal or absent. Pulmonary fibrosis, cystic changes, and cor pulmonale are end results of progressive disease.

Skin lesions (plaques, papules, and subcutaneous nodules) frequently are present in patients with chronic sarcoidosis. Nasal and conjunctival mucosal granulomas may occur. **Erythema nodosum** with fever and arthralgias is a frequent mode of onset in Europe, but less common in the USA.

Hepatic granulomas are found in 70% of patients examined by percutaneous biopsy, even if patients are asymptomatic with normal liver function tests. Hepatomegaly is noted in $< 10\%$ of patients; progressive and severe hepatic dysfunction with jaundice is rare.

Granulomatous uveitis occurs in 15% of cases; it is usually bilateral, and may cause severe loss of vision from secondary glaucoma if untreated. Retinal periphlebitis, lacrimal gland enlargement, conjunctival infiltrations, and keratitis sicca occasionally are present. **Myocardial involvement** rarely causes angina, congestive failure, or fatal conduction abnormalities. Acute **polyarthritis** may be prominent; chronic periarticular swelling and tenderness may be associated with osseous changes in the phalanges. **CNS involvement** is of almost any type, but cranial nerve palsies (especially facial paralysis)

are most common. **Diabetes insipidus** may occur. **Hypercalcemia** and **hypercalciuria** (the result of 1,25-dihydroxyvitamin D production by alveolar macrophages and sarcoid granulomas) may cause renal calculi or nephrocalcinosis with consequent renal failure, but prednisone therapy has reduced the frequency and importance of disordered calcium metabolism.

Laboratory Findings

Leukopenia frequently is present. Hypergammaglobulinemia is common among blacks. Elevated serum uric acid is not uncommon, but gout is rare. Serum alkaline phosphatase may be elevated as a result of hepatic involvement. Depression of delayed hypersensitivity is characteristic, but a negative second-strength tuberculin reaction reliably excludes complicating TB.

Pulmonary function tests show restriction, decreased compliance, and impaired diffusing capacity. CO_2 retention is uncommon, since ventilation rarely is obstructed except in patients with endobronchial disease or in late stages with severe pulmonary fibrosis. Serial measurements of pulmonary function are a guide to treatment and to the course of the disease.

Diagnosis

A clinical diagnosis may be made in asymptomatic patients with typical chest x-ray findings, but the diagnosis must be considered in the presence of the symptoms and signs described above even if (as in about 10% of patients) the chest x-ray is normal. Tissue biopsy, with microbiologic as well as histologic examination, is essential if symptoms are present and corticosteroid therapy seems indicated. When superficial or palpable lesions (eg, in skin, lymph nodes, palpebral conjunctiva) are present, biopsy is positive in 87% of specimens.

When physical examination is negative, transbronchial biopsy by fiberoptic bronchoscope is the best initial procedure for securing histologic evidence of sarcoidosis. This technic has shown granulomas in 60 to 90% of patients, whether the chest x-ray reveals pulmonary infiltration or hilar adenopathy alone.

If this approach is not available or fails to show granulomas, other possible biopsy sites include the mediastinum, which can be approached by mediastinotomy or mediastinoscopy; the lungs, approached by intercostal biopsy; or random biopsies of skeletal muscle and conjunctiva. Liver biopsy shows granulomas in 70% of cases and can be useful. Scalene fat-pad biopsy is obsolete in view of the higher yields of other methods.

Local sarcoid reactions in a single organ and granulomas due to infection or hypersensitivity must be excluded. In questionable cases, histologic evidence of granulomas should be sought in more than one site. The Kveim reaction, a granulomatous reaction appearing 4 wk after intradermal injection of extracts of sarcoid spleen or lymph node, is positive in 50 to 60% of patients, but reliable antigens are not available in the USA.

Angiotensin converting enzyme **(ACE)** is elevated significantly in sera of patients with sarcoidosis, presumably reflecting macrophage activity. Tissue levels are highest in sarcoid lymph nodes rather than in pulmonary tissues. Elevations > 2 standard deviations occur in 60% of patients with sarcoidosis, but these elevations are also seen in patients with histoplasmosis, acute miliary TB, hyperthyroidism, lymphoma, etc; therefore, elevated ACE has limited diagnostic value, but may prove useful in following the course of sarcoidosis.

Newer methods that may be helpful in special situations in diagnosing sarcoidosis or assessing its activity include **bronchoalveolar lavage** and whole-body **gallium scans**. Alveolar washings show lymphocytosis in most patients with active sarcoidosis. Since patients with hypersensitivity pneumonitis show similar lymphocytosis, this procedure is rarely indicated for diagnostic purposes. Bronchoalveolar lavage has been advocated to determine need for corticosteroid therapy, but recent studies do not support this use

of the method. Gallium scanning, a sensitive but nonspecific indicator of sarcoidal inflammation, is unnecessary in typical recent cases of sarcoidosis. It is helpful in pointing to productive extrathoracic biopsy sites in patients with normal chest x-rays or atypical presentations. The gallium scan is also useful in longstanding cases of pulmonary sarcoidosis to determine whether radiologic densities represent reversible inflammation or fibrosis. Gallium uptake is extremely sensitive to corticosteroids; a negative test in patients taking even small doses of prednisone is unreliable.

TB still must be distinguished from sarcoidosis, but aspergillosis and cryptococcosis are now more frequent complications of sarcoidosis. Hodgkin's disease also must be excluded. It is uncertain whether the typical sarcoid granulomas found in 5% of liver biopsies done for staging of Hodgkin's disease indicate 2 concurrent diseases or a sarcoid reaction to the neoplasm.

Course and Prognosis

Evaluating treatment is difficult, since spontaneous improvement or clearing is common. Massive hilar adenopathy and extensive infiltrates may disappear in a few months or years. Mediastinal adenopathy persists without change for many years in a few cases. Radiologic recovery has been observed at the end of 5 yr in 82% of Swedish patients with hilar adenopathy alone and in 57% of patients with pulmonary opacities. Clinical recovery has been observed at the end of 9-yr observations in 85% of white patients and 65% of black patients with pulmonary sarcoidosis studied in Philadelphia. The prognostic importance of race and extrapulmonary sarcoidosis is shown by these observations on the likelihood of clinical recovery of patients with pulmonary sarcoidosis: white with no extrathoracic disease, 89.4%; white with extrathoracic disease, 69.7%; black, no extrathoracic disease, 76%; black with extrathoracic disease, 46.4%. The outlook is of course better for patients who have adenopathy without radiologic evidence of pulmonary disease. The most reliable indicator of a favorable outcome of sarcoidosis is onset with erythema nodosum.

Serious disability from ocular, respiratory, or other damage is common ($\cong$ 10%), but mortality from sarcoidosis is low (< 3%). Pulmonary fibrosis leading to cardiorespiratory failure is the most common cause of death; the next most common, pulmonary hemorrhage from aspergilloma.

Treatment

No available therapeutic agents have consistently prevented tissue damage and fibrosis of the lungs. Corticosteroids accelerate clearance of symptoms, physiologic disturbances, and roentgenographic changes; but after 5 yr little difference is demonstrable between treated and untreated patients. Asymptomatic hilar or peripheral adenopathy needs no treatment. Corticosteroid therapy should be given to suppress troublesome or disabling symptoms (eg, dyspnea, severe arthralgia, fever) and should be started promptly if active ocular disease, respiratory failure, hepatic insufficiency, cardiac arrhythmia, CNS involvement, or hypercalcemia is present.

Prednisone 40 to 60 mg/day orally may be given when a prompt effect is desired, but doses of 10 to 15 mg/day by mouth usually are adequate to control the inflammatory reaction. If doses > 15 mg/day are given, alternate-day schedules should be employed. Treatment may be needed for weeks, for years, or indefinitely. Maintenance doses of 5 to 10 mg/day are surprisingly effective in controlling symptoms and radiologic changes in many chronic cases. Clinical examination, x-rays, and pulmonary function studies should be made at 2- to 3-mo intervals when dosage is being reduced or medication terminated. Serious complications of corticosteroid therapy are infrequent with low-dose therapy in this disease. Concomitant isoniazid therapy, 300 mg/day for a year, is indicated only for the few patients given corticosteroids who have positive tuberculin skin tests.

Chlorambucil is sometimes effective and occasionally results in dramatic improvement. A trial of chlorambucil is indicated when corticosteroids fail or are contraindicated.

FAMILIAL MEDITERRANEAN FEVER (FMF)

(Familial Paroxysmal Polyserositis)

An inherited disorder of unknown etiology, characterized by recurrent episodes of fever, peritonitis, and pleuritis. Arthritis, skin lesions, and amyloidosis occur occasionally.

Etiology, Epidemiology, and Pathology

Etiology is unknown, but there are intriguing data that provide 2 clues: (1) A provocative infusion of metaraminol has been reported to induce mild, typical attacks in patients with known FMF. Furthermore, the drug-induced symptoms can be prevented with prophylactic colchicine therapy. These data suggest an abnormality in the metabolic pathway of catecholamines in FMF patients. (2) Other reports relate to C5a, a fragment of complement, which is the primary chemoattractant of neutrophils. The levels of C5a-inhibitor activity in peritoneal fluid of FMF patients have been found to be very low. This deficiency may play a role in the pathogenesis of attacks. No hypothesis to connect these 2 sets of data has been formulated.

FMF occurs primarily in Sephardic Jews, Arabs, Armenians, Turks, and others who originate in the Mediterranean basin and occurs rarely in individuals of Italian, Ashkenazi Jewish, and Anglo-Saxon ancestry. About 50% of patients give no family history of FMF. Consanguinity among the parents of FMF patients is as high; 60% of patients are male.

No specific pathologic changes are found. Laparotomy shows only an acute peritonitis characterized by polymorphonuclear leukocytosis. Some patients develop amyloidosis that involves primarily blood vessels. This major complication has been reported in Israel, North Africa, and elsewhere in the Middle East, but is rare in the USA.

Symptoms, Signs, and Clinical Course

FMF usually begins between ages 5 and 15, but sometimes at much later ages or during infancy. Attacks have no rhythm or periodicity and vary considerably in the same patient. Their duration is usually 24 to 48 h, but some last 7 to 10 days. Frequency ranges from 2/wk to 1/yr, but 2 to 4 wk is the most common interval. Severity and frequency may decrease with age or with development of amyloidosis. Spontaneous remissions may last years. Fever, ranging between 38.5 C (101.3 F) and 40 C (104 F), usually accompanied by serositis, is the major manifestation and is present during most attacks. Abdominal pain occurs in > 95% of patients, and also may vary in severity in the same patient. The pain usually starts in one quadrant, then spreads to the whole abdomen. Tenderness may remain localized, with referred pain in other areas; there may be radiation to the back. The abdomen is usually distended and may become rigid; bowel sounds may be decreased or absent. Because an acute abdominal attack can closely mimic a perforated viscus, patients are often operated on unnecessarily. With diaphragmatic involvement, there may be splinting of the chest and pain in one or both shoulders. Other symptoms include acute pleuritic pain (75%), acute arthritis involving the large joints (25%), and erythematous skin lesions (25%). Rarer symptoms include recurrent pericarditis, colloid bodies in the ocular fundus, migraine, and emotional lability.

Laboratory Findings

There is no specific diagnostic laboratory test. Polymorphonuclear leukocytosis, ranging from 15,000 to 30,000 cells/μL, is usual; during acute attacks, the ESR is elevated. Other laboratory tests are normal.

Prognosis, Prophylaxis, and Treatment

Despite the severity of the symptoms during acute attacks, most patients are remarkably free of illness between attacks. Widespread use of colchicine has dramatically reduced the incidence of amyloidosis. When it does occur, the prognosis is much poorer; eg, in the past, about 25% of FMF patients in Israel were known to have amyloidosis, and it was usually fatal.

Colchicine aborts attacks and reduces recurrence. Its mechanism of action is unknown; possibly it prevents normal cellular response to inflammation. For prophylaxis, the dosage is 0.6 mg orally tid, and is reduced to bid if GI side effects develop. For acute attacks, the dosage is 0.6 mg/h orally for 4 h, then q 2 h for 4 h, then q 12 h for 48 h. Narcotics should be *avoided*, since drug addiction or habituation is a possible and serious complication.

§2. IMMUNOLOGY; ALLERGIC DISORDERS

16. INTRODUCTION

The science of immunology began with an attempt to understand resistance to infection, which was initially thought to be the only function of the immune system. Its relationship to hypersensitivity (allergy) was recognized early in this century and led to elucidation of the general biologic functions of the immune system, including a role in

immunity to cancer, prevention of tissue transplantation from one individual to another, and the capability of *causing* diseases by injuring normal tissue.

These functions are accomplished in man by a complex immune system that has emerged through the phylogenetic scale, retaining elements of all the immune responses noted in other vertebrate species. When operating normally, several immunologic processes result in very precise functions: **recognition** and **memory of, specific response to,** and **clearance of, foreign substances** (chemical and cellular antigens) that either penetrate the protective body barriers of skin and mucosal surfaces (microorganisms, transplanted tissue) or arise de novo (malignant transformation). These processes depend on (1) the development of T and B cell lymphocytes; (2) clonal proliferation of immunologically committed T and B lymphocytes; (3) plasma cell differentiation and antibody production; (4) T cell differentiation into memory, helper, cytotoxic, and suppressor cells; (5) regulation of the immune system by an intricate network of interactions between subsets of immune system cells and the production of anti-idiotype antibodies; (6) macrophages and other antigen-presenting cells (eg, Langerhans cells of the skin) required for processing most antigens; (7) phagocytosis by polymorphonuclear leukocytes and by macrophages and other cells of the reticuloendothelial system; and (8) amplification or modulation of the immune response by lymphokines, the complement system, lysosomal enzymes, vasoactive amines, and kallikreins. These same protective processes may, under special circumstances, result in injury; the result is a hypersensitivity disorder or an autoimmune disease. When the immune system fails, the result may be an immunodeficiency disease or the growth of malignant cells.

---

17. BIOLOGY OF THE IMMUNE SYSTEM

The immune response in humans is both specific and nonspecific. The **specific** processes consist of **humoral** (antibody) and **cellular** or cell-mediated (delayed immunity) components, and are discussed in detail, below. Humoral processes involve the interactions between antigens and antibodies; cellular, the interactions between antigens and certain specialized (thymus-influenced) lymphocytes, which act both directly and through the elaboration of substances other than antibody. The humoral and cell-mediated processes are considered specific for 2 reasons: (1) The lymphocytes and antibodies recognize, remember, and respond to unique pattern configurations on the surfaces of antigens; and (2) each lymphocyte and each antibody responds only to one specific antigenic configuration.

The **nonspecific** mechanisms of the immune system, such as **phagocytosis** (see under ANTIGENS, below), **mast cell degranulation**, and **complement activation** (see THE COMPLEMENT SYSTEM, below), do not involve such pattern recognition. However, these nonspecific processes often act in concert with antibodies and lymphocytes in reactions against antigenic substances.

Current concepts have evolved from study of animal models and humans and are depicted in FIG. 17–1. A primitive stem cell originates in the yolk sac, migrates through the liver and spleen, and settles in the bone marrow. These stem cells are thought to be multipotential and to develop into precursors of the lymphoid, myeloid, erythroid, and megakaryocytoid series. There is evidence to suggest that the stem-cell–derived lymphoid cells in the bone marrow are already committed to become T and B cells, and are called pro-thymocytes and pro-B cells. The pro-thymocyte migrates to the thymus where it develops the characteristics of a T cell. The pro-B cell becomes a virgin B cell in the bone marrow and peripheral lymphoid tissue.

The early development of T cells in the thymus and B cells within the bone marrow and peripheral lymphoid tissue is not antigen-driven. The subsequent differentiation of

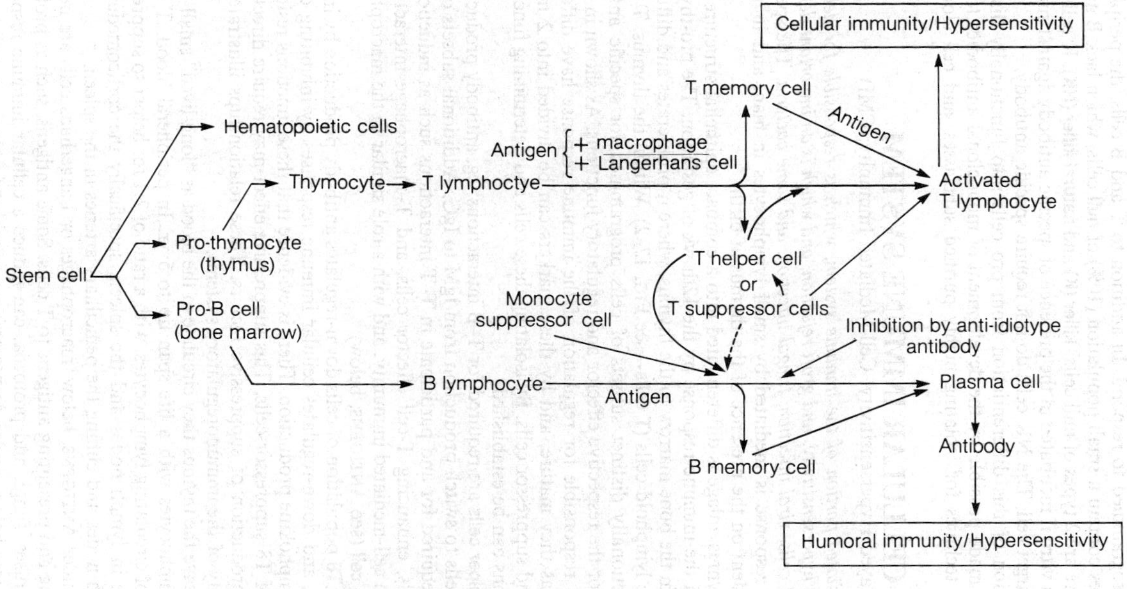

Fig. 17–1. Schematic outline of the immune system. Stem cell precursors become hematopoietic cells, pro-thymocytes, and pro-B cells. Pro-thymocytes migrate to the thymus and develop into T lymphocytes; pro-B cells become B lymphocytes, presumably in the bone marrow and peripheral lymphoid tissue. Contact with antigen induces lymphocytic differentiation; for this process, T cells require macrophage participation and most B cells require T helper cell participation. Both first and later contacts with antigen result in activated T cells or plasma cells, the mediators, respectively, of cellular and of humoral immunity and hypersensitivity.

B cells into memory and antibody-secreting cells, and T cells into helper (inducer), suppressor (cytotoxic), memory, and activated cells depends on antigen contact to which they are programmed to respond. In addition to T and B cells, the peripheral blood lymphocytes contain a small population (10%) of **null** cells, which lack B and T cell markers. There are 2 types of null cells: **killer (K)** and **natural killer (NK)**. K cells can lyse target cells in vitro if incubated in the presence of specific antibody against surface antigens of the target cell. The NK cells do not require specific antibody.

The identification of this differentiation from pro cells into functionally distinct subsets has been made possible by the development of monoclonal antibodies to cell surface markers, technics for isolating highly purified subclasses, and cell cloning.

CELLULAR IMMUNE SYSTEM

(Delayed Hypersensitivity; Cell-Mediated Immunity; CMI)

The T-cell–mediated portion of the immune system, which is responsible for delayed skin tests, delayed hypersensitivity, and graft rejection, and which is an important defense against malignant cells, viral infection, fungal infection, and some bacteria. The specific type of immune response is mediated by small lymphocytes in man, and in most animals is dependent on the presence of the thymus at birth.

In man, the thymus anlage is differentiated into a compact epithelial structure that can participate in the immune response by the 12th wk of gestation. The pro-thymocyte migrates from the bone marrow to the thymus, where it proliferates and differentiates into thymic lymphoid cells (**T cells**—see FIG. 17–2). Within the thymus, T cells diverge into functionally distinct subsets of cells programmed for specific antigen recognition and for the respective effector and regulatory functions. As shown in FIG. 17–2, the T cells responsible for regulation of the immune response have different surface antigens as they mature, and by these markers can be divided into 2 major subsets: helper and suppressor cells. By isolating these cells and determining function, further subdivisions can be established.

Different **T4 helper cells** are required for T–B interactions; eg, antibody production, and inducing B cells to switch production from IgM to IgG. Additional subsets of T4 helper cells are required for and participate in T–T interactions such as induction of suppressor T cells, enhancing T-cell effector cells, and T–macrophage interactions. Also important in cell-mediated immunity, and with a role similar to the macrophage, is the **Langerhans cell** (see ANTIGENS, below).

The **suppressor T8** population of cells down-regulates antibody production by inhibiting helper cells, and down-regulates cellular immune responses by inhibiting cytotoxic cells and lymphokine production. There is evidence that these functions reside in specific subsets of T8 suppressor cells. This suppressive effect may require direct cell contact and/or production of suppressive factors. These relationships illustrate the marked complexity of the immunoregulatory systems.

When T cells leave the thymus they circulate in the blood as "long-lived" small- and medium-sized lymphocytes with a life span up to 5 yr. In peripheral blood, T cells comprise > 70% of circulating lymphocytes, with a ratio of 2:1 for helper to suppressor cells. Some settle in lymph nodes and the spleen, specifically the corticomedullary junction of lymph nodes and cuffing the penicilliary arteries in the spleen.

As discussed under ANTIGENS, below, macrophages or Langerhans cells are necessary for processing and presenting antigens to T cells. Some antigens, such as proteins from bacteria, viruses, fungi, and protozoa, can induce a cellular immune response directly. **Haptens** (see below, under ANTIGENS) are capable of inducing a cellular immune response only after combining with carrier proteins such as tissue protein. The major histocompatibility complex (MHC) is a chromosomal region consisting of a series of genes that code for the cell surface expression of strong transplantation antigens and where the immune response (Ir) genes are located. In mice the Ia and in

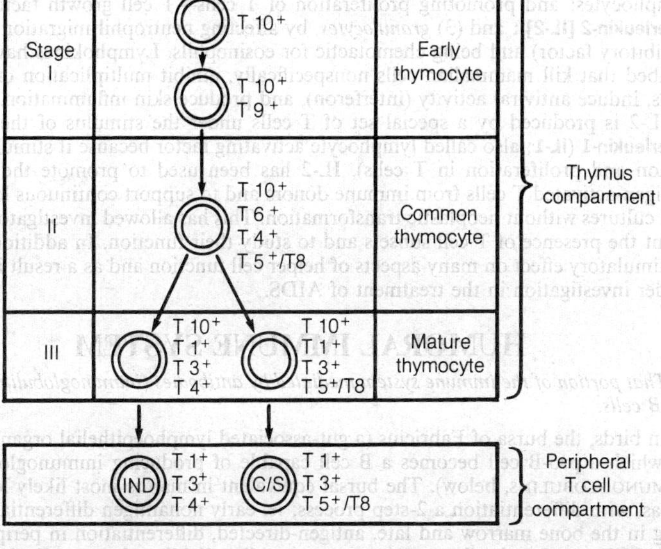

FIG. 17–2. Ontogeny of T cells with respect to markers determined by monoclonal antibodies and compartment.
IND = Inducter T cell
C/S = Cytotoxic/Suppressor T cell
(Modified from "Current Concepts in Immunology" by E. L. Reinherz and S. F. Schlossman, in *The New England Journal of Medicine* Vol. 303, No. 7, p. 371, August 14, 1980. Used with permission of *The New England Journal of Medicine* and the author.)

man the D antigens on cell surfaces are class II antigens and serve as the recognition markers that allow cell cooperation to occur for antigen processing. **On initial contact with antigen**, the T cell undergoes clonal proliferation and differentiates into sensitized lymphocytes or **committed** T cells with various functions. Some cells become **activated** and are responsible for mediating cellular immunity or resulting in injury to host tissue (hypersensitivity reactions). Others become T **memory cells,** thereby increasing the number of cells with the ability to react to specific antigen. Still others become **helper** or **suppressor cells**, regulating B cell production of antibody by concentrating antigen on B cell surfaces or releasing a local humoral factor responsible for stimulating B cells to produce antibody. Autoimmune diseases and some immunodeficiency disorders may be due to defects of suppressor T cells: autoimmune diseases representing decreased suppressor activity; immunodeficiency disorders, excessive suppressor activity. In AIDS, there is a decrease in helper cell numbers and function. If the immunogen (*a substance capable of inducing an immune response*) is a major histocompatibility antigen, then **killer cells** that are **cytotoxic T cells** for target cells bearing the antigen are generated.

The activated T lymphocyte mediates cellular immunity by a direct toxic effect, reacting directly with cell-membrane–associated antigens, or by releasing various soluble factors called **lymphokines.** Lymphokines (*the chemical mediators of cellular immunity*) affect (1) *macrophages*, by inhibiting macrophage migration inhibitory factor and causing aggregation; attracting monocytes; and causing fusion of macrophages so as to

form giant cells; (2) *lymphocytes*, by amplifying lymphokine production; promoting antibody production; suppressing T and B cell functions; attracting uncommitted lymphocytes; and promoting proliferation of T cells—T cell growth factor (TCGF; **interleukin-2 [IL-2]**); and (3) *granulocytes*, by affecting neutrophil migration (leukocyte inhibitory factor) and being chemotactic for eosinophils. Lymphokines have been described that kill mammalian cells nonspecifically, inhibit multiplication of lymphoid cells, induce antiviral activity (interferon), and produce skin inflammation.

IL-2 is produced by a special set of T cells under the stimulus of the monokine **interleukin-1** (**IL-1**; also called lymphocyte activating factor because it stimulates maturation and proliferation in T cells). IL-2 has been used to promote the growth of antigen-activated T cells from immune donors and to support continuous long-term T cell cultures without neoplastic transformation. This has allowed investigators to document the presence of T cell subsets and to study their function. In addition, IL-2 has a stimulatory effect on many aspects of helper cell function and as a result is presently under investigation in the treatment of AIDS.

HUMORAL IMMUNE SYSTEM

That portion of the immune system mediated by antibodies (immunoglobulins) produced by B cells.

In birds, the bursa of Fabricius (a gut-associated lymphoepithelial organ) is the site at which a pro-B cell becomes a B cell capable of producing immunoglobulins (see IMMUNOGLOBULINS, below). The bursal equivalent in man is most likely located in 2 areas, with differentiation a 2-step process; ie, early nonantigen differentiation occurring in the bone marrow and late, antigen-directed, differentiation in peripheral lymphoid tissue. In the bone marrow a rapidly dividing large cell type (pro-B) differentiates into a slowly dividing small cell type with a small amount of cytoplasmic, but no surface, immunoglobulin. Further differentiation into cells containing surface immunoglobulin M (IgM—see IMMUNOGLOBULINS, below) occurs in the bone marrow. The B cell leaves the bone marrow and in peripheral lymphoid tissue becomes a mature immunocompetent cell carrying both surface IgM and IgD. On encountering antigen, the B cell differentiates into either a memory or a plasma cell. This differentiation occurs by 2 mechanisms, one independent and the other dependent on T helper cells.

The characteristics of **T-independent antigens** are that they be high mol wt with linearly arranged repeating antigenic determinants or highly resistant to degradation by body enzymes. Examples are pneumococcal polysaccharides, *Escherichia coli* lipopolysaccharides, and polyvinyl pyrrolidine. The antibody response of the T-independent antigen is limited to IgM production.

Most natural antigens are T-cell–dependent and require macrophage cooperation to stimulate antibody production. Present evidence indicates that the T cell recognizes a different portion of the antigen (carrier determinant) than the B cell. During antigen stimulation of the B cells, a switch from IgM to IgG production occurs. This switch is T-helper-cell–dependent and may require different subsets of T helper cells. In addition, other switches that occur are IgM to IgA, and IgM to IgE. The role of IgD on cell surfaces has not been determined. IgD is found on a great majority of all B lymphocytes in adult animals (man included), as well as shortly after birth. Since IgD is found only in very low amounts in serum, it may be that its principal role is as a membrane receptor.

B cells, which comprise 30% of blood lymphocytes, are both short-lived (life span of 15 days) and long-lived (months to years), and are morphologically indistinguishable from T cells. **Technics distinguishing B cells** from T cells detect surface markers: (1) Immunoglobulins of the major classes can be detected on the surface with fluorescein-labeled anti-immunoglobulin (immunofluorescent technic). The largest proportion of

cells, however, bears surface IgD and IgM. (2) Receptors for the 3rd component of complement (C3 receptors) can be detected by the adherence of complement-coated RBCs to the surface of B cells, forming "rosettes." (3) Receptors for the Fc fraction of immunoglobulins (see IMMUNOGLOBULINS, below) can be detected by adherence of antigen-antibody complexes, aggregated γ-globulin to B cells, or antibody-coated sheep RBCs. B cells also can be evaluated by **histologic examination**: In the lymph node they make up the outer cortical area containing germinal centers and medullary cord; in the spleen they compose the germinal follicles and perifollicular areas.

The B cells in peripheral tissues are precommitted to respond to a limited number of antigens. The first interaction between antigen and B cells is known as the **primary immune response,** and the B cells committed to respond to this antigen undergo differentiation and clonal proliferation. Some of these become **memory cells** and others differentiate into mature antibody-synthesizing **plasma cells**. The principal characteristics of the primary immune response are a latent period before the appearance of antibody, the production of only a small amount of antibody, chiefly IgM, and, most importantly, the creation of a large number of memory cells that are capable of responding to the same antigen in the future.

The **secondary (anamnestic** or **booster) immune response** takes place on subsequent encounters with the same antigen. The principal characteristics are a rapid proliferation of B cells, a rapid differentiation into mature plasma cells, and the prompt production of large quantities of antibody. This antibody, which is chiefly of the IgG class, is released into the blood and other body tissues where it can effectively encounter and react with the antigen.

ANTIGENS

Substances capable of combining with antibody and of eliciting specific immune responses, either humoral or cell-mediated.

Antigen Structure and Antigenicity

Antibodies combine with antigens by matching combining sites on the 2 molecules, which fit together much like the pieces of a jigsaw puzzle. The antigenic combining sites that are recognized by antibody molecules are specific configurations (**epitopes** or **antigenic determinants**) present on the surfaces of large high-mol-wt molecules such as proteins, polysaccharides, and nucleic acids. The presence of at least one such epitope makes a molecule an antigen.

In fact, 2 essentials are required for a substance to be antigenic (immunogenic): (1) The sum of the antigenic determinants on the antigen's surface must make up a configuration that differs from configurations recognized by the immune system as "self." (2) The substance must be of sufficient mol wt (about 10,000 minimum). Plausibly, the larger the molecule, the more room on its surface for antigenic determinants; and the greater the number of "foreign"-looking antigenic determinants present on its surface, the greater will be its antigenicity.

A **hapten** is *a substance of lower mol wt than an antigen, which can* react *specifically with antibody but which is unable to* induce *antibody formation unless attached to another molecule,* usually a protein (the **carrier protein**). Examples of haptens are the allergenic substances in penicillin and numerous other drugs.

The combining sites of antibody and the antigen to which it is committed fit avidly together, with a strong force of attraction, because the matching areas on the surface of each molecule are relatively large. The same antibody molecule also can combine **(cross-react)** with related antigens if their surface determinants are similar enough to the determinants on the homologous (original) antigen. However, the antigen-antibody binding in such cross-reactions is weaker because smaller surface areas are in close contact, because of the differences in configuration between the immunizing antigen and the cross-reacting antigen.

The processing of an antigen by initial phagocytosis appears to be important to its antigenicity, although the role of the **macrophage** in the initial recognition of a substance as antigen is unclear. The lymph nodes and spleen are rich in phagocytic cells as well as in lymphocytes. When antigen first enters the body it is trapped and largely metabolized by these phagocytes. A small proportion of the antigen, localized on the surface of the macrophage, comes into contact with nearby T cells. These T cells will participate either in the production of cellular immunity or the production of humoral antibody by T-dependent B cells. T-cell–independent antigens do not require macrophages to stimulate antibody production (see HUMORAL IMMUNE SYSTEM, above). This processing of antigen appears to be most important in the primary immune response. In the secondary immune response, antigen interacts with antibody fixed to the surface of dendritic macrophages of cortical lymphoid follicles, and is presented to T cells.

Langerhans cells (dendritic skin cells) play a role similar to macrophages in the production of cell-mediated immunity. Langerhans cells process antigen for initiation of contact allergy and skin graft rejection. Although bone-marrow–derived, they have features distinguishing them from macrophages (eg, inability to produce interleukin-1 **[IL-1]**). In the skin, IL-1 is produced by the keratinocytes. The skin therefore should be considered immunologically active, serving as the most peripheral limb of the immune system.

IMMUNOGLOBULINS (Igs)
(Antibodies)

***Ig**: A protein produced by plasma cells, usually having antibody activity. **Antibody**: An Ig molecule with a specific amino acid sequence and tertiary surface configuration that enable it to react specifically with a matching site on the surface of a homologous antigen.*

Antibodies offer humoral protection against viruses and bacterial pathogens such as pneumococci, *Hemophilus influenzae*, streptococci, and staphylococci. IgM is the predominant antibody in the primary immune response; IgG, in the secondary immune response. Other special biologic properties of the different Ig classes are described below.

Ig Structure

Igs are remarkably heterogeneous but have a number of common properties. The γ-globulin fraction of serum is rich in antibody activity, but other globulin fractions also contain antibody.

The molecular subunits of Igs all have a similar structure: Each is composed of 4 polypeptide chains—2 identical **heavy chains** and 2 identical **light chains** (so called because of their relative mol wt)—joined into a Y shape by disulfide bonds. There are 5 major types of heavy chains, which give their name to the **5 major Ig classes** in man: IgM, IgG, IgA, IgD, and IgE (see TABLE 17–1). There are 2 types of light chains, called κ and λ; a single molecule has only 1 type of light chain, but molecules of both types are found in all 5 of the major classes. Thus, there are 10 different types of Ig molecules. IgG, IgD, and IgE each are monomers; ie, made up of 1 molecule (2 heavy and 2 light chains). IgM is a polymer of 5 units or monomers (10 heavy chains, 10 light chains), while IgA occurs in 3 forms—as a monomer and as polymers of 2 and 3 monomers.

Additional chains have been identified. **Joining (J)** chains link the 5 subunits of IgM and the 2 or 3 subunits of IgA; and secretory IgA has an additional polypeptide chain, **secretory component** (**SC**, secretory piece, transport piece), which is produced in epithelial cells and added to the IgA molecule.

Antibody Structure and Specificity

The Y-shaped Ig molecule is divided into **variable regions**, located at the distal ends of the Y arms, in which the amino acid sequence differs for the various antibody

TABLE 17–1. CHARACTERISTICS OF THE IMMUNOGLOBULINS

Immunoglobulin Class	Heavy Chains	Light Chains	Additional Chains	No. of Basic Molecules	Subclasses	Molecular Weight	Sedimentation Coefficient	Mean Survival $T^{1/2}$ (days)	Mean Serum Conc. (Adult; mg/dL)	Biologic Properties
IgM	μ	κ, λ	J	5	IgM_1, IgM_2	900,000	19S	1	45–150	Appears early in immune response; efficient agglutinator & opsonizer; fixes complement; major antibody for polysaccharides, gram-neg. bacteria
IgG	γ	κ, λ		1	IgG_1, IgG_2, IgG_3, IgG_4	150,000	7S	23	720–1500	Most abundant; found esp. in extravascular fluids; crosses placenta; subclasses 1, 2, & 3 fix complement (1 & 3 > 2); major antibody for antitoxins, viruses, bacteria
IgA	α	κ, λ	J, SC	1–3	IgA_1, IgA_2	170,000	7–15S	6	90–325	Major immunoglobulin in seromucous secretions at body surfaces
IgD	δ	κ, λ		1		180,000	7S	3	3	Not yet identified
IgE	ε	κ, λ		1		200,000	8S	2	0.03	Found in seromucous secretions; levels increased in parasitic infections; mediator of atopic allergies

J = joining chain; SC = secretory component.

molecules; and a **constant region** (proximal to the antigen-combining site), where the amino acid sequence is relatively constant for each Ig class. Electron microscopy has shown that the variable regions hold the concave **combining sites (antigen-binding sites)** of the antibody molecules. The sites also are called the hypervariable regions and contain the idiotype determinants to which **anti-idiotype antibodies** (see below under REGULATION OF CELLULAR AND HUMORAL IMMUNE RESPONSES) have been demonstrated. The great variety of possible amino acid sequences in the variable regions confers **specificity** on the antibodies, since each clone of B cells can produce its own specific amino acid sequence, and thus its own antibody configuration that is specific for a particular antigen.

The structure-function relationships of the antibody molecule were originally studied by fragmentation with proteolytic enzymes. Papain splits the molecule into 2 univalent fragments designated **Fab** (antigen-binding), which contain the variable regions and thus the combining sites, and one fragment designated **Fc** (crystallizable), which contains most of the constant region. Pepsin produces a fragment designated **$F(ab')_2$**, which retains divalent antibody activity.

Both B and T cells are capable of recognizing and responding to antigen. B cells possess small amounts of Ig bound to the cell surface, and it is assumed that these serve as specific receptors for antigen in the initiation of an immune response. The nature of the T cell receptor which binds antigen is controversial. The reputed receptor has been isolated and has amino acid sequences similar to the variable region of Igs. The receptor, however, appears to be under different genetic control than Igs and although there is 30 to 60% homology, it appears to be a different protein. In addition, there are other receptors that do not participate in antigen binding. Precursor T cells contain other receptors for the Fc fragments of Igs. Helper cells possess IgM–Fc segment receptors; suppressor cells possess IgG–Fc segment receptors; and other T cells contain receptors for the Fc segment of IgA and IgE. The role these receptors and cell surface major histocompatibility antigens play in initiating the immune response remains unknown.

Antibodies of the IgM, IgG, and IgA classes all are capable of responding to the same antigen. One hypothesis to explain this assumes that the B cells derived from a single pro-B cell may differentiate (during the process of B cell maturation described above) into a family of B cells genetically programmed to synthesize antibodies of a single antigenic specificity, while having representative cells committed to the production of each Ig class. The cells undergoing this differentiation from IgM- to IgG- to IgA-producing cells are not yet plasma cells—the development of B cells is independent of antigenic stimulation, but differentiation into plasma cells capable of synthesizing goodly amounts of antibody does require antigenic stimulation.

By use of the ultracentrifuge, sedimentation coefficients can be determined for each Ig protein. IgM has the highest sedimentation coefficient—19S; IgG is 7S. In addition to these broad classes, Ig subclasses now are recognized, termed $IgG_{1,2,3,4}$; $IgA_{1,2}$; and $IgM_{1,2}$. These distinctions may be important, since specific biologic functions are beginning to be associated with various subclasses; eg, IgG_4 does not fix complement or bind to monocytes, whereas the other 3 IgG subclasses do; IgG_3 has a half-life significantly shorter than the other 3.

Biologic Properties of Antibodies

The amino acid structure in the constant region of the heavy chain in the antibody molecule appears to determine certain biologic properties of Igs. Each Ig class has its own characteristics.

IgG, the most prevalent type of serum Ig, diffuses readily into the extravascular spaces, and is the only Ig that crosses the placenta. As the prime mediator of the secondary immune response, IgG provides the body's chief serologic defenses against bacteria, viruses, and toxins. Different subclasses of IgG neutralize bacterial toxins, fix

complement, and enhance phagocytosis by opsonization. Commercial γ-globulin is almost entirely IgG but does contain small amounts of other Igs. IgG also can inhibit other antigen-antibody interactions, and one suggested mechanism for desensitization in atopic allergies is the development of **blocking IgG antibodies,** which prevent IgE-antigen interactions.

IgM (macroglobulin) largely is confined to the bloodstream. It is the earliest Ig to appear after antigenic challenge. The large IgM molecules also fix complement and are active opsonizers, agglutinators, and cytolytics that assist the reticuloendothelial system in eliminating many kinds of microorganisms. Most antibodies to gram-negative organisms are IgM globulins.

IgA (secretory antibody) is found in the seromucous secretions of body tracts exposed to the external environment (saliva, tears, respiratory and GI tract secretions, colostrum), where IgA provides an early antibacterial and antiviral defense. Secretory IgA is synthesized in the subepithelial regions of the GI and respiratory tracts and is present in combination with locally produced secretory component **(SC)**. Few IgA-producing cells are noted in the lymph node and spleen. Most of serum IgA appears to be derived from secretory IgA, and when this is so, both should have the same antibody specificities despite structural differences between the 2 forms, serum IgA not containing SC. Serum IgA contains antibodies against brucella, diphtheria, and poliomyelitis. In order to improve mucosal IgA production, vaccines are being developed that will immunize by the mucosal route, eg, influenza vaccine.

IgD: The biologic activity is not yet known. IgD is present in serum in extremely small amounts, but is prominent on B lymphocytes. IgD's role may be that of cell-bound antigen receptor involved in triggering antibody synthesis.

IgE (reaginic, skin-sensitizing, or **anaphylactic antibody),** like IgA, is secreted chiefly in the respiratory and GI subepithelium. IgE is elevated in atopic diseases (eg, allergic asthma, hay fever, and atopic dermatitis), parasitic diseases, far-advanced Hodgkin's disease, and E-monoclonal myeloma. A beneficial role for IgE is not established, though it may be active against parasitic and respiratory infections.

Immunoglobulin Serum Assays

IgG, IgM, and IgA are present in serum in reasonably high concentrations and therefore the amounts of each can be determined by the size of precipitin rings that form in gels containing specific antibody to each. Many laboratories are now using a **nephelometer** to quantitate specific protein concentrations of many serum proteins, including Igs. It determines protein concentration, using the principle of molecular light scatter. The technic is based on the concept that antiserum to the protein to be measured will form immune complexes. These scatter an incident beam of light, and the amount of light scatter is proportional to the concentration of the antigen. **Immunoelectrophoresis** qualitatively identifies the Igs. **Electroimmunodiffusion** is more rapid and more specific, and can be quantitative. IgE is present in serum in minute quantities and may be measured by **radioimmunoassay**. A simplified modification, paper radioimmunosorbent test (PRIST), is used by most laboratories.

Monoclonal Antibodies

The heterogeneous nature of antibodies produced in animals and the contamination of such antibodies with animal serum proteins have until recently handicapped immunologists in their efforts to prepare both diagnostic antibodies and those to be used as probes in research. (For example, the specificity of the antinuclear antibody test depends in part on the antibody to human γ-globulin produced in animals. Since the strength of the diagnostic reagent may vary, titers of positive reactions will differ among laboratories and even among preparations in the same laboratory. Test differences also may occur because of different antigens these antibodies are detecting.)

Since all immunologic tests utilizing antibody, such as radioimmunoassays and nephelometry, depend on antibodies to the target material (eg, insulin), universal use of antibodies of the same specificity and strength clearly is advantageous.

The **hybridoma technic** (the procedure by which 2 cells are fused [hybrid], one an antibody-producing cell, the other a myeloma cell) now permits preparation of a continuous supply of antibody produced by a single B cell **(monoclonal antibody)**. This antibody is produced by immunizing a mouse with an antigen such as a cell preparation from a human thymus. The spleen is removed from the immunized mouse and a suspension of cells prepared. Cell fusion is then carried out with mouse myeloma cells that are in perpetual tissue culture and are not producing antibody. From this suspension of cells, individual fused cells can be isolated that are producing monoclonal antibodies. This single cell will then multiply, thereby resulting in a tissue culture preparation producing large amounts of antibody. If larger amounts of antibody are required, the cells can be injected into the peritoneum of a mouse, and extremely high concentrations of antibody obtained from the ascitic fluid. With this technic, portions of the cells can be deep-frozen, protecting against accidental losses.

Since this technology has been available, its **applications**, beyond its importance as a research tool, have included (1) routine serology to measure serum levels of proteins and drugs; (2) tissue and blood typing; (3) diagnosis of infectious agents; (4) identification of lymphocyte subsets and their appearance or disappearance during the course of a disease; (5) classification and treatment of leukemias and lymphomas; (6) identification of tumor antigens; and (7) identification of autoimmune antibody idiotypes in diabetes, myasthenia gravis, and rheumatic diseases. Future applications being considered are for passive immunization against infectious agents, removal of toxic serum levels of drugs, manipulation of the immune response, and delivery of cytoxic agents to malignant cells.

REGULATION OF CELLULAR AND HUMORAL IMMUNE RESPONSES

Immune responses vary qualitatively and quantitatively. The qualitative variation depends on the presence of immune response **(Ir)** genes, while quantitative variations have a genetic as well as a physiologic basis. The genetic control occurs with T and B cells as well as macrophage presentation of antigens to T cells. Genetic factors are therefore the most important in determining whether one will or will not respond to an antigen.

A more important question to resolve because of its therapeutic implications is the mechanism by which the Ir regulates itself so as to produce sufficient activated T cells and antibody for protection but limits the response so as not to result in unlimited production and self-destruction. Quantitative control occurs by a number of mechanisms.

Suppression by T cells: Suppressor T cells' development is stimulated by proliferating helper cells which are then suppressed, thus exerting a negative feedback. Suppressor T cells are preferentially produced in macrophage-poor areas such as occurs in Peyer's patches when antigen is given orally to animals. Suppressor T cells have 2 populations: One suppresses all thymus-dependent antibody production; the other suppresses the antibody production to specific antigens. The extent to which suppressor T cells act directly on B cells is controversial; the major effect of T cell suppression is felt to be on T helper cells.

Suppression by antibodies: Antibody of the IgG class can specifically suppress antibody, particularly IgM production. This inhibition occurs in the fetus and newborns by maternal antibodies and has been utilized to prevent Rh disease in the newborn by passive administration of IgG anti-Rh (anti-D) antibodies to the mother. Antibodies

also are formed to idiotypic (antigenic) determinants at certain portions (idiotopes) of the antigen-binding sites (variable regions) of antibody molecules: **anti-idiotype antibodies.** This phenomenon occurs because the variable portion of each antibody molecule is unique to the antibody produced by a given clone of cells. The process can be continuous; ie, anti-idiotype antibodies can themselves have idiotopes that will in turn be recognized by other anti-idiotype antibodies, etc. Anti-idiotype antibodies can suppress the production of their idiotypic antibodies by blocking receptors on B and T cells. The extent to which such regulation normally occurs is speculative but these anti-idiotypic antibodies have been used as therapeutic agents in B cell lymphomas and are being considered in the use of autoimmune diseases (eg, idiopathic thrombocytopenic purpura and myasthenia gravis) to kill antibody-producing cells with idiotype-specific markers on their surfaces.

Suppression by macrophages: The impaired immunoglobulin production observed in multiple myeloma has been demonstrated to be due in part to the presence of a monocyte or macrophage that prevents the maturation of normal B cells into immunoglobulin-secreting cells.

Production of Humoral and Cellular Immunity

Immunity can be active or passive. In **active immunization,** antibody production or cell-mediated immunity is stimulated by administration of antigen or by exposure to naturally occurring antigens such as bacteria, viruses, or fungi. In **passive humoral immunization,** pre-formed antibodies actively produced in another person or animal are given to the recipient in the form of serum or γ-globulin. The protection offered by humoral antibody may be direct, such as toxin or viral neutralization by serum IgG, or viral neutralization by secretory IgA, or may depend upon activation of the complement system.

Delayed sensitivity can be passively transferred from one individual to another with an extract prepared from immune lymphocytes **(transfer factor).** A successful transfer is demonstrated when the recipient is converted from skin-test–negative to skin-test–positive. The conversion only applies to those antigens to which the donor has a positive delayed skin test.

Measurement of Cellular and Humoral Immunity

A number of in vivo and in vitro technics are available to evaluate the presence and functional competence of T and B cells. Since these procedures often are used in the evaluation of suspected immunodeficiency disorders, they are discussed in Ch. 18. The cell-mediated phenomenon of delayed hypersensitivity is discussed in Ch. 20. See also Immunoglobulin Serum Assays, above.

The **complement fixation (CF) test** is most commonly used in the diagnosis of viral diseases by detecting the presence of specific antibody to viruses in a patient's serum. The serum is first heated to destroy its own complement activity. Subsequently, antigen (such as a virus particle) and a known amount of complement are added to the mixture. The presence of antigen and antibody in the mixture will utilize complement, thus reducing its activity. Any remaining free complement is detected by adding antibody-sensitized RBCs, which will undergo lysis in the presence of free complement. The absence of hemolysis indicates that the antigen-antibody complex has fixed all the available complement.

THE COMPLEMENT SYSTEM

The process by which antibody, combining with antigen, initiates activity of the > 18 distinct plasma proteins known as complement, through 2 pathways: ***classic*** *and* ***alternative***. These proteins react sequentially and mediate a number of biologically significant consequences. Phenomena that have been described in vitro include **immune adherence**

(adherence of antigen-antibody complexes or antibody-coated bacteria to macrophages or RBCs); **production of anaphylatoxin** (proteins that cause release of histamine from mast cells or basophils); **chemotaxis** (causing the migration of cells toward the area where complement activity is present); **phagocytosis; lysis of cells** (RBCs, nucleated cells, and many bacteria); **clearance of immune complexes**; and **modulation of the immune response** (the fragment C3a suppresses, and C5a enhances, antibody production).

The classical pathway of activation: For historic reasons the first 4 components are numbered out of order as C1, C4, C2, and C3; but the remaining 5 classical components are numbered sequentially C5 through C9. The first component of human complement is composed of 3 distinct protein molecules called C1q, C1r, and C1s, which bind together to form a macromolecule known as C1. The first stage of activation of the classical complement cascade begins when C1q recognizes antibodies and binds to them. This binding leads to activation of C1r and then C1s, which continues the complement cascade by reacting with C4. In general the activation of the components of the complement system involves enzymatic cleavage of each component into 2 fragments, the larger of which joins the preceding activated component to generate a new enzymatic activity capable of cleaving the next component.

The classical pathway of complement activation (see FIG. 17-3) begins when C1q comes in contact in vivo with antigen-antibody complexes or, in vitro, with IgM or aggregated IgG. If the antigen is a virus, viral neutralization may occur in the course of activation when the first 2 components of complement (C1 and C4) have been activated. This may be an important defense mechanism during the early phases of a viral infection when limited amounts of antibody are present.

In guinea pigs when C2 is activated, a kinin-like factor (distinct from bradykinin) is generated which no longer is believed to be the edema-producing factor in hereditary angioedema. Bradykinin, generated independently of complement activation, is now felt to be the active factor in hereditary angioedema during the active phase of the disease. In activating C3, C3a and C3b are produced. When the antigen is on a membrane, C3b may attach to the membrane receptor separate from the site of attachment of C142. The particle may then be phagocytosed. The fragment C3a also is called anaphylatoxin and is capable of releasing histamine from mast cells. C5a, which has anaphylatoxin and chemotactic properties, is generated when C5 is cleaved (not just bound). Subsequently, when C6 and C7 are activated a trimolecular complex, C567, is formed; it either fixes on the cell membrane or remains in solution and is chemotactic for leukocytes, macrophages, and probably eosinophils. When RBCs, bacteria, or nucleated target cells in tissue culture have reacted with complement components from 1 through 8, slow or partial lysis occurs. When all 9 components of complement have reacted, rapid lysis of cells occurs. Lysis depends on the membrane attack complex (C5 to C9).

An **alternative pathway** (see FIG. 17-4) for the activation of the terminal complement components from C3 to Cq also has been described. It can be activated without the requirement for antibody by the cell walls of some bacteria, viruses, tumor cells, and parasites. For this reason, it is felt to serve as one of the first mechanisms for host defense. There are 6 proteins necessary for activation of the alternative pathway: C3, Factor B, Factor D, Factor H, Factor I (C3b-inactivator), and properdin. An unusual feature is the positive feedback through C3b. The C3b resulting from activation of either the classical or alternative pathway is capable of reacting with Factor B to form the C3b complex. This factor becomes cleaved by Factor D to form C3bBb (C3 convertase) and Ba. Properdin stabilizes the C3bBb complex and it in turn activates the alternative pathway. Factor H and Factor I are inhibitors of this pathway. It would appear that the alternative pathway is constantly activated at a low rate, making available C3b to attach to cell surfaces.

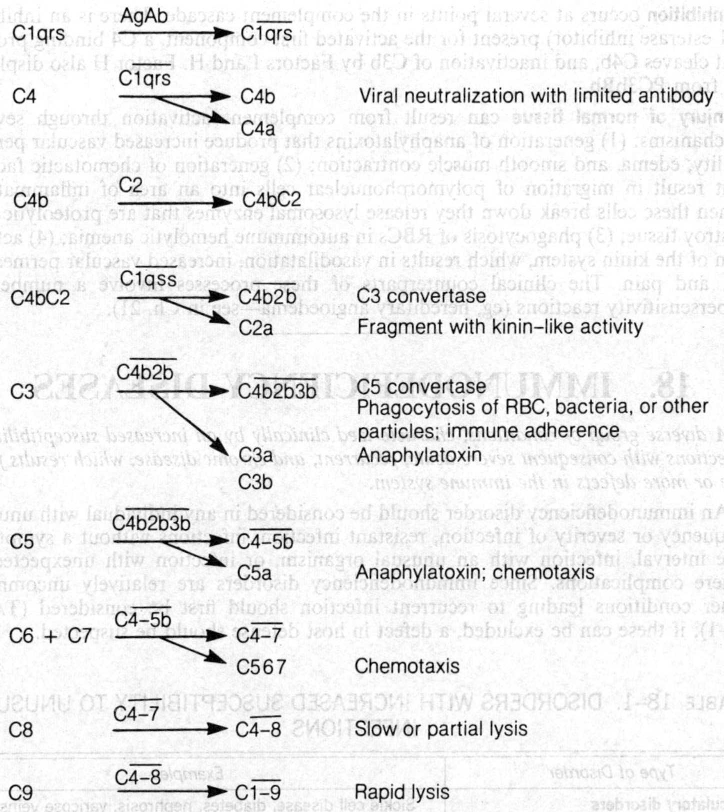

FIG. 17–3. Classical pathway of complement activation. A bar over the component indicates that the component has acquired enzymatic or other biologic activity.

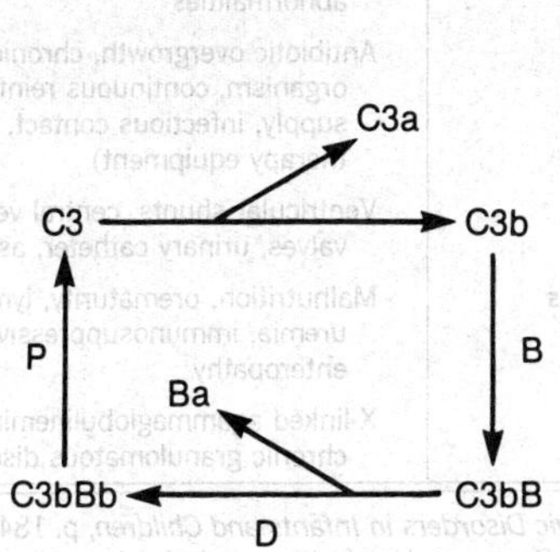

FIG. 17–4. Alternative pathway of complement activation.

Inhibition occurs at several points in the complement cascade. There is an inhibitor (C1 esterase inhibitor) present for the activated first component, a C4 binding protein that cleaves C4b, and inactivation of C3b by Factors I and H. Factor H also displaces Bb from PC3bBb.

Injury of normal tissue can result from complement activation through several mechanisms: (1) generation of anaphylatoxins that produce increased vascular permeability, edema, and smooth muscle contraction; (2) generation of chemotactic factors that result in migration of polymorphonuclear cells into an area of inflammation. When these cells break down they release lysosomal enzymes that are proteolytic and destroy tissue; (3) phagocytosis of RBCs in autoimmune hemolytic anemia; (4) activation of the kinin system, which results in vasodilatation, increased vascular permeability, and pain. The clinical counterparts of these processes involve a number of hypersensitivity reactions (eg, hereditary angioedema—see in Ch. 21).

18. IMMUNODEFICIENCY DISEASES

A diverse group of conditions, characterized clinically by an increased susceptibility to infections with consequent severe acute, recurrent, and chronic disease, which results from one or more defects in the immune system.

An immunodeficiency disorder should be considered in any individual with unusual frequency or severity of infection, resistant infection, infections without a symptom-free interval, infection with an unusual organism, or infection with unexpected or severe complications. Since immunodeficiency disorders are relatively uncommon, other conditions leading to recurrent infection should first be considered (Table 18–1); if these can be excluded, a defect in host defense should be suspected.

TABLE 18–1. DISORDERS WITH INCREASED SUSCEPTIBILITY TO UNUSUAL INFECTIONS

Type of Disorder	*Examples*
Circulatory disorders	Sickle cell disease, diabetes, nephrosis, varicose veins, congenital cardiac defects
Obstructive disorders	Ureteral or urethral stenosis, bronchial asthma, allergic rhinitis, blocked eustachian tubes, cystic fibrosis
Integumentary defects	Eczema, burns, skull fractures, midline sinus tracts, ciliary abnormalities
Unusual microbiologic factors	Antibiotic overgrowth, chronic infections with resistant organism, continuous reinfection (contaminated water supply, infectious contact, contaminated inhalation therapy equipment)
Foreign bodies	Ventricular shunts, central venous catheter, artificial heart valves, urinary catheter, aspirated foreign bodies
Secondary immunodeficiencies	Malnutrition, prematurity, lymphoma, splenectomy, uremia, immunosuppressive therapy, protein-losing enteropathy
Primary immunodeficiencies	X-linked agammaglobulinemia, DiGeorge syndrome, chronic granulomatous disease, C3 deficiency

(Modified from *Immunologic Disorders in Infants and Children,* p. 184, by E. R. Stiehm, ed. 2, 1980. Published by W. B. Saunders Company. Used with permission.)

PRIMARY AND SECONDARY IMMUNODEFICIENCY

Immunodeficiencies may be either secondary or primary. **Secondary immunodeficiencies** *occur in individuals with a previously normal immune system who as a result of an illness develop an impaired immune system.* This impairment may be reversible if the underlying condition or illness is rectified. Secondary immunodeficiencies are considerably more common than primary immunodeficiencies and occur in many hospitalized patients; indeed, nearly every prolonged serious illness interferes with the immune system to some degree. A classification of the secondary immunodeficiencies is shown in TABLE 18–2.

The primary immunodeficiencies *are classified into 4 main groups, depending on the limb of the immune system that is deficient: defects of B, T, or phagocytic cells, or complement.* An overview of the function of each limb of the immune system is given in Ch. 17, above. Over 70 primary immunodeficiencies have been described, and con-

TABLE 18–2. THE SECONDARY IMMUNODEFICIENCIES

Premature and newborn infants	Physiologic immunodeficiency due to immaturity of immune system
Hereditary and metabolic diseases	Chromosome abnormalities (eg, Down's syndrome) Uremia Diabetes mellitus Malnutrition Vitamin and mineral deficiencies Protein-losing enteropathies Nephrotic syndrome Myotonic dystrophy Sickle cell disease
Immunosuppressive agents	Radiation Immunosuppressive drugs Corticosteroids Anti-lymphocyte or anti-thymocyte globulin
Infectious diseases	Congenital rubella Viral exanthems (eg, measles, varicella) HIV infection (eg, AIDS) Cytomegalovirus infection Infectious mononucleosis Acute bacterial disease Severe mycobacterial or fungal disease
Infiltrative hematologic diseases	Histocytosis Sarcoidosis Hodgkin's disease and lymphoma Leukemia Myeloma Agranulocytosis and aplastic anemia
Surgery and trauma	Burns Splenectomy Anesthesia
Miscellaneous	Lupus erythematosus Chronic active hepatitis Alcoholic cirrhosis Aging

siderable heterogeneity may exist within each disorder. A classification of the primary deficiencies is given in TABLE 18-3. This table excludes a number of unusual variants in which only a few cases are described.

T cell defects include several disorders with associated B cell (antibody) defects, which is understandable in view of a common origin of B and T cells from a primitive stem cell, and the regulatory influences exerted by T cells on B cell function. Phagocytic diseases include disorders in which the primary defect is one of cell movement **(chemotaxis)**, and those in which the primary defect is one of microbicidal activity.

Incidence of the primary immunodeficiencies: B cell or antibody defects predominate; IgA deficiency (mostly asymptomatic) may occur in 1:400 individuals. Excluding asymptomatic IgA deficiency, B cell defects comprise 55% of the primary immunodeficiencies; T cell deficiencies, about 25%; phagocytic deficiencies, 18%; and complement deficiencies, 2%. The overall incidence of *symptomatic* primary immunodeficiency is estimated to be 1:10,000, with about 400 new cases occurring annually in the USA. Since many primary immunodeficiencies are hereditary and congenital, they occur predominately in pediatric patients (individuals under age 20 comprise about 80% of cases). Because of the X-linked nature of many of these diseases, 70% occur in males.

TABLE 18-3. CLASSIFICATION, INHERITANCE, AND ASSOCIATED FEATURES OF THE PRIMARY IMMUNODEFICIENCIES

Disorder	*Associated Findings*
B CELL (ANTIBODY) DEFICIENCIES	
X-linked agammaglobulinemia (XL)	
Immunoglobulin deficiency with hyper-IgM (XL)	Neutropenia
IgA deficiency	Usually asymptomatic, autoimmunity, allergy, sinusitis
IgG subclass deficiencies	IgA deficiency (in IgG_2 deficiency)
Antibody deficiency with normal or elevated immunoglobulins	
Immunodeficiency with thymoma	Aplastic anemia
Common variable immunodeficiency	Autoimmunity
Transient hypogammaglobulinemia of infancy	Prematurity
X-linked lymphoproliferative syndrome (XL)	Epstein-Barr virus infection
T CELL (CELLULAR) DEFICIENCIES	
Predominant T cell deficiency	
DiGeorge syndrome	Hypocalcemia, pecular facies, aortic arch abnormalities, heart disease
Chronic mucocutaneous candidiasis	Endocrinopathies
Combined immunodeficiency with immunoglobulins (Nezelof syndrome)	
Nucleoside phosphorylase deficiency (AR)	
Combined T and B cell deficiencies	
Severe combined immunodeficiency (AR or XL)	
Combined immunodeficiency with adenosine deaminase deficiency (AR)	Skeletal abnormalities
Reticular dysgenesis	Pancytopenia
Ataxia telangiectasia (AR)	Dermatitis, neurologic deterioration
Wiskott-Aldrich syndrome (XL)	Eczema, thrombocytopenia
Short-limbed dwarfism	

(*Continued*)

TABLE 18–3. CLASSIFICATION, INHERITANCE, AND ASSOCIATED FEATURES OF THE PRIMARY IMMUNODEFICIENCIES *(Cont'd)*

Disorder	*Associated Findings*
PHAGOCYTIC DISORDERS	
Defects of cell movement	
Hyperimmunoglobulinemia-E syndrome	Eczema, dermatitis
Adhesive glycoprotein deficiency (AR)	Prolonged attachment of umbilical cord, leucocytosis, periodontitis
Defects of microbicidal activity	
Chronic granulomatous disease (XL or AR)	Lymphadenopathy
Glucose-6-phosphate dehydrogenase deficiency (XL)	
Myeloperoxidase deficiency (AR)	
Chédiak-Higashi syndrome (AR)	Oculocutaneous albinism, giant granules of neutrophils
COMPLEMENT DISORDERS	
C1q deficiency	Combined immunodeficiency, SLE-like syndrome
C1r deficiency (ACD)	SLE-like syndrome, glomerulonephritis
C4 deficiency (ACD)	SLE-like syndrome, glomerulonephritis
C2 deficiency (ACD)	SLE-like syndrome, glomerulonephritis
C3 deficiency (ACD)	Pyogenic infections
C5 deficiency (ACD)	*Neisseria* infection
C5 dysfunction	Leiner's disease
C6 deficiency (ACD)	*Neisseria* infection
C7 deficiency (ACD)	*Neisseria* infection
C8 deficiency (ACD)	*Neisseria* infection
C9 deficiency (ACD)	None
C1 inhibitor deficiency (AD)	Angioedema
C3 inactivator (factor I) deficiency (ACD)	Pyogenic infections

XL = X-linked; AR = autosomal recessive; ACD = autosomal codominant; AD = autosomal dominant.

Etiology

No common cause is responsible for immunodeficiency, although a single gene defect is often implicated. The genetic defect can lead to the absence of an enzyme (eg, adenosine deaminase deficiency), absence of a protein (eg, complement component deficiencies), or developmental arrest at a specific differential stage (eg, pre-B cell arrest in X-linked agammaglobulinemia). In certain illnesses, intrauterine events may be implicated (eg, maternal alcoholism in some cases of DiGeorge syndrome); in others, drug ingestion (eg, phenytoin in IgA deficiency). The exact biologic abnormality in most of the illnesses is unknown.

Symptoms and Signs

Most manifestations of immunodeficiency result from frequent infections, usually beginning with recurrent respiratory infections. However, many immunologically normal infants have 6 to 8 respiratory infections per year, particularly when there is exposure to older siblings or other children. Further, most immunodeficient patients eventually develop one or more severe bacterial infections that persist or recur, or lead to complications. For example, sinusitis, chronic otitis, and bronchitis often follow repeated episodes of sore throat or URI. Bronchitis may progress to pneumonia, bron-

chiectasis, and respiratory failure, the most common cause of death. Infections with opportunistic organisms (eg, *Pneumocystis carinii* or cytomegalovirus) may occur, particularly in patients with T cell deficiencies.

Infection of the skin and mucous membranes also is common. Resistant thrush may be the first sign of T cell immunodeficiency. Oral ulcers also are noted, particularly in granulocytic deficiencies. Conjunctivitis occurs in many antibody-deficient adults. Pyoderma, alopecia, eczema, and telangiectasia are not uncommon.

GI symptoms are common and include diarrhea, malabsorption, and failure to thrive. The diarrhea usually is noninfectious but may be associated with *Giardia lamblia*, rotavirus, or *Cryptosporidium*. In some patients there may be exudative diarrhea with loss of serum proteins and lymphocytes.

Less common manifestations of immunodeficiency include hematologic abnormalities (autoimmune hemolytic anemia, leukopenia, thrombocytopenia) and autoimmune phenomena (vasculitis, arthritis, endocrinopathies).

Diagnosis

A **family history** should be obtained for early death, related disease, autoimmune illness, allergy, early malignancy, and consanguinity. If the family history is positive, a pedigree chart should be constructed to help identify a hereditary pattern. A **past history** of adverse reactions to immunizations or viral infections should be noted as well as prior surgery (eg, tonsillectomy or adenoidectomy), radiation therapy to the thymus or nasopharynx, and prior antibiotic and γ-globulin therapies and their apparent clinical benefit.

The type of infection may give some clue as to the nature of the immunodeficiency. Infections with major gram-positive organisms (pneumococci, streptococci) are noted in antibody (B cell) immunodeficiencies. Severe infection from viral, fungal, and other opportunistic organisms are common in cellular (T cell) immunodeficiencies. Recurrent staphylococcal and gram-negative infections are common in phagocytic deficiencies. Recurrent *Neisseria* infection is characteristic of patients with C6, C7, and C8 complement deficiencies. Certain opportunistic infections (eg, from *P. carinii*, *Cryptosporidium*, or *Toxoplasma*) may occur in several types of immunodeficiency.

The age of onset also may help in diagnosis. Patients with very early onset of diseases (< 6 mo old) usually have a T cell defect. Onset of illness around 6 mo of age suggests congenital antibody deficiency, since transplacentally acquired material antibody has disappeared by then.

Physical examination: Patients with immunodeficiency often appear chronically ill, with pallor, malaise, malnutrition, and a distended abdomen. The skin may reveal macular rashes, vesicles, pyoderma, eczema, petechiae, alopecia, or telangiectasia. Conjunctivitis is common. Cervical lymph nodes and adenoid and tonsillar tissue typically are absent in B or T cell immunodeficiency, despite a history of recurrent throat infections. This can be confirmed by a lateral pharyngeal x-ray, which may show absence of adenoidal tissue. Occasionally the lymph nodes are enlarged and suppurative. The tympanic membranes often are scarred and/or perforated. The nostrils may be excoriated and crusted, indicative of purulent nasal discharge. There may be a postnasal drip and a decreased gag reflex. Often there is a chronic cough. The liver and spleen frequently are enlarged. Muscle mass is diminished and the fat deposits of the buttocks are diminished. There may be excoriation around the anus as a result of chronic diarrhea. Neurologic examination may reveal delayed developmental milestones or ataxia.

A characteristic constellation of findings permits a tentative clinical diagnosis in a number of immunodeficiency syndromes. These include **newborns with DiGeorge syndrome** who have infections, tetany, peculiar facies, and congenital heart disease; **boys with Wiskott-Aldrich syndrome** who have pyogenic infections, eczema, and bleeding

manifestations; **children with ataxia telangiectasia** who have recurrent sinopulmonary infections, ataxia, and telangiectasia; and **redheaded girls with the Job variant of the hyper-IgE syndrome** with fair skin, eczema, and recurrent staphylococcal infections. These disorders are discussed further, below.

Laboratory tests: In all cases of immunodeficiency, selected laboratory tests are necessary to confirm or establish the diagnosis; advanced tests often are necessary to subclassify the disorder prior to rational therapy (TABLE 18–4). In general, screening

TABLE 18–4. LABORATORY TESTS IN IMMUNODEFICIENCY

Screening Tests (Office)	*Advanced Tests*	*Special Tests*
B cell deficiency		
IgG, IgM, IgA levels Isoagglutinin titers Schick test Preexisting antibody titers (eg, polio, rubella, tetanus, diphtheria)	B cell enumeration IgD and IgE levels Ab responses to vaccines (eg, typhoid, pneumococcal polysaccharide) Lateral pharyngeal x-ray	Lymph node biopsy IgG subclass levels Ig survival Secretory Ig levels In vitro Ig synthesis study Ab response to special antigens: $\phi\chi$, KLH
T cell deficiency		
Lymphocyte count and morphology Thymus size by x-ray Delayed skin tests: *Trichophyton*, mumps, *Candida*, tetanus toxoid	T cell enumeration Lymphocyte proliferative responses to mitogens, antigens, allogeneic cells T cell subset enumeration (eg, T_h/T_s ratio)	Lymphokine assays (eg, MIF, IFN) Enzyme assays (eg, ADA, NP) Cytotoxic assays (eg, NK, ADCC, CTL) Thymic hormone assays Other T cell surface antigen analysis (eg, T6, DR, etc)
Phagocytic cell deficiency		
WBC count, morphology NBT dye test IgE level	Special morphology Rebuck skin window Random mobility and chemotactic assay Quantitative intracellular killing assay	WBC response to epinephrine, steroids, polysaccharides Chemiluminescence Enzyme assays—MPO, G6PD Surface glycoprotein assays with monoclonal antibodies
Complement Deficiency		
CH_{50} activity C3 level C4 level	Classical and alternative complement activity assays Component assays—immunochemical or functional Inhibitor assays—immunochemical or functional	Serum opsonic or chemotactic activity Complement breakdown product analysis

Ab = antibody
ADA = adenosine deaminase
ADCC = antibody-dependent cellular toxicity
C = complement
CTL = cytotoxic T lymphocyte
G6PD = glucose-6-phosphate dehydrogenase
IFN = interferon
Ig = immunoglobulin
KLH = keyhole-limpet hemocyanin antigen
MIF = migration inhibitory factor
MPO = myeloperoxidase
NBT = nitroblue tetrazolium
NK = natural killer
NP = nucleoside phosphorylase
$\phi\chi$ = phage antigen
T_h = T helper
T_s = T suppressor
WBC = white blood count

tests are available in most offices and hospitals, the advanced tests are available in most large hospitals, and the specialized tests are available only in laboratories or hospitals with a sophisticated clinical immunology laboratory.

When immunodeficiency is suspected, the screening laboratory tests recommended include a CBC with differential and platelet count; IgG, IgM, and IgA immunoglobulin levels; assessment of antibody function; and infection evaluation. The CBC will establish the presence of anemia, thrombocytopenia, neutropenia, or leukocytosis. The total lymphocyte count should be noted and the presence of lymphopenia (< 2000/μL) is suggestive of T cell immunodeficiency. The peripheral smear should be examined for the presence of Howell-Jolly bodies, and other unusual red cell forms, suggestive of asplenia or poor splenic function. The granulocytes may show morphologic abnormalities such as the granules of **Chédiak-Higashi syndrome**.

Immunoglobulin **(Ig)** levels also are part of the initial screen; however, IgD and IgE levels are not done initially. Ig must be interpreted with care because of marked alterations with age; all infants aged 2 to 6 mo are hypogammaglobulinemic by adult standards. Thus levels must be compared with normal levels from age-matched controls; these are presented in TABLE 18–5. In general, Ig levels within 2 SD (standard deviation) for age are considered normal. A total Ig level (IgG + IgM + IgA) > 600 mg/dL or an IgG level > 400 mg/dL with normal screening antibody functional tests excludes antibody deficiency. A total Ig level < 200 mg/dL usually indicates significant antibody deficiency. Intermediate levels (ie, IgG levels between 200 and 400 mg/dL, and total Igs between 400 and 600 mg/dL) are nondiagnostic and must be correlated with functional antibody tests.

Screening antibody tests also are recommended for the initial screen. IgM antibody function is estimated by isoagglutinin titers (anti-A and/or anti-B). All subjects except

TABLE 18–5. LEVELS OF IMMUNOGLOBULINS IN SERA OF NORMAL SUBJECTS BY AGE*

	IgG		*IgM*		*IgA*		*Total Immunoglobulin*	
Age	*mg/dL*	*Percent of Adult Level*	*mg/dL*	*Percent of Adult Level*	*mg/dL*	*Percent of Adult Level*	*mg/dL*	*Percent of Adult Level*
Newborn	1031±200†	89±17	11±5	11±5	2±3	1±2	1044±201	67±13
1–3 mo	430±119	37±10	30±11	30±11	21±13	11±7	481±127	31±9
4–6 mo	427±186	37±16	43±17	43±17	28±18	14±9	498±204	32±13
7–12 mo	661±219	58±19	54±23	55±23	37±18	19±9	752±242	48±15
13–24 mo	762±209	66±18	58±23	59±23	50±24	25±12	870±258	56±16
25–36 mo	892±183	77±16	61±19	62±19	71±37	36±19	1024±205	65±14
3–5 yr	929±228	80±20	56±18	57±18	93±27	47±14	1078±245	69±17
6–8 yr	923±256	80±22	65±25	66±25	124±45	62±23	1112±293	71±20
9–11 yr	1124±235	97±20	79±33	80±33	131±60	66±30	1334±254	85±17
12–16 yr	946±124	82±11	59±20	60±20	148±63	74±32	1153±169	74±12
Adults	1158±305	100±26	99±27	100±27	200±61	100±31	1457±353	100±24

* The values were derived from measurements made in 296 normal children and 30 adults. Levels were determined by the radial diffusion technic, using specific rabbit antisera to human immunoglobulins.

† One standard deviation.

(From Stiehm, E. R., and Fudenberg, H. H.: "Serum levels of immune globulins in health and disease: A survey." *Pediatrics,* 37:715, 1966. Reproduced by permission of *Pediatrics.*)

young infants and individuals of blood type AB will have natural antibodies at a titer of 1:8 (anti-A) or 1:4 (anti-B) or greater. These antibodies are selectively deficient in certain immunodeficiencies (eg, Wiskott-Aldrich syndrome). In the immunized subject, antibody titers to poliovirus, rubella virus, tetanus, or diphtheria antigens can be used to estimate IgG function. An adequate antibody response to one or more of these antigens is evidence against antibody deficiency. Finally, screening should include a search for chronic infection. The ESR often is elevated, usually in proportion to the degree of infection. Appropriate x-rays (chest, sinus, etc) and cultures should be done.

If these screening tests all are normal, immunodeficiency, particularly antibody deficiency, usually can be excluded. However, if chronic infection is documented, if the history is unusually suspicious, or if the screening tests are positive, advanced tests must be done.

Tests for B cell (antibody) deficiency: If Igs are very low (total < 200 mg/dL), a diagnosis of antibody deficiency is established, and other procedures are indicated only to define the exact illness and identify other immunologic defects. If Ig levels and preexisting antibody titers are low but not absent, the antibody responses to a standardized antigen should be assessed. Antibody titers, before and 2 wk after typhoid, tetanus, or killed poliovirus vaccine series, are obtained for postvaccine titers. An inadequate response (less than a 4-fold rise in titer) is suggestive of antibody deficiency regardless of Ig levels.

If Igs are low, B cell enumeration is done by assessing the percentage of lymphocytes with surface membrane Igs by staining with fluoresceinated anti-Ig antisera. Normally, 4 to 10% of peripheral blood lymphocytes are surface membrane Ig-positive (B cells). Disorders associated with low or absent B cells are shown in TABLE 18–3.

Next, tests for IgD and IgE levels are performed. Abnormalities of IgD and IgE (both high and low levels) are not uncommon in incomplete antibody deficiency syndromes. IgE levels are high in chemotactic disorders, partial T cell immunodeficiencies, allergic disorders, and parasitism. Isolated absences of IgD and IgE are rare and not significant clinically.

Special tests for B cell deficiencies (TABLE 18–4) are indicated in certain circumstances. A lymph node biopsy (sometimes preceded by immunization in the adjacent extremity) is indicated in the presence of lymphadenopathy or to exclude malignancy. IgG subclass determinations are indicated if IgG levels are normal or near normal but antibody function is deficient. Selective deficiencies of one of the 4 subclasses may be present. If there is a suspicion of rapid IgG catabolism or IgG loss through the skin or the GI tract, an IgG survival study may be indicated, using isotope-labeled IgG; or if the patient has low levels of IgG, a large dose of IV IgG is given and the IgG levels measured daily to determine the half-life. If local infections are severe, Ig levels in secretions (eg, tears or saliva) can be done. In vitro IgG synthesis and the antibody response to special antigens such as ϕX phage or keyhole-limpet hemocyanin (KLH) are done to determine the exact location of the synthetic block.

Tests for T cell deficiency: The presence of profound and prolonged lymphopenia is suggestive of a T cell immunodeficiency; however, lymphopenia is not usually present. A chest x-ray is a useful screening test for T cell immunodeficiency in an infant. An absent thymic shadow in the newborn period is suggestive of T cell deficiency, particularly if done before the onset of infection or other stress that may shrink the thymus.

Delayed hypersensitivity skin tests are valuable screening tests for T cell deficiency. Utilized are mumps antigen, *Candida* antigen (1:100), fluid tetanus toxoid (1:10), and *Trichophyton* antigen; nearly all adults and most immunized infants and children will react to one or more of these antigens with erythema and induration (> 5 mm) at 48 h. The presence of one or more positive delayed skin tests generally indicates an intact T cell system.

The most valuable advanced test in cellular immunodeficiency is T cell enumeration, usually performed by measuring the number of lymphocytes that form rosettes with sheep erythrocytes. These erythrocyte rosette forming cells **(ERFCs)** ordinarily make up 55 to 70% of the peripheral blood lymphocytes, or > 3000/μL. In most cellular immunodeficiencies, T cells are reduced in proportion to the degree of cellular immune impairment; some patients with profound T cell immunodeficiency may have T cells < 5% of normal. Monoclonal mouse antisera (eg, Leu 1, OK-T3) are now available that react with all T cells; thus immunofluorescent procedures can be substituted for ERFC enumeration, either by microscopy or by automated fluorescent-activated cell sorting.

Monoclonal antibodies are also available that identify surface antigens of T cells that have unique properties. Leu 3 and OK-T4 monoclonal antibodies define helper/inducer T cells, and Leu 2 and OK-T8 monoclonal antibodies define suppressor/cytotoxic T lymphocytes. The ratio between helper and suppressor T cells, normally 2:1, may be characteristically altered in certain disorders and provide valuable diagnostic information. Monoclonal antibodies also are available that identify activated cells (DR), natural killer cells (Leu 11), and immature T cell (thymocyte) antigens (OK-T6).

Another useful advanced test measures the ability of the patient's lymphocytes to proliferate and enlarge (transform) when cultured in the presence of mitogens (eg, phytohemagglutinin, Concanavalin A), irradiated allogeneic leukocytes (in the mixed leukocyte reaction), or antigens to which the patient has been previously exposed. Under these stimuli, normal lymphocytes undergo rapid division; this can be assessed either morphologically or by uptake of radioactive thymidine into dividing cells. Proliferation usually is reported as an index—the ratio of counts/min **(CPM)** of stimulated cells to CPM of an equal number of unstimulated cells. Patients with T cell immunodeficiency have low or absent proliferative responses in proportion to the degree of immune impairment. The proliferative responses to mitogens (which activate all cells) are considerably higher (stimulation index 50 to 100) than the response to antigens or allogeneic cells (stimulation index 3 to 30).

Special procedures also are available to assess lymphokine production following mitogen or antigen stimulation. Although over 30 lymphokines exist, the 2 usually assayed are macrophage migration inhibitory factor **(MIF)** and gamma interferon **(γ-IFN)**. Certain patients have adequate proliferative responses but deficient lymphokine production (eg, MIF deficiency in chronic mucocutaneous candidiasis). Another group of specialized tests assesses cytotoxic function. Different types of cytotoxicity (natural killer, antibody-dependent, or cytotoxic T cell) are measured utilizing different tumor cell or viral infected target cells. Cytotoxic defects are variably present in cellular immunodeficiency. In some forms of combined immunodeficiency, enzymes of the purine pathway (adenosine deaminase, nucleoside phosphorylase) are deficient and can be assayed utilizing erythrocytes. Finally, levels of various thymic hormones (thymosin, factor thymic serique) can be assessed; these are low in certain cellular immunodeficiencies.

Tests for phagocytic and complement deficiencies: An investigation for phagocytic and complement disorders is indicated when a patient has a convincing history of immunodeficiency but has normal B and T cell immunity. A lack of pus formation at the site of inflammation or delayed umbilical cord detachment in the absence of leukopenia is a clinical clue suggestive of a **chemotactic defect**.

In addition to the blood count, initial screening should include an IgE level, which is elevated in many chemotactic disorders, and a nitroblue tetrazolium **(NBT)** dye reduction test for chronic granulomatous disease **(CGD)**, the most common phagocytic disorder. The NBT test is based on the increased metabolic activity of granulocytes during phagocytosis and killing with reduction of colorless NBT to blue formazan.

This color change, absent in CGD, can be assessed visually, microscopically, or spectrophotometrically.

The first special test is staining of the granulocytes for myeloperoxidase, alkaline phosphatase, or esterase. Absence of staining for these enzymes should be followed by quantitative assays. Next, cell movement can be assessed by a Rebuck skin window, in which the skin is superficially abraded with a scalpel and cover slips are placed over the site; these are removed and replaced at intervals, and stained for migrating cells. An initial influx of polymorphonuclear cells should occur within 2 h, and then be replaced by mononuclear cells within 24 h. A chemotactic abnormality can be confirmed by an in vitro chemotactic assay in which migration of granulocytes or monocytes is measured using either a special chemotactic chamber (Boyden) or an agarose plate; cell movement toward a chemoattractant such as opsonized zymosan is assessed.

Next, phagocytosis is assessed by measuring uptake of latex particles or bacteria by isolated granulocytes or monocytes. Microbial killing is then assessed by mixing the patient's granulocytes in the presence of fresh serum with a known number of live bacteria followed by serial quantitative bacterial assays over a 2-h period.

Other specialized tests to define phagocytic defects include assays of granulocyte mobilization following corticosteroids, epinephrine, or endotoxin administration; quantitative assays of granulocyte enzymes (myeloperoxidase, glucose-6-phosphate dehydrogenase, etc); assays for granulocyte oxidant products (chemiluminescence, superoxide); and assays of specific granulocyte proteins (cytochrome b_{245}, adhesive glycoproteins).

A **complement abnormality** is screened by measuring the total serum complement activity (CH_{50}) and serum C3 and C4 levels. Low levels of any of these should be followed by titration of the classical and alternative complement pathways and the measurement of individual complement components. These latter utilize monospecific antisera or sensitized erythrocytes and solutions that contain all components except for the one being assessed.

Antisera also are available to measure complement inhibitor proteins; hereditary angioedema is associated with deficiency of C1 inhibitor, and C3 deficiency with C3 hypercatabolism is associated with deficiency of C3 inhibitor. Assays of serum opsonic activity, chemotactic activity, or bactericidal activity measure complement function.

Principles of Treatment

Prevention of primary immunodeficiency is limited to genetic counseling in instances in which identified genetic patterns of inheritance are known. Prenatal diagnosis using cultured amniotic cells or fetal blood is feasible for a few of these disorders, including X-linked agammaglobulinemia, Wiskott-Aldrich syndrome, severe combined immunodeficiency, combined immunodeficiency with adenosine deaminase deficiency, and chronic granulomatous disease. Sex determination also can be used to exclude X-linked disorders.

General management (see also Ch. 7): Patients with immunodeficiency require an extraordinary amount of care to maintain optimal health and nutrition, prevent emotional problems related to their illness, manage infectious episodes, and cope with the financial costs of their medical care. They should be protected from unnecessary exposure to infection, sleep in their own beds, and preferably have rooms of their own. Killed vaccines should be given regularly if there is evidence of some antibody function. The teeth should be kept in good repair.

Antibiotics: Antibiotics are lifesaving in treating the infectious episodes. The choice and dose of antibiotics are identical to those used normally. However, because immunodeficient patients may succumb rapidly to infection, fevers or other manifestations of infection are assumed to be secondary to bacterial infection, and antibiotic treat-

ment is begun immediately. Throat, blood, or other cultures are obtained prior to most of therapy; these are especially important when the infection does not respond to the initial antibiotic chosen and when there is infection with an unusual organism.

Continuous prophylactic antibiotics often are beneficial in immunodeficiencies, particularly when there is the risk of sudden overwhelming infection (eg, Wiskott-Aldrich syndrome, asplenic syndromes); when other forms of immune therapy are unavailable (eg, in phagocytic disorders) or insufficient (eg, recurrent infection in agammaglobulinemia despite γ-globulin treatment); and when there is a high risk for a specific infection (eg, *P. carinii* in cellular immunodeficiency disorders).

Precautions: Patients with either B or T cell immunodeficiencies should not be given live vaccines (eg, poliomyelitis, measles, mumps, rubella, BCG) because of the risk of vaccine-induced illness. Family members of patients with immunodeficiency should not receive live poliovirus vaccine.

Patients with cellular immunodeficiency should not receive fresh blood products that may contain intact lymphocytes, because of the risk of graft-versus-host disease **(GVHD)**. Accordingly, whole blood or blood fractions (eg, red cells, platelets, granulocytes, and plasma) should be irradiated (3000 R) prior to administration to prevent GVHD. γ-Globulin or plasma usually should be avoided in patients with selective IgA deficiency because anti-IgA antibodies may develop or cause reactions. Patients with splenomegaly should avoid contact sports. Patients with thrombocytopenia should avoid IM injections such as γ-globulin. Antibiotics should be given at the time of surgery or dental work.

Gamma globulin: Human immune serum globulin **(HISG)** is effective replacement therapy in most forms of antibody deficiency. It is a 16.5% solution of IgG with trace quantities of IgM and IgA for IM injection, or a 3 to 5% solution for IV infusion. The usual loading dose is 200 mg/kg (1.4 mL/kg of the 16.5% preparation, 4 mL/kg for the 5% preparation) followed at monthly intervals by 100 mg/kg (0.7 mL/kg of the 16.5% solution, 2 mL/kg of the 5% solution). Lesser doses are therapeutically ineffective. The recommended dose of HISG only increases the serum IgG level about 200 mg/dL; larger or more frequent doses must be given to some patients. The largest IM dose at one site is 10 mL in adults, 5 mL in children; accordingly, multiple injections at various sites may be necessary. Higher doses of γ-globulin 300 to 500 mg/kg/mo can be given IV and are beneficial to some antibody-deficient patients not responding well to conventional doses.

Plasma has been used as an alternative to HISG, but because of the risk of acquiring AIDS or other viruses it is rarely indicated. Plasma does contain many factors in addition to Igs and is of particular value in patients with protein-losing enteropathy, complement deficiencies, and refractory diarrhea.

Other therapy: Immunologic-enhancing agents, including pharmaceuticals (levamisole, isoprinosine), biologic substances (transfer factor, interleukins), and hormones (thymic hormones) have been of limited value in the treatment of cellular immunodeficiencies. Fetal thymic transplants, thymic epithelial cell transplants, and fetal liver transplants occasionally are successful, particularly fetal thymic transplants in the DiGeorge syndrome. Enzyme replacement with fresh red cell transfusions has been of benefit to a few patients with adenosine deaminase deficiency.

Transplantation: Complete correction of immunodeficiency can sometimes be achieved by bone marrow transplantation (**BMT**—see also Ch. 22). In severe combined immunodeficiency and its variants, BMT from an HLA-identical, mixed leukocyte culture (MLC)-matched sibling has resulted in restoration of immunity in > 100 cases. In patients with intact or partial cellular immunodeficiency (eg, Wiskott-Aldrich syndrome), prior immunosuppression must be given to ensure engraftment. When a matched sibling donor is unavailable, a haploidentical (half-matched) BMT from a

parent may be attempted. Under these circumstances, mature T lymphocytes that will cause GVHD must be removed from the parenteral marrow prior to its administration. This can be achieved with the use of soybean lectin agglutination, lysis with monoclonal antibody and complement, or lysis with monoclonal antibody linked to ricin toxin. These are specialized procedures available in only a few centers.

SPECIFIC IMMUNODEFICIENCIES

TRANSIENT HYPOGAMMAGLOBULINEMIA OF INFANCY

A self-limited antibody deficiency occurring in both sexes, with onset at age 3 to 6 mo and persistence of the disorder usually for 6 to 18 mo. Sometimes there is an associated increased frequency of infection. The disorder results from a delay in the onset of Ig synthesis despite the presence of normal numbers of B cells. T helper cells may be reduced. Premature infants are especially prone to this disorder because of lower levels of transplacental IgG at birth. The disorder is not familial. **Treatment**: Despite low IgG levels (total < 400 mg/dL), many of these children do not require HISG injections, particularly if there is some evidence of antibody function, if the IgG levels are increasing, and if infections are absent or of a trivial nature. Patients needing HISG injections should receive full therapeutic doses for 3 to 6 mo, with recheck of the IgG levels at frequent intervals. Antibiotics are indicated with each infectious episode. The outlook is excellent for complete recovery.

X-LINKED AGAMMAGLOBULINEMIA
(Bruton's Agammaglobulinemia)

Panhypogammaglobulinemia of male infants characterized by low levels of immunoglobulins, low or absent B cells, intact cellular immunity, and onset of infections sometime after age 6 mo when maternal antibody disappears. These infants have recurrent pyogenic infections of the lungs, sinuses, and bones with such organisms as pneumococcus, hemophilus, and streptococcus. They also are susceptible to vaccine-induced poliovirus infection and chronic echovirus encephalitis. X-linked pattern of inheritance is proven in about 20% of cases. The genetic defect seems to be one of inability to form B cells from pre-B cells. **Treatment** is lifelong human immune serum globulin (HISG) injections or infusions. Prompt and adequate administration of antibiotics with each infection is crucial; continuous antibiotics are sometimes indicated. Despite these measures, many patients still develop persistent sinusitis, bronchitis, and bronchiectasis. Susceptibility to malignancy is increased.

SELECTIVE IgA DEFICIENCY

The absence or marked reduction (< 15 mg/dL) of serum IgA with normal levels of other Igs and intact cellular immunity. Selective IgA deficiency is the most common (and mildest) immunodeficiency, occurring as often as 1:400 subjects. Selective IgA deficiency usually is sporadic but occasionally is familial. It may occur as a result of phenytoin treatment and in subjects with chromosome 18 abnormalities. It also may occur in relatives of patients with common variable immunodeficiency (see below).

Most patients are asymptomatic, and their defect is noted fortuitously. Others have recurrent respiratory infections, chronic diarrhea, allergy, or autoimmune disease. Patients with IgA deficiency lack secretory IgA in their secretions, but may compensate by secreting other Igs. Patients with IgA deficiency may develop anti-IgA antibodies as a result of exposure to IgA in plasma or γ-globulin; *these antibodies can cause anaphylactic reactions when γ-globulin or blood is subsequently given.* Some patients with IgA deficiency have an associated IgG_2 subclass immunodeficiency; many such patients have recurrent infections.

Treatment is not necessary in most cases. Continuous antibiotics are needed for those with persistent respiratory infections. IgA replacement therapy is unavailable. HISG injections usually are *contraindicated*, although a few patients with IgA deficiency with IgG subclass deficiency have been given γ-globulin successfully. A few IgA-deficient patients remit spontaneously.

COMMON VARIABLE IMMUNODEFICIENCY (CVID)

(Acquired Agammaglobulinemia)

A heterogeneous disorder occurring equally in both sexes and characterized by the onset of recurrent bacterial infections in the 2nd or 3rd decade as a result of markedly decreased Ig and antibody levels. The presence of normal numbers of B cells distinguishes CVID from X-linked agammaglobulinemia. Cellular immunity usually is intact but may be impaired in some patients; and in others, T cell immunoregulatory abnormalities are described. Autoimmune abnormalities including Addison's disease, thyroiditis, and RA are not uncommon in these patients and their relatives. Diarrhea, malabsorption, and nodular lymphoid hyperplasia of the GI tract sometimes are present. Bronchiectasis often develops. Immunologic abnormalities vary in different patients; ie, excessive T suppressor activity, deficient T helper activity, intrinsic defects of B cell function, and autoantibodies to B or T cells. **Treatment**: As with X-linked agammaglobulinemia, lifelong HISG injections are required.

DIGEORGE SYNDROME

(Thymic Hypoplasia; Third and Fourth Pharyngeal Pouch Syndrome)

A congenital immunodeficiency characterized clinically by hypocalcemic tetany, congenital heart disease, characteristic facies, and increased susceptibility to infection; pathologically by absence or hypoplasia of the thymus and parathyroid glands; and immunologically by partial or complete T cell immunodeficiency but normal or near normal B cell immunity. Affected infants have low-set ears, midline facial clefts, a small receding mandible, hypertelorism, and a shortened philtrum. The onset of tetany is within 24 to 48 h of life. Boys and girls are equally affected, and genetic factors usually are not present (however, chromosome 22 abnormalities are reported in a few cases). Recurrent infections begin soon after birth. The **etiology** seems to be an interruption of normal development of pharyngeal pouch structures near the 8th wk of gestation by a number of factors, including maternal alcoholism. The degree of immunodeficiency varies considerably from patient to patient, and sometimes T cell function improves spontaneously. **Treatment**: Some success has been achieved with fetal thymic transplants. Bone marrow transplantation also has been used. The severity of the heart disease often determines the eventual prognosis. Partial deficiency is compatible with prolonged survival.

CHRONIC MUCOCUTANEOUS CANDIDIASIS

A cellular immunodeficiency characterized by persistent Candida *infection of the mucous membranes, scalp, skin, and nails, and often associated with an endocrinopathy, particularly hypothyroidism.* Onset may be in infancy with the occurrence of persistent thrush or may be delayed until late adulthood. The disorder is somewhat more frequent in females. The disease varies considerably in severity from involvement of a single nail to generalized mucous membrane and skin and hair involvement, and disfiguring granular lesions of the face and scalp. Systemic candidiasis and increased susceptibility to other infections do not occur. Several clinical patterns exist, including an autosomal recessive illness associated with hypoparathyroidism and Addison's disease (*Candida*-endocrinopathy syndrome). The characteristic immunologic findings are cutaneous anergy to *Candida*, absent proliferative responses to *Candida* antigen (but

normal proliferative responses to mitogens), and good antibody responses to *Candida* and other antigens. Associated findings in some cases include bronchiectasis, hepatitis, and biotin deficiency with carboxylase enzyme deficiency.

Treatment consists of local (nystatin, clotrimazole) or systemic (ketoconazole, amphotericin B—see in Ch. 9) antifungal drugs. Affected nails may have to be removed surgically. Immunotherapy with transfer factor, thymic epithelium, thymic hormones, or immune lymphocytes is not of permanent benefit. Bone marrow transplantation has not been attempted.

COMBINED IMMUNODEFICIENCY (CID)

A group of disorders characterized by congenital and often hereditary deficiency of both B and T cell systems, lymphoid aplasia, and thymic dysplasia; ie: **severe combined immunodeficiency (SCID); Swiss agammaglobulinemia; thymic dysplasia; CID with adenosine deaminase deficiency**; and **CID with Igs (Nezelof syndrome)**. Most patients have an early onset (within 3 mo of age) of infection with thrush, pneumonia, and diarrhea, and if left untreated, a progressive downhill course with death before age 2. Most, but not all, patients have profound deficiency of B cells and Igs. Characteristically there are lymphopenia, low or absent T cell numbers, poor proliferative response to mitogens, cutaneous anergy, an absent thymic shadow, and diminished lymphoid tissue. *P. carinii* and other opportunistic infections are common.

A number of variants of the disorder exist. In 50% of cases an X-linked or autosomal recessive pattern of inheritance can be established. About half the patients with an autosomal recessive pattern of inheritance have **adenosine deaminase (ADA) deficiency**, a purine salvage pathway enzyme which converts adenosine and deoxyadenosine to inosine and deoxyinosine respectively. ADA deficiency results in elevated quantities of deoxyadenosine triphosphate **(deoxyATP)**, which inhibits DNA synthesis. These children may be normal at birth but develop progressive immunologic impairment as deoxyATP accumulates. In **CID with Igs**, there is a profound cellular immunodeficiency but normal, near normal, or elevated levels of Igs—but with poor antibody function. The course may be only slightly less severe than in SCID. **CID with reticuloendotheliosis** is another variant with skin lesions resembling Letterer-Siwe disease, lymphadenopathy, and hepatosplenomegaly. Some of these infants may have graft-vs-host disease from maternal lymphocytes or from previous blood transfusions.

Treatment with γ-globulin and antibiotics (including *P. carinii* prophylaxis) is indicated but is not curative. The treatment of choice is bone marrow transplantation.

WISKOTT-ALDRICH SYNDROME (WAS)

An X-linked recessive disorder of male infants, characterized by eczema, thrombocytopenia, and recurrent infection. The first manifestations often are hemorrhagic (usually bloody diarrhea), followed by development of recurrent respiratory infections. Malignancy (especially lymphoma and acute lymphoblastic leukemia) is common in patients that survive beyond the first decade. The characteristic immunologic defects include poor antibody responses to polysaccharide antigens, cutaneous anergy, partial T cell immunodeficiency, elevated levels of IgE and IgA, low levels of IgM, and hypercatabolism of IgG but normal IgG levels. Because of the combined deficiency in both B and T cell function, infections occur with pyogenic bacteria, viruses, fungi, and *P. carinii*. Hematologically, these patients have small platelets and increased splenic destruction of platelets; accordingly, splenectomy may alleviate the thrombocytopenia. **Treatment** consists of splenectomy, continuous antibiotics, IV immunoglobulin (not IM, because of risk of hemorrhage), and if a matched sibling is available, bone marrow transplantation.

ATAXIA TELANGIECTASIA

An autosomal recessive progressive multisystem disorder characterized by cerebellar ataxia, telangiectasia of the conjunctiva and skin, recurrent sinopulmonary infections, and variable immunologic disease.

Both neurologic symptoms and evidence of immunodeficiency are variable in onset. Ataxia usually develops at about the time when patients begin to walk but may be delayed until age 4 yr. Its progression leads to severe disability. Speech becomes slurred, choreoathetoid movements and ophthalmoplegia occur, and muscle weakness usually progresses to muscle atrophy. Progressive mental retardation may occur. Telangiectasias develop between 1 and 6 yr of age, most prominently on the bulbar conjunctiva, ears, antecubital and popliteal fossas, and sides of the nose. The recurrent sinopulmonary infections, which result from the immunologic deficits, lead to recurrent pneumonia, bronchiectasis, and chronic obstructive and restrictive lung disease.

Endocrine abnormalities may occur, including gonadal dysgenesis, testicular atrophy, and an unusual form of diabetes mellitus characterized by marked hyperglycemia, resistance to ketosis, and a marked plasma insulin response to glucose or tolbutamide.

The disorder is associated with a high degree of malignancy (especially leukemia, brain tumors, and gastric cancer) and increased frequency of chromosome breaks, probably indicative of a defect in DNA repair. Patients often lack IgA and IgE and have cutaneous anergy and a progressive cellular immune defect. Serum α_2-fetoprotein is generally elevated. No effective **treatment** is available, and the course is one of progressive neurologic deterioration with choreoathetosis, muscle weakness, dementia, and death.

HYPER-IgE SYNDROME
(Job-Buckley Syndrome)

An immunodeficiency syndrome characterized by recurrent staphylococcal infections, particularly of the skin, and markedly elevated levels of IgE. Some patients have an autosomal recessive inheritance pattern. The staphylococcal infection may involve the skin, lung, joints, and other sites. Some patients have coarse features; some are fair and redheaded. Many have neutrophil chemotactic defects. All have exceptionally elevated IgE levels (> 1000 IU/mL). Allergic manifestations such as eczema, rhinitis, and asthma sometimes are present. Other laboratory features include subtle defects of B and T cell immunity and tissue and blood eosinophilia. The basic defect may be an immunoregulatory T cell abnormality. **Treatment** consists of intermittent or continuous antibiotic therapy. Trimethoprim/sulfamethoxazole is particularly effective as a prophylactic drug.

CHRONIC GRANULOMATOUS DISEASE (CGD)

An inherited disorder of leukocyte bactericidal function characterized by widespread granulomatous lesions of the skin, lungs, and lymph nodes; hypergammaglobulinemia, anemia, leukocytosis; and defective killing of certain bacteria and fungi. Most patients are males who have inherited the disorder as an X-linked recessive disorder; a few patients of either sex inherit the disorder as autosomal recessive. The **clinical pattern** is one of recurrent infections with catalase-producing organisms such as *Staphylococcus aureus*, *Serratia*, *Escherichia coli*, and *Pseudomonas*. These organisms do not usually cause granulomas, but because of the bactericidal killing defect, the organisms survive intracellularly.

Onset of disease usually occurs in early childhood, but may be delayed until the early teens in a few patients. Clinical characteristics are suppurative lymphadenitis, hepatosplenomegaly, pneumonia, and hematologic evidence of chronic infection. Per-

sistent rhinitis, dermatitis, diarrhea, perianal abscesses, stomatitis, osteomyelitis, brain abscess, obstructive GI tract lesions (from granuloma formation) and delayed growth also occur.

Leukocytes from CGD patients do not produce hydrogen peroxide, superoxide, and other activated oxygen species, probably because of deficient nicotinamide adenine dinucleotide phosphate (NADPH) oxidase activity. However, other granulocyte proteins (eg, cytochrome b_{245}), may also be deficient. Laboratory diagnosis is made by deficient nitroblue tetrazolium (NBT) dye reduction of granulocytes, or an in vitro bactericidal defect. **Treatment** consists of intermittent or continuous antibiotic therapy. Bone marrow transplantation also has been successful.

SPLENIC DEFICIENCY SYNDROMES

Susceptibility to infection because of splenectomy, congenital absence of the spleen, or functional asplenia due to thrombosis of splenic vessels (sickle cell disease) or infiltrative diseases (storage disorders). The spleen is a major phagocytic organ of the reticuloendothelial system with trapping of circulating organisms. The spleen also serves as a major site of antibody synthesis. Patients without a spleen, particularly young infants, are susceptible to rapid overwhelming bacterial infection with *H. influenzae*, *E. coli*, pneumococci, and streptococci, and to a lesser extent, to other infections. These patients should have continuous prophylactic antibiotics for the first 2 to 3 yr of life, and thereafter be given antibiotics at the onset of each febrile episode and with surgery. They should also receive pneumococcal polysaccharide, meningococcal, and *Hemophilus* vaccines.

PROTEIN-LOSING IMMUNODEFICIENCIES (NEPHROSIS, BURNS, ENTERITIS)

Loss of serum proteins leading to secondary antibody deficiency with striking degrees of hypogammaglobulinemia. This can be due to loss through the kidney (nephrotic syndrome), skin (severe burns or dermatitis), or GI tract (protein-losing enteropathy, intestinal lymphangiectasia). There is simultaneous loss of albumin and other serum proteins. In GI protein-loss disorders, there may also be lymphocyte loss, resulting in lymphopenia and cellular immunodeficiency. These patients are susceptible to major gram-positive infections, but since a compensatory increase of antibody production occurs, infections may be relatively uncommon despite striking hypogammaglobulinemia. Correction of the underlying disease will correct the immunodeficiency. When this is impossible, medium-chain triglycerides may be of partial benefit in decreasing the loss of immunoglobulins and lymphocytes from the GI tract.

IMMUNODEFICIENCY AND MALNUTRITION

(See also Ch. 80)

Malnutrition with immunodeficiency and infection is the world's leading cause of infant and child death. Malnutrition may be due to a deficiency of all nutrients **(marasmus)** or primarily of protein **(kwashiorkor)**, usually with superimposed vitamin and mineral deficiencies (eg, iron, zinc). When malnutrition is severe enough to reduce weight to < 80% of expected mean, some impairment of immune function is noted; when growth retardation is < 70% of expected mean, severe impairment of immune function usually is seen. Most such individuals (except anorexia nervosa patients) are extraordinarily susceptible to respiratory infection, viral disease, and gastroenteritis. These infections increase metabolic requirements and decrease appetite, leading to a vicious circle of more malnutrition and immunodeficiency. An inadequate food intake due to poverty is the most important cause of malnutrition; less often it is secondary

to ignorance (eg, strict vegetarianism), chronic disease (eg, short-gut, colitis), or psychiatric disturbance (anorexia nervosa). The immunologic defect is primarily a T cell immunodeficiency with cutaneous anergy, low T cell numbers, poor proliferative responses to mitogens and antigens, and deficiency of lymphokines (interferon) and cytotoxic activity. Secretory antibody levels may be diminished but serum antibody and Igs usually are normal or elevated, particularly IgE. The degree of immune impairment is dependent on the degree and duration of malnutrition, and underlying illness such as infection or other nutritional deficiencies. With nutritional rehabilitation, the immunologic defect is rapidly reversible.

---

19. ACQUIRED IMMUNODEFICIENCY SYNDROME (AIDS)

A secondary immunodeficiency syndrome caused by a virus and characterized by severe immune deficiency resulting in opportunistic infections, malignancies, and neurologic lesions in individuals without prior history of immunologic abnormality.

Etiology and Pathogenesis

The cause is a retrovirus that has been termed the human T-lymphotrophic virus Type III **(HTLV-III)**, lymphadenopathy-associated virus **(LAV)**, and the AIDS-associated retrovirus **(ARV)** by different laboratories. More recently, it has also been referred to as the human immunodeficiency virus **(HIV)**, the term that will be used here.

Retroviruses contain an enzyme called reverse transcriptase that can convert viral RNA in the cytoplasm into DNA, which may replicate from extrachromosomal sites or move into the cell nucleus where it becomes part of the host cell DNA. These integrated viral genes are duplicated with normal cellular genes, and all progeny of the originally infected cell will contain the viral genes. Expression of the viral genes for some retroviruses may be oncogenic, converting the cell into a cancer, or may have other pathologic effects which may alter normal cell function or produce cell death. Retroviruses have been known to cause malignant and nonmalignant diseases, and the same virus may cause different diseases in different animals; eg, bovine leukemia virus causes a B cell lymphoma in cows, a T cell lymphoma in sheep, and an immunodeficiency disorder similar to AIDS in rabbits.

There are 3 groups of retroviruses that affect humans, and all have a remarkable affinity for lymphocytes, particularly for T4 lymphocytes. HIV preferentially infects the major subset of T cells, defined phenotypically as T4 and functionally as "inducer/helper" cells, which are then depleted, resulting in a reduced ratio of T4 helper (T_h) to T8 suppressor (T_s) cells. However, the virus also is capable of infecting some nonlymphoid cells, such as macrophages and nervous tissue cells, and presumably remains present for life.

Following infection with HIV, a wide variety of qualitative defects and functional abnormalities of T cells, B cells, natural killer cells, and monocytes/macrophages may be seen; ie, all limbs of the immune system are affected. Despite the fact that cells other than T4 can be affected and regardless of whether the abnormalities seen are of cellular or humoral immunity, the complete spectrum of immunologic dysfunction in AIDS can be explained by loss of function of the critically important T4 helper lymphocytes. A variety of neurologic syndromes may occur as a result of infection or, presumably, as a result of direct injury by HIV infection of nervous system cells.

Epidemiology

HIV is not transmitted by casual contact or even the close, nonsexual contact that normally occurs at work, in school, or at home. Transmission to another person must

require transmission of body substances containing infected cells; eg, blood or plasma and plasma-containing fluids (such as saliva). Uniquely, HIV can be expected to be present in any fluid or exudate that contains lymphocytes; eg, it has been found in semen, tears, and vaginal secretions. However, transmission by tears, saliva, fomites, or air has not been reported.

Infected cells can reach target cells in a new host directly (blood transfusions, injection) or after mucous membrane exposure; ie, by close, direct contact that breaches normal body barriers. For example, chimpanzees have been infected via vaginal exposure without trauma or coexisting infection. Presumably, such mucous membrane transmission would be even easier in the presence of inflamed or traumatized tissues; eg, anorectal lesions, which are highly prevalent in homosexual men. Among humans, heterosexual transmission from men to women has been well documented. Transmission from women to men appears to be more difficult, but such instances are being increasingly reported. While transmission by accidental needle stick has occurred, transmission of HIV by this means is much more difficult and much less frequent than is hepatitis B.

The extremely low risk of transmission by casual contact deserves emphasis. In one study, nonsexual household contacts (68 children, 33 adults) of patients with AIDS or AIDS-related complex with oral candidiasis were evaluated. The contacts had lived in the same household with a patient for ≥ 3 mo and had shared household items and facilities with the patient for a median of 22 mo. Close personal interactions (eg, assisting the patient with bathing, dressing, and eating) were common. The only contact found to have signs of HIV infection was the 5-yr-old daughter of 2 IV drug abusers; the daughter had most likely been infected perinatally, rather than horizontally.

In the USA and Europe, statistical data on persons with AIDS are remarkably similar. Using data up to the beginning of 1986 from the USA, 90% of patients were 20 to 49 yr old, 93% were men, and 94% could be placed in groups that suggest a possible means of the disease acquisition: homosexual or bisexual men, 73% (8% were also IV drug users); heterosexual IV drug users, 17%; persons with hemophilia, 1%; heterosexual sex partners of persons with AIDS or at risk of AIDS (eg, spouses of persons with AIDS, prostitutes), 1%; and recipients of transfused blood or blood components, 2%. Of the 6% unassigned to a high-risk group, many could not be fully investigated.

The proportions of these relative risk groups have remained remarkably stable. However, this stability may very well change in the future. For example, while heterosexual spread of AIDS has been much less rapid than the spread among homosexual men, many experts predict that an increase in heterosexual transmission seems inevitable. Reports of prevalence can vary greatly in different groups of people and at different points in time as a result of a variety of factors. For example, the lag between infection with HIV and the appearance of AIDS distorts data. This can be illustrated by data obtained from a cohort of homosexual men who were enrolled in studies of hepatitis B from 1978 to 1980, a 10% random sample of whom was followed up in an AIDS study. By 1980 when AIDS was first diagnosed in this group, many of the men had already been infected with the virus, and the ratio of infected persons to the number of cases of AIDS was 1825:1. By 1984, a much higher percentage of this group of men had been infected, and the ratio of seropositive men to AIDS cases had fallen to 28:1.

Among persons with hemophilia, AIDS has now surpassed hemorrhage as the leading cause of mortality. The risk for seropositivity with HIV has correlated with transfusion requirements for Factor VIII concentrates and the source of plasma products. The use of commercial plasma products in the USA resulted in a very high rate of seropositivity, while in Europe, where the bulk of clotting factor material was locally produced from donors in an area where risk of AIDS was low, prevalence of seropos-

itivity was low. Fortunately, HIV can be inactivated by heating; commercial products now are heat-treated, which should substantially reduce the risk of infection.

In Africa, the incidence patterns are very different from those in the USA and Europe; eg, the sex incidence is nearly equal. Furthermore, homosexuality is generally denied, as well as sexual practices such as anal intercourse, that are considered risk factors in the USA and Europe. However, almost all African patients are in the sexually active age range.

Surprisingly, except for Australia, almost no cases have been identified in the Western Pacific region, even in cities noted for sexual tourism.

Several hundred infants and children with AIDS have been reported, most of whom are offspring of mothers with or at risk of AIDS, who received multiple blood transfusions, or who were hemophiliacs receiving blood components. It appears that HIV can be transmitted transplacentally or perinatally. The virus has been demonstrated in breast milk and, although rare, this route of transmission has been implicated. It is clear that very close, frequent, and intimate contact between infant and parent is required for transmission, as no one other than a parent in the household of children with AIDS has been reported to be infected and this has occurred only rarely and under unusual circumstances involving repeated exposure to body fluids.

The AIDS syndrome is the most severe manifestation of a spectrum of AIDS-related conditions that can occur in individuals infected with HIV (see Symptoms and Signs, below). The risk that a person infected with HIV will develop the AIDS syndrome has varied from 2 to 35%/yr in different populations studied. Because of the often long latent period between infection and the development of clinical syndromes, long-term risk data are unavailable. Furthermore, it is likely that all long-term sequelae (eg, malignancy and chronic degenerative diseases) have not yet been elucidated. Differences in rates of AIDS expression in different studies may reflect not only duration of exposure in a cohort, but also factors such as source, route, dose, and frequency of exposure; environmental factors such as other infections or immune-altering stresses; and host genetic susceptibility.

Symptoms and Signs

A broad spectrum of clinical problems may occur after infection with HIV. Immediately after infection and for an unknown period, there may be an **antibody-negative, asymptomatic carrier state,** detectable only by viral culture studies. Within 2 to 4 wk after infection, some patients have a 3- to 14-day **acute nonspecific viral syndrome** with fever, malaise, rash, arthralgias, and generalized lymphadenopathy, usually followed in 1 to 3 mo by seroconversion. Subsequently, these manifestations disappear (although lymphadenopathy may persist) and the patients may become **antibody-positive, asymptomatic carriers.** *For most patients there is no such acute viral syndrome*, and an asymptomatic, antibody-positive period follows infection with the virus that may last for years. Unless a blood specimen is found to be seropositive, diagnosis must await the presence of 1 or more manifestations of the immune defect. Among patients with transfusion-associated AIDS, the average time from infection to diagnosis is about 20 mo for children and 30 mo for adults. Among homosexual men followed from the time of seroconversion (discovery of antibodies against the virus) for up to 6 yr, about 25% developed AIDS-related conditions and up to 15% developed the full-blown AIDS syndrome.

During the asymptomatic, seropositive stage, patients may be noted to have a low T4:T8 ratio. Many of these patients develop symptoms and signs that are suggestive, but do not manifest all the secondary complications of AIDS, giving rise to several other designations.

The AIDS-related complex (ARC) is a constellation of chronic signs and symptoms manifested by persons belonging to groups with an increased incidence of AIDS, but

who do not manifest the typical opportunistic infections or Kaposi's sarcoma that characterize the full-blown syndrome. These signs and symptoms may include generalized lymphadenopathy, weight loss, intermittent fever, malaise and lethargy, chronic diarrhea, rectal condylomata, lymphopenia, leukopenia, anemia, idiopathic thrombocytopenia, immunologic abnormalities characteristic of AIDS, and oral thrush (candidiasis). A subset of ARC patients have **persistent generalized lymphadenopathy (PGL),** which describes patients with lymphadenopathy (nodes $\geq$ 1 cm) of at least 3 mo duration involving 2 or more extrainguinal sites confirmed on physical examination (in the absence of any current illness or drug use known to cause lymphadenopathy) and the presence of reactive hyperplasia in a lymph node, if a biopsy is done. A more severe manifestation of ARC is the **wasting syndrome,** which is characterized by progressive weight loss $\geq$ 15% body wt associated with fever, night sweats, oral thrush, or diarrhea persisting for $\geq$ 3 mo; full-blown AIDS is more likely to occur than in a patient whose only sign is PGL.

The full-blown AIDS syndrome consists of any of the above symptoms and signs with progression to the development of opportunistic infections and/or certain **secondary cancers** known to be associated with HIV infection (eg, Kaposi's sarcoma **[KS]**, non-Hodgkin's lymphoma, or primary lymphoma of the brain). However, some patients are first seen with an opportunistic infection or malignancy without the preceding symptoms or syndromes.

Certain symptomatic or invasive **opportunistic infections** have been particularly noted: *Pneumocystis carinii* pneumonia, chronic cryptosporidiosis, toxoplasmosis, extraintestinal strongyloidiasis, isosporiasis, candidiasis (esophageal, bronchial, or pulmonary), cryptococcosis, histoplasmosis, mycobacterial infection with *Mycobacterium avium* complex or *M. kansasii*, cytomegalovirus infection, chronic mucocutaneous or disseminated herpes simplex virus infection, and progressive multifocal leukoencephalopathy. Several other secondary infectious diseases have been noted; eg, multidermatomal herpes zoster, recurrent *Salmonella* bacteremia, nocardiosis, tuberculosis, oral candidiasis (thrush), and chronic interstitial pneumonitis. Other less specific infections may occur.

Neurologic disorders vary from acute and chronic aseptic meningitis to peripheral neuropathies with weakness and paresthesias to encephalopathy with seizures, focal deficits, hallucinations, and progressive dementia. Neurologic disorders and renal disease associated with AIDS are discussed respectively in Chs. 125 and 149.

Disease patterns vary; eg, in the USA and Europe, over 90% of AIDS patients who have KS were homosexual or bisexual men (probably because of particular cofactors in this group), and recently the incidence of KS has been diminishing in this group. Most AIDS cases in the USA and Europe (about 40%) present with *P. carinii* pneumonia, which is reported in only about 14% of patients in Africa. CNS involvement occurs in 30 to 50% of patients, the result of opportunistic infections, malignancies (primarily lymphomas), hemorrhage secondary to thrombocytopenia, and, probably, direct infection of nerve tissue. Patients are devastated by all these complications, and mortality approaches 100%, with 92% dying as a direct consequence of opportunistic infections.

Laboratory Findings and Diagnosis

The immunologic abnormalities in AIDS include anergy (demonstrated by lack of delayed hypersensitivity responses to intradermal injection of common antigens; eg, tetanus, mumps, *Candida albicans*, *Trichophyton*), poor T cell proliferative responses to mitogens (phytohemagglutinin, Concanavalin-A) and antigens, decreased numbers of T cells, polyclonal hypergammaglobulinemia, elevated immune complex levels, diminished antibody responses to both recall and new antigens, decreased natural killer function, and increased levels of α_1-thymosin, acid-labile interferon, and β_2-microglobulin. The T cell deficiency is primarily due to decreased numbers of T helper cells **(T_h)**,

while suppressor cells **(T_s)** are normal or increased. This leads to reduction of the normal T_h/T_s ratio of about 2:1 (often reversal to < 1). Patients with early AIDS or lymphadenopathy may have reduced T_h/T_s ratios as an early laboratory sign of HIV infection, but a low T_h/T_s is *not* diagnostic of AIDS, since a variety of viral infections (eg, CMV, Epstein-Barr virus, influenza, and hepatitis B) may produce transient reductions. In patients with AIDS who develop opportunistic infections, T_h/T_s ratios are usually < 0.5.

A presumptive clinical diagnosis of HIV infection may be made on the basis of the clinical manifestations described above. The isolation of HIV from serum, cells, or lymph nodes provides the most specific diagnosis of HIV infection, but current technics lack sensitivity and are not readily available. The demonstration of antibodies to HIV is also useful diagnostically.

Two tests for antibody to HIV are currently used. The first is an enzyme-linked immunosorbent assay **(ELISA)** in which beads or microtiter plate wells are coated with disrupted, inactivated HIV virus antigens and goat antihuman immunoglobulin conjugated or "linked" to an enzyme that, on incubation with the appropriate substance, will produce a color. A serum or plasma sample from the person being tested is placed in contact with the antigen-coated beads or cells. If antibody is present in the sample, it links to the antigen and is detected by the antihuman antibodies conjugated to the enzyme. Sensitivity of the test varies in different laboratories, but almost 100% of patients with AIDS and with ARC are seropositive. Antibody levels to HIV may decrease in the advanced stages of AIDS, usually after multiple opportunistic infections, and may not be detectable by ELISA; but this usually does not represent a diagnostic problem.

False-positive ELISA tests do occur, particularly in asymptomatic persons who do not belong to a high-risk group. While ELISA is a good screening test, when it is positive in an asymptomatic person, it is advisable to repeat the test. If positive a second time, the recommendation is to confirm the ELISA with a test that is more specific; ie, the **Western blot**. The Western blot is an immunoelectrophoretic procedure for identifying antibodies to proteins of specific molecular weight, in this instance those associated with HIV. It is a labor-intensive test that requires considerable skill and experience. For public health purposes, patients with repeatedly positive screening tests for HIV antibody (eg, ELISA) in whom antibody is also identified by the use of supplemental tests (eg, Western blot) should be considered infected and infective. (ELISA and Western blot are used not only to evaluate patients suspected of HIV infection, but to screen blood donors, and are major contributors to improving the safety of blood supplies.)

Finally, it should be noted that individuals in the early stages of HIV infection, who have not yet mounted an antibody response, may have negative ELISA and Western blot tests **(false negatives)**. Such individuals have been reported to remain antibody-negative while yielding positive **cultures** for several months. Efforts are in progress to develop tests that will directly measure viral antigens, rather than antiviral antibodies detected by ELISA and Western blot.

Prognosis

Although there are no complete recoveries from AIDS, some patients are long-term (> 5 yr) survivors; eg, patients with KS who do not have severe immune defects or opportunistic infections. In one large study, the median survival was determined based on the initial clinical manifestation: For patients with Kaposi's sarcoma alone, it was 125 wk; *P. carinii* pneumonia alone, 35 wk; and any other opportunistic infection, 18 wk. While about 85% of these patients survived their initial hospitalization, their quality of life was markedly compromised and about ½ spent 30 to 50% of their remaining lifetimes in the hospital. Opportunistic infection is the cause of life-threatening illness or death in > 90% of AIDS patients.

Prevention and Treatment

There is no effective treatment other than that of the opportunistic infections, neoplasms, and other complications. Clinical trials are in progress to evaluate the efficacy of potential antiviral drugs, particularly those that have been shown to inhibit the viral enzyme, reverse transcriptase. However, difficulties in finding effective drugs are enormous, exemplified by the challenges presented by an organism whose genes become part of host cell DNA and which crosses the blood-brain barrier with ease. Development of a vaccine to prevent HIV infection is being pursued actively, and studies in chimpanzees have been encouraging. Human trials will follow and it is hoped that an effective vaccine may be available in about 5 yr. However, there are many potential problems in developing a vaccine and in designing clinical trials in appropriate groups; it may take much longer or even be impossible to develop a vaccine. In the meantime, preventive measures based on knowledge of the etiology and epidemiology (see above) are essential.

Most infections occur as a result of repeated and close contact with a carrier of HIV, specifically mucous membrane contact with blood or body fluids of the carrier. Sexual relationships are the major source of such contacts, and people must be educated to modify sexual practices; eg, to avoid sexual encounters with persons in high-risk groups, reduce the number and frequency of sexual contacts, avoid high-risk practices (eg, anal intercourse), and use protective devices such as condoms. The efficacy of condoms in preventing infection with HIV is under study, but *consistent* use of condoms should reduce transmission of HIV by preventing exposure to semen and infected lymphocytes. Whether symptomatic or not, persons who know they carry the HIV virus should be counseled to avoid sexual contacts in which body fluids may be exchanged with uninfected persons.

Since HIV may be transmitted in utero or during or after birth, women carriers and those in high-risk groups should be counseled, and testing for antibody to HIV should be offered to women in high-risk groups. Women known to be HIV-positive should be advised to defer pregnancy.

Parenteral drug users need to be educated and counseled with regard to the risk of sharing needles with other drug users.

Testing for antibody to HIV should be offered on a confidential basis to anyone requesting it, but only in conjunction with pre- and post-test counseling by someone familiar with its significance. Confidentiality is necessary because the patient's job, insurability, and social life can be jeopardized. Counseling is necessary because test results require sophisticated analysis; patients need to be well informed before the tests are performed, and the results must be fully explained afterward.

HIV carriers and persons belonging to a high-risk group (*even if their HIV antibody test results are negative*) should not donate their blood (or organs for transplantation), and should inform medical and dental professionals of their status. The latter should wear gloves when examining *all* patients if contact with mucous membranes may occur, and body fluids and tissue samples should be handled in the same manner as those from patients with hepatitis B.

Accidental needle sticks of health care personnel are remarkably common and special emphasis must be placed on teaching all health care students and professionals how to avoid these potentially very dangerous accidents. While the risk of HIV transmission appears to be much less than that of hepatitis B transmission, the potential consequences are much worse.

Patients with HIV infection generally need not be isolated in the hospital, except when their complicating infections (eg, suspected or proven TB) require that other patients and hospital personnel be protected. Surfaces contaminated by blood or other body fluids should be cleaned and disinfected; HIV is readily inactivated by heat and commonly used disinfecting agents, including peroxide, alcohols, phenolics, and hypo-

chlorite. Although AIDS patients are not particularly contagious to other hospital personnel or patients, their body fluids and blood should be handled with extreme care, following the same procedures used with patients who carry hepatitis B virus.

20. HYPERSENSITIVITY REACTIONS

Pathologic processes that result from specific interactions between antigens (exogenous or endogenous) and either humoral antibodies or sensitized lymphocytes. This definition excludes disorders in which antibodies are demonstrated but have no known pathophysiologic significance (eg, the antibody to heart tissue that appears following heart surgery or myocardial infarction), even though their presence may have diagnostic value.

The gamut of diseases in which hypersensitivity phenomena may play a role ranges from hay fever (which results from hypersensitivity to an exogenous antigen, is limited to the respiratory and ocular mucosal surfaces, and lacks systemic morbidity) to SLE (a multisystem disease with significant morbidity, and which is associated with hypersensitivity to autoantigens).

Classification therefore is difficult. Some classifications are based on the time required for the appearance of symptoms or skin test reactions after exposure to antigen (such as immediate and delayed hypersensitivity), on the type of antigen (such as drug reactions), or on the nature of organ involvement. These classifications, however, do not take into account that more than one type of immune response may be occurring or that more than one type may be necessary to produce immunologic injury. The Gell and Coombs classification into 4 types of hypersensitivity reactions is used widely and continues to accommodate newer mechanisms that have been described such as receptor-specific antibody mechanisms and antibody-mediated cytotoxicity.

TYPE I HYPERSENSITIVITY REACTIONS

(Immediate-Type, Atopic, Reaginic, Anaphylactic, or IgE-Mediated Hypersensitivity Reactions)

Reactions resulting from the release of pharmacologically active substances such as histamine, leukotrienes (the active agents in slow-reactive substance of anaphylaxis [SRS-A]), prostaglandins, platelet activating factor, and eosinophilic chemotactic factor (ECF) from IgE-sensitized basophils and mast cells after contact with specific antigen. The released substances cause vasodilatation, increased capillary permeability, smooth muscle contraction, and blood and tissue eosinophilia. The consequent clinical manifestations include urticaria, angioedema, hypotension, and spasm of bronchial, GI, or uterine musculature.

The clinical conditions in which Type I reactions play a role include allergic extrinsic asthma, seasonal allergic rhinitis, systemic anaphylaxis, reactions to stinging insects, some reactions to foods and drugs, and some cases of urticaria.

Diagnostic Tests

The most convenient test to detect IgE-sensitized mast cells is the **direct skin test**. Test solutions are made from extracts of materials that are inhaled, ingested, or injected, such as wind-borne pollens from certain trees, grasses, and weeds; house dust; animal danders; molds; foods; insect venoms; horse serum; and certain drugs. The test solutions are applied either to scratches or shallow punctures of the skin or by injecting them intradermally. The former usually is safer because less antigen is introduced, and often is done initially to identify materials that may cause a systemic reaction if injected intradermally.

Scratches about 1 cm long and 2.5 cm apart are made with a needle on the forearm or back, and a drop of concentrated (1:20) test extract is placed on each scratch. Alternatively, the skin is punctured through a drop of test extract with commercially available scarifiers or a darning needle (prick technic). Control tests are performed simultaneously, using the diluent by prick and intradermally; and either histamine (0.01 mg histamine base/mL) or morphine sulfate (0.1 mg/mL), which is a mast cell degranulator, intradermally. The diluent should give a negative test result and the latter 2 substances should produce a wheal measuring 1 cm or less. The histamine and morphine tests determine the reactivity of the capillaries in the skin and the presence of mast cells capable of releasing histamine. These tests are especially important as controls when the patient has been taking drugs that are known to inhibit skin tests by blocking the effect of histamine on blood vessels (eg, antihistamines, hydroxyzine, and tricyclic antidepressants) and drugs that are mast cell degranulators (eg, codeine, meperidine, and morphine).

A positive wheal-and-flare reaction usually is obvious by 7 to 20 min after the test extract is applied. If the diameter of the wheal is > 0.5 cm larger than the diluent control wheal, the test is positive and an intradermal test should not be performed. An intradermal test can be done if the reaction is smaller than this or if the patient has dermatographia, which raises the question whether the wheal and flare are immunologically mediated.

In the intradermal test, a tuberculin syringe and short-bevel No. 26 needle are used to inject 0.02 mL of a 1:500 or 1:1000 concentration of the test extract into the skin. A wheal > 0.5 cm larger than the diluent control wheal, appearing within 15 min, is a positive reaction. The size of the skin test reaction has a rough correlation with clinical symptoms, although some patients with large reactions do not have symptoms and some patients with small intradermal skin test reactions do have symptoms. Therefore, most physicians monitor the patient with periodic clinical reevaluations to determine the significance of skin tests.

A radioallergosorbent test (RAST) may be performed when direct skin testing is not possible because of generalized dermatitis, extreme dermatographia, or the patient's anxiety. The RAST detects the presence of antigen-specific serum IgE. A known antigen, in the form of an insoluble polymer-antigen conjugate, is mixed with the serum to be tested. Any IgE in the serum that is specific for the antigen will attach to the conjugate. Adding ^{125}I-labeled anti-IgE antibody and measuring the amount of radioactivity taken up by the conjugate determine the quantity of antigen-specific IgE in the patient's circulation.

Leukocyte histamine release, another in vitro test, detects antigen-specific IgE on sensitized basophils by measuring antigen-induced histamine release from the patient's leukocytes. Though not widely used diagnostically, this test has given valuable insight into the kinetics of histamine release and has been useful in evaluating drugs for their ability to inhibit histamine release.

Provocative challenge may be performed when a positive skin test has raised a question concerning the role of the particular antigen in the production of symptoms. The antigen is applied to the eyes, nose, or lungs. **Ophthalmic testing** offers no advantage over skin testing and is rarely positive when skin tests are negative. However, it is sometimes used in testing hypersensitivity to pollens in suspected atopic conjunctivitis. A small amount of antigen (eg, dried pollen or an aqueous extract of pollen in the same concentration as used for intradermal testing) is applied to the lower conjunctival sac. An appropriate control (eg, the diluent or dried pine pollen) is used in the other eye. A positive response is characterized by burning, smarting, itching, or redness of the bulbar conjunctiva exceeding that in the control eye. Edema often follows. If a positive reaction occurs, the eye should be irrigated with isotonic saline, then a drop of epinephrine 1:1000 instilled.

Nasal challenge is performed occasionally. Numerous methods introduce the antigen—insufflating dried pollen into the nose, spraying aqueous extract from a squeeze bottle or by nebulizer, or inserting a cotton pledget soaked in aqueous extract. Response is positive if itching, sneezing, and rhinorrhea occur, accompanied by a change in the appearance of the mucosa.

Bronchial inhalation challenge has long been used by European allergists to select the antigens to be used for immunotherapy. Although bronchial challenge remains predominantly an investigative tool in the USA, some allergists use it when the clinical significance of a positive skin test is unclear or when skin test reagents are not available, to demonstrate that symptoms are related to materials to which a patient is exposed (eg, in occupationally related exposures).

Total IgE level determination also is used in evaluating patients with Type I reactions using a paper radioimmunosorbent test **(PRIST)**. Serum IgE levels may be elevated in allergic asthma, allergic bronchopulmonary aspergillosis, parasitic infections, and eczema; the levels are normal in allergic alveolitis. Very high IgE levels are seen in allergic bronchopulmonary aspergillosis and therefore may help to distinguish this form of allergic lung disease from asthma induced by pollen, dust, and mold, and from nonallergic forms of asthma. The normally wide range of IgE levels, however, limits its usefulness in separating allergic from nonallergic asthma.

Provocative food testing may be performed when regularly occurring symptoms are suspected of being food-related and skin tests are of doubtful clinical significance (see also FOOD ALLERGY AND INTOLERANCE in Ch. 21). Except for acute anaphylactic-type reactions, urticaria, rhinitis, asthma, and GI symptoms to foods, food intolerances, idiosyncrasies, and vague constitutional symptoms (fatigue, headache, insomnia) have not been demonstrably due to IgE-mediated hypersensitivity. Some adverse reactions to foods are due to nonspecific mediator releasers or to mediators themselves (such as histamine) in the food.

Food additives such as tartrazine yellow, sodium benzoate, bisulfites, and monosodium glutamate also have been demonstrated to produce Type I-like reactions. The mechanism is unknown and skin tests with these materials in general have not been helpful. Documentation of relationship of symptoms to ingestion of these additives is obtained by removing the additive from the diet and having the patient ingest them in a double-blind fashion.

Prick skin tests have been of value in selecting foods to eliminate from the diet that are suspected of causing nausea, vomiting, diarrhea, naso-ocular, asthma, and anaphylactic-like symptoms. In these IgE-mediated reactions the subjects are skin-test–positive to all foods capable of producing symptoms, and also may have positive skin tests to foods that will not produce symptoms. The clinical significance of a positive prick skin test in both adults and children must be documented by having the subject eat the food in question. In those subjects with severe anaphylaxis, provocative food testing is *not* indicated if the patient is skin-test–positive to the clinically suspected food. In other subjects provocative food challenge may not be necessary if elimination of one suspected food to which a patient is prick-test–positive results in relief of symptoms. The prick skin test only predicts symptoms that will occur within 2 h of eating a food and should be performed when symptoms suggestive of being IgE-mediated occur shortly after eating. When symptoms are relatively infrequent and food is thought to be the cause, a food diary may be useful in selecting foods to avoid. **Intradermal skin tests** to foods cause such a high frequency of positive reactions that they should not be performed in evaluating patients. The number of laboratories, lack of standardization of food antigens, and lack of quality controls has prevented a determination of the role of the radioallergosorbent test **(RAST)** in predicting its ability to detect food-related allergic symptoms. At present there is no evidence to support the use of cytotoxicity

testing or sublingual or subcutaneous provocative testing in the diagnosis of food or inhalant allergic symptoms.

In subjects suspected of having reactions to foods hours after eating, the relationship of symptoms to foods is determined by an **elimination diet** and, if symptoms improve, by reexposure to the food to determine if it is capable of inducing symptoms. All challenges are best performed by introducing the food in a fashion not recognized by the subject or known by the individual administering the challenge (double-blind); but if this is not possible, an open challenge can be performed. The basic diet is determined by eliminating foods suspected by the patient of causing symptoms or placing the patient on a diet composed of relatively nonallergic foods (see TABLE 20–1).

Commonly incriminated food allergens include milk, eggs, shellfish, nuts, wheat, peanuts, soybeans, and chocolate, and all products containing one or more of these ingredients. Most of the common allergens and all suspected foods must be eliminated from the starting diet. No foods or fluids may be consumed other than those specified in the starting diet. Eating in restaurants is not advisable, since the patient (and physician) must know the exact composition of all meals. Furthermore, one must always be certain of the purity of products used—for example, ordinary "rye" bread contains some wheat flour.

If no improvement occurs after 1 wk on a given diet, another should be tried. If symptoms are relieved, one new food is added to the diet and eaten in more than the usual amount for > 24 h or until symptoms recur. Alternatively, small amounts of the food to be tested are eaten in the physician's presence, and the patient's reactions observed. Aggravation or recrudescence of symptoms following the addition of a new food is the best evidence of allergy to that item. Such evidence should be verified by noting the effect of removing that food from the diet for several days, then restoring it.

TABLE 20–1. ELIMINATION DIETS—ALLOWABLE FOODS

Foodstuff	*Diet No. 1** (No beef, pork, fowl, milk, rye, corn)	*Diet No. 2** (No beef, lamb, milk, rice)	*Diet No. 3** (No lamb, fowl, rye, rice, corn, milk)
Cereal	Rice products	Corn products	
Vegetable	Lettuce, spinach, carrots, beets, artichokes	Corn, tomatoes, peas, asparagus, squash, string beans	Lima beans, beets, potatoes (white and sweet), string beans, tomatoes
Meat	Lamb	Chicken, bacon	Beef, bacon
Flour (bread or biscuits)	Rice	Corn, 100% rye (ordinary "rye" bread contains wheat)	Lima beans, soybeans, potatoes
Fruit	Lemons, pears, grapefruit	Peaches, apricots, prunes, pineapple	Grapefruit, lemons, peaches, apricots
Fat	Cottonseed oil, olive oil	Corn oil, cottonseed oil	Cottonseed oil, olive oil
Beverage	Tea, coffee (black), lemonade		Tea, coffee (black), lemonade, juice from approved fruit
Miscellaneous	Tapioca pudding, gelatin, cane sugar, maple sugar, salt, olives	Cane sugar, gelatin, corn syrup, salt	Tapioca pudding, gelatin, cane sugar, maple sugar, salt, olives

* Diet No. 4: Should symptoms persist when on the above 3 elimination diets, the daily diet may be restricted to an elemental diet, such as Vivonex®.

Since allergy to one or another ingredient may exist, vitamin supplements should not be added until some therapeutic response to the diet has been obtained. In severely restricted diets, a multivitamin preparation of synthetic origin may be added after the first 3 days.

TYPE II HYPERSENSITIVITY REACTIONS

(Cytotoxic, Cell-Stimulating, or Antibody-Dependent Cytotoxicity; Cytolytic Complement-Dependent Cytotoxicity)

Reactions that result when antibody reacts with antigenic components of a cell or tissue elements or with antigen or hapten that has become intimately coupled to a cell or tissue. The antigen-antibody reaction may cause opsonic adherence through coating of the cell with antibody; the reaction is then called **immune adherence,** which occurs by activation of complement components through C3 (with consequent phagocytosis of the cell); or by activation of the full complement system with consequent cytolysis or tissue damage.

Clinical examples of cell injury in which antibody reacts with **antigenic components of a cell** are Coombs-positive hemolytic anemias, antibody-induced thrombocytopenic purpura, leukopenia, pemphigus, pemphigoid, Goodpasture's syndrome, and pernicious anemia. These reactions occur in patients receiving incompatible transfusions, in hemolytic disease of the newborn, and in neonatal thrombocytopenia, and they also may play a part in multisystem hypersensitivity diseases such as SLE. For a discussion of renal effects, see Ch. 149.

The mechanism of injury is best exemplified by the effect on RBCs. In hemolytic anemias the RBCs are destroyed either by intravascular hemolysis or by macrophage phagocytosis, predominantly within the spleen. In vitro studies have demonstrated that in the presence of complement some complement-binding antibodies such as the blood group antibodies anti-A and anti-B cause rapid hemolysis; others such as anti-Le cause a slow lysis of cells; and still others do not damage cells directly but cause their adherence to and phagocytosis by phagocytes. By contrast, Rh antibodies on RBCs do not activate complement, and they destroy cells predominantly by extravascular phagocytosis.

Examples in which the antigen is a component of tissue include *early acute* (hyperacute) graft rejection of a transplanted kidney, which is due to the presence of antibody to vascular endothelium, and Goodpasture's syndrome, which is due to antibody reacting with glomerular and alveolar basement membrane endothelium. In experimental Goodpasture's syndrome, complement is an important mediator of injury, but the role of complement has not been clearly determined in the early acute graft rejection.

Examples of reactions that are due to **haptenic coupling** with cells or tissue include many of the drug hypersensitivity reactions, such as penicillin-induced hemolytic anemia and purpura.

Antireceptor hypersensitivity reactions *alter cellular function as a result of antibody binding to membrane receptors.* In a number of diseases (eg, myasthenia gravis, Graves' and Raynaud's diseases, Type B insulin-resistant diabetes, and asthma) antibodies to cell membrane receptors have been reported. In myasthenia gravis, the production of antibodies by immunization to the acetylcholine receptor in a number of animals has resulted in the typical muscle fatigue and weakness noted in humans. In humans, this antibody also is demonstrated in the serum and on muscle membranes. In addition, when serum or the IgG fraction from patients with myasthenia gravis is transfused into nonhuman primates, a self-limiting myasthenic syndrome is produced. This antibody prevents the binding of endogenously produced acetylcholine to its receptor, thereby preventing muscle activation. In some diabetics with extreme insulin resistance, antibodies to insulin receptors have been demonstrated, thus preventing insulin

binding to its receptor. In patients with Graves' disease, an antibody to the thyroid-stimulating hormone **(TSH)** receptor has been identified that simulates the effect of TSH on its receptor, resulting in hyperthyroidism. Antibodies also have been demonstrated to the β_2-adrenergic receptor in asthma and Raynaud's disease, but their role in these diseases has not been determined.

Antibody-mediated cytotoxicity (ADCC) *reactions occur when an antibody-coated cell is injured by* ***K (killer) cells.*** Technics are available to determine B and T cell subsets of circulating lymphocytes. There is also a subset that does not have B or T cell markers; these are called **null cells** and include **K** and **NK (natural killer)** cells. The K cells bind to cells coated with IgG by their Fc receptors and are capable of destroying the target cell. The NK cells do not require antibody coating of the cell for recognition and are capable of lysing tumor cells, virus-infected cells, and fetal cells. These mechanisms have been demonstrated in animal models and in vitro studies of hypersensitivity, but their role in human disease has not been established.

Diagnostic Tests

Tests to support this mechanism of immunologic injury include (1) detecting the presence of antibody or complement on the cell or on tissue, or (2) detecting the presence, in serum, of antibody to a cell surface antigen, a tissue antigen, a receptor, or a foreign (exogenous) antigen. Although complement often is required for Type II cell injury, and may be detected on the cell or in the tissue, total serum hemolytic complement activity is not depressed as it often is in immune complex (Type III) hypersensitivity reactions.

The **direct antiglobulin (Coombs')** and **anti–non-γ-globulin tests** detect antibody and complement on RBCs, respectively. These tests use rabbit antisera, one to immunoglobulin and the other to complement. When these reagents are mixed with RBCs coated with immunoglobulin or complement, agglutination occurs. Antibodies eluted from these cells have shown both a specificity for RBC blood group antigens and an ability to fix complement, thus demonstrating that they are true autoantibodies and account for the complement present on the RBCs in the direct non–γ-globulin test.

The **indirect antiglobulin test** is used to detect the presence of a circulating antibody to RBC antigens. The patient's serum is incubated with RBCs of the same blood group (to preclude false results due to incompatibility), and the antiglobulin test is then performed on these RBCs. Agglutination confirms the presence of antibody to RBC antigens.

In penicillin-induced hemolytic anemia the patient has a positive direct Coombs' test while receiving penicillin but has a negative indirect antiglobulin test using RBCs of the same type as the patient. The patient's serum, however, will agglutinate the indirect-test RBCs if they are coated with penicillin.

Fluorescent microscopy is most commonly used to detect the presence of immunoglobulin or complement in tissue (by the direct technic) and also can be used to determine the specificity of a circulating antibody (by the indirect technic). In the **direct immunofluorescent technic,** animal antibody specific for human immunoglobulin or complement is labeled with a fluorescent dye (usually fluorescein) and then layered on tissue. When the tissue is examined under the fluorescent microscope, a typical fluorescent color (green for fluorescein) indicates the presence of human immunoglobulin or complement in the tissue. Direct immunofluorescence also can be used to detect the presence of other serum proteins, tissue components, or exogenous antigen as long as specific animal antibodies to them can be produced. The technic itself does not indicate a cell-specific antigen unless the antibody can be eluted from the tissue and its specificity for tissue antigens determined.

In Goodpasture's syndrome the immunofluorescent pattern is seen as a linear fluorescence on kidney and lung basement membrane. When antibody is eluted from the kidney of a patient with Goodpasture's syndrome and layered on normal kidney or

lung, it attaches to the basement membrane and gives the same linear fluorescent pattern when tested with fluorescein-labeled antibody to human γ-globulin **(indirect immunofluorescence).**

In pemphigus the direct immunofluorescent technic reveals antibody to an antigen present in the intercellular cement of the prickle cell layer; in pemphigoid, to an antigen in the basement membrane. In both diseases serum antibody is detectable by the indirect immunofluorescent technic. The indirect immunofluorescent technic is used to detect tissue-specific circulating antibodies in many other disorders; eg, thyroiditis (antithyroid antibodies) and SLE (antinuclear antibodies, anticytoplasmic antibodies).

Antireceptor tests for detection of antibody to the acetylcholine receptors are commercially available, but tests for the insulin and thyroid receptors are not. The clinical significance of the test for detection of antibody to the β_2-adrenergic receptor has not been determined. There are no clinical situations in which the **antibody-dependent cytotoxicity test** is necessary.

TYPE III HYPERSENSITIVITY REACTIONS

(Immune Complex [IC]-Mediated, Soluble Complex, or Toxic Complex Hypersensitivity Reactions)

Reactions that result from deposition of soluble circulating antigen-antibody (immune) complexes in vessels or tissue. The ICs activate complement and thus initiate a sequence of events that results in polymorphonuclear cell migration and release of lysosomal proteolytic enzymes and permeability factors in tissues, thereby producing an acute inflammatory reaction. The consequences of IC formation depend in part on the relative proportions of antigen and antibody in the complex. With an excess of antibody, the complexes rapidly precipitate near the site of the antigen (eg, within the joints in RA) or are phagocytosed by macrophages and therefore are not toxic. With a slight excess of antigen, the complex tends to be more soluble and may cause systemic reactions by being deposited in various tissues.

Examples of clinical conditions in which ICs appear to play some role are serum sickness due to serum, drugs, or viral hepatitis antigen, SLE, RA, polyarteritis, cryoglobulinemia, hypersensitivity pneumonitis, bronchopulmonary aspergillosis, acute glomerulonephritis, chronic membranoproliferative glomerulonephritis, and associated renal disease (see Ch. 149). In brochopulmonary aspergillosis, drug- or serum-induced serum sickness, and some forms of renal disease, an IgE-mediated reaction is thought to precede the Type III reaction.

The classic laboratory examples of Type III reactions are the local Arthus reaction and experimental serum sickness.

In the **Arthus reaction** (classically a local skin reaction), animals are first hyperimmunized to induce large amounts of circulating IgG antibodies and are then given a small amount of antigen intradermally. The antigen precipitates with the excess IgG and activates complement, so that a highly inflammatory, edematous, painful local lesion rapidly appears (by 4 to 6 h), which may progress to a sterile abscess containing many polymorphonuclear cells, and then to necrosis of tissue. A necrotizing vasculitis with occluded arteriolar lumina can be seen microscopically. No lag period precedes the reaction because antibody already is present.

In **experimental serum sickness,** a large amount of antigen is injected into a nonimmunized animal. After a lag period, antibody is produced; when this reaches a critical level (10 to 14 days in man), antigen-antibody complexes form that are deposited in endothelial vessels, where they produce widespread vascular injury characterized by the presence of polymorphonuclear leukocytes. During the appearance of the vasculitis a fall in serum complement can be detected, and antigen, antibody, and complement can be found in the areas of vasculitis. The antigen-antibody complexes are not capa-

ble of inducing injury by themselves, however, but require the presence of increased vascular permeability such as occurs in IgE-mediated (Type I) reactions and when complement is activated to enhance vascular deposition of the IC.

Diagnostic Tests

Type III reactions can be suspected in human disease when a vasculitis occurs. In polyarteritis the presence of vasculitis is the only clinical evidence to support a role for ICs. Further support may be obtained by direct immunofluorescent tests (as described above), which may indicate the presence of antigen, immunoglobulin, and complement in the area of vasculitis.

In experimental studies, fluorescent microscopy shows a coarse granular deposit ("lumpy bumps") along the basement membrane when animal glomeruli are stained for the presence of immunoglobulin and complement. A similar distribution can be seen in Type III human renal diseases (see Ch. 149). The electron microscope also can be used to detect electron-dense deposits (similar to those seen in experimental serum sickness), which are felt to be the antigen-antibody complexes. Rarely, the presence of both antigen and antibody can be detected by immunofluorescence in the inflamed tissue—this has been demonstrated in the renal disease of SLE and the vasculitic lesions of hepatitis-antigen–associated serum sickness.

Further evidence in support of a Type III reaction is obtained by demonstrating the presence of circulating antibody to antigens such as horse serum, hepatitis antigen, DNA, altered IgG (rheumatoid factor), and mold spores. In SLE, for example, a rise in antibody to native undenatured, double-stranded DNA and a fall in serum complement occur during exacerbations of renal disease. If the antigen is unknown, levels of total serum complement and of the early components (C1, C4, or C2) can be tested; a depressed level indicates classic complement activation and therefore that a Type III reaction is occurring. The C4 assay is the one most readily available.

In allergic pulmonary aspergillosis an intradermal skin test with aspergillus antigen may produce an IgE wheal-and-flare reaction followed by an Arthus-like reaction.

Until recently, detection of ICs in the serum was by cryoprecipitation (using the property of some complexes to precipitate in the cold). Sophisticated equipment also could detect soluble complexes by analytic ultracentrifugation and sucrose density gradient centrifugation. Several tests detecting circulating ICs now have been developed that depend on the ability of complexes to react with complement components (such as **C1q-binding assays**) and the ability of complexes to inhibit the reaction between monoclonal rheumatoid factor and IgG. Assays such as the **Raji cell assay** are based on the interaction of ICs containing complement components with cellular receptors; eg, a C3 receptor on the Raji cell. Other assays are available, but the 3 mentioned are the most commonly used. No single test detects all ICs, and their use in clinical medicine is limited to following the activity of certain diseases.

TYPE IV HYPERSENSITIVITY REACTIONS

(Cellular, Cell-Mediated, Delayed, or Tuberculin-Type Hypersensitivity Reactions)

Reactions caused by sensitized lymphocytes (T cells) after contact with antigen. **Delayed hypersensitivity differs from other hypersensitivity reactions in that it is mediated by sensitized lymphocytes and not by antibody**. Thus, transfer of delayed hypersensitivity from sensitized to normal persons can be demonstrated with peripheral blood leukocytes or with an extract of these cells **(transfer factor)**, but not with serum.

The sensitized T lymphocyte that has been triggered or activated by contact with specific antigen may cause immunologic injury by a direct toxic effect or through the release of soluble substances **(lymphokines)**. In tissue culture, activated T lymphocytes have been demonstrated to destroy "target" cells to which they have been sensitized, when they are brought into direct contact with the target cells. The lymphokines

released from activated T lymphocytes include several factors affecting the activity of macrophages, skin-reactive factor, and a lymphotoxin.

Examples of clinical conditions in which Type IV reactions are felt to be important are contact dermatitis, allograft rejection, granulomas due to intracellular organisms, some forms of drug sensitivity, thyroiditis, and encephalomyelitis following rabies vaccination. The evidence for the last 2 is based on experimental models and, in human disease, on the appearance of lymphocytes in the inflammatory exudate of the thyroid and the brain.

Diagnostic Tests

A Type IV reaction can be suspected when an inflammatory reaction is characterized histologically by perivascular lymphocytes and macrophages. Delayed-hypersensitivity skin tests (see Tests of cell-mediated immunity in Ch. 18) and patch tests are the most readily available methods of testing for delayed hypersensitivity.

Patch tests are used to identify allergens causing a contact dermatitis, but are not performed until the contact dermatitis has cleared, in order to prevent its exacerbation. The suspected material (in appropriate concentration) is applied to the skin under a nonabsorbent adhesive patch and left for 48 h. If burning or itching develops earlier, the patch is removed. A positive test consists of erythema with some induration and, occasionally, vesicle formation. Because some reactions do not appear until after the patches are removed, the sites are reinspected at 72 h.

Blastogenesis of lymphocytes or **thymidine incorporation** following stimulation with specific antigen are in vitro tests that can be performed in a patient with a negative skin test, when the antigen is known, to determine whether the defect is an inability of the skin to react to lymphokines or an inability of T cells to produce lymphokines. The best correlate with Type IV delayed hypersensitivity, however, is the production of migration inhibitory factor and blastogenesis of lymphocytes in the mixed lymphocyte culture. (For a discussion of these tests, see Ch. 18.)

---

21. DISORDERS DUE TO HYPERSENSITIVITY

ATOPIC DISEASES

Disorders caused by IgE-mediated (Type I) hypersensitivity, resulting from the antigen-induced release of vasoactive substances by mast cells and basophils that have been sensitized by specific antibody of the IgE immunoglobulin class (**reaginic** or **skin-sensitizing antibody**). The terms **hypersensitivity** and **allergy** are often used synonymously to mean an immunologic response to an antigen, leading to host tissue damage.

The most common human allergic disorders—hay fever (seasonal allergic rhinitis), asthma (particularly in children), and some cases of urticaria and GI food reactions—are atopic diseases. Patients with these disorders and those with **atopic dermatitis** have in common an inherited predisposition to develop hypersensitivity to inhaled and ingested substances (allergens) that are harmless to 80% of people. Features similar to atopy have been identified in several mammalian species.

The predisposition to hypersensitivity in atopic diseases is characterized by the development of specific antibodies of the IgE immunoglobulin class. In most instances, these antibodies mediate hypersensitivity symptoms. Atopic dermatitis is somewhat of an exception. Although IgE-mediated food allergy does contribute to symptoms in infants and young children, the condition is largely independent of allergic factors in older children and adults, even though most patients continue to have specific allergy as detected by skin testing and measurement of serum IgE antibodies.

Diagnostic Procedures

History: Review of the symptoms, their relation to the environment and to seasonal and situational variations, and their clinical course should yield sufficient information to classify the disease as atopic. The history and clinical course are more valuable than tests in determining whether a patient is allergic, and it is inappropriate to subject the patient to extensive skin testing unless reasonable clinical evidence exists for atopy. Age of onset may be an important clue (eg, childhood asthma is much more likely to be atopic than asthma beginning after age 30). Also indicative are symptoms that are seasonal (eg, correlating with specific pollen seasons), or appear after exposure to animals, hay, or dust, or develop in specific environments (eg, at home, at work).

It is also helpful, for advising the patient, to investigate the effects of nonspecific contributory factors, such as tobacco smoke and other pollutants, cold air and cold beverages, certain drugs, and life stresses.

Tests: These are used to confirm sensitivity to an allergen when it is suspected that the patient is allergic. For details on skin tests, the radioallergosorbent test (RAST), provocative challenge tests, and leukocyte histamine release, see TYPE I HYPERSENSITIVITY REACTIONS in Ch. 20.

Nonspecific findings: Eosinophilia is often associated with some atopic conditions, particularly asthma and atopic dermatitis. **IgE levels** may be helpful in diagnosing atopic dermatitis, since they are elevated and will rise during exacerbations and fall during remissions. IgE levels usually are elevated in atopic asthma, often are normal in allergic rhinitis, but are not diagnostically useful in these conditions.

Treatment

Avoidance: Eliminating the allergen is the preferred treatment. This may require a change of diet, occupation, or residence; withdrawal of a drug; or removal of a household pet. Some locales, free of allergens such as ragweed, are havens for afflicted persons. When complete avoidance is impossible, as in the case of house dust, exposure may be reduced by removing dust-collecting furniture, carpets, and draperies; using plastic covers over the mattress and pillows; frequent wet-mopping and dusting; reducing the high humidity favorable to dust mite breeding; and installing a high-efficiency air-filtering system.

Symptomatic therapy: Relief of symptoms with drugs should not be neglected while the patient is being evaluated and specific control or treatment is being developed. The proper use of antihistamines, sympathomimetics, cromolyn, and glucocorticoids is outlined for each disease category in the discussions that follow. In general, glucocorticoids are appropriate for treatment of potentially disabling conditions that are self-limited and of relatively short duration (seasonal flares of asthma; serum sickness; infiltrative lung disease; severe contact dermatitis).

Desensitization (hyposensitization, immunotherapy): When it is not feasible to avoid an allergen or to control it sufficiently to relieve symptoms of atopic disease, desensitization can be attempted by injecting an extract of the allergen subcutaneously in gradually increasing doses. Several specific effects can be demonstrated, although there is no test that correlates absolutely with clinical improvement. The titer of blocking (neutralizing) antibody increases proportionately to the dose administered. Sometimes, particularly when high doses of pollen extract can be tolerated, the serum IgE level falls significantly. In addition, peripheral blood basophil histamine release is reduced from pretreatment levels on incubation with antigen (or an increased amount of antigen is required to release 50% of the basophil histamine). This effect may not be specific—the reduced leukocyte hypersensitivity of some patients applies to antigens not used in desensitization and to anti-IgE antibody as well.

Clinical results are most satisfactory when injections are continued year-round. Depending on the degree of sensitivity, the first dose is 0.1 mL of a dilution ranging from

1:10,000 to 1:1,000,000. The dose is increased weekly or biweekly by 75% (or less) until a maximum tolerated concentration has been reached; eg, 0.3 mL of a 1:50 dilution. For crude pollen extracts, this amounts to about 30 μg of protein nitrogen (3000 protein nitrogen u.). Once the maximum dose has been reached, it can be maintained at monthly intervals year-round. Even in seasonal allergies this **perennial method** is superior to preseasonal or co-seasonal treatment methods.

The major allergens used for desensitization are those that usually cannot be effectively avoided: pollens, house dust and dust mites, molds, and venom of stinging insects. Animal dander desensitization is ordinarily limited to those who cannot avoid exposure, such as veterinarians or laboratory workers. There is no indication for food desensitization.

Adverse reactions to desensitization: Patients often are extremely sensitive, particularly to pollen allergens, and if an overdose is given can experience constitutional reactions varying from a mild cough or sneezing to generalized urticaria, severe asthma, and anaphylactic shock. To prevent such reactions, one must (1) check that the proper dilution is used, (2) increase the dose by small increments, (3) repeat the same dose (or even decrease it) if the local reaction from the previous injection is large (2.5 cm in diameter or greater), and (4) reduce the dose when a new extract is used. Reducing the dose of pollen extract during the pollen season is often wise also. IM and intravascular injection must be *avoided.*

Despite the best precautions, reactions occur occasionally. Since the severe, life-threatening ones develop within 20 min, patients must remain under observation for that time. The first signs of an impending reaction may be sneezing, coughing, and chest tightness, or a generalized flush, tingling sensations, and pruritus. A tourniquet should be applied above the injection site at once, and the site infiltrated with 0.2 mL of epinephrine 1:1000. (The tourniquet should be released in 15 min.) If the reaction is mild or moderate, a double dose of an antihistamine can then be given orally (eg, diphenhydramine 100 mg or chlorpheniramine 8 mg); and 0.3 mL of epinephrine 1:1000 can be given s.c. in the opposite arm. However, if symptoms and signs of *shock* have developed, IV fluids should be started and epinephrine 1:100,000, 5 to 10 μg/min IV, should be given over about 10 min, and other measures instituted for treatment of anaphylaxis (see below). Glucocorticoid therapy will not help during the acute reaction, but may be helpful in preventing the late 4- to 6-h asthmatic or urticarial reaction that may develop after the patient has recovered from the first reaction and gone home.

Occasionally, a generalized reaction such as urticaria may appear 30 min to several hours after an allergen injection. This can be treated with an antihistamine alone. Following any generalized reaction, the next dose of allergen should be reduced by ⅓ or ¼, and later increments kept as small as is practicable (usually 0.03 to 0.05 mL).

ALLERGIC RHINITIS

A symptom complex including hay fever and perennial allergic rhinitis, characterized by seasonal or perennial sneezing, rhinorrhea, nasal congestion, pruritus, and often conjunctivitis and pharyngitis.

HAY FEVER
(Pollinosis)

Hay fever, the acute seasonal form of allergic rhinitis, is generally induced by wind-borne pollens. The **spring type** is due to tree pollens (eg, oak, elm, maple, alder, birch, cottonwood); the **summer type,** to grass pollens (eg, Bermuda, timothy, sweet vernal, orchard, Johnson) and to weed pollens (eg, sheep sorrel, English plantain); the **fall type,** to weed pollens (eg, ragweed). Occasionally, seasonal hay fever is due primarily

to airborne fungus spores rather than to pollens. Important geographic regional differences occur.

Symptoms and Signs

The nose, roof of the mouth, pharynx, and eyes begin to itch gradually or abruptly after onset of the pollen season. Lacrimation, sneezing, and clear, watery nasal discharge accompany or soon follow the pruritus. Frontal headaches, irritability, anorexia, depression, and insomnia may appear. The conjunctiva is injected, and the nasal mucous membranes are swollen and bluish red. Coughing and asthmatic wheezing may develop as the season progresses. Many eosinophils are present in the nasal mucus during the season.

Diagnosis

The nature of the allergic process and even the responsible allergen are often suspected from the history. Diagnosis is confirmed by the above physical findings, skin tests, and the accompanying eosinophilia in secretions.

Treatment

Symptoms may be diminished by avoidance of the allergen (see above). Most patients obtain adequate relief with oral antihistamines (eg, chlorpheniramine, in sustained-release form, 12 mg q 8 h; triprolidine 2.5 mg q 8 h). If these drugs are too sedating, a nonsedating but more expensive antihistamine may be used (terfenadine 60 mg orally q 12 h). Topical treatment is another alternative (see below). Sympathomimetics are often used in combination with antihistamines. Phenylpropanolamine, phenylephrine, or pseudoephedrine are available in many antihistamine-decongestant preparations. Ephedrine 25 mg orally q 4 h is more effective, but its central-stimulating effects limit its use. Sympathomimetic drugs taken by mouth can raise the BP, and patients with a tendency to hypertension should not use them without periodic monitoring.

If antihistaminic drugs are not satisfactory, then a nasal spray containing 4% cromolyn sodium may be used. It is delivered by means of a finger-activated pump. The dosage is one spray (5.2 mg) 2 to 6 times/day. Because cromolyn acts by blocking the reaction of allergen with tissue mast cells, it is most effective in preventing symptoms rather than in relieving acute symptoms. Because of higher cost and because its effect is limited to the nose, it usually is not the first drug to be tried for hay fever treatment.

When nasal symptoms are not relieved adequately by antihistaminic treatment, intranasal glucocorticoid spray usually is effective. Two doses bid to qid are used initially; beclomethasone dipropionate is freon-propelled from a container that delivers 0.042 mg (42 μg)/dose, and flunisolide 0.025% is delivered by a finger-activated pump, 0.025 mg/dose. When symptoms have been relieved, dosage is reduced to 1 dose bid for the remainder of the season. Severe intractable extranasal symptoms may require a short course of systemic corticosteroid treatment (prednisone 10 mg orally bid, with gradual reduction in dose; an alternate-day regimen may also be used).

Desensitization treatment (see above) is advised if drug treatment is poorly tolerated, if glucocorticoids are needed during the season, or if asthma develops. If the patient is allergic to pollens, treatment should begin soon after the pollen season has ended, in preparation for the following season.

PERENNIAL ALLERGIC RHINITIS

In contrast to hay fever, symptoms of perennial rhinitis vary in severity (often unpredictably) throughout the year. Extranasal symptoms such as conjunctivitis are uncommon, but chronic nasal obstruction is often prominent and may extend to eustachian tube obstruction. The resultant hearing difficulty is particularly common in children. The **diagnosis** of allergic rhinitis is supported by a positive history of atopic

disease, the characteristic bluish-red mucosa, numerous eosinophils in the nasal secretions, and positive skin tests (particularly to house dust, dust mites, feathers, animal danders, or fungi). Some patients have complicating sinus infections and nasal polyps.

Certain patients suffer from chronic rhinitis, sinusitis, and polyps and have negative skin tests. These patients are not atopic but often have sensitivity to aspirin and other nonsteroidal anti-inflammatory drugs, and should be evaluated also for sensitivity to tartrazine (a yellow food coloring) by a trial elimination of this food additive from the diet. Despite the negative skin tests, these patients have numerous eosinophils in their tissues and nasal secretions. A subset suffers only from chronic rhinitis. Although they are not atopic, their nasal secretions have many eosinophils. This group of patients has been given the diagnosis of **eosinophilic nonallergic rhinitis**. Some patients with mild but annoying chronic continuous nasal obstruction or rhinorrhea have no demonstrable allergy, and no polyps, infection, or drug sensitivity. Their condition is called **vasomotor rhinitis** (see Ch. 208).

Treatment

Management is similar to that for hay fever if specific allergens are identified, except that systemic glucocorticoids, even though effective, should be avoided because of the need for prolonged use. Surgery (antrotomy and irrigation of sinuses, polypectomy, submucous resection) may be necessary after allergic factors have been controlled or ruled out. The subset of patients with eosinophilic nonallergic rhinitis mentioned above usually respond best to a topical glucocorticoid. For many patients the only treatment is reassurance, antihistamine and vasoconstrictor drugs, and advice to avoid topical decongestants, which produce after-congestion and, when used continuously for a week or more, may aggravate or perpetuate chronic rhinitis **(rhinitis medicamentosa)**. Some patients with rhinitis may benefit from the frequent use of saline irrigation or nasal sprays.

ALLERGIC PULMONARY DISEASE

The lungs can be involved in known or suspected allergic reactions in several ways, depending on the nature of the allergen and its route of entry. Specific disorders are discussed in Ch. 43, and under BRONCHIAL ASTHMA in Ch. 36.

ANAPHYLAXIS

Generalized anaphylaxis is an acute, often explosive, systemic reaction characterized by pruritus, generalized flush, urticaria, respiratory distress, and vascular collapse, and occasionally by seizures, vomiting, abdominal cramps, and incontinence. It occurs in a previously sensitized person when he again receives the sensitizing antigen. This IgE-mediated reaction occurs when antigen (proteins, polysaccharides, and haptens coupled with a carrier protein) reaches the circulation. The most common causative antigens are foreign serum; parenteral enzymes; blood products; β-lactam antimicrobials and many other drugs; desensitizing injections; and insect stings. β-Adrenergic blocking drugs may aggravate anaphylactic reactions. Anaphylaxis can be aggravated or even induced de novo by exercise, and some patients suffer from recurrent symptoms for no identifiable reason. Histamine, leukotrienes (the active agents in slow-reactive substance of anaphylaxis—SRS-A), and other mediators are generated or released when the antigen reacts with IgE on basophils and mast cells. These mediators cause the smooth muscle contraction and vascular dilatation that characterize anaphylaxis. Wheezing and GI symptoms are caused by smooth muscle contraction. Vasodilatation and escape of plasma into the tissues causes urticaria and angioedema and results in a decrease in effective plasma volume, which is the major cause of shock. Fluid escapes into the lung alveoli and may produce pulmonary edema. Obstructive angioedema of the upper

airway may also occur. Arrhythmias and cardiogenic shock may develop if the reaction is prolonged.

Anaphylactoid reactions are clinically similar to anaphylaxis, but may occur after the *first* injection of certain drugs (polymyxin, pentamidine, morphine, radiographic contrast media), and have a dose-related, toxic-idiosyncratic mechanism rather than an immunologically mediated one. Aspirin and other nonsteroidal anti-inflammatory drugs can cause reactions in susceptible patients.

Symptoms and Signs

Typically, in 1 to 15 min, the patient complains of a sense of uneasiness and becomes agitated and flushed. Palpitation, paresthesias, pruritus, throbbing in the ears, coughing, sneezing, urticaria-angioedema and difficulty breathing due to laryngeal edema or bronchospasm are other typical complaints. Primary cardiovascular collapse can occur in the absence of respiratory symptoms. Nausea, vomiting, and abdominal pain are less common. The symptoms and signs of shock may develop within another 1 or 2 min, and the patient may become incontinent, convulse, become unresponsive, and die.

Prophylaxis

Patients with the greatest risk of anaphylactic reactions to a drug are those who have reacted previously to that drug, but anaphylactic deaths occur in patients with no such history. The risk of a reaction to horse serum (eg, antisera for botulism, diphtheria, or snake and black widow spider bites) is high, routine skin testing before giving the serum is *mandatory*, and prophylactic measures may be needed (see under SERUM SICKNESS, below). Routine skin testing before other drug treatment is neither practicable nor reliable, except for penicillin (tests are discussed under DRUG HYPERSENSITIVITY, Mechanisms, below).

Long-term desensitization is effective and appropriate for prevention of insect-sting anaphylaxis but has rarely been attempted in patients with a history of drug or serum anaphylaxis. Instead, if treatment with a drug or serum is essential, rapid desensitization must be carried out under carefully controlled conditions (see DRUG HYPERSENSITIVITY, below; and SERUM SICKNESS, below).

A patient with a history of a previous reaction to a radiographic contrast agent, even an anaphylactoid one, can be given an agent again with reasonable safety (if the study is essential) by pretreatment with prednisone 50 mg orally q 6 h for 3 doses, diphenhydramine 50 mg orally 1 h beforehand, and ephedrine (if no contraindication) 25 mg orally 1 h beforehand.

Treatment

Immediate treatment with epinephrine is imperative. It is a pharmacologic antagonist to the effects of the chemical mediators on smooth muscle, blood vessels, and other tissues.

For mild reactions such as generalized pruritus, urticaria, angioedema, mild wheezing, nausea, and vomiting, 0.3 to 0.5 mL of aqueous epinephrine 1:1000 should be given s.c. If an antigen injected in an extremity has caused the anaphylaxis, a tourniquet should be applied above the injection site and 0.1 to 0.2 mL of epinephrine 1:1000 also injected into the site, to reduce systemic absorption of the antigen. A second injection of epinephrine s.c. may be required. Once symptoms have resolved, an oral antihistamine should be given for 24 h.

For more severe reactions, with massive angioedema but without evidence of cardiovascular involvement, patients should be given diphenhydramine 50 to 100 mg IV (for an adult) in addition to the above treatment, to forestall laryngeal edema and to block the effect of further histamine release. When the edema is responding, 0.3 mL of an aqueous suspension of long-acting epinephrine 1:200 s.c. can be given for its 6- to 8-h

effect, and an oral antihistamine should be given for the next 24 h, and possibly a glucocorticoid to suppress the late phase of a dual reaction.

For severe respiratory reactions (eg, bronchial asthma) that do not respond to epinephrine, IV fluids should be started and aminophylline 6 mg/kg IV should be given over 10 to 20 min, followed by 0.5 mg/kg/h, more or less, to maintain a theophylline blood level of 10 to 20 μg/mL. Endotracheal intubation or tracheostomy may be necessary, with O_2 administration at 4 to 6 L/min.

The most severe reactions usually involve the cardiovascular system, causing severe hypotension and vasomotor collapse. IV fluids should be started and the patient should be recumbent with legs elevated. Epinephrine (1:100,000) should be given slowly IV (5 to 10 μg/min) with close observation for development of side effects, including headache, tremulousness, nausea, and arrhythmias. The underlying severe hypotension may be due to vasodilatation, hypovolemia from loss of fluid, myocardial insufficiency (rarely), or a combination of these. Each has a specific treatment and often the treatment of one exacerbates the others. The appropriate therapy may be clarified if central venous pressure **(CVP)** and left atrial pressure can be obtained (see also in Ch. 25). A low CVP and normal left atrial pressure indicate peripheral vasodilation and/or hypovolemia. Vasodilation should respond to the epinephrine (which will also retard the loss of intravascular fluid).

In most cases, hypovolemia is the major cause of the hypotension. The CVP and left atrial pressure are both low, and large volumes of saline must be given, with monitoring of the BP, until the CVP rises to normal. Colloid plasma expanders such as dextran are rarely necessary. Only if fluid replacement does not restore normal BP should one initiate treatment cautiously with adrenergic drugs such as metaraminol.

In the rare instance of myocardial insufficiency, both CVP and left atrial pressure will be elevated. Isoproterenol 1 mg is diluted in 500 mL of 5% dextrose and infused at a rate of 0.5 to 1 mL/min. The patient should be monitored carefully, for the isoproterenol may cause cardiac arrhythmias and hypotension due to peripheral vasodilatation.

Cardiac arrest may occur, requiring immediate resuscitation (see CARDIAC ARREST AND CARDIOPULMONARY RESUSCITATION in Ch. 27). Further therapy depends on ECG findings.

When all the above measures have been instituted, diphenhydramine (50 to 75 mg IV slowly over 3 min) and glucocorticoids may then be given for treatment of slow-onset urticaria, asthma, laryngeal edema, or hypotension. Hydrocortisone sodium succinate 100 mg (or equivalent) should be given q 1 to 2 h IV until symptoms are controlled, then q 2 to 4 h for 24 h IV, and then discontinued. Complications such as myocardial infarction and cerebral edema should be looked for and treated specifically. Patients with severe reactions should remain in a hospital under observation for 24 h following recovery to ensure adequate treatment in case of relapse.

Any person who has had an anaphylactic reaction to a stinging insect should be provided with a kit containing a pre-filled syringe of epinephrine and an epinephrine nebulizer to allow prompt self-treatment of any future reaction. Such an individual should also be evaluated for venom immunotherapy (desensitization).

URTICARIA; ANGIOEDEMA

(Hives; Giant Urticaria; Angioneurotic Edema)

Urticaria: *Local wheals and erythema in the dermis.* **Angioedema**: *A similar eruption, but with larger edematous areas that involve subcutaneous structures as well as the dermis.*

Etiology

Acute urticaria and angioedema are essentially anaphylaxis limited to the skin and subcutaneous tissues and can be due to drug allergy, insect stings or bites, desensitiza-

tion injections, or ingestion of certain foods (particularly eggs, shellfish, nuts, or fruits—see also FOOD ALLERGY AND INTOLERANCE, below). Some food reactions occur explosively following ingestion of only minute amounts. Others (such as reactions to strawberries) may occur only after overindulgence, and possibly result from direct (toxic) mediator liberation. Urticaria may accompany or even be the first symptom of several viral infections, including hepatitis, infectious mononucleosis, and rubella. Some acute reactions are unexplained, even when recurrent. If acute angioedema is recurrent, progressive, and never associated with urticaria, a hereditary enzyme deficiency should be suspected (see HEREDITARY ANGIOEDEMA, below).

Chronic urticaria and angioedema lasting more than 3 wk are more difficult to explain, and only in exceptional cases can a specific cause be found. They occur equally in nonatopic and atopic subjects. Occasionally, unsuspected chronic drug or chemical ingestion is responsible; eg, from penicillin in milk, from the use of nonprescription drugs, or from preservatives, dyes, or other food additives. Chronic underlying disease (SLE, polycythemia vera, lymphoma, or infection) should be ruled out. Though suspected frequently, controllable psychogenic factors are not often identified. Urticaria caused by physical agents is discussed in PHYSICAL ALLERGY, below. A few patients with intractable urticaria are hyperthyroid.

Symptoms and Signs

In **urticaria,** pruritus (generally the first symptom) is followed shortly by the appearance of wheals that may remain small (1 to 5 mm) or may enlarge. The larger ones tend to clear in the center, and may be noticed first as large (more than 20 cm across) rings of erythema and edema. Ordinarily, crops of hives come and go, a lesion remaining in one site for several hours, then disappearing, only to reappear elsewhere. **Angioedema** is a more diffuse swelling of loose subcutaneous tissue: dorsum of hands or feet, eyelids, lips, genitalia, mucous membranes. Edema of the upper airway may produce respiratory distress, and the stridor may be mistaken for asthma.

Diagnosis

The cause of acute urticaria is usually obvious. Even when it is not, a diagnostic workup is seldom required because of the self-limited, nonrecurrent nature of these reactions. In chronic urticaria, an underlying chronic disease should be ruled out by a careful history and physical examination and routine screening tests. Eosinophilia is uncommon in urticaria. Other tests such as stool examination for ova and parasites, serum complement, antinuclear antibody, and sinus or dental x-rays are not usually worthwhile unless there are clinical indications other than urticaria.

Treatment

Acute urticaria is a self-limited condition that generally subsides in 1 to 7 days; hence, treatment is chiefly palliative. If the cause is not obvious, all nonessential medication should be stopped until the reaction has subsided. Symptoms usually can be relieved with an oral antihistamine (eg, diphenhydramine 50 to 100 mg q 4 h, hydroxyzine 25 to 100 mg bid, or cyproheptadine 4 to 8 mg q 4 h). A glucocorticoid (eg, prednisone 30 to 40 mg/day orally) may be necessary for the more severe reactions, particularly when associated with angioedema. Topical glucocorticoids are of no value. Epinephrine 1:1000, 0.3 mL s.c., should be the first treatment for **acute pharyngeal or laryngeal angioedema**. This may be supplemented with topical treatment; eg, nebulized epinephrine 1:100, and an IV antihistamine (eg, diphenhydramine 50 to 100 mg). This usually prevents airway obstruction, but one must be prepared to entubate or perform a tracheostomy and give O_2.

In **chronic urticaria**, spontaneous remissions occur within 2 yr in about half the cases. Control of stressful life situations often helps reduce the frequency and severity of episodes. Certain drugs (eg, aspirin) may aggravate symptoms, as will alcoholic beverages, coffee, and tobacco smoking; if so, they should be avoided. When urticaria is

produced by aspirin, sensitivity to related nonsteroidal anti-inflammatory drugs and to the food- and drug-coloring additive tartrazine should be investigated (see also PERENNIAL ALLERGIC RHINITIS, above). Oral antihistamines with a tranquilizing effect are beneficial in most cases (eg, hydroxyzine 25 to 50 mg bid or cyproheptadine 4 to 8 mg q 4 h). All reasonable measures should be used before resorting to glucocorticoids, which are frequently effective but, once started, may have to be continued indefinitely.

HEREDITARY ANGIOEDEMA

A form of angioedema transmitted as an autosomal dominant trait and associated with a deficiency of serum inhibitor of the activated first component of complement. In 85% of cases, the deficiency is due to a lack of the C1 esterase inhibitor **(C1 Inh)**; in 15%, to C1 Inh malfunction. A positive family history is the rule, but there are exceptions. The edema is characteristically unifocal, indurated, painful rather than pruritic, and not accompanied by urticaria. Attacks are often precipitated by trauma or viral illness, and are aggravated by emotional stress. The GI tract is often involved, with nausea, vomiting, colic, and even signs of intestinal obstruction. The condition may cause fatal upper airway obstruction. **Diagnosis** may be made by measuring C4, which is low, even between attacks, or more specifically by demonstrating deficiency of C1 Inh by immunoassay and a functional assay if the former is unexpectedly normal.

Treatment

The edema progresses until complement components have been consumed. Acute attacks that threaten to produce airway obstruction therefore should be treated promptly by establishing an airway. Epinephrine, an antihistamine, and a glucocorticoid should be given, but there is no proof that these drugs are effective.

For short-term prophylaxis of the previously untreated patient, as before a dental procedure, endoscopy, or surgery, 2 units of fresh frozen plasma can be given. Although there is a theoretic concern that a complement substrate in the plasma might provoke an attack, this has not been observed in practice in symptom-free patients. Recently, a partially purified C1 Inh fraction of pooled plasma has been shown to be safe and effective for prophylaxis but is not yet available for general use. If time permits, though, it is preferable to treat the patient for 3 to 5 days with an androgen as described below.

For long-term prophylaxis, androgens are effective. For men, methyltestosterone (starting dose 10 mg orally tid) is preferred, being inexpensive and relatively free of side effects. One of the impeded androgens should be used for women; treatment is begun with oral stanozolol 2 mg tid or danazol 200 mg tid. Stanozolol is less expensive. Once control is achieved the doses should be reduced as much as possible to reduce the cost and, in women, to minimize masculinizing side effects. These drugs are not only effective but also have been shown to raise the low C1 Inh and C4 toward normal.

MASTOCYTOSIS

A condition of unknown etiology characterized by an excessive accumulation of mast cells in various body organs and tissues. Normally, tissue mast cells contribute to host defense by releasing potent preformed mediators (eg, histamine) from their granules and by generating newly formed mediators (eg, leukotrienes) from membrane lipids. Normal tissue mast cells also mediate the symptoms of common allergic reactions by means of IgE antibodies attached to specific surface receptors.

Mastocytosis can occur in 3 forms: **mastocytoma** (*a benign cutaneous tumor*); **urticaria pigmentosa** (*multiple small cutaneous collections of mast cells that develop as salmon-colored or brown macules and papules*, which urticate when stroked and may become vesicular or even bullous); and **systemic mastocytosis** (*mast cell infiltrates in the skin, lymph nodes, liver, spleen, GI tract, and bones*).

Symptoms, Signs, and Diagnosis

Patients with **systemic mastocytosis** have arthralgias, bone pain, and anaphylactoid symptoms. Other symptoms are caused by stimulation of H_2 histamine receptors (increased gastric acid and mucus secretion). Thus, peptic ulcer disease and chronic diarrhea are common problems. The histamine content of tissue biopsies can be extremely high, commensurate with the elevated mast cell concentration. The urinary excretion of histamine and metabolites is high in systemic mastocytosis, and plasma histamine may be elevated. Increased plasma levels of heparin, thromboxane B_2, and prostaglandin D_2 (**PGD_2**) have also been reported.

Prognosis and Treatment

Cutaneous mastocytosis usually develops in childhood. The solitary mastocytoma should involute spontaneously; and **urticaria pigmentosa** either clears completely or is substantially improved before adolescence. These conditions rarely, if ever, progress to systemic mastocytosis. Treatment of pruritus with an H_1 antihistamine (see URTICARIA, above) is usually all that is needed.

The symptoms of **systemic mastocytosis** should be treated with an H_1 antihistamine and an H_2 antihistamine (cimetidine 300 mg tid or qid; or ranitidine 150 mg bid). Because prostaglandins, especially PGD_2, are thought to contribute to mast cell-related symptoms, aspirin therapy may be tried, but cautiously; while inhibiting prostaglandin synthesis, this and similar drugs may enhance leukotriene production. If GI symptoms are not adequately controlled, oral cromolyn sodium 200 mg qid should be given. Although oral cromolyn is approved for investigational use only, it may be available from the manufacturer for treatment of the rare patient with a confirmed diagnosis and intractable symptoms. There is no effective treatment available to reduce the number of tissue mast cells.

PHYSICAL ALLERGY

A condition in which allergic symptoms and signs are produced by exposure to cold, sunlight, heat, or mild trauma.

Etiology

The underlying cause is unknown in most cases. Photosensitivity (see Ch. 253 and CONTACT DERMATITIS in Ch. 230) may sometimes be induced by drugs or topical agents, including certain cosmetics. Cold and light sensitivity in some cases can be passively transferred with serum that contains a specific IgE antibody, suggesting an immunologic mechanism involving a physically altered skin protein as antigen. An alternative mechanism is suggested by the recent finding of IgG and IgM autoantibodies in some patients with cold urticaria. The serum of a few patients with cold-induced symptoms contains cryoglobulins or cryofibrinogen; these abnormal proteins may be associated with a serious underlying disorder such as a malignancy, a collagen vascular disease, or chronic infection. Cold may aggravate asthma or vasomotor rhinitis, but cold urticaria is independent of any other known allergic tendencies. Heat sensitivity usually produces cholinergic urticaria, which is also induced in the same patients by exercise, emotional stress, or any stimulus that causes sweating. **Dermatographia (dermographism),** a wheal-and-flare reaction seen after scratching or firmly stroking the skin, is usually idiopathic but occasionally is the first sign of an urticarial drug reaction. The sensitivity of about half the idiopathic cases studied can be passively transferred by serum and appears to be IgE-mediated. Urticaria has also occurred following a persistent, vibratory stimulus (familial), after water exposure ("aquagenic"), and as an immediate or late (4 to 6 h, occasionally 24 h) reaction to pressure.

Symptoms and Signs

Pruritus and unsightly appearance are the most common complaints. Cold sensitivity is usually manifested by urticaria and angioedema, which develop most typically

after exposure to cold is terminated and during or after swimming or bathing. Bronchospasm and even histamine-mediated shock may occur in extreme cases and result in drowning. Sunlight may produce urticaria or a more chronic polymorphous skin eruption.

The skin lesions in cholinergic urticaria are small, highly pruritic, discrete wheals surrounded by a large zone of erythema. Cholinergic urticaria appears to be caused by an unusual sensitivity to acetylcholine. A skin test using methacholine 1:5000 may reproduce the lesions, but in only about 1/3 of cases. The most reliable test is to provoke symptoms with exercise, using occlusive garments to promote sweating.

Prophylaxis and Treatment

The use of drugs or cosmetics should be reviewed with the patient, particularly if photosensitivity is suspected. Protection from the physical stimulus is necessary. Management of photosensitivity is discussed in Ch. 253 and under CONTACT DERMATITIS in Ch. 230.

For relief of itching, an antihistamine with sedative effects should be given orally (diphenhydramine 50 mg qid; cyproheptadine 4 to 8 mg qid). Cyproheptadine has been noted to be the most effective in cold urticaria. Hydroxyzine 25 to 100 mg orally qid is the preferred drug for cholinergic urticaria; anticholinergic drugs are ineffective at tolerable doses. Prednisone 30 to 40 mg/day orally should be given in severe light eruptions other than urticaria to shorten the clinical course; the dose is gradually reduced as the patient improves.

ALLERGIC CONJUNCTIVITIS

(See also VERNAL KERATOCONJUNCTIVITIS in Ch. 219)

Atopic conjunctivitis of an acute or chronic catarrhal form is usually part of a larger allergic syndrome such as hay fever, but may occur alone through direct contact with airborne substances such as pollen, fungus spores, various dusts, or animal danders.

Symptoms, Signs, and Diagnosis

Itching is prominent and may be accompanied by excessive lacrimation. The conjunctiva is edematous and hyperemic. The cause is often suggested by the history and may be confirmed by skin testing. If *atopic* conjunctivitis is suspected but skin tests are equivocal, an ophthalmic challenge (see TYPE I HYPERSENSITIVITY REACTIONS in Ch. 20) occasionally will be positive. Since so few antigens can be tested in a reasonable period, ophthalmic challenge has limited application. *It should not be used for diagnosis of contact hypersensitivity.*

Treatment

An identified or suspected causative allergen should be avoided. Frequent use of a bland eyewash (eg, buffered 0.65% saline) may reduce the irritation. Contact lenses should not be worn. Oral antihistamines usually are helpful. Topical antihistamines are available (antazoline 0.5%, pheniramine 0.3, 0.5%, or pyrilamine 0.1%), but only in combination with the vasoconstrictors naphazoline 0.025 to 0.05% or phenylephrine 0.125% as ophthalmic solutions. Topical antihistamine or the preservative in the preparation may be sensitizing and most patients respond as well or better to an oral antihistamine plus a topical vasoconstrictor alone than to the topical combination. Cromolyn sodium (4% ophthalmic solution) may be helpful, particularly in preventing the development of symptoms when allergen exposure is anticipated (see HAY FEVER, above). Indications for desensitization are similar to those for hay fever. A corticosteroid ophthalmic suspension (eg, medrysone 1% or fluorometholone 0.1% applied qid) may be used as a last resort in severe cases. *Intraocular pressure should be checked before and regularly during such treatment, and treatment should be terminated as soon as possible.*

OTHER ALLERGIC EYE DISEASES

The **lids** may be involved by angioedema or urticaria, contact dermatitis, or atopic dermatitis. Contact dermatitis of the eyelids, a cellular (delayed—Type IV) hypersensitivity reaction, may be caused by various ophthalmic medications or drugs conveyed by the fingers to the eyes (eg, antibiotics by drug handlers) or by face powder, nail polish, or hair dye. The **cornea** may become involved by extension of allergic conjunctivitis or by a variant of superficial punctate keratitis, leading rarely to scarring.

Pain, photophobia, lacrimation, and circumcorneal ciliary inflammation indicate probable **anterior uveitis**. In most cases the cause is unknown; it may, rarely, be due to a specific environmental allergen, and bacterial hypersensitivity of the cell-mediated (delayed) type may be suspected. **Sympathetic ophthalmia** is felt to be a hypersensitivity reaction to uveal pigment. **Endophthalmitis phacoanaphylactica** is caused by allergy to native lens protein. The reaction, which is severe, occurs typically in the remaining lens after one lens has been removed uneventfully, though it may follow trauma or inflammation involving the lens capsule. Prompt evaluation and treatment by an ophthalmologist is required in these serious ophthalmic conditions.

GASTROINTESTINAL ALLERGY

An uncommon symptom complex due to ingestion of specific food or drug allergens, manifested by nausea, vomiting, crampy abdominal pain, diarrhea, and urticaria. Other symptoms of anaphylaxis (see above) also may occur. GI symptoms from food or drugs, however, more often represent nonspecific intolerance or are secondary to digestive enzyme defects (as in celiac disease and disaccharidase deficiency); hypersensitivity to food allergens is more commonly manifested as urticaria or angioedema. Most people prone to severe reactions can detect traces of the offending food in their mouths by the rapid onset of mucosal burning or itching.

FOOD ALLERGY AND INTOLERANCE

Food allergy: *Reproducible symptoms occurring after ingestion of a specific food, and for which an immunologic basis is proved or suspected.* **Food intolerance**: *Clinical GI reactions in which the mechanism is not immunologic or is unknown.*

Many common, probably psychophysiologic, adverse food reactions are attributed to food allergy where no convincing cause-and-effect evidence exists, at least of the type of allergy that can be evaluated by skin tests and is thus associated with specific IgE antibodies to foods. Certain claims are controversial; eg, that intolerance (or allergy) to food or food additives can be responsible for hyperactive children, the "tension-fatigue syndrome," and enuresis. Unsubstantiated claims are made blaming food allergy for arthritis, obesity, suboptimal athletic performance, depression, etc.

Occasionally, cheilitis, aphthae, pylorospasm, spastic constipation, pruritus ani, and perianal eczema have been attributed to food allergy or intolerance, but the association is difficult to prove. Recently, food intolerance was found to be responsible for symptoms of some patients with the **irritable bowel syndrome**, confirmed by double-blind food challenge. Of additional interest was the increase in rectal prostaglandin levels when a reaction occurred. Preliminary information suggests that the same phenomenon may take place occasionally in patients with chronic ulcerative colitis. **Eosinophilic enteropathy,** which may be related to specific food allergy, is an unusual illness with pain, cramps, and diarrhea that is associated with blood eosinophilia, eosinophilic infiltrates in the gut, protein-losing enteropathy, and a history of atopic disease. Rarely, dysphagia occurs, indicating esophgeal involvement.

Symptoms and Signs

True IgE-mediated food allergy usually develops in infancy, most likely in those with a strong family history of atopy. The first manifestation may be eczema (atopic dermatitis) alone or in association with GI symptoms. By the end of the first year, dermatitis usually is less of a problem as allergic respiratory symptoms begin to develop. Asthma and allergic rhinitis can be aggravated by allergy to foods that can be identified by skin testing. However, as the child gets older, foods become less important as the child reacts more and more to inhaled allergens. By the time the child with asthma and hay fever is 10 yr old, it is rare for a food to provoke respiratory symptoms, even though positive skin tests persist. If atopic dermatitis persists or appears in the older child or adult, its activity seems to be largely independent of IgE-mediated allergy, even though atopic patients with extensive dermatitis have much higher IgE levels in the serum than those who are free of dermatitis.

Some patients very sensitive to potent allergens (eg, in nuts, legumes, seeds, and shellfish) may react violently to ingestion of even a trace of such foods, with explosive urticaria and angioedema (see in that discussion, above), and even anaphylaxis. Anaphylaxis may occur in patients with a lower level of sensitivity only if they exercise after eating the offending food.

Milk intolerance is sometimes caused by an intestinal disaccharidase deficiency, and is expressed by GI symptoms. In other patients, milk causes GI, and even respiratory, symptoms for no identifiable reason. **Food additives** can produce systemic symptoms (monosodium glutamate); asthma (metabisulfite, tartrazine—a yellow dye); and possibly urticaria (tartrazine, benzoates). A few patients suffer from food-induced or aggravated migraine, confirmed by blinded oral challenge.

The effectiveness of digestion in preventing food allergy symptoms in most adults is demonstrated by allergic patients who react on inhalation or contact, but not on ingestion (eg, **bakers' asthma** —the affected workers wheeze on exposure to flour dust and have positive skin tests to wheat and/or other grains, yet have no problem eating grain products).

It is a common experience to develop urticaria after dietary overindulgence. Since the responsible food can be eaten in moderation later on with no problem, the reaction can best be classed as a toxic one, although the mechanism is unknown.

Diagnosis

Severe food allergy is usually obvious to the patient. When it is not, diagnosis is difficult and the condition must be differentiated from functional GI problems. For specific tests, see under **Provocative food testing** in TYPE I HYPERSENSITIVITY in Ch. 20.

Treatment

Except for elimination of the offending foods, there is no specific treatment. Elimination diets can be used both for diagnosis and treatment (see Ch. 20, TYPE I HYPERSENSITIVITY REACTIONS) but are often misleading. When only a few foods are involved, abstinence is preferred. Sensitivity to one or more foods may disappear spontaneously. Oral desensitization (by first eliminating the offending food for a time and then giving small, daily increased amounts) has not been proved effective nor has the use of sublingual drops of food extracts. Heating certain foods (eg, milk) may reduce their antigenicity by protein denaturation. Antihistamines are of little value except in acute general reactions with urticaria and angioedema. Oral cromolyn sodium has been used with apparent success in other countries, but the oral form has not been approved for use in the USA. Prolonged glucocorticoid treatment is not indicated except in eosinophilic enteropathy.

For treatment of the severe, potentially fatal acute attack, see URTICARIA; ANGIOEDEMA, and ANAPHYLAXIS, above.

DRUG HYPERSENSITIVITY

Drug eruptions are discussed in Ch. 237. Discussed here are other hypersensitivity reactions that can follow oral or parenteral drug administration. Contact dermatitis, which is a cellular (delayed—type IV) hypersensitivity reaction that follows topical use, is discussed in Ch. 230; and drug reactions that result from other than immunologic mechanisms are also discussed in Ch. 277.

Before attributing a given reaction to a drug, one should appreciate that *placebos* also may cause unwanted effects. Nausea, tachycardia, excessive sweating, epigastric disturbance with diarrhea, dry mouth, headache, easy fatigue, somnolence, and even skin rashes have been reported by persons taking inert substances in double-blind studies. Nevertheless, true drug reactions constitute a major medical problem. The literature on specific drugs should be consulted for the most likely adverse reactions.

With **overdosage of a drug,** toxic effects occur in direct relation to the total amount of drug in the body, and can occur in any patient if the dose is large enough. *Absolute* overdosage results from an error in the amount or frequency of administration of individual doses. *Relative* overdosage may be seen in patients who, because of liver or kidney disease, do not metabolize or excrete the drug normally.

In **drug idiosyncrasy,** the adverse reaction develops on the first use of the drug. It may be the same toxic reaction ordinarily expected at higher doses (more correctly called **intolerance**); it may be an exaggeration of a common mild side effect, such as antihistaminic sedation; or it may be unique. Reactions due to genetically determined enzyme deficiencies are being identified in increasing numbers. Hemolytic anemia, for example, develops in patients with G6PD deficiency during treatment with any of several drugs. Succinylcholine apnea and isoniazid peripheral neuropathy are other examples based on pharmacogenetics.

Most toxic and idiosyncratic reactions (eg, hyperergic reactions from anesthetic agents) differ sufficiently from allergic reactions to cause no confusion. There are a few exceptions. Toxic or idiosyncratic reactions from drugs with a direct histamine-releasing action (eg, radiographic contrast media, opiates, pentamidine, polymyxin) may present as urticaria or even as anaphylactoid reactions. Hemolytic anemia may be allergic (eg, penicillin, stibophen) or due to G6PD deficiency. Drug fever may be allergic, toxic (eg, amphetamine, tranylcypromine), or even pharmacologic (eg, etiocholanolone).

Allergic reactions have the following characteristics: (1) The reaction occurs only after the patient has been exposed to the drug (not necessarily for therapy) one or more times without incident. (2) Once hypersensitivity has developed, the reaction can be produced by doses that are far below therapeutic amounts, and usually below those levels that give idiosyncratic reactions. (3) The clinical features are restricted in their manifestations. Skin rashes (particularly urticaria), serum sickness, unexpected fever, anaphylaxis, and eosinophilic pulmonary infiltrates appearing during drug therapy are almost always due to hypersensitivity; some cases of anemia, thrombocytopenia, or agranulocytosis may be. Rarely, vasculitis develops after repeated exposure to a drug (eg, sulfonamides, iodides, penicillin), and interstitial nephritis (eg, methicillin) and liver damage (eg, halothane) have been reported in circumstances consistent with development of specific hypersensitivity.

Mechanisms of Drug Hypersensitivity

Protein and large polypeptide drugs can stimulate specific antibody production by straightforward immunologic mechanisms. Perhaps the smallest molecule that is potentially antigenic is **glucagon,** with a mol wt of about 3500. Most drug molecules are much smaller than this and cannot act alone as antigens. However, as **haptens** some bind covalently to proteins, and the resulting conjugates stimulate antibody production specific for the drug. The drug, or one of its metabolites, must be chemically

reactive with protein, and must form a stable covalent bond. The usual serum-protein binding common to many drugs is much weaker and of insufficient strength for antigenicity.

The specific immunologic reaction has been determined only for benzylpenicillin. This drug does not bind firmly enough with tissue or serum proteins to form an antigenic complex, but its major degradation product, benzylpenicillenic acid, can combine with tissue proteins to form benzylpenicilloyl **(BPO)**, the **major antigenic determinant** of penicillin. Several **minor antigenic determinants** are formed in relatively small amounts, by mechanisms that are not as well defined. IgE antibodies to the BPO determinant cause the urticaria that follows penicillin administration, while IgE antibodies to minor determinants are usually responsible for anaphylaxis as well as urticaria. In addition, IgG antibodies have been demonstrated to the major but not to the minor determinants. It is felt that these act as "blocking antibodies" to BPO, modifying or even preventing a reaction to BPO, while the lack of blocking IgG antibodies to the *minor* determinants seems to explain the ability of these determinants to induce anaphylaxis.

A BPO-polylysine conjugate (benzylpenicilloyl-polylysine), is commercially available for **skin testing**. Since the minor determinants are not available, penicillin G in a dilution of 1000 u./mL may be used. Skin testing is first performed by the prick technic. If the patient gives a history of a severe explosive reaction, the reagents should be diluted 100-fold for initial testing. Negative prick tests may be followed by intradermal testing. If skin tests are positive, the patient risks an anaphylactic reaction if treated with penicillin. Negative skin tests minimize but do not exclude the risk of a serious reaction. Although there is no evidence in man that the penicillin skin test has ever induced de novo sensitivity, it is prudent in most instances to test the patient to rule out penicillin allergy only immediately before essential penicillin therapy is begun. Since they detect only IgE-mediated reactions, skin tests will not predict the occurrence of morbilliform eruptions or hemolytic anemia.

The semisynthetic penicillins (eg, amoxicillin, carbenicillin, ticarcillin) all cross-react with penicillin, so that penicillin-sensitive patients often (though not always) react to them as well. Cross-reactions also occur with the cephalosporins, but to a lesser degree. Treatment with a cephalosporin should be started with great *caution* if the patient gives a history of a severe reaction, such as anaphylaxis, to penicillin.

Hematologic antibody-mediated (cytotoxic, Type II) drug reactions may develop by any of 3 mechanisms, examples of which are as follows: (1) In penicillin-induced anemia, the antibody reacts with the hapten, which is firmly bound to the RBC membrane, producing agglutination and increased destruction of RBCs. (2) In stibophen- and quinidine-induced thrombocytopenia (see in Ch. 99), the drug forms a soluble complex with its specific antibody. The complex then reacts with nearby platelets (the "innocent bystander" target cells) and activates complement, which alone remains on the platelet membrane and induces cell lysis. (3) In other hemolytic anemias, the drug (eg, methyldopa) appears to alter the RBC surface chemically, thereby uncovering an antigen that induces and then reacts with an autoantibody, usually of Rh specificity.

Diagnosis

Toxic-idiosyncratic and **anaphylactic reactions** are sufficiently unique in kind or in time that the offending drug is usually easily identified. **Serum-sickness–type reactions** are most often due to the penicillins, but occasionally sulfonamides, hydralazine, sulfonylureas, or thiazides are responsible. **Photosensitization** is characteristic of chlorpromazine, certain antiseptics in soaps, sulfonamides, psoralens, demeclocycline, and griseofulvin. All drugs except those deemed absolutely essential should be stopped. When **drug fever** is suspected, the most likely drug is stopped (eg, allopurinol, penicillin, isoniazid, sulfonamides, barbiturates, quinidine). Reduction in fever within 48 h

implicates that drug. If fever is accompanied by granulocytopenia, drug toxicity is more likely than allergy and is a much more serious matter (see Ch. 100).

Allergic pulmonary reactions to drugs are usually infiltrative, with eosinophilia, and can be produced by gold salts, penicillin, and sulfonamides, among others. The most common cause of an acute infiltrative pulmonary reaction is nitrofurantoin. This is probably allergic but usually not eosinophilic.

Hepatic reactions may be primarily cholestatic (phenothiazines and erythromycin estolate are most frequently involved) or hepatocellular (allopurinol, hydantoins, gold salts, isoniazid, sulfonamides, valproic acid, and many others). The usual **allergic renal reaction** is interstitial nephritis, most commonly due to methicillin; other antimicrobials and cimetidine have also been implicated.

A syndrome similar to SLE can be produced by several drugs, most commonly hydralazine and procainamide. The syndrome is associated with a positive test for antinuclear antibody and is relatively benign, sparing the kidneys and CNS. Penicillamine can produce SLE and other autoimmune reactions, most notably myasthenia gravis.

Allergic reactions in blood transfusion recipients to components in donor blood are discussed under ALLERGIC REACTIONS, in Ch. 97.

Diagnosis of any drug hypersensitivity reaction can be confirmed by challenge, ie, by readministering the drug; but reproducing most allergic reactions to confirm the relationship may be risky, and is seldom warranted.

Laboratory tests for specific drug hypersensitivity (eg, RAST, histamine release, basophil or mast cell degranulation, lymphocyte transformation) are either unreliable or remain experimental. Tests for hematologic drug reactions are an exception (see Diagnostic Tests under TYPE II HYPERSENSITIVITY REACTIONS in Ch. 20).

Skin tests for immediate-type (IgE-mediated) hypersensitivity help in diagnosis of reactions to penicillin (see under DRUG HYPERSENSITIVITY, Mechanisms, above), enzymes, xenogeneic serum, and some vaccines and polypeptide hormones, but for most drugs they are unreliable.

Treatment

It is usually necessary to stop treatment with the offending drug if the reaction appears to be allergic, in contrast to toxic reactions, where the dose often can be reduced and still be effective without causing a reaction. Most allergic reactions clear within a few days after a drug is stopped. Treatment usually can be limited to control of pain or itching. Conditions such as drug fever, a nonpruritic skin rash, or mild organ system reactions require no treatment. However, if a patient is acutely ill, with signs of multiple system involvement, or with exfoliative dermatitis, intensive glucocorticoid treatment is required (eg, prednisone 40 to 80 mg/day orally). More information on treatment of specific clinical reactions is found in the pertinent chapters throughout THE MANUAL.

Sometimes a drug that may be life-saving must be continued despite allergic manifestations; eg, treatment of bacterial endocarditis with penicillin may be continued despite the appearance of a morbilliform eruption, urticaria, or drug fever. Urticaria is treated in the usual manner, including a glucocorticoid if necessary.

Rapid desensitization to a drug may be necessary if sensitivity has been established by history and positive challenge or (for penicillin, insulin, antisera) a positive skin test, and if treatment is essential and no alternative exists. As examples, desensitization to penicillin will be described here, and foreign serum desenitization is described in the section on serum sickness. **Penicillin desensitization** is most likely to be needed to prepare an allergic person for treatment of bacterial endocarditis. This should be done if possible with the collaboration of an expert consultant. If only the intradermal skin test is positive, then the first dose should be given IV: 100 u. (or μg)/mL in a 50-mL bag. It is run in very slowly at first. If no symptoms appear, the flow rate can be

increased gradually until the bag is empty after 20 to 30 min. This is then repeated with concentrations of 1,000 and 10,000 u./mL, followed by the full therapeutic dose. If any allergic symptoms develop, the flow rate should be slowed, and the patient given appropriate drug treatment (see Anaphylaxis, above). IV desensitization is safer than s.c. or IM desensitization because not only the amount but also the rate of administration of the drug is under control. **Oral desensitization** also is safe and effective. The first dose is 100 u. (or μg); the following doses are doubled every 15 min, and symptoms are relieved with suitable anti-anaphylactic drugs if they occur. Whichever route is used, the starting dose should be a thousandfold lower if the prick test for penicillin is positive, but this practically never happens.

SERUM SICKNESS

An allergic reaction usually appearing 7 to 12 days after administration of a foreign serum or certain drugs, characterized by fever, arthralgias, skin rash, and lymphadenopathy.

Etiology

The most common cause of serum sickness is not serum, but pencillin and related drugs (see DRUG HYPERSENSITIVITY, above). Reactions from horse serum antitoxins occur in at least 5% of persons given the serum for the first time. Serum reactions have become infrequent with current active-immunization programs and antibiotics, and with the development of human immune sera for tetanus and rabies. However, horse antiserum is still used in managing diphtheria, botulism, and venomous snake and spider bites; and anti-lymphocyte or -thymocyte serum from horses and other species is used to suppress immune reactions to transplanted organs.

Injected serum is slowly excreted, so that it remains in the circulation long enough to simulate production of specific IgG antibodies that form soluble complexes with the antigen to cause an immune complex (Type III) reaction; IgE antibodies and consequently an IgE-mediated reaction also are produced. (See Ch. 20 for a discussion of the immunologic mechanisms.) Little evidence exists for an IgG immune complex mechanism in serum-sickness-type reactions caused by small-molecular-weight drugs.

Symptoms and Signs

Onset is usually several days after injection of the serum or drug but may be much sooner than the usual 7 days if the patient has been exposed previously (**anaphylaxis** or **accelerated serum sickness**). Urticaria is the usual skin manifestation. Less frequently, the rash may be multiform or morbilliform; rarely, it is scarlatiniform or purpuric. Most patients have polyarthritis or periarticular edema. Temporomandibular arthritis may be severe, and has been confused with tetanus. When fever occurs, it is mild and lasts for only 1 or 2 days. Adenopathy develops in the region draining the injection site and may become generalized. Splenomegaly is sometimes present. Occasionally, abdominal pain and diarrhea may accompany other symptoms. Myocarditis may develop but is rare. Peripheral neuritis is the only complication that may cause irreversible injury. Surprisingly, glomerulonephritis, so prominent in experimental serum sickness in animals, is rarely a problem.

Prophylaxis in Using Animal Serum to Avoid Anaphylaxis

Before giving any animal serum or animal serum product, the patient should be asked whether he has ever received serum before and whether he has a history of asthma, hay fever, urticaria, or other allergic symptoms—particularly on exposure to horses. A positive history calls for special caution to avoid acute anaphylactic reactions.

Regardless of history, any person about to receive a foreign serum *must be tested first*. Some written instructions still call for an intracutaneous test using 0.1 mL of a

1:10 dilution, but this procedure is unsatisfactory and may be dangerous: It produces many false-positive reactions and is likely to produce a generalized reaction in an allergic patient. A patient who is not atopic and who has not received horse serum previously should first be given a **prick test** with a 1:10 dilution; if this is negative, 0.02 mL of a 1:10 dilution is injected intracutaneously. A wheal more than 0.5 cm in diameter will develop within 15 min if the patient is sensitive. All patients who may have received serum previously (*whether or not they reacted*) and those with a suspected allergic history should be tested first with a 1:1000 dilution. Negative skin test results make anaphylaxis (IgE-mediated reaction) unlikely but do not predict the incidence of subsequent serum sickness.

Desensitization to foreign serum: If the skin test is positive, the risk of anaphylaxis is high. If serum treatment is essential, then desensitization is necessary first. Skin tests, using weaker concentrations prepared by serial dilution, are performed to determine the proper starting dose for desensitization, which is at the concentration that gave a weak or negative reaction. One-tenth mL of this injected s.c. or slowly IV; although not the standard method, the IV approach, as with penicillin desensitization, gives the physician control over both the concentration and rate of delivery. If no reaction occurs in 15 min, the dose is doubled every 15 min until 1 mL of undiluted serum is given. This dose is repeated IM, and if no reaction occurs in another 15 min, the full dose can be given. If a patient does react, it may still be possible to proceed cautiously by cutting back the dose, treating with an antihistamine and glucocorticoid, given as for acute urticaria, and then increasing with smaller increments.

Whenever desensitization is to be carried out, O_2, epinephrine, and resuscitation equipment must be at hand to initiate prompt treatment of anaphylaxis.

Treatment

Since the disease is self-limited, treatment of serum sickness is usually restricted to relief of symptoms. Pruritus is treated with an antihistamine as for acute urticaria; arthralgias, with salicylates (aspirin 0.6 to 1.5 gm orally q 4 h). If these are not adequate, prednisone 30 mg/day orally is almost always effective; the dose is gradually reduced to zero after symptoms have been relieved. Early, intensive glucocorticoid treatment is necessary if the rare complications of peripheral neuritis or myocarditis develop.

AUTOIMMUNE DISORDERS

Disorders in which the immune system produces autoantibodies to an endogenous antigen, with consequent injury to tissues.

Considered here are the pathogenetic immunologic mechanisms underlying autoimmune diseases (see also TABLE 21–1). Clinical aspects of the specific disorders are presented elsewhere in THE MANUAL.

Development of the Autoimmune Response

Although precise details of the autoimmune response are incompletely understood, the outcome of antigenic stimulation, whether antibody formation or activated T cells or tolerance, seems to depend on the same factors with autoantigen as with exogenous antigen. Four possible mechanisms for developing an immune response to autoantigens are recognized:

1. Hidden or sequestered antigens (eg, intracellular substances) may not be recognized as "self"; if released into the circulation they may induce an immune response. This occurs in sympathetic ophthalmia with the traumatic release of an antigen normally sequestered within the eye. Autoantibody alone may not produce disease because it cannot combine with the sequestered antigen. For example, antibodies to sperm and

TABLE 21–1. PUTATIVE AUTOIMMUNE DISORDERS

	Disorder	*Mechanism or Evidence*
Highly Probable	Hashimoto's thyroiditis	Cell-mediated and humoral thyroid cytotoxicity
	Systemic lupus erythematosus	Circulating and locally generated immune complexes
	Goodpasture's syndrome	Anti-basement membrane antibody
	Pemphigus	Epidermal acantholytic antibody
	Receptor autoimmunity	
	Graves' disease	TSH receptor antibody (stimulatory)
	Myasthenia gravis	Acetylcholine receptor antibody
	Insulin resistance	Insulin receptor antibody
	Autoimmune hemolytic anemia	Phagocytosis of antibody-sensitized erythrocytes
	Autoimmune thrombocytopenic purpura	Phagocytosis of antibody-sensitized platelets
Probable	Rheumatoid arthritis	Immune complexes in joints
	Progressive systemic sclerosis	Nucleolar and other nuclear antibodies
	Mixed connective tissue disease	Antibody to extractable nuclear antigen (ribonucleoprotein)
	Polymyositis	Non-histone ANA*
	Pernicious anemia	Anti-parietal cell, microsomes, and intrinsic factor antibodies
	Idiopathic Addison's disease	Humoral and (?) cell-mediated adrenal cytotoxicity
	Infertility (some cases)	Antispermatozoal antibodies
	Glomerulonephritis	Glomerular basement membrane antibody, or immune complexes
	Bullous pemphigoid	IgG and complement in basement membrane
	Sjögren's syndrome	Multiple tissue antibodies, a specific non-histone ANA (SS-B)
	Diabetes mellitus (some)	Cell-mediated and humoral islet cell antibodies
	Adrenergic drug resistance (some asthmatics)	β-adrenergic receptor antibody
Possible	Chronic active hepatitis	Smooth muscle antibody
	Primary biliary cirrhosis	Mitochondrial antibody
	Other endocrine gland failure	Specific tissue antibodies in some cases
	Vitiligo	Melanocyte antibody
	Vasculitis	Some cases: immunoglobulin and complement in vessel walls, low serum complement
	Post-myocardial infarction, cardiotomy syndrome	Myocardial antibody
	Urticaria, atopic dermatitis, asthma (some cases)	IgG and IgM antibodies to IgE
	Many other inflammatory, granulomatous, degenerative, and atrophic disorders	No reasonable alternative explanation

* ANA = Antinuclear antibody.

heart muscle antigens are blocked by the basement membrane of the seminiferous tubules and myocardial cell membrane, respectively. Immunologically active T cells however, may not have such restrictions and would be more effective in producing injury.

2. The "self" antigens may become immunogenic because of chemical, physical, o

biologic alteration. Certain chemicals couple with body proteins and render them immunogenic, as seen in contact dermatitis. Drugs can produce several autoimmune reactions (see DRUG HYPERSENSITIVITY, above). Photosensitivity exemplifies physically induced autoallergy: ultraviolet light alters skin protein, to which the patient becomes allergic. Biologically altered antigens are seen in New Zealand mice that develop autoallergic disease resembling SLE when persistently infected with an RNA virus known to combine with host tissues, altering them sufficiently to induce antibody.

3. Foreign antigen may induce an immune response that cross-reacts with normal "self" antigen. Examples are the cross-reaction that occurs between streptococcal M protein and human heart muscle, and the encephalitis that can follow rabies vaccination in which an autoimmune cross-reaction probably is initiated by animal brain tissue in the vaccine.

4. Autoantibody production may be a result of mutational change in immunocompetent cells. This may explain the monoclonal autoantibodies seen occasionally in patients with lymphoma.

Finally, autoimmune phenomena may be epiphenomena, and the primary pathogenesis the result of an immune response to an obscure antigen; eg, a virus.

Probably the autoimmune reaction is normally held in check by the action of a population of specific suppressor T cells. Any of the above processes could lead to, or be associated with, a suppressor T cell defect. Perhaps a perturbation in the regulation of antibody activity by anti-idiotype antibodies (antibodies to the antigen combining site of other antibodies) may play a role.

The role of other complex mechanisms demonstrable experimentally still needs clarification. For example, adjuvants such as alum or bacterial endotoxin, while not antigenic themselves, enhance the antigenicity of other substances. Freund's complete adjuvant, an emulsion of antigen in mineral oil with heat-killed mycobacteria, is usually required in order to produce autoimmunity in experimental animals.

Genetic factors play a role in autoimmune disorders. Relatives of patients with autoimmune disorders often show a high incidence of the same type of autoantibodies, and the incidence of autoimmune disease is higher in identical than in fraternal twins. Women are more often affected than men. The genetic contribution appears to be one of predisposition. In a predisposed population a number of environmental factors could provoke disease; eg, in SLE these might be latent virus infection, drugs, or tissue injury such as occurs with ultraviolet light exposure. This situation would be analogous to the development of hemolytic anemia as a consequence of environmental factors in persons with G6PD deficiency, a predisposing genetically determined biochemical abnormality.

Pathogenesis

The pathogenetic mechanisms of autoimmune reactions are, in many cases, better understood than the way in which autoimmune antibodies develop. In some autoimmune hemolytic anemias, the RBCs become coated with cytotoxic (Type II) autoantibody; the complement system responds to these antibody-coated cells just as it does to similarly coated foreign particles, and the interaction of complement with the antibody complexed to the cell surface antigen leads to RBC phagocytosis or cytolysis.

Autoimmune renal injury can occur as the result of either an antibody-mediated (Type II) or immune complex (Type III) reaction. The antibody-mediated reaction occurs in Goodpasture's syndrome, in which lung and renal disease is associated with the presence of an anti-basement membrane antibody (see Ch. 44). The best-known example of autoimmune injury associated with soluble antigen-antibody complexes (immune complexes) is the nephritis associated with SLE (see in Chs. 110 and 149 and below). Another example is a form of membranous glomerulonephritis that is associated with an immune complex containing renal tubular antigen. Although it is possible

that poststreptococcal glomerulonephritis could be due in part to streptococcus induced cross-reacting antibodies, there is as yet no proof of this.

A variety of autoantibodies are produced in **SLE** and other systemic (as opposed to organ-specific) autoimmune diseases. Antibodies to formed elements in the blood account for autoimmune hemolytic anemia (see in Ch. 96), thrombocytopenia, and possibly leukopenia; anticoagulant antibodies may cause bleeding problems. Antibodies to nuclear material result in deposition of antigen-antibody complexes, not only in glomeruli, but also in vascular tissues and in skin at the dermal-epidermal junction. Synovial deposition of aggregated IgG-rheumatoid factor **(RF)**-complement complexes occurs in **RA. RF** is usually an IgM globulin (occasionally IgG or IgA) with specificity for a receptor on the constant region of the heavy chain of autologous IgG. The IgG-RF-complement aggregates can also be found within neutrophils, where they cause the release of lysosomal enzymes that contribute to the inflammatory joint reaction. Plasma cells are also present in large numbers within the joint, and may synthesize anti-IgG antibodies. T cells and lymphokines are also found in rheumatoid joints and may contribute to the inflammatory process. The process that sets off the immunologic events is unknown; it could be a bacterial or viral infection. In SLE the low serum complement level reflects the widespread immunologic reactions taking place; in RA, by contrast, serum complement is normal but intrasynovial complement levels are low.

In **pernicious anemia,** autoantibodies capable of neutralizing intrinsic factor are found in the GI lumen. Autoantibodies against the microsomal fraction of gastric mucosal cells are even more common. It is postulated that a cell-mediated autoimmune attack against the parietal cells results in the atrophic gastritis that, in turn, reduces the production of intrinsic factor but still allows absorption of sufficient vitamin B_{12} to prevent the megaloblastic anemia. If autoantibodies to intrinsic factor should also develop in the GI lumen, however, B_{12} absorption will cease and pernicious anemia will develop.

Hashimoto's thyroiditis is associated with autoantibodies to thyroglobulin, the microsomes of thyroid epithelial cells, a thyroid cell-surface antigen, and a second colloid antigen. Tissue injury and eventual myxedema may be mediated both by the cytotoxicity of the microsomal antibody and by the activity of specifically committed T cells. Low-titered antibodies are also found in patients with primary myxedema, suggesting that it is the end result of unrecognized autoimmune thyroiditis. An autoimmune reaction is also involved in thyrotoxicosis **(Graves' disease),** and about 10% of patients eventually develop myxedema spontaneously; many more do so after ablative therapy. Other antibodies, unique to Graves' disease, are called thyroid-stimulating antibodies. They react with thyroid-stimulating hormone **(TSH)** receptors in the gland and have the same effect on thyroid cell function that TSH normally has.

---

22. TRANSPLANTATION

The transfer of living tissues or cells from one individual to another, with the objective of maintaining the functional integrity of the transplanted tissue in the recipient.

GENERAL CONSIDERATIONS

Despite surgical technics making transplantation of almost any tissue feasible, the clinical use of transplantation to remedy disease is still limited for many organ systems. The greatest obstacle is the **rejection reaction,** which generally destroys the tissue shortly after transplantation (except in special circumstances, such as most cornea and cartilage grafts, or transplants between identical twins). Nevertheless, with improved understanding of immune mechanisms and methods for preventing rejection

organ transplantation now saves many patients with otherwise fatal disease. In addition, although the cost of organ transplantation is high, it is a curative treatment for end-stage organ failure. The cost of alternative noncurative terminal care of patients with end-stage organ failure can be exorbitant.

Transplants are categorized by the site of transplantation and by the genetic relationship between donor and recipient. A tissue or organ graft is **orthotopic** if it is transferred to an anatomically normal recipient site—as in a heart transplant. If the transplant is to an anatomically abnormal site, it is **heterotopic**—as in the transplantation of a kidney into the iliac fossa of the recipient. An **autograft** is a transfer of tissue from one location to another in the same individual (eg, bone grafting for fracture stabilization). An **isograft** is a graft between identical twins; an **allograft (homograft)** is one between genetically dissimilar members of the same species. **Xenografts (heterografts)** are transplants between members of different species.

The only xenografts now performed are with fixed, nonviable material such as porcine heart valves. With rare exceptions clinical transplants are thus allografts from either living relatives or cadaveric donors. The use of living donors is only appropriate in kidney transplantation, and even for kidneys the need for organs far exceeds the number available from relatives of patients with chronic renal failure. Use of cadaveric organs has become more prevalent as the concept of brain death has gained acceptance. As the demand for cadaveric organs has increased, procedures for procuring multiple organs from a single donor have become common. Kidneys, liver (or pancreas), heart (or heart/lungs), bones, skin, and corneas can now routinely be procured at a single operative procedure.

IMMUNOBIOLOGIC PRINCIPLES

Allografts may be rejected through either a cell-mediated or a humoral immune reaction of the recipient against **transplantation (histocompatibility) antigens** present on the donor's cell membranes. The strongest antigens are governed by a complex of genetic loci and are termed **HLA** (see below); together with the major blood group **(ABO)** antigens, they are the chief transplantation antigens presently detectable in man. Because transplantation antigens can be identified by their effects in vitro, tissue typing (see TISSUE COMPATIBILITY, below) is possible.

The **lymphocyte (cell)-mediated immune reaction** against transplantation antigens (ie, the **host-vs.-graft reaction [HVGR]**) is the principal mechanism of **acute rejection**. A delayed hypersensitivity response similar to the tuberculin reaction, HVGR causes graft destruction days to months after transplantation and is characterized histologically by mononuclear cellular infiltration of the allograft, with varying degrees of hemorrhage and edema. Usually, vascular integrity is maintained; thus, cell-mediated rejection may be reversed in many cases by intensifying immunosuppressive therapy. After successful reversal of an acute episode, histologic examination shows that severely damaged elements of the graft have healed by fibrosis and that the remainder of the graft appears to be normal. After resolution of acute rejection, the allograft will commonly survive for prolonged periods, even though the immunosuppressive drug dosages have been reduced to very low levels. This process of "graft adaptation" is most likely explained by development of donor-specific suppression of the recipient's immune response.

Late graft deterioration occurs occasionally in immunosuppressed patients. This chronic type of rejection is often insidious but relentless in progression despite increased immunosuppressive measures. The pathologic picture differs from that of acute rejection. The vascular endothelium is primarily involved, with extensive proliferation that gradually occludes the vessel lumen, resulting in ischemia and fibrosis of the graft.

The role of humoral antibody in graft rejection is obvious when the recipient has been **presensitized** (by pregnancy, blood transfusion, or previous transplantation) to HLA antigens present in the graft. Transplantation in these circumstances almost invariably leads to **hyperacute rejection,** causing destruction of the graft within hours or even minutes after revascularization (see TISSUE COMPATIBILITY, below). This antibody-mediated rejection reaction is characterized by small vessel thrombosis and graft infarction and cannot be reversed by any known immunosuppressive technics (unlike lymphocyte-mediated rejection). Interestingly, liver grafts seem not to be susceptible to this form of antibody-mediated hyperacute rejection. The role of humoral antibody in more delayed graft destruction is probably also important but is still unclear.

A result similar to antibody-mediated rejection usually occurs if a graft is transplanted in defiance of the blood group barriers normally observed in blood transfusions. Therefore, **pretransplant evaluation** must include verifying the ABO compatibility between donor and recipient and the existence of a negative cross-match for tissue antibodies (lack of significant reactivity between donor leukocytes and recipient serum in vitro), as well as tissue typing for HLA compatibility.

THE HLA SYSTEM

A group of tissue antigens termed **HLA** *(for* ***h****uman* ***l****eukocyte group* **A***), governed by a chromosomal region bearing a number of genetic loci, each with multiple alleles, that have relevance to transplantation rejection reactions and that mark the prevalence of several diseases.* HLA antigens are found in varying concentrations on virtually all nucleated cells of the body. The immunologic response to these antigens is the major cause of most graft rejection episodes.

HLA antigens are controlled by a complex of genes at several closely linked loci collectively called the major histocompatibility complex **(MHC),** located on the 6th chromosome. Four distinct genetic loci (Loci A, B, C, and D) within the MHC have been identified to date. The genes are allelic; ie, a number of different forms of each gene are found in the population; all alleles are codominant. By mendelian laws, each person has 2 alleles from each locus or, possibly, a pair of identical alleles. (See FIG. 22–1.)

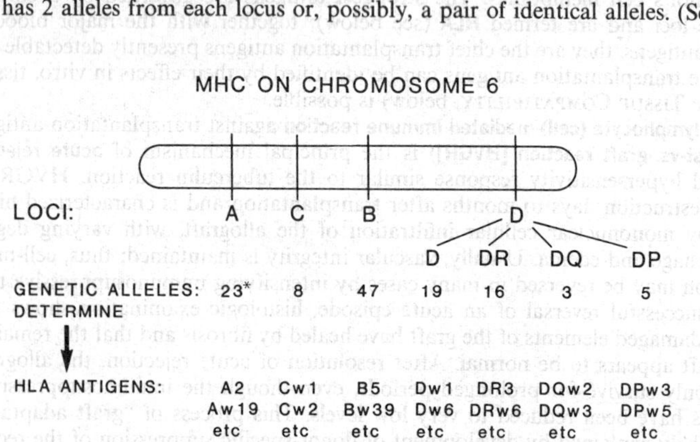

FIG. 22–1. Schematic illustration of the major histocompatibility complex (MHC) in man. Allelic genes at each of the loci determine the cell membrane antigens. The (*) denotes the number of currently recognized alleles at each locus. The cells of each individual express 2 antigens for each locus. However, because of the possibility of homozygosity at a locus, or the presence of alleles which have not yet been identified, tissue typing frequently fails to identify all the HLA antigens possessed by an individual.

Because the alleles were numbered before their loci were identified, those on Loci A and B are not numbered consecutively. The difficulties encountered in identifying and sorting out this complex allelic system led to much confusion in original nomenclature. Since 1975, the WHO committee on leukocyte nomenclature has periodically met to assign universally accepted designations to well-recognized individual alleles of each locus (eg, HLA-A1, HLA-B5, HLA-Cw1, HLA-Dw1). Those alleles that are still provisional are designated with a "w." Extensive research continues, and both the number of named specificities and understanding of the different antigens' involvement in the immune response to transplanted tissues are rapidly expanding.

The antigens encoded by the A, B, and C loci are similar biochemically and are identified serologically with relative ease. As a group they are referred to as **class I antigens** and show great homology to serologically detected transplantation antigens in other species. The D locus products are referred to as **class II antigens** and are homologous to the immune response **(Ir)** gene products of other species. These antigens are structurally dissimilar to the class I antigens and are detected serologically with some difficulty. There are several distinct subloci in the D region of the 6th chromosome. The multiple D locus products, although similar in structure, appear to differ in tissue distribution and functional significance.

In **the rejection reaction**, class I and class II antigens elicit different responses. **T lymphocytes** responding to classes I and II can be distinguished not only functionally but by **differentiation antigens** present on the surface of the responding T cells. With the development of **monoclonal antibodies** (uniformly identical antibodies produced by hybridized cells) reactive with these differentiation antigens, such antigens can be used as markers to monitor T cell subpopulations in the rejection reaction.

Class I reactive lymphocytes express T cell antigens often associated with **cytotoxic effector** and **suppressor cell** function. **Helper cell** function activity usually is provided by T cells expressing the differentiation antigens that characterize class II reactive lymphocytes. Thus, while the brunt of immune destruction of the rejection reaction may be directed at class I antigens both via anti-HLA antibodies and cytotoxic effector lymphocytes, lymphocytes that respond to the class II antigens seem to be necessary to facilitate a maximal rejection reaction. Evidence presently suggests that **immunologic tolerance** (see under IMMUNOSUPPRESSION, below) to class II antigens may be more easily produced than tolerance to class I antigens, and that abrogation of the helper function of class II reactive cells can lead to host acceptance of grafts having both class I and class II antigen incompatibilities.

Non-transplantation associations for class I and class II antigens: Evidence is accumulating that the genes encoding for these antigens (and other closely linked genes in the MHC) are of special importance to the general immune function and health of an individual. Several complement components and properdin factor B are governed by genes linked to the MHC. Also, specific HLA antigens have a statistical association with various presumed autoimmune disorders and lymphoid-cell neoplasms, although the pathogenetic meaning of such associations is unknown. For example, psoriasis incidence increases in association with B13 and Bw17, but decreases in association with B12. Ankylosing spondylitis and Reiter's syndrome have a pronounced positive correlation with the B27 genotype. DR3 and DR4 seem to be positively associated with Type I diabetes mellitus, Dw4 and DR2 with multiple sclerosis, and DR4 with RA. In contrast, persons with malignant lymphomas seem to have a markedly reduced incidence of A11. Perhaps even more intriguing in terms of transplantation is the recently postulated association of DRw6 with an Ir gene controlling the vigor of the rejection to renal allografts.

TISSUE COMPATIBILITY

The degree of similarity of the genetically determined tissue antigens on donor and recipient cells.

Histocompatibility (or tissue) typing of peripheral blood or lymph node lymphocytes is performed prior to transplantation. The goal is to identify the HLA antigens serologically and, by appropriate donor selection, to minimize the antigenic differences between donor and recipient. Histocompatibility matching of HLA-A and -B antigens has significantly improved functional survival of transplants between related individuals. Results between unrelated individuals also show definite correlations with typing tests for compatibility of class I antigens, although less clearly, since the complex histocompatibility differences in an outbred population introduce many more variables. More recent approaches have evaluated the importance of donor-recipient compatibility for class II antigens, since class II antigenic disparity seems to be necessary to generate an optimal immune response. Preliminary studies in renal allograft recipients appear to show a better survival rate in patients sharing one or two class II antigens with the donor, although this observation has not been confirmed in all clinical trials.

Detecting specific presensitization of the recipient against donor antigens is more important than matching for donor-recipient histocompatibility antigens prior to transplantation. Such presensitization most commonly results from prior blood transfusions or pregnancies and is evaluated by a lymphocytotoxic test between recipient serum and donor lymphocytes in the presence of complement. A positive cross-match usually indicates antibodies in the recipient's serum directed against donor class I antigens, commonly foreboding hyperacute rejection of the allograft and therefore generally considered to be a contraindication to transplantation. Some antibodies identified in the lymphocytotoxic cross-match are now known to be directed against HLA-D or other antigens present on the B lymphocyte (and monocyte) subpopulation of peripheral blood but not on T lymphocytes, platelets, or most other nucleated cells. The significance of a positive B cell cross-match is not clear, since transplantation in its presence does not necessarily result in early failure. Unfortunately, the length of time which some organs (ie, heart and liver) can be safely stored after procurement is very short and does not always allow for complete tissue type and cross-match testing before transplantation.

The role of blood transfusions in dialysis and renal transplantation is controversial. Historically, transfusions to patients with end-stage renal failure have been shunned to avoid sensitization of potential kidney transplant recipients. However, evidence is clear that allograft survival is improved in those recipients receiving transfusions who do not become sensitized. At first it seemed that this **transfusion effect** was simply a selection process by which individuals with a vigorous immune response were excluded from receiving transplants because of presensitization. However, careful analysis of presensitization frequency and of improved transplant survival following transfusions indicates that selection can only partially account for the improved survival rates. Some altered form (ie, suppression) of immune responsiveness seems to be induced by the transfusions.

The dilemma between risking dangerous presensitization vs. achieving a beneficial immunosuppressive effect is presently being dealt with in some transplantation centers by transfusing potential transplant recipients with buffy-coat–poor red cell preparations. The risk of presensitization may be even further reduced by using frozen washed red cell transfusions, probably because viable leukocytes are absent in these preparations. Alternatively, multiple small transfusions given with immunosuppressive drugs reduce this risk. For recipients of kidneys from cadaveric donors, random donor transfusions are used. For recipients of living-related donor kidneys, **donor-specific transfu-**

sions help in transplant survival, although they offer a greater risk of presensitization to the donor. If this occurs, a transplant with an otherwise high likelihood of success is precluded.

IMMUNOSUPPRESSION

Immunosuppressive agents are used to control the rejection reaction caused by antigenic differences remaining after tissue typing and donor-recipient matching. Since these drugs for the most part suppress all immunologic reactions, overwhelming infection is the leading cause of death in transplant recipients. Nevertheless, carefully selected and administered immunosuppressive treatment has been primarily responsible for the present success of clinical transplantation. As more selective immunosuppressive agents are introduced, optimism for further success seems warranted.

Except with isografts, immunosuppressive therapy can rarely be stopped completely after transplantation. However, intensive immunosuppression is usually required only during the first few weeks after transplantation or during rejection crises. Subsequently, the graft often seems to become accommodated and can be maintained with relatively small doses of immunosuppressive drugs and fewer adverse effects.

Prednisone or **methylprednisolone** usually is given in high doses (2 to 20 mg/kg) at the time of transplantation and then reduced gradually to a maintenance dose of 0.2 mg/kg/day given indefinitely. Late after transplantation, the drug often is administered on an alternate-day basis to reduce corticosteroid side effects, particularly important in children, where growth is desirable. This approach somewhat increases the risk of rejection. If allograft rejection occurs the dose is sharply increased, risking serious side effects, especially increased susceptibility to infection. Because prednisone causes persistent adrenal suppression, supplemental corticosteroids are needed during periods of stress such as infections, major trauma, or surgery.

Azathioprine, an antimetabolite and a key immunosuppressive drug, is given orally or IV, usually beginning at the time of transplantation. Doses of 1.5 to 3 mg/kg/day generally are tolerated indefinitely by the transplant recipient. Azathioprine's primary toxic effects are bone marrow depression and hepatitis (reactivation of viral hepatitis may be the underlying factor).

Cyclophosphamide has been substituted in patients who do not tolerate azathioprine. Equivalent doses are apparently equal in immunosuppressive activity. This alkylating agent also is used in much larger doses as one of the primary immunosuppressive drugs in bone marrow transplantation, but severe toxicity (hemorrhagic cystitis, alopecia, and infertility) is common.

Cyclosporine, a fungal metabolite, has recently been used in place of antimetabolic drugs in several transplant trials. Unlike antimetabolites, cyclosporine spares the bone marrow, acting instead more selectively to inhibit T cell proliferation and activation. The exact mechanism of its action is unknown although multiple effects seem likely, including both inhibition of **interleukin-2** (a T cell lymphokine) production, and inhibition of T cell responsiveness to this lymphokine. Interestingly, in experimental models, while helper cell activity is inhibited, activation of suppressor T cells is not.

Although cyclosporine can be given as a sole immunosuppressant, it usually is used in conjunction with prednisone, allowing a rapid reduction in corticosteroid dose and its adverse effects. At the time of transplantation, initial doses of cyclosporine are 10 to 20 mg/kg/day orally, reduced to a maintenance level of 5 to 8 mg/kg/day soon after transplantation. Rejection reactions with cyclosporine appear to be milder and more easily reversed than with other drugs. Whether, as a more selective immunosuppressant, it will lead to a decrease in infection remains to be seen. Counterbalancing optimism over cyclosporine's efficacy is its considerable toxicity. Nephrotoxicity, hep-

atotoxicity, refractory hypertension, and increased incidence of neoplasms (especially lymphomas and other lymphoproliferative lesions), as well as several less serious side effects, have been reported, especially at high doses. Although the blood level of cyclosporine can be easily measured, there is no adequate means of determining the therapeutically effective amount of cyclosporine necessary for a given patient.

Antilymphocyte globulin—ALG (antilymphocyte serum—ALS) and **antithymocyte globulin (ATG)**: Attempts to obtain more selective immunosuppression include the use of antisera to human lymphocytes or thymus cells in an effort to suppress cellular immunity while leaving the recipient's humoral immunologic response intact, preserving defenses against many bacterial infections. ALG and ATG are useful adjuncts, allowing other immunosuppressive agents to be used in lower, less toxic, doses. The use of ALG and ATG at the time of transplantation has shown only marginal benefit; however, its use to control established rejection episodes has clearly led to improved graft survival rates. Possible adverse reactions to heterologous sera include anaphylactic reactions, serum sickness, or antigen-antibody–induced glomerulonephritis; but using highly purified serum fractions, giving them IV, and combining them with other immunosuppressive agents has greatly reduced the incidence of these reactions.

Monoclonal antibodies against T cells offer a much greater concentration of specifically reactive antibody molecules and a greatly reduced amount of irrelevant serum proteins compared to polyclonal antiglobulin fractions. The monoclonal antibody, OK-T3, has been shown to reverse rejection very effectively in initial trials. This monoclonal antibody reacts with a 20-kilodalton glycoprotein which is part of the T cell antigen receptor complex. As the role of distinct T cell subpopulations in the rejection reaction is better understood, the use of monoclonal antibodies reactive with specific subpopulations will allow even greater selectivity in immune suppression. Clinical trials with monoclonal antibodies which react with antigens present only on activated T cells (sparing T cells not participating in the rejection reaction) are now in progress.

Irradiation for immunosuppression is of limited clinical use in transplantation. The graft and local recipient tissues are sometimes irradiated, either as an adjunct prophylactic immunosuppressive measure or during treatment of established rejection. The total dose (usually 400 to 600 rads) is below the threshold that might cause serious radiation injury of the graft itself. Extracorporeal irradiation of the recipient's blood or lymph as it traverses a surgically created fistula has had some success but is too cumbersome for use on a large clinical scale. In treating refractory leukemia, whole-body irradiation in 1200-rad doses combined with chemotherapy destroys the host's immunologic capability (and residual leukemic cells). Here, irradiation is followed by a bone marrow allograft.

Recently, interest in irradiation therapy has been renewed, stimulated by the observation that treatment directed (by suitable shielding such as that used for Hodgkin's disease) toward all lymphoid centers **(total lymphatic irradiation [TLI])** appears to provide a profound but relatively safe suppression of cellular immunity, possibly mediated by suppressor T cells which can be detected following TLI. Application of this technic to transplantation is experimental but promising.

Immunologic tolerance (unresponsiveness): Ultimately, transplant biologists hope to provide specific and selective suppression of the recipient's response only to the foreign antigens on the graft. Such immunologic tolerance is best exemplified by the prenatal development of a specific unresponsive state to one's own body constituents. Induction of tolerance to foreign antigens in the adult has been accomplished experimentally by careful selection of conditions, such as antigen dose, route of injection, and short-term use of other immunosuppressive agents. As stated above (see THE HLA SYSTEM), tolerance may be easier to induce to class II than to class I antigens, and tolerance to this one type of histocompatibility antigen may suffice to facilitate graft

acceptance. However, no reliable method for producing such an effect safely in patients has yet been devised.

CLINICAL TRANSPLANTATION

Rarely since the first successful kidney transplant > 25 yr ago has there been as much anticipated expansion of transplant surgery's role in treating end-stage organ failure as exists at present. Projected transplant survival rates are improved (see FIG. 22–2); transplantation of organs other than kidneys (eg, livers and hearts) has become accepted as of proved value. Instrumental in achieving this expanded role are the new, more selective immunosuppressive reagents; but improved histocompatibility typing and surgical technic, better patient selection, earlier operative intervention, earlier and more accurate detection of rejection episodes, and a better understanding of the immune rejection mechanism also have contributed.

KIDNEY TRANSPLANTATION

All patients with terminal renal failure should be considered for transplantation except those at risk from another life-threatening condition. Patient rehabilitation following successful transplantation is generally much more complete than that achieved with hemodialysis, not only because of freedom from the required prolonged treatments 3 times weekly but also because of the kidney's beneficial metabolic functions, such as erythropoietic stimulation and calcium homeostasis. Patient survival 1 yr after transplantation from a living-related donor is over 95%, with approximately 80 to 95% of the allografts functioning. Subsequently, an annual patient or graft loss of 3 to 5% is observed. The 1-yr patient survival rate following transplantation from a cadaveric donor is approximately 90%, and graft survival ranges between 50 to 85% at various centers. In subsequent years, some 5 to 8% of grafts or patients are lost annually. There are now several renal transplant recipients who have had functioning grafts for > 20 yr. Transplantation in patients over age 55 has been felt by some groups to represent an unacceptable risk to the recipient. However, with the use of more limited immunosuppression and close immunologic monitoring, allografting has proceeded in selected patients even in the 7th decade of life.

Pretransplant preparation includes hemodialysis to ensure a relatively normal metabolic state, and provision of a functional, infection-free lower urinary tract. Bladder reconstruction, nephrectomy of infected kidneys, or construction of a colon conduit for draining the allograft may be required.

Donor selection and kidney preservation: Kidney allografts are obtained from living relatives or cadaveric donors, excluding donors with a history of hypertension, diabetes, or malignant disease except possibly those with neoplasms originating in the CNS. Living donors are also carefully evaluated for emotional stability, normal bilateral renal function, freedom from other systemic disease, and histocompatibility. A living donor gives up reserve renal capacity, may have complex psychologic conflicts, and faces some morbidity from nephrectomy; yet the significantly improved long-term prognosis for a recipient of a well-matched allograft justifies the consideration of the related donor in most instances.

Over half of kidney transplants are from cadavers, in many instances from previously healthy persons who sustained brain death but maintained stable cardiovascular and renal function. Following brain death, the kidneys are removed as soon as is practical and cooled by perfusion. For simple hypothermic storage, special cooling solutions containing relatively large concentrations of poorly permeating substances such as mannitol, and electrolyte concentrations approximating intracellular levels (eg, Collins or Sachs solution), are used to flush the kidney, which is then stored in the iced

solution. Kidneys preserved by this method usually function well if transplanted within 48 h. By using the more complex technic of continuous pulsatile hypothermic perfusion with an oxygenated, plasma-based perfusate, kidneys have been successfully transplanted after ex vivo perfusion of as long as 72 h.

Transplant procedure and rejection management: The transplanted kidney usually is placed retroperitoneally in the iliac fossa. Vascular anastomoses are performed to the iliac vessels, and ureteral continuity is established. Despite prophylactic immunosup-

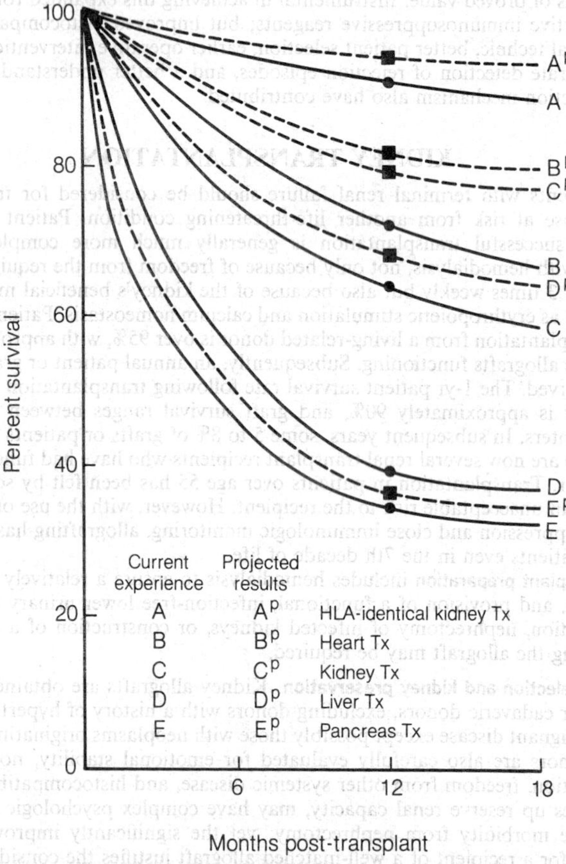

Fig. 22–2. Survival of organ transplants. The solid lines represent estimates of the survival rates of transplanted organs over the past few years at most centers. Dotted lines indicate "projected" survival rates as they are now being reported by some centers, suggesting that the overall international experience will probably rise to approach these levels in the future. The increases in survival indicated depend upon improved immunosuppressive management (including the use of cyclosporine), the judicious use of preoperative blood transfusions, and numerous other factors. In the case of liver transplants some of the surviving patients have actually received more than one liver transplant. (From "Transplantation of Solid Organs" by P. S. Russell in *Immunological Diseases,* M. Samter, ed., Little, Brown and Company, Boston. In press. Used with permission of Little, Brown and Company.)

pressive therapy (see IMMUNOSUPPRESSION, above) begun just before or at the time of transplantation, most recipients undergo one or more acute rejection episodes in the early post-transplant period. Rejection is suggested by deterioration of renal function, hypertension, weight gain, tenderness and swelling of the graft, fever, and appearance in the urine sediment of protein, lymphocytes, and renal tubular cells. If the diagnosis is unclear, percutaneous needle biopsy is performed to obtain tissue for histopathologic evaluation. In cyclosporine-treated recipients drug-induced nephrotoxicity is sometimes difficult to differentiate from rejection, even with the aid of biopsy. Rejection usually is reversed by intensified immunosuppression. If it cannot be reversed, immunosuppression is tapered, and the patient is returned to hemodialysis to await a subsequent transplant.

Most rejection episodes and other complications occur within 3 to 4 mo after transplantation, the majority of patients then returning to more normal health and activity. However, immunosuppressive medication must be maintained unless toxicity or severe infection occurs, since even brief cessation may precipitate rejection.

Late complications: Some patients suffer irreversible chronic graft rejection, with progressive hypertension and gradual deterioration of renal function that may necessitate nephrectomy and retransplantation. Other late complications include drug toxicity, recurrent underlying renal disease, prednisone side effects, and infection. In addition, the incidence of malignancy in renal allograft recipients has increased. The risk of epithelial carcinoma is 4 to 5 times higher than normal; of lymphoma, about 30 times. Management of these neoplasms is similar to that for cancer in nonimmunosuppressed patients. Reduction or interruption of immunosuppression is not generally required in treating squamous cell epitheliomas but is recommended for more aggressive tumors and lymphomas.

LIVER TRANSPLANTATION

Liver transplantation is accepted as appropriate treatment for end-stage hepatic dysfunction. Earlier poor results were due largely to technical difficulties (ie, inability to provide adequate biliary drainage) and to septic complications, but survival rates have improved markedly with advances in surgical technic and with the use of cyclosporine. One-yr survival rates have climbed from a previous 33% to 70%. Late deaths have been rare and mostly secondary to recurrent disease rather than post-transplant difficulties. The longest-surviving liver transplant recipient to date has now had his hepatic graft in place 16 yr. Most of the liver transplant procedures that have been performed have taken place within the last 5 yr, so that long-term prognosis is not yet established. However, if hepatic transplantation is successful, recipients are fully rehabilitated, returning to normal social and work activity.

In addition to direct immunosuppressant effects, cyclosporine stimulated (1) the omission of antimetabolites and the early reduction of corticosteroid dosage, resulting in better postoperative healing and greater resistance to overwhelming infection; (2) the willingness, with better results, to accept for transplantation patients with end-stage liver disease before they reach a terminal debilitated state; and (3) the demonstration that liver retransplantation is possible if a graft fails. At present, 20 to 30% of liver transplant patients are retransplanted, with a salvage rate of > 50%. Previously, these patients would have died in the early postoperative period. Improved success rates are not due to cyclosporine exclusively; one transplant center not using this drug has achieved equal success by careful patient selection and management.

Indications for liver transplantation have been mainly diseases causing chronic hepatic failure. In acute hepatic failure, prognosis is difficult to assess, time to obtain a suitable donor is often inadequate, and the risk of recurrent viral infection in the transplant liver and of transmitting infection to medical personnel is not inconsequential. End-stage chronic hepatitis and biliary cirrhosis are the most frequent indications in adults,

as are biliary atresia and inborn metabolic deficiencies in children. Primary hepatic malignancy has a relatively poor prognosis; the tumor frequently recurs following transplantation in the immunosuppressed patient, leading to a 1-yr survival rate of only about 20%. However, with hepatic carcinoma entirely confined to the liver, especially of the fibrolamellar type, long-term tumor-free survival has occurred. **Donors** of livers for transplantation must be previously normal individuals who are size- and ABO-matched to the recipient and have suffered brain death. A history of hepatic dysfunction, hypotension requiring prolonged vasopressor support, systemic infection, or evidence of liver ischemia or damage suggested by elevation of hepatic enzymes preclude organ use.

Liver preservation and transplantation procedures: Long-term extracorporeal hepatic preservation methods are not available; livers are stored after removal in cold solutions and ischemic times of only 6 to 8 h are acceptable. Tissue typing and cross-match testing usually are done retrospectively. Recipient hepatectomy, which can result in intraoperative blood loss ranging from 10 to > 100 units, is the most demanding part of the transplant procedure and is often performed in the face of portal hypertension and following previous hepatobiliary surgery. To complete the transplant, 5 anastomoses are required: suprahepatic vena cava, infrahepatic vena cava, portal vein, hepatic artery, and biliary duct (now with choledocho-coledochostomy or choledocho-enterostomy via a Roux-en-Y loop preferred). Heterotopic placement of the liver, providing an auxillary liver, obviates several technical difficulties; however, this technic has been limited to experimental situations, as results have been discouraging. Because of the shortage of donors appropriately size-matched for pediatric liver transplant recipients, some transplant centers are now attempting to use reduced-size grafts consisting of a segment of an adult liver, for extremely urgently needed transplants in children. This technic awaits further evaluation.

Immunosuppresion and rejection: Surprisingly, liver allografts are less aggressively rejected than other organ allografts, eg, kidney or heart. For example, hyperacute rejection of liver transplants does not seem to occur even when transplantation is performed in the face of subsequently proved presensitization to HLA antigens or ABO incompatibilities. Whether this is due to the anatomic uniqueness of the portal circulation, to the massive antigenic load present in the liver compared to other transplanted tissue, or to other factors is not known. Fulminant acute rejection and chronic rejection can occur, however, and when refractory to immunosuppressive therapy are treated by retransplantation.

Typical immunosuppressive therapy in an adult consists of cyclosporine usually given IV at 4 to 6 mg/kg/day starting at the time of transplantation and then 10 to 20 mg/kg/day orally when feedings are tolerated. Doses are adjusted downward with occurrence of renal dysfunction and with blood levels used as approximate measures of adequate dosage. Typically, methylprednisolone or prednisone is started at 10 mg/kg/day and reduced in a stepwise fashion to a maintenance dose of 0.2 mg/kg/day.

Mild acute rejection episodes may be self-limited, resolving without treatment. Rejection is suspected by development of hepatomegaly, light-colored bile (seen in T-tube drainage) or stools, and complaints of anorexia, right-sided pain, and fever. Jaundice and elevation in serum levels of hepatic enzymes are corroborative findings. Needle biopsy can provide pathologic confirmation. Suspected rejection episodes are treated with IV corticosteroids, antithymocyte globulin **(ATG)**, or monoclonal antibodies.

CARDIAC TRANSPLANTATION

Recent results with heart transplants have shown long-term survival rates and rehabilitation rates equal to those of patients receiving cadaveric donor renal allografts,

leading to increased use of transplantation as treatment of end-stage cardiac disease. Rehabilitation of heart transplant recipients surviving > 1 yr is excellent. Over 95% of these patients achieve a New York Heart Association Class I cardiac status, and > 70% return to full-time employment.

Common indications are cardiomyopathy and end-stage coronary artery disease. In addition, patients who could not be weaned from temporary cardiac assist devices following myocardial infarction or nontransplant cardiac surgery have received transplants successfully. **Recipient selection criteria** have been stringent; 1/4 of patients found suitable for transplantation die of their cardiac disease before a suitable donor organ becomes available. Ultimately, if an artificial heart can be perfected, its best application may be as an interim support device for patients awaiting cardiac transplantation. **Donor evaluation** includes assessment of normal cardiac function, size match, and ABO blood group compatibility.

Heart preservation and transplant procedures: Cadaveric donor hearts are preserved by simple hypothermic storage. Total ischemic time is held to < 4 to 6 h, thus excluding procurement from distant hospitals. The heart is transplanted in an orthotopic position with aortic, pulmonary artery, and pulmonary vein anastomoses. Venous return is provided by a single anastomosis joining a remnant of the recipient right atrium to that of the donor organ.

Immunosuppressive regimens are similar to those for kidney or liver transplantation, but it is in cardiac transplantation (especially in the early postoperative period) that cyclosporine's beneficial effect seems best established. One-year actuarial survival is approximately 80% for patients receiving cyclosporine, up from 60% using azathioprine. Rejection in the initial 2-mo period post-transplantation has also been reduced; approximately 40% of patients experience no rejection compared to < 10% with azathioprine.

Rejection onset may be heralded by fever, malaise, tachycardia, hypotension, and cardiac failure that is predominantly right-sided. Arrhythmias are common in more severe rejection episodes. In milder cases, rejection may be suggested by ECG changes only. With the use of cyclosporine, routine transvenous endomyocardial biopsy has been used to diagnose rejection, as other signs and symptoms are often absent and rejection may be detected prior to functional deterioration of the graft. Rejection is treated with corticosteroid and ATG if necessary. Because of the shortage of available organs and with the availability and functional success of artificial hearts being severely limited, patients with irreversible rejection often die awaiting retransplantation.

Post-transplant complications: Infection is the central concern, causing > 1/2 of all deaths secondary to cardiac transplantation. Other major causes of mortality are rejection, graft coronary artery arteriosclerosis, and malignancy, each accounting for 5 to 20% of deaths. Accelerated graft atherosclerosis is a surprising sequel to cardiac transplantation. Whether this is a result of indolent, humorally mediated chronic rejection is not clear, but it occurs in about 25% of all successful transplants and in > 80% of transplants where there is an HLA-A2 incompatibility (the most commonly observed MHC incompatibility). It now also appears that cyclosporine, which greatly increases the incidence of post-transplant hypertension, may also exacerbate coronary atherosclerosis in the graft.

BONE MARROW TRANSPLANTATION (BMT)

The objective of BMT is to provide the host with a healthy stem-cell population that will differentiate into blood cells that replace deficient or pathologic cell groups (eg, congenital immunodeficiency syndromes, severe aplastic anemia, leukemia). The use of BMT in hematopoietic or lymphoreticular disease is slowly expanding. More recently, osteopetrosis, metabolic storage diseases such as Gaucher's disease, hemoglobinopathies such as thalassemia, and even some solid tumors such as neuroblastoma have

been treated with BMT. In the common **indications** mentioned above, success rates are continually improving. BMT is being used earlier in some diseases (eg, acute leukemia in first remission but with a known poor prognosis); and nonmatched donors now are being used, in addition to HLA-identical siblings. However, long-term successful engraftment continues to be difficult to achieve; about 50 to 80% of patients with aplastic anemia and 30 to 50% with leukemia treated by BMT survive > 1 yr. **The transplantation procedure** itself is simple—aspiration of marrow from the donor and IV infusion of the marrow into the recipient.

Complicating factors include graft rejection by the host (HVGR), pancytopenia, and graft-vs.-host disease (GVHD—see below). Because of the underlying disease and the vigorous pretransplant immunosuppression, pancytopenia usually occurs before the graft begins to function, predisposing to opportunistic infection or spontaneous hemorrhage. **Chimerism** (*a long-term stable condition in which host and donor marrow cells exist compatibly*) develops if GVHD, failure of engraftment, sepsis, and recurrence of leukemia are avoided.

Graft-versus-host disease (GVHD): *A disease in which immunologically competent donor T cells react against antigens in an immunologically depressed recipient.* GVHD occurs mainly after bone marrow and fetal thymus transplantation. Even with the use of HLA-identical donors and postgraft immunosuppression, GVHD occurs in 2/3 of transplant recipients and causes many deaths after marrow engraftment. GVHD may also follow blood transfusion in some exceptional cases, since even small numbers of viable T cells can induce the reaction. Risk situations include intrauterine fetal blood transfusions and transfused immunodepressed patients, such as those with leukemia, lymphoma, neuroblastoma, or Hodgkin's disease. **Symptoms and signs** of GVHD are fever, exfoliative dermatitis, hepatitis, diarrhea or abdominal pain, ileus, vomiting, and weight loss.

Immunosuppressive preparation of the marrow recipient, for nonmalignant conditions, is directed solely to reducing immunocompetence, usually by cyclophosphamide 50 mg/kg/day for 4 days. In leukemia, therapy must also be directed at the malignant cells. Total body irradiation (see IMMUNOSUPPRESSION, above) is commonly used, in addition to cyclophosphamide. Donor marrow incubation with monoclonal antibody to T lymphocytes prior to transplantation (see IMMUNOSUPPRESSION, above) has also been used to prevent GVHD, with a decrease in the severity of GVHD but an increase in the incidence of engraftment failure. For **suppression** of GVHD, methotrexate has been given after transplantation. Recently, however, cyclosporine has been used in place of methotrexate; faster engraftment, less mucositis, and a decreased frequency of severe bacterial infections have been reported. Established GVHD has been successfully reversed with ATG or monoclonal antibodies. However, recurrent episodes on withdrawal of the medication are common. After several months of stable chimerism, immunosuppressive therapy often may be stopped without resultant graft rejection (in contrast to the situation with long-surviving allografts of other tissues) or recurrent GVH reaction.

For transfusion-induced GVHD, treatment has been unsuccessful. Effective **prevention** is by irradiation of all blood products intended for transfusion to such patients. A dosage of 1500 to 3000 rad does not damage blood components other than lymphocytes and seems to be clinically adequate.

TRANSPLANTATION OF OTHER ORGANS

Lung transplantation presents special problems, because of the risk of devastating infection in a transplanted organ continually exposed to nonsterile ambient air and dependent on the cough mechanism, which is disrupted by transplantation. Although transplanting a single lung is possible, in-block transplantation of heart and lungs is more successful. Advantages are total removal of diseased lung tissue and a tracheal

anastomosis, which receives a better blood supply than its bronchial counterpart and therefore is less prone to dehiscence. Endomyocardial biopsy has not proven as useful as initially anticipated, since rejection of the lung can proceed in the absence of any evidence of cardiac rejection. Preliminary results are promising in terms of patient survival, respiratory function, and control of infection, although the long-term effects of chronic rejection and of a graft interface exposed to unsterile environment processes are undetermined.

Indications are end-stage pulmonary hypertension and conditions leading to chronically impaired gas exchange. Donor organ procurement and recipient transplantation usually are in adjacent operating suites, as lung preservation methods are limited. **Immunosuppression** is with cyclosporine, ATG, and azathioprine initially. Corticosteroids, other than a perioperative bolus, often are avoided during the early postoperative period to avoid a detrimental effect on tracheal healing. After successful transplantation, ATG is quickly stopped, and azathioprine is later replaced with prednisone. **Rejection** in the lung remains a diagnostic dilemma. Unfortunately, lung biopsy does not always provide a clear answer. Clinically, pulmonary edema seems the earliest manifestation of rejection.

Pancreas transplantation's success rate has increased little recently. One-year graft survival so far is < 40%. However, attempts at obtaining successful engraftment continue because it offers hope of reestablishing normal carbohydrate homeostasis in diabetes and possibly preventing the development of microangiopathic lesions of the eye, kidney, and other organs.

Severe morbidity and only short-term success are due to complications arising from the exocrine portion of the gland and the demanding technical problems of the graft procedure. The most frequently employed method has been to transplant only the body and tail of the pancreas distal to the superior mesenteric vessels to an intraperitoneal or retroperitoneal site, using the splenic artery and vein for vascular attachment. Exocrine drainage approaches with this method have included duct of Wirsung ligation, reimplantation of the duct into the intestine, obliteration of the duct system with an injectable substance, or free drainage of the duct into the peritoneal cavity. None of these methods have proven uniformly satisfactory. Graft thrombosis due to inadequate vascular flow through these segmental grafts also is a frequent problem.

Transplantation of the entire pancreas with a segment of duodenum for anastomosis also has been attempted with recent renewed interest. Transplantation of the whole organ may allow for both better handling of the exocrine secretions and a more adequate vascular bed. In addition, there is greater functional islet reserve in the whole organ grafts. Detection of rejection in both segmental and whole organ pancreas grafts is difficult, as most of the graft can be destroyed by the rejection reaction before abnormalities in glucose metabolism become evident.

Islet cell allografting: Transplantation of islets alone after their isolation from donor organs has been successful in several species of small animals; however, clinical applicability, although it has received much publicity, is limited because of problems obtaining sufficient viable, purified donor islets.

Skin allografts are valuable for patients with extensive burns or other causes of massive skin loss. When insufficient donor sites negate the use of autografts alone, strips of autografts and allografts are alternated, covering the entire denuded area to reduce fluid and protein losses and discourage invasive infection. The allografts are rejected, but these secondarily denuded areas can then be re-covered with autografts taken from healed original donor sites. Allografts also serve as dressings for infected burns or wounds, which rapidly become sterile and develop well-vascularized granulations on which autografts will take readily.

Cartilage transplantation is unique in that chondrocytes are among the few types of mammalian cells that can be allografted without succumbing to the immune response,

apparently because the sparse population of cells in hyaline cartilage is protected from cellular attack by the cartilaginous matrix around the cells. In children, cartilage grafts obtained from cadaver donors may be used to replace congenital nasal or ear defects. In adults, autografts (usually from rib cartilage) are more commonly used to treat severe injuries. Utilization of cartilage allografts to resurface articular joints destroyed by arthritis has been attempted, but technical obstacles make joint replacement with prosthetic devices preferable.

Bone grafting is widely used, but, except for autografts, no viable donor bone cells survive in the recipient. However, the remaining dead matrix has a bone-inducing capacity that stimulates host osteoblasts to recolonize the matrix and lay down new bone, thus serving as a scaffolding for bridging and stabilizing defects until new bone is formed. Massive resection of malignant bone tumors and reconstruction by implantation of composite bone and cartilage allografts are practical approaches to salvaging extremities that would otherwise be amputated. Cadaveric allografts are preserved by freezing to decrease immunogenicity of the bone (which is dead at the time of implantation) and glycerolization to maintain chondrocyte viability. No postimplantation immunosuppression is used. Although these patients develop anti-HLA antibodies, early follow-up reveals no evidence of cartilage degradation.

Fetal thymus implants obtained from stillborn infants may restore immunologic responsiveness to children with thymic aplasia and consequent lack of normal development of the lymphoid system. Because the recipient is immunologically unresponsive, immunosuppression is not required; however, GVHD (see above) may be severe.

Parathyroid tissue autografts and even, rarely, allografts have been successfully performed. Parathyroid autotransplantation has been recommended by some groups for treatment of patients with hypercalcemia due to secondary hyperplasia. The technic involves removal of all parathyroid tissue from the neck, with placement of a few small slivers of tissue in a muscle pocket in the forearm, where the tissue can later easily be identified if hypercalcemia recurs. Allografts may be undertaken for patients with iatrogenic hypoparathyroidism whose course with optimal medical management is unsatisfactory. Since immunosuppression is required, this procedure is rarely indicated unless the patient also is receiving a renal allograft, for which suppression will be necessary.

---

23. TUMOR IMMUNOLOGY

The demonstration of immune responses in experimental animals to spontaneously occurring tumors, to carcinogen- or viral-induced tumors, and to transplanted tumors has stimulated interest in seeking similar immune responses in man. The availability of syngeneic strains of animals has permitted a distinction to be made between immune reactions directed against tumor-associated transplantation antigens and those against normal histocompatibility antigens also present on tumor cells.

The genetic heterogeneity of man, except in the unusual circumstance of identical twins, has made the study of human anti-tumor immunity more complex. Nevertheless, it seems likely that the presence of immunogenic surface configurations on human neoplastic cells permits their recognition by immunocompetent host cells as well as their interaction with humoral antibodies. The significance of such recognitions and reactions in the pathogenesis of tumors, and the potential for augmenting them in favor of the host, is currently the object of intensive laboratory and clinical investigation. However, after a decade of clinical trials with human cancer immunotherapy—

most of it **nonspecific** (see below)—there are major reservations concerning its efficacy. Expanded applications of **specific** immunotherapy are being investigated, using autochthonous tumor cells, cultured tumors cells, and purified tumor antigens (see below).

TUMOR-ASSOCIATED ANTIGENS (TAA)

Most induced or transplanted experimental animal tumors immunize syngeneic recipients against subsequent challenge with the same tumor but not against transplantation of normal tissues or other tumors. Such findings indicate the presence of antigens that are associated with the tumor cells but are not apparent on normal cells. These antigens are known as **TAA**.

The findings are particularly well demonstrated by chemical carcinogen-induced tumors, which tend to have individual antigenic specificity that varies from tumor to tumor, even with tumors induced by the same carcinogen; and by virus-induced tumors, which tend to show cross-reactivity between tumors induced by a given virus. Viral infections may result in "modified self"; ie, new antigens recognized along with or in context of the major histocompatibility complex.

Suggested mechanisms for the origin of such antigens include (1) new genetic information introduced by a virus; (2) alteration of genetic function by carcinogens, possibly through derepression, by which genetic material that is normally inactive, except perhaps during embryonic development, is activated and becomes expressed in the cell phenotype; (3) uncovering of antigens that are normally "buried" in the cell membrane, through the inability of neoplastic cells to synthesize membrane constituents such as sialic acid; (4) release of antigens that are normally sequestered in the cell or its organelles, through the death of neoplastic cells.

Technics to demonstrate TAA in animal tumors include standard tissue transplantation methods, immunofluorescence, cytotoxicity tests using dye uptake or radioisotope release, prevention of tumor growth in vitro or in vivo by exposing the tumor to lymphoid cells or serum from immunized donors, delayed hypersensitivity skin tests, and lymphocyte transformation in vitro.

Evidence for TAA in human neoplasms has been demonstrated with several neoplasms, including Burkitt's lymphoma, neuroblastoma, malignant melanoma, osteosarcoma, and some GI carcinomas. Choriocarcinomas in women possess paternally derived histocompatibility antigens that may serve as "tumor-specific" antigens in eliciting an immune response. The complete cure of choriocarcinomas by chemotherapy may be attributable, at least in part, to such an immune response.

HOST RESPONSES TO TUMORS

Cellular Immunity

The importance of lymphoid cells in tumor immunity has been repeatedly demonstrated in experimental animal tumor systems. In humans, the growth of tumor nodules has been inhibited in vivo by mixing suspensions of a patient's lymphocytes and tumor cells, suggesting a cell-mediated reaction to the tumor. In vitro studies have shown that lymphoid cells from patients with certain neoplasms show cytotoxicity against corresponding human tumor cells in culture. These **cytotoxic cells,** which are generally T (thymus-derived) lymphocytes, have been found with neuroblastoma, malignant melanomas, sarcomas, and carcinomas of the colon, breast, cervix, endometrium, ovary, testis. nasopharynx, and kidney. Similar antitumor cytolytic properties have been demonstrated with lymphocytes from members of the families of neuroblastoma and osteosarcoma patients, suggesting common exposure to a suspected environmental agent. The significance of such reactions in controlling tumor growth is not clear at this time. However, it seems likely that one or more types of lymphocytes,

primarily associated with T cell differentiation, are capable of damaging tumor cells in vivo. Cells with these capabilities are also found in non–tumor-bearing individuals and are termed **natural killer (NK) cells.** Some lymphoid cells require the concurrent presence of humoral antibodies directed against the tumor cells **(antibody-dependent cellular cytotoxicity).**

Humoral Immunity

Humoral antibodies that react with tumor cells in vitro are produced in response to a variety of animal tumors induced by chemical carcinogens or viruses. However, antibody-mediated protection against tumor growth in vivo has only been demonstrable in certain animal leukemias and lymphomas. By contrast, lymphoid cell-mediated protection in vivo occurs in a broad variety of animal tumor systems.

Antitumor antibodies may include the following types. **Cytotoxic antibodies** generally are complement-fixing and directed against surface antigens of relatively high density. IgM antibodies usually are more cytotoxic in transplantation systems than are IgG antibodies. **Enhancing** or **blocking antibodies** generally are IgG, possibly complexed with soluble antigen. They *favor* the growth of a tumor rather than inhibit it. The mechanisms for such immunologic enhancement are not understood but may involve (1) binding with TAA and blocking their immunogenicity (afferent enhancement); (2) reacting with and inhibiting immunologically competent cells (central enhancement); (3) coating of tumor cells and thus preventing their interaction with lymphoid cells (efferent enhancement). The enhancement of human tumors seems likely, since blocking antibodies have been demonstrated in vitro. **Unblocking factors** are not yet characterized completely, but may be antibodies. They decrease the blocking activity of enhancing antibodies or antigen-antibody complexes. They have been detected in the sera of patients following surgical removal of all clinically apparent tumor tissue. The exact relationship of cytotoxic, blocking, and unblocking factors is not yet clear; ie, whether or not the presumed antibodies involved are distinct from each other is not known.

Humoral antibodies directed against *human* tumor cells or their constituents have been demonstrated in vitro in the serum of patients with Burkitt's lymphoma, malignant melanoma, osteosarcoma, neuroblastoma, and digestive system carcinomas. Antibodies to melanoma cells and to carcinoembryonic antigen (see below) usually are found in patients *without* disseminated disease; the reasons are unknown. Perhaps a failure to produce such antibodies permits metastasis; or perhaps antibodies are formed but are promptly absorbed by the large tumor mass.

The complicated and possibly delicate balance between potentially beneficial and potentially detrimental immune responses requires clarification to assist in planning immunotherapeutic maneuvers. Shifting this balance in favor of the host by removing factors inhibiting humoral antitumor immunity is a relatively unexplored area of human immunotherapy.

Alterations of Host Immune Reactivity

Tumors that possess TAA are able to grow in vivo, which suggests a deficient host response to the TAA. Possible mechanisms include the following: (1) Specific immunologic tolerance to TAA (eg, because of prenatal exposure to the antigen, possibly viral in origin). This may involve suppressor cells in a manner not well understood at present. (2) Suppression of the immune response by chemical or viral carcinogens. A related phenomenon is seen in patients with AIDS (see Ch. 19). (3) Suppression of the immune response by treatment, especially cytotoxic chemotherapy and radiation therapy. Occurrence of > 100 times the expected incidence of tumors in patients undergoing immunosuppressive therapy for renal transplantation suggests an impairment of postulated "immune-surveillance" mechanisms, which are theorized to inhibit growth of newly transformed neoplastic cells, or an impairment of immunity to oncogenic viruses, among possible explanations. Also, tumors have been inadvertently trans-

planted to immunosuppressed human kidney recipients, and these may regress when immunosuppression is discontinued. (4) Suppression of the immune response by the tumor itself. Deficient cellular immunity can be associated with recurrence and dissemination of tumors. This has been repeatedly demonstrated with a variety of human tumors, most dramatically in Hodgkin's disease, which appears to involve a variable defect in T cell function. An immunoglobulin reacting with the host's lymphocytes appears to be associated with this defect. Deficient humoral immunity occurs in association with neoplasms involving abnormal B cell derivatives, such as multiple myeloma and chronic lymphocytic leukemia. Recent investigation implicates a macrophage-related suppressor cell in the humoral immune deficiency state of myeloma.

TUMOR IMMUNODIAGNOSIS

Many tumors release antigenic macromolecules into the circulation that eventually permit early diagnosis of neoplasms, particularly if detectable by technics appropriate for mass screening programs. These antigens also can aid in monitoring patients for tumor recurrence after therapy.

Carcinoembryonic antigen (CEA) is a protein-polysaccharide complex found in colon carcinomas and in normal fetal gut, pancreas, and liver. A sensitive radioimmunoassay permits detection of increased levels in the blood of patients with colon carcinoma, but the specificity of this technic is weak, since positive tests also occur in cirrhosis, ulcerative colitis, and with other cancers (eg, of the breast, pancreas, and bladder). Monitoring CEA levels may be useful in detection of cancer recurrences when the primary tumor was associated with elevated CEA. **α-Fetoprotein (AFP)**, an antigen migrating with the α-globulins in electrophoresis, is found in serum from patients or animals with primary hepatoma, and from certain patients with ovarian or testicular embryonal carcinoma. **β-Subunit of human chorionic gonadotropin (βHCG)** is measured by immunoassay and is a very useful marker in some patients with residual testicular choriocarcinoma or embryonal carcinoma.

The localization of tumors in vivo with radiolabeled monoclonal antibodies directed against a tumor and surface scanning is being widely studied.

IMMUNOTHERAPY OF HUMAN TUMORS

The past 15 yr have seen extensive clinical investigation of cancer immunotherapy. Varied biologic response modifiers have been used, including **specific** immunization with tumor cells or fractions thereof and **nonspecific** immunization with such materials as bacterial vaccines, thymic extracts, WBC fractions, and several chemical immunoadjuvants. These attempts at immunotherapy often have involved patients with far-advanced cancer, having large tumor-cell burdens and impaired immune mechanisms that had little chance of being effectively augmented. Investigation of these approaches with patients who have relatively poor prognoses at a time when their disease is *limited* seems justifiable at present; eg, in a patient with metastatic renal carcinoma in the lung whose primary tumor has been surgically resected. Such immunologic approaches to cancer are experimental. The possibility exists of shifting the delicate balance between factors stimulating and inhibiting immunologic defenses against a tumor in an *unfavorable* direction.

Experimental Therapeutic Methods

Large tumor masses are, if possible, reduced by prior surgery, radiotherapy, or chemotherapy to facilitate potential effectiveness of immunologic mechanisms.

Active immunization with tumor cells. Autochthonous tumors (*tumors arising in the same host*) have been used—after irradiation, neuraminidase treatment, or hybridiza-

tion with long-term cell lines in vitro—in kidney carcinoma and malignant melanoma patients, among others. Mixing the tumor cells with a bacterial adjuvant (see below) may enhance the immunogenicity of such vaccines. Clinical improvement has been seen in a minority of patients so treated, but variables such as dose and timing require additional study. Cell culture and hybridization technics help make available larger numbers of tumor cells for use in vaccines.

Allogeneic tumor cells (cells from other patients) have been used after their irradiation in acute lymphoblastic leukemia and acute myeloblastic leukemia in conjunction with BCG or other adjuvants (see below) after remission has been induced by intensive chemotherapy and radiotherapy. Prolongation of remissions or improved reinduction rates have been reported in some series but not in others. **Tumor cell extracts** and purified TAA are being studied. It is possible that the integrity of tumor cell membranes must be maintained to some extent to provide the steric configurations required for immunogenicity. **Activation of autologous lymphocytes in vitro**: Lymphoid cells, separated from peripheral blood or obtained from the thoracic duct, have been incubated with tumor cells in vitro and then reinfused. Autologous blood lymphocytes also have been activated in vitro with lymphocyte mitogens such as phytohemagglutinin and then reinfused. Recent emphasis has been on activating cytotoxic cells with interleukin-2, in vitro and in vivo, leading to so-called **lymphocyte-activated killer (LAK) cells**.

Passive immunization. Antiserum: Antilymphocyte serum has been used in chronic lymphocytic leukemia and in both T cell and B cell lymphomas, resulting in a temporary decrease in lymphocyte counts. The availability of **monoclonal antibodies** against tumor antigens has increased interest in this approach. Treatment of melanomas in this manner is being investigated. Humoral antibody, both autologous and allogeneic, might be made more effective if their interaction with soluble tumor antigens or with immunoglobulin **anti-idiotype antibodies** could be reversed or prevented. **Lymphoid cells**: Allogeneic peripheral blood leukocytes, from other cancer patients previously grafted with the recipient's tumor, have been transfused ("adoptive" immunotherapy) in studies with malignant melanoma and other tumors. Some remissions have occurred, but graft-vs.-host reactions may result, as with bone marrow transplantation.

Nonspecific immunotherapy. Interferons, derived from WBCs (α- and γ-interferons) or fibroblasts (β-interferons), or synthesized in bacteria by recombinant genetic technics, are glycoproteins which possess anti-tumor activity as well as anti-viral activity that may originate partially from immunologically mediated mechanisms. Depending on the dose administered, interferons may either enhance or decrease humoral and cellular immune functions, as well as affect macrophage and natural killer (NK) cell activity. In addition, interferons inhibit division and certain synthetic processes in a variety of cells. Human clinical trials have indicated that interferons may have anti-tumor activity in hairy cell leukemia, non-Hodgkin's lymphoma, multiple myeloma, osteogenic sarcoma, and breast and ovarian carcinomas. Considerable toxicity may be associated with their use, including fever, malaise, leukopenia, alopecia, and myalgias. **Thymosin,** an extract of bovine thymus, appears to stimulate maturation of several early stages of T cell development and to increase the ability of mature T cells to respond to antigens. Survival of certain cancer patients, including those with small-cell lung carcinoma, may be increased when receiving thymosin in addition to chemotherapy.

Skin malignancies have regressed after induction of delayed hypersensitivity to **dinitrochlorobenzene (DNCB)** and subsequent direct application of DNCB to the tumor. **Bacterial adjuvants,** such as **BCG** (attenuated tubercle bacilli), extracts of BCG such as **MER** (methanol-extracted residue), or killed suspensions of ***Corynebacterium parvum*** have been used in randomized trials, with or without added tumor antigen, in a broad variety of human cancer patients, usually in association with intensive chemotherapy or radiation therapy. Direct injection of BCG into melanoma nodules almost always

leads to regression of the injected nodules, and occasionally of distant, noninjected nodules as well. Some studies suggest that MER may help prolong chemotherapy-induced remission duration in acute myeloblastic leukemia and that BCG added to combination chemotherapy may increase survival in ovarian carcinoma and possibly in non-Hodgkin's lymphoma. Numerous other studies with these immunoadjuvants, however, have shown no beneficial effects.

Lymphokines, soluble effectors made by lymphocytes, are being tested for ability to stimulate anti-tumor activity, both through in vitro activation of cytotoxic cells (see LAK cells, above) and in conjunction with active immunization in vivo using tumor cell vaccines. **Chemical immunomodulators** such as **levamisole** (a veterinary antihelminthic agent) and **glucan** (a polyglucose) are being examined both in animal systems and in human trials. Suggestive beneficial effects have been reported in some studies but not in others, and await confirmation. The relatively low toxicity of levamisole has made it somewhat more attractive than its therapeutic effects might otherwise warrant.

In summary, nonspecific immunotherapy has resulted in very limited therapeutic benefit, if any at all. Better understanding of tumor immunity mechanisms, lymphokine action, and functions of lymphocyte subsets seems necessary for progress in tumor immunotherapy, with particular emphasis on specific immunotherapy.

§3. CARDIOVASCULAR DISORDERS

---

24. AN APPROACH TO THE CARDIAC PATIENT

Cardiovascular clinical diagnosis depends on a synthesis of information from the history, physical signs, ECG, chest x-rays, and special laboratories. Knowledge of the natural history of cardiovascular disease helps to establish both diagnosis and prognosis. Considerations may be narrowed to relatively few probabilities based upon the history alone. Specialized laboratory studies should not be ordered until the initial clinical assessment has provided a basis for judging the need for other procedures such as echocardiography, exercise testing, radionuclide imaging, cardiac catheterization, and angiographic studies. The sequence used in gathering clinical information can vary with the situation; eg, the physical examination of an infant or a young child best begins during a period of calm. Impressions gained from initial findings usually influence the objectivity with which subsequent findings are appraised. By the end of the clinical assessment, unlikely considerations should have been deemphasized or discarded, and probabilities should have been brought into sharp focus.

PHYSICAL EXAMINATION OF THE CARDIAC PATIENT

Cardiac Clues from Physical Appearance

Attention should first be directed to the *general* physical appearance, then to *detailed* deviations from normal. For example, the general appearance of chronic illness—catabolic effect of chronic heart failure—usually is readily apparent. Certain general appearances identify diseases associated with predictable types of cardiac or vascular disorders (eg, Marfan syndrome with aortic root/mitral valve abnormalities, and Down's syndrome with endocardial cushion defect). Detailed physical examination provides a host of diagnostic insights.

Eyes: Corneal arcus, *a circumferential light gray or yellowish ring around the rim of the iris,* is associated with familial hypercholesterolemia or coronary disease if it is a thick band that begins inferiorly and allows a thin rim of iris pigment to be seen between the

arcus and the sclera. The usual **arcus senilis** is not necessarily associated with hyperlipidemia. It begins superiorly and extends to the rim or limbus of the iris. Marked **xanthelasma** (*xanthomas around the eyelids*) may be associated with hypercholesterolemia.

Argyll Robertson pupil (afferent pupillary defect; ie, *reaction to accommodation but not to light*) may be noted if a luetic aortic aneurysm or aortic regurgitation **(AR)** with coronary ostial stenosis is suspected. Eversion of the lids may show conjunctival hemorrhages and petechiae when infective endocarditis is suspected. One notes the stare and exophthalmos of the thyrotoxic patient or the patient with advanced heart failure with high venous pressure. A tremulous iris **(iridodonesis)** suggests Marfan syndrome (the iris is not properly supported by the lens). These patients may have aneurysms of the aorta or pulmonary artery and prolapsed mitral valves. Blue sclera may be seen in osteogenesis imperfecta with its associated AR, or in Marfan syndrome, which may have a pulmonary or aortic aneurysm and AR, an atrial septal defect, or a prolapsed mitral valve with mitral regurgitation **(MR)**. Pallor of the everted lid may indicate anemia, which can cause cardiac symptoms if the Hct is < 50% of normal, and can induce or increase symptoms of failure in the presence of reduced myocardial function.

Funduscopic examination may show **retinal signs of arteriosclerosis:**

Grade 1. Increased light reflex width
Grade 2. Arteriovenous nicking and right-angled crossings of arteries over veins
Grade 3. Copper-wire arteries (brownish, due to thick walls and wide light streaks)
Grade 4. Silver-wire arteries (no red color)

The retinal signs of hypertension are

Grade 1. Arteriovenous ratio of < 2:3 or 3:4
Grade 2. Focal constriction or spasm of arterioles
Grade 3. Hemorrhages and exudates in addition to vascular changes
Grade 4. Papilledema

There may be oval hemorrhages near the optic disk with white spots in the center **(Roth's spots).**

Skin: Tendon xanthomas in the Achilles, patellar, and extensor tendons of the hands usually indicate Type II hyperlipoproteinemia (high cholesterol levels and premature coronary disease). Xanthomas in the palmar creases denote Type III hyperlipoproteinemia. Smooth, glossy, drum-tight skin on the fingers is seen in scleroderma, which may be associated with myocardial fibrosis or cor pulmonale. Skin warmer than normal may accompany severe anemia or thyrotoxicosis. The cold, clammy hands and feet of anxiety may explain chest pains and palpitations of neurocirculatory asthenia (**DaCosta** or **"effort" syndrome**), but these signs may also indicate the low CO of severe heart failure. If only the feet are cold, peripheral arterial obstruction may be the cause.

Cyanosis and clubbing of fingers and toes are clues to cardiac disorders. Central cyanosis (absolute blood-O_2 desaturation) is seen in both warm (tongue) or cool areas, while peripheral cyanosis alone due to the low flow of heart failure or cold temperature is seen only in cool areas (eg, nail beds, lips, nose, and earlobes). In a cyanotic patient, clubbing may be observed as an obliteration of the normal angle between the base of the nail and the proximal skin. Differential cyanosis and clubbing (the hands are pink and the feet are blue and clubbed) implies pulmonary hypertension with a right-to-left shunt via a persistent ductus. Splinter hemorrhages in the nails may accompany endocarditis. (Most splinter hemorrhages are not embolic and they move with the nail as it grows, because they are in the nail substance.) The physician should look for the brownish, muddy, skin pigmentation that may accompany either hepatic failure or hemochromatosis with cardiomyopathy due to intracellular iron deposits.

Peripheral edema is checked by pressing on the skin over a bone area for about 10 sec with at least 3 fingers spread slightly apart, then feeling for valleys between hills after release. If pitting disappears in < 40 sec, the cause is almost certainly low albumin. If edema occurs in the legs, venous pressure in the neck should be checked

immediately. If jugular venous pressure is normal and the patient has not taken a diuretic, then the edema is certainly noncardiac. Edema may be present only in the sacral area, if a patient has been in bed for some time. Edema of the face and hands tends to rule out a cardiac cause except in infants.

Extremities: Short stature and web neck characterize the patient with Turner's syndrome in whom coarctation is a common abnormality. Long slender fingers are a sign of Marfan syndrome **(arachnodactyly)**.

Chest and respiration: *Pectus excavatum* (funnel chest) may be a sign of Marfan syndrome with its mitral prolapse. Cheyne-Stokes respiration (see Ch. 31) is seen in patients with very low CO. The patient should be asked to hold his breath as long as possible; < 20 sec is abnormal and can explain dyspnea on exertion. It is usually caused by poor psychophysical control over the breathing apparatus or chronic psychogenic hyperventilation if no obvious cardiac or pulmonary fibrotic or infiltrative disease is present. (Pure chronic obstructive lung disease does not shorten the breath-holding time.)

Arterial pulses: Arm pulses are best felt by feeling the brachial with one finger or thumb, and the radial with the opposite hand (see FIG. 24–1). By feeling both simultaneously, the examination is expedited. (The radial is a lateral vessel and should be approached laterally.) If light pressure on the brachial obliterates the radial pulse, then the BP is normal; if obliteration takes no more than moderate pressure, the BP is probably between 120 and 160, but if it takes more than moderate pressure, then the BP is > 160 mm Hg.

The rate of rise of both arm and carotid pulses is noted; if there is a tapping sensation, then the rate of rise is normal. Next, the volume is noted; if it is large, disorders to consider are AR, persistent ductus, coarctation, thyrotoxicosis, severe anemia, and systolic hypertension. If the rate of rise is slow (a nudge or push rather than a tap) significant aortic stenosis **(AS)** should be considered, especially if there is a thrill on the upstroke. A dip or a notch in the carotid or brachial pulse, or a double-

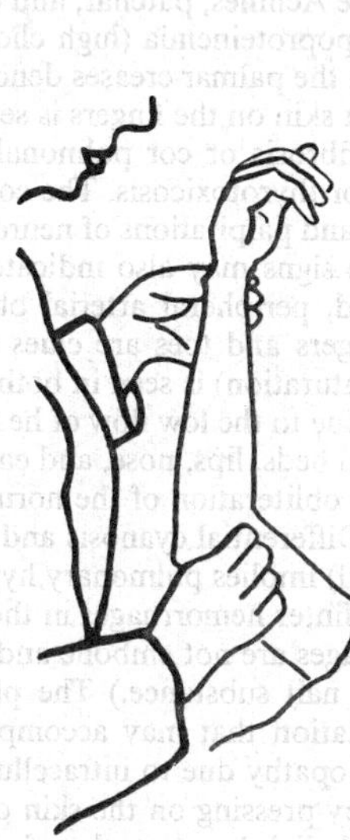

FIG. 24–1. Arterial pulses. (From *Bedside Cardiology* by Jules Constant, ed. 3, 1985. Copyright by Little, Brown and Company, Boston, 1985.)

beating (bisferiens) pulse with a normal pulse pressure suggests either a combination of AS and severe regurgitation or hypertrophic subaortic stenosis (hypertrophic obstructive cardiomyopathy). With a very rapid rate of rise and big volume (slapping pulse), it means pure, severe AR. If the carotids have a slow rise and the brachials and radials have a rapid or normal rise, this suggests a combination of AS and AR or a very mild AS. (As a pulse wave moves peripherally, the rate of rise normally increases.) A normal volume with a rapid rate of rise (brisk pulse) suggests either hypertrophic subaortic stenosis or a large ventricular volume with 2 outlets as with MR or a ventricular septal defect.

By far the most common cause of a rapidly rising bounding pulse is AR. The large carotid pulse seen at the bedside in AR is called **Corrigan's pulse**. The rapid, large volume rise and fall of the arterial pulse in AR is called a **water hammer pulse** or **collapsing pulse**. (A water hammer is a Victorian toy consisting of a tube with a vacuum and half-filled with water so that when this tube is turned, the water falls with a bang.) The word "bounding" pulse with a rapid rate of rise is probably the best term. *The loud sound (pistol shot) heard over the femorals* with the stethoscope is **Traube's sign. Duroziez's double murmur** is *the systolic flow murmur heard over the femoral artery with the stethoscope as the artery is compressed proximally, and the diastolic backflow murmur heard if the artery is compressed distally.*

The most important concept to remember in feeling the popliteals (with the patient supine) is to abolish any idea that an actual arterial pulse can be felt. Instead, an area of transmitted pulsation is sought rather than the feeling of an actual artery.

Blood Pressure

The upper normal BP in an adult should be considered to be 140/90 mm Hg. In an infant or a child the formula for systolic BP is $90 + (\text{the age} \times 5)/3$. Diastolic pressure tends to be about 60 ± 10 mm Hg in infants and children of all ages. If taken separately, 25% of normal people will have a difference of as much as 20 mm Hg in systolic pressure in each arm. About 15% of patients will have a diastolic pressure difference of about 20 mm Hg between arms. If the history suggests vertebral-basilar insufficiency and the BP is lower in one arm than in the other, a subclavian steal should be suspected. A purely high systolic pressure is due either to a large stroke volume or to a stiff aorta secondary to atherosclerosis in the elderly patient. AR tends to have a low diastolic pressure due to a reflex decrease in peripheral resistance secondary to the effect of the large pulse pressure on the carotid sinus or carotid body, as well as to the run-off backwards into the ventricle.

Method of taking and recording BP: When taking a BP, the systolic pressure is the first series of tapping sounds **(Korotkoff sounds)** heard as the BP cuff is deflated. This is phase 1 of the 5 conventional phases of Korotkoff sounds. Phase 2, which is about 10 to 15 mm lower than phase 1, is represented by a murmur that may be heard after the tap. Phase 3 is a reappearance of only the tapping sound. Phase 4 is muffling. Phase 5 is disappearance of Korotkoff sounds, which is taken as the diastolic pressure. It is unnecessary to recognize any except phases 1 and 5 unless there is > 10 mm difference between muffling and disappearance; then the muffling pressure (phase 4) must be taken as diastolic pressure. Korotkoff sounds may be difficult to hear if there is a slow rate of rise in the pulse wave, as in AS, poor blood flow to the limbs, or a small pulse pressure. To amplify the Korotkoff sounds, (1) the patient can pump his hand (clench and relax fingers) about 10 times to increase blood flow (which will not influence the actual BP level); (2) the arm can be elevated to decrease the amount of blood in the forearm; and (3) the cuff can be inflated as rapidly as possible.

BP should be recorded to the nearest 5 or zero despite the fact that manometer dials are graduated in increments of 2. Because the loudest Korotkoff sounds are actually around the central area of the cuff, the diaphragm chest piece should be slipped as far under the cuff as possible over the brachial artery. A Doppler method of taking a BP

is preferable in infants and in taking BP in the legs. For most adults, the cuff width must be ≥ 20% wider than the diameter of the arm, or ≥ 40% of the arm circumference. If less than that, the BP will be falsely high.

By hovering around systolic pressure, the listener may pick up alternating fluctuations in pulse pressure **(pulsus alternans)**; ie, in every other beat, the BP is lower. It usually occurs in patients with severe heart failure, especially in the sitting position, or after the pause of a premature beat. However, it may occur with hypertension if there is mild myocardial damage due to infarction or scarring. It may also be found in tachycardias even in the normal heart.

BP in the legs, taken with a properly sized cuff over the thigh and with the bell over the popliteal area, should not be > 20 mm higher than in the arms. BP can also be taken with a small bell over the posterior tibial with an arm cuff above the malleolus. In AR, if the cuff systolic pressure is 20 mm Hg higher in the legs than in the arms, it suggests mild regurgitation; 20 to 40 mm Hg higher is known as a **positive Hill's sign,** suggesting moderate AR. Over 60 mm Hg difference between the arms and the legs suggests severe AR.

When the BP is lower in the legs than in the arms, aortic coarctation or arterial obstruction at the iliac or femoral level should be suspected. After placing the patient's radial artery over the femoral artery, the physician can palpate the radial artery with one hand and the femoral artery with the other to note if the femoral pulse peaks are delayed. Only in coarctation or arterial obstruction is there a radial-femoral lag in peaks. In supravalvular AS the BP in the right arm is higher than that in the left by about 10 to 20 mm Hg (due to the effect of streaming).

Pulsus paradoxus is the classic sign of tamponade: It refers to *a marked fall in systolic BP ≥ 8 mm with normal respiration*. This is an exaggeration of the normal fall related to the drop in intrathoracic pressure as well as decreased filling of the left ventricle from the left atrium and lungs during inspiration. Pulsus paradoxus may be due to transmission of the increased intrapericardial pressure on inspiration to the wall of the left atrium, thus decreasing venous return from the lungs. Contributing to the decrease in left ventricular volume is a shift of the septum into the left ventricle due to the resistance of the free wall of the right ventricle to the increased volume brought in by inspiration. Severe bronchospasm (eg, in asthma or COPD) may mimic pulsus paradoxus by raising intrathoracic pressure too high during expiration due to doing Valsalva maneuvers, and decreasing intrathoracic pressure too much during inspiration due to doing **Mueller maneuvers** (*inspiratory effort against a closed glottis*). It should be noted that constrictive pericarditis does not usually produce a pulsus paradoxus.

Jugular Waves and Jugular Venous Pressure

Jugular veins can be examined both for pressure and for wave form. Only the internal jugulars should be used to measure venous pressure because external jugulars are too often unreliable. The term "distended, dilated, or engorged neck veins" should not be used to describe venous pressure, since that refers only to external jugulars. The internal jugulars may be as high as earlobe level with the patient at 45° with no distention of external jugulars whatsoever. Venous pressure is indicated by the upper level of transmitted neck pulsations caused by internal jugular movement. Examining the silhouette of the neck for pulsations is the most accurate way of finding their top level. Even slight earlobe movement should be noted; if the internal jugular pressure is very high, the earlobes may pulsate, yet neck pulsations may be almost imperceptible. The top level of internal jugular pulsations with the patient in the 45° position is a vertical level of 4.5 cm above the sternal angle. With the patient supine, the upper level is about 2 cm above the sternal angle.

Abdominal compression will cause *and maintain* a rise of ≥ 1 cm of venous pressure only if the venous pressure is relatively high (the **"hepatojugular reflux"**). The effect of

abdominal compression is more important than the absolute jugular pressure in determining whether or not venous pressure is normal or relatively high. In patients with heart failure it is probably due to increased venous volume and tone, as well as to increased volume and tone in the right atrium and right ventricle, preventing their accepting additional volume. To prevent a false increase in venous pressure due to patient discomfort, the examiner should press with warm hands or with a garment or sheet between the hand and the patient's abdomen; the fingers should be spread apart, and starting pressure should be gentle. Asking the patient to breathe through his mouth will prevent a Valsalva maneuver.

Kussmaul's sign is *the rise in height of jugular pulsations during inspiration*; it occurs typically in patients with chronic constrictive pericarditis, but it can occur with peripheral venous congestion from any cause and is also considered a sign of right ventricular infarction.

Jugular pulse contours (see FIG. 24–2): A normal jugular contour can be recognized if descents are timed, because jugular *descents*, the fastest and largest movements, are easier to see than ascents. Either internal or external jugulars may be used to analyze waves and descents. Atrial contraction and relaxation produce the A and X descents respectively. The systolic descent (X′ descent) is mostly due to the fall in pressure in the right atrium, secondary to pulling down of the floor of the atrium by right ventricular contraction (descent of the base). In most adults this is the only descent seen except for a small diastolic descent known as the Y descent. If the jugulars are normal, then the major descent will fall simultaneously with the radial pulse; when timed with the heart sounds, it will fall during systole. The peak will seem to occur with S_1 and its nadir at S_2. The C wave is due mainly to carotid artifact; by inspection of the neck it is recognized only with skill as an interruption in the systolic descent. With tricuspid regurgitation, a large V wave can completely obliterate the X′ descent; with severe tricuspid regurgitation, there is only a CV wave and Y descent. Filling of the right atrium from 2 sources (eg, an atrial septal defect or anomalous pulmonary venous connection to the right atrium) can exaggerate the Y descent and preceding V wave; these exaggerations may also be due to loss of compliance of the right atrium (eg, when sutures are placed in it secondary to open heart surgery, or, very rarely, with carcinoid disease, right atrial tumor, or pericardial calcium). The presence of an X′ descent implies in sinus rhythm that an A wave preceded this descent. In atrial fibrillation an H wave precedes the X′ descent, but the Y descent will dominate. The X descent, which is the descent produced by atrial relaxation, merges with the X′ descent in sinus rhythm.

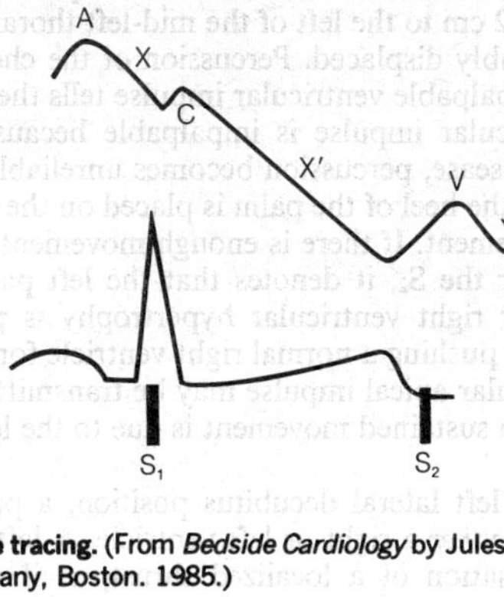

FIG. 24–2. Jugular pulse tracing. (From *Bedside Cardiology* by Jules Constant, ed. 3, 1985. Copyright by Little, Brown and Company, Boston. 1985.)

Differentiating jugulars from carotids: Jugulars have their *descents* as the fastest and largest movements, while carotid *ascents* are the fastest and largest movements. Only a carotid is easily palpable as a strong pulse; a jugular is usually either impalpable or only a faint undulation. Also, supraclavicular pressure should be able to eliminate jugular pulsations. However, if venous pressure is high, the supraclavicular pressure must be at least halfway up the neck. Abdominal compression will increase venous pulsations in amplitude or in height, but will not affect carotid pulsations.

Pulmonary stenosis exaggerates A waves and X and X′ descents; pulmonary hypertension exaggerates both A and V waves. An exaggerated A wave is known as a "giant A wave," while a large A wave produced by atrial contraction against a closed tricuspid valve due to atrioventricular **(A-V)** dissociation or retrograde P waves, is called a cannon wave. A child with rapid circulation times can have a slightly exaggerated V wave and Y descent, but the X′ descent will always be dominant.

In tamponade, the X′ descent is very deep and the Y descent is small. On the other hand, in constrictive pericarditis or effusive-constrictive pericarditis, there may be no X′ descent; if there is one, either the Y descent is deeper than the X′ or they are equal.

The wave following the V wave during diastole is called the "H wave." A rapid Y descent followed by an equally rapid rebound rise of the H wave occurs when right ventricular expansion is restricted, as in constrictive pericarditis or in restrictive cardiomyopathies such as amyloidosis. A similar rebounding type of H wave also occurs in right ventricular infarction that seems to act as a restrictive cardiomyopathy. This jugular sign reflects the "square root" sign seen in right atrial and right ventricular pressure curves during diastole.

Precordial Palpation and Movements

To look for signs of enlargement, an apex beat should be sought first with the patient sitting. In this position, the beat is palpable in about 20% of normal people over age 40, and simply feeling it in a patient with either a large chest or over age 40 suggests cardiomegaly. Vibrations of the first heart sounds should not be mistaken for an impulse or apex beat. The "point of maximum impulse" (PMI) is not a valid synonym for apex beat, because maximum precordial pulsations may be due to abnormalities (eg, a dilated pulmonary artery, or a ventricular or aortic aneurysm). With the patient in the left lateral decubitus position, however, an apex beat is palpable in 4:5 older adults, and in almost all children or young adults. The fingertips (or the palm just proximal) can best detect faint, localized movements.

The normal most lateral ventricular impulse with the patient sitting occurs at about the mid-left thorax, often described as the mid-clavicular line. It is confusing to cite in which interspace the apex beat is felt because of the oblique course of the ribs on the lateral chest wall. If it is > 2 cm to the left of the mid-left thorax, or > 10 cm from the mid-sternal line, it is probably displaced. Percussion of the chest for cardiac borders should be avoided, since a palpable ventricular impulse tells the heart size quickly and easily; and when a ventricular impulse is impalpable because of a thick chest or overaeration due to lung disease, percussion becomes unreliable.

With the patient supine, the heel of the palm is placed on the left parasternal area to detect left parasternal movement. If there is enough movement to time with the heart sounds, and if it falls after the S_2, it denotes that the left parasternal movement is sustained and, thus, either right ventricular hypertrophy is present or a huge left atrium due to severe MR is pushing a normal right ventricle forward. However, movement of a large left ventricular apical impulse may be transmitted to the left parasternal area, in which case such sustained movement is due to the left ventricle and not to the right ventricle.

With the patient in the left lateral decubitus position, a palpable impulse in the apical area may be due to *either* a right or left ventricle. A left ventricular impulse is recognized by (1) the sensation of a localized thrust, as if a ping-pong ball were

emerging between the ribs with each systole (a right ventricular impulse feels more diffuse); and (2) the presence of skin retraction medial to the impulse (medial retraction); a large right ventricular impulse at the apex area produces skin retraction lateral to the apical impulse (lateral retraction). Also in the left lateral decubitus position, cardiomegaly is suggested (1) by feeling the impulse in more than one interspace, (2) by noting the spread of the impulse in the horizontal axis over a distance of > 2 finger widths or > 3 cm, and (3) by noting a large area of medial retraction.

With the patient in the left lateral decubitus position, the apex beat should be palpated for late diastolic thrusts that feel like a double upstroke or a notch on the upstroke. This presystolic A wave is the palpable equivalent of an S_4. One should feel also for an early diastolic hump occurring at the time of an S_3.

Auscultation of the Heart (For diagramming and grading of heart sounds and murmurs, see FIG. 24–3.)

First heart sound (S_1): Heart sounds occur immediately after apposition of valve leaflets at the moment when the valve apparatus is suddenly tensed. Splitting of S_1 when narrow is probably due to mitral and tricuspid closure (M_1-T_1), especially if there is a right ventricular pressure or volume overload, as in pulmonary stenosis or atrial septal defect. When the split is wide, however, the second component is usually an aortic ejection sound, or A_1, which occurs at the moment of maximal opening of the aortic valve. A wide split may also occur in the presence of right bundle branch block **(RBBB)** because the T_1 may come late.

An aortic ejection sound, if sharp and high-pitched, may be called an ejection click whose presence in AS denotes the site of stenosis, since supra- and subvalvular stenoses do not generally have ejection clicks. It suggests congenital AS because it is not usually heard with rheumatic or calcific AS. Increased flow through a normal aortic valve or normal flow through a stiffened aortic valve (eg, in systemic hypertension) may also produce an ejection sound. In pulmonary stenosis the ejection sound is attenuated by inspiration. This does not occur with an aortic ejection sound. A pulmonary ejection click is also characteristic of pulmonary hypertension due to stiffening of the leaflets caused by the stretched pulmonary valve ring.

Loudness of S_1: The faster the ventricle contracts when it closes the mitral valve, the louder the M_1 component of the split S_1. Since the left ventricle accelerates as it contracts, the higher the left atrial pressure that has to be reached by the left ventricle before the mitral valve can be closed, the louder the M_1. Therefore in mitral stenosis **(MS)** with its high left atrial pressure, S_1 is characteristically loud. Increased contractility due to catecholamines will also cause a loud S_1. Drugs that decrease contractility as well as severe damage to the myocardium will produce a soft S_1 and it is softer also after a long P-R interval. Therefore, with A-V dissociation, as in complete A-V block or in ventricular tachycardias, the S_1 will be constantly changing due to changing P-R intervals; a short P-R producing a loud S_1, and a long P-R a soft S_1.

Second heart sound (S_2): Splitting of S_2 is due to aortic valve closure (A_2), followed by pulmonary valve closure (P_2). A_2 comes first because there is greater impedance to forward flow through the aortic than through the pulmonary valve. (Systemic resistance is 10 to 20 times pulmonary resistance.) Forward flow ceases first where there is greater impedance to forward flow. On inspiration, A_2-P_2 widens due to the following changes: In the pulmonary circuit, increased pulmonary capacity decreases impedance; the forward flow continues longer and P_2 is delayed. Ventricular volume increases on the right but decreases on the left; P_2 comes later and A_2 comes slightly earlier. (Impedance in the aortic circuit does not change with respiration.)

Loudness of S_2: Increased resistance beyond an aortic or pulmonary valve causes more elastic recoil of the great vessel beyond it and a louder S_2. Therefore, systemic and pulmonary hypertension will produce louder aortic and pulmonary components

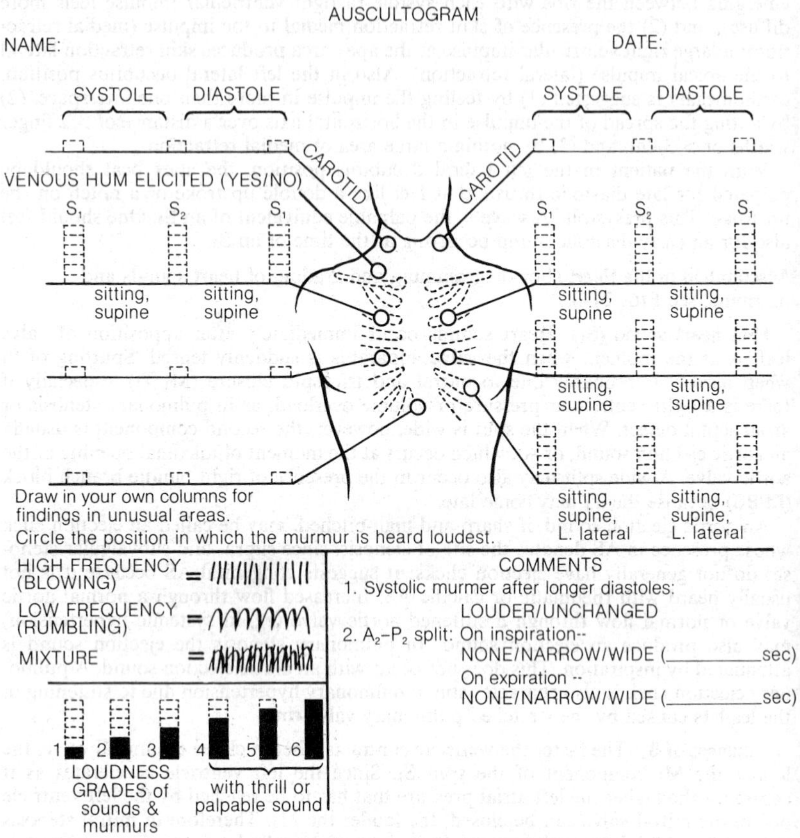

FIG. 24–3. Diagramming and grading of heart sounds and murmurs.

a. Diagramming: A graphic recording of findings develops habits of auscultation similar to those used by cardiologists. One listens separately to each component of the cycle. Height on the vertical column, divided into 6 degrees, indicates loudness and grade of sounds and murmurs. High-frequency murmurs (blowing) show as vertical parallel lines. Low-frequency murmurs use wavy lines, and those of mixed frequency use a combination of both. The only positions recorded are those where a murmur or sound is loudest. Listening and recording should be simultaneous, ie, with the stethoscope in one hand and pen in the other.

respectively. At the second left interspace A_2 is normally louder than P_2, which is contrary to common teaching. Accordingly, the second left interspace should not be called "the pulmonary area." It may be called the traditional pulmonary area but preferably simply "the second left interspace." At the apex, P_2 is normally not heard, because this is also part of the true aortic area that runs as a sash from the second right interspace to the apex. When there is systemic hypertension, there may be a ringing or drum-like quality to the S_2, which is then known as a tambour A_2. This may also be heard when there is dilation beyond the aortic valve. P_2 will also become louder when there is increased flow through the pulmonary valve, as in atrial or ventricular septal

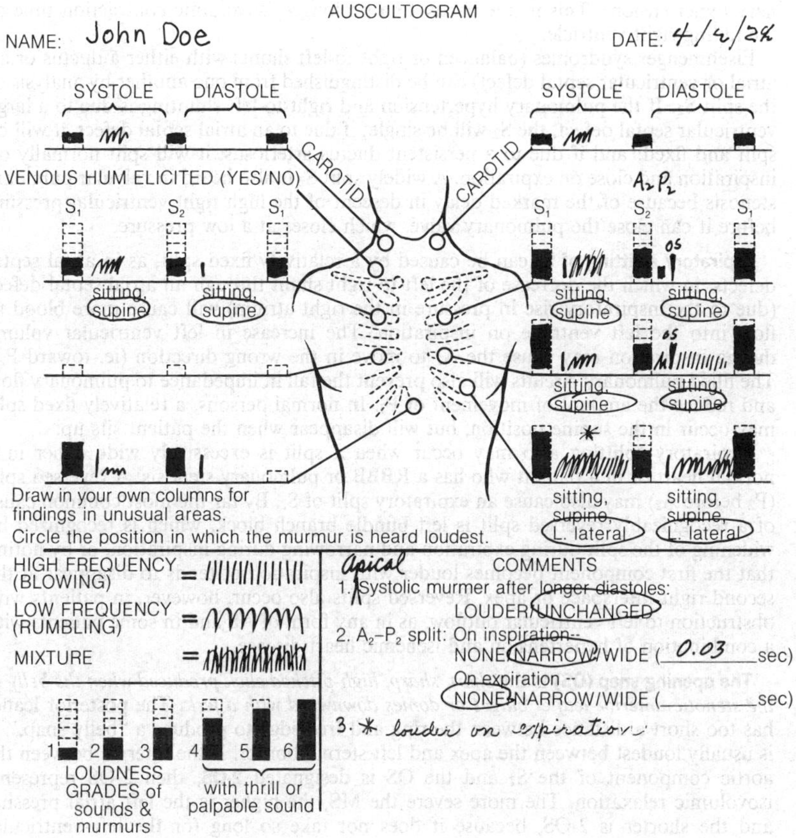

b. Grading:

Grade 1: So soft that one must know what the sound is like and concentrate to eliminate room noise.

2: Very soft; "tuning in" is unnecessary.

3: Loud, but impalpable.

4: Loud and palpable. (A palpable murmur is a thrill; a palpable sound may be called a tap.)

5: Audible with the edge of the diaphragm.

6: Audible with the stethoscope off the chest.

(From *Bedside Cardiology* by Jules Constant, ed. 3, 1985. Copyright by Little, Brown and Company, Boston, 1985.)

defects. A soft A_2 will be heard not only with a low BP, as in shock, but also with poor contractility of the myocardium and when the aortic valve is calcified and/or fibrotic, as in aortic stenosis or sclerosis.

The widely split S_2 is most commonly caused by electrical delay of right-sided events due to RBBB. Atrial septal defects, because of the large volume in the right ventricle, will often produce a widely split S_2, which is also seen with right ventricular failure, acutely (as with pulmonary embolism) or chronically (as with severe primary pulmo-

nary hypertension). This is due partly to a prolonged isovolumic contraction time of the failing right ventricle.

Eisenmenger syndromes (balanced or right-to-left shunts with either a ductus or an atrial or ventricular septal defect) can be distinguished from one another by analysis of the split S_2: If the pulmonary hypertension and right-to-left shunting is due to a large ventricular septal defect, the S_2 will be single; if due to an atrial septal defect, it will be split and fixed; and if due to a persistent ductus arteriosus, it will split normally on inspiration and close on expiration. A widely split S_2 is also heard in valvular pulmonic stenosis because of the marked delay in descent of the high right ventricular pressure before it can close the pulmonary valve, which closes at a low pressure.

Expiratory splitting of S_2 can be caused by a relatively fixed split, as in atrial septal defects, in which the decrease of the left-to-right shunt through an atrial septal defect (due to the inspiratory rise in pressure in the right atrium) will cause more blood to flow into the left ventricle on inspiration. The increase in left ventricular volume during inspiration may cause the A_2 to move in the wrong direction (ie, toward P_2). The filled pulmonary circuits will also prevent the fall in impedance to pulmonary flow and reduce the amount of movement of P_2. In normal persons, a relatively fixed split may occur in the supine position, but will disappear when the patient sits up.

Expiratory splitting also may occur when a split is excessively wide either in a normal heart or in a patient who has a RBBB or pulmonary stenosis. A reversed split (P_2 before A_2) may also cause an expiratory split of S_2. By far the most common cause of a recognizably reversed split is left bundle branch block, which is recognized by widening of the split during expiration and narrowing during inspiration, or by noting that the first component becomes louder with inspiration or tends to disappear at the second right interspace or apex. Reversed splits also occur, however, in patients with obstruction to left ventricular outflow, as in any form of AS and in some patients with a combination of hypertension and ischemic heart disease.

The opening snap (OS) is the *short, sharp, high-pitched click produced when the belly of the stenotic anterior leaflet bulges or domes downward with a jerk*. The posterior leaflet has too short a distance between the ring and free edge to produce a "belly snap." It is usually loudest between the apex and left sternal border. If the interval between the aortic component of the S_2 and the OS is designated **2-OS,** then 2-OS represents isovolumic relaxation. The more severe the MS, the higher is the left atrial pressure and the shorter is 2-OS, because it does not take so long for the left ventricular pressure to fall from aortic valve closure (A_2) pressure to mitral valve opening (OS) pressure (see FIG. 24–4). The opening snap may disappear with heavy calcification of the belly of the anterior leaflet. AR may also attenuate an OS by the regurgitant stream's holding up the belly of the anterior leaflet as it tries to come down. A narrow 2-OS is more reliable than a wide 2-OS as an indication of the degree of MS because there is not much that can narrow a 2-OS besides tight MS or tachycardia; but there are at least 5 causes besides mild MS for a wide 2-OS, one being poor myocardial function. The widest 2-OS possible is 0.1 sec, which is the time it takes to say "pa-pa" as quickly as possible.

How to tell A_2-P_2 from 2-OS: If the patient sits or stands to decrease venous return, a 2-OS will widen, but an A_2-P_2 will remain the same or even become narrower. On inspiration a P_2 will become louder while an OS will become softer. Although a tricuspid OS will increase on inspiration, it is rare to have a tricuspid OS without a mitral OS as well. On inspiration one may hear a triple second sound, the A_2-P_2, and OS.

The third heart sound (S_3) has been called a protodiastolic or ventricular gallop, but "S_3" is preferable because it specifically refers to a sound and does not require a series of sounds as gallops do. A patient with an S_3 may be said to have an S_3 gallop, although originally the word "gallop" was used only if tachycardia was present.

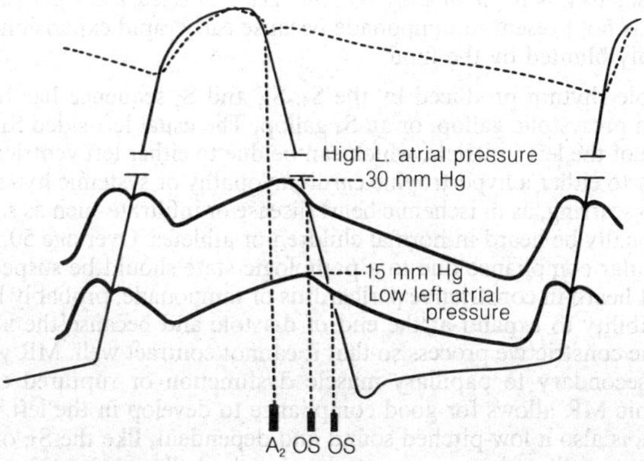

Fig. 24–4. Note that the distance between the A_2 and the OS is shorter with the higher left atrial pressure. (From *Bedside Cardiology* by Jules Constant, ed. 3, 1985. Copyright by Little, Brown and Company, Boston, 1985.)

The internal production theory of the S_3 claims that it is due to a sudden pulling short of the rapidly expanding ventricle in early diastole by unknown myocardial forces. The S_3 seems to occur at the transition between the rapid expansion and sudden change to slow expansion due to poor compliance of the dilated ventricle. The external production theory views the sound as a sudden recoil of the heart at the end of its counterclockwise rotation as viewed from the apex. This recoil in early diastole, if strong enough, may throw the heart against the chest wall structures to produce an S_3.

The physiologic S_3 can be recorded in about 1/3 of normal people under age 16 but is rarely audible or recordable in normal people over age 30. In a patient with a long P-R interval and a tachycardia, the atrial contraction may occur at the time of the physiologic S_3 and make a loud sound known as a "summation sound," and the gallop thus produced is a summation gallop. An S_3 is so dependent on volume and proximity of the stethoscope to the heart that one should listen with the patient in the left lateral decubitus position with the stethoscope bell on a palpable apex beat. The bell should be used because the S_3 is dominantly a low-frequency thud. An exaggeration of the physiologic S_3 will occur with increased flow through the mitral valve, as with MR where the systolic regurgitant flow is received back again into the left ventricle in diastole. Also, any left-to-right shunts, such as in ventricular septal defect or persistent ductus in which the extra flow goes through the mitral valve, will bring back or exaggerate a physiologic S_3.

The pathologic S_3 occurs whenever there is both loss of compliance of the left ventricle and a high left atrial pressure. This is most commonly present with cardiomyopathies of any cause. Although a pathologic S_3 is usually associated with cardiomegaly and high left atrial pressures, exceptions occur in the presence of a ventricular aneurysm or some hypertrophic cardiomyopathies with asymmetric septal hypertrophy (the septum thicker than the free wall).

A right ventricular S_3 does not occur simply with increased flow or enlargement as in atrial septal defect, but with both increased volume plus a high pressure in the right ventricle, as in primary pulmonary hypertension with tricuspid regurgitation. A right-sided S_3 always increases on inspiration.

A **pericardial knock** is *the loud early S_3 that occurs in constrictive pericarditis*. A pericardial knock is not present in tamponade because early rapid expansion of the ventricles is markedly blunted by the fluid.

S_4: The triple rhythm produced by the S_4, S_1, and S_2 sequence has been called an atrial gallop, a presystolic gallop, or an S_4 gallop. The usual left-sided S_4 is due to loss of compliance of the left ventricle, which can be due to either left ventricular hypertrophy secondary to either a hypertrophic cardiomyopathy or systemic hypertension, or it may be due to scarring, as in ischemic heart disease or infiltrate such as sarcoidosis. An S_4 can occasionally be heard in normal children or athletes. Over age 50, however, loss of left ventricular compliance due to a pathologic state should be suspected.

An S_4 is not heard in constrictive pericarditis or tamponade, probably because of the ventricle's inability to expand at the end of diastole and because the atrium may be tethered by the constrictive process so that it cannot contract well. MR will have an S_4 only if it is secondary to papillary muscle dysfunction or ruptured chordae, since primary chronic MR allows for good compliance to develop in the left ventricle.

Since the S_4 is also a low-pitched sound and dependent, like the S_3, on volume and proximity to the stethoscope, one must also use the bell and, contrary to traditional teaching, usually with firm pressure with the patient in the left lateral decubitus position. An S_4-S_1 can be distinguished from an M_1-A_1 split by knowing that it is easy to eliminate or attenuate an S_4 with maneuvers that will not much affect the M_1. Therefore an attempt should be made to eliminate the first component of the split by pressure with the diaphragm, moving the stethoscope away from the apex, and decreasing blood volume by sitting or standing the patient up. However, if S_4 is still heard under all these circumstances because it is very loud, it will then usually be palpable as an A wave or atrial hump on the apical impulse (with the patient in the left lateral decubitus position).

Murmurs

An ejection murmur is produced by *the forward flow of blood in systole through either a pulmonary or aortic valve*. The complete definition requires all the characteristics of an ejection murmur. They start with the S_1, have a crescendo-decrescendo configuration, end before the closure component of the S_2 of its side, and become louder after long diastoles. The crescendo-decrescendo is recognized by listening for a rhythm or cadence of hu–hu—duh produced by the S_1, peak of crescendo, and then S_2 (see FIG. 24–5). If the S_2 is softer than the murmur and is heard, it is an ejection murmur because only a decrescendo ending to a murmur will allow the soft S_2 to be heard. Reasons why an ejection murmur becomes louder after a long diastole follow:

(1) The long diastole stretches the left ventricle and produces a Starling effect.

(2) The long diastole allows the aortic pressure to fall to lower levels than average and creates a decrease in afterload. A decreased afterload produces an increase in contractility.

(3) If the long diastole is due to an early beat, such as a premature ventricular or atrial depolarization, then there is post-extrasystolic potentiation produced by the

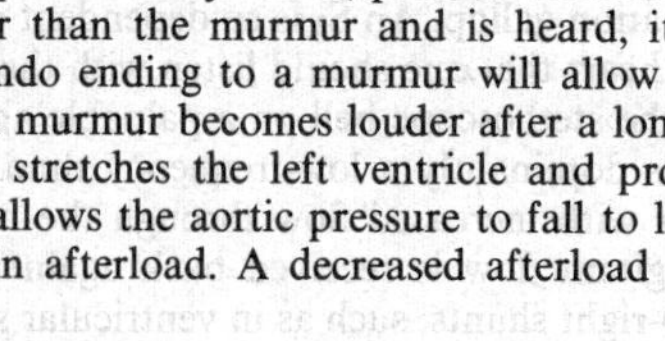

FIG. 24–5. Ejection murmur. (From *Bedside Cardiology* by Jules Constant, ed. 3, 1985. Copyright by Little, Brown and Company, Boston, 1985.)

early depolarization; ie, an early depolarization produces an inotropic effect on the heart by its effect on calcium ion flux.

Innocent ejection murmurs: Aortic valvular sclerosis in the elderly can produce a loud ejection murmur with very little gradient across the valve. Since about 50% of patients over age 50 have this murmur, it may be called the "50 over 50" murmur. Since the earlier the peak of the crescendo-decrescendo, the less the gradient, these murmurs will have an early peak at about the first third of systole.

In younger patients any increased flow across a pulmonary artery due to a hyperkinetic circulation such as in pregnancy, will also produce an innocent ejection murmur with an early peak. A humming or vibratory type of systolic ejection murmur loudest at the left sternal border that tends to disappear by puberty, known as **Still's murmur,** has an early peak to its musical quality. A very narrow posterior-anterior diameter, as with **pectus excavatum,** can produce a pulmonary ejection murmur that markedly increases in loudness with increased pressure of the stethoscope.

Ejection murmurs due to stenosis: When a murmur of mixed frequency becomes loud, as in moderate-to-severe AS, the murmur becomes harsh, rasping, or grunting. The high frequency component of an aortic ejection murmur may be transmitted to the apex and may be mistaken for MR **(Gallavardin phenomenon)**.

Ejection murmurs of pulmonary stenosis can be distinguished from those of AS because they become louder on inspiration. With pulmonary stenosis murmurs, the greater the gradient, the later the peak of the murmur; while AS murmurs, no matter how severe the obstruction, never reach a peak beyond mid-systole. AS murmurs radiate to the right clavicle and bilaterally to the neck.

The murmur of hypertrophic subaortic stenosis (**HSS**—also called hypertrophic obstructive cardiomyopathy or idiopathic hypertrophic subaortic stenosis—is best heard just medial to the apex if not at the apex. It becomes louder with any maneuver that makes the heart smaller because this increases the obstruction between the anterior mitral leaflet and the hypertrophied septum. When the septum is hypertrophied more than the free wall, this is known as asymmetric septal hypertrophy **(ASH)**. The murmur of HSS is made softer by causing the anterior mitral leaflet to move away from the septum as when squatting, which increases blood volume and peripheral resistance, or by handgrip and vasopressor agents that also increase peripheral resistance. Amyl nitrite, by decreasing peripheral resistance, will immediately make the murmur louder.

Systolic regurgitant murmurs are produced by retrograde flow from a high pressure area of the heart through some abnormal opening into an area of lower pressure such as a ventricular septal defect **(VSD)**, an incompetent mitral valve producing MR, an incompetent tricuspid valve producing tricuspid regurgitation, or an arteriovenous communication (eg, a persistent ductus). The following characteristics are common to all systolic regurgitant murmurs: If there are early components, they start with S_1. If there are late components, they always go to or beyond S_2 of the same side. When soft, they are predominantly high-pitched and blowing. They tend to remain the same after sudden long diastoles. When they go from S_1 to S_2, they are called pansystolic or holosystolic. If they go enough into diastole so that they can be recognized as going beyond S_2, they are then called continuous.

Common causes of MR are rheumatic valve damage, papillary muscle dysfunction, ruptured chordae, or prolapse of a mitral leaflet into the left atrium. Some rarer causes are left atrial myxomas, calcified mitral annulus, and endocardial cushion defects with a cleft anterior leaflet. MR is differentiated from a VSD by the site of maximum loudness. MR murmurs are always loudest at the apex, while VSD murmurs are loudest at the left sternal border. However, if the VSD is acquired, as in rupture of the muscular septum near the apex due to acute infarction, the site of maximum loudness may not be at the left sternal border but just medial to the apex beat.

Papillary muscle dysfunction murmurs: If a papillary muscle does not contract (due to infarction or fibrosis), the opposite mitral leaflet chordae-papillary muscle apparatus will be shortened during systole. Therefore, the mitral valve apparatus with the non-contracting papillary muscle will be too long, thus producing MR. If a papillary muscle is chronically shortened by fibrosis, then the opposite leaflet will bulge upwards beyond the tethered leaflet, and MR will also occur. Papillary muscle dysfunction murmurs tend to be crescendo to the S_2 and regurgitation is usually mild or moderate in degree.

Since left ventricular pressure is higher than left atrial pressure for a few milliseconds after the time of aortic valve closure, the MR murmur will go slightly beyond S_2. Therefore if the S_2 is softer than the murmur, yet still audible, it is unlikely to be an MR murmur unless one of a rare decrescendo type. Decrescendo MR murmurs usually occur only with gross MR secondary to ruptured chordae, in which case they are loud. But a soft decrescendo MR murmur may also occur with trivial MR as found in rheumatic heart disease with MS. MR associated with an S_4 is usually secondary to either papillary muscle dysfunction or ruptured chordae.

MR due to ruptured chordae: An anterior rupture tends to produce a murmur that goes posteriorly against the spine and may be heard all the way along the back from the sacrum to the top of the head. Posterior ruptured chordae tend to project a jet against the aorta and act like an aortic murmur by going up into the neck.

Quantitating the degree of MR: Since high gradients produce high frequency murmurs, and high flows produce low and medium frequencies, a purely high-pitched blow means trivial MR. MR with an unexpected S_3 is at least moderate to severe if there is no other physiologic or pathologic reason for the S_3, especially if associated with low and medium frequencies.

The prolapsed mitral valve: The typical prolapsed mitral valve regurgitation murmur is late systolic and may be preceded by a non-ejection click or series of clicks. These prolapsed mitral valve murmurs become longer and often louder when the heart is made smaller by inspiration or by having the patient sit or stand. There may be only a click, only a murmur, or both. The term **"floppy valve syndrome"** was meant to describe the most marked degree of myxomatous degeneration with elongated chordae causing severe MR and should not be used as a synonym for all patients with prolapse of the mitral valve that usually is associated with mild-to-moderate MR or no regurgitation at all. The loudest murmurs in auscultation are caused by vibrations of a prolapsed valve itself. They tend to be grade 5 or 6 "whoops" or "honks" and are occasionally audible without a stethoscope, but the degree of regurgitation is usually mild.

Tricuspid regurgitation murmurs are usually heard best at the left lower sternal border or epigastrium. They increase on inspiration **(Carvallo's sign)**. Exercise or pressure over or just below the liver can accentuate the increase of the murmur on inspiration.

Ventricular septal defect murmurs: Although the usual ventricular septal defect murmur is loudest at the left sternal border, when it is due to a ruptured septum secondary to infarction, it may be loudest near the apex, but not exactly over a palpable apex beat. It will always be at least 1 cm medial to the apex beat. This helps to distinguish it from MR murmurs due to a ruptured papillary muscle or chordae secondary to infarction since these murmurs are always loudest directly over or slightly lateral to the apex beat.

A continuous murmur is one that may go throughout all of systole and diastole, or is continuous in the sense that it goes beyond S_2 considerably into (not necessarily *all* of) diastole. The most common cause of a continuous murmur is a persistent ductus arteriosus heard best in the second left interspace; the next most common cause is

probably a coronary arteriovenous fistula. The characteristic truly continuous murmur of a persistent ductus arteriosus is a **machinery murmur** (Gibson murmur). Multiple systolic clicks or crackles, sometimes called eddy sounds, occur in the second half of systole and early diastole. They are usually heard only in large flow ducti. When pulmonary hypertension develops, the diastolic component disappears first and then only a pansystolic murmur may remain.

Venous hum is heard just above the clavicle either medial to the sternomastoid or between its insertions. It is best heard on the right side of the neck. It is never actually a hum but sounds like either a continuous roar or whine. A venous hum is elicited with the patient sitting and the head turned away from the stethoscope. Light pressure with a small bell should be used. Testing for presence of a hum is done by applying moderate finger pressure a few inches above the stethoscope. A venous hum will disappear with moderate pressure on the internal jugular vein. An unelicited venous hum, ie, without turning the head, is usually a sign of excessively rapid circulation as seen in pregnancy or hyperthyroidism unless the circulation is slowed by heart failure.

Miscellaneous continuous murmurs: Rarer causes of continuous murmurs are pulmonary arteriovenous fistulas, pulmonary artery branch stenosis, coarctation of the aorta, and the mammary souffle. In coarctation, collateral intercostal flow is the most likely cause of the continuous murmurs heard in the back. A **mammary souffle** is *an arterial murmur due to a large flow of blood in the breast during pregnancy and lactation in a minority of pregnant women.* It often starts with a delay after S_1 and spills over S_2 into early diastole.

Diastolic atrioventricular valve murmurs: Mitral stenosis (MS) diastolic murmurs begin just after the OS. The MS murmur is a low frequency rumble sounding like thunder; it typically ends with a presystolic crescendo to S_1. (The presystolic crescendo actually occurs during the beginning of ventricular contraction; ie, during the preisovolumic left ventricular contraction period. Therefore, it is not really presystolic except to the ear; ie, it occurs before S_1, which is the auscultator's onset of systole.) The presystolic crescendo in atrial fibrillation occurs only during short diastoles when a high enough left atrial pressure can create a good gradient across the mitral valve during ventricular contraction.

A soft mitral diastolic murmur is often so localized that, in order to hear it, the stethoscope must be placed exactly over the apex beat with the patient in the left lateral decubitus position. Naturally, the bell must be used with light pressure, because it is a low frequency murmur.

A left atrial myxoma may imitate rheumatic MS because the early S_3 or "tumor plop" may be mistaken for an OS and there may be a mitral diastolic rumble due to the obstruction caused by the myxoma. When an aortic regurgitant stream prevents the anterior leaflet of the mitral valve from completely opening during diastole, it creates a relative MS resulting in a diastolic rumble known as the **Austin Flint murmur**. (Austin Flint called it "presystolic" because he thought all MS murmurs should be called presystolic.)

Tricuspid diastolic flow murmurs are heard in atrial septal defects usually only during inspiration. The diastolic murmur of tricuspid stenosis is rarely ever present without some MS. The tricuspid stenosis murmur differs from the MS murmur in that in sinus rhythm it is only presystolic without any crescendo to S_1. It also always increases with inspiration.

Diastolic semilunar valve murmurs: AR murmurs begin with the aortic component of S_2 and they are decrescendo. They are high-pitched if they are mild to moderate, and usually develop low frequencies if they are moderate to severe. However, severe AR can occur with only a high-pitched murmur. Soft AR murmurs are best heard by having the patient sit up and lean forward with the breath held in expiration, while the

diaphragm chest piece is pressed firmly over the left sternal border or sternum. Loudness of an AR murmur is increased by increasing systemic resistance (eg, by having the patient squat and/or squeeze a towel [handgrip maneuver] for 30 sec).

AR murmurs may be best heard to the right of the sternum in the presence of marked post-stenotic dilation of the aorta, marked atherosclerotic tortuosity pushing the ascending aorta to the right, and when it is secondary to infective endocarditis, an aortic aneurysm, a prolapsed aortic valve, or rupture of the sinus of Valsalva. If the murmur is heard best in the mid-left thorax or at the apex or mid-axillary line, it has been called the **Cole-Cecil murmur**. The cause of this unusual radiation is unknown.

One of the major auscultatory signs of sudden, severe AR is the soft or absent S_1 and loud S_3. The soft or absent S_1 is due to the rapid and marked rise in left ventricular pressure in diastole so that the mitral valve is closed before the ventricle contracts.

In the presence of pulmonary hypertension, one hears a pulmonary regurgitation murmur (similar in pitch to the murmur of AR) caused by high pressure in the pulmonary artery **(Graham Steell murmur)**. An increase in loudness on inspiration helps to differentiate the Graham Steell murmur from the murmur of AR. When pulmonary regurgitation is present with normal pulmonary artery pressures, as in idiopathic dilation of the pulmonary artery or after surgery for pulmonary stenosis, the murmur often begins with a slight delay after P_2, tends to be short, and sounds rough due to dominant medium and low frequencies.

Pericardial friction rub sounds are caused either by 2 roughened pericardial membranes (visceral and parietal pericardium) sliding over one another, or by the overlying involved pleura rubbing against the outer layer of pericardium **(pleuropericardial friction rubs)**. A friction rub may be crunching, grating, crackling, or scratching. It often sounds creaking, like squeaky new shoes, or scraping, like pieces of sandpaper rubbed against one another. The typical friction rub has 3 components: 1 systolic and 2 diastolic. The one in early diastole occurs at the time of S_3, and may be called an S_3 rub. The one at the end of diastole occurs at the time of S_4, and may be called an S_4 rub. In systole, it may occur anywhere, and may replace S_1 or S_2 or occur only in midsystole. When a friction rub sounds like a murmur, it may be distinguished from a murmur by noting that it becomes louder on inspiration because only right-sided murmurs (relatively rare) tend to become louder on inspiration. During the course of an acute infarction, friction rubs may last for only a few minutes or a few hours.

25. SPECIAL DIAGNOSTIC PROCEDURES

NONINVASIVE PROCEDURES

RADIOLOGY

The major radiologic examinations important in the diagnosis and management of heart disorders are (1) **plain chest films** (ordinarily frontal and lateral chest x-rays; special cases may require oblique, inspiration-expiration, decubitus, or other views); (2) **fluoroscopy**; (3) **radionuclide imaging**; (4) **angiocardiography** (including coronary arteriography); and (5) cardiac ultrasonography **(echocardiography)**, see below. Angiocardiography is discussed with INVASIVE PROCEDURES, below.

PLAIN CHEST RADIOGRAPHY

Examination of frontal and lateral chest films to detect heart disease requires evaluation of 3 main aspects: (1) heart size, (2) heart shape, and (3) the lungs—especially the lung vasculature.

Heart Size

The conventional frontal chest x-ray film is made with the patient close to and facing the film holder and with the x-ray source at least 6 ft behind. This arrangement slightly magnifies (usually < 10%) the cardiac outline on the film. Although overall heart size can be determined accurately from the plain chest film, the normal and abnormal ranges overlap greatly. Factors causing wide variations in normal size include the heart rate, the phases of the cardiac cycle, the depth and phase of respiration, blood volume, and body weight and build. Overall heart size is often unequivocally normal despite the presence of severe heart disease, especially coronary artery disease, and in pressure overloads such as are caused by aortic stenosis. Thus, explicit measurement of the heart size on plain chest films is mainly helpful in statistical studies and in serial studies of the same individual. Nevertheless, certain judgments are of value, and observation of plain chest films should permit categorization of the heart size as follows: (1) **normal** (which may not exclude significant heart disease); (2) **significantly abnormal** (implying that heart disease is present); and (3) **borderline** (necessarily a large group). Some physicians estimate heart size by comparing its transverse diameter with that of the inside of the bony thorax (the ratio is usually < 1:2). Others estimate the frontal cardiac area (or, in conjunction with the lateral chest x-ray, the total cardiac volume). Serial comparisons of the same patient's heart sizes avoid many problems of normal variation and provide valuable information about the course of heart disease.

Heart Shape and Chamber Analysis

While a view of the chest may indicate an abnormality of heart shape, determining its cause may be a problem. (Mediastinal tumors and pericardial tumors or defects occasionally may be responsible for an apparently abnormal cardiac contour.) Estimating the sizes of individual chambers from a plain film is difficult; precise delineation is usually impossible since the chambers are intimately clustered and covered by other structures, such as pericardium, mediastinal fat, and diaphragm. Conventional signs of specific chamber enlargement, often dogmatically described in textbooks, are frequently difficult to apply, and in some cases are frankly misleading. However, despite these limitations, study of heart shape is worthwhile.

Analysis of the frontal cardiac silhouette is aided by noting 4 segments along the **left mediastinal (or heart) border** (see FIG. 25–1).

1. The upper or first segment is the convexity made by the lateral profile of the distal aortic arch, which tends to become more prominent as the aging aorta becomes tortuous and enlarged. Characteristically, this segment is continuous with the margin of the descending aorta on the chest film.

2. The second segment, related to the main pulmonary artery margin, becomes relatively more prominent when the main pulmonary artery enlarges in response to pulmonary hypertension, high pulmonary flow, or the poststenotic dilation of pulmonary valve stenosis.

3. The third segment, the region of the left atrial appendage, is a concave margin in most adults. When the left atrium enlarges, this segment tends to become straight or, more significantly, convex.

4. The fourth segment of the left heart border is the ventricular region, a convexity usually produced by the lateral aspects of the left ventricle, though when the right ventricle is very large, it may form this border in the frontal projection.

On the **right mediastinal (or heart) border** (see FIG. 25–1), 2 major segments should be routinely noted:

1. The upper segment in young people is usually the lateral aspect of the superior vena cava; in older people the ascending aorta more commonly produces this margin.

2. The lower convex segment on the right border is the lateral contour of the right atrium. This segment tends to become more prominent and longer with right atrial

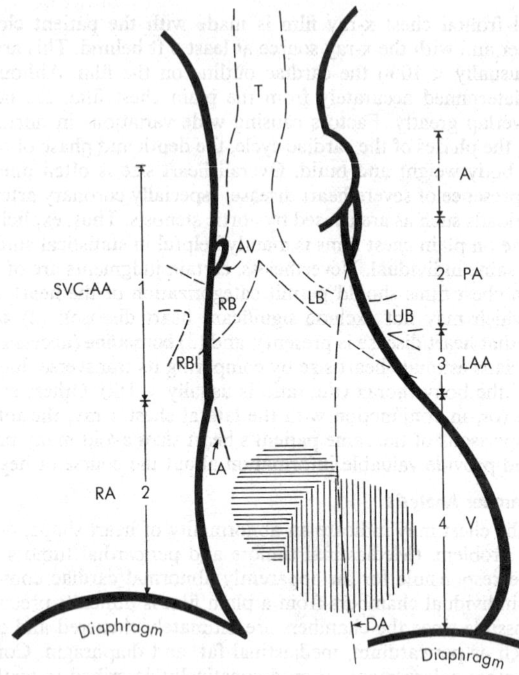

FIG. 25–1. Diagram of normal adult heart as shown on the frontal chest roentgenogram. The left border of the mediastinum is divided into 4 segments: (1) distal aortic arch segment; (2) main pulmonary artery segment; (3) left atrial appendage segment; (4) ventricular segment. The right border is divided into 2 segments; (1) the superior vena cava or ascending aortic segment; (2) right atrial segment. LA indicates the right margin of the left atrium, often seen in this region in the normal person; T, trachea; AV, azygous vein; RB, right main bronchus; RBI, right intermediate bronchus; LB, left main bronchus; LUB, left upper lobe bronchus; DA, left margin of descending aorta. The horizontally-lined area represents usual position of the aortic valve, while the vertically-lined area represents usual position of the mitral valve. The tracheal and main bronchial outlines are shown. (From *Nomenclature and Criteria for Diagnosis of Diseases of the Heart and Great Vessels*, ed. 8, 1979. Copyright 1979 by the New York Heart Association, New York, 1979. Used with permission.)

enlargement; it can also become prominent because of pericardial effusion or from right atrial displacement when other parts of the heart enlarge. The azygous vein often appears on the frontal chest film as an ovoid increase in density just lateral to the right main bronchus. This vein may dilate in response to increased venous and right atrial pressures; its size also varies greatly because of the relative pressure changes produced by respiratory effort. On a single chest film, a paratracheal lymph node may be indistinguishable from the azygous vein.

The **lateral chest film** (FIG. 25–2) is useful since the lateral dimensions and contours of the mediastinum and heart can be measured and compared. A margin of the intrathoracic inferior vena cava, concave posteriorly, is usually visible just above the right diaphragm. Typically, this margin is pushed back by a large right atrium and ventricle,

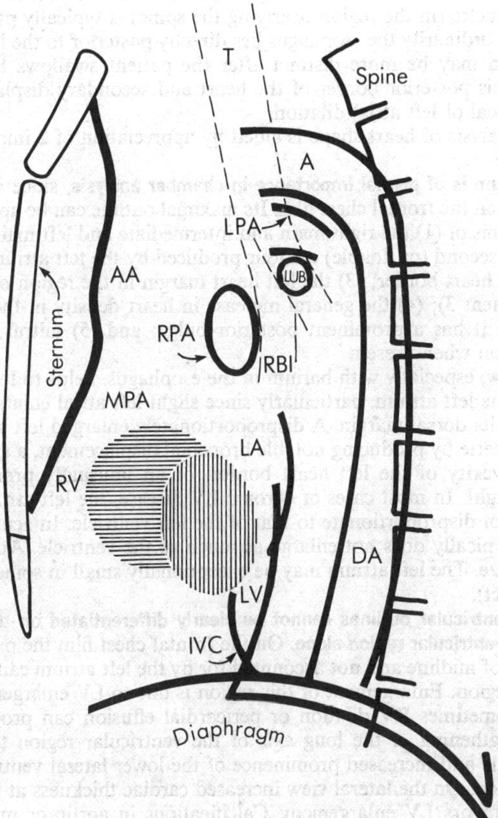

FIG. 25–2. Diagram of normal adult heart in the left lateral projection. A, aorta; LPA, left pulmonary artery at left hilus arching over LUB, circular image of left upper lobe bronchus; RPA, right pulmonary artery at right hilus; LA, dorsal margin of left atrium; LV, dorsal margin of left ventricle; IVC, dorsal margin of intrathoracic inferior vena cava; RV, ventral margin of right ventricular outflow tract; MPA, ventral margin of main pulmonary artery; AA, ventral margin of ascending aorta; RBI, right intermediate bronchus; DA, descending thoracic aorta; T, trachea. The horizontally-lined area represents usual position of the aortic valve, while the vertically-lined area represents usual position of the mitral valve. (From *Nomenclature and Criteria for Diagnosis of Diseases of the Heart and Great Vessels,* ed. 8, 1979. Copyright 1979 by the New York Heart Association, New York, 1979. Used with permission.)

but with left ventricular **(LV)** dilation, the posterior aspect of the left ventricle progressively overlaps this region. The right ventricle and the main pulmonary artery form the anterior and anterior-superior aspects of the lateral heart silhouette. Increased prominence of these margins, especially extension of the cardiac density superiorly in the retrosternal region, is a sign of right ventricular **(RV)** dilation. Such changes, however, are easily confused with the increased density in the same general region that may be caused by a dilated tortuous ascending aorta. In the lateral view the right and left hilar

arteries and major bronchi are often clearly demonstrated. The posterior upper aspect of the heart silhouette (in the region overlying the spine) is typically produced by the left atrium. Since ordinarily the esophagus lies directly posterior to the left atrium, this chamber's margin may be more distinct after the patient swallows barium sulfate. Prominence of this posterior border of the heart and secondary displacement of the esophagus is typical of left atrial dilation.

Meaningful analysis of heart shape is aided by appreciation of 2 important considerations:

1. The left atrium is of pivotal importance in chamber analysis, since its margins are usually apparent on the frontal chest film. Its maximal outline can be approximated by noting the positions of (1) the right main and intermediate and left main bronchial air shadows; (2) the second (or double) contour produced by the left atrium, usually seen close to the right heart border; (3) the left heart margin in the region of the left atrial appendage (Segment 3); (4) the general increase in heart density in the region of the left atrium when it has a prominent posterior bulge; and (5) mitral valve or valve anulus calcification when present.

The lateral view, especially with barium in the esophagus, helps to locate the posterior margins of the left atrium, particularly since slight left atrial enlargement is most impressive along its dorsal margin. A disproportionately enlarged left atrium deforms the cardiac silhouette by producing notable bronchial displacement, a straightening or especially a convexity of the left heart border, or an unusually prominent double contour on the right. In most cases of chronic LV disease, the left atrial enlargement parallels but is not disproportionate to that of the left ventricle. In acute LV dilation, the left atrium typically does not enlarge as much as the ventricle. Atrial fibrillation increases atrial size. The left atrium may be exceptionally small in some disorders (eg, atrial septal defect).

2. Individual ventricular outlines cannot be clearly differentiated on the basis of the silhouette of the ventricular region alone. On the frontal chest film the part of the heart per se to the left of midline and not accounted for by the left atrium can be considered the ventricular region. Enlargement of this region is due to LV enlargement in > 90% of adults, but sometimes RV dilation or pericardial effusion can produce the same appearance. Lengthening of the long axis of the ventricular region toward the left costophrenic angle and increased prominence of the lower lateral ventricular contour suggest LV dilation. On the lateral view increased cardiac thickness at the level of the diaphragm also favors LV enlargement. Calcifications in aortic or mitral valves, in coronary arteries, or in old myocardial infarcts, when present, help to identify the outline of the left ventricle.

Since the right ventricle seldom forms a border in the frontal projection, its dilation produces only nonspecific enlargement of the ventricular region. RV dilation does, however, tend to displace its outflow tract and the main pulmonary artery cephalad and to the left, resulting, on the lateral view, in encroachment on the retrosternal clear space from below. The value of this feature is limited in diagnosing RV enlargement since it can be mimicked by a prominent ascending aorta or even a normal thymus gland (especially if the anterior-posterior dimension of the mediastinum is small).

The Lungs and Pulmonary Vessels

FIG. 25–3 diagrams several characteristic x-ray patterns of the pulmonary vessels, which give information about many aspects of the circulatory state and, in particular, of LV function. The size of central arteries (the main pulmonary artery and its hilar branches) gives an index of the pulmonary artery pressure. The sizes of the more peripheral vessels reflect pulmonary blood volume and roughly indicate the pulmonary BP and flow. Prominence of the region of the RV outflow tract and especially dilation of the central pulmonary arteries are the most important signs suggesting RV enlargement. Dilation of the main pulmonary arteries (after discounting the effects of aging

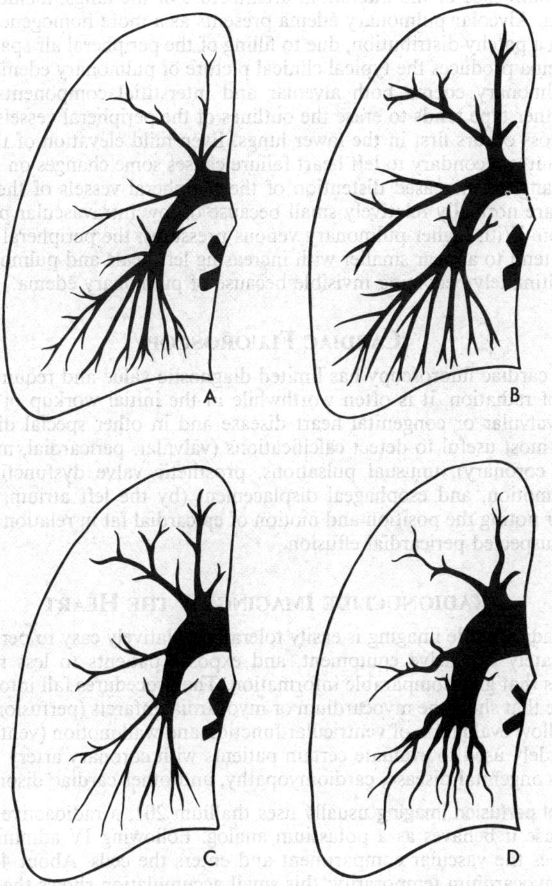

FIG. 25–3. Diagrams of the pulmonary vessels as shown on the frontal chest film in erect adult (right lung).

A. *Normal pulmonary vessels.* Note that the larger peripheral vessels are in the lower lung.

B. *General increase in prominence of pulmonary vessels.* Typical of large left-to-right shunts in congenital heart disease and high blood volume-high output states (eg, anemia, pregnancy, overhydration).

C. *Distended upper lung field vessels and relatively small lower lung field vessels* (which may not be visible in the presence of edema), typical of chronic left heart failure (eg, severe mitral stenosis).

D. *Dilated tortuous central pulmonary arteries with relatively small peripheral pulmonary arteries,* typical of acquired chronic severe pulmonary hypertension due to a high peripheral pulmonary resistance. (From *Nomenclature and Criteria for Diagnosis of Diseases of the Heart and Great Vessels,* ed. 8, 1979. Copyright 1979 by the New York Heart Association, New York, 1979. Used with permission.)

and normal variations) indicates pulmonary hypertension, poststenotic dilation, or increased pulmonary artery flow volume; RV hypertension is implied, and RV hypertrophy and/or dilation is almost certainly present.

High pulmonary capillary pressure (> 22 mm Hg) secondary to left heart dysfunction produces pulmonary edema. Interstitial edema shows as a linear pattern with

increased prominence of the interstitial architecture of the lungs, including the interlobular septa. Alveolar pulmonary edema presents as a more homogeneous lung density, often in a patchy distribution, due to filling of the peripheral air spaces with fluid. Alveolar edema produces the typical clinical picture of pulmonary edema, but in most cases of pulmonary edema both alveolar and interstitial components are present. Edema of either type tends to erase the outlines of the peripheral vessels; in left heart failure this loss occurs first in the lower lungs. Even mild elevation of the pulmonary venous pressures secondary to left heart failure causes some changes on the chest film. An early change is increased distention of the peripheral vessels of the upper lungs, where they are normally relatively small because of low intravascular pressure in the erect position. With higher pulmonary venous pressures, the peripheral vessels in the lower lungs tend to appear smaller with increasing left heart and pulmonary capillary pressures, ultimately becoming invisible because of pulmonary edema.

Cardiac Fluoroscopy

Although cardiac fluoroscopy has limited diagnostic value and requires a relatively large dose of radiation, it is often worthwhile in the initial workup of patients with perplexing valvular or congenital heart disease and in other special diagnostic situations. It is most useful to detect calcifications (valvular, pericardial, myocardial, tumorous, or coronary), unusual pulsations, prosthetic valve dysfunction, effects of respiratory motion, and esophageal displacement (by the left atrium, great vessels, etc.), and for noting the position and motion of epicardial fat in relation to the cardiac borders in suspected pericardial effusion.

Radionuclide Imaging of the Heart

Cardiac radionuclide imaging is easily tolerated, relatively easy to perform, requires only moderately expensive equipment, and exposes patients to less radiation than x-ray studies that give comparable information. The procedures fall into 2 broad categories: those that show the myocardium or myocardial infarcts (perfusion studies), and those that allow evaluation of ventricular function and wall motion (ventriculography). They are widely used to evaluate certain patients with coronary artery disease **(CAD),** valvular or congenital disease, cardiomyopathy, and other cardiac disorders.

Myocardial perfusion imaging usually uses thallium 201, a radioactive cation that is useful because it behaves as a potassium analog. Following IV administration, ^{201}Tl rapidly leaves the vascular compartment and enters the cells. About 4% of the dose enters the myocardium temporarily; this small accumulation shows the heart in relief against the low surrounding background of lung activity. After ^{201}Tl reaches its initial distribution, an equilibrium occurs between myocardial ^{201}Tl and that in the blood and other structures (eg, skeletal muscles, liver, kidneys, etc). During this equilibration, ^{201}Tl enters and leaves the myocardium at a rate roughly proportional to regional myocardial blood flow. Thus, if ^{201}Tl is injected into someone who is exercising, defects in the myocardial ^{201}Tl distribution will occur in nonviable areas (eg, infarct, scar) and in viable regions with reduced blood flow (eg, an ischemic zone distal to a hemodynamically significant coronary stenosis). Subsequently, after several hours with the patient at rest, the ^{201}Tl distribution will change. If the original ^{201}Tl myocardial defect was caused by a nonviable scar, it will appear unchanged. However, if it was an ischemic area, the late image is likely to show disappearance or diminution of the initial defect. This is the basis for detecting regions of exercise-induced ischemia by sequential ^{201}Tl studies.

Multiple views of the heart are taken with a conventional scintillation camera using video-contrast enhancement immediately after ^{201}Tl has been injected during exercise, and these views are repeated for comparison several hours later. The exercise test

usually is done on a conventional treadmill using the Bruce protocol or a similar exercise schedule with patient monitoring. If no contraindications arise, exercise is continued to at least 85% of the age-predicted maximum, and thallous chloride Tl 201 ($\cong$ 2mCi) is injected while the patient is at peak exercise. The patient is encouraged to continue at this level for an additional 30 to 60 sec to allow for distribution of radioactivity under the influence of exercise-related blood flow patterns.

Evaluation of ^{201}Tl results in patients who have coronary angiography indicate that the sensitivity of conventional ^{201}Tl imaging for significant CAD in this population is 80 to 85% and its specificity > 90%. Stress-redistribution ^{201}Tl imaging is more sensitive and specific in detecting significant coronary ischemia than ECG stress testing; when ^{201}Tl results and stress ECG findings are coupled, the sensitivity for CAD increases to > 90%. Thus, ^{201}Tl imaging can be used for initial evaluation of certain patients with chest pain (ie, mainly those with pain of uncertain origin), to determine the functional significance of coronary artery stenosis or collateral vessels demonstrated by angiography, and to follow up procedures such as bypass, transluminal angioplasty, or thrombolysis. Another important use of ^{201}Tl is to estimate prognosis after acute myocardial infarction **(MI)**, since it can reveal not only the extent of the perfusion abnormality associated with the acute MI, but also the extent of scarring from previous infarcts.

Infarct-avid imaging depends on the accumulation of technetium 99m-labeled tracers in areas of damaged myocardium. Bone scanning agents such as ^{99m}Tc pyrophosphate accumulate at these sites, probably secondary to membrane breakdown and microcalcification. Images usually become positive 12 to 24 h after an acute MI and remain positive for about 1 wk. Patients with ongoing myocardial necrosis post-MI and those who develop aneurysms may show persistently positive infarct images. These studies, when performed using conventional radionuclide imaging technics with the patient at rest, are much more likely to be positive with transmural than with subendocardial infarcts.

Multiple images are taken of the myocardial region 1 h or so after IV injection of about 20 mCi of technetium Tc 99m pyrophosphate. Views delayed from 2 to 4 h often are necessary to differentiate blood pool from myocardial activity. For this reason, much more diagnostic certainty can be attached to an image showing focal and intense ^{99m}Tc pyrophosphate accumulation (ie, greater than or equal to rib activity) than to one showing fainter or more diffuse abnormalities. As with ^{201}Tl images, computer acquisition and subsequent image enhancement seem to improve accuracy.

Overall, ^{99m}Tc pyrophosphate infarct imaging is used less than ^{201}Tl myocardial imaging, but it is useful to detect acute infarcts in patients with atypical presentations and to detect perioperative infarction after coronary bypass grafting or other types of heart surgery. The utility of the procedure for determining the infarct size is not as well established, but may be aided by single photon tomography. Such emission tomographic studies also improve detection of subendocardial infarction by ^{99m}Tc pyrophosphate imaging.

Radionuclide ventriculography evaluates cardiac performance, as evidenced by left ventricular **(LV)** and right ventricular **(RV)** function, and can be analyzed by 3 methods: first transit studies (a type of beat-to-beat evaluation), ECG-synchronized (ie, gated) imaging studies performed over several minutes, and non-imaging gated probe studies. Although first transit studies are rapid and relatively easy to do, especially when an evaluation of ventricular function both at rest and exercise is desired, gated imaging studies provide better delineation of the cardiac blood pool and ventricular-wall motion and are more widely used. Gated blood pool imaging synchronizes ^{99m}Tc RBC blood pool images with the R wave of the patient's ECG. Multiple images (usually about 14 to 28) of short, sequential portions of each cardiac cycle are taken over 5 to 10 min and stored in a computer. Later, aggregate images create an average blood pool

configuration for each portion of the cardiac cycle that was evaluated. The computer displays them in a continuous cinematic loop that resembles a beating heart, a display format that allows regional wall motion to be evaluated with great accuracy.

Numerous quantitative indices of ventricular function can be derived from gated blood pool studies, including the ejection fraction (**EF** [*the ratio of stroke volume:end-diastolic volume*]), ejection and filling rates, LV volume, and indices of relative volume overload such as LV:RV stroke volume ratios. The EF is the most frequently used index. Normal values for EF vary, based on differences in technic, but the normal resting EF is usually 50 to 75% of end-diastolic volume. EF and wall motion are measured at rest, and changes during stress can be evaluated by acquiring gated images while the monitored patient pedals an exercise bicycle. The exercise EF normally is at least 5% greater than the EF at rest (eg, 55% at rest; ≥ 60% with exercise). Ventricular dysfunction from a variety of causes (eg, valvular heart disease, cardiomyopathy, CAD) can result in a decrease in the exercise EF. The reproducibility of these rest and exercise EF measurements and other indices of ventricular function has improved with semiautomatic computer processing technics that diminish the variability of subjective operator-based analyses.

Gated blood pool imaging also is useful to detect LV aneurysms. Its sensitivity and specificity in detecting typical anterior or anteroapical true aneurysms of the left ventricle is > 90%. Inferoposterior aneurysms are more difficult to detect, because these surfaces of the left ventricle are seen less well in conventional blood pool images than its anterior and lateral aspects. Therefore, when an inferior or posterior aneurysm is suspected, steep oblique, lateral, or posterior oblique gated images of the left ventricle should be obtained. In fact, most authorities recommend that one of these additional views be obtained with all gated blood pool studies.

Because virtually no risk is associated with gated blood pool studies obtained at rest, they have been used widely for serial evaluation of RV and LV function in a variety of conditions: valvular heart disease, monitoring patients who have taken potentially cardiotoxic drugs such as doxorubicin, and in patients with CAD or infarction to assess the effects of angioplasty, coronary bypass surgery, thrombolysis, etc.

In patients with valvular disease, combined rest-exercise studies have been applied most often in patients with lesions that result in LV volume overload. In aortic insufficiency a fall in the resting EF to abnormal levels or an inability to raise the EF with exercise is a sign of deteriorating cardiac function and may be an indication for valvular repair. The radionuclide study also can be used to calculate the regurgitant fraction in patients with valvular insufficiency. Normally, the stroke volume of both ventricles is equal. In patients with left-sided valvular insufficiency, however, the LV stroke volume exceeds that of the RV by an amount proportional to the regurgitant fraction. Thus, if the right ventricle is normal, the regurgitant fraction of the left ventricle can be calculated from the ratio of the LV:RV stroke volumes.

The size of a congenital shunt can be quantified by the stroke volume ratio or during the first transit of the radionuclide by determining the ratio of abnormal early pulmonary recirculation of radioactivity to total pulmonary radioactivity. This can be done using commercially available computer programs.

The right ventricle can be evaluated by using first transit or gated blood pool technics. RV function is of special interest in patients with lung diseases and in patients with inferior LV infarcts who may have associated right-sided involvement. The semiautomatic programs that are useful in evaluating the left ventricle are not applicable to RV analysis, so computer regions of interest usually are hand-selected. The normal RVEF is lower than the LVEF, ranging from about 40 to 55% with most technics. These EF values fall to subnormal levels in many patients with advanced pulmonary hypertension and in patients who have RV infarction or RV involvement by cardiomyopathy. Idiopathic cardiomyopathy usually is characterized by biventricular dysfunc-

tion, in distinction to typical CAD, which usually shows more LV than RV abnormalities.

Other radionuclides are less widely used. Since gallium citrate Ga 67 accumulates in sites of active inflammation, it has been used to detect the presence and severity of inflammatory cardiomyopathies. Its accumulation during the active stage of myocarditis diminishes as the inflammation subsides. However, ^{67}Ga may not be an accurate monitor in the presence of steroid therapy, and is less effective than 2-dimensional echocardiography in diagnosing SBE.

Indium 111 platelet imaging of ventricular or coronary thrombogenesis, rubidium 82 myocardial imaging, and evaluation of myocardial metabolism with positron emitting radionuclides are primarily experimental. Utilization of ultra-short-lived radionuclides (which is widespread in Europe and Japan) to study myocardial function is at an early stage in the USA. Gold 195m, however, has an extremely short half-life (30.5 sec) suitable for repeat LV function studies at relatively low radiation doses, is generator-produced, and is about to be introduced in the USA for clinical trials.

ECHOCARDIOGRAPHY

The principal use of ultrasound in the diagnosis of cardiovascular disorders is **echocardiography,** which is subdivided into M-mode, two-dimensional **(2-D)**, Doppler, and contrast echocardiography. **M-mode echocardiography** uses pulsed-reflected ultrasound to visualize internal cardiac structures. The ultrasonic transducer is placed over the surface of the chest, usually along the left sternal border, and the ultrasonic beam is directed toward various portions of the heart. Occasionally the transducer will be placed in the subxiphoid or subcostal area, in the suprasternal notch, or in the supraclavicular area. Every cardiac structure that is roughly perpendicular to the ultrasonic beam will be recorded on the oscilloscope. All 4 cardiac valves can be visualized, and internal dimensions of both ventricles and the left atrium can be measured. If the structure intersected by the ultrasonic beam moves, a wavy line is inscribed on the echocardiogram. A stationary structure like the chest wall is visualized as a straight line. Ultrasound does not traverse air or bone well, and satisfactory echocardiograms are difficult to obtain in patients with emphysema or thick chests.

FIG. 25–4 shows a diagram of an echocardiogram as the ultrasonic beam is directed toward the apex of the heart (position 1) and then is gradually moved toward the base of the heart (position 4). Initially, the ultrasonic beam traverses part of the right and left ventricles in the vicinity of the posterior papillary muscle **(PPM)**. In this position, one can visualize the chest wall, the anterior right ventricular wall, a small portion of the right ventricular cavity, the interventricular septum, the left ventricular **(LV)** cavity, the PPM, the posterior LV wall, and the lung. As the beam begins to move toward the base of the heart, the PPMs become continuous with structures originating from the mitral valve. One can again see the cavities of the right and left ventricles, together with the interventricular septum and the posterior LV wall. With further movement of the ultrasonic beam toward the base of the heart, the mitral valve assumes its maximum amplitude and the anterior mitral valve inscribes a characteristic "M" appearance during diastole. The LV wall now becomes the posterior left atrial wall. Moving even further medially and superiorly, the ultrasonic beam traverses the root of the aorta and the body of the left atrium. Within the aortic root, 2 of the aortic valve leaflets produce a box-like configuration during systole. Further changes in the direction of the ultrasonic beam allow echoes from the tricuspid valve and the pulmonic valve to be recorded.

Two-dimensional (or cross-sectional) echocardiography (2-DE) provides spatially correct images of the heart and has become the dominant echocardiographic modality. These "real time" images are recorded on videotape and look much like cineangio-

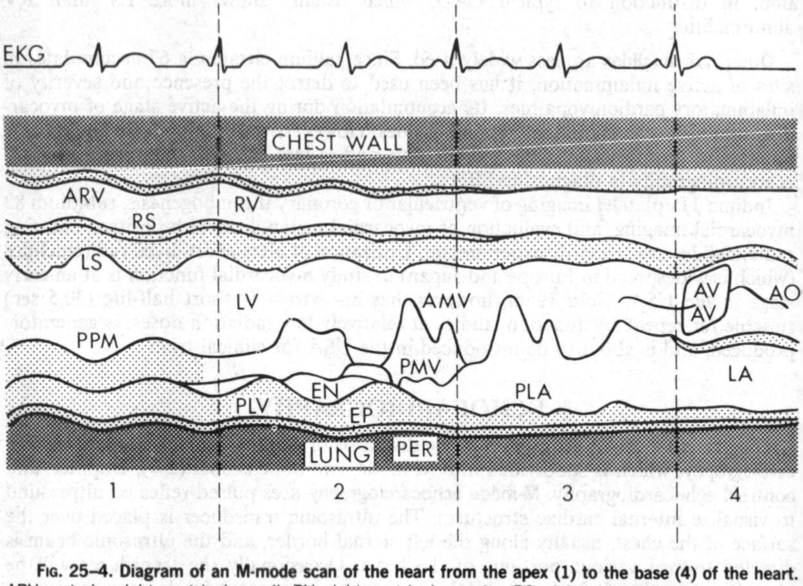

Fig. 25–4. Diagram of an M-mode scan of the heart from the apex (1) to the base (4) of the heart. ARV, anterior right ventricular wall; RV, right ventricular cavity; RS, right side of the interventricular septum; LS, left side of the interventricular septum; LV, left ventricular cavity; PPM, posterior papillary muscle; PLV, posterior left ventricular wall; EN, posterior left ventricular endocardium; EP, posterior left ventricular epicardium; PER, pericardium; AMV, anterior mitral valve leaflet; PMV, posterior mitral valve leaflet; PLA, posterior left atrial wall; AV, aortic valve, AO, aorta; LA, cavity of the left atrium. (From "Clinical applications of Echocardiography" by H. Feigenbaum, in *Progress in Cardiovascular Diseases* 14: 531–558, May 1972. Used by permission of Grune & Stratton, Inc., and the author.)

grams. Two of these frames are shown in Fig. 25–5. One can obtain multiple tomographic views of the heart and great vessels using 2-DE.

Doppler echocardiography has been increasing in importance. This technic uses ultrasound to record the flow of blood within the cardiovascular system. The Doppler signal is displayed on a strip chart recorder and provides information as to the velocity, direction, and type of flow from the area being examined. Fig. 25–6 demonstrates a Doppler examination together with a 2-DE and M-mode simultaneous recording of flow in the root of the aorta.

Contrast echocardiography is an M-mode or 2-D examination during which contrast medium is injected into the cardiovascular circulation. Almost any liquid medium that is rapidly injected into the cardiovascular space acquires microbubbles in suspension, and the bolus of microbubbles produces a cloud of echoes within the cardiac chambers. These microbubbles currently do not traverse any capillary bed.

Clinical Uses

Valvular heart disease: Echocardiography is particularly useful in assessing valvular heart disease, since all valvular abnormalities can be detected. Both M-mode and 2-DE provide direct visualization of the abnormal valves. One can use 2-DE to measure directly the valve orifice with mitral stenosis. Doppler echocardiography is valuable in assessing valvular regurgitation and also valvular stenosis, particularly aortic stenosis.

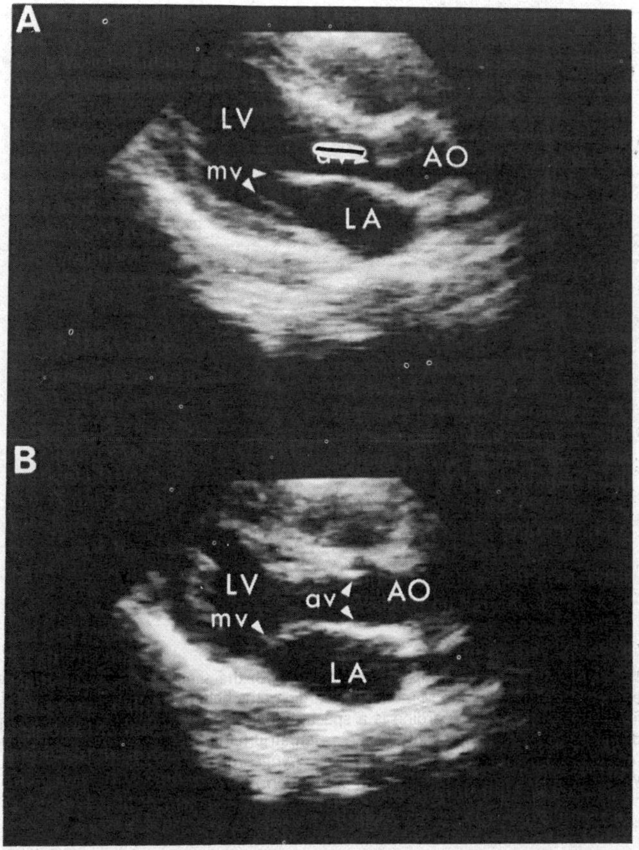

FIG. 25–5. Two-dimensional echocardiograms of a normal heart. During diastole (A) the mitral valve (mv) is open and the aortic valve (av) is closed. With ventricular systole (B) the mitral valve is closed and the aortic valve is open. The left ventricular cavity (LV) is smaller during systole (B) than in diastole (A). AO = aorta; LA = left atrium. (From "Echocardiography" by H. Feigenbaum, in *Cecil Textbook of Medicine*, edited by J. B. Wyngaarden and L. H. Smith, Jr., 1985. Copyright 1985 by W. B. Saunders. Used with permission.)

There is evidence that the velocity of blood across the stenotic valve is related to the pressure gradient. The detection of mitral valve prolapse and vegetations from bacterial endocarditis are two especially useful applications.

Evaluation of cardiac chambers: Echocardiography provides an excellent opportunity to evaluate all cardiac chambers. Although the initial quantitation of the chambers was made with M-mode echocardiography, there is increasing use of 2-DE for assessing the size and function of individual chambers.

M-mode and 2-DE can assess the location, size, shape, and motion of the interventricular septum; the latter assessment provides diagnostic information with regard to ventricular volume overload, pressure overload, and conduction abnormalities.

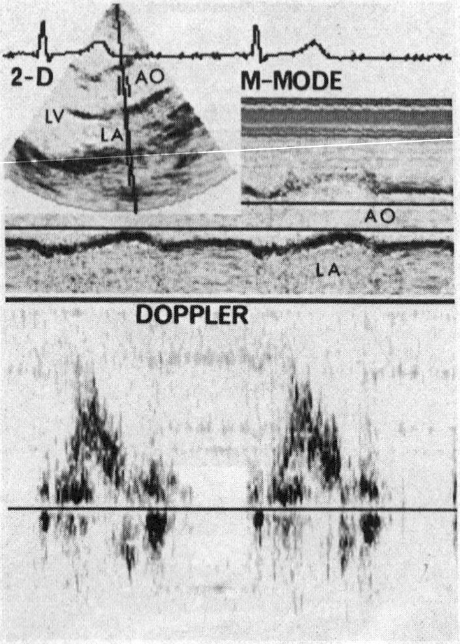

Fig. 25–6. Doppler echocardiographic examination with the sample in the root of the aorta (AO). Simultaneous two-dimensional and M-mode echocardiograms help to identify the location of the Doppler sampling site. The Doppler recording is a spectral analysis of the audible signal coming from the moving column of blood. LV = left ventricle; LA = left atrium. (From "Echocardiography" by H. Feigenbaum, in *Cecil Textbook of Medicine,* edited by J. B. Wyngaarden and L. H. Smith, Jr., 1985. Copyright 1985 by W. B. Saunders Company. Used with permission.)

Hemodynamic information: M-mode and Doppler echocardiography are particularly useful in providing hemodynamic information. The motion of the various cardiac valves gives clues as to alterations in both flow and pressure inside the heart. The pattern of motion of the mitral valve provides evidence of changes in LV diastolic pressure. The motion of the pulmonary valve will give indications of pulmonary hypertension. The amplitude and duration of opening of the various valves reflect the amount of blood flowing through the respective orifices. Doppler echocardiography gives more direct information with regard to blood flow. Technics have been described for measuring flow velocity and stroke volume. Hemodynamic measurements (eg, shunt ratios with congenital heart disease, and regurgitant fractions with valvular heart disease) have also been described with Doppler echocardiography. The blood flow velocities in the aorta can give clues to LV performance, and the blood flow pattern in the pulmonary artery provides information concerning pulmonary artery pressure.

Congenital heart disease: Echocardiographic examinations are invaluable in the diagnosis and management of patients with congenital heart disease. Two-DE provides excellent morphologic definition of anatomic abnormalities. M-mode examination provides physiologic assessment of cardiac function. Both contrast and Doppler echocardiography give precise assessment of intracardiac shunts.

Coronary artery disease: Two-DE is an excellent means of assessing regional wall motion of both left and right ventricles, making it helpful in assessing the presence and severity of coronary artery disease and in identifying the complications of myocardial infarction (eg, aneurysms, mural thrombi, ruptured interventricular septum, and papillary muscle dysfunction). Echocardiograms can be performed during or immediately after exercise to demonstrate ischemic wall motion abnormalities.

Cardiomyopathy: Hypertrophic cardiomyopathy with or without obstruction is detected readily with either M-mode or 2-DE. Both procedures are also helpful in identifying and assessing the severity of dilated congestive cardiomyopathy. The various infiltrative cardiomyopathies may produce fairly distinctive echocardiographic images.

Cardiac masses: Two-DE is the procedure of choice for evaluating cardiac masses (inflammatory, neoplastic, or thrombotic), most of which are intracavitary. Extra cardiac masses have also been detected with 2-DE.

Pericardial disease: Echocardiography is the procedure of choice for the detection of pericardial effusion. The technic is sensitive and quite reliable. Signs for cardiac tamponade have been developed. While also useful in the detection of constrictive pericarditis, reliability of ultrasonic examination is not as great as with pericardial effusion.

Diseases of the aorta: The entire aorta can be examined with 2-DE. A host of diseases, including aortic dissection, sinus of Valsalva aneurysm, or coarctation can be detected.

INVASIVE CARDIOVASCULAR PROCEDURES

VENOUS CUTDOWN AND CANNULATION

Venous cutdown and cannulation are necessary when it is impossible or hazardous to locate a vein large enough for a needle to enter percutaneously; eg, when normally accessible veins are collapsed because of volume depletion or peripheral vasoconstriction and when a patient is obese or very young. The procedure is also used when large quantities of fluid must be given rapidly (eg, in trauma). Indwelling catheters extending from the cephalic, external or internal jugular, or subclavian vein into the superior vena cava may be used to administer hypertonic solutions and to measure central venous pressure. For brief periods of cannulation, the cephalic vein in the upper arm is often used.

Percutaneous technics are replacing the surgical cutdown. One procedure uses a needle that fits snugly into a plastic catheter and projects several mm beyond the catheter tip. After the needle and catheter assembly have been introduced into the vein, the needle is withdrawn while the catheter is advanced. This method is applicable to peripheral veins. To minimize the incidence of local inflammation, the catheter should be changed q 3 days. A second approach was described by Seldinger. A wire guide is introduced into the vein and a catheter threaded over the wire. This method is primarily directed at the subclavian and internal jugular veins. It is rapid, and the catheter is well tolerated for many days. For prolonged catheter residence, to assist in parenteral nutrition, chemotherapy, or blood sampling, a flexible, Silastic® (Hickman) catheter should be used. Because of the catheter's flexibility, fluoroscopic control is usually needed to assure proper placement of its tip in the superior vena cava. The catheter is usually passed through a subcutaneous tunnel and exteriorized in the region of the 4th rib medial to the midclavicular line. Alternatively, a small chamber can be coupled to the catheter and the entire system placed s.c. One face of the chamber has a flexible membrane that can be repeatedly punctured through the skin to introduce

fluid or drugs. Such systems permit the patient added independence (eg, ability to shower) and will function for months.

Pneumothorax, a principal complication of central line placement, is noted in about 2% of patients. After intubation, a chest x-ray taken in exhalation will validate the catheter position and confirm the absence of lung collapse.

Complications: Fluid infused into an improperly placed catheter may cause hydrothorax or hydromediastinum. Infectious complications are variable, depending upon the rigidity of criteria used to define sepsis. Thus, the incidence of catheter colonization without infection may be as high as 35%, while the incidence of true septic sequelae ranges from 2 to 8%. The frequency of complications may be reduced by care in catheter placement and aseptic technic. The occasional occurrence of complications is inevitable, and must be an accepted risk in return for a large venous entry portal.

MEASUREMENT OF CENTRAL VENOUS PRESSURE (CVP)

The CVP reflects right ventricular **(RV)** end-diastolic pressure or preload. An extremely poor indicator of left ventricular **(LV)** function, it is useful in the following settings: (1) to monitor initial volume resuscitation, (2) to evaluate RV function after RV infarction, (3) tamponade, and (4) pulmonary embolism. CVP monitoring of cardiac response to blood volume changes requires extreme caution, particularly in treating heart failure. In general, a hypotensive patient with a CVP < 5 mm Hg may be given fluid safely, and fluid must be given with particular caution if the CVP is > 15 mm Hg. Because CVP is an unreliable guide to volume status or to LV function, pulmonary artery catheterization (see below) should be considered if cardiovascular instability persists after trial therapy.

Procedure and complications: The superior vena cava may be reached percutaneously or by venous cutdown via the cephalic, subclavian, or internal or external jugular vein. Percutaneous internal jugular and subclavian vein catheterization is used most often; thrombophlebitis is less likely than with external jugular or cephalic vein catheterization. Patients must be warned that sudden movements could dislodge the indwelling catheter. The risk of sepsis is always present, most often bacteremia originating from platelet-fibrin deposits on the catheter tip or local cellulitis at the entry site. Catheter damage to the tricuspid valve and bacterial endocarditis may occur (especially in burn patients).

The hazard of pneumothorax is prominent with subclavian punctures in patients with chest injury or with stiff or low-compliant lungs. Patients requiring mechanical ventilatory assistance are vulnerable and must be closely observed. Subclavian venapuncture immediately before general anesthesia and the use of positive pressure breathing exposes the patient to increased, but often unavoidable, risk. Internal jugular vein catheterization might be preferable in the perioperative period because this site leads to a reduced risk of pneumothorax, although catheter location is awkward for the patient.

CARDIAC CATHETERIZATION

A technic in which a flexible catheter is passed along veins or arteries into the heart and contiguous vessels in order to (1) obtain diagnostic data (eg, from biopsy or electrophysiologic monitoring) and (2) to perform therapeutic procedures (eg, corrective surgery, balloon angioplasty, or thrombolysis).

Indications

Congenital and acquired malformations of the heart and great vessels can be described accurately, and thus corrective surgery can be planned. Measurements of

blood-gas levels at various points may enable localization and quantification of a shunt. BP measurements at various points in the heart and great vessels, and calculation of pressure gradients across valves, as well as calculations of cardiac output **(CO)** and vascular resistance provide useful quantitative information. Infants with congenital heart disease have special needs dictated by their small size and grave illness, but many of the principles of adult catheterization apply.

Candidates for catheterization include those in whom noninvasive studies have not provided a diagnosis, those in whom more precise definition of the extent and severity of the heart lesion is sought, or those for whom surgery is contemplated; catheterizations may also be done to acquire precise data needed in clinical research.

Emergency catheterization is rarely indicated in adults. Rapid catheterization may be employed in tamponade since pericardial fluid may be demonstrated by angiography. Chest trauma with mediastinal widening is an indication for emergency aortography to define possible aortic rupture. Pulmonary embolism with hemodynamic deterioration can be rapidly diagnosed by pulmonary angiography. Bypass grafting for coronary artery disease **(CAD)** has created new indications for emergency catheterization; unstable angina (or preinfarction syndrome) and even uncomplicated myocardial infarction **(MI)** in young patients seen within 2 to 4 h of the onset of symptoms may require emergency catheterization and coronary angiography if fibrinolytic therapy, balloon angioplasty, or bypass grafting is contemplated (see also MYOCARDIAL ISCHEMIC DISORDERS in Ch. 27).

Contraindications

Coexisting disorders involving other organ systems (eg, overwhelming infection and irreversible brain damage) may contraindicate cardiac catheterization, and it should be avoided in severe heart failure unless surgery to correct the cause is contemplated.

Data

Measurements usually made during catheterization include intracardiac pressures, pressure pulse tracings, and blood-gas saturations. CO and vascular resistance can be calculated. Intracardiac electrophysiologic studies can provide a sophisticated analysis of atrial, A-V nodal, junctional, His bundle, and ventricular conduction systems. Various substances (eg, pyruvates, lactates, and citrates) can be analyzed in arterial and coronary sinus blood to evaluate myocardial metabolism.

Imaging with radiopaque dyes is discussed in this chapter in ANGIOCARDIOGRAPHY, below, and radionuclide imaging in RADIOLOGY, above.

Intracardiac and arterial pressures: BP can be measured in the atria, ventricles, and pulmonary and peripheral arteries as the catheter passes through them (see TABLE 25–1 for normal values). The **pulmonary capillary wedge pressure** is often measured during right heart catheterization (see PULMONARY ARTERY CATHETERIZATION, below).

"Pressure gradients," *differences of pressure across a valve*, are the most accurate means of evaluating valvular function. Normal pressure pulse tracings are shown in FIG. 25–7. The normal atrial pressure curve consists of (1) a small rise caused by atrial contraction (A wave), followed by a fall (Z descent); (2) a momentary rise due to valvular closure and early ventricular systole (C wave); (3) a fall with ventricular systole and "descent of the base" (moving the "floor" of the atrium downward); (4) a steady rise as blood flows in from the great veins while ventricular contraction continues (V wave); (5) a sudden fall as the atrioventricular **(A-V)** valves open (Y descent); and (6) a second steady rise as blood flows in from the great veins while the A-V valves remain open—"diastasis."

Mitral or tricuspid stenosis causes high atrial pressure, with slow fall in early diastole. In mitral or tricuspid insufficiency, ventricular systole produces a prominent

TABLE 25–1. NORMAL PRESSURES IN HEART AND GREAT VESSELS

Pressures (mm Hg)	*Average*	*Range*
Right atrium	2.8	0– 8
Right ventricle		
Peak-systolic	25	15– 30
End-diastolic	4	0– 8
Pulmonary artery		
Mean	15	9– 16
Peak-systolic	25	15– 30
End-diastolic	9	4– 12
Pulmonary artery wedge		
Mean	9	2– 12
Left atrium		
Mean	7.9	2– 12
A Wave	10.4	4– 16
V Wave	12.8	6– 21
Left ventricle		
Peak-systolic	130	90–140
End-diastolic	8.7	5– 12
Brachial artery		
Mean	85	70–105
Peak-systolic	130	90–140
End-diastolic	70	60– 90

(Modified from *Cardiac Diagnosis and Treatment* by N. O. Fowler, ed. 3, 1980, p. 11. Copyright 1980 by Lippincott/Harper & Row. Used with permission.)

atrial systolic V wave. The slow-rising "anacrotic" aortic pulse in aortic stenosis and the "collapsing" pulse in aortic insufficiency are well shown in tracings of arterial pressure.

When the heart fails as a pump, one of the earliest indices of myocardial failure may be a rise in the ventricular end-diastolic pressure to > 12 mm Hg in the left ventricle or > 8 mm Hg in the right ventricle. With continued high end-diastolic ventricular pressures, cardiac dilation eventually results. When ventricular distensibility is reduced (eg, in constrictive pericarditis or stiffened endocardium or myocardium), atrial pressure curves exhibit a W form: an early diastolic dip ("snap-open" effect), followed by a sharp dip caused by descent of the base, succeeded in turn by a plateau. With restricted ventricular filling (as may occur in constrictive pericarditis, pericardial tamponade, infiltrative myocardiopathies, and occasionally in biventricular failure), an early diastolic component of ventricular pressure tracings resembles the square root sign; ie, a sudden dip followed by a plateau.

Normally there is no significant difference between right atrial and RV diastolic pressures, but the right atrial tracing is similar to that of the right ventricle in tricuspid insufficiency. There is normally no gradient between the left ventricle and the aorta during systole; however, there is a clear difference between pressure tracings taken from the aorta and those in the systemic arteries. Distal arteries reflect a higher pulse pressure than the central aorta by 30 to 40%. These changes are usually ascribed to resonance characteristics in the peripheral arteries.

Diastolic pressures of the left ventricle along with accurate volume data may help to describe the compliance characteristics of that chamber. Without data on LV volume, however, pressure elevations cannot be ascribed solely to decreased compliance.

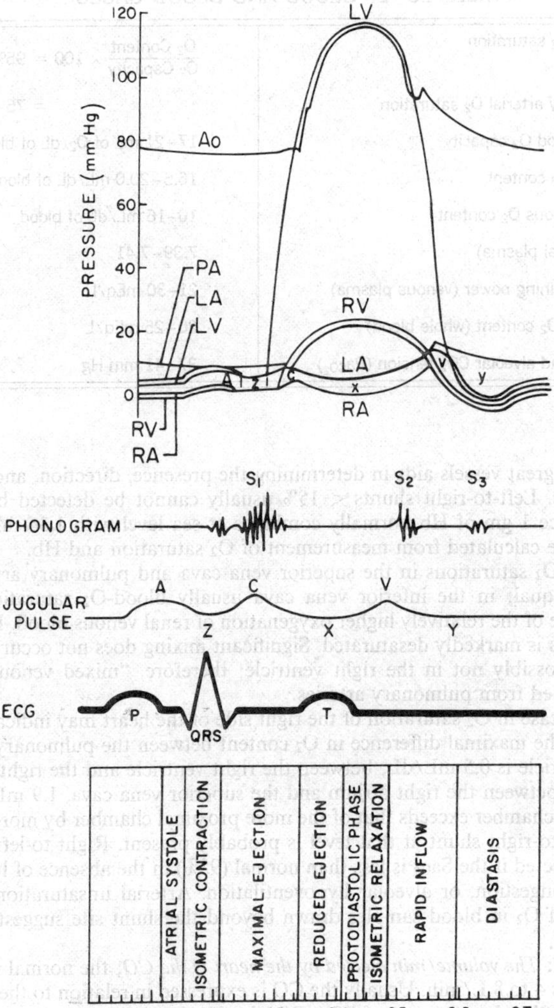

FIG. 25–7. Diagram of the cardiac cycle, showing the pressure curves of the great vessels and cardiac chambers, heart sounds, jugular pulse wave, and the ECG. Ao, aorta; PA, pulmonary artery; LA, left atrium; LV, left ventricle; RA, right atrium, RV, right ventricle. For illustrative purposes, the time intervals between the valvular events have been modified and the z point has been prolonged. (Adapted from *The Heart,* ed. 3, edited by J. W. Hurst et al, copyright 1974 by McGraw-Hill, Inc.; and *A Primer of Cardiology,* ed. 4, by G. E. Burch, copyright 1971 by Lea & Febiger. Used with permission.)

Blood gases: Normal values are shown in TABLE 25–2. A central circulatory shunt is *an abnormal communication between the pulmonary and systemic circulations*; it connects either of the 2 pairs of cardiac chambers or the great vessels. Blood may shunt in either or both directions. Determination of blood-O_2 content at various levels within

TABLE 25-2. BLOOD AND BLOOD GASES

Arterial O_2 saturation	$\frac{O_2 \text{ Content}}{O_2 \text{ Capacity}} \times 100 = 95\%$
Pulmonary arterial O_2 saturation	= 75-80%
Whole blood O_2 capacity	17-21 mL of O_2/dL of blood
Arterial O_2 content	16.5-20.0 mL/dL of blood
Mixed venous O_2 content	10-16 mL/dL of blood
pH (arterial plasma)	7.39-7.41
CO_2 combining power (venous plasma)	21-30 mEq/L
Arterial CO_2 content (whole blood)	20-25 mEq/L
Arterial and alveolar CO_2 tension (Pa_{CO_2})	37-41 mm Hg

the heart and great vessels aids in determining the presence, direction, and volume of central shunts. Left-to-right shunts < 15% usually cannot be detected by blood-O_2 sampling. Since 1 gm of Hb normally combines at sea level with 1.36 mL of O_2, O_2 content can be calculated from measurement of O_2 saturation and Hb.

The blood-O_2 saturations in the superior vena cava and pulmonary artery are approximately equal; in the inferior vena cava usually blood-O_2 saturation is much higher because of the relatively higher oxygenation of renal venous blood. Blood in the coronary sinus is markedly desaturated. Significant mixing does not occur in the right atrium and possibly not in the right ventricle; therefore, "mixed venous blood" is usually obtained from pulmonary arteries.

A 10% increase in O_2 saturation of the right side of the heart may indicate a left-to-right shunt. The maximal difference in O_2 content between the pulmonary artery and the right ventricle is 0.5 mL/dL; between the right ventricle and the right atrium, 0.9 mL/dL; and between the right atrium and the superior vena cava, 1.9 mL/dL. If the blood-O_2 in a chamber exceeds that of the more proximal chamber by more than these values, a left-to-right shunt at that level is probably present. Right-to-left shunts are strongly suspected if the Sa_{O_2} is less than normal (95%) in the absence of lung disease, pulmonary congestion, or alveolar hypoventilation. Arterial unsaturation associated with increased O_2 in blood samples drawn beyond the shunt site suggests a bidirectional shunt.

CO and flow: *The volume/min ejected by the heart is the CO*; the normal range in the resting state is 4 to 8 L/min. Usually the CO is expressed in relation to the BSA as the **cardiac index (CI)**—*L/min/sq m of BSA*. BSA is calculated from the DuBois and DuBois height-weight equation: $BSA\ sq\ m = (wt\ in\ kg)^{0.425} \times (ht\ in\ cm)^{0.725} \times 0.007184$. Various nomograms for BSA have been devised based on this equation, although the assumption that the absolute CO varies with the size of the individual is open to question. (See TABLE 25-3 for normal values for CO and related measurements.)

Various methods are used to calculate the CO: the Fick technic and indicator-dilution technics are among those most commonly used. The **Fick technic** is based on the principle that the difference between the O_2 concentrations in arterial and mixed venous blood represents the amount of O_2 taken up by each unit of blood as it passes through the lungs. Thus the CO can be calculated from the subject's O_2 uptake for a given period of time and the O_2 saturations of mixed venous and arterial blood sam-

TABLE 25–3. NORMAL VALUES FOR CARDIAC OUTPUT AND RELATED MEASUREMENTS

Measurements	*Units*	*±S.D.*
O_2 uptake	143 mL/min/sq m	14.3
Arteriovenous O_2 difference	4.1 dL	0.6
Cardiac index	3.5 L/min/sq m	0.7
Stroke index	46 mL/beat/sq m	8.1
Total systemic resistance	1130 dynes sec cm^{-5}	178
Total pulmonary resistance	205 dynes sec cm^{-5}	51
Pulmonary arteriolar resistance	67 dynes sec cm^{-5}	23

(From B. G. Barratt-Boyes and E. H. Wood, "Cardiac output and related measurements and pressure values in the right heart and associated vessels, together with an analysis of the hemodynamic response to the inhalation of high oxygen mixtures in healthy subjects," in the *Journal of Laboratory and Clinical Medicine 51:* 72–90, 1958. Used with permission.)

ples. Accurate measurement of CO by this method requires that the heart rate, respiratory rate, O_2 consumption, and respiratory exchange rate be stable for 6 to 8 min.

The **indicator-dilution technic** is based on the principle that the degree of dilution of an indicator injected into the circulation is a measure of the flow. A known amount of indicator is injected into a central vein, and its concentration in a peripheral artery is recorded. The concentration curve is divided into 3 time segments: (1) appearance (from injection to the first appearance of the indicator in the artery); (2) build-up (from the first appearance to peak concentration); and (3) disappearance (from peak concentration to a minimal value). Changes in these segments are important in detecting shunts and evaluating valvular regurgitation and heart failure.

Increased tissue demand for O_2 is met normally by both increased CO and increased O_2 extraction. In a normal subject, exercise sufficient to double the resting O_2 consumption increases the A-V O_2 difference by no more than 3 mL/dL; the CO normally increases 800 to 1500 mL/min for every dL increase in O_2 consumption with exercise. Patients with heart failure or limited cardiac reserve must meet an increased O_2 demand primarily by increasing tissue extraction, thus increasing the A-V O_2 difference. Low resting CO with an inadequate response to exercise may result from inadequate ventricular filling (as in mitral or tricuspid stenosis or constrictive pericarditis) or inadequate ventricular emptying (as in pulmonary or aortic stenosis or when myocardial contractility is impaired). High CO occurs in conditions such as anxiety, fever, severe anemia, thyrotoxicosis, beriberi, and various A-V fistulas.

Vascular resistance and valve areas: Vascular resistance, *the impedence to blood flow through a segment of the circulation*, is frequently expressed as the pressure differential across the vascular bed divided by the flow through that bed. It is difficult to define resistance adequately in terms of cardiac dynamics; a change in resistance through a given segment of the circulation does not define its cause. Resistance can be given either in absolute units (1 dyne/sq cm at a flow of 1 mL/sec, or 1 dyne sec cm^{-5}) or in resistance units (a pressure of 1 mm Hg at a flow of 1 L/min). Resistance indices calculated by using the CI rather than the CO are considered to be more comparable between individuals. (See TABLE 25–3 for normal resistance values.) Pulmonary arteriolar (or vascular) resistance is an estimation of the resistance between the main pulmonary artery and the pulmonary venous bed; it is calculated from mean pulmonary artery pressure and mean pulmonary artery wedge pressure. It is elevated in pulmonary hypertension, cor pulmonale, some cases of mitral stenosis, LV failure, and some left-to-right shunts. Total pulmonary resistance, calculated from mean pulmo-

TABLE 25–4. VALVE AREAS AND VALVE FLOWS

Measurements	Units
Aortic area	2.6 – 3.5 sq cm
Aortic valve flow	250 mL/SEP/sec
Mitral area	4 – 6 sq cm
Mitral valve flow	150 mL/DFP/sec

SEP, systolic ejection period; DFP, diastolic filling period.

nary artery pressure and LV mean diastolic pressure, includes the resistance in the pulmonary artery, the pulmonary vein, and across the mitral valve.

Total systemic resistance is an estimation of the resistance between the systemic arteries and the capillary bed. Since the capillary bed is assumed to have no pressure, total systemic resistance equals mean arterial pressure divided by CO. Normally < 20 resistance units, it is most commonly elevated in systemic hypertension.

An expression of the areas of the mitral and aortic valves can be calculated from the pressure gradients across them and the CO. Normal valve areas are given in TABLE 25–4. Clinical disability occurs with mitral valve areas of ≤ 1 sq cm and generally with an aortic valve area of ≤ 0.75 sq cm (and always when it is ≤ 0.5 sq cm). Tricuspid and pulmonary valve areas can be calculated, but are rarely used clinically. Similar formulas can figure the size of a patent ductus arteriosus or of atrial or ventricular septal defects.

Myocardial energetics: Decreased availability of O_2 for metabolism within the myocardium, or myocardial hypoxia, and the resulting shift to an anaerobic metabolism can be detected by an increased lactate/pyruvate concentration ratio in coronary sinus blood. Myocardial citrate extraction is significantly decreased in CAD. However, too much emphasis should not be placed on substrate analysis without accurate steady-state measurements of coronary flow.

Catheterization Procedure

Equipment: All fluoroscopy is done with an image intensifier and videotape recorders. Angiograms can be replayed immediately and the physician can determine whether additional views are needed. Catheters must be radiopaque, nonthrombogenic, and flexible enough to bend without becoming soft and unmanageable at body temperatures. Flow-directed catheters have a small balloon at the tip that allows venous flow to direct them into the pulmonary artery from peripheral veins. These catheters are also valuable for bedside management of seriously ill patients in intensive care units.

Oximetric devices are needed to analyze O_2 and CO_2 content of blood samples, which may be drawn anytime during the procedure. ECG monitoring is essential, and the ECG should be displayed simultaneously with other information for immediate detection of arrhythmias and for electrophysiologic studies.

ECG monitoring equipment, a DC defibrillator in perfect working order, and transvenous pacing wires should be in the catheterization laboratory at all times in case of refractory ventricular arrhythmias. Wall outlets for O_2, endotracheal tubes, a source of negative pressure for suction, and an emergency tray containing epinephrine, isoproterenol, atropine, lidocaine, morphine, and needles for intrathoracic injection should be immediately available.

Preparation: The patient should be prepared by explanation and discussion of the procedure, its purpose and risks, and specific details such as the number of needle

punctures and their sites. For children or infants, thiopental 9 mg/kg rectally is used for anesthesia.

Right heart catheterization: In an adult the femoral or antecubital vein may be used for entering the right heart. A small cutdown is usually used on the arm; a medial vein is usually more satisfactory than the lateral since the lateral circulation enters the subclavian vein at a right angle, and advancing the catheter may be difficult. The femoral vein is usually entered using the Seldinger technic (see above in VENOUS CUTDOWN AND CANNULATION).

Insertion of a Swan Ganz pulmonary arterial flow-directed catheter at the bedside or in the operating room is usually done percutaneously, also using the Seldinger approach. The subclavian and internal jugular veins are the common sites of catheter introduction. Usually no difficulty is met as the catheter advances from a peripheral vein to the right atrium, through the tricuspid valve to the right ventricle, and across the pulmonary valve into one or both pulmonary arteries. For selective catheterization of the coronary sinus, the catheter should be advanced to the tricuspid valve and turned somewhat posteriorly to enter the sinus.

Left heart catheterization: Methods of obtaining information from the left side of the circulation include (1) retrograde arterial catheterization via an arteriotomy in the right brachial artery or via percutaneous femoral artery puncture; both vessels are used with equal frequency and (2) transseptal technics. The catheter can usually cross the aortic valve into the left ventricle without difficulty in the retrograde technic, even when the aortic valve is stenotic. Transseptal catheterization involves passing a catheter from the right femoral vein to the right atrium, through the atrial septum, into the left atrium, and then across the mitral valve into the left ventricle. This technic is used infrequently.

Rarely, the left ventricle cannot be entered via retrograde or transseptal technics, and a direct percutaneous puncture is indicated. Pressures should be monitored continuously, and the needle should be kept in the chamber as briefly as possible. This procedure is relatively free of complications and is useful despite its dramatic aspects.

Complications of Cardiac Catheterization

The mortality and complication rates vary with specific procedures and medical expertise. No more than 1 death should occur per 500 catheterizations, including those performed for cardiac angiography and selective coronary angiography. Serious complications are uncommon (< 4%) in centers where at least 200 to 300/yr are performed.

Arrhythmias: Ventricular tachycardia, ventricular fibrillation, and cardiac arrest are the most serious complications. Isolated premature ventricular contractions, atrial fibrillation, or supraventricular arrhythmias are relatively easily controlled, usually short-lasting, and rarely of physiologic significance. Ventricular arrhythmias are most common during selective coronary angiography. Catheter withdrawal and/or DC cardioversion usually restore sinus rhythm and do not preclude completing the procedure. The incidence of ventricular fibrillation during coronary angiography is < 1:250 in men and somewhat higher in women; the reason for this difference is not known.

Pericardial tamponade is most often a complication of transseptal technics. Some degree of pericardial tamponade can be expected in about 25% of patients whose cardiac wall is perforated (an event that very seldom occurs).

Arterial trauma includes dissection, thrombosis, A-V fistulas, false aneurysms, and bleeding. It is slightly more common with the Seldinger technic and more frequent in patients with conditions that produce wide pulse pressures (eg, A-V fistulas, high-output states, or aortic regurgitation). The incidence of injury to the brachial and femoral arteries is about the same. Removing intra-arterial clots with Fogarty catheters at the time of arterial closure has reduced the incidence of thrombosis to between

1 and 4%. If there is no palpable distal pulse at the end of arterial closure, a vascular surgeon should explore the arterial lumen and repair the artery.

Profound **hypotension** is associated usually with an allergic reaction, or perforation of a heart chamber. Occasionally vagal episodes can produce transient but remarkable hypotension that can be corrected with small amounts of atropine. The recommended IV dose is 0.5 mg q 5 min (maximum dose 2 mg) until the heart rate equals 50 to 60 beats/min. Allergic reactions are usually related to contrast or catheter material. If there is a history of allergy to iodine-containing dyes, care should be taken during angiography. Negative reaction to a test dose does not preclude a reaction to the full dose. Resuscitation supplies and equipment should be available.

Bacterial endocarditis and **systemic sepsis** rarely follow catheterization. **Local infections** around the entry site are also rare, but may be perpetuated by sutures. These may need to be removed before the infection will clear.

Emboli can result when clots formed at the catheter tip are flushed into the bloodstream. MI, cerebrovascular accidents, and other systemic complications have been reported. Thrombophlebitis, a rare occurrence at the site of venous catheterization, has resulted in pulmonary thromboembolism and pulmonary infarction. Catheters have become knotted and broken. The lumen can become thrombosed, and the catheter will be useless and dangerous if it is left in a vessel for long without adequate flushing.

Hemorrhage may occur at a venous entry site but is more common at an arterial entry; heparin, commonly used during catheterization to prevent clotting, increases the risk. The nursing and house staff should understand this possibility as they observe the patient closely for 24 h after the procedure.

PULMONARY ARTERY CATHETERIZATION

Passage of a flow-directed catheter from a peripheral or central vein to the pulmonary artery is indicated in acutely ill patients with (1) hypotension resistant to therapy; (2) sudden respiratory failure manifested by dyspnea, tachypnea, and hypoxia; (3) failure of 2 or more organ systems; and (4) patients at high risk for cardiopulmonary failure. Catheter passage is > 95% successful.

Procedure

A 4-lumen, No. 7 French catheter is used in adults. The lumena are (1) **distal**—for measuring pulmonary artery and pulmonary arterial wedge pressure **(PAWP)** and for withdrawing blood; (2) **balloon**—for inflating with 1 mL of air to help advance the catheter and measure PAWP; (3) **proximal**—for measuring right atrial pressure or CVP and for injecting iced dextrose and water; and (4) **thermistor**—for measuring CO by using a temperature-sensing device that describes a temperature-time curve after injection of iced dextrose and water.

The catheter is inserted as described under right heart catheterization, above. Partial inflation of the balloon permits blood flow to propel the catheter after it is advanced into a major vein. The position of the catheter tip is determined by pressure monitoring using a strain gauge transducer coupled to the distal lumen. The right ventricle has been entered when the systolic pressure suddenly increases to about 30 mm Hg; diastolic pressure is similar to right atrial or vena caval pressure. When the catheter is in the pulmonary artery, the transducer characteristically shows a systolic pressure equivalent to that in the right ventricle and a narrow pulse pressure, so that the diastolic pressure is higher than RV end-diastolic pressure or CVP.

Further movement of the catheter wedges the balloon in a distal pulmonary artery. Blood samples taken in the "wedged" position are as highly oxygenated as peripheral arterial samples. Since this vascular segment no longer has blood flow, there is no

kinetic energy loss or pressure drop across the pulmonary capillary bed; the **pulmonary capillary wedge pressure** readings now reflect pressure in the pulmonary veins. This pressure is equivalent to LV end-diastolic pressure except (1) when mitral stenosis is present; (2) when high levels (> 10 cm H_2O) of positive end-expiratory pressure **(PEEP)** are used; (3) when the pulmonary artery balloon is excessively inflated (deflating the balloon produces the characteristic pulmonary arterial pressure); and (4) when severe pulmonary hypertension is present, the catheter may be impossible to wedge.

A chest x-ray should follow catheter passage to verify proper placement. The patency of the proximal and distal lumena is maintained with a slow infusion (4 mL/h) of dilute heparinized 0.9% sodium chloride solution (1000 u./L) through a filter with high resistance.

When measuring CO, the pulmonary artery catheter must not be in the wedge position. To measure the CO, 10 mL of 5% D/W at 0 C (32 F) is rapidly injected into the proximal lumen and a temperature–time curve is constructed using the thermistor located at the end of the catheter. The thermistor signal is usually electronically integrated and a direct measure of flow is obtained in < 1 min.

Complications and Precautions

When the catheter enters the right ventricle, *the ECG must be monitored and lidocaine must be available, since the catheter frequently induces ventricular irritability*. Further passage of the catheter into the pulmonary artery usually corrects the arrhythmia, but *severe arrhythmias or persistent minor ones demand termination of the procedure*. Balloon rupture is frequent if > 1 mL of air is used for inflation. Air embolism, though theoretically possible, has not been a problem. Knotting of the catheter has been infrequent as has rupture of a pulmonary artery. Pulmonary infarction may result if the catheter remains in the wedge position for more than several minutes. Strict asepsis while inserting the catheter, during repositioning and blood withdrawal, CO measurements, and pressure monitoring should prevent phlebitis and septic complications. The catheter should not stay in the pulmonary artery > 3 to 4 days.

Measurements and Their Interpretation

Hydrostatic and increased permeability or high protein pulmonary edema can be differentiated using the PAWP. The composition of mixed venous blood, particularly mixed venous O_2 tension **($P\bar{v}_{O_2}$)**, can be determined using the catheter. If the $P\bar{v}_{O_2}$ decreases to < 30 mm Hg, the prognosis is poor. Therapy may be evaluated, such as the effects of inotropic drugs, intra-aortic balloon assist, fluid infusions, or respiratory therapy. Since mechanical ventilation may depress CO, particularly when combined with high levels (> 10 cm H_2O) of PEEP, thermodilution measured flow in combination with arterial O_2 content **(C_aO_2)** measurement may be used to calculate O_2 delivery (CO × C_aO_2) and thereby determine an optimal PEEP setting. If spontaneous ventilation is possible, continuous positive airways pressure should be employed to minimize increased intrathoracic pressure. In most critically ill patients, fluid is infused until the CI (CO/BSA) is normal or slightly increased. The CI should exceed 2.5 L/min/sq m or the prognosis is poor. If flow is unsatisfactory and the PAWP < 12 mm Hg, fluid is infused. When the PAWP is > 12 mm Hg, the CI can be raised by β-agonists (eg, dopamine or dobutamine), and by correction of pH and Hct.

Other derived variables, including pulmonary vascular resistance and right and left ventricular stroke work **(LVSW)**, have clinical and research applications. Starling-type myocardial performance curves have been constructed from measurements of LVSW and PAWP during and after a rapid fluid infusion. These curves may yield information regarding cardiac function at different filling pressures, although their interpretation is often confounded by unknown changes in cardiac compliance. Thus, in many clinical settings LV end-diastolic pressure does not allow the end-diastolic volume to be pre-

dicted. However, LV filling pressure does remain a valid estimate of pulmonary capillary pressure.

Rupture of the pulmonary arterial balloon may require that pulmonary artery end-diastolic pressure be substituted for the PAWP. This may be done if pulmonary vascular resistance is normal and if the heart rate is slow. With a functioning balloon at the end of the catheter, the ratio of the pulmonary artery end-diastolic pressure to PAWP may be used as an index of pulmonary vascular resistance.

ANGIOCARDIOGRAPHY

Visualization by x-ray of contrast material injected into arteries, veins, or heart chambers to define anatomy, disease, or direction of blood flow.

Technic

Procedure: Using the technics described above for cardiac catheterization, contrast material (usually iodinated compounds) can be injected to define any heart chamber, the major vessels, or the coronary arteries.

For suspected anomalies (eg, septal defect and narrowed outlets) contrast material is injected proximal to the lesion or into the chamber with the higher pressure (see also CARDIAC CATHETERIZATION, above). In valvular incompetence the contrast material is injected into the chamber with the higher pressure distal to the valve. If technical difficulties preclude the best positioning of the catheter, the injection is made in the nearest convenient site and circulation of the contrast material filmed.

Recording: Most x-rays are taken 3 to 6 times/sec. For studies of anomalies (eg, congenital lesions), cut film provides excellent detail. Biplane angiocardiography (lateral and frontal exposures) gives a 3-dimensional perspective of the chambers and great vessels. Unlike static films, cinecardiograms can be monitored during the injection, and the injection sequence can be simultaneously recorded on videotape and instantly replayed. The resolution of details on individual cine frames is only 1/3 that of conventional x-rays, but motion, a natural expression of the heart, intensifies details that are not appreciated on still films. Digital subtraction methods have not been of value for coronary angiography.

Physiologic Effects and Complications

Contrast media, which are all hypertonic, are excreted by the kidneys. A transient sense of warmth, especially in the head and face, is universally experienced after injection. Cardiovascular responses include tachycardia, a slight fall in systemic pressure, and a rise in CO. Nausea, vomiting, and coughing are minor side effects. Major complications such as cardiac arrest, anaphylactoid reactions, shock, convulsions, cyanosis, and renal toxicity are rare. Patients with a high Hct are susceptible to clotting and the Hct should be < 65% before the angiogram is performed. Allergic reactions may include urticaria and conjunctivitis, which respond to diphenhydramine 50 mg IV. Bronchospasm, edema of the larynx, and dyspnea are potential but rare reactions. Ventricular arrhythmias are common if the catheter tip contacts the ventricular endocardium, but ventricular fibrillation is rare. Monitoring and resuscitation equipment, as described under CARDIAC CATHETERIZATION, above, must be available.

Specific Structures

Right ventricle and pulmonary valve: Direct injection of contrast material into the apex of the right ventricle records tricuspid valve competence and shows the pulmonary valve, the subvalvular region, and the proximal pulmonary arteries. The RV outflow tract shows best with the patient in a steep lateral position, which also reveals the relation of the pulmonary artery to the aorta and occasionally the presence of a ventricular septal defect or communication between the right ventricle and the aorta.

Pulmonary artery: Pulmonary angiography is the most definitive technic for the diagnosis of acute pulmonary embolism; intraluminal filling defects of arterial cutoffs are diagnostic. Contrast material is usually injected into the main pulmonary artery or RV outflow tract, but selective injection into one or both pulmonary arteries may be indicated for safety.

Left atrium: Space-occupying lesions (eg, myxoma or clots) are the usual reasons for opacifying the left atrium, although echocardiography is the procedure of choice for diagnosis. Direct injection into the left atrium may be hazardous in such cases, and the levo phase of a pulmonary angiogram is currently used to visualize it.

Left ventricle: A 30- to 45-degree right anterior oblique projection best demonstrates the long axis of the left ventricle and ventricular aneurysms or areas of asynergy of the anterior wall. This projection also permits a "side-on" view of the A-V valves and separates the left atrium from the left ventricle so that mitral regurgitation can be seen. The left anterior oblique projection defines the LV outflow area and subvalvular aortic obstruction as well as the motion of the interventricular septum and LV posterior wall. Cineangiography is valuable in assessing LV motion and performance.

After LV mass and volume are determined from single plane or biplane angiocardiograms, end-systolic and end-diastolic volumes and the ejection fraction can be calculated mathematically. Stroke volume is the difference between end-diastolic and end-systolic volumes, and the ejection fraction is the ratio of stroke volume to end-diastolic volume. When resting, the normal heart ejects 50 to 60% of its end-diastolic volume with each systole.

Aorta: Aortic regurgitation is best seen by injecting contrast material into the ascending aorta in a 60-degree left anterior oblique or left lateral projection. Aortopulmonary window, coarctation of the aorta, and patent ductus arteriosus also are commonly diagnosed from aortic angiocardiograms.

Coronary arteries: Indications for coronary arteriography include (1) chest pain refractory to medical management and probably due to CAD; (2) chest pain of uncertain etiology refractory to medical management; (3) aortic stenosis that might be corrected by aortic valve replacement, especially in patients with a history of angina or syncope; (4) unexplained heart failure possibly due to a LV aneurysm; and (5) medically uncontrolled angina pectoris when a surgical procedure is considered to relieve pain.

There are no absolute contraindications to coronary arteriography, although relative contraindications include MI within the past 3 mo (unless fibrinolytic or surgical treatment is contemplated) or debilitating disease of some other major organ system. Passing catheters into the heart and injecting contrast media in the coronary arteries is associated with recognizable hazards. Cardiac arrhythmias, ventricular fibrillation, and asystole may occur and should be treated promptly. Temporary transvenous pacemakers are routinely inserted into the right ventricle before any angiographic procedure in patients who have experienced conduction disturbances. Angina may develop and should be treated with sublingual nitroglycerin. To guard against clots that can produce MI or cerebrovascular accidents, the catheter must be kept well flushed and free from thrombi. The mortality rate of coronary angiography should not be > 1:1000 to 2:1000 (0.15%), and in centers where the procedure is done > 400 times/yr, the mortality is even lower.

PERICARDIOCENTESIS

(See Pericardial Disease in Ch. 27)

26. GENERALIZED CARDIOVASCULAR DISORDERS

ARTERIOSCLEROSIS; ATHEROSCLEROSIS

Arteriosclerosis: *A generic term for a number of diseases in which the arterial wall becomes thickened and loses elasticity.* **Atherosclerosis** is the most important; others include **Mönckeberg's arteriosclerosis** and **arteriolosclerosis.**

Incidence and Epidemiology

Because of its effects upon the brain, heart, kidneys, extremities, and other vital organs, vascular disease is a leading cause of morbidity and mortality in the USA and in most Western countries. Of a population of 226.5 million in the USA in 1980, 551,400 died of ischemic heart disease, and 169,500 died of cerebrovascular causes related to arterial disease. Ten years earlier, of a population of 203.3 million, 666,700 died of ischemic heart disease, and 207,200 of cerebrovascular diseases. Despite this improvement, atherosclerotic heart disease and stroke remain major health problems. In many societies the incidence of atherosclerosis is much lower than in ours.

The death rate from coronary heart disease among white men aged 25 to 34 is about 1:10,000; at age 55 to 64 it is nearly 1:100. This age relationship may be due to the time required for lesions to develop or to the duration of exposure to risk factors. Between ages 35 to 44 the death rate from coronary heart disease among white men is 6.1 times that among women. In nonwhites, for unknown reasons, the sex difference is less apparent.

In the past 50 yr, obliterative arterial disease, its relation to the lipidemias, and the evolution of the fatty streak and the atheroma have been intensively studied. Much has been learned about arteriosclerosis, atherosclerosis, and the lipidemias, with particular reference to cholesterol. The improvement noted in the morbidity and mortality from ischemic heart disease and stroke is believed to be, at least in part, related to changes in how people live.

Etiology

If one or more of certain biochemical, physiologic, and environmental factors, known as **risk factors,** is present in an individual, the possibility of his suffering from atherosclerosis and its complications increases. Major risk factors are (1) **hypertension** (see below), (2) **elevated serum lipids** (ie, there is convincing evidence of a reciprocal relationship between a high serum cholesterol and a low concentration of high density lipoprotein **[HDL]** in the plasma and the incidence of atherosclerosis and its complications [see in ANOMALIES IN LIPID METABOLISM in Ch. 85]), (3) **cigarette smoking,** (4) **diabetes mellitus,** (5) **obesity** (see in Ch. 83), and (6) **male sex**. Presumed risk factors include physical inactivity, increasing age, certain behavioral patterns and personality types, hardness of the drinking water, and a family history of premature atherosclerosis. Hypertriglyceridemia is commonly associated with obesity and also has a causative relationship with alcohol. Lipid metabolism is discussed under ANOMALIES IN LIPID METABOLISM in Ch. 85 and diabetic arteriosclerotic disease is discussed below.

Pathology and Pathogenesis

Arteriosclerosis is generalized. Small muscular arteries as well as large vessels develop hypertrophy of the media and subintimal fibrosis with hyaline degeneration. These changes may involve arteries or arterioles of the microcirculation. During the aging process, fibrosis and some intimal thickening develops along with weakening and

disruption of the elastic lamellae in the walls of the great arteries (eg, the aorta and its major branches). The media (smooth muscle coat) atrophies to a certain extent, and the lumen of the aorta or of one or more of its branches widens **(aneurysm, ectasia)**. Evidence is accumulating that the weakening and the consequent formation of ectasia and aneurysm may have a genetic basis.

Diffuse light calcification takes place, with overall loss of elasticity in the vessel wall. Hemodynamically, the pulse pressure widens and systolic pressure increases. In later years, spotty degeneration takes place in the smooth muscle of the media; in some areas of the bead-like calcified lesions, a bone marrow develops **(Mönckeberg's sclerosis)**. The arterial lumen is often normal or larger than normal. However, intimal injury and ulceration may develop, followed by thrombus formation, embolism, or complete thrombosis.

Because arteriosclerosis is practically universal, it is considered a process of aging and anatomic changes are commonly referred to as **involutional**.

The atheroma, or atherosclerotic plaque, is *the most important pathologic lesion of atherosclerosis*; it represents an end process that begins with deposition of lipid in the smooth muscle cells of the intima and media of the arterial wall. In the intima of the aortas of all children ≥ 3 yr old the naked eye can see fine longitudinal yellow ridges or fatty streaks and droplets that stain red, like neutral fat, with Sudan IV. These depositions seldom appear in the coronary arteries before the age of 10. The subsequent history of fatty streaks is not clear: while they are present regardless of race or geography, they disappear as streaks and are later found in some children as fibrous plaques. They finally become atheromas whose most prominent components are large amounts of lipid, mostly cholesterol and cholesterol esters. The initial lesion probably is at the intimal barrier; lesions may be produced experimentally by various important mechanisms (eg, turbulence, hypertension, and local hypoxia). Following such injury, smooth muscle cells proliferate, and some migrate to the intima where they are affected by blood elements with which they come in contact, especially platelets and lipoproteins. Platelets contain a factor that stimulates smooth muscle cell proliferation and migration. Lipoproteins, especially low-density lipoproteins **(LDL),** attach to smooth muscle cells and stimulate their growth. The uptake of LDL can convert what ordinarily would be a limited tissue response to injury into atherosclerosis by introducing cholesterol, a major component of the LDL, into the vessel wall. Smooth muscle cells also synthesize collagen, elastin, and other proteins that are present in increased amounts in the atheromatous lesion. Collagen causes accumulation of fibrous tissue that becomes laden with lipids and cellular debris.

Atherosclerosis is superimposed upon the generalized arteriosclerosis of aging vessels and involves the aorta and all of its branches, but lesions are segmentally rather than diffusely or uniformly distributed. Therefore, the aorta or a major artery may be severely involved with scattered and confluent atheromas over a short segment adjoining a portion of nearly normal vessel wall.

The atheroma obstructs circulation by protruding into the arterial lumen, which must be decreased to 20 or 25% of normal size before blood flow is significantly diminished. Subjected to the trauma of turbulent blood flow, the intima overlying the atheroma may ulcerate and form small platelet and fibrin thrombi on the ulcerated surface. If these break away from their attachments, they and the grumous contents of the atheroma (blood, crystals of cholesterol and its esters) act as microemboli. Signs and symptoms become apparent depending upon the sites of lodgment. Hemorrhage into the tumor-like atheroma may cause an abrupt interference with blood flow resulting in acute symptoms and signs that can be temporary or permanent.

Microemboli from ulcerated atheromas and acute hemorrhage into atheromas have been documented, especially those obstructing and causing transient or permanent occlusion of the internal carotid artery or its distal branches. Blood is a prominent component of atheromas, as described in lesions obtained by endarterectomy performed for an occluding event, as in the internal carotid artery.

Symptoms, Signs, and Diagnosis

Atherosclerosis is characteristically silent until stenosis, thrombosis, aneurysm, or, rarely, embolus supervenes. Symptoms and signs commonly develop gradually as the atheroma slowly encroaches upon the vessel lumen. However, when a major artery is acutely occluded by thrombosis, embolism, dissecting aneurysm, or trauma, the symptoms and signs may be dramatic. Clinical findings occur distal to the obstructive lesion in tissues whose circulation depends upon the affected artery. Specific ischemic disorders related to occlusion are described in Chs. 27, 29, 30, and 123.

Hyperlipidemia (see also in ANOMALIES IN LIPID METABOLISM in Ch. 85): Common clinical indications are the signs and symptoms of premature obliterative atheromatous arterial disease affecting the brain, heart, intestine, and lower extremities. Premature transient cerebral ischemic attacks, or stroke, intermittent claudication in men or women < 45 yr old, and angina pectoris or myocardial infarction may be indicative of increased lipid concentrations in the plasma. Xanthomas in the creases of hands and elbows, along tendon sheaths, and xanthelasma are sometimes associated with hyperlipidemia and should alert the physician to further investigation. Recurrent attacks of acute pancreatitis, with or without alcoholism, also should alert the physician to hypertriglyceridemia. A familial history of hyperlipidemia is an indication for investigation regardless of age.

Prophylaxis

Elimination or modifications of alterable risk factors in a population seems to diminish the incidence of the complications of atherosclerosis (eg, coronary disease). Prevention and treatment must start early. Diabetes mellitus and obesity should be treated early and adequately. Cigarette smoking should be limited or stopped. Regular exercise may help to prevent clinical coronary disease and may be a useful therapeutic measure. Lowering BP reduces the incidence of stroke and probably congestive heart failure, although it has not been shown to decrease the incidence of myocardial infarction. Hypertensive individuals should be identified and treated early.

In the Framingham Study, myocardial infarction occurred in individuals whose cholesterol levels were above the average for the population and whose HDL levels were in the lower range of concentrations. Reduction of total caloric intake resulting in some weight loss does not have dramatic cholesterol-lowering effects, nor is a drastic reduction in exogenous cholesterol intake impressive. A decrease of as little as 20% reduces the incidence of cardiac events and stroke. A radical reduction in dietary cholesterol achieves only a decrease of about 10 or 15% in the plasma cholesterol, but antilipidemic drugs added to the diet can increase the effect to about a 20 to 25% reduction and has decreased the morbidity and mortality from cardiac events in hypercholesterolemic patients by about 25%.

Increasing the blood levels of HDL also appears to have a beneficial relationship. Experimentally, some regression of atherosclerotic lesions has been observed when a lowering of the total plasma cholesterol by 10 to 20% has been obtained and when HDL has been increased by diet and exercise. At least the rate of progression of the atherosclerotic process is decreased.

The main step in preventing hyperlipidemia is to change dietary habits. Specific dietary steps and the use of drugs are discussed under the treatment of Type II hyperlipoproteinemia in ANOMALIES IN LIPID METABOLISM in Ch. 85.

Treatment

Treatment of atherosclerosis is directed at its complications (eg, angina pectoris, myocardial infarction, arrhythmias, heart failure, kidney failure, stroke, and peripheral arterial occlusion). These subjects are covered elsewhere in THE MANUAL.

DIABETIC ARTERIOSCLEROTIC DISEASE

In diabetes mellitus 3 types of vascular disease are seen: (1) **diabetic microangiopathy,** characterized by diffuse thickening of the capillary basement membrane and microaneurysms; (2) **arteriolar disease,** frequently associated with hypertension; and (3) **atherosclerosis,** involving primarily the medium-sized and larger arteries. This discussion is limited to atherosclerosis. Microvascular disease and other aspects are discussed under DIABETES MELLITUS in Ch. 94. No histopathologic difference between diabetic and nondiabetic atherosclerotic lesions can be demonstrated, but the incidence of atherosclerosis is higher in diabetics. Peripheral vascular disease is estimated to occur 11 times more frequently and to develop about 10 yr earlier in diabetics. Gangrene is about 50 times more frequent in diabetic men than in nondiabetic men over age 40, and 70 times more frequent in women in this age group. The incidence of coronary artery disease is greater and life expectancy is shorter among diabetic women than among nondiabetic women. In nondiabetic patients, larger vessels (eg, the aorto-iliac or femoropopliteal arteries) are most likely to be involved, with relative sparing of the leg arteries. In contrast, involvement of the peroneal, anterior and posterior tibial, and digital arteries of the legs is greater in diabetics.

Unexplained geographic differences occur in diabetic vascular disease. Diabetic patients in some groups in Israel, North Africa, and the Middle East have a low incidence of coronary artery disease, and the incidence of atherosclerosis, including peripheral vascular disease, in Japanese diabetics is small.

An abnormal glucose tolerance test has been found in about 37% of men and 42% of women with coronary artery disease who were not known to have diabetes mellitus. The high incidence of atherosclerotic disease in diabetes mellitus is unexplained, and the relationship to blood glucose appears to be independent of coexisting hypercholesterolemia or hypertension. A correlation between hyperglycemia and hypertriglyceridemia has been found in some studies, but other data are contradictory.

Symptoms and Signs

Peripheral arterial disease (arteriosclerosis obliterans) in diabetics is usually manifested by the effects of **ischemia,** which are often complicated by **neuropathy** and **infection**. The foot of the diabetic is very susceptible to all forms of trauma; the heel and the bony prominences are particularly vulnerable. The common response is infection and gangrene. Specific symptoms and signs are similar to those seen in any patient with occlusive arterial disease (see below, and in Ch. 30) except that pain is often absent.

The clinical manifestations of diabetic **neuropathy** that may complicate peripheral vascular disease include sensory disturbances, plantar ulcers, trophic skin lesions and ulcers, autonomic neuropathy (anhidrosis, vasodilation, edema, erythema, atrophy of skin and subcutaneous tissues), and the neuropathic or Charcot joint, a painless degenerative arthropathy involving chiefly the tarsometatarsal and metatarsophalangeal joints.

When **infections** occur, pyogenic organisms are frequently associated with a fungal infection. A mycotic infection frequently is the initial process, leading to wet interdigital lesions, cracks, fissures, and ulcerations that favor secondary bacterial invasion. Infections also commonly result from manipulation of an ingrown toenail, plantar corn, or callus. Infections may progress to cellulitis, lymphangitis, and involvement of the deeper soft tissues by abscess formation, osteomyelitis, and gangrene. The neuropathy renders infection and gangrene relatively painless in the diabetic. Osteomyelitis of the small bones is unlikely to heal.

HYPERTENSION

ARTERIAL HYPERTENSION

Elevation of systolic and/or diastolic BP, either primary (essential hypertension) or secondary.

Etiology and Pathogenesis

The etiology of primary or essential hypertension is unknown, and it seems improbable that a single cause will explain the diverse hemodynamic and pathophysiologic derangements described under the rubric of "essential" hypertension. Heredity undoubtedly predisposes individuals to hypertension, but the exact mechanism is unclear. Isolated, perfused kidneys from Dahl salt-sensitive rats do not excrete water or Na as rapidly as isolated perfused kidneys from Dahl salt-resistant rats, even before hypertension develops. Environmental factors (eg, dietary Na, obesity, and stress) seem to act only in genetically susceptible individuals.

Whatever the pathogenic mechanisms responsible for primary hypertension, they must lead either to increased total peripheral vascular resistance **(TPR)** by inducing vasoconstriction or to increased cardiac output **(CO)**, or both, because BP equals flow (CO) times resistance. Although it is widely claimed that expansion of intra- and extravascular fluid volume is sometimes important, it can only raise BP by increasing CO (by increasing venous return to the heart) or by increasing TPR by causing vasoconstriction, or both. It can do either, but frequently does neither. The sympathetic nervous system and the renin-angiotensin-aldosterone system have received the most attention by investigators of the pathophysiology of hypertension, since both can increase CO and TPR.

Sympathetic nervous system: Maneuvers to stimulate the sympathetic nervous system (eg, cold pressor tests, Valsalva maneuver, mental arithmetic) raise BP, usually more in hypertensive or prehypertensive patients than in normotensives. Whether this hyperresponsiveness resides in the sympathetic nervous system itself or in the myocardium and vascular smooth muscle that it innervates is not known, but it can often be detected before sustained hypertension develops. A high resting pulse rate, which can manifest increased sympathetic nervous activity, is a well-known predictor of subsequent hypertension. Some, but by no means all, hypertensives have higher than normal circulating plasma catecholamines at rest.

Drugs that depress sympathetic nervous activity are widely used to treat primary hypertension. However, this observation cannot be considered hard evidence for implicating the sympathetic nervous system as the causative factor in primary hypertension. In hypertensives the baro-reflexes tend to sustain rather than counteract hypertension, a phenomenon known as "resetting the barostats," but this could be a result, rather than a cause of hypertension. Hypertension can be induced in animals by stimulation of vasomotor centers. Some hypertensives have defective storage of norepinephrine, thus permitting more to circulate.

The renin-angiotensin-aldosterone system: The juxtaglomerular apparatus **(JGA)** is involved in volume and pressure regulations. Renin, a proteolytic enzyme formed in the granules of the JGA cells, catalyzes the conversion of angiotensinogen (a plasma protein) to angiotensin I. This inactive product is cleaved by a converting enzyme, mainly in the lung but also in the kidney and brain, to angiotensin II, which then is a potent vasoconstrictor and also stimulates release of aldosterone. Also found in the circulation, the des-ASP heptapeptide (angiotensin III) is as active as angiotensin II in stimulating aldosterone release, but has much less pressor activity.

Renin secretion is controlled by at least 4 mechanisms that are not mutually exclusive: (1) a renal vascular receptor that apparently responds to changes in tension in the afferent arteriolar wall; (2) a macula densa receptor that appears to detect changes in the delivery rate or concentration of NaCl in the distal tubule; (3) a negative feedback effect of circulating angiotensin on renin secretion; and (4) the sympathetic nervous system that stimulates renin secretion via the renal nerve mediated by β-receptors.

Plasma renin activity **(PRA)** is usually normal in patients with primary hypertension, but may be suppressed in some (about 25%) and elevated in others (about 15%). The accelerated (malignant) phase of hypertension is usually accompanied by elevated PRA. While angiotensin is generally acknowledged to be responsible for renovascular hypertension, at least in the early phase, there is no consensus regarding the role of the renin-angiotensin-aldosterone system in patients with primary hypertension, even those with high PRA.

The mosaic theory states that recruitment of multiple factors sustains elevated BP even though an aberration of only one was initially responsible; eg, the interaction between the sympathetic nervous system and the renin-angiotensin-aldosterone system. Sympathetic innervation of the JGA in the kidney releases renin; on the other hand, angiotensin II stimulates autonomic centers in the brain to increase sympathetic discharge. Angiotensin also stimulates production of aldosterone, which leads to Na retention, and an excess of intracellular Na enhances the reactivity of vascular smooth muscle to sympathetic stimulation. This is why it is so difficult to separate the relative roles of the autonomic nervous system and the renin-angiotensin-aldosterone system in the genesis of primary hypertension.

Hypertension begets hypertension. Other mechanisms become involved when hypertension due to some readily identifiable cause (eg, catecholamine release from a pheochromocytoma, renin and angiotensin from renal artery stenosis, or aldosterone from an adrenal cortical adenoma) has existed for some time. Structural changes in the arterioles resulting from prolonged hypertension reduce the caliber of the lumen, thus increasing TPR. In addition, trivial shortening of hypertrophied smooth muscle in the thickened wall of an arteriole will reduce the radius of an already narrowed lumen to a much greater extent than if the muscle and lumen were normal. This may be why the longer hypertension has existed, the less likely it is that surgery for secondary causes will restore it to normal.

Miscellaneous factors: Abnormal Na transport across the cell wall due to a defect in or inhibition of the Na-K pump (Na^+-K^+ ATPase) or because of increased permeability to the Na^+ has been described in some forms of human hypertension and also in animal studies. The net result is increased intracellular Na, which makes the cell more sensitive to sympathetic stimulation. Since Ca follows Na, it is postulated that it is the accumulation of intracellular Ca and not Na per se that is responsible for increased sensitivity to sympathetic stimulation. Na^+-K^+ ATPase may also be responsible for pumping norepinephrine back into the sympathetic neurons to inactivate it. Thus, inhibition of this mechanism could conceivably enhance the effect of norepinephrine. Defects in Na transport have been described in normotensive children of hypertensive parents.

Hypertension may result from deficiency of a vasodilator substance rather than excess of a vasoconstrictor (eg, angiotensin or norepinephrine). The kallikrein system, which produces the potent vasodilator bradykinin, is beginning to be studied. It is recognized that extracts of renal medulla contain vasodilator substances, including a neutral lipid and a prostaglandin; their absence due to renal parenchymal disease or bilateral nephrectomy would permit BP to rise. Modest hypertension sensitive to Na and water balance is characteristic of anephric animals and humans (renoprival hypertension).

Information about the role of prostaglandins in BP regulation and the development of hypertension is discussed in Ch. 284.

Secondary hypertension is associated with bilateral renal parenchymal disease (eg, chronic glomerulonephritis or pyelonephritis, polycystic renal disease, collagen disease of the kidney, or obstructive uropathy) or with such potentially curable disorders as pheochromocytoma, Cushing's syndrome, primary aldosteronism, hyperthyroidism, myxedema, coarctation of the aorta, renal vascular disease, and unilateral renal disease. It may also be associated with use of oral contraceptives and excessive ingestion of alcohol.

Hypertension associated with chronic renal parenchymal disease is due to various combinations of 2 mechanisms, one apparently renin-dependent and another volume-dependent. In most of these patients, increased renin activity cannot be demonstrated in peripheral blood, and meticulous attention to fluid balance usually controls BP.

Renovascular hypertension (caused by occlusion of a renal artery or its branches) is discussed separately in this chapter, below; **malignant hypertension (malignant nephroangiosclerosis)** is discussed in Ch. 154.

Prevalence

It is estimated that there are > 35 million hypertensives in the USA (> 20% of adults). Hypertension occurs about twice as often in blacks (37% of adults) as in whites (18%), and morbidity and mortality are greater in blacks. No consistent difference in the prevalence of diastolic hypertension has been observed between men and women, but it increases with age, at least until age 55 or 60. Prevalence of isolated systolic hypertension (≥ 160 mm Hg systolic, < 90 mm Hg diastolic) increases with age until at least age 80. If one includes persons with diastolic hypertension and isolated systolic hypertension, > 50% of blacks and whites over age 65 have hypertension. Isolated systolic hypertension is more prevalent among women than men in both races. Prevalence data, derived mainly from large screening programs, rely on one or more BP determinations made at the same encounter. Thus, these figures are greater than if BP had been measured at several visits over a period of time. Between 85 and 90% of cases are primary (essential); in 5 or 10%, hypertension is secondary to bilateral renal parenchymal disease, and only 1 or 2% of cases are due to a potentially curable condition.

Pathology

No pathologic changes occur early in primary hypertension. Ultimately, generalized arteriolar sclerosis develops; it is particularly apparent in the kidney and is characterized by medial hypertrophy and hyalinization. Nephrosclerosis is the hallmark of primary hypertension. Left ventricular hypertrophy and, eventually, dilation develop gradually. Coronary, cerebral, aortic, renal, and peripheral atherosclerosis are more common and more severe in hypertensives since hypertension accelerates atherogenesis. Tiny Charcot-Bouchard aneurysms, frequently found in perforating arteries (especially in the basal ganglia) of hypertensives, may be the source of intracerebral hemorrhage.

Malignant hypertension is characterized by widespread necrotizing arteriolitis with fibrinoid changes and proliferative endarteritis, especially in, but not confined to, the kidneys. (See Ch. 154.)

Hemodynamics

Not all patients with primary hypertension have normal CO and increased total peripheral resistance **(TPR)**. CO is increased and TPR is inappropriately normal for the level of CO in the early labile phase of primary hypertension. TPR increases and CO returns to normal after a period of time, probably because of autoregulation. Patients with high, fixed diastolic pressures often have decreased CO. The role of the large veins

in the pathophysiology of primary hypertension has largely been ignored, but venoconstriction early in the disease may contribute to the increased CO.

Plasma volume tends to decrease as BP increases, although some patients with primary hypertension have expanded plasma volumes. Hemodynamic, plasma volume, and PRA variations are evidence that primary hypertension is more than a single entity or that different mechanisms are involved in different stages of the disorder.

Renal blood flow gradually decreases as the diastolic BP increases and arteriolar sclerosis begins. GFR remains normal until late in the disease, and, as a result, the filtration fraction is increased. Coronary, cerebral, and muscle blood flow are maintained unless there is concomitant severe atherosclerosis in these vascular beds.

In the absence of cardiac failure, CO is normal or increased, and peripheral resistance is usually high in hypertension associated with pheochromocytoma, primary aldosteronism, renal artery disease, and renal parenchymal disease. Plasma volume tends to be high in hypertension due to primary aldosteronism or renal parenchymal disease and is lower than normal in pheochromocytoma.

Systolic hypertension (with normal diastolic pressure) is not a discrete entity. Often it is the result of increased CO or stroke volume (eg, labile phase of primary hypertension, thyrotoxicosis, arteriovenous fistula, or aortic regurgitation); in the elderly, with normal or low CO, it usually reflects inelasticity of the aorta and its major branches ("arteriosclerotic hypertension").

Symptoms and Signs

Primary hypertension is asymptomatic until complications develop. Symptoms and signs are nonspecific and arise from complications in target organs; they are not pathognomonic for hypertension since identical symptoms and signs can develop in normotensives. Dizziness, flushed facies, headache, fatigue, epistaxis, and nervousness are not caused by uncomplicated hypertension. Complications include left ventricular failure; atherosclerotic heart disease; retinal hemorrhages, exudates, papilledema, and vascular accidents; cerebrovascular insufficiency; and renal failure. Hypertensive encephalopathy due to severe hypertension and cerebral edema is encountered only in hypertensive patients (see also Ch. 123).

On the basis of retinal changes, Keith, Wagener, and Barker classified hypertension into 4 groups that have important prognostic implications: Group 1—constriction of retinal arterioles only; Group 2—constriction and sclerosis of retinal arterioles; Group 3—hemorrhages and exudates in addition to vascular changes; Group 4 (malignant hypertension)—papilledema.

A fourth heart sound and broad, notched P-wave abnormalities on the ECG are among the earliest signs of hypertensive heart disease. X-ray evidence of left ventricular hypertrophy may appear later. Aortic dissection or leaking aneurysm of the aorta may be the first sign of hypertension or may complicate untreated hypertension. Polyuria, nocturia, diminished renal concentrating ability, proteinuria, microhematuria, cylindruria, and N retention are late manifestations of arteriolar nephrosclerosis.

Diagnosis

Diagnosis of primary hypertension depends on (1) demonstrating that systolic and diastolic BP are usually, but not necessarily always, higher than normal and (2) excluding secondary causes. At least 2 BP determinations should be made on 3 separate days before labeling a patient hypertensive. For patients in the low hypertension range and especially for patients with markedly labile BP, more than this minimum number of determinations are desirable. The upper limit of normal BP in adults is 140/90 mm Hg; it is much lower for infants and children. A somewhat higher limit, especially for systolic pressure, is acceptable (though not normal) for patients of > 60 yr. Sporadic higher levels in patients who have been resting for > 5 min suggest an unusual lability of BP that may precede sustained hypertension.

TABLE 26–1. MINIMAL EVALUATION FOR PATIENTS WITH MILD AND MODERATE HYPERTENSION (140–180/90–115)

History and physical examination
Complete blood count
Routine urinalysis (with microscopic examination)
Serum levels of importance: BUN and/or creatinine, potassium, cholesterol, uric acid, glucose, HDL cholesterol
ECG

TABLE 26–1 lists the basic or minimal evaluation recommended for patients with mild hypertension. The more severe the hypertension and the younger the patient, the more extensive the evaluation should be. Rapid sequence IVP, chest x-ray, screening tests for pheochromocytoma, and renin-sodium profiling are not necessary routinely. Plasma renin activity has not been helpful in diagnosis, prognosis, or drug selection.

Besides elevating BP, **pheochromocytoma** usually produces symptoms (various combinations of headache, palpitations, tachycardia, excessive perspiration, tremor, and pallor) that should alert the physician to this possibility. Diagnosis depends on demonstrating increased urinary or plasma concentrations of catecholamine or increased urinary concentrations of its metabolic products, metanephrines and VMA. (The catecholamines, such as epinephrine and norepinephrine, are eventually metabolized in the body to a common product, 3-methoxy-4-hydroxymandelic acid, often called vanillylmandelic acid **[VMA].**) For a full discussion of pheochromocytoma, see Ch. 91.

Hypokalemia not due to diuretics should suggest **primary aldosteronism**. Proteinuria, cylindruria, or microhematuria with or without N retention early in the course of hypertension is strong evidence of underlying **primary renal disease**. Absent or markedly reduced femoral arterial pulsations in a hypertensive patient of < 30 yr is presumptive evidence of **coarctation of the aorta. Renovascular hypertension** is discussed below. Cushing's syndrome, collagen disease, toxemia of pregnancy, acute porphyria, hyperthyroidism, myxedema, and some CNS disorders that also must be excluded, as well as aldosteronism, are discussed in detail elsewhere.

Prognosis

An untreated hypertensive patient is at great risk of developing disabling or fatal left ventricular failure, myocardial infarction, cerebral hemorrhage or infarction, or renal failure at an early age. Hypertension is the most important risk factor predisposing to stroke. It is one of 3 important risk factors predisposing to coronary atherosclerosis. The others are cigarette smoking and hypercholesterolemia. The higher the BP and the more severe the changes in the retina, the worse is the prognosis. Fewer than 5% of patients with Group 4 or malignant hypertension characterized by papilledema and < 10% of patients with Group 3 changes in the fundus survive 1 yr without treatment. Effective medical control of hypertension will prevent or forestall all complications and will prolong life in patients whose diastolic BP is ≥ 90 mm Hg. Coronary disease is the most common cause of death among treated hypertensive patients.

Treatment

There is no cure for primary hypertension, but therapy can modify its course. It is estimated that at least 35% of the 35 million hypertensive patients in the USA are adequately controlled. Less than 25% are not aware that they have hypertension.

Nonpharmacologic therapy: Sedation, extra rest, prolonged vacations, admonitions not to worry, and half-hearted attempts at weight reduction and dietary Na restriction are poor substitutes for effective antihypertensive drug therapy. Patients with uncom-

plicated hypertension should live normal lives as long as the BP is controlled. Dietary restrictions should be imposed to control diabetes mellitus, obesity, or blood lipid abnormalities. In mild hypertension, weight reduction to ideal levels and modest dietary Na restriction may make drug therapy unnecessary; if antihypertensive drugs are prescribed, a low-salt diet (< 2 gm/day of Na) will minimize dose requirements. Prudent exercise should be encouraged and alcohol consumption should be curtailed to < 3 oz of whiskey daily. Cigarette smoking should be discouraged to reduce the risk of atherosclerotic heart disease.

Heart failure, symptomatic coronary atherosclerosis, or cerebrovascular disease and renal failure should be treated as usual and do not contraindicate judicious antihypertensive therapy. Hypertension increases both the maternal hazards of pregnancy and the fetal mortality rate. Close prenatal supervision, and judicious use of appropriate antihypertensive drugs will decrease maternal and fetal mortality. When hypertension cannot be controlled or azotemia supervenes, the pregnancy should be terminated. (See HYPERTENSION in Ch. 178.)

Antihypertensive drug therapy: Not all authorities agree that patients with diastolic BP averaging ≥ 90 mm Hg should receive antihypertensive drugs if weight control and limitations of dietary Na do not normalize BP, but many believe that unequivocal benefit of drug therapy for patients with mild hypertension has been demonstrated. When complications are present or impending, or when the diastolic BP is > 100 mm Hg, drug therapy should not be deferred while awaiting the uncertain results of dietary therapy. There are no data on the efficacy of antihypertensive therapy for borderline hypertension or for systolic ("arteriosclerotic") hypertension of the elderly. Except in patients over age 65, the goal of therapy should be to reduce BP to normal (ie, < 140/90 mm Hg) or as nearly normal as the patient and his cardiovascular system can tolerate. The 1984 report of the Joint National Committee on Detection, Evaluation and Treatment of High BP recommended reducing diastolic BP to < 90 mm Hg but added that a "reasonable further goal is the lowest diastolic pressure consistent with safety and tolerance." Usually it is advantageous to have the patient measure his BP at home.

Treatment is usually started with an oral diuretic or β-blocker when diastolic pressure is 90 to 115 mm Hg. All thiazide derivatives and their congeners are equally effective in equivalent doses (see TABLE 26–2). Metolazone and the loop diuretics, furosemide, bumetanide, and ethacrynic acid, are no more effective than the thiazides in managing hypertension, but unlike the thiazides, they are effective when renal function is impaired and hence are preferred for hypertension associated with chronic renal failure. The distal tubular diuretics (spironolactone, triamterene, and amiloride) do not cause hypokalemia, hyperuricemia, or hyperglycemia, but they are not as effective as the thiazides in controlling hypertension. K supplementation or the use of a K-sparing diuretic is recommended with kaliuretic diuretics for patients who are also receiving digitalis, have known heart disease, have an abnormal ECG, ectopy or arrhythmias, or who develop ectopy or arrhythmias while on the diuretic. As much as 100 mEq/day of potassium chloride may be needed to prevent hypokalemia, and most patients will not ingest this much. Spironolactone 50 to 100 mg/day, triamterene 50 to 200 mg/day, or amiloride 5 to 10 mg once daily can be added to the regimen instead of K supplementation. The antihypertensive action of diuretics seems to be due to a modest reduction in plasma volume and a decrease in vascular reactivity, possibly mediated by shifts in Na from intra-to extracellular loci.

If the diuretic does not adequately control the hypertension, a sympathetic depressant drug should be added to the regimen (see TABLES 26–3 and 26–4). A β-blocker is preferred because its side effects are better tolerated. Drugs such as methyldopa, reserpine, clonidine, and guanabenz, which have a central action, are more likely to produce drowsiness, lethargy, and sometimes depression than are the others. Methyl-

TABLE 26–2. ORAL DIURETIC DRUGS USEFUL AS ANTIHYPERTENSIVE AGENTS

Diuretic Agents	*Trade Name*	*Usual Daily Dose* (mg)*	*Side Effects*
Benzothiadiazine derivatives			Unpleasant taste Dry mouth Weakness Muscle cramps GI irritation Skin rash Photosensitivity (except ethacrynic acid) Hypokalemia Hyponatremia Hyperuricemia Hyperglycemia Hypercalcemia (except furosemide, bumetanide, & ethacrynic acid) Nerve deafness (ethacrynic acid, bumetanide, and furosemide only when given IV) Impotence Pancreatitis Marrow depression Purpura Azotemia
Chlorothiazide	Diuril	250–500†	
Hydrochlorothiazide	HydroDIURIL Esidrix Oretic	25–50†	
Hydroflumethiazide	Saluron	25–50†	
Bendroflumethiazide	Naturetin	2.5–5	
Trichlormethiazide	Naqua Metahydrin	2–4	
Methyclothiazide	Enduron	2.5–5	
Benzthiazide	Exna Aquatag	25–50†	
Polythiazide	Renese	2–4	
Cyclothiazide	Anhydron	1–2	
Phthalimidine derivative			
Chlorthalidone	Hygroton	25–50	
Quinazoline derivatives			
Quinethazone	Hydromox	50–100†	
Metolazone	Zaroxolyn Diulo	2.5–5	
Indoline derivative			
Indapamide	Lozol	2.5–5.0	
Anthranilic acid derivative			
Furosemide §	Lasix	40–480†	
Phenoxyacetic acid derivative			
Ethacrynic acid §	Edecrin	50–200†	
Metanilamide derivative			
Bumetanide §	Bumex	0.5–2†	
Distal tubular diuretics (potassium sparing)			
Spironolactone	Aldactone	50–100	GI irritation, gynecomastia, impotence, menstrual irregularities, lethargy, hyperkalemia, hyponatremia, dry mouth, hirsutism
Triamterene	Dyrenium	50–200	Hyperkalemia, hyponatremia, GI irritation
Amiloride	Midamor	5–10	

* Given once daily unless otherwise indicated.
† Usually divided and given twice daily.
§ Loop diuretics.

TABLE 26–3. STEPS IN THE MEDICAL TREATMENT OF HYPERTENSION

Step	*Suggested Agent*
1. Give an **oral diuretic**†	Usually a thiazide or related diuretic; use loop diuretic indapamide, or metolazone if azotemia is present; β-blocker is an option on Step 1 (see text)
2. Add a **sympathetic depressant**	β-blocker or methyldopa, guanabenz, guanadrel, clonidine, prazosin* or reserpine
3. Add a **vasodilator**	Hydralazine (minoxidil in resistant hypertension)
4. Add another **sympathetic depressant**	Guanethidine or clonidine

† In some patients a beta blocker is preferred as Step 1 (see text).
* Prazosin can also be used as an alternative to hydralazine in Step 3.

dopa, clonidine, and guanabenz reduce sympathetic nervous activity by stimulating the α_2-adrenergic receptors in the brainstem. Clonidine is available for transdermal administration in impregnated patches applied once weekly. The patches contain 2.5, 5, or 7.5 mg of clonidine, delivering 0.1, 0.2, or 0.3 mg/day. This unique dosage form seems to be as effective as the oral route with fewer side effects. Unfortunately about 20% of patients develop cutaneous reactions at the site of application, requiring discontinuation of the drug in this form. Reserpine depletes the brain of norepinephrine and serotonin and also depletes the peripheral sympathetic nerve terminal of norepinephrine. Prazosin is a postsynaptic α_1-adrenergic blocking drug that acts on veins and arterioles.

A vasodilator (hydralazine) can be added as a third agent (see TABLES 26–3 and 26–5). It is a direct vasodilator that does not act on the autonomic nervous system centrally or peripherally. Minoxidil, more potent than hydralazine, is associated with side effects including Na and water retention and hirsutism, which is poorly tolerated by women. It should be reserved for severe, resistant hypertension.

The fourth step is to add either guanethidine or clonidine (if it or another α_2-agonist has not been used in Step 2) to the regimen (see TABLE 26–3). Guanethidine blocks sympathetic transmission at the neuroeffector junction and, like reserpine, depletes tissue stores of norepinephrine. It is usually reserved for patients with severe hypertension, whose BP has not responded optimally to the drugs already mentioned. Clonidine seems more effective and better tolerated in Step 4 than guanethidine. Guanadrel is closely related to guanethidine clinically and pharmacologically, but is shorter acting and produces fewer side effects. Consequently, it can be used as a Step 2 agent.

β-Blockers are as effective but more expensive than diuretics as monotherapy for Step 1. β-Blockers are preferred to diuretics for young patients, patients with hyperkinetic circulation (resting tachycardia and cardiac awareness), patients with angina pectoris, gout, or previous myocardial infarction. However, diuretics have been shown to be more effective as monotherapy than β-blockers in elderly and black patients. If a β-blocker is used as Step 1, a diuretic should be added as Step 2 if necessary.

If the patient also has diabetes mellitus, chronic occlusive peripheral arterial disease, or chronic obstructive pulmonary disease **(COPD)**, it is preferable to use a cardioselective β-blocker (metoprolol, atenolol, or acebutolol). However, cardioselectivity is only relative and diminishes as the dose of the β-blocker increases. Even cardioselective β-blockers are contraindicated in the presence of severe asthma or COPD with a prominent bronchospastic component. In the absence of one of the above indications

TABLE 26–4. ANTIHYPERTENSIVE DRUGS THAT DEPRESS THE SYMPATHETIC NERVOUS SYSTEM

Drug	*Trade Name*	*Dose (mg)*	*Side Effects*
Central inhibition			
Methyldopa	Aldomet	250–1000 bid	Lethargy, sedation, dry mouth, impotence or loss of ejaculation, depression, abnormal liver function tests with or without hepatic necrosis, positive direct Coombs' test (hemolytic anemia rare), nasal congestion, drug fever, retroperitoneal fibrosis (rare), myocarditis (rare), skin rash, orthostatic hypotension
Clonidine Guanabenz	Catapres Wytensin	0.1–0.6 bid 4–16 bid	Drowsiness, dry mouth, impotence, constipation, hypertensive overshoot following sudden withdrawal, GI irritation
Neuroeffector blockade			
Guanethidine Guanadrel	Ismelin Hylorel	10–200/day 5–75 bid	Orthostatic hypotension worse after prolonged recumbency, exercise hypotension, nasal congestion, diarrhea, impotence or loss of ejaculation
Reserpine (single alkaloid)	Serpasil Sandril	.05–0.25/day	Lethargy, fatigue, sedation depression, activation of peptic ulcer, nasal congestion, parkinsonian-like state, impotence, diarrhea, bradycardia
Pargyline	Eutonyl	10–200/day	Orthostatic hypotension worse after recumbency, exercise hypotension, nasal congestion, bradycardia, impotence or loss of ejaculation; interactions with drugs such as tyramine, ephedrine, & amphetamines & with foods containing tyramine to produce hypertensive crisis
Receptor blockade			
Alpha			
Prazosin	Minipress	1/day*–10 bid	Orthostatic hypotension (usually with first dose or with increments in dosage), headache, tachycardia, palpitations, fatigue, nausea, weakness, impotence or loss of ejaculation

(Continued)

* Small test dose of 1 mg advisable to minimize risk of "first dose effect" (orthostatic hypotension and syncope).

TABLE 26-4. ANTIHYPERTENSIVE DRUGS THAT DEPRESS THE SYMPATHETIC NERVOUS SYSTEM *(Cont'd)*

Drug	*Trade Name*	*Dose (mg)*	*Side Effects*
Beta			
Propranolol	Inderal	40–240 bid†	Fatigue, listlessness, GI irritation, depression, bradycardia, impotence, bizarre mental aberrations, hyperglycemia, nightmares, insomnia. Precautions: congestive heart failure (impending or actual), 2° or 3° heart block, bronchial asthma, chronic occlusive arterial disease with peripheral ischemia, brittle insulin-dependent diabetes mellitus (may mask the warning symptoms of hypoglycemia)
Propranolol LA	Inderal LA	80–480/day	
Metoprolol‡	Lopressor	50–300/day	
Nadolol	Corgard	40–320/day	
Pindolol	Visken	5–30 bid	
Timolol	Blocadren	10–30 bid	
Atenolol‡	Tenormin	25–100/day	
Acebutolol‡	Sectral	200–1200/day	
Alpha and Beta blockade			
Labetalol	Normodyne Trandate	po: 200–1200 /day IV: 10–40 q 5–10 min, or follow initial injection with infusion of 2 mg/min	Bronchospasm, nausea, fatigue, dizziness, headache

† Doses up to 3 gm daily have been used in United Kingdom.

‡ Cardioselective β-blockers are less likely to aggravate asthma or peripheral ischemia than nonselective β-blockers. Nevertheless, in large doses selectivity is only relative and precautions must be observed in giving cardioselective β-blockers to asthmatics or patients with occlusive arterial disease.

for a cardioselective β-blocker, there is no advantage to using one, since there is no difference in the antihypertensive potency of selective and nonselective β-blockers.

The only advantage of β-blockers with intrinsic sympathomimetic activity (pindolol, acebutolol) in the management of hypertension is that they are less likely to produce severe bradycardia than β-blockers without this property. However, asymptomatic sinus bradycardia, even with rates in the 40s is not harmful.

For moderately severe hypertension (diastolic pressure between 115 and 130 mm Hg), it is usually advisable to start therapy with concurrent use of an oral diuretic and a sympathetic depressant. For severe hypertension (diastolic pressure > 130 mm Hg), therapy should be started with a triple drug regimen simultaneously.

Prompt BP reduction with parenteral agents is indicated for patients with hypertensive encephalopathy, acute left ventricular failure, severe hypertension accompanying unstable angina or acute myocardial infarction, or other hypertensive emergencies. Diazoxide, nitroglycerin, labetalol, or sodium nitroprusside is usually used for this purpose. These very potent agents must be given IV. Because **diazoxide** is a nondiuretic thiazide derivative that can cause fluid retention if given without a diuretic, furosemide 40 or 80 mg IV is usually given with it. Previously diazoxide 300 mg was usually given by rapid IV injection that reduced BP to normal within 3 to 5 min, and the effect of one injection lasted 12 h or more. A preferable and safer way to administer diazoxide is by rapid IV injections of 100 mg given q 5 to 10 min until the BP reaches the optimal

TABLE 26-5. ANTIHYPERTENSIVE DRUGS THAT ACT DIRECTLY ON VASCULAR SMOOTH MUSCLE

Drug	Trade Name	Dose Range	Side Effects
Hydralazine	Apresoline	25–150 mg bid	Headache, flushing, palpitation, tachycardia, fluid retention, aggravation of angina, GI irritation, lupus-like syndrome, drug fever, skin rash, psychosis
Minoxidil	Loniten	2.5–50 mg bid	Headache, flushing, palpitation, tachycardia, fluid retention, aggravation of angina, GI irritation, hirsutism, pericardial effusion
Diazoxide	Hyperstat IV	IV:100 mg injected rapidly; repeat q 5–10 min	Nausea, vomiting, hyperglycemia, tachycardia, fluid retention, hypotension
Sodium nitroprusside	Nitride Nitropress	IV:0.5–10 μg/kg/min continuous infusion; continuous monitoring	Nausea, vomiting, agitation, muscular twitching, cutis anserina, thiocyanate toxicity
Nitroglycerin*†	Tridil Nitrostat IV Nitro-BID IV Nitroglycerin injection Nitrol IV	IV: 5 μg/min–100 μg/min or more	Headache, tachycardia, nausea, vomiting, apprehension, restlessness, muscular twitching, palpitations

* Dilute for IV use.
† Need for special infusion set due to loss of drug in polyvinyl tubing.

level. Side effects include nausea, vomiting, hyperglycemia, tachycardia, and, only occasionally, hypotension (without shock).

Sodium nitroprusside 0.5 to 10 μg/kg/min given by continuous IV infusion in 5% D/W can reliably and promptly reduce BP in a hypertensive crisis, but its evanescent effect and potency require almost continuous monitoring of BP in an intensive care unit. Unlike diazoxide, it produces venodilation as well as arteriolar dilation and therefore reduces both pre- and afterload, making it especially useful for managing hypertensive patients with heart failure. Side effects include nausea, vomiting, agitation, muscular twitching, and cutis anserina if BP is reduced too rapidly. Acute psychosis from thiocyanate intoxication can result from prolonged therapy, especially in patients with renal failure. The drug should be discontinued if the serum thiocyanate concentration exceeds 12 mg/dL.

Nitroglycerin, like sodium nitroprusside, relaxes the resistance vessels as well as the large capacitance veins. Compared to sodium nitroprusside it has a greater effect on the veins than on arterioles. IV infusions of nitroglycerin have been used to manage hypertension during and after coronary bypass, heart failure, acute myocardial infarction, intractable angina pectoris, and acute pulmonary edema. (It should also be useful in managing acute hypertensive crisis associated with unstable angina.) Hemodynamic studies indicate that IV nitroglycerin is preferable to sodium nitroprusside in managing hypertension associated with severe coronary disease because it increases coronary flow whereas sodium nitroprusside tends to decrease coronary flow. The most frequent adverse reaction is headache, which occurs in about 2% of patients; tachycardia, nau-

sea, vomiting, apprehension, restlessness, muscular twitching, and palpitations have also been observed.

Labetalol, administered intermittently in doses of 20 to 40 mg IV q 10 min or as an infusion has been just as effective as nitroprusside, diazoxide, or nitroglycerine in managing hypertensive crises. Serious hypotensive episodes have not been observed when labetalol is given by this method, and side effects have been minimal. Because of its β-blocking activity, labetalol should probably not be used for hypertensive emergencies associated with acute left ventricular failure.

A convenient way to manage some hypertensive crises is to give **nifedipine sublingually.** This does not require close observation in an intensive care unit. BP begins to decrease within 1 to 2 min after the contents of a 10 mg nifedipine capsule are squeezed under the tongue.

Methyldopa or trimethaphan may be given parenterally to manage hypertensive encephalopathy, but these agents are usually less desirable than diazoxide, sodium nitroprusside, labetalol, or nitroglycerin.

Some **angiotensin II analogues** have been synthesized that block the angiotensin II receptor. One of these is sar^1-ala^8 angiotensin II (saralasin). These agents must be given IV, thus limiting their usefulness in managing hypertension. **Saralasin** has not been used extensively to control hypertensive crises, but it has been promoted to select patients with renovascular disease who are most likely to respond to surgery, because a depressor response to an infusion of saralasin indicates that the hypertension is angiotensin II dependent. Experience indicates that it is probably no more accurate in selecting patients for renovascular surgery than previous tests (see below).

Converting enzyme inhibitors (eg, **captopril, enalapril**) prevent the conversion of vasoinactive angiotensin I to vasoactive angiotensin II (see TABLE 26–6). While these agents are more effective in angiotensin II dependent hypertension, they are surprisingly effective in managing hypertension even though plasma renin activity is not elevated. Hemodynamically, these agents behave like vasodilators on arterioles and capacitance veins similar to the action of sodium nitroprusside. They are effective in managing refractory heart failure even though hypertension is not a major contributor.

In large doses captopril caused a high incidence of skin rash; nephrotoxicity and marrow toxicity (granulocytopenia) were also reported rarely. In lower doses the incidence of these side effects is much lower and within an acceptable range. Captopril and enalapril have been reported occasionally to cause angioedema, a potentially dangerous side effect. Converting enzyme inhibitors can be used at any step in the Stepped Care approach to antihypertensive therapy including Step 1 monotherapy. In double-blind studies, enalapril was as effective as hydrochlorothiazide for monotherapy.

Calcium slow channel blocking agents behave as direct vasodilators and reduce BP by decreasing total peripheral vascular resistance. They are usually used as Step 2 agents with an oral diuretic although they may ultimately prove to be useful as Step 1 drugs. Verapamil, and to a lesser extent, diltiazem have a negative inotropic effect and should

TABLE 26–6. CONVERTING ENZYME INHIBITORS

Drug	*Trade Name*	*Usual Dose (mg)*	*Side Effects*
Captopril	Capoten	12.5 bid to 150 tid on empty stomach	Acute renal failure in severe bilateral renal artery stenosis or renal artery stenosis supplying a solitary kidney. Angioedema, skin rash, dysgeusia, proteinuria, leukopenia. Volume depletion can lead to excessive hypotension. Hyperkalemia may occur if K^+-sparing diuretic is used or renal insufficiency is present.
Enalapril	Vasotec	10 to 40 daily	

not be used in patients with second or third degree heart block. Since β-blockers have similar myocardial effects, it is preferable not to use either one of these agents in the same regimen with a β-blocker. On the other hand, nifedipine has no significant cardiac effect; for this reason it can cause reflex tachycardia as hydralazine and minoxidil do, but it can be used with a β-blocker, which will prevent this side effect. Verapamil is useful in treating supraventricular paroxysmal tachycardia.

Side effects are frequent, especially with nifedipine and include GI symptoms, headache, and palpitations. All of these drugs must be given bid or tid, but longer acting Ca-channel blockers are being investigated.

Prostaglandins (see Ch. 284) may offer new possibilities in treating hypertension.

RENOVASCULAR HYPERTENSION

Acute or chronic elevation of systemic BP caused by partial or complete occlusion of one or more renal arteries or their branches, often surgically correctable.

Etiology and Pathophysiology

Stenosis or occlusion of one or both main renal arteries or their branches or an accessory renal artery or its branches can cause hypertension by inciting release of the enzyme renin from juxtaglomerular cells of the affected kidney. The area of the lumen must be decreased by at least 60% before the occlusion is hemodynamically significant.

In patients > 50 yr old (usually men), the most frequent cause of renal arterial stenosis is atherosclerosis; in younger patients (usually women), it is one of the fibrous dysplasias. Rarer causes of renal arterial stenosis or obstruction include emboli, trauma, inadvertent ligation during surgery, and extrinsic compression of the renal pedicle by tumors.

Although renovascular disease is the most frequent cause of curable hypertension (with the possible exception of oral contraceptive therapy in women), it accounts for < 2% of all cases of hypertension.

Symptoms, Signs, and Diagnosis

Renovascular hypertension should be suspected when hypertension first develops in a patient < 30 or > 50 yr old or whenever previously stable hypertension abruptly accelerates. Rapid progression to malignant hypertension within 6 mo of onset is suggestive of renal artery disease.

A systolic-diastolic bruit in the epigastrium, usually transmitted to one or both upper quadrants, is the most important physical finding. Unfortunately, about 50% of patients with renovascular hypertension do not have systolic-diastolic bruits in the abdomen. Trauma to the back or flank or acute pain in this region with or without hematuria should alert the physician to the possibility of renovascular hypertension, but these historic features are rare. Renovascular hypertension is characterized by both high CO and high peripheral resistance.

Both renovascular and primary hypertension are usually asymptomatic, and only a difference in history, the presence of an epigastric bruit, or abnormalities on an intravenous urogram **(IVU)** will distinguish them clinically. The main justification for diagnostic evaluation is to find a surgically curable lesion.

No available test for renovascular hypertension is ideal. All give false-positive and false-negative results; all are expensive; and some are hazardous. The most widely used test for screening purposes is the rapid sequence IVU, although it has been shown that nearly 20% of patients with renovascular hypertension will have a normal IVU. The renal flow scan may be as useful as urography for screening, but does not give as much anatomic information. A positive excretory urogram is indicated by a differential of > 1.5 cm in vertical axis length of the kidneys (allowing for the fact that the left

kidney is normally 0.5 cm longer than the right), and by delay of the ischemic kidney in excreting the contrast media.

Digital subtraction or Seldinger **arteriography** with selective injection of the renal arteries can establish the diagnosis of renovascular disease or is useful in determining operability and planning the best surgical approach. A normal rapid sequence urogram does not contraindicate arteriography if other indications warrant it. However, a lesion found on an arteriogram may not be responsible for the hypertension. Further study is necessary to define the probable significance of lesions and the probable response to surgical therapy (see below).

Prognosis and Treatment

Without treatment, the prognosis in renovascular hypertension is similar to untreated primary hypertension. Most investigators have found that appropriate surgery will relieve hypertension if the renal vein renin activity **(RVRA)** ratio (involved to uninvolved side) is > 1.5:1. However, many patients with RVRA ratios less than this have also been cured of hypertension by revascularization or removal of the ischemic kidney. There is evidence that short duration of hypertension (< 5 yr) and appropriate abnormalities on the rapid sequence IV urogram, when considered together, are just as reliable in predicting the outcome of surgery as is RVRA ratio. To enhance the reliability of the RVRA ratio, blood should be obtained from the renal veins under conditions of Na depletion to stimulate the release of renin. This can be accomplished by use of a 0.5-gm Na diet and oral diuretics for 48 h or by injecting 40 to 80 mg furosemide IV and obtaining blood 30 min later. Bilateral lesions, which occur in 35% of cases, make the rapid sequence urogram and the RVRA ratio less dependable. Peripheral venous renin activity is often normal in renovascular hypertension.

Revascularization of the involved kidney with a saphenous vein bypass graft is recommended for younger patients with fibrous dysplasia of the renal artery. The cure rate is 90% with proper selection, and the surgical mortality rate is < 1%. If disease in the arterial branches precludes adequate revascularization, nephrectomy may be considered, but medical treatment is preferable if the BP can be controlled.

Percutaneous transluminal angioplasty (PTA) using a balloon catheter to dilate stenotic renal arteries has been successful in some patients with renal artery stenosis with minimal risk. Recurrence of the stenosis is common in atherosclerotic lesions.

Compared to fibrous disease, atherosclerotic lesions have been found to respond less well to surgery, presumably because the patients are older and have more extensive vascular disease within the kidneys and throughout the vascular system. The hypertension may persist and surgical complications occur more commonly. Surgical mortality is higher than for young patients with fibrous dysplasia of the renal artery. Since renovascular hypertension usually responds to antihypertensive drugs as does primary hypertension (see ARTERIAL HYPERTENSION, above), medical treatment or PTA is preferable to surgery for elderly patients with atherosclerotic lesions unless the BP cannot be controlled or unless bilateral involvement or a lesion in an artery to a solitary kidney threatens renal function. The decision as to surgery must be individualized on the basis of the patient's overall status, age, the type of renal arterial disease, and prior response to medical therapy. When possible, surgery should involve repair and revascularization instead of nephrectomy.

SYNCOPE
(Fainting)

A sudden brief loss of consciousness.

Etiology and Pathophysiology

The most common pathophysiologic basis for syncope is decreased cerebral blood flow secondary to limitation of the cardiac output **(CO)**; arrhythmias are the most

frequent cause. Heart rates < 30 to 35/min and > 150 to 180/min may cause syncope; when cardiovascular disease is present, less extreme heart rate alterations may be causal. Bradyarrhythmias causing syncope include the sick sinus syndrome, with and without tachyarrhythmias, and high-grade atrioventricular block. Although bradyarrhythmias occur at all ages, they are most frequent in the elderly, with ischemia or fibrosis of the conducting system usually responsible. Digitalis, β-blockers, and other drugs may also cause bradyarrhythmias. Supraventricular or ventricular tachyarrhythmias that cause syncope may be precipitated by ischemia, heart failure, drug toxicity (quinidine syncope is the best known), preexcitation, etc. Syncope with chest pain of myocardial infarction is usually related to arrhythmia, but rarely may reflect massive myocardial damage with a reduced CO.

Many other mechanisms, often in combination, may limit CO. Diminished cerebral flow may also be caused by a decrease in systemic arterial pressure due to: (1) peripheral vasodilation; (2) decreased venous return to the heart; (3) hypovolemia; (4) cardiac outflow obstruction; and (5) cerebral vasoconstriction as that induced by hypocapnea.

Exertional (effort) syncope suggests cardiac outflow obstruction, most typically due to aortic stenosis. The exertional syncope of cardiac outflow obstruction reflects cerebral ischemia from inability to increase CO, combined with the peripheral vasodilation of exercise. Seizures may occur with prolonged syncope. Hypovolemia and positive inotropic agents (eg, digitalis) accentuate the obstruction in hypertrophic cardiomyopathy and may precipitate syncope; arrhythmias may be contributory. Effort syncope may also be due to other causes of cardiac outflow obstruction (eg, pulmonary hypertension) or obstruction to venous return (eg, intracardiac myxoma, severe pulmonic or tricuspid stenosis). The syncope due to intracardiac myxoma may also be related to postural changes. A decrease in venous return is also responsible for **cough** and **micturition syncope** and that occurring with a Valsalva maneuver; the increase in intrathoracic pressure limits venous return, decreasing CO and arterial pressure.

A decrease in systemic arterial pressure due to peripheral vasodilation explains **carotid sinus syncope** (often accompanied by a slowing of the heart rate), **postural hypotension** (including the diminished baroreceptor-mediated cardioacceleration of aging), and the **syncope after sympathectomy** or with a variety of **peripheral neuropathies** that are characterized by failure of compensatory vasoconstriction. It is also the initial mechanism of the **simple faint (vasodepressor syncope)**; the vasodilation, teleologically, is to prepare for flight after fright. When vasodilation is followed by a slowing of the heart rate (rather than the anticipated tachycardia of flight), the inadequate CO results in syncope. **Swallowing syncope** in patients with esophageal disease is usually due to vasovagal reflex mechanisms. Syncope may be due to **hypovolemia** (often diuretic or vasodilator-drug induced), particularly in the elderly; blood loss results in the same clinical picture. Characteristically the patient recovers completely from the episode of syncope once the horizontal posture is assumed.

Hyperventilation may cause syncope by hypocapnea-induced vasoconstriction, which reduces cerebral blood flow. Another benign cause is **weightlifter's syncope**; hyperventilation before lifting causes hypocapnea, cerebral vasoconstriction, and peripheral vasodilation; the Valsalva maneuver of lifting decreases venous return and CO, and squatting causes further systemic vasodilation and decreased BP.

Common noncardiovascular causes of syncope may be neurologic or metabolic. Syncope may be part of a transient ischemic attack (TIA), but typically there is an associated transient sensory or motor deficit. Syncope may occur during episodes of seizure disorders or in the postictal state. Hypoglycemia may cause syncope by altering cerebral metabolism.

Symptoms and Signs

The patient becomes unresponsive and loses postural tone. Faintness, dizziness, or lightheadedness sometimes indicates an impending loss of consciousness and more often progresses when the patient is upright.

Syncope of cardiac etiology typically occurs suddenly and ends abruptly and spontaneously; it is most commonly due to an arrhythmia. **Stokes-Adams syncope** typically occurs without warning even in a seated patient; syncope due to other arrhythmias often occurs with or after palpitations. (See also Exertional Syncope above.)

Vasovagal syncope usually is precipitated by physical or emotional stimuli (eg, pain, fright, sight of blood) and is often preceded by vagally-mediated warning symptoms—nausea, weakness, and sweating. **Orthostatic syncope** (see below), most commonly seen after prolonged bed rest in elderly patients or with a variety of drugs, occurs on assuming the upright posture.

Syncope due to seizures is associated with muscular jerking or convulsions, incontinence, and tongue biting; postictal confusion may follow; and traumatic injury may result from a seizure. Syncope also may occur in the postictal state.

Syncope due to pulmonary embolism indicates massive obstruction and is often associated with dyspnea, tachypnea, chest discomfort, cyanosis, and hypotension.

Syncope of gradual onset (with warning symptoms) suggests hypoglycemia or hyperventilation; the latter is often preceded by paresthesias and chest discomfort.

Diagnosis

The history and physical examination, with particular attention to cardiovascular and neurologic abnormalities, typically defines needed diagnostic procedures. Differentiation between syncope due to cardiovascular causes and that due to noncardiovascular causes or of unknown cause is important; the former is associated with a threefold increase in mortality and requires precise definition.

The history may suggest the etiology by defining the age at onset, relationship to posture or activity, associated diseases, premonitory symptoms, and evidence of precipitating features. However, syncope is often unwitnessed, and these key features may be difficult to ascertain. A knowledge of prior drug therapy is of value (particularly antihypertensives, diuretics, or vasodilators).

Physical examination may provide valuable clues. The patient is often described as pale, motionless, and diaphoretic, with a weak pulse, hypotension, and shallow breathing. The heart rate and BP should be determined and checked for postural changes. (In **hysterical fainting,** there is no abnormality of the heart rate or BP, and no evidence of pallor or sweating.) A carotid bruit or diminished carotid pulse suggests a cerebrovascular cause. The harsh murmur of aortic stenosis, or the systolic murmur of hypertrophic obstructive cardiomyopathy that disappears with squatting suggests outflow obstruction, but associated arrhythmias may also cause syncope. The click and murmur of mitral valve prolapse (which are heard earlier and are more prominent on standing) suggest an arrhythmic etiology. Further evaluation is needed for suspected hemorrhage, other forms of hypovolemia, or for a focal neurologic deficit.

Asking the patient to hyperventilate may mimic the clinical presentation. Carotid sinus pressure (*which should always be done with ECG monitoring*) may elicit evidence of carotid sinus hypersensitivity and may also mimic the clinical presentation.

Laboratory studies: The history and physical examination, with particular attention to cardiovascular or neurologic abnormalities, define which diagnostic procedures are needed. The 12-lead ECG may suggest arrhythmia, conduction abnormality, ventricular hypertrophy, or myocardial infarction. In the absence of any suggestive clinical clues, at least 24 h of long-term (Holter) ECG monitoring is prudent. Any arrhythmia detected must be associated with an alteration of consciousness to be implicated as etiologic. Exercise testing is less valuable, unless activity precipitated the syncope. The

role of electrophysiologic testing remains controversial, except in unexplained recurrent syncope. Echo- and/or phonocardiography may confirm suspected heart disease.

A fasting blood sugar can confirm hypoglycemia, and a Hct can detect anemia. Cardiac serum isoenzyme elevation may identify the unusual case of acute myocardial infarction presenting as syncope. The PO_2 is decreased and there may be ECG evidence of acute cor pulmonale with pulmonary embolism; perfusion/ventilation scanning is an excellent screening technic. An EEG is warranted if a seizure disorder is suspected; head and brain scanning procedures are indicated when there is a focal neurologic deficit or if an intracranial process is suspected.

Prognosis and Treatment

Characteristically, assuming the horizontal posture ends the syncopal episode and no further immediate treatment is needed. If the patient is placed upright too rapidly, syncope may recur; ill-informed bystanders sometimes aggravate the situation by propping the subject upright or carrying him in an upright position. In young people without cardiovascular disease, syncope of unknown cause has a favorable prognosis, and elaborate evaluation is rarely required.

Bradyarrhythmias respond to pacemaker insertion and tachyarrhythmias to specific drug therapy. Carotid sinus hypersensitivity may require pacemaker insertion for bradyarrhythmias; or radiation may cure the vasodepressor component. The management of volume depletion, hypoglycemia, anemia, or drug toxicity is standard. Age is no contraindication to aortic valve surgery, the most common form of heart surgery in the elderly. β-Blockade is the therapy for hypertrophic cardiomyopathy with obstruction, and the associated arrhythmias respond best to amiodarone.

As suggested above, specific therapy should be based on the diagnosis of the exact underlying cause in each case. More detailed discussion of these disorders and further therapeutic details can be found elsewhere in THE MANUAL.

ORTHOSTATIC HYPOTENSION

An excessive fall in BP on assuming the upright position. It is not a specific disease, but a manifestation of abnormal BP regulation due to a variety of causes.

Etiology and Pathophysiology

The gravitational stress of sudden standing normally causes blood to pool in the venous capacitance vessels of the legs. The subsequent transient decrease in venous return and CO results in a reduction of BP. Baroreceptors in the aortic and carotid sinus areas then activate autonomic reflexes that rapidly restore the BP and cause a transient tachycardia. These changes reflect primarily the increase in catecholamine levels that augments vasomotor tone of the capacitance vessels, increases heart rate and myocardial contractility, and thereby enhances CO; arterial vasoconstriction is mediated by similar mechanisms.

When afferent, central, or efferent portions of the reflex arc are impaired by diseases or drugs, when myocardial function is decreased, or when hypovolemia is present, these compensatory mechanisms may be inadequate to restore the decrease in BP. Decreased tissue perfusion is manifested initially by the effects of impaired cerebral blood flow.

The commonest cause of symptomatic orthostatic hypotension is the **hypovolemia** secondary to excessive use of diuretic agents (eg, loop diuretics such as furosemide, bumetanide and ethacrynic acid), and the relative hypovolemia seen with vasodilator therapy with nitrate preparations and calcium antagonist drugs (verapamil, nifedipine, or diltiazem) used to treat hypertension, angina pectoris, or heart failure. The hypovolemia caused by protracted bed rest is often etiologic, as is the **decreased baroreceptor responsiveness** seen in elderly persons.

Drugs that impair autonomic reflex mechanisms, such as excessive doses of antihypertensive drugs (methyldopa, clonidine, reserpine, and other ganglionic blocking drugs) are also frequent causes. Orthostatic hypotension is rarely due to β-adrenergic blocking drugs, but α-adrenergic blocking agents such as prazosin may be causative, especially at the initiation of therapy ("first dose effect").

Several groups of drugs reversibly interfere with autonomic reflexes and reduce BP in the standing position as an important adverse effect. These include a variety of drugs used to treat neuropsychiatric disorders such as the monoamine oxidase inhibitors (isocarboxazid, phenelzine, and tranylcypromine) used to treat depression; the tricyclic antidepressants (nortriptyline, amitriptyline, desipramine, imipramine, and protriptyline); and the phenothiazine antipsychotic drugs such as chlorpromazine, promazine, and thioridazine. Other drugs that may result in orthostatic hypotension are quinidine, L-dopa, barbiturates, and alcohol. The antineoplastic drug vincristine may produce severe long-lasting orthostatic hypotension as a sign of its neurotoxicity.

Acute or subacute severe **hypovolemia caused by disease** may produce orthostatic hypotension due to a decrease in CO, despite intact autonomic reflexes. This is seen with hemorrhage, severe vomiting or diarrhea, excessive sweating, or the osmotic diuresis in uncontrolled diabetes mellitus; these may lead to volume depletion, dehydration, and orthostatic hypotension unless there is adequate fluid and/or electrolyte replacement. The adrenocortical hypofunction of Addison's disease may lead to hypovolemic orthostatic hypotension in the absence of adequate salt intake. The effects of diuretics and vasodilators are discussed above.

Neurologic disorders that involve the autonomic nervous system interrupt the sympathetic reflex arc and impair normal adrenergic responses to standing. This is common with diabetic neuropathy, amyloidosis, porphyria, tabes dorsalis, syringomyelia, spinal cord transection, pernicious anemia, alcoholic neuropathy, Guillain-Barré syndrome (postinfectious polyneuropathy), and Riley-Day syndrome (familial dysautonomia). Surgical sympathectomy, vasospastic disorders, or peripheral vascular insufficiency (particularly severe varicose veins) may result in reduction of BP on standing. In a variety of causes of secondary systemic arterial hypertension, where BP control is not mediated by the usual homeostatic mechanisms, assuming the upright posture may cause orthostasis; this is prominent in most patients with pheochromocytoma, and is also seen with primary hyperaldosteronism; these patients, paradoxically, have hypertension in the supine position, as well as orthostatic hypotension.

Two possibly related primary neuropathic disorders commonly associated with severe orthostatic hypotension are the **Shy-Drager syndrome** and **idiopathic orthostatic hypotension.** In patients with the Shy-Drager syndrome, no increase occurs in plasma norepinephrine on standing; and in idiopathic orthostatic hypotension there appears to be depletion of norepinephrine from the sympathetic nerve endings. In these conditions, widespread lesions affect the sympathetic and parasympathetic nervous systems, basal ganglia, and spinal tracts. There is often widespread autonomic dysfunction in addition to failure of arteriolar and venous vasoconstriction; loss of sweating; bowel, bladder, and stomach atony; impotence; decreased salivation and tearing; mydriasis and impaired visual accommodation. Paradoxically, the BP in the supine position may be elevated, even when there are severe orthostatic changes, because of the loss of parasympathetic, as well as sympathetic, regulation of the cardiovascular system.

Orthostatic hypotension also occurs secondary to vasodilation during the febrile phase of falciparum malaria.

Symptoms, Signs, and Diagnosis

Patients who report faintness, lightheadedness, dizziness, and mental or visual blurring have these as evidence of a mild to moderate reduction in cerebral blood flow. With more severe restriction of cerebral perfusion, syncope and even generalized sei-

zures may occur (see also SYNCOPE above). Other phenomena that occur in association with the orthostatic hypotension usually relate to the underlying cause.

The diagnosis of orthostatic hypotension is made when symptoms suggestive of hypotension and a marked reduction in measured BP occur when the patient assumes the upright position. However, the specific etiologic diagnosis must be sought and is based on each patient's presenting circumstances and associated phenomena (eg, as described above for Shy-Drager syndrome).

Prognosis and Treatment

The prognosis depends on the underlying cause. When orthostatic hypotension is due to hypovolemia or drug excess, it is rapidly reversed by correcting these problems. The orthostasis of protracted bed rest can be lessened by allowing patients to sit up each day.

The outlook in patients with a chronic underlying disorder is determined by the management of that disease. When the etiologic disease cannot be altered, management is designed to produce peripheral vasoconstriction and/or increase CO. Often this allows BP to be maintained at an asymptomatic (although reduced) level in the standing position. However, in advanced stages of the Shy-Drager syndrome or idiopathic orthostatic hypotension, pharmacotherapy is often inadequate and some form of counterpressure or counterpulsation device may be needed: If orthostatic hypotension is related to venous pooling in the legs, fitted tailored elastic hose may enhance the CO and BP on standing. In more advanced cases, inflatable aviator-type antigravity suits may be needed to produce sufficient leg and abdominal counterpressure.

With mild orthostasis, the peripheral adrenergic agent ephedrine 25 to 50 mg orally q 3 to 4 h, when the patient is awake, may maintain the BP in an adequate range. An alternative or concurrent therapy is volume expansion, initially by increasing salt intake and subsequently by the administration of salt-retaining hormones. It is often adequate to increase the Na intake by 5 to 10 gm above the usual dietary level by liberal salting of food or by the administration of sodium chloride tablets. Fludrocortisone 0.1 to 0.5 mg/day orally is effective only when there is associated adequate salt ingestion and evidence of weight gain of 1.3 to 2.2 kg (3 to 5 lb) due to salt retention and expansion of the extracellular fluid volume. The risk of this management, particularly in patients with impaired myocardial function, is the development of congestive heart failure; occurrence of dependent edema alone, in the absence of congestive heart failure, does not contraindicate continuation of therapy. An important complication is hypokalemia, due to the K-wasting effect of mineralocorticoid administration accompanied by a high Na intake; K replacement may be needed. Propranolol has been reported to enhance the beneficial effects of salt and mineralocorticoid therapy.

A number of nonsteroidal anti-inflammatory agents may result in salt retention and the inhibition of prostaglandin synthesis; indomethacin 25 to 50 mg orally tid has been described as beneficial. However, the complications of use of these drugs include GI symptoms and unwarranted pressor reactions (described in patients who received indomethacin and sympathomimetic drugs concurrently).

SHOCK

(See also Ch. 6)

A state in which blood flow to peripheral tissues and perfusion is inadequate to sustain life because of insufficient CO or maldistribution of peripheral blood flow, usually associated with diminished peripheral circulation, hypotension, and oliguria.

Etiology and Pathophysiology

Shock may be due to insufficient intravascular volume (hypovolemic), to inadequate cardiac function (cardiogenic), to inadequate vasomotor tone (vasodilation), or to combinations of these factors. The fundamental defect is reduction in perfusion of

vital tissues so that O_2 delivery is inadequate to meet the requirements of aerobic metabolism, resulting in a shift to anaerobic respiration and a resultant increased production and accumulation of lactic acid. When shock persists, impaired organ function is followed by irreversible cell damage and death.

Hypovolemic shock: Inadequate intravascular volume (absolute or relative) produces diminished ventricular filling and a reduction in stroke volume that, unless compensated for by increased heart rate, results in a decreased CO. Acute hemorrhage following trauma is a common cause of hypovolemic shock, or hemorrhage may occur in a preexisting (often unrecognized) disease (eg, peptic ulcer, esophageal varices, or aortic aneurysm). Hemorrhage may be apparent (hematemesis or melena) or concealed (ruptured ectopic pregnancy) and should always be considered in patients presenting with shock. As shock may develop within minutes (before homeostatic hemodilution) following acute blood loss, normal Hb and Hct do not rule out hemorrhage as its cause.

In the absence of hemorrhage, hypovolemic shock may follow increased losses of body fluids. It usually takes several hours to develop and is frequently associated with a rising Hb or Hct. Fluid may be lost from the body surface following thermal or chemical injury or may be sequestered in the peritoneal cavity in response to generalized peritonitis following perforation of the GI tract or pancreatitis. Fluid may also be pooled within or lost from the GI tract due to vomiting or diarrhea from a variety of conditions including small or large bowel obstruction, paralytic ileus, or gastroenteritis. Excessive renal losses of fluid may occur in diabetes mellitus or insipidus, adrenal insufficiency, "salt-losing" nephritis, the polyuric phase following acute tubular damage, and after administration of potent diuretic agents. Intravascular fluid may also be lost to the extravascular space because of increased capillary permeability secondary to anoxia or cardiac arrest, or shock may result from acute hypersensitivity reactions.

In addition to excessive fluid loss, hypovolemic shock may be due to inadequate fluid intake, often associated with modest increases in fluid loss. Frequently, because of neurologic or physical disability, patients cannot respond to thirst by increasing fluid intake. In hospitalized patients, hypovolemia can be compounded (or worsened) if early signs of circulatory insufficiency are incorrectly ascribed to heart failure, and fluids are withheld or diuretics given for fear of precipitating pulmonary edema.

Cardiogenic shock: Because reduced CO is secondary to ventricular failure and blood volume is adequate, CO will not be significantly improved by fluid administration. Cardiogenic shock may result from mechanical interference with ventricular filling, as during tension pneumothorax and pericardial tamponade, or from interference with ventricular emptying, as in massive pulmonary embolism or prosthetic valve malfunction. In these conditions proper diagnosis and immediate specific therapy may be lifesaving. Cardiogenic shock also may result from a disturbance of heart rate or rhythm, frequently associated with preexisting cardiac disease. Inadequate myocardial contraction, a third mechanism for cardiogenic shock, is most commonly due to acute myocardial infarction **(MI)**, but may also occur in valvular heart disease, in cardiomyopathies, following administration of drugs that depress myocardial function, or in severe hypoxemia secondary to pulmonary or neurologic disease.

Vasodilation: Hypovolemic shock may be *relative* in that circulating blood volume is normal but insufficient for adequate cardiac filling. A variety of conditions may cause widespread venous and/or arteriolar dilation. If CO does not increase commensurate with reduced vascular resistance, arterial hypotension develops, and if arterial pressure falls below a critical level, vital centers will be inadequately perfused. The degree of hypotension necessary to cause the shock syndrome varies and often is related to the presence of preexisting vascular disease. Thus, a modest degree of hypotension that is tolerated well by a young, relatively healthy individual might result in severe cerebral, cardiac, or renal dysfunction in a patient who has significant arteriosclerosis in vessels supplying these organs. Widespread vasodilation may occur following severe cerebral

trauma or hemorrhage **(neurogenic shock),** hepatic failure, or ingestion of certain drugs or poisons. Shock associated with bacterial infection **(bacteremic** or **septic shock)** may be partly due to the effects of endotoxin or other chemical mediators on resistance vessels, resulting in vasodilation and decreased vascular resistance (see Ch. 6). In addition, some patients with acute MI and shock appear to have inadequate compensatory vasoconstriction in response to the decreased CO.

Symptoms and Signs

The manifestations associated with shock may be due to the shock state itself or to the underlying disease process. Findings in patients with **hypovolemic** or **cardiogenic shock** are similar. Mentation may be preserved, but lethargy, confusion, and somnolence are common. The hands and feet are cold, moist, and often cyanotic and pale. Capillary filling time is prolonged and, in extreme cases, a bluish reticular pattern may appear over large areas. The pulse is weak and rapid unless there is associated heart block or terminal bradycardia; in some instances only femoral or carotid pulses can be felt. Tachypnea and hyperventilation are present, but apnea may be a terminal event when the respiratory center fails due to inadequate cerebral perfusion. BP taken by cuff tends to be low (< 90 mm Hg systolic) or unobtainable, but direct measurement by intra-arterial cannula often gives significantly higher values.

The findings in **septic shock** (see also Ch. 6) may be similar to those in hypovolemic and cardiogenic shock, but with some significant differences. Fever, usually preceded by chills, is generally present. *Elevated* CO is associated with diminished total peripheral resistance, possibly accompanied by hyperventilation and respiratory alkalosis. Thus, early symptoms may include the onset of a shaking chill, rapid rise in temperature, warm flushed skin, a bounding pulse, and falling and rising BP **(hyperdynamic syndrome)**. Urinary flow is decreased despite the high CO. Mental status is usually markedly impaired, and mental confusion may even be a premonitory sign preceding hypotension by 24 h or more. However, these findings are variable and may not be apparent even in patients whose markedly increased CO and reduced vascular resistance are confirmed by direct hemodynamic measurement. The presence of fever and hypotension suggest septic shock; in later stages hypothermia is common.

Manifestations of the underlying disease process may be important clues to the diagnosis of shock. Acute blood or fluid loss from a ruptured aorta, spleen, or tubal pregnancy or from peritonitis can be suspected from the physical findings. Signs of generalized dehydration are helpful in recognizing hypovolemia in patients with neurologic, GI, renal, or metabolic disorders. Cardiogenic shock is suggested by engorged neck veins, signs of pulmonary congestion, and a gallop rhythm. A systolic murmur may indicate ventricular septal rupture or mitral insufficiency, either of which may result in shock after acute MI. Pericardial tamponade is suggested by jugular venous distention, muffled heart sounds, a pericardial rub, and a paradoxic pulse. Massive pulmonary embolism is suspected in patients with a parasternal lift, a loud 4th heart sound at the left sternal border, and an accentuated, widely split pulmonary closure sound. Septic shock tends to occur at the extremes of age and is more common in men than in women. The signs of preexisting pulmonary, GI, or urinary tract infection may be present, as may signs of an underlying malignancy or debilitating disease resulting in altered immunity against infection. In women of childbearing age, septic abortion was formerly a common cause of shock when the procedure was performed illegally.

Diagnosis

The diagnosis of shock requires evidence of insufficient tissue perfusion that is due to either reduced CO and/or inadequate peripheral vasomotor tone. Within the framework of those conditions known to result in the shock syndrome, most consider shock to be present in any patient who develops a significant fall in BP, a urine flow of < 30 mL/h, and a progressive increase in the arterial lactic acid concentration or increased

anion gap associated with reduced arterial P_{CO_2} and HCO_3 levels. The diagnosis of shock would be supported by the presence of signs relating to hypoperfusion of specific organs (obtundation, ECG abnormalities, peripheral cyanosis) or signs relating to compensatory mechanisms (tachycardia, tachypnea, diaphoresis). In the earliest stages of shock, especially septic shock, many of the above signs might be absent or undetected if not specifically sought. Thus, treatment might not be initiated until the shock is irreversible. None of these findings *alone* is specific for the shock syndrome; each must be evaluated in the context of the overall clinical setting. The arterial BP, in particular, may be reduced to levels commonly associated with the shock syndrome in patients who otherwise show no evidence of inadequate tissue perfusion. In such patients, reversal of hypotension with vasopressor agents might do more harm than good.

Hypovolemic shock is diagnosed by demonstrating normal or reduced ventricular filling pressure with a low CO and the shock syndrome. A right ventricular filling pressure or central venous pressure **(CVP)** < 7 cm H_2O (5 mm Hg) suggests hypovolemia; however, the CVP may be above this level when hypovolemic shock occurs with preexisting pulmonary hypertension. A better index to left ventricular **(LV)** filling is obtained by floating a balloon-tipped catheter into the pulmonary artery and measuring pulmonary end-diastolic **(PEDP)** or pulmonary capillary wedge **(PCWP)** pressure, both of which are usually closely related to the actual LV pressure during diastole. A PEDP or PCWP of < 12 mm Hg (or < 18 mm Hg in a patient with acute MI or preexisting LV disease) suggests that hypovolemia is causing or contributing to the shock syndrome.

When hypovolemia is suspected, a therapeutic trial with volume loading may help confirm the diagnosis. Hypovolemia can be assumed to be present when BP and urine flow are improved and the clinical manifestations of shock are reduced with small increments in CVP or PCWP following rapid infusion (100 mL/10 min) of a colloid (eg, dextran, plasma, or serum albumin). Right ventricular infarction, which may occasionally result in clinical shock, occasionally responds favorably to rapid volume expansion and should be considered in patients with shock following inferior wall infarction when right-sided ventricular filling pressure (CVP) is significantly elevated in the absence of markedly elevated left-sided ventricular filling pressure (PEDP or PCWP).

Cardiogenic shock is diagnosed by demonstrating reduced CO associated with an increased ventricular filling pressure. Since hypovolemia may occur with acute MI or preexisting heart disease, the shock cannot be assumed to be due entirely to myocardial damage. Pericardial tamponade, tension pneumothorax, or massive pulmonary embolism can usually be diagnosed if thought of, using available emergency diagnostic procedures (eg, echocardiography, lung scan). When myocardial damage is sufficient to result in shock, the ECG is usually diagnostic of acute MI (see in Ch. 27); however, prior infarction, left bundle branch block, or atrioventricular block with idioventricular or pacemaker rhythm may preclude an ECG diagnosis. The ECG helps also to identify arrhythmias that may, in themselves, cause shock.

Shock secondary to vasodilation is suspected in patients with cerebral trauma, sepsis, or drug intoxication, but hypovolemia, which is frequently also present, must be excluded. Myocardial dysfunction secondary to inadequate coronary perfusion or other poorly defined mechanisms may also complicate shock due to vasodilation.

Prognosis

Untreated, shock is usually fatal. Prognosis following development of shock depends on the cause, the presence of preexisting or complicating illness, time between onset and diagnosis, and adequacy of therapy. The mortality in shock due to massive MI and in elderly patients with sepsis remains extremely high.

Treatment

First aid: The patient should be kept warm and his legs raised slightly to improve venous return. Hemorrhage should be stopped, airway and ventilation checked, and respiratory assistance given, if necessary. Nothing should be given by mouth, and the patient's head should be turned to avoid aspiration, if emesis occurs. Narcotics should generally be avoided, but severe pain may be treated with morphine 2.5 to 5.0 mg IV, repeated if necessary. Anxiety may be due to cerebral hypoperfusion, and sedatives or tranquilizers should *not* be given.

Supportive therapy: Vital functions may have to be stabilized before diagnostic procedures can be carried out. Norepinephrine or dopamine may be needed (see TABLE 26–7) to reverse profound hypotension that may result in depression of respiratory function, hypoventilation, hypoxemia, worsening acidosis, and death. Assisted ventilation with high O_2 concentrations should be instituted promptly. Airways obstruction from secretions or gastric contents must be removed.

If hemorrhage is suspected, a large (16- to 18-gauge) catheter should be inserted into a peripheral vein (femoral or internal jugular) by direct skin puncture to infuse blood or other fluids and to administer drugs. Analyses of arterial pH and blood gases may be helpful. Giving sodium bicarbonate 50 to 100 mL IV of an 8.4% (1 mEq/mL) solution may help to reverse metabolic acidosis, but care to avoid pulmonary edema due to the sodium load is required in cardiogenic shock.

Monitoring: Patients in whom shock is not immediately reversed should be considered critically ill and definitive treatment should be continued in a special care area (eg, ICU, CCU). Careful monitoring should be followed: (1) ECG; (2) arterial BP—preferably by direct intra-arterial cannula; (3) ventricular filling pressure (CVP, or preferably PEDP or PCWP); (4) respiratory rate and depth; (5) urine flow (usually by indwelling bladder catheter); (6) arterial blood pH, Pa_{O_2}, and Pa_{CO_2}; (7) body temperature; and (8) clinical status including sensorium, pulse volume, skin temperature, and color. Measuring CO using thermodilution technics is also helpful in patients requiring extended treatment. A well-designed flowsheet is extremely valuable. Serial measurements of blood volume, lactic acid, plasma oncotic pressure, Hct, and EEG may also be helpful.

TABLE 26–7. INOTROPIC CATECHOLAMINES

Drug	*Route of Administration and Dosage*	*Hemodynamic Actions*
Norepinephrine	4 mg/1000 D5W continuous IV infusion at 1 mL (0.004 mg) to 4 mL (0.016 mg)/min	α-adrenergic: vasoconstriction β-adrenergic: inotropic and chronotropic*
Dopamine	400 mg/500 mL D5W continuous IV infusion at 0.3 mL (0.25 mg) to 1.25 mL (1 mg)/min 2 to 10 μg/kg/min for low dose 20 to 50 μg/kg/min for high dose	α-adrenergic: vasoconstriction† β-adrenergic: inotropic, chronotropic, and vasodilation† Nonadrenergic: renal and splanchnic vasodilation
Dobutamine	250 mg/250 mL D5W continuous IV infusions at 2.5 to 10 μg/kg/min	β-adrenergic: inotropic‡

* Effect not apparent if arterial pressure elevated too much.
† Effects depend upon dosage given and underlying pathophysiology.
‡ Chronotropic, arrhythmogenic, and direct vascular effects are minimal at lower doses.

Hypovolemic shock: Outside of the hospital or in the emergency room, temporary increase of BP may be achieved by the use of military antishock trousers (MAST suit). However, experience with this device is required if complications are to be avoided. Definitive treatment of hypovolemic shock necessitates restoring intravascular volume and eliminating the underlying cause. Rapid infusion of fluids to elderly patients may precipitate pulmonary edema; therefore, monitoring of CVP, PEDP, or PCWP is helpful during therapy even after the diagnosis of hypovolemia has been established. Generally PEDP or PCWP should not be raised > 18 to 20 mm Hg by fluid replacements. The primary measurements to follow are BP, PEDP or PCWP, and urine flow. CVP monitoring is helpful when PEDP or PCWP measurements are not available but may be misleading in patients with significant preexisting cardiac or pulmonary vascular disease. Care must also be taken when interpreting filling pressures in patients during ventilatory assistance, particularly when high levels of end expiratory pressure (> 10 cm H_2O) are being used. The precise mode and type of fluid to be given are determined by the specific circumstances and are guided by frequent determination of Hct and serum electrolytes. Sodium chloride solution (0.9%) is as good as any other solution, but large quantities may cause pulmonary edema. After approximately 40 to 50% of the calculated blood volume is replaced, whole blood or a colloid solution should be given. Whole blood should be cross-matched, but in an urgent or desperate situation, giving 1 to 2 u. of O, Rh-negative blood is an alternative. Colloid solutions include dextran, plasma, or reconstituted 5% human serum albumin, all of which lack RBCs and will dilute the Hct. Serum albumin, the most physiologic and safest, is expensive and may be unavailable. Fresh frozen plasma carries the risk of hepatitis B. Dextran is an excellent osmotic expander, but using > 1 L is not advised because it can alter coagulation and may make compatibility testing inaccurate.

Shock that fails to respond to volume replacement may be due to insufficient volume administration while bleeding or fluid loss continues or may be due to complicating factors (eg, myocardial damage or coexisting septic shock). When hypovolemia is not the probable cause or when BP does not respond promptly to volume administration, a pressor agent (norepinephrine or dopamine given by controlled IV infusion—see TABLE 26–7) may be considered to raise the systolic pressure to between 90 and 100 mm Hg. Pressor agents should be used primarily in shock patients with profound hypotension in whom it may be necessary to elevate BP acutely to establish adequate cerebral and/or coronary blood flow. Once BP is stabilized, efforts should be made to correct associated abnormalities (eg, hypoxemia, acidosis, hypovolemia, sepsis) so that pressor agent administration can be reduced or discontinued; prolonged vasoconstriction due to α-receptor stimulation can result in further impairment of visceral microcirculation as well as increased myocardial work and O_2 demand. In addition to vasoconstrictor effects, norepinephrine and dopamine (along with dobutamine) have inotropic and chronotropic effects that in the presence of heart failure and/or bradycardia will tend to improve CO and systemic perfusion. In some patients, adding a vasodilator (eg, sodium nitroprusside or phenoxybenzamine) may further improve hemodynamics. In the absence of adrenal insufficiency, the benefit of massive doses of corticosteroids (eg, hydrocortisone 2 to 10 gm IV) is unproven, but is advocated by some authorities, particularly if sepsis is considered likely. For treatment of patients with adrenal insufficiency, see Ch. 91.

Bradycardia and other arrhythmias, if due to hypoxemia, acidosis, or hypotension, often respond to the above measures, but specific antiarrhythmic drugs, cardioversion, or temporary cardiac pacing may be necessary (see CARDIAC ARRHYTHMIAS in Ch. 27).

Cardiogenic shock (see also under COMPLICATIONS OF MYOCARDIAL INFARCTION in Ch. 27) is treated by improving cardiac performance. Shock following **acute MI** should be treated by O_2 inhalation, stabilization of cardiac rate and rhythm, and volume expansion if indicated by normal or low CVP, PEDP, or PCWP. Morphine 3 to 5 mg

given IV over a 2-min period may relieve severe chest pain and help restore BP; the response must be closely monitored since morphine causes respiratory depression and is a venodilator and may cause BP to drop. The initial dose can be repeated after 10 min if there is no evidence of respiratory depression or adverse BP response. Atropine 1 mg IV is often effective in reversing the bradycardia and hypotension that frequently occur very early after the onset of symptoms, particularly in inferior-posterior infarctions. Atropine will also help prevent the undesired vagal effects of morphine. Norepinephrine or dopamine is used to maintain arterial systolic pressure at > 90 mm Hg (but not > 110 mm Hg). Because it markedly increases O_2 demand, isoproterenol is *contraindicated* in patients with shock after acute MI.

When shock is complicated by bradycardia or advanced A-V block, restoring BP with norepinephrine or dopamine and correcting acidosis usually results in an adequate ventricular rate. Temporary transvenous pacing may be necessary in patients with evidence of persisting high-grade A-V block or severe sinus node dysfunction. Short-term administration of isoproterenol (2 mg/5 dL 5% D/W at 0.001 mg to 0.004 mg/min) may occasionally be needed before pacing in patients having prolonged asystolic periods or recurrent ventricular tachycardia or fibrillation associated with severe bradycardia. Digoxin is not routinely used in shock, but may be of value in patients with supraventricular tachycardia or signs of pulmonary congestion. In the absence of severe hypotension, dobutamine infusion, or amrinone (0.75 mg/kg IV over 2 to 3 min followed by infusions of 5 to 10 μg/kg/min), may be used to improve CO and reduce LV filling pressure. Tachycardia and arrhythmias may occasionally occur during dobutamine administration, particularly at higher doses. Since amrinone is not only inotropic but has vasodilator properties, arrhythmias and hypotension may occur during its administration. Vasodilators (eg, nitroprusside and nitroglycerin), which act to increase venous capacitance and/or lower systemic vascular resistance, reduce the workload imposed on the damaged myocardium and may also be of value in patients who do not have severe arterial hypotension. Combination therapy (eg, dopamine or dobutamine with nitroprusside or nitroglycerine) may be particularly useful, but requires close monitoring of infusion rates and clinical and hemodynamic responses.

Early use of intra-aortic balloon counterpulsation appears to be extremely valuable for temporarily reversing shock in patients with acute MI, and should be considered in patients who require pressor support (norepinephrine or dopamine) for > 30 min and in patients with acute MI complicated by ventricular septal rupture or severe acute mitral regurgitation. The development of percutaneous technics for bedside insertion makes balloon counterpulsation available to community hospitals for early stabilization of patients with acute MI. Whether the early use of balloon pumping in non-shock patients with large acute infarcts complicated by persisting pain, early LV failure, or recurring arrhythmias will reduce the incidence of cardiogenic shock remains to be seen.

Emergency aorto-coronary bypass has been effective and may improve survival in selected patients with cardiogenic shock following acute MI, especially if surgery is done within the first 6 h after onset of symptoms. Such patients often require support with balloon pumping before diagnostic angiography and surgery. Surgical correction of mechanical defects (ie, ruptured intraventricular septum, pseudoaneurysm, severe mitral regurgitation, or large dyskinetic segment) may also be necessary.

The role of emergency nonsurgical myocardial revascularization in patients with cardiogenic shock following acute MI utilizing IV or intracoronary administration of thrombolytic agents and/or percutaneous transluminal coronary angioplasty has on occasion resulted in dramatic reversal of shock if performed very early (within a few hours of the onset of infarction).

Management of **shock due to vasodilation** is primarily supportive while treating the underlying cause. Isoproterenol is occasionally of value, but norepinephrine may be

necessary. Dopamine is an inotropic agent that in low dosage is less vasoconstrictive than levarterenol and causes less vasodilation than isoproterenol, but selectively improves mesenteric and renal blood flow; it may have advantages over other vasopressors in selected patients. Dobutamine, a more selective β-agonist, increases CO without vasoconstriction and thus may not be as useful in such patients. Shock due to sepsis is discussed in Ch. 6. Little can be done when shock follows massive irreversible cerebral damage.

Other considerations: Pericardial tamponade requires pericardiocentesis, and, in life-threatening situations, pericardial fluid may have to be removed at the bedside. Under less urgent circumstances surgical creation of a pericardial window or pericardectomy may be advisable to avoid recurrence. **Massive pulmonary embolism** resulting in shock is treated by supportive measures (norepinephrine, digoxin) to improve cardiac function and with IV heparin to prevent recurrent thrombosis. In patients who cannot be stabilized with these measures, emergency pulmonary angiography and surgical embolectomy should be considered. The use of urokinase or streptokinase to lyse clots already formed appears to be of value, and is preferable to attempted embolectomy unless a full surgical and pump team is on 24-h standby.

Pulmonary complications that often coexist or develop in patients with shock must not be overlooked. Massive doses of corticosteroids (eg, hydrocortisone 2 to 10 gm IV) may reduce cellular damage and have been advocated for patients with shock, especially septic shock. Repeat doses are rarely needed more than once or twice in 24 h. When given with norepinephrine and similar agents, steroids may block their adverse effects on peripheral or visceral microcirculation without hampering their inotropic effect on the heart. Mannitol (15 gm in 1 dL H_2O IV) or furosemide (40 to 80 mg IV) may help prevent renal tubular damage resulting from diminished renal perfusion.

---

27. DISEASES OF THE HEART AND PERICARDIUM

HEART FAILURE (HF)

(Congestive Heart Failure [CHF]—For HF in infants, see Ch. 187)

A common syndrome that may be caused by many different etiologies whose clinical manifestations reflect a fundamental abnormality—a decrease in the myocardial contractile state such that cardiac output **(CO)** *is inadequate for the body's needs.* Reduced cardiac function may be manifest initially only during exercise, but, with progression of disease, occurs also at rest. As the contractile properties of the heart decline, symptoms and signs of congestion due to increased ventricular filling pressures, and fatigue associated with low CO develop.

Physiology

The clinical findings and rational treatment of HF are best understood by first reviewing normal heart function and the effect of disease. At rest and during exercise, the amount of venous return, CO, and the distribution of blood flow and delivery of O_2 to tissues is delicately balanced by nervous, humoral, and intrinsic cardiac factors to meet body needs. Since the energy of cardiac muscle contraction is a function of the length of the muscle fiber before stimulation, cardiac stroke work is directly proportional to the length or degree of stretch of the myocardial fiber at end-diastole. Left ventricular outflow resistance or aortic impedance is also important in regulating pump performance. It is useful to describe cardiac function in terms of the **ventricular function curve (the Frank-Starling relationship**—see FIG. 27–1). As the figure depicts,

contractile function, which can be measured in various ways, is dependent upon the diastolic length of cardiac muscle fiber. Fiber length is not easily measured at bedside so that end-diastolic pressure is used as an index of volume or stretch with the assumption that during a given set of observations, diastolic compliance, *the stiffness of the ventricle*, is unchanged. Often this assumption is not justified, but end-diastolic pressure is easily measured, and it is useful in conceptualizing abnormal cardiac function. The axes of the ventricular function curve can be related to the symptoms of patients with heart disease. Dyspnea, congestion, and edema develop as ventricular filling pressure rises, as depicted on the abscissa. Peripheral hypoperfusion, fatigue, and peripheral cyanosis develop as CO falls, as depicted on the ordinate.

A variety of factors (eg, catecholamine level, contractility, and metabolic influences) are thought to create a family of Frank-Starling curves. Changes in muscle stretch and diastolic volume probably play a minor role in the normal heart. Myocardial disease may present either as a primary increase in ventricular diastolic stiffness or as reduced

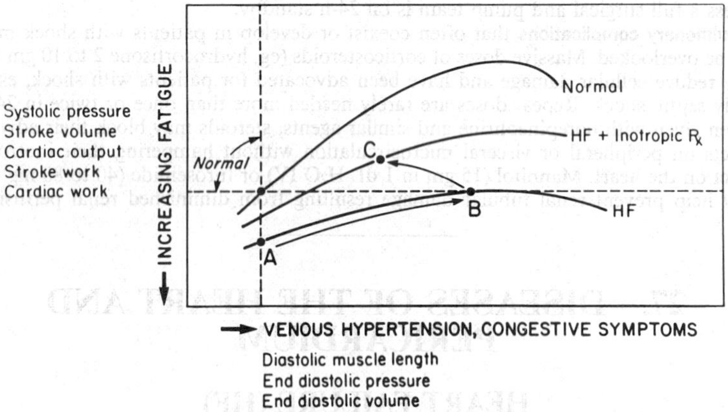

FIG. 27–1. Frank-Starling relationship. *Ordinate,* ability of ventricle to function as a pump. *Abscissa,* direct or indirect measurements of length or stretch of myocardial fiber. Dotted lines depict resting normal values; the normal curve includes point of intersection. Note that under normal conditions left ventricular systolic pressure, stroke volume, and work increase rapidly as the myocardial fiber is lengthened at end-diastole. There is a family of ventricular function curves depicting cardiac performance under normal and abnormal conditions. During heart failure consequent to reduced contractility, ventricular performance falls sharply (Point A). Reduced stroke volume causes increased end-diastolic volume with consequent stretching of diastolic muscle length. Ventricular function moves to the right on a relatively flat ventricular function curve to achieve relatively normal resting cardiac performance (Point B). Thus, adequate resting cardiac performance results from increased ventricular diastolic volume and pressure. Treatment of the failing ventricle with an inotropic agent improves the ventricular function curve (Point C), which, however, remains abnormal. Afterload reduction may have similar effects.

Note that this diagram assumes a direct relationship between diastolic muscle length, end-diastolic pressure, and end-diastolic volume, a relationship that is generally true when ventricular contractility is reduced. This relationship does not apply to HF due to increased myocardial diastolic stiffness; CO is usually normal, end-diastolic pressure is high, yet diastolic muscle length may be normal. The problem in disease causing increased diastolic stiffness is a markedly reduced myocardial compliance, hence abnormally high ventricular filling pressure and congestion with adequate ventricular emptying. (Adapted from "Recent Advances in the Understanding of Congestive Heart Failure (II)" by J. F. Spann, D. T. Mason, R. Zelis, in *Modern Concepts of Cardiovascular Disease,* Vol. 39, pp. 79–84, February 1970. Used by permission of the American Heart Association, Inc.)

myocardial contractility. **Increased diastolic stiffness** (eg, as in hypertrophic heart disease) interferes with ventricular filling, but not emptying, with resulting pulmonary congestion and a normal CO. **When contractility is reduced** by disease, however, filling pressure rises, diastolic volume increases, CO improves. It is generally assumed, but difficult to prove, that after a certain point on the curve, cardiac function progressively declines as filling pressures increase, creating a descending limb. In advanced disease, the function curve is displaced downward so that much greater stretch and higher filling pressures are required to produce a small increment in CO. Stimulation of the sympathetic nervous system or injection of catecholamines increases cardiac contractility and moves the ventricular function curve upward, but this mechanism is probably not very helpful in the presence of advanced cardiac disease. Changes in afterload or outflow resistance reduce systolic work and may be more important in controlling ventricular function in the diseased myocardium. Reduced contractility results in both congestion and a low CO. The physiologic manifestations of HF are greatly exaggerated during exercise.

Atrial contraction adds only a small volume to the ventricle, but this atrial "kick" stretches the well-filled ventricle creating a small but significant increment in ventricular end-diastolic pressure. This maximizes cardiac performance by providing optimal diastolic stretch, but minimizes mean ventricular filling pressure (ie, minimizes pulmonary venous and systemic venous pressures). In patients with decreased myocardial function, loss of the normal atrial "kick," as in atrial fibrillation, will reduce CO and arterial systolic pressure and increase mean venous pressures.

Increased **afterload** (*the resistance against which the heart contracts*), as in hypertension or aortic stenosis, causes hypertrophy of the myocardium (*an increase in cell size*). Myocardial capacity for hyperplasia (*an increase in cell number*) is negligible. Myocardial hypoxia possibly results from hypertrophy because neovascularization is deficient (multiple areas of fibrosis are commonly present in the hypertrophied ventricle).

Acute changes in myocardial contractility are largely modulated through the sympathetic nervous system. Sympathetic discharge to the heart generally has greater influence than circulating catecholamines. Sympathetic regulation of contractility is markedly reduced in CHF and advanced myocardial disease, because myocardial concentration of the neurotransmitter norepinephrine is greatly decreased and the receptors are altered or reduced in number.

Reduction in afterload, as might occur with standing or vasodilation accompanying exertion, induces more complete ventricular emptying, thus increasing the **ejection fraction** (systolic volume/end-diastolic volume). Acute increase in afterload has the opposite effect. When an individual rises from the sitting or supine position, venous inflow momentarily falls, stroke volume falls, systolic pressure declines somewhat, and the heart rate increases. Generally, CO does not fall despite the stroke volume decrease because the increased heart rate permits a constant volume/min. Within moments of continued standing, systemic arterial and venous tone increase, venous return or preload rises to the control state, stroke volume increases, and the heart rate slows. The sequence of changes reflects the critical importance of reflex adjustment, largely mediated through baroceptor mechanisms, in maintaining adequate cardiac performance. Therapeutic reduction in afterload, an important modality in treating chronic myocardial failure due to decreased contractility, reduces cardiac systolic work and often improves ventricular performance.

In some situations, the sequence of ventricular contraction may significantly influence ventricular performance. Ventricular activation is abnormal in bundle branch block. If the myocardium is diseased, ventricular function can be adversely affected. Patchy ventricular dysfunction **(dyskinesia)** is characteristic of coronary artery disease and adversely influences ventricular performance.

Recently, attention has focused on the important influence of afterload in controlling ventricular function. **Afterload** may be further defined as *those factors opposing*

ventricular emptying when the semilunar valves open at the end of isovolumic contraction. In patients with poor myocardial contractility, an increase in afterload (eg, a rise in arterial pressure) may result in increased ventricular filling pressure and a decline in CO. A reduction in afterload reduces cardiac systolic work, increases myocardial fiber shortening, and hence increases stroke volume. In the dilated ventricle with high filling pressure, reduction of afterload may significantly decrease ventricular diastolic pressures, and long-term afterload reduction with drugs may be clinically effective. It is important to recognize, however, that in the patient with a primary increase in diastolic stiffness (eg, hypertrophic heart disease and some patients with coronary artery disease) afterload reduction is *contraindicated,* since it may markedly reduce stroke volume and CO.

Ultrastructure: The fundamental contractile unit of the heart is the sarcomere, which consists of interdigitating bands of actin and myosin protein connecting through dynamic crosslinks of troponin, tropomyosin, and Ca. The fibers of actin are anchored to the intercalated discs or Z bands. According to current understanding, electrical depolarization mobilizes free Ca ions, stimulating alteration in the crosslinks so that the filaments of actin and myosin slide by each other and the muscle contracts. A direct relationship between initial sarcomere length and force of contraction has been demonstrated and Frank-Starling curves can be constructed for individual sarcomeres.

Energetics: The major determinants of myocardial O_2 need are heart rate, contractile state, and afterload or systolic tension. Pressure work is far more costly metabolically than volume work. Thus, in general, aortic stenosis engenders a greater myocardial O_2 requirement than aortic regurgitation. A rough index of myocardial O_2 demand under different loads can be calculated by multiplying the heart rate by the systolic pressure.

Because of its obligate oxidative metabolism, the heart depends on coronary blood flow and O_2 delivery for sustained normal function. It extracts more O_2 per unit of flow than any other tissue. Coronary sinus P_{O_2} is the lowest of a venous sample from any organ. Any factor that reduces coronary blood flow (eg, increased ventricular wall tension, hypotension, tachycardia, or coronary artery obstruction) may compromise ventricular function. Anaerobic metabolism can provide only about 10 to 30% of the energy needed for sustained myocardial contraction. Anaerobiosis results in increased lactate production. An important metabolic sign of myocardial hypoxia is increased lactic acid concentration in the coronary sinus.

No effective treatment to increase myocardial energy production or substrate utilization is currently available. However, methods of reducing cardiac work by reducing the heart rate, altering contractility, or decreasing systolic afterload can improve the performance of the failing ventricle. When left ventricular **(LV)** function is impaired, reflex arterial vasoconstriction increases impedance to LV ejection and reduces stroke volume. Thus, treatment with a vasodilator to reduce impedance may improve ventricular performance by reducing cardiac work to a more tolerable level and increasing stroke volume.

Exercise and cardiac reserve: Cardiac reserve may be defined as *unutilized ability of the resting heart to deliver O_2 to the tissues.* Reserve mechanisms include alterations in heart rate, systolic and diastolic volume, stroke volume, and tissue extraction of O_2. In well-trained young adults during maximal exercise, CO may increase from its resting normal value of 6 L/min to 25 L/min or more; O_2 consumption increases from 250 to 1500 mL/min or more; heart rate may increase from a sedentary 72 to 180 beats/min. The increased demand of the body for O_2 to meet metabolic requirements is met by a marked increase in CO (stroke volume $\times$ heart rate) and by greater than normal extraction of O_2 from capillary blood in the tissues. In the normal young adult at rest, arterial blood contains about 18 mL O_2/dL of blood, and mixed venous or pulmonary artery blood contains about 14 mL/dL. The arteriovenous O_2 difference (A-V_{O_2}) is thus about 4.0 $\pm$ 0.4 mL O_2/dL of blood. During exercise the increase in CO, even to

maximal levels, is insufficient to meet tissue metabolic needs; hence the tissues extract more O_2, and mixed venous blood O_2 content falls considerably. The A-V_{O_2} difference widens to 12 to 14 mL/dL.

In heart failure, stroke volume is reduced and relatively fixed so that the major components of cardiac reserve are heart rate and tissue extraction of O_2 as reflected in the A-V_{O_2} difference. Measurement of systemic A-V_{O_2} difference is one of the most sensitive indices of ventricular performance available. An increase in resting systemic arterial-pulmonary artery O_2 difference greater than normal is irrefutable evidence of compromised ventricular function. With the Swan-Ganz pulmonary artery catheterization technic and bedside measurement of blood gases, this index of cardiac function is readily available, easily interpreted, and provides valuable clinical physiologic information (see INVASIVE CARDIOVASCULAR PROCEDURES in Ch. 25).

Oxyhemoglobin dissociation: Availability of O_2 to the tissues is largely influenced by the oxyhemoglobin dissociation curve (FIG. 27–2). The position of this curve is frequently expressed as P_{50} (*the partial pressure of O_2 in blood at 50% oxyhemoglobin saturation*); normal P_{50} is 27 ± 2 mm Hg. An increase in P_{50} indicates a rightward shift of the oxyhemoglobin dissociation curve (decreased affinity of Hb for O_2). Alterations in this curve provide another reserve mechanism in heart failure. Shift of the curve to the right, downward displacement, means that for a given P_{O_2}, less O_2 is combined with Hb and the saturation is lower; at the capillary, more O_2 is released and thus available to the tissues. Increased hydrogen concentration (reduced pH) shifts the oxyhemoglobin dissociation curve to the right (Bohr effect). A major factor influencing the position of the curve is the concentration of 2,3-diphosphoglycerate **(DPG)** in Hb. Increased DPG alters the spatial relationships within the Hb molecule, reducing its affinity for O_2 and shifting the curve to the right. Increased DPG and a favorable rightward shift enhancing O_2 availability at the tissues occurs in anemia, hypoxemia, and heart failure.

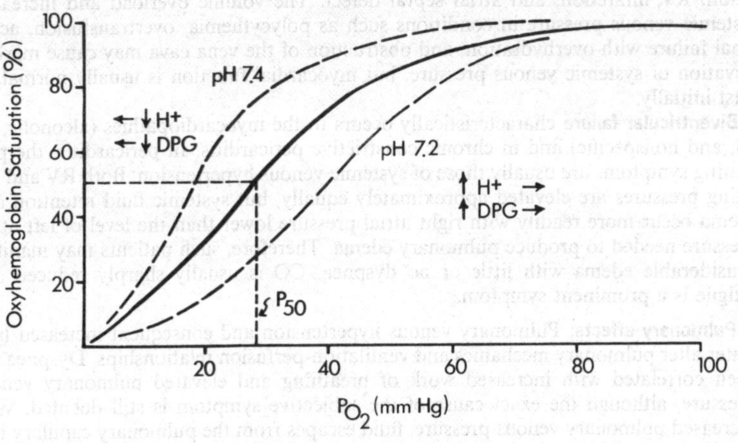

FIG. 27–2. Oxyhemoglobin dissociation curve. Arterial oxyhemoglobin saturation (ordinate) is related to partial pressure of O_2 (abscissa). P_{50} (PO_2 at 50% saturation) is normally 27 mm Hg. The dissociation curve is shifted to the right by increased H^+ concentration and increased RBC diphosphoglycerate. The curve is shifted to the left by decreased H^+ and lower RBC diphosphoglycerate. Hb characterized by rightward shifting of the curve has a decreased affinity for O_2; Hb characterized by a leftward shift of curve has an increased affinity for O_2.

Etiology and Pathophysiology

Contractile deficiency: The sequence of events leading to the clinical manifestations of heart failure in contractile deficiency begins when the myocardium cannot contract with sufficient force to maintain a normal stroke volume. Because of incomplete emptying, the ejection fraction (stroke volume/end-diastolic volume), normally > 50%, falls. End-diastolic volume increases, shifting the ventricle to the right on the Frank-Starling curve with a consequent rise in end-diastolic pressure. The increased diastolic stretch induces a more forceful systolic contraction, enabling the ventricle to maintain adequate cardiac work at the expense of greater diastolic volume and tension (see FIG. 27–1). As the process proceeds, ventricular filling pressure and hence venous pressure, pulmonary or systemic, gradually increase while CO falls and the A-V_{O_2} difference widens. Systemic arterial pressure is maintained by an increase in peripheral vascular resistance. The resultant rise in LV outflow resistance may further adversely affect myocardial performance.

In many forms of heart disease, clinical manifestations of HF are dominant in either the right or the left ventricle. **LV failure** is characterized by reduced CO and increased pulmonary venous pressure. The cardinal clinical signs are dyspnea on exertion and fatigue. Elevation of pulmonary venous pressure to the level of plasma protein oncotic pressure (about 24 mm Hg) leads to increased lung water, reduced pulmonary compliance, and a rise in the O_2 cost or work of breathing. LV failure occurs characteristically in hypertension, aortic valve disease, patent ductus arteriosus, large ventricular septal defect, mitral regurgitation, and coronary artery disease.

Right ventricular (RV) failure is most commonly associated with LV failure, which causes pulmonary arterial hypertension induced by pulmonary vascular changes and by elevated pulmonary venous pressure. RV failure is characterized by systemic venous hypertension and edema; fatigue and low CO are late manifestations. Diseases causing RV failure include any form of LV failure, mitral stenosis, primary pulmonary hypertension, multiple pulmonary embolization, pulmonary stenosis, tricuspid regurgitation, RV infarction, and atrial septal defect. The volume overload and increased systemic venous pressure in conditions such as polycythemia, overtransfusion, acute renal failure with overhydration, and obstruction of the vena cava may cause marked elevation of systemic venous pressure, but myocardial function is usually normal, at least initially.

Biventricular failure characteristically occurs in the myocardiopathies (alcoholic, viral, and nonspecific) and in chronic constrictive pericarditis. In pericarditis, the presenting symptoms are usually those of systemic venous hypertension. Both RV and LV filling pressures are elevated approximately equally, but systemic fluid retention and edema occur more readily with right atrial pressure lower than the level of left atrial pressure needed to produce pulmonary edema. Therefore, such patients may manifest considerable edema with little or no dyspnea. CO is usually sharply reduced and fatigue is a prominent symptom.

Pulmonary effects: Pulmonary venous hypertension and consequent increased lung water alter pulmonary mechanics and ventilation-perfusion relationships. Dyspnea has been correlated with increased work of breathing and elevated pulmonary venous pressure, although the exact cause of the subjective symptom is still debated. With increased pulmonary venous pressure, fluid escapes from the pulmonary capillary into the interstitial space and alveoli with consequent alveolar collapse and atelectasis. Pleural effusions of HF characteristically accumulate in the right hemithorax. Lymphatic drainage is greatly enhanced, but cannot mobilize the continual increase in lung water. Unoxygenated pulmonary arterial blood is shunted past nonaerated alveoli, decreasing mixed pulmonary capillary P_{O_2}. A combination of alveolar hyperventilation due to increased lung stiffness and reduced Pa_{O_2} is characteristic of LV failure. Thus,

arterial blood gas analysis reveals an increased pH and a reduced P_{O_2} (respiratory alkalosis) with decreased saturation reflecting increased intrapulmonary shunting. Increasing the inspired O_2 concentration will increase Pa_{O_2} and improve O_2 delivery to the tissues, but the pulmonary shunting limits the response.

Renal function: Renal blood flow and GFR are reduced in HF, and blood flow within the kidney is redistributed. The filtration fraction is reduced, and filtered Na is decreased, but tubular Na absorption is enhanced. Decreased renal blood leads to increased renin release from the juxtaglomerular apparatus, which enhances angiotensin II release from angiotensin I. Angiotensin II is a potent vasoconstrictor and also promotes aldosterone secretion from the adrenal glands. Antidiuretic hormone (ADH) may be released, if plasma volume is decreased. As a result of these complex renal changes, afterload, blood volume, total body Na, and body water are increased. These alterations are partly compensatory, since they enhance myocardial fiber stretch by increasing ventricular volume, but they also lead directly to the congestive clinical manifestations of HF.

Liver function: Reduced splanchnic blood flow and increased venous pressure characteristic of HF cause liver engorgement and decreased nutrient hepatic blood flow. Moderate hepatic dysfunction commonly occurs in systemic venous hypertension secondary to RV failure, with approximately equal elevations of conjugated and unconjugated bilirubin, increased prothrombin time, and rise in hepatic enzymes (eg, alkaline phosphatase, AST [SGOT], and ALT [SGPT]). These enzyme elevations are usually modest, but in severely compromised circulatory states with marked reduction of CO and hypotension, central liver necrosis and the manifestations of liver failure may be severe enough to suggest hepatitis with acute liver failure. In advanced HF, reduced aldosterone breakdown by the liver further contributes to fluid retention.

Other organs: Chronic severe venous hypertension has been associated with the syndrome of protein-losing enteropathy characterized by marked hypoalbuminemia. Bowel infarction, acute and chronic GI hemorrhage, and malabsorption syndromes may complicate low CO states. Peripheral gangrene in the absence of large vessel occlusion has been reported in patients with chronic markedly reduced CO. Chronic irritability and decreased mental performance may reflect severely reduced cerebral blood flow and hypoxemia in chronic low-output states.

High output failure: Certain conditions (eg, thyrotoxicosis, beriberi, chronic A-V fistula, chronic anemia, and Paget's disease) induce a high output failure. In these conditions, venous return is markedly increased due to low peripheral vascular resistance. Chronic volume overload eventually causes contractile failure in the dilated heart with high output.

Increased diastolic stiffness: It has recently been recognized that congestive symptoms due to reduced diastolic compliance despite normal systolic function occurs in a variety of settings including hypertrophic obstructive myocardiopathy, constrictive pericarditis, LV hypertrophy, the aged heart, and some patients with coronary disease. The altered compliance retards ventricular filling. Diastolic pressure may be quite high with associated venous congestion despite normal or even enhanced ventricular emptying. Inotropic agents (eg, digitalis) are not useful. Afterload reduction with vasodilators is contraindicated because the accompanying dilation of the venous capacitance bed reduces ventricular filling already compromised by the stiffness with potentially disastrous results.

Symptoms and Signs

HF may produce systemic and/or pulmonary venous congestion (presenting signs and symptoms of predominantly right- or left-sided failure, respectively), may develop gradually, or may present suddenly as with acute pulmonary edema.

LV failure (HF due to lesions altering LV function) may become apparent early with undue tachycardia, fatigue with exertion, dyspnea with mild exercise, and intolerance to cold. Paroxysmal nocturnal dyspnea and cough reflect the movement of excess fluid from the extremities to the lungs that occurs when a patient with borderline LV compensation is recumbent. Such symptoms may be important early clues. Occasionally, pulmonary venous hypertension and increased pulmonary fluid manifest primarily as bronchospasm and wheezing. In advanced HF, severe cough is prominent. Rusty tinged or brownish sputum due to blood and the presence of HF cells is common. Frank hemoptysis presumably due to ruptured pulmonary varices from bronchial veins is uncommon, but may occur, and large amounts of blood may be lost. Physical findings are influenced by the type of heart disease. Signs of LV failure from conditions that lead to LV dilation include reduced carotid pulsations, diffuse and laterally displaced apical impulse, palpable and audible 3rd and 4th heart sounds, accentuated pulmonic 2nd sound, inspiratory basilar rales, and right-sided pleural effusion.

Acute pulmonary edema is a dramatic and life-threatening manifestation of acute LV failure secondary to sudden onset of pulmonary venous hypertension. A sudden rise in LV filling pressure to high levels results in rapid movement of plasma fluid through pulmonary capillaries into the interstitial spaces and alveoli. The patient presents with extreme dyspnea, cyanosis, tachypnea, hyperpnea, restlessness, and anxiety with a sense of suffocation. Pallor and diaphoresis are common. The pulse may be thready, and the BP may be difficult to obtain although direct measurement reveals a normal central aortic pressure. Respirations are grunting and labored with inspiration; expiration is prolonged. Rales are widely dispersed over both lung fields anteriorly and posteriorly. In some patients the major manifestation is marked bronchospasm or wheezing **(cardiac asthma)**. Vigorous, noisy respiratory efforts often prevent careful examination of the cardiovascular system. Hypoxemia is severe, and cyanosis is deep. CO_2 retention is a late, ominous manifestation of secondary hypoventilation.

RV failure: The principal symptoms include increasing fatigue, awareness of fullness in the neck, fullness in the abdomen, occasionally an ache in the right upper quadrant of the abdomen, ankle swelling, and, in advanced stages, ascites. Pertinent signs include evidence of systemic venous hypertension, abnormally large A or V waves in the external jugular pulse, an enlarged and tender liver, murmur of tricuspid regurgitation, and pitting edema of the lower extremities.

Cyanosis may occur with any form of HF. The cause may be central, and reflect hypoxemia. A peripheral component due to capillary stasis with increased A-V_{O_2} difference and resultant marked venous oxyhemoglobin unsaturation may also be present. Improved color of the nail bed with vigorous massage suggests the presence of peripheral cyanosis. Central cyanosis cannot be altered by increasing local blood flow.

There are no specific **ECG** findings in HF. Abnormalities (eg, ventricular hypertrophy, acute myocardial infarction, or bundle branch block) may provide clues to the presence or etiology of the heart disease. Analysis of rhythm is often helpful; determining whether arrhythmias are primary or secondary is important; eg, the recent onset of rapid atrial fibrillation may precipitate acute LV failure and requires prompt treatment. On the other hand, frequent ventricular premature beats may be secondary and may subside when the heart failure is treated.

Chest x-rays are helpful in evaluating the presence and severity of CHF and its cause. Hilar congestion and the "butterfly" or "batwing" configuration of increased vascular markings are characteristic of pulmonary edema. Recognition of edema surrounding bronchioles, peribronchial cuffing, may help to establish that HF is the cause of pulmonary infiltrates. Kerley B lines reflect chronic elevation of left atrial pressure and represent chronic thickening of the intralobular septa from edema. Careful examination of the cardiac silhouette, evaluation of chamber enlargement, and a search for intra- or extracardiac calcifications are important x-ray clues to the etiology of the primary cardiac abnormality.

Treatment of HF Due to Decreased Myocardial Contractility

Management of HF is based on the physiologic concepts, specific etiology, and pathophysiology outlined above. Therapy includes rest, oxygenation, measures to improve myocardial contractility, correction of arrhythmias, diuresis, Na restriction, and reduction of afterload, if possible. Even in the most urgent situation, the cause of the HF must be determined, correctable conditions searched for, and contributing factors eliminated.

Rest: Reduction of heart rate and cardiac work by bed rest and sedation contributes importantly to management. The degree of restriction depends upon the severity of the HF. Sedation with diazepam 5 to 10 mg orally prn and flurazepam 15 to 30 mg orally at bedtime is often helpful. The head of the bed should be elevated and patients encouraged to sit as tolerated. Maintaining the trunk upright reduces the work of breathing and improves ventilation.

Contributing factors: An important component of management is the recognition and control of factors that may be causing increased cardiac demands or adversely affecting myocardial function (eg, hypertension, anemia, excess salt intake, excess alcohol, arrhythmias, thyrotoxicosis, fever, increased ambient temperature, or pulmonary emboli).

Rhythm: Arrhythmias should be evaluated as primary or secondary. Usually, arrhythmias are secondary to HF and improve with therapy. Frequent ventricular premature or atrial premature beats will often subside as congestion improves. However, some arrhythmias may require specific treatment (eg, in rapid atrial fibrillation, control of the ventricular rate or cardioversion may resolve the failure, persistent "sinus tachycardia" at 150/min may actually be atrial flutter with 2:1 A-V block).

Diuretics: Diuretics and Na restriction are essential to long-term management of HF. In both acute and chronic HF, the importance of reliable daily weights cannot be overemphasized for gauging the effectiveness of therapy and adjusting diuretic dosages. Ambulatory patients can weigh themselves at home at the same time of day under the same conditions and keep a daily log.

TABLE 27–1 lists details of various diuretics (see also Ch. 286). In mild HF, thiazide diuretics (eg, hydrochlorothiazide 50 mg/day or chlorothiazide 500 mg daily or bid) are useful. Increasing their dosages does not significantly increase the diuretic effect. Supplemental potassium chloride is generally needed since chronic diuresis causes hypokalemic alkalosis. Increased daily ingestion of foods with a high K content (eg, bananas and orange juice) may suffice for adequate replacement, or liquid preparations of 20 to 40 mEq potassium chloride bid to qid may be necessary. K salts other than potassium chloride are generally not useful since both K and Cl must be replaced. K-sparing diuretics (eg, triamterene 100 mg bid after meals) may be useful. The "loop" diuretics (eg, furosemide or ethacrynic acid) are highly effective. Their advantages include rapid onset of action both IV and orally and effectiveness of increasing the dose; their disadvantage is their potency. Furosemide IV has a potent venodilator action before onset of diuresis, which, by reducing venous inflow, may be effective early treatment. Overdosage may cause hypovolemia, hyponatremia, and profound hypokalemia, and they should be used cautiously. Small initial doses and careful evaluation of response is wise. Oral doses of furosemide should start with 40 mg, increasing to 80 or 160 mg daily or bid, depending on the response; higher dosages may be needed. IV doses of 20 to 40 mg can be given initially and increased as needed. In refractory cases rapid injections are more effective than slow infusion. Nerve deafness due to specific and nonreversible ototoxicity has occurred shortly following IV injection of both "loop" diuretics. Spironolactone 25 to 50 mg tid may be useful in severe HF and hypokalemia; however, it is expensive and may induce hyperkalemia. Spironolactone seems to be most effective in hyperaldosterone states, which are unusual except in severe and refractory HF.

TABLE 27–1. CLINICAL AND PHARMACOLOGIC PROPERTIES OF DIURETICS

Classification	Drugs	Relative Potency	Site of Action	Onset of Action	Advantages	Adverse Effects
Thiazides	Chlorothiazide po: 500–2000 mg/day Hydrochlorothiazide po: 50–200 mg/day Metolazone po: 2.5–10 mg/day	Moderate	Excreted into proximal tubule, inhibit Na and Cl absorption in distal segment	1–2 h	Mild, relatively nontoxic, oral administration, antihypertensive	K loss, hyperglycemia, decreases platelets, ineffective when GFR < 20 mL/min, hyperuricemia
Loop diuretics	Furosemide po: 40–200 mg 1, 2, or 3 times/day IV: 40 mg initially; may increase to 200–400 mg depending on response Ethacrynic acid IV: 50 mg initially; may increase depending on response Bumetanide po: 0.5–2.0 mg; IV or IM: 0.5–1.0 mg	High	Inhibition of Cl transport in ascending limb of loop of Henle	po: 1 h IV: 10–20 min	Rapid onset, potency, independent of acid-base balance, effective even when GFR is reduced	Excessive diuresis, hypovolemia, K loss and hypokalemia, hyperuricemia, transient or irreversible deafness with IV administration, especially when used with aminoglycoside antibiotic
Potassium sparing	Spironolactone po: 25–50 mg bid to qid	Moderate to low	Aldosterone homolog, competitive inhibition for receptor site in distal tubule Secondary: inhibition of aldosterone biosynthesis	2–3 days for maximum effect	Useful in combination with more proximal-acting diuretic to spare K	Hyperkalemia when K salts are given concomitantly or renal function is reduced markedly
	Triamterene po: 100 mg bid to tid	Moderate	Inhibition of Na resorption in distal tubule	1–2 h	Useful in combination with more proximal-acting diuretic to spare K	Hyperkalemia when K salts are given concomitantly, renal function is reduced markedly, or with ACE inhibitors

Na restriction: Reduction of salt intake is an important, but frequently neglected aspect of the management of HF; neglect of this factor is a major cause of refractoriness to treatment. Habits of salt usage in cooking and at the table vary and should be evaluated for each patient. Many patients may need to eliminate only table salt and avoid salted foods (eg, ham, bacon, peanuts, french fries). Restrictions below 2 gm of Na (87 mEq), about 5 gm of sodium chloride, may be necessary in severe cases. Advanced HF may require the combination of potent diuretics and severe restriction of Na to 0.5 to 1.5 gm/day.

Acute pulmonary edema is a medical emergency demanding prompt and effective treatment. The major aims of treatment are to reduce preload as rapidly as possible and maintain oxygenation. Unless in shock, the patient should sit upright, preferably with legs dangling. High concentrations of O_2 should be given by mask or nasal cannula. Morphine sulfate 4 to 6 mg IV or 10 to 15 mg IM reduces agitation, has transient arteriolar and venous dilating effects, decreases the respiratory rate, and may slow the heart rate; these effects reduce the work of breathing and cardiac work. Reducing preload with sublingual nitroglycerin may be highly effective by inducing venodilation and redistributing blood volume away from the chest. Occasionally, in refractory cases, IV nitroglycerin is effective. In severe cases rotating tourniquets are effective: BP cuffs are applied to 3 limbs, inflated midway between diastolic and systolic pressures, deflated and rotated q 10 to 20 min. *The BP cuffs should not be applied to the limb into which an IV infusion is running.* Occasionally phlebotomy is necessary; the rapid removal of 300 to 500 mL of blood may have a dramatic effect. Useful therapy includes the IV administration of a rapidly acting diuretic (eg, furosemide 40 mg IV or ethacrynic acid 50 mg IV) to initiate a prompt diuresis in 15 to 20 min, thus decreasing the plasma volume and ventricular filling pressure. Most patients with acute pulmonary edema can be treated successfully without digitalis, although it may be needed later to prevent further episodes. If digitalis is given, low doses are mandated because of the rapidly changing clinical situation, including aggressive diuresis. Not > 50% of the digitalizing dose should be given initially. In severe cases requiring close monitoring in intensive care units, dobutamine may be useful to improve cardiac function.

The cause of the pulmonary edema should be diligently sought. In valvular heart disease, sudden onset of a rapid arrhythmia (eg, atrial flutter or fibrillation) may precipitate pulmonary edema that responds to cardioversion. Pulmonary edema due to a hypertensive crisis or significant systolic hypertension may respond to a vasodilator (eg, apresoline or nitroprusside). Deliberate reduction of afterload with nitroprusside in refractory cases despite lack of hypertension may be useful.

Treatment of Increased Diastolic Stiffness

Symptoms of HF in patients with increased diastolic stiffness reflect high ventricular filling pressures due to abnormal myocardial relaxation or restriction of normal diastolic expansion of volume during ventricular filling. Myocardial contractility is actually increased in hypertrophic heart disease (also known as idiopathic hypertrophic heart disease). In hypertrophic heart disease, fluid retention with elevated body water is not usually a problem. Since a reduced blood volume and decreased venous return exacerbate symptoms, diuretics are usually contraindicated. A β-adrenergic blocker to reduce ventricular contractility may be effective therapy. Verapamil, a Ca- or slow channel blocker, is also useful, although the precise mechanism of action is unknown.

In myocardial involvement in hemochromatosis, amyloid, and certain other infiltrative diseases, contractility is reduced and diastolic stiffness increased. Generally these patients are treated in the same manner as those with myocardiopathy of any cause.

Digitalis is useful in treating some patients with HF. Digitalis suppresses ventricular arrhythmias, increases venous tone, increases renal blood flow, slows heart rate, prolongs A-V conduction, and, in toxic doses or the presence of hypokalemia, may induce ventricular extrasystoles. It is highly effective in the treatment of atrial fibrillation. In

management of HF, its primary purpose is usually to increase myocardial contractile force, but the effect is modest.

Since improved ventricular performance in the patient with HF may follow reduction in filling pressure (preload) by use of diuretics or reduction in preload and afterload by use of vasodilators, controversy over the role of digitalis in treatment of HF has developed. Effective treatment of HF is often possible without use of digitalis. The drug appears to be most useful in patients with large end-diastolic volumes and a 3rd heart sound.

The properties and dosages of digitalis preparations are outlined in TABLE 27-2. Familiarity with use of digoxin will suffice in most clinical situations.

TABLE 27-2. DIGITALIS PREPARATIONS—ROUTES OF ADMINISTRATION, PHARMACOKINETICS, DOSAGES

	Digoxin	*Digitoxin*	*Ouabain*
Preferred route*	Orally, IV	Orally, IV	IV
Percent GI absorption	85%	100%	
Onset of effect, IV	15–30 min	½–2 h	5–10 min
Peak effect, IV	4–6 h	6–12 h	½–2 h
Plasma half-life	30–36 h	5–7 days	18–25 h
Excretion, metabolism	Renal	Hepatic, GI	Renal, GI
Plasma level Therapeutic Toxic	 1.0–1.4 ng/mL > 2 ng/mL	 20–30 ng/mL > 40 ng/mL	
Digitalization schedule† Oral, 24 h	 0 h: 0.5 mg 8 h: 0.25 mg 16 h: 0.25 mg 24 h: 0.25 mg Thereafter, daily maintenance dose‡	 0 h: 0.6 mg 8 h: 0.3 mg 16 h: 0.2 mg 24 h: 0.1 mg Thereafter, daily maintenance dose	
Oral, 48 h	0.25 mg q 8 h × 6 Thereafter, daily maintenance dose‡	0.2 mg q 8 h × 6 Thereafter, daily maintenance dose	
Oral, gradual	0.25 mg/day (digitalization achieved in 5–7 days)‡	0.1 mg/day (digitalization achieved in 10–14 days)	
IV, 24 h	0 h: 0.5 mg 6 h: 0.25 mg 12 h: 0.125 mg 18 h: 0.125 mg Thereafter, daily maintenance dose‡	0 h: 0.6 mg 8 h: 0.3 mg 16 h: 0.2 mg 24 h: 0.1 mg Thereafter, daily maintenance dose	0 h: 0.3 mg 4 h: 0.2 mg 8 h: 0.1 mg 12 h: 0.1 mg‡
Daily maintenance dose, oral	0.25–0.375 mg/day	0.1 mg 5 times/wk to 1.5 mg/day	

* IM injections are *not* recommended because they are painful and absorption is erratic.

† Doses are designed to produce effective but prudent plasma and tissue concentrations (see text for details).

‡ Abnormal renal function prolongs plasma half-life, necessitating *reduction* in suggested dosage.

Since digitalis compounds are eliminated from the body in proportion to their concentration, large doses have traditionally been given rapidly (digitalization) for initial full therapeutic effect, followed by lower maintenance doses (see TABLE 27–2). However, digitalis has a narrow toxic-therapeutic ratio, and low dose schedules are best. When there is no urgent need, standard maintenance doses of digitalis can be given orally initially without loading doses. Digitalization will be achieved in this manner in about 5 days with digoxin and in 10 to 14 days with digitoxin. This approach is favored in elderly, ambulatory patients who do not need rapid treatment, who may be seen only intermittently, and who may be confused by changing dosages. Digitalis blood levels may be helpful in evaluating absorption when the drug is given orally and in regulating the dosage in difficult cases. The serum sample should be drawn not < 6 h after the most recent dose, or falsely high values will be obtained.

Digitalis toxicity may result from overdosage, hypokalemia, advanced degenerative heart disease associated with conduction abnormalities, or a combination of factors. Continual alertness to the possibility of K loss with diuresis and appropriate replacement with oral K salts or use of a K-sparing diuretic are important in preventing toxicity. Because digoxin is largely eliminated by the kidneys, digitoxin may be preferable in patients with actual or suspected renal disease; renal function may be considerably compromised although the BUN remains within a normal range. Although digitoxin is largely eliminated by the liver, even advanced liver failure seems to have little effect on blood level.

Systemic toxic effects of digitalis include nausea, vomiting, anorexia, diarrhea, confusion, amblyopia, and xerophthalmia. The most important toxic effects of the drug are life-threatening arrhythmias due to the drug's direct effect on the A-V node, causing a prolonged P-R time, Wenckebach phenomenon, and ultimately complete heart block. Nonparoxysmal junctional tachycardia developing in the presence of atrial fibrillation is a frequently overlooked, but serious sign of digitalis toxicity. Digitalis increases the automaticity of Purkinje fibers and may enhance reentry, resulting in coupled extrasystoles, ventricular tachycardia, or ventricular fibrillation. Bidirectional ventricular tachycardia is a pathognomonic sign of digitalis intoxication. The development of a new arrhythmia or worsening of a previous one while the patient is taking digitalis should always raise the suspicion of digitalis intoxication. Arrhythmia may be the first and only manifestation of digitalis toxicity.

The first step in treating digitalis toxicity is to discontinue the drug. The ECG should be closely monitored throughout all treatment. If the serum K is low, 80 mEq of potassium chloride IV should be given in 1 L 5% D/W at a rate of 6 mL/min (0.5 mEq/min). Ventricular arrhythmias are treated with a 50- to 100-mg rapid IV injection of lidocaine, repeated in 3 to 5 min until a therapeutic effect is obtained, a total of 300 mg is given, or CNS toxicity occurs. When the arrhythmia is controlled, a continuous infusion of 2 to 4 mg/min should be started. Alternatively, phenytoin 100 mg q 3 to 5 min can be given slowly up to a total of 1000 mg. Heart block is best treated with a temporary pervenous pacemaker. Isoproterenol is *contraindicated* in digitalis intoxication because of the increased tendency to ventricular arrhythmia. Digitalis cannot be dialyzed, since it is either protein-bound or rapidly fixed to tissues. Suicide attempts due to digitalis overdosage are especially difficult to treat because of the large amount of drug ingested. Hyperkalemia due to displacement of K^+ from cells develops. Drug-specific antibody fragments (FAB) are available from special centers in the USA for IV administration for severe cases.

Vasodilator therapy: In patients with HF, both arterial and venous constrictor tone may be inappropriately high secondary to vasoconstrictor reflexes. Ventricular response to afterload is a direct function of myocardial contractility. Inappropriately elevated ventricular filling pressures induce congestive symptoms. The clinical useful-

ness of therapeutic vasodilation rests on a solid physiologic understanding of the consequences of HF.

Vasodilators may have primarily an arteriolar or a venous (capacitance) site of action, although, in practice, most agents have mixed effects. Venodilators are similar in cardiac action to diuretics: They decrease preload or ventricular filling pressure and hence reduce congestive symptoms. It is important to recognize, therefore, that venodilators will not be effective and may have serious adverse effects in the patient with low ventricular filling pressure since they reduce preload (and hence venous return) even further. Arterial dilating agents are useful in some patients with decreased contractility or valvular regurgitation as reduction of afterload may enhance ventricular performance. CO increases, but BP is usually maintained, since the increased forward flow compensates for the fall in peripheral resistance. In clinical states associated with elevated diastolic stiffness and normal or increased contractility (eg, hypertrophic obstructive myocardiopathy), vasodilators are not helpful and may have serious consequences. Current experience suggests that acute or long-term vasodilator therapy may be useful in patients with impaired myocardial contractility who remain symptomatic with dyspnea or fatigue despite conventional therapy.

Vasodilator drugs: Sodium nitroprusside, given IV only, relaxes smooth muscle of both arteries and veins. Its effect must be monitored by pulmonary artery catheter to confirm the hemodynamic response, which usually takes place within 5 min and wears off within 10 min after the infusion is ended. Initial infusion rate is 10 μg/min, increasing 5 μg/min until the desired effect or hypotension is reached. Maximum dose is 500 μg/min. Major immediate side effects are treated by discontinuing the infusion or, if necessary, giving a vasoconstrictor (eg, phenylephrine or norepinephrine). The metabolite thiocyanate may accumulate in renal insufficiency or with large doses, leading to toxicity.

Nitrates, IV, oral, or topical, are primarily venodilators, with a lesser effect of arteriolar dilation. Side effects of all nitrates are similar: headache, postural hypotension, and, rarely, methemoglobinemia with prolonged, large doses. Tolerance may develop with some preparations. Some reflex tachycardia may be encountered. **Sublingual nitroglycerine** 0.4 mg is effective within 1 to 2 min, with maximal effect in 10 min, persisting 15 to 30 min. **IV nitroglycerine** is given initially 10 μg/min, increasing 10 μg/min about q 5 min to a maximum of 100 μg/min. **Topical nitroglycerine ointment**: a 1 to 10 cm strip (0.5 to 4 in.) on the chest has a duration of action at least 3 h. **Transdermal patches** contain various dosages and persist many hours. Recent evidence suggests tolerance with continued, 24-h administration. Thus, authorities recommend removal of the patch 4 to 6 h/day. **Isosorbide dinitrate** 2.5 to 10 mg is given sublingually q 2 to 4 h; orally 20 to 60 mg q 4 to 6 h.

Hydralazine used orally or IV dilates arterioles. Effects begin within 30 min and last up to 6 h. With doses > 400 mg/day, it may cause LE. Reflex tachycardia is occasional. Its use is most effective in patients with large hearts and very high peripheral resistance. Long-term efficacy is uncertain.

Angiotensin converting enzyme (ACE) inhibitor (eg, captopril orally—an initial dose 6.25 mg bid, is increased to 200 mg/day in divided doses) appears to be highly effective in many patients with advanced HF associated with elevated filling pressure, reduced CO and increased afterload when circulating Angiotensin II is elevated. With effective doses, filling pressures fall, CO increases, and BP is maintained without tachycardia. Comparative trials suggest improved survival when patients with advanced myocardiopathy are treated with captopril, which is probably the most effective addition to treatment of HF in many years.

Toxicity includes decreased renal function, nephrotic syndrome, dysgeusia, membranous glomerulonephritis, and leukopenia. Its effectiveness is sharply reduced in the

presence of renal failure. Enalapril, another ACE inhibitor, is available; its effectiveness and toxicity appear to be similar to captopril.

Refractory heart failure: In some patients chronic or acute HF persists despite appropriate therapy. In such cases an orderly approach is useful. Has the etiology been established? Have mitral stenosis, aortic stenosis, excess alcohol intake, thyrotoxicosis, pulmonary emboli, anemia, or other contributing factors been overlooked? Are drug doses optimal? (Some patients require very large doses of "loop" diuretics for effective diuresis.) Is the oral digitalis being absorbed? (Small bowel disorders and interference by other drugs, eg, neomycin or antacids containing magnesium trisilicate, inhibit absorption of digoxin.) Is the patient adhering to an adequate low-salt diet? Hyponatremia in the presence of an elevated venous pressure and edema must reflect excess water intake rather than low body Na and is a clue to inadequate fluid and Na restriction. When extensive edema is refractory to intensive therapy, the following is occasionally effective: metolazone followed in ½ to 1 h by an IV loop diuretic. It must be recognized, of course, that even the best medical efforts may fail in the face of advanced myocardial disease.

COR PULMONALE (CP)

Right ventricular **(RV)** *enlargement secondary to malfunction of the lungs producing pulmonary artery hypertension that may be due to intrinsic pulmonary disease, an abnormal chest bellows, or a depressed ventilatory drive.* The term does not include RV enlargement secondary to left ventricular **(LV)** failure, congenital heart disease, or acquired valvular heart disease. CP is usually chronic but may be acute and reversible.

Etiology

Several disease processes can lead to CP. The most common cause of **chronic CP** is chronic obstructive pulmonary disease (chronic bronchitis, emphysema). Other possibilities include extensive loss of lung tissue from surgery or trauma, chronic unresolved pulmonary emboli, primary pulmonary hypertension, pulmonary veno-occlusive disease, scleroderma, diseases leading to diffuse interstitial fibrosis, kyphoscoliosis, obesity with alveolar hypoventilation, neuromuscular diseases involving respiratory muscles, and idiopathic alveolar hypoventilation. **Acute CP** usually results from massive pulmonary embolization, but acute reversible exacerbations of chronic CP often occur in patients with COPD, usually during acute respiratory infections.

Pathogenesis

CP is directly caused by alterations in pulmonary circulation that lead to pulmonary arterial hypertension and thereby impose an increased mechanical load on RV emptying (afterload). **Pulmonary hypertension** (see also PRIMARY PULMONARY HYPERTENSION, below) can be caused by irreversible reduction in the size of the vascular bed, as in diseases primarily affecting pulmonary blood vessels (eg, embolization [see Ch. 39] or scleroderma) or as in massive loss of lung tissue (eg, from emphysema or surgery). However, the most important mechanism leading to pulmonary hypertension is alveolar hypoxia, which results either from localized inadequate ventilation of alveoli that are well perfused or from a generalized decrease in alveolar ventilation. Alveolar hypoxia, whether acute or chronic, is a potent stimulus of pulmonary vasoconstriction, and chronic alveolar hypoxia, in addition, promotes hypertrophy of smooth muscle in the pulmonary arterioles. These hypertrophied vessels then respond vigorously to acute hypoxia. Hypercapnic acidosis acts synergistically with hypoxemia to augment the pulmonary vasoconstriction. During chronic hypoxia, pulmonary hypertension is intensified, both by increased blood viscosity arising from secondary polycythemia and by increased CO. Even though increased pulmonary capillary pressure does not contribute per se to the pathogenesis of pulmonary arterial hypertension in CP, indepen-

dent disease of the left ventricle is often aggravated by hypoxemia and acidosis, and respiratory insufficiency in turn is intensified if LV failure induces pulmonary edema.

Symptoms, Signs, and Diagnosis

CP should be suspected in all patients with a disorder mentioned above under Etiology. Signs of right heart enlargement appear early and are readily discernible in acute CP. In chronic CP caused by pulmonary vascular disease, dyspnea may be slight or absent at rest, even when frank RV failure is present. Some patients suffer syncopal attacks on exertion, and substernal anginal pain is common. Physical signs include left parasternal systolic lift, a loud pulmonic 2nd sound, and fatigue on exertion. Murmurs due to functional tricuspid and pulmonic insufficiency may occur. Chest x-rays show RV and pulmonary arterial enlargement. ECG evidence of RV hypertrophy correlates well with the degree of pulmonary hypertension. Gallop rhythm (S_3 and S_4), distended jugular veins (with a dominant A wave unless tricuspid regurgitation is present), hepatomegaly, and edema may be seen in patients with RV failure.

In CP due to disease of the pulmonary parenchyma, clinical manifestations of the primary disease frequently overshadow those of CP. Major symptoms and signs (dyspnea, cough, cyanosis, and wheezing) are also seen in left heart failure, and differentiation may be difficult. Echocardiographic or radionuclide evaluation of LV function is an important step in the workup of CP. Arterial blood gases are helpful in such cases since appreciable hypoxemia, hypercapnia, and acidosis are unusual in left heart failure unless there is also frank pulmonary edema. Because pulmonary hyperinflation and bullae cause a realignment of the heart in these patients, the physical examination, x-rays, and ECG may be relatively insensitive indicators of RV enlargement.

Treatment

Therapy of primary lung disorders is discussed in §4. Therapy of right heart failure is discussed in HEART FAILURE, above. Phlebotomy during hypoxic CP has been suggested, but beneficial effects of decreased blood viscosity are not likely to outweigh the effects of reducing the O_2-carrying capacity of the blood; also, substantial polycythemia is uncommon in hypoxic CP. Digitalis is not effective in hypoxic CP. However, LV dysfunction may be present and clinically masked. Many patients who improve with digitalis and vasodilators may actually have LV dysfunction. Diuretics can improve pulmonary gas exchange in hypoxic CP, presumably by relieving extravascular fluid accumulation in the lungs. However, vigorous use of diuretics can lead to metabolic alkalosis, which diminishes the effectiveness of CO_2 as a respiratory stimulus. K and Cl losses must be carefully replaced when diuretics are used. Continuous use of O_2 can decrease pulmonary hypertension, prevent polycythemia in hypoxic patients, and has been shown to reduce mortality. Use of pulmonary vasodilators (hydralazine, calcium-channel blocking agents, etc) is controversial. Because of the possibility of inducing systemic hypotension or aggravating hypoxemia, individual responses should be monitored during cardiac catheterization studies before instituting long-term use of these agents. Patients with CP are at increased risk of venous thromboembolism. Should this occur, long-term anticoagulation is necessary.

PRIMARY PULMONARY HYPERTENSION (PPH)

A very uncommon obliterative disease of unknown etiology involving medium and small pulmonary arteries and terminating in right ventricular ***[RV]*** *failure or fatal syncope 2 to 5 yr after detection.* Intimal hyperplasia and consequent narrowing of the vessel lumen is always present. Areas of medial hypertrophy and hyperplasia, "plexiform" lesions, and necrotizing arteritis are seen in more advanced cases. The last two are associated with irreversibility.

Women are affected 5 times oftener than men. The median age at diagnosis is 35 yr. Progressive exertional dyspnea occurs in > 95% of cases. Precordial pain and syncope

on exertion are less common. Raynaud's phenomenon and arthralgias are present in many patients, often antedating the apparent onset of PPH by years. Physical examination shows, to a variable extent, the manifestations of cor pulmonale (see above).

Diagnosis and Treatment

Diagnosis is suspected on the basis of clinical manifestations, but requires exclusion of all known causes of cor pulmonale (see above), especially those that may be modified by therapy (eg, pulmonary embolism). Echocardiogram, ventilation-perfusion scans, pulmonary function testing, and cardiac catheterization are usually necessary to exclude other causes of pulmonary hypertension. Pulmonary angiography is risky because sudden deaths have occurred, but should be undertaken if ventilation-perfusion scans show unmatched segmental or larger perfusion defects indicative of chronic thrombotic occlusion of pulmonary arteries due to unresolved pulmonary embolism. Need for open lung biopsies in PPH is controversial.

A few patients can respond to vasodilators (eg, hydralazine, nifedipine) with drastic reductions in pulmonary artery pressure. Administration of vasodilators should always be preceded by demonstration of efficacy in the cardiac catheterization laboratory. Injudicious use of these agents has resulted in marked worsening or fatalities.

CARDIAC ARRHYTHMIAS

Physiology

Normal sinus rhythm originates within pacemaker cells of the sinoatrial (**S-A,** sinus) node (at the junction of the superior vena cava and high right atrium). These cells represent the primary electrical generator (pacemaker) for the normal human heart. Conduction within the sinus node is slow, since it must occur through cells that are automatic and partially depolarized. The sinus node depolarizes at least 80 to 120 msec before the start of the P wave on the ECG. Indirect human studies of S-A conduction suggest it to be considerably longer than previously estimated and at least part of this conduction delay is due to specialized perionodal fibers surrounding the sinus node. The P wave is inscribed on the ECG as the electrical impulse spreads first over the right and then the left atrium (FIG. 27–3). The total duration of atrial excitation is generally 80 to 100 msec and represents the normal P wave duration. The impulse travels from the S-A node to the atrioventricular **(A-V)** node preferentially via 3 specialized tracts within the atria, but may also be conducted by ordinary atrial myocardium. Conduction velocity within these specialized pathways is more rapid than in ordinary atrial myocardium, and the excitation wave enters the A-V node about 40 msec after the P wave begins.

Conduction through the A-V node is also slow, and A-V nodal refractoriness is generally longer than that of any other cardiac tissue. After the impulse has crossed the A-V node, it is still on the atrial side of the anulus fibrosus and then travels to the His bundle. The **bundle of His** conducts propagating impulses between the atria and ventricles (FIG. 27–3). It runs along the tricuspid valve ring to the area of the trigone of the tricuspid valve, penetrates the anulus fibrosus, and continues down through the membranous interventricular septum as a discrete fascicle.

At the point where membranous septum becomes muscular septum, the His bundle divides into 3 major fascicles. The **right bundle** continues down the right ventricular endocardial surface and does not branch or result in depolarization of myocardium until it reaches the anterior right ventricular papillary muscle and apex of the right ventricle. The **main left bundle** crosses the summit of the muscular interventricular septum to emerge on the left side of the heart just below the noncoronary cusp of the aortic valve. At this point it divides (at least functionally) into a **left posterior division** that cascades down the mid and posterior left side of the interventricular septum.

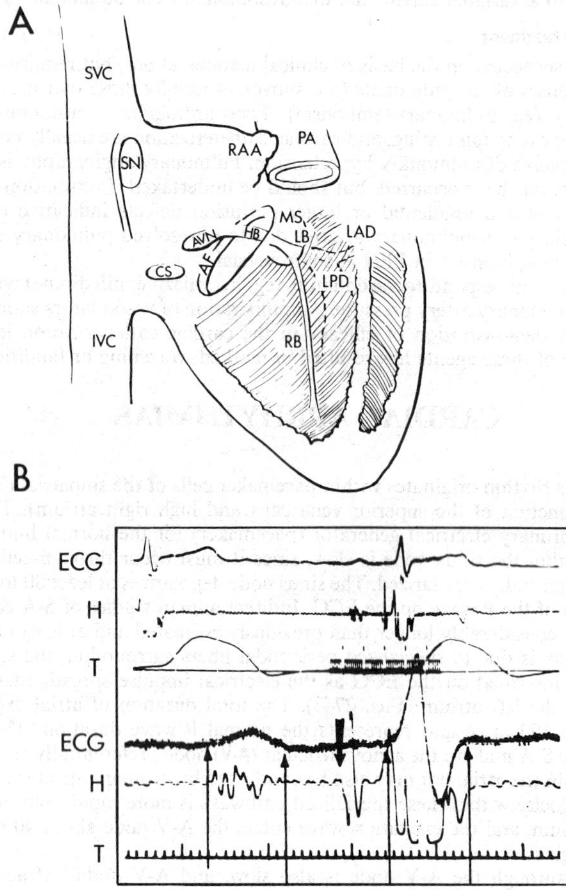

FIG. 27–3. Relationship between cardiac conduction system and ECG.

A. A schematic diagram of the human heart, labeled as follows: SVC, superior vena cava; IVC, inferior vena cava, SN, sinus node; CS, coronary sinus; RAA, right atrial appendage; PA, pulmonary artery; AF, anulus fibrosus; AVN, atrioventricular node; HB, bundle of His; MS, membranous septum; RB, right bundle; LB, left bundle; LAD, left anterior division; LPD, left posterior division.

B. Electrical events associated with cardiac excitation. The upper and lower portions (identical except that the lower portion is time-expanded) include an electrocardiogram (ECG), a His bundle electrogram (H), and time marks (T) at 10- and 100-msec intervals. In the upper portion a pressure tracing shows the recording site of the His bundle electrogram to be within the right ventricle. In the lower portion a P wave lasting 90 msec is illustrated between 2 vertical ascending arrows. A QRS of 95 msec is similarly illustrated. During the isolectric P-R segment of the surface ECG, the depolarization of the His bundle is shown by the heavier descending arrow. Conduction time from the onset of the P wave to His bundle depolarization (A-H interval) is normal at 150 msec. Conduction time within the infranodal structures (H-V interval) is slightly prolonged at 55 msec (normal = 40–50 msec).

Studies suggest that a portion of this posterior division behaves like an independent conduction fascicle and is responsible for providing input for septal depolarization. The anterior portions of the left bundle divide into a thinner, free-running **left anterior division** that runs to the anterior papillary muscle of the left ventricle before its terminal branches begin. This anterior superior fascicle of the left bundle controls the appropriate timing of activation of the anterolateral and basilar portions of the left ventricle.

The S-A node and these specialized cardiac tissues all contain cells capable of automaticity (spontaneous Phase IV diastolic depolarization) with the probable exception of the A-V node. The intrinsic rhythmicity is highest in the S-A node and the rate of each of the other latent cardiac pacemakers decreases with increasing distance from the S-A node. Thus, heart rhythm is normally controlled by the rhythmicity of the S-A node. If the sinus node, either reflexly or due to intrinsic disease, slows sufficiently, one of the other pacemaking tissues assumes its function. The intrinsic rate of the sinus node can vary from 60 to 100/min. Rates < 60/min are termed sinus bradycardias and rates > 100/min sinus tachycardias. Enhanced vagal tone can produce bradycardia with rates of 40 to 50/min, while enhanced sympathetic tone can produce sinus tachycardia with rates of 100 to 150/min. Failure to increase the sinus rate > 90/min with moderate exercise suggests sinus node dysfunction.

None of this conduction—ie, within the atrial specialized tracts, A-V node, bundle of His, 3 fascicles, and terminal His-Purkinje system—has electrical manifestations on the surface ECG, although specialized intracardiac recording technics may record some of these events (FIG. 27-3). The surface ECG depicts only depolarization of atrial (P waves) and ventricular (QRS complexes) myocardium. The relationship between depolarization of these specialized cardiac tissues and the surface ECG is depicted in FIG. 27-3.

Evaluation of Patients with Arrhythmias

Most arrhythmias are accompanied by symptoms. Some arrhythmias can be detected and correctly diagnosed by physical examination (from characteristic changes in pulse rate, rhythm, or heart sounds, or from the relationship between atrial and ventricular mechanical events), but arrhythmias are diagnosed with any degree of accuracy only with the ECG. Intracardiac recording technics have significantly augmented knowledge of normal and abnormal rhythms. A careful history, physical examination, evaluation of physical manifestations, but primarily, an understanding of the basic mechanism of any cardiac arrhythmia, are all necessary to estimate prognosis and to plan patient care.

NORMAL SINUS RHYTHM

The average adult heart at rest beats 72 to 78 times/min. However, from birth to old age, the sinus rate progressively decreases. Normal sinus rhythm in the infant (110 to 150) is sinus tachycardia in the adult. Also, heart rates < 60 may occur in as many as 33% of hospitalized men and 19% of hospitalized women. In deciding whether the sinus rate is too fast or too slow, the patient's age and the circumstances of the examination are important.

SINUS BRADYCARDIA

A slow sinus rhythm characterized on ECG by an atrial rate < 60 beats/min and by a sequence of atrial depolarization (ie, P wave morphology) that reflects initiation of the impulse from the area of the high right atrium.

Etiology

Sinus bradycardia, the result of slowed diastolic depolarization within all S-A pacemaker cells, is most often caused by increased vagal tone, which often occurs normally

during rest or sleep. It is common in athletes and young persons in vigorous health and in noncardiac conditions (eg, myxedema, jaundice, recovery from illness causing sinus tachycardia, increased vagal tone from GI disturbances), and occasionally results from drug intoxication. In patients with organic heart disease, it commonly results from digitalis excess or use of β-blockers (eg, propranolol) or Ca blockers (eg, verapamil or diltiazem).

Sinus bradycardia also commonly results from intrinsically depressed automaticity within the S-A node of elderly persons with arteriosclerotic heart disease and is benign if asymptomatic. Chronic, inappropriate sinus bradycardia—where sinus rate does not increase appropriately with exercise or emotion—is a recognized form of S-A node dysfunction and may occur in the absence of other forms of heart disease.

Symptoms and Signs

Sinus bradycardia with rates between 40 to 60/min is generally asymptomatic if the patient is sedentary or at rest, but may be severely limiting in terms of exercise tolerance. Slower sinus rates may result in fatigue even at rest. *Sinus rates < 30 beats/min may require emergency treatment if the patient is symptomatic*; due to the emergence of other cardiac arrhythmias and cerebral anoxia, < 20 beats/min may result in syncope, convulsions, and even death.

Treatment

Asymptomatic patients require no treatment.

Acute sinus bradycardia < 40 beats/min associated with symptoms should be treated first with atropine 0.5 to 1 mg IV, repeated if no effect is seen within 4 min. If atropine is ineffective (eg, in patients with the "**sick sinus syndrome**"), isoproterenol IV may be life-saving. Very small doses (0.5 to 1.0 μg/min) should be used initially, (since these patients may be extremely sensitive to IV isoproterenol) and then increased to raise the sinus rate to the desired level. Emergency percutaneous temporary pacemaker insertion may prove lifesaving. External temporary pacemakers with large electrode pads are available and may be preferable to or used while percutaneous leads are being inserted. For chronic symptomatic sinus bradycardia, permanent pacemaker therapy is the only long-term solution.

SINUS TACHYCARDIA

A sinus rhythm > 100 beats/min in an adult.

Etiology

In sinus tachycardia, neural mechanisms affect the rate of automaticity of the sinus node pacemaker cells. Typically, increased sympathetic tone results in an increased heart rate; occasionally, decreased vagal tone is the cause. Emotion, exercise, thyrotoxicosis, hypotension, hypoxia, hyperthermia, anemia, bleeding, and infections are frequent noncardiac causes. Heart failure will increase the sinus rate reflexly, and inflammatory diseases of the pericardium, myocardium, or endocardium are often accompanied by sinus tachycardia. Sympathomimetics (nicotine, caffeine, marijuana) all increase the heart rate. Habitual use of anticholinergic drugs may cause persistent sinus tachycardia.

Symptoms, Signs, and Diagnosis

There are rarely symptoms, but the patient may be aware of a fast rate and forceful contractions. Unlike paroxysmal tachycardia, sinus tachycardia does not start and stop suddenly. Rather, an episode begins gradually, with the heart rate increasing over several minutes, and tapers off in the same way.

The diagnosis is made by ECG: normal P waves precede each QRS complex by a normal interval, but their rate is between 100 and 180/min. Maneuvers that increase

vagal tone (eg, carotid sinus massage) slow the rate, but it returns to its tachycardic level as soon as the maneuver is stopped.

Prognosis and Treatment

The prognosis is that of the causative condition (eg, anemia or hypothyroidism). Sinus tachycardia is clinically significant when it results from heart failure, active myocarditis, myocardial infarction, or other primary myocardial disease.

Although β-blockers (eg, propranolol) may slow the heart rate, therapy should be directed at the cause.

SINUS ARRHYTHMIA

A common variant of regular sinus rhythm characterized by cyclic changes in heart rate due to periodic fluctuation in the discharge rate of the sinus node.

Sinus arrhythmia is the result of alternate increases and decreases in vagal and sympathetic tone. In the respiratory variety, the heart rate increases with inspiration and slows with expiration. In the nonrespiratory variety, the same phasic changes occur, but are unrelated to respiration. Sinus arrhythmia produces no symptoms.

Diagnosis and Treatment

The P wave morphology remains identical throughout, but the interval between P waves shows a phasic increase and decrease that generally varies by < 160 msec. A relationship to respiration, if present, is easily identified. Confusion between sinus arrhythmia and atrial premature depolarizations can be avoided by recognizing that sinus arrhythmia is repetitive and cyclical. No treatment is required.

SICK SINUS SYNDROME
(Sinus Node Dysfunction Syndromes)

A variety of syndromes associated with inadequate sinus node function most often resulting in cerebral manifestations of lightheadedness, dizziness, and near or true syncope.

Etiology

Coronary artery disease is the most common cause (eg, ischemia and changes in vagal stimulation after an acute right coronary artery occlusion). The 2nd most common cause is progressive degeneration of sinoatrial **(S-A)** conduction, a sclerotic process analogous to degeneration of the interventricular conduction system; these processes are frequently seen together. However, a variety of heart diseases ranging from cardiomyopathies, both dilated and infiltrative, through inflammatory myocardial disease may result in sinus node dysfunction. The syndromes are more often caused by abnormal S-A *conduction* than by abnormal sinus node pacemaker function (automaticity).

Symptoms and Signs

The most common forms of sinus node dysfunction are related to **intermittent S-A block**. Here, one sees varying degrees of block ranging from S-A Wenckebach through high-degree S-A block with what has been called "sinus arrest." The patient, basically in sinus rhythm, who has a prolonged period of S-A block, experiences symptoms related to the duration of the asystolic period—weakness, dizziness, pre- or near-syncope, or unconsciousness.

The 2nd most common sinus node dysfunction syndrome is that of **tachycardia-bradycardia syndrome,** wherein a patient with inadequate S-A conduction experiences paroxysmal atrial arrhythmias. Episodes of supraventricular tachycardia, atrial flutter, or atrial fibrillation are followed by a variable period of depression of S-A conduction; ie, a prolonged pause before sinus rhythm resumes. The length of this asystolic period

will determine the patient's symptoms, as noted above. Although occasionally aware of palpitations, most patients are unaware of cardiac irregularities accompanying or preceding the usually brief episodes described more often as "grey-out" than true loss of consciousness. Occasionally patients have **persistent sinus bradycardia** that may result in lethargy and weakness.

Diagnosis

Sinus node dysfunction may be suspected in elderly patients with episodes of presyncope or near syncope, particularly if a history of palpitations is associated. Accurate diagnosis is made only with ECG (often requiring 24-h Holter monitoring) to document the dysrhythmias described above. Electrophysiologic stimulating procedures have been used to determine the responsiveness of sinus node tissue. Single atrial premature beats are evoked or the atria are paced at rates in excess of the sinus node rate. Prolonged S-A recovery times following single premature beats or prolonged sinus node reset times following atrial pacing are highly suggestive of sinus node dysfunction, but there is a high incidence of false-negative results.

Treatment

Any symptomatic patient with sinus node dysfunction requires the implantation of a permanent demand pacemaker.

PREMATURE DEPOLARIZATION
(Premature Beats; Premature Contractions)

Depolarization of the atria, ventricles, or both, that occurs before the next expected sinus beat. Such depolarizations can arise from the S-A node, the atrial specialized conduction system, ordinary atrial myocardium, the His bundle, any of the 3 interventricular fascicles, or the terminal branches of the His-Purkinje system or ventricular myocardium. The A-V node is *not* a site of impulse formation; thus, the term "nodal premature beats" is meaningless, while the term "junctional premature beats" is too broad. Junctional premature beats arise within either the bundle of His or the 3 fascicles of the interventricular conducting system. Since the significance of premature depolarizations depends on the site of impulse formation, each is considered separately, below.

ATRIAL PREMATURE BEATS (APBs)
(Atrial Premature Depolarizations)

Although APBs may occur in normal hearts, they are more often associated with heart disease, especially rheumatic and arteriosclerotic, and with conditions that tend to increase atrial and ventricular size and filling pressures. APBs are a common result of sympathomimetic drugs, tobacco, caffeine, and CNS disturbances.

It is unresolved whether APBs represent the firing of ectopic automatic cells within the atrial myocardium or conduction pathways, or reflect reentry within localized areas of atrial myocardium. Both automaticity and re-entry are probably responsible for specific APBs. Clinical differentiation is currently impossible.

Symptoms, Signs, and Diagnosis

Most patients who complain of a skipped beat, flutter, or extra beats in the chest generally disregard them until their frequency causes alarm. Depending on the timing of the premature beat, heart sounds may be identical to or totally different from normal. Very early APBs may not allow sufficient ventricular filling to produce a palpable pulse. The diagnosis of an APB is certain if an S_4 gallop sound precedes the premature beat.

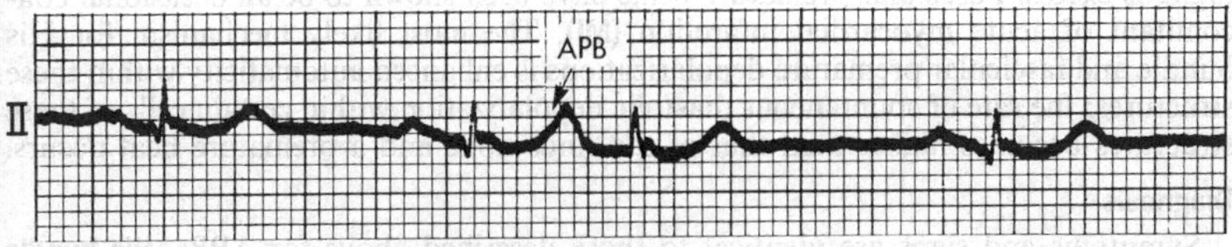

FIG. 27–4. Atrial premature depolarization (APB). ECG lead II is shown. Following the 2nd beat of sinus origin, the T wave is deformed by an APB. Since the APB occurs relatively early during the sinus cycle, the sinus node pacemaker is reset and a pause less than fully compensatory precedes the next sinus beat.

On ECG, irrespective of the site of origin, APBs interrupt sinus rhythm characteristically, producing a premature P wave (FIG. 27–4). If this wave is conducted to the ventricles, it is followed by a premature QRS complex. No QRS complex is seen if the APB occurs while the A-V node or subsidiary A-V conducting structures are refractory. The length of the cycle surrounding the APB is determined by its prematurity and by sinus node function, but finding a pause equal to, less than, or greater than fully compensatory is *not* an aid in diagnosis. In APBs late in the sinus cycle, the premature depolarization does not enter and reset the sinus node. The sinus node discharges on time, but atrial myocardium is refractory. The next sinus impulse is on time and the pause surrounding the APB is fully compensatory. APBs occurring during the midportion of the sinus cycle retrogradely enter the sinus node, discharge, and reset its dominant pacemakers. A pause less than compensatory and generally ≤ 130% of the preceding sinus cycle results. (Very prolonged sinus reset times > 150% of the preceding sinus cycle may be an indication of sinus node dysfunction.) APBs occurring very early in the sinus cycle may find S-A conduction pathways refractory and fail to enter and discharge the sinus node. The next S-A impulse is capable of re-exciting the atrium and an interpolated APB results.

The contour of the premature P wave may suggest the source of the APBs; eg, origin in the low right atrium typically produces inverted P waves on the ECG in the inferior leads II, III, and aVF. Origin in the anterior left atrium may cause inverted anterior precordial P waves. Origin within the atrium is certain if a P wave is the first event of the premature beat complex, since there is no way for a premature beat originating below the atrial level to result in atrial depolarization before depolarization of ventricular myocardium.

Treatment

Treatment of APBs is directed at the cause (eg, in heart failure, the use of **digitalis** may abolish APBs). In the absence of heart disease, mild sedation (eg, phenobarbital or diazepam) may help, and the use of caffeine and nicotine should be eliminated. Use of potent and potentially toxic antiarrhythmic drugs are seldom indicated for APBs since they are usually benign, but **procainamide** or **quinidine** may be used to suppress APBs when necessary in organic heart disease (see treatment of ventricular premature beats **[VPBs]**, below).

Propranolol may also be used to control APBs in patients intolerant to quinidine; but it is generally less effective, and its β-adrenergic blocking effect and slowing of sinus rate must be considered (see treatment of VPBs, below).

HIS BUNDLE AND FASCICULAR PREMATURE DEPOLARIZATIONS

His bundle and fascicular premature beats (formerly called **junctional** or **nodal premature beats**) may occur in normal hearts during periods of stress or of excess catecholamine production; in organic heart disease, they may result from ischemia or

digitalis excess. Fascicular premature beats have been shown to be an occasional concomitant of acute myocardial infarction **(MI)**. The most likely mechanism for His bundle and fascicular premature depolarizations is enhanced automaticity within these structures; the rate of spontaneous diastolic depolarization within certain cells of these structures becomes higher than that of the sinus node and a premature beat occurs.

Diagnosis

Symptoms and signs are identical to those described above for APBs. **His bundle premature beats** are diagnosed on ECG by the presence of a premature, but otherwise normal, QRS complex that is *not* preceded by a premature atrial complex. Although often hard to detect, there is generally a retrograde P wave within or just after the QRS complex.

Fascicular premature beats occur most commonly in acute MI, and arise within either the anterior or posterior fascicle of the left bundle branch. The normal rhythm is interrupted by a premature QRS complex whose morphology reflects right bundle branch block plus either left anterior or left posterior hemiblock, depending on the originating fascicle. The more characteristic the bundle branch block pattern, the more likely it is that the premature depolarization originates within one of the fascicles of the left bundle branch.

Treatment

The treatment of His bundle and fascicular premature depolarizations is as for APBs, except that lidocaine and phenytoin may be useful (see below). Since their incidence is not common, it is difficult to state the aggressiveness with which they should be treated. In the presence of acute MI, however, the refractoriness of the A-V node does not protect the ventricular myocardium from depolarization during its vulnerable period. This suggests that an early His bundle PB could be as ominous as an early VPB in the initiation of more life-threatening ventricular arrhythmias in the presence of a vulnerable or irritable myocardium.

VENTRICULAR PREMATURE BEATS (VPBS)
(Ventricular Premature Depolarizations)

VPBs (FIG. 27–5) may occur in normal or diseased hearts, or as a result of digitalis excess. In normal hearts, any process causing excess catecholamine release may result in VPBs. Peri-, epi-, or myocardial inflammatory states may also precipitate VPBs. Myocardial stretching (as in heart failure) or ischemia, results in a high incidence of VPBs. VPBs occur in > 90% of patients with acute MI. VPBs are common in patients with mitral prolapse.

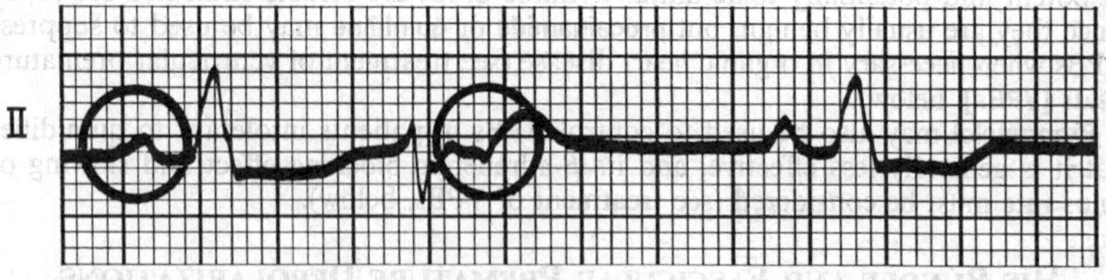

FIG. 27–5. Ventricular premature depolarization (VPB). ECG lead II demonstrates normal sinus rhythm with an upright P wave (first circle) followed by premature depolarization of the ventricles. The premature inverted P wave (second circle) following this VPB is the result of ventriculoatrial conduction (VAC). After the VPB, sinus rhythm resumes.

iagnosis

Symptoms and signs are identical to those described above for APBs. VPBs are iagnosed on ECG when the sinus rhythm is interrupted by a premature QRS complex not preceded by a premature P wave) whose morphology is distinctly abnormal. The CG patterns of VPBs originating from the distal His-Purkinje system do not resem-le any form of classic bundle branch block, and the more bizarre the QRS complex, he more distal its site of origin within the His-Purkinje system is likely to be.

Depending on their timing, each VPB may be interpolated ("sandwiched") between normal sinus beats or may cause the next sinus beat to block in the A-V node, giving ise to a fully "compensatory pause." VPBs often cause retrograde conduction to the tria and may or may not reset the sinus node, giving rise to a pause less than compen-atory. *The cycle surrounding any premature beat is not helpful in diagnosing its site of rigin.* A premature depolarization originating above the level of the A-V node could esult in ventricular depolarization prior to that of the atrium—and vice versa. Al-hough morphologic diagnostic criteria for VPBs may be helpful, the above criteria are bsolute.

reatment

In a patient without heart disease, frequent VPBs may disturb the physician more han the patient. If no evidence of valvular heart disease is found by physical examina-ion and echocardiogram, and no evidence of ischemic heart disease is elicited by istory, exercise ECG, or thallium myocardial perfusion studies, Holter monitoring hould be used to characterize the VPBs present. Probably only VPBs occurring early n the cycle (R on T VPBs), in salvos, or as ventricular tachycardia require therapy.

In patients with organic heart disease, chronic VPBs are a different problem, often equiring correction. The urgency of treatment depends upon the underlying organic eart disease and the malignancy of the ventricular arrhythmias encountered. For xample, consider a patient presenting with VPBs in whom mitral valve prolapse is ocumented both clinically and by echocardiogram as the cause of the ventricular ctopic activity. A trial with standard antiarrhythmics is indicated to suppress the 'PBs only when the quality of life is compromised or sustained ventricular tachycar-ia is seen as a cause of symptoms.

In patients with coronary artery disease or myocardiopathies with severely de-ressed left ventricular function, ventricular ectopic activity should be treated more ggressively. Prognosis is improved in patients in whom electrophysiologic-directed herapy proves to be successful. A 24-h Holter recording should be made before initi-ting antiarrhythmic therapy to determine the characteristics and severity of the ar-hythmia. Repeat recordings permit evaluation of the efficacy of drug treatment. lectrophysiologic studies using programmed stimulation may be necessary to deter-nine the efficacy of some antiarrhythmics. In patients who survive sudden death due o ventricular tachycardia **(VT)** or fibrillation **(VF)** and in patients with dilated cardio-nyopathies, 2-yr survival appears to be at least 70% when programmed stimulation ails to elicit sustained VT or VF. Drug effects that increase the risk of arrhythmia **'proarrhythmic" effects)** can also be identified by this procedure.

Although digitalis is occasionally effective in diminishing the frequency of VPBs or bolishing them completely in patients with severe left ventricular dysfunction, a spe-ific antiarrhythmic drug generally should be used. **Antiarrhythmic drugs are classified ccording to their presumed site of action: Class I agents** (also called local anesthetics or nembrane stabilizing drugs) act directly on membrane conductance of cations, espe-ially Na-channel blockade (eg, lidocaine, procainamide, quinidine, disopyramide, to-ainide, and flecanide). **Class II agents** are β-adrenergic blockers; **Class III agents**

prolong repolarization (eg, amiodarone and bretylium). **Class IV agents** are the Ca channel blockers. Not necessarily in order of preference, the following antiarrhythmi drugs should be considered:

1. Procainamide: Procainamide is a potent Class 1A antiarrhythmic useful for acut and chronic treatment of atrial and ventricular arrhythmias. It is rapidly absorbed an has a relatively short clinical half-life (**$t_{1/2}$**). Procainamide delays repolarization, pro longs the effective refractory period of atrial and ventricular muscle, decreases th slope of phase 4 depolarization, and slows the rate of automatic firing. The majo metabolite, N-acetylprocainamide (NAPA) also has antiarrhythmic effects. It prolong the action potential duration and the effective refractory period. This may be pro arrhythmic by causing early after-depolarization and triggered activity. The anticholin ergic effect of procainamide may increase sinus rate. The drug prolongs QRS duratior QT interval, and A-V conduction. It is a vasodilator and depresses myocardial con tractility, thus rapid IV administration may cause hypotension.

IV route: 100 mg is given over 1 min and repeated q 5 min until arrhythmia i controlled; the total dose should not be > 1 gm with BP, heart rate, and ECG moni tored before each dose. When the arrhythmia is controlled, antiarrhythmic plasm levels can be maintained with a constant IV infusion at 2 to 8 mg/min. Usual thera peutic plasma levels are 4 to 10 μg/mL; toxicity is common at > 12 μg/mL. A infusion may be started with the first IV dose to eliminate a possible decline in th plasma level. **Oral route**: In patients with normal elimination, doses ranging from 0.2 to 1.0 gm q 3 to 4 h may be required (to control APBs, 2 to 4 gm/day are usuall needed). In some patients, $t_{1/2}$ is prolonged, and 5- to 8-h dosing intervals may b satisfactory. To avoid toxicity when transferring from steady IV infusion to the ora route, the first oral dose is delayed until 4 h after discontinuing IV.

Toxicity: Procainamide may induce sinus arrest, A-V block, ventricular arrhythmia and hypotension. An ECG should be taken often (eg, after every other dose) durin the first 3 days of quinidine or procainamide therapy. Prolongation of the Q-T interva and QRS widening are ECG signs of toxicity; *either drug should be stopped or used ver cautiously if QRS widening is ≥ 25%.*

After several months, essentially all patients receiving oral procainamide therap will have seriologic evidence of lupus, and as many as 40% may have systemic symp toms (eg, arthralgia, fever, pleural effusion). Rapid acetylaters may have relative pro tection against drug-induced lupus. Nonspecific GI irritation is common.

2. Quinidine sulfate: Although quinidine sulfate in isolated tissue preparations be haves similarly to procainamide and is a Class 1A antiarrhythmic drug that prolong action potential duration and refractoriness, in clinical situations quinidine has bee effective in cases where procainamide has failed and vice versa. It is effective in acut and chronic atrial and ventricular arrhythmias. The drug is not used IV because c severe hemodynamic depression.

An initial oral test dose of quinidine sulfate 200 mg is given to exclude idiosyncras If, within 4 h, no tinnitus, deafness, urticaria, diarrhea, or falling BP appears, amoun of 200 to 400 mg q 4 to 6 h are generally used to suppress ventricular ectopic activit ECG and/or Holter monitoring will disclose the drug's efficacy and permit dosag adjustment so that QRS duration is < 0.14 sec (see procainamide, above). Quinidir blood levels continue to rise during the initial 72 h of therapy, so that quinidine shoul not be considered ineffective after a trial period of only 24 to 48 h. Serum quinidir levels are also readily available and should be followed to determine if a lack c efficacy is due to low serum levels or a nonresponse of the arrhythmia; the therapeut range is 2 to 6 μg/mL.

Adverse effects of quinidine occur in about 1/3 of patients. GI bloating and diarrhe are the most common side effects, but fever, liver disease, and thrombocytopenia hav

een seen occasionally. Digitalis blood levels may rise 2 to 4 times to toxic levels when uinidine is added to a previously well tolerated digoxin dosage regimen. It should be emembered that quinidine may cause a significant *increase* in ventricular ectopic ctivity and, by prolonging ventricular refractoriness (Q-T time), has even been implicated as a cause of sudden death due to ventricular fibrillation **(quinidine syncope).**

3. Lidocaine (a local anesthetic) is widely used IV for short-term management of lifehreatening ventricular arrhythmias. It is quickly metabolized and excreted. Lidocaine cts preferentially on ischemic tissue to decrease the rate of rise of the action potential nd to decrease the slow but spontaneous diastolic depolarization in Purkinje fibers. Generally, it has little effect on sinus activity, but may depress sinus node function in ome patients with sinus node disease. Although it is not effective orally, it is almost ompletely bioavailable when given IM into deltoid tissue.

Administration and dosage: For acute ventricular arrhythmia (especially in patients vith acute MI): An initial rapid IV dose is given of 1 to 2 mg/kg (the usual dose is 75 o 100 mg). For further effect, doses of 1 mg/kg IV (50 to 75 mg) may be repeated at - to 5-min intervals for 2 or 3 additional doses to a maximum of 325 to 375 mg or ntil undesirable CNS side effects occur. If the drug is effective and continued suppresion is required, it is given by continuous IV infusion at 2 mg/min. If arrhythmia eappears, small additional IV doses are required to achieve an adequate therapeutic evel, and the infusion rate may be increased gradually to 4 mg/min. Effective plasma oncentration is 2 to 5 μg/mL, although high concentrations (8 to 10 μg/mL) may ccasionally have a therapeutic effect without severe toxicity. Lidocaine should be topped and IV **procainamide** begun if signs of CNS toxicity begin to develop or VPBs re uncontrolled (see above). Although one drug will be effective in 98% of patients vith MI, in nonresponders lidocaine and procainamide may be used concurrently.

Toxicity: CNS toxicity is most common, characterized by circumoral paresthesias, ransient auditory disturbances, drowsiness, delirium, muscle twitching, and, finally, eizures. Cardiovascular toxicity is uncommon, but occasionally the drug induces sinus radycardia, A-V block, and rarely it depresses myocardial contractility. The drug is apidly cleared by the liver and metabolized by hepatic microsomes. Elimination is ensitive to alteration in hepatic blood flow; $t_{1/2}$ is prolonged in patients with MI or eart failure, or in elderly patients with reduced hepatic blood flow. In renal disease, idocaine metabolites may accumulate causing CNS toxicity.

4. Tocainide (produced by slight modification of the lidocaine molecule) is effective rally, generally to treat the same arrhythmias as lidocaine. The electrophysiologic and emodynamic effects are similar to those of lidocaine. Neither myocardial depression or hypotension appear to result from use of the drug. **Administration**: Initially 400 mg s given orally q 8 h, with cautious increase to 600 to 800 mg q 8 h. The therapeutic lasma level is 6 to 12 μg/mL. If the drug is effective, reduction to bid dosage may be ttempted. The drug appears to be well tolerated with dose-related adverse reactions imilar to those of lidocaine (see above); these effects usually occur with higher dosges and especially at the time of peak drug concentration. If the drug is given at nealtime, smaller peaks in blood concentration will result. Some patients may experince GI upset. Some reports suggest drug-induced lupus including glomerulonephritis.

5. Disopyramide is effective for chronic suppression of ventricular arrhythmia. Elecrophysiologic effects are similar to those of quinidine and procainamide. **Administraion**: A loading dose of 300 to 400 mg orally will rapidly produce therapeutic levels. he maintenance dose is 400 to 600 mg/day in divided doses, usually 100 to 150 mg q h. The therapeutic plasma level is 3 to 8 μg/mL.

Disopyramide has significant negative inotropic effects that are dose-dependent and

especially pronounced in patients with pre-existing ventricular dysfunction. Although cardiac depression is uncommon, heart failure may occur with high dosage, even in patients with apparently normal hearts. Disopyramide can markedly slow sinus rate in patients with sinus node disorders and should be used cautiously in patients with myocardiopathy. It also induces vasoconstriction, probably from a direct effect on smooth muscle. The drug has a powerful anticholinergic effect; changes in bowel habits and urinary retention are common, especially in elderly patients, and it has been associated with acute glaucoma.

6. Propranolol, the β-blocker most extensively used in treating arrhythmias, affects the ventricular myocardium both directly and reflexly. It prolongs conduction, action potential duration, and refractoriness, and also raises the threshhold for VF with significant effects on A-V nodal conduction and the incidence of ventricular ectopic activity. Propranolol is used either orally or IV to treat paroxysmal atrial tachycardia, atrial premature beats, and to slow ventricular rate in atrial fibrillation or flutter. It is not usually effective for conversion of atrial fibrillation or flutter. **Usual dosage**: Oral: 20 to 30 mg given tid or qid, may be increased to a maximum dosage of about 320 mg depending on response. IV: 0.1 mg/min is given with close hemodynamic and ECG monitoring to a total dosage of no more than 10 mg. Following therapeutic effect, maintenance is usually continued orally. **Toxic effects** largely relate to the extent of sympathetic blockade. Heart failure may be induced, limiting its use in patients with severe left ventricular dysfunction. Bradycardia is common. Prolonged A-V conduction with increased P-R time may occur. Patients with lung disease may have increased bronchospasm as a result of blockage of β_2 receptors. GI disturbance, insomnia, and nightmares may occur.

7. Phenytoin is used mainly in patients with ventricular ectopic activity caused by digitalis excess. **VPBs resulting from digitalis toxicity** should be initially treated by discontinuing digitalis and correcting the serum K if hypokalemia is present. Phenytoin 100 mg IV can be given q 5 min until CNS toxicity occurs or the VPBs are abolished. Propranolol also may help to abolish VPBs. *Hypotension should be avoided.*

Other drugs: Mexiletine, amiodarone, and flecainide have recently been approved for use in the USA; experience with them is limited, serious toxic effects may occur, and their value in the treatment of arrhythmia is yet to be determined.

Mexiletine is a congener of lidocaine with many similar properties and electrophysiologic effects. It does not interact with the autonomic nervous system. It may increase A-V nodal conduction occasionally. **Indications** include acute and chronic ventricular arrhythmias, Wolff-Parkinson-White syndrome, and it is occasionally effective in other supraventricular arrhythmias. **Administration**: 200 to 400 mg is given orally q 6 to 8 h. Its therapeutic serum level is 0.5 to 2.0 μg/mL. **Toxicity**: The drug depresses myocardial contractility, thus reducing mean arterial pressure, especially in patients with pre-existing ventricular dysfunction. It occasionally induces mild GI distress and may have CNS toxicity similar to lidocaine with high dosage. Adverse effects occur in 30% of patients and require discontinuation of drug in about 15%.

Flecainide has electrophysiologic effects similar to lidocaine and appears to be an effective agent for APBs and ventricular arrhythmia. It prolongs P-R and QRS intervals, but does not change sinus rate or prolong Q-T time. It depresses left ventricular function in experimental animals. **Administration**: 200 to 600 mg/day is given orally bid. Fewer side effects are observed with doses $\leq$ 400 mg/day. Arrhythmia suppression occurs with serum levels of 0.4 to 1.6 μg/mL. **Toxic effects** have included blurred vision, tinnitus, sleepiness, paresthesias, occasionally symptomatic bradycardia, and myocardial depression.

For amiodarone administration, see under Ventricular Fibrillation, below.

Experimental antiarrhythmic drugs available in the USA should probably be reserved for patients with malignant and life-threatening arrhythmias until clinical efficacy and toxicity are clearly established.

PAROXYSMAL SUPRAVENTRICULAR TACHYCARDIA

(Paroxysmal Atrial Tachycardia [PAT]; Paroxysmal Nodal Tachycardia)

A condition in which the heart rate suddenly increases to 100 to 200 beats/min and 1:1 A-V conduction is maintained (see TABLE 27–3).

Pathophysiology

Intracardiac electrocardiography has shown that paroxysmal atrial and paroxysmal nodal tachycardias are the same and are initiated and maintained by atrial reentry via the A-V node. The arrhythmia develops spontaneously when a single atrial depolarization enters the A-V node during a specific portion of its relative refractory period. Because the impulse is propagating very slowly toward the ventricles, this physiologically slowed conduction through the A-V node allows the impulse to be reflected back to the chamber of its origin and to reenter the atrium. Although most patients use the A-V node and perinodal tissues for both the antegrade and retrograde limbs of the reentry pathway, studies have demonstrated a variety of concealed tracts bypassing the A-V node in a retrograde direction thus suggesting a congenital basis for this electrophysiologic disorder. However conducted retrogradely, once the impulse is in the atrium, if the A-V node is again receptive, the cycle may be repeated continuously. The result is supraventricular tachycardia **(SVT).**

Any mechanism that allows A-V conduction to be significantly slowed will allow reentry within or adjacent to the A-V node and the development of paroxysmal SVT. It characteristically occurs in young persons with no evidence of organic heart disease, but may also occur in older persons with arteriosclerotic cardiovascular disease.

Symptoms and Signs

The patient with spontaneous APBs may or may not be aware of single premature beats, but at the beginning of a paroxysm the sudden, rapid, regular fluttering sensation in the chest is easily noticed. The almost simultaneous diastolic filling of atria and

TABLE 27–3. SUPRAVENTRICULAR TACHYCARDIAS

Sinoatrial reentrant tachycardia
Intraatrial reentrant tachycardia
Automatic atrial tachycardia
Atrial tachycardia with or without block (Paroxysmal atrial tachycardia)
Chaotic atrial tachycardia
Atrioventricular nodal reentrant tachycardia
Slow-fast form
Fast-slow form
Atrioventricular reentrant tachycardia
Wolff-Parkinson-White reentrant tachycardia
Concealed bypass type

ventricles or a negative atrial kick results in hemodynamic derangements far mor severe than previously recognized. Paroxysmal SVT is considerably less benign tha previously thought. Most patients feel weak and faint, but true syncope is rare. Arte rial BP falls and giant atrial waves in the neck cause a feeling of tightness and palpita tions. Shortness of breath is not uncommon, and older patients may develop angin during the paroxysm. Precordial "oppression" is a common complaint even in thos without coronary disease. Polyuria often occurs during or after attacks.

Diagnosis

The ECG (Fig. 27–6) shows an atrial rate of 150 to 214 beats/min (average, 187 where each atrial impulse is conducted to the ventricles with a normal QRS morphol ogy. When P waves are seen, they are generally inverted in the inferior leads and follov the QRS complex. More frequently, however, P waves occur simultaneously with QR complexes and are difficult to discern. Paroxysmal SVT cannot be differentiated fron paroxysmal His bundle or fascicular tachycardia by the ability to discern P wave between QRS complexes, since the tachycardias may all have the same rate; the onl difference is the degree of A-V nodal conduction delay. The diagnosis is established b observing the onset of the tachycardia on the ECG, since an APB exhibits prolonge

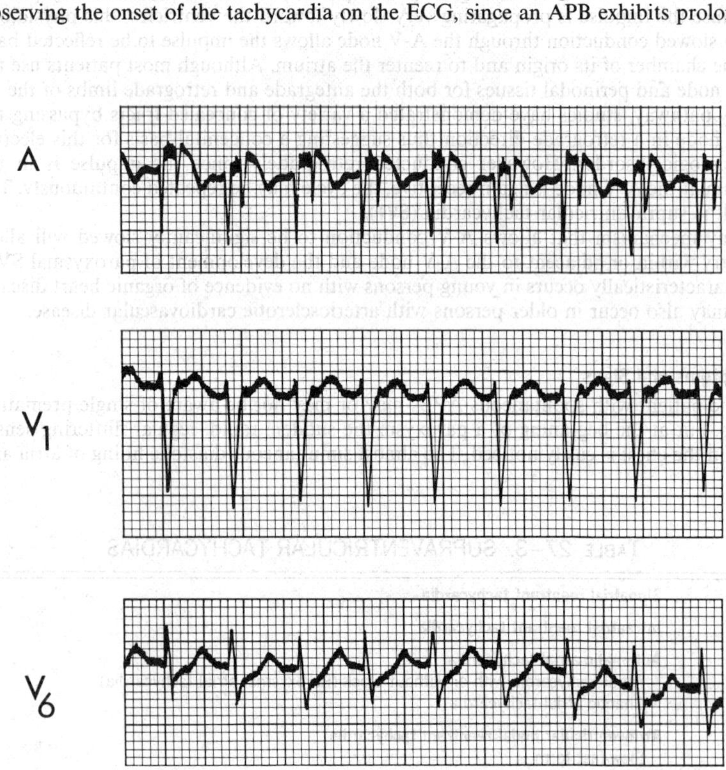

Fig. 27–6. Supraventricular tachycardia (SVT). An atrial electrogram (A) and ECG leads V_1 and V_6 a simultaneously recorded. Although P waves are not readily apparent in the ECG leads, the rapid defle tion following the QRS complex in the atrial electrogram represents the P wave. In this arrhythmia eac P wave generates the next QRS complex with a P-R interval of 240 msec.

\-V conduction and initiates SVT (FIG. 27–7), or by observing its cessation, since the ast beat of SVT is followed by a prolonged pause before the sinus rhythm resumes its lower rate (FIG. 27–8).

'reatment

In the **acute attack,** the patient should be reassured and should lie down. Significant ıypotension is the rule rather than the exception and is greatly exaggerated by the ıpright position.

Since SVT requires A-V nodal conduction for at least one limb of its re-entrant ›athway, any maneuver that prolongs or temporarily interrupts conduction via the \-V node could result in a termination of SVT. **Valsalva's maneuver** should be tried, vith ECG monitoring; gagging or vomiting may also increase vagal tone enough to nterrupt the tachycardia. In some instances, paroxysmal SVT can be simply termi-ıated with **carotid sinus massage** (providing the patient is not markedly hypotensive), .nd this should be the next therapeutic maneuver. *Atropine should always be on hand,* nd the carotid sinus should be palpated and then gently massaged before firm mas-age is applied. When carotid sinus massage is effective, the rate of the SVT slows lightly and then there is a long pause, after which sinus rhythm resumes.

If carotid sinus massage is ineffective, **verapamil,** a slow channel blocking antiar-hythmic drug that has potent effects on A-V nodal conduction, may be specific. ;tudies suggest it is effective both in patients with standard A-V nodal re-entrant SVT .s well as those with concealed bypass tracts. Given IV, it has become the treatment of hoice for rapid termination of paroxysmal SVT; 5 mg are given q 20 to 30 min, vatching for A-V block and hypotension. Up to 3 doses may be given if necessary. Iowever, long-term prophylaxis is less effective. **Edrophonium** IV is also an effective .gent to terminate SVT. Again, with atropine close at hand, a 1-mg test dose is given. f there is no idiosyncratic reaction, 10 mg IV is then given rapidly. The anticholines-erase effect of this drug allows acetylcholine to build up at the A-V node and thus nds many episodes of SVT.

When the patient is hypotensive, vagal maneuvers may be insufficient to interrupt ›aroxysmal SVT because of sympathetic nervous system overactivity. Propranolol (1 ɔ 5 mg IV) has also been advocated in the emergency therapy of SVT. Its depressant ffect on A-V nodal conduction and rapid onset of action when given IV make it an xcellent choice. Caution is advised when propranolol is given in the presence of ompromised left ventricular function or significant hypotension. Most cardiologists vould cardiovert if verapamil, edrophonium, and vagal maneuvers fail, and not go on ɔ another drug therapy.

If these emergency procedures fail, the patient may either be digitalized or treated vith cardioversion and should be hospitalized. For the younger patient whose hemo-lynamic function is not seriously compromised by a sustained rate of 180 beats/min,

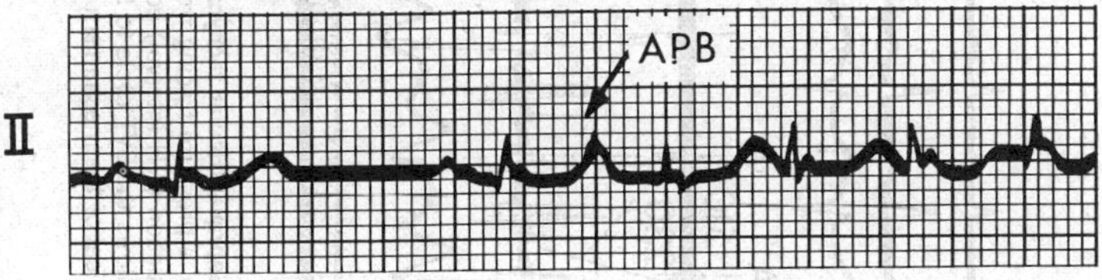

FIG. 27–7. Onset of supraventricular tachycardia (SVT). In ECG lead II, 2 normal sinus beats are ›llowed by an atrial premature depolarization (APB), which distorts the T wave of the 2nd sinus beat. 'his APB shows prolonged A-V conduction and initiates an episode of sustained SVT with a cycle length ' 340 msec (rate, 160 beats/min).

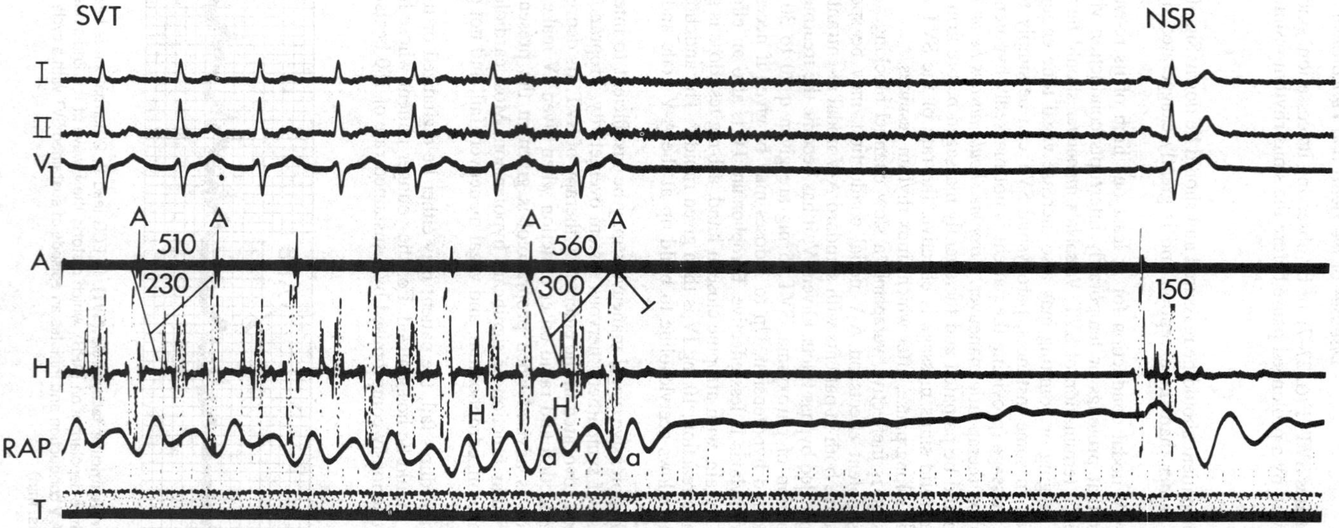

Fig. 27–8. Supraventricular tachycardia (SVT) terminated by Valsalva's maneuver. Recorded are ECG leads I, II, and V_1, an atrial electrogram (A), a His bundle electrogram (H), a pressure tracing from the right atrium (RAP), and time marks at 10-, 100-, and 1000-msec intervals. During SVT at a cycle length of 510 msec, A-V nodal conduction (A-H interval) equals 230 msec. During Valsalva's maneuver, the release of acetylcholine at the A-V node prolongs A-V nodal conduction to 300 msec and slows the SVT cycle to 560 msec, thereby terminating the arrhythmia. There is a 1.5-second pause before normal sinus rhythm (NSR) resumes. This sequence is typical of the mechanism by which any vagally mediated maneuver terminates SVT.

ligitalization is the therapy of choice. Digoxin 0.5 mg IV, followed by 0.25 mg IV q 4 o 6 h usually results in resumption of sinus rhythm. Immediate DC cardioversion is dvisable if the patient is older or hemodynamically compromised by the SVT or if schemic chest pain is present. For cardioversion, anteroposterior paddles are sugested and the amount of electrical energy required may be only 10 to 50 watt-seconds. n all patients with paroxysmal SVT, a temporary atrial pacemaker may be used to nitiate APBs, which render the A-V node refractory and thereby immediately termiate SVT. The electrical conversion of SVT by programmed atrial stimulation is uniormly successful and essentially without risk. Single atrial premature depolarizations r atrial pacing at rates in excess of SVT are equally effective. Implantable permanent acemakers with circuits designed to sense and convert episodes of SVT by prorammed stimulation have been used in patients with frequently occurring or refracory SVT.

ATRIAL ECTOPIC TACHYCARDIA (AET)

tiology and Pathophysiology

Generally nonparoxysmal, these atrial tachycardias tend to occur in persons with rganic heart disease—especially those with hypokalemia, digitalis excess (PAT with lock—see below), or myo- or pericarditis—and following overingestion of alcohol.

In contrast to paroxysmal SVTs, AETs *are* the result of a rapidly firing automatic ocus located within the atrial myocardium. Premature beats initiating these tachycarlias usually occur late in the atrial cycle and arise well outside the refractory period of he A-V node. Since their rate is totally unrelated to A-V conduction, drugs or maneuers affecting A-V nodal conduction do not stop AETs, but may produce varying legrees of A-V block.

ymptoms, Signs, and Diagnosis

Although the atrial rate of AETs is similar to that seen in paroxysmal SVT, the enerally present 2:1 A-V block tends to lessen symptoms. Patients with 1:1 A-V onduction experience symptoms identical to those of paroxysmal SVT.

A rapid, regular atrial rate of 150 to 214 is seen on the ECG. Because depolarization loes not originate within the sinus node, the P waves are abnormal in contour. Alhough occasionally difficult to diagnose, in general AET may be distinguished from VT even when 1:1 A-V conduction is present. In AET the rate is not a function of -V conduction, PR intervals tend to be < 50% of the cycle length (short), and discrete waves are seen preceding each QRS complex. In SVT atrial and ventricular depolarzations occur almost simultaneously, since the PR interval is so long (> 60% of the ycle length) and discrete P waves are rarely seen.

Absolute distinction between SVT and AET is possible using vagal maneuvers. With n AET, these will produce increasing A-V block, Wenckebach periods, and 2:1 or 3:1 -V conduction without altering the atrial rate (FIG. 27–9). The tachycardia continues nabated despite A-V block because these arrhythmias are unrelated to A-V nodal onduction.

If the ECG captures the initiating atrial premature depolarization, one can see that t occurs late in the atrial cycle, well past the relative refractory period of the A-V ode. The tachycardia then demonstrates the "warm-up" phenomenon characteristic f pacemakers, in that subsequent atrial cycles increase in rapidity until the eventual ycle length of the tachycardia is established.

reatment

AETs are unresponsive to vagal maneuvers and to therapy designed to increase A-V odal refractoriness, but they respond to drugs that suppress atrial automaticity. These

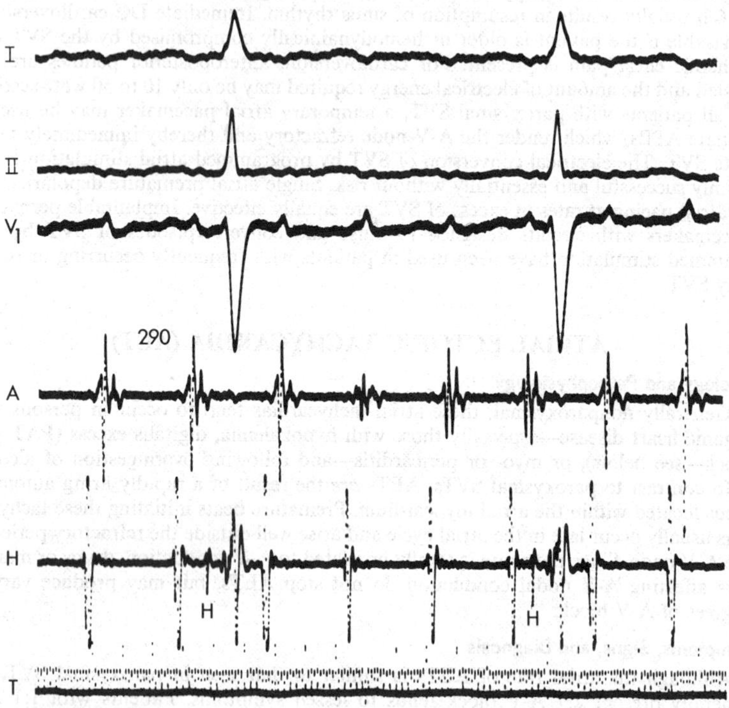

FIG. 27–9. Atrial tachycardia with block. Recorded are ECG leads I, II, and V_1, an atrial electrograr (A), a His bundle electrogram (H), and time marks at 10- and 100-msec intervals. The atrial cycle lengt is 290 msec (a rate slightly above 200 beats/min). A 4 : 1 A-V nodal block is present, since depolariza tion of the His bundle follows only every 4th atrial beat.

include quinidine, procainamide, and propranolol (given as for APBs, see above), bu not phenytoin or lidocaine. AETs can neither be initiated nor terminated by singl stimulated premature beats nor terminated by rapid atrial stimulation (eg, overdriv suppression). Although cardioversion may temporarily convert the patient's rhythm t sinus, a suppressant drug must be used to prevent AET from recurring.

ATRIAL ECTOPIC TACHYCARDIA WITH BLOCK
(PAT with Block)

All AETs may demonstrate A-V block, but the designation **PAT with block** is gener ally used when digitalis excess is the cause. Since digitalis acts to prolong A-V conduc tion, these atrial tachycardias always demonstrate at least 2:1 A-V nodal block (FIG 27–9). The mechanism and diagnosis is as described above, but **treatment** differs. Sinc the ventricular response in PAT with block is generally fairly slow, simply waiting fo the digitalis level to fall often allows the arrhythmia to end spontaneously. Giving K will speed this sequence of events. Both quinidine and procainamide (see treatment c ventricular premature beats, above) can be used if discontinuing digitalis does not en the tachycardia, but cardioversion is **contraindicated** for PAT with block since *th presence of digitalis excess may result in life-threatening ventricular arrhythmias.*

ATRIAL FLUTTER

An arrhythmia wherein continuous electrical activity within the atrium is organized into gular cyclic waves with a cycle length of about 200 msec, producing an atrial rate ·tween 240 and 400 (about 300).

iology

Atrial flutter (much less common than atrial fibrillation) may occur in any organic :art disease, but particularly in arteriosclerotic heart disease, myocardial infarction, ıeumatic heart disease, and inflammatory diseases of the atrium. In some patients rial flutter is paroxysmal, and without known cause.

ıthophysiology and Diagnosis

The mechanism of atrial flutter has long been debated, but electrophysiologic evi- :nce from both human and canine studies strongly suggests that atrial flutter is itiated by single atrial premature beats occurring during the relative refractory pe- ɔd of the atrial myocardium. As a result, the slow spread of atrial excitation through fractory muscle results in continuous atrial electrical reentry, via ordinary atrial yocardium. Direct recordings from inside the atrium demonstrate regular atrial ac- vity with a fixed periodicity and an isoelectric segment between atrial cycles. Atrial ıtter is probably independent of both the S-A and the A-V nodes for its maintenance. nce perpetration of atrial flutter requires re-entry via ordinary atrial myocardium, e atrial excitation waves in flutter must approximate the cycle length of the arrhyth- ıa itself, the ECG appearance is one of a regular saw-tooth base line, particularly in e inferior leads where continuous atrial electrical activity is usually seen (FIG. '–10). This, plus determining that an atrial rate between 240 and 400 exists with a gular cycle length, is diagnostic. Since maintenance of the arrhythmia does not de- :nd on A-V nodal conduction, some degree of A-V block is always present (FIG. '–11). This may be 2:1, 4:1, or less commonly 3:1 or 5:1. Atrial flutter with 1:1 A-V ınduction may be a life-threatening arrhythmia since ventricular rates of 300/min are ıcountered. These extremely rapid ventricular rates are generally the result of some rm of A-V nodal bypass tract. Atrial flutter with high degrees of A-V block *in the ·sence of digitalis* suggests intrinsic A-V nodal pathology, and conduction may not be ɔrmal when sinus rhythm is restored.

Since atrial flutter generally occurs at a rate of 300 and the usual degree of block in e undigitalized patient is 2:1, the ventricular response is 150. If the characteristic w-tooth does not appear on the ECG, it is difficult to distinguish sinus tachycardia, rial tachycardia with 1:1 conduction, and atrial flutter with 2:1 conduction. **Carotid ıus massage** can be useful. If the degree of A-V block can be increased from 2:1 to 1, diagnostic saw-tooth flutter waves will appear.

Symptoms, signs, and treatment are discussed below under atrial fibrillation.

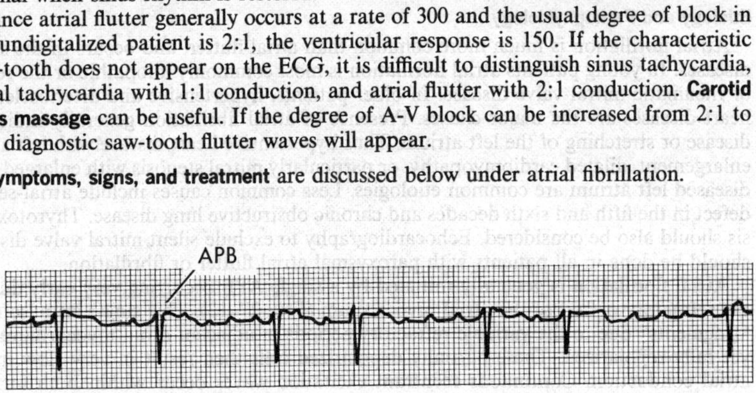

FIG. 27–10. Onset of atrial flutter. ECG lead V_1 is recorded. Following the 2nd normal sinus beat, an ·ial premature depolarization (APB) with a coupling interval of 140 msec initiates a sustained atrial ·thm with a cycle length of 200 msec (rate, 300 beats/min) and variable A-V block.

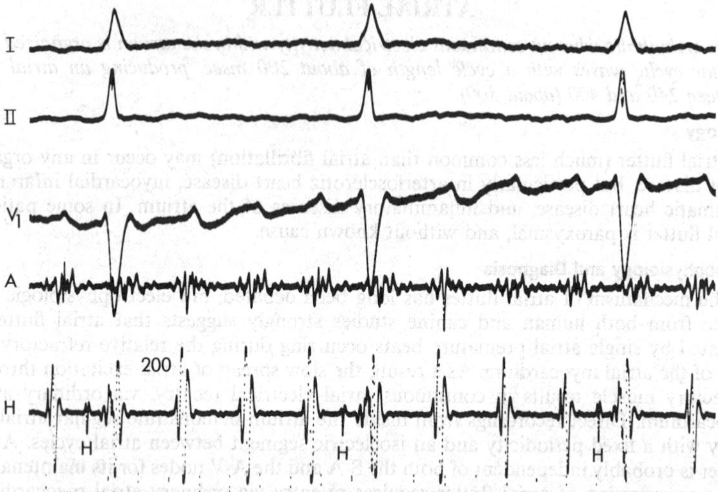

FIG. 27–11. Recordings during atrial flutter. Recorded are ECG leads I, II, and V_1, an atrial electr gram (A), a His bundle electrogram (H), and time marks at 10- and 100-msec intervals. Note the broa notched, but regular atrial depolarizations at a cycle length of 200 msec (rate, 300 beats/min); 4 A-V nodal block exists, since depolarization of the His bundle occurs only after every 4th flutter wav

ATRIAL FIBRILLATION

An arrhythmia that results from continuous, chaotic reentry of electrical impulses with the atrial myocardium. Since electrical activity is continuous and chaotic, it is difficu to discuss an atrial rate, but recordings from inside the atrium demonstrate rap activity at cycle lengths between 100 and 200 msec (FIG. 27–12).

Etiology and Pathophysiology

Atrial fibrillation is much more common than atrial flutter, and occurs in the san diseases. In young patients atrial fibrillation is most commonly idiopathic or the resu of rheumatic mitral valve disease. In older patients, hypertensive and arterioscleroti heart diseases are the major causes. Presence of atrial fibrillation generally indicat disease or stretching of the left atrium. Thus hypertensive heart disease with left atri enlargement, dilated cardiomyopathy, or particularly mitral stenosis with enlarged an diseased left atrium are common etiologies. Less common causes include atrial-sept defect in the fifth and sixth decades and chronic obstructive lung disease. Thyrotoxic sis should also be considered. Echocardiography to exclude silent mitral valve disea should be done in all patients with paroxysmal atrial flutter or fibrillation.

Atrial fibrillation is generally initiated by a single APB occurring very early duri the refractory period of the atrial myocardium (FIG. 27–13). This single impulse th "fragments" due to the variable refractory periods of adjacent atrial myocardium n yet fully repolarized. These partially depolarized cells then result in very slow intr atrial conduction. Continuous reentrant excitation waves occur within both atria excitability and refractoriness vary enough from one portion of atrial myocardium the next. The arrhythmia depends on a disparity between refractoriness and condu tion velocity in various parts of the atrium, and, therefore, significant atrial myocardi disease must exist. The mechanism is independent of S-A or A-V nodal reentry, an

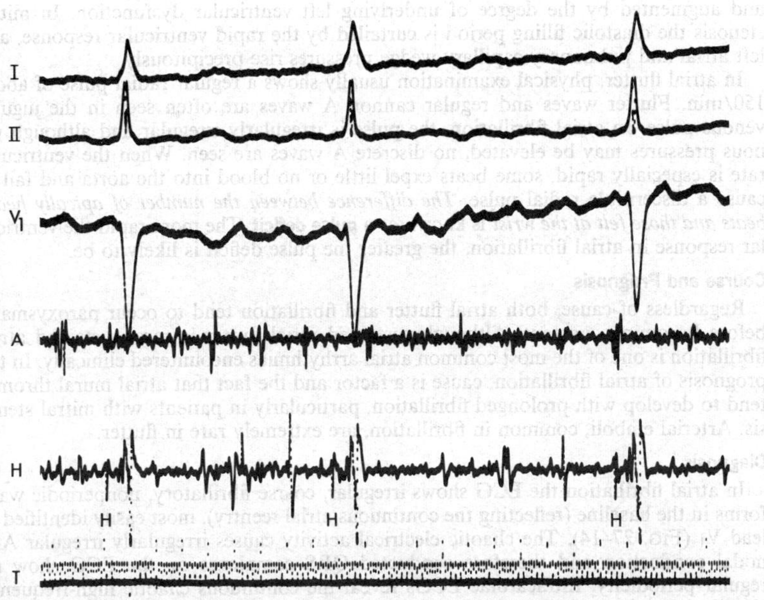

FIG. 27–12. Recordings during atrial fibrillation. Recorded are ECG leads I, II, and V_1, an atrial electrogram (A), a His bundle electrogram (H), and time marks at 10- and 100-msec intervals. Electrical activity within the atrial electrogram shows no regularity. A chaotic continuous series of wave fronts occurs within the atrium, which represents atrial fibrillation. Each QRS complex is preceded by depolarization of the His bundle, indicating the supraventricular origin of each QRS complex.

maneuvers or drugs affecting A-V nodal conduction will not change the basic rate of atrial fibrillation, although they diminish the ventricular response.

Symptoms and Signs

At the onset of both flutter and fibrillation, symptoms are generally similar to those of paroxysmal tachycardia except that the patient is frequently aware of an irregularly irregular pulse. Palpitations, near-syncope, pallor, nausea, weakness, lightheadedness, and fatigue occur in atrial fibrillation because the ventricular response is rapid and irregular. When cardiac reserve is extremely limited by left ventricular disease or in severe mitral stenosis, cardiogenic shock or acute pulmonary edema may occur. The severity of symptoms is directly proportional to the rapidity of the ventricular response

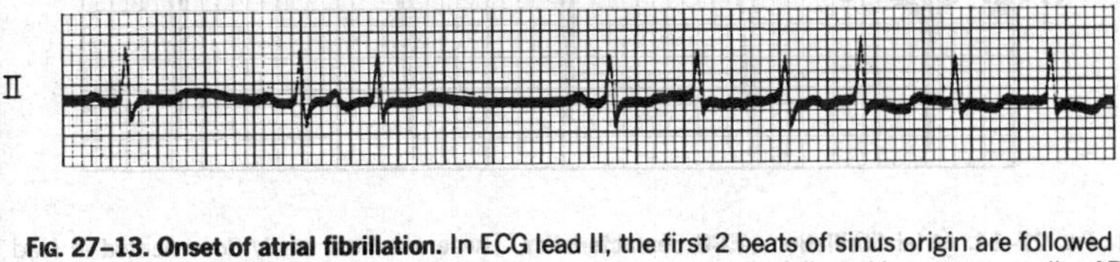

FIG. 27–13. Onset of atrial fibrillation. In ECG lead II, the first 2 beats of sinus origin are followed by a single atrial premature beat (APB). Sinus rhythm resumes only to be followed by an even earlier APB, which initiates the episode of atrial fibrillation.

and augmented by the degree of underlying left ventricular dysfunction. In mitra stenosis the diastolic filling period is curtailed by the rapid ventricular response, anc left atrial and pulmonary capillary wedge pressures rise precipitously.

In atrial flutter, physical examination usually shows a regular radial pulse of abou 150/min. Flutter waves and regular cannon A waves are often seen in the jugulai venous pulse. In atrial fibrillation, the pulse is irregularly irregular and although ve- nous pressures may be elevated, no discrete A waves are seen. When the ventriculai rate is especially rapid, some beats expel little or no blood into the aorta and fail tc cause a discernible radial pulse. *The difference between the number of apically heard beats and those felt at the wrist* is known as a **pulse deficit**. The more rapid the ventricu- lar response in atrial fibrillation, the greater the pulse deficit is likely to be.

Course and Prognosis

Regardless of cause, both atrial flutter and fibrillation tend to occur paroxysmally before becoming constant. Although sustained atrial flutter is rare, sustained atria fibrillation is one of the most common atrial arrhythmias encountered clinically. In the prognosis of atrial fibrillation, cause is a factor and the fact that atrial mural thromb tend to develop with prolonged fibrillation, particularly in patients with mitral steno- sis. Arterial emboli, common in fibrillation, are extremely rare in flutter.

Diagnosis

In atrial fibrillation the ECG shows irregular, coarse fibrillatory, nonperiodic wave forms in the baseline (reflecting the continuous atrial reentry), most easily identified in lead V_1 (FIG. 27–14). The chaotic electrical activity causes irregularly irregular A-V nodal conduction and therefore conducted QRS complexes on the ECG show no regular periodicity. Intracardiac ECGs reveal the continuous chaotic high-frequency electrical activity with no isoelectric segment (FIG. 27–12).

Treatment

The primary aim of therapy in atrial fibrillation and in atrial flutter is to slow the ventricular response, thereby increasing the CO. If the patient shows evidence of se- vere cardiac compromise (eg, shock or pulmonary edema), it is best to stop the ar- rhythmia immediately by **DC cardioversion,** but if the rapid ventricular response is wel tolerated, digitalis therapy is recommended. **Digitalis** decreases the ventricular response by slowing A-V conduction, and occasionally will convert flutter or fibrillation intc regular sinus rhythm. More often, after the patient is fully digitalized and the ventricu- lar response acceptably slowed, **quinidine sulfate** 300 to 400 mg q 6 h or **procainamide** 1 gm q 6 h is given to convert fibrillation to sinus rhythm; these drugs are effective in 50% of patients. If 3 days of such therapy does not convert the arrhythmia and the fibrillation has not been protracted, digitalis should be withheld for 24 h, and then DC

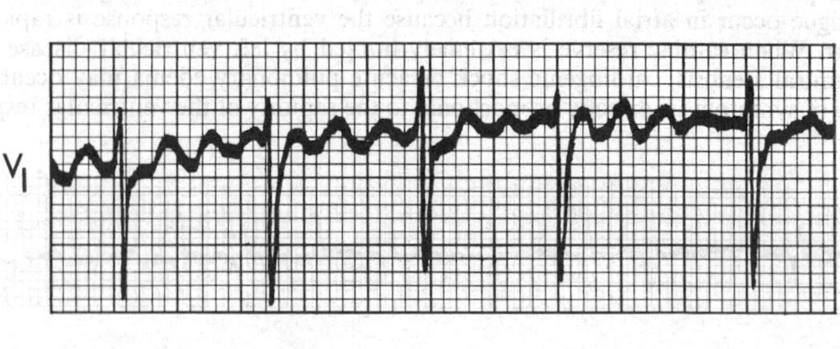

FIG. 27–14. Atrial fibrillation—ECG characteristics. These are most easily documented in lead V where irregular waves of varying amplitude and frequency demonstrate the rhythm to be due to atria fibrillation.

cardioversion should be attempted. If atrial fibrillation has been present for > 6 mo or the left atrium is large, maintenance of sinus rhythm is unlikely, and attempts to convert with drugs or DC cardioversion are unsuccessful and should not be attempted in most instances.

For the occasional patient in whom digitalis does not effectively slow the ventricular response, and if heart failure is not a therapeutic problem, **propranolol** 0.5 to 1 mg/min IV for a total dose of 2 mg generally decreases the ventricular response to a rate < 100 and occasionally converts atrial fibrillation to sinus rhythm directly. Occasionally large doses may be necessary, but monitoring for the development of high-grade A-V block is mandatory. **Verapamil** may be extremely useful in paroxysmal atrial flutter or fibrillation both because of its effects on atrial myocardium directly and also because its profound slowing of A-V nodal conduction results in a slower ventricular response when fibrillation occurs. Verapamil, however, does not usually convert atrial fibrillation to sinus rhythm but, in contrast to digoxin, will slow the ventricular rate both at rest and exercise.

Once atrial flutter or fibrillation is ended, therapy is given to prevent recurrences. Quinidine, propranolol, and procainamide, in that order, are the drugs of choice, and should be continued for as long as the underlying cause of the atrial fibrillation exists.

The hazard of releasing arterial emboli during cardioversion for atrial fibrillation is probably not significantly greater than the risk of emboli from the fibrillation itself. Because this hazard exists if fibrillation was present for > 1 wk, however, many believe that 3 wk of anticoagulant therapy should precede cardioversion, especially if the patient has had a prior arterial embolus. The need for cardioversion and for anticoagulant therapy must be determined for each patient. A maintained sinus rhythm is less likely to follow cardioversion (1) the longer the atrial fibrillation has lasted, (2) the worse the atrial myocardial disease, (3) the larger the atrial muscle mass, (4) the worse the predisposing coronary artery disease, and (5) in the presence of inflammation or infarction. The hemodynamic advantages of sinus rhythm over atrial fibrillation with a well-controlled ventricular response are generally small except in the presence of severe valvular disease when atrial transport can augment resting CO up to 20%, but in patients with atrial fibrillation the best prophylaxis against arterial emboli is conversion to and maintenance of sinus rhythm.

MULTIFOCAL ATRIAL TACHYCARDIA (MAT)

An arrhythmia that results from multiple areas of enhanced automaticity within ordinary atrial myocardium.

The underlying rhythm, generally sinus or sinus tachycardia, is interrupted by frequent atrial premature depolarizations **(APBs)** that occur singly, in pairs, or often in salvos of 3 to 15 beats. The P wave morphology varies greatly from beat to beat as does A-V conduction. These salvos occur without sequence or specific repetitive pattern and result in periods of rapid, irregular heart action. MAT is often a precursor of atrial fibrillation.

Etiology and Pathophysiology

Although MAT may occur with all forms of heart disease, it is most common in patients with severe chronic lung disease, respiratory insufficiency, and/or theophylline excess. An acute exacerbation of underlying respiratory illness is the most common predisposing factor to the development of MAT.

Atrial irritability is enhanced by pulmonary hypertension with elevated right atrial pressures and right atrial stretch. This, combined with systemic hypoxemia, the use of sympathomimetics in treating lung disease, and/or elevated theophylline levels, results in multiple areas of enhanced automaticity within ordinary atrial myocardium. These

multiple abnormal atrial pacemaker cells fire singly or in salvos, thus producing the characteristic pattern of MAT.

Symptoms, Signs, and Diagnosis

MAT is usually asymptomatic; symptoms of the underlying lung disease predominate. Sustained rapid heart rates, however, may exacerbate left ventricular dysfunction precipitated by hypoxemia, resulting in overall worsening of the cardiopulmonary status.

MAT is generally distinguishable from atrial fibrillation by finding discrete irregular and multiform atrial activity preceding each QRS complex. Irregular rates of 100 to 180 beats/min are common, and intracardiac ECGs merely reflect the varying atrial depolarization sequence engendered by various foci of abnormal atrial automaticity. Since patients with MAT generally have a high level of sympathetic nervous system activity (intrinsic or iatrogenic), vagal maneuvers generally do not result in A-V block or a slowing of ventricular response in MAT.

Treatment

The treatment of MAT should be directed at correcting its underlying cause rather than at the rhythm itself. Ventilatory assistance in patients with respiratory insufficiency, hypoxemia, and hypercapnia may be mandatory. If the patient is receiving aminophylline or a similar drug, theophylline levels should be monitored. Digitalis may be helpful in treating the overall cardiopulmonary state, but is of no specific advantage in treating MAT and may facilitate onset of atrial fibrillation. Similarly, antiarrhythmics (eg, quinidine or procainamide) are generally less effective in converting MAT than is correction of the underlying lung disease. β-Blockers are specifically to be *avoided* because of their tendency to increase bronchospasm and worsen the patient's respiratory status.

HIS BUNDLE RHYTHMS

Arrhythmias that result from sustained enhanced automaticity within the bundle of His.

Junctional rhythms of rates from 70 to 150 may arise due to spontaneous Phase IV diastolic depolarization (enhanced automaticity) within the bundle of His or the subsequent branching portions of the interventricular conducting system. These ectopic tachycardias are generally nonparoxysmal and tend to be relatively short-lasting. They result in normal impulse propagation through the ventricles and hence a QRS of normal duration and morphology. Generally, 1:1 retrograde conduction across the A-V node is present.

His bundle rhythms and tachycardia may occur in ischemic heart disease, acute myocardial infarction, rheumatic heart disease, or digitalis excess.

Symptoms, Signs, and Diagnosis

The patient may be totally asymptomatic or may be aware of a rapid beat; the sensation of palpitation is enhanced when 1:1 ventriculoatrial conduction results in cannon A waves felt in the neck. Carotid sinus massage may transiently slow, but not terminate, these rhythms.

On ECG (FIG. 27-15), His bundle rhythms and tachycardias are diagnosed by the regular QRS complexes of generally normal duration and morphology that are either dissociated from an atrial rhythm (ie, sinus rhythm, atrial flutter, or fibrillation) or are accompanied by 1:1 ventriculoatrial conduction. Under these circumstances, an inverted P wave may be seen early in the S-T segment, during the QRS complexes, or following the QRS in leads II, III, and aVF.

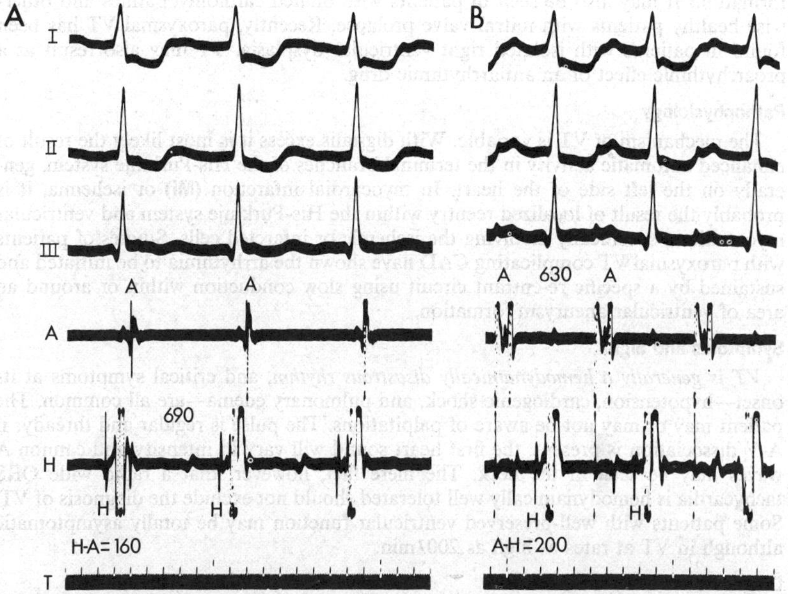

Fig. 27–15. His bundle rhythm. Recorded are ECG leads I, II, and III, an atrial electrogram (A), a His bundle electrogram (H), and time marks at 10- and 100-msec intervals.

A. A sustained rhythm with a cycle length of 690 msec is shown to originate within the bundle of His. Each QRS complex is preceded by depolarization of the His bundle and this sustained His bundle rhythm results in 1 : 1 ventriculoatrial conduction. The retrograde A-V nodal conduction time has an H-A interval of 160 msec.

B. The origin of the rhythm within the His bundle is substantiated since atrial pacing at a cycle length of 630 msec shows antegrade conduction with a normal A-H interval of 200 msec.

Treatment

Immediate cardioversion is required if His bundle tachycardias are very rapid, have resulted in cardiac compromise, and are not the result of digitalis excess. If the patient's digitalis status is unknown, or the arrhythmia is fairly well tolerated, then antiarrhythmic drugs (quinidine, procainamide, propranolol) should be given to treat and to suppress the redevelopment of these tachycardias. Correction of serum K^+ is mandatory in the presence of tachycardias. Digitalis will only increase the automatic rate of the His bundle focus and should *not* be used.

VENTRICULAR TACHYCARDIA (VT)

A regular ventricular rhythm with broad QRS complexes and a rate between 100 and 200 beats/min.

Etiology

VT may occasionally be paroxysmal in young persons without other evidence of heart disease, but it occurs most commonly in arteriosclerotic heart disease, coronary artery disease **(CAD)** with myocardial ischemia, and digitalis excess. Paroxysmal VT is generally encountered in patients with CAD complicated by ventricular aneurysm

formation. It may also be seen in patients with dilated cardiomyopathies and otherwise healthy patients with mitral valve prolapse. Recently, paroxysmal VT has been found in patients with isolated right ventricular dysplasia. VT may also result as a proarrhythmic effect of an antiarrhythmic drug.

Pathophysiology

The mechanism of VT is variable. With digitalis excess it is most likely the result of enhanced automatic activity in the terminal branches of the His-Purkinje system, generally on the left side of the heart. In myocardial infarction **(MI)** or ischemia, it is probably the result of localized reentry within the His-Purkinje system and ventricular myocardium, specifically involving the ischemic or infarcted cells. Studies of patients with paroxysmal VT complicating CAD have shown the arrhythmia to be initiated and sustained by a specific re-entrant circuit using slow conduction within or around an area of ventricular aneurysm formation.

Symptoms and Signs

VT is generally a hemodynamically disastrous rhythm, and critical symptoms at its onset—hypotension, cardiogenic shock, and pulmonary edema—are all common. The patient may or may not be aware of palpitations. The pulse is regular and thready; if A-V dissociation is present, the first heart sound will vary in intensity and cannon A waves may be seen in the neck. The mere fact, however, that a rapid wide QRS tachycardia is hemodynamically well tolerated should not exclude the diagnosis of VT. Some patients with well-preserved ventricular function may be totally asymptomatic although in VT at rates as high as 200/min.

Diagnosis

The ECG shows wide, regular QRS complexes whose rate exceeds that of the atrial rhythm (FIG. 27–16). Although ventriculoatrial conduction can occur, usually the atria remain under control of the sinus node and ⅔ of patients in VT have A-V dissociation resulting in P waves "marching through" the QRS complexes. The ventricular origin is also indicated by the presence of fusion beats (QRS morphology partly resembling the observed tachycardia and the normal) or "capture" (conduction of a dissociated P wave through the A-V node, resulting in both premature and normal ventricular depolarization). Carotid sinus massage has no effect on this tachycardia. Intracardiac ECGs demonstrate that His bundle depolarization does not precede each QRS complex, thereby establishing the more distal ventricular origin of the tachycardia.

Treatment

VT is usually a cardiac emergency. In acute MI, immediate cardioversion should be undertaken. **Lidocaine** (see in treatment of VPBs, above) is the treatment of choice if digitalis excess is a possible cause or if the patient's state of digitalization is unknown. If the VT is unresponsive to lidocaine, IV **procainamide** should be given (see treatment of VPBs, above). If VT is unresponsive to either lidocaine or procainamide, **propranolol** is given IV 1 mg q 2 to 3 min to a total dosage of 3 to 5 mg. Propranolol is *contraindicated* in bronchospastic lung disease, and, if the VT is not converted, it frequently causes a further decrease in CO and arterial BP. **Bretylium tosylate,** 300 to 600 mg IV given rapidly and 1 to 3 mg/min IV can be used for resistant VT. **Disopyramide, amiodarone, propafenone,** and **sotalol** are also effective.

In VT resulting from digitalis excess, **phenytoin** 100 mg IV q 5 min is particularly effective. (Potassium chloride and lidocaine are also useful.) Its efficacy in VT resulting from ischemia or infarction is less clear.

Once the VT has been terminated, further episodes must be prevented by continued use of a suppressive drug. Lidocaine and procainamide (in that order) are most effective in the presence of acute MI; otherwise quinidine or propranolol should be given. Several

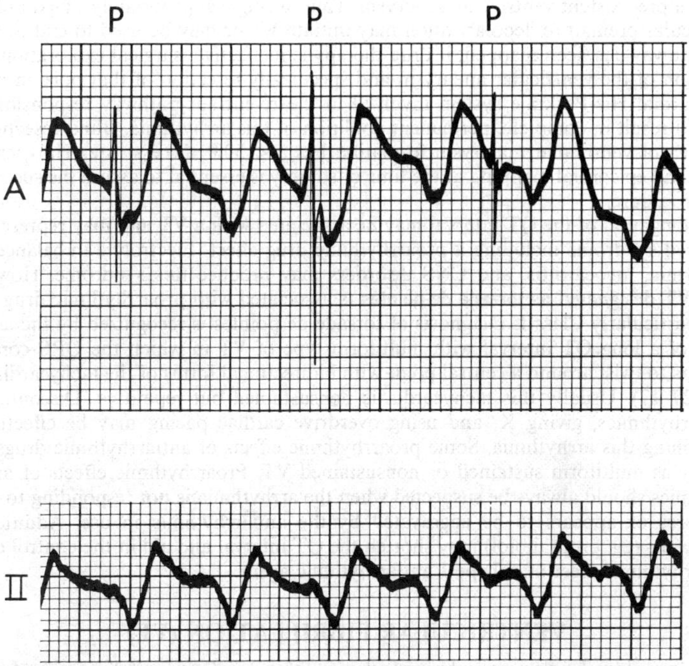

FIG. 27–16. Ventricular tachycardia—ECG characteristics. The rapid ventricular response with A-V dissociation establishes the diagnosis. An atrial electrogram (A) and ECG lead II are simultaneously recorded. Although P waves are not apparent in the ECG, the intra-atrial electrogram shows sharp spiking P waves at a regular cycle length considerably slower than those of the QRS complexes, indicating ventricular tachycardia.

new classes of antiarrhythmic drugs have recently been advocated for the treatment of paroxysmal VT unresponsive to quinidine, procainamide, or propranolol. Disopyramide phosphate may be effective, but its deleterious effect on left ventricular function must be seriously considered. Mexiletine, flecainide, tocainide, and amiodarone are Type I antiarrhythmics available for treatment of ventricular arrhythmias.

A slow channel blocking drug, **amiodarone,** has undergone extensive testing in patients with refractory VT. The agent is given orally and requires 2 to 4 wk before adequate tissue levels are achieved. An IV preparation is also available for emergency use; it is often effective in resistant cases. Its extremely slow elimination allows it to be given once/day and clinical investigations thus far show a drug efficacy far superior to any antiarrhythmic previously used on a long-term basis. *However, the drug's toxicity is potentially a serious problem* (see treatment of VF, below).

In patients with paroxysmal VT unresponsive to standard or newer antiarrhythmic drugs, serious consideration should be given to electrophysiologic investigation and cardiac surgery to correct the potentially life-threatening arrhythmias. Intracardiac electrophysiologic mapping both at the time of cardiac catheterization and heart surgery have shown that most of these patients have a specific re-entrant pathway using ordinary ventricular myocardium and a slow pathway involving the center of periph-

ery of a pre-existent ventricular aneurysm. Thus, a single appropriately timed induced ventricular premature depolarization may initiate VT or may be used to end it. Once the pathway has been mapped, if drug therapy is ineffective, surgical exploration with resection of the ventricular aneurysm and specifically resection of that portion of the endocardial His-Purkinje system involved in the re-entrant pathway responsible for VT will result in complete, permanent abolition of this arrhythmia. Blind resection of the area of ventricular aneurysm formation has a < 50% success rate. Thus, careful endo- and epicardial mapping at the time of surgery is essential to assure the success of this procedure.

Prolongation of the QT interval may be associated with a VT and may represent an acquired syndrome including a proarrhythmic drug effect. Electrolyte imbalance, hypothermia, myocarditis, and CNS disorders may produce this syndrome. However, most VT designated as **torsade de pointes** is associated with proarrhythmic drug therapy, particularly Class I. Diagnosis of torsade de pointes is recognized by the association of a long QT interval with multiform type of VT in which the QRS complex appears to twist around a central point with bidirectional forms of the tachycardia (see FIG. 27–17). Usually this tachycardia is nonsustained but repetitive. Discontinuing antiarrhythmics, giving K, and using overdrive cardiac pacing may be effective in controlling this arrhythmia. Some proarrhythmic effects of antiarrhythmic drugs also appear as multiform sustained or nonsustained VT. Proarrhythmic effects of antiarrhythmics should always be suspected when the arrhythmia is not responding to usual measures or appears to be aggravated by the antiarrhythmic in use. Addition of β-blockers (eg, propranolol) may shorten the QT interval and aid in the control of the proarrhythmic effect of a Type I antiarrhythmic agent.

VENTRICULAR FIBRILLATION (VF)

An irregular, chaotic ventricular arrhythmia with a rapid rate and disorganized spread of impulses throughout the ventricular myocardium. Since electrical activity is chaotic, ventricular systole becomes an uncoordinated event, mechanical activity cannot occur, and CO and BP fall to zero. Heart sounds become inaudible and syncope occurs,

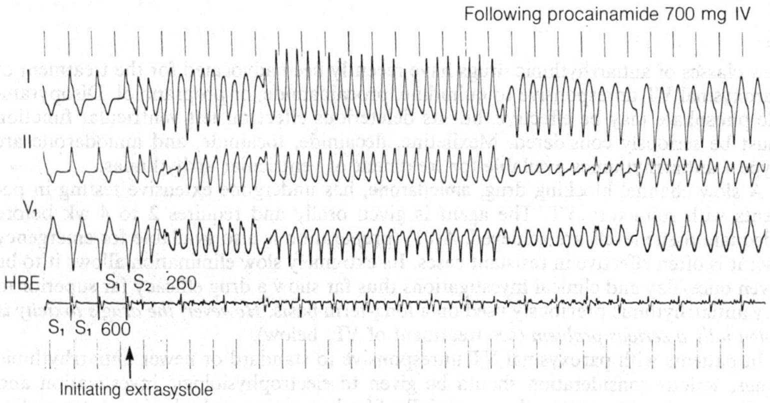

FIG. 27–17. Torsade de pointes. Following procainamide, a single extrasystole (S_2) produced a torsade.

followed within minutes by death. **VF is fatal if not immediately corrected** (see also CARDIAC ARREST AND CARDIOPULMONARY RESUSCITATION, below).

Etiology and Pathophysiology

Acute myocardial infarction **(MI)** is the most common cause although many patients with coronary artery disease have VF without a preceding infarction. VF is likely to occur within minutes and is probably the mechanism in most cases of sudden death. VF is occasionally the result of general anesthesia or of overdosage with digitalis, quinidine, or procainamide, and often accompanies drowning and electrocution.

The mechanism of VF is comparable to that of atrial fibrillation. An initiating ventricular premature beat falling during the refractory period of the ventricular myocardium results in irregular, slow, and chaotic impulse transmission throughout both ventricles. This electrical activity is maintained as multiple reentrant cycles until death supervenes (FIG. 27–18).

Diagnosis

The ECG diagnosis of VF is easy. All electrical activity is chaotic, and although the QRS complexes may initially be saw-toothed, they diminish in amplitude and increase in frequency until a wandering, erratic baseline is the only evidence of cardiac electrical activity (FIG. 27–18). If VF is not corrected, electrical activity ceases, and the ECG becomes a straight line.

Treatment

Treatment should be primarily directed at prevention, particularly in acute MI. Since VPBs herald and initiate VF, their suppression may prevent it. Prophylactic use of lidocaine may virtually abolish VF in acute MI. Should VF develop, *immediate DC defibrillation is the only effective therapy*, and must be followed by an antiarrhythmic regimen designed to prevent further episodes. **Lidocaine** and **procainamide** (see treatment of ventricular premature beats, above) are generally effective.

Bretylium tosylate has a mechanism of action unlike other antiarrhythmics and not only may prevent repetitive VF but may, under certain circumstances, chemically defibrillate the patient. Originally introduced as an antihypertensive, the drug was withdrawn because of severe side effects due to postural hypotension. It was subsequently approved by the FDA for limited use in the treatment of malignant ventricular arrhythmias; eg, refractory ventricular tachycardia or VF or in the management of difficult resuscitation in cardiac arrest. Bretylium is concentrated in the adrenergic nerve terminals resulting in initial release of norepinephrine causing a transient sympathetic effect (initial increase in sinus rate and possible proarrhythmia effect) followed by inhibition of release of neurotransmitter. The drug has no direct effect on resting action potential but does prolong the effective refractory period of ventricular muscle and Purkinje fibers. It has no direct effect on phase 4 depolarization. Bretylium increases the threshold for VF, but causes hypotension because of sympathetic block-

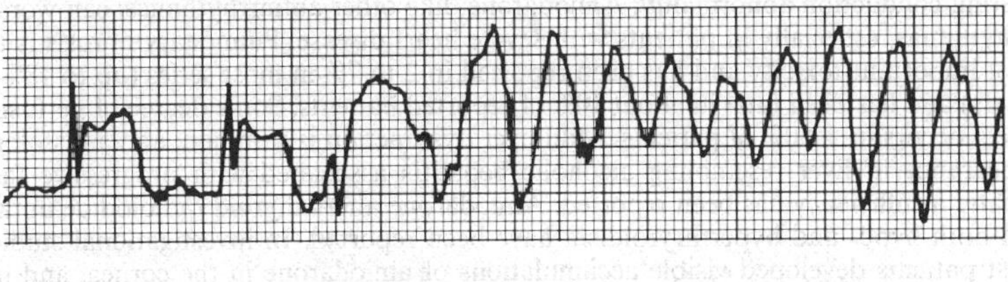

FIG. 27–18. Ventricular fibrillation. Two sinus beats in a patient with an acute inferior myocardial infarction are followed by a VPB, which initiates an episode of ventricular fibrillation.

ade, especially in upright posture. It does not depress myocardial contractility. **Administration**: Bretylium is generally given IV or IM. After an IV dose, the effect on ventricular arrhythmia may be delayed 10 to 20 min; it is usually effective within 30 min after IM injection. The initial IM dose is 5 to 10 mg/kg, which may be repeated to a total dosage of 30 mg/kg; the maintenance dosage is 5 mg/kg IM q 6 to 8 h. Given IV, the initial dose is 5 mg/kg, followed by 1 to 4 mg/min IV given as a constant infusion. Effective plasma levels are 1 to 1.5 μg/mL.

Among patients who have been revived from out-of-hospital sudden cardiac death and VF, many have not sustained an acute MI. The prognosis of this resuscitated group of patients is extremely poor; the incidence of recurrent sudden cardiac death due to VF is about 50% within 2 yr. All such patients should undergo extensive investigation of cardiac anatomy and function; echocardiography, treadmill testing, Holter monitoring, cardiac catheterization, and electrophysiologic studies with coronary arteriography are indicated. Many will demonstrate malignant ventricular ectopic activity on repeated Holter monitoring and, although not clearly established, it is suggested that they be placed on some form of antiarrhythmic therapy.

Amiodarone may be effective for the prevention of paroxysmal ventricular tachycardia, VF, and sudden cardiac death when all other drugs have failed. It is also effective for long-term treatment of recurrent paroxysmal or chronic atrial fibrillation with serious hemodynamic consequence (converts and maintains sinus rhythm) and in refractory Wolff-Parkinson-White syndrome. However, its absorption, volume of distribution, and half-life is highly variable and the half-life is extremely long (40 to 55 days in most patients), making onset and offset of antiarrhythmic activity extremely slow and unpredictable both at initiation of treatment and with dosage adjustment. Furthermore, amiodarone has the potential for very serious adverse reactions and tends to alter the kinetics of most other antiarrhythmic agents. Interactions with other drugs, particularly warfarin and digoxin, have been noted. *Because of its unpredictability, toxicity, and long half-life, amiodarone should be used only as the drug of last resort in patients with life-threatening arrhythmias.* Furthermore, it should be used only by physicians who are experienced with the drug, have access to all other available teatments for arrhythmias, and have the facilities to monitor its efficacy and toxicity.

Major antiarrhythmic action may not occur before several weeks of treatment. Amiodarone prolongs the action potential and effective refractory period of atria, ventricles, A-V node, and accessory A-V pathways. It decreases the slope of phase 4 depolarization of atrial pacemaker cells and blocks effects of sympathetic stimulation. It decreases peripheral resistance and increases coronary blood flow by direct effect, relaxing smooth muscle. Antiarrhythmic plasma levels during chronic therapy range from 1 to 5 mg/mL; steady state level may require administration for weeks. There may be active plasma metabolites. Elimination after chronic oral therapy is very slow with half-time of 40 to 55 *days*; thus, it has a long duration of action. Drug has been detected in plasma 12 mo after discontinuation. **Toxicity**: Bradycardia, A-V or bundle branch block, and severe hypotension may occur, especially in patients with preexisting conduction abnormality. Amiodarone, like other antiarrhythmics, can worsen arrhythmias, especially in patients with severe heart disease. Pulmonary fibrosis is the most important toxicity and has been reported in 2 to 7% in most series (up to 18% in others) and has been fatal in about 10% of reported patients. Some degree of perfusion defect occurs in > 50% of patients. Mild liver dysfunction is common, and a histologic appearance in liver resembling alcoholic hepatitis associated with progressive fatal hepatic insufficiency has been reported. Amiodarone alters thyroid radioiodide uptake and both hypo- and hyperthryroidism have been reported. In investigational studies, most patients developed visible accumulations of amiodarone in the cornea, and impaired vision (mostly the appearance of halos around objects) was noted in ≤ 10% of patients. Photosensitivity of the skin and blue discoloration were also common, as

were nausea, vomiting, and neurologic complaints. **Administration**: Amiodarone is usually given orally, 600 mg/day for 1 wk, followed by reduction to 200 to 400 mg/day. An initial single loading dose of 1400 mg (during the first few days of administration) may more rapidly achieve a steady state therapeutic level. Once clinical effectiveness is achieved, the aim should be to maintain the patient on the lowest possible oral dose. An IV preparation is available for emergency use; 300 to 600 mg given IV slowly over 2 to 6 h, and 300 to 600 mg IV over the next 24 h is often effective in resistant cases.

HEART BLOCK

Conditions in which the spread of cardiac electrical excitation is slowed or interrupted in a part of the normal conduction pathway.

SINOATRIAL (S-A) BLOCK

Impulse transmission is physiologically very slow in S-A node tissues (from 40 to 120 msec) because many cells within the node undergo spontaneous diastolic depolarization, and each successive cell is activated at a low resting membrane potential. Further slowing of conduction by disease results in S-A block. Impulses originating within pacemaker cells of the S-A node are initiated by normal Phase IV diastolic depolarization, but the impulse is prevented from leaving the sinus node area and exciting surrounding atrial myocardium. Thus deprived of their primary pacemaker, the atria and ventricles fail to contract unless a subsidiary pacemaker arises elsewhere within the conduction system. Subsidiary pacemakers, generally located within the bundle of His or atrial specialized conduction system, have an intrinsically slower rate of impulse generation. Depending on the degree of S-A block, either an escape beat or an escape rhythm results. Various forms of S-A block may occur and are described below.

S-A Wenckebach periods: During regular sinus rhythm, impulses emerging from the S-A node may demonstrate progressive conduction delay until one is finally blocked. Since depolarization of the S-A node is not recorded by the ECG, this form of S-A block appears as progressive shortening of the P-P interval until finally one P wave is "dropped." On ECG, 5:4, 4:3, and 3:2 Wenckebach periods may be recognized.

2:1 S-A block: The sinus node is firing at a regular rate; suddenly, alternate impulses fail to emerge from the node to excite the atrial myocardium. One sees a sudden slowing of the P wave rate, with a cycle length exactly twice that of normal sinus rhythm (FIG. 27-19). The P wave morphology must remain the same and sinus arrhythmia is minimal.

Higher degrees of S-A block: Sinus node impulses may also be blocked with a 3:1, 4:1, or 5:1 periodicity, resulting in atrial cycles 3, 4, and 5 times the length of the basic sinus rhythm.

Complete S-A block (sinus arrest): During normal sinus rhythm, P waves may suddenly stop. This condition, previously known as "sinus arrest," is much more likely to be the result of complete S-A block. Cardiac arrest will follow unless a subsidiary pacemaker (escape rhythm) develops.

Etiology

S-A block may occur in arteriosclerotic and chronic rheumatic heart disease, but is most common in patients with coronary artery disease. S-A Wenckebach periods and 2:1 S-A block are commonly the result of vagotonia or digitalis excess. The combination of digitalis and quinidine frequently gives rise to sinus node dysfunction. Hyperkalemia rarely results in S-A block, but may cause **sinoventricular rhythm**—a progressive diminution of P wave amplitude until the P waves disappear, despite the fact that pacemaker function remains within the sinus node.

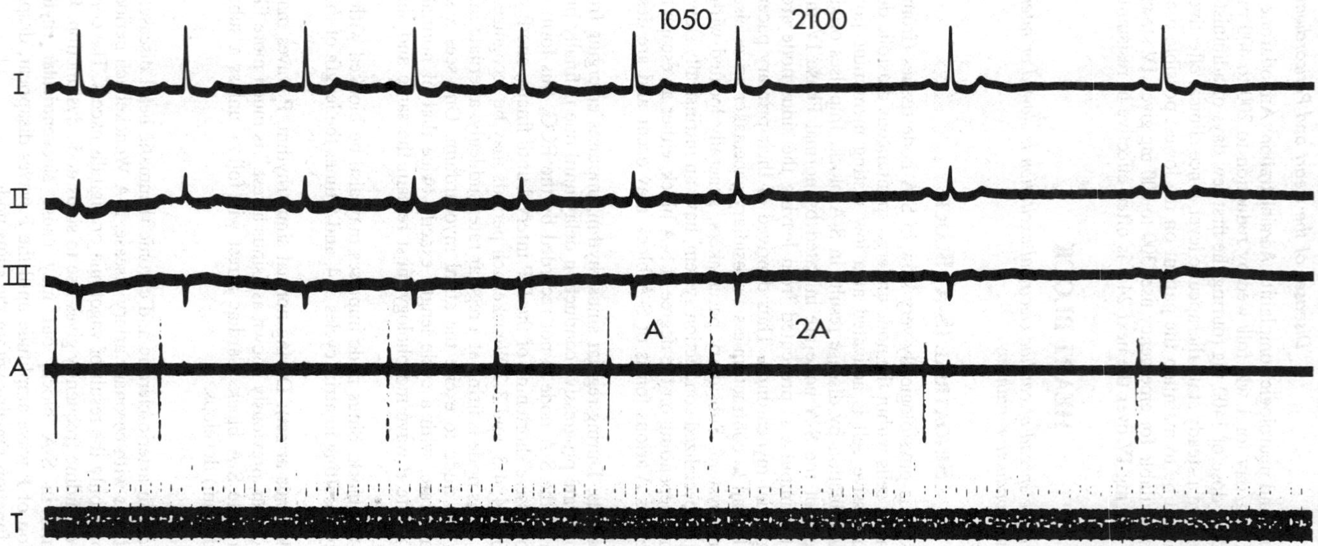

Fig. 27–19. 2:1 S-A block. Recorded are ECG leads I, II, and III, an atrial electrogram (A), and time marks at 10-, 100-, and 1000-msec intervals. During sinus bradycardia at a cycle length of 1050 msec there is a sudden doubling of the atrial cycle length to 2100 msec, as each 2nd sinus impulse fails to emerge from the sinus node.

Symptoms, Signs, and Diagnosis

S-A block is apt to be an intermittent event in elderly patients. S-A Wenckebach periods and 2:1 S-A block seldom cause symptoms, but higher degrees of S-A block may prolong cardiac asystole enough to diminish cerebral perfusion and cause dizziness, near-syncope, or, rarely, syncope and convulsions. Physical examination may reveal the rhythm change characteristic of each type of block, and the ECG shows the absence of P waves in a characteristic pattern. A normal jugular venous pulse is preserved. Paroxysmal S-A block may be an exasperatingly difficult diagnosis to establish. Most patients are elderly and complain of infrequent paroxysms of lightheadedness or near syncope. Frequently, prolonged in-hospital monitoring or repeated Holter monitors are required before a symptomatic period accompanied by S-A block is demonstrated.

Prognosis and Therapy

The prognosis of S-A block depends on its cause, frequency, and the duration of the asystolic periods. Elderly patients tend to have increasingly frequent symptomatic periods. Neither atropine, ephedrine, nor isoproterenol therapy is successful in patients with symptomatic S-A block. Permanent demand pacemaker implantation is the treatment of choice. The site of implantation (atrial, ventricular, or bifocal) depends on the physiologic state in the remainder of the A-V conduction system. If the P-R interval and QRS duration are normal, a permanent atrial pacemaker is the preferred therapy.

INTRA-ATRIAL BLOCK

Slowed conduction of the propagating cardiac impulse through the atrial myocardium. Intra-atrial block is generally the result of atrial myocardial disease (either secondary to rheumatic or coronary artery disease) or of infiltrative primary myocardial diseases.

Diagnosis is made by finding broad P waves lasting 120 msec or more on the ECG. They are frequently notched and may be of low amplitude. Intra-atrial block is, in itself, asymptomatic and **therapy** is not required. Patients with intra-atrial block and slowed atrial conduction, however, are frequently prone to the subsequent development of atrial arrhythmias (eg, flutter and fibrillation).

ATRIOVENTRICULAR (A-V) BLOCK
(A-V Nodal Block)

Prolonged or blocked impulse propagation from atrial to ventricular myocardium, resulting from abnormal conduction across the A-V node.

Etiology

A-V nodal block is usually the result of A-V nodal ischemia secondary to acute inferior myocardial infarction **(MI),** digitalis toxicity, vagal stimulation (eg, from carotid sinus hypersensitivity or parasympathomimetic drugs), or primary A-V nodal disease. It also may occur in acute rheumatic fever and congenitally.

Pathophysiology and Diagnosis

A-V nodal block may be incomplete, intermittent, or complete. In **incomplete A-V nodal block** (prolonged A-V nodal conduction), the transmission of impulses across the A-V node is prolonged, but 1:1 conduction is still present (FIG. 27–20a). The conduction delay is seen on ECG as a prolongation of the P-R interval beyond 200 msec. The contours of the P waves and QRS complexes remain normal. As the degree of block increases, A-V conduction time is prolonged until some P waves fail to reach the bundle of His and ventricular myocardium, resulting in intermittent A-V conduction.

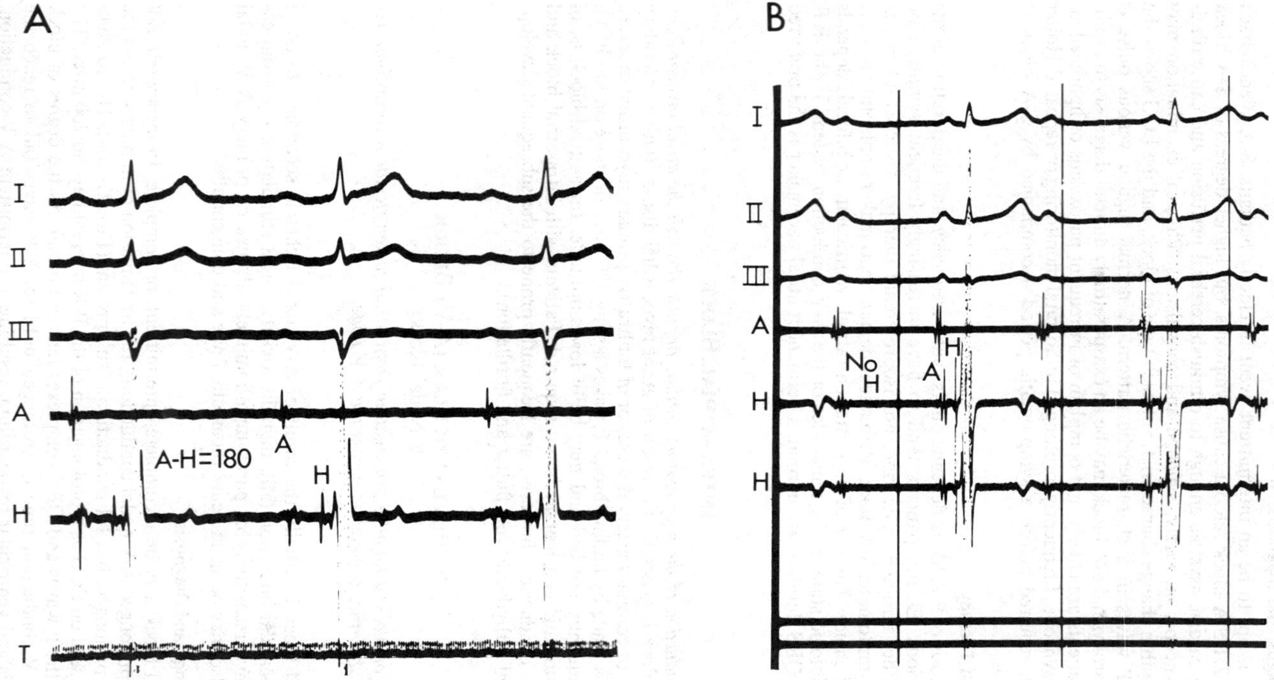

Fig. 27–20. A-V nodal block.

A. Prolonged A-V nodal conduction (first degree A-V block). Recorded are ECG leads I, II, and III, an atrial electrogram (A), a His bundle electrogram (H), and time marks at 10- and 100-msec intervals. The P-R interval is prolonged because conduction from atrium to the His bundle (A-H interval) is abnormally long (180 msec). P-R interval prolongation generally results from A-V nodal conduction delay.

B. 2 : 1 A-V nodal conduction. Every 2nd atrial depolarization of sinus origin fails to traverse the A-V node and excite the His bundle, resulting in 2 : 1 A-V block with the A-V node.

Intermittent A-V nodal block characteristically takes the form of **Wenckebach periodicity**. The P-R interval progressively lengthens until finally one P wave fails to result in a QRS complex. The cycle then repeats. A-V nodal Wenckebach periods are generally 3:2, 4:3, or 5:4 cycles, according to the number of impulses that precede the "dropped" beat. Other forms of intermittent A-V nodal conduction may also occur. Impulses may block within the A-V node in a pattern of 2:1, 3:1, or even 4:1 A-V block (FIG. 27–20b). In these higher degrees of A-V nodal block, the P waves are normal, and every second, third, or fourth wave is followed by a QRS complex of *normal* contour with a constant P-R interval.

As A-V nodal conduction becomes more abnormal, **complete A-V nodal block** may occur; none of the P waves seen on the ECG results in QRS complexes. The ventricles are controlled by a subsidiary pacemaker (escape focus), most often from the bundle of His. As a result, the P waves are entirely dissociated from the QRS complexes, and the form of the QRS complexes remains identical to that seen before block occurred. This point is important in differentiating complete A-V nodal from infranodal block. The escape focus within the bundle of His generally fires at a rate of 40 to 70 beats/min. Thus, complete A-V nodal block is only moderately symptomatic.

Symptoms and Signs

Incomplete and intermittent A-V nodal blocks usually are without symptoms. The patient may recognize complete block as a slower heart beat accompanied by weakness or fatigue. Syncope is rare, but may occur when the rate of the subsidiary pacemaker is extremely slow. Complete A-V block may be recognized on physical examination by the varying intensity of the first heart sound and the lack of correlation between jugular venous pulsations and carotid pulses. This results in characteristic cannon A waves when a P wave is superimposed upon a QRS complex and atrial and ventricular mechanical systole occur simultaneously.

A-V nodal block of any type is rarely permanent. When it is the result of inferior MI, it almost always disappears within 72 h after onset.

Therapy

Therapy is required only if the patient is symptomatic. A-V nodal block resulting from digitalis intoxication is best treated by withholding the drug. Although K or phenytoin may decrease the block, these drugs should be *avoided* in complete A-V nodal block caused by digitalis excess because they may slow the subsidiary pacemakers and increase symptoms. However, atropine or isoproterenol, even if they do not reverse the A-V nodal block, will speed the His bundle pacemaker and improve CO. Since the condition producing A-V nodal block is generally transient, permanent pacemakers are almost never required.

INFRANODAL A-V BLOCK

A type of A-V block in which impulses traverse the A-V node normally, but are blocked within the ventricular specialized conduction system; ie, within the bundle of His or all 3 fascicles of the cardiac conduction system.

Etiology

Infranodal A-V block is the result of arteriosclerotic coronary artery disease, intrinsic degeneration of the ventricular conduction system, or infiltrative diseases (eg, amyloid, syphilis, or tumor). The ventricular conduction system may also be damaged by Ca deposition in the anulus of the aortic or mitral valves. Acute myocardial infarction with occlusion of the left anterior descending coronary artery proximal to its first septal perforating branch may result in ischemia or infarction of the proximal ventricular specialized conducting system and development of complete infranodal A-V block.

Pathophysiology

Impulses traversing a normal A-V node find an infranodal conduction system in which all 3 fascicles (right bundle, and anterior and posterior divisions of the left bundle branch) are abnormal. During periods of conduction (generally 1:1), patients usually demonstrate block in one or more branches of the fascicles; ie, **bundle branch block (BBB)**. Suddenly, conduction fails in all 3 fascicles (complete infranodal A-V block), either as an isolated event or over a series of successive beats. A subsidiary pacemaker must take over cardiac excitation, or cardiac arrest and death will result. Since impulses are blocked within the fascicles, this pacemaker is distal in the His-Purkinje system and its rate is extremely slow. The inciting cause for the sudden conduction loss and its equally sudden resumption is unknown.

Symptoms and Signs

Infranodal A-V block is most common in elderly patients and results in syncope (referred to as a **Stokes–Adams attack**) with unheralded, short-lived episodes that tend to increase in frequency. The pulse is usually between 20 and 50 beats/min. Cannon A waves may also be recognized in the jugular venous pulse.

Diagnosis

Only an ECG can distinguish nodal from infranodal A-V block, but the presence of syncope suggests that it is infranodal. The ECG almost always shows intraventricular conduction disturbances during sinus rhythm. During periods of 1:1 conduction, one may find right BBB plus left anterior hemiblock, right BBB plus left posterior hemiblock, or left BBB. Left BBB with a superiorly oriented mean frontal plane axis is a more common precursor of complete A-V block than previously recognized. The P-R interval is generally normal. During the period of complete infranodal A-V block, P wave morphology is normal (FIG. 27–21). QRS complexes are wide and bizarre, with a rate between 20 and 50 beats/min, and (in contrast to those of complete A-V nodal

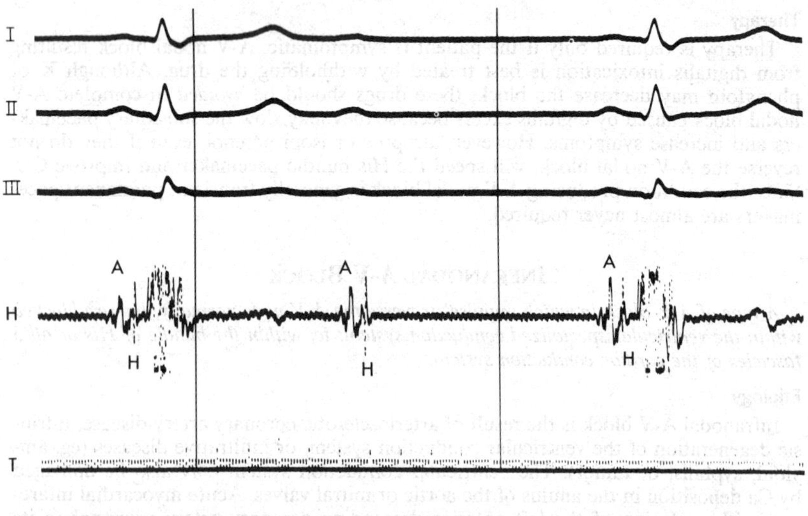

FIG. 27–21. 2 : 1 Infranodal A-V block with right bundle branch block (RBBB). Recorded are ECG leads I, II, and III, a His bundle electrogram (H), and time marks at 10- and 100-msec intervals. The ECG demonstrates RBBB on the conducted beats. Each atrial depolarization (A) is followed by depolarization of the His bundle (H), but alternate His bundle depolarizations fail to excite the ventricular muscle.

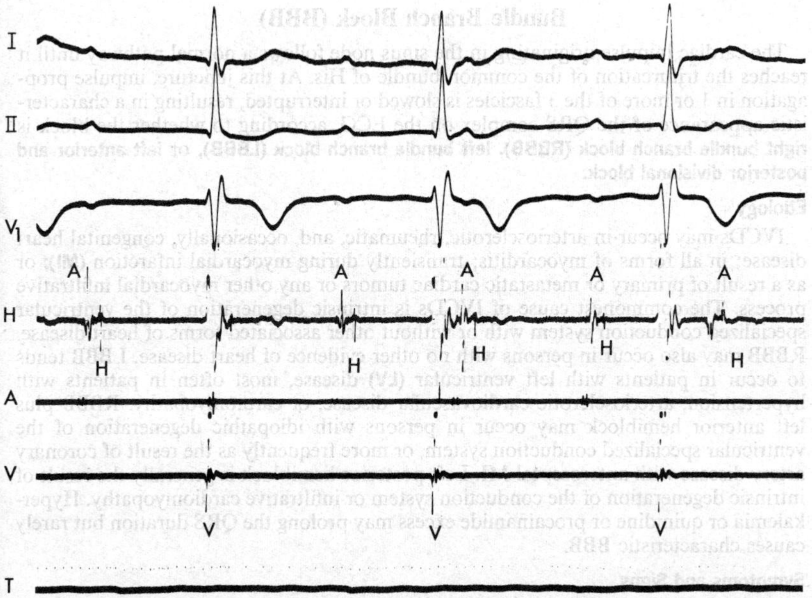

FIG. 27–22. Complete intranodal A-V block. Recorded are ECG leads I, II, and V_1, a His bundle electrogram (H), atrial electrogram (A), ventricular electrogram (V), and time marks (T). Each atrial beat of sinus origin (A) is followed by depolarization of the His bundle, but conduction proceeds no further, and QRS complexes are the result of an independent idioventricular pacemaker.

block) are entirely different from those observed during conducted rhythm. The wide QRS complexes and their very slow rate prove that the block is infranodal. Intracardiac ECGs show that each P wave propagates across the A-V node and activates the bundle of His, but is blocked distally to it (FIG. 27–22).

Therapy

Implantation of a permanent right ventricular endocardial demand pacemaker is the only therapy for intermittent complete infranodal A-V block. These have markedly reduced the former mortality rate of almost 50% over 2 yr in patients with true Stokes-Adams seizures. In the emergency situation, if the patient has lost consciousness and has a slow heart rate, the subsidiary focus may be speeded up by isoproterenol 1 to 3 μg/min IV, but implanting a temporary demand pacemaker is preferable to the use of sympathomimetics. Atropine is probably ineffective. External pacemakers that can stimulate the heart through the chest wall are available for emergency temporary pacing until a transvenous electrode can be implanted. Transthoracic pacemaker insertion has only rarely been effective and should be reserved for extreme emergencies.

INTRAVENTRICULAR BLOCK
(Intraventricular Conduction Defect; IVCD)

This includes the various bundle branch or fascicular blocks as well as other forms of IVCDs.

Bundle Branch Block (BBB)

The cardiac impulse originating in the sinus node follows a normal pathway until it reaches the trifurcation of the common bundle of His. At this juncture, impulse propagation in 1 or more of the 3 fascicles is slowed or interrupted, resulting in a characteristic appearance of the QRS complex on the ECG, according to whether the block is **right bundle branch block (RBBB), left bundle branch block (LBBB),** or **left anterior and posterior divisional block.**

Etiology

IVCDs may occur in arteriosclerotic, rheumatic, and, occasionally, congenital heart disease; in all forms of myocarditis; transiently during myocardial infarction **(MI)**; or as a result of primary or metastatic cardiac tumors or any other myocardial infiltrative process. The commonest cause of IVCDs is intrinsic degeneration of the ventricular specialized conduction system with or without other associated forms of heart disease. RBBB may also occur in persons with no other evidence of heart disease. LBBB tends to occur in patients with left ventricular **(LV)** disease, most often in patients with hypertension, arteriosclerotic cardiovascular disease, or cardiomyopathy. RBBB plus left anterior hemiblock may occur in persons with idiopathic degeneration of the ventricular specialized conduction system, or more frequently as the result of coronary artery disease with anteroseptal MI. Left posterior hemiblock is generally the result of intrinsic degeneration of the conduction system or infiltrative cardiomyopathy. Hyperkalemia or quinidine or procainamide excess may prolong the QRS duration but rarely causes characteristic BBB.

Symptoms and Signs

Patients with IVCD are asymptomatic, unless the disease has progressed enough to cause periods of complete infranodal A-V block (see above). The commonest sign of RBBB on physical examination is wide splitting of the second sound that moves but never closes with expiration. In LBBB a paradoxic splitting of the second sound may be heard.

Pathophysiology and Diagnosis

An IVCD is readily diagnosed by ECG: it exists (by definition) if the QRS duration is > 100 msec. In **RBBB,** because the right bundle impulse is conducted slowly or not at all, right ventricular **(RV)** activation occurs by muscle-to-muscle spread of the cardiac impulse. Since myocardial excitation is slower than that via the His-Purkinje system, RV activation is delayed (causing delayed and slowed terminal forces on the ECG) and is dissynchronous with LV activation. Typically, there is a large S wave in leads I and V_6 and an RR′ is present in V_1 and V_2. Vectorially, in the frontal plane, terminal forces are slowed and directed rightward, resulting in broad S waves in ECG leads I, aVL, V_6, and X. In the transverse plane, this delayed activation is seen anteriorly, corresponding anatomically to the right ventricle (FIG. 27–23). An rR′ is seen in ECG leads V_1, V_2, and Z.

The **left bundle** is responsible for activating the ventricular septum and body of the left ventricle. Most authorities agree that ventricular septal activation occurs primarily via branches of the left posterior division, and that the left anterior division activates the anterior LV papillary muscle, the LV outflow tract, and the base of the heart.

Several types of LBBB are now recognized. FIG. 27–24 demonstrates **classic LBBB.** The posterior division of the left bundle branch is so abnormal that it fails to result in normal septal activation. The interventricular septum is therefore activated from right to left and the septal Q waves generally seen in leads I, aVL, and V_6 (X on the vector) are no longer inscribed. In addition, overall LV activation is delayed and characteristic mid-to-terminal QRS notching is seen in these same leads. The normal mean QRS axis in the frontal plane (lying between +90 degrees and –30 degrees) is maintained be-

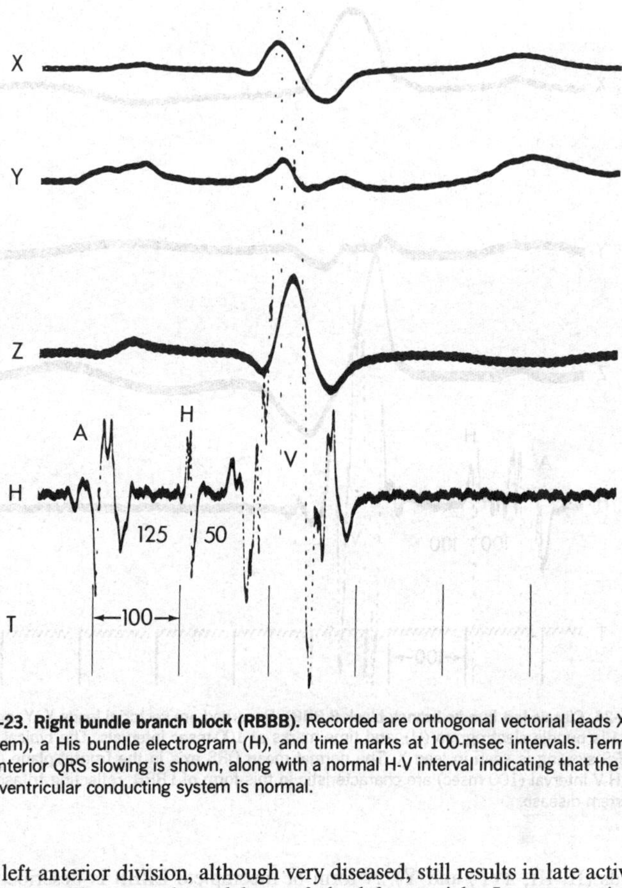

FIG. 27–23. Right bundle branch block (RBBB). Recorded are orthogonal vectorial leads X, Y, and Z (Frank system), a His bundle electrogram (H), and time marks at 100-msec intervals. Terminal rightward and anterior QRS slowing is shown, along with a normal H-V interval indicating that the remainder of the intraventricular conducting system is normal.

cause the left anterior division, although very diseased, still results in late activation of the anterior papillary muscle and base of the left ventricle. In most patients with LBBB, conduction within the right bundle is also delayed; although it is not as abnormal as conduction in the left bundle, it can prolong the H-V interval, as seen on the His bundle electrogram in FIG. 27–24.

When conduction fails within the anterior as well as the posterior division of the left bundle branch (FIG. 27–25), ventricular activation occurs solely via the right bundle branch. This situation (akin to that seen with pacemakers implanted within the RV apex) results in a superiorly directed QRS complex in the frontal plane. A QRS axis superiorly directed more than −45 degrees should suggest that both fascicles of the left bundle are no longer conducting.

When only the anterior fascicle of the left bundle fails to conduct, a characteristic ECG pattern referred to as **left anterior hemiblock (LAH)** results (FIG. 27–26). Ventricular septal activation is normal, as is RV depolarization. Since the LV anterobasal portions are activated by muscle-to-muscle excitation, their depolarization is delayed. QRS complexes are minimally widened (90 to 110 msec), but the mean QRS axis in the frontal plane is shifted superiorly and large S waves appear in the inferiorly directed

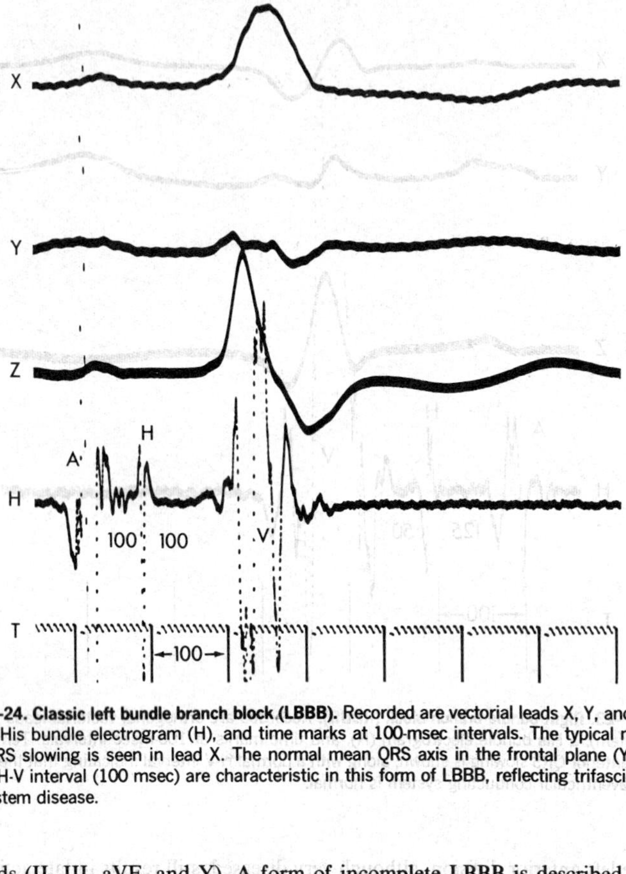

Fig. 27–24. Classic left bundle branch block (LBBB). Recorded are vectorial leads X, Y, and Z (Frank system), a His bundle electrogram (H), and time marks at 100-msec intervals. The typical mid-to-late leftward QRS slowing is seen in lead X. The normal mean QRS axis in the frontal plane (Y) and the prolonged H-V interval (100 msec) are characteristic in this form of LBBB, reflecting trifascicular conducting system disease.

ECG leads (II, III, aVF, and Y). A form of incomplete LBBB is described wherein only those portions of the left bundle responsible for septal activation fail to conduct. Only minimal QRS prolongation results but septal activation now proceeds from right to left and normal septal Q waves seen in I, L, and V_6 are lost. The H-V interval is prolonged since septal activation now occurs via the right bundle.

Although LBBB can result from disease of all 3 fascicles of the interventricular conducting system, more typically a bifascicular block is seen; ie, RBBB combined with block in either the anterior-superior or posterior-inferior division of the left bundle branch. **RBBB with LAH** results in the combined ECG features of both (Fig. 27–27). The delayed RV activation produces the typical large S waves seen in ECG leads I, aVL, V_6, and X, while the associated LAH shifts the mean QRS axis superiorly in the frontal plane, resulting in large S waves in the inferior ECG leads II, III, aVF, and Y. In almost ⅔ of patients with RBBB plus LAH, trifascicular conduction system disease is present and can be detected by characteristic H-V interval prolongation on the His bundle electrogram. Subsequent paroxysmal complete infranodal A-V block is likely.

In **RBBB combined with left posterior hemiblock,** a failure of conduction within the posterior division of the left bundle branch (Fig. 27–28), all the characteristic features

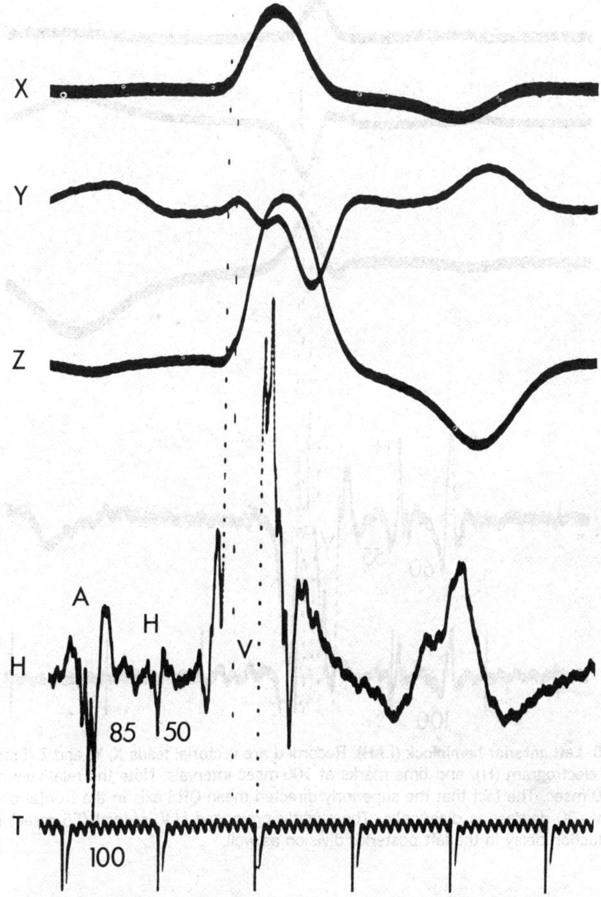

Fig. 27–25. Left bundle branch block (LBBB) with a leftward mean QRS axis. Recorded are vectorial leads X, Y, and Z (Frank system), a His bundle electrogram (H), and time marks at 100-msec intervals. The mean QRS axis in the frontal plane is terminally directed superiorly, resulting in a large S wave in lead Y. The H-V interval of 50 msec seen in this patient is the exception rather than the rule.

of RBBB are present, but the terminal rightward vector is even more exaggerated; ie, the terminal S waves in leads I, aVL, V_6, and X are even deeper. In this condition ventricular activation is occurring solely via the anterior division of the left bundle branch; virtually all of the ventricular myocardium is being activated from left to right except the anterobasal portion of the left ventricle. The initial septal vector X (usually reflected by a small Q wave in leads I, aVL, and V_6) is lost. An initial Q wave seen in the inferiorly directed ECG leads (Y) may reflect a reversal of septal depolarization or, more likely, indicate that initial ventricular activation at the termination of the left

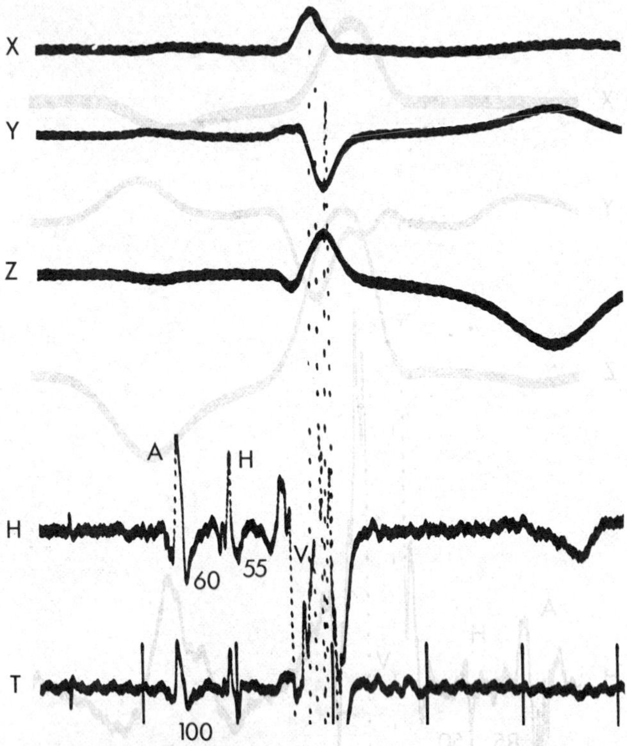

FIG. 27–26. Left anterior hemiblock (LAH). Recorded are vectorial leads X, Y, and Z (Frank system), a His bundle electrogram (H), and time marks at 100-msec intervals. Note the relatively normal QRS duration of 90 msec. The fact that the superiorly directed mean QRS axis in the frontal plane is more negative than −30 degrees is diagnostic. The slightly prolonged H-V interval (55 msec) may reflect minimal conduction delay in the left posterior division as well.

anterior division is proceeding in a superior direction. Since the base of the left ventricle is activated first, the major QRS vector is inscribed in an inferior direction. This results in a characteristic open and inferiorly inscribed vector loop in the frontal plane, which results from the muscle-to-muscle spread of electrical activity first to the apex of the left and then the right ventricle.

Nonspecific IVCDs are said to be present when the total QRS duration exceeds 100 msec and none of the criteria of classic BBB are met.

Prognosis and Treatment

Although the prognosis of any BBB is primarily that of the cardiac disease underlying it, the presence of disease in 2 of the 3 fascicles of the ventricular conduction system predisposes to the development of intermittent complete infranodal A-V block and Stokes-Adams attacks. No specific therapy is indicated for IVCDs and the incidence with which these progress to complete infranodal IV block is only 2 to 3%/yr.

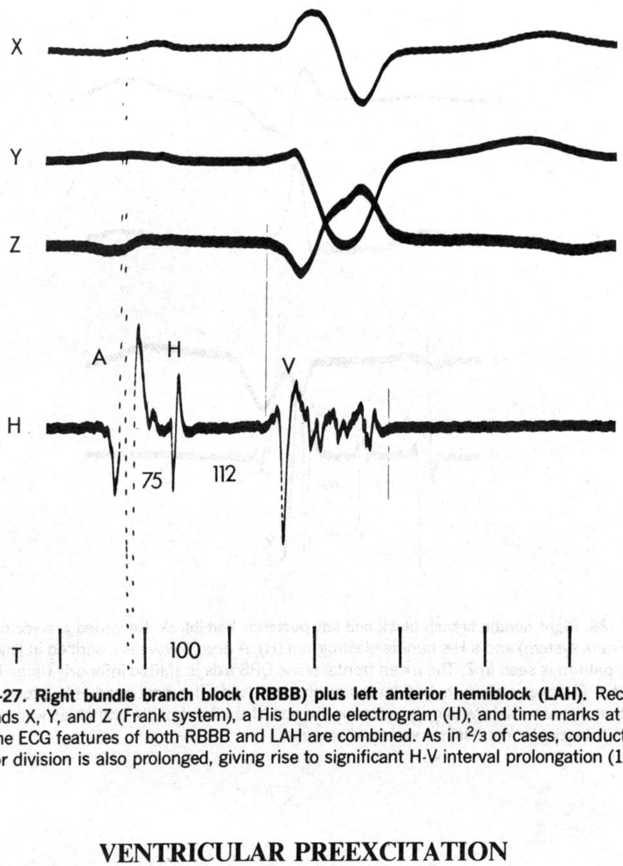

Fig. 27–27. Right bundle branch block (RBBB) plus left anterior hemiblock (LAH). Recorded are vectorial leads X, Y, and Z (Frank system), a His bundle electrogram (H), and time marks at 100-msec intervals. The ECG features of both RBBB and LAH are combined. As in 2/3 of cases, conduction in the left posterior division is also prolonged, giving rise to significant H-V interval prolongation (112 msec).

VENTRICULAR PREEXCITATION

Wolff-Parkinson-White (WPW) syndrome: *A form of accelerated A-V conduction, resulting from the existence of 2 A-V conduction pathways.* Conduction proceeds down the normal A-V nodal His-Purkinje pathway, but the ventricles are preexcited by an anomalous A-V connection between the atria and one of the ventricular muscle masses. Because 2 conduction pathways exist, QRS complexes really represent fusion complexes. The initial activation, the result of muscle-to-muscle spread, is slow, and results in a characteristic and pathognomonic delta wave at the onset of the QRS complex (Fig. 27–29a). The P-R interval is usually short (Fig. 27–29b). Although previously divided into Type A and B, electrophysiologic studies have disclosed that accessory A-V corrections may occur anywhere around the fibrous rings of both mitral and tricuspid valves. The vector of the initial ventricular pre-excitation or delta wave is determined by the site of the bypass tract. The P-R interval is a function of the relative conduction velocity down the normal as opposed to the pre-excitation path.

Lown-Ganong-Levine (LGL) syndrome: *Ventricular preexcitation in which part or all of the normal A-V nodal conduction system is bypassed by an anomalous A-V connection between atrial muscle and the bundle of His.* This results in a short P-R interval and normal QRS complexes (Fig. 27–30a).

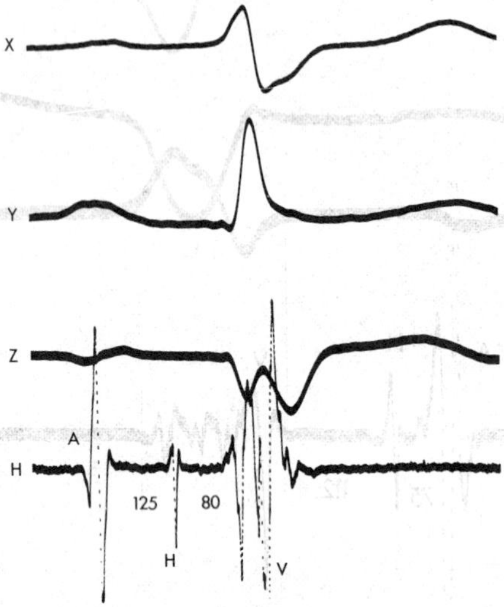

FIG. 27–28. Right bundle branch block and left posterior hemiblock. Recorded are vectorial leads X, Y, and Z (Frank system) and a His bundle electrogram (H). A deep S wave is inscribed in lead X, and the typical RR′ pattern is seen in Z. The mean frontal plane QRS axis is shifted inferiorly (large R wave in Y) and an initial Q wave is seen in this inferiorly directed lead. The prolonged H-V interval (80 msec) indicates that disease exists within the anterior division of the left bundle branch as well, and that this patient has trifascicular conduction system disease.

Symptoms, Signs, and Diagnosis

The ECG is diagnostic in both of these conditions. In ventricular pre-excitation of the WPW variety, the P-R interval is short and initial ventricular activation slowed resulting in a characteristic delta wave (FIG. 27–29). In partial A-V nodal bypass of the LGL type, the P-R interval is short but QRS duration is normal as is the initial ventricular activation sequence. They are entirely without manifestations unless accompanied by paroxysmal atrial arrhythmias. A re-entrant type of supraventricular tachycardia (SVT) is common. In this re-entrant arrhythmia, the initiating APB finds the accessory pathway refractory and conducts slowly down the normal A-V nodal conduction system. Having excited ventricular myocardium, the bypass tract has recovered excitability and is capable of conducting the impulse retrogradely to the atrium. The cycle is continued as an episode of SVT. It should be noted that because antegrade conduction proceeds down the normal A-V pathway, the delta wave is lost during episodes of SVT. Both atrial flutter and fibrillation occur in patients with both WPW and LGL syndromes. The associated manifestations may be severe in patients

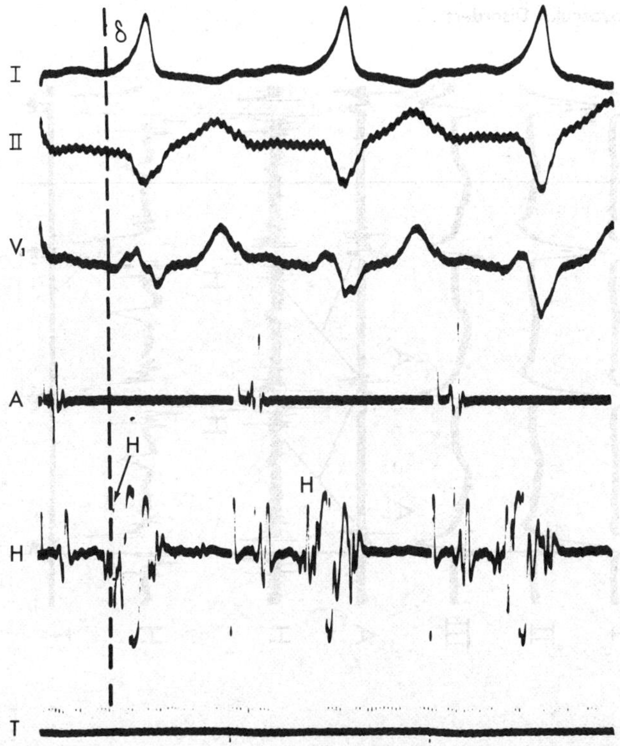

a. Recorded are ECG leads I, II, and V_1, an atrial electrogram (A), a His bundle electrogram (H) and time marks at 10- and 100-msec intervals. Depolarization of the His bundle (H) occurs during inscription of the characteristic delta wave (δ). The QRS morphology represents the result of ventricular excitation via 2 independent pathways.

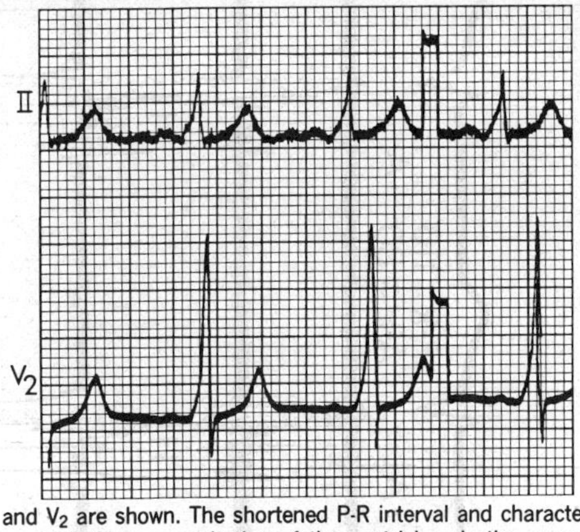

b. ECG leads II and V_2 are shown. The shortened P-R interval and characteristic initial slow ventricular depolarization result from preexcitation of the ventricles via the anomalous A-V conduction pathway.

FIG. 27–29. Wolff-Parkinson-White syndrome.

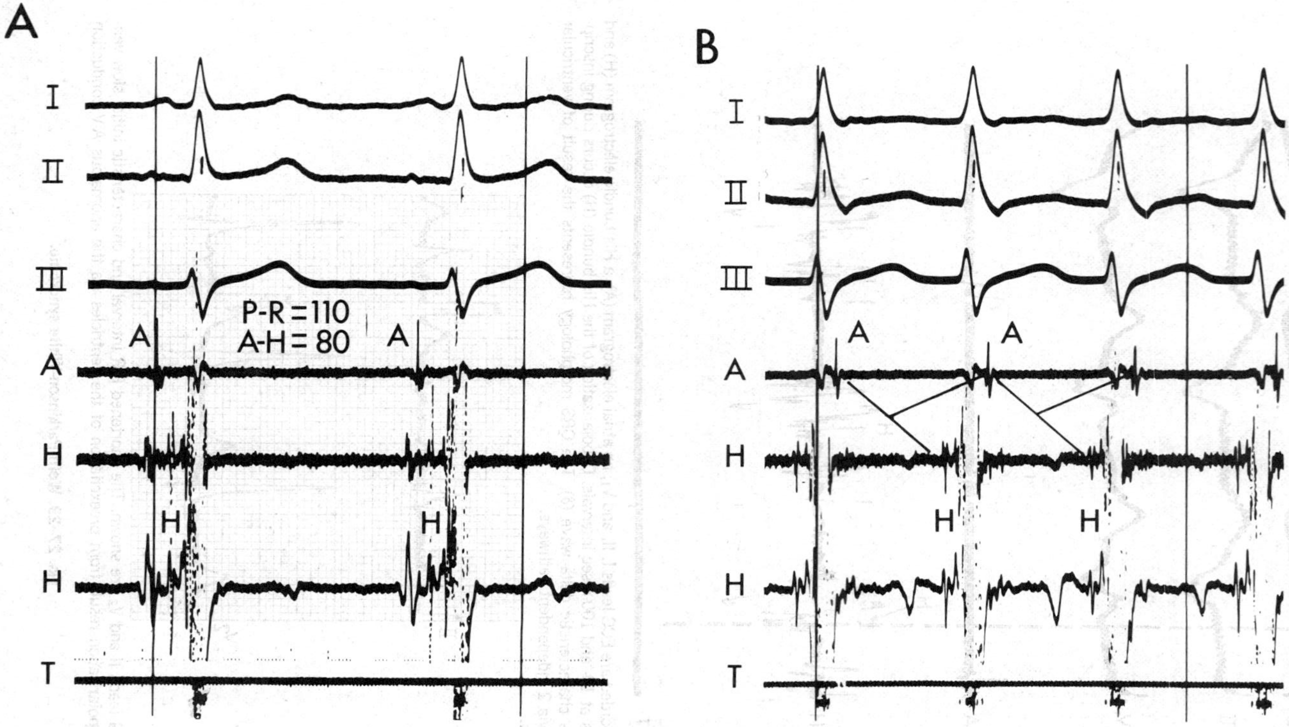

Fig. 27–30. Lown-Ganong-Levine syndrome.

A. ECG leads I, II, and III, an atrial electrogram (A), a His bundle electrogram (H), and time marks at 10- and 100-msec intervals are shown during *normal sinus rhythm.* The shortened P-R interval at 110 msec is a function of the short A-V nodal conduction time (A-H interval, 80 msec).

B. Despite the short P-R interval during sinus rhythm, prolonged A-V nodal conduction (A long A-H interval) is responsible for the sustained reentrant tachycardia

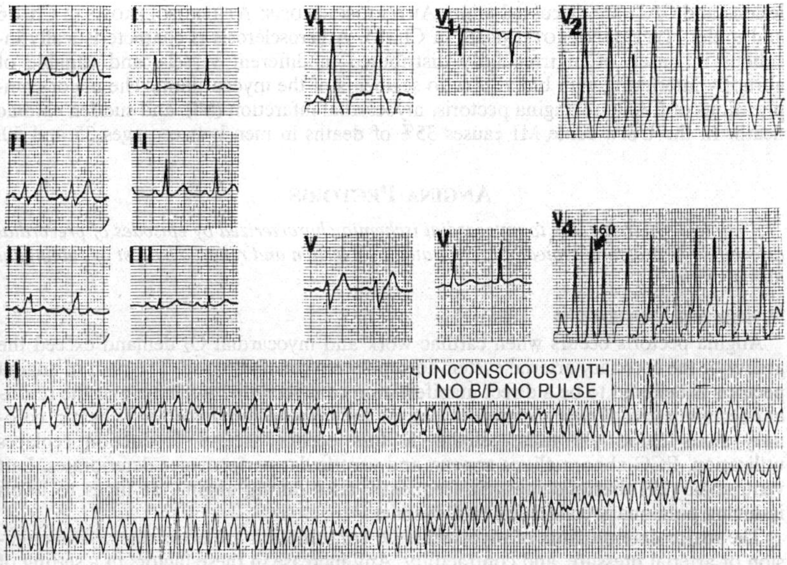

FIG. 27–31. Wolff-Parkinson-White syndrome. Leads I, II, III, V_1, V_6, wide with delta wave on left. V_2 and V_4 atrial fibrillation on right. Shortest R-R interval is 160 msec. Lead II lower strips show ventricular fibrillation.

with anomalous A-V conduction (FIG. 27–30b). It is now recognized that an anomalous, rapidly conducting bypass tract may have dire consequences in the presence of atrial flutter or fibrillation. Extremely rapid ventricular rates (200 to 300/min) have resulted in ventricular fibrillation and sudden death (see FIG. 27–31).

Therapy

Therapy is directed at preventing episodes of SVT. Quinidine sulfate 200 to 400 mg orally tid or qid is most useful; procainamide and propranolol may also be used (see treatment of ventricular premature beats **[VPBs]**, above). Amiodarone has also been an effective drug when other Class I and β-blockers are ineffective (see treatment of VPBs, above). Pacemaker therapy and surgical interruption of the anomalous pathways have been used with some success in patients with refractory and debilitating recurrent SVT. Electrophysiologic studies and surgical interruption with or without cryoablation of the bypass tract should be seriously considered when atrial fibrillation with extremely rapid ventricular responses is encountered. *Digoxin and verapamil are strictly contraindicated with WPW and atrial fibrillation.*

MYOCARDIAL ISCHEMIC DISORDERS

CORONARY ARTERY DISEASE (CAD)

Most CAD is due to subintimal deposition of atheromas in the large and medium-sized arteries serving the heart. Risk factors and the pathogenesis of atherosclerotic

lesions and CAD are discussed under ARTERIOSCLEROSIS; ATHEROSCLEROSIS in Ch. 26 and under HYPERLIPOPROTEINEMIA in Ch. 85. Atherosclerosis is characteristically insidious in onset, often irregularly distributed in different vessels, and capable of abruptly interfering with blood flow to segments of the myocardium. The major complications of CAD are angina pectoris, myocardial infarction **(MI)**, and sudden cardiac death. In the USA, acute MI causes 35% of deaths in men between ages 35 and 50.

ANGINA PECTORIS

A clinical syndrome due to myocardial ischemia characterized by episodes of precordial discomfort or pressure, typically precipitated by exertion and relieved by rest or sublingual nitroglycerin.

Etiology and Pathogenesis

Angina pectoris occurs when cardiac work and myocardial O_2 demand exceed the ability of the coronary arterial system to supply oxygenated blood. The pain of angina pectoris is believed to be a direct manifestation of myocardial ischemia and the resultant accumulation of hypoxic metabolites. As the myocardium becomes ischemic, coronary sinus blood pH falls, cellular K loss occurs, lactate production replaces utilization, ECG abnormalities appear, and ventricular performance deteriorates. Left ventricular **(LV)** diastolic pressure frequently rises during angina, at times to levels inducing pulmonary congestion and dyspnea.

The major determinants of myocardial O_2 consumption are heart rate, systolic tension or arterial pressure, and contractility. Any increase in these factors in a setting of reduced coronary blood flow may induce angina. During spontaneous angina the subjective awareness of pain is usually preceded by modest increases in heart rate and a rise in BP that may at times be marked. If the angina is not relieved, these changes represent a potentially disastrous positive biofeedback system: the higher the BP and the faster the heart rate, the greater the unmet myocardial O_2 need.

Patients with angina who die almost invariably have extensive coronary atherosclerosis and patchy myocardial fibrosis. Evidence of old MI may be present. Underlying disease other than atherosclerosis (eg, calcific aortic stenosis, aortic regurgitation, or hypertrophic subaortic stenosis) may occasionally be present, either alone or coexisting with CAD. In these conditions, myocardial work is markedly increased. An occasional patient with fatal MI is found to have anatomically normal coronary arteries. Either coronary embolus or spasm may be postulated as causative (see below).

Symptoms and Signs

The discomfort of angina pectoris, highly variable, is most commonly felt beneath the sternum. It may be a vague, barely troublesome ache, or it may rapidly become a severe, intense precordial crushing sensation. Pain may radiate to the left shoulder and down the inside of the left arm, even to the fingers. It may radiate straight through to the back, into the throat, the jaws, the teeth, and occasionally even down the right arm. Anginal discomfort may be felt in the upper or lower abdomen. Since it is seldom felt in the region of the cardiac apex, the patient who points to that precise area or describes fleeting, sharp, or hot sensations usually does not have angina.

Angina pectoris is characteristically triggered by physical activity and usually persists no more than a few minutes, subsiding with rest. The response to exertion is usually predictable, but in some persons a given exercise may be tolerated one day and may precipitate angina the next. Angina is worsened when exertion follows a meal. It is also exaggerated in cold weather, so that exertion without symptoms in the summer may induce angina in the winter. Walking into the wind or first contact with cold air on leaving a warm room may also precipitate an attack. Angina may occur at night

(nocturnal angina) or when the patient is resting quietly and seemingly without stimulation **(angina decubitus)**. Nocturnal angina is frequently preceded by a dream that may be accompanied by striking changes in respiration, pulse rate, and BP. Nocturnal angina may also be a sign of recurrent LV failure.

Attacks may vary in frequency from several/day to occasional seizures separated by symptom-free intervals of weeks, months, or years. They may increase in frequency to a fatal outcome or may gradually decrease or disappear if an adequate collateral coronary circulation develops, if the ischemic area becomes infarcted, or if heart failure supervenes.

Since the characteristics of angina are usually constant for a given individual, any change in the pattern of symptoms—increased intensity of attacks, decreased threshold of stimulus, longer duration, or occurrence when the patient is sedentary or awakening from sleep—should be viewed as serious. Such changes are termed **unstable angina pectoris, acute coronary insufficiency, preinfarction angina,** or the **intermediate syndrome.** Unstable angina is the preferred term because it implies less judgment about prognosis. Unstable angina may be prodromal to acute MI; sudden death is less common. Prospective studies suggest that about 30% of patients with unstable angina will suffer an MI within 3 mo of onset.

Variant angina (Prinzmetal's angina), usually secondary to large vessel spasm, is characterized by pain *at rest* and by S-T segment elevation, not depression, during the attack. Between episodes, the ECG may be normal or may present a stable control pattern. Arrhythmia is not uncommon and attacks tend to occur with regularity at certain times of day. Ergonovine IV has been used as a provocative test to induce spasm, but *should be done only in an experienced angiographic laboratory*. Relief is usually prompt after sublingual nitroglycerin. Prognosis is variable. Vasodilators that block slow Ca movement (eg, verapamil, nifedipine, and diltiazem) appear to be highly effective.

Physical findings: Between and even during attacks, there may be no signs of organic heart disease. However, during the attack, heart rate may increase modestly, BP is often elevated, heart sounds become more distant, and the apical impulse is more diffuse. Palpation of the precordium may reveal a localized systolic bulging or paradoxic movement reflecting segmental myocardial ischemia in noncontracting myocardium. The 2nd heart sound may become paradoxic due to more prolonged LV ejection during the ischemic episode. A 4th heart sound is common. In some persons, a mid or late systolic apical murmur, rather shrill but not especially loud, may be heard. This murmur has been ascribed to localized papillary muscle dysfunction secondary to the ischemia.

ECG: A continuous recording during an attack of chest pain is most helpful. A wide variety of changes may appear: characteristic S-T segment depression, hyperacute S-T segment elevation, decrease in R wave height, intraventricular or bundle branch conduction disturbances, and arrhythmia (usually ventricular extrasystoles). However, between episodes the ECG at rest is normal in about 30% of patients with a typical history of angina pectoris, even in extensive 3-vessel CAD.

Diagnosis

Angina pectoris is a *clinical diagnosis* based on a characteristic complaint of chest discomfort brought on by exertion and relieved by rest. Confirmation may be obtained by observing ischemic ECG changes during a spontaneous attack or by a test dose of sublingual nitroglycerin that characteristically relieves the pain within 1.5 to 3 min. Failure to obtain prompt relief casts suspicion on a diagnosis of angina.

An abnormal resting ECG alone does not establish or refute the diagnosis of angina pectoris, which must be recognized from characteristic symptoms. A positive exercise tolerance test (ie, the development of ischemic ECG changes) does not confirm the diagnosis unless the exact symptoms are produced during the exertion. Demonstration of CAD by angiography also does not establish a diagnosis of angina pectoris, since the latter is a *symptom* reflecting myocardial ischemia, and the former is an anatomic demonstration of deformed blood vessels.

Exercise tolerance tests: Determining the cardiovascular response to exercise is an important tool in evaluating patients with possible CAD, but the tests must be interpreted with due regard to reliability and specificity. Since the diagnosis of angina is essentially based on the patient's history, the major purpose of exercise testing is to determine the patient's functional response to graded stress. Thus, the *symptom-limited* test is preferred by many experts.

Maximal heart rate during exercise correlates with maximal O_2 consumption, with a linear relationship between heart rate and O_2 uptake by the body. The adequacy of an exercise test may thus be judged by the heart rate achieved during stress. (Maximal heart rate attained during exercise declines with age; tables are available relating predicted maximal heart rate during exercise to sex and age.) Exercise may be limited by dyspnea, reduced endurance, fatigue, or chest pain.

The "ischemic" ECG response during or after exercise is characterized by a flat or downward-sloping S-T segment depression $\geq$ 0.1 millivolts (1 mm) lasting $\geq$ 0.08 sec in a properly calibrated recording. J junction depression with an upward sloping S-T segment is difficult to interpret; it is associated with a high incidence of false-positive tests. Both sensitivity and specificity increase with the patient's age. Thus, abnormal tests are falsely positive in $\geq$ 20% patients under age 40, whereas over age 60 this may be reduced to < 10%. A diagnosis of ischemic heart disease due to coronary artery abnormality as a result of a positive exercise test (due to ECG change) is almost always inferential. A positive test may mean that the heart is metabolically abnormal, but coronary angiography may show the large coronary arteries to be quite normal. False-negative tests also occur. The frequency of positive tests increases with the number of coronary arteries obstructed, and greater degrees of S-T segment depression generally are correlated with more extensive disease. The test is most useful in men with chest pain suggestive of angina; specificity is 70% and sensitivity is 90%. Exercise tests are more difficult to interpret in women under age 55; a high incidence of false-positive responses reduces the specificity.

Exercise testing is increasingly performed in asymptomatic subjects as a health screening measure or to determine fitness for strenuous exercise (eg, jogging). However, in the absence of symptoms, most positive tests will be false-positives, and a positive test may engender considerable alarm and expense.

With proper indications and a closely monitored test, exercise tolerance in the patient with ischemia carries a low risk. Patients with unstable angina or those in whom a recent diagnosis of MI is suspected should not be given an exercise test. However, in patients with unstable angina or post-MI who are stable and doing well, a submaximal exercise test just prior to discharge is often performed. The response of the patient to exercise provides valuable prognostic information and helps to evaluate the need for angiography and possible bypass surgery. *A complete life support system including emergency drugs, airway, and defibrillator should always be immediately available for any patient undergoing exercise testing.*

Coronary arteriography (see also under CARDIAC CATHETERIZATION in Ch. 25) is used to determine the extent of anatomic coronary artery obstruction. Thus it is indicated when bypass surgery is being considered and to determine the extent of disease in difficult clinical situations (eg, atypical pain, survivors of sudden cardiac death, unstable angina, and selected patients post-MI).

Findings on the coronary angiogram parallel those at postmortem, but the extent of disease is usually underestimated. Vessels as small as 1 mm may be visualized with high-quality imaging. CAD is recognized by narrowing, beading, or occlusion of the vessels. Obstruction is assumed to be physiologically significant when the lumenal diameter is reduced > 70%, which correlates well with the presence of angina pectoris; lesser degrees of obstruction are unlikely to result in ischemia.

An LV angiogram to evaluate wall motion is an essential part of the study. Because of the important relationship between ventricular function and prognosis, analysis of ejection fraction provides essential information. Patients with poor ventricular function have a reduced life expectancy, but paradoxically benefit most from coronary artery bypass grafting, if they survive.

The major complications of coronary angiography are thrombosis at the arterial insertion site, MI secondary to catheter trauma, and death. Mortality rates < 1:1000 have been reported from many laboratories.

In 5 to 10% of patients with apparent angina, coronary arteries are found to be normal. This condition occurs predominantly in young women; the history may be typical or atypical. That some patients with this syndrome have ischemia cannot be doubted; lactate production during spontaneous or induced pain has been observed. The cause of ischemia in absence of CAD is not known. Disease of small arterioles or a primary metabolic defect has been postulated. Many patients are heavy smokers. Coronary spasm has been cited as the cause in some instances, sometimes as part of a general vasospastic disorder because of its apparent association with migraine or Raynaud's phenomenon. Spasm may develop in normal coronary arteries or complicate extensive coronary artery atherosclerosis. Its cause and mechanism are unknown.

Radionuclide studies are very valuable in evaluating the presence and significance of myocardial ischemia, including the size and location of infarctions and the integrity of ventricular walls and can reliably define ventricular dysfunction (see RADIONUCLIDE IMAGING OF THE HEART in Ch. 25).

Differential Diagnosis

Many conditions must be considered in the differential diagnosis (eg, abnormalities of the cervicodorsal spine, costochondral separation, and nonspecific chest wall pain). However, few truly mimic angina, and the syndrome of angina is so characteristic in most persons that errors in diagnosis are usually the result of careless history taking. Difficulties arise when the patient has atypical symptoms, especially with associated GI symptoms (eg, bloating, belching, and abdominal stress); at times belching may give relief. The symptoms are often ascribed to indigestion. Anginal discomfort felt in the upper or lower abdomen may be difficult to recognize. Peptic ulcer, hiatus hernia, and gallbladder disease may cause symptoms similar to angina pectoris or may precipitate attacks in persons with preexisting CAD. Thus, the possibility that a GI disorder and angina pectoris are both present must also be considered. Nonspecific changes in the T waves and S-T segments have been reported in esophagitis, peptic ulcer disease, and cholecystitis—observations that complicate the task of unraveling the patient's complaints.

At times angina may be confused with dyspnea. In part this is explained by the striking alteration in ventricular function with a sharp and reversible rise in LV filling pressure that often accompanies the ischemic attack. The patient's description may be imprecise, and whether he is suffering from angina, dyspnea, or both may be difficult to determine.

Silent ischemia: 24-h Holter monitoring has revealed a surprising incidence of T wave and ST segment abnormality in the absence of pain in patients with CAD. Such changes are rare in normal persons. Radionuclide studies have documented myocardial ischemia in some persons during mental stress (mental arithmetic) and during

spontaneous ECG change. Silent ischemia and classic angina may coexist in the same person. The relationship to sudden death and MI is unclear, although recent data document increased subsequent cardiac events in patients with known silent ischemia.

Prognosis

The major risks are sudden death or recurrent MI. Four major factors influence prognosis: age, extent of coronary disease (determined by angiography), severity of symptoms, and ventricular function. Clinically, an annual mortality rate of 1.4% has been reported in men with angina and no history of MI, a normal resting ECG, and normal BP. The rate rises to about 7.5% in those with systolic hypertension, to 8.4% when the ECG is abnormal, and to 12% if both risk factors are present.

Lesions of the left main coronary artery or high in the anterior descending vessel carry a particularly high risk. Although outcome correlates with number of coronary vessels involved, in stable patients the prognosis is surprisingly good even in patients with 3-vessel disease, *if ventricular function is normal.* Reduced ventricular function, often measured by analysis of ejection fraction, is a powerful factor adversely influencing prognosis, especially in patients with 3-vessel disease. The outcome also correlates with the symptoms: Patients with mild or moderate angina (Class I or II) have a better prognosis than those with severe exercise-induced angina (Class III).

Treatment

The underlying disease, usually atherosclerosis, must be delineated and risk factors reduced to the fullest extent possible (see ARTERIOSCLEROSIS; ATHEROSCLEROSIS in Ch. 26). Every effort should be made to induce smokers to stop the habit. Discontinuing smoking for ≥ 2 yr reduces the risk of MI to the level of those who never smoked. Reduction of overweight reduces cardiac demand. Hypertension should be treated diligently, since even mild diastolic hypertension increases cardiac work. Angina sometimes improves markedly with treatment of mild LV failure. Paradoxically, digitalis occasionally intensifies angina, presumably because increases in myocardial contractility raise O_2 demand in the presence of fixed coronary blood flow. An exercise program with emphasis on walking often improves the sense of well-being. Although the scientific evidence for long-term effect on prognosis is not complete, most authorities strongly recommend aggressive attempts to reduce blood total and HDL cholesterol by dietary manipulation and by treatment with lipid-lowering drugs in patients with significant blood lipid abnormality (see ANOMALIES IN LIPID METABOLISM in Ch. 85).

For stable angina pectoris, the major tenet of treatment is to prevent or reduce ischemia and minimize symptoms.

Nitrates: For the **acute episode** or for prophylactic use before exertion, nitroglycerin 0.3 to 0.6 mg sublingually is the most effective drug. Dramatic relief is usual within 1.5 to 3 min, is complete by about 5 min, and lasts up to 30 min. The dose may be repeated after 4 to 5 min 3 times, if initial relief is incomplete. Patients should carry nitroglycerin tablets with them at all times. Nitroglycerin loses potency unless stored in a tightly sealed glass container; small amounts should be obtained frequently.

Nitroglycerin is a potent smooth-muscle relaxer and vasodilator. In advanced CAD, because its major site of action is in the peripheral vascular tree, especially in the venous or capacitance system, it probably has little effect on the coronary blood vessels. It also lowers systolic pressure, thus reducing myocardial wall tension, a major determinant of myocardial O_2 need. Overall, the drug brings myocardial O_2 supply and demand into more favorable balance.

Amyl nitrite, an extremely potent vasodilator, may be effective when severe angina is unresponsive to nitroglycerin and complicated by hypertension. An ampul containing 0.3 mL is crushed and its vapor briefly inhaled; the patient should be lying down and in a well-ventilated room. Because of the drug's potency, only 2 or 3 inhalations are required.

Long-acting nitrates are available in oral and cutaneous preparations. They improve exercise tolerance for several hours in patients with angina.

(1) **Isosorbide dinitrate,** orally, is effective within 1 to 2 h, with persistent action for 4 to 6 h. Initial dosage of 10 to 20 mg qid or q 6 h may be increased, depending on response, to 40 mg qid.

(2) **Pentaerythritol tetranitrate** is an oral preparation, effective for about 6 h. The initial dosage of 10 to 20 mg qid or q 6 h may be increased, depending upon response, to 40 mg qid.

(3) **Cutaneous patches** are available in various sizes each containing a different amount of nitroglycerin; all are designed to provide prolonged therapeutic effect by slow release of drug. In patients with angina pectoris, exercise capacity is improved 4 h after patch application, but most studies fail to show sustained improvement at 18 to 24 h. Response is related to the size of the patch and the concentration of the drug. Tolerance may develop in some patients; thus, removal of patches after 14 to 18 h has been suggested. For each specific preparation, the manufacturer's brochure should be reviewed.

(4) **Nitroglycerin ointment**: The drug is well absorbed from the skin, especially in a moist environment. Dispensed as a 2% preparation (0.5 mg/2.5 cm [1 in.]), it is applied over the upper torso or arms at 6- to 8-h intervals. The initial dose is 1.25 cm (0.5 in.) increasing to 7.5 cm (3 in.) as tolerated; it should be spread evenly over the skin surface and covered with plastic. Because of possible tolerance, some authorities suggest omitting the evening or nighttime dose.

β-Adrenergic blocking agents block sympathetic stimulation of the heart and reduce systolic pressure, heart rate, contractility, and CO, thus decreasing myocardial O_2 demand and increasing exercise tolerance. Since tissue O_2 requirements are met by greater O_2 extraction from capillary blood, systemic arteriovenous O_2 difference is widened. A number of preparations are available.

Ca blockers (eg, diltiazem, nifedipine, and verapamil) are the important third arm in the triple therapy approach to angina pectoris and CAD. They are effective vasodilators and counter coronary spasm if present. They are often highly effective in variant or Prinzmetal's angina.

Antiplatelet drugs: Experimental evidence and inferences from clinical observations strongly suggest that platelet aggregation may play a pivotal role in the genesis of MI and unstable angina, although data from direct observation in patients are not yet available. However, many authorities recommend that aspirin be given prophylactically to patients with CAD in a dose of 80 to 300 mg daily.

Unstable angina is a medical emergency to be treated in a cardiac care unit **(CCU)**. Bed rest, sedation, nasal O_2, nitrates, β-blockers, and Ca antagonists may be useful. Nitroglycerin as a continuous IV drip with close monitoring of BP and heart rate has proved useful in many patients with unstable angina and recurrent pain. Both heparin in full IV therapeutic doses and aspirin have been shown to reduce the incidence of subsequent MI in unstable angina, but these 2 drugs should *not* be given concurrently; many authorities recommend giving the heparin while the patient is in the CCU.

When symptoms are unresponsive to drugs, angiography and evaluation of the patient for coronary bypass surgery or angioplasty may be indicated. Patients with continual ischemic episodes who respond poorly to aggressive medical therapy may be candidates for insertion of an intra-aortic counterpulsating balloon. This device reduces systolic afterload and increases diastolic pressure, the driving force for coronary arterial flow. It frequently relieves pain and may be used to support the patient during cardiac catheterization and before surgery.

Coronary arterial bypass surgery is highly effective. The "ideal" candidate has severe angina pectoris, a normal-sized heart, no history of MI, localized disease suitable for bypass, good ventricular function, and no adverse risk factors. In such patients, elec-

tive surgery carries a 5 to 7% risk of perioperative MI and a mortality of 1.5% or less. About 85% of such patients have complete or dramatic relief of symptoms. At the end of 1 yr about 85% of the bypass grafts remain patent. Exercise testing shows a positive correlation between patency of the graft and improvement in exercise tolerance, but some patients improve significantly despite closure of the bypass.

CAD may progress despite bypass surgery. The rate of proximal occlusion of bypassed vessels is increased. Vein graft obstruction proceeds in 2 phases: early thrombus formation and a later (several years) slow atherosclerotic degeneration of the media. Recent data suggest that treatment with aspirin and dipyridamole prolong vein graft patency. Internal mammary arteries are increasingly used for grafting because of high patency rates; after 10 yr as many as 97% remain functioning and the artery hypertrophies to accommodate increased flow to the myocardium.

The effects of bypass surgery in the prognosis of CAD continue to be debated. Patients with left main obstruction and those with 3-vessel disease and poor LV function have improved survival following bypass. This may be true also for some patients with 2-vessel disease. However, in patients with mild or moderate angina (Class I or II), 3-vessel disease, and good ventricular function, survival appears to be equally good with medical or surgical therapy. Bypass surgery does not improve prognosis in patients with 1-vessel disease. Long-term effects of bypass surgery are subject to continued evaluation.

Angioplasty: Insertion of a balloon-tipped catheter into a partially obstructive atherosclerotic lesion and inflation of the balloon can dramatically dilate the obstruction. About 20% reocclude in a few days or weeks, but most can be redilated successfully. Repeat angiography 1 yr later has revealed an apparently normal lumen in about 30% of vessels undergoing the procedure. Angioplasty is an alternative to bypass surgery in the patient with suitable anatomic lesions. The risk currently is comparable to surgery: Mortality is 1 to 3%; MI rate is 3 to 5%; emergency bypass surgery is required in < 5%; the rate of success is 85 to 90% in highly experienced hands.

MYOCARDIAL INFARCTION (MI)

Ischemic myocardial necrosis usually resulting from abrupt reduction in coronary blood flow to a segment of myocardium.

Etiology and Pathogenesis

An acute thrombus occludes the artery previously partially obstructed by an atherosclerotic plaque, which supplies the damaged area in > 90% of patients with acute MI. Altered platelet function induced by endothelial change in the atherosclerotic plaque presumably contributes to genesis of the clot. Spontaneous thrombolysis occurs in about ⅔ so that 24 h later, thrombotic occlusion is found in only about 30%. In unstable angina, ⅓ or more of patients studied angiographically have partially occluding thrombi in the vessel subtending the recurrent ischemic area. Since recognition of a thrombus on angiography may be difficult, the incidence is probably underreported.

MI is also rarely caused by arterial embolization (eg, in mitral or aortic stenosis, infective endocarditis, and marantic endocarditis). MI in patients with coronary spasm and otherwise normal coronary arteries has been reported.

MI is predominantly a disease of the left ventricle, but damage may extend into the right ventricle or the atria. Right ventricular **(RV)** infarction usually results from occlusion of the right coronary artery and is characterized by high RV filling pressure, often with severe tricuspid regurgitation. RV infarction should be considered in any patient with inferior-posterior infarction and hypotension or shock. **Transmural infarcts** involve the whole thickness of myocardium from epicardium to endocardium and are characterized by abnormal Q waves on the ECG. **Nontransmural or subendocardial infarcts** do not extend through the ventricular wall and cause only S-T segment and T

wave abnormalities. **Subendocardial infarcts** usually involve the inner 1/3 of the myocardium where wall tension is highest and myocardial blood flow is most vulnerable to circulatory changes. They may also follow prolonged hypotension of any etiology.

The ability of the heart to continue functioning as a pump is related directly to the extent of myocardial damage. Thus, autopsy studies have shown that patients who die with cardiogenic shock usually have an infarct, or a combination of scar and new infarct, of 50% or more of LV mass. Furthermore, anterior infarcts tend to be larger and have a worse prognosis than inferior-posterior infarcts. Anterior infarcts are usually due to occlusion in the left coronary arterial tree, especially the anterior descending artery. Posterior-inferior infarcts reflect right coronary occlusion or occlusion of a dominant left circumflex artery.

Symptoms and Signs

The first symptom of acute MI usually is deep, substernal, visceral pain described as aching or pressure, often with radiation to the back, jaw, or left arm. The pain is similar in character to that of angina pectoris, but is usually more severe and relieved little, or only temporarily, by nitroglycerin. However, discomfort may be very mild, and a significant percentage (perhaps 20%) of acute MIs are silent or unrecognized as illness by the patient. In severe episodes the patient becomes apprehensive and may develop a sense of impending doom. Symptoms of LV failure, pulmonary edema, shock, or significant arrhythmia may develop and dominate the clinical picture.

On examination the patient is usually restless, apprehensive, pale, diaphoretic, and in severe pain. Peripheral or central cyanosis may be apparent and the skin is usually cool. The pulse may be thready and the BP is variable, although many patients initially manifest some degree of hypertension unless cardiogenic shock is developing. Arrhythmia is common: Bradycardia or extrasystoles may be observed early in the course of MI; of those who die, 60% die of primary ventricular fibrillation *before* reaching the hospital. The heart sounds are usually somewhat distant; the presence of a 4th heart sound is almost universal. There may be a soft systolic blowing apical murmur (a reflection of papillary muscle dysfunction) at the apex. At initial evaluation, the presence of a friction rub or more striking murmurs suggests the possibility of preexisting heart disease or another diagnosis. Detection of a friction rub within a few hours after the onset of symptoms of acute MI is distinctly unusual and might suggest a diagnosis of acute pericarditis rather than MI.

Laboratory Findings

The most important laboratory procedure in the patient suspected of suffering an acute MI is analysis of the ECG. In **acute transmural MI** the initial ECG may be diagnostic, showing abnormal deep Q waves and elevated S-T segments in leads subtending the area of damage, or the ECG may be strikingly abnormal with elevated or depressed S-T segments and deeply inverted T waves without abnormal Q waves (see FIGS. 27–32 to 27–37). Serial tracings showing a gradual evolution toward a stable, more normal pattern, or the development of abnormal Q waves over the next few days tends to confirm the initial impression of acute MI. Since **nontransmural infarcts** are usually in the subendocardial or mid-myocardial layers, they are not associated with diagnostic Q waves on the ECG and commonly produce only varying degrees of S-T segment and T wave abnormality. In some patients the ECG abnormalities are less striking, variable, or nonspecific, and therefore difficult to interpret. However, a diagnosis of acute MI is probably untenable when repeated ECGs are completely normal. A normal ECG when the patient is pain free does not rule out unstable angina that may culminate in acute MI.

Routine laboratory examination reveals abnormalities compatible with tissue necrosis. Thus the ESR is increased, the WBC is usually elevated, and differential WBC count reveals a shift to the left. The most helpful laboratory findings are **serial measure-**

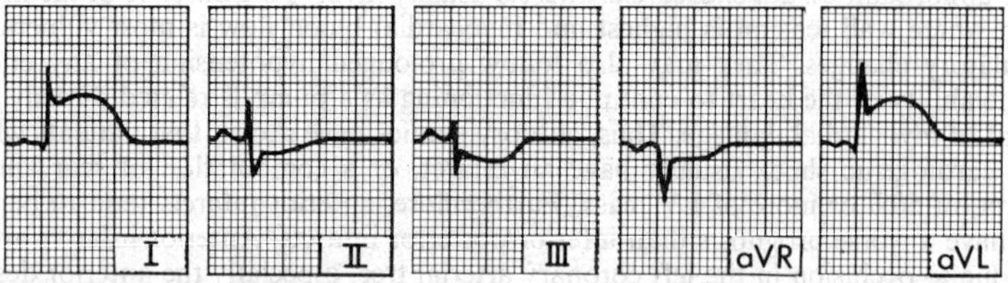

Fig. 27–32. Acute anterior left ventricular infarction—tracing obtained with a few hours of the onset reciprocal depression in the other leads.

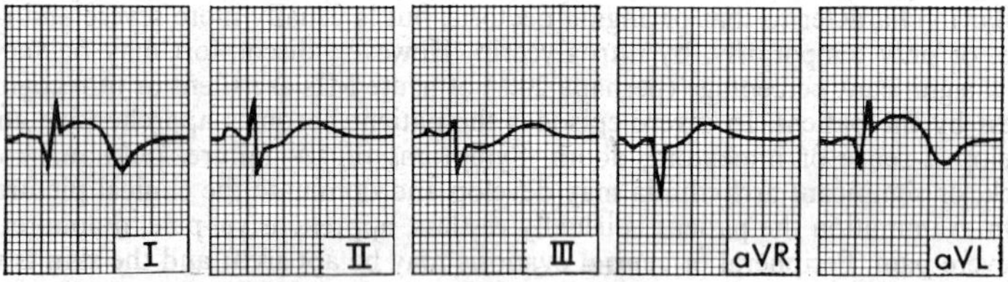

Fig. 27–33. Acute anterior left ventricular infarction—24 h later. Note that the S-T segments are less and V_6.

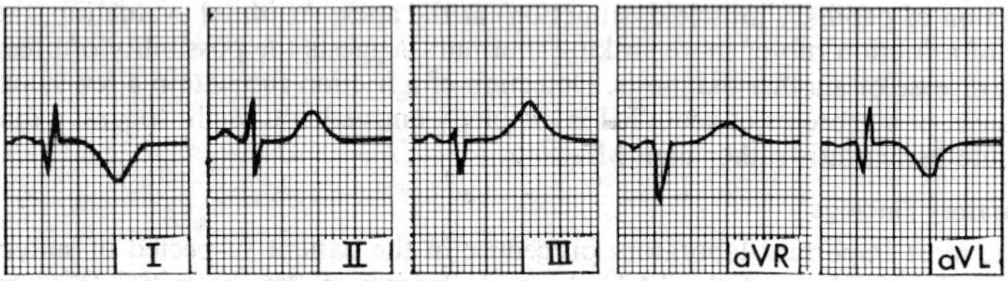

Fig. 27–34. Acute anterior left ventricular infarction—several days later. Significant Q waves and the only change slowly over the next several months.

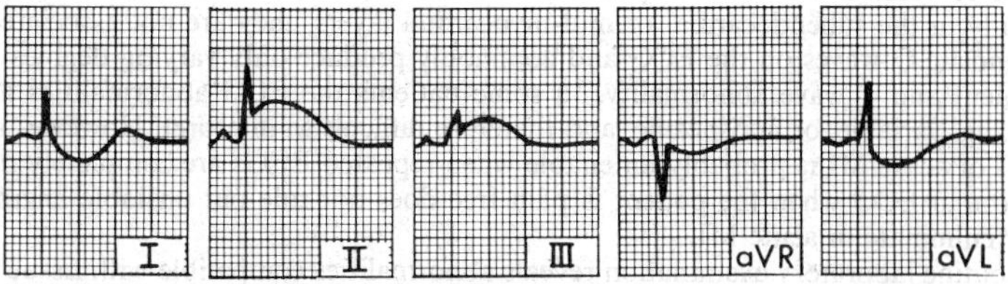

Fig. 27–35. Acute inferior diaphragmatic left ventricular infarction—tracing obtained within a few reciprocal depression in the other leads.

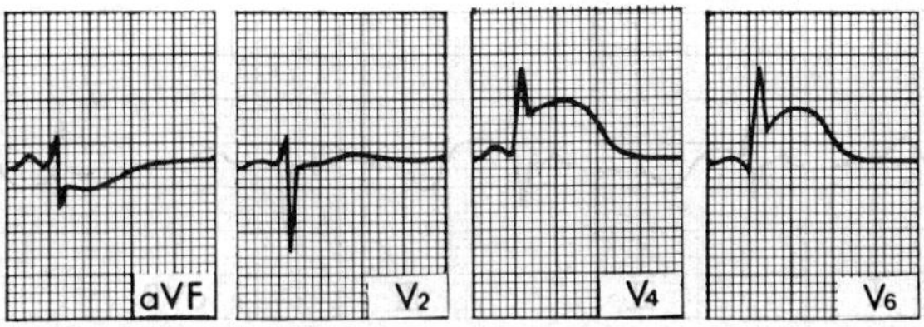

of illness. Note the striking hyperacute S-T segment elevation in leads I, aVL, V_4, and V_6, and the

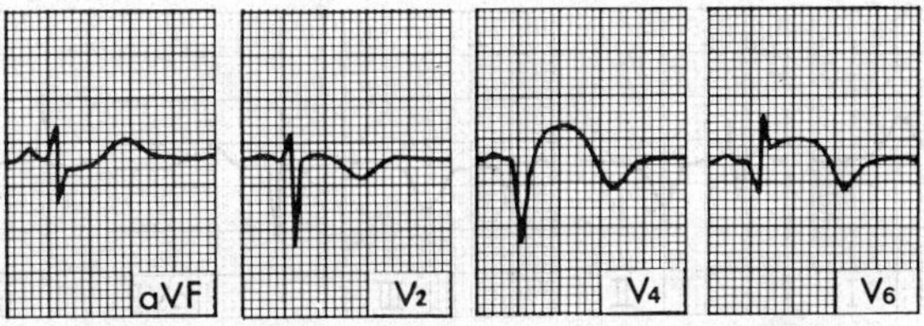

elevated; also note the development of significant Q waves and the loss of the R wave in leads I, aVL, V_4,

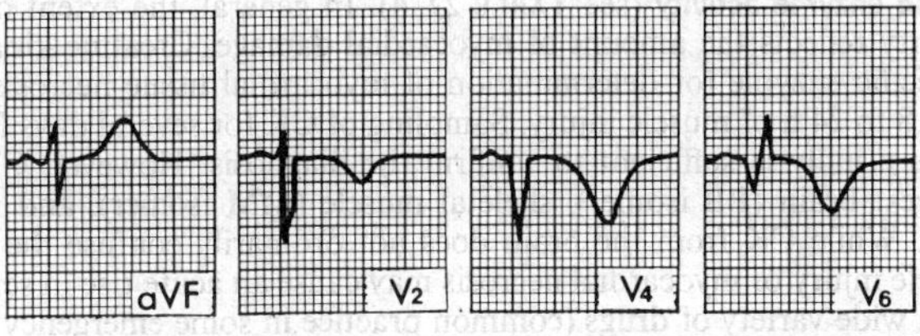

loss of the R wave voltage persist. S-T segments are now essentially isoelectric. The ECG will probably

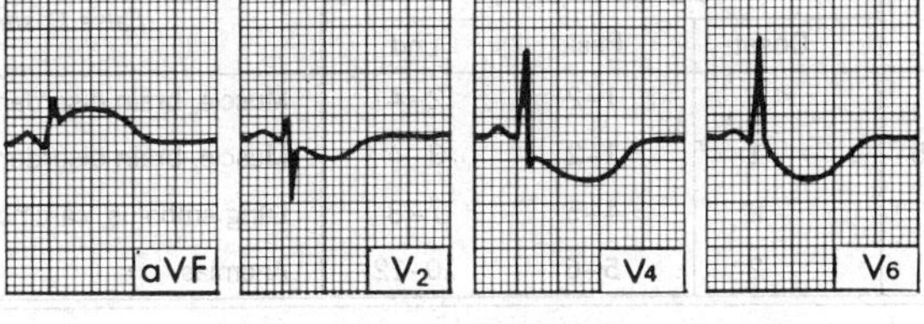

hours of the onset of illness. Note the hyperacute S-T segment elevation in leads II, III, and aVF, and the

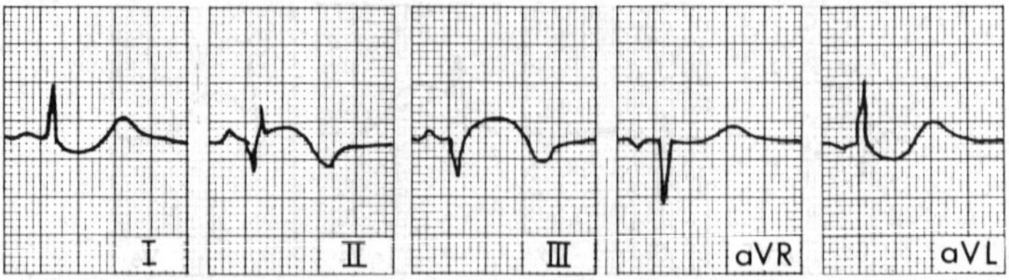

FIG. 27–36. Acute inferior diaphragmatic left ventricular infarction—after the first 24 h. Note the in the same leads.

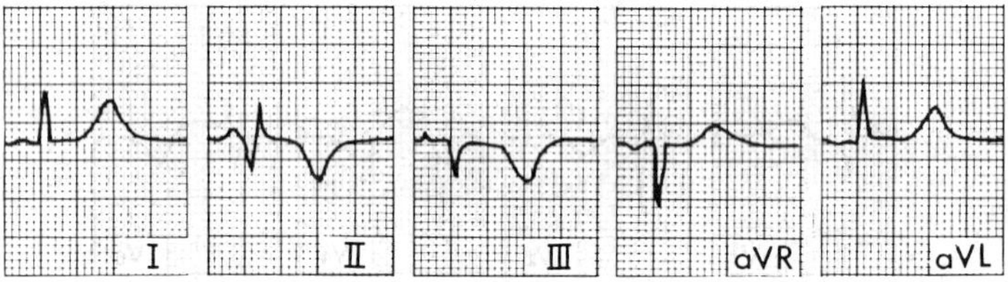

FIG. 27–37. Acute inferior diaphragmatic left ventricular infarction—several days later. S-T segments persist.

ments of blood enzyme activity (see TABLE 27–4). In general, the extent of the rise of enzyme activity reflects the amount of myocardial damage. Creatine kinase **(CK)** is a relatively specific enzyme for determination of myocardial tissue necrosis, rising to a peak within 18 to 24 h of muscle injury. Sampling of CK for several days following the acute episode usually is sufficient to confirm the diagnosis. However, CK originates from 3 sources: brain (BB isomer), skeletal muscle (MM isomer), and myocardium (MB isomer). While CK from the brain does not ordinarily confuse the issue, either skeletal muscle injury or myocardial necrosis may cause an acute rise in serum CK. IM injection of a wide variety of drugs (common practice in some emergency rooms) may cause sufficient skeletal muscle damage to increase serum CK. When the diagnosis is in

TABLE 27–4. SERUM ENZYMES IN MYOCARDIAL INFARCTION

*Normal**	*Elevations (days)*			*False Positives*
	Onset	Peak	End	
CK < 30	< 1	1–2	2–4	Muscle, brain disorders
AST (SGOT) < 45	1	1–2	3–4	Muscle, brain disorders
LDH < 600	2	4–5	7–8	Lung embolus, carcinoma, anemias
HBD < 300	2	5–6	10–12	Anemias

* CK, creatine kinase; AST, aspartate amino transferase (formerly SGOT); LDH, lactic dehydrogenase; HBD, α-hydroxybutyric dehydrogenase.

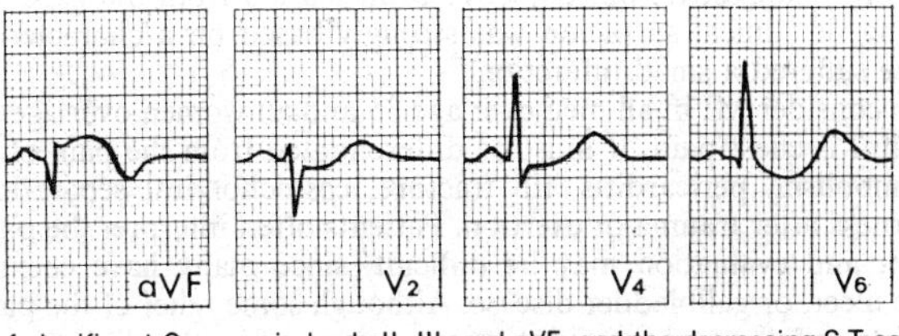

development of significant Q waves in leads II, III, and aVF, and the decreasing S-T segment elevation

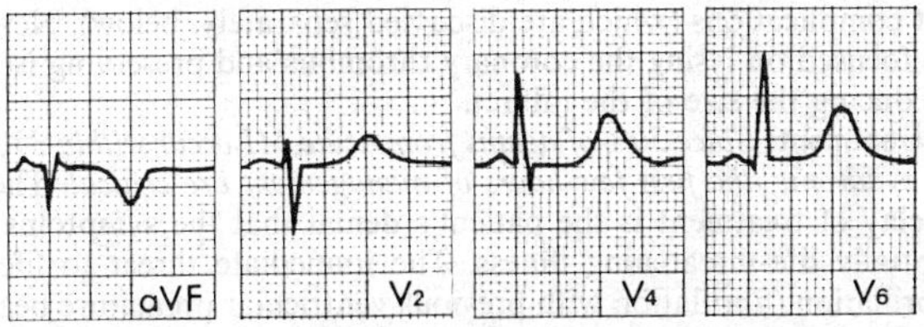

are now isoelectric. There are abnormal Q waves in leads II, II, and aVF, indicating that myocardial scars

doubt, analysis of MB-CK is often helpful, since serum does not normally contain significant MB isomer. Analysis of LDH or α-hydroxybutyric dehydrogenase activity in serum may be useful if the early peak activity of CK has been missed, since these enzymes are maximal at 4 to 5 days.

Myocardial imaging (see in RADIONUCLIDE IMAGING OF THE HEART in Ch. 25): For imaging an MI, 2 technics are available. Technetium (^{99m}Tc) pyrophosphate precipitates as Ca accumulates in recently (up to 3 to 4 days) infarcted myocardium. Thallium (^{201}Tl) accumulates intracellularly in viable myocardium in the manner of K and is distributed according to blood flow. Precordial scanning after injection of the tracer in a patient with an MI may reveal a cold spot or lack of image because of the scar or necrosis.

Cardiac catheterization (see also Ch. 25): Management of complications (eg, severe heart failure, hypoxia, or hypotension) may be aided by measurement of right heart, pulmonary artery, and wedge pressures using balloon-tipped catheters that float into position (Swan-Ganz). CO can be determined with indicator dilution technics. In acutely ill patients with MI complicated by acute mitral regurgitation or acquired ventricular septal defect, echo, radionuclide ventriculogram, or contrast angiography may be necessary to evaluate the possibility of surgical repair.

Diagnosis

In typical MI, the diagnosis is evident from the history, confirmed by the initial ECG and its subsequent evolution, and supported by the serial enzyme changes. In other instances, a definitive diagnosis may not be possible, and patients must be classified as having had a "possible" or "probable" MI; usually the clinical findings are

typical or strongly suggestive, but objective confirmation from the ECG and enzyme assay is lacking. If clinical suspicion was strongly based on a characteristic history, most will have suffered a small infarction.

It is wise to consider MI in all men over age 35 and all women over age 50 when the major complaint is chest pain. It must be differentiated from the pain of pneumonia, pulmonary embolism, pericarditis, rib fracture, costochondral separation, or chest muscle tenderness after trauma or exertion. Patients often interpret the pain of infarct as indigestion, and evaluation may be difficult, since many have coexisting hiatus hernia, peptic ulcer, or gallbladder disease. Although some relief of the pain of infarction by belching or following antacid therapy is common, such relief is usually brief or incomplete. Other conditions to be considered include acute aortic dissection, renal stone, splenic infarction, and a wide variety of abdominal disorders.

Treatment

Treatment is designed to: (1) relieve distress, (2) reduce cardiac work, and (3) prevent and treat complications (which are discussed separately, below). Newer forms of treatment are focused on lysing the coronary thrombus and preserving ischemic myocardium by reducing the size of the infarct.

Prehospital treatment: *Since 50% of deaths from acute MI occur within 3 to 4 h of onset of the clinical syndrome, the first few hours of management are critical.* The major factor causing delay of treatment is the patient's denial that the symptoms represent a serious, potentially life-threatening illness. The immediate threat to life is primary ventricular fibrillation (fibrillation with previous ventricular premature beats) or, occasionally, heart block or profound bradycardia with consequent hypotension that initiates cardiac arrest. Optimal early management includes rapid diagnosis, alleviation of pain and apprehension, stabilization of heart rhythm and BP, and transportation to a hospital with a monitoring unit.

Morphine 4 to 6 mg IV, repeated as needed, is highly effective for the pain of MI. Morphine depresses respiration, reduces myocardial contractility, and is a potent vasodilator. Hypotension and bradycardia secondary to morphine can usually be overcome by prompt elevation of the lower extremities. Other narcotics may be used (eg, ≥ 75 mg of meperidine). Continued pain may also be relieved in some patients by administration of nitroglycerine by continuous IV drip.

Extreme bradycardia with hypotension may respond to atropine sulfate 0.5 to 1 mg IV, which may be repeated after several minutes if the response is inadequate. It is best to give several small doses, because of the risk of inducing tachycardia from excessive dosage. Occasionally, a pacemaker catheter must be inserted. Ventricular premature beats are best treated with lidocaine 50 to 100 mg IV, repeated in 3 to 5 min if necessary. Lidocaine may also be given IM in a dose of 400 mg; antiarrhythmic blood levels are achieved in 10 to 15 min and maintained for as long as 1 h. Some advocate that IM lidocaine be given routinely before transporting the patient. This approach has little risk but has not been universally accepted. Moreover, skeletal muscle damage following any IM injection may confound diagnostic enzyme determinations.

Most patients are moderately hypertensive on arrival at the emergency room, and the BP gradually falls over the next several hours. Severe hypotension or signs of shock are ominous and may be treated with vasopressors before arrival at the hospital. Continued hypertension requires aggressive treatment with vasodilators, preferably IV, to lower BP and reduce cardiac work.

Treatment in the hospital: A patient suspected of having acute MI should be admitted to a hospital with a cardiac care unit **(CCU)** as rapidly as possible. The patient should have a 12-lead ECG recorded, and should be monitored on arrival in the emergency room, a reliable IV route should be established, and blood drawn for enzyme analysis. Transfer to the CCU should be accomplished without delay for further diagnostic procedures. Despite the wide variety of electronic monitoring equip-

ment available, the only function that has consistently proved useful to monitor routinely and continuously is the rate and rhythm of the heart as revealed by the ECG. Qualified nurses can interpret the ECG for arrhythmia and initiate protocols for prophylaxis or treatment with lidocaine or other agents. All professional personnel should be prepared to apply CPR at an instant's notice. (See CARDIAC ARREST AND CARDIOPULMONARY RESUSCITATION, below.)

The primary goals should be to limit myocardial loss and prevent recurrence. Steps are taken to reduce pain, to alleviate anxiety, to maintain adequate arterial PO_2, to enforce proper rest initially, to monitor closely for arrhythmia, to prevent and treat arrhythmia vigorously during the acute phase, to minimize cardiac work, to prevent further ischemia, to detect early heart failure for judicious treatment with diuretics and to treat hypotension or shock with vasopressor and inotropic drugs if it does not respond to appropriate volume loading.

Limiting the extent of ischemia: Cardiac performance after recovery depends largely on the mass of functioning myocardium surviving the acute episode. Scars from previous infarcts add to the acute damage. When the total damaged myocardium exceeds 50% of LV mass, survival is unusual. Reduction of myocardial O_2 requirements by decreasing afterload with vasodilators or reducing heart rate and contractility with β-adrenergic blockers may restrict the area of infarction. It is common practice in selected patients with elevated BP, or increased LV filling pressure to reduce afterload judiciously in the acute state of MI with vasodilators (eg, nitroglycerin, nitroprusside, or isosorbide dinitrate). A short-acting IV drug with quick onset and offset of pharmacologic effect (eg, either of the first 2 mentioned) is preferable. Some authorities prescribe β-adrenergic blockers during acute MI to reduce heart rate, cardiac work, and myocardial O_2 demand, especially in patients with prolonged ischemic pain or undue tachycardia not secondary to heart failure, fever, or other complication. These are best administered IV during the acute phase to ensure prompt onset of action and adequate dose response.

Lysis of thrombus: Recently, attention has focused on the possibility that lysis of coronary thrombi by intracoronary or IV administration of thrombolytic agents (eg, streptokinase, urokinase, or tissue plasmin activator [**TPA**]) may salvage ischemic myocardium destined to become necrotic. The subendocardial myocardium is most susceptible to ischemic damage. In transmural or Q wave infarction, thrombi generally occlude the coronary arteries subserving the area of infarction. In non-Q wave or subendocardial infarction and in unstable angina, thrombi, if present, are usually only partially occlusive. Studies are underway to determine the effect of thrombolytic therapy on the integrity of the clot, size of subsequent infarction, and prognosis. Current results indicate that, in the presence of an occlusive clot, IV streptokinase is effective in about 35% of cases, intracoronary streptokinase in about 80% and intravenous TPA (an experimental drug) in about 65%. Even if clot lysis is effective, the abnormal coronary artery persists and reocclusion will occur in 30 to 50%. Evidence suggests that intracoronary streptokinase reduces the short term mortality, especially in acute anterior transmural MI, and that IV streptokinase reduces in-hospital mortality by about 20% if given with 6 h of onset. The sooner thrombolysis is attempted after onset of MI, the more effective; 6 h seems to be about the upper limit. Currently, many authorities recommend that IV streptokinase (1 to 1.5 million units in 100 mL of 0.9% sodium chloride solution in 1 h) be administered to patients with anterior transmural MI seen within 6 h of onset of symptoms. The role of angioplasty or coronary bypass in decreasing recurrence of thrombosis and improving the blood supply to the infarcted area after clot lysis is being evaluated. Some groups advocate emergency mechanical destruction of the clot in the affected vessel followed by immediate angioplasty in patients admitted within a few hours to hospitals with suitable cardiac catheterization laboratory facilities.

Antiarrhythmics: The usefulness of giving routine prophylactic lidocaine IV remains controversial. When nursing and monitoring facilities are limited, prophylactic lidocaine is probably indicated for the first 48 to 72 h, since the drug is safe and highly effective. For details of use, see above under VENTRICULAR PREMATURE BEATS in CARDIAC ARRHYTHMIAS.

The CCU should be a quiet, calm, restful area. Single rooms are preferred and privacy consistent with monitoring function should be assured. Usually visitors are restricted during the first few days of illness, and outside influences (eg, radios, newspapers) are reduced to a minimum. A wall clock, a calendar, and an outside window help to orient the patient and prevent a sense of isolation.

Anxiety and denial are common in patients with acute MI. Depression is common by the 3rd day of illness and is almost universal at some time during recovery. After the acute phase of illness, the most important tasks are often management of depression, rehabilitation, and institution of long-term preventive programs. Overemphasis on bed rest, inactivity, and the seriousness of the illness reinforces depressive tendencies. A thorough explanation of the illness and an outline of a positive rehabilitation program in the setting of a thorough understanding of the patient's life situation and interpersonal adjustments will have an important beneficial impact.

Morphine may be given for pain as outlined above. Mood changes and apprehension during the acute illness are common, and a mild tranquilizer may be helpful (eg, diazepam 2.5 to 5 mg orally tid or qid). To maximize Pa_{O_2}, most patients are given nasal O_2 3 to 5 L/min during the first few days.

Anticoagulants are used to reduce the risk of pulmonary embolism in poor-risk patients requiring prolonged bed rest. An effective form of therapy is heparin s.c. 5000 u. q 8 or 12 h. Many authorities treat unstable angina and patients post MI with recurrent pain with full dose heparin, 5,000 to 10,000 u. given rapidly IV q 3 to 6 h or 1000 to 2000 u./h by continuous drip preceded by 5000 u. given rapidly IV to maintain PTT at twice the control. Full dose heparin is also indicated in transmural infarction with mural thrombus. The diagnosis is established by echocardiography in patients with Q-wave infarcts, especially anterior. After several days of heparin, the patient may be switched to warfarin-sodium–like anticoagulants for long-term maintenance, depending on the clinical situation.

General measures include maintenance of normal bowel function and avoidance of straining at stool. Milk of magnesia 30 mL bid is an effective laxative; dioctyl sodium sulfosuccinate 100 mg bid may be added if necessary. Urinary retention is common in older patients, especially after several days of bed rest and atropine therapy. A catheter may be required, but it usually can be removed when the patient can stand or sit to void.

Smoking should be prohibited; a sojourn in a CCU is a potent motivation to discontinue smoking, and the physician should reinforce this attitude.

Acutely ill patients have little appetite for food, although modest amounts of tasty food are good for morale. Patients usually are offered a soft diet, somewhat reduced in calories (1500 to 1800/day) with some reduction of Na (2 to 3 gm [87 to 130 mEq]). Salt restriction is not required after the first 2 or 3 days for the patient who has no evidence of heart failure.

Complications of Myocardial Infarction

Arrhythmia in some form with ventricular ectopic beats occurs in > 90% of patients with MI. Disturbances in conduction can reflect damage to the sinus node, the A-V node, or the specialized conduction tissues. Recognition and management of arrhythmia require a thorough understanding of electrophysiology, electrocardiography, and pharmacology. A scheme of management of the commonly encountered arrhythmias is outlined in TABLE 27–5, and details of commonly used drugs are presented under Treatment of specific arrhythmias above in CARDIAC ARRHYTHMIAS.

TABLE 27-5. MANAGEMENT OF ARRHYTHMIAS IN ACUTE MYOCARDIAL INFARCTION

Arrhythmia	*First Choice*	*Second Choice*	*Comments*
Atrial premature beats (APBs)	Digitalis or β-blocker	Quinidine, Verapamil	APBs are frequently forerunners of atrial fibrillation or flutter. CAUTION: *Avoid excessive dosage of digitalis because of increased susceptibility to arrhythmia in acute myocardial infarction*
Paroxysmal atrial tachycardia	Verapamil	Precordial DC shock, Digitalis	An uncommon complication of acute infarction. Verapamil IV effective 95% of cases
Atrial fibrillation	Digitalis or β-blocker	Precordial DC shock β-blocker	Arrhythmia tends to recur, hence first aim of treatment is control of ventricular rate. If patient tolerates arrhythmia poorly, needs atrial "kick," or shows low stroke volume, immediate DC conversion may be necessary. Eventual spontaneous reversion is the rule. If rate is fast, small doses of β-blocker orally or IV may increase A-V block and slow ventricular rate.
Atrial flutter	Digitalis	Precordial DC shock β-blocker	Comments above on atrial fibrillation are applicable to flutter. Some authorities recommend immediate DC shock in all instances of atrial flutter or fibrillation. If rate is fast, small doses of β-blocker orally or IV may increase A-V block and slow ventricular rate.
Paroxysmal nodal tachycardia			See atrial tachycardia. If rate is only moderately increased and associated with A-V dissociation, consider digitalis toxicity as causative.
Ventricular premature beats (VPBs)	Lidocaine	Quinidine Procainamide Disopyramide Tocainide Mexiletine Flecainide Overdriving with pacemaker	Decision to treat depends on setting. More than 5 VPBs/min, occurrence in salvos, or R on T phenomena (closely coupled) demands immediate and adequate treatment. Once VPBs are initially suppressed with IV lidocaine, a plan for long-term therapy with a longer-acting agent should be considered.
Ventricular tachycardia	Precordial DC shock or Lidocaine	Lidocaine Quinidine Procainamide Disopyramide Tocainide Overdriving with pacemaker	Forerunner of ventricular fibrillation. Best combination is immediate precordial shock followed by long-term administration of suppressive drugs. May respond to lidocaine IV. Amiodarone or bretylium may be effective in desperate situations.
Ventricular fibrillation	Precordial DC shock	Closed-chest cardiac massage Intubation and ventilatory support	When cardiac arrest occurs in the CCU, precordial shock should be administered immediately. If unsuccessful, cardiopulmonary resuscitation may be necessary. The longer fibrillation persists, the less likely is survival. Bretylium sometimes helps to convert refractory VF.

Sinus node disturbances are influenced by the origin of the artery to the sinus node (whether from the left or right coronary artery), the location of the occlusion, and the possibility of preexisting sinus node disease, especially in the elderly. Sinus bradycardia may be treated expectantly in most cases; however, a rate < 55 usually indicates treatment with IV atropine (avoiding overdosage because unwanted tachycardia may occur) or a temporary transvenous pacemaker.

Life-threatening arrhythmias, major causes of mortality in MI in the first 72 h, include tachycardia from any focus rapid enough to reduce CO and lower BP, frequent ventricular premature beats, Mobitz 2 or third degree heart block, and ventricular tachycardia and fibrillation. Complete heart block with failure of atrial impulses to capture the ventricle and slow ventricular rate is uncommon and usually denotes massive anterior infarction. Asystole is uncommon except as a terminal manifestation of progressive LV failure and shock.

Persistent sinus tachycardia is generally ominous, often reflecting LV failure and low CO. Other causes (eg, sepsis or thyroid excess) should be sought. **Atrial premature beats (APBs), atrial fibrillation**, and **atrial flutter** occur in about 10% of MI patients and may reflect LV failure or right atrial infarction. Since APBs are often a forerunner of sustained atrial arrhythmia, prompt treatment is usually in order. Frequent APBs usually respond well to digitalis. A β-adrenergic blocker or the Ca blocker verapamil may also be effective. Atrial flutter and fibrillation may be treated with digitalis or a β-blocker to slow the ventricular rate. If the rhythm persists and the patient develops heart failure or hypotension, electrical cardioversion may be indicated. It is not used as first-line treatment because these arrhythmias frequently recur during the first few days of the illness. The aim of treatment is to slow the ventricular rate to acceptable levels. After several days, these arrhythmias usually revert spontaneously to a sinus mechanism; if not, DC shock may then be used. **Paroxysmal atrial tachycardia** is uncommon and usually occurs in patients who have had previous episodes.

It is important to make an exact diagnosis by ECG of the mechanism of **atrioventricular (A-V) block.** Reversible changes in A-V conduction, Mobitz 1 conduction abnormalities with prolonged P-R time, or Wenckebach phenomenon are relatively common, particularly with an inferior-diaphragmatic infarction involving the blood supply to the posterior wall of the left ventricle with branches to the A-V node. These disturbances usually are self-limited and, if the rate is well maintained, do not merit treatment. Progression to complete heart block is unusual. True Mobitz 2 with dropped beats or A-V block with slow, wide QRS complexes is usually an ominous complication of massive anterior infarction. The rhythm and rate may be restored temporarily with isoproterenol infusion, but temporary transvenous pacemaking is the treatment of choice.

Ventricular premature beats (VPBs) occur in most patients with acute MI. VPBs, especially if closely coupled, multifocal, or in salvos, are important because they may initiate sustained ventricular arrhythmia—tachycardia or fibrillation. Treatment is required if the VPBs are frequent, multifocal, or sufficiently premature to strike the vulnerable period of the diastolic repolarization phase of the cardiac cycle (during the ascending limb of the T wave). In most CCUs, > 3 VPBs/min are routinely treated with lidocaine IV. Since constant lidocaine infusion requires several hours to reach equilibrium at therapeutic levels, treatment should be started with loading doses of 1 mg/kg by rapid injection twice at 5-min intervals. An infusion of 2 to 4 mg/min is then maintained, usually for 24 h, and then discontinued. Recurrence of VPBs requires additional rapid doses of lidocaine and an increase in the infusion rate. If ventricular arrhythmias still persist, quinidine, procainamide, disopyramide, tocainide, mexiletine, and flecainide may be indicated. When large doses of these drugs are required, monitoring their blood levels aids in avoiding toxicity. Causes of persistent arrhythmia (eg, hypoxemia, hypokalemia, ventricular aneurysm, or digitalis toxicity) should be dili-

gently sought. For details in administering these drugs, see under treatment of specific arrhythmias above, in CARDIAC ARRHYTHMIAS.

Cardiac arrest due to ventricular tachycardia or fibrillation is treated by immediate defibrillation, or if equipment must be sent for, by CPR followed by defibrillation. Equipment in perfect working order should be immediately on hand in the emergency room and the CCU. Prophylactic antiarrhythmics are usually given after resuscitation.

Heart failure occurs in about 2/3 of hospitalized patients with acute MI. LV dysfunction is usually predominant; hence the findings include dyspnea, inspiratory rales at the lung bases, and hypoxemia. Clinical signs depend upon the size of the infarction, the elevation of LV filling pressure, and the extent to which CO is reduced. The mortality rate varies directly with the severity of LV failure. It is useful to classify patients according to the presence or absence of clinical evidence of LV failure (see TABLE 27–6). Class 1 patients have a hospital mortality rate of 3 to 5%; Class 2, a rate of 6 to 10%. The rate is about 20 to 30% in Class 3, and > 80% in Class 4 patients. For further discussion, see HEART FAILURE, above.

Treatment depends on severity. Caution is urged in mild cases. Digitalis is not effective in the first few days after MI. Use of a loop diuretic (eg, furosemide 20 to 40 mg IV once or twice daily) to reduce ventricular filling pressure by inducing diuresis is often satisfactory. Treatment of pulmonary edema is discussed in detail above under HEART FAILURE.

Hypoxemia, a common accompaniment of acute MI, is usually secondary to increased left atrial pressure with alteration of pulmonary ventilation-perfusion relationships, pulmonary interstitial edema, alveolar collapse, and increased physiologic shunting. Pa_{O_2}, determined while the patient is breathing room air, is essentially normal in Class 1, slightly reduced in Class 2, and severely abnormal in Classes 3 and 4. In patients aged 50 to 70, normal Pa_{O_2} at bed rest is about 82 ± 5 mm Hg. It is reasonable to give O_2 by nasal cannula in an attempt to maintain the Pa_{O_2} at about 100 mm Hg, which may help to oxygenate the myocardium and limit the extent of the infarction or the ischemic zone. In LV failure, Pa_{O_2} before and after response to a rapidly acting diuretic (eg, furosemide 40 mg IV) may be helpful in establishing a diagnosis: the reduced Pa_{O_2} should rise following diuresis.

Hypotension in acute MI may be due to decreased ventricular filling or power failure secondary to massive infarction. Decreased LV filling is most often caused by reduced

TABLE 27–6. CLINICAL CLASSIFICATION OF ACUTE MYOCARDIAL INFARCTION (DETERMINED BY REPEATED EXAMINATION OF THE PATIENT DURING THE COURSE OF ILLNESS)

Class	*Description*
1.	No clinical evidence of left ventricular failure
2.	Mild to moderate left ventricular failure
3.	Severe left ventricular failure; pulmonary edema
4.	Cardiogenic shock: hypotension, tachycardia, mental obtundation, cool extremities, oliguria, hypoxia

(Modified from "Treatment of Myocardial Infarction in a Coronary Care Unit. A Two-Year Experience with 250 Patients" by T. Killip and J. T. Kimball, in *The American Journal of Cardiology,* Vol. 20, pp. 457–464, October 1967. Used with permission of the *Journal* and the author.)

venous return secondary to low blood volume, especially in patients receiving intensive loop diuretic therapy, but may reflect RV infarction, which is characterized by high right (but low left) atrial pressure. Determining the cause of hypotension usually requires measurement of intracardiac pressure with a percutaneously inserted Swan-Ganz floating, balloon-tipped catheter. If left atrial pressure is low in the face of systemic hypotension, a fluid challenge with crystalloid (0.9% or 0.45% NaCl solution) is in order: 200 to 400 mL may be given over 30 min as systemic arterial and left atrial pressures are monitored. If BP rises with only modest increment in left atrial pressure, a diagnosis of hypovolemia is probable and fluid replacement should be possible without left heart overload (excessive rise in left atrial pressure). In some hypovolemic patients, LV function is so compromised that adequate fluid replacement is extremely difficult because it is accompanied by sharp rise in pulmonary wedge pressure to levels associated with pulmonary edema (> 25 mm Hg), if plasma proteins are normal. A fluid challenge may be carried out without measurement of intracardiac pressure, if hypovolemia is strongly suspected. Increase in BP with clinical improvement and no signs of pulmonary congestion suggests that hypovolemia was present.

Cardiogenic shock, characterized by hypotension, tachycardia, reduced urine output, mental confusion, diaphoresis, and cold extremities carries a grave prognosis. Mortality is ≥ 80%. Cardiogenic shock is most often associated with massive anterior infarction and loss of LV functioning myocardium in excess of 50%. Drug therapy with β- or α-agonists may be temporarily effective. Dopamine, a catecholamine, is given at 0.5 to 1 μg/kg/min and the dose increased until a satisfactory response or a maximum of about 10 μg/kg/min is achieved. Higher doses induce vasoconstriction. Dobutamine, a β-agonist, may be given IV 2.5 to 10 μg/kg/min or in higher doses. Dobutamine appears to be most effective when hypotension is secondary to low CO; dopamine may be more effective when a pressor effect is also required. In refractory cases, the 2 drugs may be combined. The intra-aortic counter pulsating balloon will often temporarily support the patient. Anecdotal reports have described selected cases in which remarkable recovery of ventricular function followed intracoronary injection of a thrombolytic agent (eg, streptokinase) and lysis of the causative coronary artery clot.

Recurrent ischemia: The chest pain of MI generally subsides within 12 to 24 h. Chest pain after the first day may represent pericarditis, pulmonary embolus, and other complications (eg, pneumonia or recurrent ischemia). Usually, recurrent ischemia is accompanied by reversible ECG change in the T wave and ST segment. It may be associated with elevated BP. Recent evidence indicates that silent ischemia (ECG change without pain) may occur in as many as 1/3 of patients with recurrent pain. Continued evidence of ischemia post MI suggest further myocardial jeopardy and is treated like unstable angina. Treatment with sublingual or IV nitroglycerin is usually effective. Following vasodilator therapy, coronary angiography and the possibility of bypass surgery should be considered to salvage ischemic myocardium.

Functional papillary muscle insufficiency is common in MI, occurring in about 35% in one reported series. Frequent auscultation during the first few hours of infarction will often reveal a transient late apical systolic murmur thought to represent papillary muscle ischemia with failure of complete coaptation of the valve leaflets. In some patients mitral regurgitation is a permanent reflection of papillary muscle scar.

Myocardial rupture occurs in 3 forms: (1) **Rupture of the papillary muscle**, a rare complication, is most often associated with inferior-posterior infarcts due to right coronary artery occlusion. It produces acute, severe mitral regurgitation and is characterized by the sudden appearance of a loud apical systolic murmur and thrill, usually accompanied by pulmonary edema. Emergency replacement of the mitral valve has

been accomplished successfully. (2) **Rupture of the intraventricular septum,** while rare, is 8 to 10 times more common than rupture of the papillary muscle. Sudden appearance of a loud systolic murmur and thrill medial to the apex along the left sternal border in the 3rd or 4th intercostal space, accompanied by hypotension with or without signs of LV failure, is characteristic. Diagnosis may be confirmed with a balloon-tipped catheter and comparison of blood O_2 saturation or P_{O_2} of right atrial, RV, and pulmonary artery samples. A significant step-up in the right ventricle is diagnostic. Echo-Doppler studies are useful in establishing diagnosis and may replace hemodynamic confirmation in selected cases. Although mortality is high, surgical repair of the defect has been accomplished in a number of instances. (3) **External rupture,** characterized by sudden loss of arterial pressure with momentary persistence of sinus rhythm and often by signs of cardiac tamponade, is universally fatal.

Ventricular asynergy: The hallmark of CAD is patchy LV damage due to ischemia or infarction. Thus normal and abnormal myocardium are juxtaposed. A local noncontracting segment of left ventricle with no systolic inward motion, as revealed by angiography, is termed **akinetic. Hypokinetic** myocardium has reduced contractile excursion with partial impairment of inward motion. In an occasional patient, the myocardial hypokinesis is diffuse, and the term **ischemic myocardiopathy** is applied if presenting symptoms predominantly reflect low CO and heart failure with pulmonary congestion. A **dyskinetic** area shows systolic expansion or bulging (paradoxic motion). These changes may be recognized by 2-D echo, radionuclide ventriculogram, or at angiography, and may contribute to reduced ventricular function and long-term disability.

Ventricular aneurysm is a common complication favored by a large transmural infarct and good residual myocardium. Aneurysms may develop in a few days or in weeks or months and are most commonly associated with large anterior infarcts due to left anterior descending coronary artery occlusion. They do not rupture, but may be associated with recurrent ventricular arrhythmias and low CO. Mural thrombi and systemic embolization are distinct hazards. Diagnosis of mural thrombus may be established by echocardiography. Treatment consists of IV heparin in full doses followed by long-term administration of coumarin anticoagulants. Evidence that this therapy reduces the risk of embolus is not available. Ultrasound studies have shown that ≥ 30% of large dyskinetic areas in the left ventricle have in situ thrombus. An aneurysm is suspected when paradoxic precordial movements are seen or felt, accompanied by persistent elevation of S-T segments on the ECG or a characteristic bulge of the cardiac shadow on x-ray. Ventriculography has revealed a high incidence of unsuspected LV aneurysm. Surgical excision may be indicated when LV failure or arrhythmia persist in the presence of a functionally significant aneurysm.

Pericarditis: A pericardial friction rub may be detected in about ⅓ of patients with acute transmural MI if auscultation is frequent. It is usually heard 24 to 96 h after the onset of infarction. Hearing a friction rub earlier is unusual and suggests the possibility of other diagnoses (eg, acute pericarditis), although hemorrhagic pericarditis occasionally complicates the early phase of MI. Acute tamponade is rare. The pericarditis of MI usually subsides in 3 to 5 days. A post-pericardiotomy syndrome characterized by recurrent pericarditis develops in an occasional patient.

Postmyocardial infarction syndrome (Dressler's syndrome): In a few patients, a syndrome develops several days to weeks after acute MI and is characterized by fever, pericarditis with friction rub, pericardial effusion, pleurisy, pleural effusions, and joint pains. This syndrome is analagous to the **postpericardiotomy syndrome** and appears to be an autoimmune disorder secondary to damaged myocardium and pericardium. Differentiation from extension or recurrence of infarction may be difficult, but a significant rise in the cardiac enzymes does not occur. Patients usually respond satisfactorily

to intensive aspirin therapy, 600 to 900 mg q 4 to 6 h, but it can recur a number of times. A short, intensive course of corticosteroids or a nonsteroidal anti-inflammatory agent may be necessary in severe cases.

Treatment and Prognosis Post-Hospital Discharge

Mortality in the year after acute MI is 8 to 10%. Most fatalities occur in the first 3 to 4 mo. Clinical evaluation permits stratification into low- and high-risk groups. High risk is associated with continued ventricular arrhythmia, heart failure or poor ventricular function, and possibly recurrent ischemic pain. A 24-h Holter ambulatory ECG may reveal significant persistent ventricular arrhythmia. Treatment with potent antiarrhythmic drugs is usually recommended, but there is no definitive evidence that this approach improves prognosis. At hospital discharge or within 6 wk of the acute attack, many authorities recommend use of the symptom-limited exercise tolerance test; good exercise performance without ECG abnormality identifies patients with a favorable prognosis. Further immediate evaluation is probably not indicated. Abnormal resting or exercise performance is associated with a poor prognosis; these patients should probably have LV function evaluated noninvasively with a radionuclide technic at rest and during exercise. Many authorities proceed to coronary arteriography in the hope that bypass surgery will improve the long-term outlook, but this has not been proved by prospective randomized controlled studies.

Despite the importance of thrombosis in the genesis of MI, controversy continues over the role of anticoagulants post MI. Full-dose heparin is often given in transmural anterior MI because of the high incidence of mural clot. It may also be effective in unstable angina or in patients with recurrent ischemia post-MI. After discharge, warfarin sodium may be continued if thrombus was present for about 3 mo, then discontinued if an echocardiogram fails to demonstrate a thrombus. Many physicians also treat patients post MI with low-dose aspirin (80 to 300 mg/day) to reduce platelet aggregation. Proof of effectiveness, except in unstable angina, remains controversial.

β-Blocking agents post MI: Post-MI mortality is reduced about 25% by therapy with timolol, propranolol, or metoprolol. The effect appears to persist for up to 7 yr. Current debate focuses on whether all patients or only those at higher risk should be treated. Since the drugs are generally well tolerated, it seems reasonable to treat all patients who have minimal side effects and are willing to continue long-term therapy.

Rehabilitation: It is wise to keep the patient quiet in bed for the first 2 or 3 days until the course of the illness becomes reasonably evident. Longer bed rest results in rapid physical deconditioning with development of orthostatic hypotension, decreased work capacity, and increased heart rate during effort. Feelings of depression and helplessness are intensified. Patients without complications may be permitted chair rest, passive exercise, and a commode. Walking to the bathroom and nonstressful paperwork or reading are allowed shortly thereafter. Discharge from the hospital after 10 days to 2 wk is reasonable and without significant hazard. Physical activity is gradually increased during the next 3 to 6 wk. Factors such as age, extent of injury, arrhythmia, heart failure, occupation, and personal ambition influence the rehabilitation program. Resumption of sexual activity is often of great concern and may be encouraged in parallel with other moderate physical activities. If cardiac function is well maintained 6 wk after acute infarction, most patients can return to their full range of normal activity. A regular exercise program consistent with lifestyle, age, and cardiac status may be protective and certainly enhances general well-being.

The impact of acute illness and treatment in the CCU provides strong motivation to both physician and patient to analyze and manage risk factors. Frank discussion and thorough evaluation of the patient's physical and emotional status coupled with sound advice about smoking, diet, work and play habits, and exercise, together with effective

treatment of known risk factors may improve the patient's long-term outlook and are important obligations of the physician providing continuous medical care.

SUDDEN CARDIAC DEATH (SCD)

SCD does not have a single, uniform definition. Broadly, it is *death due to a primary cardiac cause or mechanism occurring within 24 h of the onset of acute illness in a person thought to be free of heart disease or with symptomatically mild cardiac disease.* For greater precision, the definition is frequently restricted to a narrower time-span (eg, instantaneous death, death within 1 h, 2 h, 6 h, etc, or simply prehospitalization death).

Etiology and Pathophysiology

In adults, > 90% of SCDs are due to coronary heart disease. Advanced coronary arteriosclerosis is found in 2 or 3 of the major coronary vessels in at least 75% of cases; 15% have a major narrowing of only a single coronary vessel, and < 10% are free of substantial coronary artery disease. Evidence of old myocardial infarction **(MI)** is found in 50% of patients, and 25% have small (< 1 cm in size) fibrotic scars in the myocardium. Acute coronary obstruction due to a thrombus or ruptured plaque is found in 40 or 50% of SCDs. Histologic changes of acute MI are found in only 10 or 15% of cases since a minimum of 6 to 12 h of survival after the onset of severe ischemia is required for such changes to become visible on light microscopy. However, in 5 to 10% of SCDs, the histologic age of such fresh infarcts antedates symptoms described by relatives and friends.

Ventricular fibrillation is the most common cardiac rhythm observed immediately or shortly after a victim of SCD collapses, and cardiac standstill is found with increased frequency later following collapse. Immediately antecedent rhythm disturbances include marked ectopic ventricular activity and ventricular tachycardia, though ventricular fibrillation can arise without such prior dysrrhythmia. SCD can occur without acute MI and over 1/2 of patients resuscitated from ventricular fibrillation outside the hospital do not develop clinical, ECG, or enzymatic characteristics of MI.

In addition to arrhythmias, the pathophysiologic mechanisms that can result in SCD include intrinsic pump failure due to loss of cardiac muscle or myocardial contractile performance; failure of impulse formation or conduction; coronary arterial constriction, generally in association with coronary arteriosclerosis, leading to catastrophic ischemia and arrhythmia; electromechanical dissociation; loss of valvular function due to perforation of a cusp or to rupture or incompetency of a papillary muscle; ventricular septal perforation with shunt development; extrinsic pump failure with pressure overload; cardiac rupture with or without tamponade; or emboli.

Underlying diseases, in addition to coronary heart disease, include rheumatic heart disease (especially aortic valvular disease); hypertensive heart disease; fibrotic, infiltrative, and degenerative processes involving the myocardium, sinus node, or conduction system; hypertrophic and other cardiomyopathies; myocarditis; congenital heart diseases (especially those with cyanosis or aortic stenosis) and anomalies of the coronary circulation; cor pulmonale; ball valve thrombus or myxoma obstructing flow in the left ventricle; bacterial endocarditis with cusp perforation; aneurysms with dissection or rupture; and emboli to the coronary or peripheral vessels. Ventricular fibrillation and SCD can be caused by the prolonged Q-T syndrome (which may be accompanied by deafness). Mitral valve prolapse may be associated with this fatal arrhythmia, but very rarely considering its high prevalence. Some SCD seems to be emotionally precipitated and neurally mediated, and sometimes the toxic effect of drugs prescribed to treat cardiovascular or other disease is causal.

Risk Factors

Because most SCD is due to coronary heart disease, its risk factors are basically those for arteriosclerosis (see above in ARTERIOSCLEROSIS; ATHEROSCLEROSIS). However, the most powerful risk factors are a history of MI and its severity as manifested by acute arrhythmias and heart failure and by residual arrhythmias, heart failure, cardiomegaly, and S-T segment abnormalities in the ECG at rest. When associated with heart disease, ventricular arrhythmias of increasing frequency and severity—eg, > 10/h or 2/min, multifocal or coupled premature ventricular contractions, and ventricular tachycardia—are risk factors. *However, ventricular arrhythmias without readily detectable heart disease carry little or no added risk for SCD.*

Symptoms, Signs, and Clinical Course

Questioning of the family reveals new or progressive symptoms of cardiovascular disease in perhaps 2/3 of SCD victims—over several days, or sometimes for just hours or minutes. These may be new chest discomfort, palpitations, increased anginal pain, breathlessness for no apparent reason, symptoms referred to the musculoskeletal system or GI tract, overwhelming fatigue, or depression. Such symptoms are not specific for impending SCD, and the frequency with which SCD follows them is unknown.

It is often impossible to define the onset of acute illness precisely. The symptoms are often within the range of normal experience for the victim and represent premonitory symptoms of impending SCD only in retrospect. In other instances, typical symptoms of acute MI may progress rapidly to death. Denial of the significance of symptoms and the nonspecificity of many symptoms are major impediments to early recognition and adequate medical care of those who succumb to SCD. Half of those who die of ischemic heart disease die within 1 h of the onset of the acute illness, including the 25 to 33% who drop dead instantaneously or are found dead.

Diagnosis

Diagnosis of SCD is best made from the clinical findings in association with autopsy confirmation of coronary or cardiac disease. Other illnesses must be excluded; eg, pulmonary emboli, deaths due to prescribed or "recreational" drugs, hepatic decompensation (especially with alcoholism), stroke, overwhelming infection (particularly pulmonary and CNS), and GI bleeding or perforation. Noncardiac causes must be carefully sought in victims whose death is unwitnessed or whose history is unreliable. The absence of ECG findings of MI should not negate the diagnosis of SCD nor diminish appropriate treatment for patients with symptoms of acute cardiovascular disease.

Prevention

Management of SCD includes long-term prophylaxis, early therapy of acute cardiovascular symptoms, and cardiac resuscitation for patients who develop cardiac arrest (see below). The most effective prevention of SCD is prevention of cardiac disease (eg, by avoiding smoking) and management of high blood cholesterol and hypertension.

The increased risk of SCD when ventricular irritability accompanies heart disease, and the common role of ventricular fibrillation in SCD raise the question of prophylactic antiarrhythmic therapy. Several oral drugs have become available with some effectiveness in controlling ventricular arrhythmias. However, success in reducing premature ventricular contractions should not automatically be equated with effectiveness in prophylaxis against SCD. Such drugs have not been demonstrated to save lives except in the very small number of patients with recurrent ventricular fibrillation; for such patients implanted automatic defibrillators must also be considered. These drugs may have important and possibly prohibitive side effects,including exacerbating ventricular arrhythmias. Therefore, long-term therapy is best restricted to patients who

have significant symptoms from their ventricular arrhythmias. For more details, see above under VENTRICULAR PREMATURE BEATS in CARDIAC ARRHYTHMIAS.

Following acute MI, the long-term administration of certain β-blockers to patients who have no contraindication to such therapy reduces all-cause mortality by about 1/4 (eg, from about 10 to 7.5%) over 1 to 2 yr of therapy. Favorable effects are noted for nonsudden death and nonfatal myocardial infarction, but the beneficial effect is most marked for SCD, which is reduced by about 1/3. This therapy has the greatest impact in patients whose acute MI was complicated by arrhythmias and/or heart failure, though favorable effects are also present in those who had uncomplicated MI. The beneficial effect is statistically most persuasive for timolol and propranolol; whether other β-blockers have this effect is unproven, but some β-blockers with intrinsic sympathomimetic activity, pindolol and oxprenolol, have shown the least or no apparent benefit. In patients who do not have contraindications to β-blocker therapy (eg, heart failure, bronchial asthma, second- or third-degree atrioventricular block without cardiac pacemaker), therapy can be started a few days after the onset of MI, once the patient is stabilized, and it should be continued for 12 to 18 mo and perhaps longer. In definitive trials, the doses of drugs were timolol 10 mg bid or propranolol 60 mg tid or, in some patients, 80 mg tid.

SCD may occasionally be a consequence of conduction disturbances (or disordered impulse formation—the sick sinus syndrome) discussed in CARDIAC ARRHYTHMIAS, above. Note the therapies of other etiologic conditions cited under the specific disease headings.

Those who have been resuscitated (see below) from out-of-hospital "SCD" most commonly have extensive coronary disease, though the other conditions discussed may be causative. Those resuscitated and found to have sustained an MI have a prognosis characteristic of acute MI infarction and the severity of its residua. Those in whom an accompanying MI cannot be documented have an extremely high likelihood of recurrent cardiac arrest. Such patients should be studied for the nature of the underlying cardiac condition and these are among the patients in whom the prophylactic antiarrhythmic and possibly automatic defibrillatory regimens must be most considered. Therapy and the provocative testing of its adequacy by electrical stimulation and exercise testing are discussed under CARDIAC ARRHYTHMIAS, above.

CARDIAC ARREST AND CARDIOPULMONARY RESUSCITATION (CPR)

Cardiac arrest: *Absent or inadequate ventricular contraction that immediately results in systemic circulatory failure.* Major clinical findings include loss of consciousness, rapid, shallow breathing leading rapidly to apnea, profound arterial hypotension accompanied by non-palpable pulses over major vessels, and absent heart sounds. Within several minutes the resultant arterial hypoxemia leads to progressive cyanosis and loss of the pupillary light reflex (dilated pupils). Cardiac arrest is a medical emergency taking precedence over all others except exsanguinating external hemorrhage, which should be controlled simultaneously. Cardiac arrest can result from cardiac causes (ventricular fibrillation [85%], asystole [10%], shock [5%]), or from abnormalities in ventilation leading to significant respiratory acidosis (cardiopulmonary arrest). Although either heart or lungs may fail first, the 2 events usually are closely related.

Etiology and Pathophysiology

Ventricular fibrillation (VF) is the most common cause of cardiac arrest. Although usually associated with acute myocardial infarction **(MI)** secondary to ischemic heart disease, ≅ 50% of victims of sudden death due to VF have no evidence of MI on follow-up ECG and enzyme studies.

In VF, loss of coordinated global contraction of ventricular myocardium leads to immediate loss of effective CO, resulting in circulatory shock. While focal ischemia and anoxia from acute coronary artery spasm or obstruction is common, VF can also occur in the following situations: (1) "primary" VF secondary to worsening of chronic ventricular arrhythmias; (2) low-voltage electric shock (110 to 220 volts for 2 to 3 sec); (3) ionic imbalances (especially K and Ca); (4) hemolysis from fresh water near-drowning; (5) profound hypothermia (< 28 C [82.4 F]); and (6) excessive sympathetic stimulation of ventricular myocardium sensitized by hypoxemia and vasoactive drugs (eg, dopamine, theophylline, epinephrine).

Asystole is the *complete ECG absence of electrical activities, accompanied by absent perfusion, BP, and pulse.* Causes include severe generalized myocardial ischemia and hyperpolarization of cardiac cell membranes seen in severe hyperkalemia (serum K^+ > 7 mEq/L), hypomagnesemia, or ventricular rupture.

Circulatory shock has many etiologies, but diastolic arterial hypotension is the final common denominator leading to impairment of coronary artery blood flow, myocardial electrical instability, and cardiac and respiratory arrest. Circulatory shock may be due to a decreased effective circulating blood volume (eg, hypovolemia due to massive hemorrhage, massive "third-space" fluid losses [severe burns, pancreatitis]); loss of peripheral vasomotor tone that reduces venous return (eg, sepsis, anaphylaxis, profound hypothermia, CNS damage, drug or anesthetic overdose); or obstruction to ventricular filling or to ventricular output (eg, cardiac tamponade, massive pulmonary embolus, aortic dissection).

Respiratory arrest may be *primary*, caused by airway obstruction, decreased respiratory drive or respiratory muscle weakness, or *secondary*, as a result of cardiac arrest itself. Complete respiratory arrest manifests clinically as absence of spontaneous ventilatory movement in an unconscious person, often with associated cyanosis, but may develop acutely in a conscious victim secondary to foreign body obstruction (eg, "cafe coronary"). If prolonged, cardiac arrest quickly follows as progressive hypoxemia impairs cardiac function. Impending respiratory arrest is characterized by a depressed sensorium and feeble, gasping, or irregular respirations, often with accompanying tachycardia, diaphoresis, and relative hypertension due to agitation and CO_2 accumulation. Airway obstruction may be partial or complete; the most common cause in an unconscious or collapsed person is upper airway obstruction due to posterior tongue displacement into the oropharynx secondary to a loss of muscular tone. Other causes of upper airway obstruction include blood, mucus, vomitus, foreign body; spasm or edema of the vocal cords; and pharyngolaryngeal inflammatory, neoplastic, or traumatic processes. Lower airway obstruction may occur following particulate aspiration of gastric contents, widespread severe bronchospasm, or extensive airspace-filling processes (eg, pneumonia, pulmonary edema, or pulmonary hemorrhage).

Respiratory depression implies inadequate ventilation. Suspicion of inadequate ventilation necessitates arterial blood gas analysis to confirm hypoxemia and hypercapnia (hypercarbia), since clinical estimation alone of the adequacy of ventilation is unreliable. If uncorrected, progressive CO_2 retention and hypoxemia result in systemic acidemia, which, when severe (pH < 7.2), can compromise cardiac function and can lead to cardiac arrest. Respiratory depression may be due to impairment of multiple levels of the respiratory system by several factors: (1) **CNS** (eg, drug overdose, vascular lesions, intracranial hypertension due to mass lesions or craniocerebral trauma); (2) **upper and lower airways** (eg, near-drowning, tumor, hemorrhage, strangulation, asphyxiation, aspiration); (3) **alveolar spaces or chest wall,** with impairment of the normal physiologic mechanisms of ventilation (eg, pulmonary edema, extensive lung infectious processes, pneumothorax, flail chest); or (4) **blood and circulatory system** (eg, carbon monoxide or cyanide poisoning, profound anemia, or cardiocirculatory derangements).

TECHNICS OF CARDIOPULMONARY RESUSCITATION (CPR)

In collapsed or unconscious persons, the state of ventilation and circulation must be determined immediately. A systematic approach used with greatest urgency should ensure that only seconds elapse between recognizing arrest and intervening; speed, efficiency, and proper application of CPR directly relate to successful outcomes. While tissue anoxia for > 4 to 6 min can result in irreversible brain damage or death, wide variability in prognosis exists depending on age, cause of arrest, and clinical circumstances. Therefore, CPR must be continued until the cardiopulmonary system is stabilized, the patient is pronounced dead, or resuscitation cannot be continued (rescuer exhaustion). Following profound hypothermia or prolonged cold-water submersion, CPR should be continued until the total body core is rewarmed, since patients needing as long as 3 h of CPR have recovered.

Resuscitation efforts can be divided into basic life support **(BLS)**, which is immediately available, and advanced cardiac life support **(ACLS)**, which involves drug therapy, cardiac monitoring, and other technics and equipment. The goal of BLS is to provide emergency ventilation and systemic perfusion. Thus, *after establishing unresponsiveness of the victim* (tap, shake, or shout), the rescuer calls for help, notes the exact time of arrest, and positions the victim horizontally on a hard surface. Then the initial 3 steps of the mnemonic A-B-C (see TABLE 27-7) that constitute BLS are carried out rapidly and *in sequence*. If the patient's cardiac rhythm is being monitored and VF develops, a precordial thump should be given (delivered with a clenched fist raised 10 to 30 cm [about 8 to 12 in.] above the sternum and brought down firmly). BLS and ACLS should then be immediately instituted. In an unmonitored arrest, BLS is used until ACLS is available.

(A)—(A)irway Opened

Opening the (a)irway—(A)—is the first priority in respiratory inadequacy (labored, noisy breathing) and in BLS for respiratory or cardiac arrest. Sometimes (A) is all that

TABLE 27-7. THE A-B-Cs OF CARDIOPULMONARY RESUSCITATION

FOR RESPIRATORY OR CARDIAC ARREST	
Airway obstruction	Asystole
Respiratory depression	Ventricular fibrillation
Cardiac arrest	Shock
QUICKLY EVALUATE THESE SIGNS:	
Unresponsive	
Breathing absent	
Airway patent	
Pulse absent	
AND GIVE LIFE SUPPORT:	
A — AIRWAY OPENED B — BREATHING RESTORED C — CIRCULATION RESTORED	Basic life support (BLS)
D — DEFINITIVE TREATMENT DEFIBRILLATION DRUGS DIAGNOSTIC AIDS	Advanced cardiac life support (ACLS)

is needed to restore spontaneous breathing (B) and circulation (C); in these instances cardiac compression is not needed.

In an unconscious person, the relaxed tongue and neck muscles fail to lift the tongue from the posterior pharyngeal wall, blocking the hypopharyngeal airway. This effect is accentuated with neck flexion. In contrast, tilting the head backward stretches the anterior neck structures, lifting and drawing the tongue away from the posterior pharyngeal wall. Since head tilt alone usually may not open the airway sufficiently, 1 of 3 additional measures is used: (1) **Head tilt-chin lift** is performed by tilting the head back and placing a finger of the second hand under the rim of the mandible, lifting the chin forward (vertically upwards) until the teeth are brought almost together, but that the mouth is not closed (see FIG. 27–38a). (2) **Head tilt-neck lift** is performed by placing one hand on the victim's forehead, lifting the neck straight up while tilting the head back. Either (1) or (2) can open the airway quickly; when (1) is unsuccessful, (2) should be used. (3) If neither is successful, or if the patient is breathing spontaneously with noisy respirations from partial airway obstruction, a **mandibular jaw thrust** produces additional forward displacement of tongue and neck structures. This **triple airway maneuver** includes tilting the head backward, displacing the mandible forward, and opening the mouth. With hands placed from behind on each side of the victim's head, and the rescuer's elbows resting on the surface where the victim is lying, the head is tilted backward, while the thumbs depress the mandible at the corners of the mouth. The remaining fingers of each hand grasp the lower-jaw angles and lift upwards.

Removing dentures may make a mouth-to-mouth seal more difficult during rescue breathing, and therefore they should be left in place unless initial attempts to open the airway are unsuccessful by the above methods. *Backward head tilt in the presence of cervical spine injury is absolutely contraindicated*; if cervical spine injury is a possibility (eg, a trauma victim), a modified jaw thrust can be used. The head and neck are held in a neutral position while the mandible is thrust forward. This can be combined with chin lift alone as needed.

After the airway is opened, evidence of spontaneous ventilation is sought by *watching* for the rise and fall of the victim's chest while *listening* for airflow at the mouth and *feeling* exhaled air on the rescuer's cheek. If breathlessness continues while the airway is held open, rescue breathing is begun without delay.

(B)—(B)reathing Restored

Rescue breathing (mouth-to-mouth resuscitation) is begun by placing the heel of one hand against the victim's forehead to keep the head tilted backward, while the nostrils are gently pinched shut with the thumb and index finger of the same hand to prevent escape of air (FIG. 27–38b). The rescuer opens his own mouth widely, takes a deep breath, places his mouth over the victim's (making a tight seal), and blows 2 full breaths (1 to 1.5 sec each) thereby beginning ventilation, yet avoiding trapping air in the stomach. The adequacy of these ventilatory efforts are assessed by seeing the victim's chest rise and fall and by hearing and feeling his passive exhalation.

In single-rescuer CPR, 2 breaths (about 1 to 1.5 sec each) are given to adults after each cycle of 15 cardiac compressions delivered at a rate of 80 to 100/min (see [C]irculation Restored, below). This totals about 12 to 15 breaths/min for adults. **In 2-rescuer CPR,** one ventilation (1 to 1.5 sec) should be delivered after every 5 compressions. The second rescuer should try to determine whether restoration of spontaneous circulation has occurred by instructing the first rescuer to stop compressions for no longer than 5 sec; if no pulse is present, 2-rescuer CPR is resumed with rescuers on opposite sides of the victim. In children and infants, two (1 to 1.5 sec) breaths are delivered after each 5 compressions in both single and 2-rescuer CPR.

For adults, breaths of about 1 L each—ie, twice the normal tidal volume—are adequate to maintain normal blood O_2 saturation (> 90%) and to eliminate CO_2 (Pa_{CO_2} = 20 to 40 mm Hg). Smaller breaths are required for children, and only small puffs

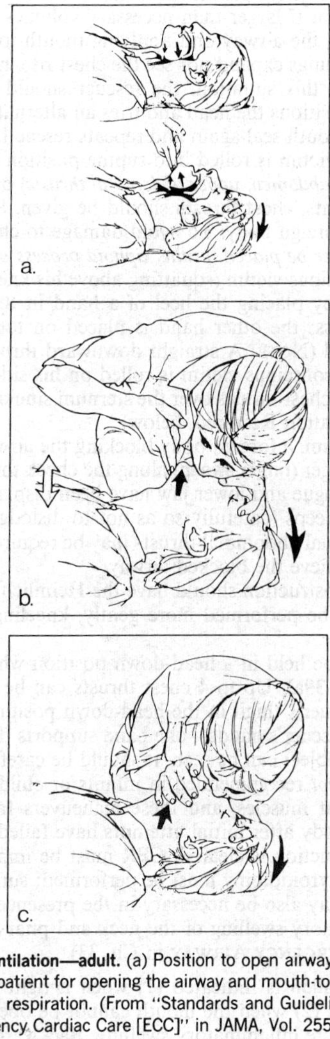

Fig. 27–38. Expired air ventilation—adult. (a) Position to open airway alone. (b) Rescue breathing: proper position of hands and patient for opening the airway and mouth-to-mouth respiration. (c) Proper positioning for mouth-to-nose respiration. (From "Standards and Guidelines for Cardiopulmonary Resuscitation [CPR] and Emergency Cardiac Care [ECC]" in JAMA, Vol. 255, pp. 2916 and 2918, June 6, 1986. Copyright 1986, American Medical Association. Used with permission of JAMA.)

from the rescuer's cheeks for infants. While inhaled air contains about 21% O_2 and trace amounts of CO_2, exhaled air contains 16 to 18% O_2 and 4 to 5% CO_2. Exhaled air values are more than adequate to maintain the victim's blood O_2 and CO_2 values at close to normal levels, if the correct rate and amplitude are used. If the rescuer develops hyperventilation alkalosis (manifested by dizziness, numbness, ringing in the ears, and paresthesias), the respiratory rate should be slowed or the amplitude of each

breath decreased. Also, excessive gastric distention with the associated risk of subsequent aspiration may occur if larger-than-necessary volumes of air are used.

In adults, after opening the airway and applying mouth-to-mouth breathing, if the rescuer does not feel the lungs expand nor see the chest rise, he should assume that **the airway is still blocked.** In this situation, the rescuer should carry out the following maneuvers: First, he repositions the head and tries an alternative head-tilt method. He makes a firm mouth-to-mouth seal again and repeats rescue breathing attempts. If the obstruction persists, the victim is rolled into supine position and the **Heimlich maneuver** (*manual thrusts to the abdomen, upper abdominal thrusts*) or, in the case of pregnant or extremely obese patients, **chest thrusts** should be given. Six to 10 thrusts may be necessary to dislodge a foreign body. To avoid damage to chest structures and to the liver, *the hand should never be placed on the xiphoid process or over the lower rib cage.* While astride the unconscious victim (squatting above his knees), the rescuer performs the Heimlich maneuver by placing the heel of a hand in the upper abdominal area below the xiphoid process; the other hand is placed on top of the first and a firm *upward* thrust is delivered (NOTE: A straight downward thrust may injure the aorta). For **chest thrusts,** the unconscious victim is rolled on his side with the hand position for the application of the chest thrusts over the sternum similar to that used for cardiac compression (see [C]irculation Restored, below).

In the unconscious victim, a foreign body blocking the airway may also be removed by sweeping the index finger **(finger sweep)** along the cheek through the victim's mouth and pharynx after the tongue and lower jaw have been displaced forward (tongue-jaw lift). Additional finger sweeps (carefully so as not to dislodge a foreign body further into the airway) and manual abdominal thrusts may be required to dislodge the foreign body completely or to relieve the blocked airway.

Children with airway obstruction should have the Heimlich maneuver performed; in small children it should be performed more gently, kneeling at the feet rather than astride.

Infants < 1 yr should be held in a head-down position while the rescuer delivers 4 back blows (see FIG. 27–39a). Up to 4 chest thrusts can be delivered by placing the infant's back on the rescuer's thigh in the head-down position. Or, the infant can be supported between the rescuer's hands—one hand supports the neck and the other the back. If the obstructing object can be seen, it should be carefully removed. Otherwise, blind finger sweeps are *not* recommended in infants or children. Progressive hypoxemia may relax the throat muscles, and these maneuvers frequently will dislodge a supralaryngeal foreign body after initial attempts have failed.

Once the airway obstruction is cleared, CPR must be implemented quickly. If obstruction persists, cricothyroidotomy must be performed; surgical establishment of an airway (tracheostomy) may also be necessary in the presence of severe orofacial injuries or massive inflammatory swelling of the neck and pharyngeal structures (see ESTABLISHMENT OF AN EMERGENCY AIRWAY in Ch. 33).

Mouth-to-nose resuscitation is indicated (1) when a tight seal around the victim's mouth is impossible, and (2) when the mouth cannot be opened because of muscular spasm, deformity, or severe inflammatory swelling. Backward tilt of the head in these instances is similar to mouth-to-mouth resuscitation but with the rescuer's other hand, the lower jaw is pushed forward, closing the mouth. A tight seal is made around the victim's nose and a deep breath is delivered. The patient's mouth should be allowed to open during passive exhalation.

Combined mouth-and-nose resuscitation is used for infants and small children when a tight mouth seal cannot be maintained. The mouth is placed over both the mouth and nose of the victim and the lungs are inflated with varying amounts of air according to the size of the child (see FIG. 27–39c). In general, in children ≥ 8 yr old of normal body size, adult CPR technics can be used.

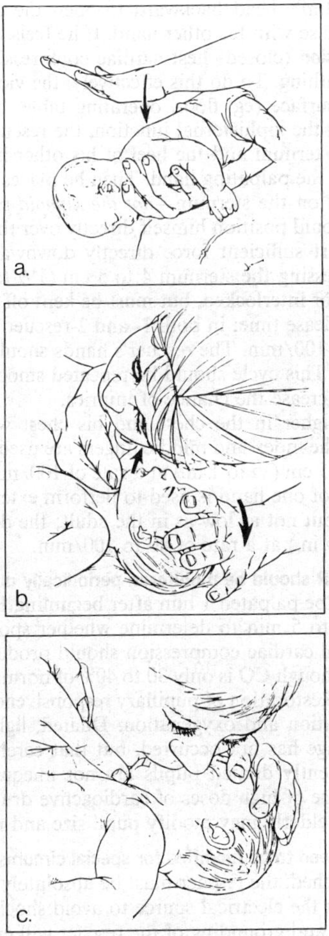

Fig. 27-39. Expired air ventilation—child. (a) Head-down position: dislodgement of foreign bodies from tracheobronchial tube. (b) Position for mouth-to-mouth respiration. (c) Combined mouth-to-nose respiration. (From "Standards and Guidelines for Cardiopulmonary Resuscitation [CPR] and Emergency Cardiac Care [ECC]" in JAMA, Vol. 155, pp. 2956 and 2959, June 6, 1986. Copyright 1986, American Medical Association. Used with permission of JAMA.)

The most common errors in performing expired-air resuscitation are (1) delays in diagnosing respiratory or cardiac arrest; (2) failure to establish a patent airway; (3) delays in instituting BLS promptly; and (4) inadequate ventilation (eg, poor seal around mouth or nose, failure to deliver the initial 2 full breaths, inadequate amount of expired pressure generated to cause chest movements). When available, adjuncts using supplemental O_2 are used as part of ACLS (see below).

(C)—(C)irculation Restored

After determining unresponsiveness, lack of respiratory activity, clearing the airway, and initiating rescue breathing, the next step is to establish pulselessness. As the

rescuer is tilting the victim's head backward to open the airway, he should gently palpate for the carotid pulse with his other hand. If he feels no pulse, he should begin **external cardiac compression** (closed-chest cardiac compression) immediately in conjunction with rescue breathing. To do this effectively, the victim must be placed horizontally on a flat hard surface (eg, floor, operating table, bedside tray, bed-board). With his middle finger in the xiphisternal junction, the rescuer places his index finger on the lower end of the sternum and the heel of his other hand on the sternum just above the index finger of the palpating hand. Then he places the heel of the palpating hand on top of the hand on the sternum—*not the xiphoid process*—and begins compressions. The rescuer should position himself directly over the victim, and keeping his arm straight, should exert sufficient force directly downward over the sternum (to avoid rib fractures) depressing the sternum 4 to 5 cm (1½ to 2 in.) in the adult. The fingers may be extended or interlocked, but must be kept off the chest wall. Compression time should equal release time; in both 1- and 2-rescuer CPR, a cardiac compression rate should be 80 to 100/min. The rescuer's hands should remain on the sternum during the release phase. This cycle should be repeated smoothly; jerky, bouncing, or irregular compressions increase the chance of injuries.

An infant's heart is higher in the chest and his chest wall is more pliable. For compression, the tips of the index and middle fingers are used over the mid-sternum to a depth of about 1.3 to 2.5 cm (½ to 1 in.) at a rate of 100/min. In children > 1 yr but < 8 yr old, only the heel of one hand is used to perform external cardiac compression over the lower sternum, but not as low as in the adult; the depth should be increased to 2.5 to 3.8 cm (1 to 1½ in.) at a rate of 80 to 100/min.

The effectiveness of CPR should be monitored periodically during resuscitation efforts. The carotid pulse should be palpated 1 min after beginning BLS, after the arrival of a second rescuer, and q 4 to 5 min to determine whether spontaneous circulation has returned. Ideally, external cardiac compression should produce a palpable pulse with each compression; even though CO is only 30 to 40% of normal, a systolic BP > 80 mm Hg should be produced. Restoration of pupillary responsiveness is an encouraging sign of adequate brain circulation and oxygenation. Dilated, light-responsive pupils may indicate that brain damage has not occurred, but that cerebral oxygenation is inadequate. However, persistently dilated pupils are not unequivocal evidence of brain damage or death, since use of high doses of cardioactive drugs, other patient medications, or cataracts in the elderly may modify pupil size and reaction.

The ABCs of BLS may need to be modified for special circumstances. When a victim of **electrical shock** is approached, the rescuer must be absolutely certain that the victim is no longer in contact with the electrical source to avoid shock to himself. Use of nonmetallic grapples or rods and grounding of the rescuer will enable safe removal of the victim, and CPR then can be started. In the case of **near-drowning**, artificial ventilation may be started in shallow water, although chest compression cannot be done effectively when the patient is not horizontal. Placing the victim on a surfboard or float may help. Several potential problems may impede optimum performance when CPR is needed in **accident victims.** A cervical spine injury requires modification of the airway-opening technique as described above. Facial injuries associated with oropharyngeal bleeding or debris may require clearing the airway before beginning ventilation. Severe facial injuries may make mouth-to-mouth resuscitation impossible without using special adjunctive devices and advanced procedures (eg, endotracheal intubation). Chest trauma, including flail chest injury or penetrating lesions of the heart or lungs may present similar obstacles. In these situations, stabilization in the field by trained medical personnel and immediate transport to a specialized facility are indicated.

When CPR is carried out in the hospital, the adequacy of ventilation must be checked by obtaining an arterial blood sample (see under Therapy of Respiratory

Failure in Ch. 34), since peripheral cyanosis is not a reliable guide because of influence by local circulation, lighting, and Hb value.

Complications of CPR

External cardiac compression can cause injuries that are minimized if properly performed. Since elevation of intrathoracic pressure by chest compression and direct cardiac compression between the sternum and spine are possible mechanisms of blood flow during CPR, efforts to depress the sternum greater than recommended levels, despite an adequate pulse, are not indicated. **Laceration of the liver** is the most serious (sometimes fatal) complication and is usually caused by pressing too low on the sternum. *Do not press down on the xiphoid process!* Delayed **rupture of the spleen** after CPR has been reported, and **rupture of the stomach** can occur (particularly if gastric distention with air has occurred) following forcible abdominal thrusts. A serious complication is regurgitation followed by **aspiration of gastric contents,** producing an aspiration pneumonitis that may be fatal. Excessive **gastric distention** during artificial ventilation can be avoided by using the recommended amounts of air required for adequate ventilation, by completely opening the airway before attempting to administer rescue breathing, and by early endotracheal or nasotracheal intubation. If marked distention develops, one should recheck the airway for patency and avoid excessive airway pressure. Attempts to relieve gastric distention should wait until suction equipment is available, since regurgitation with aspiration of gastric contents may occur. If marked gastric distention interferes with ventilation and cannot be corrected by the above methods, the victim should be positioned on his side, the epigastrium compressed, and the airway cleared. **Costochondral separation** and **fractured ribs** sometimes cannot be avoided in pressing hard enough to produce a palpable pulse. **Bone marrow emboli** to the lungs have rarely been reported after external cardiac compression, but there is no clear evidence that they contribute to mortality. External cardiac compression does not cause serious **myocardial damage** unless there is a preexisting ventricular aneurysm. **Lung damage** is rare, but pneumothorax secondary to rib fracture can occur. Overall, concern for these injuries should neither deter nor modify appropriately performed CPR.

When the exact duration of cardiac arrest is uncertain, the victim should be given the benefit of the doubt, unless he is in a terminal stage of an incurable condition. Once begun, it is the physician's responsibility to decide when to end BLS.

(D)—(D)efinitive Treatment

The D step of the A-B-C-D mnemonic (see TABLE 27–7) comprises advanced cardiac life support **(ACLS)** performed in conjunction with BLS. ACLS includes drug therapy, cardiac monitoring and dysrhythmia recognition (ECG diagnosis), adjunctive equipment, and special technics for establishing and maintaining effective oxygenation and circulation. Arrhythmia recognition and clinical circumstances dictate the specific arrest sequence to be used. VF, bradycardia, and electromechanical dissociation (**EMD,** *presence of ECG complexes without a pulse*) require prompt recognition and intervention. Therefore, **ECG monitoring** should be established in all collapsed or unconscious persons as soon as feasible. **Drugs** and **defibrillation equipment** should be prepared even before the ECG is obtained since VF causes about 85% of cardiac arrests in hospitalized patients, and empiric therapy may be lifesaving. Rapid defibrillation is the major factor determining survival following VF.

Ventricular Fibrillation

VF is treated by emergency **direct current defibrillation** using electrical countershock by placing defibrillating paddles (with conducting paste or moist saline pads placed beneath them) over the second intercostal space along the right sternal border and over the fifth or sixth intercostal space at the apex of the heart. If the development of

VF is observed in a monitored patient, an initial countershock of 200 to 300 joules should be given immediately. If unsuccessful, a second defibrillation attempt of 200 to 300 joules is then performed. A third shock of 360 joules is used if VF persists. When defibrillation is unsuccessful, BLS is continued with supplemental O_2. Lidocaine and epinephrine are repeated as indicated. An arterial blood sample should be obtained to assess pH and Pa_{O_2}. In refractory/recurrent VF unresponsive to repeated shocks, several drugs can be used. If VF recurs, the number of joules that previously converted the patient should be used. Epinephrine may increase the amplitude of VF, facilitating subsequent electrical cardioversion to more stable rhythms. Supplemental O_2 should be given to all patients during ALS, as described below (see Mechanical Resuscitative Devices).

An IV line should be immediately started; 2 lines are desirable to minimize the chance of loss of IV access because of infiltration at a critical time. During CPR, anticubital veins are the initial preferred access sites. Large volumes of fluid can be delivered through short, large-bore peripheral IV lines. Long femoral vein lines also do not require CPR to be interrupted and have less potential for lethal complications. A subclavian or internal jugular central line can then be placed by experienced personnel, if initial treatment does not restore circulation. As ACLS procedures are being used, *BLS should not be compromised* by unduly long interruptions for endotracheal tube or central line placement. The maximum time of interrupting ventilation or chest compressions for procedures should be 15 to 30 sec. In a patient with an endotracheal tube but no IV access, lidocaine, atropine, and epinephrine may be given down the endotracheal tube. Type and volume of fluids or drugs given depend on the clinical circumstances; in cardiac arrest complicating myocardial ischemia, IV fluids (5% D/W) are usually given only to keep an IV line open, whereas vigorous volume replacement (crystalloids, colloid solutions, and/or blood) may be required to expand the plasma volume in circulatory collapse resulting from volume losses.

Drugs for Ventricular Fibrillation or Tachycardia

Lidocaine (50 to 100 mg IV given rapidly q 5 min up to a total dosage of 3 mg/kg) remains the standard therapy for VF or ventricular tachycardia **(VT)** and is used with countershock to convert VF. Onset of action is immediate after rapid IV administration, but a constant infusion is required to maintain therapeutic blood levels.

Procainamide (100 mg IV no faster than 50 mg/min up to a total dosage of 1000 mg) is used to treat VF resistant to defibrillation and lidocaine and to suppress ventricular dysrhythmias predisposing to VF. (For details of dosage and administration, see Treatment of Ventricular Premature Beats under CARDIAC ARRHYTHMIAS in Ch. 27.)

Bretylium tosylate can be given when VF is unresponsive to countershock and lidocaine therapy or VT resistant to other drugs. The initial dose of 5 mg/kg is given rapidly IV for VF. Electrical defibrillation should then be repeated. CPR may need to be continued for as long as 15 to 30 min to see a response to bretylium. Persistent VF is treated by increasing the dose to 10 mg/kg and repeating it q 15 to 30 min as indicated up to a total dose of 30 mg/kg. A continuous infusion may be administered when necessary (500 mg in 250 mL 5% D/W [2 mg/mL]), at 1 to 2 mg/min for recurrent VF or VT. Bretylium may cause supraventricular tachycardia or hypotension after administration.

The effects of procainamide and bretylium may be additive with lidocaine and DC countershock in converting VF or controlling VT.

Phenytoin may be used to treat VF or VT due to digitalis toxicity that is refractory to other agents. An initial loading dose of 250 mg is given slowly (no more than 50 mg/min) in an IV running *0.9% sodium chloride solution*. Subsequent doses of 100 mg IV up to 1 gm total dose can be given at the same rate.

β-Adrenergic blockers can be used to control symptomatic supraventricular tachyarrythmias. Malignant ventricular arrhythmias can, at times, also be controlled using

β-blockers, although extreme caution must be observed in using these medications in patients with asthma, cardiac failure, or dependent on adrenergic support. Propanolol is the β-blocker that has been most extensively used (for details of dosage and administration, see TREATMENT OF VENTRICULAR PREMATURE BEATS in Ch. 27 under CARDIAC ARRHYTHMIAS).

Bradycardia, Asystole, and Electromechanical Dissociation

Asystole (*absent cardiac contraction and ECG evidence of cardiac electrical activity*) is treated by IV or intraairway administration of epinephrine (0.5 to 1.0 mg q 5 min). Atropine sulfate (0.5 to 1.0 mg) can also be given if rhythm is not restored. Temporary pacing using a transvenous electrical pacemaker passed into the right ventricle should be attempted. Transthoracic percutaneous pacing electrodes placed subcostally may also be used for temporary pacing. Electrical thresholds to sensing and pacing are determined immediately after insertion; successful temporary pacing thresholds are usually about 1 to 2 milliamperes. Maintenance electrical output should be 2 to 3 times this threshold, and the pacemaker should be set to maintain a heart rate of at least 70 to 80 beats/min. Following pacemaker insertion, epinephrine, atropine, or lead repositioning may be attempted if pacing failure occurs. *Intracardiac* injection of epinephrine is *not* recommended unless IV and/or airway routes are inaccessible, because of complications of pneumothorax, coronary artery laceration, cardiac tamponade, and prolonged interruptions of CPR.

Electromechanical dissociation (EMD) resulting in circulatory collapse may occur despite satisfactory electrical complexes on the ECG. This may be due to pump failure from extensive myocardial dysfunction, profound loss of peripheral vasomotor tone, or massive volume loss. BLS should be instituted in conjunction with volume infusions, epinephrine (0.5 to 1.0 mg IV) and other ACLS measures. A common cause is relative or absolute volume depletion and infusions of crystolloid or colloid solutions should therefore be administered (500 to 1000 mL); larger volumes may be required in the setting of anaphylaxis or massive volume loss. Dopamine and/or epinephrine infusions may be used in titrated doses to augment systemic venous return. Cardiac tamponade is an important cause of electromechanical dissociation and is readily treatable by pericardiocentesis at the bedside. (For PERICARDIOCENTESIS, see PERICARDIAL DISEASE, below.) A tension pneumothorax is another important cause that can be remedied by needle placement or chest tube insertion.

Drugs for Bradycardia, Asystole, and Electromechanical Dissociation

Epinephrine, used for cardiac asystole, EMD, and to coarsen fine VF, has combined α- and β-adrenergic receptor properties and several beneficial effects during CPR. Alpha effects may augment peripheral and coronary diastolic pressure, thereby increasing perfusion to subendocardial regions during chest compressions. This may, in turn, generate electrical activity and increase the cardiac contractility, thus increasing CO. Since good absorption of epinephrine occurs from the lungs, its administration should not be delayed if there is difficulty in starting an IV line. One mg (10 mL of a 1:10,000 solution) can be administered through an endotracheal tube. Intravenously, 0.5 to 1.0 mg (5 to 10 mL of a 1:10,000 solution) can be given q 5 min prn, but it should not be administered concurrently in the same IV line with alkaline solutions.

Atropine (0.5 to 1.0 mg IV repeated q 5 min as indicated) is a parasympatholytic that increases conduction through the A-V node and increases heart rate. It may be useful in the presence of bradyarrhythmias in the setting of myocardial ischemia (especially inferior wall) or high degree A-V nodal block.

Isoproterenol has β-sympathomimetic action and is used to increase heart rate for a slow idioventricular rhythm in the absence of effective circulation or symptomatic bradycardia unresponsive to atropine. It is given as a continuous infusion beginning at titrated doses of 2 μg/min (1 mg isoproterenol in 250 mL of 5% D/W [4 μg/mL]).

Excessive β-adrenergic activity can increase myocardial O_2 consumption and worsen ventricular arrhythmias, especially if myocardial ischemia is present. In excessive doses, arterial hypotension may result from peripheral vasodilation.

Other Drugs

Verapamil (5 to 10 mg slowly IV) may be useful in controlling symptomatic supraventricular tachycardias. However, its use has been associated with cardiovascular deterioration in the setting of sustained VT.

Sodium bicarbonate is *no longer* recommended as *initial*, automatic therapy for cardiac arrest, since recent data suggests that its use may induce paradoxical acidosis of the brain and heart, hyperosmolarity, hypernatremia or alkalemia, and inhibit the release of O_2 by the blood. Other adjuncts (eg, defibrillation, ventilation, cardiac compression, and pharmacologic agents) should be tried first unless the cause of the arrest is pre-existing acidosis, hyperkalemia, or tricyclic overdose with complex ventricular arrhythmias. When sodium bicarbonate is used, its administration should be dictated by arterial pH monitoring (q 5 min).

Calcium chloride is *no longer* recommended in the absence of hyperkalemia, hypocalcemia, or Ca^{++}-channel blocker toxicity, since high circulating levels of Ca^{++} may also have adverse effects. When necessary, Ca^{++} can be given IV (10% solution, [100 mg equals 1 mL] 1.36 mEq/mL), 2 mL can be given prn at a rate of not over 1 mL/min. Other forms of calcium may be used (calcium gluceptate [0.9 mEq/mL] 5 mL or calcium gluconate [0.45 mEq/mL] 10 mL). Caution is necessary when digitalis toxicity is a potential cause of the arrest.

Circulatory shock (*hypotension following restoration of spontaneous circulation*) after cardiac arrest is first treated by cautious IV volume infusions if left ventricular failure is not evident. For severe arterial hypotension unresponsive to volume replacement, the following drugs are useful in titrated doses by continuous infusion: (inotrope) **dopamine** 400 mg in 250 mL of 5% D/W (1.6 mg/mL) beginning at 3 to 5 μg/kg/min, (inotrope and vasoconstrictor) **epinephrine** 8 mg in 250 mL 5% D/W (32 μg/mL) at 2 to 10 μg/min; (peripheral vasoconstrictors) **norepinephrine** 8 mg in 250 mL of 5% D/W or 0.9% sodium chloride solution (32 μg/mL) at 2 to 16 μg/min; or **phenylephrine** 50 mg in 250 mL of 5% D/W (200 μg/mL) beginning at 0.1 to 1.5 μg/kg/min, with titration as needed to restore BP. Since BP cuffs may not accurately reflect BP in low output states, intra-arterial pressure monitoring is recommended to guide the response to therapy. Vasoactive drugs should be used in minimal dose necessary to achieve a satisfactory BP since they may increase vascular resistance and decrease organ perfusion, especially in the mesenteric bed. Sometimes CPR must be resumed after resuscitation and continued until adequate ventilation, palpable pulse, and acceptable BP indicate stabilized cardiorespiratory function.

Special circumstances will modify the institution of ACLS procedures. When the ECG is already under observation at the time of cardiac arrest and when defibrillators are available for immediate use, priority is given to immediate correction of dysrhythmias by a single precordial thump and DC countershock in the case of VF or VT, or electrical pacing for drug resistant symptomatic bradycardia.

Post-resuscitative care in the early post-arrest period centers on correction of predisposing factors that may jeopardize cardiovascular function, as well as standard measures to ensure optimal brain oxygenation and circulation. Blood volume should be restored and mean arterial pressure **(MAP)** should be maintained > 65 mm Hg (initial slight hypertension during coma may be beneficial—MAP 100 to 120 mm Hg. Hct, serum glucose, and electrolytes must be monitored, and fever should be reduced to decrease metabolic demands. Arterial PaO_2 should be kept at normal values (80 to 100 mm Hg) and, if mechanical ventilation is used, mild to moderate respiratory alkalosis is frequently desirable ($PaCO_2$ = 25 to 35 mm Hg). The dynamics of systemic blood

low or intravascular volume status may be uncertain following arrest and monitoring entral pressures may be necessary. After myocardial infarction, in particular, a pulmonary artery catheter capable of measuring CO, pulmonary capillary wedge pressure, and mixed venous O_2 saturation may be required to titrate therapy optimally.

In **low-output states following myocardial ischemia,** additional vasoactive drugs may be indicated: (inotropes) **dobutamine** 500 mg in 250 mL of 5% D/W (2 mg/mL), beginning at 2 to 5 μg/kg/min and **aminrone** directly increase myocardial contractility. The initial dose is 0.75 mg/kg given over 2 to 3 min, 500 mg in 250 mL of 0.9% sodium chloride solution (2 mg/mL) then by continual infusion 5 to 10 μg/kg/min. **Sodium nitroprusside** 50 mg in 100 mL of 5% D/W (500 μg/mL) with solution wrapped in aluminum foil to protect it from light exposure, beginning at 0.5 to 10 μg/kg/min as indicated by clinical and hemodynamic conditions is a preload and afterload vasodilator that can reduce pulmonary congestion and increase CO. **Nitroglycerine** IV 100 mg in 250 mL 5% D/W (400 μg/mL) is also a vasodilator that may be useful as a preload reducing agent particularly in the settings of unstable angina and congestive heart failure. These 2 agents are used optimally with full hemodynamic monitoring because of their rapid and significant hemodynamic effects.

Open-chest cardiac compression may be more effective following penetrating chest trauma, cardiac tamponade, cardiac arrest in the operating room with the patient's chest already open, and crushed-chest injury. However, this procedure *requires training and experience in the performance of thoracotomy* and is best performed only in extreme, extenuating circumstances.

The physician stops treatment and pronounces the patient dead if deep unconsciousness, absence of spontaneous respiration, circulation, and brainstem reflexes indicate that resuscitation is not possible. This implies that the patient has been refractory to standard BSL and available ACLS measures. Although evidence of neurologic function during resuscitation favors brain recovery, absence of this evidence is not a reliable indication that the brain will not recover. Therefore, failure of appropriate support procedures to re-establish effective cardiovascular function is recommended as the basis for the decision to end resuscitative efforts. As indicated above, patients with hypothermia represent a special circumstance, and CPR should be continued until warming measures have raised core body temperature to normal.

MECHANICAL RESUSCITATIVE DEVICES

Mechanical devices are adjunctive. They are not intended to nor should they replace immediate mouth-to-mouth ventilation and manual external cardiac compression during institution of BLS. They should be used only when available within seconds or to replace manual methods during sustained resuscitation, or when the patient must be moved. Specialized equipment should be used only by experienced personnel.

Airway Adjuncts

The primary purpose of airway adjuncts is to provide supplemental O_2 and ventilation during resuscitation efforts.

Bag-valve-mask devices incorporate a self-inflating bag and a nonrebreathing valve mechanism (resuscitator bags, Ambu bag). These self-inflating manual resuscitator bags should always be used with supplemental O_2 and can achieve from 60 to 100% delivered O_2 when the following principles are pursued: (1) the highest acceptable O_2 flow rate should be used, (2) the longest possible bag refill must be used, and (3) a reservoir for O_2 collection to avoid entrainment of room air should be used whenever possible.

Bag-valve-mask units are best used in association with artificial airways. However, oropharyngeal airways should be used with them only when the patient is unconscious. Airway obstruction and subsequent hypoxemia, vomiting, and resultant aspiration may occur if an airway is forced into a conscious or stuporous patient's mouth.

Cuffed endotracheal tubes are used to secure a compromised airway, prevent aspira tion, initiate mechanical ventilation, and suction the lower respiratory tract. They ar indicated in comatose patients and those in whom artificial ventilation will be re quired. Manual airway control, ventilation, and oxygenation during BLS, and supple mental O_2 by the adjuncts noted above during ACLS procedures are always indicate before attempts at tracheal intubation. Orotracheal intubation is preferable in emer gencies and it can be accomplished faster than nasotracheal intubation; suction appa ratus and necessary equipment should always be at hand before attempted passage Bag-valve-mask units with adaptors are fitted to endotracheal tubes, and the arres victim should be manually ventilated until cardiovascular stability is restored. When deformity or muscle spasm prevents opening of the oral airway, blind nasotrachea intubation may be attempted. If this is impossible, special technics to gain airwa control including transtracheal catheter ventilation and cricothyroidotomy may b required. (These procedures are described in Ch. 33.)

Double oropharyngeal airways have been used instead of mouth-to-mouth ventilatio during BLS, but are more difficult to use since the rescuer's fingers must seal th victim's lips around the tube while the thumb clamps the nose. Difficulty in openin the mouth and maintaining a patent airway, or stimulation of the victim's hypophar ynx may cause vomiting as consciousness is regained. **Esophageal obturator airway (EOA)** have been used as adjuncts in the treatment of arrest victims, but should b inserted by personnel experienced in their use who are not trained in endotrachea intubation. Complications include esophageal perforation and excessive gastric disten tion causing regurgitation. Before the EOA is removed, the patient should have a endotracheal tube inserted, be turned on his side, and suction should be availabl

Several types of face masks are available in child and adult sizes for the patient wh is breathing spontaneously. They must fit well, ideally be transparent, and be capabl of delivering an O_2 concentration of 50% with an O_2 flow rate of 10 L/min. Masks ar most effectively applied when a rescuer stands at the patient's head and ensures a fir seal of the mask while the airway is kept open during CPR by head-tilt and jaw-thrus technics. With the simple mask, O_2 is delivered to a cone-shaped face piece from whic the patient inhales O_2 (entraining varying amounts of room air through the exhalatio ports) and exhales through the exhalation ports. Commonly used flows are 6 to 1 L/min, capable of delivering O_2 concentrations of 35 to 55%. Since ventilation pattern will affect O_2 delivered with these masks, Venturi masks can be used, especially i patients with CO_2 retention and chronic lung disease. They can provide O_2 concentra tions of 24%, 28%, 31%, 35%, 40%, and 50%. A non-rebreathing mask, similar to simple mask, but with an O_2 reservoir bag and one-way exhalation valves, is capable c delivering tracheal O_2 concentrations up to 90%. Flow should be adequate (6 to 1 L/min) to prevent the reservoir bag from collapsing with each breath. Supplementa O_2 can also be given by nasal catheters in flow rates up to 5 L/min.

Mechanical Ventilators (see also Ch. 34)

Mechanical respirators, resuscitators, and anesthesia machines can provide artifici ventilation if an adequate airway is maintained. They are best used with cuffed endo tracheal tubes, although continuous positive airway pressure may be applied by seale face mask in special situations (eg, pulmonary edema with adequate ventilation bu not oxygenation). Proper positioning of the head and/or the airway is essential, an frequent checks of proper chest movement and arterial oxygenation should be do after introducing the airway. Mechanical ventilation in the hospitalized patient re quires a volume ventilator with adjustable airway pressure, tidal volume, flow rate, C concentrations, cycling rate, and appropriate alarm systems. It should produce inte mittent positive pressure ventilation with or without positive end-expiratory pressu and be capable of delivering humidified air and aerosol therapy. Since the patient

lung compliance may change during the post-resuscitation period, a volume-set timed-cycle ventilator should be used.

Adjuncts for Artificial Circulatory Support

Since many forms of cardiac arrest are accompanied by evidence of volume depletion, **medical antishock trousers (MAST)** can be used to increase central blood volume, particularly in patients with hypovolemic shock secondary to trauma and hemorrhage. They also raise peripheral resistance and therefore increase coronary blood flow. This device has separate lower extremity and abdominal compartments allowing independent inflation and compression. Compressive pressure can be adjusted for the desired effect. When in place, the garment should be deflated sequentially (abdominal compartment first) as indicated. This device may cause pulmonary congestion and heart failure when the intravascular volume is adequate and myocardial function is poor.

Intra-aortic balloon counter pulsation (IABP) has been used to assist circulation when low output circulatory states are due to significant refractory left ventricular pump failure. A catheter is usually introduced via the femoral arterial route, percutaneously or by arteriotomy, retrograde into the thoracic aorta just distal to the left subclavian artery. The pulsation augments coronary artery perfusion during diastole and decreases afterload during ventricular systole. Its primary value is during conditions of rapid hemodynamic deterioration when cardiac surgery is imminent and other measures are ineffective. Patients with cardiogenic shock subsequent to resuscitation who have lesions that are potentially remediable by surgical intervention (eg, acute myocardial infarction with acute mitral insufficiency or ventricular septal defect, severe aortic insufficiency due to acute vascular lesions) are candidates for use of IABP. Experience in inserting and monitoring the catheter is necessary for its safe use.

MYOCARDIAL DISEASE

All cardiac disease due to any cause except congenital developmental defects, valvular disease, systemic or pulmonary vascular disease, isolated pericardial disease, isolated nodal or conduction system disease, and epicardial coronary artery disease in all its forms except instances in which it results in a state of chronic diffuse myocardial dysfunction.

Because the primary etiology can be any one of myriad diseases or can occur in the absence of any identifiable disease process, a pathophysiologic classification is most useful initially. Once the diagnosis and pathophysiologic type have been identified by means of history, physical examination, and invasive or noninvasive testing, the primary etiology can be sought (see TABLE 27–8). If no etiology can be found, myocardial disease is considered primary or idiopathic.

DILATED CONGESTIVE CARDIOMYOPATHY

Disorders of myocardial function with heart failure in which ventricular dilation predominates.

Pathophysiology

The pathologic basis for this clinical state is either acute myocardial inflammation or, more often, chronic fibrosis and diffuse loss of myocardial myocytes. Many patients with chronic congestive cardiomyopathy may initially have had an acute or myocarditic phase followed by a latent period of variable duration before progressing to the undifferentiated phase of chronic fibrosis and myocyte loss. This leads to dilation, thinning, and compensatory hypertrophy of remaining myocardium (see FIG. 27–40) interspersed with fibrosis. Altered ventricular geometry leads to secondary functional mitral or tricuspid regurgitation and atrial dilation.

TABLE 27–8. CLASSIFICATION OF MYOCARDIAL DISEASE

Pathophysiology	Etiology
Dilated congestive cardiomyopathy (acute or mild)	
Diffuse (all chambers involved)	Chronic diffuse myocardial ischemia (coronary artery disease)
Nondiffuse (one or more chambers spared)	Infective agents (acute or chronic); bacteria, spirochetes, rickettsia, viruses, fungi, protozoa, helminths
	Granulomatous diseases: sarcoidosis, granulamatous or giant cell myocarditis, Wegener's
	Metabolic disorders: nutritional (beriberi, selenium deficiency, kwashiorkor), familial storage disorders, uremia, hypokalemia/hypomagnesemia, hypophosphatemia, endocrinopathy (diabetes mellitus, hyper- or hypothyroidism, pheochromocytoma, acromegaly)
	Drugs and toxins: ethanol, anthracyclines, cobalt, psychotherapeutic drugs (tricyclic, quadricyclic, and phenothiazine), catecholamines, cyclophosphamide, radiation
	Neoplasms
	Connective tissue disorders
	Heredofamilial neuromuscular and neurologic disorders
	Peripartum
Hypertrophic cardiomyopathy	
Asymmetric (obstructive, nonobstructive, and apical)	Hereditary autosomal dominant, Friedrich's ataxia, pheochromocytoma, acromegaly, neurofibromatosis
Symmetric	
Restrictive cardiomyopathy	
Diffuse (obliterative and nonobliterative)	Amyloidosis; diffuse systemic sclerosis; hemochromatosis; endocardial fibrosis, fibroelastosis, and Loffler's disease; neoplasms; Gaucher's disease
Nondiffuse	

The physiologic consequence of this pathologic process is a predominant depression of ventricular systolic function reflected by a low ejection fraction (**EF**). CO is maintained at the expense of tachycardia and a large diastolic filling volume that in turn increases wall tension and myocardial O_2 demand. Diastolic compliance and pressure become abnormal only late in the course of the disease.

Symptoms and Signs

This disorder is most often chronic, presenting with effort dyspnea and fatigability due to elevated left ventricular diastolic pressure and low CO. Because both ventricles may be affected equally, symptoms and signs of right ventricular failure also are often prominent. Less often, the onset is acute and associated with fever if an infective agent is responsible, in which case it is called **myocarditis**. Infection with coxsackie B virus is most common in the temperate zone while **Chagas' disease** due to *Trypanosoma cruzi* is most prevalent in Central and South America. For discussion of these diseases see VIRAL INFECTIONS in Ch. 191 and PROTOZOAL DISEASES in Ch. 13.

Physical examination reveals a normal or low BP, sinus tachycardia, basal rales, neck vein distention with prominent A and V waves and hepatojugular reflux, and peripheral pitting edema. In severe cases, hepatomegaly, ascites, and skeletal muscle wasting is seen. The precordium often has a diffuse parasternal lift, and a diastolic

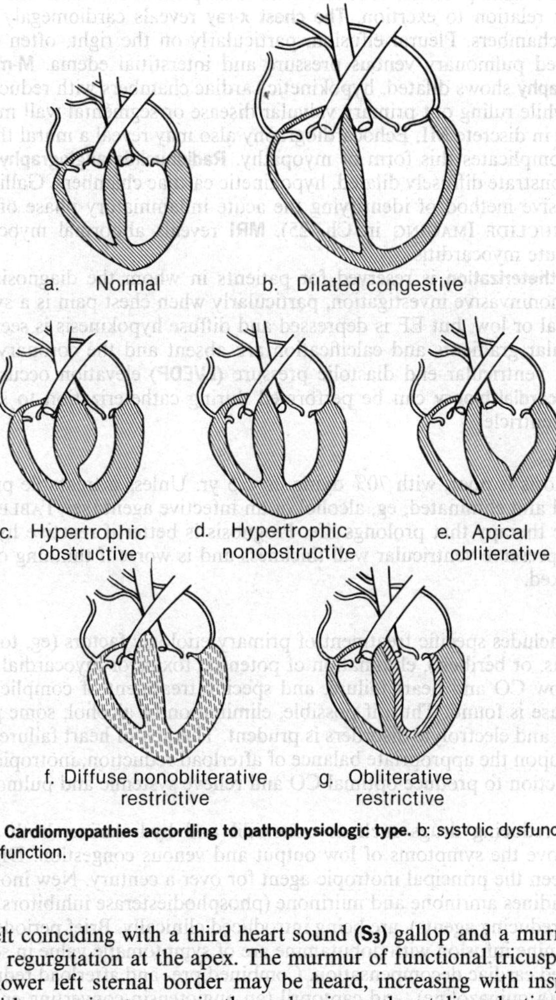

FIG. 27–40. Cardiomyopathies according to pathophysiologic type. b: systolic dysfunction; c through g: diastolic dysfunction.

impulse is felt coinciding with a third heart sound **(S_3)** gallop and a murmur of functional mitral regurgitation at the apex. The murmur of functional tricuspid regurgitation at the lower left sternal border may be heard, increasing with inspiration and associated with regurgitant waves in the neck veins and systolic pulsation of the liver. In a few patients, the pathologic process is isolated to 1 ventricle (usually the left), thus altering the clinical picture.

Diagnosis

Diagnosis depends upon the characteristic history and physical examination, and exclusion of other explanations for ventricular failure (eg, systemic hypertension, primary valvular disease, or myocardial infarction **[MI]**). **The ECG** may show sinus tachycardia, low voltage QRS, and nonspecific ST segment depression with low voltage or inverted T waves. Sometimes pathologic Q waves are present in the precordial leads simulating remote MI. In about 25% of cases of congestive dilated cardiomyopathy, differentiation from previous MI may be further complicated by chest pain that may

closely mimic angina pectoris, but most often is atypical in character and position and lacks a clear relation to exertion. **The chest x-ray** reveals cardiomegaly that usually involves all chambers. Pleural effusion, particularly on the right, often accompanies signs of raised pulmonary venous pressure and interstitial edema. **M-mode and 2-D echocardiography** shows dilated, hypokinetic cardiac chambers with reduced fractional shortening while ruling out primary valvular disease or segmental wall motion abnormalities seen in discrete MI. Echocardiography also may reveal a mural thrombus that frequently complicates this form of myopathy. **Radionuclide angiography** can also be used to demonstrate diffusely dilated, hypokinetic cardiac chambers. Gallium scanning is a noninvasive method of identifying the acute inflammatory phase of myocarditis (see RADIONUCLIDE IMAGING in Ch. 25). **MRI** reveals abnormal myocardial tissue texture in acute myocarditis.

Cardiac catheterization is reserved for patients in whom the diagnosis remains in doubt after noninvasive investigation, particularly when chest pain is a symptom. CO can be normal or low, but EF is depressed and diffuse hypokinesis is seen on angiography. Valvular gradients and calcification are absent and the coronary arteries are normal. Left ventricular end diastolic pressure **(LVEDP)** elevation occurs late in the disease. **Myocardial biopsy** can be performed during catheterization to sample tissue from either ventricle.

Prognosis

The prognosis is poor, with 70% dying in < 5 yr. Unless a treatable primary cause can be found and eliminated, eg, alcohol or an infective agent (see TABLE 27–8), there is no specific therapy that prolongs life. Prognosis is better if reactive hypertrophy is adequate to preserve ventricular wall thickness and is worse if thinning of ventricular walls is marked.

Treatment

Therapy includes specific treatment of primary etiologic factors (eg, toxoplasmosis, thyrotoxicosis, or beriberi), elimination of potential toxins or myocardial depressants, therapy of low CO and heart failure, and specific treatment of complications. Most often, no cause is found. Thus, if possible, elimination of alcohol, some psychotherapeutic drugs, and electrolyte disorders is prudent. Therapy of heart failure and low CO will depend upon the appropriate balance of afterload reduction, inotropic agents, and preload reduction to produce optimal CO and relieve systemic and pulmonary venous congestion.

Afterload reducing drugs such as minoxidil and hydralazine, both vasodilators, greatly improve the symptoms of low output and venous congestion. Digitalis glycosides have been the principal inotropic agent for over a century. New inotropic drugs, eg, the bipyridines amrinone and milrinone (phosphodiesterase inhibitors that act also as afterload reducing agents), are being introduced clinically. Brief periods (48 to 72 h) of catecholamine infusion with dobutamine are of symptomatic value in some patients with advanced cardiac decompensation. Combined pre- and afterload reducing agents, eg, prazosin (a quinazoline), and captopril (an angiotensin-converting enzyme inhibitor), often reduce the need for preload reducers, eg, diuretics and nitrates. While all are effective in treating the symptoms and signs of congestive dilated myopathy and improve the quality of life, there is no evidence that they alter long-term prognosis. Similarly, while corticosteroids, with or without azathioprine and equine antithymocyte globulin, appear to shorten the acute phase of certain inflammatory myocarditic myopathies proved by biopsy, eg, acute postviral or sarcoid myocarditis, there is no evidence that the incidence of chronic myopathy or its ultimate course is altered. Therefore, biopsy proof of active myocarditis is recommended before starting corticosteroids.

Since mural thrombus formation in any chamber is frequent once chamber dilation is significant, prophylactic oral anticoagulant therapy is used to prevent systemic or

pulmonary emboli (see Ch. 39). Cardiac arrhythmias that often complicate both acute myocarditic-phase myopathy and the late chronic dilated phase are treated with antiarrhythmic drugs as required—see CARDIAC ARRHYTHMIAS above. (CAUTION: *Most antiarrhythmics have a depressant effect upon myocardial contractility; thus, potent negative inotropic agents, eg, disopyramide and procainamide, are best avoided.*) Permanent pacemakers may be required if heart block complicates the chronic dilated phase; however, atrioventricular block during acute myocarditis often resolves and permanent pacing is not usually needed.

Since the most common identifiable cause of chronic congestive cardiomyopathy in temperate zones is diffuse coronary artery disease with diffuse ischemic myopathy, therapy for angina pectoris with nitrates, β-blockers, and Ca-blocking agents may be indicated (see MYOCARDIAL ISCHEMIC DISORDERS above). However, the benefit of β-blockers and certain Ca-channel blockers in controlling angina must be weighed against their negative inotropic effects. Serial echocardiographic or radionuclide ventriculograms will help alert one to a decline in cardiac function if these drugs are used. Some studies suggest that low-dose β-blockers may be of benefit for some patients with dilated congestive cardiomyopathy in situations in which there is a significant compensatory adrenergic response causing chronic downregulation of cardiac myocyte β-adrenoceptors, but insufficient proof of benefit is available to recommend them without hemodynamic monitoring in the early phase of their use. Similarly, nifedipine normally acts as a vasodilator and afterload reducer; in the presence of cardiac decompensation, the reflex sympathetic response to arteriolar vasodilation may already be maximal, and then the direct negative inotropic effect of the drug may manifest itself with a worsening of heart failure.

Appropriate rest, sleep, and stress avoidance are important. Curtailment of physical exercise ultimately is unavoidable because of inadequate cardiac reserve, but prolonged bed rest should be prescribed only as symptoms dictate.

Because prognosis is grim and no therapy alters mortality unless a primary etiology can be treated, these patients represent the greatest proportion of heart transplantation recipients. Patients selected should be below age 50 and without associated systemic disease, psychologic disorders, or high, irreversible pulmonary vascular resistance.

HYPERTROPHIC CARDIOMYOPATHY

Congenital or acquired disorders characterized by marked ventricular hypertrophy in the absence of an afterload demand, eg, valvular aortic stenosis, coarctation of the aorta, or systemic hypertension. Cardiac muscle is usually abnormal with cellular and myofibrillar disarray, although this finding is not universal nor specific to hypertrophic cardiomyopathy. Most often, the interventricular septum is hypertrophied to a greater degree than the left ventricular free wall **(asymmetric septal hypertrophy)**. Congenital hypertrophy is autosomal dominant in cases of asymmetric septal hypertrophy, but not in other varieties.

Pathophysiology

The major consequence of hypertrophy is that the stiff, noncompliant chamber, usually the left ventricle, resists diastolic filling, leading to an elevated end-diastolic pressure that raises pulmonary venous pressure. Angina pectoris results from an imbalance between demand for O_2 by the hypertrophied myocardium and supply via the coronary arteries, which may be compromised by the noncompliant myocardium. Effort-induced lightheadedness and syncope are caused by an increased outflow tract gradient that results from the decreased diastolic filling period related to exercise-induced sinus tachycardia. Sudden death is thought to result from ventricular tachycardia or fibrillation. Infective endocarditis can complicate hypertrophic cardiomyopathy because of the mitral valve abnormality that appears to result from the altered

ventricular geometry as well as Venturi effect produced by the rapid early systolic flow through the outflow tract. Heart block sometimes complicates the terminal years of the disease process.

Symptoms, Signs, and Diagnosis

Clinical manifestations are chest pain, syncope, palpitations, effort dyspnea, and sudden death—alone or in any combination. Chest pain is usually typical angina related to exertion. Syncope is usually exertional, due to a combination of arrhythmia, outflow tract obstruction, and poor diastolic filling of the ventricle. Dyspnea on exertion is a result of poor diastolic compliance of the left ventricle that leads to a rapid rise in LVEDP as flow increases. Systolic function is preserved and fatigability is seldom a complaint. Palpitations are produced by ventricular or atrial arrhythmias. Thus, symptoms of hypertrophic cardiomyopathy may simulate those of aortic stenosis or coronary artery disease.

Physical examination usually clarifies this differential diagnosis. Signs of raised venous pressure such as jugular venous distention, ascites, ankle edema, and pleural effusion are rare until the terminal phase. BP and heart rate are usually normal. The carotid pulse in cases with asymmetric septal hypertrophy and outflow tract obstruction has a brisk upstroke, a bifid peak due to dynamic obstruction in the latter part of systole, and a rapid downstroke. Precordial palpation reveals the apex beat in its normal position with a sustained thrust due to LV hypertrophy. Sometimes a biphasic apical thrust can be appreciated in cases with severe outflow obstruction. Systolic murmurs are usually present, but patients with only apical and symmetric hypertrophic cardiomyopathy may have no murmur. Most common is a crescendo-diminuendo ejection type murmur that does not radiate to the neck; it is best heard at the left sternal edge in the 3rd or 4th intercostal space. This murmur is caused by obstruction to left ventricular **(LV)** ejection (produced in systole when the hypertrophied interventricular septum and the anterior leaflet of the mitral valve approach each other). A mitral regurgitation murmur is heard in some patients due to distortion of the mitral apparatus. It has the characteristic blowing quality and is best heard at the apex, radiating toward the left axilla. Rarely, early or mid-systolic clicks are heard. In some patients with right ventricular **(RV)** outflow tract narrowing, a systolic ejection murmur will be heard in the second interspace at the left sternal border. An S_4, almost always present, is indicative of a forceful atrial contraction against a poorly compliant left ventricle in late diastole.

The ejection murmur of hypertrophic cardiomyopathy can be altered by maneuvers to decrease venous return so that LV diastolic volume is decreased and apposition of the anterior mitral valve leaflet with the hypertrophied interventricular septum increases. Thus, the Valsalva maneuver increases the intensity of the murmur. Maneuvers to lower aortic pressure (eg, amyl nitrite inhalation) also increase the intensity of the murmur, as will a post-extrasystolic contraction, both of which increase the outflow tract pressure gradient. Handgrip raises aortic pressure and causes the murmur to diminish in intensity.

Laboratory findings: Noninvasive tests to confirm the diagnosis have generally replaced heart catheterization (see below). **The ECG** usually shows voltage criteria for LV hypertrophy. Asymmetric septal hypertrophy is often suggested by very deep septal Q waves in leads I, aVL, V_5, and V_6. A Q-S complex sometimes occurs in V_1 and V_2 simulating previous septal infarction. The T waves are abnormal in most cases with deep symmetric T-wave inversion in leads I, aVL, V_5 and V_6 the most common finding. ST segment depression in the same leads is quite common. The P wave is often broad and notched in leads II, III, and aVF with biphasic P wave in V_1 and V_2, indicative of left atrial hypertrophy. Pre-excitation phenomenon of the Wolff-Parkinson-White syndrome type occurs more often than by chance alone and is one of the mechanisms of arrhythmia-induced palpitations.

The chest x-ray is often deceptively normal-looking, since hypertrophy occurs at the expense of the ventricular cavities. A globular LV contour within a normal-sized cardiac silhouette may be the only radiologic abnormality. Cardiac fluoroscopy will rule out aortic valve calcification.

M-mode and 2-D echocardiography is the best noninvasive diagnostic technic. Thickened ventricular walls can be seen and measured allowing differentiation of the different forms of hypertrophic cardiomyopathy (see FIG. 27–40). Outflow tract obstruction can often be quantitated by observing the degree of systolic anterior movement of the anterior leaflet of the mitral valve and its degree and duration of apposition to the hypertrophied interventricular septum. LV fractional shortening will be normal or increased. Midsystolic closure of the aortic valve is sometimes seen in patients with severe outflow tract obstruction. **Radionuclide angiography** will show a small ventricular cavity with a normal or high EF.

Cardiac catheterization is usually reserved to evaluate patients when surgical therapy is a consideration. Intraventricular pressure gradients may be found in the left and, less commonly, the right ventricle. The gradient will rise in a postextrasystolic beat, during Valsalva maneuver, and after amyl nitrite inhalation. End diastolic pressure is high due to poor ventricular compliance. EF is normal or high. Ventriculography will show characteristic chamber deformity depending upon the type of hypertrophic cardiomyopathy and will sometimes also confirm mitral valve regurgitation. The coronary arteries are usually widely patent with torrential flow.

Prognosis

Prognosis is guarded; the annual mortality rate is 4%. Sudden death is most common, with chronic heart failure occurring less often. Genetic counseling is applicable for patients with asymmetric septal hypertrophy variety, in whom the hypertrophy appears to accelerate during puberty.

Treatment

Therapy is directed primarily at abnormal diastolic compliance. β-Adrenoceptor blocking and Ca-channel blockers alone or in combination are the mainstays of treatment. Both agents decrease myocardial contractility and lead to improved diastolic ventricular function. β-Blockers have the added benefit of slowing the heart rate, allowing prolongation of the diastolic filling period, and thus decreasing outflow obstruction. β-Blockers with intrinsic sympathomimetic action (eg, pindolol and oxprenolol) are best avoided. Ca blockers vary in their negative inotropic effect and arterial vasodilator capacity. It is important to choose a weak vasodilator that has a significant depressant effect upon contractility. Verapamil is currently the Ca blocker of choice for hypertrophic cardiomyopathy.

Drugs that reduce preload (eg, nitrates or diuretics) decrease chamber size and make these patients worse. Inotropic agents such as digitalis glycosides and catecholamines worsen outflow tract obstruction and do not relieve the high end-diastolic pressure. Vasodilators make these patients worse by increasing the outflow tract gradient and produce a reflex tachycardia that further decreases ventricular diastolic function. While antiarrhythmic therapy can be prescribed for arrhythmias proved by ECG or 24-h ambulatory monitoring, there is no evidence that they alter the risk of sudden death. The antifibrillatory action of β-blockers may help to prevent sudden death, but this has not been proved. Disopyramide has been shown to have negative inotropic effect and has been used for hypertrophic cardiomyopathy both as an antiarrhythmic and as a negative inotropic agent. Amiodarone shows promise in preventing sudden death. Unfortunately, it has a high incidence of side effects, some of which are irreversible. Antibiotic prophylaxis to prevent infective endocarditis should be recommended (see INFECTIVE ENDOCARDITIS below). Competitive sports should be avoided, since many sudden deaths occur on greater than ordinary exertion.

Surgical treatment in the form of septal myotomy or myomectomy is reserved for patients with incapacitating symptoms despite medical therapy in whom outflow tract obstruction has been demonstrated by catheterization studies. It improves symptoms in most carefully selected cases, but has not been shown to alter mortality. In a few cases, mitral valve replacement has been done for severe mitral dysfunction; this coincidentally eliminates the outflow tract gradient.

RESTRICTIVE CARDIOMYOPATHY

Myocardial disorders characterized by rigid, noncompliant ventricular walls resisting diastolic filling of one or both ventricles, most commonly the left.

Etiology

Restrictive cardiomyopathy, whose etiology is usually unknown, is the least prevalent form of cardiomyopathy. It is divided into a diffuse nonobliterative variety in which the whole myocardium is infiltrated by abnormal substance (eg, amyloidosis) and an obliterative variety in which the endocardium and subendocardium are fibrosed (eg, endomyocardial fibrosis). **Löffler's disease** occurs in the tropics. It begins as thrombus formation on the endocardium, chordae, and A-V valves progressing to fibrosis. **Endocardial fibrosis** occurs in temperate zones and involves only the left ventricle. **Amyloidosis** involving the myocardium is usually systemic as is iron infiltration in **hemochromatosis. Sarcoidosis** and **Fabry's disease** involve the myocardium, and nodal conduction tissue can be involved.

Pathophysiology

Pathophysiologic consequences of the above disorders include endocardial thickening or myocardial infiltration with loss of myocytes, compensatory hypertrophy, and ultimate fibrosis. Any of these may lead to A-V valve malfunction resulting in mitral or tricuspid regurgitation. Involvement of nodal and conduction tissue results in sinoatrial node dysfunction, and various grades of heart block in some cases. Amyloidosis can involve the coronary arteries. The main hemodynamic consequence of these pathologic states is a rigid, noncompliant chamber with a high filling pressure. Systolic function may deteriorate if compensatory hypertrophy is inadequate to compensate for infiltrated or fibrosed chambers. Mural thrombosis and systemic emboli can complicate either the restrictive or obliterative variety.

Symptoms, Signs, and Diagnosis

Like hypertrophic cardiomyopathy, the main dysfunction is abnormal compliance and diastolic filling of one or both ventricles, most commonly the left ventricle. Symptoms are due to high diastolic pressure giving rise to pulmonary venous hypertension with effort dyspnea and orthopnea and peripheral edema when the right ventricle is involved. Effort limitation is a consequence of a fixed CO due to resistance to ventricular filling. Angina and syncope are uncommon, but both atrial and ventricular arrhythmias and heart block are common.

Physical examination reveals a quiet precordium, a low volume and rapid carotid pulse, pulmonary rales, and pronounced neck vein distention with a rapid Y descent. An S_4 is heard in virtually all cases and an S_3 may occur and must be differentiated from a precordial knock, but there is often no murmur. In some cases, a murmur of functional mitral or tricuspid regurgitation results from changes in chordae or ventricular geometry as a result of infiltration or fibrosis of myocardium and endocardium. Symptoms and signs thus closely mimic constrictive pericarditis from which this form of cardiomyopathy must be differentiated. Noninvasive tests may help make this differentiation, but occasionally even heart catheterization does not clearly define the diagnosis and thoracotomy is required to explore the pericardium.

Laboratory findings: The ECG is usually nonspecifically abnormal, showing ST and T wave abnormalities and sometimes low voltage. Pathologic Q waves sometimes occur without previous MI. LV hypertrophy is sometimes seen due to compensatory hypertrophy of myocardium. On chest x-ray the heart is often normal size or small but can be enlarged in late stage amyloidosis or hemochromatosis. Echocardiography shows normal systolic function. The atria are often dilated. Disease due to amyloidosis shows an unusually bright echo pattern from the myocardium. Echocardiography helps differentiate constrictive pericarditis with its thickened pericardium, but paradoxical septal motion can occur in either disorder. Myocardial hypertrophy is often seen in restrictive myopathy. MRI reveals abnormal myocardial texture in diseases with myocardial infiltration (eg, amyloid or iron).

Cardiac catheterization and myocardial biopsy are usually necessary. High atrial pressure with a prominent Y descent and an early diastolic dip followed by a high diastolic plateau in the ventricular pressure curve are found. Unlike constrictive pericarditis, LV diastolic pressure usually is a few mm Hg higher than RV. Angiography reveals normal-sized ventricular cavities with normal or decreased systolic shortening. Functional A-V valve regurgitation may be seen due to infiltration of myocardium and papillary muscles or endocardial thickening. Biopsy can demonstrate endocardial

TABLE 27–9. DISEASES OF THE MYOCARDIUM

	Dilated/Congestive	*Hypertrophic*	*Restrictive*
Clinical	Left & right heart failure Cardiomegaly Functional A–V valve regurgitation S_3 & S_4	Angina, effort dyspnea, syncope, sudden death Ejection ± mitral regurgitation murmurs S_4, bifid carotid	Effort dyspnea & fatigue Left ± right heart failure Functional A–V valve regurgitation
ECG	Nonspecific ST & T abnormality Q waves	Left ventricular hypertrophy Deep septal Q waves	Left ventricular hypertrophy or low voltage
X-ray	Cardiomegaly Pulmonary venous congestion	No cardiomegaly	No or mild cardiomegaly
Echocardiogram	Dilated hypokinetic ventricles ± mural thrombus	Hypertrophied ventricle ± mitral systolic anterior motion ± asymmetry	Increased wall thickness ± cavity obliteration
Hemodynamics	Normal EDP, low EF, diffusely dilated hypokinetic ventricles ± A–V valve regurgitation Low CO	High EDP, high EF ± outflow subvalvular gradient ± mitral regurgitation Normal or low CO	High EDP, dip & plateau diastolic left ventricular Normal CO
Pathophysiology	Systolic dysfunction	Diastolic dysfunction ± outflow obstruction	Diastolic dysfunction
Therapy	Pre- and afterload reduction, inotropic drugs, anticoagulants	β-blocker &/or Ca–channel blockers ± septal myomectomy	Endocardial resection
Prognosis	70% 5 yr mortality	4%/yr mortality	70% 5 yr mortality

A-V = atrioventricular; EDP = end-diastolic pressure; EF = ejection fraction; ± = with or without

fibrosis and thickening, myocardial infiltration with iron or amyloid, or chronic myocardial fibrosis. Coronary angiography will be normal, except in rare cases of amyloidosis involving the epicardial coronary arteries.

Careful search for primary causes of restrictive cardiomyopathy should be done (eg, rectal biopsy for amyloidosis and iron studies or biopsy for hemochromatosis).

Prognosis and Treatment

Prognosis is poor (see TABLE 27–9). It is similar to that of a dilated congestive cardiomyopathy.

There is no therapy for most patients with restrictive cardiomyopathy. Diuretics must be used with caution because of their ability to lower preload upon which the noncompliant ventricles depend to maintain CO. Digitalis helps little to alter the hemodynamic abnormality and may be dangerous in amyloidosis cardiomyopathy where extreme digitalis sensitivity is common. Afterload reducers may induce profound hypotension and usually are not of value.

Hemochromatosis may improve with regular phlebotomies to reduce the body's iron stores and cases with active biopsy-proven sarcoidosis will respond to corticosteroids. Rarely, patients with endocardial fibroelastosis or Löffler's disease improve after surgical debridement of the endocardial fibrotic and thrombotic thickening and freeing up of chordae and valve tissue. Sometimes A-V valve replacement has helped severe functional A-V valve regurgitation. In some cases of significant compensatory hypertrophy, Ca-channel blockers might be of value. Hemodynamic monitoring during initiation of such therapy to confirm its efficacy would be prudent.

VALVULAR HEART DISEASE

(See also CONGENITAL HEART DISEASE in Ch. 187)

MITRAL VALVE DISEASE

MITRAL VALVE PROLAPSE (MVP)

(Systolic Click Murmur Syndrome; Barlow's Syndrome; Click Late Systolic Murmur Syndrome; Billowing Mitral Valve Syndrome or Ballooned Valve Syndrome)

A bulging of one or both mitral valve leaflets into the left atrium during systole so that a crisp systolic sound or click and late systolic mitral regurgitation **(MR)** *murmur are commonly heard.*

Etiology, Pathology, and Physiology

Primary prolapse is associated with myxomatous transformation of the mitral valve. Complete myxomatous degeneration of the valve can lead to severe MR (floppy valve syndrome). The tricuspid valve can also show myxomatous changes and produce tricuspid valve prolapse. Marfan syndrome is commonly associated with myxomatous valves, and about 25% of patients with prolapsed valves have joint laxity, high-arched palate, or other skeletal abnormalities (eg, scoliosis, funnel chest, and straight back). Atrial septal defects commonly have an MVP. Prolapse of one leaflet can be due to disproportion between chordae tendinae and papillary muscle length, or between mitral leaflet area and valve orifice area (as in hypertrophic subaortic stenosis **[HSS]**).

The click is probably a valvular sound produced by a systolic loss of support of one leaflet by its opposing leaflet. When a click and murmur are present, the degree of MR is usually mild to moderate.

Symptoms, Signs, and Diagnosis

Although most patients do not have symptoms, when they do, symptoms often occur in common with neurocirculatory asthenia; eg, fatigue, nonanginal chest pains, dyspnea, or palpitations, the latter due to either atrial or ventricular arrhythmias. Any

maneuver that makes the left ventricle smaller, as with sitting or standing, will increase the disproportion between the leaflets and the mitral ring and cause earlier and greater prolapse and thus an earlier click and longer murmur. There may be only click or murmur, or both.

Cerebral emboli occur, but are rare. Ventricular tachycardia and sudden death (rare) may occur in patients with the complete click-murmur syndrome, which includes T-wave negativity in 2, 3, aVF, and the left precordial leads, especially with prolonged QT intervals either at rest or only with exercise. The diagnosis may be confirmed by either M-mode echocardiography in about 75% of patients, and by 2-D echocardiography in about 95%.

Prophylaxis and Treatment

Prophylaxis against endocarditis may be necessary only if MR is present either with or without maneuvers that make the heart smaller. To prevent the occasional rupture of chordae that can lead to severe MR, patients with definite clicks and murmurs should probably avoid competitive sports that require maximum effort. Excess sympathetic tone symptoms can be relieved with β-blockers, which may also raise fibrillation threshold in patients with dangerous tachycardias.

MITRAL REGURGITATION (MR)
(Mitral Insufficiency; Mitral Incompetence)

Retrograde flow from the left ventricle through an incompetent mitral valve into the left atrium.

Etiology, Pathology, and Physiology

The 4 commonest causes in the adult are rheumatic valve damage, papillary muscle dysfunction, ruptured chordae tendinae, and myxomatous degeneration of the mitral valve. Some rare causes in the adult are left atrial myxoma, an endocardial cushion defect with a cleft anterior leaflet, and markedly calcified mitral annulus (mainly in elderly women). In an infant the most likely causes are papillary muscle dysfunction secondary to an anomalous left coronary artery arising from a pulmonary artery, endocardial fibroelastosis, acute myocarditis, endocardial cushion defect with cleft mitral valve, or myxomatous degeneration of the mitral valve.

Rheumatic MR, rare today without mitral stenosis, is due to shortening not only of valve cusps but also of papillary muscles and chordae tendinae that become matted and adherent to the valve. Papillary muscle dysfunction MR is secondary to myocardial infarction, recent or old, with or without a ventricular aneurysm, and with or without papillary muscle fibrosis. Infarction of the ventricle at the base of the papillary muscles, or ischemia of that area during an anginal attack can cause marked MR even with a normal papillary muscle. If one papillary muscle is unable to contract or is attached to infarcted muscle at its base, its muscle plus chordae will be longer than the opposite contracting papillary muscle plus chordae. Thus, during systole the contracting normal papillary muscle will pull down the mitral leaflets on its side. The other leaflet will then prolapse into the left atrium because it loses support of the opposite leaflet.

Symptoms, Signs, and Diagnosis

Severe MR may cause palpitations long before heart failure symptoms develop, probably due to the frequency of ectopic beats and post-extrasystolic hyperdynamic action of the enlarged left ventricle. If MR is severe, the high left atrial pressure can produce dyspnea due to the high regurgitant wave (CV wave) even before heart failure symptoms of low CO occur.

On physical examination of moderate-to-severe MR, there is a brisk pulse, a sustained left parasternal movement due to expansion of an enlarged left atrium, and

sustained and enlarged area apical movement that is displaced to the left. On auscultation the second sound (**S_2**) is usually widely split unless severe pulmonary hypertension has developed, and it moves normally with respiration unless there is gross failure. A pansystolic murmur is loudest at the apex; if due to papillary muscle dysfunction, it may be crescendo to S_2. If it is due to an MVP, the murmur may be delayed and preceded by a click. If the murmur is due to posterior ruptured chordae, it may radiate well into the second right interspace and carotids, and mimic aortic stenosis. If the murmur is due to anterior ruptured chordae, it may radiate to the spine and even to the top of the head. An S_3 at the apex will be loud in proportion to the degree of MR. The S_3 may be followed by or even replaced by a short rumbling inflow murmur, the latter only with severe MR. If MR is trivial, the systolic murmur will be purely high-pitched or blowing. As the flow increases, the murmur will develop more low and medium frequencies. A Grade 4/6 or louder murmur (without a thrill) implies severe MR.

Chest x-rays of moderate to severe MR will show an enlarged left atrium and ventricle. The ECG will show various degrees of left atrial and left ventricular (**LV**) overload. The echocardiogram shows increased left atrial and LV dimensions and permits evaluation of LV function. Atrial fibrillation is common when the left atrium enlarges and is invariable when it is extremely large. Marked separation of the septal from the mitral valve echo is strongly suggestive of depressed LV contractility. Many etiologies of MR give diagnostic echocardiographic evidence (eg, prolapse, myxomas, ruptured chordae, and calcified annulus). Left ventriculography defines the degree of regurgitation, and right ventricular (**RV**) pressures indicate the degree of pulmonary hypertension that invariably accompanies high left atrial pressures. The highest left atrial pressures occur with ruptured chordae, because both the left atrium and ventricle are prevented from dilating with the regurgitant volume by the restricting effect of a relatively nondistensible pericardium.

Prophylaxis and Treatment

Prophylaxis against endocarditis is indicated at times of anticipated bacteremia, as with dental extraction or cleaning (see ENDOCARDITIS, below). If the diagnosis is rheumatic, and the MR is at least moderately severe, then RF prophylaxis with daily penicillin until about age 30 is recommended. RF is too rare after age 30 in most western countries to require prophylaxis. To prevent both pulmonary and systemic emboli, anticoagulation (see Ch. 39) should be used in patients with gross failure or with atrial fibrillation. If a patient is Class 3 or 4 New York Heart Association Classification (symptoms on less than ordinary exertion) on maximum medical management, then an elderly patient should have either an annuloplasty or a tissue valve, and a young patient either a prosthetic ball or disc valve.

MITRAL STENOSIS (MS)

Obstruction of flow from left atrium to left ventricle because of narrowing of the mitral orifice.

Etiology, Pathology, and Physiology

MS in the adult is almost always caused by previous RF. Infants with congenital MS rarely live beyond 2 yr. RF can cause a chronic process of valvular fibrosis and fusion, as well as calcification with shortened, thickened chordae tendinae. A left atrial myxoma can also cause obstruction at the mitral orifice.

Critical MS requiring valvotomy or valve replacement is associated with an oval orifice of $\leq 1.75 \times 0.85$ cm. High left atrial pressure leads not only to dyspnea on exertion but also can result in pulmonary arteriolar constriction of excessive degree, which obstructs circulation proximal to the pulmonary capillaries. Although this prevents dangerously high pressures in the pulmonary capillaries and left atrium, the high

pulmonary arteriolar resistance leads to decreased CO and a low output syndrome with severe fatigue as its major symptom. Ultimately, it can lead to RV failure.

Symptoms, Signs, and Diagnosis

In temperate climates the latent symptom-free period may last 10 to 20 yr; symptoms usually begin between ages 30 and 40. In tropical or subtropical climates, progress is swifter. The first symptoms of MS are usually either exertional dyspnea or fatigue. The tachycardia of exertion, fevers, or atrial fibrillation shortens diastolic filling time: insufficient flow through the mitral orifice in diastole raises left atrial pressure and decreases CO.

Frank pulmonary edema occurs with sudden elevations of left atrial pressure, as when uncontrolled atrial fibrillation produces too rapid a ventricular rate as an added insult to the loss of atrial contraction. Hemoptysis due to rupture of small pulmonary vessels as well as pulmonary edema is especially likely with the increase of blood volume due to pregnancy. Emboli can occur in as high as 15% of patients and is usually associated with atrial fibrillation, but it can occur in sinus rhythm. Left vocal cord paralysis **(Ortner's syndrome)** can cause huskiness due to paralysis of the left recurrent laryngeal nerve, which is compressed when a dilated left atrium presses against a dilated pulmonary artery.

Physical findings: On inspection and palpation there may be a Grade 2 to 3/4 left parasternal sustained movement due to either RV hypertrophy and dilation, or because a normal right ventricle may be held against the sternum by a large left atrium. There may be a diastolic thrill at the apex with the patient in the left lateral decubitus position, the S_2 may be palpable due to pulmonary hypertension, and the S_1 may be palpable at the apex.

On auscultation there will be a slightly exaggerated P_2 with a normal split. An opening snap loudest between the apex and left lower sternal border can be heard if the mitral valve is not excessively fibrosed and calcified. A loud, sharp M_1 at the apex or "closing snap" will be heard. With the patient in the left lateral decubitus position, one should listen for an apical diastolic rumbling murmur with a presystolic crescendo over a palpable apex beat. (An Austin Flint murmur [see Symptoms, Signs, and Diagnosis below, under AORTIC REGURGITATION] can imitate the diastolic murmur of MS.) A soft decrescendo diastolic murmur along the left sternal border may imply pulmonary regurgitation **(Graham Steell murmur)** secondary to severe pulmonary hypertension. The commonest cause, however, of this kind of murmur is aortic regurgitation, which often accompanies MS.

The ECG will show signs of left atrial overload in V_1 by a large area of terminal P negativity (one small square in area or one Ashman unit). There may be widely notched P waves in any leads (formerly called P mitrale, and thought to be due to left atrial overload, but now known to be due to an intra-atrial conduction block). Lead 1 will have low voltage and there may be a right axis deviation due to RV hypertrophy. However, if V_1 shows the tall R waves of RV hypertrophy, pulmonary hypertension is severe. If atrial fibrillation is present, the f waves in V_1 will usually be large, as a sign of atrial overload. However, if there is much atrial damage, the f waves may be small.

The x-ray will show straightening of the left cardiac border due to a dilated left atrial appendage. The main pulmonary artery will be prominent if there is much pulmonary hypertension. The upper lobe pulmonary veins may be dilated—a redistribution of blood flow from the lower lobes to the upper lobes due to compression of the lower lobe veins as a result of gravity plus high interstitial pressure. A double shadow of a fibrosed, enlarged left atrium is characteristic along the right cardiac border. Kerley B lines are horizontal lines in the lower posterior lung fields diagnostic of interstitial edema associated with a high left atrial pressure.

An echocardiogram will show not only the amount of valvular calcification and indicate the patient's suitability for valvotomy, but will tell the size of the left atrium,

which indicates whether the patient will profit from cardioversion. A 2-D echo can show the exact size of the mitral orifice.

Cardiac catheterization (see in Ch. 25) will give a wedge pressure determination reflecting left atrial pressure and will indicate the degree of pulmonary hypertension. The degree of MS and regurgitation can also be quantitated.

Treatment

Medical management consists of using either β- or Ca-channel blockers to slow the heart rate. In atrial fibrillation the use of a small amount of digitalis together with Ca-channel blockers and/or β-blockers is recommended. Anticoagulants are recommended for all but the mildest MS. Antiplatelet drugs (eg, sulfinpyrazone, dipyridamole, or aspirin) may be substituted for warfarin if the latter is contraindicated. Sulfinpyrazone should probably not be used without aspirin.

Surgery should be considered for patients who remain in Class 3 (symptoms on less than ordinary exertion) despite the best medical management. If echocardiography and the presence of a good opening snap indicate that the valve is not heavily calcified, open valvotomy and valvuloplasty can be done. Otherwise, valve replacement is necessary. In young patients, a porcine valve cannot be safely depended upon for long-term endurance, so a mechanical disc or ball valve should be used. Anticoagulation is needed if the patient remains in atrial fibrillation or has a prosthetic mechanical valve.

AORTIC VALVE DISEASE

AORTIC REGURGITATION (AR)

(Aortic Incompetence or Aortic Insufficiency)

Retrograde flow from aorta into the left ventricle through incompetent aortic cusps.

Etiology, Pathology, and Physiology

In adults, the commonest causes of severe chronic AR are rheumatic heart disease and endocarditis; in the child, ventricular septal defect with aortic valve prolapse. The commonest causes of *mild* adult AR are a bicuspid aortic valve (which occurs in about 2% of males and 1% of females) and severe hypertension with diastolic pressures of ≥ 110 mg Hg (probably in the presence of a bicuspid aortic valve as well). Rarely AR is found in association with ankylosing spondylitis, Reiter's syndrome, rheumatoid or psoriatic arthritis, SLE, and the arthritis associated with ulcerative colitis. Without arthritis, the rare causes are leutic aortitis, osteogenesis imperfecta, dissecting aneurysm of the aorta, supravalvular aortic stenosis, aortic arch syndrome (Takayasu's disease), rupture of a sinus of Valsalva, giant cell arteritis, and myxomatous transformation in patients with Marfan syndrome.

LV volume and LV stroke volume are increased because the left ventricle must receive blood regurgitated in diastole in addition to normal blood volumes coming from the pulmonary veins. Proportionate hypertrophy of the left ventricle always occurs with dilation to maintain pressure (LaPlace's law: pressure = tension/radius. Tension is maintained by hypertrophy.)

Symptoms, Signs, and Diagnosis

Effort tolerance usually remains remarkably good for many years even with severe AR. Finally, dyspnea on exertion, orthopnea, and paroxysmal nocturnal dyspnea develop. Palpitations may occur because of awareness of the heart due to LV enlargement. Angina pectoris occurs in only about 5% of patients, and only with gross AR. It is especially common at night, perhaps because AR increases with slow heart rates.

On inspection and palpation, there is a rapid rise of pulse with a large volume (a "slapping" pulse). The low diastolic pressure is mostly due to peripheral vasodilation (carotid sinus reflex) as well as to back flow into the left ventricle. The large pulse

pressure with its brisk rise has spawned many descriptive terms and eponyms. The tendency for the arterial pulse to be slapping and fall away rapidly is called a "**water hammer pulse**" or "**collapsing pulse.**" The sharp sound heard over the femoral pulse is called the "**pistol shot sound,**" or "**Traube's sign.**" The systolic murmur in the femoral artery distal to finger pressure and the diastolic murmur heard proximal to finger pressure on the artery are called the "**double Duroziez murmur.**" The large carotid pulsations seen in the neck are called "**Corrigan's pulse.**" The head nodding that occurs due to the ballistic force of the large stroke volume is "**DeMusset's sign.**" The pulsatile blanching and reddening of the fingernails when slight pressure is applied, is called "**capillary pulsation**" or "**Quincke's sign.**"

The systolic pressure is higher than normal, because of the large stroke volume. A positive **Hill's sign** is present when the leg BP is > 20 mm Hg higher than systolic pressure of the arm. The apex beat will be displaced, enlarged, and sustained, with a large area of medial retraction, often of the entire left parasternal area.

On auscultation, S_2 is usually single, slightly sharp or slapping, and loud due to the increased elastic aortic recoil power. If, however, the AR is gross, the S_2 may disappear. There is a pandiastolic decrescendo murmur loudest over the sternum and left lower sternal border. If the AR is severe, there may be medium and low frequencies in it. If it is trivial, it may have only high frequencies and, therefore, be blowing. If the AR is not rheumatic, but due to ruptured cusps or to an ascending aortic aneurysm, the murmur may be loudest along the right sternal border. Often the murmur is heard best near the axilla or the mid left thorax **(Cole-Cecil murmur)**. There may be an MS-like diastolic rumble at the apex due to prevention of full opening of the anterior mitral leaflet by the descending aortic regurgitant stream **(the Austin Flint murmur)**. Lowering aortic pressure and decreasing AR with amyl nitrite will attenuate or eliminate the Austin Flint murmur and make an MS murmur louder. An aortic ejection sound is especially common if there is a bicuspid aortic valve. An aortic ejection flow murmur due to excessive forward flow, which may imitate aortic stenosis, may be present. The combination of forward ejection and backward regurgitant flow murmur is called a **to-and-fro murmur**.

Treatment

Aortic valve replacement is the therapy of choice when the patient develops symptoms of heart failure or if an echocardiogram shows a reduced ejection fraction and end systolic diameter of ≤ 55 mm. Prophylaxis against endocarditis is necessary both before and after valve replacement (see ENDOCARDITIS, below). Medical management of those in failure consists of not only digitalis but also afterload reduction, because, despite the reflex peripheral vasodilation and diastolic pressures as low as 50 mm Hg, these patients seem to benefit from further peripheral vasodilation (see HEART FAILURE, above).

AORTIC STENOSIS (AS)

Narrowing of the aortic outflow tract at valvular, supravalvular, or subvalvular levels, causing obstruction to flow from left ventricle into the ascending aorta and resulting in a pressure gradient across the obstruction of ≥ 10 mm Hg.

Etiology, Pathology, and Physiology

Even in the adult, AS is considered congenital, unless there is concomitant rheumatic mitral valve disease or the patient is > 60 yr, at which time a normal aortic valve may become so sclerosed and finally calcified that it can produce significant AS. Rheumatic AS results from fibrosis of the leaflets and fusion of the commissures. No matter what the cause of valvular stenosis, whether congenital or acquired, severe calcification may make the leaflets almost unrecognizable.

Supravalvular AS occurs just above the sinuses of Valsalva (3 outpouchings or bulges at the root of the aorta) as either a discrete membranous or a diffusely hypoplastic constriction. Discrete subvalvular AS may be either a membrane or fibrous ring just beneath the aortic valve. A sporadic form of supravalvular AS is associated with a facies (high, broad forehead, hypertelorism, strabismus, upturned nose, long filtrum, wide mouth, dental abnormalities, puffy cheeks, micrognathus, and low-set ears). Hypertrophic subaortic stenosis **(HSS)** is a form of hypertrophic cardiomyopathy. It is often called "idiopathic" HSS, but this term is unnecessary. It is also called hypertrophic obstructive cardiomyopathy. It is due to a thickened septum that impinges on the anterior leaflet of the mitral valve during systole and causes outflow obstruction. It is usually associated with asymmetric septal hypertrophy; ie, the septum is hypertrophied more than is the free wall. There is usually some AR with either supravalvular, valvular, or discrete subvalvular AS.

The first response to outflow obstruction is LV hypertrophy with encroachment on the chamber volume rather than external enlargement. Only when there is myocardial damage or heart failure due to extreme obstruction does the ventricle enlarge.

Symptoms, Signs, and Diagnosis

The classic triad of AS symptoms is syncope, angina, and dyspnea on exertion. If syncope occurs on exertion, it is considered due to fixed output and represents severe AS. Syncope may, however, be due to ventricular fibrillation unrelated to exertion. Angina pectoris may be due to significant coronary atherosclerosis, but 50% is due to insufficient subendocardial arterial supply to the thick left ventricle despite normal coronary arteries.

With a fixed obstruction, the carotid pulse is slow in rising and may have a thrill on it because of transmission of the cardiac murmur via the neck vessels. When AR is present to a significant degree, there may be a **bisferiens pulse;** ie, a notch or dip in midsystole. In severe cases, BP is low and the pulse pressure is small (**pulsus parvus** and **tardus**). In mild or moderate cases, especially if there is AR, the systolic pressure may even be elevated. The apex beat is sustained (begins to fall with the S_2) and is not displaced unless there is cardiomegaly due to heart failure or to concomitant AR or MR.

The ejection murmur of AS is always a mixed frequency murmur that becomes very harsh when Grade 4/6 or more. The later the peak of the crescendo and the longer the murmur, the more severe is the stenosis. The high frequency components tend to radiate to the apex and suggest the murmur of MR. This is called the **Gallavardin phenomenon**. In the elderly patient, the murmur of calcific AS is often musical or cooing at the apex, probably because commissural fusion may be absent and allows the cusps to vibrate and produce pure frequencies.

The murmur of HSS (see HYPERTROPHIC CARDIOMYOPATHY, above) is increased by any maneuver that makes the heart smaller and thereby approximates the septum to the anterior leaflet. Any maneuver that reduces pressure in the outflow tract will make the murmur louder for the same reason. Therefore, it will be made louder by sitting or standing, and by amyl nitrite. Conversely, it will be made softer by squatting, handgrip, or a vasopressor agent. A Valsalva maneuver tends to make the murmur louder, because decreased venous return causes the heart to become smaller and also causes an increase in sympathetic stimulation and inotropism. This murmur is usually heard loudest either at the apex or between the apex and the left sternal border.

Carotid and peripheral pulses in HSS tend to be extremely rapid because obstruction does not occur until after about the first quarter of systole. After a premature ventricular contraction the pulse pressure will not increase **(Brockenbrough effect),** unlike that which occurs in patients with fixed obstruction. In supravalvular AS, the right carotid and brachial have an increased volume and pressure in comparison with

the left due to a streaming effect. An ejection sound will be present only in patients with valvular AS.

X-rays and echocardiograms may show calcification of the aortic cusps and hypertrophy of the septum and free walls. LV enlargement will be seen only if there is LV failure, myocardial damage, or a concomitant regurgitant lesion.

An ECG will show various degrees of LV hypertrophy, and if an LV strain pattern is present, it usually signifies severe AS.

Doppler echocardiography gives gradients with satisfactory accuracy, and cardiac catheterization will give the precise valvular gradient (see INVASIVE CARDIOVASCULAR PROCEDURES in Ch. 25). If angina is present, coronary angiography is necessary.

Treatment

Since a significant gradient across either an aortic or pulmonary valve is considered 70 mm Hg with normal myocardial function, and about 50 mm Hg with poor myocardial function, patients with such gradients should have activity restricted in order to avoid sudden death, and if they have any of the triad of symptoms mentioned above, surgery should be considered. Balls, discs, or tissue valves are available. Anticoagulants are not needed for tissue valves. Prophylactic antibiotics are necessary in patients with prosthetic valves to prevent endocarditis (see ENDOCARDITIS, below) if any procedure is contemplated that may produce bacteremia, especially if the patient has AR as well. Only rarely does endocarditis occur in a purely stenotic valve.

TRICUSPID VALVE DISEASE

TRICUSPID REGURGITATION (TR)

(Tricuspid Incompetence or Insufficiency)

Retrograde flow of blood from right ventricle to right atrium due to inadequate apposition of the tricuspid valves.

Etiology, Pathology, and Physiology

TR is usually secondary to a combination of dilation and high pressure due to severe pulmonary hypertension or outflow obstruction. Dilation alone, as in large atrial septal defects, or high pressure alone, as in severe pulmonary stenosis, does not produce TR. More rarely, it may be secondary to infective endocarditis or the papillary dysfunction of RV infarction. TR may occasionally be primary; ie, due to a cleft tricuspid valve, as in endocardial cushion defects, or to **Ebstein's anomaly;** ie, downward displacement of a distorted tricuspid cusp into the right ventricle, or to carcinoid disease, in which the valve may be fixed in a semi-open position. More rarely, TR is caused by a myxomatous transformation causing prolapse, usually together with MVP.

Symptoms, Signs, and Diagnosis

Aside from low output symptoms, the only specific symptom of severe TR would be the sensation of pulsations in the neck due to the high jugular regurgitant (CV) waves from the transmitted RV pressure. Atrial fibrillation or flutter, which usually occurs when the right atrium enlarges, decreases the CO still more and may precipitate sudden, severe heart failure.

The jugulars may show various degrees of V wave and Y descent, depending on the degree of TR, and this will be associated with various degrees of systolic pulsation of the liver synchronous with the V waves. A pansystolic TR murmur may be high-pitched, if trivial and secondary to pulmonary hypertension, or medium frequency, if rather gross and primary. It will be increased by inspiration **(Carvallo's sign)**. It is best heard at the 4th and 5th intercostal spaces close to the sternum or in the epigastrium but will be transmitted to the apex if the right ventricle usurps that area.

The ECG may show various degrees of RV overload, depending on the severity of the TR and whether it is secondary to pulmonary hypertension. There may be the tall peaked P waves of right atrial overload or a QR in V_1 (characteristic of a large right atrium in the presence of RV hypertrophy). X-rays will show enlargement of the superior vena cava as well as of the right atrium (enlargement of the cardiac silhouette to the right) and right ventricle (enlargement of the cardiac silhouette to the left). Lateral chest films may show also the RV enlargement. The echocardiogram shows an increased right atrial and RV dimension. Doppler and 2-D echocardiography can confirm the diagnosis. Cardiac catheterization and angiography can demonstrate the TR directly, and by measuring pressure in the right ventricle can tell whether the TR is primary or secondary (see INVASIVE CARDIOVASCULAR PROCEDURES in Ch. 25).

Treatment

Even severe TR is well tolerated for years. (The tricuspid valve is often removed for the infective endocarditis of heroin addicts.) Pulmonary hypertension and high RV pressures may be secondary to a left-sided valvular lesion (eg, MS), which may be amenable to surgery.

TRICUSPID STENOSIS (TS)

A narrowing at the tricuspid orifice obstructing flow from right atrium to right ventricle.

Etiology and Pathology

TS is nearly always rheumatic and always accompanies MS, but occasionally TS is dominant. Rarely, SLE, carcinoid, or a right atrial myxoma can also cause it. Congenital TS is even more rare. The right atrium becomes hypertrophied and distended, while the right ventricle remains underfilled and small.

Symptoms, Signs, and Diagnosis

The only symptom of severe TS apart from some fluttering discomfort in the neck caused by giant A waves in the jugular pulse is the low CO symptom of fatigue, or the discomfort of an enlarged liver.

If cardiac rhythm is normal, there is invariably a giant A wave in the jugular pulse. If there is atrial fibrillation, there will be a prominent V wave in the jugular pulse. In sinus rhythm only a presystolic murmur will be heard at the left sternal edge in the 4th interspace or epigastrium, which increases with inspiration. However, there is no crescendo to S_1, and very little or no mid-diastolic rumble as in MS. Only if the patient is in atrial fibrillation will the murmur be mid-diastolic.

The ECG will show the tall peaked P waves of right atrial overload in the inferior leads and V_1. The chest x-ray will show a dilated right atrium and superior vena cava. Cardiac catheterization will show a diastolic pressure gradient across the tricuspid valve (see INVASIVE CARDIOVASCULAR PROCEDURES in Ch. 25). An echocardiogram will show right atrial enlargement and the slow EF slope of TS.

Treatment

Only rarely is TS severe enough to require valvotomy.

PULMONIC VALVE DISEASE

(See CONGENITAL HEART DISEASE in Ch. 187)

ENDOCARDITIS

INFECTIVE ENDOCARDITIS (IE)

(Acute Bacterial Endocarditis [ABE]; Subacute Bacterial Endocarditis [SBE])

Microbial infections of the endocardium, characterized by fever, heart murmurs, petechiae, anemia, embolic phenomena, and endocardial vegetations that may result in valvu-

lar incompetence or obstruction, myocardial abscess, or mycotic aneurysm. The course may be acute or subacute and clinical findings vary greatly, depending on host age and susceptibility, underlying or associated disease, and the organism involved.

The overall incidence of IE has probably not changed significantly in the last 2 decades and men continue to be affected about twice as often as women. However, epidemiologic patterns have been changing. The median age of onset has increased from about 35 yr before antibiotics were available to about age 50. There is a higher incidence of right-sided IE associated with IV drug abuse and diagnostic procedures requiring vascular lines. Cardiac surgery and other invasive procedures have led to an increase in nosocomial endocarditis (10 to 15% in recent series), and an increasing elderly population with thickened, stiff, calcified valves constitutes a growing subset of IE patients (almost 30%). Demographic, epidemiologic, and clinical disease patterns vary greatly in different settings; eg, the picture is different in small, suburban private hospitals compared to large, urban medical centers.

Etiology

ABE is usually caused by *Staphylococcus aureus*, Group A hemolytic streptococcus, pneumococcus, or the gonococcus. Less virulent microorganisms may produce ABE in certain patients.

SBE is usually caused by streptococcal species with the viridans streptococci, microaerophilic and anaerobic streptococci, non-enterococcal Group D, and enterococci most frequently isolated. *S. aureus*, *S. epidermidis*, and fastidious *Hemophilus* sp may also produce SBE. SBE often develops on abnormal valves after asymptomatic bacteremias from infected gums, GU tract, or GI tract.

Prosthetic valvular endocarditis (PVE) develops in 2 to 3% of patients in the year following prosthetic valve placement and in 0.5%/yr thereafter, but it should be noted that the incidence is higher with aortic valve prostheses than with mitral, and porcine (heterograft) valves are less often infected than other prosthetic valves. **Early onset infections** (< 2 mo postsurgery) that result in high mortality rates occur mainly from antimicrobial-resistant organisms implanted during surgery (eg, *S. epidermidis*, *Diphtheroid* sp, coliform bacilli, *Candida* sp, and *Aspergillus* sp). A better prognosis is associated with **later onset infections** that are produced by low-virulence organisms implanted at surgery, or by transient asymptomatic bacteremias often from susceptible organisms. Late onset PVE is most often due to *Streptococcus* sp, *S. epidermidis*, diphtheroids, and the fastidious gram-negative rods—*Hemophilus* sp, *Actinobacillus actinomycetemcomitans*, and *Cardiobacterium hominis*.

Right-sided endocarditis involving the tricuspid valve and less often the pulmonary valve and artery may result from IV use of illicit drugs or infections associated with central vascular lines, which not only facilitate entry of microorganisms, but may damage the endocardium. Organisms originating from the skin (eg, *S. aureus*, *Candida* sp, or coliform bacilli) produce septic phlebitis, fever, pleurisy, hemoptysis, septic pulmonary infarction, and tricuspid regurgitation. These infections more often respond to antimicrobial therapy and have a better prognosis than left-sided IE.

Pathology

The intravascular nidus for microorganisms within the heart and blood vessels is thought to be a sterile fibrin-platelet vegetation formed when tissue factor is released by damaged endothelial cells. Microorganisms colonizing vegetations are covered by a layer of fibrin and platelets that prevents access to the site of infection by neutrophils, immunoglobulin, and complement, thus permitting the pathogens to resist host defenses. Without treatment IE is progressive and uniformly fatal. Death usually ensues from heart failure due to exacerbation of underlying heart disease or acute valve dysfunction, embolization of vegetations to vital organs producing infarction, rupture of a mycotic aneurysm, septic shock in ABE, renal failure, or complications of cardiac surgery.

IE occurs most often on the left side, involving the mitral, aortic, tricuspid, and pulmonic valves (in descending order of frequency). Congenital defects and rheumatic valvular disease are still major predisposing factors. Mural thrombi, arterio-venous fistulae, ventricular-septal defects, and patent ductus arteriosus sites may also become infected. Rheumatic valvular heart disease, bicuspid or calcific aortic valves, mitral valve prolapse, hypertrophic subaortic stenosis, and prosthetic valves predispose to IE. Infections treated with antimicrobial agents heal by endothelization of vegetations.

Symptoms and Signs

SBE has an insidious onset and may mimic other systemic illnesses with low-grade fever (< 39 C [102.2 F]), night sweats, fatigability, malaise, weight loss, and valvular insufficiency. Chills and arthralgias may be present. Emboli may produce stroke, myocardial infarction, flank pain and hematuria, abdominal pain, or acute arterial insufficiency in an extremity. Physical examination may be normal or show chronic illness with pallor; fever; a change in preexisting murmur or new regurgitant cardiac valvular murmur; tachycardia; petechiae over the upper trunk, conjunctiva, mucous membranes, and distal extremities; painful erythematous subcutaneous nodules about the tips of the digits **(Osler's nodes)**; splinter hemorrhages under the nails; or hemorrhagic retinal lesions (particularly **Roth's spots,** round or oval lesions with small white centers). With prolonged infection, splenomegaly or clubbing of the fingers may also be present.

Hematuria and proteinuria may result from embolic infarction of the kidney or a diffuse glomerulonephritis due to immune complex deposition. Manifestations of CNS involvement are common (about 35% of patients) and may range from transient ischemic attacks and toxic encephalopathy to brain abscess, subarachnoid hemorrhage from rupture of a mycotic aneurysm, and purulent meningitis in ABE.

In ABE, symptoms and signs are similar to those of SBE, but the course is more rapid. ABE can develop on normal valves and is marked by the variable presence of high fever, toxic appearance, rapid valvular destruction, valve ring abscesses, septic emboli, an obvious source of infection, and septic shock.

PVE often results in valve ring abscesses, obstructing vegetations, myocardial abscesses, and mycotic aneurysms manifested by valve obstruction, dehiscence, and cardiac conduction disturbances in addition to the usual symptoms of ABE or SBE.

Diagnosis

Since symptoms and physical findings associated with IE are nonspecific, highly variable, and may present insidiously, it is important to search actively for this infection in high-risk patients (eg, those with a history of cardiac valvular disease, those who have had recent invasive medical procedures or dental work, drug addicts). The multitude of symptoms and signs described above may all be present, but most are being seen less frequently, perhaps because of earlier diagnosis and treatment; fever and heart murmurs are the most constant. Although up to 15% of patients with IE may not have fever or a murmur initially, almost all will have both these signs eventually. Thus, any patient suspected of having a septicemia, especially those with fever and a murmur, must have blood drawn for cultures as soon as possible. Due to the continuous bacteremia seen in intravascular infections, usually 3 to 5 blood cultures of 20 to 30 mL each within 24 h suffice to isolate the etiologic agent. Identification of both the organism and its antimicrobial susceptibility are keys to appropriate management of IE, because treatment with agents lethal to the organism is required. Blood cultures may require 3 to 4 wk incubation, and certain infections (ie, *Aspergillus* sp) may not produce positive cultures; others (ie, *Coxiella burnetii*, *Chlamydia psittaci*) require serodiagnosis.

Other than positive blood cultures, there are no specific laboratory findings. Patients with bacteremias from organisms known to be frequent causes of endocarditis should

be examined carefully and repeatedly for new valvular murmurs and for signs of embolic phenomena. Two-dimensional echocardiographic studies will detect vegetations in 60 to 80% of patients with IE if they have underlying valvular heart disease. In established infections a normocytic-normochromic anemia, elevated ESR, neutrophilia, increased immunoglobulins, circulating immune complexes, and rheumatoid factors are often, but not always, present.

Patients with negative blood cultures may have suppression due to prior antimicrobial therapy, infection with organisms that do not grow in routine laboratory culture media, or may not have infective endocarditis. Nonbacterial thrombotic endocarditis (see below), atrial myxomas with embolic phenomenon, and vasculitides must be differentiated from culture-negative infective endocarditis.

Prognosis

Untreated, IE is almost always fatal. When treated, the mortality varies greatly, depending upon the patient's age and condition, severity of underlying diseases, site of infection, susceptibility of the microorganism to antibiotics, and complications. The expected mortality of viridans streptococcal endocarditis without major complications is < 10%, while virtually all patients with aspergillus endocarditis following prosthetic valve surgery die. Cardiac surgical procedures that correct acute valvular insufficiency, remove infected foreign bodies, and eliminate recalcitrant infection have significantly improved survival. Factors associated with a poor prognosis include heart failure, extreme age, aortic or multiple valve involvement, large vegetations, polymicrobial bacteremia, antimicrobial resistance, delay in initiating therapy, prosthetic valve infections, mycotic aneurysms, valve ring abscess, and major embolic events. Following cardiac surgery, early-onset IE has a higher mortality rate than late-onset IE, as noted above. Right-sided IE has a better prognosis than left-sided.

Prophylaxis

Although its value has never been proven, most physicians recommend antimicrobial prophylaxis for patients with known valvular predisposition to IE when they are exposed to procedure-related bacteremias that have been associated with subsequent development of IE. Prophylaxis is directed against viridans streptococci during oral-dental procedures, against the enterococcus for GI and GU tract infections, and against *S. aureus* and *S. epidermidis* during cardiac valvular surgery. Practical options for IE prophylaxis in the dental office are amoxicillin 3 gm orally 1 h before the procedure and 1.5 gm orally 6 h later, or erythromycin 1 gm orally 1 h before the procedure followed by 0.5 gm orally q 6 h for 4 to 8 doses. Prophylaxis for the enterococcus consists of ampicillin 1 gm plus gentamicin 1.5 mg/kg (up to 80 mg) parenterally 30 to 60 min before the procedure, followed by 2 additional doses q 8 h. Prophylaxis during cardiac surgery usually consists of cefazolin 2 gm IV during initiation of anesthesia with 2 gm IV q 8 h for 3 to 6 doses, but other antimicrobial agents may be necessary if there are frequent postoperative infections with cefazolin-resistant organisms.

Treatment

Successful treatment requires (1) administration of an effective antibiotic maintained at high serum levels and (2) surgical procedures for the management of mechanical complications and resistant organisms.

Penicillin-susceptible streptococci (penicillin G minimum inhibitory concentration < 0.1 μg/mL): This group includes most viridans streptococci, microaerophilic and anaerobic streptococci, and non-enterococcal group D streptococci. Several regimens have equivalent results: penicillin G 10 to 20 million u./day IV in divided doses q 4 h, or procaine penicillin G 1.2 million u. IM q 6 or 12 h for 4 wk. When streptomycin 7.5 mg/kg IM twice a day is administered concurrently, the length of treatment should be

reduced to 2 wk, and organisms should be tested for high level (> 2000 μg/mL) streptomycin resistance. High level resistance is rare in nonenterococcal streptococci, but, if present, gentamicin should be used instead of streptomycin to reduce the duration of treatment. In patients allergic to penicillin, cefazolin may be given cautiously if there is no history of penicillin anaphylaxis, or, alternatively, vancomycin may be given parenterally. Oral treatment programs are less reliable and should not be used without close monitoring of serum levels to be certain of adequate GI absorption.

Penicillin-resistant streptococci (penicillin G minimum inhibitory concentration > 0.1 μg/mL): Enterococcal and some other streptococcal strains (including fastidious pyridoxyl-requiring viridans streptococci) are relatively resistant to penicillin G and require the synergistic activity of a penicillin or vancomycin combined with an aminoglycoside to cure enterococcal endocarditis. About 40% of enterococcal strains with a high level (> 2000 μg/mL) resistance to streptomycin do not respond to penicillin G plus streptomycin and should be treated with penicillin plus gentamicin. Penicillin G 15 to 24 million u./day IV or ampicillin 8 to 12 gm/day IV should be given concurrently with streptomycin 7.5 mg/kg IM twice a day or gentamicin 1 mg/kg IV q 8 h for 4 to 6 wk. Patients with enterococcal infections lasting > 3 mo, with large vegetations (as seen by echocardiogram), or with vegetations on prosthetic valves should be treated for 6 wk. Persons allergic to penicillin may be desensitized or treated with vancomycin 7.5 mg/kg IV q 6 h and streptomycin or gentamicin.

Pneumococcal or Group A streptococcal endocarditis should be treated with penicillin G 10 to 20 million u./day IV for 4 wk.

S. aureus endocarditis should be treated with penicillin G 15 to 24 million u./day IV if the strain does not produce β-lactamase. Ninety percent of strains are penicillin resistant and should be treated with a penicillinase-resistant penicillin (nafcillin, methicillin, or oxacillin) 1.5 to 2 gm IV q 4 h for 4 to 6 wk. Staphylococcal strains resistant to the methicillin family of penicillins are also resistant to the cephalosporins, although this may be difficult to demonstrate with routine susceptibility testing. Methicillin-resistant staphylococci should be treated with vancomycin 7.5 mg/kg IV q 6 h. Methicillin-susceptible infections in penicillin-allergic patients may be cautiously treated with cefazolin 1 to 2 gm IV q 6 h if there is no history of penicillin anaphylaxis, or vancomycin may be given.

S. epidermidis endocarditis occurs most often in patients with prosthetic valves who may require surgery as well as antimicrobial agents to cure the infection. Penicillin- or methicillin-susceptible strains should be treated for 6 to 8 wk as outlined above for *S. aureus*. Methicillin-resistant strains should be treated with vancomycin 7.5 mg/kg IV q 6 h and rifampin 300 mg orally q 8 h for 6 to 8 wk. *Hemophilus* sp should be treated with ampicillin and gentamicin for 4 wk using the same doses as mentioned for enterococcal infections. Coliform bacillary endocardial infections are often resistant to antimicrobial infections and should be treated for a minimum of 4 wk with a β-lactam antimicrobial agent selected on the basis of susceptibility studies given concurrently with an aminoglycoside.

Cardiac valve surgery (debridement and replacement of the valve) is frequently required to eradicate infection that is uncontrolled medically, particularly in early-onset prosthetic valvular endocarditis. The timing of surgical intervention requires good clinical judgment. It may be required urgently if heart failure caused by a correctable lesion is worsening (particularly when the organism is *S. aureus*, a Gram-negative bacillus, or a fungus), but generally should be preceded by 24 to 72 h of an optimal antibiotic regimen.

Response to treatment: Patients with penicillin-susceptible streptococcal IE usually feel better and have a reduction in fever within 3 to 7 days of starting therapy. However, fever may persist for reasons other than continued active infection; eg, drug allergy, phlebitis, or infarction from emboli. Staphylococcal IE often responds more

slowly. Sterile emboli and valve rupture may occur up to a year after successful antimicrobial therapy. Relapse after therapy usually occurs within 4 wk; the patient may respond to retreatment or may require surgery and antibiotics for cure. Recrudescence of IE after 6 wk in patients without prosthetic valves usually is a new infection rather than a relapse.

NONINFECTIVE ENDOCARDITIS

(Nonbacterial Thrombotic Endocarditis [NBTE])

Formation of sterile platelet and fibrin thrombi on cardiac valves and adjacent endocardium in response to trauma, local turbulence, circulating immune complexes, vasculitis, and hypercoagulable states.

Etiology and Pathophysiology

Vegetations may be clinically undetectable, serve as a nidus to be colonized by circulating microorganisms, produce embolic episodes, or impair valvular function. Catheters passing through the right heart may injure the tricuspid and pulmonic valves resulting in the attachment of platelets and fibrin at the site on injury. The incidence of catheter-induced endocarditis in humans has been lower than would be expected from animal studies.

In SLE friable platelet and fibrin vegetations may develop along the line of valve leaflet closure. At autopsy, 40% of SLE patients dying of active disease have lesions on one or more valves. These **Libman-Sachs lesions** are not usually associated with significant valvular obstruction or regurgitation, although mild regurgitant murmurs may be detected by cardiac auscultation.

Larger valvular thrombotic lesions that produce significant emboli to the brain, kidney, spleen, mesentery, extremities, and coronary arteries have been observed in patients with chronic wasting diseases; disseminated intravascular coagulation; mucin-producing metastatic carcinomas of lung, stomach, and pancreas; and chronic infections (eg, TB, pneumonia, and osteomyelitis). These noninfective endocardial vegetations tend to form more often on abnormal cardiac valves damaged by RF or congenital heart disease; they are most common on the mitral valve, followed by the aortic valve, and combined aortic and mitral valve lesions.

Symptoms, Signs, and Diagnosis

NBTE should always be suspected when chronically ill patients develop symptoms suggestive of arterial embolism. The diagnosis may be established by examination of embolic fragments after embolectomy, or suspected when echocardiograms show valvular vegetations without atrial myxoma, and blood cultures are negative. Differentiation from culture-negative infective endocarditis may be difficult but is important, since anticoagulation of patients with infective endocarditis is associated with a high incidence of hemorrhage.

Prognosis and Treatment

The prognosis for NBTE is generally poor due to seriousness of the predisposing conditions.

Treatment of NBTE consists of anticoagulation with heparin or warfarin, and the elimination of the predisposing condition whenever possible. Results of anticoagulant therapy have not been evaluated.

PERICARDIAL DISEASE

Etiology

The pericardium may be involved by inflammation, trauma, or neoplasms. **Inflammation** follows bacterial, viral (especially echovirus and Coxsackie Group B), or fungal

infection and sometimes accompanies systemic diseases (RA, SLE, scleroderma, uremia). Pyogenic pericarditis is uncommon, but may occur with infective endocarditis, pneumonia, septicemia, penetrating trauma, after cardiac surgery, and in patients receiving immunosuppressive therapy. Most often, the etiology of acute pericarditis cannot be identified, and is referred to as nonspecific or idiopathic pericarditis, which later may be proved to be viral in some instances. Acute pericarditis occurs after pericardiotomy (postpericardiotomy syndrome) or as a consequence of myocardial infarction (postmyocardial infarction syndrome) and, occasionally, from therapy (eg, radiation or drugs such as procainamide, hydralazine, phenytoin, or anticoagulants). **Trauma** to the pericardium may be due to penetrating or nonpenetrating chest injuries and may cause hemopericardium. Saccular or dissecting aortic aneurysms may rupture into the pericardium, as may a myocardial aneurysm after infarction or trauma. Cardiac catheters occasionally penetrate the myocardium and enter the pericardial sac. **Neoplasms** affecting the pericardium include carcinoma (especially of the lung or breast), sarcoma, and lymphomas; they may be an extension of thoracic tumors or metastases with or without serous hemorrhagic effusion. Neoplastic involvement may be focal or extensive; if extensive, cardiac performance may be hindered.

Pathology

Acute pericarditis may be fibrinous, serous, sanguineous, hemorrhagic, or purulent. The amount and quality of the cellular reaction depend on the inciting cause. The pericardial sac normally contains little fluid, but effusion may develop in disease. The superficial layers of the subepicardial myocardium may be involved. **Chronic pericarditis** may be serous, fibrous, adhesive, hemorrhagic, purulent, fibrinous, or calcific.

Fibrosis of the pericardium results from infection, trauma, or hemopericardium, or it may accompany collagen disease, including rheumatic fever; often the cause is unknown. The fibrosis may be patchy or extensive and is frequently the site of calcific deposits. Pericardial fibrosis may be without hemodynamic effects, or may cause chronic constrictive pericarditis. Chronic pericarditis may take the form of pericardial effusion, with or without cardiac tamponade. Uremia, connective tissue disease, TB, myxedema, or neoplasm may be responsible. Chronic pericardial disease may also appear as cholesterol pericarditis or chylopericardium. The latter may result from trauma, neoplasm, thoracic duct obstruction or anomalous connections, but is often idiopathic. Adhesion of the visceral and parietal layers may partially or wholly obliterate the sac, or effusion may separate the 2 layers (effusive-constrictive pericarditis).

Pathophysiology

Pericardial effusions vary in amount from about 50 mL to > 1 L. Rapid but small—or slower, more massive—accumulation of pericardial fluid or decreased pericardial compliance due to fibrosis, calcification, or neoplasm may limit ventricular filling during diastole. In that case, the end-diastolic pressure in the ventricles is determined by the limiting effusion or thickened pericardium, and the diastolic pressures in the ventricles, atria, and venous beds become virtually the same. Systemic venous congestion increases and the hydrostatic pressure in systemic capillaries approaches osmotic pressure. Therefore, a further small increase in systemic venous and capillary pressure causes considerable transudation of fluid from the systemic capillaries. Signs of peripheral congestion in pericardial disease are more striking than those of pulmonary congestion, and frank pulmonary edema is uncommon.

Rising ventricular diastolic pressure, atrial, and venous pressures and falling stroke volume, CO, and ultimately systemic arterial pressure follow abrupt fluid accumulation **(cardiac tamponade)**. The resulting clinical findings are like those of shock (decreased CO and low systemic arterial pressure) and tachycardia, together with dyspnea and orthopnea, except that systemic and pulmonary venous pressures are elevated. Cardiac tamponade is nearly always accompanied by an accentuation of the normal

inspiratory decline in systemic systolic BP **(pulsus paradoxus)**. A decline of > 10 mm Hg is usually significant. The pulse may disappear during inspiration in advanced cases. Pulsus paradoxus can also occur in chronic obstructive lung disease, bronchial asthma, pulmonary embolism, right ventricular infarction, and clinical shock.

The effect of gradual pericardial scarring **(constrictive pericarditis)** differs in several respects. The only early abnormalities may be elevation of ventricular diastolic, atrial, and pulmonary and systemic venous pressures. CO and systemic arterial pressures may be maintained by tachycardia and systemic arteriolar vasoconstriction. Prolonged elevation of pulmonary venous pressure results in dyspnea and orthopnea; systemic venous hypertension produces hypervolemia, engorgement of neck veins, pleural effusion, hepatomegaly, ascites, and peripheral edema. Pulsus paradoxus occurs in the minority of instances, and is usually less severe than in tamponade.

Symptoms and Signs

Acute pericarditis may appear with pain, fever, pericardial rub, tamponade, ECG changes, or radiologic changes, or may be discovered incidentally in the course of a systemic illness. There may be dull or sharp precordial or substernal pain radiating to the neck, trapezius ridge, or shoulders. Pain varies from mild to severe and is usually aggravated by thoracic motion, cough, and respiration; it may be relieved by sitting up and leaning forward. Indolent pericarditis (often neoplastic, tuberculous, or uremic) may be painless. Usually pericardial pain can be distinguished from ischemic coronary pain, because the latter is not aggravated by thoracic motion. Tachypnea and nonproductive cough may be present; fever, chills, and weakness are common.

When present, the dominant physical finding is a systolic and diastolic precordial **friction rub**. However, it is often intermittent and evanescent or it may be present only in systole or, less frequently, only in diastole. Considerable pericardial fluid may muffle heart sounds, increase the area of cardiac dullness, and change the size and shape of the cardiac silhouette. However, cardiac tamponade may occur with normal heart sounds and no appreciable increase in cardiac dullness. The accumulation of even large amounts of fluid is usually sufficiently slow that the pericardium stretches and accommodates the fluid without interfering with cardiac performance. Other manifestations (eg, pulsus paradoxus and those due to elevated venous pressure and falling CO culminating in tamponade and shock) are described above under pathophysiology.

With acute pericarditis, leukocytosis and a rapid ESR are common. Serial ECGs early in the disorder may show abnormalities confined to the ST segments and T waves, generally involving most leads. The ST segments in 2 or 3 of the standard leads become elevated, but subsequently return to the baseline. Unlike myocardial infarction, ST segments do not show reciprocal depression (except in leads aVR and V_1), and there are no pathologic Q waves. The T waves may become flattened and then inverted throughout the ECG, except in lead aVR. With effusion, QRS voltage is usually decreased. Electrical alternans is uncommon, and is usually limited to occasional cases of cardiac tamponade. Sinus rhythm occurs in about 90% of cases. The cardiac silhouette on x-ray is not enlarged except with coexisting heart disease or effusion > 250 mL. Pleural effusion, especially on the left, is common.

Chronic pericarditis: Pericardial fibrosis or calcification is asymptomatic unless constrictive pericarditis is present; then symptoms and signs of peripheral congestion may appear along with an early diastolic sound, often best heard on inspiration **(pericardial knock),** and at times pulsus paradoxus. Pericardial calcification often is best seen in lateral chest films. The cardiac silhouette may be small, normal, or large. Nonspecific ECG changes may occur. The QRS voltage is usually low. T waves are usually abnormal. Atrial fibrillation (less commonly, atrial flutter) is present in perhaps 25% of patients with constrictive pericarditis.

Diagnosis

Acute pericarditis may be diagnosed solely from the history of pain and the characteristic ECG. A pericardial friction rub is also diagnostic. Pericarditis must be distinguished from causes of pleuritic pain and myocardial or pulmonary infarction. Pericardial effusion may be suspected by a rapid change in the cardiac silhouette on serial chest x-rays, especially when the lung fields remain clear. (When rapid changes in heart size are due to heart failure, pulmonary congestion is more likely.) The silhouette is often symmetrically enlarged, and the outlines of the individual cardiac chambers and great vessels are obliterated. Since considerable pericardial fluid may be present in myxedema or congestion secondary to ventricular failure, its presence does not necessarily imply pericarditis. Echocardiography is the best means of recognizing pericardial effusion with acute pericarditis; however, the echocardiogram may be normal when there is only fibrinous pericarditis.

Tuberculous pericarditis is insidious in onset and may exist without pulmonary involvement. The PPD skin test is usually positive. Culture of pericardial fluid or tissue may be necessary for diagnosis, or response to antituberculous therapy may confirm the diagnosis. Pericarditis from pyogenic, viral, or mycotic infections or that associated with acute RF, collagen disease, uremia, or acute myocardial infarction may be overlooked because of concern with other manifestations of the underlying disease; once recognized, its cause is usually identified.

Idiopathic pericarditis is frequently preceded by a URI. Other possible causes must be carefully excluded before idiopathic pericarditis is diagnosed. Blood cultures, skin tests for TB, examination of pericardial fluid or pericardial biopsy specimens for fungi, antinuclear antibody tests, histoplasmosis complement fixation tests, streptozyme tests, tests for neutralizing antibodies for coxsackievirus, influenza virus, and ECHO virus, and search for SLE cells in the blood should be among the diagnostic procedures. Anti-DNA and anti-RNA antibody tests may be useful. If pericardial fluid is recovered, it should be cultured and examined for tumor cells. Direct pericardial biopsy for culture and microscopic examination may be needed in recurrent or persistent pericardial effusion.

Postpericardiotomy and **postmyocardial infarction syndromes** may be difficult to identify and must be distinguished from pericardial infection following surgery and from a recent myocardial infarction or pulmonary embolus. Pain, friction rub, and fever appearing and recurring 2 wk to several months after the known insult, and their rapid response to corticosteroids aid diagnosis. Trauma to the pericardium is usually suggested by the history and a rapid accumulation of blood in the sac precipitating tamponade.

The appearance of atrial arrhythmias and evidence of tamponade or constriction in neoplastic diseases suggest pericardial involvement.

Chronic pericarditis: Fibrosis of the pericardium is recognized by the demonstration of pericardial calcification (sometimes without pericardial constriction) or manifestations of circulatory congestion. **Constrictive pericarditis** must be distinguished from myocardial or valvular disease or cirrhosis of the liver with congestion. Restrictive cardiomyopathy especially must be distinguished from constrictive pericarditis (see below).

Special diagnostic technics may be required to differentiate effusion or constrictive pericarditis from a dilated heart. **Echocardiography,** which is safe, quick, and noninvasive, has a high degree of sensitivity and specificity for the recognition of pericardial fluid. It usually shows characteristic changes with tamponade, but the changes are not specific in constrictive pericarditis. With effusion the procedure discloses 2 echoes behind the left ventricle in the region of the posterior cardiac wall: one from the epicardium and the other from the pericardium. The interval between the echoes represents the fluid. Uncommonly, angiocardiography is needed to demonstrate pericardial fluid.

Hemodynamic studies: Constrictive pericarditis may be suggested by the characteristic pressure records described below. The diagnosis may be confirmed by angiocardiography, which typically shows moderate pericardial thickening, as a thickened border between the cardiac chamber and the cardiac shadow, and straightening of the lateral right atrial border. These changes are not always present, and exploratory thoracotomy may be necessary.

The mean pulmonary wedge pressure, the pulmonary artery diastolic pressure, the right ventricular end-diastolic pressure, and the mean right atrial pressure are usually 10 to 30 mm Hg and virtually identical in tamponade or constriction. The pulmonary arterial and right ventricular systolic pressures are only modestly elevated, so that pulse pressures are small. In the presence of constrictive pericarditis, atrial pressure curves may show accentuation of the X and Y descents, and ventricular pressure curves demonstrate a diastolic dip at the time of rapid ventricular filling. These changes in the pressure curves almost always occur in congestion due to constrictive pericarditis. In cardiac tamponade, there is no early diastolic dip in the ventricular pressure record. Similar hemodynamic abnormalities may be found in severe congestive states due to cardiomyopathy. In that case, pulmonary wedge or left ventricular diastolic pressures usually exceed right atrial mean pressure and right ventricular diastolic pressure by 4 to 6 mm Hg or more. When the pulmonary wedge pressure equals the right atrial mean pressure, angiocardiograms or CT are useful to demonstrate pericardial thickening or fluid. When pericardial thickening or fluid cannot be demonstrated, the diagnosis of restrictive cardiomyopathy is favored, but not proven.

Treatment

General: Aspirin 600 mg orally, codeine 15 to 60 mg orally, meperidine 50 to 100 mg orally or IM, or morphine 10 to 15 mg IM may be given q 4 h for pain. Anxiety or insomnia may respond to diazepam 2 to 10 mg orally tid or qid or flurazepam 15 or 30 mg orally at bedtime. Anticoagulants are usually *contraindicated* in pericardial disease since they may cause intrapericardial bleeding and even fatal tamponade.

Possible causative therapeutic agents (eg, anticoagulants, procainamide, or phenytoin) should be discontinued.

Specific: Pericarditis due to bacterial or mycotic infections is treated with specific antimicrobial agents. Tuberculous pericarditis may be treated with drug therapy (see under TUBERCULOSIS in Ch. 8). The pericardial sac should be drained surgically if the pericarditis is due to a pyogenic infection.

Antibiotics are not indicated in idiopathic pericarditis nor in the postinfarction or postpericardiotomy syndromes. Indomethacin 25 to 50 mg orally tid may control pain and effusion. Prednisone 20 to 60 mg/day orally in divided doses may be given for 3 to 4 days when required to control pain, fever, and effusion. The dose is gradually reduced if the response is satisfactory and may be discontinued in 7 to 14 days in some cases, but many months of treatment may be needed.

Therapy for pericarditis in RF and the connective tissue diseases and for pericardial involvement in neoplastic diseases is directed at the underlying process. Surgical intervention is required in some instances of trauma to repair the injury and evacuate blood from the sac. Uremic pericarditis may respond to increased frequency of hemodialysis, aspiration, or systemic or local adrenal corticosteroid therapy.

Immediate **pericardiocentesis** may be required when tamponade develops; removal of even a small volume may be life-saving. Except in emergencies, pericardiocentesis, *a potentially lethal procedure*, should be performed under the supervision of a cardiologist or thoracic surgeon and in the cardiac catheterization laboratory. Thoracotomy is usually safer. Premedication with morphine 5 to 15 mg or meperidine 50 to 100 mg IM is desirable in non-urgent situations. The patient should be seated upright in a chair with his back supported. Some physicians prefer the patient recumbent with his back

supported by a pillow for the subxiphoid approach. Under antiseptic conditions, the skin and subcutaneous tissues are infiltrated with lidocaine. A 75-mm (3-in.), short-beveled, 16-gauge needle is attached via a 3-way stopcock to a 30-or 50-mL syringe. The pericardial sac may be entered via the right or left xiphocostal angle or from the tip of the xiphoid process with the needle directed inward, upward, and close to the chest wall. An alternate approach is via the 5th left intercostal space 1 to 2 cm medial to the left border of cardiac flatness with the needle directed inward and slightly medially; if a distinct apical impulse is visible, the needle may be introduced 1 to 2 cm lateral to the impulse. The subxiphoid approach may be preferable for smaller effusions, and is now generally preferred for any pericardiocentesis.

The needle is advanced with constant suction applied to the syringe. Cardiac impulses may be easily felt through the needle when the pericardial sac has been entered and fluid will be aspirated. Blood aspirated from the pericardial sac usually will not clot, while blood inadvertently aspirated from the cardiac chambers will. The needle should be clamped next to the skin to prevent it from entering farther than necessary and possibly puncturing the heart or injuring a coronary vessel. ECG monitoring is essential during the procedure to detect arrhythmias produced when the myocardium is touched or punctured. Echocardiography may be used to guide the needle. A plastic catheter may be passed through the needle into the sac and the needle withdrawn if continued drainage is needed.

Congestion due to constrictive pericarditis may be alleviated with bed rest, salt restriction, and diuretics. Digoxin is indicated in atrial arrhythmias or myocardial failure. Recurrent or persistent effusions, with or without tamponade, and constrictive pericarditis usually require pericardiectomy. With specific infections, pericardiectomy is done preferably after specific antimicrobial therapy is begun. Patients with constrictive pericarditis who have mild symptoms, heavy calcification, or extensive myocardial damage, or who are elderly may be poor candidates for pericardial resection. Patients who have constrictive pericarditis associated with radiation therapy or with connective tissue disease are especially liable to have severe myocardial damage, and may show no improvement with pericardial resection.

CARDIAC TUMORS

Primary heart tumors are rare, being found in < 1:2,000 at autopsy; secondary tumors are 30 to 40 times more common. Tumors may be epicardial, myocardial, or endocardial, and their symptoms and signs may have localizing features. However, they mimic other heart diseases and are often diagnosed either by chance or because of a strong index of suspicion. The development of cardiac signs and symptoms in a patient with an extracardiac malignancy suggests metastases to the heart.

PRIMARY CARDIAC TUMORS

Malignant cardiac tumors, which can arise from any heart tissue, are rare and occur mostly in children. Most common are sarcomas (eg, angiosarcoma, fibrosarcoma, rhabdomyosarcoma, and liposarcoma). They are associated with more acute and rapid deterioration than benign cardiac tumors. Sudden development of congestive failure, rapid accumulation of hemorrhagic pericardial effusion, often with tamponade, and various arrhythmias or heart block may herald the tumor's presence. Metastases occur to spine, neighboring soft tissues, and major organs. Prognosis is poor, and treatment is limited to radiation, chemotherapy, and management of complications.

Benign cardiac tumors, including myxomas, rhabdomyomas, fibromas, lipomas, teratomas, and pericardial cysts, may threaten life if left untreated.

Myxoma, the most common intracavity tumor, comprises 50% of primary heart tumors. Seventy-five percent are in the left atrium; the rest occur mostly in the right atrium but rarely in either ventricle. Myxomas are either semitransparent and gelatinous, with a lobular or villous surface, or appear as a round, firm mass. Myxoma cells resemble endothelial cells; they are elongated and spindle-shaped with round or oval nuclei and prominent nucleoli. Cells and vessels are embedded in an amorphous matrix rich in acid mucopolysaccharide. The tumor mass is richly supplied with thin-walled capillaries. The tumor surface is usually endothelialized and may be coated with thrombi. Atrial tumors, especially right atrial myxomas, may contain calcium deposits visible on plain chest x-ray. Left atrial myxomas usually arise from the endocardium at the border of the fossa ovalis and are pedunculated; less commonly they are broad-based, sessile tumors. They are usually solid and when pedunculated may prolapse through the mitral valve orifice in diastole.

Myxomas present the most varied clinical picture of all cardiac tumors; however, 3 major syndromes are observed: (1) embolic phenomena, (2) obstruction to blood flow, and (3) constitutional syndromes. Tumor fragments (especially from gelatinous myxomas) or thrombotic material may embolize from right- or left-sided tumors to the lungs or periphery, respectively. The diagnosis may often be made by finding tumor cells in a surgically removed embolus. Obstruction to blood flow may occur at the orifice of any valve, most commonly the mitral valve. Interference with function by the tumor mimics signs and symptoms of valvular dysfunction due to rheumatic disease. Thus, left-atrial myxomas may cause pulmonary congestion and signs of mitral stenosis including the typical murmur, opening snap, and accentuated first heart sound. Murmurs of mitral insufficiency may also be present as a result of chronic damage to the valve leaflets or to the tumor's interference with proper closure. Clinical differentiation between left atrial tumor and primary mitral valve disease may be suggested by the influence of position on symptoms such as congestive failure and syncope and on the intensity of murmurs and the opening snap. Left atrial size is likely to be disproportionately smaller in relation to severity of manifestations in patients with tumor than with valvular disease. About 25% of patients with myxomas may have friction rubs; the mechanism for this finding is not clear. Left atrial tumors can also produce a "tumor plop" sound as the pedunculated mass drops into the valve orifice during diastole. It differs from the opening snap of rheumatic mitral stenosis by its variability, timing, intensity, and character, sometimes having more than one component.

Constitutional symptoms that may be associated with myxomas are protean (see TABLE 27–10) and may mimic such disorders as bacterial endocarditis, collagen vascular disease, or occult malignancy.

Diagnosis is suspected from the symptoms and signs and usually confirmed by echocardiogram; infrequently, angiocardiography is required. Surgical removal usually is curative.

Fibromas and **rhabdomyomas** arise within the myocardium or endocardium; **rhabdomyomas** are most frequent (20% of primary tumors). Usually found in childhood or infancy, most cases are associated with tuberous sclerosis, adenoma sebaceum of the

TABLE 27–10. FINDINGS THAT MAY ACCOMPANY CARDIAC MYXOMAS

Fever	Elevated ESR
Weight loss	Elevated WBC count
Raynaud's phenomenon	Decreased platelet count
Clubbing of fingers	Positive C-reactive protein
Anemia	Abnormal serum proteins (usually increased γ-globulins)

skin, kidney tumors, and arrhythmias. These tumors are predominantly intramural and lie in the interventricular septum or free wall of the left ventricle; multiple tumor nodules are the rule. Cardiac symptoms and signs include atrioventricular and intraventricular block, paroxysmal supraventricular and ventricular tachycardias, cardiomegaly, and manifestations of outflow tract obstruction of either ventricle, such as right- or left-sided congestive failure and murmurs of pulmonary or aortic stenosis. Association of these findings with features of tuberous sclerosis should suggest the diagnosis, which can be confirmed by echo- or angiocardiography. Surgical treatment of the multiple tumor nodules is usually ineffective and the prognosis is poor beyond the first year of life. Only 15% of a collected series of patients survived 5 yr.

Teratomas of the pericardium, often attached to the base of the great vessels, are rarer than **cysts** or **lipomas** and are usually seen in infants. Generally asymptomatic, they are often discovered on routine chest x-ray. Surgery is necessary only to rule out more serious tumors.

SECONDARY CARDIAC TUMORS

Malignant tumors, including carcinomas, sarcomas, leukemias, and reticuloendothelial tumors, may metastasize to any heart tissue. Lung and breast carcinomas invade the heart most frequently. As a group, melanosarcomas have one of the highest incidences of metastasis to the heart. Cardiac involvement by systemic malignancies is suggested by sudden enlargement, bizarre changes in contour on chest x-ray, tamponade, arrhythmias, or unexplained heart failure. Therapy is palliative, as with primary malignancies.

---

28. EXERCISE AND THE HEART

THE NORMAL CARDIOVASCULAR RESPONSE TO EXERCISE

The cardiovascular response to exercise reflects the increased need for O_2 transport and utilization associated with the raised metabolic rate.

There is an increase in CO due predominantly to an increase in heart rate; stroke volume increases to a lesser extent. Additionally, there is an increased extraction of O_2 from arterial blood, with a resultant increase in the arteriovenous O_2 difference. The redistribution of blood flow shunts blood away from the skin, kidneys, and splanchnic bed, and increases the blood flow to exercising muscle. Peripheral vascular resistance decreases, and pulse pressure widens, due more to an increase in systolic than to a decrease in diastolic BP. There is a marked increase in coronary flow, and an increase in respiratory rate.

THE ATHLETIC HEART SYNDROME

The constellation of physiologic responses seen in persons trained to perform endurance exercise. Sinus bradycardia is characteristic, and biventricular cardiac enlargement is readily apparent on x-ray. This syndrome, which would be considered abnormal in an untrained person, should not be misdiagnosed as organic heart disease.

Physiology

Cardiac dilation and hypertrophy are characteristic of endurance-trained athletes, in contrast to the skeletal muscle and myocardial hypertrophy that occur in response to speed or strength (isometric) training. Hypertrophy and dilation in the endurance-trained athletes increase the pumping capability of the heart; increased O_2 delivery to

the tissues, both at rest and with exercise, is due primarily to the increased stroke volume. The increase in diastolic filling time with bradycardia further augments the stroke volume and also increases coronary blood flow, which is predominantly a diastolic event. The total Hb and blood volume of endurance-trained athletes are also increased, further enhancing O_2 transport. Both resting heart rate and the heart rate at submaximal exercise decrease progressively with endurance training, primarily due to increased vagal tone, but decreased sympathetic stimulation also plays a role. Although the increased ventricular volume results in increased left ventricular stroke work, the O_2-sparing effect of the bradycardia predominates so that myocardial O_2 consumption decreases for the same amount of external work. Cardiac enlargement and bradycardia both characteristically regress when training is discontinued.

Untrained subjects increase CO in response to exercise primarily by increasing the heart rate; the trained endurance athlete does so mainly by increasing stroke volume. Resting intracardiac pressures are normal in endurance-trained athletes, and their intracardiac pressures and pulmonary and peripheral vascular bed pressures respond normally to exercise. Ventricular work per minute is also normal.

Clinical Features

Sinus bradycardia, often with sinus arrhythmia, is characteristic. Atrial and ventricular arrhythmias may occur, and conduction and repolarization (ST-T) abnormalities are seen on the ECG. These arrhythmias are typically asymptomatic and may decrease or disappear with exercise, as the heart rate increases. QRS and T voltage are increased on the ECG, often with a prominent U wave, which is probably related to the bradycardia. Repolarization abnormalities are common. Systemic BP differs little between trained athletes and normal individuals. The heart is moderately enlarged, and the left ventricular impulse is hyperdynamic. A third heart sound is common, as is a left sternal border ejection systolic murmur and a fourth heart sound may be heard. The cardiac silhouette is enlarged on chest x-ray; at fluoroscopy, cardiac pulsations are brisk and prominent. There is no correlation between the level of training or cardiovascular performance and the extent of the bradycardia, cardiac enlargement, or ECG abnormality. At echocardiography there is an increase in left ventricular cavity dimensions and wall thickness.

There is no evidence that even the most strenuous physical activity is deleterious to the cardiovascular function of an individual with a normal heart. However, **sudden death,** both at rest and with exertion, occurs occasionally in apparently healthy young athletes, probably due to a cardiac arrhythmia. Although the increased ventricular refractory period with bradycardia favors the occurrence of ventricular ectopic rhythms, sudden death related to arrhythmia in athletes is most frequently due to previously undetected atherosclerotic coronary heart disease, hypertrophic cardiomyopathy, myocarditis, or congenital coronary artery or aortic valve anomalies.

---

29. DISEASES OF THE AORTA AND ITS BRANCHES

AORTITIS

Inflammation of the aorta may result in weakness of the aortic wall leading to aneurysm formation or obstruction of the aorta or of its major branches leading to ischemia. The adventitia is involved by chronic inflammation and fibrosis with endarteritis obliterans of the vasa vasorum. The media is involved by chronic inflammation and fibrosis, and the intima is thickened by fibroblastic proliferation.

The aortic arch syndrome accounts for most cases, although other conditions, eg, giant cell arteritis (temporal arteritis) and ankylosing spondylitis, may also involve the aorta; syphilitic aortitis is rare. Only the aortic arch syndrome will be discussed in this chapter; the other disorders are described elsewhere in the text.

THE AORTIC ARCH SYNDROME

(Pulseless Disease; Takayasu's Disease; Martorell's Disease; Reversed Coarctation; Young Oriental Female Disease)

A syndrome resulting from obliterative disease of one or more large branches of the aortic arch, commonly the innominate, left common carotid, and left subclavian arteries.

Etiology and Pathology

A variety of lesions can obliterate the great branches of the aortic arch at or near their origins, but the condition usually results from progression of arteriosclerosis and its complications. The distribution of age and sex is usually related to that of the underlying disease. The obliterative disease may affect all main arterial trunks from the aortic arch, or it may involve only one or two.

Maldevelopment of the embryonic branchial arterial arches can cause abnormal pulses in the neck and arms. Cases have been described secondary to blunt or penetrating intrathoracic trauma with contusion and intramural and perivascular hematoma. Some have been described secondary to syphilitic or arteriosclerotic aneurysms with intrasaccular thrombi extending into the orifices of the branches of the aortic arch. Atheromas with thrombi obstructing the origins of the branches of the aortic arch have been found.

In about 5% of patients, this syndrome results from a peculiar form of proliferative panarteritis of unknown etiology and is commonly referred to as **Takayasu's disease**: it occurs usually in Oriental women 15 to 30 yr old, but also in women and men of all races and ages. Obliteration of the brachiocephalic, carotid, and subclavian arteries results from a peculiar form of panarteritis, or inflammatory involvement of all layers of the vessel wall, most intensely affecting the media and adventitia. Intimal proliferation encroaches on the lumen and promotes thrombosis. Cellular infiltration by the lymphocytic series is found microscopically, and the frequency of giant cells has led to the term **"giant cell arteritis."** Elastic lamellae are disrupted, and this, with patchy necrosis of the media, weakens the wall of the aortic arch and sometimes results in aneurysm. Lesions in the media resemble those seen in temporal arteritis and syphilis. The process typically involves the aortic arch and the origins of its principal branches; more distal involvement of these branches is generally secondary to thrombosis. Involvement of the abdominal aorta and the renal, coronary, or pulmonary arteries occurs infrequently.

Symptoms and Signs

Patients present with symptoms of regional arterial insufficiency affecting the head and upper extremities, varying according to the degree and site of involvement of the arterial trunks and to the extent of collateral circulation. Other aortic branches are usually not involved. Gangrene is rare. Cerebral symptoms are common, secondary to involvement of the carotid and vertebral arteries. Syncope, sometimes with epileptiform seizures, may be a presenting symptom. Fainting related to turning of the head, as in the "carotid sinus syndrome," is often encountered. Temporary blindness, hemiplegia, aphasia, and memory loss are frequent complaints. In some cases, progressive visual impairment may be noted from early forming, rapidly maturing cataracts or corneal opacities. Occasionally, intermittent loss of visual acuity develops with muscular exercise, a steal syndrome referred to inaccurately as "intermittent visual claudication." Similarly, intermittent claudication develops in the muscles of mastication so that chewing becomes difficult. Facial signs of degeneration and atrophy appear: the

eyes are sunken, and atrophy of facial skeletal muscles produces a hollow appearance of the cheeks so that the patient looks prematurely old. Examination of the eyegrounds sometimes shows vascular changes—the perimacular arteriovenous communications that attracted Takayasu's attention. The appearance of the optic disc may suggest optic nerve atrophy.

With exercise, the patient feels aching, cramps, numbness, and paresthesias in the arms, especially when upstretched. The brachial, radial, carotid, and superficial temporal pulses are weak or absent. Arterial pulses in the lower extremities are normal. BP in the arms is low, but that in the legs is normal or elevated (hence the term reversed coarctation of the aorta). Aortic disease rarely extends peripherally into the abdominal aorta and its bifurcation; pulselessness and BP then are similar in all extremities.

Because collateral circulation develops as the obliterative disease progresses, pulsation in superficial collateral arteries may be felt. Murmurs may be audible in the supraclavicular triangles. These are frequently both systolic and diastolic ("machinery murmurs") with systolic accentuation, and are easily distinguished from venous hums. In acute phases of Takayasu's disease, systemic effects may be observed: chills, fever, leukocytosis, and an elevated ESR.

Diagnosis

The diagnosis, suggested by the symptoms and signs, can be confirmed and sites of the lesion can be identified precisely by aortic arch angiography, which is essential if surgery is contemplated.

Examination of peripheral blood shows abnormalities, especially in patients with acute and subacute panarteritis. The ESR is nearly always increased, the blood albumin and globulin may be abnormal, and LE cells may be present.

Treatment

There is no cure. Palliative therapy includes the use of vasodilators, anticoagulants, and corticosteroids, but most cases, especially those without active panarteritis, are not improved. Some success has been obtained with sympathetic denervation of the upper extremities. Endarterectomy with thrombectomy has had encouraging results in cases secondary to causes other than panarteritis, but the best results have been obtained by using synthetic grafts to bypass obstructions; resection and replacement of aortic arch aneurysms has been successful in highly selected patients.

In early stages, Takayasu's disease manifests itself as a systemic disease with chills, fever, arthralgia, myalgia, and general malaise, for which corticosteroids are most likely to bring relief. However, only about 75% of patients live > 2 yr after the onset of symptoms and average longevity is stated to be as low as 5 yr.

AORTIC AND PERIPHERAL ANEURYSMS

Aneurysm: *Localized dilation of a blood vessel, usually an artery.* **Dissecting aneurysm**: *Longitudinal cleavage of the arterial media by a column of blood; separation of medial layers usually does not completely encircle the lumen, but may involve the entire length of the vessel.*

Etiology and Classification

A **true aneurysm** contains all vessel wall layers and results from focal weakness and distention. Arteriosclerosis, often in conjunction with systolic hypertension, is commonly associated with varying degrees of elongation, tortuosity, and diffuse or localized aneurysm. The aneurysm of Marfan syndrome is associated with the first portion of the aorta, often leading to aortic valvular insufficiency. Syphilitic aneurysms most often occur in the ascending thoracic aorta. Abdominal aortic aneurysms are usually arteriosclerotic in origin, and calcification of the vessel wall may be seen on x-ray. These aneurysms, especially when luetic, press upon and erode the vertebrae dorsally,

or they may rupture laterally or ventrally. A genetic abnormality of the supporting tissues of the aortic wall has recently been proposed for some aortic aneurysms.

Congenital aneurysms of the intracranial carotid system or of the circle of Willis and its branches **(berry aneurysms)** occur often in association with other vascular anomalies (eg, coarctation of the aorta). They usually result from local weakness or absence of the arterial media. They are a common cause of subarachnoid and intracerebral hemorrhage in the adult (see SUBARACHNOID HEMORRHAGE in Ch. 123).

Mycotic aneurysms result from infection of the vessel wall in patients with bacteremia or septicemia from bacterial endocarditis, enteric infections, or trauma. These aneurysms commonly occur in peripheral arteries, rarely in the aorta.

Arteriovenous aneurysms (AVA) occur as congenital or posttraumatic malformations, "portwine stains," or cirsoid or racemose AVA that may affect the head, tongue, cheek, or intracranial vessels. Pulmonary AVA (hemangioma of the lung) may be congenital and sometimes are associated with hereditary telangiectasia. Cyanosis, dyspnea, and cardiac failure can result from large lesions. Penetrating wounds (as from bullet, knife, or needle biopsy) may lead to AVA, particularly in iliac, brachial, or carotid regions where an artery and vein are sheathed together. Arteriovenous communications are made surgically for access to hemodialysis in end-stage kidney disease. They have developed as complications after thyroidectomy and nephrectomy.

Dissecting aneurysms usually result from or are associated with atherosclerosis, especially in the elderly. In young people, they are commonly associated with cystic medial necrosis and degeneration (as in Marfan syndrome) or to necrosis with fibrotic repair, but without cystic degeneration or notable vascular proliferation (Erdheim's necrosis). Mechanisms proposed to account for the pathophysiology are (1) hemorrhage from the vasa vasorum producing an expanding intramedial hematoma or (2) spontaneous intimal rupture. Progressing dissection leads to complications and may cause death. Successful arrest of the acute process permits thrombosis and occlusion of the false lumen so that the aorta is protected from expansion or rupture. Occasionally recanalization diverts the false channel back into the normal lumen.

Clinically, dissecting aortic aneurysms are classified according to anatomic (DeBakey) and pathologic features. **Type I** dissecting aneurysms involve the ascending aorta and extend for a variable distance into the distal aorta and its terminal branches; this type is most common. **Type II** are local dissections of the ascending aorta without distal extension; this type is rarest and likely to be due to cystic medial necrosis (Marfan syndrome). **Type III dissections** begin at or just distal to the origin of the left subclavian artery and involve the descending aorta; they have the most favorable prognosis.

Symptoms and Signs

Intrathoracic aneurysms may cause cough, hoarseness (from pressure on the recurrent laryngeal nerve), dyspnea, dysphagia, and pain that is either substernal or localized in the back from irritation of thoracic vertebrae. Occasionally, bronchial or tracheal compression will cause a brassy cough that is constant, severe, and difficult to control by usual antitussive measures until the aneurysm is surgically repaired. Diagnosis may be suggested by the appearance of Horner's syndrome, deviation of the trachea, a tracheal tug, or inequality of the BP in the arms. Nonvascular tumors (eg, goiter, thymoma, neurofibroma, teratoma, bronchogenic carcinoma) may be mistaken for aneurysms because of transmitted pulsation from the adjacent aorta.

Dissecting aortic aneurysms present with a variety of symptoms, but the onset is usually associated with severe (often described as "tearing") pain, often mimicking myocardial infarction **(MI)** except for the rapid onset. A dissecting aneurysm in an arteriosclerotic aorta commonly begins in the ascending aorta and may extend proxi-

mally, distally, or in both directions. The site of pain may help to locate the dissection. If pain starts anteriorly, the aneurysm is generally in the ascending aorta; if it is in the back, the aneurysm probably arises distal to the left subclavian artery. If pain is located low in the back, the aneurysm is usually in the abdomen. Neck pain reflects dissection of the aortic arch. In some patients, dissecting aneurysms present initially with heart failure secondary to valvular involvement and aortic insufficiency or with MI due to encroachment on a coronary ostium. A few patients present in acute circulatory collapse due to rupture of the dissection into the pericardium or into the pleural space. Carotid, brachial, or peripheral pulses may disappear or become unequal, and arterial pressures in the upper and lower extremities may differ. CNS symptoms are due to involvement of the origins of vessels to the head and neck.

The pain of dissecting thoracic aortic aneurysm must be differentiated from that of MI; measurement of cardiac enzymes over several days as well as serial ECGs, may help (see MYOCARDIAL INFARCTION under MYOCARDIAL ISCHEMIC DISORDERS in Ch. 27). The low BP in the legs that occurs with dissection is seen also in aortic saddle embolism, aortic coarctation, and the Leriche syndrome.

Abdominal aortic aneurysms of arteriosclerosis commonly pass unnoticed until they become large enough to be felt (4 to 6 cm) as a pulsating mass or to cause symptoms. Pressure upon lumbar vertebrae causes excruciating boring pain in the abdomen or back. Aneurysms usually are tender to palpation. The pain from leaking or bleeding abdominal aneurysm usually is felt in the left side, but may be felt anywhere within the abdomen. Significant leaking or rupture is a frequent cause of vascular collapse and shock among the elderly.

Popliteal aneurysms endanger the life of the affected limb. They often go undiagnosed until they thrombose, become painful and tender, and compromise circulation in the leg. They may enlarge and compress adjoining nerves and veins, or they may bleed. Small emboli may move from the aneurysm to lodge in digital arteries, resulting in digital gangrene similar to embolization from subclavian aneurysms to the hands.

Arteriovenous aneurysms (AVA) in the upper or lower extremities, if congenital or acquired before epiphyseal closure, result in ipsilateral limb enlargement. The venous component of the AVA, subjected to arterial pressure, becomes hypertrophied and tortuous, and the walls may calcify. Bacterial endarteritis with bacteremia may complicate the arteriovenous communication. Congenital AVA often eventually require partial or total limb amputation.

A patient with AVA involving the carotids may be aware of a rhythmic, swishing noise synchronous with the heart beat. A large shunt will increase CO, and may lead to heart failure. This complication is the more likely the nearer the heart is to the arteriovenous communication.

Diagnostic Studies

Radiology: Plain x-rays are useful for detecting and evaluating thoracic and abdominal aortic aneurysms, since they are visible as abnormal masses with or without calcification in the wall. A mediastinal mass suggesting an aneurysm may necessitate complete visualization of the thoracic aorta with contrast material to establish the diagnosis and evaluate its resectability. To evaluate an abdominal aneurysm, more than one view is desirable; an anterior-posterior view, right and left obliques, and an appropriate lateral view should be included. Calcification in the wall of the aorta is necessary to establish the exact dimensions and location of the aneurysm; if it is not present, aortography may be required to establish the relationship of the aneurysm to visceral and renal branches of the aorta. Aortography often fails to demonstrate an aneurysm.

Invasive procedures include translumbar, retrograde femoral, or axillary aortography; vessels can be selectively catheterized by the Seldinger technic, and direct needle puncture can be used to demonstrate anatomy of single vessels. However, aortography can be misleading if the aneurysmal sac is filled with laminated clot and traversed by a lumen resembling a normal aortic channel. Selective technics can be used to visualize aortic arch vessels, intracranial arteries, arteries to the abdominal viscera, and those to lower extremities. Contrast studies are usually helpful before aortic surgery.

Ultrasound (US): Pulsed US defines the size and site of abdominal aortic aneurysms. In contrast to arteriography, US is noninvasive and can depict an aneurysmal dilation without being limited to the moving bloodstream. US images of the abdominal aorta from the level of the renal arteries to the aortic bifurcation can be made and are useful to follow the progress of an aneurysm initially considered too small (< 5 cm) to require surgery.

US imaging cannot be done for the thorax except for the heart itself. Air in the lungs interferes with imaging. However, for the abdomen, it is very useful to identify, localize, and evaluate an abdominal aortic aneurysm. Progressive enlargement in diameter of the aneurysm can be detected and recorded in serial studies, serving as an indication for its resection before spontaneous rupture.

CT permits imaging the aorta and its branches with great precision. Dimensions of aneurysms can be recorded and measured with considerable accuracy. Care has to be taken to image the aorta or major artery in cross section so as to make accurate, reproducible pictures of changes in diameter of the aorta and its major branches. Metallic objects, skin staples, and metallic prostheses in the path of x-rays make CT impossible.

Assessment of aneurysms by the technic described should be made q 6 mo, or sooner if symptoms related to the aneurysm develop. Prompt surgical correction should be considered if a diameter of 6 cm expands by 1 cm within 3 to 6 mo.

Prognosis and Treatment

All patients suspected of having a dissecting aneurysm of the aorta should be admitted to an intensive care unit. Vital signs, venous pressures, urinary output (not only volume, but also osmolarity, specific gravity, and dextrose content), and clinical condition should be monitored frequently. With a strong probability of the diagnosis, it is well to insert a Swan-Ganz catheter. Therapy is started without delay: The immediate initial goal of treatment is to reduce systolic BP and alleviate pain. Diastolic BP is less critical than systolic for propagation of the dissection.

The most useful drugs are propranolol hydrochloride, sodium nitroprusside, and trimethaphan camsylate. Propranolol, a β-adrenergic blocking agent, has a negative inotropic effect, thereby decreasing the rate of development of ventricular pressure (dv/dt) and it decreases the heart rate. In some responsive patients it can be used alone for reducing BP, but preferably it is used with a vasodilator (eg, sodium nitroprusside). Concurrent use of both drugs allows lower dosages and fewer side effects.

Propranolol is administered IV 0.5 mg as a test dose. If there is no untoward effect, 1 mg is given q 5 to 6 min until the desired hypotensive effect is attained. The total dose should not exceed 10 to 12 mg (for a 70 to 80 kg patient) or 0.15 mg/kg. The drug is then given IV 4 to 6 mg q 6 h, or as a continuous IV infusion, while carefully monitoring the BP and pulse rate.

In distal dissections (DeBakey Type III) for which surgery is not done, systolic BP can be controlled at a normal level by means of propranolol 20 to 40 mg orally tid or qid, and hydrochlorothiazide 25 mg orally bid. Doses are adjusted according to systolic BP and pulse rate responses.

Sodium nitroprusside, a vasodilator acting directly on smooth muscle of small arteries and veins, is a powerful hypotensive used IV to decrease systolic BP in the acute stage of dissecting aneurysms of all types. Its rate of administration is monitored and adjusted to a range of 15 to 200 μg/min. Use of an infusion pump is recommended. However, the drug should be used concomitantly with a β-adrenergic blocking agent, because nitroprusside often has a positive inotropic effect upon myocardium, which may raise the rate of increase of the velocity of ventricular ejection (dv/dt) and extend the dissection. This is especially important in proximal dissections (DeBakey's Types I and II), because a small proximal extension of the dissection can weaken the aortic annulus to cause regurgitation, promote erosion into the pericardium or pleural cavity, and interfere with the origins of the coronary arteries.

Propranolol itself has some untoward effects and must be used with caution in patients who, in addition to the dissection, have bladder outlet obstruction, bronchial asthma, asthmatic bronchitis, or severe coronary artery heart disease with impending failure. The drug's negative inotropic action may cause or worsen heart failure, weaken bladder detrusor activity, and decrease bronchodilation. Its metabolic effects may interfere with control of diabetes mellitus in patients taking hypoglycemic agents. Patients with atrioventricular conduction defects also need special attention since propranolol may further depress conduction. Excessive bradycardia can be treated with atropine.

Trimethaphan camsylate is a ganglionic-blocking agent effective for lowering the BP in acute aortic dissection and in selected cases of otherwise uncontrollable hemorrhage. It is not as useful as nitroprusside and propranolol because of side effects (urinary retention, heart failure, asthma, interference with control of diabetes mellitus) and the development of tachyphylaxis within about 48 h. Trimethaphan is administered by continuous IV infusion 1 to 10 mg/min according to the monitored effect on systolic BP and heart rate.

Reserpine is useful in the occasional patient with contraindications to these drugs or who respond inadequately. It will lower the BP, but may induce or worsen peptic ulcer; therefore, concomitant use of cimetidine or ranitidine hydrochloride should be considered.

When the BP reaches the desired level and the patient's condition is stable, aortography is done to determine the dissection site. Proximal lesions (DeBakey's Types I and II) are operated upon without delay. The situation with distal dissection (DeBakey's Type III) is less urgent; some patients can be treated indefinitely without repair of the dissection by controlling the BP with a long-term antihypertension regimen.

If the patient is not hypertensive on admission, the drug of choice is propranolol 20 to 40 mg orally qid. After the initial reduction of arterial pressure, emergency aortography is obtained to confirm the diagnosis and to determine whether the ascending aorta is involved.

In Marfan syndrome, survival is shortened when aortic insufficiency develops. Heart failure due to aortic insufficiency must be treated appropriately.

Long-term medical therapy with propranolol and hydrochlorothiazide is used when surgery is contraindicated because of advanced age and associated medical problems, for patients admitted to the hospital > 2 wk after the onset of symptoms of dissection, and for patients in whom the site of origin of the dissection cannot be positively identified by aortography. Mortality among patients with involvement of the ascending aorta (Types I and II) when treated surgically is about 30%, as contrasted with about 70% for medically treated patients. The mortality rates of judicious medical and surgical treatment of descending aortic dissection (Type III) range from 10 to 20%.

Hazards of medical therapy include hypotension, which may be especially dangerous for the elderly. Acute renal tubular necrosis has occurred, and patients are often confused and disoriented. Postural hypotension often develops when patients begin to ambulate, but usually can be controlled by adjusting medications. Saccular aneurysms

tend to develop late in the course of medical treatment; these may rupture spontaneously and require surgical resection.

Surgery is recommended for dissecting aneurysms of the ascending aorta and for patients admitted < 2 wk after the onset of dissection, if the origin of the dissection can be identified on angiography and the patient is otherwise a good surgical risk. Complications of dissecting aneurysm (eg, overwhelming aortic insufficiency, localized leaking or impending rupture, or compromise of a major artery) demand urgent surgical intervention. Untreated patients often survive no more than hours or a few days; 44 to 89% of patients with Types I and II dissecting aneurysms die from rupture into the pericardial space. In exceptional cases reentry of the dissection into the main aortic lumen may prolong survival for several years. Overall, > 40% of patients may require surgery after the acute dissection.

Surgical treatment for **aneurysms of the ascending aorta** requires cardiopulmonary bypass; the portion of the aorta with the intimal tear is resected, the dissected ends of the aorta are oversewn, and the resected segment of aorta is replaced with a graft. The aortic valve is replaced if necessary. Repair of the **descending aorta** is done with the patient on partial cardiopulmonary bypass.

Abdominal aortic aneurysms: Arteriosclerotic lesions progress at variable rates. Once the diameter is > 6 cm, the hazard of rapid expansion and rupture is great, and a graft is recommended.

Marfan syndrome (see in INHERITED DISORDERS OF CONNECTIVE TISSUE in Ch. 197) is a heritable abnormality of connective tissue with manifestations in the skeletal system, the eyes, and the cardiovascular system. The average age at death is 32 yr; 93% are related to cardiovascular complications (see in Ch. 24). Characteristically, heart failure follows aortic regurgitation from dilation of the aortic ring, myxomatous involvement of the aortic valve, and aneurysm and dissection of the root of the aorta. The prognosis is worse when the mitral valve is also involved. Because the disease is progressive and the prognosis poor, surgical repair of the dilating aortic ring and replacement of the aortic valve and first segment of the ascending aorta has been recommended to prevent further disintegration of the aortic ring, dissection, and aortic regurgitation, but the risk:benefit ratio is not yet established.

Luetic aneurysms are now rare. Prognosis depends on the location and progression of the luetic process. Coronary ostial stenosis or aortic insufficiency associated with cardiac symptoms reduces life expectancy, but patients with relatively stabilized lesions may survive many years. Luetic aneurysm can rupture, but never dissects. Adequate treatment of early syphilis prevents aortitis and aneurysm. However, even after an aneurysm has developed, antiluetic therapy may be helpful; procaine penicillin 600,000 u./day IM for 10 to 15 days generally suffices.

OCCLUSION OF THE ABDOMINAL AORTA AND ITS BRANCHES

Atherosclerosis of the aorta is usually asymptomatic unless occlusion occurs, plaques encroach on the ostia of one or more major branches, or embolization occurs to the periphery. Symptoms and signs relate to the organ or tissues in which clinically significant ischemia occurs and several characteristic syndromes may be seen, as indicated below. Aortic occlusive disease can also be caused by aortitis as in Takayasu's disease or syphilitic aortitis.

SPLANCHNIC ARTERY OCCLUSION

Arteriosclerotic obliterative lesions and arterial aneurysms have been described involving all major visceral branches of the abdominal aorta, in particular the celiac and

its branches, the superior mesenteric, renal, and inferior mesenteric. Obliterative lesions causing visceral ischemia can occur at the origins of these arteries or usually in their proximal portions. In most cases, when symptoms develop, all 3 arteries are partially obstructed, although lesions may predominate in one. Symptoms of visceral ischemia may also be caused by fibromuscular hyperplasia, aneurysms, and emboli, which are not uncommon, especially in the superior mesenteric artery or its branches. Rarely, partial and intermittent occlusion of the celiac and superior mesenteric arteries has been attributed to abdominal webs or bands near their origins. Embolism or acute thrombosis, often referred to as **intestinal apoplexy,** can have catastrophic results. Of all patients who develop acute ischemic intestinal necrosis, 80% have either embolism or thrombosis, each accounting for 40% of total cases.

In about 20% of patients who develop ischemic intestinal necrosis, usually fatal, no obstruction is found in the celiac or mesenteric vessels and their major branches. These patients are usually elderly and have, among other problems, arteriosclerotic heart disease and heart failure. One possible explanation is that CO temporarily has fallen, leading to a fall in pressure and collapse of the celiac and mesenteric arteries that cannot be reopened or distended to normal size when CO and BP return only to normal. (Laplace's law implies that a greater than normal pressure is required to distend an artery whose diameter has decreased.) The splanchnic vascular bed remains ischemic, and intestinal necrosis ensues.

Chronic intestinal ischemia (intestinal "claudication" or intestinal angina) : As in atherosclerotic arterial disease elsewhere, the formation of obliterative lesions in the splanchnic arteries normally is accompanied by development of collateral circulation usually adequate to fulfill basal metabolic requirements. Circulation in the GI tract is taxed by the increased work that must be performed during digestion. Meals require splanchnic circulation to be increased above basal; if this is impossible, symptoms that develop commonly include (1) postprandial (½ to 1 h) mid- or upper-abdominal cramp-like pain unrelated to the type of food eaten and unrelieved by usual therapy for peptic ulcer but often responding to nitrates; (2) changed bowel habits (commonly constipation, seldom diarrhea); (3) occasional melena; (4) progressive weight loss and failure to gain weight by dietary measures; and (5) malabsorption syndrome. Steatorrhea is rare.

Acute celiac, splenic, and mesenteric occlusion: Occlusion of the **celiac axis** may be totally asymptomatic. Acute interruption of the hepatic branch, however, can produce hepatic necrosis with chills, fever, prostration, and death. Embolism and thrombosis of the hepatic artery are rare, but occasionally the right or common hepatic artery is interrupted at surgery. Infarction of the spleen may result from acute occlusion of the **splenic artery,** and small infarcts frequently occur in the spleen by embolization of branches of the splenic artery. These can produce severe pain by parietal peritoneal irritation. Splenectomy may be necessary.

Acute occlusion of the **superior mesenteric artery** is a common cause of catastrophic abdominal emergency. The pain, difficult to control, is mid-abdominal or generalized, severe, and unrelenting, resembling that of acute hemorrhagic necrotizing pancreatitis or perforated gastric or duodenal ulcer. Nausea, vomiting, and prostration are typical. Physical examination reveals generalized abdominal spasm and shock, which is associated with hemoconcentration (instead of hemodilution as in hemorrhagic shock) and is difficult to correct by the usual means. Gross or occult blood is generally found in the stool. Abdominal x-rays can support the clinical impression of intestinal infarction in about ⅓ of patients; the presumptive diagnosis can be based on characteristic x-ray changes: (1) pneumatosis intestinalis; (2) thickening of the intestinal wall with ileus; (3) ileus with dilation of the small intestine and of the large intestine up to the splenic flexure. Fecal matter is seen in the colon in about 80% of cases with proved infarction secondary to mesenteric occlusion.

Acute occlusion and chronic obliterative disease of the **inferior mesenteric artery** are unlikely to be symptomatic except when associated with occlusive disease of the superior mesenteric and other splanchnic arteries. Branches of this artery, through the sigmoidal arcades, have ready access to branches of the mid-colic and the middle and inferior hemorrhoidal arteries for collateral circulation.

Diagnosis

Vascular disease of the celiac and mesenteric arteries must be suspected based on the symptoms and signs taken in the clinical context. Thus, in an elderly patient with a past history suggesting intestinal angina, or with extensive atherosclerotic arterial disease, the diagnosis of infarction of the intestine should be pursued aggressively (eg, with angiography) on the basis of early and inconclusive clinical and radiologic evidence. *To wait for conclusive diagnostic findings before proceeding to angiography and surgery means to wait for development of intestinal gangrene, after which mortality approaches 100% after any treatment.*

The patient is usually seriously ill: Hypotension and rapid pulse are usually noted, abdominal pain and tenderness and ileus are generally present, peristalsis is variable, and stools may be bloody. X-ray examination of the abdomen is done promptly after treating acute vital problems.

The patient is first examined in supine position for a plain film of kidneys, ureter, and bladder. The films may show calcific lesions in the aorta or in the distribution of some of its branches, edema of the bowel wall separating adjacent loops, "thumb print" loops of intestine that remain fixed in successive examinations, air within the intestinal wall (pneumatosis), and in severe cases, air within the portal system in the liver. Positive findings by x-ray are seen in 20 to 60% of patients.

When possible, an upright view is taken to demonstrate air-fluid levels in the intestine. An upright chest view is done at the same time to demonstrate fluid or free air beneath the diaphragm, or other abnormalities within the abdomen or chest. When upright examination is not feasible, a left lateral decubitus film is obtained for the same purpose.

If there is enough suspicion of actual or impending intestinal ischemia, on the basis of a history of increasing intestinal angina, time is so important for the end result that it is well to proceed directly to selective splanchnic angiography before obscuring the area with contrast material as for a barium enema or GI barium series. If one hopes to treat impending intestinal ischemia before irreversible changes have taken place, he must often do a laparotomy for diagnosis and treatment on insufficient evidence.

Selective angiography should be considered early, as it is the best objective means to demonstrate occlusive lesions of branches of the abdominal aorta: the celiac axis and its major branches, the superior mesenteric artery and its branches, the inferior mesenteric artery, and the renal arteries. Demonstration of occlusion, with precise localization, permits surgical intervention with encouraging results. Occasionally, angiography demonstrates segmental or diffuse spasm of a splanchnic vessel. The instillation of a vasodilator, especially papaverine, through the same angiographic catheter has had excellent results.

Mesenteric venous thrombosis also leads to intestinal necrosis. Symptoms and signs are similar to those of acute arterial occlusion, but are less severe and less dramatic. Intestinal necrosis is usually more limited and may be segmental. The length of intestine that must be resected is less extensive and the prognosis is better than after acute arterial mesenteric occlusion.

RENAL ARTERY OCCLUSION

Among causes of surgically correctable hypertension, occlusive disease of the renal arteries is the most common, occurring in about 5% of hypertensives. Obliterative

disease is most often unilateral and is most commonly atherosclerotic. Obstructing plaques develop at the ostia of the renal arteries in the aorta or in proximal parts of the arteries. Post-stenotic dilation of the renal artery often occurs distal to the obstructing lesion. Fibromuscular hyperplasia (or dysplasia) of the renal artery is the second most frequent arterial obstructing lesion in renal vascular hypertension. Narrowing of the renal artery is also caused by embolism or thrombosis, by renal arterial aneurysm with thrombosis or embolization, or by dissecting aneurysm. All of these lesions can cause diastolic hypertension. Their pathophysiologic relation to the hypertension can be demonstrated by determining the renin activity of venous blood differentially collected from the 2 renal veins. The kidney, its circulation, and its excretory function can be studied by pyelography, angiography, and radionuclide excretion. Angiography is the best direct means of evaluation and can often be followed immediately with balloon dilation to correct the stenosis.

OCCLUSION AT THE AORTIC BIFURCATION

Sudden occlusion at the aortic bifurcation is often dramatic, resulting in absent femoral pulses, pain, weakness, and color and temperature changes in the legs and feet. Embolism commonly is the cause and the prognosis is that of the lesion that generated the embolus. Embolectomy nearly always is indicated and can be done easily transfemorally under local anesthesia.

Gradual occlusion of the terminal aorta may cause impotence in the male and intermittent claudication in the buttocks and thighs **(Leriche syndrome)**. Claudication in the calves is due to narrowing or occlusion of the femoral arteries or their branches in addition to occlusion of the aortic bifurcation. Gangrene of the toes also can occur.

Treatment: In many cases, percutaneous transluminal angioplasty, in which a balloon is set at the obstructing lesion and distended, will effectively restore circulation. Alternatively, obliterative segments can be resected and replaced by vein grafts or prostheses.

---

30. PERIPHERAL VASCULAR DISORDERS

Vascular diseases of the extremities involve arteries, veins, and lymphatics. Since the extremities are readily accessible to examination, a correct clinical diagnosis can usually be made. Special instrumentation and angiography are rarely necessary to diagnose arterial insufficiency, but are helpful to document the location and extent of disease if surgical correction is contemplated. Noninvasive methods confirm the diagnosis and are useful to follow the patient being treated medically or after revascularization. Noninvasive tests and/or venography are usually essential to diagnose deep venous thrombosis.

OCCLUSIVE ARTERIAL DISEASES

PERIPHERAL ATHEROSCLEROTIC DISEASE

(Arteriosclerosis Obliterans)

Occlusion of blood supply to the extremities by atherosclerotic plaques (atheroma).

Most patients with occlusive arterial disease have an underlying atherosclerotic process. The incidence, pathogenesis, risk factors, and prophylaxis of atherosclerosis are discussed in Ch. 26, above. Clinical syndromes depend upon the extent of obstruction, how rapidly it progresses, what particular vessel is involved, and whether an adequate

collateral flow occurs. Various syndromes are discussed elsewhere in the text—eg, in Ch. 29, under MYOCARDIAL ISCHEMIC DISORDERS in Ch. 27, and in Ch. 123.

Patients with homozygous homocystinuria frequently have extensive thrombosis of veins and arteries. However, there is recent evidence that patients with premature (below age 50) occlusive arterial disease have an abnormally high incidence of heterozygous or mild homocystinuria as detected by an oral methionine loading test. It is believed that sustained accumulation of homocysteine, by damaging endothelial cells, predisposes to premature atherosclerosis of the aorta and its branches, the peripheral arteries and the cerebral arteries, but not the coronary arteries, for reasons unknown. The discussion here is limited to occlusive diseases of the extremities, both chronic (arteriosclerosis obliterans) and acute (thrombosis and embolism).

Symptoms and Signs

Chronic ischemia: Patients with arteriosclerosis obliterans have symptoms related to the slow, insidious development of tissue ischemia. The initial symptom is **intermittent claudication**, *a deficient blood supply in exercising muscle*. The distress is described as a pain, ache, cramp, or tired feeling that occurs on walking; it occurs most commonly in the calf but also in the foot, thigh, hip, or buttocks. Relieved quickly by rest (usually in 1 to 5 min), the patient can walk as far again before pain recurs. Sitting is not necessary to obtain relief. Distress is worsened by walking rapidly or uphill, but, by definition, claudication never occurs at rest. Progression of the disease is indicated when the distance that the patient can walk is diminishing. Similar symptoms related to exertion can occur with involvement of the upper extremity.

The occlusive disease may progress so that ischemic pain occurs at rest. **Rest pain** beginning in the most distal parts of a limb is a severe, unrelenting pain aggravated by elevation and often preventing sleep; for relief, the patient will hang his foot over the bedside or will rest in a chair with legs dependent.

If intermittent claudication is the only symptom, the extremity may appear normal, but the pulses are reduced or absent. The level of arterial occlusion and the location of intermittent claudication are closely correlated. Aortoiliac disease frequently causes claudication in the buttocks and hips in addition to the calves, and the femoral pulses are absent. In femoropopliteal disease, claudication is characteristically in the calf, and all pulses below the femoral are absent. In patients with small vessel disease (eg, Buerger's disease or diabetes mellitus) the femoral and popliteal pulses are present but foot pulses are absent. Helpful confirmatory signs of arterial insufficiency are pallor of the involved foot after 1 to 2 min of elevation, followed by rubor on dependency. Venous filling time on dependency following elevation is delayed beyond the normal limit of 15 sec.

A severely ischemic foot is painful, cold, and often numb. The skin may be dry and scaly with poor nail and hair growth. As ischemia worsens, ulceration may appear, especially after local trauma. Ulcerations are characteristically on the toes or heel or occasionally on the leg. There is usually no edema, but a severely ischemic leg may be shrunken and atrophic.

More extensive obliterative disease may compromise the viability of tissues and lead to necrosis or gangrene.

Acute ischemia is caused by sudden arterial occlusion by embolization from the heart, a proximal arteriosclerotic plaque, or an aneurysm, or by an acute thrombosis on preexisting atherosclerotic disease. The history includes sudden onset of severe pain, coldness, numbness, and pallor. The extremity is cold, either pale or cyanotic, and pulses are absent distal to the obstruction. In acute occlusion of the aorta (saddle embolus or thrombosis), all pulses in the lower extremities are absent. Characteristically, acute occlusions occur at bifurcations just distal to the last palpable pulse; thus, with occlusion at the common femoral bifurcation, the femoral pulse is palpable, and

with occlusion at the popliteal bifurcation, the popliteal pulse is present. Acute occlusion may cause severe ischemia manifested by sensory and motor loss and induration of muscles on palpation.

Laboratory Evaluation

X-ray: Plain films of the extremities have no diagnostic value in occlusive disease. Intimal calcification merely confirms the presence of atherosclerosis, and medial calcification is not correlated with the occurrence of arteriosclerosis obliterans. **Arteriography,** a prerequisite to surgical correction or percutaneous transluminal balloon angioplasty **(PTA)**, provides details of the location and extent of lesions occluding the arterial system. Angiography should be complete and include aortography and bilateral femoral arteriography, visualizing the arteries as far distally as the feet. Methods include translumbar aortography combined with bilateral femoral arteriography, a method used by many vascular surgeons, or percutaneous catheterization via femoral artery or upper extremity. **Digital subtraction angiography** simplifies imaging by angiography in selective situations. This method of image enhancement and numerical interpretation of images allows visualization of the vascular system while "subtracting" other soft tissues. Its major advantage is that it allows arteriography to be performed from a peripheral *venous* injection. Because of the limited size of the image amplifier, the best use peripherally for this technic is to visualize the aortic arch, carotid and vertebral systems, renal arteries, and the aortic and femoral bifurcations. The technic is useful in the postoperative evaluation of patients who have undergone arterial bypass grafts, PTA, and in the diagnosis of suspected pulmonary embolism. Conventional angiography is still necessary for adequate visualization of peripheral arteries from the lower aorta to the feet. Development of larger image amplifiers and moving table tops, now underway, may make digital subtraction angiography an easier, safer method to evaluate peripheral arterial occlusive disease.

Noninvasvie diagnostic instrumentation: To evaluate arterial insufficiency, a variety of noninvasive instruments are accurate, simple, portable, and relatively inexpensive. They are useful to confirm and document the arterial insufficiency found by clinical examination, to evaluate a patient for sympathectomy, revascularization, or amputation, to predict the likelihood of wound healing, and to follow the patient on conservative treatment or after surgery.

Doppler ultrasound is the most widely used method. Arterial stenosis and occlusion can be easily recognized by listening with the velocity detector (Doppler probe). The simplest method for estimating blood flow to the lower extremities is to measure the systolic BP at the level of the ankle and compare it to brachial systolic pressure. A BP cuff is applied to the ankle in the usual manner, inflated above brachial systolic pressure, and then deflated slowly. Ankle systolic pressure can be obtained accurately with a Doppler probe placed over the dorsalis pedis or posterior tibial arteries. This pressure normally is 90% or more of the brachial systolic pressure; with mild arterial insufficiency, it is between 70% and 90%; with moderate insufficiency, between 50% and 70%; and with severe insufficiency, below 50%.

If these pressure measurements are obtained before and after a standard walking exercise on a treadmill, a good estimate of the degree of disability can be made. When ankle systolic pressure is < 55 mm Hg in the nondiabetic or 70 mm Hg in the diabetic, spontaneous healing of ischemic lesions will not occur. Likewise, pressure of ≥ 70 mm Hg is necessary to heal below-knee amputations. More accurate information in regard to disability and the extent and location of arterial lesions is obtained from segmental BPs (thigh, calf, and ankle) and segmental plethysmograph recordings of pulse volume waveforms both before and after exercise. By noting pressure gradients and abnormal waveforms, isolated aortoiliac disease can be distinguished from femoropopliteal disease, below-knee disease, or any combination of these.

Treatment

Patients with intermittent claudication should walk 60 min daily, if possible; when discomfort occurs, they should stop, allow the pain to disappear, and then walk again. This mode of treatment will significantly improve the distance a patient can walk without discomfort. The mechanism by which a walking program increases walking distance is not precisely known, but could be the result of both physical training and an increase in collateral circulation as a result of muscle demand. Tobacco in all forms must be eliminated. Vasodilators are commonly prescribed, although there is no proof of their effectiveness. β-Blocking agents may worsen intermittent claudication; this effect should be anticipated in these patients. When a patient is sleeping, blocks should be used to elevate the head of the bed 4 to 6 in. Pentoxifylline 400 mg tid improves intermittent claudication, and, in some reports, rest pain, by improving blood flow and enhancing tissue oxygenation in affected areas. This agent is believed to (1) reduce blood viscosity by improving the impaired RBC membrane flexibility and deformability found in patients with occlusive arterial disease and to retard RBC and platelet aggregation. Preliminary reports seem to indicate that experimental agents (eg, Ca blockers, thromboxane inhibitors, and epoprostenol) may be clinically useful in managing patients with both occlusive and vasospastic arterial diseases.

Prophylactic foot care is especially important: (1) Patients should inspect and feel their feet daily for cracks, fissures, calluses, corns, and ulcers. (2) Feet should be washed daily in lukewarm water, using mild soap; they should be dried gently and thoroughly. (3) A lubricant, such as lanolin, should be used for dry, scaly skin. (4) Bland, nonmedicated foot powders should be used for moist feet. (5) Toenails should be cut straight across, not too close to the skin. A podiatrist should do this if the patient's eyesight is poor. (6) Calluses or corns should be treated by a podiatrist. (7) Adhesive plasters and tape should not be used on skin. (8) Harsh chemicals or corn cures should not be used. (9) Patients should change stockings daily and avoid constricting garters. (10) Loose wool stockings can keep feet warm in cold weather, but hot water bottles or electric pads must not be used. (11) Shoes should fit well; they should be wide-toed without open heels or toes and should be changed frequently. (12) Special shoes should be prescribed if there is any foot deformity (eg, previous toe amputation, hammer toe, bunion) in order to reduce trauma. (13) Walking barefoot should always be avoided.

In patients with diabetic neuropathic ulcers, weight bearing should be avoided, or if this is not possible, appropriate orthotic protection of the ulcer should be used. Since most patients with this type ulcer have little or no macrovascular occlusive disease, debridement, trimming of callus, and antibiotics frequently produce good healing. Drainage of infection may prevent major surgery later. After the ulcer has healed, appropriate inserts or special shoes should be prescribed. Refractory cases, especially if osteomyelitis is present, may require surgical removal of the metatarsal head (source of pressure), combined with amputation of the involved toe or a transmetatarsal amputation. A neuropathic joint may be satisfactorily managed with orthopedic appliances such as short leg braces, molded shoes, sponge-rubber arch supports, crutches, and prostheses. (See DIABETIC ARTERIOSCLEROTIC DISEASE in Ch. 26 for further discussion.)

In **ischemic foot lesions,** if revascularization is impossible, a therapeutic program may prevent amputation. Diabetes mellitus must be controlled as closely as possible, and complete bed rest with the head of the bed elevated on blocks is necessary. The lesion must be kept clean with daily soaks in mild soap or NaCl solution and then dressed with sterile dry dressings. A mild antibiotic ointment may be used. Irritating and sensitizing solutions should be avoided. An obvious infection should be cultured and appropriate antibiotics given systemically. Enzymatic debridement may be irritating and increase the pain. Surgical debridement when ischemia is severe does more

harm than good and is very painful. Patients should be warned that healing may take a long time.

Percutaneous transluminal angioplasty (PTA) has proven to be a useful procedure for the treatment of localized occlusive arterial lesions due to atherosclerosis. With appropriate selection of patients, which depends upon complete, adequate angiography, the success rate approaches 80 to 90%. When PTA is possible and successful, the results are gratifying, a surgical procedure is avoided, and only 1 or 2 days of hospitalization are required. Surgical backup should always be available. The technic, usually done by a radiologist, consists of dilating the diseased segment with the Grüntzig double lumen catheter, containing a balloon made of polyvinyl chloride. It can be inflated to 6 atmospheres pressure while maintaining a cylindrical balloon-shape to avoid overdilation. A postdilation arteriogram or digital subtraction angiogram is usually done at the time of the procedure. The small size of the flexible catheters allows various approaches to many arteries, such as renal, other visceral, coronary, axillary, iliac, and superficial femoral-popliteal arteries. Following dilation, to prevent reocclusion by thrombosis, the patient may be given heparin in the usual doses IV for 48 h (see under Treatment in Ch. 39). Many physicians prefer to give their patients aspirin or another antiplatelet agent. Noninvasive studies (see above) should be done before and after the dilation to document improvement and to follow-up the patient.

Indications for PTA of peripheral arteries are (1) progressive and limiting intermittent claudication that prevents the patient from working, (2) rest pain, and (3) gangrene. Various reports document success for optimal lesions in the 90% and higher range. Lesions suitable for this procedure are high-grade, short iliac stenoses and short, single or multiple stenoses of the superficial femoral-popliteal segment. Complete occlusions of the superficial femoral artery, ≤ 10 to 12 cm, have been successfully dilated, but better success results if lesions are ≤ 5 cm. An excellent indication for dilation is a short, localized iliac stenosis prior to a distal femoropopliteal bypass operation. **Contraindications** are diffuse disease, long occlusions, stenosis at the takeoff of an essential collateral, and severe arterial calcification. **Complications** that may require surgical intervention are thrombosis at the site of dilation, distal embolization, intimal dissection with occlusion by a flap, and possible complications from heparin therapy.

Reconstructive surgical procedures are well established and valuable. In properly selected patients, symptoms are relieved, ulcers healed, and amputations averted. The procedures are thromboendarterectomy, bypass graft (woven prosthetic tube or autogenous vein anastomosed end-to-side to the vessel above and below the obstruction), or resection with graft replacement (most often used in cases of abdominal aortic aneurysm and proximal atheromatous arteries that embolize peripherally). Effective surgery depends on adequate angiography (aortography and bilateral femoral arteriography) that establishes the site of occlusion and the condition of the arteries above and below.

Success of a surgical procedure is directly related to the adequacy of blood flow into the graft (run in) and out of it (run off). Autogenous veins (usually the greater saphenous) are used most often to bypass occlusive lesions of the superficial femoral, popliteal, or tibial arteries. Thromboendarterectomy is used for short, localized lesions in the aorta, iliac, common femoral, or deep femoral arteries. Woven dacron is the preferred material for an arterial prosthesis to bypass disease in the aortoiliac area. PTFE (Gortex®) is the synthetic of choice for femoropopliteal-tibial obstructions if saphenous vein is not available. The indications for surgical procedures in the aortoiliac area are incapacitating (economic or avocational) intermittent claudication or severe ischemia due to associated distal disease. Surgery for femoropopliteal and/or tibial disease is reserved for patients who have severe ischemia with rest pain, ulceration, or minor gangrene. Patients with only intermittent claudication should always be treated conservatively at first; if the disease progresses to more severe ischemia, surgery is needed.

In some cases, sympathectomy, which removes neurogenic vasoconstriction, can be very helpful and should be offered to selected patients with severe disease and those who are not candidates for revascularization. The value of revascularization procedures is well established in terms of limb salvage and relieving claudication, but reduction in mortality is small.

When **amputation** is required for uncontrolled infection, unrelenting rest pain, and progressive gangrene, it should be kept as distal as possible; it is especially important to preserve the knee for optimal use of a prosthesis.

THROMBOANGIITIS OBLITERANS

(Buerger's Disease)

An obliterative disease characterized by inflammatory changes in small and medium-sized arteries and veins.

Etiology and Incidence

Buerger's disease occurs predominantly in men aged 20 to 40 who smoke cigarettes. Only about 5% of cases occur in women. The frequency of diagnosis has decreased drastically in recent years due to better understanding of clinical and angiographic characteristics of this disease compared to arteriosclerosis obliterans. A small number of investigators doubt that the disorder is a distinct clinical and pathologic entity and believe that it is indistinguishable pathologically from occlusive disease caused by some types of atherosclerosis, systemic emboli, or idiopathic peripheral thromboses. The disagreement concerns the specificity of the pathologic lesion; however, most clinicians agree that the clinical characteristics are sufficiently distinctive to consider thromboangiitis obliterans a discrete entity. Although the etiology of the disease is unknown, the relationship of smoking to its occurrence and progression is apparent. There is no documented evidence that it occurs in nonsmokers, implicating cigarette smoking as a primary etiologic factor, perhaps a delayed type of hypersensitivity or toxic angiitis. Recent work suggests that the cause of Buerger's disease may be (1) related to the reaction to tobacco of persons with a specific phenotype, because of greater prevalence of HLA-A9 and HLA-B5 in persons with the disease; or (2) an autoimmune disorder with cell-mediated sensitivity to Types I and III human collagen, which are constituents of blood vessels.

Pathology and Pathophysiology

The disease involves small and medium-sized arteries and, frequently, superficial veins of the extremities, in a segmental pattern. Rarely, in well advanced disease, vessels in other parts of the body are affected. The pathologic appearance is that of a nonsuppurative panarteritis or panphlebitis associated with thrombosis of the involved vessels. Proliferation of endothelial cells and infiltration of the intimal layer with lymphocytes occurs in the acute lesion, but the internal elastic lamina is intact. The thrombus becomes organized and later is incompletely recanalized. The media is well preserved though it may be infiltrated with fibroblasts. Since the adventitia usually is more extensively infiltrated with fibroblasts, older lesions show periarterial fibrosis, which may involve the adjacent vein and nerve as well.

Symptoms, Signs, and Diagnosis

Onset is gradual, starting in the most distal vessels of the upper and lower extremities and progressing proximally, culminating in distal gangrene. The symptoms and signs of thromboangiitis obliterans are those of arterial ischemia and of superficial phlebitis. A history of migratory phlebitis, usually in the superficial veins of the foot or leg, is present in about 40% of cases. The patient may complain of coldness, numbness, tingling, or burning before there is objective evidence of disease. Raynaud's phenomenon is common. Intermittent claudication occurs in the involved extremity (usually

the arch of the foot or the leg, but rarely the hand, arm, or thigh). Persistent pain is felt with more severe ischemia, eg, in the pregangrenous stage and with ulceration or gangrene. Frequently, sympathetic nerve overactivity is manifested by coldness, excessive sweating, and cyanosis of the involved hand or foot probably caused by the severe, persistent pain.

Pulsations in one or more pedal arteries are impaired or absent in most cases, and in wrist arteries in about 60% of cases. Postural color changes (pallor on elevation and rubor on dependency) can frequently be demonstrated in affected hands, feet, or digits. Ischemic ulceration and gangrene, usually of one or more digits, may occur early in the disease but not acutely. Noninvasive studies show a severe decrease in blood flow and pressure in affected toes, feet, and fingers. The disease progresses proximally. The diagnosis can usually be established with clinical data. Arteriograms show segmental occlusions of the distal arteries, especially of hands and feet. Nonaffected arteries are smooth and appear normal. Collateral circulation forms around occlusions and may be more tortuous ("corkscrew" appearance) than collaterals associated with other occlusive diseases.

Prophylaxis and Treatment

Supportive care should be directed toward removal of all factors that reduce the blood supply and use all possible means to increase it. Factors to eliminate in addition to smoking include (1) thermal injury; (2) injury to tissues by chemicals such as iodine, carbolic or salicylic acids; (3) trauma, especially from poorly fitting footwear or minor surgery of digits; (4) fungal infections; and (5) vasoconstriction from exposure to cold or drugs.

The patient should walk for 15 to 30 min twice/day when there is no gangrene, ulceration, or rest pain; when these signs are present, complete bed rest is necessary. Feet should be protected by bandages with heel pads or foam rubber booties. Heat cradles should not be used unless thermostatic controls can prevent the heat from rising above body temperature. Gravity should be used to assist arterial filling by elevating the head of the bed on 6- to 8-in. blocks.

Antibiotics, corticosteroids, and anticoagulants are ineffective, and older vasodilators are of limited, if any, use. Some newer drugs, eg, pentoxifylline, Ca blockers, thromboxane inhibitors, and epoprostenol described above (see Treatment of Peripheral Atherosclerotic Disease) may be of help, especially for vasospastic manifestations.

Unremitting progression of the acute stage always occurs if the patient continues to smoke; so much tissue damage may ensue that amputation is required. The residual arterial insufficiency that is present during remissions may be ameliorated by appropriate dorsal or lumbar sympathectomy providing the patient has quit smoking. The newer drugs (described above) may be tried in those patients with less severe residual ischemia. Since large vessels such as the iliac, femoral, subclavian, and brachial arteries are rarely involved, bypass grafts are seldom applicable.

TEMPORAL ARTERITIS

(Giant Cell Arteritis; Cranial Arteritis; Granulomatous Arteritis)

A chronic generalized inflammatory disease of the branches of the aortic arch; found principally in the temporal and occipital arteries, but may develop in almost any large artery. It is rarely seen in veins. The systemic symptoms are the same as those of **polymyalgia rheumatica,** to which it may be related or identical. Most cases occur after age 50. The estimated incidence is 24:100,000; it rises considerably after age 80. While its cause is unknown, data suggest that an autoimmune reaction is involved.

Pathology

Giant cell arteritis most often involves arteries of the carotid system, particularly the cranial arteries; but segments of the aorta, its branches, the coronary arteries, and the

peripheral arteries may also be affected. The disease has a predilection for arteries containing elastic tissue. The histologic reaction is a granulomatous inflammation of the arteries; lymphocytes, epithelioid cells, and giant cells predominate. The inflammatory reaction causes marked thickening of the intimal layer with narrowing and occlusion of the lumen. The arteries may be localized, multifocal, or widespread.

Symptoms and Signs

The onset may be acute or gradual and may simulate an infection such as an influenza-like syndrome, with low-grade fever, malaise, anorexia, severe weakness, and weight loss. Polymyalgia is characterized by aching and stiffness involving mainly the trunk and proximal muscle groups such as the neck, shoulders, and the hip-pelvic area; occasionally the trunk is involved. Synovitis may occur especially in the knees. The characteristic headache, which may be uni- or bilateral, is a severe, throbbing, boring, or lancinating pain in the temporal area, with redness, swelling, tenderness, and nodulation of the temporal artery. Pulsations in the artery may be strong, weak, or absent. Serious complications include ptosis, transient blurring, diplopia, and transient or permanent blindness, stroke, coronary occlusion, and arterial insufficiency of the upper and lower extremities. Half of the patients have ocular symptoms and 40% have visual loss. When visual loss occurs, it is bilateral in 75%. Prompt recognition of the condition and early treatment may reduce the frequency of blindness to 5 to 10%. Less common symptoms include claudication of the masticatory muscles, the tongue, and the extremities. The aortic arch and its branches are involved in about 9% of cases.

Diagnosis

The ESR is always highly elevated during an active phase; levels > 100 mm/h (Westergren) are common. Leukocytosis and mild anemia may also be present. Because treatment is prolonged, the clinical diagnosis should be confirmed by biopsy of an involved artery. Multiple biopsies of the temporal artery and its branches may be required to obtain positive pathologic findings. About 40% of patients with myalgia and negative findings on clinical examination of the temporal artery have positive findings on temporal artery biopsy. The temporal arteriogram shows areas of constriction and dilation interspersed with areas that appear normal; an arteriogram may help the surgeon choose the area to be biopsied. Muscle biopsy is useless because arteries of muscles are not involved.

Treatment

To prevent blindness, treatment should start as soon as the diagnosis is suspected. High initial doses of corticosteroids control systemic and local symptoms. Prednisone 60 mg/day orally is given until symptoms and findings are gone and laboratory tests return to normal (usually 2 to 4 wk). Then the dose is reduced to 40 mg/day for 4 to 6 wk. Thereafter, 5 to 10 mg/day should be given for up to 2 yr or longer to prevent relapse. Disease activity can be monitored periodically by checking the ESR; a rise is a signal to postpone further dose reduction. Relapse is characterized by recurring symptoms of temporal arteritis or polymyalgia associated with a rise in the ESR.

FUNCTIONAL PERIPHERAL ARTERIAL DISORDERS

Peripheral vascular disorders caused by vasospasm or excessive dilation. They may be secondary to a local fault in the blood vessels or to disturbances in sympathetic nervous system activity, or they may accompany organic vascular disease.

RAYNAUD'S PHENOMENON AND DISEASE

Spasm of arterioles, usually in the digits (and occasionally other acral parts such as the nose and tongue), with intermittent pallor or cyanosis of the skin.

Etiology

Raynaud's phenomenon may be idiopathic (Raynaud's disease) or secondary to other conditions: connective tissue disorders (eg, scleroderma, RA, SLE), obstructive arterial diseases (arteriosclerosis obliterans, thromboangiitis obliterans, thoracic outlet syndrome), neurogenic lesions, drug intoxications (ergot and methysergide), dysproteinemias, myxedema, primary pulmonary hypertension, and trauma. Idiopathic Raynaud's disease is most common in young women (60 to 90% of reported cases).

Pathology and Pathophysiology

Attacks of vasospasm of the digital arteries and arterioles may last from minutes to hours, but are rarely severe enough to cause gross tissue loss. With longstanding Raynaud's disease, the skin of the digits may become smooth, shiny, and tight with loss of subcutaneous tissue **(sclerodactyly)**. Small painful ulcers may appear on the tips of the digits. Vessels are histologically normal in early stages, but in advanced cases the arterial intima may thicken and thromboses may form in small arteries. In secondary Raynaud's phenomenon, pathologic changes of the underlying disease are apparent.

Recent developments may broaden our understanding of the pathophysiology of Raynaud's phenomenon and may lead to new approaches to management. Research into prostaglandin metabolism, microcirculation, and the role of the endothelial cell are yielding promising results. Clinical association between Raynaud's phenomenon and migraine headaches, variant angina, and pulmonary hypertension suggest that there is a common mechanism for vasospasm in > 1 arterial bed. The threshold for the vasospastic response in Raynaud's disease is lowered by anything that activates sympathetic outflow or releases catecholamines (eg, emotion) in addition to local cold.

Symptoms, Signs, and Diagnosis

Intermittent attacks of blanching or cyanosis of the digits are precipitated by exposure to cold or by emotional upsets. Color changes may be triphasic: pallor, cyanosis, redness (reactive hyperemia); or biphasic: cyanosis, then reactive hyperemia. Rewarming the hands restores normal color and sensation. Color changes do not occur above the metacarpophalangeal joints and rarely involve the thumb. Pain is uncommon, but paresthesias are frequent during the attack.

Raynaud's disease is differentiated from secondary Raynaud's phenomenon by bilateral involvement, a history of symptoms for at least 2 yr without progression, and no evidence of an underlying cause. In Raynaud's disease, trophic skin changes and gangrene are either absent or present only in minimal areas. In secondary Raynaud's, the symptoms and signs of the underlying disease usually become manifest within 2 yr, occasionally longer. In Raynaud's phenomenon associated with scleroderma, there may also be tightness or thickening of the skin and telangiectases of the hands, arms, or face, difficulty swallowing, painful trophic ulcers on the fingertips, and symptoms referable to other systems.

The wrist pulses are usually present, but the **Allen test** frequently shows occlusion of the radial or ulnar artery distal to the wrist, when present. This is performed by the examiner, who faces the patient and places his thumbs over the radial and ulnar pulsations of one hand. After the patient clenches his fist to expel the blood from the hand, the examiner compresses the arteries. When the patient opens the fist, the hand is pale. The examiner then releases pressure from the radial artery, but maintains it on the ulnar artery. If the radial artery distal to the wrist is patent, the hand will pink up rapidly; if occluded, the hand will remain pale. The maneuver is then repeated by maintaining pressure on the radial artery, while releasing the ulnar artery. Noninvasive testing of the affected digits with plethysmography before and after exposure to cold has particular value in differentiating between occlusive and vasospastic disease in patients with Raynaud's phenomenon.

Treatment

Therapy of the secondary forms depends on recognition and treatment of the underlying disorder. Mild cases of Raynaud's disease may be controlled by protecting the body and extremities from cold and by using mild sedatives (eg, phenobarbital 15 to 30 mg orally tid or qid). The patient must stop smoking since nicotine is a vasoconstrictor. In a few patients, relaxation technics, such as biofeedback, may reduce vasospastic episodes. Drugs formerly used for treatment have been varied and inconsistently effective. Reserpine 0.1 mg to 0.25 mg orally bid to qid has been commonly used and may decrease the number and severity of attacks, but side effects (eg, depression) may prevent its use. Phenoxybenzamine 10 mg orally qid and methyldopa 1 to 2 gm/day orally have been tried with occasional success. The drugs of choice are the newer vasodilating agents: prazosin 1 to 2 mg orally at bedtime, and repeated in the morning, if necessary, and the Ca-channel blocker nifedipine 10 to 30 mg orally tid. Reserpine 1.0 mg in 5.0 mL of 0.9% sodium chloride solution injected into the brachial artery q 3 mo may have a beneficial effect on the healing of ulcers. Encouraging reports concerning the effectiveness of pentoxifylline 400 mg bid or tid with meals have appeared in the literature. Research with encouraging results is in progress for the use of prostaglandins (thromboxane) in the treatment of Raynaud's phenomenon. Phenoxybenzamine 10 mg orally qid may be useful. Methyldopa 1 to 2 gm/day or prazosin 4 to 8 mg/day may benefit patients with Raynaud's disease. The Ca blocker nifedipine, 10 to 30 mg tid, has been reported as being effective. *β-Blockers, clonidine, and ergot preparations cause vasoconstriction and may induce or worsen Raynaud's phenomenon and are, therefore, contraindicated.* Regional sympathectomy is reserved for patients with progressive disability; it often abolishes the symptoms, but the relief may last only 1 to 2 yr. Results from sympathectomy are generally better in patients with Raynaud's disease than in those with secondary Raynaud's phenomenon.

ACROCYANOSIS

Persistent, painless, symmetric cyanosis of the hands and, less commonly, the feet, caused by vasospasm of the small vessels of the skin. The etiology is unknown, but it may be caused by increased tone of the arterioles associated with dilation of capillaries and venules. The disorder usually occurs in women and is not associated with occlusive arterial disease. The digits and hands or feet are persistently cold, bluish, and sweat profusely; they may swell. Cyanosis is usually intensified by exposure to cold and lessened with warming. Trophic changes and ulceration do not occur, and pain is absent. **Diagnosis** is made from the persistent nature of the findings localized to the hands and feet in the presence of normal arterial pulsations. Except for reassurance and protection from cold, **treatment** is usually unnecessary. Vasodilators may be tried, but are usually ineffective. Sympathectomy is helpful but seldom warranted.

ERYTHROMELALGIA

A rare syndrome of paroxysmal vasodilation with burning pain, increased skin temperature, and redness of the feet and, less often, the hands. The etiology of primary erythromelalgia is unknown. Secondary erythromelalgia may occur in patients with myeloproliferative disorders, hypertension, venous insufficiency, or diabetes mellitus. The condition is characterized by attacks of burning pain in hot, red feet or hands. Distress is triggered by modest ambient temperatures usually varying between 29 and 32 C (84.2 and 89.6 F) in most patients. Trophic changes do not occur. Symptoms may remain mild for years or may become so severe that total disability results. **Diagnosis** is based on demonstration that the patient's complaints are related to objectively increased skin temperature. Secondary types should be differentiated from the rare pri-

mary disorder, since, in the former, correction of the underlying disorder may relieve the symptoms.

Treatment

Attacks can be avoided or aborted by rest, elevation of the extremity, and cold applications. Therapy is not always successful. Correction of the underlying disease in secondary forms is indicated. In primary erythromelalgia, modest doses of aspirin (600 mg 1 to 4 times/day) may produce prompt, prolonged relief. Avoiding factors that produce vasodilation is usually helpful, and vasoconstrictors (eg, ephedrine 25 mg orally, propranolol 10 to 40 mg orally qid, or methysergide 1 to 4 mg orally q 4 h) may also produce relief.

VENOUS DISEASES

VENOUS THROMBOSIS
(Thrombophlebitis; Phlebitis)

The presence of a thrombus in a vein.

Other than varicose veins, the most common venous disorders that bring patients to a physician are **deep venous thrombosis (DVT), thrombophlebitis,** and the sequelae of **chronic venous insufficiency**: edema, stasis pigmentation, stasis dermatitis, and stasis ulceration. These are usually readily diagnosed except for DVT of the calf, which requires venography or scanning with radioactive fibrinogen. The symptoms of acute thrombophlebitis arise over a period of hours to 1 or 2 days. The disease process is usually self-limited and lasts between 1 and 2 wk; then the acute process subsides and painful symptoms disappear.

The terms **phlegmasia alba dolens (milk leg)** and **phlegmasia cerulea dolens** are applied to extensive thrombosis of the involved extremity (depending on its color). The former term is archaic and is now referred to as **ileofemoral thrombophlebitis**. The latter term is still used and means a massive venous thrombosis often leading to venous gangrene and eventual death due to underlying disease (eg, widespread malignancy). Eponyms describe thromboses in specific anatomic areas: **Mondor's disease** refers to thrombosis of the superficial veins over the mammary gland or the adjacent chest wall; **Budd-Chiari syndrome** characterizes the results of hepatic vein thrombosis. **Phlebitis migrans** refers to recurrent venous thrombosis, mainly superficial, but occasionally in deep veins of the extremities and other areas usually due to underlying malignancy. **Effort (strain) thrombosis** occurs in the subclavian vein, secondary to trauma to the vein in the thoracic outlet during unusual physical effort in which the arm is fully abducted. **Chemical phlebitis** results from intimal injury induced by the introduction of catheters or noxious agents directly into a vein. **"Chronic thrombophlebitis"** does not exist. (Pelvic vein, mesenteric vein, portal vein, renal vein, jugular-mesenteric vein thromboses, etc., are not discussed here.)

Etiology

Many factors may contribute to venous thrombosis: (1) **injury to the epithelium of the vein,** such as occurs with indwelling catheters, injection of irritating substances, thromboangiitis obliterans, and septic phlebitis; (2) **hypercoagulability** associated with malignant tumors, blood dyscrasias, oral contraceptives, and idiopathic thrombophlebitis; and (3) **stasis** that occurs in postoperative and postpartum states, varicose thrombophlebitis, and the thrombophlebitis that complicates prolonged bedrest of any chronic illness, heart failure, stroke, and trauma. Prolonged immobilization with the legs dependent while traveling is a risk factor, even in normal, healthy persons.

It is likely that all of these factors play a role; ie, endothelial injury exposes collagen, causing platelet aggregation and tissue thromboplastin release that, when stasis or hypercoagulability is present, trigger the coagulation mechanism.

Pathophysiology

Most venous thrombi begin as platelet nidi in the valve cusps of deep calf veins. Tissue thromboplastin is released, forming thrombin and fibrin that trap RBCs and propagate proximally as a red or fibrin thrombus, which is the predominant morphologic venous lesion (the white or platelet thrombus is the principal component of most arterial lesions). Fibrin thrombi can be prevented from forming or extending by anticoagulant drugs (eg, heparin or the coumarin compounds), but the platelet portion of thrombi has not been shown to be influenced by these agents in usual therapeutic doses. Furthermore, antiplatelet agents, although under intensive study, have not been proven to be effective.

Symptoms and Signs

DVT may be asymptomatic or may be manifested over the involved area by variable combinations of tenderness, pain, edema, warmth, bluish skin discoloration, and prominent superficial veins. With deep thrombophlebitis involving the popliteal, femoral, and iliac segments, there may be tenderness and a hard cord palpable over the involved vein in the femoral triangle in the groin, the medial thigh, or popliteal space. With ileofemoral venous thrombosis, dilated superficial collateral veins usually appear over the leg, thigh, and hip areas and lower abdomen. Bedside evaluation will make the diagnosis in this clinical setting, but difficulties arise in the diagnosis of DVT of the calf. Since at least 3 main veins drain the lower leg, thrombosis in one will not cause obstruction to venous return, and there is no swelling, cyanosis of the skin, or dilated superficial vein. The patient complains of soreness or of pain on standing and walking that is usually relieved by rest with the leg elevated. On examination, deep calf tenderness can be elicited, but differentiation from muscle pain is often difficult. Pain from muscular causes will be absent or minimal on dorsiflexion of the ankle with the knee flexed, but maximal on dorsiflexion of the ankle with the knee extended or during straight leg raising **(Homans' sign),** thereby making this test an *unreliable* indication of DVT. Loss of peripheral arterial pulses may occasionally accompany massive DVT, but venous thrombosis can also be secondary to acute arterial occlusion.

Superficial thrombophlebitis: A thrombosed superficial vein always can be palpated as a linear, indurated cord; it may be associated with a variable inflammatory reaction manifested by pain, tenderness, erythema, and warmth and may need to be differentiated from acute secondary lymphedema with infection (see below). Palpation of a superficial cord in the leg reflects occlusion of a superficial vein; the inference that this finding, per se, reflects DVT is not justified, since it is seldom the case.

Chronic venous insufficiency in the leg after deep thrombophlebitis is manifested by edema and dilated superficial veins. The patient may complain of fullness, aching, or tiredness in the leg or have no discomfort. This occurs during standing or walking and is relieved by rest and elevation. There is no tenderness over the deep veins to indicate an acute thrombophlebitis, but a history of a previous deep thrombophlebitis is usual. The **stasis syndrome** occurs in patients with chronic venous insufficiency if edema is not controlled by an elastic support. With time, skin pigmentation appears on the medial and sometimes the lateral aspect of the ankle and lower leg. Further complications include **stasis dermatitis** and **stasis ulceration** in these areas. Patients with chronic venous insufficiency may develop **varicose veins,** but these are secondary to DVT, are often mild, and function as collateral vessels. They should not be excised unless severe. The symptoms and signs of varicose veins are discussed separately, below.

Diagnosis

Physical examination usually can distinguish between acute arterial and venous obstruction. If there is any question, the dilemma can be resolved by noninvasive testing or by arteriography or venography if necessary. A diagnosis of acute DVT cannot be made satisfactorily by clinical findings alone > 50% of the time; Homans' sign should not be relied upon for the diagnosis, and edema may be due to other causes. Specific limb findings (eg, edema, dilated superficial veins), evidence of pulmonary embolism, and the overall clinical setting, including the risk factors mentioned under Etiology (above), permit the physician to estimate the likelihood of a patient's having DVT. Noninvasive tests are helpful. If any doubt remains, a **venogram** should be obtained. Pulmonary embolism can be sought with lung scan or pulmonary arteriogram (see Ch. 39). Overlooking the presence of phlebitis may lead to death from pulmonary embolism, but to order anticoagulants without having demonstrated an intravascular thrombus by venography or lung scan risks serious hemorrhage.

Contrast venography, as the most accurate diagnostic procedure, is the standard of comparison for every other test. It is widely used, with infrequent complications. Procedures used to locate actively forming DVT include leg scanning, Doppler ultrasound, and plethysmography. **Scanning after injection of ^{125}I fibrinogen** is a sensitive screening test for deep calf, popliteal, and distal thigh thrombosis. Its limitations are that the thyroid gland must be blocked, which requires 24 to 36 h, and since the thrombus must be actively forming to incorporate the isotope, heparin must be withheld. Since ^{125}I fibrinogen appears in blood and exudate, the test is not reliable when healing wounds or hematomas are present in the leg, and it cannot detect thrombi in the upper thigh or pelvis.

Isotope venography is performed by injecting sodium pertechnetate Tc 99m into a peripheral vein and scanning the leg with a gamma camera. Although less painful and quick, this method does not give the resolution of conventional venography, but is a valuable alternative in the patient who is sensitive to contrast media.

Noninvasive procedures are less accurate than venography but, in combination, can be diagnostic in 90 to 95% of cases. **Doppler ultrasound** allows the examiner to hear, in various segments of an extremity, characteristic alterations in spontaneous flow sounds that occur because of recent complete obstruction of the *proximal veins* (popliteal and the veins proximal to it). The examiner listens over the femoral vein in the groin, the medial thigh, and the popliteal space. Normal sounds are like a howling wind that waxes and wanes with respirations. Below an obstruction, the respiratory phasicity disappears and abnormal sounds cannot be obliterated by Valsalva or augmented by its cessation. Above an obstruction, augmentation of the venous sound by compressing muscle distally (lower thigh or calf) is lost. For results to be reliable, this method requires considerable training. The test is not reliable in old disease with good collateral circulation. It does not detect thrombi in the calf or tributary veins since these do not cause obstruction to venous return. A negative ultrasound examination is not sufficient to exclude the diagnosis of DVT confidently in the presence of suspicious clinical findings.

Plethysmography, as with ultrasonography, can be used with acceptable accuracy to diagnose thrombotic obstruction of major proximal veins of the extremities. It cannot detect calf vein thrombosis. Reductions in venous capacitance and outflow caused by an obstructing thrombus in a proximal vein causes changes in electrical impedance as well as volume and rate of outflow. These changes can be measured with approximately 95% accuracy with instruments using these principles, ie, impedance or air plethysmography, phleborheoplethysmography, and mercury strain-gauge plethysmography. These methods are noninvasive, relatively inexpensive, require minimum cooperation from the patient, and can be performed well by a trained technician. They

are frequently used in conjunction with Doppler ultrasound, and the combination enhances the accuracy of diagnosis. Patients may be treated if either of these tests are positive. If their results are negative and the diagnosis of DVT is still suspected, venography should be done.

Prognosis

DVT is usually benign but can terminate in lethal pulmonary emboli or chronic venous insufficiency. Superficial phlebitis alone, even when recurrent, causes neither of these serious complications, although nonlethal pulmonary emboli have been rarely reported to have originated in superficial veins. The possibility of septic phlebitis exists whenever a septic process is present in the extremity distal to or at the level of the venous obstruction. Septic thrombi may form separately from the infectious focus or may occur by contiguity with the inflammatory area as part of a cellulitis.

Although there is a correlation between both superficial and deep phlebitis and cancer, the mechanism whereby malignancy may cause DVT is obscure. Most clinically recognized episodes of deep phlebitis are unassociated with cancer. However, when malignancy is the only risk factor in a patient with superficial or DVT, the malignant process is almost invariably advanced.

Prophylaxis (see Ch. 39)

Treatment

Superficial thrombophlebitis requires no specific therapy other than measures to relieve discomfort. Warm compresses over involved veins, and nonsteroidal anti-inflammatory drugs, eg, phenylbutazone 100 mg orally qid or indomethacin 25 to 50 mg orally qid are helpful. Hospitalization is unnecessary and antibiotics are not needed.

For **DVT** the objectives of therapy are to prevent pulmonary embolism (see Ch. 39) and chronic venous insufficiency. When acute DVT is diagnosed, the patient should be hospitalized, placed in bed with the foot of the bed elevated 6 in., and heparinized; then bathroom or commode privileges can be permitted. Analgesics for pain should not include aspirin or other compounds that interfere with normal platelet function. Drugs such as phenylbutazone or corticosteroids are *not* indicated routinely, and antibiotics should be used only for a specific infection. Warm moist packs are comforting but optional in patients without arterial insufficiency.

Antithrombotic therapy should be initiated immediately with **heparin** if no absolute contraindications exist. Various treatment protocols have been recommended, but a simple and effective method follows: Calculate the dose of heparin on the basis of the patient's *ideal* weight (to avoid giving too much to an obese patient), using 500 u. of heparin/kg/24 h to determine the total daily dosage. This may then be given by continuous IV drip using a pump for accuracy or it may be given in divided doses as an IV injection q 4 h (intermittent method). To guard against excessive effects, the activated partial thromboplastin time **(APTT)** is checked once a day. If the APTT is > 3 times control, the dose of heparin is lowered accordingly (but the method of administration not changed). If the PTT is < 2 to 3 times control, the dose of heparin is not changed. The duration of heparin treatment varies, but is usually 7 to 14 days. Oral therapy with **a coumarin preparation** is initiated to overlap the use of heparin; eg, warfarin sodium 10 to 20 mg/day may be given until the prothrombin time rises to a level 1.5 to 2.5 times control. When this is achieved, heparin is discontinued and the warfarin dose adjusted to maintenance level. The duration of oral anticoagulant therapy also varies, depending on the individual situation. A single episode of phlebitis subsiding clinically in 3 to 6 days in a young, active patient free of risk factors may require only 2 mo of therapy, but another patient with a demonstrable pulmonary embolus and persistent risk factors may require 6 mo of therapy.

The value of **other antithrombotic agents** (eg, snake venoms, platelet antiaggregates, and thrombolytic compounds) has not been established.

Thrombolytic therapy using streptokinase or urokinase in tandem with anticoagulants represents a significant advance in the treatment of acute DVT of the popliteal and more proximal veins. Complete or partial dissolution of thrombi will usually occur within 24 to 48 h. Successful treatment restores venous anatomy and thus prevents valvular damage and the complication of chronic venous insufficiency. Before enzymes are used, the diagnosis must be well established by venography; the contraindications and adverse effects, especially bleeding, and also the details of treatment and monitoring must be fully understood. Details of the administration of thrombolytic agents, as well as **surgical interruption of the inferior vena cava,** are discussed in detail in Ch. 39.

During the acute attack, the patient should be kept in bed with the legs elevated. Bathroom privileges are allowed once anticoagulant therapy is established. When edema subsides, the patient should be measured for a firm below-knee elastic stocking to control the edema that will occur with ambulation. This should be worn while the patient is up to prevent the **postphlebitic sequelae of chronic venous insufficiency**: pain, edema, and skin pigmentation, and subsequent stasis and ulceration. When these complications occur, treatment with an Unna boot (see under STASIS DERMATITIS in Ch. 230) or bed rest in the hospital with elevation and compression dressings will heal most ulcers. Antibiotics are usually indicated only when the ulcer is surrounded by severe acute cellulitis. Wet NaCl dressings may help to loosen superficial exudate and slough. Large, refractory or recurrent ulcers may have to be excised, the incompetent perforating veins ligated, and the area covered with a split-thickness skin graft.

VARICOSE VEINS

Elongated, dilated, tortuous superficial veins whose valves are congenitally absent or scant or have become incompetent; this condition occurs usually in the legs.

Etiology and Pathogenesis

Valved leg veins are of 3 types: (1) **deep veins** that drain venous sinusoids within the muscles, especially those of the calf, into the popliteal and femoral veins; (2) **perforator veins,** whose valves permit flow only from superficial to deep veins; and (3) **superficial veins,** forming a subcutaneous network that drains into the deep veins through perforators or the short and long saphenous veins, which enter the popliteal and femoral veins respectively. Venous flow is most efficient during muscular activity when contracting muscles compress the sinusoids and deep veins, thereby pumping blood toward the heart; the direction of flow is controlled by the venous valves. The term varicose veins refers to superficial veins that permit reversed flow in the dependent position. A family history is common.

The site of primary valvular incompetence is debated: to some the fault is valve failure at the saphenofemoral junction, permitting reflux into the saphenous vein with subsequent descending sequential valvular incompetence from the thigh to the calf. The concept of ligation of the long saphenous vein at the groin and then removing the saphenous vein by stripping is based on this theory. If this were the major factor, new varicose veins should not develop. Others believe that the primary fault is in one or more perforator veins in the lower leg, resulting in high-pressure flow and increased volume from deep to superficial veins during muscular contraction. In time, superficial veins become dilated, separation of the valve cusps prevents their apposition, and flow reverses in the affected segment. As other perforator valves become incompetent, reflux occurs at additional sites. Progression of these factors proximally in the long saphenous vein causes secondary incompetence at the saphenofemoral junction. This theory explains both the initial occurrences of varicose veins as well as the development of new ones after any form of treatment.

Other etiologic factors include congenital arteriovenous fistulas, increased hydrostatic pressure, and primary idiopathic dilation of the vein wall or secondarily due to hormonal changes during early pregnancy, pressure on the pelvic veins later in pregnancy, an abdominal tumor, or ascites. Occupations that require prolonged standing probably aggravate existing varicose veins, rather than being primary etiologic factors. Previous deep thrombophlebitis, with vein recanalization resulting in deep valve incompetency, leads to secondary incompetency of the perforator veins, and varicose veins develop.

Symptoms and Signs

Initially, superficial veins are tense and may be palpated but are not visible. Subsequently, they become visibly dilated and tortuous; the diagnosis is then obvious to the patient, who may seek medical advice. Patients with asymptomatic varicosities often seek cosmetic treatment.

Symptoms are not necessarily related to the size or degree of varicosities; severely involved legs may be asymptomatic, whereas patients may point to small visible sites as being painful. Varicose veins may be associated with aching, fatigue, or heat that is relieved by elevating the leg or by wearing compression hosiery. Symptoms tend to worsen during the menstrual period.

Diagnosis

The patient usually makes the diagnosis of varicose veins, but their extent is usually greater than can be determined by simple inspection and can be judged accurately only by palpation with the patient standing. It is essential in symptomatic patients to rule out other possible causes. Lumbar nerve root irritation can cause an aching sensation in the calf. Osteoarthritis of the hip or knee or internal derangements of the knee must be excluded. Arterial insufficiency may present with intermittent claudication or rest pain with physical findings of trophic changes in the leg and diminution or absence of one or more pulses. A burning sensation may be due to peripheral neuritis from diabetic or alcoholic neuropathy. Probably the most significant feature of the history of pain of varicose veins is that it should be relieved when the leg is elevated.

The Trendelenburg test can demonstrate retrograde flow of blood past incompetent saphenous valves in the upright position. It is done to determine if the saphenofemoral junction is incompetent and whether or not sapheno-femoral disconnection (Trendelenburg operation) is appropriate for a particular case. Testing with multiple tourniquets to determine sites of incompetent perforations is seldom necessary and is inaccurate. Venography should be reserved to confirm the presence or absence of *deep* vein thrombosis if other studies are inconclusive.

A correctly applied tourniquet in the upper thigh, with the leg elevated and the patient supine, should prevent reflux filling of the saphenous and lower superficial veins when the patient stands. Correct tightness of the tourniquet is hard to assess accurately, especially in large thighs. The test is best performed by palpating the site of the long saphenous vein in the groin with the patient standing. This is found about one finger's breadth medial to the femoral pulse. Normally it is difficult to feel and this indicates that it is not involved. It may be found more easily if, while one hand is palpating the groin with the patient standing, the other hand firmly taps the lower varicosities with the fingertips. The palpable fluid thrill at the groin identifies the long saphenous vein. The patient is now asked to lie supine while the examiner keeps 1 or 2 fingers over the long saphenous vein with *minimal* pressure so as *not* to occlude it. With the free hand the examiner raises the patient's leg to about 45° to allow the veins to empty. Firm pressure is *now* applied at the groin to occlude the saphenous vein and, while maintaining the pressure, the patient is asked to stand. If reflux from the groin into the lower veins is not significant, the lower varicosities should not be visible for at least 30 sec, at which time they would naturally fill from below. However, if pressure

on the vein is removed and rapid filling of the varicosities is seen, then retrograde filling at the sapheno-femoral junction is occurring.

Short saphenous vein incompetence can be readily determined by palpating a tense short saphenous vein at or below the popliteal fossa with the patient standing.

Complications

When pigmentation (from RBC diapedesis), eczema, edema, subcutaneous induration, and ulceration occur, these findings suggest the presence of deep vein incompetence and the terms **"postphlebitic leg"** or **"stasis syndrome"** are applied. The ulceration is usually small, superficial, and very painful because of exposure of nerve endings, if the ulcer is due to varicose veins (and not deep venous incompetence). Varicose veins may be seen or palpated close to or continuous with the ulcer. These ulcerations may start after minor trauma to an area of pigmentation, induration, eczema, or edema, and are usually chronic by the time they are seen.

Superficial thrombophlebitis presents with localized pain, cord-like induration, periphlebitis with reddish-brown discoloration, and fever; pulmonary embolism rarely occurs unless deep veins become involved. Very thin-walled **"blow-outs,"** more commonly seen in the elderly, may rupture and hemorrhage with minimal trauma. Hyperesthesia may be associated with varicose veins, and subcutaneous calcification or ossification may occur in longstanding cases.

Prognosis and Treatment

Varicose veins are incurable irrespective of the method of treatment. Veins that are *normal* at the time of the initial treatment may become varicose at any future date and are not true recurrences.

Lightweight compression hosiery for small, mildly symptomatic varicose veins are helpful and often adequate. Heavier support elastic stockings, either knee length or thigh length, may be worn for more advanced cases by patients who prefer not to have active therapy or in whom it is contraindicated. Elastic bandages should not be advocated; because patients may wrap them too tightly, especially at the calf area, producing a tourniquet effect; even if correctly applied, they rapidly loosen and become ineffectual.

Indications for surgical therapy include pain, recurrent phlebitis, skin changes, or cosmetic reasons. Since the advent of bypass grafting of the coronary and peripheral arteries, every effort is made to preserve the saphenous veins. Those who believe that surgery is the treatment of choice, recommend that the saphenous veins should be stripped only if they are diseased throughout their course from ankle to groin. Those who recommend extensive surgery strip the long and short saphenous veins and, by dissection, remove as many of the tortuous and saccular varices as possible. The patient must be forewarned that isolated persistent varices or new varices may develop; these can often be obliterated by injections of sclerosing solution (see below).

Injection sclerotherapy can be used to treat virtually all varices. Past attempts to produce fibrosis by chemical sclerotherapy were unsuccessful. Iatrogenic phlebitis and periphlebitis were painful and only a small percentage proceeded to the anticipated fibrosis required for a permanent cure. The thrombus formed in most cases, but its subsequent lysis or contraction permitted recanalization and recurrence in addition to further damage to venous valves. Additionally, with large varices, the thrombus could propagate into deep veins via perforator veins with the possibility of becoming a pulmonary embolus. Therefore, the most common therapy became surgery.

Recent studies suggest that failure occurred because the resulting thrombus prevented the apposing walls of the inflamed vein from adhering and fusing. However, in experienced hands, current methods of injection sclerotherapy, with compression, give excellent results and require no hospitalization. *Successful sclerosing therapy requires total obliteration of the vein by fibrosis.* To accomplish this, the vein should be injected while it is as empty of blood as possible during and after the injection, using one of

several "empty vein" technics. The preferred sclerosant is sodium tetradecyl sulfate in 1 or 3% solution, which damages the intima of the vein. After injection and with the leg still elevated and appropriate rubber pads placed over the injected veins to compress them and to maintain apposition of the walls, compression bandages are applied from the base of the toes to above the highest injection site. Bandages remain on for 3 wk, or longer if necessary, during which time the patient continues normal daily activities. Walking as much as possible is essential to activate the muscle pump and promote venous drainage from the lower limb. Adequate compression of the upper thigh veins may be difficult due to configuration of the thigh and the subcutaneous fat. In these cases, distal injection therapy, with compression, is combined with a Trendelenburg sapheno-femoral disconnection, under a local anesthetic, if sapheno-femoral incompetence can be demonstrated as described. The patient requires no hospitalization and remains ambulatory and active. As with surgery, isolated varices may recur and require treatment.

Complications of injection therapy are few. Allergic reactions are rare and toxic effects have not been seen. Treatment is limited to a maximum of 30 mL of 1% solution for each leg. If both are to be treated, they are done on different days to allow excretion of the material in the urine in the interim. Extravascular injection can produce a slough of the overlying skin with subsequent scarring. Deep vein thrombosis with embolism is rare. Women should avoid taking oral contraceptives for at least 6 wk before treatment because of their potential thrombogenic effect. Patients should be advised that brown pigmentation of the skin may occur; this usually fades, but may be permanent.

Idiopathic telangiectases ("spider veins") are fine intracutaneous angiectases of no serious consequence, but they may be extensive and unsightly. Although usually asymptomatic, some patients describe burning or pain, and many women find even the smallest telangiectases cosmetically unacceptable. They can usually be eliminated by intracapillary injections of 1% solution of sodium tetradecyl sulfate through a fine-bore needle. (Hypertonic saline [23.4%] also has been advocated for treating spider veins. Unlike sodium tetradecyl sulfate, this may cause fairly severe, temporary, localized pain and may require several visits to treat large areas of spider veins. However, there is no risk of allergic reactions with saline.) Care should be taken to avoid rupturing the fine capillaries and producing skin ulceration due to subcutaneous injection. Pigmentation may develop, but this subsides, often completely, and is rarely a cause for complaint. Best results are obtained by treating the whole leg at the initial visit and applying a compression bandage on the leg with ambulation, as described above, for at least 3 wk after treatment.

Small telangiectases may persist or recur after the initial treatment. Best results are obtained with subsequent treatments, as required, to residual sites until optimal results are obtained. Because they are usually small, re-compression is not usually required.

ARTERIOVENOUS FISTULA

Abnormal communication between an artery and a vein. Etiology may be congenital, in which smaller vessels are involved, or acquired due to acute, local trauma (eg, from a bullet or stab wound), or from erosion of an arterial aneurysm into the accompanying vein. It may cause symptoms of arterial insufficiency, ulceration due to embolization and ischemia, or symptoms related to chronic venous insufficiency due to the high-pressure arterial flow within the involved veins. If near the surface, a mass can be felt and the affected part is usually enlarged and warm, with distended and often pulsating superficial veins. A thrill can be palpated over the fistula, and a continuous machinery murmur with accentuation during systole can be heard with the stethoscope. The altered hemodynamics may cause heart failure if a significant portion of the CO is diverted through the fistula. The treatment of choice is surgery, if feasible.

LYMPHEDEMA

Accumulation of excessive lymph fluid and swelling of subcutaneous tissues due to obstruction, destruction, or hypoplasia of lymph vessels.

Lymphedema may be primary or secondary. The **primary type** can be present from birth (congenital lymphedema) or may occur during puberty (lymphedema praecox) or less frequently later in life (lymphedema tarda). Primary lymphedema occurs less often in men. The patient complains of swelling of the foot, leg, or entire extremity. Usually unilateral, it is worse during warm weather, before menstrual periods, and after prolonged dependency. There is usually no discomfort. On examination the edema is diffuse, causes a typical mound on the dorsum of the foot or hand, and is only partially pitting. There are usually no skin changes or evidence of venous insufficiency.

Secondary lymphedema is often a result of infection, especially dermatophytosis when it occurs in the foot. The onset is explosive, with chills, high fever, toxicity, and a red, hot, swollen leg. Lymphangitic streaks may be seen in the skin, and lymph nodes in the groin are usually enlarged and tender. These features distinguish it from acute thrombophlebitis. Secondary lymphedema in older persons may be due to malignant disease in the pelvis or groin. Obliteration of lymphatic tissue by excision or radiation therapy is another cause. The response to antistreptococcal antibiotics is rapid.

Swelling is treated by elevation or pneumatic compression, and then application of a firm elastic support to be worn while the patient is up. Occasionally diuretics are helpful.

LIPEDEMA

Lipedema is a syndrome of fatty, tender legs. The patient complains of swelling and tender tissues. Examination shows that most of the patient's fat is distributed in the hips, thighs, and legs. Although the foot is spared, fatty tissue often hangs over the ankles. Tissue tenderness is generalized and is not over the course of the veins. The only treatment is for the patient to avoid further weight gain and to try to lose weight, if obese. Unfortunately, the abnormal fat in the lower extremities cannot be mobilized and weight loss occurs in the trunk, arms, and face.

4. PULMONARY DISORDERS

31. APPROACH TO THE PULMONARY PATIENT

Diagnosis and management of pulmonary disorders requires a history and physical examination, and chest x-rays will almost always be necessary. Pulmonary function testing, arterial blood gas analysis, chemical or microbiologic tests, or special studies such as endoscopy, biopsy, or radionuclide scanning, may be needed; eg, dyspnea may lead to pulmonary function testing, or hemoptysis to bronchoscopy. These special tests and technics are discussed elsewhere in THE MANUAL.

History-taking provides essential information and it initiates understanding of the patient as a person, of the patient's environment, expectations, and fears, and is the best way to develop his understanding and collaboration. Data desired include those relating to occupational or other exposures; family, travel, and contact history; an account of previous illnesses and medications; and results of tests (eg, tuberculin skin tests or chest x-rays). Most important, however, are the clear definition of the present complaint, and both general symptoms (eg, lassitude, weight loss, or fever) and the major respiratory symptoms of cough, sputum, dyspnea, chest pain, wheeze, and hemoptysis, which are considered individually, below.

Physical examination follows history-taking in importance for most patients and for most (but not all) pulmonary diseases. Some information is absorbed almost subconsciously (general condition, demeanor, discomfort, anxiety, dyspnea on exertion as we walk with the patient from waiting-room to office), while other general and respiratory items are sought and recorded individually. The sequence of inspection, palpation,

percussion, and auscultation should be followed in examining the lungs. In some cases, physical examination of the chest may be completely negative, even in the presence of serious disease; but in others it provides information otherwise unobtainable (eg, incoordination of respiratory muscle groups, a pleural friction rub, or a localized monophonic wheeze).

COUGH

A sudden explosive expiratory maneuver that tends to clear material from the airways.

Cough is a familiar, but complex, reflex. Differences among several sites from which cough stimuli can originate may result in variations in the sounds and patterns of coughing. Cough helps protect the lungs against aspiration, and stimulation of the larynx will produce a choking type of cough without a preceding inspiration. On the other hand, a patient whose mucociliary clearance mechanisms are inadequate, as in bronchiectasis or cystic fibrosis, may develop a pattern of coughing with less violent acceleration of air, but a sequence of interrupted expirations continuing, without any intervening inspiration, down to a low lung volume. Awareness of cough varies considerably; it can be distressing when it appears suddenly, particularly if it is associated with discomfort due to chest pain, dyspnea, or copious secretions. However, if a cough develops slowly over decades (eg, in a smoker with mild chronic bronchitis), the patient may hardly be aware of it, or may consider it normal. Cough may also be denied to avoid recommendations against cigarette smoking. However, it is one of the most common presenting complaints.

Questions about cough should determine how long it has been present; whether it came on suddenly; if it has changed recently; what factors influence it (eg, cold air, talking, posture, eating or drinking, time of day); and whether it is associated with sputum production, chest or retrosternal or throat pain, dyspnea, hoarseness, dizziness, or other symptoms. The patient should be asked what he thinks causes it; sometimes he can describe "something in my lung that needs to be coughed up," or "something tickling the back of my throat." Patterns of coughing or precipitating factors may be a clue to the underlying cause of the cough, and the patient may have noted an association with work or with exercise. Cough induced by changes of posture may suggest chronic lung abscess, cavitary TB, bronchiectasis, or pedunculated tumor, while a cough associated with eating suggests a disturbance of the swallowing mechanism, or possibly even a tracheoesophageal fistula. Cough that appears on exposure to cold air or exercise may suggest asthma. A morning cough that persists until sputum is expectorated is characteristic of chronic bronchitis. Coughing associated with rhinitis, wheezing, or seasonal in its appearance may represent an allergic response.

During the interview, the alert physician will note any spontaneous coughing, because its sound can yield useful information; eg, an audible rattle of secretions, the irritable, dry, barking cough of a patient with acute tracheitis, or the low-pitched, blowing, "bovine" cough without an explosive start, heard in a patient with a paralyzed recurrent laryngeal nerve. If a patient does not cough spontaneously, he should be asked to cough after the chest examination has been completed. It is advisable to wait until then, as secretion sounds or crackles at the bases may be dispelled by a cough before being detected. It is useful to listen to the patient's lungs, and at his open mouth, both before and after the cough, since movement of secretions may alter physical findings dramatically; on the other hand, posttussive rales may appear, particularly over tuberculous lesions in the upper lobes of the lung.

Treatment of cough is mainly that of the underlying cause. Symptomatic treatment of cough is discussed in Ch. 287.

Sputum production: A major function of the cough reflex is to help clear secretions from the airways, and particularly to help expel them through the larynx. Sputum

production should be the subject of questioning while taking a patient's history; questions about cough and sputum are usually related, but occasionally a patient who denies coughing will state that he produces sputum. (In questionnaires, the proportion of responses positive for sputum production usually exceeds that for cough.) Questions should relate to its appearance and how easily it is expelled. Changes in character (eg, from clear white mucus to yellowish, green, or brown purulent material) are important indicators of infection. Blood streaking and frank hemoptysis are obviously important, and likely to be noted by the patient. Gritty material in sputum, characteristic of broncholithiasis, may be less noticeable, and a patient may commonly deny its presence on first questioning, but subsequently notice and report it.

Examination of sputum: If possible, the patient should expectorate a sputum specimen during the evaluation. Its appearance to the naked eye should be observed, and microscopic examination is simple and useful. A small drop selected from a thicker portion of freshly collected sputum (placed on a glass slide, without staining, and compressed with a cover slip) can give useful information on low power microscopic examination. Presence of squamous cells suggests that the material came from above the larynx; true sputum expelled from the airways is characterized by the presence of alveolar macrophages or histiocytes. Wright's stain will show the proportion of eosinophils, and the presence of eosinophilia suggests a probable allergic origin for sputum. Neutrophils are more often the predominant cell in purulent sputum, indicating an inflammatory and usually an infectious process. A Gram stain will confirm the presence of bacteria and begin their categorization.

DYSPNEA

An unpleasant sensation of difficulty in breathing. Dyspnea is a symptom, not a sign, and is one of several sensations that may be described by a patient aware of discomfort related to breathing.

A healthy person will note the increased ventilation required during exercise, but will not interpret it as being particularly unpleasant unless taken to an extreme. Awareness that a small amount of exercise leads to a disproportionately large increase in ventilation is a common type of dyspnea, usually described as breathlessness or shortness of breath on exertion. It may be regarded as unpleasant in part because it is limiting, or it is interpreted as a sign of disease. A normal person at high altitude will be aware of a similar disproportionately large increase in ventilation resulting from exertion, and will find it limiting, but usually not otherwise unpleasant. Comparison of sensations experienced with those expected forms a large part of this type of dyspnea, as can be elucidated by careful questioning.

Other sensations related to breathing include awareness of increased muscular effort required to expand the chest during inspiration, increased effort required to expel air from the lungs, sensations of fatigue from the respiratory muscles, awareness of delay in air leaving the lungs during expiration, the uncomfortable sensation that an inspiration is urgently needed before expiration is completed, and various sensations most often described as "tightness in the chest." The last can probably include awareness of collapse or hyperinflation of lung units; obstruction of airways; and distortion or displacement of lung, mediastinum, diaphragm, or chest wall.

Afferent impulses to the brain that generate the sensation of dyspnea come from many different sites. Some come from the lungs; others seem to originate in articulations of the rib cage and in the respiratory muscles including the diaphragm. Peripheral and central chemoreceptors provide part of the sensory input that appears to be involved in the sensation of dyspnea, either directly or indirectly, and other visceral, neural, and emotional stimuli may also participate.

Clinical Types of Dyspnea

1. Physiologic: The most common type of breathlessness (dyspnea) is that associated with physical exertion. Ventilation is increased and maintained through an augmented respiratory stimulus provided by metabolic and other undefined factors. Dyspnea is also common during acute hypoxia, as at high altitude, where the increased respiratory stimulus is, in part, the effect of arterial hypoxemia on the carotid bodies. Dyspnea is also evoked by breathing high CO_2 concentrations in a closed space, or rebreathing in a closed system without CO_2 absorption. The sensation of dyspnea in this situation is similar to that brought on by exercise, and is primarily an awareness of increased ventilation. Increased CO_2 produces different sensations from reduced O_2 in the inspired gas. For most people, hypoxemia is a much less potent stimulus to increased ventilation than is hypercapnia, and hypoxemia may produce other effects: confusion, a vague unpleasant sensation that is hard to define, or even unconsciousness. When a person enters a closed space that is devoid of O_2 (eg, containing 100% N), consciousness may be lost in about 30 sec, *before* dyspnea warns of the danger. Underwater swimmers who first hyperventilate to blow off CO_2 in order to delay the need to surface for air have lost consciousness and drowned because of hypoxemia (see Ch. 262). The sensation of dyspnea may also be minimal in CO poisoning.

2. Pulmonary: The 2 major pulmonary causes of dyspnea are a **restrictive** defect with low compliance of the lungs or chest wall or an **obstructive** defect with increased resistance to airflow. Patients with restrictive dyspnea (eg, due to pulmonary fibrosis or chest deformities) are usually comfortable at rest but become intensely dyspneic when exertion causes pulmonary ventilation to approach their greatly limited breathing capacity. In obstructive dyspnea (eg, as in obstructive emphysema or asthma), increased ventilatory effort induces dyspnea even at rest, and breathing is labored and retarded, especially during expiration.

While careful questioning about the nature of sensations as well as their pattern will help to distinguish between restrictive and obstructive dyspnea, these pulmonary function defects are commonly seen in combination, and dyspnea may show combined or transitional characteristics.

Physical examination and pulmonary function testing will add to the detailed information obtained in the history. Physical findings may reveal not only the presence of restriction by reduction in ventilatory movement, but help to show its cause (eg, in pleural effusion, pneumothorax, and some patients with interstitial lung disease). The signs of emphysema, bronchitis, and asthma are frequently helpful in defining both the nature and the severity of the underlying obstructive lung disease. Pulmonary function testing will provide numerical values to any restriction or airflow obstruction present, allowing comparison with normal values and any previous or future values for the same patient. Progression or improvement in the disease and response to therapy can be measured by repeated evaluations, the frequency of which will be determined by the tempo of the disease. Reversibility of airflow obstruction is measured by the changes, especially in the forced expiratory volume in 1 sec (FEV_1), resulting from administration of a bronchodilator. A patient with a history of episodic dyspnea may have normal pulmonary function test results if tested in remission, but challenge testing by exercise, cold air inhalation, or methacholine aerosol may reveal hyperreactivity of the airways. Such challenge testing is best conducted by physicians experienced in the technic.

Diffuse pulmonary disease, with or without hypoxia, is often accompanied by hyperventilation and lowering of the Pa_{CO_2}. Thus, it is possible to have a patient with dyspnea and a high Pa_{O_2} and a low Pa_{CO_2}, presumably due to heightened stimuli from the stretch receptors in diseased lungs.

3. Cardiac: In early stages of heart failure (see HEART FAILURE in Ch. 27), CO fails to keep pace with increased metabolic need during exercise. As a result, the respiratory drive is increased largely because of tissue and cerebral acidosis; the patient therefore hyperventilates. Various reflex factors, including stretch receptors in the lungs, may also contribute to hyperventilation. Shortness of breath is often accompanied by lassitude or a feeling of smothering or sternal oppression. In later stages of heart failure, the lungs are congested and edematous, the ventilatory capacity of the stiff lungs is reduced, and ventilatory effort is increased. Reflex factors, particularly the juxtacapillary (J) receptors in the alveolar-capillary septa, contribute to the inordinate increase in pulmonary ventilation. Noncardiogenic pulmonary edema or adult respiratory distress syndrome will produce a similar clinical picture by similar mechanisms, but more acutely. **Cardiac asthma** is *a state of acute respiratory insufficiency*. Its manifestations may be indistinguishable from other types of asthma, but it originates from left ventricular failure. The airways obstruction is accompanied by hyperventilation. **Periodic** or **Cheyne-Stokes respiration** is characterized by *regularly alternating periods of apnea and hyperpnea*, often including both neurologic and cardiologic components. In heart failure, slowing of the circulation is the predominant cause; acidosis and hypoxia in the respiratory centers contribute importantly.

Orthopnea is *the respiratory discomfort that occurs while the patient is supine, impelling him to sit up*. It is precipitated by an increase in venous return of blood to a left ventricle lacking the ability to meet the challenge of this increased preload. Of lesser importance is the increase in the work of breathing in the supine position. Orthopnea, usually a manifestation of left ventricular failure, sometimes occurs in other cardiovascular disorders (eg, pericardial effusion).

In **paroxysmal nocturnal dyspnea (PND),** *the patient awakens gasping for breath and must sit or stand to get his breath*, which may be dramatic and terrifying. The same factors that cause orthopnea interact to produce this more urgent form of respiratory distress. PND may occur in mitral stenosis, aortic insufficiency, hypertension, or other conditions affecting the left ventricle.

4. Circulatory: "Air hunger" (*acute dyspnea occurring in terminal stages of exsanguinating hemorrhage*) is a grave sign calling for immediate transfusion. Dyspnea also occurs with chronic anemia, coming on only during exertion, except when the anemia is extreme.

5. Chemical: Diabetic acidosis (blood pH 7.2 to 6.95) induces a distinctive pattern of slow, deep respirations **(Kussmaul breathing).** However, because the breathing capacity is well preserved, the patient rarely complains of dyspnea. In contrast, the uremic patient may complain of dyspnea because of severe panting brought about by a combination of acidosis, heart failure, pulmonary edema, and anemia.

6. Central: Cerebral lesions, eg, hemorrhage, are often associated with intense hyperventilation that is sometimes noisy and stertorous and occasionally unpredictably irregular periods of apnea alternating with periods in which 4 or 5 breaths of similar depth are taken **(Biot's respiration).** Hyperventilation is also frequently seen after head injury. The associated fall in Pa_{CO_2} may be beneficial by causing a reflex fall in intracranial pressure.

7. Psychogenic: Hysterical types of overbreathing are most common. In one type, there is continuous hyperventilation, sometimes leading to acute alkalosis from "blowing off" CO_2 (see also RESPIRATORY ALKALOSIS in Ch. 84), and positive Trousseau and Chvostek signs result from lowered serum calcium ion levels. Another type is characterized by deep, sighing respirations, the patient breathing at maximal depth until respiration is "satisfactory," at which time the hyperventilatory impulse subsides. This is repeated at frequent intervals.

CHEST PAIN

Chest pain is a common presenting complaint. The first task, not always an easy one, is to differentiate respiratory pain from that related to other systems. The nature of the pain and the circumstances of its appearance will usually distinguish angina or the pain of myocardial infarction; pain associated with a dissecting aneurysm may be more difficult to discern by history alone. Physical examination, x-rays, sometimes including CT or angiograms, and ECGs will usually make the distinction obvious. Esophageal pain usually has characteristics relating it to eating or acid regurgitation.

Most noncardiac chest pain arises from the pleura or the chest wall. **Pleuritic pain** is typically made worse by deep breathing or coughing and may be abolished by immobilization of the chest wall; eg, the patient may hold his side, avoid deep breathing, or suppress his cough. The patient can usually localize pleuritic pain. Over time it may move from one position to another. If a pleural effusion develops, the pain may disappear as the inflamed pleural surfaces are separated from one another. A friction rub is often associated with pleuritic pain, but either may occur alone. **Pain originating in the chest wall** may also be exacerbated by deep breathing or coughing, but can usually be distinguished by localized tenderness. Some tenderness may be present with pleuritic pain (eg, associated with pneumococcal pneumonia), but it is usually slight, poorly localized, and elicited only by deep pressure. Chest wall trauma or a broken rib can often be suspected from the history, but torn muscle fibers or even a rib fracture can result from severe coughing. A tumor infiltrating the chest wall may cause local pain or, if it involves intercostal nerves, referred pain. Herpes zoster, before the eruption appears, may present as puzzling chest pain.

Pain arising from other respiratory structures is usually less easy to characterize than pleurisy. A deep-seated, vague lung ache occurs occasionally with lung abscess, a tuberculous cavity, or a giant bulla, and may arise from stretch receptors associated with pulmonary vessels. A rapidly growing mass in the mediastinum or lung will occasionally be associated with a poorly localized ache. Physical examination and chest x-rays will usually determine the cause.

WHEEZE

Awareness of wheezing or whistling noises associated with breathing. Either the patient or relatives (eg, a parent) may be aware of wheezing as part of a chest illness. It is commonly associated with dyspnea. By its more "musical" character, wheezing should be distinguished from the noisy breathing also associated with airflow obstruction. Most (but not all) asthmatic patients wheeze during exacerbations. Asthma is the most common, but not the only cause of wheeze. In an epidemiologic study of a general population sample, the prevalence of asthma at a point in time was 6.6% and that for all forms of wheezing was 30%. Airflow obstruction at some level in the airways is a prerequisite for wheezing.

Auscultation over the chest, at the larynx, and at the open mouth will confirm the wheezing and allow more exact definition in location and pitch—or pitches, if polyphonic. A monophonic wheeze heard at one location is more likely to represent local bronchial obstruction, for example by a tumor. In asthmatics with reversible bronchospasm, bronchodilators may abolish wheezing, or lower its pitch and reduce the proportion of the respiratory cycle occupied by wheeze.

Pulmonary function testing (see below) is useful in evaluating wheezing, and chest x-ray is important to rule out such processes as tumors or foreign bodies.

HEMOPTYSIS

Coughing up blood as a result of bleeding from the respiratory tract.

Etiology

The source of hemoptysis may be either the pulmonary or bronchial circulation, or granulation tissue that contains vascular elements from both. About 95% of pulmonary blood circulation is supplied by the pulmonary artery and its branches, a low-pressure system. Bronchial circulation, a high-pressure system, originates from the aorta and usually provides about 5% of the blood to the lungs, primarily to the airways and supporting structures. Bleeding usually arises from the bronchial circulation, unless trauma or erosion by a granulomatous or calcified node or a tumor has damaged a major pulmonary vessel. Pulmonary vascular bleeding may originate in the capillaries, small vessels (usually arteries), or major large vessels. Pulmonary venous bleeding is generally modest, and occurs primarily in association with pulmonary venous hypertension, particularly in association with left heart failure. Bronchial venous bleeding occasionally complicates "tight" mitral stenosis and may be life-threatening.

Blood-streaked sputum is a rather common complaint but is usually nonthreatening (eg, a patient with a URI and bronchitis coughs up a few streaks of blood). Inflammatory causes account for 80 to 90% of hemoptysis. Acute or chronic bronchitis is probably the most common cause, since bronchitis and, to a diminishing extent, bronchiectasis cause about 50% of all cases. Recent infection in an old bronchiectatic sac, a healed cavity, or a cystic lesion causes vasodilation and engorgement of vessels and may be associated with bleeding ranging from a slow ooze to frank bleeding. Infestation of cavities by *Aspergillus* species (mycetoma, fungus ball) is an increasingly recognized cause of significant hemoptysis regardless of the cause of the cavity. TB accounts for 10 to 20% of cases. Tumors (especially carcinoma), perfused primarily by bronchial vessels, account for about 20% of cases; bronchogenic carcinoma must be strongly suspected in smokers who have hemoptysis and who are ≥ 40 yr old. Pulmonary infarction in association with thromboembolism and left heart failure (especially secondary to mitral stenosis) are less common causes of hemoptysis. Other less common causes (eg, primary bronchial adenoma, arteriovenous malformations) are disproportionately important because of their tendency to cause severe bleeding. Metastatic cancer rarely causes hemoptysis. Hemoptysis of obscure origin on rare occasion occurs at the time of menstruation. See TABLE 31–1 for conditions that may be responsible for hemoptysis.

Diagnosis

Hemoptysis, particularly if large in quantity or if recurrent, is a frightening and potentially fatal event requiring expeditious determination of the etiology, the quantity, and the precise location of the bleeding. Hemoptysis must be differentiated from hematemesis and from blood dripping into the tracheobronchial passages from the nose, mouth, or nasopharynx. The patient may be able to sense and tell the examiner where the bleeding originated, even specifying from which side of the chest. History, physical examination, and chest x-rays usually define etiologies such as trauma, tumor, TB, bronchiectasis, heart failure, or pulmonary infarct/embolism.

A lung scan and pulmonary angiogram are useful for confirming the diagnosis of pulmonary embolism; pulmonary angiography will also diagnose a pulmonary arteriovenous fistula. Aortography will demonstrate an aortic aneurysm. Endoscopic examination is crucial during or shortly after an episode of acute bleeding, especially for major bleeding. The flexible bronchoscope causes less discomfort for the patient and permits greater visualization of the bronchial tree, but the rigid bronchoscope is the instrument of choice when bleeding is profuse. When the etiology is obscure, careful examination of the upper respiratory passages using a mirror and direct visualization,

TABLE 31-1. CONDITIONS ASSOCIATED WITH HEMOPTYSIS

Larynx and Pharynx
- Lymphoma
- Carcinoma
- Tuberculous ulceration

Trachea and Large Bronchi
- Benign or malignant primary tumor
- Telangiectasia
- Erosion by an aortic aneurysm
- Bronchogenic cyst
- Broncholithiasis
- Erosion by a caseocalcific node
- Erosion by a tumor from nodes, esophagus, or other mediastinal structures
- Severe acute bronchitis
- Trauma

Cardiovascular
- Left ventricular failure
- Mitral stenosis
- Pulmonary embolism/infarct
- Primary pulmonary hypertension
- Pulmonary arteriovenous fistula
- Atrial myxoma
- Fibrous mediastinitis with pulmonary vein obstruction
- Aortic aneurysm with leakage into the pulmonary parenchyma

Smaller Bronchial Structures
- Carcinoma
- Adenoma (carcinoid or cylindromatous)
- Acute bronchitis
- Bronchiectasis
- Bronchopulmonary sequestration
- Chronic bronchitis
- Trauma

Pulmonary Parenchyma
- Primary or metastatic tumor
- Infarct
- Abscess
- Active granulomatous disease (TB, fungal, parasitic, luetic)
- Fungus ball (*Aspergillus*) in an old cavity
- Acute pneumonia
- Idiopathic hemosiderosis
- Goodpasture's syndrome
- Trauma

Clotting Defects
- Thrombocytopenia
- Vitamin K-dependent factors: prothrombin (II), Stuart factor (X), Factor VII, Christmas factor (IX)
- Diffuse intravascular coagulation
- Heparin therapy
- Fibrinolytic therapy: urokinase
streptokinase
- Miscellaneous congenital coagulation defects

bronchography, and evaluation of the clotting mechanisms are indicated. Chest CT may prove useful in evaluating recurrent hemoptysis of unclear etiology. Despite systematic and intensive search, the cause of hemoptysis will *not* be found in 30 to 40% of cases.

Treatment

The objectives are (1) to prevent exsanguination; (2) to prevent asphyxiation by exsanguinated blood; (3) to prevent blood clots from obstructing bronchi and causing segmental, lobar, or lung collapse, or hyperinflation by a check-valve mechanism of similar anatomic units; (4) to localize the area of aspirated blood as much as possible; (5) to control infection that may spread by aspiration of blood from an infected focus; (6) to stop the bleeding; and (7) to allay fear and anxiety.

Objective 1 (to prevent exsanguination) requires careful clinical monitoring of the indicators of shock (see in Ch. 26). Bleeding time, clotting time, platelet count, prothrombin time, and partial thromboplastin time should be assayed immediately to determine if there are any clotting abnormalities. *Narcotics should not be given.*

Objectives 2, 3, and 4 (to prevent asphyxiation, airways obstruction, and spread to uninvolved lung) are accomplished by removing extravascular blood from the lung. Coughing is the most efficient way to achieve this. The patient must be encouraged to cough and be shown how to clear secretions gently by slightly prolonging glottic closure before coughing. Inhalation of warm water vapor or mist helps to decrease throat irritation and ease the urge to cough explosively. The physician's reassurance,

frequently repeated, is a very effective way to keep the patient coughing efficiently. Postural drainage may be helpful if bleeding is brisk. The patient should not be immobilized but should be encouraged to move about gently, keeping the side from which the bleeding is occurring (if known) dependent. If a major bronchus becomes obstructed by a clot or if evidence of atelectasis or progressive overinflation (check-valve effect of clot) develops, bronchoscopy should be performed immediately for clearance.

Objective 5 (to prevent spread of infection) applies particularly to TB. If TB is suspected as the cause of the bleeding, therapy with at least 2 effective drugs (including INH or rifampin, or both) should be started at once. Penicillin should be given immediately if a lung abscess due to aspiration is suspected. When fungal infection is the possible cause of the bleeding, amphotericin B therapy should be considered.

Objective 6 (to stop the bleeding) requires an approach related to the cause. Bleeding from a major vessel may respond to nothing short of lung resection or ligation of the bleeding vessel, but these carry a high mortality and would be appropriate only as a last resort. Bleeding from any large vessel requires early blood replacement; this should not be withheld for fear that it will cause renewed or increased bleeding. Bleeding from smaller vessels usually stops spontaneously.

Since bleeding from bronchiectatic areas usually results from infection, treatment of the infection with appropriate antibiotics and postural drainage is essential.

If clotting abnormalities (see Ch. 99) contribute to bleeding, whole blood, specific deficient factors, or platelet transfusions are indicated.

Early resection is indicated for bronchial adenoma or carcinoma. Broncholithiasis may require pulmonary resection—*never* endobronchial removal of the stone. Hemosiderosis may require multiple blood transfusions until the bleeding stops. Bleeding secondary to heart failure or mitral stenosis usually responds to specific therapy for the heart failure. Bleeding from pulmonary infarction is rarely massive and almost always ceases spontaneously. If emboli are recurrent and bleeding persists, anticoagulation may be contraindicated, with inferior vena cava ligation or placement of an umbrella filter being the treatment of choice.

Objective 7 (to allay fear) is the most difficult for the physician, the nurse, and especially the patient. Sedatives and tranquilizers should be avoided if possible, but chlorpromazine 10 to 25 mg orally q 6 to 8 h or haloperidol may be given if absolutely necessary. Narcotics are **contraindicated.** The almost constant presence of a sympathetic and reassuring therapist is usually the best calmative.

32. PULMONARY FUNCTION TESTS

Pulmonary function testing encompasses simple spirometry as well as more sophisticated physiologic testing. Computers can free personnel from much of the mechanical work and many calculations involved, thus permitting more time with the patient to ensure maximum respiratory effort and optimal data input. This chapter surveys the major clinically applicable tests, identifies their role in clinical management, and makes recommendations for ordering them.

Physiology

Normally, the volume and pattern of ventilation are initiated by neural output from the respiratory center in the medulla of the brainstem. This output is influenced by afferent information from several sources, including higher centers in the brain, carotid chemoreceptors (Pa_{O_2}), central chemoreceptors (Pa_{CO_2}, [H^+]), and neural impulses from moving tendons and joints. Nerve impulses travel via the spinal cord and periph-

TABLE 32–1. PULMONARY FUNCTION ABBREVIATIONS

A-aD_{O_2}	Alveolar-arterial O_2 difference (gradient)
C_{STAT}	Static lung compliance
DL_{CO}	Diffusing capacity for CO (mL/min/mm Hg)
ERV	Expiratory reserve volume
$FEF_{25-75\%}$	Mean forced expiratory flow during the middle of FVC
FEV_1	Forced expiratory volume in 1 sec (L)
$FEV_{1\%VC}$	Forced expiratory volume in 1 sec as percent of FVC
FI_{O_2}	Percent of inspired O_2
FRC	Functional residual capacity
FVC	Forced vital capacity
[H+]	Hydrogen ion concentration (nanomole/L)
$MEF_{50\%VC}$	Mid-expiratory flow at 50% of FVC
MEP	Maximal expiratory pressure (cm H_2O)
$MIF_{50\%VC}$	Mid-inspiratory flow at 50% of FVC
MIP	Maximal inspiratory pressure (cm H_2O)
MVV	Maximal voluntary ventilation
PA_{O_2}	Partial pressure of alveolar O_2
PA_{CO_2}	Partial pressure of alveolar CO_2
Pa_{O_2}	Partial pressure of arterial O_2
Pa_{CO_2}	Partial pressure of arterial CO_2
P_B	Barometric pressure
P_{CO_2}	Partial pressure of CO_2
PE_{CO_2}	Partial pressure of expired CO_2
PEF	Peak expiratory flow (L/min)
PI_{O_2}	Partial pressure of inspired O_2
P_{O_2}	Partial pressure of O_2
$P\bar{v}$	Partial pressure of mixed venous (pulmonary arterial) blood
$P\bar{v}_{O_2}$	Partial pressure of mixed venous O_2
$P\bar{v}_{CO_2}$	Partial pressure of mixed venous CO_2
$\dot{Q}$	Perfusion (L/min)
R_{AW}	Airways resistance
RV	Residual volume
TLC	Total lung capacity
VC	Vital capacity
$\dot{V}$	Ventilation (L/min)
$\dot{V}_A$	Alveolar ventilation (L/min)
$\dot{V}_{CO_2}$	CO_2 production (L/min)
$\dot{V}_{O_2}$	O_2 consumption (L/min)

eral nerves to the intercostal and diaphragmatic muscles where synchronous contraction generates negative intrapleural pressure. If the resulting inspiration is transmitted through structurally sound, unobstructed airways to patent, adequately perfused alveoli, then O_2 and CO_2 are respectively added to and removed from mixed venous blood. This feedback mechanism of control of breathing is normally so sensitive that alveolar ventilation ($\dot{V}_A$) is kept proportional to the metabolic rate, and arterial blood gas tensions are maintained within a narrow range. Malfunction of the respiratory system at any point in this pathway can result in deviation from this normal range, and consequent respiratory insufficiency. A disturbance at a given point can often be specifically measured if available tests and known patterns of pathophysiologic disturbances are understood.

Static Lung Volumes (see FIG. 32–1)

Vital capacity (VC or "slow VC") is *the maximum volume of air that can be expired slowly and completely after a full inspiratory effort.* Simple to perform, it is one of the most valuable measurements of pulmonary function. It characteristically decreases progressively as restrictive disease increases in severity, and, along with the diffusing

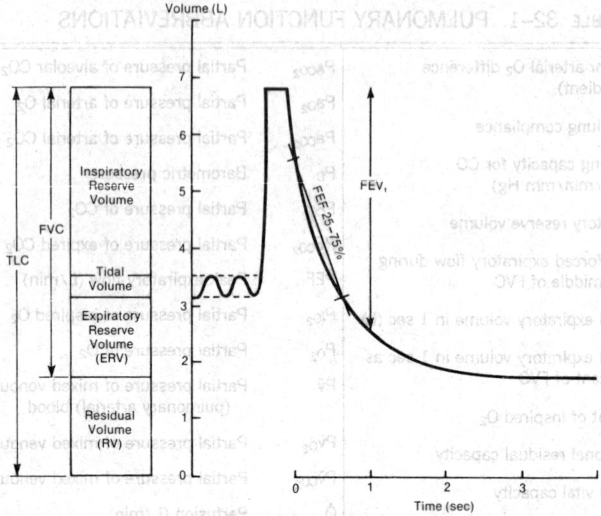

FIG. 32–1a. Normal. RV ≃ 25% of TLC; FRC ≃ 40% of TLC. FEV_1 = > 75% of FVC.

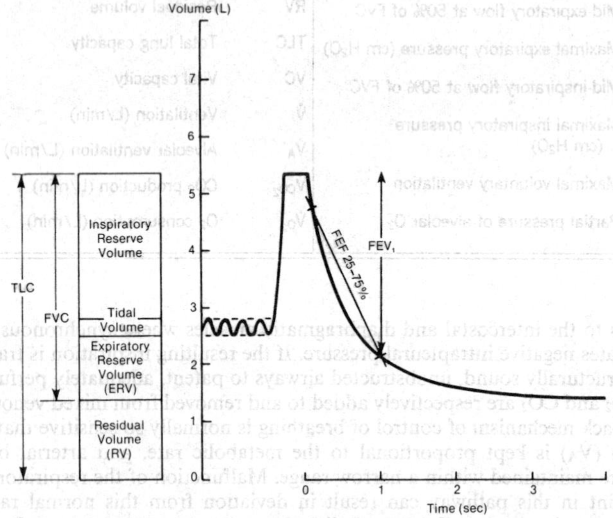

FIG. 32–1b. Restrictive disease. Lung volumes are all diminished, the RV less so than the FRC, FVC, and TLC. $FEV_{1\%FVC}$ is normal or greater than normal. Tidal breathing is rapid and shallow.

FIG. 32–1. Spirograms and lung volumes. FRC = RV + ERV. VC = TLC − RV. (*Cont'd*)

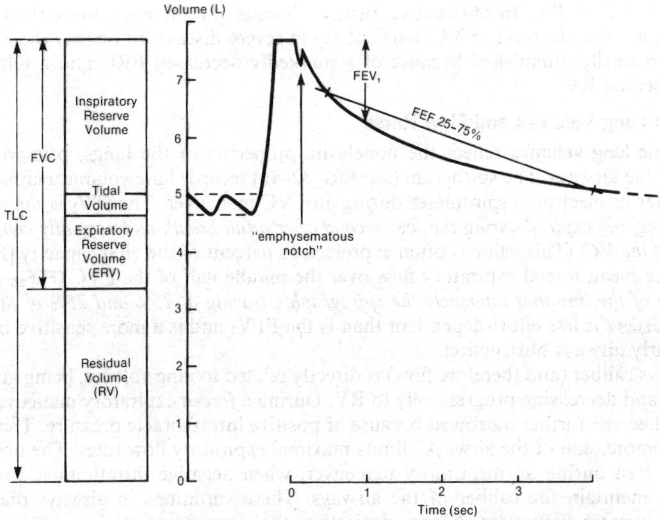

FIG. 32–1c. Obstructive disease. RV and FRC are increased. TLC is also increased, but to a lesser degree, so that VC is decreased. Expiration is prolonged. $FEV_1 = < 75\%$ of FVC. Note the "emphysematous notch."

FIG. 32–1. Spirograms and lung volumes. (*Continued*)

capacity, can be used to follow the course of a restrictive lung process and its response to therapy.

Forced vital capacity (FVC) is a similar maneuver utilizing a maximal forceful expiration. This is usually measured along with expiratory flow-rates in simple spirometry (see Dynamic Lung Volumes and Flow Rates, below).

The (slow) VC can be considerably greater than the FVC in patients with airways obstruction. During the forceful expiratory maneuver, terminal airways can close prematurely (ie, before the true residual volume is reached), and the distal gas is "trapped" and not measured by the spirometer.

Functional residual capacity (FRC) is *the volume of air in the lungs at the end of a normal expiration when all respiratory muscles are relaxed.* It is physiologically the most important lung volume because of its proximity to the normal tidal breathing range. At FRC elastic forces (stiffness) of the chest wall, which tend to increase lung volume, are balanced by those of the lungs, which tend to reduce it. These forces are normally equal and opposite at about 40% of **total lung capacity (TLC).** Changes in these elastic properties result in changes in FRC. The loss of elastic recoil of the lung seen in emphysema results in an increase in FRC. Conversely, the increased lung stiffness of pulmonary edema, interstitial fibrosis, and other restrictive processes results in a decreased FRC. Kyphoscoliosis leads to a decrease in FRC and in the other lung volumes because the stiff, noncompliant chest wall restricts lung expansion.

FRC has 2 components: **residual volume (RV),** *the volume of air remaining in the lungs at the end of a maximal expiration*, and **expiratory reserve volume** (FRC = RV + **ERV**). The RV normally accounts for about 25% of the TLC. It changes with the FRC with 2 exceptions: In restrictive lung diseases, RV tends to remain nearer to normal than other lung volumes (shown in FIG. 32–1b). In small airways diseases, presumably because premature closure of the airways leads to air trapping, RV may be elevated while FRC and FEV_1 (see below in Dynamic Lung Volumes and Flow Rates) remain normal.

TLC = VC + RV. In obstructive airways disease, RV increases more than TLC, resulting in some decrease in VC, particularly in severe disease. In obesity the ERV is characteristically diminished because of a markedly decreased FRC and a relatively well-preserved RV.

Dynamic Lung Volumes and Flow Rates

Dynamic lung volumes reflect the nonelastic properties of the lungs, primarily the status of the airways. The spirogram (see FIG. 32–1a) records lung volume against time on a water or electronic spirometer during an FVC maneuver. The **FEV_1** is *the volume of air forcefully expired during the first second after a full breath and normally comprises > 75% of the VC.* (This value is often expressed as percent of the vital capacity [$FEV_{1\%}$ VC].) The mean forced expiratory flow over the middle half of the FVC **($FEF_{25-75\%}$)** is *the slope of the line that intersects the spirographic tracing at 25% and 75% of the VC.* The $FEF_{25-75\%}$ is less effort-dependent than is the FEV_1 and is a more sensitive indicator of early airways obstruction.

Airways caliber (and therefore flow) is directly related to lung volume, being greatest at TLC, and decreasing progressively to RV. During a *forced* expiratory maneuver, the airways become further narrowed because of positive intrathoracic pressure. This "dynamic compression of the airways" limits maximal expiratory flow rates. The opposite effect is seen during an inspiratory maneuver, when negative intrathoracic pressure tends to maintain the caliber of the airways. These variations in airways diameter result in greater flow rates during inspiration than expiration during much of the breathing cycle (see FIG. 32–2a). In chronic obstructive pulmonary disease **(COPD)** and asthma, prolongation of expiratory flow rates is further exaggerated because of bronchospasm (asthma), impacted secretions (bronchitis), and loss of lung elastic recoil (emphysema). In fixed obstruction of the trachea or larynx, flow is limited by the diameter of the narrowed segment rather than by dynamic compression, resulting in *equal* reduction of inspiratory and expiratory flows (see FIG. 32–2d).

In restrictive lung disorders, increased tissue elasticity tends to maintain airways diameter during expiration so that, at comparable lung volumes, flow rates are often greater than normal. (Tests of small airways function, however, may be abnormal—see below.)

Retesting of pulmonary function after inhalation of a bronchodilator aerosol (eg, isoetharine) provides information about the reversibility of an obstructive process (ie, asthmatic component). Improvement in VC and/or FEV_1(L) of > 15% is usually considered a significant bronchodilator response. Return of these parameters to normal following inhalation of bronchodilator aerosol is diagnostic of asthma. Absence of a response to a single exposure to bronchodilator, however, does not preclude a beneficial response to maintenance therapy in patients with COPD.

Maximal voluntary ventilation (MVV) is determined by encouraging the patient to breathe at maximal tidal volume and respiratory rate for 12 sec; the amount of air expired is expressed in L/min. The MVV generally parallels the FEV_1 and can be used to test internal consistency and to estimate patient cooperation. The predicted MVV can be estimated from the spirogram by multiplying the $FEV_1(L) \times 40$. This relationship holds true in normals, as well as in patients with restrictive and obstructive disorders of most varieties.

When the MVV is disproportionately low in a patient whose cooperation seems adequate, neuromuscular weakness should be suspected. Except in advanced neuromuscular disease, most patients can generate fairly good single breath efforts (eg, FVC). The MVV is much more stressful and will demonstrate the fatigability of weakened respiratory muscles. The MVV decreases progressively with increasing weakness of the respiratory muscles and, along with maximum inspiratory and expiratory pres-

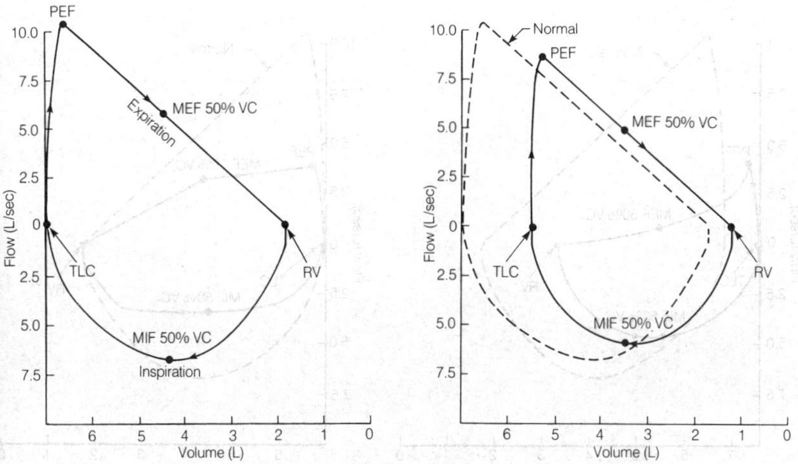

FIG. 32–2. Flow-volume loops. *(Cont'd)*

FIG. 32–2a. Normal. Inspiratory limb of loop is symmetric and convex. Expiratory limb is linear. Flow rates at mid-point of VC are often measured. $MIF_{50\%VC} > MEF_{50\%VC}$ because of dynamic compression of the airways. Peak expiratory flow is sometimes used to estimate degree of airways obstruction, but is very dependent on patient effort. Expiratory flow rates over lower 50% of VC (ie, approaching RV) are sensitive indicators of small airways status.

FIG. 32–2b. Restrictive disease (eg, sarcoidosis, kyphoscoliosis). Configuration of loop is narrowed because of diminished lung volumes, but shape is basically as in FIG. 30–2a. Flow rates are normal (actually greater than normal *at comparable lung volumes* because increased elastic recoil of lungs and/or chest wall holds airways open).

sures (see below), may be the only demonstrable pulmonary function abnormality in patients with moderately severe neuromuscular disease.

The MVV is considered important preoperatively as it reflects the severity of airways obstruction as well as the patient's respiratory reserves, muscle strength, and motivation.

Flow-Volume Loop (see FIG. 32–2)

The disadvantage of the simple measurements discussed above is that they fragment the complex dynamic interrelationships of flow, volume, and pressure into simple dimensions for arbitrary measurement. Continuous analysis of these parameters during forced respiratory maneuvers is more physiologic and can be more revealing. For the flow-volume loop the patient breathes into an electronic spirometer and performs a forced inspiratory and expiratory VC maneuver while flow and volume are displayed continuously on an oscilloscope. The shape of the loop reflects the status of the lung volumes and of the airways throughout the respiratory cycle. Characteristic changes are seen in restrictive and in obstructive disorders. The loop is especially helpful in assessing laryngeal and tracheal lesions. It can distinguish between fixed obstruction (eg, tracheal stenosis) and variable obstruction (eg, tracheomalacia, vocal cord paralysis). FIG. 32–2 illustrates some characteristic flow-volume loop abnormalities.

Lung Mechanics

Airways resistance (R_{AW}) can, with the use of a body plethysmograph, be directly measured in the laboratory by determining the pressure required to produce a given

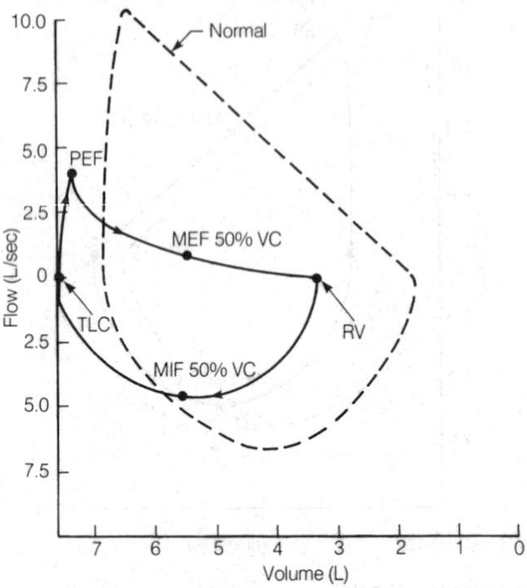

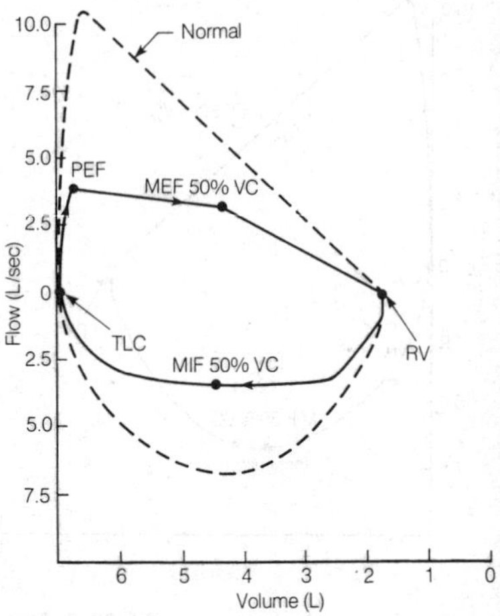

Fig. 32–2c. COPD, asthma. Though all flow-rates are diminished, expiratory prolongation predominates, and MEF ≪ MIF.

Fig. 32–2d. Fixed obstruction of upper airway (eg, tracheal stenosis, bilateral vocal cord paralysis, goiter). Top and bottom of loop are flattened so that the configuration approaches that of a rectangle. The fixed obstruction limits flow equally during inspiration and expiration, and MEF = MIF.

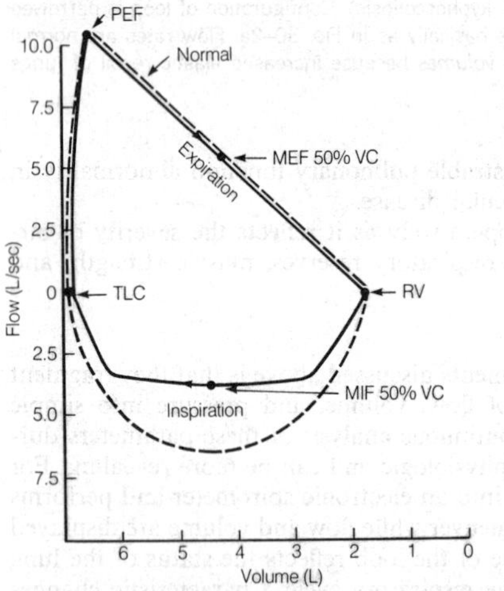

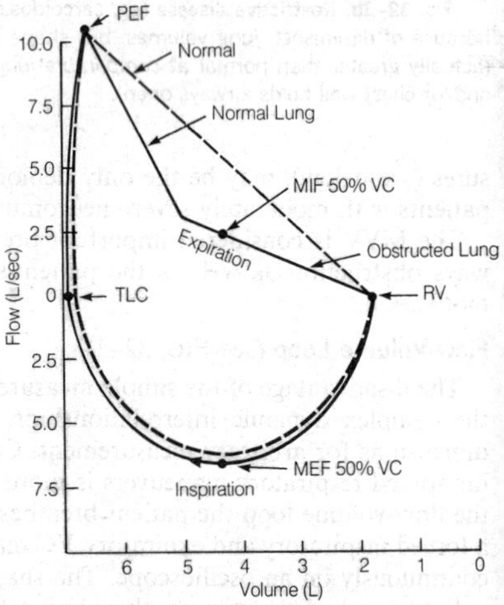

Fig. 32–2e. Variable extrathoracic obstruction (eq, vocal cord paralysis). When a single vocal cord is paralyzed, it moves passively in accordance with pressure gradients across the glottis. During a forced inspiration, it is drawn inward, resulting in a plateau of decreased inspiratory flow. During a forced expiration, it is passively blown aside and expiratory flow is unimpaired, ie, $MIF_{50\%VC} \ll MEF_{50\%VC}$.

Fig. 32–2f. Fixed obstruction of one main bronchus. Alveoli from the obstructed lung empty early, with rapid expiratory flow-rates. Latter half of expiratory limb of loop reflects the second more slowly-emptying populations of alveoli on obstructed side. This patient had a focal wheeze over left parasternal area, and was found to have a bulky carcinoma partially obstructing left main bronchus.

Fig. 32–2. Flow-volume loops. (*Continued*)

flow. More commonly, however, it is inferred from dynamic lung volumes and expiratory flow rates more easily obtainable in the clinical laboratory.

Static lung compliance (**C_{STAT}**—see FIG. 32–3) is defined as *volume-change/unit of pressure-change* and reflects lung elasticity or stiffness. This requires the use of an esophageal balloon and is seldom used. In the clinical laboratory lung compliance is inferred by the resultant changes in static lung volumes (see FIG. 32–1).

Maximal inspiratory (MIP) and expiratory (MEP) pressures reflect the strength of the respiratory muscles. These are measured as the patient forcibly inhales and exhales through a closed mouthpiece attached to a pressure gauge. Maximal pressures are reduced in neuromuscular disorders (eg, myasthenia gravis, muscular dystrophy, Guillain-Barré syndrome).

Diffusing Capacity (DL_{CO})

The **DL_{CO}** is defined as *the mL of carbon monoxide (CO) absorbed/min/mm Hg*. The single breath DL_{CO} ($DL_{CO_{SB}}$) is determined as the patient inspires maximally from RV a gas containing a known small concentration of CO, holds his breath for 10 sec, then slowly exhales to RV. An aliquot of alveolar (ie, end-expired) gas is analyzed for CO and the amount absorbed during that breath is then calculated and expressed as mL/min/mm Hg.

A low DL_{CO} probably reflects abnormal ventilation/perfusion ratios ($\dot{V}/\dot{Q}$) in diseased lungs rather than physical thickening of the alveolar-capillary membrane. The DL_{CO} is low in processes that destroy alveolar-capillary membranes (eg, emphysema and interstitial inflammatory fibrotic processes). The DL_{CO} also drops in severe anemia (less Hb is available to bind the inhaled CO) and will be artifactually lower if the patient's Hb already is occupied by CO (eg, smoking within several hours before the

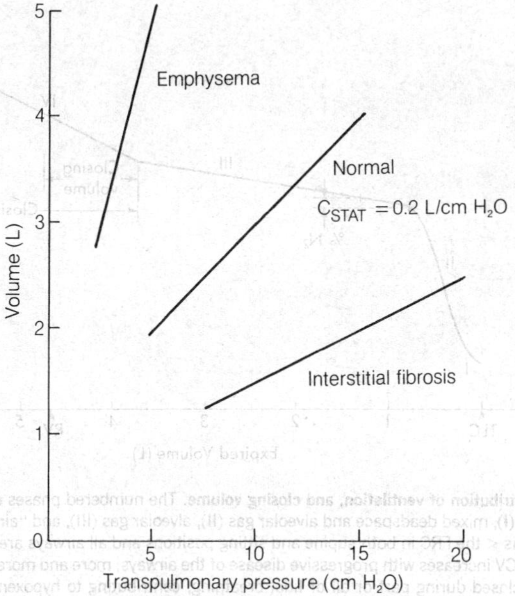

FIG. 32–3. Static lung compliance (C_{STAT}).

test). The DL_{CO} increases with increases in pulmonary blood flow as occurs during exercise and also in mild (interstitial) congestive heart failure (because of increase in blood flow to the usually poorly perfused lung apices). Also available is a steady-state technic that permits determination of the DL_{CO} during exercise, a somewhat more sensitive indicator of abnormal oxygenation.

Distribution of Ventilation

Distribution of ventilation is studied by continuously recording the concentration of expired N_2 at the mouth following a single maximal inspiration of 100% O_2 from RV. If the distribution of ventilation is normal (ie, the majority of alveoli fill and empty synchronously), there should be a < 2% increase in N_2 concentration between 750 and 1250 mL of expired breath (see FIG. 32–4). A > 2% change implies asynchronous emptying of alveoli, which most commonly is due to airways obstruction. A more direct though more complex study involves lung scanning after inhalation of radioactive xenon gas **(ventilation lung scan).**

Peripheral (Small) Airways Studies

Measurements of R_{AW} and FEV_1 primarily reflect the condition of the large airways. In the normal lung, bronchi < 2 mm in diameter comprise < 10% of the total airways resistance, yet their aggregate surface area is large. Disease primarily affecting the smaller airways can be extensive yet not affect the R_{AW} or any tests dependent on this (eg, FEV_1). This is true of early obstructive lung disease and probably also of interstitial granulomatous, fibrotic, or inflammatory disorders. The status of the small airways is reflected by the $FEF_{25-75\%}$ and by expiratory flows in the last 25 to 50% of the FVC,

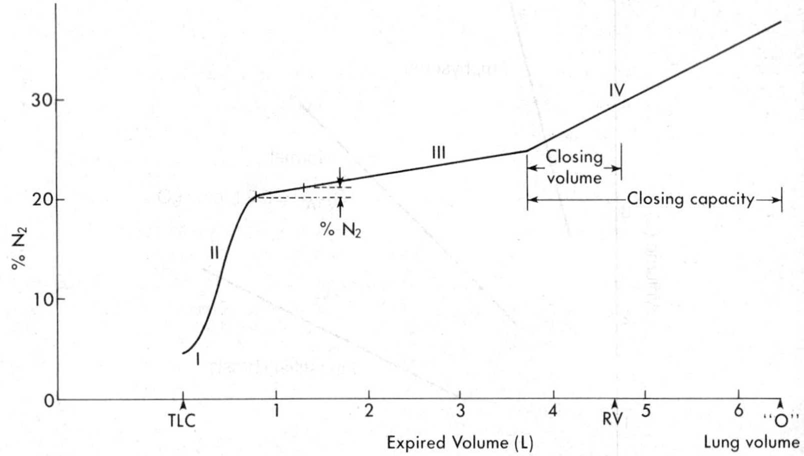

FIG. 32–4. Distribution of ventilation, and closing volume. The numbered phases of expiration refer to deadspace gas (I), mixed deadspace and alveolar gas (II), alveolar gas (III), and "airway closure" (IV). Normally, the CV is < the FRC in both supine and sitting positions and all airways are open during tidal breathing. As the CV increases with progressive disease of the airways, more and more of the dependent airways become closed during part or all of tidal breathing, contributing to hypoxemia. The % rise in nitrogen (N_2) between 750 and 1250 mL of expired gas is a reflection of the distribution of ventilation (see text).

best determined from the flow-volume loop (see FIG. 32–2a). More complex and sophisticated tests of small airways function have been devised; eg, frequency-dependent changes in lung compliance (dynamic compliance), closing volume, and closing capacity. The latter can be determined by a modification of the N_2 washout technic (see Distribution of Ventilation, above, and FIG. 32–4), but in general, measurement of these complex tests adds little to those more readily available (see above) and has little place in the clinical laboratory.

Control of Breathing

Recent emphasis on the clinical importance of obstructive sleep apnea and central hypoventilation (Pickwickian syndrome) has brought the study of the control of breathing to the clinical physiology laboratory. Hypoxic drive (function of the carotid chemoreceptors) can be studied by plotting the ventilatory response to progressive decrements in inspired O_2. CO_2 sensitivity (function of the central, medullary chemoreceptors) is reflected by the ventilatory response to progressive increments in inspired CO_2.

Central and obstructive sleep apnea can be distinguished by monitoring respiration during sleep. An ear oximeter monitors O_2 saturation. A CO_2 electrode placed in a nostril measures end-expiratory P_{CO_2} (PE_{CO_2}) and also monitors air flow. Chest wall motion is monitored by a strain gauge or by impedance electrodes. In obstructive sleep apnea, air flow at the nose ceases despite continued excursion of the chest wall, O_2 saturation drops, and PE_{CO_2} increases. In central apnea, chest wall motion and air flow cease simultaneously.

How to Order and Interpret Pulmonary Function Tests

A "complete" set of pulmonary function tests includes determination of all lung volumes (VC, FRC, RV, TLC), spirometry (FVC, FEV_1, $FEV_{1\%}$ VC, $FEF_{25-75\%}$), diffusing capacity, flow-volume loop, MVV, and maximal inspiratory and expiratory pressures. This extensive testing is tiring, time-consuming, expensive, and is usually not necessary for adequate clinical assessment.

Any physician who evaluates patients with pulmonary disorders should have access to simple spirometry, which is the backbone of pulmonary function evaluation and usually provides sufficient information. A number of inexpensive electronic spirometers are available for office use to measure VC, FEV_1, $FEV_{1\%}$ VC, and PEF. The procedure, readily learned by both patient and operator, yields permanent, reproducible, accurate data. While spirometry alone may not permit specific diagnosis, it can differentiate between obstructive and restrictive disorders and permits estimation of the severity of the process.

With a few guidelines, much useful information can be gathered from the simple spirogram. A low VC in association with normal flow rates ordinarily suggests **restrictive disease** (see FIG. 32–1b). **COPD and asthma** have the characteristic exponentially decreasing flows seen in FIG. 32–1c. In the patient with predominant emphysema, the airways can be intrinsically normal, and expiratory flow is limited by dynamic compression of the airways because of the loss of elastic supporting tissues. A finite amount of time is necessary for the airways (wide open at TLC) to snap shut after the onset of the FVC maneuver. Thus a transient rapid flow is often reflected by a notch at the beginning of the tracing. The spirogram in FIG. 32–1c shows such an "emphysematous notch," and suggests that there has been substantial loss of lung elastic recoil; ie, there is a significant component of emphysema present. In severe COPD, expiratory flow can be so prolonged as to appear almost linear on visual analysis of the spirogram. However, since lung volume is a major determinant of airways caliber, the slope of the spirogram should continuously decrease from TLC to RV. A truly linear spirogram is pathognomonic of fixed obstruction of the larynx or trachea (eg, tracheal

stenosis or tumor). The limitation to maximal flow here is no longer dynamic compression of airways but a fixed area of narrowing in the large airway.

The spirogram in asthma can occasionally mimic restrictive disease if small airways obstruction predominates. Total occlusion of small airways precludes air flow and much gas is trapped distally, thus underestimating the VC. The larger airways are patent, so the overall R_{AW} is not much increased and the $FEV_{1\%}$ VC may be normal.

The severity of COPD or asthma and the potential for response to bronchodilator can be adequately assessed by simple spirometry before and after inhalation of a bronchodilator aerosol. The response to treatment during an exacerbation of asthma can and should be monitored by portable (bedside) spirometry.

As a general preoperative screen, simple spirometry with determination of the FVC, FEV_1, $FEV_{1\%}$ VC, and MVV usually suffices and should be performed before chest or abdominal surgery in smokers > 40 yr old and in all patients with respiratory symptoms. Patients with suspected laryngeal or tracheal pathology are more adequately and specifically studied by a flow-volume loop (see FIG. 32–2d and 2e). **If weakness of the respiratory muscles is suspected,** the MVV, MIP, MEP, and FVC (sometimes collectively referred to as "lung mechanics") are the appropriate tests to order.

Full testing in the pulmonary laboratory should be requested when the clinical picture (history, physical examination, chest x-ray) does not coincide with the data obtained by simple spirometry, or when more complete characterization of an abnormal pulmonary process is desired. Such a consultation is indicated before thoracotomy or extensive abdominal surgery, (particularly in the patient with known or suspected lung impairment) and to document the severity of interstitial lung disorders. Periodic VCs and DL_{CO}s usually suffice to follow the course of interstitial lung disease.

The following tables are intended as general guides for interpreting pulmonary function tests. TABLE 32–2 illustrates several simple patterns of pulmonary function abnor-

TABLE 32–2. CHARACTERISTIC CHANGES IN PULMONARY FUNCTION IN SEVERAL DISORDERS

Test	*Restrictive Lung Diseases*	*Obstructive Airways Diseases*		*Neuromuscular Disorders*	*Obesity*
		Conventional ‡	Central, Fixed §		
VC/FVC	↓*	N† or ↓	N	N or ↓	N or ↓
TLC	↓*	↑	N	N	↓
RV/FRC	↓/↓*	↑/↑*	N/N	N/N	N/↓*
FEV_1 %VC	N or ↑	↓*	↓	N	N
FEF	↓	↓	↓	N	N
MVV	N	↓*	↓	↓*	N
$MEF_{50\%\ VC}$	N or ↓	↓	↓*	N	N
$MIF_{50\%\ VC}$	N	N	↓*	N	N
MIP, MEP	N	N	N	↓*	N
Distribution of ventilation	± abnormal	abnormal*	N*	N	N
DL_{CO}	↓*	↓ emphysema N bronchitis	N	N	N or ↓

* Distinctive features.
† N = normal.
‡ Eg, COPD.
§ Eg, tracheal stenosis.

mality. These are not necessarily mutually exclusive; a patient may have a combination of disorders (eg, restrictive and obstructive disease) that complicates the interpretation. TABLE 32–3 details the typical changes in pulmonary function expected in restrictive and obstructive disorders of varying severity.

Measurements of Arterial Blood Gases

The primary function of the lungs is to arterialize venous blood, ie, to add O_2 and eliminate CO_2. Pa_{O_2} and Pa_{CO_2} are readily determined and reflect the adequacy and the efficiency of gas exchange. The Pa_{CO_2} is normally kept within the narrow range of 35 to 45 mm Hg. An increase in $\dot{V}_{CO_2}$ results in an appropriate increase in ventilatory drive, and in $\dot{V}_A$, preventing any increase in Pa_{CO_2}. $\dot{V}_A$ and Pa_{CO_2} are inversely proportional at any given level of $\dot{V}_{CO_2}$ (ie, $\dot{V}_A \times Pa_{CO_2} = k \times \dot{V}_{CO_2}$). *The level of a patient's* Pa_{CO_2} *determines his ventilatory status; hypercapnia is synonymous with hypoventilation, and hypocapnia with hyperventilation.*

The Pa_{O_2} is considerably lower than the inspired PO_2 (**P_{IO_2}**), and somewhat lower than the P_{AO_2}. FIG. 32–5 shows the changes in P_{O_2} as inspired gas is transported to the alveoli. The P_{O_2} in inhaled gas is calculated as the fractional percent (**F_{IO_2}**) times barometric pressure (**P_B**). For room air, $P_{IO_2} = .21 \times 760$ mm Hg $= 160$ mm Hg. As inspired gas enters the upper airway, it becomes saturated with water vapor. At normal

TABLE 32–3. CHARACTERISTIC CHANGES IN PULMONARY FUNCTION IN RESTRICTIVE AND OBSTRUCTIVE DISEASE OF VARYING SEVERITY

Impairment	None	Mild	Moderate	Severe	Very Severe
	Restrictive Disease				
VC (% predicted)	>80	60–80	50–60	35–50	<35
FEV_1 %VC	>75	>75	>75	>75	>75
MVV (% predicted)	>80	>80	>80	60–80	<60
RV (% predicted)	80–120	80–120	70–80	60–70	<60
DL_{CO}	N	↓E	↓R	↓	↓↓
Pa_{O_2}	N	N	↓E	↓	↓↓
Pa_{CO_2}	N	N	↓	↓	±↑
Dyspnea (severity)	0	+	++	+++	++++
	Chronic Obstructive Pulmonary Disease				
VC (% predicted)	>80	>80	>80	↓	↓↓
FEV_1 %VC	>75	60–75	40–60	<40	<40
MVV(% predicted)	>80	65–80	45–65	30–45	<30
RV (% predicted)	80–120	120–150	150–175	>200	>200
DL_{CO}	N	N	N	↓	↓↓
Pa_{O_2}	N	↓E	↓	↓	↓↓
Pa_{CO_2}	N	N	↓	↑E	↑R
Dyspnea (severity)	0	+	++	+++	++++

N = normal; R = rest; E = exercise.

body temperature (37 C), water exerts a partial pressure of 47 mm Hg. The Po_2, after saturation with water vapor, is slightly diluted ($Po_2 = .21[760–47] = 149$ mm Hg). For practical purposes, this value (the Po_2 of inhaled gas as it enters the alveoli) can be approximated by multiplying the $F_{IO_2} \times 7$ (ie, for room air $21 \times 7 = 147$ mm Hg; for 40% O_2, $40 \times 7 = 280$ mm Hg). Since O_2 is continually removed from alveolar gas and CO_2 is continuously added, the P_{AO_2} is considerably lower and P_{ACO_2} considerably higher than inspired gas.

Since *total* gas tension in the alveoli must remain constant, the greater the amount of CO_2 entering the alveoli, the lower must be the P_{AO_2}. In a patient on a normal diet, the

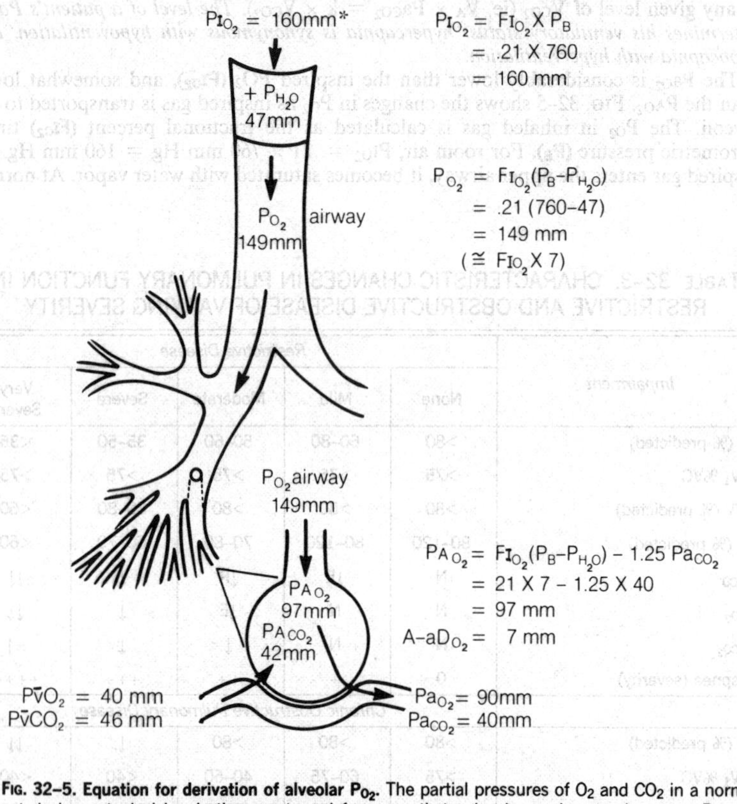

FIG. 32–5. Equation for derivation of alveolar P_{O_2}. The partial pressures of O_2 and CO_2 in a normal patient during a typical inspiration are traced from mouth to alveolus and systemic artery. P_{CO_2} of inspired gas in negligible (0.3 mm Hg). The normal mixed venous P_{O_2} ($P\bar{v}O_2$) is 35–45 mm Hg and is a very sensitive index of the adequacy of tissue-O_2 delivery. If the combination of cardiac output, Hb, and Pa_{O_2} are inadequate to meet tissue-O_2 demands, the $P\bar{v}O_2$ will fall because of the increased extraction of O_2 by the tissues.

Aliquots of pulmonary arterial blood are representative of mixed venous blood and are easily accessible via pulmonary artery catheters in the intensive care setting, permitting assessment of the adequacy of tissue O_2 delivery. Fiberoptic pulmonary artery catheters permit continuous monitoring of $P\bar{v}O_2$.

* All pressures are expressed in mm Hg.

respiratory quotient (ie, the ratio $\dot{V}CO_2/\dot{V}O_2$) is not unity, but is about 0.8, and so every mm $PACO_2$ effectively displaces 1.25 mm PAO_2. For clinical purposes, the $PACO_2$ can be assumed to equal the $PaCO_2$. From the above, it follows that the PAO_2 may be calculated by the equation

$$PAO_2 = \underbrace{FIO_2\,(BP - H_2O)}_{FIO_2 \times 7} - \underbrace{1.25 \times PACO_2}_{(PaCO_2)}$$

For room air, with a $PaCO_2$ of 40 mm Hg, the $PAO_2 = 147 - 50 = 97$ mm Hg. Normal $\dot{V}A$ is about 5 L/min, as is $\dot{Q}$ (cardiac output). If $\dot{V}A$ and $\dot{Q}$ were perfectly matched (ie, $\dot{V}/\dot{Q} = 1$) PAO_2 and PaO_2 would be equal. The overall $\dot{V}/\dot{Q}$ ratio of normal lung is, however, about 0.8. This "normal" degree of $\dot{V}/\dot{Q}$ mismatch results in a PaO_2 that is 5 to 15 mm Hg lower than the PAO_2. This is the equivalent of shunting 2% of pulmonary arterial (mixed venous) blood directly into the pulmonary venous circulation without participation in gas exchange. The difference in PO_2 between alveolus and artery **(A-aDO₂)** is a direct reflection of the degree of mismatching of $\dot{V}$ and $\dot{Q}$, ie, the severity of intrinsic lung disease.

The PaO_2 for a healthy 20-yr-old breathing room air is about 90 mm Hg. In the example in FIG. 32–5, the A-aDO_2 is 7 mm Hg. The A-aDO_2 increases progressively with age, so that the "normal" PaO_2 at age 70 is ± 75 mm Hg. The physiologic decrease in PaO_2 with age results from a decrease in lung elastic recoil **("senile emphysema")** leading to closure of small airways in the tidal volume range, with a further decrease in the overall $\dot{V}/\dot{Q}$ ratio of the lungs, and so to an increase in the A-aDO_2.

The physiologic causes of hypoxemia are listed in TABLE 32–4. This should be studied in conjunction with FIG. 32–5. Inhaling a lower than normal PIO_2 necessarily leads to hypoxemia, without any alteration in $\dot{V}/\dot{Q}$ relationships and without an increase in the A-aDO_2. It is not generally appreciated that passenger cabins of commercial aircraft are not pressurized to atmospheric pressure, but only to the equivalent of 1500 to 2400 m. The PB at 2400 m is 560 mm Hg, and the PIO_2 is 117 mm Hg (.21 × 560). This is equivalent to breathing 17% O_2 at sea level. Hypoxemia is offset some-

TABLE 32–4. PHYSIOLOGIC CAUSES OF HYPOXEMIA

Mechanism	*Examples*	*A-aDO_2*
Decreased PIO_2	Living at altitude, high-altitude aircraft	Normal
Hypoventilation	Pickwickian syndrome, sleep apnea, neuromuscular disorders, drug overdose	Normal
$\dot{V}/\dot{Q}$ imbalance (corrected by small increments in FIO_2)	COPD, asthma, most interstitial lung diseases	Increased
Right-to-left shunting (hypoxemia is resistant to increases in FIO_2)	Pulmonary edema, ARDS, atelectasis, pneumonia	Greatly increased
Impaired diffusion	? interstitial disease (probably not an important cause; most hypoxemia in interstitial disease is thought due to $\dot{V}/\dot{Q}$ imbalance)	Increased

what by hyperventilation, but Pa_{O_2}s as low as 30 mm Hg have been demonstrated in patients with COPD during commercial airline flights.

As is evident from the alveolar gas equation, hypoventilation alone can lead to hypoxemia, even without an increase in the $A\text{-}aDO_2$ (ie, without intrinsic lung disease). If the Pa_{CO_2} increases from 40 to 80 mm, as might occur with sedative overdose, the Pa_{O_2} must drop by 50 mm (ie, 40×1.25), from 90 to 40 mm. When hypoventilation is identified as the main cause of hypoxemia (ie, hypoxemia with a normal $A\text{-}aDO_2$), attention should be drawn to the diagnoses listed in TABLE 32–4. In these cases hypoxemia can be corrected by increasing ventilation, without any increase in F_{IO_2}.

By far the most common cause of hypoxemia is $\dot{V}/\dot{Q}$ imbalance (see FIG. 32–6). In patients with COPD, loss of tissue elastic recoil, bronchospasm, and inspissated secretions combine to worsen $\dot{V}/\dot{Q}$ relationships in the lungs. Areas with low $\dot{V}/\dot{Q}$ ratios result in hypoxemia; areas with high ratios lead to **wasted ventilation ("dead space")** resulting in increased work of breathing, and contributing to hypercapnia. As long as airways are not totally occluded, hypoxemia is readily corrected with small increments in F_{IO_2}, since there will be a strong gradient of diffusion to the areas of alveolar hypoxia. Characteristically, an F_{IO_2} of 24 to 28% is adequate to correct hypoxemia due to $\dot{V}/\dot{Q}$ imbalance.

Areas that are not ventilated at all (FIG. 32–7) but are still being perfused result in right-to-left shunting of blood. Shunting results in hypoxemia that is more refractory to treatment with O_2 because O_2 cannot reach the diffusing surface. Such patients must often be treated with mechanical ventilation and positive-end-expiratory pressure (PEEP) in hope of increasing the FRC and opening closed airways (see Ch. 34).

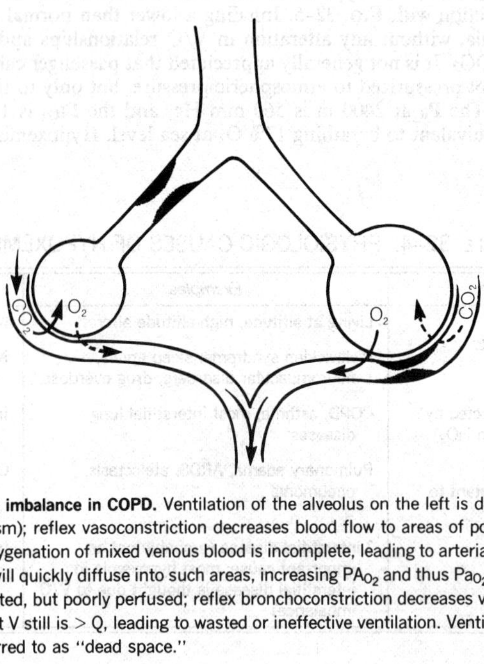

FIG. 32–6. $\dot{V}/\dot{Q}$ imbalance in COPD. Ventilation of the alveolus on the left is diminished (eg, secretions, bronchospasm); reflex vasoconstriction decreases blood flow to areas of poor ventilation, but $\dot{Q}$ still is $> \dot{V}$, and oxygenation of mixed venous blood is incomplete, leading to arterial hypoxemia. A small increment in P_{IO_2} will quickly diffuse into such areas, increasing P_{AO_2} and thus Pa_{O_2}. The alveolus on the right is well ventilated, but poorly perfused; reflex bronchoconstriction decreases ventilation to areas of poor perfusion, but V still is > Q, leading to wasted or ineffective ventilation. Ventilated areas with zero perfusion are referred to as "dead space."

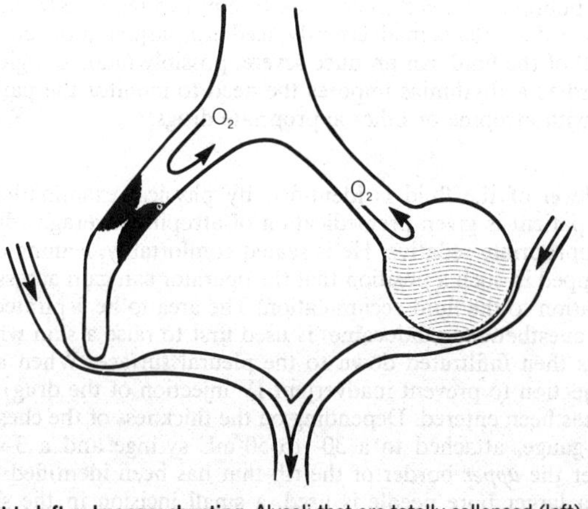

Fig. 32–7. Right-to-left pulmonary shunting. Alveoli that are totally collapsed (left) or filled with fluid (right) are incapable of contributing to oxygenation, even with large increments in $P_{I_{O_2}}$. Although alveolar hypoxemia leads to reflex vasoconstriction and some decrease in perfusion, some blood still traverses areas of zero ventilation, leading to shunting of blood and arterial hypoxemia that is refractory to O_2 administration.

Impaired diffusion across the alveolar-capillary membrane probably is of little significance as a cause of hypoxemia at atmospheric pressure.

---

33. SPECIAL PROCEDURES

CHEST IMAGING

The diagnosis of lung, mediastinal, and chest wall diseases uses the following imaging technics: conventional chest x-rays of frontal, lateral, and oblique positions; angiography and bronchography; various CT technics including injection of contrast medium to demonstrate lung parenchyma or chest wall-mediastinal structures; MRI; ultrasound, and radionuclide scanning of the lung. Thoracic applications of these technics will be described in discussions of specific diseases.

THORACENTESIS

Diagnostic indications: The presence of pleural fluid of undetermined etiology, the unanticipated recurrence of pleural fluid in the course of an illness, the occurrence of pleural fluid in patients with infectious disease when microbiologic diagnosis is not secure, the presence of pleural fluid in suspected malignant disease to help decide therapy, to establish the cell-type of a malignancy, and to uncover a pleural hemorrhage or suppuration that requires more radical intervention.

Therapeutic indications: Relief of respiratory restriction due to large quantities of pleural fluid that compress the lung or distort the mediastinum, and to introduce antineoplastic or adhesion-inducing agents into the pleural space.

Relative contraindications include bleeding diatheses, hypersensitivity to local anes-

thetics, severe pulmonary insufficiency due to emphysema (life-threatening pneumothorax may occur if a bulla is inadvertently needled), suspicion of echinococcus cyst in the pleura (spill of the fluid can produce severe, possibly fatal, allergic reactions). The presence of cardiac arrhythmias imposes the need to monitor the patient and to premedicate him with atropine or other appropriate drugs.

Procedure

The upper level of the fluid is identified by physical examination and x-ray. If necessary, the patient is given premedication of atropine (average adult dose is 1 mg s.c.) plus an appropriate sedative. He is seated comfortably, leaning on a support or, unusually, propped in such a position that the operator can gain access to a dependent position in relation to the fluid accumulation. The area to be aspirated is cleaned and draped. Local anesthetic (eg, lidocaine) is used first to raise a skin wheal; the area of the puncture is then infiltrated down to the pleural surface. When aspiration (done before each injection to prevent inadvertent IV injection of the drug) yields fluid, the pleural space has been entered. Depending on the thickness of the chest wall, a 2- to 3-in. needle, 18-gauge, attached to a 30- to 50-mL syringe and a 3-way stopcock is introduced over the *upper* border of the rib that has been identified to be below the fluid level. If a larger bore needle is used, a small incision in the skin is advisable before introducing the needle over the upper border of the rib, which avoids traumatizing the intercostal vessels and nerve located in the costal groove in the under surface of each rib. In older patients the vessels may be tortuous, making this precaution even more important.

The first 20 mL of fluid are removed through the 3-way stopcock for culture, cell count, and sp gr, with a small amount of heparin already in the collection tube. A second 15- to 20-mL sample is taken for chemical analysis and, possibly, cytology. (Examination for malignant cells is best done on either a cell block of a large quantity of fluid that has been centrifuged or on the sediment obtained by filtering a large amount of fluid through a membrane filter.) Following these collections, the bulk of the remaining fluid is drawn off either manually or with a vacuum bottle. No more than 1000 to 1200 mL are removed at one time. Even less is removed if the patient complains of pressure, dizziness, or other symptoms of distress. The pulse is monitored during this procedure. If fluid cannot be obtained despite positioning, then thoracentesis under fluoroscopic guidance is recommended. Ultrasound and/or CT imaging may be used to direct the needle position when removing fluid difficult to find. Following the procedure, posterior-anterior **(P-A)** and lateral chest x-rays are required to record the change in quantity of fluid and any possible complications.

Diagnostic thoracentesis in a very ill patient can be done with a 21- to 23-gauge needle, removing only enough fluid for the few examinations required. Minimal preparation is necessary with a simple syringe-needle setup or, in place of that, an intracatheter may be inserted into the pleural space and the fluid withdrawn through it. This eliminates the danger of injuring the expanding lung with a needle.

Complications may be prevented or recognized early by careful clinical monitoring during and after the procedure and by obtaining chest x-rays immediately following and 6 to 8 h after thoracentesis or sooner if clinically indicated. The major complication is hemorrhage from needle trauma—intrapleural, extrapleural, or intrapulmonary. Pneumothorax may occur from air leaks through the thoracentesis system or secondary to lung trauma. Air embolism from lung puncture is rare, but may be serious if large. Trauma to either liver or spleen may occur if the thoracentesis needle is inserted below or through the diaphragm. Syncope may occur from vagal reflexes (including cardiac bradyarrhythmias secondary to fear, pain, or mediastinal shift), air embolus, or kinking of vessels secondary to shift of intrathoracic structures.

CLOSED PLEURAL BIOPSY

Indications and contraindications are the same as those for diagnostic thoracentesis except that a hemorrhagic diathesis is an absolute rather than a relative contraindication. For both malignant and infectious processes, the diagnostic yield of closed pleural biopsy, when done with thoracentesis, is significantly greater than from thoracentesis alone.

Procedure

Various needles are available; use of the Abrams needle will be described here.

Local anesthesia, a small vertical incision at the insertion site at the upper border of a rib, and collection of fluid samples is performed first, as for thoracentesis (see above). The needle with a syringe attached is pushed until its aperture enters the pleural space; during insertion the needle aperture is kept open so that entry into the pleural space will be immediately recognized. The needle is angled either laterally or down and gently pulled back until the tissues are "caught" in the aperture. When the aperture is closed, a sharp blade (the occluding piece) snips the tissue sample and catches it in the barrel of the needle. The needle is then readmitted into the pleural fluid, its aperture opened with suction maintained by the syringe, and the small piece of pleura is sucked into the syringe along with a bit of pleural fluid. The procedure is repeated several times to ensure that enough tissue is taken. To prevent damage to the intercostal vessels and nerve (as noted in THORACENTESIS, above), the biopsy needle may be pushed in any direction except upward. After the biopsy, the thoracentesis may proceed as previously described. Biopsy specimens should be placed in sterile NaCl solution or on a wet sterile gauze pack in anticipation of microbiologic as well as morphologic examination. The specimen should be put into fixative as soon as microbiologic studies are accounted for. Following the procedure, P-A and lateral chest x-rays are essential.

The Cope needle is constructed with a hook that retracts into a shield; the biopsy procedure makes use of a hooking maneuver instead of the anchoring maneuver described for the Abrams needle. Otherwise, the technic follows the same directions and constraints.

Complications are the same as for thoracentesis, but the likelihood of hemorrhage or pneumothorax is greater. Careful clinical monitoring and x-ray follow-up permit early recognition and treatment of problems.

CLOSED TUBE THORACOTOMY

(Tube Drainage)

Insertion of a tube into the pleural space through a small incision.

Indications: Pneumothorax, spontaneous and traumatic, is the condition most commonly treated with tube drainage. Massive and recurrent pleural effusions (due to infection, malignancy, chylothorax, etc) unmanageable by needle aspiration also require drainage. Other indications are empyema, hemothorax, and hemopneumothorax.

Contraindications: Adhesions that may prevent introduction of the tube, clotted hemothorax, and empyema with pachypleuritis (a thick pleural membrane) preclude successful tube drainage and require a thoracotomy. A tube is required to instill antitumor drugs or sclerosing materials into the pleural space.

Procedure: The location is chosen for introduction of the tube. For pneumothorax, the anterior chest wall, 2nd or 3rd intercostal space, midclavicular line is used. For pleural effusion, hemothorax, empyema, etc, the axillary line is preferred in the 5th mid or posterior intercostal space. The skin and intercostal space are infiltrated with 2% lidocaine or similar agent, a small incision is made, the intercostal muscles are

separated, and the tube is introduced through a trocar or directly with the aid of a clamp. The tube is sutured to the skin and connected to an underwater drainage system. Sometimes drainage is promoted with a pump that can generate up to 20 cm H_2O negative pressure. A second tube is sometimes needed to achieve more complete removal of fluid or air.

Complications: Bleeding from an intercostal vessel injured by the trocar, subcutaneous emphysema if the side holes of the drainage tube are not properly placed inside the pleural space, infection of the local skin site, and pain are common.

THORACOSCOPY

Examination of the pleura through a scope under general anesthesia.

Indications: To examine and biopsy the pleura when less invasive procedures have not yielded diagnostic information, in special situations to biopsy peripheral parenchymal lung lesions, and to instill talc or other non-liquid materials into the pleural space.
Contraindications: Pleural adhesions, clotting abnormalities, and bronchopleural fistula.

Complications: Bleeding or air leak at the biopsy site are the most common complications. Infection of the pleural space in the course of the procedure is uncommon unless infected lesions are biopsied.

BRONCHOSCOPY

(Flexible Fiberoptic Bronchoscopy)

Direct visual examination of the tracheobronchial tree using a flexible tube (flexible bronchoscope; fiberbronchoscope) containing light-transmitting glass fibers that return a magnified image. Flexible bronchoscopes range in external diameter from 3 to 6 mm; the diameter used depends on the patient's size. These small calibers make it possible to enter segmental bronchi and to visualize subsegmental bronchi. The central channel of the scope permits one to aspirate secretions, give anesthetics, obtain brush or forceps biopsies, introduce bronchographic contrast material or lavage fluid (eg, NaCl solution, acetylcysteine, and heparin), and it is possible to obtain uncontaminated cultures. Cuffing the scope allows lavage of a lobe via its lobar bronchus.

Diagnostic indications: To explore the cause of an unexplained persistent cough, wheeze, or hemoptysis, or unresolved pneumonia or atelectasis, especially in a male smoker over age 30. The flexible bronchoscope is used for small hemoptysis (ie, blood-tinged sputum or small quantities of blood); for large hemoptysis, because of the blinding effect of blood on the fiberoptic lens system and the difficulty of suctioning rapidly through the 2 to 2.5 mm diameter channel, rigid bronchoscopy is used. Flexible bronchoscopy is also used to brush suspicious areas for cytologic examination, to perform transbronchial lung biopsy and/or bronchial lavage in diffuse lung disease of obscure etiology, to investigate paralysis of the recurrent laryngeal or phrenic nerves, to search for the origin of positive cytology obtained from sputum or endobronchial aspiration, for any other suggestion of lung tumor, to determine the state of the tracheobronchial tree after acute inhalation injury, to determine the anatomy of the endobronchial tree, to visualize a bronchiectatic area, and postoperatively to evaluate the stump of a resected bronchus.

Therapeutic indications include attempts to insufflate an atelectatic area or to drain an abscess; to assist a weakened patient in raising secretions; to suction extensively via an endotracheal or tracheostomy tube; to remove certain foreign bodies; to lavage the lung, especially after aspiration of a corrosive; and to identify an acute laryngeal obstruction. For removal of large amounts of secretions or foreign bodies, a rigid bronchoscope is generally preferred.

Contraindications depend, in part, on the patient's clinical state. A few conditions (eg, an intractable bleeding disorder or severe cardiopulmonary failure) are usually absolute contraindications. However, even in bleeding disorders, temporary correction of the defect by transfusion may sometimes allow enough time to visualize the airways, although biopsy is avoided. An uncooperative patient can be sedated or examined under general anesthesia. Cardiac arrhythmias, especially bradyarrhythmias, are contraindications unless they can be controlled by premedication.

Complications: The main complications include laryngospasm, cardiac arrhythmias (cardiac arrest is a particular threat in asthmatics), hemorrhage due either to biopsy or to injury of the bronchial mucosa by the bronchoscope, pneumothorax secondary to bronchial biopsy (especially after transbronchial biopsy), arterial hypoxemia due either to obstruction of a major bronchus by the bronchoscope or to spillover in the course of bronchial lavage, allergic reactions either to premedication or to anesthetic agent, urinary retention or respiratory depression due to premedication, bronchospasm due to irritation of the mucosa by the bronchoscope, and infections of the tracheobronchial tree and lung introduced during the procedure.

One complication potentially useful for cytologic or microbiologic studies is that the almost invariable mild bronchitis that follows the procedure increases sputum production for a few days.

Since the swallowing and cough reflexes are depressed, aspiration must be prevented by the patient's abstaining from eating or drinking for a few hours after the procedure.

BRONCHIAL LAVAGE

Instillation of fluid into a lung through a bronchoscope followed by aspiration of this material.

Indications: To obtain material from peripheral airways and airspaces for microbiologic, cytologic, biochemical, and immunologic examination; and to attempt to dislodge plugs of mucus or pus. A relative **contraindication** is respiratory insufficiency.

Complications: Spill of lavage fluid into adjacent areas of lung may be of no consequence unless there is borderline respiratory reserve. Hemorrhage is rare. Spread of infection is possible, but careful maintenance of wedging will prevent this.

MEDIASTINOSCOPY

Examination of the mediastinum through a scope under general anesthesia.

Indications: The prime indications are to biopsy a tumor of the upper mediastinum and to determine whether lymph node metastases have occurred. In systemic diseases (eg, Hodgkin's disease or lymphoma) both primary diagnosis and staging may be achieved by mediastinoscopy and biopsy. **Contraindications:** Superior vena cava syndrome, aneurysm of the aortic arch, and primary TB of the lung with lymph node involvement are the major contraindications, although not absolute if the need is urgent enough.

Complications are rare. Pneumothorax may occur; local bleeding may be a problem, especially if superior vena caval obstruction exists; infection is unusual; arrhythmias may occur if the pericardium and the heart are touched.

MEDIASTINOTOMY

Examination of the mediastinum through a small parasternal incision.

Indications and **contraindications** are the same as for mediastinoscopy (see above). This procedure is used to biopsy areas inaccessible by mediastinoscopy, especially the

left side of the mediastinum, the subaortic lymph nodes, and structures at or below the level of the hili. A lung biopsy may be performed through this approach.

Complications: Pneumothorax, bleeding from vessels (eg, the intercostal or internal mammary arteries), and infection occur infrequently.

SCALENE NODE BIOPSY

Excision of prescalene fat and lymph nodes.

Indications: To obtain histologic evidence of metastatic bronchogenic carcinoma or of a systemic disease (eg, sarcoidosis). **Contraindications:** Without a palpable node, the procedure is usually unrewarding. Superior vena caval obstruction and other processes that cause congestion and edema of the supraclavicular area may preclude biopsy.

Complications: Bleeding, pneumothorax, and infection are uncommon. Even more unusual is lymph accumulation in the supraclavicular space.

LUNG BIOPSY

Indications: Either open or closed lung biopsy may help deal with an unexplained diffuse process that primarily affects the interstitium or the alveoli; with an infectious process of obscure etiology, especially in immunosuppressed patients; with a pulmonary process that inexplicably worsens under treatment; and with solitary or multiple nodules when the diagnosis is unsettled.

The decision to do lung biopsy is influenced by the patient's general condition and by likelihood that the information gained may modify the outcome. However, it may be riskier to treat a pulmonary problem without a definite histologic or microbiologic diagnosis than to carry out the procedure.

Contraindications are relative, except for a bleeding diathesis. Even then, if the need is urgent, the administration of fresh blood or specific replacement therapy may make the procedure possible. Other contraindications include respiratory insufficiency, emphysematous bullae (especially in the area to be biopsied), pulmonary hypertension, uncontrollable cough (for closed procedures), uncooperative patient (for closed procedures), and lack of adequate laboratory facilities and trained personnel to handle the biopsy specimen.

Standard histologic examination is usually not enough. Microbiologic processing is routine, especially if infection is suspected, since, without culture, many infections are indistinguishable one from the other (eg, TB and histoplasmosis). Provision should be on hand for immunologic studies.

Procedure

Transbronchial biopsy is often used for diffuse lung disease, especially to diagnose lymphangitic carcinoma, diffuse granulomatous disease, *Pneumocystis carinii* pneumonia (combined with bronchoalveolar lavage) and circumscribed nodules when biplane fluoroscopy is used to guide the operator. Although the procedure can be done blindly, fluoroscopic guidance is strongly urged.

Wang needle aspiration is done through the proximal tracheobronchial tree and provides cells from masses or nodes adjacent to the bronchi. CT scan is useful in selecting a site for needle insertion. When the area to be biopsied is identified, the needle is thrust through the bronchial wall, best done with fluoroscopic guidance.

For peripheral mass lesions abutting the chest wall, drill or cutting-needle biopsies may be done. **Drill biopsy** involves pushing a trocar through the chest wall during inspiration and obtaining tissue with a high-speed trephine that simultaneously seals off blood vessels. Generally more than 1 core of tissue can be taken.

Aspiration biopsy: A "skinny" needle (22- to 24-gauge) is introduced percutaneously

into the lung when cytologic diagnosis of a peripheral nodule will be helpful, and when an infectious disease of unknown etiology urgently needs specific antibiotic therapy. Aspirated material is immediately placed on glass slides, following which cytology specimens are immersed in a fixative solution.

Open biopsy through a small incision permits the operator to inspect the lung surface, to select the biopsy site, and to obtain adequate tissue for required studies. Optimally, the biopsy is taken from an area previously identified as abnormal by means of chest x-ray, CT, or palpation at thoracotomy.

Complications: Hemorrhage, pneumothorax, cardiac arrest, and other serious vagal reflex adverse effects are possible in all of these procedures. Occasional deaths have occurred during each of these procedures except for fine needle aspiration. During closed procedures the possibility of air-embolus exists and allergic reactions to anesthetic agents occasionally occur. Postoperative pain and bronchopleural fistula with empyema are commoner after open biopsy.

TRACHEAL ASPIRATION

Indications: When the patient cannot cough up troublesome secretions or to obtain tracheobronchial secretions relatively uncontaminated by mouth, nose, and pharyngeal secretions for laboratory examination.

Clinical situations most often associated with inadequate or absent cough are deep coma with absence of protective reflexes; neuromuscular disorders (ie, cervical spine injury, myasthenia gravis, Guillain-Barré syndrome), chronic airways obstruction, bronchiectasis, cachexia; and situations in which instability of the chest wall or severe pain prevents effective coughing (eg, chest trauma, with or without rib fractures and flail chest, and postoperative pain from thoracic or abdominal surgery).

Other situations requiring tracheal aspirate for diagnosis include the immunosuppressed patient who develops a pulmonary infiltrate, the patient with a pulmonary infection who fails to respond to treatment or has a relapse while on previously effective antibiotic therapy, and life-threatening infection in the critically ill patient with pulmonary infiltrates.

Contraindications and hazards: Laryngeal edema contraindicates the use of any endotracheal instrumentation unless the need is life-threatening. Even when laryngeal edema is absent, equipment for introducing an emergency airway must always be at hand.

In the patient subject to cardiac arrhythmias, vagal stimulation during tracheal aspiration is a hazard that can be reduced by premedication with small doses of atropine (eg, 0.5 mg). $Pa_{O_2} < 60$ Torr, $Pa_{CO_2} > 50$ Torr, digitalis excess, and electrolyte imbalances exaggerate the risk.

Procedure

Tracheal aspiration through natural airways: Care is required to avoid trauma and invagination of the mucosa of the structures through which the catheter passes. Thus, it is best to use a relatively small (No. 12 to 16 for adults), flexible, sterile, disposable, plastic catheter. It should have a side vent at its proximal end or be attached to a suction source with a "Y" connector and have a round distal end-opening with 2 to 3 extra holes on the side.

In the **transnasal approach,** the patient should sit upright against a support with the neck slightly extended. The tongue is grasped with a piece of gauze and pulled forward, and the catheter with side vent open is introduced into the pharynx through the nose. No suction is applied while the catheter is being positioned in the airway. As the patient inhales, the catheter is slipped gently through the vocal cords into the trachea; usually violent coughing ensues. When it subsides, suction is applied *briefly and inter-*

mittently (for about 5 to 10 sec q 25 to 30 sec) by occluding the side vent with the finger. During suctioning, the catheter is moved gently up and down and O_2 may be given by mask.

Bronchial suctioning is usually done during tracheal aspiration. Each mainstem bronchus is aspirated selectively. The patient's head is turned to the side opposite the bronchus to be aspirated and the catheter is advanced into the bronchus. Suctioning is done while the catheter is rotated gently and withdrawn toward the trachea. Suction is released, the patient's head is turned to the opposite side, the catheter is slipped into the other bronchus, and suction is reapplied.

Suctioning episodes must be brief, since they exhaust the patient. A sterile catheter should be used each time, and, to avoid contamination of the tracheobronchial tree, the operator should wear a sterile glove on the hand holding the catheter.

The transoral approach is required when obstruction precludes nasal passage. Proper positioning is essential. The patient should sit with the head maximally extended on the neck and the neck slightly flexed on the thorax (Nefertiti sniff position) or the supine position may be used. A bite block is placed between the rear molars. The catheter is more easily dislodged by coughing during the transoral than during the transnasal approach. Bronchial suctioning is not practical in the transoral procedure.

Percutaneous transtracheal aspiration: The patient's head is extended. The skin of the anterior neck is cleansed, a local anesthetic is infiltrated, and a large-bore, thin-walled needle attached to a syringe is inserted into the tracheal lumen in the midline (with the bevel pointed down) either through the cricothyroid membrane or a high intercartilaginous space. After air has been aspirated to ensure that the needle tip is within the lumen of the trachea, the syringe is removed. A sterile 30-cm polyethylene catheter is threaded through the needle into the trachea, and the needle removed. To obtain a specimen directly, a syringe or suction is attached to the catheter and the secretions aspirated into a sterile sputum collector. A few mL of sterile NaCl solution are instilled to facilitate aspiration. In some situations (eg, postoperative chest surgery) the catheter may be left in place for 24 to 48 h to stimulate coughing until the patient can cough spontaneously.

Tracheal aspiration through an artificial airway, either an endotracheal tube or a tracheotomy, is performed using a sterile glove on the hand that holds a sterile catheter. The size of the soft plastic catheter allows 1/3 of the endotracheal tube's lumen to remain free for air passage. A few mL of sterile NaCl solution are injected through the tracheal tube, an Ambu bag is immediately applied, and the patient is given a few high-volume ventilations (using the ungloved hand) to loosen and mobilize sticky secretions. If a hypoxemic patient is being mechanically ventilated with supplemental O_2, an O_2 line should be attached to the Ambu bag and high concentrations of O_2 given for the few large-volume breaths. Immediately after this maneuver, the Ambu bag is removed and a sterile catheter inserted as deeply as possible. Suctioning is then performed by closing the side vent of the catheter, first in the trachea and then in each major bronchus while turning the patient's head to the opposite side of the bronchus to be suctioned. Use of a Teeman catheter will facilitate entering each main bronchus.

The catheter is withdrawn and the patient is ventilated. The catheter is washed through with sterile NaCl solution from a sterile cup. Each repeat suctioning is preceded by introduction of a few mL of NaCl solution and by the Ambu maneuver.

During suctioning, massive removal of air from the airway occurs, followed by reduction of lung volume and arterial hypoxemia. Cardiac arrhythmias and/or arrest are more often due to hypoxia than to heightened vagal activity in response to irritation. Each episode of suctioning is limited to 15 to 30 sec, and deep inflation with O_2 is used between episodes. Severely hypoxemic and apneic patients are suctioned through the T-opening of a swivel connector to provide a continuous flow of O_2 during the procedure.

Secretion specimens from specific parts of the bronchial tree should be obtained through the flexible bronchoscope.

Complications include laryngospasm, cardiac arrhythmias and arrest, vomiting and aspiration of vomitus, trauma to the mucosa of the entire upper respiratory area through which the catheter is introduced, and infection of the area suctioned. Rigorous coughing generally stimulated by this maneuver may result in torn muscles and other musculoskeletal problems. Equipment for introducing an emergency airway and administering atropine must be on hand.

ESTABLISHMENT OF AN EMERGENCY AIRWAY

Indications

Occlusion of the airways or cessation of breathing for any reason is a medical emergency. After 4 to 5 min of anoxia, severe or irreversible brain damage is likely. Therefore, prompt establishment of a patent airway is essential. The decision to intervene requires knowledge and experience. Personnel inexperienced in intubation technics should keep the airways open by proper positioning while ventilating the patient with a mask and bag until more experienced help can take over.

Acute respiratory arrest may occur in a variety of conditions: (1) in comatose patients, upper airways obstruction results from dropping back of the tongue, improper position of the lower jaw and head, aspiration of vomitus, secretions, or foreign body; (2) acute laryngeal edema secondary to trauma or infection, especially if one or both vocal cords are paralyzed; (3) laryngospasm; (4) severe, sudden, cardiac arrhythmia or arrest; (5) drowning or any other form of suffocation; (6) severe head trauma with acute respiratory center paralysis and coma; (7) penetrating chest trauma with consequent anoxia; (8) cervical spinal cord lesion; and (9) respiratory depression and apnea from drug overdose.

Chronic situations that require an emergency airway are (1) respiratory failure due to adult respiratory distress syndrome, (2) acute exacerbation of chronic obstructive or restrictive lung disease, (3) chronic neuromuscular diseases, (4) exhaustion from any cause for which the patient needs mechanical ventilation, (5) as protection against gastric content aspiration in a debilitated patient; and (6) to remove tracheobronchial secretions.

Contraindications: *There are no contraindications to maintaining clear airways.*

Procedures

Check first for high airways obstructions in any comatose patient. Tilt the head, lift the lower jaw, prevent the tongue from obstructing the pharynx, remove secretions, foreign bodies, vomitus or blood; these simple procedures for establishing free air passage may be lifesaving. If the patient remains apneic, **provide mechanical insufflation** using mouth-to-mouth respiration or a mask and bag. In situations where aspiration of food is suspected, the Heimlich maneuver is appropriate. It is described, along with other noninvasive maneuvers, under CARDIAC ARREST AND CARDIOPULMONARY RESUSCITATION in Ch. 27. All these noninvasive measures should last no longer than 60 sec. If they are insufficient to establish adequate air passage and ventilation, the following order of invasive procedures is suggested:

1. An oropharyngeal airway should be inserted over the tongue. The patient's head should remain tilted backwards. Insertion of a soft rubber nasopharyngeal airway through the nose may be successful in opening the airway when an oropharyngeal tube cannot be inserted. Use of any such device is only a short-term measure.

2. Endotracheal intubation is indicated for all situations in which airways control or artificial ventilation is indicated if free air passage is endangered. It remains the quickest, most efficient, and least traumatic technic for this purpose. Preparation for intubation requires the following:

1. Laryngoscope with the proper size and shape of blade. The Magill straight blade or the Macintosh curved blade can be used. For newborn infants and babies, the straight blade is preferable. Always precheck the laryngoscope light.
2. Proper size and length cuffed endotracheal tube with fitted-in connector adjusted to fit the O_2 source. Always check the integrity of the tube's cuff before use.
3. Intubation (Magill) forceps.
4. Curved wire with a stopper (a guide).
5. Water-soluble lubricant; laryngeal spray is arbitrary.
6. Proper-sized face mask.
7. Breathing bag, such as the Ambu bag.
8. O_2 source.
9. Oral airway.
10. Suction apparatus.
11. 10-mL syringe.

Intubation may be done by either the transnasal or transoral route.

Orotracheal direct vision intubation: Orotracheal intubation can be accomplished faster than nasotracheal intubation and is preferable in emergencies. This approach cannot be used in patients with anatomic problems such as a short inflexible neck, micro- or macroprognathism, rabbit teeth, or ankylosis of the temporomandibular joint; in these patients, blind nasal intubation or tracheostomy is preferable.

For orotracheal intubation to be nontraumatic, reflexes must be absent and muscles should be relaxed. These conditions, easily induced in the operating room, are difficult to arrange when emergency intubation is performed in other settings. Unless the patient is relaxed and cooperative, the upper incisors and the vocal cords can be easily traumatized during the procedure.

When using the Macintosh laryngoscope, the best position for the head is slight flexion by means of a pillow and extension of the atlanto-occipital joint (sniffing position). This position brings the mouth and the larynx into a straight line and facilitates visualization of the cords. A right-handed person holds the handle of the laryngoscope with the left hand (or switches hands) and introduces the tube with his right hand. The blade of the laryngoscope is inserted into the patient's mouth in the midline or slightly along the right side of the tongue pressing it to the left. The laryngoscope is progressively advanced over the base of the tongue in order to visualize first the uvula and then the epiglottis. The base of the epiglottis is now lifted with the distal end of the blade, avoiding pressure on the upper teeth, and the cords are recognized by their pallor and the triangular shape of the opening between them. Occasionally, if the glottis is very anterior, only its posterior part can be seen and then the tube must be inserted while fully curved by using the wire introducer. Pressure on the cricoid cartilage by an assistant brings the glottis more posteriorly to facilitate visualization.

The tube is gently passed at the right side of the laryngoscope, adjacent to the mouth angle in order to avoid blocking the view and the light, and is inserted into the larynx and trachea. If the patient is not anesthetized, the cords may be in spasm or approximated and should be allowed to relax; if forced apart, the intubation is always traumatizing and complications result. During inspiration the cords are maximally open; only then should the tube be inserted. One should not persist if the intubation is difficult but should stop, ventilate the patient with mask and bag, consider the problem, obtain help, if possible, and judge the effectiveness of noninvasive insufflation before trying

again. With the tube in position, the laryngoscope is withdrawn and a gag, airway, or any other object is placed between the teeth to prevent the patient's biting the tube.

Blind nasal intubation is indicated in all cases and may be more comfortable for a conscious patient who has to tolerate prolonged intubation. It is also less likely that the tube will dislocate after nasal than after oral intubation. Disadvantages are that a longer tube is used than for the oral route (about 2 to 3 cm more for an adult), the tube diameter is smaller, suctioning is more difficult, and the procedure is more prolonged. Blind nasal intubation may precipitate laryngospasm and vomiting; treatment facilities for these complications should be on hand.

Direct vision nasal intubation is used if blind intubation fails and a nasotracheal tube is desirable.

Flexible bronchoscope for intubation: In patients with anatomic deformities of the neck, trauma of the face, cervical spine, or any other reason that intubation using a laryngoscope is contraindicated or technically impossible, the intubation may be attempted using a flexible bronchoscope. The endotracheal tube is "run up" the bronchoscope which is inserted either through the nose or the mouth and advanced through the vocal cords into the trachea. The endotracheal tube is then "run down" the bronchoscope until it is in place in the trachea. The bronchoscope is then withdrawn. The fiberoptic stilette laryngoscope is an alternative aid when a patient is anatomically difficult to intubate.

Complications of endotracheal tubes (eg, damage to tracheal mucosa, granulomas, ulceration of the vocal cords, glottic stenosis) have been reduced by good humidification and the use of low-pressure, high residual-volume occlusive cuffs, and endotracheal tubes constructed of nontoxic materials that have been implant tested (marked I.T. or Z-79 designation). These cuffs need not be intermittently deflated. Endotracheal tubes have been left in place for several weeks without any increase in laryngeal damage.

3. The esophageal obturator airway (EOA) has proved useful for paramedics and relatively untrained medical personnel. Patients with inadequate ventilation because of upper respiratory obstruction, but with effective spontaneous breathing drive, often thrash uncontrollably and become combative. If ventilation technics and upper airways control measures are ineffective, invasive direct control will be necessary. In these patients, however, laryngoscopy and tracheal intubation may be technically impossible and surgical intervention difficult, particularly without experienced personnel. The anterior location of the larynx and its small aperture make tracheal intubation difficult, but make esophageal intubation easy. The EOA has been introduced for this purpose. This large tube, directly inserted through the mouth, tends to enter the posteriorly situated esophagus. Holes placed in the tube open into the oropharynx when the tube is properly positioned. The esophagus is "obturated" by inflating a balloon at the end of the tube. An airtight face mask is applied to the nose and mouth area; the tube is inserted into the mask by an airtight seal. Air delivered to the mask passes via the oropharynx only to the trachea, since the nose, mouth, and esophagus are completely closed off. A recent improvement in the apparatus enables venting of the distal esophageal lumen through the mask. Thus, air leakage around the esophageal balloon escapes to the atmosphere rather than to the stomach, avoiding gastric distention and vomiting. Care must be taken so that a misplaced tube does not rupture the esophagus from overinflation of the esophageal balloon or fail to produce adequate ventilation of the lungs.

4. A large-caliber needle or trocar (12- or 14-gauge) provides a rapid method of establishing an airway when the larynx is blocked. This simple method may save enough time to allow for more definitive control. A once-in-a-lifetime experience for

most persons, it is a temporary measure to be used only when all other attempts to establish and secure an airway have failed and while awaiting experienced personnel and adequate equipment.

The trachea should be located and fixed with one hand and the needle then pushed percutaneously through the cricothyroid membrane into the tracheal lumen, pointing it toward the lungs. Satisfactory artificial ventilation can be achieved via a 3-way stopcock or T-tube, connected to a 50 lb/sq in. air or O_2 source (not a flow meter). The stopcock is turned intermittently, 16 to 20 times/min to deliver gas; expiration occurs passively when the stopcock allows gas to escape. Great care must be taken not to perforate the posterior wall of the trachea into the esophagus or to permit the needle to slip into one of the adjacent large blood vessels.

5. Emergency cricothyrotomy (see FIG. 33–1): A tracheotomy is rarely necessary in an acute emergency, and initiation by an untrained person is rarely justified. An emergency cricothyrotomy can be performed by relatively untrained personnel with minimum and makeshift equipment, but it is hazardous. Since patients involved may be violent, equipment scarce, and personnel inexperienced, this approach can be advocated only as a lifesaving measure. In severe facial trauma, or if the patient's clenched jaw obviates intubation, it may be the only alternative.

After extending the patient's neck, the operator should pull the skin taut over the trachea, palpate it with the finger to locate the cricothyroid membrane (or the cricoid cartilage), and make a single vertical incision of about 0.5 cm (3/16 in.) through the membrane. The knife handle or some other blunt instrument is used to spread the edges of the incision, thereby establishing the lifesaving airway. Any small tube can be introduced through the incision to secure free air passage. As soon as this emergency airway is established and the patient is well aerated, more definitive airways control should be achieved.

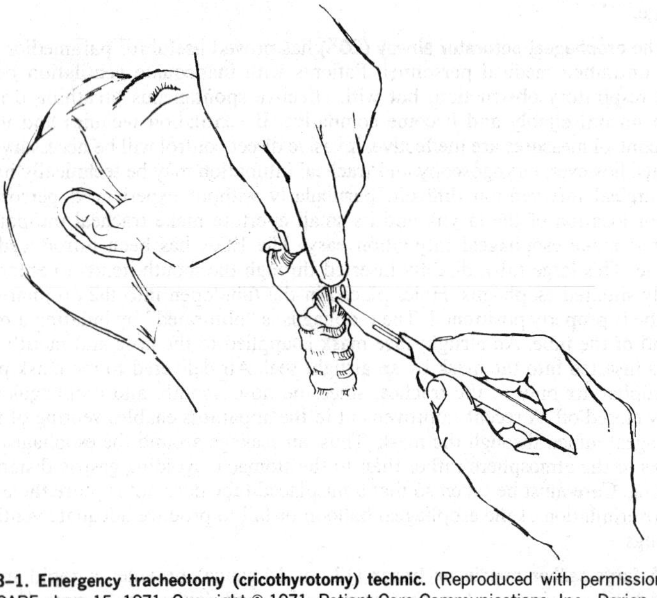

FIG. 33–1. Emergency tracheotomy (cricothyrotomy) technic. (Reproduced with permission from PATIENT CARE, June 15, 1971. Copyright © 1971, Patient Care Communications, Inc., Darien, CT. All rights reserved.)

6. Tracheostomy as an emergency procedure has been replaced by endotracheal intubation in most cases. However, emergency tracheostomy is still indicated in trauma of the upper airway or cervical spinal cord, tumors involving the mouth or vocal cords, and some laryngeal infections.

As a general rule, tracheostomy should be done electively. Though direct tracheal control of the airways by tracheostomy is appealing, complications are common (see below) and there is mortality. It is indicated to obtain *long-term* definitive airway control for ventilation of critically ill patients.

The procedure should be done with a naso- or orotracheal tube in place. The trachea is entered by vertical incision of the 2nd and 3rd tracheal rings. Lower insertion of the tracheostomy tube may traumatize the innominate artery; higher incision may damage the larynx.

A silver tracheostomy tube with an inner removable cannula is used to keep the airway open. Plastic tracheostomy tubes, with soft low pressure cuffs, are mandatory in adults if mechanical ventilatory support is needed or anticipated to relieve hypoxemia, hypercarbia, or both. In small children, cuffed tubes are not used. For a discussion of ventilatory support procedures, see Ch. 34.

Changing the tracheostomy tube during the early postoperative period should be avoided, since the tissue planes of the wound have not yet formed a sinus tract and there is a danger of inserting the replacement tube through a false route with all of the attendant complications. If it is mandatory to change the tracheostomy tube during this early postoperative period, it should be done as follows: a suction catheter No. 16 or 18 with a cut distal end is introduced into the existing tracheostomy tube providing an entry into the trachea; then the used tracheostomy tube is pulled out and replaced by the desired tracheostomy tube, which is "run down" over the catheter serving as a guide, after which the catheter is withdrawn.

Care should be taken to provide humidification, aseptic wound care, and sterile tracheal aspiration as well as to keep the tracheostomy tube in midline position and to prevent trauma to the tracheal wall from the tube's tip.

Complications

The most serious complications of artificial airways are immediate arterial hypoxemia due to airways obstruction during the procedure, cardiac arrhythmias resulting from reflex vagal stimulation via pharynx and larynx, broken teeth, traumatic bleeding from a variety of sources, and aspiration of contents contained in the throat or mouth at the time the procedure is attempted or from emesis during intubation. Other acute complications are gastric distention and subsequent regurgitation, with evident or silent aspiration, and gastric rupture that occasionally follows vigorous attempts to ventilate before the tube is in the trachea.

Further complications include injury to the vocal cords (mainly seen in prolonged intubation), ischemia, and pressure ulceration of tracheal mucosa followed within a few months by cicatricial stenosis of the trachea or larynx. This complication occurs usually at the level of the inflated cuff and is seen after endotracheal intubation as well as after tracheostomy. The use of a soft, high-compliance, low-pressure cuff minimizes, but does not preclude, this complication. In addition, the artificial airway stimulates increased tracheal and bronchial secretions. Occlusion of endotracheal and tracheostomy tubes by secretions may occur and the situation, if not quickly recognized, may be life-threatening. Proper humidification and suctioning can prevent this complication. The tracheostomy or endotracheal tube is an excellent portal of entry for microorganisms, especially in debilitated patients. Additional serious problems can arise from an infected tracheostomy wound and subsequent mediastinal suppuration.

Hazards during tracheostomy are pneumothorax, recurrent laryngeal nerve paralysis, esophageal injury, and major vessel injury. Later complications include tracheal

stenosis from an improper tracheal incision, erosive tracheoesophageal fistula, and innominate artery erosion. When the EOA is used, bleeding and gastric distention are especially likely. With the insertion of a large needle or trocar into the trachea, perforation of the esophagus can occur due to penetration of the posterior wall of the trachea. Tearing of major blood vessels next to the trachea can lead to serious hemorrhage. High flow O_2 ventilation into a perforated vessel can result in air embolism.

Most of these complications can be prevented by anticipating their occurrence. Their treatment becomes obvious as soon as the diagnosis is made.

RESPIRATORY PHYSICAL THERAPY

Respiratory physical therapy falls into 2 major categories: (1) postural drainage with clapping and vibration, and (2) deep-breathing exercises. These modalities are applied by therapists, but physicians must know the indications to initiate them.

For postural drainage, the indications are (1) inability to raise pulmonary secretions due to weakness (especially in the elderly), severe fatigue, paralysis, or postoperative respiratory complications; (2) acute respiratory infections in patients with chronic airways obstruction (chronic bronchitis/emphysema) and in acute lung abscess; and (3) chronic inability to clear secretions from the lungs (eg, in bronchiectasis, cystic fibrosis, and occasionally in patients with chronic airways obstruction without acute infections).

For deep breathing exercises, the indications are (1) before and after heart, lung, and upper abdominal operations; the exercises should be taught preoperatively and used with vigor postoperatively to prevent major pulmonary complications; and (2) in patients with chronic airways obstruction, ventilatory muscle training improves exercise tolerance, promotes a sense of well-being, and appears to be worth a trial.

Contraindications to postural drainage, clapping, and vibration are (1) a recent acute myocardial infarction; (2) a recent spine injury or unstable intervertebral disk; (3) recent rib fracture (although these generally preclude the procedure, modifications of the technics may be used when raising secretions is a serious problem); (4) recent hemoptysis, unless the bleeding is caused by active infection associated with bronchiectasis (however, some form of postural drainage with or without clapping and vibration may be helpful to promote removal of clots from the tracheobronchial tree); and (5) severe osteoporosis.

Technic

Postural drainage: *positioning of the body so that there is drainage from a specific segment of the lungs to the main bronchi.* **Clapping:** *striking the chest to promote flow of secretions from a lung segment to the main bronchi to facilitate cough and expectoration.* Cupped hands are used with fingers held together in a relaxed position. The action comes from the wrist with alternate clapping of the hands; the force applied depends on the patient's tolerance. To avoid smarting or stinging of the skin it may be advisable to put a thin towel over the skin or the patient can wear a hospital gown. **Vibration** aids in loosening tenacious secretions from the walls of the bronchi. The therapist's hands are held flat on the part being treated, and vibrations are produced with the whole arm starting at the shoulder. Electric mechanical vibrators are available and are most useful in the hands of a therapist. Treatment is given with the patient in proper postural drainage position. Clapping is done for 1 min and then vibrations are given on 5 exhalations. The patient is asked to cough if he does not do so spontaneously.

Deep-breathing exercises are used to increase distribution of ventilation and to prevent chest immobilization, with emphasis on prolonging expiration. The exercises are organized according to anatomic segments: apical areas include the upper chest, and costolateral areas include the lateral lower ribs and the diaphragm. The objective is gradually to strengthen ventilatory muscles selectively.

The therapist's hands are placed on the patient's apical area and the patient is instructed to inhale deeply through his nose expanding the upper chest only. The therapist may apply slight pressure as a stimulus. The patient is instructed to concentrate on this area only and not to use accessory neck muscles or his shoulders. He then exhales *slowly* through his mouth with slightly pursed lips. The therapist again may apply slight pressure on the area to assist in prolonging exhalation as long as possible.

The same procedure is used for costolateral areas. The lower ribs should expand laterally, but the upper chest and shoulders should not be used. For diaphragmatic breathing, the patient should flare out his anterior lower ribs. Here, also, the therapist's hands are placed on the anterior lower ribs to assist in flaring the ribs on inhalation and they give slight pressure on exhalation.

These exercises are best taught with the patient sitting in front of a mirror so that he sees himself doing them correctly. It is also helpful to have the patient put his hands on the specific segments giving slight pressure on inhalation and exhalation. Ventilatory muscle training involves 6 wk of daily sessions of sustained submaximal ventilation using the patient's established endurance as the take-off point.

Complications of postural drainage, clapping, and vibration include rib fractures from too vigorous treatment or unrecognized osteoporosis or rib metastases, dizziness and syncope, exhaustion, and dyspnea. All of these except dizziness and syncope may be prevented by monitoring the patient during the procedure or resolved by temporary discontinuation of treatment and symptomatic care.

---

34. PULMONARY INSUFFICIENCY: ACUTE RESPIRATORY FAILURE (ARF)

Pulmonary insufficiency: *Impairment of gas exchange between ambient air and circulating blood*; **acute respiratory failure** evolves when this condition becomes severe and life-threatening. ARF is characterized initially by severe hypoxemia (Pa_{O_2} is < 60 mm Hg [torr]), and eventually by progressive hypercarbia (Pa_{CO_2} is > 50 mm Hg) and acidemia requiring urgent therapy.

There are 3 pathogenic categories of diseases of the respiratory apparatus: (1) those manifested mainly by airways obstruction; (2) those largely affecting the lung parenchyma, but not the bronchi; and (3) those with defects in the regulation of ventilation caused either by abnormalities of the musculoskeletal structures of the chest wall or by primary dysfunction of the respiratory center. In this latter category the airways and lung parenchyma may be anatomically normal. These categories produce characteristic patterns of altered lung physiology despite a variety of etiologies. Certain disorders (eg, pulmonary edema, pneumonia, adult respiratory distress syndrome **[ARDS]**) appear elsewhere in THE MANUAL. TABLE 34–1 lists commonly recognized acute and chronic lung disorders that cause pulmonary insufficiency and ARF. The pathophysiology of pulmonary insufficiency and principles of management are reviewed below.

Pathophysiologic Changes in Airways Obstruction

Diseases in this category induce an abnormally high resistance to airflow in the bronchial tree due to secretions, bronchial mucosal edema, bronchial smooth muscle spasm, or structural weakness of bronchial wall supports. An abnormally high effort (and thus, energy expenditure) is required to produce the necessary pressure differences between the mouth and alveoli during expiration and inspiration. The high resistance to airflow can profoundly affect gas exchange in the alveoli by disturbing the

TABLE 34–1. DISORDERS CAUSING CHRONIC PULMONARY INSUFFICIENCY: PATHOGENIC CLASSIFICATION

Airways obstruction	
Chronic bronchitis	Cystic fibrosis (mucoviscidosis)
Emphysema	Asthma
Diffuse bronchiectasis	
Abnormal pulmonary interstitium	
Sarcoidosis	Hodgkin's disease
Pneumoconiosis	Systemic lupus erythematosus
Progressive systemic sclerosis	Histiocytosis
Rheumatoid lung	Radiation
Disseminated carcinoma	Leukemia (all cell types)
Fibrosing alveolitis (Hamman-Rich syndrome), idiopathic pulmonary fibrosis (IPF)	Pneumonia
	Adult respiratory distress syndrome
Drug sensitivity (hydralazine, busulfan, etc.)	Pulmonary edema
Alveolar hypoventilation without primary bronchopulmonary disease	
Functional: Sleep, chronic exposure to CO_2, metabolic alkalosis	
Anatomic: Abnormal respiratory center (Ondine's curse), abnormal chest cage (kyphoscoliosis, fibrothorax)	
Disordered neuromuscular function: Myasthenia gravis, infectious polyneuritis, muscular dystrophy, poliomyelitis, polymyositis	
Obesity	
Hypothyroidism	

distribution of ventilation to various parts of the lung with differing regional perfusion by mixed venous blood.

The ventilation/perfusion (**$\dot{V}/\dot{Q}$**) ratio must approach unity for Pa_{O_2} and Pa_{CO_2} to remain normal (80 ± 100 mm Hg for Pa_{O_2}; 40 ± 4 mm Hg for Pa_{CO_2}). When there is high alveolar $\dot{V}/\dot{Q}$, Pa_{CO_2} decreases. However, regional underventilation with respect to perfusion (low $\dot{V}/\dot{Q}$) causes decreased Pa_{O_2} and O_2 content of pulmonary capillary blood, a more dire occurrence. The degree of arterial hypoxemia observed in pulmonary insufficiency is determined by the quantitative contribution of blood from such underventilated regions of the lung mixing with normally oxygenated blood. A true shunt of 50% of mixed venous blood (O_2 saturation 75%) mixing with a similar proportion of fully oxygenated blood results in an Sa_{O_2} of 87% or a Pa_{O_2} of 53 mm Hg. Although CO_2 content may rise in underventilated regions, hypercarbia (*raised Pa_{CO_2}*) will not occur if there are coexisting regions of the lung that are overventilated with respect to local perfusion (high $\dot{V}/\dot{Q}$). In these regions, CO_2 is expelled from blood in large volumes and capillary P_{CO_2} is decreased. When blood from regions low in P_{CO_2} mixes with blood from underventilated regions, the net Pa_{CO_2} may be normal despite the presence of significant hypoxemia. Arterial hypercapnia occurs when total ventilation or regional ventilation is sufficiently depressed that regional hyperventilation becomes insufficient to maintain the Pa_{CO_2} at normal levels. Hypercapnia may occur with exacerbations of bronchitis, pneumonia, or status asthmaticus, or with suppression of total pulmonary ventilation due to respiratory center depression by drugs (eg, codeine, morphine, barbiturates, or other sedatives).

The characteristic changes in lung volumes and ventilatory tests in intrathoracic airways obstruction are (1) reduced vital capacity (**VC**), (2) increased residual volume (**RV**) and functional residual capacity (**FRC**) so that total lung capacity (**TLC**) may be

normal or increased, and (3) reduced maximal voluntary ventilation **(MVV),** forced expiratory volume in 1 sec **(FEV_1)**, and airflow rates on expiration at all phases of the FEV (see Ch. 32).

Diffuse Interstitial Fibrosis and Alveolitis

The pattern of physiologic abnormality in these diseases is strikingly different from that in airways obstruction. VC is reduced, usually with reduced RV, so that TLC is also reduced. However, tests of airways obstruction (eg, the FEV_1 and the MVV) are usually normal. Pa_{CO_2} is usually normal and often below normal because of hyperventilation, and is almost never raised. Pa_{O_2}, however, is mildly to moderately decreased both at rest and more markedly during exercise. In addition to $\dot{V}/\dot{Q}$ imbalance, there is impaired diffusion of O_2 from alveoli to pulmonary capillaries. This diffusion limitation is caused mainly by decreased total surface area for gas exchange and to some extent by a structurally abnormal alveolar-capillary interface. Lung diffusing capacity for CO or O_2 is characteristically decreased at rest and during exercise.

Unlike obstructive lung diseases, the major mechanical abnormality is increased lung stiffness (decreased lung compliance) with normal airways resistance. Ventilatory drive is also increased, frequently causing hyperventilation at rest and during exercise, with associated hypocapnia. Decreased lung compliance, increased ventilatory drive, and hypoxemia all contribute to dyspnea, the outstanding symptom in this group of diseases.

Alveolar Hypoventilation Without Primary Bronchopulmonary Disease

Pa_{CO_2} is proportional to CO_2 production and alveolar ventilation. CO_2 production is dependent on whole body metabolism; alveolar hypoventilation occurs when ventilation is insufficient to meet metabolic demand. The pathognomonic manifestation of this imbalance between ventilation and metabolic function is a raised Pa_{CO_2} (normal = 40 ± 4 mm Hg) and a concomitantly and proportionally decreased Pa_{O_2}. When the lung parenchyma is normal, Pa_{O_2} is dependent on the inspired O_2 concentration and the alveolar P_{CO_2} ($P_{A_{CO_2}}$), which is nearly identical to Pa_{CO_2}. The alveolar-arterial gradient for oxygen $P(A\text{-}a)_{O_2}$ in the normal lung is < 20 torr according to the equation

$$(1)\ P(A\text{-}a)_{O_2} = P_{A_{O_2}} - Pa_{O_2}$$

$$(2)\ P_{A_{O_2}} = (P_B - 47) \times F_{I_{O_2}} - Pa_{CO_2}\left[F_{I_{O_2}} + \frac{(1 - F_{I_{O_2}})}{R}\right]$$

Where P_B = barometric pressure; $F_{I_{O_2}}$ = inspired O_2 concentration; and R = respiratory quotient, assuming a normal R (.8), and that the patient is breathing ambient air at sea level, equation (2) can be simplified to $P(A\text{-}a)_{O_2} = 149 - 1.2\ Pa_{CO_2}$

When alveolar hypoventilation occurs in the absence of intrinsic lung disease (eg, in central depression of the respiratory center), Pa_{CO_2} is raised and Pa_{O_2} decreased while $P(A\text{-}a)_{O_2}$ remains normal. Frequently, however, $\dot{V}/\dot{Q}$ imbalances occur in addition to alveolar hypoventilation. Consequently, $P(A\text{-}a)_{O_2}$ increases, contributing further to arterial hypoxemia. This combination is often seen in obesity and severe kyphoscoliosis where basilar atelectasis and alveolar hypoventilation coexist.

The pathologic basis of alveolar hypoventilation in the presence of normal lung structure (see TABLE 34–1) varies from weakness or paralysis of the ventilatory muscles (as in myasthenia gravis and infectious polyneuritis) to acquired or congenital damage to the medullary respiratory center. In most cases except obesity, lung compliance and airway resistance are unimpaired and voluntary hyperventilation usually markedly improves blood gas composition. In some cases, alveolar hypoventilation leads to microatelectasis, which can reduce lung compliance.

Symptoms, Signs, and Diagnosis

Depressed arterial and tissue O_2 tensions affect the cellular metabolism of all organs and, if severe, can cause irreversible damage in minutes. Moderate alveolar hypoxia (P_{AO_2} < 60 mm Hg) over days or weeks can induce pulmonary arteriolar vasoconstriction and increased pulmonary vascular resistance leading to pulmonary hypertension, right ventricular **(RV)** hypertrophy (cor pulmonale), and eventually RV failure.

Raised arterial and tissue P_{CO_2} affect mainly the CNS and acid-base balance. Raised Pa_{CO_2}, usually > 70 mm Hg, causes changes in sensorium ranging from subtle personality changes to marked confusion and narcosis. Hypercapnia also causes cerebral vasodilation and increased CSF pressure; occasionally papilledema occurs when hypercapnia persists for several days and subsides when Pa_{CO_2} is lowered.

Ventilatory responsiveness to CO_2 as a stimulus to breathing is diminished by persistent hypercapnia. This is caused by increased CSF, blood, and tissue buffers resulting from generation of HCO_3 by the kidney in response to the raised Pa_{CO_2}. Increased buffering capacity in the CNS diminishes the decrease in pH that occurs with increases in plasma and tissue P_{CO_2}, as reflected by the relationship between pH, P_{CO_2}, and HCO_3, according to the Henderson-Hasselbalch equation. Consequently, the contribution of pH to the ventilatory stimulus of CO_2 is diminished. This effect on ventilatory responsiveness is reversed when Pa_{CO_2} returns to normal.

Sudden rises in Pa_{CO_2} occur much faster than compensatory rises in extracellular buffer base; this causes marked acidemia (pH < 7.3) that also contributes to pulmonary arteriolar vasoconstriction, reduced myocardial contractility, hyperkalemia, hypotension, and cardiac irritability. This type of acidemia is rapidly reversed by increasing alveolar ventilation by mechanical hyperventilation, if necessary, and rapidly lowering Pa_{CO_2} to normal levels.

Because the clinical symptoms and signs of ARF are nonspecific diagnostically and may be minimal in the presence of severe hypoxemia, hypercarbia, and acidemia, the detection of ARF of any cause depends on analysis of Pa_{O_2}, Pa_{CO_2}, and pH.

Treatment

The therapeutic goals in the management of ARF are the amelioration of hypoxemia and hypercarbia to maintain adequate tissue oxygenation and a normal hydrogen ion milieu. The ultimate assessment of clinical management of ARF depends on analysis of arterial blood gas data. Therapy must be directed toward maintaining patency of the airways and adequacy of both oxygenation and ventilation. All available technics for reducing airways obstruction (ie, bronchodilation, tracheal suction, moisturization, and chest physiotherapy) may be required. Ultimate recovery demands recognition of every factor leading to respiratory failure and use of therapeutic agents that can reverse these factors while the patient receives respiratory support by mechanical ventilation and high O_2 mixtures.

Intensive respiratory care is frightening, extremely uncomfortable, totally immobilizing, and severely limits the patient's ability to communicate. Accordingly, it is necessary for the physician to establish the goals of therapy before beginning such treatment and to reevaluate the possibility of achieving these goals periodically. Not every patient can be saved; those with a chance must receive maximum therapy, but dying patients should not be subjected to the unnecessary morbidity of invasive procedures when a fatal end result is evident.

During the period of critical care, patients are completely dependent and must endure great physical discomfort while feeling depressed and anxious about their chances for survival. It is vitally important that a physician expend time and effort to

establish a personal relationship with the patient and his family, and explain the nature of the therapy, the goals, and the status on at least a daily basis. This will not only prevent or relieve much distress, but help ensure cooperation in the treatment program.

Maintenance of clear airways: The lumen of the tracheobronchial tree can be compromised by retained secretions, bronchospasm, and mucosal edema.

Clearing of secretions from upper and lower airways is crucial to treating respiratory failure. If the patient's coughing efforts are ineffective, secretions have to be removed by suctioning. Upper airway secretions can be removed by a suction catheter inserted into the nose or mouth. If their amount is minimal, secretions arising from the lower airway can be removed by introducing the catheter past the vocal cords. If this is unsuccessful or if the lower airway secretions are copious, an artificial airway is required. For short-term use an oral or nasal endotracheal tube can be used; if suctioning is required for prolonged periods, a tracheostomy may become necessary (see Ch. 33). Parenteral hydration may aid in keeping secretions adequately liquefied. Occasionally mucolytic agents (eg, acetylcysteine) are used if secretions remain tenacious despite adequate hydration and humidification of inspired air.

Humidification: Since alveolar gas is 100% humidified at body temperature, any gases delivered from a tank or respirator tend to dry out mucous membranes and add to the difficulty of raising secretions. All inspired gas mixtures delivered to the patient must be fully moisturized to ensure reduced viscosity of secretions. This can be achieved by heated nebulization, which highly moisturizes the inspiratory stream.

Bronchodilators—When bronchospasm and bronchial edema are factors, airways resistance can be decreased and gas exchange improved by β-adrenergic agents administered by aerosol and by xanthines or corticosteroids given IV. Aerosols can be given by nebulizers either attached to a mechanical ventilator or held by the patient. These agents are discussed in detail in BRONCHIAL ASTHMA in Ch. 36.

Antibiotics are given to control infection.

Oxygenation: The lowest concentration of inspired O_2 that provides an acceptable Pa_{O_2} should be selected. Concentrations > 60%, which have significant toxic effects on the lung parenchyma and airways, should be avoided unless necessary for the patient's survival. Concentrations < 60% are well tolerated for long periods without manifest toxicity. Although many patients tolerate a Pa_{O_2} > 55 mm Hg, Pa_{O_2} values ranging between 60 to 80 mm Hg are desirable for adequate O_2 delivery to tissues and for the amelioration of pulmonary hypertension induced by hypoxemia. Because of the nature of the oxyhemoglobin dissociation curve, Pa_{O_2} values > 80 mm Hg do not increase significantly the O_2 content of blood. For pulmonary insufficiency caused by $\dot{V}/\dot{Q}$ imbalances and diffusion limitation (eg, obstructive lung disease), inspired O_2 concentrations of < 40% usually suffice and most of these patients receive adequate oxygenation with 25 to 35% inspired O_2. Such concentrations can be given by face masks designed to deliver specific concentrations, or by nasal cannulas. With face masks, the flow of O_2 required depends on the given percentage of O_2 and by the mask design.

With nasal cannulas, the inspired O_2 concentration delivered to the patient (F_{IO_2}) can only be estimated. Such estimates require knowledge of the total minute ventilation of the patient in room air and the duration of inspiration and expiration. If the time in both phases of ventilation is equal, only ½ the flow of 100% O_2 from the O_2 reservoir can be assumed to be delivered to the patient. Thus, for a ventilatory rate of 10 L/min and a 4 L/min flow of 100% O_2 through nasal cannulas, the O_2 concentration delivered to the patient would be estimated at $(2 \times 100\%) + (8 \times 21\%)/10\ L =$

37% O_2. If the minute ventilation rises and the O_2 flow is unchanged, the inspired concentration of O_2 decreases. Because of the uncertainties in such estimates (including the admixture of O_2 with room air, mouth breathing, varying respiratory rate), the actual Pa_{O_2} must be monitored regularly to determine the results of therapy. Ordinarily, O_2 flow rates between 2 to 4 L/min are sufficient to raise Pa_{O_2} to therapeutic levels.

When there is a significant degree of shunting (perfusion of nonventilated airspaces) to cause severe hypoxemia, high concentrations of O_2 must be administered to achieve acceptable Pa_{O_2} levels. Such a situation may occur in severe pneumonia, ARDS, and pulmonary edema, and require tight-fitting face masks capable of delivering up to 100% inspired O_2.

If O_2 concentrations of > 60 to 80% are required for prolonged periods, endotracheal intubation and mechanical ventilation usually are necessary. The patient may develop CO_2 retention because of respiratory muscle fatigue. By providing larger total volumes and more favorable $\dot{V}/\dot{Q}$ relationships, mechanical ventilation can provide adequate oxygenation with a lower concentration of inspired O_2, minimizing the risk of O_2 toxicity.

No matter which technic of O_2 delivery is used, the patient's comfort and bronchial clearance demand that inspired gas be moisturized by passing it through a humidifier.

CO_2 retention: When the ventilatory apparatus or its CNS control fails to meet CO_2 production, the end product of tissue metabolism, P_{CO_2}, rises in blood and tissue compartments. Increased Pa_{CO_2} indicates low alveolar ventilation with respect to body metabolism and reflects respiratory muscle fatigue caused by increased work of breathing and depression of the respiratory center. The principal consequence of raised Pa_{CO_2} is acidemia (*decreased pH*). When Pa_{CO_2} rises, blood and tissue buffers and renal mechanisms cause a compensatory increase in HCO_3 to maintain arterial pH near normal. A Pa_{CO_2} even to levels > 80 mm Hg is generally well tolerated as long as it is compensated by an increase of HCO_3, which keeps arterial pH near normal.

In the management of hypercarbia, attention is directed toward decreasing the work of breathing and minimizing depression of the respiratory center. During exacerbations of obstructive lung disease, removing secretions and the administration of bronchodilators, in addition to improving gas exchange, may lessen the work of breathing by decreasing airways obstruction and thereby improving alveolar ventilation. In patients with pulmonary edema, diuretics and other measures may facilitate mobilization of extravascular lung water, thereby increasing lung compliance and lessening the workload of the respiratory muscle apparatus.

A common cause of respiratory depression in the management of CO_2 retention is excessive O_2 administration. In hypercarbia the respiratory center may become insensitive to changes of P_{CO_2} and is responsive only to hypoxic stimuli. If Pa_{O_2} is raised excessively, the hypoxic ventilatory drive is obliterated and further CO_2 retention may ensue. Such a complication is prevented by judicious use of O_2 and is detected at an early stage only by arterial blood gas analysis. This underscores the importance of arterial blood gas monitoring in the management of ARF. If supplying enriched O_2 during spontaneous ventilation leads to a continuously rising Pa_{CO_2} and acidemia, mechanical assistance becomes necessary.

Mechanical ventilators cause airflow into the lungs either by delivering positive pressure during inspiration (intermittent positive pressure breathing [IPPB]) or by decreasing ambient pressure around the thorax (tank type or cuirass ventilators). These devices can be applied continuously or intermittently with or without an artifical airway, depending on the clinical circumstances. For the clinical use of ventilators, the inspired O_2 concentration, respiratory rate, and tidal volume can be adjusted to maintain Pa_{O_2} and Pa_{CO_2} at appropriate levels.

IPPB apparatus: *Devices that force air into the lungs during inspiration, but allow a return to ambient pressure during spontaneous exhalation.* Devices are available in many models.

In **pressure-preset ventilators,** the inspiratory phase of the respiratory cycle ceases when inspiratory airway pressure reaches a predetermined value. The amount of tidal volume delivered during each respiratory cycle depends on the duration of the inspiratory phase and the inspiratory flow rate. The disadvantage of this type of ventilator is that the rate of rise of inspired airway pressure is a function of the patient's lung mechanics; when lung compliance is decreased and an airway resistance raised, inspiratory airway pressure equilibrates more rapidly with the preset pressure limit, thereby decreasing the amount of tidal volume delivered to the patient's lungs.

In **volume-controlled ventilators,** a preset tidal volume is delivered to the patient regardless of the pressure required to deliver the inspiratory volume. Expiration is passive. Controls vary the inspired O_2 mixture, inspiration and expiration time, and ventilatory frequency. Humidification and nebulization are provided. These ventilators are particularly useful for maintaining adequate alveolar ventilation regardless of rapid changes in the airway resistance or pulmonary compliance while the patient is being ventilated. Volume-controlled ventilators are in general selected most commonly for ventilatory support in the setting of intensive care.

Tank- and cuirass-type body ventilators: The **tank-type body respirator** is a large cylinder into which the patient is placed with an air-tight cuff around his neck, leaving only his head outside. The push-pull action of the motor on the large diaphragm at the other end of the cylinder causes negative pressure fluctuations inside the tank and around the patient's thorax, causing air to flow into the patient's lungs. Tidal volume can be set by adjusting the excursion of the diaphragm, and the respiratory rate is set by adjusting the frequency of the motor's cycle.

The **cuirass respirator** also causes air to flow into the patient's lungs by creating negative pressure around the patient's thorax. Most of these systems use a hard shell that covers the patient's thorax. A pump removes air from within the shell in a cyclic fashion causing negative pressure fluctuations similar to that described above. Another thoracic ventilator allows the patient to lie in a flexible plastic garment extending from neck to thighs with a rigid support overlying the thorax only, leaving the arms free.

Choice of ventilator: For continuous mechanical ventilation, ordinarily a **volume preset ventilator** is used, which requires either an endotracheal tube for short periods or a tracheostomy for long-term use. This type is especially useful in clinical situations when airways resistance is markedly increased (eg, status asthmaticus) or lung compliance abnormally decreased (eg, severe pneumonia, ARDS), because high inspiratory airway pressures are required to deliver adequate tidal volumes. (In such circumstances, tank, cuirass, and pressure preset IPPB devices function suboptimally.) Furthermore, in complex situations, when lung mechanics might deteriorate, volume-preset ventilators will deliver constant tidal volumes, thus facilitating the regulation of Pa_{O_2} and Pa_{CO_2} for existing metabolic demands.

Although pressure preset ventilators at one time enjoyed wide popularity in the chronic management of obstructive pulmonary disease and in critically ill patients, their use is restricted (1) to nebulize aerosols when patients are unable to use hand nebulizers; (2) to provide intermittent respiratory muscle rest for patients with neuromuscular or musculoskeletal disorders of the respiratory apparatus (eg, severe kyphoscoliosis); and (3) to prevent postoperative atelectasis. For this latter use other modalities (eg, incentive spirometry) are gaining favor. Pressure preset ventilators can be applied by a mouthpiece with or without a noseclip or a face mask.

For patients with chronic respiratory failure due to neuromuscular disorders (eg,

amyotrophic lateral sclerosis, poliomyelitis) cuirass-type respirators can be used. Although tank-type ventilators can be used, their size is inconvenient. Furthermore, complex nursing procedures may be difficult when the patient is in a tank.

Improved oxygenation: Mechanical ventilators can raise Pa_{O_2} to acceptable levels by delivering large tidal volumes, which in diseased lungs may improve $\dot{V}/\dot{Q}$ ratios. If positive airway pressure is applied during the *entire* respiratory cycle, oxygenation can be further enhanced for a given inspired O_2 concentration. The term continuous positive pressure breathing **(CPPB)** refers to providing ventilation in this way. When the patient breathes spontaneously, he is receiving **continuous positive airway pressure (CPAP)**; the term **continuous positive pressure ventilation (CPPV)** is used when ventilation is controlled by a mechanical ventilator.

Positive end-expiratory pressure (PEEP) refers to the end-expiratory phase of CPPV. After peak pressure and tidal volume are reached, expiration proceeds unobstructed. However, exhalation ceases at a preset expiration pressure that is set by an exhalation valve sensitive to pressure and placed in the exhalation part of the ventilator. If a Pa_{O_2} of 50 to 70 mm Hg cannot be achieved with 60% inspired O_2 using inspiratory positive pressure ventilatory assistance, a continuous PEEP of 3 to 15 cm H_2O may be tried to induce further expansion of the lung and reduce shunting. Since the procedure has risks, and complications are directly related to the magnitude of the end-expiratory pressure, the lowest level of PEEP that achieves an adequate Pa_{O_2} with a safe FI_{O_2} should be applied.

Complications of Mechanical Ventilation

Any mechanical ventilator, especially if the driving pressure into the lung is high, may cause decreased venous return to the thorax, decreased CO, and a fall in systemic BP. This situation is apt to occur with high inspiratory pressure, hypovolemia, and inadequate vasomotor control due to drugs, peripheral neuropathy, or muscle weakness. Positive pressure ventilation, especially when PEEP is applied, may cause pneumothorax or pneumomediastinum, which must be treated promptly by insertion of a chest tube to re-expand the affected lung. Because of these hazards, IPPB and especially PEEP in a severely ill patient is best used by experienced personnel.

---

35. ADULT RESPIRATORY DISTRESS SYNDROME (ARDS)

(Shock Lung; Wet Lung; Pump Lung)

Respiratory failure with life-threatening respiratory distress and hypoxemia, associated with various acute pulmonary injuries.

Etiology

This important common medical emergency is precipitated by a variety of acute processes that directly or indirectly injure the lung; eg, primary bacterial or viral pneumonias, aspiration of gastric contents, direct chest trauma, prolonged or profound shock, burns, near-drowning, fat embolism, massive blood transfusion, cardiopulmonary bypass, O_2 toxicity, or acute hemorrhagic pancreatitis. The incidence of ARDS is estimated to be $>$ 30% following the "sepsis syndrome" characterized by leukocytosis or leukopenia, fever, hypotension, and a known potential source of systemic infection, whether or not blood cultures are positive for a bacterial pathogen. Patients usually have not had previous lung disease.

Pathophysiology

The pathophysiology of the initial lung injury is poorly understood. Studies in animal models suggest that activated leukocytes and platelets accumulate in capillaries, the interstitium, and airspaces; they may release products including prostaglandins, toxic O_2 radicals, proteolytic enzymes, and other mediators that injure cells, promote fibrosis, and alter bronchomotor tone and vasoreactivity.

When the pulmonary capillary endothelium and alveolar epithelium are injured, plasma and blood leak into the interstitial and intra-alveolar spaces. Alveolar flooding and atelectasis result, the latter due in part to reduced surfactant activity. Within 2 to 3 days, the second phase of lung injury is characterized by interstitial and bronchoalveolar inflammation, and by proliferation of epithelial and interstitial cells. In the third phase, collagen accumulation may progress rapidly, resulting in severe interstitial fibrosis within 2 to 3 wk. These pathologic changes lead to low lung compliance, pulmonary hypertension, decreased functional residual capacity, ventilation/perfusion maldistribution, and hypoxemia.

Symptoms, Signs, and Diagnosis

ARDS usually develops within 24 to 48 h after the initial injury or illness. Dyspnea occurs first, usually accompanied by rapid, shallow respiration. Intercostal and suprasternal retraction may be present on inspiration. The skin may appear cyanotic or mottled, and may not improve with O_2 administration. Auscultation may reveal rales, rhonchi, or wheezes, or may be normal.

Early diagnosis requires a high index of suspicion aroused by the onset of dyspnea in the presence of a known predisposition to ARDS. At this time a presumptive diagnosis can be made with an immediate ABG determination and a chest x-ray. Arterial blood gas **(ABG)** analysis initially shows acute respiratory alkalosis: a very low Pa_{O_2}, a normal or low Pa_{CO_2}, and an elevated pH. Chest x-rays usually show diffuse bilateral alveolar infiltrates similar to acute pulmonary edema of cardiac origin, except that the cardiac silhouette is usually normal. However, x-ray changes often lag many hours behind functional changes and the hypoxemia may seem disproportionately severe compared to the edema observed by chest x-ray. The extremely low Pa_{O_2} often persists despite the administration of high concentrations of inspired O_2 **(FI_{O_2})**.

After hypoxemia has been treated emergently (see Treatment, below), further diagnostic steps are indicated. When there is doubt about whether or not the syndrome is heart failure, a Swan-Ganz catheter should be passed into the pulmonary artery. A low pulmonary-arterial wedge pressure (**[PAWP]** < 15 mm Hg) is characteristic of ARDS. A high PAWP (> 20 mm Hg) is characteristic of heart failure. The clinical presentation may resemble pulmonary embolus, although widespread pulmonary edema is uncommon in pulmonary embolus. If pulmonary embolus is considered likely, appropriate diagnostic procedures (eg, pulmonary angiography) should be undertaken after the patient has been stabilized (see Ch. 39). *Pneumocystis carinii* pneumonia and occasionally other primary lung infections may mimic ARDS and should be considered, especially in immunocompromised hosts; lung biopsy may be helpful.

Complications and Prognosis

The survival rate for severe ARDS is 50% with appropriate therapy; if the severe hypoxemia of ARDS is not recognized and treated, cardiopulmonary arrest occurs in 90% of cases. Patients who respond promptly to treatment usually have little or no residual pulmonary dysfunction or disability. Those requiring prolonged ventilatory support with $FI_{O_2} > 50\%$ are more likely to develop lung fibrosis. In most cases, physiologic evidence of lung fibrosis resolves if the survivors are followed for several months, but the mechanism permitting resolution is unknown.

Secondary bacterial superinfection of the lung, multiple organ system failure (especially renal failure), and complications of invasive life-support are associated with high

morbidity and mortality. Gram-negative bacterial superinfections predominate in the lung, particularly *Klebsiella*, *Pseudomonas*, and *Proteus* spp. Tension pneumothorax associated with the placement of central venous catheters, and with the use of positive pressure ventilation **(PPV)** and of positive end-expiratory pressure **(PEEP)** may occur suddenly. Prompt recognition and treatment are necessary to prevent death. Tachycardia, hypotension, and a sudden increase in the peak inspiratory pressures required for mechanical ventilation should suggest possible pneumothorax. Pneumothorax occurring late in ARDS is an ominous sign since it is usually associated with severe lung damage and a need for high ventilatory pressures. Depression of CO due to decreased venous return resulting from PPV and PEEP without adequate replacement of intravascular volume may contribute to secondary organ system failure.

Treatment

Management principles are similar despite different etiologies. Oxygenation must be maintained and the underlying cause of acute lung injury corrected. Meticulous attention is necessary to prevent nutritional depletion, O_2 toxicity, superinfection, barotrauma, and renal failure, which may be worsened by intravascular volume depletion.

While the diagnosis is still being considered, it is essential to treat life-threatening hypoxemia with a high F_{IO_2}, followed by repeated ABG determinations to be certain that treatment is adequate. Prompt endotracheal intubation may be needed to deliver O_2 and PEEP because hypoxemia is frequently refractory to O_2 inhalation by face mask. Intravascular volume depletion frequently concurs with the onset of ARDS, because underlying sepsis is the etiology, because diuretic therapy was administered before ARDS was suspected, and because initiation of PPV decreases venous return. IV fluids should be administered if needed to restore peripheral perfusion, urine output, and BP, despite the presence of alveolar edema, and monitoring of vascular volume is crucial.

The physical examination may be difficult and misleading in critically ill patients undergoing mechanical ventilation. Both hypovolemia and overhydration are deleterious. Furthermore, in the presence of ARDS, the central venous pressure is an unreliable indicator of left ventricular filling pressures. Therefore, if severe hypoxemia persists, skin perfusion is poor, mentation is impaired, or urinary output decreases (< 0.5 mL/kg/h) a reliable index of intravascular volume is needed immediately. A Swan-Ganz catheter generally is used to determine PAWP and CO, and it can then be used for management of volume infusions, particularly if PEEP is needed (see below). A PAWP < 15 mm Hg suggests a need for increased fluids if CO is reduced; a PAWP > 18 mm Hg with a poor CO suggests heart failure and a need for infusions of an inotropic drug (eg, dopamine 5 μg/kg/min or dobutamine 5 μg/kg/min). However, vasopressors should not be used to elevate the BP without simultaneous correction of intravascular volume depletion.

If sepsis is documented or suspected as the cause of ARDS, appropriate empiric antibiotic coverage should be initiated pending culture results. Surgical drainage of closed-space infections should be undertaken. Surveillance cultures and Gram stains of sputum or tracheal aspirates are helpful to detect lung superinfection early and to guide appropriate antibiotic therapy. Hyperalimentation either by enteral or parenteral routes should be begun within 72 h. Pharmacologic doses of corticosteroids (methylprednisolone 30 mg/kg, or equivalent) have been suggested, but their value is not established, and they are rarely used to treat ARDS.

Mechanical ventilation: Most patients require endotracheal intubation and assisted ventilation with a volume-controlled mechanical ventilator. Tracheal intubation and PPV should be considered if the respiratory rate is > 30/min or if an $F_{IO_2} > 0.6$ is required by face mask to maintain a P_{O_2} in the range of 70 mm Hg for more than a few hours. A tidal volume of 10 to 15 mL/kg, PEEP of 5 cm of H_2O, F_{IO_2} of 0.6, and a patient-triggered assist-control rate is usually appropriate initially. Adjustments in the

ventilator settings are then based on ABGs and patient comfort. Sedative drugs or narcotics may improve patient comfort and promote ventilator synchrony during mechanical ventilation. PEEP is usually required to maintain oxygenation while slowly decreasing the FI_{O_2}. An $FI_{O_2} > 0.50$ for longer than 24 to 48 h may be toxic and accentuate the lung injury. An arterial P_{O_2} of 60 to 70 mm Hg ensures adequate Hb saturation, and should be the goal of therapy. Using this goal, and carefully adjusting PEEP, it is usually possible to reduce the FI_{O_2} slowly to a level < 0.50 within a few hours. PEEP of 5 to 10 cm of H_2O is usually adequate, but ≥ 15 cm may be required. PEEP may depress the CO in hypovolemic patients. Correction of hypovolemia is essential. Secondary multiple organ system failure may be unwittingly advanced by systemic hypoperfusion resulting from the combination of volume depletion and PEEP.

Weaning readiness is based on continued evidence of improved lung function, shown by a decreasing need for O_2 and PEEP, improvement of x-ray findings, and resolution of tachypnea. In patients without previous underlying lung disease, weaning can usually be accomplished smoothly; difficulty in weaning may indicate an untreated or new site of infection, overhydration, bronchospasm, or poor nutritional status causing respiratory muscle weakness. If these factors are recognized and treated, successful weaning can usually be accomplished either by decreasing the mechanical rate using intermittent mechanical ventilation or by trials of spontaneous breathing of progressively longer duration using a T-piece attached to the endotracheal tube.

---

36. AIRWAYS OBSTRUCTION

BRONCHIAL ASTHMA

A reversible obstructive lung disorder characterized by increased responsiveness of the airways.

Etiology

Bronchial asthma can occur secondarily to a variety of stimuli. The underlying mechanisms are unknown, but inherited or acquired imbalance of adrenergic and cholinergic control of airways diameter has been implicated (see Pathophysiology and Pathology, below). Persons manifesting such imbalance have hyperreactive bronchi and, even without symptoms, bronchoconstriction may be present. Overt asthma attacks may occur when such persons are subjected to various stresses, such as viral respiratory infection, exercise, emotional upset, nonspecific factors (eg, changes in barometric pressure or temperature), inhalation of cold air or irritants (eg, gasoline fumes, fresh paint and noxious odors, or cigarette smoke), exposure to specific allergens, and ingestion of aspirin or sulfites in sensitive individuals. Psychologic factors may aggravate an asthmatic attack but are not assigned a primary etiologic role.

Persons whose asthma is precipitated by allergens (most commonly airborne pollens and molds, house dust, animal danders) and whose symptoms are IgE-mediated are said to have allergic or "**extrinsic asthma.**" They account for about 10 to 20% of adult asthmatics; in another 30 to 50%, symptomatic episodes seem to be triggered by nonallergenic factors (eg, infection, irritants, emotional factors), and these patients are said to have nonallergic or "**intrinsic asthma.**" In many persons, both allergenic and nonallergenic factors are significant. Allergy is said to be a more important factor in children than in adults, but the evidence is inconclusive.

Pathophysiology and Pathology

Asthmatic attacks are characterized by narrowing of large and small airways due to spasm of bronchial smooth muscle, edema and inflammation of the bronchial mucosa,

and production of tenacious mucus. The role of inflammation in the perpetuation of the abnormal airway responses (late-phase reaction) is only now being appreciated. Airways obstruction causes hypoventilation in some lung areas, and continued blood flow to these areas leads to a ventilation/perfusion imbalance resulting in hypoxemia. Arterial hypoxemia is almost always present in attacks severe enough to require medical attention. Hyperventilation occurs early in the attack and results in a decrease in Pa_{CO_2}. As the attack progresses, the patient's capacity to compensate by hyperventilation of unobstructed areas of the lung is further impaired by more extensive airways narrowing and muscular fatigue. Arterial hypoxemia worsens and Pa_{CO_2} begins to rise, leading to respiratory acidosis. At this point, the patient is said to be in respiratory failure, stage IV of an acute attack (see TABLE 36–1).

Early in the acute attack, there may be just a modest decrease in the maximal mid-expiratory flow (**$FEF_{25-75\%}$**). As the attack progresses, the forced vital capacity (**FVC**) and the forced expiratory volume during the first second (**FEV_1**) progressively decrease; associated air trapping and increased residual volume result in hyperinflation of the lungs. Abnormalities in flow rates have been shown to persist *many weeks* after an acute attack.

Mechanisms underlying the bronchoconstriction described above are not well defined. However, an imbalance between β-adrenergic and cholinergic control of airways diameter has been proposed, based on some of the following facts: (1) Increased cholinergic responsiveness is suggested because most asthmatics respond excessively with bronchoconstriction after inhalation of cholinergic agents (eg, methacholine) and because atropine and its derivatives can often partially block irritant-induced bronchoconstriction. (2) There is biochemical evidence of decreased β-adrenergic receptor responsiveness in many asthmatics. Recent studies show decreased numbers of β-receptors in peripheral WBCs of asthmatics compared to controls. The role that treatment with adrenergic drugs may play in the pathogenesis of these findings is still

TABLE 36–1. STAGING OF THE SEVERITY OF AN ACUTE ASTHMA ATTACK

Stage	*Symptoms and Signs*	*FEV_1 or FVC*	*pH*	*Pa_{O_2}*	*Pa_{CO_2}*
I (mild)	Mild dyspnea; diffuse wheezes; adequate air exchange	50–80% of N*	N or Sl. ↑	occasionally N or most often ↓	N or ↓
II (moderate)	Respiratory distress at rest; hyperpnea; use of accessory muscles; marked wheezes; air exchange N or ↓	50% N	N or ↑	↓	generally ↓
III (severe)	Marked respiratory distress; cyanosis; use of accessory muscles; marked wheezes or absent breath sounds; check for pulsus paradoxus 20–30 mm Hg	25% N	Most often ↓	↓	N or ↑
IV (respiratory failure)	Severe respiratory distress; lethargy; confusion; prominent pulsus paradoxus 30–50 mm Hg; use of accessory muscles	10% N	↓↓	↓	↑↑

* N = normal.

unclear. (3) An asthma attack may be provoked by administration of a β-adrenergic blocker. Recently, in about 8% of asthmatics, autoantibodies to the B_2 receptor have been found that may contribute to the severity of asthma.

The observed abnormalities in adrenergic and cholinergic functions in asthma appear to be controlled by the cyclic 3′,5′-adenosine monophosphate **(cyclic AMP [cAMP])**—cyclic 3′,5′-guanosine monophosphate **(cyclic GMP [cGMP])** systems within various tissues (eg, mast cells, smooth muscle, and mucus-secreting cells). The intracellular concentration of cAMP is a principal determinant of both smooth muscle relaxation and inhibition of IgE-induced release of several chemical mediators; eg, (1) histamine, which causes bronchoconstriction (either directly or by cholinergic reflex action) and increases exocrine secretion, and (2) a low mol wt substance known as eosinophil chemotactic factor of anaphylaxis. Neutrophil chemotactic factor is a mediator of exercise-induced asthma. Leukotrienes (LTC_4, LTD_4, LTE_4), products of the lipoxygenase pathway of arachidonic acid metabolism, are potent bronchoconstrictors that also promote edema and stimulate secretion of mucus. Prostaglandins of the E series and drugs that stimulate β-adrenergic receptors lead to formation of intracellular cAMP and thus inhibit bronchoconstrictive mediator release and cause smooth muscle relaxation. Cholinergic stimulation facilitates mediator release associated with increases in intracellular cGMP.

These mechanisms explain some pathophysiologic aberrations, but the relative importance of each mediator and the degree of autonomic imbalance cannot be defined in an individual asthmatic. However, the concepts are important, because most drugs used to treat asthma have profound effects on the cyclic nucleotide systems.

Pathologic findings in patients who died of status asthmaticus frequently have shown extensive mucus plugs obstructing both large and small airways. The bronchial walls show mucosal edema, thickening of the muscularis layer and basement membrane, and infiltration with eosinophils; mast cells are decreased.

Symptoms and Signs

The symptoms of persons with asthma differ greatly in frequency and degree. Some have an occasional episode that is mild and brief; otherwise they are symptom-free. Others have mild coughing and wheezing much of the time, punctuated by severe exacerbations of symptoms following exposure to known allergens, viral infections, exercise, or nonspecific irritants. Psychosocial stress may precipitate an attack or may be additive with noxious exposures.

Children, in particular, may notice an itching sensation over the anterior neck or upper chest as an early sign of an impending attack, and dry cough, particularly at night and with exercise, may be the sole presenting symptom, especially in children. However, an asthma attack usually begins acutely with paroxysms of wheezing, coughing, and shortness of breath, or insidiously with slowly increasing symptoms and signs of respiratory distress. In either case, the patient usually first notices the onset of dyspnea, tachypnea, cough, and tightness or pressure in the chest, and may even notice audible wheezes. The episode may subside quickly or persist for hours to days. Pulmonary function abnormalities (see under Laboratory Findings, below), may persist for weeks after an acute attack, even in asymptomatic patients.

The cough during an acute attack sounds "tight" and is generally nonproductive of mucus. Except in young children, who rarely expectorate, tenacious mucoid sputum is produced as the attack subsides.

On physical examination during the acute asthmatic attack, the patient exhibits varying degrees of respiratory distress, depending on the severity and duration of the episode. Tachypnea, tachycardia, and audible wheezes are frequently present. Variable degrees of dehydration may occur during prolonged episodes because of sweating and increased insensible water loss from the lungs secondary to tachypnea. The patient

prefers to sit upright or even leans forward, uses accessory muscles of respiration, is anxious, and may appear to struggle for air. Chest examination shows a prolonged expiratory phase with relatively high-pitched wheezes throughout inspiration and most of expiration. The chest may appear quite hyperinflated due to air trapping. Although coarse rhonchi may accompany the wheezes, fine "wet" rales are not heard unless pneumonia, atelectasis, or cardiac decompensation is also present.

In more severe episodes, the patient may be unable to speak more than a few words without stopping for breath. Fatigue and severe distress are evident in rapid, shallow, ineffectual respiratory movements. Cyanosis becomes evident as the attack worsens. Confusion and lethargy may indicate the onset of progressive respiratory failure with CO_2 narcosis. In such individuals, it is not unusual to hear *less* wheezing on auscultation, because the extensive mucous plugging of airways and patient fatigue results in marked reduction of air flow and gas exchange. In an asthmatic with a quiet-sounding chest, an inexperienced examiner may incorrectly attribute the anxiety and respiratory distress to emotional factors or underestimate the severity of obstruction. Such a patient may actually have a more severe problem than a patient with audible wheezes. Extensive small airways obstruction may be present with few auscultatory findings.

Thus, the presence, absence, or prominence of wheezes does not correlate precisely with the severity of an asthma attack. The most reliable signs include the degree of dyspnea at rest, cyanosis, difficulty in talking, pulsus paradoxus of > 20 to 30 mm Hg, and the use of accessory muscles of respiration. The severity of an attack can be most precisely assessed by blood gas determinations.

Between acute attacks, breath sounds may be normal during quiet respiration. However, rales or fine wheezes may be heard during forced expiration or after the patient exercises. Low-grade to moderate wheezing may be heard at any time in some patients even when the patient claims to be completely asymptomatic. With longstanding severe asthma, especially if dating from childhood, there may be evidence of secondary effects of chronic hyperinflation on the chest wall (eg, "squared off" thorax, anterior bowing of the sternum, and depressed diaphragm).

Complications

Pneumothorax may occur during an acute asthma attack; it presents as a sudden worsening of respiratory distress, accompanied by sharp chest pains and, on physical examination, a shift of the mediastinum. X-ray examination confirms the diagnosis. **Mediastinal and subcutaneous emphysema** due to alveolar rupture and dissection of air along vessels is occasionally observed during an asthmatic attack. **Atelectasis,** usually involving the right middle lobe or even an entire lung, is more common. Unless the collapse involves a substantial amount of lung tissue, the atelectasis is usually only diagnosed as a result of x-ray examination. **Bronchiectasis** is rare. While evidence of acute **cor pulmonale** can occasionally be obtained on an ECG during a severe episode of asthma, chronic cor pulmonale secondary to asthma is rare. Contrary to popular opinion, uncomplicated asthma rarely leads to chronic obstructive emphysema, especially in a nonsmoker.

Laboratory Findings

Blood cell examination: Eosinophilia is commonly present in asthma regardless of whether allergic factors can be shown to have an etiologic role. Blood eosinophilia > 250 to 400 cells/μL is the rule; in many asthmatics, the degree of eosinophilia may correlate with the asthma's severity. The extent to which eosinophilia can be suppressed with corticosteroids (as measured by total eosinophil counts) has been used as an index of the adequacy of dosage of these agents.

Determination of **arterial blood gases and pH** is essential to the adequate evaluation of a patient with asthma of sufficient severity to warrant hospitalization. (See TABLE 36–1 and Ch. 34.)

Sputum in a patient with uncomplicated asthma is highly distinctive. Grossly, it is tenacious, rubbery, and whitish; in the presence of infection, particularly in adults, it may be yellowish. Many eosinophils are found microscopically, frequently arranged in sheets; large numbers of histiocytes and polymorphonuclear leukocytes are also present. Eosinophilic granules from disrupted cells may be seen throughout the sputum smear. Elongated dipyramidal crystals **(Charcot-Leyden)** originating from eosinophils are commonly found. When infection is present, and particularly when there is a bronchitic element, polymorphonuclear leukocytes and bacteria predominate. In uncomplicated asthma, sputum cultures rarely reveal pathogenic bacteria.

Chest x-ray findings vary from normal to hyperinflation. Lung markings are commonly increased, particularly in chronic disease. Atelectasis, most often involving the right middle lobe, is common in children and may be recurrent. Small segmental areas of atelectasis, often observed during acute exacerbations of asthma, may be misinterpreted as pneumonitis. However, the rapidity with which these areas clear suggests atelectasis rather than pneumonitis. An esophagram should be considered part of the evaluation of an infant or young child with suspected asthma to rule out congenital anomalies, which might cause symptoms and signs of airways obstruction. Inspiratory and expiratory chest x-rays are helpful to diagnose foreign-body aspiration as a cause of wheezing in children. The expiratory film will show impairment of exit of air from the affected lung. The expiratory x-rays are especially important in the case of nonopaque foreign bodies.

Pulmonary function tests (see also Ch. 32, above) are valuable in differential diagnosis, and also in known asthmatics to assess the degree of airways obstruction and disturbance in gas exchange, to measure the airways' response to inhaled allergens and chemicals (bronchial provocation testing), to quantify the response to drugs, and for long-term follow-up. Pulmonary function testing is most valuable when performed before and after giving an aerosolized bronchodilator to determine the degree of reversibility of the airways obstruction.

Static lung volumes and capacities reveal various combinations of abnormalities; no abnormalities may be detected in mild cases in remission, however. Of the tests most often used clinically, total lung capacity **(TLC)**, functional residual capacity **(FRC)**, and residual volume **(RV)** are usually increased. Vital capacity **(VC)** may be normal or decreased.

Dynamic lung volumes and capacities, an index of airways obstruction, are reduced in asthmatics and return towards normal after administration of an aerosolized bronchodilator. In mild, asymptomatic asthmatics. these tests may be normal. Since expiratory flow is determined not only by the diameter of the airways but also by the elastic recoil forces of the lung, flow at high lung volumes will exceed flow at low lung volumes. Tests that measure flow at relatively large lung volumes (forced expiratory volume in 0.5 sec **[$FEV_{0.5}$]** and peak expiratory flow **[PEF]** are, to a considerable degree, effort-dependent and are less satisfactory than tests that measure flow over a larger range of lung volume. These include FEV_1 and the mean forced-expiratory flow **($FEF_{25-75\%}$)** measured between 25 and 75% of the FVC. The $FEF_{25-75\%}$ is of particular value since it is considered to reflect small airways obstruction. Expiratory flow measurements at large lung volumes are insensitive to changes in peripheral airways resistance and reflect abnormalities principally in central airways. The expiratory flow-volume curve, in which expired lung volume is plotted against flow rate, is probably of greatest value; this curve gives a graphic picture of flow at large and small lung volumes and presumably, therefore, reveals abnormalities in both central and peripheral airways (see FIG. 32–2c above in Ch. 32). In the past, probably too much was made of these distinctions. The FEV_1 provides most of the information needed to manage a patient with asthma.

Distribution of ventilation is frequently abnormal in patients with asthma; ie, various lung units fill and empty asynchronously. This maldistribution is quantified by the

single-breath N_2 test and the 7-min N_2 washout test. Closing volume (CV) is another test for detection of small airways disease; it is increased in asthmatics. Measurements of lung elasticity (lung compliance) in asthmatics, using an esophageal balloon to estimate pleural pressure, have shown a loss of elastic recoil, which is often reversible upon remission. Diffusing capacity for CO (**DL_{CO}**) is generally normal in asthma; it is low in emphysema (in which there is loss of a functioning alveolar capillary bed with increased lung volume).

Other diagnostic tests: Assessment of etiologic factors is more difficult. Nonspecific irritant factors, particularly cigarette smoke, and evidence of infection (most often viral) should be evaluated. Exacerbations related to environmental allergen exposures, history of rhinitis, or family history of atopic disorders suggests the likelihood of extrinsic allergic factors. Confirmation is best accomplished by an allergy evaluation that includes **allergy skin testing** with extracts to detect IgE antibody to inhalants (pollens, molds, epidermals, house dust) and other allergens (eg, food) suggested by the patient's history. Bronchodilators containing adrenergic agents should be discontinued for 12 h and antihistamines for 48 h, but a corticosteroid may be continued (eg, prednisone up to 40 to 60 mg/day) without interfering with the immediate skin test response. Negative skin test responses to a suitable battery of appropriate allergens strongly rule against an allergic component. Positive skin tests indicate the presence of IgE antibody to the test allergen and represent only the *potential* for allergic reactivity to the allergens in question. Their clinical significance is determined when results are correlated with the pattern of symptoms and related to environmental exposures.

Specific IgE antibody to inhalants may also be detected by a **radioallergosorbent test (RAST)** on the patient's serum, but this test is expensive, subject to laboratory error, and offers little advantage over properly done and interpreted skin tests. Measurement of total serum IgE may be useful in establishing the atopic constitution of the patient. **Inhalational bronchial challenge testing** has been used (1) with allergens to establish the clinical significance of positive skin tests, (2) with methacholine or histamine to assess the degree of airways hyperactivity in known asthmatics, or (3) to aid in diagnosing asthma when the symptoms are atypical. **Exercise testing** using a treadmill or bicycle ergometer has been used, particularly in children, to confirm the diagnosis of asthma in equivocal cases.

Diagnosis and Staging

Asthma should be considered in anyone who wheezes; it is the likeliest diagnosis when typical paroxysmal wheezing starts in childhood or early adulthood and is interspersed with asymptomatic intervals. A family history of allergy or asthma can be elicited in > ½ of asthmatics. Difficulties in diagnosis occur with the initial presentation of asthma, particularly in adults over age 50, or when atypical symptoms (eg cough without audible wheezing), physical findings, or chest x-rays are noted. A number of other disorders may produce wheezing.

Children with **congenital malformations of the vascular system** (vascular rings and slings) and of the GI and respiratory tracts (tracheoesophageal fistula) may present with wheezing. The presence of other congenital malformations, special attention to infants whose symptoms begin before age 1 yr, x-ray studies, and a high index of suspicion will lead to a correct diagnosis.

Foreign-body obstruction must be considered, particularly in children with unilateral wheezing or sudden onset of wheezing without a history of respiratory symptoms. Opaque foreign bodies are readily visible on x-ray. With nonopaque foreign bodies the diagnosis can be established by a history of sudden onset of cough and wheezing in a previously well child, combined with asymmetric diaphragmatic movement or mediastinal shifts on inspiratory and expiratory chest x-rays.

Viral URI involving the epiglottis, glottis, and subglottis generally causes signs and

symptoms of croup (inspiratory stridor, high-pitched cough, and hoarseness) that are distinct from the lower airways signs and symptoms of asthma (see CROUP under VIRAL INFECTIONS in Ch. 191). When epiglottitis is suspected, direct examination of the epiglottis should be performed with great care and with the capability for immediate intubation if acute airways obstruction should develop during examination. Primary bacterial infection of the lower airways, in the absence of underlying predisposing disease, is rare in infants and children. On the other hand, viruses, particularly respiratory syncytial virus, can cause **bronchiolitis** with a clinical picture virtually indistinguishable from asthma during the first 2 yr of life. However, it is rare for an infant or young child to have > 1 to 2 episodes of infectious bronchiolitis, and a history of recurrent episodes of obstructive airways disease should strongly suggest the diagnosis of asthma. Since chronic bronchitis as a primary diagnosis is rare in children, underlying disorders (eg, cystic fibrosis, immunodeficiency disease, and ciliary dyskinesia syndrome) should always be considered. These may be ruled out by a careful history, sweat test, in vivo and in vitro evaluation of immunologic competence, and biopsy of respiratory mucosa with electron microscope study of cilia.

In **adults,** symptoms and signs of airways obstruction due to upper airways involvement may be clarified by determination of a flow-volume curve. Upper airway obstruction due to vocal cord dysfunction may be diagnosed by flexible bronchoscopy during an attack. Chronic obstructive pulmonary disease and heart failure are the main considerations in the differential diagnosis of wheezing, although multiple small pulmonary emboli frequently present with wheezing. Patients with hypersensitivity pneumonitis have a superficial clinical resemblance to asthmatics, but generally have more constitutional symptoms after exposure to the offending substance and typically do not wheeze, except in allergic bronchopulmonary aspergillosis, discussed below in Ch. 43. Patients with bronchial obstructions secondary to malignancy, aortic aneurysm, endobronchial TB, or sarcoidosis may occasionally present with wheezing.

Patients with allergic bronchopulmonary aspergillosis (see also ASPERGILLOSIS in Ch. 9) may present with typical asthmatic symptoms. The diagnosis of aspergillosis is confirmed by the findings of high peripheral blood eosinophilia, immediate skin test reactivity to *Aspergillus* antigen, precipitating antibodies against *Aspergillus* antigen, increased serum IgE concentrations (which appear to fluctuate with the activity of the disease), pulmonary infiltrates (transient or fixed), and a peculiar central type of bronchiectasis.

Other rare disorders that may simulate asthma include carcinoid syndrome, polyarteritis, and eosinophilic pneumonias (including tropical eosinophilia and other parasitic infestations that involve the lung during some phase of the disease). In all, the history is usually sufficiently atypical of asthma to suggest that another disorder is causing the airways obstruction.

Physical examination should search for heart failure and signs of chronic hypoxemia (clubbing of the fingers). Nasal polyposis should suggest aspirin intolerance. Unilateral wheezing should provoke a search for obstruction by a foreign body, vascular malformation, aneurysm, or tumor. In tracheal obstruction, an inspiratory wheeze is present over the upper airway.

Staging of the severity of the asthma attack is critical after the diagnosis is established. This is accomplished by a combination of evaluation of respiratory distress, monitoring of arterial blood gases, and spirometry. TABLE 36–1 illustrates one staging method.

Treatment

Treatment may be conveniently considered as management of the acute attack and day-to-day therapy. Drug therapy enables most patients to lead relatively normal lives with few adverse drug effects. The detailed approach described below is one of a

number that may be tried, but several **general principles** are important regardless of the particular drug or drugs used. (1) Staging of the severity of the attack (see above) is paramount, especially if it has been prolonged (> 12 h) or if the patient is unfamiliar to the examiner. (2) Bronchodilators should be used in orderly progression, with the patient under close observation during the initial therapy. Treatment to alleviate acute respiratory distress without maintenance follow-up treatment often results in a return of acute symptoms within 24 h. (3) Although some asthmatics may benefit from inhalation of nebulized bronchodilators, many cannot inhale the aerosol effectively and require parenteral drugs.

Drug therapy: Five classes of drugs are useful:

1. β-adrenergic agents cause bronchial smooth muscle relaxation and modulate inhibition of mediator release, at least in part by stimulating the adenylate cyclase-cAMP system. They include epinephrine, isoproterenol, ephedrine, and some more selective β_2-adrenergic agents (relatively more bronchodilatory β_2 effect and less cardiostimulatory β_1 effect). The latter commonly used β_2-adrenergic agents include metaproterenol, terbutaline, isoetharine, albuterol, and bitolterol. Fenoterol is not yet released in the USA. In general, epinephrine s.c. and one of the inhaled B_2 agents are most useful to treat the acute attack.

2. Theophylline, a methylxanthine, relaxes bronchial smooth muscle and modulates mediator release; its mechanism of action is unclear, but it acts as an adenosine antagonist and influences Ca flux across cell membranes and, to a limited extent in vivo, inhibits cAMP phosphodiesterase. Theophylline is a valuable adjunct to adrenergic drugs in the management of acute episodes; many, particularly in the USA, consider it to be the drug of choice for long-term continuous therapy.

3. Corticosteroids have multiple mechanisms of action: inhibition of attraction of polymorphonuclear leukocytes to the site of an allergic reaction, stimulation of synthesis of B_2 receptors, and blockage of leukotriene synthesis. While exceptionally effective, systemic corticosteroids are reserved for more difficult cases because of their potential for adverse effects. Short-term use in high dosage (eg, for 5 to 7 days to abort an attack) is unassociated with significant problems. The new generation of surface-active inhaled steroids are very useful for maintenance therapy.

4. Cromolyn sodium (disodium cromoglycate—**DSCG**), used prophylactically, appears to inhibit mediator release and reduce airways hyperreactivity. DSCG is primarily useful in children and some adults *for maintenance therapy only and has no place in treatment of the acute attack.* Cost and problems with patient compliance appear to have limited its use in the USA.

5. Anticholinergic agents (eg, atropine and its derivative ipratropium bromide) block cholinergic pathways that cause airways obstruction.

Treatment of the Acute Attack

Drug therapy: Patients with acute asthma presenting in Stage I or II (see TABLE 36–1) may be treated effectively with an aerosolized bronchodilator (eg, isoetharine 1% 0.5 mL or metaproterenol 5% 0.3 mL in 2 mL of 0.9% sodium chloride solution) using compressed air for nebulization. Alternatively, epinephrine 1:1000 in a dose of 0.01 mL/kg s.c. up to a maximum of 0.2 mL in children and 0.3 mL in adults, repeated once in 20 to 30 min, if indicated, may be given. Terbutaline, an alternative to epinephrine in the same dosage, is preferred in adults because of somewhat less cardiovascular effect. If there is no response after 2 adrenergic aerosol treatments and/or epinephrine injections, theophylline (as aminophylline) should be given IV.

Different schedules for administering aminophylline are used because individual patients vary in susceptibility to its beneficial or adverse effects. Maintaining serum levels of 10 to 20 µg/mL of theophylline is most effective. Most regimens start with an IV loading dose of 6 mg/kg aminophylline (25 mg/mL, diluted 1:1 with IV fluids) for children or adults given over about 20 min; then a continuous infusion is begun (0.45

mg/kg/h in adults and 1.0 mg/kg/h in children < 12 yr of age). Serum concentrations should be monitored at least q 12 h. If continuous infusion is unfeasible, then giving aminophylline 4 to 6 mg/kg IV over 20 min q 6 h is an acceptable alternative. Arterial blood gases should be obtained, especially if there is no sign of a prompt response (within about 30 min), if the patient is in severe distress or worsening, or if there is uncertainty about what stage the patient is in.

For any patient presenting in Stage III, an arterial blood gas determination should be obtained immediately and aminophylline started IV. For a patient in severe distress, continuous infusion doses may be raised to the limit of 1 mg/kg/h in young or middle-aged adults and 1.25 mg/kg/h in children. Monitoring serum theophylline concentrations is essential to prevent toxicity. Greater caution is necessary and lower dosages (by 1/3 to 1/2) should be used in patients who have heart failure or liver disease or who are elderly. O_2 at an FIO_2 of 40% should be given to correct hypoxemia.

While corticosteroids may be advantageously used in Stage II of an asthma attack, when patients present in Stage III and show no improvement or get worse despite one dose of aminophylline, IV corticosteroids are mandatory. Criteria for hospitalization vary, but definite indications are failure to improve or relapse after repeated adrenergic therapy and aminophylline, and significant decrease in PaO_2 (PaO_2 < 50 mm) or increase in $PaCO_2$ ($PaCO_2$ > 50 mm), indicating progression to respiratory failure. Far too many patients with severe asthma attacks are sent home from hospital emergency rooms.

Any patient presenting in or reaching Stage IV should immediately be given hydrocortisone sodium succinate 4 mg/kg IV q 2 to 4 h or methylprednisolone 1 to 2 mg/kg IV q 4 h. IV corticosteroids in these doses (or double the maintenance dose, whichever is greater) are also indicated immediately for any acute asthmatic attack if the patient had taken maintenance corticosteroids any time within the previous 6 to 12 wk.

Patients in Stage IV who show no favorable response to aminophylline and who show evidence of fatigue and progressive deterioration in blood gases and pH should be considered candidates for endotracheal intubation and respiratory assistance. (See Ch. 34.) Such patients should be hospitalized in an intensive care unit **(ICU).**

Children in Stage III or IV have been given isoproterenol 0.08 to 2.7 μg/kg/min by continuous IV infusion with a suitable infusion pump. This procedure requires ECG and arterial blood gas monitoring in an ICU and supervision by clinicians experienced in monitoring asthmatic children. IV albuterol has been used effectively in England and Canada. It is not available in the USA. Because of the increased potential for arrhythmias in adults, IV isoproterenol should probably not be used.

IV aminophylline and corticosteroids should be continued until the patient's condition has stabilized and there is no danger of progression to respiratory failure. Drugs given orally to a dehydrated, possibly nauseated patient may be erratically delivered to affected tissues. Nebulized bronchodilators (isoetharine or metaproterenol in 1:4 solution in 2 mL of 0.9% sodium chloride solution) may be ineffective in a patient in acute respiratory distress because of the severity of the airways obstruction, but, in some patients, they give short-term relief and may be used q 30 min prn or even more often. Use of continuous nebulization of adrenergic bronchodilators is being investigated. O_2, rather than room air, should be used as the aerosolizing gas. Sedatives and cough suppressants are **contraindicated.**

Anxiety may be extreme, because of hypoxia and the feeling of asphyxiation. Treatment of the underlying respiratory problems, including judicious use of O_2 therapy (see below), is the preferred approach, especially when conducted by calm, attentive, supportive medical personnel.

Fluid and electrolyte balance requires attention, especially when the episode lasts > 12 h, since these patients may be dehydrated. Therapy replaces previous and current fluid losses, not with an arbitrary amount/24 h, but by constant infusion of amounts

sufficient to result in a urine output adequate for the patient's age and size. Overhydration may cause pulmonary edema. Humidification of inhaled air or O_2 reduces excess respiratory tract loss.

With progressive severity and duration of the episode, respiratory acidosis may supervene; the arterial pH may drop alarmingly to ranges of pH 7 to 7.1. Most adults are intubated at this stage and started on assisted ventilation, because *the acidosis mainly reflects a respiratory mechanical problem that must be relieved.* Use of alkaline solutions (eg, sodium bicarbonate) in the IV fluid should be limited to maintain the pH between 7.2 and 7.3, since there is some evidence that adrenergic agent resistance is reversed by normalizing the pH. While there are theoretic objections to adding bicarbonate to a closed system, sodium bicarbonate has been safely and successfully used in children with status asthmaticus. It should be used only with careful blood gas and pH monitoring.

Supplemental K may need to be added to the infusion, since K shifts occur with changes in arterial and tissue pH and fluid turnover in a dehydrated patient. In addition, high doses of hydrocortisone more so than methylprednisolone given during therapy promote urinary K loss.

O_2 therapy is always indicated, since severe asthmatics are invariably hypoxemic. The inspired O_2 concentration (**F_{IO_2}**) is guided by blood gas levels; Pa_{O_2} should be maintained > 60 mm Hg, preferably in the 70 to 90 mm range, if possible. O_2 may be given effectively with nasal prongs or, if tolerated, a Venturi mask. In the occasional patient who will not tolerate a mask, use of nasal prongs with low O_2 flow (2 to 4 L/min) may achieve the same result. Since O_2 may be drying to the respiratory mucosa, it should always be humidified.

Respiratory tract infections exacerbating asthma are predominantly viral; bacterial infections rarely play a significant role, especially in children. However, if the patient expectorates yellowish, green, or brown sputum, and Wright's stain of the sputum shows a predominance of polymorphonuclear WBCs, antibacterial therapy is given empirically. This is especially appropriate in adults with a known tendency to have chronic or recurrent bronchitis. The antibiotic should be chosen according to bacteriologic findings, but ampicillin is usually most useful. If the patient is allergic to β-lactam antibiotics, erythromycin or tetracycline (the latter should not be given to young children) may be given. Gram stain of the sputum, noting intracellular bacteria, and chest x-rays are useful guides to therapy.

Although not all physicians agree, many believe that **chest x-ray** is mandatory in all hospitalized asthmatics. Spontaneous pneumothorax and subcutaneous and mediastinal emphysema are complications of acute asthma, particularly in children. A large pneumothorax requires immediate treatment. Mediastinal and subcutaneous emphysema rarely cause difficulty, even when large. Rarely, compression of the glottis may occur with extreme extravasation of air into the soft tissues of the neck.

Maintenance Therapy of Asthma

Following an acute asthma attack, oral drugs should be continued for 2 to 4 wk even if the patient is asymptomatic, because pulmonary function abnormalities and hypoxemia may persist for this long. Several types of treatment are described below with the understanding that more than one approach may be used. Patients with mild asthma and infrequent episodes of wheezing may need therapy only intermittently when symptomatic. Others with more persistent symptoms benefit from continuous around-the-clock treatment.

Cromolyn sodium, 1 capsule (20 mg) q 6 h via an inhaler, or with cromolyn solution and a pressure-driven nebulizer, is most useful in children; it may avoid the need for corticosteroids or may enable a reduction in their maintenance dosage. While some physicians use cromolyn as a first-line maintenance drug for chronic asthma, in the

USA it is often used in patients who do not respond satisfactorily to theophylline and adrenergic drugs; it should be tried before starting corticosteroids. *The drug is not a bronchodilator, has no place in treating an acute asthma attack, and is used only prophylactically.* It is effective in preventing exercise-induced asthma: Administration immediately before exercise blocks an attack (the most effective drug for this purpose is an inhaled adrenergic agent). Patients with either extrinsic or intrinsic asthma may respond favorably, although the likelihood is greater with extrinsic asthma. The drug is generally stopped during an exacerbation, since, in this instance, it may act as an airways irritant.

Bronchodilators: A variety of oral theophylline formulations are available as tablets, capsules, or liquids. Anhydrous preparations are preferred to theophylline combinations. Sustained-release **(SR)** formulations maintain serum theophylline concentration in the therapeutic range when given tid, bid, or even once/day in particularly slow theophylline metabolizers. Since children, in particular, metabolize theophylline rapidly, serum concentration peaks (which may cause toxic symptoms) and troughs (which may be therapeutically ineffective), often occur with the conventional rapidly absorbed formulations. SR formulations overcome this problem and are convenient for adults and older children. Because capsules may be opened and the pellet contents mixed with moist food, they are very useful in young children. Neither tablets nor pellets should be chewed. As with IV administration, toxic symptoms may be observed at concentrations > 20 μg/mL. Nausea, vomiting, and CNS stimulation should be watched for, serum theophylline measured, and the dosage or interval modified accordingly.

With adequate doses of theophylline, further improvement can occasionally be gained by adding one of the newer β_2-adrenergic bronchodilators. Ephedrine, formerly a mainstay of therapy, frequently caused undesirable side effects and is rarely used today. Metered dose inhalers **(MDI)** that contain terbutaline, metaproterenol, albuterol, fenoterol, or bitolterol give bronchodilator effect for 4 to 6 h. *Patients should be cautioned about overuse of MDI.* The average MDI provides 200 doses and should last 4 wk. A variety of "spacers" or holding chambers are available for use by young children or adults who are unable to use the MDIs properly. Adrenergic aerosols with a pressure-driven nebulizer can be used at home advantageously in children too young to use an MDI. Often cromolyn solution (2 mL unit dose) is mixed with the adrenergic drug (eg, 0.5 mL isoetharine) in the nebulizer. The significance of a poor, short-lived response to several inhalations of adrenergic agents must be understood by the patient as an indication to seek medical attention.

Alternatively, terbutaline 2.5 to 5 mg orally qid can be given to supplement theophylline therapy, but adverse side effects of the β_2-selective agents are more evident with oral drugs than aerosols. Hand tremor, the most commonly observed adverse β_2-effect, becomes much less troublesome with continuous administration of the drug as tolerance develops. These drugs should be used cautiously in patients with a history of cardiac arrhythmias or hyperthyroidism.

When there is no satisfactory response to theophylline and a β_2-adrenergic agent, a corticosteroid should be added; short-term use of high doses frequently relieves exacerbations. Prednisone 40 to 60 mg/day orally in adults or 1 to 2 mg/kg/day in children (either divided or given as a single dose in the early morning) should be maintained for 5 to 7 days, after which the patient is reevaluated. Some patients may require 7 days more to achieve maximum benefit; then the prednisone dosage can be reduced by 50% decrements q 2 days until the drug is discontinued or the lowest dose that maintains good control of symptoms is reached. If prednisone cannot be discontinued without the appearance of an unacceptable degree of symptoms, it may be worthwhile to attempt alternate-day therapy with prednisone or another short-acting corticosteroid, beginning with double the previous daily dose given as a single dose before 8 AM q 48 h. If the patient does well, an attempt is made to reduce the dose by 5 mg q 10 to 14

days. Side effects are minimized with alternate-day therapy, but satisfactory asthma control may be difficult to achieve in adults. Daily doses should be reinstituted during an exacerbation.

Beclomethasone, triamcinolone acetonide, and flunisolide represent a new generation of **aerosol corticosteroids** with potent surface activity and offer a major advance in long-term maintenance therapy (supplemental systemic corticosteroids are necessary for an acute attack). They control asthma, with minimal adverse effects, in doses from 400 to 800 μg/day. However, when chronic steroid-dependent asthmatics are converted to aerosols from systemic corticosteroids, *an inadequate hypothalamic-pituitary-adrenal axis response to stress may occur that may require resumption of systemic corticosteroids.* When patients are converted from oral to inhaled steroids, flaring of allergic rhinitis or eczema may occur and is further evidence of a lack of systemic effect of the aerosolized agent. *Candida albicans* has been cultured from the nasopharynx of patients on topical steroid aerosol therapy, but it rarely causes disease.

Ipratroprium bromide is being used successfully as an inhaled bronchodilator alone, or in combination with an adrenergic agent or theophylline in the management of both acute and chronic asthma. It is not yet available in the USA.

The role that **extrinsic factors** (generally animal danders, dust, airborne molds, and pollens) play in the disease should be rigorously investigated. If suspected, allergy skin tests should be done to confirm the history. Allergens that can be controlled by avoidance (animal danders, house dust mite) should be eliminated. Other allergens (dust mite, mold, and pollens) may be selected for a trial of allergy immunotherapy (formerly "hyposensitization"). Improvement should be noted within 12 to 24 mo after beginning treatment. If no significant improvement is noted within this period, therapy should be discontinued. When improvement occurs, the optimum duration of therapy is unknown, but at least 3 yr is recommended.

Nonspecific exacerbating factors (eg, cigarette smoke especially, odors, irritant fumes, and changes in temperature, atmospheric pressure, and humidity) should also be investigated and controlled when possible. Aspirin should be avoided, particularly by patients with nasal polyposis, because of a significant incidence of aspirin-induced asthma. A few aspirin-intolerant asthmatics also react adversely to indomethacin, and rarely to tartrazine (FD and C yellow No. 5). Sensitivity to sulfites (used widely as food preservatives) is suggested by asthma attacks that follow eating from a salad bar or drinking red wine or beer.

Surgical procedures should be performed when the patient's pulmonary state is optimum. Corticosteroids may be required; short-term use is less hazardous than a compromised respiratory status. Procedures involving nasal and tracheal manipulation are particularly troublesome and polypectomies in aspirin-sensitive asthmatics may require a week's pretreatment with prednisone 50 to 60 mg/day orally.

ACUTE BRONCHITIS

Acute inflammation of the tracheobronchial tree, generally self-limited and with eventual complete healing and return of function. Though commonly mild, bronchitis may be serious in debilitated patients and in those with chronic lung or heart disease. Pneumonia is a critical complication.

Etiology

Acute infectious bronchitis, most prevalent in winter, is often part of an acute URI. It may develop after a common cold or other viral infection of the nasopharynx, throat, or tracheobronchial tree, often with secondary bacterial infection. Exposure to air pollutants and, possibly, chilling, fatigue, and malnutrition are predisposing or contributory factors. Recurrent attacks often complicate chronic bronchopulmonary dis-

eases, which impair bronchial clearance mechanisms. Repeated infections may be associated with chronic sinusitis, bronchiectasis, bronchopulmonary allergy, or, in children, hypertrophied tonsils and adenoids.

Acute irritative bronchitis may be caused by various mineral and vegetable dusts; fumes from strong acids, ammonia, certain volatile organic solvents, chlorine, hydrogen sulfide, sulfur dioxide, or bromine; the environmental irritants ozone and nitrogen dioxide; or tobacco or other smoke.

Cough variant asthma, asthma in which the degree of bronchoconstriction is not sufficient to produce overt wheezing, may be caused by allergen inhalation in an atopic individual, or chronic exposure to an airways irritant when airways hyperreactivity is relatively mild. Its management is similar to that of ordinary asthma (see BRONCHIAL ASTHMA above).

Pathology and Pathophysiology

Hyperemia of the mucous membranes is the earliest change, followed by desquamation, edema, leukocytic infiltration of the submucosa, and production of sticky or mucopurulent exudate. The protective functions of bronchial cilia, phagocytes, and lymphatics are disturbed, and bacteria may invade the normally sterile bronchi with consequent accumulation of cellular debris and mucopurulent exudate. Cough, though distressing, is essential to eliminate bronchial secretions. Airways obstruction may result from edema of the bronchial walls, retained secretions, and, in some cases, spasm of bronchial muscles.

Symptoms and Signs

Acute infectious bronchitis is often preceded by symptoms of a URI: coryza, malaise, chilliness, slight fever, back and muscle pain, and sore throat. Onset of cough usually signals onset of bronchitis. The cough is initially dry and nonproductive, but small amounts of viscid sputum are raised after a few hours or days; it later becomes more abundant and mucoid or mucopurulent. Frankly purulent sputum suggests superimposed bacterial infection. In a severe uncomplicated case, fever to 38.3 or 38.9 C (101 or 102 F) may be present for up to 3 to 5 days, following which acute symptoms subside (though cough may continue for several weeks). Persistent fever suggests complicating pneumonia. Dyspnea may be noted secondary to the airways obstruction.

Pulmonary signs are few in uncomplicated acute bronchitis. Scattered high- or low-pitched rhonchi may be heard, as well as occasional crackling or moist rales at the bases. Wheezing, especially after cough, is commonly noted. Persistent localized signs suggest development of bronchopneumonia.

Serious complications are usually seen only in patients with an underlying chronic respiratory disorder. In such patients, acute bronchitis may lead to severe blood gas abnormalities (acute respiratory failure).

Diagnosis

Diagnosis is usually based on the symptoms and signs, but a chest x-ray to rule out other diseases or complications is indicated if symptoms are serious or prolonged. Arterial blood gases should be monitored when serious underlying chronic respiratory disease is present. In persons who do not respond to antibiotic therapy, or in special circumstances (eg, immunosuppression), Gram stain and sputum culture should be done to determine the causative organism.

Treatment

General: Rest is indicated until fever subsides. Oral fluids (up to 3 or 4 L/day) are urged during the febrile course. An antipyretic analgesic (eg, aspirin 600 mg q 4 to 6 h) relieves malaise and reduces fever.

Local: A cough suppressant may be used if a troublesome cough interferes with sleep, but extreme care should be used if the patient also has chronic obstructive

pulmonary disease **(COPD).** Steam inhalations may help. A vaporizer may be used for irritative cough. Bronchodilators may be indicated to relieve wheezing (see BRONCHIAL ASTHMA, above).

Antibiotics are indicated when there is concomitant COPD, when purulent sputum is present, or when high fever persists and the patient is more than mildly ill. Oral tetracycline or ampicillin 250 mg q 6 h is a reasonable first choice for most cases. When symptoms persist or recur, or in unusually severe disease, smear and sputum culture are indicated. The antibiotic is then chosen according to the predominant organism and its sensitivity.

CHRONIC OBSTRUCTIVE PULMONARY DISEASE (COPD)

(Chronic Obstructive Lung Disease [COLD])

Generalized airways obstruction, particularly of small airways, associated with varying combinations of chronic bronchitis, asthma, and emphysema. The term COPD was introduced because these conditions often coexist, and it may be difficult in an individual case to decide which is the major one producing the obstruction. **Airways obstruction** is defined as *an increased resistance to airflow during forced expiration.* It may result from narrowing or obliteration of airways secondary to intrinsic airways disease, from excessive collapse of airways during a forced expiration secondary to pulmonary emphysema, from bronchospasm as in asthma, or may be due to a combination of these factors. Although obstruction of large airways may occur in all these disorders, particularly in asthma, patients with severe COPD characteristically have major abnormalities in their small airways, namely those < 2 mm internal diameter, and much of their airways obstruction is situated in this zone. The airways obstruction is irreversible except for that which can be ascribed to asthma. The type of asthma seen is often quite persistent and refractory to ordinary bronchodilation therapy.

To avoid confusion, the following definitions are given: (1) **Chronic bronchitis** (unqualified) is *a condition associated with prolonged exposure to nonspecific bronchial irritants and accompanied by mucus hypersecretion and certain structural changes in the bronchi.* Usually associated with cigarette smoking, it is characterized clinically by chronic productive cough. The term **chronic obstructive bronchitis** is used when chronic bronchitis is associated with extensive abnormalities of the small airways leading to clinically significant airways obstruction. (2) **Pulmonary emphysema** is *enlargement of the air spaces distal to terminal nonrespiratory bronchioles, accompanied by destructive changes of the alveolar walls.* The term **chronic obstructive emphysema** is used when airways obstruction is also present and where it is clear that the major features of the disease can be explained by emphysematous changes in the lungs. (3) **Persistent asthma** is defined as *asthma which is so persistent that clinically significant chronic airflow obstruction is present most of the time despite antiasthmatic therapy.* (4) **"Chronic asthmatic bronchitis"** is used to define *patients who have elements of both chronic bronchitis with chronic productive cough as well as persistent asthma with evidence of reversibility of their airways obstruction.* This diagnosis is important to distinguish since patients often show considerable improvement with intensive therapy and appear to have a better prognosis than with other types of COPD.

Interrelationships between chronic bronchitis, pulmonary emphysema, asthma, and COPD are depicted in FIG. 36–1. Some degree of emphysematous change is very common in the general population, but not all patients with emphysema have sufficient airways obstructive problems to be considered as having COPD. Similarly, many cigarette smokers have evidence of chronic bronchitis, but only a minority have clinically significant airways obstruction, usually associated with marked changes in the small airways of the lung. Most patients with COPD have some combination of chronic bronchitis and emphysema and many have an asthmatic component as well. It

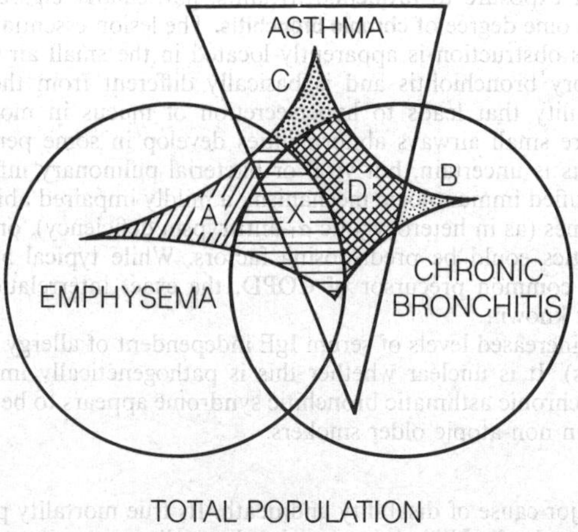

Fig. 36–1. Interrelationship of asthma, emphysema, chronic bronchitis, and persistent airways obstruction (COPD). Shaded areas represent patients with COPD. Patients with a relatively pure emphysematous-type disease (type A) are labeled A: those with a primarily bronchitic-type disease (type B) are labeled B. Group C represents patients with typical asthma, which is so persistent that there is clinically significant chronic airflow limitation. Group D are persons with chronic asthmatic bronchitis who show considerable fluctuation in the severity of the airways obstruction, but never return to normal. Persons with a totally mixed type of disease are labeled X.

is uncertain, however, whether this overlap results from a common causal factor or whether asthma, emphysema, and chronic bronchitis predispose to one another. While most asthmatics, particularly those < 40 yr old, have a totally reversible disease that cannot be considered COPD, the disease tends to become more persistent with age. Persistent airways obstruction that varies in intensity is relatively common in the elderly; this entity, which is generally accompanied by some degree of chronic cough, is conveniently classified as chronic asthmatic bronchitis.

Etiology

The development of chronic bronchitis, emphysema, and chronic airways obstruction appears to be determined by a balance between individual susceptibility and exposure to provocative agents.

The basic lesion of **emphysema** apparently results from the effect of proteolytic enzymes on the alveolar wall. Such enzymes can be released from leukocytes participating in an inflammatory process. Thus, any factor leading to chronic alveolar inflammation encourages development of emphysematous lesions. Smoking presumably has adverse effects on lung defenses and leads to low-grade inflammation with consequent recurrent or chronic release of leukocytic proteolytic enzymes. Fortunately, in most people, such enzymes are neutralized by antiproteolytic activity of the α_1-globulin fraction of serum. However, in a rare condition known as **homozygotic α_1-antitrypsin deficiency,** this activity is markedly diminished, and emphysema may develop by middle age even without exposure to substances that interfere with lung defenses. In the absence of severe deficiency of α_1-globulin in the serum, however, the factors that make some cigarette smokers more susceptible to development of emphysema than others remain uncertain. It is also uncertain why persons with similar degrees of emphysema have such varying degrees of severity of airways obstruction.

With sufficient exposure to bronchial irritants, particularly cigarette smoke, most persons develop some degree of **chronic bronchitis.** The lesion essential to development of severe airways obstruction is apparently located in the small airways. It is essentially a respiratory bronchiolitis and is basically different from the ordinary large airways abnormality that leads to hypersecretion of mucus in most smokers. The reason that severe small airways abnormalities develop in some persons exposed to bronchial irritants is uncertain, but viral or bacterial pulmonary infections in childhood, an unidentified immunologic mechanism, a mildly impaired ability to inactivate proteolytic enzymes (as in heterozygotic α_1-antitrypsin deficiency), or unidentified genetic characteristics could be predisposing factors. While typical allergic bronchial asthma is not a common precursor of COPD, the exact interrelationships of these disorders are not known.

Smokers have increased levels of serum IgE independent of allergy skin test reactivity (atopic status). It is unclear whether this is pathogenetically important, but the frequency of the chronic asthmatic bronchitic syndrome appears to be related to serum IgE levels, even in non-atopic older smokers.

Prevalence

COPD is a major cause of disability and death. Its true mortality probably exceeds that of lung cancer. In the USA, it is second to heart disease as a cause of disability in Social Security statistics, and reported mortality rates have doubled about every 5 yr. Some of this increase reflects the longer survival of patients who previously would have died of bacterial pneumonia before the COPD became known. It is estimated that COPD affects 15% of older men. Symptomatic COPD affects men more often than women, presumably because men have been heavier smokers; however, the incidence in women is increasing, while in males it is beginning to plateau.

Pathology

In patients with severe **emphysema,** the lungs are large and pale and often fail to collapse when the thorax is opened. Microscopic examination reveals "departitioning" of the lung due to loss of alveolar walls. Large bullae may be present in advanced disease. Changes may be most marked in the center of the acinus **(centrilobular emphysema)** or more diffusely scattered throughout the lobule **(panacinar emphysema).** In all forms, normal architecture is destroyed; loss of alveolar walls results in air sacs of various sizes. The number of capillaries in the remaining alveolar walls is reduced, and pulmonary arterial vessels may show sclerotic changes. These abnormalities lead not only to a reduction in the area of alveolar membrane available for gas exchange, but also to the perfusion of nonventilated areas and to the ventilation of nonperfused parts of the lung; ie, **ventilation/perfusion ($\dot{V}/\dot{Q}$) abnormalities.** They also lead to poor support of the airways, accounting for excessive collapse of airways on expiration.

In **chronic bronchitis,** the bronchial walls are thickened, there is mucus in the lumen, and the numbers of goblet cells and mucous glands are increased. There may be purulent secretions and inflammatory changes in bronchial walls and surrounding lung parenchyma if infection is present. Such large airways changes do not account for severe obstruction, however, and in patients dying of COPD, narrowing and obliteration of small airways are generally observed.

Right ventricular hypertrophy (cor pulmonale) is common in patients with advanced respiratory insufficiency.

Symptoms, Signs, and X-ray Findings

COPD is thought to begin early in life, though significant symptoms and disability usually do not occur until middle age. Mild ventilatory abnormalities may be discernible long before the onset of significant clinical symptoms. A mild "smoker's cough" is often present many years before onset of exertional dyspnea.

Gradually progressive exertional dyspnea is the most common presenting complaint. Patients may date the onset of dyspnea to an acute respiratory illness; the acute infection may only unmask a preexisting subclinical chronic respiratory disorder or it may reduce an already limited respiratory reserve. Cough, wheezing, recurrent respiratory infections, or, occasionally, weakness, weight loss, or lack of libido may also be initial manifestations. Rarely, initial complaints are related to heart failure secondary to cor pulmonale, because some patients apparently ignore cough and dyspnea prior to the onset of dependent edema and severe cyanosis.

Cough and sputum production are extremely variable. One patient may admit only to "clearing my chest" on awakening in the morning or after smoking the first cigarette of the day. Another may describe a severe disabling cough. Sputum varies from a few mL of clear viscid mucus to large bronchiectasis-like quantities of purulent material.

Wheezing also varies in character and intensity. Asthma-like episodes may occur with acute infections. A mild chronic wheeze that is most obvious on reclining may be noted. Many patients deny having any wheeze.

A history of typical episodic asthma or of marked fluctuation in disease severity should make one suspect a chronic asthmatic bronchitic type of syndrome.

Physical findings in COPD are notoriously variable, especially in early stages. A consistent abnormality is obstruction to expiratory air flow manifested by a slowing of forced expiration. To demonstrate this, the patient is asked to take a deep breath and then empty the lungs as quickly and completely as possible. Forced expiration is normally virtually complete in < 4 sec. This test, which should be part of every routine physical examination, may be abnormal even though the patient does not complain of dyspnea.

Typical findings—gross pulmonary hyperinflation, prolonged expiration during quiet breathing, depressed diaphragm, pursed-lip breathing, stooped posture, calloused elbows from repeated assumption of the "tripod position," and marked use of accessory muscles of respiration—are seen only in later stages of COPD. Other findings, including rhonchi, diminished vesicular breath sounds, tachycardia, distant heart tones, and decreased diaphragmatic motion, are not consistently present. A barrel-chested appearance is an unreliable finding often noted in elderly patients without significant respiratory problems. Late in the disease, there may be frank cyanosis from hypoxemia, a plethoric appearance associated with secondary erythrocytosis, and, in patients with severe cor pulmonale, signs of heart failure. Mild, chronic, dependent edema is quite common, but does not necessarily indicate heart failure. It may result from prolonged sitting, elevated intrathoracic pressures, and renal retention of salt secondary to blood gas abnormalities even in the absence of cor pulmonale.

Chest x-ray findings are also variable. In early stages of the disease, the x-ray is often normal. Changes indicative of hyperinflation (eg, depressed diaphragm, generalized radiolucency of the lung fields, increased retrosternal air space, and tenting of the diaphragm at the insertions to the ribs) are common and suggestive of emphysematous disease, but are not diagnostic. They may also be found in patients with asthma and occasionally in healthy persons. Localized radiolucency with attenuation of vascular markings is a more reliable indicator of emphysema.

Bullae are seen occasionally with COPD. Large bullae are generally well seen on ordinary x-rays, but small ones are more reliably detected with **planograms** or CT scans. They may occur as part of a diffuse emphysematous process or as isolated phenomena and thus do not necessarily indicate a generalized lung disease.

Bronchitis itself does not have a characteristic appearance on ordinary chest x-ray, but **bronchograms** may reveal cylindrical dilation of bronchi on inspiration, bronchial collapse on forced expiration, and enlarged mucous ducts. Frank saccular bronchiectasis is unusual and generally occurs only in patients who have had a previous severe respiratory infection. However, bronchography is not indicated to evaluate bronchitis unless severe localized saccular bronchiectasis is suspected.

In patients with recurrent chest infections, a variety of nondescript postinflammatory abnormalities may be noted on the plain chest film, such as localized fibrotic changes, honeycombing, or contraction atelectasis of a segment or lobe.

Isotopic lung scans generally demonstrate uneven ventilation and perfusion.

Diagnosis

COPD should be suspected in any patient with chronic productive cough or exertional dyspnea of uncertain etiology, or whose physical examination reveals evidence of slowing of forced expiration. Definite diagnosis depends on (1) demonstration of physiologic evidence of airways obstruction that persists despite intensive and maximum medical management, and (2) exclusion of any specific disease (eg, silicosis, TB, or upper airway neoplasm) as a cause of this physiologic abnormality.

With inhalation of a bronchodilator, a $> 15\%$ improvement in a forced expiratory volume in 1 sec **(FEV_1)** suggests a significant reversible component; it is often noted in patients with chronic asthmatic bronchitis.

RBC count may reveal erythrocytosis in chronically hypoxemic patients. A differential WBC count may show eosinophilia, which strongly suggests a chronic asthmatic bronchitic type of disease.

Spirometric testing (see also Ch. 32) reveals characteristic obstruction to expiratory air flow with slowing of forced expiration as shown by a reduced FEV_1 and a low maximum mid-expiratory flow. Slowing of forced expiration is also evident on flow-volume curves. The vital capacity **(VC)** and forced vital capacity **(FVC)** are somewhat impaired in patients with severe disease, but are better maintained than the measures of the speed of expiration. For this reason, the FEV_1/VC ratio is regularly reduced to $< 60\%$ with clinically significant COPD. This degree of abnormality should persist despite prolonged, maximal therapy before a diagnosis of COPD is considered confirmed.

Maldistribution of ventilation and perfusion occurs in COPD and is manifested in several ways. An excessive physiologic deadspace ventilation indicates that there are areas of the lung in which ventilation is high relative to blood flow (a high $\dot{V}/\dot{Q}$ ratio), resulting in "wasted" ventilation. Physiologic shunting indicates the presence of alveoli with reduced ventilation in relation to blood flow (a low $\dot{V}/\dot{Q}$ ratio) that allows some pulmonary blood flow to reach the left heart without becoming fully oxygenated, resulting in hypoxemia. In late stages, overall alveolar underventilation with hypercapnia occurs, aggravating any hypoxemia resulting from physiologic shunting. Chronic hypercapnia is usually well compensated, and pH levels are close to normal, except in acute exacerbations of disease.

The pattern of physiologic abnormality in each patient depends to some extent on the relative severity of intrinsic bronchial disease and emphysema. Diffusing capacity is regularly reduced in patients with severe emphysema, but is more variable in those with airways obstruction associated with predominant intrinsic bronchial disease. In patients with severe emphysema and a well maintained ventilatory drive, resting hypoxemia is usually mild and hypercapnia does not occur until terminal stages. In these patients, sometimes called **"pink puffers,"** CO may be quite low, but frank pulmonary hypertension and cor pulmonale usually develop late. In patients with airways obstruction associated primarily with an intrinsic bronchial disorder, severe hypoxemia and hypercapnia may be noted relatively early. Such patients, sometimes called **"blue bloaters,"** usually have a well-maintained CO and tend to develop severe pulmonary hypertension with chronic cor pulmonale. A reduced ventilatory drive or persistent sleep apnea problems also appear to contribute to the early development of cor pulmonale and the "blue bloater" syndrome. The residual volume **(RV)** and total lung capacity **(TLC)** are markedly elevated in emphysematous patients, while pulmonary hyperinflation may be relatively slight in bronchitic COPD, but the ratio of RV/TLC tends to be elevated in both types of disease.

Detailed lung function measurements help to determine the severity of emphysema and intrinsic bronchial disease in an individual case, but are rarely needed for ordinary clinical evaluation. With severe emphysema, pressure-volume curves show characteristic loss of recoil and increased compliance. Airways resistance measurements made in the body plethysmograph tend to reflect the severity of intrinsic bronchial narrowing.

In a few cases with severe emphysema but little bronchitis or with severe obstructive bronchitis but little, if any, emphysema, it is possible to distinguish **emphysematous type (Type A)** disease from **bronchial type (Type B)** disease on the basis of clinical and physiologic findings. The typical Type B disease, probably a result of persistent bronchial infection, is becoming quite rare except in persons with obvious bronchiectasis.

It is more important to recognize patients with chronic asthmatic bronchitis since these patients often show considerable improvement with corticosteroid therapy. A history of fluctuating severity of illness, a good response to bronchodilator therapy, and blood or sputum eosinophilia should make one suspect this syndrome. The characteristics of the different clinical types of COPD are summarized in TABLE 36–2.

Specific parenchymal lung diseases that may lead to airways obstruction can usually be excluded by chest x-ray. Upper airways lesions (generally associated with stridor) and localized bronchial obstructions (often associated with a localized wheeze) must also be excluded. It is particularly important to exclude primary heart disease with heart failure as a cause of respiratory insufficiency. A normal or small cardiac silhouette on chest x-ray is characteristic of COPD before development of frank cor pulmonale, but is most unusual when dyspnea results from a cardiac disorder.

TABLE 36–2. CLINICAL TYPES OF CHRONIC OBSTRUCTIVE PULMONARY DISEASES

Characteristics	*Emphysematous (Type A)*	*Bronchial (Type B)*	*Chronic asthmatic bronchitis*
Sex	Primarily male	Primarily male	Both sexes
Age at diagnosis	55 to 75	45 to 65	45 to 70
History of asthma	Uncommon	Uncommon	Frequent
Sputum	Scanty; mucoid	Copious; purulent	Scanty; often eosinophilic
Infections	Occasional	Frequent	Variable
Chest x-ray	Attenuated vessels; hyperinflation	Normal; localized fibrosis, or bronchiectasis	Normal or hyperinflation
Chronic cor pulmonale	Usually only late in disease	Common	Rare
Diffusing capacity	Low	Variable	Variable
Chronic hypoxemia	At rest only late in disease; may be noted earlier with exercise	Common; may be severe	Usually mild to moderate
Chronic hypercapnia	Usually only late in disease	Common	Unusual
Bronchodilator response	None to slight	None to slight	Usually significant
Eosinophilia	Uncommon	Uncommon	Common

Homozygotic α_1-antitrypsin deficiency should be suspected when there is a family history of obstructive airways disease, or when emphysema occurs in a woman, a relatively young man, or a nonsmoker. The diagnosis may be confirmed by measuring serum α_1-antitrypsin levels or by specific phenotyping.

Course and Prognosis

Some reversal of airways obstruction and considerable symptomatic improvement can often be obtained initially, but the long-term prognosis is less favorable in patients with persistent obstructive abnormality. After initial improvement, the FEV_1 generally falls 50 to 75 mL/yr, which is 2 to 3 times the rate of decline expected from aging alone. There is a concomitant slow progression of exertional dyspnea and disability. The course is punctuated by acute symptomatic exacerbations, generally related to superimposed bronchial infections.

Prognosis is closely related to the severity of expiratory slowing. In older studies, when the FEV_1 exceeded 1.25 L, the 10-yr survival rate was about 50%; when the FEV_1 was 1 L, the average patient survived about 5 yr; when there was very severe expiratory slowing (FEV_1 about 0.5 L), survival for > 2 yr was unusual, particularly if the patient also had chronic hypercapnia or demonstrable cor pulmonale. Newer series show better survivals, probably resulting in part from more frequent use of ambulant O_2 therapy.

The course of chronic asthmatic bronchitis is less well documented, but most clinicians believe that it is less progressive. With proper treatment most of these patients appear to die with the disease rather than from it.

Treatment

Therapy does not cure, but relieves symptoms and controls potentially fatal exacerbations. It may also slow progression of the disorder. Treatment is directed at alleviating conditions that cause symptoms and excessive disability (eg, infection, bronchospasm, bronchial hypersecretion, hypoxemia, and unnecessary limitation of physical activity). Avoidance of bronchial irritants (especially smoking cessation) is of primary importance.

Infection: An attempt should be made to clear purulent sputum with a broad-spectrum antibiotic (eg, tetracycline or ampicillin 250 mg qid for 10 days), the course repeated promptly at the first sign of recurrent bronchial infection or sputum purulence. As prophylactic therapy, regular courses of a broad-spectrum antibiotic are sometimes recommended for patients with frequent infectious exacerbations.

Bronchospasm: The degree of reversibility of airways obstruction can be assessed only by a vigorous and prolonged therapeutic trial of bronchodilators. See BRONCHIAL ASTHMA, above, for a detailed discussion of these drugs.

Corticosteroids have no role in treating the emphysematous type of COPD, but a trial of these agents may be required to prove conclusively that the airways obstruction is not due to chronic asthmatic bronchitis. This is especially true when there is a history suggesting asthma, eosinophilia, fluctuations in the severity of airways obstruction, or a positive response to inhalation of a bronchodilator. If a corticosteroid trial (eg, prednisone 30 to 40 mg every morning for 3 wk) is undertaken, its usefulness should be documented by improvement in spirometric tests before long-term corticosteroid therapy is recommended; then the lowest dose that sustains improvement is used. In some patients, alternate-day therapy or inhaled corticosteroids can be used for maintenance.

Bronchial secretions: Adequate systemic hydration is essential to prevent inspissation of secretions. In some patients bronchial hygiene may also be improved by inhalation of mist, postural drainage, and chest physical therapy, particularly following bronchodilator inhalation. Despite their wide use, IPPB machines have not been

shown to improve the patient's ability to raise secretions or to affect favorably the overall condition of ambulatory patients with COPD.

Hypoxemia: Severe chronic hypoxemia, often associated with hypercapnia, accentuates pulmonary hypertension and leads to development of cor pulmonale in patients with COPD. Around-the-clock O_2 supplementation has been shown to benefit patients with severe chronic hypoxemia (Pa_{O_2} consistently < 55 torr at rest) and to prolong survival. When instituting long-term O_2 therapy, it is important to monitor blood gas responses. No more O_2 should be given than is needed to raise the Pa_{O_2} to about 65 torr. One should also be sure that longterm O_2 therapy does not lead to a progressive rise in Pa_{CO_2} as a consequence of removing hypoxic ventilatory drive; in fact, this has rarely proved to be an important problem.

Use of O_2 for symptomatic relief of dyspnea without verification of severe hypoxemia is unjustified and potentially dangerous therapy.

Hypercapnia: Patients with rapidly developing or worsening hypercapnia require immediate hospitalization and intensive therapy (see THERAPY OF RESPIRATORY FAILURE in Ch. 34), but chronic well-compensated hypercapnia is generally well tolerated and requires no specific therapy.

Heart failure: The most important measure to control heart failure secondary to cor pulmonale is correction of hypoxemia. Diuretic therapy and controlled Na intake are important adjuncts. Digoxin must be used cautiously, if at all, since digoxin intoxication readily occurs in patients with COPD, probably as a result of fluctuating blood gas and electrolyte abnormalities.

Exercise tolerance: Prolonged inactivity leads to excessive disability. As long as there is no severe heart disease, it is important to maintain a regular exercise program that can usually be prescribed directly by the physician. If the patient is severely disabled, however, a trained physical therapist may be more effective in supervising such a program. Exercise should have a specific meaningful goal (eg, walking to the store, golfing) and should train the muscles needed for the activity. Breathing "exercises" (breathing training) may have a place in treating anxious patients who develop an excessively rapid ventilatory rate during exertion, but such exercises have not been shown to improve ventilatory capacity.

Depression: Because periods of severe depression or marked anxiety are frequent, a vigorous therapeutic program and an enthusiastic physician are most helpful. A nihilistic attitude toward management of COPD is inexcusable. The patient must understand the nature of the disease and the goals and expectations of therapy.

Exacerbations require prompt treatment; eg, if sputum becomes purulent, prescription of a course of broad-spectrum antibiotics and a more intensive program of bronchodilation and bronchial hygiene (see above). Patients with increasing hypoxemia or hypercapnia should be hospitalized promptly for intensive therapy. *Sedatives and hypnotics should always be avoided* in patients with COPD, particularly during exacerbations, since they increase the risk of acute ventilatory failure.

---

37. BRONCHIECTASIS

Irreversible focal dilation of the bronchi, usually accompanied by infection. Most often acquired, it is associated with diverse conditions, including some that are (either or both) congenital and hereditary.

Etiology and Pathogenesis

Congenital bronchiectasis: *A rare condition in which the lung periphery fails to develop resulting in cystic dilation of developed bronchi.* **Acquired bronchiectasis** results from (1)

direct bronchial wall destruction after infection, inhalation of noxious chemicals, immunologic reactions, or vascular abnormalities that interfere with bronchial nutrition or (2) from mechanical alterations secondary to atelectasis or loss of parenchymal volume leading to bronchial dilation and secondary infection.

Conditions commonly leading to bronchiectasis are severe pneumonia (especially one complicating measles, pertussis, or certain adenovirus infections in children); necrotizing infections at any age due to *Klebsiella*, staphylococci, influenza virus, fungi, mycobacteria, and perhaps mycoplasma; and bronchial obstruction from any cause (eg, foreign body, enlarged lymph nodes, mucus impaction, or lung cancer). Miscellaneous chronic fibrosing lung diseases (eg, those following aspiration pneumonia, inhalation of injurious gases or irritant or immunologically active particles [eg, silica, talc, or bakelite]) also predispose to bronchiectasis. Immunologic deficiencies and various congenital and/or hereditary abnormalities that decrease host susceptibility to infection or impair respiratory defenses and clearance of bronchial secretions are also important. Although incidence and mortality have decreased with widespread use of antibiotics and immunizations in children, bronchiectasis as a manifestation of cystic fibrosis **(CF)** is still common (see CYSTIC FIBROSIS in Ch. 193). With situs inversus and sinusitis, bronchiectasis is also a feature of **Kartagener's syndrome,** a subgroup of the "immotile cilia syndrome," in which various abnormalities in the cilial organelles result in defective mucociliary clearance that leads to suppurative bronchial infections and bronchiectasis, as well as chronic rhinitis, otitis, male sterility, corneal abnormalities, headaches, and poor sense of smell. Bronchiectasis has also been reported in patients with **Young's syndrome,** which is characterized by obstructive azoospermia, chronic sinopulmonary infections, normal spermatogenesis, dilated epididymal head filled with spermatozoa, and amorphous material without spermatozoa in the region of the corpus. Absent are ciliary ultrastructural abnormalities seen in the "immotile cilia syndrome" and the electrolyte abnormalities characteristic of cystic fibrosis. An unusual pattern of bronchiectasis occurs in allergic bronchopulmonary aspergillosis (see ALLERGIC BRONCHOPULMONARY ASPERGILLOSIS in Ch. 43): dilation occurs in the proximal portions of the segmental or subsegmental bronchi (rather than in the peripheral bronchi as in idiopathic bronchiectasis).

Pathology

Bronchiectasis may be uni- or bilateral; it is most common in the lower lobes, though the right middle lobe and lingular portion of the left upper lobe may often be involved. It may be cylindrical, varicose, or saccular. In **cylindrical bronchiectasis,** the bronchi are slightly dilated and in bronchograms appear to end abruptly instead of tapering in the usual branching pattern. The distal smaller bronchi cannot be seen on bronchograms, but can be identified pathologically and are filled with inflammatory exudate. In **varicose bronchiectasis,** the bronchi are irregularly dilated and contracted. In **saccular bronchiectasis,** the dilated bronchi are much wider and end in blind sacs, giving a ballooned appearance, because of obliteration of the bronchi and bronchioles beyond the dilated bronchi.

Microscopic examination of bronchial walls shows extensive inflammatory destruction, chronic inflammation, increased mucus, and loss of cilia. Where adjacent interstitial and alveolar areas are destroyed, tissue reorganization and fibrosis result in loss of volume. Pathologic evidence shows that bronchiectasis is associated with chronic bronchitis and/or emphysema. Extensive anastomoses between the bronchial and pulmonary arteries may be seen with markedly enlarged bronchial arteries.

Symptoms and Signs

Bronchiectasis can develop at any age; it begins most often in early childhood, but symptoms may not be apparent until much later. The severity and characteristics of symptoms vary widely from patient to patient, and from time to time in an individual

depending largely on the extent of the disease and the extent and presence of complicating chronic infection. Although a patient may be completely asymptomatic, chronic cough and sputum production are the most characteristic and common symptoms. They often begin insidiously, usually following a respiratory infection, and tend to worsen gradually over a period of years. Severe pneumonia with incomplete clearing of symptoms and residual persistent cough and sputum production is a common mode of onset. As the condition progresses, the cough tends to become more productive; it occurs with typical regularity in the morning on arising, late in the afternoon, and on retiring, but many patients are relatively free of cough during intervening hours. The sputum usually is similar to that of bronchitis and is not characteristic. Less commonly, in longstanding cases, sputum may be abundant and on standing may separate into 3 layers: frothy at the top, greenish and turbid in the middle, and thick with pus at the bottom. Hemoptysis is common and may be the first and only complaint. Recurrent pneumonia is also common; its investigation may lead to the diagnosis of bronchiectasis. Wheezing, shortness of breath and other manifestations of respiratory insufficiency (see Ch. 34) and right heart failure from cor pulmonale (see in Ch. 27) may occur in advanced cases with associated chronic bronchitis and emphysema.

Physical findings are nonspecific, but persistent rales over any part of the lungs suggest bronchiectasis. Clubbing of the fingers sometimes occurs with extensive disease and persistent chronic infection. Pulmonary functional and hemodynamic changes depend largely on the extent of accompanying pathologic changes such as diffuse chronic bronchitis, pulmonary emphysema, or pulmonary fibrosis. They may include reduction in lung volumes and airflow rates, ventilation/perfusion defects, hypoxemia, and in severe cases, pulmonary hypertension.

Diagnosis

Bronchiectasis must be suspected in anyone with the above symptoms and signs. Standard chest x-rays may show increased crowded bronchovascular markings, "tram tracking," areas of honeycombing, or cystic areas with or without fluid levels, but often they are normal. Experienced interpretation of CT of the chest may make bronchography unnecessary, but the latter is necessary to confirm the diagnosis and extent, particularly in puzzling cases or when surgery is contemplated. It should be done when the patient's state is stable and after vigorous bronchial hygiene. Excessive secretions or blood in the bronchial tree, or acute bronchopneumonia can lead to misinterpretation. The reversible dilation that occurs when there is air space consolidation, such as in pneumonia, should not be confused with true bronchiectasis. Bronchography should not be done in an iodine-sensitive patient or one with significant functional lung impairment. Chronic bronchitis and mycobacterial and fungal infections should be ruled out. When disease is unilateral or of recent onset, fiberoptic bronchoscopy is indicated to rule out tumor, foreign body, or other localized endobronchial abnormality. Fiberoptic bronchoscopy can also be combined with bronchography; dye is injected through a catheter that has been passed through the bronchoscope into the area of interest in the lung *or* a catheter is passed over a guide wire that had been first inserted and positioned through a bronchoscope. A search for associated conditions should be made, particularly CF, which is increasingly seen in adults, immune deficiencies, and predisposing congenital abnormalities.

Treatment

To control infection, therapy includes appropriate antibiotics, drugs, and physical therapy to promote bronchial drainage. Flora in the sputum usually are mixed gram-positive and gram-negative microorganisms, and anaerobes commonly inhabit bronchiectatic cysts. A broad spectrum antibiotic such as ampicillin 250 to 500 mg orally q 6 h (50 mg/kg/day in divided doses q 6 to 8 h in children weighing < 20 kg) or tetracycline 250 to 500 mg orally q 6 h is often used until the sputum is nonpurulent

and less voluminous, about 1 to 2 wk. Trimethoprim 320 mg orally and sulfamethoxazole 1600 mg orally q 12 h for 14 days has also been successful in reducing volume and eliminating pathogens. Antibiotics should be repeated at the first sign of returning infection (change in volume or increase in purulence of the sputum). If infection recurs frequently, prolonged chemoprophylaxis with ampicillin or tetracycline may be tried but is generally disappointing. In severe cases, high dose amoxicillin (3 gm orally bid), although not widely accepted, is reported to achieve higher serum and sputum concentrations than equal doses of ampicillin. For bronchopneumonia or serious respiratory infection, parenteral antibiotics guided by Gram stain, cultures, and sensitivity studies are indicated. Optimal treatment of CF complicated by bronchiectasis is controversial, but is usually directed against *Staphylococcus aureus*, *Hemophilus influenzae*, and *Pseudomonas*. Whether or not elective hospitalization, intensive parenteral antimicrobial therapy, chest physiotherapy, and/or administration of aerosol antibiotics improves prognosis or quality of life is not clear. Pneumococcal and yearly influenza virus vaccines are recommended. Patients with bronchiectasis should avoid cigarette smoke and other irritants, and refrain from using sedatives or antitussives. Postural drainage, clapping, and vibration (see under RESPIRATORY PHYSICAL THERAPY in Ch. 33) should be done regularly as tolerated. Diffuse chronic bronchitis, often accompanying bronchiectasis, should be treated accordingly (see under CHRONIC OBSTRUCTIVE PULMONARY DISEASE in Ch. 36). If asthma or allergic bronchopulmonary aspergillosis is also present, corticosteroids may be beneficial.

Surgical resection is rarely necessary, but should be considered when response to conservative management is unacceptable, as demonstrated by recurrent pneumonia, disabling bronchial infections, or frequent hemoptysis, and the disease is sufficiently localized and stable. For massive pulmonary hemorrhage, emergency resection or bronchial artery embolization has been lifesaving.

38. ATELECTASIS

A shrunken and airless state of part or all of the lung; the disorder may be acute or chronic, complete or partial, and is often accompanied by infection. The affected area often demonstrates a complex mixture of airlessness, infection, bronchiectasis, destruction, and fibrosis.

Etiology

The chief cause of **acute or chronic atelectasis** in adults is intraluminal bronchial obstruction that is often due to plugs of tenacious bronchial exudate, endobronchial tumors, or foreign bodies. Bronchial distortions or kinkings may also produce atelectasis, as can external compression of a bronchus by enlarged lymph nodes, tumor, or an aneurysm. External pulmonary compression by pleural fluid or gas (eg, due to pleural effusion, pneumothorax) may also cause atelectasis. Surfactant, a lipoprotein, covers the surface of the alveoli, reduces surface tension, and contributes to alveolar stability. Interference with its production and/or effectiveness may occur in O_2 toxicity, pulmonary edema, and other conditions that cause alveolar airlessness including the adult respiratory distress syndrome (see Ch. 35) and pulmonary embolism (see Ch. 39), and is probably important in perpetuating atelectasis.

Acute massive lung collapse is usually a postoperative complication, most often after upper abdominal procedures and cardiac surgery utilizing cardiopulmonary bypass. Large doses of opiates and sedatives, very high O_2 concentrations during anesthesia, tight dressings, abdominal distention, and immobility of the body favor development of atelectasis, because of limited respiratory movement, elevated diaphragm, accumulated viscid bronchial secretions, and suppressed cough reflex. However, other condi-

tions can lead to atelectasis if they produce a pattern of shallow breathing and interfere with cough and effective clearance of secretions. These include CNS depressive disorders, thoracic cage abnormalities, pain and muscle spasm, and neuromuscular diseases that impair respiratory function.

In the **middle lobe syndrome,** *a form of chronic atelectasis*, middle lobe collapse usually results from bronchial compression by surrounding lymph nodes. Partial bronchial obstruction in the presence of infection may also lead to chronic atelectasis and, ultimately, to chronic pneumonitis because of poor drainage of bronchial secretions. Acute pneumonia, usually with delayed and incomplete resolution, may also develop. Ineffective collateral ventilation of the right middle lobe is another predisposing factor in the pathophysiology of atelectasis in the right middle lobe, and helps to explain the occurrence of the syndrome when the right middle lobe bronchus appears patent to beyond the segmental division.

Pathology and Pathophysiology

Following obstruction of a bronchus, gas in the peripheral alveoli is absorbed by circulating blood, and consequent lung retraction produces airlessness within a few hours; lung shrinkage or collapse may be complete without infection. In early stages, blood perfuses the airless lung, with consequent arterial hypoxemia. Capillary and tissue hypoxia may result in transudation of fluid and pulmonary edema, filling alveolar spaces with secretions and cells, and preventing complete collapse of the atelectatic lung. Although distention of uninvolved surrounding lung may partially compensate for the volume loss, in cases of extensive collapse, the diaphragm may become elevated and the chest wall may flatten. Volume loss from atelectasis of an entire lung may cause the heart and mediastinum to shift to the affected side.

Hyperventilation and dyspnea are common. A decrease in Pa_{O_2} is usual and, if the atelectatic area is large, may be considerable; Pa_{O_2} often improves during and after the first 24 h, presumably as blood flow to the atelectatic area decreases. Pa_{CO_2} is usually normal or low as a result of increased ventilation of the remaining normal lung parenchyma.

If the obstruction is removed, air enters the affected area, any complicating infection subsides, and the lung returns to its normal state in a variable length of time, depending on how much infection is present. If the obstruction is not removed and infection is present, airlessness and lack of circulation initiate changes leading to fibrosis. If these conditions persist, the lung becomes fibrotic and bronchiectatic. Even in the absence of bronchial obstruction, small areas of atelectasis may ensue from inadequate regional ventilation and disturbances in surfactant formation from hypoxia, hyperoxia, or exposure to various toxins. Mild to severe disturbances in gas exchange may result. (See Ch. 35.)

Symptoms and Signs

Most symptoms and signs depend upon how rapidly the bronchial occlusion occurs, the extent of lung affected, and whether an infection is present. **Rapid occlusion with massive collapse,** particularly with infection, causes pain on the affected side, sudden onset of dyspnea and cyanosis, a drop in BP, tachycardia, elevated temperature, and shock. Chest examination reveals dullness to flatness over the involved area and diminished or absent breath sounds. Chest excursion in the area is reduced or absent and the trachea and heart are deviated toward the affected side. **Slowly developing atelectasis** may be asymptomatic or cause only minor pulmonary symptoms. The **middle lobe syndrome** is also often asymptomatic, though a severe, hacking, nonproductive cough may result from irritation in the right lower and middle lobe bronchi. Physical examination discloses the same findings as in rapid occlusion.

Chest x-rays may show an airless lung area whose size and location depend on the bronchus involved. If only segments are affected, the shadow will be triangular, with

its apex toward the hilum. When small areas are involved, surrounding tissue distention causes them to appear curiously discoid, particularly in subsegmental lower lobe atelectasis. If the atelectasis is lobar, the entire lobe is airless. The trachea, heart, and mediastinum may be deviated toward the affected area, the diaphragm on that side may be elevated, and rib spaces are narrowed.

Diagnosis and Differential Diagnosis

Diagnosis is made from clinical findings plus x-ray evidence of diminished lung size (indicated by retracted ribs, elevated diaphragm, and deviated mediastinum) and of a solid, airless mass. A cause for obstruction should always be sought regardless of the patient's age. With the fiberoptic bronchoscope it is possible to see segmental and subsegmental divisions. CT can help to clarify the mechanism of collapse; an experienced interpreter can distinguish atelectasis secondary to endobronchial obstruction from compression atelectasis due to fluid or air, and cicatrization resulting from chronic inflammation.

Spontaneous pneumothorax produces similar clinical findings, but the percussion note is tympanitic, the heart and mediastinum are pushed to the opposite side, and x-rays are diagnostic. Massive effusion may also cause dyspnea, cyanosis, weakness, flatness to percussion over the involved area, and absent breath sounds, but the heart and mediastinum are deviated away from the involved area and the chest wall is not flattened.

An unusual form of peripheral lobar collapse, rounded atelectasis, or "folded lung" is often mistaken for tumor. Most commonly a complication of asbestos-induced pleural disease, it has a characteristic appearance on x-ray that distinguishes it from tumor. The lung density is round and immediately subpleural, with an acute angle between it and the pleura, and it frequently has a "comet tail" extending toward the hilum, thought to represent compressed vessels and bronchi that enter the atelectatic area.

Prophylaxis

Acute massive atelectasis is best combated by prevention. Since pre-existing chronic bronchitis and heavy smoking increase the risk of postoperative atelectasis, preoperative cessation of smoking and measures to improve bronchial toilet (see CHRONIC OBSTRUCTIVE PULMONARY DISEASE in Ch. 36) should be encouraged. Anesthetic agents with a long period of postanesthesia narcosis should be avoided, and narcotics should be used sparingly after surgery, since they depress the cough reflex. At the conclusion of anesthesia, the lungs should be left filled with some air, not 100% O_2. The patient must not be allowed to lie in one position > 1 h. Early ambulation is important. The patient should be encouraged to cough and breathe deeply. A combined approach encouraging coughing and deep breathing along with the use of nebulized bronchodilators and aerosols of water or saline to liquefy and facilitate removal of secretions, and tracheal suctioning as necessary, is most effective. The relative merits of IPPB, incentive spirometry (in which a simple device is used to encourage voluntary maximum sustained [3 to 5 sec] inspiratory maneuvers) and the components of physical therapy (percussion, vibration, postural drainage, and deep breathing) are disputed. If it is to be effective, each modality must be used appropriately and with adjunctive measures. Chest percussion in the postoperative patient may actually enhance the risk of atelectasis if it increases pain and muscular splinting.

Treatment

Acute atelectasis (including postoperative acute massive lung collapse) requires removal of the underlying cause. When a mechanical obstruction is suspected, but relief is not obtained by coughing or suctioning and a 24-h trial of vigorous respiratory and physical therapeutic measures, or when the patient is unable to cooperate with such measures, fiberoptic bronchoscopy should be performed (see BRONCHOSCOPY in Ch.

33). Once bronchial obstruction is established, therapy is directed at the obstruction and the infection invariably present. Often mucus plugs or inspissated secretions can be removed through the bronchoscope and the involved lung will reinflate, but vigorous chest physical therapy and other measures noted above should be continued. If foreign body aspiration is suspected, bronchoscopy should be performed promptly; removal of the foreign body may require use of a rigid bronchoscope. Patients with atelectasis should (1) lie with the involved side uppermost to promote drainage of the affected area, (2) have appropriate physical therapy, and (3) be encouraged to cough. Subsequently they should be encouraged to move from side to side and breathe deeply. Frequent (q 1 to 2 h) supervised use of IPPB or an incentive spirometer may help to assure deep breaths. If the atelectasis occurred outside the hospital (eg, foreign body aspiration), a broad-spectrum antibiotic (eg, ampicillin 500 mg orally or 1 gm q 6 h parenterally) should be given at the outset. If the patient has been in the hospital and is seriously ill, antimicrobial therapy should be based on the known local pathogens and drug susceptibility profiles of the hospital. In general the regimen might include a penicillin (eg, ampicillin) or clindamycin 1200 to 2700 mg/day IV and an aminoglycoside (eg, amikacin 15 mg/kg/day IM or IV in 2 divided doses) or a second- or third-generation cephalosporin (eg, cefuroxime 0.75 to 1.5 gm q 8 h IV or cefamandol 0.5 to 1 gm q 4 to 6 h IV). If a specific pathogen is subsequently isolated from sputum or bronchial secretions, the antibiotic should be modified accordingly.

Chronic atelectasis: The longer the lung remains unexpanded, the more likely it is to develop destructive, fibrotic, bronchiectatic changes. Since secondary atelectasis usually becomes infected regardless of the cause of obstruction, a broad spectrum antibiotic such as ampicillin or tetracycline or others based on Gram stain and culture results should be given when sputum volume and purulence increase. Surgical resection of the atelectatic segment or lobe should be considered, particularly when the patient has had recurrent disabling respiratory infections and/or recurrent hemoptysis from the affected area. When a tumor is shown to cause the obstruction, its cell type and extent, the overall condition of the patient, and his pulmonary function will determine whether the obstruction can best be relieved by surgery, radiation, or chemotherapy. In selected cases, laser therapy has effectively reduced obstruction from an endobronchial lesion.

---

39. PULMONARY EMBOLISM (PE)

(Thromboembolism)

Lodgment of a blood clot in a pulmonary artery with subsequent obstruction of blood supply to the lung parenchyma. **Pulmonary infarction (PI):** *Hemorrhagic consolidation (often followed by necrosis) of lung parenchyma resulting from thromboembolic pulmonary arterial occlusion.*

Etiology and Pathogenesis

The most common type of pulmonary embolus is a thrombus that usually has formed in a leg or pelvic vein. Most of those causing serious hemodynamic disturbances form in an iliofemoral vein, either de novo or by propagation from calf vein thrombi. Thromboemboli that originate in the veins of the upper extremities or in the right cardiac chambers are infrequent. Amniotic fluid emboli and fat emboli following fractures are rarer types of PE whose primary site of vascular obstruction is the pulmonary microcirculation (arterioles and capillaries rather than pulmonary arteries); involvement of the microcirculation may initiate the so-called adult respiratory distress syndrome (see in Ch. 35).

PI is an infrequent (< 10% of cases) consequence of PE. It is sometimes due to

thrombosis in situ of the pulmonary arteries as might occur in congenital heart disease associated with severe pulmonary hypertension or in hematologic disorders (eg, sickle cell anemia).

The pathogenesis of venous thrombosis involves stasis, increased blood coagulability, and vascular wall damage (Virchow's triad). Factors predisposing to thromboembolic disease include prolonged bed rest with immobility, chronic heart failure, the postoperative state, pregnancy, hip fracture, use of oral contraceptives, chronic obstructive pulmonary disease **(COPD)**, obesity, malignancy, hematologic disorders (eg, polycythemia vera), vascular injuries resulting from minor trauma, and immobilization with stasis as may occur in chronic disease states. In many patients, no predisposing factor can be found.

Once released into the venous circulation, emboli are distributed to both lungs in about 65% of cases, to the right lung in 20%, and to the left lung in 10%. Lower lobes are involved 4 times more often than upper lobes. Most thromboemboli lodge in larger or intermediate (elastic or muscular) pulmonary arteries; 35% or fewer reach the smaller arteries.

Pathophysiology

The pathophysiologic changes that follow PE involve adjustments in pulmonary hemodynamics, gas exchange, and mechanics. The extent of change in cardiopulmonary function is determined by the extent of pulmonary arterial obstruction, which varies with the size and number of thrombi embolizing and obstructing the pulmonary arteries, and by the patient's preembolic cardiopulmonary status. A consideration of the pathophysiology of PE must include the mechanisms responsible for the following: (1) pulmonary hypertension, right ventricular failure, and shock; (2) dyspnea with tachypnea and hyperventilation; (3) arterial hypoxemia; and (4) PI.

1. Pulmonary hypertension, a most important physiologic alteration, results from increased pulmonary vascular resistance. As a consequence, the right ventricle must generate higher pulmonary artery pressure to maintain normal CO. Significant pulmonary hypertension (> 25 mm Hg mean pressure) usually occurs only when > 30 to 50% of the pulmonary arterial tree is occluded in a previously healthy lung. Pulmonary hypertension may be increased by preexisting cardiopulmonary disease (eg, mitral stenosis or obstructive lung disease).

The primary mechanism of increased resistance is obstruction of pulmonary arteries by thrombi; ie, a decrease in the total cross-sectional area of the pulmonary vascular bed. However, because some degree of pulmonary hypertension often develops with obstruction of < 50% of the vascular bed, pulmonary vasoconstriction appears to play a definite, but secondary, role. Vasoconstriction is partly mediated by hypoxemia, by serotonin release from platelet aggregates on the thrombi, and possibly by other humoral substances, including prostaglandins.

If pulmonary vascular resistance increases acutely to the extent that the right ventricle cannot generate sufficient pressure (ie, > 70 to 80 mm Hg systolic) to maintain CO, **hypotension** develops (in which the central venous and right atrial mean pressures are increased). This occurs only after massive embolization involving at least 50% and usually 75% or more of the pulmonary vascular bed without preexisting cardiopulmonary disease. With severe hypotension and **shock**, mean central venous pressure tends to fall.

2. Tachypnea, often with **dyspnea,** almost always occurs after an embolic episode. It appears to be of reflex origin, most likely due to stimulation of juxtacapillary receptors in the alveolar capillary membrane by swelling of the alveolar interstitial space. This stimulation increases vagal afferent activity that in turn stimulates medullary respiratory neurons. Consequent alveolar hyperventilation is manifested by a lowered Pa_{CO_2}.

Following occlusion of the pulmonary artery, areas of the lung are ventilated but not perfused, resulting in "wasted ventilation" (the physiologic hallmark of PE). The exis

tence of wasted ventilation in the setting of acute PE is signaled by increased arterial-alveolar CO_2 tension difference reflecting augmented physiologic deadspace, but this is not specific for PE; it occurs also with coexisting pulmonary disease, as well as systemic hypotension.

Changes tend to occur in lung mechanics as airways resistance increases and lung compliance decreases. A decrease in the maximal expiratory flow rate results from diminished lung volume and possibly from bronchoconstriction. Reduced lung volume following PE sometimes is manifested on the chest x-ray by elevation of the diaphragm due to atelectatic or infarcted segments. Heparin appears to lessen bronchoconstriction, when present, as evidenced by improved maximal expiratory flow rates. Since changes in lung mechanics are usually transient and minor, they are unlikely to be important in the genesis of prolonged dyspnea. However, they probably contribute to development of arterial hypoxemia, described below.

3. Arterial hypoxemia: Sa_{O_2} is characteristically diminished (94 to 85% or lower), but may be normal. Hypoxemia is due to right-to-left shunting in areas of partial or complete atelectasis in areas not involved by the embolic process. Characteristically this atelectasis can be partially corrected by deep breathing, either voluntary or induced by a positive pressure ventilator. Ventilation/perfusion ($\dot{V}_A/\dot{Q}$) imbalance probably also contributes to the hypoxemia. The mechanisms responsible for the $\dot{V}_A/\dot{Q}$ imbalance and atelectasis are not fully defined. One important factor relates to regional changes in compliance, which together with hyperventilation sets the stage for varying degrees of airways hypocapnia, producing nonuniform constriction of distal airways and peripheral lung units. Underventilation of the units results with respect to perfusion, and atelectasis ensues if these changes are severe. Tachypnea may augment the changes. In massive embolization, severe hypoxemia may result from right atrial hypertension that causes right-to-left shunting of blood through a patent foramen ovale.

4. Pulmonary infarction (PI): Most PE do not produce infarction. When bronchial circulation is intact and normal (ie, in the absence of heart failure or underlying chronic lung disease), PI rarely develops. This suggests that collateral circulation of the bronchial artery keeps the lung tissue viable despite blockage of the pulmonary artery. However, patients with previously abnormal pulmonary circulation are prone to develop PI. Such infarcts may heal by absorption and fibrosis, leaving a linear scar, or may resorb completely, leaving a normal lung (incomplete infarction).

Acute PE is a dynamic process. Thrombi begin to lyse immediately after reaching the lung. Usually, complete clot lysis takes place within several weeks in the absence of preexisting cardiopulmonary disease, but, in some instances, even large thrombi may lyse in a few days. The physiologic alterations lessen over hours or days as the pulmonary circulation improves. Massive emboli may cause death within minutes or hours without sufficient time for infarction to develop. Smaller emboli may produce infarction that can heal with recanalization and restored blood flow. Infrequently, embolic events recur for months or years, causing progressive pulmonary arterial obstruction with chronic pulmonary hypertension, increasing dyspnea, and cor pulmonale.

Symptoms and Signs

The clinical manifestations of PE are nonspecific. Diagnosis may be difficult without using special procedures, the most important of which are radioisotope perfusion lung scans and pulmonary arteriography (see Diagnosis, below). The symptoms and signs vary in frequency and intensity depending on the extent of pulmonary vascular occlusion, the development of PI, and the patient's preembolic cardiopulmonary function. There may be no symptoms with small thromboemboli.

Embolism without infarction is manifested by breathlessness, which may be the only symptom if infarction does not develop. Tachypnea is a consistent and often striking feature. Anxiety and restlessness may be prominent.

Pulmonary hypertension, if severe, may cause dull substernal chest discomfort due to pulmonary artery distention or possibly myocardial ischemia. It may be manifested by an increase in the intensity of the pulmonary component of the basal 2nd sound or abnormal splitting (ie, widened with less variation of splitting during inspiration) of the aortic and pulmonary components of the basal 2nd sound. If pulmonary vascular obstruction is massive, acute RV insufficiency may supervene, with distended cervical veins, RV heave, RV presystolic or protodiastolic gallop, sometimes with arterial hypotension and evidence of peripheral vasoconstriction. Lightheadedness, syncopal episodes, convulsive phenomena, and neurologic deficits may be the presenting events in a significant number of patients, usually reflecting a transient fall in CO with secondary cerebral ischemia. Cyanosis is usual in patients with massive embolism, but not with lesser obstruction.

Examination of the lungs is usually normal in the absence of PI. Wheezing is sometimes heard, particularly if underlying bronchopulmonary or cardiac disease is present.

In addition to the above symptoms and signs, the manifestations of PI include cough, hemoptysis, pleuritic chest pain, fever, and signs of pulmonary consolidation or pleural fluid. A pleural friction rub may be heard. A small, peripheral embolus may cause infarction but not obstruct the pulmonary arteries to the extent that pulmonary hypertension develops.

The manifestations of embolization usually develop abruptly in minutes; those of infarction over a period of hours. They often last several days, depending on the rate of clot lysis and other factors, but usually decrease daily in intensity. In patients with chronic, recurrent emboli, the symptoms and signs of chronic cor pulmonale tend to develop insidiously during weeks, months, or years.

Diagnosis and Differential Diagnosis

The diagnosis of PE with or without infarction is often difficult to establish. **Differential diagnosis** in patients with massive PE includes bacteremic shock, acute myocardial infarction **(MI),** peritonitis, and cardiac tamponade. Without infarction, the patient's symptoms and signs may be attributed to anxiety with hyperventilation because of the paucity of objective pulmonary findings. When infarction occurs, the differential diagnosis includes pneumonia, atelectasis, heart failure, and pericarditis. A systematic approach to diagnosis is outlined below.

1. **The clinical symptoms and signs** should suggest the diagnosis.
2. **Appropriate clinical diagnostic studies,** including chest x-ray, ECG, CBC, and serum enzyme (AST, LDH) and serum bilirubin determinations may be helpful. With infarction, the **chest x-ray** frequently shows a peripheral infiltrative lesion, often involving the costophrenic angle, with elevation of the diaphragm and pleural fluid on the affected side. Diminished pulmonary vascular markings in the embolized area may be noted in the absence of infarction. Dilation of the pulmonary arteries in the hilar area, the superior vena cava, and the azygos vein signal pulmonary hypertension and RV strain. Since **ECG changes** are characteristically transient, serial tracings are often helpful in the diagnosis and in the exclusion of acute MI. Changes most frequently seen in the ECG include P pulmonale, right bundle branch block, right axis deviation, and supraventricular arrhythmias. The sensitivity and specificity of **serum enzyme studies** have been disappointing and the studies are rarely helpful in diagnosis. The triad of elevated serum LDH and bilirubin and normal AST (SGOT) occurs in $< 15\%$ of patients with acute PE and PI. Elevated LDH may be demonstrable in as many as 85% of patients with PI, but is nonspecific, occurring also in heart failure, shock, pregnancy, renal and liver disease, anemia, pneumonia, carcinoma, and after surgical procedures. A profile of enzyme studies involving elevated LDH, normal CK, and normal hydroxybutyrate dehydrogenase (HBD) is more specific in the diagnosis of PI and may differentiate acute MI, but is of little value in diagnosing PE without PI. Blood levels of **fibrin split products** appear to rise rather consistently after PE whether PI occurs or

not, but the interval of time between this rise and the onset of symptoms, and its duration, vary considerably. The specificity of this finding is also questionable since the incidence of elevation in other diseases is not well defined.

3. Radioisotope perfusion lung scanning, sometimes combined with **ventilation scanning,** is very valuable in establishing the diagnosis. **Lung perfusion scans** follow IV injection of 20- to 50-μm particles of biodegradable albumin labeled with technetium 99m. These particles traverse the right heart and, via the pulmonary arteries, ultimately lodge in the small precapillary arterioles of both lungs. Nearly 100% of the particles remain in the lungs, except when right-to-left shunting is present either at the cardiac or pulmonic level. Regional distribution of these particles is directly proportional to regional pulmonary arteriolar blood flow. This distribution is relatively homogeneous in normal persons, but visible activity is greater at the base and gradually diminishes up to the apex, reflecting gravitational effects on perfusion when the patient is injected in the sitting position. The distribution of particles depends on the position of the patient and pulmonary blood flow distribution at the time of injection. Perfusion deficit, with reduced or absent radioactivity, may result from vascular obstruction, displacement of lung by fluid, chest masses, any condition causing pulmonary arterial or venous hypertension, or loss of lung parenchyma as in pulmonary emphysema.

The lung perfusion scan is a valuable noninvasive method of detecting **acute PE,** especially when x-rays are normal. A normal scan excludes life-threatening PE with an accuracy of > 98%. Conversely, single or multiple wedge-shaped marginal scan defects, especially in a segmental or lobar distribution, are highly suggestive evidence of vascular obstruction. Sometimes, however, acute obstructive airways disease or COPD may produce a pattern of focal perfusion abnormalities. Progressive resolution of lesions favors a diagnosis of emboli, while a static picture favors chronic preexisting changes. Serial scans over a 3- to 6-day period may resolve the issue. Edema and alveolar secretions caused by lung infection will also produce perfusion defects. Characteristic x-ray changes of pneumonia and positive microbiologic studies help differentiate pneumonia from PE.

In cases where differentiation between PE and COPD is difficult, the xenon 133 lung **ventilation scan** may be useful. Inhaled radioactive gas distributes with the respiratory air. In acute PE with large perfusion defects, the radioxenon scan usually exhibits relatively normal ventilation of these areas, with $\dot{V}/\dot{Q}$ mismatches. Areas of parenchymal disease usually show abnormalities of both perfusion and ventilation, and will demonstrate delayed ventilation and trapping of radioactive gas.

However, combined ventilation-perfusion defects may be found with PE, particularly if scanning is carried out > 24 h after the event. Similarly, small perfusion defects with ventilation mismatch have neither sufficiently high nor low probability of PE to be of diagnostic value.

Any process leading to increased pulmonary venous pressure (eg, heart failure, mitral valve disease, or veno-occlusive disease) may produce redistribution of pulmonary blood flow. Thus, in this setting, instead of normal preponderance of radioactivity at the base of the lung, basal perfusion deficits may develop without PE.

4. Pulmonary arteriography: Demonstration of emboli by angiography remains the most definitive diagnostic test and should be performed if the diagnosis is in doubt and appears urgent. The 2 primary criteria for arteriographic diagnosis of PE are intra-arterial filling defects and complete obstruction (abrupt cutoff) of pulmonary arterial branches. Other frequent findings include partial obstruction of pulmonary arterial branches with increased caliber proximal and decreased caliber distal to the stenosis, oligemic zones, and persistence of dye in the proximal portion of the artery during the late (venous) phase of the arteriograms. In those lung segments with obstructed arteries, pulmonary venous filling with contrast medium is delayed or absent.

5. Additional diagnostic studies to establish the presence or absence of iliofemoral venous thrombotic disease may be useful in the management of PE, particularly when signs of recurrent embolization despite anticoagulant therapy or contraindications to anticoagulant therapy make vena caval interruption an important therapeutic consideration. Contrast venography appears to be the most reliable means of establishing the diagnosis of iliofemoral venous thrombosis, though noninvasive measures (eg, impedance plethysmography of the leg and assessment of femoral venous flow velocity by externally applied Doppler ultrasound flow probe) have been found to be about 75 to 90% as sensitive as phlebography. Intravascular injection of technetium-labelled albumin and iodine 125-labelled fibrinogen with leg scanning may detect venous thrombi, but the latter technic is useful only in relation to deep veins of the calf.

Prognosis

Mortality following the initial thromboembolic event varies with the extent of embolization and the patient's preexisting cardiorespiratory status. A patient with markedly compromised cardiopulmonary function is at greater risk of developing thromboemboli, and the likelihood that he will die following significant embolization is high (probably > 25%). On the other hand, it is unlikely that a patient with normal cardiopulmonary status will die unless the occlusive process involves > 50% of the pulmonary vascular bed. When the initial embolic event is fatal, death often occurs within 1 to 2 h.

If a patient survives the initial embolic event but is not treated, the likelihood of a recurrent embolus is about 50%; as many as half of these recurrences may be fatal. Anticoagulant therapy reduces the rate of recurrence to about 5%; only about 20% of these will be fatal.

Prophylaxis

PE can be prevented by preventing venous thrombosis. Therefore, the reduction of factors that predispose to venous thrombosis is of great importance, particularly those that minimize venous stasis. In postoperative (particularly elderly) patients, the use of elastic stockings to augment velocity of venous return in the legs, leg exercises, and early ambulation are widely used to lower the incidence of PE, but their benefit is questioned since they have little effect on the incidence of deep calf vein thrombosis. Intra- and postoperative pneumatic leg compression and electrical calf stimulation reduce the incidence of deep calf vein thrombosis, but their effects on iliofemoral vein thrombosis and pulmonary thromboembolic complications are unknown.

Low-dose heparin administration is generally considered effective in reducing the incidence of deep vein (calf) thrombosis and PE in patients who undergo a variety of elective major surgical procedures. At a blood level about ⅕ that required for therapeutic efficacy (prevention of thrombus propagation), heparin activates antithrombin III sufficiently to inhibit Factor X, which is required to convert prothrombin to thrombin at an early stage in the coagulation sequence. This results in preventing the initiation of clot formation, but is ineffective once Factor X is activated and the process has started. Heparin should be prescribed in USP units rather than in milligrams, since different preparations vary in potency. (NOTE: There are claims that the USP heparin unit is 10 to 15% more potent than the IU used in all Canadian and European studies.) The preparation of choice is aqueous sodium heparin given s.c. The repository form is not recommended because absorption is irregular and hematomas may form at the site of injection.

Heparin 5000 u. s.c. is given 2 h preoperatively and q 8 to 12 h thereafter for 7 days. Although no laboratory monitoring is usually required, it should be recognized that heparin administered in this dosage is not entirely without risk. Bleeding, impaired wound healing, induction of a fully anticoagulated state, and thrombocytopenia have been observed. Further, its effectiveness has been demonstrated only with elective

surgery, not including orthopedic procedures or abdominal prostatectomy. The low overall incidence of fatal PE with elective surgical procedures (an order of 0.2%) does not appear to warrant its routine administration. In view of these considerations, it is recommended with elective surgery only in patients at increased risk due to prior thromboembolic disease, lower extremity paralysis, obesity, heart failure, COPD, prolonged immobilization, or chronic venous stasis of the lower extremities. It is **contraindicated** with cerebral surgery.

Heparin prophylaxis may also be used in hospitalized patients at high risk for PE with acute MI, cardiac failure, stroke, paraplegia, or other debilitating disease. The MI group at highest risk includes elderly patients, those with heart failure, hypotension or shock, obesity, and previous thromboembolism. Although a favorable impact on mortality (fatal PE) has not been established, both heparin and oral anticoagulants effectively prevent venous thrombosis in these high risk medical patients, with reduced incidence of PE in some studies. In the absence of bleeding diathesis, these patients, particularly those with MI also at risk for development of intracardiac thrombi and systemic embolization, may be considered for "moderate" dose heparin administration of 18 to 25,000 u./24 h, by continuous infusion or s.c. injection q 8 to 12 h, or full dose heparin administration (see below) sufficient to prolong the partial thromboplastin time (PTT) to 1.5 to 2.0 times the normal control. Treatment should be continued for the duration of hospitalization or until the patient becomes ambulatory. Oral anticoagulant therapy may be initiated on admission (see below), with discontinuance of heparin several days later when anticoagulation is established.

Agents to prevent platelet aggregation (aspirin, dipyridamole) have been tried to prevent venous thromboembolism, but results are inconclusive or frankly negative. Dextran appears effective in reducing the incidence of thromboembolism in postoperative patients, but requires IV administration, is no better than warfarin, has as many hemorrhagic complications, and may precipitate volume overload.

Treatment

The management of PE involves treatment of the initial thromboembolic event and prevention of further episodes.

Treatment of the initial event is supportive. Analgesics are given if pleuritic pain is severe. Though anxiety is often prominent, sedatives, especially barbiturates, should be prescribed cautiously. O_2 therapy is indicated when appreciable arterial hypoxemia ($Pa_{O_2} < 60$ to 65 mm Hg) is present, particularly if CO is also reduced. Continuous O_2 should be given, usually by mask or cannula, in a concentration sufficient to raise Pa_{O_2} and Sa_{O_2} to normal (85 to 95 mm Hg, 95 to 98%) or as near normal levels as possible (≥ 60 mm Hg).

In patients with clinical findings suggestive of pulmonary hypertension and acute cor pulmonale, particularly pending diagnostic procedures (eg, lung scanning and/or arteriography), β-adrenergic stimulation may help to maintain tissue perfusion because of its effects as a pulmonary vasodilator and cardiotonic. Isoproterenol 2 to 4 mg/L of 5% D/W may be infused at a rate sufficient to maintain systolic BP at 90 to 100 mm Hg under continuous ECG monitoring. Appropriate drugs may be useful in aborting and preventing supraventricular tachyarrhythmias. Digitalis should be avoided during acute hypoxemia unless absolutely necessary (eg, for serious arrhythmia or heart failure). When given IV, a modest initial dose is usually desirable (digoxin 0.25 to 0.5 mg; deslanoside 0.4 to 0.8 mg). Response to therapy in patients suspected of hemodynamic impairment with acute cor pulmonale may be monitored by serial measurement of arterial blood gases and hemodynamic parameters. Use of a flow-directed balloon (Swan-Ganz) catheter is valuable for determination of pulmonary artery and wedge pressures, as well as mixed venous blood O_2 saturation and/or content and thermodilution determination of CO.

Following massive PE, particularly with hypotension, or submassive PE and hypoten-

sion in patients with preexisting cardiorespiratory disease, 2 approaches to management may be considered: pulmonary embolectomy or thrombolytic therapy. In the event of cardiac arrest with massive PE, the usual resuscitative measures are ineffective due to obstruction of blood flow through the lungs. In this setting, emergency partial (femoral venoarterial) bypass, pending pulmonary embolectomy, may be life-saving. In view of the considerable potential for diagnoses other than PE, pulmonary angiography while on bypass is advisable in most cases before surgery.

Thrombolytic therapy may now be considered as an alternative to embolectomy when massive PE is uncomplicated by hypotension or when systolic BP can be maintained at 90 to 100 mm Hg on moderate vasopressor dosage. Streptokinase and urokinase, equally effective fibrinolytic activators, enhance the conversion of plasminogen to plasmin, the active fibrinolytic enzyme. **Contraindications** to thrombolytic therapy include intracranial neoplasm, stroke within 2 mo, active bleeding from any source, preexisting hemorrhagic diathesis (as in severe liver or kidney disease), pregnancy, and surgery within the preceding 10 days—the latter representing a major limitation to its use. Therapy should be carried out within 3 days of the embolic episode, as organization of the thrombus will obviate the lytic effect.

If the patient has been on heparin, the PTT should be permitted to fall to < 2 times the control before initiating fibrinolytic therapy. Premedication with hydrocortisone sodium succinate 100 mg IV and re-injection q 12 h will minimize allergic and pyrogenic reactions to streptokinase. After baseline determination of fibrinogen level or thrombin time, streptokinase 250,000 u. is given IV over 30 min, followed by continuous infusion of 100,000 u./h for 24 h. After 3 to 4 h, the fibrinogen level should be about ½ control and thrombin time 2 times or more the baseline. If significant change does not occur, the patient is resistant to streptokinase, and should be placed on urokinase or heparin therapy. A priming dose of urokinase 4400 u./kg is given over a 10-min period, followed by 4400 u./kg/h for 12 h. Following streptokinase or urokinase infusion, the PTT should be allowed to fall to 1.5 to 2.5 times the baseline value before initiation of a sustaining infusion of heparin without loading dose. All patients undergoing thrombolytic therapy have an increased bleeding risk, particularly from recent operative wounds, needle puncture sites, sites of invasive procedures, and the GI tract. Thus invasive procedures should be avoided. Pressure dressings are usually required to stop oozing; serious or catastrophic bleeding will require cessation of the thrombolytic agent, and administration of cryoprecipitate or fresh frozen plasma. In addition, aminocaproic acid 5 gm IV immediately and 1 gm/h thereafter may be effective in reversing the fibrinolytic state.

Preventing further thrombus formation with embolization then becomes the essence of treatment. Heparin may be given IV q 4 to 6 h, or by continuous IV drip with an infusion pump. However, a hemorrhagic disorder or an active bleeding site is an **absolute contraindication** to heparin therapy; septic embolization is usually taken as a contraindication. Hemorrhagic complications of heparin therapy are discussed below. They are frequent in patients over age 65, particularly women, and heparin should be given to these patients only for short periods—usually no more than several days—before changing to an oral anticoagulant. Some evidence suggests that hemorrhagic complications are reduced by continuous infusion, which obviates the peaks and troughs of blood levels with bolus injection. By either method of administration, larger dosage may be required for the first 48 h.

Following a rapid IV loading dose of heparin 100 u./kg, it is given at a rate to keep the clotting time **(CT)** at 2 to 2.5 times control or the PTT at 1.5 to 2 times control by checking the level 30 min before giving the next dose of heparin. The maintenance dose by continuous infusion is usually 10 to 50 u./kg/h. Once a therapeutic level is established with continuous infusion, CT and/or PTT need to be monitored only 1 to 2 times/day.

After 5 to 10 days, or when the patient becomes ambulatory, oral warfarin sodium is given in addition to heparin. The oral agent and heparin should overlap for 5 to 7 days, allowing the oral anticoagulant to take effect. Warfarin sodium may be given, usually in a dosage of 5 to 15 mg/day. When the prothrombin time rises to a level 1.5 to 2.5 times control, heparin is discontinued.

The duration of anticoagulation therapy is adjusted individually for each patient. In patients with a definable, reversible cause (eg, the postoperative state), anticoagulation need be continued only until the condition is corrected (eg, the patient is fully ambulatory). Otherwise, anticoagulation therapy may be continued empirically for 3 to 6 mo. A patient with a chronic medical disorder associated with high incidence of thromboembolism should be considered for long-term anticoagulant therapy.

Five to 10% of patients treated with oral anticoagulants are prone to bleeding complications, of which up to 50% may be severe. Patients taking anticoagulants should not be given any drug containing aspirin, which can further impair hemostatic mechanisms. Drugs that interfere with protein binding or metabolism of the oral anticoagulants (eg, barbiturates, quinine, phenylbutazone, clofibrate, chloral hydrate) should be used cautiously when given concurrently with warfarin.

Complications of anticoagulation: Minor bleeding manifestations (ecchymoses at the site of injections, microscopic hematuria, bleeding from gums) or a prolongation of clotting times to > 60 min can usually be controlled by withholding the next scheduled dose of heparin and reducing subsequent doses. If **major bleeding** occurs, protamine, a protein that combines with heparin to form an inactive complex, should be used to neutralize the anticoagulant effect of heparin. One ampul containing 50 mg/5 mL diluted with 20 mL of 0.9% sodium chloride solution and injected IV over a 5-min period (CAUTION: *Rapid injection may cause hypotension, dyspnea, and bradycardia*) neutralizes about 5000 u. of heparin and usually suffices to counteract overheparinization. The therapeutic effect of protamine may be checked by testing the clotting time 5 min after the injection. Blood transfusions may be required to cover major blood losses but do not reduce the anticoagulant effect of overheparinization.

Surgical venous interruption of the inferior vena cava should be considered in certain situations: (1) contraindications to anticoagulation, (2) recurrent emboli despite adequate anticoagulation, (3) septic pelvic thrombophlebitis with emboli, and (4) in conjunction with pulmonary embolectomy. Venous ligation at the femoral level is accompanied by unacceptable mortality from postoperative pulmonary embolism. The optimum site of interruption is the inferior vena cava just below the entry of the renal veins together with the spermatic or ovarian veins. Procedures used for interruption in addition to ligation include partially occluding clips or suture, as well as an umbrella device introduced into the inferior vena cava via the internal jugular vein. Patients who have had vena caval interruption require anticoagulation for at least 6 mo following the procedure. Morbidity following such procedures is significant (10 to 15%), and recurrent embolization may occur in as many as 50% of patients from the site of interruption or through large collateral (lumbar) veins if interruption is complete.

---

40. PNEUMONIA

(Pneumonitis)

An acute infection of lung parenchyma including alveolar spaces and interstitial tissue; involvement may be confined to an entire lobe ***(lobar pneumonia),*** *a segment of a lobe* ***(segmental*** *or* ***lobular pneumonia),*** *alveoli contiguous to bronchi* ***(bronchopneumonia)*** *or interstitial tissue* ***(interstitial pneumonia).*** These distinctions are generally based on x-ray observations.

Etiology and Epidemiology

The most common causes in adults are bacteria: *Streptococcus pneumoniae*, anaerobic bacteria, *Staphylococcus aureus*, *Hemophilus influenzae*, *Legionella pneumophila*, *Klebsiella pneumoniae*, and other gram-negative bacilli. *Mycoplasma pneumoniae*, a bacteria-like organism, is a particularly common cause in older children and young adults. Major pulmonary pathogens in infants and children are viruses: respiratory syncytial virus, adenovirus, parainfluenza, influenza A and B, agents of viral exanthems (eg, varicella, measles, rubella), Epstein-Barr virus, and enterovirus. These agents may also cause pneumonia in adults; however, the only potentially serious and prevalent viruses in previously healthy adults are influenza A and occasionally influenza B. Among other agents are higher bacteria including nocardia and actinomyces; mycobacteria, including typical strains (*M. tuberculosis*) and atypical strains (primarily *M. kansasii* and *M. avium-intracellulare*); fungi including *Histoplasma capsulatum*, *Coccidioides immitis*, *Blastomyces dermatitidis*, *Cryptococcus neoformans*, *Aspergillus fumigatus* and *Mucor* sp; parasites, primarily *Pneumocystis carinii* and *Toxoplasma gondii*; rickettsia, primarily *Coxiella burnetii* (Q fever); and Chlamydia, primarily *C. psittaci* (psittacosis) and *C. trachomatis*, a relatively common pathogen in infants. (For a discussion of bacterial and chlamydial pneumonias in newborns, see NEONATAL PNEUMONIA in Ch. 186.)

Predisposing factors include respiratory viral infections, alcoholism, age extremes, debility, immunosuppressive disorders and therapy, compromised consciousness, dysphagia, and exposure to transmissible agents. The usual mechanisms are either to inhale droplets small enough to reach the alveoli, or to aspirate secretions from the upper airways. Other means include hematagenous dissemination, via the lymphatics, or directly from contiguous infections.

In the USA, of about 2 million people who get pneumonia each year, 40,000 to 70,000 die; as the most common lethal infection, it ranks sixth among all disease categories as a cause of death and is the most frequent lethal hospital-acquired infection. In developing countries, lower respiratory tract infections are usually either the major cause of death or they rank second only to diarrhea. Despite this prevalence, there are few infections whose etiologic agent is so difficult to identify. Thirty to 50% of patients have no identifiable pathogen despite a clinical impression of bacterial pneumonia. Although the time-honored method to identify bacterial pathogens is to culture expectorated sputum, these specimens are often misleading due to contamination by the normal oropharyngeal flora during passage through the upper airways. The most reliable specimen sources include positive blood cultures in patients with bacteremic pneumonia, cultures of pleural fluid in patients with empyema, and of transtracheal and transthoracic aspirates collected more directly from the lower airways. Special culture technics, serologic assays, or lung biopsies are required to identify many pathogens: mycobacteria, mycoplasma, anaerobic bacteria, chlamydia, viruses, fungi, legionella, rickettsia, and parasites.

PNEUMOCOCCAL PNEUMONIA

S. pneumoniae is the most common cause of bacterial pneumonia, although it may be less prevalent in this era of chemotherapy. The disease is generally sporadic but most frequent in winter. Studies of pharyngeal flora indicate that 5 to 25% of healthy persons are carriers of pneumococci, with the highest rates noted for children and parents of children in winter. There are > 80 serotypes based on antigenically distinct capsular polysaccharides that appear to confer type-specific immunity following infection.

Pathology and Pathogenesis

Pneumococci usually reach the lungs via the upper respiratory tract by inhalation or aspiration. They lodge in bronchioles, proliferate, and initiate an inflammatory process

that begins in alveolar spaces with an outpouring of protein-rich fluid, which acts as a culture medium for the organism as well as a mechanism for spread to alveoli in contiguous segments.

The earliest stage of pneumonia is **congestion** characterized by extensive serous exudation, vascular engorgement, and rapid bacterial proliferation. The next stage is called **"red hepatization,"** reflecting the liver-like appearance of the consolidated lung: Airspaces are filled with polymorphonuclear cells, there is vascular congestion, and extravasation of RBCs provides the basis for the reddish discoloration on gross examination. The parenchyma is intact, but transformation of the usual air-containing spaces into a solid organ with a dense inflammatory response provides the anatomic basis for the term "hepatization." The next stage is **"gray hepatization"** in which an accumulation of fibrin is associated with inflammatory WBCs and RBCs in various stages of disintegration, and alveolar spaces are packed with an inflammatory exudate. The final stage is **resolution** characterized by resorption of the exudate.

Symptoms and Signs

Pneumococcal pneumonia is often preceded by a URI. The onset is usually sudden with a single shaking chill; persistent chills suggest an alternative diagnosis. This is ordinarily followed by fever, pain with breathing on the involved side (pleurisy), cough, dyspnea, and sputum production. The pain may be referred and, with lower lobe involvement, may suggest intraabdominal sepsis. The temperature rises rapidly to 38 to 40.5 C (100.4 to 105 F); the pulse is usually 100 to 140/min; and respirations accelerate to 20 to 45/min. Additional common findings are nausea, vomiting, malaise, and myalgias. The cough may be dry initially, but usually becomes productive with purulent, blood-streaked or "rusty" sputum. The features noted are typical for pneumococcal pneumonia in a previously healthy host. In many instances, especially among patients at age extremes, the disease is more insidious with relatively fewer symptoms to suggest a lower respiratory tract infection.

Findings on physical examination are variable depending on the character of the process and the stage in which the patient is evaluated. **Typical pulmonary signs of lobar pneumonia** are tactile fremitus, percussion dullness, bronchial breath sounds, and whispered pectoriloquy. With pleural effusions or empyema, there is dullness to percussion, diminished breath sounds, or a pleural rub. In bronchopneumonia the usual findings of consolidation may occur, but the most frequent observation is simply rales.

Complications

Serious, potentially lethal complications include overwhelming sepsis, sometimes associated with the adult respiratory distress syndrome and/or septic shock. Some patients develop infections at contiguous sites (eg, empyema or purulent pericarditis). Bacteremia may result in extrapulmonary foci of infections, the principle metastatic foci being septic arthritis, endocarditis, meningitis, or peritonitis (in patients with ascites). Some patients develop pulmonary superinfections; during the usual course of treatment, temporary improvement is followed by deterioration with recurrence of fever and new pulmonary infiltrates. Pleural effusions are found in about 25% of patients by chest x-ray, but only about 1% of patients have empyema.

Laboratory Findings

Laboratory studies usually show a leukocytosis with a shift to the left. There may be blood gas abnormalites due to perfusion of poorly aerated lung resulting in hypoxemia and a respiratory alkalosis.

Gram stain of exudate typically shows gram-positive lancet-shaped diplococci in short chains. With expectorated sputum there should be ≥ 10 typical morphotypes per oil immersion field. Definitive evidence that these streptococci are *S. pneumoniae* in expectorated sputum or other samples may be determined by demonstrating capsular swelling with the application of polyvalent pneumococcal antiserum; this is the **"quel-**

lung reaction," which provides immediate information, but requires an experienced observer. This technic can specify types by using a type-specific antiserum with isolated strains. Some laboratories use counterimmunoelectrophoresis **(CIE)** as an alternate antigen detection method to determine serotypes of isolated strains or for case detection using specimens of sputum, urine, or other body fluids.

X-ray Findings

A chest x-ray invariably shows a pulmonary infiltrate, although findings may be minimal or indetectable during the first several hours. Pneumococci are clearly responsible for most cases of lobar pneumonia in which the chest x-ray shows dense consolidation confined to a single lobe with typical air bronchograms. However, pneumococci are also relatively common causes of bronchopneumonia, the most frequent x-ray finding. Thus, the most frequent cause of lobar pneumonia is *S. pneumoniae*, but the most frequent x-ray pattern among all patients with pneumococcal pneumonia is a bronchopneumonia pattern.

Diagnosis

Pneumococcal pneumonia should be suspected in anyone with an acute febrile illness associated with chill, chest pain, and cough. A presumptive diagnosis can be based on the history, changes on chest x-ray, culture and Gram stains of appropriate specimens, the quellung reaction, or CIE. An absolute diagnosis requires demonstration of *S. pneumoniae* in pleural fluid, blood, or lung or transtracheal aspirate.

Prognosis

Although the morbidity and mortality of pneumococcal pneumonia have changed substantially since the advent of penicillin (no substantial changes are related to other antibiotics), antibiotics have minimal impact on mortality during the first 5 days of illness. The overall mortality rate is about 5%. Factors that herald a relatively poor prognosis include the following: age extremes, especially < 1 yr or > 60 yr; positive blood cultures; involvement of > 1 lobe; a peripheral WBC count < 5000/mL; presence of associated diseases (eg, cirrhosis, heart failure, immunosuppression, agammaglobulinemia, splenectomy or functional asplenia, and uremia); involvement with certain serotypes (especially 3 and 8), and development of extrapulmonary complications (eg, meningitis or endocarditis).

Prophylaxis

Vaccine containing 23 of the 80-plus pneumococcal type-specific polysaccharide antigens is available. These serotypes account for 85 to 90% of pneumococcal serotypes that cause serious pneumococcal infections. Most children > 2 yr old and adults show an antigenic response within 2 to 3 wk after vaccination, although measurement of antibody titers is not indicated since precise protective levels are unknown. About 50% of vaccinated patients develop erythema and/or pain at the injection site; about 1% develop fever, myalgias, or a severe local reaction; and 5:million develop an anaphylactoid or other serious reaction. Severe reactions are more frequent after revaccination. Vaccination is recommended for children > 2 yr and adults who have an increased risk for pneumococcal disease or its complications. Included are persons with chronic diseases, especially cardiovascular and pulmonary; patients with splenic dysfunction or anatomic asplenia, Hodgkin's disease, multiple myeloma, cirrhosis, alcoholism, renal failure, organ transplant, and other conditions associated with immunosuppression; children with nephrosis; older adults, especially those ≥ 65 yr who are otherwise healthy; and patients with CSF leaks. Antibody response is reduced in immunosuppressed patients, and asplenic children should receive prophylactic penicillin as well as pneumococcal vaccine. Recurrent URI in children (including otitis media and sinusitis) is not considered an indication for vaccination. The duration of protec-

tion is not known, although the period appears to be extended; revaccination is not advocated due to the increased incidence of side effects.

Treatment

Penicillin G is the preferred agent when pneumococcal pneumonia is suspected or established; alternative drugs with demonstrable efficacy include cephalosporins, erythromycin, and clindamycin. Since tetracyclines are less predictably active against *S. pneumoniae*, they *should not be used for seriously ill patients*. Pneumococcal resistance is categorized as "relative resistance" (minimum inhibitory concentration **[MIC]** 0.1 to 1.0 μg/mL) or "resistant" (MIC ≥ 1 μg/mL). The prevalence of relative resistance in clinical isolates ranges from 1 to 16%, but is usually 2%; implications for therapy are unclear, but high-dose penicillin is usually advocated. Highly resistant strains should be treated with erythromycin, chloramphenicol, tetracycline, or vancomycin. The 1 μg oxycillin disk is advocated as an appropriate method to detect resistant strains. Isolates with zone sizes of ≤ 19 mm should be tested with broth dilution.

Specific therapy: Patients who are not severely ill may be treated with penicillin G or V 250 to 500 mg orally q 6 h. Alternative oral regimens include tetracycline, erythromycin, or cephalexin 500 mg q 6 h or clindamycin 300 mg q 6 h. Regimens recommended for parenteral treatment of uncomplicated pneumococcal pneumonia are procaine penicillin 600,000 u. IM q 12 h or aqueous penicillin G 500,000 to 1 million u. IV q 4 to 6 h. Alternative parenteral regimens include cephalothin 500 mg IV q 6 h or cefazolin 500 mg IM or IV q 8 to 12 h, erythromycin 500 mg to 1 gm IV q 6 h or clindamycin 300 to 600 mg IV q 6 to 8 h.

When meningitis or endocarditis is suspected, the dose of penicillin G should be 2 million u. IV q 2 h; the alternative agent recommended for pneumococcal meningitis in patients hypersensitive to penicillins is chloramphenicol 1 gm IV q 6 h. Patients with empyema should have appropriate drainage as well as antibiotic therapy.

Supportive measures include bedrest, fluids, and analgesics for pleuritic pain. O_2 is given to patients with cyanosis, significant hypoxia, severe dyspnea, circulatory disturbances, or delirium. It must be given cautiously with frequent monitoring of blood gases, especially in patients with chronic lung disease.

Response to therapy varies: Mildly ill patients who are treated relatively early in the course will usually defervesce during the first 24 to 48 h; however, seriously ill patients and particularly those with the poor prognostic features noted above will often require ≥ 4 days to become afebrile. Therapy should not be modified if there is gradual clinical improvement and the etiology is confirmed.

Factors to consider when patients do not improve include the following: wrong etiologic diagnosis, adverse drug reaction, far-advanced or superinfection, inadequate host defenses due to associated conditions, non-compliance to the drug regimen in outpatients, antibiotic resistance of the involved strain of *S. pneumoniae*, and complications like empyema requiring drainage, or metastatic foci of infection requiring higher doses of penicillin (eg, meningitis, endocarditis, or septic arthritis). Resistance of pneumococci to penicillin has been noted recently, especially in South Africa. These strains are relatively rare in the USA; most are only "moderately resistant" with minimum inhibitory concentrations of < 1 μg/mL, so they should respond to penicillin or other β-lactam antibiotics using somewhat higher doses than those recommended (see above). Follow-up x-rays are usually advised for patients > 35 yr. Resolution of the infiltrate as seen on chest x-ray may take several weeks, especially in patients with severe disease, bacteremia, or preexisting chronic lung disease. Persistent infiltration ≥ 6 wk after therapy begins suggests possibility of an underlying bronchogenic neoplasm or TB.

STAPHYLOCOCCAL PNEUMONIA

Incidence and Epidemiology

S. aureus accounts for about 2% of community-acquired pneumonias and 10 to 15% of hospital-acquired pneumonias. These patients are at particular risk: infants, debilitated patients and the elderly; hospitalized patients, especially those with severe debility, surgery, tracheostomy, endotracheal intubation, and immunosuppression; children and young adults with cystic fibrosis; patients with a bacterial superinfection following viral pneumonias, especially influenza; patients with IV drug abuse who are prone to staphylococcal tricuspid-valve endocarditis with embolic pneumonia; patients with certain types of immunosuppression, especially those with chronic granulomatous disease of childhood, in which there is a defect in phagocytic killing of bacteria.

Symptoms and Signs

Clinical observations in general parallel those (noted above) for pneumococcal pneumonia. Staphylococcal pneumonia differs by a tendency to cause recurrent rigors, tissue necrosis with abscess formation (rare with pneumococcal pneumonia), and pneumatoceles (most common in infants and children); a fulminant course with marked prostration; and the specific settings noted above. Changes on chest x-ray are variable. The most common pattern is a bronchopneumonia with or without abscess formation or pleural effusion; lobar consolidation is infrequent. Pneumatoceles are most frequent in infants and strongly suggest this etiologic diagnosis. Embolic staphylococcal pneumonia is characterized by multiple infiltrates at discontiguous sites that tend to cavitate and suggest an endovascular source (eg, right-sided endocarditis or septic thrombophlebitis). Leukocytosis is generally present. Empyema is relatively common, often complicating a bronchopleural fistula, and *S. aureus* is especially prevalent in post-thoracotomy empyemas or empyemas complicating tube drainage of a hemothorax following chest wall trauma. Although often fulminant, staphylococcal pneumonia occurs in some patients who do not appear critically ill; occasional individuals have a rather indolent course, sometimes with chronic pneumonia or chronic lung abscess. Nevertheless, most adults with bronchopneumonia will not have these complications.

Diagnosis

The diagnosis is suspected in patients who have *S. aureus* in expectorated sputum according to Gram stain and culture and established by recovery of *S. aureus* in blood cultures, empyema fluid, or transtracheal or transthoracic aspirate. Unlike the pneumococcus, this organism is relatively easy to cultivate so that false-negative cultures are unusual.

Prognosis and Treatment

The mortality rate is generally reported at 30 to 40%. This reflects in part the serious associated conditions found in most patients, although a fulminant course with a lethal outcome is sometimes seen among previously healthy adults who develop this infection following influenza. Response to antibiotics tends to be slow and convalescence is prolonged.

Most strains of *S. aureus* produce penicillinase, and methicillin-resistance is also increasing. The recommended therapy is a penicillinase-resistant penicillin (eg, oxacillin or nafcillin 2 gm IV q 4 to 6 h). The major alternative is a cephalosporin; preferred agents are cephalothin or cefamandole 2 gm IV q 4 to 6 h. Third generation cephalosporins are somewhat less active than first or second generation agents. Another alternative that is active against 90 to 95% of strains is clindamycin 600 mg IV q 6 h.

Methicillin-resistant strains are considered resistant to all β-lactam antibiotics. These strains are particularly prevalent in large teaching hospitals, where they may account for up to 20% of all staphylococcal isolates. Vancomycin is preferred when

methicillin-resistance is suspected or established with in vitro sensitivity tests. The usual dose is 0.5 gm IV q 6 h with appropriate modifications when renal failure is present.

STREPTOCOCCAL PNEUMONIA

Lancefield's Group A β-hemolytic streptococci are a relatively rare cause of pneumonia. The largest epidemics occurred among recruits during World War I; since then even sporadic cases have been infrequent. The occasional case now seen is usually a complication of influenza, measles, chickenpox, or pertussis.

Symptoms and Signs

As with other bacterial pneumonias, the onset of fever, dyspnea, cough, and chest pain is usually abrupt. Rigors are seen less often than with pneumococcal pneumonia, possibly due to the infrequency of bacteremia. Pleurisy is highly characteristic; when present, it usually indicates pleural complications. Usual findings on chest x-ray are an interstitial bronchopneumonia with a large pleural effusion. Thoracentesis may show serous, serosanguinous, or purulent fluid. Occasionally there is a lobular pneumonia with abscess formation.

Diagnosis

Streptococcal pneumonia should be suspected in an acutely ill patient whose pneumonia is complicated by an early pleural effusion and associated with measles, chickenpox, pertussis, influenza, streptococcal pharyngitis, or scarlet fever. However, pneumonia is a rare complication of streptococcal tonsillitis, pharyngitis, or scarlet fever. A Gram stain of expectorated sputum will show many gram-positive cocci in chains that may be distinguished from *S. pneumoniae* by lack of the lancet shape, and a negative quellung reaction. However, these organisms resemble α-hemolytic streptococci, which are normal oral flora. Cultures of expectorated sputum usually yield typical hemolytic streptococci, although these may be contaminants from the upper airways and Lancefield grouping is important. Group A is the usual pulmonary pathogen and other groups that are β-hemolytic are more likely to represent oropharyngeal contaminants. Throat cultures yield hemolytic streptococci in 20 to 70% of cases, pleural fluid cultures are positive in 30 to 50%, and blood cultures are usually negative. Serologic evidence of streptococcal infection can be established by demonstrating a significant increase in the antistreptolysin-O titer with serial tests.

Treatment

In contrast to pneumococcal pneumonia, although response to therapy tends to be slow, overall mortality is very low.

Penicillin G 500,000 to 1 million u. IV q 4 to 6 h is the preferred regimen. Alternative agents are cephalosporins, erythromycin, or clindamycin. Tetracycline shows erratic activity against hemolytic streptococci and *should not be used*. Large pleural effusions are anticipated, but the fluid remains thin for a longer period so that it may usually be managed with repeated thoracentesis or closed catheter drainage. Purulent collections and loculated effusions should be drained by tube thoracostomy.

PNEUMONIA CAUSED BY *Klebsiella* AND OTHER GRAM-NEGATIVE BACILLI

Etiology

While most species of *Enterobacteriaceae* and *Pseudomonas* are implicated as pulmonary pathogens, the most frequent and best characterized is *K. pneumoniae*, which causes **Friedländer's pneumonia.** These organisms rarely cause lung infections in a previously well adult host. The usual settings are infancy and old age; pneumonia ac-

quired in hospitals or nursing homes; and debilitated or immunocompromised hosts, especially those with neutropenia. The usual pathophysiologic mechanism is colonization of the oropharynx followed by microaspiration of upper airway secretions. Gram-negative bacilli colonize the upper airways in association with serious diseases with a frequency that is directly correlated with the severity of the underlying condition. Gram-negative bacilli are most often encountered in hospital-acquired pneumonia, and gram-negative bacillary pneumonia is the most frequent lethal nosocomial infection. The usual pathogens are *K. pneumoniae*, *Pseudomonas aeruginosa*, *E. coli*, *Enterobacter* sp, *Proteus* sp, *Serratia marcescens*, and Acinetobacter.

Symptoms and Signs

Friedländer's pneumonia is characterized by frequent upper lobe involvement, sputum that looks like currant jelly, tissue necrosis with early abscess formation, and a fulminant course. While serotypes 1 to 6 are considered most virulent, experience indicates that *K. pneumoniae* lung infections tend to involve higher serotypes and that the unique features found in the classical studies are not usually present. Most patients with lung infections involving *K. pneumoniae* or other gram-negative bacilli have a bronchopneumonia similar to other bacterial lung infections except for the associated high mortality. All of these organisms may cause abscess formation, especially *K. pneumoniae* and *P. aeruginosa*.

Diagnosis

Gram-negative bacilli should be suspected in a patient with pneumonia who is in one of the risk categories noted above, especially with neutropenia or nosocomial pneumonia. Gram stains of sputum usually show large numbers of gram-negative bacilli; however, it is impossible to distinguish the various species and genera in the group on the basis of morphologic characteristics. Sputum cultures usually yield the pathogen; the major problem is false-positive cultures from organisms that colonize the upper airways, especially in patients previously treated with an antibiotic for pneumonia due to other bacteria. ("Sputum superinfection" must be distinguished from "patient superinfection.") Positive cultures from blood, pleural fluid, or a transtracheal aspirate obtained before treatment are considered diagnostic.

Prognosis and Treatment

The mortality for gram-negative bacillary pneumonia is about 25 to 50% despite availability of presumably effective antibiotics.

Antibiotic regimens are based on antimicrobial sensitivity patterns. The usual treatment is an aminoglycoside combined with a β-lactam antibiotic or a β-lactam agent used alone. Most authorities prefer drug combinations rather than aminoglycosides alone. Empirically, when this diagnosis is suspected (because of the disease setting or the sputum Gram stain), most use gentamicin or tobramycin 1.7 mg/kg IV q 8 h, or amikacin 5 mg/kg q 8 h. One of these agents is combined with a cephalosporin, a broad spectrum penicillin, or both. Cephalosporin options include cephalothin 1.5 to 2 gm IV q 4 to 6 h, cefoxitin 2 gm IV q 6 h, cefamandole 2 gm IV q 6 h or cefotaxime 2 gm IV q 6 h. Penicillins commonly selected for combination with an aminoglycoside are carbenicillin 6 gm IV q 4 h, ticarcillin 3 gm IV q 4 h or piperacillin 3 gm IV q 4 h. A broad spectrum cephalosporin such as cefotaxime may be used alone, although this is inadequate for many infections involving *P. aeruginosa* and incurs the risk of emerging resistance during treatment. Most infections involving *P. aeruginosa* are treated with an aminoglycoside combined with an antipseudomonad penicillin selected on the basis of in vitro sensitivity tests. These treatment guidelines may require modification when multiple pathogens are suspect, since expectorated sputum cultures often yield a polymicrobial flora. Optimal regimens may also require in vitro studies of synergy. Dosage recommendations noted above apply only to adults and should be modified when renal failure is present.

PNEUMONIA CAUSED BY *Hemophilus influenzae*

Etiology and Incidence

H. influenzae, erroneously implicated as a cause of influenza during the pandemic of 1889, is a relatively common cause of bacterial pneumonia, second only to *S. pneumoniae* in most studies of community-acquired lung infections. Strains containing the type b **(Hib)** polysaccharide capsule are most virulent and most likely to cause serious disease including meningitis, epiglottitis, and bacteremic pneumonia. Incidence rates of Hib disease are increased in certain high-risk groups, such as American Indians and Eskimos, blacks, individuals of lower socioeconomic status, and patients with asplenia, sickle cell disease, Hodgkin's disease, and antibody deficiency syndromes. Recent studies also have suggested that the risk of acquiring primary Hib disease for children < 5 yr of age appears to be greater for those who attend day-care facilities than for those who do not. By age 6 yr, most people have had antigenic exposure to Hib, which confers relative protection. Strains of *H. influenzae* (that commonly colonize the upper airways of adults) colonize the lower respiratory tract of patients with chronic bronchitis, and cause lung infections in adults that are usually unencapsulated or "nontypable."

Symptoms, Signs, and Diagnosis

Hib pneumonia usually occurs in children with a median age of 1 yr. Coryza precedes most cases and early pleural effusions are noted in about 50%. Most adults have infections involving non-encapsulated strains with a bronchopneumonia that resembles other bacterial pneumonias. Many patients have underlying chronic lung disease, especially bronchitis.

Gram stain of expectorated sputum shows numerous, small, gram-negative coccobacilli; the organism is relatively fastidious and frequently colonizes the upper airways so that false-negative and -positive cultures are common. In children, bacteremia and empyema are usually found with infections involving Hib.

Prophylaxis

H. influenza type b capsular polysaccharide vaccine is advocated for all children at 24 mo of age and possibly for children aged 2 to 5 yr who have not previously been immunized. Earlier vaccination (at age 18 to 23 mo) should be considered in high-risk children (eg, with sickle cell disease and clients of day care centers).

Treatment

The usual treatment is ampicillin 100 mg/kg/day IV for children < 20 kg or 250 mg to 1 gm q 6 h for children > 20 kg and adults. Alternative regimens are amoxicillin 20 to 40 mg/kg orally tid for children < 20 kg or 250 to 500 mg orally tid for children > 20 kg and adults; sulfamethoxazole/trimethoprim **(SMX/TMP)** for children (40/8) mg/kg/day orally or IV, or for adults (400 to 800/40 to 80) mg q 12 h; cefamandole 0.5 to 2 gm IV q 6 h; cefaclor 20 to 40 mg/kg/day orally for children or 500 mg orally q 6 h for adults; tetracycline 500 mg orally q 6 h (contraindicated in children ≤ 8 yr old) and chloramphenicol 50 mg/kg/day orally or IV for children or 500 mg to 1 gm q 6 h orally or IV for adults. In most areas, 20 to 30% of type b strains and 5 to 15% of non-typable strains are resistant to ampicillin. Serious infections involving resistant strains should be treated with chloramphenicol, SMX/TMP, or cefamandole.

PNEUMONIA OF LEGIONNAIRES' DISEASE

Etiology and Epidemiology

Investigation of an outbreak of acute febrile respiratory illness among members of the American Legion in Philadelphia in 1976 led to discovery of a bacterium now

called *Legionella pneumophila*. Subsequently, a variety of related organisms have been tentatively classified in this genera, and retrospective studies have identified cases of Legionellosis as early as 1943. There are now 23 proposed species of Legionella, but half of them have been isolated only from environmental sources. The most common agent of human disease is *L. pneumophila*, followed by *L. micdadei* and then *L. bozemanii*. These organisms are morphologically similar, share biochemical characteristics, and cause similar diseases. The spectrum of disease includes (1) asymptomatic seroconversion; (2) a self-limited flu-like illness without pneumonia sometimes called **Pontiac fever**; (3) Legionnaires' disease, the most serious and the most frequently recognized form of pneumonia, and (4) localized, rare soft-tissue infections.

Legionnaires' disease accounts for 0.5 to 3% of all pneumonias and about 4% of lethal nosocomial pneumonias, but these rates may increase substantially in areas or hospitals where the disease is endemic. Most cases are sporadic with a distinct predilection for occurrence in late summer and early fall. However, numerous outbreaks, analogous to the original outbreak in Philadelphia, tend to occur in buildings, especially hospitals and hotels, or in certain geographic areas. The natural habitat of *L. pneumophila* and other species is water: lakes, creeks, and rivers. Major sources in outbreaks have been aerosolized organisms from evaporative condensers of air conditioning systems or potable water with contaminated shower heads. Person-to-person transmission has not been demonstrated.

Symptoms and Signs

The usual incubation period is 2 to 10 days. Legionnaires' disease may occur at any age, but most patients have been middle-aged males. Identified risk factors include smoking, alcohol abuse, and immunosuppression, especially from corticosteroids. A characteristic feature is high fever with relative bradycardia. Most patients have a prodromal phase that may resemble influenza with malaise, fever, headache, and myalgias; they develop cough that is initially nonproductive and subsequently productive of mucoid sputum. A common associated finding is diarrhea. Altered mental status with confusion, lethargy, or delirium is less frequent.

Chest x-rays early in the course generally show a unilateral, patchy segmental or lobar alveolar infiltrate. As the disease progresses, many patients develop bilateral involvement, and pleural effusions are relatively common. Occasional patients develop lung abscesses and multiple rounded densities suggesting septic emboli. In patients with altered mental status, CSF studies are normal and in patients with diarrhea, the stool is negative for blood and leukocytes. Most patients have a moderate leukocytosis with peripheral WBC counts of 10,000 to 15,000/μL. Other common laboratory findings are hyponatremia, hypophosphatemia, and abnormal liver function tests. Occasionally, patients have microscopic hematuria, sometimes with impaired renal function.

Diagnosis

There are 3 diagnostic studies to detect Legionella: culture of the organism, a direct fluorescent antibody **(DFA)** stain of exudate, and serology using the indirect fluorescent antibody assay **(IFA)**. All are reasonably specific, but none are particularly sensitive. Numerous species within the genera are noted above (see Etiology); most have been implicated in causing a similar type of lung infection. These organisms may be recovered from expectorated sputum, transtracheal aspirates, lung biopsies, pleural fluid, or blood. The preferred media for culture of uncontaminated specimens is charcoal yeast extract agar; this agar, with antibiotics to inhibit competitive flora, may be used with expectorated sputum. Because Legionella are not part of the normal flora, positive cultures are diagnostic, but the yield with sputum culture in cases confirmed by alternative technics is only 30 to 50%. Although the DFA stain provides immediate results, the test requires considerable expertise. The serologic diagnosis is made by demonstrating a 4-fold rise in titer to at least ≥ 1:128. A single convalescent serum showing

a titer ≥ 1:256 with a compatible clinical illness is strongly supportive. The diagnostic rise in titer that is usually noted 3 to 6 wk after the onset of illness is generally unavailable when therapeutic decisions are required.

Treatment and Prognosis

Erythromycin is the preferred drug. Patients with mild illness should receive 500 mg orally q 6 h. Seriously ill patients should receive erythromycin 1 gm IV q 6 h. Alternative regimens include erythromycin combined with rifampin 600 mg bid or doxycycline 100 mg orally or IV bid with or without rifampin. Treatment should be continued for ≥ 3 wk to prevent relapses. Without treatment, mortality is 15 to 25% in cases that are community acquired, and much higher among immunosuppressed or hospitalized patients. Most patients treated with erythromycin respond, but convalescence may be slow and x-ray abnormalities usually persist ≥ 1 mo.

TULAREMIC PNEUMONIA

(See TULAREMIA in Ch. 8)

PNEUMONIC PLAGUE

(See PLAGUE in Ch. 8)

MYCOPLASMAL PNEUMONIA

(Primary Atypical Pneumonia; Eaton Agent Pneumonia; Pneumonia Caused by Pleuropneumonia-like Organisms)

Etiology

Mycoplasma pneumoniae is the most common pathogen recognized in lung infections among children and young adults from 5 to 35 yr old, but is infrequent otherwise. This transmissible agent may be responsible for epidemics that spread slowly due to the 10- to 14-day incubation period. It may involve close contacts or closed populations in schools, the military, and families.

Pathology

M. pneumoniae attaches to and destroys ciliated epithelial cells of the respiratory tract mucosa. Microscopically, there is interstitial pneumonitis, bronchitis, and bronchiolitis. Peribronchial areas are infiltrated with plasma cells and small lymphocytes; within the bronchial lumina are polymorphonuclear leukocytes, macrophages, fibrin strands, and epithelial cell debris.

Symptoms and Signs

Initial symptoms resemble influenza with malaise, sore throat, and dry cough. As the disease progresses, they increase in severity; there may be paroxysms of coughing, and cough produces sputum that is mucoid, mucopurulent, or blood-streaked. Unlike classical pneumococcal pneumonia, the disease progresses gradually. Physical examination tends to be unimpressive in contrast with the patient's complaints and x-ray changes. Acute symptoms usually persist for 1 to 2 wk followed by gradual recovery, although many patients continue to experience constitutional symptoms with fatigue and malaise for several weeks. The disease is generally mild, and spontaneous recovery is the rule. However, occasional patients have severe pneumonia, sometimes causing the adult respiratory distress syndrome. Also, a few patients have hemolytic anemia, thromboembolic complications, polyarthritis, or neurologic syndromes including meningoencephalitis, transverse myelitis, peripheral neuropathies, or cerebellar ataxia. Maculopapular rashes occur in 10 to 20% and may be important diagnostic clues when present; occasional patients develop erythema multiforme or the Stevens-Johnson syndrome. Bullous myringitis, previously thought to be almost diagnostic of mycoplasmal infection, is now regarded as a nonspecific finding in relatively few patients.

Diagnosis

M. pneumoniae may be recovered from expectorated sputum or throat cultures, but isolation and identification generally require 7 to 10 days and most hospital laboratories do not offer this test. Gram stain of expectorated sputum shows sparse bacteria, a mixture of polymorphonuclear leukocytes and macrophages, and clumps of desquamated respiratory epithelial cells. Chest x-ray changes are variable, but most commonly show a patchy bronchopneumonia in the lower lobes; lobar consolidation and pleural effusions are infrequent. The peripheral WBC is usually normal or there may be a modest elevation. The cold hemagglutinin reaction is considered positive if there is a 4-fold change in titer with sequential specimens or a single titer ≥ 1:64. However, the test is positive in only 50 to 75% of patients and is considered somewhat nonspecific. The most practical method to confirm the diagnosis is with serologic assays (most often complement-fixation) to show a 4-fold rise in titer with peak titers at 2 to 4 wk after the onset of symptoms with a titer ≥ 1:64.

Prognosis and Treatment

Because mycoplasmas are cell-wall deficient, they do not respond to cell-wall–active antibiotics including all β-lactam agents. The preferred drugs are tetracycline or erythromycin 500 mg orally q 6 h for adults or erythromycin 30 to 50 mg/kg/day for children < 8 yr old. This treatment reduces the period of fever and pulmonary infiltrates, and hastens symptomatic recovery. However, antibiotics do not cause a microbial cure, since treated patients continue to carry the organism for several weeks. Nearly all patients recover with or without treatment.

VIRAL PNEUMONIA

Etiology and Epidermiology

Many viruses may cause lower respiratory tract infections, but distinct patterns prevail according to age and epidemiologic setting. Most common among infants and children are respiratory syncytial virus, adenovirus, parainfluenza, influenza A and B and, occasionally, rhinovirus and coronaviruses. Measles continues to be an important cause of respiratory infections wherever immunization is uncommon and malnutrition is highly prevalent. Among otherwise healthy adults the only frequently recognized viral pathogens are influenza A and B. Important pathogens among the elderly include influenza, parainfluenza, and respiratory syncytial virus. Patients with compromised cell-mediated immunity frequently develop pulmonary infections from latent viruses, especially cytomegalovirus **(CMV)** or herpes simplex. With this exception, most viral infections result from exposure of a nonimmune individual to infected persons who are shedding the implicated agent.

The most important, best studied viral pathogen is influenza A, which is classified into subtypes on the basis of 2 antigenic determinants: hemagglutinin and neuraminidase antigens. Immunity to these antigens reduces the likelihood of infection and reduces disease severity among those who develop infection. However, there may be enough antigenic variation (antigenic drift) within a subtype so that infection or immunization with one strain does not necessarily confer protection to others. A major worldwide epidemic often results when a change in subtype (antigenic shift) exposes antigenically naive populations. The elderly are at particular risk for serious disease and > 90% of deaths in recent years have been in persons over age 65. Influenza B viruses show more antigen stability, and cause less serious disease, although some antigenic variation may occur with consequent outbreaks, and serious disease with high mortality rates has been noted in nursing homes.

Pathology

Viruses invade the bronchiolar epithelium causing a bronchiolitis; the infection may extend to the pulmonary interstitium and alveoli to cause pneumonia. Affected areas are congested and, at times, hemorrhagic; there is an intense inflammatory reaction composed of mononuclear cells. Alveoli may contain fibrin, mononuclear cells, and, on occasion, some polymorphonuclear leukocytes. In severe cases there may be hyaline membranes. Characteristic intracellular viral inclusions may be seen with adenovirus, cytomegalovirus, respiratory syncytial virus, or varicella virus.

Symptoms and Signs

The clinical spectrum of viral infections of the lower airways includes bronchitis, bronchiolitis, and pneumonia. Most patients have headache, fever, myalgia, and cough that usually produces mucopurulent sputum. The most common finding on chest x-ray is an interstitial pneumonia or peribronchial thickening. Lobar consolidation and pleural effusions are infrequent. The peripheral WBC count is often low, but may be normal or moderately elevated.

Diagnosis

Identification of the virus is usually difficult, but may be important during outbreaks, among seriously ill patients, and for those with treatable viruses. Findings of sparse bacteria and a dominance of mononuclear cells on smears of sputum, and failure to recover a likely bacterial pathogen support the diagnosis of viral pneumonia. Pneumonias complicating exanthematous viral infections (eg, measles, varicella, or herpes) may be tentatively diagnosed on the basis of associated clinical findings including the rash. A specific diagnosis in most viral respiratory infections requires recovery of the virus from throat washings or tissue, identification of typical inclusions in cytopathology or biopsy specimens or serologic assays. Most hospital laboratories do not have facilities for viral culture. The diagnosis of influenza is usually established by presence of typical symptoms during an outbreak of disease and serologic assays using acute and convalescent sera.

Prophylaxis

Amantadine 100 mg orally q 12 h may be given prophylactically or within 48 h of the onset of symptoms either to prevent or treat infections with influenza A. Acyclovir 5 mg/kg q 8 h for adults or 250 mg/m^2 BSA q 8 h for children is advocated for lung infections involving herpes simplex, herpes zoster, or varicella (chickenpox). Vaccine is available for prevention of influenza A and B using mixed antigen preparations based on recent experience and anticipated epidemic strains. Two doses separated by $\geq$ 4 wk are advocated for children $<$ 12 yr old. Persons $>$ 12 yr should receive a single dose since they have a higher level of immunologic priming. Vaccine efficacy varies with the host and the epidemic strain, but an overall protection rate is usually about 70%. Most patients may receive the vaccine and derive potential benefit. Target populations with the highest priority are (1) persons with chronic cardiovascular and pulmonary disease, (2) residents of chronic care facilities, and (3) medical personnel who have extensive contact with high risk patients. The next level of priority is for persons $>$ 65 and those with numerous chronic conditions, eg, metabolic diseases (as diabetes mellitus), renal dysfunction, anemia, immunosuppression, and asthma.

Some patients, especially those with influenza, have superimposed bacterial infections that require antibiotics. Major pathogens encountered in this setting are *S. pneumoniae* and *S. aureus*; less frequent superinfecting pathogens include *H. influenzae*, group A β-hemolytic streptococci and *N. meningitidis*. Prognosis varies widely with the causative organism, the patient's age, and associated diseases.

RICKETTSIAL PNEUMONIA

(See Q Fever in Ch. 10)

PSITTACOSIS

(Ornithosis; Parrot Fever)

An infectious atypical pneumonia caused by Chlamydia psittaci *and transmitted by certain birds.*

Etiology and Epidemiology

The species of *Chlamydia* (see Ch. 11) that causes psittacosis is found principally in psittacine birds (parrots, parakeets, love-birds), less often in poultry, pigeons, and canaries (often called ornithosis), and occasionally in the snowy egret and some sea-birds (eg, herring gulls, petrels, and fulmars). Human infection usually occurs by inhaling dust from feathers or excreta of infected birds, or it may be transmitted by a bite from an infected bird, and rarely by cough droplets of infected patients. Man-to-man transmission may be associated with highly virulent avian strains, or the disease may be transmitted venereally. Pathologic changes are those of a pneumonitis with a mononuclear cell exudate, as in other "primary atypical" pneumonias (see viral and mycoplasmal pneumonias above, and Q fever in Ch. 10).

Symptoms and Signs

Following a 1- to 3-wk incubation period, onset may be insidious or abrupt, with fever, chills, general malaise, and anorexia. The temperature gradually rises and cough develops, initially dry but at times becoming mucopurulent. Chest x-rays during the first week show pneumonitis radiating from the hilum; migratory lesions may be present. During the 2nd wk, pneumonia and frank consolidation may occur with secondary purulent lung infection. The temperature remains elevated for 2 to 3 wk, then falls slowly. The course may be mild or severe, depending on the patient's age and the extent of pneumonia. A progressive, pronounced increase in pulse and respiratory rates is an ominous sign. Mortality may reach 30% in severe untreated cases, and even higher rates are reported with virulent strains. A gradual convalescence may be prolonged, especially in severe cases.

Diagnosis and Laboratory Findings

Clinical differentiation from other atypical pneumonias is difficult. Initially, the disease may be confused with influenza, typhoid fever, mycoplasmal pneumonia, Legionnaires' disease, or Q fever. Psittacosis is suggested by a history of exposure to birds, and is confirmed by recovery of the agent or by serologic CF tests. In the USA, serum specimens obtained early in the disease and in late convalescence may be submitted to the Centers for Disease Control through the State Laboratory Director.

Prophylaxis

Infected pigeons in the lofts of breeders (eg, of racing or carrier pigeons) and dust from feathers and cage contents must be avoided; handling sick birds should be avoided. Spread by imported psittacine birds is controlled with a mandatory 45-day course of chlortetracycline-treated feed, which generally, but not always, eliminates causative organisms from the birds' blood and feces. This may also be useful to control the disease in turkeys raised for market. Since cough droplets and sputum may infect other persons by inhalation, strict patient isolation should be instituted when the diagnosis is suspected on clinical and epidemiologic grounds (exposure to possible sources).

Treatment

Tetracycline 1 to 2 gm/day orally in divided doses given q 6 h is effective. Fever and other symptoms usually are controlled within 48 to 72 h, but the antibiotic should be continued for at least 10 days. Strict bed rest, O_2 when needed, and cough control with codeine 15 mg orally q 3 or 4 h are indicated.

FUNGAL PNEUMONIA

Primary fungal pneumonia is most commonly caused by *Histoplasma capsulatum* or *Coccidioides immitis*, and less commonly by species of *Candida*, *Cryptococcus*, or *Blastomyces* (see Ch. 9). Fungal pneumonia also may be a complication of antibacterial therapy, especially in patients with altered host defense mechanisms due to illness or immunosuppressive therapy (see Ch. 7).

PNEUMONIA CAUSED BY *Pneumocystis carinii*

Etiology

Pneumocystis carinii, a protozoan parasite that is usually dormant in the host lung, causes disease when defenses are compromised, and there may be patient to patient transmission. Nearly all patients have immunologic deficiencies, the most common being defects in cell-mediated immunity as with hematologic malignancies, lymphoproliferative diseases, cancer chemotherapy, and about ½ of patients with AIDS develop *P. carinii* pneumonia; these patients account for most cases in recent years (see in Ch. 19).

Symptoms and Signs

Most patients have a history of fever, dyspnea, and a dry, nonproductive cough that may evolve in a subacute fashion over several weeks or acutely over several days. The chest x-ray characteristically shows diffuse, bilateral, perihilar infiltrates. Gallium scanning may be especially helpful in patients with typical symptoms and a negative chest x-ray. Arterial blood gases show hypoxemia, with a marked increase in the alveolar-arterial O_2 gradient.

Diagnosis

The diagnosis requires histopathologic demonstration of the organism with methenamine silver, Giemsa, Wright-Giemsa, modified Grocott or Gram-Weigert stains, with specimens obtained by transtracheal aspiration, transthoracic needle aspiration, open lung biopsy, or bronchoscopy. The preferred diagnostic method is bronchoscopy to obtain specimens by means of transbronchial biopsy, bronchial lavage, and brush biopsy. The highest yield is with transbronchial biopsy for fixed tissue specimens and touch imprints.

Treatment

The drug of choice is trimethoprim/sulfamethoxazole **(TMP/SMX)** TMP 20 mg/SMX 100 mg/kg/day in 4 doses IV for 14 to 21 days. The major potential side effects, especially in patients with AIDS, are skin rash and neutropenia. The alternative drug is pentamidine 4 mg/kg IM once daily for 14 days. The major limitation of pentamidine is the high frequency of toxic side effects including renal failure, hepatotoxicity, hypoglycemia, hematologic abnormalities, and pain or abscess at injection sites. The overall mortality with treatment is 20 to 30%. Patients who receive pentamidine due to failure of TMP/SMX have a very high mortality rate; those who are switched due to side effects of TMP/SMX generally do well. Supportive treatment includes O_2 therapy sometimes requiring positive end-expiratory pressure to maintain $Pa_{O_2} \geq 60$ mm Hg.

PNEUMONIA IN THE COMPROMISED HOST

Etiology

The list of potential pathogens in patients with compromised defenses is legion. However, likely etiologic agents can often be predicted on the basis of the nature of the host defect, x-ray changes, and the pattern of evolution of clinical symptoms. Probabilities based on the type of defect in host defenses are summarized in TABLE 40–1.

It should be noted that respiratory symptoms and changes on the chest x-ray may be due to a variety of processes other than infection. Other diagnostic considerations include pulmonary hemorrhage, pulmonary edema, radiation injury, pulmonary toxicity due to cytotoxic drugs, and tumor infiltrates. The rate of progression of the disease process is helpful to identify the responsible mechanism. In patients with acute symptoms, likely diagnoses are bacterial infections, hemorrhage, pulmonary edema, a leukoagglutinin reaction, or pulmonary emboli. A subacute or chronic presentation is more suggestive of fungal or mycobacterial infection, an opportunistic viral infection, *Pneumocystis* pneumonia, tumor, cytotoxic drug reaction, or radiation injury.

The pattern of changes on chest x-rays is also helpful. X-rays showing localized disease with consolidation usually indicate an infection involving bacteria, Mycobacteria, fungi, or Nocardia. An interstitial pattern is more likely to represent a viral infection, *Pneumocystis* pneumonia, drug or radiation injury, or pulmonary edema. Diffuse nodular lesions suggest Mycobacteria, Nocardia, fungi, or tumor. Cavitary disease suggests Mycobacteria, Nocardia, fungi, or bacteria.

Diagnosis

The need for an etiologic diagnosis is emphasized by the diversity of pathogens, availability of specific therapies for most infectious diseases, and the high mortality

TABLE 40–1. DIAGNOSIS OF PATHOGENS IN THE COMPROMISED HOST

Host Defect	*Example*	*Likely Pathogens*
Humoral immunodeficiency		
Hypogammaglobulinemia	Multiple myeloma	Bacteria: *S. pneumoniae, H. influenzae, N. meningiditis, P. aeruginosa*
Selective deficiency: IgA, IgG, IgM		
Defective polymorphonuclear neutrophils		
Neutropenia	Acute leukemia, aplastic anemia, cancer chemotherapy	Bacteria: gram-negative bacteria; *S. aureus;* aspergillosis
Defective chemotaxis	Diabetes	Bacteria
Defective intracellular killing	Chronic granulomatous disease	Bacteria; *S. aureus*
Defective alternative pathway	Sickle cell disease	*S. pneumoniae; H. influenzae*
C5 deficiency		S. pneumoniae; S. aureus; gram-negative bacteria
Cell-mediated immunity	Hodgkins disease, cancer chemotherapy, AIDS, corticosteroids	Mycobacteria; viruses (herpes, cytomegalovirus); Strongyloides; opportunistic fungi (Aspergillus, Mucor, Cryptococcus); *P. carinii;* Nocardia; Toxoplasma

rate associated with improper therapy. Diagnostic strategies vary according to the clinical setting and available resources. The first tests are usually stains and culture of expectorated sputum, but these are frequently inconclusive for many or most diagnostic considerations. Patients whose diagnoses remain enigmas or have other findings suggesting alternative diagnoses will often require an invasive procedure (eg, transtracheal aspiration, transthoracic needle aspiration, bronchoscopy, or open lung biopsy). A biopsy will supply tissue for both histology and culture; tissue may be obtained by means of bronchoscopy (a transbronchial biopsy) or an open surgical procedure. Although the latter usually requires general anesthesia and a chest tube after the procedure, a biopsy under direct visualization permits substantial specimens to be collected directly from involved sites; it remains the most definitive procedure with the highest diagnostic yield.

Treatment

Acutely ill patients who have suspected bacterial infections are often treated with antibiotics selected on the basis of probabilities and the findings with sputum Gram stain and culture. Treatment is adjusted on the basis of more definitive diagnostic evaluation, as described above.

POSTOPERATIVE AND POSTTRAUMATIC PNEUMONIAS

Etiology

Hypoventilation, impaired or inhibited cough reflex, bronchospasm, and dehydration may cause retention of bronchial secretions leading to segmental atelectasis and, in turn, to lung infection. The incidence of such infection is higher in winter and greatest in elderly or debilitated patients. About 60% of postoperative lung infections follow abdominal operations, and about 20% occur after operations on the head and neck. These infections have also become frequent after chest operations involving the lung or esophagus. Pneumonia occurs equally after inhalation and spinal anesthesia; only about 10% of such infections follow operations performed under local or IV anesthesia. About 40% of post-traumatic pneumonias are complications of fractured ribs or chest trauma; the rest are divided about equally among skull fractures or other head injuries, other fractures, burns, or major contusions. Postoperative pneumonia differs from aspiration pneumonia by absence of irritating gastric secretions, and anaerobic flora is not usually involved.

Bacteriologic studies of sputum and bronchial secretions show good correlations between profuse growth of pneumococci, *Hemophilus influenzae*, or both, and clinical evidence of pulmonary infection. Purulent sputum usually indicates infection, but scant or mucoid sputum with an abundance of organisms is sometimes found. Cultures yielding *S. aureus*, coliform bacilli, or both, may be obtained from patients recently treated with antibiotics; such organisms, unless found in abundance in purulent sputum along with other clinical evidence of infection in the chest, are not an indication for antibacterial therapy.

Symptoms, Signs, and Diagnosis

These are the same as for other pneumonias caused by the same bacteria. Chest x-rays may show atelectatic areas and sometimes evidence of pulmonary embolism and infarcts; the latter usually are associated with bloody sputum.

Prophylaxis

Routine use of prophylactic antibiotics preoperatively or immediately following trauma is not recommended. Nevertheless, ampicillin or, preferably, a cephalosporin may be given immediately preceding and after the operation and for not more than 48 h after operations on patients with chronic bronchitis, or following skull fractures (but

penicillin is recommended to prevent meningitis) or rib fractures with lung trauma. However, results of prolonged use of antibiotics for prophylaxis have *not* been uniformly favorable.

Prognosis and Treatment

Prognosis depends on the underlying disorder that required operation, the patient's age and prior health status, and on the nature, location, and extent of trauma. Complications resemble those of other pneumonias of the same bacterial etiology, but empyema may be more frequent in pneumonias that follow trauma or operations involving the lung and mediastinum.

ASPIRATION PNEUMONIA

Pathologic consequences of abnormal entry of fluids, particulate matter, or secretions into the lower airways. Healthy persons commonly aspirate, but the inoculum is usually readily cleared without sequelae by normal defense mechanisms. Because the nature of the inoculum dictates the pathophysiology, symptoms, and treatment, at least 3 distinct syndromes are included in this category.

Chemical pneumonitis occurs when the aspirated material is directly toxic to the lungs. The best studied and most frequent prototype is acid pneumonitis following aspiration of gastric acid **(Mendelson's syndrome).** The requirement (according to animal studies) is a relatively large inoculum of fluid with a pH < 3 that results in acute lung injury with a rapid onset and evolution of pulmonary symptoms within hours. The patient presents with acute dyspnea, tachypnea, and tachycardia. Common associated findings are cyanosis, bronchospasm, fever, and sputum that is often pink and frothy. Chest x-rays invariably show infiltrates usually involving one or both lower lobes. Arterial blood gas analysis shows hypoxemia. The most important therapeutic modality is respiratory support, usually with positive pressure breathing (see Ch. 35). Tracheal suction should be performed if the patient is seen early in the course; however, *the injury is precipitous, analogous to a "flash burn," and the acid is so rapidly neutralized by pulmonary secretions that there is minimal opportunity to reverse the chemical injury.* The major purpose of tracheal suction is to clear the airways of particulate matter that may have been aspirated (see Ch. 33). Corticosteroids and antibiotics are often given, but their efficacy is not established.

Recent studies of this form of pneumonitis show 1 of 3 patterns: (1) rapid recovery in a fashion analagous to that described by Mendelson; (2) progression to the acute respiratory distress syndrome; or (3) bacterial superinfection. Reported mortality rates have been 30 to 50%.

Bacterial infection of the lower airways is the most common form of aspiration pneumonia, primarily involving anaerobic bacteria that colonize the gingival crevice of the oropharynx. Patients usually have a more insidious onset and progression of symptoms than those with gastric acid pneumonia. Usual findings are those of a bacterial lung infection with cough, fever, and purulent sputum. Chest x-rays show an infiltrate in a dependent lung segment, determined to some extent on the patient's position during aspiration. Favored segments for aspiration in the recumbent position are the superior segment of a lower lobe or the posterior segment of an upper lobe; the lower lobes are favored segments following aspiration in the upright position. Common sequelae when anaerobic bacteria are involved include pulmonary necrosis with an empyema due to a bronchopleural fistula or a cavity (ie, lung abscess). The major therapeutic modality is antibiotics directed against the involved pathogens, and since expectorated sputum is not valid for anaerobic processing, the preferred specimen is a transtracheal aspirate. Patients who aspirate outside the hospital setting usually have an anaerobic infection, but nosocomial aspiration pneumonia tends to involve com-

plex mixtures of organisms including gram-negative bacilli and *S. aureus* as well as anaerobic bacteria. These distinctions are important in drug selection. For anaerobic infection the preferred drug is aqueous penicillin G, 4 to 10 million u./day IV in 4 doses or clindamycin 600 mg IV q 6 to 8 h. A comparative trial of penicillin vs. clindamycin in patients with putrid lung abscesses showed that clindamycin was superior. The most likely explanation is that about 25% of cases involve penicillin-resistant anaerobes (eg, *B. melaninogenicus*, *B. ruminicola*, *B. ureolyticus*, or *B. fragilis*).

Mechanical obstruction of the lower airways may be caused by aspiration of inert fluids or particulate matter (eg, in drowned victims, or patients with severely compromised consciousness who may aspirate non-acid gastric contents, oral feedings, etc). These patients may need immediate tracheal suction for acute dyspnea and cyanosis. Particulate matter can also lodge in the lower airways. The most common objects recovered are vegetal (eg, peanuts). This type of accident is usually seen in children during the oral stage of development, but it may occur in adults, especially with meat aspirated when dining—the "cafe coronary syndrome" (see Technics of CPR in CARDIAC ARREST AND CARDIOPULMONARY RESUSCITATION in Ch. 27, and TRACHEAL ASPIRATION in Ch. 33). Symptoms depend on the caliber of both object and airway. Obstruction high in the trachea may produce acute apnea, often with aphonia and rapid death. Obstruction of more distal airways results in an irritating chronic cough and sometimes with recurrent infections distal to the obstruction. Atelectasis or hyperinflation of the involved lung is best seen on chest x-rays taken during exhalation; partial obstruction causes the cardiac shadow to shift away from the abnormal lung during this phase of respiration. Another clue to this diagnosis is recurrent parenchymal infections involving the same segment of lung. Therapy consists of extracting the object, usually by bronchoscopy.

41. LUNG ABSCESS

A localized cavity with pus, resulting from necrosis of lung tissue, with surrounding pneumonitis. "Gangrene of the lung" denotes a similar though more diffuse and extensive process in which necrosis predominates. A lung abscess may be **putrid** (due to anaerobic bacteria) or **nonputrid** (due to anaerobes or aerobes).

Etiology and Pathology

Lung abscesses are usually due to aspiration of infected material from the upper airway when a patient is unconscious or obtunded from alcoholism, CNS disease, general anesthesia, or excessive sedation. Usually due to anaerobes, they are often associated with periodontal disease; sometimes multiple organisms act synergistically. Bacteria cultured from lung abscesses include common pyogenic bacteria and nasopharyngeal flora, particularly anaerobes, and less often aerobic bacteria or fungi. Bronchogenic carcinoma is an occasional cause of lung abscess in persons over age 55.

Pneumonia due to *Klebsiella pneumoniae* (Friedländer's bacillus), *Staphylococcus aureus*, *Actinomyces israelii*, *β*-hemolytic streptococcus, *Legionella* sp, or *H. influenzae* are sometimes complicated by abscess formation. Lung abscess in the compromised host is usually due to *Nocardia*, cryptococcus, *Aspergillus*, *Phycomyces*, or gram-negative bacilli. Other less common causes of lung abscess include septic pulmonary emboli, secondary infection of pulmonary infarcts, and direct extension of amebic or bacterial abscesses from the liver through the diaphragm into the lower lobe of the lung. Cavitary TB is not clinically considered a lung abscess.

Single lung abscesses are most common. Multiple abscesses usually are unilateral and may develop simultaneously or spread from a single focus. In abscesses due to

aspiration, the superior segment of a lower lobe and the posterior segment of an upper lobe are affected most frequently. The solitary abscess secondary to bronchial obstruction or an infected embolus starts as necrosis of the major portion of the involved bronchopulmonary segment. The base of the segment is usually adjacent to the chest wall, and the pleural space in the area is often obliterated by inflammatory adhesions. Hematogenous spread, which is most often due to *S. aureus* tricuspid endocarditis in persons who abuse IV drugs, is usually characterized by multiple lesions in noncontiguous sites.

The abscess usually ruptures into a bronchus and its contents are expectorated, leaving a cavity filled with fluid and air. With adequate drainage, the walls of the abscess usually collapse and contract, eventually obliterating the cavity. If drainage is inadequate, the abscess wall becomes fibrotic and rigid and healing does not occur. Occasionally, an abscess ruptures into the pleural cavity, resulting in a sudden empyema, sometimes with bronchopleural fistula.

Bronchi or large blood vessels may appear on x-ray as ridges on the cavity wall. Erosion of vessels may cause serious hemorrhage. Rarely, septic emboli migrate via pulmonary veins to the arterial system and initiate a secondary brain abscess. Bronchiectasis and amyloid disease are other late, but rare, complications.

Symptoms and Signs

Onset may be acute or insidious. Early symptoms are often those of pneumonia; ie, malaise, anorexia, sputum-producing cough, sweats, and fever. The sputum is purulent unless the abscess is completely walled off, and it is frequently blood-streaked. A putrid odor (a penetrating foul odor that may be discernible at some distance from the patient) is diagnostic of anaerobic bacterial causation and this simplifies the choice of antibiotic. However, about 40% of patients with abscesses due to anaerobes do not present a putrid odor; so its absence does not exclude this diagnosis. Severe prostration and a temperature of 39.4 C (103 F) or higher may be present. Chest pain, if present, usually indicates pleural involvement. Repeated chills in a patient with pneumonia suggest abscess formation.

Physical signs include a small area of dullness indicating localized pneumonic consolidation, and, usually, suppressed rather than bronchial breath sounds. Fine or medium moist rales may be present. If the cavity is large (unusual with current therapy), there may be tympany and amphoric breathing.

An abscess may remain unsuspected until it perforates a bronchus, when a large amount of purulent sputum, fetid or nonfetid, may be expectorated over a few hours or several days. The sputum may contain gangrenous lung tissue. Fever, anorexia, weakness, and debility are usually present but are sometimes minimal if the disease is limited or if the abscess is draining well. Dyspnea occurs when the involvement is massive.

With appropriate antibiotic therapy, signs of pulmonary suppuration generally disappear though this does not necessarily denote cure. If the abscess becomes chronic, weight loss, anemia, and hypertrophic pulmonary osteoarthropathy appear. Physical examination of the chest may be negative in the chronic phase, but rales and rhonchi are usually present.

Diagnosis

Lung abscess is suggested by the symptoms and signs described above. Chest x-rays initially show a segmental or lobar consolidation that becomes globular as it distends with pus. Following rupture into a bronchus, a cavity with a fluid level appears on x-ray. Failure of an area of pneumonia to resolve always suggests abscess formation, bronchial neoplasm, or both. The course must be followed by x-rays at 1- to 2-wk intervals in search of central areas of diminished density. If chest x-rays suggest an

underlying lesion (eg, bronchogenic carcinoma) and surgery is contemplated, tomograms or CT may permit better anatomic definition.

Sputum should be examined by smear and culture for bacteria (including mycobacteria). The attribution of disease to anaerobes usually requires a specimen of bronchial secretions obtained by transtracheal aspiration, because the mouth normally contains anaerobic organisms that contaminate sputum. Since this procedure is not completely innocuous, it should be reserved for cases with atypical presentation or that remain diagnostic enigmas.

Bronchoscopy is unnecessary if abscess resolution on x-ray is rapid and uneventful and if there is no reason to suspect a foreign body or tumor. If these must be ruled out, it can often be deferred until the patient's condition has been improved by antibiotics.

CT scan may demonstrate a persistent cavity or bronchiectatic changes despite antibiotic resolution of an acute abscess and only minimal residual shadows on routine x-ray, but these abnormalities are usually of no clinical significance in the absence of continued symptoms and signs.

Lesions that simulate lung abscess include bronchogenic carcinoma, bronchiectasis, primary empyema with secondary bronchopleural fistula, TB, coccidioidomycosis and other mycotic lung infections, infected pulmonary bulla or air cyst, pulmonary sequestration, silicotic nodule with central necrosis, and subphrenic or hepatic (amebic or hydatid) abscess with perforation into a bronchus. Repeated clinical evaluation and the procedures described above will usually differentiate these disorders from simple lung abscess.

Prognosis and Treatment

Prompt, complete healing of a lung abscess depends on adequate antibiotic treatment and drainage. Almost all patients recover without surgery.

Antibiotics should be started as soon as sputum and blood have been collected for culture and sensitivity tests. Most often, the drug of choice is penicillin G 1.2 million u. (750 mg) orally qid, or 2 to 10 million u./day IV. If there is no clinical response or defervescence in 4 to 7 days and a specific pathogen such as *Klebsiella* or *Staphylococcus* has not been isolated, clindamycin 600 mg IV q 6 to 8 h should replace the penicillin. Some physicians prefer to initiate treatment with clindamycin for abscesses presumed to be due to anaerobes. If a gram-negative organism, *Staphylococcus*, or other aerobic pathogen is isolated, the choice of an antibiotic depends on the results of sensitivity tests. Treatment should be continued until the pneumonitis has resolved and the cavity has disappeared or stabilized on serial x-rays. This usually requires several weeks or months of treatment, most of which can be accomplished with oral antibiotics on an outpatient basis.

Postural drainage may be a helpful adjunct, but it may also cause spillage into other bronchi with extension of the process or acute obstruction. If the patient is weak or paralyzed, tracheostomy and suctioning may be necessary. Rarely, bronchoscopic aspiration may be required for thick, tenacious sputum. Surgical drainage is rarely necessary, since lesions usually respond to antibiotics, even when spontaneous drainage through the communicating bronchus is initially inadequate.

Pulmonary resection is the procedure of choice for an abscess resistant to medical therapy, particularly if bronchogenic carcinoma is suspected. Lobectomy is the most common procedure; segmental resection usually suffices for small lesions. Pneumonectomy may be necessary for multiple abscesses or pulmonary gangrene refractory to medical management. The mortality rate following pneumonectomy is 5 to 10%; following lesser resections, much lower. Patients with large cavities who do not respond to medical therapy, but are too seriously ill to undergo a thoracotomy, may have drainage accomplished percutaneously.

42. OCCUPATIONAL LUNG DISEASES

Lung disorders directly related to matter inhaled from the occupational environment.

The effects of an inhaled agent depend on many factors; ie, its physical and chemical properties, the susceptibility of the exposed person, and the dose (see TABLE 42–1). A particle is a solid particulate, a mist is a liquid particulate, a vapor is the gaseous form of substance that is normally a liquid, and gas is that physical state in which a substance has no fixed volume. In some instances, the inhaled particle is deposited and retained in the lungs; if soluble, it is absorbed into the bloodstream. For the most part, the body's defenses remove insoluble particles and mists.

The physical state of the inhaled agent is of great importance. Particles are deposited in the respiratory tract mainly as the result of 3 physical processes: sedimentation, inertial impaction, and diffusion. Sedimentation depends on Stokes' law, and is dependent on the particle's density and the square of its diameter. Inertial impaction occurs in bifurcating airways when the momentum of a particle is sufficient to carry it along its original path so that it impinges on the bronchial wall. Diffusion is due to kinetic energy that is present in all small particles and causes them to move at random. Most fibers (eg, asbestos and cotton) are deposited as a result of interception—a process that usually involves long fibers straddling bifurcations. Larger particles between 6 and 25 μm are deposited by sedimentation in the nose, and to a lesser extent in the conducting airways. Since they are too large to find their way into the lung parenchyma, they are known as the nonrespirable fraction. Particles of between 0.5 and 6 μm, known as the respirable fraction, are most prone to be deposited in the gas-exchanging portions of the lung. Particles between 1 and 3 μm are most often involved in the development of pneumoconiosis. Particles below 0.1 μm are deposited in the lung parenchyma due to diffusion. Other physical properties also influence the effects of deposited particles. Thus, those asbestos fibers with the greatest penetrability are most likely to migrate to the pleura and cause mesothelioma. Chemical properties of the inhaled agent are also important. Quartz is markedly fibrogenic, but, in contrast, particles of coal, carbon, and tin oxide are relatively inert.

Individual susceptibility affects the development of occupational lung diseases (eg, the rate of clearing of particles from the respiratory tract varies markedly). The mucociliary escalator removes particles from the dead space more rapidly in some persons than in others; the clearance rate is genetically determined. Alveolar macrophages engulf particles deposited in the lung parenchyma and then are either carried to the terminal bronchioles where they catch the mucociliary escalator, or migrate into the interstitium of the lungs to the lymph nodes.

The site of deposition of the particle is of prime importance since it governs substantially the lung's response (see TABLE 42–2). Deposition of particles in the nose may lead to hay fever, which may be regarded as occupationally related in an agricultural

TABLE 42–1. FACTORS AFFECTING AN AEROSOL'S TOXICITY

Physical properties	Physical state (ie, particle, mist, or gas; solubility, shape, density, penetrability, concentration, radioactivity, size)
Chemical properties	Acidity, alkalinity, fibrogenicity, antigenicity
Individual susceptibility	Integrity of body's defenses, immunologic status; ie, atopy, HLA type, airways geometry

(Modified from *Occupational Lung Diseases*, ed.2, 1984, by W. K. C. Morgan and A. Seaton. Copyright 1984 by W. B. Saunders Company. Used with permission.)

TABLE 42–2. PARTICLE DEPOSITION SITE AND RESPIRATORY RESPONSE

Site of Deposition	*Clinical Response*
Nose	Rhinitis, hay fever, septal perforation, nasal cancer
Trachea and bronchi	Bronchoconstriction Antigen-antibody–mediated Pharmacologically induced Reflex-induced due to irritation Bronchitis Nonspecific response to inert dusts Lung cancer (radioactive dusts and gases)
Lung parenchyma	Extrinsic allergic alveolitis (organic dusts) Pneumoconiosis (mineral dusts) Acute pulmonary damage, bronchiolitis, pulmonary edema

(Modified from *Occupational Lung Diseases*, ed.2, 1984, by W. K. C. Morgan and A. Seaton. Copyright 1984 by W. B. Saunders Company. Used with permission.)

worker. Septal perforation may be seen in chrome workers, and nasal cancer in furniture workers. Deposition of particles in the trachea and bronchi may induce 3 responses: (1) There may be bronchoconstriction from an antigen-antibody reaction; eg, in some forms of occupational asthma, while in byssinosis the deposition of particles may (through pharmacologic mechanisms) cause the mast cells of the airways to produce bronchoconstrictors such as histamine and SRS-A. (2) Long-continued deposition of particles may induce mucous gland hypertrophy or bronchitis, which sometimes leads to a minor degree of chronic airflow obstruction. (3) The deposition of asbestos fibers or of dusts with adsorbed radon daughters may lead to the development of lung cancer.

If particles deposited in the lung parenchyma are organic and antigenic, they may lead to the development of extrinsic allergic alveolitis (hypersensitivity pneumonia), an acute granulomatous process involving the alveoli and respiratory bronchioles (see Ch. 43). If particles are inorganic, a fibrotic response may occur that is either focal and nodular as in typical silicosis, or diffuse and generalized as in asbestosis and berylliosis. If particles are inert (eg, tin oxide), a benign pneumoconiosis without fibrosis develops. Inhalation of certain gases and vapors (eg, Hg, cadmium, nitrogen dioxide) can cause acute pulmonary edema, acute alveolitis, and bronchiolitis obliterans.

DISEASES DUE TO INORGANIC (MINERAL) DUSTS

FIBROGENIC DUST DISEASES

SILICOSIS

A fibrogenic pneumoconiosis caused by inhaling crystalline free silica (quartz) dust; characterized by discrete nodular pulmonary fibrosis and, in more advanced stages, by conglomerate fibrosis and respiratory impairment.

Etiology

Silicosis, the oldest known occupational lung disease, usually follows long-term inhalation of small particles of free crystalline silica (silicon dioxide) in such industries as metal mining (lead, hard coal, copper, silver, gold), foundries, pottery making, and sandstone and granite cutting. Usually, 20 to 30 yr of exposure are necessary before the disease becomes apparent, though it develops in < 10 yr when the dust-dose is

extremely high, as in industries such as tunneling, abrasive soap making, and sandblasting. The present standard for free silica in the industrial atmosphere is an 8-h time-weighted average based on the percent of silica in the dust. The formula for calculating this threshold limit value **(TLV)** for respirable dust is: TLV = (10 mg per cu meter/% SiO_2) + 2.

Pathology and Pathophysiology

Alveolar macrophages engulf respirable particles of free silica (< 5 μm in diameter). When the macrophages die, hydrolytic enzymes are released, and fibrosis of the lung parenchyma occurs. The typical initial pathologic change is the formation throughout the lungs of discrete hyalinized silicotic nodules. Later, coalescence of fibrosis results in conglomerate masses, contraction of the upper lung zones, and basilar emphysema with marked distortion of lung architecture. Ventilatory and gas exchange functions are affected. What usually distinguishes the overall physiologic pattern of conglomerate silicosis from that of advanced pulmonary emphysema is reduced lung volumes. Thus severe functional impairment is found in the late stages of conglomerate silicosis. Respiratory insufficiency, its ultimate consequence, may progress along with radiographic worsening for some years even after exposure ceases.

When the dust-dose is extremely high and acute silicosis develops, more uniform pathologic findings occur in the lung parenchyma. There is a diffuse interstitial reaction and, at times, filling of the alveolar spaces with a proteinaceous material similar to that found in alveolar proteinosis.

Symptoms, Signs, and Clinical Course

Patients with **simple nodular silicosis** have no respiratory symptoms and usually no respiratory impairment. They may cough and raise sputum, but these symptoms are due to industrial bronchitis and occur as often in persons with normal x-rays. Though simple silicosis has little effect on pulmonary function, occasionally categories 2 and 3 (see under Diagnosis) lead to a slight reduction of lung volumes, but the values are seldom outside the predicted range. **Conglomerate silicosis,** in contrast, may lead to severe shortness of breath, cough, and sputum. The severity of the shortness of breath is related to the size of the conglomerate masses in the lungs; when they are extensive, the patient becomes severely disabled. As the masses encroach on and obliterate the vascular bed, pulmonary hypertension and right ventricular hypertrophy supervene and, in an advanced state, there may be physical findings of consolidation over the affected area and of pulmonary hypertension. Cor pulmonale eventually causes death.

Pulmonary function abnormalities are frequent in complicated pneumoconiosis, especially in the later stages. These consist of decreased lung volumes and diffusing capacity, airways obstruction, and frequently pulmonary hypertension and desaturation. CO_2 retention is unusual. Persons exposed to silica have 3 times the risk of developing TB; generally, the more silica in the lungs, the greater the risk. **Silicotuberculosis** resembles conglomerate silicosis on x-ray; the distinction can be made only by sputum culture. The sera of many silicotics contain lung autoantibodies and antinuclear factor.

Diagnosis

Silicosis is diagnosed from characteristic chest x-ray changes and a history of exposure to free silica. Simple silicosis is recognized by the presence of multiple, small, rounded or regular opacities in the chest film, and is subdivided into categories 1, 2, and 3 according to their profusion. Conglomerate silicosis is recognized by the development of an opacity > 1 cm in diameter on a background of category 2 or 3 simple silicosis. Numerous other diseases may resemble simple silicosis, including miliary TB, welders' siderosis, hemosiderosis, and coal workers' pneumoconiosis. However, the presence of eggshell calcification in the hilar and mediastinal lymph nodes distinguishes silicosis from other occupational lung diseases.

Prophylaxis

Effective dust control can prevent silicosis. Since dust suppression cannot reduce the risk in sandblasting, external-air–supplied hoods should be used. Such protection may not be available to personnel performing other jobs in the area (eg, painting, welding). For this reason, the substitution of other abrasive materials instead of sand is desirable. Surveillance of all exposed workers includes periodic chest x-rays q 6 mo for sandblasters and q 1 to 2 yr for other workers.

Treatment

No effective treatment is known. Persons with airways obstruction should be treated as for chronic airflow obstruction (see CHRONIC OBSTRUCTIVE PULMONARY DISEASE in Ch. 36). Those exposed to silica who have a positive tuberculin test should be given isoniazid for at least 1 yr. Some authorities recommend lifetime treatment because the function of the alveolar macrophage is permanently compromised by silica. Lifetime isoniazid prophylaxis may be indicated for those who have been treated for active pulmonary TB.

COAL WORKERS' PNEUMOCONIOSIS (CWP)

(Coal Miners' Pneumoconiosis; Black Lung Disease; Anthracosis)

Diffuse nodular deposition of dust in the lungs as a result of long-term exposure to bituminous or anthracite coal dust in coal mining.

Pathology and Pathophysiology

In **simple CWP**, coal dust is widely distributed throughout the lungs, leading to the development of "coal macules" around the bronchioles. Later on mild dilation known as focal dust emphysema also occurs; however, it does not extend to the alveoli and is not associated with airflow obstruction. Because coal is relatively nonfibrogenic, distortion of lung architecture and functional impairment are minimal. However, each year about 1 to 2% of miners with simple CWP go on to develop **progressive massive fibrosis (PMF)**, which is defined as *development of an opacity ≥ 1 cm in diameter on a suitable background of simple CWP* (ie, categories 2 or 3). Although not all PMF will progress, PMF may develop after exposure has ceased, or it may progress without further exposure. As an amorphous black mass, PMF encroaches on and destroys the vascular bed and airways (as in complicated silicosis). The development of PMF is usually unrelated to the silica content of the coal; however, as in silicosis, antinuclear antibodies and lung autoantibodies may be present in the serum.

Symptoms, Signs, and Diagnosis

CWP is not associated with respiratory symptoms. Cough and sputum occur as often when x-rays are negative for this condition. If present, airways obstruction is due either to coincident pulmonary emphysema from smoking, industrial bronchitis, or to PMF, the only disabling form of CWP. A few minor abnormalities of the distribution of inspired gas are found in simple CWP, but these are not associated with respiratory symptoms. The diagnosis depends on a history of suitable exposure, usually at least 10 yr underground, and the characteristic x-ray pattern of small rounded opacities in both lung fields (simple CWP) or, in PMF, a shadow > 1 cm in diameter occurring on a background of at least category 2 or 3 simple CWP.

Prophylaxis and Treatment

CWP can be prevented by increasing the efficiency of dust suppression at the coal face. PMF usually can be prevented by removing patients with x-ray changes typical of early simple CWP (ie, category 1) from further coal dust exposure. There is no specific treatment; therapy is similar to that for nonspecific chronic obstructive disease (see CHRONIC OBSTRUCTIVE PULMONARY DISEASE in Ch. 36).

Asbestosis and Other Asbestos-Related Thoracic Disorders

Asbestosis: *A diffuse fibrous pneumoconiosis resulting from the inhalation of asbestos dust (fibrous mineral silicates of different chemical compositions).*

Etiology

Asbestosis is a consequence of long-term inhalation of asbestos fibers in the mining, milling, manufacturing, or application (eg, of insulation) of asbestos products. The risk of developing asbestosis is related to the dose of asbestos dust to which the worker has been exposed. The incidence of lung cancer is also increased in asbestos-exposed persons. Although the risk of lung cancer is usually less in non-smokers, the risk is not limited to cigarette smokers. **Pleural or peritoneal mesotheliomas,** uncommon tumors of mesothelial lining surfaces, have been associated with asbestos exposure, although the exposure may have occurred many years earlier and may have been brief. Mesothelioma is nearly always associated with crocidolite, one of the 4 main commercial fibers. The other 3 in their order of decreasing potential for causing mesothelioma are amosite, chrysotile, and anthophyllite. Benign pleural plaques and pleural effusions may also develop after asbestos exposure.

Pathology and Pathophysiology

Asbestos fibers continually divide along their long axes, their diameter ultimately becoming $< 1\ \mu m$. These fibers can be inhaled deep into the lung parenchyma where they produce diffuse alveolar, interstitial, and pleural fibrosis, resulting in reduced lung volumes and compliance (increased stiffness), and impaired gas transfer. Uncoated and coated (with an iron-protein complex) asbestos fibers (coated fibers are called **"asbestos or ferruginous bodies"**) may be present in lung tissue, with or without associated fibrosis, and are thought to be harmless. If there is no associated fibrosis, the presence of fibers in lung tissue indicates exposure only, not disease.

Symptoms and Signs

The patient characteristically notices the insidious onset of exertional dyspnea and reduced exercise tolerance. Symptoms of airways disease (cough, wheezing) are not usual but may occur in heavy smokers with associated chronic bronchitis. The chest film reveals diffusely distributed irregular or linear small opacities, most prominent in the lower lung zones. Occasionally the chest film shows minimal changes. Diffuse or local pleural thickening, with or without parenchymal disease, may also be visible. The parenchymal fibrosis is progressive and symptoms become more severe in association with advancing x-ray and physiologic abnormalities. Ultimately, respiratory failure with marked impairment in oxygenation occurs.

Mesothelial tumors associated with asbestos exposure are invariably fatal. Bloody effusion with chest-wall pain is often present. Spread is usually by local extension or, rarely, distant metastases.

Diagnosis

The diagnosis of asbestosis requires a history of occupational exposure, and x-ray, clinical, and physiologic evidence of diffuse pulmonary fibrosis. Histologic confirmation is rarely necessary or indicated. Mesothelioma is harder to diagnose and may be confirmed only by biopsy or autopsy. While the diagnosis of bronchogenic carcinoma can be made readily, a cause and effect relationship to asbestos exposure in an individual case presents formidable medical and legal problems.

Prophylaxis and Treatment

Asbestosis is preventable, primarily by effective dust suppression in the work environment; marked reduction in asbestos exposure has reduced its incidence, and further industrial hygiene advances are likely essentially to eliminate it. Once dust is controlled to the point that asbestosis is no longer a problem, evidence suggests that the excess risk of lung cancer in asbestos workers will either disappear or almost so. The

most effective preventive measure with respect to lung cancer can be taken by the worker himself, however, by abstaining from cigarette smoking. Since brief, but usually heavy, asbestos exposure (at least 3 to 6 mo) may lead to the development of mesothelioma, its prevention cannot be confidently predicted, but the latest studies suggest that only crocidolite represents a serious hazard.

No specific therapy is available. Treatment is symptomatic. Surgical resection occasionally cures bronchogenic carcinoma, but is ineffective in treating mesothelioma.

BERYLLIOSIS
(Beryllium Disease, Poisoning, or Granulomatosis)

A generalized granulomatous disease with pulmonary manifestations, caused by inhalation of dust or fumes containing beryllium compounds and products.

Etiology

Beryllium exposure used to be common in many industries including beryllium mining and extracting, electronics, chemical plants, and the manufacture of fluorescent light bulbs. Its main use today is in the aerospace industry. Berylliosis differs from most pneumoconioses: it appears to be a hypersensitivity disease that occurs in only about 2% of those exposed. Exposure may be relatively brief, with onset of the disease delayed as long as 10 to 20 yr. A few patients reported have lived in the vicinity of beryllium refineries.

Pathology and Pathophysiology

Acute berylliosis is a chemical pneumonitis, but other tissues (eg, skin and conjunctivae) may be involved. Pathologic changes in the lung include diffuse parenchymal inflammatory infiltrates and nonspecific intra-alveolar edema. Early granuloma formation with mononuclear and giant cells may also occur. The hallmark of chronic berylliosis is a diffuse pulmonary and hilar lymph node granulomatous reaction histologically indistinguishable from sarcoidosis.

Symptoms, Signs, and Diagnosis

Patients with acute beryllium disease often have dyspnea, cough, weight loss, and a highly variable chest x-ray pattern, usually indicating diffuse alveolar consolidation. In chronic disease, patients complain of insidious and progressive exertional dyspnea. The chest x-ray shows diffuse infiltrations, often with hilar adenopathy, resembling the pattern seen in sarcoidosis. Diagnosis depends on a history of exposure and the appropriate clinical manifestations. However, in the absence of sophisticated immunologic technics, it is usually impossible to distinguish berylliosis from sarcoidosis.

Prognosis

The acute disease can be fatal, but surviving patients have an excellent prognosis. The chronic form often results in progressive loss of respiratory function. Right heart strain usually results, with death from cor pulmonale.

Prophylaxis and Treatment

Industrial dust suppression is the basis of preventing exposure to beryllium, but its efficiency is imperfect. The disease (both acute and chronic) must be promptly recognized and affected workers removed from further beryllium exposure.

Treatment of acute disease is generally symptomatic. The lungs often become edematous and hemorrhagic and mechanical ventilation is necessary in severely affected patients. The clinical manifestations in survivors are usually short-lived and completely reversible. Although steroids have been used in chronic berylliosis, the response has been in the main unsatisfactory. Marked and sustained improvement probably means that the patient had sarcoidosis rather than berylliosis. When a decision is made to use steroids, full doses of prednisone, 60 mg/day orally for a period of 2 to 3 wk

should be given, and then gradually tapered off during the next 3 or 4 wk to 10 to 15 mg/day.

LESS COMMON CAUSES OF PULMONARY FIBROSIS

Tungsten carbide and aluminum dust have been rarely associated with diffuse pulmonary fibrosis. Clinical, x-ray, and physiologic changes resemble those found in other diseases caused by dust inhalation and characterized by diffuse pulmonary fibrosis.

BENIGN PNEUMOCONIOSES

Several inert dusts, including iron oxide, barium, and tin, may produce conditions known respectively as **siderosis, baritosis,** and **stannosis.** These dusts are nonfibrogenic, and the abnormal x-rays they produce should not be regarded as indicative of disease since there are neither symptoms nor functional impairment.

DISEASES DUE TO ORGANIC DUSTS

HYPERSENSITIVITY PNEUMONITIS

(See in Ch. 43)

OCCUPATIONAL ASTHMA

Diffuse, intermittent, reversible airways obstruction caused by inhalation of irritant or allergenic particles or vapors from industrial processes.

Etiology

Numerous allergenic and nonallergenic materials in the occupational environment are recognized causes of reversible airways obstruction. Examples include castor bean, grain, proteolytic enzymes used in detergent manufacturing and beer- and leather-making industries, western red cedar wood, isocyanates, cotton, flax, formalin, epoxy resins, and hemp. The list is continually growing. (For exposure to textile dust, see BYSSINOSIS, below.)

Pathophysiology

Although it is tempting to attribute most forms of asthma to either a Type I (IgE) or Type III (IgG) mediated immunologic response, such a simplistic approach is not justified. Thus, isocyanates and western red cedar sometimes cause bronchospasm up to 24 h following exposure, and the response may recur every night for a week or more without further exposure.

Symptoms, Signs, and Diagnosis

Patients generally complain of shortness of breath, chest tightness, wheezing, and cough, often in association with such upper respiratory symptoms as sneezing, rhinorrhea, and tearing. Symptoms may develop during work hours in association with specific dust or vapor exposure, but are often not apparent until some hours after leaving work, which makes the association with occupational exposure less obvious. Often the symptoms disappear on weekends or when the worker is on holiday. Nocturnal wheezing may be the only symptom.

Diagnosis depends on recognition of causative agents in the working environment and on immunologic tests (eg, skin tests) using the suspect antigen. In difficult cases, a positive, carefully controlled inhalation challenge test performed in the laboratory confirms the etiology of the airways obstruction. Differentiation from idiopathic asthma is generally based on the pattern of symptoms and relationship to exposure to

allergens (see BYSSINOSIS, below). Pulmonary function tests that show decreasing air flow during work are further evidence that occupational exposure is causative.

Prophylaxis and Treatment

Dust suppression is essential in industries where known allergens or bronchoconstrictors have been identified; however, elimination of all instances of sensitization and clinical disease may not be possible. A highly susceptible individual must be removed from a setting known to produce asthmatic symptoms.

Treatment for asthma (generally including an oral and aerosol bronchodilator, theophylline, and, in severe cases, corticosteroids) provides symptomatic improvement (see BRONCHIAL ASTHMA in Ch. 36).

BYSSINOSIS

Bronchoconstriction occurring in cotton, flax, and hemp workers.

Byssinosis is seen almost entirely in workers who come in contact with cotton trash (ie, unprocessed, unpurified cotton); those who open bales or work in the card room are most affected. Evidence suggests that some material in the cotton bract leads to development of bronchoconstriction. Formerly, it was believed that prolonged exposure to cotton dust led to emphysema and irreversible obstruction, but this now seems unlikely in view of a series of post-mortem studies that have shown some bronchitis but no increased prevalence of emphysema and destructive changes.

Chest tightness develops on the first day after returning to work following a weekend or vacation. Many subjects who complain of chest tightness also demonstrate a drop in ventilatory capacity over the first work shift. Unlike asthma, which worsens with repeated exposure to allergens, the symptoms and chest tightness lessen with repeated exposure and usually by the end of the week the subject is symptom-free. With repeated, prolonged exposure over a period of years, there is a tendency for chest tightness to persist on Tuesday and Wednesday, and even occasionally to the end of the week.

DISEASES DUE TO IRRITANT GASES AND CHEMICALS

ACUTE EXPOSURE

Etiology

Among the important irritant gases to which workers may be exposed in an industrial accident are chlorine, phosgene, sulfur dioxide, hydrogen sulfide, nitrogen dioxide, and ammonia. Acute heavy exposures may occur due to a faulty valve or pump or during transport of the gas.

Pathology and Pathophysiology

Respiratory damage is related to various factors, including the solubility of the gas. Relatively soluble gases (eg, chlorine, ammonia) initially cause mucous membrane irritation of the upper respiratory tract, but affect the lower, deep portions of the airways and lung parenchyma only if the victim's escape from the gas source is impeded. Less soluble gases (eg, nitrogen dioxide) do not produce the warning signs of upper respiratory tract symptoms and are more likely to cause severe bronchiolitis, pulmonary edema, or both. In nitrogen dioxide intoxication (eg, a disease of **silo fillers** or **welders**), a lag of up to 12 h may occur before symptoms of pulmonary edema develop; occasionally, bronchiolitis obliterans progressing to respiratory failure is a sequel occurring 10 to 14 days after acute exposure.

Symptoms and Signs

The more soluble irritant gases cause severe burning and other manifestations of irritation of the eyes, nose, throat, trachea, and major bronchi. Marked cough, hemoptysis, wheezing, retching, and dyspnea are common, the severity of these symptoms being generally dose-related. After heavy exposure, patchy or confluent alveolar consolidation, seen on chest x-ray, indicates pulmonary edema; most persons recover fully from a heavy acute exposure. Bacterial infections, common during the acute phase, are the most serious complications.

Prophylaxis and Treatment

Care in handling gases and chemicals is the most effective preventive measure. The availability of adequate respiratory protection (eg, gas masks with self-contained air supplies) is also of great importance should accidental exposure occur.

Treatment of heavy acute exposures is directed toward maintenance of vital gas exchange with assurance of adequate oxygenation and alveolar ventilation, at times requiring mechanical ventilation through an artificial airway (eg, endotracheal tube). Bronchodilators, mild sedation, IV fluids and antibiotics, and nasal O_2 are required and may suffice in less severe cases. Adequate humidification of the inspired air must be assured. The efficacy of corticosteroid therapy (eg, prednisone 45 to 60 mg for 1 to 2 wk) is difficult to prove, but corticosteroids are frequently used.

CHRONIC EXPOSURE

Chronic, low-level, continuous, or intermittent exposure to irritant gases or chemical vapors may be an important factor that initiates or accelerates the development of chronic bronchitis, though the role of such exposures is difficult to substantiate. Exposure to carcinogenic chemicals is another important disease mechanism; the route of entry is via the lungs, and lung tumors (from exposure to bischloromethyl ether or certain metals) as well as tumors in other parts of the body may result (eg, liver angiosarcomas following vinyl chloride monomer exposure).

---

43. HYPERSENSITIVITY DISEASES OF THE LUNGS

(Allergic Pulmonary Diseases)

Hypersensitivity (allergic) diseases of the lungs include hypersensitivity pneumonitis (extrinsic allergic alveolitis), allergic bronchopulmonary aspergillosis, and many drug reactions. Other eosinophilic pneumonias and the pulmonary granulomatoses are of suspected allergic origin. Bronchial asthma is discussed in Ch. 36; OCCUPATIONAL ASTHMA, in Ch. 42.

Hypersensitivity reactions (see also Ch. 20) are classified into 4 types according to their pathogenetic mechanisms. **Type I (atopic or anaphylactic)** reactions (eg, allergic [extrinsic] bronchial asthma) result from the release of mediators (eg, histamine, leukotrienes) from IgE-sensitized basophils and mast cells after contact with antigen. **Type II (cytotoxic)** reactions (eg, Goodpasture's syndrome) involve complement-fixing antibody with consequent cell lysis or antibody-dependent cellular cytotoxicity mechanisms. **Type III (immune-complex–mediated)** reactions (eg, SLE) are associated with soluble antigen-antibody complexes, activated complement components, polymorphonuclear leukocyte chemotaxis, and subsequent vasculitis. **Type IV (cell-mediated or delayed)** reactions (eg, tuberculin skin test) result from release of lymphokines (which affect other cells and lead to tissue damage) by sensitized lymphocytes following contact with antigen.

Hypersensitivity diseases of the lungs may involve mixed, rather than single, types f hypersensitivity reactions. For example, hypersensitivity pneumonitis may involve oth Types III and IV; allergic bronchopulmonary aspergillosis, Types I and III.

HYPERSENSITIVITY PNEUMONITIS

(Extrinsic Allergic Alveolitis; Diffuse Hypersensitivity Pneumonia; Allergic Interstitial Pneumonitis; Organic Dust Pneumoconiosis)

A diffuse interstitial granulomatous lung disease caused by an allergic response after ıhalation of one of a variety of organic dusts or, less commonly, simple chemicals. **Farm-r's lung**, associated with repeated inhalation of dusts from hay containing thermo-hilic actinomycetes, is the prototype of numerous similar lung diseases that are ssociated with specific antigens.

tiology and Pathogenesis

The number of specific materials known to be capable of causing hypersensitivity ıeumonitis is increasing. The agents are most commonly either a microorganism or a ›reign animal or vegetable protein inhaled in considerable amounts. Recent reports ıdicate that simple chemicals may also be capable of causing interstitial disease. ABLE 43–1 lists the offending antigen associated with each form of the disease.

The disease is considered to be immunologically mediated. Precipitating antibodies › the offending antigen are usually demonstrated, suggesting a Type III allergic re-›onse, although vasculitis is not a common finding. Type IV hypersensitivity is sug-ested by the granulomatous primary tissue reaction and animal models.

Only a small proportion of exposed persons develop symptoms, and then only after ıe considerable period of exposure required for induction of sensitization. Chronic rogressive parenchymal disease may result from continuous or frequent low-level xposure to the antigen. A history of previous allergic disease (eg, asthma, hay fever) is ıcommon and is not a predisposing factor.

athophysiology

A diffuse granulomatous interstitial pneumonitis is characteristic. Lymphocytes and ıasma cells are present in thickened alveolar septa; the degree of fibrosis depends on ıe stage of the disease. Bronchiolitis is seen to some degree in about 50% of patients ith farmer's lung. Some cases of idiopathic pulmonary fibrosis may represent the end sult of sensitization to an organic dust.

ymptoms and Signs

In **acute disease,** episodes of fever, chills, cough, and dyspnea occur in a previously nsitized person, typically appearing 4 to 8 h after reexposure to the antigen. An-exia, nausea, and vomiting may also be present. Fine-to-medium inspiratory rales ay be heard on auscultation. Wheezing is unusual. With avoidance of the antigen, mptoms usually improve within hours, though complete recovery may take weeks ıd pulmonary fibrosis may follow repeated episodes. A **subacute form** may begin sidiously with cough and dyspnea over a period of days to weeks with progression quiring urgent hospitalization. In the **chronic form,** progressive exertional dyspnea, oductive cough, fatigue, and weight loss may occur over months to years. The dis-ıse may progress to respiratory failure.

Chest x-ray findings range from normal to diffuse interstitial fibrosis. Bilateral ıtchy or nodular infiltrates and coarsening of bronchovascular markings, or a fine inar pattern suggestive of pulmonary edema is commonly present. Hilar lymphade-›pathy is rare. Pulmonary function studies show restrictive abnormalities: decreased ng volume, decreased CO diffusing capacity, hypoxemia, and abnormal ventila-›n/perfusion ratios. Airways obstruction is unusual in acute disease, but may de-lop in chronic disease. Eosinophilia is not expected.

TABLE 43–1. SELECTED CAUSES OF HYPERSENSITIVITY PNEUMONITIS

Disease	Antigen	Source of Particles
Farmer's lung	*Micropolyspora faeni* or *Thermoactinomyces vulgaris*	Moldy hay
Bird fancier's lung; pigeon breeder's lung; hen worker's lung	Serum proteins and droppings	Parakeets; pigeons; hens
"Air-conditioner (or humidifier) lung"	*M. faeni, T. vulgaris,* etc.	Humidifiers, air conditioners
Bagassosis	*T. vulgaris* or *M. faeni*	Bagasse (sugar cane waste)
Mushroom worker's lung	*M. faeni* or *T. vulgaris*	Mushroom post-spawning compost
Suberosis (cork worker's lung)	Moldy cork dust	Moldy cork
Maple bark disease	*Cryptostroma corticale*	Infected maple bark
Malt worker's lung	*Aspergillus fumigatus* or *A. clavatus*	Moldy barley, malt
Sequoiosis	*Pullularia pullulans* or *Graphium* species	Moldy sawdust from redwood
Cheesewasher's lung	*Penicillium* species	Moldy cheese
Wheat weevil disease	*Sitophilus granarius*	Infested wheat flour
Pituitary snuff taker's lung	Bovine and porcine serum protein and pituitary antigens	Heterologous pituitary snuff
Coffee worker's lung	Coffee bean dust	Coffee beans
Thatched roof worker's lung	Unknown	Straw, reed, etc., used as roofing
Chemical worker's lung	Isocyanates (TDI, MDI), phthallic anhydride, vinyl chloride, etc.	Manufacturing of polyurethan foam, molding, insulation, synthetic rubber, meat wrapping and labeling, etc.

Diagnosis

Diagnosis depends on a history of environmental exposure, compatible clinical fe tures, chest x-ray, and pulmonary function tests. The demonstration of specific precip tating antibodies to the suspected antigen in the serum helps to confirm the diagnosi though neither their presence nor their absence is definitive. Since symptoms are r lated to exposure to the antigen, the history may give excellent clues (eg, perso exposed at work may become symptom-free every weekend or symptoms may rea pear 4 to 8 h after a reexposure). History of exposure to causative antigens may not elicited easily, particularly in air conditioner or humidifier lung, and an environment visit by the physician may prove helpful in difficult cases. In puzzling cases or tho without a history of environmental exposure, lung biopsy may be necessary. Bronch alveolar lavage is being used to aid in diagnosing interstitial lung diseases. The value this procedure in diagnosis has not been established. Increased numbers of lymph cytes, particularly T cells, have been reported in hypersensitivity pneumonitis (and sarcoidosis). The OKT8+ (suppressor/cytotoxic) T-cell subset may predominate

hypersensitivity pneumonitis, and the OKT4+ (helper/inducer) subset may constitute the majority of T cells in active sarcoidosis.

Hypersensitivity pneumonitis can be distinguished from psittacosis, viral pneumonia, and other infective pneumonias by cultures and serologic tests. Because of similar clinical features, x-rays, and pulmonary function tests, idiopathic interstitial pneumonitis or fibrosis (Hamman-Rich syndrome, cryptogenic fibrosing alveolitis, intrinsic allergic alveolitis) may be difficult to distinguish when the typical history of exposure followed by an acute episode cannot be elicited. Evidence of autoimmunity (positive antinuclear-DNA antibody or latex fixation tests; presence of a collagen vascular disease) suggests idiopathic interstitial pneumonitis. Chronic eosinophilic pneumonias are usually accompanied by peripheral blood eosinophilia. Sarcoidosis often results in hilar and paratracheal lymph node enlargement and may involve other organs. Pulmonary angiitis-granulomatosis syndromes (Wegener's and allergic granulomatosis) are usually accompanied by upper respiratory tract or renal disease. Bronchial asthma and allergic bronchopulmonary aspergillosis present with eosinophilia and are obstructive rather than restrictive pulmonary abnormalities.

Prophylaxis

Avoidance of the responsible antigen is advisable, but socioeconomic factors may make a change of environment difficult. Dust control or the use of protective masks to filter the offending dust particles in contaminated areas may be effective preventive measures. It may also be possible to prevent the growth of antigenic microorganisms (eg, in bagasse or hay) by chemical means.

Treatment

The most effective treatment is cessation of further exposure. Acute disease is self-limiting if exposure to the antigen is avoided. Corticosteroids may be useful in severe acute or subacute cases. Prednisone 60 mg/day is given orally in 4 divided doses for 1 to 2 wk, tapered over the next 2 wk to 20 mg/day in 1 dose, followed by weekly decrements of 2.5 mg until withdrawal is complete. A recurrence or progression of symptoms requires modification of this regimen. Precautions regarding the use of corticosteroids should be observed (see THE CORTICOSTEROIDS in Ch. 283). Antibiotics are not indicated unless there is a superimposed infection.

THE EOSINOPHILIC PNEUMONIAS

(P.I.E. [Pulmonary Infiltrates with Eosinophilia] Syndrome; Löffler's Syndrome)

A group of diseases of both known and unknown etiology characterized by eosinophilic pulmonary infiltration and, commonly, peripheral blood eosinophilia.

Etiology and Pathogenesis

Parasites including roundworms, *Toxocara* larvae, and filariae; drugs such as penicillin, aminosalicylic acid, hydralazine, nitrofurantoin, chlorpropamide, sulfonamides; chemical sensitizers such as nickel carbonyl inhaled as a vapor; and fungi such as *Aspergillus fumigatus* (causing allergic bronchopulmonary aspergillosis, discussed separately below) may be causative. Most eosinophilic pneumonias, however, are of unknown etiology, though a hypersensitivity mechanism is suspected. The eosinophilia suggests a Type I hypersensitivity reaction, while other features of the syndrome (vasculitis, round cell infiltrates) suggest Type III and possibly Type IV reactions.

Many patients have coexisting bronchial asthma. Eosinophilic pneumonias of unknown etiology associated with asthma can be separated into 3 general groups: (1) extrinsic bronchial asthma with the P.I.E. syndrome, which often is in fact allergic bronchopulmonary aspergillosis; (2) intrinsic bronchial asthma with the P.I.E. syndrome, frequently with peculiar peripheral infiltrates on chest x-ray; and (3) allergic

granulomatosis (Churg-Strauss syndrome, a variant of polyarteritis nodosa with a pre-dilection for the lung).

A classification of the eosinophilic pneumonias based on clinical and pathologi characteristics is given in TABLE 43–2.

Pathology

Characteristic features include alveolar filling with eosinophils and large mononu clear cells, and septal infiltration with eosinophils, plasma cells, and large and smal mononuclear cells. Mucus plugging of bronchioles and vascular infiltrations are als found.

Symptoms and Signs

Symptoms and signs may be mild or life-threatening. Simple pulmonary eosino philia **(Löffler's syndrome)** may be associated with low-grade fever, minimal (if any respiratory symptoms, and prompt recovery. With other forms of the P.I.E. syndrome there may be fever and symptoms of bronchial asthma, including cough, wheezing, an dyspnea at rest. Without treatment, chronic eosinophilic pneumonia is often progres sive and life-threatening.

Marked blood eosinophilia (between 20 and 40% and at times considerably higher is usually striking. Chest x-rays reveal rapidly developing and disappearing infiltrate in various lobes depending upon the timing and frequency of the x-rays (migrator infiltrates).

Diagnosis

Helminthic infections should be sought depending on the patient's geographic loca tion. Parasites and *A. fumigatus* may be found in the sputum. A careful drug histor should be elicited. Differential diagnosis includes TB, sarcoidosis, Hodgkin's diseas and other lymphoproliferative disorders, eosinophilic granuloma of the lung, des quamative interstitial pneumonitis, collagen vascular disease, and the hypereosinc philic syndrome. Hypersensitivity pneumonitis and Wegener's granulomatosis ar uncommonly associated with eosinophilia.

Treatment

The disease may be self-limited and benign, requiring no treatment. If the severity c the symptoms warrants it, however, treatment with corticosteroids (eg, prednisone a for HYPERSENSITIVITY PNEUMONITIS, above) is usually dramatically effective and i idiopathic chronic eosinophilic pneumonia may be lifesaving. When bronchial asthm is present, the usual therapy is indicated (see BRONCHIAL ASTHMA in Ch. 36). F helminthic infections, appropriate vermifuges should be used (see in DISEASES CAUSE BY WORMS in Ch. 13).

ALLERGIC BRONCHOPULMONARY ASPERGILLOSIS

A noninvasive form of aspergillosis occurring in asthmatic patients as an eosinophil pneumonia resulting from an allergic reaction to Aspergillus fumigatus.

Etiology, Pathology, and Pathogenesis

The presence of *A. fumigatus* growing in the bronchial lumen provokes an allerg response in the airways and parenchyma. Type I and Type III (and possibly Type IV hypersensitivity reactions are involved in pathogenesis. The alveoli are packed wit eosinophils. A granulomatous interstitial pneumonitis, showing peribronchial and a veolar septal infiltration with plasma cells, mononuclear cells, and numerous eosin phils, may be present. Bronchiolar mucous glands and goblet cells may be increased. proximal bronchiectasis develops in advanced cases.

TABLE 43–2. CHARACTERISTICS OF THE EOSINOPHILIC PNEUMONIAS

Disease	*Etiology*	*Association with Bronchial Asthma*	*Degree of Peripheral Eosinophilia*	*Systemic Involvement*	*Prognosis*
Simple eosinophilic pneumonia (including idiopathic Löffler's syndrome)	Unknown Drugs Parasites	Rare	Moderate	Rare	Excellent
Chronic eosinophilic pneumonia	Unknown Drugs Parasites	Usual	High (can be minimal or normal)	Rare	Good
Allergic bronchopulmonary aspergillosis (ABPA)	*Aspergillus fumigatus*	Always	High	None	Fair
Tropical eosinophilia	Parasites	Occasional	High	Occasional	Good
Allergic granulomatosis of Churg and Strauss	Unknown ? Drugs	Always	High	Common	Fair to poor

Symptoms and Signs

The patient usually presents with an exacerbation of bronchial asthma and may have intermittent low-grade fever and systemic symptoms. The sputum may contain brownish flecks or plugs. Signs of airways obstruction (prolonged expiration and wheezing) are found on chest examination.

Serial chest x-rays show transient shadows that may migrate from lobe to lobe. Mucus plugs may produce atelectasis. In chronic cases, bronchograms reveal bronchiectasis with a peculiar preference for proximal airways but are rarely indicated and may be dangerous in these patients. Sputum examination may reveal small yellowish or brownish plugs containing *A. fumigatus* mycelia, Curschmann spirals, Charcot-Leyden crystals, mucus, and eosinophils. Sputum cultures may be positive for *Aspergillus* but are inconsistent with occasional difficulty in demonstrating this fungus. Pulmonary function studies show an obstructive pattern with decreased flow rates. Blood eosinophilia is usually > 1000/mm^3. Serologic tests commonly demonstrate precipitating antibodies to *A. fumigatus*. IgE levels may be extremely high in both total IgE and IgE antibody specific for *A. fumigatus*. Skin testing with *Aspergillus* antigen typically results in a biphasic positive reaction with an immediate Type I wheal-and-flare reaction, followed by a late-onset reaction (erythema, edema, and tenderness that is maximum at 6 to 8 h). The significance of the late response is uncertain, however, and is both unnecessary and insufficient for the diagnosis.

Diagnosis

Diagnostic features include the presence of extrinsic bronchial asthma, usually longstanding, pulmonary infiltrates, sputum and blood eosinophilia, and hypersensitivity to *Aspergillus* as revealed by a wheal-and-flare skin test, precipitating antibody in the serum, and high levels of total (and specific) IgE. The presence of these features, the first 6 criteria in TABLE 43–3, makes the diagnosis very likely.

Presenting features mimic simple bronchial asthma and may resemble allergic granulomatosis and other chronic eosinophilic pneumonias. In hypersensitivity pneumonitis, pulmonary abnormalities are restrictive rather than obstructive, and eosinophilia is rare. Invasive forms of aspergillosis (see ASPERGILLOSIS in Ch. 9) have different clinical features. Invasive aspergillosis usually occurs as a serious opportunistic pneumonia in immunosuppressed patients or after antibacterial or antifungal therapy in patients whose bronchi have been damaged by bronchitis, bronchiectasis, or TB. Aspergillomas may also occur in old cavitary disease (eg, TB) or, rarely, in the upper lobes of patients with rheumatoid spondylitis.

TABLE 43–3. DIAGNOSTIC CRITERIA FOR BRONCHOPULMONARY ASPERGILLOSIS

Major:	Bronchial asthma Transient or fixed pulmonary infiltrates Wheal and flare skin reactivity to *Aspergillus* antigen Blood and sputum eosinophilia Serum precipitins to *Aspergillus* antigen Elevated serum IgE Proximal bronchiectasis
Minor:	*Aspergillus fumigatus* in sputum History of expectoration of brownish plugs or flecks Late onset skin reactivity to *Aspergillus* antigen

Treatment

A. fumigatus is ubiquitous and its avoidance is difficult. Treatment with corticosteroids and other antiasthmatic drugs (theophylline, sympathomimetics) is usually successful in allowing expectoration of the mucus plugs and, with them, the *Aspergillus*. The prednisone dosage regimen given above for HYPERSENSITIVITY PNEUMONITIS is appropriate, though 7.5 to 15 mg/day may be necessary for maintenance in long-term treatment and prevention of progressive, irreversible disease. The success rate for maintenance therapy with inhaled beclomethasone diproprionate is not established. Immunotherapy and fungicidal or fungistatic agents are not recommended. Hyposensitization with extracts of *A. fumigatus* is *contraindicated* since it produces bothersome local reactions and may cause symptoms to exacerbate.

A sign of successful treatment and favorable prognosis is a sustained fall in serum IgE level.

PULMONARY WEGENER'S GRANULOMATOSIS

A limited or variant form of Wegener's granulomatosis characterized by a necrotizing granulomatous angiitis involving the lungs. For a discussion of the progressive form of the disease characterized by generalized necrotizing granulomatous vasculitis involving the upper and lower respiratory tracts, the skin, the lung, and the kidneys, see WEGENER'S GRANULOMATOSIS in Ch. 110.

Etiology, Pathogenesis, and Pathophysiology

The etiology is unknown; Type III and Type IV hypersensitivity reactions may be involved. The characteristic pulmonary pathology consists of focal destruction and infiltration of veins and arteries, not explained by thromboembolism, accompanied by peripheral chronic necrotic lesions engulfed in granulation tissue containing plasma cells, lymphocytes, large mononuclear cells, and occasional epithelioid and giant cells. Limited forms of Wegener's granulomatosis involve the lung only; variant forms occur with atypical pathologic findings, including active lymphoreticular proliferation or bronchial rather than vascular localization.

Symptoms and Signs

Limited or variant forms of Wegener's granulomatosis may be asymptomatic or may present with fever, weight loss, malaise, cough, dyspnea, and chest pain. Symptoms and signs of generalized Wegener's granulomatosis are described in Ch. 110.

Chest x-rays reveal diffuse or nodular infiltrates that may resemble malignant metastases. Necrotizing lesions are usually multiple and bilateral, occur in any part of the lung, and may cavitate. Hilar adenopathy is uncommon. Eosinophilia is *not* a feature of this disease. Serum complement levels are normal or elevated.

Diagnosis and Treatment

Lung biopsy is usually necessary for definitive diagnosis when upper respiratory tract disease or typical skin lesions are absent. Differential diagnosis includes metastatic or primary neoplasm, lymphoma, infectious granulomas (eg, TB), sarcoidosis, rheumatoid nodules, pulmonary infarction, lung abscess, aspiration pneumonia, and bronchiolitis obliterans.

Although pulmonary disease may improve spontaneously, treatment is recommended as soon as the diagnosis is established since, without treatment, progression of the disease with attendant high mortality may occur. Therapy is described in Ch. 110. Limited Wegener's is reported to respond more readily to corticosteroids than does the full-blown disease, for which cyclophosphamide is the agent of choice.

44. GOODPASTURE'S SYNDROME

An uncommon Type II hypersensitivity disorder (see Ch. 20) of unknown etiology, manifested by pulmonary hemorrhage with associated severe and progressive glomerulonephritis, and characterized by circulating antiglomerular basement membrane antibodies in the blood and linear deposition of immunoglobulin and complement in the glomerular basement membrane.

Pathology

Changes observed at kidney biopsy are like those in any rapidly progressive glomerulonephritis, with epithelial cell crescents, glomerular adhesions, and interstitial inflammatory exudates. Intra-alveolar hemorrhages, hemosiderin-laden macrophages, and septal fibrosis are present in the lungs. Immunofluorescent staining demonstrates linear deposition of immunoglobulin and complement in the glomerular and, in some cases, in the alveolar-capillary basement membranes.

Symptoms, Signs, and Diagnosis

The patient, most often a young man, characteristically presents with severe hemoptysis, dyspnea, and rapidly progressive renal failure. Circulating antiglomerular basement membrane antibodies are present in the blood. Iron-deficiency anemia is usual. Hematuria and proteinuria are common, and the urinary sediment usually contains cellular and granular casts. Chest x-rays may show progressive, migratory, asymmetric, bilateral, fluffy densities.

Though the combination of pulmonary hemorrhage and renal failure can also occur in certain collagen vascular diseases (eg, SLE, RA), acute glomerulonephritis with circulatory congestion, Wegener's granulomatosis, and bacterial endocarditis, these diseases can often be excluded by their other distinguishing features and by renal biopsy. Linear deposition of immunoglobulin has been described in few cases of lupus nephritis and diabetic glomerulosclerosis, but antibody eluted from kidneys in these settings does not have antiglomerular basement membrane activity.

Prognosis and Treatment

The disease may be rapidly fatal. The management of Goodpasture's syndrome relies on the use of high-dose corticosteroids (methylprednisolone 7 to 15 mg/kg/day in divided doses IV), immunosuppression with cyclophosphamide, and repeated plasmapheresis to remove antiglomerular basement membrane antibody from the circulation. Early use of these measures in combination may result in preservation of renal function. End-stage renal disease can be managed by long-term hemodialysis or by kidney transplantation.

---

45. IDIOPATHIC INFILTRATIVE DISEASES OF THE LUNGS

A spectrum of disorders with different etiologies but similar clinical features and diffuse pathologic changes that affect primarily interalveolar interstitial tissue (see TABLE 45–1). Interstitial infiltration is characterized in its acute phase by abnormal accumulation of polymorphonuclear leukocytes, histiocytes, lymphocytes, plasma cells, and eosinophils with proteinaceous exudate in alveoli and bronchioles. Hyperplasia of bronchiolar or alveolar epithelium may be present at a later stage. If the disorder progresses, the exudate may become organized, and necrosis, scarring, and reepithelialization of alveolar septae may take place. The whole process may ultimately lead to extensive

TABLE 45–1. CLINICAL–PATHOLOGICAL CLASSIFICATION OF INTERSTITIAL LUNG DISORDERS

Stage	*Etiology*
Acute processes	Biologic agents, eg, viruses, rickettsiae, mycoplasmas, miliary TB Physical agents, eg, radiation, gases, fumes Chemical, eg, aspiration of gastric contents Immunosuppressive and antineoplastic drugs, eg, methotrexate, busulfan, cyclophosphamide
Subchronic processes	Interstitial pneumonias: interstitial pulmonary fibrosis, lymphoid, desquamative, giant-cell (rare) Eosinophilic granuloma Extrinsic allergic alveolitis Sarcoidosis
Chronic process	Interstitial fibrosis Honeycomb lung (a late stage of interstitial fibrosis)

(Table used through the courtesy of Mario J. Saldana, M.D., University of Miami School of Medicine.)

interstitial fibrosis, progressive destruction of lung and formation of cysts ("honeycombing").

When a specific etiology is defined, the disease is classified accordingly (eg, occupational and hypersensitivity diseases of the lungs are discussed elsewhere in this section; sarcoidosis is discussed in Ch. 15).

Idiopathic pulmonary fibrosis, (**IPF**; nonspecific ["usual"] interstitial pneumonia [UIP]), diffuse fibrosing alveolitis, Hamman-Rich syndrome): when the etiology leading to pulmonary fibrosis cannot be defined (about 50% of cases), the term "idiopathic" is used.

Desquamative interstitial pneumonia (DIP) resembles idiopathic pulmonary fibrosis, but the histology tends to be more uniform: the cellular infiltrate is more sparse and less pleomorphic. There is striking hyperplasia of type II pneumocytes and filling of air spaces with macrophages. It has been argued that the separation of DIP from idiopathic pulmonary fibrosis is artificial because both histologic patterns can be found frequently in the same lung (probably representing different phases of the same process). However, clinical recognition of DIP is important because the process is associated with a better prognosis and a better response to systemic corticosteroids.

Lymphoid interstitial pneumonia (LIP) involves predominantly the lower lobes. In about 30% of cases it is associated with Sjögren's syndrome and with dysproteinemia. There is preservation of normal alveolar architecture and extensive infiltration with mature lymphocytes, occasional plasma cells, and histiocytes. The clinical course is slowly progressive and may eventually lead into honeycombing. Response to corticosteroids is variable. LIP may evolve to frank lymphoma and has recently been described in association with AIDS (see in Ch. 19).

Symptoms and Signs

Symptoms and signs vary with the extent of pulmonary infiltration, its rate of progress, and with presence of complications (eg, pulmonary infections or cor pulmonale). Pulmonary symptoms may be few, but exertional dyspnea of insidious onset is almost invariably present. Cough, not usually prominent, is more likely to be present when there is secondary bronchial infection. Anorexia, weight loss, fatigue, weakness, and vague chest pains are common. Physical signs may be absent early in the course, but, as the disease progresses, tachypnea and labored breathing are observed and chest

examination reveals prominent breath sounds and end-inspiratory crackles at lung bases. With progression, cyanosis, cor pulmonale, and clubbing may appear.

Diagnosis

Diagnosis of diffuse infiltrative lung diseases is made by recognizing the clinical features, demonstrating the presence of a diffuse interstitial disorder on chest x-ray, and excluding a specific etiology. Because the amount of tissue obtained by transbronchial biopsy is frequently insufficient, open lung biopsy is recommended to identify DIP and IPF, but is not indicated when x-rays show extensive honeycombing.

Routine laboratory studies are not helpful. Erythrocytosis may be present secondary to chronic hypoxemia. **Chest x-rays** may be normal even in the presence of significant symptoms or functional abnormalities. X-ray changes tend to be more prominent at the bases and may include diffuse or patchy "ground-glass" haziness, linear markings, rounded opacities, small cystic lesions (honeycombing), evidence of reduced lung volumes, and signs of pulmonary hypertension. **Pulmonary function studies** reveal a restrictive ventilatory defect with reductions in vital capacity, total lung capacity, and residual volume. The coefficient of retraction (maximum static transpulmonary pressure/total lung capacity) can be increased. Arterial blood gases show a low Pa_{CO_2}, denoting hyperventilation at rest and a decrease in Pa_{O_2}. The abnormal increase in $P(A\text{-}a)_{O_2}$ at rest may be exacerbated during exercise. The diffusing capacity for carbon monoxide is usually reduced. These functional abnormalities can worsen as the disease progresses.

Prognosis

The outcome varies with the etiology and the rate of progression. Some patients may die within a month, while others survive many years. The mortality is smaller and the mean survival greater when histologic features of DIP are present on open lung biopsy.

Treatment

A trial of systemic corticosteroids is indicated in patients without evidence of extensive fibrosis. Prednisone 40 to 60 mg/day usually is given with gradual reduction of the dose to maintenance levels (10 to 30 mg every other day). Response to therapy is followed by serial chest x-rays and appropriate lung function tests. A few patients who do not improve on prednisone may show improvement with azathioprine 3 mg/kg/day, but experience with this agent is limited. Other treatment is supportive and palliative. O_2 in high concentrations may help relieve hypoxemia. Antibiotics are required if secondary bacterial infection occurs. Digitalis and diuretics are used to treat heart failure.

HISTIOCYTOSIS X

(Letterer-Siwe Disease; Hand-Schüller-Christian Disease; Eosinophilic Granuloma)

A group of disorders characterized by proliferation of histiocytes. Granulomatous lesions may occur in many organs, especially the lungs and bones. The etiology is unknown. Pathologically, changes begin with progressive proliferation of histiocytes and infiltration with eosinophilic granulocytes. A fibrotic phase with little cellular infiltration finally supervenes. The lungs show varying degrees of granulomatosis, fibrosis, and honeycombing. Histiocytosis X-body seen on electron microscopy is characteristic of this disorder and may be recognized on examination of alveolar lavage fluid.

Letterer-Siwe disease occurs before age 3 yr and is usually fatal. Skin, lymph nodes, bone, liver, and spleen are frequently involved. **Hand-Schüller-Christian syndrome** most often begins in early childhood, but can appear even in late middle age. The lungs and bones are most frequently involved, though other organs may be affected. A triad of bone defects, exophthalmos, and diabetes insipidus occurs rarely. **Eosinophilic granu-**

loma occurs most commonly between ages 20 and 40 and characteristically involves bone, though about 20% of patients have lung infiltration and the lungs sometimes may be involved exclusively.

Without therapy, Letterer-Siwe disease is always fatal. Patients with Hand-Schüller-Christian syndrome or eosinophilic granuloma may recover spontaneously. Death usually results from respiratory or cardiac failure. **Treatment** of the lung involvement in the 3 disorders is with corticosteroids. For therapy of bone lesions, see Ch. 115.

IDIOPATHIC PULMONARY HEMOSIDEROSIS

A rare disease of unknown etiology characterized by episodes of hemoptysis, hemorrhage into the lung, pulmonary infiltration, and secondary iron deficiency anemia. It must be distinguished from Goodpasture's syndrome (see above) and from lung hemorrhage in SLE. It is most common in young children, but can occur in adults. Diffuse infiltration with hemosiderin-containing macrophages is characteristic, though hemosiderin deposition is found in many other disorders. Pulmonary hemorrhages, which determine the clinical course, vary from mild to severe, but are most often mild and continuous. Blood in the interstitial spaces leads to pulmonary fibrosis. Patients may live for several years, developing pulmonary fibrosis and insufficiency along with chronic secondary anemia. **Treatment** is symptomatic and supportive. Death often occurs as a result of massive hemorrhage.

---

46. PULMONARY ALVEOLAR PROTEINOSIS

A rare disease of unknown etiology characterized pathologically by filling of alveolar spaces with granular, periodic acid-Schiff ***(PAS)****-positive material consisting mostly of phospholipids and proteins.* The disease occurs predominantly in previously healthy men or women who are usually from 20 to 60 yr old.

Pathology

Pathologic findings are limited to the lungs. Since the etiology is unknown, the earliest pathologic lesion is unknown. Typically, the alveolar lining and interstitial cells are normal, but the alveoli are plugged with amorphous PAS-positive granules containing lipoproteins, plasma proteins, and other blood elements. The lipid concentration in the alveolar spaces is high, possibly because of abnormal clearance of alveolar phospholipids. Interstitial fibrosis occurs rarely. The pathologic process may be diffuse or local, and may progress, remain stable, or clear spontaneously. The basal and posterior lung regions are most commonly affected; occasionally only the anterior segments are involved. The pleura is unaffected.

Symptoms, Signs, and Diagnosis

The natural history of this disease is unknown and clinical findings vary greatly. Some patients are asymptomatic; others have severe respiratory insufficiency. Most patients present with gradually progressive exertional dyspnea and cough that is only occasionally productive, especially if the patient smokes cigarettes. Sputum characteristics are generally not helpful. Secondary infections rarely develop with nonbacterial organisms such as *Nocardia*, *Aspergillus*, and *Cryptococcus*. Though the patient may recently have had a febrile illness or present with one, persistent fever is rare unless secondary infection is present. Extrapulmonary symptoms are unusual. A few cases have occurred in patients with myeloproliferative disease, but the significance of this association is unclear.

Physical findings are restricted to the lungs but may be absent despite diffuse parenchymal involvement visible on chest x-ray. Fine inspiratory rales are usually heard over the involved lung areas. On chest x-ray, the usual, though not invariable, appearance is a "butterfly" pattern of infiltrates resembling that seen in pulmonary edema; the cardiac silhouette is normal. Hilar lymph node enlargement and pleural involvement are absent.

Laboratory findings: Vital capacity, residual volume, functional residual capacity, total lung capacity, and CO single-breath diffusing capacity are usually slightly reduced. Obstructive pulmonary disease is not a feature. Hypoxemia may be present even at rest or, if disease is mild, only with mild-to-moderate exercise. The partial pressure of O_2 while breathing 100% O_2 is usually low, indicating an intrapulmonary right-to-left shunt. The serum LDH is usually elevated.

However, the specific diagnosis can be made only by examination of pathologic material from an open lung biopsy, transbronchial biopsy or segmental bronchoalveolar lavage. The latter requires special staining technics.

Prognosis and Treatment

Disability from respiratory insufficiency is common, but death rarely occurs if the patient with significant symptoms is treated with bronchopulmonary lavage.

Therapy is largely empiric. Any therapeutic regimen is difficult to evaluate because spontaneous remissions may occur and because of the limited number of cases available for any one investigator to study. Many agents have been tried with varying success, including potassium iodide, tyloxapol, and proteolytic enzymes (eg, trypsin and streptokinase-streptodornase). Systemic corticosteroids have been unsuccessful and may increase the possibility of secondary infection.

Whole lung bronchopulmonary lavage using 0.9% sodium chloride solution (see in Ch. 33), the most effective treatment, is indicated only in patients with significant symptoms and hypoxemia. With the patient under general anesthesia, 1 lung is usually lavaged at a time at 3- to 5-day intervals. Some patients require only 1 lavage and never have a recurrence of symptoms or infiltrates; others require lavage q 6 to 12 mo for many years.

Patients with minimal or no symptoms do not require treatment, but should be watched for exacerbations that may lead to respiratory failure. Secondary infections should be promptly identified and treated.

---

47. PLEURAL DISORDERS

PLEURISY

Inflammation of the pleura, often characterized clinically by pain worsened by respiration and cough.

Etiology

Pleurisy may result from (1) pleural injury by a process in the underlying lung (eg, pneumonia, infarction); (2) entry of an infectious agent or irritating substance into the pleural space (eg, as in amebic empyema or pancreatitic pleurisy); (3) transport of an infectious or noxious agent or neoplastic cells directly to the pleura by the bloodstream or lymphatics (eg, as in TB pleural effusion, uremic pleurisy, pleural carcinomatosis or collagen vascular diseases such as rheumatoid disease and SLE); (4) pleural trauma; (5) asbestos-related pleural disease in which asbestos particles reach the pleura by traversing the conducting airways and respiratory tissues; or (6) rarely, pleural effusion related to longstanding ingestion of dantrolene sodium.

Pathology

In early stages, the pleura usually becomes edematous and congested, cellular infiltration occurs, and fibrinous exudate develops on the pleural surface. Exudate may be reabsorbed or organized into fibrous tissue with resultant pleural adhesions. Some diseases (eg, pleurodynia due to coxsackie B virus) may run their course without significant exudation of fluid from the inflamed pleura, the pleurisy remaining dry or fibrinous. More often, however, following this early stage, pleural exudate develops due to an outpouring from damaged vessels of fluid rich in plasma protein. Occasionally, marked fibrous or even calcific thickening of pleura occurs without an antecedent acute pleurisy (eg, asbestos pleural plaques, idiopathic pleural calcification).

Symptoms and Signs

Onset is usually sudden. Pain, the dominant symptom of fibrinous pleurisy, may vary from vague discomfort to an intense stabbing sensation. Pain is aggravated by breathing and coughing, or may be present only when the patient breathes deeply or coughs. The visceral pleura is insensitive; pain results from inflammation of the parietal pleura. Since the latter is innervated by intercostal nerves, pain is usually felt over the pleuritic site, but may be referred to distant regions. Irritation of posterior and peripheral portions of the diaphragmatic pleura, which are supplied by the lower 6 thoracic nerves, may cause pain referred to the lower chest wall or abdomen. As a result, diaphragmatic pleurisy may simulate intra-abdominal disease. The central portion of the diaphragmatic pleura is innervated by the phrenic nerves, and involvement in this area causes pain referred to the neck and shoulder.

Respiration is usually rapid and shallow. Motion of the affected side may be limited. Breath sounds may be diminished. A pleural friction rub is the characteristic physical sign, though it is often absent and quite frequently is heard only 24 to 48 h after the onset of pain. The friction rub varies from a few intermittent sounds that may simulate crackles to a fully developed harsh grating, creaking, or leathery sound synchronous with respiration and usually heard on both inspiration and expiration. Friction sounds due to pleuritis adjacent to the heart (pleuropericardial rub) may vary with the heart beat as well as with respiration. It should be remembered that the clinical picture varies with the underlying disease.

When pleural effusion develops, pleuritic pain usually subsides. Percussion dullness, absent tactile fremitus, decreased or absent breath sounds, and egophony at the upper border of the fluid are then noticeable. The larger the pleural effusion, the more obvious the above signs. A large effusion may encroach on lung volume and produce or contribute to dyspnea.

Diagnosis

Fibrinous pleurisy is readily diagnosed because of the characteristic pleuritic pain. A pleural friction rub is pathognomonic. Diaphragmatic pleurisy may produce pain referred to the point of the shoulder. Basilar pleurisy may produce pain referred to the abdomen. Pleurisy is usually differentiated from acute inflammatory abdominal disease by x-ray and clinical evidence of a respiratory process; absence of nausea, vomiting, or disturbed bowel function; marked aggravation of pain by deep breathing or coughing; shallow rapid breathing; and tendency toward relief of pain by pressure on the chest wall or abdomen. Intercostal neuritis may be confused with pleurisy, but the pain is rarely related to respiration and there is no friction rub. With herpetic neuritis, development of the characteristic herpetic eruption is diagnostic; pain may be present for months after the herpetic eruption subsides. Myocardial infarction, spontaneous pneumothorax, pericarditis, and chest wall lesions may simulate pleurisy. The friction rub of pericarditis may be confused with that of pleurisy, but usually is heard best over the left border of the sternum in the 3rd and 4th interspaces and characteristically is a "to-and-fro" sound synchronous with the heartbeat. Unlike the pleural friction rub,

the pericardial rub is not influenced significantly by respiration, though there may be some variation in its intensity synchronous with respiration.

Chest x-rays are of limited value in diagnosing fibrinous pleurisy. The pleural lesion causes no shadow, but an associated pulmonary or chest wall lesion may. Chest x-rays are the most precise way to confirm physical findings and to diagnose the presence of pleural fluid. When there are no adhesions between the visceral and parietal pleurae, fluid seeks the most dependent portion of the thorax. Because of the recoil force of the underlying lung, the upper border of the fluid is meniscus-shaped. With the patient in an upright position, the minimum amount of detectable fluid ranges from 300 to 500 mL. However, when frontal x-rays are taken with a horizontal x-ray beam and the patient lying on the affected side, < 100 mL of fluid is easily detectable; with careful positioning, as little as 10 to 15 mL of fluid can be seen. Large pleural effusions may result in complete opacification of the hemithorax and shift of the mediastinum to the contralateral side. Adhesions between visceral and parietal pleurae may result in atypical localization of pleural fluid (loculated pleural effusions). Such collections may be confused with an intrapulmonary tumor, particularly if located in the horizontal fissure. When associated with heart failure, they have been termed "vanishing tumor" because of their disappearance following diuretics and digitalis. Obliteration of the costophrenic angle usually denotes a fibrosing and healing reaction and may remain after healing is complete. Pleural plaques due to asbestos exposure present as localized areas of pleural thickening, usually in the lower ⅔ of the thorax.

Fibrosis of the pleura: Inflammatory reactions in the pleura heal by resolution and fibrosis. Even with longstanding or severe pleural inflammations, the amount of scar tissue remaining after complete healing may be surprisingly slight. Occasionally, however, the lung becomes encased in a thick layer of fibrous tissue that limits chest wall motion, retracts the mediastinum toward the side of disease, and impairs pulmonary function. It may be impossible to differentiate localized pleural thickening from loculated pleural fluid except by thoracentesis, although characteristic differences may be present on ultrasonography.

Calcification of the pleura presents as focal, usually fenestrated, irregular plaques on the costal surfaces following intrapleural hemorrhage or infection, though a history of such an antecedent acute pleural lesion is often not obtainable. Focal plaque-like pleural fibrosis, at times with calcification, occurs many years after occupational exposure to asbestos, most often involving the diaphragmatic pleura; this may be the only evidence of low-dose, relatively brief exposure to inhaled asbestos fibers.

When pleural fluid is present, pleural thoracentesis (see Ch. 33) should almost always be performed to confirm the presence of fluid and to determine its characteristics, including color and consistency. Clear yellow fluid is described as serous; bloody or blood-tinged fluid as sanguineous or serosanguineous; and translucent or opaque, thick fluid as purulent. Specimens should be taken for chemical, bacteriologic, and cytologic examination (the latter using tubes with heparin, 3 u./mL fluid, added). Microscopic examination of gram-stained pleural fluid sediment is essential with all purulent fluids when infection of the pleural space is a possibility. Fungi or actinomycetes may also be detected during the course of such an examination. Cultures for anaerobes should be sent to the laboratory in special transport media or in a capped syringe.

It is always important to determine whether serous fluid is a transudate or an exudate. Pleural fluid **transudates** generally have sp gr values < 1.015, total protein contents < 2.5 gm/dL, with a pleural fluid to serum protein ratio < 0.5, relatively low cell counts, pleural fluid to serum LDH ratios generally < 0.6, and pleural fluid LDH concentrations < 200 IU. Whenever the extravascular fluid space is increased, as in heart failure, edematous renal disease, or myxedema, fluid tends to enter the pleural space. Peritoneal transudates may enter the pleural space more often on the right, directly through microscopic, mesothelial-lined communications that perforate the dia-

phragm. Such pleural fluid differs from that due to inflammation of the visceral or parietal pleura and subsides with control of the causative disease. Pleural **exudates** generally have sp gr values > 1.018, total protein contents > 3 gm/dL with a pleural fluid:serum protein ratio > 0.5, and pleural fluid to serum LDH ratios > 0.6.

Total and differential cell counts should be obtained routinely except on grossly purulent pleural fluids. A predominance of polymorphonuclear leukocytes **(PMNs)** suggests an underlying pneumonia and a synpneumonic effusion that is usually sterile even with bacterial pneumonia. In the early stages of bacterial infection, fluid is not visibly purulent, there are many PMNs, and bacteria may be seen in a Gram stain. Presence of many small mature lymphocytes, particularly with few mesothelial cells, strongly suggests TB. Pleural fluid is commonly bloodstained in pulmonary infarction and pleural carcinomatosis. In pulmonary infarction, there is usually a mixture of lymphocytes and PMNs, and mesothelial cells are numerous. Presence of malignant cells in Papanicolaou-stained smears of pleural fluid is diagnostic of pleural carcinomatosis. LE cells may be seen in the pleural fluid in SLE. Glucose concentrations < 10 mg/dL are rare except in rheumatoid pleural effusion. Very high pleural fluid amylase values are characteristic of pancreatitic pleural effusion; salivary amylase may gain access to the pleural space in rupture of the esophagus, but the clinical picture and acid pH (< 7.00) of the fluid are usually enough to prevent misdiagnosis. Loculated pleural effusions that complicate pneumonia tend to have pH values < 7.20. Eosinophils in the pleural fluid have little diagnostic significance, but are rarely present in a TB or malignant effusion. These laboratory tests on the pleural fluid are most useful when integrated with all of the clinical data and other appropriate tests; eg, a tuberculin skin test is the key in investigating a patient with suspected TB pleural effusion.

Needle biopsy of the parietal pleura (see Ch. 33) should be considered at the time of the initial thoracentesis or soon after, if the cause of the effusion is not readily apparent from the clinical findings and pleural fluid analysis. Culture of parietal pleural tissue in pleural TB often yields mycobacteria when the pleural fluid culture does not. Replacement of fluid by air and performance of thoracoscopy with visually directed parietal pleural biopsy using a flexible or rigid thoracoscope may permit definitive diagnosis in obscure cases.

Hemothorax, *blood in the pleural space,* occurs most often from trauma, or, rarely, following rupture of a vessel in a parietopleural adhesion associated with spontaneous pneumothorax. Spontaneous hemothorax may also rarely be a complication of a coagulation defect. Pleural blood often does not clot and may be easily withdrawn through a needle or a water-sealed tube thoracotomy.

Chylothorax, *a milky or chylous pleural effusion,* is caused by traumatic or neoplastic (most often a lymphoma) injury to the thoracic duct. The lipid content of the fluid (neutral fat and fatty acids) is high; sudanophilic fat droplets are often seen microscopically. Cholesterol content is low.

Cholesterol effusion (chyliform or pseudochylous effusion): Rarely, golden, iridescent pleural fluid (due to the presence of light-reflecting cholesterol crystals) is obtained on thoracentesis. Crystals may be seen on microscopy; high concentrations (up to 1 gm/dL) of cholesterol may be measured, but neutral fat and fatty acid concentrations are low. This type of effusion results from longstanding chronic pleural effusion, as in TB pleurisy or rheumatoid pleural effusion. The underlying disease should be carefully sought; cholesterol pleural effusion is not acceptable as a complete diagnosis.

Treatment

Treatment of the underlying disease is essential for fibrinous pleurisy and for pleural effusion. Pleural exudates due to underlying pulmonary disease (eg, pneumonia, pulmonary infarction) and effusions secondary to a systemic disease (eg, uremia or SLE) usually respond to such treatment.

Chest pain may be relieved by wrapping the entire chest with two or three 6-in. wide

nonadhesive elastic bandages. Though they must be reapplied once or twice daily, the skin irritation that results from applying adhesive strapping to the affected hemithorax is avoided and pain relief is comparable. Aspirin 0.6 gm or indomethacin 50 mg orally qid is often effective. If not, codeine 30 to 60 mg orally or s.c. may be necessary, but its cough suppressant properties must be considered.

To prevent complicating pneumonia, adequate bronchial drainage must be provided. Coughing is often facilitated if additional temporary splinting of the chest wall is provided by having the patient or an attendant hold a pillow firmly against the painful chest wall. The patient taking narcotics should be urged to breathe deeply and cough when pain relief from the drug is maximal. Antibiotic therapy and aqueous aerosol inhalation therapy with bronchodilators should be considered for treatment of any associated bronchitis.

Thoracentesis often dramatically relieves dyspnea due to a large pleural effusion. Since cardiovascular collapse may occur rarely if several liters of pleural fluid are removed too quickly, fluid removal should be limited to 1200 to 1500 mL at one time. Pneumothorax may complicate thoracentesis if the visceral pleura is punctured or if air leaks into the pleural space (which is at subatmospheric pressure) as a result of a break in the continuity of the thoracentesis system used. Ultrasonography is of great assistance in the accurate localization of loculated pleural effusions and in their drainage by guided placement of a needle.

Indolent infection in the pleural space must be treated by a long course of appropriate antibiotic therapy. For example, TB pleurisy responds to treatment with 2 simultaneously given antituberculosis drugs (eg, isoniazid and rifampin); amphotericin B is effective in coccidioidal pleural effusion. Pleural fluid in such cases usually reabsorbs spontaneously.

Empyema (*purulent exudate in the pleural cavity*) is treated with high doses of parenteral antibiotics and drainage of the pleural space. One or two needle aspirations repeated daily may be adequate for small collections of thin pus, but water-sealed tube thoracotomy is usually preferable. When the empyema cavity is lined by a thick, organizing, fibrinous exudate or cortex, open drainage over weeks or months through a rib resection or intercostal tube may be necessary to obliterate the space. If the lung is partially collapsed by a thick cortex or the empyema is loculated, thoracotomy and surgical decortication is the best way to expand the lung and obliterate the space. Decortication for a loculated empyema is best performed within the first 3 to 6 wk of the illness. Surgery may also be necessary when bronchopleural fistula complicates empyema.

Treatment of pleural effusion due to **malignant pleural implants** is often difficult. Pleural fluid occasionally does not reaccumulate after the thorax has been tapped dry with a needle, especially if systemic antitumor therapy has been started, as in metastatic carcinoma of the breast. When fluid does reaccumulate, it generally responds to obliteration of the pleural space by instillation of a pleural irritant (eg, tetracycline). Adhesion of visceral and parietal pleurae (obliterating the pleural space) may be aided if the pleural space is kept empty after instilling the irritant by using water-sealed tube drainage for a few days. Specific intrapleural chemotherapy of malignant pleural effusion with antineoplastic agents (eg, mechlorethamine) *is not recommended* because they may cause bone marrow depression and are no more effective than less toxic irritants.

For **hemothorax,** water-sealed tube drainage is generally sufficient, providing the bleeding has stopped. Fibrinolytic enzymes (streptokinase-streptodornase) may be instilled through an intercostal drainage tube to lyse fibrinous adhesions if the effusion becomes loculated, but thoracotomy and decortication may be necessary to expand the lung and obliterate the pleural space.

Treatment of **chylothorax** is directed at the underlying cause of ductal damage.

Pleural fibrosis should be minimized by appropriate early therapy of pleural disease.

Surgical decortication of pleural fibrous tissue does not usually improve lung function unless a sizable collection of air or fluid is removed simultaneously.

---

48. PNEUMOTHORAX

Free air in the pleural cavity, between the visceral and parietal pleurae.

Etiology and Pathophysiology

Traumatic pneumothorax: Normally, pressure in the pleural space is less than atmospheric because of lung recoil pressure. Following trauma, air may enter the pleural cavity in several ways. **Open pneumothorax** occurs when a penetrating chest wound creates a communication (pleurocutaneous fistula) between the outside air and the pleural space that permits air to rush in, thus causing the lung to collapse. In **closed pneumothorax,** the chest wall becomes airtight after penetration (eg, by a thoracentesis needle, by central vein percutaneous catheter placement via the subclavian veins, or after a stab wound), or it may continue to receive air (eg, when air leaks from a lung punctured by a fractured rib). Air may also leak from a ruptured bronchus or perforated esophagus into the mediastinum and then rupture into the pleural space. During thoracentesis, air may leak into the pleural space if the syringe and needle are not kept firmly sealed at all times. **Pulmonary barotrauma** is an important present-day cause of pneumomediastinum and pneumothorax in patients being mechanically ventilated. The complication occurs most often in the adult respiratory distress syndrome and is increased in frequency in patients with severe disease requiring high peak inspiratory pressure or positive end-expiratory pressure for management. Air may enter the pleural space because of breach of the parietal pleura or a pneumomediastinum may rupture through the mediastinal pleura into the pleural space.

Spontaneous pneumothorax: Air may enter the pleural space without antecedent trauma during the course of pulmonary disease or in a previously healthy person. Emphysema with rupture of a bulla is the most common underlying disorder. Asthma, eosinophilic granuloma, or lung abscess with bronchopleural fistula and empyema may also be causative. Active TB may (rarely) cause pneumothorax from perforation of a cavity into the pleural space; pneumothorax may also complicate inactive TB owing to the presence of associated emphysema. Whatever the disease process, it is usually evident before pneumothorax occurs.

The usual cause of spontaneous pneumothorax in an apparently healthy person (most often a man between 20 to 40 yr old) is rupture of an emphysematous bulla, which may be undetectable by clinical examination. Most spontaneous pneumothoraces occur without associated exertion. Some have occurred during diving or high-altitude flying, apparently in association with the ambient pressure change that is unequally transmitted to different portions of the lung. A pneumothorax may also occur as a complication of interstitial pulmonary air leak and pneumomediastinum, which may be spontaneous or may complicate other processes such as spontaneous rupture of the esophagus or traumatic rupture of the bronchus.

A **tension (positive-pressure) pneumothorax** occurs when a check-valve mechanism in a bronchopleural fistula permits air to enter, but not leave, the pleural space, causing pressure within the space to rise above atmospheric; complete collapse of the lung and shift of the mediastinum to the opposite side result.

Induced pneumothorax: Artificial pneumothorax, formerly used extensively to treat TB, is rarely used as a diagnostic procedure to outline masses or replace fluid for better x-ray visualization of intrathoracic structures.

Symptoms, Signs, and Diagnosis

Symptoms vary greatly according to the size of the pneumothorax and the extent of disease in the lung. They range from minimal disturbance to severe dyspnea, shock, and life-threatening respiratory failure and circulatory collapse. Sudden sharp chest pain, dyspnea, and, occasionally, a dry, hacking cough occur at onset. The pain may be referred to the corresponding shoulder, across the chest, or over the abdomen; it may simulate an acute coronary occlusion or an "acute abdomen." Symptoms tend to be less severe in a slowly developing pneumothorax and usually subside as accommodation to the altered physiologic state occurs.

Physical findings also depend on the size of the pneumothorax. With a small collection of air, there may be no detectable signs, or diminution of voice and breath sounds may be the only abnormality. With large or tension pneumothoraces, tympany on percussion, diminished or absent tactile fremitus, and diminished motion on the affected side occur. Shift of the mediastinum may be detectable as displacement of the cardiac dullness and apex beat away from the affected side. Hypoxemia is minimal or absent in a previously well young person with spontaneous pneumothorax, but may be severe and associated with hypercapnia in a patient with diffuse underlying lung disease.

The chest x-ray is usually characteristic, showing air without lung markings peripherally, but limited by a sharp pleural margin with lung markings medially, indicating the position of the collapsed lung. A small pneumothorax may be overlooked on a routine inspiratory x-ray, but is obvious on an expiratory x-ray. This is because the size and density of the lung (but not of the pleural air space) change during expiration. The mediastinum shifts to the contralateral side, especially with a large pneumothorax. Differential diagnosis includes emphysematous bullae and herniation of the stomach, the colon, or, much less commonly, the small bowel through the diaphragm. In patients receiving mechanical ventilation for the adult respiratory distress syndrome, pneumothorax may present subtly in loculated form in a subpulmonic or paracardiac location. Pneumomediastinum may precede the development of pneumothorax.

Prognosis and Treatment

A small spontaneous pneumothorax requires no special treatment; the air is reabsorbed in a few days. Full absorption of a larger air space may take 2 to 4 wk, during which time there is uncertainty as to whether the pleural leak is closed and whether pleural fluid and epipleural fibrinous exudate will develop. The course can be shortened by introduction of a chest tube with water-sealed drainage or a pleuro-cutaneous valve that permits egress of air from the pleura, but does not permit air to enter the space. There is a risk of reexpansion pulmonary edema following application of suction, particularly if the pneumothorax is large, longstanding, and high suction pressures are used. In both traumatic and spontaneous pneumothorax, the bronchopleural fistula usually stops leaking and heals quickly as the lung collapses. However, application of suction to a water-sealed drain may be used to effect rapid expansion of the lung if air leakage from a bronchopleural fistula persists. If there is a persistent bronchopleural fistula, it should be surgically repaired or the involved lung segment should be removed. The use of intrapleural tetracycline for persistent or recurrent pneumothorax, especially in patients who are poor risks for thoracotomy (eg, cystic fibrosis, emphysema) has been reported. If there is a large bronchopleural fistula, loculation of the pneumothorax may occur, which will make its drainage difficult.

In **tension pneumothorax,** *quick removal of air may be life-saving.* Air may be removed simply by inserting a 19-gauge or larger needle into the chest followed by use of a 3-way stopcock attached to a large syringe to withdraw air rapidly through the needle. The needle may be inserted anteriorly or laterally over a site displaying absent breath sounds and enhanced percussion note. If there is time for a chest x-ray, sites where the

lung is held to the chest wall by adhesions should be avoided. Air is alternately withdrawn from the pleural space and expelled from the syringe into the room. This procedure is continued, as determined by the patient's clinical condition, until a tube thoracostomy has been done and water-sealed drainage of the hemithorax has been accomplished. A check valve fitted to a catheter inserted into the pleural space may also be used to evacuate air from the pleural space.

Recurrent pneumothorax may cause considerable disability. Surgical intervention is generally indicated following 2 spontaneous pneumothoraces on the same side. The preferred procedures are thoracotomy with oversewing or excision of bullae and roughening of the pleura by rubbing with gauze, or, when bullous disease is extensive, parietal pleurectomy.

49. TUMORS OF THE LUNG

Etiology and Incidence

The lungs are the site of origin of benign and malignant primary tumors, as well as of metastases from primary cancers of many other organs and tissues. Primary lung carcinoma is the most common cancer in men (22%) but ranks fourth in women (10%). Even more important as a cause of cancer death, it is first in men (35%) and in women (19%). Its incidence is rising more rapidly in women. The disease is most common between ages 50 and 70.

Cigarette smoking accounts for > 90% of cases in men and about 70% in women, with a strong dose-response relationship and regression of incidence after quitting. The dose-response relationship is shown in the 3 commonest types of lung cancer: squamous cell, small cell, and adenocarcinoma; the slope of the curve is steepest for small cell carcinoma and lowest for adenocarcinoma. A small proportion of lung cancers (15% in men and 5% in women) is related to occupational agents, often overlapping with smoking: asbestos, radiation, arsenic, chromates, nickel, chloromethyl ethers, mustard (poison war) gas, and coke oven emissions. The exact role of air pollution is still uncertain. Occasional lung cancers, especially adenocarcinoma and alveolar cell carcinoma, are associated with pulmonary scars.

Pathology

Four histologic types of bronchogenic carcinoma usually are distinguished: **(1) squamous cell,** frequently arising in the larger bronchi and commonly spreading by direct extension and lymph node metastasis; **(2) undifferentiated small cell,** producing early hematogenous metastases; **(3) undifferentiated large cell,** usually spreading through the bloodstream; and **(4) adenocarcinoma,** commonly peripheral, usually spreading through the bloodstream. All types also frequently spread via the lymphatics. **Alveolar cell (bronchiolar) carcinoma** consolidates air spaces, often does not extend beyond the lungs, and, although a solitary form of the tumor exists, it is sometimes distinguished from bronchogenic carcinoma by its multifocal origin. The lungs are sometimes involved by **multifocal lymphomas.** Less common primary lung tumors include **bronchial adenoma** (sometimes malignant), **chondromatous hamartoma** (benign), **solitary lymphoma,** and **sarcoma** (malignant). **Metastases** to the lungs are common from primary cancers of the breast, colon, prostate, kidney, thyroid, stomach, testis, and bone.

Symptoms and Signs

Manifestations depend on the tumor's location and type of spread. Since most primary tumors are endobronchial, **cough** usually is present. In patients with chronic bronchitis, increased intensity and intractability of preexisting cough suggest a neoplasm. **Sputum** arising from an ulcerated bronchial tumor usually is not excessive (though it may be profuse and watery with alveolar cell carcinomas), but contains inflammatory exudate and is often blood-streaked. Copious **bleeding** (uncommon)

strongly suggests invasion of large underlying blood vessels. Bronchial narrowing may cause air trapping with **localized wheezing,** and commonly causes **atelectasis** with mediastinal shift, diminished expansion, dullness to percussion, and loss of breath sounds. **Infection** of obstructed lung produces fever, chest pain, and weight loss. Persistent localized chest pain suggests neoplastic invasion of the chest wall. Peripheral nodular tumors are asymptomatic until they invade the pleura or chest wall and cause pain or metastasize to distant organs. **Late symptoms** include weight loss and weakness.

Malignant serosanguineous **pleural effusions** are common and often large and recurrent. **Horner's syndrome** (due to invasion of the cervical thoracic sympathetic nerves) and infiltration of the brachial plexus and the neighboring ribs and vertebrae occur with apical (Pancoast) tumors. A tumor may extend directly into the esophagus, producing obstruction, sometimes complicated by a fistula. Phrenic nerve invasion may cause diaphragmatic paralysis. Superior vena cava obstruction and left recurrent laryngeal nerve paralysis (causing hoarseness) are produced by direct extension of the tumor or by extension of tumor from neighboring lymph nodes. The **superior vena cava syndrome (SVC)** obstruction of venous drainage leads to dilation of collateral veins of the upper part of the chest and neck; edema and plethora of the face, neck, and upper part of the torso, including breasts; suffusion and edema of the conjunctiva; breathlessness in the supine position; and CNS symptoms (eg, headache, visual distortion, and disturbed states of consciousness). Although a dramatic clinical situation, SVC requires urgent but not emergency care. Most importantly, a histologic diagnosis needs to be made if an undiagnosed mediastinal mass is present. Benign diseases rarely cause the syndrome; however, TB, fungal infections, and aortic aneurysms may. Malignant neoplasms, including lymphoma, small cell lung cancer, squamous cell lung cancer, and breast cancer, frequently cause a SVC syndrome. Once a histologic diagnosis is made, therapy consists of either steroids and drugs (small cell lung cancer or lymphoma) or radiotherapy (breast cancer, squamous cell lung cancer, or lymphoma).

Intrapulmonary spread of primary and secondary cancer may cause lymphangitic carcinomatosis with subacute cor pulmonale, worsening hypoxemia, and severe dyspnea. Secondary hematogenous nodular metastases within the lungs are common, but bronchial invasion is rare. Hematogenous spread of primary lung neoplasms to the liver, brain, adrenals, and bone is common and may occur early, resulting in symptoms of those sites before obvious pulmonary symptoms.

Extrapulmonary manifestations of lung cancer are numerous. In hypertrophic pulmonary osteoarthropathy (the best known), clubbing of the fingers and toes and periosteal elevation of the distal parts of the long bones occur. All levels of the nervous system may be affected—principally encephalopathy, subacute cerebellar degeneration, encephalomyelitis, and peripheral neuropathy. Polymyositis and dermatomyositis or metabolic syndromes due to production of substances with hormonal activity may develop (see Ch. 92). Small cell carcinomas may secrete ectopic ACTH (resulting in Cushing's syndrome) or ADH (with water retention and hyponatremia) and are associated with the carcinoid syndrome (flushing, wheezing, diarrhea, and cardiac valvular lesions). Squamous cell tumors may secrete parathyroid-hormone–like substances that produce hypercalcemia. Other endocrine syndromes associated with primary lung carcinomas include gynecomastia, hyperglycemia, thyrotoxicosis, and skin pigmentation. Hematologic disorders, including thrombocytopenic purpura, leukemoid reaction, myelophthisic anemia, polycythemia, and marantic thrombosis may also occur.

Peripheral benign primary tumors usually are asymptomatic. **Benign endobronchial tumors** cause obstruction with distal infection or atelectasis.

Bronchial adenoma may be benign or malignant and occurs equally in both sexes. Its course is prolonged. The endobronchial portion of the adenoma dilates and obstructs the lumen of major bronchi. Brisk bleeding from the overlying mucous membrane

often occurs. Recurrent pneumonia within the same lung zone and localized overlying pleural pain are common. Metastasis is infrequent, but may occur to regional lymph nodes.

Diagnosis

The principal sources of diagnostic information are the history, which raises the suspicion of tumor and provides early localizing information, and the chest x-ray, which visualizes and locates the lesion and demonstrates its anatomic effects. X-ray patterns depend on the site of involvement: major bronchial, segmental, and peripheral. In **asymptomatic** patients, a peripheral nodular mass is often seen. Previous x-rays are valuable to discern new growth. With smaller solitary nodules, overpenetrated x-rays and tomograms may demonstrate calcification, the amount of which must be more than a fleck to diagnose a benign tumor or a chronic granulomatous process and exclude lung cancer. CT may demonstrate small lesions invisible to other technics and may be useful in staging by suggesting the presence or absence of nodal spread.

In **symptomatic** patients, the chest x-ray may show bronchial narrowing and irregularity, parenchymal infiltration, or atelectasis. Cavitation may be visible in an obstructed area or within a peripheral tumor. Obstructive emphysema is not common. Rarely, x-rays reveal zones of infiltration or obstruction in separate lobes that cannot be explained by a single neoplastic focus but result from diffuse submucosal lymphatic permeation of the bronchial tree. Pleural effusions are often associated with infiltrating or peripheral tumors; cytologic examination of pleural fluid or pleural biopsy may confirm the cancer.

Photoscans may show metastases in the liver, brain, and bones, but are worthwhile only in the presence of abnormal clinical or laboratory findings. The presence of primary tumors and metastases may be directly established by **cytologic studies** of the sputum and by **tissue biopsy.** In rare cases, the sputum is positive for tumor cells when there is no demonstrable focus of disease.

Bronchoscopy is used to visualize and biopsy bronchial tumors. With a rigid bronchoscope, the visual field is limited to the major bronchi and their primary divisions, but the extent of the tumor can be effectively determined by carinal and random biopsy and the resistance produced by extrabronchial masses can be sensed. Using the flexible bronchoscope, the subsegmental bronchi can be explored to demonstrate and sample tumors by washings, brushings, and biopsy. Mediastinoscopy is often useful to confirm the diagnosis and to separate operable from inoperable tumors.

Exploratory thoracotomy can establish the diagnosis and resectability of the tumor, but is required in $< 10\%$ of cases. Contraindications include distant or mediastinal metastases or cardiorespiratory insufficiency. Exploration is unnecessary when metastases are demonstrated by **mediastinoscopy** or **parasternal mediastinotomy** (see above in Ch. 33), which has largely replaced scalene node exploration, or by pleural or liver biopsy. Palpable lymph nodes and skin nodules provide important diagnostic material.

Staging of lung cancer is useful from a prognostic viewpoint. It may be done clinically, but is more accurate after procedures that yield information on the extent of disease, both local and systemic, especially after thoracotomy. The **TNM (tumor, node, metastasis) system** is a standard staging classification (see CLINICAL STAGING in Ch. 105). It is also useful for comparison and selection for treatment or control.

Differential diagnosis includes foreign bodies, nonsegmental pneumonia, and endobronchial and focal pulmonary manifestations of TB, systemic mycoses, and autoimmune disease.

Prophylaxis, Prognosis and Treatment

The poor prognosis for patients with **bronchogenic carcinoma** requires emphasis on prevention. Cigarette tobacco should be avoided, and exposure to potentially carcinogenic substances in industry must be reduced below dangerous levels.

On the average, patients with untreated bronchogenic carcinoma survive 9 mo; about 25% of tumors are resectable, but the overall 5-yr survival rate is < 10%. In patients with well-circumscribed, slowly growing tumors, the 5-yr survival rate after excision ranges from 25 to 40%. Best results are obtained in patients with peripheral nodular lesions treated by lobectomy. Survivors should be followed carefully, since second lung cancers develop in 6 to 12%.

Resection is the treatment of choice for lung cancer. It should be done in the absence of contraindications, namely evidence of spread beyond the lung, location of tumor too close to the trachea, serious other conditions (eg, coronary artery disease, or the inadequate lung function of chronic obstructive pulmonary disease). Pulmonary function assessment does not provide clearcut answers to the question of operability, but there are some simple rules of thumb for thoracotomy, keeping in mind that the extent of resection can be determined only at operation, and pneumonectomy may be needed. The functional criteria for pneumonectomy are: (1) Forced expiratory volume in 1 sec **(FEV_1)** is > 2 L and equals > 50% of the observed forced vital capacity; (2) maximal voluntary ventilation is > 50% of the predicted value; and (3) residual volume is < 50% of total lung capacity. In addition, Pa_{CO_2} should be normal at rest. If any of these criteria are not met, then regional lung function should be assessed by a quantitative differential perfusion scan and, if available, a ventilation scan. (The predicted postoperative FEV_1 equals the percent of perfusion to the nonresected lung times the preoperative FEV_1.) If these studies indicate that the patient's FEV_1 will still be > 800 mL after pneumonectomy, then the risk can be considered, recognizing that the patient's activity will be limited the closer the value comes to 800 mL.

To provide a safe plane of bronchial division proximal to the tumor, central endobronchial lesions usually require pneumonectomy and removal of neighboring lymph nodes. Tumors extending into the chest wall can be removed en bloc; preoperative radiation has been reported to be beneficial, especially in apical tumors.

Postoperative radiation is used if positive hilar and/or mediastinal nodes are noted at thoracotomy, in managing painful metastases to bone, and in treating brain metastasis. Sometimes radiation is used instead of surgery when thoracotomy is contraindicated because of cardiorespiratory insufficiency or other serious disease. For 3 mo after radiation, patients should be carefully watched for x-ray and clinical signs (including cough, dyspnea, and fever) of radiation pneumonitis, which may be controlled by prednisone 60 mg/day orally for about 1 mo and then gradually tapered off.

Though some improved results with chemotherapeutic agents have been reported, no effective specific drug regimen for bronchogenic carcinoma has been established. In **small cell carcinoma,** multiple drug chemotherapy with or without radiation has yielded higher survival rates than surgery and perhaps cures (see CHEMOTHERAPY in Ch. 105).

Anxiety and persistent pain are common in patients with incurable lung cancer. Sedatives, narcotics, and other drugs in combination are required (see PAIN in Ch. 119).

Bronchodilator drugs, O_2, mechanical assistance (tracheal suction, mechanical ventilation), and physiotherapy may be needed for airways obstruction. Antibiotics are given to treat complicating infections.

Solitary or occasionally multiple metastases to the lungs have been excised after removal of the primary tumor; the 5-yr survival rate is about 10%. **Benign bronchial tumors** should be removed because of the adverse effects of location, possible growth, and potential malignant transformation. Most **benign peripheral tumors** are undiagnosed until surgical exploration and excision.

§5. GASTROINTESTINAL DISORDERS

50. DIAGNOSTIC AND THERAPEUTIC GASTROINTESTINAL PROCEDURES

(See ENDOSCOPIC RETROGRADE CHOLANGIOPANCREATOGRAPHY [ERCP], PERCUTANEOUS NEEDLE BIOPSY OF THE LIVER, AND PERCUTANEOUS TRANSHEPATIC CHOLANGIOGRAPHY [PTC] in Ch. 68)

Evaluating and caring for patients with GI disorders requires a balanced, individualized, comprehensive approach. Diagnostic evaluation now available through endoscopy, radionuclide scanning, angiography, and CT permits remarkable precision and accuracy, but at potentially great cost and increased risk of morbidity. Also, > 50% of patients presenting with GI complaints will be diagnosed to have a "functional" disorder (see Ch. 52) with no structural abnormality. Therefore, a thorough history and physical examination with consideration of both biologic and psychosocial features that may be contributing to the illness is required to minimize unneeded diagnostic studies and to develop effective treatment strategies. This section will review indications, contraindications, methods, and complications of frequently used major GI procedures.

The history and physical examination remain the bases of clinical evaluation. Information should be obtained using an interview style that initially encourages the patient to report symptoms through spontaneous associations rather than in response to direct questioning (see also Ch. 52). Facilitating questions (eg, "How can I help you?", or "Tell me more about your symptoms?") should precede clarifying questions (eg, "When did the pain begin?"; "What makes it better?"). From this information, the clinician develops diagnostic hypotheses to be modified through more specific queries (eg, "Is the pain relieved by antacid?"; "Did you vomit blood?"). Questions that elicit yes-no responses should be used only when specific diagnostic options are being considered.

A directed physical examination will refine the differential diagnosis; eg, the finding of an enlarged liver in a patient complaining of dark, tarry stools may expand the previous consideration of gastritis or peptic ulcer disease to include cirrhosis with esophageal varices, or GI carcinoma with metastases to the liver. Then, if not already obtained, further inquiry with regard to alcohol consumption or weight loss, or careful examination of the skin for spider angiomas, will allow for a more directed diagnostic evaluation.

NASOGASTRIC OR INTESTINAL INTUBATION

Indications: To decompress the stomach when there is gastric atony, ileus, or obstruction; to remove ingested toxins; to obtain a sample of gastric contents for analysis (volume, acid content, blood); to supply nutrients through tube feeding.

Several types of tubes are available: A Levin or Salem sump tube is used for gastric decompression or analysis, or rarely for feeding on a short-term basis. Balloon-tipped Hg tubes, eg, Miller-Abbott or Cantor tubes, allow for intestinal decompression or feeding. The balloon facilitates passage into the small intestine and (with the Miller-Abbott tube) is inflated when the tip of the tube enters the stomach. Very flexible Hg or tungsten-tipped tubes, eg, the Corpak®, Dobbhoff®, and Entriflex®, are used mainly for prolonged enteral feeding. **Contraindications:** Nasopharyngeal or esophageal obstruction, maxillofacial trauma, uncontrollable coagulation abnormalities, and large esophageal varices.

Procedure: The patient sits upright or lies in the left lateral decubitus position. With the head partially flexed, the lubricated tube is inserted through the nares; it is aimed back and then down to conform with the nasopharynx. As the tip reaches the posterior pharyngeal wall, the patient should sip water through a straw. (Violent coughing with flow of air through the tube during respiration indicates that the tube is misplaced in the trachea.) Aspiration of gastric juice verifies entry into the stomach. The position of larger tubes may be confirmed by instilling 20 to 30 mL of air and listening with the stethoscope under the left subcostal region for a rush of air.

Smaller, more flexible intestinal feeding tubes usually require the use of stiffening wires or stylets, and may require fluoroscopic or endoscopic assistance for passage through the pylorus.

Complications: Nasopharyngeal trauma with or without hemorrhage, pulmonary aspiration, traumatic esophageal or gastric hemorrhage or perforation, and (very rarely) intracranial or mediastinal penetration.

ESOPHAGEAL MANOMETRY

(See Ch. 51)

BERNSTEIN (ACID PERFUSION) TEST

(See Ch. 51)

GASTRIC ANALYSIS

Indications: To evaluate the possibility of hyperchlorhydria (eg, Zollinger-Ellison syndrome), or of hypochlorhydric states (eg, pernicious anemia, atrophic gastritis Ménétrier's syndrome); as part of pre- or postoperative assessment for patients with planned acid-reducing surgery; to evaluate the possibility of incomplete vagotomy in patients with recurrent peptic ulcer disease after a surgical vagotomy. **Contraindications:** Recent active bleeding or pain due to active ulcer disease.

Procedure: The Levin nasogastric tube is passed (see NASOGASTRIC INTUBATION above). Gastric contents are aspirated and discarded. Four 15-min samples of gastric juice are collected by continuous manual aspiration (Basal Acid Output **[BAO]**). Next pentagastrin (6 μg/kg) is given s.c., and again, four 15-min samples are obtained (Maximal [or Peak] Acid Output **[MAO or PAO]**). Samples are titrated with NaOH to calculate BAO and stimulated MAO secretory rates.

SECRETIN TEST

(See under PANCREATITIS in Ch. 55)

SMALL BOWEL BIOPSY AND DUODENAL ASPIRATION

Indications: To support, confirm, or exclude diseases of the small intestine (eg, celiac sprue, Whipple's disease, *Giardia lamblia* infection). **Contraindication:** uncorrectible coagulation disorder.

Procedure: The lubricated Hg-tipped Rubin-Quinton tube or Carey capsule is placed in the oropharynx and the patient swallows. When the tube enters the stomach, it is manipulated with fluoroscopic guidance through the pylorus to the third or fourth portion of the duodenum. The biopsy is obtained by producing negative pressure with a syringe while the aspiration port is open. Mucosa is suctioned through the port into the tube or capsule and then sliced off by a knife that is activated by the operator. Fluid samples for diagnosis of Giardia infection are obtained by aspirating duodenal contents.

Complications: Bleeding, entrapment of the tube in the duodenum, bacteremia, and aspiration of fluid or Hg during passage of the tube occur rarely.

FIBEROPTIC GASTROINTESTINAL ENDOSCOPY

Direct visual examination of the intestinal tract with a flexible tube containing light-transmitting glass fibers that return a magnified image. The procedure can be done diagnostically; eg, to evaluate pain or dysphagia, to identify structural abnormalities or bleeding sites, to obtain biopsies, or to inject dye for x-ray studies. Therapeutic indications include removal of polyps or foreign bodies, hemostasis by coagulation, debulking of tumors, and placement of feeding tubes or stents through obstructed areas.

UPPER GASTROINTESTINAL ENDOSCOPY

(See also COMMON DIAGNOSTIC PROCEDURES in Ch. 51)

Diagnostic indications: To establish the site of upper GI bleeding; to visually define and biopsy abnormalities seen on upper GI series (gastric ulcers, filling defects, mass lesions); to follow up treated gastric ulcers; to evaluate dysphagia, dyspepsia, abdominal pain, and gastric outlet obstruction. **Therapeutic indications:** Removal of foreign bodies or gastric or esophageal polyps, sclerosis of esophageal varices, and control of hemorrhage by coagulation.

Absolute contraindications include acute shock, acute myocardial infarction, coma (unless the patient is intubated), seizures, acutely perforated ulcer, and atlantoaxial subluxation. **Relative contraindications** must be considered with respect to the expected benefits. They include uncooperativeness, coagulopathy (prothrombin time > 3 sec over control, platelet count < 100,000/μL, bleeding time > 10 min), Zenker's diverticulum, high esophageal stricture, myocardial ischemia, and thoracic aortic aneurysm.

Procedure: The patient should have taken no food for $\geq$ 4 h. A topical anesthetic is gargled or sprayed into the pharynx, and usually a narcotic and/or diazepam is given IV for sedation. The patient is appropriately positioned and the tip of the endoscope is placed in the hypopharynx. As the patient swallows, the scope is gently guided through the cricopharyngeal muscle (upper esophageal sphincter) and then advanced under direct vision through the stomach and into the duodenum. Examination of all structures may be supplemented by photographs, cytology, and biopsy sampling. Therapeu-

tic procedures are performed as indicated; eg, sclerotherapy is done by passing a needle-tipped cannula through the endoscope and injecting the sclerosing agent into the varix.

Complications: The overall complication rate ranges from 0.1 to 0.2%; mortality rate is about 0.03%. Drug-related complications are commonest and include phlebitis and respiratory depression. Aspiration, bleeding from biopsy sites, and perforation are the commonest procedural complications. Transient bacteremia often occurs (8%), but is not associated with development of endocarditis. The patient with a coagulation disorder is more likely to experience a retropharyngeal hematoma or other bleeding complication. Procedures such as variceal sclerosis and polypectomy are associated with higher complication rates.

COLONOSCOPY

Diagnostic indications: To further evaluate an abnormality seen on barium enema; to determine the source of occult or active GI bleeding or unexplained (microcytic) anemia; to evaluate pre- or postoperatively for other lesions in patients with colonic cancer; to determine the extent of inflammatory bowel disease. **Therapeutic indications** To remove polyps; to coagulate bleeding sites; to reduce volvulus or intussusception

Absolute contraindications include acute shock, acute myocardial infarction, peritonitis, intestinal perforation, and fulminant colitis. **Relative contraindications** include poor bowel preparation or massive intestinal hemorrhage, poor patient cooperation, diverticulitis, recent abdominal surgery, history of multiple pelvic operations, or a large hernia. Patients with cardiac prostheses will need antibiotic prophylaxis to prevent endocarditis.

Procedure: Preparation involves taking cathartics and enemas, or drinking an intestinal lavage solution (eg, polyethylene glycol-electrolyte). The patient is placed in the left lateral position and is given an IV narcotic and/or diazepam for sedation. After a rectal examination, the colonoscope is gently inserted through the anal sphincter into the rectum. Under direct visualization, air is infused and the instrument is manipulated through the colon to the cecum and terminal ileum. Fluoroscopy is rarely needed The patient may experience cramplike discomfort that can be relieved by aspiration of air, rotation or retraction of the tube, or additional medication. Diagnostic evaluation is done by visualization of structures, photography, and obtaining brushings or biopsy of abnormal structures.

Polypectomy is performed by using a flexible wire loop attached to a grounded electrosurgical cautery unit. The polyp is snared around its neck and current is applied as the loop is tightened enough to cut through. Bleeding lesions are coagulated with electrocautery using a ball-tipped probe, with a heat probe, or by laser.

Complications are similar and slightly more frequent than upper endoscopy. Snare cautery of polyps is associated with a 1.7% bleeding and 0.3% perforation rate.

RIGID AND FLEXIBLE SIGMOIDOSCOPY AND ANOSCOPY

Examination of the perianal area and distal rectum can be performed with the 7 cm anoscope, the entire rectum with either the rigid 25 cm or flexible 60 cm instrument and the sigmoid colon with the flexible sigmoidoscope. Flexible sigmoidoscopy is about twice as expensive as the rigid procedure, but can be performed with the patient in the left lateral position, and readily permits photography and the obtaining of biopsy and cytology specimens.

Indications: To examine the patient with symptoms referable to the rectum or anus (eg, bright rectal bleeding, discharge protrusions, pain); to evaluate a lesion known to be within reach of the instrument; to evaluate the rectum or sigmoid colon before

anorectal surgery; to evaluate the rectum in any patient in whom a barium enema is indicated (barium enema does not adequately visualize this area). **Contraindications:** None that are absolute. Patients with cardiac arrhythmias or recent myocardial ischemia should have the procedure postponed until the condition improves, or will need cardiac monitoring. Patients with prosthetic valves may need antibiotics to prevent endocarditis.

Procedure: Flexible sigmoidoscopy is performed as described above for colonoscopy. Usually IV medication is not needed. A phosphate enema may be given to empty the rectum. Rigid sigmoidoscopy is usually performed with the patient in the knee-chest position. After the rectal examination, the perianal area is examined, and the lubricated instrument is gently inserted 3 to 4 cm past the anal sphincter. The obturator is removed and the instrument is inserted under direct vision. Considerable skill is required to pass it beyond the rectosigmoid junction (15 cm) without producing patient discomfort. Anoscopy may be performed in either position. The instrument is inserted its full length as described above for rigid sigmoidoscopy.

Complications are exceedingly rare when the procedure is properly performed.

ABDOMINAL PARACENTESIS

Indications: To evaluate the etiology of ascitic fluid (eg, metastasis, TB, pancreatic ascites); to diagnose a perforated viscus in a patient with a history of blunt abdominal trauma. This procedure may be therapeutic for patients with tense ascites causing respiratory difficulties, pain, or oliguria. **Absolute contraindications** include a disorder of blood coagulation or hemostasis, intestinal obstruction, or an infected abdominal wall. **Relative contraindications** include poor patient cooperation, surgical scarring over the puncture area, or severe portal hypertension with abdominal collateral circulation.

Procedure: CBC, platelet count, and coagulation studies are obtained before the procedure. After emptying his bladder, the patient sits in bed with the head elevated 45 to 90°. A point is located in the midline halfway between the umbilicus and the pubic bone and cleaned with an antiseptic solution and alcohol. Under sterile technic, the area is anesthetized to the peritoneum with lidocaine 1%. An 18-gauge needle attached to a 50-mL syringe is inserted through the peritoneum (generally a "pop" is noted). Fluid is gently aspirated and sent for cell count, protein or amylase content, cytology, or culture as needed.

Complications: The most frequent complication is hemorrhage. Occasionally, with tense ascites, there may be prolonged leakage of ascitic fluid through the needle site.

PERITONEOSCOPY (LAPAROSCOPY)

Indications: To evaluate intraabdominal or pelvic pathology (eg, tumor, endometriosis); for lymphoma staging; to assess operability of patients with carcinoma; to evaluate patients with acute or chronic abdominal pain; to guide liver biopsy under direct visualization. **Absolute contraindications:** Coagulation or bleeding disorder, poor patient cooperation, peritonitis, intestinal obstruction, and infection of the abdominal wall. **Relative contraindications:** Severe cardiac or pulmonary disease, large abdominal hernias, multiple abdominal operations, or tense ascites.

Procedure: CBC, coagulation studies, x-rays of the chest and the kidneys, ureters, and bladder, and typing and sensitivity testing for 2 u. of whole blood are obtained before the procedure. The laparoscopy is performed with sterile technic in a well equipped endoscopy suite or operating room. A narcotic and/or diazepam is given IV while the abdomen is sterilized with an antiseptic solution. Lidocaine 1% is injected to

the peritoneum at the site of puncture. A 5-mm surgical incision is made and the Verres pneumoperitoneum needle is inserted. Nitrous oxide is infused. The incision is extended to 10 to 15 mm and the cannula with trocar is introduced into the peritoneal cavity. The trocar is removed and the peritoneoscope is inserted through the cannula. The abdominal contents are examined and aspiration of ascitic fluid and biopsy procedures are performed as needed. When the procedure is completed, the nitrous oxide is expelled by the patient with a Valsalva maneuver and the cannula is removed. The incision is sutured. An IV line is maintained for 24 h and the patient is checked at 6 and 24 h for signs of bleeding or infection.

Complications: Bleeding, bacterial peritonitis, and perforation of a viscus.

---

51. DISORDERS OF THE ESOPHAGUS

(See also GASTROINTESTINAL DEFECTS in Ch. 187)

The human swallowing apparatus consists of the pharynx, upper esophageal (crico pharyngeal) sphincter, and the body and lower sphincter of the esophagus. The uppe ⅓ of the esophagus and structures proximal to it are composed of skeletal muscle; th distal esophagus and lower esophageal sphincter contain smooth muscle. This inte grated system transports material from the mouth to the stomach and prevents it reflux into the esophagus.

COMMON SYMPTOMS AND SIGNS

Dysphagia

A subjective awareness of difficulty in swallowing due to impaired progression of matte from pharynx to stomach. The usual complaint is that food "gets stuck" on the wa down. Dysphagia, the major symptom of esophageal transport disorders, may be ac companied by pain. Transport of liquids and solids may be impeded by organic lesion of the pharynx, esophagus, and adjacent organs, or by functional derangements of th nervous system and musculature. The cause of dysphagia, which may be a pre-esoph ageal or an esophageal abnormality, should always be carefully sought.

Pre-esophageal dysphagia: *Difficulty emptying material from the oral pharynx into th esophagus.* This symptom occurs with disorders proximal to the esophagus, most ofte in patients with neurologic or muscular disorders that affect skeletal muscles (eg dermatomyositis, myasthenia gravis, muscular dystrophy, bulbar poliomyelitis, pseu dobulbar palsy, and other CNS lesions). The patient with these disorders not infre quently presents with nasal regurgitation or tracheal aspiration followed by coughing

Esophageal dysphagia, *difficulty passing food down the esophagus,* may be the conse quence of **obstructive** or **motor disorders. Obstructive disorders** (eg, carcinoma, benig peptic stricture, and lower esophageal ring) usually produce dysphagia for solids alon by mechanically reducing the esophageal lumen. Meat and bread are often singled ou as the major offenders, but some patients can tolerate only liquids. The patient wh refers the dysphagia to the lower esophagus is usually correct, while a complaint o dysphagia in the upper esophagus may be referred from a lower lesion. In carcinom of the esophagus, the dysphagia progresses rapidly over weeks or months. In pepti stricture, dysphagia progresses over years and is preceded by a prominent history o gastroesophageal reflux. With a lower esophageal ring, dysphagia is intermittent.

Motor disorders causing esophageal dysfunction involve the smooth muscle of th esophagus. They produce *dysphagia for both solids and liquids* by impairing esophagea

peristalsis and lower esophageal sphincter function, thus interrupting the smooth esophageal transport of a bolus. Achalasia, *symptomatic diffuse esophageal spasm*, and scleroderma are the most common motor disorders. From the onset of symptoms, the presence of dysphagia for *both* liquids and solids accurately distinguishes motor from obstructive causes.

Dysphagia should not be confused with **globus hystericus** (globus sensation), *a feeling of having a lump in the throat that is unrelated to swallowing and occurs without impaired transport*. Often noted in association with anxiety or grief, globus hystericus is mainly emotional in etiology. (See also Ch. 52.)

Chest Pain of Esophageal Origin

Chest or back pain, the second major symptom complex of esophageal disease, is classified as heartburn, pain during swallowing, or spontaneous esophageal motor disorder pain.

Heartburn, caused by reflux of gastric contents into the esophagus (**gastroesophageal reflux;** see below), is a substernal burning pain that rises in the chest and may radiate into the neck, throat, or even face. It usually occurs after meals or when the patient is lying down, and is frequently accompanied by regurgitation of gastric contents into the mouth **(waterbrash).**

Pain during swallowing **(odynophagia)** may occur with or without dysphagia and may be due to mucosal destruction (eg, in esophagitis induced by gastroesophageal reflux); to bacterial, viral, or mycotic infections; to neoplasms, chemicals, or esophageal motor disorders (eg, achalasia and diffuse esophageal spasm). The patient may describe the pain as a burning sensation or a substernal tightness typically elicited by very hot or very cold food or liquid. Onset is prompt on swallowing. Severe squeezing chest pain, induced by swallowing hot or cold beverages in association with dysphagia, is characteristic of esophageal motor disorders.

Spontaneous motor disorder pain is difficult to characterize apart from other esophageal symptoms and cardiac chest pain. Spontaneous esophageal chest pain may be severe and mimic angina pectoris in every way. A definitive diagnosis of esophageal chest pain cannot be made unless the motor disorder can be recorded during manometric study concurrent with the patient's typical pain. The presence of dysphagia with chest pain may be a clue of an esophageal origin.

COMMON DIAGNOSTIC PROCEDURES

A **history** precisely detailing the patient's symptoms should establish an accurate diagnosis in about 80% of patients. The only **physical findings** in esophageal disease are (1) cervical and supraclavicular lymphadenopathy due to metastasis, (2) swellings in the neck from large pharyngeal diverticula, and (3) prolonged swallowing time (the time from the act of swallowing to the sound of the bolus of fluid and air entering the stomach, heard by auscultation with the stethoscope over the epigastrium and normally $\leq$ 12 sec). Esophageal motor disorders are associated with prolonged swallowing times. Watching the patient swallow may also be very helpful to evaluate patients with pre-esophageal dysphagia for aspiration or nasal regurgitation.

Laboratory Tests

X-ray studies: In addition to the standard barium meal, the advent of cinefluoroscopy has aided in detecting disorders (eg, esophageal webs) and in assessing motor disorders (eg, cricopharyngeal spasm and achalasia).

Esophagoscopy can be done diagnostically (eg, to evaluate pain or dysphagia, to identify structural abnormalities or bleeding sites, or to obtain biopsies). Therapeutic

indications include removal of foreign bodies, hemostasis by coagulation or sclerotherapy, and debulking of tumors.

Esophageal manometry is used to evaluate patients with dysphagia, heartburn, or chest pain. It determines the pressure in the upper and lower esophageal sphincters, the effectiveness and coordination of propulsive movements, and detects abnormal contractions. It is used in diagnosing achalasia, diffuse spasm, scleroderma, and lower esophageal sphincter hypo- and hypertension and to evaluate certain therapeutic procedures (eg, antireflex surgery, pneumatic dilation for achalasia). The use of provocative tests for esophageal spasms, with agents like edrophonium chloride, increases the sensitivity of detecting diffuse esophageal spasm in patients with noncardiac chest pain.

Esophageal pH monitoring, performed either during esophageal manometry or as a prolonged study in ambulatory patients, is discussed under GASTROESOPHAGEAL REFLUX AND ITS COMPLICATIONS, below.

The Bernstein (acid perfusion) test is done by perfusing the esophagus through a nasogastric tube with alternating solutions of isotonic saline and 0.1 N hydrochloric acid at a rate of 6 mL/min. The Bernstein test is a sensitive means of detecting the presence of esophagitis, but may be falsely negative in the patient receiving treatment.

DISORDERS ASSOCIATED WITH PRE-ESOPHAGEAL DYSPHAGIA

In **cricopharyngeal incoordination,** the cricopharyngeal muscle (the upper esophageal sphincter) remains closed or opens in an uncoordinated way. It may cause a Zenker's diverticulum (see under ESOPHAGEAL DIVERTICULA, below); repeated aspiration of material from the diverticulum may lead to chronic lung disease. The condition may be **treated** by surgical section of the muscle.

Myasthenia gravis, muscular dystrophy, Parkinson's disease, amyotrophic lateral sclerosis, pseudobulbar palsy, bulbar poliomyelitis, and the oculogyric crises associated with phenothiazine therapy are other causes of pre-esophageal dysphagia.

DISORDERS ASSOCIATED WITH ESOPHAGEAL DYSPHAGIA

OBSTRUCTIVE DISORDERS

EXTRINSIC OBSTRUCTION

Extrinsic tumors or adjacent organs may compress the esophagus. The symptom is dysphagia for solids, similar to intrinsic esophageal obstruction. Extrinsic obstruction may occur with an enlarged left atrium, aortic aneurysm, aberrant subclavian artery (see DYSPHAGIA LUSORIA below), substernal thyroid, bony exostosis, or extrinsic tumors—most commonly lung. Diagnosis is usually made on x-ray and prognosis depends upon the etiology.

CARCINOMA OF THE ESOPHAGUS

(See also Ch. 212)

Etiology and Pathophysiology

Conditions associated with an increased frequency of squamous cell carcinoma include lye stricture, achalasia, esophageal webs, and squamous cell carcinomas of the head and neck. Most patients use tobacco or ethanol to excess. Nearly all patients with

rimary adenocarcinoma of the esophagus will have **Barrett's metaplasia**, which is a ›rm used to describe columnar metaplastic epithelium that may occur in the lower sophagus following the chronic injury of peptic esophagitis. This unusual premalig-ant metaplastic condition may develop in up to 10% of patients with chronic gastro-sophageal reflux (see below).

Mechanical obstruction of the esophagus may also be caused by involvement of the sophagus by lymphoma, leiomyosarcoma, or (very rarely) metastatic carcinoma.

ymptoms, Signs, and Diagnosis

The most serious cause of dysphagia, carcinoma usually presents with progressive ysphagia for solids over several weeks, associated with marked weight loss. Carci-oma may occur anywhere in the esophagus and may appear as a stricture, mass, or laque. The tumor is best diagnosed by x-ray, followed by endoscopy with biopsy and ytology. The yield on brush cytology is > 95% positive, while biopsy may be positive ı about 70% of patients. Tumors are most often squamous cell carcinoma with about % of esophageal cancer being adenocarcinoma.

reatment and Prognosis

Leiomyoma, the most common benign tumor of the esophagus, may be multiple, but as an excellent prognosis in most patients. Otherwise, the overall prognosis is poor, ith < 5% long-term survival. Chemotherapy may prolong survival in selected pa-ents. Surgery offers the patient the most prolonged palliation when feasible. Treat-ent of squamous cell carcinoma is either surgical resection or radiation therapy; lenocarcinoma is treated by surgery. Other palliative measures include dilation pro-edures, tube prosthesis, radiation therapy, and laser photocoagulation of the intralu-inal mass.

LOWER ESOPHAGEAL RING

(Schatzki's Ring)

A 2- to 4-mm submucosal structure, probably congenital, causing a ring-like narrowing the distal esophagus at the squamocolumnar junction. Intermittent dysphagia for sol-s may occur when the narrowing is sufficient to produce obstruction, usually when e esophageal lumen is < 12 mm in diameter. The ring is usually demonstrated by ırium x-ray studies if the distal esophagus is adequately distended. Rings > 20 mm in ameter are usually asymptomatic and should not have symptoms attributed to them.

Instructing the patient to chew food thoroughly is usually the only **treatment** re-ıired, but rings may be fractured endoscopically, by dilation, or by resection.

ESOPHAGEAL WEBS

(Plummer-Vinson or Paterson-Kelly Syndrome; Sideropenic Dysphagia)

A thin, mucosal membrane that grows across the lumen of the esophagus. Webs may velop rarely in patients with untreated severe iron deficiency anemia or, even more rely, without an overt anemia. Usually in the upper esophagus, they produce dyspha-a for solids; usually missed on ordinary barium swallow, they can be shown best on efilms. The webs disappear with therapy for the anemia, but may be easily ruptured ring esophagoscopy.

DYSPHAGIA LUSORIA

Dysphagia due to compression of the esophagus by a congenital vascular abnormality sually an aberrant right subclavian artery arising from the left side of the aortic arch). ıe dysphagia may occur in childhood or may develop later due to arteriosclerotic

changes in the aberrant vessel. Esophageal x-ray studies show the extrinsic compres sion above the aortic arch, at the third thoracic vertebra. Arteriography is necessar for absolute diagnosis. Surgical correction is only rarely indicated.

MOTOR DISORDERS

ACHALASIA

(Cardiospasm; Esophageal Aperistalsis; Megaesophagus)

A neurogenic esophageal disorder of unknown etiology causing impairment of esophe geal peristalsis and of lower esophageal sphincter relaxation. The condition may be du to a malfunction of the myenteric plexus of the esophagus that results in denervatio of esophageal muscle.

Symptoms and Signs

Achalasia may occur at any age, but usually begins between ages 20 and 40. Dy phagia for both solids and liquids is the major symptom; other symptoms incluc chest pain, regurgitation, or nocturnal cough. Onset is insidious and progression gradual over many months or years. Increased pressure at the lower esophage sphincter produces obstruction with secondary dilation of the esophagus. Nocturn regurgitation of undigested food occurs in about 1/3 of the patients and may cau pulmonary aspiration with lung abscess, bronchiectasis, or pneumonia. Chest pain less common, but may occur upon swallowing or spontaneously. Weight loss is usual mild to moderate. When weight loss is pronounced, particularly in the elderly patie in whom the symptoms of dysphagia have had a rapid development, achalasia secon ary to a neoplasm of the gastroesophageal junction should be considered.

Diagnosis

X-ray studies of the esophagus demonstrate the absence of progressive peristalt contractions during swallowing. The esophagus is dilated and frequently reaches enc mous proportions, but is narrowed and beaklike at the lower esophageal sphincte Esophageal manometry shows aperistalsis, increased lower esophageal sphincter pre sure, and incomplete sphincteric relaxation with swallowing. Esophagoscopy revea dilation but no obstructing lesion. The esophagoscope usually passes readily into t stomach; difficulty doing so should raise the possibility of malignancy or stricture. A increased sensitivity of the denervated structures to pharmacologic stimuli (eg, meth choline) can usually be demonstrated manometrically, but may be associated wi adverse side effects and is rarely necessary to make the diagnosis.

Achalasia must be differentiated from a distal stenosing carcinoma and a pept stricture; this is particularly true in the patient with scleroderma in whom the esop ageal manometric study may also show aperistalsis. Scleroderma will usually be a companied by a history of Raynaud's phenomenon and symptoms of gastroesophage reflux. A retroflexed view of the gastric cardia, biopsies, and brushings for cytolo should be obtained in all patients to exclude malignancy.

Prognosis

Pulmonary aspiration and secondary carcinoma are the determining factors in prc nosis. Nocturnal regurgitation with coughing suggests possible aspiration. Pulmona complications secondary to aspiration are difficult to manage. The incidence of esop ageal carcinoma in patients with achalasia is about 5%.

Treatment

The aim of treatment is to reduce the pressure and thus the obstruction at the low esophageal sphincter. Forceful or pneumatic dilation of the sphincter with a Mosher

Browne-McHardy dilating instrument is indicated initially, since results are satisfactory in about 80% of patients; repeated dilations may be needed. Esophageal rupture and secondary mediastinitis requiring surgery occur in < 1% of patients. Nitrates (eg, nitroglycerine 0.4 mg sublingually before meals) or Ca-channel antagonists (eg, nifedipine 10 mg orally qid) will reduce lower esophageal sphincter pressure and may prolong periods between dilations. A Heller myotomy, in which the muscular fibers in the lower esophageal sphincter are cut, is usually reserved for patients who fail to respond to pneumatic dilation; its success rate is about 85%. Symptomatic gastroesophageal reflux follows surgery in about 15% of patients.

Symptomatic Diffuse Esophageal Spasm

(Spastic Pseudodiverticulosis; Rosary Bead or Corkscrew Esophagus)

A generalized neurogenic disorder of esophageal motility in which normal peristalsis is replaced by phasic nonpropulsive contractions and, in some cases, by abnormal lower esophageal sphincter function.

Symptoms and Signs

Diffuse esophageal spasm typically causes substernal chest pain in association with dysphagia for both liquids and solids. The pain may be severe and may awaken the patient from sleep. Liquids that are very hot or cold may aggravate the pain. Over many years, this disorder may evolve into achalasia.

Esophageal spasms may also produce a severe pain in the absence of dysphagia that is indistinguishable from angina pectoris. This pain is often described as a substernal squeezing pain and may occur in association with exercise.

Diagnosis

X-rays may show poor progression of a bolus and disordered, simultaneous contractions or tertiary contractions. Severe spasms may mimic diverticuli that vary in size and position with time. Esophageal scintigraphy may be a sensitive method of detecting impaired bolus transport. Esophageal manometry provides the most sensitive and specific description of the spasms. Contractions are usually simultaneous, prolonged or multiphasic, and may be of very high amplitude. In patients with nondiagnostic baseline studies, provocative tests with pharmacologic agents (eg, edrophonium chloride 10 mg IV or a meal) may disclose a propensity to symptomatic spasms. Lower esophageal sphincter pressure or relaxation pattern may be impaired in 30% of patients.

Treatment

Esophageal spasms are often difficult to treat. Anticholinergics, nitroglycerin, and long-acting nitrates have been used with limited success. Ca-channel blockers (eg, verapamil 80 mg orally tid, or nifedipine 10 mg orally qid) may be useful in selected patients. Pneumatic dilation and bougienage may be helpful. Potent analgesics are often needed, but may be habit-forming. Medical management is usually sufficient, but surgical myotomy along the full length of the esophagus may be needed in intractable cases.

Variants of Diffuse Spasm and Achalasia

Some patients show symptom complexes that fit neither typical achalasia nor typical diffuse spasm. Some have been called **"vigorous achalasia,"** since they have both the severe pain and spasm of diffuse spasm and the fluid retention and aspiration of achalasia.

SCLERODERMA

(See PROGRESSIVE SYSTEMIC SCLEROSIS in Ch. 110)

GASTROESOPHAGEAL REFLUX AND ITS COMPLICATIONS

Reflux of gastric contents into the esophagus.

Etiology

The presence of gastroesophgeal reflux indicates incompetence of the lower esophageal sphincter. Other factors that contribute to the development of esophagitis include the caustic nature of the refluxate, the inability to clear the refluxate from the esophagus, the volume of gastric contents, and local mucosal protective functions. Factors that contribute to the competence of the gastroesophageal junction include intrinsic sphincter pressure, the angle of the cardioesophageal junction, the action of the diaphragm and, when upright, gravity. Gastroesophageal incompetence was previously attributed solely to a sliding hiatus hernia, but recent evidence indicates that the cause is lower esophageal sphincter incompetence.

Symptoms and Signs

Heartburn with or without regurgitation of gastric contents into the mouth is the most prominent symptom. Complications of gastroesophageal reflux include esophagitis, peptic esophageal stricture, esophageal ulcer, and Barrett's metaplasia. Esophagitis may cause odynophagia and possibly massive, but usually limited, hemorrhage. Peptic stricture causes a gradually progressive dysphagia for solid foods. Peptic esophageal ulcers cause the same type of pain as do gastric or duodenal ulcers, but are usually localized to the xiphoid or high substernal region. They heal slowly, tend to recur, and usually leave a stricture upon healing.

Diagnosis

A careful history points to the diagnosis. X-ray studies, endoscopy, esophageal manometry, pH monitoring, and the Bernstein acid perfusion test (see above) help to confirm the diagnosis and demonstrate possible complications. X-rays taken with the patient in the Trendelenburg position may show reflux of barium from the stomach into the esophagus. Abdominal compression may be used, but radiographic maneuvers are not usually sensitive indicators of gastroesophageal reflux. X-rays taken following a barium swallow readily demonstrate esophageal ulcers and peptic strictures, but are only rarely diagnostic in patients with hemorrhage due to esophagitis. Esophagoscopy provides accurate diagnosis of esophagitis with or without hemorrhage. Esophagoscopy in conjunction with cytologic washings and direct vision biopsy is essential for distinguishing benign peptic stricture from carcinoma of the esophagus. Esophageal manometry, by determining pressure at the lower esophageal sphincter, indicates its strength and thereby distinguishes a normal from an incompetent sphincter. Esophageal pH monitoring shows the reflux of acid gastric contents into the esophagus and provides direct evidence of gastroesophageal reflux. The Bernstein test correlates closely with the presence of symptomatic gastroesophageal reflux; symptoms are promptly reproduced by acid perfusion and relieved by saline perfusion. Esophageal biopsy is an accurate indicator of gastroesophageal reflux, showing thinning of the squamous mucosal layer and basilar cell hyperplasia. These histologic changes may occur without evidence of gross esophagitis by endoscopy. A positive biopsy or a positive Bernstein test correlates best with esophageal symptoms of reflux regardless of endoscopic or x-ray findings. Endoscopic biopsy is also the only test that consistently detects the columnar mucosal changes of Barrett's metaplasia.

Treatment

Uncomplicated gastroesophageal reflux may be tolerated for many years with good response to medical therapy. Management consists of (1) elevating the head of the bed 6 in.; (2) avoiding strong stimulants of acid secretion (eg, coffee, alcohol); (3) avoiding certain drugs (eg, anticholinergics), specific foods (fats, chocolate), and smoking, all of which reduce lower esophageal sphincter competence; (4) giving an antacid 30 mL 1 h after meals and at bedtime to neutralize gastric acidity and possibly increase lower esophageal sphincter competence; and (5) use of cholinergic agonists (eg, bethanechol 25 mg orally tid or metoclopramide 10 mg orally 30 min before meals and at bedtime) to increase sphincter pressure; and (6) use of H_2 antagonists to reduce gastric acidity (eg, cimetidine 300 mg orally qid or ranitidine 150 mg orally bid).

Hemorrhage from esophagitis, unless massive, does not require emergency surgery, but it may recur.

Esophageal strictures are managed by an intensive medical regimen and by repeated dilation (eg, with Hg-filled bougies) to achieve and maintain esophageal patency. If properly dilated, they do not seriously limit what the patient can eat.

Anti-reflux operations (Belsey, Hill, Nissen) are used in patients with serious esophagitis, hemorrhage, stricture, ulcer, or intractable symptoms, whether or not a hiatus hernia was present.

Barrett's metaplasia responds inconsistently to medical or surgical therapy. Endoscopic surveillance of malignant transformation is often recommended, but has uncertain cost effectiveness.

CORROSIVE ESOPHAGITIS AND STRICTURE

(See also Ingestion of Caustics in Ch. 189)

Caustic injury to the esophagus most commonly results from accidental ingestion of cleaning solutions or as a suicidal attempt (see Ch. 201). Odynophagia and, less commonly, esophageal strictures may result when certain drugs are temporarily lodged in the esophagus by a motility disorder or anatomic variant. Potassium chloride supplements, tetracycline, and quinidine are most commonly implicated.

ESOPHAGEAL DIVERTICULA

There are several types of esophageal diverticula, each of different etiology. A **pharyngeal diverticulum (Zenker's)** is an outpouching of the mucosa and submucosa posteriorly through the cricopharyngeal muscle. It probably results from incoordination between pharyngeal propulsion and cricopharyngeal relaxation. **Mid-esophageal (traditionally called traction) diverticula** are either due to traction from mediastinal inflammatory lesions or secondary to motor disorders. An **epiphrenic diverticulum,** also probably of propulsive origin, occurs just above the diaphragm and usually accompanies an esophageal motor disturbance (achalasia, diffuse esophageal spasm).

Symptoms, Signs, and Diagnosis

A Zenker's diverticulum fills with food that may be regurgitated when the patient bends or lies down. Aspiration pneumonitis may result if regurgitation is nocturnal. Rarely, the pouch becomes large and causes dysphagia. Traction and epiphrenic diverticula are rarely symptomatic in themselves. All diverticula are diagnosed by barium-swallow x-ray.

Treatment

Specific treatment is usually not required, though surgical resection of the diverticulum is occasionally necessary.

HIATUS HERNIA

Protrusion of the stomach above the diaphragm.

Etiology and Pathology

Etiology is usually unknown, but a hiatus hernia may be a congenital abnormality or secondary to trauma. In a **sliding hiatus hernia,** the gastroesophageal junction and a portion of the stomach are above the diaphragm. One side of the herniated stomach is covered by peritoneum. In **paraesophageal hiatus hernia,** the gastroesophageal junction is in the normal location, but a portion of the stomach is adjacent to the esophagus.

Symptoms and Signs

A sliding hiatus hernia is common and may be seen by x-ray in > 40% of the population. Most patients are asymptomatic. Although gastroesophageal reflux occurs in a few patients, it is doubtful whether the hernia is the cause since reflux may also be found in patients with no demonstrable hernia on x-ray. Chest pain without gastroesophageal reflux can also occur. A paraesophageal hiatus hernia is generally asymptomatic, but, unlike a sliding hiatus hernia, may incarcerate and strangulate. Occult or massive GI hemorrhage may occur with either type of hiatus hernia.

Diagnosis

X-rays usually readily demonstrate hiatus hernia. Vigorous testing by applying abdominal compression may be required to show a sliding hiatus hernia.

Treatment

A sliding hiatus hernia usually requires no specific therapy, but any accompanying gastroesophageal reflux should be treated (see GASTROESOPHAGEAL REFLUX, above). A paraesophageal hernia should be reduced surgically because of risk of strangulation

ESOPHAGEAL LACERATION AND RUPTURE

Mallory-Weiss syndrome: *Laceration of the distal esophagus and proximal stomach during vomiting, retching, or hiccups.* GI hemorrhage from an arterial site is the usual clinical presentation. Initially described in alcoholics, the Mallory-Weiss syndrome is recognized in all types of patients. It frequently causes GI hemorrhage, comprising about 10% of patients with this disorder. **Diagnosis** is made during endoscopic evaluation or arteriography. The lesion is not seen on routine upper GI x-rays. Most episodes of bleeding stop spontaneously, but some patients require ligation of the laceration. Intra-arterial infusion of pitressin into the left gastric artery during angiography has also been shown to control bleeding.

Esophageal rupture may be iatrogenic during endoscopic procedures or other instrumentations. Spontaneous rupture, **Boerhaave's syndrome,** is a catastrophic illness with a high mortality. Esophageal perforation or rupture leads to mediastinitis and pleural effusion. Immediate surgical repair and drainage are required.

INFECTIOUS DISORDERS OF THE ESOPHAGUS

Candida albicans is a fungal organism that is a normal constituent of oral flora. When conditions favor fungal growth over that of oral bacteria, infection of monilia results. Conditions favoring fungal growth include treatment with broad-spectrum antibiotics, notably tetracycline; high salivary concentrations of glucose (eg, as in diabetes mellitus); compromised cellular immunity (eg, in leukemic states or during chemotherapy); and esophageal stasis (eg, in achalasia or scleroderma). Patients usually complain of odynophagia, and less commonly, dysphagia. Examination of th

oropharynx may reveal the typical white patches, but their absence does not exclude esophageal involvement. Barium swallow may reveal slightly raised plaques throughout the esophagus or only a motor abnormality. Culture or histology shows clusters of budding spores or hyphae. In minor cases, a nystatin suspension may be swished through the mouth and swallowed (5 mL of a 100,000 U/mL suspension qid). In more resistant cases, systemic treatment with ketoconazole or amphotericin B may be necessary (see GENERAL THERAPEUTIC PRINCIPLES in Ch. 9).

Herpes simplex virus **(HSV)** may cause severe odynophagia in patients who are immunosuppressed. Endoscopy is usually necessary to make the diagnosis with histologic or cytologic specimens showing the typical intranuclear inclusions. Treatment may not be necessary in mild cases, but when symptoms are severe or prolonged, acyclovir (ara A) given IV may be tried. In immunocompromised patients, cytomegalovirus produces esophagitis that is distinguished from HSV by biopsy, culture, and resistance to acyclovir.

52. FUNCTIONAL DYSPEPSIA AND OTHER NONSPECIFIC GASTROINTESTINAL COMPLAINTS

Symptoms referred to the GI system in which a pathologic condition is not present, is poorly established, or, if present, does not entirely explain the clinical state. Patients with such complaints are common in the primary care setting, and account for 30 to 50% of referrals to gastroenterologists. Both referring physicians and GI specialists consider these illnesses difficult to understand and treat, as they do not fit into previously learned disease categories. Uncertainty may lead to frustration, judgmental attitudes, and the ordering of inappropriate tests in a futile attempt to find a biologic cause to explain the complaints.

Although functional or nonspecific symptoms may in part derive from medical disease (eg, peptic ulcer, esophagitis), contributory psychologic or cultural factors make diagnosis difficult and medical treatment alone insufficient. More often, histopathologic abnormalities are not established. Evidence may indicate altered physiologic activity (eg, symptomatic diffuse esophageal spasm [see above], irritable bowel syndrome [see IRRITABLE BOWEL SYNDROMES in Ch. 61]), the patient may be preoccupied with normal physiologic function (eg, borborygmus in the hypochondriac), or psychologic illness may assume primary importance (conversion disorder, somatization in depression). In many patients, more than one of these factors is involved.

Regardless of etiology, the experience and reporting of symptoms vary, depending on the patient's personality, the psychologic meaning of the illness to him, and the influence of sociocultural patterns. Thus, symptoms of nausea and vomiting due to cholecystitis may be minimized or reported indirectly or even bizarrely by the severely depressed patient, but presented with dramatic urgency by the histrionic patient. Although distressing, the illness may satisfy certain psychologic needs; eg, it may serve to avoid overt mental distress or lead to benefits derived from the attention and privileges of the sick role (removal from responsibilities, disability compensation). This helps to explain why many of these patients are noncompliant, have unexpected side effects to medication, and seem resistant to improvement. Finally, cultural influences may affect the reporting of symptoms; eg, the belief that illness is derived from evil spirits may indicate a primary psychiatric disorder in an educated businessman, but be of little etiologic significance in someone from a primitive society.

Approach to the Patient

In patients with inexplicable complaints, a patient-oriented clinical approach with appreciation of the psychosocial aspects of illness should be followed:

1. The history should be obtained by an open-ended interview style. Questions that encourage spontaneous responses prevent physician bias from affecting the content of the history. The patient is then likely to present the symptoms in relation to physiologic and psychosocial events that contribute to the illness. Leading questions or those that elicit "yes" or "no" answers should be avoided. To ask directly, "Is the pain relieved by food?" may get a falsely positive response, since the patient's wish to comply to the doctor's expectations overrides his intention to be accurate. However, a query like "What makes the pain better or worse?" will minimize bias and may elicit important information that can be further developed through specific questions. The physician must identify not only the location and quality of the symptoms but also their setting, the presence of aggravating and alleviating factors, and any associated symptoms. All information is then synthesized until the complex of symptoms and related factors fit into diagnostic categories.

2. The role of psychologic stress factors must be considered. The stressfulness of a specific event varies; eg, divorce may sadden one person but relieve another. Such data rarely emerge from direct inquiry. Rather, when the patient volunteers relevant information while discussing the setting of the symptoms, he should be encouraged to elaborate. The physician must maintain a noncritical attitude.

3. A behavioral ("functional") disorder does not preclude present medical disease or its future development. Even though a history contains vague, dramatic, or bizarre symptoms, new and possibly significant complaints should not be minimized. New physical findings or "hard" data suggesting pathologic changes (eg, blood in the stool, fever, anemia, or metabolic disturbance) should prompt further evaluation. Complete objectivity must guide the approach to each clinical problem.

4. When in doubt, "don't just do something—stand there." The tendency to order excess or unnecessary studies for the insistent patient with inexplicable complaints should be avoided; patients must often be managed with incomplete or nonspecific medical data. When a problem is not critical, the wise physician will temporize rather than embark upon an uncertain diagnostic or therapeutic plan. In time, new information may lead to directed evaluation and management.

5. Diagnostic studies may not entirely explain a patient's clinical condition. Endoscopy can establish the presence of a duodenal ulcer, but cannot clarify why one patient is asymptomatic and another disabled. Furthermore, the indications for and accuracy of all procedures selected must be considered. A negative medical evaluation does not entirely exclude physical disease. The appropriate study may not have been selected, the results may have been misinterpreted, or a false-negative result may have been obtained because of limitations of the study.

6. Removal of the symptom is not always the goal of therapy. The illness may have such adaptive value to the patient that the loss from giving up its "benefits" may be greater than the gain from relief of symptoms. Pain or suffering may substitute for more distressing guilt and sadness. The attention and privileges derived from chronic illness may also be significant. When the patient overtly or covertly resists management, the illness can be assumed to fulfill certain needs. In this case, the illness must be accepted and treatment should be oriented toward improving function *despite the continuation of the symptoms*. In this approach, although the physician seemingly abandons the commitment to cure or remove disease, his frustration is reduced when the therapeutic goals are realistic, and results of this approach are often favorable.

FUNCTIONAL DYSPEPSIA

Common discomfort often described as "indigestion," gaseousness, fullness, or pain that is gnawing or burning in quality and localized to the upper abdomen or chest.

These symptoms, which are not confined to a single organ or disease process, can have many etiologies, and correlation of symptoms with pathophysiologic states is difficult. Endoscopic and x-ray detection of structural abnormalities to explain the symptoms varies so widely (14 to 87%) that estimates of incidence are meaningless. The studies may not be comparable because methods differ for population selection, analysis, and interpretation. Also, an *association* between symptoms and pathophysiologic abnormalities does not necessarily mean *causation*; eg, histologic evidence of inflammatory gastritis can be found in 15 to 50% of *asymptomatic* healthy volunteers. Radiologic or pathologic "duodenitis," pyloric dysfunction with alkaline reflux, and cholelithiasis are other commonly described conditions with uncertain relationships to clinical symptoms.

Symptoms and Signs

Belching, abdominal distention, and borborygmus are often described in addition to epigastric or substernal pain. Eating may worsen or relieve the pain. Other associated symptoms may include anorexia, nausea, and change in bowel habits. Dysphoric states such as anxiety or depression may often be found.

Differential Diagnosis

Dyspepsia may be reported in cardiac ischemia (in which exertion increases the discomfort), gastroesophageal reflux, diffuse esophageal spasm (particularly if dysphagia is present), peptic ulcer disease, and cholecystitis. Psychologic causes include anxiety with or without aerophagia, conversion disorder, somatization in depression, or hypochondriasis. Lactose intolerance may mimic these symptoms (see CARBOHYDRATE INTOLERANCE in Ch. 58). It is important to inquire about bowel habits. A history of alternating constipation and diarrhea suggests a generalized motility disorder as the etiology, eg, irritable bowel syndromes (see IRRITABLE BOWEL SYNDROMES in Ch. 61).

No preplanned method of evaluation can be recommended. The history and complete examination will determine if further studies are indicated. At a minimum, a CBC and tests for occult blood in the stool should be done. An upper GI series is usually required, particularly if the patient also has dysphagia, weight loss, vomiting, or change in the pattern of symptoms with eating. Upper esophagogastroduodenoscopy has been suggested for patients with continued unexplained symptoms and may be of additional value; it is more sensitive for detecting mucosal abnormalities. Caution is required in using any nonspecific findings obtained to explain the symptoms. Esophageal manometry is indicated only if dysphagia, regurgitation, or evidence for aspiration suggests an esophageal motor disorder. Dyspepsia without other clinical findings is unlikely to be caused by cholelithiasis. In this situation, if oral cholecystography reveals gallstones in a functioning gallbladder, cholecystectomy may not relieve the dyspepsia. However, a compatible history and objective findings also suggestive of cholecystitis or choledocholithiasis (see Ch. 78) require thorough evaluation of the biliary system and surgical intervention if disease is found.

Treatment

Dyspepsia with no evidence of underlying somatic disease usually calls first for reassurance and symptomatic management with observation over time. Treatment of reflux symptoms or epigastric discomfort may be tried for brief periods with antacids or H_2 antagonists.

Changes in the clinical state may require more extensive evaluation if new problems arise or if symptoms persist and become more disabling, but, for most patients with chronic nonspecific dyspepsia, continued observation, support, and reassurance, with minimization of diagnostic studies suffices.

PSYCHOGENIC (FUNCTIONAL) NAUSEA AND VOMITING

Nausea: *The unpleasant feeling that one is about to vomit.* It may represent the patient's awareness of afferent stimuli to the medullary vomiting center. Nausea is associated with altered physiologic activity, including the gastric hypomotility and increased parasympathetic tone that precede and accompany vomiting. **Vomiting:** *Forceful expulsion of gastric contents produced by involuntary contraction of the abdominal musculature when the gastric fundus and lower esophageal sphincter are relaxed.* Vomiting should be distinguished from **regurgitation:** *the spitting up of gastric contents without associated nausea or forceful abdominal muscular contractions.*

Etiology and Psychophysiology

Vomiting may be considered part of a regulatory mechanism that allows for expulsion of potentially harmful substances. **Psychogenic vomiting** may be self-induced or may occur involuntarily in situations perceived by the patient to be anxiety-inducing, threatening, or in some way "distasteful." Common expressions referable to the digestive system express aversion: "I can't stomach that," "This is nauseating," "You make me want to throw up," and such thoughts can have physical representation. The psychologic factors leading to vomiting may be culturally determined (eg, eating exotic food considered repulsive in one's own cultural group). Vomiting may express hostility, as when a child vomits during a temper tantrum, or may be an attempt to represent a forbidden idea or wish, as with conversion disorders. For example, vomiting soon after or on the anniversary of an abortion or a hysterectomy can often be observed when a woman has unresolved conflicts related to the lost fetus or to her identity as a woman or mother. In this example of a conversion reaction, the patient's ambivalence leads to symptoms that represent both the experience of pregnancy (to retain symbolically what was lost) and its rejection.

"Rewards" (eg, exemption from school or work) may reinforce vomiting, whatever its cause. In such situations the event removes or protects the patient, usually without his awareness, from a real or imagined threat that would otherwise produce mental distress. The physician will remain unaware of these factors unless he determines the meaning of the symptom to the patient.

Diagnosis

Elucidating the behavioral features that produce the vomiting in order to establish a psychogenic etiology may take more time than is available. Often this type of confirmation is never achieved and the physician must make inferences, working with indirect or suggestive data: (1) The history, physical examination, and initial laboratory data can often reasonably exclude significant physical disorders within the GI tract (cholecystitis, choledocholithiasis, intestinal obstruction, peptic ulcer disease, acute gastroenteritis, perforated viscus or other "acute abdomen," ingestion of noxious substances); derangements in other organ systems (eg, acute pyelonephritis, myocardial infarction, acute hepatitis); toxic or metabolic disorders (systemic infection, radiation exposure, drug toxicity, diabetic ketoacidosis, cancer); or neurogenic causes (stimulation of the vestibular center, pain, meningitis, CNS trauma, or tumor). (2) The episodes may not follow any expected physiologic pattern; eg, the vomiting may occur at the thought of food and may not be temporally related to eating. (3) Patients may have personal and family histories of functional nausea and vomiting, experiences that serve

as models for the present symptoms. (4) With encouragement to describe the setting of the episodes, many patients will relate onset to stress and will report recurrence and worsening during similar stressful periods; however, this association or even awareness of mental distress may not be acknowledged by the patient. (5) Despite the presence of symptoms for weeks or months, examination usually shows no weight loss, dehydration, or objective clinical abnormalities. However, patients with severe psychologic disturbance may develop malnutrition and metabolic abnormalities from protracted vomiting.

If history and examination do not exclude a physical disorder, further studies will depend upon clinical information already obtained. These include CBC, ESR, urinalysis, glucose, BUN, electrolytes, liver function tests, stools for blood, upper GI series with small bowel follow-through, and abdominal ultrasound. If these are normal (ie, having excluded upper GI, metabolic, and toxic diseases), psychogenic nausea and vomiting can be diagnosed with reasonable assurance.

Treatment

Comments like "Nothing is wrong" or "The problem is emotional" should be avoided. Therapeutic reassurance indicates awareness of the patient's discomfort and expresses the desire to work toward his relief, regardless of the etiology. Brief symptomatic treatment with antiemetics can be tried. Long-term management involves supportive, regular office visits, during which the patient may be helped to resolve his underlying problems.

GLOBUS SENSATION

("Lump in the Throat," Globus Hystericus)

The subjective sensation of a lump or mass in the throat. No specific etiology or physiologic mechanism has been established. Some studies suggest that elevated cricopharyngeal (upper esophageal sphincter) pressures or abnormal hypopharyngeal motility exist during the time of symptoms. The sensation may result from esophageal reflux or from frequent swallowing and drying of the throat associated with anxiety or other emotional states. Globus is probably a physiologic manifestation of certain mood states. It is not associated with a specific psychiatric disorder or set of stress factors. Certain individuals may have an inherent or learned predisposition to respond in this manner.

The sensation resembles the normal reaction of being "choked up" during events that elicit grief, pride, or even happiness from mastery of hardship; suppression of sadness is most often implicated. Clinically, chronic symptoms may occur during unresolved or pathologic grief and may be relieved by crying.

Diagnosis

Medical disorders that can be confused with globus sensation include cricopharyngeal or upper esophageal webs, symptomatic diffuse esophageal spasm, gastroesophageal reflux, skeletal muscle disorders (myasthenia gravis, myotonia dystrophica, polymyositis), or mass lesions in the neck or mediastinum causing esophageal compression. A careful history and physical examination can usually exclude these disorders. True dysphagia must be ruled out, for it would suggest a structural or motor disorder of the pharynx or esophagus. With globus, the symptoms occur during certain emotional states and do not worsen during swallowing. Food does not stick, and the symptom is often relieved with eating or drinking. There is no pain or weight loss.

If psychosocial features have been elicited and the physical examination is negative, the diagnosis is probable; if it is still in doubt, a CBC, plain or video-esophagogram, chest x-ray, and esophageal manometric study as indicated by the clinical data may exclude other disorders.

Treatment

Treatment involves reassurance and sympathetic concern. No medication is of proven benefit. Underlying depression, anxiety, or other behavioral disturbances should be managed in a supportive manner and psychiatric referral if necessary. At times, indicating the association of symptoms to the patient's mood state can be beneficial.

ADULT RUMINATION
(Merycism)

The usually involuntary regurgitation of small amounts of food from the stomach (most often 15 to 30 min after eating), rechewing the material and, in most cases, again swallowing it. It is commonly observed in the infant. The true incidence in adults is unknown, as it seems to be a private action, but in the past some persons offered public performances in which they selectively regurgitated objects swallowed at random. The pathophysiology is poorly understood. Only rarely have barium contrast studies been successful in showing the disturbance. The reverse peristalsis of animal ruminants has not been reported in humans. The few psychiatric studies available relate the act to an unconscious wish to attack or reject a threatening person or object.

Symptoms and Signs

Rumination is most often reported in patients with emotional disorders. During periods of stress, the patient may be less careful to conceal the act, and seeing it for the first time, others refer the patient to the physician. The patient reports no nausea, pain, or dysphagia.

Treatment

The general approach to the patient (see above) may disclose underlying emotional concerns. An upper GI series and esophageal manometry are necessary to exclude disorders causing mechanical obstruction, a Zenker's diverticulum, or motility disturbances. Endoscopy usually adds little to the clinical evaluation. Although drug therapy generally does not help, metoclopramide 10 mg orally qid, a stimulant of intestinal motor activity, has had varied success. Psychiatric consultation is often required when food is continually expectorated, leading to weight loss.

HALITOSIS, REAL AND IMAGINED
(See also Breath Odor in Ch. 246)

An unpleasant odor to the breath may be produced from ingested or inhaled substances that are excreted in part by the lungs, from gingival or dental disease, from fermentation of food particles in the mouth, or from an association with systemic diseases (eg, hepatic encephalopathy, diabetic acidosis, infectious or neoplastic disease of the respiratory tract). The esophagus is normally collapsed and separate from the airway. Although foul eructations may occur with gastric retention or gastric and esophageal tumors, GI disorders do not generally cause halitosis, and it is a fallacy that breath odor reflects the state of digestion and bowel function.

The response of others to halitosis is partly determined by adaptation and social factors. Thus, a person may be unaware of his or her own bad breath, and what is unpleasant to a stranger may not be to a spouse or relative.

Psychogenic halitosis, *an individual's complaint of bad breath, possibly based on psychologic factors that others do not perceive,* may occur during an anxiety state (eg, a teenager's first date). It may be reported by the hypochondriacal patient who commonly amplifies normal body sensations. At times the complaint may reflect a serious thinking disorder. The obsessional patient may have a pervading sense of uncleanliness, or the paranoid person may have the delusion that his organs are rotting.

Treatment

The removal or treatment of specific causes is effective. Extensive diagnostic evaluation should not be undertaken unless history and physical examination suggest an underlying disease. Attentive listening and reassurance help most patients with psychogenic halitosis. Persistence in this complaint despite reassurance may require psychiatric consultation.

53. GASTROINTESTINAL BLEEDING

Vomiting of blood **(hematemesis);** *passage of black tarry stool* **(melena);** *passage of gross blood per rectum* **(hematochezia).**

GI bleeding may originate anywhere from the mouth to the anus and may be overt or occult. **Hematemesis** or **"coffee ground" emesis** indicates an upper gastrointestinal **(UGI)** source of bleeding, almost always above the ligament of Treitz. Hematemesis often indicates brisk bleeding from the UGI tract, usually from an arterial source or varix. Coffee ground emesis results from bleeding that has slowed or stopped and from conversion of red Hb to brown hematin by gastric acid. **Hematochezia** usually indicates lower GI bleeding, but may result from vigorous UGI bleeding with rapid transit of blood through the intestines. **Melena** typically indicates UGI bleeding, but a small bowel or right colon bleeding source can present with melena. About 100 to 200 mL of blood in the UGI tract are required to produce melena. Melena may continue for several days after a severe hemorrhage and does not necessarily indicate continued bleeding. Black stool that is negative for occult blood may result from ingestion of iron, bismuth, or a variety of foods, and should not be mistaken for melena. Chronic occult bleeding can present as iron deficiency anemia if chronic, but may be detected by chemical testing of a stool specimen.

The common causes of GI bleeding are listed in TABLE 53–1.

Symptoms and Signs

The manifestations of GI bleeding depend upon the source, rate of bleeding, and the underlying or coexistent diseases. For example, the patient with underlying ischemic heart disease may present after brisk GI bleeding with angina or myocardial infarc-

TABLE 53–1. COMMON CAUSES OF GASTROINTESTINAL BLEEDING

Upper GI Tract			
Duodenal ulcer	(20–30%)	Mallory-Weiss tear	(5–10%)
Gastric or duodenal erosions	(20–30%)	Erosive esophagitis	(5–10%)
Varices	(15–20%)	Angioma	(5–10%)
Gastric ulcer	(10–20%)		
Lower GI tract (percentages vary with the age group sampled)			
Diverticular disease			
Colonic carcinoma			
Colonic polyps			
Inflammatory bowel disease: Ulcerative proctitis/colitis; Crohn's disease; infectious colitis			
Colitis: Radiation; ischemic			
Angiodysplasia (vascular ectasia)			
Hemorrhoids			
Anal fissures			
Small bowel lesions			
Meckel's diverticulum; neoplasm; angioma			

tion. Other important coexistent diseases may be aggravated by severe GI bleeding including heart failure, hypertension, pulmonary disease, renal failure, or diabetes mellitus. Massive bleeding may present as **shock** (see under Treatment, below, and SHOCK in Ch. 26). Lesser degrees of bleeding may be manifested as **orthostatic changes in pulse or BP,** (*a BP drop of* $\geq$ *10 mm Hg, or pulse rise* > *10/min on assuming the upright position*). Orthostatic changes can be elicited by first taking the BP and pulse in the supine position and then having the patient slowly assume the upright posture to repeat these measurements. Orthostatic changes must be interpreted with caution in patients with underlying heart disease, peripheral vascular disease, or those taking drugs known to influence peripheral vascular resistance. Patients with chronic blood loss may present with signs and symptoms of anemia (eg, weakness, easy fatigability, pallor, chest pain, or dizziness). Signs and symptoms of cirrhosis and portal hypertension may be evident. GI bleeding may precipitate **hepatic encephalopathy** (*mental status changes secondary to liver failure*) or **hepatorenal syndrome** (*kidney failure secondary to liver failure*).

Diagnosis and Differential Diagnosis

Although precise diagnoses are important, stabilization of the patient with transfusions and other treatment is essential before any diagnostic investigations. All patients require a complete history and physical examination, blood studies including coagulation studies (platelet count, prothrombin time, and partial thromboplastin time), and liver function tests (bilirubin, alkaline phosphatase, albumin, aspartate aminotransferase [AST, formerly SGOT], and alanine aminotransferase [ALT, formerly SGPT]), and repeated monitoring of Hb and Hct.

A history of epigastric abdominal pain that is relieved by food and/or antacids suggests peptic ulcer disease. However, many patients with ulcer bleeding have no history of pain. Weight loss and anorexia suggest a GI malignancy. Dysphagia suggests esophageal carcinoma or esophageal stricture. Vomiting and retching before the onset of bleeding might suggest a Mallory-Weiss tear of the esophagus, although about 50% of patients with Mallory-Weiss tears do not have this history. A history of bleeding (eg, purpura, ecchymosis, hematuria) may indicate a bleeding diathesis (eg, hemophilia). Bloody diarrhea, fever, and abdominal pain is consistent with inflammatory bowel disease (ulcerative colitis or Crohn's disease) or an infectious colitis (eg, *Shigella, Salmonella, Campylobacter*, amebiasis). Changes in bowel habits (constipation or diarrhea) with hematochezia or occult blood in the stool may be the first sign of a colon carcinoma or polyp, particularly in patients over age 45.

A drug history may reveal use of drugs that break the gastric barrier and damage the gastric mucosa (eg, aspirin and nonsteroidal anti-inflammatory agents). The amount and duration of ingestion of these substances are important. Many patients are unaware that many OTC cough remedies and analgesics contain aspirin.

Physical examination, after assessment of vital signs, includes careful examination of the nasopharynx to exclude the nose and throat as sources of bleeding. One should check for evidence of trauma, especially to the head, chest, and abdomen. Spider angiomas, hepatosplenomegaly, or ascites is consistent with chronic liver disease. Arteriovenous malformations, especially of the mucous membranes, may be associated with hereditary hemorrhagic telangiectasia (Rendu-Osler-Weber syndrome), in which multiple angiomas of the GI tract are associated with recurrent episodic bleeding.

No examination is complete without a digital rectal examination for masses, fissures, and hemorrhoids. Color of the stool (black, red, or maroon) should also be recorded. Chemical testing of a stool specimen for occult blood completes the examination.

A nasogastric aspiration and lavage should be done in all patients suspected of upper GI bleeding. **Panendoscopy** (*examination of the esophagus, stomach, and duodenum with a flexible endoscope*) offers the highest yield in making the diagnosis and

establishing the bleeding site. In acute UGI bleeding, an UGI barium x-ray series has no role. In addition to being less accurate than upper panendoscopy, the films are unable to detect which lesion is bleeding should there be more than one, and may interfere with a subsequent endoscopy or angiography, if either is necessary.

Nasogastric aspiration will usually diagnose an UGI source of bleeding and determine the rate of bleeding (coffee grounds indicate bleeding that is slow or stopped, but continuous bright red blood indicates active, vigorous bleeding). A nasogastric tube also can be helpful for continual monitoring of the bleeding status. About 10% of patients with an UGI bleeding source have a negative nasogastric aspirate.

If panendoscopy is unavailable, an UGI series can be performed after the patient is stable for ≥ 36 to 48 h. An UGI series should also be considered in a patient who has had definite evidence for UGI bleeding, but whose panendoscopy was negative or inconclusive. Adequate stabilization with restoration of blood volume should be done before the examination.

Hematochezia suggests a lower GI source of bleeding. Distal lesions (eg, hemorrhoids, inflammatory bowel disease, cancers, or polyps) are commonly seen at sigmoidoscopy, which is the usual first diagnostic test for evaluation of hematochezia. If sigmoidoscopy fails to establish a diagnosis, and active bleeding continues, further evaluation is indicated. Nasogastric aspiration should be performed to exclude an UGI source: If the aspirate is positive, an upper panendoscopy should be performed; if negative, elective or emergency colonoscopy is indicated, depending upon the severity of the hematochezia. Emergency colonoscopy in experienced hands after adequate bowel preparation (eg, oral sulfate purge to clear the gut of blood, clots, and stool) has a high yield in diagnosing colonic bleeding sites. Angiography and technetium-labeled RBC scans may be of value, but the magnitude of bleeding required to demonstrate the bleeding site limits their usefulness. If the bleeding rate is > 0.5 mL/min, angiography may show extravasation of contrast medium. In patients whose hematochezia stops, elective colonoscopy or air contrast barium enema should be performed. Colonoscopy will find lesions in about 10 to 50% of patients whose barium enema is nondiagnostic or reveals only diverticuli.

Occult bleeding often requires judicious use of GI x-rays and endoscopy to establish the diagnosis. The decision to use barium x-rays vs. colonoscopy depends upon a number of factors: local availability, expertise, and patient acceptance. Colonoscopy is generally preferred in lower GI bleeding, but the combination of contrast barium enema and sigmoidoscopy is an alternative when colonoscopy is not available or is refused by the patient. If initial study with a barium enema and sigmoidoscopy is negative or reveals only diverticula, colonoscopy should be done. If the lower GI study is negative and the patient has persistent evidence of occult bleeding from positive stool tests or symptoms suggestive of UGI disease, an UGI series or panendoscopy should be performed.

Treatment

Hematemesis, melena, or hematochezia should be considered an emergency until proven otherwise. Admission to an intensive care unit is recommended for all patients with severe GI bleeding; a team approach, including a gastroenterologist, surgeon, and skilled nurses, is essential. In all cases, a surgeon with expertise in GI surgery should be appraised of the situation, if not already consulted. A major cause of morbidity and mortality in patients with active GI bleeding is aspiration of blood with subsequent respiratory compromise, particularly in patients who have inadequate gag reflexes or who are obtunded or unconscious. To prevent this complication in such patients, endotracheal intubation should be considered to protect the airway.

Assessment and restoration of blood loss: Most GI bleeding stops spontaneously. However, major blood loss is manifested by a pulse rate > 110 beats/min, systolic BP

< 100 mm Hg (or it shows an orthostatic drop of 16 mm or more), oliguria, cold clammy extremities, and often mental status changes (confusion, disorientation, somnolence, loss of consciousness, or coma due to decreased cerebral perfusion). The Hct is a valuable index of blood loss, but may not be accurate if the bleeding has occurred over the preceding few hours, since complete restoration of blood volume by hemodilution may take several hours. Transfusions are usually given to maintain the Hct at about 30 if there is risk of further hemorrhage, if complicating vascular disease is present, or if the patient is > 40 yr old. Packed RBCs may be used instead of whole blood when heart disease makes it important not to overload the circulation. After an adequate blood volume is restored, the patient must be observed closely for such evidence of further bleeding as an increase in pulse rate, a drop in BP, vomiting of fresh blood, or a recurrence of loose, tarry stools (see also SHOCK in Ch. 26).

Continuous gastric aspiration via a nasogastric tube (preferably a Salem pump) may be used if the patient is vomiting and as a monitor of continuing or recurrent bleeding. A large (Ewald) tube may be helpful in cleaning out the stomach if there are clots, especially in preparation for diagnostic endoscopy.

Specific therapy depends upon the site of bleeding. Treatment of peptic ulcer after bleeding has been controlled is discussed in Ch. 54. Emergency operation is occasionally required to control acute bleeding or rebleeding, although endoscopic coagulation (with lasers, electrocoagulation, or heater probes) is available in some hospitals to control ulcer bleeding. Active variceal bleeding can be treated with vasopressin, esophagogastric (Sengstaken-Blakemore) or gastric (Linton) tamponade tubes, endoscopic sclerotherapy, or portal-systemic shunt surgery. No method is clearly superior. Angiography has a limited role in both the diagnosis and treatment of UGI bleeding. Should the lesion be identified, the catheter may be left in place for infusion of vasopressin or embolic therapy.

Most lower GI bleeding does not require specific emergency therapy. For severe, ongoing diverticular bleeding, surgery or angiography with intra-arterial infusion of vasopressin may be necessary. For severe bleeding from angioma of the colon, surgery or endoscopic coagulation have been used. Other lower GI bleeding lesions (eg, polyps or cancers) can be removed via colonoscopic polypectomy or laparotomy.

---

54. DISORDERS OF THE STOMACH AND DUODENUM

GASTRITIS

There is no single definition of "gastritis." The term is used by endoscopists, who base the diagnosis on appearances; by pathologists, who define it on the basis of histologic appearances; by radiologists, from gross changes in mucosal profiles; and by clinicians, using none of the objective methods, who assume the presence of gastritis when, in a suggestive clinical setting (alcoholism, taking of nonsteroidals, or serious illness), dyspepsia or upper GI bleeding occur.

Strictly defined, gastritis means *inflammation of the gastric mucosa*, and, in the first instance, gastritis should be described according to histologic criteria. By such criteria, gastritis may or may not be present when the diagnosis is suggested by clinical, radiologic, or even endoscopic means. Even given all the information, no completely satisfactory general classification exists.

The stomach is composed of (1) the metabolically active acid and pepsin secreting body and fundus, and (2) the endocrine and motor antrum. Either may be affected separately or both together in many of the categories of gastritis.

Histologically, gastritis is first divided into erosive and nonerosive; within each group the inflammation, if it exists, may be acute (polymorphonuclear infiltration) or chronic (round cell infiltration). The latter is much more common, though the 2 may coexist. Chronic nonspecific nonerosive gastritis may be superficial or deep (transmucosal), with or without gland atrophy or metaplasia. Gastritis with advancing age is so common that some consider it to be an epiphenomenon of aging.

Erosive gastritis is best diagnosed endoscopically, and clinically may be either acute erosive gastritis (stress ulcer) or chronic nonspecific erosive gastritis (aphthous ulcer).

ACUTE GASTRITIS

(Acute Erosive Gastritis; Acute Stress Erosion; Acute Gastric Ulcer; Acute Hemorrhagic Gastritis)

Superficial, mucosal lesions of the stomach that occur very rapidly in relation to a variety of stresses.

Etiology and Pathology

This condition is perhaps clinically the most important and the most serious. Typically it occurs in the setting of acute, severe trauma or illness (often in an intensive care unit **[ICU]**), and may include one or more of the following: (a) extensive trauma, especially with added shock, anoxia, sepsis, or organ failure of liver, kidneys, heart or lungs, or with diseases in which coagulation factors have failed; (b) burns, seldom with < 20% BSA, almost always with > 40% BSA burn; (c) head injury, including Cushing's ulcer; and (d) hemorrhage, rarely with bleeding requiring < 4 u. of blood for resuscitation, but frequent with > 10 u.

Symptoms, Signs, and Diagnosis

Typically, the patient may be too ill to complain of noticeable gastric symptoms, which are usually (if present) mild and nonspecific dyspepsia. The first obvious sign may be blood in the nasogastric aspirate, usually within 2 to 5 days of the major initial stress.

Diagnosis is made endoscopically; in certain patients mentioned above (burns, shock, sepsis), acute erosions may be seen within a few hours. These most often begin in the fundus as petechiae or ecchymoses that progress to irregular small ulcers varying from 2 to 20 mm. At this first stage, they seldom bleed and histologically are confined to the mucosa; they may heal rapidly upon correction or removal of stress. The lesions may progress to invade the submucosa and even perforate the serosa or, more commonly, may bleed, usually from multiple sites (both fundus and antrum may be involved). In head injury, unlike the other states, acid secretion is increased, rather than decreased, and the lesions (Cushing's ulcer) may involve the duodenum as well or exclusively.

Treatment

Once torrential bleeding occurs (in about 2% of ICU patients), the reported mortality is > 60%. Transfusion of many units of blood may further impair hemostasis. A wide variety of surgical and nonsurgical treatments have been used, but few have been shown conclusively to improve the outcome. Treatments havc included antisecretory ulcer medications, vasoconstrictors (eg, ice water lavage, intragastric levarterenol, intra-arterial vasopressin or somatostatin via angiographically placed catheters); angiographic technics (eg, arterial occlusion), or coagulation. Surgery of various types has been performed. Except for total gastrectomy, continued bleeding is common, and mortality equals that for medical treatment. Endoscopic coagulation technics temporarily halt bleeding, but bleeding recurs if the background illness is unimproved.

It is most important to try to prevent or halt the progression of acute erosions. Reports of reduction in the incidence of bleeding by preventing acidification of the

gastric lumen with antacids or H_2 histamine-receptor antagonists have led to the widespread use of around-the-clock antacid instillation and IV cimetidine or ranitidine after surgery and in most ICUs. Some authorities doubt the value of these treatments and attribute better results to great improvement in the level of critical care and an increase in the number of competently staffed ICUs. Rapid evacuation and resuscitation of injury and burn victims; prevention and treatment of shock (central venous pressure, Swan-Ganz catheter), hemoconcentration, anoxemia (frequently monitored blood gases and rapid correction), and sepsis; early and appropriate use of blood replacement in hemorrhage; monitoring and treatment of coagulopathies; improvement of controlled anesthesia; and dialysis have together greatly reduced the incidence of severe hemorrhagic erosive gastritis.

CHRONIC EROSIVE GASTRITIS

Presence of multiple punctate or aphthous stomach ulcers. Based largely on endoscopic findings, the disorder includes various entities whose etiology may be known or suspected (eg, drugs, Crohn's disease, viral infection), or idiopathic. Symptoms are nonspecific, including mild nausea, epigastric discomfort, or may even be absent (eg, in many chronic aspirin users).

Idiopathic chronic erosive gastritis presents with vague dyspeptic or ulcer-like symptoms, and endoscopy reveals erosions most often on the ridges of thickened folds in the body or antrum of the stomach, some of which may have healed and left scars. Histologically these lesions may or may not show associated gastritis (infiltration of inflammatory cells). Differential diagnosis includes the specific causes discussed below, lymphoma, and superficial cancer. Treatment is symptomatic with antacids, and avoidance of potentially etiologic drugs and foods (eg, pickles, spices). The condition may be transitory or may persist or recur, even for years. If it persists or recurs, an evaluation for systemic disease (eg, sarcoid, amyloid immune deficiency) and of diet, drugs, and drinking habits, and viral culture for herpes and cytomegalovirus (CMV) should be undertaken. (Herpes may also present as a diffuse, shaggy, generalized, exudative gastritis and concurrently involve the esophagus and duodenum.)

Specific chronic erosive gastritis: Known causes for the punctate ulcers that characterize this condition include aspirin and most nonsteroidal anti-inflammatory drugs **(NSAIDs),** more so in alcoholics; Crohn's disease; and viral infections.

Most commonly, NSAIDs produce lesions in the antrum, probably because of gravity in ambulatory patients, but ulcers also occur in the fundus, especially in recumbent patients. Patient susceptibility varies for unknown reasons. In those who consume both alcohol and aspirin, mucosal damage may be more widespread and frequently involves the body, fundus, and antrum. Lesions seldom penetrate beyond the submucosa, and inflammation and fibrosis are usually absent. The incidence of lesions is generally dose-dependent and varies from 25 to 100% in those taking ≥ 6 aspirin tablets/day. Ulcer production is thought to be due to cell damage from salicylate derived from aspirin hydrolyzed after gaining entry into the cell. The incidence of lesions is greater with mucosa exposed to aspirin directly, especially in an acid environment. Enteric-coated aspirin produces fewer lesions than uncoated aspirin.

Crohn's disease: Ulcerating lesions of Crohn's disease may occur anywhere in the GI tract mucosa. They are usually 1 to 2 mm, circular with an erythematous collar, but may be irregular in shape, and seldom number > 4 or 5. Granulomas are seen on biopsy in < 50%. Symptomatic upper GI lesions occur in about 5% of patients and may require systemic steroid treatment (see Ch. 59).

NONEROSIVE GASTRITIS

A general category of idiopathic gastritis including several manifestations based largely on histologic findings. The antrum and the body/fundus are considered separately.

The most useful classification considers inflammation, atrophy, and metaplasia. First, gastritis (inflammatory cell infiltrate) is divided into superficial and deep, or transmucosal, that involves the whole mucosa, extending to the muscularis mucosa. A second, parallel description of the mucosa includes the state of the gastric glands—preserved, with variable loss (partial atrophy) or with complete loss (gastric mucosal atrophy). A third set of conditions depends on the degree and type of metaplasia (see below). Loss of glands or metaplasia may occur with or without gastritis and vice versa.

Precision calls for careful use of the terms: (1) **gastritis** (superficial, deep), (2) **gland atrophy** (none, partial, complete), and (3) **metaplasia** (type). The 3 descriptions should be individually addressed. To be more exact, the anatomic source of the biopsy (above or below the angulus and distance from pylorus or esophagus, which wall or curvature of the stomach, and relation to chronic lesion (eg, cancer or ulcer) should be known. A definitive diagnosis depends upon finding the same appearances in more than one location.

GASTRITIS

The etiology is unknown. Only a small fraction of patients with atrophic gastritis have autoantibodies to parietal cells compared to a high proportion in pernicious anemia. Gastritis may remain stationary, recover completely, progress from superficial to deep, or may worsen, inducing gland atrophy or metaplasia.

Superficial gastritis: The predominant infiltrating cells in gastritis are round cells with an admixture of plasma cells; inflammation is superficial and may be patchy. It may involve only the fundus or the antrum or both. The condition may resolve or progress, sometimes slowly. It is usually unaccompanied by atrophy or metaplasia and has no significant medical implications. It occurs more often with advancing age and is common over age 40. There are no typical symptoms, and gastritis is frequently asymptomatic. There is also no reliable endoscopic appearance and even normal appearing mucosa may be affected.

Deep gastritis is more likely to be symptomatic (vague dyspepsia), but, again, it correlates poorly with endoscopic appearances; round cells infiltrate the entire mucosa down to the muscularis, but seldom with exudate or crypt abscesses. Lesions may be patchy and may coexist with areas of superficial gastritis. Partial gland atrophy and metaplasia may be present. Deep gastritis is almost always present in postgastrectomy gastric remnants (see below). It is always present in the vicinity of gastric ulcers and cancers and is more common in relatives of patients with gastric cancer.

ATROPHY

Fundus: Because glands in the body and fundus are abundant, the diagnosis and degree of atrophy can be reliably determined. Atrophy may follow injury of various kinds, especially gastritis. Atrophy and gastritis can be found in about 50% of persons over age 50 yr; the extent and degree increases with age. **Antrum:** Because glands are shallower and less abundant, the degree of atrophy is less easily determined. By age 40, there is partial atrophy in 1/3 of persons; the antrum is more commonly affected than the fundus.

Symptoms, Signs, Diagnosis, and Treatment

All degrees of atrophy may occur without specific symptoms. Endoscopic appearances are not definitive, and the mucosa may appear normal until atrophy is advanced, when the submucosal vascular tree may be visible. The appearance of the fundus in pernicious anemia **(PA)** is characteristic of advanced atrophy (see below).

As atrophy becomes complete, not only acid and pepsin secretion diminish, but intrinsic factor may be lost, resulting in vitamin B_{12} malabsorption. Serum gastrin (lacking feedback control) rises, but is seldom very high except in complete atrophy. Pepsinogen I in plasma derives from the fundus and declines with atrophy and loss of peptic cells. Pepsinogen II, a much smaller amount, derives from antrum, which may or may not be atrophic. If it is normal, as in PA, the ratio PG-I:PG-II, normally > 20, falls and may be < 1. Urinary pepsinogen is all PG-I and disappears in fundic atrophy.

No definitive treatment is known and symptomatic treatment is usually confined to a diet selected to avoid symptoms.

Metaplasia

Gastric mucosa may exhibit metaplasia into types of mucosa different from the original. In atrophic gastritis, metaplasia of fundic mucosa to antral type is most common. Thus, the antral mucosa appears to replace the fundic progressively, especially along the lower curvature **(antral creep)** and occurs commonly with advancing age. Gastric ulcers are said to occur most commonly at the junction of antral and fundic mucosae; whether as cause or consequence of the antrification is not clear. Later, mucosal transformation may alter the mucosa to resemble small bowel, with goblet cells, endocrine cells, rudimentary villi, and even the functional (absorptive) characteristics of small bowel mucosa. Intestinalization always occurs first in the antrum and may then extend from the antrum to the fundus. Metaplasia has not been identified as a precursor to cancer.

SPECIAL CATEGORIES OF GASTRITIS

Postgastrectomy Gastritis

Except in cases of gastrinoma, atrophic gastritis always occurs early after partial or subtotal gastrectomy, and metaplasia of the remaining fundic mucosa occurs commonly. The degree and extent of gastritis is usually greatest at the stoma (stomatitis).

Several causes are possible: (1) Vagotomy may result in a loss of vagal trophic action. (2) Bile bathing the gastric mucosa may be damaging. Bile reflux (bilious vomiting) is a mechanical problem, but surgery devised to divert bile from the stomach is often disappointing. Medical treatments are uniformly unsuccessful. (3) Loss of antral gastrin, the gastrotrophic hormone, results in greater loss of parietal than peptic cells. Thus, patients with gastrinomas who have had partial gastrectomy do not have atrophic gastritis despite the presence of both acid and bile.

Endoscopy and histologic appearance do not always coincide and symptoms usually do not match the presence or degree of gastritis. Postgastrectomy gastritis usually progresses to severe atrophy and eventual achlorhydria. Intrinsic factor may be lost and some patients may become vitamin B_{12} deficient (bacterial overgrowth in the afferent loop may contribute to B_{12} deficiency).

Pernicious Anemia (PA)

(See also in Chs. 81 and 96)

Addisonian PA may be defined as *the absence of intrinsic factor* **(IF)** *associated with complete atrophy of the fundic mucosa* and loss of parietal cells. Atrophy is usually

complete when the disease is diagnosed, generally after age 50; it is not known when the process begins, nor the stages through which PA passes. At the stage of discovery, no inflammation is present; ie, the pathologic process is one of atrophy without gastritis. The antrum is spared in > 80% of patients with PA and, because there is no acid, gastrin cells increase in number and serum gastrin is high (often 1000 to 6000 pg/mL). It is not clear whether the 20% who have atrophy of the antrum have true PA or are a subset presenting as the last stage in generalized gastritis.

Several findings point to an immunologic and inherited basis for this disease. In PA, 90% of patients have antibodies to parietal cells, compared to < 20% of non-PA patients with advanced atrophic gastritis; antibodies to intrinsic factor (either IF-blocking or -binding) are found in 60% of PA. Half of the PA patients have associated thyroid antibodies; conversely, parietal cell antibodies are found in 30% of patients with thyroiditis. Twenty percent have adrenocortical antibodies and may have Addison's disease. Vitiligo may also occur in PA. T cell antibodies occur in 85% of PA. From 10 to 20% of relatives of PA patients exhibit a PA-like gastritis and atrophy, with 65% exhibiting parietal cell antibodies and 20% intrinsic factor antibodies.

For diagnosis and treatment of PA see under ANEMIA DUE TO VITAMIN B_{12} DEFICIENCY in Ch. 96. The question of surveillance for the development of gastric cancer is not settled. The relative increase in risk (threefold over age-matched population controls) probably requires endoscopy about q 5 yr. There are no good clinical or histologic markers by which to screen such persons.

EPIDEMIC GASTRITIS

There are several reports of sudden illness with dyspepsia; malodorous breath; abdominal pain; loss of ability to secrete acid for a variable period up to a year or more; a mucoid, (perhaps alkaline) gastric secretion and elevated serum or urinary pepsinogen, (parietal cell antibodies are not found); and, in some persons, a newly developed pyloric or duodenal peptic ulcer. These cases have been reported from laboratories performing multiple gastric analyses, usually in otherwise healthy volunteers, and gastric biopsies have shown severe gastritis. Seventeen cases, including a patient with gastrinoma, occurred in one epidemic. The epidemiology suggested an infectious agent. An investigator, suspecting that the agent was *Campylobacter pyloridis*, swallowed 10^9 organisms and developed hunger upon awakening, irritability, headache, bad breath, and gastritis on biopsy, with recovery of organisms sensitive to metronidazole and bismuth citrate. He became asymptomatic after 2 wk. Epidemic gastritis may be representative of gastritis at large and other infectious agents may be capable of producing it.

UNCOMMON SPECIFIC GASTRITIS SYNDROMES

Ménétrier's disease: *A disorder of unknown cause manifested by very large, thick gastric folds; with large glands, little inflammation, and cystic dilation, occasionally involving the submucosa, and often confined to the body and fundus* (ie, the antrum is commonly spared). Characteristically, acid and pepsin secretion are decreased and there is loss of serum protein, often enough to cause hypoalbuminemic edema, which, with anorexia and epigastric pain, may be the presenting symptoms. X-ray and endoscopy show huge folds that never cross the pylorus (only lymphomatous folds do). Ménétrier's disease usually affects adults aged 30 to 60 and is usually chronic, but can be reversible. Metaplasia and loss of parietal cells may occur and adenocarcinoma develops in about 10%.

Differential diagnosis includes lymphoma, in which multiple gastric ulcers often occur, pseudolymphoma with an extensive infiltrate of lymphocytes, carcinoma (linitis plastica), hypertrophic acid-hypersecreting gastropathy (with Zollinger-Ellison, or without hypergastrinemia) and the **Cronkite-Canada syndrome,** a mucosal polypoid

protein-losing condition also affecting the bowel, with alactasia and diarrhea. A full thickness or deep snare biopsy in conjunction with the clinical state is helpful in making a diagnosis. Gastric resection may be necessary for severe hypoalbuminemia. Medical treatment is not helpful.

Eosinophilic gastritis, *a condition with extensive infiltration of the mucosa (and occasionally the full stomach wall thickness) with eosinophils, frequently involving the antrum and intestine.* It may result from nematode infestation. If obstruction of the pylorus occurs and steroids are ineffective, surgery may be required.

Plasma cell gastritis is a manifestation of **systemic mastocytosis** in which a pigmented skin rash, gastric acid hypersecretion, and diarrhea may be presenting symptoms. Treatment of the hypersecretory state with H_2 antagonists, especially ranitidine, may be sufficient to control the condition.

Pseudolymphoma, *a condition of massive lymphoid hyperplasia* resembling Ménétrier's disease has no known cause and is diagnosed by the finding of nonuniform lymphoid cell populations on monoclonal antibody staining, as opposed to a uniform population of lymphocytes in lymphoma.

For **Zollinger-Ellison syndrome,** see in CANCER OF THE PANCREAS in Ch. 55.

Other causes for gastritis include **systemic disorders** (eg, sarcoid, TB, syphilis, amyloid, and other granulomatous disease) that are rare and seldom of primary importance.

Physical causes for gastritis include ingestion of corrosives and radiation; 1600 rads will produce marked deep gastritis; 4500 rads affects antrum more than fundus, and causes gastritis with ulceration, even perforation, scarring, and permanent partial atrophy; rarely pyloric stenosis may result.

Infectious (septic) gastritis: Following ischemia, corrosives, or irradiation, bacteria may invade the gastric mucosa, causing acute phlegmonous gastritis with gas outlining the mucosa. The condition presents as an acute abdomen and carries a very high mortality. Surgery is mandatory.

Debilitated or immunocompromised hosts may develop viral or fungal gastritis with candida, histoplasmosis, mucormycosis; these diagnoses should be considered in patients found to have exudative gastritis, esophagitis, or duodenitis.

PEPTIC ULCER

A circumscribed ulceration of the mucous membrane penetrating through the muscularis mucosa and occurring in areas exposed to acid and pepsin.

Peptic ulcers occur most commonly in the first few centimeters of the duodenum, known as the duodenal bulb **(duodenal ulcers)**; they are also common along the lesser curvature of the stomach **(gastric ulcers)**. Less frequently, ulcers occur in the pyloric canal **(channel ulcers)**, in the duodenum just beyond the bulb **(postbulbar ulcers)**, or in a Meckel's diverticulum containing islets of secreting gastric mucosa. Following gastrojejunostomy, with or without partial gastrectomy, ulcers may develop in the stomach at the margin of the anastomosis **(marginal or stomal ulcers)**, or in the jejunum just beyond the anastomosis **(jejunal ulcers)**. Ulcers may also occur in the lower end of the esophagus. **Stress ulcers** appearing in severe illness or trauma are discussed in ACUTE GASTRITIS, above.

Etiology

Peptic ulcer occurs only if the stomach secretes acid. Most people secrete acid; < 1:10 develop ulcers. There appears to be a balance between ulcer-promoting factors (eg, secretion of acid or pepsin into the stomach) and factors protecting the stomach's mucosal lining (eg, mucus production, membrane barriers to permeability, and replacement of shed or damaged mucosal cells). Many influences can disturb this bal-

ance, but the immediate cause of peptic ulcer remains unknown. The causes of gastric and duodenal ulcers may differ; gastric ulcer, unlike duodenal ulcer, tends to develop later in life and is not associated with increased acid secretion. Certain drugs, (especially aspirin, other nonsteroidal anti-inflammatory drugs, and possibly corticosteroids) predispose to the formation of upper GI ulcers that tend to heal when the drug is discontinued and are unlikely to recur unless the drug is taken again. An ulcer penetrates the muscularis mucosa. If it does not, the lesion is an erosion. The drugs mentioned may be associated with erosion or ulcer.

Pathology

A single ulcer is most common, but 2 and occasionally more (duodenal, gastric, or both) are encountered. **Gastric ulcers** usually occur along the lesser curvature of the stomach where the pyloric glands border the oxyntic glands; they may vary from a few mm to several cm. Surrounding gastritis usually is present. **Duodenal ulcers,** usually found within 3 cm of the pylorus, also vary in size but tend to be smaller than gastric ulcers. They average about 1 cm in diameter.

Ulcers are usually round or oval, with sharp margins. The surrounding mucosa is often hyperemic and edematous. Ulcers penetrate into the submucosa or muscular layer. A thin layer of gray or white exudate usually covers the crater base, which is composed of fibrinoid, granulation, and fibrous tissue layers. During healing, fibrous tissue in the base contracts the ulcer and may distort the surrounding tissue. Granulation tissue fills the base, and, in the process of healing, epithelium from the edges covers its surface.

Duodenal ulcers are almost always benign, but a gastric ulcer may be malignant. Malignant degeneration within a benign gastric ulcer is a rare event. However, a malignant gastric ulcer may occasionally be mistaken for a benign gastric ulcer, even, rarely, appearing to heal on treatment.

Symptoms and Signs

The usual peptic ulcer has a chronic, recurrent course. Symptoms vary with its location and the patient's age; complaints may be atypical in children (see CHILDHOOD PEPTIC ULCER in Ch. 194) and minimal in the elderly. Some patients may not have symptoms; others report them for the first time when a complication (see COMPLICATIONS OF PEPTIC ULCER, below) develops. Only about 1/2 of patients present with the characteristic pattern of symptoms. Typical pain is described as burning, gnawing, or aching, but distress may also be described as soreness, an empty feeling, or hunger. Typical pain is steady, mild or moderately severe, located in a well-circumscribed area, almost always epigastric, and relieved by antacids or milk.

In patients with **duodenal ulcer,** typically, *the pattern of pain* tends to be consistent: It is absent when the patient awakens, but appears in mid-morning; it is relieved by food, but recurs 2 or 3 h after a meal. Pain that awakens the patient at 1 or 2 AM is common and highly suggestive of ulcer. Frequently the pain occurs once or more each day for one to several weeks, and may then disappear without treatment. However, recurrence is usual, often within the first 2 yr, occasionally after several years. Patients often learn by experience when a recurrence is likely (eg, commonly in spring and fall and during episodes of life stress).

The symptoms of **gastric ulcer** often do not follow the duodenal ulcer pattern, and eating may cause rather than relieve the pain; this is especially true for **pyloric channel ulcer.** Because of edema or scarring, pyloric ulcers also often have symptoms of obstruction (eg, bloating after eating, or nausea and vomiting). The pain of **postbulbar ulcer** may be unrelated to meals. With **esophageal ulcer** or esophagitis, pain tends to occur when the patient swallows or lies down.

Complications of peptic ulcer are discussed below.

Diagnosis and Differential Diagnosis

Diagnosis is suggested by the symptoms and confirmed by the studies described below. Gastric cancer may present with similar manifestations and is discussed below in NEOPLASMS OF THE STOMACH. Endoscopic appearances, cytology, and multiple biopsies are generally reliable ways to distinguish benign from malignant gastric ulcer. When patients present with a severe ulcer diathesis, especially when ulcers are noted in atypical locations, the presence of a gastrinoma and the Zollinger-Ellison syndrome should be considered (see CANCER OF THE PANCREAS in Ch. 55).

Endoscopy (see above in Ch. 50) usually can establish the diagnosis. Increasingly, many clinicians recommend endoscopy in preference to x-ray as the initial diagnostic procedure. However, even in experienced hands, endoscopy may overlook as many as 5 to 10% of gastric or duodenal ulcers. Thus, if the clinical picture warrants it, a negative endoscopy might be supplemented by a barium contrast study. Endoscopy is generally the only way to identify esophageal ulcers or esophagitis and acute gastric or duodenal erosions, since these lesions are usually too shallow to be identified by x-ray. Endoscopy is also more reliable in the discovery of craters in the duodenum, posterior wall of the stomach, and sites of surgical anastomosis not demonstrable by x-ray. Endoscopy in conjunction with multiple biopsies helps to identify malignant gastric ulcers. A **cytologic search** for tumor cells in gastric washings and with gastric brushing technics can be helpful in experienced laboratories to identify malignant gastric ulcers.

X-ray studies with barium: fluoroscopy is important to distinguish ulcer craters from barium trapped between gastric folds. In about ½ of patients with duodenal ulcer, a crater cannot be shown. Deformity of the duodenal bulb is suggestive, but not conclusive evidence of an active duodenal ulcer, since scarring of a healed ulcer, as well as edema and spasm secondary to an active ulcer, can cause deformity. Technics using air contrast have greatly improved the accuracy of x-ray studies.

Gastric analysis: Gastric secretory studies may be useful to demonstrate achlorhydria or hypersecretion. To obtain reliable findings, the position of the aspirating tube is checked by fluoroscopy and the adequacy of drainage (of a continuous suction machine) is also checked by hand aspiration. Achlorhydria (eg, in pernicious anemia) is diagnosed by the failure of gastric juice pH to fall below 6.5 with maximum stimulation (pentagastrin 6 μg/kg s.c.). Gastric analysis is indicated where ulcers recur frequently or respond poorly to treatment. High rates of basal and stimulated secretion may suggest Zollinger-Ellison syndrome; the diagnosis is confirmed by an elevated fasting serum gastrin associated with acid hypersecretion. All duodenal ulcer patients should have fasting serum gastrin measured if the ulcer recurs after treatment (see also CANCER OF THE PANCREAS in Ch. 55). Any patient considered for ulcer surgery should have preoperative gastric analysis.

Treatment

Treatment of gastric and duodenal ulcer is designed to neutralize or decrease gastric acidity (even though gastric acidity is usually normal in patients with gastric ulcer). If symptoms do not subside within a few days of such therapy, the diagnosis may be incorrect; the patient may have a complication—often penetration; the therapeutic regimen may not be adequate; or the patient may not be following the regimen.

Healing commonly requires from 4 to 8 wk and may require a longer time, particularly for large or longstanding ulcers. **Gastric ulcers** should be monitored by regular x-ray or endoscopic examination, preferably the latter, until healing is complete. Treatment is maintained until healing is confirmed, because otherwise the ulcer can be only presumed to be benign. If complete healing does not occur, the ulcer should be biopsied to rule out cancer.

Duodenal ulcers heal in 4 to 6 wk in about 80% of persons, but demonstration of

healing by endoscopy is less critical, since they are almost never malignant. Most patients are advised to follow the regimen for the period that experience suggests is required for healing.

Antacids give symptomatic relief, promote healing, and reduce recurrences. In general, there are 2 types: (1) **Absorbable antacids** provide rapid, complete neutralization. Sodium bicarbonate and calcium carbonate, the most potent antacids, are occasionally taken for short-term or intermittent relief, but because they are absorbable, continuous use may cause alkalosis or the **milk-alkali syndrome.** Since symptoms of this complication are not distinctive (nausea, headache, weakness), the disorder may progress unrecognized to irreversible kidney damage. These soluble antacids should generally be avoided.

(2) **Nonabsorbable antacids** (*relatively insoluble salts of weak bases*) are preferred because of fewer side effects. They interact with hydrochloric acid forming nonabsorbed or poorly absorbed salts, thereby increasing gastric pH. Pepsin activity diminishes as the pH rises above 4, and pepsin may be adsorbed by some antacids. Antacids may interfere with the absorption of other drugs (eg, tetracycline, digoxin, and iron).

Aluminum hydroxide is a relatively safe, commonly used antacid. Phosphate depletion may rarely develop as a result of binding of phosphate by aluminum in the GI tract. Symptoms include anorexia, weakness, and malaise. The risk of phosphorus depletion increases in alcoholics and patients with renal disease, including those on hemodialysis. Aluminum hydroxide may cause constipation.

Magnesium hydroxide is a more effective antacid than aluminum hydroxide and is a mild cathartic, but may cause diarrhea. Since aluminum hydroxide tends to be constipating, many proprietary antacids contain both magnesium and aluminum hydroxides; some contain aluminum hydroxide and magnesium trisilicate. The latter tends to have less neutralizing potency. With magnesium hydroxide, bowel movements will usually be regular if 4 doses of 15 to 30 mL are taken daily; > 4 doses may cause diarrhea. Since small amounts of magnesium are absorbed, magnesium preparations should be given cautiously to patients with renal damage.

Dosage regimens: Antacid preparations vary in their neutralizing capacity with the method of measurement, from patient to patient, and in the same patient from time to time. Effectiveness, cost, and patient preference determine the choice of antacid. Optimal bowel function may require titration with different antacids. The optimal regimen appears to be 15 to 30 mL of liquid or 2 to 4 tablets 1 h and 3 h after each meal and at bedtime. Tablets tend to be more convenient but less effective than liquids. If antacids are used for primary treatment of ulcer, they should be given for 6 wk for duodenal and 8 wk for gastric ulcer.

Histamine H_2 receptor blocking agents (see also in Ch. 285): Most physicians prefer these agents. The largest experience to date has been with cimetidine and ranitidine; similar drugs are under study. Cimetidine 300 mg with each meal and at bedtime or ranitidine 150 mg bid lowers gastric acidity and promotes healing of duodenal and gastric ulcer. A single bedtime dose of cimetidine 400 mg or ranitidine 150 to 300 mg may be equally effective. While symptoms are commonly relieved within 1 wk, healing may take 4 to 8 wk and occasionally longer. A fraction of duodenal (10%) and gastric (10 to 20%) ulcers do not respond. With anastomotic and stomal ulcers, promising reports need further evaluation.

Both drugs have so far proved to be safe in both short- and long-term use. However, there have been slight elevations of aminotransferase and serum creatinine, and rare cases of gynecomastia. Drowsiness, tiredness, dizziness, diarrhea, and rash, slightly more common in patients receiving cimetidine than placebo, were seen in < 2% of patients. Some abnormalities (eg, those of aminotransferase and creatinine) may clear even while the patient continues the drug. Ranitidine penetrates the blood-brain bar-

rier less readily than cimetidine and is much less likely to cause mental confusion, especially in the elderly or severely ill patient treated with cimetidine. Rare side effects of ranitidine (< 2%) include headache and diarrhea.

Dosages of other drugs being given should be reviewed because cimetidine may alter the metabolism or prolong the action of some drugs by decreasing hepatic microsomal enzyme activity (eg, diazepam, theophylline, digoxin, and warfarin). Ranitidine does not cause gynecomastia and, unlike cimetidine, does not affect the hepatic microsomal enzyme-dependent (P-450) metabolism of other drugs.

An antacid and/or an anticholinergic may be added to a cimetidine or ranitidine regimen in persons difficult to treat.

Sucralfate is a sucrose-aluminum complex reported to combine with proteins to form a protective coating in the base of the ulcer that promotes healing. Beneficial in all peptic ulcers, it offers a reasonable alternative at a cost comparable to other forms of therapy. The recommended dosage is 1 gm tid or qid. It is not absorbed, and causes no systemic effects, but may cause constipation.

Anticholinergics are used much less frequently now in ulcer treatment, except as an adjunct when H_2 antagonists fail to control disease in hypersecretors. They can cause dry mouth and blurred vision; dosage is adjusted for each patient to just below that which produces these effects. Common doses are poldine 4 mg, glycopyrrolate 1 mg, propantheline 7 to 15 mg, or isopropamide 5 mg, given orally before each meal and at bedtime. Occasionally, tincture of belladonna is used because the dose can be precisely titrated; the dosage may range from 0.6 to 1.0 mL (0.18 to 0.3 mg) qid.

Difficulty urinating, evidence of acute narrow-angle glaucoma, or gastric retention **contraindicates** the use of anticholinergics. Complete pyloric obstruction may develop in patients with partial obstruction; urinary retention and glaucoma occur most often in patients over age 50. Patients with esophageal ulcers or esophagitis should not be given anticholinergics, as they may impair the efficiency of the lower esophageal sphincter.

Certain prostaglandins seem promising because they inhibit gastric secretion and appear to protect gastric mucosa against damaging drugs (see Ch. 284). Various analogs of prostaglandin E_2 and others suitable for oral use are in clinical trials for the treatment of both duodenal and gastric ulcer.

Additional agents, mainly used outside the USA, have been reported effective. These include **sulpiride,** said to act on the hypothalamus as a neuroleptic and to diminish vagally stimulated gastric secretion, and **several bismuth-containing preparations** (including zolimidine and colloidal bismuth subcitrate) with an action similar to that of sucralfate (see above) described in Scandinavian and British literature. **Carbenoxolone** is reported to have beneficial effects on the gastric and duodenal mucosa, but it may cause Na retention, edema, hypertension, and/or hypokalemia. The extent of these aldosterone-like side effects tends to correspond with the dose and duration of treatment. Caution should be exercised in patients with cardiovascular, pulmonary, or renal impairment, and especially hypertension.

Omeprazole, a substituted benzimidazole, is a potent inhibitor of the proton (acid) pump, the enzyme H^+K^+ATPase, which is located in the apical secretory membrane of the parietal cell. It can completely inhibit acid secretion and has a long duration of action. In early reports of clinical testing in duodenal (but not gastric) ulcer, virtually 100% healing occurred within 2 to 4 wk. However, recurrences after stopping treatment were not prevented. The long-term safety of omeprazole is not established.

Other medications: Evidence of coexistent anxiety or depression should be treated appropriately, keeping in mind that the most potent "therapeutic agent" is the physician as a sympathetic listener and strong supportive figure. Sedatives or tranquilizers (eg, chlordiazepoxide 5 to 10 mg orally 1 to 4 times/day) may be helpful, but should be

prescribed only for clear nonulcer indications. Prochlorperazine 5 mg 1 to 4 times/day may be given if nausea is a problem. If nausea persists > 2 or 3 days, pyloric obstruction or another cause should be ruled out.

Aspirin and aspirin-containing drugs, other nonsteroidal anti-inflammatory agents, corticosteroids, and reserpine should be *avoided*, if possible.

Diet: No firm evidence proves that any diet speeds healing or prevents recurrence. Thus, many physicians eliminate only foods that cause the patient distress (eg, fruit juices, spicy, and fatty foods). Pepper, the only food that objective studies suggest is harmful, and coffee (even decaffeinated) may produce ulcer-like dyspepsia in some persons and should be avoided. Snacks between meals can be encouraged, but while food may neutralize acid, it also stimulates acid secretion. **Alcohol,** which can also stimulate acid secretion, is commonly restricted to dilute solutions in small amounts. **Smoking** delays or prevents ulcer healing and ulcer patients are well advised to stop smoking.

Nocturnal pain: An occasional patient awakens several hours after retiring despite control of daytime symptoms. Cimetidine 300 mg or ranitidine 150 mg given at bedtime should relieve nocturnal pain within 3 or 4 days. Also helpful may be a large dose (30 to 60 mL) of a liquid nonabsorbable antacid. Nocturnal pain not relieved by these measures suggests complications (eg, penetration or obstruction) or another diagnosis (eg, esophagitis).

Recurrences: Current antiulcer drugs partially interrupt the natural history of duodenal ulcer only as long as they are being given in adequate dosage. Prolonging the treatment to ≥ 2 yr does not reduce the risk of relapse, which amounts to 60 to 80% of patients in 1 yr after stopping therapy. This leads to 2 options: (1) to treat only symptomatic relapses for 6 wk, healing 80% during this time and accepting a relapse rate of 60 to 80% during the next 1 to 2 yr; or (2) to follow relapse with maintenance therapy with a bedtime dose of cimetidine 400 mg or ranitidine 150 mg. On this regimen, relapses occur in 45% at 1 yr and 54% at 2 yr, but with fewer episodes of bleeding and many without pain.

For those not managed adequately by conscientiously conducted and followed medical treatment, surgery should be considered. The operation with least morbidity and mortality and with acceptable results is a fundic or parietal cell vatogomy.

Hospitalization is not often necessary, but is recommended when an ambulatory regimen does not give adequate relief or when complications occur; it expedites studies to detect malignancy of a gastric ulcer, ensures an adequate therapeutic trial, can temporarily remove the patient from a stressful environment, and offers patient and physician a special opportunity to consider psychosocial problems.

Surgery: With current drug therapy, indications for surgery are becoming more restrictive and the number of patients requiring surgery has declined significantly. Indications include perforation; obstruction that does not respond to medical therapy or that recurs; 2 or more major hemorrhages; a gastric ulcer suspected of being malignant; and disabling recurrences of uncomplicated peptic ulcer.

Symptoms after gastric surgery: The incidence and type of symptom varies with the type of operation. Subtotal gastrectomy is much less commonly performed than in former years. For this discussion, gastrectomy includes antrectomy, hemigastrectomy, partial gastrectomy, and subtotal gastrectomy (ie, resection of from 30 to 90% of the distal stomach with either gastroduodenostomy—Billroth I—or gastrojejunostomy—Billroth II). Gastrectomy may or may not include vagotomy. After gastrectomy, as many as 30% of patients have significant symptoms that include weight loss due to the small stomach syndrome and maldigestion; dumping syndrome; reactive hypoglycemia; bilious vomiting; and anemia. Diarrhea is especially common after truncal vagotomy, even without a resection (pyloroplasty).

More recently, the most commonly recommended and performed operation for duodenal ulcer is highly selective or fundic vagotomy, which carries a very low mortality and avoids the morbidity associated with gastrectomy and with truncal vagotomy.

Ulcer recurrence rates of 5 to 12% have been reported after fundic vagotomy. These may be expected to respond to medical therapy based on H_2 antagonists. Ulcer recurrences of 2 to 5% are reported after gastrectomy. Diagnosis is by endoscopy. For recurrent ulcers, the completeness of vagotomy should be tested by gastric analysis and Zollinger-Ellison syndrome ruled out by serum gastrin studies. Preoperative studies of gastric secretion and serum gastrin will detect a significant proportion of Zollinger-Ellison syndrome patients.

Weight loss is common after subtotal gastrectomy; the patient may have limited food intake because of early satiety (since the residual gastric pouch is small) or to prevent the dumping syndrome and other postprandial symptoms. With a small gastric pouch, distention or discomfort may follow a meal of even moderate size and patients who have limited their intake or lost weight as a result should be encouraged to eat smaller but more frequent meals. Maldigestion and steatorrhea due to pancreatobiliary bypass, especially with Billroth II anastomosis may contribute to weight loss. Anemia is common (usually from iron deficiency, but occasionally due to B_{12} deficiency because of loss of intrinsic factor), and osteomalacia may occur. Vitamin B_{12} 100 μg IM/mo is recommended as prophylaxis for all patients with total gastrectomy, but it may also be given to patients with subtotal gastrectomy if there is reason to suspect deficiency.

A **"dumping syndrome"** may follow surgical drainage procedures, particularly with gastrectomy. Weakness, dizziness, sweating, nausea, vomiting, and palpitation occur soon after eating, especially of hypertonic foods. Another form of "dumping" (reactive hypoglycemia) results from an overshoot of the postprandial blood sugar curve because of too rapid emptying from the stomach pouch. Early high peaks of blood sugar stimulate the release of insulin. By this time (about 2 h after a meal) the food bolus has passed on and symptomatic hypoglycemia results. A high-protein diet and adequate caloric intake (in frequent small feedings) are recommended.

COMPLICATIONS OF PEPTIC ULCER

PENETRATION
(Confined Perforation)

A peptic ulcer may penetrate the wall of the stomach or duodenum and enter an adjacent confined space or organ (eg, the pancreas or liver). Adhesions prevent leakage into the free peritoneal cavity. Pain may be intense, persistent, referred to sites other than the abdomen (usually the back and, due to penetration of a posterior duodenal ulcer, into the pancreas), and modified by the patient's position. When medical therapy is unsuccessful in producing healing, surgery is required.

PERFORATION

A free perforation usually presents as an acute abdominal emergency. Ulcers that perforate into the peritoneal cavity are usually located in the anterior wall of the duodenum, less commonly in the stomach. The patient experiences sudden, intense, steady epigastric pain that spreads rapidly throughout the abdomen, often becoming prominent in the right lower quadrant and at times being referred to one or both shoulders. The patient usually lies as still as possible, since even deep breathing can worsen the pain. The abdomen is tender and rebound tenderness is intense, the abdominal muscles are rigid, and bowel sounds are diminished or absent. Liver dullness may be absent. *Symptoms and signs may be less striking in the aged, the moribund, or those on corticosteroids.*

Pain and abdominal rigidity may partially subside and the patient's condition ap-

pears to improve several hours after onset. However, peritonitis with a temperature elevation may develop and the patient's condition seriously deteriorates; shock, heralded by increased pulse rate and decreased BP and urine output, may ensue.

Diagnosis is confirmed by an upright or a lateral decubitus x-ray of the abdomen showing air under the diaphragm or in the peritoneal cavity, but it is not excluded if no air is seen. An upright chest x-ray often defines air under the diaphragm.

Perforation into the lesser sac and intermittent seepage occur rarely. They may be difficult to recognize as the condition has no characteristic clinical picture. It is most commonly recognized from barium contrast studies, but may be suspected from a double gas shadow on a plain upright x-ray of the abdomen.

Treatment: Acute perforation usually requires immediate surgery. The longer the delay, the poorer the prognosis. When surgery is contraindicated, alternatives are continuous suction (preferably in an intensive care unit) and antibiotics.

HEMORRHAGE

(See also Ch. 53)

Hemorrhage is a common complication. Symptoms include vomiting of fresh blood or "coffee ground" material; passage of bloody or tarry stools; and weakness, syncope, thirst, and sweating due to blood loss. Ulcer must be considered as a possible cause of upper GI tract bleeding even if the patient denies having ulcer symptoms. In addition to what is discussed here, management requires location of the bleeding site.

Treatment

Immediate management is discussed in Ch. 53.

Feedings of bland food (eg, milk) may be started after bleeding has been controlled and nausea and vomiting subside. **Antacids** can be given hourly; if aluminum hydroxide is given, a cathartic salt (eg, magnesium hydroxide) should be included, since aluminum hydroxide may cause fecal impaction following GI hemorrhage. Anticholinergics are usually *not* given during the acute phase, as they may alter the response of the circulatory system to hemorrhage. Sedation (eg, morphine sulfate 2 mg q 4 to 6 h) can allay apprehension and control restlessness. Cimetidine 300 mg qid or ranitidine 50 mg q 6 h is frequently given; it is given IV if the patient is nauseated or vomiting, though no clear indication for its use exists, since H_2 antagonists have not been demonstrated to help control GI bleeding.

Nonsurgical intervention: If bleeding from an ulcer persists or recurs, several choices exist. Repeat endoscopy may be done and the bleeding site coagulated by either electrocautery, heater probe coagulation, or laser (if available). Bleeding may recur, even after coagulation. Angiographic control may be accomplished by the injection of autologous clot or other means of coagulation of the branch vessel supplying the bleeding site. In patients who are poor surgical risks, these technics may be reasonable first choices. Failing nonsurgical intervention, **emergency surgery is usually indicated when** (1) pulse rate, BP, and Hct indicate a deterioration in the patient's condition despite adequate treatment and transfusions; (2) > 6 transfusions in 24 h have been needed to maintain a stable pulse and BP; and (3) bleeding stops but recurs enough to require transfusion.

OBSTRUCTION

Obstruction of the outlet of the stomach or duodenum may be due to scarring, to spasm and inflammatory swelling associated with an active ulcer, or, most commonly, to both.

Symptoms

Vomiting may occur with ulcer in the absence of obstruction, especially with pyloric channel ulcers, and is therefore only suggestive of obstruction. However, gastric reten-

tion is suggested if the vomitus is of large volume, especially at the end of the day, or contains food eaten > 6 h earlier, and is probable if it contains food from 2 or more prior meals. Bloating or fullness after eating, and loss of appetite are also suggestive. A prolonged period of vomiting may cause weight loss, dehydration, and alkalosis. Commonly, a patient will have progressively cut total food intake and even have eliminated solid foods. Thus, he may present with marked weight loss and a history of either no vomiting or vomiting of very recent onset. In other patients, as obstruction continues, vomiting will become less frequent, decreasing to once/day, but the vomitus will be large in amount. Some patients disregard or deny symptoms, coming for help only when the obstruction is quite advanced.

Diagnosis

If the patient's history suggests obstruction, physical examination, gastric aspiration, or x-ray study may provide objective evidence of retention. Gastric retention is suggested if a succussion splash persists for 6 h after a meal, or if aspiration after an overnight fast yields > 200 mL of fluid or food residue. If gastric aspiration shows marked retention, the stomach should be emptied and x-rays may be used to determine whether obstruction is present and to aid in determining the site, cause, and degree of obstruction. Obstruction is suggested if x-rays show more than a trace of barium in the stomach 6 h after its ingestion. If obstruction is severe with significant retention of barium or food for > 24 h, and particularly if the stomach is greatly enlarged, ulcer is the probable cause. Carcinoma of the stomach should be considered primarily with lesser degrees of obstruction and if there is no history of ulcer. After the stomach has been emptied, endoscopy may be helpful in demonstrating whether the pylorus or duodenum is narrowed and in identifying the responsible lesion.

Treatment

If diagnostic evaluation does not indicate whether obstruction is due primarily to scarring or to edema and spasm, a trial of therapy including IV H_2 antagonists (cimetidine 300 mg or ranitidine 50 mg q 6 h) is usually indicated. Obstruction due to edema and spasm from an active ulcer usually responds to conservative treatment. Mild retention may respond to routine ulcer therapy, but more marked obstruction requires continuous gastric suction to allow the stomach to regain its tone. Continuous suction requires monitoring of electrolytes and fluid balance and giving adequate amounts of parenteral fluids to compensate for the fluid and electrolytes aspirated as well as for normal fluid losses. Any dehydration and electrolyte depletion resulting from vomiting before treatment also must be corrected. If malnutrition is present, increasing the surgical risk, parenteral hyperalimentation may be considered.

Gastric emptying should be tested after 2 or 3 days of continuous suction by monitoring emptying of normal secretions or by a saline load test (with 0.9% sodium chloride solution). If adequate emptying is restored, hourly feedings of a liquid diet or milk can start; aspiration is performed q 4 h. Feedings may be increased if large volumes are not aspirated. The time interval between aspirations can be lengthened as evidence of retention subsides, but aspiration should continue at least once daily for several days, either at bedtime or in the morning, to determine whether retention recurs after a more liberal diet, and at further intervals until the patient eats a full, regular diet. After 5 to 7 days of therapy including full doses of H_2 antagonists (eg, cimetidine 300 mg IV q 6 h), repeat endoscopy should be performed to define the status of the pylorus and the underlying ulcer.

NEOPLASMS OF THE STOMACH

This discussion is largely concerned with carcinoma, which accounts for 95% of malignant neoplasms of the stomach; less common are lymphomas (which may be

localized primarily in the stomach) and leiomyosarcomas. The incidence of stomach cancer shows enormous differences in worldwide distribution, with extremely high levels in Japan, Chile, and Iceland. In the USA it is most common in the North, in the poor, and in blacks, but its incidence has decreased to about 8:100,000, making it the 7th most common cause of death from cancer. However, in Japan, where its incidence has also decreased, stomach cancer is still the most common malignancy. Its incidence increases with age; < 25% of patients are under age 50.

Etiology and Pathogenesis

While its cause is unknown, stomach cancer is often associated with gastritis and intestinal metaplasia of the gastric mucosa. Such findings are now generally thought to result from gastric cancer rather than representing a common precursor state. Gastric ulcer has been described as leading to cancer, but, if at all, it occurs in a very small proportion of patients, in most of whom an undetected cancer was probably present from the beginning. Gastric polyps, also cited as precursors of cancer, are uncommon, but any polyp should be viewed with suspicion and removed, usually via endoscopy. Malignancy is particularly likely in a polyp > 2 cm in diameter or if there are several polyps. Cancer of the stomach is rare among patients with duodenal ulcer.

Pathology

Gastric carcinomas can be classified according to gross appearance: **(1) protruding** (polypoid or fungating); **(2) penetrating**—the tumor has a sharp, well-circumscribed border and may be ulcerated; **(3) spreading,** either superficially along the mucosa or infiltrating within the wall—if an ulcer is present, its edge tends to be ill-defined or heaped up. If there is infiltration of the stomach wall by tumor and an associated fibrous reaction, a "leather bottle" stomach **(linitus plastica)** may be produced; **(4) miscellaneous,** showing characteristics of 2 of the other types; this is the largest group. Protruding tumors have a better prognosis than infiltrating tumors.

Another classification is based on histologic criteria: the extent to which the cells are arranged into normal-appearing tubular glands and the degree of differentiation of the cells. Grading based on these criteria correlates moderately with gross appearance and prognosis.

The Japanese Society for Gastroenterological Endoscopy (1962) developed a classification for Early Gastric Cancer; ie, cancer limited to the mucosa and submucosa. Gross morphology provides the basis of identification: **Type I,** Protruded; **Type II,** Superficial—elevated, flat, or depressed; and **Type III,** Excavated.

Symptoms and Signs

In early stages, there are no specific symptoms. Patients and physicians alike tend to dismiss symptoms present for a year or more. Careful inquiry may detect a range of provocative clues. "Fullness" or slight pain after a large meal is a likely pattern if a cancer is in the pyloric region, a common site. Symptoms may suggest peptic ulcer, especially if a cancer involves the lesser curvature. A cancer in the cardiac region of the stomach may obstruct the esophageal inlet and cause dysphagia. Such cancers may be confused with esophageal cancer, even after careful study. Adenocarcinoma or tumors of the lower esophagus indicate a gastric origin. Loss of weight or strength, usually resulting from dietary restriction, may bring the patient to the physician. Massive hematemesis or melena are uncommon, but secondary anemia may follow occult blood loss. Occasionally, the first symptoms and signs are due to metastases; the primary tumor in the stomach is "silent."

Late in the course of gastric cancer, loss of weight or a palpable mass may be present. Finally, spreading tumor or metastases may lead to an enlarged liver, jaundice, ascites, skin nodules, and fractures.

Diagnosis

Differential diagnosis commonly involves peptic ulcer and its complications, which are considered above.

Endoscopy permits direct inspection and biopsy of suspicious areas. A gastric ulcer should have multiple biopsies from the margins, in addition to brush cytology (see below) from the base and under the edges. Occasionally, a biopsy limited to the mucosa will miss tumor tissue in the submucosa.

Cytologic studies of gastric washings are helpful in some institutions; special technics (eg, spraying the surface of the tumor with a jet of water during endoscopy or using devices that abrade the surface of the tumor) may increase the yield of positive washings. In experienced hands, use of a brush, together with biopsy, improves results.

X-ray studies generally have been unreliable in finding small, early lesions. However, by using double-contrast technics that involve coating the mucosa with barium and inflating the stomach to bring out mucosal details, Japanese radiologists report carcinomas as small as 1 cm in diameter.

Gastric analysis is of limited value.

Treatment

Excision of the tumor offers the only hope of cure, and the prognosis is good if the tumor is limited to the mucosa and submucosa. In the USA results are poor, because most patients have more extensive cancer when they come to surgery. In Japan, where early cancers are detected by mass screening, the results of surgery are better. Results with primary lymphoma of the stomach are better than those with carcinoma. There may be long survivals and even "cure," particularly with lymphosarcoma. With carcinoma, patients with malignant ulcers have the best results, probably because symptoms bring them to the doctor early. Chemotherapy may have palliative value; x-ray therapy does not help.

Surgery for cancer involves removal of most or all of the stomach and adjacent lymph nodes. Metastases or extensive tumor preclude cure. The decision to perform a palliative operation (eg, gastroenterostomy to bypass a pyloric obstruction) will depend on whether the patient's quality of life can be improved by surgery.

---

55. ACUTE ABDOMEN AND SURGICAL GASTROENTEROLOGY

ABDOMINAL PAIN

(See also Pelvic Pain in Ch. 171 and Recurrent Abdominal Pain in Ch. 194)

Among the diverse symptoms associated with GI disorders, none requires more circumspection and judgment than abdominal pain and the elucidation of its cause. It is frequently difficult for patients to describe it in terms meaningful to the physician. Since pain is subjective, descriptions of its severity and quality are not reliable indices for diagnosis, but must be interpreted in light of the patient's degree of sophistication, perception, and sensitivity. Furthermore, emotional factors (eg, anxiety, depression, hysteria, and suggestibility) influence the awareness and severity of pain. Another difficulty is the overlapping innervation of several viscera by the same spinal segments as detailed below. Nevertheless, the diagnosis can usually be established by a careful analysis of the history and by its correlation with physical findings and laboratory information.

Types of Pain

Abdominal pain may be divided into (1) visceral, (2) parietal, (3) superficial, and (4) referred pain. The special features of each are of considerable diagnostic importance.

Visceral or splanchnic pain arises in abdominal organs covered by visceral peritoneum. The impulses are conducted to the spinal cord via visceral afferent pain fibers in the sympathetic and parasympathetic nerves. Visceral pain may be induced by distention or stretching, ischemia, inflammation, or, in the case of hollow viscera, by spasm. Severe visceral pain may be accompanied by restlessness and by autonomic reflex responses (eg, sweating, nausea, vomiting, tachycardia or bradycardia, hypotension, and hyperesthesia). Visceral pain is usually poorly localized because of the relative paucity of nerve endings, the multisegmental innervation of the viscera, and referral to more superficial areas. Pain from paired structures (eg, the kidneys) is perceived on the affected side. Pain from all other viscera is felt in the midline, because of bilateral innervation, unless their overlying parietal peritoneum is affected.

Parietal pain arises from impulses in the parietal peritoneum and can be localized more precisely than visceral pain. Pain impulses from the parietal peritoneum as well as from the body wall, diaphragm, and the root of the mesenteries reach the CNS via somatic afferents in the spinal nerves or phrenic nerves. Extensive peritoneal involvement, as in a perforated peptic ulcer, may be accompanied by board-like rigidity. Acute appendicitis illustrates both visceral and parietal pain. In the early stage, when the lumen is occluded and the appendix becomes inflamed, the patient complains of vague discomfort in the periumbilical area. As the appendix becomes more distended, the overlying peritoneum is involved and the pain is localized in the right lower quadrant **(McBurney's point).** Parietal pain is aggravated by movement and coughing. The tenderness on palpation diminishes when the abdominal muscles are contracted.

Superficial or abdominal wall pain is associated with injuries to or excessive exertion of abdominal muscles or inflammation of the skin or peripheral nerves, as in herpes zoster. The pain is usually sharp, constant, and superficial, and aggravated by contraction of the abdominal musculature.

Referred pain is perceived at a distance from the diseased viscus. The area of reference is usually supplied by the same spinal segment and shares central pathways for afferent neurons. All pain from deep structures is referred to more superficial areas and in some instances far away from the involved organ. For example, pain from irritation of the diaphragm by a subdiaphragmatic abscess may be felt in the shoulder. An unusual form of referred pain, "habitual pain" or "habit reference," is influenced by pain from a chronically diseased viscus, previous trauma, or a scar from an old operation; eg, a patient with repeated episodes of biliary colic, who then has a myocardial infarction, may interpret the new pain as merely another attack of colic.

Etiology

Abdominal pain may be caused not only by a great variety of GI and intraperitoneal diseases, but also because of overlapping nerve distribution by extraperitoneal disorders. Pain of intra-abdominal origin (see TABLE 55–1) may emanate from the viscera, mesentery, peritoneum, and pelvic organs, and may be caused by inflammation, ulceration, vascular disturbances, and mechanical processes, eg, obstruction, torsion, distention, and spastic contraction. (See also BOWEL OBSTRUCTION, PERITONITIS, and PANCREATITIS, below, and ACUTE AND CHRONIC CHOLECYSTITIS in Ch. 78.)

The extraperitoneal causes of abdominal pain are outlined in TABLE 55–2. Because of similar segmental distribution, pain from intrathoracic disorders may be identical to that emanating from upper abdominal diseases. Intraspinal disorders may also simulate referred pain patterns from intraabdominal pathologic conditions, but usually lack tenderness to palpation and muscular rigidity. In peripheral nerve inflammatory disorders (eg, herpes zoster), pain may be present before typical cutaneous lesions are apparent.

TABLE 55–1. PAIN OF INTRA-ABDOMINAL ORIGIN

Mechanism	*Origin*	*Pathologic Processes*
Inflammation	Peritoneum	Chemical and nonbacterial peritonitis: perforated peptic ulcer, gallbladder, ruptured ovarian cyst, mittelschmerz Bacterial peritonitis Primary: pneumococcal, streptococcal, tuberculous Perforated hollow viscus: stomach, intestine, biliary tract
	Hollow intestinal organs	Appendicitis, cholecystitis, peptic ulcer, gastroenteritis, regional enteritis, Meckel's diverticulum, diverticulitis Colitis: ulcerative, bacterial, amebic
	Solid viscera	Pancreatitis, hepatitis, hepatic abscess, splenic abscess
	Mesentery	Lymphadenitis
	Pelvic organs	Pelvic inflammatory disease, tubo-ovarian abscess, endometritis
Mechanical (obstruction, acute distention)	Hollow intestinal organs	Intestinal obstruction: adhesions, hernia, tumor, volvulus, intussusception Biliary obstruction: calculi, tumor, choledochal cyst, hematobilia
	Solid viscera	Acute splenomegaly Acute hepatomegaly: cardiac failure, Budd-Chiari syndrome
	Mesentery	Omental torsion
	Pelvic organs	Ovarian cyst, torsion or degeneration of fibroid, ectopic pregnancy
Vascular	Intraperitoneal bleeding	Rupture: liver, spleen, mesentery, ectopic pregnancy; aortic, splenic, or hepatic aneurysm
	Ischemia	Mesenteric thrombosis, splenic infarction, omental ischemia Hepatic infarction: toxemia, purpura
Miscellaneous		Endometriosis

(Modified from *Principles of Surgery*, by S. I. Schwartz, ed. 3. Copyright © 1979 by McGraw-Hill Book Company. Used with permission of McGraw-Hill Book Company and the author.)

TABLE 55–2. EXTRAPERITONEAL CAUSES OF ABDOMINAL PAIN

Origin	*Pathologic Processes*
Cardiopulmonary	Pneumonia, empyema, myocardial ischemia, active rheumatic fever
Blood	Leukemia, sickle cell anemia
Neurogenic	Spinal cord tumor, osteomyelitis of the spine, tabes dorsalis, herpes zoster, abdominal epilepsy
Genitourinary	Nephritis, pyelitis, perinephric abscesses, ureteral obstruction (calculi, tumor), prostatitis, seminal vesiculitis, epidydimitis
Vascular	Dissection, rupture, or expansion of aortic aneurysm; periarteritis
Metabolic	Uremia, diabetic acidosis, porphyria, Addisonian crisis
Toxins	Bacterial (tetanus), insect bites, venoms, drugs, lead poisoning
Abdominal wall	Intramuscular hematoma
Psychogenic	Conversion reaction, hypochondriasis, somatic delusions

(Modified from *Principles of Surgery,* by S. I. Schwartz, ed. 3. Copyright © 1979 by McGraw-Hill Book Company. Used with permission of McGraw-Hill Book Company and the author.)

Differential Diagnosis

The correct diagnosis of a disorder responsible for abdominal pain depends on specific historical information, careful analysis of physical findings and appropriate laboratory evaluation. The history should include details about the onset, duration, location, radiation, and character of the pain; factors inducing aggravation and amelioration of pain; and concurrent symptoms.

The onset of pain may be sudden or gradual. **Sudden pain** is characteristic for perforation; rupture and torsion of a viscus; hemorrhage into the peritoneum, retroperitoneum, and abdominal wall; vascular occlusion with consequent ischemia (see OCCLUSION OF THE ABDOMINAL AORTA AND ITS BRANCHES in Ch. 29) and biliary and ureteral colic. Perforation is commonly associated with gastric or duodenal ulcer, sigmoid diverticulitis, toxic megacolon, and bowel obstruction. Rupture may complicate tubo-ovarian and liver abscess, ovarian cysts, and hematomas. Torsion may involve the ovary, volvulus of the bowel or omentum, and intussusception. Hemorrhage causing sudden pain may be due to ectopic pregnancy, a leaking aneurysm, or traumatic rupture of the liver or spleen. **Pain of gradual onset** is associated with increasing distention of a hollow organ, vascular insufficiency, and peritoneal irritation.

The **duration of pain** may also be of diagnostic value. Pain lasting only a few seconds or minutes is usually due to distention or spasm of a hollow viscus. Epigastric discomfort that lasts 15 to 45 min, or until relieved by food or antacids, is characteristic of peptic ulcer disease. The duration of biliary colic is usually several hours, while pain associated with pancreatitis is measured in days. Chronic or unremitting pain for several weeks, especially if aggravated by recumbency and relieved by knee flexion, should arouse suspicion of a retroperitoneal tumor (eg, carcinoma of the pancreas or lymphoma). Chronic pain of many months or years duration is associated with addiction to narcotics, emotional disturbances, and functional disorders.

The location of pain includes the original site, subsequent loci, and areas of radiation. In general, pain emanating from the stomach, duodenum, pancreas, liver, and biliary tree is perceived in the upper abdomen, from the jejunum and ileum in the periumbilical area, from the colon in the lower abdomen, and from the rectum in the presacral

area. Although more specific localization is not always possible for reasons previousl cited, some common patterns deserve emphasis. Pain in the right upper quadrant i more frequently due to diseases of the liver and gallbladder; in the right lower quad rant to appendicitis, regional enteritis, and gynecologic disorders; in the left uppe quadrant to gastritis, splenic congestion or infarction and distention of the spleni flexure of the colon; and in the left lower quadrant due to diverticulitis and gyneco logic diseases. Pain may radiate to the right scapula in biliary colic, to the back wit acute pancreatitis and a posterior wall duodenal ulcer, and into the groin with ureter colic.

The character of pain is established by proper interpretation of patients' descriptions Burning, aching, or gnawing discomfort in the epigastrium is commonly associate with peptic ulcer disease. Cramping, intermittent, or stabbing pain is compatible wit spasm, distention, or obstruction of a hollow viscus. It is associated with both acut and chronic diarrheas, regardless of cause. Squeezing, steady, or vise-like pain is usu ally reported with biliary colic.

Physical examination is important in the diagnosis of abdominal pain. The positio assumed by the patient should be noted and the skin, eyegrounds, neck, chest, heart skeleton, and abdomen should be examined. The scrotum and inguinal canals shoul be checked for hernias. Rectal and pelvic examinations may support the diagnosis o acute appendicitis, pelvic abscess, or pelvic inflammatory disease. Gastric peristalsi (*visible waves moving from left to right across the upper abdomen*) indicate gastric outle obstruction. Visible distension of the abdomen may be due to bowel obstruction o ascites. Absent bowel sounds are compatible with ileus or peritonitis, while increase bowel sounds may be heard in the presence of partial bowel obstruction, intestina inflammation, or infection.

A number of signs suggest the specific cause of an acute abdomen. **Murphy's sign** i found in acute cholecystitis and the **psoas** and **obturator signs** may be present in acut appendicitis (see below) or pelvic abscess. A hepatic friction rub may be heard o palpated in the presence of a malignant tumor or acute infection of the liver. Retro peritoneal bleeding from hemorrhagic pancreatitis or a dissecting aneurysm may b manifested by bluish discoloration or frank ecchymoses at the costovertebral angle **(Grey-Turner's sign)** or around the umbilicus **(Cullen's sign).** A detailed description o all of the physical findings associated with abdominal pain is beyond the scope of thi chapter and the reader is referred to specific diseases for additional information.

Diagnostic Procedures

Laboratory studies for patients with abdominal pain should include Hct, WBC, di ferential and platelet counts, urinalysis, electrolytes, liver enzymes, serum bilirubi and serum amylase. In acute disorders with diarrhea, stools should be cultured f bacteria and examined for ova and parasites.

Standard x-rays of the abdomen, including supine and either upright or decubit and flat films, may identify gastric retention and bowel obstruction or perforatio **Ultrasonography** may reveal aneurysms; biliary tract calculi; hepatic and pancreat abscesses, cysts, and tumors; and dilation of bile ducts and ureters. An **IVP** may reve renal disease or ureteral obstruction or displacement. A **sigmoidoscopy** may identi infectious, inflammatory, and neoplastic conditions of the sigmoid colon and rectu A **barium enema** is useful in the diagnosis of certain inflammatory conditions, tumor fistulas, obstruction, and volvulus of the colon. It may be both diagnostic and ther peutic in pediatric intussusception. **CT** defines specific lesions and, by quantifying the density, helps to distinguish abscesses, cysts, hematomas, and solid tumors. **Angiogr phy** is helpful in determining the site of active bleeding and defining vascular diseas of the GI tract.

BOWEL OBSTRUCTION

Arrest or serious impairment to the passage of intestinal contents.

Etiology

Mechanical blockage or cessation of peristalsis can obstruct either the small or large intestine. **Mechanical blockage** occurs more often, and may result from intra- or extraluminal or intramural barriers. Fibrous bands and adhesions (congenital or following surgery or inflammatory disease) and incarceration in a hernial sac are the most frequent causes. Primary or metastatic neoplasms, impacted feces, strictures from active or previous inflammatory disease of the bowel, intestinal worms, gallstones, Hirschsprung's disease, and volvulus are additional causes.

Adynamic (paralytic) ileus, resulting from failure of normal intestinal peristalsis, is most often associated with intra-or retroperitoneal infection. Ileus may be produced by mesenteric ischemia, by arterial or venous injury, by retroperitoneal or intra-abdominal hematomas, after intra-abdominal surgery, in association with renal or thoracic disease, and by metabolic disturbances (eg, hypokalemia). Gastric and colonic motility disturbances following abdominal surgery are largely a result of abdominal manipulation. The small intestine is largely unaffected and motility and absorption are normal within a few hours after operation. Stomach emptying is usually impaired for about 24 h, but the colon may remain inert for 48 to 72 h. This is confirmed by daily plain x-rays of the abdomen taken postoperatively; they show gas accumulating in the colon but not in the small bowel. Activity tends to return to the cecum before it returns to the sigmoid colon. If gas accumulates in the small intestine, it implies that a complication (eg, obstruction or peritonitis) has developed.

Pathology

In **simple mechanical obstruction,** blockage occurs without vascular or neurologic compromise. Ingested fluid and food, digestive secretions, and gas accumulate in excessive amounts, if obstruction is complete. The proximal intestine distends and the distal segment collapses. The normal secretory and absorptive functions of the mucous membrane are depressed and the bowel wall becomes edematous and congested. Severe intestinal distention is self-perpetuating and progressive, intensifying the peristaltic and secretory derangements and increasing the risks of dehydration, ischemia, necrosis, perforation, peritonitis, and death.

Strangulation or infarction of the bowel is most commonly associated with hernia, volvulus, intussusception, or vascular occlusion. Strangulation usually begins with venous obstruction, which may be followed by arterial occlusion resulting in rapid ischemia of the bowel wall. The bowel becomes edematous and infarcted, leading to gangrene and perforation.

In **closed-loop obstruction,** a loop of bowel is obstructed both proximally and distally (eg, by a hernial sac). The same changes occur as in simple obstruction, but with a rapid rise in intraluminal pressure in the affected segment and early edema of the bowel wall, vascular occlusion produces gangrene and perforation.

Symptoms and Signs

Clinical features depend upon whether the intestinal obstruction is high or low, complete or incomplete, simple or strangulated, mechanical or paralytic. Vomiting, crampy pain, and abdominal distention occur; in general, the higher the obstruction, the less prominent the distention and the earlier and more severe the vomiting. With high obstructions of the proximal jejunum and above, vomiting causes early, substantial loss of electrolyte-rich intestinal fluid, which rapidly depletes the extracellular fluid and produces hypovolemic shock.

Complete mechanical obstruction of the small intestine causes severe, intermittent, crampy upper abdominal pain (colic) usually referred to the midline but sometimes radiating over the whole abdomen. Vomiting occurs and usually becomes malodorous and fecal smelling as a result of overgrowth of colonic bacteria. Although small amounts of feces may be passed early, constipation and failure to pass flatus are usually present, peristalsis above the obstruction may be visible, and bowel sounds are increased, high-pitched, and tinkling. Abdominal distention may not be prominent initially, but becomes conspicuous later when the obstruction is low in the small bowel. As the intestinal lumen proximal to the obstruction fills with electrolyte-containing intestinal fluid and gas, extracellular fluid dehydration develops. Increasing abdominal wall tenderness, muscle rigidity, and adynamic ileus suggest strangulation. **Partial obstruction of the small intestine** causes similar but less severe symptoms. Bowel actions may persist, usually with diarrhea.

Obstruction of the colon is usually insidious in onset. Abdominal distention with fullness of the flanks is more prominent, and is massive with volvulus of the colon. Vomiting tends to occur later in the course, and pain may be less severe than in small bowel obstruction. If the obstruction is complete, constipation and failure to pass flatus are complete. With partial obstruction, irregular bowel action may allow passage of frequent, small, or even diarrheal stools.

Paralytic ileus causes severe abdominal distention and distress. Bowel sounds are absent. The diagnosis may be overlooked since small amounts of flatus or liquid stools may be passed. Plain abdominal x-rays will show gas in the small intestine.

Strangulation may be difficult to differentiate from simple obstruction. Onset may be rapid with severe, colicky pain. The symptoms and signs are initially those of mechanical obstruction, but gradually become those of ileus and peritonitis. Bowel sounds disappear; abdominal rigidity and acute, possibly localized, tenderness accompanied by marked shock may result from gangrenous change. With closed loop obstruction, the presence of a tender mass suggests the diagnosis. The WBC count is increased. Passage of blood from the rectum may occur, especially following vascular occlusion.

Diagnosis

X-ray findings help to establish the diagnosis and locate the level of obstruction. Plain films show gaseous distention; in the small intestine this generally lies in the central area. Fluid levels are visible in x-rays taken with the patient upright. Loops of small bowel may be arranged in a stepladder pattern; mucosal folds may be prominent in the upper small bowel. The colon can be distinguished by haustral markings and by the distribution of the distended large bowel. Gas confined to the small bowel with multiple air-fluid levels ("J-loops") usually indicates a mechanical small bowel obstruction. Gas distributed throughout both the small and large intestines ("U-loops") occurs in paralytic ileus and obstruction due to vascular insufficiency. Barium enema radiography (using only 100 mL) may localize the site of a colonic obstruction or can be used when uncertainty exists in distinguishing large from small bowel gas. Barium *should not be given by mouth* until it is known that the obstruction is not in the colon

Mechanical obstruction of the small intestine may simulate many acute abdominal conditions. Appendicitis, cholecystitis, salpingitis, ureteral colic, acute peptic ulcer, and acute pancreatitis must be included in the differential diagnosis. Serum amylase concentration is elevated in the acute pancreatitis.

Finding the cause of obstruction is important. A hernia should be sought and examined for evidence of incarceration. The presence of an operative scar suggests obstruction due to adhesions. Intussusception is suggested by rectal bleeding in a young child Volvulus of the colon tends to occur later in life and is accompanied by the development of early, prominent distention.

Treatment

Obstruction must be relieved surgically at the earliest time consistent with safety; fluid, electrolyte, and hemodynamic balance must be restored; and the effects of the obstruction, including bowel distention and possible secondary infection, must be neutralized.

Nasogastric aspiration is performed by means of a Levin tube to remove intestinal contents regurgitating into the stomach. Long intestinal tubes such as the double-lumen Miller-Abbott tube or a Cantor tube may be passed to decompress the intestine directly, but they are often difficult to position, resulting in more distress to the patient. The Levin tube is almost always sufficient for this purpose. Unless the patient has low-grade partial obstruction or grave intercurrent illnesses that confer a prohibitive operative risk, intubation should be used only long enough to replace fluid and electrolyte deficits before proceeding to surgery.

Relief of intestinal obstruction usually requires surgical intervention. While celiotomy for relief of simple obstruction can usually be delayed until shock is overcome and electrolyte balance reestablished, timing is important and immediate surgery may be necessary to prevent strangulation or infarction.

Fluid and electrolyte losses require extracellular fluid replacement. The approximate loss may be gauged by the severity of vomiting and a clinical appraisal of the degree of dehydration. Pulse, BP, central venous pressure, and urine flow must be monitored. In dehydration, the Hb and Hct are elevated. The amount of fluid given depends in part on the level of the obstruction. During the first 24 h, sufficient lactated Ringer's solution or 0.9% sodium chloride solution should be given to restore urine flow and return the hemodynamic vital signs toward normal. A potassium deficit may require adding potassium chloride to the parenteral fluids after urine flow has been reestablished. Fluid balance charts should be maintained continuously and serum electrolyte levels determined daily so that fluid and electrolyte replacement can be related to losses after dehydration is corrected. Fluid replacement in patients with severe hepatic or cardiovascular disease must be done cautiously, and saline solution should usually not be given.

Once the diagnosis and course of action are clear, analgesics may be given to control pain; sedation may also be necessary. Since morphine and its derivatives cause increased segmentation of the small intestine and may intensify nausea, meperidine 50 to 100 mg IM q 4 to 6 h is probably best. Confused or comatose patients should be given sedatives and analgesics cautiously. Parenteral antibiotics are indicated if peritonitis is present.

In very occasional patients (eg, persons with terminal neoplasm in the abdominal cavity) surgery may be impossible. Some palliation can be provided with analgesia, scopolamine 0.3 to 0.6 mg sublingually to relieve colic, and an antiemetic (eg, chlorpromazine or prochlorperazine) given parenterally or by suppository.

APPENDICITIS

Inflammation of the vermiform appendix.

Etiology, Incidence, and Pathology

Acute appendicitis results from bacterial infection of the vermiform appendix. Contributory factors include intraluminal obstruction by a fecalith, lymphoid hyperplasia, and rarely parasites, or even a carcinoid tumor or a tumor in the cecum. However, mucosal ulceration with bacterial invasion but no concomitant obstruction can mimic appendicitis. The condition is most common in adolescents and young adults, with a peak incidence between ages 15 and 24, and is also a common reason for intra-abdominal surgery in infants and children.

The inflammation causes edema and ischemia in all layers of the appendix and can progress to gangrene and perforation. Polymorphonuclear leukocytes and, possibly, micro-abscesses are present in the appendiceal lumen and wall. Loops of bowel, omentum, or parietal peritoneum may become adherent and an abscess may develop, either at the site of the appendix or elsewhere in the peritoneal cavity. Perforation may occur early in the course of the disease (within 24 to 48 h) and may produce either a localized or generalized peritonitis. Subsequently, abscesses may develop in areas of the peritoneal cavity remote from the appendix (eg, pelvis, beneath the diaphragm, and the left side of the abdominal cavity). A mixed bacterial flora dominated by anaerobes and gram-negative bacilli is responsible for the infection.

Symptoms and Signs

Pain typically begins in the midepigastrium and moves to the right lower quadrant where it is persistent, steady, well localized, and accentuated by movement, deep respiration, coughing, or sneezing. Nausea and vomiting are common but not invariably present. Constipation of recent onset is characteristic, and the patient may not pass any rectal gas. A few patients have diarrhea, but this is more likely to be a sign of regional or viral enteritis. There may be mild fever (up to 39 C [102.2 F]), which appears later than other signs, and a moderate leukocytosis.

When the appendix is in the normal position, tenderness and guarding are present over the right lower quadrant, typically at McBurney's point (1/3 the distance between the anterior superior iliac spine and the umbilicus). Tenderness may be localized to a spot lying under one finger. Rebound tenderness anywhere over the abdomen indicates peritoneal inflammation. The **psoas sign** (pain on passive hyperextension of the thigh) strongly suggests appendicitis.

Since the tip of the appendix may be located almost anywhere in the abdomen, findings may vary greatly. Abdominal muscle spasm and resistance may be absent with a retrocecal appendix. An appendix low in the pelvic cavity may cause tenderness on rectal and vaginal examination, without the usual marked abdominal tenderness; an appendix high in the pelvic cavity may cause less rectal tenderness. An appendix lying near the ureter may simulate ureteral colic, with pain radiating to the genitalia and burning on urination; hematuria from ureteral inflammation is occasionally seen. Other atypical sites may result in referral of symptoms to the right hypochondrium or to the left side of the abdomen.

Pain, fever, and leukocytosis usually increase following perforation. Peritonitis causes generalized pain and tenderness; the abdomen is usually rigid and there may be protracted vomiting; ileus and subsequent shock are likely.

Appendiceal abscess usually develops 24 to 72 h following onset of symptoms; fever, leukocytosis, and local tenderness may be increased, and a mass may be palpable in the right ileal fossa.

Diagnosis and Differential Diagnosis

The diagnosis is often difficult in young children because it is a less likely age group and because vomiting may be the dominant symptom, overshadowing abdominal tenderness. Mesenteric adenitis is a common misdiagnosis in children, but pain and guarding are less prominent in this condition. Although CT scan may detect an abscess and barium enema may demonstrate a normal appendix, the potential of perforation by barium enema and the radiation exposure from either of these low-yield procedures speak against their routine use. The rate of 20 to 30% for normal removed appendices attests to the concern that demand for absolute diagnostic certainty may lead to delay in operation and to an unacceptably high rate of perforation. In the elderly and in patients receiving corticosteroids, symptoms and signs may be muted, and in the elderly there are several additional possibilities to consider.

An elevated WBC count with a shift to the left is a useful diagnostic aid, although it may be absent or less evident in elderly patients. Pelvic inflammatory disease in fe-

males can usually be excluded by the history and a pelvic examination. Nausea and vomiting are prominent in acute gastroenteritis, and pain, when it occurs, is usually more generalized than in acute appendicitis. Appendicitis can also mimic other abdominal disorders, including pancreatitis, regional enteritis, Yersinia enterocolitis, cholecystitis, pyelonephritis, spastic colon, and, in children, volvulus and intussusception. However, the wise clinician will think of appendicitis in every patient with the sudden onset of pain. Intrathoracic emergencies, including myocardial infarction and pulmonary embolus with diaphragmatic pleurisy, have occasionally been misdiagnosed as acute appendicitis.

Prognosis

With early operation, the mortality is low, the patient is usually discharged within 4 to 5 days, and convalescence is normally rapid and complete. With complications, the prognosis is more serious; if an appendiceal abscess develops, final resolution may take several weeks.

Treatment

With few exceptions, appendicitis is treated by operation. Rarely, an early attack will subside spontaneously and will not show convincing signs of inflammation. After appendectomy for acute uncomplicated appendicitis, parenteral fluids usually are not required beyond the first day, and GI function returns promptly. Ambulation is desirable as soon as the patient recovers from the anesthetic. An appendiceal abscess requires drainage with or without appendectomy. When appendectomy is deferred under these circumstances, it may be performed a number of weeks after recovery from the acute process. The presence of an abscess or diffuse peritonitis resulting from rupture of the appendix dictates treatment for peritonitis (see that chapter, below, for further discussion of treatment).

Non-surgical treatment may be required in rare situations in which the facilities and surgical team required for an operation are unavailable. In such cases, nasogastric suction, IV fluid replacement, ampicillin (IV dosages are as follows: adults, at least 500 mg q 6 h; infants < 1 wk, 50 mg/kg/day; infants of 1 to 4 wk, 100 mg/kg/day; infants and children of 4 wk to 2 yr and up, 200 mg/kg/day) or another broad-spectrum antibiotic, and analgesics should be used.

PERITONITIS

ACUTE PERITONITIS

Acute inflammation of the visceral and parietal peritoneum.

Etiology and Pathogenesis

Although chemical or mechanical stimuli can cause peritoneal irritation, the most common causes are the infecting bacteria *Escherichia coli* and *Streptococcus faecalis*; other pathogens and occasionally fungi have been identified. Organisms or irritants escape from the intestinal tract most often following perforation of the appendix or a peptic ulcer. Peritonitis may also complicate any operation in the abdominal cavity (eg, due to leakage at a GI anastomosis), or may result from the spread of pelvic infection into the peritoneal cavity (eg, from salpingitis) or from a hemoperitoneum due to injury or to rupture of an ectopic pregnancy. Cholecystitis, diverticulitis, colitis, strangulated or infarcted bowel, and penetrating wounds of the abdomen are other common causes. Occasionally, peritonitis can arise spontaneously, especially in persons with advanced liver disease.

Peritoneal inflammation may be localized or diffuse, depending on the origin of the infection and the patient's defenses. Localized peritonitis frequently occurs in diverticulitis or early appendicitis, while a ruptured appendix or perforation of the colon or

of a peptic ulcer usually causes widespread peritoneal contamination. Leakage of bile from the biliary tree produces a particularly severe peritonitis.

Symptoms, Signs, and Diagnosis

Clinical manifestations vary according to the cause and extent of the peritonitis. Onset is marked by severe localized or diffuse abdominal pain. In patients treated with steroids, pain and tenderness may be masked. In the early stages, as paralytic ileus develops, moderate abdominal distention is present, usually with nausea and vomiting and, occasionally, diarrhea. Direct abdominal tenderness, rebound tenderness, and marked muscle spasm are present; rebound tenderness may occur without direct tenderness. Later, the abdomen is silent to auscultation. Rectal examination discloses pelvic tenderness and may reveal a pelvic abscess. Plain x-rays of the abdomen may show patchy gaseous filling of the small and large bowel and the absence of well-defined loops. Free peritoneal fluid can often be seen between the coils, and the presence of intraperitoneal air is diagnostic of a perforation. A diagnostic tap or peritoneal lavage may demonstrate the type of exudate or allow culture of the bacteria. CT or sonography is useful in detecting intra-abdominal abscesses.

Fever, tachycardia, chills, rapid breathing, and leukocytosis are signs of sepsis; shallow rapid respiration suggests diaphragmatic irritation with splinting. Hiccups and shoulder pain indicate diaphragmatic involvement. Vomiting, initially of reflex origin, usually persists, indicating ileus. As ileus progresses, distention increases and extracellular fluid loss into the intestinal lumen and the peritoneal cavity produces dehydration. Early leukocytosis may be followed by leukopenia in fulminant cases. Dehydration and acidosis develop if the disease is not treated. The eyes become sunken and the mouth becomes dry; circulatory collapse can be fatal; ultimately, the abdomen is tense and distended, and the typically shrunken "Hippocratic facies" appears.

Complications

Early, acute complications of peritonitis include shock, acute renal failure, acute respiratory insufficiency, and sometimes liver failure secondary to pylephlebitis and liver abscesses. Because the infection tends to loculate, abscess formation is typical. Abscesses most commonly are subdiaphragmatic, subhepatic, peritoneal, or pelvic, but they may occur anywhere in the peritoneal cavity. Pelvic abscesses, which may be accompanied by diarrhea or increased urinary frequency, can be identified during pelvic examination by palpating a soft tender swelling that bulges into the anterior wall of the rectum. A subphrenic abscess may be obscure and may remain latent for weeks or years; it should be borne in mind, however, since severe toxemia and a high mortality rate may follow delayed treatment. Pain, which may be intermittent, is usually present in the upper abdomen; tenderness over the area of the abscess is an important localizing sign. Elevation and splinting of the diaphragm often occur, as well as small pleural effusions with basal rales. For more detailed discussion of intra-abdominal abscesses, see Ch. 5.

Treatment

The cause must be eliminated, the infection treated, and the paralytic ileus and dehydration corrected. The source of peritoneal contamination usually must be eliminated by surgery (eg, appendectomy, cholecystectomy, closure of a perforated peptic ulcer, resection of a gangrenous intestine, or exteriorization of a perforated colon).

Antibiotics (eg, gentamicin, clindamycin, and selected cephalosporins) effective against the usual bacteria should be started early and revised if necessary once results of peritoneal fluid or blood cultures are known. Parenteral administration is usually necessary. Localized abscesses should be sought continuously until all local and systemic evidence of infection subsides; abscesses should be incised and drained.

The peritonitis and associated ileus require nasogastric decompression, IV fluids,

and, when protracted, parenteral alimentation. Careful monitoring of urine flow, respiratory efficiency, and intravascular volume is necessary. Blood transfusion or plasma expanders are usually needed if the patient is in shock. The optimal initial replacement fluid is lactated Ringer's solution. Whole blood or packed RBCs are reserved for anemia. Treatment is continued until the gastric aspirate becomes clear and scanty, bowel sounds return to normal, and passage of flatus or feces occurs. Oral feedings should not be resumed too early; fully developed paralytic ileus rarely recovers within 48 h. Small doses of meperidine (10 to 20 mg IV) or morphine (2 to 4 mg IV) q 4 to 6 h may help to relieve pain.

CHRONIC PERITONITIS

Chronic inflammation of the visceral and parietal peritoneum.

Etiology and Pathogenesis

Mechanical and chemical causes of irritation producing mild chronic peritonitis are usually introduced during abdominal surgery (eg, powder from surgical gloves, or pads or sponges that are left in the abdomen). The main impact of such chronic peritonitis results from chronic abscess formation or from adhesions with consequent small bowel obstruction.

Chronic bacterial peritonitis is most often seen in patients with indwelling catheters on continuous ambulatory peritoneal dialysis **(CAPD).** This may be associated with recurring bouts of peritonitis, which under optimum conditions should occur no more than once in 2 yr. Introduction of disposable units (eg, bacterial filters and collapsible plastic bags) has contributed to a lowered incidence of infection. Factors in repeated bouts of peritonitis include breaks in the integrity of the equipment, decreased patient immune defenses, patient error in dialysis technic, and occasional intrinsic sources from the intestinal tract. The most common organisms involved with breaks in the tubing system and in technic are *Staphylococcus epidermidis* and *Staphylococcus aureus.* Enteric organisms originate from perforations of the intestinal tract. A hematogenous origin is rare and *Streptococcus viridans* and *Mycobacterium tuberculosis* are the predominant organisms.

Chronic TB peritonitis is rarely seen. TB within the abdominal cavity accounts for about 4% of extrapulmonary TB, with about 80% of these cases involving only the peritoneum rather than the GI tract per se. The pathogenesis is most likely hematogenous spread from lung to mesenteric lymph nodes of the bacilli, which then infect the peritoneal cavity.

Fungal species can produce chronic peritonitis, almost always in the immunocompromised host (eg, a patient in renal failure with peritoneal dialysis tubes, with an intrauterine device, or one with advanced malignancies). While most fungi are *Candida* varieties, *Fusarium, Drechslera,* and *Exophiala* have been reported.

Symptoms and Signs

Chronic chemical peritonitis is manifested by the usual symptoms and signs of small bowel obstruction (see BOWEL OBSTRUCTION, above). The course of chronic localized peritonitis from a retained surgical sponge may be punctuated by episodes of acute peritonitis (see above).

Chronic bacterial peritonitis is manifested by recurrent fevers, tenderness, and elevation of peripheral WBC counts. **TB peritonitis** can present with fever, vague abdominal tenderness, and the characteristic doughy-feeling abdomen. A less common presentation of TB peritonitis is the so-called "wet" form with ascites. **Chronic fungal peritonitis** can present insidiously with vague abdominal pains, mild tenderness, but little in the way of systemic manifestations.

Complications of the various types of chronic peritonitis are similar. As in acute peritonitis, one sequel of chronic peritonitis is localization of infection with resultant

abscess formation in certain areas of the abdominal cavity. Occasionally, host defenses are so depressed that a chronic, smoldering peritonitis becomes acute and the patient may exhibit systemic manifestations of infection and even hypotension. Especially in the case of candidiasis, candidemia can lead to a spread of infection and is associated with a high mortality rate unless treated. Small bowel obstruction may occur anytime after dense abdominal adhesions have formed.

Diagnosis

Microbial culture is the key to diagnosis of specific types of chronic peritonitis. In the case of peritoneal dialysis, the culture is easily obtained from dialysis fluid. An occasional patient with infection that persists in spite of appropriate antibiotic treatment may benefit from a CT scan to rule out a localized area of resistant infection. Diagnostic surgical exploration of the abdomen may be necessary as a last resort, especially in the nondialysis patient. In cases of TB, fine granular tubercles can be easily seen all along the surface of the visceral and parietal peritoneum. Peritoneal biopsy is diagnostic in about 80% of cases, compared to 50% for a fluid culture.

Prophylaxis and Treatment

Since no treatment of abdominal adhesions is effective, the emphasis in **chemical-mechanical peritonitis** should be prevention. Gentle handling of intra-abdominal tissues and cleansing of gloves with a wet pad before operation are time-honored principles.

Catheter-associated chronic **bacterial peritonitis** is usually treated initially by one of the first generation cephalosporins. These agents are about 70 to 90% absorbed from the peritoneal cavity when given through the dialysis catheter and left in place 4 to 8 h. Alternative treatment is 1 gm IM or IV. A recommended loading dose for the cephalosporin is 500 mg/L of dialysate with a daily maintenance dose of 125 to 250 mg/L for up to 40 days or until the culture has been negative for 1 wk in CAPD patients. Culture results may require a change in antibiotic coverage, based on the sensitivity of the organisms. Perhaps the most serious bacterial infection is that of methicillin-resistant *Staphylococci*. Vancomycin given at 20 mg/kg with the first exchange, 10 mg/kg at the second exchange, and 30 mg/L total/exchange thereafter until 7 days after the last positive culture (usually 2 wk) is a recommended regimen. If gram-negative organisms are suspected initially or if initial cultures are subsequently returned as positive, an aminoglycoside should be added (eg, gentamicin 1.5 mg/kg IM as a loading dose, and 4 to 8 mg/L in each exchange). If an aminoglycoside is started initially and cultures are negative, the drug should be discontinued and the appropriate antibiotic started or continued. In the case of TB peritonitis, systemic or oral isoniazid 300 mg and rifampin 600 mg/day for the 1st mo and then isoniazid 15 mg/kg and rifampin 600 mg times 2/wk for 1 mo is the recommended regimen. In patients with rifampin intolerance, isoniazide is given at the dosage above combined with ethambutol, 50 mg/kg twice/wk for 18 mo.

In **fungal peritonitis,** treatment is somewhat controversial. One regimen consists of treating candidiasis with amphotericin B, 1 to 3 mg/L of peritoneal infusion with 800 mL of dialysate left in place for 2 h. This regimen is recommended bid for 8 to 21 days. Treatment with amphotericin B, 0.5 to 1 mg/kg/day IV, is an alternative method. Ketoconazole and 5-fluorocytosine are other possible agents. 5-Fluorocytosine crosses from blood into the peritoneal fluid much more readily than does ketoconazole. The suggested oral dose is 5-fluorocytosine 15 mg/kg/day. Dose adjustments based on monitored blood levels should assure a concentration < 100 μg/mL. While there is not complete agreement concerning removal of the dialysis catheter for either bacterial or fungal peritonitis in this situation, most authorities favor early catheter removal for fungal infections. Surgical drainage or CT-guided catheter drainage must be considered for localized infections resistant to antibiotic therapy.

PANCREATITIS

Acute pancreatitis is the term usually reserved for an *acute inflammation that resolves both clinically and histologically* (eg, pancreatitis associated with biliary tract calculi). The terms **chronic pancreatitis** or **chronic relapsing pancreatitis** indicate that *histologic changes persist even after the etiologic agent (usually alcohol) has been removed.* This classification emphasizes that histologic changes in chronic pancreatitis are irreversible and tend to be progressive, leading to a serious loss of exocrine and endocrine pancreatic function. A problem with this classification is a possible discordance between the clinical and histologic components; eg, at the initial overt episode of alcoholic pancreatitis, the pancreatitis may best be described as "acute" clinically, but may already be "chronic" histologically.

ACUTE PANCREATITIS

Etiology and Pathogenesis

Biliary tract disease and alcoholism account for ≥ 80% of hospital admissions for acute pancreatitis. The remaining 20% are caused by hereditary pancreatitis, hyperlipidemia (especially Types I and V hyperlipoproteinemia), hyperparathyroidism and hypercalcemia, blunt and penetrating trauma to the pancreas, drugs (eg, azathioprine, sulfasalazine, furosemide, valproic acid), structural abnormalities of the common bile duct and ampullary region (eg, choledochal cyst and sphincter of Oddi stenosis), structural abnormalities of the pancreatic duct itself (eg, stricture, carcinoma, or pancreas divisum), surgery (particularly of stomach and biliary tract), vascular disease (especially severe hypotension), infection (eg, mumps), endoscopic retrograde pancreatography (ERP), renal transplantation, or uncertain etiology.

In biliary tract disease, attacks of pancreatitis are caused by temporary impaction of a gallstone within the sphincter of Oddi before its passage into the duodenum, but the precise pathogenetic mechanism is unclear. Alcohol intake of > 100 gm/day for several years may cause precipitation of pancreatic enzymic protein in random fashion within small pancreatic ductules. In time, deposition of protein plugs becomes more widespread and induces additional histologic abnormalities. After ≥ 3 to 5 yr, the first clinical episode of pancreatitis occurs, presumably because of premature activation of pancreatic enzymes.

Gross pathologic changes may be dominated by edema or necrosis and hemorrhage. Tissue necrosis is caused by several pancreatic enzymes including activated trypsin and activated phospholipase A. Hemorrhage is caused by pancreatic elastase, which dissolves elastic fibers of blood vessels. In edematous pancreatitis, the inflammatory response is usually confined to the pancreas, and the mortality is < 5%. In pancreatitis characterized by severe necrosis and hemorrhage, the inflammatory response is not confined to the pancreas, and the mortality is ≥ 30 to 50%. Pancreatic exudate containing toxins and activated pancreatic enzymes permeates the retroperitoneum and at times the peritoneal cavity, inducing a chemical burn and increasing the permeability of blood vessels, thereby causing extravasation of large amounts of protein-rich fluid from the systemic circulation into "third spaces" producing hypovolemia and shock. As these activated enzymes and toxins enter the systemic circulation, they cause increased capillary permeability throughout the body and may also reduce peripheral vascular tone thereby intensifying hypotension. Circulating activated enzymes may damage tissue directly (eg, injury to alveolar membranes of lungs thought to be caused by phospholipase A).

Death during the first several days of acute pancreatitis is usually caused by cardiovascular instability (with refractory shock and renal failure), respiratory failure (with hypoxemia and at times adult respiratory distress syndrome), and, occasionally, heart

failure (secondary to unidentified myocardial depressant factor). Circulating enzymes and toxins are thought to play a large role in early death.

After the first week, death is usually caused by a complication of **pancreatic necrosis.** For example: (1) secondary infection of devitalized retroperitoneal tissue (ie, **pancreatic abscess),** usually caused by gram-negative organisms. Mortality is usually 100% without extensive surgical debridement of infected retroperitoneal tissue; (2) **pancreatic pseudocyst,** *a collection of enzyme-rich pancreatic fluid and tissue debris demarcated from surrounding structures by a capsule composed of fibrous and vascular tissue.* Related deaths are caused by secondary infection, hemorrhage, or rupture.

Symptoms and Signs

Almost all patients suffer severe abdominal pain that radiates straight through to the back in about 50% of patients. Rarely, pain is first appreciated in the lower abdomen. Pain usually develops suddenly and reaches maximal intensity within minutes, is severe and often refractory to large doses of parenteral narcotics, is steady and boring in quality, and invariably persists for many hours and usually for several days without relief. Usually no change in position or maneuver appreciably reduces the level of pain, but coughing, vigorous movement, and deep breathing may accentuate it. Most patients experience nausea and vomiting, at times to the point of dry heaves.

The patient appears acutely ill and is sweating. Pulse rate is usually 100 to 140 beats/min. Respirations are shallow and rapid. BP may be transiently high or low, with significant postural hypotension. At first, the temperature may be normal or even subnormal, but increases within a few hours to 37.7 to 38.3 C (100 to 101 F). Sensorium may be blunted to the point of semi-coma. Scleral icterus is occasionally present. Lipemia retinalis with hyperlipidemia is very rare. Examination of the lungs may reveal limited diaphragmatic excursion and evidence of atelectasis. Upper abdominal distension is present in about 20% of patients, caused by gastric ileus or a large pancreatic inflammatory mass displacing the stomach anteriorly. There may be ascites. Abdominal tenderness is invariably present, often severe in the upper abdomen and less severe in the lower abdomen. There may be mild-to-moderate muscular rigidity in the upper abdomen, but rarely in the lower abdomen. It is unusual for the entire abdomen to exhibit severe peritoneal irritation in the form of a rigid board-like abdomen. Bowel sounds may be hypoactive. Rectal examination usually discloses no tenderness, and the stool is usually negative for occult blood.

Laboratory Findings and Diagnosis

Acute pancreatitis should be considered in the differential diagnosis of every acute abdomen. The differential diagnosis includes a perforated gastric or duodenal ulcer, mesenteric infarction, intestinal obstruction with strangulation, ectopic pregnancy, dissecting aneurysm, biliary colic, appendicitis, and diverticulitis. Other diagnostic possibilities include inferior wall myocardial infarction, hematoma of abdominal muscles, and hematoma of the spleen.

No laboratory test can confirm a diagnosis of acute pancreatitis. However, many tests are used to support the clinical impression. **Serum amylase and lipase concentrations** are increased on the first day of acute pancreatitis and return to normal in 3 to 7 days, but both may remain "normal" if so much acinar tissue has already been destroyed during prior episodes that insufficient amounts of enzymes can be liberated to raise serum levels. Serum amylase may also remain normal if there is coexisting hypertriglyceridemia (which may contain a circulating inhibitor that must be diluted before an elevation in serum amylase can be appreciated). Both serum amylase and lipase may be increased in renal failure and in severe abdominal conditions requiring urgent surgical therapy (eg, perforated ulcer, mesenteric vascular occlusion, and intestinal obstruction associated with ischemia). Other causes of increased serum amylase include salivary gland dysfunction, macroamylasemia, and tumors that secrete amylase.

The amylase:creatinine clearance ratio does not appear to have sufficient sensitivity or specificity to confirm a diagnosis of pancreatitis. Fractionation of total serum amylase into pancreatic type **(p-type)** isoamylases and salivary type (s-type) isoamylases is now possible in most commercial laboratories. P-type isoamylases are increased on the first day of pancreatitis and, along with serum lipase, remain increased longer than total serum amylase. However, an increase in p-type isoamylase also occurs in renal failure and (probably) in severe abdominal conditions that mimic pancreatitis.

The WBC count is usually increased to 12,000 to 20,000. The Hct may be as high as 50 to 60% as a result of third space fluid losses. Hyperglycemia may occur. Serum Ca concentration may be reduced as early as the first day, probably because of loss of serum albumin into retroperitoneal spaces as part of the chemical burn. Serum bilirubin concentration is increased in 15 to 25% of patients.

Supine and upright plain films of the abdomen may disclose a variety of abnormalities including calculi within pancreatic ducts (evidence of prior inflammation), calcified gallstones, or a localized ileus in the left upper quadrant or central abdomen (either a "sentinel loop" of small bowel, dilation of the transverse colon, or duodenal ileus). **Chest x-ray** may reveal atelectasis or a pleural effusion (usually either on the left side or bilaterally, but rarely confined to the right pleural space). **Ultrasonography** should be performed and may detect gallstones or dilation of the common hepatic duct indicating biliary tract obstruction. Edema of the pancreas may be visualized, but overlying gas frequently obscures the pancreas. **CT** usually affords much better visualization of the pancreas (unless the patient is very thin). **IV cholangiography** is no longer recommended to determine if there are calculi within the biliary tract; if impaction of a gallstone in the ampullary region is strongly suspected and requires documentation, a **percutaneous transhepatic cholangiogram** or **endoscopic retrograde cholangiopancreatography (ERCP)** can be attempted. In some medical centers, gallstones impacted in the ampulla of Vater are being removed endoscopically if the pancreatitis does not resolve quickly. The benefits of this approach require clarification.

Prognosis

The prognosis is difficult to gauge at the bedside. Pancreatitis associated with necrosis and hemorrhage has a mortality $\geq$ 30 to 50%. Features suggestive of this entity include a progressive fall in Hct, presence of hemorrhagic fluid within ascites, reduction in serum Ca, or presence of **Grey-Turner's** or **Cullen's sign** (indicating *extravasation of hemorrhagic exudate to the flanks or umbilical region respectively*).

Ranson's 11 prognostic signs alert the clinician to the presence of severe acute pancreatitis. Five signs can be documented at admission: (1) age > 55 yr, (2) serum glucose > 200 mg/dL, (3) serum lactic dehydrogenase > 350 IU/L, (4) AST (formerly SGOT) > 250 u., and (5) WBC count > 16,000/μL. The rest are determined within 48 h after admission: (6) Hct fall > 10%, (7) BUN rise > 5 mg/dL, (8) serum Ca < 8 mg/dL, (9) arterial P_{O_2} < 60 mm Hg, (10) base deficit > 4 mEq/L, and (11) estimated fluid sequestration > 6 L. If < 3 signs are positive, the mortality is < 5%; if 3 or 4 are positive, the mortality is 15 to 20%; mortality increases progressively with the number of positive signs.

Treatment

Mild edematous pancreatitis: The aims are to maintain the patient in a fasting state until signs and symptoms of acute inflammation have subsided (ie, cessation of abdominal tenderness and pain, normalization of serum amylase, and return of hunger and well-being) and to infuse sufficient IV fluids to prevent hypovolemia and hypotension. Insertion of a nasogastric tube and removal of gastric fluid and air are helpful if there is persistent nausea and vomiting or presence of ileus.

Severe acute pancreatitis: When this diagnosis is suspected, care should be given in an intensive care unit with hourly monitoring of vital signs (at times more often) and

urine output; accurate metabolic flow sheet, which is reassessed q 8 h; arterial blood gases at least q 12 h (at times q 2 to 3 h); measurements q 1 h from central venous pressure line or Swan-Ganz catheter; gastric pH determination q 2 h and appropriate neutralization with antacids; Hct, glucose, and electrolyte assessment q 6 to 8 h; and daily studies including CBC, platelet count, coagulation parameters, total protein with albumin, BUN, creatinine, Ca, Mg, amylase, and lipase.

The patient is maintained in a fasting state for at least 2 and possibly 3 to 4 wk. A nasogastric tube is usually used to counteract vomiting and intestinal ileus and as a means of instilling liquid antacids if there is a threat of stress ulcers. If intragastric contents are maintained at a neutral pH, there is probably no additional value to the use of an H_2 receptor blocking agent (eg, cimetidine or ranitidine). Additional efforts to reduce pancreatic secretion with drugs (eg, anticholinergics, glucagon, and somatostatin) have no proven benefit.

A most important component of therapy is fluid resuscitation that may require 6 to 8 L/day of replacement fluid containing appropriate electrolytes and colloid. If there is retroperitoneal hemorrhage, transfusions are required. Adequacy of fluid replacement and cardiac function should be gauged at least by a central venous pressure line and usually by measurements obtained by a Swan-Ganz catheter. If arterial blood gases reveal hypoxemia, humidified O_2 via mask or nasal prongs should be used. If hypoxemia does not respond, assisted ventilation may be required. If hypoxemia persists and wedge pulmonary artery pressure **(WPAP)** remains normal, adult respiratory distress syndrome is probably developing, and assisted ventilation with positive end expiratory pressure may be required (see Ch. 34). Severe pain should be treated with meperidine 75 to 100 mg IM q 3 to 4 h (not morphine, because it causes contraction of the sphincter of Oddi); at times, IV meperidine is required q 2 to 3 h. A serum glucose of 200 to 250 mg/dL should not be treated, but higher levels should be treated cautiously with s.c. or IV insulin and careful monitoring. Hypocalcemia is frequently corrected by administration of albumin-containing fluids. If there is neuromuscular irritability, calcium gluconate (10% solution) can be given 10 to 20 mL IV in 1 L of replacement fluid over 4 to 6 h. If there is coexisting hypomagnesemia, magnesium replacement (at least 8 mEq, the amount in a 2-mL vial of 50% magnesium sulfate) should be given q 8 to 12 h diluted as above in replacement fluid (if there is renal failure, serum Mg levels should be monitored and IV magnesium given cautiously). With restoration of Mg levels to normal, serum Ca levels should also return to normal.

Cardiac failure documented by increased WPAP should be treated by digitalization and diuretic therapy. Renal failure should be treated by intensification of fluid replacement, if there is prerenal azotemia, or by mannitol, if there is acute renal failure. Peritoneal dialysis may also be required.

The use of antibiotics is controversial. There is no evidence that antibiotic prophylaxis can prevent a pancreatic abscess. However, vigorous antibiotic therapy should be used to treat specific infections (eg, biliary sepsis, pulmonary infection, or UTI). If a pancreatic abscess is documented, antibiotic therapy should be instituted and surgical debridement performed. The value of peritoneal lavage to wash out activated pancreatic enzymes and toxins remains controversial. Despite anecdotal reports of at least temporary improvement, the value of this technic in improving survival is not confirmed.

The nutritional needs of the patient must be adequately met. A seriously ill patient should not be fed for ≥ 2 to 3 wk (often 4 to 6 wk). Thus, it is important to initiate total parenteral nutrition within the first several days (see in Ch. 79).

Surgical intervention during the first several days is clearly justified for severe blunt or penetrating trauma. Other indications for surgery include uncontrolled biliary sepsis and inability to distinguish acute pancreatitis from a surgical emergency. The value of surgery during the first several days to counteract a progressive downhill course

remains unclarified in the absence of a controlled study. There are anecdotal reports of marked improvement following pancreatic debridement.

A **pancreatic abscess** usually does not occur until after the first week of illness. An abscess should be suspected if the patient maintains a generally toxic appearance with elevated temperature and WBC count or if deterioration follows an initial period of stabilization. The diagnosis is supported by positive blood cultures and particularly by presence of air bubbles in the retroperitoneum on abdominal CT. Percutaneous aspiration of pancreatic exudate guided by abdominal CT may reveal organisms on Gram stain and/or culture, a finding that should lead to prompt surgical debridement.

A **pancreatic pseudocyst** that persists for > 4 to 6 wk, is > 5 cm in diameter, and causes abdominal symptoms (especially pain) requires surgical decompression. Within this time span, a pseudocyst that is expanding rapidly, is secondarily infected, or is associated with bleeding or impending rupture requires more urgent surgical therapy. In some instances percutaneous pigtail catheter drainage is effective in closing a pseudocyst (especially when it is infected).

When acute pancreatitis is caused by **biliary calculi,** surgical strategy is dictated by the severity of the pancreatitis. If it is mild, elective cholecystectomy can usually be performed safely later during the same period of hospitalization. If the pancreatitis is severe, but decompression of the biliary system is required, a cholecystostomy is frequently a safer choice than more lengthy surgery, eg, cholecystectomy and common bile duct exploration (see also Ch. 78).

CHRONIC PANCREATITIS

Etiology and Pathogenesis

In the USA, the commonest cause of chronic pancreatitis is alcoholism; rare causes are hereditary pancreatitis, hyperparathyroidism, and obstruction of the main pancreatic duct due to stenosis, stones, or carcinoma. Rarely, an episode of severe acute pancreatitis causes sufficient pancreatic ductal stenosis to impair drainage and result in chronic pancreatitis.

In tropical countries (eg, India, Indonesia, and Nigeria) idiopathic calcific pancreatitis occurs among children and young adults.

Symptoms and Signs

In **chronic relapsing pancreatitis,** symptoms and signs may be identical to an episode of acute pancreatitis. In chronic pancreatitis, there is occasionally no pain. However, severe epigastric pain, the etiology of which is not always clear, may last many hours or several days. Possible causes include acute inflammation that cannot be recognized by conventional tests, distension of pancreatic ducts caused by strictures or calculi, a pseudocyst, perineural inflammation, or obstruction of either the duodenum or common bile duct caused by fibrosis of the head of the pancreas. In time, when acinar cells that secrete pancreatic digestive enzymes are progressively destroyed, abdominal pain may subside. Eventually, when lipase and protease secretions are reduced to < 10% of normal, the patient develops steatorrhea and creatorrhea, and may pass greasy stools or even oil droplets. Islet cell destruction reduces insulin secretion and causes glucose intolerance.

Diagnosis

Structural abnormalities can be visualized by a plain film of the abdomen (showing pancreatic calcification, indicating the presence of intraductal stones), abdominal ultrasound or CT (showing abnormalities in size and consistency of the pancreas, pancreatic pseudocyst, or dilated pancreatic ducts), and endoscopic retrograde cholangiopancreatography (showing abnormalities of the main pancreatic duct and secondary branches).

Tests of pancreatic function assess endocrine and exocrine function. Diabetes melli-

tus is present if a 2-h postprandial serum glucose is > 200 mg/dL or 2 fasting serum glucose levels are > 120 mg. The most sensitive test of pancreatic exocrine function, the **secretin test,** is not available in most hospitals. It involves positioning a tube in the duodenum and collecting pancreatic secretions stimulated by IV secretin alone or with either cholecystokinin-pancreozymin or cerulein. Duodenal contents are collected for volume determination, HCO_3 concentration, and enzyme concentration. A collection that is of normal volume (> 2 mL/kg) and low in HCO_3 (< 90 mEq/L) suggests chronic pancreatitis; low volume (< 2 mL/kg), normal HCO_3 concentration (> 90 mEq/L), and normal enzyme concentration suggest pancreatic cancer. A 72-h test for stool fat is insensitive for pancreatic exocrine dysfunction, because steatorrhea does not occur until lipase output is < 10% of normal. Newer, more sensitive tests include measurement of serum trypsinogen, fecal chymotrypsin, and urinary p-aminobenzoic acid (the bentiromide test).

Treatment

A relapse of chronic pancreatitis may require treatment appropriate for an episode of acute pancreatitis.

Medical treatment of chronic pain is frequently unsatisfactory. The patient must eschew alcohol. At times, an interval of IV fluids and fasting proves beneficial. Dietary measures of uncertain benefit include small feedings with restriction in fat and protein (to reduce secretion of pancreatic enzymes), and either an H_2 receptor blocker or antacids (to reduce acid-stimulated release of secretin, which increases the flow of pancreatic juice). Too often, these measures do not relieve pain, and, because increasing amounts of narcotics are required, the threat of drug addiction is very real.

A complication of chronic pancreatitis may cause chronic pain, such as a pancreatic pseudocyst, which can be decompressed into a nearby structure (eg, the stomach, if it is firmly adherent to it) or a defunctionalized loop of jejunum (if it is not). If the pain is refractory and the main pancreatic duct is dilated (to a diameter > 8 mm), a lateral pancreaticojejunostomy can be expected to relieve pain in about 70 to 80% of patients. If the duct is not dilated, perineural inflammation may be responsible, and percutaneous denervation of the celiac plexus with alcohol can be attempted (with relief of pain for several months in some instances). Alternatively, a resection can be considered, eg, 50% pancreatectomy, 95% subtotal distal pancreatectomy, or Whipple operation (if the disease is most extensive at the head of the pancreas). These operative approaches may relieve pain in 40 to 70% of patients and should be reserved for patients with a nondilated duct, who have discontinued the use of alcohol, and are able to manage a diabetic condition that may be intensified by pancreatic resection.

Steatorrhea can be improved, but rarely abolished, with potent pancreatic extracts (containing lipase ≥ 5000 u./tablet or capsule) 4 to 6 tablets with meals. If the response is unsatisfactory, the effectiveness of pancreatic extracts may be enhanced by a liquid antacid 30 mL before meals and 1 h after meals (to reduce intragastric acidity and thereby protect enzymes that are denatured in an acid milieu). If antacid therapy fails, pancreatic enzymes can be protected by the use of an H_2 receptor blocking agent (cimetidine 300 mg before meals and at bedtime or ranitidine 150 mg bid). Favorable clinical response can be appreciated in terms of weight gain, reduction in number of daily bowel movements, elimination of oil droplet seepage, and improvement in general well-being. Clinical response can be quantitated by comparing tests for stool fat (see above under Diagnosis) before and after enzyme therapy. If steatorrhea is particularly severe and refractory to these measures, medium chain triglycerides can be provided as a source of fat, reducing dietary fat proportionally. At times, supplementation of fat-soluble vitamins (A, D, and K) is required.

Oral hypoglycemic agents rarely help in the treatment of diabetes mellitus caused by chronic pancreatitis. Insulin should be administered *cautiously*, since the coexisting deficiency of glucagon secretion by α-cells means that the hypoglycemic effects of

insulin are unopposed and prolonged hypoglycemia may occur. Serum glucose levels from 200 to 250 mg are acceptable and do not require treatment. Diabetic ketoacidosis rarely occurs in chronic pancreatitis; it is better to maintain the patient in a slightly hyperglycemic range than to risk hypoglycemia due to overzealous administration of insulin.

CANCER OF THE PANCREAS

EXOCRINE TUMORS

DUCTAL ADENOCARCINOMA

Symptoms and Signs

Adenocarcinomas of the exocrine pancreas arise from duct cells 9 times oftener than from acinar cells. Eighty percent occur in the head of the gland and may produce obstructive jaundice, while tumors located in the body and tail may cause splenic vein obstruction, splenomegaly, gastric and esophageal varices, and GI hemorrhage. Otherwise, symptoms are similar, regardless of the location of the cancer. Cancers appear at the mean age of 55 yr and occur 1.5 to 2 times oftener in men. At diagnosis, weight loss > 10% and abdominal pain are present in 90% of patients. Severe upper abdominal pain usually radiates to the back. Relief may be obtained by bending forward, assuming the fetal position, or using aspirin. Symptoms occur late; by the time of diagnosis, in 90% of patients the tumor has spread beyond the gland or metastasized to the liver or lung.

Diagnosis

Routine laboratory tests are often normal. If bile duct obstruction or liver metastases are present, an increased alkaline phosphatase and bilirubin may be present. Hyperglycemia occurs in 25 to 50% of patients. Of a number of immunologic and enzyme tests, carcinoembryonic antigen, pancreatic oncofetal protein, and galactosyltransferase II are the most sensitive, and are elevated in 40, 67, and 67% respectively. However, because they do not detect nonmetastatic localized pancreatic cancer and are increased in patients with nonpancreatic cancers, they are not used routinely.

The most commonly used tests to detect pancreatic cancer are ultrasound **(US)**, CT, and endoscopic retrograde pancreatography **(ERP)**. The diagnosis is usually confirmed by percutaneous CT- or US-guided needle biopsy of the tumor (75 to 95% sensitive) or percutaneous biopsy of liver metastasis. US is the recommended first test, because it is relatively inexpensive, uses nonionizing radiation, and has a sensitivity of 65 to 85%, if the pancreas can be visualized. However, if US is negative or indeterminant, CT should be done. It may be more sensitive than US and its rate of nonvisualization of the pancreas is lower. If CT is negative and clinical suspicion of pancreatic neoplasm is still high, one should do an ERP, which has a sensitivity and specificity > 90% when the pancreatic duct can be cannulated (85% success rate). In unusual situations where the clinical suspicion of pancreatic cancer remains high and all diagnostic tests are normal, an exploratory laparotomy may be indicated.

Arteriography, radioselenium pancreatic scans, and pancreatic function tests are rarely done.

Prognosis and Treatment

Overall 5-yr survival is < 2%. At operation, only 10% of patients have localized tumors. They should undergo a total pancreatectomy or Whipple procedure (pancreaticoduodenectomy) and can expect a 5-yr survival of 10%. If an unresectable tumor is found at operation and gastroduodenal or bile duct obstruction is present or pending, a double gastric and biliary bypass operation is performed. In patients with inoperable

lesions and jaundice, bile duct obstruction is relieved by nonoperative CT- or US-guided catheter or endoscopic placement of a stent to drain the liver through the bile duct into the duodenum.

Radiotherapy and chemotherapy may lengthen survival in ambulatory patients with locally unresectable tumors. Surgical implantation of 20 to 36 μCi of Iodine 125 into the tumor followed by postoperative radiation (4000 to 4500 rads), the combination of radiation and 5-fluorouracil **(5-FU)** and combinations of 5-FU, adriamycin, and mitomycin have increased survival in controlled trials. Most patients with inoperable pancreatic cancer are offered a combination of chemotherapy and irradiation.

To control pain, aspirin 0.65 gm alone or combined with codeine 30 to 120 mg orally q 4 h may be effective. Stronger oral or parenteral narcotics in dosages sufficient to relieve pain may be required. Percutaneous or operative splanchnic block can be remarkably effective. If palliative surgery has not relieved pruritus secondary to obstructive jaundice, it can be managed with cholestyramine 4 gm orally 1 to 4 times/day and phenothiazines.

Exocrine pancreatic insufficiency should be treated with pancrelipase (6 to 8 tablets with meals) and diabetes mellitus should be carefully monitored and controlled.

CYSTADENOCARCINOMA

Rare pancreatic tumor that arises as a malignant degeneration of a mucus cystadenoma and presents as upper abdominal pain and a palpable abdominal mass.

Diagnosis by US or CT scanning of the pancreas demonstrates a cystic mass with some debris within the cyst. Scans may be erroneously interpreted as demonstrating a necrotic adenocarcinoma. In contrast to ductal adenocarcinoma, cystadenocarcinoma has a relatively good prognosis. Only 20% have metastasis at the time of operation, and complete excision of the tumor by either distal or total pancreatectomy or the Whipple procedure results in a 65% 5-yr survival.

ENDOCRINE TUMORS

Pancreatic islet cell tumors have 2 general presentations. **Nonfunctioning tumors** may cause obstructive symptoms of the biliary tract or duodenum or bleeding into the GI tract, or exist as abdominal masses. Hypersecretion of a particular hormone by **functioning tumors** may cause various syndromes; these include hypoglycemia (**insulinoma** hypersecretes insulin), Zollinger-Ellison syndrome (**gastrinoma** hypersecretes gastrin), watery diarrhea, hypokalemia, and alkalosis (or WDHA syndrome) also called pancreatic cholera, (caused by hypersecretion of vasoactive intestinal peptide or of prostaglandins E and E_2), carcinoid syndrome (caused by **carcinoid tumors,** which are difficult to distinguish histologically from islet-cell tumors), diabetes (**glucagonoma** hypersecretes glucagon), and **Cushing's syndrome** (from ACTH hypersecretion). These clinical syndromes also occur sometimes in **multiple endocrine neoplasia,** *syndromes in which tumors or hyperplasia affect 2 or more endocrine glands, usually the parathyroid, pituitary, thyroid, or adrenals* (see Ch. 92).

INSULINOMA

Rare, islet-cell tumor with hypersecretion of insulin.

Symptoms and signs of hypoglycemia secondary to an insulinoma appear during fasting, are insidious, and may mimic a variety of psychiatric and neurologic disorders. CNS disturbances are characteristic: headache, confusion, visual disturbances, motor weakness, palsy, ataxia, marked personality changes, and possible progression to loss of consciousness, convulsions, and coma. Evidence of sympathetic stimulation (faint-

ness, weakness, tremulousness, palpitation, sweating, hunger, and nervousness) may occur, but is often absent.

Diagnosis

Correlation of excessive insulinemia, measured by insulin radioimmunoassay **(IRI)** with plasma glucose levels is mandatory to confirm the diagnosis. The most helpful procedure is a carefully supervised 72-h fast. Plasma insulin concentration falls progressively in normal individuals; in those with insulinoma, high insulin levels coexist with hypoglycemia. The possibility *must be considered* of surreptitious self-administration of insulin; it can be detected by demonstrating the presence of circulating insulin antibodies.

Usually within the first 24 h, hypoglycemia as the cause of the symptoms is established by **Whipple's triad:** (1) The attack comes during the fast, (2) symptoms occur in the presence of hypoglycemia (glucose < 40 mg/dL), and (3) ingestion of carbohydrates relieves the symptoms. Simultaneous hyperinsulinemia of > 6 μU/mL is diagnostic of insulin-mediated hypoglycemia.

If Whipple's triad is not observed after prolonged fasting, and the fasting plasma glucose after an overnight fast is > 50 mg/dL, the **tolbutamide test** is useful. On the day of the test, sodium tolbutamide 1 gm is given IV over a 2-min period. Persistent hypoglycemia (plasma glucose < 57 mg/dL) and hyperinsulinemia (IRI > 20 μU/mL) 2 to 3 h after tolbutamide administration is characteristic of insulinoma.

In difficult diagnostic problems, a **C-peptide suppression test** can be performed. During insulin infusion (0.1 u./kg/h) insulinoma patients fail to suppress C-peptide to normal levels ($\leq$ 1.2 ng/mL).

Angiography is the most reliable method for visualizing highly vascular insulinomas. Preoperative localization can be achieved in 90% of patients. Celiac arterial injection followed by hepatic or splenic artery injection usually permits visualization of the tumor; occasionally, selective catheterization of pancreatic vessels is required. Stereoscopic filming in association with magnification and subtraction are almost routinely used.

Treatment

A small, single **adenoma** at or near the surface of the pancreas can usually be enucleated. In the case of a single large or deep adenoma within the body or tail of the pancreas, multiple lesions of the body or tail (or both), or if no insulinoma is found (an unusual circumstance), a distal, subtotal pancreatic resection is performed. In < 1% of cases, the insulinoma is ectopically located in peripancreatic sites of the duodenal wall or periduodenal area and can be found only by diligent search. Total pancreatectomy is reserved for resectable malignant lesions of the proximal pancreas, when medical therapy is ineffective, or if a previous subtotal resection proves inadequate.

Overall surgical cure rates should approach 90%, since only 10% of tumors are malignant. When hypoglycemia continues, diazoxide orally (3 to 8 mg/kg in 2 to 3 equal doses q 8 to 12 h) in conjunction with a natriuretic can be used. The appropriate starting dose is 3 mg/kg. Subsequent doses can be adjusted according to need. The combination of streptozocin (1 gm/sq m BSA IV weekly for 4 wk), a broad-spectrum antibiotic, and 5-fluorouracil may give measurable benefit in 50% of patients. Its use requires monitoring of renal function (urine proteins, serum creatinine), hepatic function, and potential hematopoietic toxicity (CBC).

ZOLLINGER-ELLISON SYNDROME

(Z-E Syndrome; Gastrinoma)

A syndrome characterized by marked hypergastrinemia, gastric hypersecretion, and peptic ulceration. Usually there is an associated gastrin-producing tumor of the pan-

creas with cells of the non-β-type. Occasionally the tumors are at other sites, particularly in the duodenal wall. Most patients have multiple tumors, of which ½ are malignant. Usually the tumors are small (< 1 cm in diameter) and their growth and spread are slow. They may be seen in patients with other endocrine abnormalities, particularly of the parathyroids and, less often, of the pituitary and adrenal glands. This polyglandular disorder, **multiple endocrine neoplasia,** is discussed in Ch. 92.

Symptoms and Signs

The typical clinical presentation is an aggressive peptic ulcer diathesis with ulcerations occurring in atypical locations (up to 25% are located distal to the duodenal bulb) or following surgical treatment. The complications of perforation, bleeding, and obstruction can be frequent and life-threatening. However, in > 50% of patients, clinical, x-ray, and endoscopic findings are indistinguishable from ordinary peptic ulcer disease. Furthermore, Z-E ulcers may wax and wane as ordinary ulcers do and as many as 25% of Z-E patients may not have an ulcer at diagnosis. Diarrhea may be the initial symptom in 25 to 40% of patients. The diagnosis may not be suspected until after surgery and then may be more difficult to make. Therefore, serum gastrin should always be measured before any operation for peptic ulcer.

Diagnosis

Diagnosis is suspected in patients with a compatible clinical history, x-ray evidence of a duodenal or postbulbar ulcer associated with large edematous gastric and duodenal folds and large amounts of fluid in the stomach, and an excessive basal gastric acid secretory rate (> 10 mEq/h in the unoperated patient or 5 mEq/h after a previous ulcer operation and is > 60% of the amount of acid secreted after a maximal stimulating dose of histamine, ametazole, or pentagastrin). However, the most reliable test is the radioimmunoassay measurement of serum gastrin. All patients have > 150 pg/mL; markedly elevated levels of > 1000 pg/mL in a patient with compatible clinical features and gastric acid hypersecretion establishes the diagnosis. However, hypergastrinemia can be found in pernicious anemia, chronic gastritis, renal insufficiency, massive intestinal resection, and pheochromocytoma.

Provocative tests may be useful in patients without marked hypergastrinemia. In these tests, calcium (5 mg/kg/h IV for 3 h), secretin (2 u. GI hormone secretin/kg/h as a rapid IV injection), or a test meal is accompanied by measurements of serum gastrin. Characteristic responses in Z-E syndrome are marked increases in serum gastrin with Ca, a paradoxic increase with secretin, and a failure to increase > 50% after a standard meal. Patients with antral G-cell hyperplasia have increased concentrations of gastrin in antral tissue, fasting hypergastrinemia that may not increase in response to Ca^{++}, decreases with secretin, and increases markedly in response to a test meal. These patients do not have a pancreatic tumor and, following gastrectomy, fasting serum gastrin falls to normal and does not increase in response to a meal. In the usual peptic ulcer disease, there is a small increase of serum gastrin in response to Ca, no paradoxic increase in response to secretin, and a moderate increase after a test meal.

Gastrinomas are visualized < 50% of the time by arteriography, but it is the most sensitive imaging test. Because the tumors are small, abdominal ultrasonography and CT visualize the tumors in only 20 to 30% of patients.

Treatment

The advent of H_2 receptor antagonists, which markedly decrease gastric acid output, alleviate clinical symptoms, and promote healing, has greatly modified treatment of the Z-E syndrome. However, because surgical cure (resection of tumor) is possible in 20% of patients with the nonfamilial type of Z-E syndrome, these patients should undergo exploratory laparotomy. Patients with MEN-Type I or metastatic tumors should not be explored. These patients, as well as patients with unresectable tumors should be treated with cimetidine 300 mg orally qid between meals, but some patients

may require 3 to 4 gm/day in divided doses. The drug must be used indefinitely. Side effects (eg, gynecomastia and impotence) have been reported. Ranitidine is as effective and may not be associated with side effects. However, doses greater than the recommended 150 mg bid may be needed to control symptoms. In refractory patients, the addition of anticholinergics (eg, propantheline bromide 15 to 30 mg orally 30 min before meals) or antacids (eg, magnesium-aluminum hydroxide gel 30 mL orally 1 and 3 h after meals and at bedtime), or both, may also be helpful. If this treatment is unsuccessful, total gastrectomy may be necessary; this procedure in Z-E syndrome is well tolerated without crippling nutritional complications, but patients need vitamin B_{12} 100 μg/mo IM, and iron and Ca supplements daily. In patients with metastatic disease, streptozocin plus 5-fluorouracil may reduce tumor mass and serum gastrin concentration and be a useful adjunct to H_2-receptor antagonist therapy or total gastrectomy.

Omeprazole is an investigational drug available for patients with the Z-E syndrome. It inhibits H^+, K^+ adenosinetriphosphate, and markedly reduces gastric parietal cell H^+ secretion. In patients with Z-E syndrome, 20 to 100 mg/day orally will control gastric acid secretion. Somatostatin analog also dramatically reduces symptoms in patients with Z-E syndrome as well as patients with other functioning islet cell tumors (eg, carcinoid, vipoma, glucagonoma); it will likely be available soon for use in these patients.

VIPOMA SYNDROME

(Verner-Morrison Syndrome; WDHA [Watery Diarrhea, Hypokalemia, Achlorhydria]; WDHH [Watery Diarrhea, Hypokalemia, Hypochlorhydria]; Pancreatic Cholera)

A syndrome caused by non-β islet cell tumors; it may be associated with multiple endocrine neoplasia (see Ch. 92).

Symptoms and Signs

The major clinical features are prolonged massive watery diarrhea (fasting stool volume > 750 to 1000 mL/day) and symptoms of hypokalemia and dehydration. Half of the patients have relatively constant diarrhea while the rest have alternating periods of severe and moderate diarrhea. One third have diarrhea < 1 yr before diagnosis, but in 25%, diarrhea is present for 5 yr or more before diagnosis. Lethargy, muscular weakness, nausea, vomiting, and crampy abdominal pain are frequent symptoms. During attacks of diarrhea, flushing similar to the carcinoid syndrome occurs rarely.

Diagnosis

Diagnosis requires demonstration of a secretory diarrhea (stool osmolality is close to plasma osmolality and the product of twice the sum of Na and K stool concentrations accounts for all measured stool osmolality) without apparent cause. Other causes of secretory diarrhea and, in particular, laxative abuse must be excluded (see also DIARRHEA in Ch. 56). Arteriography and ultrasonography should be done, but will not visualize the tumor in 2/3 of patients. Circulating vasoactive intestinal peptide by radioimmunoassay may be elevated but many false-positive and -negative results limit its usefulness. Gastric acid secretion is usually low, but normal values do not exclude the diagnosis. Pancreatic secretion, jejunal biopsy, and stool fat are normal or only mildly abnormal. In most patients, the diagnosis is established by finding a pancreatic tumor or a neurotumor at exploration.

Treatment

Initially, fluids and electrolytes must be replaced. To avoid acidosis, bicarbonate must be given to replace fecal loss of this ion. Because fecal losses of water and electrolytes increase as rehydration is achieved, continual IV replacement may become more difficult.

Resection of the tumor results in complete cure in 1/2 of the patients. In patients with metastatic tumor, resection of all visible tumor may provide temporary relief of symptoms. The combination of streptozocin and 5-fluorouracil has also been effective in reducing diarrhea and tumor mass. In 1/2 of the patients with metastases, a corticosteroid (eg, prednisone 20 mg/day orally) controls diarrhea.

CARCINOID SYNDROME

(See Ch. 95)

GLUCAGONOMA

Pancreatic α-cell glucagon-secreting tumors are very rare but similar to other islet cell tumors in that the primary and metastatic lesions are slow-growing: 15-yr survival times are common. The average age at the onset of symptoms is 50 yr, 80% of patients have been women, and 80% of the tumors are malignant. Hypersecretion of glucagon is associated with diabetes mellitus (see GLUCAGON in Ch. 94). Frequently, weight loss and normochromic anemia are present, but the most distinctive clinical feature is a chronic eruption involving the extremities and often associated with a smooth, shiny, vermillion tongue and cheilitis. The exfoliating, brownish-red, erythematous lesion with superficial necrolysis is termed **necrolytic migratory erythema.**

Diagnosis is made by demonstrating elevated levels of circulating immunoreactive glucagon in the presence of the typical angiographic appearance of an islet-cell tumor and proven by laparotomy.

Treatment by resection of the tumor will alleviate all symptoms. In the event of unresectability, metastasis, or recurrence, the combination of streptozocin and 5-fluorouracil may cause a decrease in the levels of circulating immunoreactive glucagon and symptomatic improvement.

---

56. DIARRHEA AND CONSTIPATION

No body function is more variable and subject to extraneous influences than is defecation. Normal bowel habits vary considerably from one person to another, being modified by age, by dietary, social, and cultural patterns, and by individual physiologic factors. In an urban civilization, the normal frequency of bowel movements ranges from 2 to 3/day to 2 to 3/wk. Increased stool frequency or fecal volume, changes in stool consistency, or blood, mucus, pus, or excess fatty material (oil, grease, or film) in the stool may indicate disease.

DIARRHEA

(See also Chs. 57 and 58, and ACUTE INFECTIOUS GASTROENTERITIS in Ch. 191 and ACUTE INFECTIOUS NEONATAL DIARRHEA in Ch. 186)

Increased volume, fluidity, or frequency of bowel movements relative to the person's usual pattern.

Etiology and Pathophysiology

In healthy adults, stool weight ranges from 100 to 300 gm/day depending on the amount of nonabsorbable dietary material (mainly carbohydrate). Diarrhea occurs when stool weight is increased to > 300 gm/day, except in persons whose diet is rich in vegetable fiber, when such weight is normal. Since 60 to 90% of stool weight is water, diarrhea is mainly due to excess fecal water. Categorizing diarrhea according to the major pathophysiologic cause of the increased stool weight may facilitate etiologic investigation and choice of specific treatment.

1. Osmotic diarrhea occurs when excess nonabsorbable, water-soluble solutes are present in the bowel and retain water in the lumen. This occurs with lactose (lactase deficiency) and other sugar intolerances, and when poorly absorbed salts (magnesium sulfate, sodium phosphates) are prescribed as saline laxatives.

Ingestion of large amounts of the hexitols, sorbitol and mannitol, used as sugar substitutes in dietetic foods, candy, and chewing gum, causes diarrhea by a combination of slow absorption and rapid small-bowel motility (**"dietetic food"** or **"chewing-gum" diarrhea).** The severity of symptoms is proportional to the amount consumed and body weight; the condition disappears as soon as intake stops.

2. Secretory diarrhea: The small and large bowel normally reabsorb salts (especially sodium chloride) and water which are ingested or which reach the lumen as a consequence of digestive secretions. Diarrhea may occur when the small and large bowel secrete rather than absorb electrolytes and water. Substances that induce secretion include bacterial toxins (eg, as in cholera), enteropathogenic viruses, bile acids (eg, after ileal resection), unabsorbed dietary fat in steatorrhea, anthraquinone cathartics, castor oil, and some hormones (eg, secretin, calcitonin), drugs (eg, prostaglandins), and vasoactive intestinal peptide (VIP) from a pancreatic tumor.

3. Malabsorption (see also Ch. 58) may produce diarrhea by either of the above mechanisms. If the unabsorbed material is abundant, water-soluble, and osmotically important (ie, of low mol wt), the mechanism could be osmotic. Lipids are not appreciably water-soluble and cannot act this way; some (fatty acids, bile acids) act as secretagogues for electrolytes and water. In generalized malabsorption, as in nontropical sprue, fat malabsorption (causing colonic secretion) and carbohydrate malabsorption (causing osmotic diarrhea) can coexist.

4. Exudative diarrhea: Many mucosal diseases (eg, regional enteritis, ulcerative colitis, TB, lymphoma, and carcinoma) cause an "exudative enteropathy." Mucosal inflammation, ulceration, or tumefaction may result in an outpouring of plasma, serum proteins, blood, and mucus, thus increasing fecal bulk and fluidity. Involvement of the rectal mucosa may cause urgency and increased frequency of bowel movements because the inflamed rectum is more sensitive to distention.

5. Altered intestinal transit: Chyme must be exposed to adequate absorptive surface of the GI tract for a sufficient amount of time if normal absorption is to occur. Factors that **decrease** exposure time include resection of the small or large bowel, gastric resection, surgery on the pyloric sphincter, vagotomy, surgical bypass of intestinal segments, and drugs or humoral agents (eg, prostaglandins, serotonin) that speed transit by stimulating intestinal smooth muscle.

Malabsorption and diarrhea may also develop when the transit time of chyme through the bowel is prolonged and fecal bacteria proliferate in the small intestine. Factors that **increase** transit time and permit bacterial overgrowth include strictured segments, sclerodermatous intestinal disease, and stagnant loops created by surgery.

Complications of Diarrhea

Electrolyte loss (Na, K, Mg, organic anions, and Cl), fluid loss with consequent dehydration, and vascular collapse may occur. **Collapse** may develop rapidly in patients who are very young, elderly, debilitated, or who have severe diarrhea (eg, those with cholera). **Metabolic acidosis** may develop due to HCO_3 loss. Serum Na concentrations vary according to the composition of diarrheal losses relative to plasma. **Hypokalemia** may occur in severe or chronic diarrhea or if the stools contain excess mucus. Tetany due to **hypomagnesemia** following prolonged diarrhea has been observed.

Diagnosis

Clinical features vary greatly depending on the cause, duration, and severity of the diarrhea, on the area of bowel affected, and on the patient's general health. The history

should note the time, place, and other circumstances of onset; duration and severity; associated abdominal pain or vomiting; presence of overt or occult blood in the stool; frequency and timing of bowel movements; evidence of steatorrhea (fatty, greasy, or oily stools with a foul odor); associated changes in weight or appetite; use of dietetic products (see Osmotic diarrhea, above); and presence of rectal tenesmus.

Macro- and microscopic examination of the stools may be helpful. The fluidity, volume, and presence of blood, pus, mucus, or excess fat should be noted. Generally, in diseases of the upper gut, the stools are voluminous and watery or fatty. In colonic disease, movements are frequent, sometimes small in volume, and possibly accompanied by blood, pus, mucus, and abdominal discomfort. In diseases of the rectal mucosa, the rectum may be more sensitive to distention, and diarrhea may be characterized by frequent, small stools. Microscopy may confirm the presence of WBCs (ulceration or bacterial invasion), unabsorbed fat, meat fibers, or parasitic infestation (eg, amebiasis, giardiasis). Stool pH, normally > 6.0, is decreased by bacterial fermentation of unabsorbed carbohydrate and protein in the colon. Alkalinization of the stool reveals the pink color of phenolphthalein, a commonly abused laxative.

Evidence of vascular collapse, dehydration, electrolyte depletion, or anemia should be sought. Abdominal examination and digital and proctoscopic rectal examination should be performed. Biopsy of the rectal mucosa and rectal swabbing for microscopic examination should be considered at proctoscopy.

Treatment

Diarrhea is only a symptom and the underlying disorder should be specifically treated if possible. Symptomatic treatment may also be necessary. Intestinal tone may be increased by diphenoxylate 2.5 to 5 mg as tablets or liquid tid or qid, codeine phosphate 15 to 30 mg bid or tid, or paregoric (camphorated opium tincture) 15 mL q 4 h. Peristalsis is decreased by anticholinergics (eg, belladonna tincture, atropine, or propantheline). Bulk is provided by a psyllium or methylcellulose compound; these bulking agents, though usually prescribed for constipation, also decrease the fluidity of liquid stools when given in small doses. Kaolin adsorbs fluid.

Severe acute diarrhea may require urgent fluid and electrolyte replacement to correct dehydration, electrolyte imbalance, and acidosis. Sodium chloride, potassium chloride, glucose, and fluids to counteract acidosis (sodium lactate, acetate, or bicarbonate) may be indicated. Fluid balance and estimates of body fluid composition must be monitored carefully (see REGULATION OF WATER AND SODIUM HOMEOSTASIS in Ch. 84). Associated vomiting or GI bleeding may require additional measures.

An oral glucose-electrolyte solution may be given if nausea and vomiting are not severe. Fluids containing glucose (or sucrose, as table sugar), sodium chloride, and sodium bicarbonate are rapidly absorbed and easily prepared. Five mL (1 tsp) table salt, 5 mL (1 tsp) baking soda, 20 mL (4 tsp) table sugar, and flavoring are added to 1 L water (about 1 qt). Parenteral fluids are generally required for more severe diarrhea. If nausea or vomiting is present, oral intake should be restricted. However, when water and electrolytes must be replaced in massive amounts (eg, in epidemic cholera), oral glucose-electrolyte supplements are sometimes given in addition to the more conventional IV therapy with electrolyte (bicarbonate) fluids (see CHOLERA in Ch. 8).

CONSTIPATION

(Constipation in children is discussed in BEHAVIORAL PROBLEMS in Ch. 188)

Difficult or infrequent passage of feces. Constipation can also refer to hardness of stool or a feeling of incomplete evacuation.

Acute constipation represents a definite change *for that individual*, suggesting an or-

ganic cause. In patients complaining of constipation for only hours or a few days, mechanical bowel obstruction must be considered. A second organic cause is adynamic ileus, which often accompanies acute intra-abdominal disease (eg, localized peritonitis, diverticulitis); it may complicate a variety of traumatic conditions (eg, head injuries, spinal fractures) or may follow general anesthesia. Strong laxatives should be avoided in all of these circumstances. Less ominous, but often confusing, is the acute onset of constipation in bedridden patients (particularly the aged) or constipation related to side effects of drugs. A careful drug history should always be obtained, since constipation is caused by many agents, including those that act within the lumen (aluminum hydroxide, bismuth salts, iron salts, cholestyramine), anticholinergics, opiates, ganglionic blockers, and many tranquilizers and sedatives.

When the change of bowel habit persists for weeks or occurs intermittently with increasing frequency and/or severity, colonic tumors and other causes of partial obstruction should be suspected. Underlying causes must be identified and treated. Local anorectal conditions (eg, anal fissures) that cause pain or bleeding should be sought; plain abdominal films with upright views, proctosigmoidoscopy, and possibly a barium enema examination may be required. If no disorder is found, treatment should be symptomatic (see below).

In **chronic constipation,** the common functional causes are those that hamper normal bowel movements because the storage, transporting, and evacuating mechanisms of the colon are deranged, sometimes by systemic disorders (eg, debilitating infections, hypothyroidism, hypercalcemia, uremia, or porphyria), but more often by local neurogenic disorders—eg, irritable bowel syndromes (see in Ch. 61), inactive colon (see below), and megacolon (see HIRSCHSPRUNG'S DISEASE under GASTROINTESTINAL DEFECTS in Ch. 187). Certain neurologic disorders (eg, Parkinson's disease, cerebral thrombosis, tumor, and injury to the spinal cord) are important extraintestinal causes. Psychogenic factors are most common. (See below under psychogenic constipation and under suggested treatments for specific disorders.)

Treatment

The diet should contain enough fiber to ensure adequate stool bulk. Vegetable fiber, largely indigestable and unabsorbable, increases stool bulk; certain components of fiber also adsorb fluid into the solid phase, making stools softer and thus facilitating their passage. Fruits and vegetables are recommended, and the diet can be supplemented with cereals containing bran, taken to tolerance. Unrefined miller's bran, taken as 2 to 3 tsp on fruit or cereal bid or tid, may be preferred.

Bulking agents (eg, bran, psyllium, and methyl cellulose) are the only laxatives that should be considered for long-term use. They act slowly and gently and are the safest medications for promoting stool elimination. Proper use involves gradually increasing the dose, best taken tid or qid and with sufficient liquid (by adding 2 to 3 glasses/day of extra fluid) to prevent impaction of inspissated medication, until a softer, bulkier stool results. This approach produces natural effects and is not habit-forming. **Psyllium** may fulfill the difficult qualifications of a bi-directional normalizer: In constipation it promotes peristalsis and fecal elimination, and in diarrheal states it decreases the number of watery stools.

Laxatives and cathartics should be used with care. They may interfere with absorption of various drugs by binding them chemically (tetracycline, calcium, and phosphate) or physically (digoxin on cellulose matrices). Rapid transit of the fecal stream may rush some drugs and nutrients beyond their optimal absorptive locus. Abdominal pain of unknown etiology, inflammatory bowel disorders, intestinal obstruction, GI bleeding, and fecal impactions are **contraindications** for their use. In addition to **bulking agents** (see above), laxatives and cathartics can be divided into the following classes:

1. **Wetting agents (detergent laxatives)** soften stool by increasing the wetting ability of intestinal water. They have both hydrophilic and hydrophobic properties. They break down surface barriers, allow water to enter the fecal mass, soften it, and increase its bulk. Increased bulk may stimulate peristalsis and the softened stool moves more easily. **Mineral oil** softens fecal matter, resulting in more easily passed stool mass, but it may decrease absorption of fat-soluble vitamins. Mineral oil and detergent laxatives act slowly; either may be useful following myocardial infarction or anorectal surgery, and in situations requiring prolonged bed rest.

2. **Osmotic agents** or **saline cathartics** are used to prepare patients for some diagnostic bowel procedures and occasionally in the therapy of parasitic infestations. They contain poorly absorbed polyvalent ions (eg, phosphate, magnesium, sulfate) and/or carbohydrates (eg, lactulose, sorbitol). Since these substances remain in the bowel, intraluminal osmotic pressure increases, drawing water into the intestinal lumen. Stool volume increases and consistency decreases. The increased volume stimulates peristalsis, and the softened, watery stool moves easily through the bowel. These agents usually work within 3 h. Magnesium and phosphate are partially absorbed and may be detrimental in some conditions (eg, in renal insufficiency). Sodium (present in some preparations) may adversely affect heart failure. These drugs may also upset the fluid and electrolyte balance if patients without underlying disease ingest large or frequent doses. A novel approach to cleansing the bowel for diagnostic procedures or surgery uses large volumes of a balanced, osmotic agent (eg, polyethylene glycol-electrolyte solutions).

3. **Secretory or stimulant cathartics** (eg, senna and its derivatives, cascara, phenolphthalein, bisacodyl, and castor oil) act by irritation of the intestinal mucosa or by direct neuronal (submucosal and myenteric plexus) stimulation. Some are absorbed, metabolized by the liver, and returned to the bowel in the bile. Peristaltic movements and intraluminal fluid both increase, with cramping and passage of semisolid stool in 6 to 8 h. With continued use, melanosis coli, neuronal degeneration in the colon, "lazy bowel" syndrome, and serious fluid and electrolyte disturbances may occur. Stimulant-type cathartics are frequently helpful to cleanse the bowel for diagnostic procedures.

PSYCHOGENIC CONSTIPATION

Many persons incorrectly believe that daily defecation is integral to normalcy and complain of constipation because the frequency of their bowel movements is not what they expect. Others may be concerned with a certain appearance (thin or pelletlike, color) or consistency of stools, though sometimes the major complaint is lack of satisfaction with the act of defecation. As a result, they abuse the colon with laxatives, suppositories, and enemas. Overzealous treatment of an *imaginary* disorder can result in *real* illness—an irritable bowel syndrome. This may be accompanied by **cathartic colon** (a "pipestem" colon lacking haustra on barium enema examination, thus mimicking ulcerative colitis) and **melanosis coli** (deposits of brown pigment in the mucosa, seen endoscopically and in colonic biopsies), both caused by long-term laxative ingestion.

Obsessive-compulsive people have problems of personal belief and emotional need. They control anxiety by perfectionistic behavior, and their need to rid the body daily of "unclean" wastes may take on exaggerated importance. Failure to defecate daily may result in a sorry cycle in which depression reduces defecatory frequency and failure to defecate augments depression. Such people often become chronic cathartic users or spend excessive time on the toilet.

Treatment

Before advising or reassuring a patient concerning defecatory habits, the physician must exclude serious disease by rectal and proctoscopic examination, and by barium

enema when indicated. Extraintestinal disease also should be excluded by appropriate tests. The psychologic needs of the individual should also be considered. It is neither kind nor useful to accuse an obsessive-compulsive patient of an abnormal attitude toward defecation, as one's psychophysiologic makeup cannot be altered, although psychotherapy may help to inculcate more rational ideas. On the other hand, when the problem is due to a mistaken belief, the physician must explain that daily bowel movements are not essential, that the bowel must be given a chance to function, that laxatives or enemas taken more often than once/3 days deny the bowel that chance, and that the way to "cure a stool" that is "too thin" or "too green" is to avoid looking at it.

COLONIC INERTIA

(Atonic Constipation; Colon Stasis; Inactive Colon)

Etiology

This constipation occurs in aged or invalid patients, especially the bedridden. Feces accumulate because the colon does not respond to the usual stimuli promoting evacuation, or because accessory stimuli normally provided by eating and physical activity are lacking. Use of drugs for associated medical conditions frequently compounds the problem. It sometimes occurs in patients whose rectal sensitivity to the presence of fecal masses is dulled by habitual disregard of the urge to defecate, or by prolonged dependence on laxatives or enemas, often initiated in childhood.

Symptoms, Signs, and Diagnosis

The principal symptom, constipation, is unlike that seen in the irritable colon syndrome, since abdominal discomfort is absent or minimal and the stools are often putty-like or soft and not scybalous. Rectal examination frequently discloses an ampulla full of feces, yet the patient has no urge to defecate and is unable to do so effectively, even with effort. Proctoscopic and barium enema examinations are normal, though the contrast medium may sometimes be evacuated with difficulty and the colon may appear unusually redundant and capacious.

Fecal impaction may develop spontaneously or after barium has been given by mouth or enema. The patient has rectal pain and tenesmus and makes repeated but futile attempts to defecate. Cramps may occur and the patient may pass watery mucus or fecal material around the impacted mass, mimicking diarrhea. Rectal examination discloses a firm, sometimes rocklike, but often rubbery, putty-like mass.

Treatment

This is adapted to the patient's general status. Since abdominal distress and other signs of bowel irritability are minimal, there is no harm in treating an elderly or invalid patient with osmotic laxatives (eg, milk of magnesia 15 to 30 mL or sodium sulfate 15 gm in 1/2 glass of water). In the more chronic situation, the patient should try to have the bowel move at the same time daily, preferably 15 to 45 min after breakfast, since food ingestion stimulates colonic motility. Initial efforts at regular, unhurried bowel movements may be aided by rectal instillation of 60 to 90 mL (2 to 3 oz) of warm (43.3 C [110 F]) olive oil or isotonic saline, or glycerin suppositories may be used.

Fecal impaction is treated by enemas of warm (43.3 C [110 F]) olive oil 60 to 120 mL (2 to 4 oz) followed by enemas of small (100 mL), commercially prepared, hypertonic solutions. If these fail, manual fragmentation and disimpaction of the mass are necessary. This procedure is painful, and peri- and intrarectal application of local anesthetics (eg, lidocaine 5% ointment or dibucaine 1% ointment) is recommended. Some patients require general anesthesia.

57. GASTROENTERITIS: INFECTIVE AND TOXIC

(See also Ch. 56, ACUTE INFECTIOUS GASTROENTERITIS in Ch. 191, and ACUTE INFECTIOUS NEONATAL DIARRHEA in Ch. 186)

A group of clinical syndromes predominantly manifested by upper GI tract symptoms (anorexia, nausea, or vomiting), diarrhea of variable severity, and abdominal discomfort. Subsequent losses of electrolytes and fluids from the body may be little more than an inconvenience to an otherwise healthy adult, but can be of grave significance to persons less able to withstand the stress (eg, the aged, debilitated, or very young).

Etiology and Epidemiology

Gastroenteritis, a generic term, often implies a nonspecific, uncertain, or unknown etiology. However, certain diseases of known bacterial, viral, parasitic, or toxic etiology can be included in the clinical definition. When a specific etiology can be identified, the less specific term (gastroenteritis) can be avoided. Some types of bacterial gastroenteritis (eg, cholera, salmonellosis, and shigellosis) have established pathogenic mechanisms and can be considered prototypes for syndromes of lesser specificity.

Several viruses and subtypes have been etiologically identified: Norwalk virus, rotavirus, and adenovirus; and enteroviruses (coxsackie A1 and echo). Worldwide epidemics of diarrheas in infants, children, and adults are usually spread via water or food by the fecal-oral route (and possibly by the respiratory route). Year-round and second in prevalence only to the common cold, the **Norwalk virus** causes about 40% of nonbacterial diarrhea in children and adults. **Rotaviruses** are major causes of serious diarrheal illness during winter in temperate climates that result in hospitalization of infants and children under age 2 yr. Adults, whose infections tend to be milder, probably have some immunity. **Enteroviral** and **adenoviral infections** have also been identified worldwide, and may be associated with upper respiratory symptoms.

Pathophysiology

1. Bacterial diarrheas due to exotoxins: Certain bacterial species elaborate exotoxins (enterotoxins) that impair intestinal absorption and can provoke secretion of electrolytes and water. In some instances (eg, the enterotoxin of *Vibrio cholerae*), a chemically pure toxin has been characterized; pure toxin alone will produce the voluminous watery secretion from the small intestine seen clinically, thereby demonstrating an adequate pathogenic mechanism for diarrhea. Enterotoxins probably explain other diarrhea syndromes previously attributed to nonspecific causes (eg, *Escherichia coli* enterotoxin may cause some outbreaks of "nursery diarrhea" and "traveler's diarrhea").

2. Bacterial diarrheas due to mucosal invasion or ulceration: Some *Shigella*, *Salmonella*, and *E. coli* species penetrate the mucosa of the small bowel or colon and produce microscopic ulceration, bleeding, exudation of protein-rich fluid, and secretion of electrolytes and water. The invasive process and its results may occur whether or not the organism elaborates an enterotoxin.

Campylobacter infections are increasingly being recognized as a cause of gastroenteritis (see *Campylobacter* INFECTIONS in Ch. 8).

3. Incompletely categorized gastroenteritis syndromes: This entity includes "intestinal flu" or "grippe" and some types of "traveler's diarrhea" (eg, "turista"). Bacterial enterotoxins are the cause in some cases, viral infections in others.

Experiments with the "Norwalk agent" (a virus that causes transient symptoms in man) and with viruses isolated from the intestines of children with diarrhea show that both can cause jejunal mucosal damage and that electrolyte and fluid secretion occur in infected animals. The incubation periods and self-limited courses of these experimental viral diseases suggest a similar pathogenesis for "intestinal flu."

4. Nonbacterial food poisonings: Gastroenteritis may follow ingestion of chemical toxins contained in plants (eg, mushrooms, potatoes, garden flora), seafood (fish, clams, mussels), or contaminated food.

5. Miscellaneous causes: Inability to digest and absorb carbohydrate (eg, lactose intolerance) may cause abdominal symptoms, possibly following milk ingestion and erroneously attributed to milk allergy (see CARBOHYDRATE INTOLERANCE in Ch. 58). True food allergy is rare and poorly understood. Heavy-metal (arsenic, lead, mercury, cadmium) ingestion may cause acute nausea, vomiting, and diarrhea. Many therapeutic agents, including broad-spectrum antibiotics, have major GI side effects.

General Symptoms and Signs

The character and severity of symptoms depend on the nature and dose of the irritant, the duration of its action, the patient's resistance, and the extent of GI involvement. Onset is often sudden and sometimes dramatic, with anorexia, nausea, or vomiting; borborygmi; abdominal cramps; and diarrhea, with or without blood and mucus. Associated malaise, muscular aches, and prostration may occur.

Persistent vomiting and diarrhea result in severe dehydration and shock, with vascular collapse and oliguric renal failure. If vomiting causes excessive fluid loss, metabolic alkalosis with hypochloremia occurs; if diarrhea is more prominent, acidosis is more likely. Hypokalemia may result from either excessive vomiting or diarrhea. Hyponatremia may develop, particularly if nonelectrolyte fluids are used in replacement therapy. Severe dehydration and acid-base imbalance can produce headache and symptoms of muscular and nervous irritability.

The abdomen may be distended and tender; in severe cases, muscle guarding may be present. Gas-distended intestinal loops may be visible and palpable. Borborygmi are audible with the stethoscope, even without diarrhea (an important differential feature from paralytic ileus). The BP may be reduced, the pulse rapid, and the temperature elevated. Signs of extracellular fluid depletion (see in REGULATION OF WATER AND SODIUM HOMEOSTASIS in Ch. 84) may be present.

Diagnosis

A history of food intolerance, ingestion of potentially contaminated food or a known GI irritant, and recent travel habits may be important. An elevated total WBC count is of little diagnostic significance, but eosinophilia suggests allergy or parasitic infection. Stool examination and culture are indicated unless symptoms subside within 48 h. Sigmoidoscopy helps diagnose ulcerative colitis and amebic dysentery, though shigellosis may produce colonic lesions indistinguishable from those of ulcerative colitis. These and other differential diagnoses may require culture of food, vomitus, feces, urine, and blood; specific agglutination tests (positive after about 1 wk) may also be helpful.

The acute "surgical abdomen" is usually excluded by a history of frequent stools, a low WBC count, and lack of muscle spasm and localized tenderness. However, diarrhea may occur at times in acute appendicitis, incomplete small bowel obstruction, other acute intra-abdominal emergencies, and colonic malignancy.

General Principles of Treatment

Supportive treatment is most important. Bed rest with convenient access to a bathroom, commode, or bedpan is desirable. When nausea or vomiting is mild or ended, fluids such as warm sweetened tea, "soda pop," oral glucose-electrolyte solutions (see DIARRHEA in Ch. 56), strained broth, cereal, gruel, or bouillon with added salt are taken. Nothing is taken by mouth while vomiting is present. If vomiting persists or dehydration is prominent, IV infusions of 5% dextrose are necessary, together with appropriate electrolyte replacements. The most dramatic example and a full discussion of the role of fluid therapy in gastroenteritis is in acute cholera (see CHOLERA in Ch. 8).

Similar principles apply in other instances. Blood or a plasma expander is indicated in severe cases when shock occurs.

Vomiting can usually be helped by sedation with phenobarbital sodium 30 to 100 mg s.c. tid or qid, alone or with scopolamine 0.5 mg s.c. Injections of an antiemetic (eg, dimenhydrinate 50 mg IM q 4 h, or chlorpromazine 25 to 100 mg or more/day IM) or a prochlorperazine suppository (25 mg bid) may be beneficial. Meperidine 50 mg IM q 4 or 6 h if necessary, or an antispasmodic (eg, propantheline 5 to 10 mg IM q 6 h) may be given for severe abdominal cramps. Morphine is best avoided because it increases intestinal muscle tone and may aggravate vomiting.

When the patient tolerates warm fluids, the diet gradually includes cooked bland cereals, gelatin, jellied consommé, simple dessert, soft-cooked eggs, and other bland foods. If after 12 to 24 h, moderate diarrhea persists in the absence of severe systemic symptoms, diphenoxylate 2.5 to 5 mg in tablet or liquid form tid or qid, paregoric 5 mL orally q 4 h, codeine 15 to 30 mg orally tid or qid, or a preparation containing bismuth, belladonna, and kaolin may be given.

Antibiotic therapy: The role of antibiotics is disputed, even for specific infectious diarrheas, but most authorities recommend treating symptomatic shigellosis. Antibiotics appropriate to sensitivity testing should be given when evidence shows systemic infection. However, antibiotics do not help patients with simple gastroenteritis nor do they help asymptomatic carriers to "clear" rapidly. In fact, antibiotics may favor and prolong the carrier state of salmonellosis. Emergence of drug-resistant organisms may be related to indiscriminate use of antibiotics, which should be discouraged.

GASTROENTERITIS DUE TO BACTERIAL ENTEROTOXINS

CHOLERA AND NONCHOLERA VIBRIO DISEASE

(See Cholera and Campylobacter and Noncholeric Vibrio Infections in Ch. 8)

NURSERY DIARRHEA DUE TO *Escherichia coli*

(See under Acute Infectious Neonatal Diarrhea in Ch. 186)

STAPHYLOCOCCAL FOOD POISONING

An acute syndrome of vomiting and diarrhea caused by eating food contaminated by staphylococcal enterotoxin.

Etiology and Pathophysiology

Staphylococcal enterotoxin rather than the organism per se is one of the most common causes of food poisoning. The potential for outbreaks is high when food handlers with skin infections contaminate foods left at room temperature. Custards, cream-filled pastry, milk, processed meat, and fish provide media where coagulase-positive staphylococci grow and produce enterotoxin. There is no mucosal ulceration.

Symptoms and Signs

The incubation period is 2 to 8 h after eating food containing the toxin. Onset is usually abrupt, characteristically with severe nausea and vomiting. Other symptoms may include abdominal cramps, diarrhea, and occasionally headache and fever. Acid-base imbalance, prostration, and shock may ensue in severe cases. Stools occasionally contain blood and mucus. The attack is brief, most often lasting only 3 to 6 h, and recovery is usually complete. Rarely, fatalities occur, especially among the very young, the elderly, or those with chronic illness, as a result of fluid and metabolic stresses.

Diagnosis

Diagnosis hinges on recognizing the clinical syndrome described above. Usually, a number of persons are similarly affected, constituting a "point source" outbreak. Diagnostic confirmation requires isolating coagulase-positive staphylococci from the suspected food.

The syndrome should be distinguished from staphylococcal pseudomembranous enterocolitis arising from staphylococcal superinfection after oral administration of antibiotics (see Ch. 60).

Treatment

Treatment is supportive; see above under General Principles of Treatment. Rapid IV replacement of fluids and electrolytes often brings dramatic relief.

BOTULISM

Neuromuscular poisoning from Clostridium botulinum *toxin.* Botulism occurs in 3 forms: foodborne, wound, and infant botulism.

Etiology and Pathophysiology

The sporulating, anaerobic gram-positive bacillus *C. botulinum* elaborates 7 types of antigenically distinct toxins. Humans are usually poisoned by Type A, B, E, or F toxin. Type A and B toxins are highly poisonous proteins resistant to digestion by GI enzymes. In foodborne botulism, toxin produced in contaminated food is eaten; but in wound and infant botulism, neurotoxin is elaborated in vivo by growth of *C. botulinum* in infected tissue and in the GI tract, respectively. After absorption, the toxins interfere with release of acetylcholine at peripheral nerve endings.

C. botulinum spores are highly heat-resistant; they may survive several hours at 100 C (212 F); however, exposure to moist heat at 120 C (248 F) for 30 min will kill the spores. Toxins, on the other hand, are readily destroyed by heat, and cooking food at 80 C (176 F) for 30 min safeguards against botulism. Toxin production (especially type E) can occur at temperatures as low as 3 C (37.4 F) and does not require strict anaerobic conditions. Between 1970 and 1977 in the USA, foodborne outbreaks were caused most often by type A toxin (51%), followed by type B (21%) and type E (12%); in 16% the toxin type was not identified. Type F outbreaks are rare. Home-canned foods are the most common sources, but commercially prepared foods have been identified in about 10% of outbreaks. Vegetables, fish, fruits, and condiments are the most common vehicles, but beef, milk products, pork, poultry, and other foods have been involved. In outbreaks caused by marine products, type E accounted for about half, with types A and B causing the rest.

Botulinum toxin types are distinctively distributed in the USA: Type A is seen predominantly west of the Mississippi River, type B in the Eastern states, and type E in Alaska and the Great Lakes area.

Symptoms and Signs

In foodborne botulism, onset is abrupt, usually 18 to 36 h after ingestion of the toxin, though the incubation period may vary from 4 h to 8 days. Neurologic symptoms are characteristically bilateral and symmetrical, beginning with the cranial nerves and following with descending weakness or paralysis. Common initial symptoms include dry mouth, diplopia, diminished acuity, blepharoptosis, loss of accommodation, and diminished or total loss of pupillary light reflex. Nausea, vomiting, abdominal cramps, and diarrhea frequently precede neurologic symptoms. Symptoms of bulbar paresis (dysarthria, dysphagia, nasal regurgitation) develop. Dysphagia can lead to aspiration pneumonia. Muscles of the extremities and trunk become weak. There are no sensory disturbances and the sensorium usually remains clear until shortly before death. Fever is absent and the pulse remains normal or slow unless intercurrent infection develops.

Routine studies of the blood, urine, and CSF are usually normal. Constipation is frequent after neurologic impairment appears. **Major complications** include respiratory failure and pulmonary infections.

Wound botulism is manifested by the same symptoms of neurologic involvement as is seen in foodborne botulism, but there are no GI symptoms or epidemiologic evidence implicating food as a cause. Careful search should be made for breaks in the patient's skin.

Infant botulism, seen most frequently in infants 2 to 3 mo old, results from the ingestion of botulinal spores and their colonization in the GI tract and toxin production in vivo; unlike foodborne botulism, infant botulism is *not* caused by ingestion of preformed toxin. Constipation is present initially in 2/3 of cases and is followed by neuromuscular paralysis that begins with the cranial nerves and proceeds to peripheral and respiratory musculature. Cranial nerve deficits may be asymmetric and a spectrum based on severity may show variation from mild lethargy and slowed feeding to severe hypotonia and respiratory insufficiency. Affected infants have characteristically been normal before the onset of illness and have been either breast- or formula-fed. However, they have generally been exposed to foods other than milk, and spores are common in the environment. Cases have been related to the ingestion of honey, vacuum cleaner dust, and soil containing *C. botulinum.*

Diagnosis

The pattern of neuromuscular disturbances suggests the diagnosis of an isolated case; a likely food source provides an important clue. The simultaneous occurrence of 2 or more cases after eating the same food simplifies the diagnosis. It is confirmed by demonstrating botulinal toxin in the serum or feces of the patient or by isolating the organism from feces. Finding *C. botulinum* **toxin** in suspect food identifies the source. Pets may develop botulism from eating the same contaminated food. Botulism may be confused with the Guillain-Barré syndrome, poliomyelitis, stroke, myasthenia gravis, tick paralysis, and poisoning due to curare or belladonna alkaloids.

In infant botulism, sepsis, congenital muscular dystrophy, hypothyroidism, and benign congenital hypotonia are additional considerations. Finding *C. botulinum* toxin or organisms in the feces establishes the diagnosis.

Special Precautions

Since even minute amounts of botulinal toxin acquired by ingestion, inhalation, or absorption through the eye or a break in the skin can cause serious illness, all materials suspected of containing toxin require special handling. Only experienced personnel, preferably immunized with botulinal toxoid should perform laboratory tests. Specimens should be placed in unbreakable, sterile, leakproof containers, refrigerated (preferably not frozen), and examined as soon as possible. Wound specimens are an exception and should not be refrigerated. Further details regarding specimen collection and handling can be obtained from the Centers for Disease Control, Atlanta, Georgia 30333.

Prophylaxis and Treatment

Proper home and commercial canning and adequate heating of food before serving are essential (see Etiology and Pathophysiology, above). Food showing any evidence of spoilage should be discarded. Infants < 1 yr old should not be fed honey. Toxoids can be prepared for active immunization of persons working with *C. botulinum* or its toxins; anyone known or thought to have been exposed to contaminated food must be carefully observed. To eliminate unabsorbed toxin, induction of vomiting, gastric lavage, and purgation are recommended.

The greatest threat to life is from respiratory impairment and its complications. All patients should be hospitalized and closely supervised (eg, with serial measurements of vital capacity). Respiratory impairment requires management in an intensive care unit

where intubation, tracheostomy, and mechanical ventilators are readily available (see Ch. 34). IV alimentation may be required. Improvements in such supportive care have reduced mortality to < 10%.

Trivalent antitoxin (A, B, E) is available from the Centers for Disease Control, which also stores a polyvalent antitoxin (A, B, C, D, E, F) for specific outbreaks due to C, D, or F botulism. Antitoxin should be given as soon as possible after botulism has been diagnosed. Risks must be weighed against potential benefits. Antitoxin may be beneficial even if given several weeks after toxin ingestion, since circulating toxin has been detected in serum as late as 30 days after such ingestion. Antitoxin will not release toxin that is already bound; therefore, preexisting neurologic impairment will not be reversed; at best it will slow or halt further progression of the disease. Since these are horse serum antitoxins, there is a risk of anaphylaxis or serum sickness. The use of antitoxin in **infant botulism** has not been adequately studied, and at present is not generally recommended. For precautions in the use of horse serum antitoxin, see SERUM SICKNESS under DRUG HYPERSENSITIVITY and for treatment of reactions, see ANAPHYLAXIS under ATOPIC DISEASES, both in Ch. 21.

Guanidine is thought to increase acetylcholine release from terminal nerve endings and is advocated by some to treat patients with botulism. Reported results have been conflicting and the effectiveness of guanidine therapy for botulism remains unproven.

Clostridium perfringens FOOD POISONING

Acute gastroenteritis due to ingestion of an enterotoxin contained in food contaminated by C. perfringens.

Etiology

C. perfringens is widely distributed in feces, soil, air, and water. Contaminated meat has caused many outbreaks. The organisms form spores and generate a variably potent enterotoxin. The toxin produced by Type A strains causes a mild to moderate, self-limiting disease; that produced by Type C strains causes a severe, often fatal gastroenteritis. Some toxins are resistant and some are sensitive to heat of up to 100 C (212 F) for 1 h.

Symptoms, Signs, and Diagnosis

A mild gastroenteritis is most common, though a potentially fatal syndrome with severe diarrhea and abdominal pain, abdominal distention with gas, and collapse may occur. Diagnosis is based on epidemiologic evidence and the isolation of organisms from contaminated food.

Treatment

For supportive measures, see General Principles of Treatment at the beginning of this chapter. Penicillin (1 million u./day) may be helpful in severe cases. Necrosis of the small bowel may require surgical resection of the affected intestine.

SALMONELLOSIS

(See SALMONELLA INFECTIONS in Ch. 8)

INFECTIOUS GASTROENTERITIS DUE TO INVASIVE ORGANISMS

These syndromes are largely due to *Shigella* infection (see SHIGELLOSIS in Ch. 8). Some types of enteropathogenic *E. coli* enteritis and salmonellosis may also be associated with mucosal invasion.

Certain intestinal parasites, notably *Giardia lamblia* (see GIARDIASIS in Ch. 13), invade the jejunal mucosa and cause nausea, vomiting, diarrhea, and general malaise.

Giardiasis is endemic in many cold climates (eg, Rocky Mountains, northern USA and Europe). Large outbreaks have occurred in travelers. The disease can become chronic and can cause malabsorption syndrome (see Ch. 58).

INFECTIOUS GASTROENTERITIS OF UNCERTAIN ETIOLOGY

("Travelers Diarrhea"; "Intestinal Flu")

Sporadic cases of gastroenteritis in travelers ("turista") or of gastroenteritis affecting individuals or families ("intestinal flu," "grippe").

Etiology, Epidemiology, and Pathophysiology

Enteropathogenic *E. coli* and incompletely characterized enteric viruses (eg, "Norwalk agent") are the most probable causes. Little is known of the epidemiology, though outbreaks may be sporadic or epidemic. The pathophysiology is uncertain, though enterotoxins and histologic alterations of the jejunal mucosa by viruses, with intestinal fluid secretion, have been suggested.

Symptoms, Signs, and Diagnosis

Nausea, vomiting, borborygmi, abdominal cramps, and diarrhea occur in highly variable combinations and degrees of severity. Most cases are mild and self-limited. The diagnosis is made clinically.

Prophylaxis and Treatment

Travelers should use restaurants with a reputation for safety and avoid foods from street vendors and school cafeterias. They should eat cooked foods, fruit that can be peeled, and drink bottled carbonated beverages; salads containing uncooked vegetables should be avoided. Bismuth subsalicylate suspensions are protective but must be taken in large doses (60 mL qid), which is inconvenient. The role of prophylactic antibiotics is controversial. Trimethoprim/sulfamethoxazole is appropriate for severe, established cases, but its prophylactic use should probably be reserved for those patients particularly susceptible to the consequences of "turista."

For supportive measures, see General Principles of Treatment, at the beginning of this chapter. Symptomatic treatment for diarrhea, and a bland diet are helpful. Iodochlorhydroxyquin *should not be used*, as it may cause neurologic damage. Antibiotics are **contraindicated;** they may alter intestinal flora adversely and promote resistant organisms.

NONBACTERIAL FOOD POISONING

Poisoning due to eating plants and animals that contain a naturally occurring poison.

1. Mushroom (toadstool) poisoning: Two species of the *Amanita* genus are responsible for most cases. In **muscarine** poisoning due to *A. muscaria*, symptoms begin a few minutes to 2 h after eating. They consist of lacrimation, salivation, sweating, miosis, vomiting, abdominal cramps, diarrhea, vertigo, confusion, coma, and occasionally convulsions. Though patients may die in a few hours, complete recovery in 24 h is usual with appropriate therapy.

In **phalloidine** poisoning due to eating *A. phalloides* and related species, symptoms occur after 6 to 24 h. GI symptoms are similar to those of muscarine poisoning above, but oliguria and anuria may develop; jaundice due to liver damage is common and develops in 2 or 3 days. Remissions may occur, but eventual mortality is ≥ 50%, with death occurring in 5 to 8 days.

The potential for poisoning by mushrooms is unpredictable; it may vary within the same species, at different times of the growing season, and with cooking. Drinking of

alcohol may precipitate symptoms, because disulfiram has been identified in some mushrooms.

2. Other poisonous plants: Many wild and domestic plants and shrubs contain poisons in their leaves and fruit. Common examples include yew, morning glory, nightshade, castor bean, dieffenbachia (dumb cane), jequirity bean ("indian bean," "rosary pea"), tung nuts, horse chestnuts, and the bird-of-paradise flower (seeds or peapods). Fruit of the Koenig tree causes "vomiting sickness" of Jamaica. Green or sprouting tubers that contain solanine may produce acute nausea, vomiting, diarrhea, and prostration, usually of mild degree. The eating of fava beans by susceptible persons may precipitate acute hemolysis (favism). Ergot poisoning follows eating grain contaminated by *Claviceps purpurea*, the ergot fungus. Specialized texts provide a full listing of recognized poisonous plants.

3. Fish poisoning: Most cases are caused by eating ichthyosarcotoxic fish (ie, those that contain toxin in their musculature, viscera, skin, or mucus). The severity of attacks from ichthyosarcotoxism varies greatly, depending to some extent on the fish involved. Most important are the following: (1) **Ciguatera poisoning** can occur after eating any of > 400 species of fish from the tropical reefs of Florida, the West Indies, or the Pacific where a dinoflagellate may supply a toxin that accumulates in the marine animal's flesh; larger, older fish are more toxic. The fish's flavor is unaffected, and no known processing procedures are protective. After abdominal cramps, nausea, vomiting, and diarrhea that lasts 6 to 17 h, pruritus, paresthesias, headache, myalgia, and face pain may occur. For months after, unusual sensory phenomena may keep a person from work. (2) **Tetraodon poisoning,** from the puffer fish, causes similar symptoms and signs; death may result from respiratory paralysis. (3) **Scombroid poisoning,** from mackerel, tuna, bonito, or albacore, is due to bacterial decomposition after the fish is caught. Histamine-like, the toxin causes an immediate reaction with characteristic facial flushing. It can also cause nausea, vomiting, epigastric pain, and urticaria within a few minutes of eating an affected fish. Symptoms usually last < 24 h.

4. Paralytic shellfish poisoning: From June to October (especially on the Pacific and New England coasts), mussels, clams, oysters, and scallops may ingest a poisonous dinoflagellate ("red tide") that produces a neurotoxin resistant to cooking. Circumoral paresthesias, the earliest symptoms, appear 5 to 30 min after eating. Then nausea, vomiting, and abdominal cramps develop, followed by muscle weakness and peripheral paralysis. Respiratory failure may cause death.

Another shellfish poison, venerupin, was isolated in Japan following the eating of asari (*Venerupis semidecussata*) and oyster (*Ostrea gigas*). After a 24- to 48-h incubation period, GI symptoms, leukocytosis, retardation of blood coagulation, and liver function disturbances develop. Death occurs in about 1/3 of cases. The neurotropic effects of mussel poison are absent.

5. Contaminants: Chemical poisoning may follow the eating of unwashed fruits and vegetables sprayed with arsenic, lead, or organic insecticides; acidic liquids served in lead-glazed pottery; or food stored in cadmium-lined containers. Symptoms are described in Ch. 289, under the name of the chemical involved.

Treatment

General: Unless violent vomiting or diarrhea has occurred, or symptoms appeared several hours after the food was eaten, efforts should be made to remove the poison by gastric lavage. An emetic may be used. Apomorphine 5 mg s.c. is given only once. Alternatively, ipecac syrup 15 mL (1/2 oz) orally for children, up to 45 mL (1 1/2 oz) for adults, repeated once in 15 min if necessary, may be given, followed by about 200 mL of water. A saline cathartic (eg, sodium sulfate 15 to 30 gm orally in water) may be required. If nausea and vomiting persist, fluids containing salts and dextrose should be given parenterally to combat dehydration and acid-base imbalance. Dextran, Normal

Human Serum Albumin, or blood is indicated if shock threatens. Meperidine 50 to 100 mg IM q 4 to 6 h should be given for pain. Mechanical ventilation and intensive respiratory care may be required.

Specific: After eating an unidentified mushroom, the patient should be induced to vomit immediately; then identification of the mushroom species will aid further treatment. Atropine, 1 mg s.c. or IV q 1 to 2 h until symptoms are controlled, is a specific antagonist of parasympathetic overstimulation due to **muscarine** poisoning. In **phalloidine** poisoning, a high-carbohydrate diet (if tolerated) supplemented by IV administration of 10% dextrose and sodium chloride may help to combat the hypoglycemia of severe liver damage. In the treatment of **ergotism,** arterial spasm may be combated by amyl nitrite 0.3 mL by inhalation, nitroglycerin 0.4 mg sublingually, or papaverine 30 to 60 mg IM or IV. An anticonvulsive agent (eg, sodium amobarbital 300 to 500 mg—more if required—slowly IV) should be used when indicated. Cholinesterase reactivators have been suggested as antidotes for **fish toxins.** For poisoning due to **food contamination** with arsenic, lead, cadmium, or organic insecticides, see Ch. 289.

MISCELLANEOUS CAUSES OF GASTROENTERITIS

DISACCHARIDASE DEFICIENCY AND GLUCOSEGALACTOSE MALABSORPTION

(Alactasia)

(See CARBOHYDRATE INTOLERANCE in Ch. 58)

FOOD ALLERGY

(See GASTROINTESTINAL ALLERGY in Ch. 21)

ADVERSE EFFECTS OF DRUGS

Many therapeutic agents produce nausea, vomiting, and diarrhea as side effects. A detailed drug intake history must be obtained. In mild cases, cessation followed by reuse of the drug may establish a causal relationship. Commonly responsible agents include antacids containing magnesium as a major ingredient, antibiotics, anthelmintics, chemotherapeutic agents used in cancer therapy, colchicine, digitalis, heavy metals, laxatives, and radiation therapy. Specialized literature should also be consulted.

Iatrogenic, accidental, or intentional heavy-metal poisoning frequently produces nausea, vomiting, abdominal pain, and diarrhea.

Laxative abuse, sometimes denied by patients, may lead to weakness, vomiting, diarrhea, electrolyte depletion, and metabolic disturbances.

The **"Chinese-restaurant syndrome"** is a pharmacologic, not an allergic, phenomenon. The monosodium glutamate often used in Chinese food produces a dose-related syndrome of burning sensations throughout the body, facial pressure, and chest pain. The threshold dose varies considerably among individuals.

---

58. MALABSORPTION SYNDROMES

Syndromes resulting from impaired absorption of nutrients from the small bowel.

Symptoms and Signs

Many different diseases or their consequences can cause malabsorption, either by means of impaired digestion or impaired absorption (see TABLE 58–1).

1. Manifestations directly attributable to malabsorption: weight loss, glossitis, carpopedal spasms, absent tendon reflexes, cutaneous bruising, abdominal distention, flatu-

TABLE 58–1. DISEASE STATES ASSOCIATED WITH MALABSORPTION

	In the Presence of This Condition
Impaired digestion results from:	
Inadequate mixing	Gastroenterostomy Billroth II gastrectomy Gastrocolic fistula
Insufficient digestive agents	Chronic pancreatitis Cystic fibrosis Chronic liver failure Biliary obstruction Alactasia Sucrase-isomaltase deficiency
Improper milieu	Zollinger-Ellison syndrome (low duodenal pH) Bacterial overgrowth-blind loops (deconjugation of bile salts) Diverticula
Impaired absorption results from:	
Acute abnormal epithelium	Acute intestinal infections Neomycin Alcohol
Chronic abnormal epithelium	Celiac disease Tropical sprue Whipple's disease Amyloid Ischemia Crohn's disease
Short bowel	Intestinal resection for Crohn's disease Volvulus Intussusception Infarction
Impaired transport	Blocked lacteals—lymphoma Lymphangiectasia Addison's disease—? transport enzymes ? Abetalipoproteinemia

lence, abdominal bloating, and discomfort due to increased bulk of intestinal contents and gas production. Dermatitis herpetiformis is often associated with a mild degree of celiac-like enteropathy. Diarrhea is not always present. Sometimes steatorrhea occurs—pale, soft, bulky, malodorous stools that stick to the side of the toilet bowl or float and are difficult to flush away. This kind of stool is most likely to occur in celiac disease or tropical sprue. The stools in chronic pancreatic disease may appear greasy with free-floating globules of undigested dietary fat (triglyceride) because of pancreatic lipase deficiency. Steatorrhea can be present without florid abnormalities of the stool, and about 20% of patients may have no increase in fecal fat. Explosive diarrhea with abdominal bloating and gas after milk ingestion points to alactasia (lactase deficiency).

2. Manifestations due to deficiencies secondary to malabsorption: The range and severity of nutritional deficiencies relate to the severity of the primary disease and the area of the GI tract involved. Many patients with malabsorption are anemic, usually due to **deficiencies of iron (microcytic anemia) and folic acid (megaloblastic anemia).** Vitamin B_{12} deficiency is uncommon, partly because body stores are considerable, and partly because few disorders cause B_{12} absorption to fall below the daily requirement. For pernicious anemia, see discussion of vitamin B_{12} and folic acid deficiencies in Ch.

96; for neurologic manifestations, see COMBINED SYSTEM DISEASE in Ch. 130. **B_{12} deficiency** may occur in blind loop syndrome or many years after extensive resection of the distal small bowel or stomach. The usual 50-cm resection of the terminal ileum for ileocecal Crohn's disease seldom leads to significant B_{12} deficiency.

Ca deficiency is common and is due partly to **vitamin D deficiency** with impaired absorption and partly to Ca binding with unabsorbed fatty acids. This may cause bone pain and tetany. Infantile rickets is rare but osteomalacia may occur in severe adult celiac disease. **Thiamine (vitamin B_1) deficiency** may cause paresthesia (so does B_{12} deficiency), and malabsorption of the mainly fat-soluble **vitamin K** can lead to hypoprothrombinemia with bruising and a bleeding tendency. Severe **riboflavin (vitamin B_2) deficiency** may cause a sore tongue and angular stomatitis, but **vitamin A, C, and niacin deficiencies** seldom cause clinical problems. **Protein malabsorption** may lead to hypoproteinemic edema, usually of the lower limbs. Dehydration, K loss, and muscle weakness can follow profuse diarrhea.

Secondary endocrine deficiencies may occur, and amenorrhea (primary or secondary) is an important presentation of celiac disease in young girls.

3. Manifestations of malabsorption due to an underlying disease: Some diseases that cause malabsorption have distinctly different clinical presentations; eg, the jaundice of biliary cirrhosis and pancreatic carcinoma; the abdominal angina of mesenteric ischemia; the boring central abdominal pain of chronic pancreatitis; and the severe, persistent ulcer dyspepsia of the Zollinger-Ellison syndrome.

Diagnosis and Differential Diagnosis

The symptoms and signs described above lead to the diagnostic impression of malabsorption. Weight loss, an obvious consequence of malabsorption, is nonspecific. *Any combination of weight loss, diarrhea, and anemia should raise the suspicion of malabsorption.* Laboratory studies confirm the diagnosis.

Fecal fat excretion: Steatorrhea (literally derived from "flow of tallow"), or excess stool fat, is absolute evidence of malabsorption when it is present. The measurement of fecal fat is the most reliable single test for establishing malabsorption. For an adult eating a normal Western diet with a daily fat intake of 50 to 150 gm, a fecal fat loss of 17 mEq or more/day is abnormal. Accuracy of stool collections during a period of typical daily routine is more important than strict balance studies. It is feasible and advantageous to perform fecal fat studies on ambulant outpatients. A 3- or 4-day collection is usually adequate. There is no completely satisfactory alternative to the direct measurement of fecal fat.

Stool inspection and microscopic examination are both valuable. The typical stool appearances described above are unmistakable. The presence of fragments of undigested food suggests either extreme hypermotility or intestinal short circuits (eg, gastrocolic fistula). Greasy stools from a jaundiced patient point to pancreatic cancer or primary biliary cirrhosis. Microscopic examination showing fat globules and undigested meat fiber suggests pancreatic insufficiency. Microscopy permits identification of ova or parasites.

Absorption tests: The **oral glucose test** is not used, since a significant proportion of normal subjects shows a flat absorption curve.

D-Xylose absorption: The D-xylose test is an indirect but relatively specific measure of proximal small bowel absorption. It is nearly always abnormal in primary jejunal disease, but rarely in other causes of malabsorption. D-Xylose 5 gm is given orally to the fasting patient, and urine is collected for the next 5 h. This dose is slightly less sensitive than a larger (25-gm) dose, but it does not cause nausea or diarrhea. Provided urine output is adequate and the GFR is normal, the test is unequivocally abnormal if $<$ 1.2 gm of xylose is present in the 5-h collection. Values between 1.2 to 1.4 gm are borderline. The test is popular in pediatric practice, but because collecting complete urine samples in young children is difficult, some investigators prefer blood levels.

However, the overlap between normal and abnormal levels is considerable unless the dose is calculated as 0.5 gm/kg, and even then the urinary level is more reliable.

Lactose absorption: See CARBOHYDRATE INTOLERANCE, below.

Iron absorption: Malabsorption of dietary iron can usually be inferred if a patient whose diet is adequate, and who has no chronic blood loss or thalassemia, has an iron deficiency state, indicated by low serum iron levels and diminished iron storage noted on bone marrow evaluation. It occurs mainly in celiac disease and postgastrectomy patients.

Folic acid absorption: Malabsorption of dietary folate can usually be inferred if a patient eating an adequate diet and not consuming excessive amounts of alcohol has a low serum and/or RBC folate level. Folate malabsorption occurs mainly in celiac disease and tropical sprue.

Vitamin B_{12} absorption: The Schilling test can be used to evaluate malabsorption. Reduced urinary excretion (< 5%) of radiolabeled B_{12} indicates malabsorption of B_{12}, and when excretion is corrected to normal (> 9%) with intrinsic factor bound radiolabeled B_{12}, the malabsorption is due to loss of gastric intrinsic factor activity (often true pernicious anemia). When intrinsic factor bound B_{12} is not adequately absorbed, chronic pancreatitis, drugs, or small bowel disease (blind loops, jejunal diverticuli, or ileal disease) must be suspected.

Carbon 14 (^{14}C)-labeled glycocholic acid breath test: Excessive deconjugation of bile salts by intestinal bacteria occurs in small bowel disorders that cause stasis and bacterial overgrowth (eg, blind loops, diverticula, and scleroderma) and can be demonstrated by the oral administration of ^{14}C-labeled glycocholic acid. If bacterial growth is excessive, ^{14}C-labeled glycine is split off, absorbed, and metabolized, and the labeled carbon is measured as breath $^{14}CO_2$. The test has limited usefulness.

Radiology: X-ray appearances may be nonspecific or diagnostic. An upper GI follow-through examination of the small bowel may show dilation of bowel loops, thickening of mucosal folds, and coarse fragmentation of the barium column, but these appearances only suggest malabsorption. On the other hand, radiology may show pancreatic calcification—a sign of chronic pancreatitis—fistulas, blind loops, or various inter-enteric anastomoses; jejunal diverticulosis; superior mesenteric artery occlusion; and mucosal patterns suggestive of intestinal lymphoma, scleroderma, or Crohn's disease.

Small bowel biopsy (see TABLE 58–2): Jejunal biopsy is a routine procedure; some modification of the Crosby capsule or the Rubin tube is used. Samples of jejunal juice can be taken simultaneously for microbiologic testing of the intestinal flora. Endoscopic biopsies are also suitable but should be taken beyond the second part of the duodenum. The mucosal sample can be examined grossly by hand lens or dissecting microscope and by light or electron microscopy, and tissue homogenates can be assayed for enzyme activity. The abnormalities thus demonstrated may be specific or nonspecific. Specific diagnoses include Whipple's disease, lymphosarcoma, intestinal lymphangiectasia, and giardiasis (in which the trophozoite may be seen in close association with the villus surface). Jejunal histology is also abnormal in celiac disease, tropical sprue, and dermatitis herpetiformis. The changes may be severe (subtotal villus atrophy), moderate (partial villus atrophy), or mild.

Pancreatic function: Two kinds of pancreatic function tests are currently in use, both of which require duodenal intubation: (1) In the Lundh test pancreatic secretion is *indirectly* stimulated by oral intake of a formula diet, and lipase levels are measured in the duodenal aspirate; and (2) pancreatic secretion is *directly* stimulated by injecting secretin IV (see PANCREATITIS in Ch. 55).

An oral test for pancreatic function has recently been introduced, but its accuracy and usefulness need to be evaluated. The test is based on the cleavage of the synthetic peptide bentiromide by the pancreatic enzyme chymotrypsin. The para-aminobenzoic

TABLE 58–2. JEJUNAL HISTOLOGY IN CERTAIN MALABSORPTIVE DISORDERS

Condition	*Morphologic Characteristics*
Normal	Finger-like villi with a villous-crypt ratio of about 4:1; columnar epithelial cells with numerous regular microvilli (brush border); mild round cell infiltration in the lamina propria
Untreated celiac disease	Virtual absence of villi and elongated crypts; increased round cells (especially plasma cells) in the lamina propria; cuboidal epithelial cells with scanty, irregular microvilli
Tropical sprue	*Mild* (minimal changes in villus height; moderate epithelial cell damage) *Severe* (similar to untreated celiac disease except lymphocytes predominate in the lamina propria)
Whipple's disease	Lamina propria densely infiltrated with periodic acid–Schiff-positive macrophages; villus structure may be obliterated in severe lesions
Intestinal lymphangiectasia	Dilation and telangiectasia of the intramucosal lymphatics

acid moiety is absorbed and excreted in the urine and the amount measured by chemical titration. Accuracy depends on factors such as normal gastric emptying, normal absorption, and normal renal function, and certain drugs (eg, sulfonamides and acetominophen) can give false results.

Miscellaneous investigations: Special tests may be needed to diagnose less common causes of malabsorption; eg, serum gastrin levels and gastric acid secretion in the Zollinger-Ellison syndrome, sweat Cl in cystic fibrosis, lipoprotein electrophoresis in abetalipoproteinemia, plasma cortisol in Addison's disease.

CELIAC DISEASE

(Nontropical Sprue; Gluten Enteropathy; Celiac Sprue)

A chronic intestinal malabsorption disorder caused by intolerance to gluten, characterized by a flat jejunal mucosa with clinical and/or histologic improvement following withdrawal of dietary gluten.

Etiology and Prevalence

This hereditary congenital disorder is caused by sensitivity to the gliadin fraction of gluten, a cereal protein found in wheat and rye, and to a lesser degree in barley and oats. Gliadin, acting as antigen, combines with antibodies to form an immune complex in the intestinal mucosa that promotes the aggregation of K (killer) lymphocytes. In some way these lymphocytes cause mucosal damage with loss of villi and proliferation of crypt cells. The prevalence of celiac disease varies from about 1:300 in southwest Ireland to 1:5000 or more in North America. There is no single genetic marker for the condition.

Symptoms and Signs

Celiac disease may be symptomatic or asymptomatic. Family studies show that typical mucosal abnormalities appear in apparently healthy siblings of affected patients. The disease may present for the first time in infancy or adulthood, but it should not be assumed that an adult presentation is the first manifestation. Although the patient may have no knowledge of childhood disease, his mother may recall abdominal symptoms. If the adult patient is significantly smaller than his siblings, and has evi-

dence of mild bowing deformities of the long bones, the likelihood of latent or undiagnosed childhood disease is increased.

In **infancy,** symptoms are absent until the child eats food containing gluten. The child fails to thrive, begins to pass pale, malodorous, bulky stools, and suffers painful abdominal bloating. Iron deficiency anemia develops and, if hypoproteinemia is severe enough, edema appears. Celiac disease is strongly suspected in a pale, querulous child, with wasted buttocks and a pot belly, who has an adequate diet (thus ruling out protein-calorie malnutrition or kwashiorkor).

In **adults,** celiac disease is usually diagnosed when malabsorption is found in conjunction with a flat jejunal biopsy not due to some recognizable cause (eg, tropical sprue, neomycin intake) and gluten is shown to be of etiologic significance. Family incidence is a valuable clue. It may present, apparently for the first time, at any age. The average age of presentation in women is 10 to 15 yr earlier, because anemia in pregnancy and amenorrhea in young women may heighten clinical suspicion.

There is no single typical presentation. Many symptoms (eg, anemia, weight loss, bone pain, paresthesia, edema, and skin disorders) are secondary to deficiency states. If overt alimentary symptoms (eg, diarrhea, abdominal discomfort, and distention) also occur, the real diagnosis is unlikely to be missed. Without these direct clues, malabsorption may not be suspected.

Laboratory Findings

There tends to be iron deficiency anemia in children and folate deficiency anemia in adults. Depending on severity and duration, there can be any combination of low albumin, Ca, K, and Na, and elevated alkaline phosphatase and prothrombin time. The 5 gm D-xylose test (see Diagnostic Studies, above) will usually be abnormal, and most patients will have steatorrhea that can range from mild to massive (7 to 50 gm [20 to 150 mEq] fatty acid/day).

In the immune protein system, levels of C_3 and C_4 are low in the untreated patient and rise with gluten withdrawal. The serum C_3 level is a possible screening test for celiac disease. The serum IgA level is usually normal or increased in untreated patients, and in $1/3$ to $1/2$, the IgM level is reduced.

Diagnosis

Diagnosis is suspected on the basis of the symptoms and signs, enhanced by the laboratory and x-ray studies, and confirmed by biopsy showing a flat mucosa and clinical and histologic improvement on a gluten-free diet. Jejunal biopsy can be performed even in small infants, but to obviate the risk of bowel perforation, only an experienced investigator should do the test. If a biopsy cannot be done, the diagnosis may have to depend on the clinical and laboratory response (including xylose absorption) to a gluten-free diet.

Prognosis and Natural History

While gluten withdrawal has transformed the prognosis for celiac children and substantially improved it for adults, there is still some mortality from the disease, mainly among adults whose condition is severe from the beginning. An important cause of death is the development of lymphoreticular disease (especially intestinal lymphoma). It is not known whether this risk is diminished by scrupulous adherence to a gluten-free diet. Some patients can tolerate the reintroduction of gluten into the diet. It is not certain whether this means that some mild cases can achieve complete remission (unlikely) or whether the gluten toxicity is a nonspecific effect on a mucosa previously damaged by an acute bacterial or viral enteritis. In any case, apparent clinical remission is often associated with histologic relapse that is only detected if review biopsies are performed.

Treatment

Dietary gluten must be excluded, as ingesting even small amounts may prevent remission or induce relapse. Gluten is so widely used (eg, in commercial soups, sauces,

ice creams, hot dogs) that patients need detailed lists of food-stuffs to avoid and expert advice from a dietitian familiar with the problems of celiac disease.

Supplementary vitamins, minerals, and hematinics may be given depending on the degree of deficiency. In mild cases no supplementation may be necessary. In severe cases comprehensive replacement may be required. For adults this includes ferrous sulfate 300 mg/day, folic acid 5 to 10 mg/day, calcium gluconate 5 to 10 gm/day, and any standard multivitamin preparation, all orally. Only if the prothrombin time is abnormal should vitamin K 10 mg IM be given. Proportional pediatric doses are given to children. Sometimes children, and rarely adults, who are seriously ill on first diagnosis may require a period of IV feeding. This should be carried out in accordance with the general principles of total parenteral nutrition (see PARENTERAL NUTRITION in Ch. 79).

A few patients respond poorly or not at all to gluten withdrawal, either because the diagnosis is incorrect or because the disease has entered a refractory phase. In the latter case, a response may be induced by a period of treatment with oral corticosteroids (eg, prednisone 10 to 20 mg bid).

TROPICAL SPRUE

A disease of unknown etiology characterized by malabsorption, multiple nutritional deficiencies, and abnormalities in the small bowel mucosa.

Etiology and Incidence

Tropical sprue is an acquired disease related in some way to environmental and nutritional conditions. It occurs chiefly in the Caribbean, south India, and southeast Asia, affecting both natives and newcomers. Some suggested causes are infection (bacterial or viral), parasitic infestation, vitamin deficiency (especially folic acid), or food toxin (eg, as in rancid fats).

Symptoms, Signs, and Laboratory Findings

A common presentation is the triad of sore tongue, diarrhea, and weight loss. All features of a malabsorption syndrome (see above) may develop. Steatorrhea is common and D-xylose absorption is abnormal in > 90% of cases. Deficiencies of albumin, Ca, prothrombin, folic acid, vitamin B_{12}, and iron may occur. There is a megaloblastic anemia due to folic acid and vitamin B_{12} deficiency. Small bowel radiology shows the nonspecific changes of malabsorption—flocculation and segmentation of the barium column, with dilation of the lumen and thickening of the mucosal folds.

Diagnosis

The diagnosis should be suspected in anyone who has lived in an endemic area and who has megaloblastic anemia and manifestations of the malabsorption syndrome. Celiac disease must be ruled out. Jejunal biopsy shows a varying degree of broadening and shortening of the villi and lengthening of the crypts with changes in the surface epithelium and an inflammatory cell infiltrate of lymphocytes, plasma cells, and eosinophils. In some patients changes may be minimal or absent, while in others there is subtotal villus atrophy. Biopsies must be compared with normal tissue from individuals in the same geographic region. What is a "mild" abnormality in the intestinal mucosa of Europeans and North Americans is "normal" in areas of India, Africa, and southeast Asia. It is not yet clear whether this difference is racial or genetic, or whether it is due to environmental factors (eg, chronic infection or infestation).

Treatment

The best treatment is folic acid 10 mg/day and tetracycline or oxytetracycline 250 mg qid for 1 or 2 mo, and then in half dosage for up to 6 mo, depending on the severity of the disease and response to treatment. Other replacements are given as needed.

WHIPPLE'S DISEASE

(Intestinal Lipodystrophy)

An uncommon illness occurring predominantly in males aged 30 to 60, characterized clinically by anemia, skin pigmentation, joint symptoms (arthralgia and arthritis), weight loss, diarrhea, and severe malabsorption. Though this systemic disorder affects many organs (eg, heart, lung, brain, serous cavities, joints, eye, GI tract), the small intestinal mucosa is always severely involved and the lesions observed in mucosal biopsies are specific and diagnostic.

Symptoms, Signs, and Diagnosis

The typical presentation is malabsorption in an adult male with additional features of polyarthritis, lymphadenopathy, and abnormal pigmentation. Abdominal pain is common. Cough and pleuritic pain may be accompanied by hilar adenopathy and pleural effusion. Symptoms of cardiac, hepatic, and neuropsychiatric disease may also be present. Untreated, the disease is progressive and fatal.

Diagnosis

Lymph node or intestinal biopsy establishes the diagnosis by showing foamy macrophages containing a glycoprotein that stains with the periodic acid-Schiff (PAS) reagent. Jejunal tissue may be otherwise normal or show clubbing of the villi, dilated lymphatics, or even partial villus atrophy. Electron microscopy shows the PAS-positive material to be masses of rod-shaped bacilli.

Treatment

Many different types of antibiotics are curative (eg, chloramphenicol, tetracycline, chlortetracycline, sulfasalazine, ampicillin, and penicillin). One recommended regimen is procaine penicillin G 1,200,000 u. and streptomycin 1 gm daily for 10 to 14 days followed by tetracycline 250 mg orally qid for 10 to 12 mo. The streptomycin is often omitted. Clinical improvement occurs rapidly but histologic recovery may take up to 2 yr and recurrence is possible.

INTESTINAL LYMPHANGIECTASIA

(Idiopathic Hypoproteinemia)

A syndrome affecting children and young adults, characterized by telangiectasia of the intramucosal lymphatics of the small intestine. A congenital malformation of the lymphatics is most likely when onset occurs at birth. In acquired cases the defect may be secondary to retroperitoneal fibrosis, pancreatitis, constrictive pericarditis, and a few other causes.

Symptoms, Signs, and Diagnosis

Early manifestations include massive, often asymmetric edema, and mild intermittent diarrhea with nausea, vomiting, and abdominal pain. Chylous effusions and ascites may be present. Lymphocytopenia occurs, as well as a marked reduction of serum albumin and immunoglobulins IgA and IgG. Cholesterol may be low. A few patients have mild to moderate steatorrhea, but D-xylose absorption is normal. Intestinal protein loss can be demonstrated using Chromium 51-labeled albumin. Jejunal biopsy shows the characteristic dilation and telangiectasia of the lymphatic vessels that distinguish this condition from other protein-losing disorders (eg, Crohn's and Whipple's diseases).

Treatment

Some patients improve on a low-fat diet (< 30 gm/day), supplements of medium-chain triglycerides, and occasionally by resection, if the lesion is localized.

INFECTION AND INFESTATION

(For giardiasis, diphyllobothriasis, ascariasis, and hookworm disease, see Ch. 13.)

Acute bacterial and viral infections may cause transient malabsorption, probably due to temporary, superficial damage to the villi and microvilli. Chronic bacterial infections of the small bowel are uncommon apart from blind loops and diverticula. Intestinal bacteria may utilize dietary vitamin B_{12}, perhaps interfere with enzyme systems, and cause areas of superficial inflammation.

CARBOHYDRATE INTOLERANCE

(Lactose Intolerance; Lactase Deficiency; Disaccharidase Deficiency; Glucose-Galactose Malabsorption; Alactasia)

Diarrhea and abdominal distention caused by inability to digest carbohydrate because of a lack of one or more intestinal enzymes.

Pathophysiology

Disaccharides are normally split into monosaccharides by lactase, maltase, isomaltase, or sucrase (invertase) in the small intestine. Lactase splits lactose into glucose and galactose. Unsplit disaccharides remain in the lumen and osmotically retain fluid, causing diarrhea. Bacterial fermentation of sugar in the colon leads to gaseous, acidic stools. Since the enzymes are located in the brush border of mucosal cells, secondary deficiencies occur in diseases associated with morphologic alterations of the jejunal mucosa (eg, celiac disease, tropical sprue, acute intestinal infections, neomycin toxicity). In infants, temporary secondary disaccharidase deficiency may complicate enteric infections or abdominal surgery.

The monosaccharides glucose and galactose are absorbed by an active transport process in the small bowel (fructose is absorbed passively). The **transport system** for these monosaccharides is lacking in the small bowel in glucose-galactose malabsorption, and symptoms develop after ingestion of most kinds of sugar.

Incidence

Lactase deficiency occurs *normally* in about 75% of adults in all ethnic groups except those of northwest European origin for whom the incidence is < 20%. Although statistics are unreliable, most nonwhites of North America gradually lose the ability to digest lactase between ages 10 and 20 yr. It affects 90% of Orientals, 75% of American blacks and Indians, with a high incidence among peoples from the Mediterranean area.

Glucose-galactose intolerance is an extremely rare congenital disorder, as are deficiencies of other mucosal enzymes (eg, sucrose, isomaltase).

Symptoms and Signs

Symptoms and signs are similar, regardless of the specific enzyme deficiency. A child who cannot tolerate sugar will have diarrhea and fail to gain weight. An adult may have borborygmi, bloating, flatus, nausea, diarrhea, and abdominal cramps. Even when only lactose absorption is directly impaired by deficiency of the enzyme lactase, the resulting diarrhea may be severe enough to purge other nutrients before they can be absorbed. A clear history of milk intolerance may be obtained in patients with lactose intolerance. Some people recognize this early in life and consciously or unconsciously avoid eating dairy products, thus making a diagnostic history more obscure. In others, symptoms may simulate the irritable bowel syndrome or complicate a duodenal ulcer or gastrectomy.

Diagnosis

The diagnosis may be suspected if acidic stools (pH < 6) are passed or if after a glass of milk the patient develops abdominal bloating and watery diarrhea within 20 to 30

min. It is further substantiated by a flat oral lactose tolerance test and can be absolutely confirmed by the finding of low lactase activity in a jejunal biopsy specimen. Glucose-galactose malabsorption is also diagnosed by demonstrating a flat oral tolerance test when the affected sugar is ingested.

The **lactose tolerance test** is specific for the clinical disorder of lactose intolerance. An oral dose of 50 gm of lactose causes diarrhea with abdominal bloating and discomfort, and there is a low or flat blood glucose curve. Equivalent amounts of glucose and galactose produce a normal rise in blood glucose without diarrhea. A rise in the blood glucose level of < 20 mg/dL is abnormal.

Treatment

The disorder is readily controlled by a lactose-free diet, or often simply by avoiding milk drinks. A child who lacks the transport enzyme can absorb fructose. If a lactose-free diet is continued, oral Ca supplements should be given.

59. CHRONIC INFLAMMATORY DISEASES OF THE BOWEL

A spectrum of disorders with overlapping clinical, epidemiologic, and pathologic findings, but without a definite etiology. Both regional enteritis and ulcerative colitis (see below) are characterized by chronic inflammation at various sites in the GI tract. Certain differences in disease patterns justify a distinction at least between ulcerative colitis and regional enteritis, although groupings and subgroupings are somewhat artificial. Some cases will be difficult, if not impossible, to classify.

REGIONAL ENTERITIS

(Granulomatous Ileitis or Ileocolitis; Crohn's Disease)

A nonspecific chronic transmural inflammatory disease that most commonly affects the distal ileum and colon, but may also occur in any part of the GI tract from the mouth to the anus and perianal area.

Etiology

The etiology of this group of diseases is unknown. *Immunologic factors* have been extensively examined, but no immune mechanisms of pathogenesis or susceptibility have been definitely proven. The search for possible *infectious agents* has included various enteric bacteria, viruses, and chlamydiae, and has most recently focused on L-form (cell wall-deficient) bacteria and on atypical mycobacteria, but no specific microorganism is clearly established as the cause. *Dietary factors* including chemicals and the fiber-poor diet consumed in modern developed countries have also been considered but not proven to play a role in causing these diseases.

Epidemiology

Since its recognition as a distinct entity only several decades ago, Crohn's disease has been reported with increasing frequency, particularly in Western populations with Northern European and Anglo-Saxon ethnic derivation. The disease occurs about equally in both sexes, is more common among Jews, and shows a familial tendency that frequently overlaps with the occurrence of ulcerative colitis. Most cases begin before age 40, with the peak incidence in the 20s.

Pathology

The earliest macroscopic lesions of Crohn's disease appear to be tiny focal "aphthoid" ulcerations of the mucosa, usually with underlying nodules of lymphoid tissue. Sometimes these early aphthoid lesions regress, but in other cases, the inflammatory

process progresses to involve all layers of the intestinal wall, which becomes greatly thickened. Changes are most marked in the submucosa, with lymphedema and lymphocytic infiltration occurring first, and extensive fibrosis later. Patchy ulcerations develop on the mucosa, and the combination of longitudinal and transverse ulcers with intervening mucosal edema frequently creates a characteristic "cobblestone" appearance. The attached mesentery is thickened and lymphedematous; mesenteric fat typically extends onto the serosal surface of the bowel. Mesenteric lymph nodes often enlarge. The transmural inflammation, deep ulceration, edema, and fibrosis are responsible for obstruction, deep sinus tracts and fistulas, and mesenteric abscesses, which are the major local complications.

Segments of diseased bowel are characteristically sharply demarcated from adjacent normal bowel—thus the name "regional" enteritis. Segmental lesions may be separated by normal areas ("skip areas"). The ileum alone is involved in about 35% of cases **(ileitis);** both ileum and colon, with a predilection for the right side of the colon, are affected in about 45% **(ileocolitis);** and the colon alone is diseased in < 20% **(granulomatous colitis).** Occasionally the entire small bowel **(jejunoileitis)** is involved, and rarely also the stomach, duodenum, or esophagus.

Sarcoid-type epithelioid granulomas in the intestinal wall and occasionally in the involved mesenteric nodes are pathognomonic, but since they are absent in up to 1/2 the patients, they are not essential to diagnose Crohn's disease. Although they may represent a hidden clue to pathogenesis, they appear to have no definitive bearing on the clinical course.

Symptoms and Signs

Chronic diarrhea associated with abdominal pain, fever, anorexia, weight loss, and a right lower quadrant mass or fullness are the most common presenting features. However, many patients are first seen with an "acute abdomen" simulating acute appendicitis or intestinal obstruction, both of which must be ruled out. Four patterns of regional enteritis occur most often: (1) *inflammation*, characterized by right lower quadrant abdominal pain and tenderness, mimicking appendicitis when acute; (2) *obstruction*, in which intestinal stenosis causes recurrent partial obstruction with severe colic, abdominal distention, constipation, and vomiting; (3) *diffuse jejunoileitis,* with both inflammation and obstruction resulting in malnutrition and chronic debility; and (4) *abdominal fistulas and abscesses*, usually late developments, often causing fever, painful abdominal masses, and generalized wasting. Fistulas may be enteroenteric, enterovesical, retroperitoneal, or enterocutaneous. Obstruction, fistulization, and abscess formation are common complications of inflammation; intestinal bleeding, perforation, and small bowel cancer develop rarely. A history of perianal disease, especially fissures and fistulas, can be elicited in about 1/3 of patients. When the colon alone is affected, the clinical picture may be indistinguishable from ulcerative colitis (see below).

Extraintestinal manifestations fall into 3 principal categories: (1) Complications often paralleling the activity of the intestinal disease and possibly representing acute immunologic or microbiologic concomitants of the bowel inflammation; these include peripheral arthritis, episcleritis, aphthous stomatitis, erythema nodosum, and pyoderma gangrenosum. These manifestations may be seen in over 1/3 of patients hospitalized with inflammatory bowel disease. They are twice as common when colitis is present than when disease is confined to the small intestine. When extraintestinal manifestations occur, they are multiple in about 1/3 of patients; (2) Disorders associated with inflammatory bowel disease but running an independent course—ankylosing spondylitis, sacroiliitis, and uveitis. The genetic interrelationships among these syndromes, colitis (both ulcerative and granulomatous), and the HLA antigen B27 are discussed under the extracolonic complications of ulcerative colitis, below; (3) Complications relating directly to the disrupted physiology of the bowel itself; chief among these are

renal problems. Kidney stones result from disorders of uric acid metabolism, impairment of urinary dilution and alkalinization, and excessive oxalate absorption; urinary infections occur especially with fistulization into the urinary tract; and hydroureter and hydronephrosis may ensue from ureteral compression by retroperitoneal extension of the intestinal inflammatory process. Other bowel-related complications include malabsorption, especially in the face of extensive ileal resection or bacterial overgrowth from chronic small bowel obstruction or fistulization; gallstones, related to impaired ileal reabsorption of bile salts; and amyloidosis, secondary to longstanding inflammatory and suppurative disease.

In children, extraintestinal manifestations frequently predominate over GI symptoms. Arthritis, FUO, anemia, or growth retardation may be presenting symptoms; abdominal pain or diarrhea may be absent. Thus, evaluation of these systemic symptoms in young people must include barium studies of the small bowel and colon, since these may be the only presenting clues to the diagnosis of inflammatory bowel disease.

Diagnosis

The diagnosis of regional enteritis should be suspected in any patient with the inflammatory or obstructive symptoms described above, and in a patient without prominent GI symptoms who presents with perianal fistulas or abscesses or with otherwise unexplained arthritis, erythema nodosum, fever, anemia, or (in a child) stunted growth.

Laboratory findings are nonspecific and may include anemia, leukocytosis, hypoalbuminemia, and increased levels of acute-phase reactants reflected in elevated ESR, C-reactive protein, and/or orosomucoids.

Definitive diagnosis is usually made by x-ray. Barium enema x-ray may show reflux of barium into the terminal ileum with irregularity, nodularity, stiffness, thickening of the wall, and a narrowed ileal lumen. A small bowel series with spot x-rays of the terminal ileum usually most clearly demonstrates the nature and extent of the lesion. An upper GI series alone, without small bowel follow-through, will almost invariably miss the diagnosis. In advanced cases, the "string sign" may be seen with marked stricturing of the ileum and separation of bowel loops. In earlier cases, radiologic diagnosis may sometimes be difficult, but technics of double air-contrast barium enema and enteroclysis may demonstrate superficial aphthous and linear ulcers. In questionable cases, fiberoptic colonoscopy and biopsy may help confirm the diagnosis. Although CT is beginning to prove useful to characterize pathologic changes within the bowel wall and to identify abscesses, it is not routinely needed for initial diagnosis.

Differential Diagnosis

When disease is limited to the colon (granulomatous colitis), differentiation from chronic ulcerative colitis may be difficult, though only about 20% of patients show this strictly colonic distribution. The diagnosis of granulomatous disease is more likely when there is no x-ray or sigmoidoscopic evidence of rectal involvement ("rectal sparing") and when rectal bleeding is absent. Asymmetric involvement of the bowel wall and segmental distribution of lesions on x-ray help to confirm the diagnosis. Severe perianal disease also suggests the presence of granulomatous and not ulcerative colitis.

In diagnosing Crohn's disease in the small bowel, one must consider a number of other situations where right lower quadrant disease may resemble granulomatous ileitis. Disease of adjacent organs (eg, appendix and adnexae) may mimic regional enteritis. In the acute presentation without a history of chronic bowel symptoms, ileitis may first be diagnosed during exploration for suspected appendicitis. Pelvic inflammatory disease and ectopic pregnancy, as well as ovarian cysts and tumors, may also produce right lower quadrant inflammatory signs, and must certainly be considered when first diagnosing Crohn's disease in women.

Furthermore, other intrinsic neoplastic, vascular, and infectious diseases of the bowel may create the x-ray picture of regional enteritis. These include carcinoma of the cecum, ileal carcinoid, lymphosarcoma, systemic vasculitis, radiation enteritis, and ileocecal TB. Especially when confronted with an inflamed and edematous terminal ileum and associated mesenteric adenitis during surgery for acute right lower quadrant pain, one must exclude acute *Yersinia enterocolitica* enteritis before labeling a patient with the diagnosis of chronic regional ileitis. Although *Yersinia* enteritis is a self-limited infection without chronic intestinal sequelae, the initial clinical picture may be indistinguishable in both disorders, so appropriate serologic and bacteriologic studies are necessary. In questionable cases, a 3-mo follow-up x-ray of the terminal ileum is most valuable, since complete resolution is usually seen by this time with *Yersinia* ileitis, but not with Crohn's disease.

Prognosis

Complete recovery may follow a single isolated attack of acute ileitis. As already noted, however, this self-limited syndrome is usually unrelated to Crohn's disease and often due to *Yersinia* infection.

Established chronic regional enteritis is characterized by lifelong exacerbations. Growth retardation commonly results from disease occurring during the developmental years. The disease rarely spreads spontaneously without surgical manipulation of the bowel. Fatal complications from free perforation, sepsis, inanition, or carcinoma may occur, but are rare.

Treatment

No specific therapy is known. Anticholinergics and diphenoxylate 2.5 to 5 mg, loperamide 2 to 4 mg, deodorized opium tincture 0.5 to 0.75 mL (10 to 15 drops), or codeine 15 to 30 mg, given orally (ideally before meals) up to qid, may relieve cramps and diarrhea. Hydrophilic mucilloids (eg, methylcellulose or psyllium preparations) sometimes help to prevent anal irritation by increasing stool firmness.

Antibacterials should be reserved for bacterial complications (eg, abscesses, infected fistulas). Long-term sulfasalazine therapy is useful in suppressing or preventing relapses of chronic low-grade inflammatory activity, especially in the colon, but it is less useful in severe acute exacerbations. It has not been found helpful in preventing postoperative recurrence. (For sulfasalazine therapy, see ULCERATIVE COLITIS, below.)

Metronidazole 1 to 1.5 gm/day has been shown to be beneficial in Crohn's disease, especially with perianal involvement. Neuropathy manifested chiefly by paresthesias is a common, potentially serious side effect of long-term use, which is usually reversible when the drug is stopped. There is a high incidence of relapse of Crohn's disease after discontinuation of metronidazole therapy.

Corticosteroid therapy is useful in the acute stages of Crohn's disease. It may dramatically reduce fever and diarrhea, relieve abdominal pain and tenderness, and improve the appetite and sense of well-being. Large doses of oral prednisone, 40 to 60 mg/day, should be given initially; the dosage is gradually reduced following a satisfactory response so that, at the end of 4 wk, the daily dosage does not exceed 10 or 20 mg. Long-term corticosteroid therapy is of less obvious benefit, but as little as 5 or 10 mg/day may help to control symptoms in some individuals.

Immunosuppressive drugs: Striking responses have been reported, but their exact role in therapy is not established. One large multicenter study demonstrated no benefit from azathioprine in Crohn's disease, although a longer-term investigation has suggested that 6-mercaptopurine significantly improved patients' overall clinical status, decreased their steroid requirements, and often healed fistulas. Cyclosporin E is currently being evaluated. Other treatments that have been tried or proposed include transfer factor, levamisole, BCG vaccination, antilymphocyte globulin, plasmapheresis, interferon, and even thymectomy, but no scientific studies of these measures have

proved their efficacy. The wide variety of suggested approaches attests to the inadequacy of present-day therapy for this baffling disease.

Some patients with intestinal obstruction or fistula formation have improved on **elemental diets or hyperalimentation,** at least over a short term, and some children have achieved increased rates of growth. Thus, these measures may sometimes be valuable as preoperative or adjunctive therapy.

Surgery is usually necessary when recurrent intestinal obstruction or intractable abscesses or fistulas are present. Resection of the grossly involved bowel may result in amelioration of symptoms indefinitely, but surgery is not curative. The cumulative postoperative recurrence rate, usually at the anastomotic site, is 60 to 95%; ultimately, another operation is often required. Thus, surgery should not be performed unless specific complications or failure of medical therapy make it necessary. When operations have been required, however, most patients consider their quality of life to have been improved by surgery.

ULCERATIVE COLITIS

A chronic, nonspecific, inflammatory and ulcerative disease arising in the colonic mucosa, characterized most often by bloody diarrhea.

The term "colitis" should be applied only to inflammatory disease of the colon (eg, ulcerative, granulomatous, ischemic, or radiation colitis; bacillary or amebic dysentery). "Spastic" or "mucous" colitis is a functional disorder more properly described as "irritable bowel" (see THE IRRITABLE BOWEL SYNDROMES in Ch. 61).

Etiology and Epidemiology

The same considerations described for regional enteritis apply equally to ulcerative colitis, except that the evidence for any specific microbial etiology is even less convincing, and the familial tendency is slightly less pronounced. Like Crohn's disease, ulcerative colitis may afflict patients at any age, but the age-onset curve shows a bimodal distribution with a major peak at ages 15 to 30 and a second smaller peak at ages 50 to 70 that may include some cases of ischemic colitis.

Pathology

The disease usually begins in the rectosigmoid area and may extend proximally, eventually involving the entire colon, or it may attack most of the large bowel at once. **Ulcerative proctitis,** a very common and more benign and limited form of the disease, usually remains localized to the rectum, although it too may undergo late proximal spread in about 10% of cases.

Pathologic change begins with degeneration of the reticulin fibers beneath the mucosal epithelium, occlusion of the subepithelial capillaries, and progressive infiltration of the lamina propria with plasma cells, eosinophils, lymphocytes, mast cells, and polymorphonuclear leukocytes. Crypt abscesses, epithelial necrosis, and mucosal ulceration ultimately develop.

Symptoms and Signs

The usual manifestation is a series of attacks of bloody diarrhea varying in intensity and duration, interspersed with asymptomatic intervals. Onset of an attack may be acute and fulminant, with sudden violent diarrhea, high fever, signs of peritonitis, and profound toxemia. More often, an attack begins insidiously, with an increased urgency to defecate, mild lower abdominal cramps, and the appearance of blood and mucus in the stools.

When the ulcerative process is confined to the rectosigmoid area, the feces may be normal or hard and dry, but rectal discharges of mucus loaded with RBCs and WBCs accompany or occur between bowel movements. Systemic symptoms are mild or ab-

sent. If the process extends proximally, stools become looser and the patient may have 10 to 20 bowel movements/day, often with severe cramps and distressing rectal tenesmus, without respite at night. The stools may be watery and contain pus, blood, and mucus; they frequently consist almost entirely of blood and pus. Malaise, fever, anemia, anorexia, weight loss, leukocytosis, hypoalbuminemia, and elevated ESR may be present with extensive active colitis.

Complications

Hemorrhage is the most common local complication. In **toxic colitis,** a particularly severe local complication, transmural extension of the ulcerative process results in localized ileus and peritonitis. As the toxic colitis progresses, the colon loses muscular tone and within a matter of days or even hours begins to dilate. Plain x-rays of the abdomen show an accumulation of intraluminal gas over a long, continuous, paralyzed segment of colon, which results from loss of muscle tone. *When the diameter of the transverse colon exceeds 6 cm,* **toxic megacolon** (or toxic dilation) is said to have developed. The severely ill patient has fever to 40 C (104 F), leukocytosis, abdominal pain, and rebound tenderness. Treatment must be administered in the early stages before full blown megacolon has occurred, or else such dangerous complications as perforation, generalized peritonitis, and septicemia may ensue. The mortality rate can be held below 4% with prompt and effective treatment, but may exceed 40% if perforation has occurred.

Except for small **rectovaginal fistulas,** perirectal complications such as those seen in granulomatous colitis (eg, major fistulas and abscesses) are not associated with ulcerative colitis.

Risk of **colon cancer** is increased in patients with longstanding, extensive ulcerative colitis and such patients merit surveillance for early warning signs of carcinoma (see Prognosis, below).

Extracolonic complications include peripheral arthritis, ankylosing spondylitis, sacroiliitis, posterior uveitis, erythema nodosum, pyoderma gangrenosum, episcleritis, and, in children, severely retarded growth and development. The peripheral arthritis, episcleritis, and skin complications often tend to fluctuate in tandem with the colitis, whereas the spondylitis, sacroiliitis, and uveitis usually follow a course independent of the bowel disease. Most colitis patients with spinal or sacroiliac involvement also have evidence of uveitis, and vice versa. In fact, these conditions may precede the colitis by many years and may even occur without coexisting bowel disease in relatives of colitis patients. Moreover, both ankylosing spondylitis and uveitis, whether they occur in the presence or absence of colitis, have a very strong association with the HLA antigen B27. These observations suggest genetic overlaps among colitis, spondylitis, uveitis, and the B27 genotype.

While minor changes in liver function tests are common, clinically apparent liver disease may occur in only 1 to 3% of patients. The liver disease may manifest as fatty liver or more seriously as chronic active hepatitis, sclerosing cholangitis, or cirrhosis. Sclerosing cholangitis is a complication being recognized with increasing frequency, especially in patients who were young when the colitis began. **Cancer of the biliary tract** is another risk, though rare, appearing late in the course of ulcerative colitis, even 20 yr after colectomy.

Diagnosis

The history and stool examination permit a presumptive diagnosis that should almost always be supported by **sigmoidoscopy,** which provides a direct and immediate indication of the activity of the disease process. In early cases, the mucous membrane is finely granular and friable, with loss of the normal vascular pattern, and often with scattered hemorrhagic areas; minimal trauma causes bleeding in multiple pinpoint spots. The mucosa soon breaks down into a red, spongy surface dotted with a myriad

of tiny blood- and pus-oozing ulcerations. As the mucosa becomes progressively involved, the inflammatory and hemorrhagic processes extend into the muscular coats of the bowel. Large mucosal ulcerations with copious purulent exudate characterize severe disease. Islands of relatively normal or hyperplastic inflammatory mucosa (pseudopolyps) project above areas of ulcerated mucosa. Even during asymptomatic intervals, the sigmoidoscopic appearance is rarely normal; some mild degree of friability or granularity almost always persists, and biopsy shows evidence of chronic inflammation.

Plain films of the abdomen are sometimes helpful in judging the severity and proximal extent of the colitis, by showing loss of haustration, mucosal edema, and absence of formed stool in the diseased bowel. **Barium enema** is not usually necessary before initiation of treatment and may be hazardous in active stages because of risk of perforation; this study should be performed at some point in the course of the disease for precise delineation of colonic involvement. The contrast x-ray examination shows loss of haustration, mucosal edema, minute serrations, or gross ulcerations in severe cases. A shortened, rigid colon with an atrophic or pseudopolypoid mucosa is seen in cases of longer duration. Severe perianal disease, sparing of the rectum, absence of bleeding, and asymmetric or segmental involvement of the colon indicate granulomatous rather than ulcerative colitis.

In certain difficult cases, **colonoscopy** and **biopsy** may aid in assessing the extent of disease, in evaluating the nature of a stricture, and in distinguishing ulcerative from Crohn's colitis.

Differential Diagnosis

The importance of excluding an infectious cause of acute colitis before commencing treatment cannot be overemphasized, especially during the first attack. Stool cultures for salmonella, shigella, and campylobacter must be obtained. The presence of *Entamoeba histolytica* should be excluded by examination of fresh, still-warm stool specimens, or of colonic exudate aspirated at the time of sigmoidoscopy. Rectal biopsies and serologic titers for amebiasis should also be obtained when a parasitic infection is suspected because of epidemiologic or travel history. Prior history of antibiotic use should prompt stool assay for *Clostridium difficile* toxin (see Ch. 60). Especially in the male homosexual, specific infectious proctitis (eg, gonorrhea, herpes virus, chlamydia) should be ruled out (see Ch. 14). In women using birth control pills, one must entertain the possibility of contraceptive-induced colitis, a recently recognized entity that usually resolves spontaneously upon discontinuation of hormone therapy. In the elderly patient, especially with a history of atherosclerotic heart disease, ischemic colitis should be considered. The x-ray findings of "thumbprinting" and segmental distribution would further suggest the latter diagnosis. Colon cancer seldom produces fever or purulent rectal discharge, but must nonetheless be excluded as a cause of bloody diarrhea.

Prognosis

A rapidly progressive initial attack may be fatal in nearly 10% of patients, usually due to exsanguinating hemorrhage, perforation, or sepsis and toxemia. Patients who first develop the disease after age 60 have a particularly poor prognosis; mortality from severe attacks is > 25%. Complete recovery after a single attack may occur in another 10% of all patients; in such cases, however, there always remains the possibility of an undetected specific pathogen. Usually, the disease is chronic with repeated exacerbations and remissions.

The incidence of colon cancer is increased when the entire colon is involved and the disease lasts for > 10 yr, independent of disease activity. After 10 yr, the cancer risk of universal ulcerative colitis appears to be about 0.5 to 1%/yr among those patients remaining in the population at risk. Cancer risk increases measurably even when colitis does not involve the entire colon, but in such cases the cancers tend to develop at least

10 yr later than in patients with universal disease. There is probably no specifically higher cancer risk among patients with childhood-onset colitis, independent of their longer durations of disease. Moreover, new studies show about 50% long-term survival after diagnosis of colitis-related cancer, a figure no worse than for colorectal cancer in the general (non-colitis) population. Regular colonoscopic surveillance, preferably during periods of remission, is advised for patients whose duration and extent of disease place them at high risk of developing colon carcinoma. Endoscopic biopsies should be performed throughout the colon and submitted for review by an experienced pathologist. The finding of high-grade mucosal dysplasia, in the absence of active inflammation, is a strong indication for colectomy, since the likelihood of concomitant or imminent colorectal carcinoma in such cases may be anywhere from 30 to 80%, especially in the presence of a macroscopic dysplasia-associated lesion or mass.

Nearly 1/3 of all patients with extensive ulcerative colitis ultimately require surgery. Total proctocolectomy is permanently curative and, when performed in time, restores both life expectancy and quality of life to normal.

Patients with localized ulcerative proctitis have the best prognosis. Severe systemic manifestations, toxic complications, or malignant degeneration are unlikely, and late extension of the disease occurs in only about 10%. Surgery is rarely required and life expectancy is normal. However, since extensive ulcerative colitis may begin in the rectum and then spread proximally, it is not safe to characterize a case as limited proctitis until it has stayed localized for at least 6 mo.

Treatment

Avoidance of raw fruits and vegetables to limit mechanical trauma to the inflamed colonic mucosa may result in symptomatic improvement. A milk-free diet may decrease symptoms in 1/3 of patients, but need not be continued if no benefit is noted. Anticholinergics or low doses of diphenoxylate 2.5 mg orally bid or tid are indicated for relatively mild diarrhea; higher oral doses of diphenoxylate (5 mg tid or qid), deodorized opium tincture 0.5 to 0.75 mL (10 to 15 drops) q 4 to 6 h, loperamide 2 mg after each loose movement, or codeine 15 to 30 mg q 4 to 6 h may be required for more intense diarrhea. *All these anti-diarrheal agents must be used with extreme caution in more severe cases, lest toxic dilation be precipitated.*

Mild or moderate disease may respond to sulfasalazine. Since GI intolerance is common, the drug should be given with food, and, if necessary, in the enteric-coated form. Dosage should initially be low (eg, 0.5 gm orally bid) and gradually increased over a period of several days to 3 to 6 gm/day in divided doses. If a drug rash develops, desentization may be carried out by beginning with small doses. More serious side effects (eg, blood dyscrasias, hemolytic anemia, and rarely hepatitis) may prevent use of sulfasalazine altogether. Currently under investigation are analogs (eg, 5-aminosalicylate enemas and oral azodisalicylate), which may circumvent the systemic side effects of the sulfa moiety. Long-term sulfasalazine therapy (0.5 to 1 gm bid or tid) may help to maintain remissions and reduce the frequency of relapses.

In either **mild or moderate disease,** when the colitis does not extend proximally beyond the splenic flexure, remission may sometimes be achieved with instillation of hydrocortisone by enema instead of with oral corticosteroid therapy. Initially, hydrocortisone 100 mg in 60 mL of isotonic saline and methylcellulose is given rectally once or twice/day. It should be retained in the bowel as long as possible; instillation at night, with the patient's hips elevated, may prolong retention. Treatment, if effective, should be continued daily for about 1 wk, then every other day for 1 to 2 wk, then discontinued gradually over 1 to 2 wk. Enema preparations of steroid analogs with less systemic activity (eg, tixocortol pivalate) are currently undergoing clinical study.

Moderately severe disease in ambulatory patients usually requires systemic corticosteroid therapy. Relatively intensive therapy with oral prednisone 40 to 60 mg/day in

either single or divided doses frequently induces dramatic remission. After 1 to 2 wk, the daily dose may be gradually reduced by about 5 to 10 mg/wk. Sulfasalazine (2 to 4 gm/day in divided doses) may be added when the colitis is controlled by prednisone at a level of about 20 mg/day; very gradual tapering off and ultimate withdrawal of the corticosteroid may then be possible.

Patients with chronic fecal blood loss may require iron to prevent anemia. If oral iron is not tolerated, treatment may have to be given parenterally.

Severe disease, manifested by > 10 bloody bowel movements per day, tachycardia, high fever, or severe abdominal pain, requires hospitalization. If the patient has already been receiving steroid treatment ≥ 30 days, at the time of admission, hydrocortisone 300 mg/day should be given by continuous IV drip. In patients who have not received steroids, ACTH 75 to 120 u./day IV given by continuous drip may be the more effective initial therapy. In either event, treatment is given for 7 to 10 days while the response is monitored by recording the nature and frequency of bowel movements. An initial abdominal x-ray should be obtained to assess the extent and severity of colonic involvement and the patient must be observed closely for the development of toxic megacolon.

Unless dehydration due to diarrheal losses is imminent, it is usually advisable not to give hydrocortisone or ACTH in IV 0.9% sodium chloride solution, since edema is then a frequent complication. The addition of potassium chloride 20 to 40 mEq/L to the IV fluids usually helps to prevent hypokalemia. Patients with heavy rectal bleeding often require blood transfusions to correct anemia.

Oral prednisone 60 mg/day may be substituted after remission has been achieved with the 7- to 10-day course of parenteral treatment. The patient who remains well on the oral regimen for 3 to 4 days may leave the hospital, and corticosteroid dosage may be gradually reduced at home under close medical supervision.

Azathioprine and 6-mercaptopurine have been used in the treatment of ulcerative colitis, but their long-term risk/benefit ratios in this disease have not been clearly established.

Toxic colitis *is a grave emergency*. As soon as signs of toxic colitis or impending toxic megacolon are detected, the following steps should be instituted immediately: (1) Discontinue all antidiarrheal medication; (2) Give nothing by mouth and pass a long intestinal tube attached to intermittent suction; (3) Give aggressive IV fluid and electrolyte therapy, with 0.9% sodium chloride, potassium chloride, albumin, and blood as needed; (4) Give ACTH 120 u./day or hydrocortisone 300 mg/day by continuous IV drip; and (5) Give antibiotics (eg, ampicillin 2 gm IV q 4 to 6 h, or cefazolin 1 gm IV q 4 to 6 h).

Having the patient roll over in bed from the supine to prone position q 2 to 3 h may help redistribute colonic gas and prevent progressive distention. Passage of a soft rectal tube may also be helpful in some cases, *but must be done with extreme caution to avoid bowel perforation*.

The patient must be watched closely for signs of progressive peritonitis or perforation. Percussion over the liver is important, since loss of hepatic dullness may be the first clinical sign of free perforation, especially in the patient whose peritoneal signs are suppressed by massive corticosteroid dosage. Abdominal x-rays should be obtained at least daily to follow the course of colonic distention and to detect free air. If intensive medical measures do not produce definite improvement within 24 to 48 h, immediate surgery is required or the patient may die from perforation and attendant sepsis.

Surgery: Emergency colectomy is indicated for massive hemorrhage, fulminating toxic colitis, or perforation. In the latter 2 conditions, subtotal colectomy with ileostomy and rectosigmoid mucous fistula is usually the procedure of choice, since total proctocolectomy with abdominoperineal resection is more than most critically ill patients can tolerate.

The rectosigmoid stump may then be electively removed at a later date, or in certain highly-selected cases may be used for mucosal stripping and ileorectal "pull through" procedures with or without intrapelvic intestinal reservoirs. In any event, the intact rectal stump should not be allowed to remain indefinitely because of the risks of disease activation or malignant degeneration at a later date.

Elective surgery is indicated for high-grade mucosal dysplasia or clinically suspected carcinoma, for all symptomatic strictures even if benign, for growth retardation in children, or most commonly for intractable chronic disease resulting in invalidism or high-dose steroid dependence. Rarely, severe colitis-dependent extraintestinal manifestations (eg, pyoderma gangrenosum) may also provide an indication for surgery.

Total proctocolectomy permanently cures chronic ulcerative colitis. Permanent ileostomy is usually the price of this cure, although various alternative procedures (eg, the continent ileostomy or various endorectal "pull-through" procedures) are being performed at many centers in efforts to obviate the need for an external appliance. The cosmetic details of the surgery are less critical than the curative nature of colectomy in a disease as serious as ulcerative colitis. Nonetheless, the physical and emotional burdens imposed by any form of colon resection must be recognized, and care should be taken to see that the patient receives all the logistic instructions and psychologic support that are so necessary both before and after surgery.

---

60. ANTIBIOTIC-ASSOCIATED COLITIS

An acute inflammatory bowel disorder associated with antibiotic use that encompasses a spectrum from transient mild diarrhea to a severe colitis marked by exudative mucosal plaques ***(pseudomembranous colitis).***

Etiology and Pathology

Various antibiotics may alter the balance of normal gut flora and allow overgrowth of certain pathogenic organisms. *Clostridium difficile*, a gram-positive rod, is the most frequently recognized. This organism produces a cytopathic toxin capable of damaging the colonic mucosa. Although earlier reports attributed pseudomembranous colitis to *Staphylococcus aureus*, this organism is no longer believed to play a role in the disease.

The antibiotics implicated most frequently are clindamycin, lincomycin, ampicillin, and the cephalosporins. Other causative agents include the penicillins, erythromycin, sulfamethoxazole-trimethoprim, chloramphenicol, and tetracycline. Rarely, even antibacterials that inhibit *C. difficile* in vitro, such as metronidazole, can cause the disease. No cases have yet been definitely attributed to vancomycin, parenteral aminoglycosides, or drugs whose activity is limited to mycobacteria, parasites, or fungi. The route of administration, dosage, and duration of antibiotic therapy do not appear to be significant risk factors. Susceptibility, however, increases with age, although young adults and even children may be afflicted.

In mild cases, the colonic mucosa may show only minimal inflammation or edema, or can even appear grossly normal. More severe colitis is manifested by diffuse friability and ulceration that grossly and microscopically may simulate idiopathic ulcerative colitis. In the extreme case, raised, yellowish, exudative plaques are seen lining the colonic mucosa. Histologically, these pseudomembranes consist of fibrin, leukocytes, and sloughed, necrotic epithelial cells. Bacterial invasion of the mucosa, however, is not seen.

Pseudomembranous colitis with positive stool assays for *C. difficile* toxin may occasionally be the result of situations other than antibiotic exposure. In such cases, there is often a specific predisposing condition (eg, recent bowel surgery, uremia, intestinal ischemia, or shock).

Symptoms and Signs

Symptoms usually begin during a course of antibiotic therapy, but in 1/3 of patients they may not appear until 1 to 10 days after treatment has ceased. Indeed, the diagnosis of antibiotic-associated colitis must be considered in anyone who develops diarrhea up to 6 wk following antibiotic exposure. Clinical manifestations may range widely from simple loosening of stool to fulminant colitis with bloody diarrhea, abdominal pain, fever, and leukocytosis. In the most severe cases, dehydration, hypotension, toxic megacolon, and colonic perforation may supervene.

Diagnosis

The diagnosis is best established by endoscopic visualization of colitis, especially with pseudomembranes. Since most cases usually involve the distal colon, sigmoidoscopy is usually adequate; but colonoscopy may sometimes be required because cases occur with more proximal involvement and rectal sparing.

Plain films of the abdomen may show mucosal edema and an abnormal haustral pattern. Although barium enema examination may further outline the detail of mucosal abnormalities, the procedure is **contraindicated** in active or severe cases because of the risk of perforation.

Confirmation of the diagnosis requires stool culture for *C. difficile* or assay for its toxin. Demonstration of the toxin is usually the preferred method, because stool culture technics for *C. difficile* are relatively demanding and not available in many clinical laboratories. Tissue culture assay is positive when it identifies a cytopathic toxin neutralized by specific antitoxins. The frequency of positive toxin assay increases with severity of the colitis, ranging from 20% in the most common form of simple post-antibiotic diarrhea, without sigmoidoscopically visible inflammation, to > 90% in cases of overt pseudomembranous colitis. By contrast, healthy adults show only a 2 to 3% carrier rate of the *C. difficile* organism and virtually zero incidence of *C. difficile* toxin.

Prophylaxis

Attempts to maintain the homeostasis of fecal flora during antibiotic therapy by using oral lactobacillus preparations have been inconclusive. The best means of preventing antibiotic-associated colitis is to avoid the indiscriminate use of antibiotics and to keep any course of indicated treatment as short as possible. Since clustering of hospital cases has been reported, it is prudent to institute stool isolation precautions for affected patients.

Treatment

If significant diarrhea occurs during antibiotic administration, the antibiotic should be stopped immediately, unless its use is absolutely essential. Antiperistaltic drugs (eg, diphenoxylate) should be avoided, since they may protract the illness by prolonging contact time of the colonic mucosa with the offending agent.

Uncomplicated antibiotic-induced diarrhea, without evidence of frank colitis or toxicity, will usually subside spontaneously within 10 to 12 days once the antibiotic is discontinued; no other specific therapy is required. If mild symptoms persist, the anion exchange resin cholestyramine 4 gm orally qid may be effective, presumably by binding *C. difficile* toxin.

For most cases of frank antibiotic-associated colitis, metronidazole 250 mg orally qid is the treatment of choice, being much less expensive and usually as effective as oral vancomycin, which in the past was the recommended therapy. Oral vancomycin 500 mg qid is reserved for the most severe or resistant cases. Clinical relapses may occur in up to 20% of patients and must be retreated. However, the asymptomatic persistence of *C. difficile* toxin in stool, even for several months after resolution of symptoms, does not require further therapy.

In intractable or fulminant cases, hospitalization for supportive treatment with IV

fluids, electrolytes, and blood transfusion becomes necessary according to the same principles that govern the management of idiopathic ulcerative colitis (see ULCERATIVE COLITIS in Ch. 59). The value of systemic corticosteroids is not established. Rarely, subtotal colectomy or diverting ileostomy has been required as a lifesaving measure.

---

61. FUNCTIONAL BOWEL DISORDERS

IRRITABLE BOWEL SYNDROMES (IBS)

(Spastic Colon; Mucous Colitis)

Motility disorders involving the small intestine and large bowel associated with variable degrees of abdominal pain, constipation, or diarrhea, largely as a reaction to stress in a susceptible individual. These syndromes represent about 1/2 of all GI referrals or initial GI complaints in private and institutional care facilities. Women are more commonly affected than men, in a 3:1 ratio.

Etiology and Pathophysiology

No anatomic cause can be found. Emotional factors, diet, drugs, or hormones may precipitate or aggravate an inherent heightened sensitivity to GI motility. IBS patients are more often neurotic, anxious, or depressed than comparable patients. Periods of stress and emotional conflict, particularly those resulting in depression, frequently coincide with onset and recurrences (eg, marital discord, anxiety related to children, loss of a loved one, and obsessional worries over trivial everyday problems—see also Approach to the Patient in Ch. 52.) In addition, it appears that IBS sufferers are more prone to chronic illness behavior and that this behavior is learned.

The circular and longitudinal muscles of the small bowel and sigmoid colon are particularly susceptible to motor abnormalities. The proximal small bowel and the colon appear to be hyperreactive to ingestion of food and parasympathomimetic drugs. Transit through the small bowel is rapid in patients with spastic colon and predominant diarrhea, and slow in the constipated group. When the normal segmentation mechanism of the sigmoid colon becomes hyperreactive, so-called "spastic constipation" results. In the pelvic colon, increased frequency and amplitude of contractions are associated with spastic constipation, in contrast to diminished motor function associated with diarrheal episodes. Mucorrhea may result from excessive parasympathomimetic stimulation or increased mechanical irritation of the colon.

Patients are more aware of normal amounts of intraluminal gas and also have a heightened perception of pain in the presence of normal intestinal gas. The pain of IBS seems to be due to abnormally strong contraction of the intestinal smooth muscle or to undue sensitivity to distention of the intestine. Hypersensitivity to the hormones gastrin and cholecystokinin may also be present. A common myoelectric pattern consists in a greater frequency of basic electrical rhythm slow wave (3 cycle/min) activity. The caloric density of a meal may increase the magnitude and frequency of myoelectrical activity and motility. Fat ingestion may cause a delayed peak of motor activity that may be inhibited by a concomitant increase in proteins or amino acids. In addition, some patients may be intolerant to wheat, dairy products, coffee, tea, or citrus fruits. Rectal prostaglandin E_2 concentrations may rise after offending foods are ingested, particularly if diarrhea develops.

Symptoms and Signs

Symptoms include abdominal distress, erratic frequency of bowel action, and variation in stool consistency. Disagreeable abdominal sensations may also be associated with nonspecific symptoms; eg, bloating, flatulence, nausea, headache, fatigue, lassitude, depression, anxiety, and difficulty with mental concentration.

Two major groups or clinical types of IBS are recognized. In the first group, the **spastic colon type,** bowel movements are variable. Symptoms are commonly triggered by eating. Most patients have pain of colonic origin over one or more areas of the colon in association with either periodic constipation or diarrhea; in some patients, the two alternate. Mucorrhea occurs frequently, as does a sensation of incomplete evacuation after defecation. Proctalgia fugax, headache, and backache are commonly present. The most common location of the pain or discomfort is over the course of the sigmoid colon. The pain is either colicky and comes in bouts or is a continuous dull ache. It may be relieved by a bowel movement.

The second group primarily manifests **painless diarrhea** that is usually urgent and precipitous. It occurs immediately upon arising or, more typically, during or immediately after a meal. Incontinence may occur, but nocturnal diarrhea is unusual.

Diagnosis and Differential Diagnosis

The diagnosis of IBS is based upon identification of the clinical syndromes described above and exclusion of other disease processes. In general, the manifestations characteristic for a given patient remain consistent; variations or deviations from the usual symptoms suggest the possibility of intercurrent organic disease and should be thoroughly investigated.

On physical examination, patients with either variant of IBS generally appear to be in good health without evidence of significant organic disease. Palpation of the abdomen may reveal tenderness, particularly in the left lower quadrant, at times associated with a contracted, tender colon. Physical examination always includes digital rectal examination and, in females, a pelvic examination; commonly found are a tender rectum, empty or nearly empty rectum, or hard firm feces. Tapping the posterior rectal mucosa evokes pain in most IBS patients.

Stool examinations for occult blood should be performed, preferably a 3-day slide series. In patients with diarrhea (alone or alternating with constipation), stools should be examined for ova and parasites and cultured for bacteria. A smear of the stool or the anal mucosa should be examined for leukocytes, which suggest an inflammatory or infectious process and the need for further evaluation.

Proctosigmoidoscopy with either a rigid or flexible fiberoptic instrument should be performed. The latter is preferred, since it enables the examiner to see as far as 60 cm; ie, the area where 65 to 70% of colonic neoplasms and polyps are found. Introduction of the sigmoidoscope and air insufflation will frequently trigger bowel spasm and pain. Mild hyperemia may be noted, as well as a significant volume of mucus. The mucosal and vascular pattern will otherwise usually appear normal.

Laboratory examinations should include a CBC, ESR, 6- and 12-channel biochemical profile (SMA 6 and 12), including serum amylase, and urinalysis. An abdominal sonogram, Ba enema x-ray, and upper GI and small bowel radiography may be selectively used, based upon the findings of history, physical examination, the patient's age, and follow-up evaluations.

A major problem in the differential diagnosis of IBS is the similarity of its manifestations to organic bowel diseases. A diagnosis of IBS should never preclude suspicion of an intercurrent disease, particularly in patients over age 40. Symptoms indicative of organic disease requiring investigation include fresh blood mixed with the stool, weight loss, steady progressive worsening of symptoms, very severe abdominal pain or unusual abdominal distention, steatorrhea, or noticeably foul-smelling stools, fever and/or chills, persistent vomiting, hematemesis, or symptoms that awaken the patient from sleep (eg, pain or the urge to defecate).

Common illnesses that may be confused with IBS include lactose intolerance, diverticular disease, duodenal ulcer (with antacid therapy), biliary tract disease, abuse of cathartics, parasitic diseases (eg, amebiasis, giardiasis), campylobacter enteritis, allergic gastroenteropathy, and early ulcerative or granulomatous colitis. In patients over

age 40, particularly those with no previous history of IBS symptoms, colonic polyps and neoplasms must be excluded. In patients over age 60, ischemic enteropathy is also a consideration. Pelvic examination in women helps to rule out ovarian neoplasms and cysts or uterine fibroids, the symptoms of which may mimic IBS. In patients with diarrhea, the possibilities of hyperthyroidism, carcinoid syndrome, medullary carcinoma of the thyroid, or the Zollinger-Ellison syndrome should be considered. Patients with constipation should be evaluated for hypothyroidism or hyperparathyroidism. In selected cases, malabsorption studies should be obtained to rule out tropical and nontropical sprue.

Treatment

Therapy is supportive and palliative. The physician's sympathetic understanding and guidance are of overriding importance. Both patient and physician must be assured that no organic disease is present. The physician must explain the nature of the underlying condition and convincingly demonstrate to the patient that no organic disease is present. This requires time for listening and explaining and includes a discussion of normal bowel physiology and the bowel's hypersensitivity to stress, food, drugs, or hormones. These explanations form the foundation for attempting to reestablish regular bowel routine and the selection of individualized therapy. The prevalence and chronicity of the syndrome should be emphasized, and the need for regular follow-up evaluation mandated (both for symptom control and early detection of possible intercurrent organic disease). Psychologic stress, particularly a depressive reaction, should be sought, evaluated, and treated. Informed awareness will help the patient avoid stressful situations. Regular physical activity helps to relieve stress and assists in bowel function, particularly in patients who present with constipation.

In general, a normal diet should be followed. Patients with abdominal distention and increased flatulence may do well to reduce or eliminate eating beans, cabbage, and other foods containing fermentable carbohydrates. Less apple and grape juice, and fewer bananas, nuts, and raisins may also reduce the incidence of flatulence. Patients with evidence of lactose intolerance should reduce their intake of milk and milk products. Patients with postprandial abdominal pain may try a low-fat diet supplemented with increased protein.

In those patients presenting with spastic colon and constipation, a bland bulk-producing agent may be helpful (eg, raw bran starting with a dose of 15 mL [1 tbsp] with each meal, supplemented with increased fluid intake). Alternatively, psyllium hydrophilic mucilloid taken with 2 glasses of water tends to stabilize the water content of the bowel and provide bulk. These agents may increase the diameter of the large bowel, particularly of the sigmoid colon, thereby reducing lateral pressure. They will need to be taken for 1 to 2 mo before intraluminal pressure will change, but symptoms should be relieved sooner. In patients with diarrhea, diphenoxylate 2.5 to 5 mg (1 to 2 tablets) or loperamide 2 to 4 mg (1 to 2 capsules) may be given before meals.

Anticholinergic agents (eg, propantheline 7.5 to 15 mg) alone or in combination with a mild tranquilizer (eg, chlordiazepoxide 5 to 10 mg) or sedative (eg, phenobarbital 15 to 30 mg) tid orally 30 to 60 min before meals, may be used in combination with bulk-producing agents. These agents should be used only as a temporary expedient to relieve spastic pain; dependency upon tranquilizers should be discouraged. In depressed patients, amitriptyline 10 mg tid orally 30 to 60 min before meals has both antidepressant and anticholinergic effects and may be used without other anticholinergic therapy. Effective antidepressant therapy may require higher dosages.

For the small group of patients totally refractory to the therapeutic modalities noted above, hypnotherapy or psychotherapy may be indicated.

GAS

Physiology

Gas is present in the gut as a result of (1) swallowed air (aerophagia), (2) production in the lumen, or (3) diffusion from the blood into the lumen.

Aerophagia occurs normally in small amounts while eating and drinking, but some people unconsciously swallow repeated boluses of air at other times, especially when anxious. Most swallowed air is subsequently eructated; only a small amount passes into the small bowel, the quantity apparently being influenced by posture. The esophagus empties into the posterior, cephalad aspect of the stomach. When the person is upright, air rises above the liquid contents of the stomach, comes in contact with the gastroesophageal junction, and is readily eructated. When the person is supine, air trapped below the fluid tends to be propelled into the duodenum. Excessive salivation may also lead to increased air swallowing and may be associated with various GI disorders (eg, peptic ulcer), ill-fitting dentures, or with nausea of any etiology. Belching in many persons may be associated with use of antacids (eg, baking soda). Attributing the relief of ulcer symptoms to belching rather than to antacids, the person continues to belch to relieve distress.

Gas is produced in the lumen by several mechanisms. Bacterial metabolism yields important volumes of hydrogen (H_2), methane (CH_4), and CO_2. Nearly all H_2 is produced by bacterial metabolism of *ingested* fermentable materials (carbohydrates and amino acids) in the colon and therefore is negligible after a prolonged fast or after a meal that is completely absorbed in the small bowel. H_2 is produced in large quantities after eating certain fruits and vegetables (eg, baked beans) containing indigestible carbohydrates and by patients with malabsorption syndromes. Patients with disaccharidase deficiencies (most commonly lactose intolerance) pass large amounts of disaccharides into the colon that are fermented to H_2 (see CARBOHYDRATE INTOLERANCE in Ch. 58).

CH_4 is produced by bacterial metabolism of *endogenous* substances in the colon; the production rate is only minimally influenced by food ingestion. Some people consistently excrete large quantities of CH_4; others, little or none. Apparently familial, this trait appears during infancy and persists for life.

CO_2 may also be produced by bacterial metabolism, but a more important source is the reaction of bicarbonate and hydrogen ions in which 22.4 mL of CO_2 are released for each mEq of bicarbonate. Hydrogen ions, which may represent several hundred mEq of hydrogen ion, may be derived from gastric hydrochloric acid or the fatty acids released during digestion of the fats of a single meal. Theoretically, up to 4 L of CO_2 may be released into the duodenum following ingestion of a meal. The acid products released by bacterial fermentation of nonabsorbed carbohydrates in the colon may also react with bicarbonate to produce CO_2. Though bloating may occasionally occur, the rapid absorption of CO_2 into the blood prevents intolerable distention.

Gas diffuses between the lumen and the blood in a direction dependent upon the partial pressure difference between the two. The production of H_2, CO_2, and CH_4 may reduce the partial pressure of nitrogen in the lumen to a value far below that in the blood, possibly accounting for much of the nitrogen in the lumen.

Gas is eliminated by eructation, diffusion from the lumen into the blood with ultimate excretion by the lungs, bacterial catabolism, and passage through the anus (flatus). Antibiotics that selectively inhibit bacterial H_2 catabolism markedly increase H_2 excretion.

Symptoms, Signs, and Diagnosis

Excessive gas is commonly thought to cause abdominal pain, bloating, distention, eructation (belching), or passage of excessively voluminous or noxious flatus. However,

excessive intestinal gas has not been clearly linked to the above complaints; it is likely that many symptoms are incorrectly attributed to "too much gas." In most normal persons, 1 L of gas/h can be infused antegrade into the gut with a minimum of symptoms, while persons with gas problems often cannot tolerate much smaller quantities. Similarly, retrograde colonic distension by balloon inflation or during colonoscopy often elicits severe discomfort in patients with the irritable bowel syndrome, while causing minimal symptoms in other people. Thus, the basic abnormality in persons with gas-related problems may be a hypersensitive intestine. Altered motility may contribute further to symptoms; gas could be the inciting agent or have no role in their pathogenesis.

Repeated eructation indicates **aerophagia.** Some persons with this problem can readily produce a series of belches on command. This form of belching is due to unconscious, repeated aspiration of air into the esophagus, often in response to stress, followed by rapid expulsion. When such habitual eructation is suspected, patient education and behavior modification should be undertaken rather than extensive medical evaluation and drug therapy.

In the **splenic flexure syndrome,** swallowed air becomes trapped in the splenic flexure and may cause diffuse abdominal distention. Left upper quadrant fullness and pressure radiating to the left side of the chest may result. There is increased tympany in the extreme left lateral aspect of the upper abdomen. Relief occurs with defecation or passage of flatus.

Flatulence: Among those who are flatulent, the quantity and frequency of gas passage shows great variability. As with bowel frequency, persons who complain of flatulence often have a misconception of what is normal. In a study of 8 normal men aged 25 to 35 yr, the average number of gas passages was 13 ± 4 in one day with an upper limit of 21/day, which overlapped with many persons who complained of excess flatus. On the other hand, one study noted a person with daily flatus frequency as high as 141, including 70 passages in one 4-h period. Hence, objectively recording flatus frequency should be the first step in evaluating a complaint of excessive flatulence. In persons who pass increased amounts of rectal gas, high concentrations of H_2 and CO_2 are usually present. These gases, not significantly present in swallowed air, are usually the product of fermentation by colonic bacteria of unabsorbed carbohydrates. Thus, lactase deficiency, sprue, pancreatic insufficiency, and other cases of carbohydrate malabsorption should be considered in the setting of excess colonic gas (see above in Ch. 58). Furthermore, studies show that even normal persons incompletely absorb carbohydrates in certain common foods (eg, wheat, corn, and potato flour). The normally indigestible polysaccharides in fruits and vegetables (eg, fiber and raffinose) may also be a source of excess gas. Finally, poorly understood factors (eg, differences in colonic flora and motility) may also account for variations in gas production.

Because "excessive gas" symptoms are so nonspecific and commonly overlap with the irritable bowel syndrome (see above) as well as with organic disease, a careful history is essential to guide the extent of medical evaluation. Longstanding symptoms in a young person who is otherwise well and has not lost weight are unlikely to be caused by serious organic disease. The older person, especially with the onset of new symptoms, merits more thorough examination before "excessive gas," real or imagined, is treated.

Treatment

Belching, bloating, and distention are difficult to relieve, since most complaints are due either to unconscious aerophagia or to exaggerated sensitivity to normal amounts of gas. An attempt must be made to reduce aerophagia. Since aerophagia may be due to excessive salivation, one must exclude habits like excessive gum chewing or smoking, upper GI tract diseases (eg, peptic ulcer) that may cause reflex hypersalivation,

and disorders that may cause nausea and reflex salivation. When belching is associated with use of carbonated beverages or antacids (eg, baking soda), these should be eliminated. The mechanism of repeated eructation should be explained and demonstrated. When aerophagia is troublesome, clamping a pencil or other object between the teeth may decrease the amount of involuntary or habit swallowing and break the cycle of aerophagia-discomfort-belch-relief.

Foods containing nonabsorbable carbohydrates can be avoided. Milk-containing products should be excluded from the diet of patients with lactose intolerance.

There are few well-controlled studies demonstrating clear-cut benefit from any drug. Simethicone, an agent that breaks up small gas bubbles, has been incorporated into several preparations, and a variety of anticholinergic drugs have also been used, all with variable results. Some persons with dyspepsia and postprandial upper abdominal fullness have benefited from antacids, metoclopramide (10 mg 30 min before meals), or bethanechol (5 to 25 mg 30 min before meals). These drugs work by increasing the rate of gastric emptying or increasing lower esophageal sphincter tone. Complaints of excessive flatus are treated with similar measures to try to minimize the volume of gas in the gut. Roughage (eg, bran or psyllium seed) may be added to the diet to try to increase colonic transit rate; however, in some patients, worsening of symptoms may result.

In general, symptoms of functional bloating, distention, and flatus run an intermittent, chronic course that is only partially relieved by therapy. Reassurance that these problems are not detrimental to health is important.

62. DIVERTICULAR DISEASE

DIVERTICULOSIS

Diverticula, *small, saccular, mucosal herniations through the muscular wall of the colon,* occur anywhere in the colon, but most frequently in the sigmoid. Varying in diameter from 3 mm to > 3 cm, they are present in 30 to 40% of persons over age 50, and their incidence increases with each subsequent decade of life. The diverticular wall consists of only thin layers of mucosa and serosa. Diverticula are occasionally responsible for severe rectal bleeding; they often become inflamed, causing diverticulitis.

Etiology and Pathogenesis

Evidence suggests that a highly refined low-residue diet plays an important role in the formation of diverticula. Lack of dietary bulk is associated with spasm of the colonic musculature, especially in the sigmoid. When intraluminal pressure builds up, the mucosa can eventually push through the muscular coat at weak points, usually where colonic blood vessels pierce the muscle to supply the mucosa. Diverticula can become filled with inspissated feces, and ulceration of the attenuated mucosa and serosa may occur. Severe rectal hemorrhage may result if a small ulcer at the neck of the diverticulum erodes a branch of the colonic artery. Diverticula in the cecum or ascending colon are fewer but more likely to ulcerate and bleed than those in the descending colon or sigmoid.

Symptoms, Signs, and Diagnosis

Most patients with diverticula are asymptomatic. When a barium enema shows diverticula in a patient with nonspecific abdominal distress (pain, flatulence) and disturbed bowel function, other causes should be excluded before symptoms are attributed to the diverticula. If rectal bleeding occurs, proctoscopy should be done; if

negative, a barium enema is indicated to rule out cancer in the proximal colon. If bleeding persists, colonoscopy may reveal a polyp missed on the barium enema. The bleeding, although less common, is usually more profuse than with cancer (see DIVERTICULITIS, below).

Treatment

A bland diet is *not* indicated for persons with diverticula. For normal colonic function, the diet should include a sufficient intake of fluid and roughage (eg, from whole wheat bread, bran cereal, fruits, and vegetables). With local heat application, rest, a diet with adequate bulk, and a drug (eg, diazepam 5 mg orally occasionally, to relieve nervous tension and stress, or bid to qid), symptoms usually subside. Small doses of phenobarbital (30 mg orally bid) or an anticholinergic and sedative combination may relieve abdominal distress.

All patients with bleeding should have a trial of conservative treatment; minor bleeding permits a persistent search for its cause. If severe bleeding occurs, immediate hospitalization, blood transfusions, and close observation are necessary. Surgery is occasionally required to prevent fatal hemorrhage. Since many diverticula are usually scattered throughout the colon, pinpointing the one responsible for the bleeding may be difficult. Colonoscopy, followed, if necessary, by radionuclide scan and angiography can usually locate the source of persistent bleeding; resecting that segment of the colon controls the life-threatening complication. When the bleeding source cannot be determined, total colectomy is the safest procedure, since patients have died from secondary hemorrhage when only the sigmoid colon was removed. A subtotal colectomy may be considered if there are few diverticula in only one segment or if the patient is a poor risk. The operative risk in an elderly, rapidly bleeding patient can be reduced by staging the procedure. The colon is removed down to the low sigmoid to stop the bleeding; the ileum is exteriorized as an ileostomy and the low sigmoid colon as a colostomy; and intestinal continuity is later restored by ileorectal anastomosis.

DIVERTICULITIS

Inflammation of one or more diverticula, potentially leading to obstruction or perforation, and to abscess and fistula formation.

Pathogenesis and Complications

A small, even minute, perforation of a thin-walled diverticulum due to inflammation or high colonic pressure leads to bacterial or possibly fecal contamination of the pericolic tissues. A small abscess develops; it may be absorbed, may drain back into the bowel lumen, or may enlarge. The inflamed bowel segment (usually the sigmoid) often adheres to the bladder or other nearby pelvic organs (eg, the vagina, especially after a hysterectomy), and a fistula may develop. With repeated inflammation, the colonic wall thickens, the lumen narrows, and acute obstruction may occur. One of the most dangerous complications is perforation into the free peritoneal cavity, resulting in leakage of purulent or fecal material and generalized peritonitis.

Symptoms and Signs

Pain and localized tenderness occur most commonly in the left lower quadrant (since diverticula are most numerous in the sigmoid colon), but at times in the suprapubic area or low in the right lower quadrant where they mimic acute appendicitis. Pain is occasionally severe and associated with signs of spreading peritonitis. Crampy pain with abdominal distention suggests large or small bowel obstruction due to adherent jejunum or ileum. Pain aggravated by urination suggests adhesion of the inflamed bowel to the bladder. A change in bowel function to constipation (often interrupted by periods of diarrhea) is frequent. A mass is often palpable in the left lower quadrant. Fever and leukocytosis are usually present.

Diagnosis

Pain and tenderness in the lower abdomen associated with disturbed bowel function and, perhaps, rectal bleeding suggest not only diverticulitis, but also *colon carcinoma, which must be ruled out before a diagnosis of diverticulitis is made.* Fiberoptic sigmoidoscopy must be performed to exclude carcinoma of the rectum and sigmoid colon, particularly if rectal bleeding has occurred. A barium enema is usually still done to rule out carcinoma of the rest of the colon and to demonstrate diverticula and the presence of perforation, obstruction, or fistula. Proctoscopy and an initial barium enema do not exclude cancer in 15 to 20% of patients; if fiberoptic colonoscopy does not rule out malignancy, but a definite lesion is present, complete surgical removal is indicated. Crohn's disease of the colon should be suspected when clinical signs of diverticulitis are associated with persistent or recurrent anorectal disease, especially fistulas.

Prognosis

Morbidity and mortality (higher than they should be) can be reduced (mortality to < 3%) by early surgery before a serious complication develops, and by the use of a 2- or 3-stage operative procedure when primary resection is hazardous, particularly in elderly, poor-risk patients.

Treatment

For patients with acute diverticulitis, conservative therapy (hospitalization, bed rest, IV fluids, and nothing given orally) should be tried first; about 2/3 of patients will do well. IV hyperalimentation may also be used to put the diseased bowel "at rest." If the patient is febrile and has evidence of abscess formation, antibiotics (oral or IV) to cover gram-positive cocci and gram-negative bacilli (aerobic and anaerobic) are indicated. Metronidazole with ampicillin or gentamicin are commonly used. Pain may be severe and can usually be relieved with 50 to 100 mg of demerol IM q 3 to 4 h.

Surgical consultation should be obtained when the patient is admitted to the hospital to avoid later delay if an operation is needed. The inflammatory process usually subsides, but signs of continued inflammation and spreading peritonitis must be anticipated and sought. If these continue beyond 24 to 48 h, the segment of colon containing the perforation must be removed immediately. If the perforation is high enough in the colon to permit it, exteriorization of the perforated segment of bowel, with a proximal and distal colostomy should be done. If the involved segment is too low to be exteriorized, it is resected, the proximal colon brought out as a colostomy, and the rectal segment closed. Resection, with primary anastomosis, may be done safely if the peritoneal contamination is limited or contained in a small localized abscess. In any situation where there is concern about the integrity of the anastomosis, it is wise to provide a temporary proximal colostomy.

In elderly or poor risk patients, or when distended colon, large abscesses, or peritonitis make resection and anastomosis hazardous, diversion of the fecal stream by a proximal transverse colostomy is carried out first. Usually, inflammation gradually subsides, and the diseased bowel can be resected with little risk 4 to 6 wk later, followed by closure of the temporary colostomy. Similar management is indicated when a fistula (eg, colovesical) results in a severe pelvic inflammatory reaction.

In patients with recurrent diverticulitis or with symptoms suggesting an increasing degree of obstruction or early bladder involvement, early surgery often precludes the morbidity associated with 2 or 3 operative procedures and weeks of hospitalization. An adequate elective resection, done when the disease is quiescent and the colon is well prepared, is associated with little risk and few complications.

63. NEOPLASMS OF THE BOWEL

TUMORS OF THE SMALL INTESTINE

BENIGN TUMORS

Neoplasms of the jejunum and ileum comprise 1 to 5% of GI tumors. Predominantly benign, they include leiomyomas, lipomas, neurofibromas, and fibromas; all may cause symptoms requiring surgery. Polyps occur in the small bowel but are more common in the colon (see below). Vascular tumors are multicentric in the small bowel in 55% of cases. **Hereditary hemorrhagic telangiectasia (Rendu-Osler-Weber syndrome)** is *an inborn progressive tendency to form dilated endothelial spaces.* Hemangiomas may bleed or intussuscept. Angiodysplasias or arteriovenous malformations, consequences of aging, tend to occur in the distal small bowel or cecum. Arteriography or technetium bleeding scans may help to locate bleeding points; enteroclysis may identify mass lesions of the small bowel. If a surgeon must operate without knowing the bleeding site, transillumination of the bowel or intraoperative endoscopy may help the search. Electrocautery, thermal obliteration, or laser phototherapy may be alternatives to resection.

MALIGNANT TUMORS

Adenocarcinoma is uncommon. It usually arises in the proximal jejunum and causes minimal symptoms. Adenocarcinomas of the small bowel occur more frequently in patients with Crohn's disease of the small intestine where the tumors tend to occur distally and in bypassed or inflamed loops of small bowel. **Primary malignant lymphoma** arising in the ileum may produce a long, rigid segment. Small intestinal lymphomas arise frequently in a setting of celiac sprue. The small bowel, particularly the ileum, is the second commonest site (after the appendix) of **carcinoid tumors.** Multiple tumors occur in 50% of cases. Of those > 2 cm in diameter, 80% have metastasized by the time of operation. About 30% of small bowel carcinoids cause symptoms of obstruction, pain, bleeding, or the carcinoid syndrome (see Ch. 95). Treatment is best accomplished by surgical resection; repeated operations may be required.

TUMORS OF THE LARGE BOWEL

POLYPS OF THE COLON AND RECTUM

Polyp (a clinical term without pathologic significance) refers to *any mass of tissue that arises from the bowel wall and protrudes into the lumen.* Polyps may be sessile or pedunculated and vary considerably in size. Such lesions are classified histologically as tubular adenomas, tubulovillous adenomas (villoglandular polyps), villous (papillary) adenomas (with or without adenocarcinoma), hyperplastic polyps, hamartomas, juvenile polyps, polypoid carcinomas, pseudopolyps, lipomas, leiomyomas, or other rarer tumors.

Incidence ranges from 7 to 50%; the higher figure includes very small polyps of 6 mm or less (usually hyperplastic polyps or adenomas) found at autopsy. Polyps are detected in about 5% of patients by routine barium enemas, and more often by flexible fiberoptic sigmoidoscopy, colonoscopy, or air contrast barium enema. Polyps are often multiple, occur most commonly in the rectum and sigmoid colon, and in decreasing frequency toward the cecum. About 25% of patients with cancer of the large bowel also have "satellite" adenomatous polyps.

The cancer risk of tubular adenomas is controversial, but the preponderance of evidence suggests that they can become malignant. Risk of malignancy is related to size; a 1.5 cm tubular adenoma has a 2% risk. As its size increases, its glands develop

villous features. When > 50% of a tubular adenoma's glands are villous, it is called a villoglandular polyp; its malignancy potential is still that of a tubular adenoma. When > 80% of the glands are villous, the polyp is considered a villous adenoma and these become malignant in about 35% of cases. The risk of malignancy for villous adenomas also increases with size, and for a lesion of any given size, is greater than that of a tubular adenoma.

Symptoms, Signs, and Diagnosis

Most polyps are asymptomatic. **Rectal bleeding** is the most frequent complaint. Cramps, abdominal pain, or obstruction may be signs of a large lesion. Large, villous adenomas may be associated with profuse watery diarrhea that may result in hypokalemia. Occasionally a polyp on a long pedicle will prolapse through the anus.

Rectal polyps may be palpable by digital examination, but are discovered usually by endoscopy. Since polyps are often multiple and may coexist with cancer, complete investigation of the colon with colonoscopy is mandatory even if a lesion is found by flexible sigmoidoscopy. On barium enema x-rays, a polyp appears as a rounded filling defect. Double contrast (pneumocolon) examination is of great value, but fiberoptic colonoscopy is the most reliable diagnostic method.

Treatment

Polyps should be removed completely with a snare after total colonoscopy; *electrocautery (excisional snaring or fulguration) should not be performed in the unprepared bowel due to the explosion risk of hydrogen and methane* produced by colonic bacteria. Large villous adenomas have a high malignant potential and must be excised completely. Laparotomy should be considered if a polyp is sessile or if colonoscopic removal is unsuccessful. Colon resection may be advisable if the polyp contains cancer that has invaded the muscularis mucosa.

Follow-up procedures and their timing after polypectomy are controversial. Most authorities recommend 2 annual inspections of the entire colon with colonoscopy or barium enema with removal of any newly discovered lesions. Thereafter, colonoscopy or barium enema is recommended every 2 to 3 yr.

FAMILIAL POLYPOSIS

A heterozygous, autosomal dominant, heritable disease of the colon in which 100 or more adenomatous polyps carpet the colon and rectum. Malignancy develops before age 40 in nearly all untreated patients. Total proctocolectomy eliminates this risk, but since rectal polyps often regress after abdominal colectomy and ileorectal anastomosis, that operation is favored initially by many authorities. Subtotal colectomy requires reinspection of the rectal remnant every 3 to 6 mo; new polyps must be excised or fulgurated. If new ones appear so rapidly or prolifically that they cannot be extirpated, the rectum should be removed and a permanent ileostomy established. Careful follow-up of the index patient and family is essential; genetic counseling is indicated.

Gardner's syndrome is *a variant of a familial polyposis associated with desmoid tumors, osteomas of the skull or mandible, and sebaceous cysts*; other rarer variants involve multiple colonic adenomas and other lesions. **Peutz-Jeghers syndrome** is *an autosomal dominant, congenital disease in which multiple hamartomatous polyps appear in the stomach, small bowel, and colon.* Affected individuals have melanotic pigmentation of the skin and mucous membranes, especially about the lips and gums.

OTHER POLYPS

Juvenile polyps occur in children, are usually non-neoplastic, and often outgrow their blood supply and autoamputate at puberty. Treatment is required only for uncontrollable bleeding or intussusception. **Hyperplastic polyps,** also non-neoplastic, are common

in the colon and rectum. **Pseudopolyps** that occur in chronic ulcerative colitis are discussed in Ch. 59. Inflammatory polyps and pseudopolyps also occur in Crohn's disease of the colon.

CANCER OF THE COLON AND RECTUM

In Western countries the colon and rectum account for more new cases of cancer each year than any other anatomic site except the lung. In the USA approximately 60,000 people will die of this disease in 1986. About 70% of these cancers occur in the rectum and sigmoid colon, and 95% are adenocarcinomas. Cancer of the colon and rectum is the second most frequent cause of death among visceral malignancies that affect both sexes. The incidence increases with age, beginning to rise at age 40 and reaching a peak at 60 to 75 yr. Carcinoma of the colon is more common in females; carcinoma of the rectum is more common in males. Synchronous colonic cancers (more than one cancer) are found in 5% of patients.

There is a low genetic predisposition to cancer of the large bowel, but "cancer families" and "colon cancer families" are described in which colorectal cancer occurs across several generations, usually presents before age 40, and occurs more commonly in the right colon. Other predisposing factors include chronic ulcerative colitis, granulomatous colitis, and familial polyposis; in these disorders, the risk of cancer is related to the age of onset and duration of the underlying disease.

Populations with a high incidence of colorectal cancer consume diets containing less fiber and more animal protein, fat, and refined carbohydrates than populations with a low incidence of the disease. Although carcinogenic substances may be ingested in the diet, it seems more likely that carcinogens are produced from dietary substances or from biliary or intestinal secretions, probably by bacterial action. The exact carcinogenic mechanism is unknown.

Cancer of the colon and rectum spreads by (1) direct extension through the wall of the bowel, (2) hematogenous metastases, (3) regional lymph node metastases, (4) perineural extension, and (5) intraluminal metastases.

Symptoms, Signs, and Diagnosis

Adenocarcinoma of the colon and rectum has a slow growth rate and a correspondingly long interval before reaching symptom-producing size. During this asymptomatic phase, diagnosis depends on routine examination. When symptoms develop, they depend on the location of the lesion, its type, extent, and complications. The **right colon** has a large caliber, a thin wall, and a liquid consistency of its contents; carcinomas here are usually fungating. Tumors here may grow large and even be palpable through the abdominal wall. Fatigue and weakness due to severe anemia may be the only complaints. Bleeding is usually occult. Because of the liquid consistency of stool, obstruction is a late event. The **left colon** has a smaller lumen, the feces are semisolid and cancer here tends to encircle the bowel, causing alternating constipation and frequency of bowel movements. Partial obstruction with colicky abdominal pain or complete obstruction may be the presenting picture. The stool may be streaked or mixed with blood. In cancer of the **rectum** the most common presenting symptom is the passage of blood with a bowel movement. Whenever rectal bleeding occurs, even with obvious hemorrhoids or known diverticular disease, coexisting cancer must be ruled out. There may be tenesmus or a sensation of incomplete evacuation. Pain is noticeably absent until perirectal tissue is involved.

Simple, inexpensive testing of the stool for occult blood may be done by asymptomatic patients as part of screening and high risk surveillance programs. When tests are positive, further studies should be done.

About 65% of cancer of the colon and rectum are within reach of the flexible fiberoptic sigmoidoscope. Fiberoptic sigmoidoscopy should be performed in every patient with

suspected cancer of any portion of the bowel, and in every patient with symptoms referable to the colon. If a lesion is detected on sigmoidoscopy, total colonoscopy and complete removal of all colonic lesions should be undertaken. Fractional endoscopic biopsies may be misleading 25% of the time, and a "negative" biopsy does not completely exclude the possibility of cancer. If a lesion is sessile or not removable at colonoscopy, surgical excision should be strongly considered.

Barium enema x-ray examination is unreliable to detect rectal cancer, but is the most important initial step to diagnose colonic cancer. Air contrast examination may visualize more small lesions (< 6 mm) than full column barium enema, but pneumocolon can miss large lesions (> 2 cm) with surprising frequency (20 to 30%). The essential ingredient of any barium examination of the colon is a well-prepared bowel, often requiring cathartics, oral lavage, or multiple enemas. Barium should not be given orally when an obstructing colonic lesion is suspected, since resorption of water from the barium suspension by the colon may precipitate barium sulfate and produce complete large-bowel obstruction. Colonoscopy should be done even when x-ray diagnosis is reasonably sure; 30% of tumors and 40% of polyps are missed by barium enema, but colonoscopy will identify synchronous lesions, which may dictate the amount of bowel to be resected.

Elevated serum carcinoembryonic antigen **(CEA)** is not specifically associated with colorectal cancer, but CEA levels are high in 70% of patients. If CEA is high preoperatively and low after removal of a colonic tumor, monitoring CEA may help to detect recurrence.

Treatment and Prognosis

Primary treatment of colon cancer consists of wide surgical resection of the lesion and its regional lymphatic drainage after preparation of the bowel. The choice of operation for rectal cancer depends upon its distance from the anus and gross extent. Abdominoperineal resection of the rectum requires a permanent sigmoid colostomy. Low anterior resection, with anastomosis of the sigmoid colon to the rectum, is the curative procedure of choice only if a 5 cm margin of normal bowel can be resected below the lesion and if the operation is technically possible. The use of a stapler has permitted low anterior resection and anastomosis closer to the rectum with rectal sparing for more patients.

An attempt at surgical cure is possible in 70% of patients. The best 5-yr survival rate after curative operation with cancer limited to the mucosa approaches 90%; with penetration of the muscularis propria, 80%; with positive lymph nodes, 30%. When the patient is an unacceptable surgical risk, some tumors can be controlled locally by electrocoagulation. Preliminary results from studies of adjuvant radiation therapy after "curative" rectal cancer surgery suggest that recurrence can be delayed among patients with limited lymph node involvement, but survival benefit is uncertain. Chemotherapy and immunotherapy have not proven effective as surgical adjuvants in properly controlled clinical trials of colon or rectal cancer.

The frequency of follow-up after curative surgery for colorectal cancer is controversial. Most authorities recommend 2 annual inspections of the remaining bowel with colonoscopy or x-rays, and if negative, repeat evaluations at 2- to 3-yr intervals thereafter.

When surgery is not curative, limited palliative surgery may be indicated; median survival is 7 mo. The only drug with proven efficacy for advanced colorectal cancer is 5-fluorouracil **(5-FU)** given IV 1500 mg/m² BSA/wk or for 5 days q 4 to 5 wk; 15 to 20% of patients receiving it experience demonstrable tumor shrinkage and prolongation of life. Other single drugs and combinations with or without 5-FU have not demonstrated better results.

When metastases are confined to the liver, ambulatory hepatic artery infusion with floxuridine via an implantable subcutaneous pump or an external pump worn on the

belt may offer more benefit than systemic chemotherapy; this form of treatment is expensive, and its value awaits confirmation. When metastases are extrahepatic as well, infusion pumps offer no advantage over systemic chemotherapy.

---

64. ANORECTAL DISORDERS

Introduction

The anal canal is derived from an invagination of the ectoderm, the rectum from entoderm. The resultant anatomic differences are important considerations in evaluating and treating anorectal disorders. The **lining** of the rectum consists of red, glistening glandular mucosa; the anal canal is lined with anoderm, a continuation of the external skin. For their **nerve supply,** the anal canal and adjacent external skin are generously supplied with somatic sensory nerves and are highly susceptible to painful stimuli; the rectal mucosa has an autonomic nerve supply and is relatively insensitive to pain. **Venous drainage** above the anorectal juncture is through the portal system; the anal canal is drained through the caval system. The area of the anorectal junction can drain into both the portal and caval systems. **Lymphatic return** from the rectum is along the superior hemorrhoidal vascular pedicle to the inferior mesenteric and aortic nodes, but the lymphatics from the anal canal pass to the internal iliac nodes, the posterior vaginal wall, and the inguinal nodes. The venous and lymphatic distributions determine how malignant disease and infection spread.

At the superior boundary of the anal canal is the anorectal juncture (pectinate line, mucocutaneous juncture, or dentate line) where there are 8 to 12 anal crypts and 5 to 8 tiny papillae. Anorectal abscesses and fistulas originate in relation to the crypts.

The sphincteric ring encircling the anal canal is composed of the fusion of the internal sphincter, longitudinal muscle, the central portion of the levators, and the components of the external sphincter. Anteriorly it is more vulnerable to trauma which can result in incontinence. The puborectalis forms a muscular sling around the rectum for support and assistance in defecation.

In diagnosing anorectal disorders, the **history** should include the details of bleeding pain, protrusion, discharge, swelling, abnormal sensations, bowel actions, nature of the stool, use of cathartics and enemas, and abdominal and urinary symptoms. **Examination** should be gentle and requires good lighting. It consists of external inspection perianal and intrarectal digital palpation, rectovaginal bi-digital palpation (in women) anoscopy and rigid or flexible sigmoidoscopy to 25 to 60 cm above the anal verge, as well as examination of the abdomen. Inspection, palpation, and anoscopy and sigmoidoscopy are best done with the patient in the left lateral Sims' or knee-chest position, or inverted on a tilt-table. With painful anal lesions, topical, regional, or even general anesthesia may be required. If required, a cleansing phosphate enema can be given to facilitate sigmoidoscopy. Biopsies, smears, and cultures may be taken and x ray examination ordered if indicated.

HEMORRHOIDS

(Piles)

Cushions of tissue that line the lower rectum and serve to produce complete closure of the anal canal. External hemorrhoids are located below the dentate line and are covered by squamous epithelium. Internal hemorrhoids are located above the dentate line. Hemorrhoids typically occur in the right anterior, right posterior, and left lateral positions. Since hemorrhoids occur universally in adults and children, they should not be considered abnormal.

Symptoms, Signs, and Diagnosis

Symptoms due to the hemorrhoid are bleeding, protrusion, and pain. Rectal bleeding should be attributed to hemorrhoids only after other more serious conditions have been excluded. Hemorrhoidal bleeding, which typically occurs following defecation and is noted on toilet tissue, rarely leads to anemia or an acute exsanguinating hemorrhage. Either external or internal hemorrhoids can protrude and then regress spontaneously or be reduced manually. Hemorrhoids are painful only when they are ulcerated or thrombosed. A thrombosed hemorrhoid presents as a perianal protrusion in which pain may be nonexistent, or severe and incapacitating. Ulcerated edematous strangulated hemorrhoids ("the acute attack of piles") can cause severe pain. Less common symptoms due to internal hemorrhoids are mucus discharge and a sensation of incomplete evacuation, and of external hemorrhoids, difficulty in cleansing the anal region. Pruritus ani is *not* a symptom of hemorrhoids.

Diagnosis of external or thrombosed hemorrhoids and the acute attack of piles can be readily made on inspection of the rectum. Examination following straining at stool or a phosphate enema often will reveal the extent of the patient's hemorrhoidal pathology. Anoscopy is essential in evaluating hemorrhoids that are not painful.

Treatment

Correction of constipation and straining by means of stool softeners or psyllium seed may be effective. Bleeding hemorrhoids, after other possible causes have been excluded, can be treated by injection sclerotherapy with 5% quinine and urea hydrochloride, or 5% phenol in vegetable oil. Bleeding should cease at least temporarily.

Larger hemorrhoids or those that fail to respond to injection sclerotherapy are treated by means of rubber-band ligation: A 1/4" diameter elastic band is dilated up to about 3/8"; the internal hemorrhoid is grasped in an area that is insensible to pain and withdrawn through the band, which is then released to ligate the hemorrhoid, resulting in its necrosis and sloughing. One hemorrhoid is ligated q 2 wk and a total of 3 to 6 treatments may be required. Operative hemorrhoidectomy is rarely performed for bleeding hemorrhoids.

If protruding hemorrhoids are internal, they are treated by rubber-band ligations. With mixed internal and external hemorrhoids, the internal component should be rubber-band ligated. If there is no significant internal component, operative hemorrhoidectomy or cryosurgical hemorrhoidectomy (freezing) is required. Painful hemorrhoids, if due to a thrombosed hemorrhoid, can be treated with reassurance, warm Sitz baths, topical anesthetic ointments, or witch hazel compresses.

The acute attack of piles can be managed similarly, since rapid resolution of pain and swelling can be anticipated and the thromboses are reabsorbed over 4 to 8 wk. Severe incapacitating pain may be treated (1) by the introduction of local anesthetic containing hyaluronidase with resolution of the acute process followed by rubber-band ligation of the internal hemorrhoids and multiple thrombectomies or (2) formal operative hemorrhoidectomy may be required.

Mucus discharge and a sensation of incomplete evacuation of the rectum are usually due to internal hemorrhoids, which are ideally treated by rubber-band ligation.

ANAL FISSURE

(Fissure in Ano; Anal Ulcer)

An acute longitudinal tear or a chronic ovoid ulcer in the stratified squamous epithelium of the anal canal.

Etiology, Symptoms, and Signs

The exact etiology of anal fissures is unknown. They are believed to be due to a traumatic laceration from a hard or large stool, with secondary infection. The fissure rests on the internal sphincter and causes it to go into spasm, which is believed respon-

sible for perpetuating the fissure. Infants may develop acute fissures. The fissure usually lies in the posterior midline, but may occur in the anterior midline. An external skin tag (the **"sentinel pile"**) may be present at the lower end of the fissure and an enlarged ("hypertrophic") papilla at the upper end. Chronic fissures must be differentiated from carcinoma, primary lesions of syphilis, TB, and ulceration associated with Crohn's disease.

Fissures cause pain and bleeding with defecation. The pain typically occurs with or shortly following defecation, lasts for several hours, and then subsides until the next bowel movement. Examination must be gentle and may only require spreading the anus apart, revealing the fissure in its midline location.

Treatment

Fissures often respond to conservative measures (eg, stool softeners or psyllium seed laxatives) that minimize trauma during bowel movements. Healing often results from use of bland suppositories (eg, glycerin) that melt, lubricate the lower rectum, and act as an emollient. Warm (not hot) sitz baths for 10 or 15 min after each bowel movement or prn to ease discomfort will give temporary relief. When conservative measures fail, surgery is required.

ANORECTAL ABSCESS

(See also Ch. 5)

Etiology, Symptoms, and Signs

Anorectal abscess results from bacterial invasion of the pararectal spaces, originating in an intermuscular (intersphincteric) space into which an anal crypt has penetrated. A mixed infection usually occurs; *Escherichia coli*, *Proteus vulgaris*, streptococci, staphylococci, and bacteroides are predominant causes. The abscess may be subcutaneous, ischiorectal, retrorectal, submucous, pelvirectal (supralevator), or intramuscular.

Superficial abscesses are the most painful; swelling, redness, and tenderness are characteristic. Deeper abscesses cause toxic symptoms, but localized pain is less severe. External swelling may not occur, but digital rectal examination reveals tender swelling. High pelvirectal abscesses may cause no rectal symptoms and may be associated with lower abdominal pain and FUO. It must be remembered that inflammatory bowel disease (eg, Crohn's disease, especially of the colon) is sometimes found in association with anorectal abscess.

Treatment

Prompt incision and adequate drainage are required; one should not wait until the abscess points externally. Suppuration is almost always present when the diagnosis is made. Antibiotics are of limited value. Persistent anorectal fistula may occur following drainage.

ANORECTAL FISTULA

(Fistula in Ano)

A tube-like tract with one opening in the anal canal and the other usually in the perianal skin.

Etiology

Fistulas usually arise spontaneously or occur secondary to drainage of a perirectal abscess. Predisposing causes include Crohn's disease and TB. Usually there is no recognized predisposing cause. Most fistulas originate in the anorectal crypts; others may result from diverticulitis, neoplasm, or trauma. Fistulas in infants are congenital and are more common in boys. Rectovaginal fistulas may be secondary to Crohn's disease, obstetric injuries, radiotherapy, or malignancy.

Symptoms, Signs, and Diagnosis

A history of recurrent abscess followed by intermittent or constant discharge is usual. On inspection, one or more secondary openings can be seen. A cord-like tract can often be palpated. A probe can be inserted into the tract to determine its depth and direction. Anoscopy of the crypts may reveal the primary opening. Sigmoidoscopy is required. Hidradenitis suppurativa, pilonidal sinus, dermal suppurative sinuses, and urethroperineal fistulas must be differentiated from cryptogenic fistulas.

Treatment

The only effective treatment is surgical. The primary opening and the entire tract are unroofed and converted into a "ditch." Partial division of the sphincters may be necessary. Some degree of incontinence may occur if a considerable portion of the sphincteric ring is divided. Fistulotomy is inadvisable in the presence of diarrhea, active ulcerative colitis, or active granulomatous enterocolitis since delayed wound healing may present a severe problem.

PROCTITIS

(See also Chs. 14 and 59)

Inflammation of the rectal mucosa.

Increasing in incidence, proctitis may result from rectal gonorrhea, nonspecific sexually transmitted infection, candidiasis, and syphilis, usually secondary. The patient complains of rectal bleeding or passage of mucus per rectum. The diagnosis is made by proctoscopy or sigmoidoscopy, which may reveal an inflamed rectal mucosa. Diagnosis is by smears, culture of material from the rectal wall, or biopsy and by STS. The underlying cause should be treated. Specific proctitis in which the underlying cause can be identified can be treated by appropriate antibiotics. The treatment of nonspecific proctitis includes topical corticosteroids in the form of steroid enemas or steroid foam, bid for 3 wk, or sulfasalazine 500 to 1000 mg orally qid for 3 wk or more. A small percentage of patients with nonspecific proctitis will evolve into chronic ulcerative colitis (see Ch. 59).

PILONIDAL DISEASE

Acute abscess or chronic draining sinuses in the sacrococcygeal area.

Pilonidal disease usually occurs in young, hirsute whites, and is more common in males. One or several midline or eccentric pits or sinuses occur in the skin of the sacral region and may lead to a cavity, often containing hair. The lesion is usually asymptomatic unless it becomes acutely infected.

Treatment of acute abscesses is by incision and drainage. As a rule, one or more chronic draining sinuses persist and must then be surgically extirpated by excision and primary closure or, preferably, by an open technic (eg, cystotomy or marsupialization).

RECTAL PROLAPSE AND PROCIDENTIA

Protrusion of the rectum through the anus.

Transient, minor **prolapse** of just the rectal mucosa frequently occurs in otherwise normal infants. In adults, however, mucosal prolapse is persistent and may progressively worsen.

Procidentia consists of complete prolapse of the entire thickness of the rectum. Abnormal anterior displacement of the rectum due to elongation of the mesorectum is probably the primary cause. Most patients are women over age 60.

The patient should be examined while standing or squatting, and straining, to determine the full extent of the prolapse. Diminished anal sphincter tone is usually present.

Sigmoidoscopy and barium enema x-rays of the colon must be done to search for intrinsic disease. Primary neurologic disorders must be ruled out.

Treatment

In infants and children conservative treatment is most satisfactory. Underlying nutritional disorders should be corrected and causes of straining eliminated. Strapping the buttocks together firmly between bowel movements usually facilitates spontaneous resolution of the prolapse. For simple mucosal prolapse in adults, the excess mucosa can be excised or rubber-band ligated (see HEMORRHOIDS, above). For complete procidentia, an abdominal operation with elevation and posterior fixation of the rectum to the sacrum to correct its anterior displacement or a low anterior resection has been most successful. In patients who are very old or in poor general condition, a wire loop can be inserted to encircle the sphincteric ring (Thiersch procedure).

MALIGNANT TUMORS OF THE ANORECTUM

(See also Chs. 63 and 105)

Epidermoid (squamous cell) carcinoma of the anorectum comprises 3 to 5% of rectal and anal cancers. Leukoplakia, lymphogranuloma venereum, chronic fistulas, and irradiated anal skin are predisposing causes. Metastasis is along the lymphatics of the rectum as well as in the inguinal lymph nodes. Basal cell carcinoma, Bowen's disease (intradermal carcinoma), extramammary Paget's disease, cloacogenic carcinoma, and malignant melanoma are less common. Wide local excision is often satisfactory treatment for perianal carcinomas. Combination chemotherapy and radiation therapy has been successfully used for tumors in this region. Abdominoperineal resection may be indicated.

FECAL INCONTINENCE

Loss of voluntary control of defecation.

The history attempts to elucidate the etiology. Anal incontinence may result from injuries or diseases of the spinal cord, congenital abnormalities, accidental injuries to the rectum and anus, procidentia, senility, diabetes, fecal impaction, extensive inflammatory processes, tumors, following obstetric injuries, and following operations involving division or dilation of the anal sphincters.

Physical examination should evaluate gross sphincter function and perianal sensation and exclude the presence of a fecal impaction. Other useful studies are pelvic floor electromyography and anorectal manometry.

Treatment includes a bowel management program that attempts to develop a predictable pattern of defecation. This includes adequate fluid intake and provision of sufficient dietary bulk. Defecation is encouraged by positioning the patient on a commode along with other defecatory stimulants customary for him (eg, a cup of coffee). A suppository (eg, glycerine or bisacodyl) or a phosphate enema also may be used. If a regular defecatory pattern does not develop, a low residue diet may reduce the frequency of defecation. Loperamide will have this effect and also may enhance sphincter function.

Simple perineal exercises in which the patient repeatedly contracts the sphincters, perineal muscles, and buttocks may serve to strengthen and hypertrophy these structures and may contribute to continence, particularly in mild cases. Biofeedback, used to train the patient to use the sphincters maximally and to better appreciate physiologic stimuli, should generally be considered before recommending surgery.

Several operations are used. A postanal repair is useful when the sphincter mechanism is basically intact without gaps, which are common in women with spontaneous

onset of incontinence at or over age 60. Increasing the anterior angulation of the rectum augments a factor that normally contributes to continence.

Direct suture of the sphincter is performed when there is a defect in it. When there is insufficient residual sphincter to repair directly, particularly in patients under age 50, a gracilis muscle transposition can be used. Where that is impossible, anal encircling procedures with Thiersch wire or other materials can be used. When all else fails, a colostomy can be considered.

PRURITUS ANI

Anal and perianal itching.

Etiology

The perianal skin has a maximum "readiness to itch," and pruritus ani has many causes: (1) **dermatologic disorders** (eg, psoriasis, atopic dermatitis); (2) **allergic reactions** (eg, contact dermatitis due to local anesthetics—"-caine" preparations), various ointments, or aromatic and other chemicals used in soap; and eczema following ingestion of certain foods (it is doubtful, however, that true allergy is a causative agent); (3) **microorganisms** such as fungi (eg, dermatophytosis, candidiasis) and bacteria (secondary infection due to scratching); (4) **parasites** (pinworms and, less commonly, scabies or pediculosis); (5) **oral antibiotics** (especially tetracyclines); (6) **disease processes** such as systemic diseases (eg, diabetes mellitus, liver disease), proctologic disorders (eg, skin tags, cryptitis, draining fistulas), and neoplasms (eg, Bowen's disease, extramammary Paget's disease); (7) **hygiene,** either poor with residual irritating feces or overmeticulous with excessive use of soap and rubbing; (8) **warmth and hyperhidrosis,** due to tight body stocking, jockey shorts, warm bed clothing, obesity, climate; and (9) **psychogenic response** (the importance of the anxiety-itch-anxiety cycle varies from trivial to overwhelming). Hemorrhoids do not cause pruritus ani.

Skin changes may be characteristic or minimal and may be masked by excoriation due to scratching and secondary infection.

Treatment

Spices, citrus fruits, vitamin C tablets, coffee, beer, and cola can all be associated with pruritus ani and the effect of eliminating them from the diet should be determined. Clothing should be loose and bed clothing light. After bowel movements, the anal area should be cleansed with absorbent cotton, moistened, if necessary, with plain water. Liberal, frequent dusting with nonmedicated talcum powder may combat moisture. Hydrocortisone acetate 1% in emulsion base, applied sparingly qid, is usually most effective. Topical fungicides (eg, amphotericin B) may be used. Systemic causes and parasitic infestations must be treated specifically. Biopsies should be taken in refractory lesions to detect malignancy. X-ray treatment and surgery or injections to create permanent local anesthesia are rarely if ever indicated.

FOREIGN BODIES IN THE RECTUM

Swallowed foreign bodies, including toothpicks, chicken bones, fish bones, gallstones, or fecaliths, may lodge at the anorectal juncture. Urinary calculi, vaginal pessaries, or surgical sponges or instruments may erode into the rectum. Foreign bodies, some bizarre, may be introduced intentionally; enema tips and thermometers, broken or intact, are among the most common.

Sudden, excruciating pain during defecation should arouse suspicion of a penetrating foreign body, usually lodged at the anorectal juncture. Other manifestations depend upon the size and shape of the foreign body, its duration in situ, and the presence of infection or perforation.

The foreign body usually becomes lodged in the midrectum where it is unable to negotiate the anterior angulation of the rectum. It can be felt on digital examination. Abdominal examination and chest x-rays may be necessary to exclude the possibility of an intraperitoneal rectal perforation.

Treatment

If the object can be palpated, local anesthesia is given by means of s.c. and submucosal injections of ½% lidocaine or bupivacaine containing hyaluronidase 150 u./15 mL. The anus can then be dilated with a rectal retractor, the foreign body grasped, deflected anteriorly, and removed. If the object cannot be palpated, the patient should be hospitalized. Peristalsis generally brings the foreign body down to the mid-rectum and the above routine can be followed. Removal via a sigmoidoscope or proctoscope is rarely successful and sigmoidoscopy usually results in forcing the foreign body into a proximal position delaying its extraction. Infrequently, regional or general anesthesia will be necessary and, rarely, laparotomy with milking of the foreign body toward the anus, or colotomy and extraction of the foreign body. After the extraction, sigmoidoscopy should be done to rule out significant rectal trauma or perforation.

65. BEZOARS AND FOREIGN BODIES

BEZOARS

Concretions of hair or vegetable matter, bezoars are rare, but attract preternatural interest. Balls made up of shellac or even bubble gum have been reported, but hair or wool, oranges or persimmons are the stuff of most true bezoars. A true bezoar should be distinguished from a pseudobezoar, a radiologic phenomenon simulated by food or other gastric contents in the patient who has not fasted for a barium meal.

Etiology

Delayed gastric emptying favors bezoar formation. Therefore, they are not uncommon after operations on the stomach that, like vagotomy, delay gastric emptying, and they are also more likely in the patient with diabetic gastroenteropathy. Bezoars also occur in the otherwise normal stomach, usually of persons gluttonous for persimmons.

Symptoms, Signs, and Diagnosis

Most bezoars probably cause no symptoms, even if postprandial fullness, nausea and vomiting, abdominal pain or peptic ulcer, and GI bleeding have been ascribed to them. Usually they are detected at x-ray when they may be mistaken for tumors. At endoscopy, bezoars display an unmistakable irregular surface, often gray-black or green. They can also be shown by imaging studies (eg, ultrasound or CT).

Treatment

A pseudobezoar requires only patience. Many true bezoars probably also could be ignored, but the usual approach is to try to dissolve them with papain (commercial meat tenderizer) 5 mL (1 tsp) in a glass of water qid or cellulase 30 mL (2 tbsp) pulverized in a glass of water after meals tid and then to give metoclopramide 10 mg IM q 3 to 4 h for 1 to 2 days to try to eject the fragments from the stomach through the pylorus. Before that, however, the endoscopist called in to evaluate the lesion usually will have tried to break it up by a jet spray of water or with forceps. Very rarely, operative removal at gastrotomy will prove necessary. In children, metoclopramide dosage should be adjusted for age; usually not > 0.5 mg/kg/day should be given to avoid extrapyramidal effects. For children under age 6 yr, the dosage is 0.1 mg/kg/day.

FOREIGN BODIES

From time to time foreign bodies are swallowed by children, deranged persons, or those who have drunk too much alcohol; denture-wearers are prone to swallow chicken or fish bones. Probably most foreign bodies that have gotten into the stomach could be ignored, but the temptation to retrieve an object from the esophagus, stomach, or duodenum will prove irresistible to most endoscopists. There can be little quarrel with the attempt to remove an object from as far down as the duodenum if only to forestall further x-ray surveillance. Sharp objects should be retrieved, if possible, but small round ones (eg, coins) can probably be watched without undue apprehension.

Foreign objects that have passed into the small intestine usually traverse the GI tract without problem, even if they take weeks or months to do so. They tend to hold up at the ileum, just before the ileocecal valve or at any site of narrowing, as in Crohn's disease. Drug smugglers, who sometimes swallow rubber balloons filled with drugs to escape detection, have developed intestinal obstruction as the balloons come up against a stricture. Sometimes objects like toothpicks remain within the GI tract for many years, only to turn up in a granuloma or abscess, particularly at a clinicopathologic conference.

§6. HEPATIC AND BILIARY DISORDERS

66. INTRODUCTION

The liver, the largest and metabolically most complex organ in the body, consists of myriads of individual microscopic functional units. These have traditionally been called lobules, bounded by portal triads and central veins. Rappaport's concept of the hepatic acinus, however, is more physiologic. This perceives the portal triad as the center, not the periphery, of a functional microvascular unit or acinus. Each acinus is divided into 3 zones based upon distance from the feeding vessels; the traditional centrizonal region of the lobule is in reality the periphery (zone 3) of 2 or more acini.

The liver has a remarkable capacity for regeneration in response to injury. Even extensive patchy necrosis usually resolves completely, as in acute viral hepatitis. Incomplete regeneration with fibrosis, however, results from confluent necrosis that bridges entire acini, or from less pronounced but ongoing chronic damage.

For clinical purposes the liver can be considered in terms of blood supply, hepatocytes, Kupffer cells, and biliary passages. Specific diseases tend to affect these components in predictable patterns, often with characteristic clinical and biochemical consequences. Symptoms of liver disease usually reflect hepatocellular necrosis or impaired bile secretion. Fibrosis by itself causes no symptoms; clinical manifestations are due to any resultant portal hypertension (see Ch. 76).

The liver receives its **blood supply** from both the portal vein and the hepatic artery; the former provides about 75% of the total 1500 mL/min flow. Small branches of each vessel, the terminal portal venule and terminal hepatic arteriole, enter each acinus at the portal triad (zone 1 of Rappaport). The pooled blood then flows through sinusoids between plates of hepatocytes. Nutrients are exchanged across the spaces of Disse, which separate hepatocytes from the porous sinusoidal lining. Sinusoidal flow from adjacent acini merges at the terminal hepatic venule (central vein, zone 3). These tiny vessels coalesce and eventually form the hepatic vein, which carries all efferent blood into the inferior vena cava. A rich supply of lymphatic vessels also drains the liver. Interference with the hepatic blood supply is common in cirrhosis and other chronic diseases and is usually manifested by portal hypertension (see Ch. 76).

Hepatocytes (parenchymal cells) comprise the bulk of the organ. These polygonal cells lie next to the blood-filled sinusoids and are arranged in sheets or plates that radiate from each portal triad toward adjacent central veins. Hepatocytes carry out exquisitely complex metabolic processes and are responsible for the liver's central role in metabolism. Their more important functions include formation and excretion of bile; regulation of carbohydrate homeostasis; lipid synthesis and secretion of plasma lipoproteins; control of cholesterol metabolism; formation of urea, serum albumin clotting factors, enzymes, and numerous other proteins; and metabolism or detoxifica-

tion of drugs and other foreign substances. In most liver diseases, hepatocellular dysfunction occurs to some degree and produces various clinical and laboratory abnormalities (discussed below).

Kupffer cells line the hepatic sinusoids and are an important part of the body's reticuloendothelial system. These spindle-shaped cells filter out minute foreign particles, bacteria, and gut-derived toxins, and play a role in immune processes involving the liver. Other endothelial cells of less certain function also line the hepatic sinusoids. Because of its Kupffer cells and rich blood supply, the liver is often secondarily involved in infections and other systemic illnesses.

Biliary passages begin as tiny bile canaliculi formed by adjacent hepatocytes. These microvilli-lined structures progressively coalesce into ductules, interlobular bile ducts, and larger hepatic ducts. Outside the porta hepatis, the main hepatic duct joins the cystic duct from the gallbladder to form the common bile duct, which drains into the duodenum. Interference with the flow of bile anywhere along this route produces the characteristic clinical and biochemical picture of cholestasis (see Ch. 67).

67. CLINICAL FEATURES OF LIVER DISEASE

Symptoms and signs of hepatic dysfunction are numerous; only the major clinical features are discussed here. Some abnormalities occur only in chronic disease; others are seen in either acute or chronic disorders.

JAUNDICE

A yellow discoloration of the skin, sclerae, and other tissues due to excess circulating bilirubin. Serum bilirubin is normally < 1 mg/dL, with the conjugated or direct-reacting fraction not > 0.3 mg/dL when measured by standard diazo technics; more sophisticated technics show no conjugated bilirubin in normal sera. Jaundice becomes apparent if levels exceed 2 to 2.5 mg/dL. Mild jaundice is best seen by examining the sclerae in natural light.

DISORDERS OF BILIRUBIN METABOLISM

(See also Hyperbilirubinemia in Premature Infant and Postmature Infant and Metabolic Problems in the Newborn in Ch. 186)

Bilirubin Metabolism

The catabolism of heme yields bile pigments; sources include the Hb of degenerating RBCs, RBC precursors in the marrow, and heme proteins of liver and other tissues. There is no evidence for the direct synthesis of bilirubin from heme precursors. Bilirubin is a pigmented organic anion closely related to porphyrins and other tetrapyrroles. As an insoluble waste product, it must be converted to water-soluble forms for excretion. This transformation is the overall purpose of bilirubin metabolism, which takes place in 5 major steps:

1. Formation: About 250 to 350 mg of bilirubin forms daily; 70 to 80% is derived from the breakdown of senescent RBCs. The remaining 20 to 30%, the **early-labeled bilirubin**, comes from other heme proteins located primarily in the bone marrow and liver. The heme moiety of Hb is degraded to iron and the intermediate product biliverdin by the enzyme heme oxygenase. Biliverdin is converted to bilirubin via another enzyme, biliverdin reductase. These steps occur primarily in cells of the reticuloendothelial system.

Enhanced destruction of RBCs (hemolysis) is the most important cause of increased bilirubin formation. Increased production of early-labeled bilirubin occurs in some hematologic disorders with ineffective erythropoiesis, but usually is not clinically important.

2. Plasma transport: Bilirubin, which is insoluble in water because of internal hydrogen bonding, is transported in the plasma bound to albumin. The binding weakens under certain conditions (eg, acidosis) and there is competition for the binding sites (eg, by certain antibiotics and salicylates). Because this circulating **unconjugated** ("indirect-reacting") bilirubin cannot cross cell membranes except those in the liver, it does not appear in urine.

3. Hepatic uptake: The details of bilirubin uptake by the liver have not been worked out. The process is rapid and probably involves active transport, but does not include uptake of the attached serum albumin. The importance of intracellular binding proteins (eg, ligandin or Y protein) is still unclear.

4. Conjugation: Free bilirubin is concentrated in the liver, then conjugated with glucuronic acid to form bilirubin diglucuronide or **conjugated** ("direct-reacting") bilirubin. This reaction, catalyzed by the microsomal enzyme glucuronyl transferase, renders the pigment water-soluble. Controversial evidence suggests that glucuronyl transferase forms only bilirubin monoglucuronide, with the second glucuronic acid moiety being added at the bile canaliculus via a different enzyme system. This latter reaction is not widely accepted, however. Bilirubin conjugates other than the diglucuronide are also formed, but their significance is uncertain.

5. Biliary excretion: Conjugated bilirubin is secreted into the bile canaliculus with other bile constituents. Other organic anions or drugs can affect this complex process. In the gut, bacterial flora deconjugate and reduce the pigment to various compounds called **stercobilinogens.** Most of these are excreted in the feces and lend the stool its brown color; substantial amounts are absorbed and re-excreted in the bile, and small amounts reach the urine as **urobilinogen.** The kidney can also excrete bilirubin diglucuronide, but not unconjugated bilirubin. This explains the dark urine characteristic of hepatocellular or cholestatic jaundice, whereas urinary bile is absent in hemolytic jaundice.

Abnormalities at any of the above steps can result in jaundice. Increased formation, impaired hepatic uptake, or decreased conjugation all cause **unconjugated hyperbilirubinemia.** Impaired biliary excretion produces **conjugated hyperbilirubinemia.** In practice, hepatic disease and biliary obstruction create multiple defects, resulting in a **mixed hyperbilirubinemia.** Moreover, when conjugated bilirubin builds up in plasma, a portion becomes tightly covalently bound to serum albumin. This protein-bound fraction is not measurable by routine technics, but is often a major component of circulating bilirubin, especially during the recovery phase of jaundice. Thus, in most patients with obvious hepatobiliary disease, standard bilirubin fractionation is of little diagnostic value, and in particular will not differentiate hepatocellular from obstructive jaundice. Fractionation is useful only if one of the disorders discussed below is suspected; these produce jaundice in the absence of demonstrable liver disease.

Unconjugated Hyperbilirubinemia

Hemolysis: Although the normal liver can metabolize supranormal quantities of bilirubin, the increased bilirubin formation that occurs in hemolysis may even exceed this capacity. Because the hyperbilirubinemia is unconjugated, bile is absent from the urine. Even in brisk hemolysis, serum bilirubin rarely exceeds 3 to 5 mg/dL unless liver damage is also present. However, the combination of modest hemolysis and mild liver disease may result in surprisingly severe jaundice; in these circumstances the hyperbilirubinemia is mixed, since canalicular excretion becomes impaired. Hemolytic anemia is discussed in Ch. 96.

Gilbert's syndrome: *Mild unconjugated hyperbilirubinemia is the only significant abnormality, which is important clinically only because it is often misdiagnosed as chronic hepatitis.* The disorder, presumably lifelong, is most often detected in young adults with vague nonspecific complaints. Previously considered rare, but the most common of the benign chronic hyperbilirubinemias, it may affect as many as 3 to 5% of the population. Some family members may be affected, but a clear genetic pattern is often difficult to establish. Its pathogenesis is uncertain. There appear to be complex defects in the hepatic uptake of bilirubin, which usually fluctuates between 2 and 5 mg/dL and tends to increase with fasting and other stresses. In addition, glucuronyl transferase activity is low; therefore, the disorder may be related to the much rarer Type II Crigler-Najjar syndrome (see below). Many patients also have mildly diminished RBC survival, but this is insufficient to explain the hyperbilirubinemia.

Gilbert's syndrome can be easily differentiated from hepatitis by normal ranges of liver function tests, absence of urinary bile, and characteristic bilirubin fractionation. Hemolysis is differentiated by the absence of anemia or reticulocytosis. Liver histology is normal, but biopsy is not needed to make the diagnosis. Patients should be reassured that they do not have liver disease.

Crigler-Najjar syndrome: *A rare inherited disorder associated with glucuronyl transferase deficiency.* It occurs in 2 forms: Patients with autosomal recessive Type I (complete) disease have severe hyperbilirubinemia and usually die of kernicterus within the first year of life. Patients with autosomal dominant Type II (partial) disease have less severe hyperbilirubinemia (< 20 mg/dL) and usually survive into adulthood without neurologic damage. Phenobarbital, which induces the partially deficient glucuronyl transferase, can diminish the jaundice.

Primary shunt hyperbilirubinemia is a rare, familial benign condition associated with overproduction of early-labeled bilirubin.

Noncholestatic Conjugated Hyperbilirubinemia

Dubin-Johnson syndrome: Asymptomatic mild jaundice characterizes this rare autosomal recessive disorder. The basic defect involves *impaired excretion of various organic anions as well as bilirubin,* but bile salt excretion is not impaired. In contrast to Gilbert's syndrome, the hyperbilirubinemia is conjugated and bile appears in the urine. The liver is deeply pigmented due to an intracellular melanin-like substance, but is otherwise histologically normal. The cause of the pigment deposition is unknown. Aminotransferase and alkaline phosphatase levels are usually normal. For unknown reasons, a characteristic derangement in urinary coproporphyrin excretion may accompany this syndrome.

Rotor syndrome: This rare disease is similar to the Dubin-Johnson syndrome, but the liver is not pigmented and there are other subtle metabolic differences.

CLINICAL APPROACH TO JAUNDICE

The differential diagnosis of jaundice involves asking specific questions to narrow the possibilities. The first question should be whether the jaundice is due to hemolysis or an isolated disorder of bilirubin metabolism (uncommon), hepatocellular dysfunction (common), or biliary obstruction (intermediate). If hepatobiliary disease is present, other important questions follow: Is the condition acute or chronic? Is it due to primary liver disease or to a systemic disorder involving the liver? Are alcohol or other drugs responsible? Is cholestasis of intra- or extrahepatic origin? Will surgical therapy be needed? Are complications present? These questions are approached by clinical, functional, and morphologic assessment.

Diagnostic errors usually result from an inadequate history and physical examination with undue reliance on laboratory data.

Symptoms, Signs, and Diagnosis

Jaundice without dark urine suggests unconjugated hyperbilirubinemia due to hemolysis or Gilbert's syndrome rather than hepatobiliary disease. See other signs and symptoms below for clinical features that suggest a hepatocellular or cholestatic disorder. Ascites, signs of portal hypertension, or cutaneous and endocrine features usually imply a chronic rather than an acute process. Patients frequently notice dark urine before skin discoloration, and its onset therefore provides a better guide to the duration of jaundice. Sudden nausea and vomiting preceding jaundice most often indicate acute hepatitis or common duct obstruction by stone; abdominal pain or rigors favor the latter. More insidious anorexia and malaise occur in many conditions, but particularly suggest alcoholic liver disease or chronic hepatitis.

A systemic disorder rather than primary liver disease should be considered. For example, distended jugular veins are an important clue to heart failure or constrictive pericarditis in a patient with hepatomegaly and ascites. Cachexia and an unusually hard or lumpy liver are more often due to metastases than to cirrhosis. Diffuse lymphadenopathy suggests infectious mononucleosis in an acutely jaundiced patient and lymphoma or leukemia in a chronic illness. Hepatosplenomegaly without other signs of chronic liver disease may be due to an infiltrative disorder (eg, lymphoma or amyloidosis), though jaundice is usually minimal or absent in such disorders; schistosomiasis and malaria commonly give this picture in endemic areas.

Other diagnostic features and the approach to cholestatic jaundice are discussed below.

Laboratory Findings

Liver function tests and x-rays are discussed in more detail in Ch. 68.

Mild hyperbilirubinemia with normal aminotransferase and alkaline phosphatase levels usually reflects hemolysis or Gilbert's syndrome rather than liver disease; bilirubin fractionation usually settles the issue. By contrast, the depth of jaundice and bilirubin fractionation does not help to differentiate hepatocellular from cholestatic jaundice. Striking aminotransferase elevations (> 500 u.) suggest a hepatitis or an acute hypoxic episode, and disproportionate increases of alkaline phosphatase a cholestatic or infiltrative disorder. In the latter, bilirubin is typically normal or only slightly increased. Bilirubin levels > 25 to 30 mg/dL are usually due to hemolysis or to renal dysfunction superimposed on severe hepatobiliary disease, as the latter alone rarely causes such deep jaundice. Low albumin and high globulin levels indicate chronic rather than acute liver disease. Improvement of an elevated prothrombin time after vitamin K administration (5 to 10 mg IM for 2 to 3 days) favors a cholestatic over a hepatocellular process. This fact, however, has limited diagnostic value since patients with hepatocellular disease may improve when given vitamin K. Radiologic procedures are of greatest value in the diagnosis of infiltrative and cholestatic disorders. Abdominal ultrasound and CT scanning often detect metastatic and other focal liver lesions, and have largely replaced radionuclide scanning for this purpose. MRI, also valuable, is confined to a few centers. These procedures are less helpful in diffuse hepatocellular disorders (eg, cirrhosis), since findings are usually nonspecific. The crucial role of radiology in the investigation of cholestatic jaundice is discussed below.

Morphologic Evaluation

Percutaneous liver biopsy has great diagnostic value but is not usually required in jaundice. **Peritoneoscopy** (laparoscopy) permits direct inspection of the liver and gallbladder without the trauma of a full laparotomy, and is useful in selected patients. Rarely, **diagnostic laparotomy** may be needed in some patients with cholestatic jaundice or unexplained hepatosplenomegaly. These procedures are discussed more fully in Chs. 50 and 68.

CHOLESTASIS

A clinical and biochemical syndrome that results when bile flow is impaired. The term "cholestasis" is preferred to "obstructive jaundice" because a mechanical obstruction is not always present.

Etiology

Bile flow may be impaired at any point from the liver cell canaliculus to the ampulla of Vater. For clinical purposes a distinction between intra- and extrahepatic causes is crucial.

The most common **intrahepatic** causes are viral or other hepatitis (see Ch. 71), drugs (see Ch. 72), and alcoholic liver disease (see Ch. 73). Less common etiologies include primary biliary cirrhosis (see Ch. 70), cholestasis of pregnancy (see HEPATIC DISORDERS in Ch. 178), metastatic carcinoma, pericholangitis secondary to ulcerative colitis, and numerous uncommon disorders.

Extrahepatic cholestasis is most often due to a common duct stone or pancreatic carcinoma. Less often, benign stricture of the common duct (usually related to previous surgery), ductal carcinoma, pancreatitis or pancreatic pseudocyst, and sclerosing cholangitis are causes.

Cholestasis in infants, caused by the neonatal hepatitis-biliary atresia spectrum, is discussed under GASTROINTESTINAL DEFECTS in Ch. 187.

Pathophysiology

Cholestasis reflects **bile secretory failure;** the mechanisms are complex, even in mechanical obstruction. Contributing factors may include interference with microsomal hydroxylating enzymes, which leads to the formation of poorly soluble bile acids; impaired activity of Na^+, K^+-ATPase, which is necessary for canalicular bile flow; interference with the function of microfilaments, thought to be important for canalicular function; and enhanced ductular reabsorption of bile constituents.

The pathophysiologic effects of cholestasis reflect backup of bile constituents into the systemic circulation plus their failure to enter the gut for excretion. Bilirubin, bile salts, and lipids are the most important constituents affected. Bilirubin retention produces mixed hyperbilirubinemia with spillover of conjugated pigment into the urine; stools are often pale because less bilirubin reaches the gut. High levels of circulating bile salts are traditionally blamed for causing pruritus, but correlation is poor and the pathogenesis of itching remains unclear. Since bile salts are needed for absorption of fat and vitamin K, impairment in biliary excretion of bile salts can produce steatorrhea and hypoprothrombinemia. If cholestasis is longstanding, concomitant Ca and vitamin D malabsorption may eventually result in osteoporosis or osteomalacia. Cholesterol and phospholipid retention produces hyperlipidemia, though increased hepatic synthesis and decreased plasma esterification of cholesterol also contribute; triglyceride levels are largely unaffected. The lipids circulate as a unique, abnormal low-density lipoprotein called lipoprotein-X.

Symptoms and Signs

Jaundice, dark urine, pale stools, and generalized pruritus are the clinical hallmarks of cholestasis. Chronic cholestasis may produce muddy skin pigmentation, excoriations from pruritus, a bleeding diathesis, bone pain, and cutaneous lipid deposits (xanthelasma or xanthomas). These features are independent of the etiology. Any abdominal pain, systemic symptoms (eg, anorexia, vomiting, fever), or additional physical signs reflect the underlying cause rather than cholestasis itself, and therefore provide valuable etiologic clues.

Diagnosis

Intra- and extrahepatic cholestasis must be differentiated. A detailed **history** and **physical examination** are especially important, since most diagnostic errors result from

inadequate clinical judgment and over-reliance on laboratory data. Intrahepatic cholestasis is favored by symptoms of hepatitis, heavy alcohol ingestion, recent use of potentially cholestatic drugs, or signs of chronic hepatocellular disease (eg, spider nevi, splenomegaly, or ascites). Extrahepatic cholestasis is suggested by biliary or pancreatic pain, rigors, or a palpable gallbladder.

Laboratory tests are of limited diagnostic value. The most characteristic abnormality is a disproportionately high serum alkaline phosphatase level; this is primarily due to increased hepatic synthesis rather than impaired excretion, but does not help clarify the cause. Serum bilirubin levels similarly reflect the severity but not the cause of cholestasis, and fractionation will not help distinguish an intrahepatic from an extrahepatic disorder. Aminotransferase levels largely depend on the underlying cause, but are usually only modestly elevated. Marked elevations suggest a hepatocellular process, but are occasionally seen in extrahepatic cholestasis, especially with acute obstruction due to a common duct stone. High serum amylase levels usually indicate extrahepatic obstruction. After vitamin K is given, an improved prothrombin time favors an extrahepatic blockage, but hepatocellular disorders may also respond. The presence of antimitochondrial antibody strongly favors primary biliary cirrhosis over other etiologies.

Imaging studies of the biliary tract are essential; abdominal ultrasound and CT scanning have rendered oral cholecystography and IV cholangiography obsolete in the investigation of cholestasis. Ultrasound is faster, cheaper, and more widely available than CT, and in most modern centers is the primary study for cholestasis. Both procedures are noninvasive and reliably reveal dilated bile ducts, which implies mechanical obstruction; however, absence of this sign does not necessarily indicate intrahepatic cholestasis, especially in acute situations. The underlying cause of the obstruction may also be revealed; in general, gallstones are more reliably shown by ultrasound, and pancreatic lesions by CT.

Transhepatic cholangiography or endoscopic retrograde cholangiopancreatography **(ERCP)** provide direct radiologic visualization of the biliary tree, but require specialized expertise and involve some risk to the patient. If available, these tests are especially useful preoperatively to define extrahepatic obstruction.

Liver biopsy usually clarifies the diagnosis in intrahepatic cholestasis; however, errors may arise, especially with inexperienced interpreters, and early extrahepatic obstruction may simulate an intrahepatic problem. Biopsy is safe in most cholestatic patients, but more hazardous with severe or longstanding extrahepatic obstruction, which should therefore be excluded by ultrasound or CT before biopsy is undertaken.

Except in patients with suppurative cholangitis, cholestasis is not an emergency. The approach to diagnosis should be based on clinical judgment plus the local availability of specialized technics. If the diagnosis is initially uncertain, ultrasound (or CT scan) should first be obtained. Mechanical obstruction can be safely diagnosed if this shows dilated bile ducts, especially in a patient with progressing cholestasis; further delineation by direct cholangiography (transhepatic or ERCP) can then be considered. If biliary dilation is not apparent on ultrasound, an intrahepatic problem is highly likely and liver biopsy should therefore be considered.

In centers lacking the above special tests, **diagnostic laparotomy** should be considered if clinical judgment points to mechanical obstruction and cholestasis progressively worsens. Care should be taken, however, to avoid operation on patients with cholestatic, viral, or alcoholic hepatitis.

Treatment

Extrahepatic biliary obstruction usually requires surgical therapy. In specialized centers, recent technical advances now permit nonoperative biliary drainage via trans-

hepatically-placed stents in selected patients with malignant obstruction (see Ch. 78), and endoscopic papillotomy in selected patients with retained common duct stones.

Laparotomy is contraindicated in intrahepatic cholestasis; treating the underlying cause usually suffices. Pruritus in irreversible disorders such as primary biliary cirrhosis usually responds to cholestyramine 4 to 16 gm/day in 2 divided doses, which binds bile salts in the intestine. Unless severe hepatocellular damage is present, hypoprothrombinemia usually improves after vitamin K_1 5 to 10 mg/day IM for 2 to 3 days. Supplements of Ca and fat-soluble vitamins A and D may be needed in longstanding cases, and severe steatorrhea can be minimized by partial replacement of dietary fat with medium-chain triglycerides.

HEPATOMEGALY

Enlargement of the liver indicates either primary or secondary liver disease, but absence of hepatomegaly does not exclude a serious disorder. When the liver is palpable, its upper border should be percussed to ensure that the organ is not merely low-lying. The lower border of a normal liver is often palpable at or slightly below the right costal margin. Serial determinations of liver size may be of prognostic value; eg, a rapidly shrinking liver in fulminant hepatitis implies a poor outcome, as does a rapidly enlarging organ in metastatic carcinoma.

Equally as important as liver size is its quality on palpation. The normal liver has a rubbery-soft, sharp, smooth edge. This consistency is often maintained in enlargement due to acute hepatitis, fatty infiltration, passive congestion, and early biliary obstruction. The cirrhotic liver edge is usually firm, blunt, and irregular; individual cirrhotic nodules are rarely palpable, and discernible lumps suggest malignant infiltration. Audible friction rubs or bruits over the liver, though rare, are other valuable clues to tumor.

Hepatic tenderness is overdiagnosed, usually because of the patient's anxiety when the liver edge is palpated. True tenderness, a deep-seated aching sensation, is best elicited by punch percussion or compression of the rib cage. It is most often felt in acute hepatitis, passive congestion, and malignancy. Spontaneous right upper quadrant discomfort is usually minimal in these disorders, but, occasionally, severe pain and tenderness may mimic an acute surgical condition.

ASCITES

The presence of free fluid in the peritoneal cavity.

Etiology

In liver disease, ascites indicates a chronic or subacute disorder and is not seen in acute conditions (eg, uncomplicated viral hepatitis, drug reactions, or biliary obstruction). The most common cause is cirrhosis, especially from alcoholism. Other hepatic causes include chronic active hepatitis, severe alcoholic hepatitis without cirrhosis, and hepatic vein obstruction. Portal vein thrombosis does not usually produce ascites unless hepatocellular damage is also present.

Nonhepatic causes of ascites include generalized fluid retention due to systemic disease (eg, heart failure, nephrotic syndrome, severe hypoalbuminemia, or constrictive pericarditis) and intra-abdominal causes (eg, carcinomatosis or TB peritonitis). Hypothyroidism occasionally causes marked ascites, and pancreatitis rarely produces surprisingly large amounts of fluid ("pancreatic ascites"). Patients with renal failure, especially those on hemodialysis, occasionally develop unexplained intra-abdominal fluid ("nephrogenic ascites").

Pathophysiology

Mechanisms that produce ascites are complex and incompletely understood. Two important factors in liver disease are (1) low serum osmotic pressure due to hypoalbu-

minemia and (2) high portal venous pressure; these appear to act synergistically by altering the Starling forces that govern fluid exchange across the peritoneal membrane. Hepatic lymphatic obstruction may also be involved. Circulating blood volume is usually normal or high, yet the kidney behaves as if it were low and avidly retains Na; urinary Na concentration is typically < 5 mEq/L. This has led to the concept that renal Na retention is due to decreased "effective" circulating volume secondary to the ascites. However, other evidence suggests that the kidney plays a primary role in initiating the process, perhaps by a neural or humoral mechanism, and that ascites is a result rather than the cause of Na retention (the "overflow" theory of ascites). Increased circulating aldosterone probably contributes to renal Na retention and is due both to enhanced production and to decreased metabolism. The pathogenetic role of antidiuretic hormone, kinins, prostaglandins, and atrial natriuretic factor remains uncertain.

Symptoms, Signs, and Diagnosis

Nonspecific abdominal discomfort and dyspnea may occur with massive ascites, but lesser amounts are usually asymptomatic. Diagnosis is made by detecting shifting dullness on abdominal percussion. In advanced cases the belly is taut, the umbilicus is flat or everted, and a fluid wave can be elicited. Differentiation from obesity, gaseous distention, pregnancy, or ovarian tumors and other intra-abdominal masses usually is easily made by clinical examination, but abdominal ultrasound or diagnostic paracentesis may occasionally be required. In liver disease or in intra-abdominal disorders, ascites is usually isolated or out of proportion to peripheral edema; in systemic disease, the reverse is usually true.

If the cause is uncertain, a **diagnostic paracentesis** (see in Ch. 50) should be done. From 50 to 100 mL of fluid is removed and, as clinically indicated, is assessed for gross appearance, protein content, blood cells, cytology, culture, acid-fast stain, or amylase. In most disorders the fluid is clear and straw-colored. Turbidity and a high WBC count (> 300 to 500 cells/mL) suggest infection, while sanguineous fluid usually signals neoplasm or TB. The rare milky (chylous) ascites is most common with lymphoma. A protein concentration of < 3 gm/dL favors liver disease or a systemic disorder; a higher protein content suggests an exudative cause such as tumor or infection, but ascitic protein in cirrhosis occasionally exceeds 4 gm/dL.

Cirrhotic ascites, especially in alcoholics, occasionally becomes infected without an apparent source **("spontaneous bacterial peritonitis")**. Clinical diagnosis may be difficult, as the fluid masks signs of peritonitis. Thus, early diagnostic paracentesis and culture should be done in cirrhotics with unexplained deterioration and fever, especially if abdominal discomfort is present; presence of > 300 WBCs/mL of fluid justifies therapy. Survival depends on early, vigorous antibiotic therapy.

Treatment

Bed rest and dietary Na restriction are the mainstays of therapy. A 20- to 40-mEq/day Na diet, though unpalatable, usually initiates diuresis within a few days and rarely causes serious electrolyte derangements. Diuretics should be used if rigid Na restriction fails. Spironolactone 100 to 300 mg/day orally in 2 or 3 divided doses is usually effective without causing the marked K loss often associated with thiazides or related diuretics. If this proves insufficient, a thiazide or loop diuretic should be added (eg, hydrochlorothiazide 50 to 100 mg/day or furosemide 40 to 160 mg/day orally in divided doses). Fluid restriction is not needed unless serum Na falls below 130 mEq/L. Unless massive ascites causes respiratory embarrassment, therapeutic paracentesis is best avoided, because it depletes the body of needed protein and may impair circulating volume; recent evidence suggests that paracentesis can be effective and safe if combined with IV albumin infusions, but this requires more study. Technics for th

autologous infusion of ascites (eg, the LeVeen peritoneovenous shunt) are associated with complications; their role in managing resistant ascites is controversial.

Changes in body weight and urinary Na determinations measure response to treatment. Weight loss of about 0.5 kg/day is optimum, as the ascitic compartment cannot be mobilized much more rapidly. Harsh diuresis produces fluid loss at the expense of the intravascular compartment and may cause renal failure or electrolyte imbalance (eg, hypokalemia) that may precipitate hepatic encephalopathy. Inadequate dietary Na restriction is the usual reason for persistent ascites.

PORTAL–SYSTEMIC ENCEPHALOPATHY

(Hepatic Encephalopathy; Hepatic Coma)

A neuropsychiatric syndrome due to liver disease and usually associated with portal-systemic shunting of venous blood. The term "portal-systemic encephalopathy" is more descriptive of the pathophysiology than "hepatic encephalopathy" or "hepatic coma," but clinically all 3 are used interchangeably.

Etiology

Portal-systemic encephalopathy may be seen in fulminant hepatitis due to viruses, drugs, or toxins, but more commonly occurs in cirrhosis or other chronic disorders where extensive portal-systemic collaterals have developed. The syndrome also follows portacaval shunt or similar portal-systemic anastomoses.

In patients with chronic liver disease, encephalopathy is usually precipitated by specific, potentially reversible stresses (eg, GI bleeding, infection, electrolyte imbalance—especially hypokalemia, and alcoholic debauches) or iatrogenically by tranquilizers, sedatives, analgesics, and diuretics.

Pathogenesis

The liver metabolizes and detoxifies digestive products brought from the gut by the portal vein. In liver disease these products escape into the systemic circulation if portal blood bypasses parenchymal cells or if the function of these cells is severely impaired. The resulting toxic effect on the brain produces the clinical picture.

The offending toxic substances are not precisely known, and the syndrome is probably multifactorial. Ammonia, a product of protein digestion, probably plays an important role, but biogenic amines, short-chain fatty acids, and other enteric products may also be responsible or may act with ammonia. Aromatic amino acid levels in serum are usually high and branched chain levels low, but this is probably not causal. The pathogenesis of the cerebral toxicity is also uncertain. Alterations in cerebrovascular permeability and cellular integrity may play a role, especially in fulminant hepatitis. In patients with liver disease, the brain appears abnormally sensitive to metabolic stresses. Interference with cerebral energy metabolism and inhibition of neural impulses by toxic amines acting as false neurotransmitters may occur. Recent evidence implicates γ-aminobutyric acid **(GABA),** the principal cerebral inhibitory neurotransmitter; synthesis appears increased and there may be an increased number of GABA receptors in the brain.

Pathologic changes are usually confined to hyperplasia of astrocytes with little or no neuronal damage, but in fulminant hepatitis, cerebral edema is common.

Symptoms, Signs, and Diagnosis

Personality changes (eg; inappropriate behavior, altered mood, and impaired judgment) are common early manifestations and may antedate any apparent change in consciousness. Sophisticated psychomotor tests can often detect such abnormalities not suspected clinically. Usually, **impaired consciousness** occurs. Initially, subtle sleep pattern changes or sluggish movement and speech may be present. Drowsiness, confusion, stupor, and frank coma indicate increasingly advanced encephalopathy. **Construc-**

tional apraxia, in which the patient cannot reproduce simple designs (eg, a star) is a characteristic early sign. A typical musty sweet odor of the breath, **fetor hepaticus,** frequently occurs. A peculiar and characteristic flapping tremor, **asterixis,** is elicited when the patient holds his arms outstretched with wrists dorsiflexed; as coma progresses, this sign disappears and **hyperreflexia** and the **Babinski response** may be seen. **Agitation** or **mania** may occur in fulminant cases and in children, but is otherwise uncommon. **Seizures** and **localizing neurologic signs** are also uncommon. Their presence should suggest another cause of coma (eg, subdural hematoma).

The diagnosis should be made on clinical grounds. There is no correlation with liver function tests. An **EEG** shows diffuse slow-wave activity even in mild cases, and may be useful in questionable early encephalopathy. The **CSF** is unremarkable except for mild protein elevation. **Blood ammonia levels** are usually elevated, but values correlate poorly with clinical status; bedside judgment is a better guide.

Prognosis

Encephalopathy due to chronic liver disease usually responds to treatment, especially if the precipitating cause is reversible. In most such cases the syndrome completely regresses without permanent neurologic sequelae. Some patients, especially those with surgical portacaval shunts, require continuous therapy, and irreversible extrapyramidal signs or spastic paraparesis may eventually develop; this is rare. Coma associated with fulminant hepatitis is fatal in up to 80% of cases despite intensive therapy, and patients with advanced chronic liver failure often die in hepatic coma.

Treatment

Precipitating causes should be sought; treating the cause may be sufficient in mild cases. Eliminating toxic enteric products is the other main therapy: (1) The bowels should be cleared with enemas. (2) Dietary protein should be eliminated (20 to 40 gm/day may be allowed in mild cases), and oral or IV carbohydrate will supply lost calories. (3) Oral neomycin, 4 to 6 gm/day in 4 divided doses, helps to minimize bacteria-formed toxins, and can be tube-fed in liquid form to comatose patients. Parenteral antibiotics are usually ineffective. (4) Oral lactulose is a useful alternative to neomycin, especially in cases of mild or chronic encephalopathy. This synthetic disaccharide syrup alters colonic pH and flora, and also acts as an osmotic cathartic. The initial dosage, 30 to 45 mL tid, should be adjusted to maintain 2 or 3 soft stools daily.

Sedation deepens the coma and should be avoided, even if the patient is agitated. Treating coma due to fulminant hepatitis by high-dose corticosteroids or by exchange transfusion and other complex procedures designed to remove circulating toxins has not proved effective. Instead, meticulous nursing care and careful attention to associated complications give the best chance of survival. Other treatment under study includes L-dopa, a precursor of normal neurotransmitters; bromocriptine, a dopamine agonist; infusions of branched chain amino acids or of keto-analogs of essential amino acids; and development of an "artificial liver." To date, none has proven effective.

PORTAL HYPERTENSION

(See Ch. 76)

OTHER SYMPTOMS AND SIGNS OF LIVER DISEASE

SYSTEMIC ABNORMALITIES

Anorexia, fatigue, and weakness are common features of liver disease due to hepatocellular dysfunction. Fever may occur, especially in viral or alcoholic hepatitis, but rigors are rare and in a jaundiced patient suggest biliary obstruction with cholangitis

Profound anorexia and nausea are especially common in viral and alcoholic hepatitis. Marked deterioration of general health and development of a "cirrhotic habitus" with wasted extremities and protuberant belly often signal advanced cirrhosis.

SKIN AND ENDOCRINE CHANGES

Patients with chronic liver disease can develop several cutaneous abnormalities. Spider nevi (vascular spiders), palmar erythema, and Dupuytren's contractures are common, especially in alcoholic cirrhosis. In hemochromatosis, deposition of iron and melanin makes the skin slate gray or bronze. Chronic cholestasis often causes muddy skin pigmentation, excoriations from constant pruritus, and cutaneous lipid deposits (xanthelasmas or xanthomas).

Endocrine derangements are common. Glucose intolerance, hyperinsulinism, insulin resistance, and hyperglucagonemia are often present in cirrhosis; the elevated insulin levels reflect decreased hepatic degradation rather than increased secretion, while the opposite is true for glucagon. Thyroid function tests must be interpreted with caution because of altered hepatic handling of thyroid hormones and changes in plasma binding proteins.

Complex derangements occur in the metabolism of sex hormones. Amenorrhea and decreased fertility are common in women with chronic liver disease. Male cirrhotics, especially alcoholics, often demonstrate both hypogonadism (testicular atrophy, impotence, decreased spermatogenesis) and feminization (gynecomastia, female body habitus). The biochemical basis is incompletely understood. Gonadotrophin reserve of the hypothalamic-pituitary axis is often blunted. Circulating testosterone levels are low, due mainly to decreased synthesis, but also to increased peripheral conversion to estrogens. The levels of minor estrogens are usually increased, but estradiol levels are variable and correlate poorly with clinical feminization. These changes are more prevalent in alcoholic liver disease than in cirrhosis of other etiologies; evidence indicates a direct toxic effect of ethanol on the testis.

HEMATOLOGIC DISTURBANCES

Multiple hematologic abnormalities are associated with liver disease. Anemia is frequent. Its pathogenesis may involve blood loss, nutritional folate deficiency, hemolysis, marrow suppression by alcohol, and chronic liver disease per se. Leukopenia and thrombocytopenia often accompany splenomegaly in portal hypertension, while leukocytosis is seen in cholangitis, tumor, alcoholic hepatitis, and fulminant liver necrosis.

Coagulation disturbances are common and complex. Impaired hepatic synthesis of clotting factors is frequent and may be due to hepatocellular dysfunction and/or to inadequate absorption of vitamin K, which is required for the hepatic synthesis of factors II, VII, IX, and X. An abnormal prothrombin time results and, depending on the severity of hepatocellular dysfunction, may respond to parenteral phytonadione (vitamin K_1) 5 to 10 mg/day given for 2 to 3 days. Thrombocytopenia, disseminated intravascular coagulation, and dysfibrinogenemia also contribute to clotting disturbances in many patients.

RENAL AND ELECTROLYTE ABNORMALITIES

Renal and electrolyte disorders are common, especially in chronic disease with ascites. **Hypokalemia** is caused by excess urinary K loss from increased circulating aldosterone, renal retention of ammonium ion in exchange for K, secondary renal tubular acidosis, and diuretic therapy. Management consists of giving oral potassium chloride supplements and avoiding K-losing diuretics. The kidney may avidly retain Na (see

under Ascites, above). Nevertheless, **hyponatremia** is common; it usually reflects advanced hepatocellular disease and is difficult to correct. Total body Na depletion is much less often responsible than relative **water overload;** K depletion may also contribute. Appropriate water restriction and K supplements may be helpful; use of diuretics that increase free water clearance is controversial. Intravenous NaCl solution is rarely useful unless hyponatremia is life-threatening or good evidence exists for total body Na depletion; it should be avoided in cirrhotics with fluid retention, as it exacerbates ascites and has only a transitory effect on serum Na levels. Variable metabolic and respiratory derangements may produce **alkalosis** or **acidosis** in advanced liver failure. **Blood urea concentrations** are often low because of impaired hepatic synthesis; superimposed GI bleeding causes elevations because of an increased enteric load rather than true renal impairment, since creatinine values usually remain normal.

Kidney failure in hepatic disease may reflect (1) disease directly affecting both organs (eg, carbon tetrachloride toxicity—rare); (2) circulatory failure with decreased renal perfusion; or (3) functional renal failure, often called **"hepatorenal syndrome."** This is a progressive disorder with no apparent anatomic abnormality in the kidney, and usually occurs in fulminant hepatitis or advanced cirrhosis with ascites. Its unknown pathogenesis probably involves neural or humoral alterations of renocortical blood flow. Insidiously progressive oliguria and azotemia herald its onset. A low urinary Na concentration and benign sediment usually distinguish it from tubular necrosis, but prerenal azotemia may be more difficult to differentiate; in doubtful cases, response to a volume load should be assessed. Once established, renal failure is almost invariably progressive and fatal. Terminal hypotension with tubular necrosis may complicate the picture, but the kidneys are characteristically unremarkable at autopsy.

CIRCULATORY CHANGES

A hyperkinetic circulatory state with increased cardiac output and tachycardia may accompany acute liver failure or advanced cirrhosis. Cirrhotic patients with collateral anastomoses may also develop arterial desaturation and clubbing of the fingers. Hypotension often occurs in advanced liver failure and may contribute to the development of renal dysfunction. The pathogenesis of these circulatory derangements is poorly understood.

Specific disorders of hepatic circulation (eg, Budd-Chiari syndrome, portal hypertension) are discussed in Ch. 76.

---

68. LABORATORY EVALUATION OF THE LIVER AND BILIARY SYSTEM

It is impractical to try to isolate hepatocytic, mesenchymal, and biliary tree functions, since they are so interdependent in this complex organ. Because of this, and because interpretation of most biochemical studies used in the routine investigation of liver disorders is so imperfect, no attempt will be made to categorize or isolate the various functions and the tests that may or may not reflect their disorders. In general, too many laboratory tests are available and too few are interpreted adequately; relatively few improve patient care.

Useful tests that should be part of the routine evaluation of liver disease include serum bilirubin, alkaline phosphatase, aminotransferases, and prothrombin time determinations. Other tests are practical in particular circumstances: various viral antigens and antibodies in patients suspected of having viral hepatitis; serum copper and ceruloplasmin in suspected cases of Wilson's disease; serum protein electrophoresis in

possible α_1-antitrypsin deficiency; serum mitochondrial antibodies in possible primary biliary cirrhosis **(PBC)**; dye elimination studies in some patients with congenital hyperbilirubinemia; and α-fetoprotein levels in possible hepatocellular carcinoma. Most other biochemical tests are either redundant or applicable only to research. Numerous radiologic tests may be useful. Discussion here is limited to the practical application of tests in evaluating liver disorders.

Tests Useful for Routine Evaluation

Serum bilirubin: Hyperbilirubinemia is discussed in detail in JAUNDICE in Ch. 67. Determination of the serum bilirubin is a necessary part of the routine evaluation of liver disease. Fractionation into total- and direct-reacting bilirubin is performed much too frequently in light of its clinical value. Estimation of the reserve bilirubin binding capacity of the serum can be important in the attempt to prevent kernicterus (see METABOLIC PROBLEMS IN THE NEWBORN in Ch. 186).

Serum enzymes: Increase in the serum activity of certain enzymes of hepatobiliary origin is common in all kinds of liver disorders.

Aminotransferases: The enzyme most widely studied is the aspartate aminotransferase **(AST)**, formerly SGOT. Elevations of its activity are found in myocardial infarction, heart failure, muscle injury, CNS disease, and other nonhepatic disorders. While nonspecific, this test is reliable and economical to use in routine screening for liver disorders. Values of 500 SI/L (> 400 u./mL) are highly suggestive of acute viral or toxic hepatitis.

The alanine aminotransferase **(ALT)**, formerly SGPT, is equally sensitive and possibly more specific for liver disease than the AST, but since it usually adds nothing to one's understanding of underlying liver disorders, it is not recommended in addition to the AST. The same advice applies to the lactic and isocitric dehydrogenases.

γ-Glutamyl transpeptidase: Estimation of the serum activity of this enzyme provides a very sensitive index of alcohol and drug hepatotoxicity, of infiltrative lesions of the liver, and of biliary tract obstruction. It is normal in the presence of bone disease; thus it renders the rather complex estimation of alkaline phosphatase isoenzymes unnecessary in most of the few cases where confusion may exist. Although perhaps more sensitive than some other routine tests, it too is nonspecific. Therefore, its precise contribution remains undefined.

Alkaline phosphatases: Alkaline phosphatase is elevated in diseases of the liver, pancreas, lung, and bone; in some malignancies without metastases; and in pregnancy. It is composed of a group of enzymes that hydrolyze organic phosphate ester bonds in vitro, at alkaline pH. The physiologic function of these enzymes is unknown.

In the first 4 wk of life, alkaline phosphatase activity rises rapidly to 5 or 6 times above normal adult values. It then decreases slowly until puberty, when there is another increase, followed by a decrease to adult levels at age 16 to 20 yr. It is slightly increased in older people. The level rises twofold during the 3rd trimester of pregnancy, threefold during labor, and returns to normal 2 to 3 wk after delivery.

Alkaline phosphatase may be fractionated by physiochemical technics into **bone, intestinal, liver, and placental fractions.** Such fractionation is sometimes useful in establishing the existence of metastatic malignancy or defining the site of otherwise unappreciated disease.

There are many conditions, drugs, and chemicals that affect alkaline phosphatase determinations. It is therefore important to collect and prepare the specimen carefully, and to interpret the result in the light of the patient's clinical and therapeutic drug history.

Alkaline phosphatase is elevated in a wide variety of liver diseases, but such elevation tends to be most pronounced in the presence of cholestatic disease, space-occupying lesions of the liver, and granulomatous hepatitis (see Ch. 75).

5′-Nucleotidase: The 5′-nucleotidases are phosphatases that differ from the alkaline phosphatases because they are inhibited by nickel ions. They are apparently restricted to the plasma membranes of the liver cell. Determination of their activity in the serum can be useful in distinguishing between increased alkaline phosphatase activity of hepatic and nonhepatic origin. In practice the test is useful only in assessing the anicteric patient.

Prothrombin time: Although the liver manufactures most of the plasma coagulation factors and influences blood coagulation by several other mechanisms, bleeding is rarely the direct cause of death in liver failure. More frequently the multifactorial coagulation abnormalities in liver disease serve only to increase blood loss from the GI tract or elsewhere, or to prevent diagnostic procedures (eg, liver biopsy).

The test is of little diagnostic use in the detection of mild hepatocellular function, because most of the analytical procedures involved are relatively insensitive to small reductions in the concentration of the vitamin K-dependent coagulation factors. However, because the biologic half-lives of the proteins involved are relatively short, a matter of hours to a very few days, hypoprothrombinemia can be the first sign of *fulminant hepatic failure*. Determining the prothrombin time after excluding vitamin K deficiency is the single most useful test to follow the patient with severe acute viral or toxic hepatitis.

Tests Useful in Special Circumstances

Serum albumin is a transport vehicle for numerous substances and the main determinant of plasma osmotic pressure. Its concentration in the serum is determined by its distribution between the intra- and extravascular beds, by the relative rates of its synthesis and degradation, and by plasma volume. Although the normal human liver produces 10 to 15 gm (0.2 mM)/day of this important protein, determination of its serum concentration is usually of little value as an index of hepatocellular function in acute liver disease, because the biologic half-life of the protein is about 20 days. The test itself is insensitive and nonspecific.

The concentration of serum albumin is frequently decreased in patients with advanced chronic liver disease. This does give some quantitative information about hepatocellular function in these patients, but there is poor correlation between its rate of synthesis and its concentration in the serum. Serum albumin is also decreased in some renal diseases, chronic infections, intestinal malabsorption, third-degree burns, and water intoxication. The decrease is due, respectively, to urinary loss of albumin, impaired hepatic synthesis of albumin, direct loss of albumin through the burned skin, or dilution of albumin by hydration.

Serum immunoglobulins: Most of the serum γ-globulins consist of immunoglobulins produced in response to specific antigenic stimulation. Serum γ-globulin levels can rise in acute liver disease and are usually raised in chronic liver disease, regardless of etiology. Knowledge of the serum γ-globulin concentration adds little to the evaluation of most patients. While serum IgM may be elevated in acute viral hepatitis A and in PBC, IgA in alcoholic liver disease, and IgG in chronic active hepatitis, the response is both variable and nonspecific; thus, quantitation of the individual serum immunoglobulins is of little diagnostic value.

Viral antigens and antibodies: (See VIRAL HEPATITIS in Ch. 71.) Other viruses (eg, the Epstein-Barr virus) can produce hepatitis (see INFECTIOUS MONONUCLEOSIS in Ch. 202).

Mitochondrial antibodies are present in > 90% of patients with PBC. The test is particularly valuable because needle biopsy of the liver may not provide diagnostic tissue. Although there is some overlap with chronic active hepatitis, and a low titer of antibodies can be found in some cases of drug-induced hepatotoxicity, a high titer of mitochondrial antibodies in the appropriate clinical situation is usually accepted as

diagnostic of PBC. (Further refinement in the diagnosis of PBC can be expected as the exact nature of the PBC-specific mitochondrial antigens becomes defined.)

Other antibodies: Smooth muscle, microsomal, and nuclear antibodies are in widespread use for the diagnosis of "autoimmune" chronic active hepatitis. In practice, they are nonspecific, of little diagnostic value, and unnecessary when properly interpreted liver biopsies are available.

α-Fetoprotein, normally synthesized by the hepatocytes, can be elevated in the newborn, in the patient with hepatocellular carcinoma, and in the patient recovering from massive hepatic necrosis. However, judging from reports of its secretion by nonhepatic primitive mesenchymal cell tumors, the response cannot be considered specific. Testing for α-fetoprotein is probably of value in screening patients for hepatocellular carcinoma and may prove of prognostic value in the patient with fulminant hepatic failure. Immunoelectrophoresis appears to be an adequate method for screening, but the considerably more sensitive radioimmunoassay may be necessary in certain clinical situations involving response to therapy.

Dye elimination tests: Tests that measure the removal of various endogenous and exogenous substances from the blood are too sensitive for routine clinical use; furthermore, they are nonspecific and tend to be both complex and time-consuming.

The **BSP retention test** is not quantitative, need not be done if the patient has evidence of liver disease, is *not without danger*, and is rarely indicated in clinical practice. It can play a role in the evaluation of **Gilbert's syndrome,** in which it is usually normal, and of the **Dubin-Johnson syndrome,** when regurgitation of conjugated dye into the bloodstream can be demonstrated at 90 to 120 min.

Indocyanine green, metabolized differently than BSP, has been less studied. Although measurable by ear-piece densitometry, apparently less toxic than BSP, and not subject to extrahepatic uptake, renal excretion, or an enterohepatic circulation, the dye is unlikely to gain widespread use. It is expensive and shares the same limitations as BSP in terms of clinical practice.

Bile acid studies: Bile acid metabolism is extremely complex and methods available for analyses are undergoing rapid evolution. Measurement of serum bile acids may prove useful to monitor liver function, but further comparisons with more conventional tests are needed. It is possible that serum can be used instead of duodenal bile to monitor patients undergoing bile acid therapy for gallstone disease. Analysis of fecal and urine bile acids is difficult, of undetermined clinical value, and restricted to special research units.

Bile pigment excretion: The study of bile pigments in the urine is simple and of some clinical importance. Bilirubinuria can be the earliest sign of hepatobiliary disease; commercially prepared tablets that detect bilirubin provide the most sensitive and satisfactory test for evaluating the anicteric patient.

Normal urine contains trace amounts of urobilinogen and no bilirubin. While the urobilinuria can increase with hemolysis and hepatobiliary disease, the test for urobilin is too sensitive, and the response too nonspecific to be of any diagnostic value. Quantitative analysis of urine pigments is of no diagnostic significance; the value of their quantitative evaluation in feces is restricted to research units.

The quantitative estimation of coproporphyrin I and III is also restricted to research units and will likely remain so. The diagnostic significance of coproporphyrin isomer excretion in hepatobiliary disease is probably limited to study of the Dubin-Johnson syndrome. Analysis of δ-aminolevulinic acid and porphobilinogen is required for evaluating certain metabolic diseases of the liver.

Breath tests: The precise role of the aminopyrine demethylation and other breath tests in the evaluation of patients with liver disease has not yet been defined.

X-rays of the Liver and Biliary Tree

Plain x-ray of the abdomen is of limited clinical usefulness; however, calcifications of the liver, hemochromatosis, opaque dye deposits, the presence of air in the biliary tree, and radiopaque biliary calculi can be identified. This examination usually provides an accurate assessment of spleen size, as the lower margin of the spleen is almost always visible. An enlarged spleen causes downward displacement of the splenic flexure of the colon and medial displacement of the fundus of the stomach.

Oral cholecystogram: This examination is simple, reliable, and relatively undemanding of the patient. Side effects are common, but usually mild; iodine sensitivity reactions and acute renal failure are the only serious ones reported.

This test is indicated in the diagnosis of cholelithiasis, chronic cholecystitis, and tumors of the gallbladder. It is useful in the differential diagnosis of opacities or masses in the right upper quadrant of the abdomen. Although ultrasound (see below) has largely replaced cholecystography as the primary procedure to detect gallbladder disease, the latter will continue to have a role in the evaluation of gallbladder function.

In 95% of properly prepared patients without vomiting, diarrhea, pyloric obstruction, malabsorption, or significant hepatocellular dysfunction, failure to visualize the gallbladder indicates gallbladder disease, usually with stones. If the results are not definite, a repeat examination with the same or greater dose of contrast agent is carried out the following day.

IV cholangiography is restricted to patients with symptoms suggestive of biliary duct disease to provide anatomic information.

The common bile duct will be visualized in > 90% of noncholestatic, anicteric patients, but in only about 10% of those with a serum bilirubin > 80 μmol/L. Small calculi can easily be missed; intrahepatic calculi are rarely seen. The indications for IV cholangiography have been sharply reduced since the advent of ultrasonography and endoscopic retrograde cholangiography (see below).

Operative cholangiography: A direct approach to the biliary tree with injection of dye into the cystic duct or common bile duct at laparotomy provides excellent visualization of the duct system and is both quicker and more accurate than IV cholangiography. While indications remain controversial, this procedure is recommended in any patient who is jaundiced on the basis of calculus disease of the biliary tree or who gives a history suggestive of choledocholithiasis. This diagnostic approach will be less used as operative choledochoscopy becomes more widely available.

Endoscopic retrograde cholangiopancreatography (ERCP) involves passing a side-viewing endoscope as for upper gastrointestinal endoscopy (see Ch. 50) and identifying the Ampulla of Vater on the medial aspect of the second portion of the duodenum. A catheter is passed through the scope into the ampullary orifice, and radiographic contrast material is injected. Spot x-rays are taken when the ducts are visualized. The biliary and pancreatic ducts may both fill with a single injection, or may need to be cannulated separately. Therapeutic procedures are done as indicated. Usually postprocedure x-rays are taken to ensure adequate drainage of contrast material. This technic (see also Ch. 78) provides precise definition of biliary and pancreatic anatomy, and with its associated surgical technics, it may substantially reduce the morbidity, mortality, and economic cost of biliary tract disease.

The initial endoscopic examination often provides information concerning upper GI tract pathology and can identify ampullary and periampullary pathology. The pancreatogram may identify a pancreatic neoplasm or pancreatitis. It will also define pancreatic duct anatomy, providing information that may be useful when subsequent biliary tract manipulation is attempted. The cholangiogram will visualize the intrahepatic and entire extrahepatic biliary tree. Cystic duct obstruction, stones, strictures, and tumors will be identified.

Therapeutically, pus can be drained, small common bile duct stones disrupted or flushed from the bile duct, and a large common bile duct stone removed by basket extraction or endoscopic papillotomy. Strictured bile ducts can be drained through endoscopic placement of tubes or stents.

In addition to the contraindications for endoscopy in general, ERCP should not be performed in the patient with significant bleeding or with acute pancreatitis unless the pancreatitis persists and a stone is considered responsible. The therapeutic procedures are contraindicated if there is evidence of a coagulation or bleeding disorder. Although hemorrhage and pancreatitis have been encountered, the incidence of significant side effects is remarkably low. The immediate future of endoscopic biliary surgery is secure.

Percutaneous transhepatic cholangiography (PTC): This technic is useful in defining the site, and possibly the nature, of mechanical obstruction to the biliary tree **(obstructive jaundice)**. The technic is usually used after ultrasound **(US)** examination has identified mechanical obstruction on the basis of dilated intra- or extrahepatic bile ducts. PTC is simpler and less expensive than ERCP and the complication rates of the two procedures are essentially the same. PTC is indicated when ERCP cannot or should not be done (Billroth II gastrojejunostomy, severe pancreatitis).

The basic technic is similar to that of liver biopsy. Coagulation parameters must be checked and prophylactic antibiotics are recommended. Either an anterior subcostal or lateral intercostal approach is used. The liver is punctured under fluoroscopic or US control with a thin 15- to 20-cm–long plastic-sheathed needle. The needle is removed and the sheath then slowly withdrawn while suction is maintained. When bile is aspirated, withdrawal is stopped and water-soluble radiopaque material is injected under fluoroscopic control. If no bile is aspirated on 4 to 6 passes into the liver, the bile ducts are probably not dilated and no mechanical obstruction exists. False positive results can be obtained if the contrast medium fails to mix well with stagnant viscous bile.

Sepsis is the major complication with intraperitoneal bile leakage and hemorrhage (subcapsular, intraperitoneal, retroperitoneal) also occurring in 1 to 1.5% of cases. The study does not have to be performed immediately preoperatively when the thin needle approach is used.

Therapeutically, the technic is used to introduce decompressing catheters into the biliary tree in a particularly useful adjunct to management of complete mechanical biliary tract obstruction. A modification of the technic is currently under investigation for the introduction of gallstone-dissolving agents directly into the gallbladder.

Radionuclide scanning: IV-injected Technetium 99 m sulfur colloid suspensions are taken up primarily by the reticuloendothelial system. In health the uptake of the colloid is greater by the liver than the spleen and there is essentially no colloid uptake by the bone marrow, lungs, and other tissues. Such radionuclide scanning can determine the size, shape, and location of the liver, follow liver function during the course of therapy, define right upper quadrant masses, direct the approach for liver biopsy, and investigate space-occupying lesions of the liver. Colloid scanning is used mainly to demonstrate liver tumors and, while lesions < 2 cm in diameter may be missed, the diagnostic precision of colloid scanning in combination with US approaches that of CT scanning.

The colloid scan of the cirrhotic liver features changes in the size and shape of the liver, heterogeneous uptake of colloid by the liver, and increased uptake of colloid by the spleen and bone marrow. Increased uptake of colloid by the caudate lobe can be found in the Budd-Chiari syndrome (see below).

Although colloid liver scans lack specificity and have relatively low limits of resolution, they remain in widespread use as a screening procedure in the investigation of liver disease, because they are rapid, simple, convenient, economical, and relatively noninvasive.

Technetium-labeled imino diacetic acid (IDA derivatives) are taken up by the parenchymal cells of the liver and rapidly secreted into bile. In such *dynamic scans* the liver usually is visible within 2 min after IV injection of the agent. In normal subjects the biliary tree is visible in 12 to 15 min. The appearance of a normal gallbladder virtually excludes the diagnosis of acute calculous cholecystitis and this is the primary use of these scans. They are also used effectively in the detection of intrahepatic stones, choledocholithiasis, perforation of the gallbladder, intrahepatic bile leaks, and in the postoperative evaluation of biliary-digestive anastomoses.

Biliary tree scanning, using radiolabeled IDA derivatives, may play a useful clinical role in evaluating cholestasis in infants. A definitely positive or negative test is definitive. Too often, however, the test is indeterminate even when duodenal aspirates and/or stools are analyzed for radioactivity. In the presence of hyperbilirubinemia, liver biopsy is still the preferred diagnostic approach to the infant with cholestasis.

Hepatocellular function aside from bile production has been evaluated by studying the uptake of radioactive selenomethionine and vitamin B_{12}, while radionuclide rapid sequence flow studies and blood pool images are used to assess hepatic blood flow and especially the vascularity of space-occupying lesions.

Ultrasound (US)

US uses non-ionizing sound waves and demonstrates echoes from the interfaces between tissues of different densities and elasticities. This technic is exceptionally useful in evaluating lesions of the abdomen. Real time systems permit sequential presentation of images as moving structures. US data are morphologic and independent of physiologic and pathologic considerations.

US is useful in evaluating cholestatic jaundice. The bile ducts stand out as echo-free tubular structures. The technic is > 95% accurate in differentiating surgical from medical jaundice. US can locate the site of biliary obstruction in 85% of cases and can determine the cause in 50% of cases of obstructive jaundice.

US defines cystic lesions of the liver, bile ducts, and pancreas as echo-free lesions with sharp borders and strong posterior echoes. Abscesses and hematomas can be defined and the technic is about 90% accurate in detecting liver tumors. US is more accurate than radionuclide scanning in detecting liver tumors, more specific in differentiating solid from cystic lesions, and has a lower false-positive rate. Because lesions can be localized accurately in 3 dimensions, aspiration or biopsy needles can be precisely guided.

US will not detect about 25% of common bile duct stones and is not particularly sensitive to changes resulting from diffuse hepatocellular disease. It may show parenchymal changes in advanced disease, can detect small amounts of ascites, and can define some vascular abnormalities associated with portal hypertension. By integrating the cross-sectional areas of serial planes of analysis, one can determine the volume of the liver and spleen with reasonable accuracy. US will probably become the initial diagnostic approach to lesions of the gallbladder and biliary tree. It is already the screening procedure of choice for pancreatic disease. The normal pancreas can be visualized in 70% of examinations and its overall accuracy in designating a normal pancreas from one with an abnormality approaches 90%. Although limited by fat, bone, and intestinal gas, and dependent upon the expertise of the operator and interpreter, US is an increasingly valuable technic. It is easy, noninvasive, versatile, and economical.

Computerized Tomography (CT)

Using x-rays to demonstrate the density of tissues has proved useful in the clinical evaluation of the liver, biliary tree, and pancreas. CT is noninvasive and it provides excellent definition of the anatomy. It is not limited by intestinal gas, bone, or fat, and it is much less dependent than US on operator and interpreter expertise. However, the

current accuracy of CT is not significantly greater than that of gray scale US, CT uses radiation and highly complex equipment, has its versatility restricted by its planes of scanning, is much more expensive than US, and is less widely available. CT may succeed where US fails because of intestinal gas or obesity, and it complements US in investigating abdominal lesions, especially those of the distal common bile duct and head of the pancreas. CT is of most use in the detection and follow-up of space-occupying lesions and especially those that are peripheral or in the left lobe of the liver. The simultaneous use of contrast medium helps to differentiate isodense structures and to define the vasculature and biliary tree.

Percutaneous Liver Biopsy

This provides valuable diagnostic and prognostic information at relatively small risk. Done at the bedside under local anesthesia, the procedure usually causes minimal patient discomfort. The Menghini aspiration technic is simple and safe to use, but requires a trained operator. US guidance can aid the biopsy of focal lesions. In expert hands the incidence of serious complications is about 0.2%. Electron microscopy of liver biopsies has greatly advanced the knowledge of hepatic pathophysiology, but is of little diagnostic value clinically.

Indications include (1) hepatosplenomegaly of unknown cause, (2) unexplained liver function abnormalities, (3) diagnosis and staging of alcoholic liver disease (findings are usually characteristic, and the extent of irreversible fibrosis vs. reversible inflammation can be determined), (4) atypical hepatitis (biopsy is not needed in ordinary acute viral hepatitis but should be done if the diagnosis is uncertain or the clinical course atypical), (5) evaluation of chronic hepatitis (biopsy is essential for diagnosis and follow-up; unsuspected alcoholic liver disease and other alternate disorders are detected often enough to justify biopsy in most patients with chronic hepatocellular disease), (6) differential diagnosis of cholestasis if evidence points to an intrahepatic cause, (7) suspected malignancy (biopsy under US guidance detects metastatic carcinoma in at least ⅔ of cases and may establish the diagnosis despite negative scanning technics; cytologic examination of the biopsy fluid yields positive findings in about 10% more cases. Results are less valuable in lymphoma and correlate poorly with the clinical impression of hepatic involvement), and (8) fever of unknown origin (obscure cases are often clarified, especially if the alkaline phosphatase or other liver chemistry tests are abnormal; biopsy is particularly valuable in detecting TB and other granulomatous infiltrations).

Limitations of the procedure include (1) need for a skilled interpreter (many pathologists have little experience with needle specimens), (2) sampling error (collecting tissue from a nonrepresentative area of the liver seldom occurs in hepatitis and other diffuse conditions but may be a problem in cirrhosis and malignancy), (3) inability to differentiate hepatitis etiologically (eg, viral vs. drug-induced), and (4) occasional errors or uncertainty in cases of cholestasis.

Relative contraindications include a clinical bleeding tendency or a coagulation disorder (prothrombin time > 3 sec over control values despite administration of vitamin K, bleeding time > 10 min), severe thrombocytopenia, severe anemia, peritonitis, marked ascites, high-grade biliary obstruction, and subphrenic or right pleural infection.

Procedure: The patient should not eat past midnight; a CBC is obtained, and blood is typed and held the night before. The biopsy site is identified and marked, then cleansed with a disinfectant solution and alcohol. Under sterile technic, the site is anesthetized from skin to liver capsule with lidocaine 1% solution. After sounding with an appropriate probe, the Klatskin or Menghini (16 gauge) needle, which is attached to a 10 mL syringe filled with 0.9% sodium chloride solution, is inserted along the back of the probe to the liver capsule. The patient is instructed to maintain expiration; with negative pressure placed on the syringe, the needle is inserted 2 to 3 cm further and

then rapidly removed. The specimen is sent for pathology and cytology, and often for culture. The procedure may be repeated. When completed, the patient is instructed to remain on the right side for 2 h and at bed rest with frequent observation of vital signs for 24 h. A Hct is obtained 6 h after the procedure. There is an increasing tendency to perform liver biopsies on outpatients.

Complications occurring most frequently are intra-abdominal bleeding and bile peritonitis. These hazards are minimized by appropriate selection of cases, preliminary coagulation studies, blood typing, and bed rest with observation for several hours post biopsy. Rare complications include hemobilia, intrahepatic hematoma, transient bacteremia, and hepatic arteriovenous fistula.

Peritoneoscopy (Laparoscopy)

This procedure is described in Ch. 50. It allows direct inspection of the peritoneum, liver, and other organs, and biopsy can be done under direct vision. However, peritoneoscopy is more complex than percutaneous biopsy, and requires more skill. Adhesions from previous surgery may preclude adequate visualization.

Laparotomy

Surgical wedge or needle biopsy provides better specimens and less sampling error than percutaneous needle specimens. Unexplained hepatosplenomegaly, fever of unknown origin, and lymphoma may require laparotomy for clarification. Laparotomy establishes the cause of extrahepatic cholestatic jaundice when simpler tests fail. Diagnostic laparotomy should be avoided in patients with severe hepatocellular dysfunction because of the risk of precipitating acute liver failure.

---

69. FATTY LIVER

The abnormal accumulation of fat in hepatocytes, said to occur in 25% of all persons and to be the commonest response of the liver to injury.

Etiology

Diffuse fatty change of the liver, often zonal in distribution, is associated with many clinical situations. In the neonatal period it can occur in a familial or idiopathic manner, in Wolman's disease (see under LIPIDOSES in Ch. 85), in cystic fibrosis of the pancreas, and in association with inborn errors of glycogen, galactose, tyrosine, and homocystine metabolism. Later it can be found in Reye's syndrome, phytanic acid storage disease (Refsum's disease), Wilson's disease, hemochromatosis, abetalipoproteinemia, obesity, and diabetes. It can be a complication of a diet deficient in proteins or involving amino acid imbalances and it can be caused by a wide variety of chemicals and drugs, including alcohol, corticosteroids, tetracyclines, valproic acid, carbon tetrachloride, and yellow phosphorus. Diffuse fatty metamorphosis can complicate both small-bowel bypass surgery and pregnancy.

Focal fatty change is much less common and less well recognized. Occurring in nodular form and usually subcapsular in location, focal fatty change can be important in the differential diagnosis of space-occupying lesions of the liver.

Pathology

If lipid deposition is marked, the liver tends to be grossly enlarged, smooth, and pale. Microscopically, the general architecture can be normal. In the form of triglycerides, the fat tends to appear as large droplets that coalesce and displace the cell nucleus to the periphery. In Wolman's disease, triglyceride collects with cholesterol esters in lysosomes that do not fuse. Lipid accumulation, presumably as triglyceride, also occurs in small droplet form in tetracycline and aflatoxin hepatotoxicity. Fat that

gathers as free fatty acids, cholesterol, cholesterol esters, and phospholipids tends to collect in a microvesicular form in secondary lysosomes that do not fuse. The hepatocytes feature a foamy cytoplasm and a central nucleus.

Free fatty acids collect in acute fatty liver of pregnancy and probably in Reye's syndrome. Cholesterol esters gather in familial high density lipoprotein deficiency (Tangier disease), cholesterol ester storage disease, and Wolman's disease. Phospholipids accumulate under the influence of certain drugs and in several rare inborn errors of phospholipid metabolism.

With hepatotoxins primarily affecting protein synthesis or with protein malnutrition, the lipid tends to collect in Zone I. With other hepatotoxins and with diets deficient in factors other than amino acids, the fat tends to collect in Zone 3. In acute fatty liver of pregnancy, the fine droplet fatty change is diffuse, but usually spares those hepatocytes in Zone I immediately around the portal tracts. In contrast, the fat accumulation in Reye's syndrome is predominantly in Zone I.

Unusual lysosomes, called lipolysosomes, featuring a limiting membrane, containing fat, and exhibiting acid phosphatase activity are usually associated with the fatty liver and may play a major role in metabolizing storage lipid.

Pathogenesis

The liver occupies a central position in lipid metabolism. Nonesterified fatty acids **(NEFA),** absorbed from the diet or released into the blood from chylomicrons or adipose sites, comprise a small but rapidly used pool that accommodates almost all energy requirements of a fasting animal. Some NEFA are taken up by the liver to join the hepatic pool of free fatty acids, a portion of which is synthesized by the liver. Some hepatocytic NEFA are oxidized for energy, but most are rapidly incorporated into complex lipids (eg, triglycerides, phospholipids, glycolipids, cholesterol, and cholesterol esters). Some of these complex lipids enter a slowly used pool that comprises the structural lipids of the cell and their storage site. The remaining complex lipids enter an active pool that is used to synthesize lipoproteins. Most lipoproteins are secreted into the plasma where they provide the main source of lipid for the peripheral tissues in a fasting animal.

Except for specific inborn errors of lipid metabolism and for poorly understood conditions (eg, acute fatty liver of pregnancy and Reye's syndrome) the lipid that collects in the liver is mainly triglyceride. This is so because hepatic triglycerides have the highest turnover rate of all hepatic fatty acid esters and because no feedback inhibition regulates fatty acid uptake by the liver.

Triglyceride accumulation in the liver results from either increased synthesis or decreased elimination of triglyceride from the hepatocytes. Increased triglyceride synthesis may be associated with an increase in the activity of triglyceride synthetase or an increased concentration of NEFA as a result of increased uptake, increased synthesis from acetyl CoA, or decreased oxidation by the hepatocytes. Decreased elimination of NEFA may involve decreased hydrolysis by lysosomal lipases, decreased lipoprotein secretion, or decreased synthesis of lipids other than triglycerides.

The several possible mechanisms involved in the pathogenesis of the fatty liver may operate alone or together. Increased hepatic uptake of NEFA seems to contribute to the fatty liver induced by carbon tetrachloride, phosphorus, isopropanol, and various inhibitors of protein synthesis. Increased synthesis of NEFA from acetyl CoA seems to contribute to the fatty liver caused by essential fatty acid deficiency, acute ethanol poisoning, and phenobarbital treatment. Decreased oxidation of fatty acids may contribute to the fatty liver induced by carbon tetrachloride, phosphorus, hypoxia, and certain vitamin deficiencies (niacin, riboflavin, and pantothenic acid). A block in the hepatocytic production and secretion of lipoproteins is often the main cause of triglyceride accumulation in the liver. A block in apolipoprotein synthesis appears to be the most important pathogenetic factor in several types of toxic fatty liver and in the fatty

liver produced by diets deficient in protein (kwashiorkor) or imbalances in amino acids. Toxic inhibition of protein synthesis can lead to a fatty liver through inhibition of mRNA synthesis (aflatoxin, amanita phalloides toxins, D-galactosamine and dimethylnitrosamine), through inhibition of amino acyl transfer RNA synthesis, or binding to ribosomes (puromycin, tetracycline), through inhibition of mRNA translation (cycloheximide, emetine) or through inhibition of initiation of protein synthesis (carbon tetrachloride, phosphorus). In spite of much research, the pathogenesis of most cases is very complex and remains poorly understood.

Symptoms, Signs, and Diagnosis

Fatty liver most often is discovered on physical examination as nontender hepatomegaly and is usually asymptomatic. However, it can present with right upper quadrant pain and jaundice or can be the only physical abnormality found after sudden, unexpected, and presumably metabolic death.

There is a poor association between fatty liver and abnormalities of the commonly used biochemical tests for liver disease. The diagnosis of fatty liver can be made only on histologic grounds.

Fatty liver is potentially reversible and usually is not in itself harmful. However, since it may indicate the action of a hepatotoxin or the presence of an unrecognized disease or metabolic abnormality, the diagnosis calls for further evaluation of the patient.

Treatment

No specific therapy is known except to eliminate the cause or treat the underlying disorder. Anabolic steroids can augment the release of hepatic triglycerides from the fatty liver, but their use is rarely indicated.

70. FIBROSIS AND CIRRHOSIS

FIBROSIS

Excess fibrous tissue in the liver resulting passively from collapse and condensation of preexisting fibers or actively through the synthesis of new fibers by fibroblasts.

Etiology

Fibrosis is a common response to hepatocyte injury induced by a wide variety of agents, including numerous chemicals and drugs (eg, alcohol, methotrexate, arsenicals, isoniazid, oxyphenisatin, methyldopa, polyvinylchloride, and thorium dioxide). Associated with fibrosis is deposition in the liver of endogenous and exogenous substances, as in myeloid metaplasia, Gaucher's disease, certain glycogen storage diseases, Wilson's disease, and the iron overload syndromes. Various infections of the liver (viral, bacterial, spirochetal, and parasitic) can cause hepatic fibrosis, as can chronic obstruction to bile flow and various disturbances of the hepatic circulation.

Pathogenesis

Active fibroplasia is usually associated with inflammation. It may be located around hepatocytes, proliferated bile ductules, or macrophages, and in the portal tracts. Many cell types appear to be capable of collagen synthesis, but in the liver, interest has focused mainly on the myofibroblasts and on the lipocytes or Ito cells, which lie in the perisinusoidal recesses and which may represent inactive fibroblasts. Collagen can be removed as well as synthesized; regression of liver fibrosis is possible after removal of the offending agent.

The influence of fibrosis on hepatic structure and function depends upon its localization: Pericellular fibrosis leads to hepatocellular atrophy; fibrosis around the terminal hepatic venules leads to venous outflow block; periportal fibrosis leads to portal hypertension on the basis of portal venous inflow block; and periductular fibrosis leads to cholestasis. Extensive fibrosis can result in the formation of septa that can interfere significantly with hepatic circulation. Congenital hepatic fibrosis, a variant of congenital cystic liver disease, features excess portal and periportal connective tissue that is mature and interferes with portal venous blood flow. The condition presents as portal hypertension with excellent hepatocellular function and no cirrhosis.

Diagnosis

The fibrosis that accompanies many hepatic disorders is rarely the main characteristic of the disease. The diagnosis depends upon histologic examination of the liver. Aniline blue or trichrome stains are particularly useful. Silver impregnation of the reticulin can be used to distinguish passive from active fibrosis.

Treatment

Management includes treating the underlying cause and complications of fibrosis (eg, portal hypertension) and is discussed below in relation to these subjects. New therapeutic approaches focus on inhibiting collagen synthesis and maturation by proline analogs, colchicine, penicillamine, and lathyrogenic agents.

CIRRHOSIS

The disorganization of liver architecture by widespread fibrosis resulting in nodule formation. The nodules are portions of parenchyma demarcated by connective tissue; in cirrhosis all parts of the liver must be involved, but large nodules can contain intact architecture. Fibrosis is not synonymous with cirrhosis; nodule formation with fibrosis is not cirrhosis.

Partial nodular transformation of the liver and the solitary hyperplastic nodule or **focal cirrhosis** are not examples of a true cirrhosis. These lesions consist of isolated areas of fibrosis and nodularity in an otherwise normal organ.

Etiology and Incidence

Cirrhosis is exceeded only by cardiovascular disease and cancer as a cause of death in the 45 to 65 age group in the USA; by far the majority of cases are secondary to chronic alcohol abuse. In many parts of Asia and Africa, cirrhosis due to chronic viral hepatitis B is a major cause of death.

Cirrhosis can be induced by **chemicals** (eg, alcohol, methotrexate, and oxyphenisatin) or caused by **infections** (eg, Type B or Non A-Non B viral hepatitis and congenital syphilis). Cirrhosis can develop after **intestinal bypass operations; intra-or extrahepatic biliary obstruction;** or prolonged **passive congestion** of the liver associated with tricuspid insufficiency, constrictive pericarditis, or hepatic vein thrombosis. In many instances, no etiology can be established, and the term **cryptogenic cirrhosis** is applied. Primary biliary cirrhosis is discussed separately below.

Pathology

Each cirrhotic liver has a different configuration, the end result of the interplay of many factors, and the lesion of cirrhosis is not static. The initiating lesion in portal cirrhosis is usually in Zone 3, and all cirrhosis follows cellular necrosis and inflammatory change. The activity, stage of development, and complications of the disease process are most important, and a current tendency avoids classifying cirrhosis and accepts a morphologic description of the pathology. However, to accommodate those committed to classifications, the following one is reasonably practical:

Micronodular cirrhosis is characterized by thin, regular bands of connective tissue and by small nodules that vary little in size and, characteristically, terminal hepatic

veins or portal spaces cannot be identified. **Macronodular cirrhosis** is characterized by connective tissue bands of varying thickness and by nodules that vary in size and contain portal spaces and terminal hepatic veins. The concentration of portal spaces in the fibrous scars demonstrates previous collapse. **Mixed cirrhosis** combines the features of micro- and macronodular cirrhosis.

Pathogenesis

Cirrhosis is the end product of the reaction of the liver to certain types of injury. The morphology of the cirrhosis is related not so much to the injurious agents as to the form of the injury and the liver's reaction to it. The liver may be injured severely and all at once (as in submassive necrosis with hepatitis), moderately over months or a few years (as in biliary tract obstruction and chronic active hepatitis), or modestly, but continuously and chronically (as in alcohol abuse). Fibrosis and parenchymal regeneration result as the natural, but modifiable, reactions to this injury.

Restoration of intrahepatic circulatory pathways is an essential part of the repair process. New vessel formation follows intact pathways to connect hepatic artery and portal vein with the hepatic venules. The interconnecting vessels, contained in fibrous sheaths around the surviving parenchymal nodules, receive the sinusoidal flow of these nodules. However, these new passageways provide a high-pressure, relatively low-volume sinusoidal drainage system that is much less efficient than normal. The result is an increase in portal vein pressure **(portal hypertension).** Disordered blood flow to the nodules and compression of hepatic venules by regenerating nodules also contribute to portal hypertension.

Symptoms and Signs

Many patients with cirrhosis are asymptomatic and well-nourished, making the diagnosis difficult and somewhat surprising. Generalized weakness, anorexia, malaise, weight loss, and loss of libido are common. In the malnourished patient, other problems may exist (eg, paresthesias and glossitis). Patients may also present with symptoms of portal systemic encephalopathy (see in Ch. 67), with pruritus caused by cholestasis, or with other nonspecific symptoms associated with hitherto undetected chronic liver disease.

A palpable, firm, smooth liver with a blunt edge is characteristic. Cirrhotic nodules are rarely palpable. Evidence of collateral venous circulation, ascites, and splenomegaly may occur with portal hypertension. Clubbing of the fingers, Dupuytren's palmar contracture, and hepatic fetor are common. Other clinical signs may suggest chronic liver disease, but none is specific: muscular wasting, palmar erythema, vascular spiders, gynecomastia, parotid gland enlargement, hair loss, testicular atrophy, and peripheral neuropathy.

Laboratory Diagnosis

None, any, or all of the routine biochemical tests used to assess liver integrity and function may be abnormal. A prolonged prothrombin time, decreased serum albumin, and increased serum γ-globulin suggest cirrhosis. Anemia and various morphologic abnormalities of the erythrocytes are common and usually multifactorial in origin.

Scintiscanning characteristically reveals decreased uptake of isotope with an irregular pattern of labeling in the liver and uptake of label by the spleen and bone marrow. Ultrasound examination is not particularly helpful in uncomplicated cirrhosis. The diagnosis of cirrhosis is a pathologic one and needle biopsies are usually diagnostic (see PERCUTANEOUS LIVER BIOPSY in Ch. 68).

Complications

Most of the severe complications of cirrhosis are secondary to portal hypertension, since it leads to the development of collateral flow from the portal system to the systemic circulation. Collateral vessels form and those lining the stomach and esopha-

gus (gastric esophageal varices), are particularly hazardous. GI hemorrhage (see also Ch. 53) from esophageal, gastric, or other varices is caused in part by high pressure in the portal circulation. Rarely, severe hemorrhoidal disease occurs. In addition, jaundice, ascites, renal failure (see Ch. 67), and portal-systemic encephalopathy can occur because of the portal hypertension and/or the portal-systemic shunting (see also PORTAL HYPERTENSION in Ch. 76).

In addition to complications secondary to portal hypertension, hepatocellular carcinoma frequently complicates cirrhosis, especially that associated with chronic viral hepatitis B and hemochromatosis.

Prognosis and Treatment

If the patient has experienced major complications such as hematemesis, hepatic coma, ascites, and jaundice (see above), the prognosis is grave; eg, a 1-yr survival of < 50% can be expected in such a patient with alcohol-induced liver disease who continues to drink alcohol excessively. However, even with severe signs, a patient may respond to treatment, especially if the offending agent can be removed.

Treatment of cirrhosis is based upon the etiology involved and the management of specific complications. Abstinence from alcohol, and a nutritious diet (see Ch. 79) with or without vitamin supplements are indicated for the patient with alcohol-induced cirrhosis. Withdrawal of any incriminated drug or chemical is indicated. The use of corticosteroids, azathioprine, penicillamine, and antiviral agents remains controversial, but may aid the treatment of chronic active hepatitis, even when cirrhosis has developed. The treatment of cirrhosis is discussed further under specific etiologic diseases (see Etiology, above), and its complications (eg, ascites, portal-systemic encephalopathy) are discussed in Ch. 67.

BILIARY CIRRHOSIS

PRIMARY BILIARY CIRRHOSIS (PBC)

A disease of unknown etiology that initially affects the intrahepatic bile ducts and that is characterized by chronic cholestasis. It is commonly associated with autoimmune disorders, but the precise significance of this association is not yet known.

Pathogenesis

The early course of PBC features a chronic nonsuppurative destructive inflammation of the intrahepatic bile radicles. Only later does a true cirrhosis develop.

Although 4 typical stages in its evolution have been defined, the disease is focal with considerable overlap between the stages in any one case. **Inflammation of the medium-sized bile ducts** (the initial lesion) is associated with chronic inflammation of the portal tracts. Granulomas may be found. In the smaller portal tracts, bile ducts may be conspicuously absent. Parenchymal changes are minimal and histologic cholestasis unusual. As destruction of the medium-sized bile ducts progresses, the portal tracts become distorted, inflammation spreads into the parenchyma, bile ducts proliferate intensely, and **periportal fibrosis develops.** By this time most portal tracts are affected. **Progressive scarring** continues with less bile duct proliferation and less inflammation. Fibrous bands link the portal tracts, and Zone I cholestasis and Mallory hyaline can become evident. Although often slow, progression is usual, with the end product **a firm, regular, intensely bile-stained cirrhosis.** It can be difficult to distinguish PBC from other cirrhotic processes microscopically in the absence of granulomas and the pathognomonic bile duct lesions.

Symptoms and Signs

Although it can affect both sexes and a broad age spectrum, PBC most commonly affects females aged 35 to 60. It usually presents insidiously. At least 30% of patients

are asymptomatic at presentation, drawn to medical attention by abnormalities of serum chemistry detected during routine screening. Pruritus and/or nonspecific fatigue are the initial symptoms in about 50% of patients and can precede clinical signs by months or even years. About 50% of patients will present with an enlarged, firm, nontender liver and 25% with splenomegaly. About 15% will present with skin xanthomas or xanthelasma and 10% will be hyperpigmented; < 10% will present with jaundice as the only clinical evidence of the condition. Other possible developments include clubbing, metabolic bone disease, peripheral neuropathy, renal tubular acidosis, and steatorrhea. As the disease progresses, all the features and complications of cirrhosis can develop. PBC is associated with many other conditions, especially the collagen diseases (eg, RA, scleroderma, sicca complex, and autoimmune thyroiditis).

Laboratory Findings

Early laboratory findings feature cholestasis with elevation of the alkaline phosphatase disproportionately greater than any increase in the serum bilirubin and aminotransferases. In fact, the serum bilirubin is often normal early in the course of the disease. The concentration of serum bile acids and the activity of the serum γ-glutamyl transpeptidase are elevated. The serum cholesterol concentration may be increased and the serum total lipids usually are increased. The serum lipoproteins are increased mainly because lipoprotein-X is present. Serum albumin is normal early in the course of the disease, but the globulins usually increase, the serum IgM often to very high values. Antibodies against a component of the inner membrane of mitochondria are present in 85 to 95% of patients and are of considerable diagnostic value. Because such antibodies can also be found in some patients with HBsAg-negative chronic active hepatitis, sometimes it can be very difficult to distinguish between them.

Diagnosis

The differential diagnosis includes extrahepatic biliary obstruction, chronic active hepatitis, primary sclerosing cholangitis, drug-induced cholestasis, and the cholangitic lesions associated with inflammatory bowel disease. Potentially curable extrahepatic biliary obstruction must be ruled out early. Liver biopsy can be diagnostic but is often nonspecific. IV cholangiography is often negative because of cholestasis. Retrograde cannulation of the biliary tract **(ERCP)** is currently the most satisfactory method for ruling out extrahepatic bile duct obstruction. Ultrasound examination of the liver and percutaneous transhepatic cholangiography provide alternate approaches. Diagnostic laparotomy is rarely necessary.

Prognosis

The course of PBC involves a broad spectrum. In some patients the disease compromises neither the quality nor the duration of life. Fewer than 50% of patients who present without symptoms will demonstrate clinical evidence of liver disease over the ensuing 15 yr. The slow progress of the disease is compatible with prolonged survival. A rising serum bilirubin, associated autoimmune disorders, and advanced histologic changes indicate a poor prognosis. The natural history of PBC is still being written, at least in part because of the trend to earlier diagnosis.

Treatment

No specific treatment is known. Pruritus may be controlled with cholestyramine 6 to 12 gm/day orally in divided doses. Bile salt insufficiency associated with steatorrhea may require supplements with Ca and with vitamins A, D, and K to prevent deficiencies. The complications of PBC are treated as in other types of cirrhosis.

Corticosteroids have been used but not subjected to controlled clinical trials. Most authorities consider such treatment contraindicated because of the metabolic bone disease associated with PBC. Azathioprine has been used in clinical trials, but the results to date have not been encouraging. Penicillamine therapy has been shown to

improve survival in randomized controlled clinical trials, but beneficial effects are small and adverse effects have been common and sometimes serious. PBC is one of the best indications for liver transplantation.

PRIMARY SCLEROSING CHOLANGITIS (PSC)

A rare disease of unknown etiology characterized by progressive cholestasis due to fibrosing inflammation of the intrahepatic and/or extrahepatic bile ducts.

The diagnosis of PSC is reserved for patients with disorders of cholestasis that are not associated with biliary calculi, previous bile duct surgery, bile duct carcinoma, or other bile duct disease. It primarily affects young males. PSC tends to be associated with inflammatory bowel disease, retroperitoneal fibrosis, autoimmune thyroiditis, and other conditions. The pathogenetic significance of this association, if any, is unknown. PSC presents with fatigue, jaundice, and a cholestatic biochemical profile similar to that found in PBC (see above). It tends to progress steadily to cirrhosis and death from liver failure.

PSC features abnormal copper metabolism, tests of which may be of prognostic value. Hepatic copper accumulates and urinary copper excretion increases as PSC advances.

Cholangiography, direct or endoscopic, can show a characteristic picture with diffuse irregular strictures of the bile ducts. However, the diagnosis must be established by liver biopsy, which will demonstrate a fibrosing, nonsuppurative destructive cholangitis and loss of bile ducts leading to secondary biliary cirrhosis.

There is no specific treatment for PSC; liver transplantation should be considered.

---

71. HEPATITIS

An inflammatory process in the liver characterized by diffuse or patchy hepatocellular necrosis affecting all acini.

The major causes of hepatitis are viruses Types A, B, and non-A, non-B; alcohol; and drugs. Rarer etiologies include other viruses (eg, infectious mononucleosis, yellow fever, and cytomegalovirus **[CMV]**) and leptospirosis.

Parasitic infections (eg, schistosomiasis, malaria, and amebiasis) affect the liver, but do not cause a true hepatitis. Pyogenic infections and abscesses are also generally considered to be separate problems. Involvement of the liver with TB and other granulomatous infiltrations is sometimes called **"granulomatous hepatitis"** but produces different clinical, biochemical, and histologic features than diffuse hepatitis (see Ch. 75).

A variety of systemic infections and other illnesses may produce small focal areas of hepatic necrosis and inflammation. This nonspecific **reactive hepatitis** causes minor liver function abnormalities, but is usually asymptomatic.

Noninfectious hepatitis and some hepatic infections are described under their specific topic headings, and in part are summarized in TABLE 71–1, below. Hepatitis due to drugs and alcohol is discussed in Chs. 72 and 73, respectively.

ACUTE VIRAL HEPATITIS

(See also NEONATAL HEPATITIS B VIRUS INFECTION in Ch. 186)

Diffuse hepatocellular inflammatory disease caused by at least 3 different viral agents.

This is a common, important worldwide disease. Older terms that should be abandoned include infectious hepatitis (IH) and short-incubation hepatitis for Type A

TABLE 71–1. SELECTED INFLAMMATORY CONDITIONS OF THE LIVER

Disease or Organism	Comments
Viruses	
Epstein-Barr	Infectious mononucleosis. Clinical hepatitis with jaundice, 5–10%; subclinical liver involvement in remainder. Important cause of acute hepatitis in young adults.
Yellow fever	Jaundice with systemic toxicity, bleeding. Liver necrosis with little inflammatory reaction.
Cytomegalovirus	*Neonatal:* hepatomegaly, jaundice, congenital defects. *Adult:* mononucleosis-like illness with hepatitis; may occur posttransfusion.
Other	Hepatitis occasionally, from herpes simplex, ECHO, coxsackie, rubeola, rubella, varicella.
Bacteria	
Tuberculosis	Hepatic involvement common. Granulomatous infiltration. Usually subclinical; jaundice rare. Disproportionate ↑ alkaline phosphatase. Liver biopsy valuable.
Actinomycosis	Granulomatous reaction with progressive necrotizing abscesses.
Pyogenic abscess	Serious infection acquired via portal pyemia, cholangitis, hematogenous or direct spread. Various organisms, especially gram-negative & anaerobic. Patient ill, toxic, yet only mild liver dysfunction. Differentiate from amebic abscess, drain surgically or aspirate under ultrasonic guidance.
Other	Minor focal hepatitis common in numerous systemic infections. Usually subclinical.
Fungi	
Histoplasmosis	Granulomas in liver & spleen, usually subclinical; heal with calcification.
Other	Granulomatous infiltration sometimes in cryptococcosis, coccidioidomycosis, blastomycosis, etc.
Protozoa	
Amebiasis	Important disease, often without obvious dysentery. Usually large single abscess with liquefaction. Patient ill, tender hepatomegaly, surpisingly mild liver dysfunction. Differentiate from pyogenic abscess.
Malaria	Major cause of hepatosplenomegaly in endemic areas. Jaundice absent or mild unless active hemolysis.
Toxoplasmosis	Transplacental infection. Neonatal jaundice, CNS & other systemic manifestations.
Kala-azar	Infiltration of reticuloendothelial system by parasite. Hepatosplenomegaly.
Helminths	
Schistosomiasis	Important disease. Periportal granulomatous reaction to ova with progressive hepatosplenomegaly, "pipestem" fibrosis, portal hypertension, varices. Hepatocellular function preserved; not true cirrhosis.
Clonorchiasis	Biliary tract infestation; cholangitis, stones, cholangiocarcinoma.
Fascioliasis	*Acute:* tender hepatomegaly, fever, eosinophilia. *Chronic:* biliary fibrosis, cholangitis.
Echinococcosis	One or more hydatid cysts, usually calcified rim. May be large but often asymptomatic; liver function preserved. Can rupture into peritoneum or biliary tract.
Ascariasis	Biliary obstruction by adult worms, parenchymal granulomas from larvae.
Toxocariasis	Visceral larva migrans syndrome. Hepatomegaly with granulomas, eosinophilia.

(*Continued*)

TABLE 71–1. SELECTED INFLAMMATORY CONDITIONS OF THE LIVER *(Cont'd)*

Disease or Organism	*Comments*
Spirochetes	
Leptospirosis	Acute fever, prostration, jaundice, bleeding, renal injury. Liver necrosis often mild despite severe jaundice.
Syphilis	*Congenital:* neonatal hepatosplenomegaly, fibrosis. *Acquired:* variable hepatitis in secondary stage, gummas with irregular scarring in tertiary stage.
Relapsing fever	Borrelia infestation. Systemic symptoms, hepatomegaly, sometimes jaundice.
Unknown	
Sarcoidosis	Granulomatous infiltration common. Usually subclinical; jaundice rare. Occasionally progressive inflammation with scarring, portal hypertension. Liver biopsy valuable.
Idiopathic granulomatous hepatitis	Active chronic granulomatous inflammation not due to known causes (sarcoid variant?). Systemic symptoms may dominate with fever, malaise. Corticosteroids suppress symptoms.
Ulcerative colitis Crohn's disease	Spectrum of hepatic disease, especially in ulcerative colitis. Includes periportal inflammation ("pericholangitis"), sclerosing cholangitis, cholangiocarcinoma, ↑ incidence of chronic active hepatitis. Poor correlation with activity or treatment of bowel disorder.

disease; and serum hepatitis (SH), posttransfusion hepatitis, and long-incubation hepatitis for virus B infection.

Etiology and Viral Characteristics

At least 3 distinct viruses are responsible—viruses A, B, and non-A, non-B; the latter is probably more than one agent. Liver infections due to other specific viruses (eg, CMV and yellow fever virus) are considered separate disorders and are not included in general usage of the term *acute viral hepatitis.*

Hepatitis B virus (HBV) is the most thoroughly characterized. The infective ("Dane") particle consists of an inner core plus an outer surface coat. The former contains DNA and DNA polymerase, and replicates within the nuclei of infected hepatocytes. Surface coat is added in the cytoplasm, and for unknown reasons is produced in great excess; it can be detected in serum by immunologic means as hepatitis B surface antigen (see below).

HBV is associated with a wide spectrum of liver disease, from a subclinical carrier state to acute hepatitis, chronic hepatitis, cirrhosis, and hepatocellular carcinoma. It also has a poorly understood association with several primarily nonhepatic disorders including polyarteritis nodosa and other collagen vascular diseases, membranous glomerulonephritis, essential mixed cryoglobulinemia, and papular acrodermatitis of childhood. The pathogenetic role of the virus in these disorders is not clear, but in some patients tissue deposition of immune complexes contains viral antigen.

At least 4 distinct antigen-antibody systems are intimately related to the HBV: (1) HBV surface antigen (**HBsAg,** Australia antigen) is associated with the viral surface coat; its presence in serum usually provides the first evidence of acute B infection and implies infectivity of the blood. (Several antigenetic subtypes of HBsAg are of epidemiologic interest, but little clinical significance.) It characteristically appears during the incubation period, usually 1 to 6 wk before clinical or biochemical illness develops, and disappears during convalescence. The corresponding antibody (anti-HBs) appears

weeks or months later, after clinical recovery, and usually persists for life; thus, its detection implies past HBV infection and relative future protection. In up to 10% of patients, HBsAg persists following acute infection and anti-HBs does not develop; these patients usually develop chronic hepatitis or become asymptomatic carriers of the virus.

(2) Core antigen **(HBcAg)** is associated with the viral inner core. It can be found in infected liver cells, but is not detectable in serum except by special technics that disrupt the Dane particle. Antibody to the core (anti-HBc) is thought to reflect active viral replication and generally appears at the onset of clinical illness, with gradually diminishing titer thereafter, usually for years. Its presence with anti-HBs has no special significance beyond indicating previous HBV infection. It is also regularly found in chronic HBsAg carriers, who do not mount an anti-HBs response. In this situation, anti-HBc is of the IgG class, whereas in acute infection, IgM anti-HBc predominates. Occasionally the latter may be the only marker of recent HBV infection, reflecting a "window" period between disappearance of HBsAg and appearance of anti-HBs.

(3) The e antigen **(HBeAg)** is closely associated with virus B, and may be a constituent of the viral core. Found only in HBsAg-positive serum, its presence is associated with greater infectivity of the blood and a greater likelihood of progression to chronic liver disease. In contrast, presence of the corresponding antibody (anti-HBe) points to lesser infectivity and usually portends a benign outcome.

(4) The **delta agent** (δ, hepatitis D virus, **HDAg)** is a unique, defective RNA virus that can replicate only as a co-infecting agent in the presence of HBV, but never alone; infected hepatocytes contain δ-particles covered by a coat of HBsAg. Prevalence of the agent varies widely geographically, with endemic pockets in several countries. Drug addicts are at relatively high risk, but the virus has not yet widely permeated the homosexual community. Clinically, delta infection is typically manifest either by unusually severe acute hepatitis (up to 50% of fulminant HBV infections may be delta-associated), an acute "exacerbation" in chronic HBV carriers, or a relatively aggressive course of chronic hepatitis B.

Hepatitis A virus (HAV), an enterovirus-like RNA virus, is a smaller particle than HBV. Viral antigen (HAAg) is found in serum, stool, and liver only during acute infection. IgM antibody appears early in the disease, but disappears within a few weeks, followed by the development of IgG antibody that persists, probably for life (anti-HA). Thus IgM antibody is a marker of acute infection, while IgG anti-HA indicates previous exposure to HAV and immunity to recurrent infection. Unlike HBV, there is no known chronic carrier state, and HAV appears to play no role in the production of chronic active hepatitis or cirrhosis.

Non-A, non-B virus(es): Little is known about the identity of these agents, though evidence points to at least 2 separate viruses. In general, the biologic and clinical behavior appears akin to that of HBV, although at least one agent can produce hepatitis epidemics.

Epidemiology

HAV spreads primarily by fecal-oral contact; blood and secretions are also possibly infectious. Fecal shedding of the virus occurs during the incubation period and usually ceases a few days after symptoms begin; thus infectivity often has already passed when the diagnosis is made. Water- and food-borne epidemics are common, especially in underdeveloped countries. Eating of contaminated raw shellfish can be responsible. Sporadic cases are usually due to person-to-person contact. Most infections are subclinical or unrecognized, and population surveys of anti-HA have revealed remarkably widespread exposure that varies with age, socioeconomic class, geography, and other factors. In some countries > 3/4 of the adults appear to have been exposed.

HBV is often transmitted parenterally, typically by transfusion of contaminated blood or blood products, and often through needles shared by drug abusers. An in-

creased risk to patients in renal dialysis and oncology units has also been identified, as well as to hospital personnel in contact with blood. Nonparenteral spread can also occur between both heterosexual and male homosexual partners and in closed institutions (eg, those for the mentally retarded and prisons), but infectivity is far lower than for HAV, and the means of acquisition is often unknown. The role of transmission by insects that bite is unclear. Many cases of acute hepatitis B occur sporadically without a known source. Surveys of anti-HBs have shown that unrecognized infection with HBV is common, though much less widespread than with HAV.

A worldwide HBV reservoir is provided by chronic carriers. Prevalence varies widely with geographic and other factors from < 0.5% of the population in North America and northern Europe to > 10% in some regions of the Far East. Vertical transmission from mother to infant is partly responsible, especially in regions of high prevalence (see HEPATIC DISORDERS in Ch. 178).

Relatively little is known about the epidemiology of non-A, non-B viruses. They can be transmitted parenterally, especially by blood and blood products, and are responsible for many cases of sporadic acute hepatitis. A chronic carrier state also exists, though its prevalence is unknown. Small outbreaks and occasional large-scale waterborne epidemics of non-A, non-B hepatitis are probably produced by a different agent or agents than those responsible for sporadic disease.

Non-A, non-B hepatitis accounts for 80 to 90% of cases of posttransfusion hepatitis. HBV is responsible for most of the rest. A few cases are due to CMV and Epstein-Barr virus. HAV is now deemed a rare cause.

HAV infection has an incubation period of about 2 to 6 wk; HBV about 6 to 25 wk; and virus(es) non-A, non-B from < 2 wk to about 25 wk (average 7 to 8 wk). All age groups are affected, though HAV is most common in children and young adults.

Pathology

All liver acini are affected by patchy necrosis and mononuclear inflammatory infiltrate. Even in early cases, histologic evidence of regeneration is also present. The underlying reticulin framework is usually preserved and complete histologic recovery occurs unless extensive necrosis bridges entire acini. In most instances, the histopathology is similar regardless of the specific virus; HBV can occasionally be diagnosed by the presence of "ground glass" hepatocytes (due to HBsAg-packed cytoplasm) and by special immunologic stains for the viral components. However, these findings are paradoxically rare in acute hepatitis B, but much more typical of chronic HBV infection. Non-A, non-B causation can sometimes be inferred by subtle morphologic clues.

Symptoms and Signs

Hepatitis varies from a minor flu-like illness to fulminant, fatal liver failure, depending on the patient's immune response and other poorly understood virus-host factors. The following applies to a typical case; variants are discussed below.

The **prodromal phase** begins suddenly with anorexia, malaise, nausea and vomiting, and fever. Distaste for cigarettes is a characteristic early manifestation of profound anorexia. Urticarial eruptions and arthralgias may occur, especially in HBV infection. After 3 to 10 days dark urine appears, followed by jaundice (the **icteric phase**). Systemic symptoms typically regress at this point, and the patient feels better despite worsening jaundice. Features of cholestasis may develop. Jaundice usually peaks within 1 to 2 wk, then fades during a 2- to 4-wk **recovery phase.**

Physical examination shows variable jaundice. The liver is usually enlarged and often tender, but the edge remains soft and smooth. Mild splenomegaly is present in 15 to 20% of patients. Signs of chronic liver disease are not seen in uncomplicated cases.

Laboratory Findings

Striking aminotransferase elevations are the hallmark of the disease. High values appear early in the prodromal phase, peak before jaundice is maximal, and fall slowly

during the recovery phase. The aspartate aminotransferase (**AST**, SGOT) and alanine aminotransferase (**ALT**, SGPT) are typically 500 to 2000 u., but correlation with clinical severity is poor. The ALT is typically more elevated than the AST, but this is only of limited value in differentiation from alcoholic or obstructive liver disease. Urinary bile appears before jaundice; its early detection provides a valuable clue to the diagnosis. The degree of hyperbilirubinemia is variable and fractionation is of little clinical value. Alkaline phosphatase is only modestly raised unless cholestasis is severe. Major prolongation of the prothrombin time is not common, and, if present, portends a severe illness. The WBC count is usually low-normal, and blood smear often shows a few atypical lymphocytes.

Diagnosis and Differential Diagnosis

In the prodromal phase, hepatitis mimics a variety of flu-like illnesses and is difficult to diagnose. (For the approach to jaundice, see Ch. 67). Drug or toxic hepatitis is distinguished primarily by history. Prodromal sore throat, diffuse adenopathy, and marked atypical lymphocytosis favor infectious mononucleosis. Alcoholic hepatitis is suggested by a history of drinking, more gradual onset of symptoms, and presence of spider nevi or other signs of chronic hepatocellular disease. In addition, aminotransferase values rarely exceed 300 u., even in severe cases, and unlike viral hepatitis, AST is typically higher than ALT. Extrahepatic obstruction and neoplasm are usually easily distinguished from hepatitis but occasionally are more difficult to rule out. Liver biopsy is not usually needed, but should be considered if the diagnosis is uncertain; if the clinical course is atypical or unduly prolonged; if spider nevi, palmar erythema, or other clues to chronic liver disease are present; or if complications develop (eg, encephalopathy or fluid retention).

For specific etiology, HBV is diagnosed by identifying HBsAg in serum, with or without concomitant anti-HBc. Failure to detect HBsAg does not entirely exclude HBV, as antigenemia may be transient; in such cases the isolated presence of anti-HBc of the IgM class may establish the diagnosis. HAV is diagnosed indirectly by detecting antibody of the IgM type; better routine tests should soon be available. Non-A, non-B causation is currently diagnosed by exclusion.

Prognosis

Hepatitis usually resolves spontaneously after a 4- to 8-wk illness. Atypical courses are discussed below. A favorable prognosis is less certain in HBV than in HAV infection, especially in the elderly and in posttransfusion hepatitis, when mortality may reach 10 to 15%. Non-A, non-B hepatitis is more likely to have a fluctuating clinical course, sometimes with "roller coaster" aminotransferase fluctuations for several months.

Progression to chronic hepatitis is rare with HAV and is invariably of the benign persistent type (see below); aggressive chronic disease or cirrhosis does not develop. Chronicity occurs in 5 to 10% of HBV infections: Mild persistent hepatitis, full-blown chronic active hepatitis with eventual cirrhosis, and a subclinical chronic carrier state all occur. The latter is especially prone to lead ultimately to hepatocellular carcinoma (see Ch. 77). Non-A, non-B hepatitis has the highest likelihood of chronicity, which occurs in up to 50% of infections acquired via transfusion and about 20% of sporadic cases, even though the initial illness usually seems relatively mild. Usually the resultant chronic hepatitis is benign and often subclinical, but cirrhosis sometimes develops.

Prophylaxis

Personal hygiene helps to prevent spread of HAV. Blood of patients with acute hepatitis must be handled with care, and in HAV disease, stool should also be considered infectious. However, isolation of patients has been overemphasized; it does little to prevent spread of HAV and is of no value in HBV or non-A, non-B disease. Posttransfusion infection is minimized by avoiding unnecessary transfusions, using volunteers rather than paid donors, and screening all donors for HBsAg. The latter is

now almost universally available and has significantly decreased, though not eliminated, iatrogenic hepatitis B. Some cases of posttransfusion non-A, non-B hepatitis can be prevented by screening donor blood for ALT elevations, but the cost-benefit is debated and the practice is not widespread.

The value of **passive prophylaxis** with γ-globulin preparations is debated; variable antibody titers underlie much of the uncertainty. Standard **immune globulin (IG,** formerly immune serum globulin or ISG) provides protection against clinically apparent HAV and should be given to household contacts of index cases and to travelers planning a prolonged visit to endemic areas; 0.02 mL/kg given IM is generally recommended, but some experts advise 0.06 mL/kg (3 to 5 mL for adults). IG is less clearly effective against non-A, non-B hepatitis, but should be given at the higher dosage after accidental "needle-stick" exposure to infected blood, and perhaps to regular sexual contacts of index cases; other household contacts need not be treated. **Hepatitis B immune globulin (HBIG)** contains much higher antibody titers against HBV. However, it is uncertain how much better it is clinically than IG, and high cost limits its use. HBIG should be given to persons with accidental "needle stick" exposure to HBsAg-positive blood (0.06 mL/kg IM within 24 h and again a month later), and perhaps to regular sexual contacts of index cases (0.06 mL/kg IM within 2 wk of last contact); vaccination should also be considered (see below). HBIG has also proven about 70% effective in preventing chronic HBV infection in infants born of HBsAg-positive mothers; current recommendations advise 0.5 mL IM within 12 h of birth, coupled with active prophylaxis by vaccination (see below).

Vaccination against HBV gives an almost universal anti-HBs response in normal recipients and dramatic reduction of about 90% in incidence of hepatitis B infection; dialysis patients and other immunocompromised recipients respond less well. Initial fears regarding vaccine safety appear unfounded and side effects are minimal.

Vaccination policies are currently influenced by limited supplies and high cost. **Post-exposure** vaccination is recommended for newborn infants of HBsAg-positive mothers (in conjunction with HBIG; see above). It should also be considered after "needle-stick" exposure to known HBsAg-positive blood (along with HBIG), and for spouses or regular sexual contacts of index cases. Vaccination is ineffective for eliminating established HBV infection. **Pre-exposure** vaccine prophylaxis is advised for selected individuals at increased risk of contacting hepatitis B; eg, patients and staff in hemodialysis units, medical and other health care personnel exposed to blood, dentists and dental hygienists, residents and staff of institutions for the mentally retarded, and male homosexuals.

Genetic engineering technics hold promise for yielding abundant supplies of lower-cost vaccine. This should enable widespread vaccination in geographic regions with a high prevalence of hepatitis B, thereby having a major worldwide impact on the disease and eventually diminishing hepatocellular carcinoma, which is associated with chronic HBV infection (see Ch. 77).

Vaccination against HAV virus is not yet available. Active prophylaxis against non-A, non-B hepatitis must await identification of the responsible agent or agents.

Treatment

In most cases no special treatment is required. Appetite usually returns after the first several days, and patients need not be confined to bed. Undue restrictions on diet or activity are without scientific basis. Vitamin supplements are not required. Corticosteroids are contraindicated in ordinary cases. Most patients may safely return to work after jaundice completely resolves, even if AST or ALT are not entirely normal.

VARIANTS OF ACUTE VIRAL HEPATITIS

Anicteric hepatitis, a minor flu-like illness without jaundice, may be the only clinical manifestation of acute hepatitis, especially in children. There is evidence that this far

exceeds "typical" hepatitis in frequency, but the diagnosis is usually overlooked unless the characteristic elevations in AST and ALT are sought.

Recrudescent hepatitis occurs in a minority of patients during the recovery phase. The prognosis remains good and chronic hepatitis rarely follows. Repeated recrudescences and aminotransferase fluctuations are relatively common in non-A, non-B hepatitis, however, often with progression to chronicity (see above).

Despite general regression of the inflammatory process, **cholestatic hepatitis** occasionally persists with jaundice, elevated alkaline phosphatase, and pruritus. Clinical differentiation from extrahepatic biliary obstruction may be difficult. Eventual resolution is the rule. Cholestyramine 8 to 16 gm/day orally can relieve itching.

Fulminant hepatitis, a rare syndrome, is usually seen in infection with HBV, non-A, non-B virus, or drug injury; HAV is rarely responsible. Rapid clinical deterioration with the onset of hepatic encephalopathy presages a serious illness; in some cases coma develops within hours. There is massive necrosis of liver parenchyma and a decrease in liver size ("acute yellow atrophy"). Bleeding is common, resulting from hepatocellular failure and disseminated intravascular coagulation. Increasing prothrombin time is a bad prognostic sign. Functional renal failure often develops and usually portends a fatal outcome.

Survival in adults is uncommon despite heroic measures; the prognosis for children is less grim. Meticulous nursing care and careful management of specific complications provide the best hope for recovery. Therapeutic measures such as massive doses of corticosteroids or exchange transfusions have not proved effective. Remarkably, survivors usually recover completely without permanent liver damage.

Bridging necrosis, an uncommon variant, is characterized histologically by zones of collapse that bridge adjacent portal and/or central areas. It is mainly a pathologic entity, and clinically it may be indistinguishable from ordinary viral hepatitis; but it is suggested by an insidious rather than sudden onset and by the development of fluid retention or mild encephalopathy. The prognostic implication of bridging is debated; patients with chronic active hepatitis may largely arise from this subgroup, though most patients with bridging do recover fully. Corticosteroid therapy is controversial.

CHRONIC HEPATITIS

A spectrum of disorders merging between acute hepatitis and cirrhosis. Hepatitis lasting for 6 mo is generally defined as "chronic," though this is arbitrary. Complex terminology has created confusion; however, most chronic hepatitis can be classified as chronic persistent or chronic active forms.

Chronic Persistent Hepatitis (Persistent Hepatitis)

This *benign* disorder usually follows typical acute hepatitis, but may be detected de novo. Persistently high aminotransferase values with vague or no symptoms are characteristic. Other liver function tests are usually unremarkable and jaundice is uncommon. Clinical signs of chronic liver disease are absent.

The **diagnosis** depends on needle biopsy, which shows portal mononuclear infiltrate without significant fibrosis or acinar disarray. Overlap with chronic active hepatitis occurs, but is uncommon. Occasionally, diffuse lobular inflammation is superimposed, with features of persisting acute hepatitis **(chronic lobular hepatitis).** Eventual recovery is usual, though the disorder may persist for years. Treatment is not necessary, and neither diet nor activity should be restricted.

Chronic Active (Aggressive) Hepatitis

This *serious* disorder often results in liver failure and/or cirrhosis. It is best regarded as a group of closely related conditions rather than a single disease. The **etiology** varies

HBV causes a minority of cases, but HAV is not thought responsible; non-A, non-B virus(es) cause some cases, but their overall role in "idiopathic" disease is unknown. Drugs (eg, methyldopa, isoniazid, nitrofurantoin, and possibly acetaminophen) are occasionally responsible. Wilson's disease may present as chronic active hepatitis and should be considered in children and young adults with the disorder. Most cases, however, are of unknown etiology; many of these idiopathic cases have prominent "immune" features. The **pathogenesis** is obscure, but considerable evidence favors an abnormal immune response to the causative agents. Some cases appear to have antibodies directed against a liver membrane antigen, but firm proof of a true autoimmune mechanism is still lacking.

Clinical features vary. About 1/3 of the cases follow acute hepatitis, but most develop insidiously de novo. Nonspecific malaise, anorexia, and fatigue often dominate the clinical picture. Jaundice is variable and is not always present. Signs of chronic liver disease (eg, splenomegaly, spider nevi, and fluid retention) usually eventually develop. Multisystemic or "immune" manifestations often occur, especially in young women whose disease is of idiopathic origin. These can affect virtually any body system and include acne, amenorrhea, arthralgia, ulcerative colitis, pulmonary fibrosis, nephritis, and hemolytic anemia.

Laboratory abnormalities are those of an active hepatitis (predominant AST and ALT elevations, with variable bilirubin and alkaline phosphatase levels), plus the frequent presence of "immune" abnormalities. These may include high γ-globulin levels (especially IgG), antinuclear factor, LE cells, and smooth-muscle antibodies. HBsAg, if present, indicates HBV as the etiology and is usually not associated with the above "immune" manifestations.

Diagnosis: The disorder must be differentiated from alcoholic liver disease, recrudescent viral hepatitis, chronic persistent hepatitis, and primary biliary cirrhosis. Clinical and laboratory features are helpful but *liver biopsy is essential for definitive diagnosis.* Biopsy shows periportal necrosis with lymphocytic and plasma cell infiltrates (so-called "piecemeal necrosis"); the acinar architecture is usually distorted by zones of collapse and fibrosis, and frank cirrhosis often coexists with the signs of ongoing hepatitis. Cases due to HBV can often be distinguished by the presence of "ground glass" hepatocytes and special stains for HBV components.

Treatment includes cessation of causative drugs, management of complications, and the use of corticosteroids with or without azathioprine. These drugs suppress the inflammatory reaction and may play some role in altering the immune response to causative agents. Controlled trials have demonstrated clinical, biochemical, and histologic improvement in patients with non-viral chronic active hepatitis, especially if immune features are prominent. Dosage adjustment should be supervised by a specialist. In contrast, HBsAg-associated cases tend to respond relatively poorly to corticosteroid therapy, and viral proliferation may be enhanced. Thus, on present evidence this patient subgroup should be treated only if a relentlessly downhill course is evident. To date, therapy with antiviral agents (eg, acyclovir, adenine arabinoside, and interferons) has not given impressive results.

Prognosis is highly variable. With drug etiology, the disease may regress completely when the offending agent is withdrawn. Cases associated with HBsAg tend to progress, and as noted above are usually relatively resistant to therapy. Idiopathic cases generally improve with treatment, especially if autoimmune features are present. With adequate therapy patients usually live several years, but hepatocellular failure, cirrhosis, or both eventually develop in most cases.

72. DRUGS AND THE LIVER

The liver metabolizes many drugs and toxins, most commonly by oxidation, reduction, or conjugation. Interaction between drugs and the liver can be divided into 3 basic categories: (1) hepatic enzyme induction; (2) effects of liver disease on drug metabolism; and (3) liver damage due to drugs.

Enzyme Induction (See also Ch. 276)

Hepatic enzymes responsible for drug transformation are often induced (stimulated) by the agents they metabolize; hence many drugs stimulate their own catabolism. This effect is usually nonspecific so that transformation of other drugs is also enhanced. Important clinical consequences may result; eg, a patient on both oral anticoagulants and phenobarbital may suddenly bleed if the latter, a potent enzyme inducer, is discontinued. Ethanol likewise acts as a drug, which accounts for the well-known tolerance of alcoholics to sedatives and other agents.

In contrast, hepatic drug metabolism is inhibited by the H_2-receptor antagonist cimetidine. Clearance of various other drugs is thereby impaired, including benzodiazepines, theophylline, warfarin, propranolol, and phenytoin. This interaction can be clinically important, especially when cimetidine is either started or discontinued. Ranitidine,an equally useful H_2-receptor antagonist, does not have this effect.

Influence of Liver Disease on Drug Metabolism

Complex effects on drug clearance and biotransformation can occur in liver disease, depending on alterations in plasma binding capacity, hepatic blood flow, extraction capacity, cellular transformation pathways, biliary excretion, etc. Cerebral sensitivity to narcotics and sedatives is often enhanced, so that seemingly small doses may precipitate encephalopathy. Net results for an individual drug are unpredictable and do not correlate well with the type of liver damage, its severity, or liver function tests. Thus, no general rules can be used to modify drug dosage in patients with liver disease.

Liver Damage Due to Drugs

Drugs are an important cause of hepatic disease. The mechanisms are variable, complex, and in most instances poorly understood. Some agents act as direct cellular toxins; injury from these is generally predictable, dose-related, and characteristic for the particular agent. Others produce damage only rarely in susceptible individuals, but the injury is generally unpredictable and not dose-related. Although the latter is often termed a hypersensitivity, evidence for a true allergic reaction is usually lacking; idiosyncratic response is a preferable term. Moreover, the distinction between direct toxicity and idiosyncrasy seems less clear than previously thought. For example, in susceptible patients some drugs previously considered allergens appear to damage cell membranes directly via toxic intermediate metabolites.

No classification of drug jaundice is completely satisfactory, but most acute cases can be divided into hemolytic, hepatocellular, cholestatic, and miscellaneous reactions. Some drugs can produce chronic damage, including neoplasms.

Hemolysis: Drugs cause hemolysis by a variety of mechanisms. Mild jaundice may result from unconjugated hyperbilirubinemia, but no true hepatic damage occurs and liver function tests are normal.

Hepatocellular necrosis is conceptually divided into direct toxicity and idiosyncrasy, though as noted above this distinction may be artificial.

Direct toxicity: Most direct hepatotoxins produce dose-related liver necrosis, often with effects on other organs (eg, the kidneys). Damage can take several forms; eg, carbon tetrachloride and related hydrocarbons cause severe centrizonal necrosis and fatty infiltration; phosphorus produces primarily periportal damage; ingestion of var-

ious *Amanita* mushrooms results in fatal hemorrhagic necrosis; and high-dose IV tetracycline, especially in pregnant women, produces diffuse fine-droplet fatty infiltration with a hepatitis-like clinical picture.

Acute overdosage of the mild analgesic **acetaminophen (paracetamol)** is an important cause of fulminant liver failure in Great Britain and is becoming increasingly common in North America. Doses exceeding 10 to 15 gm deplete the liver of glutathione, which normally detoxifies the drug by binding potentially hazardous intermediate metabolites. When this mechanism is saturated, the resulting free intermediates bind to liver macromolecules and produce centrizonal necrosis. Liver damage is often not apparent until 2 to 5 days after ingestion, when the picture of acute hepatic failure develops. Mortality climbs as ingestion exceeds 25 gm; in alcoholics, much lower doses can be fatal. Early treatment with N-acetylcysteine, which repletes glutathione, will prevent liver necrosis and can be lifesaving, but therapy must be started within 10 to 12 h of poisoning; delay beyond 16 h renders treatment ineffective. N-acetylcysteine is nontoxic and can be given either orally (140 mg/kg followed by 70 mg/kg q 4 h for 3 days) or IV (300 mg/kg infused over 20 h, with ½ the dose given in the first 15 min). Evidence also incriminates acetaminophen in chronic liver damage (see below).

Idiosyncrasy: Drugs can produce acute hepatocellular necrosis that is clinically, biochemically, and histologically indistinguishable from viral hepatitis. This type of reaction appears to differ from the above forms of toxic necrosis and is generally considered idiosyncratic; however, the mechanism is uncertain and probably varies with the specific drug. Offending agents are numerous and include isoniazid **(INH),** methyldopa, monoamine oxidase inhibitors, indomethacin, propylthiouracil, phenytoin, and the anesthetic agent halothane. Of these, INH and halothane have been most thoroughly studied.

INH causes minor, usually transient aminotransferase elevations in up to 20% of patients. Frank hepatitis occurs in 1 to 2% and can be fatal. Persons over age 35 and those in whom rapid acetylation occurs seem more susceptible. Unlike most similar drug hepatitis, which appears within a few weeks of starting the agent, INH injury may be delayed up to a year and by then the association may be overlooked. Chronic active hepatitis and cirrhosis can develop if the drug is not stopped. Whether the reaction is due to a hypersensitivity mechanism or to hepatotoxic metabolites is debated, but most evidence favors the latter.

The rare **halothane-related hepatitis** tends to occur after repeated exposure to the anesthetic at relatively short intervals; unexplained postoperative fever after the preceding exposure may provide a warning signal. The mechanism of injury is still unclear. Obesity seems a risk factor, possibly because halothane metabolites are stored in adipose tissue. Hepatitis typically develops within a few days to 2 wk after operation, is heralded by fever, and is often severe. Distinction from posttransfusion viral hepatitis is aided by a shorter latent period, absence of hepatitis antigens in serum, occasional presence of eosinophilia or skin rash, and sometimes subtle histologic differences. Mortality is high, but surviving patients usually recover completely. Methoxyflurane and enflurane, related anesthetic agents, can produce the same syndrome.

Cholestasis: A variety of agents can produce a primarily cholestatic reaction. In most instances the pathogenesis is poorly understood, but there are at least 2 clinically distinct forms of cholestatic injury.

The **phenothiazine type** is a periportal inflammatory reaction often associated with acute clinical onset, fever, and high aminotransferase as well as alkaline phosphatase levels. Differentiation from extrahepatic obstruction may be difficult, even by liver biopsy. The reaction seems due to individual idiosyncrasy, and in some cases eosinophilia and other evidence of a sensitivity reaction occurs. Other evidence, however, points to a direct toxic action on hepatic canaliculi, possibly via interference with membrane ATPase. This type of cholestasis occurs in about 1% of patients given

chlorpromazine, less often with other phenothiazines. Complete resolution is usual, though progression to a chronic biliary cirrhosis-like illness can occur rarely, even if the drug is withdrawn. A similar picture can be produced by tricyclic antidepressants, chlorpropamide, phenylbutazone, erythromycin estolate, and other drugs, though these have been less thoroughly studied and progression to chronic liver damage has not been established.

The **steroid type** is a pure cholestatic reaction with little or no hepatocellular inflammation. Gradual onset of cholestasis without systemic symptoms is usual. Alkaline phosphatase is elevated but aminotransferase levels are usually unimpressive, and liver biopsy shows only centrizonal bile stasis with little portal reaction or hepatocellular disarray. Complete resolution follows cessation of the offending steroid. This type of cholestasis is produced by oral contraceptives, methyltestosterone, and related drugs, most of which are C-17 alkylated steroids. About 1 to 2% of women taking oral contraceptives develop the syndrome; figures vary around the world, possibly because of genetic factors. The reaction appears to be an exaggeration of the physiologic effect of sex hormones on hepatic bile formation, rather than an immunologic sensitivity or membrane cytotoxicity. Interference with canalicular water flow and microfilament function may be responsible, although the exact mechanism of impaired bile transport is uncertain. The syndrome is closely related to cholestasis of pregnancy (see Ch. 178); women with the latter condition often develop cholestasis when given oral contraceptives, and vice versa.

Miscellaneous reactions: Some drugs produce mixed forms of hepatic dysfunction, a granulomatous reaction, or other variants of liver injury that are difficult to classify. Responsible agents include aminosalicylic acid (PAS), sulfonamides, several other antibiotics, quinidine, allopurinol, valproic acid, aspirin, and numerous other agents. Many anti-neoplastic drugs also cause hepatic damage; mechanisms vary.

Chronic Liver Disease

Ongoing liver damage indistinguishable from chronic active hepatitis can be produced by INH, methyldopa, and nitrofurantoin. In some instances the illness begins as an acute hepatitis, in others more insidiously; progression to cirrhosis may occur. A chronic active hepatitis-like picture with scarring has also been reported in patients using acetaminophen long-term in doses as low as 3 gm daily; alcohol abusers appear particularly susceptible. The cardiac drugs perhexilene maleate and amiodarone occasionally produce chronic liver injury that histologically mimics alcoholic liver disease, including the presence of Mallory bodies.

As noted above, chlorpromazine can rarely produce chronic cholestasis with biliary fibrosis. Methotrexate induces insidiously progressive hepatocellular damage and scarring, typically with unremarkable liver function tests; occasional biopsy is advisable in patients on long-term use of the drug, usually for psoriasis or RA. Arsenicals can produce non-cirrhotic hepatic fibrosis with portal hypertension, and chronic scarring is also occasionally seen in health faddists who ingest enormous amounts of vitamin A or niacin. In many tropical and subtropical countries, chronic liver disease and hepatocellular carcinoma are believed to result from ingestion in food of fungal products known as aflatoxins.

In addition to the cholestasis noted above, considerable evidence associates the use of oral contraceptives with the occasional development of benign hepatic adenomas, and very rarely, hepatocellular carcinoma (see Ch. 77). Focal nodular hyperplasia, an adenoma-like hamartomatous lesion, may also expand under the influence of oral contraceptives. Adenomas and focal nodular hyperplasia are usually subclinical but may present with sudden intraperitoneal rupture and hemorrhage requiring emergency laparotomy. Hepatic vein thrombosis with Budd-Chiari syndrome may also occur in women on oral contraceptives, as part of a general increased clotting tendency. These

drugs also enhance the lithogenicity of bile, with a resultant increased incidence of gallstones.

---

73. LIVER DISEASE DUE TO ALCOHOL

(See also DEPENDENCE ON ALCOHOL in Ch. 138)

A spectrum of clinical syndromes and pathologic changes in the liver caused by alcohol. It constitutes a major and potentially preventable health problem.

Pathogenesis

In general, a linear correlation exists between the severity of liver damage and the intensity of alcohol abuse as measured by duration and dose. However, the mechanisms by which alcohol damages the liver have not yet been defined.

By providing calories without essential nutrients, decreasing the appetite, and causing malabsorption through its toxic effects on the gut and pancreas, ethanol promotes malnutrition. Ethanol is also a hepatotoxin whose metabolism creates profound derangements of the liver cell. Apparent variations in the susceptibility of individuals and the greater susceptibility of females to alcoholic liver disease suggest that other factors are also significant. Family clustering of alcoholic liver disease occurs frequently enough that the influence of genetic factors cannot be dismissed. Although controversial, there are data to suggest that one's immunologic status may play a role in determining susceptibility to alcohol.

Metabolism of Ethanol

Ethanol is readily absorbed from the GI tract and > 90% of it is metabolized by the liver through oxidative mechanisms involving mainly alcohol dehydrogenase and certain microsomal enzymes. Acetaldehyde, the major product of oxidation, is in turn oxidized. Although details of its subsequent metabolism are not entirely clear, acetaldehyde itself may be implicated in some of the untoward effects of alcohol on the liver and other organs. The conversion of ethanol to acetaldehyde and of the latter to either acetate or acetyl coenzyme A involves the production of reduced nicotinamide adenine dinucleotide **(NADH)**. Therefore, ethanol metabolism promotes a reduced intracellular state that interferes with carbohydrate, lipid, and other aspects of intermediary metabolism. The oxidation of ethanol is coupled with the reduction of pyruvate to lactic acid, which promotes hyperuricemia, hypoglycemia, and acidosis (see HYPOGLYCEMIA in Ch. 94). Ethanol oxidation is also coupled with the reduction of oxaloacetic acid to malate. This may explain the reduced activity of the citric acid cycle, reduced gluconeogenesis, and increased fatty acid synthesis associated with ethanol metabolism. An increase in α-glycerophosphate after ethanol administration is well documented; the glycerol thus produced may promote increased triglyceride synthesis. Although O_2 consumption is normal after ethanol, there is a metabolic shift from O_2 consumption during the breakdown of fatty acids to that consumed during the oxidation of alcohol to acetate. This shift may explain the reduced lipid oxidation and increased ketone formation recorded after ethanol ingestion. There is also evidence that alcohol metabolism induces a local hypermetabolic state in the liver, promoting hypoxic damage in Zone 3, that area around the terminal hepatic venules.

Although the hypothesis that alcoholics metabolize ethanol differently than nonalcoholics remains under study, there is no doubt that chronic ingestion of ethanol leads to adaptation by the liver with hypertrophy of the smooth endoplasmic reticulum and increased activity of the hepatic drug metabolizing enzymes. This fact is of clinical importance, since the alcohol abuser develops an increased tolerance to alcohol and to a variety of drugs including sedatives, tranquilizers, and antibiotics. Individual suscep-

tibility to ethanol and the complex interactions between drugs, other chemicals, and ethanol have been clarified by recent identification of a component of the drug metabolizing system of the liver, which is modulated specifically by ethanol.

Pathology

The spectrum of hepatic pathology associated with prolonged alcohol consumption ranges from the simple accumulation of neutral fat in hepatocytes to cirrhosis and hepatocellular carcinoma. The widely accepted fatty liver-alcoholic hepatitis-cirrhosis spectrum is a concept of convenience. The findings usually overlap and many patients present features of the entire spectrum. The key lesion may well be fibrosis around the terminal hepatic venules. From the pathologic point of view, it is better to make a diagnosis of alcoholic liver disease and describe the specific findings in each patient.

Fatty liver appears to be the initial change and is the most common hepatic abnormality in hospitalized alcoholics. Usually asymptomatic, it may produce painful, tender hepatomegaly or even intrahepatic obstructive jaundice. It has also been associated with portal hypertension and acute hepatocellular failure. Its pathogenesis is not clear. Fat droplets of varying size are found in most hepatocytes except in regenerating areas. The droplets tend to coalesce, forming large globules that frequently occupy the entire cytoplasm. Fatty cysts probably represent late stages of the fatty change. These cysts are usually located periportally and ultrastructural evidence suggests that they form through fusion of the fat content of several hepatocytes (see also Ch. 69).

Hydropic change is prevalent in the early stages of alcoholic liver injury. Although insufficiently explained, ethanol does affect the membrane transport of cations, increasing intracellular Na and water. It can also be associated with the intracellular accumulation of excess protein. Giant spherical mitochondria, visible even by light microscopy, can be found in about 30% of patients with alcoholic liver disease.

Mallory's alcoholic hyaline is a fibrillar protein of uncertain origin and significance. It appears as dense acidophilic masses of variable size and shape near the nuclei of cells containing little or no fat. These cells, which have characteristic ultrastructural morphology and enzymatic activities, undergo hyaline degeneration, but need not be irreversibly damaged. Mallory's alcoholic hyaline is characteristic of alcoholic liver disease, but it is also found in some cases of Wilson's disease, Indian childhood cirrhosis, the cirrhosis that follows small-intestine bypass surgery, primary biliary cirrhosis, hepatocellular carcinoma, focal nodular hyperplasia, and other conditions. In association with this hyaline change, one usually finds a laying down of connective tissue in the sinusoids and around individual hepatocytes, especially in Zone 3 of the liver acinus.

A subgroup of patients have prominent sclerosis around the terminal hepatic venules. This lesion, called **sclerosing hyaline necrosis** or **central hyaline sclerosis,** can lead to portal hypertension *before* the development of cirrhosis, and may be one of the earliest manifestations of the tendency to develop cirrhosis. The importance of sinusoidal myofibroblasts in the pathogenesis of the fibrosis is increasingly appreciated.

Focal liver necrosis is frequently found in biopsy specimens; these patients have no specific clinical or laboratory abnormalities. However, patients with **diffuse inflammation and necrosis** have **alcoholic hepatitis.** They have enlarged, smooth, yellow livers that microscopically feature necrosis, inflammation, and sclerosis. Progression of alcoholic hepatitis to cirrhosis has been documented. About 20% of heavy drinkers will develop *cirrhosis* in which the liver is finely nodular with its architecture disorganized by fibrous septa and nodules. If drinking stops and the liver undergoes a constructive regenerative response, the picture can be that of a mixed cirrhosis (see Ch. 70).

Increased liver **iron** is seen in alcoholics with normal, fatty, or cirrhotic livers, but the incidence is $< 10\%$. The underlying mechanisms are obscure, but there appears to be no relationship with the amount of iron consumed in the alcohol or with the length of drinking history. The distribution of iron found in hepatocytes and Kupffer cells is not

pathognomonic. This iron elicits a meager inflammatory response and its role in hepatocellular damage is controversial.

Symptoms, Signs, and Diagnosis

Variations in drinking patterns, individual susceptibility to hepatotoxic effects of alcohol, and the many kinds of tissue damage noted above promote a highly variable clinical picture. For a long time, there may be no symptoms and no signs referable to the liver. In general, symptoms can be related to the amount of alcohol ingested and the overall duration of alcohol ingestion. Thus, symptoms usually become apparent in patients during their 30s and severe problems tend to appear in the 40s.

Patients with only a fatty liver are usually asymptomatic, but may have an enlarged, smooth, and occasionally tender liver. Routine biochemical studies are often within normal limits.

Alcoholic hepatitis can be suspected on clinical grounds, but the diagnosis is a pathologic one and the histologic lesion can be found in all parts of the clinical spectrum of alcoholic liver disease. Patients with alcoholic hepatitis may present with fever, jaundice, right upper quadrant pain, leukocytosis, and hepatomegaly, but so also may patients with sepsis, cholecystitis, or mechanical extrahepatic biliary obstruction. Patients with alcoholic liver disease who have cirrhosis, portal hypertension, portal systemic encephalopathy, or hepatocellular carcinoma often present clinical features of these problems (see elsewhere in THE MANUAL under the appropriate headings).

Laboratory Findings

The laboratory can be remarkably *un*helpful in establishing the diagnosis of alcoholic liver disease. Although sometimes suggestive, routine hematologic and biochemical tests are nonspecific and do not permit a definitive diagnosis. In alcoholic liver disease there can be various abnormalities of RBC morphology, including target cells, macrocytes, spur cells, and stomatocytes. The mean corpuscular volume **(MCV)** is usually elevated and this can be a useful marker of alcohol abuse, because the MCV returns quite slowly to normal after cessation of drinking. The activity of the serum alanine transferase (ALT, formerly SGPT) is depressed relative to that of the serum aspartate transferase (AST, formerly SGOT). The activity of the serum γ-glutamyl transpeptidase **(γ-GT)** may be helpful in detecting alcohol consumption, the value of the enzyme lying not in its specificity, but in its sensitivity to changes in liver status. The MCV, γ-GT, and alkaline phosphatase appear to provide the best combination of routine laboratory tests in the identification of chronic alcohol abuse. Liver scans and ultrasound examinations are frequently performed and sometimes helpful. In the final analysis, one depends on the assessment of the liver morphology, and a blind needle biopsy (see Ch. 68) is usually sufficient, since the lesion is diffuse.

Prognosis and Treatment

With abstinence, nonfibrotic liver damage may be reversed and the survival of patients with alcoholic hepatitis, fibrosis, and cirrhosis improves. The significance of alcoholic hepatitis appears to be determined by the degree of associated fibrosis and liver cell necrosis. The reversibility of sclerosing hyaline necrosis is under study.

In theory, the treatment of this condition is simple and straightforward; in practice, it is difficult: *the patient must stop drinking alcohol.* Following severe bouts of illness and major adverse social consequences (eg, job loss, family unit breakdown) and a review of the facts by a physician who has established rapport, many will stop drinking. It helps to point out that much of alcoholic liver disease is reversible. Otherwise, management is nonspecific and focuses on general supportive care. One should wait for delirium tremens to develop. The attempt to prevent this problem, which may not develop, may do more harm than good in the patient prone to encephalopathy (see also DEPENDENCE ON ALCOHOL in Ch. 138).

Although still controversial, it is unlikely that corticosteroids have any role to play in the treatment of alcoholic liver disease. There is much interest in therapeutic measures directed against hepatic fibrogenesis, but the use of colchicine, penicillamine, and proline analogs must still be restricted to carefully designed and executed clinical trials. The same comment must be applied to propylthiouracil. The value of this drug, after ethanol has been withdrawn, has not been established. Trauma, infection, malignant degeneration, GI bleeding, nutritional deficiencies, fluid retention, and portal systemic encephalopathy require specific attention.

74. POSTOPERATIVE LIVER DISORDERS

Mild liver function derangements sometimes occur after major surgery and reflect poorly understood effects of anesthetic and operative stress. Patients with underlying liver disease may develop more severe dysfunction postoperatively; eg, in the patient with viral or alcoholic hepatitis, laparotomy may precipitate acute liver failure.

Postoperative jaundice in patients without previous liver disease can take several forms. The most frequent is a **multifactorial mixed hyperbilirubinemia** due to a complex interaction between enhanced bilirubin load and diminished hepatic clearance. This is most often seen following major surgery or trauma requiring multiple transfusions. Hemolysis, sepsis, resorption of hematomas, and blood transfusions can all contribute to increased pigment production; at the same time, hepatic function is impaired by hypoxemia, circulatory failure, and other poorly understood factors. The result is variable, but severe jaundice with nondescript aminotransferase and alkaline phosphatase elevations often occurs. Frank liver failure is rare and the syndrome typically resolves slowly, but completely.

Transient hypotension during anesthesia or from perioperative shock can cause acute centrizonal liver necrosis, manifested by a rapid and dramatic increase in aminotransferase levels (often > 1000 u./L). Jaundice is usually mild. This so-called **ischemic hepatitis** is not a true inflammatory necrosis and characteristically resolves within a few days unless complicating factors are present.

True hepatitis postoperatively is usually due to viral transmission via transfusion, especially non-A, non-B hepatitis, and must be differentiated from the above abnormalities. The latter are usually maximal within a few days of operation, whereas viral hepatitis rarely develops before 2 wk. Anesthesia with halothane or related agents may also produce postoperative hepatitis and should be suspected if hepatitis develops within 10 days of surgery, especially if preceded by unexplained fever (see Ch. 72).

Cholestatic reactions are most often due to biliary obstruction from intra-abdominal complications or to drugs prescribed postoperatively (see Ch. 72). Obscure intrahepatic cholestasis occasionally develops in patients who have undergone major surgery, especially abdominal or cardiovascular procedures **("benign postoperative intrahepatic cholestasis")**. The pathogenesis is unknown, but the disorder usually slowly resolves spontaneously; ultrasound helps to differentiate it from mechanical obstruction. Patients receiving prolonged total parenteral nutrition **(TPN)** perioperatively may also develop a progressive cholestatic syndrome, usually with a component of hepatocellular inflammation **("TPN cholestasis")**. This is rarely seen with < 3 wk of TPN, but the risk then increases with the duration of therapy; infants appear particularly susceptible. Despite intense study, the pathogenesis is still uncertain. Liver biopsy usually shows a nonspecific mixed cholestatic-inflammatory picture, sometimes with progressive fibrosis. The syndrome regresses with discontinuation of TPN, but can otherwise lead to liver failure or irreversible scarring.

75. HEPATIC GRANULOMAS

A multifactorial infiltrative liver disorder with or without additional hepatic inflammation and fibrosis. The term **"granulomatous hepatitis"** is often used, but the condition is not a true hepatitis. Hepatic granulomas are found in about 3 to 10% of liver biopsies. They may be insignificant incidental findings, but more often reflect clinically relevant disease—usually a systemic disorder rather than primary liver disease.

Etiology

The causes of liver granulomas are legion. **Infectious disorders** are the most important: bacterial (eg, TB and other mycobacterial infections, brucellosis, tularemia, actinomycosis); fungal (eg, histoplasmosis, cryptococcosis, blastomycosis); parasitic (eg, schistosomiasis—the most important worldwide, toxoplasmosis, visceral larva migrans); viral infections, which are less common (eg, infectious mononucleosis, cytomegalovirus); and numerous others (eg, Q fever, syphilis).

Sarcoidosis is the most important noninfectious cause; liver involvement occurs in about 2/3 of patients and occasionally is the dominant clinical manifestation. A variety of **drugs** can be responsible (eg, quinidine, sulfonamides, allopurinol, phenylbutazone). Hepatic granulomas can also occur in polymyalgia rheumatica and other **collagen-vascular diseases;** in **Hodgkin's disease,** sometimes without other morphologic evidence of the lymphoma; and in a host of other systemic conditions.

Granulomas are less common in primary liver disease. Of these, **primary biliary cirrhosis** is the only important cause; periportal granulomas are typical in this disorder, especially in the early stages. Small granulomas are occasionally seen in various other liver diseases, most often associated with fat droplets **("lipogranulomas"),** but are of no clinical significance.

In many cases no etiology can be established. A few such patients have a syndrome of recurrent fevers, myalgias, fatigue, and other systemic symptoms, often occurring intermittently for years. Whether this **"idiopathic granulomatous hepatitis"** is a specific syndrome or a variant of sarcoidosis is debated.

Pathophysiology

Granuloma formation is incompletely understood. The lesions are regarded as a host attempt to protect against poorly-soluble exogenous or endogenous irritants. Immunologic mechanisms convert cells of the mononuclear phagocytic system into the typical collection of epithelioid cells that comprise a granuloma; multinucleated giant cells are believed to derive from fusion of macrophages.

In the liver, granulomas often incite little or no hepatocellular reaction and merely serve as the morphologic clue to some underlying process; hepatic disease is not apparent clinically and liver function is well preserved. However, when granulomas are part of a broader inflammatory reaction involving the liver (eg, drug reactions, infectious mononucleosis), clinical and biochemical evidence of hepatocellular dysfunction is usually present. Sometimes an aggressive inflammatory response ensues around the granulomas, resulting in progressive hepatic fibrosis and portal hypertension. This is typical of schistosomiasis and occasionally occurs in extensive sarcoidal infiltration.

Symptoms, Signs, and Laboratory Findings

Clinical features reflect the underlying etiology. Granulomas themselves are typically subclinical; even extensive infiltration usually produces only minor hepatomegaly and little or no jaundice. Fever, malaise, and other systemic symptoms are the usual presenting manifestations of an infective etiology; prolonged FUO is especially common in TB and fungal infections. The history is critical in establishing a drug etiology. Various systemic features may provide the clue to sarcoidosis, collagen-vascular dis-

ease, lymphoma, and other etiologies. Signs of primary liver disease are usually lacking, and hepatosplenomegaly is typically absent or mild except in schistosomiasis.

In most situations, liver function test results are only mildly deranged, usually with a disproportionate elevation of alkaline phosphatase. Bilirubin levels are typically normal or only mildly elevated. Enzyme values may simulate viral hepatitis if extensive hepatocellular necrosis is present (eg, in infectious mononucleosis or a drug reaction). A predominant cholestatic reaction suggests primary biliary cirrhosis, especially if longstanding. Other laboratory abnormalities depend on the specific cause.

Diagnosis

Liver biopsy is essential for diagnosis and should be considered whenever a systemic granulomatous disorder is suspected, even in the absence of apparent hepatic involvement. Biopsy demonstrates granulomas and may provide histologic evidence of the specific etiology (eg, schistosomal ova, caseation of TB, fungal organisms, primary biliary cirrhosis). However, the morphologic pattern is often nonspecific and the diagnosis must be pursued with appropriate studies (eg, cultures, skin tests, laboratory and x-ray studies, and other tissue specimens). Infective etiologies are especially important to establish in patients with FUO; this task often proves challenging. A portion of the fresh biopsy specimen should be sent for culture; special stains for acid-fast bacilli, fungi, and other organisms can sometimes prove the cause.

Prognosis and Treatment

Hepatic granulomas of infective or drug etiology regress completely after appropriate therapy. Sarcoid granulomas may disappear spontaneously or persist for years, usually without clinically important hepatic disease, but progressive fibrosis and portal hypertension occasionally develop (sarcoidal cirrhosis). In schistosomiasis, progressive portal scarring is the rule ("pipestem fibrosis"); hepatic function usually remains well preserved, but increasing portal hypertension leads to marked splenomegaly and risk of variceal hemorrhage.

Treatment depends on the underlying etiology. Without an etiologic diagnosis, it is generally best to follow the patient rather than blindly treat with antibiotics or other therapies. Antituberculous therapy may be justified in a patient with prolonged fever, a compatible clinical picture, and a downhill systemic course. Patients with progressive hepatic sarcoidosis may benefit from corticosteroid therapy, though it remains unclear whether this prevents hepatic fibrosis; corticosteroids are not indicated for most patients with sarcoidosis and should be given only if TB and other infective disorders can confidently be excluded. Corticosteroids usually suppress the recurrent fevers in patients with the syndrome of idiopathic granulomatous hepatitis.

---

76. VASCULAR LESIONS OF THE LIVER

Thrombotic, occlusive, and inflammatory lesions of arteries and veins within and adjoining the liver.

LESIONS OF THE HEPATIC ARTERY

Congenital anomalies of the hepatic artery are common; 45% are variations on the conventional textbook picture. The main variants are replacement of the left or right hepatic artery, an accessory left or right hepatic artery, or a common hepatic artery originating from the superior mesenteric artery. Usually of no clinical significance, these anomalies can be important to the surgeon and interesting to the angiographer.

Hepatic artery occlusion is usually caused by thrombosis, embolism, or surgical ligation. The occlusion may produce an ischemic infarct of the liver, but results are unpre-

dictable because of individual differences in hepatic vasculature and the extent of collateral circulation. The underlying problem is usually part of a systemic process. The hepatic artery and its branches are involved in about 60% of cases of polyarteritis nodosa, and thrombotic occlusion leading to hepatic infarction has been documented in 15% of cases. A necrotizing hepatic arteritis has been described in drug addicts. Hepatic artery occlusion is used therapeutically in treating certain malignancies involving the liver.

Aneurysms of the hepatic artery are not rare. They are usually saccular and often multiple. When sufficiently large, they can produce extrahepatic mechanical bile duct obstruction. Without treatment, and with high mortality, up to 75% of hepatic artery aneurysms rupture into the common bile duct, peritoneum, or adjacent hollow viscera. The lesions usually are secondary to infection, arteriosclerosis, trauma, and polyarteritis nodosa. The diagnosis can be suspected on the basis of other x-ray technics, but can be made reliably only by arteriography. When identified, these aneurysms should be embolized using transarterial catheter technics; if this approach fails, then direct surgical ligation of the hepatic artery is indicated.

LESIONS OF THE HEPATIC VENOUS SYSTEM

Veno-occlusive disease (VOD): *an obliterative lesion of the hepatic venules and small tributaries of the hepatic venous system; the larger branches of the hepatic veins are not involved. The lesion leads to ischemia, hepatocellular necrosis, and sinusoidal cell damage.* The lesion has been produced experimentally by alkaloids from Crotalaria and Senecio plants, by other hepatotoxins (dimethylnitrosamine, aflatoxin, and azathioprine), by radiation, and as a part of the graft-vs.-host reaction. It has also been reported in a family featuring immune deficiencies.

VOD is endemic in Jamaica, where tea is made from Senecio leaves, and it is reported from many other countries. VOD presents acutely with the sudden onset of ascites and tender, smooth hepatomegaly. Although all age groups are affected, it involves primarily children of ages 1½ to 3 yr. Typically, the patient recovers promptly with or without treatment, but some die with acute hepatic failure, and others present at a later date with portal hypertension with or without cirrhosis. There is no specific therapy apart from withdrawal of any offending toxin. Treatment of the associated portal hypertension is similar to that for the Budd-Chiari syndrome (see below).

BUDD-CHIARI SYNDROME

A rare syndrome resulting from thrombosis of the major hepatic veins. It affects both sexes and all age groups, but especially those between ages 20 and 40 yr.

Etiology

Congenital absence of the hepatic venous ostia has caused the Budd-Chiari syndrome, but usually the problem is acquired and no cause is confirmed. An underlying condition with a thrombogenic tendency is commonly associated with the Budd-Chiari syndrome. Hence this syndrome may develop in patients with polycythemia vera and other myeloproliferative disorders, sickle cell disease, paroxysmal nocturnal hemoglobinuria, and pregnancy. An underlying thrombogenic tendency may also be involved in cases associated with oral contraceptives, abdominal trauma, suppurative lesions of the liver, and malignant disease in the region of the hepatic veins, especially primary hepatocellular carcinoma and renal cell carcinoma.

Pathology

Hepatic vein occlusion occurs either in the intrahepatic portion of the inferior vena cava, or more often in the large hepatic veins near their entrance to the inferior vena cava. The obstruction is usually caused by thrombi, sometimes by fibrous cords, webs,

or membranes that presumably are the residue of thrombi. Hepatic veins may be obscured by surrounding fibrosis, and the parenchyma of the liver features severe sinusoidal congestion, atrophy, and/or destruction of the hepatocytes in Zone 3. In chronic cases, perivascular fibrosis develops, and nodular regeneration with subsequent loss of normal architecture may occur. Portal hypertension develops with splenomegaly and portal systemic anastomoses. Secondary portal vein thrombosis occurs in about 20% of patients, and spontaneous rupture of the liver has been reported.

Symptoms and Signs

Patients usually present with abdominal pain, tender smooth hepatomegaly, gross ascites resistant to therapy, and mild jaundice. The onset can be acute and devastating, but it is usually subacute, with a delay of weeks or months before portal hypertension and liver cell failure become apparent. The prognosis is poor; < 1/3 of patients survive for 1 yr.

Diagnosis

Routine biochemical testing is of little value, but hepatic scintiscanning can be diagnostic. The isotope becomes concentrated in the caudate lobe, which is drained by veins that empty directly into the vena cava and which are often unaffected in patients with thrombosis of the main hepatic veins. Hepatic venography defines the extent of the thrombosis and any involvement of the vena cava. Liver biopsy can reveal the changes mentioned above.

Treatment

Side-to-side portacaval decompressive surgery should be considered early in the treatment of patients with a patent portal vein and normal pressures in a patent vena cava. Hepatic transplantation has a definite role in treatment and should be considered early. Hepatoatrial anastomosis has recently been presented as an effective form of treatment for this syndrome. Conservative management using anticoagulants or fibrinolysins should be reserved for patients with incomplete obstruction of the hepatic veins. It should be continued only if clinical improvement is rapid and clearing of the thrombus is demonstrated.

LESIONS OF THE PORTAL VEIN

Congenital anomalies of the portal vein include aplasia and stricture, which result from abnormal obliteration of the vitelline veins and their ventral anastomoses. **Cavernous transformation of the portal vein** may represent a congenital malformation, but is usually the end result of postpartum thrombosis followed by recanalization and new vessel formation.

Portal vein aneurysms are extremely rare.

Portal vein thrombosis may occur at any point in its course. No etiologic factor can be identified in > 1/2 of patients, but it may be associated with inflammatory processes (eg, suppurative pyelophlebitis, cholangitis, adjacent suppurative lymphadenitis, and hepatic abscess). It occurs in 10% of patients with cirrhosis and especially those with hepatocellular carcinoma. It occurs in pregnancy, especially in eclampsia and in conditions causing portal vein stasis (eg, hepatic venous obstruction, chronic heart failure, and constrictive pericarditis). Encasement of the portal vein by pancreatic, gastric, and other malignancies can lead to portal vein thrombosis.

While the diagnosis can be made on the basis of ultrasound or CT scanning, the diagnosis is most reliably and definitively established by angiography (eg, splenoportography, venous phase of superior mesenteric or splenic arteriography).

The clinical effect of portal vein thrombosis depends on the location and extent of

the thrombosis, the rapidity with which it develops, and the nature of any underlying liver disease. It may lead to infarction of the liver **(Zahn's infarct)** or segmental atrophy; ie, left lobe atrophy. If associated with mesenteric vein thrombosis, it is acutely fatal. If the portal vein thrombosis develops slowly, then collaterals may form and portal vein recanalization occurs. Nevertheless, **portal hypertension** is the end result (see below).

The major clinical problem is bleeding varices. Recurring hemorrhage tends to be well tolerated because liver cell function is so often normal. Management should be conservative with endoscopic obliteration of the varices being the first choice of definitive therapy. If this approach fails and the splenic vein is patent, a splenorenal shunt is the surgical treatment of choice. Failing this, a mesocaval shunt should be performed. Since small veins promote shunt thrombosis, shunting procedures in a child should be delayed as long as possible. Staplegun transection of esophageal varices has also been advocated.

LESIONS OF THE SINUSOIDS

Sinusoidal portal hypertension with normal portal veins and without clinical evidence of postsinusoidal portal hypertension has been reported. Pathologically, the liver features marked Kupffer cell hypertrophy with narrowing of the sinusoidal lumena and perisinusoidal fibrosis with obliteration of the space of Disse.

Peliosis hepatis: *an uncommon lesion characterized by multiple small blood-filled cystic spaces distributed in an apparently random manner in the liver parenchyma.* Its pathogenesis remains obscure, but focal parenchymal cell necrosis with hemorrhage is the generally accepted concept. Peliosis hepatis is associated with chronic wasting disorders (especially advanced pulmonary TB), with a number of different malignant neoplasms, and with the use of anabolic androgenic steroids and oral contraceptives. Although it is usually asymptomatic, benign, and diagnosed incidentally, peliosis can cause liver failure and the lesions can rupture.

Sinusoidal dilation without peliosis has been associated with the use of corticosteroids and oral contraceptives and has been observed near space-occupying lesions of the liver. In the latter case, the lesion may reflect local mechanical obstruction of the microcirculation.

PORTAL HYPERTENSION

Increased portal vein pressure caused by extrahepatic portal vein obstruction, increased hepatic blood inflow, or increased resistance to hepatic blood outflow. The veins of the portal venous system carry all blood from the abdominal GI tract, spleen, pancreas, and gallbladder back to the heart through the liver. The portal vein is formed posterior to the head of the pancreas at the level of the 2nd lumbar vertebra by union of the splenic and superior mesenteric veins. At the porta hepatis it divides into 2 main branches; its intrahepatic distribution is segmental, with terminal portal venules draining into the sinusoids. The portal vein carries about 1 to 1.2 L of blood/min and 70% of the O_2 supplied to the liver. The portal venous system is valveless; its pressure, produced and maintained by the volume of inflow and resistance to outflow, is normally < 13 mm Hg. Portal venous inflow includes everything up to the level of the sinusoids. It is controlled by the sympathetic nervous system and is therefore responsive to certain vasoactive drugs and hormones. The venous outflow tracts, the hepatic venules and veins, are passive conduits unreactive to neurogenic and other stimulation. The normal portal vein pressure is therefore chiefly controlled by variations in inflow.

Portal hypertension depends on increased inflow and/or increased resistance to outflow. However, the response of the portal venous pressure to increases in hepatic

blood flow is not linear. Furthermore it is limited, and the portal vein pressure does not usually rise above 25 mm Hg. Therefore, most cases of portal hypertension not caused by extrahepatic portal vein obstruction are thought to be caused by increased resistance to hepatic blood outflow.

Pathogenesis

The creation of arteriovenous or venous-venous anastomoses, the creation of abnormal and conflicting inflow currents, and mechanical compression and distortion of effluent channels by fibrous septa and parenchymal nodules are sufficient to explain the portal hypertension of cirrhosis (see Ch. 70). However, the basis for the postsinusoidal portal hypertension of partial nodular transformation, biliary cirrhosis, the late stages of a hepatic artery-portal vein fistula, or the late stages of schistosomiasis remains unexplained.

Most consequences of portal hypertension are associated with the development of portal-systemic anastomoses formed in order to return splanchnic blood to the heart. These collateral vessels develop along the falciform ligament and into the left renal vein via the splenic, diaphragmatic, or pancreatic veins, where protective epithelium adjoins absorptive epithelium, as in the cardia of the stomach, and where abdominal organs contact retroperitoneal tissues or adhere to the abdominal wall. Thus, blood returns to the heart via the azygos-hemiazygos system, the inferior vena cava, or the pulmonary veins. The metabolic effects of this collateral circulation are not yet fully understood: they include the development of portal-systemic encephalopathy (see Ch. 67); reduced uptake of O_2, nutrients, metabolites, and drugs by the liver; and the production of antibodies against gut-derived antigens, which would normally be degraded in the liver.

Symptoms, Signs, and Diagnosis

Clinically, portal hypertension is most often associated with cirrhosis and therefore, in this situation, the patient can present with splenomegaly, ascites, GI bleeding, or portal-systemic encephalopathy.

A plain x-ray of the abdomen may show splenomegaly. Ultrasound of the abdomen may show an enlarged portal vein and portal-systemic collaterals. Esophageal varices may be visualized by radiologic technics or endoscopy, and a combined approach is often used.

In any candidate for portal surgery, the patency of the portal vein and other relevant vascular anatomy should be determined by angiography.

Portal venous pressure can be measured by several approaches. **Intrasplenic pressure** can be measured by percutaneous insertion of a catheter into the red pulp of the spleen. This procedure is simple, safe, and repeatable. **Pressure in the portal vein** itself can be measured at operation or by omphaloportography. **Intrahepatic pressure,** obtained by percutaneous liver puncture, also reflects portal vein pressure, but is rarely used. The **wedged hepatic vein pressure,** obtained by insertion of a catheter into a hepatic vein until it can be advanced no further, is easy, safe, and reliable, but does not usually provide information concerning the patency of the portal vein. The sinusoidal or postsinusoidal pressure thus obtained reflects the portal venous pressure in most cases of chronic liver disease.

Portal hypertension can be classified as prehepatic, hepatic, or posthepatic, according to the site of vascular obstruction. Furthermore, the combination of the wedged hepatic vein pressure and one of the prehepatic measurements of portal vein pressure permits classification of intrahepatic portal hypertension into presinusoidal and postsinusoidal categories. In **presinusoidal portal hypertension,** only the prehepatic portal vein pressure is elevated; in **postsinusoidal portal hypertension,** both the prehepatic portal vein and the wedged hepatic vein pressures are elevated. **Prehepatic portal hypertension**

results from a block in the splenic or portal vein. **Intrahepatic presinusoidal portal hypertension** can occur in the early stages of schistosomiasis, congenital hepatic fibrosis, granulomatous infiltrations, myeloproliferative disease of the liver, acute alcoholic fatty liver, and acute viral hepatitis. **Intrahepatic postsinusoidal portal hypertension** is associated with the later stages of schistosomiasis, veno-occlusive disease **(VOD)** of the liver, partial nodular transformation of the liver, and almost all cases of cirrhosis. **Posthepatic portal hypertension** is caused by hepatic vein outflow block and can be found with prolonged tricuspid insufficiency, constrictive pericarditis, and obstructive diseases of the hepatic venous system (eg, the Budd-Chiari syndrome, VOD, and sickle cell disease).

Treatment

The patient with portal hypertension presenting with an acute upper GI hemorrhage should be hospitalized regardless of the size of the hemorrhage (see also Ch. 53). Encephalopathy should be anticipated and no sedatives administered. The patient should be given a reduced protein intake, neomycin or lactulose orally, cleansing enemas, and blood transfusions as clinically indicated. Vitamin K_1, though often ineffective in the presence of severe parenchymal cell disease, should be given parenterally to the patient.

Vasopressin lowers the portal pressure at least temporarily in many cases and in general it is the initial routine treatment of bleeding esophageal varices. It can be given as 20 u. in 1 dL glucose IV over 10 min with the patient sitting on a bedpan and forewarned of abdominal pain. A satisfactory response in terms of bleeding is not specific for variceal bleeding, since erosive gastritis and peptic ulceration can also respond to the mesenteric vasoconstriction induced by vasopressin. Reduction in hepatic artery flow is undesirable, but at present no alternative method of lowering portal pressure is available. Furthermore, vasopressin causes coronary vasoconstriction, and evidence of myocardial ischemia is a *contraindication* to its use. Vasopressin may be repeated q 3 to 4 h if rebleeding occurs, but its efficacy usually diminishes with continued use. Glypressin (triglycyl lysine vasopressin) produces fewer side effects and may prove to be more effective. The use of vasopressin and its analogs in the management of acute variceal bleeding remains controversial. Somatostatin probably acts in a manner similar to vasopressin and its analog, but its use needs further investigation. That these agents ultimately fail to control hemorrhage reflects the degree of liver failure rather than the treatment.

Esophageal tamponade by means of a Sengstaken-Blakemore tube should be attempted if vasopressin fails, but its use is associated with such a high complication rate that it should be restricted to specialized centers. Esophageal tamponade will control variceal bleeding most effectively, but rebleeding occurs in up to 60% of cases. Complications, most relating to faulty technic, include aspiration pneumonia, esophageal rupture, and asphyxia.

Endoscopic sclerotherapy, used initially in the 1930s, but neglected for decades, is becoming increasingly used as the treatment of choice in patients whose variceal bleeding has been brought under control by nature, vasopressin, or balloon tamponade. However, 40% of patients will rebleed, overall mortality may not be reduced, the complication rate can be as high as 40%, and at least 50% of patients experience recurrence of varices. In spite of these figures, sclerotherapy may prove to be safer and more effective than the alternative technics available for the long-term management of varices that have bled.

From the time of admission to the hospital, every patient with an upper GI hemorrhage should be under the care of a surgeon as well as a physician. Most centers still prefer to submit the patient with cirrhosis complicated by variceal bleeding to elective rather than emergency surgery. Insufficient evidence exists to justify the claim that the

selective decompression of gastroesophageal varices achieved through a distal splenorenal shunt provides somewhat better long-term results than either the classic portacaval or splenorenal shunt. Complications associated with portal decompressive surgery include deterioration of liver function, the development of disabling portal-systemic encephalopathy, and hemosiderosis. Portacaval decompression usually prevents repeat hemorrhage from the varices; other long-term benefits to the patient remain to be established. Patients in whom portal diversion produces a low residual intrahepatic venous pressure can be identified. The potentially valuable observation that these patients experience either early death or chronic encephalopathy after portal decompressive surgery of any kind has not yet been confirmed.

Widespread dissatisfaction with the safety and efficacy of portal decompressive surgery has led to the introduction of other approaches to variceal hemorrhage. These approaches, none of them studied in a prospective and adequately controlled manner, include transhepatic obliteration of the varices, laser coagulation of the varices, and esophageal transection. These approaches have also involved the use of propranolol, a nonselective adrenergic β-blocker that can reduce portal pressure. Unfortunately, the results of trials to date have been contradictory, and it is clear that many patients do not respond satisfactorily.

The relative merits of sclerotherapy, decompressive surgery, and drugs (eg, propranolol) in the long-term treatment of patients with portal hypertension who have experienced variceal bleeding have not yet been clarified.

VASCULAR DISORDERS OF THE LIVER ASSOCIATED WITH SYSTEMIC DISEASE

Circulatory Failure

In **acute heart failure,** ischemic changes of the liver are common. Histologically, the liver features necrosis of the hepatocytes and congestion in Zone 3. The inflammatory response is usually modest and the lobular architecture retained.

With **chronic heart failure** the liver is usually firm. Its nutmeg appearance on cross-section is produced by the association of dark, congested Zone 3 areas and pale, sometimes fatty, Zone I areas. Fibrosis is frequent, but cirrhosis is rare; its pathogenesis requires repeated, prolonged episodes of heart failure. Histologically one finds congestion and loss of hepatocytes in Zone 3. The areas of necrosis can join and in severe cases Zone 3 to Zone 3 bridging can be found. The lobular reticulin framework can be destroyed and new collagen forms around the terminal hepatic veins.

Diagnostically, acute cardiac decompensation can present with elevations of the aminotransferases to ranges suggesting acute hepatitis. **Therapeutically,** efforts are directed toward the underlying heart disease.

Sickle Cell Disease (see Ch. 96)

Liver damage due to impaired sinusoidal blood flow is common in sickle cell disease. Aggregates of erythrocytes and thrombi obstruct the sinusoids, especially in Zone 3 and lead to sinusoidal congestion and focal necrosis. The Kupffer cells are enlarged and contain ceroid, hemosiderin, and phagocytosed erythrocytes. While primarily an ischemic lesion, the clinical presentation can mimic acute viral or toxic hepatitis. Sickle cell disease can be associated with the Budd-Chiari syndrome (see above).

Rendu-Osler-Weber Disease (see Ch. 99)

In hereditary hemorrhagic telangiectasia one may find telangiectasia, hemangioma, fibrosis, and cirrhosis of the liver. The associated arteriovenous shunting can produce an enlarged liver with a palpable thrill and continuous bruit. High output cardiac failure can be severe and can further compromise the integrity of the liver.

77. NEOPLASMS OF THE LIVER

(See also Ch. 105)

BENIGN NEOPLASMS OF THE LIVER

Benign liver tumors are relatively common, but most are subclinical. Many are detected incidentally by ultrasound **(US)** or other scanning technics. Others are discovered because of hepatomegaly, right upper quadrant discomfort, or intraperitoneal hemorrhage. Liver function tests are normal or only trivially elevated. The diagnosis is often established only at laparotomy, although scanning technics and arteriography may provide preoperative clues.

Hepatocellular adenoma is the most important benign neoplasm of the liver. Seen primarily in women of childbearing age, its prevalence has increased due to the widespread use of oral contraceptives, which appear to play a role in pathogenesis (see also Chs. 72 and 174). Most are asymptomatic, but it may present as an acute surgical abdominal problem due to abrupt rupture and bleeding into the peritoneal cavity. Though not generally precancerous, a few cases with malignant transformation have been described. Contraceptive-related adenomas often regress if the drug is stopped. **Focal nodular hyperplasia** is a similar localized tumorlike disorder that histologically may resemble macronodular cirrhosis and is a hamartoma rather than a true neoplasm. Oral contraceptives have been implicated in enhancing the size of the lesion, but are probably not causative. Related variants exist, and histopathologic overlap with adenoma may occur.

Asymptomatic small **hemangiomas** are relatively common in adults and often have a characteristic appearance on US or CT scan; they should be left alone. In infants, large hemangiomas occasionally become apparent because of associated consumption coagulopathy or hemodynamic disturbances. **Bile duct adenomas** and a variety of rare **mesenchymal neoplasms** also occur.

HEPATIC CYSTS

Hepatic cysts are not neoplasms, but are conveniently considered with benign tumors. **Isolated cysts** are commonly detected incidentally on abdominal US or CT scan, and have no clinical significance. The rare **congenital polycystic liver** produces progressive lumpy hepatomegaly, sometimes of giant proportions, in adults. Nevertheless, hepatocellular function is remarkably well preserved and portal hypertension does not develop. In contrast, the related **congenital hepatic fibrosis** is characterized by cystic proliferation of microscopic bile ducts, hepatic fibrosis, and progressive portal hypertension; the condition is often misdiagnosed as cryptogenic cirrhosis. Both variants are commonly associated with polycystic disease of the kidneys and other organs (see CYSTIC DISORDERS in Ch. 156). Other cystic lesions of the liver include **hydatid cysts** (see DISEASES CAUSED BY WORMS in Ch. 13); the rare **Caroli's disease,** characterized by segmental cystic dilation of intrahepatic bile ducts (often complicated by stone formation and cholangitis); and true cystic neoplasms (rare).

MALIGNANT NEOPLASMS OF THE LIVER

METASTATIC CARCINOMA OF THE LIVER

This is by far the most common form of hepatic tumor. The liver provides a fertile bed for bloodborne metastases; lung, breast, colon, pancreas, and stomach are the most frequent primary sites, though virtually any source may be responsible. Hepatic spread is not uncommonly the initial clinical manifestation of cancer elsewhere.

Clinically, nonspecific evidence of malignancy is frequent (eg, weight loss, anorexia, and fever). The liver is characteristically enlarged and hard, and may be tender; massive hepatomegaly with easily palpable lumps signifies advanced disease. Hepatic bruits and pleuritic-like pain with an overlying friction rub are uncommon but characteristic signs. Splenomegaly is occasionally present, especially with a primary pancreatic cancer. Concomitant ascites is frequent, but jaundice is usually absent or mild until the late stages unless biliary obstruction by tumor coexists. Alkaline phosphatase, and sometimes LDH, typically increase earlier or to a greater degree than other liver function tests. Bilirubin and aminotransferase levels are variable.

Diagnosis of hepatic metastases is usually easy in the late stages, but often difficult in patients without advanced disease. Various scanning technics are widely used in diagnosis (see also Ch. 68 and SPECIFIC ORGAN IMAGING TECHNICS in Ch. 266); though often highly suggestive, they cannot detect small metastases or reliably discriminate tumor from cirrhosis and other benign causes of an abnormal appearance. In general, however, US and CT scanning are more accurate than radionuclide scans; most centers now use US as the primary investigation. Routine screening for metastases by means of US and liver function tests is widely practiced in patients with known malignancy; this is reasonable when treatment depends on whether spread has occurred, but low sensitivity and specificity limit the value.

Liver biopsy provides the definitive diagnosis and should be done if doubt exists or histologic proof is required for therapeutic decisions. Biopsy gives positive results in about ⅔ of cases; another 10% can be identified by cytologic examination of aspirated fluid, and the yield can be increased by US-guided biopsy. Some authorities prefer biopsy under direct vision through a laparoscope, though this is more complex.

Treatment of hepatic metastases is usually futile.

Systemic chemotherapy may cause temporary shrinkage and prolong life, depending on the primary, but will not cure the disease. Radiotherapy to the liver is occasionally helpful for severe pain, but is not otherwise warranted. Some surgeons will resect isolated metastases, especially from a colonic primary, though this is not widely accepted. Most patients with extensive disease are best managed by palliative therapy.

PRIMARY CANCERS OF THE LIVER

HEPATOCELLULAR CARCINOMA
(Hepatoma)

Hepatocellular carcinoma is much less common than metastatic disease in most areas of the world, but is an important cause of death in certain areas of Africa and Southeast Asia where it is the most common internal malignancy. Chronic hepatitis B virus **(HBV)** infection is largely responsible for the high prevalence of the tumor in endemic areas; the risk is several hundred-fold higher among HBV carriers, and tumor incidence generally parallels HBV prevalence geographically. In HBV carriers, most of whom are asymptomatic, viral DNA eventually becomes incorporated into the host genome of infected hepatocytes. In time this leads to malignant transformation, though the precise mechanism is unknown. Environmental carcinogens may also play a role; eg, ingestion of food contaminated with fungal aflatoxins is believed by many to contribute to the high incidence of hepatoma in subtropical regions.

In North America, Europe, and other areas of low prevalence, at least half the patients have underlying cirrhosis: Alcoholic, postnecrotic, and especially hemochromatotic cirrhosis all have a propensity to malignant transformation, though primary biliary cirrhosis curiously does not. As noted above, malignant transformation of hepatic adenomas can occur, but this is rare. The remaining patients have no apparent underlying hepatic disorder.

Symptoms and Signs

Abdominal pain, weight loss, a right upper quadrant mass, or unexplained deterioration in a previously stable patient with cirrhosis are the most common clinical presentations. Fever is relatively frequent and may simulate infection. Occasionally the first manifestation is an acute abdominal emergency due to rupture or hemorrhage of the tumor. Interesting systemic metabolic manifestations sometimes occur, including hypoglycemia, erythrocytosis, hypercalcemia, and hyperlipidemia.

Findings on physical examination are usually nondistinctive. Painful or growing hepatomegaly, a hepatic friction rub, or a bruit should suggest the diagnosis, especially in patients with known cirrhosis or in endemic areas.

Diagnosis

Except for the presence of α-fetoprotein in serum, biochemical tests are of little diagnostic help. This is a fetal protein that disappears soon after birth; its presence in the adult signifies dedifferentiation of hepatocytes and is thus most characteristically seen in hepatocellular carcinoma. Values > 400 ng/mL are typical and are otherwise rare except in teratocarcinoma of the testis, a much less common tumor. Lower values are less specific and occur with hepatocellular regeneration (eg, in hepatitis). Most hepatomas in endemic geographic areas are associated with markedly elevated α-fetoprotein levels; high levels are less frequent in low-prevalence areas.

Abdominal US and CT scanning are useful diagnostic aids and can sometimes detect subclinical carcinomas; US screening of chronic HBV carriers is now done for this purpose in some high-prevalence areas (eg, Japan). Scanning technics are less valuable in patients with underlying cirrhosis, because results are more difficult to interpret. Hepatic arteriography often gives characteristic findings of tumor and should be considered if the diagnosis is strongly suspected, and to outline the vascular anatomy when surgery is planned.

Liver biopsy proves the diagnosis and has a high yield, especially when done under US guidance; the risk is generally low, but is increased if the tumor is highly vascular or necrotic.

Prognosis and Treatment

The prognosis for hepatocellular carcinoma is usually grim, and treatment is generally unsatisfactory. Surgical resection provides the best hope, but is suitable in only a minority of cases. Occasional patients with localized small tumors have prolonged survival after resection, but in most patients the diagnosis is established late, and death occurs within a few months. The tumor is not radiosensitive, and results of chemotherapy are usually unimpressive even when given by hepatic artery infusion. An uncommon histologic variant, fibrolamellar carcinoma, tends to afflict younger patients without underlying liver disease, and has a generally better prognosis.

Other Primary Malignancies of the Liver

Cholangiocarcinoma, tumor arising from intrahepatic biliary epithelium, is common in the Orient where underlying infestation with liver flukes is believed partially responsible. Elsewhere it is less frequent than hepatocellular carcinoma. Histologic overlap between the two may occur. Patients with longstanding ulcerative colitis occasionally develop cholangiocarcinoma. **Hepatoblastoma** is one of the more common cancers of infants; it occasionally presents with precocious puberty due to ectopic gonadotropin production, but is usually detected because of failing systemic health and a right upper quadrant mass. The rare **angiosarcoma** has recently attracted attention because of an association with industrial exposure to vinyl chloride. For all these tumors, diagnosis is based on histologic assessment. Therapy is usually of little value, and the prognosis is poor.

HEMATOLOGIC MALIGNANCIES AND THE LIVER

Hepatic involvement in **leukemia** and related disorders is common, due to infiltration with the abnormal cells. The diagnosis is usually apparent from hematologic assessment, and liver biopsy is not needed. Diagnosing **hepatic lymphoma**, especially Hodgkin's disease, is more complex. Knowledge of liver involvement is important for staging and therapeutic decisions, but unfortunately there is poor correlation among clinical, biochemical, and histologic findings. Hepatomegaly and abnormal liver function tests may reflect a nonspecific reaction to Hodgkin's disease elsewhere rather than true liver involvement, and biopsy often shows nondescript focal mononuclear infiltrates or granulomas of uncertain significance. The role of periteonoscopy or open biopsy is still debated.

---

78. EXTRAHEPATIC BILIARY DISORDERS

Physiology of Bile Acid Metabolism

Bile is formed in the liver as an isosmotic solution of bile acids, electrolytes, bilirubin, cholesterol, and phospholipids. Of these constituents, the quantity of bile acids best correlates with total volume output of bile.

The liver synthesizes bile acids from cholesterol, although precise mechanisms and regulation are incompletely understood. Cholic and chenodeoxycholic acids are the 2 primary bile acids formed in the liver in a ratio of about 2:1, and constitute 80% of bile acids in man. After virtually complete conjugation in the hepatocyte with both glycine and taurine, conjugated bile acids are excreted in bile. Bile then flows from the intrahepatic collecting system into the proximal or common hepatic duct. About 50% of bile secreted in the fasting state passes into the gallbladder via the cystic duct; the rest flows directly into the distal or common bile duct. Up to 90% of water in gallbladder bile is absorbed as an electrolyte solution, principally via gallbladder mucosal intracellular pathways. Bile remaining in the gallbladder is thus a concentrated solution primarily of bile acids and Na.

During fasting, bile acids are concentrated in the gallbladder, and there is little bile-acid–dependent bile flow from the liver. When food enters the duodenum, an exquisite hormonal and neural sequence is set in motion. Cholecystokinin and perhaps other GI hormone peptides (eg, gastrin-releasing peptide) are released from duodenal mucosa; cholecystokinin stimulates the gallbladder to contract and the biliary sphincter to relax. Bile flows into the duodenum to mix with food contents and carry out its several functions: (1) Bile salts, the water-soluble excretory products of cholesterol, remove more cholesterol as they form mixed micelles. (2) Bile acids increase the solubility of dietary fats to facilitate their absorption and that of fat-soluble vitamins. (3) Bile acids induce water secretion by the colon as they enter that organ, and thus promote catharsis. (4) Bilirubin is excreted in bile as a mixture of degradation products of heme compounds from worn out RBCs.

When food enters the duodenum, gallbladder contraction releases a large proportion of the total body pool of bile acids into the small intestine. Bile acids are poorly absorbed by passive diffusion in the proximal small intestine, but most of the pool reaches the terminal ileum, where 90% is absorbed into the portal venous circulation by an active transport process. Bile salts are efficiently extracted by the liver and then promptly modified and secreted back into bile. The fraction of bile acids cleared by the liver remains relatively constant and independent of the concentrations presented to it. The rise in hepatic excretion of bile salts following each meal is thus a function of the increased concentration of portal vein bile acids coming from the ileum.

The total body pool normally contains 3 to 4 gm of bile acids, which undergo an

interplay between forces for and against nucleation, which include the action of specific proteins or apoproteins, gallbladder mucin, or gallbladder stasis.

Virtually all gallstones form within the gallbladder. With rare exceptions, stones form behind biliary duct strictures due to stasis, or in bile ducts after cholecystectomy.

Symptoms and Signs

Virtually all possibile clinical consequences of gallstone formation occur, though with what frequencies is often unclear. Most patients remain asymptomatic for long periods, frequently for life. Stones may traverse the cystic duct with or without symptoms of obstruction. Transient cystic duct obstruction results in colicky pain, while persistent obstruction usually produces inflammation and acute cholecystitis (see below). Most obstructive events are transient, producing biliary colic lasting up to several hours. Pain location varies, but most often is in the epigastrium or right upper quadrant, radiating to the right lower scapula. The typical pain is constant, progressively rising to a plateau and falling gradually. Nausea and vomiting are frequently associated. Fever and chills are absent in uncomplicated gallbladder colic. The patient or physician may note some right upper quadrant tenderness.

Calculi that pass from the gallbladder into the common bile duct may remain there quietly and indefinitely or may pass into the duodenum with or without symptoms. Silent common duct stones are often undetected until they obstruct the biliary or pancreatic ducts producing severe disease: pain, jaundice, pancreatitis, or infection **(cholangitis).** Finally, large stones that erode through the gallbladder wall may rarely obstruct the small intestine **(gallstone ileus).** Acute cholecystitis and the rarer complications of pancreatitis or cholangitis rarely occur as the first manifestation of gallstone disease; they are usually preceded by recurrent episodes of colic. Complications increase when the patient is acutely ill, has serious disease in other organ systems, or is subjected to other procedures (eg, common duct exploration). These risk factors require careful evaluation in individual patients, in relation to the severity of disease being considered for treatment.

Symptoms of dyspepsia and fatty food intolerance are often inaccurately ascribed to gallbladder disease. Belching, bloating, fullness, or nausea are associated about equally with gallstones, peptic ulcer disease, or functional distress. Such symptoms may disappear after cholecystectomy, but should not comprise the only indication for operation. Postprandial fatty food intolerance is more likely due to gallstones if symptoms include right upper quadrant pain.

Diagnosis

Methods of evaluating calculi in the gallbladder or in the common duct have improved and increased in recent years. Few calculi escape detection. The relative accuracy, ease, safety, and cost of diagnostic methods are subject to change, to debate, and to local availability and skills.

Real time ultrasonography is the diagnostic method of choice for evaluating possible gallbladder calculi. Static B mode sonography and **oral cholecystography** are also sensitive and specific. Sensitivity (*diagnosis of disease present*) is 98%; specificity (*not making a diagnosis when disease is not present*) is satisfactory, usually approaching 90%. Further information on US can be found in Ch. 68.

Treatment

Asymptomatic gallstones: Since they are often discovered during evaluation of other problems, the question arises whether to recommend observation or elective gallbladder removal for cholelithiasis. Neither choice will fit all circumstances. While the natural history is unpredictable in any individual with asymptomatic gallstones, there is a cumulative chance (about 1 to 2%/yr) of developing symptoms. Most patients with clinically silent gallstones will decide that the discomfort, expense, and risk of purely elective surgery is not worth the potential gain of removing an organ that may never

enterohepatic circulation 10 to 12 times/day. During each pass, a small amount of primary bile acids reach the colon where anaerobic bacteria containing 7α-hydroxylase form secondary bile acids. Cholic acid is converted to deoxycholic acid, which is largely reabsorbed and conjugated, acting much like its primary predecessor. Chenodeoxycholic acid conjugates are converted in the colon to their secondary bile acid form, lithocholic acid. This insoluble secondary bile acid is partially reabsorbed; the rest is lost in the feces.

Anatomy of the Biliary Tract

Other than absorptive functions of the normal gallbladder and storage mediation by the sphincters, the extrahepatic ductal system is a passive conduit. There are no functional smooth muscle fibers in the biliary duct walls. Ductal secretions stimulated by secretin contain a high concentration of bicarbonate and contribute variably to total bile volume.

The Vaterian segment consists of the terminal intramural segments of both biliary and pancreatic ducts and the 2 or 3 sphincter segments and soft tissue surrounding them. The sphincter of Oddi surrounds both ducts or their common channel and each duct has its separate (inconstant) sphincter. The sphincters have a basal "tone" of up to 10 mm Hg and a phasic spike activity that is independent of duodenal smooth muscle activity. These muscles are responsive to extremely small amounts of hormones, GI peptides, anticholinergics, and other drugs. Much is being learned about these important and exquisitely tuned structures located at the nutritionally important confluence of bile, pancreatic juice, and food. Normal sphincter function results in timely release of bile and pancreatic enzymes during food passage; during fasting, however, gallbladder filling is facilitated. The 2 systems normally remain independent; ie, bile does not flow retrograde into the pancreatic duct.

BILIARY CALCULI

(Gallstones)

Presence of calculi in the gallbladder **(cholelithiasis)** *or in the biliary ducts* **(choledocholithiasis)**.

Most clinical disorders of the extrahepatic biliary tract are related to gallstone problems, which are more frequent in women and in some ethnic groups (eg, North American Indians) and increase with age. In the USA, 20% of persons over age 65 have gallstones and each year > 500,000 undergo cholecystectomy. Other factors that increase the probability of gallstones include obesity, a Western diet, and a family history of gallstones.

Pathophysiology

Cholesterol, the major component of most gallstones, is highly insoluble in water. By incorporation into micelles, cholesterol is tremendously solubilized, and thus normally excreted in bile. Bile salt micelles are *aggregates of bile salts in which water-soluble (ionic) regions of the molecule face outward into aqueous solution, while the water-insoluble (nonpolar) steroid nuclei face inwards.* Cholesterol is soluble in the interior of these spheroid micelles, and their cholesterol-carrying ability is further enhanced by the additions of lecithin, a polar phospholipid.

Why do some persons develop gallstones while others do not? Supersaturation of cholesterol in native bile solution is a necessary condition, but not a sole cause, of cholesterol gallstone formation, since supersaturation is frequent in bile of fasting persons without gallstones. The other critical factor in determining whether gallstones form is the regulation of the initiating process, cholesterol monohydrate crystal formation. In gallbladder bile that is lithogenic, there is supersaturation of cholesterol and also relatively rapid nucleation of cholesterol crystals. There may normally be dynamic

cause clinical illness although the potential complications represent serious disease. However, if symptoms appear, active therapy is clearly advisable.

Symptomatic gallstones: Biliary colic recurs with very irregular, pain-free intervals of days or months. Symptoms are often not progressive in severity or frequency, but neither do they cease altogether. With development of symptoms the patient is at increased risk of developing complications. Diets and drugs are not helpful substitutes for cholecystectomy, which is indicated for most patients. If cholecystectomy is performed for disease clearly of gallbladder origin, symptoms may confidently be expected to cease. Nonspecific symptoms of postprandial dyspepsia also remit in patients who have had colic. Colic recurring, even years later, should prompt an evaluation for possible common duct stones. Cholecystectomy does not result in nutritional problems and no dietary limitations are required postoperatively. When the gallbladder is removed by a trained surgeon during an elective period free of complications, the procedure is relatively safe with a mortality of 0.1 to 0.5%.

Drug therapy: Gallbladder calculi may sometimes be dissolved in vivo by giving bile acids orally for many months. The bile salt usually given is chenodiol 15 mg/kg/day, which acts in part by reducing hepatic synthesis and biliary secretion of cholesterol. Cholesterol saturation of bile is reduced and cholesterol-containing stones may slowly dissolve. Gallstones may dissolve completely in 30 to 40% of patients at this dose, but recurrence of stones and colic after cessation of drug is usual. Ursodeoxycholic acid (an investigational drug) may be used (10 mg/kg/day) with the same clinical expectations, but without the diarrhea or disturbed liver function seen in occasional patients on the earlier drug.

Potential candidates for this therapy must have stones readily visible in a gallbladder that opacifies on cholecystography. Progress is checked by periodic cholecystography and/or ultrasound studies. Bile acid therapy is continued for 2 yr during which time symptoms of colic often continue. Indications for drug therapy are unclear at present. Treatment is ineffective or contraindicated in the presence of (1) stones that are calcified, very large, or made up of bile pigment; (2) pregnancy; (3) liver disease; (4) a nonfunctioning gallbladder; and (5) obesity. The place of dissolution therapy is presently a minor one, although further developments may be expected.

CHOLECYSTITIS

CHRONIC CHOLECYSTITIS

A pathologic term for a thick-walled, fibrotic, contracted gallbladder; clinically, it is used to describe chronic gallbladder disease characterized by symptoms that include recurrent colic. The mucosa may be ulcerated and scarred and the lumen contains mud or stones, frequently obstructing the cystic duct. One is tempted to ascribe these findings to the ravages and repair of previous episodes of acute cholecystitis, but the clinical history may not include any record of such events. Poor correlation exists between clinical and pathologic manifestations. Both are nearly always associated with calculi in the gallbladder.

ACUTE CHOLECYSTITIS

Acute inflammation of the gallbladder wall, usually as a response to cystic duct obstruction by a gallstone.

Although this is the most common consequence of cholelithiasis, the pathophysiologic events are not completely understood. Secretion of fluid by the gallbladder mucosa against an obstructed cystic duct may regularly occur. Constituents of bile,

including bile salts, lysolecithin, and even cholesterol, may be altered, thus inducing mucosal inflammation. Arterial occlusion and ischemia may be late changes. Acute cholecystitis is not due to bacterial infection except in rare instances, and intraoperative gallbladder bile cultures taken during the first few days of illness are positive in < 1/3 of cases. Acute cholecystitis is accompanied by gallbladder stones in at least 95% of patients.

When acute cholecystitis occurs in the absence of calculi, **(acute acalculous cholecystitis)**, it is a serious disease that tends to occur in adults and children already ill after trauma, operations, burns, sepsis, or critical illness. Prolonged use of total parenteral alimentation predisposes to bile stasis and acute acalculous cholecystitis. Prior symptoms suggesting gallbladder disease are usually absent. Symptoms and signs are typical of cholecystitis, although the clinical course is often fulminant, with gangrene or perforation. Surgical management is urgently indicated. The pathology includes intense vascular injury, edema, and focal necrosis, principally involving the muscularis and serosa.

Symptoms and Signs

Acute cholecystitis begins with acute colicky pain, which 75% of patients have previously experienced. Pain becomes severe, localizing to the right upper quadrant and often radiating around to the right lower scapular. Nausea and vomiting are usual. Within a few hours physical findings include involuntary guarding of right-sided abdominal muscles, without rebound tenderness at first. The gallbladder becomes palpable in < 1/2 of cases. Painful splinting of respiration during deep inspiration and right upper quadrant palpation **(Murphy's sign)** is frequently present. Fever is low grade at first and neutrophilic leukocytosis is modest.

A typical episode of acute cholecystitis improves in 2 to 3 days and resolves within a week. Failure to do so suggests serious complications. High fever, leukocytosis, rigors, taken with findings of rebound tenderness or ileus suggest empyema, gangrene, or perforation, which require urgent surgical management. When acute cholecystitis is suspected, jaundice or cholestasis suggest partial common duct obstruction by calculi or by contiguous inflammation. Amylase elevation suggests, but is not diagnostic of gallstone pancreatitis.

Diagnosis

Clinically suspected acute cholecystitis is most accurately confirmed by hepatobiliary scintigraphy and ultrasound. Iminodiacetic acid compounds labeled with technetium 99m are rapidly taken up and excreted by the normal liver after IV injection. Using isotope scanning technics, the liver, extrahepatic bile ducts, gallbladder, and duodenum are sequentially visualized. Nonvisualization of the gallbladder with normal visualization of liver and bile ducts virtually always indicates cystic duct obstruction, and this finding supports a clinical diagnosis of acute cholecystitis with 95% sensitivity. Real-time ultrasonography is valuable for confirming the presence of cholelithiasis, and demonstration of gallbladder wall thickening is helpful when present.

The clinical diagnosis of acute cholecystitis may be difficult when findings are atypical, and cholangitis, pancreatitis, appendicitis, peptic ulcer, or pleurisy may be considered. Each has distinguishing clinical features, and hepatobiliary scanning and ultrasound provide strong evidence for acute cholecystitis.

Treatment

Management includes rehydration with IV fluids and electrolytes. No oral feedings are given, and nasogastric suction is instituted. Antibiotics may be indicated later in the course of complicated disease.

Cholecystectomy is indicated for management of acute cholecystitis. When the diagnosis is clear and the patient is a standard surgical risk, operation may be scheduled as

an early but elective procedure during the first day or two of the illness. When further management of other system (usually cardiorespiratory) disease is likely to reduce surgical risk, cholecystectomy may be deferred and medical management continued. If the acute illness subsides, subsequent or late cholecystectomy may be planned at least 6 wk later. Whenever complications of empyema, gangrene, or perforation are suspected, urgent surgical management is indicated. Cholecystectomy cures acute cholecystitis and biliary colic in nearly all patients.

Postcholecystectomy pain: After cholecystectomy a small percent of patients experience new or recurrent biliary colic-like pain. Although the pathogenesis and clinical course are poorly understood, **papillary stenosis** has been defined as *a structural or functional disorder of the Vaterian segment involving the terminal ducts and sphincters, causing pain from impedance to flow of biliary and/or pancreatic secretions.* Rarely, demonstrable **papillary fibrosis** of the sphincter area is present, perhaps due to prior inflammation or operative trauma. In the remainder of patients with **sphincter dysfunction,** no structural abnormality is evident, although disturbed function and symptoms are clearly present periodically. Both groups of patients experience periodic colicky pain with variable associated findings of transient elevation of bilirubin or liver enzymes suggesting cholestasis, or elevation of serum amylase levels. The biliary tree, and less often the pancreatic duct, may be dilated on direct cholangiography and pancreatography, with delayed drainage (> 45 min and 15 min respectively). Sphincter pressures may be elevated when measured during direct endoscopic ductal studies. Thus, findings from endoscopic retrograde cholangiopancreatography and perhaps sphincter manometry are most useful diagnostically. Small residual calculi will be discovered in some patients. Treatment by endoscopic sphincterotomy is curative in many patients, and selection criteria are being evaluated.

CHOLEDOCHOLITHIASIS

Stones in bile ducts, although present less often than in the gallbladder, are the most common cause of extrahepatic obstructive jaundice, potentially leading to serious or lethal infection (cholangitis), pancreatitis, or chronic liver disease. An obstructed biliary tree rather quickly becomes colonized, usually with gram-negative bacteria. The resulting cholangitis becomes an important potential source of bacteremia and systemic infection. Early surgical or endoscopic decompression is usually indicated.

As noted under BILIARY CALCULI, above, ductal calculi may pass quietly into the duodenum, may remain silent for long periods in the duct, or may at some time partially obstruct the terminal duct, producing either transient or persistent pain, jaundice, and infection. Patients (usually elderly) whose gallbladder stones have never caused cholecystitis or colic may experience ductal obstruction as their *initial* disease. Many common duct stones are discovered and removed during an operation for gallbladder disease. Of those missed despite assiduous search during surgery, most will clinically obstruct in ensuing months or years.

Diagnosis

Diagnostic considerations of choledocholithiasis are essentially those of extrahepatic obstructive jaundice, whether due to stones, malignancy, or benign strictures. Abdominal pain, jaundice, and chills and fever **(Charcot's triad)** are most often seen (with variations) in calculus obstruction. The diagnosis may be accurately suspected clinically, but usually requires confirmation before deciding on management.

Several methods provide diagnostic information of varying detail and accuracy, including endoscopic retrograde cholangiopancreatography **(ERCP),** percutaneous transhepatic cholangiography **(PTC),** CT, and ultrasound **(US).** Choices depend on local skill and availability, and all have their advocates. Extrahepatic obstruction is virtually always detected by a successful direct cholangiogram, and calculi are reliably

detected when present. Direct cholangiography by either ERCP or PTC has a small but definite incidence of sepsis and of failure. US and CT reliably detect ductal dilation as evidence of obstruction; however, stones obstruct undilated ducts with significant frequency.

How should an expeditious, cost effective evaluation proceed? A clinical impression of extrahepatic obstruction is usually rather accurate, based on history, physical examination, and simple laboratory tests, and can be used to dictate further definitive evaluation. Before deciding on surgical or endoscopic management, whenever extrahepatic obstruction is likely, the biliary tree and its contents should usually be visualized by direct cholangiography. US is often indicated as the initial study when the clinical picture is less clear. Results of US may suggest need for liver biopsy to evaluate intrahepatic cholestasis, and may obviate more invasive tests, at least initially.

Treatment

Despite their varied behavior, common duct stones are a potential source of major disease and should be removed when discovered. They may be removed surgically or endoscopically after initiation of antibiotic therapy and reversal of sepsis or shock.

Endoscopic retrograde sphincterotomy (ERS) is a therapeutic application of ERCP in which soft tissues and sphincter fibers of the papilla and intraduodenal duct are divided with electrocautery to permit release of ductal calculi into the duodenum. Successful emptying of the duct is expected in 90% of attempted procedures, following which patients are observed for 1 or 2 days and discharged. Mortality (0.3 to 1.0%) and morbidity (3 to 7%) are lower than reported surgical experience. Immediate morbidity is due to bleeding, pancreatitis, perforation, and cholangitis. A late 2 to 6% complication rate includes restenosis and reformed stones in open ducts.

For older patients with choledocholithiasis and prior cholecystectomy, ERS is the procedure of choice if available. When these patients present with acute cholangitis or gallstone pancreatitis, endoscopic decompression usually results in dramatic clinical improvement, as seen with surgical decompression. Patients with calculus duct obstruction and intact gallbladders should be managed by operation when there is a history of cholecystitis or colic. Differences of opinion exist with respect to a patient with calculus duct obstruction and an asymptomatic intact gallbladder. If patients are observed for 2 yr after ERS, 10 to 14% will develop symptoms that require cholecystectomy; this is probably acceptable management for patients who are at increased risk for biliary surgery.

Retained stones: When calculi remain in the bile ducts after surgery despite maximal efforts to find them, they often are discovered as cholangiography is performed postoperatively via an externally draining T-tube. Reoperation is rarely necessary.

If the T-tube diameter is > 14 mm, it may be left in place for 4 to 6 wk while the tract matures. Small stones may pass spontaneously, and remaining stones can be mechanically extracted safely at that time. ERS is reserved for mechanical extraction failures, for large stones, or for patients with small diameter T-tubes.

NEOPLASMS OF BILE DUCTS

(See also Ch. 105)

Nearly 50% of patients with extrahepatic biliary obstruction have some noncalculous cause, of which malignancy is the most frequent. Most originate in the head of the pancreas, through which the distal common duct normally courses (see CANCER OF THE PANCREAS in Ch. 55). Less common tumors may originate in the ampulla, the bile duct, gallbladder, or liver. Even less commonly, ducts may be obstructed by metastatic tumor or nodes of lymphoma. Benign tumors, most usually papilloma or villous adenoma, also occur in bile ducts and may cause obstruction.

Symptoms, Signs, and Diagnosis

Obstructive signs and symptoms are usually progressive: jaundice, variable abdominal discomfort, anorexia, weight loss, pruritus, and palpable mass or gallbladder. Fever and chills are unusual.

Diagnosis of malignant ductal obstructions is made by findings from US, CT, or direct cholangiography. Specific cytology can be obtained safely in 85% of pancreatic tumors by directed transabdominal "skinny needle" aspiration of the tumor. Needle biopsy of the liver usefully establishes the presence of metastases at times.

Treatment

Individual findings and circumstances will dictate the best management approach. Surgical exploration is the most direct means of determining resectability and specific histology, and also of providing suitable internal bypass of bile flow. Malignancies are usually not resectable for cure, with the occasional exception of primary ampullary carcinoma. Neither are they significantly responsive to radiation therapy. Recently applied chemotherapy regimens offer hope for palliation.

Alternatives to surgical management include the endoscopic placement of flexible prostheses across malignant ductal strictures to provide internal drainage of bile. Similar results are obtained by placement of relatively large prostheses across malignant strictures or external drainage of bile by a transhepatic approach. These nonsurgical drainage procedures are specifically reserved for symptomatic relief of pruritus, sepsis, or pain. Many patients with malignant obstruction mercifully never experience these problems.

NONNEOPLASTIC CAUSES OF EXTRAHEPATIC OBSTRUCTION

Conditions other than stones or neoplasms occasionally obstruct the extrahepatic ducts. Duct trauma as a result of surgery or complicated biliary disease heads the list. *Ascaris lumbricoides* rarely inhabit the biliary tree, but in the Orient, *Clonorchis sinensis* is an important cause of obstructive jaundice with intrahepatic ductal inflammation, proximal stasis, stone formation, and cholangitis (see Ch. 13).

CHOLESTEROLOSIS OF THE GALLBLADDER

Deposition of cholesterol esters in macrophages of the gallbladder lamina propria, as evident small yellow specks against the red bile-stained mucosa **(strawberry gallbladder)**; *if lipid deposition continues, polypoid excrescences may project into the lumen.* The incidence and cause of cholesterol deposition are unknown. It is not associated with supersaturation of bile or with hypercholesterolemia, but cholesterol stones are formed in 50% of patients. Oral cholecystography usually demonstrates a functioning gallbladder. Polyps may be single or multiple, occur anywhere in the gallbladder, and do not change with position of the patient. Stones may coexist. Pain is irregularly attributed to this condition and cholecystectomy may be considered for patients with convincing symptoms and/or cholelithiasisis.

DIVERTICULOSIS OF THE GALLBLADDER
(Adenomatosis)

Rokitansky-Aschoff sinuses, normally small finger-like invaginations of the gallbladder mucosa, become more evident with age, and may extend into the muscular or serosal layers as variably cystic spaces. Their appearance on cholecystogram varies from fine generalized serrations to local large outpouchings. An association may exist with chronic cholecystitis and attendant increased luminal pressures. Indication for cholecystectomy is acute or chronic cholecystitis.

§7. NUTRITIONAL AND METABOLIC DISORDERS

79. NUTRITION—GENERAL CONSIDERATIONS

NUTRITION

Nutriment, that part of food which nourishes the body, consists of micro- and macronutrients. **Micronutrients** (see TABLE 79–1) include **vitamins** and some **elements.** They are essential for health, generally are consumed in small amounts (< 1 gm/day), usually are absorbed unchanged, and many have catalytic functions. **Vitamins** are classified as fat-soluble (A, D, E, and K) or water-soluble (B group and C). The former and vitamin B_{12} tend to be stored in the body.

Many **elements** present in food are essential for health (see Ch. 82). Some, such as calcium, phosphorus, and potassium, occur in the body in concentrations > 0.005%. Others, termed **trace elements,** such as iron, zinc, and iodine, occur in much smaller concentrations (< 0.005%). Some elements (eg, barium, strontium) are suspected of being essential, but definite proof is lacking. Other elements found in the body (eg, gold, silver) have no known metabolic role.

TABLE 79–1. THE PRINCIPAL MICRONUTRIENTS (VITAMINS AND MINERALS)

Micronutrient	*Principal Sources*	*Functions*	*Effects of Deficiency and Toxicity*	*Usual Therapeutic Dosage*
Vitamin A	Fish liver oils, liver, egg yolk, butter, cream, vitamin A-fortified margarine, green leafy or yellow vegetables	Photoreceptor mechanism of retina; integrity of epithelia; lysosome stability; glycoprotein synthesis	*Deficiency:* Night blindness; perifollicular hyperkeratosis; xerophthalmia; keratomalacia *Toxicity:* Headache; peeling of skin; hepatosplenomegaly; bone thickening	10,000–20,000 μg (30,000–60,000 IU/day; see Ch. 81 for higher dosage)
Vitamin D	Ultraviolet irradiation of the skin is the major source; fortified milk is main dietary source; fish liver oils, butter, egg yolk, liver	Calcium and phosphorus absorption; resorption, mineralization, & collagen maturation of bone; tubular reabsorption of phosphorus (?)	*Deficiency:* Rickets (tetany sometimes associated); osteomalacia *Toxicity:* Anorexia; renal failure; metastatic calcification	*Primary Deficiency:* 10–40 μg (1400–1600 IU)/day *Metabolic Deficiency:* 1–2 μg/day 1,25-$(OH)_2D_3$ or 1α-$(OH)D_3$
Vitamin E group	Vegetable oil, wheat germ, leafy vegetables, egg yolk, margarine, legumes	Intracellular antioxidant; stability of biologic membranes	*Deficiency:* RBC hemolysis; creatinuria; ceroid deposition in muscle *Toxicity:* Interferes with enzymes, increased infection (?)	30–100 mg/day
Vitamin K (activity) **Vitamin K_1** (phytonadione) **Vitamin K_2**	Leafy vegetables, pork, liver, vegetable oils, intestinal flora after newborn period	Prothrombin formation; normal blood coagulation	*Deficiency:* Hemorrhage from deficient prothrombin *Toxicity:* Kernicterus	In situations conducive to neonatal hemorrhage, 2–5 mg during labor or daily for 1 wk prior; or 1–2 mg to newborn (see Ch. 81)

(Continued)

TABLE 79–1. THE PRINCIPAL MICRONUTRIENTS (VITAMINS AND MINERALS) *(Cont'd)*

Micronutrient	*Principal Sources*	*Functions*	*Effects of Deficiency and Toxicity*	*Usual Therapeutic Dosage*
Essential fatty acids (linoleic, linolenic, arachidonic acids)	Vegetable seed oils (corn, sunflower, safflower); margarines blended with vegetable oils	Synthesis of prostaglandins, membrane structure	Growth cessation, dermatosis	Up to 10 gm/day
Thiamine (vitamin B_1)	Dried yeast; whole grains; meat (especially pork, liver); enriched cereal products; nuts; legumes; potatoes	Carbohydrate metabolism; central & peripheral nerve cell function; myocardial function	Beriberi; infantile & adult (peripheral neuropathy, cardiac failure; Wernicke-Korsakoff syndrome) Dependency states (see Ch. 81)	30–100 mg/day
Riboflavin (vitamin B_2)	Milk, cheese, liver, meat, eggs, enriched cereal products	Many aspects of energy & protein metabolism; integrity of mucous membranes	Cheilosis; angular stomatitis; corneal vascularization; amblyopia; sebaceous dermatosis	10–30 mg/day
Niacin (nicotinic acid, niacinamide)	Dried yeast, liver, meat, fish, legumes, whole-grain enriched cereal products	Oxidation-reduction reactions; carbohydrate metabolism	Pellagra (dermatosis, glossitis, GI & CNS dysfunction)	Niacinamide 100–1000 mg/day
Vitamin B_6 group (pyridoxine)	Dried yeast, liver, organ meats, whole-grain cereals, fish, legumes	Many aspects of nitrogen metabolism, e.g., transaminations, porphyrin & heme synthesis, tryptophan conversion to niacin. Linoleic acid metabolism	Convulsions in infancy; anemias; neuropathy; seborrhea-like skin lesions Dependency states (see Ch. 81)	25–100 mg/day
Folic acid	Fresh green leafy vegetables, fruit, organ meats, liver, dried yeast	Maturation of RBCs; synthesis of purines & pyrimidines	Pancytopenia; megaloblastosis (especially pregnancy, infancy, malabsorption)	1 mg/day

Vitamin B_{12} (cobalamins)	Liver; meats (especially beef, pork, organ meats); eggs; milk & milk products	Maturation of RBCs; neural function; DNA synthesis, related to folate coenzymes; methionine & acetate synthesis	Pernicious anemia; fish tapeworm & vegan anemias; some psychiatric syndromes; nutritional amblyopia Dependency states (see Ch. 81)	For usual therapeutic dosage see Anemia due to vitamin B_{12} deficiency in Ch. 96
Biotin	Liver, kidney, egg yolk, yeast, cauliflower, nuts, legumes	Carboxylation & decarboxylation of oxalocetic acid; amino acid & fatty acid metabolism	Dermatitis, glossitis Dependency states (see Ch. 81)	150–300 μg/day
Vitamin C (ascorbic acid)	Citrus fruits, tomatoes, potatoes, cabbage, green peppers	Essential to osteoid tissue; collagen formation; vascular function; tissue respiration & wound healing	Scurvy (hemorrhages, loose teeth, gingivitis)	100–1000 mg/day
Sodium	Wide distribution—beef, pork, sardines, cheese, green olives, corn bread, potato chips, sauerkraut	Acid-base balance; osmotic pressure; pH blood; muscle contractility; nerve transmission; sodium pumps	*Deficiency:* Hyponatremia; confusion, coma *Toxicity:* Hypernatremia; confusion, coma	See in Ch. 84
Potassium	Wide distribution—whole and skim milk, bananas, prunes, raisins	Muscle activity, nerve transmission; intracellular acid-base balance and water retention	*Deficiency:* Hypokalemia; paralysis, cardiac disturbances *Toxicity:* Hyperkalemia; paralysis, cardiac disturbances	See in Ch. 84
Calcium	Milk and milk products, meat, fish, eggs, cereal products, beans, fruits, vegetables	Bone and tooth formation; blood coagulation; neuromuscular irritability; muscle contractility; myocardial conduction	*Deficiency:* Hypocalcemia and tetany; neuromuscular hyperexcitability *Toxicity:* Hypercalcemia; GI atony; renal failure; psychosis	10–30 mL 10% calcium gluconate soln IV in 24 h

(Continued)

TABLE 79–1. THE PRINCIPAL MICRONUTRIENTS (VITAMINS AND MINERALS) *(Cont'd)*

Micronutrient	*Principal Sources*	*Functions*	*Effects of Deficiency and Toxicity*	*Usual Therapeutic Dosage*
Phosphorus	Milk, cheese, meat, poultry, fish, cereals, nuts, legumes	Bone and tooth formation, acid-base balance, component of nucleic acids, energy production	*Deficiency:* Irritability; weakness; blood cell disorders; GI tract & renal dysfunction *Toxicity:* Hyperphosphatemia in renal failure	Potassium acid and dibasic phosphate parenteral 600 mg (18.8 mEq)/day
Magnesium	Green leaves, nuts, cereal grains, seafoods	Bone and tooth formation; nerve conduction; muscle contraction; enzyme activation	*Deficiency:* Hypomagnesemia; neuromuscular irritability *Toxicity:* Hypermagnesemia; hypotension, respiratory failure, cardiac disturbances	2–4 mL 50% magnesium sulfate soln/day IM
Iron	Wide distribution (except dairy products)—soybean flour, beef, kidney, liver, beans, clams, peaches Much unavailable (<20% absorbed)	Hemoglobin, myoglobin formation, enzymes	*Deficiency:* Anemia; dysphagia; koilonychia; enteropathy *Toxicity:* Hemochromatosis; cirrhosis; diabetes mellitus; skin pigmentation	Ferrous sulfate or gluconate 300 mg orally tid
Iodine	Seafoods, iodized salt, dairy products Water variable	Thyroxine (T_4) & triiodothyronine (T_3) formation and energy control mechanisms	*Deficiency:* Simple (colloid, endemic) goiter; cretinism; deaf-mutism *Toxicity:* occasional myxedema	150 μg iodine/day as potassium iodide added to salt 1:10–40,000 ppm

Fluorine	Wide distribution—tea, coffee Fluoridation of water supplies with sodium fluoride 1.0–2.0 ppm	Bone and tooth formation	*Deficiency:* Predisposition to dental caries; osteoporosis (?) *Toxicity:* Fluorosis, mottling, pitting of permanent teeth; exostoses of spine	Sodium fluoride 1.1–2.2 mg/day orally
Zinc	Wide distribution—vegetable sources Much unavailable	Component of enzymes and insulin; skin integrity; wound healing; growth	*Deficiency:* Growth retardation; hypogonadism; hyogeusia; in cirrhosis; acrodermatitis enteropathica	30–150 mg zinc sulfate/day orally
Copper	Wide distribution—organ meat, oysters, nuts, dried legumes, whole-grain cereals	Enzyme component; hemopoiesis; bone formation	*Deficiency:* Anemia in malnourished children; Menkes' kinky hair syndrome *Toxicity:* Hepatolenticular degeneration; some biliary cirrhosis (?)	0.3 mg/kg/day copper sulfate, orally
Cobalt	Green leafy vegetables	Part of vitamin B_{12} molecule	*Deficiency:* Anemia in children (?) *Toxicity:* Cardiomyopathy	20–30 mg/day cobaltous chloride, orally
Chromium	Wide distribution—brewer's yeast	Part of glucose tolerance factor (GTF)	*Deficiency:* Impaired glucose tolerance in malnourished children; some diabetics (?)	200 μg/day chromium chloride, orally
Selenium	Meats and other animal products reliable sources; Soil concentration influences plant content	Component of glutathione peroxidase	*Deficiency:* Cardiomyopathy of Keshan disease (?) *Toxicity:* Loss of hair and nails, dermatitis, polyneuritis (?)	100 μg/day sodium selenite, orally

Carbohydrates, fats, and **proteins** are **macronutrients** and upon digestion yield, respectively, glucose and other monosaccharides, fatty acids and glycerol, and peptides and amino acids. Macronutrients are interchangeable sources of energy; fat yields 9 kcal/gm, protein or carbohydrate yields 4 kcal/gm, and ethanol yields 7 kcal/gm.

Carbohydrate and fat spare tissue protein. If sufficient nonprotein calories are not available, from either dietary sources or tissue stores (particularly of fat), efficient use of protein for tissue maintenance, replacement, or growth does not occur and considerably more dietary protein is required for positive nitrogen balance.

The polyunsaturated fatty acids, **linoleic** (9,12-octadecadienoic), **linolenic** (9,12,15-octadecatrienoic), and **arachidonic** (5,8,11,14-eicosatetraenoic), are termed **essential fatty acids (EFA)** and unlike all other lipids must be provided by the diet. Arachidonic acid can be made in the body from linoleic acid. The EFA are precursors of prostaglandins, and vitamin B_6 is involved in their metabolism.

Dietary requirements depend on age, sex, height, weight, and activity (metabolic and physical). The objective of a proper diet is to achieve and maintain the desirable body

TABLE 79–2. RECOMMENDED DAILY
FOOD AND NUTRITION BOARD, NATIONAL ACADEMY

	AGE (yr)	WEIGHT kg (lb)	HEIGHT cm (in.)	PROTEIN (gm)	FAT-SOLUBLE VITAMINS		
					VITAMIN A ACTIVITY (RE) †	VITAMIN D (μg) ‡	VITAMIN E§ (mg α T.E.)
Infants	0.0–0.5	6 (13)	60 (24)	kg × 2.2	420	10	3
	0.5–1.0	9 (20)	71 (28)	kg × 2.0	400	10	4
Children	1–3	13 (29)	90 (35)	23	400	10	5
	4–6	20 (44)	112 (44)	30	500	10	6
	7–10	28 (62)	132 (52)	34	700	10	7
Males	11–14	45 (99)	157 (62)	45	1000	10	8
	15–18	66 (145)	176 (69)	56	1000	10	10
	19–22	70 (154)	177 (70)	56	1000	7.5	10
	23–50	70 (154)	178 (70)	56	1000	5	10
	51+	70 (154)	178 (70)	56	1000	5	10
Females	11–14	46 (101)	157 (62)	46	800	10	8
	15–18	55 (120)	163 (64)	46	800	10	8
	19–22	55 (120)	163 (64)	44	800	7.5	8
	23–50	55 (120)	163 (64)	44	800	5	8
	51+	55 (120)	163 (64)	44	800	5	8
Pregnant				+30	+200	+5	+2
Lactating				+20	+400	+5	+3

* The allowances are intended to provide for individual variations among most normal persons a[s] they live in the USA under usual environmental stresses. Diets should be based on a variety of commo[n] foods in order to provide other nutrients for which human requirements have been less well define[d].

† Retinol equivalents. 1 Retinol equivalent = 1 μg retinol or 6 μg β carotene.

‡ As cholecalciferol. 10 μg cholecalciferol = 400 IU vitamin D.

§ α-tocopherol equivalents. 1 mg d-α-tocopherol = 1α T.E.

** The folacin allowances refer to dietary sources as determined by *Lactobacillus casei* assay afte[r] treatment with enzymes ("conjugases") to make polyglutamyl forms of the vitamin available to the te[st] organism.

†† 1 N.E. (niacin equivalent) is equal to 1 mg of niacin or 60 mg of dietary tryptophan.

composition. Recommended dietary allowances (which include a significant safety factor) are given in TABLE 79-2. For some micronutrients for which there is less information, estimated safe and adequate daily dietary intakes have been recommended and are given in TABLE 79-3. In adults, body weight in relation to height, frame, and sex is useful as an indication of overall nutritional status. Generally, up to about age 25, body weight progressively increases.

A wide variety of foods in the diet tends to ensure adequate intake of all essential nutrients. Persons on a "general" diet should be encouraged to include at least a minimum of certain types of foods recommended in a basic dietary plan (see TABLE 79-4, below). The remainder of the diet can be built freely around these foods, with caloric values as needed. Supplemental vitamin, mineral, and caloric requirements, associated with increased physiologic need, may be met by additional portions from the food groups listed in the table or by taking extra nutrients in concentrated or pure form. Intake of foods supplying only energy should be limited.

Prenatal diets are discussed in Ch. 176 and **diets for infants** in NUTRITION in Ch. 182.

DIETARY ALLOWANCES,* REVISED 1980
OF SCIENCES—NATIONAL RESEARCH COUNCIL

WATER-SOLUBLE VITAMINS							MINERALS					
ASCORBIC ACID (mg)	FOLACIN ** (µg)	NIACIN †† (mg N.E.)	RIBOFLAVIN (mg)	THIAMINE (mg)	VITAMIN B_6 (mg)	VITAMIN B_{12} (µg) ‡‡	CALCIUM (mg)	PHOSPHORUS (mg)	IODINE (µg)	IRON (mg)	MAGNESIUM (mg)	ZINC (mg)
35	30	6	0.4	0.3	0.3	0.5	360	240	40	10	50	3
35	45	8	0.6	0.5	0.6	1.5	540	360	50	15	70	5
45	100	9	0.8	0.7	0.9	2.0	800	800	70	15	150	10
45	200	11	1.0	0.9	1.3	2.5	800	800	90	10	200	10
45	300	16	1.4	1.2	1.6	3.0	800	800	120	10	250	10
50	400	18	1.6	1.4	1.8	3.0	1200	1200	150	18	350	15
60	400	18	1.7	1.4	2.0	3.0	1200	1200	150	18	400	15
60	400	19	1.7	1.4	2.2	3.0	800	800	150	10	350	15
60	400	18	1.6	1.4	2.2	3.0	800	800	150	10	350	15
60	400	16	1.4	1.2	2.2	3.0	800	800	150	10	350	15
50	400	15	1.3	1.1	1.8	3.0	1200	1200	150	18	300	15
60	400	14	1.3	1.1	2.0	3.0	1200	1200	150	18	300	15
60	400	14	1.3	1.1	2.0	3.0	800	800	150	18	300	15
60	400	13	1.2	1.0	2.0	3.0	800	800	150	18	300	15
60	400	13	1.2	1.0	2.0	3.0	800	800	150	10	300	15
+20	+400	+2	+0.3	+0.4	+0.6	+1.0	+400	+400	+25	§§	+150	+5
+40	+100	+	+0.5	+0.5	+0.5	+1.0	+400	+400	+50	§§	+150	+10

‡‡ The RDA for vitamin B_{12} in infants is based on average concentration of the vitamin in human milk. The allowances after weaning are based on energy intake (as recommended by the American Academy of Pediatrics) and consideration of other factors such as intestinal absorption.

§§ The increased requirement during pregnancy cannot be met by the iron content of habitual American diets nor by the existing iron stores of many women; therefore the use of 30–60 mg of supplemental iron is recommended. Iron needs during lactation are not substantially different from those of nonpregnant women, but continued supplementation of the mother for 2–3 months after parturition is advisable in order to replenish stores depleted by pregnancy.

(Reproduced from "Recommended Dietary Allowances," 9th ed., 1980, by permission of the National Academy Press, Washington, D.C.)

TABLE 79–3. RECOMMENDED DIETARY ALLOWANCES, REVISED 1980
FOOD AND NUTRITION BOARD, NATIONAL ACADEMY OF SCIENCES—NATIONAL RESEARCH COUNCIL
(Estimated Safe and Adequate Daily Dietary Intakes of Selected Vitamins and Minerals*)

		Vitamins			Trace Elements**						Electrolytes		
	Age (yr)	*Vitamin K (μg)*	*Biotin (μg)*	*Panto-thenic Acid (mg)*	*Copper (mg)*	*Manga-nese (mg)*	*Fluoride (mg)*	*Chromium (mg)*	*Selenium (mg)*	*Molyb-denum (mg)*	*Sodium (mg)*	*Potassium (mg)*	*Chloride (mg)*
Infants	0–0.5	12	35	2	0.5–0.7	0.5–0.7	0.1–0.5	0.01–0.04	0.01–0.04	0.03–0.06	115–350	350–925	275–700
	0.5–1	10–20	50	3	0.7–1.0	0.7–1.0	0.2–1.0	0.02–0.06	0.02–0.06	0.04–0.08	250–750	425–1275	400–1200
Children	1–3	15–30	65	3	1.0–1.5	1.0–1.5	0.5–1.5	0.02–0.08	0.02–0.08	0.05–0.1	325–975	550–1650	500–1500
and	4–6	20–40	85	3–4	1.5–2.0	1.5–2.0	1.0–2.5	0.03–0.12	0.03–0.12	0.06–0.15	450–1350	775–2325	700–2100
Adolescents	7–10	30–60	120	4–5	2.0–2.5	2.0–3.0	1.5–2.5	0.05–0.2	0.05–0.2	0.1 –0.3	600–1800	1000–3000	925–2775
	11+	50–100	100–200	4–7	2.0–3.0	2.5–5.0	1.5–2.5	0.05–0.2	0.05–0.2	0.15–0.5	900–2700	1525–4575	1400–4200
Adults		70–140	100–200	4–7	2.0–3.0	2.5–5.0	1.5–4.0	0.05–0.2	0.05–0.2	0.15–0.5	1100–3300	1875–5625	1700–5100

* Because there is less information on which to base allowances, these figures are not given in TABLE 79-2 and are provided here in the form of ranges of recommended intakes.

** Since the toxic levels for many trace elements may be only several times usual intakes, the upper levels for the trace elements given in the table should not be habitually exceeded.

(Reproduced from "Recommended Dietary Allowances," 9th ed., 1980, by permission of the National Academy Press, Washington, D.C.)

TABLE 79–4. BASIC DAILY DIETARY PLAN*

Milk group: (Whole milk unless skim is desirable)	
Children to age 12	3 to 4 cups
Teenagers	4 cups
Adults	2 cups
Pregnant women	4 cups
Nursing mothers	6 cups
(Cheese, ice cream, and other milk products can replace all or part of the fluid milk. Butter and margarine and other fats and oils are included, consistent with caloric requirements.)	
Meat group: 2 or more servings	
Beef, veal, pork, lamb, poultry, or fish (3 oz edible portion = 1 serving); eggs, preferably not > 4/wk; nuts and dried beans or peas as alternates (1 cup, cooked = 1 serving)	
Vegetable-fruit group: 4 or more servings ($3^1/_2$ oz or $^1/_2$ cup = 1 serving)	
A dark green or deep yellow vegetable (important source of vitamin A) at least every other day	
A citrus fruit or other fruit or vegetable rich in vitamin C daily	
Other fruits and vegetables including potatoes	
Bread-cereal group: 4 or more servings (bread, 1 slice = 1 serving; cereals, cooked or prepared, 1 cup = 1 serving)	
Whole-grain, enriched, or restored products	

* Provides approximately 1600 kcal.

Fiber, mainly a complex mixture of indigestible carbohydrate material, is a natural and hitherto much-neglected component of the normal diet. The typical Western diet is low in fiber (about 20 gm/day), due to the prevailing consumption of highly refined wheat flour and a low intake of fruit and vegetables. The role of fiber in the prevention of constipation and the management of diverticular disease (see Ch. 62) is well established. Other possible effects of fiber being investigated include an influence on the development of cardiovascular disease through modification of bile acid metabolism; a relationship to carcinoma of the colon; and a satiety-producing effect and the control of obesity.

The body is about 60% water and balance is vital for normal metabolism (see Ch. 84).

NUTRITION IN CLINICAL MEDICINE

The importance of nutrition in clinical medicine is being increasingly acknowledged. This is partly due to the recognition that malnutrition frequently occurs in prolonged illness and may accompany acute injury and complicated surgical and medical procedures. Many genetic metabolic disorders require special diets for their management. There is also an increased understanding of the role of nutritional factors in degenerative disorders. Deficiency states such as marasmus, kwashiorkor, and xerophthalmia continue to form a major part of clinical practice in developing countries, but these and other deficiencies may occur anywhere under conditions of deprivation.

Recognition of the frequency with which nutrition is compromised in systemic disease and the serious consequences that this may have on outcome has led many centers to establish a multidisciplinary nutrition team approach involving physicians, surgeons, nurses, dietitians, pharmacists, and laboratory services. A patient suspected of requiring nutritional support should have his nutritional status assessed and monitored. If an adequate intake cannot be maintained orally, then the decision should be made on clinical grounds to institute either enteral or parenteral nutrition.

Assessment of Nutritional Status

Specific micronutrient deficiencies are uncommon in clinical practice (see Chs. 81 and 82). Most commonly encountered is some degree of protein-calorie malnutrition **(PCM)**. Data indicative of nutritional depletion in common use include:

1. Recent weight loss > 10%
2. Serum albumin < 35 gm/L
3. Serum transferrin < 2 gm/L
4. Triceps skinfold thickness < 10 mm males; < 13 mm females
5. Upper-arm circumference < 23 cm males; < 22 cm females
6. Lymphopenia < 1.2×10^9/L
7. Skin anergy to a battery of antigens: candida, mumps, streptokinase, streptodornase, dermatophytin, PPD.

These indicators have been used in a variety of combinations. One of the best tested of these is the **prognostic nutritional index (PNI)**, a linear predictive model of increased morbidity and mortality following surgery. In this model serum albumin gm/dL **(A)**; triceps skinfold thickness mm **(TSF)**; serum transferrin mg/dL **(TFN)**; and delayed hypersensitivity response **(DH)** are used in the formula:

$$\text{PNI \%} = 158 - 16.6(\text{A}) - 0.78(\text{TSF}) - 0.2\,(\text{TFN}) - 5.8(\text{DH})$$

Thus, a well-nourished patient with, eg, 4.8 gm/dL (A); 14 mm (TSF); 250 mg/dL (TFN); and 2 (DH) has a PNI of 158.0 - 152.2 or a 5.8% chance of complications. A malnourished patient with all indices abnormal, eg, 2.8 (A); 9 (TSF); 180 (TFN); and 1 (DH) has a PNI of 158 - 95.3 or a 62.7% chance of complications.

NUTRITIONAL SUPPORT

ENTERAL NUTRITION

Oral supplementation with energy and protein-rich foods is indicated for patients on modified consistency diets, the chronically ill with anorexia, and those with chronic inflammatory and malignant disease. In practice, commercial products provide a more reliable and acceptable method of supplementation than table foods (see TABLE 79–5).

Enteral tube alimentation may be used in patients with a functioning GI tract to supplement oral feeding or to replace it entirely. The latter is indicated for patients requiring intensive protein and calorie support, who are unable or unwilling to take oral supplementation. It is safer and cheaper than TPN (see below) and is the preferred route when the integrity of the GI tract is preserved. General indications include prolonged anorexia, existing severe PCM, trauma to the head and neck or neurologic disorders preventing satisfactory oral feeding, coma or depressed mental state, and serious illnesses (eg, burns) in which metabolic requirements are high. Specific indications may include preparation of the bowel for surgery in seriously ill or malnourished patients, closure of enterocutaneous fistulas, small bowel adaptation following massive intestinal resection, and malabsorption disorders such as Crohn's disease.

The technic consists of directly installing the nutrient mixture into or just proximal to the upper end of the small bowel through a nasogastric or nasoduodenal tube or less commonly through a gastrostomy or jejunostomy. The choice of route depends on individual circumstances, but availability of a variety of small caliber, soft tubes for nasogastric and nasoduodenal feeding has made these preferred routes.

In addition to high energy, high protein supplements, **elemental (chemically defined) diets** are frequently given by this route. They provide essential nutrients in a readily assimilated form, require little or no active digestion, and have minimal residue. Components of a selection of elemental diets are listed in TABLE 79–6.

TABLE 79–5. CLASSIFICATION OF VARIOUS COMMERCIALLY AVAILABLE PROTEIN AND CALORIE ORAL SUPPLEMENTS BY THEIR PRINCIPAL USE

	Calorie supplement						
Protein supplement							
		Nutritionally complete					
				Low fat (≤ 15 g/1000 kcal)			
Casec Powder	Lonalac	Carnation Instant Breakfast*	ProSobee‡	Precision LR	Citrotein	Hy-Cal	Controlyte
Gevral		Enfamil†‡	Renu	Precision NH		Polycose	Lipomul-Oral
		Ensure	Similac*‡	Vital†		Sumacal	MCT Oil
		Ensure Plus	Slender*	Vivonex†		Cal Plus	Microlipid
		Flexical†	SMA*†	Vivonex HN†		Moducal	
		Isomil‡	Sustacal	Sustagen*			
		Lolactene*	Sustacal HC	Sego*			
		Magnacal	Sustacal pudding	Travasorb STD†			
		Meritene*	Travasorb	Travasorb HN†			
		Nutramigen†‡	Travasorb MCT				
		Nutri–1000*	Vipep†				
		Nutri–1000 LF	Vitaneed				
		Portagen					
		Precision Isotonic					
		Presgestimil†‡					

* Contains lactose alone or when prepared in the usual way; all others are lactose free.
† Contains hydrolyzed proteins and/or amino acid as the protein source (the "elemental" diets).
‡ Intended for infant use.

(Adapted from *Manual of Nutritional Therapeutics*, p. 207, by D. H. Alpers, R. E. Clouse, W. F. Stenson. Copyright Little, Brown & Company, Boston, 1983. Used with permission.)

TABLE 79–6. COMPARISON OF COMPONENTS OF ELEMENTAL OR CHEMICALLY DEFINED DIETS

Component	*Vivonex®*	*Vivonex HN®*	*Vital®*	*Precision LR®*	*Precision HN®*	*Precision Isotonic®*	*Flexical®*
Carbohydrate							
gm/1000 kcal	230	211	188	223	205	150	152
% cal	90.5	86.5	74	89.2	82.2	59.9	61
Type	Glucose Oligosaccharides	Glucose Oligosaccharides	Hydrolyzed corn syrup solids Sucrose	Maltodextrin Sucrose citrate	Maltodextrin Sucrose citrate	Glucose Oligosaccharides Sucrose citrate	Corn syrup solids Modified tapioca starch
Lactose	None	None	None	None	None	None	None
Fat							
gm/1000 kcal	1.5	0.9	10.8	1.4	1.2	31.3	34
% cal	1.3	0.8	9.3	1.3	1.1	28.1	30
Type	Safflower oil	Safflower oil	Med. chain triglycerides Safflower oil	Med. chain triglycerides Soy oil	Med. chain triglycerides Soy oil	Soy oil	Soy oil MCT oil
Essential fatty acids (% total fat)	80	80					26.5
Amino acids							
gm/1000 kcal	20.6	43.3	41.7	24	41.7	30	22.5
% cal	8.2	17.7	16.7	9.5	16.7	12	9
Type	Pure crystalline amino acids	Pure crystalline amino acids	Hydrolyzed soy, whey, & meat. Free amino acids.	Egg albumin (pasteurized egg white solids)	Egg albumin (pasteurized egg white solids)	Egg albumin (pasteurized egg white solids) Sodium caseinate	Hydrolyzed casein plus free amino acids—Met., Try., Trp.
Osmolality							
mOsm/kg (at standard dilution)	550	810	460	525 (Orange)	557	300	550 (Plain)

(Modified from *CLINICAL NUTRITION: A physiologic approach*, by M. H. Overton and B. P. Lukert. Copyright © 1977 by Yearbook Publishers, Inc., Chicago. Used with permission.)

Nasogastric or nasoduodenal feeding is usually started with a 25% wt/vol solution; 1 kcal/mL is fed at a rate of 50 mL/h and increased by 25 mL/h to a total of 125 mL/h (3000 kcal/24 h). Jejunostomy feeding is started with a 10% wt/vol solution at 50 mL/h and increased by 25 mL/h up to the daily fluid requirements. Concentration is thereafter increased by 5% wt/vol/day until maximum tolerance is achieved (usually 20% wt/vol concentration; 0.8 kcal/mL, at 125 mL/h for 2400 kcal/day).

Complications of enteral feeding are usually neither common nor serious and can be overcome by careful monitoring. Diarrhea and GI discomfort may occur in up to 20% of patients from intolerance of the intestine to a major nutrient component or to the osmotic fluid load of the formula. Esophagitis is uncommon with small bore soft tubes, and tracheobronchial aspiration, a serious complication, may be avoided by careful attention to details of technic. Electrolyte disturbances, volume overload, and hyperosmolarity syndrome must be guarded against by daily monitoring of water balance, electrolytes, osmolality, and blood urea.

PARENTERAL NUTRITION

Partial parenteral nutrition: *Nutritional support given IV that supplements oral intake and provides only part of the daily requirements.* Many hospitalized patients receive dextrose or amino acid solutions by this method as part of their routine care.

Total parenteral nutrition (TPN): *The IV administration of all the patient's daily nutrient requirements.* A peripheral vein may be utilized for short periods, but its use with concentrated solutions to achieve positive energy and nitrogen balance and also to provide adequate daily volume of fluids can readily lead to thrombosis. Therefore, **central venous access** (see Procedure below) is usually required. In addition to long-term TPN administration by this route in hospital, many who have lost small bowel function are now able to lead useful lives at home maintained on **home parenteral nutrition (HPN).**

Indications: Severely malnourished patients can be prepared for surgery, radiation, or chemotherapy for cancer and also maintain their nutritional status thereafter. In major surgery, severe burns, multiple fractures, especially in the presence of sepsis, subsequent morbidity and mortality are improved, tissue repair is promoted, and the immune response enhanced. Prolonged coma and anorexia often require TPN after intensive enteral feeding in the earlier stages. Conditions necessitating complete bowel rest, such as some stages of Crohn's disease, ulcerative colitis, severe pancreatitis, and pediatric GI disorders, such as congenital anomalies and protracted nonspecific diarrhea, often respond well to TPN.

Basic requirements (see TABLES 79–7 and 79–8)

TABLE 79–7. BASIC REQUIREMENTS FOR TOTAL PARENTERAL NUTRITION

	In kg/body weight/day
Water mL	30–40
Energy kcal*	
Medical patient	30
Postoperative patient	30–45
Hypercatabolic patient	45–60
Nitrogen gm (× 6.25 = protein)	0.11–0.20
Medical patient	0.20–0.31
Postoperative patient	0.35–0.60
Hypercatabolic patient	
Vitamins and essential minerals (See Table 79–8)	

* These requirements are increased by 12% per °C fever.

TABLE 79–8. RECOMMENDED DAILY INTAKE OF PARENTERAL MINERALS AND VITAMINS FOR AN ADULT

Sodium	100 mEq	Ascorbic acid	100 mg
Potassium	100 mEq	Thiamine	3 mg
Chloride	130 MEq	Riboflavin	3.6 mg
Acetate/gluconate	90 mEq	Niacin	40 mg
Calcium	15 mEq	Pantothenic acid	15 mg
Magnesium	20 mEq	Pyridoxine	4 mg
Phosphorus	300 mg	Biotin	60 μg
Zinc	5 mg	Folic acid	400 μg
Copper	1.5 mg	Cobalamin	5 μg
Iodine	120 μg	Vitamin A	4000 IU
Selenium	100 μg	Vitamin D	400 IU
Chromium	15 μg	Vitamin E	15 mg
Manganese	2 mg	Vitamin K	200 μg

(Modified from "Guidelines for Essential Trace Element Preparations for Parenteral Use" by the AMA Department of Foods and Nutrition, in *JAMA*, Vol. 241, May 11, 1979, pages 2051–2054. Copyright 1979 by the American Medical Association. Used with permission.)

Procedure: Solutions must be prepared aseptically under a laminar-flow filtered-air hood. Insertion of a central venous catheter is never done as an emergency and requires full aseptic conditions and adequate assistance. Subclavian placement is standard, using a silastic Broviac or Hickman catheter. The catheter is burrowed through the subcutaneous tissue in the anterior chest wall and exits away from the site of subclavian puncture. A chest x-ray is always obtained after catheter insertion or position change to confirm the location of the tip. The TPN line should not be used for any other purpose. External tubing should be changed q 24 h with the first bag of the day. In-line filters are not recommended. Special occlusive dressings are an essential part of catheter maintenance and are usually changed q 48 h with full aseptic and sterile precautions.

Precautions to be observed during administration include: starting slowly at 50% calculated patient requirements, making up the balance of fluid with 5% dextrose; giving energy and nitrogen sources simultaneously; giving regular insulin (added directly to the TPN solution) depending on blood sugar estimations—if blood glucose is normal (fasting 70 to 110 mg/dL) the usual starting dose is 5 to 10 u. regular insulin/L TPN fluid containing 25% dextrose in the final concentration; and guarding against rebound hypoglycemia after discontinuing high concentrations of dextrose.

Formulations: A great variety are in common use; samples for the average patient and those requiring base solution modification are given in TABLE 79–9.

Special modifications of the formulation are necessary for patients with organ failure. These relate in particular to amino acid composition for patients with renal or hepatic failure; volume (liquid) limitations for those in heart failure; and avoidance of increased CO_2 production in patients with respiratory failure by providing most of the nonprotein calories by lipid emulsion. Pediatric patients have special nutrient requirements; additionally, they may not tolerate lipid emulsions well.

Monitoring: The following should be monitored daily: weight, urea, glucose (several times daily until stable), CBC, blood gases, accurate fluid balance, and a 24-h urine and electrolytes. When the patient becomes stable, the frequency of these tests can be considerably reduced. Liver function tests, plasma proteins, prothrombin time, plasma and urine osmolality, and calcium, magnesium and phosphate (not to be measured

during glucose infusion) should be measured twice weekly. Progress should be followed on a flow chart. Nutritional assessment and C3 complement should be repeated at 2-wk intervals.

Complications may be metabolic—those relating to the nutritional formula—or nonmetabolic—due to faults in delivery technics. In many institutions, complications are the greatest deterrent to the use of TPN. Where the team approach has been adopted, complications have been reduced to < 5%.

Metabolic complications: Hyperglycemia and hyperosmolality should be avoided by careful monitoring and the administration of insulin. Hypoglycemia is precipitated by sudden discontinuation of constant concentrated dextrose infusion. Treatment consists of peripheral infusion of 5 or 10% dextrose for 24 h before resuming central line feeding. Abnormalities of serum electrolytes and minerals should be detected by monitoring before symptoms and signs occur. Treatment involves appropriate modification of subsequent infusions, or appropriate peripheral vein infusions if more urgent correction is required. Vitamin and element deficiencies are most likely to occur during long-term TPN (see Chs. 81 and 82). Elevation of BUN not infrequently occurs during TPN, and may result from hyperosmolar dehydration that can be corrected by free water given as 5% dextrose via a peripheral vein. Hyperammonemia is not a problem in adults with currently available amino acid solutions. In infants, signs include lethargy, twitching, and generalized seizures; correction consists of arginine supplementation at a total of 0.5 to 1.0 mmol/kg/day. Metabolic bone disease, resulting in severe periarticular, lower extremity and back pain in some patients on long-term TPN is associated with low serum $1,25(OH)_2D$. Temporary or permanent discontinuance of TPN is the only treatment known. Liver dysfunction, evidenced by elevations of transaminases, bilirubin, and alkaline phosphatase, is common with the initiation of TPN, but these elevations are usually transitory. Detection is by regular monitoring. Delayed or persistent elevations may relate to the amino acid infusion, and protein delivery should be reduced. Painful hepatomegaly suggests fat accumulation and the carbohydrate load should be reduced. Adverse reactions to lipid emulsions are uncommon, but they may occur early, as evidenced by dyspnea, cutaneous allergic phenomena, nausea, headache, back pain, sweating, and dizziness. Temporary hyperlipidemia occurs and is especially common in renal and hepatic failure. Delayed adverse reactions include hepatomegaly, mild elevation of liver enzymes, splenomegaly, thrombocytopenia, leukopenia, and alterations in pulmonary function studies, especially in premature infants with hyaline membrane disease. Temporary or permanent cessation of lipid emulsion infusion may be indicated.

Nonmetabolic complications: Pneumothorax and hematoma formation are the most common, but damage to other structures and air embolism have been reported. Proper placement of the catheter tip in the superior vena cava must always be confirmed by chest x-ray prior to infusion of TPN fluid. Complications related to central catheter placement should be < 5%. Thromboembolism and catheter-related sepsis are the most common serious complications of TPN therapy. The more common organisms include: *S. aureus*, *Candida* sp, *Klebsiella pneumoniae*, *Pseudomonas aeruginosa*, *S. albus*, and *Enterobacter*. Fever during TPN should be systematically investigated. If no other cause is found, and if the temperature remains elevated for > 24 to 48 h, central catheter infusion should be stopped. Before removing the catheter, blood for culture should be drawn directly from the central catheter and the catheter infusion site. On withdrawal, 2 to 3 in. of the catheter tip should be cut off with a sterile scalpel or scissors and sent for bacterial and fungal culture in a dry, sterile culture tube. Volume overload may occur when high daily energy requirements necessitate large fluid volumes. Weight should be monitored daily; gain of > ½ lb/day suggests volume overload, and daily fluid delivery should be reduced.

TABLE 79–9. SAMPLE FORMULATION OF STANDARDIZED CENTRAL VEIN TPN BASE SOLUTIONS FOR THE AVERAGE PATIENT AND FOR PATIENTS REQUIRING BASE SOLUTION MODIFICATION

Additives	*Standard Solution*			*Heart Failure Solution (low volume–low Na+)*			*Low K+–Low Na+ Solution*			*Renal Failure Solution*		
	From Additives	*Provided* by Amino Acid Solution*	*Final Content*	*From Additives*	*Provided* by Amino Acid Solution*	*Final Content*	*From Additives*	*Provided* by Amino Acid Solution*	*Final Content*	*From Additives*	*Provided by Amino Acid Solution*	*Final Content*
Crystalline amino acid 8.5%	500 mL		4.25%	300 mL		3.18%	500 mL		4.25%			
Nephramine 5.4%			—			—			—	500 mL		338%
Dextrose 50%	500 mL		25%			—	500 mL		25%			—
Dextrose 70%			—	500 mL		44%			—	300 mL		26%
Sodium (mEq)	35	5	40	—	3	3	—	5	5†	‡	3	3
Potassium (mEq)	40	—	40	40	—	40	—	—	—	‡	—	—
Chloride	35	—	35	—	—	0	—	—	0	‡	—	—
Calcium§ (mEq)	4.6	—	4.6	4.6	—	4.6	4.6	—	4.6	‡	—	—
Phosphorus** (mmol)	7	5	12	7	3	10	6	5	11	‡	—	—
Magnesium†† (mEq)	8.1	—	8.1	8.1	—	8.1	8.1	—	8.1	‡	—	—
Sulfate‡‡ (mEq)	8.1	—	8.1	8.1	—	8.1	8.1	—	8.1	‡	—	—
Gluconate‡‡ (mEq)	4.6	—	4.6	4.6	—	4.6	4.6	—	4.6	‡	—	—
Acetate‡‡ (mEq)	30	37	67	30	22.2	58.2	—	37	37	‡	22	22
Approximate total volume			1050 mL			830 mL			1015 mL			800 mL
Grams amino acids			42.5			25.4			42.5			27.0
Grams nitrogen			6.5			3.9			6.5			3.2
Grams protein equivalent§§			41			24			41			20
Nonprotein calories (kcal)***			850			1190			850			714
Caloric concentration (kcal mL)			0.81			1.4			0.84			0.89

* Based on electrolyte content of FreAmine® III 8.5%.
† Additional sodium can be added as sodium chloride.
‡ Additives only as indicated by serum levels.
§ Added as calcium gluconate 0.46 mEq/mL.
** Added as potassium phosphate: K^+ 4.4 mEq/mL, phosphorus 3 mmol/mL.
†† Added as magnesium sulfate 4.06 mEq/mL.
‡‡ Not ordered by the physician; these anions balance the ordered cations.
§§ Based on 6.25 gm protein per gm nitrogen.
*** Dextrose monohydrate provides 3.4 kcal/gm.

(Adapted from *Manual of Nutritional Therapeutics*, p. 252, by D. H. Alpers, R. E. Clouse, W. F. Stenson. Copyright Little, Brown & Company, Boston, 1983. Used with permission.)

NUTRIENT-DRUG INTERACTIONS

Nutritional deficiency may impair the metabolism of drugs. Energy and protein deficiencies reduce tissue levels of enzymes and impair drug response by reducing absorption and causing liver dysfunction. Response to drugs may be affected by impaired absorption due to changes in the GI tract and by disturbed liver function. Deficiency of minerals such as Ca, Zn, and Mg impairs drug metabolism. Potassium depletion from the use of diuretics, especially the thiazides, and corticosteroids increases the risk of digitalis-induced cardiac arrhythmias. Vitamin C deficiency is associated with decreased activity of drug-metabolizing enzymes. The frequency of adverse drug reactions in the elderly may be related to their frequently low vitamin C status.

Many drugs affect appetite and absorption, and glucose, lipid and protein metabolism. Some of the most important of these are listed in TABLE 79–10. Those drugs that are used specifically to produce such an effect are not included.

Other drugs affect mineral metabolism. Potassium depletion may also result from the regular use of purgatives. Na and water retention is marked, at least temporarily, with cortisol, deoxycorticosterone, and aldosterone; much less with prednisone, prednisolone, and the newer steroid analogs. It also occurs with estrogen-progestogen oral contraceptives and phenylbutazone. Non-heme iron absorption is either impaired or facilitated by a number of dietary substances. Other effects include impaired thyroid uptake or release of iodine by sulfonylureas, phenylbutazone, cobalt, and lithium; lowered plasma Zn and elevated Cu by oral contraceptives; and osteoporosis from prolonged use of adrenal steroids, the cause of which is unclear.

The metabolism of many vitamins is affected. Ethanol impairs thiamine absorption and isoniazid is a niacin and pyridoxine antagonist. Complaints of depression in

TABLE 79–10. EXAMPLES OF SIDE EFFECTS OF DRUGS ON NUTRITIONAL STATUS

Effect	*Drugs*
Appetite increased	Alcohol, insulin, steroids, thyroid hormone, sulfonylureas, psychotropic drugs, antihistamines
Appetite decreased	Bulk agents (methyl cellulose, guar gum), glucagon, indomethacin, morphine, cyclophosphamide, digitalis
Malabsorption	Neomycin, kanamycin, chlortetracycline, phenindione *p*-aminosalicylic acid, indomethacin, methotrexate, liquid paraffin
Glucose metabolism	
Hyperglycemia	Narcotic analgesics, phenothiazines, benzothiadiazine diuretics, probenecid, phenytoin, coumarins
Hypoglycemia	Sulfonamides, aspirin, phenacetin, β-adrenergic blockers, monoamine oxidase inhibitors, phenylbutazone, barbiturates
Lipid metabolism	
Plasma lipids reduced	Aspirin and *p*-aminosalicylic acid, L-asparaginase, chlortetracycline, colchicine, dextrans, fenfluramine, glucagon, phenindione, sulfinpyrazone, trifluperidol
Plasma lipids increased	Oral contraceptives (estrogen-progestogen type), adrenal corticosteroids, chlorpromazine, ethanol, thiouracil, growth hormone, vitamin D
Protein metabolism decreased	Tetracycline, chloramphenicol

women taking oral contraceptives are usually associated with high progestogen content. These patients have a disturbance of tryptophan metabolism that is responsive to 20 mg pyridoxine tid. The disturbance is due to induction of tryptophan pyrrolase, a rate-limiting enzyme affecting niacin metabolism, resulting in the use of pyridoxine for niacin synthesis at the expense of 5-hydroxytryptamine neurotransmitter formation. Folic acid absorption is inhibited by ethanol and oral contraceptives. Most patients receiving phenytoin, phenobarbital, primidone, or phenothiazines for long-term anticonvulsant therapy develop low serum and erythrocyte folate levels and occasionally megaloblastic anemia, probably as an effect on hepatic microsomal drug metabolizing enzymes. Administration of folic acid interferes with the anticonvulsant action, but regular yeast tablet supplements raise folate levels without this effect. Vitamin B_{12} malabsorption has been reported with aminosalicylic acid, slow-release potassium iodide, colchicine, trifluoperazine, ethanol, and oral contraceptives. Anticonvulsant-induced vitamin D deficiency is well-recognized.

FOOD ADDITIVES AND CONTAMINANTS

The addition of chemicals to foodstuffs to facilitate their processing, preserve them, or to enhance their analeptic properties, and for the elimination or control of natural and artificial contaminants of food are subject to increasingly stringent legislation and control. Only those additives that have been passed as safe at specified "action levels" after exacting laboratory testing are permitted. Poisonous or deleterious contaminants, such as pesticide residues, are subject to similar control. Long-term effects of additives and contaminants on health are difficult to assess.

The use of additives reduces the wastage of foods and food raw materials, prevents spoilage of many perishable foods, and provides the public with a greater variety of attractive foods than would otherwise be possible. Against these benefits have to be set the known risks. The issues involved are frequently difficult to resolve. The use of nitrite in cured meats may be taken as an example of the complexity of the problem. Nitrite inhibits the growth of *C. botulinum* and imparts a desired flavor. However, there is evidence that nitrite is converted in the body to nitrosamines, which are known carcinogens in animals. This issue is not fully resolved. Another example is sweetening agents. Cyclamates have been banned because they are carcinogenic in high doses in animals. The intense sweeteners saccharin and aspartame are currently permitted. Bulk sweeteners, such as fructose, sorbitol, and xylitol have the same caloric content as sucrose and consumption of large amounts (30 to 50 gm/day) may cause abdominal pain or diarrhea.

There is current concern about the production of food intolerance and allergy in a few susceptible individuals by some additives, especially permitted coloring agents. However, most of these reactions are caused by natural food (see FOOD ALLERGY AND INTOLERANCE under GASTROINTESTINAL ALLERGY in Ch. 21).

The complete elimination of contaminants from certain foodstuffs cannot be achieved without damaging the foodstuff. Action levels are set which may vary for different foodstuffs. Thus the residual tolerance for aldrin and dieldrin is 0.03 ppm for eggs but 0.3 ppm for butter, fish (smoked, frozen, canned), and milk. Aflatoxin, a known liver carcinogen in animals, has a residual tolerance level of 20 ppb for peanuts and peanut products but 0.5 ppb for milk. A level of 0.5 ppm has been set for lead in evaporated milk and of 1.0 ppm for mercury in fish, oysters, clams, mussels, and wheat.

In summary, demonstrated health problems arising from food additives have been trivial except for isolated incidents.

80. UNDERNUTRITION

NUTRITIONAL DISORDERS

Early Detection

Deviations from normal nutritional status arise from an imbalance between the nutrient supply to tissues, whether from inappropriate dietary intake or defective utilization by the body, and the requirements for that nutrient. When imbalance is established, syndromes of deficiency, toxicity, or dependency (in the case of some vitamins) result. Early detection of this imbalance poses considerable problems as symptoms (eg, fatigue or anorexia), if present, are vague. Apart from some falling off in growth rate in children or slight occasional weight loss in adults, clinical signs are absent at this stage.

The evolution of nutrient deficiency follows a steady progression from tissue depletion (a lengthy process in the case of nutrients that are stored, such as energy sources, protein, and some vitamins and elements), to biochemical changes, reduction in blood or urinary levels, functional changes, early histologic changes, and finally the appearance of clinical signs.

The key to early detection is **awareness of high risk** in certain sets of circumstances. For example, undernutrition is particularly associated with poverty and deprivation, and newly arrived immigrant families from third world countries may be especially vulnerable. In all communities, high-risk groups comprise: infants and young children who are not thriving; adolescents who are undergoing rapid growth spurts; pregnant and lactating women; the elderly; those on fad or crash slimming diets; those practicing some forms of vegetarianism; patients with an alcohol or drug problem; those receiving drug treatment that may impair nutrition (see NUTRIENT DRUG INTERACTIONS in Ch. 79); and patients with chronic diseases of the GI, hepatic, and renal systems that may interfere with nutrient absorption and utlization.

Inquiry should be made about the regular consumption of the main food groups—cereals and cereal products, vegetables and fruit, dairy products and eggs, and meat and fish. If the inquiry reveals some evident inadequacy, the services of a dietitian should be sought. Precise dietary intake data by any method are extremely difficult to obtain, especially for young children. The patient should also be questioned about self-medication with vitamin or trace element supplements.

A thorough physical examination should reveal any underlying disease. The presence of physical signs attributable to nutritional disorders indicates that the early detection phase has passed. Biochemical tests are available for most micronutrients in specialized rather than in routine hospital or commercial laboratories, and are indicated only if the history and examination arouse suspicion concerning specific nutrients. Broad vitamin screening is not recommended and the practice of carrying out trace element profiles on hair samples is to be condemned.

Energy status is best estimated in office practice by assessment of the fat stores by the use of skinfold calipers. These should be spring-loaded, and not those of the simple plastic variety, and considerable practice is required for their accurate use. Standards for men and women of different ages are shown in TABLE 80–1. Changes in body weight from one day to the next can be quite considerable, amounting to as much as 1 to 2 kg in a study of a group of young men. Persistent weight loss of 2 to 3 kg over about 3 mo merits investigation, but is unlikely to be due to primary nutritional deficiency.

Estimates of **protein status** can be made for the somatic and visceral compartments separately. The mid-arm muscle circumference is an indication of the somatic compartment. It is derived from the formula:

Mid-arm muscle circumference (mm) = mid-arm circumference (mm) – (triceps skinfold [mm] × 3.14)

TABLE 80–1. STANDARD FAT STORES IN MEN AND WOMEN

The equivalent fat content, as a percentage of body weight, for a range of values for the sum of four skinfolds (biceps, triceps, subscapular, and suprailiac) of males and females of different ages

Skinfolds (mm)	*Percentage Fat*							
	Males (age in years)				*Females (age in years)*			
	17–29	*30–39*	*40–49*	*50+*	*16–29*	*30–39*	*40–49*	*50+*
15	4.8				10.5			
20	8.1	12.2	12.2	12.6	14.1	17.0	19.8	21.4
25	10.5	14.2	15.0	15.6	16.8	19.4	22.2	24.0
30	12.9	16.2	17.7	18.6	19.5	21.8	24.5	26.6
35	14.7	17.7	19.6	20.8	21.5	23.7	26.4	28.5
40	16.4	19.2	21.4	22.9	23.4	25.5	28.2	30.3
45	17.7	20.4	23.0	24.7	25.0	26.9	29.6	31.9
50	19.0	21.5	24.6	26.5	26.5	28.2	31.0	33.4
55	20.1	22.5	25.9	27.9	27.8	29.4	32.1	34.6
60	21.2	23.5	27.1	29.2	29.1	30.6	33.2	35.7
65	22.2	24.3	28.2	30.4	30.2	31.6	34.1	36.7
70	23.1	25.1	29.3	31.6	31.2	32.5	35.0	37.7
75	24.0	25.9	30.3	32.7	32.2	33.4	35.9	38.7
80	24.8	26.6	31.2	33.8	33.1	34.3	36.7	39.6
85	25.5	27.2	32.1	34.8	34.0	35.1	37.5	40.4
90	26.2	27.8	33.0	35.8	34.8	35.8	38.3	41.2
95	26.9	28.4	33.7	36.6	35.6	36.5	39.0	41.9
100	27.6	29.0	34.4	37.4	36.4	37.2	39.7	42.6
105	28.2	29.6	35.1	38.2	37.1	37.9	40.4	43.3
110	28.8	30.1	35.8	39.0	37.8	38.6	41.0	43.9
115	29.4	30.6	36.4	39.7	38.4	39.1	41.5	44.5
120	30.0	31.1	37.0	40.4	39.0	39.6	42.0	45.1
125	30.5	31.5	37.6	41.1	39.6	40.1	42.5	45.7
130	31.0	31.9	38.2	41.8	40.2	40.6	43.0	46.2
135	31.5	32.3	38.7	42.4	40.8	41.1	43.5	46.7
140	32.0	32.7	39.2	43.0	41.3	41.6	44.0	47.2
145	32.5	33.1	39.7	43.6	41.8	42.1	44.5	47.7
150	32.9	33.5	40.2	44.1	42.3	42.6	45.0	48.2
155	33.3	33.9	40.7	44.6	42.8	43.1	45.4	48.7
160	33.7	34.3	41.2	45.1	43.3	43.6	45.8	49.2
165	34.1	34.6	41.6	45.6	43.7	44.0	46.2	49.6
170	34.5	34.8	42.0	46.1	44.1	44.4	46.6	50.0
175	34.9					44.8	47.0	50.4
180	35.3					45.2	47.4	50.8
185	35.6					45.6	47.8	51.2
190	35.9					45.9	48.2	51.6
195						46.2	48.5	52.0
200						46.5	48.8	52.4
205							49.1	52.7
210							49.4	53.0

(From Durnin, J. V. G. A. and Womersley, J., in *British Journal of Nutrition,* 32:77, 1974. Copyright 1974 by Cambridge University Press. Reprinted with permission of Cambridge University Press.)

Standards for men and women of different ages are shown in FIG. 80–1. A visceral component deficit is reflected by serum albumin values (gm/dL) as follows: severe < 2.5; moderate < 3.0 to 2.5; mild < 3.5 to 3.0; or serum transferrin values (mg/dL) as follows: severe < 160; moderate < 180 to 160; mild < 200 to 180.

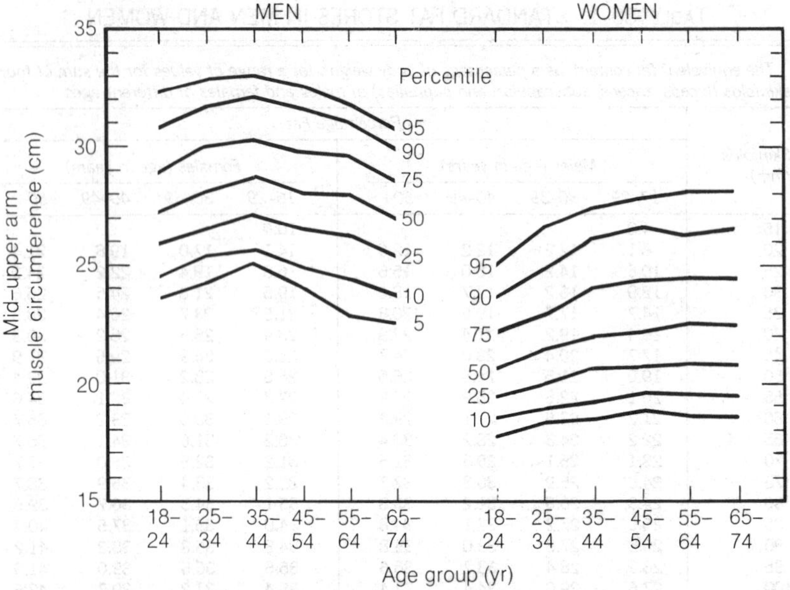

FIG. 80–1. Apparent changes in the mid-upper arm muscle circumferences of American adults with advancing age. (From C. W. Bishop et al in the *American Journal of Clinical Nutrition* 1981; 34: 2530–9. Copyright *American Journal of Clinical Nutrition,* American Society for Clinical Nutrition. Used with permission.)

Detection of Nutritional Disorders in Infants and Children (see in Ch. 195)

Eating Disorders in Adolescents (see in Ch. 202)

Nutritional Disorders in Pregnant and Lactating Women

Requirements for all nutrients are increased. Aberrations of diet are especially common in pregnancy, including pica (see IRON DEFICIENCY ANEMIA in Ch. 96) and anemia should be prevented (see ANEMIA in Ch. 177). Exclusively breast-fed infants have developed vitamin B_{12} deficiency when the mothers were vegans and folic acid deficiency when the mothers were taking estrogen-progesterone contraceptive pills.

Nutritional Disorders in the Elderly and the Chronically Ill

Old age, loneliness, physical and mental handicap, immobility, and chronic illness all militate against adequate dietary intake. Absorption is reduced and may contribute to iron deficiency, osteoporosis (also related to calcium intake), and osteomalacia (contributed to also by lack of exposure to sunlight and drug treatment)—see Ch. 113 and VITAMIN D DEFICIENCY—RICKETS AND OSTEOMALACIA in Ch. 81.

With aging, independent of disease or dietary deficiency, there is progressive loss of lean body mass, amounting to about 10 kg in men and 5 kg in women. This accounts for the fall in basal metabolic rate, total body weight, and skeletal mass and height, and for the rise in mean body fat (as percent of body weight) from about 20 to 30% in men and from 27 to 40% in women. These changes, together with the reduction in physical activity, result in a decrease in both energy and protein requirements as compared with younger adults. (See also Ch. 264.)

In patients with chronic disease, malabsorption states (including those resulting from surgery) tend especially to impair the absorption of fat-soluble vitamins, vitamin B_{12}, Ca, and Fe. Liver disease impairs the storage of vitamins A and B_{12} and interferes with the metabolism of protein and energy sources. Patients with renal disease, including those on dialysis, are prone to develop deficiency of protein, iron, and vitamin D. The increasing number of patients on long-term home parenteral nutrition (see PARENTERAL NUTRITION in Ch. 79), most commonly following total or near-total resection of the gut, living active and productive lives constitutes a triumph of technologic medicine. The development of trace element deficiencies should be especially guarded against.

Nutritional Disorders in Vegetarians

Most people will not eat the meat of certain animals (eg, horse) or certain organs (eg, brain); some eat fish and dairy produce but not meat. These practices carry no nutritional risk. The most common form of true vegetarianism is **ovo-lacto vegetarianism** in which meat and fish are eschewed. Iron deficiency is the only risk. Ovo-lacto vegetarians tend to live longer and to suffer less from chronic disabling conditions than their meat-eating peers. However, they also usually abstain from alcohol and tobacco and take regular exercise as part of their lifestyle. **Vegans** consume no animal products and are susceptible to vitamin B_{12} deficiency. Yeast extracts and fermented foods of oriental origin provide this vitamin. Ca, Fe, and Zn intakes tend to be low. A **fruitarian diet** consists solely of fruit, is deficient in protein, salt, and many micronutrients and cannot be sustained for long.

Nutritional Disorders and Fad Diets

A plethora of commercial diets purporting to enhance well being or reduce weight are in vogue and the physician should be alert to the development of early evidence of nutrient deficiency or toxicity states in patients adhering to them. Frank vitamin, mineral, and protein deficiency states and cardiac, renal, and metabolic disorders have been induced by these diets and some deaths have resulted. Some trace element supplements have induced toxicity. Most of these dietary practices are nutritionally unsound and many have been condemned by the American Medical Association.

Nutritional Disorders in Patients with Alcohol or Drug Dependency

Patients with alcohol or drug problems are notoriously unreliable when questioned about the practices they indulge in. It may be necessary to make judicious inquiry of relatives or acquaintances. Addiction leads to a disturbance of lifestyle in which adequate nourishment is neglected. Absorption and metabolism of nutrients are impaired. Alcoholics frequently put on weight, due to the high energy content of alcohol (7 kcal/gm) while drug addicts are usually emaciated. Alcoholism is the most common cause of thiamine deficiency in the West (see THIAMINE DEFICIENCY in Ch. 81), but any nutrient deficiency can develop in either of these groups (see also Ch. 138).

STARVATION —INANITION

Structural and functional changes due to inadequate intake of nutrients and energy sources.

Etiology

Exogenous inanition results from inadequate intake of all nutrients as in famine and other circumstances of privation, such as anorectic disease, voluntary fasting, and anorexia nervosa.

Endogenous inanition may be caused by (1) impaired digestion in gastric and pancreatic disease; (2) disordered absorption in malabsorption syndromes; (3) impaired uti-

lization in endocrine dysfunction, metabolic disorders, prolonged infections, or malignant disease leading to anorexia; (4) increased nutritional requirements in thyrotoxicosis, surgical procedures, injuries, burns, and convalescence; and (5) loss of body fluids as in hemorrhage, burns, draining wounds, large-scale removal of fluids from body cavities, transudation from traumatized tissue, or of protein in protein-losing enteropathy and nephrosis.

Symptoms and Signs

Weight loss is characteristic and may reach 50% in adults and even more in children. The loss is greatest in the liver and intestines, moderate in the heart and kidney, and least in the nervous system. Emaciation is most obvious where normally prominent fat depots and muscle masses waste and bones protrude. The skin becomes thin, dry, inelastic, pale, and cold. A patchy brown pigmentation may occur. Perifollicular keratosis is not infrequent. The hair is dry and sparse and falls out easily.

Most systems are affected. Achlorhydria and diarrhea are frequent, the latter often being terminal. Heart size and output are reduced. There is bradycardia and lowered systolic, diastolic, and venous pressure. Respiratory rate, minute volume, and vital capacity are all reduced. The main endocrine disturbance is gonadal atrophy with loss of libido (there is amenorrhea in the female). Intellect remains clear but apathy and irritability are common. Work capacity is diminished due to muscle destruction and eventual anemia and cardiorespiratory failure. Hypothermia frequently contributes to death. Anemia is usually mild, normochromic, and normocytic. In famine edema, serum proteins are normal, but due to loss of fat, extracellular water is relatively increased, tissue tension is low, and the skin is inelastic.

For a discussion of how the immune system is affected by malnutrition, see IMMUNODEFICIENCY AND MALNUTRITION in Ch. 18.

Laboratory Findings

Plasma levels of total amino acids and fatty acids are elevated, indicating catabolism of tissue protein and triglyceride, respectively. Individual amino acids follow different patterns; eg, alanine falls progressively; glycine shows a delayed rise; and valine rises over 10 days and then progressively falls. Plasma insulin is low, glucagon may be high, and albumin is usually only slightly depressed, insufficient to account for the commonly occurring dependent edema, the cause of which is still poorly understood. Urinary nitrogen excretion progressively falls, mainly due to diminished urea output.

Treatment

In the early stages of rehabilitation, food intake must be limited until GI function has been restored. Food should be bland and feedings limited initially to about 100 mL to avoid diarrhea. A recommended formula consists of 42% dried skim milk, 32% edible oil, 25% sucrose plus electrolyte, mineral, and vitamin supplements. In the absence of signs of specific deficiencies of micronutrients these should be provided at about twice the respective RDAs (see Ch. 79). For treatment of specific deficiencies see Chs. 81 and 82. Intake is gradually increased until about 5000 kcal/day may be consumed and weekly weight gain of 1.5 to 2.0 kg attained. If diarrhea persists in the absence of infections, temporary lactose intolerance may be suspected. Yogurt, in which lactose is partially hydrolyzed to glucose and galactose, is well tolerated. Debilitated patients may require feeding by nasogastric tube and parenteral nutrition is indicated if malabsorption is severe (see Ch. 79).

Detailed dietary instruction, not merely a prescribed balanced diet, is needed for correction of deficiencies that are often multiple. When the diet is inadequate because of such factors as allergy, GI disease, dietary fads, or poor eating habits, or when there is impaired utilization of, or abnormal requirement for, one or more nutrients, nutritional supplements are needed.

PROTEIN-CALORIE MALNUTRITION (PCM)
(Protein-Energy Malnutrition)

Classification and Etiology

PCM is classified according to *degree* of severity as 1st (mild), 2nd (moderate), or 3rd (severe). Mild PCM is characterized by growth failure in the child or wasting in the adult; moderate PCM by superimposed biochemical changes (see Laboratory Findings, below); and severe PCM by the development of additional clinical signs.

Meeting energy requirements is basic to survival, and the ways in which this is accomplished from protein or nonprotein sources determines the *type* of severe PCM produced. A diet adequate in nonprotein calories, from starch, sugar, and fat, but deficient in total protein and essential amino acids, results eventually in protein deficiency or **kwashiorkor**. Severe inadequacy of energy intake from all sources causes total inanition, which in young children is called **marasmus,** but does not differ in essence from semistarvation in adults. Intermediate forms are termed **marasmic-kwashiorkor**.

Epidemiology

Marasmus is the predominant form of PCM throughout most developing countries. It is associated with the early abandonment or failure of breast feeding and with consequent infections, most notably those causing infantile gastroenteritis. These infections result from lack of hygiene and proper knowledge of infant rearing that are prevalent, especially in the rapidly growing third-world slums.

Protein deficiency is less common and is usually manifest as the intermediate marasmic-kwashiorkor state. It tends to be confined to those parts of the world (rural Africa, the Caribbean and Pacific islands) where staple and weaning foods such as yam, cassava, sweet potato, or green banana are protein deficient.

Pathophysiology

In marasmus, energy intake is insufficient to match requirements and the body draws on its own stores. Liver glycogen is exhausted within a few hours and skeletal muscle protein is then utilized by gluconeogenesis to maintain adequate plasma glucose. At the same time, triglycerides in fat depots give rise to free fatty acids that contribute to the energy needs of most tissues except the nervous system. In prolonged starvation, fatty acids are incompletely oxidized to ketone bodies that can be utilized by the brain as an alternative energy source. Thus in the severe energy deficiency of marasmus, adaptation is facilitated by high cortisol and growth hormone levels and depression of insulin and thyroid hormone secretion.

In kwashiorkor there is a failure to adapt to protein deficiency. Consequently, serum amino acid patterns are distorted (see Laboratory Findings, below) and protein synthesis is impaired. The resulting hypoalbuminemia causes dependent edema; and the impaired β-lipoprotein synthesis produces fatty liver. In the absence of hypoglycemic stress, plasma cortisol and growth hormone levels in kwashiorkor are maintained within normal limits. As in marasmus there is poor insulin response to a glucose load, possibly due to chromium deficiency (see under OTHER TRACE ELEMENTS in Ch. 82).

Total body protein synthesis is about 300 gm/day in the average adult male. The daily obligatory loss is only about 30 to 90 gm, as 80 to 90% is reutilized. The daily allowance of protein recommended for an adult is about 0.8 gm/kg body wt (see TABLE 79–2). Of this dietary protein, about 20% of the constituent amino acids should be essential amino acids (see TABLE 80–2), since these cannot be synthesized in adequate amounts by the body and must be present in the diet. The degree to which the essential amino acid pattern of the dietary protein approximates that of the body's requirement determines **protein quality.**

In protein deficiency, adaptive enzyme changes occur in the liver, amino acid synthetases increase, and urea formation diminishes, thus conserving nitrogen and reduc-

TABLE 80–2. ESTIMATED ESSENTIAL AMINO ACID REQUIREMENTS

Amino Acid	Daily Requirements (mg/kg)		
	Adult	Infant	Child (10–12 yr)
Histidine	16	26	19
Isoleucine	13	46	28
Leucine	19	93	44
Lysine	16	66	44
Methionine & cystine	17	42	22
Phenylalanine & tyrosine	19	72	22
Threonine	9	43	28
Tryptophan	5	17	9
Valine	13	55	25

(Modified from Energy and Protein Requirements; Report of a Joint FAO/WHO *Ad Hoc* Expert Committee. *WHO Technical Report Series* No. 724. Copyright 1985 by FAO and WHO. Used with permission.)

ing its loss in the urine. Homeostatic mechanisms initially operate to maintain the level of plasma albumin. The rate of synthesis and catabolism soon decrease. Albumin shifts from the extravascular to the intravascular compartment. Eventually plasma albumin concentration falls, leading to reduced oncotic pressure and edema. Growth, immune response, repair, and production of enzymes and hormones are all impaired in severe protein deficiency.

Symptoms and Signs

Mild and moderate PCM may be classified by calculating weight as a percentage of expected weight/length (normal, 90 to 110%; mild PCM, 85 to 90%; moderate, 75 to 85%; severe, < 75%) using international standards.

Marasmic infants show gross weight loss, growth retardation, and wasting of subcutaneous fat and muscle. Kwashiorkor is characterized by generalized edema, "flaky paint" dermatosis, thinning and decoloration of the hair, enlarged fatty liver, and petulant apathy in addition to retarded growth.

Laboratory Findings

Mild or moderately severe cases of PCM may show slight depression of plasma albumin and a lowering of the urinary excretion of urea, due to decreased protein intake, and of hydroxyproline, reflecting impaired growth. Increased urinary 3-methylhistidine reflects muscle breakdown. In both marasmus and kwashiorkor the percent body water, extracellular water, and plasma volume are increased. Electrolyte depletion (especially K and Mg), anemia (usually Fe deficiency), low levels of some enzymes and circulating lipids, falling blood urea, and metabolic acidosis are also present. Diarrhea is sometimes related to intestinal disaccharidase deficiency, especially lactase. Kwashiorkor is characterized by low plasma levels of albumin (10 to 25 gm/L), transferrin, essential amino acids (especially the branched-chain), β-lipoprotein, and glucose, and an "overflow" aminoaciduria. Plasma cortisol and growth hormone levels are high, but insulin secretion is depressed.

Diagnosis

Differential diagnosis includes secondary growth failure due to malabsorption, congenital defects, or deprivation. The skin changes of kwashiorkor differ from those of pellagra in which they occur on parts exposed to light and are symmetrical. Edema in nephritis, nephrosis, and cardiac failure is accompanied by features of these diseases. Hepatomegaly from disorders of glycogen metabolism and cystic fibrosis must be differentiated.

Treatment

Fluid and electrolyte balance should be restored and maintained. All but the most severely ill respond to a diet based on milk; dilute milk feedings can usually be introduced after 24 h. For treatment of shock superimposed on established dehydration, see SHOCK in Ch. 26.

Low-lactose formulas have been helpful in some cases in controlling excessive diarrhea caused by lack of disaccharidases. Lactic acid-fortified milk (0.125 mL/oz of milk) is preferred by some. Sufficient milk should be given to infants and small children to supply 2 to 5 gm of protein/kg/day. At this stage, more calories in the form of sugar and cereal may be added to the milk diet to provide 150 to 250 kcal/kg/day. Increased dietary allowances soon become possible and the diet is supplemented with high-energy foods such as candies, cake, puddings, meats, eggs, and fruit juices. Prepared nutritional supplements are available commercially. Bulky or low-caloric vegetables or fruits should be avoided and those containing 10 to 20% carbohydrate used. Supplementary vitamins may be advisable. Small, frequent feedings around the clock are tolerated best in the early stages of recovery. Antibiotics may be indicated. Unless urgent, treatment of malaria or other parasitic infections should be postponed until the patient is clinically improved. Anemia is usually mild and will respond to oral protein, iron, and folic acid supplements. If severe (Hb < 6 gm/dL), transfusion is indicated with packed RBCs (15 to 20 mL/kg) given slowly to avoid circulation overload as evidenced by rise in venous pressure, tachycardia, hypotension, tachypnea, pulmonary edema, and cyanosis.

Prognosis

Mortality varies between 15 and 40%. Death in the first days of treatment is usually due to electrolyte imbalance, infection, hypothermia, or circulatory failure. Stupor, jaundice, petechiae, low serum Na, and low serum vitamin A are ominous signs. Recovery is more rapid in kwashiorkor than in marasmus; disappearance of apathy, edema, and anorexia are favorable signs.

Long-term effects of malnutrition in childhood are not fully understood. In the adequately treated case the liver probably recovers fully without subsequent cirrhosis, but some GI malabsorption and pancreatic deficiency may remain. Persistent chromosomal breaks observed in malnourished children have not been shown to be due to the malnutrition per se. Humoral immunity is usually unimpaired. Cell-mediated immunocompetence is markedly compromised in the acute phase but is restored with recovery. Behavioral development may be markedly retarded in the severely malnourished child. The degree of mental impairment is related to the duration of malnutrition and to the age of onset. The infant with marasmus is more severely affected than the older child with kwashiorkor. Prospective studies suggest that a relatively mild degree of mental retardation persists into school age.

81. VITAMIN DEFICIENCY, TOXICITY, AND DEPENDENCY

In technologically advanced societies vitamin deficiency mainly results from food fadism, misuse of drugs (see NUTRIENT-DRUG INTERACTIONS in Ch. 79), chronic alcoholism, or prolonged parenteral feeding.

Megavitamin therapy is a not infrequent cause of toxicity. Vitamin dependency usually relates to those vitamins with coenzyme function and results from an apoenzyme abnormality that can be overcome by administration of doses of the appropriate vitamin that are many times the RDA. Numerous vitamin dependency states have been described.

VITAMIN A (RETINOL) DEFICIENCY

(Night Blindness; Xerophthalmia; Keratomalacia)

Vitamin A (retinol) is fat-soluble and is found mainly in fish liver oils, liver, egg yolk, butter, and cream. Green leafy and yellow vegetables contain **β-carotene** and other provitamin carotenoids that undergo central fission of the molecule in the mucosal cells of the small intestine to form retinol, which is then esterified. Most of the body's vitamin A is stored in the liver as **retinyl palmitate**. It is released into the circulation as retinol, bound to a specific protein, retinol-binding protein **(RBP)**, and is also attached to prealbumin (transthyretin). The 11-*cis* isomer of retinal (vitamin A_1 aldehyde), combined with a protein moiety, forms the prosthetic group of photoreceptor pigments in the retina that are involved in night, day, and color vision. Vitamin A is also concerned with the maintenance of normal epithelial tissue. TABLES 79–1 and 79–2 give sources and recommended daily allowances. Equivalents, for diets with different proportions of retinol and β-carotene, are as follows: 1 USP u. equals 1 IU; 1 IU equals 0.3 μg of retinol; 1 μg of β-carotene equals 0.167 μg of retinol; other provitamin carotenoids are half as active as β-carotene. Inadequate intake or utilization of vitamin A can impair dark adaptation and cause night blindness; xerosis of the conjunctiva and cornea; xerophthalmia and keratomalacia; keratinization of lung, GI tract, and urinary tract epithelia; and increased susceptibility to infections. Defective taste and smell, and anemia that may be masked by hemoconcentration have also been reported.

The possible protective role of β-carotene and retinol against certain cancers is under intense investigation.

Etiology

Primary vitamin A deficiency is usually caused by prolonged dietary deprivation. It is endemic in areas such as southern and eastern Asia where rice, devoid of carotene, is the staple. Secondary deficiency may be due to inadequate conversion of carotene, or to interference with absorption, storage, or transport of vitamin A. Interference with absorption or storage is likely in celiac disease, sprue, cystic fibrosis, operations on the pancreas, duodenal bypass, congenital partial obstruction of the jejunum, obstruction of the bile ducts, giardiasis, and cirrhosis of the liver. Vitamin A deficiency is common in protein-calorie malnutrition (marasmus or kwashiorkor) not only because the diet is deficient but also because vitamin A storage and transport are defective. Liver stores are depleted in deficiency before plasma levels begin to fall, followed later by retinal dysfunction, and finally by epithelial structural changes.

Symptoms and Signs

The severity of the effects of vitamin A deficiency is inversely related to age. Growth retardation is a common sign in children. Increased susceptibility to infection occurs at all ages. Pathognomonic changes are confined to the eye (see KERATOMALACIA in Ch. 220). Perifollicular hyperkeratosis of the skin is nonspecific and sporadic. The earliest, rod dysfunction, can be detected by dark adaptometry, rod scotometry, or electroretinography. These tests require cooperative subjects. Xerosis of the bulbar conjunctiva consists of drying, thickening, wrinkling, and muddy pigmentation. In advanced deficiency, **Bitot's spots** (superficial, foamy patches composed of epithelial debris and secretions on the exposed bulbar conjunctiva) are most likely due to vitamin A deficiency when they are large and occur in young children with other evidence of hypovitaminosis A. The cornea becomes xerotic, infiltrated, and hazy at an early stage. Keratomalacia rapidly supervenes with liquefaction of part or all of the cornea, leading to rupture, with extrusion of the eye contents and subsequent shrinking of the globe **(phthisis bulbi)**, or to anterior bulging **(corneal ectasia** and **anterior staphyloma)**, and blindness. Mortality in advanced cases is high (50% or more).

Diagnosis and Laboratory Findings

Evidence of depletion is unobtainable in the preclinical stage except for a history of inadequate intake. Plasma retinol levels fall when liver stores are exhausted. The normal range is 20 to 50 μg/dL; 10 to 19 μg is low, and < 10 μg is deficient. Mean plasma RBP is 47 μg/mL for adult males and 42 μg for females. Up to the age of 10 yr the range is 20 to 30 μg. Plasma vitamin A and RBP fall in deficiency and in acute infections. Other causes of night blindness (eg, retinitis pigmentosa) must be excluded. Secondary infection may complicate the corneal changes. Trial with therapeutic doses of vitamin A will assist in the diagnosis.

Prophylaxis

Xerophthalmia remains the major cause of blindness in young children in most developing countries, where prophylactic doses of 200,000 IU (66,000 μg) of oily vitamin A palmitate orally once every 3 to 6 mo are advised for all children 1 to 4 (half the dose for those under 1). The diet should include green leafy vegetables. Bread, sugar, and monosodium glutamate are being fortified with vitamin A. Vitamin A supplements should be given routinely in secondary deficiency. Infants suspected of being allergic to milk should receive adequate vitamin A in the substitute formula.

Treatment

The cause should be corrected, and vitamin A given in therapeutic doses at once, followed by maintenance doses as required. Eye lesions and accompanying systemic changes are a threat to vision and to life. Vitamin A palmitate in oil given orally 200,000 IU (66,000 μg) daily for 2 days and once before discharge from hospital after 7 to 10 days is usually effective. In the presence of vomiting or malabsorption, water-miscible vitamin A must be given IM, as oil preparations are not utilized by this route. Thereafter, 25,000 to 50,000 IU/day (8,000 to 16,000 μg) may be given orally until response is adequate. Maintenance therapy, or treatment of mild or suspected deficiency, includes 10,000 to 20,000 IU (3000 to 6000 μg)/day orally in 3 divided doses as cod-liver oil, red palm oil, or other concentrate. Prolonged daily administration of large doses, especially to infants, is to be **avoided** as hypervitaminosis (see below) may result. During pregnancy and lactation prophylactic doses should not exceed the RDA in order to avoid possible damage to the fetus.

HYPERVITAMINOSIS A

Excessive intake of vitamin A may be either acute or chronic. **Acute toxicity** in children has resulted from taking large doses (> 300,000 IU or 100,000 μg) and manifests as increased intracranial pressure and vomiting. Recovery is spontaneous with no residual damage; no fatalities have been reported. Arctic explorers, after ingesting several million units of vitamin A in polar bear or seal liver, have developed drowsiness, irritability, headache, and vomiting a few hours later, with subsequent peeling of the skin. Tablets containing vitamin A, sold for the prevention and relief of sunburn, have occasionally induced acute hypervitaminosis even when taken in accordance with the manufacturer's directions.

Chronic poisoning in older children and adults usually develops after doses above 100,000 IU (33,000 μg)/day have been taken for months. Infants may develop evidence of toxicity within a few weeks when given 20,000 to 60,000 IU (6,000 to 20,000 μg)/day of water-dispersible vitamin A. Regular consumption of beef liver is not an infrequent cause in adults in the USA. Birth defects have been reported in the offspring of women receiving 13-*cis*-retinoic acid (isotretinoin) for skin conditions during pregnancy (see DRUGS IN PREGNANCY under PRENATAL CARE in Ch. 176).

Clinical Findings

Sparse coarse hair, alopecia of the eyebrows, dry rough skin, and cracked lips are early signs. Severe headache, **pseudotumor cerebri,** and generalized weakness are

prominent later. Cortical hyperostoses and arthralgia are common, especially in children. Hepatomegaly and splenomegaly may occur.

Excessive ingestion of carotene does not cause hypervitaminosis A but produces high carotene blood levels (> 250 μg/dL) **(carotenemia)** which, while usually asymptomatic, may lead to **carotenosis** wherein the skin (but not the sclera) becomes deep yellow, especially on the palms and soles. Carotenosis may also occur in diabetes mellitus, myxedema, and anorexia nervosa possibly from a defect in conversion of carotene to vitamin A.

Diagnosis

Normal plasma vitamin A values range from 20 to 50 μg/dL. In hypervitaminosis A, fasting blood levels may exceed 100 μg/dL and have been as high as 2000 μg/dL. Differential diagnosis may be difficult as symptoms are varied and bizarre.

Prognosis and Treatment

Prognosis is excellent. Symptoms and signs usually disappear within 1 to 4 wk after stopping vitamin A ingestion.

VITAMIN D DEFICIENCY AND DEPENDENCY

(Rickets and Osteomalacia)

This fat-soluble vitamin occurs mainly in 2 forms: **ergocalciferol** (activated ergosterol, calciferol, **vitamin D_2**), found in irradiated yeast; and **cholecalciferol** (activated 7-dehydrocholesterol, **vitamin D_3**), formed in human skin by exposure to sunlight (ultraviolet radiation) and found chiefly in fish liver oils and egg yolks. Milk is fortified with both forms. Synthesis in the skin is normally the major source. For recommended daily allowances see TABLE 79–2; 1 μg vitamin D equals 40 IU.

Vitamin D can be considered to be a prohormone with several active metabolites that behave as hormones. In the skin previtamin D_3 is synthesized photochemically from 7-dehydrocholesterol and is slowly isomerized to vitamin D_3, which is removed by vitamin D-binding protein. Vitamin D_3 is converted in the liver to 25-(OH)D_3, the major circulating form. It undergoes enterohepatic circulation and is reabsorbed from the gut. In the kidney it is further hydroxylated to the much more metabolically active form 1,25-$(OH)_2D_3$ (1,25-DHCC; calcitriol) whose main function is to increase Ca absorption from the intestine and promote normal bone formation and mineralization. The critical 1-hydroxylation of 25-(OH)D_3 is strongly stimulated by parathyroid hormone **(PTH)** and, independently of PTH, by hypophosphatemia. Other metabolites, which may also have hormonal function, have been identified.

Metabolic bone disease resulting from vitamin D deficiency is called **rickets** in children and **osteomalacia** in adults. These diseases result from common pathogenetic factors but differ in their clinical and pathologic expression owing to differences between growing and formed bones.

Inadequate exposure to sunlight and poor dietary intake are usually necessary for clinical vitamin D deficiency to develop. Rickets is not uncommon in the tropics, due to swaddling of infants and confinement of women and children to the home. Nutritional rickets is rare in the USA, but is not uncommon in Asian immigrants to Britain, where lack of sunlight, chelation of calcium by consumption of traditional cereal diet, and low intake of milk are probably responsible. Very low intakes of calcium or phosphorus may rarely be the cause.

All the features of rickets and osteomalacia may become evident when the supply of vitamin D is inadequate, its metabolism is abnormal, or tissues are resistant to its action (see TABLE 81–1). The actions of vitamin D and its metabolites are summarized in TABLE 81–2.

TABLE 81–1. CLASSIFICATION OF RICKETS AND OSTEOMALACIA

Deficiency of vitamin D	
	Dietary lack, high phytate or phosphate intake, lack of sunlight, malabsorption syndromes
Defects related to production of 25-$(OH)D_3$	
	Liver disease (advanced parenchymal and cholestatic disease)
	Anticonvulsants (prolonged use of phenobarbital, phenytoin), enzyme induction, impaired absorption (?)
Defects related to action of 1,25-$(OH)_2D_3$	
	Vitamin D-dependent (pseudo-vitamin D deficiency) rickets, type I (? defective 1-hydroxylation)
	Vitamin D-dependent rickets, type II (at least 2 types, receptors for 1,25$(OH)_2D_3$ absent or defective)
Other forms	
	Familial hypophosphatemic (vitamin D-resistant) rickets (renal tubular defect in phosphate transport); chronic renal failure (renal osteodystrophy); Fanconi syndrome; renal tubular acidosis; diabetes mellitus (increased incidence of osteopenia, osteoporosis, and some fractures); pseudohypoparathyroidism

Familial hypophosphatemic (vitamin D-resistant) rickets, an X-linked dominant disorder, is discussed under ANOMALIES IN KIDNEY TRANSPORT in Ch. 187.

Etiology

An etiologic classification of rickets and osteomalacia is important in relation to the manifestations of disease and to effective treatment. Some diseases interfere with the absorption of vitamin D or with the formation of its active metabolites. In these circumstances, the manifestations of these diseases will be superimposed upon those described below. If there is deficiency of vitamin D metabolites, vitamin D-resistant states occur that may be overcome to a varying extent (but often with undesirable side

TABLE 81–2. ACTIONS OF VITAMIN D AND ITS METABOLITES

Intestine	
	Enhances Ca transport (absorption), the main function of 1,25-$(OH)_2D_3$
	Enhances PO_4 transport (absorption)
Bone	
	Stimulates mineralization
	Mobilizes Ca to bone fluid compartment (PTH-like effect)
	Promotes biosynthesis and maturation of collagen
Muscle	
	Maintains integrity (through Ca and P transfer?)
Parathyroid glands	
	Inhibits PTH secretion (?)
Lymphomedullary system	
	Antitumor activity

effects) by massive doses of vitamin D. Some of these states are now better treated with very small doses of metabolite or synthetic analog (see below).

Pathology

Changes in children include defective calcification of growing bone and hypertrophy of the epiphyseal cartilages. Epiphyseal cartilage cells cease to degenerate but new cartilage continues to form, so that the epiphyseal cartilage becomes irregularly increased in width. Calcification then stops and osteoid material accumulates around the capillaries of the diaphysis. The cancellous bone of the diaphysis and of cortical bone may be resorbed in chronic deficiency.

Adequate treatment with vitamin D permits Ca and PO_4 deposition through degeneration of the cartilage cells within 24 h and penetration by a vascular network within 48 h. Osteoid material at the diaphysis ceases to form, and normal endochondral production of new bone is resumed. The changes in adults are similar but not confined to the ends of the long bones.

Symptoms and Signs

In the neonatal period metaphyseal lesions and tetany accompany maternal osteomalacia. Young infants are restless, sleep poorly, and have reduced mineralization of the skull **(craniotabes)** away from the sutures. In older infants, sitting and crawling are delayed and there is bossing of the skull, costochondral beading **(rachitic rosary)** and delayed fontanelle closure. From 1 to 4 yr, there is enlargement of epiphyseal cartilages at the lower ends of the radius, ulna, tibia, and fibula; delay in walking; bowlegs, and kyphoscoliosis. In older children and adolescents there is pain on walking, and the development of such deformities as bowlegs and knock-knees in extreme cases.

Rachitic tetany is caused by hypocalcemia and may accompany either infantile or adult vitamin D deficiency. The clinical findings are discussed under HYPOCALCEMIA in DISTURBANCES IN CALCIUM METABOLISM in Ch. 84.

X-ray changes precede clinical signs, becoming evident in the 3rd or 4th mo of life—even at birth if the mother is vitamin D-deficient. Bone changes in rickets are most evident at the lower ends of the radius and ulna. The diaphyseal ends lose their sharp, clear outline, are cup-shaped, and show a spotty or fringy rarefaction. Later, the distance between the ends of the radius and ulna and the metacarpal bones appears increased, since the true ends are noncalcified and invisible. The shadows cast by the shaft decrease in density, and the network formed by laminas becomes coarse. Characteristic deformities are produced by bending of the bones at the cartilage-shaft junction due to weakness in the substance of the shaft. As healing begins, a thin white line of calcification appears at the epiphysis, becoming denser and thicker as calcification proceeds. Later, calcium salts are deposited beneath the periosteum, the shaft casts a denser shadow, and the lamellas disappear.

In adults, demineralization **(osteomalacia)** occurs, particularly in the spine, pelvis, and lower extremities; the fibrous lamellas become visible by x-ray, and incomplete ribbon-like demineralizations appear in the cortex (pseudofractures, Looser's zones, Milkman's fractures). As the bones soften, weight may cause bowing of the long bones, vertical shortening of the vertebrae, and flattening of the pelvic bones, which contracts the pelvic outlet. The use of vitamin D in the treatment of **renal osteodystrophy** caused by chronic renal failure is discussed in Ch. 147.

Laboratory Findings

With identification of specific binding proteins for vitamin D metabolites, 25-$(OH)D_3$ and other vitamin D sterols may be measured in plasma. Reported values for healthy subjects are 25 to 40 ng/mL for 25-$(OH)D_3$ and 20 to 45 pg/mL for 1,25-$(OH)_2D_3$. In nutritional rickets and osteomalacia 25-$(OH)D_3$ values are very low and 1,25-$(OH)_2D_3$ is undetectable. A low serum phosphorus (normal 3.0 to 4.5 mg/dL) and a high serum alkaline phosphatase are characteristic. The serum Ca is low or normal

depending on the effectiveness of the secondary hyperparathyroidism in restoring the serum Ca to normal. The serum PTH is elevated, and urinary Ca is low in all forms of the disease except those associated with acidosis. In hereditary forms of the disease laboratory findings vary (see below).

Diagnosis

A history of inadequate vitamin D intake suggests rickets and helps to distinguish it from infantile scurvy (see in Ch. 195) and other conditions. Congenital syphilis can be identified by serologic and other tests; chondrodystrophy, by the large head, short extremities, and thick bones, and by normal serum Ca, P, and phosphatase values.

Osteogenesis imperfecta, cretinism, congenital dislocation of the hip, hydrocephalus, and poliomyelitis should be readily distinguishable. Manifest tetany in infantile rickets must be differentiated from convulsions due to other causes. Rickets refractory to vitamin D may be caused by severe renal damage or occurs in renal tubular acidosis, sex-linked hypophosphatemia, and Fanconi's syndrome.

Osteomalacia must be differentiated from other causes of widespread bone decalcification (eg, hyperparathyroidism, senile or postmenopausal osteoporosis, the osteoporosis of hyperthyroidism, Cushing's syndrome, multiple myeloma, and atrophy of disuse). Serum Ca, PO_4, alkaline phosphatase, and 25-$(OH)D_3$ levels, together with x-ray findings, confirm the diagnosis.

Treatment

With adequate calcium and phosphorus intake, adult osteomalacia and uncomplicated rickets can be cured by intake of vitamin D 1600 IU (40 μg)/day. Serum 25-$(OH)D_3$ and 1,25-$(OH)_2D_3$ begin to rise within 1 or 2 days. Serum P rises in about 10 days, followed in the 3rd wk by x-ray signs of Ca and P deposition in the osseous tissues. After about 1 mo of therapy, the dose can be reduced gradually to normal levels. If tetany is present, treatment should be supplemented during the 1st wk with IV calcium salts (see HYPOCALCEMIA under DISTURBANCES IN CALCIUM METABOLISM in Ch. 84).

Those forms of rickets and osteomalacia that result from defective production of vitamin D metabolites (see TABLE 81–1) do not respond to the usual doses effective in nutritional rickets. Some of these conditions respond to massive doses (600 to 1200 μg vitamin D_2 or D_3 daily) but toxicity may result. In some of the conditions in which there is evidence of defective 25-$(OH)D_3$ production, 50 μg/day of 25-$(OH)D_3$ will augment plasma levels and result in clinical improvement.

Hereditary Vitamin D-Dependent Rickets

Type I (pseudo-vitamin D deficiency) is an autosomal recessive syndrome, characterized by severe rickets, normal 25-$(OH)D_3$ and subnormal 1,25-$(OH)_2D_3$ plasma levels, low or normal serum Ca, hypophosphatemia, and generalized aminoaciduria. This disorder responds to physiologic quantities of 1,25-$(OH_2)D_3$ (1 to 2 μg/day) IV or orally. **Type II vitamin D-dependent rickets** exists in at least 2 forms—in one, receptors for 1,25$(OH)_2D$ are absent or defective with a high ineffective plasma 1,25$(OH)_2D$, and a second form in which receptors are present but unable to induce 24(OH)D following exposure to 1,25$(OH)_2D$. A number of cases have been described with a defect in 1α-hydroxylase in the kidney resulting in high plasma 25(OH)D and negligible 1,25$(OH)_2D$. Some patients have responded to very high doses of 1,25-$(OH)_2D_3$ (10 to 40 μg/day); a few have responded to high doses of 25-$(OH)D_3$; others have not responded at all.

Prophylaxis

Health education, including dietary advice, should be given to susceptible communities. Fortified cow's milk contains 1.0 μg/dL, about 10 times that present in breast milk. A weekly capsule of vitamin D 3000 IU (75 μg) gives complete protection.

Vitamin D fortification of unleavened chapati flour (125 μg/kg) has proved effective among Asian immigrants in Britain. In adolescents, a single IM dose of 100,000 IU (2.5 mg) ergocalciferol in the fall has produced a substantial rise of plasma 25(OH)D until spring.

HYPERVITAMINOSIS D

Vitamin D 40,000 IU (1000 μg)/day produces toxicity within 1 to 4 mo in infants; toxic effects have been observed in adults receiving 100,000 IU (2500 μg)/day for several months. Elevated serum Ca levels of 12 to 16 mg/dL are a constant finding when toxic symptoms occur (normal values are 8.5 to 10.5 mg/dL). *Frequent determinations of serum calcium (weekly at first and then monthly) should be made in all patients receiving large doses of vitamin D.*

The first symptoms are anorexia, nausea, and vomiting, followed by polyuria, polydipsia, weakness, nervousness, and pruritus. Renal function is impaired, as evidenced by low specific gravity urine, proteinuria, casts, and azotemia. Metastatic calcifications may occur, particularly in the kidneys. Plasma 25-$(OH)D_3$ and 1,25-$(OH)_2D_3$ are usually within the normal range.

A history of excessive vitamin D intake is critical in differentiating this condition from all other hypercalcemic states. Vitamin D toxicity occurs commonly during the treatment of hypoparathyroidism. So-called "**hypercalcemia in infancy, with failure to thrive**" has been seen with daily vitamin D intakes less than 2000 IU or 50 μg (as low as 1000 IU or 25 μg); in these cases there may be hypersensitivity to the vitamin. **Williams syndrome** consists of transient hypercalcemia in infancy with the triad of supravalvular aortic stenosis, mental retardation and elfin facies. Plasma levels of 1,25$(OH)_2$D during the hypercalcemic phase are 8 to 10 times normal. Most cases are due to an unidentified defect in vitamin D metabolism rather than to excessive intake. As the new, highly active forms of vitamin D are being increasingly used, possible toxic effects of long-term therapy will need to be watched for.

Treatment consists of discontinuing the vitamin, a low-calcium diet, keeping the urine acidic, and corticosteroids. If kidney damage or metastatic calcification has occurred, it may be irreversible. Diuretics and forced fluids are not helpful.

VITAMIN E (TOCOPHEROL) DEFICIENCY AND TOXICITY

The vitamin E group includes the α, β, γ, and δ tocopherols; α is the most active. Tocopherols act as antioxidants to prevent lipid peroxidation of polyunsaturated fatty acids in cells and maintain membrane integrity. Vitamin E has close metabolic relationships with selenium (see in Ch. 82). Deficiency in man causes RBC hemolysis, creatinuria, and deposition of ceroid in muscle. Neurologic changes consisting of cerebellar ataxia, posterior column dysfunction, and peripheral neuropathy have been described (see in Ch. 120). Retrolental fibroplasia (see RETINOPATHY OF PREMATURITY under GESTATIONAL AGE AND BIRTH WEIGHT in Ch. 186) may improve with vitamin E therapy, as may some cases of intraventricular and subependymal hemorrhage in the newborn. (For sources and daily allowances, see TABLES 79–1 and 79–2.)

Etiology

Primary deficiency may occur in early infancy, especially with infant formulas high in unsaturated oils. Protein-calorie malnourished children often have low vitamin E status. Adult males have required many months on experimental diets to evidence vitamin E deficiency. Secondary deficiency may be expected in any malabsorption syndrome, especially with steatorrhea (as in sprue, celiac disease, cystic fibrosis, or biliary atresia), cholestasis, and in abetalipoproteinemia due to transport dysfunction.

Diagnosis and Laboratory Findings

Shortened length of RBC life has been attributed to vitamin E deficiency in adults. Edema and flaky dermatitis have been associated with low plasma E as has increased peroxide hemolysis in premature infants on formulas containing vegetable oil. The deficiency state may be diagnosed when the plasma tocopherol level is low (< 0.8 mg/dL in the adult; < 0.4 mg/dL in the child). RBC susceptibility to hydrogen peroxide is increased with levels < 0.5 mg/dL. Excessive creatinuria and increased plasma creatine phosphokinase levels are present on a creatine-free diet.

Treatment

If there is malabsorption in overt deficiency, vitamin E 30 to 100 mg/day should be given IM as *dl-α*-tocopheryl acetate (1 mg = 1 IU). For infants, who are especially susceptible, a minimum daily allowance of 0.5 mg/kg (the amount usually obtained from human milk) is recommended. Much larger doses (up to 100 mg/kg/day by mouth in divided doses) are required for the early treatment of neuropathy or to overcome the defect in abetalipoproteinemia.

Toxicity

Large doses of vitamin E (100 mg/kg/day) in low-birth weight infants are suspected of increasing the incidence of necrotizing enterocolitis and sepsis, probably by causing a decrease in the oxygen-dependent intracellular killing ability of lymphocytes and macrophages. A new IV vitamin E product has caused the death of several premature infants with pulmonary deterioration, thrombocytopenia, and liver and renal failure.

VITAMIN K DEFICIENCY

Vitamin K activity is present in 2-methyl-1,4-naphthoquinones substituted at the 3 position with a phytyl group (phylloquinone or vitamin K_1 including synthetic **menadione** and **phytonadione**) or a multiprenyl side chain (the menaquinone or vitamin K_2 series). Vitamin K controls the formation in the liver of factors II (prothrombin); VII (proconvertin); IX (Christmas factor, plasma thromboplastin component **[PTC]**); and X (Stuart-Prower factor). They all contain the previously undescribed amino acid, γ-carboxylglutamic acid, as do proteins of similar structure isolated from plasma, bone, skeletal muscle, and kidney, suggesting a possibly wider function for vitamin K. Deficiency causes *hypoprothrombinemia, manifested by defective coagulation of the blood and hemorrhage.* The adult daily requirement is about 2 mg.

Etiology

Vitamin K is usually formed in the body from intestinal bacterial synthesis. Lack of intestinal bacterial flora probably in part explains the hypoprothrombinemia observed during the first 3 to 5 days of life. Low levels of factors II, VII, IX, and X may reflect hepatic immaturity; as protein synthesis increases vitamin K becomes limiting. Therapy with nonabsorbable sulfonamides or oral antibiotics may interfere with vitamin K synthesis in the intestines.

Secondary deficiency often results from impaired absorption due to lack of bile salts in patients with external biliary fistulas or obstructive jaundice and other GI conditions causing malabsorption. Excessive amounts of mineral oil taken orally may also prevent absorption. Severe liver disease may inhibit prothrombin synthesis, a condition unresponsive to vitamin K therapy. Coumarin anticoagulants suppress synthesis of the 4 vitamin K-factors in the liver, since they act as competitive inhibitors of vitamin K. Enteral feeds may contain high amounts of vitamin K and result in resistance to oral anticoagulants. Deficiency due to dietary lack or prolonged total parenteral nutrition has been described.

Symptoms and Signs

Symptoms are those of hypoprothrombinemia superimposed on the conditioning disease. In obstructive jaundice, hemorrhage, if it occurs, usually begins after the 4th to 5th day. It may begin as a slow ooze from a surgical wound, the gums, nose, or GI mucosa, or it may be massive into the GI tract. Some intracranial hemorrhages at birth and other hemorrhagic disorders are traceable to the hypoprothrombinemia of the first few days of life. Breast-fed infants who have not received vitamin K are especially susceptible, as human milk is a poor source of the vitamin. In the USA and Britain, there has recently been an increased incidence of intracranial hemorrhage from this cause in breast fed infants aged 4 to 6 wk.

Laboratory Findings

All vitamin K-dependent plasma glycoproteins—factors II, VII, IX, X, and a fifth, recently discovered—are significantly depressed. Reduction of quantitative prothrombin to 80% of normal or below is abnormal, and reduction to 20% or less is associated with an increasing incidence of active bleeding. Bleeding and coagulation times are usually not altered significantly until the prothrombin level has fallen to below 20%. Abnormal prothrombin is present in plasma.

Laboratory findings identical to those of vitamin K deficiency will also be found in rare, psychiatrically disturbed patients who ingest oral anticoagulants surreptitiously and then seek medical help for abnormal bleeding.

Clinical significant vitamin K deficiency always lengthens the prothrombin time **(PT),** primarily because of depression of factor VII. *Therefore, a normal PT rules out vitamin K deficiency as a cause for bleeding and giving vitamin K to a bleeding patient with a normal PT will have no effect upon bleeding.* The partial thromboplastin time **(PTT)** will be normal initially because prothrombin, factor IX, and factor X levels fall more slowly than factor VII levels. Moreover, the PTT sometimes remains within a laboratory's normal range because elevation of factor VIII (an acute phase protein) in a sick patient may counterbalance the effect upon the PTT of the fall of the vitamin K-dependent factors.

Diagnosis

Hypoprothrombinemia may result from anticoagulant or salicylate therapy, failure to absorb vitamin K, severe liver damage, or an unknown cause. Liver pathology can usually be ruled out if 2 to 5 mg of water-soluble synthetic vitamin K, given IV, produces a significant increase in prothrombin levels within 2 to 6 h. Many diseases, such as scurvy, allergic purpura, leukemia, and thrombocytopenia, can produce hemorrhagic symptoms without hypoprothrombinemia.

Treatment

Phytonadione (vitamin K_1) is the preparation of choice. It may be used in any hypoprothrombinemia, particularly that caused by the vitamin K antagonists derived from coumarin or indandione. Menadione sodium bisulfite is not effective against these antagonists. Whenever possible, phytonadione should be given s.c. or IM. The usual adult dose is 10 mg IM. *In emergencies,* from 10 to 50 mg of phytonadione dissolved in 5% dextrose or 0.9% sodium chloride should be given IV **at a rate not to exceed 1 mg/min.** This may be repeated in 6 to 8 h if the prothrombin time has not been shortened satisfactorily. The counteractive effect is detectable within an hour or 2 and, in most cases, is effective within 3 to 6 h. Oral phytonadione 5 to 20 mg is indicated for nonemergency control of hypoprothrombinemia in patients taking anticoagulants. Beneficial effects are usually apparent within 6 to 10 h after starting oral therapy.

Prophylaxis

Phytonadione (vitamin K_1) 0.5 to 1 mg IM is routinely recommended for the newborn (CAUTION: *Large doses may cause toxicity; see* HYPERVITAMINOSIS K *below*) to prevent hypoprothrombinemia, to reduce the incidence of intracranial hemorrhage incidental to birth trauma, and prophylactically when surgery is contemplated. Recommended alternative procedures are: (1) vitamin K_1 given to the mother in prophylactic dosages (2 to 5 mg orally/day) for 1 wk prior to expected confinement, or (2) vitamin K_1 solution (2 to 5 mg IM) given to the mother 6 to 24 h before delivery. Pregnant women on anticonvulsants should receive vitamin K 20 mg/day for 2 wk prior to delivery to prevent fetal hemorrhage. Low breast milk content is due to deficient consumption that can be prevented by eating some fresh green leafy vegetables daily.

HYPERVITAMINOSIS K

Menadione and its water-soluble analogs can cause hemolysis in persons with G6PD deficiency and in others when large doses are used. **In the newborn,** large doses of menadione have produced anemia with Heinz bodies, hyperbilirubinemia, and kernicterus (especially in premature infants with erythroblastosis). The dose should be limited: 2 to 5 mg for women in labor; 1 to 2 mg for newborn babies.

ESSENTIAL FATTY ACID DEFICIENCY

Full-term babies fed a skim-milk formula low in linoleic acid suffered growth failure and a dermatosis; the condition was reversed when linoleic acid was added. Deficiency is unlikely to occur on natural diets, although cow's milk has only about 1/4 the amount present in human milk. While total fat intake in many developing countries is very low, much of it is of vegetable origin and rich in linoleic acid. Essential fatty acid deficiency has been a hazard of long-term fat-free parenteral nutrition in the past, but fat emulsions, now in general use, prevent this (see PARENTERAL NUTRITION in Ch. 79). A 10% soybean oil emulsion contains about 56 gm/L linoleic acid. A single case report of deficiency has claimed response of a neurologic syndrome to linolenic, but not linoleic, acid.

Early in deficiency, plasma levels of linoleic and arachidonic acids are low and the abnormal presence of 5,8,11-eicosatrienoic acid occurs from lack of inhibition of its synthesis from oleic acid. An upper limit of normalcy of the ratio of eicosatrienoic acid to eicosatetraenoic (arachidonic) acid in plasma of 0.2 has been suggested.

Requirements of essential fatty acids are 1 to 2% of dietary calories for adults and 3% for infants.

THIAMINE (VITAMIN B_1) DEFICIENCY

(Beriberi)

The coenzyme thiamine pyrophosphate **(TPP)** participates in carbohydrate metabolism through decarboxylation of α-keto acids. Thiamine also acts as coenzyme to the apoenzyme transketolase in the pentose monophosphate pathway for glucose. (For sources and daily allowances of thiamine, see TABLES 79–1 and 79–2.) Deficiency causes **beriberi** with peripheral neurologic, cerebral, and cardiovascular manifestations.

Etiology

Primary thiamine deficiency arises from inadequate intake, particularly in people subsisting on highly polished rice. Milling removes the husk, which contains most of the thiamine, but boiling before husking disperses the vitamin throughout the grain, thus preventing its loss. **Secondary deficiency** arises from (1) increased requirement, as

in hyperthyroidism, pregnancy, lactation, and fever; (2) impaired absorption, as in long-continued diarrheas; and (3) impaired utilization, as in severe liver disease. A combination of decreased intake, impaired absorption and utilization, increased requirements, and possibly an apoenzyme defect occurs in alcoholism. Frequent, long-continued, or highly concentrated dextrose infusions, coupled with low thiamine intake, may precipitate thiamine deficiency.

Pathology

The most advanced neural changes occur in the peripheral nerves, particularly of the legs. The distal segments are characteristically affected earliest and most severely. Degeneration of the medullary sheath has been demonstrated in all tracts of the cord, especially in the posterior columns and in the anterior and posterior nerve roots. Changes are noted also in the anterior horn and posterior ganglion cells. Lesions of hemorrhagic polioencephalitis occur in the brain when deficiency is severe.

The heart is dilated and enlarged; muscle fibers are swollen, fragmented, and vacuolized, with interstitial spaces dilated by fluid. Edema and serous effusions may develop, even in patients without congestive heart failure.

Symptoms and Signs

Early deficiency produces fatigue, irritation, poor memory, sleep disturbances, precordial pain, anorexia, abdominal discomfort, and constipation.

Peripheral neurologic changes (dry beriberi) are bilateral and symmetric, involving predominantly the lower extremities, and are ushered in by paresthesias of the toes, burning of the feet (particularly severe at night) calf muscle cramps, and pains in the legs. Calf muscle tenderness, difficulty in rising from a squatting position, a quantitative diminution in the vibratory sensation in the toes, and plantar dysesthesia are early signs. A diagnosis of mild peripheral neuropathy can be made when ankle jerks are absent. Continued deficiency causes loss of knee jerk, loss of vibratory and position sensation in the toes, atrophy of the calf and thigh muscles, and finally foot-drop and toe-drop. The arms may become involved after leg signs are well established.

Cerebral beriberi (Wernicke-Korsakoff syndrome; acute hemorrhagic polioencephalitis) results from severe and acute deficiency superimposed on chronic deficiency. Mental confusion, aphonia, and confabulation constitute the early stage called **Korsakoff syndrome** (see in THE AMNESIAS under FOCAL DISORDERS OF HIGHER FUNCTION in Ch. 118). Cerebral blood flow is markedly reduced and vascular resistance increased. Nystagmus, total ophthalmoplegia, coma, and death in the untreated case is **Wernicke's encephalopathy** (see in Ch. 120).

Cardiovascular (wet) beriberi takes 2 forms—the more common high output state or the rare low output state **(Shoshin disease)**. In the former, before heart failure supervenes, there is tachycardia, a wide pulse pressure, sweating, and warm skin. With heart failure orthopnea, pulmonary and peripheral edema, and peripheral vasoconstriction causing cold and cyanosed extremities, occur. The low output state is characterized by severe hypotension, lactic acidosis, very low systemic vascular resistance, and absence of edema.

Infantile beriberi occurs in infants breast-fed by thiamine-deficient mothers, usually between the 2nd and 4th mo of life. Cardiac failure, aphonia, and absent deep tendon reflexes are characteristic.

Laboratory Findings

Elevated blood pyruvate and diminished urinary thiamine excretion ($< 50\ \mu g/day$) are consistent but late changes. Erythrocyte transketolase activity diminishes before and increases after addition of thiamine pyrophosphate (**TPP** effect), and is more sensitive. Variations in apoenzyme levels in some diseases may complicate interpretation.

Diagnosis

A form of polyneuropathy, which does not respond to thiamine, occurs in uncontrolled or long-continued diabetes mellitus and is clinically similar to that of thiamine deficiency. Other forms of bilateral symmetric polyneuropathy beginning in the legs are infrequent. Single-nerve neuritides and those beginning elsewhere are unlikely to be due to thiamine deficiency.

Edema of cardiovascular beriberi responds to bed rest as well as or better than the edema of most other forms of heart disease but responds poorly to digitalis or diuretics. Response to a therapeutic trial of thiamine in uncomplicated cardiovascular or cerebral beriberi is usually prompt and complete. Diagnosis is difficult when complicated by hypertensive, degenerative, or infectious heart disease.

Treatment

In mild polyneuropathies, 10 to 20 mg/day of thiamine is given in divided doses. The dose is 20 to 30 mg/day in moderate or advanced neuropathy. In cardiovascular beriberi and in Wernicke-Korsakoff syndrome, 50 to 100 mg IM or IV bid is usually given; these doses should be continued until a therapeutic response is obtained or until a strong odor of thiamine in the urine indicates saturation. Basic therapy should then be resumed. Rarely, fatal anaphylactic reactions unrelated to dose size have followed IV injection. The possibility of such reactions must be considered, particularly in patients who have previously received thiamine parenterally, if an interval has elapsed without treatment.

Thiamine deficiency is often associated with other B complex deficiencies, and multiple water-soluble vitamin therapy usually is advisable.

Magnesium, a cofactor for transketolase, should be given as magnesium sulfate (1 to 2 mL IM of a 50% solution) with thiamine to correct thiamine resistance and frequently accompanying hypomagnesemia. Hyponatremia should be corrected *slowly* as rapid correction may cause central pontine myelinosis.

Recovery is often incomplete in neurologic beriberi and in cerebral forms central pontine myelinolysis may be residual.

Thiamine Dependency

Several inborn errors of metabolism respond to pharmacologic doses of thiamine (5 to 20 mg/day). These include a megaloblastic anemia of unknown mechanism, lactic acidosis due to low activity of liver pyruvate carboxylase, and ketoaciduria due to low activity of branched-chain keto acid dehydrogenase and lack of TPP in neural tissue.

RIBOFLAVIN (VITAMIN B_2) DEFICIENCY

Riboflavin, as flavin mononucleotide or flavin adenine dinucleotide, serves as an essential coenzyme in many oxidation-reduction reactions involved with carbohydrate metabolism. Sources and recommended daily allowances are listed in TABLES 79–1 and 79–2. Deficiency results in oral, ocular, cutaneous, and genital lesions.

Etiology

Primary riboflavin deficiency is associated with inadequate consumption of milk and other animal protein. Conditioned deficiencies are most frequent in chronic diarrheas, liver disease, chronic alcoholism, and when postoperative nutrient infusions lack supplementary vitamins.

Symptoms, Signs, and Laboratory Findings

The most common signs consist of pallor and maceration of the mucosa in the angles of the mouth **(angular stomatitis)** and vermilion surfaces of the lips (cheilosis), followed by superficial linear fissures that may leave scars on healing. When these lesions are infected by *Candida albicans*, grayish white exuberant lesions, termed **perlèche,** result. The tongue may have a magenta hue. **Cutaneous manifestations** usually

affect the nasolabial folds, alae nasi, ears, eyelids, scrotum, and labia majora. These areas become red, scaly, and greasy, and sebaceous material accumulates in hair follicles, producing **dyssebacea** or **shark skin**.

The **eye** may rarely show neovascularization of the cornea and epithelial keratitis, resulting in lacrimation and photophobia. Nutritional amblyopia may respond to riboflavin.

Urinary excretion of < 30 μg of riboflavin/gm of creatinine is associated with clinical signs of riboflavin deficiency. Increased activation of RBC glutathione reductase by riboflavin is an early sign of deficiency.

Diagnosis

The lesions described are not found solely in riboflavin deficiency. Cheilosis may result from vitamin B_6 deficiency, edentulism, or ill-fitting dentures. Seborrheic dermatitis and ocular lesions may be produced by a number of conditions. Therefore, diagnosis of riboflavin deficiency cannot depend on the history and presence of suggestive lesions alone. Laboratory tests, elimination of other causes, and a therapeutic trial may be necessary.

Treatment

Riboflavin 10 to 30 mg/day orally in divided doses is given until a response is evident; then 2 to 4 mg/day until recovery. Riboflavin can be given IM 5 to 20 mg/day in single or divided doses.

NIACIN (NICOTINIC ACID) DEFICIENCY

(Pellagra)

This water-soluble B vitamin is found in many foods that also contain thiamine (see TABLE 79–1). Through the role of nicotine-adenine dinucleotide (**NAD**, coenzyme I) and nicotine-adenine dinucleotide phosphate (**NADP**, coenzyme II) in oxidation-reduction reactions, niacin derivatives play a vital function in cell metabolism. (For daily allowances, see TABLE 79–2.)

Etiology

Severe niacin deficiency is a principal cause of **pellagra**. **Primary deficiency** usually occurs in areas where maize (Indian corn) forms a major part of the diet. Bound niacin, found in maize, is not assimilated in the intestinal tract unless it has been previously alkali-treated (as in the preparation of tortillas). Corn protein is also deficient in tryptophan, a precursor from which the body can synthesize niacin. Amino acid imbalance may also play a part, as pellagra is common in India among those who eat a millet with a high leucine content. **Secondary deficiencies** are seen in diarrheal disease, cirrhosis of the liver, and alcoholism, and following extensive postoperative use of nutrient infusions lacking vitamins. Pellagra may also complicate prolonged isoniazid (INH) therapy (the drug replaces niacinamide in NAD); malignant carcinoid tumor (tryptophan is diverted to form 5-hydroxytryptamine); and Hartnup disease (see in ANOMALIES IN KIDNEY TRANSPORT in Ch. 187).

Symptoms and Signs

Pellagra is characterized by cutaneous, mucous membrane, CNS, and GI symptoms. The complete syndrome of advanced deficiency includes scarlet stomatitis and glossitis, diarrhea, dermatitis, and mental aberrations. Symptoms may appear alone or in combination.

Four types of cutaneous lesions, usually bilaterally symmetric, are recognized: (1) acute, consisting of erythema followed by vesiculation, bullae, crusting, and desquamation; secondary infection is common, notably following exposure to sunlight (actinic trauma); (2) intertrigo, also an acute lesion, characterized by redness, maceration,

abrasion, and secondary infection in the intertriginous areas; (3) chronic hypertrophy, in which the skin is thickened, inelastic, fissured, and deeply pigmented over pressure points; secondary infection often develops, and the lesion shows a sharply defined pearly border of regenerating epithelium when healing begins; and (4) chronic atrophic lesions, with dry, scaly, inelastic skin too large for the part it covers (seen in older pellagrins). Distribution of the above lesions, which occur at trauma points, is more characteristic than their form. Sunlight causes **Casal's necklace** and butterfly-shaped lesions on the face.

Changes in the mucous membranes primarily involve the mouth but may also affect the vagina and urethra. Scarlet glossitis and stomatitis are characteristic of acute deficiency. The tip and margins of the tongue and the mucosa around Stensen's duct are affected first. As the lesion progresses, the entire tongue and oral mucous membranes become a bright scarlet color, followed by sore mouth, increased salivation, and edema of the tongue. Ulcerations may appear, especially under the tongue, on the mucosa of the lower lip, and opposite the molar teeth. They are often covered by a grayish slough containing Vincent's organisms.

Gastrointestinal symptoms, which are indeterminate in early cases, include burning of the mouth, pharynx, and esophagus, and abdominal discomfort and distention. Later, nausea, vomiting, and diarrhea may occur. Diarrhea, often bloody because of gastrointestinal hyperemia and ulceration, is serious.

CNS involvement includes (1) **organic psychosis**, characterized by memory impairment, disorientation, confusion, and confabulation (excitement, depression, mania, and delirium predominate in some patients; in others, the reaction is paranoid), and (2) **"encephalopathic syndrome,"** characterized by clouding of consciousness, cogwheel rigidity of the extremities, and uncontrollable sucking and grasping reflexes. Differentiation from the CNS changes in thiamine deficiency is difficult.

Diagnosis

Niacin deficiency must be distinguished from other causes of stomatitis, glossitis, diarrhea, and dementia. Diagnosis is easy when the clinical findings include skin and mouth lesions, diarrhea, delirium, and dementia. More often, the condition is less fully developed. In these cases, history of a diet lacking niacin and tryptophan is significant. Urinary excretion of N′-methylniacinamide and pyridone is decreased.

Treatment

Multiple deficiencies of B vitamins and protein often occur together; therefore, the diet should be balanced. Supplemental niacinamide 300 to 1000 mg/day should be given orally in divided doses. In most cases, 300 to 500 mg is sufficient. Niacinamide is generally used in deficiency states, since niacin can cause flushing, itching, burning, or tingling sensations and niacinamide does not; however, niacinamide does not possess hypolipidemic or vasodilating properties as does niacin. When oral therapy is precluded, due to lack of patient cooperation or diarrhea, 100 to 250 mg should be injected s.c. 2 to 3 times/day. In encephalopathic states, 1000 mg orally plus 100 to 250 mg parenterally is recommended. Other B-complex vitamins should also be given in therapeutic dosages.

VITAMIN B_6 (PYRIDOXINE) DEFICIENCY AND DEPENDENCY

Vitamin B_6 comprises a group of closely related compounds: **pyridoxine, pyridoxal,** and **pyridoxamine.** They are phosphorylated in the body to pyridoxal phosphate, which functions as a coenzyme in many reactions, including decarboxylation and transamination of amino acids, deamination of hydroxyamino acids and cysteine, conversion of

tryptophan to niacin, and metabolism of fatty acids. Consequently, the vitamin complex is important in blood, CNS (see in Ch. 120), and skin metabolism. (For sources and daily allowances, see TABLES 79–1 and 79–2.)

Etiology

Primary deficiency is rare, since most foods contain the vitamin, but an outbreak of convulsions in infants did follow the destruction of vitamin B_6 in artificial milk. **Secondary deficiencies** may result from malabsorption, chemical inactivation by drugs (eg, isonicotinic acid hydrazide, hydralazine, DL-penicillamine), excessive loss, and increased metabolic activity.

Symptoms and Signs

Deficiency: The vitamin B_6 antagonist deoxypyridoxine produces seborrheic dermatosis, glossitis, cheilosis, peripheral neuropathy, and lymphopenia. Vitamin B_6 deficiency can cause convulsions in infants and anemia in adults (usually normoblastic but occasionally megaloblastic).

Dependency: Several recessive or X-linked states have been described, affecting different apoenzymes and producing symptoms such as convulsions, mental deficiency, and cystathioninuria; iron overload anemia, urticaria, and asthma; and xanthurenicaciduria.

Diagnosis and Laboratory Findings

At present there is no generally accepted test of vitamin B_6 status. Whole blood pyridoxal phosphate is a better indicator than the level in plasma. Erythrocyte glutamic pyruvate and oxaloacetic transaminase activities are increased but are nonspecific changes.

Treatment

Deficiency in the adult usually responds to pyridoxine 50 to 100 mg/day orally. Underlying causes such as use of pyridoxine inactivating drugs (anticonvulsants, corticosteroids, estrogens, isoniazid, penicillamine, and hydralazine) or malabsorption should be corrected. Conditions that increase metabolic demand require amounts in excess of the recommended allowance. In **dependency in the infant** the daily requirement (normally 0.4 mg) is increased many times (up to 10 mg). As much as 200 to 600 mg daily of pyridoxine may be needed for treatment of adults.

Type I primary hyperoxaluria has responded to pyridoxine 25 mg/day orally, possibly by increasing transaminase activity responsible for the conversion of gloxylate, the immediate oxalate precursor, to glycine.

Vitamin B_6 Toxicity

The ingestion of megadoses (2 to 6 gm/day for 2 to 40 mo) of pyridoxine has recently been blamed for progressive sensory ataxia and profound lower limb impairment of position and vibration sense. Touch, temperature, and pain were less affected. The motor and central nervous systems were unimpaired. Recovery was slow and only partial following cessation of pyridoxine ingestion.

FOLIC ACID DEFICIENCY

Many plant and animal tissues contain folic acid **(pteroylglutamic acid, folacin)** as reduced methyl or formyl polyglutamates. They are unstable, and 50 to 90% may be destroyed by boiling or canning. (See TABLES 79–1 and 79–2 for sources and daily allowances.) In the tetrahydro form, folates act as coenzymes for processes in which there is transfer of a one-carbon unit, as in purine and pyrimidine nucleotide biosynthesis, amino acid conversions such as histidine to glutamic acid through formiminoglutamic acid, and generation and use of formate.

Absorption takes place in the small intestine. In the epithelial cells polyglutamates are reduced to dihydro- and tetrahydrofolates. They are bound to protein and transported as methyl tetrahydrofolate. Plasma levels vary from 3 to 21 ng/mL and closely reflect dietary intake. Red cell folate (normal 160 to 640 ng/mL whole blood, corrected to packed cell volume of 45%) is a better indicator of status. The total body folate is about 70 mg, 1/3 of which is found in the liver. About 20% of ingested folate is excreted unabsorbed together with 60 to 90 μg/day not reabsorbed from bile.

Folate deficiency causes megaloblastic anemia and other hematologic changes (see ANEMIA DUE TO FOLIC ACID DEFICIENCY under MEGALOBLASTIC ANEMIAS in Ch. 96). Infertility and GI disturbances such as glossitis, stomatitis, and intestinal malabsorption also occur. Deficiency has been reported in association with the following conditions but has not been proved to be their cause: abortion, abruptio placentae, neural tube defects, neuropathy, and psychiatric disorders. Possible causes of folic acid deficiency are given in TABLE 81–3. The usual therapeutic dosage is 1 mg/day orally. (CAUTION: In megaloblastic anemia, it is important to rule out vitamin B_{12} deficiency [pernicious anemia] before treating with folate, which would alleviate the anemia, but permit the associated neurologic damage to progress.)

Folic Acid Dependency

A disorder characterized by homocystinemia and hypomethioninemia, due to a biosynthetic defect affecting tetrahydrofolic acid coenzyme, has been described. Dosage of folic acid treatment has not been standardized.

VITAMIN B_{12} DEFICIENCY

The vitamin B_{12} molecule consists of the nucleotide 5,6-dimethylbenzimidazole linked at right angles to a four-pyrrole ring with a cobalt atom (the corrin nucleus). Several different **cobalamins,** which vary only in the ligand attached to the cobalt atom, occur in nature. (See TABLES 79–1 and 79–2 for sources and recommended daily allowances.) Strict vegetarians may obtain cobalamin from legume nodules where it is synthesized by microorganisms.

Intrinsic factor, secreted by parietal cells of the gastric mucosa, probably has two binding sites: one for free cobalamin and the other for ileal microvilli, which require a neutral pH and the presence of free calcium and are readily saturated. Vitamin B_{12}

TABLE 81–3. CAUSES OF FOLIC ACID DEFICIENCY

Primary deficiency

Poor diet: lacking fresh, slightly cooked food; chronic alcoholism; total parenteral nutrition

Secondary deficiency

Inadequate absorption: malabsorption syndromes (esp. celiac disease, sprue), drugs (phenytoin, primidone, barbiturates, cycloserine, oral contraceptives?), specific malabsorption for folate (congenital, acquired), blind loop syndrome

Inadequate utilization: folic acid antagonists (methotrexate, pyrimethamine, triamterene, diamidine compounds, trimethoprim), anticonvulsants?, enzyme deficiency (congenital, acquired), vitamin B_{12} deficiency, alcohol, scurvy

Increased requirement: pregnancy, infancy, malignancy (esp. lymphoproliferative), increased hematopoiesis (esp. thalassemia major), increased metabolism

Increased excretion: vitamin B_{12} dependency?, liver disease?

(Modified from V. Herbert: "The Five Possible Causes of all Nutrient Deficiency: Illustrated by Deficiencies of Vitamin B_{12} and Folic Acid," in the *American Journal of Clinical Nutrition,* Vol. 26, pp. 77–86, Jan. 1973. Copyright American Society for Clinical Nutrition. Used with permission of the Society and the author.)

alone passes into the mucosal cell. Little cobalamin is absorbed passively throughout the length of the GI tract.

Vitamin B_{12} is present in plasma as methylcobalamin, 5′-deoxyadenosylcobalamin, and hydroxocobalamin bound to specific proteins, transcobalamin I and II. The normal range of vitamin B_{12} plasma concentration is 150 to 750 pg/mL, which represents only about 0.1% of the total body content, most of which is in the liver. Excretion is mainly through the bile and to a lesser extent via the kidneys. The total daily loss is 2 to 5 μg. Vitamin B_{12} and folic acid are both involved in nucleoprotein synthesis, probably facilitating the reduction of the ribose moiety of uridylic acid, before methylation of uracil to thymine in the synthesis of DNA.

Because of its slow rate of utilization and considerable stores, vitamin B_{12} deficiency (a fall in tissue stores below 0.1 mg and a plasma level below 100 pg/mL) usually takes many months to appear. However, hematologic and neurologic changes have been reported recently in the breast-fed babies of vegan mothers. The hematologic changes due to vitamin B_{12} deficiency are discussed in Ch. 96; the neurologic changes of combined system disease are discussed in Ch. 130. Psychoses and optic atrophy may also occur. In one form of the latter, **tobacco amblyopia,** the cyanide in tobacco smoke may be detoxified by hydroxocobalamin that is converted to the more readily excreted congener cyanocobalamin, thereby causing a deficiency in vitamin B_{12}. It is also postulated that vitamin B_{12} deficiency could result in deficiency of a sulfur donor, necessary for the conversion of cyanide to thiocyanate, by its known role as methylcobalamin in the transmethylation of homocysteine to methionine. TABLE 81–4 lists the main causes of vitamin B_{12} deficiency. For the usual therapeutic dosage see ANEMIA DUE TO VITAMIN B_{12} DEFICIENCY in Ch. 96.

VITAMIN B_{12} DEPENDENCY

Several specific disorders of cobalamin-dependent metabolism have been reported. In each there is some defect either in (1) cellular uptake of the vitamin precursor, (2) conversion of the vitamin to the coenzyme form, or (3) coenzyme-apoenzyme interaction. The metabolism of methylmalonic acid is usually affected, with large amounts excreted in the urine. These disorders usually respond to massive doses of vitamin B_{12} (1000 μg/day IM).

TABLE 81–4. CAUSES OF VITAMIN B_{12} DEFICIENCY

Primary deficiency

Inadequate diet: veganism, infants breast-fed by vegan mothers, chronic alcoholism (rare), dietary faddism

Secondary deficiency

Inadequate absorption: lack of intrinsic factor (pernicious anemia, destruction of gastric mucosa, endocrinopathy), intrinsic factor inhibition, small intestine disorders (celiac disease, sprue, malignancy, drugs, specific malabsorption for vitamin B_{12}), competition for vitamin B_{12} (fish tapeworm, blind loop syndrome)

Inadequate utilization: antagonists, enzyme deficiencies, organ disease (liver, kidney, malignancy, malnutrition), transport protein abnormality

Increased requirement: hyperthyroidism, infancy, parasitic infestation, α-thallasemia

Increased excretion: inadequate binding in serum, liver disease, renal disease

(Modified from V. Herbert: "The Five Possible Causes of all Nutrient Deficiency: Illustrated by Deficiencies of Vitamin B_{12} and Folic Acid," in the *American Journal of Clinical Nutrition,* Vol. 26, pp. 77–86, Jan. 1973. Copyright American Society for Clinical Nutrition. Used with permission of the Society and the author.)

BIOTIN DEFICIENCY AND DEPENDENCY

Biotin is a coenzyme that is essential to the metabolism of both fat and carbohydrate. Raw egg white contains a biotin antagonist, avidin, and high and prolonged consumption has resulted in dermatitis and glossitis responding rapidly to 150 to 300 μg biotin daily. Deficiency has occurred during longterm total parenteral nutrition.

Dependency: Retarded physical and mental development, alopecia, keratoconjunctivitis, and defects in T cell and B cell immunity have been reported in children with deficiencies of biotin-dependent carboxylases. Urinary excretion of various organic acids assists diagnosis; response has been complete to large doses of biotin (10 mg) daily.

PANTOTHENIC ACID DEFICIENCY

Pantothenic acid is a vitamin widely distributed in foodstuffs and is an essential component of coenzyme A, which functions as an acyltransfer cofactor for many enzymatic reactions.

In adult volunteers on a deficiency diet, malaise, abdominal discomfort, and "burning feet" associated with paresthesias occurred. In clinical practice these symptoms rarely respond to the vitamin. Adults probably require about 4 to 7 mg/day, corresponding to a whole blood level of 100 to 180 μg/dL, but no RDA has been set.

CARNITINE DEFICIENCY

L-Carnitine is contained in the normal western diet and is also synthesized from methionine and lysine by the liver. It is required for the transport of activated long-chain fatty acids into the matrix compartment of mitochondria of tissues for subsequent oxidation.

Deficiency may occur in various genetic disorders (eg, carnitine palmitoyltransferase deficiency, methylmalonic aciduria, propionic acidemia, and isovaleric acidemia) and has been corrected by L-carnitine 25 mg/kg/6 h orally. It may also result from diminished synthesis in severe liver disease or excessive loss from dialysis in chronic renal failure. Symptoms of hypoglycemia and skeletal muscle weakness, associated with biochemical evidence of carnitine deficiency during long term total parenteral nutrition, have been reversed by carnitine therapy.

VITAMIN C (ASCORBIC ACID) DEFICIENCY

(Scurvy)

(See also INFANTILE SCURVY in Ch. 195)

Vitamin C is essential to collagen formation and helps to maintain the integrity of substances of mesenchymal origin, such as connective tissue, osteoid tissue of bone, and dentin of teeth. It is essential for wound healing and facilitates recovery from burns. It is a strong reducing agent and is reversibly oxidized and reduced readily in the body, functioning as a redox system in the cell. It is involved in the metabolism of phenylalanine and tyrosine and, as a reductant (with oxygen, ferrous iron, and a 2-ketoacid) activates enzymes that hydroxylate protocollagen proline and lysine to collagen hydroxyproline and hydroxylysine. Synthesis of an elastin, which becomes increasingly deficient in hydroxyproline, occurs in scorbutic animals. Vitamin C protects folic acid reductase, which converts folic acid to folinic acid. It may participate in the release of free folic acid from its conjugates in food and it facilitates the absorption of iron. Severe deficiency results in **scurvy,** *an acute or chronic disease characterized by hemorrhagic manifestations and abnormal osteoid and dentin formation.* (For sources and daily allowances of vitamin C, see TABLES 79–1 and 79–2.)

Etiology

In adults, primary deficiency is usually due to food idiosyncrasies or improper diet. Deficiencies occur in GI disease, especially when the patient is on an "ulcer diet." Pregnancy, lactation, and thyrotoxicosis increase vitamin C requirements. Diarrhea increases fecal loss, and achlorhydria decreases the amount absorbed. Acute and chronic inflammatory diseases, surgery, and burns can significantly increase the body requirements. Cold or heat stress increases urinary excretion of vitamin C. Heat (eg, sterilization of formulas, cooking) can destroy vitamin C in food.

Pathology

Formation of intercellular cement substances in connective tissues, bones, and dentin is defective, resulting in weakening of capillaries with subsequent hemorrhage and defects in bone and related structures. Hemorrhagic areas are organized avascularly, so that wounds heal poorly and break open easily. Bone lesions result from cessation of endochondral growth due to failure of the osteoblasts to form osteoid tissue. Instead, a fibrous union is formed between the diaphysis and the epiphysis, and costochondral junctions enlarge. Densely calcified fragments of cartilage are embedded in this fibrous tissue. Small ecchymotic hemorrhages within or along the bone, or large subperiosteal hemorrhages due to small fractures just shaftward of the white line, complicate these lesions.

Symptoms and Signs

In adults, scurvy remains latent for 3 to 12 mo following onset of severe vitamin C deficiency. Overt scorbutic symptoms are preceded by lassitude, weakness, irritability, weight loss, and vague myalgias and arthralgias. Multiple splinter hemorrhages may form a crescent near the distal ends of the nail and are more extensive than those in bacterial endocarditis. The gums become swollen, purple, spongy, and friable, and bleed readily in extreme deficiency. Secondary infection, gangrene, and loosening of teeth eventually occur. Gum changes occur only with natural teeth or hidden roots. Old scars break down, new wounds fail to heal, and spontaneous hemorrhages may occur in any part of the body, especially as perifollicular petechiae and ecchymoses into the skin of the lower limbs. (These changes in old age are not necessarily scorbutic.) Bone lesions, except for subperiosteal hemorrhage, do not occur.

Other symptoms and signs of scurvy include bulbar conjunctival hemorrhage, femoral neuropathy from hemorrhage into femoral sheaths, oliguria, edema of the lower extremities, impaired vascular reactivity, and arthritis resembling rheumatoid arthritis. Bleeding gums are not the most characteristic feature of scurvy. The hyperkeratotic hair follicle with surrounding hyperemia or hemorrhage is almost pathognomonic.

Laboratory Findings

Usually the plasma ascorbic acid content is nearly nonexistent in manifest scurvy, but this is not always diagnostic; low levels may also be found in nonscorbutic persons. *Ascorbic acid levels in the WBC-platelet layer of centrifuged blood are more significant*; levels < 0.1 mg/dL are closely correlated with scurvy. When vitamin C stores are depleted, little appears in the urine following a test dose. A positive capillary fragility test is an almost constant finding, and anemia not due to blood loss is common. Bleeding, coagulation, and prothrombin times are normal.

Diagnosis

Adult scurvy must be differentiated from arthritis, hemorrhagic diseases, and gingivitis. Joint symptoms are due to bleeding around or into the joint. The presence of hemorrhage elsewhere, plus blood studies, aids in diagnosis.

Prophylaxis

Vitamin C 100 mg/day orally is fully protective. Most nutritionists believe that huge doses of vitamin C (about 10 gm/day) do not decrease the incidence or severity of the

common cold (see in Ch. 12) or influence the progress of malignant disease and may predispose to oxalate urinary calculi and iron overload.

Treatment

For **adult scurvy,** ascorbic acid 250 mg qid orally is recommended until signs have disappeared. The usual maintenance doses can then be given. When parenteral therapy is required, sodium ascorbate can be given at the same dosage. Ascorbic acid 300 to 500 mg/day orally in divided doses should be given for several months in chronic scurvy with gingivitis, repeated hemorrhagic manifestations, or joint symptoms. Superimposed infection and calcareous deposits prevent rapid response in chronic scorbutic gingivitis.

82. ELEMENT DEFICIENCY AND TOXICITY

There are 13 trace elements presently recognized as necessary for warm-blooded animals. They occur in concentrations $< 0.005\%$ body wt. In order of demonstrated need, they are iron, iodine, copper, manganese, zinc, cobalt, molybdenum, selenium, chromium, fluorine, silicon, nickel, and arsenic. The status of tin and vanadium is unclear. Nickel and arsenic are not known to be important in human nutrition and are not considered here. Disturbances in metabolism of the macroelements sodium, potassium, calcium, and magnesium are considered in Ch. 84.

Except for iron and iodine, it is uncommon for element deficiencies to develop spontaneously in man, however bizarre the diet. The introduction of synthetic diets as treatment for inborn errors of metabolism, the development of IV feeding, and the advent of renal dialysis present iatrogenic risks that emphasize the nutritional importance of these elements. As methods for their assay have been developed and their physiology studied, new errors of metabolism have been discovered. With increasing pollution and development of synthetic foods, excessive intake may occur, producing signs of toxicity only after many years. Many lay periodicals and "health food" stores promote dolomite as a good source of calcium and magnesium, and it is widely used. However, recent reports indicate that dolomite may also contain potentially toxic metals, including iron, chromium, phosphorus, nickel, silicon, zinc, and cadmium.

PHOSPHATE (PO_4) DEPLETION

The risk of PO_4 depletion has increased following chronic hemodialysis (in which patients may be dialyzed with PO_4-free solutions while ingesting large amounts of PO_4-binding antacids), chronic renal failure, and renal transplantation. Total parenteral nutrition regimes may be low in PO_4, as may be the diet in chronic alcoholism.

As in other hypophosphatemic states (see also Chs. 81 and 84), there is osteomalacia; blood Ca is normal or raised and there is marked parathyroid hyposecretion. Renal clearance of PO_4 is markedly reduced; of Ca, greatly elevated.

Symptoms involving several organ systems, not seen in other conditions with low plasma PO_4, include confusion, dysarthria, parasthesias, peripheral neuropathy; muscle weakness, true myopathy; red cell rigidity and overt hemolytic anemia, impaired O_2 release due to red cell deficiency of 2,3-diphosphoglycerate; abnormal liver function tests; profound anorexia, nausea and vomiting; and renal tubular dysfunction (see TABLE 79–1).

DISTURBANCES IN IRON (Fe) METABOLISM

The total body Fe in healthy adult males is about 3.45 gm and in females about 2.45 gm. About 61% in males and 71% in females is found in Hb; 10 and 12% respectively

is found in tissues as myoglobin and enzymes; and 29% in males and 16% in females is as storage Fe in liver, spleen, and bone marrow. Serum ferritin accurately reflects Fe stores (normal male 94 ng/mL, female 34 ng/mL).

The main features of Fe metabolism are described in FIG. 82–1 and its legend. Dietary non-heme Fe is reduced to the ferrous state and released from conjugation by gastric and other secretions. The absorption of non-heme Fe in any food is affected by the composition of the meal; for example, when eggs and bread were eaten separately, absorption was 1 to 2% and 30% respectively, but 5 and 5.3% respectively when eaten together. Phytate reduces absorption, as do Ca and PO_4 together; tea forms insoluble Fe tannate complexes. EDTA (ethylenediaminetetraacetic acid) is added to food to prevent oxidation by free metals. FDA regulations permit EDTA in certain foods at levels ranging from 25 to 800 mg/kg. Diets containing as much as 50 to 100 mg of EDTA have been shown to cause significant reduction of non-heme Fe absorption. Conversely, ascorbic acid maintains Fe in a reduced, more soluble form and greatly enhances non-heme Fe absorption. Dosing with 200 mg/day increases Fe absorption 2- to 3-fold. The long-term effect on Fe status of these and larger doses of ascorbic acid used for prophylaxis against the common cold (see Ch. 12) deserves further study.

A smaller fraction of dietary Fe is in the form of heme. This is absorbed as an intact porphyrin complex into the mucosal cell and absorption is neither inhibited nor enhanced by the substances mentioned above. Regular consumption of meat may account for as much as 1/3 of the total Fe absorbed daily. Dual radioiron tags are available to measure Fe absorption from a complete meal. In one study in males, non-heme Fe averaged 5.3% absorption and heme Fe 37%.

Daily Fe requirements (see TABLE 79–2) are 10 mg for men and 18 mg for women. In health, average intakes are 16 mg for men and 11 mg for women. Absorption in men was 0.9 mg (6%) but 1.3 mg (12%) in women.

IRON DEFICIENCY

Etiology, pathophysiology, symptoms and signs, diagnosis, and treatment are dealt with under HYPOCHROMIC MICROCYTIC ANEMIA in Ch. 96.

Prevention

Fe is absorbed with difficulty and most people barely meet their daily requirements. Additional losses due to menstruation (mean 0.5 mg/day), pregnancy (0.5 to 0.8 mg/day), lactation (0.4 mg/day), and blood loss due to disease or accident readily lead to Fe deficiency. Proposals by the FDA to increase the level of Fe fortification of food (at present 33 mg/kg) to protect these vulnerable groups have met with strong opposition on the grounds that those segments of the population not requiring additional Fe may be put at risk of developing Fe overload. The conflict is unresolved. It is clear that an available Fe salt will have the same absorption as the non-heme Fe of the diet, regardless of the vehicle. However, some presently employed salts are less well absorbed. Ferrous sulfate and reduced Fe of small particle size are the best.

IRON OVERLOAD

(Hemosiderosis; Hemochromatosis)

For acute Fe poisoning, see TABLE 289–4. Chronic Fe overload is characterized by greater than normal focal or generalized deposition of Fe within body tissues **(hemosiderosis)**. When such deposition is associated with tissue injury, with total body Fe > 15 gm, it is known as **hemochromatosis**. TABLE 82–1 presents a classification of these conditions. Differential diagnosis is difficult but depends on the history of Fe administration, examination of relatives, degree of Fe overload, and presence or absence of localizing signs.

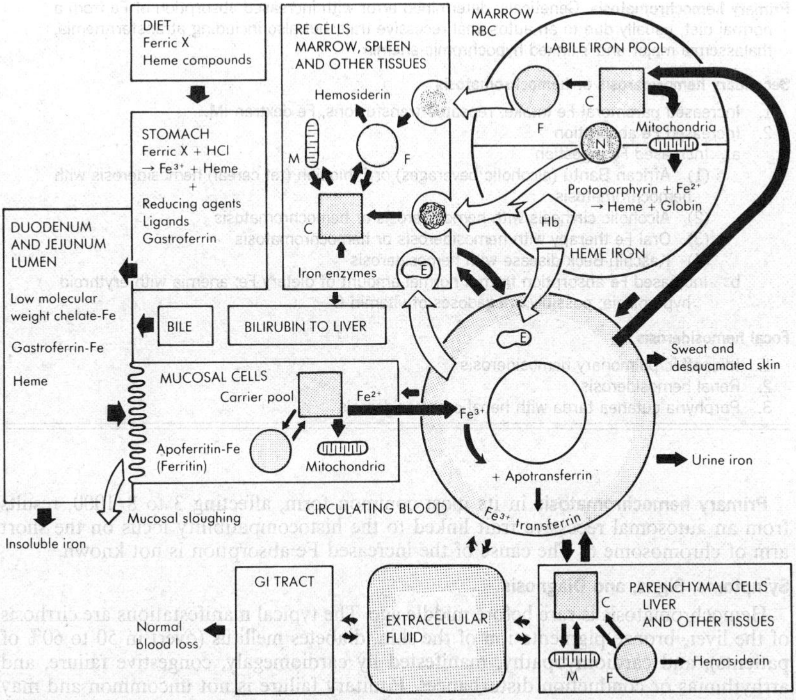

FIG. 82–1. Iron metabolism. Ingested heme compounds and organic chelates, when subjected to the action of hydrochloric acid (low pH) in the stomach, are broken down to form heme molecules and ferric ions. The ferric ions react with reducing agents, ligands, and gastroferrin. Only iron kept soluble, either as heme molecules or by binding to low-molecular-weight chelates or gastroferrin, can undergo absorption, which occurs chiefly in the duodenum and proximal jejunum. Luminal iron incorporated into the mucosal cell enters the carrier pool (C). Most of this iron is deposited as ferritin (F) or utilized by mitochondria (M) for enzyme synthesis and then is lost by sloughing. The remainder is absorbed by being transferred from the carrier pool to the plasma, where it is bound tightly in the ferric state to the β_1-globulin transferrin. Iron leaves the plasma primarily by entering the labile iron pool of the erythroid series, from which there is considerable feedback of iron into the plasma, mainly via reticuloendothelial (RE) cells. Within the developing erythroid cells of the bone marrow, ferrous ions combine with protoporphyrin to form the porphyrin heme, which in turn combines with globulin to form hemoglobin. Hemoglobin is released into the circulation within circulating red cells (E) that have an average life span of 117 days. At the time of their disintegration, these cells are removed from the circulation by the spleen and other reticuloendothelial tissues with excretion of the split prophyrin as bilirubin in the bile and conservation of almost all the iron, which reenters the plasma and is bound once more to transferrin. These phagocytic RE cells normally are the chief source of iron entering the plasma. About 2/3 of normal total body iron loss (1.0 mg/day) occurs as the result of the GI blood loss of 1.2 mL/day (0.6 mg Fe/day). About 18% of the iron leaving and entering the plasma does so in equilibration with extracellular fluid transferrin; the formation and breakdown of myoglobulin and the heme enzymes; iron absorption; and iron storage. Arrows are not quantitative. (From J. B. Stanbury, J. B. Wyngaarden, and D. S. Fredrickson, *The Metabolic Basis of Inherited Disease,* ed. 4, 1978. Copyright © by McGraw-Hill, Inc. Used with permission of McGraw-Hill Book Co.)

TABLE 82–1. CLASSIFICATION OF HEMOCHROMATOSIS AND HEMOSIDEROSIS

Primary hemochromatosis. Genetically determined error with increased absorption of Fe from a normal diet, usually due to an autosomal recessive trait, but also including atransferrinemia, thalassemia major and Y-linked hypochromic anemia

Secondary hemosiderosis or hemochromatosis

1. Increased parenteral Fe intake; repeated transfusions, Fe dextran IM.
2. Increased Fe absorption
   a. Increased Fe ingestion
      (1) African Bantu (alcoholic beverages) or Ethiopian (tef cereal) hemosiderosis with hemochromatosis
      (2) Alcoholic cirrhosis with hemosiderosis or hemochromatosis
      (3) Oral Fe therapy with hemosiderosis or hemochromatosis
      (4) Kaschin-Beck disease with hemosiderosis
   b. Increased Fe absorption from a normal amount of dietary Fe; anemia with erythroid hyperplasia; possibly, megadoses of vitamin C

Focal hemosiderosis

1. Idiopathic pulmonary hemosiderosis
2. Renal hemosiderosis
3. Porphyria cutanea tarda with hepatic hemosiderosis

Primary hemochromatosis in its most common form, affecting 3 to 8/1000, results from an autosomal recessive trait linked to the histocompatibility locus on the short arm of chromosome 6. The cause of the increased Fe absorption is not known.

Symptoms, Signs, and Diagnosis

Hemochromatosis is rare before middle age. The typical manifestations are cirrhosis of the liver, bronze pigmentation of the skin, diabetes mellitus (overt in 50 to 60% of patients), and cardiomyopathy, manifested by cardiomegaly, congestive failure, and arrhythmias or conduction disturbances. Pituitary failure is not uncommon and may be the cause of the frequently observed testicular atrophy and loss of libido. Abdominal pain, arthritis, and chondrocalcinosis occur less often. Presumably, all of these changes are due to parenchymal Fe deposition, although an increased familial incidence of diabetes mellitus suggests that factors other than pancreatic siderosis may play a role. Hepatomas occur with increased frequency in patients with longstanding hemochromatosis.

The plasma Fe is > 200 μg/dL and the transferrin saturation is > 70%. Urinary Fe excretion is markedly increased (> 2 mg/24 h) by the chelating agent deferoxamine 500 to 1000 mg IM. Demonstration of hepatic siderosis and cirrhosis by liver biopsy confirms the diagnosis. Family members should be screened by human leukocyte antigen typing. Determination of homozygosity for hemochromatosis in a population is done equally well by measuring serum Fe, total Fe binding capacity, or serum ferritin.

Treatment

Phlebotomy removes excess Fe from the body and improves survival, though without altering the incidence of hepatoma. Phlebotomy should be instituted prior to the development of advanced liver disease. About 500 mL of blood (about 250 mg Fe) is removed weekly until plasma Fe levels are normal, then every 3 to 4 mo as necessary to maintain plasma Fe below 150 micrograms/dL. Repeat liver biopsy may be a more reliable way of monitoring tissue Fe deposits. Anemia occasionally develops during venesection treatment. In such cases, deferoxamine 20 mg/kg/24 h either as a slow s.c. or IV infusion given overnight by a small portable pump may permit further reduction

of Fe stores without producing anemia. Diabetes mellitus, cardiac abnormalities, and other secondary manifestations are treated as indicated.

Focal hemosiderosis chiefly occurs in the lungs and kidneys. Pulmonary hemosiderosis due to recurrent pulmonary hemorrhage occurs as an idiopathic entity, as part of Goodpasture's syndrome, and in mitral stenosis. Occasionally the Fe loss into the lungs is severe enough to cause iron-deficiency anemia. Renal hemosiderosis results from extensive intravascular hemolysis due to trauma (eg, fragmentation of RBCs in association with prosthetic aortic valves) or in paroxysmal nocturnal hemoglobinuria. Free Hb is filtered at the glomerulus, and renal Fe deposition occurs with saturation of haptoglobin. No damage to the renal parenchyma occurs, but unusually heavy hemosiderinuria may cause Fe deficiency.

Treatment is predominantly supportive. In acute episodes, blood transfusion may be required, but otherwise anemia responds to oral Fe. Results with splenectomy and with ACTH or corticosteroids have been variable.

IODINE (I)

Nearly 80% of the total iodine present in the body is found in the thyroid, almost all as **thyroglobulin,** the storage form of thyroid hormone (see THYROID HORMONE FORMATION in Ch. 89). Marine foods are rich dietary sources. Drinking water, which supplies a relatively small proportion of the intake, reflects the soil content of locally grown foods.

Iodine deficiency results in colloid or endemic goiter, and when severe, cretinism, which occurs in 2 forms: myxedematous, which improves with thyroid hormone (see EUTHYROID GOITER in Ch. 89), and neurologic, including deaf mutism, which does *not* respond. Iodine deficiency should be corrected with iodized salt, not with Lugol's solution (see TABLE 79–1).

Chronic toxicity results when daily requirements are exceeded about 20-fold (> 2000 μg). Increased uptake of iodine by the thyroid leads to inhibition of organic iodine formation **(Wolff-Chaikoff effect),** and eventually iodide-goiter or myxedema especially in patients with pre-existing Hashimoto's thyroiditis.

FLUORINE (F)

Bones and teeth contain most of the body's F. Sea fish and tea are rich sources, but intake is mainly from drinking water. Fluoridation of water that contains less than the ideal level of 1 ppm significantly reduces the incidence of dental caries in the community. Prevention of osteoporosis with sodium fluoride 60 mg/day orally is presently restricted to investigative studies.

Excess accumulation of F **(fluorosis)** occurs in teeth and bone in proportion to the level and duration of intake. Communities with drinking water containing > 10 ppm are commonly affected. Fluorosis is most evident in permanent teeth that develop during high F intake. Deciduous teeth are affected only at very high levels of intake. The earliest changes, chalky-white, irregularly distributed patches on the surface of the enamel, become infiltrated by yellow or brown staining, giving rise to the characteristic "mottled" appearance. Severe fluorosis weakens the enamel, resulting in surface pitting. Bony changes, characterized by osteosclerosis and exostoses of the spine and genu valgum, usually are seen only after prolonged high intake in adults.

ZINC (Zn)

The body contains 1 to 2.5 gm of Zn, found mainly in bones, teeth, hair (which can be used to assess Zn status), skin, liver, muscle, and testes. In the plasma, ⅓ is attached loosely to albumin, and about ⅔ is firmly bound to globulins. Plasma levels

relate closely to dietary intake, but various diseases may cause low levels. Zn is also present in RBCs, mainly as carbonic anhydrase, and in WBCs and platelets. For estimated dietary requirements, see TABLE 79–2.

Deficiency: Chelation of dietary Zn by high fiber and phytate content of whole-meal bread, geophagia, and parasitism may be factors leading to reduced absorption and deficiency problems. In several studies in the USA and elsewhere a small proportion of children over age 4 yr had low Zn status, associated with poor appetite, poor growth, and impaired taste (hypogeusia). With Zn treatment, appetite improved, taste became normal, and catch-up growth occurred. High milk consumption, poor in Zn, may have been responsible. A syndrome of dwarfism and hypogonadism with low Zn status, seen in the Middle East, has been shown to respond to Zn supplementation. Cell-mediated immunity and wound healing are frequently impaired. Hepatic encephalopathy has responded to oral zinc acetate 600 mg/day in divided doses probably through improved enzymatic conversion of ammonia to urea. Maternal deficiency may cause anencephaly in the offspring. Secondary deficiency occurs in liver disease, malabsorption states, and during prolonged parenteral nutrition. Night blindness and mental lethargy may be features.

Acrodermatitis enteropathica, an autosomal recessive, previously fatal disorder has been shown to result from malabsorption of Zn. The defect appears to be in the tryptophan metabolizing pathway proximal to the synthesis of picolinic acid. Symptoms usually begin after the infant is weaned from breast milk. It is characterized by psoriasiform dermatitis, hair loss, paronychia, growth retardation, and diarrhea. Zinc sulfate 30 to 150 mg/day orally results in complete remission.

Toxicity: Ingestion of Zn in large amounts, usually from an acid food or drink from a galvanized container has caused vomiting and diarrhea. **Metal fume fever** is an industrial hazard caused by inhalation of zinc oxide fumes and results in neurologic damage. It is also called **brass founders' ague** or **zinc shakes.**

DISTURBANCES IN COPPER (Cu) METABOLISM

The normal adult body contains about 100 to 150 mg of Cu, 90% of which is found in muscle, bone, and liver. In the blood, more than 90% is found in the plasma associated with the α_2-globulin **ceruloplasmin,** with the remainder bound to albumins to a newly described protein, transcuprein, and in the RBCs. The plasma Cu concentration is elevated during pregnancy and estrogen therapy because the rise in plasma protein levels includes ceruloplasmin.

The Cu content of an ordinary diet is about 2 to 5 mg/day. Absorption occurs mainly in the proximal small intestine and is regulated by bodily needs and affected by dietary form. Some Cu may be complexed and rendered unavailable. Albumin-bound Cu is transported to the liver, bone marrow, and other sites. It is readily dissociable, making free Cu available for excretion in the urine. The major route of excretion, however, is by way of the bile. Cu is removed from the blood by hepatic uptake, partially excreted in the bile (35 to 205 μg/dL), and partially returned to the blood associated with ceruloplasmin, which is synthesized in the liver.

Cu is a component of mitochondrial (eg, cytochrome oxidase), cytoplasmic (eg, tyrosinase), and nuclear enzyme systems. Cu-deficient animals exhibit diminished activity of such cuproenzymes. Ceruloplasmin has enzyme activity.

COPPER DEFICIENCY

Cu deficiency is a rare cause of anemia in adults, although hypocupremia is found in states characterized by depressed serum protein levels, such as kwashiorkor, sprue, and nephrotic syndrome. In "dysproteinemia" of infancy, hypocupremia is associated with some features similar to Cu deficiency in animals (eg, anemia associated with de-

pressed serum Fe—see Ch. 96). Anemia, skin and bone lesions, and psychomotor retardation occurred in a newborn on long-term total parenteral nutrition.

Menke's kinky (steely) hair disease is a sex-linked abnormality caused by a defect in intestinal Cu absorption. Affected infants have low levels of Cu and ceruloplasmin that lead to progressive cerebral degeneration, retarded growth, abnormally sparse and brittle hair, arterial lesions, and scurvy-like bone changes. Parenteral Cu in various forms has given only temporary improvement and the outcome is fatal.

COPPER TOXICITY

Acute intoxication usually from ingestion of > 15 mg of elemental Cu is manifest by nausea, vomiting, abdominal pain, diarrhea, and diffuse myalgias. In some instances, abnormal mental states progressing to coma and death are associated with profound metabolic acidosis and necrotizing pancreatitis. However, the most consistent feature is severe hemolytic anemia, associated with increased Heinz bodies, abnormal autohemolysis, Hb thermolability, and depressed levels of RBC G6PD and glutathione reductase. Direct damage to the RBC membrane may contribute to the hemolysis, the severity of which correlates better with the erythrocyte (whole blood) level than with the serum Cu level.

Treatment involves gastric lavage and, if the dose ingested is very high, oral penicillamine 1 gm/day in adults is administered.

WILSON'S DISEASE
(Hepatolenticular Degeneration)

Etiology and Pathogenesis

This rare, often familial, progressive disease commonly occurs in male or female siblings, but not parents or children, suggesting autosomal recessive inheritance. The observed alterations result from progressive accumulation of Cu within the body tissues, particularly in the erythrocytes, kidney, liver, and brain. One primary defect appears to be failure to incorporate Cu into apoceruloplasmin resulting in low plasma ceruloplasmin (normal 150 to 400 mg/L), but a small proportion of cases have values within the normal range, and some asymptomatic heterozygotes have low ceruloplasmin values. There is also defective biliary excretion of Cu, but absorption appears normal.

Symptoms and Signs

Asymptomatic hepatic Cu accumulation proceeds for several years before hepatic Cu binding sites are saturated. Thereafter Cu is released from the liver, and an early feature is often **acute hemolytic anemia** that may be severe and recurrent, due to rapid uptake of Cu into erythrocytes. In 30 to 50% of patients **chronic active hepatitis** develops producing cirrhosis with ascites, edema, and progressive hepatic failure. Five to 10% present with evidence of liver disease, usually in their first or second decades of life. Alternatively, the hepatic manifestations may resolve. The serum Cu is usually depressed (< 70 μg/dL in adults; < 25 μg/dL in children); ceruloplasmin levels usually are decreased (< 15 mg/dL). Hypercupriuria frequently is present (> 50 μg/day). The **Kayser-Fleischer ring** (a golden-brown or gray-green pigment ring at the corneal limbus due to Cu deposition in Descemet's membrane) is present in about 50% of patients. Radiating brownish spokes of copper carbonate on the anterior or posterior lens capsule less commonly form the characteristic **sunflower cataract**. Some patients survive the early stages to become asymptomatic.

The **neurologic syndrome** usually occurs a decade or so after evidence of liver damage, but the patient may present with behavior disturbance, and liver dysfunction may only be revealed by a history of hepatitis or jaundice and an investigation. The globus

pallidus and especially the putamen (collectively the lenticular nucleus) are markedly damaged by Cu accumulation, but other basal ganglia at the cerebral cortex are also affected. The most common features include tremor of one or both upper extremities (volitional at first, and later at rest as well), choreoathetoid movements, rigidity of skeletal muscles (occasionally resulting in permanent contractures), dysarthria, and personality changes progressing to dementia. In this stage, the triad of cirrhosis, basal ganglia disease, and Kayser-Fleischer rings is found. The serum Cu and ceruloplasmin levels are abnormally low in association with hypercupriuria.

Many patients also exhibit **renal dysfunction** due to intrarenal Cu deposition. While GFR may be reduced, the most common abnormalities are tubular. Proximal tubular dysfunction results in Fanconi's syndrome with generalized aminoaciduria, glycosuria, hyperuricosuria, and phosphaturia. Distal renal tubular acidosis may produce medullary nephrocalcinosis, and a urinary concentrating defect may be present. Osteomalacia may result from phosphate wasting.

Diagnosis

Detection as early as possible is vital in this eminently treatable disease. Asymptomatic siblings of patients should have periodic determinations of serum Cu and ceruloplasmin and urinary Cu, but hypercupriuria may occur in other liver diseases and any condition associated with proteinuria. In some patients with Wilson's disease all these values are within the normal ranges. Specialized studies of the metabolism of radioactive Cu may assist in diagnosis, but normally in these circumstances, unless there are contraindications, liver biopsy should be performed. Liver Cu > 250 mg/gm wet liver is diagnostic.

Children or young adults presenting with any form of dyskinesia or akinetic-rigid syndrome or with unexplained liver disease should undergo tests of liver function for aminoaciduria, hemolytic anemia, and slit-lamp examination for Kayser-Fleischer ring, which is always present in the neurologic form. If all of these tests and those for serum Cu, ceruloplasmin, and urinary Cu are negative, liver biopsy should be performed for liver Cu.

Treatment

The untreated disease is invariably fatal, with death usually resulting from hepatic failure or infection. Prevention of further Cu accumulation is achieved by avoiding foods high in Cu (organ meats, shellfish, nuts, dried legumes, chocolate, whole-grain cereals, etc). With the added use of the oral Cu binder penicillamine, a negative Cu balance may be achieved in treating asymptomatic patients, either in the early hepatic accumulation stage or after reduction of tissue Cu stores.

D-Penicillamine 250 mg once/day orally is given initially, with increments every 1 or 2 wk up to a maintenance dose of 2 to 4 gm/day given in divided doses on an empty stomach. With clinical improvement (usually after several months) or with return of serum Cu to normal levels, the dose is reduced to 1.5 gm/day. Pyridoxine 25 to 50 mg/day is given to prevent pyridoxine deficiency due to chelation; serum Fe concentrations should be monitored, since Fe may also be chelated. Acute toxic reactions to penicillamine (eg, fever, rash, leukopenia, or thrombocytopenia) occur in about 1/3 of patients, but often it is possible to discontinue the drug temporarily and restart therapy with concomitant administration of corticosteroids. Platelet and WBC counts should be obtained every 1 to 2 wk for several weeks, with monthly counts thereafter. Occasionally, the start of treatment exacerbates neurologic symptoms, but these usually subside with temporary cessation of the drug. Chronic administration rarely is associated with toxic side effects other than easily preventable or correctable vitamin B_6 and Fe deficiency. Proteinuria usually does not occur during penicillamine treatment. However, frequent urinalyses should be obtained during therapy, as penicillamine may rarely precipitate Goodpasture's syndrome. Penicillamine therapy is

contraindicated during pregnancy, but there is some amelioration of the disease as serum Cu and ceruloplasmin rise. Although not accepted universally, prevailing opinion is that lifelong penicillamine therapy is indicated in conjunction with a low-copper diet.

When treatment with penicillamine is not possible because of intolerable or life-threatening side effects, **trientine hydrochloride** 750 to 1250 mg/day for adults and 500 to 750 mg/day for children ≤ 12 yr may be taken orally in divided doses (bid, tid, or qid) at least 1 h before or 2 h after meals and at least 1 h apart from any other drug, food, or milk—it is important that trientine be given on an empty stomach. Dosage may be increased to a maximum of 2 gm/day in adults and 1.5 gm/day in children when the clinical response is not adequate or the concentration of free serum copper is persistently > 20 μg/dL.

Iron deficiency and systemic lupus erythematosus have been reported in patients with Wilson's disease who were on therapy with trientine. Because of the potential for contact dermatitis, any skin exposed to the capsule contents should be promptly washed with water. For the first month of treatment, patients should have their temperature taken nightly, and should be asked to report any symptoms such as fever or skin eruption.

Recently the use of **oral zinc sulfate** 200 to 300 mg/day, which competes with Cu for the transport and storage of protein metallothioneine, resulted in the increased excretion of Cu and has proved to be effective and safe.

Indian childhood cirrhosis is a rapidly progressive disorder and an important cause of death in the Asian subcontinent. A recent study there demonstrated prolific orcein-staining material in hepatocytes, suggesting accumulation of copper-binding protein as in Wilson's disease. Similar deposits have been reported in liver and renal tubules in an infant of Asian immigrants to Britain. The usual cause appears to be the practice of feeding animal milk contaminated by boiling and storing in brass and Cu pots.

OTHER TRACE ELEMENTS

Cobalt

The significance of cobalt in health and nutrition is confined, as far as is known, to its presence in the cobalamin (vitamin B_{12}) molecule. Rare cases of anemia associated with geophagia in areas with soil deficient in cobalt have been reported to respond to the element.

Cobaltous chloride in large doses (20 to 30 mg/day) has been advocated in addition to Fe in the treatment of iron-deficiency in chronic renal failure, but should be used only if cobalt deficiency is suspected, as it is potentially toxic. Overdosing in infants may cause hypothyroidism and congestive heart failure. A cardiomyopathy with a high mortality has been described after industrial exposure, during maintenance dialysis, and following consumption of large quantities of beer contaminated during processing.

Chromium

In addition to being part of several enzyme systems, chromium is associated with a low-molecular weight organic complex termed **glucose tolerance factor (GTF)** that acts with insulin in promoting normal glucose utilization. Brewer's yeast, which is rich in GTF, has been shown to improve glucose tolerance, lower serum cholesterol and triglycerides in some elderly subjects, and to reduce insulin requirements in some diabetics. Glucose tolerance is usually impaired in protein-calorie malnutrition, especially in kwashiorkor, and some cases have shown a dramatic response to trivalent chromium. One patient after several years of home total parenteral nutrition developed sudden weight loss, peripheral neuropathy, and glucose intolerance that were reversed by chromium therapy.

Selenium

Selenium is involved in the reoxidation of reduced glutathione and has close metabolic interrelationships with vitamin E. It is part of the enzyme glutathione peroxidase, which is thought to destroy peroxides derived from unsaturated fatty acids. Deficiency has occurred in patients on long-term parenteral feeding. Muscle pain and tenderness, and whitening of the fingernail beds in one child, have responded to selenium therapy (100 μg/day selenious acid). Several cases of a fatal cardiomyopathy have been attributed to selenium deficiency. In China, a childhood cardiomyopathy known as **Keshan disease**, after the province in which it has been studied, has been attributed to selenium deficiency and protection claimed for prophylactic dosing with 150 μg selenium/day as selenomethionine.

Selenium toxicity **(endemic selenosis)** has long been recognized in animals and has been suspected in some human communities. The most convincing evidence has recently been reported from China. The most common signs were loss of hair and nails. Skin lesions and polyneuritis were less certainly attributable to selenium toxicity. It has been reported from the taking of "health store" tablets.

Manganese

Manganese is a component of several enzyme systems and is essential for normal bone structure. Intake varies greatly, depending mainly upon the consumption of rich sources such as unrefined cereals, green leafy vegetables, and tea. One case of human deficiency has been reported; a volunteer, who received a purified diet from which the element was inadvertently omitted, developed weight loss, transient dermatitis, nausea and vomiting, and changes in color and slow growth of hair. Manganese poisoning is usually limited to those who mine and refine ore; prolonged exposure causes neurologic symptoms resembling parkinsonism or Wilson's disease.

Molybdenum

In a patient on prolonged total parenteral nutrition, deficiency appeared to be responsible for tachycardia, tachypnea, central scotomas, night blindness, and irritability proceeding to coma. These were reversed by ammonium molybdate 300 μg/day orally. The neurologic abnormalities were similar to those in a case of deficiency of the molybdenum cofactor.

Silicon

Human deficiency has not yet been reported, but in animals it causes retarded growth, and bone, cartilage, and connective tissue defects. **Toxicity** has resulted in the formation of silicate urinary calculi after many years of antacid therapy with magnesium trisilicate.

83. OBESITY

The excessive accumulation of body fat. Except for heavily muscled persons, a body weight 20% over that in standard height-weight tables is arbitrarily considered obesity. As with hypertension, obesity represents one arm of a distribution curve of body fat or body weight, with no sharp cut-off point. Obesity may be classified as **mild** (20 to 40% overweight), **moderate** (41 to 100% overweight), and **severe** (> 100% overweight). See TABLE 83–1. Treatment is required to prevent the many complications of obesity (see below).

Etiology

The cause of obesity is unknown but the mechanism is simple—consuming more calories than are expended. At least 7 factors may contribute to obesity. How these

factors interact to determine the body weight of any individual is unknown, but it is not a haphazard process. It is believed that the body weight of many people including the obese is subject to **physiologic regulation** and that elevation of the regulatory level or **"set point"** is responsible for obesity. This set point theory is currently in vogue as an explanation of the difficulty obese people experience in losing weight and in maintaining the loss.

Recent research has outlined a neurophysiologic basis for the regulation of body weight and for the level of a body weight set point. The traditional view of the catecholamines and indolamines as mediators of hunger and satiety, respectively, has been greatly refined and an array of new agents affecting food intake has been discovered. Thus endogenous opiates have been shown to stimulate eating, while several gut hormones—cholecystokinin, neurotensin, and bombesin, in particular—have been found to initiate satiety. These discoveries not only are laying a basis for a better understanding of hunger and satiety, but hold out hope for a more rational pharmacologic control of appetite.

Social factors are very important determinants of obesity, particularly among women. For example, obesity is 6 times more prevalent among lower-class than among upper-class women. This social class relationship is more than correlational; it is also causal. The social class of one's parents is almost as closely linked to obesity as is one's own. Although obesity influences one's social class (lowering it), it cannot have influenced that of one's parents, suggesting that the social class into which a person is born is a powerful determinant of obesity. Obesity is far more common among lower-class than upper-class children; significant differences are apparent by age 6. Economic and other social factors, particularly ethnic and religious, are also closely linked to obesity. The mechanisms appear to be multiple and complex, but differences in life style, and particularly dietary and exercise patterns, probably play a major role.

Endocrine and metabolic factors are usually the consequences rather than causes of obesity. An exception is adipose tissue proliferation in hyperadrenocorticism, in which corticosteroid excess leads to increased gluconeogenesis and a correspondingly greater demand for insulin, which stimulates lipogenesis. Even in this condition the proximate cause of weight gain is the same: more calories are consumed than are expended as energy.

Psychologic factors: The influence of psychologic factors on obesity remains obscure; while many obese persons overeat when emotionally upset, so do many nonobese persons. For a small number of obese persons psychopathology may be linked to their obesity, especially in obese young women of upper and middle socioeconomic classes who have been obese since childhood. They may manifest disordered eating patterns and are at high risk for another troublesome syndrome—disparagement of the body image. Characteristically, they feel that their bodies are grotesque and loathsome and that others view them with hostility and contempt. This results in self-consciousness and impaired social functioning.

Two deviant eating patterns apparently precipitated by stress and emotional disturbance, however, may contribute to the obesity of a few persons. **Bulimia** is *the sudden, compulsive ingestion of very large amounts of food in a very short time, usually followed by agitation, self-condemnation, and often by self-induced vomiting.* The **night-eating syndrome** *consists of morning anorexia, evening hyperphagia, and insomnia.* Attempts at weight reduction in these 2 conditions are usually unsuccessful and may cause the patient unnecessary distress.

Genetic factors: Obesity runs in families: 80% of the offspring of 2 obese parents are obese, compared with 40% of 1 obese parent and only 10% of 2 nonobese parents. At least part of this familial aggregation of obesity is genetically determined. Twin studies

and a recent adoption study have provided strong evidence for the role of genetic factors in human obesity.

Developmental factors: Increased adipose tissue mass can result from an increase in the size of fat cells **(hypertrophic obesity)**, an increase in the number of fat cells **(hyperplastic obesity)**, or an increase in both **(hypertrophic-hyperplastic obesity)**. Obesity beginning in adult life is hypertrophic; patients have larger fat cells, but no increase in number. Juvenile-onset obesity, on the other hand, is more likely to be of the hyperplastic type, usually of the combined hypertrophic-hyperplastic type. Such persons may have up to 5 times as many fat cells as persons of normal weight or those with hypertrophic obesity. As a result, they may achieve a normal body weight only by marked depletion of the lipid content of each fat cell. Such depletion, and particularly the associated events at the cell membrane, may set a biologic limit to their weight reduction possibly explaining their difficulty in reducing to normal weight and their proclivity to regain weight. Thus, there are compelling anatomic as well as psychologic reasons for preventing childhood obesity.

With aging, there is a tendency to accumulate body fat and the prevalence of obesity more than doubles between the ages of 20 and 50.

Physical activity: Decreased physical activity in affluent societies is often cited as a major factor in the rise of obesity; eg, the prevalence of obesity in the USA has more than doubled since the turn of the century, despite a 10% decrease in daily caloric intake.

Caloric requirements are lower with a sedentary life style, and animal experiments suggest that physical inactivity contributes to obesity also by a paradoxic effect on food intake. Although food intake increases with increasing energy expenditure, food intake may not decrease proportionately when such activity falls below a minimum level; restricting physical activity may actually increase food intake in some people.

Brain damage, particularly to the hypothalamus, can lead to obesity, although it is a very rare cause in humans. Its major significance is as a reminder that whatever the social and metabolic determinants of obesity, the final common pathway to caloric balance lies through behavior mediated by the CNS.

Symptoms and Signs

The signs of obesity are an increase in body weight and the evident mass of fatty tissue. Pressure on the thorax from the encompassing sheath of fatty tissue combined with pressure on the diaphragm from below by large intra-abdominal accumulations of fat may occasionally be life-threatening. The resulting reduced respiratory capacity may produce dyspnea on even minimal exertion. In the massively obese this condition may progress to the **Pickwickian syndrome**, characterized by hypoventilation, retention of CO_2 leading to decreased effects of CO_2 as a respiratory stimulant, and resultant hypoxia and somnolence (see also SLEEP APNEA in Ch. 122).

Obesity may lead to a variety of orthopedic disturbances, including low back pain, aggravation of osteoarthritis, particularly of the knees and ankles, and often huge calluses on the feet and heels. Even mild degrees of obesity may be associated with amenorrhea and other menstrual disturbances. BP is frequently elevated and hypertension is commoner in the obese. However, masses of subcutaneous tissue between the BP cuff and the brachial artery can cause false elevated readings when a standard size cuff is used. The remedy is to use a wide cuff long enough to completely encircle the arm with the bladder containing air. Skin disorders are particularly common among the obese. Their lower ratio of body surface to body mass results in impaired heat loss and an increase in sweating, particularly after meals. Sweat, trapped with skin secretions in the thick folds of skin, produces a culture medium particularly conducive to bacterial growth and infections. Motion produces friction between the skin folds that further macerates the skin and adds to pain and discomfort. Mild to moderate edema of the feet and ankles is common.

Diagnosis

Obesity is apparent on observation and can be quantified by weight and height measurements. Although the measurement of skinfold thickness has been widely used in epidemiologic studies, clinicians have generally not found it helpful and it is infrequently used in current practice. Attention should be paid to special distributions of fat; eg, a truncal distribution with a buffalo hump is suggestive of hyperadrenocorticism, although generalized obesity is also seen in this disease. The peculiar accumulation of fluid of the hypothyroid patient should be kept in mind, since mild obesity can be confused with hypothyroidism.

Complications

Obesity adversely affects morbidity and mortality, primarily through cardiovascular complications. The death rate from many diseases, from accidents, and from surgery, is significantly higher among the obese, increasing with the magnitude of the obesity. Sudden death is also more common. The risks increase with overweight in excess of 35% or with any degree of obesity among diabetics and hypertensives.

A common problem in obesity is impaired glucose tolerance and fasting hyperglycemia. Obesity is associated with marked resistance to the action of insulin, increasing insulin requirements and resulting in hyperinsulinism. Histologic examination of the pancreatic islets shows an increased number of enlarged islets. Blood immunoreactive insulin assays demonstrate not only increased fasting levels of insulin, proportional to the degree of obesity, but also excessive responses to glucose or amino acid challenges. This hyperinsulinism responds well to weight reduction, disappearing completely, unless diabetes is present.

Three of the most potent risk factors for coronary artery disease—hypertension, adult-onset diabetes, and hyperlipidemia—are far more prevalent among the obese than among slim subjects. Furthermore, these conditions are markedly improved by weight reduction, suggesting that obesity plays a role in their genesis. Weight reduction may allow 75% of adult-onset diabetics to discontinue medication, and the BP of most hypertensives will be reduced.

Prognosis and Treatment

The prognosis for obesity is poor; untreated, it tends to progress. Attempts to lose weight may cause complications; symptoms of anxiety and depression may appear in as many as half of patients undergoing medical treatment for obesity. Treatment is still only modestly effective, but progress has been made in recent years.

The aim of all therapy for obesity is to establish a caloric deficit by reducing the number of calories ingested as food below the number of calories expended as energy. Methods to achieve this deficit vary widely, and the variety of treatments may seem confusing. Some order has been brought to this confusion by the simple new classification of obesity given above and shown in TABLE 83–1.

TABLE 83–1. CLASSIFICATION OF OBESITY

Type	*Severe*	*Moderate*	*Mild*
Percentage overweight	> 100%	41–100%	< 40%
Prevalence (among obese women)	0.5%	9.0%	90.5%
Pathology	Hypertrophic Hyperplastic	Hypertrophic Hyperplastic	Hypertrophic
Complications	Severe	Conditional	Uncertain
Treatment	Surgical	Diet and behavior therapy (medical)	Behavior therapy (lay)

Severe obesity: The basis of treatment is **surgery,** which can produce large weight losses that are often well maintained. Such surgery is not without risk, and should be confined to those with severe obesity who have repeatedly failed at conservative treatment.

The first extensively-used surgical procedure was jejunoileal bypass, but complications resulted in its replacement by gastric restriction procedures that reduce stomach volume. The currently favored procedure is vertical-banded gastroplasty, in which a 25-mL vertical pouch oriented along the lesser curvature of the stomach is constructed, leading to a stoma 1.5 cm in diameter that is reinforced by a plastic mesh collar.

Weight loss after surgery is at first quite rapid, slowing gradually over 2 yr; about half of the total weight loss occurs during the first 6 mo. The amount of weight lost is directly proportional to the extent of overweight and usually varies between 40 and 60 kg. This loss is accompanied by marked improvement in the medical complications of obesity noted above. Patients also benefit psychosocially, with improvement in mood, self-esteem, body image, activity levels, sexual and marital relations, and interpersonal and vocational effectiveness.

The psychosocial benefits of surgery are often striking and have been underestimated. For example, anxiety and depression, which occur frequently during attempts at weight loss by the usual therapies (eg, diet and drugs), are infrequent among surgically treated patients.

Surgery produces earlier onset of satiety and shifts patients' food preferences away from high calorie foods. Binge-eating, night-eating, excessive snacking, and difficulty in stopping eating are also reduced. Surprisingly, during rapid weight loss, patients who had stopped eating breakfast, began again.

The many favorable results of surgery are so profound as to suggest that they result from major changes in the biology of the patient, such as a lowering of a set point around which body weight is regulated.

Moderate obesity afflicts about 9% of the obese population. Standard treatment with diet and medication appears to be enhanced by the addition of behavior modification technics.

Diet: The primary goal of diet therapy is to establish the largest caloric deficit that can be safely and comfortably tolerated. Conventional reducing diets of 1200 to 1500 kcal/day are safe and comfortable but may produce too slow a weight loss to be practical. For some patients, a very low calorie diet, also called the **protein-sparing-modified-fast,** may be indicated. These diets provide from 400 to 700 kcal/day, largely or exclusively as protein, either as formula or as natural foods such as fish, fowl, or lean meat. As contrasted with "liquid protein" diets, which were associated with a number of fatalities, these diets appear safe when administered under medical supervision for up to 3 mo.

The principal problem in all diet therapy of obesity is maintenance of weight loss, which is poor following very low calorie diets, as most patients regain the lost weight.

Medication: Previously, appetite suppressants were more commonly used for obesity therapy, but the tendency of patients to regain lost weight following termination of drug therapy has lessened the attractiveness of this modality. A rationale for this tendency in terms of the "set point" theory of obesity proposes that medications lower a body weight set point, thereby facilitating patient control of food intake. Medications *do* suppress appetite, but this effect tends to be lost when medication is discontinued. For this reason and because of the addictive potential of some agents they are less used today than in the past (see GENERAL CNS STIMULANTS AND ANOREXIANTS in Ch. 281).

Behavior modification is based upon behavioral analysis, which considers the **behavior to be changed,** its **antecedents,** and its **consequences**. The primary behavior to be changed is eating. Next, great emphasis is placed upon changing the antecedents of eating behavior, from those that are relatively remote (eg, shopping for food) to closer

ones (eg, the ready availability of high-calorie food). The consequences are rewards for behaviors that increase control. Procedures used in changing behavior include self-monitoring—record-keeping—to determine what aspects of behavior should be modified, to develop programs to modify them, and to monitor the effectiveness of these programs; nutrition education; increased physical activity, which raises caloric expenditure and probably limits the fall in metabolic rate caused by dieting, and which decreases appetite and food intake among sedentary, obese persons; and cognitive restructuring, designed to overcome the self-defeating and maladaptive attitudes toward weight reduction and toward themselves that many obese persons experience.

Mild obesity is the most common weight disorder, afflicting over 90% of obese persons. Treatment combines diet with behavior modification and is increasingly being utilized by lay groups.

Diet: The mildly obese should use diets that are less restrictive than the very low calorie diets appropriate for the moderately obese—about 1200 kcal for women and 1500 kcal for men. In recent years there has been a change in what is viewed as appropriate dietary treatment and even the concept of "dieting" has been criticized on psychological grounds: *going on* a diet implies *going off* it and the resumption of old eating habits and former caloric intakes.

The most effective diet involves a gradual change in eating patterns that includes increasing the intake of complex carbohydrates (particularly fruits, vegetables, and cereals) and decreasing the intake of fats and concentrated carbohydrates. Sensible eating habits do not require medical monitoring and may be effectively taught by lay organizations.

Behavior modification, as described above, is easy to teach and learn. The key elements are described in manuals and can be administered by laymen. While a growing number of physicians are enlisting the help of psychologists, nutritionists, and nurses to conduct weight loss groups in their practices, far more obese persons (at least a million a week) are being treated by lay groups; eg, TOPS (Take Off Pounds Sensibly), the largest non-profit group, and Weight Watchers,® the largest commercial group. Their effectiveness is hard to assess because of very high drop-out rates—as high as 50% in 6 wk. Reports of weight loss based upon a select sample of treatment of those who continue treatment should be regarded with caution. Nevertheless, the low cost and ready availability of lay groups make them an important resource and physicians should encourage their patients to join and remain in such groups.

---

84. WATER, ELECTROLYTE, MINERAL, AND ACID-BASE METABOLISM

(See also Ch. 185)

In health, the composition and volume of body fluids remain remarkably constant despite wide ranges of dietary intake and metabolic activity. The mechanisms responsible for maintaining this homeostasis are closely interrelated. Thus many disorders of water, electrolyte, and acid-base metabolism are mixed disturbances. This discussion summarizes aspects of the pathophysiology, recognition, and management of commonly encountered fluid and electrolyte abnormalities.

REGULATION OF WATER AND SODIUM HOMEOSTASIS

Water

The total body water **(TBW)** content of adult men varies from 55% of body wt in the obese to 65% in thin individuals. Values for adult women average about 10% less.

About 2/3 of TBW is intracellular and 1/3 extracellular. The plasma volume comprises about 1/4 of the total **extracellular fluid (ECF)**. TBW content is normally regulated by a combination of factors, including the thirst mechanism, elaboration of antidiuretic hormone **(ADH)** by the posterior pituitary gland, and the kidneys. The major physiologic controls for thirst and ADH secretion are the osmolality and volume of TBW. Normally, body fluid osmolality is maintained within narrow limits, a 2% increase (or decrease) leading to release (or complete suppression) of ADH. However, when the volume of body fluid is sufficiently reduced, ADH release may lead to water conservation at the expense of tonicity. Pain, stress, and drugs such as narcotics and barbiturates may also cause ADH secretion.

In addition to ingested water, another 200 to 300 mL/day is formed in the body by tissue catabolism. Water losses via the kidney can be reduced to as little as 300 to 500 mL/day in the absence of renal disease or other factors affecting the renal concentrating mechanism. Insensible water losses, via expired air and the skin (without sweating), constitute about 0.4 to 0.5 mL/h/kg body wt or about 650 to 850 mL/24 h in a 70-kg man. In the presence of fever, an additional 50 to 75 mL/day may be lost for each degree of temperature elevation above normal. Losses via sweat vary from negligible to large amounts. GI water losses are negligible in health but can be significant in diarrhea or vomiting.

Since cell membranes in general are freely permeable to water, the osmolality of the ECF (290 mOsm/kg water) is about equal to that of the **intracellular fluid (ICF)**. Therefore, the serum osmolality is a convenient and accurate guide to intracellular osmolality. One may *approximate* body fluid osmolality by using the formula

Serum osmolality (mOsm/kg) =

$$2\,([Na] + [K])\text{ serum} + \frac{[BUN]}{2.8} + \frac{[Glucose]}{18}$$

where sodium **(Na)** and potassium **(K)** are given as mEq/L and blood urea nitrogen **(BUN)** and glucose concentrations are in mg/dL.

Serum hypertonicity (hypernatremia) indicates cellular dehydration, and **serum hypotonicity (hyponatremia)** indicates cellular swelling. This relationship may not hold with significant azotemia, hyperglycemia, or hyperlipidemia. Urea penetrates readily into cells; since the intracellular urea concentration equals the extracellular urea concentration, no significant change in cell volume occurs. Thus, in azotemia, although the serum osmolality is increased, the "effective" serum osmolality is not changed and approximately equals twice the serum sodium concentration. In marked hyperglycemia, ECF osmolality rises and exceeds ICF osmolality (since glucose penetrates cell membranes slowly), prompting a shift of water from ICF to ECF. Thus, the serum Na concentration falls in proportion to the dilution of the ECF, declining 1.6 mEq/L for every 100 mg/dL increment in the serum glucose level above the normal. Finally, apparent hyponatremia with normal serum osmolality may occur in hyperlipidemia and extreme hyperglobulinemia, since the lipid or protein forms a significant part of the serum taken for analysis, but the Na concentration/L of serum water is normal.

Sodium

The total body Na content is regulated by a balance between dietary intake and renal Na excretion. Because renal Na excretion can be adjusted to wide ranges of Na intake, significant Na depletion does not occur unless renal Na conservation is abnormal (eg, from primary renal disease or adrenal insufficiency) or when extrarenal losses (eg, GI losses) are combined with inadequate intake. Similarly, Na overload implies defective renal Na excretion.

Renal Na excretion is controlled by a number of variables, which include (1) glomerular filtration rate **(GFR)** and the filtered load of Na, (2) the rate of adrenal gluco-

corticoid and mineralocorticoid (primarily aldosterone) secretion, and (3) a complex of hemodynamic and possibly humoral adjustments. The latter (known as "third factor") diminishes proximal tubular Na reabsorption in response to ECF volume expansion. Recently, an atrial natriuretic factor has been identified (see in Ch. 286). The role of "third factor" and atrial natriuretic factor in disorders characterized by Na retention and edema formation remains uncertain.

The ECF volume is regulated by the total body Na content. Thus disorders of Na balance are manifested by changes in the ECF and intravascular volume, and the best clinical guide to Na needs is the ECF volume. In contrast, the serum Na concentration and osmolality best reflect water balance with respect to body fluid solute. Serum Na levels are usually determined by flame photometry or by the use of an ion-specific electrode.

Water metabolism here refers to *excretion or retention of water independent of Na.* Although isotonic fluid losses constitute the loss of both water and Na, the clinical manifestations of such disorders are referable primarily to ECF volume depletion and resultant hemodynamic disturbances. In contrast, both hypotonicity and hypertonicity of body fluids are manifested primarily as mental disturbances. The term **"disorders of water balance"** is restricted here to *disturbances in osmolality*. It should be noted that mixed disorders of salt and water homeostasis are frequent. Thus depletion of total body fluid content due to renal losses of Na and water may be found in adrenal insufficiency, and a disorder of water balance exists only if body fluid osmolality is altered (ie, if hyponatremia or hypernatremia is present).

CLINICAL DISORDERS OF WATER AND SODIUM METABOLISM

Although conditions of pure Na depletion or excess and water depletion (dehydration) or excess can exist, most clinical disturbances of Na and water balance are mixed. Deficits or excesses of water are shared by the ICF and ECF in approximate proportions of $^2/_3$ ICF and $^1/_3$ ECF. As a result, clinical signs of ECF and intravascular volume alteration usually are absent or not prominent. Instead, abnormalities of the CNS (due to osmotically mediated changes in brain cell volume) are the most frequent clinical changes. These vary from subtle changes in mental status and personality to irritability, hyperreflexia, seizures, coma, and death.

In contrast, Na depletion is characterized by signs of ECF and intravascular volume depletion. When mild, the only alterations may be diminished skin turgor or intraocular tension; both are unreliable signs. When ECF volume has diminished by about 5% or greater, evidence of intravascular volume deficit is present in the form of orthostatic tachycardia and/or hypotension (decrease of systolic pressure of 10 mm Hg or greater) and decreased central venous pressure **(CVP)**. The latter often can be estimated by observing the height of the internal jugular venous pulsation above the 2nd intercostal space; this height in cm + 5 is approximately equal to the CVP. Accurate measurement of the CVP by means of a central venous catheter in the right atrium or superior vena cava provides reliable information regarding intravascular volume status except in the presence of pericardial tamponade or restriction, or acute left ventricular failure (eg, acute myocardial infarction). ECF volume depletion usually is readily distinguished clinically from states of ECF volume overload with low effective circulating intravascular volume (eg, congestive heart failure or cirrhosis with ascites). However, when acute left ventricular failure is present, the pulmonary capillary wedge pressure provides a more accurate assessment of the intravascular volume and effective left ventricular filling pressure. Na excess expands the ECF volume and, when severe, causes edema. About 3 L of fluid must accumulate in an average 70-kg man before edema becomes evident. If local causes of edema are excluded, its presence is a reliable

sign of Na excess. Additional manifestations of Na excess depend largely upon cardiac status and the distribution of ECF between the vascular and interstitial spaces.

PRINCIPLES OF FLUID THERAPY

Fluid and electrolyte therapy consists of providing maintenance requirements and replacing any deficits and ongoing abnormal losses. The approximate composition and volume of some common losses are given in TABLE 84–1. In the presence of normal renal function, the provision of maintenance and other requirements is quite simple, since the kidney retains what is needed and excretes any excess. When renal function is abnormal and/or when there are large abnormal losses, it is necessary to measure the volume and electrolyte content of all significant losses and to tailor administered fluids to the individual patient. Deficits of Na may be estimated initially from the change in body wt. In any event, it is best to monitor volume parameters carefully (BP, pulse, Hct, and CVP or pulmonary capillary wedge pressure) during the administration of saline solutions, especially if large amounts of fluid are given rapidly or if renal or cardiac disease is present. The type of solution given to replace ECF volume deficits depends upon the presence or absence of CNS symptoms and the initial serum Na concentration. If the latter is < 115 to 120 mEq/L, 3% or 5% sodium chloride is given (see Treatment under HYPONATREMIA, below). Likewise, if there is severe hypernatremia, salt replacement must consist of hypotonic solutions, eg, 0.45% sodium chloride.

In states characterized by renal retention of Na, intake must be restricted, based upon the rate of renal Na excretion and the degree of ECF volume expansion.

Water needs are determined by estimates of maintenance requirements and the serum Na concentration. If renal function is seriously impaired or if a disturbance of water metabolism is present, major adjustments must be made in water intake. For

TABLE 84–1. FLUID LOSSES IN ADULTS

Type of Loss	Composition		Volume/24 h
Maintenance (predicted needs in absence of disease)			
Insensible	Water		12 mL/kg body wt
Sweat	Na^+	50 mEq/L	Variable; should be estimated when sweating is severe
	K^+	7 mEq/L	
	Cl^-	40 mEq/L	
Urine	Variable; average 24-h loss of:		Variable; average volume, 1000–1500 mL
	Na^+	75–170 mEq*	
	K^+	40– 60 mEq	
	Cl^-	115–145 mEq	
Abnormal losses			
Nasogastric suction	Na^+ varies directly with pH:	20–116 mEq/L (60)**	Measure
	K^+	5– 32 mEq/L (9)	
	Cl^-	50–154 mEq/L (100)	
Diarrheal stool	Na^+	50–100 mEq/L	Measure
	K^+	20– 40 mEq/L	
	Cl^-	40– 80 mEq/L	

* Note that urinary Na content normally varies directly with dietary Na intake.
** Numbers in parentheses indicate average values.

example, when severe hyponatremia exists due to water retention, restriction of water intake to 1000 mL or less/24 h may be mandatory. Additional modifications of electrolyte content must be made in the presence of disturbances of acid-base and K metabolism, which will be discussed separately.

As a rule of thumb, ½ of calculated deficits, plus maintenance and projected losses, may be given during the first 24 h of treatment. About ½ of the total 24-h volume is given in the first 8 h. In shock, it may be necessary to give fluid at faster rates, and careful attention must be given to volume parameters and the K content of such fluids.

COMBINED SODIUM AND WATER DEFICITS

A loss of sodium and water, producing extracellular fluid volume depletion.

Losses of Na from the body are always combined with water losses. The end result of Na depletion is ECF volume depletion; whether it is hypotonic, isotonic, or hypertonic depends largely upon the route of loss (eg, GI, renal) and the type of fluid ingested by or given to the individual. Other factors, such as the activation of ADH secretion or impaired solute delivery to the distal tubule with resultant water retention, may also affect the final serum Na concentration. The common causes of ECF volume depletion are listed in TABLE 84–2.

Symptoms, Signs, and Diagnosis

ECF volume depletion should be suspected in patients with a history of inadequate fluid intake (especially in comatose or disoriented patients), vomiting, diarrhea (or iatrogenic GI losses; eg, nasogastric suction, ileostomy, or colostomy), diuretic therapy, symptoms of diabetes mellitus, or renal or adrenal disease. A history of weight loss over a short period of time is useful. Physical signs, such as diminished skin turgor, intraocular tension, and dry shrunken tongue, are often unreliable, especially in the elderly or "mouth-breathers." More reliable signs include a low CVP (measured or estimated from the neck veins), postural hypotension, or tachycardia (the last 2 signs may occur in bedridden patients without ECF volume depletion). When depletion is severe, disorientation and overt shock may be present. The Hct is often increased but is valueless unless the baseline level is known or it is disproportionately high for the underlying disease (eg, renal failure).

If renal function is sufficiently intact and losses are extrarenal, the urine Na concentration is usually < 10 to 15 mEq/L, fractional excretion of Na **(FeNa)** < 1% (FeNa = [urine Na/serum Na divided by the urine creatinine/serum creatinine] × 100), and urine osmolality is often elevated. In the presence of metabolic alkalosis the urine Na

TABLE 84–2. PRINCIPAL CAUSES OF ECF VOLUME DEPLETION

I. Extra-renal
  - A. GI: vomiting, diarrhea, GI suction
  - B. Skin: sweating
  - C. Dialysis: hemodialysis, peritoneal dialysis
  - D. Third space losses

II. Renal/Adrenal
  - A. Chronic renal failure; salt-wasting renal disease (medullary cystic disease; Interstitial nephritis; less frequently, pyelonephritis, myeloma)
  - B. Acute renal failure: recovery phase
  - C. Diuretic therapy
  - D. Diabetes mellitus with ketoacidosis or extreme glucosuria
  - E. Bartter's syndrome
  - F. Adrenal disease: Addison's disease (glucocorticoid deficiency), hypoaldosteronism

concentration may be high; a low urine chloride concentration (< 10 mEq/L) indicates ECF volume depletion in this instance. If the Na loss is due to renal disease or adrenal insufficiency, the urine Na concentration generally exceeds 20 mEq/L. Significant ECF volume depletion frequently produces mild to moderate rises in the BUN and plasma creatinine levels (prerenal azotemia).

Treatment

Mild to moderate ECF volume depletion may be corrected by increased oral intake of Na and water in the conscious patient with no GI dysfunction. Correction of the underlying cause is always appropriate and often consists of simple measures such as discontinuation of diuretic therapy. When depletion is severe and accompanied by hypotension or when oral fluid administration is impractical, IV sodium chloride is infused, following the precautions outlined under PRINCIPLES OF FLUID THERAPY, above. When renal excretion of water is normal, Na and water deficits may be safely replaced with 0.9% sodium chloride. When there is an associated disturbance in water metabolism, replacement fluids are modified as discussed in the following sections.

HYPONATREMIA

A decrease in the serum sodium concentration below the normal range (136 to 145 mEq/L), usually indicative of hypo-osmolality of body fluid due to an excess of water relative to solute.

The principal causes of hyponatremia are shown in TABLE 84–3. With the exception of the artifactual (hyperlipidemia) and osmotic varieties, hyponatremia usually results from renal retention of water. In Na-depleted patients, the manifestations are primarily those of ECF volume depletion, unless water intake is excessive and resultant hyponatremia severe.

Dilutional hyponatremia with expansion of TBW usually is associated with an elevated total body Na content. In edematous states (eg, congestive heart failure, cirrhosis, nephrotic syndrome, and idiopathic edema syndrome), the kidney is unusually salt-acquisitive, presumably because of a diminished effective circulating blood volume. The kidney responds by retaining salt and water as if the individual were intravascular volume-depleted; this renal response may be further heightened by superimposed therapy with diuretics or, possibly, cyclooxygenase inhibitors (eg, nonsteroidal anti-inflammatory drugs). The urine Na concentration generally is very low (< 10 mEq/L) and the urine osmolality elevated in the absence of diuretics. Hyponatremia may result

TABLE 84–3. PRINCIPAL CAUSES OF HYPONATREMIA

I. Sodium depletion in excess of water depletion or replacement of sodium losses with water alone (may occur in many of conditions listed in TABLE 84-2)

II. Dilutional hyponatremia (water intake in excess of output; always implies impaired water excretion)
   - A. Primary dilutional hyponatremia: renal failure; states characterized by elevated output of ADH, e.g., postoperative narcotic administration; syndrome of inappropriate ADH secretion (SIADH), e.g., with pulmonary neoplasms or infections (tuberculosis), CNS infections (meningitis, encephalitis), trauma, acute intermittent porphyria
   - B. Neuroendocrine: adrenal and pituitary insufficiency, myxedema
   - C. Associated with sodium retention and edema (congestive heart failure; hepatic cirrhosis; renal sodium acquisitive states such as nephrotic syndrome, toxemia of pregnancy)
   - D. Osmotic hyponatremia: severe hyperglycemia
   - E. Thiazide diuretics

from volume-mediated or angiotensin-stimulated ADH release, direct impairment of renal water excretion by angiotensin, diminished delivery of Na to the distal tubular diluting site, or in part from stimulation of thirst by angiotensin. The clinical features are those of the underlying disease plus low urinary Na excretion and, frequently, a concentrated urine with respect to serum.

Dilutional hyponatremia may also result from excessive water intake without Na retention in the presence of renal failure, Addison's disease, myxedema, or nonosmotic ADH secretion (eg, stress, postoperative states, and drugs such as chlorpropamide or tolbutamide, opioids, barbiturates, vincristine, clofibrate, and carbamazepine). All involve defective water excretion. Certain drugs, such as cyclophosphamide or chlorpropamide, potentiate the renal effect of endogenous ADH, while others such as oxytocin have a direct ADH-like effect on the kidney. Rarely, massive water ingestion ($>$ 20 to 25 L/day) may produce hyponatremia in the presence of normal renal water excretion.

The **syndrome of inappropriate ADH secretion (SIADH)** occurs in association with oat cell carcinoma of the lung, a variety of pulmonary and CNS disorders, the Guillain-Barré syndrome, or acute intermittent porphyria; or it may be idiopathic. It is due to sustained ADH elaboration that is inappropriate with respect to body fluid osmolality. Typically, there are (1) inappropriately hypertonic urine with respect to serum (the urine osmolality should be $<$ 130 mOsm/kg when hyponatremia is present; therefore, a urine osmolality that is less than the serum osmolality but is $>$ 130 mOsm/kg is inappropriately concentrated in the face of hyponatremia); (2) normal GFR; (3) hyponatremia and hypo-osmolality of body fluids; (4) isovolemia or expansion of TBW without edema; and (5) urinary Na wasting that increases with salt-loading. The syndrome is identical to that produced by chronic administration of exogenous vasopressin in individuals allowed free access to water. Both the hyponatremia and urinary Na wasting can be corrected by water restriction. This syndrome must be distinguished from other hyponatremic states with identifiable causes of ADH secretion, especially Addison's disease.

Thiazide diuretics may cause hyponatremia by several mechanisms. Most frequently, diuretic-induced losses of salt produces hypovolemia and water retention as the result of volume-mediated ADH secretion and impaired delivery of filtrate to the distal diluting site. Less commonly, thiazides may produce hyponatremia, hypokalemia, and metabolic alkalosis in the absence of detectable ECF volume contraction. In this circumstance, hyponatremia presumably is due to intracellular uptake of Na and exaggerated volume receptor release of ADH in response to the diuretic-induced salt losses. This effect of the drug may last for up to 2 wk after cessation of therapy; however, hyponatremia will usually respond to replacement of potassium and volume deficits, along with judicious restriction of water intake until the drug effect dissipates. Elderly patients may be especially susceptible to thiazide-induced hyponatremia, particularly if there is a preexisting defect in renal water excretion. Such patients infrequently may develop severe, life-threatening hyponatremia within a few weeks after the initiation of a thiazide diuretic. Here, the mechanism appears to involve an exaggerated natriuresis and impaired urinary diluting capacity, but not hypokalemia or ADH production.

Water intoxication may result when the effective serum osmolality falls to 240 mOsm/kg or less, irrespective of the underlying cause. However, the rate of fall of osmolality may be as important as the absolute magnitude of the decrease; symptoms may occur at somewhat higher serum osmolalities if the change is rapid. Experimentally, brain water content is elevated both in acute and chronic hyponatremia. However, as a result of decreased brain electrolyte content (primarily K) in the chronic setting, the increase in brain water content is less than would be expected from the level of serum osmolality. The development of subtle changes in mental status, lethargy, and confusion in a clinical setting associated with impaired water excretion

suggests water intoxication. If intoxication is progressive, stupor, neuromuscular hyperexcitability, convulsions, prolonged coma, and death may result. Evidence of volume expansion is not prominent unless there is an associated disturbance of Na metabolism, since the expansion of body water is predominantly (2/3) intracellular.

Treatment

Management of hyponatremia depends upon its severity and the underlying cause. The presence of hyponatremia, hyperkalemia, and hypotension should suggest adrenal insufficiency and the need for IV glucocorticoid administration (100 to 200 mg of soluble hydrocortisone in 1 L of 5% glucose in 0.9% sodium chloride is given rapidly over 4 h in acute adrenal insufficiency). When adrenal function is normal, the correction of hyponatremia associated with ECF volume depletion usually requires 0.9% sodium chloride administration alone. If the underlying disorder is slow to respond or hyponatremia is marked, water restriction (500 to 1500 mL/24 h, depending on the severity of the disturbance) is prudent. If the syndrome of inappropriate ADH release is present, severe water restriction is required; ie, 25 to 50% of maintenance. Lasting correction depends upon successful correction of the basic disease. In cases where the ADH excess is untreatable (tumor, some idiopathic cases), the use of the tetracycline derivative demeclocycline 900 to 1200 mg/day has been helpful. However, nephrotoxicity has resulted from demeclocycline administration to patients with hepatic cirrhosis. Prudence dictates that the drug be avoided in patients with cirrhosis and used with caution in other settings.

When symptoms of water intoxication are present or imminent (eg, serum Na < 120 mEq/L; effective osmolality < 240 mOsm/kg), it is necessary to give hypertonic (3% or 5%) sodium chloride. A 3% sodium chloride solution provides 0.51 mEq of Na/mL; a 5% solution, 0.86 mEq/mL. Sufficient Na to raise the serum concentration to about 120 to 125 mEq/L is given over 12 to 24 h with water restriction. In general, the serum Na concentration should be raised by no more than 2 mEq/L/h in order to avoid CNS complications or congestive heart failure. The amount of Na required to raise the serum Na level to 125 mEq/L can be approximated by multiplying the deficit (125 mEq/L less the measured serum value in mEq/L) by the TBW. Although the Na given will remain in the extracellular compartment, it will behave as if it were distributed in the TBW, owing to its osmotic effect. In patients with concomitant ECF volume expansion (including those with SIADH), the administration of a potent loop diuretic such as furosemide or ethacrynic acid may be combined with isotonic or hypertonic saline plus potassium chloride to replace diuretic-induced K losses. The use of captopril, in combination with a loop diuretic, has effectively corrected the hyponatremia of patients with congestive heart failure and may be efficacious in other ECF volume expanded states characterized by increased activity of the renin-angiotensin axis (eg cirrhosis or nephrotic syndrome). The dose of captopril must be titrated carefully (initial dose, 12.5 mg orally q 8 to 12 h) to avoid hypotension and resultant diminished renal perfusion. If the diuretic response is small, or if the hyponatremia is severe (eg serum Na < 105 mEq/L), dialysis against a bath with an appropriate Na concentration may correct hyponatremia without expanding the ECF volume.

HYPERNATREMIA

An elevation of the serum sodium concentration above the normal range (136 to 14 mEq/L), indicative of a deficit in body water relative to sodium.

Pathogenesis

Hypernatremia generally results when water losses exceed Na losses in conjunctio with inadequate water intake. Usually, this implies either an impaired thirst mechanism or limited access to water. Water losses may be due to abnormal renal wate conservation and/or excessive extrarenal losses. Since impaired renal water conserva

tion and impaired thirst are common in the elderly, they may be particularly prone to develop hypernatremia. Rarely, hypernatremia may result from a grossly elevated Na intake (without concurrent water loss) in association with limited access to water (eg, in infants or unconscious adults). The principal causes of hypernatremia are listed in TABLE 84–4. Pituitary ADH deficiency, or central diabetes insipidus **(DI)**, most often results from surgical hypophysectomy or cranial trauma (see under POSTERIOR LOBE DISORDERS in Ch. 88). It occurs less frequently in association with intracranial tumors or infiltrative disorders of the CNS (eg, sarcoidosis or histiocytosis), as a hereditary syndrome, or idiopathically. Depending on the level of pituitary stalk interruption, central DI may be transient (below the median eminence) or permanent (above the median eminence). In some individuals, there is inadequate production of ADH, while in others there is adequate production but impaired hormone release in response to osmotic stimuli. In the latter group, however, ADH release is stimulated by a 7 to 10% reduction in the intravascular volume, and may also occur in response to drugs such as clofibrate or carbamazepine.

Nephrogenic (ADH-unresponsive) diabetes insipidus (NDI) may be congenital but is most often acquired and results from drugs such as demethylchlortetracycline, volatile fluorocarbon anesthetics (particularly methoxyflurane and, less commonly, halothane), amphotericin B, and lithium carbonate (see in ANOMALIES IN KIDNEY TRANSPORT in Ch. 187). A transient form of NDI may occur late in pregnancy and remit postpartum. ADH-unresponsive polyuric states also may result from osmotic diuresis, or impairment of the renal concentrating mechanism by parenchymal disease (eg, sickle cell nephropathy, chronic interstitial renal disease) or electrolyte abnormalities (eg, hypokalemia, hypercalcemia).

Symptoms, Signs, and Diagnosis

As in pure water excess, the major clinical feature of water deficit is CNS dysfunction resulting from brain cell shrinkage. Confusion, neuromuscular excitability, seizures, or coma may result. Experimentally, brain solute is elevated in response to chronic hypernatremia (due to the accumulation of "idiogenic" osmoles). Excretion of a large volume of hypotonic urine is characteristic of patients with abnormal renal water conservation. When losses are extrarenal, the route of water loss is often evident (eg, vomiting, diarrhea, excessive sweating) and the urine is highly concentrated and of

TABLE 84–4. PRINCIPAL CAUSES OF HYPERNATREMIA

I. Abnormal renal wasting of water with inadequate intake of water
    - A. Diabetes insipidus
        1. Pituitary ADH deficiency
        2. Nephrogenic (ADH unresponsive)
    - B. Osmotic diuresis: marked glycosuria, mannitol diuresis, urea diuresis due to high-protein tube feedings (high sodium load contributory), chronic renal failure
    - C. Recovery phase of acute renal failure
    - D. Hypercalcemia, hypokalemia, sickle cell anemia

II. Water depletion with normal renal conservation of water but inadequate intake of water
    - A. Excessive sweating and insensible losses (often infants, comatose or disoriented patients without access to water)
    - B. Diarrheal disorders (especially in children)
    - C. Disordered thirst mechanism

III. Grossly excessive intake of sodium with limited access to water

IV. Water loss due to peritoneal dialysis

low volume. In the absence of severe renal impairment, osmotic diuresis, or early metabolic alkalosis, the urinary Na concentration will be low if concomitant Na depletion exists. However, the diagnosis of Na depletion or excess is made clinically.

The syndrome of hyperglycemic (hyperosmolar) nonketotic coma is recognized by the combination of marked hyperglycemia, hyperosmolality, and absence of ketosis, usually associated with combined Na and water depletion. Water depletion can be recognized in this syndrome by correcting the serum Na for the level of the serum glucose concentration.

Treatment

The initial aim is water replacement and, in those patients with associated Na depletion, restoration of ECF volume. Water replacement can be accomplished orally in the conscious patient without GI disturbance, or by IV infusion in patients unable to swallow. Although most patients may be given 5% D/W, too rapid infusion may produce glycosuria, thereby increasing salt-free water excretion and increased hypertonicity of body fluids. However, in patients with the **hyperglycemic hyperosmolar syndrome,** or associated Na deficits, 0.45% sodium chloride is preferable. When severe acidosis ($pH < 7.20$) is present, a hypotonic sodium bicarbonate solution is substituted for 0.45% sodium chloride. If volume disturbances are severe enough to produce shock, colloid and isotonic (0.9%) sodium chloride may be required before turning to hypotonic saline. The hypernatremia should be corrected over a period of 24 to 48 h (ie, the serum Na should be lowered no more rapidly than 2 mEq/L/h) in order to avoid cerebral edema due to the presence of excess brain solute. The amount of water necessary for replacement of existing deficits may be estimated by the formula:

$$\text{Deficit} = \text{TBW} - \frac{140 \text{ mEq/L (TBW)}}{\text{actual serum Na}}$$

where TBW is in liters, and Na concentration in mEq/L. In patients with excess total body Na, a loop diuretic is given and urine losses are replaced with 5% D/W plus potassium chloride; such replacement is in addition to that of existing water deficits.

In pituitary DI, administration of vasopressin stops the renal water loss. The type and route of vasopressin administration depends upon the severity of the hypernatremia and the clinical state of the patient. When hypernatremia is moderate and the patient is alert, desmopressin acetate, 0.1 to 0.4 mL q 12 to 24 h, may be given intranasally. When hypernatremia is severe (serum Na > 155 mEq/L), or if CNS impairment is present, 5 to 10 u.of aqueous vasopressin are administered s.c. The short duration of action of aqueous vasopressin may be advantageous and allow more controlled reduction of the serum Na in severely ill patients, particularly when water deficits are large. Chronic management of pituitary DI is discussed in Ch. 88.

In nephrogenic DI, administration of a thiazide diuretic along with modest Na restriction reduces free water loss.

Patients with **hyperglycemic hyperosmolar coma** should receive regular insulin in an initial dose of 0.22 to 0.33 u./kg body weight IM, and 5 to 7 u./h IM thereafter or until the blood glucose falls below 250 mg/dL. Alternatively, an initial dose of 0.33 to 0.44 u./kg body weight of regular insulin is given IV and, thereafter, a continuous IV infusion of 7 u./h is given in saline until the blood glucose falls below 250 mg/dL. The blood glucose concentration should be measured q 2 h during treatment.

DISTURBANCES IN POTASSIUM METABOLISM

Potassium **(K)** is primarily an intracellular cation, only about 2% of total body K being extracellular. Since most intracellular K is contained within muscle cells, total

body K is roughly proportional to lean body mass. A 70-kg man contains about 3500 mEq of K. In health, and in states of simple K deficiency or excess, the serum K level provides a reasonable clinical estimate of total body K content with respect to capacity; that is, serum K rises when total K content exceeds capacity and falls when total body K is depleted with respect to intracellular capacity. Serum K levels may be determined by flame photometry or by the use of an ion-specific electrode.

Assuming no change in pH, a 1 mEq/L decrease in serum K concentration, when the initial level is 4 mEq/L or greater, indicates a deficit of 100 to 200 mEq of K. A fall in serum K to < 3 mEq/L indicates a deficit in total body K of about 200 to 400 mEq. However, when disease states alter membrane function (permeability or active transport), when acid-base disturbances exist, and when lean body mass is significantly diminished (as in prolonged starvation), the serum K level is an unreliable guide to total body K content.

The serum K concentration is affected significantly by the serum bicarbonate concentration and serum pH. Acidosis is associated with movement of K from cells into the extracellular space, and alkalosis with transfer of K in the opposite direction, independent of the total body K/capacity relationship. In this regard, it appears that changes in the serum bicarbonate concentration may be more important than the change in pH. While a rule of thumb is that a 0.1 u. change in pH results in about a 0.6 mEq/L inverse change in serum K concentration, this relationship is highly variable and the change in serum K level may range between 0.3 and 1.3 mEq/L. Nevertheless, serum K increases with acute acidosis and falls with acute alkalosis; this implies that a low or normal serum K level in the presence of significant acidosis indicates K depletion.

Dietary intake of K normally varies between 40 and 150 mEq/day. In the steady state, urinary and fecal K excretion equals K input into the ECF and chronic K balance is regulated chiefly by renal K excretion. When the ingested or administered K load increases acutely, only about 50% of the acute K load appears in the urine after several hours. The rise in serum K concentration is minimized as most of the retained K transfers into the intracellular compartment. The internal distribution of K in response to an acute K load is controlled by insulin secretion, sympathetic nervous system activity (cellular K uptake is promoted by β_2 receptor activation and opposed by α receptor stimulation), and by adrenal production of aldosterone. If elevated intake continues, renal K excretion rises (K adaptation), probably due to K-stimulated aldosterone secretion. In addition, stool K content may rise. The renal response to K restriction is relatively slow in developing, and when urinary K excretion is reduced to 10 mEq/24 h, significant K depletion is present. Thus, the renal conservation mechanism for K is far less efficient than that for Na.

Most of the K filtered at the glomerulus is reabsorbed in the proximal tubule and loop of Henle; excreted K is secreted into the filtrate in the distal tubule and collecting duct. K excretion is regulated by aldosterone, acid-base status, the electrical potential difference in the distal and collecting tubules, and the rate of urine flow. Aldosterone secretion leads to kaliuresis, and aldosterone deficit or suppression impairs renal K excretion. Acute acidosis impairs K excretion while chronic acidosis and acute alkalosis lead to kaliuresis. The relationship of K and hydrogen ion excretion is discussed further under DISTURBANCES IN ACID-BASE METABOLISM, below. Actions that increase the luminal negativity of the distal tubule favor secretion of K; a similar change in the collecting tubule also increases K secretion and limits back-diffusion of K into the renal interstitium. Physiologically, the most important variable governing luminal negativity is the presence of Na ions. Thus, states characterized by diminished distal Na delivery (eg, severe congestive failure) may be attended by impaired K excretion. Conversely, increased distal Na delivery may be associated with increased K excretion. In such conditions, however, the rate of flow of filtrate along the distal nephron may be the most important factor as K excretion is highly flow dependent.

POTASSIUM DEFICIT AND HYPOKALEMIA

Etiology and Pathogenesis

K depletion usually is due to excessive losses of K in the urine or stool. **Renal K wasting** and profound hypokalemia are found in Bartter's syndrome, an uncommon disorder of uncertain cause and characterized by sodium wasting, excessive production of renin and aldosterone, and normotension. More often, kaliuresis occurs in adrenal steroid excess (particularly mineralocorticoid excess); in association with diuretics (eg, thiazides, furosemide, ethacrynic acid, but not spironolactone or triamterene); in hypomagnesemia; in osmotic diuresis (eg, diabetic ketoacidosis); in renal tubular disease, such as renal tubular acidosis, Fanconi's syndrome, and, rarely, pyelonephritis; with excessive licorice ingestion; and with antipseudomonal penicillins (eg, carbenicillin) or high-dose penicillin treatment. **Gastrointestinal losses** usually are due to diarrhea, chronic laxative abuse or clay ingestion, vomiting or gastric suction (renal K wasting with developing metabolic alkalosis is of primary importance), and bowel diversion. Villous adenoma of the colon is a rare cause of K loss from the GI tract. The **transfer of extracellular K into cells** may also cause hypokalemia, as in glycogenesis (total parenteral nutrition or enteral hyperalimentation, or administration of insulin to patients with diabetes mellitus), familial periodic paralysis, and acute alkalosis. β_2-Adrenergic agonists such as albuterol or terbutaline may produce hypokalemia due to cellular K uptake. Similarly, hypokalemic thyrotoxic periodic paralysis may result from excessive β-sympathetic stimulation. **Other causes** include decreased intake, as in starvation and failure to give K in IV solutions, and losses in sweat, as in cystic fibrosis.

Symptoms, Signs, and Diagnosis

Severe hypokalemia (serum K < 3 mEq/L) may produce muscular weakness and lead to paralysis and respiratory failure. Muscular malfunction may result in respiratory hypoventilation, paralytic ileus, hypotension, muscle twitches, and tetany. K nephropathy impairs the concentrating mechanism, producing polyuria and decreased maximal urinary concentrating ability with secondary polydipsia.

Cardiac effects usually are minimal until serum K levels are < 3 mEq/L, *except in patients receiving digitalis*. The characteristic ECG changes of S-T segment depression, increased U wave amplitude, and T wave amplitude < U wave amplitude (in same lead) are shown in FIG. 84–1. Severe hypokalemia may produce premature ventricular and atrial contractions and ventricular and atrial tachyarrhythmias, as well as advanced disturbances of atrioventricular conduction in patients not receiving digitalis. Similar disturbances occur at less severe degrees of hypokalemia in the presence of digitalis.

Laboratory Findings

The serum K level is < 3.8 mEq/L. Metabolic alkalosis is often present unless the hypokalemia results from diarrhea or renal tubular acidosis, both of which cause metabolic acidosis. Severe depletion of K impairs the response of the tubule to ADH and may result in isosthenuria or a state resembling nephrogenic diabetes insipidus. Generally, the creatinine clearance and serum creatinine are normal and urine sediment changes are nonspecific. The concentrating defect is reversible with repletion of K.

Treatment

Correction of the underlying cause may suffice when hypokalemia is minimal. When deficits and hypokalemia are more severe (serum K < 3 mEq/L) or when continued therapy with K-depleting agents is necessary, potassium chloride is given orally (10% KCl) or IV. Usually 20 to 80 mEq/day in excess of losses given in divided doses is sufficient to correct deficits over a period of several days. However, K retention and the need for K supplementation may continue for several weeks during refeeding after prolonged starvation. Enteric-coated K preparations should be *avoided* as they ma

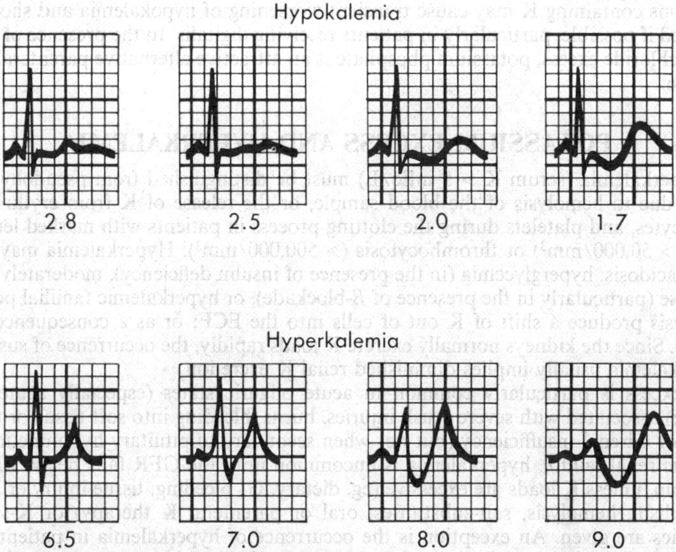

Fig. 84–1. EGG patterns in hypokalemia and in hyperkalemia. (Serum potassium in mEq/L.)

lead to small-bowel ulceration. A wax impregnated KCl preparation containing 8 mEq/tablet appears to be a safe alternative to 10% KCl. One should attempt to ensure that oral food intake contains sufficient quantities of K.

Routine K replacement is not necessary in most patients receiving diuretics. However, avoidance of hypokalemia and K depletion in patients receiving digitalis (increased risk of arrhythmias), in asthmatic patients receiving β_2 agonists, and in type II diabetics (worsening of glucose intolerance) is particularly important. Such patients should receive the lowest effective dose of a diuretic of moderate duration of action, their dietary Na intake should be restricted (eg, 2 gm/day), and their serum K should be monitored closely. Should hypokalemia develop, K supplementation is indicated and the diuretic should be discontinued if possible. Addition of triamterene 100 mg/day or spironolactone 25 mg qid may be useful in occasional patients who become hypokalemic with diuretic therapy, but should be avoided in patients with renal failure, diabetes, or other interstitial renal diseases associated with hyporeninemic hypoaldosteronism. Correction of K deficiency should be carried out with particular care in patients with renal insufficiency.

When K deficits must be replaced parenterally, the rate of correction of hypokalemia is limited because of the slow rate of transfer of K from the extra- to intracellular compartments. If serum K is high (states of acidemia) even though total body K is low, one should wait until the serum K starts to fall before administering IV K. Even when K deficits are severe, it is rarely necessary to give > 80 to 100 mEq of K in excess of continuing losses in a 24-h period. In most situations, the K concentration of IV solutions should not exceed 40 mEq/L and infusion rates should not exceed 10 mEq/h. Rarely, it may be necessary to give K solutions IV at a more rapid rate in order to prevent progressive severe hypokalemia. Infusion of > 40 mEq potassium chloride/h should be undertaken *only with continuous monitoring of the ECG and hourly serum K determinations in order to avoid severe hyperkalemia and cardiac arrest*. Glucose

solutions containing K may cause transient worsening of hypokalemia and should be avoided if possible, particularly in patients receiving digitalis. In the presence of acidosis or chloride excess, potassium phosphate is an attractive alternative parenteral preparation.

POTASSIUM EXCESS AND HYPERKALEMIA

Hyperkalemia (serum K > 5 mEq/L) must be distinguished from pseudohyperkalemia due to hemolysis of the blood sample, or the release of K from erythrocytes, leukocytes, and platelets during the clotting process in patients with marked leukocytosis (> 50,000/mm³) or thrombocytosis (> 500,000/mm³). Hyperkalemia may occur when acidosis, hyperglycemia (in the presence of insulin deficiency), moderately heavy exercise (particularly in the presence of β-blockade), or hyperkalemic familial periodic paralysis produce a shift of K out of cells into the ECF; or as a consequence of K excess. Since the kidneys normally excrete K loads rapidly, the occurrence of sustained hyperkalemia usually implies diminished renal K excretion.

K excess is particularly common in acute oliguric states (especially acute renal failure) associated with severe crush injuries, burns, bleeding into soft tissue or the GI tract, or adrenal insufficiency (but not when secondary to pituitary hypofunction). In chronic renal failure, hyperkalemia is uncommon until the GFR falls below 10 to 15 mL/min, unless K loads are excessive (eg, dietary, GI bleeding, tissue injury or hypercatabolism, hemolysis, salt-substitutes, oral or parenteral K therapy) or K-sparing diuretics are given. An exception is the occurrence of hyperkalemia in patients with diabetic nephropathy (or interstitial renal disease), hyporeninemia, and hypoaldosteronism despite creatinine clearances often > 10 mL/min. Such patients may be more susceptible to development of hyperkalemia with the administration of β-blockers or inhibitors of prostaglandin synthesis. If sufficient potassium chloride is ingested orally, or rapidly given parenterally, severe hyperkalemia may result, even with normal renal function.

Symptoms, Signs, and Diagnosis

Although flaccid paralysis occasionally occurs, hyperkalemia is usually asymptomatic until cardiac toxicity supervenes (FIG. 84–1). The earliest ECG changes are shortening of the Q-T interval and tall, peaked T waves (serum K > 5.5 mEq/L). Progressive hyperkalemia produces nodal and ventricular arrhythmias, widening of the QRS complex (serum K > 6.5 mEq/L), P-R interval prolongation and disappearance of the P wave, and, finally, degeneration of the QRS complex to a sine wave pattern and ventricular asystole or fibrillation.

Laboratory Findings

The serum K level is > 5.0 mEq/L. Artifactual hyperkalemia is recognized by the finding of a normal K level in plasma or in a nonhemolyzed blood sample. Other laboratory abnormalities reflect any underlying disease.

Treatment

Mild hyperkalemia may respond to diminished K intake or discontinuance of drugs such as K-sparing diuretics, β-blockers, or angiotensin converting enzyme inhibitors (eg, captopril). The rare patient with hyperkalemic familial periodic paralysis may be treated effectively with inhaled albuterol. A serum K of 6 mEq/L requires aggressive therapy. However, in acute or chronic renal failure (especially in the presence of hypercatabolism or tissue injury), treatment should be initiated when the serum K level exceeds 5 mEq/L.

If no ECG abnormalities are present and the serum K is < 6 mEq/L, sodium polystyrene sulfonate, a sodium-cycle cation exchange resin, is given in 70% sorbitol to ensure rapid passage through the GI tract; 15 to 30 gm for adults (1 gm/kg/day in

divided doses for infants or young children) in 30 to 70 mL of 70% sorbitol may be given orally q 4 to 6 h. Patients unable to take oral medications because of ileus or other reasons may be given similar treatment by rectal retention enema. About 1 mEq of K is removed/gm of resin given. Resin therapy is slow and often fails to lower serum K significantly in hypercatabolic states. Since Na is exchanged for K when sodium polystyrene sulfonate is used, Na overload may be iatrogenically produced.

In emergencies (*cardiac toxicity or serum K level > 6 mEq/L*) the following measures are instituted immediately and followed by sodium polystyrene sulfonate therapy:

1. IV administration of 10 to 20 mL of 10% calcium gluconate over 15 to 30 min (hazardous in patients on digitalis) in adults may reverse the ECG changes without changing serum K level. When the ECG has deteriorated to a sine wave or worse, the calcium gluconate may be given rapidly IV (5 to 10 mL over 2 min). **In infants and young children,** myocardial contractility is stabilized by giving 0.25 mL/kg of calcium gluceptate over 2 to 3 min with ECG monitoring.

2. Sodium bicarbonate 88 to 176 mEq is given to adults by rapid IV push and repeated as needed, especially if the patient is acidotic. **In infants and young children,** sodium bicarbonate 3 mEq/kg may be given over 30 to 60 min.

3. IV administration of 100 to 300 mL of 50% glucose containing 1 u. of regular insulin/3 gm glucose over a 30-min period may lower serum K for 4 to 6 h. Effects may not occur for 30 to 60 min. In extreme emergencies 15 u. of regular insulin may be given by IV push and covered with 50% glucose or continuous infusion of 10% D/W. **In infants and young children,** similar effects may be accomplished by giving a continuous infusion of 10 or 20% glucose to which is added 0.5 u. of insulin/gm of glucose.

4. Hemodialysis should be instituted promptly after emergency measures in patients with renal failure or if emergency treatment is not effective. peritoneal dialysis is relatively inefficient with respect to K removal but may benefit the acidotic patient, especially if volume overload is likely to occur with sodium bicarbonate.

DISTURBANCES IN CALCIUM METABOLISM

Normal serum calcium **(Ca)** levels range between 8.8 and 10.4 mg/100 mL. Approximately 40% of the total blood Ca is bound to serum proteins (about 0.8 mg Ca bound/gm protein) while the remaining 60% is ultrafilterable and includes ionized Ca plus Ca complexed with phosphate and citrate. The ionized Ca fraction (about 50% of the total blood Ca) is influenced by pH changes. Acidosis is associated with decreased protein-binding and increased ionized Ca and alkalosis with a fall in ionized Ca due to increased protein-binding. These pH-induced changes in ionized Ca occur independently of any change in total blood Ca concentration.

In the laboratory determination of serum Ca, only total serum Ca is usually measured (atomic absorption spectrophotometry is the most accurate method). Ideally, the ionized serum Ca should be determined, since it is the physiologically active form, but such a test is not available for routine use. However, development of ion-specific electrodes for Ca has facilitated the determination of ionized Ca.

Maintenance of the blood Ca level is partially dependent upon dietary Ca intake (0.5 gm to 1 gm/day), GI absorption of Ca, and renal Ca excretion. The major factor preserving the constancy of the blood Ca concentration is the bone Ca reservoir. About 99% of body Ca is in bone, of which 1% is freely exchangeable with ECF.

Parathyroid hormone (PTH), an 84-amino acid, single-chain polypeptide (mol wt 9500), is secreted by the parathyroid glands. PTH and vitamin D (now also considered to be a hormone) are the principal regulators of Ca and phosphorus **(P)** homeostasis; their metabolic actions are interrelated. PTH promotes renal formation of the active metabolite of vitamin D. Conversely, with a deficiency of the vitamin or any resistance to its action, some of the effects of the hormone are blunted.

The most important actions of PTH are (1) rapid mobilization of Ca and phosphate from bone and the long-term acceleration of bone resorption, (2) increasing renal tubular reabsorption of Ca, (3) increasing intestinal absorption of Ca (mediated by an action on the metabolism of vitamin D), and (4) decreasing renal tubular reabsorption of phosphate **(PO_4)**. These actions account for most of the important clinical manifestations of PTH excess or deficiency.

In periods of Ca balance, the amount of Ca added to the ECF from the gut and the skeleton is equal to the amount of calcium excreted in the urine. The percentage of dietary Ca absorbed via the intestine increases with a fall in Ca intake and decreases when dietary Ca is increased. The mechanism is vitamin D-dependent. The most active metabolite of vitamin D (1,25-dihydroxycholecalciferol; 1,25-DHCC) enhances small-intestine Ca transport in part by mediating synthesis of mucosal Ca-binding proteins. PTH also enhances intestinal Ca absorption, but this action appears to be due to PTH-mediated formation of 1,25-DHCC in the kidney. Renal Ca excretion generally parallels Na excretion and is influenced by many of the factors that govern Na transport in the proximal tubule. Independently of Na (and vitamin D), PTH enhances renal distal tubular Ca absorption and increases renal PO_4 excretion. PTH causes an efflux of Ca (presumably from the labile Ca pool) into the ECF within minutes after glandular release. The mechanism is not clear. Long-term increases in PTH secretion inhibit osteoblast function and promote osteoclastic osteolysis. PTH activates adenyl cyclase in bone and kidney, leading to formation of cAMP. The role of cAMP in the target organ effects of PTH is not entirely clear. The physiologic effects of PTH upon bone are signifcantly influenced by normal levels of vitamin D. In vivo, both hormones function as important regulators of bone modeling and remodeling (ie, bone growth and turnover). See VITAMIN D DEFICIENCY AND DEPENDENCY in Ch. 81.

Physiological tests of parathyroid function largely have been supplanted by the measurement of circulating PTH levels in the plasma or serum by radioimmunoassay **(RIA)**, and by the measurement of total or nephrogenous cAMP excretion in the urine.

PTH is secreted into the circulation by the parathyroid glands as the intact hormone and as carboxy-terminal (C-terminal) fragments. The intact hormone has a very short half-time (< 10 min), whereas that of the C-terminal fragment is considerably longer. It is not clear whether amino-terminal (N-terminal) fragments circulate as such, but some evidence suggests that N-terminal fragments, released by the liver after hepatic uptake of intact hormone, are taken out of the circulation by bone. While intact PTH is cleared by hepatic (60%) and renal (40%) mechanisms, the kidneys are the sole route of elimination for C-terminal fragments. Clinically available RIAs for PTH utilize antibodies that detect the C-terminal segment and intact hormone, the mid-portion of the intact hormone, or the N-terminal segment and intact hormone. Biologic activity appears to reside in the intact hormone and the N-terminal fragment; the C-terminal segment is biologically inactive. Nonetheless, N-terminal assays have generally failed to distinguish reliably between hyperparathyroid and normal subjects, perhaps due to the short half-time of the fragment in the circulation. N-terminal assays have been more suitable for detecting rapid changes in PTH secretion in response to acute changes in ionized Ca. C-terminal assays correlate highly with the number of osteoclasts and are useful in the diagnosis of primary hyperparathyroidism. Since C-terminal fragments accumulate in the plasma with declining renal function, PTH levels measured by a C-terminal assay will increase progressively with decreasing renal function, limiting the usefulness of the assay. However, assays directed at both the C-terminal or the intact, mid-region portion of the PTH molecule have reflected the long-term activity of the parathyroid glands in patients on chronic dialysis. Whatever the RIA utilized, clinical interpretation of the PTH level is possible only in the context of the concomitantly measured serum Ca level.

Cyclic AMP excreted in the urine is derived both from filtered cAMP and tubular secretion of cAMP in response to PTH (any component due to physiologic concentra-

tions of ADH is negligible). The nephrogenous component of urinary cAMP constitutes up to 50% of the total urinary cAMP excreted. Total urinary cAMP (or nephrogenous cAMP) excretion per 100 mL of glomerular filtrate, particularly when related to acute changes in the ionized Ca level, has been proposed as an alternative to PTH RIA. However, diagnostic superiority over currently available clinical RIAs for PTH remains to be established. Furthermore, since the excretion of total and nephrogenous cAMP may be increased in many patients with humoral hypercalcemia of malignancy (with normal or suppressed levels of immunoreactive parathyroid hormone **[iPTH]**), the measurement of urinary cAMP must be coupled with the determination of circulating iPTH in the evaluation of hypercalcemia. Urinary excretion of cAMP may be elevated in pheochromocytoma and is an unreliable index of parathyroid hormone activity when the GFR is < 20 to 25 mL/min.

HYPOCALCEMIA

(Hypocalcemia in neonates is discussed under METABOLIC PROBLEMS IN THE NEWBORN in Ch. 186)

Total serum calcium < 8.8 mg/dL in the presence of normal serum proteins.

Etiology and Pathogenesis

Hypocalcemia is an infrequent laboratory finding. It occurs as the result of:

(1) **Deficiency or absence of parathyroid hormone:**

Hypoparathyroidism *(a tendency to hypocalcemia, often associated with chronic tetany, resulting from hormone deficiency, characterized chemically by low serum calcium and high serum phosphorus levels)* usually follows accidental removal of or damage to several parathyroid glands during thyroidectomy. Although transient hypoparathyroidism is common following subtotal thyroidectomy, the disease occurs permanently in < 3% of expertly performed thyroidectomies. Manifestations usually begin about 24 to 48 h postoperatively but may first occur after months or years. Parathyroid deficiency is more common after radical thyroidectomies for cancer.

Idiopathic hypoparathyroidism, in which the parathyroids are absent or atrophied, is uncommon. It may occur sporadically as an isolated or inherited condition, or in association with the DiGeorge syndrome. It also occurs as part of a genetic syndrome of hypoparathyroidism, Addison's disease, and mucocutaneous candidiasis. Although antiparathyroid antibodies may be detectable, there is no evidence that such antibodies are responsible for the hypoparathyroidism.

Pseudohypoparathyroidism (PHP) differs from the postoperative and idiopathic forms and is characterized not by deficiency of PTH but by target organ (bone and kidney) unresponsiveness to its action. The inheritance of these uncommon disorders is uncertain but may involve both autosomal dominant and recessive mechanisms. In Type I PHP, patients may be normocalcemic or hypocalcemic, and fail to exhibit a phosphaturic response or increased urinary cAMP after administration of PTH. Many of these patients demonstrate deficiency of a guanine nucleotide-binding regulatory protein (N-protein or G-unit) in erythrocytes and other tissues, including kidney. Patients with deficient N-protein activity usually have associated abnormalities of shortened metacarpal and metatarsal bones, short stature, round facies, and mental retardation, as well as mild hypothyroidism and other subtle endocrine abnormalities. Even less common is Type II PHP, in which the urinary cAMP (but not the phosphaturic) response to exogenous PTH is normal. In some patients with hypoparathyroidism and pseudohypoparathyroidism, subnormal formation of 1,25-DHCC may contribute to the relative refractoriness of hypocalcemia to correction by vitamin D.

(2) **Vitamin D deficiency,** due to inadequate dietary intake, decreased exposure to sunlight, hepatobiliary disease, or intestinal malabsorption and associated with rickets or osteomalacia. Functional vitamin D deficiency may occur during prolonged anti-

convulsant therapy with barbiturates and phenytoin presumably the result of increased catabolism of 25-(OH)D_3. (See VITAMIN D DEFICIENCY AND DEPENDENCY in Ch. 81.)

(3) **Vitamin D dependent rickets,** in which the formation of 1,25-DHCC is defective (Type I), or there is marked resistance of target organs to the effects of 1,25-DHCC and other vitamin D metabolites (Type II), and familial hypophosphatemic (vitamin D-resistant) rickets.

(4) **Renal tubular disease,** including the Fanconi syndrome due to nephrotoxins (eg, heavy metals) and distal renal tubular acidosis.

(5) **Renal failure,** where diminished formation of 1,25-DHCC coupled with hyperphosphatemia produces hypocalcemia.

(6) **Magnesium depletion** occurring with intestinal malabsorption or dietary deficiency, which causes hypocalcemia by relatively deficient secretion of PTH, as well as end-organ resistance to its action.

(7) **Acute pancreatitis,** which lowers serum Ca levels when Ca is chelated by lipolytic products.

(8) **Hypoproteinemia** of any cause with reduction in protein-bound Ca (eg, nephrotic syndrome, cirrhosis, protein-losing enteropathy). Hypocalcemia due to diminished protein-binding is asymptomatic, since the ionized Ca fraction is unaltered and the effects of Ca upon membrane excitability are produced by the ionized fraction.

(9) **During periods of increased Ca utilization** coupled with inadequate intake (eg, after surgical correction of hyperparathyroidism with healing bone lesions), hypocalcemia can also develop. It may also develop in oxalic acid poisoning and during sodium edetate therapy.

Although excessive secretion of calcitonin might be expected to cause hypocalcemia, low serum Ca levels are rare in patients with medullary carcinoma of the thyroid, a tumor that typically secretes large amounts of calcitonin.

Symptoms, Signs, and Diagnosis

Hypocalcemia is frequently asymptomatic and is often suggested by the clinical manifestations of the underlying disorder (eg, cataracts, basal ganglia calcification, and chronic moniliasis in some patients with **idiopathic hypoparathyroidism**).

The clinical manifestations of hypocalcemia are primarily neurologic. Slowly developing, insidious hypocalcemia may produce mild, diffuse encephalopathy and thus should be suspected in any patient with unexplained dementia, depression, or psychosis. Papilledema occasionally may be present and cataracts may develop after prolonged hypocalcemia. Severe hypocalcemia (serum Ca < 7 mg/dL) may cause laryngospasm and generalized convulsions.

The most characteristic syndrome is **tetany,** resulting from severe hypocalcemia or a reduction in the serum ionized Ca fraction without marked hypocalcemia (eg, in respiratory or metabolic alkalosis). Tetany is characterized by (1) sensory symptoms consisting of paresthesias of the lips, tongue, fingers, and feet; (2) carpopedal spasm, which may be prolonged or painful; (3) generalized muscle aching; and (4) spasm of facial musculature. Tetany may be overt (spontaneous symptoms) or latent. In **latent tetany** (generally present at serum Ca levels of 7 to 8 mg/dL), the neuromuscular instability frequently is brought out by provocative tests. **Chvostek's sign** is contraction of the facial muscles, elicited by a light tapping of the facial nerve. It occasionally is present in normal individuals and is often absent in chronic hypocalcemia. **Trousseau's sign** is carpopedal spasm caused by reduction of the blood supply to the hand when a tourniquet or blood pressure cuff above systolic pressure is applied to the forearm for 3 min. It also occurs in alkalotic states, hypomagnesemia, hypokalemia, and hyperkalemia, and in about 6% of normal persons. Latent tetany may become overt due to hyperventilation or administration of sodium bicarbonate or Ca-depleting

diuretics (eg, furosemide). All of the manifestations of hypocalcemic tetany may be masked by concomitant hypokalemia. The ECG typically shows prolongation of the Q-T interval.

Diagnosis

The serum Ca level is < 8.8 mg/dL and is usually 7 mg/dL or less when tetany is present (unless it is induced by alkalosis). The characteristic abnormalities of metabolic and respiratory alkalosis are discussed in DISTURBANCES IN ACID-BASE METABOLISM, below. **Parathyroid deficiency** is characterized by low serum Ca, high serum PO_4, normal alkaline phosphatase, and low or absent urinary Ca. Immunoreactive circulating PTH is inappropriately low for the serum Ca level or, less frequently, undetectable in patients with idiopathic hypoparathyroidism. This disorder becomes manifest in childhood and may be associated with Addison's disease, steatorrhea, and moniliasis. Hyperphosphatemia is present when hypocalcemia results from hypoparathyroidism or renal failure. The 2 are easily differentiated by the presence of marked azotemia in renal failure. **Type I pseudohypoparathyroidism** can be distinguished by the frequent presence of some skeletal abnormalities (most frequently shortening of the 1st, 4th, and 5th metacarpals), the absence of phosphaturia, the failure of plasma and urinary cAMP to increase normally following injection of parathyroid extract, and the presence of immunoreactive hormone in the circulation.

Increased stool weight and fat content, along with a low serum carotene level, are characteristic of **intestinal malabsorption**. Steatorrhea frequently is associated with **hypomagnesemia** (eg, < 1.6 mEq/L). In **osteomalacia** or **rickets**, typical skeletal abnormalities may be present, the serum PO_4 level often is mildly reduced, and alkaline phosphatase elevated. Measurement of serum vitamin D levels, including 25-(OH)D_3 and 1,25-DHCC, may help distinguish vitamin D deficiency from vitamin D dependent states. Familial hypophosphatemic rickets is recognized by the associated renal PO_4 wasting.

Treatment

Acute severe hypocalcemic tetany is treated initially with IV infusion of Ca salts. Ten mL of 10% calcium gluconate may be given IV over 15 to 30 min, but the effect lasts for only a few hours. Therefore, it may be necessary to repeat infusions and/or to add 20 to 30 mL of 10% calcium gluconate to 1 L of 5% D/W and infuse it over 12 to 24 h. Infusions of Ca are *hazardous in patients receiving digitalis and should be given slowly with continuous ECG monitoring.* Calcium chloride causes thrombophlebitis when given IV and is highly irritating if extravasated. IM injection of calcium gluconate likewise is contraindicated because it can cause local necrosis. When tetany is due to hypomagnesemia, it may respond transiently to Ca or K administration but is permanently relieved by magnesium repletion (see HYPOMAGNESEMIA, below).

In **transient hypoparathyroidism after thyroidectomy or excision of a parathyroid adenoma,** supplemental oral Ca may be sufficient to prevent hypocalcemia. However, hypocalcemia may be particularly severe and prolonged following subtotal parathyroidectomy in patients with chronic renal failure. The marked hypocalcemia and elevated serum alkaline phosphatase in such settings may be due to the rapid uptake of Ca into bone. Prolonged parenteral administration of Ca may be necessary to avoid serious hypocalcemia in the postoperative period; as much as 1 gm of Ca/day may be required for 5 to 10 days, before oral Ca and vitamin D are sufficient to maintain adequate blood Ca levels.

In **chronic hypocalcemia,** as in hypoparathyroidism or renal failure, Ca usually is given orally with vitamin D. Ca may be given as calcium gluconate (1 gm $\cong$ 90 mg Ca) or calcium carbonate (1 gm $\cong$ 400 mg Ca) to provide 1 to 2 gm of Ca/day. Although any vitamin D preparation may suffice, 1-hydroxylated compounds such as calcitriol (1,25-DHCC), and "pseudo" 1-hydroxylated analogs such as dihydrotachysterol

(DHT), offer the advantage of more rapid onset of action and more rapid clearance from the body. Calcitriol is particularly useful in renal failure, since it requires no metabolic alteration; it is the drug of choice in Type I vitamin D dependent rickets, which responds to physiological doses of 0.25 to 0.5 μg/day orally. Patients with hypoparathyroidism and pseudohypoparathyroidism usually respond, respectively, to calcitriol in oral dosages of 0.5 to 2 μg and 1 to 3 μg/day. Two to 4 mg of dihydrotachysterol may be given for 2 days, followed by 1 mg or less/day depending on serum Ca response.

In all instances, *vitamin D intoxication with severe symptomatic hypercalcemia can be a serious complication.* Adequate dietary or supplemental Ca (1 to 2 gm/day) and phosphorus must be supplied. Effective therapy is indicated by absence of symptoms and normal or near-normal Ca. The latter should be checked frequently (eg, weekly) at first, and at 1- to 3-mo intervals after the patient's condition has stabilized. In most instances, the maintenance dose of calcitriol or DHT will decrease with time.

Treatment of hypocalcemia in patients with renal failure must be combined with dietary phosphorus restriction and phosphate-binding agents, such as aluminum hydroxide gel, in order to prevent hyperphosphatemia and metastatic calcification. Unfortunately, the accumulation of aluminum in bone and brain, respectively, has been associated with the development of osteomalacia resistant to 1,25-DHCC and the syndrome of dialysis dementia. Therefore, emphasis should be placed upon dietary restriction of phosphorus, and aluminum hydroxide gel should be used only if dietary restriction and the lesser phosphate-binding effect of calcium carbonate fail to keep the serum PO_4 level below 6 mg/dL. *Vitamin D administration is hazardous in renal failure* and should be limited to individuals with symptomatic osteomalacia unrelated to aluminum or secondary hyperparathyroidism (serum Ca < 11 mg/dL) or to patients with postparathyroidectomy hypocalcemia. The efficacy and relatively short duration of action of calcitriol (and other 1-hydroxylated analogs that may become available in the future) makes it the drug of choice in such patients. Simple osteomalacia may respond to as little as 0.25 to 0.5 μg/day (unless it is due to aluminum in which case removal of aluminum with desferoxamine may be necessary), while correction of postparathyroidectomy hypocalcemia may require prolonged administration of as much as 2 μg of calcitriol/day and 2 gm or more of Ca/day.

Vitamin D-deficiency rickets responds to as little as 400 IU/day; in **osteomalacia** 5000 IU/day of vitamin D_2 or D_3 is given for 6 to 12 wk and then reduced to 400 IU/day. Provision of 2 gm of Ca/day is desirable, at least during the early stages of treatment. **Vitamin D-resistant, familial and nonfamilial, hypophosphatemic rickets** are treated with inorganic phosphate (1 to 3.5 gm/day) and calcitriol (0.25 to 1 μg/day). Treatment with vitamin D requires monitoring of the serum Ca level; although hypercalcemia may result, it generally responds quickly to adjustment in the dose of calcitriol. **Alkalosis-induced tetany** is treated by correction of the underlying disturbance.

HYPERCALCEMIA

Total serum calcium > 10.5 mg/dL.

The principal causes of hypercalcemia are listed in TABLE 84–5. Most frequently, hypercalcemia is due to excessive bone resorption with respect to new bone formation and release of Ca into the ECF.

Primary hyperparathyroidism is *a generalized disorder resulting from excessive secretion of parathyroid hormone by one or more parathyroid glands; it is usually characterized by hypercalcemia, hypophosphatemia, and excessive bone resorption.* While asymptomatic hypercalcemia is the most frequent presentation, nephrolithiasis is common, particularly when hyperparathyroidism and hypercalciuria are of long duration. Primary hyperparathyroidism probably is the most common cause of hypercalcemia in the general

TABLE 84–5. PRINCIPAL CAUSES OF HYPERCALCEMIA

I. Excessive osteolysis
   A. Parathyroid hormone excess; eg, primary hyperparathyroidism, parathyroid carcinoma, hypercalciuric hypocalcemia, advanced secondary hyperparathyroidism (especially after renal transplantation)
   B. Humoral hypercalcemia of malignancy; eg, malignancy with calcemia in absence of bone metastases
   C. Malignancy with bone metastases; eg, carcinoma, leukemias, lymphomas, myeloma
   D. Hyperthyroidism
   E. Vitamin D intoxication
   F. Immobilization (in patients with rapid bone remodeling—eg, young, growing individuals or those with Paget's disease; elderly patients with osteoporosis)

II. Excessive GI calcium absorption and/or intake
   A. Milk-alkali syndrome
   B. Vitamin D intoxication
   C. Sarcoidosis and other chronic granulomatous diseases

III. Elevated concentration of plasma proteins

IV. Uncertain mechanism
   A. Myxedema, Addison's disease, postoperative Cushing's disease
   B. Thiazide diuretic treatment
   C. Infantile hypercalcemia

V. Artifactual
   A. Prolonged venous stasis while obtaining blood sample
   B. Exposure of blood to contaminated glassware

population. It occurs with increased frequency in women and with aging and is found in both nonfamilial and familial forms. The 2 most common familial forms are major components of **multiple endocrine neoplasia—Types I and II** (see Ch. 92). Histologic examination reveals a parathyroid adenoma in about 90% of patients, although it is sometimes difficult to distinguish an adenoma from a normal gland when the hypercalcemia is mild (ie, < 12 mg/dL). The other 10% of cases are due to hyperplasia of 2 or more glands (7%) or parathyroid cancer (3%).

The syndrome of **familial hypocalciuric hypercalcemia** is transmitted as an autosomal dominant trait with 100% penetrance. It is characterized by persistent hypercalcemia, often from an early age, elevated levels of PTH, and hypocalciuria. The hypercalcemia is usually asymptomatic, renal function is well-maintained, and nephrolithiasis unusual. However, severe primary hyperparathyroidism may occur in infants of affected kindreds and, occasionally, severe pancreatitis may be seen. Although parathyroid hyperplasia is consistently found, the response to subtotal parathyroidectomy generally is unsatisfactory.

Secondary hyperparathyroidism refers to hypocalcemia caused by conditions that can lower the serum Ca, such as renal insufficiency and intestinal malabsorption syndromes in which increased secretion of the hormone represents an adaptive response to a normal stimulus. These disorders are characterized by hypocalcemia or, less often, normocalcemia. When secondary hyperparathyroidism has been established for some time, parathyroid sensitivity to Ca may be diminished due to pronounced glandular hyperplasia and elevation of the calcium-set point (ie, the amount of Ca necessary to reduce secretion of PTH by 50%). Thus, hypersecretion of PTH may continue in the face of normocalcemia or even hypercalcemia (ie, **tertiary hyperparathyroidism**).

Malignancies may cause hypercalcemia by several mechanisms, each of which ultimately results in bone resorption. Hematologic cancers, most often myeloma but also

certain lymphomas and lymphosarcomas, cause hypercalcemia by elaboration of an osteoclast activating factor leading to osteoclastic bone resorption with osteolytic lesions and/or diffuse osteopenia. Most frequently, hypercalcemia of malignancy occurs in the setting of solid tumors (eg, breast cancer and squamous cell tumors of the lung) with bone metastases. Breast cancer with bone metastases accounts for > 50% of patients with malignancy-associated hypercalcemia. In these instances, hypercalcemia results from local elaboration of osteoclast activating factor or prostaglandins, and/or direct bone resorption by tumor cells.

Less frequently, hypercalcemia may occur in association with squamous carcinomas of any organ, hypernephroma, or ovarian cancer, but without detectable bone metastases **("humoral hypercalcemia of malignancy")**. Many such occurrences were formerly attributed to ectopic production of PTH; however, the frequency of ectopic hyperparathyroidism remains controversial. Immunoreactive PTH levels, as measured by some C-terminal assays, are elevated in up to 25% of patients with malignancy-associated hypercalcemia. In contrast, other RIAs usually yield undetectable or markedly suppressed levels of PTH in similar patients, although there may be associated hypophosphatemia, phosphaturia, and elevated levels of urinary or nephrogenous cAMP. Although the precise factor(s) responsible for these events remains uncertain, the variable immunoreactivity of utilized antibodies to PTH must play a role. Recent evidence suggests that some tumors produce substances that bind to PTH receptors and mimic some of the effects of the hormone. In any event, osteoclastic bone resorption is the main cause of hypercalcemia in these patients and may result from PTH-like substances or other tumor-elaborated factors (eg, transforming growth factors).

Vitamin D in pharmacologic doses produces excessive bone resorption as well as increased intestinal Ca absorption and hypercalciuria. (See HYPERVITAMINOSIS D in Ch. 81.) **Sarcoidosis** is associated with hypercalcemia in up to 20% of patients and hypercalciuria in about 40%. The cause appears to be increased synthesis of 1,25-DHCC by mononuclear cells in the sarcoid granulomas. Similarly, hypercalcemia and hypercalciuria have been described in other granulomatous diseases (eg, tuberculosis, berylliosis, histoplasmosis, and coccidioidomycosis). It is tempting to speculate that the mechanism is similar to that in sarcoidosis; indeed, a single patient with silicone-induced granulomas, hypercalcemia, and hypercalciuria, was found to have elevated serum levels of calcitriol. In addition to primary hyperparathyroidism and familial hypocalciuric hypercalcemia, **hypercalcemia in infancy** may be due to a group of idiopathic disorders, all of which are associated with increased intestinal absorption of Ca and may result from vitamin D intoxication or increased sensitivity to vitamin D.

In the **milk-alkali syndrome,** excessive amounts of Ca and absorbable alkali are ingested, usually during peptic ulcer therapy, resulting in increased Ca absorption and hypercalcemia.

Symptoms and Signs

The underlying cause of hypercalcemia (see TABLE 84–5) is often apparent from the history and associated clinical findings (eg, excessive ingestion of Ca and alkali, widespread malignancy, or overt Addison's disease). Radiographic evidence of bone disease may suggest the diagnosis (eg, hyperparathyroidism, Paget's disease, osteolytic or osteoblastic lesions in myeloma).

Many patients with mild hypercalcemia are asymptomatic, and the condition is discovered accidentally during routine laboratory screening. The clinical manifestations of hypercalcemia include constipation, anorexia, and nausea and vomiting with abdominal pain and ileus. Reversible impairment of the renal concentrating mechanism leads to polyuria, nocturia, and polydipsia. More severe elevation of serum Ca (usually > 12 mg/dL) is associated with emotional lability, confusion, delirium, psychosis, stupor, and coma. Neuromuscular involvement may cause prominent skeletal

muscle weakness. Seizures are rare. Hypercalciuria with nephrolithiasis or urolithiasis is common. Less often, prolonged or severe hypercalcemia may produce reversible acute renal failure or irreversible renal damage, due to precipitation of Ca salts within the kidney parenchyma **(nephrocalcinosis)**. Peptic ulcers and pancreatitis may also be associated with hyperparathyroidism, but the relationship between these conditions and the parathyroid dysfunction remains obscure. The Q-T interval in the ECG is shortened in severe hypercalcemia. Renal damage may result in azotemia and hypertension. Hypercalcemia that exceeds 18 mg/dL may result in shock, renal failure, and death.

Osteitis fibrosa cystica, in which increased osteoclastic activity causes rarefying osteitis with fibrous degeneration, the formation of cysts, and the development of fibrous nodules in the affected bone, may develop when hyperparathyroidism is severe or of long duration. Once common, osteitis fibrosa cystica is now rarely seen, except in chronic dialysis patients with secondary hyperparathyroidism, and only a few patients show one or more features of bone disease that are readily recognized by x-ray examination (bone cysts, "salt-and-pepper" appearance of the skull, subperiosteal resorption of bone in the phalanges and distal clavicles). Hyperparathyroid bone disease often is associated with increased serum alkaline phosphatase.

Laboratory Findings and Diagnosis

In **hyperparathyroidism** the ionized serum Ca concentration is elevated, although the level may fluctuate. A low serum PO_4 level suggests some form of hyperparathyroidism, especially when coupled with an elevated PO_4 clearance (depressed tubular reabsorption of PO_4) and mild hyperchloremia (with or without acidosis). It may be difficult to distinguish primary from secondary hyperparathyroidism in the presence of renal insufficiency. A high serum Ca and normal serum PO_4 suggest primary hyperparathyroidism, especially in the nondialyzed patient.

Hypercalcemia of malignancy may be associated with similar changes in PO_4, but there is often metabolic alkalosis, hypochloremia and hypoalbuminemia as well. The serum Ca is rarely > 12 mg/dL in primary hyperparathyroidism. A serum Ca > 12 mg/dL usually is due to tumors or other causes of hypercalcemia. Circulating PTH (C-terminal or intact, mid-region assay) usually is elevated for the simultaneous level of ionized Ca in patients with hyperparathyroidism, and is suppressed in patients with most other causes of hypercalcemia.

Familial hypocalciuric hypercalcemia is distinguished from primary hyperparathyroidism by the early age of onset, the frequent occurrence of hypermagnesemia, and the presence of hypercalcemia without hypercalciuria in other family members. The fractional excretion of Ca (ratio of Ca clearance to creatinine clearance) is low (ie, < 1%) in patients with familial hypocalciuric hypercalcemia; it is almost always elevated (ie, 1 to 4%) in primary hyperparathyroidism.

Idiopathic hypercalcemia of infancy is recognized by the combination of suppressed levels of PTH, hypercalciuria, and, in some severely affected patients, the somatic abnormalities of **Williams syndrome** (eg, supravalvular aortic stenosis, mental retardation, and an elfin facies).

The **milk-alkali syndrome** is recognized by history and by the combination of hypercalcemia, metabolic alkalosis, and, frequently, azotemia with hypocalciuria. With cessation of Ca and alkali ingestion, the blood Ca level rapidly returns to normal.

Myeloma should be suggested by the syndrome of anemia, azotemia, and hypercalcemia. This diagnosis is confirmed by bone marrow examination or finding a monoclonal gammopathy or free light chains in the serum or urine on immunoelectrophoresis.

In **other endocrine causes** of hypercalcemia (eg, thyrotoxicosis, Addison's disease), the typical laboratory findings of the underlying disorder help to establish the diagnosis.

Hypercalciuria is found in most disorders causing hypercalcemia, except familial hypocalciuric hypercalcemia, milk-alkali syndrome, Addison's disease, thiazide therapy, and renal failure.

Circulating PTH (C-terminal assay) usually is elevated in patients with hyperparathyroidism, and is suppressed in patients with vitamin D intoxication, the milk-alkali syndrome, and sarcoidosis. Detectable iPTH secreted by a tumor may be immunologically different from iPTH produced in ordinary hyperparathyroidism. Immunoassays capable of detecting such differences may differentiate primary hyperparathyroidism from humoral hypercalcemia of malignancy **(HHM)**. However, the majority of patients with HHM have suppressed or undetectable iPTH. Since many such individuals will have phosphaturia, hypophosphatemia, and elevated urinary cAMP excretion/dL GFR, the additional finding of suppressed iPTH will distinguish these patients from those with primary hyperparathyroidism (iPTH elevated).

Treatment

The management of hypercalcemia depends upon the severity of Ca elevation and the underlying cause. When the blood Ca is < 11.5 mg/dL, correction of the underlying disturbance often is sufficient.

When the serum Ca exceeds 15 mg/dL, or when severe clinical signs of hypercalcemia are present at lower levels of Ca, *rapid reduction is necessary.* The mainstay of therapy in patients with relatively normal renal function is extracellular volume expansion with IV saline to promote calciuria. The aim is to attain a urine volume of 3 L/day. Preexisting volume deficits should be replaced prior to beginning the diuresis with the infusion of isotonic (0.9%) sodium chloride and administration of furosemide in patients with sufficient renal function. One to 2 L of 0.9% sodium chloride IV are followed by furosemide 80 to 100 mg IV q 2 h for 24 h. Urine losses are replaced with 0.9% sodium chloride and 5% D/W in a ratio of 4:1 plus sufficient potassium chloride (20 mEq/L) to prevent hypokalemia. Fluid intake and output and serum and urine electrolytes must be monitored carefully.

While there is no completely satisfactory and reliable means by which severe hypercalcemia can be corrected in patients with renal insufficiency, acute hemodialysis (with low or calcium-free dialysis fluid) is probably the safest and most reliable method. *A more hazardous approach* is the IV administration of 1 L of disodium and monopotassium phosphate (0.081 mole disodium phosphate + 0.019 mole monopotassium phosphate to provide a solution of pH 7.4). Each liter contains 3.1 gm of phosphorus. No more than 0.5 to 1.0 gm should be given IV in 24 h; usually 1 or 2 doses in 2 days are sufficient to lower serum Ca for 10 to 15 days. Lowering of serum Ca with such treatment is associated with diminished urinary Ca content. Soft-tissue calcification is the major complication, and acute renal failure may occur. *In view of the high morbidity associated with IV PO_4 infusion in this setting, it should be used only when hypercalcemia is life-threatening and acute hemodialysis is not possible.* The IV infusion of sodium sulfate decahydrate is even more hazardous and less effective than phosphate infusion and *should not be utilized.*

Recent evidence suggests that administration of salmon calcitonin (4 to 8 IU/kg s.c. q 12 h) and prednisone (30 to 60 mg/day orally in 3 divided doses) may control severe hypercalcemia associated with malignancies within 12 h, even in patients with renal disease in whom prior stabilization with IV saline is not possible (see also discussion of calcitonin below).

Long-term control of hypercalcemia may be achieved by oral administration of neutral phosphate. The equivalent of 1 to 3 gm/day of elemental phosphorus may be given in divided doses. The risk of metastatic calcification is related to the level of serum phosphate; therefore, it should not be used in patients with renal insufficiency. Otherwise, diarrhea is the usual limiting factor in oral phosphate therapy.

The addition of prednisone 20 to 40 mg/day orally will effectively control hypercalcemia in most patients with vitamin D intoxication, idiopathic hypercalcemia of infancy, and sarcoidosis. Some patients with myeloma, lymphoma, leukemia, or metastatic breast cancer respond to 40 to 60 mg/day of prednisone. However, since the response to glucocorticoids takes several days and since > 50% of patients with hypercalcemia due to such malignancies fail to respond to glucocorticoids, it is usually necessary to seek other treatment modalities.

In patients with skeletal metastases or humoral hypercalcemia of malignancy, plicamycin (mithramycin) 25 μg/kg body wt IV in 50 mL of 5% D/W is extraordinarily effective, producing a prompt, reliable lowering of serum Ca. However, the duration of the calcium-lowering effect of plicamycin is variable (ie, several days to 3 wk) and rebound hypercalcemia may be rapid and severe. Long-term therapy with plicamycin can be accomplished but is often limited by toxicity and an interval of at least 72 h between doses should be observed. Plicamycin produces thrombocytopenia, a qualitative platelet defect (bleeding diathesis with normal platelet count), hepatotoxicity, and renal damage. Other agents are preferred in patients with preexisting abnormalities of hematopoiesis, hepatic, or renal function. If the drug must be used in such settings, it may be advisable to reduce the dose to 12.5 μg/kg body wt.

Calcitonin (thyrocalcitonin): *The rapidly acting peptide hormone of the parafollicular cells (thyroid "C" cells) of ultimobranchial origin.* The ultimobranchial bodies, which fuse with the thyroid in mammals, remain as separate structures in lower species. Calcitonin is secreted in response to hypercalcemia, which it reduces by inhibiting osteoclastic activity and thus the rate of Ca release from bone. Human, porcine, and piscine preparations differ structurally and immunologically.

A commercial preparation of salmon calcitonin is available; it is most useful in the treatment of Paget's disease, but its usefulness in the treatment of hypercalcemia has been limited by its short duration of action. The combination of salmon calcitonin and prednisone may provide control of serum Ca in some patients with malignancy for up to several months; although escape from the effects of the drug combination may occur after 4 to 6 days of continual therapy, discontinuance of calcitonin for 2 days (while prednisone is continued) may be followed by lowering of the serum Ca once again when calcitonin administration is resumed. Other agents, such as diphosphonates and indomethacin have been used for long-term control of malignancy-associated hypercalcemia. However, effective diphosphonates are not yet available and most patients fail to respond to indomethacin (150 mg/day).

In **hyperparathyroidism,** treatment is surgical if the disease is symptomatic or progressive. The outcome of surgery depends on successful removal of all excess functioning tissue and on reversibility of renal damage; renal insufficiency may progress despite cure of the underlying disease. Abnormally functioning parathyroid glands may be found in unusual locations and experience is required to find them. Preoperative localization of parathyroid tissue is possible by ultrasound or CT scan, and abnormal function may be confirmed by immunoassay of the thyroid venous drainage. Such procedures are mandatory in all patients having had previous unsuccessful parathyroid surgery.

The indications for surgery in patients with mild, asymptomatic primary hyperparathyroidism are yet to be clarified. Current data suggest that such patients be managed conservatively in the absence of progressive hypercalcemia or other complications. Similarly, conservative management is indicated for patients with familial hypocalciuric hypercalcemia, unless pancreatitis or severe neonatal primary hyperparathyroidism should occur. In such cases, total parathyroidectomy is the operation of choice.

When hyperparathyroidism is mild, no special postoperative precautions are required. The elevated serum Ca level drops to just below normal within 24 to 48 h after surgery. In patients with severe osteitis fibrosa cystica, prolonged symptomatic hypo-

calcemia may occur and require large doses of Ca together with vitamin D, usually for 1 to 3 mo (see HYPOCALCEMIA, above).

HYPOPHOSPHATEMIA

The incidence of hypophosphatemia (*serum phosphorus concentration < 2.5 mg/dL*) in hospitalized patients ranges between 2 and 10%. Most (85%) of the 500 to 700 gm of body phosphorus is contained in bone; the remainder is predominantly intracellular. Phosphorus is an important component of nucleic acids and cellular and subcellular membranes and is intimately involved in aerobic and anaerobic energy metabolism. Phosphate **(PO_4)** is a major intracellular anion.

The causes of hypophosphatemia are many, but clinically significant hypophosphatemia commonly occurs in relatively fewer settings. Chronic hypophosphatemia most often results from a fall in renal PO_4 reabsorption and is not associated with intracellular PO_4 depletion. Causes include hyperparathyroidism, hormonal disturbances, renal tubular defects (intrinsic and acquired, as with hypomagnesemia and hypokalemia), and chronic diuretic administration. Though hypophosphatemia usually is asymptomatic, muscle weakness and osteomalacia can occur if PO_4 depletion is present.

Similarly, chronic starvation, malabsorption, or deficient dietary intake of phosphorus may cause hypophosphatemia but are uncommon as sole causes of PO_4 depletion. Mild chronic hypophosphatemia of any etiology may predispose to the development of severe acute or chronic hypophosphatemia. Severe chronic hypophosphatemia usually results from a prolonged negative PO_4 balance and leads to PO_4 depletion, anorexia, muscle weakness, and osteomalacia with bone pain. Causes include chronic starvation or malabsorption, especially if combined with vomiting or copious diarrhea, or chronic ingestion of large amounts of aluminum hydroxide antacid. The latter is particularly prone to produce PO_4 depletion when combined with decreased dietary intake and dialysis losses of PO_4 in patients with chronic renal failure.

Acute severe hypophosphatemia (*serum phosphorus < 1 to 1.5 mg/dL*) is most often due to transcellular shifts of phosphorus, often superimposed upon chronic hypophosphatemia and PO_4 depletion. Serious neuromuscular disturbances may occur, including progressive encephalopathy, coma, and death. Profound muscle weakness may be accompanied by rhabdomyolysis, especially in acute alcoholism. Hematological disturbances include hemolytic anemia, decreased release of O_2 from Hb, and impaired leukocyte and thrombocyte function. These acute syndromes presumably result from depletion of intracellular ATP or decreased red cell 2,3-diphosphoglycerate and diminished delivery of O_2 to tissues. The most common clinical settings of acute severe hypophosphatemia include the recovery phase of diabetic ketoacidosis and acute alcoholism, total parenteral nutrition **(TPN)**, the recovery phase after severe burns, and severe respiratory alkalosis.

Treatment

Treatment is empiric and is dictated by the underlying cause and the severity of hypophosphatemia. In mild to moderate chronic PO_4 depletion, supplemental phosphorus (0.08 to 0.16 mM/kg body wt, bid to tid) may be given as oral phosphate but usually is poorly tolerated due to diarrhea. Ingestion of 1 qt of low fat or skim milk will provide 1 gm of phosphorus (32 mM) and may be more acceptable. Removal of the cause of hypophosphatemia (eg, cessation of phosphate-binding antacids or diuretics, correction of hypomagnesemia) is preferable when possible.

When hypophosphatemia is anticipated, as in diabetic ketoacidosis, acute alcoholism and TPN, the IV administration of phosphorus as monobasic potassium phosphate in appropriate dosage is relatively safe as long as renal function is well preserved. The usual maintenance dose in TPN is 15 mM/day, while alcoholics may require up to 30

mM/day during the course of parenteral nutrition. In diabetic ketoacidosis, 50 mM of phosphorus or more may be required in the first 24 h; supplemental PO_4 is discontinued when oral intake is resumed. In each instance, but particularly when PO_4 is given IV or to patients with impaired renal function, it is advisable to monitor serum Ca and phosphorus levels during therapy. Sodium phosphate preparations generally should be used in patients with impaired renal function.

When the serum phosphorus concentration falls below 1.0 to 1.5 mg/dL, PO_4 (as monobasic potassium phosphate) should be given IV in larger amounts. In most cases, no more than 0.25 mM/kg of body wt (17.5 mM for a 70 kg adult) of phosphorus should be given over 6 h. Hypocalcemia, hyperphosphatemia, metastatic calcification, and hyperkalemia may be avoided by careful monitoring and avoidance of more rapid rates of PO_4 administration.

DISTURBANCES IN MAGNESIUM METABOLISM

Magnesium **(Mg)** is the 4th most plentiful cation in the body (total body content about 2000 mEq in a 70-kg man), but only 1% exists in the ECF. About 50% of the total body Mg is found in bone and is not readily exchangeable with Mg in ECF; the remainder is intracellular. Serum Mg concentration is maintained between 1.6 and 2.1 mEq/L. Observations in Mg-depleted individuals suggest that maintenance of serum Mg concentration largely is a function of dietary intake and extremely effective renal and intestinal conservation, possibly regulated in part by PTH. Within 7 days of initiation of a Mg-deficient diet, renal and fecal Mg excretion fall to about 1 mEq/24 h each. The intestinal response is impaired if dietary intake of Ca and PO_4 is high.

About 70% of serum Mg is ultrafilterable (roughly 55% free or ionized); the remainder is bound to protein. Like Ca, protein-binding of Mg is pH-dependent. Serum Mg concentration and either total body Mg or intracellular Mg content are not closely related. However, severe serum hypomagnesemia may reflect diminished body stores of Mg.

A wide variety of enzymes including phosphatases (eg, adenosine triphosphatase and alkaline phosphatase) are Mg-activated or -dependent. Mg is required for thiamine pyrophosphate cofactor activity and appears to stabilize macromolecular structure (eg, DNA and RNA). Mg is also related to Ca and K metabolism in an intimate but poorly understood fashion (see HYPOMAGNESEMIA, below).

HYPOMAGNESEMIA

Serum magnesium concentration < 1.6 mEq/L.

Severe hypomagnesemia often is equated with Mg depletion. However, serum Mg concentration, even if free Mg ion is measured, may not reflect the status of intracellular or bone Mg stores.

Etiology and Pathogenesis

Magnesium depletion usually results from inadequate intake plus impairment of renal or gut absorption. It has been described in association with (1) **prolonged parenteral feeding,** usually in combination with loss of body fluids via gastric suction or diarrhea; (2) **lactation** (increased requirement for Mg); and (3) **conditions of abnormal renal conservation** of Mg, such as hypersecretion of aldosterone, ADH, or thyroid hormone, hypercalcemia, diabetic acidosis, and diuretic therapy.

Clinically significant Mg deficiency most commonly is associated with (1) **malabsorption syndromes** from all causes, in which elevated fecal Mg is probably related to the level of steatorrhea rather than to deficient bowel absorptive sites per se; (2) **protein-calorie malnutrition** (eg, kwashiorkor); (3) **parathyroid disease,** in which hypomagnesemia is seen after removal of a parathyroid tumor, especially if severe osteitis fibrosa is

present (presumably, Mg is transferred to rapidly mineralizing bone and Mg deficiency may account for the resistance of hypocalcemia to correction with vitamin D in occasional patients with hypoparathyroidism); (4) **chronic alcoholism,** in which hypomagnesemia probably is due to both inadequate intake and excessive renal excretion; and (5) chronic diarrhea.

Neonatal hypomagnesemia occurs in normal premature infants, in DiGeorge's syndrome, in familial hypoparathyroidism, after exchange transfusion, and in infants of mothers having diabetes mellitus, toxemia, hyperparathyroidism, and Mg deficiency. It often is associated with hypocalcemia and hypophosphatemia.

Symptoms, Signs, and Diagnosis

The disorders associated with Mg deficiency are complex and usually accompanied by multiple metabolic and nutritional disturbances. Furthermore, since the curare-like action of Mg ion is well known, response of neuromuscular irritability to Mg administration is not necessarily proof that Mg deficiency caused the neuromuscular irritability.

The clinical manifestations of Mg deficiency are most reliably described by experimental Mg depletion in human volunteers. In this setting, anorexia, nausea, vomiting, lethargy, weakness, personality change, tetany (eg, positive Trousseau's or Chvostek's sign, or spontaneous carpopedal spasm), tremor, and muscle fasciculations may be present. The neurologic signs, particularly tetany, correlate with the development of hypocalcemia and hypokalemia. Myopathic potentials are found on electromyography. Any changes in the ECG are also compatible with hypocalcemia or hypokalemia. Although not observed experimentally, it is likely that severe hypomagnesemia may produce generalized tonic-clonic seizures, especially in children.

Laboratory Findings

Hypomagnesemia is often present when Mg depletion is severe. Hypocalcemia and hypocalciuria are common in patients with steatorrhea, alcoholism, or other causes of Mg deficiency. In these settings, hypocalcemia responds to Mg repletion and is resistant to Ca administration. Hypokalemia, with increased urinary K excretion and metabolic alkalosis, may be present. Thus, the presence of unexplained hypocalcemia and hypokalemia should suggest the possibility of Mg depletion.

Treatment

Treatment with Mg salts (sulfate or chloride) is indicated when Mg deficiency is symptomatic or associated with severe, persistent hypomagnesemia (eg, < 1 mEq/L). In such settings, a deficit of 1 to 2 mEq/kg may exist. The amount given should be twice the estimated deficit (if renal function is normal), since about 50% of the administered Mg will be excreted in the urine. **In emergencies** (eg, seizures) or when serum Mg is < 1 mEq/L, magnesium sulfate heptahydrate is given IV at a rate not exceeding 1.5 mL of a 10% solution/min (magnesium sulfate heptahydrate contains about 8.1 mEq of Mg/gm of the salt). Usually, half of the deficit is given in the first 24 h and the remainder over the next several days. Alternatively, magnesium chloride 2 mEq/kg body wt may be given IV over 4 h. In less severe instances, gradual repletion is achieved by parenteral administration of 0.25 to 0.5 mEq/kg/day. Mg salts also may be given orally and are well tolerated, even in patients with steatorrhea. During Mg therapy, the serum Mg level should be monitored frequently, particularly in patients with renal insufficiency. Treatment is continued until a normal serum Mg level is achieved.

In emergencies involving neonates, 0.25 to 1 mL of 50% magnesium sulfate injection IM or IV is given over 10 to 15 min with careful ECG monitoring. This dose may be repeated 2 to 3 times/day. Close monitoring of the serum Mg and the patient's clinical status is essential.

HYPERMAGNESEMIA

Serum magnesium > 2.1 mEq/L.

Symptomatic hypermagnesemia is common in patients with renal failure who receive Mg salts or ingest Mg-containing drugs such as antacids or purgatives.

Hypermagnesemia leads to generalized impairment of neuromuscular transmission, probably as the result of inhibition of acetylcholine release at the neuromuscular junction. At serum concentrations of 5 to 10 mEq/L, the ECG shows prolongation of the P-R interval, widening of the QRS complex, and increased T wave amplitude. Deep tendon reflexes disappear as the serum Mg level approaches 10 mEq/L; hypotension, respiratory depression, and narcosis develop with progression of the hypermagnesemia. Cardiac arrest may occur as the result of a high blood Mg concentration (about 25 mEq/L).

Treatment of severe Mg intoxication consists of circulatory and respiratory support, with IV administration of 10 to 20 mL of 10% calcium gluconate. The latter may reverse many of the Mg-induced changes, including the respiratory depression. The administration of IV furosemide or ethacrynic acid increases Mg excretion, if continuous and adequate hydration is maintained and renal function is adequate. Hemodialysis may be of value in severe hypermagnesemia if BP can be maintained, since a relatively large fraction (about 70% of blood Mg) is ultrafilterable. When hemodialysis is impractical, peritoneal dialysis may be effective.

DISTURBANCES IN ACID–BASE METABOLISM

The pH of ECF in health is maintained at about 7.40 (range, 7.35 to 7.45). Acute changes in pH due to acid or alkali loads (or deficits) are immediately damped by interaction with extracellular and intracellular buffer systems. In the absence of pulmonary disease, respiratory compensation further diminishes pH aberrations. Ultimately, however, the kidneys maintain pH homeostasis by excretion or retention of hydrogen ions and regeneration of lost buffers.

The bicarbonate **(HCO_3^-)** buffer system, one of several body buffers, is of singular importance. The **Henderson-Hasselbalch** equation, expressed in terms of the HCO_3^- system, reads:

$$pH = 6.1 + \log \frac{HCO_3^-}{\alpha(Pa_{CO_2})}$$

where α = .03 mM/L/mm Hg at 38 C

At a pH of 7.4, the ratio of HCO_3^- to α (Pa_{CO_2}) is 20:1. Their *ratio*, rather than their concentrations, determines blood pH. The physiologic importance of this buffer system derives from the fact that 2 mechanisms (renal and respiratory) exist for adjusting the ratio of this major ECF buffer pair, and thus the pH of the ECF. The denominator $\alpha(Pa_{CO_2})$ can be modified rapidly by changes in respiratory minute ventilation, while the numerator (HCO_3^-) is subject to renal regulation.

Renal regulation of the HCO_3^- concentration of ECF is accomplished in several ways. Hydrogen **(H)** ion may be secreted into the renal tubular lumen in exchange for Na; for each H ion secreted, a HCO_3^- ion is added to the ECF. Thus, net reabsorption of filtered HCO_3^- occurs. Since the pH of the fluid leaving the proximal tubule is about 6.5, most filtered HCO_3^- is reabsorbed in the proximal tubule. In the distal tubule, H ion secretion is partially dependent upon aldosterone-mediated Na reab-

sorption and can lower the pH to as low as 4.5 to 5. Throughout the nephron, secreted H ion is buffered by urinary buffers such as PO_4 (titratable acid) and ammonia. In this manner, filtered HCO_3^- operationally is reabsorbed, and also new HCO_3^- can be generated to replace that lost in body buffer reactions. Since filtered Na is reabsorbed either in association with an anion (ie, chloride) or by cationic exchange (ie, with H ion and, to a lesser extent, K), the total Na reabsorbed approximates the sum of the chloride reabsorbed and H ion secreted. Thus, there is an inverse relationship between chloride reabsorption and H ion secretion. This relationship is highly dependent upon the existing level of Na reabsorption.

Renal HCO_3^- reabsorption also is influenced by body potassium stores. There is a general reciprocal relationship between intracellular potassium content and hydrogen ion secretion. Thus, potassium depletion is associated with increased hydrogen ion secretion and attendant HCO_3^- generation, leading to an HCO_3^- increase in ECF and metabolic alkalosis. Finally, renal HCO_3^- reabsorption is influenced by the Pa_{CO_2} and the state of ECF volume. An increased Pa_{CO_2} leads to increased HCO_3^- reabsorption, and a decreased ECF volume leads to increased Na reabsorption and HCO_3^- generation; eg, in the proximal tubule.

Clinical disturbances of acid-base metabolism classically are defined in terms of the HCO_3^- buffer system (see Henderson-Hasselbalch equation, above). Rises or falls of the numerator (HCO_3^-) are termed, respectively, **metabolic alkalosis** or **acidosis;** rises or falls in the denominator ($\alpha[Pa_{CO_2}]$) define, respectively, **respiratory acidosis** and **alkalosis. Simple disturbances** include both the primary alteration and the expected compensation (eg, in metabolic acidosis there is a primary fall in the HCO_3^- concentration of the ECF and a secondary fall in the Pa_{CO_2} due to compensatory hyperventilation). Compensation may be classified as uncompensated, partial, or complete. **Mixed disturbances** are more complex disorders in which 2 or more primary alterations coexist (eg, respiratory acidosis with superimposed diuretic-induced metabolic alkalosis).

It may be necessary to refer to a nomogram in order to distinguish simple from mixed disorders. However, measurement of the pH of arterial (or arterialized venous) blood, the Pa_{CO_2}, and the CO_2 content of venous blood (or calculation of HCO_3^-) along with recognition of a disease entity known to produce an acid-base derangement and knowledge of the expected responses of the blood gases and buffers, including compensatory changes, are usually sufficient to correctly identify most clinical acid-base problems (see TABLE 84–6).

METABOLIC ACIDOSIS

A primary fall in extracellular fluid bicarbonate concentration; pH and carbon dioxide content are reduced.

Etiology and Pathogenesis

The principal causes of metabolic acidosis are shown in TABLE 84–7.

Excessive acid production or ingestion: A common form is diabetic ketoacidosis with increased production of acetoacetic and β-hydroxybutyric acid. Occasionally, diabetic acidosis may be associated with an altered NADH/NAD ratio leading to lactic acidosis and elevated levels of β-hydroxybutyric acid. The serum ketone level is not increased when measured by the usual methods that detect only acetoacetic acid. Lactic acidosis may develop in any state of diminished tissue oxygenation (eg, vascular shock), with hepatic dysfunction (and diminished conversion of lactate to glucose), or ethanol ingestion. Rarely it occurs idiopathically. In salicylate, methanol, or ethylene glycol poisoning, interference with normal intermediary metabolism or accumulation of exogenous organic anions may cause metabolic acidosis.

Impaired renal excretion of acid occurs in acute or advanced chronic renal failure due to reduced hydrogen ion excretion. In chronic renal failure, the major defect is insuf-

TABLE 84–6. CHEMICAL FINDINGS IN THE PLASMA OF PATIENTS WITH ACID-BASE DISTURBANCES

Disturbance	*pH*	*Pa_{CO_2}*	*CO_2 Content*
Normal	7.34–7.38 (venous) 7.38–7.42 (arterial)	43 mm Hg (venous) 40 mm Hg (arterial)	21–28 mEq/L
Metabolic alkalosis	↑	↑**	↑*
Metabolic acidosis	↓	↓**	↓*
Respiratory alkalosis	↑	↓*	↓**
Respiratory acidosis	↓	↑*	↑**
Mixed metabolic and respiratory acidosis	↓	↑	↓
Mixed metabolic and respiratory alkalosis	↑	↓	↑
Mixed metabolic acidosis and respiratory alkalosis	↑↓	↓	↓
Mixed metabolic alkalosis and respiratory acidosis	↑↓	↑	↑

* Primary change
** Compensatory change

ficient ammonia production (and thus decreased ammonium ion excretion) as the result of progressive diminution in functioning renal mass. In renal tubular acidosis **(RTA)** with a relatively normal filtration rate, the defect is either proximal tubular HCO_3^- wasting (proximal RTA) or an inability to generate an acid urine (gradient-limited or distal RTA).

TABLE 84–7. PRINCIPAL CAUSES OF METABOLIC ACIDOSIS AND METABOLIC ALKALOSIS

I. Metabolic Acidosis
- A. With elevated "anion gap"
  1. Renal failure
  2. Diabetic ketoacidosis
  3. Lactic acidosis
  4. Exogenous poisons (ethylene glycol, salicylates, methanol, paraldehyde)
- B. With normal "anion gap"
  1. GI alkali loss (diarrhea, ileostomy, colostomy)
  2. Renal tubular acidosis
  3. Interstitial renal disease (e.g., "selective hypoaldosteronism")
  4. Ureterosigmoid loop, uncommonly, ureteroileal conduit
  5. Ingestion of acetazolamide or ammonium chloride

II. Metabolic Alkalosis
- **A. Diuretic therapy (thiazides, ethacrynic acid, furosemide)**
- **B. Vomiting or gastric drainage**
- **C. Hyperadrenocorticism (Cushing's syndrome, aldosteronism, exogenous corticosteroid administration)**

Symptoms, Signs, and Diagnosis

The major symptoms and signs of acidosis are often obscured by or difficult to separate from those of the underlying disease. Mild acidosis may be asymptomatic or may be accompanied by vague lassitude, nausea, and vomiting. The most characteristic finding in severe metabolic acidosis (eg, pH < 7.2 and CO_2 content < 10 mEq/L) is hyperpnea, manifested by an early increase in depth and, later, frequency of respiration (Kussmaul breathing). Signs of ECF volume depletion may also be present, especially in patients with diabetic acidosis or GI alkali loss. Severe acidosis may cause circulatory shock, due to impaired myocardial contractility and peripheral vascular response to catecholamines, and progressive obtundation.

Laboratory Findings

The urine pH is < 5.5 when the plasma HCO_3^- concentration falls to low levels with severe acidosis. The blood pH is < 7.35 and CO_2 content < 21 mEq/L. In the absence of pulmonary disease, the Pa_{CO_2} is < 40 mm Hg. In simple metabolic acidosis, the Pa_{CO_2} may be expected to fall approximately 1.0 to 1.3 mm Hg for each mEq/L reduction in the plasma HCO_3^-. A greater than expected decline in the Pa_{CO_2} suggests the coexistence of primary respiratory alkalosis.

Many forms of metabolic acidosis are characterized by an **abnormal anion gap** (TABLE 84–7). The anion gap (representing undetermined serum anions) is estimated by subtracting the sum of the chloride concentration and CO_2 content from the serum Na concentration (normal up to 15 mEq/L). When metabolic acidosis is associated with the accumulation of unmeasured anions, such as sulfate in renal failure, ketones in diabetic or alcoholic ketoacidosis, lactate or exogenous toxins such as ethylene glycol or salicylates, the anion gap is > 15 mEq/L. Metabolic acidosis associated with a normal anion gap (hyperchloremic metabolic acidosis) usually results from primary bicarbonate loss, either via the GI tract or in the urine (eg, renal tubular acidosis). **Diabetic acidosis** usually is characterized by the presence of hyperglycemia and ketonemia. In diabetic patients with hyperglycemia and nonketotic acidosis, blood lactic acid and/or β-hydroxybutyric acid levels are elevated. **Ethylene glycol** poisoning should be suspected in individuals having unexplained acidosis and oxalate crystals in the urine. **Salicylate poisoning** is characterized early by respiratory alkalosis with metabolic acidosis developing later; blood levels of salicylate are usually > 30 to 40 mg/dL.

Since volume depletion often accompanies acidosis, mild azotemia (BUN 30 to 60 mg/dL) is common. Greater elevations of the BUN, especially in conjunction with hypocalcemia and hyperphosphatemia, suggest renal failure as the cause of the acidosis. Changes in the serum K during acidosis were discussed earlier in this chapter.

Treatment

Therapy of chronic renal acidosis is discussed under ANOMALIES IN KIDNEY TRANSPORT in Ch. 155.

The treatment of metabolic acidosis consists of therapy of the underlying disease (eg, insulin in diabetic acidosis) and IV administration of sodium bicarbonate when acidosis is severe (pH < 7.2). This can be given by adding varying amounts of sodium bicarbonate (44 to 88 mEq) to either 5% D/W or hypotonic (0.45%) sodium chloride solution, or by using 5% sodium bicarbonate solutions, depending on the clinical setting and attendant water and volume disturbances. The goal of HCO_3^- therapy is to raise the CO_2 content to about 10 to 12 mEq/L. The amount of sodium bicarbonate necessary can be approximated by the formula:

$$\text{mEq of } NaHCO_3 \text{ required} = (CO_2 \text{ content desired} - CO_2 \text{ content observed}) \times 25\% \text{ TBW}$$

The apparent distribution space of HCO_3^- is > 25% of TBW, due to continuing transfer of intracellularly buffered H ion out of cells into the ECF. However, it is best to raise the pH of the ECF only to a safe level, such as 7.2, while other measures are instituted to correct the cause of the acidosis, thereby averting some of the **complications of alkali treatment**. These include volume overload in patients with cardiac and renal disease and the precipitation of acute tetany in patients with renal failure. Too rapid correction of acidosis may also result in a rise in the Pa_{CO_2} at a time when CSF bicarbonate levels are still low, thus inducing a "relative CSF acidosis." Occasionally, this may be associated with obtundation, coma, or death. In patients with marked overproduction of H ions (eg, lactic acidosis), it may be necessary to give very large quantities of sodium bicarbonate IV in conjunction with dialysis to minimize ECF volume expansion.

RESPIRATORY ACIDOSIS

A primary increase in arterial carbon dioxide pressure; pH is low and carbon dioxide content increases if renal function is intact.

Etiology and Pathogenesis

Respiratory acidosis is the result of alveolar hypoventilation leading to pulmonary CO_2 retention. It occurs with (1) depression of the central respiratory center caused by drugs, anesthesia, neurologic disease, abnormal sensitivity to CO_2 (eg, cardiopulmonary obesity syndrome); (2) abnormalities of the chest bellows (eg, poliomyelitis, myasthenia gravis, Guillain-Barré syndrome, crush injuries of the thorax); (3) severe reduction of alveolar surface area for gas exchange (conditions characterized by ventilation/perfusion imbalance; eg, chronic obstructive pulmonary disease [emphysema, chronic bronchitis], severe pneumonia, pulmonary edema, asthma, or pneumothorax); and (4) laryngeal or tracheal obstruction. Neurologic changes with CO_2 retention may depend upon the development of CSF acidosis or intracellular acidosis in the brain. Hypoxemia and metabolic alkalosis frequently accompany respiratory acidosis and may contribute to the neurologic abnormalities.

Symptoms, Signs, and Diagnosis

The most characteristic change is metabolic encephalopathy with headache and drowsiness progressing to stupor and coma. It usually develops slowly with advancing respiratory failure, but abrupt, full-blown encephalopathy may be precipitated by sedatives or pulmonary infection in patients with advanced respiratory insufficiency. Asterixis and multifocal myoclonus are generally present; in some patients, dilation of retinal venules and papilledema result from increased intracranial pressure. The encephalopathy may be reversible if hypoxic brain damage has not occurred.

Laboratory Findings

In acute respiratory acidosis, the low pH is due to the acute elevation in Pa_{CO_2}. The CO_2 content may be normal or slightly increased. In acute respiratory acidosis, an abrupt increase in the Pa_{CO_2} is associated with a rise in plasma HCO_3^- of no more than 3 to 4 mEq/L as the result of cellular buffering. When renal compensation is fully developed, as in chronic respiratory acidosis, the fall in pH is blunted due to renal HCO_3^- retention and elevation of the CO_2 content. The expected compensatory rise in the plasma HCO_3^- is approximately 0.3 to 0.4 mEq/L for each mm Hg increment in the Pa_{CO_2}. A greater than expected increase in plasma HCO_3^- indicates the coexistence of primary metabolic alkalosis. If diuretic therapy (eg, for chronic cor pulmonale) causes superimposed metabolic alkalosis, the high Pa_{CO_2} may be associated with a high CO_2 content, hypochloremia, and a normal or alkaline blood pH.

Treatment

The treatment must improve the underlying pulmonary disturbance. Severe respiratory failure with marked hypoxemia often requires mechanically assisted ventilation. Sedative drugs (narcotics, hypnotics) should be avoided except as necessary to facilitate mechanical ventilation. Although most patients with chronic CO_2 retention and hypoxia tolerate modest O_2 enrichment of inspired air, some patients respond with a significant fall in respiratory minute volume and further acute elevation of the Pa_{CO_2}. Presumably, such patients have adapted to chronic hypercapnia (CO_2 narcosis) so that their major respiratory stimulus is hypoxemia. Therefore the lowest O_2 concentration required to elevate the Pa_{O_2} to acceptable levels (> 50 mm Hg) should be given. This can be accomplished with O_2 administration by a Ventimask®, beginning with a 24% O_2 concentration. The Pa_{CO_2} should be carefully monitored and, if it rises to dangerous levels (> 50 to 55 mm Hg), mechanical ventilation must be considered.

If mechanical ventilation is used in patients with chronic respiratory failure, the Pa_{CO_2} should be lowered slowly, especially if concomitant metabolic alkalosis (high CO_2 content and normal or alkaline pH) is present. Rapid lowering of the Pa_{CO_2} will cause severe metabolic alkalosis (pH > 7.5). The resultant leftward shift of the oxyhemoglobin dissociation curve and cerebral vasoconstriction may lead to seizures and death. Providing adequate inspired O_2, lowering the Pa_{CO_2} more slowly, and repairing potassium or chloride deficits will prevent such neurologic consequences.

METABOLIC ALKALOSIS

A primary increase in blood bicarbonate; pH and carbon dioxide content are elevated.

Etiology and Pathogenesis

Metabolic alkalosis develops as the consequence of loss of acid from the ECF; eg, loss of acid-containing gastric juice, loss of acid via the urine or stool, transfer of H ions into cells, excessive loads of HCO_3^- (eg, alkali administration to patients with renal failure), or rapid contraction of the extracellular space (eg, with potent diuretics). Whatever the cause, the kidney tends to correct the alkalosis rapidly by excreting excess HCO_3^-, unless other factors, such as volume contraction, result in both a Na-acquisitive state and increased HCO_3^- reabsorption. Thus, a diminished effective arterial volume, K deficiency, and persistent adrenal steroid excess are common clinical settings for chronic metabolic alkalosis (TABLE 84–7). Perhaps the most frequent and important of these settings is ECF volume contraction and avid renal sodium reabsorption.

Diuretics cause metabolic alkalosis by several mechanisms, including (1) acute contraction of the ECF volume (sodium chloride excretion without HCO_3^-), thereby increasing the concentration of HCO_3^- in the ECF; (2) diuretic-induced K and chloride depletion, and (3) secondary aldosteronism. Continued use of the diuretic or either of the latter 2 factors may maintain the alkalosis.

The loss of gastric hydrochloric acid by suction or vomiting produces metabolic alkalosis that is perpetuated by concomitant ECF volume contraction (sodium chloride loss in gastric juice) and development of K deficiency, due to secondary aldosteronism (ie, renal K wasting) and K loss in gastric juice.

In states of persistent adrenal steroid excess, alkalosis results from steroid-mediated reabsorption of Na in the distal tubule in exchange for H ion. Sodium chloride reabsorption in the distal tubule leads to ECF volume expansion and decreased proximal Na reabsorption. Thus, a continuing supply of Na is delivered distally for exchange with H and K ions. Potassium depletion then leads to persistence of the alkalosis.

Symptoms, Signs, and Diagnosis

Metabolic alkalosis should be suspected in the above clinical settings. The most common clinical manifestations are irritability and neuromuscular hyperexcitability.

perhaps due to hypoxia from a transient leftward shift of the oxyhemoglobin dissociation curve. When severe, the ionized Ca fraction may fall low enough to provoke tetany, although total serum Ca is unchanged (see HYPOCALCEMIA, above). Muscular weakness, impaired GI motility (eg, gastric retention, ileus), and polyuria should suggest K depletion.

Laboratory findings: The blood pH and CO_2 content are elevated. Striking increases in the Pa_{CO_2} to levels as high as 50 to 60 mm Hg may occur with compensatory hypoventilation, especially in patients with mild renal insufficiency. The expected rise in the Pa_{CO_2} equals 0.4 to 0.7 mm Hg for each mEq/L increment in the plasma HCO_3^-. A greater than anticipated increase in the Pa_{CO_2} suggests a mixed disorder with coexistent primary respiratory acidosis. The urine is alkaline except in the presence of severe K depletion, in which case it may be acid **("paradoxic aciduria")**. Hypochloremia and hypokalemia are usual. When metabolic alkalosis is associated with ECF volume depletion, the urine chloride is almost always low (< 10 mEq/L), while the urine Na may exceed 20 mEq/L in the early stages. Conversely, metabolic alkalosis associated with primary adrenal steroid excess and volume expansion is characterized by high urine chloride.

Treatment

Correction of the underlying disturbance is desirable, when possible. Metabolic alkalosis usually resolves when ECF volume deficits are replaced with oral or IV sodium chloride. However, when K deficiency is severe, or in patients with adrenal steroid excess, the alkalosis cannot be corrected until the K deficit is repaired **(saline-resistant alkalosis)**. In the post-hypercapnic state, persistent metabolic alkalosis responds to chloride, given as potassium chloride, sodium chloride (if volume depletion is present), or ammonium chloride. When mild, metabolic alkalosis usually requires no specific therapy. It should be corrected promptly, however, in patients with myocardial irritability and those with neuromuscular hyperexcitability. In such instances, ammonium chloride administration may be desirable along with other measures (eg, correction of hypokalemia).

RESPIRATORY ALKALOSIS

A primary decrease in carbon dioxide pressure; blood pH is raised and carbon dioxide content is reduced.

Etiology and Pathogenesis

Hyperventilation, leading to excessive loss of CO_2 in expired air, results in respiratory alkalosis. The Pa_{CO_2} and cerebral tissue P_{CO_2} fall, and both plasma and cerebral tissue pH rise. Cerebral vasoconstriction results and, along with the Bohr effect, may produce cerebral hypoxia and the characteristic symptom complex. The common causes are anxiety **("hyperventilation syndrome")**, overventilation of patients on assisted ventilation, primary CNS disorders, salicylism, hepatic cirrhosis, hepatic coma, hypoxemia, fever, and gram-negative septicemia.

Symptoms, Signs, and Diagnosis

Obvious hyperventilation is usually present, particularly when respiratory alkalosis is due to cerebral or metabolic disorders. The breathing pattern in the anxiety-induced syndrome varies from frequent, deep, sighing respirations to sustained, obvious rapid, deep breathing. Patients tend to complain of anxiety, often expressing fear of cardiac disease, and are often surprisingly unaware of their hyperventilation. When symptoms are referable to respirations, the complaint is usually of inability to "catch my breath" or "get enough air," despite the fact that unimpaired overbreathing is taking place. Tetany, circumoral paresthesias, acroparesthesias, giddiness or lightheadedness, and syncope may occur. In such patients, the symptoms often can be reproduced by volun-

tary overventilation. Blood lactate and pyruvate levels increase and ionized calcium falls. In all situations, the diagnosis of hyperventilation is confirmed by finding a low $Paco_2$.

Laboratory findings: In acute respiratory alkalosis, a rapid decline in the $Paco_2$ to 20 to 25 mm Hg is associated with a drop in plasma HCO_3^- of no greater than 3 to 4 mEq/L, due to cellular buffering. In chronic respiratory alkalosis, the plasma HCO_3^- may be expected to decline by approximately 0.4 to 0.5 mEq/L for each mm Hg reduction of the $Paco_2$. A greater than expected fall in the plasma HCO_3^- suggests coexistent primary metabolic acidosis.

Treatment

Respiratory alkalosis due to anxiety resolves with reassurance. Rebreathing expired CO_2 from a *paper* bag (plastic bags may cause accidental suffocation) may occasionally be helpful. Other measures are aimed at amelioration of the anxiety (see ANXIETY NEUROSIS in Ch. 140). Overventilation with mechanical respirators can be corrected by diminishing minute ventilation, when excessive, or by adding dead space. When hyperventilation is due to hypoxemia, O_2 enrichment of inspired air and treatment aimed at correction of abnormal pulmonary gas exchange is appropriate. Correction of respiratory alkalosis by increasing the inspired CO_2 concentration may be dangerous in patients with CNS disturbances (which may be associated with a low CSF pH). The treatment of salicylism is given in Ch. 189.

---

85. METABOLIC ANOMALIES

ANOMALIES IN PIGMENT METABOLISM

THE PORPHYRIAS

A group of inborn errors of metabolism caused by mutations in genes that code for various enzymes of the heme biosynthetic pathway. One type of porphyria (porphyria cutanea tarda) can also be caused by certain toxic agents such as hexachlorobenzene.

The specific enzymes affected by the mutations and the diseases that are caused by each mutation are best understood after examination of the heme biosynthetic pathway, shown in FIG. 85–1. The pathway can be considered to consist of 8 basic steps, starting with the condensation of glycine and succinyl coenzyme A **(CoA)** to form δ-aminolevulinic acid **(ALA),** the aliphatic precursor of heme. The ALA undergoes self-condensation to form porphobilinogen **(PBG)** in step 2, which is followed by polymerization of PBG to uroporphyrinogen III in steps 3 and 4. This intermediate is the reduced (hexhydro-) form of uroporphyrin and differs from the porphyrin in that it is colorless, non-fluorescent, and nonphotosensitizing (it is readily oxidized to the porphyrin in the presence of light and O_2). In step 5, the four acetic acid side chains are sequentially decarboxylated to form methyl groups, and in the process uroporphyrinogen III is converted to coproporphyrinogen III. Both propionic acid side chains of pyrrole rings A and B undergo oxidative decarboxylation to vinyl groups in the conversion of coproporphyrinogen III to protoporphyrinogen in step 6. Protoporphyrinogen is then oxidized to protoporphyrin by removal of 6 hydrogen atoms. The final step involves chelation of ferrous iron by protoporphyrin to form heme, which is then utilized in various hemoproteins.

Mutations that decrease enzyme activity have been described for all enzymes of the heme biosynthetic pathway except ALA synthetase. The diseases that correspond to the various mutations are presented in TABLE 85–1. The classification of the porphyr

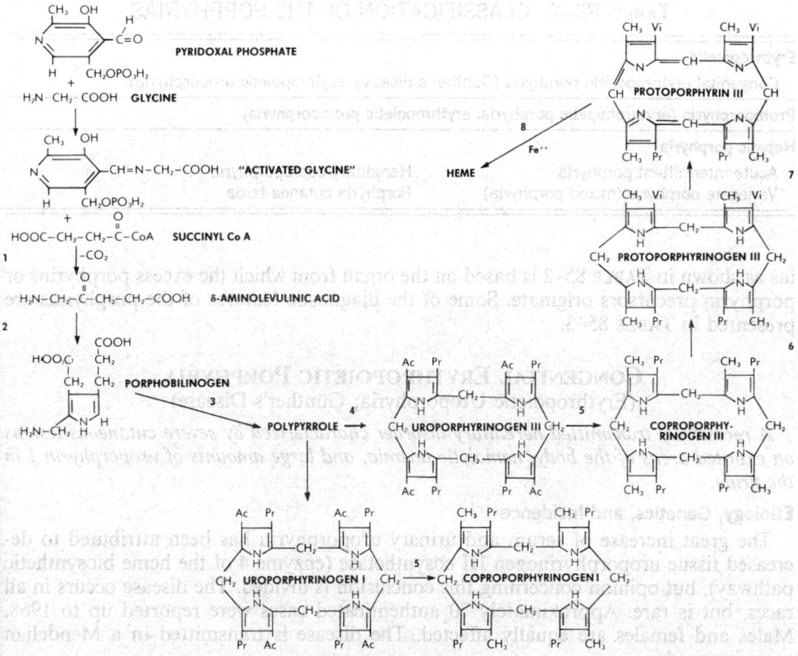

Fig. 85–1. Heme biosynthetic pathway. (From *Metabolic Control and Disease* [formerly *Duncan's Diseases of Metabolism*], ed. 8, 1980, edited by P. K. Bondy and L. E. Rosenberg. Copyright 1980 by W. B. Saunders Company. Used with permission.)

Table 85–1. DISEASES THAT CORRESPOND TO VARIOUS MUTATIONS IN HEME SYNTHESIS

Step of Pathway Affected by Mutation	*Name of Enzyme Involved*	*Name of Disease*	*Genetic Mode of Transmission*
2	ALA dehydrase	No disease in heterozygotes	See text
3	Uroporphyrinogen I synthetase	Acute intermittent porphyria	Dominant
4	Uroporphyrinogen III cosynthetase	Congenital erythropoietic porphyria	Recessive
5	Uroporphyrinogen decarboxylase	Porphyria cutanea tarda	Dominant or acquired
6	Coproporphyrinogen oxidase	Hereditary coproporphyria	Dominant
7	Protoporphyrinogen oxidase	Variegate porphyria	Dominant
8	Ferrochelatase	Protoporphyria (erythrohepatic porphyria; erythropoietic protoporphyria)	Dominant

TABLE 85–2. CLASSIFICATION OF THE PORPHYRIAS

Erythropoietic	
Congenital erythropoietic porphyria (Günther's disease, erythropoietic uroporphyria)	
Protoporphyria (erythrohepatic porphyria; erythropoietic protoporphyria)	
Hepatic porphyria	
Acute intermittent porphyria	Hereditary coproporphyria
Variegate porphyria (mixed porphyria)	Porphyria cutanea tarda

ias as shown in TABLE 85–2 is based on the organ from which the excess porphyrins or porphyrin precursors originate. Some of the diagnostic features of the porphyrias are presented in TABLE 85–3.

CONGENITAL ERYTHROPOIETIC PORPHYRIA
(Erythropoietic Uroporphyria; Günther's Disease)

A recessively transmitted hereditary disorder characterized by severe cutaneous lesions on exposed areas of the body, hemolytic anemia, and large amounts of uroporphyrin I in the urine.

Etiology, Genetics, and Incidence

The great increase of serum and urinary uroporphyrin has been attributed to decreased tissue uroporphyrinogen III cosynthetase (enzyme 4 of the heme biosynthetic pathway), but opinion concerning this conclusion is divided. The disease occurs in all races, but is rare. Approximately 70 authenticated cases were reported up to 1968. Males and females are equally affected. The disease is transmitted in a Mendelian recessive mode.

Symptoms and Signs

This disease is manifested by cutaneous lesions and hemolytic anemia. The onset of symptoms is often in the first year and almost always before age 5. Skin lesions appear as vesicles or bullae on exposed portions of the body. Ulceration and sometimes secondary infection, followed by healing, leads to scarring. This ultimately may produce severe deformities of the nose, ears, eyes, and fingers, with areas of alopecia, pigmentation, and depigmentation. Hypertrichosis may develop on the limbs and face. The skin lesions are related to the photosensitizing action of the excess porphyrin, but the cause of the hypertrichosis remains unknown. Most patients experience hemolysis and ineffective erythropoiesis, but some compensate sufficiently by increased RBC production to prevent the normochromic anemia that occurs in others. Splenomegaly develops in some patients and occasionally thrombocytopenia, which has been attributed to hypersplenism. With rare exceptions, these patients have not survived beyond middle age. The cause of death is not always clear, but some have died of renal failure, hepatic failure, or bleeding of uncertain etiology.

Laboratory Findings

The basic defect causes a huge increase of uroporphyrin I and an increase of coproporphyrin I (produced by the non-enzymatic oxidation of the corresponding porphyrinogens) that produce a red ("port wine") urine. Uroporphyrin excretion may reach 50 mg/day, ie, more than 1000 times the normal excretion rate. Fecal coproporphyrin I is increased but fecal protoporphyrin is usually not significantly increased. Plasma and erythrocyte uroporphyrin I and coproporphyrin I levels are increased. Erythrocyte free protoporphyrin levels usually do not exceed those seen in other hemolytic anemias. Urinary porphyrin precursor excretion is not increased, and the Watson-Schwartz test (for porphobilinogen) is negative.

TABLE 85–3. DIAGNOSTIC FEATURES OF THE PORPHYRIAS

Disease	*Skin*	*Neurologic* (Includes abdominal pain)	*Urinary* PBG (±ALA)	Uro	*Fecal* Copro	Proto	*RBC* Proto	Enzyme
Congenital erythropoietic porphyria	+	−	−	+	−	−	−	−
Protoporphyria	+	−	−	−	−	±	+	−
Acute intermittent porphyria								
Latent	−	−	±	±	−	−	−	+
Active	−	+	+	±	−	−	−	+
Variegate porphyria								
Latent	±	−	±	+	−	+	−	−
Active	±	+	+	+	−	+	−	−
Hereditary coproporphyria								
Latent	−	−	±	−	+	−	−	−
Active	±	+	+	+	+	−	−	−
Porphyria cutanea tarda	+	−	−	+	−	−	−	+*

This table is a simplified guide to the major diagnostic findings in the porphyrias. The + symbol indicates findings that are of primary importance in the diagnosis. The − symbol indicates that changes are small or do not occur and are not of primary diagnostic value. The symbol ± indicates that values may be increased or normal, not that changes are necessarily slight. Enzyme tests that are either not possible in erythrocytes or too complex to be readily available are included in the − symbol. PGB = porphobilinogen; Uro = uroporphyrin; Copro = coproporphyrin; Proto = protoporphyrin; ALA = δ-aminolevulinic acid.

*Applies to the familial type only.

Normoblastic hyperplasia is usually seen in marrow samples. Fluorescence microscopy shows fluorescent normoblasts (the nucleus is most evident). In the peripheral blood, some of the circulating red cells fluoresce and reticulocytosis is often seen. There may be poikilocytosis, anisocytosis, and polychromatophilia.

Diagnosis

The appearance of dark urine and severe cutaneous photosensitivity in early life, usually accompanied by hemolytic anemia and erythrodontia, suggests the diagnosis. This is confirmed by demonstration of high levels of uroporphyrin I (by direct measurement) and fluorescence of red cells and marrow normoblasts. If erythrodontia is not obvious, red fluorescence of the teeth should be sought by examination with an ultraviolet (Wood's) light.

Treatment

The skin should be shielded from light by means of protective clothing. The creams and lotions used for sunburn prophylaxis are of little value in this disease, because they do not absorb the Soret band of wavelengths (those in the violet portion of the spectrum [about 400 nm]) that are absorbed by porphyrins and cause the skin damage. Beta-carotene, taken orally, has been used successfully to protect against acute photosensitivity reactions in protoporphyria (see details below). Preliminary studies of patients with congenital erythropoietic porphyria suggest that β-carotene has some value

in this disorder. Another approach has been the topical application of dihydroxyacetone and lawsone (Duoshield®, Rowell Labs, Inc., Baudett., Minn.), which produces a sun-screen filter that is chemically induced in the skin.

Hemolysis can augment photosensitivity, since stimulation of erythropoiesis by hemolysis also increases porphyrin production (which is responsible for the photosensitivity). Splenectomy has sometimes been followed by decreased hemolysis and porphyrin excretion, but some patients have experienced recurrence of anemia. Likewise, steroid (prednisone) therapy has produced variable results in treatment of the hemolysis. Transfusions have decreased urinary porphyrin excretion as much as 90%, presumably by suppressing erythropoiesis. Recent investigations have shown IV hematin administration to diminish red cell, plasma, and urinary uroporphyrin levels. Further studies are necessary to determine the possible value of hematin therapy in this disease.

PROTOPORPHYRIA

(Erythrohepatic Porphyria; Erythropoietic Protoporphyria)

A dominantly transmitted disorder characterized by acute photosensitivity reactions, no urine abnormalities, and, in some patients, serious liver disease.

Etiology, Genetics, and Incidence

A deficiency of ferrochelatase (the final enzyme of the heme biosynthetic pathway) has been shown in bone marrow, peripheral blood reticulocytes, liver, and fibroblasts, resulting in accumulation of protoporphyrin. The measured enzyme activity usually ranges between 8 and 25% of normal. Enzyme and other chemical studies show that one parent is normal and the other bears the mutation. This is in keeping with the dominant mode of inheritance of the disease, but measurements showing the enzyme decrease to greatly exceed 50% of normal constitute an unexplained paradox. The fact that the genetically affected parent is sometimes asymptomatic, along with other considerations, has raised some question concerning a simple mendelian dominant mode of transmission of this disease. The exact prevalence is not known, but is probably 4 or higher per 100,000 population, as high or higher than acute intermittent porphyria.

Symptoms and Signs

Cutaneous symptoms almost always begin before age 13 and usually involve (in decreasing order of frequency) burning, swelling, itching, and redness of the skin. Itching and burning may occur without redness, swelling, and scarring. This lack of objective findings may suggest psychiatric problems. Since window glass transmits the Soret band of wavelengths that are responsible for the photosensitization, the burning can occur indoors, as well as outdoors. Symptoms may begin after just a few minutes of exposure or may require hours. The burning may be mild or severe and persist for days. Some patients develop erythema and edema of the involved areas; the edema occasionally persists for weeks. Bullae and purpura may occur in children and occasionally in adults. These lesions may produce crusts and heal with superficial scars. There may be chronic skin lesions with thickening and scarring of the skin of the nose, cheek, and back of the hands and fingers. These are usually mild, but in tropical areas papular thickening of the skin may produce a "cobblestone" appearance. The erythrondontia and fluorescence of teeth, characteristic of congenital erythropoietic porphyria, are *not* seen in this disease. Hirsutism and hyperpigmentation are rare in protoporphyria.

There is an increased incidence of gallstones, sometimes at an early age, with high levels of protoporphyrin in the gallstones. Deposition of protoporphyrin in the liver is thought to be the basis for the development of liver disease. Liver function tests are generally normal until shortly before clinical evidence of hepatic disease appears. Jaundice is followed by a downhill course over a period of months. At least 16 deaths

from liver failure have been reported. Jaundice, increased serum transaminase levels, BSP retention, hepatosplenomegaly, hepatic encephalopathy, and portal hypertension with bleeding esophageal varices have been reported during the liver failure of protoporphyria. Some patients have a mild to moderate microcytic and normochromic anemia. Occasionally a mild hemolytic anemia occurs.

Laboratory Findings

Urinary porphyrins and porphyrin precursors are not increased. The **3 patterns of chemical abnormalities** seen in patients or their asymptomatic relatives are (I) increased protoporphyrin in erythrocytes, plasma, and feces, (II) increased erythrocyte protoporphyrin with no increase of fecal protoporphyrin, and (III) increased fecal protoporphyrin with no increase of erythrocyte protoporphyrin. Pattern III is unusual and has been seen in some asymptomatic relatives of symptomatic patients; some increase of coproporphyrin occurs with the increased protoporphyrin. The increase of red cell protoporphyrin is usually not accompanied by an increased fecal protoporphyrin excretion and hence pattern II above is the most commonly observed finding in symptomatic patients.

Although morphology of the marrow is normal, there is fluorescence of a variable fraction of normoblasts and circulating red cells. A brown pigment, which has been identified as protoporphyrin, is present in the cytoplasm of hepatocytes, the lysosomes of Kupffer cells, portal histiocytes, and sometimes in bile ducts and canaliculi. Micronodular cirrhosis is seen in some patients. A distinctive finding by polarization microscopy is the birefringence of the porphyrin crystals observable as Maltese crosses.

Diagnosis

A history of acute photosensitivity reactions and increased red cell protoporphyrin levels are the most important findings for the diagnosis. Increased erythrocyte protoporphyrin levels occur in other disorders, such as iron deficiency, lead intoxication, and hemolysis, but these do not cause photosensitivity. Since photosensitivity occurs in other conditions, neither acute photosensitivity nor increased erythrocyte protoporphyrin alone is sufficient to prove the diagnosis. If other causes of increased erythrocyte protoporphyrin levels are ruled out, the diagnosis is justified in the presence of the 2 basic findings characteristic of the disease. A positive family history is helpful, but may be negative. If liver disease is evident or suspected, fluorescence and polarization microscopy is valuable in demonstrating protoporphyrin crystals in liver biopsy samples. The most definitive diagnostic test for this disease is demonstration of decreased tissue levels of ferrochelatase, but this complicated measurement is available only in certain research laboratories at present.

Treatment

Administration of beta-carotene 15 to 180 mg/day orally usually increases tolerance to light, beginning 1 to 2 mo (sometimes 3 mo) after initiation of therapy. Blood levels of 400 to 600 μg/dL are usually adequate, but if these do not provide sufficient protection, beta-carotene can be administered in a dose of 180 mg/day for 3 mo before considering this agent a failure. At these doses blood levels are often in the range of 800 μg/dL. Some patients have been treated with doses of 250 mg/day without apparent toxicity. This agent can produce skin discoloration, but no serious side effects have been reported in these patients. While beta-carotene can provide protection against photosensitivity, it does not alter the fundamental biochemical abnormalities, since red cell, plasma, and fecal porphyrin levels are unaffected.

Although prevention and treatment of liver disease are important considerations in this disorder, experience is limited in treatment and nonexistent in prevention. Both the erythron and liver may be sources of excess protoporphyrin in this disorder. A high carbohydrate intake has been shown to lower fecal protoporphyrin excretion in some

patients, presumably by repression of hepatic ALA synthetase. Accumulation of hepatic protoporphyrin may result from flux through the liver of protoporphyrin originating in the erythron, as well as that originating in the liver. The latter component might be decreased by a high carbohydrate intake in patients in whom excess protoporphyrin originates in the liver. Attempts to diminish hepatic protoporphyrin by interrupting its enterohepatic circulation with cholestyramine and by repression of hepatic ALA synthetase using IV hematin are being studied.

Acute Intermittent Porphyria

A dominantly transmitted inherited disorder that can exist in latent form indefinitely or acute attacks of neurologic dysfunction can be precipitated by various environmental and endogenous factors. It does not produce cutaneous disease.

Etiology, Genetics, and Incidence

The basic enzyme defect in this disease is a 50% decrease of uroporphyrinogen I synthetase (enzyme 3 of the heme biosynthetic pathway). This defect is transmitted by an autosomal dominant mode of inheritance. The manifest disease is more frequent in women and occurs in all races. The prevalence in the USA is probably 5 to 10 per 100,000 population.

The disease exists in latent form until an attack of acute neurologic dysfunction is precipitated. Four groups of precipitating factors have been described: drugs, starvation, sex hormones, and infection. Some attacks of acute porphyria occur in individuals in whom no exogenous precipitating factor can be found. **Drugs that have been implicated in precipitating attacks of acute porphyria include** barbiturates, sulfonamides, griseofulvin, phenytoin, methsuximide, chlordiazepoxide, meprobamate, isopropylmeprobamate, dichloralphenazone, glutethimide, amidopyrine, antipyrine, isopropylantipyrine, dipyrone, methprylon, imipramine, ergot preparations, methyldopa, chloramphenicol, chlorpropamide, pentazocine, eucalyptol, and danazol.

Safe and probably safe drugs include morphine, codeine, methadone, hyoscine, chloral hydrate, meperidine, penicillins, streptomycin, tetracyclines, nitrofurantoin, mandelamine, corticosteroids, rauwolfia alkaloids, guanethidine, diphenhydramine, promethazine, promazine, chlorpromazine, trifluoperazine, prochlorperazine, meclizine, digoxin, mersalyl, atropine, prostigmine, neostigmine, tetraethylammonium bromide, propoxyphene, diazepam, ketamine, propanidid, acetylsalicylic acid, ether, nitrous oxide, dicumarol, and propranolol.

Starvation and crash dieting have precipitated attacks of porphyria. In animals, a high carbohydrate intake decreases and starvation increases experimental porphyria caused by certain compounds. The effects of diet relate to the ability of glucose and certain other carbohydrates to block the induction of hepatic ALA synthetase.

Female sex hormones have been implicated in precipitating acute attacks of porphyria as evidenced by the facts that (a) biochemical and clinical manifestations almost always occur after puberty, (b) the manifest disease is more frequent in females, and (c) a certain fraction of women with this disease experience a cyclic pattern of recurrent attacks in relation to menstrual periods, often beginning about 3 days before menstruation. Pregnancy has also been implicated in precipitating some attacks of acute porphyria, but probably less than 5% of women with known latent acute intermittent porphyria will experience significant activity of the disease during pregnancy, particularly if they avoid the known precipitating factors.

Both **bacterial and viral infections** have been followed by acute attacks of porphyria, but the mechanism is unknown.

Symptoms and Signs

Symptoms of the acute attack result from nervous system damage. *Any part of the nervous system can be involved and the specific clinical findings depend on which areas are*

affected. The outcome of the acute attack can vary through a spectrum from death to complete recovery. Some patients who recover may retain varying types of neurologic deficit.

Autonomic neuropathy is common and causes abdominal pain, which may be mild or severe. The pain may be localized or general and is often accompanied by vomiting and constipation. It may be constant or colicky and may be accompanied by abdominal tenderness. Low grade fever and mild leukocytosis, along with the pain, can suggest a number of other diagnoses. Other autonomic manifestations include labile hypertension, sinus tachycardia, postural hypotension, sweating, and vascular spasm in the retina or skin of the extremities.

Peripheral neuropathy may be sensory or motor. Low back and leg pain may occur as a chronic pain syndrome without other significant neurologic manifestations or it may precede motor neuropathy. Paresthesias are occasionally seen, but sensory neuropathy is usually not accompanied by objective findings. All motor nerves are subject to porphyric neuropathy, which may be asymmetric and may progress at a highly variable rate. Flaccid paralysis may develop within days or weeks.

CNS involvement can produce an organic brain syndrome (hallucinations, coma, etc.), seizures, cerebellar and basal ganglion manifestations, hypothalamic dysfunction, and bulbar paralysis. Respiratory paralysis may require assisted respiration and is associated with a high mortality rate.

Hyponatremia, which may be profound (serum Na < 100 mEq/L), develops in some patients during acute attacks. This may be caused by GI loss of Na, inappropriate release of ADH, and probably primary renal loss of Na. Some patients who have many of the classical findings of inappropriate ADH release are found to be hypovolemic and probably are experiencing primary renal loss of Na. Thus, hypothalamic pathology may cause hyponatremia, but the other causes should also be considered carefully, since treatment for inappropriate ADH release differs from that for primary Na loss.

Psychiatric manifestations most often are are depression and an organic brain syndrome. In patients who are not experiencing other activity of the disease, it is difficult to estimate the role of porphyria in producing depression.

Laboratory Findings

The characteristic finding of this disease is increased porphyrin precursor excretion in the urine. During asymptomatic periods some patients do not excrete increased amounts of either ALA or PBG, some excrete increased amounts of PBG with no increase of ALA, and others excrete increased amounts of both precursors. During the acute attack, however, all patients excrete increased amounts of PBG. Since the mutation of this disease causes a decrease of the enzyme that converts PBG to uroporphyrinogen, there is no increase of enzymatically produced porphyrins. However, when urine PBG excretion is high, an increase of urinary uroporphyrin may be evident. This is thought to result from polymerization of PBG, particularly in acid urine.

BSP retention, increased thyroxin-binding globulin, hypercholesterolemia, and hyperbetalipoproteinemia may be found in some patients.

Diagnosis

Abdominal pain of obscure origin, unexplained peripheral neuropathy, or unexplained cerebral lesions should raise the question of an attack of porphyria. Tachycardia, hypertension, dark urine, and a positive family history are further helpful findings. However, the diagnosis of an attack of acute intermittent, variegate, or hereditary coproporphyria cannot be made with certainty unless increased urinary PBG is demonstrated. This can be done by the qualitative Watson-Schwartz or Hoesch tests or by quantitative chromatographic methods, which should always be used to confirm positive qualitative tests. Lead intoxication can be mistaken for acute porphyria and vice versa, but lead intoxication is accompanied by increased ALA excretion without a significant increase in PBG excretion.

Measurement of erythrocyte uroporphyrinogen I synthetase has provided an enzyme test for acute intermittent porphyria. This is useful in detecting the presence of the mutation, but is not capable of distinguishing between the acute attack and asymptomatic periods. Furthermore, while the mean value of the enzyme in a population of patients with acute intermittent porphyria is ½ the mean of a non-porphyric population, there is some overlap in the range of values of the 2 groups, producing a "gray zone" of values, which are not diagnostic.

Differentiation of acute intermittent porphyria from variegate and hereditary coproporphyria is largely academic, since each can produce the same types of neurologic disease. However, the latter 2 disorders can produce cutaneous lesions, which are not seen in acute intermittent porphyria. In addition to the enzyme test, acute intermittent porphyria is distinguished from the other porphyrias by a characteristic pattern of metabolite excretion. Porphyrin precursor excretion is usually, but not always, increased during asymptomatic periods and increases with attacks of acute intermittent porphyria. Although urinary coproporphyrin may be increased, freshly voided urine may not contain increased amounts of uroporphyrin.

There is no major increase of fecal protoporphyrin, as seen in variegate porphyria (see below) during both remission and active phases of the disease, and no great increase of fecal coproporphyrin, as usually seen in hereditary coproporphyria.

Treatment

Management involves prevention of attacks, treatment of symptoms, and attempts to reverse the fundamental disease process. **Prevention of attacks** entails instructing the patient to avoid the known precipitating factors as listed above. An example would be avoidance of sodium thiopental for oral or other surgery. This is very important and can be lifesaving. Other members of the patient's family should also be tested, first by urine measurements and then, if urine tests are negative, by the enzyme test.

Pain control is the first step in the management of symptoms. In some patients, phenothiazines are useful for control of abdominal pain, presumably by their effect on decreasing autonomic outflow. The dose required varies with each patient and should be started at low levels and increased until abdominal pain is controlled. In some patients meperidine is also required. An extrapyramidal syndrome produced by phenothiazines should not be confused with activity of porphyria.

Hyponatremia requires careful analysis of its physiologic mechanism to determine the optimum treatment. Propranolol has been useful in treating tachycardia and hypertension. Management of infections and other complications that are not specific for porphyria are discussed elsewhere in THE MANUAL.

To reverse the basic disease process, many methods have been used but only 2 will be discussed. The first involves a **high carbohydrate intake** of 300 to 400 or more gm/day. Liquid supplements containing sugar are useful. There is a spectrum of responsiveness that varies from a large decrease of porphyrin precursor excretion and dramatic clinical improvement to no significant response biochemically or clinically. The reason for this variation is unknown. Since there is virtually no risk in this treatment, it should be attempted in all patients experiencing an acute attack. A second approach utilizes **IV hematin,** which lowers porphyrin precursor excretion. Although its value in reversing the clinical manifestations of acute attacks has not been proved by double blind studies, many clinicians feel that it is useful, particularly if started early in the acute attack. As might be expected, established neuropathy does not respond to hematin. Treatment protocols have varied. One group of patients were given 3 to 4 mg/kg once a day for 3 to 13 days. Another group was given 4 mg/kg bid for 3 days, at which time each patient was reevaluated. Each dose was given over 15 min. Doses considerably higher than the above have produce reversible anuria. Hematin affects the clotting mechanism and caution should be exercised in patients receiving anticoagulants or with clotting deficiencies.

In women experiencing regular cyclic attacks related to menstrual periods, oral contraceptives (given cyclically) have been valuable in preventing the attacks. Some of the new preparations are too low in estrogen content and require additional estrogen supplements. Experience with the cyclic pattern of attacks is limited and patients suffering from them must be carefully supervised. Patients who do not have the cyclic pattern of attacks should not receive hormone therapy.

Variegate Porphyria

A disorder clinically identical to acute intermittent porphyria (see above) but capable of also producing cutaneous disease on exposed portions of the body.

Etiology, Genetics, and Incidence

Although there have been claims of decreased ferrochelatase activity in this disease, recent studies show a decrease of protoporphyrinogen oxidase as the fundamental defect. Variegate porphyria is transmitted as an autosomal dominant disorder. It probably has a lower prevalence than acute intermittent porphyria in the USA, but in South Africa it has been estimated at 300 per 100,000 in the white population.

Symptoms and Signs

This disease can produce neurologic and cutaneous disease, either simultaneously or separately. The skin lesions resemble those of porphyria cutanea tarda (see below). There may be bullae, erosions, scarring, and pigmentation, involving skin that is exposed to light. Acute photosensitivity is uncommon, and increased skin fragility is of much greater significance. Hypertrichosis may be evident. The acute attack of neurologic dysfunction is similar to that of acute intermittent porphyria described above.

Laboratory Findings

Fecal protoporphyrin is increased during both asymptomatic periods and acute attacks of neurologic disease. Porphyrin precursor excretion is often normal or slightly increased during asymptomatic periods, but increases during acute attacks. Increased urinary PBG can be detected by the Watson-Schwartz or Hoesch tests, but should be confirmed by a quantitative determination. Urine uroporphyrin and coproporphyrin are increased, with coproporphyrin usually exceeding uroporphyrin during asymptomatic periods. During acute attacks, uroporphyrin increases and usually exceeds coproporphyrin.

Diagnosis

The differential diagnosis of the acute attack (*in which increased PBG excretion must be demonstrated*) is the same as that for acute intermittent porphyria. If typical skin lesions on the exposed portions of the body are or have been present, a diagnosis of variegate porphyria should be considered. Increased fecal protoporphyrin excretion must be demonstrated along with the characteristic urinary findings before the diagnosis is certain. Although the enzyme defect has been demonstrated in cultured fibroblasts, no practical diagnostic enzyme test is available at present.

Treatment

The acute attack is treated as described for acute intermittent porphyria (see above). In preliminary studies, carotenoid therapy for the cutaneous lesions has been disappointing.

Hereditary Coproporphyria

Etiology, Genetics, and Incidence

A decrease of about 50% of coproporphyrinogen oxidase activity is the fundamental defect in this disease. It is transmitted as an autosomal dominant disorder. The incidence is unknown, but data on at least 111 cases have been reported by one author.

Symptoms, Signs and Laboratory Findings

The disease can produce neurologic dysfunction as in acute intermittent porphyria, and also can cause photosensitivity, which usually does not extend beyond the acute attack.

During asymptomatic periods the urine may be normal or there may be an increase of urinary coproporphyrin. Fecal coproporphyrin is increased during both symptomatic and asymptomatic periods. During acute attacks porphyrin precursor excretion is increased.

Diagnosis and Treatment

Findings are similar to those of acute intermittent porphyria. The diagnosis of an acute attack must be substantiated by demonstration of increased urinary PBG. A positive Watson-Schwartz or Hoesch test should be confirmed by quantitative determination of urinary PBG. The high fecal coproporphyrin excretion differentiates this disease from acute intermittent porphyria. The high fecal protoporphyrin in variegate porphyria differentiates it from acute intermittent porphyria and hereditary coproporphyria. **Treatment** of the acute attack is the same as for acute intermittent porphyria (see above).

PORPHYRIA CUTANEA TARDA

A type of porphyria that may be inherited or acquired that produces cutaneous lesions on exposed portions of the body, but no neurologic disease. Liver disease occurs in some patients.

Etiology, Genetics, and Incidence

The basic defect is a decrease of uroporphyrinogen decarboxylase activity, which is transmitted as an autosomal dominant defect. The decreased enzyme activity is demonstrable in circulating RBCs of patients with the genetically mediated form of the disease, but not in those with the acquired form, where the activity (but not the amount) of the hepatic enzyme is decreased. The prevalence is not known, but the disease is probably as common or more common than acute intermittent porphyria.

The factors that can activate this disease are alcohol, excess iron intake, and estrogen or oral contraceptives. Iron overload appears to be a major activating factor. This disease was formerly very uncommon in menstruating women, but as ingestion of all of the above precipitating factors increases, a number of young menstruating women are now victims of the active disease. In men, most cases occur after age 35. The effect of estrogen in men is seen in the number of cases of porphyria cutanea tarda that are reported in men receiving estrogen for carcinoma of the prostate.

Symptoms and Signs

The cutaneous manifestations begin as areas of erythema with vesicles or bullae that occur on exposed portions of the body, usually following minor trauma. Crusts and scabs develop, followed by scarring. Hirsutism, areas of pigmentation and depigmentation, and sclerodermoid changes may be evident as chronic lesions. The vesicles and bullae are usually most evident in sunny weather, particularly in late summer and autumn. Acute photosensitivity reactions are not common in this disease. In severe untreated cases, disfiguring changes can occur in the ears, nose, and fingers.

Liver disease is present in some patients with porphyria cutanea tarda. Histologically, the most frequent findings are siderosis and evidence of recurring liver damage. Some patients have frank cirrhosis. Liver fluorescence may be demonstrable. Chloroquine produces a reaction in this disease that can include fever, headache, malaise, abdominal pain, vomiting, and red urine. The latter results from a great increase of uroporphyrin excretion.

Laboratory Findings

Urinary uroporphyrin is considerably increased. Coproporphyrin is also increased in the urine, but usually not to the level seen with uroporphyrin. Some increase of ALA may occur, but there is no increase of PBG excretion. Porphyrins with 7, 6, and 5 carboxyl groups are also demonstrable in the urine. In recent years a group of tetracarboxylated porphyrins, the isocoproporphyrins, have been demonstrated in the feces in this disorder. In some patients there is an increase of serum iron and abnormal liver function tests.

Diagnosis

Vesicles, bullae, erosions, crusting, and chronic changes on exposed portions of the skin should raise the possibility of porphyria cutanea tarda. The skin lesions cannot be distinguished clinically from those of variegate porphyria. A high urinary uroporphyrin (which usually exceeds coproporphyrin) is present in porphyria cutanea tarda, and levels in this disease (untreated) are usually higher than the urinary uroporphyrin levels in patients with only cutaneous manifestations of variegate porphyria (where coproporphyrin often exceeds uroporphyrin). *Because treatment and prophylaxis of these diseases are different*, it is important to make the distinction between them. Variegate porphyria is accompanied by a high fecal protoporphyrin, which is not seen in porphyria cutanea tarda. Increased urinary PBG rules out porphyria cutanea tarda, but a slight increase of ALA does not. Two other measurements are specific for porphyria cutanea tarda, but are not yet widely available. These are decreased erythrocyte uroporphyrinogen decarboxylase (in the genetic form of the disease, but not the acquired form) and increased fecal isocoproporphyrin.

Treatment

The disease responds clinically and biochemically to iron removal by phlebotomy. If there are no contraindications to phlebotomy, 300 to 500 mL of blood can be removed about every 3 wk while Hb and urine porphyrin levels are monitored. If Hb decreases to < 11 gm/dL, phlebotomy is stopped until the level increases. Phlebotomy is then continued until urine uroporphyrin excretion is < 500 to 600 μg/day. In one study the mean amount of blood that had to be removed in order to produce a remission was 6.8 L (range: 2 to 14 L). Remissions usually last for years; recurrences can be retreated.

Since chloroquine can mobilize tissue porphyrins, it has been used to treat this disease. Only low doses can be used (125 mg twice a week) over a long time period (8 to 18 mo) because of the acute reaction to chloroquine described above. Occasionally, after a year of this drug therapy, the dosage must be doubled to 250 mg twice a week in order to achieve a remission. Phlebotomy is quicker in producing a remission and is the preferred method of treatment. Patients should be urged to avoid the precipitating factors mentioned above.

ALA Dehydrase Deficiency

A 50% decrease of ALA dehydrase (enzyme 2 of the heme biosynthetic pathway) has been described in a few asymptomatic individuals. Two unrelated male patients who experienced symptoms of an acute attack of porphyria were recently shown to have a profound (98 to 99%) deficiency of ALA dehydrase. A 50% decrease of activity was demonstrable in their parents. Since ALA dehydrase is normally present at levels that greatly exceed the rate limiting level for heme biosynthesis, it is likely that heterozygous (50%) deficiency of the enzyme will not produce disease, unless complicated by lead intoxication, whereas rare instances of homozygous deficiency may produce acute attacks of porphyria. The urine findings in this disorder are similar to those of lead intoxication, ie, increased ALA and coproporphyrin.

ANOMALIES IN AMINO ACID METABOLISM

(See Ch. 196)

GENETIC ABNORMALITIES OF CARBOHYDRATE METABOLISM

(See Ch. 196)

ANOMALIES IN LIPID METABOLISM

Abnormal levels of blood or tissue lipids resulting from metabolic disorders that may be inborn or due to endocrinopathy, specific organ failure, or external causes.

HYPERLIPOPROTEINEMIA

(Hyperlipidemia)

The major plasma lipids, including cholesterol and the triglycerides, do not circulate free in solution in the plasma, but are bound to proteins and transported as macromolecular complexes called lipoproteins. The major lipoprotein classes—chylomicrons, very low-density (prebeta) lipoproteins **(VLDL)**, low-density (β-) lipoproteins **(LDL)**, and high-density (α-) lipoproteins **(HDL)**—although closely interrelated, usually are classified in terms of their physicochemical properties, such as electrophoretic mobility, and density when separated in the ultracentrifuge. Triglycerides are the major lipids transported through the blood; between 70 and 150 gm enter and leave the plasma each day as compared to 1 to 2 gm of cholesterol or phospholipid. Chylomicrons, the largest lipoproteins, carry exogenous glyceride from the intestine via the thoracic duct to the venous system. In the capillaries of adipose tissue and muscle, 90% of chylomicron glyceride is removed by a specific group of lipases. Fatty acids and glycerol, derived from hydrolysis of chylomicrons, enter the cells for energy utilization or storage. The remnant chylomicron particles are then removed by the liver. VLDL carry endogenous glyceride primarily from the liver to the same peripheral sites for storage or utilization and are quickly degraded by lipases similar to those that act on chylomicrons. This endogenous VLDL rapidly becomes a lipoprotein of intermediate density **(IDL)** shorn of much of its glyceride and surface apoproteins. Within 2 to 6 h this IDL is degraded further through the removal of more glyceride to LDL which, in turn, has a plasma half-life of 3 to 4 days. VLDL is the main source of plasma LDL. The fate of LDL is unclear, but about 60% is removed by the liver, and active receptor sites have been found on the surface of fibroblasts and other cells that specifically bind to the major protein of LDL (which is apolipoprotein B) and remove most of the remainder from the circulation. A small, but important, portion of LDL appears to be removed from the circulation by nonreceptor mechanisms; eg, by ingestion of scavenger macrophages that may migrate into arterial walls, where their cholesterol contributes to the formation of "foam cells" of the atherosclerotic plaque.

Hypercholesterolemia can result from increased conversion of VLDL to LDL or defective clearance of LDL. Increased secretion of VLDL from the liver may be the result of obesity, diabetes mellitus, or a genetic disorder and each can result in increased LDL and cholesterol levels, frequently associated also with hypertriglyceridemia. Defective clearance of LDL may be due to diminished LDL receptors or their abnormal function. The degree of hypercholesterolemia that results depends on the severity of the abnormal activity of the LDL receptors.

Dietary cholesterol goes to the liver where the elevated concentrations suppress the synthesis of LDL receptors, reducing their number and resulting in increased plasma LDL and cholesterol levels. Saturated fatty acids also are known to increase plasma LDL and cholesterol levels; the mechanism of action is unknown, but is believed to be

related to reduced activity of LDL receptors. In the USA, dietary cholesterol and saturated fatty acid intake is high and is thought to account for almost 50 mg/dL of higher average blood levels of LDL—enough to significantly increase the risk of CHD. LDL receptor function abnormalities are also possible on the basis of molecular defects in the protein structure of the receptors which interferes with LDL binding; this is the mechanism of the genetic disorders described below.

Normal Levels of Serum Cholesterol and Triglycerides

It is difficult to define a normal level of serum cholesterol, since prospective studies have shown that the incidence of coronary heart disease **(CHD)** rises in linear fashion with the level of serum cholesterol, and values that are generally accepted as normal in the USA are higher than those found among comparable individuals in populations with a low incidence of atherosclerosis.

The optimal serum cholesterol for a middle-aged American man is probably 200 mg/dL, or less. For practical purposes hypercholesterolemia is defined as a value above the 95th percentile for the population, which in Americans ranges from 210 mg/dL in individuals < 20 yr old, to > 280 in individuals > 60 yr old. However, these limits are clearly excessive because of the known cardiovascular risk of cholesterol values at these levels, and a convenient rule of thumb is that any level of serum cholesterol > 180 mg/dL plus the person's age should be considered abnormal. Even these limits may be too high. (NOTE: In women, values are slightly higher [by 10 mg/dL] after the reproductive years and slightly lower in the 3rd through 5th decades. Mean values are lower among children before age 10 [125 to 190 mg/dL for boys and 130 to 195 mg/dL for girls].) The optimum recommendation may be to aim for levels ≤ 200 mg/dL.

In contrast to serum cholesterol, it is not clear that serum triglycerides are independent risk variables. Triglyceride levels, like cholesterol, vary with age and a serum triglyceride concentration of > 250 mg/dL is considered abnormal. While hypertriglyceridemia has not clearly been related to coronary artery disease risk, elevated triglycerides have been associated with diabetes, hyperuricemia, and pancreatitis.

As indicated below, even more information can be obtained about coronary risk by viewing the plasma cholesterol in terms of the units of lipid transport—the lipoproteins—than by a simple measurement of total cholesterol. Sixty to 75% of total plasma cholesterol is transported on LDL, the levels of which are directly related to cardiovascular risk. HDL, which normally accounts for 20 to 25% of the total plasma cholesterol, is *inversely* associated with cardiovascular risk. HDL levels are positively correlated with exercise and moderate alcohol intake and inversely related to smoking, obesity and the use of progestin-containing contraceptives.

Studies show CHD prevalence at HDL levels of 30 mg/dL to be more than double that at 60 mg/dL and familial excesses of HDL or deficiency of LDL have been associated with decreased CHD risk. These findings provide a cogent reason to determine whether elevated cholesterol levels are due to increases in LDL or to "benevolent" HDL. However, in countries where LDL levels are low, concentrations of HDL usually are also low, and yet the risk for CHD is low. Thus, the development of atherosclerosis appears to depend on high levels of LDL; HDL levels apparently are not as important when LDL levels are low.

Laboratory Methods

A useful clinical appraisal of lipids can usually be made by determining total serum cholesterol, HDL-cholesterol, and triglyceride levels for a serum sample obtained from a patient who has fasted for ≥ 12 h. The specimen should also be observed for a milky chylomicron layer after standing overnight in a refrigerator at 40 C.

Serum cholesterol may be determined by colorimetric, gas-liquid chromatographic, or enzymatic methods. Other automated "direct" methods have been developed. Enzymatic methods are usually most accurate.

TABLE 85–4. CHARACTERISTICS OF

Type	Other Names	Genetic Form	Plasma Cholesterol Level	Plasma Triglyceride Level
I	Exogenous hypertriglyceridemia Familial hyperglyceridemia Familial chylomicronemia Fat-induced hyperlipidemia Hyperchylomicronemia	Autosomal recessive; rare	Normal or slightly increased	Very greatly increased
II	Familial hypercholesterolemia Familial hyperbetalipoproteinemia Familial hypercholesterolemic xanthomatosis	Autosomal dominant; common	Greatly increased	(a) Normal (b) Slightly increased
III	Broad beta disease Familial dysbetalipoproteinemia Floating betalipoproteinemia	Mode of inheritance unclear; uncommon but not rare	Greatly increased	Greatly increased
IV	Endogenous hypertriglyceridemia Familial hyperprebetalipoproteinemia Carbohydrate-induced triglyceridemia	Common, often sporadic when familial; genetically heterogeneous	Normal or slightly increased	Greatly increased
V	Mixed hypertriglyceridemia Combined exogenous and endogenous hypertriglyceridemia Mixed hyperlipemia	Uncommon but not rare; genetically heterogeneous	Normal or slightly increased	Very greatly increased

Serum triglyceride usually is measured as glycerol either colorimetrically, enzymatically, or fluorometrically after hydrolysis of triglyceride to glycerol and formaldehyde.

LDL cholesterol is difficult to measure directly, but can be estimated from the following formula: LDL cholesterol = total cholesterol − HDL cholesterol − 1/5 triglyceride.

Lipoprotein electrophoresis is only useful when hyperlipidemia exists and should be preceded by serum triglyceride and cholesterol measurements. Electrophoretic methods should be used only when triglycerides or cholesterol are elevated or abnormally low, and not for routine screening.

Translating Hyperlipidemia to Hyperlipoproteinemia

Hyperlipidemia is the manifestation of a heterogeneous group of disorders differing in clinical features, prognosis, and therapeutic response. An excess in the serum level of any lipoprotein can result in hypercholesterolemia. Similarly, hypertriglyceridemia may result from increased levels of chylomicrons, VLDL, or both. This lack of speci-

THE PRIMARY HYPERLIPOPROTEINEMIAS

Risk for Atherosclerosis	*Major Secondary Causes*	*Clinical Presentation*	*Treatment*
Risk not increased	SLE; dysgammaglobulinemia; insulinopenic diabetes mellitus	Pancreatitis Eruptive xanthomas Hepatosplenomegaly Lipemia retinalis	Dietary: low intake of fat; no alcohol
Very strong risk, especially for coronary atherosclerosis	Excess dietary cholesterol; hypothyroidism; nephrosis; multiple myeloma; porphyria; obstructive liver disease	Accelerated atherosclerosis Xanthelasma Tendon and tuberous xanthomas Juvenile corneal arcus	Dietary: low-cholesterol, low-fat diet Drugs: cholestyramine; colestipol; niacin; probucol Possible surgery
Very strong risk for atherosclerosis, especially in peripheral and coronary arteries	Dysgamma-globulinemia; hypothyroidism	Accelerated atherosclerosis of coronary and peripheral vessels Planar xanthomas Tuboeruptive and tendon xanthomas	Dietary: reduction to ideal weight; maintenance of low-cholesterol, balanced diet Drugs: niacin; clofibrate
Possible risk, especially for coronary atherosclerosis	Excess alcohol consumption; oral contraceptives; diabetes mellitus; glycogen storage disease; pregnancy; nephrotic syndrome; stress	Possible accelerated atherosclerosis Glucose intolerance Hyperuricemia	Weight reduction; low-carbohydrate diet; no alcohol Drugs: niacin, gemfibrozil
Risk of athero-sclerosis not clearly increased	Alcoholism; insulin-dependent diabetes mellitus; nephrosis; dysgamma-globulinemia	Pancreatitis Eruptive xanthomas Hepatosplenomegaly Sensory neuropathy Lipemia retinalis Hyperuricemia Glucose intolerance	Weight reduction; low-fat diet; no alcohol Drugs: niacin, gemfibrozil

ficity makes translation of hyperlipidemia into hyperlipoproteinemia **(HLP)** useful. TABLE 85–4 describes 5 types of hyperlipoproteinemia. Each represents a shorthand or jargon term for the lipoproteins increased in the plasma. Since each lipoprotein class has a relatively fixed composition with respect to cholesterol and triglycerides, and since the 2 largest (chylomicrons and VLDL) refract light and cause plasma turbidity, hyperlipoproteinemia can be defined by observing a standing plasma sample, after 24 h storage at 4 C, followed by a more precise cholesterol and triglyceride assay. Electrophoresis usually is *not* required for the translation of hyperlipidemia into HLP.

Defining the lipoprotein pattern does not conclude the diagnostic process, since no HLP can be regarded as unique. Each may be *secondary* to other disorders that must be ruled out, such as hypothyroidism, alcoholism, and renal disease, or may be *primary* (usually familial), in which case family screening should be performed to identify other (often asymptomatic) hyperlipoproteinemic subjects.

In evaluating lipid or lipoprotein measurements, one must be aware of the follow-

ing: (1) The concentrations of lipids and lipoproteins increase with age. A value acceptable for a middle-aged adult might be alarmingly high in a child of 10. (2) Chylomicrons normally appear in the blood 2 to 10 h after a meal; therefore, a fasting specimen (12 to 16 h) should be used. (3) Lipoprotein concentrations are under dynamic metabolic control and are readily affected by diet, illness, drugs, and weight change. Lipid analysis should be done during a steady state. If abnormal, at least 2 confirmatory samples should be taken before selecting therapy (always dietary first). (4) When HLP is secondary to another disorder, treatment of that disorder usually will correct the HLP.

TYPE I HYPERLIPOPROTEINEMIA

(Exogenous Hypertriglyceridemia; Familial "Fat-Induced" Lipemia; Hyperchylomicronemia)

A relatively rare disorder due to a congenital deficiency of either lipoprotein lipase **(LPL)** *activity or of the lipase-activating protein apolipoprotein C-II. In either case the ability to remove or "clear" chylomicrons from the blood is impaired.*

Symptoms, Signs, and Diagnosis

This disease is manifested in children or young adults by pancreatitis-like abdominal pains; pinkish-yellow papular cutaneous deposits of fat (eruptive xanthomas), especially over pressure points and extensor surfaces; lipemia retinalis; and hepatosplenomegaly.

Symptoms and signs are exacerbated by increased dietary fat that accumulates in the circulation as chylomicrons, sometimes causing spectacular plasma triglyceride levels with marked lactescence. Chylomicrons not only refract light and produce lactescence, but also accumulate as a floating cream layer on standing overnight in the refrigerator. This cream layer overlying an otherwise clear plasma is often diagnostic, as is the failure of the lipoprotein lipase activity to increase after injection of IV heparin (**PHLA,** post-heparin lipolytic activity).

Prognosis

Pancreatitis is the principal sequela. Recurrent bouts of abdominal pain during periods of fat indulgence may be marked by severe and sometimes fatal hemorrhagic pancreatitis. Avoidance of dietary fat will prevent serious sequelae and allow for an otherwise normal life. There is no evidence that this form of HLP predisposes to atherosclerosis.

Treatment

The goal is reduction of circulating chylomicrons to avoid episodes of acute pancreatitis. Since hypertriglyceridemia is promoted by ingesting fat, whether it is saturated, unsaturated, or polyunsaturated, a diet markedly restricted in *all* common sources of fat is effective. Calories can be supplemented and diet palatability enhanced by using 20 to 40 gm of medium chain (C_{12} or less) triglycerides a day. These fatty acids are not transported via chylomicron formation, but are bound to albumin and pass directly through the portal system to the liver.

TYPE II HYPERLIPOPROTEINEMIA

(Familial Hypercholesterolemia; Hyperbetalipoproteinemia; Familial Hypercholesterolemic Xanthomatosis)

A genetic disorder of lipid metabolism characterized by elevated serum cholesterol in association with xanthelasma, tendon and tuberous xanthomas, arcus juvenilis, accelerated atherosclerosis, and early death from myocardial infarction. This disorder occurs most frequently with a familial distribution in the pattern of a dominant gene with complete penetrance. It appears to be caused by absent or defective LDL cell receptors resulting

in delayed LDL clearance, increased levels of plasma LDL, and accumulation of LDL cholesterol over joints, pressure points, and in blood vessels.

Symptoms, Signs, and Diagnosis

The patient may be asymptomatic or any of the aforementioned manifestations may be present. Xanthomas are usually in the Achilles, patellar, and digital extensor tendons. A family history of premature coronary heart disease (before age 55) may be present.

The serum cholesterol elevation in the presumed heterozygote may be as much as 2 to 3 times normal, all secondary to increased LDL. The plasma is usually translucent, since LDL does not refract light, regardless of its concentration, and triglyceride levels are normal or slightly increased. In the rare presumed homozygote with this disorder, cholesterol levels of 500 to 1200 mg/dL occur and are usually associated with xanthomas before age 10. A normal free cholesterol to cholesterol ester ratio and phospholipid level differentiate this disorder from the marked hypercholesterolemia (with clear plasma) seen in obstructive liver disease (see below and in CHOLESTASIS in Ch. 67).

Prognosis

The incidence of xanthomas and other external stigmas will increase with each decade in the presumed heterozygote with this disorder. Sometimes, especially in females, an Achilles tendonitis will recur. Atherosclerosis, especially of the coronary vessels, is markedly accelerated, particularly in males. One of 6 Type II males will have had a heart attack by age 40, and by age 60 the ratio increases to 2 of 3. Homozygotes with this disorder may develop and succumb to coronary atherosclerosis and its sequelae before age 20.

Treatment

With effective cholesterol lowering, an unsightly xanthoma will cease growing and regress or disappear. However, the major reason to treat with diets and cholesterol-lowering drugs is to decelerate the premature development of atherosclerosis and lessen the likelihood of an acute myocardial infarction.

Diet: The most effective dietary means of lowering serum LDL levels (cholesterol) has been strict avoidance of foods containing cholesterol and saturated fatty acids. The total amount of saturated fat in the diet of the average adult should be limited to 50 to 60 gm/day, accounting for < ⅓ of the 24-h calorie intake. Meat (especially organ meats and obvious fat), eggs, whole milk, cream, butter, lard, and other saturated cooking fats are eliminated and replaced with foods low in saturated fat and cholesterol (eg, fish, vegetables, poultry) and supplemented when necessary with polyunsaturated oils and margarines and mayonnaise made with polyunsaturated oils. Most vegetable oils (eg, corn oil, safflower oil) are poor in saturated fat and relatively rich in polyunsaturated fat, but some (eg, coconut and palm oils) are relatively rich in saturated fat.

Cholestyramine and colestipol, bile acid sequestrants, effectively lower serum cholesterol, especially when coupled with diet. A dosage of 12 to 32 gm orally in 2 to 4 divided daily doses will lower LDL levels (by increasing LDL removal) by 25 to 50%. Side effects, such as constipation and unpalatability, may limit general patient acceptance. Cholesterol reduction with cholestyramine reduces the number of cardiovascular events. **Niacin** may also be useful in Type II HLP, but the high dosage required (3 to 9 gm/day orally in divided doses with meals) coupled with its side effects of gastric irritability, hyperuricemia, hyperglycemia, flushing, and pruritus, often restricts its use. Niacin is most effective when combined with cholestyramine in the Type II homozygote or severe heterozygote. **Probucol** 500 mg orally bid may lower LDL levels 10 to 15% when added to diet, but it often has the additional undesirable side effect of lowering HDL levels. Thyroid analogs like **D-thyroxine** effectively lower LDL levels but are contraindicated in patients with suspected or proved heart disease. **Clofibrate** has

little effect on serum cholesterol or LDL levels in this disorder, may produce gallstones and other metabolic problems, and usually is not indicated. Other agents are generally less effective than strict dietary management.

Newer agents that enhance LDL receptor activity by competitively inhibiting the rate limiting enzyme for cholesterol biosynthesis (HMG CoA reductase) are promising but still investigational.

SECONDARY HYPERCHOLESTEROLEMIA

Hypercholesterolemia is common in **biliary cirrhosis,** as is a marked increase in the serum phospholipids and an abundant free cholesterol to cholesterol ester ratio. The serum is not lactescent because the overabundant lipoproteins (lipoproteins-x) are small and do not scatter light. Planar xanthomas and xanthelasma are common with prolonged and severe lipemia.

Hypercholesterolemia due to increased concentrations of LDL may be associated with **endocrinopathies** (hypothyroidism, hypopituitarism, diabetes mellitus) and usually is reversed by hormone therapy. Hypoproteinemias as seen in the **nephrotic syndrome,** metabolic aberrations such as **acute porphyria,** or **dietary excesses** with cholesterol-rich foods may also produce hyperbetalipoproteinemia. Cholesterol levels may be elevated secondary to increased concentrations of HDL in postmenopausal women or younger females taking oral contraceptives primarily containing estrogen.

TYPE III HYPERLIPOPROTEINEMIA

(Broad Beta Disease; Dysbetalipoproteinemia)

A less common familial disorder characterized by the accumulation in serum of a beta-migrating very low-density lipoprotein, rich in triglycerides and cholesterol, associated with tuboeruptive and pathognomonic planar (palmar) xanthomas and a marked predisposition to severe premature atherosclerosis. It is often associated with abnormalities of apolipoprotein E and defective conversion and removal of VLDL from the plasma. Though usually familial this type of HLP may be seen in dysproteinemias and hypothyroidism.

Symptoms, Signs, and Diagnosis

The disorder usually appears in early adulthood in males and is further delayed 10 to 15 yr in females. Peripheral vascular disease manifested by claudication or tuboeruptive xanthomas on the elbows and knees may be the first symptoms.

Serum may be cloudy to grossly turbid, often with a slight chylomicron layer. Both cholesterol and triglyceride levels are elevated, often equally. Precise definition of this abnormality requires ultracentrifugation and electrophoresis with the demonstration of a cholesterol-rich, beta-migrating VLDL. A mild abnormality in glucose tolerance and hyperuricemia may be present.

Prognosis

There is a marked predilection for early and severe coronary and peripheral artery disease. With treatment, hyperlipidemia can nearly always be reduced to normal and the peripheral vessel disease may abate.

Treatment

Weight reduction to ideal body weight and restriction of dietary cholesterol saturated fat and carbohydrate may suffice to reduce both cholesterol and triglyceride levels and result in marked regression of xanthomas. For those who do not respond adequately the addition of niacin 2 to 3 gm/day orally or clofibrate 2 gm/day orally is most effective and usually normalizes blood lipid levels.

Type IV Hyperlipoproteinemia

(Endogenous Hypertriglyceridemia; Hyperprebetalipoproteinemia)

A common disorder, often with a familial distribution, characterized by variable elevations of serum triglycerides, contained predominantly in very low-density (prebeta) lipoproteins and a possible predisposition to atherosclerosis. Depending on the level of endogenous triglyceride used to define Type IV HLP, the disorder is common in adult American middle-aged males.

Symptoms, Signs, and Diagnosis

This lipemia is frequently associated with mildly abnormal glucose tolerance curves and obesity, and may be exaggerated when dietary fat is restricted and carbohydrate added reciprocally (with caloric intake kept constant). Serum is turbid and triglyceride levels disproportionately elevated. Cholesterol may be normal or slightly increased (frequently secondary to stress, alcoholism, and dietary indiscretion) and may be associated with hyperuricemia.

Prognosis

The prognosis is uncertain. The disorder may be associated with premature coronary artery disease.

Treatment

Weight reduction, when applicable, is the most effective treatment and will often normalize the blood lipid levels. Maintenance of proper body weight and dietary restriction of carbohydrate and alcohol are important. Niacin 3 gm/day orally or gemfibrozil 0.6 to 1.2 gm/day orally in divided doses will further reduce the lipemia in those not controlled by diet.

Type V Hyperlipoproteinemia

(Mixed Hypertriglyceridemia; Mixed Hyperlipidemia; Hyperprebetalipoproteinemia with Chylomicronemia)

An uncommon disorder, sometimes familial, associated with defective clearance of exogenous and endogenous triglycerides and the risk of life-threatening pancreatitis.

Symptoms, Signs, and Diagnosis

This disorder usually first appears in early adulthood with showers of eruptive xanthomas over the extensor surfaces of the extremities, lipemia retinalis, hepatosplenomegaly, and abdominal pain. Symptoms are exacerbated by increased ingestion of dietary fats. Serum triglyceride levels usually are markedly elevated with only modest elevations in cholesterol. Serum is turbid to cloudy with a distinct cream layer on top. Levels of lipoprotein lipase are usually normal. Hyperuricemia, glucose intolerance, and obesity are common. This pattern may be secondary to alcoholism, nephrosis, starvation with refeeding, or severe insulinopenic diabetes.

Prognosis

The main risk is pancreatitis. Recurrent bouts may occur with fat indulgence and lead to pseudocyst formation, hemorrhage, and death. Peripheral neuropathy characterized primarily by dysthesia may occur and together with pancreatitis can usually be prevented by fat restriction. This form of HLP, like Type I, shows little predilection to atherosclerosis.

Treatment

Weight reduction is extremely effective, as in Types III and IV, and should be followed with a maintenance diet restricting all fats to < 50 gm/day together with alcohol restriction. Niacin 3 to 6 gm/day orally is effective. Gemfibrozil 1.2 gm/day orally may also be helpful.

SECONDARY HYPERTRIGLYCERIDEMIA

The most common forms of hypertriglyceridemia seen in clinical practice are not the primary (familial) types but those secondary to other disorders such as acute alcoholism, chronic severe uncontrolled diabetes mellitus (diabetic lipemia), nephrosis, and glycogenosis, and to drugs (estrogens, oral contraceptives, thiazides, corticosteroids, etc.). Any of the familial lipoprotein abnormalities may be mimicked or exacerbated. **Treatment** depends on reversal of the underlying disorder or withdrawal of the offending drug.

FAMILIAL LECITHIN CHOLESTEROL ACYLTRANSFERASE DEFICIENCY
(LCAT Deficiency)

A rare inheritable disorder, transmitted as a recessive trait, characterized by absence of the enzyme that normally esterifies cholesterol in the plasma, and manifested by marked hypercholesterolemia and hyperphospholipidemia (free cholesterol and lecithin), together with hypertriglyceridemia. Renal and liver failure, anemia, and lens opacities are common. **Treatment** with a fat-restricted diet reduces the concentration of lipoprotein complexes in plasma and may be of value in preventing kidney damage. Renal transplantation has been successfully performed for renal failure.

HYPOLIPOPROTEINEMIA
(Hypolipidemia)

Low lipoprotein levels in the serum seen as rare familial disorders, or secondary to hyperthyroidism, anemia, malabsorption, and malnutrition.

HYPOBETALIPOPROTEINEMIA

A rare inheritable disorder transmitted as a simple mendelian dominant trait and characterized by reduced levels of beta-lipoprotein (LDL). There are usually no signs or symptoms. Serum lipids are low with plasma cholesterol levels in the 70 to 120 mg/dL range despite normal food intake. Absorption of fat is normal. In the extremely rare homozygous forms of this disorder most of the symptoms and signs described for abetalipoproteinemia (see below) are applicable. Familial hypobetalipoproteinemia and familial hyperalphalipoproteinemia (also transmitted as a simple mendelian dominant trait) are associated with a decreased incidence of coronary artery disease and other atherosclerotic sequelae and have been referred to as the "longevity syndromes." No treatment is required.

ABETALIPOPROTEINEMIA
(Acanthocytosis; Bassen-Kornzweig Syndrome)

A rare congenital disorder usually transmitted as a recessive trait and characterized by the complete absence of beta-lipoproteins and by steatorrhea, acanthocytes (erythrocytes with spiny projections of the membrane), retinitis pigmentosa, ataxia, and mental retardation. Absorption of fat is markedly impaired. Neither chylomicrons or VLDL are formed. All serum lipids are significantly reduced and no postprandial lipemia can be demonstrated. There is no specific **treatment**. Parenteral and oral administration of massive doses of vitamins E and A may delay or retard the neurologic sequelae. (See also SPINOCEREBELLAR DEGENERATIONS in Ch. 128.)

TANGIER DISEASE
(Familial Alpha-Lipoprotein Deficiency)

A rare familial disorder characterized by recurrent polyneuropathy, lymphadenopathy, orange-yellow tonsillar hyperplasia, and hepatosplenomegaly (storage of cholesterol esters

in reticuloendothelial cells) associated with a marked decrease in high-density lipoproteins. Serum cholesterol is very low; triglycerides are normal or elevated. The disorder may manifest in adult life with hepatosplenomegaly or recurrent polyneuropathy. There is no treatment.

LIPIDOSES

GAUCHER'S DISEASE
(Glucosyl Cerebroside Lipidosis)

A familial disorder of lipid metabolism resulting in an accumulation of abnormal glucocerebrosides in reticuloendothelial cells, and manifested clinically by hepatosplenomegaly, skin pigmentation, skeletal lesions, and pingueculae. Although uncommon, it is the lipidosis most frequently seen by physicians.

Etiology and Pathology

The underlying defect appears to be a lack of glucocerebrosidase activity, which normally hydrolyzes glucocerebroside to glucose and ceramide. Inheritance is recessive. The condition usually appears in childhood, but onset may be in infancy or adult life. The characteristic pathologic finding is widespread reticulum cell hyperplasia. The cells are filled with glucocerebroside and a fibrillar cytoplasm, vary in shape, and have one or several small eccentrically placed nuclei. They are found in the liver, spleen, lymph nodes, and bone marrow.

Symptoms, Signs, Diagnosis, and Prognosis

Splenomegaly is the outstanding finding. Hepatomegaly and occasionally lymphadenopathy occur. Bone involvement may result in pain, and swelling of adjacent joints sometimes appears. Pingueculae and brown pigmentation of the skin may be present. Onset is more acute in infants (cerebral form); nuchal rigidity and opisthotonos may be noted. Splenic and marrow involvement frequently leads to pancytopenia. Epistaxis or other hemorrhages due to thrombocytopenia may occur. X-rays show flaring of the ends of the long bones and thinning of the cortex. Diagnosis is based on demonstration of the characteristic cells in bone marrow, splenic aspiration, or liver biopsy specimens, and may be confirmed by demonstrating the absence of glucocerebrosidase activity in cell culture. There are 3 major clinical forms due to differential cellular enzyme deficiency: Type I, the **adult** chronic nonneuronopathic form, which is the most common, manifest primarily by hypersplenism, splenomegaly, and bone lesions; Type II, the acute **infantile** neuronopathic form, associated with splenomegaly and severe neurologic abnormalities; and Type III, the **juvenile** form which may occur anytime in childhood, and combines the features of the adult chronic form with slowly progressive but usually milder neurologic dysfunction. Infants usually die within a year. Patients who survive to adolescence may live for many years.

Treatment

Splenectomy may be indicated in cases with anemia, leukopenia, or thrombocytopenia, or when the size of the spleen causes discomfort. Blood transfusions may be given for the anemia. Enzyme replacement by administration of glucocerebrosidase may be useful; however, this procedure is still under study.

NIEMANN-PICK DISEASE
(Sphingomyelin Lipidosis)

A familial disorder of lipid metabolism in which sphingomyelin (ceramide phosphorylcholine) accumulates in the reticuloendothelial cells. There are at least 5 different forms of this lipidosis characterized by different levels of sphingomyelinase. The enzyme is absent in the severe juvenile form. Demyelination and neurologic symptoms may be

seen. The infantile and juvenile forms are inherited as recessive traits, appearing most often in Jewish families. Patients may show xanthomas, pigmentation, hepatosplenomegaly, lymphadenopathy, and mental retardation. Pancytopenia is common. Diagnosis may be made by tissue biopsy and confirmed by enzyme assay. Absence of the sphingomyelin-cleaving enzyme can be demonstrated in both biopsy specimens and tissue culture. Serum lipids usually are normal. **Treatment** at present is supportive; there is no specific therapy.

FABRY'S DISEASE
(Angiokeratoma Corporis Diffusum Universale; α-Galactosidase Deficiency)

A rare, familial, sex-linked disorder of lipid metabolism in which glycolipid (galactosylgalactosylglucosyl ceramide) accumulates in many tissues. The metabolic abnormality is due to the absence of the lysosomal enzyme α-galactosidase A needed for the normal catabolism of trihexosyl ceramide. Clinical recognition in males results from characteristic skin lesions (angiokeratomas) over the lower trunk. Patients may have corneal opacities, febrile episodes, and burning pain in the extremities. Death results from renal failure, or cardiac or cerebral complications of hypertension or other vascular disease. Heterozygous females may exhibit the disorder in an attenuated form and are most likely to show corneal opacities. Enzymatic replacement of the deficient enzyme by transfusion is being explored and may have potential therapeutic value. Treatment is otherwise supportive, especially during periods of pain and fever.

WOLMAN'S DISEASE
(Acid Cholesteryl Ester Hydrolase Deficiency)

A familial autosomal recessive disease characterized by hepatosplenomegaly, steatorrhea, and adrenal calcification manifested in the first weeks of life. Large amounts of neutral lipids, particularly cholesteryl esters and glycerides, accumulate in the body tissues. Deficiency of an acid lipase has been described. There is no specific therapy, and death usually occurs by 6 mo of age.

CHOLESTERYL ESTER STORAGE DISEASE

An extremely rare familial autosomal recessive disease characterized by hepatomegaly and accumulation of cholesteryl esters and triglycerides mainly in lysosomes in the liver, spleen, lymph nodes, and other tissues. Hyperbetalipoproteinemia is common and premature atherosclerosis may be severe. A deficiency in cholesteryl ester hydrolase has been described. Patients may be asymptomatic. Diagnosis is made by liver biopsy. There is no treatment.

CEREBROTENDINOUS XANTHOMATOSIS
(van Bogaert's Disease)

A rare recessive familial disorder characterized by progressive ataxia, dementia, cataracts, and tendon xanthomas. Cholestanol (dihydrocholesterol), which is usually barely detectable in the body, is found in increased concentrations in the nervous system, lungs, blood, and xanthomas. The underlying defect involves a deficiency of a hepatic enzyme that catalyzes the 24S hydroxylation of an intermediate sterol in the bile acid synthetic pathway. Though plasma cholesterol levels are usually low or normal, premature atherosclerosis also occurs. Disability is progressive, though often not manifested until after age 30. Treatment with chenodiol (0.5 to 1.5 gm/day), which inhibits normal bile acid synthesis, reduces plasma cholesterol and may prevent further progression of the disease.

β-Sitosterolemia and Xanthomatosis

A rare recessive familial disease characterized by the accumulation of plant sterols in the blood and tissues and by the occurrence of tendon and tuberous xanthomas, premature atherosclerosis, and abnormal RBCs. Increased intestinal absorption of dietary β-sitosterol has been demonstrated. Treatment consists in reducing the intake of foods rich in plant sterols (such as vegetable oils), and administering cholestyramine resin to promote sterol excretion.

Refsum's Syndrome
(Phytanic Acid Storage Disease)

A rare recessive familial disorder of phytanic acid metabolism characterized clinically by peripheral neuropathy, cerebellar ataxia, retinitis pigmentosa, and bone and skin changes. The disorder is due to a deficiency of phytanic acid hydroxylase, an enzyme that metabolizes phytanic acid. It is associated with marked accumulation of phytanic acid in the plasma and tissues. (See also Table 128–1 in Ch. 128.) A diet deficient in phytanic acid ("chlorophyll free") is beneficial. Serial plasmapheresis may help keep plasma phytanic acid levels down.

Other Lipidoses

Several rare inheritable lipidoses have been demonstrated using sophisticated technics of tissue culture and enzyme analysis. The more common ones are described.

Tay-Sachs disease (G_{M2} gangliosidosis) is characterized by very early onset, progressive retardation in development, paralysis, dementia, blindness, cherry red retinal spots, and death by age 3 or 4. This recessive disorder is most common in families of Eastern European Jewish origin and is caused by deficiency of the enzyme hexosaminidase A, resulting in accumulation of gangliosides (complex sphyngolipids) in the brain. An infantile disorder often fatal by age 2 is **generalized (G_{M1}) gangliosidosis** in which the ganglioside G_{M1} accumulates in the nervous system. In **sulfatide lipidosis (metachromatic leukodystrophy)** there is a deficiency of the enzyme cerebroside sulfatase, causing metachromatic lipids to accumulate in the white matter of the CNS, peripheral nerves, kidney, spleen, and other visceral organs. It is characterized by progressive paralysis and dementia usually beginning before age 2 and fatal by age 10. **Galactosyl ceramide lipidosis,** also known as **Krabbe's disease** or **globoid leukodystrophy,** is a fatal infantile disorder characterized by progressive retardation, paralysis, blindness, deafness, and pseudobulbar palsy. This familial condition is secondary to a deficiency of galactocerobroside β-galactosidase. **Diagnosis** of these disorders may be made *prenatally* from amniotic fluid. No specific therapy is known.

ANOMALIES IN KIDNEY TRANSPORT
(See in Ch. 187)

---

86. AMYLOIDOSIS

Accumulation in the tissues of the fibrillar protein amyloid usually in amounts sufficient to impair normal function.

Pathophysiology and Classification

The cause of amyloid production and its deposition in tissues is unknown. Immunologic derangements have been implicated—B cell activation, T cell suppression, mac-

rophage involvement—but all such abnormalities have been nonspecific. In the different biochemical types of amyloid, etiologic mechanisms may vary. For example, in secondary amyloid (see below), a defect in the metabolism of the precursor protein may exist, while in hereditary amyloid a genetically variant protein appears to be present. Under light microscopy amyloid is a homogeneous, highly refractile substance with an affinity for Congo red dye, both in fixed tissues and in vivo. On electron microscopy amyloid consists of 100 Å fibrils; on x-ray diffraction it has a cross beta pattern.

Biochemically, however, 3 major types of amyloid and several less common forms have been defined. One has an N-terminal sequence that is homologous with a portion of the variable region of an immunoglobulin light chain termed AL and is seen in patients with primary amyloidosis, and that associated with multiple myeloma. The second has a unique N-terminal sequence of a non-immunoglobulin protein called AA protein and is seen in patients with secondary amyloidosis. The third type, which is associated with familial amyloid polyneuropathy, is a prealbumin molecule that appears to have a single amino acid substitution. The chemical structure of amyloid associated with aging in skin, and with endocrine organs may represent other biochemical forms of amyloid. Chemical analyses relating to various forms of amyloidosis may lead to a more refined classification.

At present, 2 major clinical forms are recognized, though differentiation is not always clearcut. Amyloidosis is classified as **primary** when there is no associated disease and **secondary** or **acquired** when associated with chronic diseases, either infectious (tuberculosis, bronchiectasis, osteomyelitis, leprosy) or inflammatory (rheumatoid arthritis, granulomatous ileitis). Amyloid is also found in association with multiple myeloma, Hodgkin's disease, other tumors, and familial Mediterranean fever. Amyloid may accompany aging and appear in familial forms unassociated with other disease, often with distinctive types of neuropathy, nephropathy, and cardiopathy. Amyloid is found in the histopathologic lesions of Alzheimer's disease.

In **primary amyloidosis,** the heart, lung, skin, tongue, thyroid gland, and intestinal tract may be involved. Localized amyloid "tumors" may be found in the respiratory tract or other sites. Parenchymal organs (liver, spleen, kidney) and the vascular system are frequently involved.

Secondary amyloidosis shows a predilection for the spleen, liver, kidney, adrenals, and lymph nodes. However, no organ system is spared and vascular involvement may be widespread. The liver and spleen are often enlarged, firm, and rubbery. The kidneys are usually enlarged. Spleen sections show large, translucent, waxy areas where the normal malpighian bodies are replaced by pale amyloid, producing the **"sago" spleen.**

Amyloid associated with certain malignancies (eg, multiple myeloma) tends to be widespread and present in nontumorous organs; with others (eg, medullary carcinoma of the thyroid gland) it may have a strictly local occurrence in association with the tumor, although it may occur in metastases. It has a high association in the pancreas with adult onset diabetes mellitus.

Symptoms and Signs

Manifestations are nonspecific, determined by the organ or system affected and often are obscured by the underlying disease, which may be fatal before secondary amyloidosis is suspected. The nephrotic syndrome is the most striking manifestation. In the early stages only slight proteinuria may be noted; later the distinctive symptom complex develops with anasarca, hypoproteinemia, and massive proteinuria. Amyloid disease of the liver produces hepatomegaly, but rarely jaundice. Liver function tests usually are normal, although abnormal BSP excretion or elevated alkaline phosphatase may be observed. Occasionally, portal hypertension may occur with esophageal varices and ascites. Massive hepatomegaly (liver weight > 7 kg) has been reported. Skin le-

sions may be waxy or translucent; purpura may result from amyloidosis of small cutaneous vessels. Cardiac involvement is common and may manifest itself as cardiomegaly, intractable heart failure, or any of the common arrhythmias. Atrial standstill has been found in several kinships. GI amyloid may cause esophageal motility abnormalities, gastric atony, small and large intestinal motility abnormalities, malabsorption, bleeding, or pseudo-obstruction. Macroglossia is common in primary and myeloma-related amyloid. A firm, symmetric, nontender goiter resembling Hashimoto's or Riedel's struma may result from amyloidosis of the thyroid gland. Amyloid arthropathy may mimic RA in some cases of multiple myeloma. Peripheral neuropathy is common in some familial amyloidoses, and is also seen in some cases of primary or myeloma-associated amyloid. Lung involvement may be characterized by focal pulmonary nodules, tracheobronchial lesions, or diffuse alveolar deposits.

Diagnosis

Amyloidosis is suspected on the basis of symptoms and signs described above, but can be diagnosed only by biopsy. Subcutaneous abdominal fat pad aspiration or biopsy of rectal mucosa are the best screening tests. Other useful biopsy sites are gingiva, skin, nerve, kidney, and liver. Tissue sections should be stained with Congo red dye and observed with a polarizing microscope for the characteristic green birefringence of amyloid.

Prognosis

In secondary amyloidosis, prognosis depends on successful treatment of the underlying disease. All forms of renal amyloidosis carry a poor prognosis, but with supportive therapy (eg, eradication of pyelonephritis), patients may remain stable and even improve. Amyloidosis associated with multiple myeloma has the poorest prognosis, early death within 1 to 2 yr being common. Localized amyloid tumors may be removed without recurrence. Myocardial amyloidosis is the commonest cause of death, primarily due to arrhythmias or intractable cardiac failure. Prognosis in familial amyloidoses varies with each kinship.

Treatment

Therapy is directed first to the underlying cause. If this can be controlled, amyloidosis may be arrested. Management of amyloidosis itself is generally symptomatic. Kidney transplantation has been performed in a few patients with renal amyloid; however, it is technically difficult due to the potential for bleeding. Amyloid will ultimately recur in a donor kidney, but several recipients have done very well and lived up to 10 yr. Corticosteroids or immunosuppressive agents are not of proven value. Digitalis should be used with care in amyloid heart disease, since it may precipitate arrhythmias. Colchicine has been used to prevent the acute attacks of familial Mediterranean fever, and it has been suggested that patients so treated develop no new amyloid. Clinical trials are in progress to determine if colchicine alleviates primary or secondary amyloid.

§8. ENDOCRINE DISORDERS

---

87. HYPOTHALAMIC-PITUITARY RELATIONSHIPS

The pituitary gland (hypophysis) can no longer be considered the "master gland." The hypothalamus is the final common pathway directing input to the pituitary, and it in turn receives input from virtually all other areas of the CNS.

The hypothalamus modulates the activities of the anterior and posterior lobes of the pituitary in 2 distinct ways. Neurohormones synthesized in the hypothalamus reach the **anterior pituitary (adenohypophysis)** directly through a specialized portal vascular system. These neurohormones regulate the synthesis and secretion of the 6 major peptide hormones of the anterior pituitary; the pituitary hormones in turn regulate peripheral endocrine glands (thyroids, adrenals, gonads) as well as growth and lactation. No direct neural connection exists between the hypothalamus and the anterior pituitary. In contrast, the **posterior pituitary (neurohypophysis)** is composed of axons originating in neuronal cell bodies located in the hypothalamus. These axons serve as storage sites for 2 peptide hormones synthesized in the hypothalamus that act in the periphery to regulate water balance, milk ejection, and uterine contraction.

It appears that virtually all hormones produced by the hypothalamus and the pituitary are secreted in a pulsatile or burst-like fashion with brief periods of inactivity and activity interspersed. In addition, some of the hormones (eg, ACTH, growth hormone, prolactin) have definite circadian or diurnal rhythmicity with increased secretion during specific hours of the day; other hormones (eg, LH and FSH during the menstrual cycle) have still longer ultradian rhythms.

Neurohypophyseal (Posterior Pituitary) Function

The posterior pituitary secretes **antidiuretic hormone (ADH, vasopressin)** and **oxytocin.** Each contains 9 amino acids and is synthesized in separate cells in both the supraoptic and paraventricular nuclei of the hypothalamus. Each peptide is synthesized as part of a larger precursor protein and remains bound to a portion of the precursor, termed **neurophysin,** with which it is transported down the axons and stored in secretory granules in nerve terminals in the posterior pituitary. ADH and oxytocin are secreted in response to neural impulses, rapidly dissociate from their neurophysins, and are rapidly cleared from the circulation with half-lives of about 10 min. Any functions for the neurophysins are unknown.

The major action of ADH is to promote water conservation by the kidney. At high concentrations it also causes vasoconstriction. Like aldosterone, ADH plays an important role in maintaining fluid homeostasis and vascular and cellular hydration. The main stimulus to ADH release is increased osmotic pressure of body water, sensed by osmoreceptors in the hypothalamus. Volume depletion, sensed by baroreceptors in the left atrium, pulmonary veins, carotid sinus, and aortic arch, is the second major stimulus to ADH secretion, and is transmitted to the CNS through the vagus and glossopharyngeal nerves. ADH release is also stimulated by pain, stress, exercise, hypoglycemia cholinergic agonists, β-adrenergic agonists, angiotensin, prostaglandins, etc. Alcohol, α-adrenergic agonists, glucocorticoids, etc, *inhibit* ADH secretion.

Diabetes insipidus results either from lack of ADH **(central diabetes insipidus)** or from inability of the kidney to respond normally to ADH **(nephrogenic diabetes insipidus)** These disorders are discussed further in Ch. 88. Hypophysectomy (removal of the pituitary gland) does not usually result in permanent diabetes insipidus, because a number of ADH-containing neurons terminate in the median eminence of the hypothalamus and continue to function.

The 2 major targets for oxytocin are the myoepithelial cells of the breast, which surround the alveoli of the mammary gland, and smooth muscle cells of the uterus. In response to oxytocin stimulated by suckling, the myoepithelial cells contract and milk is moved from the alveoli to large sinuses for ejection (ie, the milk "letdown" reflex of nursing mothers). Oxytocin stimulates contraction of uterine smooth muscle cells and uterine sensitivity to oxytocin increases throughout pregnancy, but plasma concentrations do not increase sharply during parturition and the role of oxytocin in the initiation of labor is unclear.

Hypothalamic Control of the Anterior Pituitary (Adenohypophysis)

Upon reaching the anterior pituitary through the portal vascular system, the various **releasing** and **inhibiting hormones** secreted by the hypothalamus bind to specific cell membrane receptors and initiate sequences of metabolic steps stimulating or inhibiting release of pituitary hormones into the general circulation. Thus far, 6 hypothalamic neurohormones have been identified (see TABLE 87-1). With the exception of the biogenic amine dopamine, all are small peptides. Several are produced in the periphery as well as in the hypothalamus and also function in local paracrine systems, especially in the GI tract. These neurohormones may control release of more than 1 pituitary hormone, but are quite specific in their effects. Regulation of most anterior pituitary hormones depends on positive stimulatory signals from the hypothalamus; only prolactin is primarily under inhibitory control (see below).

Thyrotropin-releasing hormone (TRH) stimulates synthesis and secretion of both **thyroid-stimulating hormone (TSH)** and **prolactin (PRL).** It is not known if the release of PRL by TRH is physiologic. Under pathologic conditions TRH may also stimulate growth hormone **(GH)** production and release.

Gonadotropin-releasing hormone (GnRH), also known as **luteinizing-hormone releasing hormone (LHRH),** stimulates secretion of both **luteinizing hormone (LH)** and **follicle-stimulating hormone (FSH)** physiologically and when administered exogenously in a pulsatile fashion. When exogenous GnRH is administered as a continuous infusion, LH and FSH release are stimulated initially but are soon inhibited due to down regulation of GnRH receptors by the GnRH. This observation has led to the development of long-acting agonists of GnRH that have great potential use in clinical situations where "medical castration" might be warranted (see PRECOCIOUS PUBERTY in Ch. 202). GnRH may also stimulate PRL release in certain situations.

Somatostatin exerts *negative* control over both GH and TSH synthesis and secretion. GH release is stimulated by **growth hormone-releasing hormone (GRH)** and inhibited by somatostatin, with the rate of GH production depending on the relative strength of these 2 stimuli.

Corticotropin-releasing hormone (CRH) stimulates release of ACTH from the pituitary.

TABLE 87-1. HYPOTHALAMIC NEUROHORMONES

Neurohormone	*Structure*	*Hormones Affected*	*Effect*
Thyrotropin releasing hormone (TRH)	Peptide with 3 amino acids	TSH PRL	Stimulate Stimulate
Gonadotropin releasing hormone (GnRH)	Peptide with 10 amino acids	LH FSH PRL (?)	Stimulate* Stimulate* Stimulate (?)*
Dopamine	Biogenic amine	PRL LH FSH TSH	Inhibit Inhibit Inhibit Inhibit
Corticotropin releasing hormone (CRH)	Peptide with 41 amino acids	ACTH	Stimulate
Growth hormone-releasing hormone (GRH)	Peptide with 40–44 amino acids	GH	Stimulate
Somatostatin	Peptide with 14 amino acids	GH TSH	Inhibit Inhibit

*Under physiologic conditions and when administered exogeneously in intermittent pulses (see text).

Dopamine appears to be the primary factor regulating PRL release and is inhibitory. Under certain circumstances dopamine can also inhibit LH, FSH, and TSH release.

Many hypothalamic abnormalities (including neoplasms, encephalitis, and other inflammatory lesions) may alter secretion of hypothalamic neurohormones and thus affect pituitary function. Clinical syndromes that occur as a result of such lesions present as aberrations of pituitary hormone function and are discussed in detail in Ch. 88. Since the various neurohormones are synthesized in different centers within the hypothalamus, it is not uncommon for only one or some of the neuropeptides to be affected. In **Kallmann's syndrome,** for example, a deficiency in hypothalamic GnRH leads to hypogonadism (see SECONDARY HYPOGONADISM in THE TESTES in Ch. 196). However, hypothalamic lesions may decrease secretion of all hypothalamic neurohormones, producing secondary panhypopituitarism with hyperprolactinemia and galactorrhea (due to decreased release of dopamine). Hypothalamic lesions can also lead to *hyper*secretion of neurohormones and may be responsible for some cases of precocious puberty and Cushing's syndrome.

Anterior Pituitary Anatomy and Function

The pituitary gland, which weighs about 500 mg, is located in a bony cavity, the sella turcica, in the base of the skull, and is composed of functionally and anatomically distinct **anterior** and **posterior lobes.** An **intermediate lobe** located between the anterior and posterior lobes is present in some species and during fetal development in humans but appears to be largely vestigial in adults. Expansion of the pituitary due to tumor formation can occur superiorly, compromising the optic chiasm and leading to visual loss, or laterally, with compression of the cavernous sinuses containing cranial nerves. The cells of the anterior lobe, which comprises 80% of the pituitary by weight and is derived from an outpouching of oral ectoderm, synthesize and release several protein hormones that are necessary for normal growth and development and also stimulate the activity of several target glands.

Adrenocorticotropic hormone (ACTH) is a single chain polypeptide containing 39 amino acids. Biologic activity resides in its N-terminal 20 amino acids. CRH is the primary agent that simulates ACTH release, and ACTH stimulates the adrenal cortex to secrete cortisol and several weak androgens. The CRH-ACTH-cortisol axis is central to the response to stress, and in the absence of ACTH, the adrenal cortex atrophies and secretion of cortisol virtually ceases.

Several peptide hormones are derived from a common precursor, **pro-opiomelanocorticotropin (POMC),** which gives rise to **ACTH, β-lipotropin (β-LPH), α-** and **β-melanocyte stimulating hormone (MSH), enkephalins,** and **endorphins.** POMC is present in both the anterior and pituitary lobes of the pituitary and in the hypothalamus, but the active hormones formed from this precursor differ in each site where it is present, depending on variations in enzymatic processing. Thus, ACTH and β-LPH (with a small amount of additional processing to form α-LPH and β-endorphin) are the predominant hormones synthesized in the anterior lobe, while almost all β-LPH is cleaved to form α-LPH and β-endorphin, and ACTH is cleaved to form **corticotropin-like intermediate lobe peptide (CLIP,** corresponding to ACTH 18–39) and α-MSH (corresponding to ACTH 1–13) in the intermediate lobe. In addition, the formation of POMC within the intermediate lobe appears to be regulated primarily by dopamine and serotonin, while CRH is the important regulatory agent in the anterior lobe. POMC and MSH can cause hyperpigmentation of skin and are only significant in disorders in which ACTH levels are markedly elevated (ie, Addison's disease and Nelson's syndrome). Enkephalins and endorphins are considered endogenous opioids and bind to and activate opioid receptors throughout the CNS.

The pituitary glycoprotein hormones—TSH, LH, and FSH—and the placental hormone **human chorionic gonadotropin (HCG),** are each composed of α and β subunits.

The α subunits of all these hormones are identical, whereas the sequences of the β subunits differ.

TSH regulates the structure and function of the thyroid gland and stimulates synthesis and release of thyroid hormones. TSH synthesis and secretion are controlled by the hypothalamic hormone, TRH, and by circulating thyroid hormone from the periphery.

Synthesis and secretion of both LH and FSH are stimulated by a single hypothalamic neurohormone, GnRH (or LHRH). In women, LH and FSH are necessary to stimulate ovarian follicular development and ovulation, as discussed in Ch. 169. In males, FSH acts on Sertoli cells and is essential for spermatogenesis and LH acts on the Leydig cells of the testis to stimulate testosterone biosynthesis. These actions are discussed in Ch. 196.

Human GH is a single chain polypeptide that is structurally similar to the placental hormone **human chorionic somatomammotropin (hCS)** and less similar to PRL. GRH is the major stimulator and **somatostatin** is the major inhibitor of the synthesis and secretion of GH. The major actions of GH are stimulation of somatic growth and regulation of metabolism. Growth is mediated in large part by **somatomedins,** insulin-like growth factors whose synthesis is controlled by GH. The metabolic effects of GH are biphasic. Acutely, GH exerts insulin-like effects, increasing glucose uptake in muscle and fat, stimulating amino acid uptake and protein synthesis in liver and muscle, and inhibiting lipolysis in adipose tissue. Several hours after GH administration, these effects disappear and the more profound metabolic effects of GH occur. These later effects, which persist with prolonged elevations in plasma GH, are antiinsulin-like. Glucose uptake and utilization are inhibited, causing plasma glucose to rise, and lipolysis increases, causing plasma free fatty acids to rise. GH, which rises during fasting, is important in the body's adaptation to lack of food. Along with cortisol, epinephrine, and glucagon, GH maintains blood glucose for CNS use and mobilizes fat as an alternative metabolic fuel.

Lactotrophs producing PRL constitute approximately 30% of the cells of the anterior pituitary. The pituitary doubles in size during pregnancy largely because of hyperplasia and hypertrophy of lactotrophs. In humans the major function of PRL is regulation of milk production. Although PRL has many other effects in other species, it is not clear that it has any other significant actions in humans. **Dopamine,** which inhibits its synthesis and release, is the major regulator of PRL. When the pituitary stalk (connecting the pituitary to the hypothalamus) is severed, PRL secretion increases whereas secretion of all other anterior pituitary hormones decreases. PRL is the most frequent hormone produced in excess by pituitary tumors.

88. PITUITARY

Relationships between the hypothalamus and the pituitary gland, as well as pituitary structure and function, are discussed in Ch. 87.

Patients with hypothalamic-pituitary disorders present with some combination of (1) symptoms of a mass lesion (ie, headaches, visual field defects), (2) hypersecretion of one or more pituitary hormones, or (3) hyposecretion of one or more pituitary hormones. Other hypothalamic functions may be affected as well. Syndromes of hypo- or hyperpituitary secretion are the most common presenting complaints of patients with pituitary or hypothalamic neoplasms, but may be based on other etiologies. A mass involving the hypothalamus or pituitary also should be suspected if the sella turcica is enlarged on skull x-ray or if neurologic symptoms and signs suggestive of compression of the optic chiasm are present (especially bilateral hemianopsia). The chance finding of an enlarged sella turcica on skull x-ray obtained for other reasons is not uncommon.

If there is no endocrine or visual disorder, the enlarged sella may represent the

empty sella syndrome. Diagnosis can be confirmed by CT scan. Pituitary functions in such patients are most frequently normal. The typical patient with this syndrome is female (over 80%), obese (about 75%), hypertensive (30%), and may have benign intracranial hypertension (10%) and rhinorrhea (10%). Occasionally, affected patients may have small coexisting pituitary tumors secreting growth hormone, prolactin, or ACTH. No specific therapy is needed for an empty sella alone.

ANTERIOR LOBE DISORDERS

HYPOFUNCTION OF THE ANTERIOR PITUITARY

(Hypopituitarism in children [pituitary dwarfism] is discussed in Ch. 196)

Hypopituitarism in the Adult

Endocrine deficiency syndromes due to partial or complete loss of anterior lobe pituitary function. The more common causes are listed in Table 88–1.

Symptoms and Signs

The symptoms and signs of hypopituitarism relate to the underlying cause and to the specific pituitary hormones that are absent. The onset is most often insidious and may not be recognized as abnormal by the patient but occasionally may be sudden or dramatic. Gonadotropins are usually lost first, followed by GH, and finally by TSH and ACTH. ADH deficiency is rare in primary pituitary disease but is common with stalk and hypothalamic lesions. The function of all target glands will decrease when all hormones are deficient **(panhypopituitarism).** Lack of LH and FSH in women leads to amenorrhea, regression of secondary sexual characteristics, and infertility; few if any symptoms result in castrate or postmenopausal women. Lack of the gonadotropins in men results in impotence, testicular atrophy, regression of secondary sexual characteristics, and decreased spermatogenesis with consequent infertility. GH deficiency is generally not clinically detectable in adults. TSH deficiency leads to hypothyroidism, and ACTH deficiency results in hypoadrenalism with attendant fatigue, hypotension, and intolerance to stress and infection. In **Sheehan's syndrome,** as a result of pituitary necrosis from hypovolemia and shock in the immediate peri-partum period, lactation may not develop postpartum, the patient may complain of fatigue, and loss of pubic and axillary hair may occur. **Isolated pituitary hormone deficiencies** are usually identified in childhood or in the teenage years because of failure to grow or failure to achieve pubescence.

Diagnosis

Hypopituitarism must be established with certainty before committing the patient to a lifetime of hormonal replacement therapy. Evidence of structural pituitary abnormalities and of hormonal deficiencies should be sought. X-rays of the sella turcica and formal visual field testing will demonstrate tumors. High resolution CT scanning with contrast media as required is the procedure of choice in the diagnosis of pituitary adenomas. Polytomography of the sella turcica remains a primary diagnostic tool where high resolution CT is unavailable. Cerebral angiography is indicated only when dynamic CT scanning suggests the possibility of perisellar vascular anomalies or aneurysms. A simple coned down lateral x-ray of the sella turcica remains a reasonable screening procedure for macroadenomas of the pituitary with a diameter of > 10 mm where modern neuroradiologic facilities are unavailable.

When panhypopituitarism is suspected, initial evaluation should be aimed at detecting TSH and ACTH deficiencies, as both are potentially life-threatening.

To evaluate the patient for hypothyroidism, T_4, T_3, and TSH levels can be determined by radioimmunoassay. All should be low since elevated TSH levels indicate a primary

TABLE 88–1. CAUSES OF HYPOPITUITARISM

I. Causes Primarily Affecting the Pituitary Gland (Primary Hypopituitarism)

- A. Pituitary tumors
  1. Adenomas
  2. Craniopharyngiomas
- B. Infarction or ischemic necrosis of the pituitary
  1. Shock, especially postpartum (Sheehan's syndrome), or in diabetes mellitus or sickle cell anemia
  2. Vascular thrombosis or aneurysms, especially of the internal carotid artery
  3. Sarcoidosis
- C. Inflammatory processes
  1. Meningitis (tubercular, fungal, malarial)
  2. Pituitary abscesses
- D. Infiltrative disorders
  1. Hand-Schüller-Christian Disease (histiocytosis X)
  2. Hemochromatosis
- E. Isolated or multiple pituitary hormone deficiencies
- F. Iatrogenic
  1. Irradiation
  2. Surgical extirpation
- G. Autoimmune dysfunction of the pituitary

II. Causes Primarily Affecting the Hypothalamus (Secondary Hypopituitarism)

- A. Hypothalamic tumors
  1. Pinealomas
  2. Meningiomas
  3. Ependymomas
  4. Metastatic neoplasms
- B. Inflammatory processes, such as sarcoidosis
- C. Trauma
- D. Isolated or multiple neurohormone deficiences of the hypothalamus
- E. Surgical transection of the pituitary stalk

abnormality of the thyroid gland (see Ch. 89). The administration of 200 to 500 μg protirelin (synthetic TRH) given IV over 15 to 30 sec may help to identify those patients with hypothalamic as opposed to intrinsic pituitary dysfunction. Peak levels of TSH in response to TRH are generally observed 30 min after injection. A delayed rise in plasma TSH levels may be seen in individuals with hypothalamic disease. Unfortunately, some patients with primary pituitary disease also will have such an abnormal TSH response.

Evaluation of ACTH secretion begins by collecting a 24-h urine sample for measurement of urinary free cortisol and 17-OHCS. Both values should be low in hypopituitarism. Unfortunately basal cortisol secretion is often normal, even though the ability to release ACTH is diminished in early or partial hypopituitarism. Thus, evaluation of ACTH secretory reserve is of practical significance. Cosyntropin 0.25 mg given IV over 15 to 30 sec should elicit a distinct increase in plasma cortisol of at least 7 μg/dL or to a level > 20 μg/dL 1 or 2 h after injection if the adrenal cortex is intact. The response to this stimulus is blunted in **primary adrenal insufficiency (Addison's disease).** However, the response of cortisol also may be blunted in longstanding ACTH deficiency. Therefore, the most reliable method for evaluating ACTH, (as well as GH and PRL) reserve is by means of the **insulin tolerance test.** Regular insulin at a dosage of 0.1 u./kg body weight is given IV over 15 to 30 sec and venous blood samples are obtained for determination of GH, cortisol, and glucose at zero time (prior to insulin administration) and at 20, 30, 45, 60, and 90 min later. If test results do not show at least a 50% fall in serum glucose levels to values < 40 mg/dL, the test should be repeated. *This test*

is hazardous in patients with severe documented panhypopituitarism, diabetes mellitus, and in the elderly, and is contraindicated in the presence of ischemic heart disease or epilepsy. A medical attendant should be present during the test. Usually only transient perspiration, tachycardia, and nervousness occur. Should the patient complain of palpitations, lose consciousness, or have a seizure, the test should be terminated promptly by giving 50% glucose solution IV.

An insulin tolerance test alone will not differentiate between primary (Addison's disease) and secondary (hypopituitary) adrenal insufficiency unless ACTH as well as cortisol is measured. Unfortunately accurate measurement of plasma ACTH concentrations is rarely available.

In the **metyrapone test,** plasma cortisol levels are reduced by blocking the 11-hydroxylation of the cortisol precursors with metyrapone. In the normal individual, the decreased cortisol stimulates increased secretion of ACTH and leads to increased production of cortisol precursors, particularly 11-deoxycortisol, secreted in the urine as 17-OHCS. Since metyrapone tests only steroid-suppressible ACTH secretion, certain stresses such as surgery, which are nonsuppressible, may cause release of ACTH even in patients who fail to respond to metyrapone. Urine samples are taken over 24 h for 2 consecutive days and baseline determinations made of 17-OHCS. On the 3rd day, metyrapone 750 mg orally (300 mg/m² BSA for children) is given at 8 AM and q 4 h thereafter for a total of 6 doses or 4.5 gm in adults. Failure of the urinary 17-OHCS to double or the plasma 11-deoxycortisol to exceed 10 μg/dL on the last day of treatment (the 4th day) or the day following treatment is abnormal. Dizziness and nausea commonly occur and are alleviated in part by bedrest. Since failure to respond to metyrapone can indicate either hypothalamic-pituitary insufficiency or adrenal failure, it is often helpful to perform an ACTH stimulation test on the 4th day.

The response to metyrapone is generally reduced or absent in patients with hypoadrenalism or hypopituitarism. However, some patients with hypothalamic or pituitary disease have normal responses. Responses may also be abnormal in normal individuals who metabolize metyrapone at an increased rate and in patients with hyperthyroidism, some pregnant women, and in patients taking phenytoin or estrogens.

Corticotropin-releasing hormone (CRH) test: The recent discovery and synthesis of CRH may provide a better tool for evaluating hypothalamic-pituitary-adrenal function than any test described thus far, but at present its use is investigational. A dose of 1 μg/kg given IV over 20 sec appears to elicit maximal responses of both ACTH and cortisol. Plasma ACTH levels rise within 2 min and peak initially within 10 to 15 min of CRH administration. After the initial peak, ACTH concentrations fall but rise to a 2nd peak at 3 h. Plasma cortisol levels rise more slowly, beginning 10 min or more after injection and reaching peak values at 30 to 60 min.

Patients with primary adrenal insufficiency have markedly increased responses to CRH, presumably because of the absence of immediate glucocorticoid negative feedback inhibition of CRH action on the pituitary. Individuals with secondary adrenal insufficiency may either have little or no ACTH responses (presumably due to primary pituitary ACTH deficiency) or have exaggerated and prolonged responses (presumably due to primary hypothalamic CRH deficiency). Although there are simpler and more direct approaches to diagnosing primary adrenocortical insufficiency, further studies may document that CRH is of value in distinguishing hypothalamic from pituitary causes of secondary adrenal insufficiency.

PRL levels are not regularly depressed in patients with panhypopituitarism. In fact elevated levels may be present in hypothalamic disorders freeing the pituitary lactotrophs of the inhibitory effects of dopamine.

GH measurements are only helpful when performed after one of several provocative stimuli and, since GH responses are generally abnormal in individuals with diminished thyroid or adrenal function, testing should be conducted only after adequate hormon

replacement therapy. The insulin tolerance test is the most effective stimulus to GH release. Less dangerous, but also less reliable, are tests of GH release using arginine infusion (500 mg/kg given IV over 30 min), oral L-dopa (500 mg to adults; 10 mg/kg to children), sleep, or 20 min of vigorous exercise. Clonidine (4 μg/kg orally) is another potent stimulator of GH secretion and holds promise as an alternative to insulin. Side effects include only sleepiness and a minimal fall in BP. Generally, any GH determination > 10 ng/mL or any response of > 5 ng/mL following a stimulus is sufficient to rule out GH deficiency. Increases in GH of < 5 ng/mL or to levels < 10 ng/mL are difficult to interpret. What constitutes a normal response is arbitrary, and all provocative tests of GH secretion occasionally produce misleading results. Since no single test is 100% effective in eliciting GH release, at least 2 different tests should be performed in the absence of GH response. GH levels will generally peak 30 to 90 min following administration of insulin and the onset of arginine infusion, 30 to 120 min after L-dopa, 60 to 120 min after the onset of sleep and clonidine, and after 20 min of vigorous exercise.

The utility of exogenous GRH in evaluating GH secretion is not yet established. A dose of 1 μg/kg GRH administered IV over 15 to 30 sec results in maximal but variable release of GH, typically reaching a peak about 60 min after GRH injection. Presumably absent or diminished increases in GH in response to GRH will identify individuals with GH deficiency, but whether the pattern of response will distinguish primary hypothalamic from pituitary disease is unclear.

Measurement of serum LH and FSH levels in the basal state is most helpful in the evaluation of hypopituitarism in postmenopausal women not taking exogenous estrogens in whom circulating gonadotropin concentrations are normally high (> 40 mIU/mL). Basal LH and FSH levels are less helpful in other patients. Although gonadotropin levels will be low in panhypopituitarism, overlap exists with the normal ranges for LH and FSH. LH and FSH should increase in response to gonadorelin HCl (synthetic GnRH) 100 μg IV, with LH peaking about 30 min and FSH 40 min after GnRH administration. However, normal, diminished, or absent responses to GnRH may occur in hypothalamic-pituitary dysfunction. Normal increases in LH and FSH in response to GnRH are quite variable. In addition, administration of exogenous GnRH has not been helpful in distinguishing primary hypothalamic from primary pituitary disorders.

The testing of pituitary reserve for several hormones simultaneously is the most efficient method of evaluating pituitary function. Insulin (0.1 u./kg reg), TRH (200 μg), and GnRH (100 μg) may be administered together IV over 15 to 30 sec. Glucose, cortisol, GH, TSH, prolactin, LH, FSH, and ACTH are measured at frequent intervals for the ensuing 180 min. Alternatively, insulin can be given alone followed by simultaneous administration of TRH and GnRH 120 min later. It has been suggested that GRH (1 μg/kg) and CRH (1 μg/kg) be given IV together with TRH and GnRH and that insulin is no longer necessary as a part of a combined anterior pituitary function test. The usefulness of these recently available releasing hormones in pituitary testing remains to be established. In any case, the normal responses are the same as those delineated earlier.

Panhypopituitarism also must be differentiated from a number of other disorders, including anorexia nervosa, chronic liver disease, and myotonia dystrophica. The clinical features in anorexia nervosa (which generally occurs in females) are usually diagnostic. They include cachexia, abnormal ideation regarding food and body image, and the maintenance of secondary sexual characteristics despite amenorrhea. Patients with anorexia nervosa generally have increased basal levels of GH and cortisol as well. Because hypothalamic lesions can disturb centers controlling appetite, x-ray evaluation of the sella turcica is not unreasonable in suspected patients. (See also ANOREXIA NERVOSA in Ch. 202.) Hypopituitarism is often suspected in men with alcoholic liver

disease or hemochromatosis when testicular atrophy is combined with general debility. However, in most cases, the underlying primary disease can be recognized and hypopituitarism can be ruled out by laboratory testing. Morphologic evidence of extensive pituitary dysfunction is rarely found at necropsy in these diseases. Individuals with myotonia dystrophica complain of progressive muscular weakness, develop premature balding and cataracts, and have facial features suggesting accelerated aging; men may develop testicular atrophy. Hypopituitarism is excluded by endocrine testing.

Treatment

Treatment is directed toward replacing the hormones *of the hypofunctioning target glands* as discussed in the pertinent chapters in this section and elsewhere in THE MANUAL. When hypopituitarism is due to a pituitary tumor, specific treatment must be directed to the tumor as well. Controversy exists as to the appropriate management of such neoplasms. If the tumor is small, most favor transsphenoidal removal of the neoplasm. Supervoltage irradiation of the pituitary may be used as well. With larger tumors and suprasellar extension, resection of the entire neoplasm, either transsphenoidally or transfrontally, may not be possible and adjunctive supervoltage irradiation may be warranted. Both surgery and irradiation may be followed by the loss of other pituitary hormone functions. Irradiated patients may lose endocrine function slowly over years and may also develop visual difficulties related to fibrosis of the optic chiasm. Therefore, post-treatment hormonal status should be evaluated at frequent intervals, preferably at 3 and 6 mo, and yearly thereafter. How complete such evaluation should be is open to question, but it must include assessment of thyroid and adrenal function, as well as sellar x-ray evaluation and visual field examination.

SELECTIVE PITUITARY HORMONE DEFICIENCIES

It is important to remember that selective deficiencies of pituitary hormones may represent an early stage in the development of more generalized hypopituitarism. Patients must be observed for signs of other pituitary hormone deficiencies, and the sella turcica should be evaluated radiographically at intervals to look for signs of pituitary tumors.

Isolated growth hormone (GH) deficiency is responsible for many cases of pituitary dwarfism (see in Ch. 196).

Isolated gonadotropin deficiency occurs in men and women and mainly must be distinguished from primary hypogonadism. A eunuchoid habitus will be present in both disorders if they arise in childhood. Patients with primary hypogonadism have elevated levels of luteinizing hormone **(LH)** and follicle-stimulating hormone **(FSH)** while those with gonadotropin deficiency have low or unmeasurable levels. Although most cases of hypogonadotropic hypogonadism have deficiencies of both LH and FSH, there are rare cases in which the secretion of only a single gonadotropin is impaired. Isolated gonadotropin deficiency must also be distinguished from hypogonadotropic amenorrhea secondary to exercise, diet, or psychologic stress. Although the history may be helpful, differential diagnosis may be impossible in some cases. Treatment is discussed in Ch. 170. In **Kallmann's syndrome** the specific lack of gonadotropin-releasing hormone **(GnRH)** is often associated with midline facial defects, including anosmia, color blindness, and cleft lip or palate (see in SECONDARY HYPOGONADISM in THE TESTES in Ch. 196).

Isolated ACTH deficiency is a rare clinical entity. Symptoms of weakness, hypoglycemia, weight loss, and decreased axillary and pubic hair suggest the diagnosis. Plasma and urinary steroid levels are low and rise to normal after ACTH treatment. Clinical and laboratory evidence of other hormonal deficiencies is absent.

Isolated thyroid-stimulating hormone (TSH) deficiency is likely when clinical features of hypothyroidism exist, plasma TSH is not elevated, and there are no other pituitar

hormone deficiencies. Plasma TSH, as measured by immunoassay, is not always lower than normal, suggesting that the TSH secreted is biologically inactive. Administration of bovine TSH will increase thyroid hormone levels (see also HYPOTHYROIDISM in Ch. 89).

Isolated prolactin (PRL) deficiency has been noted rarely in patients who fail to lactate after delivery. Basal PRL levels are low and there is no increase in response to provocative stimuli.

HYPERSECRETION OF ANTERIOR PITUITARY HORMONES

ACROMEGALY AND GIGANTISM

Syndromes of excessive secretion of growth hormone **(GH)**, *nearly always due to a pituitary adenoma of the somatotrophs.* A few cases of ectopic GH-producing tumors, especially of pancreas and lung, have also been described.

Symptoms and Signs

Rarely, GH hypersecretion begins in childhood, prior to closure of the epiphyses, and leads to the exaggerated skeletal growth termed **pituitary gigantism.** GH excess can begin at any age but most commonly starts between the 3rd and 5th decades of life. In children growth velocity is increased but there is little bony deformity. However, there is soft tissue swelling and the peripheral nerves are enlarged. Delayed puberty or hypogonadotropic hypogonadism is also frequently present, resulting in an eunuchoid habitus. When GH hypersecretion begins after epiphyseal closure, the earliest clinical manifestation is coarsening of the facial features and soft-tissue swelling of the hands and feet. The appearance of the patient changes, and there is a need for larger rings, gloves, and shoes. Photographs are important in delineating the course of the disease. The increase in dimension of the acral parts has led to the term **acromegaly.**

Other changes in affected adults occur as well. Coarse body hair increases, and the skin thickens and frequently darkens. The size and function of sebaceous and sweat glands increase such that patients frequently complain of excessive perspiration and an offensive body odor. Overgrowth of the mandible leads to protrusion of the jaw (prognathism). Cartilaginous proliferation of the larynx leads to a deep husky voice. The tongue is frequently enlarged and furrowed. In longstanding acromegaly, costal growth leads to a barrel chest. Articular cartilaginous proliferation occurs early in response to GH excess, with the articular cartilage possibly undergoing necrosis and erosion. Joint symptoms are common and crippling degenerative arthritis may occur.

Peripheral neuropathies are common, due to compression of nerves by adjacent fibrous tissue as well as to endoneural fibrous proliferation. Because of the pituitary tumor, headaches are also common and bitemporal hemianopsia may develop if there is suprasellar extension involving the optic chiasm. The heart, liver, kidneys, spleen, thyroid, parathyroid glands, and pancreas are also larger than normal. GH increases tubular reabsorption of phosphate and leads to mild hyperphosphatemia. Impaired glucose tolerance is present in nearly half the cases of acromegaly as well as in gigantism, but clinically significant diabetes mellitus occurs in only about 10% of patients.

Galactorrhea occurs in some women with acromegaly, usually in association with hyperprolactinemia. However, lactation may occur with GH excess alone, because GH itself is a potent lactogenic hormone. Decreased gonadotropin secretion often occurs in association with GH-secreting tumors. As noted, sexual immaturity is common in gigantism. About 1/3 of men with acromegaly develop impotence, and nearly all women develop menstrual irregularities or amenorrhea.

Diagnosis

Diagnosis can be made from the characteristic clinical findings, described above. Skull x-rays disclose cortical thickening, enlargement of the frontal sinuses, and en-

largement and erosion of the sella turcica. X-rays of the hands show tufting of the terminal phalanges and soft tissue thickening. Glucose tolerance is usually abnormal, and serum phosphate levels are generally elevated.

Plasma GH levels measured by radioimmunoassay are typically elevated in acromegaly and are the simplest way to assess GH hypersecretion. Blood should be obtained in the basal state before breakfast; in normal individuals basal GH levels are < 5 ng/mL. Transient elevations of GH occur in normal individuals and must be distinguished from pathologic hypersecretion. Secretion in normal individuals is suppressed to < 5 ng/mL 90 min after administration of 75 gm of glucose orally. Levels between 5 and 10 ng/mL are indeterminant, and higher values support the diagnosis of GH excess. Most acromegalics have substantially higher values. Basal plasma GH levels are also of value in monitoring the response to therapy. Plasma somatomedin C (also known as insulin-like growth factor I, IGF-I), measured by radioimmunoassay, is generally elevated in active acromegaly.

Treatment

Ablative therapy with surgery or radiation is generally indicated. **Transphenoidal resection** of the tumor is currently preferred, but choices vary at different institutions. **Supervoltage radiation,** delivering about 5000 R to the pituitary, is used, but GH levels may not fall to normal for several years. However, the treatment generally does not induce hypopituitarism, and damage to cranial nerves and hypothalamic tissues is rare. Treatment with accelerated protons **(heavy particle radiation)** permits delivery of larger doses of radiation (equivalent to 10,000 R) to the pituitary; however, there is a higher risk of cranial nerve and hypothalamic damage, hypopituitarism is common, and such therapy is only available in a few centers. Because radiation damage is cumulative, proton beam therapy should *not* be used following conventional gamma irradiation. A combined surgery/radiation approach is indicated in patients with progressive extrasellar involvement by a pituitary tumor and in those in whom the entire tumor cannot be resected.

It is often difficult to lower GH levels to normal even with both surgical and radiation therapy. In such instances, **bromocriptine mesylate** up to 15 mg/day orally in divided doses may be effective in further lowering GH levels in a small percentage of affected individuals.

Cushing's Syndrome

(See under Adrenal Cortical Hyperfunction in Ch. 91)

Galactorrhea

Lactation in men, or in women who are not breast-feeding an infant.

Etiology

In both sexes, **prolactinomas** are the most common secretory tumors of the pituitary, producing excessive quantities of PRL. The majority of tumors in women are microadenomas (< 10 mm in diameter), but a small percentage are macroadenomas (> 10 mm) at the time of diagnosis. The frequency of microadenomas is much lower in men perhaps because of later recognition.

Hyperprolactinemia and galactorrhea also may be caused by ingestion of several drugs, including phenothiazines, certain antihypertensives (especially α-methyldopa) and opioids. Primary hypothyroidism also must be ruled out, since increased TRH stimulates increased secretion of both TSH and prolactin. It is unclear why hyperprolactinemia is associated with hypogonadotropinism and hypogonadism. Causes of hyperprolactinemia are listed in Table 88–2.

TABLE 88–2. CAUSES OF HYPERPROLACTINEMIA

I. Physiologic
- A. Nipple stimulation in men and women
- B. Pregnancy
- C. Postpartum
- D. Stress
- E. Food ingestion
- F. Sexual intercourse in some women
- G. Sleep
- H. Hypoglycemia
- I. Early infancy (up to 3 months)

II. Pathologic
- A. Hypothalamic disorders
  1. Hypothalamic tumors
  2. Non-tumorous hypothalamic infiltration
     a. Sarcoidosis
     b. Hand-Schüller-Christian disease (histiocytosis X)
  3. Post-encephalitis
  4. Idiopathic galactorrhea (presumed abnormality in dopamine secretion)
- B. Prolactin-secreting pituitary tumors
- C. Surgical pituitary stalk section and other stalk lesions
- D. Primary hypothyroidism
- E. Chronic renal failure
- F. Ectopic production of prolactin
  1. Bronchogenic carcinoma (not squamous cell; mostly small cell undifferentiated)
  2. Hypernephroma
- G. Chest wall lesions
  1. Surgical scars
  2. Trauma
  3. Neoplasms of the chest wall
  4. Herpes zoster

III. Pharmacologic
- A. Psychotropic drugs
  1. Phenothiazines
  2. Tricyclic antidepressants
  3. Butyrophenones (haloperidol)
  4. Benzamides (metoclopramide, sulpiride)
- B. Antihypertensive drugs
  1. Reserpine
  2. α-Methyldopa
  3. Oral contraceptives
  4. TRH

(Modified from R. W. Rebar, "Practical Evaluation of Hormonal Status" in *Reproductive Endocrinology: Physiology, Pathophysiology and Clinical Management,* edited by S. S. C. Yen and R. B. Jaffe, p. 493. Copyright by W. B. Saunders Company, 1978. Used with permission.)

Symptoms, Signs, and Diagnosis

Amenorrhea is commonly associated with the galactorrhea in women. Three subsets of **galactorrhea-amenorrhea syndrome** have been described: (1) persistent galactorrhea-amenorrhea after pregnancy **(Chiari-Frommel syndrome),** (2) galactorrhea-amenorrhea unassociated with pregnancy **(Ahumada-del Castillo syndrome),** and (3) galactorrhea-amenorrhea caused by a chromophobe adenoma of the pituitary **(Forbes-Albright syndrome).** The first 2 of these syndromes also may be associated with pituitary tumors. Men with PRL-secreting pituitary tumors typically present complaining of headaches or visual difficulties. About 2/3 of affected men note loss of libido and potency.

Women with galactorrhea-amenorrhea frequently complain of symptoms of estrogen deficiency, including hot flushes and dyspareunia. However, estrogen production may also be normal and signs of androgen excess have been observed in some hyperprolactinemic women. Furthermore, hyperprolactinemia may be associated with other menstrual cycle disturbances besides amenorrhea, including infrequent or oligo-ovulation and corpus luteum dysfunction.

The first diagnostic objective should be to document the presence of hyperprolactinemia in the basal state. In general, basal PRL levels seem to correlate with size of a pituitary tumor and can be used to follow patients over time. Serum gonadotropin and estradiol levels are either low or in the normal range in hyperprolactinemic women. Primary hypothyroidism is easily ruled out in the absence of elevated TSH. Although a single lateral coned-down view of the sella turcica can be used to exclude large pituitary neoplasms, high resolution CT scanning is the method of choice to identify individuals with microadenomas. Visual field examination is indicated in all patients with macroadenomas and in any patient who elects medical treatment or surveillance only.

Treatment

The treatment of pituitary tumors associated with hyperprolactinemia is controversial. Patients with PRL levels < 100 ng/mL and with normal CT scans or who have microadenomas only can be treated with bromocriptine or kept under surveillance. Because hyperprolactinemic women are often hypoestrogenic and appear to be at increased risk of developing osteoporosis, treatment (with bromocriptine) of even those with no neoplasm is preferred. Bromocriptine should be recommended to patients desiring pregnancy and to those with embarrassing galactorrhea. Bromocriptine is also the preferred treatment for patients with a microadenoma. Periodic monitoring of basal PRL levels and radiographic evaluation of the sella turcica are indicated in all individuals with hyperprolactinemia. How extensive such monitoring should be is controversial. Patients should be evaluated at least quarterly and should undergo repeat CT scanning annually for at least an additional 2 yr. The frequency of sellar x-rays can then be reduced if there is no increase in basal PRL levels.

Individuals with macroadenomas should be treated with surgery, radiotherapy, or bromocriptine only after thorough endocrine testing of pituitary function and consultation with an endocrinologist, neurosurgeon, and radiotherapist. Bromocriptine is frequently used with some success (prior to surgery) to reduce tumor size. The mode of therapy selected varies among medical centers and remains controversial. Frequent (at least yearly) monitoring of endocrine status and evaluation of the sella turcica are indicated for the remainder of a patient's life following therapy of a macroadenoma.

POSTERIOR LOBE DISORDERS

DIABETES INSIPIDUS (DI)

(Central Diabetes Insipidus; Vasopressin-Sensitive Diabetes Insipidus)

A temporary or chronic disorder of the neurohypophyseal system due to deficiency of vasopressin (antidiuretic hormone, ADH) and characterized by excretion of excessive quantities of very dilute (but otherwise normal) urine and by excessive thirst.

Central or **vasopressin (ADH)-sensitive diabetes insipidus,** which is a hypothalamic/pituitary disorder, will be referred to in this discussion as **DI** to distinguish it from **nephrogenic diabetes insipidus (NDI),** in which the kidney is ADH-resistant (see in ANOMALIES IN KIDNEY TRANSPORT in Ch. 155). Polyuria may result from DI (a deficiency of ADH), NDI, or compulsive (psychogenic) water drinking (physiologic suppression of ADH).

Etiology and Pathophysiology

DI may be complete, partial, permanent, or temporary. All of the pathologic lesions associated with DI involve the supraoptic and paraventricular nuclei of the hypothalamus or a major portion of the pituitary stalk. Simple destruction of the posterior lobe of the pituitary leads to temporary, unsustained DI. The posterior lobe is the major site for ADH storage and release, but ADH is synthesized within the hypothalamus. Newly synthesized hormone can still be released into the circulation as long as the hypothalamic nuclei and part of the neurohypophyseal tract are intact. Only about 10% of neurosecretory neurons must remain intact to avoid central DI.

DI may be (1) **primary (idiopathic),** in which there is a marked decrease in the hypothalamic nuclei of the neurohypophyseal system, or (2) **secondary (acquired),** due to a variety of pathologic lesions, including (1) hypophysectomy; (2) cranial injuries, particularly basal skull fractures; (3) suprasellar and intrasellar neoplasms (primary or metastatic); (4) histiocytosis X (Hand-Schüller-Christian disease); (5) granulomas (sarcoidosis or tuberculosis); (6) vascular lesions (aneurysm and thrombosis); and (7) infections (encephalitis or meningitis).

Symptoms and Signs

Onset may be insidious or abrupt and may occur at any age. The only symptoms in the idiopathic form are polydipsia and polyuria. In acquired forms of DI, symptoms and signs of the associated lesions are also present. Enormous quantities of fluid may be ingested and large volumes (3 to 30 L/day) of a very dilute urine (sp gr usually < 1.005 and osmolality < 200 mOsm/L) are excreted. Nocturia is almost always present in DI and in NDI. Dehydration and hypovolemia may develop rapidly if urinary losses are not continuously replaced.

Diagnosis

DI must be differentiated from other causes of polyuria (TABLE 88–3). All tests for DI are based on the principle that increasing the plasma osmolality in normal individuals will lead to decreased excretion of urine with increased osmolality.

The **water deprivation test** is the simplest and most reliable test, but *should only be performed with the patient under constant supervision.* For patients with DI the test may be hazardous, while those who are compulsive water drinkers may be unable to avoid drinking unless prevented from doing so. The test is started in the morning by weighing the patient, obtaining venous blood to determine electrolyte concentrations and osmolality, and measuring urinary osmolality. Voided urine is collected hourly and its sp gr or osmolality (preferable) is measured. Dehydration is continued until (1) orthostatic hypotension and postural tachycardia appear, (2) 5% or more of the initial body

TABLE 88–3. COMMON CAUSES OF POLYURIA

- **I. Vasopressin-sensitive polyuria**
  - A. Decreased *synthesis* of ADH* (idiopathic or acquired diabetes insipidus)
  - B. Decreased *release* of ADH (compulsive polydipsia)
- **II. Vasopressin-resistant polyuria**
  - A. Congenital nephrogenic diabetes insipidus
  - B. Acquired nephrogenic diabetes insipidus
    1. Chronic renal disease
    2. Systemic or metabolic disease (e.g., myeloma, amyloid, hypercalcemic or hypokalemic nephropathy, sickle cell disease)
  - C. Osmotic diuresis
    1. Glucose (diabetes mellitus)
    2. Poorly resorbed solutes (mannitol, sorbitol, urea)

*Antidiuretic hormone (vasopressin).

weight has been lost, or (3) the urinary concentration does not change > 0.001 sp gr or 30 mOsm/L in sequentially voided specimens. At this point, serum electrolytes and osmolality are again determined, and 5 u. of *aqueous* vasopressin are injected s.c. Urine for sp gr or osmolality is collected one final time 60 min post injection and the test is terminated.

A **normal response** is one in which the maximum urine osmolality after dehydration (often > 1.020 sp gr or 700 mOsm/L) exceeds the plasma osmolality and does not increase more than an additional 5% after injection of vasopressin. Patients with **DI** are generally unable to concentrate urine to greater than the plasma osmolality and increase their urine osmolality by > 50% following vasopressin. Patients with **partial DI** are often able to concentrate urine to above the plasma osmolality but show a rise in urine osmolality of > 9% after vasopressin administration. Patients with **NDI** are unable to concentrate urine to greater than the plasma osmolality and show no additional response to vasopressin administration.

Compulsive (psychogenic) water drinking may present a difficult problem in differential diagnosis. Patients may ingest and excrete up to 6 L of fluid/day and are often emotionally disturbed. Unlike patients with DI and NDI, they usually do not have nocturia, nor does their thirst awaken them at night. The polydipsia leads to increased water intake and suppression of endogenous ADH with resultant polyuria. Since chronic water intake diminishes medullary tonicity in the kidney, resistance to ADH also develops. Although some patients have a normal response to water deprivation, in others urine osmolality increases to hypertonic, but submaximal, levels, ie, a response similar to patients with partial DI. In contrast, however, the compulsive water drinker, like the patient with NDI, will not show any further response to exogenous vasopressin after water deprivation. Continued ingestion of large volumes of water in this situation can even lead to life-threatening hyponatremia. After prolonged restriction of fluid intake to 2 L or less/day, normal concentrating ability returns, although this may take several weeks.

Hypertonic saline infusion has also been used to test DI. The patient drinks a 20 mL/kg load of water. One hour later 2.5% sodium chloride is given IV at a rate of 0.25 mL/kg/min for 45 min. Urinary and plasma osmolality are measured in at least one urine specimen before and in one immediately following the saline infusion to determine the ability of the kidney to excrete a hypertonic urine. However, this test is dangerous in patients unable to tolerate a saline load (eg, those with limited cardiac reserve) and is uninterpretable in patients developing salt diuresis. Consequently, it cannot be recommended.

Measurement of circulating vasopressin concentrations by radioimmunoassay offers potentially the most direct method for diagnosing DI. However, the test is difficult to perform and not available routinely. In addition, water deprivation is so accurate as to make direct measurement of vasopressin unnecessary.

Treatment

Hormonal therapy: Central DI can be treated by hormonal replacement, but such therapy should be preceded or accompanied by specific treatment of the organic cause for the DI. *In the absence of appropriate management of DI, permanent renal damage can result with time.* Because vasopressin is a small peptide, it is ineffective when administered orally. **Aqueous vasopressin** can be given s.c. or IM in doses of 5 to 10 u. to provide an antidiuretic response that usually lasts 6 h or less. Thus, this agent has little use in chronic treatment but can be used in the initial therapy of unconscious patients and in affected individuals undergoing surgery. Synthetic vasopressin (Pitressin®) may also be administered 2 to 4 times/day as a nasal spray with the dosage and interval designed for each patient. **DDAVP® (desmopressin acetate,** 1-desamino-8-D-arginine vasopressin), a synthetic analog of arginine vasopressin, has prolonged antidiuretic activity lasting for 12 to 24 h in most patients and may be administered

intranasally, s.c., or IV. DDAVP is the preparation of choice for both adults and children. The drug is generally administered via a calibrated nasal catheter in 2 daily divided doses with the dosage determined for each individual patient. The nightly dose is the lowest dose required to prevent nocturia. Response is estimated by determining if urinary output is adequate but not excessive. The morning and evening doses should be adjusted separately for an adequate diurnal rhythm to water turnover. The usual dosage range in adults is 0.1 to 0.4 mL (10 to 40 μg) with most requiring 0.2 mL/day in 2 divided doses. For children age 3 mo to 12 yr, the usual dosage range is 0.05 to 0.3 mL/day. Overdosage can lead to fluid retention and decreased plasma osmolality, possibly even resulting in convulsions in small children. In such instances, furosemide may be used to induce diuresis. Headache may be a troublesome side effect but generally disappears if the dosage is reduced. Infrequently, DDAVP may cause a slight increase in BP. Absorption from the nasal mucosa may be erratic, especially in the presence of an URI or allergic rhinitis. When intranasal delivery of DDAVP is inappropriate, it may be administered s.c. with the comparable antidiuretic dose of the injection being about 1/10 the intranasal dose. DDAVP may also be used IV in acute situations. **Lypressin** (lysine-8-vasopressin), a synthetic agent, is given by nasal spray as required at 3- to 8-h intervals. **Vasopressin tannate in oil** can be given IM in a dose of 0.3 to 1 mL (1.5 to 5 u.) and may control symptoms for up to 96 h.

Nonhormonal therapy: Two types of drugs have been found useful in reducing polyuria: (1) various diuretics, primarily thiazides, and (2) ADH-releasing drugs such as chlorpropamide, carbamazepine, and clofibrate. These agents have been particularly useful in *partial* DI and avoid the hypersensitivity reactions and potential vascular consequences of exogenous ADH. The thiazide drugs paradoxically reduce urine volume in partial and complete DI and NDI, primarily as a consequence of reducing ECF volume and increasing proximal tubular resorption. Urine volumes may fall by 25 to 50% during the daily administration of customary doses of thiazides (eg, 15 to 25 mg/kg of chlorothiazide).

Chlorpropamide, carbamazepine, and clofibrate are capable of reducing or eliminating the need for vasopressin in some patients with partial DI when residual ADH is present. None are effective in NDI. Chlorpropamide (3 to 5 mg/kg orally once or twice/day) not only causes some release of ADH but also potentiates the action of ADH on the kidney. Clofibrate 500 to 1000 mg orally bid or carbamazepine 100 to 400 mg orally bid is recommended for adults only. Because the effects of chlorpropamide, carbamazepine, and clofibrate differ from those of the thiazides, the use of one of these agents with a diuretic may show additive effects and complement each other therapeutically. Hypoglycemia may be a significant side effect of chlorpropamide therapy. Significant hypersensitivity reactions (especially jaundice) have been observed with chlorpropamide, hematologic disturbances including aplastic anemia have been seen with carbamazepine, and an association of malignancy in rodents has been noted with clofibrate. Such adverse reactions mandate that these agents be used with caution.

---

89. THYROID

THYROID HORMONES

The general scheme of thyroid hormone biosynthesis is depicted in FIG. 89–1. Iodide, ingested in food and water, is actively concentrated by the thyroid gland, converted to organic iodine by peroxidase, and incorporated into tyrosine in **thyroglobulin.** The tyrosines are iodinated at either one (monoiodotyrosine, MIT) or two (diiodotyrosine, DIT) sites and then coupled to form the active hormones (diiodotyrosine +

diiodotyrosine → tetraiodothyronine **[thyroxine, T_4]**; diiodotyrosine + monoiodotyrosine → **triiodothyronine [T_3]**). Thyroglobulin, a glycoprotein containing T_3 and T_4 within its matrix, is taken up as colloid droplets by the thyroid cells. Lysosomes containing proteases cleave T_3 and T_4 from thyroglobulin, resulting in release of free T_3 and T_4. The iodotyrosines (MIT and DIT) are also released from thyroglobulin but do not reach the bloodstream. They are deiodinated by intracellular deiodinases and their iodine utilized by the thyroid gland.

Although some of the free T_3 and T_4 is deiodinated in the thyroid gland with the iodine reentering the thyroid iodine pool, most diffuses into the bloodstream where it is bound to certain serum proteins for transport. The major thyroid transport protein is **thyroxine-binding globulin (TBG),** which normally accounts for about 80% of the bound thyroid hormone. Other thyroid-binding proteins, including **thyroxine-binding prealbumin (TBPA)** and **albumin,** account for the remainder of the bound serum thyroid hormone (20%). About 0.05% of the total serum T_4 and 0.5% of the total serum T_3 remain free but in equilibrium with the bound hormone.

All reactions necessary for T_3 and T_4 formation are influenced and controlled by pituitary **thyrotropin (thyroid-stimulating hormone, TSH).** TSH binds to its thyroid plasma membrane receptor on the external cell surface and activates the enzyme adenylate cyclase, increasing the formation of cyclic AMP, the nucleotide that serves as a

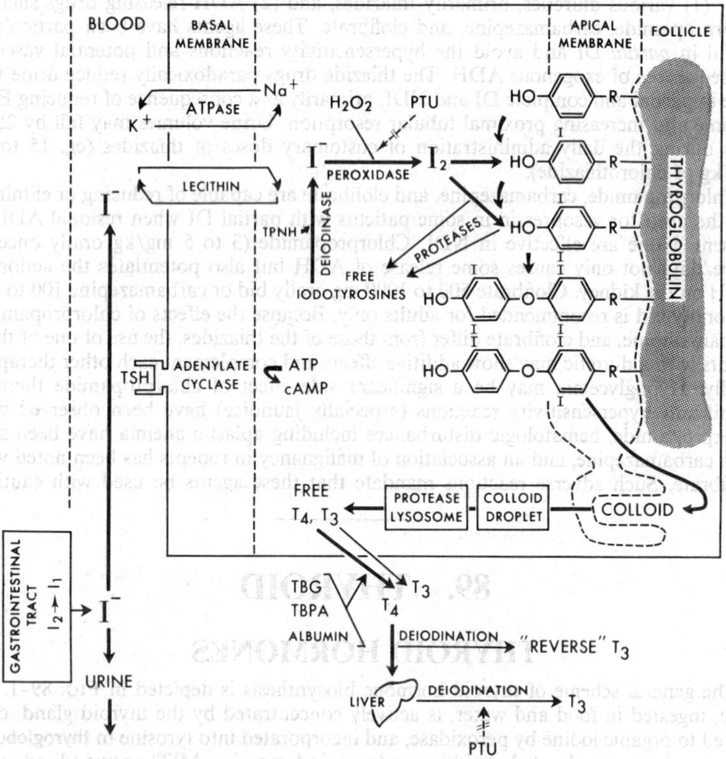

Fig. 89–1. Biosynthesis of thyroid hormones.

messenger to mediate the intracellular effects of TSH. Pituitary TSH secretion is controlled by a negative feedback mechanism modulated by the circulating level of free T_3 (and probably free T_4). Increased levels of free T_3 and free T_4 inhibit TSH secretion by the pituitary, whereas decreased levels of free T_3 or free T_4 increase TSH release from the pituitary. TSH secretion is also influenced by **thyrotropin-releasing hormone (TRH),** a 3-amino acid peptide synthesized in the hypothalamus. TRH, released into the portal system between the hypothalamus and pituitary, binds to the thyrotropic cells of the anterior pituitary and causes the subsequent release of TSH. The precise regulation of TRH synthesis and release has not been completely elucidated.

About 15% of the circulating T_3 is produced by the thyroid. The remainder is produced by monodeiodination of the outer ring of T_4, mainly in the liver. Monodeiodination of the inner ring of T_4 also occurs in hepatic and extrahepatic sites including kidney, to yield 3,3′,5′-T_3 **(reverse T_3 or rT_3).** This compound has minimal metabolic activity but is present in normal human serum and thyroglobulin. In many instances where serum T_3 levels decline (eg, chronic liver and renal disease, acute illness, starvation, and carbohydrate-deficient diets), rT_3 levels increase, suggesting that peripheral deiodination pathways shift to produce rT_3.

Observations pertaining to rT_3 metabolism in fetal life are of great importance. Total amniotic T_4 and T_3 are low, in contrast to levels in maternal serum. Fetal rT_3 levels in amniotic fluid are much higher than the corresponding values in maternal serum throughout pregnancy (15 to 42 wk). These data imply that rT_3 derives primarily from the fetus and that it may be possible to diagnose fetal hypothyroidism as early as the 15th wk of pregnancy, utilizing radioimmunoassay for rT_3. These levels appear to decrease after 30-wk gestation and may serve as a useful index of pregnancies of < 30 wk duration.

Physiologic Effects of Thyroid Hormone

Thyroid hormones have 2 major physiologic effects: (1) they increase protein synthesis in virtually every body tissue (the mechanism has not been precisely defined, but it is known that T_3 and T_4 enter cells, bind to discrete nuclear receptors, and influence the formation of mRNA); and (2) they increase O_2 consumption by increasing the activity of the Na-K ATPase (Na pump), primarily in tissues responsible for basal O_2 consumption (ie, liver, kidney, heart, and skeletal muscle). The increased activity of Na-K ATPase is secondary to increased synthesis of this enzyme; therefore, the increased O_2 consumption is also probably related to the nuclear binding of thyroid hormone.

Laboratory Testing of Thyroid Function

1. Protein-bound iodine (PBI): The measurement of PBI permits an estimate of the circulating thyroid hormone level, but direct measurement of T_3 and T_4 is more accurate and has replaced the PBI test. However, it may be useful in Hashimoto's thyroiditis.

2. Serum total T_4 (serum total thyroxine) is measured by **radioimmunoassay (RIA)** involving a specific antigen-antibody reaction. A double antibody technic is used. RIA measures total T_4, both bound and free. It may also be measured by competitive protein-binding or by column chromatography. The tests are simple, inexpensive, and rapid. Total T_4 is a direct measurement of thyroxine, unaffected by contaminating non-T_4 iodine. However, changes in serum-binding protein levels produce corresponding changes in total T_4, even though the physiologically active free T_4 is unchanged. Thus, a patient may be physiologically normal but have an abnormal total T_4. **TBG is increased** in pregnancy, by estrogen therapy or oral contraceptives, in the acute phase of infectious hepatitis, in cirrhosis, hypothyroidism, carcinoma of the breast, acute intermittent porphyria, and prolonged perphenazine therapy. TBG may also be increased genetically or idiopathically. **TBG is decreased** by large protein losses (as in the

nephrotic syndrome), by anabolic steroids including testosterone, by cortisol, and by the growth hormone excess in acromegaly. TBG may also be decreased genetically or idiopathically. Finally, large amounts of drugs such as phenytoin and aspirin displace T_4 from its binding sites on TBG, thereby falsely lowering the serum total T_4 level.

3. T_3 resin uptake circumvents the problem of variations in serum TBG levels and reflects the **unsaturated** thyroid hormone-binding sites on TBG. It is *not* a measurement of circulating T_3. In normal subjects, 25 to 35% of the TBG binding sites are occupied by thyroid hormone. When $^{125}I-T_3$ is added to the patient's serum, in vitro, a portion binds to unoccupied TBG sites. After equilibration, a resin is added which binds the remaining unbound $^{125}I-T_3$. The value obtained is expressed as a ratio or percentage; some laboratories report as % unbound, while others report as % bound.

Thus, in hypothyroidism, characterized by decreased levels of circulating thyroid hormone, there are less occupied and more unoccupied TBG binding sites. More $^{125}I-T_3$ is bound to TBG, resulting in *less* uptake of $^{125}I-T_3$ by the resin. The converse pertains in hyperthyroidism. The T_3 resin uptake test is most useful when there is a stable change in the TBG level and the concentration of free thyroxine is unchanged. For example, when TBG is increased (as in pregnancy), *both* occupied and unoccupied binding sites on TBG are increased. The total of T_4 is increased because the TBG sites tend to remain 25 to 35% occupied regardless of the TBG level. Since 99.5% of circulating T_4 is bound to transport proteins, total T_4 is increased if TBG rises in a euthyroid patient with a normal free T_4. However, the T_3 resin uptake reflects the unoccupied sites on the increased amount of TBG, therefore more $^{125}I-T_3$ is bound, resulting in a *decreased* resin uptake. Thus, when TBG is increased in the euthyroid patient, the total T_4 is increased and the T_3 resin uptake is decreased; when TBG is decreased in the euthyroid patient, the total T_4 is decreased and the T_3 resin uptake is increased.

Performance of the serum total T_4 assay and the T_3 resin uptake test permits a valid interpretation of thyroid status in virtually all patients (see TABLE 89–1).

4. Free thyroxine (T_4) index: The product of the value of the T_3 resin uptake and the serum total thyroxine concentration is known as the free thyroxine index and provides an estimate of the concentration of free T_4.

5. Free thyroxine: Theoretically, this determination is the optimum test, since it most accurately reflects thyroid status. However, the measurement of free thyroxine is difficult, has many technical pitfalls, and is not readily available.

6. Serum total T_3 (serum total triiodothyronine) measurement is performed by RIA. Since T_3 is also bound to circulating serum proteins such as TBG, TBPA, and albumin, alterations in serum proteins change the total T_3 levels in a manner identical to that observed for T_4.

7. Serum thyroid-stimulating hormone (TSH) is measured by RIA and is the best test available for demonstrating primary hypothyroidism and for distinguishing between primary and secondary hypothyroidism. In primary hypothyroidism TSH is elevated, whereas in secondary hypothyroidism it is usually undetectable. Some patients, following partial thyroidectomy or ^{131}I treatment, have increased serum TSH but may have sufficient thyroid secretion to maintain a normal T_4.

8. Thyrotropin-releasing hormone (TRH) test: Serum TSH is determined before and after an IV injection of 500 μg of synthetic TRH. Normally, there is a rapid rise in TSH of 5 to 25 $\mu U/ml$, reaching a peak in 30 min and returning to normal by 120 min. The rise is exaggerated in primary hypothyroidism. The TRH test is useful in distinguishing pituitary from hypothalamic hypothyroidism. Hypothyroid patients secondary to a pituitary deficiency do not release TSH in response to TRH. It is assumed that patients with a hypothalamic disorder having deficient TRH reserve and a normal pituitary reserve will usually release TSH in response to TRH. However, it is not certain that this is always the case and probably depends on other associated hormonal

TABLE 89–1. LABORATORY EVALUATION OF THYROID FUNCTION IN VARIOUS THYROID DISORDERS

Physiologic State	*Serum T_4 (Thyroxine)*	*Serum T_3 (Triiodo-thyronine)*	*Resin T_3 (Triiodothyro-nine Uptake)*	*24-h Radio-iodine Uptake (Thyroid)*	*Basal Metabolic Rate*
Hyperthyroidism, untreated	High	High	High	High	High
Hyperthyroidism, T_3 toxicosis	Normal	High	Normal	Normal	High
Hypothyroidism, untreated	Low	Low	Low	Low	Low
Euthyroid, on iodine	Normal	Normal	Normal	Low	Normal
Euthyroid, on exogenous thyroid hormone	High, on T_4 Low, on T_3	High, on T_3 Normal, on T_4	Normal	Low	Normal
Euthyroid, on estrogen	High	High	Low	Normal	Normal
Euthyroid, on phenytoin	Low	Low	High	Normal	Normal

abnormalities. The TRH test is also useful in the diagnosis of hyperthyroidism *where TSH release remains suppressed, even in response to injected TRH*, because of the inhibitory effects of the elevated free T_4 and free T_3 on the pituitary thyrotroph cell.

9. Radioactive iodine uptake (RAI): This test has disadvantages in cost, time, patient inconvenience, and radiation exposure. It is of value in the diagnosis of hyperthyroidism in which the RAI uptake is elevated, but is useless in the diagnosis of hypothyroidism, since the normal 24-h RAI uptake may be as low as 1% due to the large iodine intake in our diet. RAI uptake is particularly useful in the context of a T_3 suppression test and in calculating the dose when ^{131}I is used as the treatment modality.

10. Thyroid scanning with radioiodine or ^{99m}technetium is not a routine test. It is useful in delineating structural abnormalities of the thyroid; eg, to distinguish Graves' disease from multinodular goiter and a single toxic adenoma or to determine the functional state of a single nodule ("hot" vs "cold"). For a discussion of radioisotope scanning of the thyroid see SPECIFIC ORGAN IMAGING PROCEDURES in Ch. 266.

EUTHYROID SICK SYNDROME (ESS)

The presence of abnormal thyroid-function tests in clinically euthyroid patients suffering from severe nonthyroidal systemic illness.

It has recently been recognized that patients with a variety of acute or chronic *nonthyroidal* illnesses or other stresses may have abnormal thyroid function tests, in large part secondary to decreased peripheral conversion of T_4 to T_3, increased conversion of T_4 to reverse T_3, and decreased binding of thyroid hormones to TBG. The patients are euthyroid and the clinical setting and laboratory features have been named ESS. The characteristic thyroid function abnormalities found in ESS include a decreased total serum T_3, increased serum reverse T_3, increased T_3 resin uptake, normal or decreased serum total T_4, and a normal serum TSH. Examples of conditions commonly associated with this syndrome include fasting, starvation, protein-calorie malnutrition, general surgical trauma, myocardial infarction, chronic renal failure, diabetic ketoacidosis, anorexia nervosa, cirrhosis, thermal injury, and sepsis. The interpretation of thyroid function test abnormalities observed in ESS are further complicated by the effects of a variety of drugs including iodinated contrast agents,

propranolol, and amiodarone, which impair the peripheral conversion of T_4 and T_3.

Diagnosis

The diagnostic dilemma is whether the patient is hypothyroid or has ESS. The most sensitive indication of hypothyroidism due to primary thyroid gland failure is a marked elevation of serum TSH (see in Laboratory evaluation under HYPOTHYROIDISM, below). In contrast, patients with ESS have normal levels of serum TSH or, in some patients with cirrhosis, modest increases. Coexistent hypothyroidism in the patient with an acute or chronic systemic illness is also suggested by a low or low normal serum reverse T_3 level.

Alteration of T_4 metabolism in acute illness may also obscure the laboratory diagnosis of hyperthyroidism by lowering the serum total T_3 concentration. Thus, the physician must frequently rely on clinical judgment based on a meticulous history and physical examination when attempting to interpret abnormalities in thyroid function tests in the acutely or chronically ill patient.

Treatment is that of the underlying disorder.

HYPERTHYROIDISM

(Thyrotoxicosis; Toxic Diffuse Goiter; Graves' Disease; Basedow's Disease; Toxic Nodular Goiter; Plummer's Disease)

See TABLE 89–2 for types of hyperthyroidism.

Graves' Disease (Toxic Diffuse Goiter)

Graves' disease *consists of hyperthyroidism, but also is characterized by one or more of the following: goiter, exophthalmos, and pretibial myxedema.* The cause of the hyperthyroidism is not completely understood but is probably immunologic. Patients with Graves' disease have circulating thyroid stimulators in their serum known as **thyroid stimulating immunoglobulins (TSI)** or **thyroid stimulating antibodies (TSAb),** which are 7S IgG immunoglobulins. TSI are of particular interest because they are antibodies directed against the TSH receptor and specifically stimulate the activity of the thyroid. The antibodies presumably arise secondary to a defect in suppressor T-lymphocytes that permits a clone of helper T-lymphocytes to interact with specific thyroid antigens, proliferate, and interact with B-lymphocytes producing TSI. TSH is *not* a cause of Graves' disease.

Symptoms and Signs

Many symptoms and signs are associated with hyperthyroidism. They are the same for all hyperthyroidism with some exceptions, such as infiltrative ophthalmopathy and dermopathy, which are confined to Graves' disease. The clinical presentation may be dramatic or subtle. **The more common signs are:** (1) goiter; (2) tachycardia; (3) widened pulse pressure; (4) warm, fine, moist skin; (5) tremor; (6) eye signs (see below); and (7) atrial fibrillation. **The most frequent symptoms are:** (1) nervousness and increased activity, (2) increased sweating, (3) hypersensitivity to heat, (4) palpitations,

TABLE 89–2. TYPES OF HYPERTHYROIDISM

Most Common	*Very Rare*
Graves' disease (toxic diffuse goiter)	TSH-producing tumor of the pituitary
Toxic multinodular goiter	Metastic embryonal carcinoma of the testis
Toxic adenoma	Choriocarcinoma
Thyrotoxicosis factitia	Struma ovarii
Subacute thyroiditis	
Silent thyroiditis	

(5) fatigue, (6) increased appetite, (7) weight loss, (8) tachycardia, (9) insomnia, (10) weakness, and (11) frequent bowel movements (occasionally diarrhea). Many symptoms of hyperthyroidism are similar to those of adrenergic excess. There is a marked increase in adrenergic activity in hyperthyroidism, and many agents that block stimulation of the adrenergic nervous system relieve the symptoms of hyperthyroidism (see Treatment). However, the mechanism of the augmented adrenergic activity in hyperthyroidism is uncertain and further puzzling, since serum catecholamine levels are decreased. Older persons, particularly those with toxic nodular goiter, may present atypically with **apathetic** or **masked** (monosymptomatic) hyperthyroidism (see Ch. 264).

Eye signs noted in patients with thyrotoxicosis include stare, lid lag, lid retraction, and mild degrees of conjunctival injection or edema-producing symptoms including orbital pain, lacrimation, irritation, and photophobia. These eye signs are largely due to excessive adrenergic stimulation and remit promptly upon successful treatment of the thyrotoxicosis. **Infiltrative ophthalmopathy** is a more serious development and is specific for Graves' disease. It is characterized by increased retro-orbital tissue, producing exophthalmos, and by lymphocytic infiltration of the extraocular muscles, producing a spectrum of ocular muscle weakness frequently leading to blurred and double vision. The pathogenesis of infiltrative ophthalmopathy is poorly understood. It may occur before the onset of hyperthyroidism or as late as 15 to 20 yr afterwards and frequently worsens or improves independent of the clinical course of hyperthyroidism. Infiltrative ophthalmopathy results from autoimmune phenomena distinct from those initiating Graves'-type hyperthyroidism, and in the presence of normal thyroid function is known as **euthyroid Graves' disease.**

Infiltrative dermopathy, also known as pretibial myxedema (a confusing term, since myxedema suggests hypothyroidism), is characterized by nonpitting infiltration of mucinous ground substance, usually in the pretibial area. The lesion is very pruritic and erythematous in its early stages and subsequently becomes brawny. Like ophthalmopathy, infiltrative dermopathy may appear years before or after the hyperthyroidism. TSI are invariably present. Topical steroids can sometimes relieve the pruritus. The dermopathy usually spontaneously remits after months or years.

Other Forms of Hyperthyroidism

Thyroid storm is characterized by abrupt onset of more florid symptoms of thyrotoxicosis, with some exacerbated symptoms and signs atypical of uncomplicated Graves' disease. Included are fever; marked weakness and muscle-wasting; extreme restlessness with wide emotional swings; confusion, psychosis, or even coma; and hepatomegaly with mild jaundice. The patient may present with cardiovascular collapse and shock. Thyroid storm, which is rare in children, results from untreated or inadequately treated thyrotoxicosis and may be precipitated by infection, trauma, surgery, embolism, diabetic acidosis, fright, toxemia of pregnancy or labor, discontinuance of antithyroid medication, or radiation thyroiditis. *Thyroid storm is a life-threatening emergency requiring prompt and specific treatment* (see Treatment and TABLE 89–5, below).

T_3 toxicosis: Both T_3 and T_4 are regularly increased in patients with hyperthyroidism. Increases in serum T_3 are usually somewhat greater proportionally compared to T_4, probably because of both increased thyroidal secretion of T_3 and increased peripheral conversion of T_4 to T_3. In some thyrotoxic patients, only T_3 is elevated; this condition is called "T_3 toxicosis."

T_3 toxicosis may be seen in any of the natural disorders producing hyperthyroidism, including Graves' disease, multinodular goiter, and the autonomously functioning solitary thyroid nodule. If T_3 toxicosis continues untreated, the patient eventually develops the typical laboratory abnormalities of hyperthyroidism; ie, elevated T_4 and ^{131}I

uptake. This suggests that T_3 toxicosis is an early manifestation of ordinary hyperthyroidism and should be treated as such.

It is difficult to diagnose T_3 toxicosis because T_3 is not measured by the ordinary thyroid function tests, but requires a specific RIA. The criteria to establish the diagnosis are (1) symptoms and signs of hyperthyroidism, (2) normal T_4 and ^{131}I uptake, (3) nonsuppressible ^{131}I uptake, (4) failure to release TSH in response to TRH (see TRH test, above), or (5) elevated serum T_3 in the presence of normal T_4.

Toxic adenoma and toxic multinodular goiter (Plummer's disease): One or more thyroid nodules occasionally hyperfunction autonomously for unknown reasons. The excess T_3 and T_4 inhibit the hypothalamic-pituitary axis, stopping TSH production and decreasing production of hormone in the rest of the thyroid. RAI uptake in the hyperfunctioning nodule is increased while, in the rest of the gland, it is decreased. Multinodular goiter with or without hyperthyroidism is more common in older people. Neither toxic multinodular goiter nor toxic adenoma is associated with TSI, exophthalmos, or the pretibial myxedema found in Graves' disease. Since nodules often produce selective increases in T_3 levels, determination of serum total T_3 should be included in the thyroid function tests selected for evaluation of nodular goiter.

Toxic adenoma and multinodular goiter are treated surgically or with radioiodine.

Thyrotoxicosis factitia: This syndrome of hyperthyroidism results from self-administration of thyroid hormone; patients (commonly medical or paramedical personnel) may be surreptitiously taking T_4 or T_3. Laboratory evaluation will vary accordingly. If the disorder is caused by ingestion of preparations containing T_4, the serum T_4 will be elevated. When ingestion of T_3 is the cause, serum T_4 will be below normal. In either case, serum T_3 levels will be increased, particularly when preparations containing T_3 are the causative agents; there will be no goiter.

The various forms of thyroiditis commonly have a hyperthyroid phase. These are discussed separately below.

Secondary hyperthyroidism through overproduction of thyroid hormone can result from excess TSH secreted by a pituitary tumor. Hyperthyroidism secondary to metastatic embryonal carcinoma or choriocarcinoma is due to the TSH-like properties of human chorionic gonadotropin (hCG). **Struma ovarii** is a generally benign ovarian teratoma containing predominantly thyroid tissue. Approximately 5% of the patients with struma ovarii develop hyperthyroidism. Treatment involves removal of the teratoma.

Diagnosis

The diagnosis of hyperthyroidism is usually straightforward and depends on a careful clinical history and physical examination, a high index of suspicion, and routine thyroid hormone determinations. A serum T_4 assay and a T_3 resin uptake test are a highly accurate combination of initial tests for assessing thyroid status and are relatively inexpensive. Occasionally, a serum T_3 determination is required (see above, T_3 Toxicosis). The determination of free thyroxine is less often required and is not as easily available. If the diagnosis of hyperthyroidism remains unclear after these initial tests, more expensive, sophisticated, and time-consuming tests may be required. For example, a TRH test may have to be performed.

Treatment of Hyperthyroidism

A number of approaches are utilized for the treatment of hyperthyroidism (see TABLE 89–3).

Iodine in pharmacologic doses inhibits the release of T_3 and T_4 within hours and inhibits the organification of iodine, a transitory effect lasting from a few days to a week. It is used for the emergency management of thyroid storm, for thyrotoxic patients undergoing emergency surgery, and (since it also decreases the vascularity of the

TABLE 89–3. TREATMENT OF HYPERTHYROIDISM

Iodine
Propylthiouracil and methimazole
Radioactive iodine
Surgery
Propranolol—adjunctive, usually not used alone except for special, short-term circumstances

thyroid gland) for the preoperative preparation of thyrotoxic patients selected for subtotal thyroidectomy. Iodine is generally *not* used for routine treatment of hyperthyroidism. The usual dosage is 2 to 3 drops of a saturated potassium iodide solution tid or qid orally (300 to 600 mg/day) or 0.5 gm sodium iodide in 1 L 0.9% sodium chloride solution given IV slowly q 12 h. Complications of iodine therapy include inflammation of the salivary glands, conjunctivitis, skin rashes, and induction of hyperthyroidism **(Jod-Basedow phenomenon).**

Propylthiouracil and methimazole are antithyroid agents that decrease organification and impair the coupling reaction. There is no "escape" phenomenon as there is with iodine. Although reports vary, it appears that 16 to 40% of the patients will enter remission anywhere from 1 mo to 2 yr after induction of the euthyroid state with antithyroid drugs. At the present time there is no clear benefit in using high doses of antithyroid drugs concomitantly with replacement doses of thyroid hormone.

Propylthiouracil (but not methimazole) also inhibits the peripheral conversion of T_4 to T_3. The usual starting dosage for propylthiouracil is 100 to 150 mg orally q 8 h, and for methimazole 10 to 15 mg orally q 8 h. When the patient becomes euthyroid the dosage is decreased to the lowest effective amount, usually 100 to 150 mg propylthiouracil or 10 to 15 mg methimazole daily in 2 or 3 divided doses. In general, control can be achieved within 6 wk to 3 mo. More rapid control can be achieved by increasing the dose of propylthiouracil to 450 to 600 mg/day (at the risk of increasing the incidence of side effects). Doses of propylthiouracil of this magnitude or greater (800 to 1200 mg/day) are generally reserved for the more seriously ill patients including those with thyrotoxic storm. Maintenance doses can be continued for one year or many years depending on the clinical circumstances. **Carbimazole,** which is used widely in Europe, is rapidly converted in vivo to methimazole. The usual starting dosage is 10 to 15 mg orally q 8 h; maintenance dosage is 10 to 15 mg/day. The incidence of agranulocytosis appears to be higher for carbimazole than for either propylthiouracil or methimazole.

Adverse effects include allergic reactions, nausea, loss of taste, and, in < 1% of patients, a reversible agranulocytosis. If the patient is allergic to one agent, it is acceptable to switch to the other. In case of agranulocytosis, it is *unacceptable* to switch to another agent, and more definitive therapy should be invoked, such as radioiodine or surgery.

The disappearance or marked decrease in gland size and the redevelopment of suppressible thyroid function, as determined by T_3 suppression test or TRH test, may be evidence that the patient is undergoing remission.

Radioactive sodium iodine ^{131}I is generally used in patients past their childbearing years, because it is not clear what the effects may be on their progeny. There has been no proven increased incidence of tumors, leukemia, or carcinoma of the thyroid and some use this therapy in younger patients. Radioiodine is the treatment of choice for Graves' disease in patients > 40 yr of age. Dosage of ^{131}I is difficult to gauge and the response of the gland cannot be predicted. If enough ^{131}I is given to produce euthyroidism, 1 yr later 25% of the patients will have hypothyroidism, and the incidence continues to increase at a regular rate for up to 20 yr or more thereafter. On the other

hand, if smaller doses are used, there is a high incidence of recurrence of hyperthyroidism.

Surgery is used in patients < 21 yr who should not receive radioiodine; in individuals who cannot tolerate other agents because of hypersensitivity or other problems; in patients with very large goiters (100 to 400 gm [normal thyroid weighs 20 gm]), and in some patients with toxic adenoma and multinodular goiter.

Surgery offers a good prospect for recovery of normal function. In expert hands, postoperative recurrences vary between 2 and 9%; hypothyroidism occurs in about 3% of patients the first year and in about 2% with each succeeding year. Vocal cord paralysis and hypoparathyroidism are uncommon complications, but difficult to treat. Iodine is used in preparing the patient for surgery. Saturated solution of potassium iodide 3 drops orally tid (about 300 to 500 mg/day) should be given for 2 wk before the operation to reduce the vascularity of the gland and facilitate surgery. Propylthiouracil must also be given prior to surgery, since the patient should be euthyroid before surgery. Surgical procedures are more difficult in patients who previously have undergone thyroidectomy or radioiodine therapy.

β-Adrenergic blocking drugs: Symptoms and signs of hyperthyroidism due to adrenergic stimulation may respond to these agents. Propranolol has had the greatest use. Phenomena that improve and that do not improve with propranolol are shown in TABLE 89–4. Propranolol is not as useful for stare and lid retraction as once thought, suggesting that these may be predominantly α-effects (or at least a mixture of α- and β-effects). It should be noted that propranolol decreases myocardial contractility through a non-β-adrenergic mechanism. Because propranolol is a direct myocardial depressant, there are some difficulties that accompany its use (see below).

Propranolol is indicated in thyroid storm. It rapidly decreases heart rate, usually within 2 to 3 h when given orally, and in minutes when given IV. It may bring about rapid defervescence of fever in thyroid storm. Propranolol is also indicated for the prompt management of troublesome tachycardia found in other forms of hyperthyroidism (including thyroiditis) and especially in older patients with no history of congestive heart failure, since it ordinarily takes several weeks to get relief from antithyroid agents. However, propranolol should not be used routinely in all types of hyperthyroidism. For details concerning propranolol therapy see β-Blockers under ARTERIAL HYPERTENSION in Ch. 26.

A treatment regimen for **thyroid storm** listing all of the above-mentioned therapies is shown in TABLE 89–5.

TABLE 89–4. EFFECTS OF PROPRANOLOL ON SYMPTOMS AND SIGNS OF HYPERTHYROIDISM

Phenomena Improved	*Phenomena Not Improved*
Tachycardia	Oxygen consumption—although excess catecholamines (as in patients with pheochromocytoma) increase O_2 consumption, the major stimulus to O_2 consumption is thyroid hormone increase of $Na^+ \cdot K^+ \cdot$ATPase activity
Tremor	Goiter
Mental symptoms	Bruit
Heat intolerance and sweating (occasional)	Circulating thyroxine levels
Diarrhea (occasional)	Weight loss (may be stabilized, but not improved)
Proximal myopathy (occasional)	Exophthalmos
Serum T_3 (decreased about 50%)	Myocardial contractility

TABLE 89–5. TREATMENT OF THYROID STORM

Iodine—30 drops Lugol's solution/day orally in 3 or 4 divided doses; or 1 to 2 gm sodium iodide slowly by IV drip
Propylthiouracil—900 to 1200 mg/day orally or by gastric tube
Propranolol—160 mg/day orally in 4 divided doses; or 1 to 2 mg *slowly* IV q 4 h under careful monitoring
IV glucose solutions
Correction of dehydration and electrolyte imbalance
Cooling blanket for hyperthermia
Digitalis if necessary
Treatment of underlying disease such as infection
Adrenal steroids—100 to 300 mg hydrocortisone/day IV or IM
Definitive therapy after control of the crisis consists of ablation of the thyroid gland with ^{131}I or surgery.

HYPOTHYROIDISM

(Myxedema)

The characteristic reaction to thyroid hormone deficiency in the adult.

Primary hypothyroidism, the most common form, is probably an autoimmune disease, usually occurring as a sequel to Hashimoto's thyroiditis. It results in a shrunken fibrotic thyroid gland with little or no function. The second most common form is **post-therapeutic hypothyroidism,** especially following RAI therapy or surgery for hyperthyroidism. Hypothyroidism during therapy with propylthiouracil, methimazole, and iodides usually abates after cessation of therapy.

Most patients with goiters are either euthyroid or have hyperthyroidism, but **goitrous hypothyroidism** may occur in endemic goiter. Iodine deficiency decreases thyroid hormonogenesis; TSH is released, the thyroid gland enlarges under the TSH stimulus and traps iodine avidly, and goiter ensues. If iodine deficiency is severe, the patient becomes hypothyroid, but this disease is virtually extinct in the USA since the advent of iodized salt. **Endemic cretinism** may occur in the offspring of parents with endemic goitrous hypothyroidism.

Rare inherited enzymatic defects can also alter the synthesis of thyroid hormone and cause goitrous hypothyroidism. (See also CONGENITAL GOITERS in Ch. 196.)

Secondary hypothyroidism occurs when there is failure of the hypothalamic-pituitary axis, either due to deficient secretion of TRH from the hypothalamus or lack of secretion of TSH from the pituitary.

Symptoms and Signs

The symptoms and signs of primary hypothyroidism are generally in striking contrast to those of hyperthyroidism and may be quite subtle and insidious in onset. The facial expression is dull; there is puffiness and periorbital swelling caused by infiltration with the mucopolysaccharides, hyaluronic acid and chondroitin sulfate; eyelids droop because of decreased adrenergic drive; hair is sparse, coarse, and dry; and the skin is coarse, dry, scaly, and thick. Patients are forgetful, and show other evidence of intellectual impairment with a gradual change in personality. There may be frank psychosis **("myxedema madness").**

There is often carotenemia, particularly notable on the palms and soles, caused by deposition of carotene in the lipid-rich epidermal layers. Deposition of mucinous ground substance in the tongue may produce macroglossia. There is bradycardia due to a decrease in both thyroid hormone and adrenergic stimulation. The heart is enlarged due, in large measure, to accumulation of a serous effusion of high protein

content in the pericardial sac. There may also be pleural or abdominal effusions. The pericardial and pleural effusions develop slowly, and only infrequently result in respiratory or hemodynamic distress. Patients generally note constipation, which may be severe. Paresthesias of the hands and feet are common, due to carpal-tarsal tunnel syndrome caused by deposition of mucinous ground substance in the ligaments around the wrist and ankle, producing nerve compression. The reflexes may be very helpful diagnostically because of the brisk contraction and the slow relaxation time. There is often menorrhagia, in contrast to the hypomenorrhea of hyperthyroidism. Hypothermia is commonly noted if the temperature is measured rectally. Anemia is often present, usually normocytic normochromic in character and of unknown etiology; but it may be hypochromic due to menorrhagia, and sometimes is macrocytic because of impaired B_{12} absorption related to decreased intrinsic factor synthesis. In general, the anemia is rarely severe (Hb > 9 gm/dL). As the hypometabolic state is repaired, the anemia subsides. Complete repair may require 6 to 9 mo.

Myxedema coma, a life-threatening complication of hypothyroidism, is extremely rare in warm climates but not uncommon in cold areas. Its characteristics include a background of longstanding hypothyroidism, coma with extreme hypothermia (temperatures 24 to 32.2 C [75.2 to 90 F]), areflexia, seizures, CO_2 retention, and respiratory depression caused by decreased cerebral blood flow. Severe hypothermia may be missed unless special low-reading thermometers are used. Rapid diagnosis (based on clinical judgment, history, and physical examination) is imperative because early death is likely. Precipitating factors include exposure to cold, infection, trauma, and drugs that suppress the CNS. See below for treatment.

Diagnosis of Primary vs. Secondary Hypothyroidism

It is important to differentiate secondary from primary hypothyroidism, because, while secondary hypothyroidism is not common, it often involves other endocrine organs affected by the hypothalamic-pituitary axis. The clues to secondary hypothyroidism are a history of amenorrhea rather than menorrhagia in a woman with known hypothyroidism and some suggestive differences on physical examination. In secondary hypothyroidism, the skin and hair are dry but not as coarse; skin depigmentation is often noted; macroglossia is not as prominent; breasts are atrophic; the heart is small without accumulation of the serous effusions in the pericardial sac; BP is low; and hypoglycemia is often found because of concomitant adrenal insufficiency or growth hormone deficiency.

Laboratory evaluation shows a *low* level of circulating TSH in secondary hypothyroidism, whereas in primary hypothyroidism there is no feedback inhibition of the intact pituitary and serum levels of TSH are *very high.* The serum TSH is the most simple and sensitive test for the diagnosis of primary hypothyroidism. Serum cholesterol is generally low in secondary hypothyroidism, but high in primary hypothyroidism. Other pituitary hormones and their corresponding target tissue hormones may be low in secondary hypothyroidism.

The **TRH test** (see thyroid function testing, above) is useful in distinguishing between hypothyroidism secondary to pituitary failure and hypothyroidism due to hypothalamic failure. In the former, TSH is not released in response to TRH, whereas in the latter TSH is released.

The **TSH stimulation test** was used to distinguish between primary and secondary hypothyroidism before the serum TSH immunoassay became available but is only occasionally used today. The test is performed by carrying out an initial RAI uptake for a 24-h period. On the next 3 days, 5 USP units of TSH are given IM. On the 4th day, the 2nd RAI uptake is performed. Patients with primary hypothyroidism will not respond; patients with secondary hypothyroidism will have a brisk response unless they have had longstanding secondary hypothyroidism (eg, for 15 or 20 yr). The test

has 3 disadvantages: (1) it requires administration of radioactive iodine on two occasions, with its associated radiation exposure; (2) it is expensive and time-consuming for the patient; and (3) allergic reactions to the bovine TSH used in the test are not infrequent. There are also certain risks associated with TSH stimulation. If the patient has arteriosclerotic heart disease, a sudden increase in heart rate may lead to angina or myocardial infarction. Patients with secondary hypothyroidism may have adrenal insufficiency, and an increase in metabolic rate can precipitate adrenal crisis unless glucocorticoid therapy is given. Finally, in rare cases, there may be enlargement of the thyroid as a result of TSH stimulation which, if the gland is located substernally, may result in respiratory distress.

The **determination of serum total T_3 levels** in hypothyroidism deserves special mention. Other conditions are characterized by decreased circulating levels of total T_3 besides primary and secondary hypothyroidism; these include decreased serum TBG, drugs (see above) and the euthyroid sick syndrome found in patients with chronic liver and renal disease, acute and chronic illness, starvation, and low carbohydrate diets (see above for discussion of euthyroid sick syndrome).

Generally, both serum T_3 and T_4 levels are decreased in hypothyroidism. Curiously, perhaps as many as 25% of patients with primary hypothyroidism (elevated serum TSH, low serum T_4) may have normal circulating levels of T_3. This remains unexplained, but may result from sustained TSH stimulation of the suboptimally functioning thyroid and incorporation of the trapped iodine preferentially into the pathway responsible for synthesizing the more potent thyroid hormone, T_3.

Treatment of Hypothyroidism

A variety of thyroid hormone preparations are available for replacement therapy, including synthetic preparations of thyroxine, liothyronine (triiodothyronine), combinations of the 2 synthetic hormones, and desiccated animal thyroid. **Synthetic preparations of T_4 (L-thyroxine)** are preferred; the *average* maintenance dosage is 150 to 200 μg/day orally. Absorption is fairly constant at about 60% of the dose. T_3 is generated from the T_4 by the liver. In infants and young children the average maintenance dose of T_4 is 2.5 μg/kg/day. The dose used should be the minimum that restores TSH levels to normal (though this criterion cannot be used in patients with secondary hypothyroidism).

T_3 (liothyronine sodium) should not be used alone for long-term replacement because its rapid turnover requires that it be taken bid or tid. T_3 is occasionally used mainly in starting therapy because the rapid excretion is useful in the initial titration of a patient with longstanding hypothyroidism in whom cardiac arrhythmias may occur early in replacement therapy. In addition, administering standard replacement amounts of T_3 (25 to 75 μg/day) results in rapidly increasing serum T_3 levels to between 300 and 1000 ng within 2 to 4 h; these levels return to normal by 24 h. Therefore, when assessing serum T_3 levels in patients on this particular regimen, it is important for the physician to be aware of the time of prior administration of the hormone. Additionally, patients receiving T_3 are chemically hyperthyroid for at least several hours a day and thus are exposed to greater cardiac risks. Similar patterns of serum T_3 concentrations are seen when mixtures of T_3 and T_4 are taken orally, although the peak levels of T_3 are somewhat lower. Replacement regimens with synthetic preparations of T_4 reflect a different pattern of serum T_3 response. Increases in serum T_3 occur gradually over weeks, finally reaching a normal value about 8 wk after starting therapy.

Treatment of myxedema coma is with large doses of T_4 (500 μg IV bolus) or T_3, if available (40 μg IV), because TBG must be saturated before any free hormone is available for response. The maintenance dose for T_4 is 50 μg/day IV, and for T_3, 10 to 20 μg/day IV until T_4 can be given orally. The patient should *not* be rewarmed rapidly because of the threat of cardiac arrhythmias. If alveolar ventilation is compromised, immediate mechanical ventilatory assistance is required.

THYROIDITIS

HASHIMOTO'S THYROIDITIS

(Chronic Lymphocytic Thyroiditis; Hashimoto's Struma; Autoimmune Thyroiditis)

A chronic inflammation of the thyroid with lymphocytic infiltration of the gland generally thought to be caused by autoimmune factors. This disorder is believed to be the most common cause of primary hypothyroidism. It is more prevalent (8:1) in women than men and most frequent between the ages of 30 and 50. A family history of thyroid disorders is common and incidence is increased in patients with chromosomal disorders, including Turner's, Down's, and Klinefelter's syndromes. Histologic studies reveal extensive infiltration of lymphocytes in the thyroid.

Patients complain of painless enlargement of the gland or fullness in the throat. On examination there is a nontender goiter, smooth or nodular, firm, and more rubbery in consistency than the normal thyroid; 20% of patients have hypothyroidism when first seen. Other forms of autoimmune disease are common, including pernicious anemia, RA, SLE, and Sjögren's syndrome. Frequent coexistence with other endocrine disorders, including Addison's disease (adrenal insufficiency), hypoparathyroidism, and diabetes mellitus, all of which may be autoimmmune in nature, is also observed. There may be an increased incidence of thyroid neoplasia, particularly papillary carcinoma, possibly because of increased TSH stimulation.

Laboratory findings early in the disease consist of a normal T_4 but an increased PBI (due to production of abnormal iodinated proteins) and high titers of antithyroid antibodies. Similarly, RAI uptake is increased early because of a defect in organification in conjunction with a gland continuing to trap iodine. Late in the disease, the patient develops hypothyroidism with a decrease in T_4 and in RAI uptake. Antibodies in this stage are usually no longer detectable.

Treatment of Hashimoto's thyroiditis requires lifelong replacement with thyroid hormone to correct and prevent hypothyroidism. The average oral replacement dose with L-thyroxine is 150 to 200 μg/day.

SUBACUTE THYROIDITIS

(Granulomatous, Giant-Cell, or DeQuervain's Thyroiditis)

An acute inflammatory disease of the thyroid probably caused by a virus. Frequently, there is a history of mumps, and the disease has been described following a wide variety of URIs. Histologic studies do not show lymphocyte infiltration of the gland, as in Hashimoto's disease, but there is a characteristic giant-cell infiltration.

Clinical features are the sudden onset of "sore throat" (in reality, neck pain) with progressive tenderness in the neck and low-grade fever (37.8 to 38.3 C [100 to 101 F]). The neck pain shifts characteristically from side to side and finally settles in one area, frequently radiating to the jaw and ears. It is often confused with dental problems, pharyngitis or otitis, and is aggravated by swallowing or turning the head. Hyperthyroidism is common early in the disease because of hormone release from the markedly inflamed gland. Also, there is lassitude and prostration not seen in other thyroid disorders. On physical examination, the thyroid is asymetrically enlarged, firm, and tender. Subacute thyroiditis is self-limiting, generally subsiding in a few months; occasionally it recurs, and only rarely results in hypothyroidism.

Laboratory findings early in the disease include an increase in T_4, a decrease in RAI uptake (often 0), leukocytosis, and a high ESR. After several weeks, the T_4 is decreased and the RAI uptake remains low. Full recovery is the rule; rarely, patients may become hypothyroid.

Treatment consists of aspirin 600 mg q 4 h and, only as a last resort, glucocorticoids such as prednisone 5 mg orally q 6 h. On discontinuance of the latter, there is often a severe rebound in symptoms.

SILENT THYROIDITIS

A subacute disorder occurring most commonly in women, often in the postpartum period, characterized by a variable but mild degree of thyroid enlargement, absence of thyroid tenderness, and a self-limited hyperthyroid phase of several weeks to several months, often followed by transient hypothyroidism but with eventual recovery to the euthyroid state.

Although the etiology of silent thyroiditis is obscure, recent evidence suggests an autoimmune component. In the postpartum period, this disorder comprises the vast majority of cases of postpartum hypothyroidism.

Diagnosis: Biopsies reveal lymphocytic infiltration as is seen in Hashimoto's thyroiditis. Human antithyroglobulin antibodies measured by a RIA are sometimes elevated in silent thyroiditis and may remain so for up to 9 mo; thus, this disorder would appear to be a variant of Hashimoto's thyroiditis. However, unlike the hyperthyroidism occasionally seen with Hashimoto's thyroiditis or with Graves' disease, the elevated thyroid hormone levels of silent thyroiditis occur in association with a very low RAI uptake. The combination of a high serum thyroid hormone concentration and a low RAI uptake can also be seen with subacute thyroiditis, factitious hyperthyroidism, and iodine ingestion. The WBC count is normal and the ESR normal or slightly elevated. Eye signs and pretibial myxedema do not occur.

Treatment: Since silent thyroiditis is a self-limited transient disorder of one to several months, treatment is conservative, usually only requiring β-adrenergic blockade with propranolol (see above). Surgery and radioactive iodine therapy are contraindicated. Although the transient phase of hypothyroidism may require thyroid hormone replacement therapy, most patients recover normal thyroid function; therefore, their thyroid status should be reevaluated in 6 mo to 1 yr. Overall, 10% of patients may experience relapses within 3 yr. Therefore, follow-up for at least 3 yr is advisable.

EUTHYROID GOITER

(Simple, Endemic, Nontoxic Diffuse, or Nontoxic Nodular Goiter)

An enlargement of the thyroid gland due to diminished thyroid hormone production but without clinical hypothyroidism. If the deficiency is caused by inadequate dietary intake of iodine, it is called **endemic (colloid) goiter.** Euthyroid goiter is the most common form of thyroid enlargement and is frequently noted at the onset of puberty, during pregnancy, and at menopause. Numerous other causes include intrinsic thyroid hormone production defects or the ingestion of goitrogens (such as turnips) that contain antithyroid substances similar to thiouracil. Many drugs, including aminosalicylic acid, sulfonylureas, lithium, and even iodine in large doses, may block the synthesis of thyroid hormone. Compensatory TSH elevations occur, preventing hypothyroidism, but the TSH stimulation results in goiter formation. Recurrent cycles of stimulation and involution may result in nontoxic nodular goiters.

Symptoms, Signs, and Diagnosis

In the early stages, diagnosis depends on the presence of a soft, symmetric, smooth goiter. There may be a history of low iodine intake or ingestion of goitrogens. Thyroidal RAI uptake may be normal or high, with a normal thyroid scan. The serum T_4 level and the T_3-resin uptake are usually normal. Later, multiple nodules and cysts may appear.

Treatment

The cause should be identified. Iodine deficiency is rare in the USA today, but if present, iodine is given. If a goitrogen is being ingested, it should be discontinued. In other instances, suppression of the hypothalamic-pituitary axis with thyroid hormone will block the TSH stimulation that leads to goiter formation. Full replacement doses are necessary; ie, sodium levothyroxine 150 to 200 μg/day orally. Large goiters occasionally require surgery to prevent interference with respiration or to correct cosmetic problems.

THYROID CANCERS

Usually, either the patient or the doctor notices an otherwise symptomless lump in the neck. Rarely, metastases from a small thyroid cancer may lead to presenting complaints due to lymph node enlargement, pulmonary symptoms, or a destructive bone lesion. Most thyroid nodules are benign and, as a rule, thyroid cancers are not highly malignant and generally are compatible with normal life expectancy, *if treated properly*. There are 4 types of thyroid cancer: papillary, follicular, mixed (most common), medullary (solid, with amyloid struma), and anaplastic (rare).

The suspicion that the patient has cancer is increased by the following factors: (1) age (the young are more susceptible); (2) sex, if the patient is a man (more women have thyroid cancer by a ratio of 2:1, but women have more thyroid disease by a ratio of about 8:1; thus, a man with a nodule should be regarded with greater suspicion); (3) a solitary nodule (multinodular lesions are usually multinodular goiter); (4) a cold nodule on RAI uptake scanning (hot nodules are seldom cancer); (5) a history of radiation exposure to the head, neck, or chest (eg, for an enlarged thymus or tonsils, for acne or Hodgkin's disease); (6) if there is radiographic evidence of fine, stippled "psammomatous" calcification (papillary carcinoma) or dense, homogeneous calcification (medullary carcinoma); (7) recent or rapid enlargement; and (8) "stony-hard" consistency. Needle aspiration biopsy is of some use in distinguishing benign from malignant nodules when one has the technic available and an experienced pathologist to read the samples. The diagnosis can only be firmly established by histologic or cytologic examination of the neoplastic tissue.

Papillary carcinoma is the most common thyroid malignancy (60 to 70% of all thyroid cancers). Females are affected 2 to 3 times more often than males. It is more frequent in the young, but it takes a more malignant course in the elderly. It is often associated with a history of radiation exposure and spreads via the lymphatics. Lateral aberrant thyroid rests may be found that are actually occult metastases with a benign histologic appearance. These well-differentiated cancers are highly TSH-dependent and may develop in hypothyroid glands secondary to Hashimoto's thyroiditis. Many papillary cancers contain follicular elements but this does not alter the basic biology of the tumor. **Treatment** for small (< 1.5 cm), encapsulated tumors localized to one lobe is lobectomy and isthmusectomy. Thyroid hormone in suppressive doses is given to minimize chances of regrowth or produce regression of any microscopic remnants of papillary carcinoma, surgery is almost always curative. Large (> 1.5 cm) or diffusely spreading tumors require total or near-total thyroidectomy with postoperative radioiodine ablation of residual thyroid tissue with 150 mCi ^{131}I administered when the patient is hypothyroid. Replacement doses of L-thyroxine are given afterwards at an average oral dose of 150 to 200 μg/day.

Follicular carcinoma accounts for about 15% of thyroid cancer and is more common in the elderly. It is more malignant than papillary carcinoma, spreading hematogenously with distant metastases. It also is occasionally associated with a history of radiation exposure and is more frequent in females than in males. **Treatment** for follicular cancer of any size requires near-total thyroidectomy with postoperative radioi-

odine ablation of residual thyroid tissue similar to the patient with papillary cancer. Metastases appear to be more amenable to radioiodine therapy.

Anaplastic carcinoma accounts for 10% or less of thyroid cancer and occurs mostly in elderly patients, females slightly more than males. The tumor is characterized by rapid and painful enlargement and about 80% of patients die within 1 yr of diagnosis.

Medullary (solid) carcinoma of the thyroid may occur as a sporadic form (usually unilateral) or as a familial form (frequently bilateral), transmitted as an autosomal dominant. Patients are usually > 15 yr of age. Pathologically there is a proliferation of parafollicular cells ("C" cells) that produce excessive calcitonin, a hormone that can lower serum Ca and PO_4, and there are characteristic amyloid deposits that stain with Congo red. Metastases are via lymphatics to cervical and mediastinal nodes, but there may also be metastases to liver, lungs, and bone, with dense calcifications.

Medullary carcinoma of the thyroid may have a dramatic biochemical presentation when it is associated with ectopic production of hormones such as ACTH, prostaglandins, and serotonin. This tumor is a component of **Sipple's syndrome** which presents with medullary carcinoma of the thyroid, pheochromocytoma, and hyperparathyroidism (see MEN II in Ch. 92). All 3 disorders are not always present in the same patient. Pheochromocytoma is present in 50 to 75%; hyperparathyroidism, in 50%. Additional findings not regularly present with this syndrome include disorders of the neural ectoderm, including mucosal neuromas; megacolon; pectus excavatum; poorly developed musculature; and marfanoid appearance, with long arms and fingers. When these associated conditions occur, the syndrome is classified as MEN, type IIb; hyperparathyroidism is not present in this subset.

Laboratory evaluation: RAI scan shows a nonfunctioning, cold nodule that does not concentrate radioiodine (see also SPECIFIC ORGAN IMAGING PROCEDURES in Ch. 266). X-rays may show a dense, homogenous, conglomerate calcification. The best diagnostic test for medullary carcinoma is assay for excess calcitonin, since only rarely is the serum level normal. A challenge with calcium (15 mg Ca/kg over 4 h IV), glucagon, or pentagastrin (0.5 μg/kg IV in 5 sec) provokes output of abnormal amounts of calcitonin. Precise figures for calcitonin levels vary in different laboratories. The histaminase level is increased in 50% of patients and usually indicates metastatic disease. Increased histaminase levels occasionally may be found without metastases and also may be seen in pregnancy, subacute thyroiditis, and after heparin injection. As a clinical test, intradermal injection of histamine is used; in medullary carcinoma patients, no flare occurs. Inhibitors of histaminase have no effect on the tumor.

Treatment of medullary carcinoma consists of total thyroidectomy, even if bilateral involvement is not obvious. Lymph node and radical neck dissection may also be performed if metastases are found. If hyperparathyroidism is present, removal of hyperplastic or adenomatous parathyroids is required. If pheochromocytoma occurs, it is usually bilateral; therefore, an anterior abdominal approach is preferred for the surgery. Because of the danger of provoking hypertensive crisis during surgery, pheochromocytomas should be removed before thyroidectomy.

Owing to the familial incidence of medullary carcinoma of the thyroid, it is important to screen relatives by periodically determining the levels of serum calcitonin, Ca, PO_4, and urinary catecholamines. Screening is most sensitive if a Ca or pentagastrin stimulus is used.

Implications for Thyroid Cancer of External Irradiation to the Head, Neck, and Upper Thorax in Infancy and Childhood

External irradiation to the head, neck, or upper thorax was administered in the past to treat a variety of minor conditions, including recurrent tonsillitis, adenoiditis, acne, tinea capitis, and thymic enlargement as well as serious diseases such as Hodgkin's

disease and leukemia. The thyroid was incidentally irradiated by these procedures.

Although not appreciated at the time, relatively small doses of radiation during infancy and childhood increase the risk of developing benign and malignant thyroid neoplasms. It requires about 5 yr after exposure to develop a thyroid abnormality, but the patient remains at increased risk for at least 30 to 40 yr after exposure. Probably no more than 1/3 of those irradiated develop a thyroid neoplasm; most are benign. However, about 7% of the irradiated group develop thyroid carcinoma; most are papillary, mixed follicular-papillary, or follicular, and are generally slow-growing and relatively nonaggressive. The tumors are frequently multicentric and a thyroid scan does not always reflect areas of involvement. In a number of instances microscopic foci of cancer have been observed in areas considered normal.

Initial evaluation of all patients having received external irradiation to the thyroid gland should include examination of the thyroid gland for any palpable abnormality and a radioisotope scan, preferably using ^{99m}technetium in combination with a gamma counter and a pinhole collimator. In the absence of any abnormality, many physicians recommend physiologic replacement therapy with thyroid hormone with the aim of suppressing thyroid function and thyrotropin secretion to decrease the chance of developing a thyroid neoplasm. The presence of a scan abnormality in the absence of a palpable abnormality requires clinical judgment as to whether a period of suppressive therapy with thyroid hormone is required or whether there should be surgery. Unless the nodule disappears within 3 to 6 mo, it should be biopsied or excised. Additionally, all patients should have a determination of thyroid autoantibodies in the initial evaluation, since diffuse or irregular enlargement of the thyroid gland may be due to Hashimoto's (lymphocytic) thyroiditis. Physical examination of the neck should be performed yearly. Scanning is *not* repeated routinely.

Near-total thyroidectomy is the treatment of choice when operative intervention is required, followed by ablation of residual thyroid tissue with radioiodine if a cancer is found. The operation must be performed by a surgeon with proven expertise in thyroid surgery because of the risks inherent in such a procedure, including hypoparathyroidism and destruction of the recurrent laryngeal nerve.

90. PARATHYROID

(See DISTURBANCES IN CALCIUM METABOLISM in Ch. 84)

91. ADRENAL

The adrenal cortex produces androgens, glucocorticoids (eg, cortisol), and mineralocorticoids (eg, aldosterone). The effects of the adrenocortical hormones and the physiology of the pituitary-adrenal system are described in Chs. 87 and 88. The distinct clinical syndromes produced by **hypofunction** or **hyperfunction** of the cortex are discussed below.

ADRENAL HYPOFUNCTION

ADDISON'S DISEASE

(Primary or Chronic Adrenocortical Insufficiency)

An insidious and usually progressive disease resulting from adrenocortical hypofunction.

Etiology and Incidence

About 70% of cases are due to idiopathic atrophy of the adrenal cortex, the remainder to destruction of the gland by granuloma (eg, tuberculosis), neoplasm, amyloidosis, or inflammatory necrosis. The incidence is about 4:100,000. Addison's disease occurs

in all age groups, about equally in each sex, and tends to become clinically apparent during metabolic stress or trauma.

Pathophysiology

The principal hormones produced by the adrenal cortex are cortisol (hydrocortisone), aldosterone, and dehydroisoandrosterone (dehydroepiandrosterone). Adults secrete about 20 mg of cortisol, 2 mg of corticosterone (which has similar activity), and 0.2 mg of aldosterone daily. Although considerable quantities of androgens (primarily dehydroisoandrosterone and androstenedione) are normally produced by the adrenal cortex, these exert their chief physiologic activity after conversion to testosterone and dihydrotestosterone.

In Addison's disease, there is increased excretion of Na and decreased excretion of K chiefly in the urine, which is dilute, and also in the sweat, saliva, and GI tract. Low blood concentrations of Na and Cl and high serum K result. Inability to concentrate the urine, combined with changes in electrolyte balance, produce severe dehydration, increased plasma concentration, decreased circulatory volume, hypotension, and circulatory collapse.

Cortisol deficiency contributes to the hypotension and produces disturbances in carbohydrate, fat, and protein metabolism, and severe insulin sensitivity. In the absence of cortisol, insufficient carbohydrate is formed from protein; hypoglycemia and diminished liver glycogen result. Weakness, due in part to deficient neuromuscular function, follows. Resistance to infection, trauma, and other stress is diminished because of reduced adrenal output. Myocardial weakness and dehydration cause reduced cardiac output and circulatory failure can occur. Reduced cortisol blood levels result in increased pituitary ACTH production and an increase in β-lipotropin, which has melanocyte-stimulating activity and produces the hyperpigmentation of skin and mucous membranes characteristic of Addison's disease.

Symptoms and Signs

Weakness, fatigue, and orthostatic hypotension are early symptoms. Pigmentation is usually increased except in adrenal insufficiency secondary to pituitary failure. Increased pigmentation is characterized by diffuse tanning of both exposed and nonexposed portions of the body, especially on pressure points (bony prominences), skin folds, scars, and extensor surfaces. Black freckles over the forehead, face, neck, and shoulders; areas of vitiligo; and bluish-black discolorations of the areolas and of the mucous membranes of the lips, mouth, rectum, and vagina are common. Weight loss, dehydration, hypotension, and small heart size are characteristic in the later stages of the disease. Anorexia, nausea, vomiting, and diarrhea often occur. Decreased cold tolerance, with hypometabolism, may be noted. Dizziness and syncopal attacks may occur. The ECG may show decreased voltage and prolonged P-R and Q-T intervals. The EEG shows a generalized slowing of the α-rhythm.

An **adrenal crisis** is characterized by profound asthenia; severe pains in the abdomen, lower back, or legs; peripheral vascular collapse; and, finally, renal shutdown with azotemia. Body temperature may be subnormal, though severe hyperthermia due to infection is often seen. Crisis is precipitated most often by acute infection (especially with septicemia), trauma, operative procedures, and salt loss due to excessive sweating during hot weather.

Laboratory Findings

A low serum Na level (< 130 mEq/L), a high serum K level (> 5 mEq/L), and an elevated BUN, together with a characteristic clinical picture, suggest the possibility of Addison's disease (see TABLE 91–1).

Diagnostic Tests

Adrenal insufficiency can be specifically diagnosed by demonstrating failure to increase plasma cortisol levels, or urinary 17-hydroxycorticosteroid **(17-OHCS)** or 17-

TABLE 91–1. LABORATORY FINDINGS SUGGESTING ADDISON'S DISEASE

Blood chemistry	Low serum Na* (< 130 mEq/L)
	High serum K* (> 5 mEq/L)
	Ratio of serum Na:K (< 30:1)
	Low fasting blood sugar (< 50 mg/dL)
	Decrease in plasma bicarbonate (< 28 mEq/L)
	Elevated BUN (> 20 mg/dL)
Hematology	Elevated hematocrit
	Low WBC count
	Relative lymphocytosis
	Increased eosinophils
X-ray	Evidence of:
	Small heart
	Calcifications in the adrenal areas
	Renal tuberculosis
	Pulmonary tuberculosis

* Na = sodium; K = potassium.

ketogenic steroid **(17-KGS)** excretion, upon administration of corticotropin **(ACTH)**. Urinary 17-KGS or 17-OHCS excretion, in the absence of endogenous ACTH stimulation, is unreliable as an index of adrenocortical functional capacity, since baseline excretion does not adequately separate low-normal from the abnormally low value. A single determination of plasma cortisol or 24-h urinary 17-OHCS or 17-KGS excretion is not useful and may be misleading in diagnosing adrenal insufficiency. However, if the patient is severely stressed or in shock, a single depressed plasma cortisol determination is highly suggestive. An elevated plasma ACTH level in association with a low plasma cortisol level is highly diagnostic.

Testing for adrenal insufficiency is performed as follows: Cosyntropin 0.25 mg is injected IV. Normal pre-injection plasma cortisol ranges from 4 to 25 μg/dL and doubles at 60 to 90 min. Patients with Addison's disease have low or normal values that do not rise.

To distinguish between primary and secondary adrenal insufficiency: The plasma ACTH concentration is high (50 pg/mL or more) if adrenal failure is caused by adrenal disease. Patients with pituitary failure have a low ACTH concentration. If ACTH determination is not available, a **metyrapone test** should be done. The best and simplest method is to administer metyrapone 30 mg/kg orally at midnight with a little food to avoid gastric irritation. The plasma cortisol at 8:00 AM the following morning should be < 10 μg/dL, and the plasma 11-deoxycortisol ("compound S") should be 7 to 22 μg/dL. Patients with primary adrenal failure will have low levels of both; those with hypopituitarism will respond to ACTH but not to metyrapone. It may be necessary to prime the patient with long-acting ACTH 20 u. IM bid for several days before doing the test, to prevent failure of adrenal response because of atrophy in patients with pituitary failure. A new test, which may distinguish hypothalamic from pituitary failure, is based on response to **corticotropin releasing factor (CRF).** After 100 μg (or 1 μg/kg) IV, the normal response is a rise of plasma ACTH of 30 to 40 pg/mL; patients with pituitary failure do not respond, but those with hypothalamic disease may respond.

Plasma and urinary cortisol levels are usually determined by radioimmunoassay. Urinary 17-OHCS may be determined by reacting phenylhydrazine with C-21 adrenocorticoids having the dihydroxyacetone group (17,21-dihydroxy-20 ketone). This is known as the **Porter-Silber reaction.** This reaction does not measure all of the 17-

hydroxycorticoids, and thus a more inclusive method may be used by converting 17-oxygenated C-21 steroids to C-19 17-ketosteroids that are then measured as 17-KGS.

Diagnosis

The diagnosis is suspected on the basis of symptoms and signs and confirmed by laboratory tests as described above, keeping in mind the fact that many patients with some adrenal function but limited reserves appear well until stress precipitates acute adrenal insufficiency.

Addison's disease is usually suspected following the discovery of hyperpigmentation, although in some patients this may be minimal. In the early stages of the disease, weakness, although prominent, is benefited by rest, unlike neuropsychiatric weaknesses that are often worse in the morning than after activity. Most myopathies can be differentiated by their distribution and the lack of pigmentation and characteristic laboratory findings. Patients with hypoglycemia due to oversecretion of insulin may have attacks at any time, usually have increased appetite with weight gain, and have normal adrenal function. Patients with adrenal insufficiency develop hypoglycemia following fasting, due to their decreased ability to carry out gluconeogenesis. The low serum Na must be differentiated from edematous patients (particularly those on diuretics), the dilutional hyponatremia of inappropriate ADH syndrome, and the rare salt-losing nephritis. These patients are not likely to show hyperpigmentation, hyperkalemia, and increased BUN, which are characteristic of adrenal insufficiency. Hyperpigmentation due to bronchogenic carcinoma, ingestion of heavy metals such as iron or silver, chronic skin conditions, or hemochromatosis should be considered. The characteristic pigmentation of the buccal and rectal mucosa seen in Peutz-Jeghers syndrome should not cause confusion. The frequent presence of vitiligo in association with hyperpigmentation may be a helpful indication, although it may also occur with hyperpigmentation due to other causes.

Prognosis

With continued substitution therapy, the prognosis is excellent and a patient with Addison's disease should be able to lead a full life.

Treatment

In addition to appropriate treatment of complicating infections (eg, tuberculosis), therapy should include the following.

Treatment of acute adrenal insufficiency: Therapy should be instituted immediately once a provisional diagnosis of adrenocortical failure has been made. If the patient is acutely ill, confirmation by an ACTH response test should be postponed until recovery is achieved. Hydrocortisone 100 mg as a water-soluble ester (usually the succinate or phosphate) is injected IV over 30 sec, followed by an infusion of 1 L of a 5% dextrose in 0.9% sodium chloride solution containing 100 mg hydrocortisone ester given over 2 h. Additional 0.9% sodium chloride is given until dehydration and hyponatremia have been corrected. Hydrocortisone therapy is given continuously to a total dosage in 24 h of > 300 mg. Mineralocorticoids are not required when high-dose hydrocortisone is given. Restoration of BP and general improvement may be expected within 1 h or less after the initial dose of hydrocortisone. Vasopressor agents may be needed until the full effect of hydrocortisone is apparent. An IV infusion of metaraminol bitartrate, 100 mg in 500 mL of sodium chloride injection, may be given at a rate adjusted to maintain BP. (CAUTION: *In acute addisonian crisis, a delay in instituting corticosteroid therapy may result in the patient's death, particularly if hypoglycemia and hypotension are present.*) A total dose of hydrocortisone 150 mg is usually given over the second 24-h period if the patient is markedly improved, and 75 mg is given on the third day. Maintenance oral doses of hydrocortisone (30 mg) and fludrocortisone acetate (0.1 mg) are given daily thereafter, as described under treatment of chronic adrenal insuffi-

ciency, below. Recovery depends upon treatment of the underlying cause (eg, infection, trauma, metabolic stress) and adequate hydrocortisone therapy.

Recognition of patients with Addison's disease is not difficult. However, a significant number of patients with "limited" adrenocortical reserve who appear healthy experience acute adrenocortical insufficiency when under stress. Shock and fever may be the only signs observed. Treatment should not be delayed until the diagnosis is certain, but hydrocortisone should be given as described above. Salt and water requirements may be considerably less than in cases with total deficiency.

Treatment of complications: These include hyperpyrexia and psychotic reactions. Fever > 40.6 C (105 F) orally occasionally accompanies the rehydration process. Except in the presence of a falling BP, antipyretics (eg, aspirin 600 mg) may be given orally with caution q 30 min until the temperature begins to fall. If psychotic reactions occur after the first 12 h of therapy, hydrocortisone dosage should be reduced to the lowest level consistent with maintenance of BP and good cardiovascular function.

Treatment of chronic adrenal insufficiency: Normal hydration and absence of orthostatic hypotension are criteria of adequate replacement therapy. Adequacy of mineralocorticoid replacement can also be checked by restoration of elevated levels of plasma renin activity to normal. Hydrocortisone 20 mg orally is usually given in the morning and 10 mg in the afternoon. A daily dosage of 40 mg may be required. Night doses should be avoided, as they may produce insomnia. Normally, hydrocortisone is secreted maximally in the early morning hours, little being secreted at night. Additionally, fludrocortisone 0.1 mg to 0.2 mg orally once/day is recommended. This mineralocorticoid replaces aldosterone that is normally secreted in healthy individuals. It is often necessary to reduce the dose of fludrocortisone to 0.05 mg every 2nd day on initial institution of therapy because of ankle edema, but the patient usually adjusts and can then take the larger doses. Fludrocortisone produces hypertension in some patients. This should be treated by reducing the dosage rather than using diuretics. Intercurrent illnesses (eg, infections) should be regarded as potentially serious and the patient should double his hydrocortisone dosage until he is well. If nausea and vomiting preclude oral therapy, medical attention should be sought immediately and parenteral therapy started. Patients living or traveling in areas where medical care is not readily available should be instructed in self-administration of parenteral hydrocortisone.

In **coexisting diabetes mellitus and Addison's disease,** hydrocortisone dosage usually should not be > 30 mg/day; otherwise, insulin requirements are increased. Complete control of glycosuria is often difficult in this syndrome. In coexisting thyrotoxicosis and Addison's disease, definitive therapy should be given early. **Following total bilateral adrenalectomy** for hyperadrenocorticism, carcinoma of the breast, or hypertension, the patient should be maintained on oral hydrocortisone 20 to 30 mg/day. In addition, a mineralocorticoid may be given as described above.

SECONDARY ADRENAL INSUFFICIENCY

Adrenal hypofunction due to a lack of ACTH may occur in panhypopituitarism, in patients receiving corticosteroids, or for a period of time after discontinuing corticosteroid therapy. Panhypopituitarism occurs most commonly in women with Sheehan's syndrome, but may also occur secondary to chromophobe adenomas, craniopharyngioma in younger persons, and a variety of tumors, granulomas, and, rarely, infections or trauma that lead to destruction of pituitary tissue. Patients receiving corticosteroids for > 4 wk, or who have discontinued their use after a period of weeks to months, may have insufficient ACTH secretion during metabolic stress to stimulate the adrenals to produce adequate quantities of corticosteroids; or they may have atrophic adrenals that are unresponsive to ACTH. These problems may persist for up to 1 yr after

steroid treatment is terminated. Isolated ACTH deficiency is idiopathic and extremely rare.

Symptoms and Signs

Patients with secondary adrenal insufficiency are not hyperpigmented as are those with Addison's disease. They have relatively normal electrolyte values. Hyperkalemia and elevated BUN are generally not present because of the near-normal secretion of aldosterone in these patients. Hyponatremia may occur on a dilutional basis. Those with panhypopituitarism, however, have depressed thyroid and gonadal function and hypoglycemia, and coma may supervene when symptomatic secondary adrenal insufficiency occurs. Tests to differentiate primary and secondary adrenal insufficiency are discussed under Addison's disease, above.

Treatment

Treatment of secondary adrenal insufficiency is similar to that described above for Addison's disease. Each case varies with regard to the type and degree of specific adrenocortical hormone deficiencies. Generally, fludrocortisone is not required, since aldosterone is produced. These patients may do better on lower doses of hydrocortisone than patients with primary insufficiency. During acute febrile illness or following trauma, patients receiving corticosteroids for nonendocrine disorders may require supplemental doses to augment their endogenous hydrocortisone production. In panhypopituitarism, other pituitary deficiencies should be treated appropriately (see under ANTERIOR LOBE DISORDERS in Ch. 88).

ADRENAL CORTICAL HYPERFUNCTION

Hypersecretion of one or more adrenocortical hormones produces distinct clinical syndromes. Excessive production of androgens results in adrenal virilism; hypersecretion of glucocorticoids produces Cushing's syndrome; and excess aldosterone output results in aldosteronism. These syndromes frequently have overlapping features. Adrenal hyperfunction may be compensatory as in congenital adrenal hyperplasia, or may be due to acquired hyperplasia, adenomas, or adenocarcinomas.

CONGENITAL ADRENAL HYPERPLASIA

(See Ch. 196)

ADRENAL VIRILISM

(Adrenogenital Syndrome)

Any syndrome, congenital or acquired, in which excessive output of adrenal androgens causes virilization. The effects depend on the sex and age of the patient when the disease begins and are more marked in women than men. In adult women, this syndrome is caused by adrenal hyperplasia or by an adrenal tumor. In either case, symptoms and signs include hirsutism, baldness, acne, deepening of the voice, amenorrhea, atrophy of the uterus, clitoral hypertrophy, decreased breast size, and increased muscularity. An increase in libido may occur. Hirsutism (see in CHRONIC ANOVULATORY DISORDERS in Ch. 170) may be the only feature in mild cases.

Delayed virilizing adrenal hyperplasia is a variant of congenital adrenal hyperplasia and both are caused by a defect in hydroxylation of cortisol precursors. Urinary 17-KS are elevated, pregnanetriol excretion is often increased, and cortisol or 17-OHCS excretion is diminished. Plasma testosterone and androstenedione are elevated. Suppression of 17-KS excretion with dexamethasone 0.5 mg orally q 6 h confirms the diagnosis. Dexamethasone 0.5 to 1 mg orally at bedtime is the recommended treatment, but even these small doses may produce signs of Cushing's syndrome in some

patients. Cortisol (25 mg) or prednisone (5 to 10 mg) daily can also be used. Though most symptoms and signs of virilism disappear, the hirsutism and baldness disappear slowly and the voice may remain deep.

With **virilizing adenomas** or **adenocarcinomas,** in contrast to adrenal hyperplasia, dexamethasone administration either does not suppress or only partially suppresses androgen excretion. The tumor site may be determined by CT scan. **Treatment** requires adrenalectomy. In some cases, the tumor secretes both excess androgens and cortisol, resulting in Cushing's syndrome with suppression of ACTH secretion and atrophy of the contralateral adrenal. If this is the case, hydrocortisone should be given pre-and postoperatively as described below. Mild hirsutism and virilization with hypomenorrhea and elevated plasma testosterone may be seen in the **polycystic ovary (Stein-Leventhal) syndrome.**

CUSHING'S SYNDROME

A constellation of clinical abnormalities due to chronic exposure to excesses of cortisol (the major adrenocorticoid) or related corticosteroids.

Etiology

Hyperfunction of the adrenal cortex may be ACTH-dependent or it may be independent of ACTH regulation, eg, production of cortisol by an adrenocortical adenoma or carcinoma. The administration of supraphysiologic quantities of exogenous cortisol or related synthetic analogs suppresses adrenocortical function and mimics ACTH-independent hyperfunction. ACTH-dependent hyperfunction of the adrenal cortex may be due to (1) hypersecretion of ACTH by the pituitary, (2) secretion of ACTH by a nonpituitary tumor such as an oat cell carcinoma of the lung (the **ectopic ACTH syndrome**), or (3) administration of exogenous ACTH. While the term **Cushing's syndrome** has been applied to the clinical picture resulting from cortisol excess regardless of the cause, hyperfunction of the adrenal cortex resulting from pituitary ACTH excess has frequently been referred to as **Cushing's disease,** implying a particular physiologic abnormality. Patients with Cushing's disease may have a basophilic adenoma of the pituitary, or a chromophobe adenoma. In some cases, no histologic abnormality is found in the pituitary despite clear evidence of ACTH overproduction. Microadenomas, which are difficult to visualize even by CT scan, are often the cause.

Symptoms and Signs

Clinical manifestations include rounded "moon" facies with a plethoric appearance. There is truncal obesity with prominent supraclavicular and dorsal cervical fat pads (buffalo hump); the distal extremities and fingers are usually quite slender. Muscle wasting and weakness are present. The skin is thin and atrophic, with poor wound healing and easy bruising. Purple striae may appear on the abdomen. Hypertension, renal calculi, osteoporosis, glucose intolerance, and psychiatric disturbances are common. Cessation of linear growth is characteristic in children. Females usually have menstrual irregularities. An increased production of androgens, in addition to cortisol, may lead to hypertrichosis, temporal balding, and other signs of virilism in the female.

Diagnosis

Plasma cortisol is normally 10 to 25 μg/dL in the early morning hours (6 to 8 AM) and declines gradually to < 10 in the evening (6 PM and later). Patients with Cushing's syndrome usually have elevated morning cortisol levels and lack the normal diurnal decline in cortisol production, so that evening plasma cortisol levels are above normal and total 24-h cortisol production is elevated. Single cortisol samples may be difficult to interpret due to the episodic secretion that produces the wide range in normal values.

About 1/3 of the secreted cortisol is metabolized to 17-OHCS that are measured in

the urine. Urinary 17-OHCS are influenced by body size and weight; obese patients may have relatively elevated values. Normal urinary 17-OHCS range between 3 and 10 mg/24 h. Urinary 17-KGS measure a somewhat larger proportion of cortisol metabolites; normal excretion is 5 to 16 mg/24 h. Patients with Cushing's syndrome have higher values. Urinary 17-KS may also be elevated to > 20 mg/24 h in men and to > 15 in women. The most specific test is measurement of free urinary cortisol, which is elevated and less subject to increase in obese patients (normal 10 to 100 μg/24 h).

Dexamethasone test: The administration of 1 mg of dexamethasone orally at 11 to 12 PM with measurement of plasma cortisol at 7 to 8 AM the following morning is a good screening test for Cushing's syndrome. Most normal patients will suppress their morning plasma cortisol to 5 μg/dL or less following this procedure, whereas most patients with Cushing's syndrome will continue to secrete undiminished quantities of cortisol.

Giving oral dexamethasone 0.5 mg q 6 h for 2 days to normal subjects leads to inhibition of ACTH secretion. Consequently, urinary 17-OHCS will usually decrease to < 3 mg/24 h on the 2nd day. In patients with Cushing's disease, pituitary ACTH secretion is relatively resistant to suppression and therefore urinary 17-OHCS will not decrease in a normal fashion. In patients with adrenal tumors, cortisol production is independent of ACTH and therefore dexamethasone will have no suppressive effect. In patients with the ectopic ACTH syndrome, the production of ACTH by the nonpituitary tumor is almost always unaffected by dexamethasone; hence urinary 17-OHCS remain unchanged. The production of ACTH by the pituitary in Cushing's disease is only *relatively* resistant to suppression. Hence, when the oral dose of dexamethasone is increased to 2 mg q 6 h for 2 days, urinary 17-OHCS will usually decrease by at least 50% from the baseline values. In contrast, urinary 17-OHCS or cortisol will not be suppressed in most patients with an adrenal tumor or with the ectopic ACTH syndrome. This test distinguishes patients with a pituitary abnormality from other forms of Cushing's syndrome.

If the dexamethasone test points to an adrenal tumor or the ectopic ACTH syndrome, these 2 possibilities can be separated by determining the plasma ACTH concentration. The plasma ACTH level will be markedly elevated in the ectopic ACTH syndrome (usually > 200 pg/mL) and will be unmeasurable in Cushing's syndrome due to an adrenal tumor. Patients with Cushing's disease usually have moderately elevated plasma ACTH values (75 to 200 pg/mL).

The overnight **metyrapone test** will often give useful information in determining the etiology of the Cushing's syndrome. Patients with pituitary dependent Cushing's disease have a marked increase in plasma substance S (11-desoxycortisol), but patients with adrenal tumors, or the ectoric ACTH syndrome, fail to show this increase. The total amount of steroid produced (as metyrapone blocks 11-hydroxylation of cortisol) must be determined. Therefore, total cortisol and substance S levels are measured to see that an increase in total steroid has occurred, and not just that 11-desoxycortisol has replaced cortisol in the plasma.

A less useful test in evaluating patients with Cushing's syndrome is the **ACTH stimulation test.** Infusion of ACTH 50 u. over an 8-h period produces a 2- to 5-fold increase in urinary 17-OHCS in patients with Cushing's disease, where the adrenals show bilateral hyperplasia and hyperresponsiveness due to chronic endogenous ACTH excess. In about 50% of cases of adrenal adenoma, ACTH stimulation will produce a clear and sometimes marked increase in plasma cortisol and urinary 17-OHCS. Adrenal carcinomas are generally unresponsive to ACTH.

Although it is still too early to be certain, it seems likely that the **CRF test** (see above in Diagnostic Tests, under ADDISON'S DISEASE) may distinguish between hyperadrenocorticism associated with the ectopic ACTH secretion and hypersecreting adrenal tumors, in which no response occurs, and the pituitary form of Cushing's disease, in which the response is normal or increased.

The evaluation of the patient with Cushing's syndrome, after adrenal hyperfunction is established, should also include a CT scan for a pituitary tumor and a careful search for signs of a nonpituitary, ACTH-producing neoplasm. An IVP may show depression of a kidney by an adrenal tumor. Adrenal scanning, after ingestion of iodinated cholesterol, may differentiate hyperplasia and adenoma or carcinoma; however, a CT scan of the adrenal region is the procedure of choice if biochemical tests suggest the presence of an adrenal tumor.

Treatment

Therapy is directed at correcting the hyperfunction of the pituitary gland or the adrenal cortex; the precise approach depends on the underlying abnormality.

Initially, the patient's general condition should be supported by appropriate administration of potassium and a high protein intake. If clinical manifestations are severe, it may be reasonable to block steroid secretion with aminoglutethimide. When the pituitary is the source of excessive ACTH secretion, the standard approach is to perform a **transphenoidal exploration of the pituitary** and excise a tumor, if one is found. This surgical procedure is demanding and should be performed only in experienced centers, since results are unsatisfactory in inexperienced hands. If no tumor is found, some proceed to hypophysectomy, but most feel that the next step is **supervoltage irradiation** of the pituitary, delivering 4000 to 5000 rad. In special centers, heavy particle beam irradiation, providing about 10,000 rad, is also often successful. Response to irradiation may require several months. **Bilateral adrenalectomy** is reserved for patients who fail to respond to both pituitary exploration (with possible adenomectomy) and irradiation, which usually restore pituitary function to normal. Adrenalectomy requires steroid replacement for the remainder of the patient's life, in the same pattern as that required for patients with primary adrenal failure, and also carries a serious risk of developing **Nelson's syndrome,** which occurs in 5 to 10% of patients who have undergone adrenalectomy for Cushing's disease. The pituitary gland continues to expand, causing a marked increase in ACTH and β-MSH secretion, resulting in severe hyperpigmentation. Although irradiation may arrest continued pituitary growth in these patients, many also required hypophysectomy, the indications for which are the same as for any pituitary tumor—an increase in size such that it encroaches upon surrounding structures, producing visual field defects, pressure upon the hypothalamus, or other complications. Routine irradiation after hypophysectomy is often carried out.

Adrenocortical neoplasms are treated by surgical removal of the tumor. Patients must receive supplementary cortisol during surgery and the postoperative period, since their nontumorous adrenal cortex will be atrophic and suppressed. Where possible, treatment of the ectopic ACTH syndrome consists of removing the nonpituitary tumor producing the ACTH. However, in most cases, the tumor is disseminated and cannot be excised. Adrenal inhibitors such as metyrapone 250 mg qid combined with aminoglutethimide 250 mg bid orally, increasing to a maximum of no more than 2 gm/day; or mitotane (*o,p'*-DDD) 0.5 gm qid orally, increasing to a maximum total dose of 8 to 12 gm/day, will usually control severe metabolic disturbances (eg, hypokalemia) resulting from hyperfunction of the adrenal cortex. When mitotane is used, 20 mg/day of cortisol should be added to the regimen to protect the patient against the effects of complete abolition of corticosteroid secretion.

HYPERALDOSTERONISM

Aldosterone is the most potent mineralocorticoid produced by the adrenals. It causes Na retention and K loss. In the kidney, aldosterone causes transfer of Na from the lumen of the distal tubule into the tubular cells in exchange for K and H. The same

effect occurs in the salivary glands, sweat glands, and cells of the intestinal mucosa, and in exchanges between intra- and extracellular fluids.

Aldosterone secretion is regulated by the **renin-angiotensin mechanism,** and to a lesser extent by ACTH. Renin, a proteolytic enzyme, is stored in the juxtaglomerular cells of the kidney. Reduction in blood volume and flow in the afferent renal arterioles induces secretion of renin. Renin causes transformation of **angiotensinogen** (an α_2-globulin) in the liver to **angiotensin I,** a 10-amino acid polypeptide, which is converted to **angiotensin II,** an 8-amino acid polypeptide. Angiotensin II causes secretion of aldosterone and, to a much lesser extent, of cortisol and desoxycorticosterone. The Na and water retention resulting from increased aldosterone secretion increases the blood volume and reduces renin secretion. Aldosterone is measured by radioimmunoassay.

Primary aldosteronism (Conn's syndrome) is due to an adenoma, usually unilateral, of the glomerulosa cells of the adrenal cortex or, more rarely, to an adrenal carcinoma or hyperplasia. Hypersecretion of aldosterone may result in hypernatremia, hyperchlorhydria, hypervolemia, and a hypokalemic alkalosis manifested by episodic weakness, paresthesias, transient paralysis, and tetany. Diastolic hypertension and a hypokalemic nephropathy with polyuria and polydipsia are common. Aldosterone excretion on a high Na intake (> 10 gm/day) is usually > 200 μg/day if a tumor is present. Deprivation of Na causes K retention. Personality disturbances and hyperglycemia and glycosuria are occasionally seen. In many cases, the only manifestation may be mild to moderate hypertension.

A helpful test is to give spironolactone 200 to 400 mg/day orally, which reverses the manifestations of the disease, including hypertension, within 5 to 8 wk (this may also occur in patients with hypertension not due to increased aldosterone). Measurement of plasma renin is helpful in the diagnosis. This is usually carried out by determining the plasma renin value in the morning with the patient recumbent, giving furosemide 80 mg orally, and then repeating the renin determination after the patient has remained upright for 3 h. Normal individuals will have a marked increase in renin in the upright position, while the patient with hyperaldosteronism will not. About 20% of patients with essential hypertension, who do not necessarily have hyperaldosteronism, have a low renin that does not respond to the upright position. Measurements of plasma aldosterone, either peripherally or following catheterization of the adrenal veins, may be helpful. Diagnosis is thus dependent upon demonstrating elevated secretion of aldosterone in urine or blood, expansion of the extracellular space as demonstrated by lack of increase in plasma renin in the upright posture, and the K abnormalities noted. A CT scan will often demonstrate a small adenoma in these cases.

Secondary aldosteronism, an increased production of aldosterone by the adrenal cortex caused by stimuli originating outside the adrenal, mimics the primary condition and is related to hypertension and edematous disorders (eg, cardiac failure, cirrhosis with ascites, the nephrotic syndrome). Secondary aldosteronism seen with the accelerated phase of hypertension is believed to be due to renin hypersecretion secondary to renal vasoconstriction. Hyperaldosteronism is also seen in hypertension due to obstructive renal artery disease (eg, atheroma, stenosis). This is caused by reduced blood flow in the affected kidney. Hypovolemia, which is common in edematous disorders, particularly during diuretic therapy, stimulates the renin-angiotensin mechanism with hypersecretion of aldosterone. Secretion rates may be normal in cardiac failure, but hepatic blood flow and aldosterone metabolism are reduced so that circulating levels of the hormone are high.

The principal differences between primary and secondary aldosteronism are shown in TABLE 91–2.

Treatment

Once the diagnosis of primary aldosteronism is made, both adrenal glands should be explored for possible multiple adenomas. It may be necessary to dissect the gland to

TABLE 91–2. ALDOSTERONISM—DIFFERENTIAL DIAGNOSIS

Clinical Finding	*Primary Aldosteronism*		*Secondary Aldosteronism*	
	Adenoma	*Hyperplasia*	*Hypertension*	*Edema*
Blood pressure	↑↑	↑	↑↑↑↑	N,↑
Edema	0	0	0	++
Serum Na+	N,↑	N	N,↓	N,↓
Serum K+	↓	N,↓	↓	N,↓
Plasma renin activity*	↓↓	N,↑	↑↑	↑
Aldosterone	↑	↑	↑↑	↑

* When corrected for age. Older individuals have lower mean renin activities.

↑↑↑↑ = very greatly increased; ↑↑ = greatly increased; ↓↓ = greatly decreased; ↑ = increased; ↓ = decreased; 0 = absent; N = normal; ++ = present.

demonstrate a tumor. The prognosis is good in overt aldosteronism when a solitary adenoma can be defined. Following removal of an aldosterone-producing adenoma, all patients have lowering of BP; complete remission occurs in about 70%. With adrenal hyperplasia and hyperaldosteronism, about 70% remain hypertensive although there is reduction of BP in most patients. Hyperaldosteronism in these patients can usually be controlled by spironolactone. Bilateral adrenalectomy is rarely necessary. In normokalemic aldosteronism, diagnosis and definition are difficult, and surgical exploration may be unrewarding.

PHEOCHROMOCYTOMA

A tumor of chromaffin cells that secrete catecholamines, causing hypertension. In about 80% of cases, pheochromocytomas are found in the adrenal medulla, but may also be found in other tissues derived from neural crest cells (see Pathology, below). They appear equally in both sexes, are bilateral in 10% of cases (20% in children), and are usually benign (95%). Although pheochromocytomas may occur at any age, the maximum incidence is between the third and fifth decades.

Pathology

Pheochromocytomas vary in size but average only 5 to 6 cm in diameter. They usually weigh 50 to 200 gm but tumors weighing several kilograms have been reported. Rarely, they are large enough to be palpated or cause symptoms due to pressure or obstruction. The tumor is usually a well-encapsulated nest of chromaffin cells that appear malignant upon microscopic examination. The cells have multiple bizarre shapes with pyknotic, large, or multiple nuclei. The tumor may be considered benign if it has not invaded the capsule and if no metastases are found. In addition to the adrenals, tumors may be found in the paraganglia of the sympathetic chain, retroperitoneally along the course of the aorta, in the carotid body, in the organ of Zuckerkandl (at the aortic bifurcation), in the GU system, in the brain, and in dermoid cysts.

Pheochromocytomas are part of the **syndrome of familial multiple endocrine adenomatoses—Type II (Sipple's syndrome),** and may be found along or associated with medullary thyroid carcinoma and parathyroid adenomata (see Ch. 92). A **Type III syndrome** has been described which includes pheochromocytoma, mucosal (oral and ocular) neuroma, and medullary thyroid carcinoma. There is a significant association (10%) with **neurofibromatosis (von Recklinghausen's disease)** and it may be found with hemangiomas, as in **von Hippel-Lindau disease.**

Symptoms and Signs

The most prominent feature is hypertension, which may be paroxysmal (45%) or persistent (50%) and is rarely absent. It is due to secretion of one or more of the catecholamine hormones or precursors: norepinephrine, epinephrine, dopamine, or dopa. Additionally, tachycardia, diaphoresis, postural hypotension, tachypnea, flushing, cold and clammy skin, severe headache, angina, palpitation, nausea, vomiting, epigastric pain, visual disturbances, dyspnea, paresthesias, constipation, and a sense of impending doom are common; some or all of these symptoms and signs may occur in any patient. Paroxysmal attacks may be provoked by palpation of the tumor, postural changes, abdominal compression or massage, induction of anesthesia, emotional trauma, β-adrenergic blocking agents, and, rarely, micturition.

Physical examination, except for the common finding of hypertension, usually is normal, unless performed during a paroxysmal attack. The severity of retinopathy and cardiomegaly is often less extensive than might be expected for the degree of hypertension present.

Diagnosis

The principal urinary metabolic products of epinephrine and norepinephrine are the **metanephrines** and **vanillylmandelic acid (VMA).** Normal persons excrete only very small amounts of these substances in the urine. Normal values for 24 h are: free epinephrine and norepinephrine < 100 μg; total metanephrine < 1.3 mg; and VMA < 10 mg. In pheochromocytoma and neuroblastoma, there is an intermittent increased urinary excretion of epinephrine, norepinephrine, and their metabolic products. Excretion of these compounds may also be elevated in coma or extreme stress states. All of these compounds may be measured in the same urine specimen. The methods for detection of VMA and metanephrines depend upon the conversion to vanillin, the extraction of vanillin into toluene, and the final spectrophotometric determination of vanillin at 360 mμ. These values may be exceeded in patients being treated with rauwolfia alkaloids, methyldopa, or catecholamines, or following ingestion of foods containing large quantities of vanilla, especially if renal insufficiency is present.

Catecholamines (mainly epinephrine and norepinephrine) are measured fluorimetrically after extraction and adsorption on alumina gel. Interference from epinephrine-like drugs, antihypertensives (eg, methyldopa), and other drugs that produce fluorescence (eg, tetracycline and quinine) must be considered in the evaluation of abnormal results. Radioenzymatic procedures are also available.

Plasma catecholamine determinations are usually valueless unless collected during a paroxysm or following a drug such as glucagon that is known to provoke the release of catecholamines.

Because of their hyperkinetic states, these patients may have an elevated BMR despite being euthyroid. Although the BMR is rarely measured, these patients appear hyperkinetic. Blood volume is reported to be constricted. Hyperglycemia, glucosuria, or overt diabetes mellitus may be present with elevated fasting levels of plasma free fatty acid and glycerol. Plasma insulin concentrations are inappropriately low for the simultaneously collected plasma glucose values.

Provocative tests with histamine or tyramine *are hazardous and should not be used.* Glucagon (0.5 to 1 mg injected rapidly IV) will provoke a rise in blood pressure exceeding 35/25 mm Hg within 2 min in normotensive patients with pheochromocytoma. *Phentolamine mesylate must be available to terminate any hypertensive crisis.*

If a patient with pheochromocytoma is hypertensive, phentolamine 5 mg injected IV will cause a fall in blood pressure exceeding 35/25 mm Hg within 2 min. False-positive results occur in patients with uremia, stroke, and malignant hypertension, and in those taking certain pharmacologic agents. A modification of this test has been developed which takes advantage of catecholamine inhibition of insulin release. An IV infusion

of 10% glucose in water is begun (2 mL/min) 30 min prior to the injection of phentolamine (blood is sampled twice for measurement of glucose and insulin prior to the injection). Following the administration of phentolamine, each time the BP is measured, blood is again sampled. Pheochromocytoma is present if there is a significant fall in BP, a fall in glucose exceeding 18 mg/dL, or a rise in insulin exceeding 13 μu./mL.

A new test using oral clonidine has been described. Forty-eight hours after discontinuing all drugs that act on the sympathetic nervous system, the patient is given 0.3 mg of clonidine. Blood is drawn for plasma catecholamine determinations prior to and 3 h following the administration of clonidine. The normal response is a fall of plasma norepinephrine values to normal (< 400 ng/mL) and a fall of at least 40% from basal values. Patients with pheochromocytoma maintain elevated values.

Attempts to localize tumors by x-ray should be limited to multiple views of the chest and abdomen and IV pyelography with tomography of the perirenal areas. Phlebography has been recommended by certain radiologists as safe and effective in the localization of these tumors; others feel that phlebography, aortography, and retroperitoneal gas insufflation are contraindicated as they may induce a serious or fatal paroxysm. Localization of the level of the tumor by repeated sampling of plasma catecholamine concentrations during catheterization of the vena cava has been accomplished, but is also a potentially dangerous procedure. CT scanning can localize tumors exceeding 2 cm in diameter. Recently radiopharmaceuticals have been used to localize pheochromocytomas with nuclear imaging technics. The most studied compound is metaiodobenzylguanidine (MIBG) containing ^{131}I. 0.5 mCi is injected IV and the patient scanned on day 1, 2, and 3. Normal adrenal tissue rarely picks up this isotope but 90% of pheochromocytomas do. Lastly, digital subtraction angiography may have an important place in localizing pheochromocytomas. Although this procedure is only modestly invasive, proper blockade of the patient should be achieved prior to testing.

Treatment

Surgical removal of the tumor is the treatment of choice. It is usually possible to delay operation until the patient is in optimum physical condition by the use of a combination of α- and β-adrenergic blocking agents (phenoxybenzamine 40 to 160 mg/day and propranolol 30 to 60 mg/day, respectively, orally in divided doses) and the infusion of trimethaphan camsylate or sodium nitroprusside. When adrenergic-blocking agents are used, the α-compounds are usually begun first.

Metyrosine may be used alone or in combination with an α-adrenergic blocking agent (phenoxybenzamine); the optimally effective dosage of metyrosine should be given for at least 5 to 7 days before surgery.

An anterior abdominal approach should be used by the surgeon, even if the tumor has been localized in the renal area, so that a search for other pheochromocytomas can be made. It is essential that BP be continuously monitored via an intra-arterial catheter and that central venous pressure be continuously measured to avoid a fall in blood volume. Anesthesia should be induced with a nonarrhythmogenic agent, such as a thiobarbiturate, and continued with enflurane. During surgery, paroxysms of hypertension should be controlled with direct IV injections of phentolamine 1 to 5 mg, and tachyarrhythmias with propranolol 0.5 to 2 mg IV. Ventricular ectopy should be treated with lidocaine; 50 to 100 mg are given by rapid IV injection followed by an infusion of 2 to 4 mg/min as required. If a muscle relaxant is needed, pancuronium, which does not release histamine, is the agent of choice. The use of atropine preoperatively should be *avoided*. Blood should be given prior to the removal of the tumor; the patient should receive 1 to 2 u. (500 to 1000 mL) in anticipation of probable operative loss. A levarterenol infusion of 4 to 12 mg/L should be started any time hypotension appears. Some patients whose hypotension responds poorly to levarterenol may benefit by the addition of hydrocortisone 100 mg IV.

Malignant metastatic pheochromocytoma should be treated with α- and β-adrenergic blocking agents and with metyrosine. The latter agent inhibits tyrosine hydroxylase, which catalyzes the first transformation in catecholamine biosynthesis. Thus, levels of VMA and blood pressure fall. It is possible to control the blood pressure even though the tumor growth continues and will eventually cause death.

NONFUNCTIONAL ADRENAL MASSES

The most common problem is unexpected detection of **adrenal adenomas** on CT scan of the abdomen for some unrelated reason. These are usually nonfunctional and require no special treatment. **Spontaneous neonatal adrenal hemorrhage** may produce large suprarenal masses, simulating neuroblastoma or Wilms' tumor. Adrenal insufficiency is rarely observed unless both glands are involved. **Benign adrenal cysts** are observed in the elderly and may be due to cystic degeneration, vascular accidents, bacterial infections, or parasitic infestations (*Echinococcus*). Rare **nonfunctional adrenal carcinoma** produces a diffuse and infiltrating retroperitoneal process that usually manifests as metastatic disease and is not amenable to surgery, though mitotane may afford chemotherapeutic control when used in association with supportive exogenous corticosteroids. **Tuberculosis of the adrenal** is a blood-borne disease which may cause calcification and adrenal insufficiency (Addison's disease).

---

92. MULTIPLE ENDOCRINE NEOPLASIA (MEN) SYNDROMES

(Multiple Endocrine Adenomatosis [MEA]; Familial Endocrine Adenomatosis)

A group of genetically distinct familial diseases involving adenomatous hyperplasia and malignant tumor formation in several endocrine glands. Three distinct syndromes have been identified; all 3 appear to be inherited as an autosomal dominant trait with a high degree of penetrance, variable expressivity, and significant pleiotropism. The relationship between the genetic abnormality and the pathogenesis of the various tumors is not understood. Clinical manifestations may be noted as early as the 1st or as late as the 7th decade of life. The clinical features depend upon the type of endocrine tumors present. Proper management includes the early identification of affected members within a kindred and surgical removal of the tumors where possible. Although the various syndromes are generally considered to be distinct entities, significant overlap has occasionally been noted.

MULTIPLE ENDOCRINE NEOPLASIA, TYPE I (MEN-I)

(Multiple Endocrine Adenomatosis, Type I [MEA-I]; Wermer's Syndrome)

The MEN-I syndrome is characterized by tumors of the parathyroid glands, pancreatic islets, and the pituitary.

Hyperparathyroidism is present in almost 90% of affected patients. Asymptomatic hypercalcemia is the commonest manifestation; about 25% of patients have evidence of nephrolithiasis or nephrocalcinosis. In contrast to sporadic cases of hyperparathyroidism, diffuse hyperplasia or multiple adenomas are found more frequently than solitary adenomas.

Islet cell tumors of the pancreas have been reported in about 80% of affected patients. About 40% of these islet cell tumors originate from the β-cell, secrete insulin, and are associated with fasting hypoglycemia. In about 60% of cases the islet cell tumors are derived from non-β-cell elements. Gastrin is the hormone most commonly

secreted by the non-β-cell tumors and is associated with intractable and complicated peptic ulceration (**Zollinger-Ellison syndrome** —see under ENDOCRINE TUMORS in Ch. 55). Over 50% of affected MEN-I patients have peptic ulcer disease; in the majority of cases the ulcers are multiple or atypical in location and the incidence of hemorrhage, perforation, and obstruction is correspondingly high. The extreme hypersecretion of gastric acid in these patients may be associated with inactivation of pancreatic lipase, resulting in diarrhea and steatorrhea. In patients presenting initially with the Zollinger-Ellison syndrome, further investigation commonly reveals evidence of the MEN-I complex.

In other cases, non-β-cell islet tumors have been associated with a severe secretory diarrhea that results in fluid and electrolyte depletion. This complex, referred to as the "watery diarrhea, hypokalemia, and achlorhydria syndrome" (**WDHA; pancreatic cholera;** —see VIPOMA SYNDROME under ENDOCRINE TUMORS in Ch. 55) has been ascribed to vasoactive intestinal peptide (**VIP**) in some patients, although other intestinal hormones or secretogogues, including prostaglandins, may contribute. Many patients with pancreatic islet cell tumors appear to have increased levels of pancreatic polypeptide, which may eventually prove useful in diagnosing the MEN-I syndrome; but the clinical manifestations associated with overproduction of this hormone have not been clearly defined. Hypersecretion of glucagon and the ectopic secretion of ACTH (with the production of Cushing's syndrome) have also been noted in some patients with non-β-cell tumors.

Both the β- and non-β-cell tumors are usually multicentric in origin, and multiple adenomas or diffuse islet cell hyperplasia commonly occur. In about 30% of cases the islet cell tumors are malignant, with local or distant metastases. The incidence of malignancy appears to be higher in the non-β-cell tumors. Malignant islet cell tumors within the MEN-I syndrome often follow a more benign course than sporadic islet cell carcinomas.

Pituitary tumors have been noted in about 65% of patients with the MEN-I syndrome. About 25% of those with pituitary tumor have acromegaly, which is clinically indistinguishable from the sporadic form of the disease. The remainder appear to have chromophobe adenomas, which initially were believed to be nonfunctioning, but recent evidence suggests that many secrete prolactin. Local expansion of the tumor may cause visual disturbance and headache as well as *hypo*pituitarism.

Adenomas and adenomatous hyperplasia of the thyroid and adrenal glands have been described less often in patients with the MEN-I syndrome. These have rarely been functional and their significance within the MEN-I complex is uncertain. **Carcinoid tumors,** particularly those derived from the embryologic foregut, have been reported in isolated cases of the MEN-I syndrome. Multiple subcutaneous and visceral **lipomas** may be associated as well.

Diagnosis

The clinical features of the MEN-I syndrome depend upon the pattern of tumor involvement in the individual case. About 40% of reported cases have had tumors of the parathyroids, pancreas, and pituitary. Almost any combination of tumors and symptom complexes outlined above is possible. A patient in an affected kindred manifesting any one of the classic features of the syndrome is at risk for the development of the other associated tumors. *Periodic screening of both affected individuals and unaffected relatives is, therefore, essential.* This should usually include the following: review of the history for symptoms suggestive of peptic ulcer disease, diarrhea, nephrolithiasis, hypoglycemia, and hypopituitarism; physical examination for features of acromegaly and subcutaneous lipomas; x-ray of the sella turcica; and measurement of serum Ca, PO_4, gastrin, and prolactin. The diagnosis of insulin-secreting β-cell tumor of the pancreas is established by demonstrating fasting hypoglycemia in conjunction with an elevated plasma insulin level; gastrin-secreting non-β-cell tumor of the pancreas is

established by demonstrating elevated basal plasma gastrin levels, an exaggerated gastrin response to infused Ca, and a paradoxic rise in gastrin level after infusion of secretin. The diagnosis of acromegaly is established by elevated growth hormone levels that are not suppressed by glucose administration.

Treatment

Treatment of the parathyroid and pituitary lesions is primarily surgical, although in some cases pituitary irradiation may suffice. Islet cell tumors are more difficult to manage, since the lesions are often small and difficult to find and multiple lesions commonly exist. If a single tumor cannot be found, total pancreatectomy may be required for adequate control of hyperinsulinism. Diazoxide and/or streptozocin may be useful therapeutic adjuncts in the treatment of hypoglycemia. The therapy of gastrin-secreting non-β-cell tumors is complex. An attempt to localize and remove the tumor should be made in all cases. If this is impossible, symptomatic treatment with H_2 receptor-antagonists will frequently provide symptomatic relief from peptic ulcer disease, although higher doses than usual may be required.

MULTIPLE ENDOCRINE NEOPLASIA, TYPE II (MEN-II)

(MEN-IIA; Multiple Endocrine Adenomatosis, Type II [MEA-II]; Sipple's Syndrome)

The MEN-II syndrome is characterized by medullary carcinoma of the thyroid, pheochromocytoma, and hyperparathyroidism. The clinical features of MEN-II depend upon the type of tumor present. A chromosomal deletion on the short arm of chromosome 20 has been noted in several kindreds.

Medullary carcinoma of the thyroid is a malignant neoplasm derived from the calcitonin producing parafollicular or C cells. The tumors contain and secrete large amounts of calcitonin, which is useful in establishing the diagnosis and following the course of the disease. Almost all patients with the MEN-II syndrome will have medullary carcinoma of the thyroid. The usual presentation is that of an asymptomatic thyroid nodule, although many cases are now diagnosed during routine screening of affected MEN-II kindreds before a palpable tumor develops. Diarrhea may be present in advanced cases, presumably on the basis of a humoral product such as calcitonin or ectopically produced substances such as kallikreins, serotonin, or prostaglandins. Ectopic production of ACTH with Cushing's syndrome has been noted as well. Medullary carcinoma of the thyroid begins as C-cell hyperplasia, is almost always bilateral and multicentric, and may be associated with the local production of amyloid; fibrosis and calcification within the tumor are commonly noted. Although very high levels of calcitonin are the rule in advanced medullary carcinoma of the thyroid, hypocalcemia is extremely rare. Occasionally, symptoms secondary to metastatic disease lead to diagnosis. The tumor metastasizes to cervical lymph nodes, liver, lung, and bone, and although metastases may occur early, long-term survival is common with ⅔ of affected patients alive at the end of 10 yr.

Pheochromocytoma occurs in about 50% of affected patients within an MEN-II kindred and in some kindreds accounts for 30% of the deaths. As compared with sporadic cases of pheochromocytoma, the familial variety within the MEN-II syndrome begins with adrenal medullary hyperplasia and is multicentric and bilateral in > 50% of cases; extra-adrenal pheochromocytomas are rare in conjunction with MEN-II. The pheochromocytomas are usually epinephrine-producing and increased epinephrine excretion may be the only abnormality early in the course of the disease. Hypertensive crisis secondary to pheochromocytoma is a common presentation, and many of the reported kindreds have first come to medical attention after the diagnosis of bilateral pheo-

chromocytomas in the proband. The hypertension in patients with pheochromocytoma in MEN-II syndrome is more often paroxysmal than sustained, in contrast to the usual sporadic case. The pheochromocytomas are almost always benign, but a tendency for local recurrence has been noted in some of the reported kindreds.

Hyperparathyroidism is present less commonly than medullary carcinoma of the thyroid or pheochromocytoma. About 25% of affected patients within an MEN-II kindred have clinical evidence of hyperparathyroidism (which may be longstanding), with hypercalcemia, nephrolithiasis, nephrocalcinosis, or renal failure. In an additional 25%, without clinical or biochemical evidence of hyperparathyroidism, parathyroid hyperplasia is noted incidentally during thyroid surgery for medullary carcinoma. As in the MEN-I syndrome, the hyperparathyroidism frequently involves multiple glands either as diffuse hyperplasia or multiple adenomas.

Although islet cell tumors of the pancreas are not part of the MEN-II syndrome, an association of islet cell tumors (frequently non-functional) with bilateral pheochromocytoma (frequently familial) has been reported in patients without other manifestations of the MEN-II complex.

On rare occasions clinical features typical of MEN-I, such as the Zollinger-Ellison syndrome, may appear in patients with the MEN-II syndrome.

Diagnosis

Since pheochromocytoma may be asymptomatic in MEN-II patients, excluding pheochromocytoma with certainty may be difficult. Measurement of free catecholamines in a 24-h urine specimen with a specific analysis for epinephrine is the most sensitive way of establishing the diagnosis. VMA excretion is often normal early in the course of disease. CT scan is useful in localizing the pheochromocytoma or establishing the presence of bilateral lesions. Medullary carcinoma of the thyroid is diagnosed by measurement of plasma calcitonin after provocative infusion of pentagastrin and calcium. In most patients with palpable thyroid lesions basal calcitonin levels are elevated; in those with early disease the basal levels may be normal and the medullary carcinoma can be diagnosed only by an exaggerated response to calcium and pentagastrin. Hyperparathyroidism is diagnosed by hypercalcemia, hypophosphatemia, and increased parathormone level.

Family members in affected kindreds should be screened periodically as follows: the history for paroxysmal symptoms suggestive of pheochromocytoma (headache, sweating, palpitations) and renal colic should be reviewed; the BP should be checked; and the thyroid carefully palpated. Laboratory studies are performed as described above for suspected probands. Early diagnosis of medullary carcinoma in the children of affected kindreds is particularly important so that the tumors may be removed while still localized to the thyroid.

Treatment

Pheochromocytoma should be removed first, since, even if asymptomatic, it greatly increases the risk of surgery for medullary carcinoma or hyperparathyroidism. Since medullary carcinoma of the thyroid is ultimately fatal if untreated, *any patient within an MEN-II kindred displaying pheochromocytoma or hyperparathyroidism should have a total thyroidectomy* even if the diagnosis of medullary carcinoma of the thyroid cannot be established preoperatively.

MULTIPLE ENDOCRINE NEOPLASIA, TYPE III (MEN-III)

(MEN-IIB; Multiple Endocrine Adenomatosis, Type III [MEA-III]; Mucosal Neuroma Syndrome)

MEN-III consists of multiple mucosal neuromas, medullary carcinoma of the thyroid, and pheochromocytoma, often associated with a marfanoid habitus. Although about 50%

of the reported cases have been sporadic rather than familial, it is not clear that families were thoroughly screened in all the reported cases; the true incidence, therefore, of sporadic MEN-III syndrome is unknown. In distinction to MEN-I or II, hyperparathyroidism does not appear to be a feature of the MEN-III syndrome. Many MEN-III kindreds appear to possess the same chromosomal deletion noted in MEN-II patients, suggesting a close genetic relationship between the 2 syndromes.

The distinctive feature of this syndrome is the presence of mucosal neuromas in most, if not all, affected subjects. The neuromas present as small glistening bumps about the lips, tongue, and buccal mucosa. The eyelids, conjunctiva, and cornea are also commonly involved. Thickened eyelids and diffusely hypertrophied lips are also characteristic. Although the neuromas and facial characteristics are often present at an early age, the syndrome is often not recognized until the presentation of medullary carcinoma of the thyroid or pheochromocytoma in later life. GI abnormalities related to altered motility (constipation, diarrhea, and, occasionally, megacolon) are common, and are thought to result from diffuse intestinal ganglioneuromatosis. In addition to the marfanoid habitus, skeletal abnormalities of the spine (lordosis, kyphosis, scoliosis), pes cavus, and talipes equinovarus, are frequently present.

About half the reported cases show the complete syndrome with mucosal neuromas, pheochromocytomas, and medullary carcinoma of the thyroid. Less than 10% have neuromas and pheochromocytomas alone, while the remainder have neuromas and medullary carcinoma of the thyroid without pheochromocytoma.

Medullary carcinoma of the thyroid and pheochromocytoma resemble the corresponding disorders in the MEN-II syndrome; both tend to be bilateral and multicentric. Medullary thyroid carcinoma in the MEN-III syndrome, however, tends to be particularly aggressive, and may be present in very young children. The implications for diagnosis, family screening, and treatment are the same as described above for the MEN-II syndrome. The early diagnosis of medullary carcinoma within the pediatric age group is particularly important. *All affected patients should have a total thyroidectomy as soon as the diagnosis is established.* Pheochromocytoma, if present, should be removed prior to the medullary carcinoma.

93. POLYGLANDULAR DEFICIENCY SYNDROMES

(Autoimmune Polyglandular Syndromes; Polyendocrine Deficiency Syndromes)

Concurrent subnormal function of several endocrine glands.

Etiology and Pathogenesis

Endocrine deficiency can be caused by infection, infarction, or tumor destroying all or a large part of the gland. However, the activity of an endocrine organ is most often depressed as a result of an autoimmune reaction that produces inflammation, lymphocyte infiltration, and partial or complete destruction of the gland. Autoimmune disease affecting one organ is frequently followed by impairment of other glands, resulting in multiple endocrine failure. Two major patterns of failure have been described (see TABLE 93–1).

In Type I, onset usually occurs in childhood and hypoparathyroidism is the most frequent manifestation, followed by adrenal cortical failure. Chronic mucocutaneous candidiasis is also commonly present, and diabetes mellitus seldom occurs. This pattern is not associated with any specific HLA type. The pattern of inheritance is not clear, but some kinships appear to have an autosomal recessive pattern.

TABLE 93–1. CHARACTERISTICS OF TYPE I AND TYPE II POLYGLANDULAR DEFICIENCY SYNDROMES

	Type I	*Type II*
Age at onset	Childhood (peak 12 yr)	Adult (peak 30 yr)
HLA types	No predominance	Primarily B8, DW3, DR3; others in specific diseases
Female/male	1.4/1.0	1.8/1.0
Clinical manifestations (% involved)		
Addison's disease	67%	100%
Thyroid disease*	10–11%	69%
Pernicious anemia	13–15%	<1%
Diabetes mellitus	2–4%	52%
Gonadal failure	12–17%	3.5%
Hypoparathyroidism	82%	Not seen
Vitilligo	8–9%	4.5%
Chronic mucocutaneous candidiasis	73–78%	Not seen
Chronic active hepatitis	11–13%	Not seen
Alopecia	26–32%	Not seen
Malabsorption	22–24%	Not seen
Celiac disease and myasthenia gravis	Not seen	Incidence uncertain

* Usually chronic lymphocytic thyroiditis, but includes also Graves disease.

(Adapted from D. L. Trence et al, *American Journal of Medicine, 77*:107–116, 1984. Copyright 1984 by the *American Journal of Medicine.* Used with permission.)

In Type II, glandular failure generally occurs in adults, with peak incidence at age 30. It always involves the adrenal cortex and frequently also the thyroid gland **(Schmidt's syndrome)** and the pancreatic islets, producing insulin-dependent diabetes mellitus **(IDDM).** Antibodies against the target organs are frequently present, but their role in producing glandular damage is unclear. Some patients have thyroid-stimulating antibodies and initially present with the clinical picture of hyperthyroidism. The glandular destruction seen in these patients is chiefly a result of cell-mediated autoimmunity, probably because of depressed suppressor T cell function. In addition, reduced cell-mediated immunity is frequently present, manifested by poor response on skin testing to standard antigens such as candida, trichophyton, and tuberculin. Depressed reactivity is also found in about 30% of first-degree relatives with normal endocrine function. There is a characteristic HLA pattern, and it has been suggested that the specific HLA types in Type II are associated with susceptibility to certain viruses that induce the destructive reaction.

An additional group, **Type III,** occurs in adults and does not involve the adrenal cortex, but includes at least 2 of the following: IDDM, pernicious anemia, vitiligo, and alopecia. Since the diagnosis of the Type III pattern depends on the absence of adrenocortical insufficiency, it may merely be a wastebasket of combined disease that is converted to Type II if adrenal failure develops.

Symptoms, Signs, and Diagnosis

The clinical appearance of patients with polyglandular deficiency syndromes is the sum of the picture of each of the individual deficiencies. There is no specific sequence for appearance of individual glandular damage. Measurement of the levels of circulating antibody against the endocrine organs or their components does not appear to be useful, since such antibodies may persist for years without development of clinical endocrine failure. However, the presence of antibodies is clearly helpful in differentiat-

ing autoimmune from tuberculous hypoadrenalism and determining the cause of hypothyroidism. The presence of multiple endocrine deficiencies may raise a question of hypothalamic-pituitary failure. In almost all instances, elevated plasma levels of pituitary tropic hormones will demonstrate the peripheral nature of the defect; but rare instances of hypothalamic-pituitary insufficiency have also been reported as a part of the Type II syndrome (see Ch. 87).

Treatment

Treatment of the various glandular deficiencies is the same as for sporadic examples of the individual diseases and are discussed elsewhere in THE MANUAL, but the interaction of multiple deficiencies (eg, adrenal cortical insufficiency combined with diabetes mellitus) may complicate clinical management. Patients manifesting hypofunction of one organ should be observed during follow-up over a period of years for development of additional defects. Gonadal failure does not respond, and chronic mucocutaneous candidiasis is usually resistant to treatment.

Suppression of cell-mediated immunity may be useful in preventing development or progression of some of these diseases, and clinical trials of cyclosporin as a preventive of IDDM are currently being carried out. Whether such therapy will be useful for preventing diabetes or for other manifestations of these disease complexes is unknown at present.

94. DISORDERS OF CARBOHYDRATE METABOLISM

DIABETES MELLITUS (DM)

A syndrome resulting from a variable interaction of hereditary and environmental factors, and characterized by abnormal insulin secretion, inappropriately elevated blood glucose levels, and a variety of end organ complications including nephropathy, retinopathy, neuropathy, and accelerated atherosclerosis.

DM has no distinct etiology, pathogenesis, invariable set of clinical findings, specific laboratory tests, or definitive and curative therapy, although it is nearly always associated with fasting hyperglycemia and decreased glucose tolerance. The complete clinical syndrome of DM involves hyperglycemia, large-vessel disease, microvascular disease (retina and kidney), and neuropathy.

Current DM classification distinguishes the following subclasses: (1) **Insulin-dependent diabetes mellitus (IDDM** or **Type I)** defines a group of patients who are literally dependent on exogenous insulin to prevent ketoacidosis and death. This type of diabetes is associated with certain histocompatibility antigens (HLA) on chromosome 6, with autoimmunity directed against the islet, and possibly with a predisposition to viral infections. Viruses of several types are some of the environmental agents that may induce IDDM in genetically susceptible persons, perhaps involving cell-mediated immune mechanisms. (2) **Noninsulin-dependent diabetes mellitus (NIDDM** or **Type II)** refers to patients who may or may not use insulin for symptom control but who do not need it for survival. This subclass of diabetes has been subdivided into **obese NIDDM** and **nonobese NIDDM.** (3) **Diabetes associated with certain conditions and symptoms** such as pancreatic disease, changes in other hormones besides insulin, the administration of various drugs and chemical agents, insulin receptor abnormalities, genetic syndromes, and malnourished populations. (4) **Gestational diabetes,** where glucose intolerance develops or is discovered during pregnancy (often during the 2nd or 3rd trimester) is considered as a separate class. It usually disappears or becomes subclinical following

the end of the pregnancy. (See DIABETES MELLITUS in Ch. 178.) (5) **Impaired glucose tolerance (IGT)** is present when individuals have plasma glucose levels intermediate between normal and those considered diabetic. Terms such as chemical, latent, borderline, subclinical, and asymptomatic diabetes should be abandoned in clinical practice, since the use of the term diabetes invokes social, psychologic, and economic sanctions that are unjustified in light of the lack of severity of the glucose intolerance.

Pathophysiology

Hyperglycemia: A relative or absolute lack of insulin secretion associated with an excess of circulating stress hormones (including glucagon, catecholamines, and cortisol) is responsible for inappropriate elevation of blood glucose and associated alterations in lipid metabolism characterizing the metabolic syndrome. Depending upon the severity of insulin secretion impairment, patients usually can be categorized as IDDM or NIDDM. The differing characteristics of these 2 categories are listed in TABLE 94–1.

Large vessel disease (see DIABETIC ARTERIOSCLEROTIC DISEASE under ARTERIOSCLEROSIS; ATHEROSCLEROSIS in Ch. 26): Diabetics have an increased incidence, earlier onset, and increased severity of atherosclerosis in the intima and calcification in the media of the arterial wall. DM usually is present when such calcification is seen in patients under 40. A diabetic has a risk of cardiovascular death 3.5 times that of a nondiabetic of the same age. About 30% of all diabetics eventually develop peripheral vascular disease. Leg and foot amputations are 5 times more frequent in diabetic than in nondiabetic persons, and a significant majority of these amputees have a history of smoking.

Microvascular disease: The capillaries of diabetics demonstrate, among other changes, an abnormality of the basal lamina (basement membrane) characterized by added layers and consequent increased thickness of the lamina. This is easily demonstrable in the major capillary beds of skin and skeletal muscle. It is not a diffuse generalized process but is regional (eg, more frequent in the legs than the abdominal wall) and focal (involving one segment of a capillary but not the next). Clinically, the most important sites of microvascular involvement are the retina and the renal glomeruli. The process is also observed in the renal medulla, nervous system, pancreas, and heart, but apparently spares the lungs. A similar process involving capillaries is seen in aging, though to a lesser degree.

Neuropathy: Segmental injury to nerves, associated with demyelination and Schwann cell degeneration, involves sensory and motor peripheral nerves, nerve roots, the spinal cord, and the autonomic nervous system. It is characterized by temporary changes with nerve repair evident both microscopically and clinically. Affected nerves show basal lamina thickening similar to the capillary abnormalities. Clinical neuropathy may precede symptoms or signs of carbohydrate or vascular abnormalities, and the presence of unexplained neuropathy should lead to investigations of other components of the syndrome.

Ketoacidosis: Important physiologic aspects are discussed below.

Symptoms and Signs

The earliest symptom of elevated blood glucose is polyuria from the osmotic diuretic effect of glucose. Continued hyperglycemia and glucosuria may lead to thirst, hunger, and weight loss. Glucosuria is also associated with an increased incidence of monilial vaginitis and itching. It is uncertain whether the incidence of other infections (eg, pyelonephritis, cystitis) is increased as a *direct* result of hyperglycemia. Accelerated fat catabolism in the untreated insulin-dependent patient produces ketoacidosis leading to anorexia, nausea, vomiting, air hunger, and, if untreated, coma and death. Onset tends to be abrupt in children and insidious in older patients.

The symptoms and signs of large-vessel atherosclerosis in the diabetic are the same

TABLE 94–1. GENERAL CHARACTERISTICS OF TWO MAJOR CLINICAL TYPES OF DIABETES MELLITUS

Characteristic	*Insulin-Dependent (Type I)*	*Non-Insulin-Dependent (Type II)*
Age of onset	Often < 30	Often > 30
Body build	Almost always lean	90% are obese
Ketoacidosis develops without exogenous insulin	Yes	No
Endogenous insulin secretion	Insulinopenia	Variable insulin levels associated with insulin resistance
Predominant vascular disease	Microangiopathy	Atherosclerosis
Specific histocompatibility antigens (HLA DR3/DR4) and islet cell antibodies	Present	Decreased with different distribution
Family history	Minor (10% DM in parent or sibling)	Marked
Twin concordance	Low	High
Islet cell morphology	Loss of B cells, often with hyperplasia of other islet cells	Hyperplasia, usually with decreased mass

as in nondiabetic patients. The symptoms and signs of microvascular disease are those of renal failure if the glomerular capillaries are involved, or visual loss if the retinal capillaries are affected. Proteinuria usually is the first indication of nephropathy, and it may reach nephrotic levels. The greater the proteinuria, the more rapid is the development of renal failure. Renal failure is seen in 50% of IDDM patients after 20 to 30 yr of diabetes. Diabetic retinopathy is usually first detected 5 yr or more after the diagnosis of DM is made and is present to some degree by 10 yr in 50% of patients (see Ch. 223).

A bilateral, comparatively symmetric, distal polyneuropathy (predominantly sensory) is the most frequent form of diabetic neuropathy. Symptoms generally appear earlier and more severely in the feet, occasionally with sensory loss in a "glove and stocking" distribution or with the appearance of painless penetrating plantar ulcers. Nerve involvement may be characterized by lancinating pain in the distribution of a single dermatome, or the posterior columns of the spinal cord may be affected, producing loss of position sense and deep tendon reflexes with a positive Romberg sign. Major nerve trunks may be involved, with pain, sensory loss, motor weakness, and deprivation of sympathetic innervation in the distribution of a major spinal or cranial nerve. The 3rd and 6th cranial nerves are most often involved.

Diabetic amyotrophy is found characteristically in elderly men, producing severe pain and muscle weakness around the hip and upper leg. While the appearance resembles other neuropathies and myopathies, these symptoms in diabetics may be reversible, often improving within 1 to 2 yr. The autonomic nervous system may be involved diffusely, and autonomic insufficiency often occurs early as sweating disturbances or postural hypotension with significant symptoms. Sexual impotence in the male may be the most common symptom (50 to 60%) of neuropathy in DM; over a period of 6 mo to 1 yr, there is a gradual onset of decreasing firmness of erection. While constipation is perhaps the most common intestinal manifestation of diabetic autonomic neuropathy, it tends to be overshadowed by diarrhea, which is usually intermittent, watery,

and frequently worse at night. Severe continuous steatorrhea suggests the possibility of coexisting celiac disease or pancreatic carcinoma.

Clinical course: Some diabetics deteriorate rapidly with a course complicated by episodes of ketoacidosis and/or vascular manifestations, while others go through life with mild nonprogressing glucose intolerance and few other manifestations of the syndrome. The presence of large- and small-vessel disease, as well as neuropathy, seems unrelated to the degree of glucose intolerance or to the amount of insulin required. The only reliable direct correlate with serious vascular manifestations is the duration of DM. The longer the disease is present, the more likely are such manifestations.

Diagnosis of Diabetes Mellitus

Despite the importance of neuropathy, microangiopathy, and large-vessel disease to the diabetic syndrome, they do not conclusively establish the diagnosis. The absence of a precise diagnostic marker for DM continues to be a problem. The diagnosis should be based on (1) unequivocal elevation of plasma glucose concentration, together with the typical symptoms of polyuria, polydipsia, ketonuria, and rapid weight loss; or (2) fasting plasma glucose concentration ≥ 140 mg/dL on more than one occasion (without the presence of other factors such as fasting, complicating illness, pregnancy, certain drugs or stress that are known to elevate plasma glucose); or (3) elevated plasma glucose concentration after an oral glucose challenge on more than one occasion.

Although glucose tolerance testing has been used in an attempt to detect the diabetic syndrome at an early stage, many factors that elevate fasting glucose levels (eg, stress, starvation, drugs, or hormones—see TABLE 94–2) can alter glucose tolerance. Erroneous diagnoses of DM may be made in patients who demonstrate hyperglycemia, glucosuria, and abnormal glucose tolerance when hospitalized with severe stress such as is associated with stroke, myocardial infarction, or systemic infection. Such patients may even require insulin temporarily to control hyperglycemia, but they become normoglycemic as the stressful situation subsides.

An **oral glucose tolerance test (OGTT)** is not required to diagnose most cases of DM. It is primarily useful for diagnosing (1) postprandial reactive hypoglycemia (see under HYPOGLYCEMIA, below), (2) DM in pregnancy, when special measures may affect fetal survival (see DIABETES MELLITUS in Ch. 178 and METABOLIC PROBLEMS IN THE NEWBORN in Ch. 186), (3) DM in the presence of other metabolic abnormalities (eg, hyperlipidemia or hyperuricemia) that might be helped by treatment of hyperglycemia, and (4) DM in the unexplained presence of neuropathy, retinopathy, or peripheral vascular disease. In addition, an abnormal test may help persuade a coronary-prone patient to lose weight or stop smoking. When the fasting plasma glucose concentration is in the diabetic range more than once, an OGTT is not necessary for the diagnosis.

If one of the rare indications for an OGTT is present, the test should be performed in the morning after at least 3 days of unrestricted diet (≥ 150 gm/day carbohydrate) and normal physical activity. The subject should then fast for at least 10 h but no more than 16 h (water is permitted). During the test the subject should remain seated and not smoke, and the adverse influences of the drugs and hormones listed in TABLE 94–2 must be avoided. The dose of glucose administered should be 1.75 gm/kg ideal body weight but not more than 75 gm. A commercially prepared carbohydrate load equivalent to this dose is also acceptable.

A fasting blood sample is then collected, after which glucose, in a concentration not exceeding 25 gm/dL in flavored water, is drunk in about 5 min. Zero time is when drinking starts, and blood samples are collected at 30-min intervals for 2 h. DM is diagnosed (by the OGTT) in nonpregnant adults and children if, after the glucose load, both the 2-h sample and another sample within the 2-h period show a venous

TABLE 94–2. DRUGS AND HORMONES ASSOCIATED WITH IMPAIRED GLUCOSE TOLERANCE

Diuretics and antihypertensive agents	**Psychoactive agents**
Chlorthalidone	Chlorprothixene
Clonidine	Haloperidol
Diazoxide	Lithium carbonate
Ethacrynic acid	Phenothiazines
Furosemide	Tricyclic antidepressants
Metolazone	**Neurologically active agents**
Thiazides	Phenytoin
Hormones and hormonally active agents	Isoproterenol
Catecholamines	Levodopa
Danazol	**Antineoplastic agents**
Mineralocorticoids	Alloxan
Progestins } Oral contraceptives	Cyclophosphamide
Estrogens } Oral contraceptives	L-Asparaginase
Growth hormone	Streptozocin
Glucagon	**Miscellaneous**
Glucocorticoids (natural and synthetic)	Cimetidine
Ritodrine hydrochloride	Clofibrate
Thyroid hormones (toxic levels)	Isoniazid
	Niacin
Analgesic, antipyretic, and anti-inflammatory agents	Amiodarone
Indomethacin	Verapamil hydrochloride (toxic levels)

plasma glucose ≥ 200 mg/dL. Impaired glucose tolerance is present if values are between these and normal glucose levels (see TABLE 94–3).

Gestational DM is diagnosed in pregnant women, who were not diabetic before pregnancy, whose plasma glucose levels meet or exceed the levels in TABLE 94–3 for 2 or more values following a 100-gm oral glucose load.

Diagnosis of Ketoacidosis and Hyperosmolar Coma

The possibility of ketoacidosis is suggested by (1) changes in sensorium, at times manifest by confusion or coma; (2) air hunger (an attempt to compensate for metabolic acidosis); (3) fruity acetone odor on the breath; (4) nausea and vomiting (almost always present); (5) abdominal tenderness, a complaint of nearly 1/3 of patients, which, with nausea and vomiting, may mimic viral gastroenteritis or an acute abdomen; (6) extreme thirst and dry mucous membranes, reflecting water depletion; (7) weight loss; and (8) a diabetic history, present in about 90% of patients.

Differentiation of ketoacidotic coma from insulin shock (hypoglycemia), and rapid bedside confirmation of a clinical impression without delaying treatment is possible by confirming the patient's blood glucose level at the bedside using commercially available blood glucose test strips with or without a reflectance meter. A rough quantitation of plasma or serum ketones can be made using either Ketostix® reagent strips or Acetest® reagent tablets. Serum or plasma is serially diluted with tap water using test tubes and a syringe providing 1 in 2, 1 in 4, 1 in 8, and 1 in 16 dilutions. The presence of hyperglycemia plus a "large" amount of ketones in the serum 1 in 2 dilution confirms the diagnosis of diabetic ketoacidosis, and therapy can be started at once. Occasionally, lactic acid and β-hydroxybutyric acid can contribute significantly to the low pH without reacting to the ketone strips or tablets. Determinations of serum bicarbonate, pH, serum electrolytes, and BUN help in the patient's management but are not necessary for initial diagnosis and emergency treatment.

Ketoacidosis also occurs in **nondiabetic alcoholic patients.** There is chronic heavy

TABLE 94–3. DIAGNOSTIC CRITERIA OF THE NATIONAL DIABETES DATA GROUP

	Criteria for Diagnosis of Diabetes Mellitus and Impaired Glucose Tolerance (All plasma glucose values in mg/dL)						*Criteria for Diagnosis of Gestational Diabetes* (100 gm OGTT)**
	Normal		*Diabetes Mellitus*		*Impaired Glucose Tolerance*		*Venous Plasma Glucose*
	Adult	Child	Adult	Child	Adult	Child	Fasting ≥ 105 mg/dL
FPG*	< 115	< 130	≥ 140	≥ 140	115–139	130–139	1 h ≥ 190 mg/dL 2 h ≥ 165 mg/dL
OGTT**	< 140	< 140	≥ 200	≥ 200	140–199	140–199	3 h ≥ 145 mg/dL

* Fasting Plasma Glucose
** Oral Glucose Tolerance Test (at least 2 values)

(From "Classification and Diagnosis of Diabetes Mellitus and Other Categories of Glucose Intolerance," by the National Diabetes Data Group, M. Harris et al, in *Diabetes*, Vol. 28, page 1049, December 1979. Reproduced with permission of the American Diabetes Association, Inc., and the National Institutes of Health.)

drinking until 1 to 3 days before presentation when persistent anorexia, abdominal pain, nausea, and vomiting commence with consequent food abstention. Hydrogen ion formation by alcohol metabolism leads to increased production of β-hydroxybutyrate (not measurable by the standard nitroprusside, Acetest®, or Ketostix® tests), increased lactate formation, and decreased gluconeogenesis. Metabolic acidosis with variable plasma glucose levels (hypoglycemic to mildly hyperglycemic) in a patient with a history of alcoholism suggests the diagnosis. Alcoholic diabetics may present with a complex mixture of alcohol and diabetic acidosis. (For treatment of ketoacidosis, see below).

Hyperglycemic-hyperosmolar nonketotic coma occurs in the setting of insulin deficiency and renal and cerebral impairment, largely in elderly, mildly obese patients who often present a history of previous mild DM. Hyperglycemia from insulin deficiency leads to osmotic diuresis and decreased renal perfusion, which exaggerates the hyperglycemia and hyperosmolality. Cerebral impairment decreases fluid intake, which again exacerbates the dehydration, renal impairment, and hyperosmolality culminating in frank coma, acute renal shutdown, thrombosis, vascular collapse, and lactic acidosis. **Lactic acidosis** occurs in about 10% of patients with diabetic ketoacidosis, 40 to 60% of patients with hyperglycemic-hyperosmolar nonketotic coma, and, of course, all patients with cardiogenic, septic, or hypovolemic shock. Diagnosis is inferred by serum pH < 7.3 with decreased serum bicarbonate, an increased serum anion gap, and the absence of serum ketones, uremia, or a history of ingesting salicylates or methanol. Definitive diagnosis is based on an arterial or free-flowing venous plasma lactate concentration in excess of 5 mM. The patient's serum osmolality, either directly measured or reflected by combined elevation of the serum Na and glucose, exceeds 360 mOsm/L. (For treatment see below.)

Treatment of Diabetes Mellitus—General Considerations

The primary objective is to achieve the patient's optimal health and nutrition. An integrated index of long-term blood glucose control is now available through the use of *stable glucosylated Hb* determinations. Normally about 7% of HbA molecules are modified during erythrocyte synthesis. Since the half-life of this cell and its Hb is 60 days, the percent of stable glucosylated Hb reflects the mean blood glucose concentration over the preceding 2 mo. With the removal of the labile glucosylated Hb fraction

prior to assay, the final result is not significantly influenced by recent or transient glucose fluctuations. Determinations of glucosylated Hb are helpful in judging the degree of chronic glucose control in both IDDM and NIDDM patients and in judging efficacy of changes in therapy.

Whether treatment of asymptomatic hyperglycemia decreases morbidity and mortality is unknown, and there is significant risk of hypoglycemia in proportion to the tightness of blood glucose control in elderly patients given oral hypoglycemic agents or insulin therapy. Therefore, it appears best not to use drug therapy in elderly patients with impaired glucose tolerance or asymptomatic fasting hyperglycemia.

Whether a more physiologic approach to insulin replacement will significantly reduce morbidity and mortality from DM in patients taking insulin is still unknown. To approach the answer to the question of whether normalizing blood glucose levels helps to prevent or ameliorate diabetic complications, the National Institutes of Health has organized a 21 Center Diabetes Control and Complication Trial **(DCCT)** to study 1000 patients with IDDM over an 8- to 10-yr period. These patients are being randomly assigned to a "standard" group approximating therapy that most IDDM patients are now receiving, or an "experimental" group on a regimen designed to achieve and maintain as near normal blood glucose control as possible without significant hypoglycemia.

Approaches to more normal blood glucose levels can include the use of an insulin pump worn on the belt that constantly infuses a low dose of rapid-acting (regular or crystalline zinc) insulin s.c. with additional doses of insulin pumped in immediately prior to meals. Alternatively, 3 daily premeal injections of rapid-acting insulin may be given through an indwelling subcutaneous needle in addition to a low daily dose of intermediate or long-acting insulin (see Intensified Insulin Therapy, below). It is hoped that an attempt to emulate normal pancreatic function will be associated with a clearly demonstrable improvement in the morbidity and mortality from the vascular and neural manifestations of diabetes, but the situation is still unclear, and the final results of the DCCT will be awaited with interest.

The objectives of symptom control are (1) to avoid ketoacidosis and (2) to control symptoms resulting from hyperglycemia and glucosuria. Through the use of **self blood glucose monitoring (SBGM)** technics involving reagent test strips with or without a reflectance meter, more normal blood and urine glucose levels have become a realistic goal for many patients with diabetes. Such monitoring is more reliable than urine glucose tests for detection of hyperglycemia and enables swift confirmation of episodes of hypoglycemia for patients on insulin therapy. All of the available products include the use of a reagent strip that develops a color reaction to the glucose in the patient's blood. The use of a spring-powered lancet for finger prick is recommended. After the color develops on the strip, it is either compared to a color chart by the patient or it can be read by a reflectance meter that electronically provides a numerical value for blood glucose concentration. SBGM involves patients in the management of their disease. With proper instructions, they can be taught to make adjustments in the therapy based on test results. One approach is to have a patient measure his blood glucose 7 times a day—before each meal, 1 h after each meal, and at bedtime. Such a profile is obtained no more frequently than twice a week and may be needed rarely with a stable, well-controlled patient. Generally, the resulting improved patient motivation and understanding of the disease result in reduced blood glucose levels.

Urine glucose determinations are indirect, yet at times useful measurements of glucose control. They are easily done using commercially available tablets (Clinitest®) or paper strips containing glucose-specific enzymes (Tes-Tape®, Diastix®, or Clinistix®).

Types of Insulin Available

The 7 forms of insulin currently available in the USA have different rates of onset of effectiveness and duration of action. These insulins may be classified as rapid-, inter-

mediate-, and long-acting; their properties are listed in TABLES 94–4 and 94–5. All are available in 10-mL bottles, at concentrations of 100 u. and 40 u./mL. Syringes for U-100 and for U-40 insulin indicate directly on the syringe the number of insulin units. To simplify insulin use and to reduce patient error, only U-100 insulin should be prescribed, with U-40 given rarely for patients on low doses. Insulins are available in 2 series: Lente (Lente®, Semilente® and Ultralente®) and protamine (crystalline-zinc,

TABLE 94–4. INSULINS SOLD IN THE UNITED STATES, 1986

Brand Name	*Maker*	*Species*	*Concentration*
Rapid acting			
Standard			
Regular Iletin® I	Lilly	Beef and pork	U40, U100
Regular Insulin	Squibb-Novo	Pork	U100
Semilente® Iletin® I	Lilly	Beef and pork	U100
Semilente®	Squibb-Novo	Beef	U100
Purified			
Regular Iletin® II	Lilly	Pork or beef	U100 (U500*)
Actrapid	Squibb-Novo	Pork	U100
Velosulin®	Nordisk	Pork	U100
Humulin® R**	Lilly	Human	U100
Novolin® R	Squibb-Novo	Human	U100
Purified Semilente®	Squibb-Novo	Pork	U100
Intermediate-acting			
Standard			
NPH Iletin® I	Lilly	Beef and pork	U40, U100
Lente® Iletin® I	Lilly	Beef and pork	U40, U100
NPH Insulin	Squibb-Novo	Beef	U100
Lente®	Squibb-Novo	Beef	U100
Purified			
NPH Iletin® II	Lilly	Pork or beef	U100
Lente® Iletin® II	Lilly	Pork or beef	U100
Protaphane NPH	Squibb-Novo	Pork	U100
Lentard®	Squibb-Novo	Pork and beef	U100
Monotard®	Squibb-Novo	Pork	U100
Insulatard® NPH	Nordisk	Pork	U100
Mixtard®	Nordisk	Pork	U100
Humulin® N**	Lilly	Human	U100
Novolin® L**	Squibb-Novo	Human	U100
Novolin® N	Squibb-Novo	Human	U100
Humulin® L	Lilly	Human	U100
Long-acting			
Standard			
Ultralente® Iletin® I	Lilly	Beef and pork	U100
PZI Iletin® I	Lilly	Beef and pork	U40, U100
Ultralente®	Squibb-Novo	Beef	U100
Purified			
PZI Iletin® II	Lilly	Pork or beef	U100
Ultratard®	Squibb-Novo	Beef	U100

* The U500 concentration is available as pork insulin only.

** The abbreviations R, N, and L (for Humulin and Novolin insulins) refer to regular, NPH, and Lente, respectively.

(Adapted from J. H. Karam, "Insulins 1983: Overview and Outlook," *Clinical Diabetes* 1983; 1[July/August], pp. 1–10. Used with permission of the American Diabetes Association, Inc., and the author.)

NPH, and protamine zinc). Sources of insulin in the USA are pork and beef pancreas and synthetic human insulin (see TABLE 94–4).

All insulin preparations available in the USA are extremely pure, with generally < 10 parts per million **(ppm)** of the commonly measured pancreatic impurity proinsulin. Some insulins have < 1 ppm, but whether the increased purity is worth the additional cost is unclear. A trial of purer insulin is suggested when insulin allergy, insulin resistance, or lipoatrophy is encountered (see Complications of Insulin Treatment, below). *Care must be taken in switching to a purer insulin preparation,* as patients may require lower or higher doses. An initial dosage reduction of 20% at the time of switching will usually prevent hypoglycemia. Monospecies pork insulins and synthetic human insulins (as opposed to beef or beef/pork insulins) are less immunogenic in humans and are indicated for patients with insulin allergy, lipoatrophy, or severe insulin resistance due to insulin antibodies.

Regular insulin (crystalline-zinc insulin, insulin injection, Humulin® R, Novolin® R) and Semilente® (prompt insulin zinc suspension) have a rapid onset and short duration of action. *Regular insulin (insulin injection) is the only insulin that may be given IV* and is the insulin used for the initial emergency treatment of diabetic ketoacidosis and marked hyperglycemia. Both of the rapid-acting insulins are used when early onset of action is desired, generally supplementing intermediate-acting insulins.

Intermediate-acting insulins include **isophane insulin suspension** (NPH insulin, Insulatard®, Novolin® N, Humulin® N) and **insulin zinc suspension** (Lente®, Novolin® L, Humulin® L). These preparations have sufficiently rapid onset of action to control post-breakfast blood glucose levels, and activity lasts long enough to continue control to the following morning. Patients requiring insulin treatment are best regulated as outpatients, since insulin requirements during hospitalization often differ from those required during customary daily activities. In the absence of ketoacidosis or other acute complications, most diabetics can be controlled with a single daily injection of 20 to 60 u. of an intermediate-acting insulin given s.c. before breakfast. Initially, 10 to 20 u./day may be given. Thereafter, self blood glucose monitoring, glucose determinations on pre-meal, double-void urine samples (empty the bladder and then collect a test sample 20 to 30 min later), and symptoms of hypoglycemia are used to adjust the dose by 2 to 10 u./day until satisfactory control is obtained. As optimum control is approached, it is advisable to continue a given dose for 3 successive days before changing it. If adequate control cannot be obtained with a single daily dose of an intermediate-acting insulin, the addition of a small amount of rapid-acting insulin of the same series to the morning injection may be required. Alternatively, the dose of intermediate-acting insulin may be divided; approximately ⅔ of the total dose can be given in the morning, and the remainder just before the evening meal.

TABLE 94–5. TIME COURSE OF ACTION OF INSULIN PREPARATIONS*

Insulin Preparation	*Onset of Action*	*Peak Action (Hours)*	*Duration of Action (Hours)*
Rapid-acting regular	15–30 min	2–4	6–8
Rapid-acting Semilente® (Prompt insulin zinc suspension)	1½–2 h	4–9	10–16
Intermediate-acting (NPH and Lente®)	1–3 h	6–12	18–26
Long-acting (Ultralente® and PZI)	4–8 h	14–24	28–36

* Extreme variability between different persons accounts for the broad ranges indicated.

Ultralente® (extended insulin zinc suspension) and **protamine zinc insulin suspension** (PZI-Iletin®) are long-acting insulins that are occasionally given as a single daily dose 30 to 90 min before breakfast to some patients with mild to moderately severe stable DM. Alternatively, administration of long-acting insulins once or twice daily may represent replacement of basal insulin secretion with additional preprandial short-acting insulin doses permitting the assimilation of ingested carbohydrates. Since stability of the patient is difficult to achieve with long-acting preparations, they are nearly always used in combination with short-or intermediate-acting insulins.

Intensified Insulin Therapy

Recently, efforts have been made to improve on the traditional methods of prescribing 1 or 2 daily insulin injections. One approach has been the use of **intensified conventional therapy**. Baseline pancreatic low-level insulin release has been duplicated by using long- or intermediate-acting insulin to which are added variable premeal doses of rapid-acting insulin to cover postprandial hyperglycemia. A second approach is through the use of one of the available **electromechanical pump** devices similarly to mimic the natural pattern of insulin release. The pump delivers, through a subcutaneous needle, a continuous, variable, small supply of insulin, augmented by extra insulin doses prior to eating. The management of diabetes and pregnancy is one of the clear indications for intensive insulin regimens (see DIABETES MELLITUS in Ch. 178). In other areas of diabetes management, however, it remains to be shown that the use of intensified insulin therapy will delay or prevent the onset of vascular or neural complications. With the use of a pump, problems are seen with infections and abscess formation at the infusion site, local allergic skin reactions, diabetic ketoacidosis due to undetected mechanical obstruction to insulin delivery, or hypoglycemia. Moreover, there is a marked variability among people in the time course of their response to exogenous insulin. Intensive insulin regimens require hard work on the part of all involved—patients, physicians, and nurses.

Management of Difficult-to-Control ("Brittle") Diabetics

Some insulin-requiring patients demonstrate rapid swings between heavy glucosuria and symptomatic hypoglycemic reactions. This frequently results from altered or defective hypoglycemia counterregulation involving glucagon and epinephrine. Glucagon secretory response usually becomes deficient early in the course of IDDM. If epinephrine also becomes ineffective in raising the plasma glucose, as a feature of diabetic autonomic (adrenergic) neuropathy, or as the result of the use of β-adrenergic antagonist therapy for hypertension or ischemic heart disease, the patient can become defenseless against hypoglycemia. Seven principles are helpful in approaching glucose control in such patients:

1. Patient self monitoring of a profile of blood glucose levels at home (see above), may help both patient and physician analyze the precise nature of the "brittleness" and take appropriate steps towards its correction.

2. The patient's dietary, insulin, and emotional baselines should be stabilized and daily exercise should remain relatively constant. The time of day and caloric content of breakfast, lunch, dinner, and additional scheduled snacks should be stable from day to day.

3. On the basis of a self-monitored blood glucose profile, the morning insulin dose may be adjusted and supplemented with either the rapid- or long-acting preparation of the same series, as indicated. Under these circumstances, the Lente series of insulins are a little easier to use; protamine zinc insulin added in the same syringe to isophane or insulin injection inordinately prolongs the effect of the combination.

4. Between-meal and bedtime snacks, representing a shift in mealtime calories but not an increase in total daily caloric intake, match caloric intake more closely to the intermediate insulin action curves.

5. Giving ⅓ of the total daily insulin dose before the evening meal is helpful.

6. Rarely, unstable ketoacidosis-prone patients require multiple injections of rapid-acting insulin. The insulin is given in divided portions before meals based on the results of blood tests.

7. Some diabetics demonstrate brittleness, with wide swings of plasma glucose from daytime hyperglycemia and glucosuria to nighttime hypoglycemic reactions. It is important to document such swings with blood glucose self-monitoring. Such patients often benefit by having their insulin dose reduced by 30 to 70%, and then gradually increased over several days; they often stabilize at a lower dose level. Should a patient regularly demonstrate defective glucose counterregulation due to impaired secretion of glucagon and epinephrine or the need for β-adrenergic antagonist therapy, the therapeutic goal of euglycemia may be unreasonable.

Complications of Insulin Treatment

Insulin shock (hypoglycemia) may occur if too much insulin or too little food is taken. (See HYPOGLYCEMIA, below, for diagnosis and therapy.) All patients receiving insulin, and their families, must be instructed concerning the symptoms and immediate treatment of hypoglycemia. A patient receiving insulin should always carry sugar or candy to be eaten immediately if epinephrine-like symptoms are felt (see Symptoms and Signs under HYPOGLYCEMIA, below). Carrying an identification card or engraved metallic emblem on a bracelet or necklace (Medic Alert Foundation, Turlock, California 95380) stating that the patient has DM and is taking insulin will help in case of accident or emergency illness.

Local reactions to insulin injections, often occurring during the first few weeks of insulin therapy, most commonly consist of stinging or itching at the injection site, possibly followed by heat, induration, erythema, and an urticarial reaction. The new more purified insulin preparations may reduce the incidence of local reactions. Treatment may consist of switching from the beef-pork insulin combination to human or pure pork (or occasionally pure beef) insulin. Systemic allergic reactions are uncommon; they include hives, urticaria, cardiopulmonary or GI symptoms, and, rarely, anaphylaxis. Systemic treatment with antihistamines, corticosteroids, and even epinephrine injection may be required.

Patients occasionally develop **insulin resistance** and require > 200 u. daily to control hyperglycemia. Shifting to a human or more purified pork insulin preparation may lower insulin requirements, as may the *cautious* addition of tolbutamide or other sulfonylurea to the insulin regimen. Lilly's concentrated regular pork insulin preparation (Iletin II®, U-500) is designed for insulin-resistance patients.

The s.c. injection of insulin in certain susceptible patients may rarely result in either atrophy or hypertrophy of the local fat tissue. Nearly all patients with atrophy show improvement when their daily dose of one of the newer purified insulins is injected directly into the affected area. No specific treatment for injection site hypertrophy is effective; careful injection site rotation is recommended.

Oral Hypoglycemic Agents

Several sulfonylureas that can lower the blood glucose level when given orally may be used to treat selected patients. These drugs are listed in TABLE 94–6. Oral agents should not be used as a substitute for insulin in the insulin-dependent patient; although their mechanisms of action are not clear, they are not oral forms of insulin. Their biologic half-lives following oral administration cannot be measured accurately, making the selection of dose and timing of administration somewhat haphazard.

The **University Group Diabetes Program (UGDP)** attempted to evaluate various types of therapy in noninsulin-dependent diabetic patients, comparing tolbutamide or phenformin (a biguanide, since withdrawn from general use in the USA) treatment with diet alone and with 2 insulin treatment regimens. The study led to 2 major conclusions: (1) The combination of diet and tolbutamide or diet and phenformin therapy in

TABLE 94–6. CHARACTERISTICS OF SULFONYLUREA AGENTS

Generic Name	Brand Name	Daily Dosage Range (mg)	Duration of Action (h)	Tablet Size (mg)	Doses/day
Tolbutamide	Orinase®	500–3000	6–12	250, 500	2–3
Chlorpropamide	Diabinese®	100–750	60	100, 250	1
Acetohexamide	Dymelor®	250–1500	12–18	250, 500	1–2
Tolazamide	Tolinase®	100–1000	12–24	100, 250, 500	1–2
Glyburide	Diabeta® Micronase	2.5–30	Up to 24	5	1–2
Glipizide	Glucatrol®	5–40	Up to 24	5	1–2

(Modified from "The Clinical Pharmacology of Glipizide" by A. Melander in *American Journal of Medicine* 1983: 75 (Supplement 5B): pp 41–45; and from "The Pharmacology of Sulfonylureas" by T. G. Skillman and J. M. Feldman in *American Journal of Medicine,* Feb. 1981, 70:363. Used with permission of the *Journal* and the authors.)

the treatment of mild noninsulin-dependent diabetics is no more effective than diet alone in prolonging life, at least in the dosages of phenformin and tolbutamide that were used. (2) Tolbutamide plus diet, or phenformin plus diet, may be less effective than diet alone or than diet plus insulin in minimizing cardiovascular mortality.

The UGDP study raised controversy about whether increased cardiovascular mortality is associated with the use of sulfonylureas. However, after 17 yr, the investigators reported that, in their NIDDM patients, there was no evidence that insulin, or any other drug that lowered plasma glucose levels, altered the course of vascular complications. Furthermore, only a variable insulin dose program showed reliable and sustained reduction of plasma glucose levels.

For the symptomatic noninsulin-dependent patient, who cannot physically administer or receive insulin injections (eg, the arthritic or blind) the sulfonylureas may lower plasma glucose levels and control symptoms. Such a situation accounts for a very small number of NIDDM patients. For the remaining symptomatic patients, insulin is indicated. For asymptomatic NIDDM patients, management should focus first on control of weight and hypertension, reduction of other atherosclerotic risks, and control of the progression of complications (eg, through foot care, training programs, and regular eye evaluation by an ophthalmologist experienced in laser therapy).

Acute toxic effects following the use of oral hypoglycemic agents appear to be relatively rare. Following either an initial dose or months of therapy with one of the sulfonylureas, cholestatic jaundice or severe hypoglycemia has occurred. The latter at times may last for several days. Chlorpropamide and, to a lesser extent, tolbutamide have been associated with symptomatic hyponatremia and water intoxication due to potentiation of antidiuretic hormone action on renal tubules.

If a sulfonylurea is tried, a given dose should be continued for 4 to 6 wk before determining that the drug is a success or failure at symptom control. Sustained improvement in hyperglycemia should be monitored with glucosylated Hb determinations q 2 or 3 mo. Doses of the sulfonylureas should not exceed the maximum listed in TABLE 94–6.

Treatment of Ketoacidosis

Ketoacidosis is associated with 5 physiologic abnormalities that must be immediately evaluated and corrected. (1) **Hyperglycemia:** With normal renal circulation, blood glucose concentrations rarely exceed 400 mg/dL. With fluid loss and compromised renal perfusion, however, higher values are found. (2) **Acidosis** is the result of lipid

mobilization and breakdown of free fatty acids in the liver to acetoacetic and β-hydroxybutyric acids. (3) **Low blood volume** is due to loss of both fluid and electrolytes. Hct, postural BP changes, neck vein observation, and central venous pressure can reflect the severity of this depletion. (4) **Hyperosmolality** is also a potential contributing factor in coma as a result of renal water loss and water depletion due to sweating, nausea, and vomiting. Significant osmolal elevation generally is reflected by hyperglycemia > 500 mg/dL and suggests inadequate renal perfusion. Occasionally hyperosmolality alone can cause hyperglycemic-hyperosmolar nonketotic coma (see above). (5) **Potassium loss:** Although total body K is depleted, the serum K in the presence of acidosis is often deceptively sustained in the normal range.

Immediate treatment: The cornerstones of ketoacidosis therapy, required in all patients, are insulin and IV fluids. **Insulin** is given immediately. The choice of insulin regimen should be based on the experience of the therapeutic team; the objective in all approaches is to achieve optimally effective levels of circulating insulin and maintain them until there is evidence of biochemical recovery. An ideal rate of blood glucose lowering is 75 to 100 mg/dL/h. A more rapid drop may lead to osmotically induced fluid shifts, manifested by confusion or other evidence of CNS deterioration. One approach is to give a continuous IV infusion of insulin injection in 0.9% sodium chloride at a rate of 10 u./h or, alternatively, to give the same dose via intermittent IM (not s.c.) injection. Because circulatory insufficiency is common in ketoacidosis, absorption from s.c. sites is unpredictable; therefore, insulins other than regular insulin (crystalline-zinc insulin or insulin injection) are never used. The IV infusion can be administered through an infusion pump or a pediatric infusion set. This "low-dose" approach is as safe and effective as previous high-dose regimens and provides greater ease in avoiding hypoglycemia and hypokalemia. Any method of treatment, however, requires close clinical supervision.

IV fluids should also be started at once. The first liter of isotonic saline (0.9% sodium chloride) should be given over 20 to 60 min, depending upon the severity of extracellular volume depletion. Hypotonic solutions are less effective in restoring renal perfusion. Glucose solutions do not help correct the electrolyte and pH disturbances and are withheld until plasma glucose falls below 250 mg/dL. Low blood volume and shock usually respond to vigorous infusion of saline but may require plasma or plasma expanders (see SHOCK in Ch. 26). If serum K is low, addition of KCl to the first or second bottle of IV fluid must be considered.

Two other immediate measures which may be required include **nasogastric intubation** (for intractable vomiting, abdominal distention, and gastric dilation, or to avoid aspiration in a comatose patient) and **bladder catheterization** (to monitor urine output in severely ill or comatose patients).

Continuing treatment: Hourly blood glucose determinations and semiquantitation of serum ketones by serum serial dilution will reflect patient improvement. Patients without a 10% drop in plasma glucose after 2 h should have the insulin dose doubled each hour until a response occurs. After the blood glucose falls to 250 mg/dL, an infusion containing glucose helps to avoid late hypoglycemia.

Bicarbonate may be added to the IV solution during the first 2 or 3 h *only* if acidosis is severe (blood pH < 7.1, bicarbonate < 10 mEq/L). It is seldom required, and the administration rate should not exceed 100 mEq/h. Excessive bicarbonate therapy may be paradoxically associated with CSF acidosis and inhibition of hemoglobin O_2 transport and tissue oxygenation.

Potassium loss is estimated from the serum K level interpreted in light of the degree of acidosis. Initially, serum K should be measured hourly; *failure to assess K accurately is the most common cause of death during treatment of ketoacidosis.* As soon as the urine flow is adequate, K can be added to the infusion at the rate of 20 mEq/h or less. Faster rates in the presence of severe depletion require extreme caution with careful monitor-

ing to avoid hyperkalemic cardiac arrest. If the initial serum K is very low, replacement should be started even before adequate urine flow is confirmed.

Marked improvement should occur within 8 h. Reevaluation at that time of the 5 areas of physiologic abnormalities (listed above) should direct therapy to any significant remaining imbalances. Treatment is continued until the patient is able to take fluid freely by mouth. As soon as food is tolerated, oral fluids followed by the patient's diet and insulin therapy should be resumed.

An underlying cause for the ketoacidosis must always be sought; common problems include omitted insulin dose, infection, GI upset, alcoholism, myocardial infarction, CVA, or previously undiagnosed diabetes mellitus. Since a leukocytosis of 15,000 to 30,000 is common in ketoacidosis, this is not helpful in indicating infection.

Treatment of **alcoholic ketoacidosis** is by IV infusion of glucose in saline or water. Insulin may also be required if hyperglycemia suggests DM is present. **Hyperglycemic-hyperosmolar nonketotic coma** is treated by giving 1 or 2 L of 0.9% sodium chloride IV initially to restore intravascular volume and BP followed by 5 or 6 L of 0.45% sodium chloride over the next 24 h to replace free water loss. The patient's clinical state (hypotension vs. edema) will determine the exact volume and rate of administration. IV regular insulin is administered cautiously (10 to 30 u. regular insulin q 2 to 3 h as a bolus or by constant infusion—5 to 10 u./h) until plasma glucose approaches 250 mg/dL. *In contrast to diabetic ketoacidosis, these patients are often very sensitive to insulin*. Lower values during the first 24 to 48 h may cause or aggravate cerebral edema. Supplements of K are also indicated as in the treatment of ketoacidosis. In spite of attentive therapy, mortality is 40 to 70%, with ⅓ of the deaths occurring within the first 24 h.

Treatment of lactic acidosis consists of the administration of large volumes of saline and bicarbonate. In patients with plasma glucose > 250 mg/dL, giving small doses of insulin may be helpful even in the absence of ketoacidosis or severe hyperosmolality.

Treatment to Prevent or Control Vascular Complications

Diabetic retinopathy (see under VASCULAR RETINOPATHIES in Ch. 223).

Diabetic renal disease: Four conditions precipitate or exacerbate renal impairment. **Hypertension** should be controlled with the recognition that antihypertensive drug side effects have special problems in diabetes—eg, male sexual impotence associated with diuretics or sympathetic inhibitors may be erroneously attributed to diabetic neuropathy; β-adrenergic blockers may delay recovery from insulin-induced hypoglycemia and blunt hypoglycemia symptoms (see Management of Difficult-to-Control ["Brittle"] Diabetics, above). **Neurogenic bladder** from diabetic neuropathy can accelerate renal failure following urinary retention or obstructive nephropathy. **Repetitive urethral instrumentation** increases the risk of infection and injury, accelerating renal azotemia. **Dye contrast radiographic studies** are associated with increased incidence amd acceleration of renal failure in diabetics. Since there is no known effective therapy, such studies should be performed only after careful consideration of alternative procedures.

When the diabetic's serum creatinine reaches 3 mg/dL, referral to a nephrologist should be considered and evaluation for dialysis or transplantation initiated with a creatinine of 5 mg/dL.

Diabetic foot problems: Foot lesions in diabetics commonly result from a combination of diabetic peripheral neuropathy and peripheral vascular disease, with the primary event being the development of an insensitive foot.

Prevention of foot problems starts with stressing that patients who smoke have a *very* significant reversible risk in addition to their diabetes for peripheral circulatory problems. A history of smoking is nearly always present in diabetics who require foot or leg amputations. Further, alcoholic peripheral neuropathy may worsen diabetic neuropathy. The importance of foot care is best stressed for all diabetic patients b

having the physician personally conduct a thorough examination of the patient's feet *at least annually*. The potential hazard of heat, cold, new shoes, constricting or mended socks, and going barefoot should be emphasized (see also PERIPHERAL ATHEROSCLEROTIC DISEASE under OCCLUSIVE ARTERIAL DISEASE in Ch. 30).

PREGNANCY IN THE DIABETIC PATIENT

DM is associated with increased maternal, fetal, and neonatal morbidity and mortality. These problems and their management are discussed in Chs. 178 and 186.

CARE OF THE INSULIN-REQUIRING DIABETIC DURING SURGERY

The aim of diabetic treatment is to prevent ketoacidosis and minimize osmotic diuresis and hypoglycemic reactions. Because of the insulin-antagonizing action of high plasma cortisol levels associated with surgical stress, it is safe to give 1/3 to 1/2 of the patient's normal daily dose of insulin in the morning prior to the operation. Five percent glucose in either water or 0.9% sodium chloride solution is infused during the operation and continued postoperatively to provide 50 gm of glucose q 8 h until oral feeding is resumed. After the patient begins to recover from anesthesia, the preoperative insulin dose may be repeated. Serum glucose and ketone levels should be obtained at least 4 h and 8 h postoperatively, although bedside monitoring of blood glucose with reagent strips and a reflectance meter may be carried out easily with greater frequency. Additional insulin injection is indicated only if hyperglycemia is > 250 mg/dL or if ketone concentration becomes "large" in the undiluted serum specimen. Serum glucose levels < 100 mg/dL indicate a need for more glucose infusion. As oral feeding is tolerated and activity increases, the patient may, over a few days, resume his preoperative insulin dose. Emergency nonelective surgical procedures with greater associated stress, or patients who develop early postoperative complications, require more frequent monitoring of serum glucose and ketones.

Patients who normally do not require insulin can usually be managed without supplemental insulin, but some may temporarily require small doses of regular insulin (10 to 12 u. once or twice/day) to control the hyperglycemia and glucosuria associated with surgical stress.

DIET FOR DIABETES

Beyond the basic requirements to provide adequate calories and necessary nutrients to achieve desirable weight and sustain normal growth and development, 2 factors in diabetic patients require specific dietary adjustments. **Insulin-treated patients** require day-to-day consistency of intake of calories (carbohydrate, protein, and fat) and the timing of meals. This often is effectively achieved by telling adult patients to "eat about the same amount of food at similar times daily." Extra food may be needed for unusual exercise or to treat, abort, or prevent hypoglycemia. Patients treated with sulfonylureas usually do not require meticulous dietary adjustment. **Obesity** is the other factor requiring dietary treatment. Decreased caloric intake with even moderate (15 lb) weight reduction will lower fasting plasma glucose, lipid, and insulin levels toward normal as insulin resistance is decreased. An exchange list system involves grouping foods with similar fat, carbohydrate, and protein content into lists, allowing the exchange of a portion of one food on a list for another on the same list when composing a menu. Such a system has been prepared by committees of the American Diabetes Association and the American Dietetic Association in cooperation with the National Institutes of Health, and published in 1976. This system, of necessity, includes a limited number of foods, but may be helpful for some patients in their efforts to maintain

a varied diet while losing weight or maintaining consistency of food intake. Current information, however, fails to demonstrate that diet programs emphasizing adhering to a specific "diabetic" diet or avoiding specific foods can reverse or prevent the disabling manifestations of diabetes.

Complicated dietary problems, especially attempts at weight loss, can benefit from guidance provided by a registered dietitian or other qualified diet counselor who will work closely with the individual patient. Many physicians lack adequate background and time to instruct a patient properly about diet. Furthermore, single encounters between a diet counselor and patient cannot alter lifelong habits, nor can generalized preprinted meal lists and diets be effective in meeting the challenge. A single lesson in diet or in any other principle of diabetic management is useless. The educational plan for the diabetic must be a continuing lifelong process. Most successful educational programs for diabetics involve a team including a dietitian, nurse, and physician in which each member of the team educates the patient in his or her area of expertise. The patient's role with the team must be emphasized, for without the patient's cooperation, even the best plans will fail.

HYPOGLYCEMIA

An abnormally low blood glucose level.

Etiology

The causes of hypoglycemia may be divided into 2 categories: (1) reactive hypoglycemia in response to a meal, specific nutrients, or drugs, and (2) spontaneous hypoglycemia in the fasting state.

Reactive hypoglycemia following a meal is the most common type and is characterized by the development of symptomatic hypoglycemia 2 to 4 h after eating. A very rapid absorption of glucose into the circulation and a subsequent outpouring of a corresponding excess of insulin appear in **alimentary or postgastrectomy hypoglycemia,** often, but not always, seen after gastric resection. A similar reactive hypoglycemia due to delayed insulin response is seen in some mild maturity-onset diabetic patients after a carbohydrate load and may be one of the first indications of DM. Another type of reactive hypoglycemia which follows a carbohydrate load is known as **"functional" hypoglycemia** and its mechanism is unknown.

Other types of reactive hypoglycemia may be caused by the administration of excess insulin, less frequently by oral hypoglycemic agents, and in some patients after ingestion of alcohol or other drugs (see TABLE 94–7).

Alcohol-induced hypoglycemia is metabolically related to alcoholic ketoacidosis (see above) and either may occur separately or together in alcohol abusers. Neither requires impaired liver function and both occur 1 to 3 days after anorexia, nausea and vomiting, and consequent starvation have terminated a period of chronic alcohol abuse. Hypoglycemia results from a combination of starvation and impaired hepatic gluconeogenesis.

Spontaneous hypoglycemia in the fasting state may be due to failure of glucose production (extensive hepatic disease) or, rarely, the inability of normal production to keep up with excessive glucose consumption (vigorous exercise or pregnancy). Hypoglycemia in the fasting state can also result from excess glucose utilization through insulin overproduction from an islet cell tumor or, rarely, from an extrapancreatic neoplasm. Occasionally a large tumor such as a sarcoma may consume enormous amounts of glucose, leading to hypoglycemia. Other less common causes of hypoglycemia are included in TABLE 94–7.

Symptoms and Signs

The symptoms and signs of hypoglycemia may be grouped into 2 categories: (1) faintness, weakness, tremulousness, palpitation, diaphoresis, hunger, and nervousness,

TABLE 94–7. CLINICAL CLASSIFICATION OF HYPOGLYCEMIC DISORDERS

I. Reactive causes (following administration of exogenous factors)

A. Meals (carbohydrate)

1. Excessive insulin action or defective counter-regulatory response to normal insulin action
   a. Alimentary (postgastrectomy) hypoglycemia
   b. Late hypoglycemia of early maturity-onset diabetes mellitus
2. Mechanism unknown (probably similar)
   a. "Functional" hypoglycemia (essential, idiopathic)

B. Specific nutrients (inhibit hepatic glucose output)

1. Fructose: hereditary fructose intolerance (fructose-1-phosphate aldolase deficiency)
2. Galactose: galactosemia (galactose-1-phosphate uridyl transferase deficiency)
3. Leucine: leucine hypersensitivity of infancy and childhood; branched-chain ketonuria (maple syrup urine disease)

C. Drugs

1. Excess glucose utilization
   a. Exogenous insulin administration (factitious, iatrogenic)
   b. Insulin plus:
      Beta-adrenergic receptor blocking drugs
      Oxytetracycline
      EDTA (ethylenediaminetetraacetic acid)
      Mebanazine* (monoamine oxidase inhibitor)
      Manganese
   c. Sufonylurea
   d. Sulfonylurea plus:
      Sulfisoxazole
      Dicumarol
      Phenylbutazone
      Alcohol
   e. Phenformin*
   f. Pentamidine
   g. Disopyramide
   h. Quinine
2. Deficient glucose production
   a. Alcohol
   b. Unripened ackee fruit ("Jamaican vomiting sickness")
   c. Salicylates
   d. Aminobenzoic acid
   e. Haloperidol
   f. Propoxyphene
   g. Chlorpromazine

II. Spontaneous causes (endogenous metabolic processes) producing hypoglycemia in the fasting state

A. Excessive glucose utilization

1. Excessive insulin effect
   a. Insulinoma
   b. Deficiency of contrainsulin hormones:
      Glucagon, Epinephrine
      Cortisol, Thyroid hormones
      Growth hormone
   c. Neonatal hypoglycemia in infants of diabetic mothers
   d. Treated erythroblastosis fetalis in neonates
2. Other mechanisms increasing glucose utilization
   a. Exercise
   b. Fever
   c. Pregnancy
   d. Renal glycosuria
   e. Large tumor (e.g., sarcoma)

* Not used in USA.

(Continued)

TABLE 94–7. CLINICAL CLASSIFICATION OF HYPOGLYCEMIC DISORDERS *(Cont'd)*

B. Deficient glucose production
  1. Diffuse liver disease (hepatomas, acute necrosis—rarely cirrhosis)
  2. Specific hepatic enzyme defects for:
     a. Glycogen mobilization (glycogen storage disease)
     b. Glucose release (glucose-6-phosphatase deficiency)
     c. Gluconeogenetic renewal of glucose-6-phosphate from smaller fragments (fructose-1, 6-diphosphatase deficiency)
  3. Nonpancreatic neoplasms—release substance(s) inhibiting hepatic glucose production (occasionally tumors demonstrate excessive glucose utilization)
  4. Ketotic hypoglycemia of childhood (deficient gluconeogenetic substrate alanine)

* Not used in USA.

such as may result from epinephrine administration (acute hypoglycemia with epinephrine-like symptoms indicates that endogenous epinephrine-induced glycogen mobilization has already started), and (2) a pattern of CNS symptoms including headache, confusion, visual disturbances, motor weakness, palsy, ataxia, and marked personality changes. These CNS disturbances may progress to loss of consciousness, convulsions, and coma. With recurring episodes of hypoglycemia in the same patient, the symptoms may be repetitive, although the tempo and severity of an attack may vary.

Symptoms of anxiety, including sweating, headaches, hunger, tachycardia, weakness, and occasionally seizures and coma may suggest hypoglycemia, but most patients with such symptoms are not hypoglycemic.

Diagnosis

The documentation of low plasma glucose (< 50 mg/dL) specifically associated with objective signs or subjective symptoms, which are relieved by the ingestion of sugar or other food, are the essentials for diagnosing hypoglycemia. Lower plasma glucose levels are often seen in normals. While normal men fasting for 72 h rarely drop their plasma glucose levels below 55 mg/dL, normal women demonstrate lower levels during a similar fast, more than half showing levels < 50 mg/dL. During 5-h OGTT, 25% of normal individuals demonstrate plasma glucose levels < 50 mg/dL at some time following glucose ingestion, and occasional individuals have values below 35 mg/dL without symptoms.

Once hypoglycemia has been diagnosed, careful consideration of onset time and symptom pattern leads rapidly to appropriate tests to establish the cause. The first factor for diagnostic discrimination is to determine whether the hypoglycemia occurs within 4 h of a meal (carbohydrate load) or other causative agent or whether it is brought on by a fast, either overnight or more prolonged. Epinephrine-like symptoms are more typically associated with the former, reactive category.

In fasting hypoglycemia, it is important to rule out an **islet cell tumor (insulinoma)** which may be surgically correctable. Symptoms from insulinoma hypoglycemia usually appear insidiously and can mimic a variety of psychiatric and neurologic disorders. The symptoms are characterized by CNS disturbances (eg, headache, confusion and coma), while evidence of sympathetic stimulation is often absent. Since excessive insulin release is a manifestation of this disease, the correlation of the **insulin radioimmunoassay** with plasma glucose levels is mandatory in confirming the diagnosis. A carefully supervised fast, which in normal individuals is associated with a progressive fall in plasma insulin concentration, will reveal inappropriately high tumor-sustained

insulin levels in the presence of hypoglycemia. The ratio of immunoreactive insulin (μU/mL) to glucose (mg/dL) in the plasma rarely exceeds 0.3 in the absence of an insulinoma. Where elevated insulin levels are associated with hypoglycemia, however, the possibility that the insulin was exogenously given rather than endogenously produced must be considered. Measurement of C-peptide, a by-product of endogenous insulin production and absent in exogenous insulin, may aid in differentiation of these 2 causes of hypoglycemia.

Treatment

Acute or severe episodes of hypoglycemia with epinephrine-like or CNS symptoms may be relieved by ingestion of oral glucose or sucrose. In an attack characterized primarily by CNS symptoms (suggesting that the corrective action of epinephrine is inoperative), glucose should be given promptly. One convenient method is to stir 2 or 3 tbsp of granulated sugar into a glass of fruit juice or water. If the patient is unable to swallow, the immediate parenteral administration of glucagon (see under GLUCAGON, below) will often arouse the patient from coma and permit oral therapy. Failing this, IV glucose must be given.

The treatment of spontaneous hypoglycemia in the fasting state involves removing or controlling the cause whenever possible. An operable insulinoma must be ruled out. Hypoglycemic symptoms from inoperable tumors may be controlled with drugs such as diazoxide or streptozocin. Reactive hypoglycemia following ingestion of drugs or specific nutrients is similarly treated by avoiding or controlling the causative agent.

Treatment of hypoglycemia following meals, on the other hand, is often complex. "Functional" hypoglycemia may occasionally be treated successfully by relieving emotional stress. The single most useful treatment regimen for all 3 reactive hypoglycemias that follow meals is a diet high in protein and restricted in carbohydrate. Not all patients will be completely relieved on this regimen, but many will have amelioration of their attacks.

Diabetic patients taking insulin should always carry sugar lumps or candy with them, and the patient's family and friends should be instructed in recognizing the symptoms of hypoglycemia and in giving the emergency treatment mentioned above.

Before a patient receives definitive treatment for hypoglycemia (excluding emergency treatment), *all* of the following should be present: (1) documented occurrence of low blood glucose level; (2) symptoms shown to occur when the blood glucose is low; (3) demonstration that the symptoms are relieved specifically by the ingestion of sugar or other food; and (4) identification of the particular type of hypoglycemia that is causing the symptoms.

GLUCAGON

Glucagon is a single-chain polypeptide hormone produced by alpha cells in the pancreatic islets of Langerhans and in the wall of the stomach and duodenum. The plasma concentration of alpha-cell glucagon can be measured by radioimmunoassay (**RIA**). The GI tract and probably other sites also secrete several other substances with glucagon-like immunoreactivity, but these differ in physicochemical and biologic properties from alpha-cell glucagon. While these substances interfered with the earlier RIA determinations, the development of a more specific antiserum for circulating alpha-cell glucagon now allows more precise measurement.

Glucagon has a hyperglycemic action. It mobilizes glucose and raises the blood glucose level by both stimulating glycogenolysis and augmenting glucose formation from amino acids. It also accelerates free fatty acid release from adipose tissue. Thus, glucagon is a regulator of nutrient mobilization, as insulin is a regulator of nutrient storage.

Glucagonomas are infrequently occurring glucagon-secreting tumors of the islet alpha cells (see CANCER OF THE PANCREAS in Ch. 55).

Glucagon is used pharmacologically primarily to counteract severe hypoglycemic reactions in diabetic patients taking insulin. It has also been used in psychiatric patients during insulin shock therapy. The ability of glucagon to counteract hypoglycemia depends upon the availability of liver glycogen. It is virtually useless in starvation, adrenal insufficiency, or chronic hypoglycemia, and may be ineffective in a number of diabetic patients with hypoglycemia severe enough to require hospitalization. However, it is the drug of choice for the initial urgent counteraction of hypoglycemia in comatose patients unable to take oral glucose solution and for whom IV glucose is not immediately available. Insulin-requiring diabetics with a tendency toward hypoglycemic reactions should have glucagon available in their home for family members to administer in case of a hypoglycemic emergency. The home diagnosis of hypoglycemia is facilitated by the use of blood glucose monitoring strips with or without an electronic meter. Instruction in the preparation and parenteral administration of glucagon should be given before an emergency arises.

Glucagon is available commercially in vials containing 1 mg of dried powder accompanied by a vial of diluting solution for parenteral administration. It can be stored as a powder without refrigeration for 4 or 5 yr and up to 3 mo after reconstitution if refrigerated. The usual dose is 0.5 to 1 mg, which may be given s.c. (using an insulin syringe), IM, or IV. There is generally no advantage in giving > 1 mg of glucagon. If the patient does not awaken from coma within 20 min, IV glucose must be given immediately and the diagnosis of the cause of coma must be reconsidered. Oral carbohydrate should be given as soon as the patient responds. The most frequent side effects are nausea and vomiting.

A diabetic in coma from acidosis rather than from insulin reaction is characterized by hyper- rather than hypoglycemia on blood glucose monitoring strips and thus will not respond to glucose or glucagon, but will require immediate appropriate therapy as indicated in DIABETES MELLITUS, above.

GENETIC ABNORMALITIES OF CARBOHYDRATE METABOLISM

(See Ch. 196)

95. CARCINOID SYNDROME

A syndrome of episodic cutaneous flushing, cyanosis, abdominal cramps, diarrhea, and valvular heart disease (and less commonly, asthma and arthropathy), usually caused by metastatic intestinal carcinoid tumors that secrete excessive amounts of vasoactive substances, including serotonin, bradykinin, histamine, prostaglandins, and polypeptide hormones.

Etiology and Pathophysiology

Functioning tumors of the diffuse peripheral endocrine or paracrine system (as described by Feyrter) produce various amines and polypeptides, with corresponding clinical presentations. The carcinoid syndrome is usually associated with functioning malignant tumors that produce serotonin and arise from enteroendocrine cells in the ileum, but can occur with comparable tumors elsewhere in the GI tract, pancreas, gonads, or bronchi. Rarely, certain highly malignant tumors, including oat cell carcinoma of the lung, islet cell carcinoma of the pancreas, and medullary carcinoma of the thyroid may also be responsible. The intestinal carcinoid does not ordinarily produce the syndrome unless hepatic metastases have occurred, since metabolic products released by the tumor are rapidly destroyed by blood and liver enzymes in the portal

circulation—serotonin, for example, by hepatic monoamine oxidase. Hepatic metastases, however, release these substances via the hepatic veins directly into the systemic circulation. Primary pulmonary and ovarian carcinoid products bypass the portal route and may similarly induce symptoms, as can rare intestinal carcinoids with only intra-abdominal spread, but draining directly into the systemic circulation or the lymphatics. Serotonin acts on smooth muscle to produce diarrhea, colic, and malabsorption; histamine and bradykinin, through their vasodilator effects, cause flushing. The role of prostaglandins and of the various polypeptide hormones, which may be produced by paracrine cells, awaits further investigation; however, human chorionic gonadotropin and pancreatic polypeptide are occasionally elevated with carcinoid tumors. Certain carcinoid symptoms such as flushing have been relieved by somatostatin (which inhibits release of most hormone secretions) without lowering urinary 5-hydroxyindoleacetic acid or gastrin.

Symptoms and Signs

The most common and often earliest manifestation is an uncomfortable cutaneous flushing, typically of the head and neck, often precipitated by emotion or the ingestion of food, hot water, or alcohol; striking color changes ranging from pallor or erythema to cyanosis may occur. Abdominal cramps with recurrent diarrhea develop and are often the major complaint. A malabsorption syndrome has been documented in some. Many patients develop right-sided endocardial fibrosis, leading to pulmonary stenosis and tricuspid regurgitation; left heart lesions, which have been reported with bronchial carcinoids, are rare because serotonin is destroyed during passage through the lung. A few patients have asthmatic wheezing and some have decreased libido and impotence; pellagra has developed rarely.

Diagnosis

Most appendiceal carcinoids are benign, asymptomatic, and discovered incidentally following appendectomy. Functioning carcinoids are suspected by the symptoms and signs, and diagnosis is confirmed by demonstrating increased urinary excretion of the serotonin metabolite, 5-hydroxyindoleacetic acid **(5-HIAA).** A colorimetric test is carried out after the patient has abstained from serotonin-containing foods (such as bananas, tomatoes, plums, avocados, pineapples, eggplant, and walnuts) for 3 days to avoid false-positive results. Certain drugs, including guaifenesin, methocarbamol, and phenothiazines, also interfere with the test. On the 3rd day a 24-h urine sample is collected for assay. Normal excretion of 5-HIAA is < 10 mg/day; in patients with carcinoid syndrome it is usually > 50 mg/day.

Provocative tests with calcium gluconate, catecholamines, pentagastrin, or alcohol have been used to induce flushing. These may aid in the diagnosis in some patients, but must be carried out with care. A liver scan may be sufficient to demonstrate metastases, but localization of the tumor may require an extensive evaluation, including laparotomy. The rarer tumors mentioned above must be excluded by appropriate examinations.

Treatment

Curative resection of primary lung carcinoids is possible. For patients with hepatic metastases, surgery is diagnostic or palliative only, and radiation therapy is unsuccessful, in part because of the poor tolerance of the normal hepatic tissue. Despite metastatic disease, 10- to 15-yr survivals are not unusual. No effective chemotherapeutic regimen is established, but streptozocin with 5-fluorouracil is most widely used. Tamoxifen has been infrequently effective in anecdotal case reports; leukocyte interferon has produced temporary symptomatic benefits. Niacin and an adequate protein intake are needed to prevent pellagra, because dietary tryptophan is diverted to serotonin by the tumor. Diarrhea may be controlled by codeine phosphate 15 mg orally q 4 to 6 h, tincture of opium 0.6 mL q 6 h, or diphenoxylate 2.5 mg orally 1 to 3 times/day, or by

peripheral serotonin antagonists such as cyproheptadine 4 to 8 mg orally q 6 h, or methysergide 1 to 2 mg orally qid. Enzyme inhibitors that prevent the conversion of 5-hydroxytryptophan to serotonin include methyldopa 250 to 500 mg orally q 6 h, or phenoxybenzamine 10 mg/day.

Flushing may be treated with phenothiazines (eg, prochlorperazine 5 to 10 mg or chlorpromazine 25 to 50 mg orally q 6 h). Histamine H_2 receptor antagonists (eg, cimetidine, ranitidine) may also be used. Phentolamine 5 to 15 mg (an α-adrenergic blocking agent) has prevented experimentally induced flushes. Anti-inflammatory corticosteroids (eg, prednisone 5 mg orally q 6 h) may be useful for the severe flushing caused by bronchial carcinoids.

§9. HEMATOLOGY AND ONCOLOGY

96. ANEMIAS

Decreases of RBC or Hb content because of blood loss, impaired production, or RBC destruction.

General Considerations

The term anemia has been used incorrectly as a diagnosis; more properly, it denotes a complex of signs and symptoms, and defining its pathophysiologic mechanism is required to understand its essential nature and plan appropriate therapy. Ignoring the need to investigate even a mild anemia is a serious error; its presence indicates an underlying disorder, and its severity offers little information about its genesis or true clinical significance.

The clinical expression of anemia results from tissue hypoxia, and its specific symptoms and signs represent cardiovascular-pulmonary compensatory responses to the severity and duration of that hypoxia. Severe anemia can be associated with weakness vertigo, headache, tinnitus, spots before the eyes, ease of fatigue, drowsiness, irritability, and even bizarre behavior. Amenorrhea, loss of libido, GI complaints, and sometimes jaundice and splenomegaly can occur. Finally, heart failure or shock can result (See TABLE 96-1, below.)

General diagnostic patterns can be used to expedite the differential diagnosis. Anemia results from one or more combinations of 3 basic mechanisms: blood loss, decreased production, or increased destruction (hemolysis). Blood loss should be the first consideration. Once it is ruled out, only the other 2 mechanisms remain. Since RBC survival is 120 days, maintenance of steady populations requires renewal of 1/120 of the cells each day. Complete cessation of RBC production results in a decline of about 10%/wk of the control value. Production defects result in a relative or absolute reticulocytopenia. When RBC values fall at a rate > 10% (ie, 500,000 RBC/μL) without hemorrhage, hemolysis is established as a causative factor.

A convenient approach to most anemias that result from production defects is to examine cellular changes. Thus, microcytic-hypochromic RBCs (see LABORATORY EVALUATION, below) provide evidence that the production defect results from defects in heme or globin synthesis (eg, Fe deficiency, thalassemia and related Hb-synthesis defects, or the anemia of chronic disease). By contrast, normochromic-normocytic anemias with defective production pose a hypoproliferative or hypoplastic mechanism. Finally, some anemias are characterized by large RBCs or macrocytes, which suggest a defect in DNA synthesis. These are usually due either to defective vitamin B_{12} or folate metabolism, or to an interference with DNA synthesis by cytoreductive chemotherapeutic agents. Adequate marrow response to anemia is evidenced by reticulocytosis or polychromatophilia.

Similarly, a few common mechanisms of increased destruction such as sequestration by spleen, antibody-mediated destruction, defective RBC membrane function, and an abnormal Hb provide a rapid focus for differential diagnosis of hemolytic anemias.

A critical tenet in the management of anemias is that *therapy should be specific*, and this infers that a specific diagnosis be made. Indeed, the response to therapy corroborates the diagnosis. While treatment with multiple agents (ie, "shotgun therapy") may at times provide transient repair of the anemia, because it risks serious sequelae, such therapy is not justifiable. RBC transfusion provides a form of "instant" repair that should be reserved for patients with cardiopulmonary symptoms or signs, active uncontrollable bleeding, or some form of hypoxemic end-organ failure. Transfusion procedures and blood components are discussed in detail below in Ch. 97.

A detailed discussion of the anemias follows a discussion of laboratory tests used in their diagnosis and an outline of their etiologic classification.

LABORATORY EVALUATION

Laboratory tests quantitate the degree of the anemia and provide data to aid in understanding its cause. The basic evaluation requires a CBC, which includes RBC indices, reticulocyte count or estimate of polychromatophilia, platelet count, and a review of cellular morphology on the peripheral blood smear.

Blood specimen collection: Blood is preferably collected by venipuncture, though fingertip puncture with a sterile lancet may sometimes suffice. The tests to be performed determine which anticoagulant, if any, should be in the collection tubes. Vacuum tubes are available that have double-ended needles for ease in specimen collecting and that contain suitable amounts of anticoagulants appropriate for most routine hematologic procedures. However, most commercially available vacuum tubes are nonsterile; any backflow of blood from the filled tube to the vein may permit the entry of bacteria. Efforts to avoid such infections include the following: (1) Removing the tourniquet well before blood flow into the tube stops, preferably before the tube stopper is completely punctured; (2) Moving the patient's arm during sampling should be avoided; even a few centimeters' elevation after the tube draw is complete may lower venous pressure sufficiently to produce backflow; and (3) No pressure should be exerted on the stopper end of the tube. Whenever possible, sterile tubes or needle and tube arrangements that have a check valve in the system should be used.

Table 96–1. CHARACTERISTICS OF COMMON ANEMIAS

Etiology or Type	Morphologic Changes	Special Features
Acute blood loss	Normochromic, normocytic; marrow hyperplastic	In severe hemorrhage may be nucleated RBCs & left shift of WBCs; also leukocytosis
Chronic blood loss	*See* Anemia Due to Iron Deficiency; may show features of acute blood loss if recent severe hemorrhage has supervened	
Iron deficiency	Hypochromic, microcytic, aniso- & poikilocytosis; marrow hyperplastic, with delayed hemoglobinization	Achlorhydria, smooth tongue, & spoon nails may be present; stainable marrow iron absent; serum iron low; total iron-binding capacity increased; low serum ferritin; absent marrow iron
Vitamin B_{12} deficiency	Oval macrocytes; megaloblastic marrow; granular leukocytes hypersegmented	Serum B_{12} level < 150 pg/mL; frequent GI & CNS involvement; Schilling test positive; indirect serum bilirubin elevated
Folic acid deficiency	Same as vitamin B_{12} deficiency	Serum folate < 5 ng/mL; nutritional deficiency & malabsorption (sprue, pregnancy, infancy, alcoholism)
Marrow failure	Normochromic, normocytic; marrow aspiration often fails or may show hypoplasia of erythroid series or of all elements	Occasionally idiopathic, but usually a history of exposure to toxic drugs or chemicals (eg, chloramphenicol, atabrine, hydantoins, insecticides)
Vitamin B_6-responsive anemia	Usually hypochromic; rarely normocytic or macrocytic; marrow hyperplastic, with delayed hemoglobinization; siderocytes may be present	Inborn or acquired metabolic defect; stainable marrow iron plentiful; response to B_6 partial, rarely complete
Acute hemolysis	Normochromic, normocytic; marrow, normoblastic hyperplasia	Increased serum bilirubin (indirect) & increased stool & urine urobilinogen; hemoglobinuria in fulminating cases

Chronic hemolysis	Normochromic, normocytic; marrow, normoblastic hyperplasia; basophilic stippling (especially in lead poisoning)	Survival studies show shortened RBC life span; radio-iron turnover increased
Hereditary spherocytosis (congenital hemolytic jaundice)	Spheroidal microcytes in smear	Erythrocytes show increased osmotic fragility; shortened survival of labeled RBCs, radioactivity of spleen progressively increases and exceeds that in liver.
Paroxysmal nocturnal hemoglobinuria	Normocytic (may be hypochromic due to iron deficiency)	Dark morning urine; hemosiderin present; positive acid hemolysis & sugar-water tests; reticulocytes may be decreased
Paroxysmal cold hemoglobinuria	Normocytic, normochromic	Follows exposure to cold; due to a cold agglutinin. Often associated with syphilis or other infections.
Sickle cell anemia	Aniso- & poikilocytosis; some sickle cells in smear; all sickle in wet preparation	Largely limited to blacks; electrophoresis shows S Hb; painful crises & leg ulcers may occur; bony changes shown by x-ray
Thalassemia	Hypochromic, microcytic; thin cells; target cells; basophilic stippling; aniso- & poikilocytosis; nucleated RBCs in homozygotes	Decreased osmotic fragility; often elevated A_2 & F Hb; commonly Mediterranean ancestry; homozygotes anemic from infancy; splenomegaly; bony changes on x-ray
Infection or chronic inflammation	Normochromic, normocytic early, then hypochromic, microcytic; marrow normoblastic; iron plentiful	Serum iron decreased; total iron-binding capacity decreased; normal serum ferritins; normal marrow iron content.
Marrow replacement (myelophthisis)	Aniso- & poikilocytosis; nucleated RBCs; early granulocyte precursors; marrow aspiration may fail, or show leukemia, myeloma, or metastatic cells	Liver and spleen may be enlarged; bone changes may be demonstrable; radio-iron uptake greater over spleen and liver than sacrum; reticulocytes may be slightly increased if many normoblasts in blood

EDTA (ethylenediaminetetraacetic acid) is the preferred anticoagulant for blood counts, since morphology is less distorted and platelets are better preserved. It can be added to clean test tubes, or vacuum tubes containing EDTA may be obtained commercially. Slides should be prepared within 3 to 4 h after obtaining blood, or within 1 to 2 h for platelet counts.

For small amounts of blood or when venipuncture is unfeasible, the finger, earlobe, or, in infants, the plantar surface of the heel is punctured quickly with a sterile disposable lancet, piercing deeply enough to ensure spontaneous flow of blood. Undue pressure that might cause tissue fluids to dilute the blood should be avoided while collecting the specimen.

Complete blood count (CBC): The CBC is a basic evaluation that usually includes Hb, Hct, WBC count, WBC differential count, estimation of platelet number, and a description of the blood smear, including RBC morphology and an estimation of platelet number and polychromatophilia. An RBC count is frequently included, especially when calculation of RBC indices is desired. Anemia, erythrocytosis, inflammation, leukemia, bone marrow failure, and adverse drug reactions may be detected.

A blood smear examination can aid in detecting other abnormalities (eg, thrombocytopenia, malarial parasites, significant rouleau formation, and the presence of nucleated RBCs or immature granulocytes) that may occur despite normal counts. It is important in evaluating RBC morphology and abnormal WBCs.

Blood counts are normally made by diluting a measured volume of blood with an appropriate diluent or lysing agent and counting in a chamber under the microscope. Hb can be measured colorimetrically after treatment with dilute hydrochloric acid or with Drabkin's reagent, which permits colorimetric or spectrophotometric comparison with standards of hematin or cyanmethemoglobin, respectively. The Hct is measured by centrifuging a volume of blood and determining the percentage of RBCs. The WBC differential count is made by spreading a small drop of blood on a glass slide and staining with Wright's stain. The smear is examined by oil immersion microscopy and a count kept of each type of WBC identified. A minimum of 100 cells are counted and each type is reported as a percentage. Automated equipment is available to do differential counts by computerized pattern recognition. The platelet number is estimated.

Normal values for the total WBC count range between 4,300 and 10,800/μL; normal values for the **differential leukocyte count** are: segmented neutrophils 34 to 75%, band neutrophils 0 to 8%, lymphocytes 12 to 50%, monocytes 3 to 15%, eosinophils 0 to 5%, and basophils 0 to 3%.

RBCs: The normal range at sea level is 5.4 million/μL (± 0.8) for men and 4.8 million (± 0.6) for women. At birth, this count is slightly higher; by the 3rd mo it falls to levels of about 4.5 million (± 0.7), slowly increasing after age 4 through puberty.

The normal Hb level for men is 16 (± 2) gm/dL and 14 (± 2) gm/dL for women. The Hct, which is the volume of packed RBCs, is 47% (± 5) for men and 42% (± 5) for women.

The diagnostic criteria for anemia in men are an RBC < 4.5 million/μL, a Hb < 14 gm/dL, or a Hct < 42 gm/dL; for women these criteria are an RBC < 4 million/μL, Hb < 12 gm/dL, or a Hct < 37 gm/dL.

The normal life span of an RBC is 120 days; therefore, 1/120 of the total RBC mass must be replaced daily. This newly released population (40,000 to 50,000/μL) represents 0.5 to 1.5% of the total RBC count and can be identified as **polychromatophilic cells** on routine stains (eg, Wrights' or Giemsa stain will color remnants of RNA) or "reticulocytes" when supravital staining technics are used that recognize the endoplasmic reticular material within them. Since reticulocytes represent a young cell population, it is an important criterion of marrow activity that can be considered a response to a need for RBC renewal. Reticulocytes in numbers above normal are evidence of

restoration response following acute blood loss or after specific therapy in anemias of decreased production (ie, vitamin B_{12}, folic acid, and iron **(Fe)**-deficient anemias). Reticulocytosis is particularly prominent in hemolytic anemias and in acute and severe bleeding. It may indicate the onset of remission in aplastic anemia or leukemia. A "normal" reticulocyte count in anemia indicates failure of the bone marrow to respond appropriately.

Reticulocyte count: A few drops of blood are initially stained with fresh methylene blue, counterstained with Wright's stain, and then counted under oil immersion. One thousand consecutive RBCs are counted and the number having a blue-staining reticulum are expressed as a percentage. The normal range is 0.5 to 1.5%. These may also be counted using automated differential counters.

Other features of circulating RBCs help to indicate the type of anemia present. The **RBC indices** (the mean corpuscular volume **[MCV]**, mean corpuscular Hb **[MCH]**, and mean corpuscular Hb concentration **[MCHC]**) derived from the quantitative data, denote the volume and character of the Hb content. Thus, RBC populations with MCVs < 80 fL (femtoliter = μm^3) are termed **microcytic** and those with MCV > 95 fL are termed **macrocytic.** The term **hypochromia** refers to populations of cells with MCH content < 27 pg/RBC or a MCHC < 30%. These quantitative relationships can usually be recognized on a peripheral blood smear, and, *together with the indices, permit a classification of anemias that correlates well with etiologic classification (see* TABLE *96–1) and greatly aids diagnostic evaluation.*

By most automated technics, the Hb, RBC count, and MCV are electronically measured. The Hct, MCH, and MCHC, by contrast, are calculated from the electronically measured data. Therefore, the MCV has become the most important RBC index in the differential diagnosis of anemias, and use of the less reliable derived figures of the Hct and MCHC has declined. Automatic-flow cytometric methods provide a new parameter in differential diagnosis: A histogram or picture of variation in cell size (formerly expressed as anisocytosis) can be expressed as *the coefficient of variation of the volume distribution width* (**RDW**—see TABLE 96–2).

In addition to variations in size **(anisocytosis)**, variations in shape **(poikilocytosis)** may be seen. Evidence of RBC injury may be identified directly from RBC fragments or portions of disrupted cells **(schistocytes)**, as well as evidence of significant membrane alterations from oval-shaped cells **(ovalocytes)** or spherocytic cells. **"Target" cells,** which have either insufficient Hb or excess membrane, are thin with a central dot of Hb.

Bone marrow aspiration and biopsy provide direct observation of erythroid activity, status, and character of the maturation of the RBC precursors, abnormalities (dyspoiesis) of the cells, and semiquantitation of amount and cellular pattern of Fe content. It is helpful in anemias, other cytopenias, unexplained leukocytosis, thrombocytosis, or when leukemia or myelophthisis is suspected.

Bone marrow aspiration and biopsy are not difficult and should therefore be done early in suspected hematologic diseases. In general, both can be done as 1 simple procedure. Since the biopsy requires adequate bone depth, it is usually performed on the posterior (or less commonly anterior) iliac crest. After the biopsy needle is inserted, a small amount (preferably < 0.5 mL) of marrow is aspirated into a syringe. A few drops are smeared directly onto slides to be stained with metachromatic stains (eg, May-Grünwald, Giemsa, Wrights') and examined under the microscope. The remainder can be placed in heparin for subsequent study or permitted to clot and handled as a surgical tissue. The core biopsy can then be obtained with the needle inserted for aspiration; it must be decalcified and handled as a surgical tissue. If only an aspiration is sought, the sternum or dorsal lumbar vertebral spine may be used. One should avoid

aspirating > 1 mL of marrow, since dilution with peripheral blood makes interpretation difficult.

RBC fragility (osmotic fragility): A series of 12 small test tubes containing sodium chloride **(NaCl)** solutions varying from 0.28 to 0.5% in 0.02% increments is prepared. A drop of the patient's blood is placed in each of these tubes and the blood of a normal control is added to another series of tubes. The percent of NaCl at which hemolysis begins and the first tube showing complete hemolysis are noted. Normal blood begins to hemolyze at ≤ 0.44% NaCl. The process is usually complete at about 0.32% NaCl. Normal values may vary by ± 0.04%. If many spherocytes are present, as in familial hemolytic jaundice, hemolysis will appear at higher concentrations. If the predominating cell is abnormally thin, as in thalassemia major, hemolysis will appear first at lower concentrations and in some cases may never be complete.

Other tests are discussed below under specific anemias and bleeding disorders. For **bleeding time, clot retraction and observation, fibrin/fibrinogen degradation products,** and **partial thromboplastin time and prothrombin time,** see Laboratory Tests in Ch. 99.

Classification of Anemias

I. Anemias Due to Bleeding
  A. Acute Posthemorrhagic Anemia
  B. Chronic Posthemorrhagic Anemia
II. Anemias Due to Deficient Erythropoiesis
  A. Hypochromic-Microcytic Anemias
    1. Iron-Deficiency Anemia
    2. Iron-Transport–Deficiency Anemia (Atransferrinemia)
    3. Iron-Utilization Anemias (Sideroblastic Anemias)
    4. Iron-Reutilization Anemias (Anemia of Chronic Disease)
  B. Normochromic-Normocytic Anemias
    1. Hypoproliferative Anemias
      a. Anemia of Renal Disease
      b. Anemia of Endocrine Failure (Hypothyroidism and Hypopituitarism)
      c. Anemia of Protein Depletion
    2. Hypoplastic (Aplastic) Anemias
    3. Myelophthisic Anemias
  C. Megaloblastic Anemias
    1. Anemia Due to Vitamin B_{12} Deficiency
    2. Anemia Due to Folic Acid Deficiency
    3. Anemia Due to Copper Deficiency
    4. Anemia Due to Vitamin C Deficiency
III. Anemias Due to Excessive RBC Destruction—Hemolytic Anemias
  A. Hemolytic Anemias Due to Defects Extrinsic to the Red Cell
    1. Anemias Due to Reticuloendothelial Hyperactivity
        Hypersplenism-Congestive Splenomegaly
    2. Anemias Due to Immunologic Abnormalities
      a. Isoimmune (Isoagglutinin) Hemolytic Anemia
      b. Autoimmune Hemolytic Anemia
        (1) Warm-Antibody Hemolytic Anemia (Coombs-Positive Hemolytic Anemia)
        (2) Cold-Antibody Disease
          (a) Cold Agglutinin Disease
          (b) Paroxysmal Cold Hemoglobinuria
      c. Complement-Sensitive Associated Anemia
          Paroxysmal Nocturnal Hemoglobinuria

3. Anemias Due to Mechanical Injury
   a. Traumatic Hemolytic Anemias (Microangiopathic Hemolytic Anemia)
   b. Hemolysis Due to Infectious Agents

B. Hemolytic Anemias Due to Intrinsic Red Cell Defects
1. Anemias Due to Alterations of Red Cell Membrane
   a. Congenital Red Cell Membrane Disorders
      (1) Congenital Erythropoietic Porphyria
      (2) Hereditary Elliptocytosis
      (3) Hereditary Spherocytosis
   b. Acquired Red Cell Membrane Disorders
      (1) Stomatocytosis
      (2) Anemia Due to Hypophosphatemia
2. Anemias Due to Disorders of Red Cell Metabolism (Hereditary Enzyme Deficiencies)
   a. Embden-Meyerhof Pathway Defects
   b. Hexose Monophosphate Shunt Defects (Glucose-6-Phosphate Dehydrogenase Deficiency)
3. Anemias Due to Defective Hemoglobin Synthesis (Hemoglobinopathies)
   a. Sickle Cell Anemia
   b. Hemoglobin C Disease
   c. Hemoglobin S-C Disease
   d. Hemoglobin E Disease
   e. Thalassemias
   f. Hemoglobin S-Beta Thalassemia Disease

ANEMIAS DUE TO BLEEDING

ACUTE POSTHEMORRHAGIC ANEMIA

Anemia caused by rapid massive hemorrhage.

Etiology and Pathogenesis

Since the marrow reserve is limited, anemia may result from any massive hemorrhage, which may be due to spontaneous or traumatic rupture or incision of a large blood vessel, erosion of an artery by lesions (eg, peptic ulcer or a neoplastic process) or failure of normal hemostatic processes. Immediate effects depend on the duration and amount of hemorrhage. Sudden loss of ⅓ of the blood volume may be fatal, but as much as ⅔ may be lost slowly over 24 h without such risk. Symptoms are due to a sudden decrease in blood volume and to subsequent hemodilution, with a decrease in the O_2-carrying capacity of the blood.

Symptoms and Signs

The pace of the anemia determines the degree of symptoms. Faintness, dizziness, thirst, sweating, weak and rapid pulse, and rapid respiration (at first deep, then shallow) may occur. Orthostatic hypotension is common. BP may at first rise slightly because of reflex arteriolar constriction, then gradually fall. If bleeding continues, BP may fall and death may ensue (see also SHOCK in Ch. 26).

Laboratory Findings

During and immediately after hemorrhage, the RBC count, Hb, and Hct are deceptively high because of vasoconstriction. Within a few hours, tissue fluid begins to enter the circulation, resulting in hemodilution and a drop in the RBC count and Hb pro-

…al to the severity of bleeding. The resultant anemia is normocytic. Polymorpho-…ear leukocytosis and a rise in platelet count may occur within the first few hours. Several days after the bleeding event, evidence of regeneration appears: blood smears may disclose polychromatophilia, reticulocytosis, slight macrocytosis; if hemorrhage was massive and acute, occasional normoblasts and immature WBCs may be seen.

Treatment

Immediate therapy consists of hemostasis, restoration of blood volume, and treatment of shock (see also SHOCK in Ch. 26). Blood transfusion, the only reliable means of rapidly restoring blood volume, is indicated for severe bleeding with threatening vascular collapse. Plasma is presently the most satisfactory temporary substitute for blood. Trials with chemicals (primarily perfluorochemicals) capable of transporting O_2 have shown significant promise; at least one such agent (FLUOSOL-DA®) is in clinical trials and may be able to provide O_2-carrying capacity for up to 72 h. Saline or dextrose infusions effect only transient benefit. Absolute rest, oral fluids as tolerated, and other standard measures for treating shock are indicated. Subsequent therapy can include Fe to replace that lost with bleeding.

CHRONIC POSTHEMORRHAGIC ANEMIA

A hypochromic-microcytic anemia caused by prolonged moderate blood loss, as from a chronically bleeding GI tract lesion (eg, peptic ulcer or hemorrhoids) or urologic or gynecologic site. The clinical features and treatment of this condition are discussed below, under IRON-DEFICIENCY ANEMIA.

ANEMIAS DUE TO DEFICIENT ERYTHROPOIESIS

HYPOCHROMIC-MICROCYTIC ANEMIAS

Deficient or defective heme or globin synthesis produces a hypochromic-microcytic RBC population. However, early changes may be minimal. Differential diagnosis includes Fe-deficiency anemia, defects of Fe transport (atransferrinemia), Fe-utilization and Fe-reutilization anemias, which are discussed below, and the thalassemias, which are discussed with ANEMIAS DUE TO DEFECTIVE HEMOGLOBIN SYNTHESIS.

Laboratory Evaluation

Fe and Fe-binding capacity: Both tests should be performed, since the relationship between their values is important. A variety of assay methods exist and the range of normal relates to the method used; however, generally the normal serum Fe is between 75 to 150 µg/dL for men and 60 to 140 µg/L for women; the total Fe-binding capacity is 250 to 450 µg/dL. Serum Fe concentration has a diurnal pattern. It is low in Fe lack and in the anemia of chronic disease; it is elevated in hemolytic states and in Fe-overload syndromes (hemochromatosis; hemosiderosis). Patients on oral Fe therapy may have a normal serum Fe in spite of existent deficiency; in such circumstances a valid assay requires cessation of Fe therapy for 24 to 48 h. The Fe-binding capacity (or transferrin) is increased in Fe lack, but reduced in the anemia of chronic disease.

Serum ferritin: Ferritin is an Fe-storage glycoprotein known to exist as tissue-specific isoferritins and measurable in the serum by radioimmunometric methods. The range of normal in most laboratories is 30 to 300 ng/mL and the geometric mean is 88 in men and 49 in women. Serum ferritin concentrations are closely correlated with total body-Fe stores. Therefore, low serum-ferritin levels occur only in the Fe-deficient state. Elevated serum levels occur in Fe-overload states. In liver injury (ie, hepatitis) or in

association with some neoplasms (especially acute leukemia, Hodgkin's disease, GI tract) where the ferritins may be likened to a carcinofetal antigen, serum ferritin levels are elevated also. Specific erythrocyte ferritin concentrations can be used to characterize body iron stores in these latter circumstances.

Free erythrocyte protoporphyrin (FEP): FEP is measurably increased in circumstances of altered heme synthesis (eg, Fe lack, lead intoxication). It has limited usefulness because it does not differentiate Fe deficiency from a common diagnostic problem, that of the anemia of chronic disease.

IRON-DEFICIENCY ANEMIA

(Anemia of Chronic Blood Loss; Hypochromic-Microcytic Anemia; Chlorosis; Hypochromic Anemia of Pregnancy, Infancy, and Childhood)

Chronic anemia characterized by small, pale RBCs and depletion of Fe stores.

Etiology (See also DISTURBANCES IN IRON METABOLISM in Ch. 82)

Fe deficiency, the commonest cause of anemia, may be due to increased Fe requirement, diminished Fe absorption, or both. Fe deficiency is likely during the first 2 yr of life if dietary Fe is inadequate for the demands of rapid growth. Adolescent girls may become Fe-deficient from inadequate diet for growth requirements plus the added loss from menstruation. In adult males, the most frequent cause is chronic occult bleeding, usually from the GI tract. The chief lesson concerning Fe deficiency is that hemorrhage must be the foremost consideration in any adult. In women, pregnancy causes Fe deficiency unless supplemental Fe is given.

Other bases for anemia may be decreased absorption of Fe after gastrectomy, upper small-bowel malabsorption syndromes, and occasionally some forms of pica (primarily clay), but such mechanisms are rare compared to bleeding. Most forms of pica (starch, ice, etc) are associated with decreased intake due to caloric substitution rather than with decreased absorption. In circumstances of chronic intravascular hemolysis (eg, paroxysmal nocturnal hemoglobinuria, chronic disseminated intravascular coagulation, etc), RBC fragmentation (recognizable on a peripheral smear) may produce Fe lack by chronic hemoglobinuria and hemosiderinuria.

Pathophysiology

Stage 1: Fe loss exceeds the gain, storage Fe (represented by bone marrow Fe content) is progressively depleted, but Hb and plasma Fe remain normal. As storage Fe decreases, there is a compensatory increase in absorption of dietary Fe and in the concentration of transferrin (represented by a rise in Fe-binding capacity).

Stage 2: Exhausted stores have insufficient Fe available to meet the needs of the erythroid marrow. While the plasma-transferrin level increases, the plasma-Fe concentration declines, leading to a progressive decrease in Fe available for RBC formation. When plasma Fe falls to < 50 μg/dL and transferrin saturation to < 16%, erythropoiesis is impaired.

Stage 3 is defined by an anemia with normal appearing RBCs and indices.

Stage 4: Microcytosis precedes hypochromia.

Stage 5: Symptoms and signs of Fe deficiency appear in the tissues.

Symptoms and Signs

In addition to the usual manifestations, in chronic, severe Fe deficiency, a person may crave dirt or paint **(pica)** or ice **(pagophagia)**, have **glossitis, cheilosis,** and **koilonychia,** and, in rare advanced cases, have dysphagia associated with a postcricoid esophageal web (**Plummer-Vinson syndrome** [see in Ch. 51]. Glossitis and cheilosis, which are not specific for Fe-deficiency anemia, will develop only with severe anemia.) Finally, fatigue and loss of stamina can occur through a separate effect on the tissues (perhaps cellular enzyme dysfunction).

Diagnosis

Although pica and especially pagophagia suggest Fe lack as the mechanism in the differential diagnosis of the hypochromic-microcytic states, actually no specific symptoms or signs exist. Therefore, laboratory characteristics (see TABLE 96–2) serve as critical diagnostic features. The classical criterion of Fe-deficient erythropoiesis is absence of marrow-Fe stores. Other laboratory findings follow a predictive pattern of the pathophysiologic stages. Serum-ferritin concentration provides a useful measure of body-Fe stores. A low serum-ferritin concentration (< 12 ng/mL) identifies Fe deficiency and currently represents the best noninvasive test of Fe status. Unfortunately, ferritin values are elevated in the presence of liver injury and in some neoplasms and must be interpreted with care.

Treatment

Fe therapy without pursuit of its cause is poor practice; a mild degree of anemia must never be used as an excuse for failure to seek the bleeding site.

Fe can be provided by ferrous sulfate or ferrous gluconate, best given orally between meals since food or antacids may reduce absorption. Oral Fe is safer than parenteral Fe; the rate of response is the same with either route. Parenteral Fe should be reserved for those who do not tolerate or will not take oral Fe, or for patients who lose large amounts of blood steadily due to capillary or vascular disorders (eg, hereditary hemor-

TABLE 96–2. DIFFERENTIAL DIAGNOSIS OF THE HYPOCHROMIC–MICROCYTIC STATES

	Deficiency	*Transferrin Defect*	*Defect in Iron Utilization*	*Defect in Iron Re-utilization*
Peripheral Blood				
Microcytosis (***M***) vs. hypochromia (***H***)	M > H	M > H	M > H	M < H
Polychromatophilic targeted cells	Absent	Absent	Present	Absent
Stippled red cells	Absent	Absent	Present	Absent
RDW*	Increased	Increased	Increased	Normal
Serum Iron				
Serum iron: Iron-binding capacity	↓ : ↑	↓ : ↓	↑ : Normal	↓ : ↓
% Saturation of Transferrin	< 10%	0	> 50%	> 10%
Serum ferritin (normal 30–300 ng/mL)	< 12	(No data available)	> 400	30–400
Bone marrow				
Erythrocyte-granulocyte ratio (normal 1:3 to 1:5)	1:1—1:2	1:1—1:2	1:1—5:1	1:1—1:2
Marrow iron	Absent	Present	Increased	Present
Ringed sideroblasts	Absent	Absent	Present	Absent

* RDW = Red blood cell volume distribution width expressing the degree of anisocytosis (ie, variation in cell size)

(Adapted from "The Differential Diagnosis of the Hypochromic Microcytic States," by E.P. Frenkel, in *The Medical Journal of St. Joseph Hospital* [now *Houston Medical Journal*], Vol. 11, June, 1976. Copyright by the Houston Medical Journal. Used with permission of the *Journal* and the author.)

rhagic telangiectasia). Fe in enteric-coated capsules is not well absorbed and has no place in therapy.

A maximal reticulocyte response usually occurs 7 to 10 days after Fe replacement begins. For 2 wk, the Hb rises little, but thereafter the rise should be 0.7 to 1 gm/100 mL/wk in severe anemia. A subnormal response may result from continued hemorrhage, underlying infection or malignancy, insufficient intake of Fe, or, very rarely, malabsorption of oral Fe. As the Hb approaches normal, its pace tapers; the anemia should be corrected within 2 mo. Therapy should continue for ≥ 6 mo to replenish tissue stores.

IRON-TRANSPORT–DEFICIENCY ANEMIA
(Atransferrinemia)

This exceedingly rare anemia appears when Fe cannot move from storage sites (mucosal cells, liver, etc) to the erythron (developing RBCs). The presumed mechanism is either absence of the Fe-transport protein transferrin or the presence of a defective transferrin molecule. In addition to anemia, hemosiderosis of lymphoid tissue, especially along the GI tract, is prominent.

IRON-UTILIZATION ANEMIAS
(Sideroblastic Anemias)

These anemias are due to inadequate or abnormal utilization of intracellular Fe for Hb synthesis, despite adequate or increased amounts of Fe within the mitochondria of the developing RBC precursors. This defect includes 2 clinical subgroups: first, hemoglobinopathies, primarily of the thalassemic type; and, second, sideroblastic (or Fe-overload) anemias. Since other clinical-laboratory characteristics help define circumstances of thalassemia, the term sideroblastic is generally applied to the second subset.

Although sideroblastic anemia is commonly microcytic and hypochromic, a high RDW results from the dimorphic (both large- and small-sized) population of circulating cells; the cellular heterogeneity is recognizable on examination of the peripheral blood smear. An important clue to defective heme synthesis in the peripheral blood is the presence of polychromatophilic stippled, targeted RBCs. Other laboratory features include increases in serum-Fe and serum-ferritin concentrations and saturation of transferrin. Erythroid hyperplasia is present in the bone marrow; Fe stain reveals the pathognomonic morphologic feature of Fe-engorged paranuclear mitochondria in the developing RBCs called ringed sideroblasts.

These anemias are particularly characterized by evidence of ineffective erythropoiesis, which is defined clinically as *anemia and a relative or absolute reticulocytopenia in the presence of erythroid hyperplasia.* Radiolabeled Fe transfers rapidly from plasma transferrin to the marrow, but it fails to reappear normally in circulating RBCs at a normal rate. Ferrokinetic studies provide evidence of ineffective erythropoiesis, inferring that abnormal erythroid maturation results in increased intramedullary death of RBCs.

Etiology and Pathophysiology

Clinical correlates (TABLE 96–3) have been made in some cases of sideroblastic anemia, but clear etiologic and pathophysiologic mechanisms are unknown. The list of diseases known to be associated occasionally with sideroblastosis is formidable and virtually all of them commonly produce other more typical defects in RBC production.

Treatment and Prognosis

The best results follow recognition and removal of a specific cause (especially alcohol). Although rare congenital cases have responded to vitamin B_6 50 mg tid orally, complete correction of the anemia does not result. Similar trials in acquired cases have

TABLE 96–3. TYPES OF IRON–UTILIZATION DEFECTS

Defects in hemoglobin synthesis	Thalassemias Other related hemoglobinopathies

Sideroblastic anemias	Congenital
	  Sex-linked
	    Pyridoxine responsive
	    Non-pyridoxine responsive
	  Autosomal
	Acquired
	  Primary (Idiopathic)
	  Secondary
	    Drugs (eg, anti-TB agents, chloramphenicol)
	    Alcohol
	Occasional incidence (eg, granulomatous diseases, neoplasms, RA)

(Adapted from "The Differential Diagnosis of the Hypochromic Microcytic States," by E.P. Frenkel, in *The Medical Journal of St. Joseph Hospital* [now *Houston Medical Journal*], Vol. 11, June, 1976. Copyright by *The Houston Medical Journal.* Used with permission of the *Journal* and the author.)

had weak responses. Rare responses to androgens also are recorded. In general, idiopathic cases must be managed supportively. If anemia produces cardiopulmonary symptoms, packed RBC transfusions may be necessary. Because of the already significant Fe burden, such transfusions hasten the advent of clinical symptoms secondary to hemosiderosis, and Fe-chelation therapy should be considered.

A subset of idiopathic cases progresses to frank leukemia (usually acute granulocytic leukemia). Early occurrence of leukopenia and thrombocytopenia seems to suggest such a likelihood. Since the leukemic transition may take up to 10 yr and since early therapy (with currently available cytoreductive agents) of the pre-leukemic phase does not result in improved survival, no special therapy is indicated.

IRON-REUTILIZATION ANEMIA
(Anemia of Chronic Disease)

This is the second commonest form of anemia in the world. Early, the RBCs are normocytic; with time they become microcytic (see TABLE 96–2). The major issue is that the marrow erythroid mass fails to expand appropriately in response to the anemia.

Etiology and Pathogenesis

This type of anemia was thought to occur as part of a chronic disorder of which infections, inflammatory disease (especially RA), and cancer are most frequently identified. However, the underlying disease need not be chronic, since the pathophysiologic features of this anemia appear during virtually any infection or inflammation. The induced defect is one of decreased RBC production. With an RBC loss of about 1%/day, anemia is not clinically evident before 1 to 3 wk. The pathophysiologic mechanism is that senescent RBC Fe fails to be released by the reticulum cells for Hb synthesis by the erythron. Man uses about 25 mg/day of Fe for normal erythropoiesis. Only 1 to 2 mg of Fe is available from the diet, but highly efficient recycling of Fe derived from senescent RBCs provides a critical Fe-balance mechanism. In chronic disease, reticulum cells tenaciously retain Fe from senescent RBCs, making it unavailable for reuse. In some respects, the circumstance has the pattern of an "internal" Fe deficiency to which the normal compensatory responses are blunted. There is a reticulocytopenia and a failure to compensate for the anemia with erythroid hyperplasia. A

decrease in erythropoietic activity may be a partial factor in the anemia. Fe studies are as shown in TABLE 96–2 with the failure of compensatory production of transferrin. Thus, the primary pattern is one in which a barrier or defect in the movement of storage Fe (in reticuloendothelial cells) to plasma (and hence the erythron) exists and in which the usual compensatory mechanisms fail to generate a response. That some potential for response exists has been documented by the ability to generate RBC production following hemorrhage or hypoxia; ie, circumstances of markedly enhanced erythropoietic production.

Symptoms, Signs, and Laboratory Findings

Clinical findings are usually those of the underlying disease (whether infectious, inflammatory, or neoplastic). Laboratory findings are shown in TABLE 96–2. Anemia is generally moderate, rarely with a Hb < 8 gm/dL unless a secondary complicating mechanism is also present. The serum-ferritin determination helps to differentiate Fe deficiency from the anemias of chronic disease. If Fe deficiency is present in addition to the anemias of chronic disease, the serum ferritin does not increase (generally remaining < 60 to 65 ng/mL). Thus, in the clinical setting of infection, inflammation, or cancer, such a value suggests Fe deficiency combined with the anemia of chronic disease.

Treatment

The only therapy is that of the underlying disease. Hematinics have no value. Since these mild anemias generally do not progress, blood transfusions are rarely required.

NORMOCHROMIC-NORMOCYTIC ANEMIAS

Decreased RBC production, termed bone-marrow failure, results in normochromic-normocytic anemias. The mechanisms involved are **hypoproliferation,** in which normal humoral stimulus (erythropoietin) is lacking; **hypoplasia,** in which RBC precursors are lost, either from a defect in stem cell pool or an injury to the microenvironment that supports the marrow, and **myelophthisis,** in which the normal marrow space is infiltrated and replaced by abnormal or nonhematopoietic cells.

HYPOPROLIFERATIVE ANEMIAS

Normochromic-normocytic anemias are characterized by a normal RDW and reticulocytopenia (ie, decreased delivery of cells) and failure of the erythroid mass to expand in response to the anemia. Studies with radiolabeled Fe reveal sluggish production of RBCs. The pathophysiologic mechanism appears to be a relative or absolute decreased production of erythropoietin or a hypometabolic state with resultant failure to respond to erythropoietin. As noted above, the anemias of Fe deficiency and lack of Fe reutilization are also hypoproliferative, since they have restricted erythroid hyperplasia and decreased erythropoietinemia; nonetheless, the primary mechanistic defect is altered Fe metabolism, and the proliferative failure appears to be an epiphenomenon of unknown basis. Hypoproliferation is commonly associated with anemias of renal disease, of hypometabolic states (eg, myxedema), and of protein deprivation, which may cause hypometabolism.

Anemia of Renal Disease

The severity of anemia that occurs in renal failure correlates roughly with the extent of renal dysfunction. Thus, the secretory function of the kidney in producing the hormone erythropoietin in general parallels the excretory function, and anemia occurs when the creatinine clearance falls to < 45 mL/min. Decreased erythropoietin production, resulting in inadequate humoral stimulus of RBC production, is expressed as a peripheral reticulocytopenia and a subnormal marrow response (absence of erythroid

hyperplasia). Renal lesions primarily in the glomerular region (eg, amyloidosis, diabetic nephropathy) generally result in the most severe anemia for their degree of excretory failure.

Other mechanisms may compound the severity of this disorder. In uremia, a mild added hemolytic component (a shortened RBC survival) is common; its basis is uncertain, but it is related to the retained "metabolic debris of uremia" that somehow injures RBCs. Less common, but more easily recognizable, is anemia associated with RBC fragmentation, called microangiopathic hemolytic anemia, that occurs when the renal vascular endothelium is injured (eg, in malignant hypertension, polyarteritis nodosum, or acute cortical necrosis). In children, this can be an acute, often fatal illness called the hemolytic-uremic syndrome (HUS—see under THROMBOCYTOPENIA in Ch. 99). Recognition of these hemolytic mechanisms helps in the clinical approach to the renal lesion as well as the anemia; the term *anemia of renal failure* applies only to the hypoproliferative hypoerythropoietinemic mechanism.

Laboratory findings: No specific features identify this form of hypoproliferative anemia (see above). A superimposed, microangiopathic hemolysis can be recognized on peripheral blood smear by RBC fragmentation and (usually) thrombocytopenia.

Therapy is directed at the underlying renal disease. If adequate renal function is reestablished, anemia is relieved. In patients on long-term dialysis, increased erythropoiesis has been seen, but it rarely reverts to normal. Androgens have been used to stimulate erythropoiesis; in general, they raise the peripheral venous Hct about 10%, a degree almost too modest to warrant their problems and risks. Transfusions are rarely indicated, except when cardiopulmonary symptoms or signs develop.

Anemia of Endocrine Failure

(See HYPOTHYROIDISM in Ch. 89)

Anemia of Protein Depletion

Clinical and laboratory findings mimic those in the hypometabolic states. Its mechanism has been related to general hypometabolism without actual supportive data. In animals, protein depletion results in decreased erythropoietin production. The exact role of protein in hematopoiesis in man is not clear.

HYPOPLASTIC (APLASTIC) ANEMIAS

Anemias with decrease of marrow mass, often with borderline high MCV values. "Hypoplastic (aplastic) anemia," a term commonly used, implies a panhypoplasia of the marrow with associated leukopenia and thrombocytopenia. That confusion in nomenclature has led to the term *pure red cell aplasia* to define the selective marked reduction or absence of erythroid precursors.

Etiology and Pathogenesis

True aplastic anemia is an uncommon event; about 1/2 of cases are idiopathic; they are most common in adolescents and young adults. In the rest, the cause can be a chemical agent (eg, benzene, inorganic arsenic), radiation, or drugs (eg, antineoplastics). Many drugs (eg, antibiotics, anti-inflammatory drugs, anticonvulsants) have been implicated in individual cases. The mechanism of such events is unknown, but a selective (perhaps genetic) hypersensitivity appears to be the basis. A very rare form of aplastic anemia, **Fanconi's anemia** (a type of familial aplastic anemia with bone abnormalities, microcephaly, hypogenitalism, and brown pigmentation of skin), occurs in children with abnormal chromosomes. Finally, it should be noted that marrow hypoplasia may be found in the elderly. Stress (acute infections or inflammatory events) may result in peripheral cytopenias because of their limited marrow reserve. With

clearing of the interval event, peripheral values return to normal in spite of the reduced marrow mass.

Pure RBC aplasia, on the other hand, implies a mechanism selectively destructive to the erythroid precursors; other hematopoietic elements are unaffected. Clinical correlations exist with some cases of RBC aplasia but the pathophysiologic mechanisms are unknown. Thus, acute erythroblastopenia is well known to be a brief reversible disappearance of RBC precursors in the marrow during a variety of acute viral illnesses, especially in children. Indeed, this may be recognized fortuitously, since the sequela of aplasia (ie, anemia) requires a duration longer than usually exists with the acute episode. **Chronic RBC aplasia** has been associated with thymomas, immunologic injury, and less often with drugs (tranquilizers, anticonvulsants, etc), toxins (organic phosphates), riboflavin deficiency, and chronic lymphocytic leukemia. A rare congenital form, Blackfan-Diamond syndrome, is described. Erythroid aplasia may occur transiently during various infections and hemolytic disorders (aregenerative crisis, acute erythroblastopenia), and in association with tumors of the thymus.

Symptoms and Signs

Although the clinical onset is usually insidious, often occurring over weeks or months after exposure to a toxin, occasionally it is explosive. Signs vary with the severity of the pancytopenia. General symptoms of anemia are usually severe. Waxy pallor of skin and mucous membranes is characteristic. Chronic cases may show considerable brown skin pigmentation.

In aplastic anemia severe thrombocytopenia may occur, with bleeding into the mucous membranes and skin. Hemorrhages into the ocular fundi are frequent. Agranulocytosis with life-threatening infections is common. Splenomegaly is absent, unless induced by transfusion hemosiderosis.

The clinical presentation of pure RBC asplasia is generally milder. Symptoms relate to anemia, or to the underlying disorder.

Laboratory Findings

RBCs are normochromic and normocytic (rarely macrocytic). A WBC count ≤ 1500 is common, the reduction occurring chiefly in the granulocytes. Platelets are often markedly reduced. Reticulocytes are decreased, even when coexistent with hemolysis. The aspirated bone marrow is acellular. The serum Fe is elevated. In pure RBC aplasia, the marrow cellularity and maturation may be normal except for a complete absence of erythroid precursors.

Treatment

Bone marrow transplantation from an identical twin or an HLA-compatible sibling is a proven treatment for aplastic anemia, particularly for those under age 30. Thus, at diagnosis siblings should be evaluated for HLA compatibility. Because blood transfusions represent a risk to the subsequent successful transplant, blood products should be used only when essential.

Recent experience with equine antithymocyte globulin ([**ATG**] 15 mg/kg diluted in 500 mL saline and infused over 4 to 6 h for 10 consecutive days) has yielded responses in about 60% of patients; it has become the treatment of choice for older patients or those without a compatible donor. Because this is a biologic product, allergic reactions and even serum sickness may occur; all patients require concomitant corticosteroids (prednisone 40 mg/m^2/day beginning on day 7 for 10 days or until symptoms subside). Androgens have been used, but a defined response is rare. Trials with cyclosporin suggest value for ATG failures.

Pure RBC aplasia has been successfully managed with immunosuppressives (prednisone and cyclophosphamide), especially when an immunologic basis is implicated. Recent trials with cyclosporine suggest significant efficacy. Since patients with a

thymoma-associated pure RBC aplasia improve following thymectomy, presence of such a lesion should be sought by CT imaging, and surgery considered when found.

MYELOPHTHISIC ANEMIAS

In addition to being normochromic, the hallmarks of these anemias are anisocytosis, poikilocytosis, and the presence of nucleated RBCs in the smear. Immature myeloid cells are also seen. These findings occur when there is replacement of the marrow by infiltrative neoplasms, granulomatous diseases, (lipid) storage disease, or fibrosis.

Etiology and Pathogenesis

An attractive but unproved hypothesis is that this form of anemia is the logical sequela of a decreased amount of functioning hematopoietic tissue. A metabolic fault related to the underlying disease and, in some cases, erythrophagocytosis have also been considered pathogenetic factors, but never demonstrated.

The most common cause is carcinoma metastasizing to bone marrow from primary tumors, most often located in the breast, prostate, kidney, lung, or adrenal or thyroid gland. Another frequent cause is myelofibrosis, which may be of undetermined origin, or sometimes appears in a late stage of polycythemia vera or chronic granulocytic leukemia. In children a rare cause is marble-bone disease of Albers-Schönberg.

Unfortunately, the terms are confusing: **Myeloid metaplasia** refers to *extramedullary hematopoiesis in the liver and spleen that may accompany myelophthisis from any cause.* **Myelofibrosis,** *replacement of marrow by fibroblastic cells*, may be idiopathic or secondary. An old term, **agnogenic myeloid metaplasia**, indicates *primary myelofibrosis and extramedullary hematopoiesis*, but myelofibrosis may be present with little or no extramedullary hematopoiesis. In some cases, **myelosclerosis** (*new bone formation*) occurs.

Symptoms and Signs

In severe cases, the usual symptoms of anemia may be present, as well as symptoms of the underlying disease. Symptoms of pressure from splenomegaly may be the presenting complaint; sometimes massive splenomegaly occurs, and associated hepatomegaly is common.

Laboratory Findings

Anemia, usually moderately severe, is characteristically normocytic, but may be slightly macrocytic. Measurements of RBC production rates have yielded normal or increased values in some cases. RBC life span is often reduced. Changes in the erythrocyte morphology may show extreme variation in size and shape; also prominent in the peripheral blood are nucleated RBCs (mostly normoblasts) and immature WBCs. **Leukoerythroblastic** is the term applied to this cellular pattern, which results from either disruption of the marrow sinusoids or hematopoiesis in extramedullary sites. Polychromatophilia and reticulocytosis are often present. Reticulocytosis that may be due to premature release of reticulocytes from the marrow or extramedullary sites is not necessarily an index of increased blood regeneration. The WBC count may be normal, reduced, or increased. The platelet count is often low, and giant, bizarre-shaped platelets may be seen.

Kinetic studies with labeled Fe may indicate hematopoietic activity in the spleen and the liver. The marrow may be difficult to obtain by aspiration; findings vary according to the underlying disease. Marrow trephine biopsy is usually necessary to establish the diagnosis.

X-rays of the skeletal system may disclose bony lesions (myelosclerosis) characteristic of longstanding myelofibrosis or other osseous changes (ie, lytic lesions of a neoplasm) suggesting the cause of anemia.

Treatment

Therapy is that of the underlying disorder. In idiopathic cases, management is supportive. Transfusions are indicated if anemia produces cardiovascular symptoms. In primary myelofibrosis, androgens and corticosteroids have been used in an attempt to increase RBC production or decrease their destruction; modest responses have been observed.

MEGALOBLASTIC ANEMIAS

Megaloblastic states result from defective DNA synthesis. RNA synthesis continues, resulting in an increase in cytoplasmic mass and maturation. The circulation receives macro-ovalocytic RBCs and all cells have disordered maturation (dyspoiesis) in which cytoplasmic maturity is greater than nuclear maturity, producing the "megaloblast" in the marrow. Interference with normal cellular maturation increases intramedullary cell death (ineffective erythropoiesis) with resultant indirect hyperbilirubinemia and hyperuricemia. Because all cell lines are affected, leukopenia and thrombocytopenia may occur with anemia. Another hallmark includes reticulocytopenia from defective RBC production. Hypersegmentation of polymorphonuclear leukocytes is a standard finding in megaloblastic states; the mechanism of their production is unknown. In addition to the morphologic recognition of the megaloblastic changes, a test termed "deoxyuridine suppression" can be used to demonstrate the presence of defective DNA synthesis at the biochemical level.

Mechanisms that cause megaloblastic states most often include deficiency or defective utilization of vitamin B_{12} *or* folic acid; cytotoxic agents (generally antineoplastics or immunosuppressives) that interfere with DNA synthesis; and a rare autonomous form, the **Di Guglielmo syndrome**. Identifying both the etiology and pathophysiologic mechanisms of megaloblastic anemias is crucial.

ANEMIA DUE TO VITAMIN B_{12} DEFICIENCY

(Pernicious Anemia [PA])

(See also in Ch. 81 and under NONEROSIVE GASTRITIS in Ch. 54)

Vitamin B_{12} is available in meat, animal protein foods, and legumes. Its absorption (in the terminal ileum) requires the presence of **intrinsic factor**, *a secretion of parietal cells of the gastric mucosa*, to transport the vitamin across the intestinal mucosa. B_{12} stores in the liver are normally sufficient to sustain physiologic needs for 3 to 5 yr.

Etiology and Pathophysiology

Decreased B_{12} absorption is the major pathophysiologic mechanism that may be due to one of several factors (see also VITAMIN B_{12} DEFICIENCY in Ch. 81, in Ch. 58, and under NONEROSIVE GASTRITIS in Ch. 54). In PA, the most common cause of B_{12} deficiency, the atrophic gastric mucosa fails to secrete intrinsic factor. Gastrectomy, chronic atrophic gastritis, and myxedema may also cause similar deficient secretion, and, rarely, it is congenital. Endocrine deficiencies, especially of the thyroid and adrenal glands, if they are associated with PA, suggest an autoimmune basis for gastric mucosal atrophy. Hypogammaglobulinemia may be associated with PA. Competition for available B_{12} and cleavage of the intrinsic factor may occur in the blind loop syndrome (because of bacterial utilization of B_{12}) or in fish-tapeworm infestation. Ileal absorptive sites may be congenitally absent or destroyed by inflammatory regional enteritis or surgical resection. Less common causes of decreased B_{12} absorption include chronic pancreatitis, malabsorption syndromes, and administration of certain drugs (eg, oral calcium-chelating agents, aminosalicylic acid, biguanides). Inadequate B_{12} intake in vegans, or, very rarely, increased metabolism of B_{12} in longstanding hyperthyroidism may also be causes.

Symptoms and Signs

Anemia usually develops insidiously and progressively as the large hepatic stores of B_{12} are depleted. It is often more profound than would be expected from the symptoms, because its slow evolution can elicit physiologic adaptation. Splenomegaly and hepatomegaly may occasionally be seen. Various GI manifestations may be present, including anorexia, intermittent constipation and diarrhea, and poorly localized abdominal pain. Glossitis, usually described as "burning of the tongue," may be an early symptom. Considerable weight loss is common. Among rare signs may be fever of unknown origin that responds promptly to B_{12} therapy.

Neurologic involvement (see also COMBINED SYSTEM DISEASE in Ch. 130) may be present *even in the absence of anemia.* The most common involvement is that of peripheral nerves. Next is spinal cord involvement beginning in the dorsal column with loss of vibratory sensation in the lower extremities, loss of position sense, and ataxia; lateral column involvement follows, with spasticity, hyperactive reflexes, and a Babinski's sign. Some also have irritability, mild depression, or actual paranoia (megaloblastic madness). Yellow-blue color blindness occurs rarely.

Laboratory Diagnosis

The anemia is macrocytic, with an MCV > 100. The smear shows macro-ovalocytosis, aniso- and poikilocytosis, and basophilic stippling of RBCs. As expected, the RDW is high. Howell-Jolly bodies (residual fragments of the nucleus) are common. Unless the patient has been treated, there is a reticulocytopenia. Hypersegmentation of the granular leukocytes is one of the earliest findings; leukopenia develops later. Thrombocytopenia is observed in about ½ of severe cases, and platelets are often bizarre in size and shape. Bone marrow shows erythroid hyperplasia and megaloblastic changes. Serum bilirubin may be elevated because of ineffective erythropoiesis.

The commonest method to establish B_{12} deficiency as the cause of megaloblastosis is by serum vitamin B_{12} assay with either microbiologic or radioisotopic method. The former is specific but tedious, subject to interference by a variety of drugs, and now rarely done. Radioisotopic assays have suffered from problems in specificity. In general, low values (< 150 pg/mL) are reliable indications of B_{12} deficiency. In borderline circumstances (150 to 250 pg/mL), clinical judgment and other tests must supplement the radioassay. Tissue deficiency of B_{12} results in methylmalonic (and propionic) aciduria. Autoantibodies to gastric parietal cells can be identified in 80 to 90% of patients with PA and antibodies to intrinsic factor can be found in the sera in most of these patients.

Achlorhydria is present in most patients with PA. Gastric analysis demonstrates a small volume of gastric secretions (achylia gastrica) with a pH > 6.5; achlorhydria is confirmed if the pH rises to between 6.8 and 7.2 following histamine administration. Absent secretion of intrinsic factor is the cardinal basis of typical PA; it should be assayed in the gastric secretions collected regardless of pH, since discordant secretion of acid and intrinsic factor may occur.

The **Schilling test** measures the absorption of radioactive B_{12} with and without intrinsic factor. It is particularly useful to establish the diagnosis in patients who have been treated and are in remission. The test is done by the oral administration of radiolabeled B_{12} followed in 1 to 6 h by a parenteral "flushing" dose (1000 μg) of B_{12} to delimit hepatic storage; the percentage of radiolabeled material found in the 24-h urine collection is then measured. Reduced urinary excretion (in the presence of the required normal renal function) supports decreased absorption of vitamin B_{12}. This test, called Schilling I, can then be repeated using the radiolabeled cobalt attached to (hog) intrinsic factor. Correction of the previously reduced excretion by this Schilling II supports the absence of intrinsic factor as the pathophysiologic mechanism for the

low B_{12}. Finally, failure to correct excretion suggests a GI mechanism of malabsorption. Schilling III can be done after a 2-wk trial of oral tetracycline. Normally each labeled urine collection will contain > 9% of the administered dose. Decreased excretion of radiolabeled B_{12} (< 5%) and normal excretion of labeled B_{12} bound to intrinsic factor establishes a defect in intrinsic factor production (generally PA). Subnormal absorption of B_{12}, uncorrected by intrinsic factor, is seen in sprue and other malabsorption syndromes. Since the test provides B_{12} repletion, it should be performed after completion of all studies and planned therapeutic trials.

Because of the increased incidence of gastric cancer in patients with PA, GI x-rays are advisable at diagnosis. These may also disclose other causes of megaloblastic anemia (eg, intestinal diverticula or blind loops, or abnormal small-bowel patterns characteristic of sprue). Subsequent x-rays should be done when clinical findings (ie, symptoms, positive test for occult blood in the stool, etc) suggest a change in the status of the stomach.

Treatment

The amount of B_{12} retained by the body is in proportion to the amount given. Calculation of the specific amount of therapeutic B_{12} required is difficult, since repletion must include restoration of liver stores, normally 3,000 to 10,000 μg, and B_{12} retention declines as restoration of stores is achieved. Vitamin B_{12} 1000 μg is given IM 2 to 4 times/wk until hematologic abnormalities are corrected, and then is given once monthly. Although hematologic correction usually occurs within 6 wk, neural improvement may take up to 18 mo. Folic acid administration (instead of B_{12}) to anyone in the B_{12}-deprived state is *contraindicated*, since it may result in fulminant neurologic deficit. Oral Fe therapy is given if Fe deficiency is diagnosed by an absence of stainable Fe in the bone marrow or other parameters before treatment with B_{12}.

B_{12} maintenance therapy must be given for life unless the pathophysiologic mechanism for the deficiency is corrected.

Anemia Due to Folic Acid Deficiency

Etiology and Pathophysiology

The metabolism, several pathophysiologic mechanisms, and causes of folate deprivation are also discussed in Ch. 81.

Long-term cooking destroys folic acid, which is abundant in foods such as green leafy vegetables, yeast, liver, and mushrooms. Folate is absorbed in the duodenum and upper jejunum. Liver stores provide only a 2- to 4-mo supply in the absence of intake. Borderline dietary intake of folic acid is common. Alcohol interferes with its intermediate metabolism and probably absorption as well. Thus, persons subsiding on a marginal diet ("tea-and-toasters" and chronic alcoholics) are prone to develop macrocytic anemia from folic acid deficiency, as are those with chronic liver disease. Infants deficient in vitamin C may have "megaloblastic anemia of infancy." Since the fetus obtains folic acid from maternal supplies, pregnant women are susceptible to developing a megaloblastic anemia.

Intestinal malabsorption is another common cause of folate deficiency (see in Ch. 58). In tropical sprue, since malabsorption is secondary to the atrophy of intestinal mucosa resulting from lack of folic acid, even minute doses will usually correct both anemia and steatorrhea. Folic acid deficiency may develop in patients on long-term anticonvulsant therapy or oral contraceptives due to decreased absorption, or antimetabolites (methotrexate) and antimicrobial agents (eg, trimethoprim/sulfamethoxazole) that interfere with folate metabolism. Finally, increased demand for folate occurs in pregnancy and lactation, with long-term dialysis, chronic hemolytic anemias, and psoriasis.

Diagnosis

Clinical features are those of anemia. Folate deficiency is indistinguishable from B_{12} deficiency in regard to peripheral blood and bone marrow findings, but neurologic lesions (as seen in B_{12} deficiency) do not occur. The primary laboratory feature that differentiates this from other forms of megaloblastic anemia is measurable folate depletion. Serum folic acid levels < 5 ng/mL suggest a deficiency; low RBC folate levels (normal, 225 to 600 ng/mL) are diagnostic. (The range of "normal" depends upon the laboratory method used.)

Treatment

Folic acid 1 mg/day orally is given to replenish tissues. The patient must understand that about 50 μg of folate is required daily, with 2 to 3 times that amount required in pregnancy and childhood. (CAUTION: *In myeloblastic anemia, it is important to rule out vitamin B_{12} deficiency [pernicious anemia] before treating with folate, which would alleviate the anemia, but permit the associated neurologic damage to progress.*)

ANEMIA DUE TO COPPER DEFICIENCY

(See DISTURBANCES IN COPPER METABOLISM in Ch. 82)

ANEMIA DUE TO VITAMIN C (ASCORBIC ACID) DEFICIENCY

(See also VITAMIN C DEFICIENCY in Ch. 81)

Vitamin C deficiency is often associated with anemia that is hypochromic, but may be normocytic or microcytic (with chronic blood loss). When it is occasionally macrocytic, investigation will demonstrate associated folic acid deficiency, and then correction requires both vitamin C (500 mg/day) and folic acid (as noted above).

ANEMIAS DUE TO EXCESSIVE HEMOLYSIS

At the end of their normal life span (about 120 days), RBCs are removed by components of the reticuloendothelial system, principally in the spleen, where Hb catabolism takes place. The essential feature of hemolysis is a shortened RBC life span; hemolytic anemia results when bone marrow production can no longer compensate for RBC destruction. General aspects of hemolytic anemias will be discussed below, followed by a description of specific disorders.

Pathogenesis

Most hemolysis occurs **extravascularly;** ie, in phagocytic cells of the spleen, liver, and bone marrow. Hemolysis usually stems (1) from intrinsic abnormalities of RBC contents (Hb or enzymes) or membrane (permeability, structure, or lipid content), or (2) from problems extrinsic to the RBC (serum antibodies, trauma in the circulation, or infectious agents). The spleen is usually involved, and if splenomegaly results, it reduces RBC survival by destroying mildly abnormal RBCs or warm antibody-coated cells. Severely abnormal RBCs or those with cold antibodies or complement coating are destroyed within the circulation or in the liver, which (because of its large blood flow) can remove damaged cells efficiently.

Intravascular hemolysis is uncommon; it results in hemoglobinuria when the Hb released into plasma exceeds the Hb-binding capacity of plasma haptoglobin. Hb is reabsorbed into renal tubular cells where Fe is converted to hemosiderin, part of which is assimilated for reutilization and part of which reaches the urine when the tubular cells slough.

Symptoms and Signs

Systemic manifestations resemble those of other anemias. Hemolysis may be acute, chronic, or episodic. Acute severe hemolysis **(hemolytic crisis)** is uncommon; it may be accompanied by chills, fever, pain in the back and abdomen, prostration, and shock.

Severe hemolysis is also accompanied by increased RBC destruction (jaundice, splenomegaly, and, in certain types of hemolysis, hemoglobinuria, and hemosiderinuria), and increased RBC production (reticulocytosis and hyperactive bone marrow). Anemia in chronic hemolytic states may be exacerbated by a temporary failure of RBC production **(aplastic crisis)**; this is usually related to an infection.

Laboratory Findings

Jaundice occurs when the conversion of Hb to bilirubin exceeds the liver's capacity to form bilirubin glucuronide and to excrete it into bile (see also JAUNDICE in Ch. 67). Thus, unconjugated (indirect) bilirubin accumulates. Increased pigment catabolism is also manifested by increased stercobilin in the stool and urobilinogen in the urine. Pigment gallstones frequently complicate chronic hemolysis. Hemolysis can usually be identified by the simple criteria described. Nevertheless, the definitive criterion of the hemolytic process is a measure of RBC survival, preferably with a nonreutilizable label such as radiochromium (^{51}Cr). The measured survival of radiolabeled cells establishes not only the hemolytic state but, with surface counting, one can also identify sites of RBC sequestration, thereby providing diagnostic and therapeutic implications. In general, a half-life (for ^{51}Cr-labeled RBCs) of $\geq$ 18 days (normal 28 to 32 days) indicates hemolysis mild enough that a normally responsive marrow should be able to maintain normal RBC values. When the marrow responds appropriately, producing near-normal RBC values, the term **"compensated" hemolytic anemia** is used. Selective splenic sequestration with expected repair following splenectomy can be anticipated when surface count ratios reveal a spleen to liver ratio in excess of 3:1 (normal 1:1).

Other tests of RBC destruction (increased indirect hyperbilirubinemia, increased fecal urobilinogen or CO production) or evidence of repair (reticulocytosis) support but do not establish the hemolytic state.

Morphologic examination may show evidence of RBC destruction (eg, fragmentation, spherocytes) or erythrophagocytosis; these help establish the diagnosis and the mechanism. Other tests of hemolytic mechanisms include Hb electrophoresis, RBC enzyme assays, osmotic fragility, Coombs' test, cold agglutinins, and acid hemolysis or sucrose lysis tests.

Diagnosis and Differential Diagnosis

Morphologic clues, so important in diagnosing most anemias, are of limited value in the hemolytic anemias. Spherocytes, when identified, serve as the best evidence of active RBC destruction since these cells have already lost membrane mass. Spherocytes are common features of transfused blood or warm-antibody hemolytic anemia as well as the uncommon congenital spherocytosis. An unusually elevated MCHC may clue to the presence of spherocytes. A high MCHC (and MCV) is also seen in cold-antibody hemolytic anemia; these numbers decline to normal when the blood is warmed.

The common classification into intrinsic RBC defects and lesions extrinsic to the RBC is sometimes difficult to apply clinically, because a battery of tests is often involved. Another approach to the differential diagnosis is to consider the population at risk (ie, geographic, genetic, underlying disease, etc) and then proceed through the likely potential mechanisms. In general, these can be divided into (1) RBC sequestration due to alterations in vascular complex (ie, hypersplenism); (2) immunologic injury (warm- or cold-antibody mediated); (3) mechanical injury (RBC fragmentation); (4) alterations of RBC structure (abnormal membranes) or metabolism (enzymopathies); and (5) abnormal Hbs.

Treatment

Treatment is individualized to specific hemolytic disorders. Hemoglobinuria may necessitate Fe replacement therapy. Splenectomy is beneficial when the RBC defect is associated with selective splenic sequestration.

HEMOLYTIC ANEMIAS DUE TO DEFECTS EXTRINSIC TO THE RED CELL

Donor cells are destroyed at a rate equal to autologous cells. No abnormality of the RBC can be identified or implicated in RBC destruction.

ANEMIAS DUE TO RETICULOENDOTHELIAL HYPERACTIVITY

Hypersplenism-Congestive Splenomegaly

(See also HYPERSPLENISM in Ch. 104)

Hypersplenism is characterized by a mechanism that produces splenomegaly with associated increased filtering and phagocytic function. Often other cytopenias (leukopenia, thrombocytopenia) occur with the anemia. Although the primary mechanism is a mechanical sieve-like action resulting in RBC sequestration, another mechanism compounding the degree of anemia is that splenomegaly is associated with plasma volume expansion resulting in a dilutional component. In addition, in some immune-mediated conditions, the spleen may serve not only to sequester RBCs, but may also produce antibodies, thereby superimposing an immune basis upon that of congestion.

Etiology and Pathogenesis

In general, the degree of anemia relates to the size of the spleen. Thus, diseases associated with reticuloendothelial hyperplasia and splenomegaly are most likely to produce hypersplenism, but any disease that can produce splenomegaly can produce hypersplenism. The term indicates the presence of peripheral cytopenia(s) with bone marrow hyperplasia of the elements reduced in the circulation as due to splenic overfunction and by implication repairable by splenectomy. The anemia is primarily due to splenic sequestration with an added dilutional component. Radiolabeled autologous or donor RBCs can be shown to be sequestered in the spleen.

Symptoms and Signs

Clinical findings are usually based upon the underlying disease state causing the congestive splenomegaly. Unless other mechanisms coexist to compound their severity, anemia and other cytopenias are modest and asymptomatic. Splenomegaly is the hallmark of hypersplenism and spleen size correlates directly with the degree of anemia.

Laboratory Findings

Since the anemia is produced by splenic sequestration, no particular RBC morphology exists. The diagnosis may be suggested by presence of other cytopenias (platelet counts range between 50,000 to 100,000/mL; WBC in range of 2500 to 4000/mL with normal WBC differential count). ^{51}Cr-radiolabeled RBC survival studies show accelerated destruction and selective splenic sequestration. A measurable expanded plasma volume is common.

Treatment

Therapy is directed at the cause of congestive splenomegaly. Since anemia is mild, splenectomy is rarely indicated.

ANEMIAS DUE TO IMMUNOLOGIC ABNORMALITIES

Isoimmune (Isoagglutinin) Hemolytic Anemia

(See HEMOLYTIC REACTIONS under COMPLICATIONS OF TRANSFUSION in Ch. 97)

Autoimmune Hemolytic Anemia

Autoimmune hemolytic anemia affects women more often than men, and most commonly those < 50 yr old. Splenomegaly is usual and the potentially lethal anemia is

usually severe. A thrombotic tendency often accompanies the hemolysis. Since RBCs are destroyed primarily in the spleen, hemoglobinuria and hemosiderinuria are rare. A direct Coombs' (antiglobulin) test demonstrates antibody coating the RBC surface. The blood smear frequently reveals spherocytes.

Warm-antibody hemolytic anemias: RBCs coated with IgG (auto-) antibodies are removed by the reticuloendothelial system. These antibodies may arise spontaneously, or in association with certain diseases (SLE, lymphoma, chronic lymphocytic leukemia), or after stimulation by a drug (eg, α-methyldopa, L-dopa). *The laboratory hallmark is a positive Coombs' (antiglobulin) test,* and the autoantibodies may be related to a portion of the Rh locus. High-dose penicillin or cephalosporins may result in an antibody directed against an antibiotic-RBC membrane complex; cessation of the drug results in disappearance of accelerated destruction.

Therapy in all drug-induced hemolytic anemias includes withdrawal of the drug, which decreases the hemolytic rate. With α-methyldopa and related drugs, hemolysis usually ceases within 3 wk; however, the positive Coombs' test may persist for > 1 yr. Corticosteroids occasionally are used if hemolysis is very severe. With penicillin and analogous drugs, hemolysis ceases as soon as the drug is cleared from the plasma.

Idiopathic anemia responds to corticosteroids, but may relapse on withdrawal of the steroid; splenectomy is frequently required to control hemolysis. Immunosuppressives have been used in patients refractory to steroids and splenectomy.

Cold-antibody disease (cold-agglutinin disease): Patients with lymphoproliferative diseases, infectious mononucleosis, or *Mycoplasma pneumoniae* may develop IgM antibodies directed against the I or i antigen of RBCs. Agglutination occurs at low temperatures, but only minimally > 30 C (86 F). With agglutination, complement fixation results. Intravascular hemolysis is seldom enough to cause hemoglobinuria and hemosiderinuria, but their presence is an important diagnostic aid. In general, hemolysis is mild.

No underlying cause is found in some patients. This idiopathic form is generally seen in older people. *Mycoplasma pneumoniae* is a common cause in younger people. Regardless of cause, the primary site of destruction is the liver.

Therapy is of only modest effect. Avoidance of cold exposure is often quite helpful. Splenectomy is of no value. Immunosuppressive agents have often been effective. Transfusions should be given cautiously with the blood warmed via an on-line warmer. Autologous cell survival may be better than that of transfused cells because administered blood becomes antibody-coated; autologous cells have already "survived" the antibody effect on the RBCs, and effete complement fragments (C3d) on their surface do not affect RBC survival.

Paroxysmal cold hemoglobinuria (PCH; Donath-Landsteiner syndrome): In this rare disease, hemolysis occurs minutes to hours after exposure to cold; exposure may be localized (eg, drinking cold water, handwashing in cold water). Intravascular hemolysis is caused by an autohemolysin that unites with RBCs at low temperatures and lyses them only after warming. The cold hemolysin is a 7S immunoglobulin. PCH due to such a cold-activated autohemolysin occurs in some patients with congenital or acquired syphilis, and antisyphilitic therapy may cure the PCH. Most however, occur after a nonspecific "viral" illness or in patients previously well.

Symptoms include severe pain in the back and legs, headache, vomiting, diarrhea, and passage of dark brown urine. Findings include hemoglobinuria, mild anemia, and moderate reticulocytosis. There may be temporary hepatosplenomegaly. Mild hyperbilirubinemia may follow the attack.

Therapy consists of strict avoidance of exposure to cold. Splenectomy is of no value. Immunosuppressive therapy has been effective, but its trial should be restricted to nonlimited or idiopathic cases.

Complement-Sensitive Associated Anemia

Paroxysmal nocturnal hemoglobinuria (PNH; Marchiafava-Micheli syndrome): This rare disorder is characterized by episodes of hemolysis and hemoglobinemia, the latter accentuated during sleep. The cause is unknown, but PNH may be an acquired membrane defect with unusual sensitivity to normal complement in plasma. PNH is most common in men in their 20s, but it occurs at any age. Crises may be precipitated by infection, administration of Fe or vaccines, or menstruation.

Abdominal and lumbar pain may occur, along with splenomegaly, hemoglobinemia, hemoglobinuria, and symptoms of severe anemia that is normocytic and normochromic. Protracted urinary Hb loss may result in Fe deficiency even though some organs, particularly the kidneys, may be saturated with hemosiderin. Leukopenia and thrombocytopenia are common. Gross hemoglobinuria is common during crises, and the urine may contain hemosiderin. Affected patients are strongly predisposed to both venous and arterial thrombi, a common cause of death.

Diagnostic tests include the acid hemolysis test **(Ham test)**: Hemolysis usually occurs if blood is acidified with CO_2, incubated for 1 h, and centrifuged. Also useful is the sugar-water test of Hartman that depends on enhanced hemolysis of complement-dependent systems in isotonic solutions of low ionic strength. Bone marrow hypoplasia may be present.

Treatment is symptomatic. Empiric use of corticosteroids (prednisone 20 to 40 mg/day) has resulted in controlling symptoms and stabilizing RBC values in > 50% of patients. Transfusions containing plasma (complement) should be avoided, but saline-washed RBCs may be given during crises. Heparin should be used cautiously, since it may accelerate hemolysis, but its use in thrombotic disease appears warranted. Oral Fe supplements are useful. Most patients can be managed by these supportive measures for years to decades. Some progress to bone marrow hypoplasia and have all of the complications of patients with aplastic anemia.

ANEMIAS DUE TO MECHANICAL INJURY

Traumatic Hemolytic Anemias
(Microangiopathic Hemolytic Anemias)

When exposed to excessive shear or turbulence in the circulation, odd-shaped RBC fragments (triangles, helmet shapes, etc) appear in the peripheral blood and provide the diagnosis. Because of the fragments, the MCV may be low and the RDW, reflecting the anisocytosis, high. Trauma may originate (1) outside the vessel, eg, in march hemoglobinuria, karate, or bongo playing; (2) within the heart, as in calcific aortic stenosis and with faulty aortic valve prostheses; (3) in arterioles, as in malignant hypertension and some malignant tumors; or (4) in end arterioles as in thrombotic thrombocytopenic purpura and disseminated intravascular coagulation **(DIC)**. Coagulation factor deficits occur in DIC (see Ch. 99). **Treatment** is directed toward the underlying process. Fe-deficiency anemia occasionally is superimposed on hemolysis as a result of chronic hemosiderinuria, and, when demonstrated, may respond to Fe therapy.

Hemolysis Due to Infectious Agents

Infectious agents may produce hemolytic anemia by the direct action of toxins (eg, from *Clostridium perfringens*, α- or β-hemolytic streptococci, or meningococci), or by invasion and destruction of the RBC by the organism (eg, *Plasmodia* and *Bartonellae*).

HEMOLYSIS DUE TO INTRINSIC RED CELL DEFECTS

ANEMIAS DUE TO ALTERATIONS OF RED CELL MEMBRANE

Congenital Red Cell Membrane Disorders

Congenital erythropoietic porphyria: (See in ANOMALIES IN PIGMENT METABOLISM in Ch. 85).

Hereditary elliptocytosis (ovalocytosis): *A rare disorder (inherited as an autosomal dominant trait) in which RBCs are oval or elliptical; hemolysis is usually absent or slight, with little or no anemia; and splenomegaly is often present.* The abnormality in the RBC appears to be due to altered membrane proteins. Splenectomy relieves hemolysis, but is required only in patients with anemia or a clinical complex as seen in hereditary spherocytosis. The clinical features are similar to those seen in the more common hereditary spherocytoses.

Hereditary spherocytosis (chronic familial icterus; congenital hemolytic jaundice; chronic acholuric jaundice; familial spherocytosis; spherocytic anemia): *A chronic disease, inherited as a dominant trait, characterized by hemolysis of spheroidal RBCs, anemia, jaundice, and splenomegaly.* Although usually one or more family members have had jaundice, anemia, or splenomegaly, one or more generations may be skipped because of variations in the degree of penetrance of the gene.

Etiology and Pathogenesis

In hereditary spherocytosis the cell membrane surface area is decreased out of proportion to the intracellular content. There are now several different RBC membrane protein abnormalities that result in spherocyte change. The decreased surface area of the cell impairs the flexibility needed to traverse the spleen's microcirculation and RBCs are trapped in the spleen and destroyed.

Symptoms and Signs

Symptoms and signs are usually mild. Moderate jaundice and symptoms of anemia are present in severe cases. Aplastic crises due to intercurrent infection may exacerbate the anemia. Splenomegaly is almost invariable and, rarely, may cause abdominal discomfort. Hepatomegaly may be present, and cholelithiasis is common. Congenital skeletal abnormalities, such as tower-shaped skull and polydactylism, are seen occasionally.

Laboratory Findings

Anemia varies greatly in degree. The RBC count, usually between 3 and 4 million, may fall during an aplastic crisis to < 1 million and the Hb level drops proportionately. Since RBCs are spheroidal and the MCV is normal, the mean corpuscular diameter is somewhat below normal, and RBCs resemble microspherocytes. Reticulocytosis of 15 to 30% and leukocytosis are common.

The osmotic fragility of RBCs is characteristically increased, but in mild cases it may be normal unless sterile defibrinated blood is first incubated at 37 C (98.6 F) for 24 h. Coombs' test is negative. Glucose can correct an increased autohemolysis.

Prognosis and Treatment

Splenectomy, the only treatment, is indicated in patients under age 45—especially when anemia exists, episodes of jaundice or biliary colic occur, or if the patient has had episodes of erythroblastopenia (aplastic crisis). At surgery a gallbladder with stones or evidence of disease should be removed. After splenectomy, symptoms usually abate, the RBC count rises, and the reticulocyte count returns to normal; since spherocytosis persists, the osmotic fragility of the blood is still increased, but the patient is improved without the removal moiety (spleen) for these abnormal cells.

Acquired Red Cell Membrane Disorders

Stomatocytosis: *Condition of RBCs in which a mouth-like or slit-like pattern replaces the normal central zone of pallor*. These cells are associated with both congenital and acquired hemolytic anemia.

The rare congenital form is best characterized and can be used to describe some aspects of this anemia in the acquired form; it has autosomal inheritance. The RBC membrane is considered very "leaky" with hyperpermeability to monovalent cations; movement of divalent cations and anions is normal. Circulating RBCs (20 to 30%) are stomatocytic; osmotic fragility is increased, as is autohemolysis with inconstant correction with glucose. Splenectomy results in amelioration of the anemia in some.

Acquired stomatocytosis with hemolytic anemia occurs primarily with recent excessive alcoholism. Stomatocytes in the peripheral blood and the accelerated RBC destruction disappear within 2 wk of alcohol withdrawal.

Anemia due to hypophosphatemia: RBC pliability depends upon intracellular ATP, Ca, and Mg levels. Since red cell ATP content is related to the serum phosphorus concentration, hypophosphatemia (serum levels < 0.5 mg/dL) results in erythrocyte ATP depletion; this in turn causes RBC membrane rigidity, and hemolysis occurs.

Severe hypophosphatemia may occur in alcoholic withdrawal states, diabetes mellitus, the recovery (diuretic) phase after severe burns, hyperalimentation, severe respiratory alkalosis, or in uremic patients on dialysis being treated with antacids.

The metabolic sequelae of hypophosphatemia are complex and include red cell ATP and 2,3-DPG depletion, a shift in the O_2 dissociation curve to the left, decreased glucose utilization, and lactate production. The resultant rigid, nonyielding RBCs are susceptible to injury in the capillary circulatory bed, leading to a hemolytic anemia with membrane injury and microspherocytosis.

Since these changes are prevented or reversed if cellular ATP is maintained with phosphate supplements, therapy should be directed toward protection against hypophosphatemia in the potential clinical setting and phosphate administration when depletion is recognized.

ANEMIAS DUE TO DISORDERS OF RED CELL METABOLISM
(Hereditary Enzyme Deficiencies)

The prime energy source for RBCs is glucose. After it enters the RBC, glucose is converted to lactate either by anaerobic glycolysis (the Embden-Meyerhof pathway) or via the hexose monophosphate shunt. Hemolytic anemias may result from hereditary deficiencies in the enzyme systems involved in these metabolic pathways.

Embden-Meyerhof Pathway Defects

Embden-Meyerhof pathway defects are relatively rare and share the following characteristics: The trait is autosomal recessive, and hemolytic anemia occurs only in homozygotes; spherocytes are absent, but small numbers of crenated spheres may be present; and hemolysis and anemia persist after splenectomy, though there may be some improvement. The most common form is that of pyruvate kinase deficiency due to a deficient or defective enzyme. Deficiencies in virtually every enzyme reaction are associated with a congenital hemolytic anemia. The exact mechanism of RBC destruction is unknown. In general, assay of ATP and diphosphoglycerate help identify presence of a metabolic defect and assist in localizing the sites in the pathway for further biochemical characterization.

Hexose Monophosphate Shunt Defects

The only important defect in this pathway is that due to glucose-6-phosphate dehydrogenase **(G6PD)** deficiency. In some cases this is due to a genetic abnormality of

the enzyme, a form of genetic polymorphism. Clinically, the most common form is that of the drug-sensitive type.

G6PD deficiency—drug-sensitive variety: This X-linked disorder (see also in Ch. 276) is fully expressed in males and homozygous females and variably expressed in heterozygous females. It occurs in about 10% of American black males and fewer black females, and in low frequency among people from the Mediterranean basin (eg, Italians, Greeks, Arabs, and Sephardic Jews).

In affected blacks and most affected whites, hemolysis occurs in older RBCs after exposure to drugs or other substances that produce peroxide and cause oxidation of Hb and RBC membranes. These include primaquine, aspirin, sulfonamides, nitrofurans, phenacetin, naphthalene, some vitamin K derivatives, and, in some whites, fava beans. Acute viral and bacterial infections and diabetic acidosis also may precipitate hemolysis. Anemia, jaundice, and reticulocytosis develop. Heinz bodies may be seen early during the hemolytic episode, but they do not persist in patients with spleens, since they are removed by the spleen. Often the best diagnostic clue is the presence in the peripheral blood of RBCs that appear to have had one or more bites (1 μm in size) taken from the cell periphery **("bite cells")**, possibly as a result of Heinz body removal by the spleen. Since older cells are selectively destroyed, in most episodes, hemolysis is self-limited, affecting < 25% of the RBC mass in blacks. However, in whites, the deficiency is more severe, and profound hemolysis may lead to a sufficient intravascular component with hemoglobinuria and acute renal failure. Whether the patient will develop a compensated hemolytic state or lethal hemolysis if the offending drug is continued depends on the degree of G6PD deficiency in the patient and the oxidant potential of the drug. Chronic congenital hemolysis in the absence of drugs occurs in some whites.

Many screening tests for G6PD are available. Following hemolysis, false-negative results may be obtained due to the absence of older, more deficient RBCs and the presence of reticulocytes rich in G6PD. Specific enzyme assays are the best diagnostic tests. Affected patients should be advised to eliminate drugs or substances that initiate this deficiency.

ANEMIAS DUE TO DEFECTIVE HEMOGLOBIN SYNTHESIS
(Hemoglobinopathies)

Genetic abnormalities of the Hb molecule shown by changes in chemical characteristics, electrophoretic mobility, or other physical properties.

The normal adult Hb molecule (Hb A) consists of 2 pairs of polypeptide chains designated α and β. Fetal Hb (Hb F, in which γ chains replace the β chains) is present at birth, but gradually decreases in the first months of life until it makes up < 2% of total Hb in adults. In certain disorders of Hb synthesis and in aplastic and myeloproliferative states, Hb F may be increased. Normal blood also contains ≤ 2.5% of Hb A_2 (composed of α and δ chains).

The types of chains and the chemical structure of individual polypeptides in the chains are controlled genetically. Defects may result in Hb molecules with abnormal physical or chemical properties; some result in anemias that are severe in homozygotes but mild in heterozygous carriers. Some persons may be heterozygous for 2 such abnormalities and show an anemia with characteristics of both traits.

Abnormal Hbs, distinguished by electrophoretic mobility, are designated by letters; the first was sickle cell Hb, named Hb S. Since then designations follow the alphabet in order of discovery; thus, C, D, E, G, H, etc. Structurally different Hbs with the same electrophoretic mobility are named also by the city where they were discovered (eg, Hb C_{Harlem}, Hb $S_{Memphis}$). In the USA, important hemoglobinopathies are those due to Hb

S, Hb C, and the thalassemias; recent immigration of Southeast Asians has led to the common recognition of Hb E in clinical practice.

Sickle Cell Anemia

(Hb S Disease; Drepanocytic Anemia; Meniscocytosis)

A chronic hemolytic anemia occurring almost exclusively in blacks and characterized by sickle-shaped RBCs due to homozygous inheritance of Hb S.

Etiology, Incidence, and Pathogenesis

Homozygotes have sickle cell anemia (about 0.3% of blacks in the USA); heterozygotes (8 to 13% of blacks) are not anemic, but the sickling trait (sicklemia) can be demonstrated in vitro.

In Hb S, valine is substituted for glutamic acid in the sixth amino acid of the β-chain. This decreases its electrical charge and makes it move more slowly toward the anode than Hb A on electrophoretic analysis. Deoxy-Hb S is much less soluble than deoxy-Hb A; it forms a semisolid gel of rodlike tactoids, thus causing RBCs to sickle at sites of low P_{O_2}. Distorted but inflexible RBCs plug small arterioles and capillaries, which leads to occlusion and infarction. Because sickled RBCs are too fragile to withstand the mechanical trauma of circulation, hemolysis occurs when they are released into the circulation.

Symptoms and Signs

In homozygotes, clinical manifestations are due both to anemia and to tissue ischemia and infarction. Anemia is usually severe, but highly variable from patient to patient; most have mild jaundice with bilirubin from 2 to 4 mg/dL. Anemia may be exacerbated in children by acute sequestration of sickled cells in the spleen. More common is the "**aplastic crisis**" in both children and adults occurring when marrow RBC production slows during acute infections (especially viral). Episodes of arthralgia with fever may occur, and aseptic necrosis of the femoral head is common. Chronic punched-out ulcers about the ankles are a recurrent problem. Episodes of severe abdominal pain with vomiting may simulate severe abdominal disorders; such **painful crises** are usually associated with back and joint pain. Hemiplegia, cranial nerve palsies, and other neurologic disturbances may result from occlusion of major intracranial vessels. Infections, particularly pneumococcal, are common, especially in early childhood and are associated with a high mortality rate. Progressive decreases in pulmonary and renal function may be seen in older patients.

Patients may be poorly developed and often have a relatively short trunk with long extremities and a tower-shaped skull. Chronic overactivity of the marrow causes bone changes that can be seen on x-ray; widening of the diploic spaces of the skull and the "sun-ray" appearance of the diploic trabeculations are characteristic. The long bones frequently show cortical thickening, irregular densities, and evidence of new bone formation within the medullary canal. Hepatosplenomegaly is common in children, but because of repeated infarctions and subsequent fibrosis, the spleen in adult patients is rarely palpable. The heart is usually enlarged, with a prominent pulmonary conus. Heart murmurs may simulate rheumatic or congenital heart disease. Cholelithiasis is common.

In the heterozygous state, affected individuals are normal and do not experience hemolysis, painful crises, or thrombotic complications. Hyposthenuria is common. Unilateral hematuria occurs but is self-limited and should never be treated by nephrectomy. Recognition of the heterozygous sickle cell state should lead to identification of its unilateral ureteral basis and thereby avoid needless nephrectomy.

Laboratory Findings and Diagnosis

RBCs are normocytic with the count usually between 2 and 3 million and Hb reduced proportionately. Dry stained smears may show only a few sickled cells. The pathognomonic finding is sickling (crescent-shaped RBCs, often with elongated or pointed ends) in an unstained drop of blood that has been prevented from drying or has been treated with a reducing agent (eg, sodium metabisulfite). It may also be produced by reduced O_2 tension. Sealing a drop of blood under a cover slip with petroleum jelly provides such an environment, which may be viewed microscopically. A rapid tube test that depends upon the differential solubility of Hb S is widely used for screening.

Normoblasts are frequently seen in the peripheral blood, and a reticulocytosis of 10 to 40% or more is common. Leukocytosis may rise to 25,000 with a shift to the left during either crisis or bacterial infection. Platelets are usually increased. Bone marrow is hyperplastic, with normoblasts predominating; it may become aplastic during sickling crises or severe infections. Serum bilirubin is usually elevated, and fecal and urinary urobilinogen values are high. The ESR is low.

Diagnosis of the homozygous state is made by demonstrating only Hb S with a variable amount of Hb F by electrophoresis. The heterozygote is recognized by the presence of both Hb A and S (with more Hb A than Hb S) on electrophoresis. Hb S must be distinguished from other Hbs that migrate similarly by electrophoresis. This is accomplished by the sickling phenomenon that is negative with other Hbs of similar electrophoretic mobility. This difference is important for genetic counseling.

Prognosis and Treatment

The lifespan of homozygous patients has steadily increased to well beyond age 40. Common causes of death are intercurrent infections, multiple pulmonary emboli, occlusion of a vessel supplying a vital area, or renal failure.

Therapy is symptomatic. Splenectomy and hematinics are valueless. Transfusions should be given only for anemia that is more severe than usual (eg, during aplastic crises accompanying severe infections); there is little reason to use them in treating painful crises. In general, crises should be managed with vigorous oral or IV hydration and analgesics, including narcotics if needed to control pain. Accepted indications for transfusions include cardiopulmonary symptoms (particularly when Hb is < 5 gm/dL) or signs (eg, high output cardiac failure or hypoxemia with P_{O_2} < 65 mm Hg) or where other life-threatening events exist and improved O_2 delivery would be of benefit (eg, sepsis, severe infections, cerebrovascular accidents, organ failure). Transfusions are also recommended prior to general anesthesia and surgery. Finally, chronic transfusion programs appear beneficial following cerebrovascular accidents (for a minimum of 3 yr), recalcitrant leg ulcers, and probably during pregnancy. Since the goals of such programs should be to achieve sickle cell concentrations < 30% with a Hct not to exceed 46%, partial exchange transfusions are usually the best procedure. A partial exchange or hypertransfusion may break a cycle of closely spaced painful crises. Urea orally or parenterally is of no value and may be harmful. Cyanate therapy has toxic side effects when given directly, but its extracorporeal use has some promise and is currently being tested.

Prophylactic antibiotics, pneumococcal vaccine (see PNEUMOCOCCAL INFECTIONS in Ch. 8), early identification and treatment of serious bacterial infection and general prophylaxis have reduced mortality, particularly during childhood. A recent study demonstrated a marked reduction in the occurrence of pneumococcal septicemia in infants given prophylactic penicillin starting by age 4 mo, suggesting that this should become standard procedure.

Hemoglobin C Disease

A moderately severe anemia due to an inherited abnormality of Hb formation. From 2 to 3% of American blacks show the trait. Heterozygotes are usually not anemic. Symptoms in homozygotes are due to the anemia. The spleen is usually enlarged, and arthralgia is common. There may be abdominal pain but the abdominal crises of sickle cell anemia do not occur. The patient may be mildly jaundiced.

In the homozygote, anemia is normocytic, with 30 to 100% target cells, associated spherocytes, and rarely, crystal-containing RBCs seen in the smear. Reticulocytes are increased slightly, and nucleated RBCs may be present. The RBCs do not sickle. Electrophoresis shows that all the Hb is type C. Serum bilirubin is slightly elevated, and urobilinogen is increased in the stools and urine. There is no specific treatment. Anemia is usually not severe enough to require blood transfusion. **In the heterozygote,** the only finding is many normochromic cells with central targets.

Hemoglobin S–C Disease

Since 10% of blacks carry the Hb S trait, the incidence of the heterozygous S-C combination is much greater than that of the homozygous Hb C disease. Many cases of anemia in patients with sicklemia may represent undetected examples of the S-C combination. The anemia in Hb S-C disease is like that of Hb C disease, but milder; some patients even have normal Hb levels. Most symptoms are those of sickle cell anemia, but they are usually less frequent and less severe. However, gross hematuria, retinal hemorrhages, and aseptic necrosis of the femoral head are common. Stained blood smears show target cells and a rare sickle cell. All cells sickle in a sickling preparation.

Hemoglobin E Disease

Hb E ($\alpha_2\beta_2^{26glu \rightarrow lys}$) is the 3rd most prevalent Hb worldwide (after A and S), primarily in Southeast Asian (> 15%) and black populations, but rarely in Chinese.

In the heterozygote (Hb AE) no peripheral blood abnormalities are found. Hb electrophoresis reveals about 30% E (found near origin where A_2, C, and O_{Arab} occur) and 70% A. On agar gel electrophoresis at acid pH, E comigrates with A, thereby separating it from C and O_{Arab}. The relative percent of E decreases in association with α-thalassemia or in presence of Fe deficiency. Homozygous E is associated with a mild hypochromic-microcytic anemia with prominent targeting. Double heterozygotes for E and β-thalassemia have a hemolytic disease severer than S-thalassemia.

Thalassemias

(Mediterranean Anemia; Hereditary Leptocytosis; Thalassemia Major and Minor)

A group of chronic, inherited, microcytic anemias characterized by defective Hb synthesis and ineffective erythropoiesis; they are particularly common in persons of Mediterranean, African, and Southeast Asian ancestry.

Etiology and Pathogenesis

Thalassemia results from unbalanced Hb synthesis due to defective production rates of one or more of the normal globin polypeptide chains (α, β, γ, δ). β-Thalassemia results from decreased synthesis of β-polypeptide chains. This trait is autosomal dominant: Heterozygotes (thalassemia minor) have asymptomatic mild-to-moderate microcytic anemia; the typical symptoms occur in homozygotes (thalassemia major). Since genetic control of α-chain synthesis involves 2 pairs of structural genes, the inheritance pattern for α-thalassemia, which results from decreased α-chain synthesis, is more

complex. Heterozygotes for a single gene defect ("α-thalassemia-2 [silent]") are usually free from clinical abnormalities. Heterozygotes for a double gene defect or homozygotes for a single gene defect ("α-thalassemia-1 [trait]") tend to manifest a clinical picture similar to heterozygotes for β-thalassemia. Inheritance of both a single gene defect and a double gene defect results in a more severe impairment of α-chain synthesis. The deficiency of α-chains results in the formation of tetramers of excess β-chains (Hb H), or, in infancy, γ-chains (Bart's Hb). Homozygosity for the double-gene defect is lethal, since Hb lacking α-chains does not transport O_2.

Symptoms and Signs

Clinical features of all thalassemias are similar but vary in severity. Symptoms of severe anemia occur in **β-thalassemia major (Cooley's anemia)**. Clinical features result from anemia, markedly expanded marrow space, and transfusional and absorptive Fe overload. Patients are jaundiced, and leg ulcers and cholelithiasis occur as in sickle cell anemia. Splenomegaly is common, and the spleen may be huge. If splenic sequestration develops, the survival time of transfused, normal RBCs is shortened. Bone marrow hyperactivity causes thickening of the cranial bones and malar eminences, producing "hemolytic facies." Pathologic fractures are common. Growth rates are impaired and puberty may be significantly delayed or absent. Fe deposits in heart muscle may cause dysfunction and ultimately heart failure. Hepatic siderosis occurs typically, leading to functional impairment and cirrhosis. Patients with Hb H disease often have symptomatic hemolytic anemia and splenomegaly.

Laboratory Findings (see TABLE 96–4)

In thalassemia major, anemia is severe, often with Hb of 6 gm/dL or less. The RBC count is elevated. *The blood smear is virtually diagnostic,* with large numbers of nucleated erythroblasts, target cells, small pale RBCs, and punctate and diffuse basophilia.

Serum bilirubin is increased and the serum-Fe and -ferritin levels are well above normal. The bone marrow reveals florid erythroid hyperplasia. In thalassemia minor (β or α) the usual finding is mild-to-moderate microcytic anemia. Serum-Fe and -ferritin determinations will demonstrate the absence of Fe deficiency.

Diagnosis

Quantitative Hb studies are used for diagnosis, and the abnormality depends on the type of thalassemia. In homozygous β-thalassemia, Hb F is usually increased, sometimes to as much as 90%; Hb A_2 is also usually elevated to > 3%. Elevation of the Hb A_2 is the diagnostic test for heterozygous β-thalassemia. The percentages of Hb A_2 and

TABLE 96–4. CHARACTERISTICS OF THE THALASSEMIAS

Category	*Anemia*	*MCV*	*% Hb A_2*	*% Hb F*
β Thalassemia				
Heterozygous	Mild	↓	↑	Variable
Homozygous	Severe	↓	Variable	↑ up to 90%
β-δ Thalassemia				
Heterozygous	Mild	↓	N or ↓	> 5%
Homozygous	Moderate-severe	↓	Absent	100%
α Thalassemia				
Single gene defect	None	N—↓	N	N
Double gene defect	Mild	↓	N—↓	< 5%
Triple gene defect	Moderate	↓	N—↓ (Hb H or Bart's present)	Variable

F are generally normal in the α-thalassemia syndromes and the diagnosis often is one of exclusion of other causes of microcytic anemia. Hb H disease can be diagnosed by demonstrating the fast-migrating Hb H or Bart's fractions on Hb electrophoresis.

In β-thalassemia homozygotes, skeletal x-rays show findings characteristic of chronic overactivity of the marrow. The cortices of the skull and the long bones are thinned, and the marrow space is widened. The diploic spaces in the skull may be accentuated, with the trabeculae giving a "sun ray" appearance. In the long bones, areas of osteoporosis may occur. The vertebral bodies and the skull may have a granular or "ground glass" appearance. The phalanges may lose their normal shape and appear rectangular or even biconvex.

Prognosis

The outlook varies. Some patients with β-thalassemia major live to puberty or beyond. Life expectancy is normal for persons with thalassemia minor.

Treatment

Children with thalassemia major should receive as few transfusions as possible, since Fe overload can ultimately result. However, suppression of abnormal hematopoiesis by chronic RBC hypertransfusion may be valuable in severely affected patients; to prevent or delay hemochromatosis, excess (transfusional) Fe must then be removed (eg, by chronic Fe-chelation therapy). Transfusing relatively younger fractions of RBCs appears to provide a further advantage at decreasing the rate of Fe overload. Splenectomy may help patients with splenomegaly where superimposed hemolysis of RBCs may occur at that site; the benefit is primarily a decrease in transfusion requirements. Thalassemia minor requires no treatment.

Hemoglobin S-β-Thalassemia Disease

Because of the increased frequency of both Hb S and β-thalassemia genes in similar population groups, inheritance of both defects is not uncommon. Clinically, the disorder produces symptoms of moderate anemia and many signs of sickle cell anemia, which are usually less frequent and less severe.

Laboratory findings are mild-to-moderate microcytic anemia, some sickled RBCs on stained blood smears, and reticulocytosis. The Hb A_2 is $> 3\%$. Hb S predominates on electrophoresis and Hb A is decreased or absent. Hb F increase is variable.

Treatment is the same as for sickle cell anemia, although most patients will generally have a milder clinical course.

---

97. BLOOD TRANSFUSION

Blood is a living tissue; transfusion of it or of its cellular components from a donor to a recipient is a form of transplantation. About 11 to 12 million transfusions are given yearly in the USA, and the number is steadily increasing. The decision to transfuse is a *clinical* judgment that requires weighing the possible benefits and known hazards with alternative treatments. A transfusion not specifically indicated is contraindicated.

PREPARATION OF DONOR AND RECIPIENT BLOOD AND ITS COMPONENTS

Collection and Storage of Blood and Its Components

In the USA, regulations for collecting, storing, and transporting blood and its components are established by the FDA, and sometimes also by state or local health

authorities. The American National Red Cross and American Association of Blood Banks also have standards affecting their respective systems. Screening a donor includes a health interview, testing for Hb, and taking the temperature, pulse rate, and BP. **Causes for disqualification** are history of (1) hepatitis, (2) heart disease, (3) cancer (other than mild treatable forms, such as small skin cancers), (4) severe asthma, (5) bleeding disorder, (6) convulsions, and (7) acquired immunodeficiency syndrome **(AIDS)** or of being in an AIDS-risk group (see Ch. 19). **Temporary deferments** are for (1) malaria, (2) exposure to malaria, (3) exposure to hepatitis, (4) pregnancy, (5) major surgery, (6) hypertension, (7) hypotension, (8) anemia, and (9) the use of certain drugs (eg, patients receiving isotretinoin should not donate blood for 30 days after using it). Some of these criteria protect would-be donors from possible ill effects of donation; others protect the recipient. Donation is limited to once every 2 mo.

Paid donation is discouraged because of abuses inherent in the "skid row" blood banks in big cities, because blood from such banks has 5 to 10 times the usual rate of hepatitis infectivity, and because of a desire to encourage voluntary donation and thus broaden the donor base.

The standard donation is 450 mL, taken into a plastic bag containing adenine-supplemented Citrate Phosphate Dextrose **(CPDA-1)**. CPDA-1 blood may be stored for 35 days. Heparin is a poor preservative but is occasionally used, mostly for pediatric heart surgery or exchange transfusion. Stored whole blood differs considerably from circulating blood. Changes that occur during refrigerated storage are collectively referred to as the **"storage lesion."** Some changes (see TABLE 97–1) may affect certain recipients.

Before use, blood must be classified for suitability. This includes ABO and Rh typing (see below), antibody screening, STS, a test for hepatitis B surface antigen (HBsAg), and tests to detect antibodies to the virus that causes AIDS. The container label and the federally required Circular of Information give the results of these tests and important information and cautions and should be consulted by physicians using blood transfusions.

TABLE 97–1. RBCs AND WHOLE BLOOD STORED IN CPDA-1 ANTICOAGULANT

Weeks in Storage	*0*		*5*	
	RBCs	*WB**	*RBCs*	*WB*
RBC survival at 24 h after transfusion (%)	100	100	71	79
ATP (% of initial value)	100	100	49	57
2, 3-diphosphoglycerate (% of initial value)	100	100	3	5
Plasma K (mEq/u.)**	0.4	1.3	5.5	8.2
Plasma Na (mEq/u.)**	11.8	50.1	7.8	46.5
Plasma Hb (mg/u.)**	5.5	24.6	461	138.3
Total citrate (gm/u.)**	0.43	1.86	—	—
pH	7.55	7.6	6.71	6.98

* Whole blood. ** Assuming 300mL plasma/u.WB, or 70mL/u. RBCs.

(Data in part from G.L. Moore et al: "Some properties of blood stored in anticoagulant CPDA-1 solution. A brief summary," in *Transfusion* Vol. 21, No. 2, March/April 1981. Copyright by J.B. Lippincott Company. Used with permission.)

When conditions permit, the safest blood for transfusion is the patient's own: **autologous transfusion**. As many as 7 or 8 units of blood can be collected from some patients in the few weeks preceding elective surgery, and can then be used for blood replacement during or after surgery. Special procedures are also available for the collection and autotransfusion of blood shed following trauma and during surgical procedures.

The various **components of blood** can be separated, concentrated, and stored individually for precise replacement of patient needs. TABLE 97–2 shows some characteristics of blood and components as ordinarily prepared by the blood bank, not including purified manufactured derivatives that are essentially pharmaceutical rather than blood bank items.

Anticoagulants used to protect RBCs in whole blood storage are not optimal for other components. Labile components are best stored after separation from whole blood. Demand for components such as platelets, antihemophilic factor **(AHF)**, and fresh plasma for fractionation is so high that blood banks must separate fresh components from most blood donations. Whole blood, now considered more of a raw material than a transfusion medium, is used only selectively (see below). For anything other than simple RBC transfusion, consulting the blood bank physician before writing orders allows proper individualization and provides optimal choices and service.

Certain components, particularly granulocytes and some platelet preparations, are prepared by **cytapheresis**. This involves passing a donor's blood through a centrifugal blood cell separator, which harvests the desired component and returns unneeded components (eg, RBCs and plasma) to the donor. Large quantities of WBCs and/or platelets may be collected from an individual donor.

Indications for Clinical Use of Blood and Its Components

RBCs are transfused to replace Hb or O_2 carrying capacity, including blood lost at surgery, and to prime extracorporeal circuits. When volume expansion is required, other fluids can be used concurrently or separately (see SHOCK in Ch. 26).

Frozen-thawed RBCs are costly and mainly used for patients who have multiple blood group antibodies or antibodies to high frequency antigens.

Washed RBCs (by continuous-flow washing) are free of almost all traces of plasma and of most WBCs and platelets. They are suitable for patients who have severe reactions to plasma (eg, severe allergies or IgA immunization), or for those who have leukocyte antibodies and repeated febrile transfusion reactions. Less thorough washing is suitable for patients with heart failure and hypervolemia, or for pediatric heart surgery (to avoid citrate). **Leukocyte-poor RBCs,** prepared by inverted centrifugation, have largely given way to washed RBCs.

Platelet concentrates are used for severe thrombocytopenia (platelet count $< 10{,}000/\mu L$) or for bleeding related to less severe thrombocytopenia (eg, counts between 10,000 and $50{,}000/\mu L$). They are sometimes necessary for surgical patients who tend to bleed following massive transfusion or prolonged periods on extracorporeal circulation. Since a single fresh platelet concentrate in an adult usually causes a rise of about 12,000 in the platelet count, 6 to 8 concentrates are usually needed. A purpuric patient often shows no rise in count because the transfused platelets are immediately consumed. Patients who have had multiple pregnancies and/or previous transfusions may fail to respond to platelet transfusions because they have become alloimmunized to platelet antigens. Such patients may respond to platelets collected by cytapheresis (platelet apheresis) from blood relatives or from donors selected to match the patient's HLA type.

Cryoprecipitated AHF, (factor VIII) is a concentrate prepared by rapid freezing and slow thawing of fresh plasma. It is used mostly for hemophiliacs, in a dosage depending on the patient's size and degree of AHF deficiency. Cryoprecipitate may also be used in von Willebrand's disease (see under PLATELET DISORDERS in Ch. 99), and in

Table 97–2. BLOOD COMPONENTS AS PREPARED FROM CPDA–1* WHOLE BLOOD

Component	*Storage Period*	*Storage Temperature (C)*	*Hct (%)***	*Vol/unit (mL)***	*Remarks*
RBCs	35 days	4 to 6	70	300	
Frozen glycerolized RBCs	2 or more yr	−85 (high glyc.) −190 (low glyc.)	n.a.* n.a.	n.a. n.a.	There are several different freeze-thaw protocols having somewhat different characteristics
Thawed deglycerolized RBCs	24 h	4 to 6	70 to 90	200 to 300	
Washed RBCs	24 h	4 to 6	70 to 90	200 to 230	
WB	35 days	4 to 6	40	513	
WB, heparinized	48 h	4 to 6	40 to 45	477	Deteriorates during 2nd 24 h
Platelet concentrate	5 days	20 to 24	n.a.	30 to 50	Best given fresh. Must be agitated continuously during storage
Cryoprecipitated AHF*	1 yr	below −18	0	10	Contains (/unit) about 100 u. AHF and 250 mg fibrinogen
Fresh frozen plasma	1 yr	below −18	0	220	Contains all clotting factors except platelets, but unconcentrated
Cytapheresis products: Platelets Granulocytes	24 h 5 to 7 days for platelets in some systems	20 to 24	0 to 20	200 to 450	Several technics, giving concentrates of varying characteristics

* CPDA-1 = adenine-supplemented citrate-phosphate-dextrose; RBCs = red blood cells; WB = whole blood; AHF = antihemophilic factor; n.a. = not applicable.
** Approximate.

disseminated intravascular coagulation **(DIC)**. Each concentrate usually contains about 100 u. AHF plus about 250 mg **fibrinogen** and can also be used as a source of the latter, since fibrinogen concentrates are not otherwise available.

Fresh frozen plasma is an unconcentrated source of all clotting factors except platelets. It can be used to correct a bleeding tendency of unknown cause or one associated with liver failure and can supplement RBCs when whole blood is unavailable for exchange transfusion.

Granulocytes were used increasingly in hematology-oncology centers in conjunction with chemotherapy for cancer or leukemia when sepsis occurred during a period of bone marrow ablation. With improved antibiotic therapy, this use has sharply declined.

Whole blood is used for rapid massive blood loss and exchange transfusions. Whole blood also may be necessary if a component is unavailable; conversely, RBCs and other fluids or components can be used instead of whole blood. **Heparinized whole blood,** nearly out of use, is requested for some cases of pediatric heart surgery, primarily to eliminate citrate. RBCs subjected to a single saline wash may be substituted. Heparinized blood has also been used in exchange transfusions for adults with fulminant hepatitis and for infants with severe hemolytic disease.

Immunohematology

Clotted blood samples are optimal for determining antigens on RBCs and antibodies in the serum. Blood from a skin puncture may be added directly to isotonic saline for RBC typing. Washed, resuspended RBCs from anticoagulated blood (citrate, oxalate, or EDTA) may also be used. Cells are tested against antisera, and serum against test RBCs of known type, and the presence or absence of agglutination or hemolysis is recorded. To avoid potentially catastrophic errors, scrupulous attention to technical and clerical details is vital. Reagent manufacturers' instructions should be followed.

ABO and Rh typing: The 4 ABO blood types are determined by testing for the presence or absence of A and B antigens on the RBCs using Anti-A and Anti-B reagents (forward or cell typing), and by testing for Anti-A and Anti-B in the serum using A and B reagent RBCs (serum or reverse typing). Confirmatory cell typing with anti-A,B is also advised. See TABLE 97–3 for the test results seen in each group. Both cell typing and serum typing are done routinely, because results occasionally disagree, and required identification of the true type is done by testing with additional reagents before proceeding with a transfusion. Cell typing is done in test tubes or on slides.

TABLE 97–3. CHARACTERISTICS AND REACTIONS OF THE FOUR ABO BLOOD TYPES

ABO type	*Red Cells*				*Serum*		
	Antigens present	Reactions with reagents			Antibody present	Reactions with reagents	
		Anti-A	*Anti-B*	*Anti-A, B*		*A Cells*	*B Cells*
O	Neither	–	–	–	Anti-A & -B	+	+
A	A	+	–	+	Anti-B	–	+
B	B	–	+	+	Anti-A	+	–
AB	A&B	+	+	+	Neither	–	–

Reverse typing should be done by a tube technic because, with the less sensitive slide method, weakly agglutinating Anti-A and Anti-B may lead to misclassification.

As a rule, blood selected for transfusion must be of the same ABO type as the recipient. In urgent situations, type O RBCs may be used for patients of other blood types, or *either* A or B RBCs may be used for AB recipients (*not* both together).

Rh typing should be done routinely when ABO typing is done, to determine whether the Rh factor $Rh_o(D)$ is present (Rh-positive) or absent (Rh-negative) on the RBCs.

Rh_o variant (D^u) test: Occasionally, RBCs that have a weakly reacting Rh factor, called Rh_o Variant (D^u), will react negatively in the Rh typing test but will be agglutinated by Anti-$Rh_o(D)$ if the more sensitive indirect antiglobulin method is used. Persons positive for D^u are considered Rh-positive. If an apparently Rh-negative blood specimen is from a donor or a pregnant woman or her mate, the test for Rh_o Variant (D^u) should always be done. If the Rh-negative blood specimen is from a prospective recipient of a transfusion, the Rh_o Variant (D^u) test need not be done.

Except for life-threatening emergencies when Rh-negative blood may not be available, Rh-negative patients should always receive Rh-negative blood. Rh-positive patients may receive either Rh-positive or Rh-negative blood.

Screening for unexpected RBC antibodies is done routinely on each specimen submitted for blood grouping; ie, blood from donors, recipients, and prenatal patients. Unexpected antibodies are specific for RBC blood group antigens other than A and B, such as $Rh_o(D)$, Kell (K), Duffy (Fy^a), and hr′(c). Early detection of such antibodies is important because they can cause hemolytic disease of the newborn and serious transfusion reactions, and they greatly complicate and delay compatibility testing **(crossmatching)** and procurement of compatible blood. Serum is screened for the presence of such an antibody by multiple agglutination tests including the sensitive indirect antiglobulin technic, using Group O human reagent RBCs. This reagent is a pool of carefully selected Group O Rh-positive and Rh-negative RBCs that are jointly positive for most important RBC antigens.

Antibody identification: Once an unexpected antibody is demonstrated by screening, its identity should be determined by testing the serum against a panel of Group O reagent RBCs of known antigenic composition. Further studies may be required (eg, antibody elution and absorption and subtyping of the patient's RBCs). Knowing the identity of an irregular RBC antibody is helpful for future transfusion therapy or for prognosis and management of hemolytic disease of the newborn, if such an antibody were found in the serum of a pregnant woman.

Antibody titration: When an irregular RBC antibody, especially of Rh specificity, is identified in the serum of a pregnant woman, it should be titrated to estimate its strength, even though there is poor correlation between the maternal antibody titer and the severity of hemolytic disease in the incompatible fetus. A significant rise in antibody titer means that the fetus carries the antigen and may be affected. In such cases, repeated spectrophotometric examination of the amniotic fluid for bilirubin is the only direct way to monitor the condition of the fetus.

Antiglobulin testing: The **direct antiglobulin (Coombs') test** detects antibodies that coat the patient's RBCs. Washed RBCs are treated with antihuman serum and observed for agglutination. The test is done on the cord blood of infants of Rh-negative mothers, or of any infants suspected of having hemolytic disease of the newborn caused by maternal antibody. This test is also used to investigate anemias. If positive, it suggests an autoimmune hemolytic anemia that may be spontaneous or indicative of underlying lymphoma or SLE.

The **indirect antiglobulin test** aids in the recognition of a serum antibody; it is done by in vitro incubation of normal RBCs with the unknown serum. The test RBCs are then washed in saline and antihuman serum is added: agglutination indicates the

presence of an antibody (adsorbed from the unknown serum) coating the cells. This part of the routine for compatibility testing and antibody detection is sometimes positive in autoimmune hemolytic anemias.

Compabitility testing ("cross-matching"): After determining the ABO and Rh type and doing antibody screening on both prospective recipient and donor bloods, compatibility testing must be done to ensure that the recipient's serum does not contain clinically significant antibodies that will react with the transfused RBCs. Tests are able to detect IgG as well as IgM antibodies. A high-protein procedure or enzyme-modified RBCs may be used, but the indirect antiglobulin test is generally considered essential.

Even if the antibody screening test on the patient's serum is negative, an incompatibility may still be found on testing, since the donor RBCs may have an antigen not present in the reagent RBCs used for screening, or may have an antigen in a more reactive form. If the recipient has a positive screening test, his antibody should be identified and prospective donor blood should be pretested with the corresponding reagent antiserum, if it is available and if there is time, to select blood donor units negative for the RBC antigen concerned. In an emergency, units already tested for compatibility may be transfused before such identification and donor testing have been completed.

As a rule, testing must show compatibility before a transfusion is given. The few exceptions usually concern patients with autoantibodies.

Donor whole blood with an irregular antibody is not usually used for transfusion, but it is suitable for use as frozen thawed or washed RBCs.

Modified testing for compatibility: To reduce costs and simplify pretransfusion testing, several modifications of traditional compatibility tests have been introduced. **Type and Screen** is done when transfusion will probably not be needed; the patient's blood is typed and an antibody screen is done. If the screen is negative and the patient needs blood, RBCs may be released without prior compatibility testing. Of course, if an unexpected antibody is present, blood selection and such testing are required.

A related system is the **Surgical Blood Order Schedule**, whereby the surgeons and the blood bank together define the number of RBC units to be ready routinely for each surgical procedure (zero units would require only a Type and Screen). Experience indicates that both systems work well, effect savings in time and materials, and introduce no significant hazard to patients.

A controversial trend in some large hospitals is to omit the antiglobulin phase of compatibility testing, thus leaving detection of clinically significant IgG antibodies to the antibody screening test. The abbreviated testing will still detect ABO incompatibility, which is the most important. Eliminating the antiglobulin phase is not yet generally recommended, except possibly in large hospitals able to exert careful control over antibody screening technics.

Rh immune globulin: $Rh_o(D)$ immune globulin must be given to every Rh-negative mother immediately after every abortion or delivery (live or stillborn) unless the infant is $Rh_o(D)$- and D^u-negative, unless the mother's serum already contains Anti-$Rh_o(D)$, or unless the mother refuses.

Preparatory testing is done on dual specimens: (1) **Cord blood** is analyzed for ABO and Rh type, including Rh_o Variant (D^u); and a direct antiglobulin test is done. (2) **Maternal blood** drawn immediately postpartum is analyzed for ABO group and Rh type, including Rh_o Variant (D^u), and antibody screening and identification are done. An apparent maternal D^u-positive result may indicate a feto-maternal hemorrhage and should be interpreted cautiously. A truly D^u mother is Rh-positive, but can in rare cases produce anti-Rh. For this reason, some obstetricians recommend giving Rh immune globulin to D^u mothers, although evidence of its effectiveness in these circumstances is lacking.

Genotyping of mates: The mate of every Rh-negative woman should be Rh-typed. If he is also Rh-negative, Rh hemolytic disease in the newborn is most unlikely, although the possibility of other antigens' causing the disease should be borne in mind. If he is Rh-positive, his zygosity for the Rh factor (Rh genotype) should be determined for purposes of genetic counseling, to estimate prognosis, and to plan management if maternal anti-Rh appears during a pregnancy. The probable zygosity is determined by testing the mate's RBCs with the common Rh reagents, anti-Rh_o(D), anti-rh′(C), anti-rh″(E), anti-hr′(c), and anti-hr″(e), and evaluating the results statistically. *If the mate of an Rh-sensitized woman is homozygous Rh-positive, every fetus will be affected with Rh hemolytic disease*; if he is heterozygous, there is a 50% chance that each fetus will be Rh-negative and therefore free from hemolytic disease.

TRANSFUSION TECHNIC

CAUTION: *Before starting any transfusion, both label and report of compatibility testing must be checked to make sure that the blood is indeed for the patient concerned, that it is compatible, and that the component is correct.*

An 18-gauge needle, or larger, is desirable. Smaller needles may have to be used in young people, but hemolysis may occur if excess pressure is necessary. Since most transfusions are RBCs, which are more viscous than whole blood, 50 to 100 mL of 0.9% sodium chloride solution are allowed to run into the RBCs before starting. A Y blood-administration set with a filter should be used, with the RBCs attached to one limb and isotonic saline to the other. *No IV solution other than 0.9% sodium chloride solution should be allowed into the blood bag or in the same tubing with blood, since many solutions exert deleterious effects* (eg, D/W causes clumping and decreased survival of RBCs; Ringer's solution causes clotting).

Transfusion of a single unit of RBCs should not ordinarily take > 2 h. Close observation is important during the first 15 min, since most severe reactions will be evident by then. The patient should be kept warm and well covered to prevent chills that might otherwise be interpreted as a reaction. Elective transfusions at night should be discouraged, since observation of the patient is more difficult and sleep is disturbed.

If any untoward reaction appears to be related to transfusion (see COMPLICATIONS OF TRANSFUSION, below), the transfusion should be stopped and the blood bank notified so that an investigation can begin. *That unit should not be restarted.* Unless the clinical situation is urgent, it is best to delay further transfusions until the cause of the reaction is known.

Prolonged or divided transfusions (1/2 one day, 1/2 the next) should be avoided, since this increases the hazard of bacterial growth. When incipient heart failure or hypervolemia is a concern, washed RBCs should be used and a whole unit given in the usual way. Otherwise, to prevent overload, some of the patient's own blood may have to be removed as RBCs are given. For small pediatric transfusions, the blood bank can provide blood or RBCs in multiple interconnected bags that can be subdivided safely.

COMPLICATIONS OF TRANSFUSION

Reactions that accompany or follow IV administration of blood or blood components. The more serious reactions occur during the transfusion.

HEMOLYTIC REACTIONS

Reactions accompanied by hemolysis of the recipient's or the donor's RBCs—usually the latter—during or following the administration of solutions, plasma, blood, or blood components. The most severe reaction occurs when donor RBCs are hemolyzed by antibody in the recipient's plasma.

Etiology

Hemolysis can result from blood group incompatibility, incompatible plasma or serum, hemolyzed or fragile RBCs (eg, by overwarming stored blood or contact with inappropriate IV solutions), injections of distilled water or nonisotonic solutions, or instillation of water into the bladder during prostate or urinary bladder operations.

Incompatibility is the most frequent cause of hemolysis despite advances in blood typing and testing. Human error (eg, mislabeling or mixing up the samples or blood containers) is usually responsible. Poor laboratory technic, including inadequate compatibility testing or incorrect identification of the ABO group or Rh type of both donor and recipient, is less common.

Antibodies against blood group antigens other than ABO or Rh may occur naturally or may be acquired as a result of transfusion or pregnancy. They can cause a hemolytic transfusion reaction or fetal erythroblastosis. The most important of these are anti-Kell (K) and anti-Duffy (Fy^a). Recipients who have formed any clinically significant blood group antibody must *always* receive blood negative for the antigen in question. Although compatibility testing will detect almost all such antibodies, occasionally a patient will have a hemolytic reaction despite negative pretransfusion tests.

Group O whole blood, the plasma of which contains Anti-A and Anti-B of the hemolytic or IgG (incomplete) form, may be dangerous when given in emergencies to a recipient with another blood group. The plasma containing most of the antibody should be removed first, which means that *Group O RBCs should be used rather than whole blood.* Tests to determine dangerous levels of Anti-A and Anti-B are unreliable. Adding specific A and B substances to Group O blood is *not* recommended, since the dangerous IgG antibodies are not neutralized and the material itself may cause anaphylactic reactions.

Symptoms, Signs, and Diagnosis

Hemolytic reactions vary in severity depending on the degree of incompatibility, the amount of blood given, the rate of administration, and the integrity of the kidney, liver, and heart. Onset is usually acute and may occur during or immediately following a blood transfusion; rarely, later. The patient complains of discomfort and anxiety, or may have no symptoms. He may have difficulty in breathing, precordial oppression, a bursting sensation in the head, flushing of the face, and severe pain in the neck, the chest, and especially the lumbar area. Evidence of shock may appear, with a rapid feeble pulse, cold clammy skin, dyspnea, fall in BP, nausea, and vomiting. This acute phase usually develops within 1 h. Free Hb may be found in the plasma and urine, followed by an elevated serum bilirubin and clinical jaundice.

After the acute phase, one of several courses may follow: (1) no further symptoms; (2) temporary oliguria with mild N retention, then complete recovery; (3) more persistent oliguria, then possibly anuria and uremia, with death in 5 to 14 days unless adequate treatment is instituted in the early phases (see below). Prolonged oliguria is a sign of poor prognosis. When recovery occurs, it is usually marked by diuresis with elimination of retained nitrogenous wastes.

Hemolytic reactions may occur under general anesthesia, when most of the symptoms are masked. The only evidence may be uncontrollable bleeding at the site of incision and from mucous membranes, caused by an associated DIC syndrome. An important quick aid to diagnosis is to take a blood sample from the patient immediately, centrifuge it, and examine it visually for serum Hb. Significant hemolysis will be clearly visible as a pink to dark red color.

For medicolegal reasons, pretransfusion specimens and post-transfusion samples of both donor and patient blood should again be typed and tested for compatibility to check on possible technical or clerical errors or mislabeling of the initial samples

Prognosis

This depends primarily on the amount of blood given, the degree of incompatibility, and the patient's condition. Shock during the reaction is a grave sign. Diuresis is usually a happy sign. Significant permanent kidney damage is unusual.

Prophylaxis

Hemolytic reactions may be avoided by meticulous identification and indelible labeling of patient blood samples intended for compatibility testing, by equally careful identification of patient and donor blood at the time of transfusion, by allowing 15 min to give the first 50 mL, and by scrupulous adherence to the advice given under TRANSFUSION TECHNIC, above.

Treatment

The transfusion should be stopped immediately. Blankets may be used to relieve chills. To establish osmotic diuresis, an infusion of 20 gm of mannitol (eg, 100 mL of 20% solution) should be started at once and continued at 10 to 15 mL/min until 1000 mL have been given. Consultation with a nephrologist should be sought at the earliest possible stage.

If diuresis ensues, the mannitol infusion should be continued to a maximum of 100 gm/day, or volume may be maintained with other IV fluids until hemoglobinemia and hemoglobinuria have cleared. Rather than mannitol, some authorities recommend the administration of furosemide, with a starting dose of 80 to 120 mg, then further doses if the urinary flow falls below 30 mL/h. An anuric patient should be treated for acute renal failure (see Ch. 147).

FEBRILE REACTIONS

Reactions consisting of chills, fever with a rise of at least 1 C, and sometimes headache and back pain, rarely progressing to cyanosis and shock.

In some patients, after many transfusions or pregnancies, leukocyte antibodies appear in response to antigens of transfused or fetal WBCs. These antibodies may react with the WBCs in succeeding transfusions to produce a reaction. When symptoms occur repeatedly with the use of otherwise compatible blood, further transfusions should be of washed RBCs. The rare problem of febrile reactions caused by bacterial pyrogens in solutions or tubing is almost eliminated by using disposable equipment.

ALLERGIC REACTIONS

Reactions due to hypersensitivity of the patient to an unknown component in donor blood are common, usually due to allergens in donor plasma, or, less often, to antibodies from an allergic donor. Immunized IgA-deficient patients may react violently (anaphylaxis) to IgA in donor plasma.

Symptoms and Signs

Allergic reactions are usually mild, with urticaria, edema, occasional dizziness, and headache during or immediately after the transfusion. Less frequently, dyspnea, wheezing, and incontinence may be present, indicating a generalized spasm of smooth muscle. Rarely, anaphylactic shock may occur.

Prophylaxis and Treatment

In a patient with a history of known allergies or an allergic transfusion reaction, an antihistamine may be given immediately before or at the beginning of the transfusion (eg, diphenhydramine 50 mg orally or IM). *It must never be mixed with the blood.*

The transfusion is stopped immediately. An antihistamine is usually sufficient in mild cases (eg, diphenhydramine 50 mg IM). For more severe reactions, epinephrine 0.5 to 1 mL of 1:1000 solution s.c. (or, in extreme emergencies, 0.05 to 0.2 mL diluted and injected slowly IV) should be given. A parenteral corticosteroid (eg, dexamethasone sodium phosphate, 4 to 20 mg IV) may occasionally be required.

CIRCULATORY OVERLOADING

In heart disease with anemia, when cardiac reserve is likely to be deficient, transfusions may raise the venous pressure and cause congestive heart failure.

Prophylaxis: When such patients must be transfused, *whole blood is contraindicated.* A rise in venous pressure can be avoided by infusing packed RBCs at a slow-to-moderate rate. The patient should be observed for signs of increased venous pressure or pulmonary congestion. If possible, direct observation of venous pressure during the infusion is a useful precaution. Prolonged transfusions pose a hazard of bacterial growth because blood quickly reaches room temperature. If packed RBCs cause congestion, or must be given at > 2 h/u., it is better to use washed RBCs.

Treatment: The transfusion should be discontinued, and treatment for heart failure should begin immediately (see in discussion of acute pulmonary edema associated with left ventricular failure under HEART FAILURE in Ch. 27).

AIR EMBOLISM

Transmission of large amounts of air into a vein can cause foaming of blood in the heart with consequent inefficiency of pumping, leading to heart failure. It is largely a complication of pressure infusion of blood from rigid glass bottles, but can also happen when an IV set is changed or a plastic blood bag is erroneously vented.

Prophylaxis consists of guarding attentively against air in tubing with any pressure infusion and when changing IV sets. **Treatment** involves turning the patient on his left side, head down, to allow the air to escape a little at a time from the right atrium.

MICROAGGREGATES

Standard transfusion sets include a filter that traps the few visible clots and fibrin shreds present in stored blood units. In proportion to the duration of storage, blood also forms microaggregates—microscopic collections of platelets, leukocytes, and fibrin. These microaggregates can be detected in the lungs after massive transfusions and have been incriminated as a cause of the syndrome of post-traumatic pulmonary insufficiency, though direct evidence is lacking.

This hazard is avoided by using special filters that remove particles as small as 20 to 40 μm. Their use is advised only for patients likely to receive large amounts of blood that has been stored > 5 or 6 days. (CAUTION: *These filters may also remove platelets and should not be used for platelet transfusions.*)

EFFECTS OF COLD

Rapid transfusion of cold blood can chill the patient's heart and cause arrhythmia or arrest. This is avoided by using an IV set that includes a heat exchange device to warm blood gently during delivery. However, blood should not be warmed above 37 C (98.6 F). Warming devices applied to the blood container itself (eg, microwave warmers) are contraindicated because (1) a high incidence of hemolysis occurs, (2) any interruption in transfusion may encourage bacterial growth in unused warmed blood and (3) the blood bank will not know if unused blood has been warmed and rechilled

COMPLICATIONS OF MASSIVE TRANSFUSION

Deleterious effects of storage on donor blood may become important (though such complications seldom occur) when a patient receives > 20 u./day of stored blood, and his own blood is in effect "washed out."

Bleeding tendency is manifested by abnormal oozing and continued bleeding from raw and cut surfaces, because the patient has lost platelets and stored blood does not contain useful numbers. Since clotting factors other than platelets are seldom involved, platelet concentrates should be given; 4 concentrates are usually enough for an adult. If they are unavailable, very freshly collected RBCs or whole blood will usually be effective, but neither component should be given to a patient on extracorporeal circulation until the pump has been discontinued.

Citrate and K: Patients with liver failure may be unable to metabolize citrate; those with chronic renal disease may have a problem with elevated K. These overrated hazards are reduced by removal of plasma from donor blood. K accumulation is insignificant in blood stored < 1 wk (see TABLE 97–1).

OXYGEN AFFINITY

Older stored blood has an increased affinity for O_2, caused by a decrease in RBC 2,3-diphosphoglycerate **(DPG)**, resulting in slower release of O_2 to the tissues. With the possible exception of exchange transfusions in erythroblastotic infants and some patients with severe cardiac deficiency, little clinical evidence shows that DPG deficiency has a significant effect on the recipient; in fact, it is rapidly restored after transfusion. RBCs collected in CPDA-1 have adequate DPG during the first 2 wk of storage.

INVESTIGATION AND REPORTING OF REACTIONS

All transfusion reactions, even those that seem inconsequential, should be investigated and reported in writing. The investigation can be minimal in minor reactions (eg, allergic), but should be full and complete for any suspected hemolytic reactions. A scheme of investigation is given in TABLE 97–4. The report may omit laboratory details, although the blood bank should keep a permanent record of these, but it should include an interpretation of results as well as recommendations regarding the handling of future transfusion therapy.

GRAFT VERSUS HOST DISEASE (GVHD)

GVHD usually is caused by the engraftment of immunocompetent lymphocytes from bone marrow transplants to an immunodepressed patient (see Ch. 22). The syndrome consists of fever, skin and GI lesions, and pancytopenia, and is often fatal. However, even small numbers of viable lymphocytes in blood or blood component transfusions are capable of spontaneous division and can cause the disease. Patients at risk are those receiving chemotherapy or radiotherapy for neuroblastoma, Hodgkin's or non-Hodgkin's lymphoma, some acute leukemias, patients with severe immune deficiencies, fetuses receiving intrauterine transfusions, and possibly some premature newborns. Effective prevention is by irradiation of all blood products intended for transfusion to such patients. A dosage of 1500 to 3000 rad does not damage blood components other than lymphocytes and seems to be clinically adequate.

DISEASE TRANSMISSION

Hepatitis: Virus hepatitis may follow the infusion of whole blood, plasma, or other products prepared from human blood, notably AHF and factor IX concentrate. Serum

TABLE 97–4. SCHEDULE OF INVESTIGATION OF REPORTED TRANSFUSION REACTIONS

I. All reported reactions

A. Specimens needed:
  1. Pretransfusion blood of recipient
  2. Posttransfusion blood of recipient

B. Investigation (numbers refer to specimens listed above)
  Check donor and patient identification and crossmatch report
  Repeat ABO and Rh typing (2)
  Direct antiglobulin test (2)
  Examine for visible hemolysis (2); if necessary, compare (2) with (1)

If these procedures reveal no evidence of incompatibility or hemolysis and if there is no additional information to arouse suspicion, no further investigation is needed. Otherwise, proceed as follows:

II. If there is evidence of hemolysis or incompatible transfusion*

A. Specimens needed:
  1. Pretransfusion blood of recipient
  2. Posttransfusion blood of recipient
  3. Pilot samples of donor blood
  4. Blood from container implicated in reaction
  5. Posttransfusion urine

B. Immunologic investigation
  Repeat ABO, Rh, and direct antiglobulin test (1,3,4)
  Repeat crossmatch (1,2,3,4 if indicated—major; minor only if indicated)
  Repeat antibody screen (1,2,3—special, sensitive technics if necessary)
  Identification of any unexpected antibody or incompatibility

C. Other procedures as indicated
  Serum haptoglobin (1,2)
  Bacteriologic smear and culture (4)
  Serum urea and bilirubin (1,2)
  Urine hemoglobin (5)
  Urine hemosiderin (5)
  Nonimmune causes of hemolysis

* The procedures and specimens listed are generally applicable. Different approaches may be needed for particular cases.

(From *Practical Blood Transfusion*, p. 266, by D. W. Huestis, J. R. Bove, and S. Busch, ed. 3, 1981. Used with permission of Little, Brown and Company.)

albumin and plasma protein fractions that have been heated to 60 C for 10 h during preparation are, with rare exceptions, noninfectious. Depending on the geographic area and the methods used for testing, **hepatitis B surface antigen** (HBsAg) is detectable in the blood of 0.05% to 2% of donors. In pooled human plasma products such as antihemophilic factor, it is disseminated in accordance with the size of the pool. It is active in freshly frozen and liquid plasma.

Laboratory tests for HBsAg (required on all donor blood) detect 30 to 60% of carriers; the remainder are undetectable by present methods. This test will not detect **hepatitis A (infectious)** or the non-A–non-B virus or viruses that now cause most cases of post-transfusion hepatitis. Avoidance of unnecessary transfusions and of donor populations with a higher prevalence of hepatitis (eg, drug addicts, commercial donors) are important preventive measures.

Acquired immune deficiency syndrome (AIDS): The causative agent of this condition has been identified as human immunodeficiency virus **(HIV)**; epidemiologic evidence indicates that it is infectious and blood-borne. A few patients with AIDS, not belonging to any of the known high-risk groups, have a history of receiving blood products

and their disease is considered "transfusion-associated." AIDS cases among hemophiliacs apparently fall into this category. Responsible authorities recommend that prospective blood donors be given a statement pointing out the high-risk groups who might be AIDS carriers, and that members of such groups (eg, men with homosexual exposure) be given an opportunity unobtrusively and confidentially to disqualify themselves or to indicate that their blood not be used for transfusion.

Since March 1985, virtually all blood banks in the USA have been testing all blood donations for the presence of anti-HIV. Six months experience with the use of this antibody screen and the discarding of blood with a positive result has led to the conclusion that the test has markedly reduced the number of potentially AIDS-infectious blood units in the blood supply (see Ch. 19).

Cytomegalovirus (CMV) can be transmitted by leukocytes in transfused blood. Usually its effects are either absent or mild, and need cause no concern. However, CMV may cause serious or even fatal disease in immunocompromised patients who lack CMV antibody (eg, transplant recipients, newborns weighing < 1250 gm). CMV risk varies considerably in different geographic areas. Where there is evidence of significant CMV risk, CMV-seronegative patients of the types specified above should probably receive CMV-seronegative blood products. At this time, only some blood banks have this service available, and CMV testing is not required by federal regulations or accrediting authorities.

Bacterial infection: Despite careful preparation, from 2 to 5% of all blood drawn contains a few bacteria, presumably from the donor's skin. Most organisms will not grow in properly refrigerated blood (4 to 10 C), but some will, mainly gram-negatives of the coliform or aerogenes groups. Transfusion of heavily contaminated blood may be fatal. Procedures that allow blood to reach room temperature (prolonged transfusions or warming blood) may greatly accelerate the growth of any bacteria, and are potentially hazardous.

Malaria is transmitted easily by infected donor blood. Many donors are unaware that they have malaria, certain varieties of which may be latent and transmissible for 10 to 15 yr. All prospective donors must be asked whether they have ever had malaria or have been in a region where it is prevalent. Donors who have had malaria or suppressive antimalarial therapy are disqualified for 3 yr; those who have been exposed to malaria without suppressive therapy should be deferred for 6 mo. Storage does not render blood safe.

Syphilis may be transmitted by fresh blood from a donor with the disease, but the incidence is very rare. Storing the blood for 96 h or more at 4 to 10 C kills the spirochete. Federal regulations require an STS on all donor blood, but infective donors are often in a seronegative phase.

---

98. MYELOPROLIFERATIVE DISORDERS

A group of disorders characterized by abnormal proliferation by 1 or more hematopoietic cell lines or connective tissue elements. Four disorders are generally included: (1) polycythemia vera, (2) myelofibrosis (agnogenic myeloid metaplasia), (3) chronic myelogenous leukemia **(CML)**, and (4) primary (essential) thrombocythemia. Some hematologists also include acute leukemia, especially erythroleukemia, and paroxysmal nocturnal hemoglobinuria; most argue that these clonal disorders are sufficiently different from the basic 4 to omit them.

Each disorder is identified according to its predominant feature or site of proliferation (see TABLE 98–1). Despite overlap, each has a somewhat typical constellation of clinical features, laboratory findings, and course. Although proliferation of 1 particular

TABLE 98–1. CLASSIFICATION OF MYELOPROLIFERATIVE DISORDERS

Predominant Finding	*Diagnosis*
Erythrocytosis	Polycythemia vera (Vaquez disease)
Granulocytosis	Chronic myelogenous (granulocytic) leukemia
Thrombocytosis	Essential thrombocythemia (hemorrhagic thrombocythemia)
Marrow fibrosis with extramedullary hematopoiesis	Myelofibrosis (and/or myelosclerosis) with myeloid metaplasia (agnogenic myeloid metaplasia)

cell line may dominate the clinical picture, by using cytogenetic markers and isoenzyme studies, each disorder has been shown to be caused by a clonal proliferation arising at the level of a pluripotent stem cell, causing varying degrees of abnormal proliferation of erythroid, myeloid, and megakaryocytic precursors in the bone marrow. Peripheral RBCs, granulocytes, and platelets all arise from the abnormal clone. The bone marrow fibroblast is not part of this abnormal clone. All myeloproliferative disorders have a variable tendency to terminate in acute leukemia.

POLYCYTHEMIA VERA (PV)

(Primary Polycythemia; Vaquez Disease)

A chronic myeloproliferative disorder of unknown cause characterized by an increase in Hg concentration and RBC mass (erythrocytosis).

Etiology, Incidence, and Pathophysiology

PV occurs in about 5:million persons, and more often in Jews and males (abou 1.4:1). At time of diagnosis, the mean age is 60 yr (with a range from 15 to 90 yr, bu rarely in childhood); 5% of patients are < 40 at age of onset.

The bone marrow sometimes appears normal, but usually is hypercellular; hyperpla sia involves all marrow elements and replaces marrow fat. There is increased produc tion and turnover of RBCs, neutrophils, and platelets. Increased megakaryocytes ma be present in "clumps". Marrow iron is absent in > 90% of patients, even whe phlebotomy has not been done.

By studying female patients with PV who are heterozygous at the X-chromosome linked locus for G6PD, it has been shown that RBCs, granulocytes, and platelets al have the same G6PD isoenzyme, supporting a clonal origin of this disorder at a plur ipotent stem cell level. The cause of this proliferation is unknown.

Eventually, about 25% of patients have a reduction in RBC survival, with a failure t increase further erythropoiesis adequately; anemia and myelofibrosis develop. Extra medullary hematopoiesis takes place in the spleen, liver, and other sites with th potential for blood cell formation.

Symptoms and Signs

Complaints usually can be attributed to the expanded blood volume and hypervi cosity, which may manifest as weakness, headache, lightheadness, visual disturbance fatigue, or dyspnea. A bleeding diathesis is common. Pruritus is a frequent complain particularly after a hot bath. The face may be red, and the retinal veins engorge Hepatomegaly is frequent, and > 75% of patients have splenomegaly (which may b massive, extending to the pelvic brim), and following splenic infarction, a friction ru may be heard. Patients may present initially with one of the medical problems fr quently associated with PV, including peptic ulcer disease, thrombosis, Budd-Chia syndrome, and bone pain. Complications of hyperuricemia (including gout and ren calculi) tend to occur later in PV. Some patients are asymptomatic and are first su pected on routine blood examination.

TABLE 98–2. CRITERIA FOR DIAGNOSIS OF POLYCYTHEMIA VERA

Major Criteria	*Minor Criteria*
Increased RBC mass ≥ 36 mL/kg in a man ≥ 32 mL/kg in a woman **Arterial O_2 saturation ≥ 92%** **Splenomegaly**	Thrombocytosis > 400 × $10^3/\mu L$ Leukocytosis > 12 × $10^3/\mu L$ Leukocyte alkaline phosphotase activity > 100 (no fever or infection) Serum B_{12} > 900 pg/mL or unsaturated B_{12}-binding capacity > 2200 pg/mL

Diagnosis is polycythemia vera if patient has all 3 major criteria *or* the first 2 major criteria plus any 2 minor criteria.

(From "The Management of Polycythaemia Vera" by L. R. Wasserman, in *British Journal of Haematology,* Vol. 21, 1971. Published by Blackwell Scientific Publications Ltd. Used with permission of the publisher and the author.)

Eventually, erythroid activity in the marrow decreases. Immature WBCs and RBC precursors are found in the peripheral blood. There is marked aniso- and poikilocytosis with microcytes, elliptocytes, and teardrop cells. Increasing leukocytosis and thrombocytosis may be seen. The bone marrow shows increased reticulin, and progressive splenomegaly due to extramedullary hematopoiesis may be found. Increased numbers of immature WBCs and RBCs, and teardrop RBCs may be present in the blood. During this "spent phase", anemia and thrombocytopenia may eventually develop.

Problems with hemostasis frequently occur due to abnormalities of platelet function. Since surgical procedures may be hazardous, elective surgery should be postponed until the disease is under control (Hct < 42%, platelets < 600,000).

Diagnosis and Differential Diagnosis

PV must be considered in any man with a Hct > 54% and any woman with a Hct > 49%. Since PV is a panmyelosis, its diagnosis is clear in patients with elevations of all 3 peripheral blood components, splenomegaly, and no evidence for secondary polycythemia. Diagnostic guidelines are shown in TABLE 98–2.

Since the Hct is a ratio between the number of circulating RBCs per unit volume of whole blood, an elevated Hct may be caused by a decreased plasma volume. Thus, true erythrocytosis is based on demonstrating an increased RBC mass. When measured with radioactive chromium (**^{51}Cr**)-labeled erythrocytes, a RBC cell mass > 36 mL/kg in men (normal 28.3 ± 2.8 mL/kg) and 32 mL/kg in women (normal 25.4 ± 2.6 mL/kg) is considered abnormal. In relative (spurious) erythrocytosis, the RBC mass is normal and the elevated Hct is caused by a decreased plasma volume (see TABLE 98–3). This is also referred to as stress polycythemia or **Gaisböck's syndrome**.

TABLE 98–3. CLASSIFICATION OF ERYTHROCYTOSIS

Type	*Etiology*
Primary	Polycythemia vera
Secondary	Decreased tissue oxygenation: lung disease; high altitude; intracardiac shunts; hypoventilation syndromes; abnormal Hbs, including carboxyhemoglobinemia Aberrant erythropoietin production: tumors, cysts
Relative (spurious)	Hemoconcentration: diuretics; burns; diarrhea "Stress" (Gaisböck's syndrome)

TABLE 98–4. LABORATORY EVALUATION OF A PATIENT WITH ABSOLUTE ERYTHROCYTOSIS

Platelet count	B_{12} and B_{12}-binding capacity
WBC count and differential	Urinalysis
Arterial blood gas	Renal sonography, IVP, or CT
Carboxyhemoglobin	P_{50} (partial pressure of O_2 at which Hb becomes 50% saturated
Leukocyte alkaline phosphatase	

When an elevated RBC mass has been established, other causes for erythrocytosis must be sought. Possibilities are numerous (see TABLE 98–3). Most commonly encountered are the secondary erythrocytosis caused by lung disease, smokers' polycythemia caused by elevated carboxyhemoglobin (**HbCO**) levels, and tumors producing erythropoietic substances. Laboratory tests for differential diagnosis are outlined in TABLE 98–4, and suggested steps in the evaluation of erythrocytosis in FIG. 98–1.

If the arterial hemoglobin O_2 concentration is < 92%, tissue hypoxia may underlie the erythrocytosis. The leukocyte alkaline phosphatase (**LAP**) score is a histochemical stain for a neutrophil enzyme. The LAP score is elevated in 75% of patients with PV, but is usually normal in patients with other causes of erythrocytosis. However, because fever, infection, or inflammation can elevate the LAP score, it is confirmatory only in the absence of these stimuli. Urinalysis may detect microscopic hematuria, and renal sonography, IVP, or CT may reveal a renal lesion causing secondary erythrocytosis. The P_{50} (*the partial pressure of O_2 at which Hb becomes 50% saturated*) is a measure of the affinity of Hb for O_2 and is used to exclude a high affinity Hg as the cause of erythrocytosis.

Patients with PV have low or undetectable serum erythropoietin levels; those with hypoxia-induced erythrocytosis have elevated serum erythropoietin levels, whereas patients with tumor-associated erythrocytosis have normal or elevated erythropoietin

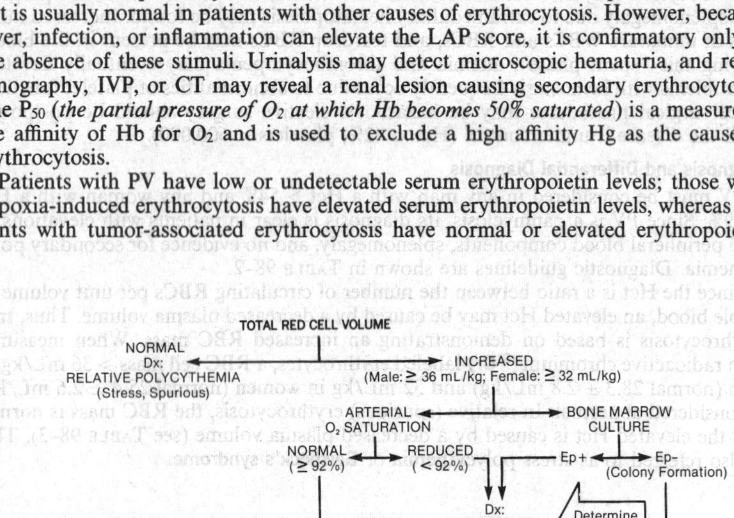

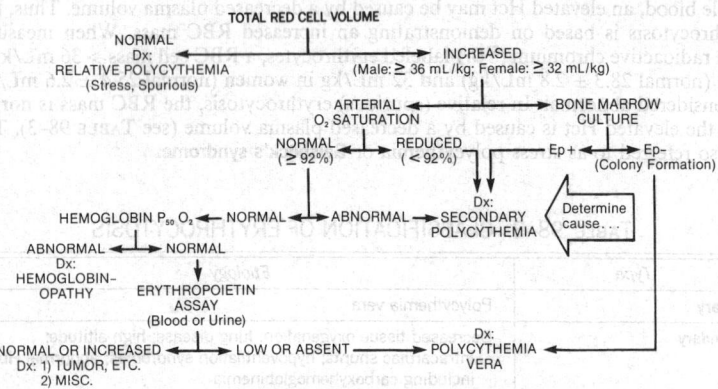

FIG. 98–1. Decision tree: evaluation of erythrocytosis. Ep = erythropoietin; Dx = diagnosis. (Mo- fied by N. I. Berlin and L. R. Wasserman from "Diagnosis and Classification of the Polycythemias" N. I. Berlin in *Seminars in Hematology*, Vol. 12, No. 4, October 1975. Published by Grune & Stratt Inc. Used with permission.)

levels. Bone marrow from patients with PV has the autonomous capacity to form endogenous erythroid colonies in culture; ie, there is no requirement for added erythropoietin. In contrast, in healthy patients or those with secondary polycythemia, the marrow requires added erythropoietin for erythroid colony formation.

Other laboratory abnormalities may occur in PV: Hyperuricemia and hyperuricosuria occur in ≥ 30% of patients, qualitative abnormalities in platelet function may be present, and vitamin B_{12} and B_{12}-binding capacity are frequently elevated.

Prognosis

Untreated, 50% of patients die within 18 mo of diagnosis. With therapy, median survival ranges from 7 to 15 yr. Thrombosis is the most common cause of death, followed by complications of myeloid metaplasia, hemorrhage, and development of leukemia.

The incidence of transformation into an acute leukemia is greater in patients treated with radioactive phosphate (**^{32}P**) or alkylating agents than those treated with phlebotomy alone, and these patients are more resistant to induction chemotherapy than those with de novo leukemia.

Treatment

Since PV is the only form of erythrocytosis for which myelosuppressive therapy may be indicated, accurate diagnosis is critical. Therapy must be individualized according to age, sex, medical status, clinical manifestations, and hematologic findings.

Phlebotomy is an integral part of all therapeutic regimens and may be the only therapy. It is the treatment of choice for women in the childbearing age and patients under age 40, since it is not mutagenic and symptoms of hypervolemia are eliminated. Patients should initially be phlebotomized 300 to 500 mL every other day until the Hct is < 45%. Elderly patients and those with cardio- or cerebrovascular disease should be phlebotomized more cautiously (200 to 300 mL twice/wk). Once the Hct is normal, the patient should be seen monthly and phlebotomized if the Hct is > 45%. Emergency surgery should be preceded by sufficient phlebotomy to reduce the RBC volume to normal. If necessary, intravascular volume can be maintained with crystalloid or colloid solutions.

Myelosuppressive therapy may be indicated in patients with platelet counts > 1 $\times 10^6/\mu L$, with discomfort from visceral enlargement, with thrombosis, with symptoms from hypermetabolism or uncontrolled pruritus, and in elderly patients or those with cardiovascular disease who do not tolerate phlebotomy well.

^{32}P, used for > 30 yr, has a success rate of 80 to 90%. Remissions may last 6 mo to several years. It is well tolerated and requires fewer follow-up visits when disease control is achieved. However, ^{32}P is associated with an increased incidence of acute leukemic transformation, and this form of therapy requires careful patient selection (eg, with patients > 60 to 70 yr old).

After phlebotomizing the patient to a normal Hct (40 to 45%), ^{32}P 2.7 mCi/sq m BSA is given IV, the total dose not exceeding 5 mCi. This dose usually normalizes the platelet count and Hct within 4 to 8 wk. After 3 mo, if control has not been achieved and the platelet count is > 100,000 and the WBC count > 3500, ^{32}P can be repeated and the dose increased by 25% to a total not to exceed 7 mCi. After an additional 3 mo, if remission has not been achieved, a further dose may be given up to the maximum dose of 7 mCi. If there is no response after 3 injections during the first year of therapy, the patient should be managed with either phlebotomy or hydroxyurea.

Because alkylating agents are recognized to be leukemogenic, they should be avoided. However, **hydroxyurea,** which acts by inhibiting the enzyme ribonucleoside diphosphate reductase, has been used successfully in younger patients when myelosuppressive therapy is indicated and is not currently known to be leukemogenic. Patients are phlebotomized to a normal Hct (40 to 45%) and placed on hydroxyurea 10 to 15

mg/kg/day. The patient is monitored with a weekly blood count. When a steady state is achieved, the interval between blood counts is lengthened to 2 wk and then 4 wk. If the WBC falls to < 4,000 or the platelet count to < 100,000, hydroxyurea is withheld and reinstituted at 50% of the dose when the blood count normalizes. For poorly controlled patients who require frequent phlebotomies or are thrombocythemic (platelet counts > 600,000), the dose can be increased by 5 mg/kg/day at monthly intervals with frequent monitoring until control is achieved. Acute toxicity is minimal; occasionally patients develop a rash, GI complaints, or fever. Long term effects are unknown.

Hyperuricemia can be managed with allopurinol orally (300 mg/day). Pruritus may be managed with antihistamines, but is frequently difficult to control. After bathing, the skin should be dried gently. Oral doses of cholestyramine 4 gm tid, cyproheptadine 4 to 16 mg qid, or cimetidine 300 mg qid have also been used successfully. For erythromelalgia (tender, inflamed toes), aspirin has been shown to provide symptomatic relief.

SECONDARY ERYTHROCYTOSIS

(Secondary Polycythemia)

Smoking may cause reversible polycythemia. Carboxyhemoglobin **(HbCO)** is a result of inhaling tobacco smoke. Erythrocytosis is caused by (1) tissue anoxia (since Hb bound to CO is incapable of transporting O_2) and (2) impaired unloading of O_2 from Hb to the tissues shown by the left shift of the HbO_2 dissociation curve.

Arterial hypoxemia: Patients with chronic lung disease or right to left intracardiac shunts with hypoxemia may develop erythrocytosis. With prolonged exposure to high altitudes (see Ch. 263), or in central hypoventilation syndromes, the RBC mass may also increase. **Therapy** for patients with lung disease is aimed at improving pulmonary function. O_2 therapy may be required, and judicious phlebotomy will decrease viscosity and improve the patient's sense of well being.

High O_2 affinity hemoglobinopathies: This diagnosis is suggested if there is a family history of erythrocytosis; it is established by measuring the P_{50} (see above) and, if possible, determining the complete HbO_2 dissociation curve. Standard Hb electrophoresis usually will not disclose an abnormal Hb band, and cannot be relied on to exclude this cause of erythrocytosis.

Tumor-associated erythrocytosis: Due to increased erythropoietin secretion, renal tumors and cysts can be associated with polycythemia. Removal of the lesion may be curative. Hepatomas, cerebellar hemangioblastomas, and uterine leiomyomas can also cause a paraneoplastic erythrocytosis.

MYELOFIBROSIS

(Agnogenic Myeloid Metaplasia)

A chronic, usually idiopathic disease characterized by bone marrow fibrosis, splenomegaly, and a leukoerythroblastic anemia with teardrop erythrocytes.

Etiology and Pathogenesis

The cause of myelofibrosis is unknown. It may complicate chronic myelogenous leukemia **(CML)** and be seen in 15 to 30% of patients with polycythemia vera **(PV)** if they survive long enough. Syndromes similar to idiopathic myelofibrosis **(IMF)** have been observed in association with a variety of neoplasms and infections, as well as after exposure to certain toxins (see TABLE 98–5). Malignant or acute myelofibrosis, an unusual variant, has a more rapidly progressive downhill course.

The typical syndrome of IMF has a peak incidence between 50 and 70 yr, with a median survival of 10 yr from estimated onset. Studies based on G6PD isoenzymes

TABLE 98–5. CONDITIONS ASSOCIATED WITH MYELOFIBROSIS

Malignant disease: Leukemias, polycythemia vera, multiple myeloma, Hodgkin's disease, non-Hodgkin's lymphoma, carcinoma
Infection: TB, osteomyelitis
Toxin: x- or γ-radiation, benzene

and chromosome abnormalities suggest that clonal proliferation of an abnormal myeloid stem cell has occurred. Since marrow fibroblasts do not arise from the same hematopoietic clone, as confirmed by analysis of marrow fibroblasts after marrow transplantation, it is believed that a major feature of the disease, the myelofibrosis, is a complicating, reactive feature of the primary disease process.

Symptoms and Signs

In early stages the patient may be asymptomatic. Splenomegaly or abnormal blood findings may be discovered on routine examination. With time, general malaise, weight loss, and symptoms attributed to splenic enlargement or infarction may occur. Hepatomegaly is found in 50% of patients. Lymphadenopathy is not typical, although it may be found.

Diagnosis

Changes in the blood cells are variable. Anemia is usual and generally increases over time. RBCs are normocytic, normochromic with mild poikilocytosis, reticulocytosis, and polychromatophilia. Nucleated RBCs may be found in peripheral blood. In advanced cases, RBCs are severely misshapen and tear-shaped; their appearance is sufficiently abnormal to suggest the diagnosis.

WBC counts are highly variable, being either normal, decreased, or most frequently increased. Granulocyte immaturity is found in most patients, and the presence of myeloblasts is not necessarily indicative of conversion to acute leukemia. Platelets may also initially be high, normal, or decreased in number; however, thrombocytopenia tends to supervene as the disease progresses.

Bone marrow aspiration may be dry. A bone marrow biopsy is required to show fibrosis. Since fibrosis may not be uniformly distributed, a repeat biopsy should be done from a different site in patients suspected of having IMF if the first biopsy is nondiagnostic.

Treatment

There is no therapy to reverse or control the underlying pathologic process. Therapy is directed at management of complications. Androgens, splenectomy, chemotherapy, and radiation therapy have sometimes been used for palliation. Androgens may be tried for severe anemia (oxymetholone orally 2 to 4 mg/kg/day). However, if there is no response in 3 to 6 mo, they should be discontinued.

PRIMARY THROMBOCYTHEMIA

(Essential Thrombocythemia)

A disease characterized by an increased platelet count, megakaryocytic hyperplasia, and a hemorrhagic or thrombotic tendency.

Etiology and Pathogenesis

As with other myeloproliferative disorders, primary thrombocythemia is a clonal abnormality of a multipotent hematopoietic stem cell. It usually occurs between 50 and 70 yr of age and affects males and females equally. Markedly elevated platelet

TABLE 98–6. CAUSES OF SECONDARY THROMBOCYTHEMIA

Chronic inflammatory disorders: RA, inflammatory bowel disease, TB, sarcoidosis, Wegener's granulomatosis
Acute infection
Hemorrhage
Iron deficiency
Hemolysis
Neoplasm: Carcinoma, Hodgkin's disease, non-Hodgkin's lymphoma
Postoperative: Splenectomy

counts are the result of an increase in platelet production. Platelet survival is usually normal, although it may be decreased due to splenic sequestration. In older patients, increased platelet number combined with degenerative vascular disease may lead to serious bleeding or thrombosis.

Thrombocythemia can also be seen as a reactive process. Causes of secondary thrombocytosis are listed in TABLE 98–6.

Symptoms and Signs

The most frequent symptoms are weakness, hemorrhage, nonspecific headache, paresthesias, and dizziness. Bleeding is usually mild, manifested by epistaxis, easy bruisability, or GI bleeding. Paresthesias of the hands and feet or digital ischemia may be seen. Splenomegaly is found in 60% of patients, usually not extending > 3 cm below the left costal margin. Hepatomegaly may also be found.

Diagnosis and Differential Diagnosis

The platelet count is usually $> 1 \times 10^6/\mu L$, although counts between $750{,}000/\mu L$ and $1 \times 10^6/\mu L$ may occur.

In the peripheral smear, platelet aggregates, giant platelets, and megakaryocyte fragments may be found. The bone marrow shows megakaryocytic hyperplasia, with an abundance of platelets being released. Marrow iron is usually present.

Primary thrombocythemia should be differentiated from other myeloproliferative diseases associated with an elevated platelet count. Diagnostic requirements for primary thrombocythemia include a normal RBC mass (increased in polycythemia vera [PV]), absence of the Philadelphia chromosome (found in chronic myelogenous leukemia), and absence of teardrop RBCs or significant increase in bone marrow fibrosis (seen in IMF).

Usually in secondary thrombocytosis the platelet count is $< 1 \times 10^6/\mu L$, and the cause may be obvious on the basis of the history or clinical examination; platelet function tests are usually normal. However, in the myeloproliferative disorders, abnormalities of platelet aggregation occur in about 50% of patients.

Treatment

Treatment of secondary thrombocythemia is that of the underlying disorder. When appropriate therapy can be instituted, the platelet count usually returns to normal. Indications for therapy in primary thrombocythemia are less clear, although in patients with platelet counts above $1 \times 10^6/\mu L$, and in those with hemorrhage or thrombotic complications, most authorities believe that definitive therapy is indicated.

Myelosuppressive therapy consists of hydroxyurea 10 to 15 mg/kg/day. Initial weekly blood counts are mandatory. The dosage can be adjusted as discussed above in

therapy for PV. ^{32}P has also been used successfully in the treatment of primary thrombocythemia (2.7 mCi/sq m IV, but not to exceed 7 mCi). The aim of therapy is a platelet count < 600,000 without significant clinical toxicity or suppression of other marrow elements.

Because of the relatively long time for therapeutic effects of either hydoxyurea or ^{32}P (2 to 6 wk), plateletpheresis has been used where available when an immediate reduction in the platelet count is required, as in serious hemorrhage or thrombosis, or before an emergency surgical procedure.

---

99. HEMORRHAGIC DISORDERS

Disorders characterized by a tendency to bleed.

Physiology of Hemostasis

Hemostasis, *the process whereby bleeding from an injured blood vessel is arrested,* requires the combined activity of vascular, platelet, and plasma factors as well as counterbalancing mechanisms to limit the accumulation of platelets and fibrin to the area of vessel wall injury. Abnormalities of hemostasis can lead to excessive bleeding or to thrombosis.

Vascular factors reduce blood flow at a site of trauma (1) by local vasoconstriction (an immediate reaction to injury) and (2) by compression of injured vessels by blood extravasated into surrounding tissues.

Platelet hemostatic plugs: *Adherent masses of platelets that accumulate at a site of vessel wall injury making up a key element of the hemostatic seal.* Platelets also release factors that augment vasoconstriction (serotonin, thromboxane A_2) and initiate vessel wall repair (platelet-derived growth factor), and they provide surface membrane sites and components for formation of enzyme/cofactor complexes of blood coagulation reactions.

Circulating platelets are nonadherent to normal endothelium or to each other, but when the endothelial lining of the vessel is broken, the platelets adhere to exposed subendothelial collagen **(platelet adhesion).** This is the first step in the formation of hemostatic plugs. It requires participation of a protein made by endothelial cells called von Willebrand **(vW)** factor, which is found both in the vessel wall and in plasma, and which binds during platelet adhesion to a receptor present on a glycoprotein **(GP)** of the platelet surface membrane called GP Ib.

Next, platelets are activated in reactions initiated by collagen and by the first thrombin formed at the injury site. These stimuli activate phospholipase C, an enzyme that hydrolyzes a membrane phospholipid called phosphatidyl inositol triphosphate. Products of this reaction activate protein kinase C and also increase the Ca concentration of platelet cytosol. As a result, a series of progressive, overlapping events ensue:

1. Platelets change shape and develop long pseudopods.
2. A receptor is assembled on the platelet surface membrane from GP IIb and GP IIIa. Fibrinogen and other adhesive proteins bind to this receptor causing platelets to stick to each other **(platelet aggregation).**
3. Arachidonic acid is liberated from membrane phospholipids and undergoes oxidation to products that include (1) prostaglandin H_2 **(PGH_2)**, which serves as an important cofactor for collagen-induced platelet activation, and (2) thromboxane A_2, that can act in itself as an additional platelet activator.
4. Contents of platelets are secreted; one material, ADP, can also stimulate platelet activation and recruit new platelets into the growing hemostatic plug.

5. The platelet surface membrane undergoes a reorganization that exposes procoagulant phospholipids needed for enzyme/cofactor complexes of blood coagulation to form on the platelet surface. Secretion of platelet factor V from platelet α-granules provides another key component for one of the enzyme/cofactor complexes. As a result, thrombin is generated in increasing amounts on the platelet surface, and clots fibrinogen, with formation of fibrin strands that radiate outward from aggregated platelets helping to secure the platelet plug to the site of injury.

6. A mechanism within the platelets is activated with the resultant contraction of platelet actinomyosin. This compresses and consolidates the platelet plug, further securing it to the site of injury.

Blood coagulation reactions form a second key element of the hemostatic seal—the fibrin clot (see FIG. 99–1). Spreading outward from and anchoring the platelet plugs, the fibrin clot adds bulk needed for the hemostatic seal. A nomenclature of Roman numerals, letters, and eponyms is currently used for components of the blood coagulation reactions (see TABLE 99–1).

Coagulation may be thought of as occurring in steps: (1) Sequences of reactions in at least 2 pathways (described below) activate serine protease proenzymes with resultant formation of a prothrombin activator. The activator is a complex of an enzyme, factor Xa, and 2 cofactors (factor Va and procoagulant phospholipid) present on the surface of activated platelets or of tissue cells. (2) The prothrombin activator cleaves

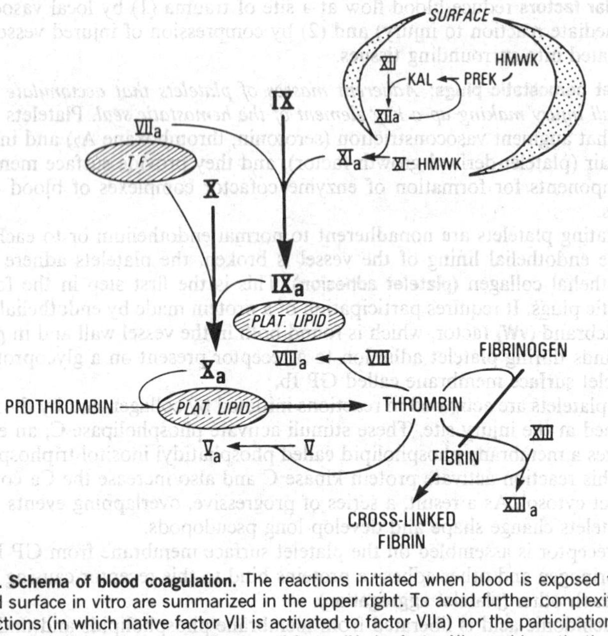

FIG. 99–1. Schema of blood coagulation. The reactions initiated when blood is exposed to a negatively charged surface in vitro are summarized in the upper right. To avoid further complexity, neither feedback reactions (in which native factor VII is activated to factor VIIa) nor the participation of Ca^{++} (in the formation of all complexes, in activation of factor IXa by factor XIa, and in activation of factor XIII) is shown.

HMWK = high mol wt kininogen; **KAL** = kallikrein; **PLAT. LIPID** = platelet procoagulant phospholipid; **PREK** = prekallikrein; **TF** = tissue factor

(From S. I. Rapaport in *Physiological Basis of Medical Practice*, 11th ed., 1985, edited by J. B. West. Copyright by The Williams and Williams Co., Baltimore, 1985. Used with permission.)

TABLE 99–1. COMPONENTS OF BLOOD COAGULATION REACTIONS*

Material	*Comments*
PLASMA FACTORS	
I. Fibrinogen	Precursor of fibrin
II. Prothrombin	Precursor of the serine protease thrombin, which converts fibrinogen to fibrin, activates factors V, VIII, and XIII, and, when bound to thrombomodulin, activates protein C. Vitamin K dependent.
V. Proaccelerin, labile factor, accelerator globulin	When activated to factor Va, serves as a cofactor for the enzyme factor Xa in a factor Xa/Va/phospholipid complex that activates prothrombin. Also present in platelet alpha granules. Inactivated by protein Ca.
VII. Proconvertin, convertin, stabile factor	Enzymatic component of a factor VII/tissue factor complex that activates factor X and IX. Many times more enzymatically active after activation to factor VIIa by factor Xa. Vitamin K dependent.
VIII. Antihemophilic globulin, AHG	When activated to factor VIIIa, serves as a cofactor for the enzyme factor IXa in a factor IXa/VIIIa/phospholipid complex that activates factor X. Inactivated by protein Ca. Has common properties with factor V. Circulates in plasma bound to von Willebrand factor.
IX. Christmas factor, plasma thromboplastin component	When activated to factor IXa, functions as the enzyme of a factor IXa/VIIIa/phospholipid complex that activates factor X. Vitamin K dependent.
X. Stuart Prower factor, Stuart factor	When activated to factor Xa, functions as the enzyme of a factor Xa/Va/phospholipid complex that activates prothrombin. Vitamin K dependent.
XI. Plasma thromboplastin antecedent, PTA	When activated to factor XIa, activates factor IX in a reaction requiring no cofactor except calcium ions. Circulates as a biomolecular complex with high mol wt kininogen.
Fletcher factor: Prekallikrein	Participates in a reciprocal reaction of contact activation in which it is activated to kallikrein by factor XIIa and the kallikrein then catalyzes further activation of factor XII to factor XIIa. Circulates as a biomolecular complex with high mot wt kininogen.
Fitzgerald factor: High mol wt kininogen	Circulates as a bimolecular complex with either factor XI or prekallikren. When absorbed onto a negatively charged surface, brings down Factor XI and prekallikrein onto the surface.
XII. Hageman factor, contact factor	When activated to factor XIIa by negatively charged surfaces or kallikrein, activates prekallikrein and factor XI in the intrinsic pathway and also factor VII in the extrinsic pathway.
XIII. Fibrin stabilizing factor	When activated by thrombin, catabolizes formation of peptide bonds between fibrin monomers, thus helping to stabilize the clot.

(Continued)

* The letter (a) designates the active form of the factor.

TABLE 99–1. COMPONENTS OF BLOOD COAGULATION REACTIONS* *(Cont'd)*

Material	*Comments*
Protein C	When activated to Protein Ca by thrombin bound to thrombomodulin, inhibits by proteolysis the cofactor activity of factors VIIIa and Va in a reaction requiring protein S and phospholipid as cofactors. Vitamin K dependent.
Protein S	Exists in plasma as free protein S and as protein S bound to the C4b binding protein of the complement system. The free form functions as a cofactor for protein S. Vitamin K dependent.
CELL SURFACE FACTORS	
Tissue factor: Tissue thromboplastin	A lipoprotein found on the surface of fibroblasts, smooth muscle cells, glial cells, and trophoblasts. Also develops on the surface of injured endothelial cells and activated monocytes and macrophages. Present on some tumor cells. Functions as a cofactor for factor VII.
Platelet factor 3: Procoagulant phospholipid	Acidic phospholipid present on the surface of activated platelets and other tissue cells. Functions as a component of the factor IX/VIIIa/phospholipid activator of factor X and of the factor Xa/Va/phospholipid activator of prothrombin. Also can function as the lipid moiety of the tissue factor lipoprotein.
Thrombomodulin	An endothelial cell surface binding site for thrombin. When bound to thrombomodulin, thrombin readily activates protein C.

* The letter (a) designates the active form of the factor.

prothrombin into 2 fragments, 1 of which is the enzyme thrombin. (3) Thrombin, by cleaving small peptides from the α- (fibrinopeptide A) and β- (fibrinopeptide B) chains of fibrinogen, gives rise to an altered molecule (fibrin monomer) that then polymerizes to form insoluble fibrin (fibrin polymer). Thrombin also activates factor XIII, an enzyme that catalyzes formation of covalent bonds between fibrin molecules, cross-linking the molecules to form a clot resistant to dissolution.

Ca ions are required for most reactions leading to generation of thrombin, which is why Ca-chelating agents (eg, citrate or oxalate) are used as anticoagulants to prevent clotting in vitro. A number of serine protease proenzymes contain residues of an unusual amino acid called γ-carboxyglutamic acid that contains, not 1, but 2 carboxy groups attached to the γ carbon of glutamic acid. The extra carboxy group creates binding sites for Ca. Vitamin K is needed for the reactions attaching the added carboxy group to glutamic acid, and the proteins containing γ-carboxyglutamic acid residues are, therefore, called vitamin K-dependent clotting factors. When synthesized in the absence of vitamin K, these proteins, lacking γ-carboxyglutamic acid residues, cannot bind Ca normally and so cannot function normally in blood coagulation.

Reactions that lead to generation of the prothrombin activator complex may be initiated in vitro (1) by exposing plasma to a negatively charged surface such as glass or certain diatomacious earth powders **(intrinsic pathway)** or (2) by adding a lipoprotein activity from tissues called tissue factor to plasma **(extrinsic pathway)**. In the intrinsic pathway, factor XII, high mol wt kininogen **(HMWK)**, prekallikrein, and factor XI come down onto a negatively charged surface where they react (contact activation reactions) to give rise to activated factor XI. Factor XIa then activates factor IX. An

intrinsic factor X activator then forms as a complex of the enzyme, factor IXa, and 2 cofactors, factor VIIIa and procoagulant phospholipid, present on the surface of activated platelets or of tissue cells.

Persons with a hereditary deficiency of factor XII, HMWK, or prekallikrein do not bleed abnormally, whereas those with hereditary factor XI deficiency have a mild bleeding disorder. Therefore, an unidentified mechanism for activating factor XI that bypasses factor XII, prekallikrein, and HMWK must exist in vivo. Patients lacking factor IX (hemophilia B) or factor VIII (hemophilia A) bleed severely, which means that formation of the intrinsic factor X activator is essential for normal hemostasis.

In the extrinsic pathway, adding tissue factor to plasma provides a cofactor for factor VII. A factor VII/tissue factor complex initiates activation of factor X. The first factor Xa formed back-activates factor VII and the resultant factor VIIa/tissue factor complex becomes a many-fold more efficient activator of factor X. The factor VIIa/tissue factor complex can also activate factor IX. Thus, since factor IXa is the enzyme of the intrinsic factor X activator complex, exposure of plasma to tissue factor results in both a direct activation of factor X by the factor VIIa/tissue factor complex and an indirect activation of factor X by the factor IXa/factor VIIIa, phospholipid complex. Both routes of activation are thought to be important for normal hemostasis, in which blood contacts only a limited number of tissue factor sites present on the surface of damaged endothelial cells, smooth muscle cells, and fibroblasts at a site of vessel wall injury. (In an important laboratory test called the prothrombin time **[PT]**, plasma is clotted with an unphysiologically high concentration of tissue factor. Then, the factor VIIa/tissue factor complex directly activates factor X so rapidly that its indirect activation through an initial activation of factor IX becomes unimportant. This is why patients with either hemophilia A [factor VIII deficiency] or hemophilia B [factor IX deficiency] have a normal PT result.) Since factor VII participates only in the extrinsic pathway, the serious bleeding of patients with severe factor VII deficiency establishes that the coagulation reactions initiated by exposure of blood to tissue factor are essential for normal hemostasis.

One important feedback reaction of blood coagulation, the activation of factor VII by factor Xa, has been mentioned. Other important feedback reactions are (1) activation of factor VIII by a trace concentration of thrombin or by a higher concentration of factor Xa; and (2) activation of factor V by a trace concentration of thrombin. Such activation is essential for the effective participation of factors VIII and V as cofactors of blood coagulation.

Regulatory mechanisms normally exist to prevent the blood coagulation reactions, once activated, from proceeding unchecked to cause either local thrombosis or disseminated intravascular coagulation **(DIC)**. These include (1) cellular clearance of activated clotting factors, particularly as blood flows through the liver, and (2) mechanisms within the blood itself for neutralizing the enzymes and activated cofactors of blood coagulation.

Protease inhibitors in plasma that can neutralize blood coagulation enzymes include antithrombin III, α_2-macroglobulin, heparin cofactor II, and α_1-antiprotease. The most important is **antithrombin III**, which is the primary inhibitor of the key enzymes—thrombin, factor Xa, and factor IXa. Adding the therapeutic anticoagulant heparin to blood in vitro converts antithrombin III from a slow to an instantaneous inhibitor of these enzymes. (This is the mechanism for heparin's therapeutic effect.) It is now known that heparin chains are present on the luminal surface of vascular endothelium and enhance the function of antithrombin III in vivo. Heterozygotes for hereditary antithrombin III deficiency with 50% of normal antithrombin III levels have an increased risk for thrombosis, which attests to the importance of this protease inhibitor in regulating blood coagulation. Homozygotes have not been identified, presumably because it would be lethal in utero.

Inhibition of the cofactors, factors VIII and Va, involves 2 newly described vitamin K-dependent proteins, protein C and protein S. Thrombin, when bound to a receptor on endothelial cells called **thrombomodulin**, acquires the ability to cleave a small peptide from and so activate protein C. Protein Ca is a serine protease, which with protein S and procoagulant phospholipid as its cofactors, catalyzes a proteolysis of factors VIIIa and Va that destroys their cofactor function. Heterozygotes for hereditary protein C or protein S deficiency, who have levels of these factors in the 50% of normal range, are also at increased risk for thrombosis. Infants born with homozygous protein C deficiency may die in the newborn period with fatal thrombosis **(neonatal purpura fulminans)**. These clinical observations establish the physiologic importance of the protein C/protein S mechanism for regulating blood coagulation.

The **fibrinolytic system** is activated by deposition of fibrin. By dissolving fibrin, this system helps keep open the lumen of an injured blood vessel. A balanced deposition and lysis of fibrin maintains and remolds the hemostatic seal during the several days required for an injured vessel wall to be repaired.

When fibrinogen is converted to fibrin, lysine residues become available on the molecule to which plasminogen, the plasma precursor of plasmin, can bind tightly. It does so through sites on plasminogen called lysine binding sites. An activator released from endothelial cells (tissue plasminogen activator) is a poor activator when free in solution, but once it is bound to fibrin, activates plasminogen efficiently. Activation results from cleavage of a single peptide bond that converts inert plasminogen into the powerful proteolytic enzyme, plasmin, which degrades fibrin first into large fragments called X and Y and then into smaller fragments called D and E. These soluble fragments, referred to collectively as **fibrin degradation products (FDP),** are swept into the circulation.

Tissue plasminogen activator is thought to be the primary physiologic activator of intravascular fibrin, although endothelial cells also release small amounts of a second activator called urokinase. Epithelial cells lining excretory ducts of the body (eg, renal tubules, mammary ducts) also secrete urokinase, which is thought to be the physiologic activator initiating lysis of any fibrin that may be deposited in these channels. Three enzymes involved in the contact activation reactions of the intrinsic pathway of coagulation—factor XIIa, kallikrein, and factor XIa—can also activate plasminogen, but they are weak activators of questionable physiologic significance. Streptokinase, a bacterial product not normally found in the body, is a potent activator of plasminogen and has been used to induce fibrinolysis therapeutically in patients with acute thrombotic disorders.

Several factors operate to prevent excessive fibrinolysis. These include the increased affinity of plasminogen for binding to fibrin rather than to fibrinogen, and the increased ability of tissue plasminogen activator to activate plasminogen when it is bound to fibrin. Both mechanisms localize fibrinolysis to the fibrin clot, preventing formation of circulating plasmin that would degrade fibrinogen and other clotting factors. Moreover, plasma contains a protease inhibitor called α_2-antiplasmin that can rapidly inactivate plasmin escaping from a fibrin clot.

Rarely, patients have been identified with a hereditary deficiency of α_2-antiplasmin. They experience severe bleeding after minor tissue injury, which establishes that α_2-antiplasmin is a key regulator of normal fibrinolytic activity. An analog of lysine, ε-aminocaproic acid **(EACA)**, by binding to the lysine binding site of plasminogen, can prevent the binding of plasminogen to fibrin and, therefore, its subsequent activation on fibrin to plasmin. It is used therapeutically in selected circumstances to inhibit fibrinolysis in patients.

Laboratory Tests

Laboratory tests are divided into categories: (1) **Screening tests** reflect the combined effect of several factors influencing a particular phase of the hemostatic process (eg,

bleeding time). (2) **Specific assays** measure the level or function of a single hemostatic factor (eg, factor VIII assay). (3) **Tests may measure a product or effect** of a pathologic in vivo activation of platelets, coagulation, or fibrinolysis (eg, level of FDP). In diagnosis, one uses the pattern of screening test results plus knowledge of the patient's basic clinical disorder as guides to selecting more specific tests. The principal tests in current use are summarized in TABLE 99–2.

Each phase of hemostasis can be evaluated: (1) formation of hemostatic plugs (eg, the platelet count, appearance of platelets on the blood smear, and a bleeding time); (2) generation of thrombin (eg, partial thromboplastin time **[PTT]** for the intrinsic pathway, and the prothrombin time **[PT]** for the extrinsic pathway); and (3) the thrombin-fibrinogen reaction and stability of the fibrin clot (eg, thrombin time, stability of a plasma clot after incubation in physiologic saline and in 5 M urea).

TABLE 99–2. LABORATORY TESTS OF HEMOSTASIS

Phase of Hemostasis	*Test*	*Comments*
Formation of hemostatic plugs	Platelet count (or estimate)	Quantitates platelet number
	Bleeding time	Screens for overall adequacy of formation of hemostatic plugs, independent of blood coagulation reactions
	vW* antigen	Measures total concentration of plasma vW protein by height of "rocket" on electroimmunoassay
	vW multimer composition	Evaluates distribution of sizes of vW factor in plasma. (Largest multimers are specifically missing in type II variants of vW disease.) Most abnormalities can be identified from shape of arc on crossed immunoelectrophoresis. Precise further evaluation requires specialized technics.
	Ristocetin agglutination	Screens for presence of intermediate multimers of vW factor. Measures change in light transmission due to clumping of platelets in platelet-rich plasma after adding ristocetin
	Ristocetin cofactor activity	Quantitative assay for intermediate-sized multimers of vW factor. Measures rate of change of light transmission after adding ristocetin to standard platelet preparation in the presence of different dilutions of a test plasma as the source of vW factor
	Platelet aggregation	Evaluates adequacy of platelet responsiveness to physiologic stimuli activating platelets. Measures change in light transmission due to platelet aggregation induced by physiologic stimuli (eg, collagen, ADP, epinephrine, and sodium arachidonate). Abnormal patterns may be found in hereditary or acquired platelet functional disorders.

(Continued)

* vW = von Willebrand

TABLE 99–2. LABORATORY TESTS OF HEMOSTASIS *(Cont'd)*

Phase of Hemostasis	*Test*	*Comments*
Formation of fibrin	Partial thromboplastin time (PTT)	Screening test of intrinsic pathway of coagulation (fibrinogen, prothrombin, factors V, VIII, IX, X, XI, XII, prekalikrein, and high mol wt kininogen)
	Prothrombin time (PT)	Screening test of extrinsic pathway (fibrinogen, prothrombin, factors V, VII, and X)
	Thrombin time	Screening test of the last step of coagulation, the thrombin-fibrinogen reaction. Prolonged when plasma antithrombin activity is increased as when plasma contains heparin. Also prolonged in conditions resulting in qualitative abnormalities of fibrinogen or hypofibrinogenemia
	Specific functional assays for prothrombin and factors V to XII	Activity of a specific factor is determined as % of normal by comparing the ability of a test plasma and dilutions of a normal reference plasma to shorten the clotting time (in a PTT- or PT-based 1-stage assay system) of a substrate plasma deficient in the specific factor being measured
	Fibrinogen level	Determined as mg/dL, usually indirectly from a procedure based upon measuring clotting time after adding a large excess of thrombin to plasma
Stability of fibrin and fibrinolytic activity	Clot stability on 24 hr incubation in saline and in 5 M urea	Clot will lyse in saline if fibrinolytic activity is excessive. Clot will lyse in 5 M urea if factor XIII is deficient
	Euglobulin lysis time	Shortened when blood contains increased plasminogen activator or plasmin activity
	Plasminogen activity	Determined from the plasmin activity generated (as measured with a chromogenic substrate) after adding a plasminogen activator to plasma
	α_2-antiplasmin	Determined by measuring residual activity of plasmin incubated briefly with the plasma being tested
Regulation of blood coagulation	Antithrombin III	Can be measured as antigen by immunological assay or as activity by assay measuring rate of inactivation of of thrombin added to plasma in presence of heparin
	Protein C Protein S	Measured as antigen by height of "rocket" obtained in electroimmunoassay. Activity assays not generally available

(Continued)

TABLE 99–2. LABORATORY TESTS OF HEMOSTASIS *(Cont'd)*

Phase of Hemostasis	*Test*	*Comments*
Activation of hemostasis in vivo	Platelet factor 4 assay β-thromboglobulin assay	Reflects release of platelet alpha-granule contents into the plasma secondary to platelet activation in vivo
	Plasma protamine paracoagulation test	Positive when plasma contains fibrin monomer, ie, when thrombin has been generated in vivo. Sensitivity low
	Fibrin degradation products	Measured immunologically as nonclottable material persisting in serum that reacts with an antibody made against fibrinogen fragments. Increased levels found when pathologic amounts of plasmin have been generated in vivo

Additional tests for screening selected patients include euglobulin lysis time for patients with suspected excessive fibrinolysis, plasma paracoagulation test for fibrin monomer, and a test for FDP if DIC is suspected.

The **bleeding time** should be done with a BP cuff on the upper arm inflated to 40 mm Hg, which makes hemostatic plugs hold against a back pressure. A convenient, disposable, spring-loaded bleeding time device is commercially available to make a 9 mm by 1 mm incision on the volar aspect of the forearm. Blood is absorbed onto the edge of a piece of filter paper at 30-sec intervals until bleeding has stopped. The upper limit of normal for bleeding time by this method is 7½ min.

Aspirin, by irreversibly inactivating an enzyme in platelets called cyclooxygenase, needed for oxidation of arachidonic acid to endoperoxides and thromboxane A_2, can prolong bleeding time to an upper limit of 12 min in normal persons. Since this effect may persist for days, one must know whether a patient has taken an aspirin-containing drug within 5 to 7 days of a bleeding time test to interpret the result. Aspirin 0.6 gm may sometimes be given 2 h before the bleeding time to detect a mild disorder of platelet hemostatic plug formation that may not prolong the bleeding time in the absence of aspirin. *However, an aspirin-sensitized bleeding time should not be done when a patient is actively bleeding at the time of examination or when surgery is contemplated within the next few days.* Thrombocytopenia, disorders of platelet function, and vW disease prolong the bleeding time, but it is not prolonged in coagulation-phase disorders.

Partial thromboplastin time (PTT) screens for abnormalities of the blood coagulation reactions triggered by exposure of plasma to a negatively charged surface (ie, the intrinsic pathway of coagulation). Plasma is incubated for 3 min with a reagent supplying procoagulant phospholipid and a surface-active powder (eg, kaolin). Calcium is then added and the clotting time is noted. Because commercial reagents and instrumentation vary widely, each laboratory should determine its own normal range (28 to 34 sec is typical). **The activated PTT (APTT)** is sensitive to deficiencies below about 30 to 40% of normal of all clotting factors except factors VII and XIII. With rare exceptions, a normal test rules out hemophilia. A prolonged test time can stem from a deficiency of 1 or more coagulation factors or from presence of an inhibitor of a plasma clotting factor (eg, a factor VIII anticoagulant) or an inhibitor of procoagulant phospholipid (lupus inhibitor). If an inhibitor is present, mixing the patient's plasma 1:1 with normal plasma will fail to shorten the APTT test result to within about 5 sec of the time obtained with normal plasma alone. Assays for specific coagulation factors are usually indicated to pinpoint the cause for a prolonged APTT, if it is not readily explainable

by the patient's other clinical findings. The APTT is frequently used to monitor heparin therapy.

In the **prothrombin time (PT) test,** plasma is recalcified in the presence of a high concentration of a tissue factor reagent (tissue thromboplastin). The test thus screens for abnormalities of factors involved in the extrinsic pathway of coagulation (factors V, VII, X, prothrombin, and fibrinogen). The normal PT varies between 10 to 12 sec, depending upon the particular tissue factor reagent used and other technical details. A PT that is 2 sec or more longer than a laboratory's normal control value should be considered abnormal and requires explanation. PT is a valuable screening test for disordered coagulation in a variety of acquired conditions (eg, vitamin K deficiency, liver disease, DIC). PT is also used to monitor therapy with the coumarin anticoagulants.

Thrombin time: Test plasma and a normal control plasma are clotted by adding a bovine thrombin reagent diluted to give a clotting time of about 15 sec for the control plasma. Since the test is independent of the reactions involved in generation of thrombin, it screens specifically for abnormalities affecting the thrombin-fibrinogen reaction: heparin, large fibrin degradation products (FDP), qualitative abnormalities of fibrinogen. It is particularly useful to establish that a plasma sample contains heparin (eg, residual heparin not neutralized after an extracorporeal bypass procedure or heparin contaminating plasma obtained from blood drawn from a line kept open with heparin flushes). In plasma that contains heparin, the thrombin time will be prolonged, but when the test is repeated, substituting for thrombin the reagent batroxobin (a snake venom enzyme insensitive to heparin that directly converts fibrinogen to fibrin), the test will be normal.

Fibrin clot stability is tested by clotting 0.2 mL plasma with 0.2 mL calcium chloride and incubating one clot in 3 mL NaCl solution and another clot in 3 mL of 5 M urea for 24 h at 37 C. Lysis of the clot incubated in urea indicates factor XIII deficiency. Lysis of the clot incubated in NaCl solution or lysis of both clots indicates excessive fibrinolysis. A normal test, however, does not rule out a milder yet potentially clinically significant abnormality of fibrinolysis (eg, a reduced plasma α_2-antiplasmin level in the 10 to 30% of normal range).

The **plasma protamine paracoagulation (3P) test** can be used as a screening test for soluble fibrin monomer in plasma in patients with suspected DIC. One-tenth volume of 1% protamine sulfate is mixed with plasma, which, after a brief incubation at 37 C, is examined for precipitated strands of fibrin. A positive test adds support to the diagnosis of DIC, but a negative test does not rule it out. A false positive test may result from difficulty with venipuncture or from inadequate anticoagulation of a blood sample.

Normal serum may contain small amounts ($< 10\ \mu g/mL$) of **residual nonclottable fibrin or FDP.** Increased amounts may be present in conditions in which fibrin deposited intravascularly is lysed (eg, DIC, diffuse vasculitis, formation of a clot in a large arterial aneurysm). Serum to be tested for FDP is prepared by clotting blood in a tube containing added thrombin (to be sure that no residual unclotted fibrinogen remains in the serum) and a trypsin inhibitor (to prevent fibrin degradation in vitro). FDP are quantitated by immunologic technics. In one commonly used test, dilutions of a test serum are mixed with latex particles coated with antisera to human fibrinogen fragments, and the mixtures are observed for agglutination of the latex particles. Agglutination with a 1:20 dilution of serum indicates presence of FDP at a concentration $\geq 40\ \mu g/mL$.

EHLERS-DANLOS SYNDROME AND OTHER HEREDITARY CONNECTIVE TISSUE DISORDERS

(See also INHERITED DISORDERS OF CONNECTIVE TISSUE in Ch. 197)

Ehlers-Danlos syndrome: *A group of hereditary connective tissue disorders producing hyperextensible, friable tissues.* One form is associated with excessive bleeding secondary to a deficiency of vascular and perivascular collagen. Patients have skin that may be stretched for several inches and lax, hypermobile joints. Subcutaneous ecchymoses are the major manifestation of the bleeding tendency, but bleeding may also occur (eg, after dental extraction, and in the GI tract). Elective surgery should be avoided because of excessively friable tissues, increased bleeding, and poor wound healing.

Other rare hereditary connective tissue disorders in which hemorrhage may result from defective vessels include pseudoxanthoma elasticum, osteogenesis imperfecta, and Marfan syndrome (see in INHERITED DISORDERS OF CONNECTIVE TISSUE in Ch. 197).

ALLERGIC PURPURA

(Henoch-Schönlein or Anaphylactoid Purpura)

An acute or chronic vasculitis primarily affecting small vessels of the skin, joints, GI tract, and kidney. The disease primarily affects young children, but older children and adults with allergic purpura are also seen. An acute respiratory infection precedes the purpura in a high proportion of affected young children. Less commonly, a drug appears to be the inciting agent, and a drug history should be obtained in every case.

Pathology and Pathogenesis

The serum frequently contains immune complexes in which the immunoglobulin component is IgA. Biopsy of an acute skin lesion reveals an aseptic vasculitis with fibrinoid necrosis of vessel walls and perivascular cuffing of vessels with polymorphonuclear leukocytes. Granular deposits of immunoglobulin reactive for IgA and of complement components may be seen on immunofluorescent study. Therefore, deposition of IgA-containing immune complexes with consequent activation of complement is thought to represent the pathogenetic mechanism for the vasculitis. The typical renal lesion is a focal, segmental proliferative glomerulonephritis.

Symptoms, Signs, and Clinical Course

The disease begins abruptly with the sudden appearance of a purpuric skin rash involving primarily the extensor surfaces of the feet and legs, a strip across the buttocks, and the extensor surfaces of the arms. Lesions may start as small areas of urticaria that progress to become indurated, palpable, purpuric spots. Crops of new lesions may appear over days to several weeks. Most patients also have fever and polyarthralgia with associated periarticular tenderness and swelling affecting the ankles, knees, hips, wrists, and elbows. Many patients also develop edema of the hands and feet. GI findings are common and include colicky abdominal pain, abdominal tenderness, and melena or stool tests positive for occult blood. From 25 to 50% of patients develop hematuria and proteinuria. The disease usually remits after about 4 wk but often recurs one or more times after a disease-free interval of several weeks. In most patients the disorder then subsides without serious residual consequences; however, in some patients the renal lesion progresses to chronic renal failure.

Diagnosis, Prognosis, and Treatment

The diagnosis is largely based on recognition of the clinical findings. **Prognosis**: Renal biopsy may help define the prognosis of the renal lesion. The finding of diffuse glomerular involvement or of crescentic changes in the majority of glomeruli predicts progressive renal failure.

A **euglobulin lysis time** is also often part of a screening evaluation, if increased fibrinolytic activity is suspected. Euglobulins are precipitated by dilution and acidification of plasma. The euglobulin fraction, which is relatively free of inhibitors of fibrinolysis, is then clotted with thrombin and the time for the clot to dissolve is measured. Normal lysis time is > 90 min. A shortened lysis time indicates increased plasma plasminogen activator activity (eg, as in some patients with advanced liver disease). A reduced plasma fibrinogen concentration, by yielding a smaller clot to be dissolved, may also result in a shortened time.

VASCULAR DISORDERS

Vascular disorders may cause petechiae, purpura, and bruising, but seldom lead to serious blood loss. Laboratory tests of hemostasis are usually normal. The diagnosis is made from other clinical findings.

PURPURA SIMPLEX
(Easy Bruising)

The most common vascular bleeding disorder, manifested by increased bruising, and representing increased vascular fragility. The patient, usually a woman, complains of bruises that develop without known trauma on the thighs, buttocks, and upper arms. The history usually reveals no other abnormal bleeding, but there may be easy bruising in other family members. The platelet count and tests of platelet function, blood coagulation, and fibrinolysis are all normal. No drug is effective in preventing the bruising; the patient is often advised to avoid aspirin and aspirin-containing drugs, but there is no evidence that the bruising is related to its use. The patient should be reassured that the condition is not serious.

SENILE PURPURA

A disorder affecting older patients, particularly those who have been exposed excessively to the sun, in whom deep purple ecchymoses, characteristically confined to the extensor surfaces of the hands and forearms, persist for a long time, and may leave a brownish discoloration due to deposits of hemosiderin. New lesions appear without known trauma. The skin and subcutaneous tissue of the involved area often appear thinned and atrophic. No treatment helps. Although cosmetically displeasing, the disorder has no serious consequences.

HEREDITARY HEMORRHAGIC TELANGIECTASIA
(Rendu-Osler-Weber Disease)

A hereditary disease of vascular malformation transmitted as an autosomal dominant trait affecting both men and women. **Diagnosis** is made on physical examination by the discovery of characteristic small, red-to-violet telangiectatic lesions on the face, lips, oral and nasal mucosa, and the tips of the fingers and toes. Similar lesions may be present throughout the mucosa of the GI tract and result in major episodes of GI bleeding. Patients also experience repeated, profuse nosebleeds. Some patients may have associated pulmonary arteriovenous fistulas. **Laboratory studies** are usually normal except for evidence of an iron-deficiency anemia in most patients.

Treatment is nonspecific. Accessible lesions may be treated with pressure, styptics, and topical hemostatics. Blood transfusions may be needed for acute hemorrhage. Most patients require continuous iron therapy to replace iron lost in repeated mucosal bleeding (see Treatment under IRON DEFICIENCY ANEMIA in Ch. 96).

Treatment, except for the elimination of a possible offending drug, is primarily symptomatic. Corticosteroids (eg, prednisone 2 mg/kg up to a total of 50 mg/day) may help to control edema, joint pain, and abdominal pain, but have no effect upon the course of acute renal involvement. Immunosuppressive therapy with azathioprine has been used with questionable benefit in patients who develop chronic renal disease.

VASCULAR PURPURAS DUE TO DYSPROTEINEMIAS

Hyper(gamma)globulinemic purpura: *A syndrome primarily affecting women and characterized by a polyclonal increase in IgG (broad-based or diffuse hypergammaglobulinemia on serum protein electrophoresis) and recurrent crops of small, palpable purpuric lesions on the lower legs.* These leave small residual brown spots. Vasculitis is seen on biopsy. Many patients have manifestations of an underlying immunologic disorder (eg, Sjögren's syndrome or SLE).

Cryoglobulinemia: *Gelling of immunoglobulins when plasma is cooled.* Monoclonal immunoglobulins made in macroglobulinemia of Waldenström or in multiple myeloma occasionally behave as cryoglobulins, as may mixed IgM-IgG immune complexes formed in some chronic infectious and collagen vascular disorders. Precipitation of cryoglobulins as blood cools while flowing through the skin and subcutaneous tissues of the extremities can lead to small vessel damage and resultant purpura. Cryoglobulinemia may be recognized by clotting blood at 37 C, incubating the separated serum at 4 C for 24 h, and examining the serum for a gel or precipitate.

Hyperviscosity of blood resulting from a markedly elevated plasma IgM concentration may also result in purpura and other forms of abnormal bleeding (eg, profuse epistaxis) in patients with macroglobulinemia of Waldenström.

In **amyloidosis,** deposits of amyloid within vessels in the skin and subcutaneous tissues produce increased vascular fragility and associated purpura. Appearance of periorbital purpura or a purpuric rash that develops in a nonthrombocytopenic patient after gentle stroking of the skin should arouse suspicion of amyloidosis.

Autoerythrocyte sensitization (Gardner-Diamond syndrome): *An uncommon disorder of women characterized by local pain and burning preceding painful ecchymoses that are found primarily on the extremities.* Intradermal injection of 0.1 mL of autologous erythrocytes or erythrocyte stroma may result in pain, swelling, and induration at the injection site. This suggests that escape of RBCs into the tissues is involved in the pathogenesis of the lesion. However, most patients also have associated severe psychoneurotic symptoms, and psychogenic factors seem somehow related to the pathogenesis of the syndrome.

Scurvy: Hemorrhage may be a prominent feature of scurvy. Perifollicular petechiae distributed over the thighs and buttocks is a characteristic finding. Large intramuscular hemorrhages also occur as well as periosteal hemorrhages in children. For details concerning bleeding as well as therapy see VITAMIN C DEFICIENCY in Ch. 81.

PLATELET DISORDERS

Platelet disorders may cause defective formation of hemostatic plugs and bleeding because of decreased platelet numbers **(thrombocytopenia)** or because of decreased platelet function despite adequate platelet numbers **(platelet dysfunction).**

THROMBOCYTOPENIA

Thrombocytopenia may stem from failure of platelet production, splenic sequestration of platelets, increased platelet destruction, increased platelet utilization, or dilution of platelets (see TABLE 99–3). Severe thrombocytopenia of any etiology causes bleeding into the skin in the form of multiple petechiae, often most evident on the

TABLE 99–3. CLASSIFICATION OF THROMBOCYTOPENIC DISORDERS

Mechanism of Thrombocytopenia	*Conditions*
Failure of production	
Diminished or absent megakaryocytes in marrow	Leukemia, aplastic anemia, paroxysmal nocturnal hemoglobinuria (some patients)
Abnormal production despite presence of marrow megakaryocytes (ineffective thrombopoiesis)	Alcohol-induced thrombocytopenia, thrombocytopenia in megaloblastic anemias, some myelodysplastic (preleukemic) syndromes
Platelet sequestration in enlarged spleen	Cirrhosis with congestive splemomegaly, myelofibrosis with myeloid metaplasia, Gaucher's disease
Increased platelet destruction, and/or utilization	
Removal of antibody-coated platelets by mononuclear phagocytes	Idiopathic thrombocytopenic purpura, post-transfusion purpura, drug-induced thrombocytopenia, neonatal thrombocytopenia, secondary to chronic leukemia, lymphoma, and SLE
Thrombin-induced platelet damage	States with intravascular coagulation: complications of obstetrics, metastatic malignancy, gram-negative septicemia, traumatic brain damage
Complex, multiple, and poorly understood mechanisms	Thrombotic thrombocytopenic purpura, hemolytic-uremic syndromes, thrombocytopenia in adult respiratory distress syndrome, severe infections with septicemia
Damage by foreign surfaces	Extracorporeal circulation (cardiac surgery)
Dilution	Massive blood replacement or exchange transfusion (platelets lose viability in stored blood)

lower legs, and scattered small ecchymoses at sites of minor trauma. Thrombocytopenia also causes mucosal bleeding (epistaxis; GI tract, GU, and vaginal bleeding) and excessive bleeding after surgery. Heavy GI bleeding and bleeding into the CNS may be life-threatening manifestations of thrombocytopenic bleeding. However, thrombocytopenia does not cause massive bleeding into tissues or hemarthroses, such as may occur in bleeding secondary to plasma coagulation factor deficiencies (eg, hemophilia).

A thorough drug history must be taken to rule out exposure to drugs known to cause increased platelet ingestion in sensitive individuals (eg, quinidine, sulfa preparations, oral antidiabetic agents, gold salts, rifampicin, and heparin). An increased prevalence of idiopathic thrombocytopenic purpura (**ITP**—see below) has recently been noted in homosexuals. Other important points in a history may be a blood transfusion within 10 days (possible post-transfusion purpura), heavy alcohol consumption (possible alcohol-induced thrombocytopenia), and symptoms (eg, arthralgia, Raynaud's phenomena, unexplained fever) suggestive of an underlying immunologic disease. The presence or absence of fever is an important point of differential diagnosis: It is usually present in thrombocytopenia secondary to infection or active SLE and in thrombotic thrombocytopenic purpura (**TTP**), but absent in ITP and in drug-related thrombocytopenias. Size of the spleen on physical examination is a second important diagnostic point. The spleen is not palpably enlarged in most thrombocytopenia caused by increased platelet destruction (eg, ITP, drug-related immune thrombocytopenias, TTP), whereas it will be palpably enlarged in patients with thrombocytopenia secondary to splenic sequestration of platelets, and often in patients with thrombocytopenia secondary to a lymphoma or a myeloproliferative disorder.

TABLE 99–4. PERIPHERAL BLOOD FINDINGS IN THROMBOCYTOPENIC DISORDERS

Normal RBCs and WBCs	Idiopathic thrombocytopenic purpura Drug-related thrombocytopenic purpura Post-transfusion purpura
RBC fragmentation	Thrombotic thrombocytopenic purpura Hemolytic-uremic syndromes Metastatic tumor emboli
WBC abnormalities	Immature cells in leukemia Markedly diminished granulocytes in aplastic anemia Hypersegmented polys in megaloblastic anemias

Laboratory findings: The **peripheral blood count** is a key examination not only to establish the presence and severity of thrombocytopenia, but also for clues to its cause (see TABLE 99–4). The platelets' sizes should be noted; an increased proportion of large platelets (determined by scanning the blood smear or by measuring mean platelet volume with an electronic blood counter) suggests compensatory increased platelet production and is often found in thrombocytopenias secondary to increased destruction or utilization of platelets. Since the **bleeding time** will be substantially prolonged in severe thrombocytopenia of any cause, it gives no added information, but may provide useful information in the patient with a moderate thrombocytopenia (eg, a platelet count of 50,000/μL). A very long bleeding time suggests that the process causing the thrombocytopenia (eg, coating of platelets with antibody) has also impaired the function of platelets still circulating. Other screening tests of hemostasis (see above) will be normal unless the thrombocytopenia is associated with another condition affecting hemostasis (eg, liver disease or DIC).

Bone marrow aspiration is used to evaluate the number and appearance of megakaryocytes and to confirm the impression gained from the peripheral blood smear of the presence or absence of disease causing marrow failure (eg, leukemia). Measurement of platelet-associated IgG may also be of value in selected patients.

Management of thrombocytopenia secondary to decreased production is directed towards attempting to correct its cause (eg, to induce a remission in a patient with acute leukemia). Platelet concentrates can be given to raise the platelet count temporarily, but, since with repeated use their effectiveness is lost due to development of platelet alloantibodies, they should be used prophylactically with discretion. If rapid correction of bone marrow failure is not expected, platelet transfusions are often reserved for treatment of an active bleeding episode. Corticosteroids have not proven beneficial in the management of patients with thrombocytopenia secondary to bone marrow failure.

IMMUNOLOGIC (IDIOPATHIC) THROMBOCYTOPENIC PURPURA (ITP)

(Purpura Hemorrhagica; Werlhof's Disease)

In children, usually a self-limited disorder that follows a viral infection; in most adults, a chronic disorder with no apparent predisposing cause. In childhood ITP, viral antigen is thought to trigger synthesis of antibody that may react with virus antigen that has come down onto the platelet surface or that may come down onto the platelet as viral antigen-antibody immune complexes. In contrast, adult ITP usually results from development of an antibody directed against a structural platelet antigen (an autoantibody). In both forms, physical examination is negative except for petechiae, purpura, and mucosal bleeding, which may be either minimal or extensive. Peripheral blood is

normal except for reduced numbers of platelets with a relative increase in large forms. Bone marrow examination usually reveals increased numbers of megakaryocytes in an otherwise normal marrow.

Treatment in the adult is usually begun with large doses of an oral corticosteroid (eg, prednisone 40 mg bid). In the patient who responds, the high dosage is maintained several weeks and then gradually tapered. Unfortunately, most patients either fail to respond adequately initially or relapse as the adrenal steroid is tapered. Splenectomy can achieve a remission in 50 to 60% of those who fail to respond to adrenal steroid therapy or who relapse after a steroid response. Administration of a synthetic androgen, danazol, or immunosuppressive therapy with azathioprine, vincristine, or cyclophosphamide has been variably effective in patients refractory to steroids and splenectomy. Platelet concentrates are of limited usefulness because of the short survival of platelets in ITP. However, they are usually given for whatever temporary effectiveness they may have to patients with active or imminent, life-threatening bleeding.

OTHER FORMS OF THROMBOCYTOPENIA

Drug-related immune thrombocytopenias have identical findings to ITP except for the history of ingestion of a drug capable of stimulating antibodies that together with the drug can bind to the platelet surface. When the drug is stopped, the platelet count begins to increase within 7 to 10 days. (An exception is gold-induced thrombocytopenia, since injected gold-salts may persist in the body for many weeks.) A small number of patients given heparin develop thrombocytopenia secondary to a heparin-related antibody. This differs from other drug-induced immune thrombocytopenia in that the platelets aggregate intravascularly. As a consequence, platelet-fibrin thrombi may form and can lead, in an occasional patient, to a serious thromboembolic occlusive event.

Other disorders producing thrombocytopenia similar to ITP include immune thrombocytopenias **secondary to a collagen disorder** (eg, SLE) or to **lymphoproliferative disease.** Steroids and splenectomy are often effective in these forms of thrombocytopenia. The clinical findings in **posttransfusion purpura** also closely resemble ITP except for a history of a blood transfusion within the preceding 7 to 10 days. The patient, usually a woman, lacks a platelet antigen (PLA-1) present in most people. The PLA-1-positive platelets in transfused blood stimulate formation of anti–PLA-1 antibodies, which apparently can also react with an epitope on the patient's own PLA-1–negative platelets. Severe thrombocytopenia results that takes 2 to 6 wk to subside. Plasmapheresis has been recommended to hasten recovery.

Thrombocytopenia secondary to sequestration of platelets in an enlarged spleen **(hypersplenism)** can occur in a variety of disorders that produce splenomegaly (see Ch. 104, below). It is an expected finding in patients with congestive splenomegaly due to advanced cirrhosis. In contrast to immune thrombocytopenias, the platelet count usually does not fall below about 50,000/μL unless the disorder producing the splenomegaly also impairs the marrow production of platelets (as may occur in myelofibrosis with myeloid metaplasia). Splenectomy will correct the thrombocytopenia, but is usually not indicated in the patient with moderate thrombocytopenia. Patients with **gram-negative sepsis** frequently develop thrombocytopenia. Its severity often parallels the severity of the infection. The thrombocytopenia has multiple causes: DIC, formation of immune complexes that can come down onto the platelets, activation of complement, and deposition of platelets on damaged endothelial surfaces. Patients with **adult respiratory distress syndrome** also may become thrombocytopenic, possibly secondary to deposition of platelets in the pulmonary capillary bed.

DISORDERS WITH THROMBOCYTOPENIA, FRAGMENTED RBCs, AND HEMOLYSIS

Disorders in which loose strands of fibrin are deposited in multiple small vessels; they include TTP and the hemolytic-uremic syndrome. Platelets and RBCs are damaged as blood flows past the fibrin strands. Platelet consumption within multiple small thrombi also contributes to the thrombocytopenia.

Thrombotic Thrombocytopenic Purpura (TTP)

An acute, potentially fatal disorder characterized by (1) severe thrombocytopenia, (2) fragmented RBCs on the blood smear (helmet cells, triangular-shaped RBCs, distorted-appearing RBCs), (3) evidence of hemolysis (a falling Hb level, polychromasia on the blood smear, elevated reticulocyte count, elevated level of plasma LDH), (4) fever, and (5) changing manifestations of ischemic damage to multiple organs. These last include varying, bizarre CNS findings; fluctuating jaundice (with elevation of both direct and indirect bilirubin because of the combination of hemolysis and hepatocellular damage); and proteinuria, hematuria, and mild elevation of the BUN as evidence of renal damage. Patients may also experience episodes of abdominal pain and changing heart rhythms due to myocardial damage. These findings are associated with a characteristic pathologic lesion involving vessels in multiple organs—bland, platelet-fibrin thrombi (without the infiltrations of granulocytes within and around vessel walls characteristic of vasculitis) localized primarily to arteriolocapillary junctions.

The etiology of TTP is unknown. A factor inducing aggregation of normal platelets in vitro has been demonstrated in the plasma of a high proportion of patients. Addition of the IgG fraction from normal plasma to TTP plasma will inhibit the platelet-aggregating activity of TTP plasma.

Untreated TTP is almost always fatal. Treatment consists of repeated administration of large volumes of normal plasma. Repeated plasmapheresis and plasma exchange (eg, a 5 L/day exchange for many days) may be needed to supply enough normal plasma to a patient to induce and maintain a remission. Corticosteroids are also usually given and some patients have been given antiplatelet drugs (eg, dipyridamole in large doses and aspirin) with questionable benefit. Administration of plasma is continued until all evidence of disease activity has subsided.

Hemolytic-Uremic Syndrome (HUS)

A disorder characterized by the sudden onset of thrombocytopenia and hemolysis with fragmented RBCs, and acute anuric renal failure.

HUS occurs primarily in infants and small children and pregnant or postpartum women; it is occasionally seen in older children and nonpregnant adults. Its pathogenesis is debated. In some patients, gram-negative infection (eg, an episode of diarrheal illness due to a gram-negative organism [ie, *E. coli* 0157:H7]) appears to be an initiating event, and then the syndrome may represent a clinical equivalent of the generalized **Shwartzman's reaction**; ie, endotoxemia may trigger an episode of DIC that results in deposition of fibrin within the glomerular capillary bed and the onset of acute renal failure.

Pathogenesis: Although HUS resembles TTP, it differs in that the kidney is primarily affected with the resultant sudden onset of anuria. Evidence of damage to other organs is minimal or lacking. A characteristically focal renal lesion is found whose major feature is evidence of fibrin thrombi in glomerular arterioles and capillaries. This may lead to fibrinoid necrosis of afferent glomerular arterioles and to areas of frank cortical necrosis. Marked fibrosis of glomerular arterioles may be noted in older

lesions. Fibrin thrombi in vessels of other organs are rare. Since the initiating episode of DIC is transient, blood coagulation tests indicative of continuing intravascular coagulation are not found when the usual patient is first seen. This concept of the pathogenesis of HUS does not preclude a role for local factors (eg, glomerular endothelial cell damage as a consequence of fibrin deposition) in the progression of HUS. Fibrin thrombi in small vessels in organs other than the kidneys are rare in HUS.

Prognosis: Most infants and children with HUS will recover with conservative management including dialysis therapy. The prognosis for recovery in adults is less certain; in particular, women who develop HUS postpartum may not recover renal function. Because some features of HUS resemble TTP, plasmapheresis and plasma exchange has also been tried, but clear evidence of its efficacy is lacking.

ABNORMALITIES OF PLATELET FUNCTION

In some conditions the platelets may be normal in number yet be unable to form hemostatic plugs normally. Then, the platelet count will be normal, but the bleeding time will be long. Impaired platelet function may stem from an *intrinsic platelet defect* or from an *extrinsic factor* that alters the function of otherwise normal platelets. Defects may be hereditary or acquired. Acquired causes include some commonly used drugs. Tests of the coagulation phase of hemostasis (eg, PTT and PT) are normal in most (but not all) circumstances (eg, see vW disease, below).

HEREDITARY DISORDERS OF PLATELET FUNCTION

When a patient's childhood history reveals easy bruising, and bleeding after tooth extractions, tonsillectomy, or other surgical procedures, the finding of a normal platelet count but a prolonged bleeding time suggests a hereditary disorder affecting platelet function. The cause will be either (1) von Willebrand **(vW)** disease, which stems from an abnormality of the plasma protein, vW factor, and is among the most common of the hereditary hemorrhagic diseases or (2) a hereditary intrinsic platelet disorder, which is less common. Special studies not available in many laboratories (eg, measurement of vW antigen, platelet aggregation studies) may be needed to establish the diagnosis. It is important to do so because treatment differs. Bleeding in vW disease is managed with infusions of desmopressin and cryoprecipitate to replace vW factor. Serious bleeding in a patient with an intrinsic platelet disorder may require transfusion of platelet concentrates. Whatever the cause of platelet dysfunction, drugs that may further impair platelet function should be avoided—particularly aspirin and other nonsteroidal anti-inflammatory agents used in arthritis. Acetaminophen may be used for analgesia, as it does not inhibit platelet function.

von Willebrand's Disease

(Angiohemophilia; Pseudohemophilia; Vascular Hemophilia)

An autosomal dominant bleeding disorder resulting from a quantitative (type I) or qualitative (type II variants) abnormality of vW factor, a plasma protein secreted by endothelial cells that circulates in plasma in multimers of up to 14,000,000 daltons in size. vW factor has 2 known hemostatic functions: (1) The very large multimers are required for platelets to adhere normally to collagen at sites of vessel wall injury; ie, for the initial step in the formation of hemostatic plugs. (2) Multimers of all sizes form complexes in plasma with factor VIII; formation of such complexes is required to maintain normal plasma factor VIII levels. (Note, therefore, that 2 hereditary disorders may cause factor VIII deficiency: hemophilia A, described below, in which the factor VIII molecule is not synthesized normally, and vW disease, in which the vW factor molecule is not synthesized normally.)

Symptoms and Signs

A typical person with vW disease may be of either sex with a positive maternal or paternal history. Bleeding manifestations will be mild to moderate and include easy bruising, bleeding from small skin cuts that may stop and start again over hours, increased menstrual bleeding (in some women), and abnormal bleeding after surgical procedures (eg, tooth extraction and tonsillectomy). Screening coagulation tests will reveal a long bleeding time and, usually, a slightly prolonged PTT reflecting a moderately reduced plasma factor VIII level.

Hormonal changes associated with stress or pregnancy and an acute phase response to inflammation or infection elevate the plasma vW factor level. In persons with mild vW disease, plasma level variation may cause screening tests to be normal on some occasions and abnormal on others, making diagnosis difficult. An aspirin-sensitized bleeding time may prove useful in this circumstance to bring out the bleeding time abnormality.

Diagnosis

A definitive diagnosis requires measuring (1) total plasma vW factor antigen as the height of the "rocket" obtained on electrophoresis of plasma through agarose containing an antibody to vW factor; (2) the ability of the plasma to support agglutination of normal platelets by ristocetin (ristocetin cofactor activity), which is a phenomenon dependent upon the presence of the intermediate-sized multimers of vW factor; and (3) the plasma factor VIII level. In patients with the common type I form of vW disease, results will be *concordant*; ie, vW antigen, ristocetin cofactor activity, and factor VIII coagulant activity will all be depressed to the same extent. The degree of depression will vary in different patients between about 15 to 60% of normal and determines the severity of a patient's abnormal bleeding.

Patients with type II variants of vW disease synthesize an abnormal vW molecule with a resultant selective deficiency of the very large multimers of vW factor. A type II variant is suspected when tests for vW antigen do not fit with results of a screening test of agglutination of the patient's plasma with different concentrations of ristocetin. Diagnosis may be confirmed by demonstrating an abnormal precipitin arc on crossed immunoelectrophoresis due to a selective deficiency of the large multimers.

Treatment

Replacement of vW factor by infusing the single donor plasma concentrate, cryoprecipitate, is effective in the control or prevention of bleeding in either the type I variant or the type II variants of vW disease. Dosage is often selected empirically (eg, 1 bag/10 kg q 8 to 12 h for several days to prevent excessive bleeding after major surgery). Lyophilized factor VIII concentrate should not be used as replacement therapy for vW factor, because of its variable content of the very large multimers of vW factor.

Desmopressin, a synthetic analog of vasopressin, stimulates release of vW factor from endothelial cell stores. It has a place in the treatment of type I vW disease but not in the treatment of type II variants, where it may have paradoxic deleterious effects. When given in a dose of 0.3 μg/kg in 50 mL 0.9% sodium chloride solution IV over 15 to 30 min, it may cause plasma levels of vW factor and factor VIII to rise sufficiently for the patient with mild type I vW disease to undergo tooth extraction or minor surgery without the need for replacement therapy. Levels of vW factor and factor VIII will revert to baseline according to an intravascular half-time of about 8 to 10 h. -Aminocaproic acid **(EACA)** 4 gm orally qid should also be given to suppress fibrinolysis. About 48 h must elapse for new endothelial stores of vW factor to accumulate and so permit a second injection of desmopressin to be as effective as an initial dose. In some instances combining the use of desmopressin and cryoprecipitate may substantially reduce the amount of cryoprecipitate needed to control or prevent bleeding.

HEREDITARY PLATELET DISORDERS

The most common of the hereditary platelet disorders are a group of mild bleeding disorders that may be considered *disorders of amplification of platelet activation*. They may result from a decreased content of ADP in the platelet dense granules (storage pool deficiency), from an inability to generate thromboxane A_2 from arachidonic acid released from the membrane phospholipids of stimulated platelets, or from an inability of platelets to respond normally to thromboxane A_2. They present with a common pattern of platelet aggregation test results: (1) impaired to absent aggregation following exposure to collagen, epinephrine, and a low concentration of ADP, and (2) normal aggregation following exposure to a high concentration of ADP. Aspirin and other nonsteroidal anti-inflammatory agents may produce the same pattern of platelet aggregation test results in normal individuals. Since aspirin's effect can persist for several days, it must be ascertained that a patient has not taken aspirin for several days before being tested to avoid confusion with a hereditary platelet defect.

Thrombasthenia and the Bernard-Soulier syndrome are other rare but important hereditary platelet defects that affect platelet surface membrane glycoproteins. Persons with **thrombasthenia** may experience severe mucosal bleeding (eg, nosebleeds that stop only after nasal packing and transfusions of platelet concentrates). Their platelets, which lack 2 surface membrane glycoproteins (**GP IIb** and **GP IIIa**) fail to bind fibrinogen during platelet activation and thus fail to aggregate. Characteristic laboratory findings are (1) failure of platelets to aggregate with any physiologic aggregating agent including a high concentration of exogenous ADP, (2) absence of clot retraction, and (3) single platelets without small platelet aggregates on a peripheral blood smear made from capillary blood obtained from a finger stick.

Bernard-Soulier syndrome: *A rare disorder in which unusually large platelets are found that do not agglutinate with ristocetin but aggregate normally with the physiologic aggregating agents ADP, collagen, and epinephrine.* A surface membrane glycoprotein that contains a receptor for vW factor is missing from the platelet surface membrane in this disorder. Therefore, the platelets do not adhere normally to collagen despite normal plasma vW factor. Large platelets associated with functional abnormalities also may be found in the **May-Hegglin anomaly,** a thrombocytopenic disorder with abnormal leukocytes, and in the **Chédiak-Higashi** syndrome.

ACQUIRED PLATELET DYSFUNCTION

Acquired abnormalities of platelet function, relatively common, may be found in a wide variety of clinical disorders (eg, myeloproliferative and myelodysplastic disorders, uremia, macroglobulinemia and multiple myeloma, cirrhosis, and SLE). Drugs may also induce platelet dysfunction. Coating of platelets by penicillin derivatives or newer cephalosporin antibiotics may impair formation of hemostatic plugs with a resultant prolonged bleeding time and increased bleeding tendency. Aspirin, which modestly prolongs the bleeding time of normal subjects, may markedly increase the bleeding time of patients who have an underlying second cause for platelet dysfunction or who have a severe disturbance of blood coagulation (eg, patients who have been given therapeutic doses of heparin or who have severe hemophilia). Platelets may be activated, discharge their granule contents, and so become "exhausted" and dysfunctional as blood circulates through a pump oxygenator during cardiac surgery. Therefore, regardless of the level of the platelet count, patients who are bleeding excessively after cardiac surgery and who have a long bleeding time should be given platelet concentrates.

Lengthening of the bleeding time in *uremia* has been attributed to retention of a low mol wt substance in uremic blood that impairs platelet function. Bleeding time usually shortens after vigorous dialysis. Moreover, administration of cryoprecipitate or infu

sion of desmopressin also shortens the bleeding time and decreases the bleeding tendency in uremia. The mechanism is unknown since these are measures whose only known effect upon the bleeding time stems from increasing plasma vW factor level, which is normal or elevated in uremia.

In many disorders causing acquired platelet dysfunction, varying degrees of thrombocytopenia may also occur. The platelet dysfunction can be recognized because the bleeding time will be prolonged disproportionately for the level of the platelet count.

HEREDITARY COAGULATION DISORDERS

THE HEMOPHILIAS

Most common of bleeding disorders due to hereditary clotting factor deficiencies. The 2 forms, hemophilia A (factor VIII deficiency) and hemophilia B (factor IX deficiency) have identical clinical manifestations, screening test abnormalities, and sex-linked genetic transmission. Specific factor assays are required to distinguish the two. About 4:5 hemophiliacs have hemophilia A.

Genetic Manifestations (see also Ch. 203)

Because it is transmitted as a defect on the X chromosome, hemophilia affects only males. All daughters of hemophiliacs will be obligatory carriers, but all sons will be normal. Each son of a carrier will have a 50% chance of being either normal or a hemophiliac and each daughter will have a 50% chance of being either normal or a carrier. By measuring factor VIII level and comparing it with the level of vW factor antigen, it is usually (but not always) possible to determine whether a person is a true carrier of hemophilia A. Similarly, measuring the factor IX level will often identify the carrier of hemophilia B. Rarely, random inactivation of 1 of the 2 X chromosomes in early embryonic life will result in a carrier's having a low enough factor VIII or IX level to experience abnormal bleeding.

Symptoms and Signs

Different abnormal allelic hemophilic genes exist and support different levels of factor VIII or IX activity. The patient with a factor VIII or IX level < 1% of normal will have severe bleeding episodes throughout his lifetime. The first bleeding episode will usually occur before age 18 mo. Minor trauma can result in extensive tissue hemorrhages and hemarthroses, which, if not properly managed, can result in crippling musculoskeletal deformities. Bleeding into the base of the tongue with airway compression may be life-threatening and requires prompt and vigorous replacement therapy. Even a trivial blow to the head requires prophylactic replacement therapy to prevent intracranial bleeding.

Patients with factor VIII or IX levels in the 5% of normal range have mild hemophilia. They rarely have "spontaneous" hemorrhages; nevertheless they will bleed seriously (and even fatally) after surgery if not managed correctly. Occasional patients have even milder hemophilia with a factor VIII or IX level in the 10 to 25% of normal range. Such patients may also bleed excessively after surgery or dental extraction.

Laboratory Findings

Typical screening test findings in hemophilia are a prolonged PTT, a normal bleeding time, and a normal PT. Specific assays of factors VIII and IX will determine the type and severity of the hemophilia. Since factor VIII levels may also be reduced in vW disease (see above), vW antigen should also be measured in patients with newly discovered hemophilia A, particularly the patient with mild hemophilia A in whom a family history of sex-linked transmission cannot be obtained.

After transfusion therapy about 15% of patients with hemophilia A develop factor VIII antibodies that act as anticoagulants inhibiting the coagulant activity of further

factor VIII administered to the patient. Patients should be screened for factor VIII anticoagulant activity (eg, by measuring the degree of shortening of the PTT immediately after mixing the patient's plasma with equal parts of normal plasma and after incubation for 1 h at room temperature) especially before an elective procedure that requires replacement therapy.

Treatment

A list of special treatment centers, other information about hemophilia care, and other hereditary bleeding problems can be obtained from the National Hemophilia Foundation, 19 West 34th Street, New York, NY 10001.

Patients with hemophilia should avoid the use of aspirin. Acetaminophen is recommended for analgesia. In some patients disabling pain from musculoskeletal complications may require judicious use of the nonsteroidal anti-inflammatory agent ibuprofen, which has a lesser and more transient effect than aspirin upon platelet function. Prophylactic dental care on a regular basis is essential to prevent tooth extractions and other dental surgery. All drugs should be given either orally or IV; IM injections can cause large hematomas.

As described above for vW disease, use of desmopressin may temporarily raise factor VIII levels in the patient with mild hemophilia A (basal factor VIII levels of 5 to 10%) and such patients should be tested for the response of their factor VIII plasma level to desmopressin. Its administration to a responsive patient after minor trauma or before elective dental surgery may obviate or reduce the need for replacement therapy. Desmopressin is uniformly ineffective in severe hemophilia A.

Preparations used for replacement therapy: Fresh frozen plasma contains both factor VIII and IX. However, unless plasma exchange is done, sufficient whole plasma cannot be given to patients with severe hemophilia to raise factor VIII or IX concentrations to levels that effectively prevent or control bleeding episodes. Plasma concentrates have therefore been developed. Two concentrates are available for treatment of hemophilia A: cryoprecipitate, and lyophilized factor VIII concentrate. For treatment of hemophilia B, a single concentrate, prothrombin complex concentrate, which contains not just factor IX but all of the vitamin K-dependent clotting factors, is available.

Cryoprecipitate is prepared from single donors by a freeze-thaw technic that removes the thawed plasma before the last ice crystals (which contain factor VIII, von Willebrand factor, and fibrinogen) are dissolved. Bags of cryoprecipitate are stored frozen and their contents dissolved in 10 mL of 0.9% sodium chloride solution before use. Factor VIII activity is expressed in units, with 1 u. being defined as the amount of factor VIII in 1 mL of normal plasma. Although the concentration of factor VIII in individual bags varies, a bag may be assumed to contain 80 u. of factor VIII in calculating the number of bags needed for replacement therapy.

Lyophilized factor VIII concentrate, prepared from plasma pools of up to 5000 donors, is packaged in bottles supplying from 250 to 1000 factor VIII units. The powder is dissolved in 10 to 100 mL of sterile diluent before use. Because of its convenience, lyophilized factor VIII concentrate has received widespread use, particularly in home care programs in which patients inject themselves with concentrate at the first indication of bleeding.

Calculation of dosage for replacement therapy: The factor VIII or IX level should be raised transiently to about 0.3 u. (30%) to protect against bleeding after dental extraction or to abort a beginning joint hemorrhage; to 0.5 u. (50%) if major joint or IM bleeding is already evident; and to 1.0 u. (100%) in life-threatening bleeding or before major surgery. Repeat infusions at 50% of the initial calculated dose should be given q 8 to 12 h to keep trough levels above 0.5 u. (50%) for several days in a life-threatening bleeding episode or after surgery.

For factor VIII replacement, dosage is calculated by multiplying the patient's weight in kg by 44 and by the level in units desired (eg, to raise the factor VIII level of a man who weighs 68 kg (150 lb) from essential zero to 1 u./mL, the dosage needed would be 68 × 44 × 1 or about 3000 u.). For an unknown reason only about ½ the number of factor IX units listed on a bottle of prothrombin complex concentrate are recovered after infusion. Therefore, when prothrombin complex concentrate is given for factor IX replacement therapy, an amount double that calculated as necessary is given. Because prothrombin complex concentrate may contain variable amounts of activated clotting factors, patients receiving repeated doses of factor IX concentrate are, paradoxically, at increased risk for thrombosis. For this reason, heparin 5 to 10 u. are often added to each mL of reconstituted prothrombin complex concentrate.

The antifibrinolytic agent ε-aminocaproic acid **(EACA)** 2.5 gm qid for 1 wk should be given to prevent late bleeding after dental extraction or other causes of oropharyngeal mucosal trauma (eg, tongue laceration). However, because prothrombin complex concentrate may contain activated clotting factors, EACA should not be given immediately after prothrombin complex, but only after 10 h has elapsed. EACA may also be useful in selected patients with other types of bleeding, but should not be given to patients with hematuria because of the possibility of forming clots within the GU system resistant to lysis.

Treatment of patients displaying factor VIII inhibitors: Treatment of hemophiliacs who are bleeding with a factor VIII inhibitor is difficult and should be undertaken in consultation with someone experienced in such care. If possible, musculoskeletal bleeding is managed without giving factor VIII, since it will stimulate further antibody production and a rise in plasma titer of antibody within 3 to 4 days. In patients with serious bleeding and a low initial antibody titer, a large dose of factor VIII, calculated to overcome the inhibitor and temporarily raise plasma factor VIII concentration, may be given. If this does not control the bleeding, further factor VIII infusion will be useless because of the rapid rise in antibody titer that the initial infusion induces. Prothrombin complex concentrate contains variable amounts of a poorly characterized activity that bypasses the role of factor VIII in coagulation; therefore, these concentrates are used to manage serious bleeding in patients with a high titer inhibitor. Special preparations of prothrombin complex concentrate with increased amounts of this activity are available, but expensive. A porcine factor VIII preparation insensitive to the inhibitor has been used experimentally with reported good results.

Safety of blood products: Since blood products can transmit AIDS, their use in hemophilia poses serious problems. Over 50 hemophiliacs in the USA developed AIDS by 1985. Most patients who have received replacement therapy either with factor VIII concentrate or large amounts of cryoprecipitate have antibody in the plasma to the human immunodeficiency virus **(HIV)** causing AIDS. It is unknown at this time which antibody-positive patients will subsequently develop AIDS. Because pooled plasma preparations have a much higher risk of transmitting infection than single donor preparations, it is recommended that bleeding episodes in infants and small children with newly diagnosed hemophilia A be managed with cryoprecipitate, since few units should be needed to control even a major bleeding episode. However, major surgery in an adult could well require use of 300 u. of cryoprecipitate, which, if prepared from blood drawn in many large cities of the USA, would entail a real risk for transmission of AIDS. Preliminary data suggest that heat treatment of factor VIII concentrate to diminish the risk of transmitting hepatitis may inactivate the HIV. If these observations are confirmed, then heat-treated factor VIII concentrate should be the preferred concentrate for use in all patients with hemophilia A. Physicians treating hemophiliacs must keep up-to-date on new developments and recommendations to reduce the risk of transfusion-induced AIDS.

Because experience with prothrombin complex concentrates is more limited, reliable data are not yet available on the association of positive tests for antibody to HIV with the use of this concentrate.

OTHER HEREDITARY HEMORRHAGIC DISORDERS

Other hereditary clotting factor deficiency states are summarized in TABLE 99–5. Most are rare, autosomal recessive conditions producing disease only in the homozygote. To this list one must also add a rare but important hereditary bleeding disorder resulting not from a deficiency of a clotting factor, but from a deficiency of a plasma protease inhibitor, the major physiologic inhibitor of plasmin, α_2-antiplasmin. A homozygote for **hereditary α_2-antiplasmin deficiency** will bleed as severely as a hemophilic patient after trauma or surgery. The only abnormal screening test will be lysis of the plasma clot on incubation overnight in saline. A euglobulin lysis time will be normal. A specific α_2-antiplasmin assay will reveal values in the 1 to 3% of normal range. Use of EACA will correct the bleeding tendency—5 gm IV over 1 h initially and then 1 gm/h by continuous IV to prevent surgical bleeding or 5 gm orally q 6 h to abort tissue bleeding after minor trauma. A heterozygote, with an α_2-antiplasmin level in the 30 to 40% of normal range, can also experience excessive surgical bleeding, if an untoward event (eg, a hypotensive episode) triggers an unusual degree of fibrinolytic activity.

TABLE 99–5. HEREDITARY DISORDERS OF BLOOD COAGULATION FACTORS

Deficiency	*Screening Test Results*	*Comments*
Factor XII **HMWK** **PK**	PTT long PT normal	Test tube abnormality without clinical bleeding. Must be distinguished by specific assays from factor XI deficiency in which post-operative bleeding may occur.
Factor XI	PTT long PT normal	Autosomal recessive. Increased frequency in Ashkenazic Jews. No excess bleeding after trauma. May have negative bleeding history after earlier surgery yet still bleed excessively after next surgery. Diagnosis by specific assay. Therapy for bleeding: Keep factor XI level > 30% with fresh frozen plasma 5–20 mL/kg/day.
Factor VIII **Factor IX**	PTT long PT normal	Factor VIII deficiency = hemophilia A; factor IX deficiency = hemophilia B. Sex-linked transmission. Severe bleeding. For therapy, see text.
Factor VII	PTT normal PT long	Autosomal recessive, rare. Severe deficiency (< 2%) associated with serious bleeding including CNS bleeding. Levels > 5% associated with mild or no bleeding. Therapy: plasma 3–5 mL/kg or prothrombin complex concentrate for life-threatening bleeding

(Continued)

HMWK = high mol wt kininogen; PK = prekallikrein; PTT = partial thromboplastin time; PT = prothrombin time

TABLE 99–5. HEREDITARY DISORDERS OF BLOOD COAGULATION FACTORS *(Cont'd)*

Deficiency	*Screening Test Results*	*Comments*
Factor V, X, or prothrombin	PTT long PT long	Autosomal recessive, rare. Bleeding may be mild or severe. Heavy menstrual flow in women. Distinguish by specific assays. Therapy of Factor V deficiency: fresh plasma, platelet concentrates (supplies platelet factor V). Therapy of factor X or prothrombin deficiency: fresh plasma or prothrombin complex concentrate for life-threatening bleeding.
Fibrinogen	In afibrinogenemia (fibrinogen < 10 mg/dL) no clotting in PTT, PT because machine endpoint not triggered. In hypofibrinogenemia (fibrinogen 70–100 mg/dL) PT often ~ 2 sec prolonged, PTT normal, thrombin time long	Severe bleeding in afibrinogenemia (homozygous state), minimal early bleeding after surgery in hypofibrinogenemia (heterozygous state). Therapy: cryofibrinogen (4gm fibrinogen as 16 bags of cryofibrinogen).
Dysfibrinogenemia	Thrombin time long PTT often normal PT slightly prolonged	Manifestations vary: may be excessive bleeding, tendency to thrombosis, wound dehiscence. Fibrinogen low by clotting assay, but normal by immunologic assay.
Factor XIII	PTT normal PT normal Thrombin time normal Clot dissolves in 5 M urea	Autosomal recessive, rare. May have severe bleeding with hemarthrosis, delayed postsurgical bleeding, poor wound healing. Spontaneous abortions in women. Therapy: plasma (One unit is effective, due to long half-life of factor XIII.
Protein C **Protein S**	PTT normal PT normal Thrombin time normal	Heterozygote state (~ 50%) associated with increased tendancy for venous thrombosis. Homozygous protein C deficiency causes neonatal purpura fulminans. Diagnosis: usually by immunoassay of plasma antigen level.

HMWK = high mol wt kininogen; PK = prekallikrein; PTT = partial thromboplastin time; PT = prothrombin time

ACQUIRED COAGULATION DISORDERS

The major causes of acquired coagulation disorders are (1) vitamin K deficiency, (2) liver disease, (3) disseminated intravascular coagulation, and (4) development of circulating anticoagulants, which are usually antibodies to hemostatic factors.

VITAMIN K DEFICIENCY

(See Ch. 81)

LIVER DISEASE

Liver disease may disturb hemostasis through impaired clotting factor synthesis, increased fibrinolysis, associated thrombocytopenia, and, in patients with fulminant

hepatitis or acute fatty liver of pregnancy, consumption of clotting factors in intravascular clotting. These disorders are discussed elsewhere in THE MANUAL.

DISSEMINATED INTRAVASCULAR COAGULATION (DIC)

(Consumption Coagulopathy; Defibrination Syndrome)

Generation of fibrin in the circulating blood. DIC usually results from entrance into or generation within the blood of material with tissue factor activity, which initiates blood coagulation by way of the extrinsic pathway. DIC usually arises in 1 of 3 clinical circumstances: (1) In complications of obstetrics, uterine material with tissue factor activity gains access to the maternal circulation (eg, in abruptio placentae, a saline-induced therapeutic abortion, retained dead fetus syndrome, and the initial phase of amniotic fluid embolism). (2) Infection is present, particularly with gram-negative organisms. Adding gram-negative endotoxin to blood in vitro causes generation of tissue factor activity on the plasma membrane of monocytes. This presumably represents a prime mechanism for endotoxin-induced DIC, since depletion of blood monocytes in rabbits by administration of the alkylating agent, nitrogen mustard, protects the animals from developing DIC after injection of endotoxin. Exposure to endotoxin will also result in generation of tissue factor activity on the surface of endothelial cells in culture, and this could be a second mechanism for initiating endotoxin-induced intravascular coagulation in vivo. (3) Malignancy is present: particularly mucin-secreting adenocarcinomas of the pancreas and prostate and a form of acute leukemia, acute promyelocytic leukemia, in which hypergranular leukemic cells are thought to release material from their granules with tissue factor activity.

Other less common causes of DIC include severe head trauma that breaks down the blood-brain barrier and allows exposure of blood to brain tissue with potent tissue factor activity; complications of prostatic surgery that allow prostatic material with tissue factor activity to enter the circulation; and venomous snake bites in which enzymes activating factor X, prothrombin, or directly converting fibrinogen to fibrin may enter the circulation.

Symptoms and Signs

Subacute DIC may be associated with thromboembolic complications of hypercoagulability including venous thrombosis, thrombotic vegetations on the aortic heart valve, and arterial emboli arising from such vegetations. Abnormal bleeding is uncommon.

Acute DIC: In contrast, thrombocytopenia and depletion of plasma clotting factors of acute, massive DIC creates a serious bleeding tendency that is worsened by secondary fibrinolysis with resultant formation of large amounts of fibrin degradation products that interfere with platelet function and with normal fibrin polymerization. If secondary fibrinolysis is extensive enough to deplete plasma α_2-antiplasmin, then a loss of control of the fibrinolytic process adds to the bleeding tendency. When such massive DIC occurs as a complication of surgery leaving raw surface (eg, prostatectomy) or of delivery, major hemorrhage results. Invasive procedures (eg, arterial puncture for blood gas studies) will give rise to persistent bleeding from puncture sites. Ecchymoses form at sites of parenteral injections. Serious GI bleeding may occur from sites of gastric mucosal erosion.

Acute DIC may also cause fibrin to be deposited in multiple small blood vessels. If secondary fibrinolysis fails to lyse the fibrin rapidly, hemorrhagic tissue necrosis may result. The most vulnerable organ is the kidney, where deposition of fibrin in the glomerular capillary bed may lead to acute, anuric renal failure. This is reversible if the necrosis is limited to the renal tubules (acute renal tubular necrosis) but is irreversible if the glomeruli are also destroyed (renal cortical necrosis). Fibrin deposits may also result in mechanical damage to RBCs with hemolysis (see discussion of HUS, above).

Occasionally, fibrin deposited in the small vessels of the fingers and toes leads to gangrene and loss of digits.

Laboratory Findings

Laboratory findings vary with the intensity of the DIC. A **subacute form** of DIC may be seen in patients with malignancy and occasionally also in an obstetric patient with a retained dead fetus or with retained placental remnants. In this slower, often more chronic form of DIC, the findings are thrombocytopenia, a normal to minimally prolonged PT, a *short* PTT, a normal or moderately reduced fibrinogen level, and an increased level of fibrin degradation products. (Since illness stimulates increased fibrinogen synthesis, a fibrinogen level in the lower portion of the normal range [eg, 175 mg/dL] is not normal in a sick patient and raises the possibility of impaired production due to liver disease or increased consumption due to intravascular coagulation.)

Acute, massive DIC produces a striking "global" constellation of screening laboratory test abnormalities consisting of (1) thrombocytopenia, (2) a very small clot (sometimes no visible clot at all) when blood is allowed to clot in a glass tube and inspected for clot size, (3) a markedly prolonged PT and PTT (the plasma contains insufficient fibrinogen to trigger the end point of coagulation instruments and test results are often reported as more than some value [eg, > 200 sec], which is the interval before the automated instrument shifts to the next sample in the machine), (4) a markedly reduced plasma fibrinogen concentration, (5) a positive plasma protamine paracoagulation test for fibrin monomer, and (6) a very high level of fibrin degradation products in the serum. Specific clotting factor assays will reveal low levels of multiple clotting factors, but particularly factors V and VIII (which are inactivated due to generation of activated protein C during DIC).

One other condition, massive hepatic necrosis, can produce laboratory abnormalities resembling acute DIC; measurement of factor VIII level helps to distinguish them. Reduced in DIC, the factor VIII level will be elevated in hepatic necrosis, because factor VIII is an acute phase protein and is the only plasma clotting factor not made by the hepatocyte.

Diagnosis

Overt DIC is suspected when bleeding occurs in clinical settings known to predispose (see above) and is confirmed by laboratory studies, as described above. Occult DIC is best anticipated with prospective monitoring of fibrinogen, platelets, FDP, and blood cultures.

Treatment

The guiding principal of therapy of DIC is to identify and correct its underlying cause without delay (eg, prompt broad-spectrum antibiotic treatment of suspected gram-negative sepsis, evacuation of the uterus in abruptio placentae). Once this is accomplished, DIC should subside quickly. If the patient is bleeding seriously, replacement therapy is indicated; platelet concentrates to correct thrombocytopenia (and also as a source of factor V in platelets); cryoprecipitate to replace fibrinogen and factor VIII; fresh frozen plasma to increase levels of factor V, other clotting factors, and as a source of antithrombin III, which may also be depleted secondary to DIC.

Heparin is usually not indicated to stop intravascular coagulation, if the underlying disorder can be brought under control quickly. However, giving heparin may be necessary when clinical findings suggest developing thrombotic complications (eg, when progressive oliguria despite adequate BP and vascular volume raises the possibility of progressive deposition of fibrin in the glomerular capillary bed or when increasing cyanosis and coldness of the fingers and toes raises the possibility of incipient gangrene of the digits). In patients with DIC secondary to malignancy, rapid control of the underlying process is not possible. Use of anticoagulants to prevent the DIC may then be indicated, particularly if the patient has a malignancy in which therapy could

induce a remission (eg, previously untreated metastatic prostatic carcinoma, acute promyelocytic leukemia). In metastatic prostatic carcinoma a combination of DIC and extensive secondary fibrinolysis may require heparin and ε-aminocaproic acid **(EACA)** to be given together to control bleeding (eg, at starting doses of heparin 500 IU and EACA 1 gm/h continuously IV, with efficacy being monitored by clinical observations of bleeding, platelet counts, and fibrinogen determinations). Heparin should never be used in DIC secondary to head injury or if CNS bleeding for any other reason is suspected.

CIRCULATING ANTICOAGULANTS

Endogenous substances that inhibit blood coagulation. They are usually antibodies that neutralize the activity of a clotting factor (eg, an antibody against factor VIII or factor V) or the activity of the procoagulant phospholipid used in certain coagulation test systems (the lupus anticoagulant). Rarely, circulating anticoagulants are not antibodies but glycosaminoglycans with heparin-like anticoagulant activity arising from their ability to increase antithrombin III reactivity. These heparin-like anticoagulants are found mainly in patients with multiple myeloma or other hematologic malignancies.

Occasionally, antibodies arise that are not circulating anticoagulants, since they do not neutralize the activity of a clotting factor, but that, nevertheless, cause bleeding. These are usually antibodies that bind prothrombin. Although the prothrombin-antiprothrombin complex retains its coagulant activity in vitro, it is rapidly cleared from the blood in vivo, with resultant acute hypoprothrombinemia.

FACTOR VIII ANTICOAGULANTS

Plasma containing a factor VIII antibody will have the same coagulation test abnormalities as plasma from a patient with hemophilia A (see above) except that adding normal plasma or another source of factor VIII to the patient's plasma will not correct the hemostatic abnormality. Instead, the antibody in the patient's plasma will neutralize the coagulant activity of the added factor VIII.

Antibodies to factor VIII develop in about 15% of patients with hemophilia A as a complication of replacement therapy. Transfused factor VIII is treated as a foreign, immunogenic agent and antibodies are made against it. Factor VIII antibodies also arise in nonhemophilic patients (1) occasionally in a postpartum woman, (2) as a manifestation of underlying systemic autoimmune disease or of a hypersensitivity reaction to a drug, or (3) as an isolated phenomenon without evidence of other underlying disease. Patients with a factor VIII anticoagulant are at risk of life-threatening hemorrhage. Immunosuppressive therapy with cyclophosphamide and corticosteroids has been successful in suppressing antibody production in a number of nonhemophiliacs, and, with the possible exception of the postpartum woman whose antibody may disappear spontaneously, immunosuppression should be attempted in all nonhemophiliacs. However, since immunosuppressives do not seem to influence antibody production in hemophiliacs, they are not recommended. Other facets of management are discussed above (see THE HEMOPHILIAS).

THE LUPUS ANTICOAGULANT

This is a common anticoagulant, first described in patients with SLE and therefore called the lupus anticoagulant, but subsequently discovered in patients with a variety of disorders, often as an unrelated finding. The phenomenon results from production of antibodies that react with epitopes on phospholipids, including the phospholipid used in the PTT and in specific clotting factor assays based upon the PTT technic. The following pattern of laboratory test results is found: a prolonged PTT that fails to correct with a 1:1 mixture of patient's and normal plasma, a normal or minimally

prolonged PT, and a nonspecific depression of those clotting factors measured by a PTT technic (factors XII, XI, IX, and VIII). Some patients will also have a false-positive VDRL test for syphilis, in which the phospholipid cardiolipin is used as the antigen, and most patients will have evidence of antibodies reacting with cardiolipin by a more sensitive radioimmunoassay technic.

Although the anticoagulant interferes with the function of procoagulant phospholipid in clotting tests in vitro, patients with only the lupus anticoagulant do not bleed excessively. Apparently, the anticoagulant does not interfere with the function of procoagulant phospholipid on cell surfaces in vivo. Paradoxically, however, patients with the lupus anticoagulant are at increased risk for thrombosis, which may be either venous or arterial. The reason is as yet unknown, but the association between the lupus anticoagulant and thrombosis is real. If a patient with the lupus anticoagulant experiences a thrombotic episode, long-term anticoagulant therapy should be seriously considered as prophylaxis against recurrent episodes. Repeated abortions in the 1st trimester of pregnancy have also been reported in occasional women with the lupus anticoagulant, possibly related to thrombosis of placental vessels.

A subset of patients with the lupus anticoagulant develop a second antibody, the non-neutralizing antibody to prothrombin described earlier that induces hypoprothrombinemia, and these patients do bleed abnormally. Hypoprothrombinemia is suspected when the screening tests reveal a long PT in addition to the long PTT and is confirmed by a specific assay. Treatment with corticosteroids is indicated and often results in a rapid return of the PT to normal.

---

100. LEUKOPENIA; NEUTROPENIA

Leukopenia: *A reduction in the circulating WBC count to < 4000/μL.* Usually leukopenia is due to a reduced number of blood neutrophils, although reduced lymphocytes, monocytes, eosinophils, or basophils may also contribute to the decreased total cell count. **Neutropenia (granulocytopenia; agranulocytosis)**: *A reduction in the blood neutrophil (granulocyte) count often leading to an increased susceptibility to bacterial and fungal infections.*

Neutropenia may be classified on the basis of granulocyte count (total WBC × % granulocytes) and the relative risk of infection: mild (1000 to 2000/μL), moderate (500 to 1000/μL), or severe (< 500/μL). Acute, severe neutropenia due to impaired production is often life-threatening and therefore of greatest clinical consequence.

Etiology (see also Ch. 7)

Neutropenia occurs because of impaired cell production, increased margination with redistribution of cells in the blood, and accelerated utilization or cell turnover. Neutropenia can be acute (occurring over a few days) or chronic (lasting months or years). It occurs as the sole hematologic abnormality in some cases (eg, chronic idiopathic neutropenia) or as part of a broad hematologic abnormality (eg, aplastic anemia).

The most common cause of neutropenia is impairment of cell production by drugs (eg, cytoreductive cancer chemotherapeutic agents, antithyroid drugs, phenothiazines, anticonvulsants, penicillins, sulfonamides, and chloramphenicol). Some antineoplastic drugs (eg, alkylating agents and antimetabolites) cause neutropenia as a predictable side effect. Other drugs cause neutropenia as an idiosyncratic reaction, ie, not predictably dose- or duration-related.

Diminished neutrophil production also occurs in rare hereditary and congenital diseases (eg, infantile genetic agranulocytosis, familial neutropenia, cyclic neutropenia, pancreatic insufficiency with neutropenia, and several disorders combining impaired

neutrophil production and severe immune deficiency). Impaired production occurs because of marrow replacement or involvement (eg, malignancies, granulomatous diseases, myelofibrosis) and as a common feature of severe vitamin B_{12} and folate deficiency.

Neutropenia due to increased margination or accelerated cell turnover is a less frequent clinical problem than neutropenia due to impaired production. Increased margination occurs in the acute phase of some infectious diseases, in some autoimmune disorders (eg, SLE, RA) and in some conditions associated with splenomegaly (eg, Felty's syndrome, malaria, and sarcoidosis). Accelerated neutrophil utilization or turnover occurs with acute bacterial infections and is the mechanism in neonatal isoimmune neutropenia and in drug-induced immune neutropenia associated with aminopyrine, penicillins, and perhaps diphenylhydantoin, gold salts, and sulfonamides.

In many patients with neutropenia, a combination of the mechanisms cited above are probably involved. In others, the etiology and mechanism cannot be ascertained.

Pathogenesis

Neutrophils, like erythrocytes, megakaryocytes, and other leukocytes, are derived from pluripotential hematopoietic stem cells. A number of proliferative and maturational steps occur before the cells mature, leave the marrow, and enter the blood. Drugs and other toxic agents can impair cell proliferation in the marrow. Immunologic injury to neutrophils can occur in the marrow during the maturation process or in the circulation. Neutrophils have distinctive cell-surface antigens that can react with autoantibodies and lead to immune-mediated cell destruction similar to the mechanisms of autoimmune hemolytic anemia (see Ch. 96).

Increased margination of neutrophils occurs because of an increased adhesiveness of the cells to the vascular endothelium and because excessively adhesive cells are trapped in the lungs and spleen. Activation of the complement system, a feature of many inflammatory states, can contribute to increased adhesiveness. Neutropenia with extracorporeal circulation for hemodialysis is attributed to increased margination because of complement activation with exposure of the blood to foreign surfaces. In bacterial infections, once neutrophils migrate from the blood and bone marrow to the tissues for phagocytosis, they do not reenter the circulation. Severe infections can divert enough neutrophils to cause neutropenia, especially in patients whose neutrophil production is already impaired.

Symptoms and Signs

There are no specific symptoms of neutropenia; manifestations are those of the infections that are present and generally depend upon the severity, duration, and cause of the neutropenia. In acute neutropenia, fever and painful mucosal ulcers of the mouth and perirectal area are common, as is bacterial pneumonia. Bacteremia and septic shock are further consequences in untreated patients. Chronic neutropenia often has a far more benign outlook, particularly when the neutropenia is only mild to moderate, the monocyte count is normal, and other immune functions (eg, immunoglobulins, complement, lymphocyte function) are intact.

Diagnosis

Neutropenia should be suspected when a patient presents with fever, chills, and mucosal ulceration, or other evidence of a severe infection and a reduced neutrophil count. Repeated total and differential WBC counts should be made to determine if the neutropenia is acute or chronic. As patients with severe acute neutropenia improve, often there is an "overshoot" in the count before it returns to normal levels. In rare patients with regularly recurring symptoms, serial count measurements will show cyclic fluctuations leading to the diagnosis of **cyclic neutropenia**.

Bone marrow aspiration and biopsy provide the most helpful laboratory evaluation. Marrow involvement by leukemia or infiltrative disorders can be detected. If early neutrophil precursors are morphologically normal but severely reduced in numbers, production of cells will be impaired for several days. If the marrow shows many precursors but no mature cells, it may be recovering from an acute interruption of cell production, the mature cells of the marrow may have been abruptly released to the circulation, or intramedullary destruction may be ongoing. Serial blood counts and a repeat marrow examination in 5 to 7 days will define the underlying mechanism.

Establishing the precise cause of neutropenia is often difficult. A specific drug etiology is usually made by inference, since methods to study the reactions of drugs with neutrophils and their precursors are generally not available. Accurate measurement of neutrophil antibodies can be done by specialized laboratories. Measurement of cell distribution and turnover using radioisotopically labeled cells is performed in some research centers. Other diagnostic studies are based on clarifying the underlying or associated disorders described above.

Treatment

Acute neutropenia (see also under CHEMOTHERAPY in Ch. 105): Patients with acute and severe neutropenia (< 500/μL) and infection generally should be hospitalized and treated promptly with broad-spectrum antibiotic therapy (eg, a penicillinase-resistant penicillin or cephalosporin plus an aminoglycoside such as gentamicin or tobramycin). If there is any suspicion that the acute neutropenia is drug induced, the potential offending agent should be stopped immediately. Cultures for bacteria and fungi should be obtained from areas of inflammation and the blood; if cultures are positive, antibiotic therapy is adjusted to match the sensitivities of the organisms and usually is continued for at least 7 to 10 days. If cultures are negative and the patient remains severely neutropenic and febrile, antibiotics should be continued until the patient becomes afebrile for 24 to 48 h, or the diagnosis and prognosis are clear.

Antibiotic therapy is usually sufficient, but, in patients with acute nonlymphocytic leukemia and severe neutropenia (expected to last 7 to 10 days or more), neutrophil transfusions can improve prognosis in severely ill neutropenic patients with serious infections. In other circumstances their use is questionable. Precise matching of donors and recipients is difficult, sensitization occurs rapidly, and transfusions are very expensive. Prophylactic transfusions generally are not warranted. Further details on the management of cancer patients who develop neutropenia and fever are discussed under side effects of treatment in Chs. 101 and 105.

Stimulation of bone marrow to produce more neutrophils with glucocorticosteroids, androgenic steroids, vitamins, and other agents is usually unsuccessful. The recovery of blood neutrophil counts after chemotherapy can be accelerated with lithium carbonate 300 mg orally tid, but the magnitude of the benefit is small.

Saline or hydrogen peroxide gargles every few hours or anesthetic lozenges (benzocaine 15 mg q 3 to 4 h) may relieve the discomfort associated with oropharyngeal ulcerations. Oral thrush (see STOMATITIS in Ch. 247) is treated with nystatin mouthwashes (400,000 to 600,000 u. qid). A semi-solid or liquid diet may be necessary during acute mucositis.

Chronic neutropenia: Many patients with moderately reduced neutrophil counts (ie, > 500/μL) have few if any symptoms related to neutropenia and no therapy is indicated. Patients with mild-to-moderate neutropenia as the sole hematologic abnormality rarely develop more severe hematologic diseases. Therapy should be expectant; patients should be taught to seek prompt medical attention when they develop fever and signs of infection, and they should be treated promptly with antibiotics targeted as precisely as possible for the specific infection. In some patients with accelerated neutrophil turnover due to autoimmune disorders, corticosteroids, generally prednisone

0.5 to 1.0 mg/kg/day orally, will improve the blood neutrophil count. This improvement can often be maintained with alternate day therapy. Splenectomy will raise the neutrophil count in most patients with splenomegaly and splenic sequestration of neutrophils (eg, Felty's syndrome, hairy cell leukemia); this therapy should be reserved for those with severe neutropenia (ie, < 500/μL) and serious problems with infections.

LYMPHOCYTOPENIA

An acute or chronic reduction in blood lymphocytes due to abnormal development of the lymphoreticular system, suppression of lymphocytopoiesis, or increased lymphocyte turnover.

Etiology

Chronic impairment of lymphocyte production is a feature of several rare primary immunologic diseases, eg, Swiss-type agammaglobulinemia, thymic alymphoplasia, DiGeorge syndrome, Wiskott-Aldrich syndrome, Bruton-type agammaglobulinemia, thymoma, ataxia telangiectasia, and severe combined immunodeficiency syndrome (see in Ch. 18). Acute or chronic impairment of production also occurs with a variety of acquired conditions (eg, acute neutropenia or agranulocytosis, aplastic anemia, sarcoidosis, renal failure, SLE, leukemia, carcinomatosis, Hodgkin's disease, lymphosarcoma, multiple myeloma). Lymphocytopenia is a very common feature of AIDS caused by HTLV-III infection of T lymphocytes. Lymphocytopenia also occurs with acute stress, corticosteroid and alkylating agent therapy, radiation, and in Cushing's syndrome. Excessive loss of lymphocytes may result from thoracic duct or intestinal drainage, intestinal lymphangiectasia, and some other conditions associated with severe edema and intestinal leakage.

Pathology and Pathogenesis

Most patients with thymus-mediated (T cell) immunologic deficiency disorders have underdeveloped central and paracortical areas in lymph nodes, severe lymphocytopenia involving the larger lymphocytes, and altered cell-mediated immunity (see Ch. 17 and 18). Those with B-cell–type disorders are deficient in the development of the germinal centers in lymph nodes and plasma cells of the bone marrow. They have modest lymphocytopenia involving smaller lymphocytes and demonstrate impaired humoral antibody responses. The lymphocytopenia is generally permanent and progressive in these disorders. Lymphocytopenia caused by drugs, hormones, or radiation generally depletes both blood and tissue lymphocytes and impairs both T and B cell function.

Lymphocytopenia associated with malignant transformation of lymphocytes (eg, some cases of acute and chronic lymphocytic leukemia, lymphoma) results from perturbation of stem cell proliferation and the maturation of these cells. Excessive lymphocyte loss due to external drainage or leakage may be associated with secondary hyperplasia of lymphoid tissues.

Chronic lymphocytopenia is often associated with reduced serum immunoglobulins, abnormal delayed hypersensitivity responses, and/or decreased lymphocyte proliferation in in vitro culture systems. These changes may result in increased susceptibility to bacterial, viral, mycotic, and parasitic infections and to development of autoimmune disorders, malignancies, and impaired homograft rejections.

Symptoms, Signs, and Diagnosis

Lymphocytopenia generally causes no symptoms per se and is usually detected in the process of diagnosing other illnesses. It should be suspected in patients with recurrent viral, fungal, or parasitic infections.

Lymphocytopenia is present when the absolute lymphocyte count is < 1500/μL in adults and < 3000/μL in children. Lymphocyte subpopulations (ie, B, T, T4, T8, and

Null cells) can be measured using fluorescein-labeled monoclonal antibodies and specialized cell counting methods. Further definition of immunologic deficiency disorders is covered in Ch. 18.

Treatment

Lymphocytopenia associated with stress, corticosteroid administration, chemotherapy, and radiation usually remits with elimination of exposure to these factors. Effective treatment of the underlying cause of the disorders associated with lymphocytopenia (eg, infections, and inflammatory and malignant diseases) generally leads also to an increase in the WBC count. In patients with B lymphocyte dysfunction and hypogammaglobulinemia, IgG therapy is frequently indicated (see Prophylaxis in Ch. 7). Some forms of primary immune deficiency disorders can be corrected by bone marrow transplantation. Generally lymphocytopenia with T or Null cell deficiency is a much more difficult therapeutic problem than B cell deficiency (see Ch. 18).

---

101. THE LEUKEMIAS

Malignant neoplasms of the blood-forming tissues.

Etiology and Pathogenesis

Although viruses cause several forms of animal leukemia, the cause of human leukemia is undefined; only 2 viral associations are identified: The Epstein-Barr virus, a DNA virus, is associated with Burkitt's lymphoma (see in Ch. 102), and the human T-cell lymphotrophic virus, an RNA retrovirus, has been linked to some T cell leukemias and lymphomas. Exposure to ionizing radiation, and certain chemicals (eg, benzene and some antineoplastic drugs) is associated with an increased risk of leukemia. Some genetic defects (eg, Down's syndrome) and some familial disorders (eg, Fanconi's anemia) predispose to leukemia.

Whatever the etiologic agent, transformation to malignancy appears to occur in a single cell through 2 or more steps with subsequent proliferation and clonal expansion. In some leukemias, specific chromosomal translocations have been identified with consistent leukemia cell morphology and special clinical features (eg, translocations of 9 and 22 in chronic myelocytic leukemia, and of 15 and 17 in acute promyelocytic leukemia). Usually, transformation occurs at the pluripotential stem cell level, but sometimes may involve a committed stem cell with capacity for more limited differentiation. The clone tends to be genetically unstable with features of heterogeneity and phenotypic evolution. In general, leukemia cell populations divide with longer cell cycle times and smaller growth fractions than normal bone marrow cells. Clonal growth advantage occurs because of the accumulation of leukemic cells defective in differentiation and maturation. Clinical and laboratory features of leukemia are caused by suppression of normal blood cell formation and organ infiltration. Inhibitory factors produced by leukemic cells or replacement of marrow space may suppress normal hematopoiesis, which results in anemia, thrombocytopenia, and granulocytopenia. Organ infiltration results in enlargement of the liver, spleen, and lymph nodes, with occasional kidney and gonadal involvement. Meningeal infiltration results in clinical features associated with increasing intracranial pressure.

Classification

Leukemias have been defined as acute or chronic. Although the original basis for this separation was life expectancy, these terms are now applied on the basis of cellular maturity. Thus, acute leukemias are predominantly undifferentiated cell populations and chronic leukemias more mature cell forms.

TABLE 101–1. CLASSIFICATION OF ACUTE LEUKEMIAS

Cell lineage	Description
Acute lymphoblastic leukemia	
Functional classification	
B cell	Immunoglobulin gene rearrangements
Undifferentiated	CALLA*-negative
Common	CALLA*-positive
Pre-B	CALLA*-positive cytoplasmic immunoglobulin (CIg)
B	Surface immunoglobulin (SIg), FAB** L 3 morphology
T cell	
Pre-T	T-antigen-positive, sheep-erythrocyte-receptor-negative
T	T-antigen and sheep-erythrocyte-receptor-positive
FAB** classification	
L 1	Lymphoblasts with uniform, round nuclei and scant cytoplasm
L 2	More variability of lymphoblasts; nuclei may be irregular with more cytoplasm than L 1
L 3	Lymphoblasts have finer nuclear chromatin and blue to deep blue cytoplasm with cytoplasmic vacuolization
Acute nonlymphoblastic leukemia	
Fab** classification	
M 1	Undifferentiated myeloblastic; no cytoplasmic granulation
M 2	Differentiated myeloblastic; a few to many cells may have sparse granulation
M 3	Promyelocytic; granulation typical of promyelocytic morphology
M 4	Myelomonoblastic; mixed myeloblastic and monocytoid morphology
M 5	Monoblastic; pure monoblastic morphology
M 6	Erythroleukemic; predominately immature erythroblastic morphology, sometimes megaloblastic appearance
M 7	Megakaryoblastic; a newer classification with cells having shaggy borders that may show some budding

* Common-acute-lymphoblastic-leukemia antigen
** French-American-British

Acute leukemias are divided into **lymphoblastic (ALL)** and **non-lymphoblastic (ANLL)** types. They may be further subdivided by their morphologic and cytochemical appearance according to the French-American-British **(FAB)** classification or according to their type and degree of differentiation (see TABLE 101–1). The currently available panel of specific B- and T-cell and myeloid-antigen monoclonal antibodies are most helpful for classification, especially with the availability of flow cytometry for analysis. In some patients, progressive bone marrow failure is associated with a smaller proportion of blast cells insufficient for a definite diagnosis of ANLL. These patients are classified as having myelodysplastic syndromes or refractory anemias with excess blasts. In time, a frankly leukemic picture may develop.

Chronic leukemias are also described as being **lymphocytic (CLL)** or **myelocytic (CML)**. CLL is characterized by the appearance of mature lymphocytes in blood, bone mar-

TABLE 101–2. FINDINGS AT DIAGNOSIS IN THE FOUR MOST COMMON TYPES OF LEUKEMIA

	Acute Lymphocytic	*Acute Nonlymphocytic*	*Chronic Myelocytic*	*Chronic Lymphocytic*
Peak age incidence	Childhood	Any age	Young adulthood	Middle and old age
Leukocyte concentration	H* in 50%; N* or L* in 50%	H in 60%; N or L in 40%	H in 100%	H in 98% N or L in 2%
Differential WBC count	Many lymphoblasts	Many myeloblasts	Entire myeloid series	Small lymphocytes
Anemia	In > 90%, severe	In > 90%, severe	In 80%, but mild	In about 50%, mild
Platelets	L in > 80%	L in > 90%	H in 60%; L in 10%	L in 20–30%
Lymphadenopathy	Commonly seen	Occasionally seen	Infrequently seen	Commonly seen
Splenomegaly	60%	50%	Usual and severe	Usual and moderate
Other features	50% CNS occurrence after 1 yr	Rare CNS occurrence	Leukocyte alkaline phosphatase low; Ph** chromosome positive in 85%	Occasional hemolytic anemia and hypogamma-globulinemia

* L = low; N = normal; H = high.
** Ph = Philadelphia.

row, and lymphoid organs. Most CLL patients have clonal expansion of lymphocytes with B-cell characteristics; occasionally CLL of the T-cell type is found. In CML the characteristic feature is the predominance of granulocytic cells of all stages of differentiation in blood, bone marrow, liver, spleen, and other organs. While the granulocytic series predominates in the expression of this leukemia, RBCs, platelets, monocytes, and even some lymphocytes can be demonstrated to be produced by the same stem cell clone. Orderly differentiation of the granulocytic series is a feature of the early phase of CML with acceleration of the disease process and eventual blast transformation as the result of clonal evolution.

The diagnosis and appropriate classification of leukemia are usually simple. General features of the 4 common forms are shown in TABLE 101–2. (For details regarding clinical and laboratory features, see specific leukemias, below).

Treatment Principles

The very nature of hematopoietic cancer necessitates using systemic chemotherapy as the primary treatment modality. Drugs selected according to sensitivities of specific leukemias are usually given in combination. Radiation therapy may be used as an adjunct to treat local accumulations of leukemic cells. Surgery is rarely indicated as a primary treatment modality, but may be used in managing some complications. Bone marrow transplantation from an HLA-matched sibling is sometimes indicated. For details, see specific headings below.

The goals for treatment of acute leukemias are to eradicate leukemic cell populations and to restore normal hematopoiesis. For patients with chronic leukemias, the intensity of therapy needed to eradicate the leukemic cell population carries a great risk with no evident survival benefits. Therefore, the goals for treating chronic leuke-

mias are to limit the size of the leukemic clone and to maintain the patient in an asymptomatic state for as long as possible.

In addition to specific therapy designed to destroy leukemic cells and limit their growth, general supportive therapy is needed as described below under treatment of the acute leukemias.

THE ACUTE LEUKEMIAS

(Acute Lymphoblastic Leukemia [ALL];
Acute Nonlymphoblastic Leukemias [ANLL])

Usually rapidly progressing forms of leukemia characterized by replacement of normal bone marrow by blast cells of a clone arising from malignant transformation of a hematopoietic stem cell. Classification as to cell type—ALL as opposed to ANLL—is critical in treatment planning and prognosis. Other names are sometimes used for ALL (eg, acute lymphocytic leukemia) and ANLL (eg, acute myelocytic, myelogenous, myeloblastic, myelomonoblastic).

Incidence

ALL is predominantly a childhood disease with peak incidence from ages 3 to 5 yr. It is the most common childhood malignancy, occurring also during adolescence, and less commonly among adults.

ANLL occurs at all ages and is the more common acute leukemia among adults; it is the form usually associated with irradiation as a causative agent and occurring as a second malignancy following cancer chemotherapy.

Pathology

Leukemic cells accumulate in the bone marrow, replace normal hematopoietic cells, and spread to the liver, spleen, lymph nodes, CNS, kidneys, and gonads. Since the cells are blood-borne, they can accumulate in and affect any organ or site. The accumulation can often be identified with specific types of acute leukemia (eg, T cell ALL often involves the CNS; acute monoblastic leukemia, the gums; acute myeloblastic leukemia, localized collections in skin or around the head and neck **[chloromas]**). Leukemic infiltration appears as sheets of undifferentiated round cells with usually minimal disruption of organ function except for the CNS and bone marrow. Meningeal infiltration results in increasing intracranial pressure, and replacement of normal hematopoiesis in the bone marrow causes anemia, thrombocytopenia, and granulocytopenia.

Symptoms and Signs

The presenting findings in acute leukemia usually represent the consequences of failure of normal hematopoiesis with bleeding, pallor, and fever. Bleeding is usually manifested by petechiae and easy bruisability with mucus membrane hemorrhage (eg, epistaxis). Hematuria and GI bleeding are uncommon. Initial CNS involvement may be associated with headaches, vomiting, and irritability. Sometimes bone and joint pain may be the dominant complaint. Granulocytopenia may be associated with an obvious bacterial infection; more commonly, the cause of fever that may be present cannot be found. Sometimes the disease has an insidious onset associated with progressive weakness, lethargy, and pallor.

Diagnosis

Diagnosis is established by laboratory findings. Some degree of anemia and thrombocytopenia is almost always found. The total WBC count may be decreased, normal, or increased. Leukemic blast cells are inevitably found in the blood smear unless the WBC count is markedly decreased. Although the diagnosis can usually be made from the blood smear, a bone marrow examination should always be done for confirmation. Sometimes a bone marrow aspiration yields such a hypocellular specimen that a needle biopsy is required. Biopsy specimen examination should include both touch prepara-

tions for cytology and sections for cellularity. Aplastic anemia should be considered in the differential diagnosis of severe pancytopenia, but bone marrow biopsy should be definitive, and an experienced observer will not confuse the atypical lymphocytes of infectious mononucleosis with leukemic cells. It is important to distinguish the blasts of ALL from ANLL. In addition to smears with the usual stains, para-aminosalicylic acid (PAS), myeloperoxidase, Sudan Black B, and specific and nonspecific esterase histochemical stains are frequently helpful.

Prognosis

Before treatment was available, the average patient survived about 4 mo after diagnosis. It is important to realize that now the treatment goal for both ALL and ANLL should be cure.

Several features help to predict the prognosis of patients with ALL. Favorable factors include an age of 3 to 7 yr, total WBC counts < 25,000/μL, FAB L-1 morphology, a leukemic cell karyotype with > 50 chromosomes and no CNS disease at diagnosis. Unfavorable factors include total WBC counts > 25,000/μL, a leukemic cell karyotype with chromosomes that are normal in number but abnormal in morphology (pseudodiploid), age of > 20 yr, and leukemic blast cells with cytoplasmic immunoglobulin.

Regardless of risk factors, the likelihood of initial remission is ≥ 90% in ALL patients. Fifty percent of children should have continuous disease-free survival for 5 yr. Depending on the presence of risk factors mentioned above, expectations might be better or worse. Most regimens select patients with poor risk factors for greater intensity of therapy with the understanding that the greater risk from treatment is outweighed by the increased risk of treatment failure.

For patients with ANLL, reported remission induction rates range from 50 to 85%. Failure to achieve remission can be related to drug resistance or death because of infection or bleeding during the period of hypoplasia. The FAB classification has not proven useful in predicting risk of failure. The most important prognostic clinical feature is age; patients > 50 yr have less likelihood of achieving remission.

In recent chemotherapy trials, long-term disease-free survival is reported to occur in 20 to 40% of patients. Bone marrow transplantation is reported to result in 40 to 50% long-term disease-free survival. Patients who develop ANLL following chemotherapy and irradiation have the poorest prognosis. It is clear that some patients with ANLL can achieve long-term disease-free survival and probably cure, which should be the therapeutic goal for all patients.

Treatment

The first goal of treatment is to achieve complete remission, which is associated with resolution of abnormal clinical features, return to normal blood counts, and hematopoiesis in the bone marrow with < 5% blast cells. Biologically, remission is associated with disappearance of the leukemic clone and restoration of normal polyclonal hematopoietic proliferation. It is only possible here to give a general outline for the treatment of acute leukemia to achieve and maintain remission. Concepts of both specific and supportive therapy are constantly being revised and improved. Treatment programs and clinical situations are complex; and for optimal outcome, require a group experienced in caring for patients with acute leukemia. The responsible physician should be knowledgeable and aware of current treatment opportunities. Ideally, patients should be treated at specialized medical centers, particularly during critical phases of therapy.

It is important to take full advantage of available laboratory studies to characterize leukemic cells. In addition to the histochemical studies mentioned above that help delineate ALL and ANLL, the subclassification of ALL according to cell type and the observations of leukemic karyotype can further identify the patient as being standard

or high risk for treatment failure. In general, high-risk patients are assigned to more intensive treatment regimens.

Although the basic principles in treating ALL and ANLL are similar, details of the regimens and drugs used are quite different. Treatment of ANLL usually requires an initial phase of marrow hypoplasia that is more intense and of longer duration before normal hematopoiesis recovers. A greater degree of supportive therapy is therefore needed.

Supportive care requires blood bank, pharmacy, laboratory, and nursing services. Bleeding, usually the consequence of thrombocytopenia, generally responds to platelet administration. In acute promyelocytic leukemia, disseminated intravascular coagulation **(DIC)** may occur as leukemic cell lysis releases procoagulant; in some centers, heparinization is routine during beginning therapy. Fever in the neutropenic patient has been mentioned; it requires prompt administration of combination antibiotic therapy after appropriate studies and cultures are obtained. Anemia is treated with packed RBC transfusions unless caused by massive bleeding in which case whole blood transfusions may be indicated to restore blood volume. Neutropenic patients with gram-negative sepsis may be helped with granulocyte transfusions. Prophylactic granulocyte transfusions are of no benefit. In the leukemic patient who is at risk also from opportunistic infections associated with chemotherapy-induced immunosuppression, prophylactic administration of trimethoprim/sulfamethoxazole (TMP/SMX [5/20] mg/kg/day for 1 mo) has proven effective in preventing *Pneumocystis carinii* pneumonia in the immunosuppressed patient.

Infections are serious in the neutropenic, immunosuppressed patient. The febrile, neutropenic patient should have appropriate studies and cultures according to clinical findings. For patients with neutrophil counts $< 500/\mu L$, combination antibiotic treatment should begin after cultures are obtained even without clinical evidence of infection because of the likelihood of an inapparent bacterial sepsis. The antibiotic regimen usually should include a semi-synthetic penicillin and an aminoglycoside. Fungal infections may be difficult to diagnose and in some situations empiric treatment with fungicidal agents is indicated. In the patient with pneumonitis, the diagnosis of *Pneumocystis carinii* should be suspected and confirmed, then treated with trimethoprim/sulfamethoxazole (TMP/SMX [20/100] mg/kg/day in 4 divided doses orally, or parenterally, if needed). Too little experience with newer antiviral agents is available to know their specific roles.

In patients undergoing rapid lysis of leukemic cells associated with the beginning of therapy, metabolic abnormalities may occur including hyperuricemia, hyperphosphatemia, and hyperkalemia. If rapid cell lysis is anticipated, then careful attention to hydration, urine alkalinization, and electrolyte balance must be maintained to avoid the complication of uric acid nephropathy. To minimize hyperuricemia, the administration of allopurinol, a xanthine oxidase inhibitor, before starting chemotherapy, can reduce the conversion of xanthine to uric acid.

ALL: Several regimens emphasize early introduction of an intensive multiple drug regimen. Remission can be induced with daily oral prednisone and weekly IV vincristine with the addition of a third agent, either an anthracycline or L-asparaginase. Other drugs and combinations that may be introduced early in treatment are cytarabine (Ara-C) and etoposide; cyclophosphamide and doxorubicin; and L-asparaginase. In some regimens, IV methotrexate is given in an intermediate dose with leucovorin rescue. The combinations of agents and the intensity of their administration is modified according to the presence of factors predicting for a high risk of treatment failure. An important site of leukemic infiltration is the meninges; treatment may include intrathecal methotrexate plus cranial irradiation or intermediate dose IV methotrexate. CNS prophylaxis is usually administered after completion of remission induction.

Most treatment regimens then include maintenance therapy for continued suppression of leukemic cells and reduction of their numbers to a point consistent with cure. Treatment usually lasts from 2½ to 3 yr. Some regimens that are more intensive in earlier phases may use shorter total therapy durations. For the patient who has been in continuous complete remission for 2½ yr, the risk for relapse after cessation of therapy is about 20%, usually within 1 yr. Thus, when therapy can be stopped, most patients are cured.

Relapse most often occurs in the bone marrow, but may also happen in the CNS or testes. Bone marrow relapse is an ominous event. Although remissions can be reinduced in 80 to 90% of patients, subsequent remissions tend to be brief and patients usually have already been exposed to the most effective drugs. If an HLA-matched sibling is available, bone marrow transplantation is advocated for patients in second remission. A small proportion of patients who have bone marrow relapses, however, can achieve long disease-free second remissions, and may even be cured. CNS disease may be the first evidence of relapse even in those who have had effective CNS prophylaxis. Treatment includes intrathecal injection of methotrexate (with or without Ara-C) 1 or 2 times/wk until all signs disappear. Most regimens include systemic chemotherapy in the form of a reinduction regimen because of likelihood of systemic spread of blast cells. The role of continued intrathecal medication or CNS irradiation is not clear. Testicular relapse may be evident clinically with painless firm swelling of the testis or it may be identified on routine biopsy. Clinical evidence of unilateral testicular involvement should always be an indication to biopsy the apparently uninvolved testis. Treatment is by irradiation and administration of systemic reinduction therapy as noted above for isolated CNS relapse.

ANLL: The initial approach to therapy, the prompt induction of a remission, is identical to ALL. The major difference in treatment of ANLL compared to ALL is that the latter responds to a wider variety of drugs, some of which are not particularly myelosuppressive. In ANLL, treatment usually results in significant myelosuppression; thus, patients often get clinically worse before they improve. The period of myelosuppression before marrow recovery requires meticulous anticipatory and supportive care. The basic induction regimen includes cytarabine given by continuous IV infusion or s.c. q 12 h for 5 to 7 days. Daunorubicin is given IV for 3 days during this time. Some regimens include 6-thioguanine or vincristine and prednisone but their contribution is unclear. The acridine derivative, amsacrine (M-AMSA) is a newer agent with some apparent activity. After remission is achieved, many regimens contain a phase of intensification with these or other agents. CNS prophylaxis is usually not given because it has no demonstrated contribution to remission duration or survival. With better systemic disease control, CNS leukemia might become a more frequently observed complication. There is no demonstrated role for maintenance therapy in ANLL. Extramedullary sites are infrequently involved in isolated relapse. Bone marrow transplantation early after a remission has been achieved would be recommended for younger patients with HLA-matched siblings. As mentioned above, ANLL of the acute promyelocytic type should be carefully observed for DIC. Most centers would recommend prophylactic heparinization before beginning therapy.

CHRONIC MYELOCYTIC LEUKEMIA (CML)

(Chronic Myeloid, Chronic Myelogenous, or Chronic Granulocytic Leukemia)

Clonal myeloproliferation caused by malignant transformation of a pluripotent stem cell and characterized clinically by striking overproduction of granulocytes. The disease may occur at any age; it is uncommon < 10 yr of age, but occurs most often in adults with a median age of 45. There is no significant sex preponderance.

Pathology

CML is characterized by excessive production of granulocytes primarily in the bone marrow but also in extramedullary sites (eg, spleen and liver). Although granulocyte production predominates, the neoplastic clone includes erythrocyte, megakaryocyte, monocyte, and even some T- and B-lymphocyte production. Normal stem cells are retained and can emerge following chemotherapy suppression of the CML clone. The bone marrow is hypercellular but in 40% of patients, myelofibrosis will be found at some stage. The CML clone is genetically unstable; in most patients it progresses to an accelerated phase and final blast crisis. At this time, myeloblast (chloroma) tumors can develop in other extramedullary sites (eg, bone, CNS, lymph nodes, and skin).

Symptoms and Signs

In some asymptomatic patients the diagnosis may be made during an incidental CBC. In other patients, the insidious onset of nonspecific symptoms (eg, fatigue, weakness, anorexia, weight loss, fever, night sweats, or a sense of abdominal fullness) may prompt a visit to the physician. At diagnosis, pallor, bleeding, and easy bruisability are unusual. On physical examination, splenomegaly is usually moderate but may be extreme. Lymphadenopathy may be found. With disease progression, splenomegaly may become extreme, pallor and bleeding occur, and fever, marked lymphadenopathy, and skin involvement are ominous developments.

Laboratory Findings

In the symptomatic patient at diagnosis the total WBC count is usually about 200,000/μL, but may reach 1,000,000/μL. In the asymptomatic patient the WBC count is increased but usually < 50,000/μL. The platelet count is normal or moderately increased and the Hb concentration is usually > 10 gm/dL. On blood smear, all stages of differentiation of the granulocytic series are seen, although in patients with total counts < 50,000/μL, immature granulocytes may be uncommon. The absolute eosinophil and basophil concentrations are strikingly increased, the absolute number of lymphocytes and monocytes may be normal. A few nucleated RBCs may be present. Morphology of the blood cells is normal. The bone marrow is hypercellular both on aspirate and biopsy. Even at diagnosis, some patients may have a degree of myelofibrosis. The leukocyte alkaline phosphatase score is low. In 90% of patients, chromosomal analysis will demonstrate the **Philadelphia (Ph,** formerly termed Ph^1) **chromosome**. Although chromosome 22 is often referred to as the Ph chromosome, the correct finding is a translocation of a piece of chromosome 9 containing the oncogene c-abl to chromosome 22 where fusion to another gene bcr results in a fusion product. (The translocation is reciprocal, because a piece of chromosome 22 is translocated to chromosome 9.) The abnormal environment of c-abl on chromosome 22 results in an altered expression of this gene. The specific gene sites at which breakpoints occur appear to be important in the pathogenesis and expression of the disease.

During the accelerated phase of disease progression, anemia and thrombocytopenia develop. In the granulocytic series, basophils may increase in the presence of pseudo Pelger-Huët cells, and the proportion of immature cells as well as the neutrophil alkaline phosphatase score may increase. In the bone marrow, myelofibrosis may develop and sideroblasts may be seen. Evolution of the clone may be associated with development of new abnormal karyotypes.

Further evolution may lead to a blast crisis in which myeloblasts are most frequent (60%) with lymphoblasts (30%) and megakaryocytoblasts (10%) also occurring. Rarely, other blast forms may predominate. In 80% of these patients, additional chromosomal abnormalities will occur.

Diagnosis

CML is relatively easy to diagnose because of the association of splenomegaly, leukocytosis with immature granulocytes and absolute increases in numbers of baso-

phils and eosinophils, low leukocyte alkaline phosphatase levels, and presence of the Ph chromosome. In differential diagnosis, the leukocytosis of patients with myelofibrosis is usually associated with nucleated RBCs, tear-shaped RBCs, anemia, and thrombocytopenia. Myeloid leukemoid reactions resulting from cancer or infection are not associated with the absolute eosinophilia and basophilia and will have an increased leukocyte alkaline phosphatase score. In troublesome cases, presence of the Ph chromosome is definitive.

Prognosis

Median survival is from 3 to 4 yr after clinical onset. About 10% of patients die of other causes; the rest die either in blast crisis or during an accelerated phase of the disease. Except for some patients receiving bone marrow transplantation, current treatment methods do not cure. Five to 10% of patients die within 1 yr following diagnosis, 15 to 20% during the second year, and about 25% in subsequent years. Median survival after blast crisis is about 2 mo but extended to about 8 to 12 mo if remission can be achieved. For the 10% of CML patients who are Ph negative, the prognosis is worse; clinical responses are less likely and survival duration is shorter.

Treatment

The goal of treatment is palliation, not cure. With chemotherapy, usually the patient may be kept asymptomatic for long periods by maintaining the total WBC count < 50,000/μL; a true remission is not achieved because the Ph-positive clone persists in the bone marrow. Attempts to eliminate or reduce this population with intensive chemotherapy has not resulted in cures and only modest improvement in survival duration. Bone marrow transplantation from an HLA-matched sibling during the early phase of the disease may result in long disease-free periods and perhaps permanent disappearance of the Ph-positive clone. Bone marrow transplantation during the accelerated or blast crisis phase has been less successful.

Antineoplastic drugs: Busulfan is the most commonly used drug for treatment of the chronic phase. The beginning adult dose is 4 to 6 mg/day orally with subsequent adjustments according to patient variability. The WBC count will begin to decrease usually within 2 to 3 wk. Busulfan is continued until the WBC count reaches 20,000/μL. Therapy is then stopped; the WBC count will continue to decrease, usually for 1 mo more. Once the decrease in WBC count begins, subsequent changes can usually be predicted by plotting the WBC count on the vertical axis of a semilogarithmic graph against time on the horizontal axis. After several early points have been plotted, it is possible to approximate how long therapy will be necessary by extrapolating the line to the value of 20,000/μL. This predictability is useful to plan office visits and the need for WBC counts. Busulfan therapy is similarly reintroduced when the WBC count becomes > 50,000/μL. In general, symptoms and physical findings are directly related to the WBC count; therefore, maintenance of a total WBC count < 50,000/μL generally assures an asymptomatic patient. Maintenance therapy with busulfan contributes nothing to disease control and carries a risk of hyperpigmentation, bone marrow aplasia, and pulmonary fibrosis.

Hydroxyurea is a useful secondary agent that is sometimes effective when the disease becomes resistant to busulfan. It has a short duration of action and no known cumulative toxicity. The drug needs to be given continuously because of its short duration of action. Increasing WBC counts are usually seen shortly after the drug is stopped. The starting dosage is 20 to 40 mg/kg orally in a single daily dose. Blood counts should be followed weekly and the dose adjusted accordingly.

Other myelosuppressive agents have been used to treat chronic phase CML including 6-mercaptopurine, 6-thioguanine, melphalan, and cyclophosphamide. Since no studies demonstrate their superiority, they are not recommended in preference to busulfan and hydroxyurea.

Splenic irradiation has a secondary role in therapy. Total dosage is in the range of 600 to 1000 rads delivered in daily fractions of 25 to 200 rads. Treatment should begin with very low doses and careful evaluation of the WBC count. Radiation therapy may control leukocytosis and splenomegaly for several months, but the disease becomes resistant after several courses of irradiation. It may be used in refractory cases of CML or in terminal phase patients with marked splenomegaly.

Splenectomy may alleviate abdominal discomfort, and improve thrombocytopenia and transfusion requirements when splenomegaly cannot be controlled with chemotherapy or irradiation. There is no evidence that splenectomy during the chronic phase plays a significant role in disease control.

Treatment of the terminal phase: The accelerated phase and blast transformation occurs in about 80% of CML patients. Of patients who have lymphoblastic transformation, a response to chemotherapy can be achieved in about 50%. The attempt at remission induction is with vincristine and prednisone as for ALL (see above). Remissions and survival durations tend to be brief. For patients with myeloblastic transformation, treatment with ANLL regimens usually is unsuccessful in producing remissions, and survival durations are brief.

CHRONIC LYMPHOCYTIC LEUKEMIA (CLL)

(Chronic Lymphatic Leukemia)

Clonal expansion of mature-appearing lymphocytes involving lymph nodes and other lymphoid tissues with progressive infiltration of bone marrow and circulation in blood. This leukemia is a disease of older persons with 75% diagnosed at the average age of 60. It is 2 to 3 times commoner in males than females. The etiology is unknown, but some are familial. The disease is rare in Japan and China and does not seem to increase among Japanese expatriots in the USA, suggesting that genetic factors are important.

Pathology

Clonal expansion in most CLL patients is by cells with B-lymphocyte characteristics and surface immunoglobulin **(SIg)**. The clonal SIg is usually IgM in type with either κ or λ light chains. In a few patients the SIg is of the IgG variety, again with either κ or λ light chains. In < 5% of CLL patients, the lymphocytes have T cell characteristics.

Accumulation of lymphocytes probably begins in lymph nodes and spreads to other lymphoid tissues. The liver and spleen become moderately enlarged and the bone marrow is progressively infiltrated by lymphocytes. Abnormal hematopoiesis results in anemia, agranulocytosis, and thrombocytopenia. There are immunoregulatory problems involving immunoglobulin production. Most patients develop hypogammaglobulinemia and impaired antibody response. In some patients this appears to be related to increased activity of T-suppressor cells. Another immunoregulatory abnormality is susceptibility to autoimmune disease characterized by immunohemolytic anemias, thrombocytopenia, vasculitis, and such clinical syndromes as RA and thyroiditis. There is an increased risk of second and even third malignancies, which are attributed to failure of immune surveillance.

Symptoms and Signs

Onset is usually insidious and initial findings may be asymptomatic lymphadenopathy. In some patients, the disease is discovered from an incidental blood count. In the symptomatic patient, nonspecific complaints are usual and may include fatigue, anorexia, weight loss, dyspnea on exertion, and a sense of abdominal fullness from an enlarging spleen. At diagnosis, usual findings include generalized lymphadenopathy and minimal-to-moderate enlargement of liver and spleen. With progressive disease, there may be pallor and petechiae. Skin infiltration may be a feature of T-cell CLL

patients. A predisposition to bacterial infection occurs because of hypogammaglobulinemia and granulocytopenia. Bacterial, viral, and fungal infections feature advancing CLL.

Laboratory Findings

The hallmark of the disease is a sustained, absolute lymphocytosis (> 5,000/μL) and an increase of lymphocytes in the bone marrow. At diagnosis, there may be moderate anemia and thrombocytopenia because of bone marrow infiltration and abnormal hematopoiesis. Accelerated blood cell destruction may occur because of splenomegaly or because of immunohemolytic anemia and thrombocytopenia. Most patients will have hypogammaglobulinemia, and occasionally a monoclonal serum immunoglobulin spike of the same type present on the leukemic cell surface can be seen.

Diagnosis

The diagnosis may be made from abnormal blood counts in an otherwise asymptomatic person. Otherwise, CLL should be suspected in the patient presenting with the insidious onset of the nonspecific features mentioned above who has generalized lymphadenopathy. The diagnosis is then confirmed by CBC and bone marrow aspiration. Reactive lymphocytosis associated with viral infections can be differentiated by the clinical picture and the presence of atypical lymphocytes on blood smear. Lymphocytic lymphomas with a leukemia phase are associated with circulating cells (larger than those seen in CLL) with distinctive notched nuclei. The cells of the **Sézary syndrome** and **hairy cell leukemias** are also quite distinctive, with cerebriform nuclei in the former, and cytoplasmic projections in the latter.

Clinical staging is useful in decisions for therapy and anticipating prognosis: Stage 0 patients have an absolute lymphocytosis of > 10,000/μL in blood and ≥ 40% lymphocytes in the bone marrow; in Stage I, enlarged lymph nodes are also found; Stage II adds hepatic and splenic enlargements; in Stage III, these findings are accompanied by anemia with Hb < 11 gm/dL; and in Stage IV, patients also have thrombocytopenia with platelet counts < 100,000/μL.

Prognosis

Median survival of CLL patients from diagnosis until death from all causes is about 6 yr. About 15 to 20% of these deaths are from causes unrelated to CLL. Median survival of patients dying from CLL or its complications is about 10 yr. A patient in Stage 0 to II at diagnosis may survive for 5 to 20 yr without treatment. A patient in Stage III or IV is more likely to die within a few years of diagnosis. Early rapid progression to bone marrow failure is usually associated with short survival. Patients with CLL are also more likely to develop second malignancies that may cause death.

Treatment

Although the disease is progressive, some patients may be asymptomatic for years; therapy is *not* indicated until active progression or symptoms occur. Supportive treatment includes transfusion of packed RBCs for anemia, platelet transfusions for bleeding associated with thrombocytopenia, and antibiotics for bacterial infections. The latter are usually associated with neutropenia and agammaglobulinemia; therefore, antibiotic therapy must be bactericidal and include a semisynthetic penicillin and an aminoglycoside. Specific therapy includes irradiation, antineoplastic drugs, and a corticosteroid. Treatment does not prolong survival, and may be associated with significant side effects. *Overtreatment is more dangerous than undertreatment.*

Antineoplastic drugs: Chlorambucil is the drug of choice for most patients. The recommended starting dose is 0.1 to 0.2 mg/kg/day with the total dose ranging from 6 to 12 mg/day; as the total WBC count decreases by ½, the dose is reduced usually by ½. When the total WBC count reaches 15,000 to 25,000/μL, chlorambucil may be

stopped until there is another indication to resume it. Cyclophosphamide is also effective but has a greater range of side effects. *Antineoplastic drugs should be used cautiously in patients who already have bone marrow failure with anemia and thrombocytopenia.*

Corticosteroid therapy: Prednisone in doses of 1 mg/kg/day may result in striking and rapid improvement in patients with advanced CLL. The period of response is usually brief. Prednisone has the advantage of lacking bone marrow toxicity, but the metabolic complications and increasing rate and severity of infections warrant caution in its prolonged use. Immunohemolytic anemia and thrombocytopenia are indications for corticosteroid therapy.

Radiation therapy: Local irradiation may be given to areas of lymphadenopathy, liver, and spleen for symptomatic palliation. The exact dose cannot be specified because the radiosensitivity of lymphocytes varies. A tumor may show response after as little as 100 to 200 rads. Total body irradiation in small doses has also been successful.

102. LYMPHOMAS

A heterogeneous group of neoplasms arising in the reticuloendothelial and lymphatic systems. The major types are Hodgkin's disease and non-Hodgkin's lymphoma. Rarer forms include Burkitt's lymphoma and mycosis fungoides.

HODGKIN'S DISEASE

A chronic disease with lymphoreticular proliferation of unknown cause that may present in localized or disseminated form. Effective treatment is based upon definitive evaluation and staging (see below).

Incidence and Etiology

Annually in the USA, 5000 to 6000 new cases are diagnosed. The male:female ratio is 1.4:1. Rare before age 10, a binodal age distribution exists with one peak at ages 15 to 34 and another after age 54. Epidemiologic studies find no evidence of horizontal spread. Hodgkin's disease resembles a low-grade graft-versus-host reaction. Recent evidence of tumor-associated antigens in Hodgkin's tissue is consistent with this interpretation. A number of infectious agents, including viruses, are postulated as causes.

Pathology

Diagnosis depends upon identification of large multinucleated reticulum cells **(Reed-Sternberg cells)** in lymph node tissue or other sites. Hodgkin's infiltrates are heterogeneous and consist of abnormal reticulum cells, histiocytes, lymphocytes, monocytes, plasma cells, and eosinophils. The 4 histopathologic classifications are (1) **lymphocyte predominance**—few Reed-Sternberg cells and many lymphocytes; (2) **mixed cellularity**—a moderate number of Reed-Sternberg cells with a mixed infiltrate; (3) **nodular sclerosis**—generally like (2) except that dense fibrous tissue, which shows characteristic birefringence with polarized light, surrounds nodules of Hodgkin's tissue; and (4) **lymphocyte depletion**—few lymphocytes, numerous Reed-Sternberg cells, and extensive fibrosis or abnormal reticulum cell infiltrate.

Symptoms and Signs

Most patients present with cervical and mediastinal adenopathy, but without systemic complaints. Despite apparent localized or regional disease (clinical stage), further studies are needed to define accurately the pathologic stage (see below). The following discussion considers the range of possible symptoms and signs, which usually do not all occur in the same patient.

A variety of manifestations develop as the disease spreads through the reticuloendothelial system. Its rate of progression varies greatly: (a) relatively slow or quiescent (lymphocyte predominance or, occasionally, in the nodular sclerosis type); (b) intermediate or moderately progressive (nodular sclerosis or mixed cellularity); or (c) aggressive (mixed cellularity or lymphocyte depletion type). Intense pruritus may occur early; fever, night sweats, and weight loss occur frequently when internal nodes (bulky mediastinal or retroperitoneal), viscera (liver), or bone marrow are involved. The **Pel-Ebstein fever** pattern (a few days of high fever regularly alternating with a few days to several weeks of normal or subnormal temperature) occasionally is seen. An unexplained symptom that may provide an early clue to diagnosis is immediate pain in diseased areas after drinking alcoholic beverages.

Bone involvement may produce pain with vertebral osteoblastic lesions ("ivory" vertebra) and, rarely, osteolytic lesions with compression fracture. Pancytopenia is occasionally due to bone marrow invasion, usually by lymphocyte-depleted types. Epidural invasion that compresses the spinal cord may result in paraplegia. Horner's syndrome and laryngeal paralysis may result from pressure on the cervical sympathetic and recurrent laryngeal nerves, respectively. Neuralgic pains follow nerve root compression. Intracranial, gastric, and cutaneous lesions occur rarely.

Intra- or extrahepatic bile duct obstruction by tumor masses produces jaundice. Congestion and edema of the face and neck can result from pressure on the superior vena cava (superior vena cava or superior mediastinal syndrome). Leg edema may follow lymphatic obstruction in the pelvis or groin. Tracheobronchial compression can cause severe dyspnea and wheezing. Infiltration of lung parenchyma may simulate lobar consolidation or bronchopneumonia and may result in cavitation or lung abscess. Ureteral compression from pelvic lymph nodes may interfere with urinary flow and cause secondary renal damage.

Most patients have a slowly progressive defect in delayed or cell-mediated immunity (T cell function) that contributes in advanced disease to common bacterial and unusual fungal, viral, and protozoal infections (see Ch. 7). Humoral immunity (antibody production) or B cell function is depressed in far-advanced disease. Evidence of cachexia is present. Patients frequently die from sepsis.

Laboratory Findings

A slight-to-moderate polymorphonuclear leukocytosis may be present. Lymphocytopenia may occur early and become pronounced with advancing disease. Eosinophilia is present in about 20% of patients, and thrombocytosis may be observed. Anemia, often hypochromic and microcytic, usually develops with advanced disease. In the latter setting, defective iron reutilization is characterized by low serum iron, low iron-binding capacity, and increased bone marrow iron. Hypersplenism may appear, but mainly in patients with marked splenomegaly. Elevation of serum alkaline phosphatase usually indicates bone marrow or liver involvement, or both. Increases in leukocyte alkaline phosphatase, serum haptoglobin, ESR, and serum copper usually reflect active disease.

Diagnosis

The symptom complex of lymph node enlargement (especially cervical) and mediastinal adenopathy, with or without fever, night sweats, and weight loss highly suggests Hodgkin's disease, but the diagnosis can be proved only by biopsy and demonstration of Reed-Sternberg cells in a characteristic histologic setting. In the absence of lymphadenopathy, the diagnosis can sometimes be established by biopsy of bone marrow, liver, or other parenchymal tissue.

The differential diagnosis of Hodgkin's disease from lymphadenopathy due to infectious mononucleosis, toxoplasmosis, cytomegalic inclusion disease, leukemia, or non-Hodgkin's lymphoma (see below) may be difficult. The clinical picture can also be

simulated by bronchogenic carcinoma, sarcoidosis, and TB, and by various diseases with splenomegaly as their outstanding feature (see Ch. 104).

Clinical Staging of Hodgkin's Disease

Radiotherapy, chemotherapy, and combinations of the two are curative, but to achieve this goal, the extent or the "pathologic stage" needs to be delineated. Successful therapy critically requires documentation of the extent of the disease, which may be localized initially (Stage I or II) in 50% of patients. The Ann Arbor staging system is commonly used: **Stage I**: Limited to 1 anatomic lymph node region. **Stage II**: Two or more anatomic lymph node regions on the same side of the diaphragm. **Stage III**: Disease on both sides of the diaphragm involving lymph nodes or spleen. **Stage IV**: Extranodal involvement (eg, bone marrow, lung, or liver). **Subclassification E**: Extranodal involvement adjacent to an involved lymph node; eg, disease of cervical nodes and hilar adenopathy with adjacent lung infiltration is classified as Stage IIE, not Stage IV.

These stages are classified as clinical **(CS)** or pathologic **(PS)** and further defined by the absence **(A)** or the presence **(B)** of constitutional symptoms (weight loss, fever, or night sweats); B findings are generally consistent with a greater net mass of disease.

A variety of procedures provide the data for appropriate staging. Clinical staging assessed by noninvasive procedures includes ultrasound and CT scans of the abdomen and pelvis, and, in selected cases, gallium body scans and bone scans. The role of MRI is being evaluated. Bipedal lymphangiograms are generally performed in patients with nodal disease, which is not readily seen on abdominal and pelvic CT scan. Since clinical and lymphangiographic studies attempting to detect disease below the diaphragm are false-positive or -negative in 25 to 33% of patients, laparotomy including splenectomy, biopsy of mesenteric and retroperitoneal lymph nodes (especially those enlarged on lymphangiograms), and core biopsy of the bone marrow and liver should be considered as a definitive pathologic staging procedure in most patients who do not have unequivocal Stage IIIA, IIIB, or IV disease.

Treatment

Curative chemotherapy and radiotherapy are available for most patients. With nodal disease, 3500 to 4000 rads in 3 to 4 wk can eradicate Hodgkin's tissue within the treated field > 95% of the time. In addition, irradiation of adjacent uninvolved nodes **(extended field)** is standard practice, since the disease spreads by lymphatic contiguity in about 2/3 of patients. Patients with subclassification E as well as those with a comparable degree of lymph node involvement only may respond to radiotherapy. The following treatment is based upon surgically staged patients (PS).

Stage I, IIA, and IIB disease can be treated with radiotherapy alone by an extended field to include a full mantle (all lymph-node–bearing areas above the diaphragm) and in most cases the periaortic lymph nodes to the aortic bifurcation. Such treatment cures about 90% of patients. In patients with bulky mediastinal disease (> 1/3 the chest diameter) radiotherapy combined with chemotherapy results in a prolonged relapse-free survival in 80 to 85% of patients.

Stage III disease can be subdivided into III_1, which defines or denotes involvement of the spleen, celiac, or portal nodes, or III_2, which includes more extensive spread into the mesenteric, para-aortic, iliac, or femoral nodes with or without upper abdominal disease. For **Stage $IIIA_1$ disease,** total nodal irradiation (mantle, periaortic, and inverted "Y") results in an overall survival of 85 to 90% with disease-free survival of 65 to 75%. In selected cases, lesser radiotherapy (omission of the inverted "Y") has been equally effective. For **Stage $IIIA_2$ disease,** combination chemotherapy (see below) is generally used with or without radiotherapy of selected nodal sites. Cure rates of 75 to 80% have been achieved.

Since radiotherapy alone may not cure **Stage IIIB** Hodgkin's disease, either combination chemotherapy alone or such therapy combined with radiotherapy is needed. Survival ranges from 70 to 80%.

In extranodal Hodgkin's disease **(Stage IVA and B)**, combination chemotherapy, particularly with mechlorethamine, vincristine, procarbazine, and prednisone ("MOPP" program), has produced a complete remission in 70 to 80% of patients, with > 50% remaining disease-free and probably cured at 5 to 10 yr. Another multiagent chemotherapy program with equal efficacy but different toxicity is ABVD (adriamycin, bleomycin, vinblastine, and dacarbazine). Other effective chemotherapeutic agents include nitrosoureas, streptozocin, cis-platinum, and epipodophyllotoxin (VP-16).

MALIGNANT LYMPHOMAS: NON-HODGKIN'S LYMPHOMA (NHL)

A heterogeneous group of diseases, consisting of neoplastic proliferation of lymphoid cells that usually disseminate throughout the body. The old terms lymphosarcoma and reticulum cell sarcoma have been replaced by nomenclature more consistent with the biologic status (see below). Their courses vary from rapidly fatal to indolent and initially well tolerated. A leukemia-like picture may develop in up to 50% of children and about 20% of adults with some types of NHL.

Incidence and Etiology

NHL occurs more frequently than Hodgkin's disease. Annually in the USA, 7000 or 8000 new cases are diagnosed. It occurs in all age groups, the incidence increasing with age. Its cause is unknown, although, as with the leukemias, substantial experimental evidence suggests a virus. Close association of a human **type C retrovirus** with some adult leukemias and lymphomas comprised of peripheral T cells has been recently demonstrated. The virus, called **HTLV-I** (human T-cell leukemia-lymphoma virus) has been isolated from several patients and appears to be endemic in Japan, the Caribbean, South America, and certain regions of the USA.

Pathology

Histopathologic classification systems, although complex and transitional, offer reasonable means to distinguish clinical subgroups with different prognoses and provide guidelines for management. In general, longer survival is related to a follicular or nodular nodal architecture and smaller lymphoid cell size; larger cell types or undifferentiated cells are usually diffuse and have a poorer prognosis.

The Rappaport classification for the histopathology of NHL is based on the degree of differentiation of the tumor, and on the presence or absence of nodules. Large immature cells are designated as "histiocytes" and smaller ones as "lymphocytes" or "undifferentiated cells." NHL is classified as (1) malignant lymphoma, undifferentiated Burkitt's type, or non-Burkitt's (pleomorphic type); (2) malignant lymphoma, histiocytic; (3) malignant lymphoma, mixed lymphocytic-histiocytic; (4) malignant lymphoma, lymphocytic (well differentiated or poorly differentiated); or (5) malignant lymphoma, lymphoblastic. All classes are further divided into nodular or diffuse except for (1) and (5), which occur only in a diffuse pattern. Nodular involvement is characterized by fibrous strands that separate the lymphoma infiltrate into nodules.

The Lukes and Collins classification, based upon the cell of origin, divides NHL into **T cell** (thymus-derived) types that include immunoblastic sarcoma and convoluted cell lymphoma, similar to lymphoblastic lymphoma (about 15% of all cases), or **B cell** (bone marrow-derived) types that include well-differentiated lymphocytic, plasmacytic, follicular center cell (small and large cleaved and non-cleaved cell type) lymphomas, and a B-cell immunoblastic sarcoma (about 75% of cases). A third category

includes rare cases of "true" **histiocytic (or monocytic) origin** (5%), while a fourth category includes **unclassifiable cases** (5%).

The new **International Panel Working Formulation** separates NHL into 3 categories, each incorporating the above classifications and having therapeutic implications, as follows (NOTE: *The prognostic designations are based on untreated disease and may not accurately reflect outcomes in patients undergoing modern therapy*, as discussed under Treatment, below):

I. **Low grade or favorable-prognosis lymphomas**: diffuse, well differentiated; nodular, poorly differentiated lymphocytic; and nodular-mixed types.

II. **Intermediate-grade or -prognosis lymphomas**: nodular histiocytic; diffuse, poorly differentiated, lymphocytic; and diffuse-mixed types.

III. **High grade or unfavorable-prognosis lymphomas**: diffuse histiocytic lymphoma (diffuse large cell, cleaved, non-cleaved, and immunoblastic types); diffuse undifferentiated (Burkitt's and non-Burkitt's type); and lymphoblastic T cell lymphoma.

IV. **Miscellaneous lymphomas**: composite lymphomas, mycosis fungoides, true histiocytic, other, and unclassifiable types.

Immunoclonal antibodies allow for subtyping of B and T cell lymphomas. However, data are inconclusive as to their role in planning treatment strategy.

Symptoms and Signs

While a variety of clinical manifestations exist, many patients present with asymptomatic adenopathy involving cervical or inguinal regions, or both. Enlarged lymph nodes are rubbery and discrete and later become matted. Local disease is apparent in some patients, but most have multiple areas of involvement. Various disease patterns follow. The tonsils are occasional sites of involvement. Mediastinal and retroperitoneal lymphadenopathy may cause pressure symptoms on various organs. Extranodal sites may dominate the clinical picture (eg, gastric involvement can simulate GI carcinoma, and intestinal lymphoma may cause a malabsorption syndrome). The skin and bones are initially involved in 15% of patients with histiocytic lymphoma and 7% of patients with lymphocytic lymphoma. Histiocytic lymphoma rarely remains localized to bone. When extensive abdominal or thoracic disease is present, about 33% of patients develop chylous ascites or pleural effusion respectively due to lymphatic obstruction. Weight loss, fever, night sweats, and asthenia indicate disseminated disease.

Anemia is initially present in about 33% of patients and eventually develops in most. It may be due to bleeding from GI involvement or low platelet levels, hemolysis due to hypersplenism or Coombs-positive hemolytic anemia, bone marrow infiltration by lymphoma, or marrow suppression by drugs or irradiation. A leukemic phase develops in 20 to 40% of lymphocytic lymphomas and 10% of histiocytic lymphomas. Hypogammaglobulinemia due to progressive decrease in immunoglobulin production occurs in 15% of patients and may predispose to serious bacterial infection.

In children, NHL may be of the undifferentiated, diffuse histiocytic or lymphoblastic type. These childhood lymphomas present different problems and require different management approaches than those seen in adults. The lymphoblastic type represents a variation of acute lymphoblastic leukemia (T cell type), since both have a predilection for marrow, peripheral blood, skin, and CNS involvement, and patients frequently present with mediastinal adenopathy (Sternberg sarcoma) and superior vena cava syndrome. Nodular histologies are rarely seen in children.

Diagnosis

NHL must be differentiated from Hodgkin's disease, acute and chronic leukemia, infectious mononucleosis, TB (especially primary TB with hilar adenopathy and TB adenitis), and other causes of lymphadenopathy, including pseudolymphoma due to phenytoin. Diagnosis can be made only by histologic study of excised tissue. Destruction of normal lymph node architecture and invasion of the capsule and adjacent fat

by characteristic neoplastic cells are the usual histologic criteria. Immunologic studies to determine B, T, or other cell of origin will identify specific subtypes and help to define prognosis, and may be of value in management decisions (see below).

Staging and Prognosis

Localized NHL does occur, but the disease is disseminated in about 90% of nodular histology and 70% of diffuse histology cases when first recognized. Clinical staging procedures similar to those for Hodgkin's disease are indicated, except that laparotomy and splenectomy are rarely required. CT scans of the abdomen and pelvis are usually carried out for staging and sequential comparison. Lymphangiograms do not often add information, but may be useful in selected patients. The final staging is more often based upon clinical findings than in Hodgkin's disease where pathologic stage is critical for management decisions.

Initially, constitutional symptoms tend to be less common in NHL than in Hodgkin's disease and do not alter prognosis in most patients. Organ infiltration is more widespread, and the bone marrow and peripheral blood may be involved. Bone marrow biopsy to determine marrow involvement should be done in all patients.

The prognosis and the response to treatment are significantly influenced by histopathology, stage of disease, and, in some reports, results of surface marker studies. Patients with "favorable prognosis" types (see above) have median survivals of > 5 to 7.5 yr, but unfortunately, most patients eventually die from the disease. Patients with "intermediate-prognosis" lymphomas have median survivals of 1 to 3 yr. Those with "unfavorable-prognosis" or high-grade lymphomas usually die within 1 yr, unless intensive treatment is carried out, in which case the prognosis may be good. Patients with T cell lymphomas generally have a worse prognosis compared to B cell types, although results of recent intensive treatment programs lessen these differences. Other factors that adversely affect prognosis are age > 70, elevated LDH level, "bulky" tumor masses > 10 cm in diameter, and > 2 extranodal sites of disease.

Treatment

Treatment of early disease (Stages I and II): With low- and intermediate-grade lymphomas, patients rarely present with localized disease, but, when they do, regional radiotherapy offers long-term control and sometimes cure. Those with high-grade lymphomas are generally treated with combination chemotherapy (see below) with or without regional radiotherapy. Cure rates vary from 40 to 60%.

Treatment of advanced disease (Stages III and IV): Treatment varies considerably in patients with low-grade or "favorable-prognosis" histologies. A "watch and wait" approach, treatment with a single alkylating agent, or 2- and 3-drug programs may be used. Interferon as well as other biologic response modifiers has resulted in some encouraging remissions. While survival may be prolonged, relapse eventually occurs and cure rates are generally < 20 to 25% and thus prognosis paradoxically is not favorable.

In patients with intermediate-grade lymphomas, combinations of cyclophosphamide, vincristine, prednisone, with or without adriamycin (COP, CVP, CHOP, C-MOPP) result in complete regression of disease in 50 to 70% of patients. A pattern of continuous late relapse usually occurs, however, and only 20 to 30% are cured.

Patients having lymphomas with "unfavorable-prognosis" histology (diffuse "histiocytic" or large cell types) usually have rapid tumor growth (high grade), but modern intensive combination chemotherapy programs have dramatically reversed the previously poor cure rate of < 10%. Use of 4-, 5-, and 6-drug programs with acronyms (eg, BACOP, CHOP-Bleo, M-BACOD, COMLA, PROMACE-MOPP, COP-BLAM, MACOP-B) that use the above drugs plus others (bleomycin, methotrexate with leucovorin rescue, cytosine arabinoside, procarbazine) has resulted in complete remission

rates of 50 to 75% with about 40 to 60% of all patients being cured. Thus, the previous designation of "unfavorable" is changed to "favorable." Newer, effective drugs include cis-platinum, epipodophyllotoxin (VP-16), and large doses of cytosine arabinoside.

With highly specific monoclonal antibodies and improved technics in bone marrow preservation, new intensive treatment programs are under investigation in selected patients who relapse from standard treatment programs. Thus, autologous marrow (from the patient) or allogeneic marrow (from an HLA matched sibling or donor) can be processed and preserved for reinfusion (rescue) after high dose chemotherapy and total body radiotherapy (designed to eradicate recurrent lymphoma).

Patients with T-cell–type lymphoblastic lymphoma are managed in similar fashion to those with acute childhood T-cell lymphocytic leukemia with intensive chemotherapy regimens including prophylactic treatment of the CNS. Results are encouraging, with an estimated 50% cure rate.

BURKITT'S LYMPHOMA

A highly undifferentiated B cell lymphoma that tends to involve sites other than the lymph nodes and reticuloendothelial system.

Etiology

Burkitt's lymphoma, unlike other lymphomas, has a specific geographic distribution. Rare in the USA, it is most common in Central Africa, where its distribution appears to be determined by climatic factors, suggesting an unidentified insect vector and an infectious agent. Strong, but unverified, evidence points to the herpes-like Epstein-Barr virus (see also INFECTIOUS MONONUCLEOSIS in Ch. 202).

Symptoms and Signs

Burkitt's lymphoma occurs in all age groups, but is rare in adults. It is more commonly seen in children and young adults, particularly in male patients. Most patients present with large abdominal masses due to involvement of the bowel or retroperitoneum. Other presenting features include adenopathy or painful jaw masses (especially in African patients). Anemia may be present due to bone marrow involvement. In all patients, the disease is rapidly progressive.

Diagnosis

Lymph node or other tissue biopsy reveals characteristic small-to-intermediate–sized non-cleaved cells that have a high nuclear-cytoplasmic ratio and mitotic count. Nuclei are immature and contain prominent nucleoli while the cytoplasm is basophilic with several conspicuous vacuoles. Under low power magnification a "starry-sky" pattern is evident in virtually all cases due to the presence of background foamy histiocytes. Immunologic studies show the presence of B cell markers (usually IgM, either κ or λ light chain) while cytogenetic studies reveal a translocation between chromosomes 8 and 14.

Staging and Treatment

Stages A and B indicate single or multiple extra-abdominal sites. Stage C is defined by intra-abdominal disease including kidneys or gonads. Stage D disease is similar to C but with involvement of extra-abdominal sites including bone marrow or CNS. Prognosis is improved when bulk abdominal tumor can be resected.

Intermittent intensive chemotherapy (high doses of cyclophosphamide alone or lower doses combined with methotrexate and vincristine) produces long-term disease-free survival in 70 to 80% of patients with Stage A or B disease and in 30 to 40% of patients with Stage C and D disease. New treatment programs include intensive chemotherapy with or without bone marrow transplantation.

MYCOSIS FUNGOIDES

An uncommon chronic T cell lymphoma primarily affecting the skin and occasionally internal organs.

The disease is rare compared to Hodgkin's disease, and, unlike most other lymphomas, is insidious in onset. It may appear as a chronic, pruritic rash that is difficult to diagnose. Initially plaquelike, it may spread to involve most of the skin, become nodular, and eventually have systemic involvement. Lesions may become ulcerated. Pathologic diagnosis is delayed because sufficient quantities of lymphoma cells appear in the skin lesions only very gradually. Most patients are over age 50 by the time of diagnosis. From then until death, even without treatment, the time span is much longer than for the other lymphomas. Average life expectancy is about 7 to 10 yr after diagnosis. In some cases, a leukemic phase called **Sézary's syndrome** is characterized by the appearance of small T lymphocytes with cerebriform nuclei in the peripheral blood.

Treatment: Electron beam radiotherapy, in which most of the energy is absorbed in the first 5 to 10 mm of tissue, and topical nitrogen mustard have proved highly effective in controlling the disease. Plaques may also be treated with sunlight and topical steroids. Systemic treatment with alkylating agents and folic acid antagonists produces transient tumor regression.

---

103. PLASMA CELL DYSCRASIAS (PCDS)

(Monoclonal Gammopathy)

A group of clinically and biochemically diverse disorders characterized by the disproportionate proliferation of one clone of cells normally engaged in immunoglobulin synthesis, and the presence of a structurally and electrophoretically homogeneous (monoclonal) immunoglobulin or polypeptide subunit in serum or urine. The disorders vary from asymptomatic and apparently stable conditions to progressive, overtly neoplastic disorders such as multiple myeloma. The classification of PCDs appears in TABLE 103–1. Both clinical and immunochemical criteria must be used to diagnose these disorders.

Structural features of immunoglobulin molecules and development of the major immunoglobulin classes are outlined in Ch. 17. Normally, production of immunoglobulins is heterogeneous, with individual clones of plasma cells producing the different immunoglobulins (IgG, IgM, IgA, IgD, or IgE). Each plasma cell clone secretes only one class of heavy chain (gamma [γ], mu [μ], alpha [α], delta [δ], or episilon [ε]) and one class of light chain (kappa [κ] or lambda [λ]) at any one time in its lifespan. A slight excess of light chains is normally produced, and small amounts of free polyclonal κ and λ chains (up to 40 mg/24 h) are excreted in the urine of normal subjects. A disproportionate proliferation of one clone results in a corresponding increase in the serum level of its secreted molecular product. This monoclonal immunoglobulin protein (the M-component) is readily detected as a tall symmetric spike with α_2, β, or γ mobility on cellulose acetate electrophoresis of serum or urine, but immunoelectrophoresis is required to identify the heavy and light chain class of the protein. The magnitude of M-component is related to the number of cells in the body producing that component; thus these proteins are valuable markers in diagnosing and managing patients with PCDs.

The etiology of PCDs is unknown. Most of the monoclonal immunoglobulins (M-components) synthesized and secreted by plasma cells are not qualitatively abnormal; rather, they appear to be normal products of a single clone that has undergone intense proliferation. The main exceptions are seen in the "heavy-chain" diseases, described below. Some of these M-proteins show antibody activity, most frequently

TABLE 103–1. CLASSIFICATION OF PLASMA CELL DYSCRASIAS (PCDs)

	Disorder	*Comments and Examples*
Malignant (PCDs) Symptomatic, progressive	Multiple myeloma	IgG, IgA, light chains (Bence Jones) only, IgD, IgE, nonsecretory
	Waldenström's macroglobulinemia	IgM
	Primary systemic amyloidosis (AL)	Usually light chains (Bence Jones) only, but occasionally intact immunoglobulin molecules (IgG, IgA, IgM, IgD)
	Heavy chain diseases	IgG heavy chain (γ-chain) disease IgA heavy chain (α-chain) disease IgM heavy chain (μ-chain) disease IgD heavy chain (δ-chain) disease
Plasma cell dyscrasias of unknown significance (PCDUS) Asymptomatic, most nonprogressive	Associated with lymphoreticular neoplasms	Leukemia, lymphoma
	Associated with nonlymphoreticular neoplasms	Especially carcinomas of the colon, biliary tree, and breast
	Associated with chronic inflammatory conditions	Especially chronic cholecystitis
	Associated with various other disorders	Lichen myxedematosus, liver disease, thyrotoxicosis, pernicious anemia, myasthenia gravis, Gaucher's disease, etc.
	In apparently healthy individuals; age-related incidence	

directed toward autoantigens and bacterial antigens. Serum levels of normal immunoglobulins are commonly reduced.

Serum M-components are usually identifiable in patients with malignant PCD (multiple myeloma, Waldenström's macroglobulinemia, primary systemic amyloidosis, or the various heavy chain diseases). Serum M-components are also found in a few asymptomatic, apparently healthy persons; the incidence is age-related—1% of persons over age 25 and 4% of those over age 70. Although many asymptomatic cases remain unchanged for years and are therefore seemingly benign, a few (< 10%) represent incipient or **"premyeloma"** fortuitously discovered on routine serum protein electrophoresis. It is impossible to predict the course in any individual patient, and clinically symptomatic myeloma may not evolve for as long as 20 yr. The designation **plasma cell dyscrasia of unknown significance (PCDUS)** is therefore preferred for asymptomatic individuals with monoclonal serum components. Patients with PCDUS usually have low serum levels of M-components (< 3.0 gm/dL) that are stable with time, and show only mild marrow plasmacytosis, normal levels of other serum immunoglobulins, and no lytic bone lesions or Bence Jones proteinuria. PCDUS also occurs in association with a variety of other diseases (TABLE 103–1). No treatment for the PCD

is recommended in this circumstance; patients should be observed for change in clinical and immunochemical status at 4- to 6-mo intervals.

MULTIPLE MYELOMA

(Plasma Cell Myeloma; Myelomatosis)

A progressive neoplastic disease characterized by marrow plasma cell tumors and overproduction of an intact monoclonal immunoglobulin (IgG, IgA, IgD, or IgE) or **Bence Jones protein** *(free monoclonal κ or λ light chains), and often associated with multiple osteolytic lesions, hypercalcemia, anemia, renal damage, and increased susceptibility to bacterial infections.* The impaired normal immunoglobulin production observed in multiple myeloma may be due to the presence of a monocyte or macrophage that inhibits the maturation of normal B lymphocytes into antibody-secreting plasma cells. Persons over the age of 40 are most commonly affected.

Pathology

The pelvis, spine, ribs, and skull are most frequently involved. Skeletal x-rays may show diffuse osteoporosis or discrete osteolytic lesions due to replacement by expanding plasma cell tumors or a factor (osteoclast-activating factor) secreted by malignant plasma cells. Usually multiple, the osteolytic lesions occasionally occur as a solitary intramedullary mass. Extraosseous plasmacytomas are unusual, but diffuse plasma cell infiltrates may occur in any organ. Extensive cast formation in the renal tubules, atrophy of tubular epithelial cells, and interstitial fibrosis may result in renal failure **(myeloma kidney)**. Amyloid deposits (see in Ch. 86) occur in 10% of myeloma patients and are especially likely in those with Bence Jones proteinuria (amyloid AL).

Plasma cell tumors produce IgG in about 55% of myeloma patients and IgA in about 20%; 40% of these IgG and IgA patients also have Bence Jones proteinuria. About 20% of patients have "light chain" myeloma; their plasma cells secrete *only* free monoclonal light chains (κ or λ Bence Jones protein) and serum M-components are usually absent on cellulose acetate electrophoresis. The light chain subgroup tends to have a higher incidence of lytic bone lesions, hypercalcemia, renal failure, and amyloidosis than do other myeloma patients. IgD myeloma accounts for about 1% of cases; serum levels are often relatively low, and heavy Bence Jones proteinuria (80 to 90% type λ) is characteristic. Only a few cases of IgE myeloma have been reported. Nonsecretory myeloma (no identifiable M-component in serum or urine) is very rare (< 1% of cases).

Symptoms and Signs

Persistent unexplained skeletal pain (especially in the back or thorax), renal failure, or recurrent bacterial infections, especially pneumococcal pneumonias, are the most common presentations. Anemia with weakness and fatigue predominates in some patients, and a few have manifestations of the hyperviscosity syndrome (see in MACROGLOBULINEMIA, below). Pathologic fractures and vertebral collapse are common; the latter may lead to spinal cord compression and paraplegia. Lymphadenopathy and hepatosplenomegaly are unusual.

Diagnosis

Physical examination usually is not helpful unless bone pain or pallor is present. Laboratory findings include a normocytic normochromic anemia with rouleau formation evident on peripheral smear. The WBC and platelet counts usually are normal. The ESR is often markedly elevated (> 100 mm/h, Westergren), and BUN, serum creatinine, and serum uric acid are frequently elevated. A low "anion gap" is present in some patients and may be a helpful diagnostic clue. Hypercalcemia occurs in about 1/3 of patients.

Proteinuria is common because of excess synthesis and secretion of free monoclonal light chains (Bence Jones protein). Significant albuminuria rarely occurs in myeloma; its presence suggests coexisting amyloidosis. A quantitative 24-h urinary protein determination is best for detecting significant proteinuria. Chemical paper strip tests of urine do *not* reliably detect Bence Jones protein, and the heat test is often misleading, but sulfosalicylic acid and toluene sulfonic acid are useful screening tests. Serum protein electrophoresis will show a tall, narrow, homogeneous M-spike in about 80% of cases; the mobility of the spike may lie anywhere from the α_2 to the slow γ region. The remaining 20% of patients synthesize free monoclonal light chains (Bence Jones protein) only, and their serum electrophoretic patterns display hypogammaglobulinemia without a monoclonal spike. However, in essentially all patients with light chain myeloma, a homogeneous M-spike is demonstrable on protein electrophoresis of concentrated urine. Immunoelectrophoresis employing monospecific antisera identifies the immunoglobulin class of the monoclonal spike in either serum or urine.

X-ray of the bones may show typical punched-out lytic lesions or diffuse osteoporosis. Osteoblastic lesions are rare and thus radionuclide bone scans are usually not helpful. The bone marrow usually contains increased numbers of plasma cells at various stages of maturation; rarely is the number of plasma cells normal. Plasma cell morphology does not correlate with the class of immunoglobulin synthesized. Although sheets and clusters of plasma cells are diagnostic of marrow tumors, myeloma is a patchy disease and often only modest nonspecific plasmacytosis is observed.

Prognosis

The disease is progressive, but optimal management improves both the quality and duration of life. Life expectancy is related to the extent of disease at diagnosis, adequacy of supportive measures, and response to chemotherapy. About 60% of treated patients show objective improvement; median survival for responding patients is 2 to 3 yr. High levels of M-protein in serum or urine, diffuse bone lesions, hypercalcemia, pancytopenia, and renal failure are unfavorable signs.

Treatment

General measures: Maintenance of ambulation is vital. Analgesics and palliative doses of radiotherapy (1000 to 2000 rads) to localized areas of symptomatic bone involvement relieve pain significantly. Adequate hydration is also essential. *(Dehydration before an IVP may precipitate acute oliguric renal failure in patients with Bence Jones proteinuria.)* Even patients with prolonged heavy Bence Jones proteinuria (10 to 30 gm/day or even more) may have little evidence of renal functional impairment if they are well hydrated (urine output > 2000 mL/day). Prednisone 60 to 80 mg/day orally is useful to control the hypercalcemia, and allopurinol 300 mg/day orally controls hyperuricemia. Antibiotics are indicated for documented bacterial infection, but prophylactic antibiotics are not recommended. Transfusion of packed RBCs is indicated for symptomatic anemia.

Chemotherapy: Objective improvement (as documented by a 50% or greater reduction in serum or urine M-component) usually follows the use of oral alkylating agents (melphalan or cyclophosphamide). Median survival may be extended three- to sevenfold. Melphalan may be given intermittently (0.25 mg/kg/day for 4 days every 4 to 6 wk) or continuously (0.09 to 0.14 mg/kg/day for 8 to 10 days followed by 0.03 mg/kg/day in a 70-kg man for maintenance). Prednisone given intermittently (1 mg/kg/day for 4 days every 6 wk) may improve the response to melphalan. Cyclophosphamide (200 mg/day for 5 to 7 days, then 50 to 100 mg/day for maintenance) appears to be as effective as melphalan. Because leukopenia and thrombocytopenia develop with these agents, dosage must be titrated in each patient. WBC levels of 2500/μL and platelet counts > 90,000/μL are usually safe. Various multiple drug regimens are being assessed for nonresponding or relapsing patients; occasional re-

sponses have been reported. The use of such regimens for initial treatment as well as the optimal duration of therapy remain controversial. Interferon appears to be a promising experimental agent in myeloma.

MACROGLOBULINEMIA

(Primary or Waldenström's Macroglobulinemia)

A plasma cell dyscrasia involving B cells that normally synthesize and secrete IgM. Macroglobulinemia, a clinical entity distinct from myeloma and other PCDs, resembles a lymphomatous disease. Many of its clinical manifestations are due to the large amount of high mol wt macroglobulin circulating in plasma. Some of these monoclonal IgM proteins are antibodies directed to autologous IgG (rheumatoid factors) or to the I red cell antigen (cold agglutinins). Cryoglobulinemia may be identified. The cause is unknown.

Twelve percent of all individuals with monoclonal gammopathy have macroglobulinemia. Small monoclonal IgM components are found in the sera of about 5% of patients with B cell non-Hodgkin's lymphoma; this circumstance has been termed **"macroglobulinemic lymphoma."**

Symptoms and Signs

The patient is usually elderly, with symptoms of the **hyperviscosity syndrome**: fatigue, weakness, skin and mucosal bleeding, visual disturbances, headache, and a variety of other changing neurologic manifestations. When cardiopulmonary abnormalities predominate, they are associated with an increased plasma volume that also contributes to circulatory impairment. A history of cold sensitivity or Raynaud's phenomenon may be associated with the presence of a cryoglobulin or cold agglutinin. Recurrent bacterial infections are a major problem in some patients. Examination may disclose modest generalized lymphadenopathy, purpura, hepatosplenomegaly, and "sausaging" of retinal veins (see Diagnosis, below). Amyloidosis occurs in 5% of patients.

Laboratory Findings

Moderate anemia with profound rouleau formation and a very high ESR are characteristic. Leukopenia, relative lymphocytosis, and thrombocytopenia occasionally occur. Cryoglobulins, rheumatoid factor, or cold agglutinins may be present; in the last instance the direct Coombs' test usually is positive. A variety of coagulation and platelet function abnormalities may be present. Results of routine blood studies may be spurious if a cryoprotein is present or if viscosity is markedly increased. Relative serum viscosity is usually > 4.0 (normal 1.4 to 1.8) in patients with the hyperviscosity syndrome.

Diagnosis

A typical M-spike on serum protein electrophoresis that proves to be IgM by immunoelectrophoresis establishes the diagnosis. Immunoelectrophoretic studies of concentrated urine frequently demonstrate a monoclonal light chain (usually κ), but gross Bence Jones proteinuria is unusual. X-rays of bones may show osteoporosis, but lytic lesions are rare. The marrow shows a variable increase in plasma cells, lymphocytes, and intermediate forms (plasmacytoid lymphocytes). Periodic acid-Schiff-positive material may be present in lymphoid cells and mast cells may be increased. Lymph node biopsy is frequently interpreted as diffuse well-differentiated or plasmacytoid lymphocytic lymphoma. The **hyperviscosity syndrome** can be diagnosed by the findings of marked retinal venous engorgement and localized narrowing that gives the veins a sausage-like appearance. Retinal hemorrhages, exudates, microaneurysms, and papilledema indicate far-advanced stages.

Prognosis and Treatment

The course is variable but tends to be more benign than in myeloma. Many patients survive for > 5 yr. If hyperviscosity is present, initial management consists of reducing the serum viscosity by plasmaphereses, which effectively and rapidly reverse bleeding and neurologic abnormalities caused by high IgM levels. Repeated plasmaphereses can be used to control viscosity.

Long-term chemotherapy with oral alkylating agents is necessary in some patients. Chlorambucil (0.03 to 0.09 mg/kg/day) is the treatment of choice. Melphalan and cyclophosphamide, given as for multiple myeloma, are alternative agents.

PRIMARY SYSTEMIC AMYLOIDOSIS

(See Ch. 86)

HEAVY CHAIN DISEASES

Neoplastic plasma cell dyscrasias characterized by overproduction of homogeneous gamma (γ), alpha (α), mu (μ), or delta (δ) immunoglobulin heavy chains. Most monoclonal proteins are structurally similar to normal antibody molecules. By contrast, the heavy chain diseases are unusual disorders in which incomplete monoclonal immunoglobulins (true **"paraproteins"**) occur. Abnormal lymphocytes or plasma cells secrete the various heavy chain components. The clinical picture is more like lymphoma than multiple myeloma. Most heavy chain proteins are fragments of their normal counterparts with internal deletions of variable length; these deletions appear to result from structural mutations. Epsilon (ε) heavy chain disease is yet to be described.

IgG Heavy Chain (γ-chain) Disease

More than 60 cases have been reported, primarily in elderly men, with a few reported in children. Associated chronic disorders include RA, Sjögren's syndrome, SLE, TB, myasthenia gravis, hypereosinophilic syndrome, autoimmune hemolytic anemia, and thyroiditis. The clinical picture resembles that of a malignant lymphoma, with lymphadenopathy and hepatosplenomegaly as usual findings. Anemia, leukopenia, thrombocytopenia, eosinophilia, and circulating atypical lymphocytes or plasma cells are common findings. Fever, recurrent infections, and reductions in normal immunoglobulin levels are also seen. Palatal edema is present in about ¼ of patients. The course is variable—from a few months to > 5 yr. Death usually results from bacterial infection or progressive malignancy.

Diagnosis is based on immunoelectrophoretic demonstration of free homogeneous heavy chain fragments of IgG in serum and urine. Evidence of associated monoclonal light chain production is absent. Fifty percent of patients have monoclonal serum components (often appearing broad and heterogeneous) in excess of 1 gm/dL, and 50% have proteinuria > 1 gm/24 h. Heavy chain proteins belonging to each of the 4 IgG subclasses have been reported, but the G3 subclass is especially common. The bone marrow and lymph node histopathology is variable. Lytic lesions are absent on bone x-rays in most patients. Amyloid deposits have rarely been found at autopsy. **Therapy** with alkylating agents or corticosteroids and radiotherapy may yield transient remissions.

IgA Heavy Chain (α-chain) Disease

This is the most common heavy chain disease and tends to appear in young persons, most being between the ages of 10 and 30 yr. It is geographically concentrated in the Middle East and bears a close relationship to "Mediterranean lymphoma" or "immunoproliferative small intestinal disease." The disorder occasionally has been described in the Western Hemisphere. The clinical picture is strikingly uniform, almost all patients presenting with diffuse abdominal lymphoma and malabsorption syn-

drome. Histopathologic examination discloses villous atrophy and massive infiltration of the lamina propria of the intestine with lymphocytes, plasma cells, and/or immunoblasts. The cellular infiltrate may be pleomorphic and not overtly malignant by histopathologic criteria. Mesenteric lymph nodes may show a similar lymphoplasmacytic infiltration, but peripheral nodes, marrow, liver, and spleen usually are not involved. No osteolytic lesions are seen on bone x-rays. A discrete M-spike may not be observed on serum protein electrophoresis, but free α-chains are demonstrable by immunoelectrophoresis in 80% of cases; special immunochemical technics are required to make the diagnosis in the remainder. The abnormal protein is usually present in intestinal secretions and may be found in concentrated urine. Bence Jones proteinuria is absent.

Several well-documented instances of prolonged remission have been reported following corticosteroid, cytotoxic drug, and broad spectrum antibiotic therapy. In view of the responses to antibiotics alone and the peculiar geographic incidence of the disorder, α-chain disease may represent an aberrant immune response to a parasite or other microorganism, which is not, in all cases, neoplastic. A respiratory-tract form of the disease has been reported rarely.

IgM Heavy Chain (μ-chain) Disease

The clinical picture in this rare disorder usually has been that of longstanding chronic lymphocytic leukemia or other lymphoproliferative disorder. Affected patients have primarily visceral organ involvement (spleen, liver, abdominal lymph nodes) with little peripheral lymphadenopathy. Vacuolated plasma cells are present in the bone marrow in $^2/_3$ of patients. Bence Jones proteinuria (type κ), pathologic fractures, and amyloidosis may occur. Routine serum protein electrophoresis usually is normal or shows hypogammaglobulinemia.

Diagnosis is made by the finding of a rapidly migrating serum component that reacts with antiserum to μ-chains but not with antisera to light chains. Free μ-chains are only rarely found in the urine. However, as noted, κ-Bence Jones proteinuria usually is present (10 of 15 patients). The monoclonal κ-light chains are not structurally linked to the μ-chains even though they appear to be synthesized by the same cells; the reason for this failure of assembly is unclear, but may be due to the nature of the deletion in the abnormal heavy chains.

IgD Heavy Chain (δ-chain) Disease

A single case has been reported. The patient was an elderly man with a clinical picture similar to multiple myeloma. Marked marrow plasmacytosis and osteolytic lesions in the skull were present. A small M-component was evident on serum protein electrophoresis that reacted with monospecific anti-IgD antiserum, but not with other antisera of heavy or light chain specificity. Proteinuria was absent. Death occurred due to renal failure. The principal histopathologic finding in the kidney was a thickening of the glomerular basement membrane, presumably resulting from deposition of the abnormal protein.

---

104. THE SPLEEN

Analysis of the structure and function of the spleen reveals that it is actually comprised of 2 organs—an immune one, the **"white pulp,"** consisting of periarterial lymphatic sheaths and germinal centers, and a reticuloendothelial one, the **"red pulp,"** consisting of phagocytic macrophages and granulocytes lining vascular spaces (the cords and sinusoids).

The functions of the white pulp include (1) generation of humoral antibodies to circulating antigens: under abnormal conditions, inappropriate autoantibodies to circulating blood elements may be synthesized, as in immune thrombocytopenic purpura **(ITP)**

or Coombs-positive, immune hemolytic anemias; and (2) production and maturation of B and T lymphocytes and plasma cells as in other lymphoid organs.

Functions of the red pulp include (1) removal of unwanted particulate matter such as bacteria or senescent blood elements: in immune cytopenias (ITP, Coombs-positive hemolytic anemias, and in some neutropenias) phagocytosis of antibody-coated cells by red pulp macrophages and granulocytes underlies their destruction; (2) a reservoir for blood elements, especially for leukocytes and platelets; (3) "culling and pitting" to remove inclusion bodies in RBCs (eg, Heinz bodies, Howell-Jolly bodies, and whole nuclei from RBCs): after splenectomy, circulating nucleated RBCs or cells with pieces of nuclei (Howell-Jolly bodies) are commonly encountered; and (4) a hematopoietic function: under abnormal conditions the spleen may replace bone marrow as a blood-forming organ. Normally hematopoiesis occurs in the spleen only during fetal life; with marrow damage, as by fibrosis or scarring (myelofibrosis), hematopoietic stem cells may repopulate the adult spleen and liver **(myeloid metaplasia).**

HYPERSPLENISM

Various disorders in which blood cytopenia is associated with splenomegaly. The cardinal features of the syndrome are (1) splenomegaly; (2) a reduction of one or more blood cell elements, resulting in anemia, leukopenia, thrombocytopenia, or any combination thereof in association with hyperplasia of the marrow precursors of the deficient cell type; and (3) correction of the cytopenias by splenectomy.

Etiology

Abnormalities of the spleen are almost always secondary to other primary disorders. Some causes of hypersplenism are summarized in TABLE 104–1. Lymphoproliferative, myeloproliferative, and connective tissue diseases are the most commonly encountered causes in temperate climates, while infectious diseases (eg, malaria and kala-azar) predominate in the tropics. Unsuspected hepatic cirrhosis or portal or splenic vein thrombosis resulting in congestive splenomegaly is uniformly distributed and a frequent cause of "idiopathic" splenomegaly.

Pathogenesis

Hypersequestration of blood in large spleens is the predominant mechanism for cytopenia in hypersplenism. The following evidence supports this conclusion: (1) Major decreases in leukocyte and platelet counts occur in splenic venous (compared to arterial) blood. (2) Inordinate accumulation of radio-chromium (^{51}Cr)-labeled RBCs or platelets occurs in enlarged spleens, indicating preferential trapping. (3) Typical hypersplenism can be induced in animals injected with metabolically inert polymers (eg, methylcellulose). (4) Viable spleen transplants placed in diffusion chambers in the peritoneal cavity of splenectomized animals have no effect on blood cell counts, which argues strongly against the existence of a splenic humerol moiety as the factor in hypersplenism. (5) Administration of epinephrine to laboratory animals leads to splenic shrinkage and concurrent elevations of peripheral leukocyte and platelet counts; this response is greatly enhanced in hypersplenic humans, suggesting that excessively sequestered blood elements can be released by the drug.

The fact that splenomegaly occurs in most chronic hemolytic anemias suggests that spleen growth may be stimulated by an increase in its "work load"—in this case, the work of trapping and destroying abnormal RBCs. The commonly observed vicious spiral of hemolysis in many chronic hemolytic states (eg, hereditary spherocytosis and thalassemia) may reflect this "work hypertrophy," and splenectomy may be of marked clinical benefit in such cases. In addition, splenic tissue, when stimulated to become hyperplastic by chronic hemolysis, may not be discriminating in its hyperfunction; thus thrombocytopenia and leukopenia are common features of many chronic hemo-

TABLE 104–1. ETIOLOGIES OF SECONDARY HYPERSPLENISM

Disease Category	*Disease*
Lympho- and myeloproliferative diseases	Lymphomas—including Hodgkin's disease Leukemias—especially chronic lymphocytic and chronic myelocytic Polycythemia vera Myelofibrosis with myeloid metaplasia
Inflammatory diseases	Acute infections—including infectious mononucleosis, infectious hepatitis, SBE, psittacosis Chronic infections—including miliary TB, malaria, brucellosis, kala-azar, syphilis Sarcoidosis Amyloidosis Connective tissue diseases—including SLE and Felty's syndrome
Reticuloendothelioses	Lipoid—including Gaucher's, Niemann-Pick, and Schüller-Christian diseases Nonlipoid—Letterer-Siwe disease
Chronic, usually congenital, hemolytic anemias	Red cell shape abnormalities—including hereditary spherocytosis, hereditary elliptocytosis Hemoglobinopathies—including thalassemias, sickle Hb variants (eg, Hb S-C disease), congenital Heinz body hemolytic anemias Red cell enzymopathies—eg, pyruvic kinase deficiency
Congestive splenomegaly	Cirrhosis of the liver External compression or thrombosis of portal or splenic veins
Splenic cysts	Usually due to resolution of previous intrasplenic hematoma

(Modified from *Hematology*, by W. J. Williams et al. Copyright 1976 by McGraw-Hill, Inc. Used with permission of McGraw-Hill Book Company.)

lytic diseases. Similarly, common transient and nonspecific blood cytopenias may occur in patients with acute splenomegaly provoked by circulating microorganisms. Such infections are diverse and include SBE, miliary TB, infectious hepatitis, psittacosis, and infectious mononucleosis.

Symptoms and Signs

Most of the presenting symptoms and signs relate to the underlying disease. Besides palpable splenomegaly, the following may be encountered: (1) Left upper quadrant abdominal pain and/or splenic friction rub suggests splenic infarction. (2) Epigastric and splenic bruits secondary to inordinate blood return from massively enlarged spleens may presage bleeding esophageal varices. (3) Early feeding satiety may be caused by encroachment on the stomach by the enlarged spleen. (4) Purpura and manifestations of mucosal bleeding may occur, although total platelet mass (the circulating pool plus that sequestered in the enlarged spleen) may be normal. Even though the excessive splenic pool can be mobilized by epinephrine, mild hemorrhagic diatheses may be seen. Significant prolongation of bleeding time may be found, but severe hemorrhage is rare; its occurrence suggests additive effects of an underlying primary disease (eg, leukemia).

Diagnostic Approach to Splenomegaly

The sequence of diagnostic procedures is generally determined by formulation of the data from the history and physical examination.

1. Peripheral blood smear. (a) Excessive basophils, eosinophils, or nucleated or teardrop RBCs suggest myeloproliferative disorders. (b) Lymphocytosis may occur in lymphoproliferative disorders. (c) Abnormality in RBC shape may suggest hereditary spherocytosis or a hemoglobinopathy (eg, Hb S or C, or thalassemia).

2. Special blood chemistries. (a) **Serum electrophoresis**: monoclonal gammopathy or decreased immunoglobulins suggest lymphoproliferative disorders or amyloidosis; diffuse hypergammaglobulinemia may be noted in chronic infections (eg, malaria, kala-azar, brucellosis, TB) or in cirrhosis with Banti's syndrome, sarcoidosis, and collagen vascular diseases. (b) **Uric acid**: Elevations occur in myeloproliferative and lymphoproliferative disorders. (c) **Leukocyte alkaline phosphatase** and **serum vitamin B_{12}**: elevated in myeloproliferative disorders. (d) **Liver function tests**: Diffusely abnormal in Banti's syndrome associated with cirrhosis; a solitary elevation of **serum alkaline phosphatase** suggests hepatic infiltration as in myeloproliferative and lymphoproliferative disorders and miliary TB.

3. Bone marrow examination. (a) General cellular hyperplasia with peripheral cytopenia is often found in hypersplenism syndromes. (b) Lymphocyte infiltration is found in lymphoproliferative disorders. (c) Hyperplasia of myeloid elements suggests myeloproliferative disorders. (d) Blast cell increase is found in leukemias. (e) Fibrosis occurs in myeloid metaplasia. (f) Periodic acid-Schiff staining clumps are present in amyloidosis. (g) Lipid-laden macrophages occur in Gaucher's and related storage disease.

4. ^{51}Cr-labeled RBC and platelet survival and splenic uptake studies are useful in assessing the degree of hypersequestration of these elements for splenectomy decision.

5. Splenic scan with technetium-labeled colloid. The spleen scan is a reliable noninvasive method to identify a left upper quadrant mass as spleen, and it may identify extrasplenic pathology. Reticuloendothelial cells in the spleen will trap technetium 99m sulfur colloid in a manner similar to the liver. In normal individuals, the apparent concentration of activity in liver and spleen are about equal. Marked reduction in spleen uptake compared to liver uptake indicates either splenic arterial obstruction or pathologic infiltration. An increase in spleen uptake is seen with decrease in hepatic portal blood flow accompanying parenchymal liver disease; it may also result from increased blood flow in acute splenitis. Primary neoplasms of the spleen are unusual, but splenic involvement in the presence of leukemia, lymphoma, or melanoma is not. Patients with Hodgkin's disease may have diffuse splenic enlargement. Spleen imaging after abdominal trauma is very helpful when splenic rupture or subcapsular hematoma is suspected. Focal scan defects in the spleen are uncommon and are mostly due to infarcts or small abscesses; they may suggest injury.

6. Iron 59 kinetics with splenic scanning. Early uptake of label (within 24 h) is observed in myeloid metaplasia.

7. Esophagogram and splenic venography. Varices and dilated splenic (or portal) veins suggest congestive splenomegaly (Banti's syndrome or splenic vein thrombosis).

8. Lymphangiography and CT (or echo) scanning of abdomen. Abnormal abdominal nodes occur in lymphoproliferative disorders.

The spleen appears as a low echo area on the gray-scale echogram and changes in size and position can be readily estimated. By integrating the cross-sectional area of ultrasonic serial scans taken at 1-cm intervals, the total splenic volume can be determined. These calculated volumes range within about ± 12% when compared with displacement volume measurements of surgically removed spleens. Measurement of splenic size can be important in obese patients where palpation is difficult and for

TABLE 104–2. HELPFUL CLINICAL FEATURES IN EVALUATING COMMON SPLENIC DISORDERS

Disease	*Spleen Size*	*Bone Marrow Findings*	*Blood Smear Findings*	*Special Studies*
Myeloproliferative disorders: polycythemia vera (PV); myeloid metaplasia (MM); chronic myelogenous leukemia (CML)	Moderate (PV); massive (MM & CML)	Hyperplastic (PV & CML); fibrotic (MM)	↑*All blood cells (PV); pancytopenia (MM); ↑blasts (CML)	^{59}Fe splenic accumulation (MM); leukocyte alkaline phosphatase—↑(PV & MM), ↓*(CML)
Lymphoproliferative disorders	Moderate	Lymphoid infiltration; Reed-Sternberg cells (Hodgkin's Disease); amyloid deposits	↑Lymphs (chronic lymphocytic leukemia)	Abnormal serum immunoglobulins
Lipid-storage diseases (e.g., Gaucher's)	Massive	Lipid-filled macrophages	Pancytopenia (if hypersplenism is severe)	Enzyme studies for glycolipid metabolic defects

* ↑ = increased; ↓ = decreased

monitoring splenic size during chemotherapy. Of diagnostic importance is the anteriorly placed spleen that is often palpable, but not enlarged.

Some of these diagnostic clues are summarized in TABLE 104–2.

Treatment of Splenic Disorders

Most patients with splenomegaly require therapy of the underlying disease, not splenectomy. Since asplenic individuals have increased susceptibility to serious systemic infections with encapsulated bacteria (eg, *H. influenzae*, pneumococci), **indications for splenectomy or radiation therapy should be strict,** and include (1) hemolytic syndromes in which the shortened survival of intrinsically abnormal RBCs is further curtailed by the additive effect of splenomegaly, as in hereditary spherocytosis and thalassemia; (2) severe pancytopenia associated with enormous splenic enlargement (up to 30 times normal has been recorded in lipid-storage diseases); (3) vascular accidents involving the spleen—either chronic infarctions or bleeding esophageal varices associated with excessive splenic venous return; (4) mechanical encroachment on other abdominal organs (eg, stomach with early satiety, or left kidney with calyceal obstruction); and (5) intolerable hemorrhagic tendency, if definitely related to hypersplenic thrombocytopenia.

SOME SPECIFIC SPLENOMEGALIC SYNDROMES

Myeloproliferative disorders: In polycythemia vera, myelofibrosis with myeloid metaplasia, myelogenous leukemia, and essential thrombocythemia (collectively referred to as "myeloproliferative syndrome") the spleen becomes enlarged, particularly with myelofibrosis in which bone marrow is obliterated and the spleen assumes an increasing hematopoietic function. Splenomegaly may be massive, and if it is associated with infarcts, esophageal varices, or early satiety, splenectomy may be beneficial.

Lymphoproliferative disorders: The spleen is enlarged in chronic lymphocytic leukemia and the lymphomas (including Hodgkin's disease); see Chs. 101 and 102, above.

Splenomegaly is usually associated with lymphadenopathy, immunoglobulin abnormalities, and lymphocyte dysfunction (eg, anergy). Finding invasion of bone marrow by lymphoid elements is helpful in diagnosis.

Lipid-storage diseases: Glucocerebroside (in **Gaucher's disease**) or sphingomyelin (in **Niemann-Pick disease**) may accumulate in splenic reticuloendothelial cells, leading to spleen enlargement. In Gaucher's disease hypersplenism may be the only significant problem; splenectomy may be beneficial, although glycolipid accumulation in liver and bones may worsen after surgery. The finding of typical lipid-laden macrophages in bone marrow preparations frequently aids the diagnosis, and the specific glycolipid metabolic error can be identified by enzyme assay of peripheral leukocytes. (See also ANOMALIES IN LIPID METABOLISM in Ch. 85.)

Collagen vascular disorders: In both SLE and RA, splenomegaly and leukopenia may coexist. In the latter, often termed **Felty's syndrome**, leukopenia may be severe and associated with frequent infections. The pathogenesis of splenomegaly in this syndrome is unknown, and splenectomy is only beneficial in about 50% of cases. Splenic amyloidosis should also be considered in RA with splenomegaly.

Congestive splenomegaly (Banti's syndrome): Chronically increased splenic venous pressure may result from hepatic cirrhosis, portal or splenic vein thrombosis, or certain malformations of the portal venous vasculature. Associated bleeding from esophageal varices may be worsened by the superimposed thrombocytopenia induced by splenomegaly. Splenic venography, which may demonstrate or exclude extrahepatic portal obstruction, aids in diagnosis. Depending on etiology, surgical shunting procedures for venous obstructions or medical management of cirrhosis will be appropriate.

SPLENIC DEFICIENCY DISORDERS

(See SPLENIC DEFICIENCY SYNDROMES in Ch. 18)

105. ONCOLOGY

Cancer: *A cellular malignancy whose unique characteristic—loss of normal controls—results in unregulated growth, lack of differentiation, and ability to invade local tissues and metastasize.*

Cancer can develop in any tissue of any organ at any age. Most cancers detected at an early stage are potentially curable; thus, physicians need a heightened awareness of predisposing inherited and environmental factors. A complete history and physical examination are prerequisites to early diagnosis, and may also allow staging of a patient's cancer (see below). Specific questions about familial cancer, environmental exposure, and prior illness (eg, autoimmune diseases or chronic osteomyelitis) must be asked. A review of systems is important, especially addressing symptoms of fatigue, weight loss, cough, hemoptysis, hematemesis or hematochezia, change in bowel habits, persistent pain, skeletal pain, fevers, and sweats. On examination, particular attention should be focused to lymph node regions, the lungs, breasts, abdomen, and to the rectal and vaginal examination. The patient should participate actively in recognizing early signs of malignancy; cooperation in self-examination and in acceptance of diagnostic tests and therapy is essential for optimal end results.

Physicians are responsibile to support their patients with cancer through treatment-related complications. Supportive care and aggressive therapy of complications related to cancer often mean the difference between cure and palliation. Psychologic support from the physician and the health care team, which should include a psychiatrist and a social worker, helps patients through therapy (see also COMPLICATIONS, below).

Physicians must be truthful, yet convey a sense of optimism. The patient should feel that all members of the health care team are concerned and available to answer questions.

Patients with terminal cancer, often grasping at straws, need to be informed and wary of those who falsely promise quick cure. The local American Cancer Society or the National Cancer Institute will furnish a list of reputable physicians.

ETIOLOGY

Age has the most significant impact on the incidence and mortality of cancer. In the USA, the incidence doubles q 5 yr after age 25 yr. Certain cancers (eg, of the prostate, stomach, and colon) reach a peak incidence between ages 60 to 80 yr; other diseases (eg, acute lymphoblastic leukemia) have a peak incidence from birth to 10 yr. The differential diagnosis of a mediastinal mass in a 20-yr-old patient includes Hodgkin's disease, non-Hodgkin's lymphomas, and mediastinal germ-cell tumors, but in a 50-yr-old patient would include lung cancer, non-Hodgkin's lymphomas, and thymoma.

Geographic differences are linked to cancer incidence, give clues to etiologies, and prompt the study of migrant populations. Gastric cancer has decreased fourfold in the USA since 1930. Incidence of colon cancer and breast cancer is low in Japan; however, in Japanese immigrants to the USA, the incidence increases and eventually equals that of the native population, presumably reflecting dietary changes. Lung cancer in the USA has increased from 5:100,000 in 1930 to 50:100,000 in 1980 and certainly reflects smoking habits.

The etiology of cancer is not clearly defined, but several mechanisms that can result in malignant transformation are described below.

Genetic Susceptibility (see in Ch. 203)

Increased incidence of malignancies in certain families follows Mendelian principles of single-gene transmission (see inherited cancers and preneoplastic states in TABLE 105–1). Several of these disorders are discussed elsewhere in THE MANUAL: **retinoblas-**

TABLE 105–1. INHERITED CANCERS AND PRENEOPLASTIC STATES

Neoplasm
Retinoblastoma
MEN,* Type I (pituitary adenoma, parathyroid adenoma, islet cell tumors of the pancreas)
MEN, Type IIa (medullary thyroid carcinoma, pheochromocytoma, parathyroid hyperplasia)
MEN, Type IIb (Type IIa plus mucosal neuromas)
Gardner's syndrome
Polyposis coli
Nevoid basal cell carcinoma syndrome
Trichoepithelioma
Premalignant state
Hamartoma: Neurofibromatosis, tuberous sclerosis, Peutz-Jeghers syndrome, von Hippel-Lindau disease, multiple exostoses
Genodermatosis: Xeroderma pigmentosum, albinism, polydysplastic epidermolysis bullosa
Immune deficiency syndrome: Ataxia telangiectasia, Wiskott-Aldrich syndrome, x-linked agammaglobulinemia
Chromosome breakage or polyploidy: Bloom's syndrome, Fanconi's syndrome, Down's syndrome

* MEN=Multiple Endocrine Neoplasia

toma (see in Ch. 192), **multiple endocrine neoplasia,** type I, IIa, and IIb (see Ch. 92), **Gardner's syndrome** and **polyposis coli** (see in Ch. 63), and **immune deficiency syndromes** (see in Ch. 18).

The **nevoid basal cell carcinoma syndrome,** in which the incidence of ovarian tumors and medulloblastoma is higher than normal, consists of skin pits on the palms and soles, hypertelorism, jaw cysts, and basal cell skin cancers.

Inherited premalignant states include the **hamartomatous syndromes or phacomatoses**: von Recklinghausen's neurofibromatosis, tuberous sclerosis, von Hippel-Lindau disease, and Peutz-Jeghers syndrome. Associated malignant tumors include neurofibrosarcoma, meningiomas, pheochromocytoma, acoustic neuroma and gliomas (von Recklinghausen's), brain tumors (tuberous sclerosis); hypernephroma, ependymomas (von Hippel-Lindau disease); and malignant degeneration of intestinal polyps and ovarian cancer (Peutz-Jeghers syndrome).

Genodermatoses, *genetic disorders that involve the skin*, are autosomal recessive. Risk of cancer increases with exposure to ultraviolet radiation; eg, in xeroderma pigmentosum, which begins in childhood, skin cancers develop as a result of exposure to sunlight. These skin cancers include basal and squamous cell carcinomas, melanomas, and sarcomas. Defective DNA repair mechanisms are believed responsible. Albinos are prone to develop squamous cell and basal cell carcinoma.

Chromosome Breakage Disorders

In the following congenital diseases, affected children are at high risk of developing acute leukemia due to chromosomes' breaking easily: In **Bloom's syndrome** (a rare autosomal recessive disorder), dwarfism, a photosensitive telangiectatic facial erythema, and characteristic facies are found. An increased incidence of both acute leukemia and solid tumors occur in patients under age 30 yr. Features of **Fanconi's syndrome** include a constitutional aplastic anemia terminating in acute nonlymphocytic leukemia, growth retardation, hyperpigmentation, genitourinary abnormalities, and ear and skeletal deformities. **Down's syndrome** patients (see Ch. 203) have a twelve- to twenty-fold increased incidence of acute leukemia. Abnormalities of chromosome 21 also occur with increased frequency in de novo acute myelogenous leukemia.

Viruses

The murine and feline leukemia viruses and the avian leukosis virus are RNA viruses of the *Oncorna* genus known to cause malignancies in animals. Viruses linked with human malignancies include **herpesvirus type 2** (cervical carcinoma), **cytomegalovirus** (Kaposi's sarcoma), and the **Epstein-Barr virus** (Burkitt's lymphoma and nasopharyngeal carcinoma). **Retroviruses** have been linked to T cell lymphomas, which have a predilection for skin involvement and hypercalcemia and frequently manifest a "leukemic" phase. These retroviruses are believed to induce neoplastic transformation by insertion of viral genome into DNA; the cell then loses the regulatory mechanisms to control growth and differentiation. Human T-lymphotropic virus Type III **(HTLV-III)** is pathogenically linked to AIDS (see Ch. 19) and patients with AIDS are predisposed to Kaposi's sarcoma and lymphoma. HTLV is not a single virus, but a family of related T cell retroviruses. HTLV-I has been linked to endemic T cell lymphoma/leukemia in southern Japan, the Caribbean, and southeastern USA. The association of hepatitis B virus and the occurrence of hepatic carcinoma have been demonstrated recently; vaccination to prevent occurrence of the hepatitis may constitute the first prevention of a human cancer by vaccination.

Environmental Factors

Known chemical carcinogens include aromatic hydrocarbons and amines, alkylating agents, tobacco and wood products, nickel, asbestos, chromates, thorium dioxide, senecio alkaloids, aflatoxin, diethylstilbestrol, and oxymetholone. These agents directly induce malignant transformation, presumably by generation of the highly reactive "carbonium ion" and subsequent DNA damage.

Chemical carcinogenesis is influenced by age, endocrine status, diet, other exogenous agents, and immunologic status. In Africa, aflatoxin is suspected of being etiologically linked to hepatocellular carcinoma, which occurs 4 to 5 times oftener in men. Youth is associated with an increased susceptibility to chemical carcinogens, with fetuses the most susceptible. Exposure of fetuses to diethylstilbestrol in the 1st trimester is associated with vaginal carcinoma in postpubertal women.

Ultraviolet radiation plays an unequivocal role in the etiology of skin cancers (ie, basal and squamous cell carcinomas, melanoma, and in patients with xeroderma pigmentosa—see above in Genodermatoses under Genetic Susceptibility).

Exposure to ionizing radiation is carcinogenic; eg, survivors of Hiroshima and Nagasaki have a higher-than-expected incidence of leukemia. Similarly, when ionizing radiation in the form of γ rays is used to treat nonmalignant disease (facial acne, thymic enlargement, and ankylosing spondylitis), the incidence of cancer increases: Malignancies include leukemias, acute and chronic; lymphomas, Hodgkin's and non-Hodgkin's; multiple myeloma; aplastic anemia terminating in acute nonlymphocytic leukemia; myelofibrosis; and thyroid cancer. Industrial exposure (eg, to uranium by mine workers) is linked to development of lung cancer after a 15- to 20-yr latent period. Long-term exposure to occupational irradiation or to internally deposited thorium dioxide predisposes persons to develop angiosarcomas and acute nonlymphocytic leukemias.

Chronic trauma to skin leads to chronic dermatitis and on rare occasions ultimately to squamous cell carcinoma.

Parasites (eg, *Schistosoma hematobium*) have been linked to bladder cancer that usually develops after chronic inflammation and fibrosis. *Clonorchis sinensis* has been linked to carcinoma of the pancreas and bile ducts.

Immunologic Disorders (see also Ch. 18)

Patients with immunologic disorders are predisposed to lymphoreticular neoplasia and should be monitored periodically; development of new or suspicious lymphadenopathy should be excised. In **ataxia telangiectasia**, the incidence of acute lymphoblastic leukemia, brain tumors, and gastric cancer exceeds that of the normal population. Patients with **Wiskott-Aldrich syndrome** and **X-linked agammaglobulinemia** are also at high risk for lymphoma and acute lymphoblastic leukemia.

Patients with **acquired immune deficiency** as a result of immunosuppressive drugs used in renal transplantation are at risk for a diffuse large cell histiocytic lymphoma of the brain. Patients with **SLE, RA,** and **Sjögren's syndrome** are also at risk for development of lymphoma, usually the B cell type. A tenable hypothesis is that chronic antigenic stimulation leads to expansion of the B lymphocyte line and ultimately an autonomous B lymphocyte clone.

PATHOGENESIS AND PATHOPHYSIOLOGY

While the cellular and molecular events that lead to malignant transformation are poorly understood, some insights are emerging. Although phenotypic heterogeneity occurs with any malignant neoplasm, genotypically a given cancer is believed to arise from a clone of transformed cells. This theory is supported by the nonrandom chromosomal abnormalities found in patients with certain cancers; eg, about 80% of patients with chronic myelogenous leukemia **(CML)** have been found to have a Philadelphia chromosome (see under CHRONIC MYELOCYTIC LEUKEMIA in Ch. 101—its presence confers an overall better prognosis than when it is absent). Further evidence for clonality in CML is provided by the observation that only a *single* G6PD isoenzyme is present in RBCs and WBCs of patients with CML, while fibroblasts from these same patients contain both isoenzymes.

While cancers represent a clonal growth, there is nonetheless tumor cell heterogeneity; eg, in B-16 melanoma, certain cells have an affinity for the lung that others lack (see Metastases, below). In human cancers, cell suspensions made from a single tumor nodule characteristically show cell populations that are sensitive to drugs as well as others that are resistant.

Other examples of nonrandom chromosomal abnormalities associated with specific cancers are shown in TABLE 105–2. Chromosomal analysis of cancer cells also provides prognostic and, at times, therapeutic information; eg, patients with acute myelogenous leukemia and a normal chromosomal analysis have a better prognosis than those with abnormal chromosomes. Similarly, patients with a 15/17 chromosome translocation always have acute promyelocytic leukemia **(APL),** and identification of these patients is important: Typically, a bleeding diathesis (disseminated intravascular coagulation) develops and heparin therapy is required. Patients with APL must be treated and supported aggressively, because they are potentially curable.

Oncogenes

Viral oncogenes (v-onc) are found in certain RNA retroviruses that induce tumors; the retroviruses consist of 3 genes that code for internal viral core proteins, reverse transcriptase, and envelope protein. A fourth gene, designated as a v-onc, induces malignant transformation.

Cellular oncogenes (c-onc) homologous to v-onc are normal genetic components of all vertebrate cells; related genes have been found in invertebrates. They may play a role

TABLE 105–2. CHROMOSOMAL ABNORMALITIES ASSOCIATED WITH NEOPLASMS

Neoplasm	*Abnormality*	*Chromosome number*
Myeloid leukemia		
Chronic myelogenous leukemia	Translocation	9 and 22
Acute myelogenous leukemia with maturation (M_2)	Translocation	8 and 21
Acute promyelocytic leukemia	Translocation	15 and 17
Acute nonlymphocytic leukemia with increased basophils	Translocation	6 and 9
Acute monocytic leukemia	Loss of long arm	11
Acute myelomonocytic leukemia with eosinophilia	Inversion	16
Malignant lymphoma		
Burkitt's	Translocation	8 and 14
Non-Hodgkin's	Extra chromosome	6
Lymphocytic leukemia		
Acute lymphoblastic leukemia	Extra chromosome	6
Chronic lymphocytic leukemia	Extra chromosome	12
Myeloproliferative diseases	Extra chromosome	1
Small cell lung cancer	Loss of small arm	3
Wilms' tumor	Loss of small arm	11
Ewing's tumor	Translocation	11 and 22
Retinoblastoma	Deletion	13

in cellular proliferation. Like v-onc, c-onc encode for proteins, which may act (1) as enzymes to add phosphate groups to amino acid residues (phosphorylation); (2) as proteins to enhance DNA binding; or (3) as proteins to act as cellular growth factors. Thus, c-onc, like v-onc, may induce malignant transformation by (1) insertion of an as-yet-unidentified oncogene near another c-onc, allowing for its activation, or by (2) environmental factors that induce DNA damage and ultimately allow activation of a c-onc.

C-onc have been localized to certain human chromosomes; eg, the c-onc MYC is found on chromosome 8. Thus, in many nonrandom chromosomal changes involving chromosome 8 (see TABLE 105–2), the MYC c-onc may be activated. In Burkitt's lymphoma, the portion of chromosome 8 translocated to the long arm of chromosome 14 contains the c-onc MYC, which is adjacent to the immunoglobulin synthesis region of chromosome 14. Not surprisingly, immunoglobulin synthesis is 5 to 20 times higher in Burkitt's lymphoma cells than in normal lymphocytes.

Cellular Kinetics

All human cells capable of replication (bone marrow and GI tract) enter the **cell cycle** (see FIG. 105–1). Daughter cells either enter a variable resting phase or reenter the cell cycle, which may be as brief as 24 h or may last many days. Malignant cells usually have a cell cycle of many days. **Generation time** is *the time it takes for malignant cells to enter the cycle and give rise to 2 daughter cells.* Many drugs are effective only if cells are in cell cycle, and some work only during a specific phase of the cycle.

A tumor may be thought of as having compartments of cells (see FIG. 105–2). At any point in tumor growth, cells may be in cell cycle, resting, or may move from a resting state into cell cycle and vice versa. Another nonproliferating compartment of cells accounts for tumor bulk. Small tumors have a greater percentage of cells in cycle and thus a greater potential to proliferate. In contrast, large tumors have fewer cells in cycle and a much lower proliferative activity. Tumor growth occurs in a Gompertzian fashion; ie, initial exponential tumor growth is followed by a plateau phase when cell death equals the rate of formation of new daughter cells.

Metastases

Local tissue invasion can result from local tumor pressure on normal tissues that can lead to inflammation, or the tumor may elaborate substances (eg, collagenase) that lead to enzymatic destruction. Almost at inception, a tumor sheds cells into the circulation. Using animal models, it has been estimated that a 1-cm tumor sheds > 1 million

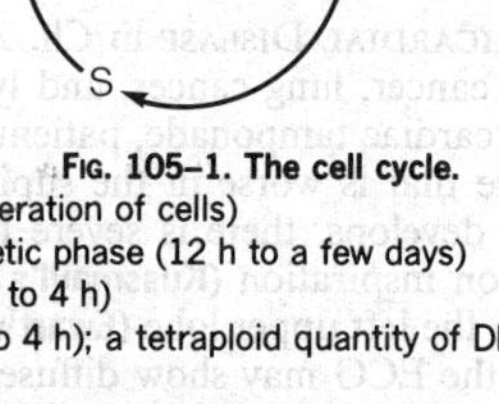

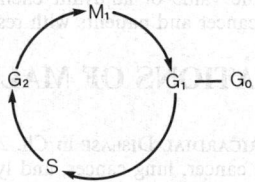

FIG. 105–1. The cell cycle.

G_0 = resting phase (nonproliferation of cells)
G_1 = Variable pre-DNA synthetic phase (12 h to a few days)
S = DNA synthesis (usually 2 to 4 h)
G_2 = post-DNA synthesis (2 to 4 h); a tetraploid quantity of DNA is found within cells
M = Mitosis (1 to 2 h)

(Modified from *Radiobiology for the Radiologist,* ed. 2, 1978, p. 114, by E. J. Hall. Copyright ©1978 by Harper & Row, Publishers, Inc. Used with permission.)

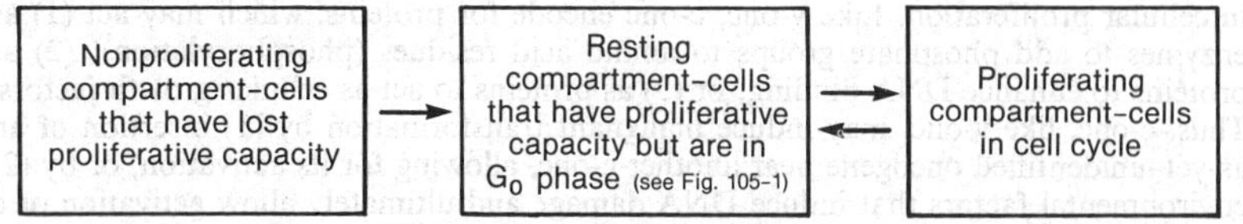

FIG. 105–2. Schematic representation of cell compartments within a malignant tumor mass.

cells/24 h into the venous circulation. In humans, circulating tumor cells have been identified in patients with early stage breast cancer and colon cancer. However, identification of circulating tumor cells in human malignancies does not predict early recurrence or limited survival; the probability that a single circulating tumor cell will become a metastatic nodule is estimated as 1 million:1. In animals, circulating tumor cells usually die as a result of trauma within arterial and venous circulation. The longer the tumor cell spends in the circulation, the greater the chance of its death.

Metastasis develops as a result of a tumor cell's adhering to the vascular endothelium. As a tumor grows, nutrients are provided by direct diffusion from the circulation; local pressure and collagenase lead to destruction of normal tissues. Subsequently, the synthesis of tumor angiogenesis factor causes formation of an independent vascular supply to the tumor nodule. As it continues to grow, cells are shed within the efferent circulation; a small number survive pressure forces and trauma and are then capable of starting *an independent tumor nodule*, a **metastasis**. The sequence of tumor growth is then resumed.

Within an individual tumor, certain cells are attracted to specific sites and not others. As the number of metastases increases, metastatic nodules can give rise to other metastases. Experiments suggest that metastasis is *not* a random event and that the primary tumor exerts an inhibitory effect on the growth of metastatic nodules (eg, in hypernephroma, the rate of growth, as measured by the labeling index, is similar in both the primary and metastatic nodules). Removal of a primary tumor will result in an explosion of metastases within a short period of time.

Since ability to metastasize occurs early in tumor development, it is clear that cancer is often a systemic disease. In mice, surgical removal alone of an implanted tumor rarely led to cure; however, when surgery (local therapy) and a single drug (to treat systemic micrometastases) were combined, a significant proportion of animals remained relapse-free and cured. With a decreasing interval between surgery and "adjuvant chemotherapy," there was an increasing number of cures. Clinical trials in human cancer clearly demonstrate the value of adjuvant chemotherapy in premenopausal patients with stage II breast cancer and patients with resectable gastric cancer.

COMPLICATIONS OF MALIGNANCY

Oncologic Emergencies

Cardiac tamponade (see PERICARDIAL DISEASE in Ch. 27) occurs precipitiously. The commonest causes are breast cancer, lung cancer, and lymphoma. Since a malignant pericardial effusion antedates cardiac tamponade, patients usually give a history of ill defined chest pain or pressure that is worse in the supine position and better when sitting up. When tamponade develops, there is severe breathlessness. Physical signs include neck vein distention on inspiration **(Kussmaul's sign)** and occasionally bronchial breath sounds audible in the left upper lobe **(Ewart's sign)**. The chest x-ray shows an enlarged cardiac shadow; the ECG may show diffuse low voltage. An echocardiogram demonstrates the presence of pericardial fluid. For diagnostic and therapeutic purposes, a pericardiocentesis (see PERICARDIAL DISEASE in Ch. 27) must be done an

a pleuropericardial window should be formed. Additional therapy depends on the underlying malignancy.

Pleural effusions, if present, should be drained and observed for reaccumulation. If the effusion reaccumulates rapidly, thoracostomy tube drainage and sclerosing agents should be used (see Ch. 33). **Spinal cord compression** requires immediate attention if patients are to be spared morbidity (see in Ch. 130). **Hypercalcemia,** caused by malignant neoplasms, is discussed under HYPERCALCEMIA in Ch. 84. **Superior vena cava syndrome (SVC),** a dramatic clinical situation, requires urgent but not emergency care (see Ch. 49). **Pain** in patients with metastatic cancer frequently results from bone metastases, nerve or plexus involvement, or pressure exerted by a tumor mass or effusion. Treatment of such pain is discussed in Ch. 119.

Paraneoplastic Syndromes (see also under extrapulmonary manifestations in Ch. 49; HYPERCALCEMIA in Ch. 84; and in Ch. 126)

The paraneoplastic syndromes may be a result of biologically active proteins, immune complexes, ectopic receptor production, release of physiologically active compounds, or unknown causes. **Endocrine paraneoplastic syndromes** include ectopic ACTH and ADH (small cell and non-small cell lung cancer); ectopic parathyroid hormone (PTH) production (squamous cell lung cancer, bladder cancer), ectopic calcitonin production (breast cancer and small cell lung carcinoma), ectopic production of thyroid-stimulating hormone (medullary thyroid carcinoma), insulin production (islet cell carcinoma), or serotonin (islet cell carcinoma). The symptoms vary with the type of ectopic hormone produced. Thus symptoms and signs include Cushingoid facies, changes in mental status (ectopic ADH or glucagon), hypercalcemia, gynecomastia, or hypoglycemia (insulinoma). Some paraneoplastic syndromes have not yet been clearly shown to be due to excess secretion of hormones (eg, hypoglycemia may also occur in the presence of liver metastases or large retroperitoneal tumors). Successful treatment consists of controlling the underlying malignancy; if it is untreatable, symptoms can be palliated with drugs, eg, minocycline (ectopic ADH), cyproheptadine (carcinoid syndrome), or mithramycin and steroids (hypercalcemia).

Neurologic paraneoplastic syndromes are of unknown cause and include subacute cerebellar degeneration, amyotrophic lateral sclerosis, sensory or sensory-motor peripheral neuropathy, Guillain-Barré syndrome, dermatomyositis, polymyositis, myasthenia gravis, and the **Eaton-Lambert syndrome** (*a myasthenia-like syndrome with weakness usually affecting the limbs and sparing the ocular and bulbar muscles*). These neuropathies can antedate, occur concurrently, or develop after a diagnosis of cancer. The Eaton-Lambert syndrome occurs most often with small cell lung cancer and often responds to guanidine. The other carcinomatous polyneuropathies are of unknown cause, and except for myasthenia gravis, which can be treated with neostigmine or prednisone, they have no specific therapy.

Hematologic paraneoplastic syndromes are hypoproliferative anemia, granulocytosis, thrombocytosis, eosinophilia, basophilia, and disseminated intravascular coagulation. In addition, idiopathic thrombocytopenic purpura and a Coombs-positive hemolytic anemia can complicate the course of patients with chronic lymphatic leukemia and Hodgkin's disease.

Renal paraneoplastic syndrome (membranous glomerulitis) has been described; eg, in patients with colon cancer, ovarian cancer, and lymphoma as a result of circulating immune complexes.

Pigmented skin lesions or keratoses associated with malignancy include acanthosis nigricans (GI malignancy), generalized melanosis (lymphoma, melanoma, hepatoma), Bowen's disease (lung, GI, and GU malignancy), and large multiple seborrheic keratoses ([Leser-Trélat] lymphoma and GI malignancy).

Other miscellaneous paraneoplastic syndromes include fever, lactic acidosis (leukemia, lymphoma), hyperlipidemia (myeloma), hypertrophic pulmonary osteoarthropathy (lung cancer or lung metastases from renal cancer, thymoma, sarcoma, and Hodgkin's disease).

METASTATIC CARCINOMA OF OCCULT PRIMARY MALIGNANCY (OPM)

A biopsy-proven metastatic malignancy for which a primary site cannot be found. These patients constitute 0.5 to 7% of all cancer patients. Except for those with germ-cell neoplasms and diffuse histiocytic lymphoma (**DHL**), OPM patient survival is generally poor (median survival, 3 to 4 mo).

The approach to patients with OPM includes a detailed history and physical examination with particular attention to the breasts and pelvic examination in women, prostate in men, and rectum in both sexes. Laboratory tests should include a CBC, urinalysis, stool examination for occult blood, and multichannel serum chemistries (including an acid phosphatase in males). X-rays should be limited to a chest x-ray, IVU, and mammography. An upper GI series and barium enema should not be done in the absence of symptoms or physical signs.

The differential diagnosis in patients with *undifferentiated* malignant tumors includes metastatic undifferentiated carcinoma, undifferentiated sarcoma, DHL, and metastatic melanoma. Metastatic undifferentiated sarcoma or melanoma cannot be cured or palliated with either chemotherapy or radiotherapy. The clinician should try to exclude beyond a doubt the possibility of DHL or an extragonadal germ-cell tumor, because each can be cured or palliated with chemotherapy. Immunoperoxidase staining for immunoglobulin and electron microscopy is helpful in diagnosing DHL. In young males, immunoperoxidase staining for α-fetoprotein or the β-subunit of human chorionic gonadotropin is helpful in diagnosing metastatic germ-cell carcinoma. A repeat biopsy may be necessary to obtain the additional histologic material required to perform the necessary immunoperoxidase and electron microscopic studies. Even if a precise histologic diagnosis cannot be made, patients with poorly differentiated carcinomas and predominant involvement of the mediastinum, retroperitoneum, or the lymph node areas should receive 2 cycles of cisplatin-based chemotherapy; patients with responses should be given a total of 3 to 4 cycles. Up to ½ have been reported to respond favorably, some with long-term disease-free intervals.

Patients with metastatic *adenocarcinoma* of OPM are a subset of OPM patients and should be approached in a limited manner, searching for neoplasms that may be palliated. Metastatic adenocarcinoma of the ovary, breast, and prostate can be palliated with chemotherapy (ovary and breast) or hormonal therapy (breast and prostate) Therefore, the pathologic investigation of metastatic tissue should include an estrogen and progesterone receptor assay and immunoperoxidase staining for acid phosphatase If the primary is not found, current treatment approach is to institute chemotherapy early. Doxorubicin and mitomycin are active in metastatic adenocarcinoma of OPM although responses tend to be short-lived.

DIAGNOSIS AND STAGING

Screening Tests

Routine use of the **Papanicolaou (Pap) smear** has led to a significant decrease i mortality from cervical carcinoma in the USA. Women with early sexual promiscuity multiparity, and herpes simplex virus type 2 infections are at increased risk for cervica cancer, which is fatal if untreated, but 100% curable if diagnosed early. **Breast sel examination** may lead to an earlier diagnosis of breast cancer and hope for more cure Preliminary data on **mammography** show that its routine use can reduce mortality fro

breast cancer about 30%, but data must be confirmed before mammography is used in a routine manner. Information from long-term studies on **stool testing for occult blood** as a screening procedure for colon cancer is not yet available, but testing should lead to earlier diagnosis of colon cancer. For screening procedures recommended by the American Cancer Society, see TABLE 105–3.

Diagnosis

Under no circumstances should cancer therapy proceed without an unequivocal histopathologic diagnosis of cancer; eg, by excisional biopsy, aspiration cytology or biopsy, endoscopic biopsy, or bone marrow biopsy.

Clinical Staging

Once an unequivocal diagnosis is made, clinical or pathologic staging determines appropriate treatment decisions and may also provide prognostic information. No single system is applicable to all cancers. In clinical staging, currently used classifications are based on knowledge of the natural history and pathophysiology of particular tumors, combined with data from the patient's history, physical examinations, and noninvasive studies. Staging of specific neoplasms is detailed under appropriate headings elsewhere in THE MANUAL.

Noninvasive staging procedures used to determine extent of disease are summarized in TABLE 105–4. Some procedures (eg, liver-spleen and bone scans) are common to the staging of any malignancy; others (eg, gallium 67 scans) are used to stage lung cancer and lymphomas, but play no role in staging a GI cancer.

Multiscreening serum chemistries and enzymes: The elevation of liver enzymes, alkaline phosphatase, LDH, and alanine aminotransferase (ALT [SGPT]) suggests the presence of liver metastases, which can be confirmed with either a liver-spleen scan or

TABLE 105–3. STATEMENT OF THE AMERICAN CANCER SOCIETY REGARDING SCREENING PROCEDURES

Procedure	*Position Statement*
For ♂* and ♀ of any age:**	
Chest x-ray	Not recommended on a routine basis
Sputum cytology	Not recommended on a routine basis
For ♂ and ♀:	
Stool examination for occult blood	Yearly after age 50
Rectal examination	Yearly after age 50
Proctoscopic examination	Every 3 yr after age 50
For ♀:	
Pelvic examination	Every 3 yr between ages 20–40; then yearly
Papanicolaou (Pap) smear	Every 3 yr between ages 20–65
Breast self-examination	Monthly after age 20
Breast physical examination	Every 3 yr between ages 20–40; then yearly
Mammography	Initial "baseline" examination between ages 35–40; q 1–2 yr from age 40–49; and yearly after age 50.

* ♂ = man; ** ♀ = woman

(Modified from *CA—A Cancer Journal for Clinicians,* p. 199, Vol. 35, No. 4, July/August 1985. Used with permission of the American Cancer Society, Inc.)

TABLE 105–4. STAGING PROCEDURES OF ORGAN–SPECIFIC NEOPLASIA

Organ System	*Lesion*	*Clinical Testing*	*Tissue Diagnosis*	*Special Procedures*	*Testing: Clinical/Pathologic*
Lung	Solitary nodule	History & physical Chest x-ray CT	Sputum cytology Bronchoscopy + biopsy Percutaneous needle aspiration cytology	Lung biopsy Pleural biopsy (if effusion present)	Gallium scan Mediastinoscopy
	Multiple mass	History & physical with rectal examination	Percutaneous needle aspiration cytology	Lung biopsy	Metastatic no further staging required
		History & physical Mammogram if palpable lesion present			
Breast	Single mass	History & physical Mammogram Xerogram	Needle aspiration excisional biopsy	Estrogen receptor Progesterone receptor	Liver scan Bone scan Brain CT scan
Lymphoid	Adenopathy	History & physical Chest x-ray (hilar/mediastinal nodes) Abdominal flat plate (splenomegaly)	Excisional biopsy		US Gallium scan IVU Abdominal CT scan Liver-spleen scan Bone scan Bone marrow biopsies *and* aspiration Laparoscopy Laparotomy + splenectomy
	Splenomegaly	History & physical Blood counts	Bone marrow aspiration + biopsies		Proceed as above Peripheral blood for B+T lymphocyte Total protein Serum protein electrophoresis

G1	Esophageal mass or stricture	Chest x-ray Barium swallow	Esophagoscopy with brushing, cytology and biopsy		CT scan Bronchoscopy Mediastinoscopy
	Gastric mass	Upper GI barium series (double contrast)	Gastroscopy with brushing cytology and biopsy		Liver scan Chest x-ray
	Pancreatic mass	US CT scan	Duodenal drainage for cytology; Cannulation of ampulla of Vater for cytology	Percutaneous cholangiogram; ERCP	Liver scan Arteriogram Laparotomy + biopsy
	Liver mass	Liver scan α-fetoprotein	Percutaneous biopsy	Peritoneoscopy and biopsy	Arteriogram Laparotomy
	Liver: Multiple masses	Liver scan Chest x-ray Mammogram if palpable mass present Pancreatic US	Percutaneous biopsy	Peritoneoscopy and biopsy	Laparotomy
Testis	Mass	Chest x-ray IVU α-fetoprotein β-human chorionic gonadotropin	High inguinal orchiectomy	α-fetoprotein β-human chorionic gonadotropin	IVU Lymphangiogram Abdominal CT scan Laparotomy
Pelvis (cervix endometrium, ovaries)	Mass	Pelvic examination under anesthesia Pelvic US Barium enema CT scan	Laparotomy	CEA Bast Antigen (CA-125) for ovarian cancer	Laparotomy Abdominal CT Scan

liver ultrasonography. An elevation in the alkaline phosphatase and serum Ca may be the first evidence of bone metastases. An elevated acid phosphate (tartrate inhibited) suggests extracapsular extension of prostate carcinoma. Hypoglycemia (more specifically, fasting hypoglycemia) may indicate an insulinoma, hepatoma, or retroperitoneal sarcoma. An elevated BUN or creatinine may indicate an obstructive uropathy secondary to either a pelvic mass, intrarenal obstruction from tubular precipitation of myeloma protein, or a uric acid nephropathy from lymphoma or other cancers. An elevated uric acid level often occurs in myeloproliferative and lymphoproliferative disorders. Special tests that may be useful in certain neoplasms include α-fetoprotein (hepatomas, testicular carcinomas), CEA-S (colon cancer), β-HCG (choriocarcinoma, testicular carcinoma), and serum immunoglobulins (multiple myeloma).

Ultrasonography (US) is a noninvasive, easily applied technic to study orbital, thyroid, cardiac, pericardial, hepatic, pancreatic, renal, and retroperitoneal areas. Percutaneous biopsies guided by US can be carried out easily. Renal sonography and arteriography can differentiate a benign renal cyst from a malignant renal cell carcinoma.

Radiologic studies: CT can be used to detect metastases to brain, lung, or abdominal viscera including the adrenal glands, retroperitoneal lymph nodes, and spleen. CT of the brain, associated with less morbidity than arteriograms, is the procedure of choice in evaluating brain tumors.

A lymphangiogram reveals enlarged pelvic and low lumbar lymph nodes and is useful in the clinical staging of patients with Hodgkin's disease and testicular carcinoma.

Radioisotopic scans: Liver-spleen scans can identify metastases to the liver or find splenomegaly that is not palpable. Bone scans are extremely sensitive in identifying metastases before they are evident on x-ray; however, scans are seldom helpful in multiple myeloma, and radiographs of bone are the study of choice. Gallium scans are helpful in staging patients with Hodgkin's disease, the non-Hodgkin's lymphomas, and lung cancer.

Pathologic Staging

Pathologic staging requires tissue specimens and is useful to further define the extent of disease. **Mediastinoscopy** (see in Ch. 33) is valuable in the staging of non–small cell lung cancer, as it helps to identify patients who would not usually benefit from a thoracotomy and lung resection. A mediastinoscopy that shows contralateral mediastinal lymph node involvement would spare the patient an unnecessary thoracotomy.

A **bone core biopsy** is useful to differentiate bone marrow metastases from malignant lymphoma or small cell lung cancer. In 50 to 70% of patients with malignant lymphoma (poorly differentiated lymphocytic nodular or diffuse), a bone core biopsy will be positive; and it will detect marrow involvement in 15 to 18% of patients with metastases from small cell lung cancer.

When a **modified radical mastectomy** is performed, the axillary lymph nodes are removed and examined. Axillary lymph node metastases indicate a high risk for recurrence and the potential for benefit from adjuvant chemotherapy.

A **staging laparotomy** with **splenectomy** is an integral part of the staging of certain patients with Hodgkin's disease when management decisions are required (see Ch. 102).

In colon carcinoma, a **laparotomy** allows for therapeutic intervention and operative staging that yields prognostic information and is helpful in making treatment decisions. Pathologic staging helps identify those patients at high risk for recurrent disease: tumor penetration into the serosa (stage B_2), or lymphatic involvement (stage C). Patients with microscopic hepatic involvement (stage D) are also identified.

TREATMENT AND PROGNOSIS

Successful cancer therapy must be directed to the primary tumor and to metastases whether clinically apparent or microscopic. Thus, local and regional therapy, surgery

or radiotherapy must be integrated with systemic therapy (eg, chemotherapy). If cure is impossible, the aim is to palliate symptoms and to improve the quality of life.

The first step toward cure is **complete remission or complete response (CR**—*disappearance of all clinical evidence of disease*). A **partial response ([PR]** > *50% reduction in the size of a tumor mass or masses*) leads to significant palliation and may prolong life, but tumor regrowth is inevitable. Unfortunately, a patient may have **no response.** If a patient has CR and ultimately relapses, *the interval between complete disappearance of the cancer to the time of relapse* is **the disease free survival; survival** measures *the time of CR to the time of death.* Similarly, in patients who achieve palliation with a PR, the **duration of response** is measured *from the time of PR to the time of progression.*

Surgery

Surgery is the oldest, most effective form of cancer therapy. In 1985, about 1,300,000 persons developed cancer; of those, about 400,000 patients had cancer either of the skin or cervix and about 900,000 patients had life-threatening cancers. Of the 900,000 patients, 64% had operable lesions. It is estimated that surgery was performed in 576,000 patients, with a cure rate of 62%.

The cancers curable in early stages with surgery alone **(oral cavity, larynx, lung, colon, prostate, kidney, testis, bladder, ovary, endometrium, cervix, and breast)** are listed in TABLE 105–5. The principles of an en bloc resection are applied in each instance. For example, in hypernephroma, a radical nephrectomy is usually performed via a flank incision; perinephric fat, kidney, and a variable length of ureter are removed. Hypernephromas that do not penetrate Gerota's fascia have a cure rate of 67%.

Surgical therapy in early breast cancer (lesion < 2 cm with no palpable lymph nodes) involves a modified radical mastectomy with en bloc dissection of axillary lymph nodes. There is no role for an internal mammary node dissection for medial quadrant or outer quadrant lesions. Current surgical trials are examining the role of quadrant resection or tylectomy and axillary nodal dissection and radiotherapy. Results of these trials at 5 yr appear comparable to a modified radical mastectomy.

Colon cancer is best staged intraoperatively (see above); the resection carried out is a right or left hemicolectomy, depending on the location of the lesion. In early colon cancers (stage A or B), the cure rate is excellent.

Radiotherapy

Radiotherapy plays a key role in the cure of Hodgkin's disease, early stage non-Hodgkin's lymphomas, squamous cell carcinoma of the head and neck, mediastinal germ-cell tumors, seminoma, prostate cancer, early stage breast cancer, early stage non–small cell lung cancer, medulloblastoma, and as an adjunct to chemotherapy in acute lymphoblastic leukemia. Radiotherapy can be used as palliative therapy in prostate cancer and breast cancer when bone metastases are present, in multiple myeloma, advanced stage lung and esophagopharyngeal cancer, gastric cancer, and sarcomas, and in brain metastases. **Cancers that are curable with radiotherapy alone are listed in TABLE 105–5**; the rate of cure for *early* lesions of the larynx and prostate is identical to that of surgery, as indicated.

Ionizing radiation causes ejection of an orbital electron during its absorption, which requires a large transfer of energy that directly affects the cell contents. During the energy transfer, interaction with water may produce short-lived free radicals that in turn alter DNA. O_2 prolongs the life of reactive free radicals, but sulfhydryl compounds reduce them and shorten their life span. The effects of ionizing radiation are random: cellular death, unusual aberrant cellular forms, functional cells incapable of division, or functional cells that are unaltered.

Radiation repair refers to *a cell's ability to function despite exposure to sublethal radiation.* Repair mechanisms account for the "shoulder" noted in radiation survival curves. An enhanced radiation effect is present in a well-oxygenated cell, but cells

TABLE 105–5. 5–YEAR DISEASE–FREE SURVIVAL RATES FOR CANCER CURED BY A SINGLE MODE OF THERAPY

Therapy	*Site*	*Stage*	*5-yr Disease-free Rate (%)*
Surgery	Cervix	I	94
	Breast	I	82
	Bladder	O + A	81
		B_1	66
	Colon	A	81
		B	64
		C	27
	Prostate	A + B	80
	Larynx	I + II	76
	Endometrium	I	74
	Ovary	I	72
	Oral cavity	I + II	67–76
	Kidney	I + II	67
	Testis (nonseminomatous)	I	65
	Lung (non–small cell)	I	50–70
		II	37
Radiotherapy	Non-Hodgkin's lymphoma (nodular)	Pathologic Stage I	60
	Non-Hodgkin's lymphoma (diffuse)		90
	Hodgkin's disease	" " IA	88
		" " IIA	83
		" " IIIA	71
	Testis (seminoma)	II + III	84
	Prostate	A + B	80
		C	67
	Larynx	I + II	76
	Cervix	II + III	60
	Nasopharynx	I, II, III	35
	Nasal sinuses	I, II, III	35
	Breast	III	29
	Esophagus		10
	Lung	III_{MO} (excluding Pancoast)	9
Chemotherapy	Choriocarcinoma	All Stages	95
	Testis (nonseminomatous)	III	88
	Hodgkin's disease	III B + IV A + B	74
	Diffuse large cell lymphoma	II, III, IV	64
	Burkitt's lymphoma	I, II, III	44–74
	Leukemia (childhood, ANLL)		54
	Leukemia (< 40 yr, ANLL)		40
	(> 40 yr, ANLL)		16
	Lung (small cell)	"Limited"	16

within hypoxic and anoxic regions of tumors resist the effects of ionizing radiation after a single lethal dose, the hypoxic cells survive. As the tumor is reoxygenated, th hypoxic cells return to their pretreatment value. Thus, radiation therapy of malignar neoplasms incorporates the principle that a fractionated dose of radiation allows fo gradual reoxygenation.

Therapeutic radiation is usually administered with megavoltage equipment using a radioactive cobalt source; roentgen rays produced are in the 2 to 35 million electron-volt (MeV) range. With megavoltage equipment, there is less scatter of the target tissue. Adverse effects experienced during a course of radiation depend on the region being radiated and on normal tissue tolerance to the effects of radiation; eg, radiotherapy administered to the head and neck region often causes oropharyngeal mucositis, and abdominal radiotherapy often causes gastritis (upper abdominal) and enteritis resulting in diarrhea.

ANTINEOPLASTIC CHEMOTHERAPY

The ideal antineoplastic drug would destroy cancer cells without adverse effects or toxicities on normal cells, but no such drug exists. However, despite the narrow therapeutic index of many drugs, treatment and even cure are possible in some patients. A review of the pharmacology of antineoplastics follows (see FIG. 105–3).

Alkylating Agents

Alkylating agents, compounds often chemically similar to mustard gas (eg, nitrogen mustard, cyclophosphamide, melphalan, and chlorambucil), attack electron-rich regions of molecules adding alkyl groups to O_2, N, and sulfur. Within the cell, proteins and nucleic acids are alkylated when exposed to such compounds. If DNA is alkylated, the single DNA strands that comprise the double helix are unable to uncoil and replicate themselves. This disruption of cellular metabolism leads to cellular death.

Nitrogen mustard is an active compound when given IV, but cyclophosphamide is inert and must undergo metabolic conversion within the liver to its active forms, aldophosphamide and phosphamide mustard. The half-life (**$t_{1/2}$**) of nitrogen mustard and cyclophosphamide is about 15 to 20 min, and they are eliminated by the kidneys.

Alkylating agents play an integral role in the treatment of Hodgkin's disease, the non-Hodgkin's lymphomas, multiple myeloma, chronic myelogenous leukemia, chronic lymphocytic leukemia, acute lymphoblastic leukemia, breast cancer, small cell cancer of the lung, non–small cell lung cancer, and prostate cancer. **Toxicities** include nausea, vomiting, alopecia, hemorrhagic cystitis, leukopenia, thrombocytopenia, anemia, the syndrome of inappropriate ADH, pulmonary fibrosis, and an increased risk of acute nonlymphocytic leukemia.

Antimetabolites

A broad group of drugs consisting of purine, pyrimidine, and folate antagonists (see FIG. 105–3). They are cycle and phase specific; ie, to promote antitumor effects, they require cells to be in cell cycle and in S phase (see FIG. 105–1).

The purine antagonists 6-mercaptopurine and 6-thioguanine inhibit de novo purine synthesis and the interconversion of purines. Both are given orally to treat acute lymphocytic and nonlymphocytic leukemia. Oral absorption is incomplete and variable and both drugs are excreted by the kidneys. The major metabolite of 6-thioguanine is thiouric acid. 6-Mercaptopurine may undergo metabolic conversion to 6-thioguanine. Toxicities include alopecia and myelosuppression.

The pyrimidine antagonists are cytarabine **(CA)**, 5-fluorouracil, and 5-floxuridine; all are given parenterally. CA acts to inhibit DNA synthesis by inhibition of deoxycytidylate kinase and DNA polymerase. Cytosine deaminase, an enzyme that resides in endothelial cells and liver, converts CA into an inactive compound, arabinosyluridine. CA has a very short plasma $t_{1/2}$; it penetrates into the CNS with levels about 30 to 50% of plasma levels. CA plays an integral role in treating acute nonlymphocytic leukemia and diffuse histiocytic lymphoma. **Toxicities** include nausea, vomiting, alopecia, myelosuppression, skin rash, and diarrhea; in high dosage, adverse effects are conjunctivitis and cerebellar ataxia.

Use of a substitution group (R): Mustards

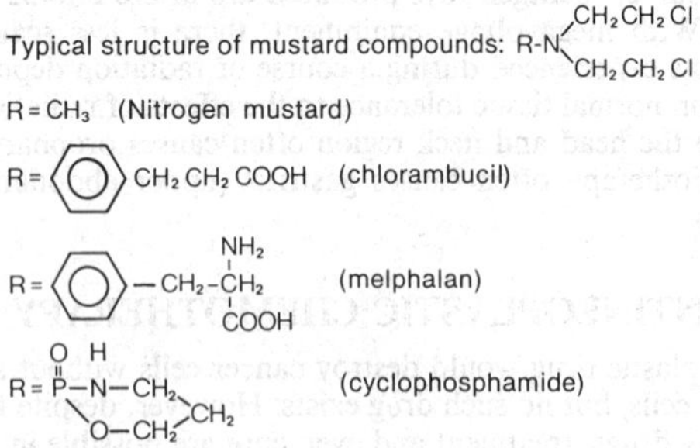

Antimetabolites
- Purine antagonists: 6-mercaptopurine, 6-thioguanine
- Pyrimidine antagonists: cytarabine, 5-fluorouracil, floxuridine
- Folate antagonists: methotrexate

Plant alkaloids
- Vincas: vincristine, vinblastine
- Podophyllotoxins: etoposide, teniposide

Antitumor antibiotics
- Intercalators of DNA: dactinomycin, daunorubicin, doxorubicin
- Scission of DNA: bleomycin
- Covalent binding of DNA: mitomycin

Other agents: Inorganic ions (cisplatin)

Biologic response modifiers: interferons

Enzymes: L-asparaginase

Endocrine therapy

Fig. 105–3. Antineoplastic drugs.

5-Fluorouracil (5-FU) and **5-floxuridine (5-FUdR)** are *substituted pyrimidine analogs that inhibit DNA by the inhibition of thymidylate synthetase.* Their therapeutic effect can be inhibited when reduced folate stores are depleted, and both are rapidly converted to CO_2; the plasma $t_{1/2}$ is about 10 to 15 min following parenteral administration. Antitumor activity for 5-FU is reported in breast cancer, colon cancer, gastric cancer, and adenocarcinoma of the lung, and when used with other drugs in squamous cell carcinoma of the head and neck. 5-FUdR, when given as an intrahepatic arterial infusion, is reported to have activity in colon cancer with hepatic metastases. **Toxicities** include nausea, vomiting, alopecia, mucositis (oropharyngeal and enteral), myelosuppression, and cerebellar dysfunction at high dose. Chemotherapy given by continuous infusion alters the toxicities of many drugs. This is especially true for anthracyclines and antimetabolites (eg, 5-FU and 5-FUrD).

Methotrexate (MTX) is *a folate antagonist that binds tightly with the intracellular enzyme dihydrofolate reductase.* It inhibits the formation of tetrahydrofolic acid, the reduced and active form of folic acid. After exposure to MTX , cell death results from inability to synthesize pyrimidines. By giving tetrahydrofolinic acid (leucovorin), one can bypass the enzymatic blockade caused by MTX. "Rescue" with leucovorin allows high doses of MTX to be given without lethal toxicity. Resistance to MTX may be a

result of decreased intracellular transport or elevated dihydrofolate reductase levels. Amplification of the dihydrofolate reductase gene has been demonstrated in a small cell carcinoma cell line resistant to MTX. Drugs that decrease cellular uptake of MTX include hydrocortisone, methylprednisolone, cephalothin, and L-asparaginase; in contrast, vincristine and vinblastine increase cellular uptake of MTX. When 5-FU is given after MTX, there is sequential enzymatic blockade and a synergistic antitumor effect. MTX is rapidly absorbed from the GI tract, and 50 to 60% of the drug present within the blood is protein bound. MTX is eliminated unchanged in urine; its clearance is dependent on glomerular filtration and active tubular secretion. MTX is widely distributed within the body, including the CSF and effusions.

MTX has a wide spectrum of antitumor activity, including squamous cell carcinoma of the head and neck, breast cancer, non-Hodgkin's lymphomas, acute lymphoblastic leukemia, small cell lung cancer, ovarian carcinoma, transitional carcinoma of the bladder, and osteogenic sarcoma. **Toxicities** include myelosuppression, anemia, leukopenia, thrombocytopenia, nausea, vomiting, anorexia, stomatitis, pharyngitis, hepatocellular injury, erythematous rashes, folliculitis, hyperpigmentation, alopecia, renal failure (especially in high doses), chills, fever, and pulmonary fibrosis.

Plant Alkaloids

The vinca alkaloids, podophyllotoxins, and colchicine act by mitotic arrest. The vinca alkaloids (vincristine, vinblastine) and colchicine inhibit mitosis by crystallization of microtubular proteins. Podophyllotoxins (etoposide and teniposide) do not crystallize spindle tubular protein, and their exact mechanisms of action are unknown. The podophyllotoxins inhibit both DNA synthesis and RNA- and RNA-dependent protein synthesis. At low doses the effect on mitosis is reversible. At high concentrations the inhibition is irreversible.

Vincristine and **vinblastine** are given rapidly IV and are rapidly cleared from the circulation. The plasma $t_{1/2}$ is 15 min for vincristine and 35 min for vinblastine. Vinblastine is partially metabolized by the liver, and both drugs are excreted in bile. Their antitumor activity includes acute lymphoblastic leukemia, breast cancer, Ewing's sarcoma (vincristine), Wilms' tumor (vincristine), Hodgkin's and non-Hodgkin's lymphomas, testicular carcinoma (vinblastine), and renal cell carcinoma (vinblastine). **Toxicities** include nausea, vomiting, alopecia, myelosuppression (vinblastine), peripheral neuropathy (vincristine), ileus, myopathy (vincristine), and syndrome of inappropriate antidiuretic hormone secretion (SIADH).

Etoposide and **teniposide** are given slowly IV. *When given rapidly IV, they precipitate severe hypotension.* Both drugs are protein bound; minimal amounts cross the blood-brain barrier. The $t_{1/2}$ of etoposide is 11.5 h; that of teniposide is 45 min. Etoposide is eliminated via the biliary tract with ½ the dose being a fecally excreted metabolite. In contrast, teniposide is dependent upon urinary excretion; in patients with renal insufficiency, teniposide has a longer $t_{1/2}$, and these patients tend to experience greater hematologic toxicity.

Etoposide is used to treat Hodgkin's disease and non-Hodgkin's lymphomas, small cell lung cancer, and testicular cancer. Teniposide is used in Hodgkin's disease, non-Hodgkin's lymphomas, and primary brain tumors. Their toxicities include nausea, vomiting, alopecia, myelosuppression, and peripheral neuropathy.

Antitumor Antibiotics

Chromatogenic compounds obtained from fermentation of Streptomyces *species* (**dactinomycin, doxorubicin,** and **daunomycin**—see FIG. 105-3). These compounds prevent cell replication by positioning themselves between planar base pairs of DNA, thus preventing the unwinding of the double helix. Dactinomycin also inhibits the synthesis of DNA-dependent RNA. Doxorubicin and daunorubicin inhibit DNA polymerase and thus ultimately interfere with nucleic acid synthesis. Doxorubicin and daunorubicin

are tetracyclic molecules (anthracyclines) that differ only by a single hydroxyl at the carbon number 14 of the alkyl side chain. The anthracycline moiety is linked at the B-ring to the amino sugar daunosamine.

Dactinomycin, doxorubicin, and daunorubicin are all given rapidly IV and *all cause tissue necrosis if extravasation occurs.* When doxorubicin and daunorubicin are given rapidly IV, there is rapid dispersement throughout tissues and plasma. The α $t_{1/2}$ is 30 min, with detectable plasma levels of doxorubicin up to 15 h. Both doxorubicin and daunorubicin are extensively metabolized by the liver, yielding active and inactive metabolites.

Dactinomycin and daunorubicin have limited antitumor activity. Dactinomycin is effective in testicular carcinoma and sarcomas. Daunorubicin is effective in treating acute leukemia. In contrast, doxorubicin is one of the most active antineoplastics ever identified: It is used to treat acute leukemia, Hodgkin's disease and non-Hodgkin's lymphomas, small cell and non–small cell lung cancer, cancers of the breast, ovaries, stomach, thyroid, and bladder, osteogenic and soft tissue sarcomas, and malignant melanoma. **Toxicities** include nausea, vomiting, alopecia, myelosuppression, and dose-dependent cardiotoxicity (> 550 mg/m^2).

Bleomycin, *an antibiotic produced by fermentation of* Streptomyces verticillus, causes scission of both single- and double-stranded DNA and is cycle and phase specific with its major effect in G_2 and M phase (see FIG. 105–1). It can be infused directly into a body cavity or can be given IM, IV, or s.c.; the peak blood level when given IM or s.c. occurs in about 30 min. The IV $t_{1/2}$ of bleomycin is 20 min, with detectable levels up to 2.5 h; since it is excreted by the kidney, it should be given cautiously in patients with renal failure.

Bleomycin is active in treating squamous cell cancer of the head and neck, cancer of the cervix, skin, penis, and rectum, Hodgkin's disease, the non-Hodgkin's lymphomas, testicular cancer, and lung cancer. **Toxicities** include anaphylactoid reactions, fever, chills, anorexia, skin changes, and a dose-dependent pulmonary fibrosis (> 200 mg/m^2).

Mitomycin is *an antibiotic that inhibits DNA synthesis by acting as a bifunctional alkylating agent.* This action is not cell cycle or phase specific; however, the kinetic effects are maximized if cells are treated in late G_1 and early S phase (see FIG. 105–1). The drug is given by slow infusion through a well-running IV line. *Local tissue necrosis occurs upon extravasation of the drug.* It is cleared from the vascular compartment with only about 10 to 30% of the dose being excreted in the urine; most is eliminated by hepatic metabolism.

Mitomycin is used in gastric adenocarcinoma, colon, breast, and lung cancer, and transitional cell carcinoma of the bladder. **Toxicities** include myelosuppression (with leukopenia and thrombocytopenia occurring 4 to 6 wk after administration), alopecia, lethargy, fever, and renal toxicity as manifested by a hemolytic-uremic syndrome.

Cisplatin, one of the inorganic salts, is a bifunctional alkylating agent as well as an intercalator and thus inhibits DNA synthesis. The drug is not cycle or phase specific; when given as a slow IV infusion, it is cleared from the plasma in 25 to 79 min (α $t_{1/2}$) followed by a slower secondary phase (β $t_{1/2}$) of 58 to 73 h. Cisplatin is protein bound and excreted by the kidneys. It is used in germ-cell neoplasms, lymphomas, ovarian carcinoma, and squamous cell carcinoma of the head and neck. The major dose-limiting toxicity is dose-related nephrotoxicity that can be overcome with vigorous hydration, mannitol, or furosemide. Other toxicities include peripheral neuropathy, ototoxicity, nausea and vomiting, anemia, and mild myelosuppression.

Enzymes

L-Asparaginase is an enzyme used to treat acute lymphoblastic leukemias **(ALL)**. Unlike normal cells, ALL cells cannot synthesize the essential amino acid asparagine and

thus require exogenous sources. L-Asparaginase depletes exogenous asparagine and thus inhibits cellular metabolism. **Toxicities** include anaphylactic reactions, anorexia, nausea, vomiting, and inhibition of protein synthesis.

Endocrine Therapy

Additive or ablative endocrine therapy can influence the course of human cancer; eg, diethylstilbestrol **(DES)** can palliate patients with prostate cancer and can alter its natural history, and sterol-binding receptors on the surface of tumor cells facilitate the effects of physiologic doses of sterols on breast cancer cells. Estrogen and progesterone receptors are present in breast cancer cells, and estrogen receptors have also been identified in adenocarcinoma of the ovary, endometrium, and fallopian tube, and in malignant melanoma. Prostate cancer cells have both estrogen and testosterone receptors. Acute lymphoblastic leukemia **(ALL)** cells and chronic lymphatic leukemia **(CLL)** cells have glucocorticoid receptors. The presence of receptors allows the use of hormones (eg, corticosteroids in ALL and CLL; DES, megestrol acetate, tamoxifen, and fluoxymesterone in disseminated breast cancer; and megestrol acetate and DES in prostate cancer).

Management of Adverse Effects of Therapy

Cytopenias (anemia, leukopenia, and thrombocytopenia) may develop during the course of cancer therapy. Transfusion of packed RBCs should be used to maintain a Hct at 30% to allow for adequate tissue oxygenation. Platelet transfusions should be given when the platelet count is $< 20,000/\mu L$ or if the platelet count is $< 50,000/\mu L$ and there is evidence of bleeding or petechiae. The platelet packs should be freshly pooled and given rapidly, as the number of viable platelets will decrease if given slowly or left sitting on the shelf. The $t_{1/2}$ of transfused random platelets is 5 to 6 days. Antibodies to platelets rarely develop; however, when they do, HLA-matched platelets are an option. Patients treated either with chemotherapy or radiation therapy for lymphomas or solid tumors may develop profound neutropenia (< 500 granulocytes); however, it usually lasts only 1 wk. The value of treatment with WBC transfusions is questionable, except in patients with acute nonlymphoblastic leukemias who have an infection.

Patients who receive systemic chemotherapy or extensive radiotherapy may develop leukopenia and granulocytopenia (see Ch. 100). When granulocyte counts fall to $< 1000/\mu L$, patients are at increased risk for infections. *Fever > 38 C (100.4 F) in a granulocytopenic patient must be treated as an emergency*. Patients should be hospitalized and started on broad-spectrum antibiotics after cultures of the blood, sputum, urine, and any suspicious skin lesions are obtained. If diffuse pulmonary infiltrates are present, the physician must include *Pneumocystis carinii* pneumonia in the differential diagnosis. This is particularly true in patients with leukemia or lymphoma.

The history and physical examination of the patient with granulocytopenia and fever should give particular attention to the rectum, tympanic membranes, and retina. If diffuse pulmonary infiltrates are present, the antibiotic regimen should include trimethoprim/sulfamethoxazole, an aminoglycoside antibiotic, and a cephalosporin. In patients without infiltrates, the initial antibiotic regimen should be an aminoglycoside and a cephalosporin. If fever continues after 24 h, a semisynthetic penicillin (eg, ticarcillin) should be added and, in patients with pulmonary infiltrates, a transbronchial biopsy or open lung biopsy (if thrombocytopenia is present) should be performed. If fever continues unabated at 72 h, amphotericin B should be added. Patients with hairy cell leukemia are at increased risk for atypical mycobacterial infections and in this setting an open lung biopsy with sampling of hilar lymph nodes is necessary.

Other common side effects of drugs and radiotherapy can be prevented or abated with judicious use of antiemetics (eg, metoclopramide, prochlorperazine) or dexametha-

sone. Enteritis from abdominal radiotherapy can be alleviated with antidiarrheals. Mucositis from radiotherapy can preclude substantial oral intake and lead to malnutrition and weight loss. Simple measures (eg, use of analgesics and topical lidocaine before meals, a bland diet without citrus food or juices, and avoidance of temperature extremes) can allow the patient to eat and to maintain weight. If these simple measures fail, enteral alimentation with a flexible plastic tube (Dobhoff) may be considered as long as the small intestine is functionally normal. In case of mucositis and diarrhea or an abnormally functioning bowel, parenteral alimentation may be substituted.

Neoplasms Responsive to Chemotherapy (see TABLE 105–5)

Acute lymphoblastic leukemia (ALL) and **acute nonlymphoblastic leukemias (ANLL)** are potentially curable (see in Ch. 101). **Hodgkin's disease and certain non-Hodgkin's lymphomas** are curable in both children and adults, but precise *pathologic* staging is mandatory (see Ch. 102). **Diffuse large cell lymphoma** (diffuse histiocytic lymphoma **[DHL]**), **Burkitt's lymphoma,** and **lymphoblastic lymphoma** are all curable. Regimens of cyclophosphamide, doxorubicin, vincristine (with or without methotrexate, cytarabine, or bleomycin), yield complete response rates of about 80%; the 5-yr survival rate is 42 to 48%.

Stage III (advanced) testicular carcinoma is curable with a 3-drug regimen of cisplatin, vinblastine, and bleomycin (PVB). Complete remission is attained in > 90% of patients; however, poor prognostic factors include high LDH, endodermal sinus tumors, and bulky retroperitoneal disease. Mediastinal germ-cell tumors are treated with either the PVB regimen or a regimen containing cisplatin, etoposide, and bleomycin (PEB), with radiation therapy and, in some cases, surgery following chemotherapy.

Combined Modality Therapy and Adjuvant Therapy

Tumors cured with combined modality therapy are shown in TABLE 105–6. The adjunctive therapy may be x-ray or drugs. Adjunctive chemotherapy has a definite role in the treatment of patients with **breast cancer** and axillary lymph node involvement; a survival benefit is seen in both pre- and postmenopausal women who receive adequate doses (75%) of adjuvant chemotherapy. Similarly, adjuvant chemotherapy with 5-FU and lomustine improves survival in patients with **gastric cancer**.

Preoperative radiotherapy plays a definite role in treating **advanced-stage bladder cancer**. Use of low dosage radiotherapy to a pelvic portal increases the cure in patients with stage B_2 and C bladder cancer.

Patients with stages II and III mucinous and serous papillary **ovarian carcinoma** can be cured with resection and chemotherapy (see Ch. 173).

Small cell lung cancer was at one time the most aggressive and lethal form of lung cancer; today, small cell lung cancer whose extent is limited (stage III_{MO}) can be cured with drugs. "Standard" regimens include cyclophosphamide, doxorubicin, vincristine, or etoposide; when they are used alone or with radiation therapy, 16 to 20% of patients will achieve long-term cure. Whole brain radiotherapy is necessary for patients with limited small cell lung cancer, to prevent brain relapse.

Squamous cell carcinoma of the rectum has been successfully treated with new protocols including mitomycin, 5-FU, and radiotherapy to a pelvic portal.

Advanced stages III and IV squamous cell carcinoma of the head and neck is potentially curable, as shown in TABLE 105–6. If cure cannot be attained, palliation of symptoms can be readily achieved. The treatment includes high-dose cisplatin and continuous infusion 5-FU. Following 3 courses of cisplatin and 5-FU, radiotherapy may be used or a surgical resection performed; cure is attainable in 20 to 40% of patients.

Finally, surgery, radiotherapy, and chemotherapy play definite roles in treating Wilms' tumor and embryonal rhabdomyosarcomas. **In Wilms' tumor (nephroblastoma),**

TABLE 105–6. FIVE–YEAR DISEASE–FREE SURVIVAL RATES FOR CANCERS TREATED WITH COMBINED THERAPIES

Therapies	*Site*	*Stage*	*5-yr Disease-free Survival*
Surgery and radiotherapy	Testis (seminoma)	I	94
	Endometrium	II	62
	Bladder	B_2 + C	54
	Oral cavity	III	36
	Hypopharynx	II + III	33
	Lung	III_{MO} Pancoast	32
Surgery and chemotherapy	Breast	II	62
	Stomach		54
	Prostate	C	50–68
	Ovary (carcinoma)	III	28–40
Radiotherapy and chemotherapy	CNS (medulloblastoma)		71–80
	Ewing's sarcoma	All stages	70
	Rectum (squamous cell carcinoma)		40
	Lung (small cell cancer)	"Limited"	16–20
Surgery, radiotherapy, and chemotherapy	Wilms' tumor	All stages	80
	Embryonal rhabdomyosarcoma	All stages	80
	Lung	III_{MO} Pancoast	32
	Oral cavity, hypopharynx	III + IV	20–40

a childhood renal cancer, the goal of surgery is to remove the primary tumor even if distant metastases are present. During surgery, care must be taken to avoid rupture of the tumor and to see that the primary is removed with a long segment of ureter. Retroperitoneal lymph nodes should be sampled and the contralateral kidney inspected. Chemotherapy is initiated at surgery with dactinomycin daily for 6 days and vincristine weekly for 12 wk once normal GI motility resumes. Dactinomycin therapy is continued q 6 to 8 wk/24 mo. Radiation therapy is administered to an abdominal portal or to the flank; the dosage is 2400 to 2600 rads/2½ to 3 wk. Areas of gross residual disease can be boosted with additional local radiotherapy.

Neoplasms for which Conventional Drugs and Radiotherapy Have No Proven Benefit

To date, no evidence suggests that chemotherapy alone or with radiotherapy prolongs the survival of patients with non–small cell lung cancer, esophageal, gastric, or pancreatic cancer, cancer of the colon, carcinoma of the small intestine, soft tissue sarcomas, primary or metastatic brain tumors, or malignant melanoma. However, radiotherapy is an effective form of *palliation* for painful bone metastases, brain metastases, or retroperitoneal masses for any cancer.

Newer Methods Currently Under Investigation

Hyperthermia: Cancer cells are susceptible to heat at a temperature of 41 C (105.8 F); normal body cells are not. Clinical trials use regional and whole body hyperthermia.

Neutron beam radiotherapy, which does not require O_2 to achieve its effect, can kill many hypoxic or anoxic cells. There is a therapeutic advantage with neutron and conventional photon radiotherapy in advanced stage carcinoma of the cervix and in squamous cell carcinoma of the head and neck.

Hydrazine sulfate may play a role in decreasing the anorexia associated with cancer; however, further testing is required.

Interferons (biologic-response modifiers): *Biologic proteins synthesized by leukocytes when invaded by viruses.* These proteins play important roles in the immune response. Interferons may be subclassified as α (leukocyte) interferon, β (fibroblast) interferon, and γ (lymphocyte) interferon. Their roles are under investigation; however, activity has been observed in therapy of breast cancer, myeloma, the non-Hodgkin's lymphomas, hairy cell leukemia, and renal cell carcinoma. **Toxicities** include nausea, alopecia, leukopenia, chills, fever, and myalgias.

§10. MUSCULOSKELETAL AND CONNECTIVE TISSUE DISORDERS

---

106. INTRODUCTION

In less than 2 generations the field of arthritis, rheumatic disorders, and connective tissue diseases has reached maturity. The 1940 7th Edition of THE MERCK MANUAL contained 2 categories of the most common types of arthritis: atrophic or inflammatory (later called rheumatoid arthritis **[RA]**), and hypertrophic arthritis or degenerative joint disease, which became known as osteoarthritis **(OA).** The 7th Edition also discussed other entities such as gout and gonorrheal arthritis. In this 15th Edition the specifically identifiable conditions exceed 100, including recently recognized ones such as Lyme disease, eosinophilic fasciitis **(EF),** polymyalgia rheumatica, and Kawasaki disease.

Increasingly effective drugs have been introduced. Fifty years ago, colchicine for gouty arthritis and salicylates for arthritis generally completed the list of available drugs except for 3 minor agents discussed below. In the late 1940s, corticosteroids and probenecid were discovered. Cortisone was initially recommended for management of RA, while probenecid, designed to inhibit penicillin excretion during its use in infectious diseases, was serendipitously found to have excellent uricosuric properties, highly valuable in treating primary and secondary intercritical (*between attacks*) gout. Later, indomethacin emerged as an improved aspirin substitute, a nonsteroidal anti-inflammatory drug **(NSAID),** soon to be followed by ibuprofen, naproxen, tolmetin, fenoprofen, sulindac, meclofenamate, and piroxicam, each selectively helpful for RA, OA, and nonspecific symptoms associated with musculoskeletal disorders.

Meanwhile, 3 agents from the 1930s were rediscovered and reintroduced into clinical practice. Gold salts, which had been promoted in Europe but not in the USA, found new friends on both continents, especially now that they can be taken orally. Bee or snake venom was supplanted, in the 1970s, by the venom of the fiery ant. And chloroquine and hydroxychloroquine were used by some rheumatologists to manage both systemic lupus erythematosus **(SLE)** and RA.

During the past 20 yr, corticosteroids have lost favor in treating RA, except for intra-articular injection. However, relatively large doses of corticosteroids have been found to be highly effective for fulminating symptoms of acute dermatomyositis, SLE, progressive systemic sclerosis, periarteritis nodosa, polymyalgia rheumatica, EF, and other related conditions. Furthermore, as other unusual connective tissue diseases became recognized, so were a number of associated, probably pathogenically significant, immunologic features. Treatment with immunosuppressive or cytotoxic drugs followed; eg, cyclophosphamide, azathioprine, methotrexate, and D-penicillamine. Methotrexate also was found to be especially helpful in certain patients with refractory psoriatic arthritis, Reiter's syndrome, and RA. Recently, levamisole has been promoted, especially in RA, because of its immunostimulating (rather than immunosuppressive) property.

A xanthine oxidase inhibitor, allopurinol, has been effective in treating intercritical gout, while patients with Paget's disease respond selectively to calcitonin, plicamycin (mithramycin), or diphosphonates. Other treatment modalities, although nonspecific, have emerged for Sjögren's, Felty's, and Reiter's syndromes, as well as sarcoidosis, hemochromatosis, ochronosis, and Lyme disease.

Managing joint disease, regardless of diagnosis, usually involves specific or nonspecific drugs plus medical-surgical procedures that alleviate in varying degrees joint, tendon, and muscle distress. These procedures include rest, heat, cold, splinting, exercise, elastic supports, massage, hydrotherapy, canes, crutches, walkers, ultrasound, traction, transcutaneous electrical nerve stimulation (TENS), biofeedback, psychotherapy, acupuncture, and reconstructive orthopedic surgery, particularly of the hips and knees but also of other large and small joints.

Much is yet to be learned and better therapies are needed, but the advances of the past 40 yr are impressive and warrant optimism for continuing growth and success.

107. APPROACH TO THE PATIENT WITH JOINT DISEASE

A complete history and physical examination are important because joint symptoms may be part of a systemic disease. Laboratory and x-ray data are usually of only supplementary help. Even mildly inflammatory or noninflammatory arthritis may be the first indication of SLE, hypertrophic pulmonary osteoarthropathy due to bronchogenic carcinoma, or a metabolic disease such as hemochromatosis. Conditions easily misinterpreted as arthritis by the patient include phlebitis, arteriosclerosis obliterans, cellulitis, edema, neuropathy, vascular compression syndromes, the stiffness of Parkinson's disease, periarticular stress fractures, myositis, and fibromyositis.

Extra-articular findings can be significant (eg, tophi in gout, nodules in RA, and pustular rash in gonococcemia). Coexisting periarticular disease also may facilitate diagnosis. For example, tendinitis commonly coexists with gonococcal arthritis, RA, and other systemic diseases; popliteal cysts due to knee arthritis cause local popliteal pain, venous compression, or rupture into the calf; prominent tenderness of bones adjacent to joints and joint effusions occur in sickle cell disease and hypertrophic pulmonary osteoarthropathy.

TABLE 107–1 contains a classification of rheumatic diseases. Many times, the arthritis is transient and does not fulfill the criteria for any of these diseases, or it resolves without diagnosis. A final diagnosis should not be forced. A tentative diagnosis is made for treatment, with other possibilities kept in mind. A systemic disease should be considered in all atypical and undiagnosed conditions.

Certain problems require immediate attention and prompt treatment. Hemorrhagic fluid suggests fracture or malignancy. Intensely inflammatory effusions suggest pyogenic infection requiring immediate antibiotic therapy and aspiration drainage to prevent joint destruction.

Physical Examination of the Musculoskeletal System

A sequence of **inspection, palpation,** and **determination of the range of motion** of each involved joint area is followed. In most cases, this determines the presence of joint disease and establishes whether the joint, the adjacent structures, or both are involved. Involved joints should be compared with their uninvolved opposites or with those of the examiner. Information is recorded objectively and quantitatively; eg, by using a numbered grading system and by measuring the range of motion in degrees.

Joint motion, generally painful in joint disease, may not be in periarticular, bone, or soft tissue disease. **Swelling** is an important finding. All swollen joints should be palpated. The examiner should then ballotte the joint to (1) elicit the presence of fluid; (2) differentiate between simple effusion, synovial thickening, and capsule or bony enlargement; and (3) determine whether the swelling is confined to the joint or is periarticular. Tenderness or swelling at only one joint margin may actually be arising in

TABLE 107–1. CLASSIFICATION OF THE RHEUMATIC DISEASES

I. Diffuse connective tissue diseases
- A. Rheumatoid arthritis
- B. Juvenile arthritis
  - 1. Systemic onset
  - 2. Polyarticular onset
  - 3. Oligarticular onset
- C. Systemic lupus erythematosus
- D. Progressive systemic sclerosis
- E. Polymyositis/dermatomyositis
- F. Necrotizing vasculitis and other vasculopathies
  - 1. Polyarteritis nodosa group (includes hepatitis B-associated arteritis and Churg-Strauss allergic granulomatosis)
  - 2. Hypersensitivity vasculitis (includes Henoch-Schönlein purpura and others)
  - 3. Wegener's granulomatosis
  - 4. Giant cell arteritis
    - a. Temporal arteritis
    - b. Takayasu's arteritis
  - 5. Mucocutaneous lymph node syndrome (Kawasaki's disease)
  - 6. Behçet's syndrome
- G. Sjögren's syndrome
- H. Overlap syndromes (includes mixed connective tissue disease)
- I. Others (includes polymyalgia rheumatica, erythema nodosum, relapsing polychondritis, and others)

II. Arthritis associated with spondylitis
- A. Ankylosing spondylitis
- B. Reiter's syndrome
- C. Psoriatic arthritis
- D. Arthritis associated with chronic inflammatory bowel disease

III. Degenerative joint disease (osteoarthritis, osteoarthrosis)
- A. Primary (includes erosive osteoarthritis)
- B. Secondary

IV. Arthritis, tenosynovitis, and bursitis associated with infectious agents
- A. Direct
  - 1. Bacterial
    - a. Gram-positive cocci (staphylococcus and others)
    - b. Gram-negative cocci (gonococcus and others)
    - c. Gram-positive rods
    - d. Mycobacteria
    - e. Treponemes
    - f. Others
  - 2. Viral
  - 3. Fungal
  - 4. Parasitic
  - 5. Unknown, suspected (Whipple's disease)
- B. Indirect (reactive)
  - 1. Bacterial (includes acute rheumatic fever, intestinal bypass, postdysenteric—shigella, yersinia, and others)
  - 2. Viral (hepatitis B)

(Continued)

(Modified from the American Rheumatism Association Classification, in *Primer on the Rheumatic Diseases*, ed. 8, 1983, edited by G. P. Rodnan and H. R. Schumacher. Copyright 1983 by the Arthritis Foundation. Used by permission of the Arthritis Foundation.)

TABLE 107–1. CLASSIFICATION OF THE RHEUMATIC DISEASES *(Cont'd)*

V. Metabolic and endocrine diseases with rheumatic states
- A. Crystal-induced conditions
  1. Monosodium urate (gout)
  2. Calcium pyrophosphate dihydrate (pseudogout, chondrocalcinosis)
  3. Hydroxyapatite
- B. Biochemical abnormalities
  1. Amyloidosis
  2. Vitamin C deficiency (scurvy)
  3. Specific enzyme deficiency states (includes Fabry's, alkaptonuria, Lesch-Nyhan, and others)
  4. Hyperlipidemias (types II, IIa, IV)
  5. Mucopolysaccharides
  6. Hemoglobinopathies (HbS disease and others)
  7. True connective tissue disorders (Ehlers-Danlos, Marfan, pseudoxanthoma elasticum, and others)
  8. Others
- C. Endocrine diseases
  1. Diabetes mellitus
  2. Acromegaly
  3. Hyperparathyroidism
  4. Thyroid disease (hyperthyroidism, hypothyroidism)
- D. Immunodeficiency diseases
- E. Other hereditary disorders
  1. Arthrogryposis multiplex congenita
  2. Hypermobility syndromes
  3. Myositis ossificans progressiva

VI. Neoplasms
- A. Primary
- B. Metastatic

VII. Neuropathic disorders
- A. Charcot's joints
- B. Compression neuropathies
  1. Peripheal entrapment (carpal tunnel syndrome and others)
  2. Radiculopathy
  3. Spinal stenosis
- C. Reflex sympathetic dystrophy
- D. Others

VIII. Bone and cartilage disorders associated with articular manifestations
- A. Osteoporosis
  1. Generalized
  2. Localized (regional)
- B. Osteomalacia
- C. Hypertrophic osteoarthropathy
- D. Diffuse idiopathic skeletal hyperostosis (includes ankylosing vertebral hyperostosis)
- E. Osteitis
  1. Generalized (osteitis deformans—Paget's disease of bone)
  2. Localized (osteitis condensans ilii; osteitis pubis)
- F. Avascular necrosis
- G. Osteochondritis (Legg-Calvé-Perthes disease, Scheuermann's disease)
- H. Congenital dysplasia of the hip
- I. Slipped capital femoral epiphysis
- K. Osteolysis and chondrolysis

(Continued)

TABLE 107–1. CLASSIFICATION OF THE RHEUMATIC DISEASES *(Cont'd)*

IX. Nonarticular rheumatism
- A. Myofascial pain syndromes
  - 1. Generalized (fibrositis, fibromyalgia)
  - 2. Regional
- B. Low back pain and intervertebral disk disorders
- C. Tendinitis (tenosynovitis) and/or bursitis
  - 1. Subacromial/subdeltoid bursitis
  - 2. Bicipital tendinitis, tenosynovitis
  - 3. Olecranon bursitis
  - 4. Epicondylitis, medial or lateral humeral
  - 5. DeQuervain's tenosynovitis
  - 6. Adhesive capsulitis of the shoulder (frozen shoulder)
  - 7. Trigger finger
- D. Ganglion cysts
- E. Fasciitis
- F. Chronic ligament and muscle strain
- G. Vasomotor disorders
  - 1. Erythromelalgia
  - 2. Raynaud's disease or phenomenon
- H. Miscellaneous pain syndromes (includes weather sensitivity, psychogenic rheumatism)

X. Miscellaneous disorders
- A. Disorders frequently associated with arthritis
  - 1. Trauma (the result of direct trauma)
  - 2. Lyme disease
  - 3. Pancreatic disease
  - 4. Sarcoidosis
  - 5. Palindromic rheumatism
  - 6. Intermittent hydrarthrosis
  - 7. Villonodular synovitis
  - 8. Hemophilia
- B. Other conditions
  - 1. Internal derangement of joints (includes chondromalacia patellae, loose bodies)
  - 2. Familial Mediterranean fever
  - 3. Eosinophilic fasciitis
  - 4. Chronic active hepatitis
  - 5. Other drug-induced rheumatic syndromes

adjacent ligaments, tendons, or bursae; findings from several approaches to the joint substantiate articular involvement. **Increased heat** over the joint should be noted and carefully localized. **Crepitus** may arise from intra-articular structures or from tendons; the crepitus-producing motions should be determined. At the knee, for example, crepitus may arise from patellofemoral "grinding" or from femorotibial motion. **Monarthritis** always suggests infection, crystal-induced arthritis, trauma, or tumor.

Small joints, such as the acromioclavicular near the shoulder, the tibiofibular at the knee, and the radioulnar at the elbow can be the source of pain initially believed to be in the major joint.

The hand: The main differential features of **osteoarthritis** and **rheumatoid arthritis** are outlined in TABLE 107–2. Subluxations producing "swan neck" or "boutonnière" deformities occur in more chronic RA. In **psoriatic arthritis,** the distal interphalangeal joints **(DIP)** are commonly affected, psoriasis often is evident around the adjacent nail, and other joint involvement is more asymmetric than in RA. In **Reiter's syndrome,** synovial, periarticular, and periosteal changes can be present in a few DIP, proximal interphalangeal **(PIP),** or metacarpophalangeal **(MCP)** joints, and there is asymmetric

TABLE 107–2. THE HAND IN RHEUMATOID ARTHRITIS AND IN OSTEOARTHRITIS

Criteria	*Rheumatoid Arthritis*	*Osteoarthritis*
Character of swelling	Synovial, capsular, "soft tissue;" bony only in late stages	Bony with irregular spurs; occasional soft cysts
Tenderness................	Usual	None or mild except during occasional acute onset
Distal interphalangeal (DIP) involvement..............	Not usual, except thumb	Characteristic
Proximal interphalangeal (PIP) involvement..............	Characteristic	Frequent
Metacarpophalangeal (MCP) involvement..............	Characteristic	Rare, except thumb
Wrist involvement...........	Usual or common	Rare, except base of thumb

(Modified from P. J. Bilka, *Bulletin on the Rheumatic Diseases*, Vol. 20, pp. 596–599, March 1970. Copyright 1970 by The Arthritis Foundation. Used with permission of The Arthritis Foundation and the author.)

finger joint involvement. Asymmetric and DIP joint involvement also occurs in chronic **gout,** in which irregular peri- or extra-articular tophaceous deposits occur, some of which can be seen under the skin as cream-colored spots. Changes in the hand are more generalized in the **shoulder-hand syndrome** (reflex dystrophy), with diffuse edema and mottled, mildly cyanotic skin. In **progressive systemic sclerosis,** the skin is thickened, flexion contractures often develop, and the history is positive for Raynaud's phenomenon. Findings in **hypertrophic pulmonary osteoarthropathy** include clubbing of the fingertips and bony tenderness of the distal radius and ulna due to underlying periostitis. Joint synovitis similar to that seen in RA occurs in **SLE** and, less often, in **dermatomyositis,** though arthralgias and sore painful hands lacking demonstrable pathologic joint changes are more typical of both these disorders. Finger deformities resembling RA can occur in SLE but are due to soft tissue disease, not advanced erosive arthritis. Raynaud's phenomenon can be present in SLE, and erythema may be found over the extensor joint surfaces in dermatomyositis.

The elbow: Synovial swelling and thickening due to joint disease is sought in the lateral area between the radial head and olecranon, where it produces a bulge. Fluid or thickening in the olecranon bursa, rheumatoid nodules, and epitrochlear nodes should also be sought. Full 180° extension of the joint should be attempted. Though full extension is possible with nonarthritic or extra-articular lesions, its loss is an early change in **arthritis.** In **tennis elbow,** sharply localized pain is elicited by firm pressure over the lateral epicondyle.

The shoulder: Limitation of motion, weakness, pain, and disturbed mobility can be screened for by having the patient raise both arms above his head. Muscle atrophy and neurologic changes should be sought. Though swelling is not common, a bulge in the anterior or lateral superior area of the shoulder is occasionally present in **RA** as a result of forward dissection of glenohumeral synovitis. Careful palpation of the relaxed shoulder may allow one to identify inflammation of bursae or tendons, a common condition occurring primarily in the subacromial area or the long head of the biceps tendon. Exact localization may permit aspiration and injection of a corticosteroid-lidocaine solution for relief of acute **tendinitis** and confirmation of the diagnosis.

The foot and ankle: Since weight-bearing may elucidate certain abnormalities, part of the examination should be performed with the patient standing. In the normal ankle joint, 15° dorsiflexion and 40° plantar flexion are possible. Swelling just below and in front of the malleoli is characteristic of synovial or intra-articular disease. In **RA,** palpation of tender, rubbery swelling below, in front of, and behind the malleoli demonstrates synovitis of the ankle joint. Ankle edema, which is associated with normal ankle joint subastragalar motion, can be differentiated from true joint swelling by its diffuse, superficial, pitting, and nontender character. Metatarsophalangeal joints are very commonly swollen and tender in RA. Interphalangeal synovitis, not common in the feet in RA, may indicate **Reiter's syndrome, psoriatic arthritis,** or **gout.** In **gout,** the first metatarsophalangeal or bunion joint is most commonly affected, but the mid tarsal or ankle areas can also be involved. Diffuse erythema is striking in an acute attack of gout.

The knee: Such gross deformities as swelling (eg, popliteal cysts), quadriceps muscle atrophy, and joint instability may be more obvious when the patient stands and walks. Careful palpation of the knee, especially noting the presence of joint fluid, synovial thickening, and local tenderness, helps detect arthritis. Tender extra-articular bursae and true intra-articular disturbances should be differentiated.

Detection of small knee effusions is a common problem in joint evaluation and is best done using the "bulge sign." The knee is extended and the leg is slightly externally rotated while the patient is supine with muscles relaxed. The medial aspect of the knee is stroked to express any fluid away from this area. The examiner places one hand on the suprapatellar pouch and then strokes or presses gently on the lateral aspect of the knee, creating a fluid wave or bulge visible medially.

Full 180° extension of the knee should be attempted to detect knee flexion contractures. With **meniscus tears** or **collateral ligament injuries,** forceful lateral or medial bending while extending the leg produces pain by compressing the meniscus and simultaneously stretching the opposite collateral ligament. The joint line can be located by medial and lateral palpation while slowly flexing and extending the knee. A displaced meniscus is painful on firm pressure; a collateral ligament injury is tender in a longitudinal direction. The intactness of the cruciate ligaments can be determined by grasping the leg with the knee flexed at 90° (best done with the patient sitting on a table edge with his legs dangling) and estimating the amount of posterior-anterior movement (which should be minimal). The patella should be tested for free, painless motion. To gauge excess mobility of the knee, especially lateral instability, the thigh is firmly fixed and an attempt is made to rock the relaxed, almost extended, knee from side to side.

The hip: A limp is common in patients with significant hip **arthritis.** It may be due to pain, shortening of the leg, flexion contracture, or muscle weakness. Loss of internal rotation, flexion, extension, or abduction can usually be demonstrated. One hand should be placed on the patient's iliac crest to detect pelvic movement that might be mistaken for hip movement. Flexion contracture can be identified by attempting extension of the leg with the opposite hip maximally flexed to stabilize the pelvis. Tenderness over the femoral greater trochanter indicates local **bursitis** rather than arthritis.

The vertebral column: Cervical and lumbar motion should be measured. Inability to reverse the normal lumbar lordosis on flexion occurs in **degenerative arthritis.** Limited lumbar flexion is characteristic of **ankylosing spondylitis.** Neck motion can be limited by either degenerative arthritis or ankylosing spondylitis. The effect of movement on pain should be noted. Pain and limitation can be due to soft tissue disease as well as to arthritis. Palpation and firm percussion over each vertebra and sacroiliac joint may elicit superficial or deep bone tenderness that should be distinguished from muscle spasm. Localized bone pain suggests such disorders as **osteomyelitis, leukemia, primary or metastatic cancer, compression fracture,** or **herniated disk.** The examiner should note

psychogenic ("touch-me-not") reactions and muscular "trigger points." Chest expansion should be measured, as it is typically impaired in **ankylosing spondylitis.**

Diagnostic Studies

Laboratory studies are useful in diagnosing the specific type of arthritis present. Specific tests are discussed in the chapters for each disease. An elevated Westergren sedimentation rate suggests inflammatory disease. Serum uric acid levels are elevated by low doses of aspirin, by diuretics, other drugs, diet, or alcohol, which lower urate clearance, and in gout. Latex fixation tests for rheumatoid factor are often highly positive in RA but may also be positive in cirrhosis, sarcoidosis, SBE, TB, and other diseases. Antinuclear factors may be positive in RA, Sjögren's syndrome, progressive systemic sclerosis, SLE, and other diseases. Serum CK and AST (SGOT) are elevated in peripheral muscle disease, including certain forms of muscular dystrophy, crush injury, and in dermatomyositis. CK can be elevated in hypothyroidism.

X-rays are important in the initial evaluation of relatively localized unexplained complaints to detect possible primary or metastatic tumors, osteomyelitis, bone infarctions, periarticular calcifications, or other changes in deep structures that may escape physical examination. X-rays also are especially useful in examination of the spine. CT scans, MRI, and tomograms can help define puzzling lesions.

Other studies useful in selected patients include needle or surgical synovial biopsy, ultrasound, arthroscopy, arthrography, bone and marrow scans, electromyography, nerve conduction times, thermography, and muscle or bone biopsy. Evaluation of synovial fluid is discussed below.

Differentiating Inflammatory and Noninflammatory Joint Disease

Inflammatory and noninflammatory processes must be differentiated once joint involvement has been established. Among the typical local signs of inflammation, increased heat and erythema are most helpful in this differentiation. Erythema should not be expected over the chronically inflamed joints in RA. Fever and an elevated ESR tend to occur with severe inflammatory arthritis, but may also be due to an inflammatory process elsewhere in the body. Soft tissue swelling tends to favor an inflammatory process, but aspiration of any effusion is essential to determine its nature. Preparation for handling the fluid obtained is critical so that the studies most pertinent for each patient can be properly performed. Not all tests need to be done on each fluid.

Synovial fluid measurements that allow classification are shown in TABLE 107–3. These differentiate most effusions as normal, "noninflammatory," inflammatory, and septic. Effusions can also be hemorrhagic. So-called "noninflammatory" fluids actually are mildly inflammatory but tend to suggest diseases with less inflammatory mechanisms. Each type of effusion suggests certain joint diseases, as shown in TABLE 107–4.

Microscopic examination of a wet synovial fluid smear for crystals (even a few drops of fluid or washings from a joint can be used for culture or examination of crystals), using polarized light, is essential for definitive diagnosis of gout. By placing an inexpensive polarizer over the light source and another between the specimen and the examiner's eye, crystals with a shiny white birefringence will be visible. Compensated polarized light is provided by inserting a first-order red plate, as in commercially available microscopes. One can also reproduce the effects of a compensator by placing 2 strips of clear adhesive tape on a glass slide and placing this slide over the lower polarizer. Sodium urate crystals then appear strongly *negatively* birefringent; ie, yellow parallel to the axis of slow vibration marked on the compensator (or the long axis of the slide). Calcium pyrophosphate dihydrate **(CPPD)** crystals appear weakly *positively* birefringent; ie, blue in the direction that urates are yellow. Sodium urate crystals tend to be needle- or rod-shaped; CPPD crystals are rhomboid or rod-shaped. Calcium oxalate crystals are bipyramidal and birefringent in some patients with renal failure. Cholesterol, recently injected intra-articular corticosteroids, oxalate or other anticoagulants, fibrils from lens paper, and dirt also appear crystalline or as birefringent objects and

TABLE 107–3. CLASSIFICATION OF SYNOVIAL EFFUSIONS

	Normal	*Noninflammatory*	*Inflammatory*	*Septic*
Gross examination:				
Viscosity	High	High	Low	Variable
Color	Colorless	Yellow	Yellow	Variable
Clarity*	Transparent	Transparent	Translucent	Opaque
Routine laboratory examination:				
WBC**	< 200/μL	200 to 2,000/μL	2,000 to 100,000/μL	> 100,000/μL
PMNs**	< 25%	< 25%	> 50%	> 75%
Culture	Negative	Negative	Negative	Often positive
Glucose (AM fasting)	≅ to simultaneously drawn blood	≅ to simultaneously drawn blood	< 50 mg/dL lower than simultaneously drawn blood	> 50 mg/dL lower than simultaneously drawn blood

* Extremely cloudy or opaque effusions can also be produced by crystals, tissue fragments, amyloid, or "rice bodies," as well as by leukocytes.

** WBC and % PMNs (polymorphonuclear leukocytes) in septic arthritis will be less if organism is less virulent or partially treated.

(Modified from R. A. Gatter and D. J. McCarty, "Synovianalysis," in *Rheumatism*, Vol. 20, pp. 2–6, Jan. 1964. Used with permission.)

TABLE 107–4. DIFFERENTIAL DIAGNOSIS BASED ON SYNOVIAL FLUID CLASSIFICATION (PARTIAL LISTING)

<table>
<tr><th>Noninflammatory</th><th>Inflammatory</th><th>Septic</th><th>Hemorrhagic</th></tr>
<tr><td>Osteoarthritis
Trauma
Osteochondritis dissecans
Neurogenic (neuropathic) arthropathy
Sickle cell disease
Osteochondromatosis
Subsiding or early inflammation
Hypertrophic pulmonary osteoarthropathy
Ehlers-Danlos syndrome
Amyloidosis
Metabolic diseases causing osteoarthritis</td><td>Rheumatoid disease
Reiter's syndrome
Psoriatic arthritis
Ankylosing spondylitis
Ulcerative colitis
Regional enteritis
Acute crystal synovitis (gout and pseudogout)
Partially treated or less virulent bacterial infections</td><td rowspan="2">Bacterial infections</td><td rowspan="2">Trauma with or without fracture
Pigmented villonodular synovitis
Neurogenic (neuropathic) arthropathy
Hemangioma
Hemophilia
Anticoagulant treatment
Scurvy
Thrombocytopenia
Tumor</td></tr>
<tr><td colspan="2">Systemic lupus erythematosus
Rheumatic fever
Progressive systemic sclerosis</td></tr>
</table>

(Modified from R. A. Gatter and D. J. McCarty, "Synovianalysis," in *Rheumatism*, Vol. 20, pp. 2–6, Jan. 1964. Used with permission.)

may be confused with the crystals. Clumps of apatite crystals are not birefringent with polarized light but appear as shiny, slightly irregular "coinlike" particles. They can be stained with alizarin red S to confirm that they are calcium-containing.

LE cells formed in vivo, marrow spicules (due to fracture), brown cartilage fragments (due to ochronosis), Gram stains or acid-fast stains showing specific organisms, Congo-red-staining amyloid fragments, sickled erythrocytes (due to sickle-cell hemoglobinopathies), or iron in large mononuclear synovial cells on Prussian blue stain (due to hemochromatosis or villous pigmented synovitis) may also be found in the synovial fluid, yielding a specific diagnosis.

Comparing synovial fluid and serum complement levels may be helpful. The synovial fluid complement tends to be < 30% of the serum complement level in RA, but is often higher in gout, Reiter's syndrome, and infectious arthritis. Synovial fluid complement levels will be low in normal and noninflammatory effusions in which little protein is present. Both serum and synovial fluid complement levels may be low in SLE. **Measurements of rheumatoid factor** in synovial fluid can give misleading false-positive or false-negative results.

---

108. ARTHRITIS; RELATED DISORDERS

RHEUMATOID ARTHRITIS (RA)

(JUVENILE RHEUMATOID ARTHRITIS is discussed in Ch. 197)

A chronic syndrome characterized by nonspecific, usually symmetric inflammation of the peripheral joints, potentially resulting in progressive destruction of articular and periarticular structures; generalized manifestations may also be present.

Etiology and Incidence

Etiology is unknown. The immunologic changes (see also in Ch. 21, AUTOIMMUNE DISORDERS) may be initiated by multiple factors. About 1% of all populations are affected, women 2 to 3 times more commonly than men. Onset may be at any age, but most often occurs between 25 and 50.

Pathology

In chronically affected joints, the normally delicate synovial membrane develops many villous folds and thickens because of increased numbers and size of synovial lining cells and colonization by lymphocytes and plasma cells. The lining cells produce a variety of materials, including collagenase, interleukin-1, and prostaglandins. The colonizing cells, initially perivenular but later forming lymphoid follicles with germinal centers, synthesize rheumatoid factor **(RF)** and other immunoglobulins. Fibrosis and necrosis also are present. These findings are typical but not diagnostic. Hyperplastic synovial tissue (pannus) may erode cartilage, subchondral bone, articular capsule, and ligaments. Polymorphonuclear leukocytes are not prominent in the synovium, but often predominate in the synovial fluid.

The **rheumatoid nodule,** seen in 30 to 40% of patients, usually found subcutaneously at sites subject to trauma, is the most characteristic pathologic lesion. It is a nonspecific necrobiotic granuloma consisting of a central necrotic area surrounded by "palisaded" mononuclear cells with their long axes radiating from the center, all enveloped by lymphocytes and plasma cells. Nodules and **vasculitis** have been found at necropsy in many visceral organs in severe cases of RA, but are clinically significant in only a few cases.

Symptoms and Signs

Onset may be abrupt, with simultaneous inflammation in multiple joints, or (more frequently) insidious, with progressive joint involvement. Tenderness in nearly all "ac-

tive" (inflamed) joints is the most sensitive physical sign. Synovial thickening, the most specific physical finding, eventually occurs in most active joints. Symmetric involvement of small hand joints (especially the proximal interphalangeal and metacarpophalangeal), feet, wrists, elbows, and ankles is typical, but initial manifestations may occur in any joint. Stiffness lasting more than 30 min on arising in the morning or after prolonged inactivity is common; early afternoon fatigue and malaise also occur. Deformities may develop rapidly, particularly flexion contractures. Ulnar deviation of the fingers with slippage of the extensor tendons off the metacarpophalangeal joints is typical. The carpal tunnel syndrome can result from wrist synovitis. Ruptured popliteal cysts can mimic deep venous thrombosis.

Subcutaneous rheumatoid nodules, though not usually an early manifestation, can be a major aid in diagnosis; they should be biopsied to differentiate gouty tophi, amyloid, and other nodules. Visceral nodules, vasculitis causing leg ulcers or mononeuritis multiplex, pleural or pericardial effusions, lymphadenopathy, and Sjögren's syndrome or episcleritis are other extra-articular manifestations. Fever may be present and is usually low-grade, except in the adult-onset **Still's disease,** a seronegative RA-like polyarthritis.

Laboratory and X-ray Findings

A normochromic or slightly hypochromic, normocytic anemia, typical of other chronic diseases, is found in 80% of cases; the Hb is usually > 10 gm/dL, but may rarely be as low as 8 gm/dL. Superimposed iron deficiency or other causes of anemia should be sought if the Hb is < 10 gm/dL. Neutropenia is found in 2% of cases, often with splenomegaly **(Felty's syndrome).** Mild polyclonal hypergammaglobulinemia and thrombocytosis may be present.

The ESR is elevated in 90% of cases. Antibodies to altered γ-globulin, the so-called **rheumatoid factors (RFs),** as detected by agglutination tests (such as the latex fixation test) that show IgM RF are found in about 70% of cases. Though RFs are not specific for RA and are found in many diseases (including granulomatous diseases, chronic liver disease, and subacute bacterial endocarditis), a high RF titer provides helpful confirmation when the typical clinical syndrome is present. The **latex** and **bentonite tube dilution tests,** utilizing human IgG adsorbed to particulate carriers such as latex or bentonite, are less specific but more sensitive than the sensitized sheep cell test using animal (rabbit) IgG. In most laboratories, a latex fixation tube dilution titer of 1:160 is considered the lowest positive value for a diagnosis of RA. A high RF titer suggests a worse prognosis and is often associated with progressive disease, nodules, vasculitis, and pulmonary involvement. The titer can be influenced by treatment or spontaneous improvement and often falls as inflammatory joint activity decreases.

The **synovial fluid,** always abnormal during active joint inflammation, is cloudy and sterile, has reduced viscosity, and usually contains 3000 to 50,000 WBCs/cu mm. Polymorphonuclear cells typically predominate, but more than ½ of the cells may be lymphocytes and other mononuclear cells in very early disease and some other cases. Leukocyte cytoplasmic inclusions may be seen on a wet smear, but are also present in other inflammatory effusions. Synovial fluid complement is often < 30% of the serum level. Crystals are absent, excluding gout and pseudogout.

Radiologically, only soft tissue swelling is seen in the first months of the disease. Subsequently, periarticular osteoporosis, joint space (articular cartilage) narrowing, and marginal erosions may be present. The rate of radiologic deterioration, like the rate of clinical deterioration, is highly variable.

Diagnosis

The American Rheumatism Association has established criteria for the diagnosis of "possible," "probable," "definite," and "classic" RA (see TABLE 108–1). While primarily intended as a communication aid for those in clinical research, these criteria can serve as a guide to clinical diagnosis. Almost any other disease that causes arthritis

TABLE 108–1. DIAGNOSTIC CRITERIA FOR RHEUMATOID ARTHRITIS

A. Classic Rheumatoid Arthritis

This diagnosis requires 7 of the following criteria. In criteria 1 through 5 the joint signs or symptoms must be continuous for at least 6 wk.

1. Morning stiffness.
2. Pain on motion or tenderness in at least 1 joint (observed by a physician).
3. Swelling (soft tissue thickening or fluid, not bony overgrowth alone) in at least 1 joint (observed by a physician).
4. Swelling (observed by a physician) of at least 1 other joint (any interval free of joint symptoms between the 2 joint involvements may not be more than 3 mo).
5. Symmetric joint swelling (observed by a physician) with simultaneous involvement of the same joint on both sides of the body (bilateral involvement of proximal interphalangeal, metacarpophalangeal, or metatarsophalangeal joints is acceptable without absolute symmetry). Terminal phalangeal joint involvement will not satisfy this criterion.
6. Subcutaneous nodules (observed by a physician) over bony prominences, on extensor surfaces, or in juxta-articular regions.
7. X-ray changes typical of rheumatoid arthritis (which must include at least bony decalcification localized to or greatest around the involved joints and not just degenerative changes). Degenerative changes do not exclude patients from any group classified as rheumatoid arthritis.
8. Positive agglutination test—demonstration of the rheumatoid factor by any method which, in 2 laboratories, has been positive in not > 5% of normal controls.
9. Poor mucin precipitate from synovial fluid (with shreds and cloudy solution). An inflammatory synovial effusion with > 2000 WBC/μL and no crystals can be substituted for this criterion.
10. Characteristic histologic changes in synovial membrane with 3 or more of the following: marked villous hypertrophy; proliferation of superficial synovial cells; marked infiltration of chronic inflammatory cells (lymphocytes or plasma cells predominating), with tendency to form "lymphoid nodules"; deposition of compact fibrin either on surface or interstitially; foci of cell necrosis.
11. Characteristic histologic changes in nodules showing granulomatous foci with central zones of cell necrosis, surrounded by a palisade of proliferated mononuclear cells, peripheral fibrosis, and chronic inflammatory cell infiltration.

B. Definite Rheumatoid Arthritis

This diagnosis requires 5 of the above criteria. In criteria 1 through 5 the joint signs or symptoms must be continuous for at least 6 wk.

C. Probable Rheumatoid Arthritis

This diagnosis requires 3 of the above criteria. In at least 1 of criteria 1 through 5 the joint signs or symptoms must be continuous for at least 6 wk.

D. Possible Rheumatoid Arthritis

This diagnosis requires 2 of the following criteria and total duration of joint symptoms must be at least 3 wk.

1. Morning stiffness.
2. Tenderness or pain on motion (observed by a physician) with history of recurrence or persistence for 3 wk.
3. History or observation of joint swelling.
4. Subcutaneous nodules (observed by a physician).
5. Elevated ESR or C-reactive protein.
6. Iritis (of dubious value as a criterion except in the case of juvenile rheumatoid arthritis).

(Modified from Criteria for the Classification of Rheumatoid Arthritis, in *Primer on the Rheumatic Diseases,* ed. 8, 1983, editied by G. P. Rodnan and H. R. Schumacher. Copyright 1983 by the Arthritis Foundation. Used by permission of the Arthritis Foundation.)

must be ruled out by exclusion. These exclusions should be considered relative, since 2 diseases causing arthritis occasionally coexist.

RA shares many features of other collagen vascular diseases, particularly SLE, but the latter usually can be distinguished by the characteristic skin lesions on light-exposed areas, temporal-frontal hair loss, oral and nasal mucosal lesions, joint fluid with a WBC count often < 2000/μL (predominantly mononuclear cells), positive antibodies to double-stranded DNA, renal disease, and low serum complement. LE cells, positive antinuclear factors, and visceral organ involvement are found in about 5% of otherwise typical RA patients, giving rise to the term "overlap syndrome." Some of these cases may represent severe RA; others have associated SLE or other collagen disease. Polyarteritis, progressive systemic sclerosis, and dermato(poly)myositis may have features that resemble RA.

Sarcoidosis, amyloidosis, Whipple's disease, and other systemic diseases may involve joints; biopsy of appropriate tissues often differentiates these conditions. **Acute rheumatic fever** is differentiated by a migratory pattern of joint involvement and evidence of antecedent streptococcal infection (culture or changing antistreptolysin-O **[ASO]** titer). Changing cardiac murmurs, chorea, and erythema marginatum are much less common in adults than in children. Infectious arthritis usually is monarticular or asymmetric. Diagnosis depends on identification of the causative agent. *Infection can be superimposed on a joint affected by RA.* **Gonococcal arthritis** usually presents as a migratory arthritis involving tendons around the wrist and ankle and finally settling in 1 or 2 joints. **Lyme disease** can occur without the classical history of tick bite and rash; it can be screened for serologically (see below). **Reiter's syndrome** is characterized by asymmetric involvement of the heel, spine, sacroiliac joint, and large joints of the leg and by urethritis, conjunctivitis, iritis, painless buccal ulcers, and balanitis circinata or keratodermia blennorrhagica on the soles and elsewhere. Serum and joint fluid complement levels are elevated. **Psoriatic arthritis** tends to be asymmetric and is not usually associated with rheumatoid factor, but differentiation may be difficult in the absence of characteristic nail or skin lesions. **Ankylosing spondylitis** may be differentiated by its predilection for males, spinal and axial distribution of joint involvement, absence of subcutaneous nodules, and negative rheumatoid factor test. **Gout** may be mono- or polyarticular with complete recovery between acute attacks early in the disease. Chronic gout may mimic RA. Typical negatively birefringent sodium urate crystals are present in the synovial effusion and can be seen by compensated polarized light. Hyperuricemia does not establish gout as the diagnosis. Response to colchicine is highly suggestive of gout, but other diseases may also subside with colchicine, or spontaneously. **Chondrocalcinosis** may produce mono- or polyarticular acute or chronic arthritis, but the presence of weakly positively birefringent calcium pyrophosphate dihydrate crystals in joint fluid and x-ray evidence of articular cartilage calcification differentiate this condition. **Osteoarthritis (OA)** often involves the proximal and distal interphalangeal joints, first carpometacarpal and first metatarsophalangeal joints, knees, and spine. Symmetry of involvement, prominent joint swelling with signs of inflammation, joint instability, and subchondral erosions on x-ray may prove confusing; the absence of rheumatoid factor, rheumatoid nodules, and systemic involvement, and the characteristic OA pattern of joint involvement permit differentiation from RA.

Treatment

As many as 75% of patients improve with conservative treatment during the first year of disease; 5 to 10% are eventually disabled despite full treatment.

Rest and nutrition: Complete bed rest is occasionally indicated for a short period during the most active painful stage of severe disease. Although symptoms and signs often subside with little other treatment, they will probably recur unless anti-inflammatory drugs are given. In less severe cases, regular rest periods should be prescribed and carefully explained. Splints provide local joint rest. An ordinary nutritious diet is

generally sufficient. Rare patients have food-associated exacerbations. Fish oil currently is under investigation and may provide amelioration of symptoms. Food and diet quackery is common and should be discouraged.

Nonsteroidal anti-inflammatory drugs (NSAIDs). See also Ch. 282. Physiologic mechanisms of NSAIDs and prostaglandins are discussed in Ch. 284; NSAID renal toxicity is discussed in Ch. 152.

Salicylates are relatively safe, inexpensive, analgesic, and anti-inflammatory, and are the cornerstone of drug therapy in RA. Aspirin (acetylsalicylic acid) is prescribed *in writing.* Dosage is begun with 0.6 to 1.0 gm (2 to 3 five-grain tablets) qid with meals and a bedtime snack. Dosage is then adjusted upward until achieving a maximally effective or mildly toxic dose (eg, tinnitus, diminished hearing). The final dose may vary from 3 to 7.5 gm (about 10 to 25 five-grain tablets). The average dose is 4.5 gm (14 tablets) per day. Antacids between meals can be taken for mild GI symptoms without discontinuing the aspirin. Enteric-coated and buffered tablets offer some advantage in patients with concomitant peptic ulcer or hiatus hernia. Sustained-release tablets provide longer relief for some patients and may be given at bedtime. Patients awakened at night by severe pain may take a dose at 2 or 3 AM. Salicylates such as sodium salicylate, salsalate, and choline magnesium salicylate seem to have better GI tolerance than aspirin and do not impair platelet adhesiveness, but may not be as effective anti-inflammatory agents.

Other NSAIDs are available for patients who do not tolerate sufficient aspirin to obtain a good effect or for whom less frequent dosing offers a major advantage. Usually only one agent is given at a time.

Indomethacin 25 mg is given orally tid with food or immediately after meals. If the response is inadequate, the daily dosage is increased by 25 mg at daily to weekly intervals depending on disease severity until the response is satisfactory or a dosage of 150 to 200 mg/day has been reached. After the acute phase of the disease is controlled, it is often possible to reduce the dosage gradually to a maintenance level of 75 to 100 mg/day. A 75-mg sustained-release capsule is also available for bid dosage.

The most frequent adverse reactions are headache, dizziness, lightheadedness, and GI disturbances (eg, nausea, anorexia, vomiting, epigastric distress, abdominal pain, diarrhea). GI effects may be minimized by giving the drug immediately after meals or with food. The drug should be **stopped** if GI bleeding occurs. Indomethacin **should not be given** to patients with active peptic ulcer, gastritis, or ulcerative colitis, and should be used with caution if there is a history of these disorders. Fluid retention and renal toxicity occur occasionally. CNS effects often are transient and disappear with continued treatment or after dosage reduction; occasionally, they are of such severity that therapy must be discontinued. Patients just beginning treatment with the drug or showing significant CNS symptoms should not operate automotive equipment or engage in hazardous occupations.

Ibuprofen 400 to 800 mg qid can be given; the larger dose usually is needed. **Naproxen** often requires only a 250-mg tablet bid; a total of 1000 mg/day may be used. **Fenoprofen** is given 300 to 600 mg qid; daily dose should not exceed 3200 mg. **Tolmetin** usually is initiated with 400 mg tid; the maximum recommended daily dose is 2000 mg. **Sulindac** is given 200 mg bid. **Meclofenamate** is given 200 to 400 mg/day. **Ketoprofen** can be given 150 to 300 mg/day. **Piroxicam** has a single recommended dosage of 20 mg once/day.

Though often less irritating to the GI tract than aspirin, these other NSAIDs can produce gastric symptoms and GI bleeding. Other possible side effects include CNS symptoms, edema, and decreased platelet adhesiveness. As with aspirin, liver enzymes can be mildly elevated. Creatinine levels can rise because of inhibition of prostaglandins; less frequently, interstitial nephritis can occur. Sulindac may be less likely to have renal side effects. Patients with urticaria, rhinitis, or asthma from aspirin can have the same problems with the other nonsteroidal agents.

Slowly acting drugs: If aspirin or other nonsteroidal drugs are not beneficial after 3 to 4 mo of treatment, addition of one of the slow-acting agents such as gold, penicillamine, or hydroxychloroquine should be considered.

Gold compounds usually are given in addition to salicylates or other nonsteroidal drugs if aspirin or 1 or 2 other NSAIDs do not provide sufficient relief. Gold is effective only against active joint inflammation. It is not analgesic but can produce remission and is the drug of choice after aspirin. Gold may also decrease the formation of new bony erosions. Gold sodium thiomalate or gold thioglucose (aurothioglucose) can be used. Gold is given IM at weekly intervals: 10 mg the first week, 25 mg the second, and 50 mg/wk thereafter until a total of 1 gm has been given or significant improvement is apparent. When maximum improvement is achieved, dosage is gradually decreased to 50 mg every 2 to 4 wk. Relapse usually occurs in 3 to 6 mo if no further gold is given following remission. Remissions often can be sustained with prolonged maintenance administration.

Gold compounds are **contraindicated** in patients with hepatic or renal disease, or blood dyscrasia. **Before receiving gold,** the patient should have a urinalysis, hemoglobin, total and differential WBC count, and an estimate of the number of platelets on the smear, with a count if they seem scarce. These tests should be repeated before each injection during the first month and every 1 to 2 wk thereafter. Presence of the HLA antigen DR3 may predict an increased risk of renal and possibly other side effects from both gold and penicillamine. Toxic reactions to gold include pruritus, dermatitis, stomatitis, albuminuria with or without a nephrotic syndrome, agranulocytosis, thrombocytopenic purpura, and aplastic anemia. Other less common side effects include diarrhea, hepatitis, pneumonitis, and neuropathy. Gold should be **discontinued** when any of the above manifestations appear. Eosinophilia > 5% and pruritus may precede appearance of a rash and are possible danger signals. Dermatitis usually is pruritic and ranges in severity from a single eczematous patch to generalized and fatal exfoliation.

Minor toxic manifestations (eg, mild pruritus or minor rash) may be eliminated by temporarily withholding gold therapy, then resuming it cautiously after the rash has been gone about 2 wk. However, if toxic symptoms progress, gold should be withheld and the patient given a corticosteroid. A topical corticosteroid or oral prednisone 15 to 20 mg/day in divided doses is given for mild gold dermatitis; larger doses may be needed for hematologic complications. A gold chelating agent, dimercaprol 2.5 mg/kg body wt, may be given IM up to 4 to 6 times/day for the first 2 days and then bid for 5 to 7 days after a *severe* gold reaction. A transient **nitritoid reaction** with flushing, tachycardia, and faintness can occur several minutes after injections of gold sodium thiomalate. This occurs more often if the gold is not stored in the dark. If these reactions occur, aurothioglucose can be used, as this does not seem to cause them.

An **oral gold compound, auranofin,** 3 mg bid or 6 mg once daily may be tried for at least 6 mo and, if necessary and tolerated, increased to 3 mg tid for 3 more months. If the response is not favorable, auranofin should be discontinued. Unlike with injectable gold, diarrhea and other GI symptoms are prominent side effects. Renal and mucocutaneous side effects appear to be fewer than with IV gold, but long-term effects of auranofin are not known. Urinalysis, hemoglobin, and leukocyte, differential, and platelet counts should be done at least monthly.

D-Penicillamine given orally has a beneficial effect similar to that of gold and may be used in some cases if gold fails or produces toxicity in patients with active RA. Suggested doses start at 250 mg/day for 30 to 90 days; the dose is then increased to 500 mg/day for another 30 to 90 days and, if definite improvement does not occur, may be increased to 750 mg/day for 60 days. When the patient starts to respond, further increases should *not* be made. The dose should be kept to the minimally effective level. Before therapy and every 2 to 3 wk during treatment, platelets must be checked and urinalysis and CBC performed. Side effects requiring discontinuation are more common than with gold. This drug can cause marrow suppression, proteinuria, nephrosis,

other serious toxic effects (including myasthenia gravis, pemphigus, Goodpasture's syndrome, polymyositis, or a lupuslike syndrome), or a rash and a foul taste, all of which require discontinuation. Fatalities due to D-penicillamine have been reported. *The drug must be monitored carefully*, and should be given by, or with guidance from, one experienced with its use.

Hydroxychloroquine can also control symptoms of mild to moderate active RA. Toxic effects usually are mild and include dermatitis, myopathy, and generally reversible corneal opacity. However, irreversible retinal degeneration has been reported. Ophthalmologic evaluation with testing of visual fields using a red test object is required before, and every 3 to 6 mo during, treatment. An initial dosage of 200 mg is given orally bid with breakfast and the evening meal; therapy is continued at that dosage for 3 to 6 mo. The drug should be discontinued if the patient fails to improve after 3 to 6 mo. If definite improvement is achieved, the dosage can be decreased to 200 mg/day and continued as long as effective. Frequent eye examinations must be continued.

Corticosteroids (see also Ch. 283) are the most dramatically effective short-term anti-inflammatory drugs. RA, however, is usually active for years, and clinical benefit from corticosteroids often diminishes with time. They do not prevent the progression of joint destruction. Furthermore, when the disease is active, severe rebound phenomena follow their withdrawal. Because of their side effects, corticosteroids should be given only after careful and usually prolonged evaluation of less potentially hazardous drugs. Corticosteroids suppress clinical manifestations and may be used to maintain joint function and allow continued performance of customary duties, but the patient should be cautioned about complications occurring with long-term use. Dosage should not exceed 7.5 mg of prednisone/day except for patients with severe systemic manifestations of RA such as vasculitis, pleurisy, or pericarditis. Large "loading doses" followed by rapid dosage reduction are *not recommended*, nor is alternate-day therapy, since RA usually is too symptomatically active the days corticosteroids are not given. Relative contraindications to the use of corticosteroids include peptic ulcer, hypertension, untreated infections, diabetes mellitus, and glaucoma. TB should be ruled out before corticosteroid therapy is begun.

Intra-articular injections of corticosteroid esters may temporarily help to control local synovitis in 1 or 2 particularly painful joints. Triamcinolone hexacetonide may suppress inflammation for the longest period; prednisolone tertiary-butylacetate also is effective. The 21-phosphate preparations of prednisolone or dexamethasone are *not recommended*, because of rapid clearance from the joint and very short duration of action. Overuse of the recently injected, less painful joint may accelerate joint destruction. Since corticosteroid esters are crystalline, local inflammation transiently increases within a few hours in about 2% of injections.

Immunosuppressive drugs such as cyclophosphamide, methotrexate, and azathioprine are increasingly used in management of severe, active RA. They can suppress inflammation and may allow reduction of corticosteroid doses. Major side effects occur with these drugs, however, including liver disease, bone marrow suppression, and, possibly, increased risk of malignancy following long-term use. Patients should be fully informed of these potential side effects and are generally advised to be under the supervision of a specialist. Of these agents, only azathioprine is marketed in the USA as approved for RA. Methotrexate, in recent years widely used to treat RA, can be given 2.5 to 15 mg in a single dose once weekly. Liver function must be monitored, and a liver biopsy may be needed if the patient continues to use this agent. Other experimental therapies such as lymphopheresis and total lymphoid radiation are being studied.

Exercise, physiotherapy, and surgery: Flexion contractures can be prevented and muscle strength restored most successfully after the inflammation is suppressed. Joint splinting reduces local inflammation and may relieve symptoms. Before the acute

inflammatory process is controlled, passive exercise to prevent contracture is given carefully and within the limits of pain. Active exercise to restore muscle mass and preserve the normal range of joint motion is desirable as inflammation subsides, but should not be fatiguing. Self-help devices have enabled many patients with severe debilitating RA to perform activities essential to daily living. Orthopedic shoes, modified to fit individual needs, are frequently helpful; metatarsal bars placed posteriorly to painful metatarsophalangeal joints decrease the pain of weight-bearing.

Established flexion contractures may require intensive exercise, serial splinting, or orthopedic measures. Though synovectomy provides only temporary relief of inflammation, it may be used in key joints to help preserve joint function if anti-inflammatory drugs have been unsuccessful. Arthroplasty with prosthetic replacement of joint parts is indicated if the degree of joint damage severely limits function. Total hip replacement is the most consistently successful of available prosthetic procedures. Total knee replacement is somewhat less successful but useful. Prosthetic hips and knees cannot be expected to tolerate resumption of activities such as vigorous athletics. Excision of subluxated painful metatarsophalangeal joints may greatly aid walking. Surgical procedures must always be considered in terms of the total disease. Deformed hands and arms limit crutch use during rehabilitation; seriously affected knees and feet prevent full benefit from hip surgery. Reasonable objectives for the patient must be determined and function must be considered before appearance. Surgery may be undertaken while the disease is active.

PSORIATIC ARTHRITIS

A rheumatoid-like arthritis associated with psoriasis of the skin or nails and a negative test for rheumatoid factor; HLA-B27 antigen is present in some patients, especially when the spine is involved.

Symptoms, Signs, and Diagnosis

Psoriasis of the nails or skin may precede or follow joint involvement. Patients with seronegative inflammatory polyarthritis should be examined for unrecognized or minimal psoriasis as well as nail pitting, and should be questioned about a family history of psoriasis.

The distal interphalangeal joints (fingers and toes) are especially affected. Asymmetric involvement of large and small joints, including the sacroiliacs and the spine, is common. Rheumatoid nodules are not present. Exacerbations and remissions of joint and skin symptoms may coincide. Arthritic remissions tend to be more frequent, rapid, and complete than in RA, but progression to chronic arthritis and severe crippling may occur. X-ray findings include distal interphalangeal involvement, resorption of terminal phalanges ("sausage toes"), arthritis mutilans, and extensive destruction and dislocation of large and small joints.

Treatment

Treatment is directed at control of skin lesions and joint inflammation. Drug therapy is similar to that for RA, except for the use of antimalarials. They are of only mild benefit, and anecdotal evidence suggests they may cause exfoliative dermatitis or may aggravate the underlying psoriasis. Benefit may be gained from gold; toxic reactions may occur. Etretinate 0.5 to 1.0 mg/kg/day orally in 2 divided doses is effective in severe psoriasis, and some studies have shown that the arthritis is helped also. Side effects may be severe: hypervitaminosis A, teratogenicity, and liver toxicity. *Because of etretinate's teratogenic potential and long-term retention in the body, patients should not become pregnant while taking the drug or for at least 1 yr afterwards.* Photochemotherapy using oral methoxsalen and long-wave ultraviolet-A light (psoralen with UV-A—**PUVA**) appears to be highly effective for the skin lesions and beneficial for peripheral arthritis, but not for spine involvement. Folic acid antagonists and immu-

nosuppressive agents, especially methotrexate (CAUTION: *Highly toxic*), used under rigidly controlled conditions, have relieved psoriatic lesions and joint symptoms. Treatment of psoriasis is further discussed in Ch. 236.

ANKYLOSING SPONDYLITIS (AS)

(Marie-Strümpell Disease)

A heterogeneous and systemic rheumatic disorder characterized primarily by inflammation of the axial skeleton and large peripheral joints.

Three times more frequent in men than in women, AS begins most often between the ages of 20 and 40. Familial clustering and the higher than expected frequency of the HLA-B27 tissue antigen among patients support a genetic basis for this disease, although environmental factors also appear to be operative. Calculations based on 2 American surveys, one of B27-positive blood donors and another of B27-positive tissue donors, indicate that the risk of spondylitis developing in individuals with HLA-B27 may be 20%.

Symptoms and Signs

The most frequent presenting symptom is back pain, but disease can begin atypically in peripheral joints, especially in children and women, and rarely even with acute iritis (anterior uveitis). Whatever the mode of onset, recurrent back pain that is often nocturnal and of varying intensity is an eventual complaint, as is early morning stiffness that is characteristically relieved by activity. Patients automatically ease back pain and paraspinal muscle spasm by adopting a flexed or bent-over posture. Consequently, in the untreated patient, some degree of kyphosis is common. Another early sign is diminished chest expansion that results from diffuse costovertebral involvement. Additional early symptoms are fever, fatigue, anorexia, weight loss, and anemia.

Systemic manifestations include recurrent attacks of acute iritis that affect 1/3 of patients but usually are self-limiting. Only rarely are bouts of iritis protracted and severe enough to impair vision. Neurologic signs result from compression radiculitis or sciatica, vertebral fracture or subluxation, and the cauda equina syndrome. The latter produces impotency, nocturnal urinary incontinence, diminished bladder and rectal sensation, and absence of ankle jerks. Cardiovascular manifestations include angina, pericarditis, electrocardiographic conduction abnormalities, and rarely aortic insufficiency. A rare pulmonary finding is upper lobe fibrosis, occasionally with cavitation that may be mistaken for TB and may be complicated by infection with *Aspergillus*. Tuberculous spondylitis is discussed in Ch. 8.

Prognosis: AS is characterized by mild or moderate flares of active spondylitis alternating with almost, or totally, inactive periods, so that with proper treatment minimal or no disability results and patients lead full, productive lives. Rarely, the course is severe and progressive so that patients end up with pronounced and largely incapacitating deformities. The prognosis also is bleak for patients with refractory iritis and the rare patient who develops secondary amyloidosis.

Diagnosis

Laboratory and x-ray findings: The ESR is elevated in most patients with active disease, as are other acute phase reactants such as serum IgA levels. Notably negative are tests for both IgM rheumatoid factor and antinuclear antibodies. A positive test for HLA-B27 is the best single laboratory clue, but its absence does not preclude AS.

Diagnosis must be confirmed by x-ray. The earliest abnormalities occur in the sacroiliac joints and include pseudowidening or narrowing of these articulations from subchondral erosions and sclerosis. Early changes in the spine are diffuse vertebral squaring and demineralization as well as spotty ligamentous calcification and 1 or 2 evolving syndesmophytes. The classic "bamboo spine" with its prominent syndes-

mophytes and diffuse paraspinal ligamentous calcification, the usual textbook illustration, is *not* useful for early diagnosis. These advanced changes occur in a minority of patients and take an average of 10 yr to develop.

Differential diagnosis: One of the most important disorders to be differentiated is a **herniated intervertebral disk.** This latter condition is limited to the spine and has no systemic manifestations such as fatigue, anorexia, or weight loss; all laboratory tests, including the ESR, are normal. The only confirmation of a herniated disk is by myelography or CT scan.

The **DISH syndrome** (**d**iffuse **i**diopathic **s**keletal **h**yperostosis) is a more difficult differential diagnosis. It occurs primarily in men > 50 yr and may resemble AS clinically and on x-ray. Patients may have spinal pain, stiffness, and insidious loss of spine motion. X-ray findings include ligamentous calcification most often affecting the cervical and lower thoracic spine. However, the sacroiliac and spinal apophyseal joints are not involved; the ESR is normal; and there is no link to HLA-B27.

Treatment

The patient's joint discomfort must first be relieved with antirheumatic drugs; long-range planning then begins—to prevent, delay, or correct deformity. To promote proper posture and joint motion, daily exercises and other supportive measures (eg, postural training or therapeutic exercise) are vital. The objective is to build up muscle groups that oppose the direction of potential deformities; ie, to strengthen extensor rather than flexor muscle groups. Long-range planning also must include the psychosocial and rehabilitative needs of the patient.

Nonsteroidal anti-inflammatory drugs (NSAIDs) facilitate exercise and other supportive measures by suppressing articular inflammation, pain, and spasm. The drugs listed in TABLE 108–2 should be considered first, since these are of proven value in AS. While aspirin or other salicylates may be tried first, they are seldom adequate and in no way comparable to the effectiveness of the other NSAIDs in the table. Tolerance or potential toxic risks rather than marginal differences in efficacy dictate drug choice. Patients should be monitored and warned of potential adverse reactions (see the NSAID discussion in RHEUMATOID ARTHRITIS, above). Patients receiving phenylbutazone or oxyphenbutazone should be routinely screened for rare but serious renal or hematopoietic

TABLE 108–2. DRUG THERAPY* OF ANKYLOSING SPONDYLITIS (AS)

Drug	Daily Dosage: Average	Daily Dosage: Range
Salicylates	4 gm	3–6 gm
Phenylbutazone† and	300 mg	100–400 mg
Oxyphenbutazone†	300 mg	100–400 mg
Indomethacin‡	100 mg	25–200 mg
Naproxen	750 mg	250–1000 mg
Sulindac	300 mg	100–400 mg

* The only nonsteroidal anti-inflammatory drugs with FDA approval for AS in the USA.

† Currently recommended only after other drugs have been tried first. Oxyphenbutazone is still available while supplies last, but manufacturing of the drug was stopped in the USA in mid 1985

‡ Also available as a sustained-release preparation of 75 mg; the range of daily dosage is 75 to 150 mg.

(Modified from "Sustained-Release Indomethacin in the Management of Ankylosing Spondylitis" by J. J. Calabro, p. 44, in *The American Journal of Medicine,* Vol. 79(4c), October 25, 1985. Used with permission.)

adverse reactions, including fatal aplastic anemia; ie, complete blood and platelet counts as well as a urinalysis must be performed weekly for the initial 2 mo and monthly thereafter. The daily dose of NSAIDs should be as low as possible. However, complete drug withdrawal should be attempted only slowly and after all systemic and articular signs of active disease have been suppressed for several months.

Corticosteroids have limited therapeutic value, and their long-term use is associated with many serious adverse effects (see also Ch. 283). For acute iritis, topical corticosteroids (and mydriatics) usually are adequate; oral corticosteroids are rarely indicated. Intra-articular corticosteroids may be beneficial, particularly when 1 or 2 peripheral joints are more severely inflamed than others, compromising exercise and rehabilitation.

Radiotherapy to the spine, while an effective form of therapy, is recommended only as a last resort; the risk of subsequently developing acute myelogenous leukemia is tenfold. The **slow-acting (remittive) drugs** used in RA, such as IM gold, are not effective for AS. **Narcotics,** strict analgesics, and muscle relaxants should be prescribed only for short periods to control severe back pain and spasm, since they lack anti-inflammatory properties.

SJÖGREN'S SYNDROME (SS)

A chronic, systemic inflammatory disorder of unknown etiology, characterized by dryness of the mouth, eyes, and other mucous membranes and often associated with rheumatic disorders sharing certain autoimmune features (eg, RA, scleroderma, and SLE) and in which lymphocyte infiltration into affected tissues is seen. An association has been found between HLA-DR3 antigen and **primary SS** (*without associated connective tissue disease*—see below). The syndrome is more common than SLE but less common than RA.

Pathophysiology, Symptoms, and Signs

In some, SS affects only the eyes or mouth **(primary SS; sicca complex; sicca syndrome);** in others, there is an associated generalized collagen vascular disease **(secondary SS).**

Ocular symptoms occur when atrophy of the secretory epithelium of the lacrimal glands causes desiccation of the cornea and conjunctiva (**keratoconjunctivitis sicca,** discussed in Ch. 219). In advanced cases, the cornea is severely damaged and epithelial strands hang from the corneal surface **(keratitis filiformis).**

One third of SS patients develop **enlarged parotid glands** that are usually firm, smooth, fluctuating in size, and mildly tender. Chronic salivary gland enlargement is rarely painful. Intraductal cellular proliferation in the parotid gland causes luminal narrowing and eventual formation of compact cellular structures termed epimyoepithelial islands. When salivary glands atrophy, saliva diminishes, and the resulting extreme dryness of the mouth and lips **(xerostomia)** inhibits chewing and swallowing and promotes tooth decay and calculi formation in the salivary ducts. Taste and smell faculties may be lost.

Desiccation may also develop in the skin and in mucous membranes of the nose, throat, larynx, bronchi, vulva, and vagina. Alopecia may occur. Dryness of the respiratory tract often leads to lung infections and sometimes to fatal pneumonia.

Other manifestations: GI effects are associated with mucosal or submucosal atrophy and diffuse infiltration by plasma cells and lymphocytes. Chronic hepatobiliary disease is often associated with SS, as is pancreatitis (exocrine pancreatic tissue is similar to that of salivary glands). Fibrinous pericarditis is the commonest cardiovascular feature. Sensory neuropathy is common, especially of the 2nd and 3rd divisions of the 5th cranial nerve. Approximately 20% of SS patients have renal tubular acidosis; in many, renal concentrating ability is decreased. Interstitial nephritis is frequent; glomerulone-

phritis unusual. Patients with parotid enlargement, splenomegaly, and lymphadenopathy may develop pseudolymphoma or malignant lymphoma. The incidence of lymphoma is increased 44-fold for SS patients, who are also at increased risk for Waldenström's macroglobulinemia.

Diagnosis and Prognosis

One suspects SS with dryness of the eyes and mouth; joint inflammation completes the classic triad. Arthritis occurs in about 33% of patients and is similar in distribution to that seen in RA; however, joint symptoms in SS tend to be milder and rarely lead to destruction. Some patients with undiagnosed SS who have rheumatic symptoms may not complain spontaneously of sicca complex; SS is then defined by laboratory evaluation.

When bilateral parotid enlargement occurs in conditions such as hyperlipoproteinemia, malnutrition, cirrhosis, or diabetes mellitus, the glands are soft and puffy, in contrast to the firm glands of SS; oral dryness is absent.

Diagnostic procedures and laboratory findings: The **Schirmer test** measures the quantity of tears secreted in 5 min in response to irritation from a filter paper strip placed under a lower eyelid. A young person normally moistens 15 mm of the paper strip. Since hypolacrimation occurs with aging, 33% of normal elderly persons may wet only 10 mm in 5 min. Most persons with SS moisten < 5 mm/5 min, although about 15% of test results are false-positive and 15% false-negative. **Ocular staining** with a drop of **rose bengal solution** into the eye is highly specific. In SS, the portion of the eye filling the palpebral aperture takes up the dye, and red triangles with their bases toward the limbus are seen. **Tear breakup time, tear lysozyme concentration,** and **slit-lamp examination** are also useful.

Salivary glands are evaluated by **salivary flow, sialography,** and **salivary scintiscan. Biopsy** of the readily accessible labial salivary glands confirms the diagnosis when foci of lymphocytes and plasma cells associated with atrophy of acinar tissue are seen.

Remarkable immunologic reactivity, detected in blood serum, is characteristic of SS; most patients have elevated levels of antibodies against γ-globulin, nuclear protein, and many tissue constituents. Precipitating antibodies to nuclear antigens (identified by immunodiffusion analysis), termed SS-B antibodies, are highly specific for primary SS. Rheumatoid factor is present in > 70% of cases; the LE cell preparation is positive in 15 to 20%. The VDRL test is negative. ESR is elevated in 70% of patients. One third of patients have anemia; 1/4, leukopenia and eosinophilia. Urinalysis may show proteinuria, reflecting interstitial nephritis.

Prognosis in SS is often related to the associated connective tissue disorder, although death may also result from pulmonary infection and, rarely, renal failure or lymphoma.

Treatment

For care of **ocular symptoms** see KERATOCONJUNCTIVITIS SICCA in Ch. 219.

Oral complications: Dryness that promotes ductal calculi and rampant dental caries may be avoided by sipping fluids throughout the day, chewing sugarless gum, and using a 2% solution of methylcellulose as a mouthwash. Drugs that decrease salivary secretion, such as decongestants and antihistamines, should be avoided. Fastidious oral hygiene and regular dental supervision are essential. Calculi must be promptly removed, preserving viable salivary tissue. The temporary pain of suddenly enlarged salivary glands is best treated only with analgesics.

Connective tissue involvement usually is mild and chronic; therefore, corticosteroids and immunosuppressive agents are indicated only occasionally, eg, in a patient with severe vasculitis or visceral involvement. Irradiation and drugs that increase the risk of lymphoproliferative disorders and infections should be avoided.

LYME DISEASE
(LD; Lyme Arthritis)

A tick-transmitted, spirochetal, inflammatory disorder best recognized clinically by an early skin lesion, erythema chronicum migrans **(ECM),** *that may be followed weeks to months later by neurologic, cardiac, or joint abnormalities.*

Etiology, Epidemiology, and Pathophysiology

The illness is caused by a newly discovered spirochete, *Borrelia burgdorferi*, transmitted by the minute tick *Ixodes dammini* and related ticks. The disease was recognized in 1975 because of close geographic clustering of cases in the small community of Lyme, Connecticut. It has since appeared in over half the states in the USA, especially in foci along the northeastern coast from Massachusetts to Maryland, in Wisconsin, and in California and Oregon. It also has appeared abroad. Onset usually is in the summer and early fall and occurs at any age and in either sex, although most patients are children and young adults living in heavily wooded areas. LD is now the most commonly reported tickborne illness in the USA.

B. burgdorferi has been cultured from the blood, skin (ECM), and spinal fluid of LD patients. The spirochete enters skin at the site of a tick bite. After an incubation period of 3 to 32 days, the organism migrates outward in the skin (ECM), is spread in lymph (regional adenopathy), or is disseminated in blood to organs or other skin sites. The spirochete has been seen in secondary skin lesions, and in inflamed synovia.

LD is associated with characteristic immune findings. Over 85% of patients with subsequent arthritis have, in the prearticular (ECM) phase, serum cryoglobulins containing IgM (reflecting high serum IgM levels), compared to < 15% of patients without subsequent arthritis. Besides having prognostic value, these differences may represent different ways of responding to an immune stimulus, and may be determined genetically. In preliminary studies, patients have an increased frequency of the B cell alloantigen HLA-DR2 but not of HLA-B27 (as in the spondyloarthropathies).

More direct evidence for circulating immune complexes (eg, abnormal C1q-binding activity) is found in sera of most patients with ECM. These complexes tend to persist in the circulation of patients who develop neurologic or cardiac abnormalities. By the time arthritis appears, immune complexes are no longer evident in most sera but are found systematically in synovial fluid, and in higher titer than in concomitant sera.

Synovial membrane from affected joints may be indistinguishable from that of RA (see above). Nonspecific findings include villous hypertrophy, vascular congestion, and colonization with lymphocytes and plasma cells that may resemble early lymphoid follicles and, as in RA, are presumably capable of producing antibody locally. In addition, there may be an obliterative endarteritis and (rarely) demonstrable spirochetes. Pannus formation and erosion of cartilage and bone may occur.

The histology of ECM resembles that of an insect bite—epidermal and dermal involvement at the center (which is often indurated), dermal in the periphery. All layers of the epidermis are heavily infiltrated with mononuclear cells around blood vessels and skin appendages. At the center there is edema of the papillary dermis, and intra- and extracellular edema and a thickened keratin layer in the epidermis.

Symptoms, Signs, and Course

ECM begins as a red macule or papule, usually on the proximal portion of an extremity or on the trunk (especially the thigh, buttock, or axilla), that expands, often with central clearing, to a diameter as large as 50 cm. At least 75% of patients with Lyme disease have this early lesion. Of these individuals, about 25% report having been bitten at that site by a minute tick 3 to 32 days before onset of ECM. Soon after onset of ECM, nearly half the patients develop multiple, usually smaller, lesions without indurated centers. ECM generally lasts for a few weeks; evanescent lesions may

appear during resolution. Former skin lesions may reappear faintly, sometimes before recurrent attacks of arthritis. Mucosal lesions do not occur.

The most common symptoms accompanying ECM (or preceding it by a few days) are malaise and fatigue, chills and fever, headache, and stiff neck. Myalgias and arthralgias are common, but frank arthritis is rare at this stage. Less common are backache, nausea and vomiting, sore throat, lymphadenopathy, and splenomegaly. Symptoms are characteristically intermittent and changing, but malaise and fatigue may linger for weeks.

Frank neurologic abnormalities develop in about 15% of patients within weeks to months of ECM (often before arthritis occurs), commonly last for months, and usually resolve completely. They include lymphocytic meningitis (about 100 cells/μL) or meningoencephalitis, chorea, cerebellar ataxia, cranial neuritis (including bilateral Bell's palsy), motor and sensory radiculoneuritis, mononeuritis multiplex, and myelitis. **Myocardial abnormalities** occur in about 8% of patients within weeks of ECM. They include fluctuating degrees of atrioventricular block (first degree, Wenckebach, or 3rd degree) and, less commonly, myopericarditis with reduced left ventricular ejection fractions and cardiomegaly.

Arthritis occurs in about half of patients with ECM within weeks to months of the onset of ECM; the interval has been as long as 2 yr. Intermittent swelling and pain in several large joints, especially knees, typically recur for several years. The knees commonly are much more swollen than painful, often hot, rarely red. Baker's cysts may form and rupture. Those symptoms accompanying ECM, especially malaise, fatigue, and low-grade fever, also may precede or accompany recurrent attacks of arthritis. About 10% of patients develop chronic (unremitting for 6 mo or more) knee involvement. Other late findings (years) associated with this infection include additional antibiotic-responsive skin lesions—*acrodermatitis chronica atrophicans* and some cases of *lymphocytoma benigna cutis*—and chronic neurologic abnormalities.

Laboratory and X-ray Findings

Recovery of *B. burgdorferi* from blood, ECM, or CSF is so far rare, difficult, and slow (weeks). Specific anti-spirochetal antibodies in significant titer—first IgM, then IgG—appear within weeks of ECM. IgG titers are higher later in the illness when arthritis is present.

Cryoprecipitates and circulating immune complexes are often seen early in the illness (see Pathophysiology, above). The ESR may be elevated when patients feel ill; the Hct, WBC, and differential counts usually are normal. Rheumatoid and antinuclear factors rarely are present. The Venereal Disease Research Laboratory (VDRL) test is negative. Serum complement components either are normal or elevated during active disease (but see Pathophysiology, above). The urinalysis and serum creatinine usually are normal; AST (SGOT) and LDH levels may be slightly abnormal when ECM is present.

Synovial fluid findings vary, but typically show about 25,000 white cells/μL (range, 500 to 110,000), mostly granulocytes; about 5 gm/dL of protein; and C3 and C4 levels usually > 1/3 those of serum.

Radiologic findings usually are limited to soft tissue swelling, but a few patients have had erosion of cartilage and bone.

Differential Diagnosis

In children, LD must be distinguished primarily from juvenile RA; in adults, from Reiter's syndrome and atypical RA. The distinguishing features of LD described above may occur in any combination. Important negative findings include absence (usually) of morning stiffness, subcutaneous nodules, iridocyclitis, mucosal lesions, rheumatoid factor, and antinuclear antibodies. Acute rheumatic fever is considered in the occasional patient with migratory polyarthritis and either an increased P-R interval or

chorea (as a manifestation of meningoencephalitis). However, patients with LD rarely have heart murmurs or evidence of a preceding streptococcal infection. Spondyloarthropathies with peripheral joint involvement can be distinguished from LD by the lack of axial involvement in the latter. LD may mimic idiopathic Bell's palsy and multiple sclerosis or other causes of lymphocytic meningitis and neuropathy.

Treatment

For adults, the drug of choice for early LD is tetracycline 250 mg qid for at least 10 days and for up to 20 days if symptoms persist or recur. Second choice is penicillin V 500 mg qid and third choice is erythromycin 250 mg qid, in each instance for 10 to 20 days. Some physicians give higher oral doses. In children or pregnant women, penicillin V is recommended rather than tetracycline. For neurologic abnormalities, penicillin G 20 million u./day IV in divided doses for 10 days is recommended. That regimen also cures about half the patients with established arthritis, but optimal therapy for this problem and for later neurologic complications is not yet clear. For symptomatic relief, aspirin (90 mg/kg/day [1.5 grains/kg] in children) or other nonsteroidal anti-inflammatory agents may be used. For tense knee joints due to effusions, aspiration of fluid and the use of crutches may be helpful. If the patient has marked functional limitation, synovectomy may be performed for chronic knee effusions (6 mo or more despite therapy), but spontaneous remission can occur after more than a year of continuous knee involvement.

INFECTIOUS ARTHRITIS

Arthritis resulting from infection of the synovial tissues with pyogenic bacteria or other infectious agents.

Etiology and Pathogenesis

Any pathogenic microbe may infect a joint. **Bacteria** are most often the etiologic agents, typically producing an acute arthritis. In young children, the predominating pathogens are staphylococci, *Hemophilus influenzae*, and gram-negative bacilli. Older children and adults are most commonly infected with gonococci (see also Ch. 14), staphylococci, streptococci, or pneumococci. Acute arthritis at any age may be associated with **viral infections** (eg, rubella, mumps, human parvovirus, or hepatitis B). Chronic arthritis may be caused by *Mycobacterium tuberculosis* (see TUBERCULOSIS OF BONES AND JOINTS in Ch. 8) and other **mycobacteria or fungi** such as *Sporothrix schenckii, Coccidioides immitis, Blastomyces dermatitidis*, and *Candida albicans*.

Microbes usually reach the joint hematogenously; however, direct inoculation of bacteria or fungi into the joint may occur during surgery or drug injection, or secondary to trauma. Patients with RA and chronically inflamed joints are particularly susceptible to bacterial arthritis.

Symptoms and Signs

An infant with septic arthritis is irritable and has a fever. Examination usually reveals failure to move a limb spontaneously, tenderness, or pain with passive motion of the involved joint. Older children and adults with nongonococcal bacterial arthritis complain of acute joint (most often the knee, followed by the shoulder, wrist, hip, phalanges, and elbow) pain and stiffness. On examination, the joint is warm, tender, and swollen, with evidence of effusion. Other signs of infection, such as fever, chills, or leukocytosis, usually are present. However, patients receiving anti-inflammatory drugs may show little systemic or local response. A history of recent urethritis, salpingitis, or hemorrhagic vesicular skin lesions suggests gonococcal arthritis (see under GONORRHEA in Ch. 14). Mycobacterial and fungal arthritides are typically chronic and monarticular.

Diagnosis

The diagnosis requires a high index of suspicion, particularly in patients with underlying chronic joint disease. *Even the remote possibility that a joint might be septic demands aspiration of synovial fluid from the involved joint and a search for the infecting organism by Gram stain and culture.* Since acute bacterial arthritis is often a manifestation of bacteremia, cultures should be taken from all likely sources of infection, such as blood, sputum, spinal fluid, and abscesses. For patients with nongonococcal bacterial arthritis, the synovial fluid culture is almost always positive unless antibiotics have recently been taken. For patients with gonococcal arthritis, the organism often is *not* recovered early in the synovial fluid; blood cultures are positive in only about 20% of cases. For those patients in whom an infecting agent is not recovered early, diagnosis of infectious arthritis may be supported by the following joint fluid characteristics: WBC count > 10,000/μL; > 90% polymorphonuclear leukocytes; synovial fluid/blood glucose ratio < 0.5; poor mucin clot; and absence of uric acid or calcium pyrophosphate dihydrate crystals.

Mycobacterial and fungal agents should be considered in any case of chronic monarticular arthritis. These agents are difficult to isolate from synovial fluids, and successful diagnosis often depends on their demonstration by microscopic examination and culture of synovial biopsy tissue.

Treatment

Acute bacterial arthritis is a medical emergency; the joint may be destroyed if not promptly treated. Successful therapy depends on **early and appropriate antibiotic use,** which may have to be started before isolating the infecting organism and evaluating its antimicrobial sensitivity pattern. Early antibiotic choice depends on an estimate of the likely infecting organism—eg, penicillin for a sexually active healthy young person; broad-spectrum antibiotics for an elderly, immunocompromised person. The appropriate antimicrobial (see TABLE 108–3) should be given parenterally, since absorption of oral antimicrobials may be inadequate. Intra-articular antimicrobials may cause synovitis and are rarely indicated.

Treatment should be continued for at least 2 wk after all symptoms and signs of inflammation have disappeared. **The joint should be aspirated and cultured daily or more often** to confirm sterilization of the joint fluid and to remove accumulated pus. If a clinical response and sterilization of the joint fluid are not apparent after 48 h of therapy, the choice and dose of antimicrobials should be adjusted until bactericidal activity of the joint fluid against the infecting organism can be demonstrated at a dilution of 1:8 or greater. **Surgical drainage** is indicated when needle aspiration of the

TABLE 108–3. INITIAL ANTIMICROBIAL PROGRAMS RECOMMENDED FOR ACUTE BACTERIAL ARTHRITIS

Gram Stain	*Antimicrobial*
Gram-positive cocci	Nafcillin 30 mg/kg q 4 h IV
Gram-negative cocci	Penicillin G 50,000 u./kg q 4 h IV
Gram-negative bacilli	Gentamicin 1.5 mg/kg q 8 h IM plus Piperacillin 50 mg/kg q 4 h IV
No organism present	
Gonococcal infection suspected	Penicillin as above
Other bacterial possibilities	Nafcillin and gentamicin as above

joint is difficult, as in hip infections, or if the infection is not controlled after 48 h. **Splinting** is useful for pain relief during the acute stage. Physical therapy is indicated during convalescence to assure optimal return of function.

Antimicrobial therapy for mycobacterial or fungal arthritis is the same as for other serious infections with these agents (see appropriate chapters in §1). Viral arthritis is usually self-limited and responds to symptomatic therapy.

REITER'S SYNDROME (RS)

Arthritis associated with nonbacterial urethritis or cervicitis, conjunctivitis, and mucocutaneous lesions. RS is classified with the seronegative spondyloarthropathies, along with ankylosing spondylitis, enteric arthritis, and psoriatic arthritis. Epidemiologically, RS, like rheumatic fever, is an example of **reactive arthritis** (*syndromes characterized by sterile inflammation of joints from infections originating at nonarticular sites*).

Etiology and Incidence

Two forms are recognized: sexually transmitted and dysenteric. The former occurs primarily in young men between ages 20 and 40. Genital infections with *Chlamydia trachomatis* are most often implicated. RS is less common in women, children, and the elderly, who usually acquire the dysenteric form following enteric bacterial infections, primarily due to shigella, salmonella, yersinia, and campylobacter. The unusually high frequency of the HLA-B27 tissue antigen in 63 to 96% of patients with RS, as compared with 6 to 15% of healthy controls, supports a genetic predisposition. Thus, individuals with the HLA-B27 genetic marker are at increased risk for developing RS after sexual contact or being exposed to certain enteric bacterial infections.

Symptoms, Signs, and Course

In typical RS, nonbacterial urethritis develops 7 to 14 days after sexual exposure or dysentery; low-grade fever, conjunctivitis, and arthritis develop over the next few weeks. The **urethritis** in men is less painful and productive of purulent discharge than that seen with acute gonorrhea, and may be associated with hemorrhagic cystitis or prostatitis. In women, **urethritis and cervicitis** may be mild (with dysuria or a slight vaginal discharge) or entirely asymptomatic, making diagnosis difficult. **Conjunctivitis** is the most common eye lesion. It usually is mild, except when keratitis and anterior uveitis coexist.

Arthritis usually is the 2nd or 3rd feature of RS and may be mild or severe. Joint involvement generally is asymmetric and polyarticular, occurring in the large joints of the lower extremities as well as the toes. Back pain may occur, usually with more severe disease. **Enthesopathy** (*inflammation at tendinous insertion into bone*) is common in RS and other seronegative arthritides; eg, plantar fasciitis, digital periostitis, Achilles tendinitis. **Mucocutaneous lesions**—small, painless superficial ulcers—are commonly seen on the oral mucosa, tongue, and glans penis (balanitis circinata). Patients may also develop hyperkeratotic skin lesions of the palms and soles and around the nails **(keratoderma blennorrhagica).**

The initial illness typically resolves in 3 to 4 mo, but 50% of patients experience transient recurrences of arthritis and/or other components of the syndrome over a period of several years. Joint deformity and ankylosis as well as sacroiliitis and/or spondylitis may occur with chronic or recurrent RS.

Diagnosis

Diagnosis of RS requires peripheral arthritis occurring in association with urethritis and/or cervicitis lasting > 1 mo. Since the various manifestations may occur at different times, diagnosis may require several months. Positive gonococcal cultures and a rapid response to penicillin therapy differentiate acute gonococcal arthritis from RS in a sexually active young patient. In patients who develop the chronic form of the

syndrome, the arthritis and/or skin lesions may resemble those seen in psoriatic arthritis, ankylosing spondylitis, or Behçet's syndrome.

Prognosis and Treatment

Only a few patients are disabled by chronic or recurrent disease. Because RS following sexual exposure often is associated with *C. trachomatis* infection, treatment of patients and their sexual partners with tetracycline or erythromycin 500 mg orally qid for 10 days is recommended (see also SEXUALLY TRANSMITTED CHLAMYDIAL AND UREAPLASMAL INFECTIONS in Ch. 14). No treatment is necessary for conjunctivitis and mucocutaneous lesions, although iritis may require ophthalmic glucocorticosteroids. Arthritis is treated with anti-inflammatory agents such as aspirin or indomethacin in doses similar to those used for RA (see above). If these fail, phenylbutazone 100 mg orally qid may be effective. Local injection of corticosteroids for enthesopathy may be indicated. Systemic corticosteroids have not been of value. Physical therapy is helpful during the recovery phase. Methotrexate or the folic acid antagonists may be required for patients with severe and protracted illness; *however, because of their toxicity, they are not warranted in the vast majority of patients with RS.*

BEHÇET'S SYNDROME

A multisystem, inflammatory, relapsing, and chronic disorder that may include mucocutaneous, ocular, genital, articular, vascular, CNS, and GI involvement. Etiology is unknown; however, histopathologic vasculitic changes are common to all involved organs. Immunologic, including autoimmune, and viral causes and an HLA-related immunogenetic predisposition have been suggested. The syndrome generally begins in the 3rd decade and occurs twice as often in men as in women. Some cases have been reported in children. Although uncommon in the USA, Behçet's syndrome must be considered frequently in differential diagnosis.

Symptoms and Signs

Almost all patients have recurrent painful oral ulcers resembling those of aphthous stomatitis, and in most patients, these ulcers are the first manifestations of the disease. Similar ulcers occur on the penis and scrotum, where they are painful, or on the vulva and vagina, where they may be asymptomatic. Other symptoms follow in days to years. Ocular disease occurs in most cases: The most common is a relapsing iridocyclitis, sometimes with hypopyon and often initially presenting as pain, photophobia, and hazy vision. The posterior segment also may be involved, with choroiditis, retinal vasculitis, and papillitis. Untreated posterior uveitis may cause blindness. Various skin lesions occur in 80% of cases: papules, pustules, vesicles, and folliculitis. Particularly suggestive are erythema-nodosumlike lesions and (in about 40% of patients) inflammatory reactions to minor trauma, eg, needle punctures. A relatively mild, self-limiting, and nondestructive arthritis involving the knees and other large joints occurs in 50% of patients. Recurrent superficial or deep migratory thrombophlebitis develops in 25%, and may lead to vena caval obstruction. Arterial damage may cause aneurysms or thrombosis. CNS involvement (18%) may present as chronic meningoencephalitis, benign intracerebral hypertension, or life-threatening brainstem and spinal cord lesions. GI manifestations vary from nonspecific abdominal discomfort to a syndrome resembling regional enteritis (Crohn's disease). The generalized vasculitis also may involve the kidneys in the form of a usually asymptomatic focal glomerulonephritis. The lungs rarely are involved, with vasculitis and aneurysms of the pulmonary arteries.

Diagnosis

Diagnosis is clinical, and detection of manifestations may require months. Differential diagnosis includes the following diseases, discussed elsewhere in THE MANUAL: Reiter's syndrome, Stevens-Johnson syndrome, SLE, regional enteritis (Crohn's dis-

ease), ulcerative colitis, ankylosing spondylitis, and herpes simplex infection, especially with recurrent aseptic meningitis. Behçet's syndrome has no specific findings that exclude all alternative possibilities, but often is distinguished by the relapsing course and multiple organ involvement.

Laboratory abnormalities are nonspecific but characteristic of inflammatory disease (elevated ESR and α_2- and γ-globulins, and mild leukocytosis). Numerous immunologic abnormalities may be detected, including the presence of autoantibodies to affected tissues, and circulating immune complexes.

Prognosis and Treatment

The syndrome generally is benign, but with periods of remission and relapse that may last from weeks to years and even extend over several decades. Blindness, vena caval obstruction, and paralysis may complicate the course; the occasional fatalities usually are associated with neurologic, vascular, and GI involvement. Symptomatic therapy of the various manifestations is reasonably successful. Needle punctures should be avoided when possible, since they provoke inflammatory skin lesions. Topical corticosteroids may provide temporary symptomatic relief for ocular and oral disease. However, topical or systemic corticosteroids do not alter the frequency of relapses. Occasional patients with severe uveitis or CNS involvement will respond to high doses of systemic corticosteroids (prednisone 60 to 80 mg/day). Immunosuppressive drugs have been used with some success in patients with severe disease (eg, chlorambucil 0.1 to 0.2 mg/kg/day to prevent blindness in cases of posterior uveitis). Other agents that have been used include cyclophosphamide and azathioprine.

Treatment efficacy is difficult to determine because of the remitting nature of Behçet's syndrome.

RELAPSING POLYCHONDRITIS (RP)

An episodic, inflammatory, and destructive disorder involving cartilaginous and other connective tissues including the ear, joints, nose, larynx, trachea, eye, heart valves, and blood vessels. An autoimmune etiology is suggested by the frequent association with RA, systemic vasculitis, SLE, and other connective tissue diseases. RP occurs with equal frequency in men and women; onset typically is in middle age.

Symptoms, Signs, and Course

The most common presentation is acute pain, erythema, and swelling of the cartilaginous portions of both external ears, with an associated arthritis. The arthropathy varies from arthralgias to symmetric arthritis involving both large and small joints, with a predilection for the costochondral joints. Inflammation of the nasal cartilage is the next most common manifestation, followed in decreasing order of frequency by inflammation of the eye (conjunctivitis, scleritis, iritis, or chorioretinitis); cartilaginous tissues of the larynx, trachea, or bronchi; the internal ear; the cardiovascular system; and the skin. The course is characterized by bouts of acute inflammation, healing over a few weeks, with recurrences over several years. Destruction of supporting cartilaginous tissues becomes prominent in the later stages of the illness and is manifested as floppy ears, saddle nose, and visual, auditory, and vestibular abnormalities. Mortality after a 5-yr illness approaches 30%, and is usually due to collapse of laryngeal and tracheal cartilaginous supporting structures, or to cardiovascular involvement in the form of large vessel aneurysm, cardiac valvular insufficiency, or systemic vasculitis.

Diagnosis

Diagnosis is made on clinical grounds, and is considered established if over a period of time the patient develops 3 or more of the following: (1) bilateral chondritis of the external ear; (2) inflammatory polyarthritis; (3) nasal chondritis; (4) ocular inflammation; (5) respiratory tract chondritis; (6) auditory or vestibular dysfunction. Biopsy of

involved cartilaginous tissue may confirm the diagnosis, or help rule out alternative diagnoses such as Wegener's granulomatosis. The only laboratory abnormalities are those that accompany chronic inflammation; eg, anemia, leukocytosis, and elevated ESR.

Treatment

Mild cases may respond to symptomatic treatment with aspirin, indomethacin, or other nonsteroidal anti-inflammatory agents. More severe cases are usually treated with daily doses of 30 to 60 mg of prednisone with rapid tapering of the dose as soon as there is a clinical response. Very severe cases may require the addition of immunosuppressive agents such as cyclophosphamide (see also RHEUMATOID ARTHRITIS, above). None of the above-mentioned therapies have been tested in controlled trials, and it does not appear that they alter RP's ultimate course.

OSTEOARTHRITIS (OA)

(Degenerative Joint Disease; DJD; Osteoarthrosis; Hypertrophic Osteoarthritis)

Primarily a disorder of hyaline cartilage and subchondral bone, though all tissues in and around involved joints are hypertrophic.

Incidence: OA, the most common form of all articular disorders, first appears asymptomatically in the 2nd to 3rd decades and becomes universal by age 70. Almost all persons by age 40 have some pathologic changes in weight-bearing joints, although relatively few people are symptomatic. Men and women are equally affected, but onset is earlier in men. OA is found in all climates.

Phylogeny: OA occurs in almost all vertebrates, suggesting that it appeared with the evolutionary arrival of the bony skeleton. OA occurred in ancient animals, fish, amphibia, reptiles (dinosaurs), birds, mammoths, and cave bears. It is seen in whales, dolphins, and porpoises, animals that live supported by water, but not in 2 mammals that hang upside down: bats and sloths. This universality suggests an ancient paleozoic mechanism of repair, rather than a disease in the usual sense.

Classification

Traditionally OA is classified in 2 broad groups, primary (idiopathic) and secondary (some known causative factor or disease state). **Primary** OA includes peripheral joints, notably the distal interphalangeal and proximal interphalangeal (producing **Heberden's** and **Bouchard's nodes);** 1st carpal metacarpal joint; cervical and lumbar spine; 1st metatarsal phalangeal joint (big toe); hips; knees; intervertebral disks and zygapophyseal joints in the spine; and several variant subsets (eg, erosive, inflammatory OA; chondromalacia patellae —*a mild OA of patellar cartilage in young people not affecting the principal weight-bearing site, with mild to moderate pain and stiffness*; and a variant, diffuse idiopathic skeletal hyperostosis).

Secondary OA: see Etiology, below.

Etiology

Etiology is unknown. OA appears to be the result of a complex system of interacting mechanical, biologic, biochemical, and enzymatic feedback loops; when one or more fails, the clinical events follow. Many mechanisms can initiate the cellular and tissue events that constitute a final common pathway; eg, anything that changes the microenvironment of the chondrocyte. This includes congenital joint abnormalities; genetic defects (primary generalized OA); infectious, metabolic, endocrine, and neuropathic diseases; virtually any disease process that alters the normal structure and function of hyaline cartilage (eg, RA, gout, chondrocalcinosis); and acute or chronic trauma (including fracture) to the hyaline cartilage or tissue surrounding it (eg, involving prolonged overuse of a joint or group of joints, as in certain occupations—foundry work,

coal mining, and bus driving). Peculiarly, pneumatic hammer drillers and long-distance running champions have no increase in OA compared with age- and sex-matched controls.

Pathophysiology

Normal joints have a coefficient of friction so low that without very unusual overuse and trauma, they cannot wear out. **Hyaline cartilage** is avascular, aneural, and alymphatic. Only 5% of the cartilage volume is occupied by cells. Nevertheless, hyaline cartilage lesions can and do heal. **Chondrocytes** divide and increase their rates of both synthesis and degradative processes, but they have the longest cell cycle in the body (similar to CNS cells and muscle cells), never dividing unless some alteration occurs in the microenvironment. Cartilage health depends on the pumping action (compression and release) of weight-bearing and use; ie, on compression, to discard used fluid and materials, which move into the joint space and then into venules; and on release, to reexpand, hyperhydrate, and absorb the nutrients necessary for chondrocyte health and function.

The most probable **initial event** in OA is mitosis of the chondrocyte with increased synthesis of the proteoglycans and type II collagen, the principal structural elements of cartilage. The earliest triggering event is a decrease in concentration of proteoglycan in the immediate neighborhood of the chondrocyte. The **second event** is increased synthesis of bone by osteoblasts in the subchondral bone, presumably by intercellular communication between chondrocyte and osteoblast in the subchondral bone cells. With increased bone formation in the subchondral area, physical properties change, the bone becomes stiffer, and microfractures occur. With microfractures come callus formation and hence more stiffness and more microfracture. The **third event** is metaplasia of the peripheral synovial cells resulting in formation of **osteochondrophytes** (the tissue is not only bone but a mixture of connective tissues with a coating of fibrocartilage and sometimes islands of hyaline cartilage on the surface) around the periphery of the joint, in the path of least resistance. The degree of formation of these "spurs" varies from joint to joint and in some proportion to underlying causative mechanisms. The **fourth event** is the formation of bony cysts **(pseudocysts)** in the marrow below the subchondral bone. The mechanism is that of extrusion of joint fluid through the hyaline cartilage clefts into the marrow with a fibroblastic, osteoblastic cellular reaction around the synovial fluid.

The **gross pathology** is that of a roughening or loss of surface of the hyaline cartilage, pitting, and irregularities, proceeding to gross ulceration with at first focal, then diffuse areas of loss of cartilage surface. Proliferation of new bone, capsule, tendon, cartilage, and synovium (all the structural elements of the joint) occurs. Basically, this is remodeling of movable joints, characterized by 2 pathologic processes: deterioration and loss of a bearing surface, and proliferation of all osteoarticular tissue at the margins of the joint and under the detached joint surface. By the time symptoms appear, virtually all cases have active synovial proliferation and synovitis.

Symptoms and Signs

Initially, OA is noninflammatory and onset is subtle and gradual, usually involving one to only a few joints. Pain is the earliest symptom, usually made worse by exercise. Morning stiffness follows inactivity but lasts < 15 to 30 min, improved with exercise. Acute episodes of severe synovitis may occur in those who have gout or pseudogout (monosodium urate or calcium pyrophosphate dihydrate crystal deposition disease as primary initiating mechanisms of OA). As the disease progresses, joint motion becomes diminished, flexion contractures occur, tenderness and crepitus or grating sensations appear. Joint enlargement induced by the proliferative reactions of cartilage, bone, ligament, tendon, capsules, and chronic synovial proliferation and inflammation is ultimately characteristic of OA.

As ligaments become lax, the joint has increasing instability with more local pain and the clinical appearance of a limp. Tenderness on palpation and pain on passive motion are late signs, and muscle spasm and contracture add to the pain. Mechanical block by osteophytes or loose bodies occurs. Deformity and subluxations are a consequence of loss of cartilage volume, subchondral bone collapse, osteochondrophytes, muscle atrophy, and pseudocysts.

OA of the cervical and lumbar spine is common. In the cervical spine, symptoms may be related to radiculitis by compression of nerve roots secondary to the proliferative osteochondrophytes; ie, pain from intervertebral disks, Luschka's joints, or zygapophyseal joint lesions; functional compromise of the vertebral artery, neuromyopathy secondary to compression; sometimes spinal cord infarcts (spinal "stroke") or esophageal compression due to pressure by anterior bony projections. Ligamentous structures, capsules, muscles, tendons, and periosteum are all pain-sensitive; there is an increase in venous pressure within the subchondral bone marrow, also a source of pain.

Diagnosis

Diagnosis is usually based on symptoms and signs, as described above, or by x-ray in asymptomatic patients.

Laboratory and x-ray studies: The ESR is normal or moderately increased. Blood studies are mainly of value to rule out other causes of arthritis (eg, gout, RA) or to detect other primary disorders (see above). Synovianalysis often discloses joint fluid characteristics of OA (see TABLES 107–3 and 107–4 in Ch. 107). The **radiologic criteria** are (1) irregular or asymmetric narrowing of the joint space; (2) increase in radiologic density of the subchondral bone; (3) formation of osteochondrophytes at the periphery of the joints; (4) formation of pseudocysts in the subchondral marrow. Isotope scanning procedures often identify active inflammation, and may help to separate OA from other disorders.

Differential diagnosis: While diagnosis is usually straightforward, other common rheumatic diseases require consideration (ie, RA, ankylosing spondylitis, psoriatic arthritis, the seronegative spondyloarthropathies, and calcium pyrophosphate crystal deposition disease). OA occurring outside of the usual joint sites of involvement suggests further consideration regarding etiology; eg, endocrine, metabolic, and neoplastic disorders affecting bone.

Prognosis and Treatment

Though the pathophysiology usually proceeds to the appearance of symptoms and signs, varying degrees of disability, and functional compromise, occasionally but with no predictability arrest or even reversal occurs.

Treatment includes **rehabilitation,** which implies preventing dysfunction, attempting to begin management before the disability develops, and decreasing the severity or duration of disability. Primary considerations are the stage and magnitude of tissue changes in the specific patient, the number of joints involved, the pain cycle of the patient, considering whether the pain is due to biomechanical defects or inflammation, and the patient's lifestyle.

Treatment also includes **patient education** regarding the nature of the problem (physiology and biomechanics), the prognosis (usually benign), the necessity for cooperation, and achieving and maintaining an optimum level of overall physical fitness. **Exercise** (range of motion, isometric, isotonic, isokinetic, postural, strengthening) maintains healthy cartilage and range of motion and develops the stress-absorbing tendons and muscles. A balance must be kept between rest (q 4 to 6 h in the daytime to rehydrate the cartilage) and exercise and use. **Activities of daily living** should receive attention: instructing the patient to avoid soft chairs or recliners and pillows under the knees; sit in a straight chair with no slumping; use a firm bed with a bed board and a

car seat designed to be most comfortable; perform postural exercises; and continue employment, physical activity, and intellectual functioning.

Drugs: Aspirin is the drug of choice for both anti-inflammatory and analgesic reasons. Other nonsteroidal anti-inflammatory drugs **(NSAIDs)** may be used (see also in RHEUMATOID ARTHRITIS, above; and Ch. 282), as they also inhibit prostaglandins by blocking lipo-oxygenase conversion of cell membrane lipids to arachidonic acid. **Muscle relaxants** include diazepam, cyclobenzaprine, carisoprodol, methocarbamol (usually in low doses).

Oral corticosteroid therapy usually is *not* indicated. **Intra-articular corticosteroids** are helpful with evidence of inflammation, usually needed only intermittently. The corticosteroid preparations themselves are crystalline and regularly induce a transient synovitis. Pure **analgesic drugs** occasionally may be useful, and **tricyclic antidepressants** may be helpful for depressed patients.

Surgery: Laminectomy, osteotomy, and total joint replacement should be considered when all conservative therapy has failed. In spinal OA or cervical spine fracture, various supports, specific exercise programs, and transcutaneous nerve stimulation are occasionally useful.

NEUROGENIC ARTHROPATHY

(Neuropathic Arthropathy; Charcot's Joints)

A destructive arthropathy with impaired pain perception or position sense.

Etiology

Impaired deep pain sensation or proprioception affects the joint's normal protective reflexes, often allowing trauma (especially repeated minor episodes) and small periarticular fractures to pass unrecognized. Also, increased bone blood flow from reflex vasodilatation, resulting in active bone resorption, may produce fractures and joint damage and repair. For conditions associated with Charcot's joints, see TABLE 108–4. Intra-articular deposition of calcium pyrophosphate dihydrate crystals and the consequent inflammatory reaction may accelerate joint destruction due to other conditions. Local joint infection associated with leprosy and diabetes mellitus may be a causative factor. Muscle hypotonia, ligamentous laxity, and distention of the joint capsule by an effusion are contributory factors tending to accelerate disease progression.

TABLE 108–4. CONDITIONS UNDERLYING NEUROGENIC ARTHROPATHY

Diabetes mellitus	Gigantism with hypertrophic neuropathy
Tabes dorsalis	Impaired pain sensitivity due to use of: Intra-articular and systemic corticosteroids
Syringomyelia	Phenylbutazone
Spina bifida with meningomyelocele (in children)	Indomethacin Excessive amounts of ethyl alcohol
Leprosy	Congenital insensitivity to pain
Tumors and injuries of the peripheral nerves and spinal cord	Familial-hereditary neuropathies: Peroneal muscular atrophy (Charcot-Marie-Tooth disease)
Degenerative spinal disease with nerve root compression	Hereditary sensory neuropathy Hypertrophic interstitial neuropathy (Déjérine-Sottas disease)
Subacute combined degeneration of the spinal cord	Familial dysautonomia (Riley-Day syndrome)
Amyloid neuropathy (secondary amyloid)	Familial amyloid polyneuropathy

Symptoms, Signs, and Diagnosis

In its early stages, the condition is often confused with osteoarthritis **(OA).** Some pain, a prominent—often hemorrhagic—effusion, and subluxation and instability of the joint are usually present. Acute joint dislocation sometimes occurs at this stage. Neurogenic arthropathy progresses much more rapidly than OA. Onset of arthropathy may be long delayed from onset of the neurologic condition, but once the arthropathy starts it can be rapidly progressive and lead to complete joint disorganization in a few months.

In a fully developed Charcot joint, hypertrophic or destructive changes may predominate, or findings may be mixed. Pain is often absent or less severe than would be expected from the degree of joint destruction, but may be severe if the disease has progressed rapidly and periarticular fractures or tense hematomas exist. The joint is swollen from bony overgrowth and massive synovial effusion. Deformity results from fracture with displacement, or dislocation following destruction of articular surfaces, ligamentous laxity, and muscular hypotonia. Fractures and bony metaplasia will cause many loose bodies (pieces of cartilage or bone) to slough into the joint, producing a coarse, grating, often audible crepitus usually more unpleasant for the observer than for the patient. The joint may feel like "a bag of bones."

Though most joints can be involved, the knee is affected as often as the sum of all other joints. Distribution depends largely on the underlying disease. Thus, in tabes dorsalis and diabetes mellitus, the lower limbs are affected (knee and hip in tabes; foot in diabetes). In syringomyelia, the upper limb joints are most commonly affected, especially the elbow and shoulder. Frequently, only one joint is affected; usually not more than 2 or 3 (except for the small joints of the feet), in an asymmetric distribution.

The **diagnosis** should be considered in a patient with an appropriate neurologic disorder who develops a destructive but relatively painless arthropathy. A lapse of several years from the onset of the underlying neurologic condition to the onset of the arthropathy is usual. An abnormal gallium scan is described in uncomplicated neurogenic arthropathy.

X-rays show a swollen joint with synovial effusion and subluxation of the articular surfaces. Sclerosis of the bone ends, usually present, may be absent in advanced destructive disease. The bones are deformed, and new bone formation usually is evident adjacent to the cortex, starting within the joint capsule and often extending well up the shaft of a long bone. Calcification and ossification occur in the soft tissues, on rare occasions leading to bony bridging across the joint. However, this may be transient, and even extensive soft-tissue calcification may disappear on a subsequent radiograph. Large, bizarrely shaped osteophytes are seen at the joint margins; these may break off to form the numerous intra-articular loose bodies that characterize this condition. Radiologic evidence of spinal involvement (the characteristic "parrot's beak" osteophytes) is frequently found in the absence of any clinical suggestion of disease at this site.

Complications include septic arthritis and compression of adjacent structures such as blood vessels, nerves, or spinal cord. Local signs are difficult to interpret but systemic manifestations (eg, malaise and fever) indicate that the joint should be aspirated and synovial fluid cultured.

Prophylaxis and Treatment

Prevention of onset of arthropathy is important in a patient at risk (eg, with severe tabes). Early diagnosis and immobilization of an often painless fracture may stop evolution of the neuroarthropathy. An unstable joint should be protected by splints, special boots, or calipers. Arthrodesis using internal fixation, a compression technic, and an adequate bone graft may be successful in a grossly disorganized joint. A total hip replacement still functioning well after 7 yr has been described in a patient with a

Charcot joint whose tabes did not result in an ataxic gait. In the past, prostheses have loosened and dislocated, but this case suggests the possibility of better results. Successful treatment of the underlying neurologic condition may slow progression of the arthropathy and, if joint destruction is still in the early stages, reverse the process.

GOUT

A recurrent acute arthritis of peripheral joints which results from deposition, in and about the joints and tendons, of crystals of monosodium urate from supersaturated hyperuricemic body fluids; the arthritis may become chronic and deforming. Not all hyperuricemic persons develop gout. The greater the degree and duration of hyperuricemia, the greater the chance of crystal deposition and of acute attacks of gout.

Pathophysiology

The normal range for serum urate levels depends on the method used for determination. The upper limit in most men is < 7 mg/dL of serum; for women, about 1 mg/dL lower until after menopause, when it may approach that of men. This difference correlates with the clinical observation that only 5% of gouty patients are women, most of them postmenopausal.

Limited solubility of uric acid and its salts in biologic fluids accounts for the major pathologic findings. Monosodium urate crystals are deposited in and about the joints and tendons and in the tubules or the interstitial tissue of the renal parenchyma. An inflammatory reaction to the deposits is basic to the acute attack of gout. Continued accretion of the crystals produces the characteristic gouty tophi responsible for erosive joint damage and chronic disability. In the urinary tract, because of the lower pH of urine, free uric acid is precipitated and forms calculi with an incidence 1000 times that of the general population. Fewer than 5% of patients with gout slowly develop progressive, fatal renal dysfunction.

Hyperuricemia may be caused by various abnormalities of purine metabolism, genetic and acquired. Excessive purine synthesis is the most common; diminished renal clearance of uric acid, the other major factor. Medical disorders associated with hyperuricemia and gout include proliferative hematopoietic diseases, psoriasis, myxedema, hypo- and hyperparathyroidism, hypertension, myocardial infarction, advanced primary renal diseases, obesity, and various hereditary diseases including Down's syndrome and glycogen storage disease, Type I. A rare but well-defined example is sex-linked uricaciduria with a deficiency of the enzyme hypoxanthine-guanine phosphoribosyltransferase. It is associated with excessive uric acid production, a tendency to develop uric acid kidney stones, and severe gouty arthritis and nephropathy at an early age. A spectrum of clinical neurologic symptoms may be present, which correlate with the severity of the enzyme deficiency (the **Lesch-Nyhan syndrome** —with choreoathetosis, spasticity, and mental retardation—is the extreme example; see also in Ch. 203). Hyperuricemia and gouty arthritis also can develop secondary to acquired lead poisoning or diuretic therapy (usually with thiazides).

Symptoms and Signs

Acute gouty arthritis appears without warning. It may be precipitated by minor trauma, overindulgence in food or alcohol, surgery, fatigue, emotional stress, infection, or administration of penicillin, insulin, or mercurial diuretics. Acute mono- or polyarticular pain, often nocturnal, is usually the first symptom. The pain becomes progressively more severe and is described as throbbing, crushing, or excruciating. Examination shows signs resembling an acute infection, with swelling, warmth, redness, and exquisite tenderness. The overlying skin is tense, hot, shiny, and a dusky red or purplish color. The metatarsophalangeal joint of the great toe is frequently involved **(podagra),** but the instep, ankle, knee, wrist, and elbow are common sites. Initially, only a single joint may be affected; in later attacks, several joints can be affected

simultaneously or sequentially. Systemic reactions may include fever, tachycardia, chills, malaise, and leukocytosis.

The first few attacks usually last only a few days, but later untreated attacks may persist for weeks. Local symptoms and signs eventually regress and joint function returns. Asymptomatic intervals vary but tend to become shorter as the disease progresses. Without prophylaxis (see below) several attacks may occur each year and **chronic joint symptoms** develop, with permanent erosive joint deformity. Limitation of motion often involves multiple joints of the hands and feet; rarely, the shoulder, sacroiliac, sternoclavicular joints, or the cervical spine are involved. Urate deposits are common in the walls of bursae and tendon sheaths. Enlarging tophi on the hands and feet may erupt and discharge chalky masses of urate crystals.

Diagnosis

The clinical features of acute gouty arthritis are so distinctive that a tentative diagnosis usually can be made by history and physical examination. An elevated serum urate content (> 7 mg/dL) supports the diagnosis but is not specific. Demonstration in tissue or synovial fluid of needle-shaped urate crystals that are free in the fluid or engulfed by phagocytes, and a therapeutic response to colchicine within 12 to 48 h are pathognomonic. The crystals, identified in the light microscope, are *negatively* birefringent when viewed under crossed polarizing filters attached to a microscope. These findings are helpful in establishing the diagnosis in atypical gout.

Radiologic examination of the affected joints may show punched-out lesions in subchondral bone, commonly in the first metatarsophalangeal joint. The urate deposits must reach 5 mm in diameter before becoming visible on x-ray. Such lesions are not specific or diagnostic.

In patients with non-urate crystalline deposit disease (chondrocalcinosis—see below), the acute synovitis is due to *positively* birefringent calcium pyrophosphate dihydrate crystals of various shapes; in addition, radiopaque calcium deposits are present in articular cartilage (particularly the knee), and the clinical course is milder than in gout. An acutely septic joint may be confused with an acute gouty joint, but the absence of regional lymphadenopathy in gout and the serum uric acid content help differentiate. Microscopic examination and culture of the synovial fluid provide proof by demonstrating either urate crystals or bacteria. Acute rheumatic fever with joint involvement and polyarticular rheumatism may simulate gout in young persons. In RA, joint involvement tends to be symmetric; the duration of an acute attack is longer and the onset more gradual than in acute gout. Heberden's nodes of OA may resemble gouty tophi but are seldom associated with acute symptoms.

Prognosis

Current therapy permits most patients to live a normal life, if the diagnosis is made early and permanent medical supervision and prophylactic medication are accepted by the patient. For those with advanced disease, some reconstitution of joint structure can be achieved. Tophi can be resolved, joint function improved, and renal dysfunction arrested. Gout is more severe in patients whose initial symptoms appear before age 30. Almost 10 to 20% of patients with gout develop urolithiasis. Complications include obstruction and infection, with secondary tubulointerstitial disease. Untreated progressive renal dysfunction, usually related to coexisting hypertension, diabetes mellitus, or some other cause of nephropathy, leads to further impairment in the excretion of urate, accelerating the pathologic process in the joints, and is also the greatest threat to life.

Treatment

Objectives are (1) termination of the acute attack with an anti-inflammatory drug, (2) prevention of recurrent acute attacks by daily use of colchicine, and (3) prevention

of further deposition of monosodium urate crystals and resolution of existing tophi (achieved by lowering the urate concentration in body fluids). A preventive maintenance program should aim at averting both the disability resulting from erosion of bone and joint cartilage and the renal damage. Specific treatment depends on the stage and severity of the disease.

Acute attack: Colchicine remains the preferred drug when the diagnosis is in doubt. The response usually is dramatic. Joint pains generally begin to subside after 12 h of treatment and are gone within 36 to 48 h. The dose of colchicine is 1 mg orally q 2 h until a response is obtained or until diarrhea or vomiting appears. Severe episodes may require from 4 to 7 mg (average, 5 mg). Because of the toxic effects of colchicine overdosage, not more than 7 mg should be taken in 48 h for a given attack. When treatment causes diarrhea, paregoric 5 mL orally q 2 to 4 h is helpful. Colchicine may also be given IV if the GI tract is intolerant of oral medication. Colchicine 2 mg is diluted with 0.9% sodium chloride to a value of 20 mL and injected slowly; not more than 4 mg are given in 24 h.

Nonsteroidal anti-inflammatory drugs **(NSAIDs)** are effective in acute attacks of established gout, and are especially useful for patients intolerant of colchicine. Daily doses for 2 or 3 days are usually taken with food. The NSAIDs include indomethacin, ibuprofen, naproxen, tolmetin sodium, piroxicam, and sulindac. Corticosteroids can produce rapid and complete remission but generally are used only when other drugs are contraindicated. In an effusion of the knee, withdrawal of fluid followed by instillation of prednisolone tebutate 25 mg usually brings relief.

In addition to specific therapy, rest, abundant fluid intake to combat dehydration and decrease urate precipitation in the kidneys, and a soft diet are indicated. To control the pain, codeine 30 to 60 mg or meperidine 50 to 100 mg orally q 4 h may be needed.

Treatment with drugs that lower the serum urate concentration should be deferred until acute symptoms have subsided.

Intercritical period: The frequency of acute attacks is reduced by daily colchicine 0.6 mg orally bid to qid (depending on tolerance and severity). An extra 1 or 2 mg of colchicine taken at the first suggestion of an attack will abort most.

Colchicine does not retard the progressive joint damage produced by tophi. It can be prevented, however, and many tophaceous deposits resolved, by lowering the serum urate concentration to the normal range and maintaining it indefinitely, either by increasing uric acid excretion with a uricosuric drug or by blocking uric acid production with allopurinol, or, in tophaceous gout, by using both drugs daily. Such hypouricemic therapy is indicated for gouty patients with tophaceous deposits, a serum urate concentration consistently > 9 mg/dL, persistent joint symptoms despite only a modest increase in serum urate, or impaired renal function.

Control of hyperuricemia should be started in conjunction with daily colchicine treatment during a quiescent phase, because all such therapy is associated with an increased tendency to develop acute attacks during the first few weeks or months of treatment. Periodic determination of serum urate concentration is a helpful guide to drug effectiveness. The dosage and selection of the drug should be adjusted to achieve a significant reduction in serum urate concentration. Resolution of susceptible tophi may take months or years.

In uricosuric therapy, either 0.5-gm tablets of probenecid or 100-mg tablets of sulfinpyrazone are given orally; the dose is adjusted to maintain a serum urate concentration in the normal range. The starting dose should be ½ tablet bid, gradually increasing the dosage over 10 days to up to 4 tablets/day. Sulfinpyrazone has a greater uricosuric effect than does probenecid, but is more toxic. Salicylates antagonize the uricosuric effect of either drug and should be **avoided**. Acetaminophen provides a comparable analgesic effect without interfering with the uricosuric action.

Inhibition of uric acid synthesis by allopurinol, 200 to 600 mg/day in divided doses, also controls serum urate concentration. In addition to blocking the enzyme (xanthine oxidase) responsible for uric acid formation, it corrects excessive purine synthesis. It is especially helpful in managing patients who repeatedly pass uric acid calculi or who have severe renal dysfunction. Established calculi may be dissolved by allopurinol. Adverse effects of allopurinol include mild GI distress, skin rash, and drowsiness. Where available, use of extracorporeal sound wave lithotripsy may be considered to disintegrate calculi.

Adjuncts to treatment: A high fluid intake of at least 3 L/day is desirable for all gouty patients and especially those who are chronic uric acid stone formers. Alkalinization of the urine with sodium bicarbonate or trisodium citrate 5 gm tid is recommended also. Drugs are so effective in lowering the serum urate concentration that rigid restriction of the purine content of the diet usually is unnecessary. Weight reduction in obese patients should be undertaken during a quiescent phase of the disease.

Surgical correction of severely damaged joints or removal of tophi to relieve tendon entrapment or for cosmetic reasons should be deferred until the disease and the serum urate concentration have been controlled medically. Large tophi should be removed surgically; all others except those walled off by extensive fibrosis should resolve under adequate prophylactic therapy.

Idiopathic Hyperuricemia

Hard data regarding specific treatment of non-gouty asymptomatic hyperuricemia are few. Until this deficiency is corrected, it is suggested that either probenecid, sulfinpyrazone, or allopurinol be given daily only to those persons under age 40 with a persistent hyperuricemia of 12 mg/dL or greater, whose urinary excretion in a 24-hour sample is < 1000 mg.

CHONDROCALCINOSIS

(Pseudogout; Calcium Pyrophosphate Dihydrate [CPPD] Crystal Deposition Disease)

A joint disease with protean manifestations which may include intermittent attacks of acute arthritis; a degenerative arthropathy that is often severe but can be asymptomatic; and x-ray evidence of calcinosis of the articular cartilage in characteristic sites.

Etiology and Incidence

The cause is unknown. Frequent association with other conditions such as trauma (including surgery), amyloidosis, myxedema, hyperparathyroidism, gout, and hemochromatosis suggests that the deposits of CPPD in the cartilage are secondary to degenerative or metabolic changes in cartilage. Symptomatic disease usually appears in maturity. The incidence of calcinosis of the cartilage in persons over age 50 is appreciable, reaching nearly 50% by age 90. Both sexes are affected equally.

Symptoms and Signs

Acute or subacute attacks of arthritis **(pseudogout)** occur, usually in the larger peripheral joints. Such attacks sometimes follow the pattern of uric acid gout but are less severe. There may be complete freedom between attacks, or distress may continue, with low-grade symptoms similar to RA. These patterns tend to persist for life. Asymptomatic calcinosis has been observed by x-ray in the intervertebral cartilages and in the symphysis pubis.

Diagnosis

Identifying CPPD crystals in a drop of synovial fluid is diagnostic (see Differentiating Inflammatory and Noninflammatory Joint Disease in Ch. 107). Crystals may be seen engulfed in leukocytes or floating free. They are weakly *positively* birefringent in

contrast to the strongly *negatively* birefringent sodium urate crystals. The x-ray finding of linear calcification in articular cartilage, especially fibrocartilages, supports the diagnosis.

Prognosis and Treatment

The prognosis usually is excellent, but severe destructive arthropathy resembling neuropathic (Charcot's) joints may occur. Colchicine is effective if given 1 mg IV followed by 1 mg in 12 h if pain persists. (IV administration of colchicine is also discussed in GOUT, above.) An acute synovial effusion should be drained, the fluid inspected for crystals, and a corticosteroid microcrystalline suspension instilled into the joint. Indomethacin 75 to 150 mg daily is helpful during the acute attack.

109. NONARTICULAR RHEUMATISM

BURSITIS

Acute or chronic inflammation of a bursa. Bursae are saclike cavities filled with synovial fluid and located at tissue sites where friction occurs, such as where tendons or muscles pass over bony prominences. Bursae facilitate normal movement and minimize friction between moving parts. Deep bursae may communicate with joints. Most bursitis occurs in the shoulder (subacromial or subdeltoid bursitis), but other common forms exist: olecranon (miner's elbow), pre- or suprapatellar (housemaid's knee), retrocalcaneal (Achilles), iliopectineal (iliopsoas), ischial (tailor's or weaver's bottom), trochanteric, and first metatarsal head (bunion). The **etiology** of most bursitis is unknown, though it may be caused by trauma, chronic overuse, acute or chronic infection, inflammatory arthritis, gout, RA, or pyogenic organisms, particularly *Staphylococcus aureus*. Tuberculous organisms rarely cause bursitis.

Symptoms and Signs

Subacromial bursitis (subdeltoid bursitis or supraspinatus tendinitis) presents with localized pain and tenderness of the shoulder, particularly in abduction in an arc from 50° to 130°. Calcific subacromial bursitis and calcific supraspinatous tendinitis may be indistinguishable clinically and radiographically. The former may result from partial or complete tears; the latter, from crystal release. **Bicipital tendinitis** results from inflammation of the tendon sheath surrounding the long head of the biceps which originates on the supraglenoid tubercle and extends through the articular capsule of the shoulder joint along the bicipital groove of the humerus to insert on the radius. Tenderness is noted over the bicipital groove of the humerus and the local pain is aggravated by resisted flexion and supination of the forearm.

Acute bursitis is characterized by pain, localized tenderness, and limitation of motion. The bursal wall secretes a serous effusion when inflamed. Swelling and redness are frequently present if the bursa is superficial (eg, prepatellar, olecranon). Chemical (eg, crystal-induced) or bacterial inflammation is particularly painful, red, and warm.

Chronic bursitis may follow previous attacks of bursitis or repeated trauma. Acute symptoms may develop following unusual exercise or strain. The bursal wall is thickened, with proliferation of the synovial lining. The bursa eventually may develop adhesions, villus formation, tags, and calcareous deposits. Pain, swelling, and tenderness may result in muscle atrophy and limitation of motion. Subdeltoid calcific deposits may be demonstrated radiographically, particularly in the supraspinatus tendon of the rotator cuff. Attacks may last from a few days to several weeks, with multiple recurrences. In gout, crystals may be isolated in the olecranon and prepatellar bursae during acute attacks of inflammation.

Diagnosis

Periarticular tendon or muscle tears, pyogenic bursitis, synovitis, osteomyelitis, and cellulitis must be ruled out. Pathologic processes may simultaneously involve a communicating bursa and joint. Localized tenderness over the particular bursa or inflamed tendon should be elicited, or swelling or synovial fluid from superficial bursae (eg, olecranon or prepatellar) demonstrated. Infection should be excluded in cases of particularly painful, red, and warm swellings.

Treatment

For noninfected acute bursitis, immobilization and high doses of nonsteroidal anti-inflammatory agents (eg, indomethacin, ibuprofen, or naproxen) accompanied by narcotic analgesics, if necessary, may be helpful. If not, aspiration and intrabursal injection of depot corticosteroids for soft-tissue injections, 1 or 2 mL (triamcinolone acetonide as 10 mg/mL or 40 mg/mL) mixed with a similar volume of local anesthetic, following infiltration with 1% local anesthetic is the treatment of choice. The depot corticosteroid dose and volume of mixture is gauged to the size of the bursa. The smallest-gauge needle should be used to inject tendon sheaths, but the larger needles used in aspiration may serve for bursal injections. Infectious agent etiology should be excluded. Reaspiration and injection may be required with resistant inflammatory processes. Systemic corticosteroids (prednisone 15 to 30 mg/day or equivalent for 3 days) are indicated in resistant acute cases in which infection or gout has been excluded. Rest and splinting are effective in the early active stages. Voluntary movement should be increased as pain subsides. Pendulum exercises are particularly helpful for the shoulder joint.

Chronic bursitis is treated as acute bursitis, except that splinting and rest are less likely to be helpful. Surgical removal or large-needle aspiration of radiologically demonstrated calcium in chronic calcific supraspinatus tendinitis may rarely be necessary if corticosteroid injections are not helpful. Disabling adhesive capsulitis of the shoulder may require repeated local corticosteroid injections and intensive physical therapy. Manipulation under anesthesia does not improve the long-term results unless other measures mentioned to correct adhesive capsulitis are followed. Muscle atrophy should be corrected by exercises to reestablish range of motion and strength. Infection requires proper antibiotics and drainage or excision therapy. Bursitis may be recurrent if the underlying cause (eg, RA, gout, or chronic occupational strain) is not corrected.

TENDINITIS AND TENOSYNOVITIS

Inflammation of the lining of the tendon sheath (tenosynovitis) and of the enclosed tendon (tendinitis) usually occur simultaneously. The synovial-lined tendon sheath usually is the site of maximum inflammation, but the inflammatory response may involve the enclosed tendon (eg, as a result of calcium deposit). Tendinitis and bursitis are terms which may be used interchangeably to describe the same process, since bursae (see above) are often located near tendons; eg, the subacromial bursa and rotator cuff tendons of the humerus.

Etiology

The etiology is often unknown, but most instances occur in middle and older ages as the vascularity of tendons attenuates and repetitive microtrauma may result in greater injury. Repeated or extreme trauma (short of rupture), strain, or excessive (unaccustomed) exercise is most frequently causative. The tendon sheaths may also be involved in systemic diseases (most commonly RA, progressive systemic sclerosis, gout, Reiter's syndrome, and amyloidosis) and when blood cholesterol levels are elevated (hyperlipoproteinemia, Type II). In younger adults, particularly females, disseminated gonococcal infection may cause a migratory tenosynovitis, with or without localized synovitis. The most common sites of inflammation are the shoulder capsule and associated ten-

dons, flexor carpi ulnaris, flexor digitorum, hip capsule and associated tendons, hamstrings, and Achilles tendons, as well as the abductor pollicis longus and extensor pollicis brevis, which share a common fibrous sheath **(De Quervain's disease).**

Symptoms and Signs

The involved tendons are usually painful on motion; their sheaths may be visibly swollen because of fluid accumulation and inflammation, or may remain dry but cause friction rubs felt on movement of the tendon in its sheath or heard with a stethoscope. Along the tendon, localized tenderness of variable severity is present; it may be severe and associated with disabling pain on movement. Calcium deposition in the tendon and its sheath may be seen by x-ray.

Treatment

Symptomatic relief is provided by immobilization (splint or cast) or rest of the part, application of heat or cold (whichever benefits the patient), analgesic agents locally, and nonsteroidal anti-inflammatory agents **(NSAIDs)** systemically; ie, full doses of aspirin, indomethacin, or comparable drugs qid for 7 to 10 days. Colchicine or NSAIDs may be helpful (see GOUT in Ch. 108 for dosage regimens) if urate deposits are responsible. Controlled exercise several times daily (becoming progressively more active with tolerance) is indicated, especially to prevent "frozen shoulder," after acute inflammation is controlled.

Injection into the tendon sheath of a depot corticosteroid indicated for soft-tissue injection, such as dexamethasone acetate, methylprednisolone acetate, or hydrocortisone acetate, 1 or 2 mL mixed in equal volume with 1% local anesthetic, depending on severity and site, may be helpful. Following infiltration with 1% lidocaine, a 27- or 25-gauge needle with bevel down is angled toward the tendon. As it reaches the space between tendon and sheath, resistance is low and the injectate is felt to balloon along the tendon sheath as it enters the synovial space. The injection is made blindly at the site of maximum tenderness if the specific inflammation site cannot be identified. Care should be taken not to inject the tendon, as it can weaken and rupture in active persons. Reexamination of a less inflamed site 3 or 4 days later often discloses the specific lesion, and a second injection can be made with greater precision. Rest of the injected part is advisable to diminish risk of tendon rupture.

The patient should be warned of the infrequent occurrence of a "post-injection flare," which is probably a form of crystal (depot corticosteroid)-induced synovitis. This may occur within several hours after injection, usually does not last longer than 24 h, and responds to cold application plus short-term analgesics.

Injections and symptomatic therapy may be required every 2 or 3 wk for 1 or 2 mo for resolution. Surgical exploration and removal of inflamed or calcific deposits, followed by graded physical therapy, may be considered in persistent cases. Surgery is rarely necessary, except for release of fibro-osseous tunnels (as in **De Quervain's disease**) or for tenosynovectomy of chronic inflammation, as in RA.

TENNIS ELBOW
(Lateral Humeral Epicondylitis)

A strain of the lateral forearm muscles (extensors of the digits and wrist) or their tendinous attachments near their origin on the lateral epicondyle of the humerus. Medial humeral epicondylitis (golfer's elbow) is a comparable syndrome involving forearm fibers—pronators and their attachments. These complaints are common but their etiology or pathogenesis is uncertain. Lateral humeral epicondylitis may be caused by repetitive strenuous supination of the wrist against resistance, as in manual screwdriving, or by violent extension of the wrist with the hand pronated, as in tennis. The disorder can be disabling. It must be differentiated from that involving the radiohumeral joint. The middle-aged athlete or worker is at greatest risk for this condition.

Symptoms and Signs

Pain directly over the lateral epicondyle of the humerus may be severe and radiate to the outer side of the arm and forearm. It is aggravated by dorsiflexion and supination of the wrist against resistance or by resisted extension of the fingers while the elbow is extended. Point tenderness is present just distal to the lateral epicondyle. Weakness of the dorsiflexed wrist may be pronounced. X-rays are negative. Infiltrating the area around the lateral epicondyle at the site of maximal tenderness with 1 to 2 mL of 1% lidocaine, using the narrowest gauge needle, relieves symptoms and signs and establishes the diagnosis in doubtful cases. Differential diagnosis includes radiohumeral joint inflammation; eg, in RA or gout, and referred pain from cervical spine disease.

Treatment

Management depends on severity. In mild cases, avoiding the pain-producing movement results in gradual improvement, often requiring weeks or months to abate. A 4-inch strap worn tightly around the forearm just distal to the elbow may be used which transfers the origin of the affected muscles and splints the sprained area, relieving symptoms. To prevent recurrences, the strap should be worn during the aggravating activity. Hydrocortisone acetate 20 to 40 mg (mixed with equal volumes of local anesthetic) may be injected into the tender soft tissues down to the periosteum, following infiltration of 1 to 2 mL of 1% local anesthetic, if strapping, decreasing stresses, and strengthening exercises are unsuccessful. Surgical release of part of the origin of the extensor muscles from the lateral epicondyle is indicated and usually successful if symptoms repeatedly recur or are not alleviated after 3 or 4 injections precisely localized into the point of maximum tenderness. The proximity of the ulnar nerve should be noted when medial humeral epicondylitis (golfer's elbow) is injected. Modulation or correction of the aggravating activities (ie, recreational or occupational) is advised.

DUPUYTREN'S CONTRACTURE

Painless thickening and contracture of the palmar fascia due to fibrous proliferation, resulting in flexion deformities and loss of function of the fingers.

Etiology and Incidence

The etiology is unknown, but repeated microtrauma may play a role. Histologically, a low-grade inflammatory fibrosis is seen in the palmar fascia and surrounding the adjacent digital flexor tendon sheaths. Similar lesions may occur in the plantar fascia. There is some familial association, and men are far more often affected than women. The incidence increases progressively after age 40 and is higher in chronic invalids, alcoholics, epileptics, and patients with pulmonary TB, diabetes mellitus, and liver disease. The disorder may appear as a late sequel to the **shoulder-hand syndrome** (reflex sympathetic dystrophy syndrome) following myocardial infarction. Usually it appears spontaneously.

Symptoms, Signs, and Diagnosis

One or both hands may be affected; the right hand is more frequently affected when involvement is unilateral. The ring finger is involved most often, followed in order by the little, middle, and index fingers. **Diagnosis** is by inspection and palpation. Initially, a small, painless, indurated plaque or nodule develops in the palmar fascia and eventually extends into a longitudinal cordlike band. The skin adheres to the fascia and becomes puckered; flexion contracture of the fingers gradually follows. Nodules may be palpated under the skin pucker or over the surface of the joints. Extension of the affected fingers is impossible in advanced cases. When the shoulder-hand syndrome is involved, the hands may resemble those affected by scleroderma or Raynaud's disease. The disorder progresses at a variable and unpredictable rate. The fibrosis may not

advance for months or years and may remain confined within the distal palmar crease. The process is benign.

Treatment

No effective treatment is known other than excision of the affected fascia in advanced cases. Local corticosteroid injection into the affected tendon sheaths, analgesics, and physiotherapy are, as a rule, ineffective. Advanced flexion contractures usually require surgery. Subcutaneous fasciotomy, limited fasciectomy, or radical fasciectomy is performed according to the extent of the deformity. Amputation of a finger may be indicated for severe deformity. Whirlpool baths, passive and active exercises, and posterior extension splints may be helpful postoperatively. Recurrence is possible.

FIBROMYALGIA

(Myofascial Pain Syndrome; Fibromyositis)

A group of common nonarticular rheumatic disorders characterized by pain, tenderness, and stiffness of muscles, areas of tendon insertions, and adjacent soft-tissue structures. These may be primary and generalized or secondary to another underlying condition, or localized and often related to overuse or microtrauma factors.

The term **myalgia** indicates muscular pain. In contrast, **myositis** is due to inflammation of muscle tissues and is an inappropriate term for fibromyalgia, where such inflammation is absent. **Fibromyalgia** indicates pain in the fibrous connective tissue components of muscles, tendons, ligaments, and other "white" connective tissues. Various combinations of these conditions may occur together as "muscular rheumatism." Any of the fibromuscular tissues may be involved, but those of the low back **(lumbago)**, neck **(neck spasm)**, shoulders, thorax **(pleurodynia)**, and thighs **(aches and "charleyhorses")** are especially affected. There is no specific histologic abnormality, and the absence of cellular inflammation justifies the preferred terminology of fibromyalgia rather than the older terms of fibrositis or fibromyositis.

Etiology

The conditions may be induced or intensified by physical or mental stress, poor sleep, trauma, exposure to dampness or cold, and occasionally by a systemic, usually rheumatic, disorder. A viral infection or sometimes toxemia from a remote bacterial infection may precipitate the syndrome in an otherwise predisposed host. The **primary fibromyalgia syndrome (PFS)** is particularly likely to occur in healthy young women who tend to be tense, depressed, anxious, and striving, but may also occur in children or in older adults, often associated with minor changes of vertebral osteoarthritis. Men are more likely to develop localized fibromyalgia in association with a particular occupational or recreational strain. A minority of cases may be associated with significant psychogenic or psychophysiologic manifestations. Symptoms can be exacerbated by environmental or emotional stress or by a physician who does not give proper credence to the patient's concerns, and discharges the matter as "all in your head."

Symptoms, Signs, and Diagnosis

Onset of stiffness and pain frequently are gradual, diffuse, and of an "achy" character in PFS. In localized forms symptoms are more often sudden and acute. The pain is aggravated by straining or overuse. Tenderness may be present, sometimes localized to specific small zones; ie, "tender points." There may be local muscle spasm, though it cannot be regularly demonstrated by electromyography. Inflammation is not characteristic and only occurs with an underlying systemic condition. Diagnosis of PFS is by recognition of the typical pattern of diffuse fibromyalgia and nonrheumatic symptoms (eg, poor sleep, anxiety, fatigue, irritable bowel symptoms) and by exclusion of other systemic diseases (eg, early onset of RA, polymyositis, polymyalgia rheumatica, or

other connective tissue disease), and (most difficult of all) of psychogenic muscle pain and spasm. PFS, like irritable bowel syndrome, is a well-defined entity, readily diagnosed by its characteristic manifestations and simple screening tests to exclude underlying conditions. Occult rheumatic disease and hypothyroidism in the middle-aged female should be excluded. Screening tests are normal. Nonspecific and mild histopathologic changes may be present in the muscles.

Prognosis and Treatment

Fibromyalgia may disappear spontaneously with decreased stress, but can become chronic or recur at frequent intervals. Relief may be obtained from important supportive measures such as reassurance and explanation of the benign nature of the syndrome, as well as stretching exercises, improved sleep, local applications of heat, gentle massage, low-dose tricyclic agents at bedtime (eg, amitriptyline 10 or 25 mg) to promote deeper sleep, aspirin 650 mg orally q 3 to 4 h, or other NSAIDs in full dosages. Areas of focal tenderness may be injected with 1% lidocaine solution, 1 or 2 mL alone or in combination with a 40-mg hydrocortisone acetate suspension. A tricyclic antidepressant drug should be used in the lowest effective dose and may be continued indefinitely with monitoring of side effects, if any. If drowsiness occurs with one product, an alternative (in low dose) may be prescribed. Prognosis is favorable with a comprehensive, supportive program.

110. COLLAGEN VASCULAR DISEASES

VASCULITIS

Inflammation of blood vessels, which is often segmental and may be generalized or localized, constituting the basic mechanism of the production of lesions in a variety of rheumatic diseases and syndromes.

The large number of diseases characterized by or strongly associated with vasculitis include the collagen vascular diseases, discussed in the subchapters below, where specific symptoms, signs, and treatment are described. (Also, the rheumatoid nodule and other lesions of the rheumatic diseases appear to have central foci of vasculitis as their pathogenetic mechanism.) Much of SLE pathophysiology can be ascribed to vasculitis with or without secondary vascular occlusion. The polymyositis or dermatomyositis of childhood frequently includes an element of vasculitis not only in the obvious muscular target organs but also at extramuscular and extracutaneous sites. Even the bland-appearing and extensive intimal proliferation of small arteries typifying progressive systemic sclerosis may be a postinflammatory event. Other syndromes dominated by serious vasculitis and adequately characterized so as to permit diagnosable clinical profiles include polyarteritis nodosa and Wegener's granulomatosis.

Pathology

Vasculitis may follow a variety of pathogenetic mechanisms, but the histologic abnormalities are limited. Inflammation of a blood vessel may be acute or chronic: In acute lesions, the predominant inflammatory cells are polymorphonuclear leukocytes; in chronic lesions, lymphocytes. Moreover, the inflammatory process is often segmental, so that major portions of the vascular tree may be normal yet contain scattered focal areas of intense inflammation. At the affected sites, variable degrees of cellular infiltration and necrosis or scarring within one or more layers of the vessel wall are seen. Thus, the inflammatory process may be most intense within the media or the adventitia, with or without an intimal or periadventitial fibrous scar reaction. Inflammation within the media of a muscular artery tends to destroy the internal elastic lamina. Inflammation at any point in the vessel wall tends to resolve by fibrosis and

intimal hypertrophy. On occasion, certain distinguishing histologic events are seen, such as the development of numerous giant cells, or patchy areas of fibrinoid necrosis where complete sections of the vessel wall have undergone inflammatory destruction and liquefaction. Wherever inflammation of a vessel wall is seen, secondary occlusion of the lumen due to intimal hypertrophy and/or intraluminal thrombus formation may be expected. In addition, once the integrity of the vessel wall is breached, RBCs and fibrin may leak into the surrounding perivascular connective tissue.

Any type and size of vessel may be involved in an inflammatory response—arteries, arterioles, veins, venules, or capillaries. However, most of the versatile and variable pathophysiology resulting from vasculitis can be ascribed to arterial inflammation with the potential for total or partial vascular occlusion and subsequent tissue necrosis. Although the primary inflammatory process of a blood vessel is invariably a segmental or focal event, biopsy of even clinically suspected tissue may not always provide definitive histologic evidence of vasculitis. However, the intimal and periadventitial fibrous response to a focus of intense vessel wall inflammation frequently extends up and down the vessel from the primary insult, so that the histologic appearance of intimal hypertrophy and fibrosis or perivasculitis would imply the presence of an adjacent area of vasculitis.

Classification

In categorizing the numerous vasculitic disorders (see also individual discussions elsewhere in THE MANUAL), classification according to the size of the predominant vessel involved is most useful. This often reflects the depth of the lesions beginning from the integument and working viscerally. Thus, predominant inflammation of a postcapillary venule with neutrophilic infiltration leads to the typical histologic appearance of leukocytoclastic angiitis manifesting clinically as palpable purpura, and best typified by **Henoch-Schönlein syndrome** or ***Pseudomonas* septicemia.** The vascular inflammation of the deep dermal panniculus, mediated mainly by septal perivascular lymphocytes and presenting clinically as tender, deep, indurated red bumps on the arms and legs, is typical of **erythema nodosum.** Inflammation of medium-sized muscular arteries with the histologic features of a pleomorphic transmural infiltrate, fibrinoid necrosis, destruction of the internal elastic lamina, and postinflammatory aneurysm formation is exemplified by **polyarteritis nodosa.** When a similar type of process is largely confined to the extracranial carotid tree and is associated with a lymphocytic infiltrate and the formation of giant cells clustered around the luminal aspect of the disrupted elastic lamina, severe headaches may result and **giant-cell arteritis** is recognized. Finally, when inflammation of the largest central vessels such as the aorta and its branches is evident, mainly mediated by adventitial and/or medial lymphocytic infiltration and fibrous scarring with a tendency to postinflammatory stenosis, the loss of major pulses may become clinically evident and **Takayasu's arteritis** is recognized.

DISCOID LUPUS ERYTHEMATOSUS

(DLE; Cutaneous LE; Chronic Discoid LE)

A chronic and recurrent disorder primarily affecting the skin and characterized by sharply circumscribed macules and plaques displaying erythema, follicular plugging, scales, telangiectasia, and atrophy.

The cause is unknown. Exposure to sunlight frequently precedes the initial appearance of lesions (50% of patients have a history of photosensitivity). The disease is more common in females, appearing most often during their 30s.

Symptoms and Signs

Active lesions may persist or recur for years. Initially, they are erythematous, round, scaling papules 5 to 10 mm in diameter, with follicular plugging. They appear most frequently on the malar prominences, bridge of the nose, scalp, external auditory

canals, and the remainder of the pinnae. The lesions may be generalized over the upper portion of the trunk and extensor surfaces of the extremities. Mucous membrane involvement may be prominent—especially mouth ulcers. The lesions of untreated DLE gradually extend peripherally, while the center atrophies. The residual scars are noncontractile. A "carpet tack" invagination of the scales into the dilated follicles may be seen in heavily scaled lesions. Alopecia of the scalp may be widespread, scarring, and permanent. Leukopenia and mild and transitory systemic manifestations, such as arthralgias, are common.

Patients with extensive skin lesions are more likely to have internal manifestations suggestive of systemic lupus erythematosus **(SLE)**. Though the disease is limited to the skin in 90% of patients with typical DLE, approximately 10% eventually develop varying degrees of systemic manifestations; approximately 5% develop SLE even when an initial study does not suggest systemic disease. A small number of patients with DLE develop chronic synovitis as the sole "systemic" manifestation.

Diagnosis

Since the cutaneous lesions of DLE and SLE may be identical, a patient presenting with typical discoid lesions must be evaluated to determine whether systemic involvement is present. A medical history and physical examination are required. Occurrence in a patient younger than age 30 suggests the possibility of an early cutaneous manifestation of SLE. Diagnostic studies should include biopsy from the active margin of the lesion, CBC, ESR, tests for antinuclear factors, and renal function studies. Skin biopsy will not differentiate DLE and SLE, but will rule out other disorders. Antibodies against double-stranded DNA (eg, DNA-binding test) are almost invariably absent in DLE, a finding of raised titers strongly suggesting systemic involvement.

In differential diagnosis, the lesions of rosacea are characterized by the absence of pustules and the presence of atrophy. The lesions of seborrheic dermatitis are never atrophic and frequently involve the nasolabial area, which is rarely affected by DLE. Lesions caused by photosensitivity are not atrophic and usually disappear when direct sunlight is avoided. Lymphoma or plaques of sarcoidosis may mimic DLE; biopsy should make the diagnosis. When the lips and oral mucosa are involved, lichen planus and leukoplakia must be ruled out.

Treatment

Early treatment is advisable, before atrophy is permanent. Exposure to sunlight (or ultraviolet light) should be minimized. If necessary, a sunscreen preparation should be applied (see Ch. 253).

It is usually possible to effect involution of small lesions by applying topical corticosteroid ointments or creams tid to qid; eg, triamcinolone acetonide 0.1% or 0.5%, fluocinolone 0.025% or 0.2%, flurandrenolide 0.05%, betamethasone valerate 0.1%, or betamethasone dipropionate 0.05%. The latter may be most effective. Plastic tape coated with flurandrenolide frequently helps with resistant lesions. Individual recalcitrant plaques may respond to intradermal injection of 0.1% suspension of triamcinolone acetonide, but secondary atrophy frequently follows. Excessive use of topical steroids is to be avoided.

Antimalarials, such as hydroxychloroquine 200 mg/day, are very useful in the management of DLE (see SYSTEMIC LUPUS ERYTHEMATOSUS, below). In resistant cases, higher doses (eg, 400 mg/day) or combinations (eg, hydroxychloroquine 200 mg/day plus quinacrine [mepacrine] 50 to 100 mg/day) may be required for a few months.

SYSTEMIC LUPUS ERYTHEMATOSUS

(SLE; Disseminated LE)

An inflammatory connective tissue disorder of unknown etiology occurring predominantly in young women, but also in children; 90% of cases occur in women. The sera of

most patients contain antinuclear antibodies, including anti-DNA antibodies. Their presence not only facilitates recognition of SLE in its milder forms but also suggests that SLE is an autoimmune disorder. The pathogenetic mechanisms of autoimmune reactions are discussed in Ch. 21. Increased awareness of mild forms of SLE has resulted in a worldwide rise in reported cases. In some countries, the prevalence of SLE rivals that of RA.

Pathology, Symptoms, and Signs

Clinical findings vary with the acuteness of the disease and the distribution of the lesions. SLE may begin abruptly with fever, simulating acute infection, or may develop insidiously over months or years with only episodes of fever and malaise. Manifestations referable to any organ system may appear. As many as 90% of patients complain of **articular symptoms** ranging from intermittent arthralgias to acute polyarthritis, some for years before other manifestations appear. A past history of "growing pains" in childhood is not uncommon. In longstanding disease, tendon contractures and secondary joint deformity may occur without x-ray evidence of erosion **(Jaccoud's arthritis)**.

A characteristic malar "butterfly" erythema is one of several **cutaneous lesions** that may occur; others include the discoid lesions described above under DLE, and erythematous, firm, maculopapular lesions of the face, exposed areas of the neck, upper chest, and elbows. Blistering and ulceration are rare, though ulcers on mucous membrane (particularly the central portion of the hard palate near the junction of the hard and soft palate, the buccal and gum mucosa, and the anterior nasal septum) are common. Generalized alopecia is frequent during active phases of the disease. Mottled erythema of the sides of the palms with extension onto the fingers, periungual erythema with edema, and macular reddish-purple lesions on the volar surfaces of the fingers also may occur. Purpura may develop secondary to thrombocytopenia or necrotizing angiitis of small vessels. Photosensitivity occurs in 40% of patients.

Recurrent pleurisy, with or without effusion, is frequent. Lupus pneumonitis is rare, though minor pulmonary function abnormalities are common. **Pericarditis** often is present. A more serious complication in occasional patients is **pulmonary hypertension.**

Generalized adenopathy is frequent, particularly in children, young adults, and blacks. **Splenomegaly** occurs in 10% of patients. Histologically, the spleen may show periarterial fibrosis ("onionskin" lesion). **CNS involvement** can cause headaches, personality changes, epilepsy, psychoses, and organic brain syndrome. Cerebral thrombosis, though rare, is now known to be associated with anticardiolipin antibodies (see below).

Renal involvement may be benign and asymptomatic or relentlessly progressive and fatal. The most common manifestation is proteinuria. The histopathology of the renal lesion varies from a focal, usually benign, glomerulitis to a diffuse membranoproliferative glomerulonephritis. Since milder cases have been increasingly detected, the incidence of clinically significant renal disease has dropped.

Laboratory Findings

The screening test for SLE is the fluorescent test for **antinuclear antibodies (ANA);** positive ANA tests (usually in high titer) are found in over 98% of SLE patients. A positive ANA test should lead to the more specific test for **anti-DNA antibodies** (measured by Farr test, or by the slightly less sensitive crithidia slide method). High titers of anti-DNA antibodies are almost specific for SLE.

A variety of other antinuclear, and also anticytoplasmic, antibodies (eg, Ro, La, Sm, RNP, Jo-1) are diagnostically valuable in connective tissue diseases. As Ro is predominantly cytoplasmic, anti-Ro antibodies may be found in occasional ANA-negative SLE patients.

False-positive STS may be seen in 5 to 10% of SLE patients. They are associated with the lupus anticoagulant. Both those tests measure antiphospholipid antibodies such as **anticardiolipin antibodies.** These are associated with a tendency to thrombosis, abortion,

and thrombocytopenia. Serum complement levels usually are depressed in active disease and are usually (though not necessarily) lowest in patients with active nephritis. C-reactive protein levels are strikingly low in SLE, even in the face of ESR elevations > 100 mm/h. The ESR is elevated almost uniformly during active disease. Leukopenia is the rule, notably lymphopenia in active SLE. Hemolytic anemia may occur.

Kidney damage can become evident at any time, even when other features of SLE are absent. **Kidney biopsy** usually is not necessary for diagnosis but may be helpful to evaluate the course of renal disease and to guide medical therapy. **Urinalysis** may be repeatedly normal despite early renal involvement confirmed by biopsy, but should be repeated at 4- to 6-mo intervals while monitoring patients in apparent remission. Red cell and granular casts suggest more active nephritis.

Diagnosis

Recognition of SLE is obvious when a patient (particularly, a young woman) has a febrile disease with an erythematous skin rash, polyarthritis, evidence of renal disease, intermittent pleuritic pain, leukopenia, and hyperglobulinemia with anti-DNA antibodies. SLE can be difficult to differentiate from other connective tissue disorders in its early stages; eg, be mistaken for RA if arthritic symptoms predominate. Meticulous evaluation and long-term observation may be required before the diagnosis is established. Migraine, epilepsy, or psychoses may be initial findings. Patients with discoid lesions must be evaluated to differentiate discoid from systemic LE. Some drugs (eg, hydralazine, procainamide, and β blockers) produce positive ANA tests and, occasionally, a lupuslike syndrome. These features disappear if the drug is withdrawn promptly.

The American Rheumatism Association has proposed criteria for the **classification** (but *not* for diagnosis) of SLE; 4 of the following are required: (1) malar rash; (2) discoid rash; (3) photosensitivity; (4) oral ulcers; (5) arthritis; (6) serositis; (7) renal disorder; (8) leukopenia (< 4000/μL), lymphopenia (< 1500/μL), hemolytic anemia, or thrombocytopenia (< 100,000/μL); (9) neurologic disorder; (10) positive LE cell or anti-DNA or anti-S_m antibody or a false-positive STS; (11) antinuclear antibodies in raised titer.

Mixed connective tissue disease (MCTD) is a syndrome with clinical features of SLE overlapping with those of progressive systemic sclerosis and polymyositis/dermatomyositis. The disorder is discussed separately, below.

Prognosis

This varies widely, depending on the organs involved and the intensity of the inflammatory reaction. The course of SLE is commonly chronic and relapsing, often with long periods (years) of remission. During the past 2 decades the prognosis has improved markedly. Provided the initial acute phase is controlled, the long-term prognosis is good. Flares are rare after the menopause. The 10-yr survival in most western countries is > 95%. This very improved prognosis underlines one lesson: In SLE, making the diagnosis is of paramount importance.

Treatment

Management of idiopathic SLE depends on the location and severity of the disease. To simplify therapy, SLE should be classified as **mild** (fever, arthritis, pleurisy, pericarditis, headaches, or rash) or **severe** (life-threatening disease; eg, hemolytic anemia, thrombocytopenic purpura, massive pleural and pericardial involvement, significant renal damage, acute vasculitis of the extremities or GI tract, or florid CNS involvement). The course is totally unpredictable. The following drugs and dosages are for adults, unless otherwise specified.

Mild or remittent disease may require little or no therapy. Arthralgias usually are controlled with nonsteroidal anti-inflammatory agents. Aspirin is useful, but high doses in SLE may cause liver toxicity. Antimalarials help, particularly where joint and

skin manifestations are prominent. Regimens vary, but hydroxychloroquine 200 mg/day is preferred. Some advocate a loading dose of 400 mg/day, but this may cause diplopia, raising fears of ocular toxicity in the patient. Alternatives are chloroquine 250 mg/day or quinacrine (mepacrine) 50 to 100 mg/day. Combinations of these drugs are sometimes used. Ophthalmologic examination usually is advised at 6-mo intervals, though on these modest doses, this practice may be excessively cautious.

Severe disease requires immediate corticosteroid therapy. The suggested doses are for adults, but children may require almost as much. **Starting prednisone dosages** for specific manifestations are as follows: **Hemolytic anemia**—60 mg/day. **Thrombocytopenic purpura**—40 to 60 mg/day. Platelets may not rise for 4 to 6 wk. **Severe polyserositis**—40 to 60 mg/day. Response begins within days.

Renal damage—60 mg/day. Improvement does not usually occur for 4 to 12 wk and may not be evident until corticosteroid dosage is reduced. A combination of prednisone with immunosuppressive agents now is recommended in active SLE or lupus nephritis. Azathioprine 2.5 mg/kg/day or cyclophosphamide 2.5 mg/kg/day is most used, though there is a trend toward the use of intermittent immunosuppressives such as cyclophosphamide 500 mg IV, repeated as the blood count allows.

Acute vasculitis and **severe CNS lupus**—the same regimens are used as for renal damage, above. In CNS lupus, methylprednisolone, 1000 mg by slow (1-h) IV infusion on 3 successive days often is the initial form of treatment, together with IV cyclophosphamide, as above.

In both mild and severe disease, after the inflammatory process is controlled, the minimal dose of corticosteroids and other agents necessary to suppress tissue inflammation must be determined. This usually is done by decreasing the dose by 10% at intervals (depending on how fast clinical improvement occurs). For example, if fever and arthritis are the initial active manifestations, the dose is reduced at weekly intervals; if thrombocytopenia or renal disease (both of which respond more slowly to initiation of therapy) are problems, reductions are made every 2 to 4 wk. Rebound (temporary flare) and relapse tend to occur in the system with the most recent exacerbation. Response to therapy is measured by relief of symptoms and signs or improvement in laboratory tests. A return of low serum complement toward normal may or may not occur with treatment, as may a return of anti-DNA antibody titers to normal. Clinical rather than serologic features are all-important in determining therapy. Below 15 mg of prednisone daily, a gradual change to alternate-day dosage may be possible. The majority of SLE patients can ultimately be weaned off prednisone.

General medical management: Intercurrent infection, often complicating the disease and easily mistaken for some of its manifestations, should be treated vigorously. The usual measures to combat heart failure and renal insufficiency must be taken in addition to using anti-inflammatory agents. Close medical supervision is imperative during surgical procedures and pregnancy. Hypersensitivity rashes are common with sulfonamides, trimethoprim/sulfamethoxazole, and penicillin. Flares may occur with oral contraceptives, but are rare. Provided that renal and cardiac functions are adequate, pregnancy is not contraindicated in SLE; however, spontaneous abortion and post partum disease flares are frequent. The latter usually are easily controlled, given increased vigilance in the puerperium.

Perhaps the greatest change in the management of SLE during the past decade has been in attitude—the realization that for the majority of patients, the disease can be controlled without recourse to heroic doses of corticosteroids.

PROGRESSIVE SYSTEMIC SCLEROSIS

(PSS; Scleroderma)

A chronic disease of unknown cause, characterized by diffuse fibrosis; degenerative changes; and vascular abnormalities in the skin **(scleroderma),** *articular structures, and*

internal organs (especially the esophagus, intestinal tract, lung, heart, and kidney). PSS is about 4 times more common in women than men, and is comparatively rare in children. The disease varies in severity and progression, its features ranging from generalized cutaneous thickening (PSS with diffuse scleroderma) with rapidly progressive and often fatal visceral involvement, to a form distinguished by restricted skin involvement (often just the fingers and face) and prolonged passage of time, often several decades, before full manifestation of characteristic internal manifestations (**CREST syndrome: C**alcinosis, **R**aynaud's phenomenon, **E**sophageal dysfunction, **S**clerodactyly, **T**elangiectasia). In addition, overlap syndromes exist; eg, **sclerodermatomyositis** (*tight skin and muscle weakness indistinguishable from polymyositis*); **mixed connective tissue disease** (**MCTD**—discussed briefly here and in a separate subchapter below); and the recently described chemically induced **toxic oil syndrome (TOS)** which occurred in Madrid in 1981, and has affected approximately 20,000 people.

Symptoms, Signs, and Diagnosis

Initial complaints: The most common are Raynaud's phenomenon and insidious swelling of the acral portions of the extremities with gradual thickening of the skin of the fingers. Polyarthralgia also is a prominent early symptom. GI disturbances (eg, heartburn and dysphagia) or respiratory complaints (eg, dyspnea) occasionally are the first manifestations of the disease.

The skin: Induration is symmetric and may be confined to the fingers **(sclerodactyly)** and distal portions of the upper extremities, or affect most or all of the body. As the disease progresses, the skin becomes taut, shiny, and hyperpigmented; the face becomes masklike; telangiectases appear on the fingers, chest, face, lips, and tongue. Subcutaneous calcifications develop (calcinosis circumscripta), usually on the fingertips and over bony eminences. Biopsy of indurated skin shows an increase in compact collagen fibers in the reticular dermis, epidermal thinning, loss of rete pegs, and atrophy of dermal appendages. There may be variably large accumulations of T-dependent lymphocytes in the dermis and subcutis (which also may be the seat of extensive fibrosis).

Musculoskeletal system: Friction rubs develop over the joints (particularly the knees), tendon sheaths (tendinitis), and large bursae, because of fibrin deposition on synovial surfaces. Flexion contractures of the fingers, wrists, and elbows result from fibrosis of the synovium and periarticular structures. Trophic ulcers are common, especially on the fingertips and overlying the finger joints.

GI tract: Esophageal dysfunction is the most frequent visceral disturbance and eventually occurs in most patients. Dysphagia, acid reflux due to lower esophageal sphincter incompetence, and peptic esophagitis with possible ulceration and stricture are common. Hypomotility of the small intestine may be associated with malabsorption resulting from anaerobic bacterial overgrowth. Pneumatosis cystoides intestinalis may occur following degeneration of the muscularis mucosa and entry of air into the submucosa of the intestinal wall. Characteristic large-mouthed sacculations develop in the colon and ileum because of atrophy of the smooth muscle of these segments. **Biliary cirrhosis** has occurred in individuals with the CREST syndrome.

Cardiorespiratory system: Lung fibrosis, with exertional dyspnea its most prominent symptom, is associated early with an impairment in gas exchange. Pleurisy and pericarditis with effusion may occur. Pulmonary hypertension may develop as a result of longstanding interstitial and peribronchial fibrosis or intimal hyperplasia of small pulmonary arteries; the latter is associated with the CREST syndrome. Cardiac arrhythmias, conduction disturbances, and other ECG abnormalities are common. Cardiac failure may develop either because of pulmonary hypertension and secondary cor pulmonale or because of diffuse fibrous replacement of cardiac muscle. The cardiac failure tends to be chronic and to respond poorly to digitalis.

The kidneys: Severe renal disease may occur as a consequence of intimal hyperplasia of interlobular and arcuate arteries, and usually is heralded by the abrupt onset of accelerated or malignant hypertension. If untreated, this is soon followed by rapidly progressive and irreversible renal insufficiency—a major cause of death.

Laboratory findings: Rheumatoid factor tests are positive in 1/3 of PSS patients; serum antinuclear and/or antinucleolar antibodies are present in 90% or more of cases. An antibody that reacts with centromeric protein is found in the serum of a high proportion of patients with the CREST syndrome (anti-centromere antibody).

Localized forms of scleroderma occur as circumscribed patches (morphea) or linear sclerosis of the integument and immediately subjacent tissues without systemic involvement; antinuclear antibodies often are found in the latter condition. **Overlap syndromes:** The most distinct is MCTD (see in this chapter [COLLAGEN VASCULAR DISEASES] below), in which scleroderma and other evidence of PSS such as Raynaud's phenomenon and esophageal dysfunction occur in association with clinical and serologic features of SLE, polymyositis, and/or RA. Patients with MCTD have extremely high titers of a serum antibody that reacts with nuclear ribonucleoprotein.

Prognosis

The course is variable and unpredictable. It is often only slowly progressive. Most patients eventually show evidence of visceral involvement. Prognosis is poor if cardiac, pulmonary, or renal manifestations are present early. However, the disease may remain limited and nonprogressive for long periods in patients with the CREST syndrome; other visceral changes (including pulmonary hypertension due to vascular disease of the lung, and a peculiar form of biliary cirrhosis) eventually develop, but the course of this form of PSS often is remarkably benign.

Treatment

No drug has significantly influenced the natural history of PSS, but numerous agents are of value in treating specific symptoms or organ systems. Corticosteroids may be helpful for disabling myositis or MCTD. Studies indicate that prolonged administration (> 1.5 yr) of D-penicillamine (0.5 to 1.0 gm/day) reduces skin thickening and may delay the rate of new visceral involvement. However, penicillamine is poorly tolerated by many patients, and long-term benefits are equivocal at best. Colchicine and various immunosuppressive agents also are under trial in PSS, but the results to date are variable. Nifedipine 20 mg qid may help control Raynaud's phenomenon. Reflux esophagitis is relieved by frequent small feedings, antacids, and cimetidine (300 mg qid—30 min before meals and at bedtime), and by having the patient sleep with the head of the bed elevated. Esophageal strictures may require periodic dilatation; successful correction of gastroesophageal reflux by gastroplasty has been reported. Tetracycline 1 gm/day orally, or another broad-spectrum antibiotic, suppresses intestinal flora and may alleviate intestinal malabsorption symptoms. Physiotherapy may help preserve muscle strength but is ineffective in preventing joint contractures.

For kidney disease, angiotensin-converting enzyme inhibitors, which inhibit the formation of angiotensin (eg, captopril), are the drugs of choice. Other vasodilators (eg, minoxidil) or β-adrenergic blockers also have been used with some success. All of these agents are effective in controlling hypertension and can preserve renal function. When end-stage renal disease is unpreventable, dialysis and transplantation can be used, although the mortality still is high.

EOSINOPHILIC FASCIITIS (EF)

EF is a recently recognized variant of an autoimmune scleroderma-like disorder characterized by symmetric and painful inflammation, swelling, and induration of the hands, arms, legs, and feet. EF occurs mostly in middle-aged men. The **etiology** is not known.

Symptoms and signs: Strenuous physical activity often precipitates symptoms in those who previously led a sedentary life. The initial features are pain, swelling, and inflammation of the skin, followed by induration creating a characteristic orange-peel configuration most evident over the anterior (volar) surfaces of the extremities. The face and trunk also may be involved, with changes resembling scleroderma (see above). Carpal tunnel syndrome may be present.

The symptoms usually appear insidiously, with gradual restriction of arm and leg movement. Contractures commonly evolve, secondary to induration and thickening of the fascia. Fatigue and weight loss are common. Although muscle strength is unimpaired, myalgia and arthritis may occur. Sjögren's syndrome and cardiac abnormalities have been reported and, rarely, aplastic anemia and thrombocytopenia. The absence of Raynaud's phenomenon and delayed esophageal motility are key points in ruling out progressive systemic sclerosis **(PSS)**.

Laboratory studies show eosinophilia, elevated ESR, and a polyclonal IgG hypergammaglobulinemia. Unlike PSS, antinuclear antibodies and rheumatoid factor are absent.

The **diagnosis** is confirmed by biopsy of affected skin and fascia deep enough to include adjacent muscle fibers. The dermis may show cellular infiltration. The subdermal fascia is greatly thickened, with collagenous hypertrophy. Marked cellular infiltrates within the fascia include histiocytes, plasma cells, lymphocytes, and in some cases, eosinophils.

Treatment and Prognosis: Most patients respond to high initial doses of prednisone, 40 to 60 mg/day, with rapid reduction to 5 to 10 mg/day that may be required for 2 to 5 yr. Alternatively, cimetidine 400 mg tid may be used. Although the long-term outcome is unknown, in many patients EF is self-limited and uncomplicated.

POLYMYOSITIS/DERMATOMYOSITIS

*A systemic connective tissue disease characterized by inflammatory and degenerative changes in the muscles—**polymyositis** (and frequently also in the skin—**dermatomyositis**), leading to symmetric weakness and some degree of muscle atrophy, principally of the limb girdles.* Certain clinical findings are shared with progressive systemic sclerosis **(PSS)** or, less frequently, SLE or vasculitis.

Classification of the types of myositis includes primary idiopathic polymyositis; childhood dermatomyositis (or polymyositis); primary idiopathic dermatomyositis in adults; dermatomyositis (or polymyositis) associated with malignant neoplasms; polymyositis or dermatomyositis associated with various connective tissue disease overlap syndromes, including mixed connective tissue disease (discussed below) and sclerodermatomyositis.

Etiology and Incidence

The etiology is unknown. The disease may be caused by an autoimmune reaction; deposits of IgM, IgG, and the 3rd component of complement have been found in the blood vessel walls of skeletal muscle (with particularly high frequency in childhood dermatomyositis). A cell-mediated immune reaction to muscle plays a role. Viruses may participate: Picornavirus-like structures have been found in muscle cells, and tubular inclusions resembling paramyxovirus nucleocapsid have been identified by electron microscopy in myocytes and endothelial cells of vessels in the skin and muscle. The association of a malignant tumor with dermatomyositis suggests that the neoplasm may incite myositis as the result of an autoimmune reaction directed against a common antigen in muscle and tumor.

The disease is not rare; it is less common than SLE or PSS, but more frequent than polyarteritis nodosa. The female:male ratio is 2:1. The disease may appear at any time from infancy through age 80, most commonly from age 40 to 60, or, in children, from age 5 to 15.

Pathology

Microscopic examination of the skin may show epidermal atrophy, basal cell liquefaction and degeneration, vascular dilatation, and lymphocytic infiltration of the dermis. Structural changes in affected muscle vary greatly. The most frequent abnormalities consist of necrosis; phagocytosis; regenerative activity reflected by basophilia, large vesicular nuclei, and prominent nucleoli; atrophy and degeneration of muscle fibers, especially in a perifascicular distribution; internal migration of nuclei; vacuolation; fiber-size variation; and a lymphocytic infiltrate, often most prominent in a perivascular location. There is an increase in endomysial and later perimysial connective tissue. In childhood, there may be widespread ulceration and infarction in the GI tract related to necrotizing arteritis. Intimal proliferation and thrombosis of small arteries and veins follow.

Symptoms and Signs

Onset may be acute or insidious. Symptoms in children and adults are similar, the only distinction being that childhood onset is more likely to be very acute, and adult onset more insidious. An acute infection may precede or incite the initial symptoms, which consist of proximal muscle weakness, muscle pain, rash, polyarthralgias, Raynaud's phenomenon, dysphagia, and constitutional complaints, most notably fever and weight loss. The **muscle weakness** may appear suddenly and progress over weeks to months. Patients may have difficulty raising the arms above the shoulders, climbing steps, or arising from a sitting position, and be unable to raise the head from the pillow. Patients may become wheelchair- or bedridden because of weakness of pelvic and shoulder girdle muscle groups. The flexors of the neck may be severely affected. Weakness of the laryngeal musculature is responsible for dysphonia. Involvement of the striated muscle of the pharynx and upper portion of the esophagus leads to dysphagia and regurgitation. A diminution in peristaltic activity and dilatation of the lower esophagus and small intestine may be indistinguishable from that found in PSS. (The diagnosis in patients with such GI changes who are described as having minimal or mild scleroderma may in fact be PSS with CREST syndrome—see above.) The muscles of the hands, feet, and face escape involvement. Contractures of limbs may develop late in the chronic stage.

The **cutaneous eruption** tends to be dusky and erythematous and to have an SLE-like butterfly distribution on the face. Periorbital edema with a heliotrope hue is pathognomonic. The skin rash may be slightly elevated and smooth or scaly, and may appear on the forehead, V of the neck and shoulders, chest and back, forearms and lower legs, elbows and knees, medial malleoli, and dorsum of the proximal interphalangeal and metacarpophalangeal joints. The base and sides of the fingernails may be hyperemic. The skin lesions frequently fade completely but may be followed by brownish pigmentation, atrophy, scarring, or vitiligo. Muscular pain, tenderness, and induration tend to be associated with the rash. The skin changes suggest scleroderma in a few patients. Subcutaneous calcification may occur, particularly in childhood: This is similar in distribution to that encountered in PSS, but tends to be more extensive **(calcinosis universalis)**, particularly in untreated or undertreated disease.

Polyarthralgia, accompanied at times by swelling, joint effusions, and other evidence of nondeforming arthritis, occurs in approximately 1/3 of patients. These rheumatic complaints tend to be mild and respond well to corticosteroids. Raynaud's phenomenon occurs, with particularly high frequency in those patients in whom polymyositis coexists with other connective tissue disorders.

Visceral involvement (with the exception of the pharynx and esophagus) is relatively uncommon in polymyositis compared to the high frequency of internal changes in other connective tissue diseases, such as SLE and PSS. Interstitial pneumonitis (manifested by dyspnea and cough) occurs and may precede myositis and dominate the clinical picture. Cardiac involvement, detected chiefly in the ECG (arrhythmias, con-

duction disturbances, abnormal systolic time intervals), has been reported with increasing frequency. Acute renal failure as a consequence of severe rhabdomyolysis with myoglobinuria (crush syndrome) has been reported. Sjögren's syndrome occurs in some patients. Abdominal symptoms, commoner in children, may be associated with hematemesis or melena from GI ulcerations that may progress to perforation and require surgical intervention.

An associated malignancy occurs in approximately 15% of men (and a smaller proportion of women) over age 50. There is no characteristic type or site.

Laboratory Findings

Laboratory studies are helpful but nonspecific. The ESR frequently is elevated. Antinuclear antibodies and/or LE cells are found in a few patients, most often those with another connective tissue disease. The muscle enzymes, especially the transaminases, creatine kinase **(CK),** and aldolase, usually show elevated serum levels; the most sensitive and useful is CK. Periodic enzyme determinations are helpful in monitoring treatment: elevated levels decrease with effective therapy. However, these enzymes may be normal despite active disease in patients with chronic myositis and widespread muscle atrophy.

Diagnosis

Five major criteria are useful in diagnosis: proximal muscle weakness; a characteristic skin rash; elevated muscle enzymes in the serum; a characteristic triad of electromyographic abnormalities; and muscle biopsy changes. Electromyography usually shows (1) spontaneous fibrillations and positive sharp potentials, with increased insertional irritability; (2) polyphasic short potentials during voluntary contraction; and (3) bizarre, repetitive, high-frequency discharges during mechanical stimulation. The preferred sites for biopsy are the muscles that show electrical abnormalities, usually the deltoid and quadriceps femoris, but on the opposite extremities in order to avoid sites previously explored.

Any adult with dermatomyositis should be studied for a malignancy.

Prognosis

Relatively satisfactory and long remissions, even apparent recovery, have been reported, especially in children. Death in adults follows severe and progressive muscle weakness, dysphagia, malnutrition, aspiration pneumonia, or respiratory failure with superimposed pulmonary infection. Polymyositis tends to be more severe and resistant to treatment in those individuals with cardiac or pulmonary involvement. Death in children usually is a result of vasculitis of the bowel. The prognosis for patients with malignancy-associated myositis generally is determined by the malignancy prognosis.

Treatment

The patient's activities should be curtailed until the inflammation subsides. Corticosteroids are the drugs of choice initially. For acute disease, prednisone is given 40 to 60 mg or more/day, together with antacids and potassium supplements. Serial measurements of muscle enzyme activity in serum provide the best guide of therapy effectiveness, with enzyme reduction moving toward or reaching normal values in a majority of patients in 4 to 6 wk. This is followed by an improvement in muscle strength. Once the enzyme levels have returned to normal, the dose of prednisone is reduced slowly; if muscle enzymes rise, the dose is increased. In adults, maintenance therapy with prednisone (10 to 15 mg/day) usually is necessary indefinitely. Occasional patients treated chronically with high doses of corticosteroids become increasingly weak because of a superimposed **corticosteroid myopathy.** Under these circumstances, the corticosteroids must be discontinued and another agent (eg, an immunosuppressant) substituted. In childhood, it may be possible to discontinue prednisone after a year or more, with apparent remission. Immunosuppressive agents, including methotrexate, cyclophos-

phamide, chlorambucil, and azathioprine have been beneficial in patients who fail to respond to corticosteroids alone. Some patients have received methotrexate for 5 yr or longer for the control of this disease. Malignancy-associated myositis often remits spontaneously if the tumor is removed. The myositis associated with nonresectable tumors or metastatic disease usually is more refractory to corticosteroids.

POLYMYALGIA RHEUMATICA (PMR)

Severe pain and stiffness in proximal muscle groups without permanent weakness or atrophy. A number of patients (15 to 30%) have an associated **giant cell arteritis** that may affect all medium-size arteries (eg, coronary and cranial) and not just the temporal arteries (see in Ch. 30). PMR occurs in patients > 50 yr, where its prevalence may equal that of RA. The female-to-male ratio is 2:1. Pathogenesis is unknown.

Symptoms and Signs

Onset may be sudden or gradual; pain and stiffness may appear symmetrically in the neck, shoulder, or pelvic girdle muscles. Morning stiffness is marked. Some patients find it difficult to get out of bed. Fever, anorexia, malaise, weight loss, and apathy may be present. In spite of the painful symptoms, there is no muscle weakness, unlike polymyositis. A nonhemolytic anemia with Hct as low as 30% may be present. When temporal arteritis is present, *headache, scalp tenderness, blurred vision, jaw claudication, or irreversible blindness may develop rapidly.*

Diagnosis

The ESR is elevated; values over 100 mm/h are common and suggest the diagnosis. Differentiation from RA is made by a negative RF and by the absence of symmetric proximal interphalangeal and metacarpo-phalangeal joint swelling. In PMR, there may be swelling of *only* one or 2 joints (not generalized joint swelling as in RA). Lymphocytic infiltration may be seen in synovia on biopsy, and joint scintigrams with ^{99m}technetium pertechnetate have shown evidence of synovitis. PMR is distinguished from polymyositis by a normal muscle biopsy and EMG as well as normal serum muscle enzyme levels (CPK, aldolase); from osteoarthritis, by the elevated ESR; and from multiple myeloma, by a normal protein electrophoresis and bone marrow examination. Biopsy of an asymptomatic temporal artery may show giant cell arteritis.

Treatment

The disease responds so well to corticosteroids that a prompt and favorable therapeutic response (within 24 to 36 h) confirms the diagnosis. Treatment should be started immediately upon diagnosis, with prednisone 30 to 40 mg/day orally, which is reduced promptly as symptoms subside and the ESR returns to normal. Prednisone at 5 to 10 mg/day should be continued as long as symptoms persist; in some, this may be required for years. If temporal arteritis is probable, prednisone, at least 60 mg/day for 1 mo or longer, should be taken under joint supervision with an ophthalmologist.

POLYARTERITIS NODOSA

(Polyarteritis; Periarteritis Nodosa)

A disease characterized by segmental inflammation and necrosis of medium-sized muscular arteries, with secondary ischemia of the tissue supplied by the affected vessels.

Etiology and Incidence

The cause is unknown, but hypersensitivity appears to be involved. The variety of clinical and pathologic features suggest multiple pathogenic mechanisms. Arterial lesions like those found in spontaneously occurring polyarteritis are seen in hyperimmunized human volunteers, in animals with experimental serum sickness, and in patients developing allergic reactions. Drugs (eg, sulfonamides, penicillin, iodide, thiouracil,

bismuth, thiazides, guanethidine, methamphetamine), vaccines, bacterial infections (eg, streptococcal or staphylococcal), and viral infections (eg, serum hepatitis, influenza) have been associated with disease onset. Usually no predisposing antigen is incriminated.

Onset generally is between ages 40 and 50, but occurs in every age group. The male:female ratio is 3:1.

Pathology

Segmental, necrotizing inflammation of media and adventitia characterizes the lesion. The pathologic process most commonly occurs at points of vessel bifurcation, beginning in the media and extending into the intima and adventitia of medium-size arteries, often disrupting the internal elastic lamellae. Lesions usually are seen in all stages of development and healing. Early lesions contain polymorphonuclear leukocytes and occasionally eosinophils; later ones, lymphocytes and plasma cells. Immunoglobulin, complement components, and fibrinogen are deposited in the lesions; the significance is unclear. Intimal proliferation with secondary thrombosis and occlusion leads to organ and tissue infarction. Weakening of the muscular vessel wall may cause small aneurysms and arterial dissection. Healing can result in nodular fibrosis of the adventitia.

Renal, hepatic, cardiac, and GI involvements are most frequent. Renal lesions are of 2 types: large-vessel (the renal lesion is a tubular infarction, and renal failure is uncommon) and microvascular, including the glomerular afferent arterioles (the lesion is diffuse, and renal failure is common and occurs early). Half of all patients with massive hepatic infarction have polyarteritis.

Several polyarteritis-associated syndromes are separated from typical polyarteritis by pathogenic or clinical differences: hypersensitivity angiitis; **Churg-Strauss syndrome** (the vasculitis includes lung involvement, eosinophilia, necrotizing granulomas, and severe asthma); **Cogan's syndrome** (the disease begins as interstitial keratitis and inner ear infarction); pure mesenteric polyarteritis (recognized in IV methamphetamine addicts); Kawasaki's disease (mucocutaneous lymph node syndrome in infants and children complicated by coronary arteritis); and necrotizing arteritis associated with hepatitis B infection (either acute hepatitis or chronic active liver disease). The interrelationships of polyarteritis and these forms of arteritis are unclear.

Symptoms and Signs

Polyarteritis mimics many diseases. The course may be that of an acute and prolonged febrile illness, or subacute and fatal after several months; or may be insidious, presenting as a chronic debilitating disease. The location and severity of the arteritis and the extent of secondary circulatory impairment largely determine symptoms, which can be referable to any organ system or combination thereof.

The most common initial complaints are fever (85%); abdominal pain (65%); symptoms of peripheral neuropathy, often a mononeuritis multiplex (50%); weakness (45%); weight loss (45%); and asthma (20%). Hypertension (60%), edema (50%), and oliguria and uremia (15%) may be present in the 75% of patients with renal involvement; proteinemia and hematuria are early manifestations. Diffuse or localized abdominal pain, nausea, vomiting, and bloody diarrhea may mistakenly suggest an acute surgical abdomen. Acute ischemia of the gallbladder or intestines may cause perforation and peritonitis. Hemorrhage from the GI tract or into the retroperitoneal space may occur. Precordial pain occurs in 25% of patients, though ECG evidence indicates coronary disease in 45%. CNS disease produces headache (30%), convulsions (10%), and organic psychosis. Myalgias and arthralgias are common; frank arthritis is not. Dermal lesions, including palpable subcutaneous nodules along the course of the affected artery and irregular areas of skin necrosis, are seen in a few patients.

Laboratory Findings

Leukocytosis of 20,000 to 40,000/μL (80% of patients), proteinuria (60%), and microscopic hematuria (40%) are the most frequent abnormalities. Transient or permanent eosinophilia is unusual but may occur in patients with an extended clinical course, pulmonary involvement, or asthmatic attacks. Frequently found are thrombocytosis, an elevated ESR, anemia due to blood loss or renal failure, hypoalbuminemia, and elevated serum immunoglobulins. Autoantibodies, though often encountered in other collagen vascular diseases, are rarely present.

Diagnosis (For some polyarteritis-associated syndromes, see Pathology, above)

Polyarteritis is a possible diagnosis when unexplained fever, abdominal pain, renal failure, or hypertension is present, or when a case simulating nephritis or a cardiac disorder is accompanied by eosinophilia or by unexplained symptoms such as arthralgia, muscle tenderness or weakness, subcutaneous nodules, purpuric skin rashes, pain in the abdomen or extremities, or rapidly developing hypertension. The diagnosis usually is suggested by a confusing combination of clinical and laboratory features, especially when other causes of a febrile, multisystem illness have been excluded. A systemic illness associated with peripheral, usually multiple, neuritis involving major nerve trunks (eg, radial, peroneal, sciatic) in a bilaterally asymmetric or symmetric fashion **(mononeuritis multiplex)** suggests polyarteritis, as does any of the above clinical profiles when seen in a previously healthy middle-aged male.

Since no serologic tests for polyarteritis are specific, diagnosis depends on demonstrating necrotizing arteritis on **biopsy of typical lesions,** or **angiographic display of the typical aneurysms on medium-size vessels.** Biopsies of skin, subcutaneous tissue, sural nerve and/or muscle are obtained when such tissues display an acute inflammatory reaction; blind biopsy of clinically uninvolved tissue usually is futile. Biopsy may be negative because of the disease's focal nature. Electromyography and nerve conduction studies may help select the site of muscle or nerve biopsy in the absence of clinical findings. The gastrocnemius muscle should *not* be biopsied unless it is the only symptomatic muscle, because of the risk of postoperative venous thrombosis. Testicular biopsy, advocated because microscopic lesions at this site are frequent, should be *avoided* if other suspected sites are accessible. Renal biopsy in patients with evidence of nephritis, and liver biopsy in those with grossly abnormal liver function tests, may be appropriate if other sites fail to provide diagnostic material. Even without a firm tissue diagnosis, **selective angiography** is diagnostic if small aneurysms are seen in renal, hepatic, and celiac vessels.

Prognosis

Acute or chronic, the untreated disease usually is fatal, often ending in failure of the heart, kidneys, or other vital organs, or in GI catastrophes or ruptured aneurysm. Without therapy, only 33% of patients survive for 1 yr; 88% are dead within 5 yr. Glomerulonephritis with renal failure occasionally responds to therapy, but anuria and hypertension are ominous findings; renal failure is the cause of death in 65% of patients.

Treatment

Therapy is vigorous and many-faceted. The offending antigen (including drugs) is sought and avoided. **Corticosteroids** in high dosage (eg, prednisone 60 mg/day in divided doses) may prevent progression, and appear to induce a partial or near-complete remission in about 30% of patients. Because long-term therapy is necessary, corticosteroid side effects, including hypertension and hypercalciuria (which may accelerate preexisting renal damage), often intervene, and the risk of supervening infection is enhanced. The daily corticosteroid dose should be reduced upon improvement; eg, reduction of fever, fall in ESR, improved cardiac and renal function, improved nerve

conduction velocity, disappearance of cutaneous lesions, and diminished pain. Some manifestations of long-term hyperadrenocorticism can be minimized by giving corticosteroids in a single morning dose every other day. This regimen may be adequate as maintenance therapy but is rarely successful in early treatment stages.

Immunosuppressive drugs, either alone or initially with corticosteroids, are used empirically with some success when corticosteroids alone are inadequate. Cyclophosphamide 2 to 3 mg/kg/day orally may be given to patients who do not respond to corticosteroids during the first few weeks of therapy or for whom prohibitively high doses of corticosteroids appear to be necessary to maintain disease control (by these criteria, the majority of patients would qualify). The drug dose should be adjusted to maintain the peripheral blood white cell count between 2000 and 3500/cu mm. (CAUTION: *Immunosuppressive drugs impose risks*, including those of microbial infections, which must be promptly treated.)

Other measures based on specific problems include antihypertensive therapy, careful fluid management, attention to renal impairment, and digitalization. Surgical intervention is required if GI involvement leads to intussusception or mesenteric artery thrombosis and bowel or viscous infarction.

WEGENER'S GRANULOMATOSIS

(See also PULMONARY WEGENER'S GRANULOMATOSIS in Ch. 43)

An uncommon disease that begins as a localized granulomatous inflammation of upper and lower respiratory tract mucosa and usually progresses into generalized necrotizing granulomatous vasculitis and glomerulonephritis.

Etiology and Incidence

The etiology is unknown. Though the disease resembles an infectious process, no causative agent has been isolated. Because of the characteristic histologic tissue changes, hypersensitivity has been postulated as the basis for the disease. The male-to-female ratio is 2:1. The disease can occur at any age.

Pathology

Biopsy of the inflamed and granular material in the nose and nasopharynx discloses granulomatous tissue containing epithelioid cells, Langhans' cells, and foreign-body giant cells. Pulmonary and skin biopsies show inflammatory perivascular exudate and fibrin deposition in small arteries, capillaries, and venules. Renal biopsy shows a focal and segmental glomerulonephritis of varying degrees of severity, occasionally with necrotizing vasculitis. Immunohistochemical studies of the kidney biopsy show extensive deposits of fibrin in blood vessels and glomeruli. Fibrin deposition in glomeruli suggests a partial activation of a clotting factor (Hageman). Immune complexes precipitated by C1q have been found and shown to disappear on therapy with cyclophosphamide and prednisone. Dense subepithelial deposits suggestive of an immune complex reaction are detectable by electron microscopy on the epithelial side of the basement membrane. Immunofluorescence may show scattered deposits of complement and IgG.

Symptoms, Signs, and Laboratory Findings

Onset may be insidious or acute. **Presenting complaints usually are referable to the upper respiratory tract** and include severe rhinorrhea, paranasal sinusitis, nasal mucosal ulcerations (with consequent secondary bacterial infection), serous or purulent otitis media with hearing loss, cough, hemoptysis, and pleuritis. Patients usually present with a granulomatous process of the nose often mistaken for chronic sinusitis. The nasal mucous membrane has a red, raised granular appearance and is friable and bleeds easily. **Other initial symptoms include** fever, malaise, anorexia, weight loss, migratory polyarthropathy, skin lesions, and ocular manifestations with nasolacrimal duct

obstruction and proptosis. Chondritis of the ear, myocardial infarction from vasculitis, and aseptic meningitis and nonhealing granulomas of the CNS may occur.

After a few weeks or months, a disseminated vascular phase develops and is associated with necrotizing inflammatory skin lesions, pulmonary lesions with cavitation, diffuse vasculitis, and focal glomerulitis that may progress to generalized glomerulonephritis with hypertension and uremia. Renal involvement is the hallmark of generalized disease. Urinalysis shows proteinuria, hematuria, and RBC casts. Functional renal impairment is inevitable without immediate appropriate therapy. Occasionally, the disease is limited to pulmonary involvement (see in Ch. 43). Anemia may be present.

Serum complement levels are normal or elevated. The ESR is elevated. Leukocytosis is present. Antinuclear antibodies and LE cells are not present.

Diagnosis

Early diagnosis and treatment are important, since a high remission rate is now possible (see below), including the avoidance or lessening of the critical renal complications. Diagnosis is established by the characteristic clinical and pathologic findings. Renal biopsy determines the extent of renal involvement and is vital in early detection of renal dissemination. Clusters of densely packed atypical cells may be found in the sputum of patients with pulmonary involvement. Differential diagnosis includes polyarteritis, the vascular renal phase of SBE, rapidly or slowly progressive glomerulonephritis, SLE, and lethal midline granuloma. RA may be simulated for as long as a year before the diagnosis becomes apparent. Polyarteritis is ruled out by biopsy of the skin lesions and by pathologic localization of the vascular lesions. Eosinophilia, not a feature of Wegener's granulomatosis, is often present in polyarteritis; nasal and pulmonary granulomatous inflammation is absent. Characteristic blood cultures and changing cardiac murmurs are present in SBE. In SLE, antinuclear antibodies and LE cells are present in the serum, and the serum complement level is depressed. Vasculitic granulomatous inflammation is absent in lethal midline granuloma.

Course, Prognosis, and Treatment

The complete syndrome usually progresses rapidly to renal failure once the diffuse vascular phase begins. Patients with the limited form of the disease may have only nasal and pulmonary lesions with little or no systemic involvement. Pulmonary manifestations may improve or may worsen spontaneously.

Prognosis, once fatal, has been improved by treatment with immunosuppressive cytotoxic agents. Cyclophosphamide (1 to 2 mg/kg/day orally) is the drug of choice, affecting the granulomatous lesions. Corticosteroids, which reduce the vasculitis, are given concurrently (prednisone 1 mg/kg/day orally). After 2 to 4 mo, prednisone is given in 60-mg doses on alternate days, then gradually decreased until the patient is maintained solely on cyclophosphamide. This drug is given at least a full year after a clinical remission of the disease. The dose then is tapered by a 25-mg decrease q 2 to 3 mo. Azathioprine is less effective but may be used as an alternative or adjunct to cyclophosphamide for those who cannot tolerate cyclophosphamide.

Side effects of cyclophosphamide include leukopenia, leading to risk of infections; hemorrhagic cystitis; gonadal dysfunction; and some hair loss, reversible on discontinuing the drug. Long-term complete remission can be achieved with therapy, even with advanced disease. Kidney transplantation has been successful in renal failure. A report of one patient who received a cadaver kidney implant is interesting in that typical renal lesions of Wegener's granulomatosis developed.

MIXED CONNECTIVE TISSUE DISEASE (MCTD)

A rheumatic disease syndrome characterized by overlapping clinical features similar to those of systemic lupus erythematosus **(SLE)**, *scleroderma, and polymyositis/dermatomyositis, and by very high titers of circulating antinuclear antibody to a nuclear ribonucleoprotein* **(RNP)** *antigen.*

Etiology, Pathogenesis, and Prevalence

The etiology is unknown, but certain findings suggest that immune injury may be involved in the pathogenesis: (1) marked hypergammaglobulinemia; (2) persistence of extremely high titers of RNP antibody; (3) mild to moderate hypocomplementemia in 25%; (4) circulating immune complexes during active disease; (5) specific deposition of IgG, IgM, or complement within the walls of blood vessels or muscle fibers and along the glomerular basement membrane; (6) RNP antibodies may penetrate live human mononuclear cells through Fc receptors, and suppressor T cell function may be abnormal in active disease; and (7) chronic inflammatory infiltration by lymphocytes and plasma cells in various tissues.

Whether MCTD is a distinct clinical entity still has not been resolved, but a number of features support this assumption: (1) overlapping clinical features suggesting several connective tissue diseases; (2) extremely high titers of RNP antibody, usually in the absence of significant titers of other antinuclear antibodies; (3) normal reticuloendothelial system clearance of immune complexes in most MCTD patients, in contrast to SLE; (4) abnormalities of immunoregulatory T cell circuits in MCTD that differ from those found in other rheumatic diseases; (5) frequent pulmonary hypertension and associated proliferative vasculopathy with minimal fibrosis; and (6) other pathologic changes which may be restricted to MCTD.

Prevalence is unknown; MCTD appears to be seen more commonly than polymyositis/dermatomyositis and less frequently than SLE. Approximately 80% of patients are female. The age range is from 5 to 80 yr with a mean of 37 yr.

Symptoms, Signs, and Pathology

The **typical clinical syndrome** is characterized by Raynaud's phenomenon, polyarthralgia or arthritis, swollen hands, inflammatory proximal myopathy, esophageal hypomotility, and pulmonary disease. Raynaud's phenomenon may precede other disease manifestations by years, and frequently the initial findings suggest early SLE, scleroderma, polymyositis/dermatomyositis, or RA. Whatever the initial presentation, there is a tendency for more limited disease to progress and become widespread and for transitions in the clinical pattern to occur over time.

The most frequent **skin finding** is swelling of the hands resulting in a sausage appearance of the fingers. Diffuse scleroderma-like changes and ischemic necrosis or ulceration of the fingertips, common in scleroderma, are much less frequent in MCTD. Other skin findings include lupuslike rashes, erythematous patches over the knuckles, violaceous discoloration of the eyelids, diffuse nonscarring alopecia, and squared telangiectasia over the hands and face.

Almost all patients have **polyarthralgias,** and 75% have frank **arthritis.** Often the arthritis is nondeforming, but erosive changes and deformities may be present, suggesting RA. **Proximal muscle weakness** with or without tenderness is common. Electromyograms are typical of **inflammatory myopathy,** and muscle biopsies show degeneration of muscle fibers and interstitial and perivascular infiltrates of lymphocytes and plasma cells.

Esophageal abnormalities including decreased lower sphincter pressure, decreased amplitude of peristalsis in the distal ⅔, and a decrease in upper sphincter pressure occur in 80% of patients, including 70% of asymptomatic patients. **Pulmonary involvement** also occurs in about 80%, and significant abnormalities of diffusing capacity may develop before the disease is clinically apparent. Chest x-rays may show pleuritis and/or diffuse interstitial infiltrates. In some patients, pulmonary involvement becomes the predominant clinical problem, leading to exertional dyspnea and/or pulmonary hypertension. Pulmonary hypertension and proliferative vascular lesions, which usually develop insidiously, represent serious complications for some. Recent studies using in vivo widefield nailfold microscopy have revealed severe capillary abnormalities characteristic of scleroderma in patients who subsequently developed pulmonary

hypertension. Lung biopsies have revealed interstitial mononuclear infiltrates, fibrosis, and vascular intimal proliferation and medial hypertrophy severe enough in some cases to cause vascular obliteration.

Pericarditis is the most frequent cardiac finding. **Myocarditis** also may be present, leading to heart failure. Mitral valve prolapse was identified in 26% of MCTD patients in a recent series. **Renal disease** occurs in only about 10% of patients, often is mild, but occasionally becomes a major clinical problem; patients have died with progressive renal failure. Renal biopsies usually show mesangial hypercellularity, focal glomerulitis, and membranous glomerulonephritis, while membranoproliferative glomerulonephritis and proliferative vascular lesions are much less frequently seen. Serious **neurologic abnormalities** including organic mental syndrome, aseptic meningitis, seizures, multiple peripheral neuropathies, and cerebral infarction or hemorrhage occur in only about 10% of patients. A trigeminal sensory neuropathy appears to be seen much more frequently in MCTD than in other rheumatic diseases.

Other findings that may be present in patients with MCTD include Sjögren's syndrome, Hashimoto's thyroiditis, fever, lymphadenopathy (often of massive proportions), splenomegaly, hepatomegaly, intestinal involvement similar to that seen in scleroderma, and persistent hoarseness.

Laboratory Findings

Almost all patients with MCTD have high titers (often > 1:1000) of fluorescent antinuclear antibodies **(ANA),** which produce a speckled pattern. Antibodies to extractable nuclear antigen **(ENA)** are usually detected at very high titers (> 1:100,000) by hemagglutination. The ANA and hemagglutination reactions are typically eliminated by digestion with ribonuclease **(RNase),** since the ENA component to which antibodies are directed in MCTD is an RNase-sensitive nuclear ribonucleoprotein **(RNP)** antigen. By immunodiffusion it can be confirmed that antibody to RNP is present, while antibody to the RNase-resistant Sm component of ENA is usually absent.

Antibodies to native DNA and LE cells are infrequent in MCTD. Rheumatoid agglutinins are frequently positive and titers often are high. The ESR is frequently elevated, and 75% of patients have diffuse hypergammaglobulinemia often ranging from 2 to 5 gm/dL. Levels of serum complement are slightly to moderately reduced in only about 25% of patients. Serum levels of creatine kinase and aldolase usually are elevated when active myositis is present.

Moderate anemia and leukopenia occur in 30 to 40% of patients with MCTD. Clinically significant Coombs-positive hemolytic anemia and thrombocytopenia are uncommon. However, in one report of childhood MCTD severe thrombocytopenia was more common, and 2 children required splenectomy because they were only partially responsive to corticosteroids. Hematuria, casts, and proteinuria are detected on urinalysis when glomerulonephritis occurs.

Diagnosis

MCTD should be considered when additional overlapping features are present in patients appearing to have SLE, scleroderma, polymyositis, RA, juvenile RA, Sjögren's syndrome, vasculitis, idiopathic thrombocytopenic purpura, lymphoma, or "viral pericarditis." MCTD occasionally may present as a fever of unknown origin. Since the characteristic serologic finding of high titers of antibody to RNP only is much more frequently associated with MCTD than with other rheumatic diseases, detection of RNP antibody permits a presumptive diagnosis early in the evolution of the disease when clinical manifestations are limited. If RNP antibody is detected at a high titer, a thorough evaluation of the muscle, esophageal, and pulmonary systems (especially diffusing capacity) frequently will reveal abnormalities even when the patients are asymptomatic with respect to these systems.

Prognosis

The overall mortality in 5 reports (194 patients) was 13%, with the mean disease duration varying from 6 to 12 yr. Causes of death have included proliferative vascular lesions with pulmonary hypertension, renal failure, myocardial infarction, colonic perforation, disseminated infection, and cerebral hemorrhage. Sustained remissions for several years on little or no maintenance corticosteroid therapy have now been observed in some patients.

Treatment

General medical management and drug therapy are similar to the approach used in SLE. Most patients are responsive to corticosteroids, particularly if treated early in the course of the disease. Mild disease often is controlled by salicylates, other nonsteroidal anti-inflammatory drugs, antimalarials, or very low doses of corticosteroids. Severe major organ involvement usually requires larger doses of corticosteroids; eg, an initial dose of 1 mg/kg of prednisone. Even in patients whose disease is progressive and widespread, more prolonged high-dose corticosteroid therapy, sometimes in combination with cytotoxic drugs, may be associated with clinical improvement. However, with disease of longer duration resulting in greater functional impairment, the response may not be so complete, and drug toxicity may contribute to serious and sometimes fatal complications. In general the scleroderma-like features of MCTD are the least likely to respond to treatment.

---

111. REGIONAL MUSCULOSKELETAL PAIN

SPASMODIC TORTICOLLIS
(Wryneck)

Tonic or intermittent spasm of the neck muscles, causing rotation **(torticollis)** *and tilting* **(anterocollis)** *of the head.*

Etiology

Etiology varies and often cannot be defined. **The congenital variety** is often associated with injury to the sternocleidomastoid muscle on one side at the time of birth during a difficult delivery, and the muscle's transformation into a fibrous cord that cannot lengthen with the growing neck. Minimal deformity may be seen at birth but, within a few weeks, a firm swelling occurs in one sternocleidomastoid muscle, which then contracts. Neck muscle contraction in children may also be secondary to ocular muscle imbalance or defects of the cervical spine or musculature. Underlying psychologic disturbance, basal ganglia disease, CNS infections, or tumors in the bones or soft tissues of the neck may occasionally be implicated in this syndrome, especially with onset in older age, which precludes congenital torticollis.

Symptoms, Signs, and Course

Onset may occur at any age, but most frequently in adults between the 3rd and 6th decades; it may be sudden or (more likely) gradual. Both sexes are equally affected. Intermittent or continuous painful spasms of the sternomastoid, trapezius, and other neck muscles usually occur unilaterally and cause turning (torticollis) and tilting (anterocollis) of the head. Sternomastoid muscle contraction causes rotation of the head to the opposite side and flexion of the neck to the same side. The condition varies from being one of mild or occasional episodes to one that is difficult to treat, may recur often or persist for life, and may result in minimal movement and postural deformity

Diagnosis

In infants, the neck should be inspected for asymmetry, abnormal structures, or masses. A hematoma of the sternomastoid muscle may be seen within several days after delivery (usually breech) and may become fibromatous in subsequent months. Similarly, other pathologic processes in the neck must be ruled out by history of trauma, dysfunction, and by radiologic studies of the cervical spine, including x-rays, CT scan, or MRI. A history of encephalitis or evidence of extrapyramidal disease may be present. Electromyographic, neurologic, and psychologic studies usually are negative.

Prognosis and Treatment

Prognosis is good for correctable pathologic processes in the neck or head; neurologic and psychiatric processes are more difficult to treat. The spasm can sometimes be temporarily inhibited by physical therapy and massage modalities; eg, applying slight tactile pressure to the same side of the jaw as the head rotation (sensory biofeedback technics). In general, however, medical remedies are useless. Relapses after thalamic surgical procedures and anterior cervical rhizotomy are common. Psychiatric treatment is indicated if there is clear evidence of an emotional problem; prognosis is best if onset is directly related to exogenous stress. **Congenital torticollis** should be treated within the first few months of life, initially with intensive physical therapy measures, including daily passive stretching of the shortened muscle for at least 1 yr. If physical therapy is started later in infancy or is not successful, operative division of the contracted sternocleidomastoid muscle and surrounding soft tissues may be indicated.

NECK, SHOULDER, AND UPPER LIMB PAIN

Pain in these regions is common and may be due to a single pathologic process or combined abnormalities. The head, neck, shoulders, and upper limbs are all highly mobile and regularly involved in very complex movements that also often require heavy weight-bearing or the use of great force. Soft tissues (nerves, blood vessels, muscles, ligaments, and capsules) of this region are compressed into tight compartments, increasing their susceptibility to stress.

Pathologic processes producing symptoms may be local (eg, inflammation of a joint, a capsule, or adjacent ligaments, muscles, or nerves), may be distant and cause radiation along the course of neurovascular bundles or brachialgia beginning anywhere from the spinal cord to the end of the extremity, or may be referred pain from diseased intrathoracic or upper abdominal organs. Symptoms also include paresthesias, muscle weakness, and reflex and sensory losses. Accordingly, diagnostic considerations involve good clinical evaluation that, in turn, requires an understanding of inflammatory processes such as the arthritides of either the shoulder or acromioclavicular joints, bursitis (eg, subacromial), tendinitis (eg, supraspinatus syndrome, epicondylitis of the elbow), synovitis, capsulitis, fibromyalgia, vascular and neurologic disorders (the latter being further subdivided into those originating in the spinal cord, nerve roots, or peripheral nerves from cervical disk protrusion, cervical spondylosis, etc), and a wide variety of intrathoracic and some abdominal processes that can refer pain to these areas. Discussions can be found in Ch. 129 and under specific designations elsewhere in THE MANUAL.

LOW BACK PAIN AND SCIATICA

Low back pain *is felt in the low lumbar, lumbosacral, or sacroiliac region.* It is often accompanied by ***sciatica,*** *pain radiating down one or both buttocks and/or legs in the distribution of the sciatic nerve.*

Etiology

Most low back pain is related to acute ligamentous (sprain) or muscular (strain) problems, which tend to be self-limited, or to the more chronic osteoarthritis **(OA)** or ankylosing spondylitis of the lumbosacral area. The incidence of these conditions tends to increase with age, reaching 50% in persons > 60 yr. Other causes of chronic low back pain are (1) back strain due to poor posture or poor conditioning and aggravated by mechanical factors (eg, overuse, obesity, or pregnancy); (2) fibromyalgia; (3) a protruding or ruptured intervertebral disk with subsequent herniation of the nucleus pulposus into the spinal canal, causing inflammatory or direct mechanical nerve root pressure; (4) traumatic ligament rupture, stress fracture of the pars interarticularis, or paraspinous muscle tear; (5) fracture, infection, or tumor involving the back, pelvis, or retroperitoneum; (6) commonly occurring, mild congenital defects of the low lumbar and upper sacral spine (eg, abnormal intervertebral facets, sacralization of L-5 transverse processes); (7) bilateral loss of substance in the pars interarticularis and subsequent slipping forward of a vertebra upon the one below (spondylolisthesis); (8) narrowed spinal canal from spinal stenosis, often superimposed on a congenitally diminished canal space, due to various degeneratiave and acquired processes; and (9) nonmechanical pain due to adjacent visceral disease.

Any type of back pain may be influenced by psychosocial problems and conflicts; these factors regularly alter the patient's perception and reporting of structurally mediated pain, as well as the resultant degree of disability and response to therapy.

Symptoms, Signs, and Diagnosis

Differential diagnosis may be difficult. It begins with **careful definition of the character and precise location of the pain,** which may be *localized* (felt at the site of pathology and associated with point tenderness), as in fibromyalgia; *diffuse* (arising from deeper-lying tissue), eg, lumbago from chronic OA of the lumbar spine; *radicular*, as in sciatica (see below); or *referred* (due to visceral or spinal disease that shares the same spinal segment distribution as the site where the pain is perceived), eg, pyelonephritis or osteomyelitis. **Mechanisms that intensify the pain** are also important diagnostically: Limitation of back motion because of pain and tenderness of the paravertebral muscles is common in all conditions affecting the musculoskeletal and neural systems (mechanical pain) but may be absent in visceral referred pain (nonmechanical pain). Visceral referred pain is typically not affected by motion or relieved by rest; it is usually constant and worse at night. Increased pain following Valsalva maneuver (straining, coughing, or sneezing), limitation of straight-leg raising, loss of reflexes, and sensory change are more characteristic of conditions affecting spinal nerve roots and the sciatic nerve.

Sciatica (*pain radiating along the course of the sciatic nerve, most often into the buttock and the posterior aspect of the leg*) may accompany low back pain, but may be more severe and may occur alone. It is most commonly caused by peripheral nerve root compression from intervertebral disk protrusion or intraspinal tumor. Compression may be within the spinal canal or intervertebral foramen by tumor or bony irregularities such as spondylolisthesis or OA. The nerves can also be compressed outside the spinal cord, in the pelvis or buttock. Toxic or metabolic causes (eg, due to alcoholism diabetic neuropathy) are rare. Such processes are confirmed by the presence of sensory and/or motor deficits, findings that are discussed further under NERVE ROOT DISORDERS in Ch. 131.

Spinal stenosis is *an uncommon form of sciatica that results from lumbar spinal canal narrowing, causing pressure on the roots (or rarely the cord) prior to their exit from the foramina, and mimics vascular disease by simulating intermittent claudication*. It involves the sciatic nerve roots and is manifested by pain in the buttocks, thighs, or calves on walking, running, or climbing stairs. The pain is not relieved by standing still, but by

flexing the back or by sitting. Walking up hills is easier than walking down. Evaluation will not disclose the anticipated vascular insufficiency unless it exists independently. The disorder occurs in middle-aged or elderly patients. A narrowed spinal canal space may be due to OA, Paget's disease, or spondylolisthesis with edema of the cauda equina. Severity of the pain is relieved by rest and flexion of the back (although paresthesias may continue). Decompression laminectomies at several levels may be required for definitive therapy when conservative measures fail (eg, improved posture, weight loss, and abdominal muscle strengthening). This type of pseudoclaudication can be differentiated from vascular intermittent claudication by the presence of a neurologic deficit and by the pain persisting for hours after resting and not coming on rapidly when exercise is begun. The pulses are normal with good skin nutrition.

Congenital bony defects, degenerative disease, or **bony instability** may be demonstrated by radiography, including oblique views showing the intervertebral facet joints. **Ruptured disk** (see in Ch. 131), **ligamentous sprain,** and **muscle tear** are suggested by sudden onset. Symptoms usually begin within 24 h after heavy lifting. Localized tenderness and muscle spasm over a particular area are significant and suggest a process in the back itself rather than in the pelvis or retroperitoneal area. Examination by CT scan or MRI is proving valuable in outlining axial spatial deformations. **Fracture** and **fracture dislocation** are ruled out by the history, nature of the trauma, and x-rays. **Chronic arthritis** of the posterior facet joints is usually associated with degenerative disk disease. The former is characterized by the usual clinical and radiologic findings in OA, and the latter by associated nerve root irritation findings. Hyperextension usually aggravates pain derived from involved posterior facet joints. **Underlying skeletal defects** such as **spondylolisthesis** or **spondyloarthropathy** (eg, ankylosing spondylitis or sacroiliitis) are suggested by gradual onset of low back pain in younger adults; onset in adolescence is highly suggestive of spondyloarthropathy. **Intrapelvic** and **retroperitoneal conditions** may be suggested by the presence of associated symptoms and by the absence of localizing signs in the back. **Tumors** and **infections** are more difficult to diagnose and may mimic a ruptured disk. A space-occupying tumor is frequently diagnosed by CT scan, MRI, or myelography. CSF examination does not always differentiate ruptured disk from tumor, since spinal fluid protein may be elevated in both conditions. CSF examination is indispensable in the diagnosis of spinal meningitis and other infections.

Fibromyalgia (see in Ch. 109) may cause chronic low back pain and stiffness as part of a localized or diffuse syndrome and may be recognized by its association with muscle strain, fatigue, nonrestorative sleep, anxiety or stress, discrete tender points, and absence of inflammation or radiographic abnormalities.

In some psychologically disturbed persons, a history of trivial trauma commonly is followed by disproportionately severe, disabling pain and no evidence of injury or significant, appropriate underlying disease. Additionally, predisposing anxiety or depression usually is present, with persistence of these affects not fully explained on the basis of the low back pain. While any organic disorder may be mimicked, carefully obtained descriptions of the pain and findings on examination tend to be vague or inconsistent with any known neuroanatomic pathways or disease process. In many cases, an organic disorder might reasonably account for the symptoms, but **psychogenic pain** becomes evident when symptoms and disability persist or worsen after the signs of injury or disease have cleared. Monetary considerations, such as worker's compensation or other insurance, rarely cause the problem but commonly facilitate its perpetuation. **Malingering** is less common than psychogenic pain and is difficult to prove. When suspected, it can only be established by garnering evidence that the patient is faking. Inconsistent historical and physical findings on sequential examinations may make one suspicious of this diagnosis. Direct evidence of malingering may best be acquired by someone other than the physician.

Prognosis and Treatment

Recovery from a single acute attack of low back pain is common, but attacks may recur or symptoms may become chronic in all conditions.

Acute low back pain following unusual strain or activity is the most common form and is characterized by prominent muscle spasm and negative neurologic examination. It is treated first by relieving muscle spasm with bed rest in a comfortable position with hips and knees flexed, local heat, massage, oral analgesics (aspirin up to a total of 3.6 gm/day or comparable dose of a NSAID, codeine up to 60 mg q 4 h, or meperidine up to 100 mg q 4 h), and oral muscle relaxants (methocarbamol 1 to 2 gm qid for 48 to 72 h; for maintenance, 1 gm qid; carisoprodol 350 mg tid to qid; meprobamate 400 mg tid to qid; or diazepam 10 mg tid). Traction is not usually needed, since bed rest (with bathroom privileges) is equally effective. Manipulation may be helpful if the pain is due to muscle spasm alone. However, caution must be exercised, since manipulation may aggravate an arthritic joint or further rupture a disk. Diathermy (deep heat) modalities may be helpful in reducing muscle spasm and pain after the acute stage.

A patient with chronic ligamentous muscle strain (ie, an obese or pregnant patient) may walk wearing a lumbosacral corset after the initial muscle spasm has subsided. When symptoms permit, abdominal muscle-strengthening exercises and lumbosacral flexion exercises (maneuvers that lessen lumbar lordosis and increase intra-abdominal pressure) are indicated to strengthen the supporting structures of the back and prevent the condition from becoming chronic or recurrent.

Chronic low back pain treatment is directed toward alleviating the cause; eg, weight reduction in the obese, improving muscle tone and strength, and improving posture. Analgesics may relieve pain; narcotics should be **avoided.** A low-dose tricyclic antidepressant (eg, 10 or 12 mg at bedtime) may improve sleep and help chronic muscle spasm. Intervertebral joint arthritis may respond to proper bracing and abdominal muscle-strengthening exercises. Lumbosacral flexion exercises may increase symptoms. Depending on the cause, surgical procedures may be necessary to relieve intractable pain or other neurologic involvement from disk disease or spinal stenosis. Such patients usually have positive neurologic findings. A trial of comprehensive conservative therapy should usually precede surgery.

Obese patients with longstanding ligamentous or muscle strain or postpartum women with stretched abdominal muscles may benefit from wearing a corset to splint the affected muscles until their strength is regained through exercises. Significant weight loss may be required first. Spinal fusion is indicated if there is instability or severe, well-localized arthritic changes in 1 or 2 interspaces.

Soft tissue injection with dexamethasone acetate, methylprednisolone acetate, hydrocortisone acetate, or triamcinolone acetonide 1 mL (various concentrations), suitable for IM injection, and combined with 2 to 3 mL of 1% local anesthetic can be most effective in relieving disabling tender points. Proper technic should include use of narrowest gauge needle for tissue density and radial (fan-like) infiltration, after initial infiltration with local anesthetic alone, for patient comfort.

Managing psychosocial factors may be direct or very difficult. Such factors must be identified as etiologic or complicating issues early in the illness. When the key problems are acute anxiety or trauma, prompt and firm reassurance following a careful history and physical examination often will suffice. Otherwise, the most important management principles involve what *not* to do. The physician should not behave indecisively or in an accusatory manner; he should not delay appropriate studies (eg x-rays, ESR, electromyography) or demanding procedures (eg, myelography, laminectomy); prescriptions should not be given for narcotics. It is best to be thorough, kind and firm, providing support by permitting the patient to talk about concerns, offering nonaddictive medications and physical therapy, and patiently awaiting improvement

If improvement does not occur in a reasonable period, the problem should be privately discussed with a psychiatric colleague in consideration of referral.

112. PAGET'S DISEASE OF BONE

(Osteitis Deformans)

A chronic disorder of the adult skeleton in which localized areas of hyperactive bone are replaced by a softened and enlarged osseous structure.

Etiology and Incidence

Etiology is unknown. A familial incidence has been observed but the specific genetic pattern is unclear. A "fingerprint" pattern in pagetic osteoclastic nuclei suggests a viral infection. About 3% of persons > age 40 have Paget's disease, with a 3:2 male predominance. The disease is more common in Eastern and Western Europe, England, Australia, and New Zealand.

Pathophysiology

Bone turnover is active at involved sites. Excessively active osteoclasts are often large, contain many nuclei, and may show an osteolytic wedge on x-ray. Osteoblastic repair is also active, producing coarsely woven thickened lamellae and trabeculae giving the x-ray appearance of osteoblastic bone; when separated by areas of fibrosis the x-ray shows a characteristic coarse trabeculation. The mosaic layering of collagen results in structurally enlarged and weakened bone, even though heavily calcified. Any bone can be involved; those most commonly affected, in order, are the pelvis, femur, skull, tibia, vertebrae, clavicle, and humerus.

Symptoms and Signs

Most often the disorder is asymptomatic. Onset is insidious when symptoms occur, which include pain, stiffness, fatigability, deformity, headaches, decreasing auditory acuity, and increasing skull size. Pagetic bone pain is aching, deep, and occasionally severe, and may be accentuated at night. Pain also may arise from compression neuropathy or associated osteoarthritis **(OA)**. Signs of the disease may be bitemporal skull enlargement with frontal "bossing," dilated scalp veins, nerve deafness or otosclerosis in one or both ears, angioid streaks in the fundus of the eye, a short kyphotic trunk with simian appearance, hobbling gait, and anterolateral bowing of the thigh or leg with warmth and periosteal tenderness. Hearing loss, spinal stenosis, paresis, or paraplegia may reflect compression neuropathy. High-output cardiac failure may occur, since the pagetic lesions are metabolically active and highly vascular. Deformities may develop from bowing of the long bones or OA of adjacent joints. Pathologic fractures may be the presenting finding. About 1% of patients develop sarcomatous degeneration, often suggested by increasingly severe pain.

Diagnosis

Diagnosis often is discovered incidentally, on the basis of x-ray or laboratory tests performed for other reasons (eg, elevated alkaline phosphatase). **Characteristic x-ray findings** of involved bones include increased density, abnormal architecture, cortical thickening, bowing, and overgrowth. Microfractures may be seen in the tibia or femur. **Characteristic findings on laboratory studies** include elevated serum alkaline phosphatase and increased urinary excretion of total peptide hydroxyproline. Serum calcium and phosphorus levels usually are normal. **Radionuclide bone scans** using technetium-labeled phosphonates show increased nuclide uptake at the pagetic sites.

Paget's disease may be confused with hyperparathyroidism, bone metastasis (especially from prostatic or breast carcinoma), multiple myeloma, and fibrous dysplasia.

Treatment

Localized and asymptomatic disease requires no treatment. **Salicylates** and **nonsteroidal anti-inflammatory agents** may reduce the pain. **Orthoses** help correct abnormal gait caused by bowed lower extremities. Some patients require **orthopedic surgery;** eg, to replace a diseased hip or to decompress a stenosed spinal canal.

Chemotherapy influences mineral ion fluxes and suppresses bone cell activity. It is indicated (1) when pain is clearly related to the pagetic process and not another source, such as OA; (2) when orthopedic surgery is anticipated, to prevent or reduce bleeding during surgery; and (3) to prevent or retard progression of complications; eg, paraparesis or paraplegia related to vertebral Paget's disease in a poor surgical candidate.

Medications available: **Etidronate disodium** 5 to 10 mg/kg/day orally in a single dose for 6 mo, repeated after a 3- to 6-mo interim, if needed; higher doses (20 mg/kg/day orally for 3 mo) may be required in markedly active disease; **synthetic salmon calcitonin** 50 to 100 Medical Research Council **(MRC)** IU (0.25 to 0.5 mL)/day s.c.; after the initial response, often after 1 mo of therapy, the drug may be tapered to 50 MRC IU every other day and perhaps to intervals of twice or once weekly; **plicamycin (mithramycin)** 10 to 25 μg/kg/day IV for 10 days—a cytotoxic drug usually reserved for severely affected and refractory patients.

---

113. OSTEOPOROSIS

A generalized, progressive diminution in bone tissue mass (ie, a reduced amount of bone) causing weakness of skeletal strength, even though the ratio of mineral to organic elements is unchanged in the remaining morphologically normal bone. Bone resorption is increased; bone formation appears to be normal, though some believe it may be defective. A greater proportional loss of trabecular than of compact bone accounts for the primary complications of the disease; ie, vertical compression, or **crush fractures** of the vertebrae (which consist primarily of trabecular bone), and fractures of the neck of the femur and distal end of the radius (which consist of both cortical and trabecular bone).

Etiology and Incidence

The etiology of **primary osteoporosis** probably is multifactorial. Important factors include failure to develop sufficient bone mass during young adult life, accentuation of age-related bone loss, increased sensitivity to endogenous parathyroid hormone, defective intestinal calcium absorption, and menopause. Possible environmental factors include smoking, excessive alcohol consumption, and decreased exercise. Primary osteoporosis is much more common in women than in men (though it is rare in premenopausal women), in older than in middle-aged individuals, and in whites than in blacks. **Secondary osteoporosis** may be produced by a number of medical disorders, most commonly hypercortisonism, hypogonadism, multiple myeloma, and subtotal gastrectomy.

Symptoms, Signs, and Diagnosis

Patients with uncomplicated osteoporosis may remain asymptomatic or have aching pain in the bones, particularly the back. Vertebral **crush fractures** develop with minimal or no trauma, usually in weight-bearing vertebrae (T-8 and below). The pain is acute, usually does not radiate, is aggravated by weight-bearing, may be associated with local tenderness, and generally subsides in a few days or weeks. Multiple compression fractures may cause dorsal kyphosis and exaggerated cervical lordosis, and complaints of chronic, dull, aching pain (because of abnormal stress on the spinal muscles and ligaments) particularly prominent in the lower thoracic and lumbar area. Hip and Colles' fractures are more common in the elderly, because of preexisting osteoporosis.

Serum calcium, phosphorus, and alkaline phosphatase levels, serum protein electrophoresis, and ESR are normal in primary osteoporosis. Abnormal biochemical findings suggest secondary osteoporosis.

On **x-ray examination,** the vertebrae show decreased radiodensity from loss of trabecular structure. Reliance on subjective impressions of bone density may be misleading. The loss of horizontally oriented trabeculae results in increased prominence of the cortical endplates and of the remaining vertically oriented, weight-bearing trabeculae of the vertebrae. Anterior wedging in the thoracic region and ballooning of the vertebral interspaces in the lumbar area are characteristic of vertebral fractures. Although the cortices of long bones may be thin because of excessive endosteal resorption, the periosteal surface remains smooth (in contrast to hyperparathyroidism). **Corticosteroid-induced osteoporosis** is likely to produce radiolucency of the skull, rib fractures, and exuberant callus formation. **Osteomalacia** (see in Ch. 81) may be radiologically confused with osteoporosis, but can be distinguished by abnormal serum biochemical findings and by bone biopsy.

Dual photon absorptiometry and **quantitative CT** are becoming increasingly available to measure bone density of the lumbar spine, useful in diagnosis and in following treatment response.

Treatment

Treatment is preventive as well as symptomatic and inhibitory. Preventive treatment comprises recognition of high-risk patients plus exercise and supplementary calcium and, in selected postmenopausal women, estrogen replacement therapy. (See also Ch. 171.)

Severe acute back pain from vertebral crush fracture should be treated with an orthopedic support, analgesics, and (when muscle spasm is prominent) heat and massage. Chronic backache may be helped by an orthopedic garment or, more physiologically, by hyperextension exercises to strengthen flabby paravertebral muscles. Avoiding heavy lifting or accidental falls is important. However, since exercise is vital for healthy bone, immobilization should be minimized and a consistent exercise regimen encouraged.

Supplementary calcium and sex hormones decrease bone resorption and may arrest or decrease disease progression. At least 2 glasses of milk/day and a small daily supplement (1000 IU) of vitamin D are recommended. Large doses of oral calcium are well tolerated. For milder disease, calcium carbonate tablets 600 mg 4 to 6 times/day (equivalent to 1 to 1.5 gm of calcium/day) are given. With more severe or progressive disease, sex hormones should be given in addition to calcium. **Women** are given an estrogen such as conjugated estrogen 0.625 to 1.25 mg/day (omitting 5 consecutive days of each month to prevent uterine endometrial hyperplasia). Estrogen produces withdrawal menstrual bleeding in about half the postmenopausal women thus treated and may increase the risk of uterine cancer. A progestin such as medroxyprogesterone acetate, given 10 mg/day for the last 10 days of the cycle, decreases the risk of endometrial cancer but increases the occurrence of withdrawal bleeding, produces an unfavorable serum lipid profile, and may increase the risk of coronary and cerebrovascular thrombosis. For women who are unable to tolerate estrogen because of side effects, or in whom estrogen therapy is contraindicated, salmon calcitonin 100 IU (MRC—Medical Research Council)/day by s.c. injection can be used. **Osteoporotic men** are given supplements of calcium 1 to 1.5 gm/day; when there is evidence of decreased calcium absorption (assessed by urinary calcium of < 100 mg/day), vitamin D 50,000 IU/day are also given.

Combined therapy with sodium fluoride 50 mg/day and at least 1 gm of supplementary elemental calcium appears to increase bone mass, but the FDA has not yet approved sodium fluoride for this use.

114. OSTEOMYELITIS

An infection of bone, usually caused by bacteria, but sometimes by fungi or mycobacteria.

Pathogenesis

Hematogenous osteomyelitis may arise from a clinically evident infection or from an unknown source via bacteremia. This osteomyelitis usually develops in bones with a good blood supply and a rich marrow. In children the most common sites are the long bones, particularly near the epiphyseal plate at the end of the shaft. Because fat replaces the marrow in these sites during adolescence and the vasculature substantially diminishes, hematogenous osteomyelitis of the long bones in adults is rare. Instead, vertebrae are the most common location. Especially predisposed to hematogenous osteomyelitis are hemodialysis patients and drug abusers, in whom the osteomyelitis occasionally occurs in other sites, such as the pubic bone or the clavicle.

Infection spread to bone from adjacent soft tissue suppuration: Typically, the infection has persisted for several days to weeks in an area damaged by trauma, radiation therapy, malignancy, or other causes. In patients with diabetic or atherosclerotic arterial insufficiency of the lower extremities, organisms usually reach the bone by entering the soft tissues through a cutaneous foot ulcer. Osteomyelitis of the skull typically arises from sinus or dental infections.

Organisms enter the bone directly with open fractures, surgical reduction of closed fractures, penetrating trauma, or operative procedures for nontraumatic bone and joint disorders. Most infections of orthopedic prostheses occur from bacterial contamination during surgery.

Because of the rigidity of bone, inflammation in the medullary cavity causes increased intracavitary pressure, leading to diminished vascular flow, ischemia, vascular thrombosis, and bone necrosis. *Fragments of devitalized bone* are called **sequestra.** The infection may extend through the cortex to cause subperiosteal suppuration and may perforate the periosteum to form soft tissue abscesses or draining sinuses through the skin. With persistent infection in the long bones, the periosteum may form new bone **(involucrum)** around the inflammation.

Symptoms, Signs, and Radiographic Findings

In children, acute hematogenous osteomyelitis appears as pain in the affected bone and fever. There may be a history of preceding trauma in the area. Sometimes the fever precedes the pain by several days. Tenderness and soft tissue swelling over the bone may develop, accompanied by pain on motion. Elevated WBC count and ESR are usual. Except in infants, radionuclide scanning with technetium phosphate is nearly always positive, even early in the disease, while x-ray changes of bone destruction usually take 3 wk or more to appear.

Vertebral osteomyelitis usually has an insidious onset and a gradually progressive course of persistent back pain unrelieved by rest, heat, or analgesics, and worsened by movement. Fever typically is minimal or absent. Tenderness to palpation and percussion over the affected bone, paravertebral muscle spasm, and guarding and splinting on motion are the usual physical signs. The WBC count typically is normal, but the ESR nearly always is elevated, a feature that distinguishes vertebral osteomyelitis from many other causes of back pain. Radionuclide scans with technetium phosphate are positive early in the disease, but tumors, fractures, and other conditions also may give positive results. Indium-labeled leukocyte scans, however, usually are positive in infection and negative in the other disorders. The major x-ray changes, appearing several weeks after the infection begins, include erosion of the subchondral bony plate, narrowed intervertebral disk space, and bony destruction with loss of vertebral height.

Tuberculous spondylitis (Pott's disease) is discussed in Ch. 8.

Posttraumatic osteomyelitis and **osteomyelitis from a contiguous source** cause, in varying combinations, local pain, draining sinuses, and soft tissue inflammation or abscesses overlying the affected bone. Fever commonly is absent, and the WBC count and ESR usually are normal. In patients with infected orthopedic prostheses, persistent pain and loosening of the appliance typically are present. X-ray changes in these forms of osteomyelitis include bony destruction with formation of radiolucent areas, radiopaque sequestra, and involucra. Injection of contrast material into a sinus may delineate the location and extent of the infection. An infected prosthesis may show radiographic evidence of loosening. Radionuclide imaging with technetium phosphate commonly is unhelpful, since it accumulates in many noninfectious circumstances, such as fracture site, uninfected nonunions of fractures, periosteal new bone, overlying cellulitis, and aseptic loosening of prostheses. Scans with indium-labeled leukocytes appear to be much more specific.

With unsuccessful treatment of acute osteomyelitis, **chronic osteomyelitis** may develop, usually causing episodic bone pain, intermittent or persistent drainage from sinus tracts, or overlying soft tissue infections. Acute exacerbations of pain and the development of subcutaneous abscesses may occur when closure of the sinuses obstructs the drainage.

Diagnosis and Treatment

Diagnosis requires isolation of the responsible organisms. In **acute hematogenous osteomyelitis in children,** blood cultures often are positive. Other sources include pus from soft tissue abscesses or synovial fluid aspirated from an affected adjacent joint. If these tests are unrevealing or not indicated, the child should receive antibiotics, such as oxacillin or nafcillin, effective against *Staphylococcus aureus,* the usual pathogen. (Usual dosages of antibiotics are given in Ch. 3.) Parenteral therapy is advisable initially, but most of the 4- to 6-wk course can be with oral agents if the clinical response is rapid. Surgery usually is unnecessary with prompt antibiotic administrations; the main indication is drainage of subperiosteal or subcutaneous abscesses.

In **vertebral osteomyelitis,** blood cultures occasionally are positive, but diagnosis usually requires needle aspiration of the appropriate intervertebral disk space if it appears infected, percutaneous needle biopsy of the infected bone, or open biopsy at surgery. Although *S. aureus* is the most common isolate, enteric gram-negative rods also are frequent. Moreover, fungal and tuberculous vertebral osteomyelitis may be indistinguishable from a pyogenic cause except by culture results. The treatment of vertebral osteomyelitis is bed rest and 6 to 8 wk of an appropriate antimicrobial agent. Surgery is reserved for drainage of paravertebral or epidural abscesses or stabilization of an unstable cervical spine.

In patients with **chronic osteomyelitis, posttraumatic osteomyelitis,** or **osteomyelitis from a contiguous site of infection,** the diagnosis depends on both aerobic and anaerobic cultures of bone, tissue, or pus from a deep abscess. These infections commonly are polymicrobial. Material obtained from draining sinuses is unreliable because the tract may harbor skin organisms not present in the deep sites. The main treatment for these forms of bone infection is a combination of surgery and antimicrobials. Antibiotics alone rarely are curative. Surgical goals include removal of all devitalized tissue and elimination of dead space, achieved by (1) open packing, allowing granulation tissue to fill the defect; (2) packing the cavity with cancellous bone grafts; (3) transfer of a pedicle of skeletal muscle into the cavity; (4) skin grafting directly onto the granulating bone surface; and (5) transfers of vascularized bone segments from the fibula or iliac crest. The patient usually receives a minimum of 3 wk of antimicrobial therapy following surgery.

Infection of a prosthesis generally requires its removal, thorough debridement, and appropriate antibiotic administration. With indolent infections, a new appliance may be implanted at the same operation. With active infection, a period of intense antibi-

otic treatment precedes replacement of the prosthesis. Alternatively, the patient may require arthrodesis or, in certain cases, amputation.

In **osteomyelitis associated with vascular insufficiency,** cure almost always requires amputation of the involves bones. The usual organisms are a combination of anaerobic and aerobic bacteria, including enteric gram-negative bacilli. Antimicrobial therapy should include agents effective against these pathogens, such as cefoxitin or a combination of an aminoglycoside and clindamycin. Most patients require only a short perioperative course.

115. NEOPLASMS OF BONES AND JOINTS

(See also Chs. 23 and 105)

Any persistent or progressive pain of the trunk or extremities, particularly if associated with a mass, must be considered to be due to a bone tumor until proved otherwise. The most common problem in diagnosing and treating bone tumors is failure to suspect their presence. Symptomatic treatment of joint or extremity pain (even when distress follows trauma) without pretreatment diagnostic x-rays can lead to tragedy. Hence, it is imperative to suspect a tumor and obtain x-rays in 2 planes before proceeding with biopsy and specific treatment.

Host-tumor immunologic factors play a role in the clinical course of malignant lesions. Both humoral and cellular expressions of immunoincompetence in patients with sarcomas have been reported. A correlation has been shown between the degree of general depression of immunologic responsiveness and the subsequent clinical progression of disease. However, the use of immunologic monitoring remains experimental; its clinical usefulness is unknown.

Sophisticated approaches to adjunctive chemotherapy are being used in a number of clinical trials; their efficacy is unproved.

Diagnosis

X-rays: Certain x-ray signs help to distinguish benign from malignant lesions, but none are infallible. X-rays help primarily in determining a tumor's location; eg, Ewing's tumor commonly appears first in the shaft of the long bone, while osteogenic sarcoma usually appears in the metaphysis toward the end of a long bone. Giant-cell tumor usually affects the epiphyseal end of a long bone. An aneurysmal bone cyst may be seen in any bone, but is usually located in the metaphyseal portion of a long bone. Similarly, CT and MRI also may help to define the location and extent of a lesion, but rarely provide specific diagnostic information. Chest x-rays are needed to rule out pulmonary metastatic involvement. Skeletal surveys and radioisotopic bone scans should be performed in a search for multicentric or metastic lesions.

The **patient's age** is helpful. In children, primary bone tumors prevail; metastatic tumors are rare. In adults, the incidence of metastatic bone tumors is about 20 times that of primary malignant tumors. A **general medical examination** is required once a bone lesion has been discovered and a neoplasm is suspected.

Biopsy is essential for diagnosis. However, histopathologic diagnosis of bone tumors is difficult and requires an adequate amount of tissue from a representative portion of the tumor. Open incisional biopsy is preferred. Blind needle aspiration biopsy should be reserved for large, easily accessible lesions when only metastatic confirmation is required, or, occasionally, for investigation of a vertebral lesion. The pathologist should be given pertinent details of the clinical history and x-ray findings. Since almost all bone tumors have soft portions that can be sectioned and examined for immediate diagnosis by fresh-frozen technic, and since these portions usually are the best material for diagnosis, an immediate, accurate, definitive diagnosis is possible in more than 90%

of bone tumors. Facilities should be available to proceed immediately with appropriate definitive treatment of malignant tumors that are best treated by ablative surgery, which can then be carried out under the same anesthetic as for the biopsy.

BENIGN TUMORS OF BONE

Osteochondromas (osteocartilaginous exostoses) are the most common benign bone tumors, occur most often in persons aged 10 to 20, and may be single or multiple. Each osteochondroma is covered by a cartilaginous cap. A strong familial tendency to multiple osteochondromas may exist. Secondary malignant chondrosarcoma (see below) appears in > 10% of patients with multiple osteochondromas.

Benign chondromas are located centrally within a bone (ie, within the marrow cavity) and occur most commonly in persons aged 10 to 30. On x-ray, they may appear as lytic lesions with areas of stippled calcification.

Chondroblastoma is a rare benign neoplasm arising in an epiphysis. It is most common in persons aged 10 to 20.

Chondromyxofibromas occur before age 30. Their x-ray appearance (usually eccentric, sharply circumscribed, lytic, and located near the end of long bones) suggests the diagnosis.

Osteoid osteoma is a benign lesion which may occur in any bone, but is most common in long bones. The characteristic appearance on x-ray is a small radiolucent zone surrounded by a large sclerotic zone. Technetium-99 bone scans are valuable in helping to identify and localize this lesion. Pain relieved by small doses of aspirin is a classic feature. Treatment is surgical; permanent relief is obtained only if the small radiolucent zone is located and removed.

Giant-cell tumors occur most commonly in the 20s and 30s. The lesions occur in the epiphyses of long bones and produce a lytic appearance on x-ray. They may erode the parent bone and produce soft tissue extensions. Treatment for small lesions usually consists of complete exteriorization, excision by curettage, and bone grafting. For larger lesions, complete excision of the lesion may be necessary. Giant-cell tumor is notorious for its tendency to recur, which may make surgical management difficult. A sarcoma eventually develops and complicates the course in < 10% of cases.

Fibromatous lesions may affect the long bones. The nature of these lesions can be ascertained only by biopsy. Not true neoplastic growths, the lesions probably result from faulty ossification. Many of them regress spontaneously without treatment.

PRIMARY MALIGNANT TUMORS OF BONE

Osteogenic sarcoma (osteosarcoma), except for myeloma, is the most common primary bone tumor and is highly malignant, with a tendency to metastasize to the lungs. Osteosarcoma is most common in persons aged 10 to 20, though it can occur at any age. About half the lesions are located in the region of the knee but can be found in any bone. Pain and a mass are the usual symptoms. X-ray findings vary greatly, with no characteristic appearance, and the tumor may be predominantly sclerotic or lytic. Accurate diagnosis rests on pathologic examination of representative biopsy tissue.

With chemotherapy and surgery, > 50% of patients survive for 5 yr or longer. Preoperative chemotherapy is often used. With adjuvant chemotherapy, it may be possible to preserve a limb using various limb salvage procedures as an alternative to amputation. The efficacy of various adjunctive treatments is under study.

Fibrosarcomas have the same characteristics as osteogenic sarcomas, above, and pose the same problems.

Malignant fibrous histiocytoma behaves clinically in a manner similar to osteosarcoma and fibrosarcoma. Treatment is the same as for osteosarcoma.

Chondrosarcomas, malignant tumors of cartilage, are clinically, therapeutically, and prognostically *unlike* osteogenic sarcomas. They develop in > 10% of patients with multiple benign osteochondromas. However, 90% of chondrosarcomas are primary, arising de novo. **Diagnosis** can be made only by biopsy. Many chondrosarcomas can be graded from 1 to 4 histologically. Grade 1 lesions are slow-growing with a good prognosis for cure; grade 4 lesions grow more rapidly and are much more likely to metastasize. Regardless of grade, the outstanding feature is their ability to "seed" or implant in surrounding soft tissues.

Treatment is total surgical resection. Neither radiation nor chemotherapy is effective in either primary or adjunctive treatment. Because of the potential to seed, the biopsy wound should be closed and ablative surgery carried out meticulously. Care must be taken to avoid entry into the tumor and spillage of tumor cells into the soft tissues of the wound, since recurrence is inevitable if this happens. With no spillage of tumor contents, the cure rate is ≥ 50%, depending on the grade of the tumor. When surgical ablation with maintenance of function is impossible, amputation is obligatory.

Mesenchymal chondrosarcoma is a rare but histologically distinct type of chondrosarcoma with a great potential for metastasizing; the cure rate is low.

Ewing's tumor (Ewing's sarcoma) is a radiosensitive round-cell bone tumor. Males are affected more frequently than females. Ewing's tumor appears at a younger age than any other primary malignant bone tumor, with a peak incidence between 10 and 20 yr. Most of the tumors develop in the extremities, but any bone may be involved. Microscopically, the lesion consists of solidly packed, small round cells. Pain and swelling are the most common symptoms. Ewing's tumor tends to be extensive, sometimes involving the entire shaft of a long bone. Generally, more of the bone is pathologically involved than is apparent from the x-rays. Lytic destruction is the most common finding, but there may be multiple layers of subperiosteal reactive new bone formation, giving the onionskin appearance once considered a classic diagnostic sign. **Diagnosis** depends on biopsy, since many other malignant bone tumors produce an identical appearance. **Treatment** includes various combinations of surgery, multimodal chemotherapy, and radiation therapy. At the present time, about 50% of patients with primary localized Ewing's sarcoma of bone may be cured by this multimodal approach.

Malignant lymphoma of bone is a small round-cell tumor that affects adults, usually in their 40s and 50s. It may arise in any bone. While the lesion may be referred to as **reticulum cell sarcoma,** a mixture of reticulum cells, lymphoblasts, and lymphocytes is common in these neoplasms. When malignant lymphoma involves bone, one of 3 clinical conditions may be found: (1) The lymphoma may be primary in bone, without evidence of disease elsewhere. (2) In addition to the bone lesion, similar disease may be found in other osseous or soft tissue sites. (3) A patient with known soft tissue lymphomatous disease may subsequently have metastatic spread into any bone.

Pain and swelling are the usual symptoms. On x-ray, bone destruction is predominant. Depending on the stage, the involved bone may be mottled or patchy, or, in more advanced disease, the entire outline of the affected bone may be lost. Pathologic fracture is common.

When malignant lymphoma is primary in bone and no disease is present elsewhere, the prognosis is better than in any other primary malignant bone tumor; the 5-yr survival rate is at least 50%. The tumors are radiosensitive. Combination radiation and chemotherapy is as effective in achieving cure as amputation or other extensive ablative surgery. Amputation is only indicated when function is lost because of pathologic fracture or extensive soft tissue involvement.

Multiple myeloma (see also Ch. 103) is a tumor of hematopoietic derivation and is the most common bone neoplasm. The neoplastic process is regularly multicentric and often involves the bone marrow so diffusely that bone marrow aspiration usually is diagnostic.

Malignant giant-cell tumor is rare; even its existence is controversial. The lesion usually is located at the extreme end of a long bone. The classic features of malignant destruction (predominantly lytic; cortical destruction; soft tissue extension; pathologic fracture) are seen on x-ray. To be sure of diagnosis, zones of typical benign giant-cell tumor must be demonstrated in a malignant neoplasm or in previous tissue obtained from the neoplasm. A sarcoma that develops in a previously benign giant-cell tumor is characteristically radioresistant. The same prinicples of treatment apply as in osteogenic sarcoma, above, but the cure rate is low.

Many other types of primary malignant bone tumors exist, most of them so rare as to be medical curiosities. **Chordoma** develops from the remnants of the primitive notochord. It has a predilection for the ends of the spinal column and usually is located in the sacrum or near the base of the skull. Pain is a virtually constant feature of a chordoma located in the sacrococcygeal region. When located in the base of the occipital region, the symptoms may be referred to any of the cranial nerves, but symptoms resulting from involvement of the nerves to the eye are most common. The duration of symptoms varies from months to several years before diagnosis. A chordoma is seen on x-ray as an expansile, destructive bone lesion that may be associated with a soft tissue mass. Hematogenous metastasis is rare. Local recurrence is more troublesome than metastatic spread. Chordomas located in the spheno-occipital region usually are inaccessible to surgery, but may respond to radiation therapy. In the sacrococcygeal region they may be cured by radical en bloc excision.

CONDITIONS THAT COMMONLY SIMULATE PRIMARY TUMORS OF BONE

Many non-neoplastic conditions of bone may simulate bone tumors, either clinically or radiologically. **Heterotopic ossification (myositis ossificans)** or **exuberant callus** after fracture may be mistakenly interpreted as a malignant neoplasm; histopathologic tissue examination differentiates the conditions.

Simple **unicameral bone cysts** occur in the long bones in children. Most come to the clinician's attention when pathologic fracture occurs. Small ones heal and may obliterate themselves in the process of fracture healing. Larger ones may require evacuation and bone grafting.

Fibrous dysplasia is a cystic bone lesion probably resulting from an anomaly in bone development. The lesion may appear in one or several bones during childhood. When several bones are involved and cutaneous pigmentation and endocrine abnormalities are present, the condition is called **Albright's syndrome.** On x-ray, the lesions appear cystic and may be extensive and deforming. The lesions commonly stop growing at puberty. Spontaneous malignant degeneration is rare. Treatment should be conservative, though deformity in the long bones may require surgical correction.

Aneurysmal bone cyst is a cystic lesion of unknown cause that usually appears before age 20. The cyst may occur in the metaphyseal region of the long bones, but almost any bone may be affected. Pain and swelling occur. The lesion may be present for a few weeks to a few years before diagnosis. It tends to increase slowly in size until therapy is begun. The appearance on x-ray often is characteristic: The rarefied area usually is well circumscribed, eccentric, and associated with soft tissue extension pro-

duced by periosteal bulging. Periosteal new bone formation tends to delimit the periphery of the tumor. Surgical removal of the entire lesion is the most successful treatment, but complete regresssion after incomplete removal sometimes occurs. Radiation is the treatment of choice only in surgically inaccessible vertebral lesions that are compressing the spinal cord, since postirradiation sarcomas occasionally occur.

Histiocytosis X (Letterer-Siwe disease, Hand-Schüller-Christian disease, eosinophilic granuloma) is also discussed in Ch. 45. Solitary or multiple reticuloendothelial osseous lesions occur and are usually well defined on x-ray. When the lesion is solitary with periosteal new bone formation, the x-ray may suggest a malignant bone tumor; diagnosis depends on biopsy. When only one or a few osseous lesions are present, local radiation therapy can produce cure, but the prognosis is ominous in patients < 3 yr old or at any age with more than 8 bones involved, and particularly in those with hemorrhagic manifestations and enlarged spleens. More extensive involvement, particularly skull lesions, may occur, and extreme widespread involvement may produce fulminating, rapidly fatal disease with death usually the result of respiratory or cardiac failure.

MALIGNANT METASTATIC LESIONS OF BONE

Any cancer may metastasize to bone, but metastases from carcinomas are the most common, particularly those arising in the breast, lung, prostate, kidney, and thyroid. Any bone may be involved, but metastatic osseous lesions distal to the knees and elbows are uncommon. Any patient being treated for cancer or known to have had cancer and presenting with skeletal complaints should be evaluated for the possibility of metastatic lesions with skeletal x-ray surveys. Whole-body bone scintigrams, using a radioisotope, occasionally demonstrate metastatic lesions before they are apparent on x-ray. The origin may be obscure, but biopsy may give clues to the location of the primary tumor. The symptoms representing a bony metastasis occasionally occur before a primary tumor is suspected.

Treatment depends on the type of primary tissue involved and the organ of origin. Radiation, combined with selected chemotherapeutic or hormonal agents, is the most common modality. When pathologic fracture is imminent or present, surgical technics can be used to avoid amputation. When the primary cancer has been removed and only a single osseous metastasis remains, excision combined with radiation, chemotherapy, or both may be curative.

---

116. COMMON FOOT DISORDERS

EXAMINATION OF THE FOOT AND ANKLE

Diagnosis and management of the patient's complaint depend on a working knowledge of foot anatomy, to determine the structures involved (ie, tendon, nerve, ligament, or bone) and whether the problem is articular or extra-articular. If more than one site is involved, the patient should be asked to indicate the location of greatest discomfort and grade the amount of pain elicited by palpation at each site. Certain areas of the foot normally are tender to palpation; eg, the sinus tarsi and the distal aspect of the ball between the metatarsals.

Once the problem is localized, its cause is considered: whether it is a local process, the result of trauma or an abnormality in foot structure or function, or a sign of systemic disease.

Examination of the ankle region: To check for tenderness or edema, the skin is first examined by moving it side to side and distally to proximally over the ankle. The skin

is compressed, using the fingers of both hands to determine if the problem rests in the skin. Below the skin, the sensory branches of the superficial peroneal nerve can be visualized and palpated by plantar flexing and inverting the foot. Tapping these nerves, which are commonly tender following trauma to the foot and ankle, may elicit pain, discomfort, or tingling **(Tinel's sign).** At this level, anterior and lateral to the medial malleolus, the great saphenous vein is observed for signs of injury, and palpated for tenderness. Below this level, the extensor tendons are examined by placing the patient's foot at a right angle, with the forefoot twisted out in abduction, and asking the patient to hold the foot in that position while the examiner plantar flexes it against resistance. This maneuver accentuates the slips of the long extensor tendons. Each slip is examined individually and palpated for tenderness, pain, or swelling. The anterior tibial tendon can be similarly examined by dorsiflexing and inverting the foot as counter-resistance is applied. **Tenosynovitis** may occur because of overuse, infection, or arthropathy (eg, RA).

The ankle joint is then examined by deep palpation medial and lateral to the extensor digitorum longus tendon. Tenderness at the anterior lateral aspect of the ankle joint between the lateral malleolus and talus is common following inversion sprains of the anterior talofibular ligament (see Sequelae of Inversion Ankle Sprains, below). Swelling below and anterior to the lateral malleolus suggests effusion from the ankle joint. Such effusions are found in intra-articular disease; eg, trauma causing osteoarthritis, ball and socket ankle joints due to abnormal frontal motion in the ankle, or ankle diastasis. Swelling over the anterior talofibular mortise, usually larger, bilateral, and symmetric, may also be caused by juxta-malleolar lipoma, common in menopausal women. These swellings are usually larger, bilateral, and symmetric, and may be painful because of entrapment of the intermediate dorsal cutaneous branch of the superficial peroneal nerve. Swelling behind one or both malleoli, usually painful, suggests tenosynovitis. Swelling of the entire ankle as opposed to localized swelling usually represents venous disease, lymphedema, or the edema of congestive heart failure. Edema tends to accumulate at the ankle because of shoe compression.

The heel is examined with the foot at a right angle to the leg. Pain, as described by the patient or elicited by palpation, usually can be localized, thus aiding in the diagnosis. In the discussion below, heel disorders are described in groups based on such localization. Deep, firm palpation to the center of the heel will elicit pain in patients with biomechanical abnormalities, fascial problems, and heel spur syndromes. Pain at the medial and lateral margins of the heel in children is a symptom of epiphysitis of the calcaneus (Sever's disease). Pain anterior to the Achilles tendon at the retromalleolar space may suggest bursitis (retromalleolar bursitis, Albert's disease), or posterior tibial neuralgia. Pain posterior to the Achilles tendon may result from an enlarged posterior-superior aspect of the calcaneus (Haglund's deformity), a common finding in children and adults whose subtalar joint functions in an inverted position, associated with painful adventitious bursae between the tendon and the skin. Tenderness at the calcaneal insertion of the Achilles tendon may be a sign of an overuse syndrome in athletes or a tight heel chord secondary to abnormal foot structure and function.

Occasionally, inflammatory arthropathies affect the heel (eg, ankylosing spondylitis, Reiter's syndrome); and the heel is second only to the first metatarsophalangeal joint for gouty arthritis. RA commonly is the cause of heel pain from inflammatory erosion at the posterior aspect of the calcaneus. These arthropathies, usually distinguishable from local causes of heel pain by the presence of moderate to severe heat and swelling, are discussed elsewhere in THE MANUAL.

HEEL PAIN

PAIN ON THE PLANTAR SURFACE OF THE HEEL

Calcaneal Spur Syndrome

The spur is a bony exostosis that originates at the inner weight-bearing tuberosity of the calcaneus and extends forward horizontally in the direction of the plantar fascia. The spur results from strain injuring the periosteal attachment of the plantar fascia to the heel bone. Spurs usually are present bilaterally and are more or less uniform in shape. They are commonly found with limited ankle joint flexion due to contracted heel chords.

Symptoms, signs, and diagnosis: Calcaneal spurs do not always cause symptoms; eg, heel pain is not necessarily due to an existing spur. Asymptomatic spurs commonly are discovered incidentally in an x-ray taken for other reasons. An existing spur may be asymptomatic for many years, with pain then developing suddenly as a result of movement that produces obliquely downward pressure on the tissues and cutaneous nerves in the area. Pain is experienced only on weight-bearing or directly applied digital pressure, and is most pronounced just anterior to the inner weight-bearing tuberosity of the calcaneus but can radiate to other parts of the heel and sometimes forward to the foot. Inferior calcaneal bursitis with mild heat and swelling also may be seen. Physical examination may demonstrate pain in the central portion of the heel, but this may represent only a strain in the plantar fascia. In a few persons with a very thin fat pad, the spur may be palpated. An x-ray is the only certain means of diagnosis. Locomotion should be biomechanically evaluated to determine its importance as a factor causing plantar fascial strain.

Treatment: Symptoms can be controlled with a corticosteroid/lidocaine injection (1 mL of triamcinolone acetonide [10 mg/mL] with 1.5 mL of 2% lidocaine with 1:100,000 epinephrine) given perpendicular to the medial border of the heel pointing toward the painful trigger point located at the central portion of the heel. Strapping alleviates tension along the plantar fascia; orthotic devices control abnormal elongation of the foot, causing strain along the plantar fascia.

PAIN LOCATED AT THE MARGINS OF THE HEEL

Epiphysitis of the Calcaneus (Sever's Disease)

A painful condition of the heel affecting children. The calcaneus is the only bone in the tarsus that develops from 2 centers of ossification: one from the body of the calcaneus and one from its epiphysis, which later forms the posterior part of this bone. Ossification of the body of the calcaneus begins at birth. Ossification of the epiphysis usually does not begin before the 8th yr. At the age of 16 and sometimes somewhat later, complete ossification with union of the body and the epiphysis of this bone usually has taken place. Between the ages of 8 and 16, before bony union has been effected, the 2 parts of the bone are connected by cartilage. Excessive strain on the epiphysis by jumping or other athletic activities sometimes results in breaking the cartilaginous union between the 2 bones or fibers of the tendinous insertion at the epiphysis. Children who are unable to dorsiflex their foot normally are more prone to this condition. Heat and swelling occasionally are present. The disorder may take several months to become asymptomatic, with healing taking place by fibrous or fibrocartilage replacement.

Diagnosis is based on the age of the patient, a history of athletic involvement, and the typical location of pain along the margins of the growth centers. X-rays are not helpful. Other causes of heel pain in children, such as RA, should be ruled out.

Treatment is often disappointing. Heel pads placed within the shoe are used to alleviate the pull of the Achilles tendon on the heel. Immobilization of the foot in a plaster cast is sometimes effective. Reassurance is important to the patient and the parents.

PAIN LOCATED CHIEFLY AT OR ENTIRELY ABOVE THE POSTERIOR PART OF THE HEEL

Haglund's Deformity (Posterior Achilles Tendon Bursitis)

Inflammation of a bursa between the skin and the Achilles tendon occurring above the tendon insertion and over the posterior-superior lateral aspect of the calcaneus, as a result of variations in heel position and function. This problem is seen mostly in young females but can occur in men. The heel then tends to function in an inverted position throughout the gait cycle, excessively compressing the soft tissue between the posterior lateral aspect of the calcaneus and the shoe counter (the stiff, formed heel portion). This aspect of the calcaneus becomes prominent, can be palpated easily, and often is mistaken for an exostosis.

Symptoms and signs: In early stages only a small erythematous, slightly indurated tender area is seen at the posterior-superior aspect of the heel; patients often place adhesive tape over the area to reduce shoe pressure. When the inflamed bursa enlarges, it appears as a painful red lump over the tendon. Sometimes swelling extends to both sides of the tendon, depending on the type of shoegear the patient wears. In chronic cases the bursa becomes fibrotic permanently.

Treatment: Foam rubber or felt heel pads elevate the heel, eliminating shoe counter pressure. Stretching of the counter or opening the back seam of the shoe may relieve inflammation in a small percent of cases. Padding placed around the bursa often relieves pressure. Infiltration of a soluble corticosteroid with a local anesthetic reduces inflammation. An orthosis constructed for the shoe also is indicated to control abnormal heel motion. When conservative therapy is ineffective, surgical excision of the posterior lateral aspect of the calcaneus may be indicated.

PAIN AT THE RETROCALCANEAL SPACE

Fracture of the Posterior Lateral Tubercle of the Talus

The fracture develops as a result of a plantar flexion injury in which forces are applied to the talar tubercle by the posterior inferior lip of the tibia. Toe walkers who have elongated lateral talar tubercles (Stieda's processes) seem more prone to this injury. Occasionally, this tubercle may be connected by a cartilaginous bar to the talus, representing a separating center for ossification known as an ostrigonum. This separation often is mistaken for a fractured tubercle on x-ray. At times, fracture of this cartilage juncture occurs, usually as a result of a sudden jump on the ball of the foot or toes in such sports as basketball and tennis. Similarly, the trauma can occur by stepping backward off a chair with force.

Symptoms, signs, and diagnosis: Pain and swelling located behind the ankle (at the retrocalcaneal space, between the Achilles tendon and the calcaneus), as well as difficulty in walking downhill or downstairs, is common. Persistent swelling may be present with no obvious history of an injury. Heat may or may not be present depending on the chronicity of the injury; if present, it is mild. Plantar flexing the foot on the leg reduplicates the patient's pain, and at times dorsiflexing the hallux is said also to do the same, although this maneuver is questionable. Lateral x-rays of the ankle are necessary to confirm the diagnosis. Bilateral x-rays are ordered to rule out an ostrigonum.

Treatment: Immobilization in a plaster cast for 4 to 6 wk is indicated. If pain persists and soft tissue inflammation is present, infiltrations of corticosteroid/anesthetic combinations may be effective. If conservative therapy is ineffective, surgical excision of the lateral tubercle is indicated.

Albert's Disease (Anterior Achilles Tendon Bursitis)

Inflammation of the bursa lying between the Achilles tendon and the calcaneus where the tendon attaches to the bone occurs as a result of trauma and also in association with inflammatory arthritis (usually RA). Any condition causing increased strain of the tendon can be responsible, as can factors such as a rigid or high shoe counter. When the bursitis is due to trauma, its onset is rapid; when caused by systemic disease, it usually develops gradually. Inflammatory changes in this bursa may cause erosive changes in the calcaneus.

Symptoms, signs, and diagnosis: Pain, swelling, and heat in the retrocalcaneal space and difficulty walking or wearing shoes are common symptoms. Initially, the swelling is localized just anterior to the Achilles tendon but in time extends medially and laterally. Swelling and heat contiguous to the tendon, with pain located primarily within the soft tissue, differentiates this condition from a fractured posterior lateral tubercle. X-rays should be ordered to rule out fracture or rheumatoid erosive calcaneal changes.

Treatment: Intrabursal injection of a soluble corticosteroid with lidocaine (1 mL of dexamethasone phosphate [4 mg/mL] with ½ mL of 2% lidocaine with 1:100,000 epinephrine) relieves symptoms. Warm compresses may help.

Posterior Tibial Nerve Neuralgia

At the level of the ankle the posterior tibial nerve passes through a fibro-osseous canal within the laciniate ligament. At its exit it terminates into medial and lateral plantar nerves. **Tarsal tunnel syndrome** refers to compression of the nerve within this fibro-osseous canal, but this diagnosis has been loosely used to label neuralgia of the posterior tibial nerve due to varied causes. Synovitis of the flexor tendons of the ankle caused by either abnormal foot function or inflammatory arthritis may on occasion cause secondary pressure neuralgia of the posterior tibial nerve. Occasionally, phlebitis of the communicating veins of the ankle and, in a small percentage of cases, abnormal foot structure and function associated with excessive subtalar eversion may cause the condition.

Symptoms and signs: Patients complain of pain, usually of a burning and tingling quality, in and around the ankle and often extending to the toes. Difficulty in standing, walking, and wearing various types of shoes may be present. The pain is worse during ambulation and is relieved by rest.

Diagnosis: Tapping the posterior tibial nerve at a site of compression or injury will often produce distal tingling (Tinel's sign). Palpating the nerve may also elicit the patient's syndrome. These objective signs along with the classic complaints of burning pain and tingling in and around the ankle will suggest the possibility of posterior tibial neuralgia. When there is swelling in the area of the nerve, attempts should be made to determine its cause; eg, rheumatic disease, phlebitis, or fracture. Electrodiagnostic testing often will confirm the diagnosis and should be performed in all patients undergoing foot surgery for decompression.

Treatment: When there is no true compression of the posterior tibial nerve within the fibro-osseous canal, local infiltration of insoluble corticosteroids (¼ mL of triamcinolone acetonide [40 mg/mL] with 2 mL of 1% lidocaine with 1:100,000 epinephrine) may be effective. Strapping the foot in neutral position or slight inversion or constructing an orthotic device for the shoe that keeps the foot in an inverted position will reduce tension on the nerve. Surgery should be reserved for those cases that are recalcitrant to conservative therapy.

DISORDERS ASSOCIATED WITH METATARSALGIA

Metatarsalgia, a general term used to describe *pain over the ball of the foot,* usually is the result of injury to the interdigital nerves or of trauma to the metatarsal-phalangeal articulations.

Interdigital Nerve Pain

The interdigital nerves of the foot travel beneath and between the metatarsals, extending distally over the ball of the foot to innervate the toes. The 3rd plantar interdigital nerve is composed of a branch of the medial and lateral plantar nerves. Neuroma formation usually occurs here **(Morton's neuroma),** although neuromas or neuralgia not uncommonly develop at other interdigital nerves. Neuroma formation is more often uni- than bilateral, and is more common in women than in men.

Symptoms and signs: In early stages, patients may only complain of a mild ache or discomfort in the area of the 4th metatarsal head. Occasionally, a burning sensation or tingling may be experienced. These symptoms are more pronounced with one type of shoe than with others. As the condition progresses, the sensations become more specific, often causing constant burning that radiates to the tips of the toes. Symptoms can appear with all forms of shoe gear; patients feel as if a marble or a pebble were inside the ball of the foot.

Diagnosis is established by eliciting the characteristic history and by palpation of the interdigital space plantarly. Pressure is exerted with the thumb between the heads of the 3rd and 4th metatarsals; when neuroma is present, this maneuver often causes pain.

Treatment: Lidocaine often provides lasting relief for simple neuralgia. Otherwise, perineural infiltrations of long-acting corticosteroids with a local anesthetic (eg, 1/8 to 1/4 mL of triamcinolone acetonide [40 mg/mL] with 1 mL of 2% lidocaine with 1:100,000 epinephrine) often are effective. Injection is at a 45° angle with the foot, into the interspace at the level of dorsal aspect of the metatarsal-phalangeal joints. Injections may have to be repeated 2 or 3 times. Concomitant use of foot orthoses is helpful. When conservative therapy is ineffective, surgical excision of the neuroma often brings complete relief.

Metatarsal-Phalangeal Articulation Pain (Lesser Toes)

Pain involving the metatarsal-phalangeal joint is a common occurrence, and is almost entirely due to malalignment of the joint surfaces, causing subluxations and capsular and synovial impingement with eventual destruction of joint cartilage (degenerative joint disease). Such subluxations are seen in patients who exhibit rigidity and stiffness of the forefoot, and who have hammer toe deformities, cavus or highly arched feet, excessive eversion of the subtalar joint (*rolling-in of the ankles [pronation]*), and hallux valgus deformity **(bunion).** As a result of an overriding hallux, patients with bunions usually have traumatic subluxations and pain in the second metatarsal-phalangeal articulations. Painful subluxation of the metatarsal-phalangeal articulation also can be caused by arthropathies such as RA.

Symptoms, signs, and diagnosis: The absence of significant heat and swelling over the joint generally rules out inflammatory arthropathies, but a rheumatic disease work-up is helpful. Joint pain can be differentiated from neuralgia or neuroma of the interdigital nerves by the absence of burning, numbness, and tingling. Palpating the joint and moving it through its range of motion usually reveals tenderness of the dorsal and plantar aspects of the joint; in neuralgia, symptoms usually are limited to the plantar surface.

Treatment should correct the initiating cause. With excess subtalar eversion, a device to control this motion should be made for the shoes. In highly arched feet or hammer toe deformities, the cause is sought; a weak anterior tibial muscle, tight heel chord,

neurologic disease such as Friedreich's ataxia, Charcot-Marie-Tooth disease, or post-stroke toe contractures should be ruled out. Orthoses are prescribed to redistribute and relieve pressure from the affected articulations. Injections of local anesthetics with or without soluble corticosteroids may be needed weekly for 2 to 3 wk, but can yield dramatic results lasting for a few months.

Hallux Rigidus

Osteoarthritis of the first metatarsal-phalangeal joint is extremely common. Most often it is the result of variations in position of the 1st metatarsal due to excessive rolling-in of the ankles (pronation), lateral deviation of the hallux (hallux valgus), dorsiflexion of the 1st metatarsal (metatarsal elevatus), or increased length or medial deviation of the first metatarsal. Occasionally, trauma is a factor.

Symptoms and signs: Initially, the only sign may be slight swelling of the joint due to capsular thickening. The joint is tender to the touch, and shoes irritate the condition further. As the condition worsens, pain increases and exostosis formation begins to limit joint motion; the patient no longer bends the joint during walking. Motion now appears to be taking place at the distal interphalangeal joint, and an accentuated skin crease is seen at this joint. Although increased heat in the area usually is absent, it may develop late in the disorder as a result of secondary impingement of the synovial membrane.

Diagnosis is established by observing an enlarged 1st metatarsal-phalangeal joint with limitation of its motion, pain on palpation of the joint capsule (particularly at its lateral aspect), and resulting increased dorsiflexion of the distal phalanx. Dorso-plantar x-rays reveal spurs laterally, and lateral x-rays may show a dorsal exostosis extending from the metatarsal head in advanced cases.

Treatment initially aims to increase joint motion using passive exercises and toe traction. Lidocaine infiltrations (1.5 mL of a 2% solution with 1:100,000 epinephrine) periarticularly relieve pain, decrease muscle spasm, and thereby increase motion. Early biomechanical control of the foot restores proper position and function of the metatarsal. In cases recalcitrant to conservative therapy, limitation of motion may be advised to decrease pain. This is accomplished by prescribing a foot orthosis with a Morton's extension; a steel splint extending from the end of the toe to the heel between the inner and outer sole or a metatarsal bar also may be prescribed. Surgery may be indicated.

ANKLE SPRAINS

Classification

Ankle sprains can be classified according to the extent of soft tissue damage.

Grade 1: Mild or minimal sprain with no ligamentous tear. Mild tenderness with some swelling may be present.

Grade 2: Moderate sprain consisting of incomplete or partial rupture with obvious swelling, ecchymosis, and difficulty in walking.

Grade 3: A complete tear of a ligament with swelling, hemorrhage, ankle instability, and inability to walk.

Etiology and Pathogenesis

The ankle is supported laterally by 3 ligaments: the anterior talofibular, fibulocalcaneal, and posterior talofibular. In ankle sprain, the anterior talofibular ligament usually is ruptured first. Only after this ligament is ruptured can the fibulocalcaneal ligament divide. The posterior talofibular ligament rarely ruptures. Therefore, if the anterior talofibular ligament is intact, one can surmise that the fibulocalcaneal ligament also is intact; conversely, if the anterior talofibular ligament is ruptured, examination for concomitant rupture of the lateral fibulocalcaneal ligament must be done. In a study of 321 ligamentous injuries of the ankle, 64% of cases injured the anterior talofibular ligament alone, and 17% also injured the lateral fibulocalcaneal ligament.

Predisposing influences leading to ankle sprain may be present. Individuals with ligamentous laxity who have extensive subtalar inversion ranges are often more prone to inversion episodes. Prophylactic control of rear foot motion in these patients using functional foot orthoses is indicated. Occasional weakness of the peroneals (which are responsible for normal subtalar joint eversion) occurs with lumbar disk disease involving L5/S1 nerve root or other causes of peripheral neuropathy involving the peroneal nerve. These persons are candidates for sprained ankles. Forefoot valgus, a condition in which the forefoot tends to function in an everted manner during the gait cycle, causing the subtalar joint to compensate by inversion, may be a predisposing factor in ankle sprain. Some individuals inherit a tendency to develop inverted subtalar joints (subtalar varus) and are predisposed to ankle sprain.

Examination

Foot structure and function are examined to rule out predisposing influences as described above. Topographic examination determines the site of the ligamentous injury, by simple palpation of the ligaments around the lateral ankle. Classification of the ankle sprain usually can be made clinically. The **Drawer sign** is useful to determine anterior talofibular rupture. This ligament prevents the talus from subluxing anteriorly on the tibia. When the ligament is ruptured, anterior displacement of the talus becomes possible. The patient sits on the side of a table with legs dangling. With the left hand of the examiner placed in front of the patient's lower leg, the right hand grasps the patient's heel posteriorly and attempts to move the talus anteriorly.

Stress x-rays of the ankle may help to determine the extent of ligamentous injury. Mortise views of the ankle consisting of an anteroposterior x-ray taken with 15° internal rotation are ordered. Both ankles are inverted to maximum (local anesthesia may be indicated) and the degree of lateral tilt of the talus is noted. If a talar tilt difference of 5° or more can be demonstrated, functional impairment should be considered. If the difference is > 10°, symptoms increase significantly and an unstable ankle often results.

Arthrography of the ankle helps to determine the exact site and extent of ligamentous injury. This procedure offers few complications but is indicated only when surgical correction of a ruptured ligament is contemplated. To be useful, the technic must be performed within the first days of trauma, since delay technically nullifies the procedure.

Treatment

Grade 1: Strapping with elastic bandages, tape, or Unna boot immobilization; elevation, followed by gentle exercise and walking.

Grade 2: Below-knee walking-cast immobilization for 3 wk.

Grade 3: Cast immobilization or surgery. Surgery is controversial because the extreme fragmentation of ligaments makes surgical repair difficult. Some surgeons cast solitary anterior talofibular ruptures but recommend surgical repair if the fibulocalcaneal ligament is torn.

Sequelae of Inversion Ankle Sprains

Meniscoid body: *A small nodule of the anterior talofibular ligament.* Impingement between the lateral malleolus and talus of this synovial-lined capsular ligament, caused by Grade 2 or 3 injuries to the ligament, results in persistent synovitis and, in time, fibrotic swelling and permanent induration. Immobilization at this time has little value. Infiltration of insoluble corticosteroids (1/4 mL of triamcinolone acetonide [40 mg/mL] with 3/4 mL of 2% lidocaine with 1:100,000 epinephrine) between the talus and the lateral malleolus often yields dramatic and lasting improvement. Surgery rarely is indicated.

Neuralgia of the intermediate dorsal cutaneous nerve: This nerve, a sensory branch of the superficial peroneal nerve, crosses over the anterior talofibular ligament and is

often injured as a result of inversion sprains. Tapping the nerve frequently elicits Tinel's sign. Local anesthetic nerve blocks often are effective treatment.

Peroneal tenosynovitis: *Chronic swelling below the lateral malleolus resulting from tenosynovitis of the peroneal tendons* is due to compensation for painful inversion sprains by chronic eversion of the subtalar joint while walking. In a few cases, dislocated peroneal tendons resulting from severe ankle sprains also may cause swelling and tenderness.

Sudeck's posttraumatic reflex atrophy: *Painful swelling of the foot associated with spotty osteoporosis* may result from angiospasms secondary to ankle sprain. The edema often is confusing, and is sometimes viewed as swelling resulting from a ligamentous injury. Characteristically, in Sudeck's atrophy the pain appears out of proportion to the clinical findings. Multiple trigger points of pain moving from one site to another associated with spotty osteoporosis help characterize the condition.

Sinus tarsi syndrome, *a persistent pain at the sinus tarsi following ankle sprains*: The pathogenesis is unclear. Partial rupture of the interosseous talocalcaneal ligament or stem of the inferior cruciate ligament of the ankle may be implicated. Diagnosis should be reserved for persistent pain in the sinus tarsi and pain on palpation. Since the sinus tarsi normally is tender, both ankles should be examined. Because the anterior talofibular ligament is tender near the sinus tarsi, patients with persistent pain over the anterior talofibular mortise often are misdiagnosed as having sinus tarsi pain. **Treatment** consists of infiltration of 1/4 mL of triamcinolone acetonide [40 mg/mL] with 3/4 mL of 2% lidocaine with 1:100,000 epinephrine into the sinus tarsi.

§11. NEUROLOGIC DISORDERS

117. APPROACH TO THE PATIENT

Faced with the intricacies of the nervous system, persons without special training can find neurologic complaints initially intimidating. Yet headache, dizziness, insomnia, back pain, weakness, and fatigue occur frequently in the practice of medicine, and the trivial must be separated from the potentially serious as causes of neurologic symptoms and signs. Other neurologic problems require emergency action and must be acted upon before neurologic consultation can be obtained. The following principles applied throughout the history-taking, examination, and test selection procedures may be helpful, regardless of the magnitude of the problem: First define the locus of the lesion (which reduces the diagnostic possibilities to a manageable number); and second, determine the pathophysiology and immediate lifesaving treatment.

Symptoms and signs that relate to specific locations and pathophysiologic processes in the nervous system are discussed in detail in the appropriate chapters elsewhere in this section. Evaluation of the unconscious patient is discussed in Ch. 118.

THE HISTORY

The history often is the most informative part of the neurologic evaluation. The patient should be made to feel at ease and be allowed to tell his story in his own words. Questions should clarify specific points and maintain a focused conversation. If not

volunteered, specific information is sought about the quality, intensity, distribution, duration, and frequency of a symptom. Any dysfunction is described in quantitative terms and its impact on the patient's life noted. How daily routines are performed often is more revealing than the patient's expostulations or denials concerning a deficit. The physician also must distinguish between the patient's perceptions and those that others around him (eg, family and medical staff) consider relevant. One should determine rapidly whether the history is reliable and not waste time with tangential and contradictory statements.

A **localizing diagnosis** is the interview's goal. Does a lesion of the nervous system exist? Some complaints can be nonspecific or elaborated by a frightened patient, and the nervous system may not be directly involved by structural disease. This often is true for the psychiatric patient, whose neurologic complaints may lack consistency and objective verification. On the other hand, one must beware of too readily dismissing complaints as "functional" or "psychotic" when described with greater than usual exuberance. Elaborated deficits often occur in the context of organic disease. Such distortions require careful evaluation, but should not by themselves trigger a host of unnecessary consultations and procedures.

Accepting that the patient has a true neurologic symptom or abnormality, the next step is to *localize the functional defect to muscle, nerve, spinal cord, or brain*. This requires a working knowledge of neuroanatomy as well as some familiarity with the major neurologic disorders described in the following pages. Not infrequently, even a novice can define a discrete anatomic localization after a thoughtful analysis.

A complete systems review is essential, as neurologic dysfunction is common in systemic illness; eg, alcoholism, cancer, and vascular disease each can produce a spectrum of neurologic deficits. **The family history** is important because many metabolic and degenerative disorders are inherited. **A social and travel history** gives information about exposure to toxins and infectious agents that can afflict the nervous system.

THE NEUROLOGIC EXAMINATION

The neurologic examination begins with careful observation of the patient's ordinary behavior and proceeds to specific tests that help to define the anatomic disturbance. For example, the physician should appreciate the speed, symmetry, and coordination of movement taken in the simple task of getting to a chair; eg, there is little mistaking the stooped posture, bradykinesia, en bloc turning, and shuffling gait underlying Parkinson's disease. The patient's demeanor and dress yield information about mood and social adaptation. Thus, the neatly groomed, unassertive individual, amused over his failing memory, may be self-sufficient at home, yet suffering in a larger world the early limitations of a dementing illness such as Alzheimer's disease. This may not be readily appreciated if the patient presents with a non-neurologic problem. Errors of language, speech, or praxis; neglect of space; unusual posturing; and other disorders of movement can occur at any point in the evaluation and should be observed and recorded.

The formal neurologic examination often confirms what the history and initial observation already suggest. Regional anatomy and pathophysiology determine which components of the examination to expand and which to delete. For the less skilled observer, a full neurologic screen may be useful to detect an unsuspected abnormality and to gain a greater appreciation for normal findings. To help avoid omissions and save the patient frequent postural changes, the examination should be a systematic series of tests on different systems, as discussed below.

The Mental Status Examination (see also Ch. 134)

Mental status testing, unless made obvious by the clarity of the history, includes asking about **orientation to time, place, and person**. The latter is lost only in severely

obtunded, delirious, or demented individuals, and its isolated absence should suggest malingering. A **normally attentive** grammar school graduate should be able to repeat 7 random digits forward and 4 in reverse order, to spell WORLD backwards, and to perform simple calculations (nickles in 1.35 dollars; serial sevens). **Immediate recall** is tested by asking a patient to remember 3 unrelated items for a period of 3 or 5 min. Whether a patient can describe news events or yesterday's breakfast yields information about **recent memory. Remote memory** can be checked by asking the patient what make and color of car he first purchased, or the color of his suit on his wedding day. **Ability to abstract** is checked with proverb interpretation and analogies. **Insight into illness** should be determined, since its absence complicates management. **Fund of knowledge** will reflect the patient's level of education; most persons should be able to name the last 5 presidents and know their state capitals. **Affect and mood** are evaluated as described in Ch. 141.

A patient should be able to follow a simple 3-component command involving peripheral and central body parts and to discriminate between right and left (eg, "put your right thumb over your left ear and stick out your tongue"). **Language function**: Naming of simple objects and body parts, reading, writing, and repetition are assessed; if disturbed, further tests of aphasia are initiated (see FOCAL DISORDERS OF HIGHER FUNCTION in Ch. 118). **Cortical sensory function** is tested by examining the ability to identify small objects in the hand and numbers written on the palm, and to discriminate 2 points from one, at the palm and fingers (stereo perception). Facility with **spatial relationships** can be checked at the bedside by asking the patient to imitate simple and complex finger constructions, and to draw a clock, a cube, or a house. The effort expended frequently is as informative as the final result and may identify impersistence or perseveration, as well as neglect of one side of space. **Praxis** can be checked by asking the patient to use a toothbrush or to take a match out of a box and strike it.

Cranial Nerve Examination

An abnormality of one cranial nerve requires meticulous scrutiny of its anatomic neighbors. Isolated dysfunction of 2 adjacent cranial nerves arises more often from compression by an extrinsic mass (eg, tumor, aneurysm) than from an intrinsic lesion (eg, demyelination, infarction). If the ipsilateral motor or sensory pathways are disturbed as well, the brainstem is likely to be involved. Such distinctions become urgent, for example, when brainstem ischemia must be distinguished from a rapidly expanding aneurysm producing cranial nerve paralysis.

The completeness of the cranial nerve examination depends on the site of the suspected lesion. Smell **(1st cranial nerve)** is not generally tested in patients with muscle disease but always should be investigated in suspected lesions of the anterior fossa. The patient is asked to identify characteristic odors (eg, soap, coffee, cloves) presented to each nostril. Alcohol and other irritants are avoided, except to detect the malingerer, since these test the nonolfactory receptors of the 5th (trigeminal) nerve.

The 2nd (optic), 3rd (oculomotor), 4th (trochlear), and 6th (abducens) cranial nerves are part of the visual system (see VISION AND EYE MOVEMENT DISORDERS in Ch. 119; and Ch. 225). Visual acuity (corrected for refractive error) and the visual fields are examined, and funduscopy done. The shape and size of the pupils, their reactivity to light and accommodation, and the extraocular eye movements are noted.

The 5th (trigeminal) nerve's 3 sensory divisions (ophthalmic, maxillary, and **mandibular)** are tested for sensation with a pin, and the **corneal reflex** is elicited by stroking the lower limbus with a wisp of cotton. If the patient has sensory loss over the face, the angle of the jaw particularly is examined, since this area is innervated by C2 and C3 and should be spared in trigeminal dysfunction. A weakened blink from facial weakness (eg, 7th cranial nerve paralysis) should not be misinterpreted as a depressed corneal response. Supranuclear corneal hyposensitivity (usually associated with hypalgesia of body as well as face) must be distinguished from infranuclear. **Trigeminal**

motor function, mediated only through the mandibular division, is tested by palpating the masseter muscles with the teeth clenched, and asking the patient to open his jaw against resistance. The jaw will deviate to the side of a weakened pterygoid muscle.

The 7th (facial) cranial nerve (see also FACIAL NERVE DISORDERS in Ch. 131): The patient is examined for facial weakness during spontaneous conversation. Asymmetry of facial movements often is more obvious when the patient smiles or (if he is obtunded) grimaces at a noxious stimulus. One looks for a depressed nasolabial fold and a widened palpebral fissure on the side of weakness. If furrowing of the forehead is preserved, facial weakness probably has a central rather than a peripheral basis. Taste in the anterior ⅔ of the tongue can be examined by stroking either side of the tongue with a sweet, sour, salty, or bitter solution.

The 8th (vestibulocochlear, acoustic) cranial nerve carries auditory and vestibular input, and is discussed in Ch. 204. See also ACOUSTIC NEURINOMA in Ch. 207.

The 9th (glossopharyngeal) and **10th (vagus) nerves** usually are examined together. The palate should elevate symmetrically, and gag is elicited by touching each side of the posterior pharynx with a tongue blade. Bilateral absence of the gag reflex is common in the normal population and has no significance. In the unresponsive, intubated patient, suctioning the endotracheal tube should trigger coughing. The vocal cords are inspected if hoarseness is evident.

The 11th (spinal accessory) nerve supplies the sternocleidomastoid muscle and the upper trapezius. The former is tested by having a patient turn his head against resistance supplied by the examiner's hand, while the active (opposite to the turned head) muscle is palpated by the examiner's free hand.

The 12th (hypoglossal) nerve innervates the tongue, which is inspected for atrophy, fasciculations, and weakness (deviation toward the side of the lesion).

Examination of the Motor System (see also MOTOR WEAKNESS in Ch. 119)

The limbs and shoulder girdle should be fully exposed and inspected for atrophy, fasciculations, and asymmetric development. Passive flexion and extension of the limbs in a relaxed patient gives information concerning muscle tone. Increased resistance followed by relaxation, the so-called "clasp-knife phenomenon" of spasticity, is seen with upper motor neuron lesions. Basal ganglia disorders usually produce a "cogwheel rigidity." Any involuntary movements (eg, chorea, athetosis, myoclonus, tremor) are noted. **Grading muscle strength** is outlined under MOTOR WEAKNESS in Ch. 119.

Examination of Coordination, Stance, and Gait (see also CEREBELLAR AND SPINOCEREBELLAR DISORDERS in Ch. 128)

Normal coordination, stance, and gait require the integrity of the motor, vestibular, and proprioceptive pathways. A lesion of any one of these systems produces characteristic deficits. A patient with cerebellar ataxia may widen his gait for stability; another with drop foot elevates his leg (steppage gait); pelvic muscle weakness may lead to waddling, a spastic leg to circumduction. Impaired proprioception may require the individual to continuously observe where his feet are.

Sensory Testing

Efforts to complete all aspects of the sensory examination often are frustrating and unnecessary, especially when there are no symptoms of pain, paresthesias, or numbness. A quick examination with a clean pin includes the face, torso, and 4 limbs; inquiry as to whether the patient perceives the pin the same on both sides avoids the vagaries of subtle distinctions. If there is a difference, can the patient distinguish dull from sharp, and has temperature sense been affected? One arm of a tuning fork, rubbed warm with the palm, can be applied to the patient's skin and compared with the colder arm. Alternatively, heat and cold are tested with water in test tubes. Joint position is tested by moving the terminal phalanges of the fingers, then the toes, up or

down. If the patient fails to identify these movements with his eyes closed, the other joints are tested in a distal to proximal direction. Gross loss often produces pseudoathetotic movements of the outstretched arms and an inability to locate a limb in space without visual cues. If postural sense is deranged, the patient will be unable to stand with his feet together and eyes closed **(Romberg test).**

The patient's vibration sense can be compared to the examiner's by pressing the ventral surface of the examiner's finger against the patient's finger and touching the dorsum of the latter with a lightly tapped, 128-cycle tuning fork. The maneuver transmits vibration through the patient's terminal phalangeal joint. Both patient and examiner should note the end of vibration at about the same time. Loss requires the more proximal joints to be checked. Light touch can be checked with a cotton wisp. **Stereognosis** and **graphesthesia** require tests of higher cortical function described above under The Mental Status Examination.

If sensation is disturbed, its anatomic pattern should be established: peripheral nerve (stocking-glove), particular nerves (mononeuritis multiplex), nerve roots (radiculopathy), spinal cord (a level below which sensation is aberrant), or brain (hemisensory loss). (See FIGS. 117–1a and 117–1b.) One then determines whether motor weakness and reflex change follow a similar pattern, so as to confirm the anatomic localization of the lesion.

Reflex Testing

Deep tendon (muscle stretch) reflex testing gives information about the afferent nerve, the synaptic connections within the spinal cord, and the motor nerves, as well as the descending motor pathways. The biceps reflex takes its innervation from C5–6; radial from C6–7; triceps from C7–8; quadriceps knee jerk from L2-L3, 4; and ankle jerk from L5, S1–2. Asymmetric increase or depression is noted. Absent reflexes are verified by reinforcement (eg, in testing the patellar reflex, the patient vigorously locks

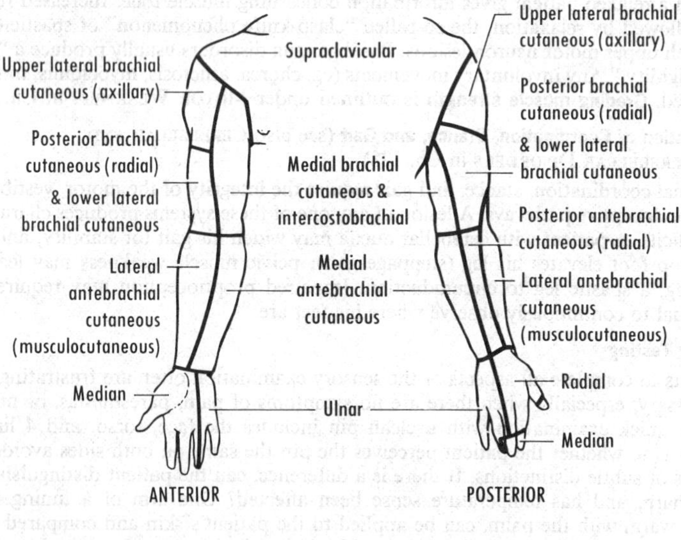

FIG. 117–1a. Cutaneous nerve distribution: upper limb. (Redrawn from E. Gardner, D. J. Gray, and R. O'Rahilly, *Anatomy*, ed. 4, 1975. Copyright 1975 by W. B. Saunders Company. Used with permission.)

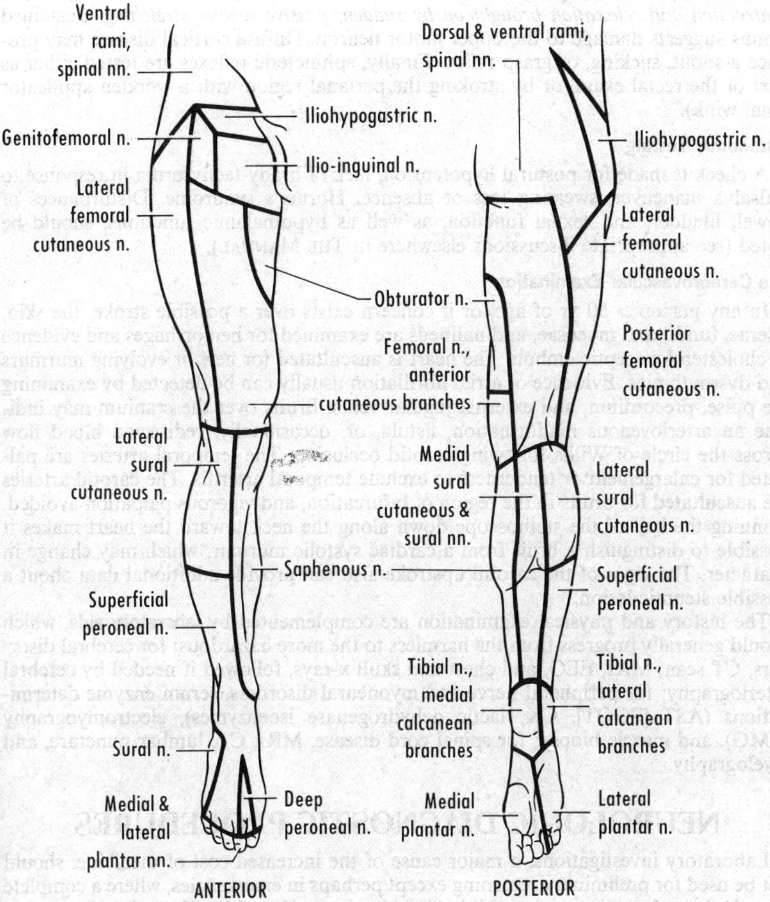

FIG. 117–1b. **Cutaneous nerve distribution: lower limb.** (Redrawn from E. Gardner, D. J. Gray, and R. O'Rahilly, *Anatomy,* ed. 4, 1975. Copyright 1975 by W. B. Saunders Company. Used with permission.)

his hands and pulls just before the tendon is percussed). Lower motor neuron lesions (eg, anterior horn cell, spinal root, motor nerve) depress the reflexes, whereas upper motor neuron lesions (ie, non–basal-ganglia disorders anywhere above the anterior horn cell) increase the reflexes. The superficial abdominal reflex is elicited by lightly stroking the 4 quadrants of the abdomen with a pin. These are diminished with most central lesions but also by obesity or lax skeletal muscles, eg, after pregnancy.

The plantar response may take several forms. There may be a quick voluntary withdrawal, which must be distinguished from the slower **Babinski's sign** (*extension of the great toe with fanning of the other toes, often in conjunction with flexion of the knee and hip*). Only the latter is of spinal reflex origin and attests to an upper motor neuron lesion. Care must be taken to stroke the lateral aspect of the sole, as a more medial

stimulus may induce a grasp reflex. **Clonus** is *the rhythmic, rapid, alternating muscle contraction and relaxation brought on by sudden, passive tendon stretching.* Sustained clonus suggests damage to the upper motor neuron. Diffuse cortical disease may produce a snout, sucking, or grasp reflex. Finally, sphincteric reflexes are tested either as part of the rectal exam, or by stroking the perianal region with a wooden applicator (anal wink).

Autonomic Testing

A check is made for postural hypotension, lack of brady-tachycardia in response to Valsalva maneuver, sweating loss or absence, Horner's syndrome. Disturbances of bowel, bladder, and sexual function, as well as hypothalamic functions, should be noted (see appropriate discussions elsewhere in THE MANUAL).

The Cerebrovascular Examination

In any person > 50 yr of age, or if concern exists over a possible stroke, the skin, sclerae, fundi, oral mucosae, and nailbeds are examined for hemorrhages and evidence of cholesterol or septic emboli. The heart is auscultated for new or evolving murmurs and dysrhythmias. Evidence of atrial fibrillation usually can be detected by examining the pulse, precordium, and external jugular veins. Bruits over the cranium may indicate an arteriovenous malformation, fistula, or, occasionally, redirected blood flow across the circle of Willis following carotid occlusion. The temporal arteries are palpated for enlargement or tenderness to exclude temporal arteritis. The carotid arteries are auscultated for bruits in the region of bifurcation, and vigorous palpation avoided. Running the bell of the stethoscope down along the neck toward the heart makes it possible to distinguish a bruit from a cardiac systolic murmur, which may change in character. The vigor of the carotid upstroke also can provide additional data about a possible stenotic lesion.

The history and physical examination are complemented by **laboratory aids**, which should generally progress from the harmless to the more hazardous: for cerebral disorders, CT scan, MRI, EEG, and chest and skull x-rays, followed if needed by cerebral arteriography; for peripheral nerve and myoneural disorders, serum enzyme determinations (AST [SGOT], CK, lactic dehydrogenase isoenzymes), electromyography (EMG), and muscle biopsy; for spinal cord disease, MRI, CT, lumbar puncture, and myelography.

NEUROLOGIC DIAGNOSTIC PROCEDURES

Laboratory investigations, a major cause of the increased cost of medicine, should not be used for preliminary screening except perhaps in emergencies, where a complete neurologic evaluation is not possible. A rational search to identify regional anatomy and pathophysiology should guide the choice of tests. For example, if symptoms and signs point to a structural intracranial abnormality, a CT scan or MRI of the brain is obtained. The need for a CT contrast study depends on the suspected pathophysiology. An apoplectic onset raises the possibility of hemorrhage, and a CT without contrast is indicated; the results determine whether a second CT with contrast is needed. A more gradual evolution of deficits, on the other hand, dictates the use of contrast on the first scan to eliminate the possibility of tumor or abscess. A negative study then obviates the need for a noncontrast CT.

Lumbar Puncture (LP)

Tapping of the lumbar subarachnoid space provides important information about intracranial pressure and allows a diagnostic analysis of the CSF (see TABLE 117–1). LP also is used to administer radiopaque material for myelography and to give medications intrathecally. Infection near the puncture site and coagulation disorders are **relative contraindications**. Since increased intracranial pressure sometimes can produce

TABLE 117–1. CSF ABNORMALITIES IN VARIOUS CONDITIONS*

	Pressure	*Cells/cu mm*	*Predominant Cell Type*	*Glucose*	*Protein*
Normal	100–200 mm	0–3	L	50–100 mg/dL	20–45 mg/dL
Acute bacterial meningitis	↑	500–5000	PMN	↓	About 100 mg/dL
Subacute meningitis (tuberculous, cryptococcal, sarcoid, leukemic, carcinoma)	N or ↑	100–700	L	↓	↑
Viral infections	N or ↑	100–2000	L	N	N or ↑
Brain abscess or tumor	N or ↑	0–1000	L	N	↑
Lead encephalopathy	↑	0–500	L	N	↑
Meningismus	N or ↑	N	L	N	N or ↓
Acute syphilitic meningitis	N or ↑	25–2000	L	N	↑
Paretic neurosyphilis	N or ↑	15–2000	L	N	↑
Guillain-Barré syndrome	N	0–100	L	N	>100 mg/dL
Cerebral hemorrhage	↑	Bloody	RBCs	N	↑
Cerebral thrombosis	N or ↑	0–100	L	N	N or ↑
Cord tumor	N	0–50	L	N	N or ↑

* N= normal; ↑ = increased; ↓ = decreased; PMN = polymorphonuclear; L = lymphocyte; RBCs = red blood cells.

NOTE: Figures given for pressure, cell count, and protein are approximations; exceptions are not infrequent. Similarly, PMNs may predominate in conditions usually characterized by lymphocyte response, especially early in the course of viral infections or tuberculous meningitis. Alterations in glucose are less variable and more reliable.

transtentorial or cerebellar tonsillar herniation, one hesitates to perform LP without a prior CT scan. When meningitis is suspected, however, LP should be done without delay, as it can provide definitive diagnosis. A fine bore (gauge 22 or at most 24) needle should be used. If herniation is a serious concern, preparation should be made for its treatment (mannitol 50 gm IV or intubation to reduce the P_{CO_2}). Absence of papilledema or focal neurologic deficits makes such complications highly unlikely. In many subarachnoid hemorrhages, the CT is diagnostic and obviates the need for LP. TABLE 117-1 gives the CSF formula for several major diseases.

Examination of CSF (see TABLE 117-1)

CSF appearance: Normal CSF is clear and colorless; 300 or more cells/μL produce haziness or turbidity. Bloody fluid requires distinguishing between a traumatic tap and subarachnoid hemorrhage. The former occurs frequently (when the needle enters the venous plexus in the anterior spinal wall) and is distinguished by gradual clearing of the CSF (confirmed by cell count in the 1st and 4th tubes of CSF) and lack of xanthochromia (heme dipstick) in a centrifuged sample. Intrinsic subarachnoid blood, on the other hand, remains uniformly bloody throughout CSF collection and, if several hours have passed after ictus, red cell lysis produces xanthochromia. Faintly yellow fluid also can arise from senile chromogens, old blood, severe jaundice, or an increased protein content (> 100 mg/dL).

The **cell count** and **differential glucose and protein** can provide useful information about a number of neurologic conditions (see TABLE 117-1).

If infection is suspected, the CSF centrifuged sediment is stained for bacteria (Gram stain), for TB (acid-fast or immunofluorescent staining), and for cryptococcus (India ink). Larger amounts of fluid (10 mL) improve the chances for detecting the pathogen, especially acid-fast bacilli **(AFB)**, in both stains and cultures. A patient with early meningococcal meningitis or severe leukopenia may have an insufficiently elevated CSF protein for bacterial adherence to the glass slide during Gram staining. Mixing a drop of aseptic serum to the CSF sediment eliminates this potentially false-negative result. A wet mount is used to search for amebas, if hemorrhagic meningoencephalitis occurs in the summer. **Counterimmunoelectrophoresis** (*an antigen-antibody precipitate reaction made more rapid and sensitive through electrophoresis*) is useful for the rapid identification of bacterial agents, especially when stains and cultures are negative (eg, partially treated meningitis). **CSF should be cultured** both aerobically and anaerobically, for AFB and fungi. Viruses seldom are isolated from the CSF. When appropriate, CSF samples should be sent for Venereal Disease Research Laboratory (VDRL) and cryptococcal antigen detection.

The normal **CSF/blood glucose** ratio is approximately 0.6, and except with severe hypoglycemia the CSF glucose generally is maintained above 50 mg/dL. An increase in CSF **protein** (> 50 mg/dL) is a sensitive but nonspecific index for the presence of disease. Increases of > 500 mg/dL are uncommon, except in purulent meningitis, complete block by spinal cord tumor, or bloody fluid. **Special examinations** for γ-globulin (normally < 15%), oligoclonal banding, and myelin basic protein are helpful in diagnosing demyelinating disease.

Computed Tomographic X-Ray (CT Scan)

CT provides rapid, noninvasive imaging of a variety of the body's soft tissues and, especially, the brain, spinal cord, and their bony enclosures. The technic passes a series of collimated x-ray beams through the region of interest and measures their attenuation by the various tissue densities within a transverse plane. A computer transforms these measurements into a 2-dimensional image of high resolution that resembles an anatomic "slice." Cerebral sulci, the ventricles, grey and white matter, and bony and calcified structures are readily visualized.

CT can detect many kinds of anatomic deviations from the normal pattern, including hydrocephalus, cortical atrophy, porencephalic cysts, and distortions produced by mass effect. A decrease in tissue density may accompany edema, infarction, demyelination, cyst formation, and abscess. An increase in density is characteristic of recent hemorrhage as well as of calcified lesions (eg, craniopharyngioma). IV infusion of an iodinated contrast agent permits visualization of blood vessels, vascular malformations, vascular tumors, and regions in which the blood-brain barrier is injured. The skull and spine can be examined for congenital anomalies, fractures, osteoarthritic impingement, and bony erosion by tumor. With intrathecal metrizamide, CT can outline abnormalities encroaching on the brainstem, spinal cord, or spinal nerve roots (eg, meningeal carcinomatosis, herniated disk) and may detect a syrinx in the spinal cord (although MRI—see below—provides superior images of syringomyelia). CT may guide therapy (eg, excluding hemorrhage before initiating anticoagulation in acute stroke) or monitor its effectiveness (eg, intraventricular shunting in hydrocephalus, radiotherapy of cerebral metastasis, antimicrobial treatment of brain abscess). With such widespread application and minimal risk, CT has revolutionized the practice of neurology.

Magnetic Resonance Imaging (MRI)

MRI yields extraordinary resolution in imaging neural structures without any known risk to the patient. The head or body is placed in a strong magnetic field to align the hydrogen protons in the direction of the field. An additional, specific radiofrequency pulse then "flips" the aligned intra- and extracellular protons into a higher energy state. When the radiopulse is turned off, the protons "relax" back into their original alignment, and the energy emitted gives information on the chemical makeup of the tissue (eg, tightly bound protons in solids such as bone give a very weak signal, whereas liquids produce a strong signal). The relaxation process is described by the interaction of the aligned protons with other nearby nuclei (spin-lattice relaxation time, or T1) and by the influence of other protons (spin-spin relaxation time, or T2). The regional relaxation times are used to compute an anatomic image in virtually any plane desired (eg, sagittal, transverse, coronal).

MRI is particularly helpful in identifying brainstem lesions and other abnormalities of the posterior fossa, as CT through this region often contains bony streak artifacts. MRI is also useful for detecting demyelinating plaques, subclinical brain edema, cerebral contusions, abnormalities of the craniocervical junction, and syringomyelia. The major disadvantages are its expense, slowness of imaging, and the need for special and spacious housing. MRI cannot be used to examine patients who have metallic prostheses or are dependent on respirators.

Echoencephalography

Graphic tracing produced by echoes from sound waves that are directed toward selected parts of the brain. This bedside procedure is useful in detecting hemorrhage and hydrocephalus in children < age 2 yr, especially in the neonatal intensive care unit. CT scanning has largely supplanted its use in older children and adults.

Positron Emission Tomography (PET)

A research tool using the uptake of tracer amounts of radioisotopes to measure blood flow, glucose, and O_2 metabolism in the living brain. Presently it has little place in clinical diagnosis. (See also Ch. 266.)

Radionuclide Imaging

The use of injected radioactive chemicals to scan the brain has been supplanted by CT and MRI, both of which provide far more structural detail.

Cerebral Angiography

The use of injected contrast media and x-rays to picture arterial circulation in the brain. With the advent of CT and MRI, cerebral angiography has increasingly become a supplementary technic for delineating the site and vascularity of intracranial lesions. It remains the method of choice to diagnose stenotic or occluded arteries, congenitally absent vessels, aneurysms, arterial venous malformations, and dural sinus thromboses.

Procedure: After mild sedation and local anesthesia, a flexible catheter is introduced via the femoral, axillary, or brachial artery and threaded into the aortic arch. Injection of a contrast dye outlines the arch and origin of the major vessels (during which the patient feels a sense of hot discomfort in the face/head). Individual carotid and vertebral arteries can be cannulated to assess patency, anatomy, and flow through the neck and into the cranium. Vessels as small as 0.1 mm can be distinguished by an experienced observer.

The incidence of complications varies with different operators and institutions but should not exceed 2 or 3%. Transient neurologic deficits can follow vertebral artery injection, and atheroma can be dislodged and embolized through any major vessel. Patients with congestive heart failure or renal failure may not tolerate the dye load. A previous history of sensitivity to contrast material requires special preparations or avoidance of the procedure.

Digital Intravenous Subtraction Angiography (DISA)

Use of rapid IV injection of radiocontrast material to provide sequential x-ray images that are displayed (about 1/sec) on a video terminal, digitized, and stored on magnetic tape. DISA does not offer the resolution of direct arteriography but sometimes is performed on an outpatient basis for screening purposes. **Procedure**: After an IV catheter is placed near or in the left atrium, 40 mL of contrast dye is injected and a series of x-ray exposures are processed by computer to produce the angiographic image. Some centers have found this study sufficient for evaluating carotid stenoses or plaques prior to endarterectomy. However, swallowing artifacts, poor patient positioning, insufficient spatial resolution, and other methodologic difficulties limit its usefulness. Dye reactions and, occasionally, heart failure can occur with a frequency that approaches that of arterial studies. DISA, however, can exclude aneurysm in patients with a pituitary mass. Intra-arterial DSA (in contrast to IV DSA) has some advantages over conventional arteriography: It can reduce the amount of contrast, film, time, and cost without sacrificing resolution.

Noninvasive Measurement of Extracranial Arterial Disease

Doppler ultrasonic scanning can assess the carotid bifurcation for dissection, stenosis, occlusion, and ulceration. Although not providing the detail of angiographic technics, the method is safe and can be rapidly performed on an outpatient basis. It is therefore useful for screening purposes and for following an abnormality over time.

Myelography

X-ray of the spinal cord after injection of a contrast medium into the subarachnoid space. Metrizamide introduced into the subarachnoid space by lumbar puncture **(LP)** can visualize the contents of the entire spinal canal. Intrinsic and extrinsic cord tumors, herniated disks, and spondylytic bars are readily diagnosed. Metrizamide, being a water-soluble dye, need not be removed, can provide increased resolution (especially of the spinal roots), and in conjunction with CT scanning can clarify otherwise problematic lesions (eg, syrinx vs. cord tumor). Contraindications to myelography are the same as for LP (see above). Generalized seizures infrequently occur following the use of metrizamide but can be avoided if the patient is kept in Fowler's position after the test. Myelography may worsen the effects of a complete spinal block, especially if too much fluid is removed too rapidly. *The radiologist always should be alerted to the possibility of a complete block.*

Electroencephalography (EEG)

Voltage (μV)-vs.-time (Hz) recording of electrical currents in the brain. EEG can detect electrical brain alterations associated with epilepsy, sleep disturbances, and metabolic and structural encephalopathies.

Procedure: Twenty electrodes are distributed symmetrically over the brain (plus a vertex electrode), and the voltage between individual leads is measured in various montages. The normal awake EEG shows 8- to 12-Hz, 50-μV sinusoidal *alpha* waves that wax and wane over the occipital-parietal lobes, > 12-Hz, 10- to 20-μV *beta* waves frontally, with 4- to 7-Hz *theta* waves interspersed. The record is examined for asymmetries between the 2 hemispheres (suggesting structural disease), for excessive slowing (appearance of 1- to 4-Hz, 50- to 350-μV *delta* waves, as seen in depressed consciousness, encephalopathy, and dementia), and abnormal wave patterns.

Some abnormal wave patterns are nonspecific (epileptiform sharp waves) and others are diagnostic (eg, 3-Hz spike and wave of petit mal epilepsy, 1-Hz periodic sharp waves of Creutzfeldt-Jakob disease). The EEG is particularly useful in appraising altered consciousness that is episodic and of uncertain etiology. If epilepsy is suspected and the routine record is normal, maneuvers that electrically "activate" the cortex (hyperventilation, photic stimulation, sleep, and sleep deprivation) sometimes can elicit evidence of a seizure disorder. Nasopharyngeal leads sometimes can detect a temporal lobe seizure focus when the EEG is otherwise uninformative.

Evoked Responses

Visual, auditory, or tactile stimuli that activate their corresponding neuroanatomic tracts and result in a cortical potential. Ordinarily these small potentials are lost in the background noise of the EEG, but computer averaging of a series of stimuli, time-locked to the EEG, cancels out the noise to reveal a wave form. The latency, duration, and amplitude of the evoked responses reflect the physiologic integrity at various levels of the tested sensory pathway.

This approach is particularly useful for detecting cryptic lesions in demyelinating disease, appraising sensory systems in uncooperative infants, quantifying deficits in histrionic patients, and following the subclinical course of disease. For example, **visual evoked responses** may reveal unsuspected optic nerve involvement by multiple sclerosis (see Ch. 127). When clinical uncertainty exists over the integrity of the brainstem, **brainstem auditory evoked responses** (see in Ch. 204) can provide an objective test. **Somatosensory evoked responses** may pinpoint the physiologic disturbance when multiple levels of the neuraxis are affected by structural disease (eg, metastatic carcinoma invading both plexus and spinal cord).

Electromyography (EMG) and Nerve Conduction Velocities

When weakness is clinically difficult to attribute to nerve, muscle, or neuromuscular junction, electrical studies can be done that are often diagnostic and can establish topographically which nerves and muscles are affected either clinically or subclinically. In **EMG,** *the recording of the electrical properties of muscle* is displayed on an oscilloscope (and heard through a loudspeaker) during needle insertion, with the muscle at rest, and during contraction. Normal resting muscle is electrically silent; and with minimal contraction, single motor unit action potentials appear. With increasing contraction, they increase in number to form an "interference" pattern. Denervated muscle fibers are recognized by their increased insertional and abnormal spontaneous activity (fibrillations and fasciculations). Fewer motor units are recruited with contraction (reduced interference pattern) and giant action potentials appear (surviving axons branch to innervate adjacent muscle fibers, and by doing so enlarge the motor unit). In muscle disease, individual fibers are affected without regard to their motor units; their amplitude is thus diminished, but the interference pattern remains full.

Nerve conduction velocities: A peripheral nerve can be stimulated with electric shocks at several points along its course to a muscle, and the time to initiation of contraction can be recorded. The time required to traverse the segment nearest the muscle is known as the distal latency. The time for an impulse to travel a measured length of nerve determines the conduction velocity. Similar measurements can be made for sensory nerves. When weakness is due to muscle disease, nerve conduction remains normal. In neuropathy, conduction often is slowed, and the response pattern may show a dispersion of potentials due to unequal involvement of myelinated and unmyelinated axons. Repetitive stimulation of a nerve can assess the neuromuscular junction for fatigability (eg, a progressive decremental response occurs in myasthenia gravis).

Electronystagmography (see CLINICAL EVALUATION OF THE VESTIBULAR APPARATUS in Ch. 204)

118. DISORDERS OF THE CEREBRAL HEMISPHERES AND HIGHER BRAIN FUNCTIONS

Disease or dysfunction of the cerebral hemispheres can be **organic** (ie, of known structural, chemical, or metabolic mechanism); or **nonorganic** (of unknown cause). The major psychoses and many behavioral disorders fit into the latter category.

Organic cerebral dysfunction is either **focal** or **global-diffuse** in distribution. Most focal dysfunction is caused by structural abnormalities such as space-occupying lesions, trauma, maldevelopment, or scars; by contrast most global dysfunction is due to metabolic-chemical disorders or disseminated structural lesions such as diffuse inflammation, vasculopathy, or disseminated malignancy. The clinical expression of most focal cerebral lesions usually reflects principles of cortical localization and physiology. Global-diffuse abnormalities, however, in addition to altering multiple dimensions of cerebral sensory and behavioral function, also often affect subcortical systems, interfering with either the activation of the level of consciousness or the normal integration of conscious thought. Diseases that begin focally can cause local dysfunction if they extend to disrupt these subcortical mechanisms. Coma and stupor represent primarily acute disturbances of the level of arousal, while dementia reflects chronic disruptions of integrated thought and its expression. Delirium and confusional states stand between, and consist of a mixture of varying degrees of impaired arousal and disordered thought and perception.

FOCAL BRAIN DISORDERS

The cerebral cortex contains proportionately small **primary sensory and motor areas** (FIG. 118–1) which, respectively, directly receive somesthetic, auditory, visual, and olfactory stimuli from peripheral receptors and transmit motor signals to the striated muscles to regulate voluntary body movement. The remainder of the cortical mantle consists of **association cortex** and **limbic system areas,** which together integrate sensory perceptions with instinctual and acquired memories to create learning and thought and their expression, behavior. A glance at the figure indicates the large ratio of the integrative association cortex to primary cortex.

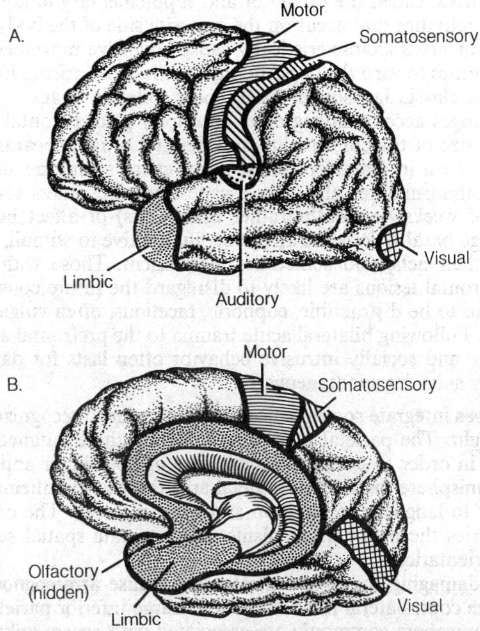

FIG. 118–1. A. The primary sensory and motor areas mapped on the cerebral surface. B. The limbic-association cortex.

The clinical effects of focal injuries on the brain depend mainly on the anatomy of the damage and the degree of adaptation, redundancy, and plasticity possessed by the rest of the cerebrum. In adult humans, the primary cortical receiving areas and pathways for somatic and visual function, as well as for motor control, are strongly lateralized with little redundancy. Their direct damage at any age usually leaves at least some permanent effects. In the adult, language functions and parietal lobe spatial functions become increasingly lateralized and also nonredundant as age progresses. By contrast to these exclusive representations, auditory signals from either ear reach both sides of the temporal lobe cortex. Furthermore, many separate areas of association cortex serve somewhat overlapping functions. Their **redundancy** allows for these loci to **adapt** to slowly acquired lesions which, accordingly, may produce few detectable signs or symptoms in their early stages. Certain areas of the brain even can alter their function given the proper stimulation and the age of the person. This **plasticity** includes the hippocampal processes that throughout normal life convert new concepts and percepts into permanent memory. Plasticity, however, is most prominent in the developing brain; eg, where the right hemisphere can assume near normal language capacities if severe damage strikes the dominant left hemisphere language areas < 8 yr of age.

SYNDROMES OF THE CEREBRAL HEMISPHERES

The frontal lobes influence 2 principal behavioral functions, learned motor activity and the planning and organizing of future expressive behavior. The prerolandic-precentral gyrus on one side of the cerebrum plus the immediately more anterior areas

of frontal lobe cortex, called the premotor and supplementary motor regions, regulate skilled muscular activities that occur on the opposite side of the body. Seizures involving these premotor areas characteristically cause adversive movements of head, eyes, trunk, and extremities toward the opposite side, while those arising from the precentral gyrus produce the classic Jacksonian focal motor epileptic attack.

Behavioral changes accompanying more anteriorly placed frontal lobe lesions vary according to the size of the abnormality and the rate of its appearance. Small unilateral lesions of < 2 cm in diameter almost never cause symptoms unless they induce seizures. Larger abnormalities also may escape attention unless they evolve rapidly (over a period of weeks or months rather than years) or affect both frontal lobes. Patients with large basal lesions are apathetic, inattentive to stimuli, indifferent to the implications of their acts, and sometimes incontinent. Those with frontal polar or anterior lateral frontal lesions are likely to disregard the future consequences of their behavior and tend to be distractible, euphoric, facetious, often vulgar, and indifferent to social niceties. Following bilateral acute trauma to the prefrontal areas, boisterously talkative, restless, and socially intrusive behavior often lasts for days or weeks. The syndrome usually subsides spontaneously.

The parietal lobes integrate somesthetic stimuli in order to recognize and recall form, texture, and weight. The parietal lobes also integrate these cutaneous percepts with other sensations in order to create self-awareness of both inner and outer worlds. In the dominant hemisphere the inferior parietal area transacts mathematical functioning and links closely to language recognition and word memory. The nondominant right parietal lobe carries the major mechanisms that integrate spatial self-awareness and extracorporeal orientation.

Small lesions damaging the post central cortex cause **astereognosis** (*loss of tactile recognition*) in the contralateral hand and body. Large inferior parietal lobe lesions in the dominant hemisphere commonly are associated with severe aphasia. Lesser damage to this area can cause apraxia, difficulty in calculating, and sometimes right-left disorientation and agraphia. Large, nondominant parietal lobe injury acutely causes a patient to ignore the serious nature of his illness **(anosognosia)** and to neglect or even deny the presence of the paralysis affecting the side of the body opposite to the injury. The inattention can spread to involve the entire extracorporeal world that plays into the right cerebral hemisphere. Confusion or delirium sometimes accompanies these agnosias. Dressing and other apraxias are common.

Temporal lobes: Visual recognition, auditory perception, memory, and emotion are critically served by temporal lobe structures. Patients with acquired unilateral damage to the right temporal lobe commonly lose acuity for nonverbal auditory and other memory, including that of spatial configurations. Left temporal lobe injury interferes severely with the recognition, memory, and formation of language (see APHASIA, below). Patients with epileptogenic foci lying in the medially placed, limbic-emotional parts of the temporal lobe commonly have seizures characterized by uncontrollable feelings, together with expressions or distortions of autonomic, cognitive, or emotional functions. Personality changes of humorlessness, philosophical religiosity, obsessiveness, and, in the male, hyposexuality occur in many temporal lobe epileptics between attacks.

FOCAL DISORDERS OF HIGHER FUNCTION

APHASIA

A defect or loss of language function, in which the comprehension or expression of words (or nonverbal equivalents of words) is impaired as a result of injury to the language centers in the cerebral cortex.

Language function resides predominantly in the left hemispheres of most persons, including the left-handed; more specifically, in the posterosuperior temporal lobe, the adjacent parietal lobe, the inferolateral frontal lobe, and the deep connections between those regions. Damage to any part of this roughly triangular area (eg, by infarct, tumor, trauma, or degeneration) interferes with some aspect of language function, resulting in an aphasia.

Many classifications describe aphasia, all having in common the recognition that damage to the language areas in the posterior superior temporal and adjacent parietal lobes produces disorders in comprehending words, in recognizing their auditory, visual or tactile symbols, and in recognizing or remembering them. These **sensory aphasias** have several subtypes, including **Wernicke's aphasia** (*normal words are spoken fluently but with neither semantic meaning nor recognition of the person's own word salad*). **Alexia** is *the selective acquired inability to comprehend written words.*

Injury to the inferior frontal gyrus just anterior to the facial and lingual areas of the motor cortex (Broca's area) produces an **expressive,** or **motor, aphasia** in which the patient's comprehension and ability to conceptualize are relatively preserved, but his ability to form language and express himself is impaired. Usually, the impairment affects both speech **(dysphasia)** and writing **(agraphia, dysgraphia). Anomia,** *the inability to name objects*, may be receptive or expressive. **Dysarthria** (*the inability to articulate words properly*) is not an aphasia; it is a motor disorder.

Brain lesions large enough to damage language function seldom produce pure defects; thus an isolated receptive or expressive aphasia is rare. Large frontal-temporal lesions cause **global aphasia** with severe defects in both the expression and comprehension of language.

APRAXIA

Inability to execute purposeful learned motor acts, despite the physical ability and willingness to do so. Typically, the patient is unable to follow a motor command even though he understands it and is physically able to execute the individual component movements. The defect is apparently a lesion in the neural pathways that retain the memory of learned patterns of movement, so that the patient cannot conceptualize the necessary movement patterns nor translate them into purposive action. Apraxia is common in many metabolic and structural diseases that involve the brain diffusely, particularly those that seem to impair frontal lobe function. Selective apraxias with loss of specific movements (eg, **constructional apraxia,** an inability to draw or build simple constructions; or an apraxia for getting dressed) may occur in dementia or, occasionally, with parietal lobe lesions.

AGNOSIA

An uncommon psychologic abnormality in which a person is unable to recognize a tactile or visible stimulus despite being able to recognize the elemental sensation of the stimulus. Language defects must be absent. Specific sensory agnosias can occur when the connections are interrupted between the primary cortical receptor region for a stimulus and the memory of that abstraction (eg, see parietal lobes, above). A typical example includes the incapacity to recognize the identity of familiar faces despite perceiving the existence of the face.

THE AMNESIAS

Disorders involving the partial or total inability to recall past experiences.

Memory can be divided into 3 major psychologic components: **immediate,** covering the past few seconds; **intermediate,** covering the period from a few seconds past to a

few days before; and **remote** or long-term, extending further back in time. Childhood memories are stored more strongly than adult ones, perhaps reflecting the inherent plasticity of the young brain. Learning is impossible without memory, so that the severity of brain injuries sometimes is judged by the extent of both retrograde and anterograde amnesia from the time of the accident.

Amnesia can result from either diffuse cerebral impairment or bilateral focal lesions, since specific neuroanatomic pathways in the cerebrum take part in the complex, poorly defined processes of memory storage and recall. The pathways underlying memory are found in the **limbic system,** extending along the hippocampal formation of the medial temporal lobes, fornix, and mamillary bodies, to the anterior nuclei of the thalamus, cingulum, septal area, and the orbital surface of the frontal lobes. Among these, the hippocampal gyri and dorsomedial thalamic nuclei seem critical. There is a close connection between the hypothalamic-mamillary area and the brainstem reticular formation (see IMPAIRED CONSCIOUSNESS, below), suggesting a close relationship in the memory process. Recent memory and the ability to form new memories are profoundly impaired by bilateral lesions involving the limbic memory route, most often occurring in the temporal lobes (from trauma, stroke, herpes simplex encephalitis) or in the mamillary bodies and medial thalamus (from thiamine deficiency, hypothalamic neoplasms, and ischemia).

Retrograde and **post-traumatic amnesias** for the periods immediately preceding and following concussion or more severe head trauma also appear to result from an interruption of limbic function, although more diffuse cerebral processes involved in memory storage and recall are probably also affected, as they are in many of the diffuse dementia-producing diseases.

Many aging persons develop gradually more noticeable difficulties in memory, at first for names, then for events, and sometimes even occasionally for spatial relationships. This widely experienced so-called **benign forgetfulness** bears no proved relationship to degenerative dementia but may be a forewarning, since some of the similarities are hard to overlook. The most common causes of severe memory loss are the degenerative dementias, severe head trauma, brain anoxia or ischemia, alcoholic-nutritional disease, and various drug intoxications.

Korsakoff's syndrome is *a severe amnesic state in which the inability to record new memory traces may lead to confabulation and a seemingly paradoxic situation in which the patient can carry out complex tasks learned before his illness but cannot learn the simplest new skills.* **Etiology** is most frequently alcoholic-nutritional disease (see also ALCOHOL DEPENDENCE in Ch. 138; and Ch. 120), subarachnoid hemorrhage, head injury, acute necrotic encephalitis (herpes simplex), invasive cerebral tumors, or neurosurgical interference. Mamillary body or dorsal medial thalamic involvement occurs in chronic alcoholism and often is associated with an initial attack of **Wernicke's disease,** or **encephalopathy** (see Ch. 120).

Symptoms and signs: In pure cases of Korsakoff's syndrome the memory defect is highly characteristic. Since memory for new information is severely affected but memories for distant events are less so, the patient's previous experience is available to guide his actions; there may be little apparent intellectual loss. Memory of events since the onset of the illness—and often, for unknown reasons, for a period of weeks or months before it—is severely or totally disturbed. Disorientation in time is inevitable. **Confabulation** often is a striking early feature, associated with the defect in recent memory. Confabulation is less apparent in more chronic cases. The bewildered patient substitutes imaginary or confused experiences for those he cannot recall, and may be so convincing that the doctor is deceived into seeing the patient's mental state as normal. Since other cognitive functions must be preserved to allow confabulation to develop, this symptom is absent or poorly developed in dementia.

Emotional changes usually develop; these include apathy, blandness, or mild euphoria with little or no response to environmental events, including fear-inducing situations.

Course and prognosis: The course, which reflects the cause, often is transient. The prognosis is good in head injury and subarachnoid hemorrhage. In alcoholism, acute necrotic encephalitis, and other conditions where destruction is irreversible, the prognosis is poor and prolonged institutional care may be required. However, improvement may occur for as long as 12 to 24 mo after onset, and one must beware of premature institutionalization. **Treatment** is that of the underlying condition.

Transient global amnesia: *The sudden appearance of severe forgetful confusion lasting from as little as 30 to 60 min to as long as 12 h or more* is a striking syndrome. During severe attacks there is total disorientation except for self, combined with a deficit in retrograde memory that can extend back for several years but gradually resolves as the attack subsides. Total recovery is the rule; convulsive or other abnormality is lacking. The cause in most instances is the result of transient ischemia affecting the posteromedial thalamus and hippocampus bilaterally. Migraine may be a cause in young persons.

Factitious (psychogenic) amnesia can impair either recent or remote recall, usually in recognizable ways; tends to be maximal for emotional crises; affects remote memories as much as or more than recent ones; and sometimes even includes a professed lack of self-recognition. By contrast, organic memory loss shows disorientation that is worse for time, less for place and persons, less for emotionally charged issues, and never, except for delirium, for self.

Treatment

Treatment of amnesia of all kinds involves management of the underlying cause. Most patients with acute acquired organic amnesia improve spontaneously. For those who do not, no specific measures can hasten the process or improve the end result.

GLOBAL-DIFFUSE DISORDERS OF THE CEREBRUM

IMPAIRED CONSCIOUSNESS—STUPOR AND COMA

The alert state with normal mentation requires an intact interaction between the cognitive functions of the cerebral hemispheres and the arousal mechanisms of the **reticular formation**, the extensive network of nuclei and interconnecting fibers found throughout much of the diencephalon, midbrain, pons, and medulla. The **reticular activating system** is a functional, not a morphologic, unit located along the central core of the diencephalon and upper brainstem. It receives afferent impulses from many somatic, visceral, auditory, and visual sensory pathways, and relays the impulses to the thalamic reticular nucleus which in turn activates areas widely distributed throughout the cerebral cortex.

Impairment of consciousness may be brief or prolonged, mild or profound. Brief unconsciousness occurs with syncope (see in Ch. 26). With a convulsive seizure, unconsciousness may last somewhat longer; in concussion, up to 24 h. Prolonged unconsciousness usually results from severe intracranial or metabolic disorders. **Obtundation** is *reduced alertness*, usually combined with hypersomnia. **Stupor** is *unresponsiveness from which the patient can be aroused only briefly and by vigorous and repeated stimulation*. **Coma** is *unarousable unresponsiveness*; in deep coma, even primitive avoidance reflexes may be absent.

Hypersomnia (*excessively long or deep sleep from which the patient can be awakened only by energetic stimulation*) and **delirium** and **confusional states** (see below) also are states of impaired consciousness.

Etiology

A clouded or depressed state of consciousness implies dysfunction of the cerebral hemispheres, the upper brainstem, or both areas. Initially, **focal lesions in supratentorial structures** may extensively damage both hemispheres or may produce so much brain swelling that the hemispheres compress the diencephalic activating system and midbrain (**transtentorial herniation**—see under INTRACRANIAL NEOPLASMS in Ch. 126), causing brainstem damage. **Primary subtentorial (brainstem or cerebellar) lesions** may compress or directly damage the reticular activating system anywhere between the level of the midpons and (by upward pressure) the diencephalon. **Metabolic or infectious diseases** may depress hemispheric and brainstem function by a change in blood composition or a direct toxic effect. Impaired consciousness may also be due to **reduced blood flow** (as in syncope or infarction) or a **change in electrical activity** (as in epilepsy). Either inadequate blood flow or a chemical change may alter the electrical activity. **Concussion** and **psychologic disturbances** impair consciousness without detectable structural changes in the brain. TABLE 118–1 lists the major disorders that produce sustained unconsciousness.

TABLE 118–1. THE MOST FREQUENT CAUSES OF IMPAIRED CONSCIOUSNESS

Supratentorial mass lesions

- Epidural hematoma
- Subdural hematoma
- Cerebral infarct or hemorrhage
- Brain tumor
- Brain abscess

Subtentorial lesions

- Brainstem infarct
- Brainstem tumor
- Brainstem hemorrhage
- Cerebellar hemorrhage
- Brainstem trauma

Diffuse and metabolic cerebral disorders

- Trauma (concussion; cerebral lacerations or contusions)
- Anoxia or ischemia (syncope; cardiac arrhythmia; pulmonary infarct; shock; pulmonary insufficiency; carbon monoxide poisoning; collagen vascular disease)
- Epilepsy
- Postictal states (following epileptic seizure)
- Infection (meningitis; encephalitis)
- Subarachnoid hemorrhage
- Exogenous toxins (ethyl alcohol; barbiturates; glutethimide; morphine; heroin; methyl alcohol; hypothermia)
- Endogenous toxins and deficiencies (uremia; hepatic coma; diabetic acidosis; hypoglycemia; hyponatremia)
- Psychomotor status epilepticus

Psychiatric disorders

- Malingering
- Hysteria
- Catatonia

(Adapted from *The Diagnosis of Stupor and Coma,* ed. 3, by F. Plum and J. B. Posner. Copyright 1980 by F. A. Davis Company. Used with permission.)

Diagnosis

The cause of unconsciousness often is not immediately evident, and diagnosis requires an orderly approach. The airway must be patent and BP supported before a detailed history or examination is undertaken. The patient may be wearing a tag or carrying a diagnostic card in his wallet. Observers or relatives should be questioned about the mode of onset or injury; ingestion of drugs, alcohol, or other toxic substances; infections, convulsions, headache, and previous illnesses (eg, diabetes mellitus, nephritis, heart disease, hypertension). Police can help in locating relatives or associates. Containers suspected of having held food, alcohol, drugs, or poisons should be examined and saved (for chemical analysis and as possible legal evidence). Signs of hemorrhage, incontinence, and cranial trauma should be sought. The patient's age may be significant: epilepsy and systemic infection are frequently responsible in those < 40 yr; cardiovascular disease (especially stroke), metabolic disorders (diabetes mellitus, hypoglycemia), and uremia are more common after 40.

Physical examination should note (1) **rectal temperature;** (2) **skin**: color, evidence of trauma or hypodermic injections (narcotics, insulin), rashes, petechiae; (3) **scalp**: contusions or lacerations; (4) **eyes**: pupil size and reaction to light, ocular palsy, corneal reflex, oculocephalic reflex ("doll's eye" response to head rotation), fundic signs of papilledema, vascular sclerosis, or diabetic or uremic retinitis; (5) **ENT**: escape of CSF or blood, scarred or bitten tongue, breath odor (alcohol, acetone, paraldehyde, bitter almonds [cyanide]); (6) **respiratory pattern**: hyperventilation; Cheyne-Stokes (periodic) breathing; (7) **cardiovascular signs**: apical rate and rhythm, character of the pulse, BP in both arms, signs of cardiac decompensation, sclerosis in peripheral vessels, cyanosis or clubbing of the fingers and toes; (8) **abdomen**: spasm, rigidity; (9) **neurologic signs**: paresis, stiff neck, reflexes, muscular twitching, convulsions.

The neurologic appraisal provides the key to whether the disease is supratentorial, subtentorial, or metabolic. **Breathing** is Cheyne-Stokes (periodic) with hemispheric disease and irregularly irregular with pontomedullary disease; hyper- or hypoventilation occurs with metabolic disease. The **pupils** are small and reactive to light with hypothalamic and pontine disease or narcotic poisoning, fixed in midposition with midbrain damage or severe glutethimide overdosage, light-reactive with metabolic disorders, dilated with anoxia or 3rd nerve compression, and normally reactive with hemispheric disease or psychogenic unresponsiveness. **Oculovestibular responses** to caloric stimulation show bilateral tonic conjugate deviation with hemispheric depression, are absent or dysconjugate with brainstem impairment, and are normal with psychogenic unresponsiveness. **Motor responses** to painful stimuli are hemiplegic with hemispheric lesions. **Decerebrate rigidity** (neck, back, and limbs extended; jaws clenched) occurs with diencephalic-midbrain dysfunction; flaccidity, with pontomedullary brainstem dysfunction. **Symmetric motor abnormalities,** often including asterixis or a multifocal myoclonus, occur with metabolic diseases, and motor signs and reflexes are normal with psychogenic unresponsiveness.

Characteristically, neurologic signs and symptoms in supratentorial mass lesions causing stupor or coma first indicate involvement of one cerebral hemisphere. Then, because of enlargement of the mass and consequent shifts in brain tissues as a result of pressure changes, signs show progressive rostral-caudal deterioration indicating involvement first of the diencephalon and finally of the brainstem (see Complications of Head Trauma in Ch. 124). With unconsciousness from a primary brainstem lesion, pupillary and oculomotor signs are abnormal from the start.

Laboratory studies: In coma of unknown cause, and where hypoglycemia is possible, the first step is to **draw blood** for glucose determination and then to give hypertonic glucose 50 mL IV. Other blood determinations should include Hct, respiratory gases, WBC, BUN, sodium, potassium, bicarbonate, chloride, alcohol, and bromide content,

and spectroscopy for sulfhemoglobin and methemoglobin. **Urine** should be collected by catheterization and examined for sugar, acetone, albumin, and sedative drugs. **Gastric lavage** is required for diagnosis and treatment in suspected poisoning, with care to avoid esophageal or gastric perforation if the poison may have been corrosive (see also Ch. 289). For patients in deep coma, endotracheal intubation should precede lavage to prevent pulmonary aspiration. Skull x-rays are substantially less useful than **CT scanning** when diagnosis is in doubt. In urgent undiagnosed cases, **lumbar puncture** to detect infection should be performed as soon as possible, unless increased intracranial pressure from an expanding lesion is suspected.

The principal diagnostic points for some of the more common causes of unconsciousness are as follows (further details are discussed in the appropriate chapters elsewhere).

Acute alcoholism: Alcoholic breath; patient usually stuporous, not comatose, responding to noxious stimuli; face and conjunctivae hyperemic; temperature normal or subnormal; pupils moderately dilated, equal, and reactive to light; respirations deep and noisy, not stertorous; blood alcohol > 200 mg/dL.

Cranial trauma: Onset of coma sudden or gradual; often local evidence or history of injury, perhaps with edema of scalp over fractures; bleeding from ear, nose, or throat; temperature normal or elevated; pupils usually unequal and sluggish or inactive; respirations variable, often slow or irregular; pulse variable, rapid initially and then slow; BP variable; reflexes frequently altered, often with incontinence and evidence of paralysis; CSF possibly bloody and under increased pressure; possible fracture lines or pineal displacement on skull x-rays.

Stroke: Patient usually over 40, with cardiovascular disease or hypertension; onset sudden, with signs of brainstem dysfunction; face often asymmetric; temperature, pulse, and respirations variable; pupils usually unequal and inactive; focal neurologic signs common, including hemiplegia; CSF often bloody or xanthochromic with increased pressure.

Epilepsy: History of previous "fits"; onset sudden and convulsive; incontinence common; temperature, pulse, and respirations usually normal, but possibly elevated after repeated convulsions; pupils reactive; tongue bitten or scarred from previous attacks.

Diabetic acidosis: Onset gradual; skin dry, face flushed; breath odor fruity; temperature often subnormal; eyeballs may be soft; air hunger (hyperventilation); glucosuria, ketonuria, hyperglycemia; metabolic acidosis in blood.

Hypoglycemia: Onset possibly acute, with convulsions, but usually preceded by lightheadedness, sweating, nausea, vomiting, pallor, palpitations, headache, abdominal pain, hunger; skin moist and pale; hypothermia; pupils reactive; deep reflexes exaggerated; positive Babinski sign; hypoglycemia during attack.

Syncope: Onset sudden, often associated with emotional crisis or heart block; coma seldom deep or prolonged; pallor; pulse slow at onset, later rapid and weak. In supine position, prompt reawakening.

Depressant drug or narcotic poisoning causes 70 to 80% of acute "coma of unknown cause." See Ch. 289 for specific agents.

Treatment

Immediate findings may call for **emergency measures**: Control of hemorrhage, cardiopulmonary resuscitation, airway maintenance (by intubation or tracheostomy), treatment of shock, O_2 administration (for the hypoxia that complicates nearly all unconsciousness), catheterization, fluid or electrolyte replacement, and chemotherapy. Temperature, pulse, respirations, and BP should be checked at frequent intervals. If the diagnosis is not immediately evident, glucose infusion may be started once blood has been drawn for blood sugar determination. Nothing should be given by mouth because of the danger of aspiration. Stimulants should be avoided. Morphine depresses respiration and is *contraindicated.* Parenteral feeding and prevention of decubitus ulcers are essential in protracted unconsciousness.

Brain death: The capacity of ventilators to perpetuate cardiopulmonary functions for long periods of time has led to widespread legal and societal acceptance of total cessation of integrated brain function as death of the person. To declare brain death, a structural or known metabolic cause of brain damage must be present; *and potentially anesthetizing or paralyzing drugs, especially self-intoxication, must be ruled out.* Hypothermia below 30 C (86 F) must be corrected. The following must be **absent** for at least 12 h: behavioral or reflex motor functions above the neck, including pupillary reflexes, oculomotor reflexes to caloric testing jaw reflex, gag reflex, response to noxious stimuli, and any spontaneous respiratory movement despite 10 min inhaling O_2 with the ventilator disconnected (apneic oxygenation). Purely spinal motor reflexes can remain. If time is critical for purposes of organ transplant, the observation period can be shortened to 6 h, but the clinical criteria should be supplemented by finding either an isoelectric EEG (no electrical activity) for 30 min, absent brainstem auditory evoked responses, or an absent cerebral circulation by angiographic examination.

Locked-in syndrome or **state** describes a condition in which patients remain awake and sentient but because of motor paralysis in all parts of the body cannot communicate except possibly by coded eye movements. Several diseases can cause the condition, which results from bilateral interruption of the corticospinal tracts between the midbrain and pons, or from severe peripheral movement of either the lower motor neurons or muscles.

The **vegetative state,** sometimes called **cerebral death,** describes a circumstance wherein overwhelming damage or dysfunction of the cerebral hemispheres removes the capacity for self-aware mental activity; but sparing of the diencephalon and brainstem leads to preservation of autonomic and motor reflexes as well as a return of natural sleep–wake cycles. The condition appears transiently following several kinds of diffuse brain injuries. A persistent or chronic vegetative state is most frequent after severe head injury or global anoxia (eg, from cardiac arrest) and can last for many years. Few such patients improve once the condition has lasted for more than a few months, and none fully recover after that time.

DELIRIUM AND CONFUSIONAL STATES

DELIRIUM

A condition characterized by extreme disturbances of arousal, attention, orientation, perception, intellectual function, and affect, most commonly accompanied by fear and agitation.

Etiology

Delirium most often occurs with acute widespread toxic or structural brain disease. It is seen especially during withdrawal from intoxication in chronic abusers of alcohol or barbiturate-like drugs, in acute inflammatory disorders such as encephalitis or meningitis, and occasionally with large right hemispheric parietal occipital infarcts in the elderly.

Symptoms and Signs

Disorientations, sometimes total (including absence of self-recognition), are characteristic, as are irritability, fear, perceptual delusions, visual hallucinations, and usually intermittently impaired arousal but sometimes sustained insomnia. Many delirious patients have fever, most are tremulous, and those with drug-alcohol withdrawal are especially likely to convulse. The severe agitation, disorientation, and occasional presence of auditory rather than visual hallucinations sometimes can be confused with

severe functional psychosis. Paranoid behavior may become prominent; such patients must be restrained to prevent injury to self or others.

Differential Diagnosis

The acute or organic reaction must be distinguished from functional disorders before ascertaining the cause. As a rule, defects in orientation, recent memory, simple calculations, and other intellectual tests identify the organic nature. Fever or evidence of drug use or systemic disease is prominent in delirium and absent in functional psychoses. Past psychiatric history for uncontrollable outbursts, manic-depressive illness, or schizophrenic reactions is crucial. Among organic disturbances to be considered are the senseless chatter and occasional agitation of acute Wernicke's fluent aphasia.

Treatment

Delirium is a dangerous, sometimes fatal condition that requires direct therapy beyond that of the underlying disease. Fluids must be restored and electrolytes closely monitored. Infusions should contain prophylactic thiamine and other B-complex vitamins. Fever should be controlled below 39 C (102.2 F). Severe agitation and tremulousness are best controlled acutely using diazepam given slowly IV in 5- to 10-mg doses q 10 to 15 min until the patient is calm but not asleep. Requirements sometimes are considerable, often exceeding 100 mg/day. With less severe agitation, haloperidol 5 to 10 mg tid to qid may suffice. Convulsions should be prevented, but if they occur, treated vigorously with diazepam. In chronic barbiturate withdrawal, severe tremulousness that continues for > 72 h should be treated by giving sufficient pentobarbital to stop the tremors, then slowly decreasing the dose over a matter of days, ceasing only when severe tremulousness stops.

CONFUSIONAL STATES

Less florid than delirium, characteristically having a less abrupt or dramatic onset, and usually marked by less severe disorientation and more subtle motor signs. **Etiology and incidence**: Mild confusional states are common, especially among elderly patients exposed to hospital care, including the trauma of major surgery. Metabolic encephalopathy due to systemic organ failure, excessive medication, nutritional insufficiency, or systemic infection with fever often adds to underlying traumatic, vascular, or senile cerebral insufficiency, precipitating a confusional state. **Symptoms and signs**: Apathy and drowsiness often are prominent. Disorientation is most marked for time, less for place, and almost never for self. Concentration is impaired and misperceptions occur, as do thinking errors. Motor abnormalities are common and consist of accentuated physiologic tremor, asterixis, and difficulty in motor relaxation.

Treatment in most instances is directed at the underlying systemic problem and correcting identifiable metabolic errors as soon as possible. All unnecessary drugs should be withheld; even necessary agents should be evaluated for adequacy of dose (eg, digitalis is a well-known cause of confusion or hallucinations in the elderly). Clinical improvement can lag behind correction of metabolic errors, especially in patients > 70 yr.

DEMENTIA

A structurally caused permanent or progressive decline in several dimensions of intellectual function that interferes substantially with the individual's normal social or economic activity. One million Americans are presently incapacitated by dementia, which can occur at any age and follow any injury severe enough to impose widespread damage on the cerebrum's association cortical areas.

Etiology and Classification

Static dementia is fixed in its degree of impairment and usually follows a single major injury (or the last of several), such as severe head trauma, cardiac arrest, or cerebral hemorrhage. **Progressive dementia** can accompany several major brain disorders. Some are discussed below. Others are discussed elsewhere in THE MANUAL; eg, chronic drug-alcohol-nutritional abuse, brain tumor, Huntington's disease, dementia paralytica, Creutzfeldt-Jakob disease, and several degenerative illnesses including Wilson's disease, parkinsonsim, multiple sclerosis, and amyotrophic lateral sclerosis.

Alzheimer-type dementia is due to a degenerative process, with a large loss of cells from the cerebral cortex and other brain areas. Acetylcholine-transmitting neurons and their target nerve cells are particularly affected. The brain shows marked atrophy with wide sulci and dilated ventricles. Senile plaques and neurofibrillary tangles are present. Memory loss is the most prominent early symptom. Disturbances of arousal do not occur early in the course. **Alzheimer's presenile** and **senile onset dementias** are similar in both clinical and pathologic features, with the former commonly beginning in the 5th and 6th decades and the latter in the 7th and 8th decades, sometimes earlier, rarely later. The dementia usually progresses steadily, becoming well advanced in 2 to 3 yr. **Pick's disease** also presents in the presenile period and shows a similar clinical picture. The primary difference is pathologic: Circumscribed convolutional atrophy affects mainly the frontal and temporal lobes. Some cases of dementia occurring in the presenile period are hard to classify and are sometimes labelled **idiopathic,** or **simple presenile dementia.**

Multi-infarct dementia is more common in men and begins most frequently in the 7th decade. Small and large cerebral infarcts of varying ages are present. Hypertensive patients are most susceptible; but hypertension, although frequently associated, is not an essential precursor. Because the pathologic process involves infarction, the dementia tends to progress in a steplike manner, each step accompanied by intellectual worsening and perhaps the development or aggravation of neurologic signs. In the early stages of the illness, personality and insight tend to be better preserved than in senile dementia. Depressive symptoms are common, and suicide is possible. As the condition advances, neurologic features may develop, especially hemiplegias, pseudobulbar palsy, with pathologic laughing and crying, or other signs of extrapyramidal dysfunction. Treatment is similar to that of other forms of cerebral ischemic disease (see Ch. 123). Control of hypertension (if present) is especially important.

Chronic communicating hydrocephalus with "normal" pressure can cause an insidiously developing dementia in mid to late middle age, affecting men more than women. Such patients are slow and slovenly, in contrast to the more alert behavior characterizing Alzheimer's disease. The gait is unsteady, slow, and shuffling, and many patients have episodes of urinary incontinence. Pathogenesis is based on impeded CSF circulation and absorption. There may have been a previous attack of meningitis, encephalitis, or head injury, and a few cases have tumors, particularly of the midbrain. CT scanning shows large dilated ventricles with little or no cortical atrophy. The CSF pressure is normal or high normal. Some improvement may follow the introduction of a ventriculoatrial shunt, especially when gait disorders precede or outweigh mental decline.

A severe head injury may cause sufficient brain damage to result in nonprogressive dementia. With repeated head injury, as in boxers, progressive dementia accompanied by extrapyramidal features **(chronic progressive traumatic encephalopathy)** may develop even though boxing may be abandoned.

Symptoms, Signs, and Course

Depression, paranoia, anxiety, or any of several other psychologic symptoms may be the predominant presenting feature. Early symptoms differ widely from patient to patient. The most common clinical picture is slow disintegration of personality and intellect due to impaired insight and judgment and loss of affect. Usually, progression of the disease is more painful to the family than to the patient. Interests become restricted, outlook rigid, and conceptual thinking more difficult; some poverty of thought becomes apparent. Familiar tasks may be performed well, but acquiring new skills is difficult. Initiative is diminished, and the patient may become distractible. Eventually, with progressive dementia a global defect develops, involving all aspects of higher cortical function. Along with the cognitive dysfunction, specific disturbances of speech (aphasia), motor activity (apraxia), and recognition of perceptions (agnosia) may be discernible. Spatial disorientation sometimes is prominent. Memory impairment increases, beginning with problems recalling recent events or finding names; the impairment varies greatly from time to time and often from moment to moment. Remote memory impairment can be circumvented at first, but also is progressive as the defect increases.

In some patients, cognitive dysfunction is preceded by modifications in their usual behavior and emotional responses. Typically, affect is blunted, but in early stages it may be excessive. Normal personality traits may become exaggerated or caricatured; an obsessive patient may be unbearably pedantic and rigid (organic orderliness), or a sociable extrovert may be facile and inappropriately jocular. The initial affective change may be dominated by irritability, with periods of anger and violence. Depression is common. If the mood change (depression, anxiety, or elation) is sustained, the disorder may be misdiagnosed as a primary affective condition. Affect becomes more and more shallow and evanescent as the condition progresses, and finally gives way to severe blunting, masked perhaps by a fatuous euphoria without depth. Habits deteriorate, and the patient becomes slovenly, dirty, and eventually incontinent, culminating with the need for total nursing care in later stages of the illness.

Coexisting neurologic features depend on the distribution and nature of the brain lesions, and these in turn on the etiology. They are marked in some syndromes as described above, but in others (eg, senile dementia) they are unusual despite the widespread atrophic process.

While dementia tends to run an insidious and progressive course, it is quite common for patients who have subtle, borderline, or mild signs of dementia to become acutely and severely confused and disturbed. This is usually due to a sudden stress; eg, acute illness of any kind, treatment with brain-affecting medications, sudden changes in environment and psychosocial stresses (particularly loss of a close relationship with another person). Typically, the stresses are multiple, as when an elderly person fractures a hip, is hospitalized, and has anesthesia, surgery, medications for pain, frequent changes of personnel, and a move to a nursing home. Time and judicious care may result in substantial improvement.

Diagnosis

Diagnosis is a matter of clinical judgment. A neuropsychologic diagnosis of dementia should *not* be accepted if the clinical evaluation is dubious, especially in patients who appear depressed or who may have other primary psychiatric disorders. Psychometric test results can be depended on only when the patient is freely communicative. Muteness or a failure to supply complete answers can result from depression as easily as from dementia. CT studies also should be correlated with the clinical state. Cerebral cortical "atrophy" increases with age in persons with normal mental status, and CT scan provides no reliable indication of intellectual impairment. The EEG is almost always pathologically slow in organic dementia.

Because dementia is sometimes secondary to a treatable condition, adequate investigations must be made unless the etiology is obvious. These should include a CBC, lumbar puncture, serum vitamin B_{12} level, tests of thyroid function, chest x-rays, CT scan, and serologic tests for syphilis.

Differentiating dementia from delirium seldom is difficult. The delirious patient usually has a brief history and a more florid illness. An EEG may be helpful in difficult cases, as when a confused patient is seen with no accompanying informant; the EEG disturbance is generally greater in delirium.

Distinguishing dementia from a primary psychiatric disorder may be more difficult. **Pseudodementia,** a reversible disorder if treated, can closely mimic neuropathologically caused disorders. Though most common in depressed elderly individuals, it can occur in patients with schizophrenic or personality disorders as well as in persons chronically intoxicated with sedatives or other medications. Diagnosis comes from a careful history and mental status examination. Accurate identification of drugs or other toxic factors may require discussion with the family. Depressed patients eat little, are constipated, sleep less than normally, and behave best at night; severely depressed patients tend to complain of memory loss disproportionate to their examination. By contrast, patients with functionally impairing dementia seldom complain of memory problems. Patients with depression give slow answers, but when they do respond, the content often is accurate; they rarely forget major current events or matters of great personal importance; they may be semi-mute, but when they do talk, they are not aphasic. Their neurologic examinations are unremarkable and their EEGs usually are normal.

Chronic barbiturate or bromide intoxication, vitamin deficiency states, and myxedema all are potentially treatable conditions that may mimic dementia.

Prognosis

Dementia generally is an insidious, slowly progressive, untreatable condition. However, the rate of progression varies widely and depends on the cause. The disorder may not be progressive, as after a head injury. Removal of alcohol in patients with alcoholic dementia can lead to substantial long-term improvement. In depressed, demented individuals, antidepressants can substantially (though transiently) improve function.

Treatment

The initial management of acute dementia should involve noting whether a prominent recent worsening has occurred in the patient's mental status. This is particularly true when the dementia has suddenly become worse because of stress. Such patients benefit from improvement in a precipitating illness, withdrawal of known toxic drugs, and minimal use of drugs that affect brain metabolism. They require time to adjust to and become familiar with new surroundings, routines, and people.

Quiet, dark private rooms should be avoided. The room should be reasonably bright and provide sensory stimuli such as a night light and a radio or television set to assist the patient in remaining oriented and in focusing his attention. Excessive stimuli, however, should be avoided. Familiar people in attendance, and frequent visits by medical personnel, encourage the patient to relate. Explanations should be precise and simple, and nonessential procedures omitted. Orientation to time is helped by using large calendars and clocks and routinizing daily activities; orientation to person, by medical personnel wearing large name tags and repeatedly introducing themselves.

Patients with dementia should be as much as possible in familiar surroundings with minimal variation in environmental stimuli, yet should be encouraged to continue with performable tasks. Major problems develop when awareness of their difficulties causes them to feel an acute sense of frustration, loss of self-esteem, and, at times, overwhelming anxiety **(catastrophic reaction)**. The family should be counseled and should encourage the patient in activities that promote a sense of participation and accomplishment.

As the disease progresses and uncontrollable agitation develops, carefully adjusted doses of haloperidol 0.5 to 1 mg as needed usually provide calming without excessive drowsiness. Hospitalization or institutionalization may be necessary for advanced deterioration.

119. MAJOR NEUROLOGIC SYMPTOMS AND THEIR TREATMENT

PAIN

Classification

Pain is a complex subjective phenomenon comprised of a sensation indicating real or potential tissue damage and the affective response this generates. Classifying pain is the first step in organizing a therapeutic approach; many schema are possible. First is the distinction between acute and chronic pain. **Acute pain** is an essential biologic signal of the potential for or the extent of injury. It is usually short-lived and is associated with hyperactivity of the sympathetic nervous system; eg, tachycardia, increased respiratory rate and BP, diaphoresis, and pupillary dilation. The concurrent affect is anxiety. Treatment involves removal of the underlying etiology if possible and the use of analgesic drugs. The pain is usually readily ameliorated.

Chronic pain is defined as pain persisting > 6 mo. Pain of this duration loses its adaptive biologic role. Vegetative signs gradually develop; eg, lassitude, sleep disturbance, decreased appetite, loss of taste for food, weight loss, diminished libido, and constipation. A depressed affect predominates. In many patients, organic disease may be insufficient to explain the degree of pain or may be altogether absent. In these patients, as well as in many with organic disease, the psychologic factors become the primary contributor to impairment. Therapy is often difficult and prognosis is guarded.

Chronic pain states can be classified in several ways. One broad classification distinguishes **somatogenic pains,** those explicable in terms of physiologic mechanisms, from **psychogenic pains,** those better understood in psychologic terms. A related taxonomy attempts to further distinguish pains by their presumed pathogenesis (see TABLE 119–1). **Nociceptive pain** is due to activation of pain-sensitive nerve fibers, either somatic or visceral. When somatic nerves are involved, the pain is typically experienced as aching or pressure-like; eg, most instances of cancer pain. **Deafferentation pain** is due to nerve tissue damage that results in interruption of afferent pathways and can be further differentiated on the basis of response to sympathetic nerve blockade. This chronic neuropathic pain is discussed further below. Finally, **psychogenic pains** are those occurring in the absence of an organic lesion sufficient to explain the degree of pain and disability (see below).

Pain can also be classified into specific pain syndromes, the etiology of which may be multifactorial. For example, cancer pain usually has a prominent nociceptive component, but may also include deafferentation states caused by damage to nerves by tumor or its treatment and psychologic processes related to loss of function and fear of disease progression. Typically nociceptive pain occurs in patients with arthritis, sickle cell anemia, and hemophilia. Pain evaluation is basic to management of these patients including a continual assessment of the treatability of the underlying painful lesion. A distinction between continuous and recurrent acute pain (as in sickle cell anemia) also is important, since the treatment plan will be different.

TABLE 119–1. PHYSIOLOGIC CLASSIFICATION OF PAIN

Type	*Subtypes*	*Example*	*Comment*
Nociceptive	Somatic Visceral	Bone metastasis Intestinal obstruction	Due to activation of pain-sensitive fibers; usually aching or pressure
Deafferentation	Peripheral Central Somatic Visceral Sympathetic dependent Nonsympathetic dependent	Causalgia Thalamic pain Causalgia Visceral pain in paraplegics Postherpetic pain Phantom pain	Due to interruption of afferent pathways. Pathophysiology poorly understood, with most syndromes probably involving both peripheral and central nervous system changes. Usually dysesthetic, often burning and lancinating
Psychogenic	Somatization disorder Psychogenic pain Hypochondriasis Specific pain diagnoses, with organic contribution	Failed low back Atypical facial pain Chronic headache	Does not include factitious disorders; ie, malingering or Munchausen's syndrome

Damage to the peripheral or CNS can produce a variety of chronic pain states, some of which may be nociceptive (eg, compression neuropathies or neuroma formation) and some due to changes in central pain pathways resulting in deafferentation pain syndromes. Pain in which psychologic processes predominate is also common, and many pain diagnoses (eg, failed low back, atypical facial pain, and chronic pelvic pain) can be included in this category. The management of these diverse patients has much in common.

Several specific pain syndromes are difficult to classify. **Myofascial pain syndrome** (also called **fibromyalgia, fibromyositis**), for example, is a controversial entity presumably due to chronic injury to muscle and surrounding connective tissue. Its prevalence is unknown and it is often misdiagnosed. The sine qua non is the identification of trigger points in muscle; pain can be managed by inactivation of these by injection or careful stretching (see also FIBROMYALGIA in Ch. 109 and MYOFASCIAL PAIN-DYSFUNCTION SYNDROME in Ch. 250). **Chronic headache** is also difficult to classify pathogenetically and in most patients probably involves a complex interaction between nociceptive perturbations in muscles and blood vessels and psychologic factors.

Evaluation of Patients with Pain

Though the etiology of chronic pain in individual patients varies remarkably, the rigorous evaluation each deserves has many elements in common. In all cases, a detailed history of pain should assess severity, location, quality, duration and course, timing (including frequency of remissions and degree of fluctuation), exacerbating and relieving factors, and associated symptoms (with emphasis on psychologic state and vegetative symptoms). Medication use, its efficacy and adverse effects, should be queried and other treatments detailed. Ongoing litigation should be identified. A personal or familial history of chronic pain can often illuminate the current problem and should be evaluated. Finally, a detailed assessment of the patient's level of function is neces-

sary. This should focus on family life (including sexual relationships), social network, and employment or avocations. In all spheres, the history should attempt to reveal the role played by the patient's pain in his or her interactions with others and attempts at normal living. Through this comprehensive interview, the issue of secondary gain is assessed, an evaluation is made of current and premorbid psychopathology, the role of family pathology is clarified, and a sense of the overall degree of abnormal illness behavior is obtained.

The pain history should also try to identify the meaning of pain descriptors to the patient. It is more socially acceptable to report pain than anxiety or depression, and proper therapy often depends on sorting out these similarly described, but divergently experienced, perceptions. Similarly, the distinction between pain and suffering should be clarified. This is especially salient in the cancer patient, whose suffering may be due as much to loss of function and fear of impending death as to pain.

Physical examination is used to assist in identifying underlying causes and to further evaluate the degree of functional impairment. Laboratory and radiographic examinations should be obtained as warranted. Organic etiologies always should be vigorously sought, since pain is best managed by removing the underlying cause; the likelihood of a prominent psychologic contribution to the pain should not preclude this search. The corollary is also true: Once an organic explanation has been appropriately ruled out, the patient is ill-served by additional useless tests. The sense of activity they provide for both physician and patient is illusory progress, actually perpetuating maladaptive behaviors and impeding a return to more normal function.

Regardless of the underlying disease mechanism, pain management depends on the understanding that the perception of pain can represent more than the pathology intrinsic to the disease. The principles discussed below can be applied to patients with known painful medical disease, whose pain fails to respond to the usual measures or whose level of disability appears out of proportion to the degree of impairment.

CANCER PAIN

Cancer-related pain can be caused by the tumor itself or by cancer therapy. Many cancer pain syndromes have been identified (see TABLE 119–2). Tumor can invade

TABLE 119–2. CANCER PAIN SYNDROMES

Associated with Tumor Infiltration	*Associated with Cancer Therapy*
Bone	**Postsurgical syndromes**
Local pain due to bone metastasis	Postthoracotomy
Base-of-skull syndromes	Postmastectomy
Vertebral body syndromes	Postradical neck
Sacral syndrome	Phantom limb and stump pain
Nerve	**Postchemotherapy syndromes**
Peripheral neuropathy	Peripheral neuropathy
Brachial or lumbosacral plexopathy	Aseptic necrosis of the femoral head
Radiculopathy	Steroid pseudorheumatism
Leptomeningeal metastasis	**Postradiation therapy syndromes**
Epidural spinal cord compression	Radiation fibrosis of brachial or lumbosacral plexus
Hollow viscus	Radiation myelopathy
	Radiation necrosis of bone
	Radiation-induced second primary tumors

bone or soft tissues, compress or infiltrate nerves or blood vessels, or obstruct a hollow viscus. Surgery, chemotherapy, or radiation therapy can be followed by pain. Accurate diagnosis of the underlying process is essential; pain management is immeasurably simplified by specific treatment.

Pain should be adequately treated while the search for its etiology is underway. Pharmacologic treatment with analgesic drugs generally is the primary mode of management, using a stepwise approach. The first step, often effective for mild to moderate pain, utilizes nonopioid analgesics, specifically acetaminophen and the nonsteroidal anti-inflammatory drugs **(NSAIDs)**—see TABLE 119–3. A large number of NSAIDs are available, differing to some extent in their cost, duration of action, and side effect spectrum. In contrast to the opioids, these drugs do not produce physical dependence or tolerance. All share a ceiling effect, which may be higher than the usually recommended starting doses for these drugs; if initial doses are tolerated but provide inadequate analgesia, a higher dose is warranted. If additional analgesia occurs but is still inadequate, the ceiling dose is not yet apparent and doses can be increased further. This process is empiric, and must be tempered by evidence of a dose-related rise in toxicities.

If nonopioid analgesics alone are ineffective, the 2nd step is initiated by adding an opioid, usually propoxyphene, codeine, or oxycodone, since these are available commercially as combination products (eg, aspirin/oxycodone or acetaminophen/codeine). These drugs are given around the clock until the maximum amount of the nonopioid drug is being administered (eg, 2 tablets of acetaminophen 325 mg/oxycodone 5 mg q 3 h). If this is inadequate, a potent opioid is prescribed separately and its dose increased until either effect or intolerable side effects occur.

The pharmacology of the opioid analgesics is described in Ch. 281. Selection of a potent opioid is empiric. Morphine is most widely available, but another drug may be preferred based on favorable prior experience, lower cost (methadone is least expensive), or limited availability. Pharmacokinetic factors should be considered; opioids with short half-lives (morphine and hydromorphone) should be used as first-line agents in the elderly, since the risk of accumulation in plasma is greater in this population. Meperidine use is limited by CNS hyperactivity (eg, tremulousness, myoclonus, and seizures) and dysphoria from accumulation in plasma of a toxic metabolite, normeperidine. Agonist/antagonist drugs (pentazocine, nalbuphine, and butorphanol)

TABLE 119–3. NONSTEROIDAL ANTI-INFLAMMATORY DRUGS

Chemical Class	*Specific Drug*
1. Para-aminophenol derivatives	Acetaminophen*
2. Salicylates	Aspirin* Diflunisal* Choline magnesium trisalicylate
3. Propionic acids	Ibuprofen* Naproxen*
4. Indoles	Sulindac
5. Oxicams	Piroxicam
6. Fenamates	Mefenamic acid
7. Pyrazoles	Phenylbutazone

NOTE: Classes 1-5 are often used as analgesics, and those drugs with (*) are specifically approved for this indication. If a trial with one at adequate dose for at least a month is ineffective, a switch to an alternate class is advisable.

also play a limited role; pentazocine is the only drug with an oral preparation, but has prominent psychotomimetic effects, and all drugs in this class are capable of inducing an acute abstinence syndrome in patients already physically dependent on opioid drugs.

Knowledge of the equianalgesic doses of the opioid drugs (see TABLE 119-4) is essential when switching medications or routes of administration. Cross-tolerance between drugs is incomplete and a change from one to another should be accompanied by a reduction in the equianalgesic dose by 50%. The duration of analgesia of the different opioids varies little, despite the variability in their plasma half-lives, and most need to be started on a q 3 to 4 h basis. It must be recognized that steady-state levels are not approached until 4 to 5 half-lives have passed, and that long half-life drugs (eg, levorphanol and methadone) carry the risk of delayed toxicity during the period of rising plasma levels. Therefore, it is prudent to begin dosing with these long half-life drugs on an as-needed basis, changing to regular dosing only after steady state is reached. Close monitoring is particularly important during the titration period.

If possible, medications should be given orally to prolong effect and avoid rapid fluctuations in plasma level. One efficient dosing technic involves the use of **"rescue doses."** In addition to regular doses around the clock, an extra dose q 2 h is offered as needed. The medication used for the rescue should be a drug of short half-life, identical to the one given on a regular basis if possible. The size of the rescue dose is empiric and based on the standing dose (eg, 15 mg morphine orally q 2 h as needed for a standing order of 30 mg orally q 4 h). The standing dose can be increased every day if rescue doses continue to be needed or if pain persists.

Other technics and routes of opioid administration have been developed in an attempt to increase analgesia and limit side effects. Slow-release morphine tablets permit q 8 to 12 h dosing, greatly preferred by some patients. Repetitive parenteral doses can be given if the oral route is unavailable; IV administration often provides greater patient comfort. Continuous s.c. or IV infusion should be considered if repetitive parenteral doses produce a prominent bolus effect; ie, toxicity at peak levels early in the dosing interval or later breakthrough pain at trough levels. **Epidural and intrathecal administrations of opioids** are recent innovations requiring special expertise. They may, via activation of opioid receptors at a spinal level, provide analgesia with fewer side effects. However, supraspinal redistribution of the drug with delayed toxicity and the

TABLE 119-4. EQUIANALGESIC DOSES OF THE OPIOID ANALGESICS FOR SEVERE PAIN

Drug	*IM (mg)*	*Orally (mg)*
Morphine	10	60*
Oxymorphone	1	—
Hydromorphone	1.5	7.5
Levorphanol	2	4
Methadone	10	20
Oxycodone	15	30
Meperidine	75	300
Codeine	130	200
Pentazocine	60	180
Nalbuphine	10	—
Butorphanol	2	—

Equivalences are based on single dose studies.

* An IM:oral ratio of 1:2–3 for repetitive dosing has been suggested from clinical series.

development of tolerance and cross-tolerance with systemic opioids are major concerns with these technics. Their precise role in cancer pain management remains controversial.

Tolerance (*the need for increasing doses to maintain effects*) occurs commonly with opioids and is first suggested by a reduced duration of analgesia. Tolerance indicates the need for higher doses to maintain effect.

The distinction between physical dependence and psychologic dependence is fundamental. **Physical dependence** is a pharmacologic process marked by the occurrence of an abstinence (withdrawal) syndrome after abrupt discontinuation of an opioid drug or administration of an antagonist. **Psychologic dependence** (or **addiction**) refers to a behavioral syndrome in which there is overriding concern with the use and acquisition of the drug, resulting in drug hoarding, diversion, and unapproved escalation in dose. While physical dependence occurs in virtually all patients treated for pain who take opioids chronically, psychologic dependence is extremely rare and should *not* be considered in the decision to begin or to increase doses in patients with cancer pain.

Adjuvant medications are used to treat side effects or provide additive analgesia. **Constipation** is common and should be managed by increasing the fiber content of the diet to > 10 gm/day and prescribing a stool softener (eg, docusate sodium 100 mg bid to tid), with or without a contact laxative (eg, senna). The dose of senna begins low but can be increased if necessary. If constipation persists, it can be managed with a periodic (q 2 to 3 days) dose of an osmotic laxative (eg, magnesium citrate) or with chronic administration of lactulose (eg, 15 mL bid). **Sedation** can be treated specifically with dextroamphetamine 2.5 to 10 mg orally 1 to 3 times/day. **Nausea** can be treated with hydroxyzine 25 to 50 mg orally q 6 h or with an antiemetic phenothiazine (eg, prochlorperazine 10 mg orally q 6 h). **Respiratory depression** is rare in patients on chronic dosing, since tolerance to this effect develops quickly; should it occur, a contributing pathologic process should be sought. If it requires treatment, dilute solutions of naloxone (0.4 mg diluted in 10 mL 0.9% sodium chloride) should be given slowly IV, titrated to respiratory rate, not alertness, *with caution to avoid an abstinence syndrome.*

To provide additive analgesia, a NSAID generally should be added to the opioid regimen. There is evidence that bone pain is particularly responsive to treatment with the NSAIDs (eg, aspirin 650 mg q 4 h or ibuprofen 600 to 800 mg tid to qid). Many other medications whose primary indication is *not* analgesia can also augment pain relief in certain settings; eg, corticosteroids (eg, dexamethasone 4 mg q 6 h orally or more) are also useful for severe bone pain and may be very helpful in pain due to infiltration of neural structures. For nonlancinating neuropathic pain, a tricyclic antidepressant (eg, amitriptyline or doxepin 10 to 25 mg orally at bedtime to start, increasing to 75 to 150 mg orally at bedtime over 1 to 2 wk) may be useful. Higher doses may be needed, especially if depression is prominent. A lancinating component to the pain may respond to treatment with an anticonvulsant or baclofen (see TABLE 119–5). With

TABLE 119–5. DRUGS USED IN THE MANAGEMENT OF LANCINATING NEUROPATHIC PAIN

Drug	Usual Dosage Range (Mg/Day Orally)
Carbamazepine	200–1000
Phenytoin	100–300
Clonazepam	1–10
Valproate	750–2250
Baclofen	10–40

NOTE: Except for phenytoin, initial doses should be low and increased slowly. Serum drug levels should be followed.

TABLE 119–6. NONPHARMACOLOGIC METHODS OF PAIN CONTROL

Treatment	Example	Indication
Cognitive-behavioral technics	Distraction Relaxation Hypnosis Biofeedback	Prominent depression or anxiety; muscle spasm; predictable pain
Psychotherapy (usually behavioral and/or cognitive)	—	Abnormal illness behavior; secondary gain; coexistent psychopathology
Physiatric	Physical or occupational therapy Prosthetics or orthotic devices	Incident pain; skeletal instability; disuse
Neuroaugmentative	TENS* Counterirritation	Localized pain; neuropathic pain
Anesthetic	Trigger point injections	Myofascial pain

* Transcutaneous electrical nerve stimulation

these drugs, except phenytoin, doses should begin low and be increased gradually. Phenytoin should be started at the usual maintenance dose (eg, 300 mg/day orally) or given first as a loading dose (eg, 500 mg orally q 6 h for 2 doses, then 300 mg/day). Though a relationship between analgesic effect and blood levels has not been determined, monitoring serum concentration may be useful to assess compliance and record a baseline effective concentration for future reference.

Nonpharmacologic analgesic therapies applicable by the nonspecialist may also be useful in selected patients with cancer pain (see TABLE 119–6).

A variety of other, **specialized anesthetic, neurosurgical, and invasive neuroaugmentative technics** are also available (see TABLE 119–7). No controlled studies of these adju-

TABLE 119–7. ANESTHETIC, NEUROSURGICAL, AND INVASIVE NEUROAUGMENTATIVE PROCEDURES USED IN THE MANAGEMENT OF CANCER PAIN

Site	Procedures		
	Anesthetic	Surgical	Neuroaugmentative
Peripheral nerve	Temporary and neurolytic block	Neurectomy	Percutaneous electrical stimulation; acupuncture
Nerve root	Temporary and neurolytic block	Rhizotomy	—
Spinal cord	—	Dorsal root entry zone lesions; cordotomy; myelotomy	Dorsal column stimulation
Brainstem	—	Mesencephalic tractotomy	—
Thalamus	—	Thalamotomy	Deep brain stimulation
Cortex	—	Lobotomy: cingulumotomy	—
Pituitary	Chemical hypophysectomy	Transphenoidal hypophysectomy	—

vant technics have been done, but large series have been reported suggesting their efficacy. The precise role each plays in the management of pain in the cancer patient is not yet defined and special expertise, which may be available only in certain centers, is required for their safe application. These technics are most useful for localized pain and should be considered only if routine noninvasive measures fail. A notable exception to this latter generalization is the anesthetic technic of celiac plexus neurolytic block for midabdominal pain, in which the benefits of early treatment appear to outweigh the potential risks.

DEAFFERENTATION PAIN

Chronic pain can develop after injury to any level of the nervous system, peripheral or central. A variety of specific syndromes have been identified. Their incidence and prevalence is not known and the pathogenesis of each remains obscure. The occurrence of these pain states appears to be low relative to the injuries that precede them, except for phantom limb pain. Of the pain states due to nervous system damage, those following deafferentation (ie, *partial or complete damage to afferent nerve pathways*) form a unique and difficult subgroup. These syndromes are complex, and though presumably related pathogenetically, vary substantially from each other. For example, a lesion in the thalamus causing pain without autonomic or trophic changes and which is unresponsive to manipulation of the sympathetic nervous system, is clearly distinct from a lesion producing reflex sympathetic dystrophy, in which all of these characteristics may be present. Nevertheless, all are believed to involve reorganization of central pain pathways.

Though deep aching may accompany nerve injury, common in such disorders as compression of nerve roots by a herniated nucleus pulposus (nociceptive pain), the deafferentation pain states tend to produce a spontaneous burning pain, often with a superimposed lancinating component. Other sensations (eg, hyperesthesia, hyperalgesia, allodynia [pain from a non-noxious stimulus], and hyperpathia [particularly unpleasant, exaggerated pain response]) may also occur.

Principles of Treatment

1. Accurate diagnosis is essential. In particular, deafferentation pain from peripheral nerve damage must be distinguished from other forms of neuropathic pain in which an ongoing, potentially treatable, pathologic process involves a peripheral nerve by compression or neuroma formation. For example, phantom limb pain must be distinguished from stump pain, since the latter suggests a different pathophysiology (neuroma). Additional evaluation (to rule out infection, hypertrophic scar, bone fragments) and unique treatments (injection or resection of the neuroma) may be indicated. Even central pains may be caused by a remediable process (eg, tumor or syrinx) and should be fully assessed. *A practical aspect of diagnosis concerns the distinction between pains that may be ameliorated by manipulation of the sympathetic nervous system (eg, reflex sympathetic dystrophy and postherpetic neuralgia) and those that are not.* Initial management often depends on this categorization, as outlined below.

2. Mobilization of the painful part. Particularly in peripheral nerve lesions, the development of trophic changes, compounded by disuse atrophy and joint ankylosis, can be a devastating complication, ultimately increasing both pain and disability. Vigorous rehabilitative therapy should be given. The goals are maintaining full motion at affected joints, improving muscle strength and tone, further desensitizing the painful extremity by repeatedly stimulating it, and retaining functional use of the limb as much as possible.

3. Constant consideration of psychologic factors, beginning at the start of therapy. Profound psychologic impairment may be present in these disorders. Anxiety and

depression must be addressed directly and treated appropriately. Social isolation is common and reintegration into the family and society at large should be prominent therapeutic goals. Loss of function beyond that explained by the neurologic deficit should be vigorously managed with psychologic and rehabilitative technics (see below).

These principles of treatment provide a backdrop against which pharmacologic and other nonpharmacologic methods of pain control can be instituted. Pain therapies applied without concern for diagnosis, rehabilitation, and psychosocial issues have a limited chance of success.

REFLEX SYMPATHETIC DYSTROPHY
(Sudeck's Atrophy; Minor Causalgia and Posttraumatic Neuralgia)

This prototype deafferentation syndrome occurs following injury to bone and soft tissue. The diagnosis depends on the association of pain with autonomic changes (eg, sweating or vasomotor abnormalities) and/or dystrophic changes (eg, atrophy of skin or bone, loss of hair, joint contractures). Radionuclide bone scan (increased uptake), radiographs of the extremity (bone loss), and thermography (decreased skin temperature) may be useful confirmatory tests, but none need be positive for the pain syndrome to exist.

Causalgia may be viewed as *a subtype of reflex sympathetic dystrophy*. In this syndrome, injury, usually partial, to a nerve trunk (typically the median nerve above the elbow or sciatic nerve above the knee) produces severe, burning pain in the extremity. The pain usually occurs soon after the injury, if not immediately, and in time becomes associated with the autonomic and trophic changes described above.

Postherpetic neuralgia is a dermatomal deafferentation pain that occurs as a sequela to herpes zoster (see in Ch. 12).

Treatment

Combined with physical therapy, **anesthetic or pharmacologic blockade of sympathetic nerve function** is the most important aspect of therapy. Sympathetic nerve block should be used. Transient relief after temporary blocks suggests the need for surgical or chemical sympathectomy. Intravenous regional sympathetic blockade with guanethidine or reserpine is a specialized anesthetic technic that may be useful in selected patients. The sympatholytic drugs prazosin (1 to 8 mg/day orally in divided doses) and phenoxybenzamine (40 to 120 mg/day orally in divided doses) have been reported in uncontrolled series to be of benefit. Other suggested drugs include nifedipine (10 to 30 mg tid), corticosteroids (eg, prednisone 60 to 80 mg/day orally tapered over 2 to 4 wk), tricyclic antidepressants (see above), and anticonvulsants (see TABLE 119–5, above). Anecdotal reports in postherpetic neuralgia and other neuropathic pain states also suggest benefit from selected neuroleptics (eg, fluphenazine 1 to 2 mg tid). Chronic treatment with opioid analgesics is controversial, but may occasionally be useful in reliable patients; such therapy should be considered only after all other approaches have failed and if close physician follow-up is possible. Guidelines for opioid maintenance therapy are listed in TABLE 119–8.

Physical therapy is essential during all phases of therapy. If myofascial trigger points are found, they should be injected. Transcutaneous electrical nerve stimulation **(TENS)** may be helpful, and a prolonged trial at multiple locations and stimulation parameters should be attempted. Alternative methods of nervous system stimulation (neuroaugmentation) include counterirritation (brisk rubbing of the affected part) and acupuncture. No studies have established that one form of neuroaugmentative therapy is superior to another or that patient response to other forms will be poor if one type is unsuccessful. Therefore, treatment remains empiric.

TABLE 119–8. GUIDELINES FOR THE MANAGEMENT OF OPIOID MAINTENANCE THERAPY IN PATIENTS WITH NONMALIGNANT PAIN

Used only after all nonopioid therapies are exhausted.
Formal consent required, specifically noting possibilities of side effects, minimal risk of addictive behaviors developing, and physical dependence of newborns in women who deliver while on therapy
Agreed-upon period of titration, aiming for at least partial relief of pain
After titration, agreed-upon monthly quantity of drug, with some leeway in daily dose but return to maintenance dose by the month's end
Monthly visits
Return of function should continue to be major emphasis
Drug hoarding, diversion, or acquisition elsewhere should not be tolerated; if they occur, opioid drugs should be tapered and maintenance therapy stopped.
Rapid escalation, or escalation without subsequent decrement, suggests need for hospitalization

Psychologic therapies are described below, under PSYCHOGENIC PAIN SYNDROMES.

Finally, a recent surgical innovation, the **dorsal root entry zone lesion,** can be considered for disabling pain unresponsive to conservative measures.

OTHER NEUROPATHIC SYNDROMES

The remaining deafferentation nerve injury syndromes are distinguished from those above by lack of observed long-term efficacy of sympathetic blockade. These include **phantom limb pain, root avulsions, painful polyneuropathy, central pain syndromes** (potentially caused by virtually any lesion at any level of the nervous system), and postoperative syndromes, such as **postmastectomy syndrome, postthoracotomy syndrome,** and **stump pain.**

Treatment

Drug treatment with tricyclic antidepressants, anticonvulsants, and/or neuroleptics may be useful (see above). Diphenhydramine in relatively high doses (eg, 400 to 600 mg/day in divided doses) and both 5-hydroxytryptophan (up to 800 mg/day in divided doses) and L-tryptophan (2 to 3 gm/day in divided doses) have been anecdotally reported to be salutary in central pain states. All the other nonpharmacologic therapies described for reflex sympathetic dystrophy, above, may be tried, *excluding those that block sympathetic nerve function.*

Patients can exhibit profound functional and psychologic impairment. These lesions can produce severe pain, but there is wide individual variation in the ability to cope with this situation and continue a semblance of normal existence, especially in the face of repeated therapeutic failures. The development of abnormal illness behavior, with prominent social withdrawal, familial disruption, and progressive inactivity is not inevitable, but patients who develop these aberrant behaviors begin to resemble those with no or insufficient explanation for pain; ie, those with the chronic nonmalignant pain syndrome. The development of psychologic and social dysfunction must be recognized and treated. When this pattern is entrenched, patients may benefit from the comprehensive approach provided by a pain clinic.

PSYCHOGENIC PAIN SYNDROMES

Chronic pain with either insufficient or no organic explanation is a common problem. Typical syndromes include chronic headache, failed low back, atypical facial pain,

and abdominal or pelvic pain of unknown etiology. The experience of pain for most of these patients is like that of organic disease; ie, the pain is not factitious. However, while accepting that the pain is real, it is better understood as a psychologic, rather than physical, disorder.

The taxonomy of this type of pain has been debated and psychologic hypotheses are as varied as the different schools of thought from which they originate. A recent classification divides patients into (1) those *with* organic pathology but in whom a psychologic disorder is the predominant influence on the intensity of pain complaints and degree of disability and (2) those with **psychogenic pain** (referred to by psychiatrists as **somatoform disorders**—see also Ch. 140), in which *no* organic pathology is seen. Most chronic pain patients fall into the former category; some of those in the latter can be further diagnosed as **somatization disorder** (numerous, and often dramatic, physical symptoms, including pain, typically involving several organ systems) or **hypochondriasis** (pathologic preoccupation with minor symptoms).

These patients often develop a pattern of inactivity, social withdrawal, rumination about physical health, and inappropriate utilization of health care which has been described as abnormal illness behavior. In patients without cancer, these behaviors are often referred to as the **chronic nonmalignant pain syndrome**. A subset of these patients, sometimes labeled the **chronic intractable pain syndrome,** display a profound psychologic and social impairment marked by depressed affect and a virtual lack of function (see TABLE 119–9).

Without denying the validity of other theoretical frameworks, the nonpsychiatric specialist is usually best able to understand the chronic pain patient in terms of learning theory—specifically, operant conditioning. From this viewpoint, the pain behaviors manifested by the patient (including pain complaints and dysfunctional behavior) can often be seen to be reinforced by a variety of factors in the patient's environment, including behaviors of family or close associates.

Treatment

Though the degree of physical disease contributing to the patient's disability should be clearly identified, and periodic reevaluation should be done when this factor is not static, primary therapy must be directed at maintaining and improving function and in treating the psychologic disorder. Analgesic therapies can be pursued, but if used exclusively, will undoubtedly fail, because pain per se is not the only, or even the major, cause of disability. Rather, from the start and during all analgesic treatments, psychologic and social issues should be explored.

While psychologic consultation is often needed, the nonspecialist can organize a behavioral program that pursues improved patient function *even in the absence of*

TABLE 119–9. CHRONIC INTRACTABLE PAIN SYNDROME

Persistent, often multiple, pains
Often history of chronic pain
History of multiple failed treatments, medical and surgical
Often history of polydrug use, sometimes drug abuse or addiction
Depressed affect common
Rumination about physical ills
Limited insight into nature of pain
Vegetative signs typical, particularly sleep disturbance and lassitude
Inability to work and loss of interest in avocations
Disturbed family relationships
Social withdrawal

successful pain reduction. Patients should keep a diary of daily activities in order to pinpoint areas amenable to change. Specific recommendations for gradually increasing physical activity and social engagement should be made and (especially those for physical activity) should be time-contingent, rather than pain-contingent. That is, activities should be prescribed in gradually increasing units of time; pain should *not*, if at all possible, be allowed to abort this commitment to greater function. Activities increased in this way often will be accompanied by reduced pain complaints. A variety of **cognitive technics of pain control** may be useful, including relaxation training, distraction technics, hypnosis, and biofeedback. Any physician can teach patients a simple method of relaxation involving repeated and systematic contraction and relaxation of different muscle groups. Similarly, instructing patients on the use of distraction by guided imagery (organized fantasy evoking calm and comfort; eg, imagining resting on a beach or lying in a hammock) also occasionally can be helpful. Other cognitive-behavioral approaches require special expertise. Attempts also should be made to reduce behaviors within the family or at work that reinforce pain behaviors; eg, constant inquiries about the patient's health or insistence that the patient perform no chores. The physician also should avoid engaging in such patterns, and should instead disapprove of maladaptive behaviors while applauding progress, and provide pain treatments while emphasizing return of function.

Nonpharmacologic methods of pain control should be stressed, including TENS and counterirritation, trigger point injection and spray and stretch, and physical therapy.

Drug treatment is sometimes useful; it includes the nonsteroidal anti-inflammatory drugs (see TABLE 119–3) and the tricyclic antidepressants. Doses of the latter may be increased (eg, amitriptyline 200 to 300 mg at bedtime) if there are indications of coexistent depression. Responsible patients can occasionally benefit from opioid drugs (see above and TABLES 119–4 and 119–8), though their use remains controversial.

Reputable **pain clinics** provide a multidisciplinary, comprehensive approach to patients with pain, which is most appropriate for the patient with chronic nonmalignant pain syndrome. Referral to such a center is often useful for patients with marked functional impairment or failure to respond to a reasonable attempt at management by the individual physician.

HEADACHE
(Cephalalgia)

Etiology and Diagnosis

Headache is a common manifestation of acute systemic or intracranial infection, intracranial tumor, head injuries, severe hypertension, cerebral hypoxia, and many diseases of the eye, nose, throat, teeth, and ear. However, such conditions account for only a few patients who consult a physician because of headache. The remainder usually suffer from muscle tension headache, migraine, or head pain for which no structural cause can be found.

The first task when a patient complains of headache is to determine precisely what hurts. Headaches may result from stimulation or traction of, or pressure on, any of the pain-sensitive structures of the head: all tissues covering the cranium; the 5th, 9th, and 10th cranial nerves and the upper cervical nerves; the large intracranial venous sinuses; the large arteries at the base of the brain and the large dural arteries; and the dura mater at the base of the skull. Dilation or contraction of blood vessel walls stimulates nerve endings, causing headache.

Diagnosis

TABLE 119–10 gives salient features of the history, physical findings, and special studies in conditions commonly associated with headache. The frequency, duration, nature, location, and severity of the headache help to identify the cause. Infrequent

TABLE 119–10. DIFFERENTIAL DIAGNOSIS OF HEADACHE

Cause	*Typical History*	*Physical & Neurologic Findings*	*Special Studies Indicated*
ORGANIC DISEASE:			
A. Intracranial (increased pressure) 1. Expanding lesions Brain tumor	Headache: mild to severe, localized or generalized, intermittent. Slowly progressive weakness on one side, convulsions, visual changes, aphasia, vomiting, mental changes	Papilledema, visual field changes, aphasia, paralysis, mental changes	CT scan often diagnostic. Other studies such as chest x-rays, lumbar puncture, or arteriogram can follow.
Brain abscess	As above; history of ear disease, sinusitis, bronchiectasis, lung abscess, rheumatic or congenital heart disease	As above; evidence of local or distant infective focus; temperature need not be elevated, pulse may be slow	As above; cultures from infection site, CSF, and blood
Subdural hematoma	As above; history of trauma, fluctuating changes in consciousness	As above; signs of recent head injury	As above for non-infective lesions
2. Meningeal irritation Meningitis, acute	Headache: recent, severe, generalized, constant, radiates down neck. Malaise, fever, with vomiting. Preceding sore throat or respiratory infection	Patient usually acutely ill and fabrile; may be confused, irrational, excited; may have stiff neck, positive Kernig's sign	Blood culture, lumbar puncture, smear & culture of CSF
Meningitis, chronic Syphilis Tuberculosis Cryptococcosis Sarcoid Cancer	Headache: dull to severe, generalized or over vertex. Moderate fever. History of syphilis or tuberculosis	Signs of meningeal irritation less marked than in acute form; cranial nerve palsies, delirium or confusion	Lumbar puncture with smear & culture of CSF; CSF protein, blood counts, & sugar; chest x-ray. Blood & spinal fluid STS
Subarachnoid hemorrhage	Headache: sudden onset, severe & constant. Prodromal pain in & about one eye; ptosis	Patient drowsy or comatose; stiff neck, positive Kernig's sign, bilateral Babinski's sign, third nerve paralysis; elevated BP	Lumbar puncture, arteriogram
B. Cranial (changes in skull) 1. Metastatic neoplasms	Headache localized; symptoms of primary cancer elsewhere; often neurologic symptoms	Scalp mass; cranial nerve signs; evidence of primary lesion or metastases elsewhere	X-ray of skull & other bones

2. Paget's disease	Headache: mild, burning, intermittent or constant, localized or generalized. History of increasing size of skull; pain in back, limbs	Skull tender; suggestive configuration of skull; evidence of compression of brain & cranial nerves	Skull x-ray, serum alkaline phosphatase
C. Involvement of sensory nerves of scalp	Headache: radiates along course of nerve. Pain of herpes zoster may be constant	Nerve may be tender on pressure, occasionally cutaneous hyperalgesia along distribution of nerve; vesicles or scars in herpes	
D. Vascular disturbances 1. Migraine	Headache: usually generalized, but may be unilateral, throbbing, beginning in & about eye, spreading to involve one or both sides; accompanied by anorexia, nausea, & vomiting. Similar periodic attacks over extended period. Family history frequently positive. Prodromata: changes in mood, anorexia, scintillating scotomas, occasionally hemiparesis	Examination negative between attacks; some cases may disclose transient neurologic findings during an attack	If in doubt and recent, CT scan. Otherwise,trial with a vasoconstrictor (dihydroergotamine or methysergide)
2. Toxic states; infections; alcoholism; uremia; lead, arsenic, morphine, carbon monoxide poisoning; encephalitides	Headache: moderate, generalized, pulsating, constant. History of exposure to toxins, or of other symptoms produced by causative agent	Other signs produced by causative agent	Studies applicable to the agent suspected; lumbar puncture, blood & urine studies
3. Hypertension	Headache: throbbing, paroxysmal, occipital or vertex. History of cardiovascular or renal disease	Elevated BP, retinal changes, cardiac findings, edema	Blood chemistry, renal studies
4. "Cluster" headaches	Headache: paroxysmal 1-h attacks, severe, unilateral, involving eye, temple, neck, and face. Symptoms of vasodilation on same side as pain, edema below eye, rhinorrhea, lacrimation. Periods of remission	Ipsilateral facial vasodilation, pupillary constriction, tenderness on pressure of external & common carotid arteries, injection of conjunctiva.	Therapeutic trial of methysergide or vasoconstrictor drugs. Corticosteroid trial. Indomethacin

(Continued)

TABLE 119–10. DIFFERENTIAL DIAGNOSIS OF HEADACHE *(Cont'd)*

Cause	*Typical History*	*Physical & Neurologic Findings*	*Special Studies Indicated*
ORGANIC DISEASE: *(Cont'd)* **E. Extracranial** 1. Lesions of eye (eyestrain, iritis, glaucoma)	Headache: frontal or supraorbital, moderate or severe pain, frequently worse after use of eyes. Pain in eye	Changes in appearance of iris; increased intraocular tension; errors of refraction	Ophthalmic examination
2. Lesions of middle ear (otitis media, mastoiditis)	Headache: temporal or aural, unilateral, intermittent, stabbing sensations. Feeling of fullness in ear, increasing deafness, tinnitus, otorrhea, general malaise with fever & acute illness	Acutely ill; tender over mastoid; red, congested, or retracted drum on affected side. Fever. Signs of meningeal irritation in children	Otoscopic examination, mastoid x-ray
3. Lesions of nasal sinuses	Headache: frontal, dull or severe, usually worse in morning, improved in afternoon; worse in cold, damp weather. History of preceding URI, pain in one part of face. Purulent nasal discharge	Evidence of nasal obstruction, swollen mucous membranes, tenderness on compression over affected sinus	X-ray of sinuses, transillumination
4. Lesions of oral cavity (teeth, tongue, pharynx)	Headache: bilateral or unilateral, variable in intensity, periodic. Pain in mouth, jaw, or throat	Lesion in oral cavity. Tenderness on tapping affected teeth or pain on syringing with ice water	Dental evaluation, including x-ray study
POST-TRAUMATIC	Headache: localized to site of injury or generalized, variable in intensity, frequency, duration. Made worse by emotional disturbances. Vertigo, worse on change of position. History of trauma, irritability, insomnia, inability to concentrate, inability to tolerate alcohol	Usually normal physical and neurologic examination	CT scan, thorough psychologic study, settle damage cases promptly
PSYCHOGENIC: 1. Conversion hysteria, anxiety states	Headache: frequently bizarre, bitemporal, constant, generalized, vise-like pain over vertex, made worse by emotional disturbance. Pain all day, every day, with no physical abnormalities	Appearance may be bland or apprehensive. Tachycardia, elevated systolic pressure, moist palms, hyperactive reflexes. Examination often normal	Studies to rule out organic disease. Evaluation of psychologic factors and personality
2. Muscle tension	Headache: intermittent, moderate, fronto-occipital or general, feeling of tightness or stiffness	Muscles may be tender, otherwise normal	As above

headaches can usually be related to acute causes such as fatigue, fever, or alcohol ingestion. The cause of chronic or recurrent headaches is often difficult to diagnose. Headache of recent origin especially requires careful attention. Useful tests include blood count, blood serology, serum chemistry profile, CSF examination, and visual tests (acuity, visual fields, refraction). Specific nasal symptoms call for sinus x-rays. If the source of recent headache is not immediately clear, a CT scan is in order, especially with any hint of abnormal neurologic signs.

Recurrent headaches associated with disease of intra- or extracranial structures are characterized by remissions lasting hours or days. Headaches from brain tumors or other intracranial lesions are usually of recent origin. They tend to be intermittently persistent for several hours each day, and may be precipitated or relieved by change of posture. The headache at first may be localized in the region of the tumor, but it tends to become generalized as intracranial pressure increases.

Headache associated with emotional tension tends to be chronic or continuous, and commonly arises in the occipital or bifrontal region and spreads over the entire head. It is described usually as a pressure sensation or as a viselike constriction of the skull. Febrile illnesses, arterial hypertension, and migraine usually cause throbbing pain in any part of the head.

Treatment

Besides attention to the cause, symptomatic analgesic therapy usually is indicated. Many headaches are trivial, of short duration, and require no further treatment. Management of chronic psychogenic, post-traumatic, or migrainous headaches is a common and more difficult problem. Both psychotherapy and pharmacotherapy are necessary (see also PSYCHOGENIC PAIN SYNDROMES, above).

Psychotherapy need not be extensive in most cases. An understanding, reassuring physician who accepts the pain as real, not imaginary, helps greatly. The patient should be seen at regular intervals and encouraged to discuss his emotional difficulties. The physician should reassure the patient that no organic lesion is present and explain the emotional basis of the headache. Environmental readjustments, removal of irritants and stresses, and reeducation, including urgings that the patient resume or continue a fully active life, may help.

The **pharmacotherapy** of chronic headache includes a variety of drugs. Those used for migraine are discussed under that topic below. In psychogenic and post-traumatic headache, simple analgesics are most effective. Aspirin 300 to 600 mg orally q 4 h may be given alone, with acetaminophen 325 mg and caffeine, or with phenobarbital. In chronic or recurrent headache, many physicians empirically supplement analgesia with tricyclic antidepressants (eg, amitriptyline 50 to 125 mg/day) or tranquilizers (eg, diazepam 2 to 5 mg orally qid). Tranquilizers or sedatives taken chronically invite habituation and intensify illness behavior. The value of drug therapy in most chronic headache depends less on the particular medication than on concomitant psychotherapy and the quality of the associated doctor-patient relationship.

MIGRAINE

A paroxysmal disorder characterized by recurrent attacks of headache, with or without associated visual and GI disturbances.

Etiology and Incidence

The cause is unknown, but evidence suggests a genetically transmitted functional disturbance of cranial circulation. Prodromal symptoms may be due to intracerebral vasoconstriction, and the head pain to dilation of scalp arteries. Migraine may occur at any age but usually begins between ages 10 and 30, more often in women than in men. Remission after age 50 is not uncommon. A family history is obtained in > 50% of cases.

Symptoms and Signs

Headache may be preceded by a short period of depression, irritability, restlessness, or anorexia, and in some patients by scintillating scotomas, visual field defects, paresthesias, or (rarely) hemiparesis. These symptoms may disappear shortly before the headache appears or may merge with it. Pain is either unilateral or generalized. Symptoms usually follow a pattern in each patient, except that unilateral headaches may not always be on the same side. The patient may have attacks daily or only once in several months.

Untreated attacks may last for hours or days. Nausea, vomiting, and photophobia are common. The extremities are cold and cyanosed, and the patient is irritable and seeks seclusion. The scalp arteries are prominent, and their amplitude of pulsation is increased. Intracranial vascular malformations are a rare cause of migrainous headaches.

Diagnosis

This is based on the symptom patterns described above in a patient who shows no evidence of intracranial pathologic changes. The diagnosis is more probable with a history of family migraine or of visual prodromata (classic migraine).

Prophylaxis

Various nonspecific medical and surgical procedures have been recommended for decreasing the frequency of attacks; their effectiveness depends largely on the patient's confidence in, and the enthusiasm of, the physician. The most effective prophylaxis is supportive psychotherapy. Methysergide 4 to 8 mg/day orally is effective but can cause retroperitoneal fibrosis and should not be used for periods > 3 mo at a time, with rest periods in between. It is **contraindicated** in pregnancy or in occlusive vascular disease.

Propranolol 10 to 20 mg orally 3 to 4 times/day has received a few successful trials in migraine prophylaxis but has only limited usefulness. Limited recent reports describe relief using the calcium channel blocker verapamil 80 mg tid or qid. Some patients are now being helped with biofeedback approaches in which they are ostensibly taught to control vascular tone; the long-term effect is uncertain.

Treatment of the Acute Attack

Aspirin or codeine may alleviate mild attacks. In severe attacks, only ergot derivatives and codeine or stronger analgesics offer relief and usually only if taken before the headache has lasted 2 h. Immediately after onset, for severe headaches (especially with nausea), suppositories containing ergotamine tartrate 2 mg should be taken and repeated, if necessary, in 2 h. For milder headache, sublingual or oral ergotamine tartrate and caffeine preparations are often more effective and require a smaller immediately absorbed dose of ergot: 2 mg plus 200 mg caffeine, then 1 mg plus 100 mg caffeine q 30 min if necessary, to a maximum of 6 mg ergotamine—or 10 mg in any week.

HICCUP

(Hiccough; Singultus)

Repeated involuntary spasmodic contractions of the diaphragm, followed by sudden closure of the glottis, which checks the inflow of air and produces the characteristic sounds.

Etiology

The condition, which is more common in men, follows irritation of afferent or efferent nerves or of medullary centers controlling the muscles of respiration, particularly the diaphragm. The cause of transient and even some prolonged episodes may never become apparent. With most prolonged or recurrent attacks the cause can be determined. Afferent nerves may be stimulated by swallowing hot or irritating sub-

stances. Hiccups accompanying diaphragmatic pleurisy, pneumonia, uremia, alcoholism, or abdominal surgical procedures are not infrequent. Abdominal causes include disorders of the stomach and esophagus, bowel diseases, pancreatitis, pregnancy, bladder irritation, hepatic metastases, or hepatitis. Thoracic and mediastinal lesions or surgery may be responsible. Posterior fossa tumors or infarcts may stimulate centers in the medulla oblongata.

Treatment

High blood CO_2 inhibits hiccups; low CO_2 accentuates them. Numerous simple measures may be tried: increasing Pa_{CO_2} and inhibiting diaphragmatic activity by a series of deep breath-holdings or by rebreathing deeply into a paper bag (CAUTION: *Not a plastic bag, as it may cling to the nostrils*). Vagal stimulation may work: drinking a glass of water rapidly; swallowing dry bread or crushed ice; inducing vomiting; traction on the tongue; pressure on the eyeballs. Carotid sinus compression (massage) may be tried with proper precautions (see PAROXYSMAL SUPRAVENTRICULAR TACHYCARDIA under CARDIAC ARRHYTHMIAS in Ch. 27). Strong digital pressure may be applied over the phrenic nerves behind the sternoclavicular joints.

Other maneuvers include gastric lavage, galvanic stimulation of the phrenic nerve, or esophageal dilation with a small bougie. Gastric overdistention can be relieved by continuous suction. Inhalation of 5% CO_2 in O_2 is of value, particularly in postoperative patients. In diaphragmatic pleurisy, tight adhesive support of the lower chest may help. The list of drugs for control of persistent hiccup includes scopolamine, amphetamine, prochlorperazine, chlorpromazine, phenobarbital, and narcotics. Metoclopramide 10 mg orally bid to qid appears to help some patients. Nevertheless, the very length of the above list implies that success often eludes the therapist.

When simpler methods fail, the phrenic nerve may be blocked by small amounts of 0.5% procaine solution, caution being taken to avoid respiratory depression and pneumothorax. Even bilateral phrenicotomy does not cure all cases.

DISORDERS OF SMELL AND TASTE

Disorders of smell and taste rarely are incapacitating or a threat to life and consequently often fail to receive close medical attention. Nevertheless, considerable distress can be allayed by proper diagnosis and treatment, and several systemic and intracranial disorders should be eliminated before dismissing symptoms as harmless.

Taste and smell are physiologically interdependent, and dysfunction of one often disturbs the other. Distinct flavors depend much on aroma stimulating the olfactory chemoreceptors. Loss or reduction of smell probably is the most common abnormality (but often goes unrecognized if limited to one nostril) and frequently is accompanied by **ageusia** (*lost taste*), even though the tongue retains its ability to discriminate between sweet, sour, salty, and bitter. The olfactory defect is confirmed by presenting a variety of nonirritating odorous stimuli (see Cranial Nerve Examination in Ch. 117). **Anosmia** (*loss of the sense of smell*) is discussed in Ch. 208.

Hyperosmia (*increased sensitivity to odors*) usually reflects a neurotic or histrionic personality. **Dysosmia** (*disagreeable or distorted smell*) may occur with infection of the nasal sinuses, partial damage to the olfactory bulbs, or psychologic depression. Some cases, accompanied by a disagreeable taste, arise from poor dental hygiene. Uncinate fits can produce brief, vivid, unpleasant olfactory hallucinations. Rarely, idiopathic **dysgeusia** and **hypogeusia** (*distortion and blunting, respectively, of the sense of taste*) and dysosmia are said to respond to zinc supplementation.

Drying of the oral mucosa from heavy smoking, Sjögren's syndrome, radiation therapy of the head and neck, and desquamation of the tongue each can impair taste. **Hyposmia** (*diminished sense of smell*) and hypogeusia can follow acute influenza. Various drugs alter taste (eg, amitriptyline, vincristine). In all instances, the gustatory

receptors are diffusely involved. When limited to one side of the tongue (eg, Bell's palsy), loss of taste rarely attracts subjective notice. Whether brainstem disease (involvement of the nucleus tractus solitarius) can produce disorders of taste and smell is uncertain, since other neurologic signs and symptoms usually are overshadowing.

VISION AND EYE MOVEMENT DISORDERS

Diverse elements of the central and peripheral nervous systems combine to produce vision. Consequently, examination of the visual system yields information about many parts of the nervous system and is especially useful for localizing lesions. For example, characteristic visual field defects distinguish lesions in the retina, optic nerve, chiasm, optic tract, geniculocalcarine radiations, and visual cortex (see Ch. 225). Disease in the brainstem, cranial nerves 2 through 8, or cerebellum may lead to specific disturbances in ocular motility and pupillary reactivity (see TABLE 119–11). The autonomic system may be affected. For example, ptosis and loss of pupillary dilatation (eg, Horner's syndrome) can arise from dysfunction of the sympathetic pathways in the diencephalon, brainstem, spinal cord, spinal root, or peripheral nerve. Finally, funduscopic examination of the retina provides direct visualization of neural tissue in health and disease, by which analogous changes in the brain may be inferred (eg, necrotizing arteriolitis). Funduscopy offers clues concerning the progression or resolution of certain local, systemic, and neurologic diseases (eg, raised intracranial pressure from tumor). Cerebrovascular disease may declare itself by amaurosis fugax (ie, carotid stenosis), hypertensive retinal changes, or retinal arterial emboli (eg, cholesterol). Most of the testing can be done easily and does not require specialized equipment.

Visual acuity is checked with a standard wall chart or convenient hand-held chart. Each eye is tested individually. Because from a neurologic standpoint the best possible vision must be ascertained, the patient's glasses are used. To minimize an uncorrectable refractive problem, the patient can read through a pinhole in a card. If the vision cannot be quantitated by these means, some statement of acuity is noted, such as the ability to count fingers at a certain distance or the ability to perceive light. The baseline is established, as sudden changes in acuity can occur in some disorders, particularly those involving the vascular system or compressive lesions of the optic nerve.

Assessment of visual fields is performed by confrontation examination. The examiner faces the patient who, with one eye covered, fixes his gaze on the examiner's eye. The examiner can slowly bring wiggling fingers from the periphery into each of the 4 visual quadrants; the patient reports when the finger first becomes visible. The examiner notes when he is able to see the fingers in his own field, and is thereby able to estimate the area of the patient's deficit. This gross test, however, misses subtle visual field defects. Using smaller targets (eg, red or blue match heads) is better; if this is done carefully, even the normal physiologic blind spots can be detected. If defects are seen or suspected, more careful mapping of the visual fields with quantitative perimetric studies should be done.

Extraocular eye movements are checked by having the patient fix on the physician's finger, which is moved to the extreme gaze horizontally, upward, and downward, and then in diagonal directions to either side. The extent of all these movements is noted, and the patient is asked if he sees double. **Diplopia** (*double vision*) may be present with minimal nerve or muscle involvement; the oculomotor defect often is not apparent by external observation. If diplopia is reported in one direction, the eyes are individually occluded, and the patient is asked which of the 2 images disappears, the peripheral or the near one. The following 2 rules apply to ascertain the weak muscle or affected nerve: (1) the objects increase their separation when moving in the direction of the affected movement; and (2) the image seen with the defectively moving eye always is the most peripheral. For example, if moving the finger horizontally to the patient's left

TABLE 119–11. NYSTAGMUS AND DISORDERS OF OCULAR MOTILITY

Type of Disorder	*Clinical Characteristics*	*Etiology*
Nystagmoid jerks	Unsustained	Normal
Pendular nystagmus	Rapid equal oscillations, increased with upgaze	Lost central vision in early age; multiple sclerosis; spasmus nutans: head-bobbing and wryneck in infancy
Jerk nystagmus		
Vestibular (Labyrinthine)	Nystagmus can be horizontal, vertical, or oblique, often with rotatory component; fast component away from side of lesion. Nystagmus increases on gaze toward normal side. Associated hearing loss and tinnitus, as well as vertigo, nausea, vomiting, past-pointing, staggering	Acute inflammatory or destructive labyrinthitis
Brainstem	Nystagmus coarse, gaze-dependent, horizontal, or vertical; inconstant vertigo. Nystagmus absent when eyes closed. Other brainstem signs	Multiple sclerosis; cerebrovascular accident in tegmentum of pons (upbeat nystagmus); Arnold-Chiari malformation; tumor of cervicomedullary junction (downbeat nystagmus); drugs (eg, phenytoin, barbiturates)
Convergence nystagmus	Slow abduction followed by quick adduction	Parinaud's syndrome; pineal tumor; lesion of upper midbrain tegmentum
Optokinetic nystagmus	Slow pursuit of moving stripes involuntarily interrupted by fast saccades in the opposite direction	Nystagmus disappears in lesions of pursuit pathways or opposite temporal-parietal lobes
Ocular bobbing	Fast downward jerk; slow upward return to midposition	Extensive pontine destruction or dysfunction
Ocular dysmetria	Gaze overshoot followed by several oscillations	Disease of cerebellar pathways
Ocular flutter	Rapid oscillations about a point of fixation	Disease of cerebellar pathways
Opsoclonus	Rapid, conjugate, chaotic movements, often present with widespread myoclonus	Many etiologies: postanoxic encephalopathy; occult neuroblastoma; ataxia telangiectasia

results in an increasing separation of the fingers, the conclusion is that either the left lateral rectus or the right medial rectus is involved. If, on occluding the left eye, the most peripheral image disappears, the fault is with the left lateral rectus. Also, the patient tends to turn or tilt his head in the direction of the faulty eye movement so that diplopia is minimized.

While checking eye movements, the presence or absence of **nystagmus** (*involuntary rapid oscillation of the eyeballs in a horizontal, vertical, or rotary direction*) is noted.

Nystagmus on extreme lateral gaze which fatigues quickly usually is physiologic. If nystagmus is sustained, it should be described in regard to (1) the direction of fast and slow component; (2) its character—eg, regular, irregular, rotatory; and (3) the degree of involvement of either eye. (See also TABLE 119–11 and below, under VERTIGO; CLINICAL EVALUATION OF THE VESTIBULAR APPARATUS in Ch. 204; and Ch. 207).

Opticokinetic nystagmus is *induced by looking at a striped pattern (such as telegraph poles) moving in front of the eyes.* Various tapes are available for this purpose, but a standard tape measure provides the needed regular sequence pattern. The patient is asked to count the numbers on the tape as it is rapidly passed in front of his field of vision. The tape is moved from left to right and right to left, and vertically. Patients with field defects, for example, have decreased opticokinetic nystagmus when the tape is moving from the affected to the intact visual field. The test also is helpful to rule in or out hysterical blindness.

Pupillary size, equality, and regularity are noted, as well as **pupillary reactions to light and accommodation.** The **swinging flashlight test** is used routinely to detect an afferent lesion of the optic nerve. The lighted flashlight is swung slowly from one eye to the other, noting the pupillary light response. Normally, the pupils react by constriction promptly and equally on both sides. If there is an afferent lesion of one optic nerve, a paradoxic dilatation can affect that pupil as the light is directed upon it. This occurs because escape from the consensual light reflex is still progressing and the direct light reflex in the presence of even a very slight optic nerve lesion is not great enough to overcome it; hence, the paradoxic dilatation.

If **ptosis** is present, it should be quantitated by noting the width of the palpebral fissures. In oculosympathetic paresis **(Horner's syndrome)** one pupil is small, and minor degrees of ptosis may be noted.

Exophthalmos can be detected by looking down on the head to inspect the eyes from above. Checking the **corneal response** and noting ability to blink the eyes provides information about the 5th and 7th nerves. The first sign of 7th-nerve involvement often is a decrease in blinking on the affected side.

Neuro-ophthalmologic tests in checking brainstem function in a patient with depressed responsiveness are valuable and simple. Instillation of 5 mL ice water into the ear canal should elicit forced deviation of the eyes conjugately to the same side, implying that the nerve pathway from the labyrinth through the brainstem to the nuclei controlling those eye movements, and the peripheral mechanism responsible for those eye movements, are intact. Similarly, rapid turning of the head results in a lag of eye movement as if the gaze were fixed, followed by a slow drift back to central fixation. Known as the **"doll's eye" response,** its presence implies intact brainstem mechanisms.

Funduscopic examination includes observations of the optic nerve, blood vessels, and appearance of the retina to detect papilledema, optic atrophy, vascular disease, retinitis, or other disorders. Papilledema usually implies an increase in intracranial pressure and shows up as blurring and disappearance of the disk margins, elevation of the nerve head, absence of retinal vessel pulsation, and, occasionally, hemorrhages and exudates. Surveying the retinal vessels in cases of stroke is important, as small emboli often can be seen. Other characteristic findings in various disorders are included in specific disease sections of THE MERCK MANUAL.

HEARING LOSS; VERTIGO; DIZZINESS

HEARING LOSS

The differentiation of sensory and neural hearing loss is fully discussed in Ch. 204. However, it should be noted here that neural hearing loss can occur as a complication of neurologic illness. In childhood, the 8th nerve can be damaged by mumps, rubella,

meningitis, and inner ear infection. In adults, tumors of the cerebellopontine angle produce sensorineural hearing loss, usually accompanied by adjacent cranial nerve dysfunction and brainstem compression. Cochlear nerve fibers entering the brainstem can be injured by a demyelinating plaque, glioma, infarction, or other lesion to produce deafness. Certain hereditary illnesses feature deafness with other neurologic abnormalities (eg, Refsum's disease). Other causes of sensorineural deafness are discussed in Ch. 207.

VERTIGO
("Dizziness")

A disturbance in which the individual has a subjective impression of movement in space ***(subjective vertigo)*** *or of objects moving around him* ***(objective vertigo)****, usually with a loss of equilibrium.*

Etiology

True vertigo, as distinguished from faintness, lightheadedness, or other forms of "dizziness," results from a disturbance somewhere in the equilibratory apparatus: vestibule; semicircular canals; 8th nerve; vestibular nuclei in the brainstem and their temporal lobe connections; and eyes. These structures may be affected by any of a large variety of disorders: (1) **otogenic**: Meniere's syndrome, myringitis, otitis media, acute vestibular neuronitis, herpes zoster oticus, labyrinthitis, middle ear or labyrinthine tumors, petrositis, otosclerosis, obstructed external auditory canal or eustachian tube; (2) **toxic**: alcohol, streptomycin, opiates; (3) **psychogenic**: hysteria; (4) **environmental**: motion sickness; (5) **ocular**: diplopia; (6) **circulatory**: transient vertebrobasilar ischemic attacks; (7) **neurologic**: multiple sclerosis, skull fracture, temporal lobe seizures, encephalitis; (8) **neoplastic**: tumors of the pons, cerebellopontine angle, or 8th nerve; (9) **hematogenic**: leukemia involving the labyrinth.

Stimulation of proprioceptors in muscles, joints, and tendons may induce a sense of dysequilibrium, but this is not true vertigo.

Diagnosis

Nystagmus, past-pointing, inability to walk a straight line, and persistent deviation to one side when walking all indicate a disturbance of the labyrinthine vestibular apparatus or its CNS connections (see below and also under Clinical Evaluation of the Vestibular Apparatus in Ch. 204). Determining whether the vertigo is **peripheral** (*arising from the labyrinth or vestibular nerve*) or **central** (*arising from the vestibular nuclei or their higher connections*) is the first step in establishing the cause.

Peripheral nystagmus is conjugate, horizontal, or horizontal-rotary, is maximal towards the affected labyrinth, and has its fast component away from the side of the lesion. **Central nystagmus** can be horizontal or vertical, characteristically has its fast component in the direction of gaze to either side, and may be pendular or unequal in the 2 eyes. Pronounced rotary, unidirectional upgaze or downgaze nystagmus always arises from central abnormalities.

Paroxysmal, episodic, or severe attacks of vertigo separated by normal interludes indicate a peripheral etiology. Persistent vertigo or dysequilibrium accompanied by nystagmus and gait disturbance usually indicates CNS disease. Unilateral deafness and tinnitus indicate cochlear nerve involvement and are reliable indicators of a peripheral nerve lesion. Labyrinthine disease produces more intense symptoms than does involvement of vestibular nuclei. Headache is more common with central lesions; and other findings such as double vision, slurred speech, incoordination of an extremity, or unilateral weakness are not seen with peripheral lesions.

Vestibular function tests (see in Ch. 204) are important—absence of the caloric response indicates a dead labyrinth. Audiograms may differentiate between cochlear and neural hearing loss. Special studies of the vestibular apparatus and CNS often are

necessary. Skull x-rays with special views and tomography of the petrous pyramids, CSF examination, and EEG help to exclude pathologic CNS changes. CT scan, MRI, or cerebral angiography may be indicated.

Sudden, episodic attacks of vertigo, tinnitus, and progressive deafness, accompanied by nausea and vomiting and persisting for minutes to hours, are characteristic of **Meniere's disease** (see also Ch. 207). Vertigo persisting for days or weeks may be due to **vestibular neuronitis** (see also Ch. 207). This diagnosis is made from the nonrecurrent nature of the attack, preservation of hearing, and absence of any neurologic signs except nystagmus and equilibratory disturbance. In patients with **postural hypotension** who become vertiginous on changing from recumbent to upright position, examination before and after this shift in posture demonstrates the exaggerated fall in BP. However, vertigo with sudden change in body or head position—eg, on rising from a recumbent posture, or on rolling over in bed (**postural** or **positional vertigo**; see Ch. 207)—is more often due to labyrinthine disturbance, as occurs after skull fracture or frequently in older persons for unknown reasons. Vertigo that occurs on sudden turning or, more often, strong extending of the head rarely may be due to **vertebral artery insufficiency** or **tumors of the floor of the 4th ventricle.**

True vertigo is not a symptom of psychoneurosis, but giddiness and fear of losing one's balance while walking may be symptoms of an anxiety neurosis or depression. Diagnosis is established by absence of objective findings, by negative laboratory tests, and by psychologic evaluation.

Treatment

Treatment depends on determining and eliminating the cause. Treatment of Meniere's disease and other otogenic causes of vertigo is discussed in Ch. 207. CNS disorders causing vertigo—posterior fossa tumors, cerebellar disorders, and multiple sclerosis—are discussed elsewhere in this section.

Symptomatic relief may be obtained by bed rest and dimenhydrinate 50 to 100 mg orally q 4 to 6 h, perphenazine 4 to 8 mg orally or 5 mg IM tid, or meclizine 25 mg orally tid. All these drugs are moderately effective against both intermittent and continuous vertigo in ambulatory patients.

MOTOR WEAKNESS

Weakness is common to many disorders ranging from muscular to psychiatric. A precise characterization of the complaint is important (weakness may have various meanings to the patient, including fatigue, clumsiness, or numbness); ie, the exact location, time of occurrence, precipitating and ameliorating factors, and associated symptoms and signs. Examination of muscles is only part of the neurologic examination which, in turn, is only a part of the general examination. Isolated muscle testing without a complete examination leads to grave diagnostic and therapeutic errors.

Synthesizing data from the history, physical examination, and pertinent laboratory tests should differentiate between upper and lower motor neuron disease. In the latter, the disorder can be localized at the anterior horn cell, peripheral nerve, neuromuscular junction, or within the muscle itself. To make these distinctions, knowledge about associated sensory findings, muscle tone, cerebellar function, and tendon reflexes is necessary. Specific examination of muscles includes observation, palpation, and strength testing. TABLES 119–12 and 119–13 summarize some of the main differentiating elements.

Observation of muscles provides information about the presence or absence of atrophy, hypertrophy, and extraneous movements. While the patient is seated and with the extremities in the resting position, the muscles are examined for bulk, contour, and fasciculations. **Atrophy** is evident by decreased muscle bulk, but with large or concealed muscles this may not be obvious until quite advanced. When the atrophy is

TABLE 119–12. MUSCLE WEAKNESS: UPPER VS. LOWER NEURON DISEASE

	Upper Motor Neuron Disease (UMN)	*Lower Motor Neuron Disease (LMN)*
Reflexes	Hyperactive	Diminished or absent
Atrophy	Absent	Present
Fasciculations	Absent	Present
Tone	Increased	Decreased or absent

bilateral, it may not be obvious when comparing one side with the other; in older people, some loss of muscle bulk is common. **Hypertrophy** occurs when one muscle works harder substituting for another; **pseudohypertrophy**, when muscle tissue is replaced by excessive fibrous tissue or some storage material. The most common extraneous movements are **fasciculations** (*brief, fine, irregular twitches of the muscle visible under the skin*). Fasciculations usually indicate disease of the lower motor neuron but sometimes can occur in normal muscle, particularly in the calf muscles of older people. **Myotonia,** *the decreased relaxation of muscle following a sustained contraction or direct percussion of the muscle itself*, is particularly seen in myotonic dystrophy and may cause a disability due, for example, to inability to relax and quickly open the closed hand.

Palpation of muscle may reveal atrophy, fasciculations, tenderness, or an abnormal consistency.

Assessment of muscle strength is essential to establish weakness, localize it, and quantitate it for subsequent changes. The patient extends his arms, and next his legs, to be inspected for weakness (a weak limb soon begins to sag) and for tremor or other involuntary movements. Strength of specific muscle groups may be tested against resistance. Pain in a muscle or involved joint may preclude an active contraction, which complicates testing. Hysterical weakness or malingering may be difficult to evaluate, but usually there is a "giveaway" reaction in which resistance to movement may be quite normal, but the subject suddenly gives way. The absence of atrophy and the presence of normal reflexes also help in these diagnoses.

Grading muscle strength often is difficult when weakness is incomplete. One scale assigns 0 to no movement; 1 to trace movement; 2 to movement with the aid of gravity; 3 to movement against gravity, but not resistance; 4 to movement against resistance supplied by the examiner; and 5 to normal strength. The difficulty with this and similar scales is the large range in strength between grades 4 and 5.

A better picture of the disability often is provided by **functional testing:** having the patient perform various maneuvers, noting any deficiencies, and quantitating these as far as possible (eg, the number of squats performed or steps climbed). Arising from a squatting position or stepping onto a chair gives good indication of proximal leg

TABLE 119–113. MUSCLE WEAKNESS: NEUROGENIC VS. MYOGENIC

Neurogenic Weakness	*Myogenic Weakness*
Wasting out of proportion to weakness	Weakness out of proportion of wasting
Fasciculations	No fasciculations
Reflexes often absent with minimal weakness (amyotrophic lateral sclerosis is an exception)	Reflexes often present with severe weakness
May have sensory changes	No sensory changes

strength; standing on the heels, then the toes, tests distal strength. Hand grip strength also should be noted. A patient with quadriceps weakness has to push off with the arms to get out of a chair. Some patients with weakness of the shoulder girdle swing their bodies to move the arms passively to other positions. Patients with weakness about the pelvic girdle characteristically arise from the supine position by first turning prone, then kneeling and slowly pushing themselves erect by standing bent forward and using the arms to climb up the thighs.

Subtle weakness may produce a depressed arm-swing while walking, a pronator drift of the outstretched arm, decreased spontaneous use of a limb, or an externally rotated leg. Rapid alternating movements may be slowed and fine dexterity impaired (eg, ability to button, open a safety pin, remove a match from its box). Coordination can be further tested with finger-to-nose or knee-to-shin maneuvers, which are useful to detect ataxic movements (cerebellar pathways—see also CEREBELLAR AND SPINOCEREBELLAR DISORDERS in Ch. 128).

120. NUTRITIONAL NEUROLOGIC DISORDERS

Lack of essential dietary nutrients can damage the brain, spinal cord, and peripheral nerves; eg, food faddism, intestinal malabsorption, systemic illness, certain hereditary diseases, and anorectic states. The common malnourished states that arise in chronic alcoholism, debilitating disease, and starvation are particularly important, since nervous system complications of these are treatable.

The process by which malnutrition causes neurologic injury is not always straightforward. There is often a lack of one or more vitamins that are essential cofactors for various enzymes of intermediary metabolism. However, since vitamin deficiencies usually do not occur in isolation, the vitamin responsible for a deficit may not be evident. Also, vitamin deficiency is not always the direct cause of neurologic dysfunction, as when a limb with insufficient subcutaneous fat and connective tissue becomes prone to compressive neuropathy. In scurvy, hemorrhage into the femoral nerve sheath may produce weakness of the quadriceps muscle. Furthermore, not every individual with a similar degree of malnutrition develops neurologic complications, suggesting that environmental and perhaps genetic factors contribute to disease expression (for example, see Wernicke's disease, below). Finally, protein-calorie malnutrition can exert a deleterious effect on the nervous system that may not be readily apparent (eg, retarded mental development in children). Major neurologic nutritional disorders are described below.

Wernicke-Korsakoff Syndrome

The coexistence of **Wernicke's disease (Wernicke's encephalopathy, cerebral beriberi**—*acute onset of mental confusion, nystagmus, ophthalmoplegia, and gait ataxia, due to thiamine deficiency) with* **Korsakoff's syndrome** *(a gross disturbance in recent memory, sometimes compensated for by confabulation*—see in THE AMNESIAS in Ch. 118; and Ch. 138).

Etiology, symptoms, and signs: The enzyme transketolase (hexose monophosphate pathway) binds its cofactor thiamine less avidly in patients with **Wernicke's disease** than in controls. This trait may be hereditary, leaving certain individuals more susceptible to thiamine deficiency, especially when challenged with a large carbohydrate load. Wernicke's disease is principally seen in the chronic alcoholic, but also can follow hyperemesis gravidarum or the prolonged use of vitamin-free infusions. Chronic alcohol intake does not result in the disease if thiamine intake is adequate. With

varying severity, nystagmus, lateral rectus weakness, and gaze paralysis arise from involvement of the vestibular, 3rd, and 6th nerve nuclei. A lesion of the superior cerebellar vermis accounts for the ataxic gait and is indistinguishable from alcoholic cerebellar degeneration (see below). Mental confusion is global (eg, apathy, impaired awareness, spatial disorientation), or may show a profound impairment of retentive memory (**Korsakoff's syndrome**—seen in 80% of surviving Wernicke patients) while other cognitive abilities are relatively spared. Korsakoff's syndrome may persist when the other features of Wernicke's disease have subsided.

Other clinical deficits are common in Wernicke patients and arise from lack of vitamins besides thiamine (eg, sensory neuropathy from folate deficiency) or from medical complications (eg, sepsis, liver cirrhosis). Autonomic dysfunction may appear either in the form of sympathetic hyperactivity (eg, delirium tremens) or hypoactivity (hypothermia, postural hypotension, and syncope responsive to thiamine). Cardiovascular dysfunction occurs without overt cardiac beriberi.

Prognosis and treatment: *Wernicke's disease is a medical emergency, since any delay in treatment can lead to necrosis of brain parenchyma with permanent deficits and, rarely, to coma and death.* Thiamine 50 to 100 mg IM or IV should be given without delay and continued orally on a daily basis. The ocular abnormalities improve within hours or days, whereas the amnesic disorder may be permanent in many patients. All alcoholics and malnourished patients, symptomatic or not, should be supplemented with thiamine and other B vitamins. *Thiamine should precede any IV infusions of dextrose solutions, since the additional carbohydrate can precipitate Wernicke's disease.*

Alcoholic or Nutritional Cerebellar Degeneration

The pathologic and clinical features of this disorder are probably identical to the cerebellar involvement by Wernicke's disease. Ataxia of stance and gait evolves over weeks or months, but can appear acutely as well. CT shows atrophy of the superior vermis and anterior cerebellar lobes. The disorder is not restricted to alcoholics, but appears in the setting of malnutrition and is ameliorated with thiamine given in conjunction with other B vitamins.

Nutritional Polyneuropathy

Peripheral neuropathy is frequent among alcoholics and the malnourished. Wasting and symmetric weakness of the distal extremities usually is insidious but can progress rapidly and is variably accompanied by sensory loss, paresthesias, and pain. Aching, cramping, coldness, burning, and numbness in the calves and feet may be worsened by touch. It is suggested that a primary axonopathy leads to secondary demyelination and axonal destruction in the longest and largest nerves. Whether this stems from thiamine deficiency or the lack of some other vitamin, such as pyridoxine, pantothenic acid, or folate is unclear. **Treatment**: Administration of a complement of vitamins is appropriate when etiology is obscure.

Nutritional Amblyopia

Severe malnutrition that damages the papillomacular bundle of the optic nerve producing symmetric central and cecocentral scotomas and resulting in permanent optic atrophy. Visual dimness, photophobia, and ocular discomfort appear over days to weeks. Nutritional amblyopia may occur with other nutritional disorders (eg, **Strachan syndrome** — polyneuropathy and orogenital dermatitis). Reversibility requires **treatment** with oral or parenteral B vitamins before amblyopia becomes severe.

Central Pontine Myelinolysis

Demyelination of the central basal pons can appear in chronically ill patients subjected to sudden fluxes in electrolyte and water metabolism, especially when hyponatremia is too rapidly corrected. Quadriparesis, weakness of lower face and tongue, can evolve over a few days or weeks. The lesion may extend dorsally to involve sensory

tracts and leave the patient with a "locked-in" syndrome (an awake and sentient state in which the patient, because of motor paralysis in all parts of the body, cannot communicate except possibly by coded eye movements). Prognosis is poor, since damage often is permanent and systemic complications intervene.

Marchiafava-Bignami Disease

A rare demyelination of the corpus callosum that occurs in chronic alcoholics, predominantly males. Patients become agitated and confused and show progressive dementia with frontal release signs. Some patients recover over several months; in others, seizures and coma may precede death. Although originally attributed to a crude red wine in Italy, the disorder occurs in many other countries and with many other alcoholic beverages. A nutritional etiology has been postulated but remains to be defined.

Pyridoxine (Vitamin B_6) Deficiency and Toxicity (see also Ch. 81)

Peripheral neuropathy from pyridoxine deficiency is largely restricted to individuals taking isoniazid for TB. Convulsions can occur in infants found to be deficient or dependent on B_6. **Homocystinuria,** which can present with strokes, mental retardation, and psychosis, appears to respond to massive doses of pyridoxine. Excessive ingestion of pyridoxine (> 2 gm/day) produces a **sensory neuropathy** in some adults which is reversible on cessation of pyridoxine.

Pellagra (see Ch. 81)

Vitamin B_{12} Deficiency (see Ch. 81; and under COMBINED SYSTEM DISEASE in Ch. 130)

Vitamin E Deficiency (see also Ch. 81)

Children with chronic liver disease, celiac disease, cystic fibrosis, and abetalipoproteinemia malabsorb fat-soluble vitamins and may have persistently low serum vitamin E levels despite supplementation. Over months to years, there is a progressive loss of proprioceptive and vibratory sensation, areflexia, ataxia, and gaze paresis. The few autopsy studies have revealed degeneration of the posterior columns and spinocerebellar tracts as well as patchy demyelination of peripheral nerves. The neurologic deterioration can be reversed or at least partly arrested with vitamin E supplementation.

Neurocomplications in Short-Bowel Syndromes

Intestinal resection or bypass (for morbid obesity) can be complicated by a variety of disorders with neurologic manifestations. Inadequate caloric intake and the malabsorption of B_{12} and other vitamins can result in severe malnutrition with the neurologic deficits elaborated above. Severe calcium and magnesium deficiency can lead to encephalopathy, tetany, and convulsions. Carbohydrate can escape the small intestine to be fermented by colonic bacteria to L- and D-lactic acid. Since the latter is not readily metabolized upon reaching the blood, the resulting D-lactic acidosis can cause irritability, bizarre neurologic dysfunction, or a frankly encephalopathic state. Before ascribing a patient's peculiar behavior to stress or emotional maladjustment, these metabolic complications should be kept in mind.

---

121. SEIZURE DISORDERS

(Epilepsy)

Epilepsy: *A recurrent paroxysmal disorder of cerebral function characterized by sudden, brief attacks of altered consciousness, motor activity, sensory phenomena, or inappropriate behavior.* **Convulsive seizures,** the most common form of attacks, begin with loss of consciousness and motor control, and tonic or clonic jerking of all extremities, but any recurrent seizure pattern may be termed epilepsy.

Seizure disorders in the newborn are also discussed in Ch. 186.

Etiology

Epilepsy is classed etiologically as symptomatic or idiopathic, **symptomatic** implying that a probable cause has been identified that at times permits a specific course of therapy. No obvious cause can be found in about 75% of adults and a smaller percentage of children under age 3. Some authorities believe that **idiopathic** epilepsy is due to a microscopic scar in the brain resulting from birth trauma or other injury, and, indeed, many patients classed during life as idiopathic show evidence of a causative lesion at autopsy. However, it is more likely that unexplained, predominantly inherited metabolic abnormalities underlie most idiopathic cases.

Idiopathic epilepsy generally begins between ages 2 and 14. Seizures before age 2 are usually related to developmental defects, birth injuries, or a metabolic disease affecting the brain; those beginning after age 25 are usually secondary to cerebral trauma, tumors, or other organic brain disease. Focal diseases of the brain can cause seizures at any age.

Convulsive seizures may be associated with a variety of cerebral or systemic disorders, as a result of a focal or generalized disturbance of cortical function. These include **hyperpyrexia** (acute infection, heat stroke), **CNS infections** (meningitis, encephalitis, brain abscess, neurosyphilis, rabies, tetanus, falciparum malaria, toxoplasmosis, cysticercosis of the brain), **metabolic disturbances** (hypoglycemia, hypoparathyroidism, phenylketonuria), **convulsive or toxic agents** (camphor, pentylenetetrazol, strychnine, picrotoxin, lead, alcohol), **cerebral hypoxia** (Adams-Stokes syndrome, carotid sinus hypersensitivity, anesthesia, carbon monoxide poisoning, breath-holding), **expanding brain lesions** (neoplasm, intracranial hemorrhage, subdural hematoma in infancy), **brain defects** (congenital, developmental), **cerebral edema** (hypertensive encephalopathy, eclampsia), **cerebral trauma** (skull fracture, birth injury), **anaphylaxis** (foreign serum or drug allergy), and **cerebral infarct or hemorrhage**. Convulsions may also occur as a **withdrawal symptom** after chronic use of alcohol, hypnotics, or tranquilizers. **Hysterical patients** occasionally simulate convulsive attacks.

The seizures are only transient in many of these conditions and do not recur once the illness ends. However, convulsions may recur at intervals for years or indefinitely if there is a permanent lesion or scar in the CNS, in which case a diagnosis of epilepsy is made.

Pathogenesis

Convulsive seizures result from an acute focal or generalized disturbance in cerebral function. Though this disturbance can usually be demonstrated by EEG, the cause is not known. Apparently, a small focus of diseased tissue in the cerebrum discharges abnormally in response to certain endogenous or exogenous stimuli, and spread of the discharge to other portions of the cerebrum results in convulsive phenomena and loss of consciousness. Whether seizures that are generalized from the outset can begin as a diffuse abnormal discharge or must originate focally is not known.

Given a sufficient stimulus (eg, convulsant drugs, hypoxia, hypoglycemia), even the normal brain can discharge in a diffusely synchronous fashion and produce a seizure. In susceptible persons, seizures may occasionally be precipitated by exogenous factors (sound, light, cutaneous stimulation).

Classification and Incidence

Epileptic seizures can be classified according to several different criteria. TABLE 121–1 gives a current internationally agreed-upon classification. **Partial seizures** begin focally with a specific sensory, motor, or psychic aberration that reflects the affected part of the cerebral hemisphere where the seizure originates. TABLE 121–2 gives some of the characteristic manifestations and their sites of origin. **Auras** are *focal manifestations that immediately precede generalized convulsions* and that also reflect where the seizure begins. Sometimes a focal lesion of the hemispheres activates deeper parts of the brain so rapidly that it produces a generalized grand mal seizure before any focal

TABLE 121–1. INTERNATIONAL CLASSIFICATION OF EPILEPTIC SEIZURES

I. Partial seizures (seizures beginning locally)
   A. Partial seizures with elementary symptomatology (generally without impairment of consciousness)
      1. With motor symptoms (includes jacksonian seizures)
      2. With special sensory or somatosensory symptoms
      3. With autonomic symptoms
      4. Compound forms
   B. Partial seizures with complex symptomatology (generally with impairment of consciousness) (temporal lobe or psychomotor seizures)
      1. With impairment of consciousness only
      2. With cognitive symptomatology
      3. With affective symptomatology
      4. With "psychosensory" symptomatology
      5. With "psychomotor" symptomatology (automatisms)
      6. Compound forms
   C. Partial seizures secondarily generalized
II. Generalized seizures (bilaterally symmetrical and without local onset)
   1. Absences (petit mal)
   2. Bilateral massive epileptic myoclonus
   3. Infantile spasms
   4. Clonic seizures
   5. Tonic seizures
   6. Tonic-clonic seizures (grand mal)
   7. Atonic seizures
   8. Akinetic seizures
III. Unilateral seizures (or predominantly)
IV. Unclassified epileptic seizures (due to incomplete data)

(Modified from "Clinical and electroencephalographical classification of epileptic seizures," by H. Gastaut, in *Epilepsia* 11:102–113, 1970. Used with permission of Elsevier Science Publishers B.V. (Biomedical Division), Amsterdam, and the author.)

sign appears. **Generalized seizures** usually affect both consciousness and motor function from the outset. The seizure itself is initiated in the deeper part of the brain and frequently has a genetic or metabolic cause.

Epilepsy affects about 2% of the population; chronically recurring seizures are perhaps 1/4 that frequent. Most patients have only 1 type of seizure; about 30% have 2 or more types. About 90% experience grand mal seizures, either alone (60%) or in combination with other seizures (30%). Absence (petit mal) attacks occur in about 25% (4%

TABLE 121–2. FOCAL MANIFESTATIONS OF PARTIAL SEIZURES AND SITES OF THE ASSOCIATED CEREBRAL DYSFUNCTION

Focal Manifestation	*Site of Dysfunction*
Localized twitching of muscles (jacksonian seizure)	Frontal lobe (motor cortex)
Localized numbness or tingling	Parietal lobe (sensory cortex)
Chewing movements or smacking of lips	Anterior temporal lobe
Olfactory hallucinations	Antero-medial temporal lobe
Visual hallucinations (formed images)	Temporal lobe
Visual hallucinations (flashes of light)	Occipital lobe
Complex automatic behaviorisms	Temporal lobe

alone, 21% in combination). Psychomotor attacks occur in 18% (6% alone, 12% in combination).

Symptoms and Signs

Partial or focal seizures begin with specific motor, sensory, or psychomotor focal phenomena. Common manifestations are given in TABLE 121–2. In **jacksonian seizures** (*focal motor symptoms begin in one hand or foot and then "march" up the extremity, or spread similarly from a corner of the mouth*), the dysfunction may remain localized or may spread to other parts of the brain, with consequent loss of consciousness and generalized convulsive movements.

Partial seizures with complex symptoms are characterized by a variety of patterns of onset (see TABLE 121–1). In most instances, the patient has a 1- to 2-min loss of contact with the surroundings. The patient at first may stagger, perform automatic purposeless movements, and utter unintelligible sounds. He does not understand what is said and may resist aid. Mental confusion continues for another 1 or 2 min after the attack is apparently over. **Psychomotor attacks** may develop at any age and are usually associated with structural lesions, most often in the temporal lobe. **Status psychomotor epilepsy** may occur, in which affected subjects act in a slow, bewildered, and sometimes confused state for hours or, rarely, days.

Partial seizures of temporal lobe origin rarely are characterized by unprovoked aggressive behavior. If restrained, however, such a patient occasionally may lash out at the person restricting his movement. No satisfactory evidence suggests that complex acts of premeditated or unprovoked aggression can ever be attributed to attacks of temporal lobe epilepsy.

Patients with temporal lobe epilepsy experience a significantly higher incidence of interictal psychiatric disorders than do either the normal population or patients with other forms of epilepsy. Selection factors in evaluation make exact figures difficult to be sure of, but some studies show as many as 33% of patients with temporal lobe epilepsy having substantial psychopathologic difficulties, with up to 10% showing symptoms of schizophreniform or depressive psychoses. The behavioral abnormalities are slightly more frequent among patients with left temporal lobe epileptic foci. Neither anticonvulsant medication nor surgical treatment has shown a predictably favorable effect on these psychiatric disorders.

Generalized seizures can be minor or major in their manifestations. **Absence (petit mal) attacks** are *brief generalized seizures manifested by a 10- to 30-sec loss of consciousness, with eye or muscle flutterings at a rate of 3/sec, and with or without loss of muscle tone*. The patient suddenly stops any activity in which he is engaged and resumes it after the attack. Petit mal seizures are genetically determined and occur predominantly in children: they never begin after age 20. The attacks are likely to occur several or many times a day, often when the patient is sitting quietly. They are infrequent during exercise. Petit mal attacks rarely indicate gross brain damage, and many patients are highly intelligent.

Infantile spasms *are characterized by sudden flexion of the arms, forward flexion of the trunk, and extension of the legs*. The attacks last only a few seconds but may be repeated many times a day. They are restricted to the first 3 yr of life, often to be replaced by other forms of attacks. Brain damage is usually evident.

Tonic-clonic (grand mal) seizures *occasionally begin with a sinking or rising sensation in the epigastrium (the* **aura**) *followed by an outcry; the seizure continues with loss of consciousness; falling; and tonic, then clonic contractions of the muscles of the extremities, trunk, and head*. Urinary and fecal incontinence may occur. The attack usually lasts 2 to 5 min. It may be preceded by a prodromal mood change, and may be followed by a **postictal state,** with deep sleep, headache, muscle soreness or, at times, focal motor or sensory phenomena. The attacks may appear at any age.

Akinetic seizures are *brief, generalized seizures seen in children.* The child falls or pitches to the ground, so that attacks carry the risk of serious trauma.

Isolated epileptic auras describe *sensory or psychic partial seizures that are confined to a single symptom.* The disturbances appear in partially treated patients or those subject to more complex seizures and can include paroxysmal attacks of abdominal pain (rare), brief somatosensory sensations, or brief, intense psychic symptoms like dream fragments. Sustained periods of mental cloudiness may last for several hours and generally represent psychomotor status or the close fusion (ie, status) of petit mal attacks.

In **status epilepticus,** *motor, sensory, or psychic seizures follow one another with no intervening periods of consciousness.* Grand mal status epilepticus may persist for hours or days, and may be fatal. It may occur spontaneously or result from too rapid withdrawal of anticonvulsants. **Partial continuous epilepsy** is a form of rare focal (usually hand or face) motor seizures in which the attacks recur at intervals of a few seconds or minutes, lasting from days to weeks at a time.

Diagnosis

Idiopathic epilepsy must be distinguished from symptomatic epilepsy. The type of seizure seen in the newborn is not helpful in distinguishing between structural and metabolic causes. In older children and adults, focal seizures or focal postictal symptoms generally imply a focal structural lesion in the brain, while generalized seizures are more likely to have a metabolic cause.

The history should include an eyewitness account of a typical attack and information on the frequency of seizures and the longest and shortest intervals between attacks. A history of prior **trauma** (eg, cranial injury producing unconsciousness, birth trauma), **infection** (eg, meningitis, encephalitis, pertussis), or **toxic episodes** (eg, excessive alcohol or drug consumption and its relation to seizures) must be sought and evaluated. A family history of convulsions or neurologic disorders is significant.

Fever and stiff neck accompanying convulsions of recent onset should suggest meningitis or subarachnoid hemorrhage. Focal cerebral symptoms and signs in association with seizures suggest brain tumor, cerebrovascular disease, or residual traumatic abnormalities. Grand mal seizures, particularly in an adult, always require a diagnostic search for an unsuspected focal lesion.

Appropriate studies include serum glucose and calcium, and EEG. If these are focally abnormal, and in all cases of adult-onset seizures, CT or MRI is indicated.

The interictal EEG in grand mal attacks is characterized most often by relatively symmetric bursts of sharp and slow, 4- to 7-sec, activity. Unilateral or focal discharges also may occur. In petit mal, spikes and slow waves appear at the rate of 3/sec. Interictal temporal lobe foci (spikes or slow waves) are frequent with psychomotor epilepsy. The presence of a focal EEG abnormality may aid in the differential diagnosis of brain disease, as may the presence of a characteristic centrencephalic abnormality. Since an EEG taken during a seizure-free interval is normal in about 15% of patients, one normal EEG does not exclude epilepsy. In rare cases even repeated EEGs may be normal and the diagnosis of epilepsy as opposed to a behavioral disorder may have to be made on clinical grounds.

Prognosis

Drug therapy can completely control grand mal seizures in 50% of cases and greatly reduce the frequency of seizures in another 35%, can control petit mal seizures in 40% and reduce the frequency in 35%, and can control psychomotor attacks in 35% and reduce the frequency in 50%. Newer anticonvulsant agents promise to improve these results even more.

Most patients with epilepsy are normal between attacks, although overuse of anticonvulsants can dull alertness. Progressive mental deterioration is usually related to an

accompanying neurologic disease that itself caused the seizures; only rarely do seizures per se impair mental abilities. The outlook is better when no brain lesion is demonstrable. About 70% of noninstitutionalized patients with epilepsy are mentally normal, 20% show a slight reduction in intellect, and 10% have a moderate to pronounced impairment.

Management and Treatment

1. General principles: In idiopathic epilepsy, treatment is primarily control of seizures. In symptomatic epilepsy, the associated disease must be treated as well; continued anticonvulsant treatment is usually needed after surgical removal of cerebral lesions.

A normal life should be encouraged. Moderate exercise is recommended; such sports as swimming and horseback riding are permitted with proper safeguards. Movies, dancing, and other social activities should be encouraged. Most state licensing agencies permit driving after seizures have stopped for 1 yr. Alcoholic beverages are **contraindicated.**

Members of the family must be taught a commonsense attitude toward the patient's illness. Instead of overprotection and oversolicitude, sympathetic support should be directed against feelings of inferiority, self-consciousness, and other emotional handicaps, and emphasis placed on preventing invalidism. Vocational rehabilitation may help. Institutional care is advisable only for patients with severe mental retardation or with attacks that are frequent, violent, and not controlled by medication.

2. Management of a convulsion, whatever its etiology, is limited to preventing injury. A firm but reasonably soft object (eg, a folded handkerchief) should be inserted between the teeth, but attempts to protect the tongue should not be too vigorous or teeth may be damaged. A finger should *not* be inserted to straighten the tongue; this is dangerous and unnecessary. Clothing about the neck should be loosened, and a pillow placed under the head. A responsible fellow worker may be trained to give emergency aid if the patient agrees.

3. Elimination of causative or precipitating factors: The first rule in treating seizure disorders is to seek and treat progressive organic lesions of the brain (eg, tumors and abscesses). Cortical scars from trauma, vascular lesions, or birth injuries can sometimes be excised when focal attacks resist medical therapy. After surgical removal of organic lesions, continued medical treatment usually is necessary. Physical disorders (eg, infections and endocrine abnormalities) should be corrected.

4. Drug therapy: New drugs are available for previously intractable seizure types, and the widespread availability of accurate estimations of drug levels has made clinical management more secure and effective.

No single drug controls all types of seizures, and different drugs are required for different patients. Furthermore, some patients may require several drugs. For the newly diagnosed patient with a seizure disorder, the single first drug of choice for the particular type of epilepsy is selected, starting with relatively low doses and increasing over a week or so to the standard therapeutic dose. After about a week at such dosage, **blood levels** are obtained to determine the individual's pharmacokinetic response and, if appropriate, whether the effective therapeutic level has been reached. If seizures continue, the daily drug dosage is increased by small increments as doses rise above the usual. If toxic blood levels or symptoms are encountered before seizures are controlled, a second anticonvulsant is added slowly, again guarding against toxicity, since interaction between agents can interfere with their rate of metabolic degradation. Once seizures are brought under control, medication should be continued *without interruption* at least 5 seizure-free years.

The most effective **anticonvulsants** for chronic use in children and adults are given in TABLE 121–3. Therapeutic and toxic blood levels are reasonably well established for

TABLE 121–3. DRUGS USED IN EPILEPSY

Drug	Indications	*Daily Dose Levels*		*Blood Levels*		Toxicity
		Child	*Adult*	*Therapeutic*	*Toxic*	
Phenytoin	Generalized motor, partial motor seizures, partial complex	5–10 mg/kg	300–500 mg	10–20 μg/mL	>25 μg/mL	Nystagmus, ataxia, dysarthria, lethargy, megaloblastic anemia, gingival hyperplasia Idiosyncratic: rash, exfoliative dermatitis, grand mal convulsions (rare)
Phenobarbital	Generalized motor, partial motor seizures	<4 yr: 5–10 mg/kg	5 yr to adult: 2–5 mg/kg	10–30 μg/mL	>35 μg/mL	Sedation, nystagmus, ataxia, learning difficulties Idiosyncratic: anemia, rash, hyperkinesis
Primidone	Partial complex, generalized motor seizures	10–20 mg/kg Increase slowly	750–1500 mg Increase slowly	5–12 μg/mL	> 15 μg/mL	See phenobarbital
Carbamazepine	Partial complex, partial motor, generalized motor seizures	6–12 yr: 20–30 mg/kg Increase slowly	800–1200 mg Increase slowly	4–12 μg/mL	>10 μg/mL	Nystagmus, diplopia, dysarthria, lethargy, nausea Idiosyncratic: granulocytopenia, thrombocytopenia, liver toxicity

Ethosuximide	Petit mal	20 mg/kg	500 mg qid (Maximum 1500 mg except with strict monitoring)	40–100 μg/mL	>100 μg/mL	Nausea, lethargy, dizziness, headache Idiosyncratic: leuco- or pancytopenia, dermatitis, SLE
Trimethadione	Petit mal	<6 yr: 300 mg bid >6 yr: 300 mg tid	600 mg tid (Maximum)	≥ 700 μg/mL (dimethadione)		Sedation, nausea Idiosyncratic: hemeralopia, neutropenia, aplastic anemia, dermatitis, SLE
Clonazepam	Petit mal, atypical petit mal, myoclonus, akinetic seizures; infantile spasms	Initial: 0.005–.01 mg/kg tid Maintenance: 0.03–0.06 mg/kg tid	Initial: 0.5 mg tid Maintenance: up to 5–7 mg tid	20–80 ng/mL (preliminary)		Drowsiness, ataxia, behavorial abnormalities Serious reaction rare, but partial or complete tolerance to beneficial effects usual in 1–6 mo
Valproate	Petit mal, myoclonus, generalized motor, akinetic, partial motor seizures, infantile spasms	15–30 mg/kg (Total given in divided doses tid. Start slowly, especially if other drugs are being taken.)	1000–1500 mg/day	50–100 μg/mL (before A.M. dose)	>100 μg/mL	Nausea and vomiting, transient drowsiness, transient neutropenia, hyperammonemic encephalopathy

phenytoin, phenobarbital, primidone, and ethosuximide, and are given in TABLE 121-3. The table also gives standard dose responses for other anticonvulsants, but it is not presently known if these levels are therapeutically optimal. Estimates of drug concentrations in blood are useful (1) to indicate the particular response to specific drugs (individuals can vary widely); (2) if abnormally high, to warn against toxicity in susceptible individuals; and (3) if abnormally low, to reflect the patient's noncompliance in taking medication. Despite these potential advantages, management must give first attention to the patient's epilepsy. Once the drug response is known, blood levels become substantially less useful to follow than the clinical course.

For generalized motor (grand mal) or **partial motor (focal) seizures,** phenytoin or carbamazepine is the drug of choice. For adults, phenytoin 300 mg/day orally can be given in divided doses or at bedtime. If seizures continue, doses can be increased cautiously to 500 mg/day with blood level monitoring. Carbamazepine 200 mg qid to 400 mg tid can be given but should be started slowly. Phenobarbital 100 mg/day at bedtime or primidone up to 1500 mg/day can be added *slowly* to minimize drowsiness.

For partial complex (psychomotor) seizures, treatment of choice begins with phenytoin, carbamazepine, or primidone. Primidone is particularly effective but is not the first choice because it may cause drowsiness. Carbamazepine appears even more effective but requires hematologic supervision. Clonazepam has produced results superior to valproate, but in many patients the drug loses its effectiveness within a few months.

For absence (petit mal) seizures, ethosuximide orally is preferred. Valproate and clonazepam orally also are effective, but the latter shows a high incidence of tolerance. Trimethadione 300 mg to 2 gm/day orally in divided doses, or acetazolamide 250 mg tid, is reserved for otherwise refractory cases. A ketogenic diet may be helpful but is difficult to maintain.

Akinetic seizures, myoclonic seizures, and infantile spasms are difficult to treat. Valproate is preferred, followed (if unsuccessful) by clonazepam. Ethosuximide sometimes is effective, as is acetazolamide (in dosages as for petit mal). Phenytoin has only limited effectiveness. For infantile spasms, corticosteroids, given for a total of 8 to 10 wk, are often effective. Prednisone 2 mg/kg orally is given for 4 wk, then reduced to about half this amount for maintenance. ACTH 20 to 60 u./day IM may also be used.

For status epilepticus, diazepam 5 to 10 mg (for adults) is given IV, followed by phenobarbital 200 to 400 mg IV; alternatively, diazepam 10 mg IV q 10 to 15 min for up to 1 h may be given, in amounts up to 40 mg/h for adults and 0.3 mg/kg for children. To prevent recurrence, in adults 500 mg to 1 gm of phenytoin may be given IV at a rate of 50 mg/min for the first 500 mg and 100 mg/30 min thereafter. Smaller doses should be used for children, according to weight. Giving the full amount in one successively administered "loading" dose produces better results than do divided doses. Anesthetic doses of pentobarbital (IV or rectally) may be necessary in some refractory cases; hypothermia may be beneficical in others. In such instances, intubation and O_2 therapy are desirable to prevent hypoxemia.

Acute convulsive seizures from febrile illnesses, ingestion of alcohol or other toxins, or acute metabolic disturbance require emergency therapy, especially for the causative condition as well as for the convulsion. Status epilepticus should be treated at once. If there has been only one seizure, both phenytoin and phenobarbital should be given in full dosages (see TABLE 121-3) for 7 to 10 days. Anticonvulsants are of little value in preventing alcoholic withdrawal seizures.

Whether children with a *single* febrile convulsion should receive long-term anticonvulsant therapy is not settled. There is little evidence to support this approach, although some physicians favor it. It is more conservative to give drugs for a short interval only, unless the EEG is grossly abnormal or seizures recur in the absence of infection. Children with *recurrent* generalized febrile convulsions should be treated as for grand mal epilepsy.

Undesirable side effects of drug therapy: Phenobarbital frequently causes incapacitating drowsiness and, in < 1% of cases, an allergic scarlatiniform or morbilliform rash. When a rash appears in a patient taking phenobarbital and phenytoin, the latter is more often responsible. In high doses phenytoin may also cause hypertrophy of the gums; and in toxic doses produces drowsiness, irritability, nystagmus, nausea, vomiting, unsteady gait, and confusion. Adenopathy is a rare complication. Megaloblastic anemia (responsive to folic acid) and aplastic anemia have also been reported with the hydantoins. Tri- and paramethadione can cause a generalized rash, photophobia, blurred vision, leukopenia, and, rarely, severe anemia, agranulocytosis, or nephrosis. Because the methadiones may be teratogenic, another anticonvulsant (eg, ethosuximide) is indicated in pregnancy. Carbamazepine commonly lowers the WBC to 3000 to 4000. Values below this level call for discontinuation.

Patients receiving carbamazepine, paramethadione, trimethadione, or mephenytoin should have a CBC once/month for the first year of therapy. If the WBC or RBC counts decrease significantly with the latter 3 drugs, they should be **discontinued immediately**. LE cells in the blood can appear with either para- or trimethadione. Another drug should be substituted if this happens. The blood should be examined for LE cells whenever suggestive symptoms appear.

When an overdose reaction occurs, one reduces the amount of drug until the intoxication subsides. When more serious acute poisoning occurs, the patient is given ipecac syrup or, if obtunded, is lavaged. After emesis or lavage, activated charcoal is administered, followed by a saline cathartic such as magnesium citrate. The suspect drug should be discontinued and a new anticonvulsant substituted at the same time.

---

122. SLEEP DISORDERS

Disturbances of sleep that affect the ability to fall and/or stay asleep, which involve sleeping too much or result in abnormal behavior associated with sleep. These disorders occur frequently.

Although sleep is necessary for survival, its precise homeostatic contribution is unknown. Individuals vary widely in their requirements, which are influenced by a number of factors including the current emotional state. The 2 types and varying depths of sleep are marked by characteristic EEG and other changes, including eye movements. A non-rapid-eye-movement **(NREM)** type (75 to 80% of total sleep time) initiates sleep, is characterized by slow waves on the EEG, and ranges in depth through stages 1 to 4 (deepest level)—with commensurate difficulties in arousal. Muscle tone, heart and respiratory rates, and BP are lowered. The second type (**REM**—rapid-eye-movement) occupies the remainder of sleep time. It is accompanied by EEG low-voltage fast activity and occurs 5 to 6 times during a normal night's sleep. In REM sleep, both rate and depth of respiration are increased but muscle tone is depressed, even further than in NREM. REM sleep follows NREM and ends each sleep cycle.

Some evidence implicates norepinephrine pathways in the brainstem with REM sleep and serotoninergic pathways with slow wave or NREM. Most dreaming occurs during REM and stage 3 (NREM); most night terrors, sleep walking, and sleep talking, in NREM stages 3 and 4. Selective interruption of REM sleep produces hyperactive and emotionally labile behavior in experimental subjects, but this relationship has not been observed under natural circumstances.

Sleep disorders are discussed below and in BEHAVIORAL PROBLEMS in Ch. 188. Nocturnal enuresis also is discussed in BEHAVIORAL PROBLEMS.

Night terrors (*fearful, screaming, flailing episodes interrupting NREM stage 4*) are more frequent in children than adults, often are accompanied by sleep walking, and

may represent hypnagogic phenomena (see NARCOLEPSY, below) during partial arousal from deep sleep. In adults, night terrors often are associated with psychologic difficulties or alcoholism; diazepam 2 to 5 mg at bedtime sometimes is preventive.

Nightmares (*frightening dreams*) frequently affect adults and (especially) children. They occur during REM sleep and are more common during fever, with excess fatigue, or after alcohol ingestion. Treatment is directed at the underlying conflicts or disorder.

During **somnambulism** (*sitting, walking, or other complex behavior during sleep*), the eyes usually are open but without evidence of recognition. Patients may mumble repetitiously, and some injure themselves on obstacles or stairs. There is no accompanying dream, and the concurrent EEG looks more like wakefulness than sleep. Treatment is to protect the subject against injury and deal with any underlying disorder.

Sleep paralysis: See under NARCOLEPSY, below.

Reversals of the sleep rhythm usually reflect jet lag, or disease or damage to the hypothalamic region of the diencephalon, as occurs following severe head injury or encephalitis. Sedative misuse or irregular night-shift working hours sometimes can induce such reversals (see under INSOMNIA, below).

INSOMNIA

Difficulty in sleeping, or disturbed sleep patterns leaving the perception of insufficient sleep. Insomnia is a common symptom, and may be due to several emotional and physical disorders.

With advancing age, the total amount of sleep tends to shorten. Stage 4 can disappear; sleep becomes more interrupted. These changes may be subjectively distressing and lead to requests for treatment. There is no evidence, however, that such insomnia interferes with health. **Initial insomnia** *(difficulty in falling asleep)* commonly is associated with an emotional disturbance such as anxiety, a phobic state, or depression; other symptoms of the emotional problem will be present.

In **early morning awakening,** the patient falls asleep normally but awakens several hours before his usual time and either cannot fall asleep again or drifts into a restless, unsatisfying sleep. This pattern is a common phenomenon of aging, but sometimes is associated with depression and should be investigated. Tendencies to anxiety, self-reproach, and self-punitive thinking often are magnified in the morning.

An **inverted sleep rhythm** (see also above) may develop in elderly persons because of inappropriate use of sedatives, often prescribed for insomnia. Patients become drowsy in the morning, sleep or doze much of the day, and have fitful and interrupted sleep at night. If sedation is increased, restlessness and wandering in a clouded or confused state may occur at night. When sedation is withdrawn from a patient who regularly takes heavy doses of hypnotics, a rebound wakefulness commonly ensues, which the patient interprets as a recurrence of his insomnia.

Diagnosis

Some normal persons sleep less than others, and insomnia may be **primary** (ie, longstanding and with little apparent relationship to immediate somatic or psychic events) or **secondary** to some acquired pain, anxiety, or depression. Insomnia of recent onset usually is due to current anxieties; eg, marital strife, problems at work, guilt over sexual conflicts, or concerns about health. If no such personal difficulties or symptoms of an emotional disturbance emerge, a physical cause should be considered. Substantial amounts of alcohol consumed in the evening can shorten sleep and lead to withdrawal effects in the early morning so that the patient awakens restless or, if he is severely dependent, fearful and tremulous. Insomnia unresponsive to simple measures often is due to a severe emotional disturbance, especially depression.

Treatment

This depends on the underlying cause. Many patients respond to reassurance that their sleeplessness is a result of normal anxieties or a treatable physical disorder. Providing an opportunity to ventilate anxieties often eases distress and helps to reestablish normal sleep patterns. Elderly patients experiencing a normal change in sleep patterns require reassurance, encouragement to take more exercise during the day, and instruction in relaxation. Warm milk helps some patients sleep.

For insomnia due to emotional disturbance other than depression, and in refractory cases due to more common causes, hypnotic medication may be required (see SEDATIVES AND HYPNOTICS, below), especially if the sleeplessness impairs the patient's efficiency and sense of well-being. Patients who awaken because of pain should be given aspirin 325 to 650 mg (5 to 10 grains) at bedtime. **For insomnia accompanying depression**, a tricyclic antidepressant taken about 1 h before bedtime usually suffices (see Ch. 141).

All hypnotics should be prescribed for short-term (2 to 4 wk) or interrupted use, and the patient encouraged to do without them as soon as possible. All depressed patients represent the risk of suicide attempts by overdosage with any hypnotic.

SEDATIVES AND HYPNOTICS

Terms such as sedative, hypnotic, antianxiety agent, minor tranquilizer, and anxiolytic are ambiguous and often used interchangeably. A single drug frequently is useful in more than one therapeutic category, depending on the dosage (for a discussion of nonhypnotic use of these drugs see ANTIANXIETY AGENTS in Ch. 281).

All of the available hypnotics involve some risk of overdose, habituation, tolerance, and addiction, as well as withdrawal symptoms that include temporary recurrence of sleeplessness. Ambulatory patients given these drugs should avoid postingestion activities requiring mental alertness, judgment, and physical coordination (eg, driving a vehicle or operating machinery). Hypnotic drugs should be used with special caution in patients with severe pulmonary insufficiency. For other potential problems of hypnotic drug use see Chs. 138 and 144.

Adverse effects (see also under specific drug discussions, below): Drowsiness, lethargy, and hangover are observed commonly after excessive intake of certain sedative-hypnotics. Rarely, skin eruptions (eg, urticaria, angioneurotic edema, and bullous erythema multiforme) and GI disturbances (eg, nausea and vomiting) may be seen. With any sedative (even small doses), the elderly may exhibit restlessness, excitement, or exacerbations of symptoms of organic brain disorders.

Many patients take higher doses of hypnotics than they admit, and slurring of speech, incoordination, tremulousness, and nystagmus should arouse suspicion of overdosage. Serum levels of many drugs can be determined in the laboratory.

Sedative-hypnotics are additive in effect with other CNS depressants (eg, alcohol, antianxiety agents, opiates, antihistamines, phenothiazines, and antidepressants). Doses should be reduced when these drugs are given concurrently. Sudden withdrawal following prolonged ingestion may precipitate severe tremors or convulsions and should be avoided. Barbiturates, chloral hydrate, chloral betaine, and glutethimide can interact with coumarin anticoagulants (see also Alteration of Metabolism in DRUG INTERACTIONS, in Ch. 276).

Commonly Used Hypnotic Drugs

Triazolam, flurazepam, temazepam, and nitrazepam (investigational in the USA), benzodiazepine derivatives can each have a marked hypnotic effect. Triazolam and flurazepam have minimal suicidal risk, minimally alter REM sleep, and do not cause REM rebound. Triazolam is the least toxic of the hypnotics. Its short, nonhangover action makes it the agent of choice for most acute insomnia, including jet lag. Flurazepam is

converted to a slowly active metabolite that can cause subsequent drowsiness or ataxia, limiting its desirability for regular use. Bedtime oral doses of triazolam 0.125, 0.25, or 0.5 mg or flurazepam 15 to 30 mg suffice for insomnia in most cases; smaller doses may be used for the elderly.

These compounds have much less addiction potential than other hypnotics, and overdoses rarely are fatal. The dosage that induces serious respiratory and vital center depression is considerably greater than with barbiturates and most other nonbarbiturate sedative-hypnotics. However, the benzodiazepines (like the others) may increase the neurologic depression caused by alcohol, and serious CNS depression may result if they are taken together. Occasional patients report an increase in daytime anxiety following the repeated use of benzodiazepine sedatives.

Chloral hydrate is a relatively weak but safe hypnotic. The usual oral dose is 1 to 2 gm; in elderly patients, 0.5 to 1 gm—if necessary, an additional 0.5 gm may be given after 1 h. Chloral hydrate is available in capsules and in solutions that have a pungent, unpleasant taste. Chloral hydrate, like the barbiturates, can cause tolerance, addiction, and induction of hepatic drug-metabolizing enzymes.

Barbiturates, though effective and cheaper than the newer agents, may cause tolerance, habituation, and drug dependence. Also, the suicide risk is higher than with other hypnotics. Attempts by the patient to discontinue the drug may lead to withdrawal symptoms, reinforcing his belief that he needs the barbiturate. Often a patient can be gradually weaned from the drug; if not, a different drug can be tried.

Barbiturates are contraindicated in patients with porphyria, since these drugs may provoke an acute episode. They also induce hepatic drug-metabolizing enzymes that can adversely interact with other drugs.

Glutethimide and **methyprylon** are related hypnotics. They have a fairly long duration of action and, like barbiturates, can produce tolerance and addiction. They are not recommended. *Overdosage with glutethimide is particularly dangerous because the toxic dose is not much larger than the hypnotic dose.* Perhaps because the drug is recycled through the GI tract, blood levels fluctuate and produce cyclic changes in the depth of coma. If hemodialysis is used to counteract an overdose of glutethimide, a nonpolar solvent used as the dialysate may enhance removal of the drug from the bloodstream.

NARCOLEPSY

A rare syndrome of recurrent attacks of sleep, sudden loss of muscle tone (cataplexy), sleep paralysis, and hypnagogic phenomena, with a characteristic initial REM sleep pattern. About 10% of narcoleptics show the full tetrad of symptoms.

Etiology and Incidence

The cause is unknown and the condition blends into normal physiologic experiences. No pathologic changes are seen in the brain. Symptoms usually begin in adolescents or young adults with no previous illness, and persist throughout life; longevity is unaffected. Narcolepsy is 4 times more common in men than women; some patients give a family history of the disorder.

Symptoms and Signs

All symptoms and signs are intensifications of normal phenomena.

Sleep attacks: *Frequent, often untimely, and almost instantaneous REM sleep (with no preceding NREM phase).* This pattern differs from normal sleep, in which NREM, usually lasting about 60 min, precedes REM. Outwardly, normal sleep is resembled except in frequency and untimely occurrence.

The sleep attacks vary from few to many in a single day, and may last minutes or hours. The desire to sleep can be resisted only temporarily, but the patient can be roused from narcoleptic sleep as readily as from normal sleep. Attacks are apt to occur

in the monotonous conditions conducive to normal sleep, but also may occur in hazardous circumstances; eg, while driving. The patient may feel refreshed on awakening, yet fall asleep again in a few minutes. Whether the total amount of sleep is actually increased is debatable. The frequent sleep episodes during the day make it seem so, but nocturnal sleep may be unsatisfactory and interrupted by vivid, frightening dreams.

Cataplexy (*momentary paralysis occurring in association with sudden emotional reactions, such as mirth, anger, fear, or joy*): An element of surprise seems important. Weakness may be confined to the limbs (eg, the patient may drop the rod when a fish strikes his line) or may cause a limp fall (when the patient laughs heartily or is suddenly angry). These attacks resemble the loss of muscle tone that occurs in REM sleep or to a lesser degree in many persons who become "weak with laughter."

Sleep paralysis (*occasional episodes in which, just when falling asleep or immediately on awakening, the patient wants to move and finds that for a moment he cannot*): Although these episodes resemble the motor inhibition that accompanies REM sleep, they also are common in normal children and in some normal adults.

Hypnagogic phenomena: *Particularly vivid auditory or visual illusions or hallucinations* may occur at the onset of sleep or, less often, on awakening, and are difficult to distinguish from intense reverie. These are somewhat similar to vivid dreams occurring in normal REM sleep. Hypnagogic phenomena occur commonly in young children and occasionally in adults who do not have narcolepsy or other sleep disorders.

No specific laboratory abnormalities are seen, except that in EEG records during an attack, the low-voltage fast record of REM sleep often appears immediately.

Diagnosis

The history of typical sleep attacks is characteristic, and other symptoms of the clinical tetrad should be sought. Occasional patients have sleep attacks only, and also lack the typically prompt appearance of REM sleep. Many otherwise normal individuals experience occasional episodes of sleep paralysis or hypnagogic phenomena but recognize them as benign and do not seek medical assistance. Patients with intracranial mass lesions, encephalitis, or metabolic encephalopathy may be hypersomnolent; this, however, is apt to be recent in origin and progressive, and does not occur in attacks. The periodic hypersomnia of the **Kleine-Levin syndrome** seen in adolescent boys is accompanied by overeating; the somnolence of the **sleep apnea syndrome** is discussed below. Exhaustion, sleepiness, and neurotic fatigue are differentiated by evaluation of personality, circumstances of sleep, and lack of cataplexy.

Treatment

Stimulant drugs may help; the dosage is regulated according to individual need: ephedrine 25 mg, amphetamine 10 to 20 mg, or dextroamphetamine 5 to 10 mg—orally q 3 to 4 h during the day. Methylphenidate 60 to 120 mg/day orally in divided doses may be even more successful. Though directed primarily against sleep attacks, these drugs also seem to lessen the attacks of cataplexy. The recommended doses are tolerated without serious untoward effects. The last dose must be taken early enough to avoid interfering with nocturnal sleep. Imipramine and monoamine oxidase inhibitors have been found somewhat useful in treating narcolepsy; *they must not be combined with an amphetamine.*

SLEEP APNEA

A potentially lethal disorder in which breathing stops during sleep for 10 sec or more, sometimes > 300 times/night.

Etiology and Clinical Features

Sleep apnea can be **obstructive** (*upper airway blockage despite airflow drive*), **central** (*decreased respiratory center output*), or **mixed**. The most frequent cause is airway ob-

struction, discussed below. Rarely, sleep apnea is due to primary brainstem medullary failure caused by neurologic medullary depression, such as from poliomyelitis, tumors of the posterior fossa, or idiopathic (primary) central hypoventilation (eg, **Ondine's curse,** in which the patient does not breathe adequately or at all except by an act of will). Mixed apnea starts as central but is quickly followed by thoracoabdominal movements with upper airway obstruction. Mixed apnea occurs more often than central but less often than the obstructive type.

Obstructive sleep apnea (the **Pickwickian syndrome**) occurs most often in obese patients, with secondary pulmonary insufficiency. The obesity, perhaps combined with a constitutional defect, leads to pulmonary failure, resulting hypercapnia, and upper airway narrowing. Eventually, the combination of hypoxia and hypercapnia may induce central apnea as well. Repeated nocturnal obstruction may cause further respiratory failure and repeated awakenings, and result in a continuous cycle of night and day episodes of sleep, obstructive choking, startled awakening with gasping, and drowsiness. Similar but less pronounced sequences occasionally occur in nonobese subjects, presumably due to congenital abnormalities of the upper airway. **Complications** include cardiac abnormalities (eg, sinus arrhythmias, extreme bradycardia, atrial flutter, and ventricular tachycardia).

Snoring (*partially obstructive breathing during sleep*), 3 times more common in obese persons, ranges from being an annoying social problem to its exaggerated form in obstructive sleep apnea. Heavy snorers should have a thorough examination of the nose, mouth, palate, throat, and neck.

Treatment and Prognosis

For the Pickwickian syndrome, weight reduction, when possible, reduces episodes of sleep apnea and improves blood gases and daytime drowsiness. Nocturnal positive pressure air flow sometimes is effective. A few patients require tracheostomy. Relief of the obstruction usually reverses the commonly associated pulmonary and systemic hypertension and cardiac arrhythmias.

For snoring: Mild symptoms may be helped by avoiding alcoholic beverages, tranquilizers, sleeping pills, and antihistamines before retiring; sleeping on one's side; tilting the head of the bed upwards. Treatment for heavy snorers may range from relieving a nasal infection or allergy to corrective surgery of obstructive conditions in the nose, pharynx, or uvula. Tracheostomy is seldom justified.

---

123. CEREBROVASCULAR DISEASE

(Stroke; Cerebrovascular Accident; CVA)

Cerebrovascular disease is the most common cause of neurologic disability in Western countries. Although vascular injury to the brain can occur as part of a number of relatively rare diseases, most cerebrovascular illnesses are secondary to atherosclerosis, hypertension, or a combination of both. The major *specific* types of cerebrovascular disease are (1) **cerebral insufficiency** due to transient disturbances of blood flow or, rarely, to hypertensive encephalopathy; (2) **cerebral infarction,** due either to embolism or to thrombosis of the intra- or extracranial arteries; (3) **cerebral hemorrhage,** which includes hypertensive parenchymal hemorrhage and subarachnoid hemorrhage from congenital aneurysm; and (4) **cerebral arteriovenous malformation,** which can cause symptoms either of a mass lesion, infarction, or hemorrhage. The vernacular terms **cerebrovascular accident** and **CVA** lack specificity and are commonly applied to the clinical syndromes that accompany either ischemic or hemorrhagic lesions. **Stroke** has by common usage come to designate ischemic lesions.

Both ischemic stroke and cerebral hemorrhage tend to develop abruptly, with hemorrhage generally having the most catastrophically acute onset. Symptoms and signs in cerebrovascular disease reflect the area of brain that is damaged and not necessarily the specific artery that is affected. Occlusion of either the middle cerebral artery or internal carotid artery, for example, can produce a similar clinical neurologic abnormality. Nevertheless, cerebral vascular injuries generally conform to fairly specific patterns of arterial supply, and a knowledge of these distributions is important in distinguishing stroke from space-taking lesions such as brain tumor or abscess.

The most important step in accurate diagnosis of cerebral vascular lesions consists of an accurate history. The most important step in treatment consists of identifying patients with potential or impending strokes so that measures can be attempted to prevent brain damage.

ISCHEMIC SYNDROMES

Cerebrovascular disorders caused by insufficient cerebral circulation.

Etiology and Pathophysiology

Normally, an adequate blood flow to the brain is ensured by an efficient collateral system: from one carotid to the other; from one vertebral artery to the other and to the carotids via the anastomoses at the circle of Willis; and via collateral circulation at the level of the hemispheres. Congenital anomalies and the vascular changes of atherosclerosis impair these compensatory mechanisms, so that **brain ischemia** and consequent neurologic symptoms can result from an intra- or extracranial interruption in arterial blood flow. Thrombosis or emboli from an atherosclerotic plaque or other causes (eg, arteritis, rheumatic heart disease) commonly produce the ischemic arterial obstruction. If the blood supply is promptly restored, brain tissues recover and symptoms disappear, but if ischemia lasts for more than a few minutes, **infarction** results and neurologic damage is permanent.

Atheromas, which underlie most thromboses, may affect any of the major cerebral arteries. Large atheromas are more commonly **extracranial,** affecting the common carotid and vertebral arteries at their origins, the cervical bifurcation of the internal carotid, the carotid siphon, and the basilar artery just proximal to the origin of the posterior cerebral artery. Occlusions can occur in these large extracranial arteries or in any of the smaller intracranial arteries. An occlusion may be partial or complete, and in the extracranial vessels is sometimes bilateral. Whether ischemia and infarction occur depends on the efficiency of collateral circulation; eg, a concomitant stenosis of the vertebral arteries, by compromising collateral circulation, may intensify the effects of carotid lesions. **Intracranial thrombosis** may occur in one of the large arteries at the base of the brain, in a deep perforating artery, or in a small cortical branch, but the main trunk of the middle cerebral artery and its branches are the most common sites.

Less frequently, thrombotic occlusion is secondary to **vascular inflammation,** as in a collagen vascular disease, acute or chronic meningitis, or syphilis. Very rarely, **arterial compression** is due to bony vertebral projections (osteophytes). Cerebral thrombosis in young women is rare but quadruples in incidence when oral contraceptives are used.

Cerebral emboli usually derive from atheromas in extracranial vessels or (in children as well as adults) from thrombi in damaged hearts. The fragments, which may lodge temporarily or permanently anywhere in the cerebral arterial tree, may come from an accumulation of platelets, fibrin, and cholesterol on the surface of ulcerated plaques in atherosclerosis; from vegetations on the heart valves in bacterial, mycotic, or marantic endocarditis; from mural thrombi in atrial fibrillation (particularly in rheumatic heart disease) or following myocardial infarction; or from clots following open-heart surgery. Rarely, cerebral emboli may originate as fat (from fractures of the long bones),

air (caisson disease), or venous clots that pass from the right to the left side of the heart through a patent foramen ovale (paradoxical embolus).

Physiologic circulatory insufficiency is a relatively uncommon cause of ischemia and infarction. The diminished perfusion may occur alone or be superimposed on an already existing partial occlusion. Many processes may reduce perfusion. Profound anemia or carbon monoxide poisoning, by reducing the O_2-carrying capacity of the blood, and severe polycythemia, by increasing the blood's viscosity, can contribute to cerebral vascular problems. A pronounced, sustained fall in arterial pressure is ordinarily needed in order to cause a severe compromise in regional blood flow, but in the presence of arterial disease, hypoxemia, or hypertension, a lesser fall in BP can cause local ischemia and infarction. Orthostatic hypotension, acute blood loss, myocardial infarction, or, less often, cardiac arrhythmias are common mechanisms producing a fall in BP. Hypersensitivity to carotid sinus compression (eg, from sudden turning of the head) usually causes bradycardia and syncope; it is doubtful whether it can cause transient ischemia or an infarction in atherosclerotic patients.

TRANSIENT ISCHEMIC ATTACKS (TIAS)

Focal neurologic abnormalities of sudden onset and brief duration (usually minutes, never more than a few hours) that reflect dysfunction in the distribution of either the internal carotid–middle cerebral or the vertebral–basilar arterial system. The attacks are often recurrent and at times presage a stroke. Most TIAs are due to cerebral emboli arising from plaques or atherosclerotic ulcers involving the carotid or vertebral arteries in the neck, less often from mural thrombi in a diseased heart. Attacks are most common in the middle-aged and elderly, but occasionally occur in children in whom severe cardiovascular disease produces emboli or greatly increased Hct.

Hypertension, atherosclerosis, heart disease, diabetes mellitus, and polycythemia are predisposing. Some TIAs may be due to a brief reduction in blood flow through stenosed arteries. A rare variation is the **subclavian steal syndrome,** in which a subclavian artery stenosed proximal to the vertebral artery takeoff "steals" reverse-flow blood from the vertebral artery to supply the arm during exertion. Theoretically, at least, the process may produce symptoms of vertebrobasilar insufficiency (see below).

Symptoms, Signs, and Course

TIAs appear suddenly, last from 2 or 3 min to 30 min or more (seldom $>$ 1 or 2 h), and then abate without neurologic residua. Consciousness remains intact throughout the episode.

Symptoms depend on the arterial system affected. **With carotid artery involvement,** symptoms generally are unilateral. Ipsilateral blindness and contralateral hemiparesis, often with paresthesias, is classic, but less complete symptoms are more frequent. Aphasia indicates involvement of the dominant hemisphere. **When the vertebrobasilar system is involved,** symptoms reflect brainstem dysfunction. Confusion, vertigo, binocular blindness or diplopia, and unilateral or, more often, bilateral weakness, and paresthesias of the extremities may be present. **Drop attacks** (falling without loss of consciousness) may result from bilateral leg weakness. Slurred speech (dysarthria) may occur with either carotid or vertebrobasilar involvement.

Patients may have several attacks daily, or only 2 or 3 over several years. The symptoms usually are similar in repeated carotid attacks, but vary somewhat in successive vertebrobasilar attacks. How often TIAs presage a completed stroke is unknown. In some patients, especially those with carotid artery involvement, stroke eventually occurs; in others, TIAs occur shortly before a stroke; in still others, symptoms repeatedly appear without sequelae.

Diagnosis

Differentiation from convulsive seizures, neoplasms, migraine, Meniere's disease or other forms of vertigo, or hyperinsulinism in diabetics is sometimes necessary. Noninvasive ultrasonography or angiography can confirm the presence of stenosis and identify the involved artery and is needed to identify potentially operable lesions in the carotid arteries. With associated subclavian artery occlusion, the brachial BP in the affected arm is significantly lower than in the opposite arm.

Treatment

In addition to treating the atherosclerosis, hypertension, or other underlying disorder, vascular surgery or anticoagulants may be indicated. In patients with carotid TIAs, if an obstruction of > 70% or an ulcerated plaque can be identified in the ipsilateral carotid artery, endarterectomy or resection and prosthetic replacement of the lesion may be beneficial: No benefit has been demonstrated for surgical treatment of asymptomatic stenoses or those that do not correspond directly with the patient's symptoms.

If the obstruction is intracranial or vertebrobasilar, or if vertebral and carotid arteries are affected, and if the patient is not hypertensive, therapy consists of platelet inhibitors or anticoagulants. Surgical anastomosis between the external carotid and middle cerebral artery (EC-MCA bypass) has been shown to have no benefit. Heparin is used acutely if attacks are of recent origin and occur daily; a warfarin derivative can be used when attacks are frequent but occur less often. Once started, duration of anticoagulant therapy is difficult to specify. Most authorities continue anticoagulants for 2 to 3 mo; a trial without therapy may then be attempted. For patients with only occasional TIAs, most authorities now give a trial of aspirin therapy before starting anticoagulants. Unless specifically contraindicated, therapy with drugs that inhibit platelet aggregation should be continued indefinitely. At present, aspirin 1300 mg/day is the agent of choice. Relative values of sulfinpyrazone, dipyridamole, or clofibrate have not been established.

STROKE IN EVOLUTION AND COMPLETED STROKE

Stroke in evolution: *The clinical condition manifested by neurologic defects that increase over a 24- to 48-h period, reflecting enlarging infarction, usually in the territory of the middle cerebral artery.*

Completed stroke: *The clinical condition manifested by neurologic deficits of varying severity, usually abrupt in onset and either fatal or showing variable improvement, resulting from infarction of brain tissue due to arteriosclerotic or hypertensive stenosis, thrombosis, or embolism.*

Symptoms, Signs, and Course

In **stroke in evolution,** unilateral neurologic dysfunction (often beginning in one arm) increases painlessly and without headache or fever over several hours or a day or two to involve progressively more of the body ipsilaterally. The progression is usually stepwise, interrupted by periods of stability, but may be continuous. **Acute completed stroke** is by far the more common condition. Symptoms develop rapidly, and typically are maximal within a few minutes. By convention, **completed stroke** also refers to the patient's condition, after either evolving or acute stroke, once symptoms have ceased to progress and are either stable or improving.

In either evolving or acute completed large strokes, deficits may worsen and consciousness may become clouded during the next few days because of cerebral edema or, less often, from extension of the infarct. Severe cerebral edema can cause a potentially fatal shift in intracranial structures (transtentorial herniation; see under INTRACRANIAL NEOPLASMS in Ch. 126). However, early improvement in function is common

unless severe infarction has occurred. Further improvement is then gradual over days, weeks, or months.

Specific neurologic symptoms are determined by the *site* of the brain infarct. The involved artery can often be inferred from the symptom pattern, although the correlation is not exact. Occlusion of several arteries can cause symptoms described under several of the following categories.

The distribution of the **middle cerebral artery** or one of its deep penetrating branches is most commonly involved. Occlusion of the proximal part of the artery, which supplies large portions of the frontal, parietal, and temporal lobe surfaces, results in contralateral hemiplegia, usually severe, with hemianesthesia and a homonymous hemianopia. Aphasia occurs when the dominant hemisphere is affected; apraxia or sensory neglect, when the nondominant hemisphere is involved. A contralateral hemiplegia of the face, arm, and leg, sometimes with hemianesthesia, also results from occlusion of one of the deep branches, which supply the basal ganglia, internal and external capsules, and thalamus. Motor or sensory impairment may be less severe when terminal branches are involved.

Internal carotid artery occlusion leads to infarction in the central-lateral portion of the cerebral hemisphere, with symptoms indistinguishable from those of middle cerebral artery occlusion.

Anterior cerebral artery occlusion is uncommon, but affects portions of the frontal and parietal lobes, corpus callosum, and sometimes the caudate nucleus and internal capsule. Contralateral hemiplegia, especially affecting the leg, may be seen. A grasp reflex and urinary incontinence may occur. Bilateral occlusion may cause emotional disturbances with apathy, confusion, and occasional mutism, plus spastic paraparesis.

Posterior cerebral artery occlusion can affect areas in the temporal and occipital lobes, internal capsule, hippocampus, thalamus, mamillary and geniculate bodies, choroid plexus, and upper brainstem. Contralateral homonymous hemianopia, hemisensory loss, spontaneous thalamic pain, or sudden hemiballism may occur; alexia may follow an infarct in the dominant hemisphere.

The vertebrobasilar system supplies the brainstem, cerebellum, and portions of the temporal and occipital lobes. Branch occlusions cause combinations of cerebellar, corticospinal, sensory, and cranial nerve signs. Complete occlusion of the basilar artery usually causes ophthalmoplegia, pupillary abnormalities, bilateral corticospinal signs (tetraparesis or tetraplegia), and changes in consciousness. Pseudobulbar manifestations (dysarthria, dysphagia, emotional instability) occur frequently. The course is often fatal.

Diagnosis

Stroke usually can be diagnosed clinically, especially in a patient over age 50 with hypertension, diabetes mellitus, or signs of atherosclerosis, or in any patient with a known source of emboli. Clinical diagnosis seldom is difficult. In the unusual case, differentiation from a rapidly growing or suddenly symptomatic tumor is aided by a negative skull x-ray or by a CT scan (which is sometimes negative for as long as several days after an acute infarction). Arteriography is limited to patients in whom the diagnosis is in doubt or a remedial vascular obstruction is suspected.

Determining the immediate cause of a stroke may be difficult. Onset during sleep or on arising suggests infarction; onset during exertion, hemorrhage. Headache, coma or stupor, marked hypertension, and convulsive seizures are more likely with hemorrhage.

Localized carotid vascular bruits and thrills in the neck may be present and suggest the presence of stenosis and plaque formation in an extracranial vessel, while the neurologic symptoms and signs can suggest the artery involved.

A stroke due to a large embolus tends to be an acute completed stroke, sudden in onset, with focal disorders that are maximal within a few minutes. Headache may precede it. Thrombosis is less frequent and is suggested by a slower onset, or a gradual

progression of symptoms, as in evolving stroke. However, the distinction is not entirely reliable. Concomitant signs of myocardial infarction, atrial fibrillation, or vegetative heart disease further suggest embolization.

Studies should be done to identify hypertension and to rule out anemia, polycythemia, and infections. Plasma lipids should be determined. A chest x-ray should be taken to search for a primary lung tumor and cardiovascular disorders, and an ECG should be performed.

Laboratory findings are nonspecific. The CSF in all forms of ischemic stroke is usually normal, but leukocytes may be transiently increased to 500/μL, sugar may be slightly reduced, and protein may be elevated to 80 mg/dL. The CSF is usually clear after an infarct, but bloody, with increased pressure, after intracranial hemorrhage. Red cells may be present due to infarction, but are far fewer than the number seen in hemorrhages. Angiography is sometimes needed to identify the site of arterial occlusion or narrowing (eg, when surgery is contemplated). A CT scan helps to differentiate an ischemic stroke from intracerebral hemorrhage, hematoma, or tumor.

Prognosis

During the early days of either evolving or completed stroke, neither progression nor ultimate outcome can be predicted. About 35% of patients die in the hospital; the mortality rate increases with age.

The eventual extent of neurologic recovery depends on the patient's age and general state of health as well as on the site and size of the infarction. Impaired consciousness, mental deterioration, aphasia, or severe brainstem signs all suggest a poor prognosis. Complete recovery is uncommon, but the sooner improvement begins, the better the prognosis. About 50% of patients with moderate or severe hemiplegia, and most of those with lesser deficits, recover functionally by the time of discharge and are ultimately able to care for their basic needs, have a clear sensorium, and can walk adequately, although use of an affected limb may be limited. Any deficit remaining after 6 mo is likely to be permanent, although some patients continue to improve slowly. Recurrence of cerebral infarction is common, and each recurrence is likely to add to the neurologic disability.

Treatment

Immediate care of a comatose patient includes airway maintenance, adequate oxygenation, or IV fluids to maintain nutritional and fluid intake, attention to bladder and bowel function, and measures to prevent decubitus ulcers. Corticosteroids have no value.

Heart failure, cardiac arrhythmias, severe hypertension, and intercurrent respiratory infection must be treated. IV spasmolytic agents such as sodium nitroprusside are preferable in malignant hypertension. Barbiturates and other sedatives are *contraindicated*, as they increase the risk of respiratory depression and subsequent pneumonitis. Passive movements, particularly of paralyzed limbs, and breathing exercises, if possible, should be begun early.

Heparin may stabilize symptoms in evolving stroke, but anticoagulants are useless (and possibly dangerous) in acute completed stroke and are *contraindicated* in hypertensive patients because of the increased possibility of hemorrhage into the brain or other organs.

Vascular surgery is not indicated as an emergency measure and is pointless after complete hemiplegic stroke or when atheromatous stenosis is widespread. Thromboendarterectomy or resection and prosthetic replacement may sometimes help to prevent recurrent neurologic episodes in patients with partial, isolated carotid occlusion who have had small strokes or TIAs. No evidence favors surgical treatment for asymptomatic carotid bruit.

Rehabilitation and aftercare: Early and repeated appraisals of the patient's status by physician, physiotherapist, and nursing staff allow a remedial program to be designed.

Elaborate programs are unnecessary, and the value of speech therapy is unproved. Younger age, limited sensory and motor deficit, intact mental function, and a helpful home environment favorably influence rehabilitation. Early treatment, continuing encouragement, and orientation toward the outside environment are important. The patient and his relatives and friends must understand the nature of his disabilities and the likelihood that progress will occur but will take time, patience, and perseverance. Mood changes may be the result of the infarct as well as a reaction to the situation; they should be expected, and treated by reassurance and understanding; tranquilizers or antidepressants may be helpful after the patient's condition has stabilized. Occupational and physical therapy should emphasize using affected limbs and achieving proficiency in eating, dressing, toilet functions, and other basic needs. Appliances such as hearing aids and walking frames often are needed; in the living quarters, handbars (eg, at tub and toilet) and ramps can be of great help (see also Ch. 265).

HYPERTENSIVE ENCEPHALOPATHY

An acute or subacute condition occurring in patients with severe hypertension marked by headache, obtundation, confusion or stupor, and convulsions. Modern hypertensive treatment has made the condition rare. Although both ischemic and hemorrhagic stroke are more common in hypertension, hypertensive encephalopathy is an additional, specific cerebral disorder confined to patients with severe hypertension. Often, one finds rapidly changing neurologic abnormalities, including cortical blindness, hemiparesis, and hemisensory defects. BP always is elevated, usually with diastolic pressures > 110 to 140 mm Hg. Grade 3 or 4 retinopathy usually is present and the CSF pressure commonly is > 200 mm with a CSF protein content usually > 60 mg/dL. The pathogenesis is believed to involve either multifocal areas of hypertensive-induced arteriolar spasm or perhaps blood-brain barrier leakage adjacent to an area of loss of vascular autoregulation.

Diagnosis depends on the characteristic clinical picture and the exclusion of other possible illnesses. Clinically, the picture most resembles uremia, from which it is differentiated by a BUN < 100 mg/dL. Other metabolic encephalopathies must also be excluded but are less of a problem, since most are not particularly associated with an elevated BP.

Treatment (see also ARTERIAL HYPERTENSION in Ch. 26) consists of deliberate (not abrupt) but progressive reduction of BP to more nearly normal ranges. When more conventional antihypertensive drugs fail, sodium nitroprusside should be used.

HEMORRHAGIC SYNDROMES

Cerebrovascular disorders caused by bleeding into brain tissue or meningeal spaces

Intracranial hemorrhage may occur into the brain substance, the epi- or subdura spaces, the subarachnoid space, or a combination of these sites. Epidural and subdura hemorrhage are often the consequence of head trauma, and are discussed in Ch. 124

INTRACEREBRAL HEMORRHAGE

Etiology and Pathogenesis

Intracerebral hemorrhage usually results from rupture of an arteriosclerotic vess either long exposed to arterial hypertension or made ischemic by local thrombus fo mation. Less often, the cause is a congenital aneurysm or other vascular malformatio Mycotic aneurysms, brain infarct, blood dyscrasias, collagen diseases, and other sy temic diseases are occasional causes. Hypertensive or aneurysmal cerebral hemorrhag is usually large and single; hemorrhages from most other causes are apt to be sma and diffusely scattered.

Intracerebral hemorrhages, as shown by CT scan, can arise almost anywhere in the brain. Most clinically destructive are those located in the region of the basal ganglia, internal capsule, thalamus, cerebellum, and brainstem.

The hematoma dissects, compresses, and displaces adjacent brain tissue and, if large, increases intracranial pressure. Pressure from supratentorial hematomas and the accompanying edema may cause transtentorial herniation (see under INTRACRANIAL NEOPLASMS in Ch. 126), compressing the brainstem and often causing secondary hemorrhages in the midbrain and pons. If the hemorrhage ruptures into the ventricular system, blood may reach the subarachnoid space. Cerebellar hematomas can expand to block the ventricular system, causing acute hydrocephalus, or dissect into the brainstem. Either course can produce stupor or coma.

Symptoms and Signs

Cerebral hemorrhage characteristically begins abruptly with headache, followed by steadily increasing neurologic deficits. Large hemorrhages produce hemiparesis when located in the hemispheres, and symptoms of cerebellar or brainstem dysfunction (conjugate eye deviation or ophthalmoplegia; stertorous breathing, pinpoint pupils, and coma) when located in the posterior fossa. Loss of consciousness is common; it may occur within a few minutes after onset or develop gradually. Nausea, vomiting, delirium, and focal or generalized seizures also are common. Large hemorrhages are fatal within a few days in > 50% of patients. In those who survive, consciousness returns and neurologic deficits gradually diminish as the extravasated blood is resorbed. Some degree of impairment usually remains, including some dysphasia if the dominant hemisphere was affected, but many patients make a reasonable degree of functional recovery, especially from hemorrhages in silent areas.

Smaller hemorrhages cause focal deficits like those seen in ischemic stroke; as with infarcts, the deficits reflect the site of the damage (see above).

Diagnosis and Treatment

It is often difficult clinically to distinguish small cerebral hemorrhages from ischemic stroke. CT scanning is the diagnostic procedure of choice. Lumbar puncture must be done cautiously, if at all, when patients are unconscious or symptoms are worsening, since the consequent change in CSF pressure may precipitate transtentorial or cerebellar herniation. With large hemorrhages, the CSF is almost always bloody (Hct > 1%) and under increased pressure. Other distinguishing features are given above under diagnosis of ischemic stroke.

Therapy following hemorrhage is similar to that for ischemic stroke (see above), except that anticoagulants are **contraindicated** in hemorrhage. Codeine 60 mg q 4 h may be needed to relieve headache, and diazepam will relieve anxiety. Hypnotic sedatives are contraindicated, as in ischemic stroke. Nausea or vomiting may require IV fluid administration and prochlorperazine 2.5 to 5 mg during the first few days. Surgical decompression of large hemorrhages producing brain displacement is sometimes attempted, but severe neurologic deficits almost always follow, since aspiration inevitably removes some brain as well as clot.

SUBARACHNOID HEMORRHAGE

Sudden bleeding into the subarachnoid space.

Etiology and Pathology

Secondary bleeding into the subarachnoid space is most commonly due to head trauma. Spontaneous or primary subarachnoid hemorrhage usually results from a ruptured congenital intracranial aneurysm. Less frequently it may be due to mycotic or arteriosclerotic aneurysm, arteriovenous **(A-V)** malformation, or hemorrhagic disease. It may occur at any age, but is most common from age 25 to 50.

Hemorrhage from aneurysm usually arises from outpouchings at the bifurcations of arteries at or near the base of the brain, points where the muscular coat is poorly developed, thus predisposing to aneurysm formation; arteriosclerosis and hypertension probably also play a role. Most aneurysms are located along the middle or anterior cerebral arteries or the communicating branches of the circle of Willis.

A secondary increase in intracranial pressure is common after subarachnoid hemorrhage and may last for days or a few weeks. The associated communicating hydrocephalus may contribute to headache or the posthemorrhage delirium.

Symptoms and Signs

Before rupture, most aneurysms are asymptomatic. A few may manifest themselves as a result of pressure on adjacent structures. Ocular palsies, diplopia, squint, and facial pain due to pressure on the 3rd, 4th, 5th, and 6th cranial nerves may be present. Visual loss and a bitemporal field defect signify pressure on the optic chiasm. Pressure on the optic tract produces a noncongruent homonymous hemianopia.

Following rupture, there usually is acute severe headache, often followed or accompanied by at least brief syncope. Some patients remain in coma, but more often the patient is merely obtunded. The mixture of escaping blood and CSF irritates the meninges and increases intracranial pressure, producing headache, vomiting, dizziness, and alterations in pulse and respiratory rates. Convulsions occasionally occur. Stiffness of the neck usually is not present initially unless the cerebellar tonsils are herniated downwards. Within 24 h, however, moderate to marked stiffness of the neck, Kernig's sign, and bilateral Babinski's signs develop. The temperature may be elevated during the first 5 to 10 days, and the patient often continues to have headaches and confusion during this time. Focal signs, generally including hemiplegia, are present in about 25% of cases, as a result of bleeding into the brain substance or associated vasospasm and ischemia.

Diagnosis

Spinal puncture is indicated for diagnosis and at first yields a bloody CSF under increased pressure; after 6 h or more, a xanthochromic supernatant is found. Once active hemorrhage ceases, the CSF gradually clears, and the pressure usually returns to normal in about 3 wk.

Acute subarachnoid hemorrhage occasionally simulates myocardial infarction because of the associated syncope and neurogenic abnormalities on the ECG. In cases with obvious neurologic signs, subarachnoid hemorrhage must be differentiated from parenchymatous cerebral hemorrhage, bleeding from A-V malformation, cerebral contusion and laceration, subdural hematoma, and sometimes brain tumor with hemorrhage. CT scanning plus cerebral angiography is necessary for differential diagnosis and as a guide to surgical therapy. All 4 cerebral vessels should be inspected, because several aneurysms may be present. Skull x-rays may show calcification in the wall of an aneurysm.

Prognosis

The mortality rate with first hemorrhages is about 35%, and an additional 15% of patients die from a subsequent rupture within a few weeks. A second rupture after 6 mo occurs at a rate of about 5/yr. In general, the prognosis is grave with cerebral aneurysm, better with bleeding from A-V malformations, and best when no lesion is discovered with 4-vessel arteriography, presumably because the bleeding source was small and sealed itself.

Treatment

Underlying vascular disease, blood dyscrasia, cardiac disease, or syphilis should be treated appropriately. Exertion should be avoided. Bed rest is mandatory until bleeding has stopped. Fluid balance and nutrition should be maintained, parenterally if necessary. Diazepam may be used for restlessness, and codeine or meperidine 25 to 5

mg parenterally may be required to relieve headaches. Constipation induces straining and should be prevented. Anticoagulants are **contraindicated.**

The desirability of spinal puncture to reduce intracranial pressure depends on the patient's reaction to the initial diagnostic puncture. If he improves, amounts of CSF may be cautiously removed at intervals, in order to reduce the intracranial pressure to normal.

In experienced hands, surgery that succeeds in trapping or obliterating an aneurysm reduces the risk of subsequent fatal bleeding and lowers long-term mortality. Procedures include extirpating or clipping the aneurysm, ligating the proximal carotid artery, inducing thrombosis, or covering the aneurysmal sac with plastic, gauze, or muscle. Surgical mortality is unjustifiably high in patients operated on when in stupor or coma. In less neurologically damaged patients, the best timing for surgery is controversial. Arteriography should be carried out as soon as practicable after the initial bleeding episode. Early surgery carries a high chance of postoperative vasospasm and infarction, while an operation delayed for 10 days or so minimizes these risks but permits a higher rebleeding rate.

Even with surgical treatment, subarachnoid hemorrhage leaves many patients with residual neurologic damage. In a few patients, obtundation, confusion, and delayed motor recovery continue for weeks after subarachnoid hemorrhage, because of a secondary communicating hydrocephalus. Cerebral ventricular shunting sometimes helps this condition.

ARTERIOVENOUS (A-V) MALFORMATIONS

Abnormal, tangled collections of dilated blood vessels that result from congenitally malformed vascular structures in which arterial afferents flow directly into venous efferents without the usual resistance of an intervening capillary bed. The result is a progressively enlarging vascular anomaly that can produce neurologic abnormalities either because of its size, because it compresses neural tissue in its interstices, or because it bleeds. The malformations are particularly likely to arise at junction points between cerebral arterial beds and are found most frequently within the cerebral parenchyma in the frontal-parietal region, in the frontal lobe, or in the lateral cerebellum or overlying occipital lobe.

Clinical Syndromes

A-V malformation produces 3 relatively distinct neurologic disorders. Most often, perhaps half the time, they bleed to produce the clinical picture of **parenchymal** or **subarachnoid hemorrhage**. Little or nothing distinctive identifies A-V malformations as the source except that such hemorrhages tend to be less neurologically devastating than those due to hypertensive or congenital aneurysm and they have a high frequency of recurrence over the years. The other 2 syndromes include **focal epilepsy,** with the nature of the focus related to the site of the malformation (see TABLE 121-2 in Ch. 121), and **progressive focal neurologic sensory-motor deficit** due to the enlarging malformation acting as a mass or progressive ischemic lesion.

Diagnosis and Treatment

Specific diagnosis of A-V malformations is difficult except by laboratory means. Some patients have arterial bruits, detectable on the overlying cranial vault. CT generally outlines malformations exceeding 1.5 cm in diameter, but arteriography is required for definitive diagnosis and to determine if the lesion is operable.

Treatment includes anticonvulsants to control seizures (see Drug Therapy in Ch. 121). Surgical removal can be attempted and, if all the arterial feeders can be identified and ligated, sometimes produces a cure. Intravascular thrombosing via intra-arterial catheters and coagulation with focused proton beams have also been attempted.

THORACIC OUTLET OBSTRUCTION SYNDROMES

(Neurovascular Compression Syndromes of the Shoulder Girdle; Scalenus Anticus Syndrome; Cervical Rib Syndrome)

A group of somewhat inconsistent disorders characterized by subjective complaints of pain and paresthesias in the hand, neck, shoulder, or arms. They are most often distributed medially in the members and sometimes extend into the adjacent anterior chest wall. The conditions are more common in women than men and most frequent between ages 35 and 55. Many patients have minor to moderate degrees of sensory impairment in the C8 to T1 distribution on the painful side, and a few will have prominent vascular-autonomic changes in the hand including cyanosis, swelling and, rarely, Raynaud's phenomenon or distal gangrene. The pathogenesis is believed to be due to compression of the subclavian vessels and, sometimes, the lower or medial trunks of the brachial plexus against a cervical rib, an abnormal 1st thoracic rib, or a putatively abnormal insertion or position of the scalene muscles.

Symptoms, Signs, and Diagnosis

More accurate imaging methods and the development of specific tests for nerve and root function have removed from this category the frequent offenders; namely, carpal tunnel compression of the median nerve and spondylitic nerve root compression. The true neurovascular condition can be suspected by the distribution of symptoms, and diagnosis is supported by the finding of obliteration of the pulse with elevation of the arm and turning of the head to the opposite shoulder **(Adson's maneuver)**. Also helpful are the auscultation of bruits at the clavicle or the apex of the axilla, or the finding of a cervical rib by x-ray. Some patients will show kinking or partial obstruction of axillary arteries or veins on angiography, but these are not incontrovertible evidence of disease.

Treatment

Most patients respond to physical therapy and exercises. Except when obvious cervical ribs or subclavian artery obstructions can be identified, surgical treatment is best avoided or left to the experienced specialist.

---

124. TRAUMA OF THE HEAD AND SPINE

HEAD INJURY

Head injury causes more deaths and disability than any other neurologic cause in subjects under age 50. Mortality in severe injury approaches 50% and is only little reduced by treatment. Damage results from penetration of the skull or from rapid acceleration or deceleration of the brain, which injures tissue at the point of impact, at its opposite pole (contrecoup), and also diffusely along the frontal and temporal lobes. Nerve tissue, blood vessels, and meninges are sheared, torn, and ruptured, resulting in neural disruption, intra- and extracerebral ischemia or hemorrhage, and cerebral edema. Hemorrhage or edema acts as an expanding intracranial lesion, causing increased intracranial pressure that can lead to fatal herniation of brain tissue through the tentorial opening. Skull fractures may lacerate meningeal arteries or large venous sinuses, producing epidural or subdural hematoma. Infectious organisms may reach the meninges even when a fracture is not clearly evident, especially when it involves the paranasal sinuses (see Ch. 208). Few head injuries occur in isolation, and most cases require simultaneous attention to other seriously traumatized parts of the body

Symptoms, Signs, and Diagnosis

Concussion is characterized by post-traumatic loss of consciousness lasting < 24 h (usually much less), without structural lesions in the brain. Although unconscious, the patient with concussion rarely is deeply unresponsive. Pupillary reactions and other signs of brainstem function are intact; thus, extensor plantar responses may be present, but not hemiplegia or decerebrate postural responses to noxious stimulation (see Motor Responses under IMPAIRED CONSCIOUSNESS—STUPOR AND COMA, Diagnosis, in Ch. 118). Lumbar puncture reveals a clear CSF.

Cerebral contusion, lacerations, and edema constitute more severe injuries. They often are accompanied by severe surface wounds and by fractures located at the base of the skull or having depressed bone fragments (see also FRACTURES OF THE TEMPORAL BONE in Ch. 207). Respiration often is labored because of pulmonary congestion (or chest trauma). Hemiplegia, decorticate rigidity (arms flexed and adducted; legs and often trunk extended), or decerebrate rigidity (jaws clenched, neck retracted, all limbs extended) is common. Lumbar puncture reveals bloody CSF, usually under increased pressure. Pupils may be unequal. Increased intracranial pressure, particularly when associated with compression or distortion of the brainstem, may produce a rising BP coupled with a slowing of the pulse and respiratory rates.

The cerebral hemispheres and underlying diencephalon generally are more exposed and susceptible to the effects of trauma than is the brainstem. **Signs of primary brainstem injury** (coma, stertorous breathing, fixation of the pupils to light, loss of oculovestibular reflexes, or diffuse motor flaccidity) almost always imply severe injury and have a poor prognosis.

Since severe head injuries frequently are accompanied by thoracic damage, the neurologic problems created by the injury often are complicated by pulmonary edema (some of which is undoubtedly neurogenic), hypoxia, and an unstable circulation. Damage to the cervical spine, also a common accompaniment, can cause fatal respiratory paralysis or permanent quadriplegia from cord injury; other cord damage can be almost as disastrous.

Complications of Head Trauma

Acute subdural or **intracerebral hematomas** are common in severe head injury and, ogether with severe **brain edema,** are present in most fatal cases. All 3 conditions cause igns of progressive rostral-caudal neurologic deterioration: deepening coma, widening ulse pressure, dilated pupils, spastic hemiplegia with hyper-reflexia, quadrispasticity, upillary fixation to light, decorticate rigidity, decerebrate rigidity (see Symptoms and igns, above). CT or MRI scans usually are diagnostic, but bilateral burr holes over he parieto-occipital and temporal regions provide a more rapid and equally effective iagnostic approach.

Epidural hematomas most often have a temporal location (middle meningeal artery), ss often occipital (venous sinus). Symptoms—increasing headache, deterioration of onsciousness, motor dysfunction, pupillary changes—develop 24 to 96 h after trauma. n epidural hematoma is uncommon but important, because continue[illegible] for nger than 24 h may cause potentially fatal compression of brain ti[illegible] acture lines suggest the diagnosis, but may not be present. CT o[illegible] ngiograms should be made or burr holes drilled promptly for diag[illegible] ion of the clot.

Chronic subdural hematoma is a late complication that may not d[illegible] eeks after trauma. Although diagnosis in early cases (2 to 4 wk af[illegible] ggested by a clinical course of delayed neurologic deterioration, [illegible] fficult because of the time lapse between the injury and the ons[illegible] gns. Most patients are over age 50, and the head injury may [illegible] vial, even forgotten. Increasing daily headache, fluctuating [illegible]

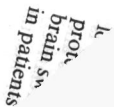

changes, and mild to moderate hemiparesis are typical. Pupillary abnormalities occur in only 10% of patients, and lumbar puncture may be normal in longstanding cases. Brain scans become abnormal in 80% of cases; these or angiograms are diagnostic.

Posttraumatic epilepsy, with seizures beginning as late as 24 mo after trauma, follows about 10% of severe closed head injuries and 40% of penetrating head wounds. To reduce the risk, patients with such injuries should receive prophylactic anticonvulsants (eg, phenytoin 100 mg orally tid) for up to 3 yr.

The worst complication of severe head injury is that of near-complete damage to forebrain functions with sparing of the brainstem. Such patients fortunately are rare, but may exist in a **chronic vegetative state** for many years if they survive. Few cases recover from the vegetative state when it lasts as long as 2 mo after injury.

Treatment

Immediate management: Multiple injuries are likely when an accident has caused severe head injury. At the accident site, once a clear airway is secured (with an oral or endotracheal tube if possible) and acute bleeding controlled, the accident victim is moved en bloc, with particular care to avoid displacing the spine or other bones and thereby injuring the spinal cord or blood vessels. Splinting can be confined to supporting the entire body for transport to a medical facility. For care of the victim with possible cord injuries, see SPINAL CORD INJURY below. Morphine and other depressants are *contraindicated.*

In the hospital, once the airway is secured (by tracheostomy when injuries are severe), fluids are started, and internal bleeding and other emergency complications are evaluated and treated.

A careful assessment is made of the state of consciousness, breathing pattern, pupil size and reaction to light, and motor activity in the limbs. These functions, BP, pulse, and temperature should be recorded at least hourly, since any deterioration demands prompt attention. Once the baseline data are obtained, x-rays should be taken and checked, particularly for skull fracture lines that could affect blood vessels, and for associated cervical spine fractures. When extensive injury is obvious, lumbar puncture is unnecessary and may be hazardous, since it can precipitate tentorial herniation. CT or MRI scans are valuable for detecting potentially operable intracranial hematomas. If CT or MRI is unavailable, cerebral angiograms are indicated when specific complications (eg, subdural or epidural hematoma) are suspected; radioactive scans and EEG are of little diagnostic help in the immediate post-trauma situation. Some trauma centers use continuous intracranial pressure measurements to monitor patient progress, but their specific advantages are unproved.

Patients should be protected against heat loss, fluid depletion, and airway obstruction, and should be monitored closely for signs of deterioration. Patients with concussion should be kept under close supervision for at least 48 h to be certain no complications arise.

Skull fractures, if aligned, require no treatment. Depressed fractures are best handled by a neurosurgeon, and may require emergency management of lacerated blood vessels. Antibiotic prophylaxis is avoided, since it only encourages drug-resistant strains.

To protect against complications, arterial hypoxemia is minimized by partial (40% oxygenation, combined if necessary with IPPB. Fever is controlled with cooling blankets. Blood and fluid loss are replaced promptly. One must prevent hypo- or hyperthermia and be alert for acute renal failure. Anticonvulsants (eg, phenytoin given as ·ding dose of 50 mg IV/min to a total of 1 gm followed by 300 to 400 mg/da ·t against seizures. Osmotic diuretics (urea, mannitol, glycerol) given IV redu ·lling but should be reserved for deteriorating patients or for preoperative u ·ith hematomas. No benefit from corticosteroids has been shown.

Restlessness occurring during improvement from coma may require sedation (eg, with chlorpromazine 50 mg IM or haloperidol 2 to 5 mg IM). If unconsciousness begins to improve within 1 wk, the outlook for reasonable recovery is good.

Convalescence after any severe head injury is marked by **amnesia** for the periods both immediately preceding and following loss of consciousness. **Retrograde amnesia** usually is brief; the duration of **posttraumatic amnesia** (measured until the restoration of complete, continuous awareness) gives a good estimate of the extent of brain damage in closed head injuries. Giddiness, attention difficulties, anxiety, and headache (**postconcussion syndrome** —see below) occur for a variable period after concussion, but seldom persist or require more than reassurance unless lawsuits are pending—in which case careful assessment of psychosocial factors is needed.

Objective assessment of residual disability is important after severe head injury, when subjective complaints may be fewer precisely because of the residual effects. Personality changes from frontal lobe damage and memory deficits from temporal lobe damage, unless tested for, may go unnoticed at first, yet cause problems later at work and at home. Focal deficits, including damage to cranial nerves, are more obvious. Anosmia is permanent; other cranial nerve deficits usually recover spontaneously but sometimes are permanent. Hemiparesis and aphasia usually recover well, except in the elderly or after severe cerebral laceration.

Most recovery after severe head injury occurs in the adult within the first 6 mo, with smaller adjustments continuing for perhaps as long as 2 yr. Children fare better, showing both better immediate recoveries from even very severe injuries and continuing improvement for longer periods of time.

POSTCONCUSSION SYNDROME

A syndrome including a wide variety of symptoms such as headaches and complaints of impaired memory, although no defect can be demonstrated objectively.

After a mild head injury, headache, dizziness, difficulty in concentration, depression, apathy, and perhaps anxiety are more common than after severe head injuries. These symptoms can cause a considerable disability. The part played by brain damage is unclear; the postconcussion syndrome is more common in patients with a premorbid neurotic disposition, though recent experimental studies indicate that even mild trauma can cause neuronal damage. Epidemiologic studies suggest that postconcussion syndrome is not more common when compensation for the injury is possible. The results of treatment with drugs or psychotherapy vary, and symptoms commonly persist after compensation claims are settled.

SPINAL CORD INJURY

Loss of neurologic function after a spinal injury can result briefly from concussion or more lastingly from compression of the spinal cord due to contusion or hemorrhage, as well as permanently from lacerations or transection. In **contusion**, rapid edematous swelling of the cord with a rise in intradural pressure can cause severe dysfunction for several days. This is followed by spontaneous improvement, but some residual disability may remain. **Hemorrhage** usually is confined to the central gray matter **(hematomyelia)** and produces signs of lower motor neuron damage (muscle weakness and wasting, fasciculations, diminished tendon reflexes) that usually are permanent. The motor weakness often is proximal rather than distal and accompanied by selective impairment of pain and temperature sensations. **Extradural, subdural,** or **subarachnoid hemorrhage** also can occur. **Lacerations** or **transection** inevitably leave permanent dysfunction.

Symptoms, Signs, and Diagnosis

An acute transverse cord lesion causes immediate flaccid paralysis and loss of all sensation and reflex activity (including autonomic functions) below the level of injury **(spinal shock)**. The flaccid paralysis gradually changes, over hours or days, to spastic paraplegia due to exaggeration of the normal stretch reflexes. Later, if the lumbosacral cord is intact, extensor or flexor muscle spasms appear, and deep tendon reflexes and autonomic reflexes return (see also NEUROGENIC BLADDER in Ch. 158).

Less complete lesions cause partial motor and sensory loss. Voluntary movement becomes disordered. Sensory loss depends on the tracts affected: posture, vibration, and light touch, if the posterior columns; pain, temperature, and light or deep touch, if the spinothalamic tracts. Hemisection of the cord results in ipsilateral spastic paralysis and loss of postural sense, and contralateral loss of pain and thermal sense **(Brown-Séquard's syndrome)**.

Clinical clues identify the level of cord damage. (Abbreviations here refer to vertebrae; one must remember that the cord is shorter than the spine, so that as one descends the spine, the cord segments and vertebral levels are increasingly out of alignment.) Lesions above C-5, if serious, cause respiratory paralysis and are often fatal. Lesions at or above C-4 to C-5 cause complete quadriplegia; with a lesion between C-5 and C-6, the arms can abduct and flex. Damage between C-6 and C-7 paralyzes the legs, wrists, and hands but allows shoulder movement and elbow flexion. Transverse lesions above T-1 cause miotic pupils; lesions at C-8 to T-1 cause **Horner's syndrome** (*constricted pupil, ptosis, facial anhidrosis*). Lesions between T-11 and T-12 affect the leg muscles above and below the knee; lesions at T-12 to L-1 cause paralysis below the knee. Trauma to the cauda equina causes hypo- or areflexic paresis of the lower extremities and, usually, pain and hyperesthesia in the distribution of the nerve roots. Damage to the 3rd, 4th, and 5th sacral nerve roots or to the conus medullaris at L-1 causes complete loss of bladder and bowel control.

Prognosis

Severed or degenerated nerve processes in the cord cannot recover, and damage is permanent, while compressed nerve tissue usually recovers its function. Return of a movement or sensation during the first week after injury heralds a favorable recovery; any dysfunction remaining after 6 mo is likely to be permanent.

Severe cord injury above C-5 usually is fatal. Cauda equina lesions seldom are complete, and motor or sensory loss therefore is likely to be partial; but reflex arcs controlling micturition, sexual activity in men, and bowel function are in the conus medullaris, and if they are destroyed even reflex micturition cannot be established. Damage to the cauda equina anywhere in the lumbar or sacral spine may cause permanent impotence and loss of sphincter control for bladder, bowel, or both, as will any permanent cord injury at a higher level.

Treatment

Immediate management: To protect the cord from further damage, any accident victim suspected of having a spinal injury, especially in the cervical region, must be handled with the utmost care. Until the extent of injury is known, all spinal injuries should be treated as potentially unstable. Either flexion or extension of the spine can contuse or transect the cord if an intervertebral disk has ruptured or the spine is fractured. Getting accident victims out of damaged cars can present a risk of quadriplegia or even death from cervical cord damage. The patient should be moved en bloc and be transported on a firm, flat board or door, with careful padding to stabilize his position without excessive pressure; proper alignment of the spine by traction is critical. Those with thoracic or lumbar spine injuries are carried prone or supine; those with cervical cord damage are likely to have respiratory difficulties and are carried

prone, with attention to a patent airway and any possible constrictions around the chest.

When the spine is stable, injuries are treated by rest until swelling and local pain have subsided. Unstable injuries must be immobilized, until bone and soft tissues have healed, with traction to ensure proper alignment. Surgery with internal fixation occasionally is needed. It is doubtful whether surgical decompression favorably influences traumatic cord injuries, but osmotic diuretics to reduce edema (as with head injuries) may be indicated.

Nursing care includes prevention of urinary infection, moving the paralyzed patient q 2 h (on a Stryker frame when necessary), and other measures to prevent bedsores. Exercises and rehabilitative measures should begin as soon as possible. Aids for the disabled patient are discussed in Ch. 265.

Emotional care of a person with spinal cord injury aims to combat the depersonalization that can occur in hospital settings and should provide (1) explanations to the patient of what is being done and why; (2) reassurance that he is not alone and will be helped; (3) recognition of the *person* he has always been by noting his previous interests and hobbies, providing comforting objects from home, and recognizing his feelings about privacy, body image, sexuality, and loss of dignity and self-esteem; (4) understanding of the intense emotions he is experiencing, including directly asking about fears; (5) the thoughtful presence of those treating him—eg, by preventing a dry mouth or running of tears, and by providing personal care such as shampoos, shaves, makeup, fingernail polish, or hair combing before visiting hours; (6) awareness that the patient's behavior, even if abrasive or manipulative, may be adaptive for him. Compromises can be reached; ie, the patient's need to control his environment can be channeled into negotiable areas such as physical therapy time, meal choices, visitors.

Honesty, understanding, and caring by the treating personnel make an incalculable difference in the patient's outcome.

125. CNS INFECTIONS

Meningitis: *Inflammation of the meninges of the brain or spinal cord.* The brain as well as the meninges can be involved; the cerebral manifestations of bacterial invasion are termed **cerebritis**; those of viral agents, **encephalitis.**

Most bacteria cause an acute meningitis, but tuberculous and syphilitic meningitis are subacute. Viral infections cause an **acute aseptic meningitis,** while fungal infections, disseminated malignancies, and chemical reactions to certain intrathecal injections usually cause a **subacute aseptic meningitis.**

Tuberculous meningitis is discussed in Ch. 8.

ACUTE BACTERIAL MENINGITIS

(See also under NEONATAL INFECTIONS in Ch. 186)

Etiology and Incidence

Although many bacteria can induce meningitis, 3 account for about 80% of all cases: *Neisseria meningitidis*, *Hemophilus influenzae*, and *Streptococcus (Diplococcus) pneumoniae*. Factors such as age, head trauma, and compromised immunity help identify the organism involved.

Meningococcus is found in the nasopharynx of about 5% of the population and is spread by respiratory droplets and close contact. For unknown reasons, only a small fraction of carriers develop meningitis. Meningococcal meningitis occurs most often in the first year of life. It is also apt to occur in epidemics in closed populations (eg,

military barracks, boarding schools). *H. influenzae* accounts for most meningitis in children > 1 mo old, but not in adults unless there is a predisposing factor (eg, head trauma, immune compromise). Pneumococcus is the most common cause of adult meningitis. Especially at risk are individuals with alcoholism, chronic otitis, sinusitis, mastoiditis, closed head injury, recurrent meningitis, pneumococcal pneumonia, sickle cell anemia, and asplenism.

Gram-negative meningitis (most often *Escherichia coli* and *Klebsiella-Enterobacter*) is seen after CNS surgery or trauma, bacteremia (eg, genitourinary manipulations in the elderly), and nosocomial infections, and in the immune-compromised. Staphylococcal meningitis occurs after penetrating head wounds (often as part of a mixed infection), bacteremia (eg, from endocarditis), or neurosurgery. *Listeria* meningitis is found in patients with chronic renal failure.

The **incidence** of meningitis is highest during the 1st mo of life with most infections due to *E. coli* and group B streptococcus. The relative incidence of meningitis for children remains high in the first 2 yr of life.

Pathophysiology

Bacteria reach the meninges by hematogenous spread, by extension from nearby infected structures (eg, sinusitis, epidural abscess), and by communication of CSF with the exterior (eg, myelomeningocele, spinal dermal sinus, posthypophysectomy CSF rhinorrhea). Covered with purulent exudate, the brain becomes congested, edematous, and susceptible to infarction from **venous stasis** and **thrombophlebitis**. The exudate (especially dense in the basal cisterns) can damage cranial nerves and obliterate the CSF pathways, producing **hydrocephalus**. The latter can occur late in the course or even after resolution of the infection.

Symptoms, Signs, and Complications

A prodromal respiratory illness or sore throat often precedes the fever, headache, stiff neck, and vomiting that characterize acute meningitis. Adults may become desperately ill within 24 h; the course can be even shorter in children. In older children and adults, changes in consciousness progress through irritability, confusion, drowsiness, stupor, and coma. Seizures and cranial neuropathies may be present. Dehydration is common and vascular collapse may lead to shock **(Waterhouse-Friderichsen syndrome)**, especially in meningococcal septicemia. Hemiparesis and other focal deficits can result from cerebral infarction, but their early occurrence is relatively uncommon and should suggest, for example, bacterial endocarditis or Todd's postictal paralysis.

In infants between 3 mo and 2 yr of age, symptoms and signs are less predictable. Fever, vomiting, irritability, convulsions, a high-pitched cry, and a bulging or tight fontanel are commonly present; stiff neck may be absent. **Subdural effusions** may develop after several days in infants and young children; typical signs are seizures, persistent fever, or enlarging head size. Subdural taps through the coronal sutures show a high protein content in the subdural fluid. Hydrocephalus and thrombophlebitis (see in Pathophysiology, above) also may complicate meningitis.

Diagnosis

Since acute bacterial meningitis, especially meningococcal, can be lethal in hours, accurate diagnosis and treatment are urgent. Any unexplained fever in infants between 3 mo and 2 yr of age warrants close monitoring and, if necessary, lumbar puncture. The other clinical features and risk factors outlined above should raise the suspicion of meningitis. *When bacterial meningitis is seriously suspected, antibiotics should not await the results of diagnostic tests.*

The head, ears, and skin of all patients should be inspected for sources of infection. A petechial or purpuric rash can occur in generalized septicemia, but its presence with meningeal signs indicates meningococcal meningitis until proven otherwise. The skin over the entire spine should be inspected for dimples, sinuses, nevi, or tufts of hair,

which may indicate a congenital anomaly communicating with the subarachnoid space. The joints may be involved in meningococcal or *H. influenzae* infections.

Abrupt neck flexion in the supine patient results in involuntary flexion of the knees **(Brudzinski's sign)**. Attempts to extend the knee from the flexed-thigh position are met with strong passive resistance **(Kernig's sign)**. Both signs are thought to be due to irritation of motor nerve roots passing through inflamed meninges as they are brought under tension. Unilateral or bilateral **Babinski's sign** may be present. Cranial nerve abnormalities (oculomotor or facial nerve palsy, and occasionally deafness) may be seen.

Laboratory findings: Lumbar puncture **(LP)** should be performed without delay and the CSF examined (see TABLE 117-1 and Ch. 117, which also discusses relative contraindications to LP, and use of prior CT scans). If the infectious agent is not readily seen on the CSF smear, a rapid diagnosis can sometimes be made by counterimmunoelectrophoresis (CIE) or other serologic detection of bacterial antigens in the CSF (in some laboratories, up to 80% positive in meningococcal, *H. influenzae b*, and pneumococcal meningitis). Search for an infectious source should also include cultures of blood, nasopharynx, respiratory secretions, urine, and any skin lesion. Disseminated intravascular coagulation commonly complicates meningitis and is characterized by elevations in the prothrombin and partial thromboplastin times, thrombocytopenia, decreased fibrinogen, and increased fibrin degradation products. Electrolytes should be monitored for possible syndrome of inappropriate antidiuretic hormone (SIADH).

The CT scan may be normal or show small ventricles, effacement of the sulci, and contrast enhancement over the convexities. Films should be scrutinized for evidence of sinus or mastoid infection, skull fracture, and congenital anomalies. Later, venous infarctions or communicating hydrocephalus may be seen.

Differential diagnosis: A number of disorders resemble bacterial meningitis. Acute cerebellar hemorrhage or infarction can produce tonsillar herniation and consequent nuchal rigidity followed by obstructive hydrocephalus, stupor, coma, and death. The presence of fever may be confusing. Neurologic deficits referable to the posterior fossa are diagnostic clues. If meningitis is the result of a large, ruptured brain abscess, the physician should be wary of transtentorial (uncal) herniation following LP. In these instances, measures to reduce intracranial pressure should be taken and an emergency CT obtained prior to LP if possible.

Viral infections: Differentiation of viral from bacterial CNS infections often is difficult and is based chiefly on CSF findings (see TABLE 117-1 in Ch. 117). However, partially treated meningitis presents a problem. The widespread use of antibiotics to treat minor respiratory infections has made the diagnosis of subsequent bacterial meningitis more difficult, since doses may be sufficient to partially reverse or obscure clinical meningeal symptoms and signs, and the CSF may be more nearly normal, as in a viral infection. This also poses a therapeutic dilemma, as discussed below.

Nonspecific infections in infants: LP should be performed with little hesitation if FUO is present in young children, especially infants, since clinical signs of meningitis are less likely to be present.

Subacute meningitis: The slowly evolving symptoms and the CSF findings usually differentiate subacute meningitis from acute bacterial meningitis. Other diagnostic points are discussed under SUBACUTE MENINGITIS, below.

Meningismus (**meningism** —*all the symptoms and signs of meningitis, without demonstrable meningeal infection*): This diagnosis requires that the CSF be normal. Meningismus is especially common in young children with pneumonia or shigella infections.

Lead encephalopathy: The clinical findings may mimic bacterial meningitis although onset usually is less explosive and fever is uncommon. CSF glucose usually is normal. Other symptoms, signs, and tests diagnostic of plumbism are discussed in Ch. 189.

Chemical meningitis can occur when either an epidermoid tumor or craniopharyngioma leaks its irritative contents into the CSF. Fever generally is not present. An iatrogenic source (eg, intrathecal chemotherapy) sometimes is responsible.

Subacute bacterial endocarditis (see also ENDOCARDITIS in Ch. 27) can produce fever, discrete skin lesions, focal embolic infarcts, and pleocytosis of the CSF. The apoplectic onset of neurologic deficits suggests embolism rather than venous infarction, whose evolution is not so abrupt.

Mollaret's meningitis is a rare, self-limiting, and often recurrent illness characterized by large "endothelial" cells in the CSF. Polymorphonuclear cells may be present, and later replaced by lymphocytes. Some cases are due to cryptic intracranial epitheliomas.

Prognosis and Prophylaxis

Antibiotics have reduced the fatality rate of acute bacterial meningitis to < 10% in cases recognized early. However, when meningitis is diagnosed late or occurs in neonates or the elderly, it is still frequently fatal. A low WBC count is a bad prognostic sign. Persistent leukopenia, delayed therapy, and development of the Waterhouse-Friderichsen syndrome diminish the chances of survival. Survivors occasionally show signs of cranial nerve damage, evidence of cerebral infarction, recurrent convulsions, or mental retardation. **Meningococcal vaccine** is used mainly in epidemic outbreaks and closed populations where epidemic spread is feared. Close contacts of patients with meningococcal meningitis should receive prophylactic therapy with rifampin over 2 days (adult, 600 mg bid; children 10 mg/kg bid; infants, 5 mg/kg bid). Minocycline for chemoprophylaxis is less desirable because of reported vestibular side effects. A vaccine for *H. influenzae b* has been found protective in older children, but not in children < 18 mo. Children 3 yr and younger who have had close contact with patients with *H. influenzae b* meningitis may benefit from rifampin (20 mg/kg/day taken orally for 4 days).

Treatment

1. Initial therapy should be guided by clinical circumstances and CSF results. The Gram stain usually can discriminate between meningococcus, hemophilus, pneumococcus, staphylococcus, and gram-negative organisms (see TABLE 125-1 for specific antibiotic therapy and TABLE 186-4 on p. 1892 for dosages in neonates). If the organism cannot be positively identified on smear, a combination of ampicillin (or penicillin) and chloramphenicol is given; it should be started immediately after the CSF, blood, and other pertinent body fluids have been cultured; it should never await the results of various other tests (eg, CT) when the patient is desperately ill.

Treatment decision problems arise when CSF pleocytosis, normal glucose content, and the absence of bacteria make it difficult to determine whether viral meningitis, partially treated bacterial infections, or early bacterial meningitis is the diagnosis. Counterimmunoelectrophoresis capabilities vary between laboratories, and a negative result does not exclude bacterial meningitis. Since antibiotics can cause anaphylactic reactions, drug fever, and difficulty in evaluating the response to therapy, it may be advisable, *if the patient's condition permits it*, to withhold antibiotics and examine the CSF in 8 to 12 h, or sooner if his condition deteriorates. If CSF glucose remains normal and no organisms grow on culture, it is best to continue without antibiotics on the assumption that the infection is not bacterial. However, if the patient's condition is serious, and especially if he has already received antibiotics that may hinder the growth of organisms on culture, a bacterial infection must be assumed and treatment begun with ampicillin or another appropriate antibiotic.

2. Specific therapy: (For dosages, see TABLE 125-1.) Once the organism is identified, penicillin G may be substituted for ampicillin in infections caused by meningococci, pneumococci, β-hemolytic streptococci, and susceptible staphylococci. Penicillinase-producing staphylococci should be treated with oxacillin or nafcillin. Because an in-

TABLE 125–1. ANTIBIOTIC THERAPY FOR ACUTE BACTERIAL MENINGITIS

Organism	Antibiotic	Total Daily Dose (Pediatric Doses in Parentheses)	Frequency of Fractional Dosage
Unknown:			
Infant < 1 mo	Ampicillin	100 mg/kg IV (0–7 days old)	q 12 h
		150–200 mg/kg IV (> 7 days old)	q 6 h
	and Gentamicin	5 mg/kg IV	q 8 h
	or Tobramycin	5 mg/kg IV	q 8 h
	or Amikacin*	15 mg/kg IV	q 8 h
	or Cefotaxime	200 mg/kg IV	q 6 h
Child < 10 yr	Ampicillin	300–400 mg/kg IV	q 4 h
	and Chloramphenicol†	100 mg/kg IV	q 6 h
Adult	Chloramphenicol†	4–6 gm IV	q 6 h
	and Penicillin G	24 million u. IV	q 2 h
	or Ampicillin	12–14 gm IV	q 3–4 h
Gram-negative Rods in CSF (Unidentified)	Cefotaxime	12 gm IV (200 mg/kg IV)	q 4–6 h
	and Gentamicin	(doses as above)	
	or Tobramycin	(doses as above)	
	or Amikacin*	(doses as above)	
Meningococcus	Penicillin G	24 million u. IV (400,000 u./kg IV)	q 2 h
H. influenzae	Ampicillin and Chloramphenicol†	(doses as above)	
Streptococcus (Pneumococcus)	Penicillin G or Ampicillin	(doses as above)	
Staphylococcus	Oxacillin	12 gm IV (300 mg/kg IV)	q 4 h
	or Nafcillin	12 gm IV (300 mg/kg IV)	q 4 h
	or Vancomycin§	2 gm IV (60 mg/kg IV)	q 6 h

(Continued)

* In areas where gentamicin resistance is common. Because CSF penetration is poor, aminoglycosides may have to be administered intrathecally or via an Ommaya reservoir, especially with *Pseudomonas* meningtis.

† Until antibiotic sensitivities are known, after which cefotaxime or another 3rd-generation cephalosporin may be substituted.

§ Penicillin allergy.

TABLE 125–1. ANTIBIOTIC THERAPY FOR ACUTE BACTERIAL MENINGITIS (INCLUDING COMMON ENCEPHALITIDES) *(Cont'd)*

Organism	*Antibiotic*	***Total Daily Dose*** *(Pediatric Doses in Parentheses)*	*Frequency of* ***Fractional*** *Dosage*
Listeria	Ampicillin or Penicillin G	(doses as above) (doses as above)	
E. coli	Cefotaxime or Gentamicin and Chloramphenicol†	(doses as above) (doses as above) (doses as above)	
Pseudomonas	Azlocillin	18 gm IV (300 mg/kg IV)	q 4 h
	or Piperacillin	18 gm IV (300 mg/kg IV)	q 4 h
	or Carbenicillin	30–40 gm IV (200 mg/kg IV; 0–7 days old) (300–400 mg/kg IV; infant) (400–500 mg/kg IV; child)	q 2 h q 2 h q 2 h
	or Ticarcillin	200–300 mg/kg IV (150–225 mg/kg IV; 0–7 days old) (225–300 mg/kg IV; > 7 days old)	q 3 h q 8–12 h q 4–6 h
	with Gentamicin or Tobramycin or Amikacin*	(doses as above) (doses as above) (doses as above)	
Proteus	Chloramphenicol† with Gentamicin† or Tobramycin or Amikacin*	(doses as above) (doses as above) (doses as above) (doses as above)	

creasing number of *H. influenzae* strains are resistant to ampicillin, both chloramphenicol and ampicillin should be given for initial treatment of bacterial meningitis in children. Subsequent therapy can be modified in accordance with culture results and susceptibility testing. Cefotaxime and cefuroxime may be effective alternatives, especially in penicillin-allergic patients (if patients are allergic to cephalosporins, chloramphenicol may substitute).

If gram-negative rods are seen in the CSF, therapy should begin with cefotaxime, which covers many gram-negative organisms (but not *Pseudomonas* and *Acinetobacter*). Cefotaxime and other "third-generation" cephalosporins appear to be as active as the

aminoglycosides without their nephro- and ototoxicity. *Pseudomonas* coverage can be achieved by concurrent use of azlocillin, piperacillin, carbenicillin, or ticarcillin with gentamicin, tobramycin, or amikacin. Amikacin should be used in hospitals where gentamicin resistance of enteric organisms is common.

Antibiotics should be continued for at least 1 wk after fever subsides and the CSF returns to normal. Drug dosages should not be reduced too early, since drug penetration in many instances will decrease as the meninges become less inflamed.

3. Supportive therapy: Dehydration and electrolyte disorders require correction (see Chs. 84 and 185). Care must be taken not to overhydrate individuals with cerebral edema. Convulsions and status epilepticus are treated appropriately (see Ch. 121, and SEIZURE DISORDERS IN THE NEWBORN in Ch. 186).

Vascular collapse and shock (Waterhouse-Friderichsen syndrome): Although attributed to adrenal insufficiency, loss of tissue fluid may be equally important, and the value of ACTH and corticosteroids remains controversial.

Cerebral edema, severe enough to produce central or transtentorial herniation, can be treated with controlled hyperventilation, osmotic agents, and dexamethasone.

In infants with subdural effusion, the fluid usually subsides with repeated daily subdural taps through the sutures. To avoid sudden shifts in the intracranial contents, not more than 20 mL/day of CSF should be removed from one side. If the effusion persists after 3 to 4 wk of taps, surgical exploration is indicated.

ACUTE VIRAL ENCEPHALITIS AND ASEPTIC MENINGITIS

Encephalitis: *An acute inflammatory disease of the brain due to direct viral invasion or to hypersensitivity initiated by a virus or other foreign protein.* **Encephalomyelitis**: *The same disorder affecting spinal cord structures as well as the brain.* **Aseptic meningitis**: *A febrile meningeal inflammation characterized by CSF pleocytosis, normal glucose, and an absence of bacteria on examination and culture.*

Etiology

Virus infection may cause encephalitis as a primary manifestation or as a secondary complication. Viruses causing **primary encephalitis** may be epidemic (arbo-, polio-, echo-, and coxsackie viruses) or sporadic (herpes simplex, herpes zoster). Arbovirus encephalitides (St. Louis, Eastern and Western equine, and California) are mosquito-borne and infect man only during warm weather. (These agents are also discussed in Ch. 12.)

Most cases of **secondary encephalitis** occur as a complication of viral infection and are considered to have an immunologic mechanism. Examples are the encephalitides following measles, chickenpox, rubella, smallpox vaccination, vaccinia, and many other less well defined virus infections. These **parainfectious** or **postinfectious encephalitides** typically develop 5 to 10 days after onset of illness and are characterized by perivascular demyelination in the brains of patients who succumb; a virus has rarely been isolated from the brain. (The condition is sometimes referred to as **acute disseminated encephalomyelitis** and is classified with the primary demyelinating diseases—see in Ch. 127.) In mumps, both primary and postinfectious CNS involvement may occur.

Meningitis with CSF findings of pleocytosis, normal glucose, and no evidence of bacterial organisms (hence, **"aseptic"**) may be due not only to viral infections (see also ENTEROVIRAL DISEASES in Ch. 191) but also to other organisms and noninfectious causes (see TABLE 125–2).

Very rarely, encephalitis or other encephalopathies occur as a late consequence of viral infections. The best known of these are **subacute sclerosing panencephalitis** (**SSPE**—see in Ch. 191), associated with the measles virus; **kuru**, a "slow virus" infec-

TABLE 125–2. CAUSES OF ASEPTIC MENINGITIS (INCLUDING COMMON ENCEPHALITIDES)

Infectious

Virus: Mumps, echovirus, poliovirus, coxsackievirus, lymphocytic choriomeningitis, herpes simplex, herpes zoster, Eastern and Western equine, St. Louis, infectious hepatitis, infectious mononucleosis

Postinfectious: Measles, rubella, varicella, smallpox, vaccinia

Bacterial: Tuberculosis, syphilis, partially treated bacterial meningitis

Miscellaneous infections: Leptospirosis, toxoplasmosis, torulosis, trichinosis, syphilis, coccidioidomycosis, mycoplasma, lymphogranuloma venereum, cat-scratch disease

Noninfectious

Parameningeal disease: Brain tumor, stroke, multiple sclerosis, abscess, chronic sinusitis or otitis

Reaction to intrathecal injections: Air, serum, antibiotics, iophendylate and other dyes

Poison: Lead

Vaccine reactions: Many, especially rabies, pertussis, smallpox

Meningeal disease: Sarcoidosis, meningeal leukemia, meningeal carcinomatosis

tion seen in New Guinea, and **Creutzfeldt-Jakob disease**, a rare dementia of middle age. (The latter 2 encephalitides are discussed in SLOW VIRUS INFECTIONS in Ch. 12.)

Pathology

Cerebral edema is present, and numerous petechial hemorrhages are scattered throughout the hemispheres, brainstem, cerebellum, and occasionally the spinal cord. Direct viral invasion of the brain is likely to be associated with neuron necrosis, and, frequently, with visible inclusion bodies. In para- and postinfectious encephalomyelitis, perivenous demyelinating lesions are characteristic.

Symptoms and Signs

CNS viral infections may take 3 forms: (1) **Asymptomatic**, with no symptoms; or fever and malaise may be present with no meningeal clinical manifestations. The CSF, however, may be abnormal, with lymphocytic pleocytosis, and a virus may be isolated from the CSF. (2) **Meningitis**: Fever, headache, vomiting, malaise, and stiff neck and back may be the predominant symptoms. (3) **Encephalitis**: Meningitis may be associated with evidence of cerebral dysfunction (alteration in consciousness, personality change, seizures, paresis) and cranial nerve abnormalities. The distinction between aseptic meningitis and encephalitis is based on the extent and severity of cerebral dysfunction, independent of signs of meningeal inflammation.

Diagnosis

Viral CNS infections must be differentiated from nonviral and noninfectious causes (see TABLE 125–2), but the major diagnostic problem is differentiation from acute or partially treated bacterial meningitis (see ACUTE BACTERIAL MENINGITIS above, and TABLE 117-1 in Ch. 117). Diagnosis usually is based on the CSF characteristics, including normal glucose and failure to grow bacteria on culture. Viruses occasionally are isolated directly from the CSF or from other tissues, but even under ideal circumstances, viruses causing aseptic meningitis and encephalitis are identified in fewer than half the cases. A precise diagnosis usually requires the use of paired sera documenting a rise in antibodies. Since many forms of encephalitis and aseptic meningitis have important public health implications, serum should be drawn and preserved whenever

the diagnosis of encephalitis or aseptic meningitis of uncertain etiology is first suspected. Information regarding more precise viral diagnosis can be obtained from local departments of health.

Although **herpes simplex encephalitis** is clinically similar to other viral encephalitides, repeated seizures occurring early in the course, and localizing signs indicating temporal or frontal lobe involvement, strongly suggest herpes simplex as the cause. The presence of erythrocytes in the CSF following an atraumatic spinal tap also suggests herpes simplex infection. The virus is rarely present in the CSF, and serologic tests are not sufficient to implicate herpes simplex virus, since antibody levels normally fluctuate even in healthy persons. Diagnosis is certain only upon demonstration of the virus (by recovery of the virus or immunologic technics) in cerebral tissue obtained by brain biopsy or at postmortem examination.

Prognosis and Treatment

Even desperately ill patients may recover completely. The mortality rate varies with the etiology, and epidemics with the same virus vary in severity in different years. Permanent cerebral disorders are more likely to occur in infants, but young children show improvement over a longer period than adults with similar infections.

Treatment of herpes simplex encephalitis is discussed in ANTIVIRAL DRUGS in Ch. 3. Supportive therapy is as for acute bacterial meningitis (see above). Fluid balance should be maintained but overhydration avoided.

SUBACUTE MENINGITIS

Meningitis in which the duration of the disease, in the absence of antibiotics, is > 2 wk but < 3 mo.

Etiology

Subacute meningitis may occur with systemic fungal infections; TB; dissemination of malignant cells, as in leukemia, metastatic carcinoma (especially of lung and breast), or primary brain tumors such as gliomas; syphilis; sarcoidosis.

A marked increase in fungal CNS infections has paralleled the decline of TB and accompanied the increase in immunosuppressive therapy. *Cryptococcus* is the most common offender; *Coccidioides*, Mucorales, *Candida*, *Actinomyces*, and *Aspergillus* are encountered occasionally. Cryptococcal meningitis may be a complication of Hodgkin's disease or other lymphomas.

Neoplastic meningitis with diffuse leptomeningeal involvement is a continuing problem in acute lymphoblastic leukemia, especially in leukemic children being treated with antileukemic drugs, which do not cross the blood-brain barrier. Neoplastic meningitis also may occur with gliomas (particularly glioblastoma, ependymoma, or medulloblastoma) or with carcinoma metastatic to the brain. Rarely, the first sign of malignant disease may be a subacute meningeal inflammation.

Symptoms and Signs

Manifestations are similar to those in acute meningitis, but the illness evolves more slowly—over a period of weeks rather than days. Fever may be minimal. Chronic communicating hydrocephalus may be a complication. In neoplastic meningitis, headache, dementia, and cranial and peripheral nerve palsies are common, and the course is progressive; death occurs within a few weeks or months after the onset of symptoms.

Diagnosis

Because of the slow evolution of cerebral symptoms, the differential diagnosis includes structural lesions such as brain tumors, abscesses, and subdural effusions. Active TB elsewhere in the body or a known malignancy suggests the etiology, but the CSF must be examined to establish a diagnosis unless contraindicated by evidence of

increased intracranial pressure from an expanding lesion. The CSF cell count is generally < 1000/μL with lymphocytes predominant; glucose frequently is low except in syphilis, and protein may be high. Besides lymphocytic pleocytosis, CSF findings in neoplastic meningitis include low glucose, slightly elevated protein, and, frequently, elevated pressure; at times, tumor cells may be found. Microscopic examination or culture of the CSF is needed to identify malignant cells or a causative organism. Fungi frequently can be identified by examination of a centrifuged sediment; TB can be identified by acid-fast or immunofluorescent staining. In syphilis, CSF pressure, cell count, and protein resemble findings in other subacute meningitides but the CSF glucose usually is normal; CSF and blood Venereal Disease Research Laboratory (VDRL) tests and STS are positive in most patients. Since most causative infections must be treated over a prolonged period with highly specific drugs, precise identification of the organism is essential before therapy is begun.

Treatment

Tuberculous meningitis: See EXTRAPULMONARY TUBERCULOSIS in Ch. 8. **Syphilitic meningitis**: See Ch. 14. **Lyme disease**: See Ch. 108. **Leukemic meningitis**: See THE ACUTE LEUKEMIAS in Ch. 101.

Sarcoid meningitis: Prednisone 80 mg/day orally is given for 3 wk, then decreased by 5 mg/day every 3 days.

***Actinomyces* meningitis**: The drug of choice is penicillin G, 20 million u./day IM or IV (200,000 u./kg/day for children), given for at least 6 wk. Treatment may be continued for an additional 2 to 3 mo with penicillin V, 1 to 2 million u./day orally (proportionately less for children).

Mycotic meningitis: Amphotericin B is the drug of choice for all fungi and yeasts. Starting at 50 mg/day, amphotericin B is given by slow IV infusion in gradually increasing doses as tolerated. (CAUTION: *Daily dosage should not exceed 1.5 mg/kg for adults and 1 mg/kg for children. See General Therapeutic Principles in Ch. 9 for other information on administration and other precautions.*) A total of 4 to 6 gm usually is given, but the optimal total dose is uncertain. Treatment duration need not exceed 10 wk if the blood level of amphotericin B can be maintained at a concentration at least twice that needed to inhibit growth of the fungus in culture. Although hazardous, intrathecal or intraventricular (via Ommaya reservoir) amphotericin B sometimes is necessary to eradicate the infection.

BRAIN ABSCESS

An intracerebral encapsulated collection of pus.

Etiology and Pathology

As in meningitis, a brain abscess can arise from direct extension of a cranial infection (eg, osteomyelitis, mastoiditis, sinusitis, subdural empyema), from penetrating head wounds, or from a blood-borne source (eg, bacterial endocarditis, bronchiectasis, congenital heart disease with right to left shunt, repeated IV drug abuse).

The brain parenchyma shows a poorly localized, inflammatory response (cerebritis) that subsequently becomes necrotic and encapsulated by glia and fibroblasts. Days or weeks later, edema around the abscess gives rise to increased intracranial pressure with signs and symptoms resembling those seen in brain tumor. The bacteria isolated from abscesses usually are anaerobic (*pus should be cultured under anaerobic conditions*), not uncommonly mixed, and often include anaerobic *Streptococcus* or *Bacteroides*. Fungal abscesses occur as well.

Symptoms, Signs, and Diagnosis

Headache, nausea, vomiting, papilledema, lethargy, seizures, and focal neurologic deficits develop over days to weeks. Fever, chills, and leukocytosis may subside once

the infected brain is encapsulated. Clinical suspicion should be raised whenever an antecedent infection or risk factor is present.

CSF findings commonly include increased pressure, mild pleocytosis (average, 135 cells/μL), and mild elevation of protein. CSF glucose usually is not decreased, and bacteria can only occasionally be cultured from the CSF. If the abscess is well encapsulated and remote from CSF pathways, the CSF may be normal.

Primary or metastatic brain tumor, subdural effusion, cerebrovascular disease, subacute and chronic meningitis, and degenerative diseases must be excluded.

Treatment

Brain abscess is fatal unless treated. Antibiotics should include penicillin G 24 million u./day IV and chloramphenicol 4 gm/day IV, if a penicillin-resistant organism is suspected. Response to antibiotics can be followed by serial CT scanning, and surgical drainage used in those patients who fail therapy or threaten to develop transtentorial herniation. Antibiotics should be continued for a minimum of 4 to 8 wk.

NEUROLOGIC COMPLICATIONS OF ACQUIRED IMMUNODEFICIENCY SYNDROME (AIDS)

For the major discussion of AIDS, see Ch. 19. Neurologic symptoms not infrequently are the first manifestation of AIDS and commonly occur during its course. Infections, neoplasms, vascular complications, aseptic meningitis, and neuropathy are among the more prominent sequelae.

CNS infections: The most common treatable neurologic illness is **toxoplasma encephalitis**. Headache, lethargy, confusion, seizures, and focal signs evolve over days to weeks. Chorioretinitis may be present from toxoplasma (or cytomegalovirus); cotton wool retinopathy also occurs. CT findings include ring-enhancing lesions with a predilection for basal ganglia. Serologic tests (eg, Sabin-Feldman) may be positive but do not always provide conclusive proof. The CSF shows a mild to moderate pleocytosis and elevated protein content. Brain biopsy can be diagnostic. Treatment is with pyrimethamine and sulfadiazine (or clindamycin if the patient is allergic to sulfa). Prognosis is at best guarded, since recurrence is possible and other complications of AIDS are likely. **Cryptococcal and tuberculous meningitides** (*Mycobacterium avium–intracellulare*) also occur in AIDS. Progressive multifocal leukoencephalopathy and infections with *Candida*, *Aspergillus*, and gram-negative organisms occur less frequently.

The most common neurologic complication is a lethal **subacute encephalitis** whose etiology is presumed to be infectious. The gray matter exhibits nodular collections of "microglial cells" without other inflammatory infiltrates. Intranuclear and intracytoplasmic inclusions, similar to those seen with cytomegalovirus infection, have been observed within the nodules. Small, poorly defined foci of perivenular demyelination are found in white matter. Memory loss, confusion, psychomotor retardation, myoclonus, seizures, and dementia progressing to coma are typical findings spanning weeks to months prior to death. Moderate cortical atrophy on CT, CSF pleocytosis and elevated protein, and a diffusely abnormal EEG are often, albeit inconsistently, found, but are nonspecific. No treatment exists.

Neoplasms: Primary CNS lymphoma is a frequent intracranial mass lesion in AIDS. It may be clinically silent or produce focal signs consistent with its anatomic location. CT usually shows a contrast-enhancing mass that cannot always be distinguished from abscess or other lesions; in these cases, MRI may be more discriminating.

Systemic lymphomas occur in AIDS, and often spread to the CNS. Metastases to the skull, brain, epidural space, and meninges produce complications. Kaposi's sarcoma rarely involves the CNS.

Vascular complications: Nonbacterial endocarditis, usually with neoplasm or severe infection, can produce transient ischemic attacks and focal ischemic stroke. Cerebral

hemorrhage can occur in thrombocytopenic states (eg, lymphoma, idiopathic thrombocytopenic purpura).

Aseptic meningitis: Rapid onset of headache, fever, stiff neck, and sometimes 7th nerve paralysis may be associated with a CSF mononuclear pleocytosis, elevated proteins, slightly depressed or normal glucose, and consistently negative cytologies and cultures. The episodes are transient, but can be recurrent.

Peripheral neuropathy: Painful dysesthesias, moderate distal sensory loss (stocking-glove), depressed ankle reflexes, distal weakness, and atrophy can occur in varying degrees, and can coincide with rapid weight loss from poor nutrition; no metabolic etiology has been identified. A Guillain-Barré type of neuropathy has been reported.

Myopathy similar to polymyositis is seen rarely in AIDS.

Treatment: Most CNS complications of AIDS respond poorly to treatment or not at all, since the primary immune defect remains uncorrected. The prognosis is poor.

---

126. CNS NEOPLASMS

INTRACRANIAL NEOPLASMS
(Brain Tumors)

An expanding intracranial lesion may be a granuloma, parasitic cyst, hemorrhage (intracerebral, extradural, or subdural), aneurysm, abscess, or neoplasm (metastatic or primary). Neoplasms are common and are frequently misdiagnosed.

Primary intracranial neoplasms are divided into 6 classes: tumors of (1) the skull (osteoma, hemangioma, granuloma, xanthoma, osteitis deformans); (2) the meninges (meningioma, sarcoma, gliomatosis); (3) the cranial nerves (glioma of the optic nerve, schwannoma [neurilemoma] of the 8th and 5th cranial nerves); (4) the supportive tissue (gliomas); (5) the pituitary or pineal body (pituitary adenoma, pinealoma); and (6) congenital origin (craniopharyngioma, chordoma, germinoma, teratoma, dermoid cyst, angioma, hemangioblastoma).

Secondary metastases may involve the skull or any intracranial structure.

Pathology and Incidence

CNS changes result from invasion and destruction by the tumor and from its secondary effects (increased intracranial pressure, cerebral edema, and compression of brain tissue, cranial nerves, and cerebral vessels).

Brain tumors are found in about 2% of routine autopsies. They may occur at any age but are most common in early adult or middle life. **Common primary childhood tumors** are cerebellar astrocytomas and medulloblastomas, ependymomas, gliomas of the brainstem and optic nerve, germinomas (pinealomas), and congenital tumors. The most **common metastatic invaders in childhood** are neuroblastoma (usually epidural) and leukemia (meningeal). **Primary adult tumors** include meningiomas, schwannomas, gliomas of the cerebral hemispheres (particularly the malignant glioblastoma multiforme, anaplastic astrocytoma, and the more benign astrocytoma and oligodendroglioma). **Metastatic tumors in adults** arise most commonly from bronchogenic carcinoma, adenocarcinoma of the breast, and malignant melanoma.

The relative frequency of various types of intracranial tumors is gliomas 45%, pituitary adenomas 15%, meningiomas 15%, schwannomas 7%, congenital tumors 3%, metastatic and other types 15%. Overall incidence in males and females is about equal, but cerebellar medulloblastoma and glioblastoma multiforme are more common in males; meningioma and schwannoma, in females.

Symptoms and Signs

1. General symptoms and signs result from increased intracranial pressure. This may be due to the space-occupying tumor mass itself or to associated cerebral edema, obstructed flow of CSF (occurring early in 3rd ventricle or posterior fossa tumors), obstructed dural venous sinuses (especially by bony or extradural metastatic tumors), or obstructed CSF absorption mechanisms (as in leukemic or carcinomatous involvement of the meninges). Headache and vomiting result, as may mental symptoms. Papilledema develops in about 25% of patients with brain tumor and may not be an early sign; its absence does not rule out a tumor or elevated intracranial pressure. In young children, elevated intracranial pressure may enlarge the head. Intracranial pressure is usually normal in patients with small tumors of the cerebral hemispheres, pituitary adenomas, or brainstem tumors that do not obstruct the aqueduct of Sylvius. Changes in temperature, pulse or respiratory rate, or BP are unusual except terminally.

Convulsive seizures, either focal or generalized, occur with cerebral hemisphere tumors and may precede other symptoms by months or years. They are more frequent with meningiomas and slowly growing astrocytomas than with malignant gliomas. Focal seizures help to locate the tumor.

Mental symptoms (eg, drowsiness, lethargy, obtuseness, personality changes, disordered conduct, impaired mental faculties, psychotic episodes) may appear at any time. They are the initial symptoms in 25% of malignant brain tumors.

2. Special (focal) symptoms and signs are due to localized destruction or compression of nervous tissue or to altered endocrine function, and depend on the location of the tumor.

A. Tumors of the cerebral hemispheres: Frontal lobe tumors (commonly meningiomas or gliomas) involving the frontal convexity are characterized by progressive hemiplegia, focal or generalized seizures, and mental changes. Expressive aphasia may accompany a tumor of the dominant hemisphere. A tumor at the base of the frontal lobes (particularly meningioma of the olfactory groove) produces ipsilateral anosmia. A tumor on the medial surface of a frontal lobe may cause precipitate urination. Mental changes (especially inattention and loss of motivation) and ataxic gait are common when the tumor spreads across the corpus callosum to both frontal lobes. Meningioma of the tuberculum sellae may compress the optic chiasm, producing a visual field defect similar to that of a pituitary adenoma (see Tumors of the Pituitary and Suprasellar Region, below). Meningioma of the inner third of the sphenoid ridge may cause exophthalmos and unilateral amblyopia. Meningioma of the outer part of the sphenoid ridge may invade the temporal lobe (see Temporal lobe tumors, below).

Parietal lobe tumors may produce either generalized convulsions or sensory focal seizures. Cutaneous tactile, pain, and temperature senses are unimpaired, but stereognosis and the cortical sensory modalities (position sense, 2-point discrimination) are impaired contralaterally. Contralateral homonymous hemianopia, apraxia, and anosognosia (nonrecognition of bodily defects) may also be present. Denial of illness is characteristic, especially if obtundation is present. Speech disturbances, agraphia, and finger agnosia may occur when the tumor involves the dominant hemisphere.

Temporal lobe tumors, particularly in the nondominant hemisphere, are often relatively "silent" except when they cause convulsive seizures. A tumor deep in the temporal lobe may cause contralateral hemianopia, psychomotor seizures, or convulsive seizures preceded by an olfactory aura or visual hallucinations of complex formed images. Tumors involving the surface of the dominant temporal lobe produce mixed expressive and receptive aphasia or dysphasia, chiefly anomia.

Occipital lobe tumors usually cause a contralateral quadrant defect in the visual field or a hemianopia with sparing of the macula. Associated convulsions may be preceded by an aura of flashing lights, but not formed images.

Subcortical tumors commonly involve the internal capsule and produce contralateral hemiplegia. They may invade any of the lobes of the hemisphere, producing corresponding symptoms. Thalamic invasion produces contralateral cutaneous sensory impairment. Invasion of the basal ganglia usually does not produce parkinsonian symptoms, but athetosis, bizarre tremors, or dystonic postures are occasionally present.

Cranial, extradural, or subdural metastatic tumors, by compressing or invading the underlying cortex, may produce the same localizing signs as those caused by a primary cortical tumor.

Herniation syndromes may be produced as lesions enlarge and brain tissue is displaced through the fixed intracranial openings. Thus, the medial surface of a hemisphere may be forced beneath the falx cerebri. **Transtentorial herniation** occurs with displacement of brain tissue through the tentorial notch. In **central herniation,** there is symmetric bilateral tissue displacement, while **temporal lobe herniation** is an asymmetric displacement of a cone of temporal lobe tissue through the tentorial notch. Both types of herniation compress vital brainstem structures. Central herniation leads to coma, mid-position fixed pupils, altered respiration, loss of oculocephalic and oculovestibular reflexes (failure of the eyes to move in response to head rotation or to caloric stimulation, respectively), and bilateral motor paralysis (decerebrate rigidity or flaccidity). Temporal lobe herniation may produce an early 3rd nerve palsy (unilateral dilated fixed pupil and extraocular paralysis) in addition to the central signs. Less commonly, a cerebellar cone may be forced through the foramen magnum, producing respiratory and cardiac arrest.

False localizing signs may accompany prolonged elevated intracranial pressure. They include uni- or bilateral lateral rectus palsy from 6th nerve compression, hemiplegia on the same side as the tumor from compression of the opposite cerebral peduncle against the tentorium, and visual field defect on the same side as the tumor from compromise of the opposite posterior cerebral artery.

B. Tumors of the pituitary and suprasellar region: Pituitary adenomas may present as intrasellar secretory or nonsecretory masses, or masses with extrasellar extension. Secretory adenomas produce hormones that cause specific endocrinopathies. Traditionally, adenomas with particular histologic staining characteristics have been associated with specific endocrinopathies: Eg, **acidophilic adenoma** overproduces growth hormone, leading to gigantism prior to puberty, acromegaly after puberty; **basophilic adenoma** overproduces ACTH, leading to Cushing's syndrome. **Chromophobe adenomas** were thought not to secrete hormones, but are now known to be responsible for most of the endocrinopathies caused by pituitary tumors. The most common endocrine hypersecretion is prolactin, producing amenorrhea and galactorrhea in women and, less frequently, impotence and gynecomastia in men. Many secretory tumors are microadenomas, found only after an endocrine abnormality is discovered (see under GALACTORRHEA in Ch. 88).

Enlarging pituitary adenomas cause headache. As the tumor grows out of the sella, it compresses the optic chiasm, nerves, or tracts, and the hypothalamus. The common visual field defect is bitemporal hemianopia, but unilateral optic atrophy, contralateral hemianopia, or any combination of the 3 may occur. Hypothalamic compression usually causes diabetes insipidus from injury to the supraoptic-pituitary tract. The tumor may destroy functioning glandular tissue and cause pituitary deficiency. X-rays show a characteristic balloon-shaped appearance of the sella, but microadenomas may only cause laterally placed focal bulging of the sella floor, visible only on tomograms.

Other tumors in the region of the sella turcica (eg, meningiomas, craniopharyngiomas, metastases, dermoid cysts) or aneurysms may compress the optic chiasm, invade the sella, and produce symptoms similar to those of chromophobic adenoma.

C. Pineal tumors (usually germinomas) occur at any age, but are most common in childhood. Precocious puberty may result, especially in boys. The tumor compresses the aqueduct of Sylvius, causing hydrocephalus, papilledema, and other signs of increased intracranial pressure. The pretectum rostral to the superior colliculi is also compressed, resulting in paralysis of upward gaze, ptosis, and loss of pupillary light and accommodation reflexes.

D. Tumors of the brainstem: Gliomas of the brainstem are usually astrocytomas. Common symptoms, resulting from destruction of nuclear masses, are unilateral or bilateral paralysis of the 5th, 6th, 7th, and 10th cranial nerves, and paralysis of lateral gaze. Damage to the motor or sensory pathways causes hemiplegia, hemianesthesia, or cerebellar disturbances (ataxia, nystagmus, intention tremor). Increased intracranial pressure appears late in brainstem tumors.

E. Posterior fossa tumors: Tumors of the 4th ventricle and cerebellum (usually medulloblastomas, gliomas, ependymomas, or metastases) interfere with CSF circulation, and symptoms of increased intracranial pressure appear early. Ataxic gait, intention tremor, and other signs of cerebellar dysfunction follow.

Cerebellopontine angle tumors, particularly neurilemomas (acoustic neurinomas, schwannomas), are characterized by tinnitus, unilateral hearing impairment, and, sometimes, vertigo. Pressure on the adjacent cranial nerves, brainstem, and cerebellum produces loss of corneal reflex, facial palsy and anesthesia, palatal weakness, signs of cerebellar dysfunction, and, rarely, contralateral hemiplegia or hemianesthesia. Loss of vestibular response to caloric stimulation, enlargement of the porus acusticus as shown by x-ray, and high CSF protein content suggest an acoustic neurilemoma (see also ACOUSTIC NEURINOMA in Ch. 207).

F. Meningeal neoplasm: See SUBACUTE MENINGITIS in Ch. 125.

Diagnosis

A brain tumor should be considered and neurologic consultation requested for patients with slowly progressive signs of focal cerebral dysfunction, focal or generalized convulsions, headaches of recent onset, or other evidence of increased intracranial pressure (eg, vomiting, papilledema).

Studies should include a complete neurologic examination, testing of visual acuity and visual fields, audiometric tests, a CT scan, and x-rays of the chest (for a source of metastases). MRI may detect low-grade astrocytomas before they are visible on CT scanning. Cerebral angiography may be necessary as a preoperative measure, less often for diagnosis.

CSF examination is unnecessary if the diagnosis is obvious but may be useful if the diagnosis or the nature of the lesion is not clear after preliminary studies; it is essential in the diagnosis of chronic or subacute neoplastic meningitis or benign intracranial hypertension (**pseudotumor cerebri**—see below). Lumbar puncture is **contraindicated** in the presence of papilledema if an expanding lesion is suspected, since the sudden pressure change in such instances can precipitate a herniation syndrome.

Treatment

Treatment of brain tumor is surgical excision or irradiation. Firm, encapsulated tumors (eg, meningiomas, schwannomas) and congenital tumors are potentially benign and not affected by irradiation. Except in older patients where meningiomas fail to enlarge over long periods of time, they should be excised if at all possible at the time of diagnosis. Infiltrating gliomas cannot be completely extirpated surgically; partial removal should be followed by x-ray therapy. If the tumor is inaccessible, as in the thalamus or brainstem, irradiation is the primary therapy. Pituitary tumors may be removed by trans-sphenoidal microsurgery or craniotomy. They may also be treated by irradiation alone or irradiation after surgery. Surgery is indicated if vision is threat-

ened, but the method of treatment of microadenomas is controversial. Treatment of pituitary adenomas is discussed in Ch. 88. The treatment of meningeal carcinomatosis remains investigational, but usually includes radiation therapy and intrathecal chemotherapy, often via an indwelling intraventricular reservoir.

If neurologic or neurosurgical consultation is not readily available, temporary measures may be necessary to relieve increased intracranial pressure and prevent herniation. Mannitol 25 to 100 gm infused IV is given to relieve pressure immediately, and should be accompanied by a corticosteroid (eg, dexamethasone 16 mg/day orally or parenterally, or prednisone 60 to 80 mg/day orally, in divided doses) to maintain the reduced pressure. Lumbar puncture is **contraindicated** for reduction of intracranial pressure accompanying brain neoplasms.

PSEUDOTUMOR CEREBRI

(Benign Intracranial Hypertension)

A disorder characterized by increased intracranial pressure in the absence of any evidence of intracranial space-occupying lesion, obstruction of the ventricular or subarachnoid pathways, infection, or hypertensive encephalopathy. Etiology in most instances is unknown; the syndrome undoubtedly includes several disorders of different causes. Generally, however, both onset and eventual disappearance are spontaneous. The condition is more common in women between ages 20 and 50, and especially affects those who are overweight. Symptoms consist of headache of varying severity (often mild), papilledema, and the appearance of generally good health. Partial or complete monocular visual loss occurs in about 5% of patients, and is the only serious neurologic sign. On the other hand, the blind spots are frequently enlarged. CT scans generally are normal, or show a somewhat small ventricular system. EEG is normal. The lumbar puncture pressure is elevated, and the fluid is normal. A similar picture can be the result of occlusion of an intracranial venous sinus involving the posterior third of the sagittal sinus or one of the circumflex sinuses; increased intracranial pressure secondary to chronic CO_2 retention and hypoxia; and other less well established abnormalities, including iron-deficiency anemia and hypoparathyroidism. In children, pseudotumor can follow corticosteroid withdrawal or the excessive ingestion of vitamin A or tetracycline. **Treatment** varies according to the cause, but once the diagnosis is made, the syndrome generally has no serious consequences and can be managed symptomatically. However, visual loss, if it occurs, may be permanent regardless of treatment. Pseudotumor recurs in about 10% of cases.

SPINAL CORD NEOPLASMS

Lesions that compress the spinal cord or its roots, arising from the cord parenchyma, roots, meninges, or vertebrae.

Pathology and Incidence

Primary neoplasms of the spinal cord are much less common than intracranial tumors and are rare in childhood or old age. Only about 10% of spinal tumors are intramedullary. Meningiomas and neurofibromas account for about 2/3 of all primary spinal tumors; others include gliomas and sarcomas. Extradural metastatic lesions are not uncommon; they may accompany carcinoma of the lung, breast, prostate, kidney, or thyroid, or lymphoma (Hodgkin's disease, lymphosarcoma, and reticulum cell sarcoma).

Symptoms and Signs

Extramedullary neoplasms: The first symptoms are usually from compression of nerve roots—pain and paresthesias followed by sensory loss, muscular weakness, and wasting along the distribution of the affected roots. Tumor growth leads to cord com-

pression, causing progressive spastic weakness and impaired cutaneous and proprioceptive sensation below the level of the lesion. Sphincter control may be affected. Depending on the location and nature of the tumor, cord symptoms may be mild or severe and are often asymmetric. Occlusion of spinal vessels by the tumor may cause myelomalacia with symptoms of cord transection (see SPINAL CORD INJURY in Ch. 124).

Intramedullary neoplasms (gliomas, ependymomas) frequently extend over several spinal segments and clinically may mimic syringomyelia. A tumor localized in one segment may clinically resemble an extramedullary tumor, but pain is usually less prominent and sphincter symptoms occur earlier.

Diagnosis

Spinal neoplasms must be differentiated from other diseases of the spinal cord (eg, vascular malformations, syphilis, multiple sclerosis, syringomyelia, pernicious anemia, amyotrophic lateral sclerosis, anomalies of the cervical spine and base of the skull, cervical spondylosis, and ruptured intervertebral disk).

X-rays of the spine may show bone destruction, widening of the vertebral pedicles, or distortion of paraspinal tissues. The CSF protein concentration is usually increased and manometric examination shows subarachnoid block. Myelography is the definitive diagnostic test for tumors and may provide the first clue that the offending lesion is an arteriovenous malformation; this can then be identified by selective arteriography.

Treatment

Extramedullary compressive growths may be removed surgically; the prognosis depends on the damage already done. For intramedullary and nonexcisable extramedullary tumors, radiotherapy is used, either alone or following surgical decompression. The tumor may be arrested; reversal of the clinical syndrome occurs in about 1/2 of patients. Corticosteroid hormones may reduce spinal cord edema and preserve function.

PARANEOPLASTIC SYNDROMES

Remote neurologic effects of cancer in which, uncommonly, nervous system dysfunction develops without evidence of direct invasion of tumor into neural tissues or of infectious or vascular complications. Paraneoplastic syndromes occur in < 7% of cancer patients, mostly those with carcinoma of the lung (usually oat cell) or ovary. The diagnosis is one of exclusion and should not be accepted until metastatic or nonmetastatic causes are ruled out. **Etiology** is unknown, although an autoimmune mechanism has been proposed, since circulating antibodies against nervous system tissue have been found in some patients. The syndromes are classified by location.

Cerebral remote effects are characterized by progressive dementia, alterations of mood, seizures, and, less commonly, focal motor or sensory signs. Pathologically, lymphocytic collections in the medial temporal lobe (limbic encephalitis) occur in some patients, while in others few abnormalities are found. Occasionally, dementia may be part of the cerebellar degeneration syndrome with or without brainstem signs (see below). The differential diagnosis includes metabolic brain disease, meningeal carcinomatosis, and progressive multifocal leukoencephalopathy. There is no specific treatment.

Cerebellum: Subacute cerebellar degeneration associated with cancer has a characteristic clinical picture. There is subacute onset of progressive bilateral leg and arm ataxia, dysarthria, and sometimes vertigo and diplopia. Associated nervous system signs may include dementia, ophthalmoplegia, nystagmus, and extensor plantar signs. The CSF occasionally demonstrates a mild lymphocytic pleocytosis. Cerebellar degeneration may precede the discovery of the cancer by weeks to years. The CT scan may

demonstrate cerebellar atrophy, especially late. The course of the illness usually is progressive over weeks to months, often leaving the patient profoundly disabled. Characteristic pathologic changes include widespread loss of Purkinje cells and lymphocytic cuffing of deep blood vessels. The disorder is differentiated from alcoholic cerebellar syndrome by the cancer-associated syndrome's greater involvement of the arms and prominence of dysarthria. There is no specific treatment, but some improvement may follow successful treatment of the cancer.

Opsoclonus (*spontaneous, chaotic eye movements*) is a rare cerebellar syndrome that may accompany childhood neuroblastoma. It is associated with cerebellar ataxia and myoclonus of the trunk and extremities. The syndrome often responds to therapy of the tumor and to corticosteroid hormones.

Spinal cord: Subacute motor neuropathy is a rare disorder of painless lower motor neuron weakness of upper and lower extremities in patients with Hodgkin's disease or other lymphomas. Pathologically, there is neuronal degeneration of spinal anterior horn cells. Spontaneous improvement usually occurs. **Subacute necrotic myelopathy** may rarely affect gray and white matter of the spinal cord, with rapid ascending sensory and motor loss to the point of clinical paraplegia. The disorder is akin to idiopathic subacute necrotic myelopathy. Myelography is required to rule out epidural compression from metastatic tumor, the much more common cause of rapidly progressive spinal cord dysfunction in patients with cancer.

Peripheral nerves: Perhaps the most common remote effect of cancer on the nervous system is a distal sensorimotor **polyneuropathy** that produces mild motor weakness, sensory loss, and absent distal reflexes. The syndrome is indistinguishable from that accompanying many chronic illnesses and may be due to nutritional deprivation and not be specific for cancer. The syndrome responds poorly to vitamin therapy, however. A more specific but rare peripheral nerve disorder is a **subacute sensory neuropathy** that may precede the cancer's appearance. There is degeneration of the dorsal root ganglia. The patients develop progressive sensory loss with ataxia but little motor weakness; the disorder may be disabling and there is no treatment. Guillain-Barré polyneuropathy is more common in Hodgkin's disease than in the general population.

Neuromuscular junction: See the **myasthenic syndrome** (Eaton-Lambert) in Ch. 131.

Muscle: The incidence of both **dermatomyositis** and **polymyositis** (see in §10) has been thought to be increased in cancer patients, especially in those over age 50 yr. Typically there is progressive proximal muscle weakness with pathologically demonstrable muscle inflammation and necrosis. A dusky and erythematous butterfly rash may develop on the face, and there may be periorbital edema with a heliotrope hue. Improvement may follow treatment with corticosteroid hormones.

RADIATION INJURY OF THE NERVOUS SYSTEM

Injury of the nervous system can occur as a complication of radiation therapy when tissue dosage has been excessive. Both acute and subacute transient symptoms may develop early, but progressive, permanent, and often disabling nervous system damage may not be evident for months to years after routine radiation therapy. The total radiation dose, the size of the fractions, the duration of therapy, and the volume of nervous tissue irradiated—all influence the likelihood of damage. Furthermore, considerable individual susceptibility complicates the effort to determine predictably safe doses for all patients.

Acute encephalopathy consisting of headache, nausea and vomiting, somnolence, and worsening neurologic signs may accompany the first or second radiation fraction, particularly when there is increased intracranial pressure and the patient has not been

given adequate corticosteroid preparation for several days. The encephalopathy becomes less severe with subsequent fractions and after treatment with corticosteroid hormones. **Early-delayed encephalopathy** occurs in the first 2 to 4 mo after therapy. In children a "somnolence" syndrome may follow prophylactic whole-brain irradiation for leukemia; it improves spontaneously over several days to weeks and may subside more rapidly with corticosteroid treatment. In adults, the syndrome must be distinguished by CT scan from worsening or recurrent brain tumor. **Early-delayed radiation myelopathy** follows radiation therapy to the neck or upper thorax and is characterized by **Lhermitte's sign** (*an electric-shock–like sensation radiating down the back and into the legs on flexion of the neck*). The syndrome resolves spontaneously.

Late-delayed radiation damage of the brain appears months to years after either prophylaxis for leukemia in childhood or prophylaxis or treatment of brain tumors in adults. Progressive dementia without focal signs is characteristic, although adults often develop unsteady gait. CT scan demonstrates cerebral atrophy. A different syndrome may follow irradiation of extracranial tumors or high-dose irradiation of intracranial tumors. The symptoms and signs are more focal and the CT demonstrates a hypodense mass that may enhance after contrast. Excisional biopsy often ameliorates the symptoms and distinguishes the cause from recurrent tumor. **Late-delayed radiation myelopathy** follows therapy of extra-spinal tumors (eg, Hodgkin's disease) by months to years. It is characterized by progressive weakness and sensory loss often of a **Brown-Séquard** type (*weakness and proprioceptive sensory loss on one side of the body and loss of pain and temperature sensation on the other side*). The course varies in its rapidity but most patients become paraplegic. **Late-delayed radiation neuropathy** may produce a brachial neuropathy after treatment for breast or lung cancer.

Rarely, radiation may produce gliomas, meningiomas, or peripheral nerve sheath tumors years after therapy.

---

127. DEMYELINATING DISEASES

The myelin that sheaths many nerve fibers is a complex of lipoprotein layers formed in early life by the oligodendroglia in the CNS and by the Schwann cells peripherally (see also in Ch. 131). The two myelins differ chemically and immunologically, but serve the same function: to promote transmission of the neural impulse along the axon.

Many congenital metabolic disorders (eg, phenylketonuria and other aminoacidurias; Tay-Sachs, Niemann-Pick, and Gaucher's diseases and Hurler's syndrome; Krabbe's disease and other leukodystrophies) affect the developing myelin sheath, mainly of the CNS. Unless the innate biochemical defect can be corrected or compensated for, permanent and often widespread neurologic deficits result.

Demyelination in later life is a feature of many neurologic disorders, and it can occur as a result of neuronal damage as well as damage to the myelin itself, whether due to local injury, ischemia, toxic agents, or metabolic disorders. Extensive myelin loss usually is followed by axonal degeneration and often by cell body degeneration, and may be irreversible. However, in many instances remyelination occurs, and repair, regeneration, and complete recovery of neural function can take place rapidly. This often is seen, for example, following the segmental demyelination that characterizes many peripheral neuropathies, and may explain the exacerbations and remissions of multiple sclerosis.

Central demyelination occurs as the predominant finding in several disorders of uncertain etiology that have come to be known as the **primary demyelinating diseases**. Of these, **multiple sclerosis (MS)** is the most prominent, and is discussed in detail below. Brief descriptions of the others follow.

Acute disseminated encephalomyelitis (**postinfectious encephalitis** —see also ACUTE VIRAL ENCEPHALITIS in Ch. 125) a perivascular CNS demyelination that can occur spontaneously but usually follows a viral infection or inoculation (or, very rarely, a bacterial vaccine), suggesting an immunologic cause. The "neuroparalytic accidents" and peripheral neuropathies that can follow rabies vaccination with brain tissue preparations, and the Guillain-Barré syndrome (discussed under PERIPHERAL NEUROPATHY in Ch. 131) are similar demyelinating disorders with the same presumed immunologic pathogenesis.

In **optic neuromyelitis,** the demyelination selectively and acutely affects the optic nerves and (usually a short time later) the spinal cord at a thoracic or, less often, a cervical segment. The optic demyelination produces acute visual loss or central scotoma; spinal cord involvement results in the same symptoms and signs as are seen in MS. The syndrome may follow febrile diseases, may occur as a feature of MS, or apparently may occur spontaneously. Early **treatment** with ACTH or corticosteroids to control the assumed inflammation has been used empirically.

Adrenoleukodystrophy (formerly called **Schilder's disease**) is a rare, sex-linked recessive metabolic disorder that occurs in boys and is characterized by adrenal atrophy and widespread, diffuse cerebral demyelination. It produces mental deterioration, corticospinal tract dysfunction, and cortical blindness. There is laboratory evidence of adrenal cortical dysfunction. Death invariably occurs in 1 to 5 yr.

MULTIPLE SCLEROSIS (MS)

(Disseminated Sclerosis)

A slowly progressive CNS disease characterized by disseminated patches of demyelination in the brain and spinal cord, resulting in multiple and varied neurologic symptoms and signs, usually with remissions and exacerbations.

Etiology and Incidence

The cause is unknown but an immunologic abnormality is suspected, with few clues presently indicating a specific mechanism. Postulated etiologies include infection by a slow or latent virus, and myelinolysis by enzymes. IgG is elevated in the CSF of most patients with MS, and elevated titers have been found to a variety of viral agents, including measles. The full significance of these findings and of variously reported associations with HLA allotypes and altered numbers of T cells in the blood is presently unclear, and the evidence somewhat conflicting. An increased family incidence suggests that genetic factors may influence susceptibility. Women are affected somewhat more often than men. Environmental factors seem to be present. MS is more common in temperate climates (1:2000) than in the tropics (1:10,000). Although age of onset generally is from 20 to 40 yr, MS has been linked to the location where a patient's first 15 yr are spent. Relocation after age 15 does not alter the risk.

Pathology

Plaques, or islands, of demyelination with destruction of oligodendroglia and perivascular inflammation are disseminated through the CNS, primarily in the white matter, with a predilection for the lateral and posterior columns (especially in the cervical and dorsal regions), the optic nerves, and periventricular areas. Tracts in the midbrain, pons, and cerebellum also are affected, and gray matter in both cerebrum and cord may be invaded. Cell bodies and axons usually are preserved, especially in early lesions. Later, axons may be destroyed, especially in the long tracts, and a fibrous gliosis gives the tracts their "sclerotic" appearance. Both early and late lesions may be found simultaneously. Chemical changes in lipid and protein constituents of myelin have been demonstrated in and around the plaques.

Symptoms and Signs

The disease is characterized by various complaints and findings of CNS dysfunction with remissions and persistently recurring exacerbations. Onset usually is insidious

The most frequent presenting symptoms are paresthesias in one or more extremities, in the trunk, or on one side of the face; weakness or clumsiness of a leg or a hand; or visual disturbances, such as partial blindness and pain in one eye **(retrobulbar optic neuritis),** diplopia, dimness of vision, or scotomas. Other common early symptoms are a fleeting ocular palsy, transient weakness of one or more extremities, slight stiffness or unusual fatigability of a limb, minor gait disturbances, difficulties with bladder control, vertigo, or mild emotional disturbances—all evidence of scattered involvement of the CNS and often occurring months or years before the disease is recognized. Excess heat may accentuate symptoms and signs.

Findings on examination are many and varied:

Mental: Apathy, lack of judgment, or inattention may occur. Emotional lability is common and, along with the widespread mild signs, can lead to the initial impression of hysteria. Euphoria occurs in many patients, but in some a reactive depression is present. Sudden weeping or forced laughter (concomitants of pseudobulbar palsy) indicates that corticobulbar pathways of emotional control are involved. Convulsive seizures may occur. Severe changes such as mania or dementia are uncommon and occur late in the disease. **Scanning speech** (*slow enunciation with a tendency to hesitate at the beginning of a word or syllable*) is common in advanced disease. Aphasia is rare.

Cranial nerve: In addition to the initial optic neuritis (see above), one or more of the following ocular signs usually are present at some time: partial atrophy of the optic nerve with temporal pallor; changes in the visual fields (central scotoma or general narrowing of the fields); transient ophthalmoplegia with diplopia (from involvement of the brainstem tracts connecting the 3rd, 4th, and 6th nerve nuclei). Choked disks are found with optic neuritis, but pupillary changes, Argyll Robertson pupils, or total blindness are rare. Nystagmus, a common finding, may be due to cerebellar or vestibular nucleus damage.

Other evidence of cranial nerve involvement is uncommon, and when present usually is due to brainstem injury in the area of the cranial nerve nuclei. Deafness is rare, but vertigo is not. Numbness on one side of the face, or pain resembling trigeminal neuralgia, is seen occasionally.

Motor: Deep reflexes (eg, knee and ankle jerks) are generally increased; Babinski's sign and clonus often are present. Superficial reflexes, particularly upper and lower abdominals, are diminished or absent. Often, the patient complains of unilateral symptoms but examination elicits signs of bilateral corticospinal tract involvement. Intention tremor from cerebellar lesions is common, and continued purposeful effort accentuates it. The motion is ataxic: shaky, irregular, tremulous, and ineffective. Static tremor, especially obvious when the head is unsupported, may be seen. Muscular weakness and spasticity from corticospinal damage produce a stumbling, weaving, drunken gait; later, a combination of spasticity and cerebellar ataxia may be totally disabling. The cerebral lesions may result in hemiplegia, sometimes the presenting symptom. Muscular atrophy or painful flexor spasms in response to sensory stimuli (eg, bedclothes) may appear in late stages.

A combination of nystagmus, intention tremor, and scanning speech is a common cerebellar manifestation in advanced disease. Mild dysarthria may result from cerebellar damage, disturbance of cortical control, or injury to the bulbar nuclei.

Sensory: Complete loss of any form of cutaneous sensation is rare, but paresthesias, numbness, and blunting of sensation such as hemianesthesia to pain or disturbances of vibratory or position sense may occur and often are localized; eg, to the hands or legs. The objective changes are fleeting and often are elicited only with careful testing.

Autonomic: Urinary urgency or hesitancy, partial retention of urine, or slight incontinence is common with spinal cord involvement, as are sexual impotence in men and

genital anesthesia in women. Bladder and rectal incontinence may occur with severe advanced involvement.

Course

The course is highly varied and unpredictable and in most patients, remittent. At first, months or years of remission may separate episodes, especially when the disease begins with retrobulbar neuritis, but usually the intervals of freedom grow shorter, and eventually permanent and progressive disablement occurs. Life span in most cases probably is not shortened. The average duration of illness probably exceeds 25 yr, but variability is great. Remissions have lasted longer than 25 yr. Some patients, however, have frequent attacks and are rapidly incapacitated; in a few, particularly when onset is in middle age, the course is progressively and unremittingly downhill, and occasionally the disease is fatal within a year.

Diagnosis

Diagnosis is indirect, by deduction from clinical and laboratory features. Typical cases usually can be diagnosed confidently on clinical grounds. A firm diagnosis, however, usually cannot be made during the first attack, although it can be suspected. Later, a history of remissions and exacerbations and clinical evidence of CNS lesions disseminated in more than one area are highly suggestive. The firm diagnosis should be made only after considering all other possibilities.

Differential diagnosis must include small cerebral infarctions, syringomyelia, amyotrophic lateral sclerosis, syphilis, pernicious anemia, arthritis of the cervical spine, ruptured intervertebral disk, basilar impression, SLE, and the hereditary ataxias. CNS tumors, abscesses, or other mass lesions, vascular malformations of the brain or spinal cord, and anomalies of the spine or base of the skull must be ruled out by the clinical findings. If these are not clear, CT or MRI and CSF examination may be required. Particular attention should be paid to the area about the foramen magnum, since treatable lesions at the junction of the spinal cord and medulla (eg, subarachnoid cyst, foramen magnum tumors) occasionally cause a variable and fluctuating spectrum of motor and sensory symptoms.

Laboratory findings: The CSF is abnormal in > 55% of cases. Gamma globulin may be > 13%, and cells (lymphocytes) and protein content may be slightly increased, but these findings are not pathognomonic. Oligoclonal bands may be found on agarose electrophoresis of the CSF of up to 90% of patients with MS, but their absence does not rule out the disease. CSF concentration of myelin basic protein may be elevated during active demyelination.

Magnetic resonance imaging is the most sensitive imaging technic available to diagnose MS; it may show many plaques. Lesions also may be visible on contrast-enhanced **CT scans**; the sensitivity of CT imaging may be increased by giving twice the dose of iodine and delaying the scanning ("double-dose delayed CT scan").

Evoked potentials (see also Ch. 117) are recorded electrical responses to stimulation of a sensory system. Pattern-shift visual, brainstem auditory, and somatosensory evoked potentials may be abnormal early in the disease.

Treatment

There is no specific therapy. Spontaneous remissions make any treatment difficult to evaluate. Many authorities believe that prednisone 60 mg/day for 5 to 7 days may hasten recovery in acute attacks (eg, retrobulbar neuritis), especially if given very early in the episode. Long-term corticosteroid therapy rarely is justified. The use of immunosuppressive agents remains investigational. Intrathecal corticosteroid therapy has no value and may cause secondary arachnoiditis. Hyperbaric O_2 or plasma exchange has no value.

The patient should maintain as normal and active a life as possible, but should avoid overwork and fatigue. Massage and passive movement of weakened spastic limbs make patients more comfortable. Muscle training is physically and psychologically benefi

cial. Encouragement and reassurance are essential; a hopeless outlook should be avoided. Invalidism may be prevented by prompt treatment and in late stages can be postponed by physiotherapy and prompt treatment of infections and urinary difficulties. Decubitus ulcer and UTIs should be prevented in bedridden patients. Intermittent catheterization is useful to maintain low bladder residual volume. This may be taught for self-use at home. Several drugs reduce spasticity by inhibiting the spinal cord reflexes; baclofen 40 to 80 mg/day in divided doses is preferred. While the short-term toxicity of these agents appears to be minimal (usually lethargy), their long-term effects are largely unknown. Cautious and judicious use is required because reducing spasticity in MS patients often exacerbates weakness, thus further incapacitating the patient.

ACUTE TRANSVERSE MYELITIS

(See under DEMYELINATING CORD DISORDERS in Ch. 130)

128. DISORDERS OF MOVEMENT: EXTRAPYRAMIDAL AND CEREBELLAR DISORDERS

Voluntary movement is the end product of a complex sequence of neural and neuromuscular events. There are 3 major components of the motor system: (1) the **corticospinal (pyramidal) tracts,** which connect the cerebral cortex to lower motor centers of brainstem and spinal cord, passing through the medullary pyramids; (2) the **basal ganglia** (caudate nucleus, putamen, globus pallidus, and substantia nigra—**extrapyramidal system**), consisting of a group of interrelated structures lying deep in the forebrain whose output is directed mainly rostrally through the thalamus to the cerebral cortex rather than passing caudally directly through the pyramidal tract; and (3) the **cerebellum,** the center for motor coordination that lies on the dorsal surface of the brainstem. The contributions of these motor system components toward producing movement are shown by the abnormal movement patterns that remain when a component is damaged or diseased.

Lesions of the corticospinal system result in weakness or total paralysis of predominantly distal voluntary movement, Babinski's sign, and, often, **spasticity** (*increased muscle tone and exaggerated deep tendon reflexes*). The increase in muscle tone of spasticity is proportional to the rate and degree of stretch placed upon a muscle up to a point at which resistance suddenly melts away: the so-called **"clasp-knife phenomenon."** Troublesome spasticity resulting from disorders such as spinal cord injury or multiple sclerosis often can be effectively reduced by the drug baclofen 30 to 120 mg/day or diazepam, 6 to 20 mg/day. However, this does not improve voluntary power.

Disorders of the basal ganglia (extrapyramidal disorders) do not cause weakness or reflex changes; the hallmark is **involuntary movement,** resulting in excesses **(hyperkinesia)** or poverty **(hypokinesia)** of movement, and changes in muscle tone and in posture.

Cerebellar disorders cause abnormalities in the range, rate, and force of movement. Strength is little affected.

HYPERKINETIC MOVEMENT DISORDERS

TREMOR

Rhythmic, alternating, oscillatory movements produced by repetitive patterns of muscle contraction and relaxation. Tremors are classified according to their rate (slow—3 to 5

Hz; rapid—6 to 12 Hz); rhythm; distribution; and whether they occur at rest **(resting tremor)** or during muscular activity **(sustention, action,** or **intention tremors)**.

Etiology

Physiologic tremor: Most individuals under certain conditions exhibit a fine, rapid tremor of the outstretched hands. **Enhanced physiologic tremor** may be produced by anxiety, stress, fatigue, or metabolic derangements such as alcohol withdrawal or thyrotoxicosis, or by certain drugs including caffeine and other phosphodiesterase inhibitors, β-adrenergic agonists, and adrenal corticosteroids. **Benign hereditary (essential) tremor** is a fine-to-coarse slow tremor usually affecting the hands, head, and voice. The tremor, which may be unilateral, is minimal or absent at rest; is brought out by performing skilled acts; and may be intensified by any of the factors that intensify physiologic tremor. It tends to increase with age and occasionally mistakenly is called **senile tremor.** Inheritance appears to be via an autosomal dominant trait in 50% of cases. In some families a marked suppression of tremor by drinking small amounts of alcohol is noted. The **resting tremor** of **Parkinson's disease** is discussed below in this chapter.

Tremor of cerebellar disease: **Intention tremor** (as occurs in multiple sclerosis and other cerebellar outflow diseases) results from the oscillation of a limb as it approaches a target; **sustension tremor** is a coarse rotatory tremor of the proximal musculature most prominent on attempting to maintain a fixed posture or on weight bearing; **titubation** is a gross tremor of the head and body and is a form of sustention tremor evident on assuming the upright position and disappearing with recumbency. Both sustention tremor and titubation are characteristic of cerebellar disease. **Hepatolenticular degeneration** (Wilson's disease—see Ch. 82): Both intention and resting (parkinsonian) tremors may be seen. The most characteristic is a rhythmic "flapping" or "wing-beating" tremor of the distal or proximal limbs, respectively. **Asterixis** ("liver flap") is a coarse, slow, nonrhythmic tremor seen in the outstretched hands of patients with hepatic (portal-systemic) and other largely metabolic encephalopathies. Asterixis results from episodic electromyographic silence in the antigravity muscles during attempted postural fixation.

Treatment

The treatment of enhanced physiologic tremor depends on its cause. The tremors of thyrotoxicosis and of alcohol withdrawal respond to treatment of the underlying condition. Judicious use of benzodiazepine anxiolytics tid or qid (eg, diazepam 2 to 10 mg, lorazepam 1 to 2.5 mg, or oxazepam 10 to 30 mg) may be useful for tremor associated with chronic anxiety states. Habituation to such agents should be avoided. Propranolol 20 to 80 mg qid often is effective in treating benign essential tremor as well as enhanced physiologic tremor due to drugs and acute anxiety states (eg, stage fright). Primidone 50 to 250 mg tid may be tried in situations where propranolol is ineffective or poorly tolerated. Treatment of parkinsonian tremor is discussed below. Treatment of portal-systemic encephalopathy is discussed in Ch. 67. No effective drug treatment is available for cerebellar tremor; physical measures such as weighting of the affected limbs or educating patients to brace the proximal limb during activity sometimes are useful.

DYSKINESIAS

Involuntary, nonrepetitive, but occasionally stereotyped movements affecting distal, proximal, and axial musculature in varying combinations. Most dyskinesias represent basal ganglia disorders. Although precise neuroanatomic correlates usually are lacking the various dyskinesias can be thought of as forming a continuum of symptoms from the lightning-like flickers of myoclonus to the slow, writhing patterns of dystonia

MYOCLONUS

A brief, lightning-like contraction of a muscle or group of muscles. Myoclonus may occur in normal individuals as they fall asleep. **Etiology** includes metabolic derangements such as uremia; various degenerative and "slow virus" diseases including Alzheimer's and Jakob-Creutzfeldt diseases; progressive myoclonus epilepsy; and subacute sclerosing panencephalitis (SSPE). Myoclonus arising following closed head trauma or hypoxic-ischemic brain injury may increase with intended movements; hence it has been termed **action myoclonus. Palatal myoclonus,** a continuous, rhythmic contraction of the posterior phyaryngeal muscles, is a form of tremor and occurs as a result of a lesion in the dentato-olivo-cerebellar circuit.

Treatment should begin with correction of any underlying metabolic abnormalities. Clonazepam 0.5 to 2 mg tid often is effective; other anticonvulsants also may be tried. Many forms of myoclonus respond to the serotonin precursor L-5-hydroxytryptophan (L-5HTP). However, this drug, which must be used with the decarboxylase inhibitor carbidopa, is still investigational.

TICS

Brief, rapid, involuntary movements, often resembling fragments of normal behavior. Tics are stereotyped and repetitive, but not rhythmic.

Simple tics (eg, eye blinking) often begin as nervous mannerisms in childhood or later and disappear spontaneously.

Gilles de la Tourette syndrome (*hereditary multiple tic disorder*) begins in childhood with simple tics but progresses to multiple, complex movements including respiratory and vocal tics. The latter may begin as grunting or barking noises and evolve into compulsive utterances. In 50% of patients **coprolalia** (*involuntary, scatologic utterances*) occurs. The tics and coprolalia may be severe enough to be physically and socially disabling.

Diagnosis and Treatment

Tics tend to be more complex than myoclonus and less flowing than choreic movements, from which they must be differentiated. Tics also may be voluntarily suppressed by the patient for seconds or even minutes.

Simple tics may respond to benzodiazepine anxiolytics. For Gilles de la Tourette syndrome, haloperidol 0.5 to 40 mg/day is the drug of choice. Side effects of dysphoria, parkinsonism, and akathisia may be limiting. Clonidine 0.1 to 0.6 mg/day or pimozide 1 to 20 mg/day may be as effective as haloperidol in some patients. Clonidine lacks the potential for causing tardive dyskinesias with long-term use. The limiting side effect of clonidine is hypotension. Intermediate-acting benzodiazepines such as lorazepam 0.5 to 2.5 mg tid or qid may be useful as adjuvant treatment.

CHOREA AND ATHETOSIS

Chorea: *Brief, purposeless, involuntary movements of the distal extremities and face.* **Athetosis**: *Writhing, proximal, often alternating postures which blend continuously into a flowing stream of movement.* Choreic movements may merge imperceptibly into purposeful or semi-purposeful acts that serve to "cover up" the involuntary motion. Chorea and athetosis often occur together **(choreoathetosis)**.

Pharmacologically, chorea and athetosis are the antithesis of Parkinson's disease, and are considered to be manifestations of dopaminergic overactivity in the basal ganglia. The role of cholinergic and other systems in the pathophysiology of the dyskinesias is less clear than in Parkinson's disease.

Huntington's disease or **chorea** (progressive hereditary chorea—see also in Ch. 203) is *an autosomal dominant disorder usually beginning in middle age (35 to 50 yr) characterized by choreiform movements and progressive intellectual deterioration.* Both sexes are affected equally. Pathologically there is atrophy of the caudate nucleus with degeneration of the small-cell population and decreases in levels of the neurotransmitters γ-aminobutyric acid **(GABA)** and substance P (an 11-amino acid peptide also called substance preparation or SP). This degeneration results in characteristic "boxcar ventricles" seen on CT scan. **Symptoms and signs**: Onset is insidious. Psychiatric disturbances, ranging from personality changes of apathy and irritability to full-blown manic-depressive or schizophreniform illness may precede the onset of the movement disorder or develop during its course. Motor manifestations include flicking movements of the extremities, a lilting gait, and motor impersistence (the inability to sustain a motor act such as tongue protrusion).

Prognosis and treatment: The course of the illness is inexorably progressive; no treatment is known. Patients ultimately lose the ability to care for themselves both physically and mentally. Walking becomes impossible, swallowing difficult, and dementia profound. The choreic movements and agitated behaviors may be suppressed, but usually only partially, by phenothiazine (chlorpromazine 100 to 900 mg/day) or butyrophenone neuroleptics (haloperidol 10 to 90 mg/day) or reserpine, beginning with 0.1 mg/day and increasing until side effects of lethargy, hypotension, or parkinsonism supervene. Therapeutic strategies aimed at replacing brain GABA stores have been ineffective.

Genetic counseling is extremely important, since ½ the offspring of an affected parent are at risk, the disorder does not present clinically until after the childbearing years, and no diagnostic test is available for presymptomatic detection.

Senile chorea occurs in elderly patients and affects predominantly the oral-buccal-lingual muscles. Though hereditary, it is not associated with the devastating intellectual and personality changes of Huntington's chorea. **Treatment** consists of the use of dopamine-blocking agents (eg, chlorpromazine or haloperidol) when chorea is unsightly or disabling.

Sydenham's chorea nowadays occurs rarely as a sequela of streptococcal infections in children (see Ch. 198).

Chorea gravidarum (*choreiform movement occurring during pregnancy*): Patients often have a history of rheumatic fever. Symptoms usually begin during the first trimester and resolve spontaneously by or following delivery. **Treatment** consists of sedation with barbiturates, because of the potential harmful effects of other drugs on the fetus. A similar disorder occurs rarely in women taking oral contraceptives.

Other causes of chorea include thyrotoxicosis, SLE affecting the CNS, and drugs (see DRUG-INDUCED MOVEMENT DISORDERS, below).

Hemiballismus (*violent continuous proximal flinging movements confined to one side of the body, usually affecting the arm more than the leg, caused by a lesion, usually an infarct, in the region of the contralateral subthalamic nucleus of Luys*): Differential diagnosis includes acute **hemichorea**, usually due to tumor or infarct of the caudate nucleus, and focal seizures. Although disabling, hemiballismus usually is self-limited, lasting 6 to 8 wk. **Treatment** with phenothiazine or butyrophenone neuroleptics often is effective.

DYSTONIA

Sustained abnormal postures and disruptions of ongoing movement resulting from alterations in muscle tone. Dystonias may be either generalized or focal.

Generalized dystonia (torsion dystonia; dystonia musculorum deformans): *A rare progressive syndrome, usually beginning in childhood, characterized by dystonic movements that result in sustained, often bizarre postures.* Symptoms usually begin with inversion and plantar fixation of the foot while walking, or with **torticollis (wryneck).** Two hereditary patterns have been described: autosomal recessive, occurring in Ashkenazi Jewish families; and dominant, occurring in families of northern European extraction. "Unaffected" relatives may exhibit "formes frustes" as focal dystonia (see below). The disorder is relentlessly progressive; in advanced stages the patient is twisted into fixed postures "like a pretzel." Mentation usually is preserved. The pathoanatomic basis is unknown.

Adult onset focal dystonia usually affects 1 or occasionally 2 contiguous body regions, and rarely progresses to generalized dystonia. **Meige syndrome** (blepharospasm-oromandibular dystonia) consists of involuntary blinking, jaw-grinding movements, and grimacing, usually with onset in late middle age. Meige syndrome must be differentiated from the buccal-lingual-facial movements of tardive dyskinesia. **Torticollis** often begins with a pulling sensation followed by sustained torsion and deviation of the head and neck. In early stages patients can voluntarily overcome the dystonia. **Occupational dystonia** consists of dystonic spasms initiated by performing skilled acts. These include writer's cramp, typist's cramp, etc. **Other causes of dystonia** include metabolic or degenerative diseases of the CNS; eg, Wilson's and Hallervorden-Spatz diseases, various lipidoses, and cerebral palsy.

Treatment

Treatment often is unsatisfactory. High-dose anticholinergics (trihexyphenidyl 6 to 30 mg/day; benztropine 3 to 15 mg/day) and the dopamine-depleting drug reserpine 0.1 to 0.6 mg/day are most often used. Levodopa and carbamazepine have benefited a few patients. Neuroleptics should be *avoided* because of possible superimposition of drug-induced movement disorders on the underlying problem.

DRUG-INDUCED MOVEMENT DISORDERS

The widespread use of phenothiazine, thioxanthine, and butyrophenone neuroleptics and antiemetics, all of which block CNS dopamine receptors, has resulted in the emergence of a number of drug-related syndromes mimicking almost all spontaneously occurring basal ganglia disorders. **Parkinsonism** is discussed below; **acute dystonia, tardive dyskinesia,** and **neuroleptic malignant syndrome** are discussed in ANTIPSYCHOTIC DRUGS in Ch. 281.

HYPOKINETIC MOVEMENT DISORDERS

PARKINSON'S DISEASE

(Paralysis Agitans; Shaking Palsy)

An idiopathic, slowly progressive, degenerative CNS disorder with 4 characteristic features: slowness and poverty of movement, muscular rigidity, resting tremor, and postural instability.

Etiology and Pathophysiology

There is loss of the pigmented neurons of the substantia nigra, locus ceruleus, and other brainstem cell groups. The loss of substantia nigra neurons which project to the caudate nucleus and putamen results in depletion of the neurotransmitter dopamine in these areas. The region of the midbrain containing the substantia nigra is destroyed by an inflammatory process in postencephalitic cases (see below). Onset generally is after age 40, with increasing incidence in older age groups.

Secondary parkinsonism results from the loss of or interference with the action of dopamine within the basal ganglia, due to idiopathic degenerative disease, drugs, or exogenous toxins. The most common cause of secondary parkinsonism is ingestion of neuroleptic drugs or reserpine. All such drugs (except thioridazine, which has potent anticholinergic activity) produce parkinsonism through their dopamine-receptor-blocking properties. Neuroleptics with the least anticholinergic activity (haloperidol) produce the greatest incidence of parkinsonism. Coadministration of an anticholinergic drug such as benztropine 0.5 to 2 mg tid or amantadine 100 mg bid may ameliorate the condition.

Less common etiologies include carbon monoxide or manganese poisoning, hydrocephalus, structural lesions (tumors, infarcts involving the midbrain or basal ganglia), subdural hematoma, degenerative disorders including striatonigral degeneration and olivopontocerebellar degeneration or multiple systems atrophy (see under SPINOCEREBELLAR DEGENERATIONS, below). Recently n-MPTP (n-methyl-1,2,3,4 tetrahydropyridine), a byproduct of the synthesis of a type of street heroin, has caused parkinsonism in a number of IV drug abusers.

Symptoms and Signs

Parkinson's disease often (50 to 80% of patients) begins insidiously with a resting 4- to 8-Hz "pill-rolling" tremor of one hand. The tremor is maximal at rest, diminishes during movement, and is absent during sleep; it is enhanced by emotional tension or fatigue. The hands, arms, and legs usually are most affected in that order. Jaw, tongue, forehead, and eyelids may be involved as well, although the voice is not. Many patients display only rigidity and never manifest tremor. Progressive rigidity, slowness and poverty of movement **(bradykinesia),** and difficulty in initiating movement **(akinesia)** follow. Rigidity and hypokinesia may contribute to muscular aches and sensations of fatigue. The face becomes masklike and open-mouthed, with diminished blinking. The posture becomes stooped. Patients find it difficult to start walking; the gait becomes shuffling with short steps, and the arms are held flexed to the waist and fail to swing with the stride. The steps may inadvertently quicken and the patient may break into a run to keep from falling **(festination).** A tendency to fall forward **(propulsion)** or backwards **(retropulsion)** when the center of gravity is displaced results from the loss of postural reflexes. Speech becomes hypophonic, with a characteristic monotonous, stuttering dysarthria. Hypokinesia and impaired control of distal musculature results in micrographia and increasing difficulties with activities of daily living.

On examination, passive movement of the limbs is met with a plastic, unvarying **"lead-pipe" rigidity;** superimposed tremor bursts may give a ratchet-like **"cogwheel"** quality. Although the sensory examination usually is normal, vague sensory complaints are not uncommon. Formally tested muscle strength usually is normal, although useful power may be diminished and the ability to perform rapid successive movements is impaired. The reflexes are normally present but may be difficult to elicit in the presence of marked tremor or rigidity. Dementia occurs in approximately 50% of patients; depression also is common. In some patients dementia and depression constitute major aspects of the disability.

In **postencephalitic parkinsonism,** which occurred following the epidemic of von Economo encephalitis in 1918–24 but rarely appears nowadays, **oculogyric crises** (*forced, sustained deviation of the head and eyes*), other dystonias, autonomic instability, and personality changes were common.

Diagnosis

Early clues include infrequent blinking and lack of facial expression, poverty of movement, impaired postural reflexes, and the characteristic gait abnormality. Tremor may be absent in about 30% of cases initially and often becomes less prominent as the disease progresses, but this should not obscure the diagnosis. Although rigidity is occasionally minimal or lacking, tremor without the above features is seldom due to

Parkinson's disease. Patients with essential tremor (see TREMOR, above), the disorder most commonly confused with Parkinson's disease, have animated facies, normal rates of movement, and no gait impairment. Elderly individuals with reduced spontaneity of movement, short-stepped or rheumatic gait, and mild depression and/or dementia may be more difficult to distinguish from Parkinson's disease. Other etiologies of parkinsonism may be discerned from history or lack of salutary response to medication, which may occur following degeneration of postsynaptic basal ganglia elements.

Treatment

Levodopa, the metabolic precursor of dopamine, crosses the blood–brain barrier into the basal ganglia where it is decarboxylated to form dopamine, replacing the missing neurotransmitter. Bradykinesia and rigidity are the symptoms helped most, although there is often substantial reduction in tremor. Mildly affected patients may return to nearly normal. Bedridden patients may become ambulatory. Extensive peripheral metabolism of the drug has 2 consequences; the drug must be given in very large doses, and side effects such as nausea, palpitations, and flushing may be severe. Coadministration of the peripheral decarboxylase inhibitor, **carbidopa,** lowers dosage requirements by preventing catabolism, thus decreasing side effects and allowing more efficient delivery of levodopa to the brain. **Carbidopa/levodopa** is available in fixed-ratio preparations of 10/100, 25/100, and 25/250 mg.

Treatment is begun with a single 10/100 or 25/100 tablet tid. The dose is gradually increased every 4 to 7 days according to patient tolerance until maximum benefit is reached. Side effects may be minimized by gradually and carefully increasing the dose and by giving the drug with or after meals. (However, large amounts of protein may interfere with absorption of levodopa.) Most patients require 400 to 1000 mg/day of levodopa in divided doses 2 to 5 h apart. A minimum of 100 mg/day of carbidopa is necessary to minimize peripheral side effects. Hence, the 25/100-mg tablets are useful for patients with lower dosage requirements or in whom therapy is being initiated. Some patients may require up to 2000 mg of levodopa (and 200 mg of carbidopa) a day.

Involuntary movements (dyskinesias) in the form of oral–facial or limb chorea or dystonia are often the dose-limiting side effects of levodopa therapy. The threshold for their emergence seems to decrease with length of treatment. In some patients effective reduction of parkinsonism cannot be achieved except at the price of some degree of dyskinesia. After 2 to 5 yr of treatment, > 50% of patients begin to experience fluctuations in their response of levodopa **("on-off" effect)**. The duration of improvement following each dose of medication shortens, and superimposition of dyskinetic movements may result in swings from intense akinesia to uncontrollable hyperactivity. Such swings can be minimized by keeping the individual doses of levodopa as low as possible, employing dosing intervals as short as q 1 to 2 h, and using adjuvant drugs. Other side effects of levodopa include orthostatic hypotension, hallucinations, and occasionally toxic delirium. The latter 2 are most common in elderly, demented individuals.

Amantadine 100 to 300 mg/day is sometimes useful in treating early, mild parkinsonism or to augment the effects of levodopa later in the illness. Its mechanism of action is uncertain; it may act through augmentation of dopaminergic activity, anticholinergic effects, or both. Amantadine often loses its effectiveness after a period of months when used as a single agent. Side effects include lower extremity edema, livedo reticularis, and confusion.

Bromocryptine and other ergot alkaloids possess antiparkinsonian activity by virtue of their ability to directly activate dopamine receptors in the basal ganglia. Bromocryptine 5 to 60 mg/day is sometimes useful in the late stages of illness when response to levodopa diminishes or the "on-off" effect is prominent, but its usefulness is limited by a high incidence of side effects including nausea, orthostatic hypotension, confusion, and delirium.

Anticholinergic medications were the mainstay of antiparkinsonian treatment before dopaminergic drugs. Currently they are used alone in the early stages of treatment and later to supplement levodopa. Commonly used anticholinergics include benztropine 0.5 to 2 mg tid and trihexyphenidyl 2 to 5 mg tid. As with levodopa, initial dosage should be small and dosage should be increased as tolerated. Adverse effects include dry mouth, urinary retention, constipation, and blurred vision. Particularly troublesome in older patients are confusion, delirium, and impaired thermoregulation due to decreased sweating. **Antihistamines** with anticholinergic action including diphenhydramine 25 to 100 mg/day and orphenadrine 50 to 200 mg/day are useful in treating tremor and as mild sedatives.

Tricyclic antidepressants such as amitryptiline, used in low doses such as 25 to 50 mg at bedtime, often are useful as nighttime sedatives and as adjuvants to levodopa, in addition to their effectiveness in treating depression. **Propranolol** 10 mg (bid) to 40 mg (qid) occasionally is helpful when parkinsonian tremor is accentuated rather than quieted by activity or intention.

The time to start dopaminergic therapy in Parkinson's disease is controversial. Some authorities believe that early levodopa therapy hastens the advent of problems such as dyskinesias and the "on-off" effect and prefer to withhold levodopa as long as possible, relying on anticholinergic medications or amantadine, reserving levodopa until the latest possible moment. Others regard the appearance of these phenomena as part of the course and severity of the underlying disease and start levodopa with carbidopa early to obtain maximal improvement in the quality of life. The precise role of dopamine agonist ergots in early treatment of Parkinson's disease is yet to be established.

PROGRESSIVE SUPRANUCLEAR PALSY

(Steele-Richardson-Olszewski Syndrome)

A rare disorder of late middle age manifested by loss of voluntary, but preservation of reflexive, eye movements; bradykinesia; muscular rigidity with progressive axial dystonia; **pseudobulbar palsy** *(spastic weakness of the pharyngeal musculature causing dysphagia and dysarthria with emotional lability); and dementia.* The oculomotor disturbance often begins with abnormality of vertical gaze. Etiology is unknown. Pathologically, there is degeneration of neurons in the basal ganglia and the brainstem. **Treatment** is unsatisfactory, but occasionally dopamine agonist drugs and amantadine provide partial relief of rigidity. A somewhat similar clinical picture can be produced by multiple small strokes (lacunes) in the basal ganglia and in the deep white matter of the hemispheres: **lacunar state,** which is differentiated by the history of a stepwise progression of deficits characteristic of strokes.

CEREBELLAR AND SPINOCEREBELLAR DISORDERS

Disorders of the cerebellum and its inflow or outflow pathways produce deficits in the rate, range, and force of movement. Anatomically, the cerebellum has 3 subdivisions. The phylogenetically oldest, the **archi-** or **vestibulocerebellum** comprises the flocculonodular lobe, is concerned with the maintenance of equilibrium and eye-head-neck movements, and is closely interconnected with the vestibular nuclei. The midline **vermis (paleocerebellum)** helps coordinate movement of the trunk and legs. Vermis lesions result in abnormalities of stance and gait. The lateral hemispheres, which comprise the **neocerebellum,** exert control over both ballistic and finely coordinated limb movements, predominantly of the upper extremities.

The signs of cerebellar disease are **ataxia** (*reeling, wide-based gait*); **dysmetria** (*inability to control range of movement*); **dysdiadochokinesia** (*inability to perform rapid alternating movements*); **hypotonia** (*decreased muscle tone*); **decomposition of movement**

(*inability to sequence properly fine, coordinated acts*); **tremor,** which may occur with intention or with sustention; **dysarthria** with slurring, inappropriate phrasing, and lack of modulation of speech volume **(scanning speech)**; and **nystagmus,** with the fast component maximal toward the side of the cerebellar lesion.

STRUCTURAL LESIONS OF THE CEREBELLUM

Vascular lesions (infarcts) and tumor deposits producing symptoms and signs appropriate to their locus within the cerebellum. Infarcts, hemorrhages, or tumors as they enlarge may acutely cause hydrocephalus or increased intracranial pressure with papilledema because of obstruction of CSF outflow pathways. The midline cerebellum is the most common site of primary brain tumors (medulloblastoma, cystic astrocytoma) in childhood. Demyelinating plaques of multiple sclerosis may arise anywhere in the cerebellar white matter and can give rise to a variety of cerebellar deficits. The Arnold-Chiari malformation and platybasia/basilar impression also cause cerebellar symptoms and signs.

Alcoholism with nutritional deprivation (see Ch. 120) can cause degeneration of the vermis and anterior cerebellum with profound gait ataxia. Other acquired cerebellar syndromes include those caused by hypothyroidism, various toxins (carbon monoxide, heavy metals, phenytoin), hyperpyrexia, and repeated head trauma. Rarely, reversible pancerebellar dysfunction may follow viral infections in children. A rare, profound cerebellar degeneration may accompany certain malignancies in adults.

SPINOCEREBELLAR DEGENERATIONS
(Hereditary Ataxias)

A group of degenerative disorders characterized by progressive ataxia due to degeneration of the cerebellum, brainstem, spinal cord, and peripheral nerves, and occasionally the basal ganglia. Many of these syndromes are hereditary; others occur sporadically. The spinocerebellar degenerations can be thought of in 3 broad groups: the predominantly spinal ataxias, the cerebellar ataxias, and multiple systems degenerations (see TABLE 128–1). Patterns of clinical involvement usually breed true but great variability may be found among affected members of ataxic kindreds. There is no treatment.

Friedreich's ataxia is the prototype spinal ataxia. Gait unsteadiness begins between the ages of 5 and 15 followed by upper extremity ataxia and dysarthria. Tremor, if any, is a minor feature. Patients are areflexic and there is loss of large-fiber sensory modalities. Pes cavus and scoliosis are common, as is progressive cardiomyopathy. Inheritance is autosomal recessive. Although **Bassen-Kornzweig syndrome** (abetalipoproteinemia, vitamin E deficiency) and **Refsum's disease** (phytanic acid storage disease) share some clinical features with Friedreich's ataxia, the metabolic basis of the latter remains unknown.

Cerebellar cortical degenerations generally begin between ages 30 and 50. Clinically, only signs of cerebellar dysfunction can be detected, and pathologic changes are restricted to the cerebellum and occasionally the inferior olives. Both sporadic and dominantly inherited cases have been reported.

In the **multiple systems degenerations (olivopontocerebellar atrophies),** ataxia occurs in young to middle adult life in varying combinations with spasticity and extrapyramidal, sensory, lower motor neuron, and autonomic dysfunction. Optic atrophy, retinitis pigmentosa, ophthalmoplegia, and dementia occur in some kindreds. These syndromes include Menzel's dominant disorder (with cranial nerve findings and spasticity); the Dejerine–Thomas sporadic or recessive syndrome in which parkinsonism is prominent; and Azorean motor systems degeneration (Machado-Joseph disease). Cerebellar ataxia with autonomic insufficiency (Shy-Drager syndrome) is discussed below.

TABLE 128–1. CLINICAL FEATURES OF SPINOCEREBELLAR DISORDERS

Syndrome	Weakness & Atrophy	Extra-pyramidal	Cranial Nerve	Sensory Loss	Are-flexia	Peripheral Neuropathy	Optic Atrophy	Retenitis Pigmentosa	Skeletal Changes	On-set†	Hered-ity*	Miscellaneous
Spinal ataxia												
Friedreich's ataxia	+	−	−	+	+	+	±	−	+	J	R	Cardiomyopathy, pes cavus
Cerebellar cortical degenerations												
Holmes	−	−	−	−	−	−	±	−	−	A	D	Hypogonadism
Marie (LCCA)‡	−	−	−	−	−	−	−	−	−	A	R/S	
Multiple systems degenerations												
Menzel	−	±	±	−	−	−	±	−	−	A	D	
Dejerine-Thomas	−	±	−	−	−	±	−	−	−	A	R/S	
Shy-Drager	±	±	±	−	−	−	−	−	−	A	S	Automatic insufficiency
Machado-Joseph	+	±	±	−	−	−	−	−	−	A	D	
Systemic disorders												
Refsum's disease	+	−	−	+	+	+	±	+	−	J	R	Icthyosis ↓ Phytanic acid
Abetalipoproteinemia	−	−	−	+	+	+	±	+	+	J	R	Steatorrhea
Ataxia telangiectasia	+	±	−	−	+	−	−	−	−	J	R	Telangiectasias ↓ IgA, infections
Mitochondrial multi-system disorder	+	−	±	−	−	−	−	±	−	J/A	S	Opthalmoplegia, heart block, "ragged red fibers"

* R = Recessive; D = Dominant; S = Sporadic.
† J = Juvenile; A = Adult.
‡ LCCA = Late cortical cerebral atrophy.
+ = Always present; − = Absent; ± = Variable

Miscellaneous disorders: Ataxia also may occur in systemic disorders of unknown pathogenesis. **Ataxia telangiectasia** is discussed in Ch. 18. In the **mitochrondial multisystem disorders,** ataxia is seen in varying combinations with ophthalmoplegia, heart block, and myopathy. Muscle biopsy reveals characteristic "ragged red fibers." The cause is unknown.

IDIOPATHIC ORTHOSTATIC HYPOTENSION; SHY-DRAGER SYNDROME

(See also ORTHOSTATIC HYPOTENSION in Ch. 26)

Autonomic insufficiency occurs in a number of nervous system disorders. When due to CNS disease it may be part of a spectrum of illnesses. Symptoms and signs of autonomic failure in addition to orthostatic hypotension include impotence, urinary retention and fecal incontinence, decreased sweating, iris atrophy, and decreased tearing and salivation. **Idiopathic orthostatic hypotension** is *a syndrome in which symptoms are confined to the autonomic nervous system;* pathologically there is degeneration of postganglionic sympathetic neurons. Absent pressor responses to tyramine infusion and supersensitivity to infused norepinephrine support the notion of peripheral denervation. The **Shy-Drager syndrome** is *a multiple systems degeneration in which signs of more widespread neurologic damage occur*: autonomic dysfunction with cerebellar ataxia, parkinsonism, corticospinal and corticobulbar tract dysfunction, and amyotrophy. Bulbar dysfunction and laryngeal stridor may prove fatal. Occasionally, the physical and pathologic findings are only those of Parkinson's disease with extension to involve the intermediolateral cell columns of the spinal cord.

Treatment involves intravascular volume expansion with fludrocortisone given 0.1 to 0.6 mg/day orally, salt supplementation, the application of constrictive garments to the lower body (including the abdomen), and α-adrenoreceptor stimulation with ephedrine 25 to 50 mg tid (see also ORTHOSTATIC HYPOTENSION in Ch. 26). Maintaining a head-up body position at night may reduce morning orthostasis. Metoclopramide 30 to 60 mg/day, parenteral dihydroergotamine, and indomethacin 25 mg tid to qid have been reported to be effective in some patients. Metoclopramide may exacerbate parkinsonian symptoms in patients with multiple systems degeneration.

---

129. CRANIOCERVICAL JUNCTION ABNORMALITIES

Developmental or acquired abnormalities in bone at the skull base or upper cervical spine that decrease the potential space for the lower brainstem and cervical cord, resulting in cerebellar, lower cranial nerve, and spinal cord symptoms. The spinal cord is flexible and therefore susceptible to intermittent compression. In consequence, several types of lesions at this level can cause symptoms that vary from patient to patient and may come and go.

Fusion of the atlas and foramen magnum produces symptoms of cervical myelopathy when the anterior-posterior diameter of the spinal canal behind the odontoid process declines to < 19 mm. **Platybasia** is *an asymptomatic flattening of the skull base* (the angle formed by the intersection of the plane of the clivus and the plane of the anterior fossa is > 135°). Patients with **basilar invagination** (*protrusion of the odontoid process into the foramen magnum*) have short necks and combinations of cerebellar, spinal cord, brainstem, and lower cranial nerve signs. The **Klippel-Feil** malformation (*fusion of cervical vertebrae*) usually is asymptomatic except for a neck deformity with

limited range of motion. **Atlantoaxial dislocation** (*displacement of the atlas anteriorly in relation to the axis*) causes acute or chronic spinal cord compression.

Etiology

Congenital abnormalities are present at birth. There is an increased incidence of associated neurologic defects including syringomyelia (see below) and the Arnold-Chiari malformation (cerebellar tonsils descend into the cervical spinal canal—see under NEUROLOGIC DEFECTS in Ch. 187). In Morquio syndrome (mucopolysaccharidosis IV) hypoplasia of the odontoid causes atlantoaxial subluxation and spinal cord compression.

Trauma to the cervical cord may cause acute atlantoaxial dislocation and acute cervical myelopathy. RA and metastatic disease to the cervical spine are other acquired causes of atlantoaxial dislocation. Paget's disease may result in platybasia, basilar invagination, or spinal cord compression from progressive bone disease. A slowly growing tumor (eg, a meningioma or a chordoma) at the craniocervical junction also decreases the potential space for the brainstem and the spinal cord, producing similar myelopathic symptoms.

Symptoms and Signs

Axons of upper motor neurons in the decussation of the pyramids may be affected, often causing weakness, spasticity, and hyperactive reflexes in one upper or both lower extremities. Lower motor neuron involvement may cause muscular atrophy and weakness in the arms and hands. Involvement of sensory fibers may cause occipital and neck pain; diminished touch, vibration, or position sensation in the limbs, singly or in combination; and may be bilateral, ipsilateral, or contralateral, or even ipsilateral at one level and contralateral at another. Dysarthria and dysphagia may occur because of pressure on brainstem and lower cranial nerves. Some patients describe a tingling down the back on neck flexion **(Lhermitte's sign)**. Involvement of the median longitudinal fasciculi in the cervical cord or, most likely, ischemia due to vertebral artery compression at the foramen magnum may cause nystagmus or an internuclear ophthalmoplegia with horizontal nystagmus on lateral gaze. Downbeat nystagmus (fast component downward) is characteristic of craniocervical junction lesions. Atlantoaxial dislocation compresses the cervical cord producing spastic quadriparesis. Neck movement may increase pain and weakness.

Diagnosis

Congenital abnormalities, Paget's disease, metastatic carcinoma, RA, and fracture dislocations all can be diagnosed from cervical spine films and skull x-rays. Myelography is necessary to determine the level and extent of any associated epidural lesions and may outline a slowly growing tumor. MRI well defines tumor masses in this area, as well as associated defects; eg, Arnold-Chiari malformation or syrinx.

Treatment

Surgical decompression of the posterior fossa and upper cervical cord is indicated for progressive neurologic signs in congenital and acquired disorders. Radiation therapy and a hard cervical collar often improve the course of metastatic disease. Calcitonin should be given to patients with Paget's disease.

130. SPINAL CORD DISORDERS

The spinal cord extends caudally from the medulla at the foramen magnum to terminate at the upper lumbar vertebrae. In the **white matter** at the periphery are the ascending and descending tracts of myelinated sensory and motor nerve fibers. The **central**

H-shaped gray matter is composed of cell bodies and nonmyelinated fibers. The **anterior (ventral) horns of the H** contain lower motor neuron cells that receive their impulses from the motor cortex via the descending corticospinal tracts; the axons of the anterior horn cells become the efferent fibers of the spinal nerves. The **posterior (dorsal) horns** contain afferent sensory nerve fibers whose cell bodies lie in the dorsal root ganglia. The **gray matter of the cord** also contains many internuncial neurons that carry motor, sensory, or reflex impulses from dorsal to ventral nerve roots, from one side of the cord to the other, and from one level of the cord to another.

The **segments of the cord** are conceptual, not actual, divisions, and correspond approximately to the attachments of the 31 pairs of spinal nerves. In spinal cord disorders, the integrity of individual segments is assessed clinically by examining the reflexes and the sensory and motor responses in the distribution of the segments (see SPINAL CORD INJURY, Symptoms, Signs, and Diagnosis in Ch. 124).

SPINAL CORD COMPRESSION

Many diseases affect the spinal cord by mechanical compression, which often presents in a stereotyped fashion and can be treated effectively if caught early.

Acute spinal cord compression usually is traumatic, presenting as flaccid paraplegia or quadriplegia ("spinal shock"—see SPINAL CORD INJURY in Ch. 124).

Subacute cord compression usually is caused by an extramedullary neoplasm (see also SPINAL CORD NEOPLASMS in Ch. 126) or an epidural abscess or hematoma (see below). Patients present with local back pain, often in a radicular distribution. Reflex changes from corticospinal tract dysfunction (hyperreflexia, Babinski's signs) follow, then weakness (often proximal) of the lower extremities, sensory loss, and loss of sphincter control. The phase of back pain and mild weakness may last hours to days, but the transition to total loss of function caudal to the lesion may take only minutes.

Chronic spinal cord compression is a consequence of bony or cartilaginous protrusions into the spinal canal (eg, from osteophytes, spondylosis, or a herniated nucleus pulposus, especially in patients with congenitally narrow spinal canals—these are discussed in Ch. 131); or of slow-growing extramedullary neoplasms (neurofibroma, meningioma—see SPINAL CORD NEOPLASMS in Ch. 126). Chronic compression follows the course outlined for subacute compression except that pain may be dull, both motor and sensory abnormalities may evolve at the same time, and spasticity is found in the lower limbs.

Diagnosis is based on the clinical signs—spine tenderness, paraparesis, sensory deficits of the legs and trunk, and corticospinal reflex changes. Spine x-rays may disclose erosion, collapse, fracture, or subluxation at the level of the lesion. A myelogram is necessary to confirm compression of the cord and to fully define the level of the lesion.

Treatment depends on the underlying illness. Management of acute injuries and of conditions causing chronic compression is discussed in the chapters referred to above.

Prompt intervention in subacute compression cannot be overemphasized. Many patients, if treated before weakness becomes marked, recover full neurologic function, whereas few do well once paraplegia or autonomic deficits have occurred. Corticosteroids (dexamethasone 100 mg/day for 3 days) are given promptly. If the tissue type of a compressing metastatic neoplasm is known, immediate radiation therapy is as effective as rapid surgical decompression. Immediate surgery is performed if a tissue diagnosis is needed or for epidural hematoma or abscess. Patients having surgery for epidural metastases should receive radiotherapy, starting 5 days postoperation.

EPIDURAL ABSCESS AND HEMATOMA

Spinal epidural abscess usually occurs in a patient with an underlying infection, either remote (eg, a furuncle or dental abscess) or contiguous (eg, vertebral osteomyeli-

tis, decubitus ulcer, or retroperitoneal abscess). About 1/3 of cases, however, arise spontaneously. *Staphylococcus aureus* is the most common causative organism, followed by *Escherichia coli* and mixed anaerobes. Rarely, a tuberculous abscess may develop in conjunction with Pott's disease of the thoracic spine. **Spinal epidural hematoma** may result from back trauma, during anticoagulant therapy, or after lumbar puncture in patients with bleeding diathesis.

Either condition begins with local back pain and tenderness, usually thoracic or lumbar, which often are severe; the pain may radiate in a root distribution. Compression of the cord leads to weakness in a paraplegic pattern which progresses over hours to days with abscess, but within minutes to several hours with hematoma. Whether sensory or sphincter deficits occur depends on the site and size of the lesion. With an abscess, patients usually are febrile and the CSF has a high protein content and a lymphocytic pleocytosis; x-rays of the spine show osteomyelitic findings in about 1/3 of cases.

Both conditions are **diagnosed** and localized with myelography, with or without accompanying CT. If the lumbar epidural space is the suspected site, it is preferable to instill the contrast medium into the subarachnoid space via a cisternal needle puncture to avoid traversing the abscess or hematoma.

Treatment of compressing hematoma and most epidural abscesses is by prompt surgical decompression and removal, although successful medical treatment of the latter is increasingly reported. In suspected abscess, cultures of blood and of focal infections should be obtained before surgery, and treatment should be started with a penicillinase-resistant penicillin. Any pus found at operation should be gram-stained and cultured. Patients with suspected hematoma who are taking coumarin anticoagulants should be given vitamin K_1 2.5 to 10 mg s.c., and fresh frozen plasma. Thrombocytopenic patients need platelets.

SYRINGOMYELIA; SYRINGOBULBIA

A fluid-filled neuroglial cavity ***(syrinx)*** *within the substance of the spinal cord* ***(syringomyelia)*** *or brainstem* ***(syringobulbia).*** About half the lesions are congenital, but for unknown reasons they often expand during the teens or young adult years. The remainder arise in association with intramedullary tumors. Usually irregular and longitudinal, the **spinal syrinx** is paramedian and commonly begins in the cervical area, but may extend across or virtually the length of the spinal cord. It may be associated with an additional congenital anomaly such as the Arnold-Chiari malformation (in which cerebellar tissue extends into the spinal canal) or dysraphic syndromes; eg, encephalocele, myelomeningocele. (See also Neurologic Defects in Ch. 187.) About 30% of spinal cord tumors have an associated syrinx. **Syringobulbia** usually occurs as a slitlike gap within the lower brainstem that may affect the lower cranial nerves or ascending sensory or descending motor pathways by disruption or compression.

Symptoms and Signs

The **syrinx,** being paramedian, first interrupts fibers crossing from one side of the spinal cord to the other. Since these are predominantly pain and temperature fibers, and usually cervical, the patient may first notice a lack of sensation for noxious stimuli in his fingers (eg, a painless burn or cut). Other sensory losses follow. A capelike sensory defect over the shoulders and back is common. Impairment of corticospinal tracts leads to spasticity and weakness of the lower extremities. Anterior horn cells may be involved at the level of the syrinx, causing segmental muscular atrophy and fasciculations. **Syringobulbia** may cause vertigo, nystagmus, uni- or bilateral facial sensory impairment, lingual atrophy, dysarthria, dysphagia, and, at times, more distal sensory or motor dysfunction due to medullary compression.

Diagnosis

Syringomyelia must be distinguished from neoplasms and vascular malformations, and an associated parenchymal cord neoplasm always must be sought. Myelography followed by delayed computerized CT scanning may aid in diagnosis if dye fills and outlines the cavity. MRI outlines the syrinx, often the neoplasm, if present, and associated abnormalities at the craniocervical junction.

Treatment

Surgical drainage of the syrinx, plugging of the obex in the 4th ventricle, or section of the spinal cord (and central canal) at the filum terminale have been advocated by some; however, benefits are hard to appraise, since the course of symptoms and signs in syringomyelia is variable. Radiation therapy has proved useless.

DEMYELINATING CORD DISORDERS

MULTIPLE SCLEROSIS

(See in Ch. 127)

ACUTE TRANSVERSE MYELITIS

A syndrome, not a disease, in which an acute spinal cord transection of unknown cause affects both gray and white matter in one or more adjacent thoracic segments. Some cases are associated with viral illness, vasculitis, or the IV use of heroin or amphetamine, but usually no cause is found. Sudden local back pain is followed by sensory symptoms and motor weakness ascending from the feet. The defect may progress over several days and is severe, usually with global sensory-motor paraplegia below the lesion, urinary retention, and loss of bowel control. Occasionally, posterior column functions are spared, at least initially. The syndrome occasionally recurs.

Diagnosis

The condition must be differentiated from anterior spinal artery occlusion and acute cord compression, particularly from an epidural abscess, hematoma, or tumor. The CSF may show mononuclear leukocytes and a slightly increased protein content. Myelography may demonstrate swelling of the cord, occasionally even producing a subarachnoid block at the level of the lesion, but no epidural lesion is seen. CT scanning following the myelogram may help in this differentiation. Supine and prone myelography should be done to rule out a vascular malformation. Blood serologies are abnormal in the rare case with collagen vascular disease. Cases associated with a viral meningoencephalitis usually can be differentiated by their more subacute onset, associated viral symptoms, and a lymphocytic pleocytosis.

Treatment

None is specific, and except for those with a viral meningoencephalitis, most patients are left with considerable disability. Corticosteroids are of no proven benefit. Treatment is symptomatic.

VASCULAR DISORDERS

The vascular supply of the spinal cord originates superiorly from the vertebral arteries, and in the low thoracic area from a branch of the aorta. Branches of the anterior spinal artery supply the anterior ⅔ of the cord, and branches of the posterior spinal artery supply the posterior ⅓.

INFARCTION

Because the spinal circulation is supplied by 2 or 3 major arterial branches, the cord is especially vulnerable to infarction (with resultant softening—**myelomalacia**) in the "watershed" area between the connection of these branches, around the 2nd to 4th thoracic segments. Infarction is uncommon, however, and more often is due to vascular compression (from tumors, acute disk compression) or to remote causes (eg, aortic surgery, dissecting aneurysm) than to intrinsic disease of the spinal arteries. Rarely, polyarteritis nodosa may cause occlusion of spinal arteries.

Symptoms and Signs

Sudden pain in the back and in the distribution of the affected segment is followed by bilateral flaccid weakness and a dissociated sensory loss with impaired pinprick and temperature sensation below the level of the infarct. The distribution of the anterior spinal artery usually is involved, so that touch, proprioception, and vibration sense are likely to be spared, since they are conducted in posterior tracts of the cord. As with all infarcts, the deficit is most marked during the first few days and may partially resolve with time.

Diagnosis and Treatment

Transverse myelitis, cord compression by a tumor or other mass, and demyelinating disease cause similar findings and must be excluded. Treatment is symptomatic, with frequent turning and skin care (see Ch. 240), attention to pulmonary toilet, and physical and occupational therapy. If urinary bladder function is compromised, intermittent catheterization with rigorous attention to antisepsis is preferable to an indwelling catheter (see also NEUROGENIC BLADDER in Ch. 158).

ARTERIOVENOUS (A-V) MALFORMATIONS

Large, tortuous veins predominate in A-V malformations of the cord. The malformations may be small and localized or may involve up to ½ the cord. They may, like a mass lesion, compress or even replace normal parenchymal tissue; or may rupture, causing a focal or generalized hemorrhage. The most common location is on the posterior aspect of the cord at the thoracic level. A cutaneous angioma sometimes overlies the spinal one.

Symptoms, Signs, and Diagnosis

Hemorrhage can provoke sudden pain in the area and loss of neurologic function below the level of the hemorrhage; fever and nuchal rigidity may result from blood in the subarachnoid space. Malformations that compress or infiltrate the cord cause subacute myelopathy or signs of intrinsic cord disease with a dissociated sensory loss and segmental weakness. Diagnosis is suggested by a "bag of worms" appearance on myelogram (with the needle removed and the patient supine) and is confirmed by selective arteriography, injecting thoracic branches of the aorta until the branch that feeds the malformation is found.

Treatment

Surgery, using specialized microtechnics, is indicated if spinal cord function is threatened, but special experience is required. Occlusion of feeder arteries by embolization through an arterial catheter is practiced in a few large medical centers.

COMBINED SYSTEM DISEASE

(Subacute Combined Degeneration of the Spinal Cord)

The neurologic manifestations of pernicious anemia. The hematologic and GI features are discussed in ANEMIA DUE TO VITAMIN B_{12} DEFICIENCY in Ch. 96; and Ch. 58.

Pathology

The descriptive names (above), which antedate discovery of vitamin B_{12} deficiency as the cause, refer to the degenerative changes seen in the posterior columns and corticospinal tracts. These changes, which are also seen in the cerebral white matter and peripheral nerves, involve both axons and myelin sheaths; the peripheral nerve abnormality usually precedes the spinal cord changes. There may be degeneration of cortical neurons as well, but neuronal changes are minor in comparison to those in myelinated tracts. Occasionally, the optic nerves are involved.

Symptoms and Signs

The neurologic symptoms occasionally precede the hematologic abnormalities (or occur in their absence if folic acid has been taken). Onset is gradual, with peripheral pins-and-needles paresthesias and weakness, progressing to leg stiffness, unsteadiness due to proprioceptive difficulties, lethargy, and fatigue. Delirium or confusion, spastic ataxia, and at times postural hypotension are seen in advanced cases.

Examination in the early stages shows peripheral loss of position and vibration sense in the extremities, accompanied by mild to moderate weakness and reflex loss. Later in the course, spasticity, Babinski's responses, more severe loss of proprioceptive and vibratory sensations in the lower extremities, and ataxia emerge. Tactile sensation may be impaired, but involvement of pain and temperature sensations usually is minor. The upper extremities are involved later and less consistently.

Diagnosis and Treatment

These are described in Ch. 96. The condition must be differentiated from compressive cord lesions and multiple sclerosis, as well as from other anemias. Early diagnosis is important, since the neurologic defects become irreversible if allowed to persist for months or years. (CAUTION: *Folic acid therapy without vitamin B_{12} corrects the hematologic abnormalities, but can aggravate the neurologic manifestations; therefore, it is* **contraindicated.**)

TABES DORSALIS

(See SYPHILIS in Ch. 14)

131. DISORDERS OF THE PERIPHERAL NERVOUS SYSTEM

The peripheral nervous system consists of the cranial and spinal nerves from their point of exit from the CNS to their terminations in peripheral structures. By convention, the olfactory and optic nerves, though not true nerves but CNS tracts, are also included.

The **cranial nerves** (except for the olfactory, optic, and a part of the spinal accessory) leave the CNS from the brainstem. Their motor nuclei lie deep within the brainstem; their sensory nuclei in ganglia just ouside it. The 31 pairs of **spinal nerves** each emerge from a segment of the spinal cord as an anterior (ventral) motor root and a posterior (dorsal) sensory root. The efferent motor fibers originate as anterior horn cells in the gray matter of the cord; the afferent sensory fibers originate in dorsal root ganglia. The ventral and dorsal roots combine to form the nerve, which exits via an intervertebral foramen. Because the cord is shorter than the spine, the foramina lie progressively farther from the original cord segment, so that in the lumbosacral region the nerve roots from the lower cord segments descend within the spinal column in a near-vertical sheaf (the **cauda equina**).

The spinal nerves anastomose peripherally into the cervical, brachial, and lumbosacral **plexuses** (the intercostal nerves remaining segmental), and then branch into the

nerve trunks that terminate (as much as 3 ft distant) in peripheral structures. By convention, the term **peripheral nerve** often is used to connote this portion of a spinal nerve, lying peripheral to the roots and plexuses.

The peripheral nerves are bundles of nerve fibers that range in diameter from 0.5 to 22 μm. The larger fibers convey motor or touch and proprioceptive impulses; the smaller fibers convey pain and autonomic impulses. The supporting satellite **Schwann cells** envelop each nerve fiber in a thin cytoplasmic tube, covered by the **neurilemma (sheath of Schwann)**. Within the neurilemma, the Schwann cells further wrap the larger fibers in a multilayered insulating membrane, the **myelin sheath**, which enhances conduction of neural impulses, so that large fibers tend to be fast conductors, and small fibers, slow conductors.

Peripheral nerve dysfunction may result from damage to the nerve fibers, cell body, or myelin sheath. When ischemic or traumatic injury stops the flow of axoplasm down the nerve fiber, the nerve process dies distally **(wallerian degeneration)**. When metabolic injury to the cell body alters the axoplasmic nutrients, the most distal part of the cell process is affected first, and axonal degeneration ascends proximally, producing the distal-to-central pattern of symptoms characteristic of the metabolic neuropathies. Injury to the myelin sheath, either directly or from Schwann cell or neuronal damage, results in **demyelination** with a consequent slowing of nerve conduction. Each Schwann cell maintains the myelin sheath along one segment of the nerve fiber, so that selective Schwann cell damage results in **segmental demyelination**, a pathologic finding characteristic of many neuropathies.

After a crush injury, nerve fiber regrowth proceeds within the Schwann cell tube at about 1 mm/day. Regrowth may be misdirected, causing **aberrant innervation** (eg, of fibers in the wrong muscle; of a touch receptor at the wrong site; of a temperature instead of a touch receptor). The myelin sheath can regenerate rapidly, especially after segmental demyelination, with complete recovery of function unless axonal destruction also has occurred.

CRANIAL NERVE DISORDERS

OLFACTORY NERVE DISORDERS

(See ANOSMIA in Ch. 208)

OPTIC NERVE DISORDERS

(See Ch. 225)

OPHTHALMOPLEGIA

(See VISION AND EYE MOVEMENT DISORDERS in Ch. 119)

TRIGEMINAL NEURALGIA

(Tic Douloureux)

A disorder of the sensory nucleus of the trigeminal nerve producing bouts of severe, seconds-long lancinating pain in the distribution of one or more divisions, most often the superior mandibular or maxillary. The cause is unknown, and no pathologic changes can be found. Older patients usually are affected. The pain is often set off by touching a trigger point or by activity such as chewing or brushing the teeth. Pain is intense, and although each bout is brief, successive bouts may incapacitate the patient.

Diagnosis

The history usually is typical and diagnostic. No signs, clinical or pathologic, occur with trigeminal neuralgia, so that finding a sensory abnormality or cranial nerve dys-

function rules out trigeminal neuralgia as the cause of pain. If trigeminal dysfunction is found, a neoplasm or other lesion impinging on the nerve or its distribution in the brainstem should be sought. Pontine lesions usually result in sensory and motor dysfunction; a medullary lesion causes a dissociated loss of pain and temperature with loss of the corneal reflex. **Differential diagnosis** includes a neoplasm, vascular malformation of the brainstem, a demyelinating lesion, or a vascular insult. Postherpetic pain is differentiated by its typical antecedent rash, scarring, and predilection for the ophthalmic division. Trigeminal neuropathy may occur in Sjögren's syndrome or RA, but with a sensory deficit that is often perioral and nasal. Patients with migraine and atypical facial pain also have a normal examination, but their pain is more prolonged and burning or throbbing in character. Chronic meningitis or acute polyneuropathy occasionally causes a trigeminal defect by catching exiting fibers in the subarachnoid space.

Treatment

Carbamazepine 200 to 1600 mg/day is generally effective and the benefit often sustained; liver and hematopoietic functions should be monitored. **Phenytoin** 300 to 600 mg/day or **baclofen** 15 to 40 mg/day is effective in some cases. Peripheral block or section of the 5th nerve branches seldom is beneficial. **Surgical approaches** to treatment include the separating away of structures (especially arteries) pressing against the trigeminal root in the posterior fossa (Jennetta procedure) and creating electrolytic lesions of the Gasserian ganglion via a percutaneous stereotaxically positioned needle. Occasionally, to relieve intractable pain, surgical section of 5th nerve fibers proximal to the Gasserian ganglion, at the brainstem level, is resorted to.

GLOSSOPHARYNGEAL NEURALGIA

A rare syndrome characterized by recurrent attacks of severe pain in the posterior pharynx, tonsils, back of the tongue, and middle ear. The cause is unknown, and no pathologic changes can be found, except in the rare case due to a tumor in the cerebellopontine angle or the neck. Men are affected more commonly than women; the syndrome usually appears after age 40.

Symptoms and Signs

As in trigeminal neuralgia, intermittent attacks of brief, severe, excruciating pain occur paroxysmally, either spontaneously or precipitated by movement (eg, chewing, swallowing, talking, sneezing). The pain, lasting seconds to a few minutes, usually begins at the base of the tongue and radiates to the ears or down the neck anterolaterally. Occasionally, increased activity of the vagus nerve causes cardiac sinus arrest with syncope. Attacks may be separated by long intervals.

Diagnosis

The location of the pain, precipitation of an attack on swallowing or by touching the tonsils with an applicator, and temporarily eliminating the pain with 0.15% tetracaine applied locally (after which the pain cannot be evoked by stimulation), will distinguish glossopharyngeal neuralgia from trigeminal neuralgia involving the mandibular division. Tonsillar, pharyngeal, and cerebellopontine angle tumors as well as metastatic lesions in the anterior cervical triangle must be ruled out.

Treatment

As in trigeminal neuralgia, carbamazepine is the drug of choice. If ineffective, cocainization of the pharynx may provide temporary relief, and surgery may be necessary. When pain is restricted to the pharynx, the nerve in the neck may be avulsed; it must be sectioned intracranially if pain is widespread.

FACIAL NERVE DISORDERS

(See also Cranial Nerve Examination in Ch. 117)

Unilateral facial weakness is a common neurologic sign. Of the many disorders that can affect the facial nerve and cause facial weakness, only the most common, Bell's palsy, is discussed here; other causes are mentioned under diagnosis of that condition.

BELL'S PALSY

Idiopathic unilateral facial paralysis of sudden onset. The cause is unknown, but the mechanism is presumed to involve swelling of the nerve due to immune or viral disease, with ischemia and compression of the facial nerve in the narrow confines of its course through the temporal bone.

Symptoms, Signs, and Course

Pain behind the ear may precede the facial weakness, which develops, sometimes to complete paralysis, within hours. The involved side is flat and expressionless, and patients may complain about the seemingly twisted intact side rather than the involved side. In severe cases the palpebral fissure is wide, and the patient cannot close his eye. Examination may show an area of decreased pinprick sensation along the distribution of Arnold's nerve behind the involved ear. A lesion just proximal to the nerve branches may affect salivation, taste, and lacrimation, and may cause hyperacusis.

Prognosis depends on the extent of nerve damage. Complete recovery within several months invariably follows partial facial paralysis. The results after total paralysis are variable. The likelihood of complete recovery is 90% if the nerve proximal in the face retains normal excitability to supramaximal electrical stimulation, but it is only about 20% if electrical excitability is absent. Misdirected regrowth of nerve fibers may innervate lower facial muscles with periocular fibers and vice versa, resulting in contraction of unexpected muscles on voluntary facial movements **(synkinesia)**, or "crocodile tears" during salivation. Facial muscle contractures may follow chronic weakness.

Diagnosis

The weakness of the entire half of the face distinguishes Bell's palsy from supranuclear lesions (eg, stroke, cerebral tumor), in which the weakness is partial and most prominent below the eye. Abrupt-onset facial palsy rarely provides a diagnostic problem. However, Bell's palsy must be differentiated from unilateral facial weakness due to other disorders of the facial nerve or its nucleus, chiefly geniculate herpes **(Ramsay Hunt syndrome)**, middle ear or mastoid infections, fractures of the petrous bone, carcinomatous or leukemic invasion of the nerve, chronic meningeal infections, or cerebellopontine angle or glomus jugulare tumors. Skull x-rays and CT scans are negative in Bell's palsy but may reveal a fracture line, bony erosion by infection or neoplasm, or internal auditory canal expansion from a cerebellopontine angle tumor. CT scans may show the contrast-enhancing mass in angle or glomus tumors.

Treatment

Methylcellulose drops or temporary patching may suffice to protect the exposed eye; tarsorrhaphy may be needed when eye closure weakness is prolonged. Corticosteroids (eg, prednisone 60 to 80 mg/day orally beginning soon after onset and given for 1 wk, then decreased gradually over the 2nd wk) are not of proven benefit, but seem to decrease acute pain. Faradic stimulation of the nerve and physical therapy are useful only to provoke motion and prevent contractures in paralyzed muscles. Hypoglossal-facial nerve anastomosis may partially restore facial function if none has returned in 6 to 12 mo.

EIGHTH NERVE DISORDERS

(See DIFFERENTIATION OF SENSORY [COCHLEAR] AND NEURAL [8TH NERVE] HEARING LOSSES in Ch. 204; and VERTIGO in Ch. 119)

DISORDERS OF THE MOTOR UNIT

A **motor unit** consists of *a single anterior horn cell; its efferent root, peripheral nerve fiber, and terminal arborization in the motor endplate at the neuromuscular junction; and the 10 to 600 muscle fibers that the neuron innervates.*

It is convenient to classify the disorders involving the motor unit according to the segment principally affected (see TABLE 131–1). Thus, in the **motor neuron diseases (muscular atrophies),** the major defect is a loss of efferent innervation at the level of the anterior horn cell. In some of these diseases, the nuclei of upper motor neurons in the

TABLE 131–1. CLASSIFICATION OF MOTOR UNIT DISORDERS

I. Neurogenic Muscular Atrophies
   A. Anterior horn cell degeneration
      1. Amyotrophic lateral sclerosis (including progressive spinal muscular atrophy and progressive bulbar palsy)
      2. Infantile spinal muscular atrophy
      3. Juvenile spinal muscular atrophy
   B. Anterior root and peripheral nerve involvements
      1. Peroneal muscular atrophy
      2. Hypertrophic interstitial neuropathy
      3. Guillain-Barré syndrome
      4. Metabolic neuropathies

II. Neuromuscular Junction Disturbance
   A. Myasthenia gravis
   B. Myasthenic syndrome
   C. Drug-induced cholinesterase inhibition (eg, from neostigmine, insecticides)

III. Disorders of Muscle Fibers
   A. Muscular dystrophies
      1. Pseudohypertrophic muscular dystrophy (Duchenne's)
      2. Limb-girdle muscular dystrophy
      3. Facioscapulohumeral muscular dystrophy
      4. Myotonic muscular dystrophy (see Myotonic myopathies, below)
      5. Rare forms: distal muscular dystrophy; ocular myopathy; benign juvenile muscular dystrophy
   B. Myotonic myopathies
      1. Myotonia dystrophy
      2. Myotonia congenita, Thomsen's disease
   C. Inflammatory myopathies
      1. Dermatomyositis, polymyositis
      2. Trichinosis
   D. Glycogen and lipid storage diseases of muscle (McArdle's, Tarui's, and Pompe's diseases)
   E. Familial periodic paralysis
      1. Hypokalemic type
      2. Hyperkalemic type
      3. Normokalemic type
   F. Endocrine myopathies (eg, in thyroid, parathyroid, adrenal disorders; hypercalcemia; hypophosphatemia)

motor cortex or axons in the brainstem (corticobulbar tracts) or spinal cord (corticospinal tracts) are also involved; in others, cranial nerve motor nuclei in the brainstem (bulbar nuclei) are affected (bulbar palsies).

In **myasthenia gravis,** the **myasthenic syndrome,** and **drug-induced cholinesterase inhibition,** the defect is at the neuromuscular junction.

In the **myopathies,** the major involvement is at the level of the muscle fibers. By convention, certain hereditary progressive myopathies are known as **muscular dystrophies.** Other myopathies may result from inflammation or from an endocrine or metabolic abnormality. Those that are hereditary are discussed here; other disorders that can cause myopathy or muscular weakness (polymyositis, dermatomyositis, trichinosis, thyroid and adrenal disorders, hypercalcemia, hypophosphatemia) are discussed elsewhere in THE MANUAL.

MOTOR NEURON DISEASES

(Neurogenic Muscular Atrophies)

Disorders characterized by muscle weakness and wasting due to denervation.

AMYOTROPHIC LATERAL SCLEROSIS (ALS); PROGRESSIVE SPINAL MUSCULAR ATROPHY; PROGRESSIVE BULBAR PALSY (PBP)

Motor neuron disease of unknown etiology characterized by progressive degeneration of corticospinal tracts and anterior horn cells or bulbar efferent neurons. The symptoms and descriptive designation vary according to the part of the nervous system most affected. Onset generally is after age 40, and the incidence is greater in males. Five to 10% of cases are familial, with an autosomal dominant inheritance.

Symptoms and Signs

Amyotrophic lateral sclerosis (ALS): Muscular weakness and atrophy, evidence of anterior horn cell dysfunction, often begin distally and asymmetrically. Forty percent of cases begin in hand muscles. Cramps are common and may precede weakness. Visible muscle fasciculations, spasticity, hyperactive deep tendon reflexes, and extensor plantar reflexes, evidence of corticospinal tract involvement, soon accompany the lower motor neuron signs. Dysarthria and dysphagia are due to involvement of brainstem nuclei and pathways. Sensory systems, voluntary eye movements, and urinary sphincters are spared. Death usually occurs in 2 to 5 yr, but 20% of patients survive 5 yr.

Progressive spinal muscular atrophy (Aran-Duchenne muscular atrophy) is a variant in which anterior horn cell involvement outpaces corticospinal involvement, and the condition is more benign. Muscle wasting and marked weakness begin in the hands, progress to the arms, shoulders, and legs, and are eventually generalized. Fasciculations are readily seen in the limb muscles, rarely in the tongue. Onset can be at any age, and survival for 25 yr or more is possible.

Progressive bulbar palsy (PBP, labioglossolaryngeal paralysis): In this variant, the muscles innervated by cranial nerves and corticobulbar tracts are predominantly involved, so that chewing, swallowing, and talking become increasingly difficult. A pseudobulbar emotional response, with labile and inappropriate emotions, may be seen. Because of the dysphagia the prognosis is particularly poor, and death in 1 to 3 yr (often from respiratory complications) is common.

Diagnosis

Diagnostic features of the ALS and PBP varieties include an onset during middle or late adult life with progressive and generalized motor involvement unaccompanied by

sensory abnormalities. Nerve conduction velocities are normal until late in the disease. Electromyography can support the diagnosis. Fibrillations, positive waves, and fasciculations are seen along with giant motor units even in clinically uninvolved limbs. Myopathies, atrophy due to cervical spondylosis, ruptured intervertebral disk, spinal cord tumor, syringomyelia, congenital malformations of the cervical spine, and multiple sclerosis must be excluded as causing the muscular atrophy.

Treatment

There is no specific treatment. Physiotherapy may help to maintain muscle function. Patients with pharyngeal weakness should be fed with extreme care, and may require a gastrostomy. Baclofen may help reduce spasticity and cramps. Anticholinergic agents decrease saliva production (atropine 0.4 to 0.6 mg orally bid). Pyridostigmine 30 to 60 mg orally tid has initially helped some patients with bulbar weakness. Surgical efforts to improve swallowing in bulbar cases have had limited success.

INFANTILE AND JUVENILE SPINAL MUSCULAR ATROPHIES

(Werdnig-Hoffmann Disease; Wohlfart-Kugelberg-Welander Disease)

Disorders beginning in infancy or childhood, characterized by skeletal muscle wasting due to progressive degeneration of cells in the anterior horn and medulla. Fifty percent of cases are inherited. Three variants are recognized.

Symptoms and Signs

The acute infantile form (Werdnig-Hoffmann disease) is an autosomal recessive disorder, symptomatic by 4 mo of age; 1/3 of babies are hypotonic at birth. All infants have delayed motor milestones by 6 mo.

In the **chronic infantile form,** babies are symptomatic by age 2, and most at about 6 to 12 mo. Fewer than 25% learn to sit, and none walk or crawl. Regardless of the age of onset, children are hypotonic with flaccid muscle weakness, absent deep tendon reflexes, and fasciculations (which may be hard to see in young children). Dysphagia may be present. The disease often is fatal early in life, frequently from respiratory complications. However, spontaneous arrest can occur, leaving the child with a chronic, static (nonprogressive) weakness.

Juvenile spinal muscular atrophy (Wohlfart-Kugelberg-Welander disease) begins between 2 and 17 yr of age with similar pathologic findings and mode of inheritance, but a slower evolution and longer life expectancy. Weakness and wasting are most evident in the legs, with onset in the quadriceps and hip flexors. Later, the arms are affected. Weakness often progresses from proximal to distal parts. Some familial cases may be secondary to specific enzyme defects (eg, hexosaminidase A deficiency).

Diagnosis and Treatment

Diagnosis usually is made by demonstrating denervation without peripheral nerve involvement, chiefly by clinical appraisal, electromyography, and nerve conduction velocity studies (usually normal). Muscle biopsy occasionally is used. Serum enzymes (CK, aldolase) may be mildly increased. The disorders cannot be diagnosed by amniocentesis.

There is no specific treatment. Physical therapy, bracing, and special appliances benefit static or slowly progressive cases, to prevent scoliosis and contractures.

NERVE ROOT DISORDERS

Nerve root dysfunction, which is usually secondary to chronic pressure or invasion of the root, causes a characteristic radicular syndrome of pain and segmental neurologic deficit. **Ventral (motor) root involvement** causes weakness and atrophy of muscles innervated by that particular root. **Dorsal (sensory) root abnormalities** produce sensory

impairment in a dermatomal distribution. The corresponding segmental deep tendon reflexes are depressed or absent. Large mass lesions in the cervical, thoracic, or lumbar levels, especially in patients with narrow canals, may compress both the root and spinal cord, adding a myelopathy to a root syndrome (see also Ch. 111).

Radicular pain is precipitated by movement of the spine, coughing, or sneezing, or with Valsalva maneuvers. Lower lumbar and high sacral roots, which form the sciatic nerve, produce pain in the buttocks and posterior lateral thigh and calf **(sciatica).** Lesions of the **cauda equina,** which involve multiple lumbar and sacral roots, cause radicular symptoms in both legs as well as impaired sphincter and sexual function. **Thoracic lesions** result in bandlike dysesthesias around the thorax or flank. **Cervical root** pain radiates into the arm, shoulder, or the occiput, depending on its particular level.

Etiology

Herniated intervertebral disks (see below), with or without associated degenerative spine disease, are the most common causes of a root syndrome. Less commonly, chronic meningitis, especially carcinomatous meningitis, produces patchy multiple root dysfunction. Epidural abscesses and tumors can present with radicular symptoms. Spinal cord meningiomas and neurofibromas may begin as isolated radicular problems (see Ch. 126). Diabetes mellitus causes a painful thoracic or extremity radiculopathy. Bone changes in RA, especially in the cervical region, may compress isolated nerve roots. Herpes zoster infection causes a painful radiculopathy with a dermatomal sensory loss and a characteristic rash.

Diagnosis

Plain spine films show degenerative arthritis or metastatic disease. CT scanning defines the dimensions of the bony canal and lateral recess encroachment. Myelography outlines soft tissue planes and delineates the level of a disk protrusion or an intramedullary or extramedullary mass lesion. Nodularity of nerve roots may be seen with meningeal disease. CSF cytology, protein, glucose, and culture differentiate neoplastic from other chronic meningitides. Electromyography and evoked potentials can be helpful in localizing the level and severity of root lesions. Nerve conduction velocities are normal, but spontaneous activity (positive waves and fibrillations) and decreased motor recruitment will be seen in muscles innervated by one or more injured roots. F-wave latencies may be prolonged, and H-reflexes are absent in S1 radiculopathies. Evoked potentials may show delay at the level of root entry after repetitive stimulation of the median, peroneal, or posterior tibial nerves.

Treatment

Specific therapy depends on the etiology of the radicular syndrome. Patients with epidural or meningeal tumor should be treated with radiation therapy to symptomatic levels and corticosteroids (dexamethasone 8 to 16 mg/day orally). Intrathecal methotrexate is being used in larger centers to try to slow tumor progression in cases with diffuse meningeal seeding. Epidural abscesses require immediate surgical drainage and 6 to 8 wk of antibiotic therapy. Diabetes mellitus is best treated with better glucose control. Severe herpes zoster infections should be treated with antiviral agents (acyclovir, vidarabine). Corticosteroids in patients > 50 yr of age may decrease the incidence of postherpetic neuralgia. Meningiomas and neurofibromas require surgical excision.

HERNIATED NUCLEUS PULPOSUS

(Herniated, Ruptured, or Prolapsed Intervertebral Disk; Disk Syndrome)

Etiology

Cartilaginous disks, consisting of an outer anulus fibrosus and an inner nucleus pulposus, separate the spinal vertebrae. Degenerative changes, with or without trauma, result in protrusion or rupture of the nucleus through the anulus fibrosus in the lumbo-

sacral or cervical area; the nucleus moves posterolaterally or posteriorly into the extradural space. Symptoms result when the herniated nucleus compresses or irritates the nerve root. Posterior protrusion can compress the cord or cauda equina, especially in patients with developmentally narrow spinal canals (spinal stenosis).

In the lumbar area, > 80% of disks affect L5 or S1 nerve roots. Severe L5 radiculopathies cause foot drop with weakness of the anterior tibial, posterior tibial, and peroneal muscles. S1 radiculopathies cause weakness of the medial gastrocnemius muscle and loss of the ankle jerk. In the cervical area, C5 to C6 and C6 to C7 herniations are most common. Chronic C5 radiculopathy may result in a frozen shoulder. Severe C8 radiculopathies interfere with fine hand movement or result in painful **shoulder–hand syndromes.**

Symptoms and Signs

Pain in the distribution of the compressed root may begin suddenly and severely, or insidiously. It is worse on movement and may be exacerbated by the Valsalva maneuver (coughing, laughing, straining at stool, etc), since this transmits pressure to the disk through the subarachnoid space. Paresthesias or numbness in the sensory distribution of the root may occur. Deep tendon reflexes in the root distribution are depressed. With a lumbosacral herniation, straight leg raising, which stretches the roots, may produce back pain (see Ch. 111); neck flexion is similarly painful with herniated cervical disks. Muscles supplied by the impaired root eventually become weak, wasted, and flaccid and may show fasciculation. Cervical cord compression may cause spastic paraparesis of the lower limbs, and cauda equina compression often results in urine retention or incontinence from loss of sphincter function; *these occurrences signal a situation requiring urgent care and close supervision.*

Diagnosis

Symptoms and signs suggest the diagnosis. Plain spine films usually reveal disk space narrowing. CT scanning defines the dimensions of the canal and may show the disk protrusion. Myelography best defines the size and location of the disk herniation. Electromyography may help to define the particular root involved.

Treatment

Treatment should be conservative, first with 2 wk of strict bed rest—supine on a firm surface. **For lumbar radiculopathies** traction with immobilization may help but does not remove pressure on the nerve. Analgesics and mild tranquilizers help relieve pain. Corticosteroids (prednisone 80 mg orally tapered over 10 days) have been advocated by some, but results are uncertain. If objective neurologic findings persist or get worse (weakness, sensory deficit), decompressive laminectomy should be performed. Any lesion acutely compressing the spinal cord or cauda equina (eg, urine retention or incontinence) requires immediate surgery.

In cervical root lesions, traction as well as a cervical collar is recommended as it effectively relieves muscle spasm, even when severe nerve root involvement and motor weakness are present. It is usually applied at home for 15 min 3 to 4 times/day, using static weights. The required amount of pull varies according to the individual's size and body type, but is usually between 5 and 15 lb. Neck position during traction is important: The most comfortable straight or mildly flexed position is used; *extension should be avoided.* The traction is applied through a head halter, with the weight attached on a rope put through a pulley that is placed above and slightly in front of the patient to ensure that the neck is pulled in flexion. The traction should relieve the pain, and relief should begin to last beyond the traction periods within a few days. The frequency of treatments may be decreased as symptoms subside.

If static home traction does not provide relief, intermittent traction using a motorized device in a physical therapy facility is indicated. Hospitalization for further evalu-

ation is indicated if motor weakness progresses or does not rapidly subside. Surgical decompression occasionally is necessary to prevent further deterioration, especially in C5 or C8 root lesions.

CERVICAL SPONDYLOSIS

A condition in which degenerative changes in both the intervertebral disk and the anulus, as well as the formation of bony osteophytes, narrow the cervical canal. A progressive myelopathy characteristically results, especially with development of a spastic gait, because of spinal cord compression. Patients with a congenitally narrow canal are at increased risk. Although patients usually lack a history of painful cervical root syndrome, radicular signs often betray the dermatome where the most significant compromise has occurred. This is usually between C-5 and C-6, and C-6 and C-7. Arm weakness and atrophy with segmental reflex loss occurs in combination with hyperreflexia, increased tone, vibratory impairment, and plantar extensor responses in the legs.

Diagnosis

Spine films reveal degenerative changes with osteophytes and disk space narrowing. If the sagittal diameter of the cervical canal is < 10 mm, compression of the cord is likely. CT defines the diameter of the canal. Myelography shows the level of the epidural block.

Treatment

Occasionally, signs improve or stabilize spontaneously. Conservative therapy includes a soft collar and physical therapy. If signs are progressive, decompressive laminectomy is conventional therapy to halt the progression or, occasionally, improve the myelopathy. The preferred (anterior or posterior) operative procedure is controversial.

PLEXUS DISORDERS

Diseases of the **brachial** or **lumbosacral plexuses** cause a mixed motor and sensory disorder of the corresponding limb. The pattern does not fit the distribution of individual roots or nerves. Disorders of the rostral brachial plexus produce disability about the shoulder, and those of the caudal brachial plexus produce dysfunction in the hand. In infants they may be caused by traction during birth; in adults, by invasion of metastatic cancer (typically breast or lung carcinoma in brachial plexus disorders and bowel or genitourinary neoplasms in the lumbosacral plexus). After radiation therapy, a plexopathy may occur from fibrosis, if the plexus was in the radiation port (eg, breast carcinoma). Diabetics develop a painful upper lumbar plexopathy associated with weight loss. A hematoma may compress the lumbosacral plexus in patients receiving anticoagulation therapy.

Acute brachial neuritis occurs mainly in men, more young than old, and produces supraclavicular pain, weakness and diminished reflexes in the distribution of the brachial plexus, and minor sensory abnormalities. Profound weakness develops within a day to a week or so of onset, then regresses over the next few months. The rostral plexus and therefore proximal muscles are involved in ⅔ of cases. The **etiology** is unknown, although viral or immunologic inflammatory processes are suspected.

Laboratory Data and Diagnosis

CT scanning of the brachial or lumbosacral plexus may reveal a mass lesion in patients with cancer or hematomas. In complete plexus lesions from cancer, extension of tumor into the epidural space may be seen on myelography. Electromyography and nerve conduction velocities help to localize plexus lesions. Slowing of nerve conduction

velocities is associated with denervation in muscles innervated by particular divisions of the plexus. Evoked potential recording after median nerve stimulation reveal delay at the Erb's point potential in metastatic lesions to the brachial plexus. Principal differentiation in inflammatory cases must be from acute nerve root compression.

Treatment

Metastatic lesions should be treated with radiation therapy with or without chemotherapy. Good glucose control is helpful in diabetic plexopathies. Corticosteroids for acute brachial neuritis have no proven benefit.

PERIPHERAL NEUROPATHY

(Peripheral Neuritis)

A syndrome of sensory, motor, reflex, and vasomotor symptoms, singly or in any combination, produced by disease of a single nerve **(mononeuropathy),** *2 or more nerves in separate areas* **(multiple mononeuropathy),** *or many nerves simultaneously* **(polyneuropathy).** Sensory loss, muscle weakness, atrophy, and decreased deep tendon reflexes are the hallmarks of peripheral nerve disease. Either the axon (diabetes, uremia, toxic agents) or the myelin sheath and Schwann cell (acute and chronic inflammatory polyneuropathy, leukodystrophies) may be the primary site of injury. Small myelinated fibers, causing primary loss of temperature and pain sensation, or large fibers, causing motor or somatosensory defects, may be affected. Some neuropathies (lead, dapsone, tick, porphyria, Guillaine-Barré) primarily involve motor fibers, whereas others mainly affect the dorsal root ganglia or sensory fibers producing sensory symptoms (dorsal root ganglionitis of cancer, leprosy, diabetes, and chronic pyridoxine intoxication). Occasionally, cranial nerves also are involved (Guillain-Barré, diabetes mellitus, diphtheria). Knowing the particular modalities involved helps the physician determine the etiology, although some neuropathies remain undiagnosed.

Etiology

Trauma is the most common cause of a localized injury to a single nerve. **Pressure** paralysis usually affects superficial nerves (ulnar, radial, peroneal) at bony prominences (eg, during sound sleep or anesthesia in thin or cachectic persons and frequently in alcoholics) or at narrow canals (eg, in entrapment neuropathies, such as the median nerve in the carpal tunnel syndrome). Pressure palsies also may result from tumors, bony hyperostosis, casts, crutches, or prolonged cramped postures (eg, from gardening). **Violent muscular activity or forcible overextension of a joint** may produce a mechanical neuritis, as may repeated small traumas such as those encountered by engravers through tight gripping of small tools, or by air-hammer operators through excessive vibration. **Hemorrhage** into a nerve, and **exposure to cold or to radiation,** may cause neuropathy. **Volkmann's ischemic paralysis** occurs when occlusion of a major artery affects nerves with a common blood supply in one limb.

Multiple neuropathy usually is secondary to collagen vascular conditions (polyarteritis nodosa, SLE, scleroderma, sarcoidosis, and RA), metabolic diseases (diabetes mellitus), or infectious agents (Lyme disease).

Microorganisms may cause mononeuritis by direct invasion of the nerve (eg, in leprosy or TB; the facial nerve in mastoiditis; the dorsal root in herpes zoster). Polyneuritis with acute febrile diseases may be due to a toxin (diphtheria), direct invasion of multiple nerves (malaria), or a probable autoimmune reaction (virus infections, the Guillain-Barré syndrome); the polyneuritis that sometimes follows immunizations also is probably immunologic (see also Ch. 127 and ACUTE VIRAL ENCEPHALITIS in Ch. 125).

Toxic agents generally cause a polyneuropathy, but sometimes a mononeuropathy. They include emetine, hexobarbital, barbital, chlorobutanol, sulfonamides, phenytoin,

nitrofurantoin, the vinca alkaloids, heavy metals, carbon monoxide, triorthocresylphosphate, orthodinitrophenol, many solvents, and other industrial poisons.

Nutritional deficiency and metabolic disorders usually cause a polyneuropathy—deficiency of B vitamins (alcoholism, beriberi, pernicious anemia, isoniazid-induced pyridoxine deficiency, malabsorption syndromes, psychoses, and hyperemesis gravidarum). Polyneuropathy also occurs in hypothyroidism, acute porphyria, sarcoidosis, amyloidosis, and in many uremic patients receiving dialysis. Diabetes mellitus causes several forms of neuropathy: a sensorimotor distal polyneuropathy (most common), a vascular mononeuritis multiplex, and an isolated mononeuritis (often of the oculomotor or abducens cranial nerves).

Malignancy may cause a polyneuropathy secondary to a monoclonal gammopathy (multiple myeloma, lymphoma) or amyloid invasion of the nerves themselves, and/or nutritional deficiencies.

Symptoms, Signs, and Clinical Forms

Mononeuropathy, both single and multiple, is characterized by pain, weakness, and paresthesias in the distribution of the affected nerve. Multiple mononeuropathy is asymmetric, and all the affected nerves may be involved from the outset or progressively. Extensive involvement of many nerves may simulate a polyneuropathy.

Compression and entrapment neuropathies result from mechanical compromise of a nerve. **Ulnar nerve palsy** is caused by trauma to the nerve in the ulnar groove of the elbow by repeated leaning on the elbow or by asymmetric bone growth after a childhood fracture ("tardy ulnar palsy"). There are paresthesias and sensory deficit in the 5th and lateral 4th fingers plus weakness and atrophy of the thumb adductor, 5th finger abductor, and interossei muscles. Severe, chronic ulnar palsy produces a "clawhand" deformity. The **carpal tunnel syndrome** results from compression of the median nerve in the volar aspect of the wrist between the longitudinal tendons of forearm muscles that flex the hand and the transverse superficial carpal ligament. This compression produces paresthesias in the radial-palmar aspect of the hand plus pain in the wrist, in the palm, or sometimes proximal to the compression site in the forearm. Sensory deficit in the palmar aspect of the first 3 digits and/or weakness of thumb opposition may follow. The syndrome is relatively common, may be uni- or bilateral, and is seen more often in women. It is associated with acromegaly, myxedema, fluid changes of pregnancy, and also with occupations that require repeated forceful wrist flexion. The chief distinction to be made is from C6 root compression due to cervical osteoarthropathy.

Peroneal nerve palsy is caused by compression of the nerve against the lateral aspect of the fibula. It is most common in emaciated bedridden patients and in thin people who habitually cross their legs. Weakness of foot dorsiflexion and eversion (foot drop) are present. Occasionally, a sensory deficit is found on the dorsal aspect of the web between the 1st and 2nd metatarsals. **Radial nerve palsy** ("Saturday night palsy") is caused by compression of the nerve against the humerus—eg, as the arm is draped over the back of a chair during intoxication or deep sleep. Symptoms include weakness of wrist and finger extensors (wrist drop) and occasionally a sensory loss on the dorsal web between 1st and 2nd metatarsals.

The site of local nerve damage can be identified by **Tinel's sign,** a distal paresthesia in the distribution of the nerve that is elicited by percussion over the site of compression. Electrical nerve conduction studies help in localization.

Polyneuropathy is relatively symmetric, and sensory, motor, and vasomotor fibers often are involved simultaneously. An acute, rapidly progressive form, the Guillain-Barré syndrome, and hereditary neuropathies are discussed separately below. The most common form of polyneuropathy is seen with metabolic diseases such as diabetes

mellitus, renal failure, or malnutrition. This form develops slowly, often over months or years, and frequently begins with sensory abnormalities in the lower extremities. Peripheral tingling, numbness, burning pain, or deficiencies in joint proprioception and vibratory sensation often are prominent. Pain is frequently worse at night and may be aggravated by touching the affected area or by temperature changes. In severe cases, objective signs of sensory loss can be demonstrated, characteristically with stocking-and-glove distribution. The Achilles and other deep tendon reflexes are diminished or absent. Painless ulcers on the digits or Charcot's joints may be seen when sensory loss is profound. Sensory or proprioceptive deficits may lead to gait abnormalities. Motor involvement results in distal muscle weakness and atrophy.

The autonomic nervous system may be additionally or selectively involved, leading to nocturnal diarrhea, bladder and bowel incontinence, impotence, or postural hypotension. Vasomotor symptoms (hyperemia, sweating, and bullae) are more common in partial lesions; complete lesions generally produce pallor, dry skin, and osteoporosis. Trophic changes are common in severe and prolonged cases.

Uncommonly, an exclusively sensory polyneuropathy is seen, which begins with peripheral pains and paresthesias and progresses centrally to a loss of all forms of sensation. This occurs as a remote effect of carcinoma, especially bronchogenic, after megadose intoxications with pyridoxine (B_6), and has been reported after high-dose penicillin therapy. The dorsal root ganglia are the sites of injury.

Diagnosis

Neuropathy is a symptom complex rather than a disease entity, and the cause must be sought. Clues to a systemic disorder may be found on physical examination or from the history. These include hypertension, rash, skin ulcers, Raynaud's phenomenon, weight loss, fever, lymphadenopathy, or mass lesions.

Laboratory findings often are helpful. A CBC may show the megaloblasts of pernicious anemia, the stippled RBCs of lead poisoning, or polyarteritic eosinophilia. Abnormal liver function tests and alkaline phosphatase may suggest an underlying malignancy. Blood creatinine and glucose may suggest a diagnosis of renal failure or diabetes mellitus. Urine should be checked for porphyrinogens, porphobilinogens, and heavy metals. Serum protein and immunoelectrophoresis support a diagnosis of a neuropathy associated with multiple myeloma or a monoclonal gammopathy. Cryoglobulins or complement fixations should be checked in appropriate settings. Thyroid function should be evaluated, including thyroid-stimulating hormone, in every patient with carpal tunnel syndrome. CSF is normal or shows an elevated protein.

Electromyography and **nerve conduction velocity tests** help confirm neuropathy, and document isolated nerve involvement and the predominant type of fiber involved (sensory, motor). Demyelinating lesions slow nerve conductions, and focal demyelinating blocks may be documented. An axonal process causes spontaneous activity in distal muscles and low amplitude evoked responses, with relatively preserved conduction velocities. In the carpal tunnel syndrome, conduction slows under the carpal ligament, prolonging the latency to the hallux or blocking it altogether. The distal sensory latency is similarly lengthened. Ulnar motor and sensory distal latencies must be normal in the same arm. **Muscle biopsy** may sometimes provide specific diagnoses (trichinosis, sarcoidosis, polyarteritis). Sural nerve biopsies rarely are indicated.

Prognosis and Treatment

Treatment of the systemic disorder (diabetes, renal failure, multiple myeloma, or tumor) may halt progression and improve symptoms, but recovery is slow. Traumatic lesions with complete transection of the nerve require surgical apposition. Entrapment neuropathies may require surgical decompression. Physical therapy and splints avoid contractures.

GUILLAIN-BARRÉ SYNDROME

(Acute Polyneuropathy; Acute Polyradiculitis; Infectious or Acute Idiopathic Polyneuropathy [AIP]; Landry's Ascending Paralysis; Acute Segmentally Demyelinating Polyradiculoneuropathy)

An acute, usually rapidly progressive form of polyneuropathy characterized by muscular weakness and mild distal sensory loss that about half the time begins 5 days to 3 wk after a banal infectious disorder, surgery, or an immunization. Guillain-Barré syndrome is the most frequently acquired demyelinating neuropathy. **Etiology** is unknown. Histologically, focal areas of segmental demyelination with perivascular and endoneurial infiltration of lymphocytes and monocytes are scattered along the peripheral nerves, roots, and cranial nerves. In severe lesions, axonal degeneration accompanies the segmental demyelination.

Symptoms and Signs

Relatively symmetric weakness usually begins in the legs and progresses to the arms, accompanied by paresthesias. Weakness always is more prominent than sensory symptoms or signs, and may first be most prominent proximally. Deep tendon reflexes are lost. Sphincters usually are spared. More than 50% of severely involved patients have weakness of facial and oropharyngeal muscles, and 5 to 10% require intubation for respiratory failure. Autonomic dysfunction, including BP fluctuations, inappropriate ADH secretion, cardiac arrhythmias, and pupillary changes occur in more severely involved patients. The respiratory paralysis and the autonomic defects may be life-threatening. Despite advances in respiratory care, 1.5 to 8% of patients die; 90% of patients reach their maximal degree of weakness in 3 wk, most in the first 2 wk.

In a variant of acute idiopathic polyneuropathy, the **Miller-Fisher syndrome,** patients develop only ophthalmoparesis, ataxia, and areflexia. Patients generally fully recover.

Diagnosis

Diagnosis is based on the clinical syndrome. Laboratory studies including increased protein without cells in the CSF and electrophysiologic abnormalities support the diagnosis, but the latter are hardly necessary in typical cases. Two-thirds of patients will have slow nerve conduction velocities and evidence of segmental demyelination at the time of onset. F-wave latencies, evidence of proximal demyelination, tend to be prolonged. Antecedent mononucleosis, or cytomegalovirus infections, mumps, or rubella can be excluded by appropriate serologic tests but do not change the prognosis.

Differential diagnosis includes toxins which act at the neuromuscular junction, such as organic phosphates, and botulism (see OTHER DISORDERS OF NEUROMUSCULAR TRANSMISSION, below; and Ch. 57). Acute poliomyelitis occurs in epidemics and produces fever, malaise, and pleocytosis in the CSF. Serologic studies are available. Tick infestation of the scalp causes an acute ascending motor neuropathy, mainly in children. Deep tendon reflexes are lost; sensation is normal. Removal of the tick results in resolution of all symptoms.

Prognosis and Treatment

Severe acute polyneuropathy represents a medical emergency, requiring constant monitoring and vigorous support of vital functions. The airway must be kept clear, and vital capacity should be measured frequently, so that respiration can be assisted if necessary. Fluid intake should be sufficient to maintain a urine volume of at least 1 to 1.5 L/day; serum electrolytes should be monitored to prevent water intoxication. The extremities should be protected from trauma and from pressure of bedclothes. Immobilization may cause ankylosis and is to be avoided. Heat helps in pain relief and

permits early physical therapy. Passive full-range joint movement should be started immediately and active exercises begun when acute symptoms subside.

The effect of corticosteroids is controversial, but controlled studies have shown that, if anything, they *worsen* outcome. Because of their side effects and lack of efficacy, they should not be used. Plasmapheresis has been used in large medical centers and may decrease recovery time and apparently halt progression of motor weakness. More experience is needed.

Considerable improvement over a period of months is usual, although approximately 30% of adults have residual weakness at 3 yr; the percentage is higher in children. Residual defects may require retraining, orthopedic appliances, or corrective surgery.

About 10% of patients relapse after initial improvement and enter a chronic state **(chronic relapsing polyneuropathy)**. Pathology and laboratory data are similar to acute cases, but the weakness may be more asymmetric and progress more slowly. Nerves eventually become palpable from repeated episodes of segmental demyelination and remyelination. Corticosteroids improve weakness, and prolonged therapy may be necessary. Immunosuppressive agents and plasmapheresis benefit some patients.

HEREDITARY NEUROPATHIES

Hereditary neuropathies are now classified as either hereditary sensory-motor neuropathies **(HSMN)** or hereditary sensory neuropathies **(HSN)**. Neurofibromatosis, a distinct hereditary neuropathy with prominent skin involvement, is discussed below. The most common HSMN, previously known as peroneal muscular atrophy, or Charcot-Marie-Tooth disease, is described below. Other less common HSMN begin from birth, and patients are more disabled. HSN are rare. Loss of distal pain and temperature modalities are more prominent than vibratory and position loss. The main problem in these patients is mutilation of their feet due to insensitivity to pain with frequent infections and osteomyelitis. Good foot care is mandatory.

PERONEAL MUSCULAR ATROPHY; HYPERTROPHIC INTERSTITIAL NEUROPATHY

(Charcot-Marie-Tooth Disease; Dejerine-Sottas Disease)

Peroneal muscular atrophy (Charcot-Marie-Tooth disease) is a relatively common hereditary disorder of the peripheral nervous system characterized by weakness and atrophy, primarily in peroneal and distal leg muscles. Autosomal dominant inheritance is usual. Other degenerative diseases, such as Friedreich's ataxia, may be present in these patients or in the same family pedigrees.

Symptoms and Signs

Type 1 patients present in middle childhood with foot drop and slowly progressive distal muscle atrophy producing "stork leg deformity." Intrinsic muscle wasting in the hand begins later. A stocking-glove decrease in vibration, pain, and temperature is present. Deep tendon reflexes are absent. Foot deformities, high pedal arches, and club feet may be the only manifestations in less affected family members who carry the trait. Type 1 patients have slow nerve conduction velocities with prolonged distal latencies. Pathologic specimens show segmental demyelination and remyelination. Enlarged peripheral nerves may be palpated. The disease progresses slowly and is compatible with a normal life span. Clinically, patients with Type 2 involvement usually develop weakness later in life, and the process is slower in evolution. They have relatively normal nerve conduction velocities but low amplitude evoked potentials, and biopsies reveal wallerian degeneration.

Hypertrophic interstitial neuropathy (Dejerine-Sottas disease), a rare autosomal recessive disorder of the peripheral nerves, presents in childhood with progressive weakness and sensory loss with absent deep tendon reflexes. Initially resembling Charcot-Marie-Tooth disease, motor weakness progresses at a faster rate. This is also a demyelinating-remyelinating disorder with enlarged peripheral nerves and "onion bulbs" on biopsy.

Diagnosis and Treatment

The characteristic distribution of motor weakness, foot deformities, family history, and electrophysiologic abnormalities confirm the diagnosis.

No specific treatment is available for these disorders. Vocational counseling, anticipating progression of the disease, may be useful in young patients. Bracing helps correct foot drop; orthopedic surgery to stabilize the foot may be of value.

NEUROFIBROMATOSIS
(von Recklinghausen's Disease)

A hereditary (autosomal dominant) disorder that produces pigmented spots and tumors of the skin, tumors of peripheral, optic, and acoustic nerves, and subcutaneous and bony deformities.

Symptoms, Signs, and Diagnosis

One third of patients with neurofibromatosis are asymptomatic and discovered on routine examination. In 1/3 of patients cosmetic problems are the initial complaints. Characteristic skin lesions, apparent at birth or in infancy in > 90% of patients, are medium-brown (café-au-lait) patches distributed most commonly over the trunk, pelvis, and flexor creases of elbows and knees. The presence of 6 or more of these freckle-like lesions with one larger than 1.5 cm is diagnostic of neurofibromatosis. Multiple cutaneous tumors, flesh-colored and of variable size and shape, appear in late childhood. There may be only a few or thousands of these lesions. Subcutaneous nodules or amorphous overgrowth of subcutaneous tissues **(plexiform neuromas)** and underlying bone may produce grotesque deformities, but this happens only rarely. Skeletal anomalies include absence of the greater wing of the sphenoid bone (posterior orbital wall) with consequent pulsating exophthalmos, fibrous dysplasia, subperiosteal bone cysts, vertebral scalloping, scoliosis, and tibial pseudoarthrosis.

The remaining 1/3 of patients present with neurologic problems. **Neurofibromas** (tumors of Schwann cells and nerve fibroblasts), which rarely appear before puberty, can be felt along the course of subcutaneous peripheral nerves. These tumors may involve spinal nerve roots, characteristically growing through an intervertebral foramen to produce intraspinal and extraspinal masses ("dumbbell" tumor). The intraspinal component may cause spinal cord compression. Plexiform neuromas may involve peripheral nerves producing deficits distal to the lesion. Tumors of cranial nerves may produce progressive blindness (optic glioma) or dizziness, ataxia, and deafness (acoustic neuroma). Bilateral acoustic neuromas are characteristic of neurofibromatosis (become symptomatic at approximately 20 yr of age), and gliomas and meningiomas are abnormally frequent. One study of patients with neurofibromatosis showed a 40 (male) to 87 (female) times increase in risk for neural tumors vs. the general population. The various tumors occur in 5 to 10% of all patients with neurofibromatosis.

Treatment

Deep tumors are treated by appropriate surgical removal or radiation. The underlying cellular disorder is unknown and no general treatment is available. Genetic counseling is advisable.

DISORDERS OF NEUROMUSCULAR TRANSMISSION

MYASTHENIA GRAVIS

A disease characterized by episodic muscle weakness, chiefly in muscles innervated by cranial nerves; and characteristically improved by cholinesterase-inhibiting drugs.

The disease is caused by an autoimmune attack on the acetylcholine receptor of the postsynaptic neuromuscular junction. The initiating event leading to antibody production is unknown. This antibody attack results in loss of acetylcholine receptors and jeopardizes normal neuromuscular transmission. The disease most commonly presents between 20 to 40 yr of age, predominantly in women, but may occur at any age.

Neonatal myasthenia is a syndrome of generalized muscle weakness seen in 12% of infants born to myasthenic mothers because of passive transfer of antibodies through the placenta. Symptoms resolve as the antibody titer declines in days to weeks. **Congenital myasthenia** is a rare autosomal recessive disorder of neuromuscular transmission beginning in childhood, usually with ophthalmoplegia. Acetylcholine receptor antibodies are absent and the condition is not regarded as an autoimmune disease.

Symptoms and Signs

The most common symptoms are ptosis, diplopia, and fatigability of muscles following exercise. Ocular muscles are affected first in 40% of cases and eventually in 85%. Dysarthria, dysphagia, and proximal limb weakness are common. Sensory modalities and deep tendon reflexes are normal. The symptoms and signs fluctuate in intensity over the course of hours to days. Severe generalized quadriparesis may develop, especially during relapses. Some patients present with bulbar symptoms; eg, alteration in voice, nasal regurgitation, choking, or dysphagia. Life-threatening respiratory muscle involvement **(myasthenic crisis)** occurs in approximately 10% of patients. **Ocular myasthenia** is a subclass of the generalized disease that remains limited to extraocular muscle involvement.

Diagnosis

Too often, the diagnosis is missed or only made after a patient has suffered a long time or presents in dire crisis—probably because the condition is rare and symptoms may be vague and passed off as unimportant. The possibility of myasthenia gravis is suggested by any of the symptoms and signs described above and is confirmed by improvement with anticholinesterase drugs. **Edrophonium** has a short duration of action (< 5 min) and is used in testing for myasthenia gravis and for differentiating between myasthenic and cholinergic crisis. **For the diagnostic test,** a syringe is loaded with 10 mg of edrophonium; 2 mg is given IV and if no reaction occurs within 30 sec, the rest is injected. In myasthenics there is a sudden, though short-lasting, improvement in muscle function. When the test is performed to differentiate between myasthenic and cholinergic crisis, the effect on muscle function and general condition indicates the diagnosis; a myasthenic crisis improves and a cholinergic crisis worsens. *Dangerous respiratory depression can occur and facilities to maintain respiration and atropine (as an antidote) must be available during the test.*

Electrophysiologic tests and serologic abnormalities substantiate equivocal diagnoses. In 90% of affected patients, neuromuscular transmission studies show a decremental response in the amplitude of the compound muscle action potential with repetitive nerve stimulation at 3 or 5 Hz, especially if 3 or more nerve-muscle groups are studied. Single-fiber electromyography may slightly improve the yield. Acetylcholine receptor antibodies are found in the sera of 85 to 95% of patients if human muscle

is used as the test antigen. The level of antibody titer does not correlate with disease severity. CT scans of the mediastinum show any associated thymoma.

Treatment

Treatment is with cholinesterase inhibitors, thymectomy, corticosteroids, and immunosuppressive agents and plasmapheresis. Anticholinesterases and plasmapheresis treat current symptoms; while thymectomy, corticosteroids, and immunosuppressives may alter the disease course by interfering with the autoimmune pathogenosis.

Pyridostigmine 60 to 240 mg orally q 3 to 4 h or **neostigmine** 15 to 60 mg orally q 3 to 4 h are the most commonly used anticholinergic drugs. Dosage must be carefully adjusted to individual requirements, and mild exacerbations may require an increase in dosage. Long-acting capsules are available for nighttime use by patients with severe dysphagia who otherwise would find it difficult to swallow medication in the morning. For some patients, abdominal cramps and diarrhea are less troublesome with pyridostigmine. Atropine 0.4 to 0.6 mg orally bid to tid or propantheline 15 mg tid to qid may be given for GI side effects. When parenteral therapy is necessary (eg, with dysphagia), neostigmine 0.5 mg IV or 1.5 mg IM may be substituted for 15 mg orally. The cholinergic drugs may not relieve all symptoms, especially extraocular muscle paralysis, in which case ephedrine 25 mg orally tid or qid may be tried as an adjunct. Patients require careful monitoring of their drugs and clinical symptoms.

Excessive neostigmine or pyridostigmine dosage causes weakness that cannot be differentiated clinically from myasthenia itself. Patients may also become refractory to the medication. Thus, if a patient who has been doing well should deteriorate, the cause must be determined. Edrophonium IV should be given; if the patient's weakness improves, the maintenance dose has been inadequate. If the weakness worsens, either the dose was too large or the patient's illness is refractory. Patients with respiratory paresis who are unresponsive to medication require complete respiratory support in a respiratory care unit.

Thymectomy should be considered in patients with generalized myasthenia, since approximately 80% of patients without a thymoma remit at some time subsequently (25% of patients remit spontaneously). If a thymoma is found, surgical excision is advised to prevent spread within the mediastinum. **Plasmapheresis** may be useful to prepare patients for thymectomy and during respiratory crisis. Some patients reduce daily drug doses by adding frequent plasmapheresis treatments. Large doses of prednisone 100 mg every other day orally and/or azathioprine or cyclophosphamide 150 to 200 mg/day orally are used in patients still seriously ill after thymectomy.

Myasthenia gravis can be a difficult problem to manage well, so that most patients with even moderately severe disease do best if treated by an experienced specialist.

OTHER DISORDERS OF NEUROMUSCULAR TRANSMISSION

The Eaton-Lambert syndrome is a presynaptic disorder that appears to be due to inadequate release of acetylcholine from nerve terminals. It occurs most commonly in patients with an underlying malignancy, especially men with intrathoracic tumors (eg, oat cell carcinoma of the lung). Patients complain of fatigability, weakness and sometimes pain in proximal limb muscles, peripheral paresthesias, dry mouth, impotence, and ptosis. Deep tendon reflexes are lost. The **diagnosis** is confirmed by finding an incremental response to repetitive nerve stimulation with the amplitude of the compound muscle action potential increasing > 200% at rates > 10 Hz (the opposite of myasthenia gravis). **Treatment** is first directed against the underlying malignancy. Guanidine (35 mg/kg), which facilitates acetylcholine release, often improves symptoms but may depress bone marrow. Corticosteroids and plasmapheresis have benefited some patients.

Botulism (see Ch. 57) also is due to decreased release of acetylcholine from presynaptic terminals (caused by the toxin produced by *Clostridium botulinum* spores, which destroys terminal cholinergic nerve twigs). An incremental response to repetitive nerve stimulation is seen.

DRUG-INDUCED NEUROMUSCULAR JUNCTION BLOCK

Cholinergic agents, used to treat myasthenia gravis, organophosphate insecticides, and most nerve gases block neuromuscular transmission by depolarizing postsynaptic receptors by excessive acetylcholine. Miosis, bronchorrhea, and myasthenic-like weakness occurs. Aminoglycoside and polypeptide antibiotics decrease both presynaptic acetylcholine release and sensitivity of the postsynaptic membrane to acetylcholine. Especially at high serum levels these antibiotics may increase neuromuscular block in patients with latent or manifest defects in neuromuscular transmission. Long-term D-penicillamine treatment may cause a reversible syndrome that clinically and electrically resembles myasthenia gravis.

Treatment: Patients with drug-induced or toxic neuromuscular blockade should receive respiratory support if needed, and intensive nursing care. Atropine 0.4 to 0.6 mg orally tid decreases the bronchial secretions in patients with cholinergic excess. Another antibiotic should be substituted for patients with aminoglycoside neuromuscular toxicity.

---

132. MUSCULAR DYSTROPHIES AND OTHER MYOPATHIES

Muscular Dystrophies

A group of inherited, progressive muscle disorders of unknown etiology. The different types are distinguished on clinical grounds.

Pseudohypertrophic (Duchenne) muscular dystrophy (see also HETEROZYGOTE DETECTION under GENETIC COUNSELING IN HEREDITARY DISORDERS, in Ch. 203) is the most common form, *a sex-linked recessive disorder typically presenting in boys aged 3 to 7 yr as proximal muscle weakness causing waddling gait, toe-walking, lordosis, frequent falls, and difficulty in standing up and climbing stairs*. The pelvic girdle is affected first, then the shoulder girdle. Serum enzymes, notably CK, are markedly elevated, especially early in the disease or during the first year of life, even before symptoms develop. Progression is steady and most patients are confined to a wheelchair by age 10 or 12. Flexion contractures and scoliosis ultimately occur, and most patients die by age 20 yr. A firm pseudohypertrophy of the calves is due to fatty and fibrous infiltration of the muscle. About 50% of patients have a lower IQ than their genetic expectation would suggest. There is no treatment, but all females on the maternal side of the family tree of an affected boy should be examined for possible elevations of CK or LDH enzymes on several occasions. Women with such elevations should be advised that they are possible carriers and counseled accordingly about childbearing.

Facioscapulohumeral (Landouzy-Dejerine) muscular dystrophy is *an autosomal dominant form characterized by weakness of the facial muscles and shoulder girdles*, usually beginning in early adolescence. Difficulty with whistling, eye closure, and elevation of the arms are early symptoms in adolescence. Life expectancy is normal. Anterior tibial and peroneal weakness develops in some kindreds, and although foot drop develops, ambulation is rarely lost.

Limb-girdle muscular dystrophy is a term used to describe *patients with weakness of pelvic* **(Leyden-Moebius [pelvifemoral] type)** *and shoulder* **(Erb [scapulohumeral] type)** *gir-*

dles. This is a mixed population, involving myopathic and neurogenic pedigrees, usually presenting in adults.

Ocular myopathy (*slowly progressive ptosis and ophthalmoplegia*) also is a heterogenous group, with some kindreds having spinocerebellar degeneration and others having, in muscle biopsies, mitochondria that stain red with trichrome stain (ragged red fibers). Most cases begin in late adolescence or early adulthood.

Congenital myopathies have been named by their characteristic findings on muscle biopsy **(central core disease, centronuclear myopathy, nemaline myopathy).** These children present with *delayed walking and mild proximal muscle weakness that is not progressive*. The biochemical defect is unknown.

Diagnosis depends on characteristic clinical findings, age of onset, and family history, supported when necessary by electromyography and muscle biopsy findings. Nerve conduction velocities are normal; electromyography reveals rapidly recruited myopathic motor units without spontaneous activity. Muscle biopsy shows necrosis, and variation in muscle fiber size. Later, fibrous tissue and fat replace muscle tissue.

Treatment: There is no specific therapy. Exercise should be encouraged as long as possible, and corrective surgery considered in slowly progressive forms. Passive exercises may extend the period of ambulation in severely affected patients. The added burden of obesity should be avoided; caloric requirements are likely to be less than normal.

Genetic counseling is indicated, especially for severe forms. Amniocentesis in Duchenne's dystrophy identifies male fetuses of carrier mothers.

Myotonic Myopathies

A group of conditions characterized by abnormally slow relaxation after contraction of voluntary muscle, due to an abnormality of the muscle membrane.

Myotonic muscular dystrophy (Steinert's disease, myotonia atrophica) is *an autosomal dominant disorder that combines dystrophic muscular weakness with myotonia*. It occurs at any age and is variable in severity. Myotonia is prominent in the hand muscles, and ptosis is common even in mildly affected individuals. Severe cases show marked peripheral muscular weakness associated with a high incidence of cataracts, testicular atrophy, premature balding, cardiac muscle conduction defects, and endocrine abnormalities. Mental retardation or dementia is relatively common. Death occurs in the early 50s in severely affected families.

Myotonia congenita (Thomsen's disease, ataxia muscularis) is *a rare, autosomal dominant myotonia that can begin anywhere between the neonatal period and about 10 yr of age, and is not associated with progressive muscle weakness*. Muscles may become hypertrophied, but muscle stiffness is the most important problem.

Diagnosis usually is established by demonstrating the myotonia by percussion of muscles and noting the slow relaxation after contraction or electromyography. Family pedigrees are important.

Treatment: In myotonia congenita, oral therapy with phenytoin 5 mg/kg/day; quinine sulfate 300 to 600 mg bid or tid; or procainamide, beginning with small amounts and increasing to 4 to 6 gm/day, may diminish the muscle stiffness and cramping. However, in myotonic dystrophy quinine or procainamide may increase cardiac conduction defects. The weakness of myotonic dystrophy does not respond to therapy, but active and passive exercises, as in other dystrophies, may be helpful.

Glycogen Storage Diseases of Muscle (see also Genetic Abnormalities of Carbohydrate Metabolism in Ch. 196)

Rare autosomal recessive diseases, characterized by abnormal accumulation of glycogen in skeletal muscle due to a specific biochemical defect in carbohydrate metabolism.

These diseases can be clinically mild or severe. The more severe **Pompe's disease** (absence of α-1,4-glucosidase or acid maltase), is evident in the first year of life and fatal by age 2. Glycogen accumulates in muscle, nerve, and heart tissue. In a less severe form, adult patients may present with proximal limb weakness and respiratory involvement causing hypoventilation. Myotonia is seen electrically but not on physical examination.

Four other enzyme deficiencies (see TABLE 196–3 in Ch. 196) are relatively mild in their clinical impact. After exercise, painful cramps develop followed by myoglobinuria. The diagnosis is supported by an ischemic exercise test and confirmed by demonstrating a specific enzyme abnormality. Diuresis is important during episodes of myoglobinuria to prevent renal failure. Most patients learn to limit their activities and to drink fluids after exercise.

Familial Periodic Paralysis

A rare group of inherited disorders of unknown cause characterized by episodes of flaccid paralysis with loss of deep tendon reflexes and failure of the muscle to respond to electrical stimulation. There is no alteration in consciousness. **Hypokalemic** and **hyperkalemic forms** have been described. (**Normokalemic** is probably the same as the hyperkalemic form.)

Symptoms and signs: In the **hypokalemic** variety, attacks usually begin at adolescence. The patient often awakens with weakness the day after vigorous exercise. This may be mild and limited to certain muscle groups or involve all 4 limbs. Oropharyngeal and respiratory muscles are spared. Serum and urine K are decreased. Weakness lasts 24 to 48 h. In the **hyperkalemic** form, the attacks often begin at an earlier age and usually are shorter, more frequent, and less severe. They often are accompanied by myotonia. (Myotonic lid lag may be the only symptom in asymptomatic family members.)

Diagnosis: The best clue is a history of the typical attack. During an episode, documentation of serum K level is important. Attacks can be provoked by glucose and insulin (hypokalemic form) or potassium chloride (hyperkalemic form), but this should be done only by experienced physicians in medical centers, since respiratory paralysis or cardiac conduction abnormalities may occur. The differential diagnosis includes persistent hypokalemia from any cause and hyperthyroidism, especially in Oriental males.

Treatment: Acetazolamide 250 to 1000 mg/day orally may prevent both hyper- and hypokalemic attacks, perhaps by inducing a mild metabolic acidosis. Potassium chloride 65 to 130 mg orally should be given during hypokalemic attacks.

Malignant Hyperthermia (see PHARMACOGENETICS in Ch. 276)

§12. PSYCHIATRIC DISORDERS

133. INTRODUCTION

Psychiatry, a branch of medicine, is responsible for the study, diagnosis, treatment, and prevention of human behavior disorders. Abnormal behavior may be determined or modified by genetic, physicochemical, psychologic, and social factors.

The psychiatrist must master the knowledge and skills not only of objective observation but of subjective, participant, and self observation. His background in natural science has fostered objective observation, but as he learns other types he finds this differentiation of his role function is necessary for understanding the relationship to his patient and for growth in his capacity for human intimacy. Only then can the general notion of personality and its underlying principles be learned: the genetic and ontogenic factors in growth, development, and decline; recognition of unconscious and preconscious factors as determinants of behavior; the idea that the personality is integral and indivisible; and recognition that man is a social animal and that the emerging stages of the life cycle reflect coordination between the evolving individual and his social environment.

Recent Historical Developments

The introduction of rauwolfia and the phenothiazines in the early 1950s contributed to the effective treatment and symptomatic management of many severely psychotic patients, reduced the duration of hospital stays, and increased the percentage of patients discharged from hospitals after acute episodes, making deinstitutionalization (see below) possible.

Concern increased that psychotic patients (including those chronically disabled) be cared for properly in the hospital or community, and that they be viewed as family and community members. Awareness increased concerning the reciprocal relations between patient and family that may enhance health or provoke illness. The patient's family became more involved in therapy, and the family physician's important role in rehabilitation has been recognized. In hospitals, new psychosocial methods have led to the avoidance of seclusion and restraint and to earlier discharge. Attempts to break down administrative and other barriers between hospital and community have increased, as have attempts to reform the internal social organization within the hospital.

Other developments include large-group technics, such as the therapeutic community; upgrading of the education of nonprofessionals; and movement toward greater precision in diagnosis (see Classification of Mental Disease, below), better understanding of genetic factors in psychopathology, and more exactness in the appropriate use of psychoactive drugs—neuroleptics, antidepressants, anxiolytics, and lithium. Pharmacologic investigation of the neuroleptic drugs has led to biochemical studies of the neurotransmitters and their possible role in the cause or course of mental illness.

Deinstitutionalization has increased, reinforced by more stringent legal mechanisms required to institutionalize a person against his wishes or, in hospitalized patients, to administer therapy. These measures protect against abuse of civil rights, but they also make it more difficult to provide treatment to patients who may be very irrational. Psychiatrists must understand and cope with the complexity of these issues, the sometimes competing demands for protection of individual rights vs. optimum therapy, and the need to assist society in developing better means of resolving these issues.

A new role for psychotherapy has emerged; ie, as an aid in coping with the travails of ordinary life rather than only as a way to deal with deep, crippling psychologic conditions. Persons are being helped who do not fit into the traditional diagnostic categories of neurosis and psychosis; ie, normal persons seeking therapy for life problems which may not be of their own making (eg, employment problems, bereavement, or family illness). Methods of short-term therapy have developed in which the therapist is more active than was the case in traditional psychoanalysis.

Hypnosis in medicine has had a resurgence of interest. In selected patients, hypnotic methods are valuable in managing pain, as an alternative or adjunctive method of anesthesia, and in treating psychosomatic disorders. Hypnotic approaches range from direct symptom modification procedures to investigations of psychodynamic issues.

The cult movement (see also Ch. 136) must interest psychiatrists, who need to understand how cult members are recruited, what happens to persons when they are in

cults (ie, methods of indoctrination), and how to understand and treat the problems of former members and their families. Clinical studies have identified specific cult-related emotional problems with which ex-members must cope during their reentry into society.

Self-help/mutual-aid groups have been with us for about 50 yr, although in a broader sense they are quite ancient—mutual aid has been practiced since families first existed. Each of us requires a social network to satisfy our needs to be accepted, cared for, and emotionally supported, particularly in times of stress.

In this century social changes have diminished this traditional support, and today the help, support, and information not always provided by natural or professional support systems is supplemented or complemented by mutual-aid groups: eg, self-care groups for those suffering from physical or mental illness, reform groups for addiction behaviors, and advocacy groups for certain minorities (handicapped, elderly, homosexuals, etc). Although professionals have launched many groups, most are not dependent on (but can and do work well with) professionals or professional agencies. Psychiatrists can help group leaders to avoid the risks of excessive hope or unrealistic goals, and also to learn more about the essential psychologic mechanisms of inspiration and hope inherent in the help movement.

In spite of these real advances, understanding of the basic causes of mental illness has yet to be achieved and requires continued and vigorous research in all fields relevant to the determinants of abnormal human behavior.

Classification and Diagnosis of Mental Disease

In all medical disciplines, classifications of disease are a dynamic process, ever changing to incorporate new knowledge. Access to the brain and technics for measuring and evaluating its functions, particularly mental activities, are still limited; thus, our understanding of the etiology and pathogenesis of mental disorders is scant. Nevertheless, attempts to categorize mental illness for the past half century have included theoretical concepts of causality, mixed with descriptive criteria. As a result, terminology and definitions of terms have varied widely among different psychiatrists and in different places. Since diagnosis implies prognosis and determines choices of therapy, and since commonality of diagnostic categories is essential to research design, the need for revision of psychiatric nomenclature and classification has been great.

The American Psychiatric Association started such a revision in 1974 and introduced a new *Diagnostic and Statistical Manual of Mental Disorders*, Third Edition **(DSM-III)** in March 1980. This classification attempts to rely entirely on descriptions of symptoms and signs; ie, what the patient says and does as indicators of how he thinks and feels. Specific diagnostic criteria (based on current clinical impressions and not yet fully validated) are suggested for the various disorders. DSM-III also inaugurated a 5-axis evaluation system for coding information. The first 3 axes comprise the diagnostic assessment. Axis I codes the clinical syndromes and some additional codes; Axis II, personality disorders and specific developmental disorders; Axis III, potentially relevant physical disorders and conditions. Axis IV codes the severity of psychosocial stressors; axis V, the highest level of functioning during the past year.

Often patients have multiple problems. A multiaxial system helps assure that some f these are not overlooked, and that the presenting problem does not shut out awareness of other important issues; eg, the presence of schizophrenia or depression should not preclude awareness of important personality or physical illnesses.

In this edition of THE MERCK MANUAL, most of the contributions use DSM-III terminology.

134. THE PSYCHIATRIC INTERVIEW

Although detail and emphasis in psychiatric and medical interviews differ, the purposes and technics are similar: to establish a therapeutic doctor-patient relationship, upon which accurate data collection and effective treatment depend. The initial interview is therefore a particularly significant encounter.

Approach to the Patient

Sources of clinical data include the patient's verbal content (what he says), manner of speaking (how he says it), and nonverbal communication (body language) and associated somatic clues, as well as the interviewer's own emotional responses. Often overlooked but important data are dress, posture, gait, facial expression, complexion, weight, and movement. These different sources of data are evaluated simultaneously in the psychiatric interview, a difficult but rewarding process that improves with the physician's increasing experience and sophistication. A mental posture of free-floating attention to the entire gestalt of the patient-interviewer interactions is the most effective way to obtain information from all levels. That is, while listening carefully to the patient's words, the interviewer is equally observant of the patient's facial expressions, gestures, postural changes, etc, and is aware of his own emotional reactions toward the patient. Data at one level will often augment, modify, or even contradict data at another level; eg, the patient who shifts position or fidgets with his watch while verbally denying concern about the item of history being discussed. Blushing, blanching, perspiring, increase in respiratory rate, and increase in tics or mannerisms all indicate emotional arousal. Often a subtle cue, a shift of gaze or slight change of expression, suggests covert emotions, fantasies, or impulses. Body language may communicate more eloquently than words the pain of a deep depression, the terror of acute anxiety, or the eroticism of seductive behavior.

The patient's behavior is determined by the reality of the present situation, his past experiences, his personality, and his outlook on life. Commonly, he will initially have mixed feelings; while he usually acknowledges his need for help and is relieved to share his concern with a potentially helpful professional, he may also be fearful of rejection, criticism, or humiliation. Thus, his perceptions of and reactions to the interviewer contain both rational and irrational elements, and his behavior may appear inconsistent, puzzling, or inappropriate. With psychotic illness or severe organic brain syndrome, these aberrations of perception and behavior may be extreme.

A spouse, relative, or friend often accompanies a patient, who usually is seen first. Sometimes, however (eg, when there is an organic problem or language difficulty, or when the patient is aged or a child), seeing the relative first or even both together may be profitable; but permission must be obtained from the patient. The opportunity to interview someone who knows the patient should not be missed, since it will add valuable perspective, but the confidentiality of each source must be respected.

The physician's attitude, while attentive, friendly, and encouraging, should retain an appropriate objectivity in relation to the patient and his problem. Total emotional neutrality is neither possible nor desirable, but the physician should be especially aware of feelings of irritability, impatience, or special attraction toward the patient. Other emotions that may be experienced are anxiety, sadness, sympathy, indifference, or resentment. Recognizing these emotions, learning what in the patient's behavior elicited them, and preventing them from disrupting the interview are essential.

The temptations to outdo the patient by recounting personal experiences, to moralize about the patient's behavior, to give gratuitous advice, or to provide dogmatic opinions should be resisted. Questions generally should be turned back to the patient ("Well, what do you think yourself?"), although at times it is beneficial to answer a question directly and promptly return the interview focus to the patient.

Interview Setting, Direction, and Length

The tone for the entire interview is established within the first few minutes. While not always available, a quiet, comfortable, and private **setting** lends dignity to the encounter and encourages free discussion. Regardless of the setting, the interviewer should communicate professionalism, concern, and willingness to take the necessary time. The physician greets the patient by name, performs introductions, indicates the purpose of the interview, and inquires regarding the patient's comfort at the moment.

Direction of the interview is next established. Needless controversy has existed concerning interviewing technic, with the two extremes represented by an entirely doctor-directed interview and a totally open-ended interview directed entirely by the patient. The important points are that doctor and patient are constantly cueing each other (verbally and nonverbally) and every interview is "directed"; the style of direction by the doctor may vary, and he should be aware of what is going on. No technic is uniformly successful under all circumstances, since the time available, the specific purpose of the interview, and the patient's clinical state will require appropriate modifications. Open-ended questions that permit the patient to respond in his own words have the virtue of eliciting unexpected information and often the most reliable data. Specific questions, as in a system review, provide important data that might not otherwise be obtained; eg, re sexual behavior, alcohol and drug abuse, suicidal ideas and plans, and hallucinations. The approach described below under Obtaining the History usually is applicable and productive.

The interview length must be appropriately flexible. With some patients 15 min are ample, as in cases of severe delirium, psychosis, or dementia. Conversely, an hour may be insufficient in a complex case where the patient is articulate and cooperative. In crisis situations with an acutely agitated patient, or when the patient is otherwise incapable of supplying a complete history, the interview goals must be realistically limited. Time constraints include the patient's tolerance for fatigue and anxiety and the physician's own time limits. However, a too-brief interview may prevent establishment of the relational bond necessary for the patient to communicate openly. At least 30 min usually are required for the initial psychiatric interview; more often, 45 or 60 min. When time constraints are inflexible, the patient should be assured of further opportunity to complete the assessment.

Termination of the interview usually is straightforward, although a loquacious or demanding patient may require firm interruption. The patient's questions should be encouraged and answered truthfully. Overly optimistic reassurance or unjustified guarantees of treatment efficacy should be avoided; the attempt to provide comfort and hope must be tempered with realism.

Obtaining the History

Inquiry should begin by asking the patient to identify the problem (in broad outline) for which he is seeking help. Questions such as "What has been the problem that brought you here?" or "Please tell me what has led you to come to see me today" are useful. Comments such as "Um-humm" or "Tell me more about that" at this stage encourage the patient to talk freely, as does repeating with a questioning inflection a key word or phrase spoken by the patient. As the patient talks, clarification is sought of key words such as depression, panic, nervousness, and anxiety, since these terms mean different things to different people. However, premature efforts to determine the exact details and their chronologic order at the very beginning of the interview may inhibit and distract the patient, and actually reduce the information available to the interviewer. In this early phase of the interview, the major focus is to learn what is significant to the patient himself, how he narrates his story, what emotions are manifest, and what nonverbal cues he communicates, as well as areas of vagueness, inconsistency, or confusion. Exceptions to this approach occur in some psychotic and organic states,

TABLE 134–1. FORMAT FOR RECORDING THE PSYCHIATRIC HISTORY

Category	*Pertinent Details*
Identifying characteristics	Name, age, sex, race, marital status, occupation, source of referral
Presenting problems	A brief verbatim statement
History of present illness	Chronologic account of the current symptoms and behavioral changes, together with coincident life events and their relationships Events are dated as accurately as possible Symptoms are recorded in the patient's own words, with qualifying details Previous treatments and responses to them are noted, and the present degree of disability estimated
Personal history	Birth and infancy Nature of delivery; temperament and habits; ages at passing milestones (walking, talking, toilet training) Childhood Emotional adjustment; neurotic symptoms; physical illnesses; relationships with peers and siblings Education Duration and details of schooling; achievements, attitudes, and adjustment Work record List of jobs; reasons for changing; achievements; adjustments Sexual maturation Date of menarche or puberty Growth of sexual interest and practice Courtship, marriage, and children Emotional and sexual compatibility with mate
Previous medical history	Physical and psychiatric illnesses
Personality and social patterns prior to illness	Social relationships within the home, at work, and in the community Individual and social activities and interests Predominant moods Character traits, strengths and weaknesses, coping style, methods of handling challenge and stress, temperament Religious and moral standards Ambitions and aspirations Habits, including drinking, drug use, smoking
Family history	Details of each parent and sibling re age, health, occupation, personality, relationship with the patient Familial diseases, including psychiatric illness For a deceased relative, the date and cause of death are recorded

where it is obvious immediately that the patient needs structure and direction in order to furnish useful information.

Once the patient has related his difficulties in his own words, a more structured approach is used to **follow up leads** in the original narrative and to **open up new areas** for discussion. Again, questions should be initially open-ended in order to encourage

TABLE 134–2. RECORDING OF MENTAL STATUS

Category	*Pertinent Details*
Appearance and behavior	Dress; posture; facial expression; motor activity such as agitation; impulsivity; mannerisms; retardation; relationship to the interviewer
Stream of talk (Thought processes)	Poverty or rigidity of thought Pace and progression of speech Whether speech is logical and to the point or confusing and irrelevant Presence of thought disorder, flight of ideas, obsessional qualification, distractibility The stream of talk is recorded verbatim if relevant
Thought content	Special preoccupations, obsessional ideas, misinterpretations, ideas of reference or influence, delusions, derogatory or grandiose ideas
Perceptual abnormalities	Auditory, visual, or tactile hallucinations Depersonalization Derealization
Affect	Happiness, elation, sadness, depression, irritability, anger, suspicion, perplexity, fear, anxiety Blunting or incongruity of affect Lability or reactivity of mood Appropriateness to context
Cognitive functions	Sensorium (level of consciousness) Memory and orientation: immediate recall; memory for recent and remote events; digit span; orientation in time, place, person Concentration: serial sevens; months of the year in reverse order General information: the Presidents, capitals, distances, etc Intelligence: Compatibility of school and work records with current performance; interpretation of proverbs; general vocabulary; calculations Insight and judgment, especially in regard to present illness and future plans Psychometric testing may be necessary

elaboration by the patient. For each problem area, one must clarify the time and mode of onset and get a detailed description of the symptoms or situations, chronology of events, aggravating and alleviating factors, and associated elements or manifestations. Progressively more directed, specific questions are required to obtain all pertinent information, including queries re some symptoms merely to establish that the patient does not have them, eg, hallucinations or suicidal thoughts.

Personal and family histories are obtained next, to provide a background against which the illness can be viewed and to find clues to the genesis of the illness and to possible therapeutic approaches. **Work history, social relationships, other interests,** and **future goals** complete this section of the interview. The interviewer must observe evidence of emotional arousal or conflict in the patient during this review and encourage further elaboration in sensitive areas.

Recording the History

In contrast to the flexibility used in obtaining a history, a particular format should be followed to record the history. The schema shown in TABLE 134–1 is commonly

used (alternatively, the developmental approach is acceptable, starting at birth or with the family history so that the illness is described in the perspective of the patient's life story).

Mental Status Examination

The distinction between history and examination is even more blurred in psychiatry than in general medicine. Most (and frequently all) of the mental status examination is carried out while the history is being obtained. It is insulting and pointless to demand from an intelligent, coherent patient the names of the last six heads of state, a recitation of long sequences of numbers, or the interpretation of proverbs and fables. However, when a specific mental status test is *required* to document the patient's mental state, the interviewer tactfully requests cooperation and is not deterred because of possible embarrassment.

The formal mental status examination is described in Ch. 117, and may be recorded as shown in TABLE 134–2.

Formulation

Essential to the psychiatric evaluation is *a concise statement of the interviewer's understanding of and plans for the case*: the formulation. It begins with a summary of the relevant data from the history and mental status examination organized as an explanatory hypothesis of the patient's condition. Included is an assessment of the patient's personality strengths and vulnerabilities, as well as identification of those factors contributing to the illness's origin and evolution. A differential diagnosis, necessary further investigations, an outline of an initial treatment plan, and a statement of prognosis complete the formulation.

135. PSYCHIATRY IN MEDICINE

PSYCHIATRIC CONSIDERATIONS IN THE MEDICAL INTERVIEW

Relating a patient's complaints and disabilities to his personality helps to form a sound clinical judgment about the nature and causes of the disorder. **To form a picture of the individual patient's personality,** the physician has to listen attentively and show interest in the patient as a person (see also Ch. 134). A rigid interview conducted hastily and in an emotionally indifferent way will more likely prevent the patient from revealing relevant information than help him divulge it. While tracing the history of the presenting illness with open-ended questions that permit the patient to tell his story in his own words, it is important to note comments that describe associated social circumstances and emotional reactions, as well as attitudes toward physicians and medicines.

Attention then should turn to the patient's social background, previous medical and psychiatric history, and adjustment at different stages of his life. Parental characteristics and the family atmosphere during his childhood are important because personality features that influence the way a person will handle illness and adversity are partly determined early in life. The way the patient has handled different family and social roles provides important clues. His schooling, manner of handling puberty and adolescence, stability and effectiveness at work, sexual adaptation, and the pattern of his social life and quality and stability of his marriage provide information valuable in appraising his personality. Use or abuse of alcohol and tobacco, behavior in driving, and any tendencies to antisocial conduct should be tactfully inquired after. The patient's responses to the usual vicissitudes of life—failures, setbacks, losses, previous

illnesses—are important; he may have endured stresses and misfortunes with courage and resilience or his history may suggest a poor capacity for tolerating frustration.

The personality profile that emerges from these inquiries may reveal traits such as narcissism, immaturity, excessive dependency, anxiety, tendencies to deny illness, histrionic behavior—or conscientiousness, modesty, and adaptability. In particular, the history may reveal patterns of repetitive behavior that the patient exhibits under stressful conditions; ie, whether distress is expressed in somatic symptoms (eg, headache, abdominal pain) or in psychologic symptoms (eg, phobic behavior, depression) or whether the expression is in social behavior, such as withdrawal or rebelliousness. With this information the physician can better interpret the patient's complaints, anticipate his reactions to his illness, and plan appropriate therapy.

Observation during the interview also provides valuable data. A patient may be depressed and pessimistic, or cheerful, facile, and prone to deny illness; he may be friendly and warm, or reserved, cold, and suspicious. Nonverbal communication may reveal attitudes and affects denied by the patient's words. For example, a patient who "chokes up" or becomes tearful when discussing a parent's death is revealing that it was a significant loss; the possibility that unresolved grief is still troubling him should occur to the physician. A tear in the eye, overt weeping, or other such manifestations of emotion should be considered as **physical signs** and should be recorded as such in the patient's chart.

Similarly, when a patient denies being angry, anxious, or depressed while his posture, gestures, and facial expression reveal these emotions, further inquiry may reveal stresses and emotionally depressing circumstances possibly related to the evolution of the present illness. However, the physician should be cautious and remember the possibilities of error in such inquiries. Discriminating and experienced judgment is needed to assess whether psychologic conflicts are highly significant, of limited importance, or perhaps merely coincidental to the patient's physical illness.

Referral for a psychiatric opinion: About 10% of patients admitted to a hospital are referred for a psychiatric consultation. Many of these patients have attempted suicide, and a substantial proportion have other conspicuous psychologic disturbances requiring appraisal and treatment. Particularly important are delirium, dementia, and functional psychiatric syndromes due to organic or metabolic brain disorders (see Ch. 118). In or out of the hospital, awareness of each patient's personality and its relation to his somatic complaints will aid in managing physically ill patients and increase the physician's awareness of psychiatrically ill or disturbed persons. Many of these patients will suffer from complex, difficult, or refractory problems that will require referral to a psychiatrist.

An infrequently used, but very helpful, procedure is for the primary care physician to discuss the situation with a psychiatric colleague *before* making a referral. Advice obtained in such an exchange may obviate the need for referral or help to make the referral in the most appropriate manner. When referral is planned, it should be discussed openly and sensitively with the patient.

PSYCHOSOMATIC MEDICINE

(Biopsychosocial Medicine)

Psychologic factors may contribute directly or indirectly to the etiology of some physical disorders; in others, psychiatric symptoms may be a direct expression of a lesion involving neural or endocrine organs. Psychologic symptoms also may occur as a reaction to the physical illness. The use of the term "psychosomatic" to encompass all these possibilities is a diffuse concept, but it draws attention to the ubiquity of emotional disturbances and psychologic interrelationships with somatic disease and disability throughout the entire field of medicine.

In a more limited sense, "psychosomatic" refers to conditions in which psychologic factors have some etiologic importance. Even in these disorders, however, the etiology is always complex and multifactorial, and psychologic factors are *not* the only contributors to the illness. It is useful to consider a *necessary* **biological** component (eg, the genetic tendency to diabetes mellitus) which, when combined with **psychologic** reactions (eg, depression) and **social** stress (eg, loss of a loved person), results in a set of conditions *sufficient* to produce the illness; hence, the term **biopsychosocial**. The stressful environmental events and psychologic reactions may be viewed as triggers or precipitants of illness. These reactions are *nonspecific* and have been noted in association with a wide variety of diseases, such as diabetes mellitus, SLE, leukemia, and multiple sclerosis. Furthermore, the importance of psychologic factors is relative and varies widely in different patients with the same illness (eg, asthma, in which inheritance and allergy and infection, as well as the patient's personality, interact to varying degrees).

The fact that psychologic stress can precipitate or alter the course of even major organic diseases has long been apparent, but very difficult for physicians to accept and comprehend. It is easy to understand how emotions can affect the autonomic nervous system and, secondarily, cardiac rate, sweating, or bowel peristalsis. But can a reaction affecting the mind (brain) alter immune responses mediated by lymphocytes and lymphokines? And if so, what are the mechanisms? The answer to the first question is becoming clear. **Psychoimmunology** is now an established area of scientific research, and both animal and human studies have demonstrated the interrelationship. For example, the immune response of mice has been clearly reduced in response to conditioned stimuli; and in humans the ability to reduce the delayed hypersensitivity skin response and even in vitro stimulation of lymphocytes to varicella zoster has been demonstrated. The pathways and mechanisms by which the brain and immune system interact remain to be elucidated.

Psychologic factors may influence the development of physical disease in other ways. For example, a patient's need to deny illness (or, more subtly, to deny the seriousness of an illness) may lead to noncompliance with medical regimens or refusal to accept therapeutic recommendations. Common examples are patients with hypertension or epilepsy, who fail to take medication, and patients who reject diagnostic procedures or operations.

Increasingly, physicians are dealing with disorders that result in chronic disability or that are liable to recurrence; eg, myocardial infarction, hypertension, cerebrovascular disease, diabetes mellitus, malignancy, RA, and chronic respiratory illness. Psychologic and social stress are entwined with these disorders; however, cause and effect are difficult to disentangle in investigating such associations. Psychosocial pressures contribute to the clinical course of these disorders in interaction with numerous other factors, including the individual's hereditary predisposition, personality features, and the autonomic and endocrine effects that arise in response to individual vicissitudes.

Psychologic Factors as Indirect Etiologic Agents

Although research has uncovered some of the most lethal etiologic agents of disease, the knowledge often proves difficult to apply in practice. Cigarette smoking and overeating are socially sanctioned forms of addiction, and smoking is also encouraged and reinforced by vast and subtle advertising campaigns that link the habit with assertiveness and virility. The roots of dependence on tobacco or excessive eating, as in other addictions, lie in the individual's personality, his reaction to his psychosocial environment, and his susceptibility to stress and to the relief of anxiety and tension provided by the addicting agent. Any attempt to control these conditions is likely to fail unless the individual psychologic determinants are appreciated, sought out through psychologic appraisal, and dealt with effectively.

Indirect effects of psychologic factors may arise in a variety of illnesses. In diabetes for example, a patient may become depressed over his endless dependence on insulin

injections and careful dietary management, resulting in neglect of his therapy. Unless his needs for independence are dealt with, medical treatment for this type of "brittle diabetes" may be frustrated.

Somatic Symptoms Reflecting Psychic States

Psychosocial stress producing conflict and requiring an adaptive response may appear *disguised in somatic form* with what appear to be symptoms of organic disease. The emotional disturbance is often overlooked or even denied by the patient and sometimes by the doctor. The mechanisms responsible for such symptoms are unclear, although they are generally ascribed to tension, acting directly (eg, increased muscle tension) or through a conversion process.

Conversion is *the unconscious process of transforming psychic conflict and anxiety into a somatic symptom.* The term was traditionally linked to hysterical (histrionic) behavior (see HYSTERICAL NEUROSIS in Ch. 140), but in primary care medicine it should be considered separately, as it occurs in both sexes and all types of patients. This type of symptom formation is seen virtually every day in a busy primary care practice but unfortunately is seldom recognized as such and is poorly understood. As a result, patients may be subjected to multiple, tedious, expensive, and sometimes dangerous investigations in a search for an elusive organic illness.

Virtually any symptom that can be imagined by a patient may become a conversion symptom, and the history usually reveals how the patient "selected" his particular symptom. Commonly, the patient will have **previously experienced the symptom on an organic basis;** eg, a painful fracture, angina pectoris, or a ruptured lumbar disk. Then, at a time of psychosocial stress, the symptom reappears (or persists following adequate treatment) as a psychogenic symptom. Alternatively, the patient may "borrow" the symptom from another person; eg, the medical student who imagines his lymph nodes are swollen while caring for a patient with lymphoma, or the person who presents with chest pain after an associate or relative has a myocardial infarction. In each case, the patient has **identified with someone else who had the symptom.** Finally, the symptom may have been unconsciously selected because of its **value as a metaphor** for his psychosocial condition; eg, the patient with chest pain following rejection by a lover ("broken heart"), or the patient with back pain who feels that his burdens are too difficult to carry. While literally any symptom may be a conversion symptom, *pain* of one sort or another is most common; eg, atypical facial pain, vague headaches, poorly localized abdominal discomfort and colic, backache or nuchal pain, limb pain that sometimes simulates intermittent claudication, dysuria, dyspareunia, or dysmenorrhea.

Anxiety and **depression** are commonly seen affects caused by psychic stress and may be expressed as symptoms in any body system. No diagnostic difficulties are encountered if several body systems are involved and the patient also describes his personal anguish and apprehension. But if the patient's symptoms are expressed through a single system and he fails to emphasize emotional discomfort, diagnostic problems are created. Such cases are often described as **masked depression,** although in some instances **masked anxiety** would be a more appropriate term. Dysphoria and depressive symptoms such as insomnia, self-disparagement, psychomotor retardation, and a pessimistic outlook are common; but the patient may deny actual depression of mood or attribute it to his alleged physical disorder. Alternatively, the patient may acknowledge the presence of depression (or anxiety), but insist that it is secondary to some elusive physical condition.

Psychologic Reactions to Physical Disease

Patients with differing personalities will respond differently to being ill, and it is wise to keep in mind the psychologic effects of chronic illnesses, the effect of the patient's knowledge or lack of understanding of the diagnosis, and the patient's re-

sponse to the physician's attitudes and communications. Individual responses to the side effects of drugs are also highly variable.

Many patients with recurrent or chronic physical disorders experience depression that frequently aggravates the disability and sets up a vicious circle. The gradual decline in well-being due to the physical disorder in Parkinson's disease, cardiac failure, or RA creates a depressive reaction that in turn lessens the sense of well-being still further. Antidepressive treatment in these cases often promotes improvement.

Patients with major losses of function or of body parts (eg, stroke, amputation, spinal cord injury) are particularly difficult to evaluate. A subtle distinction needs to be made between a reactive clinical depression that requires traditional psychiatric treatment and dysphoric emotional reactions that may be extreme, but are appropriate to devastating physical illness. The latter are mood disorders or a constellation of grief, demoralization, withdrawal, and regression. They do not respond favorably to psychotherapy or antidepressant drugs, but tend to fluctuate with the patient's clinical state and improve over time if rehabilitation is successful or if the patient adapts to his changed status. In rehabilitation hospitals, it is not unusual for staff to diagnose "depression" when that is not the problem or to miss the diagnosis when it is present. Differential diagnosis is very difficult in this situation, and it is most helpful to have a physician trained in psychiatry, but experienced in dealing with patients with somatic disorders, as a consultant.

MUNCHAUSEN'S SYNDROME

(Pathologic Malingering; Chronic Fictitious Illness; Hospital Hobos)

Repeated fabrication of illness, usually acute, dramatic, and convincing, by a person who wanders from hospital to hospital for treatment. Many of the medical disorders may be closely mimicked; eg, individual patients have produced the clinical picture of myocardial infarction, hematemesis or hemoptysis, acute abdominal conditions, or a fever of unknown origin—all mimicked with uncanny skill. A patient's abdominal wall may be a criss-cross of scars, and a digit or a limb may have been amputated. Fevers are often due to self-inflicted abscesses, and the culture, usually *Escherichia coli*, clearly indicates the source of the infecting organism.

In a bizarre variant of the syndrome, *a child may be used as a surrogate patient*. (This has been referred to as "Munchausen by proxy.") The parent falsifies history and may injure the child with drugs, add blood or bacterial contaminants to urine specimens, etc—all in order to simulate disease.

Patients with Munchausen's syndrome initially and sometimes interminably become the responsibility of medical or surgical clinics. Nevertheless, the disorder is primarily a psychiatric problem, is more complex than simple dishonest simulation of symptoms, and is associated with severe emotional difficulties. The patient's personality may show prominent histrionic features, but these individuals are usually quite intelligent and resourceful. They not only know how to mimic disease, they are sophisticated with regard to medical practices. Their deceits and simulations are conscious, but the motivations for their forgery of illness and quest for attention are largely unconscious.

Commonly, there is an early history of emotional and physical abuse. Patients appear to have problems with their identity, intense feelings, inadequate impulse control, a deficient sense of reality, brief psychiatric episodes, and unstable interpersonal relationships. The need to be taken care of is at odds with the inability to trust authority figures, who are manipulated and continually provoked or tested. Feelings of guilt and the associated need for punishment and expiation are obvious.

Factitious illnesses of various sorts bear a modicum of similarity to Munchausen's syndrome. Patients may consciously produce the manifestations of a disease (eg, dermatoses), either by traumatizing the skin or by exposing themselves to an allergen to which they know they are sensitive. They then present themselves for medical care, but

sabotage therapy with self-induced or self-perpetuated disease. These patients, however, are quite different from those with Munchausen's: They tend to simulate only one disease; this is done only at a time of major psychosocial stress; they do not tend to wander from one hospital or doctor to another. Most important, they usually can be successfully and rather easily treated. They should be confronted with the diagnosis in a manner that avoids suggesting guilt or reproach. The status of legitimate illness must be preserved, while the physician indicates that he and the patient can cooperatively resolve the underlying problem. Often this will involve another member of the family, but it is best then to discuss the problem as an illness, not as a deception; ie, the family is not told the precise mechanism of the disease.

Treatment

In these patients with psychopathology of psychotic proportions encompassed within a characterologic disorder, successful treatment is rare. Acceding to the patients' manipulations will relieve their tension, but their provocations escalate, ultimately surpassing what physicians are willing or able to do. Refusal to meet treatment demands or confrontation results in angry reactions, and the patient generally moves on to another hospital. Psychiatric treatment is usually refused or circumvented, but consultation and follow-up care may be accepted, at least to help resolve a crisis. However, management is generally limited to early recognition of the disorder and avoidance of risky procedures and excessive or unwarranted medication.

136. GROUP PSYCHODYNAMICS

The processes of influence that occur among individuals, the interactional structures that emerge, and the impact that these group processes have upon individual personality functioning.

The Learning of Behavior

We live in the most rapidly changing and complex environment that has ever existed. To cope daily with many and complex social judgments, we often rely on automatic, learned responses. However, because no one person has the knowledge and experience to deal with every decision that arises, we allow our behavior to be influenced at times by others and by what is happening around us. Since we are social creatures—born dependent on others, living our lives interacting with others—we are prepared for group living by learning the language, demeanor, beliefs, attitudes, cultural norms, and social values of those around us.

Social behavior reflects both conscious and unconscious learning, presumably through 4 prime modes: **(1) Observational learning (modeling),** in which we watch others' behavior and then copy it. **(2) Classical (Pavlovian; respondent) conditioning,** in which the pairing of a conditioned stimulus (bell) with an unconditioned stimulus (meat powder) elicits an unconditioned response (salivation). Repetition produces a conditioned reflex in which the bell alone elicits the salivation. **(3) Operant (Skinnerian; instrumental) conditioning,** where learning occurs as a consequence of reinforcement. (If a response is reinforced, its frequency will increase; if it is punished, its frequency will decrease.) **(4) Cognitive social learning;** ie, thoughts, feelings, images, and memories—the person's inner experiences—are crucial factors in learning.

Recently, theories of learning have become more **interactional,** seeing acquired or inherited behavior, internal cognitive factors, and environmental influences operating as reciprocal determinants of each other (ie, behavior affects the environment and cognitions; cognitions affect the environment and behavior; and the environment influences behavior and cognitions).

Modifying Behavior

Historically, the power of certain persons to dramatically influence others was considered supernatural; ie, the influencer was a magician or witch with secret potions and arcane knowledge, or had godlike qualities. Some people have always attained compliance and influence through coercion, brutality, or the wielding of religious, political, or financial power.

Compliance is produced by 3 general methods of persuasion—reason, coercion, or subterfuge—used singly or in various combinations; and these can be roughly arranged on an imaginary continuum. At the left end are those efforts to persuade that are characterized by **reason** and open exchange, in which each side looks at all the evidence and attempts to persuade the other. This is the approved method in a democratic society. Moving across the continuum, varying amounts of pressure are applied by the persuader to have his opinion prevail; eg, forms of advertising are followed by propaganda. At the far right end of the continuum would be placed fascism in Germany and Italy under Hitler and Mussolini and, in the USA, the Ku Klux Klan and neo-Nazi organizations. Here also are the cultic groups in which the persuader resorts to social, psychologic, or physical **coercion.** Since coercive methods make the process of persuasion obvious, **subterfuge** often is used. The persuader tries to keep his subject unaware of the intention to elicit compliance and less than fully aware of being moved along a preplanned course of action.

We are all influenced to some extent by advertising; or find ourselves "going along with the group" without realizing how influenced we are by merely being in a crowd (eg, at a rock concert or sporting event), or how our behavior is swayed by a political orator. But there is an almost universal uneasiness about admitting that one is persuaded or influenced by other persons to any marked extent. Such thoughts mobilize unacceptable feelings of powerlessness and dependency. Most persons like to think that their own minds and thought processes, their opinions, values, and ideas, are inviolate and totally self-regulated—although "other persons" may be weak-minded and easily influenced.

Vulnerability to persuasion tactics: Everyone is influenced and persuaded daily in various ways, but the vulnerability to influence varies. The ability to fend off persuaders is reduced when one is rushed, stressed, uncertain, lonely, indifferent, uninformed, distracted, or fatigued. Alternatively, a person with a sense of clarity and sureness about his own beliefs and values, with a feeling of being embedded in meaningful relationships with other persons, and with a sense of having a role in life that gives him support is much less likely to be vulnerable to persuasion.

Also affecting vulnerability are the status and power of the persuader. Further, certain persons and groups have been termed "compliance professionals"—high pressure salespersons, con artists, advertisers, fund raisers, and other people who have become skillful at employing some fundamental psychologic principles that underlie the influence process.

CULTS

(Thought Reform Programs; Intense Indoctrination Programs; Intense Resocialization Programs; New Age Groups; New Movement Groups)

Groups with religious, political, psychologic, and other ideologies at their core, which almost universally offer as their central theme a special, new psychologic awareness handed down by an indisputable and arbitrary authority that uses the technic of ***thought reform (intense indoctrination or resocialization, coercive persuasion, brainwashing*** *—ie, the systematic manipulation of social and psychologic influence, distinguished from other forms of social learning by the conditions under which it is conducted and by the technics of environmental and interpersonal manipulation employed to suppress certain behavior and to train others).* The views of cults range from new psychologic theories of conduct

sold commercially as training programs, to indoctrinations about religious beliefs, philosophies, politics, and health and eating practices. The groups vary in content, but appear to share certain contextual social and psychologic traits. Several million persons (in the USA, > 3 million young people) in the past decade have participated in cultic group experiences.

Most cults reject modern medicine, even considering physicians as enemies, because the leaders usually do not want to relinquish any control over their followers. However, physicians receive requests for help from persons traumatized by their cult experiences, or from relatives of cult members puzzled by what has happened. Understanding the social and psychologic features of group influences and their effects on individuals can help in responding to these requests and obtaining assistance from other knowledgeable persons.

Worldwide examples of intense indoctrination experiences in the past 50 yr highlight how easily human conduct can be manipulated under certain circumstances. During the Russian purge trials in the 1930s men were maneuvered into both falsely confessing and falsely accusing. The early 1950s saw the effects of the revolutionary universities in China; an entire nation was subjected to a thought reform program in which millions were induced to espouse new philosophies and exhibit new conduct through psychologic, social, and political coercion technics. In the Korean War, United Nations prisoners of war were subjected to an indoctrination program based on methods growing out of the Chinese thought reform program and combined with other social and psychologic influence technics. At that time the term **brainwashing** was introduced into our vocabulary. Since there were no Turkish-speaking brainwashers available, Turkish prisoners of war were left to themselves and hence acquired the reputation of being resistant to brainwashing.

Later, the world was shocked by Charles Manson's influence and control over a small group of middle-class young Californians whom he sent out on a murderous rampage. Soon after, the Symbionese Liberation Army **(SLA),** a small self-styled revolutionary group in California, kidnapped Patricia Hearst and manipulated and controlled her behavior to the extent that she appeared with them in a bank robbery and feared returning to society, having been convinced by the SLA that the police and FBI would shoot her. By the mid 1970s thousands of families in the USA and Europe were beginning to be puzzled and alarmed as they saw the impact on their offspring of an array of mind manipulators. When Jim Jones led 912 followers to mass suicide in a Guiana jungle on November 18, 1978, attention was called dramatically to the extent of control one man could exert over his followers.

Factors in Cult Development in the USA

Throughout history cults have arisen when there have been breakdowns in societies' structures and rules. This kind of setting occurred in the USA during the social and political changes of the late sixties (breakdowns in family life, the sexual revolution, the drug culture, civil-rights protest marches, anti-Vietnam demonstrations, the war itself, civil disobedience, and student rebellions). Cults that emerged tended to appeal primarily to the young, who felt disillusioned and estranged from their families and "the establishment." These cults offered father or god figures to youth needing such identification. Each self-appointed messiah claimed a simple solution for the complex problems of life and called for commitment, sacrifice, and zeal.

Youth communes flourished briefly but soon faded, for they did not provide the promised security, hope, and structure. Concomitantly, psychologic awareness, the consciousness expansion, and the human potential movement were strongly influencing our values. Youth were told that "mind trips" would bring nirvana. The first wave of cults drew heavily upon Eastern philosophies, in which meditation, yoga, and exotic practices were prominent. Soon these were supplanted by neo-Christian, political, and psychologically based groups. Recently, as the economy has tightened, "prosperity

groups" have emerged, which state that positive thinking coupled with psychologic awareness will bring prosperity.

The cult personality (see also "Vulnerability to persuasion tactics," above): No one type of person is prone to become involved with cults. About 2/3 of those studied have been normal young persons induced to join groups in periods of personal crises; eg, broken romances or failure to get the job or college of their choice. Vulnerable, the young person affiliates with a cult offering promises of unconditional love, new mental powers, and social utopia. Since modern cults are persistent and often deceptive in their recruiting, many prospective group members have no accurate knowledge of the cult and almost no understanding of what eventually will be expected of them as long-term members.

Technics for Changing Behavior in Intense Indoctrination Situations

The behavioral change technics of **thought reform** are applied to induce the learning of any set of information or behaviors under certain circumstances. If the sets of information and behaviors are sufficiently large, the effects of a thought reform program cause personality changes; ie, suppression of old views and conduct and expression of the behaviors that management wants.

In general, a thought reform program depends on (1) controlling an individual's social and psychologic environment, especially the person's time; (2) placing an individual in a position of powerlessness within a high-control, authoritarian system; (3) relying usually on a closed system of logic, which permits no feedback and refuses to be modified except by executive order; (4) relying on unsophistication of the person being manipulated; ie, he is pressed to adapt to the environment in increments that are sufficiently minor so that he does not notice changes; (5) eroding the confidence of a person's perceptions; (6) manipulating a system of rewards, punishments, and experiences to promote new learning or inhibit undesired previous behavior. Punishments usually are social ones (more effective in producing wanted behavior than beatings and death threats, although these do occur); ie, shunning, social isolation, and humiliation (removal of status and privilege, forced nakedness, etc).

Effects of Cult Membership

Unaware of the orchestration of the psychologic and social forces being applied to change him, in a completely controlled atmosphere with loss of privacy and sleep and nonreinforcement of former habits, and with an extremely narrowed focus of attention, the cult member absorbs new information very rapidly and becomes dependent on his changed "reality." He then dissociates from much of his past belief system, his social ties, and his own emotions. Anxiety and distress are evoked when old thoughts reappear and threaten to break through the new facade of demeanor. Those who know the person well note that he seems more rigid and inflexible and is repetitive in his communications, keeping his remarks within a narrow band of contents. The person appears to be a mentally and emotionally constricted version of his former self.

Aftereffects: No long-term, large-sample studies of carefully followed groups of persons harmed or helped by their participation in intense indoctrination programs are yet available. Most researchers agree that traumatic experiences occur; a number of cult participants are visibly harmed; and the more confrontational and domineering the leader, the more likely it is that casualties will occur. The symptoms of **stress disorder** (see also in Ch. 140) may be present (eg, recurrent nightmares, temporary reexperiencing of some of the events, diminished responsiveness to the outside world, guilt, depression, anxiety, sleep disturbances, or problems with memory or concentration). Persons leaving cults not only face the realization that they have given up productive years of their lives (and perhaps possessions) to the guru or leader, but they leave with ambition quenched, unable to make decisions.

Treatment

Understanding the myriad groups, both small and local and large and international, requires help from generalists who have studied them as a whole and specialists who know in depth about specific groups or types of groups. Psychiatrists, psychologists, social workers, clergy, lawyers, and lay persons in the community may have knowledge and experience to share and may provide referral sources and reading materials.

Contact by the patient, even if brief, with knowledgeable professionals is needed, as is participation in a network of other persons with similar experiences. Most often, optimum treatment helps the patient understand the cult's indoctrination procedures and the psychologic and social pressures that overwhelmed him. He and his relatives must learn how the intense indoctrination program produced the effects that contributed to his changed behavior and occasional breakdowns. He needs to see that the behavior change or breakdown does not doom him to a life of fragility or to a view of himself as a weak or mad creature. This perspective has been effective in working with victims of other kinds (eg, natural disasters, kidnapping and other crimes of violence) who have developed stress disorder. These persons also need to see that intense stressors lay behind their symptoms and that they were not uniquely fragile in the face of the duress.

The above approach is different from that taken in traditional psychotherapy, in which therapists wittingly or unwittingly assume that inherent, intrapersonal weaknesses of either a psychologic or constitutional nature cause breakdowns or behavioral changes. That therapy format demonstrates to the patient that problems stem from internal needs and defects, and it directs the patient to seek hidden motivations and weak internal properties of the self without properly conceptualizing the context, external factors, and system within which the breakdown or behavior change occurred.

---

137. PERSONALITY DISORDERS

Disordered patterns of behavior characterized by relatively fixed, inflexible, and stylized reactions to stress, representing the individual's way of dealing with other people and external events regardless of existing realities. **Personality traits** also are patterns of perceiving and relating to the environment and oneself; but the **disorders** are rigid and maladaptive, and damage social, interpersonal, and work relationships. The characteristic patterns of maladjustment are evident from childhood and through much of the life span.

Without environmental frustration, persons with personality disorders tend to show little anxiety or mental or emotional symptoms, and they feel that their behavior patterns are "normal" and "right." Rarely seeking help because of their own anxiety and discomfort, they more often are referred by their families or by social agencies because of the difficulties their maladaptive behavior causes others. If help is sought, usually after environmental frustrations, these patients will view their difficulties as *outside* of themselves, unlike neurotic persons, whose defense mechanisms trouble the user but not the observer.

Personality disorders are medically and psychiatrically important for three reasons: (1) These persons' externalization of internal conflicts often leads to clashes with others in ways that bring the patient under medical observation. The result often is a maladaptive doctor-patient relationship, with the patient refusing to take appropriate responsibility and the doctor blaming, distrusting, and ultimately rejecting the patient. (2) Persons with severe personality disorders are at high risk of becoming addicted to alcohol or drugs, of behaving in a self-destructive manner, of pursuing sexually deviant

lives with which they cannot cope, and of clashing with society and its mores. (3) These individuals are susceptible to breakdown on exposure to stress. The type of personality disorder may or may not determine the kind of psychiatric illness that complicates it; eg, a person with a hysterical personality may respond to excess emotional stress by hysterical conversion or dissociative symptoms, or a suicidal depression.

Diagnosis

Diagnosis is based on recognition of the typical rigid behavior patterns and the patient's lack of insight and resistance to change—his apparent inability to learn from experience. Certain **mental coping mechanisms** (see below) are used unconsciously at times by most people. The maladaptive behavior patterns seen in personality disorders tend to be exaggerations of these mechanisms, some of which, when used chronically and maladaptively, may result in the diagnosis of a personality disorder. Although these mechanisms may not be breached by reason or interpretation, they respond to improved interpersonal relationships and to supportive but forceful confrontation in prolonged psychotherapy or peer encounters.

(1) **Dissociation** (neurotic denial) effects temporary but drastic modification of one's personality or one's sense of personal identity. These modifications can include fugues, hysterical conversion reactions, short-term denial of responsibility for one's acts or feelings, trance states, chance-taking, and pharmacologic intoxication to numb unhappiness. (2) **Projection** allows one to attribute one's own *un*acknowledged feelings to others; it leads to prejudice, rejection of intimacy through paranoid suspicion, overvigilance to external danger, and injustice-collecting. (3) **Schizoid fantasy** is a tendency to use imaginary relationships and private belief systems for the purpose of conflict resolution and relief from loneliness. It is associated with eccentricity and global avoidance of interpersonal intimacy. In contrast to the psychotic person, the user of schizoid fantasy who has a personality disorder does not fully believe in or insist on acting out his or her fantasies. Unlike dissociation, the use of fantasy remakes the outer, not the inner, world. (4) **Hypochondriasis** (see also Ch. 140) transforms reproach toward others (which may have arisen from bereavement, loneliness, or anger) into unremitting somatic complaints, as an expression of the entrenched belief that some organic disease is present. In contrast to neurotic conversion reaction where distress is muted and the doctor fascinated, in hypochondriasis the patient's distress is exaggerated, he is resistant to logical reassurance and treatment, and the physician feels helpless and resentful. (5) **Turning against the self** allows aggression toward others to be expressed indirectly and ineffectively through passivity. It includes failures and illnesses that affect others more than oneself, and silly, provocative clowning. The mechanism underlies most sadomasochistic relationships. (6) **Acting out** is the direct, often impersonal, behavioral expression of an unconscious wish or impulse in order to avoid being conscious of the affect—painful or pleasurable—that accompanies it. It includes many delinquent, impulsive, and deviant acts that seem motiveless because the actor is unaware of his or her own feelings. (7) **Splitting** allows the user to divide people regarded ambivalently in his past life and/or current medical setting into all-good, idealized saviors and all-bad, devalued malefactors. Splitting avoids the discomfort of loving and being angry at the same person. Either the loved or hated facet is inappropriately transposed to another person.

Classification

The following classification largely reflects the nomenclature suggested in the American Psychiatric Association's *Diagnostic and Statistical Manual of Mental Disorders*, Third Edition **(DSM-III)**.

1. Paranoid personalities are characterized by projection of their own hostilities and conflicts onto others. These persons are markedly sensitive to interpersonal relationships and tend to find hostile and malevolent intentions behind trivial, innocent, or

even kindly acts by others. Often their suspicious attitudes lead to aggressive feelings or behavior or bring about rejection by others, which seems to justify their original feelings; however, they are unable to see their own roles in this cycle. Their behavior may be designed to prove their adequacy, while their sense of superiority becomes exaggerated and is accompanied by belittlement of others. In many spheres these persons may be highly efficient and conscientious, although envious and inflexible. They may be litigious, especially when they feel a sense of righteous indignation.

Paranoid tendencies are especially likely to develop among those who feel particularly inferior because of a defect or handicap that makes them feel noticeably different from their peers. Likewise, sensory impairment, particularly chronic deafness, has a similar effect since it reduces their capacity for reality testing and thus leads to the misinterpretation of being talked about or laughed at.

2. Schizoid personalities are introverted, withdrawn, solitary, emotionally cold, and distant. They are most often absorbed with their own thoughts and feelings and are fearful of closeness and intimacy with others. They are reticent, given to daydreaming, and prefer theoretic speculation to practical action. This personality pattern is found in about 40% of schizophrenic patients before they become ill. However, many schizoid people do not develop schizophrenia or other mental disorders. Fantasy (see above) is a common coping mechanism. Schizophrenia is discussed in Ch. 142.

3. Schizotypal personalities display oddities of thinking, perception, communication, and behavior that suggest schizophrenia but are never severe enough to meet the criteria for that disorder (see Ch. 142). These oddities in cognition may be expressed as magical thinking, ideas of reference, and paranoid ideation, and by definition are more marked than those found in schizoid (see No. 2, above) and avoidant (see No. 8, below) personalities.

4. Histrionic (hysterical) personalities are conspicuously egocentric. Since winning the esteem and admiration of others is important to them, attention-seeking and theatrical behavior tends to be characteristic. Their emotional immaturity is expressed with an exaggerated, childish, emotional response to any wounding of their vanity. Inconsistencies in behavior arise because the histrionic personality can adopt whatever pattern of conduct will place him or her in a favorable light or boost self-esteem. In our culture this form of personality disorder is noted more often in women but also is seen in men.

A histrionic person's lively manner lends itself to easily established superficial relationships, but these persons are rarely deeply involved emotionally. They may combine provocativeness or sexualization of nonsexual relationships with sexual dysfunction or fears. Their relationships are affected by a seemingly insatiable need for affection, and behind their sexually seductive behavior lies a childlike wish for nonsexual affection and protection; ie, they tend to be dependent. Promiscuous entanglements with many partners are possible because of the histrionic person's lack of real involvement with any of them. The crises that arise from these relationships are managed with manipulative behavior that may include suicidal threats and shrewd exploitation of emotional susceptibilities in other people. Insight fails to develop in histrionic persons because they can easily repress or forget unpleasant or discreditable experiences; responsibility for misfortunes and failures usually is ascribed to others. Dissociation (see above and in Ch. 140) is a commonly used coping mechanism.

5. Narcissistic personalities have an exaggerated sense of self-importance, are absorbed by fantasies of unlimited success, and exhibitionistically seek constant attention. Extreme swings between overidealization and devaluation characterize the relationships of these persons, who also display marked entitlement, interpersonal exploitiveness, and oversensitivity to failure. The primary care physician often is frustrated by these patients' incessant and frequently urgent demands relating to what he views as minor problems. As in the case of the hypochondriacal patient, the com-

plaints and entitlement of the narcissistic patient may be caused by genuine but assiduously concealed emotional pain and unhappiness. Like the dependent personality (see below), the narcissistic personality is seen so commonly in the other personality disorders that treating it as an independent disorder may prove inappropriate.

Some patients with narcissistic personalities also are characterized by a tendency to complain of multiple somatic symptoms. These patients have been referred to under a variety of terms including **histrionic (hysterical) personality disorder, primitive hysteric,** or **somatization disorder (Briquet's syndrome).** This last disorder is discussed in Ch. 140.

6. Antisocial personalities (previously used designations: **psychopathic, sociopathic)** characteristically act out their conflicts and flout normal rules of social order. These individuals are impulsive, irresponsible, amoral, and unable to forego immediate gratification. They cannot form affectionate relationships with others, but their charm and plausibility may be highly developed and skillfully used for their own ends. They tolerate frustration poorly, and opposition is likely to elicit hostility, aggression, or serious violence. Their antisocial behavior shows little foresight and is not associated with remorse or guilt, since these people seem to have a keen capacity for rationalizing and for blaming their behavior on others. Failure and punishment rarely modify their behavior or improve their judgment and foresight. A person with an antisocial personality may attempt suicide if his aggressions are turned inward instead of being directed against others.

This personality type often is associated with a history of alcoholism, drug addiction, sexual deviation, promiscuity, occupational failure, or imprisonment. In our culture men are more often labeled as antisocial and women as histrionic personalities, but the two patterns have much in common. In families of patients with both patterns, there may be antisocial and histrionic male and female relatives, and in both patterns a history of parental strife and severe emotional deprivation in the formative years frequently is found. Life expectancy is diminished, but among those surviving there is some tendency to stabilization after age 40. The effects of either severe cerebral injury or undiagnosed alcoholism may closely simulate the picture of an antisocial personality. Unless repetitive antisocial behavior is observed before age 15, the diagnosis of antisocial personality must be doubted.

7. Borderline personalities are unstable in several areas, including interpersonal relationships, behavior, mood, and self-image. Characteristics include frequent mood shifts, impulsivity, inappropriate and frequently uncontrolled intense anger, uncertainty concerning identity. These persons are extremists for whom the world is either black or white, hated or loved—never neutral. To some extent, the borderline personality has features of all the personality disorders listed above and at times their reality testing is so poor that they resemble psychotic patients. For example, brief but frank delusions and hallucinatory experiences are common. Unlike the schizoid personality, however, interpersonal relationships are far more dramatic and intense; unlike the antisocial personality, there is more disturbance of formal thought processes, and aggression is more often turned against the self; and unlike the histrionic personality, there is greater expression of overt anger and greater confusion over sexual identity. Borderline personalities are commonly seen in primary care medical practices, where they tend to appear frequently with vague somatic complaints, often do not comply with therapeutic recommendations, and tend to be very frustrating to their physicians. Splitting and projection (see above) are common coping mechanisms.

8. Avoidant personalities usually are hypersensitive to rejection, and fear starting relationships without being very sure of uncritical acceptance; there is, however, a strong desire for affection and acceptance. Unlike schizoid personalities, these individuals are openly distressed by their lack of ability to relate comfortably with others.

9. Dependent personalities surrender responsibility for major areas of their lives to others and permit the needs of those on whom they are dependent to supersede their own needs. They lack self-confidence, and feel intense discomfort when alone for more than brief periods. The features of this syndrome are commonly seen in other personality disorders and are frequently obscured by the more obvious aspects of them. For example, histrionic behavior patterns are quite striking and may mask severe underlying dependency. Therefore, use of the syndrome as a discrete diagnosis may prove untenable.

10. Compulsive personalities (obsessive-compulsive) are conscientious and have high levels of aspiration, but they also tend to be perfectionistic and often are unable to gain adequate satisfaction from their achievements. They are reliable, dependable, orderly, and methodical, but their inflexibility often makes them incapable of adapting to changed circumstances. They are cautious and weigh all aspects of a problem; consequently, making decisions may be difficult for them. They bear responsibilities seriously but may suffer much anxiety over them. They pay attention to every detail and are therefore in danger of becoming entangled with means and forgetting the main purposes of their tasks. Compulsiveness is in tune with Western cultural standards, and when the disorder is not too marked, these people often are capable of high levels of achievement, especially in the sciences and academic fields where order is desirable. On the other hand, they often feel a sense of isolation and have difficulties with interpersonal relationships, in which their feelings are less under strict control, events are less predictable, and they must rely on others.

11. Passive-aggressive personalities are characterized by helplessness, clinging dependency, and procrastination. The apparent passivity is designed to gain attention and affection, to avoid responsibility, or to control or punish others covertly. Passive-aggressive behavior is characterized by obstinacy, inefficiency, and sullenness, often disguised under a superficial compliance. Frequently, individuals with this disorder agree to perform a task and then proceed to subtly undermine its completion with complaints and passive obstructionism. They also may be provocative and argumentative, especially with those in authority. Such behavior usually serves to deny or conceal marked dependency needs. The behavior is maladaptive in that, ironically, it drives others away and prevents the individual from receiving even a normal amount of support. In most cases sadomasochism is seen as a variant of passive-aggressive behavior, but some clinicians believe that masochism should be classified as a separate personality disorder. Hypochondriasis and turning against the self (see above) are common coping mechanisms.

12. Cyclothymic personalities (see also Ch. 141) fluctuate in their moods between states of high-spirited buoyancy and states of gloom and pessimism, each sustained for weeks or longer. Characteristically, the rhythmic mood changes are regular and predictable and occur either without external cause or in response to trivial events. In one common variant of this disorder, the mood is predominantly marked by elation, energy, an infectious gaiety, and optimism; the depressive phases are relatively short-lived and unnoticed. In other individuals the depressive phase is the predominant one. It is uncertain whether the cyclothymic personality disorder lies on a continuum with manic-depressive illness or is a different entity. Many gifted and creative individuals have personalities conforming to a cyclothymic pattern.

Treatment

While specific technics of treatment and problems encountered with the various personality disorders may differ, several general concepts can be considered. Motivation for therapy often comes from someone other than the person involved, and the patient often feels that the reasons for therapy are foreign to him or that he is being

victimized. The doctor's job is to contain the patient's externalization through setting limits, confrontation, and avoiding his own tendency to become overinvolved—first to rescue and then to condemn. The temptation of both doctor and patient to hope that drugs will relieve the patient's distress must be recognized and rejected. Over the long term, the anxiety and depression of personality disorders are rarely abolished by pharmacotherapy, while drug abuse and suicide attempts are common complications of prescribing drugs to these individuals.

Commonly, therapeutic gains are made only in the setting of a long-term relationship with another person, who must be flexible, reassuring, and usually more active than passive. Patients need to be confronted with the way their behavior affects other people. Frequently, limits on behavior need to be set and reality issues dealt with. In many cases the family should be involved, since group pressure seems to be effective. Group and family treatment, group living situations, therapeutic social clubs, milieu hospital therapy—all can be valuable in treatment. The patient's self-esteem must be supported while his maladaptive modes of behavior are confronted. It is also important that those undertaking treatment be aware of the difficulties and avoid the disappointment, annoyance, and moral judgments that tend to creep in. The middle years tend to bring maturation for those with personality disorders, and this process can sometimes be given a helping hand.

138. DRUG DEPENDENCE

(Substance Use Disorders; Drug Addiction; Drug Abuse; Drug Habituation)

A single definition for drug dependence is neither desirable nor possible. The term **drug dependence of a specific type** emphasizes that different drugs have different effects, including the type and hazard of the dependence they produce. **Addiction** refers to a style of living that includes drug dependence, generally both physical and psychologic, but mainly connotes continuing compulsive use and overwhelming involvement with a drug. Addiction additionally implies the risk of harm and the need to stop drug use, whether the addict understands and agrees or not.

Drug abuse is definable only in terms of societal disapproval and involves different types of behavior: (1) experimental and recreational use of drugs; (2) use of psychoactive drugs to relieve problems or symptoms; (3) use of drugs at first for the above reasons but development later of dependence and continuation at least partially to prevent the discomfort of withdrawal.

Recreational drug use has increasingly become a part of our culture, although in general not sanctioned by society and often illegal. Users who apparently do not suffer harm tend toward episodic use involving relatively small doses, precluding clinical toxicity and the development of tolerance and physical dependence. The drugs used are often "natural"; ie, close to plant origin and containing a mixture of compounds, and are not isolated psychoactive chemicals (eg, crude opium, alcoholic beverages, marijuana products, coffee and other caffeine-containing beverages, hallucinogenic mushrooms, and coca leaf). The drugs are most often taken orally or are inhaled. The use of active potent compounds administered by injection is seldom easily controllable. Recreational use is also often accompanied by ritualization with a set of observed rules and is seldom practiced alone. Most drugs used in this fashion are psychostimulants or hallucinogens designed to obtain the "high" rather than to relieve psychic distress; depressant agents are seldom used in this controlled manner.

Two general aspects are common to most types of drug dependence: (1) **Psychologic dependence** involves *feelings of satisfaction and a desire to repeat the administration of the drug to produce pleasure or avoid discomfort.* This mental state is a powerful factor involved in chronic use of psychotropic drugs, and with some drugs psychologic de-

pendence may be the only factor involved in intense craving and compulsive use. (2) **Physical dependence** is defined as *a state of adaptation to a drug accompanied by development of tolerance and manifested by a withdrawal or abstinence syndrome.* **Tolerance** is defined as *the need to increase the dose progressively in order to produce the effect originally achieved by smaller amounts.* Physical dependence and tolerance do not accompany all forms of drug dependence. A **withdrawal syndrome** is characterized by *untoward physiologic changes that occur when the drug is discontinued or when its effect is counteracted by a specific antagonist.*

Drugs that produce dependence act on the CNS and have one or more of the following effects: reduced anxiety and tension; elation, euphoria, or other mood changes pleasurable to the user; feelings of increased mental and physical ability; altered sensory perception; and changes in behavior. These drugs may be divided into (1) those causing chiefly psychic dependence and (2) those causing both psychic and physical dependence. Important drugs in the first category are cocaine, marijuana, amphetamine, bromides, and the hallucinogens, such as lysergic acid diethylamide (LSD), methylene dioxyamphetamine (MDA), and mescaline. A major stereotyped abstinence syndrome does not follow withdrawal of these drugs, but some cause tolerance; and in some cases reactions following withdrawal resemble an abstinence syndrome (eg, depression and lethargy following withdrawal of cocaine or amphetamine; characteristic changes in the EEG with amphetamine). TABLE 138–1 lists some commonly used psychoactive drugs and their potential for various types of dependence.

TABLE 138–1. COMMONLY USED SUBSTANCES WITH POTENTIAL FOR DEPENDENCE

Drug	Physical Dependence	Psychologic Dependence	Tolerance
CNS Depressants			
Opioids	++++	++++	++++
Synthetic narcotics	++++	++++	++++
Barbiturates	+++	+++	++
Glutethimide	+++	+++	++
Methyprylon	+++	+++	++
Ethchlorvynol	+++	+++	++
Methaqualone	+++	+++	++
Alcohol	+++	+++	++
Minor Tranquilizers			
Meprobamate	+++	+++	+
Benzodiazepines	+	+++	+
Stimulants			
Amphetamine	?	+++	++++
Methamphetamine	?	+++	++++
Cocaine	0	+++	0
Hallucinogens			
LSD	0	++	++
Mescaline, peyote	0	++	+
Marijuana			
(low-dose Δ-9 THC)	0	++	0
(high-dose Δ-9 THC)	0	++	?

Abbreviations: LSD, Lysergic acid diethylamide; THC, tetrahydrocannabinol; 0, no effect; +, slight, to ++++, marked, effect.

In the USA, the Comprehensive Drug Abuse Prevention and Control Act of 1970 and subsequent changes require the drug industry to maintain physical security and strict record-keeping over certain types of drugs, and divide controlled substances into 5 schedules (or classes) on the basis of their potential for abuse, accepted medical use, and accepted safety under medical supervision. Substances included in Schedule I are those with a high potential for abuse, no accepted medical use, and a lack of accepted safety. Those in Schedules II through V decrease in potential for abuse. Placing a drug into one of these schedules determines the nature of control that must be exercised. Prescriptions for drugs in all these schedules must bear the physician's Federal Drug Enforcement Administration (DEA) license number.

Etiology

The development of drug dependence is complex and unclear. At least 3 components require consideration: the addictive drugs, predisposing conditions, and the personality of the user. The psychology of the individual and drug availability determine the choice of addicting drug and the pattern and frequency of use.

Drug dependence is partly related to cultural patterns and socioeconomic classes; the progression from experimentation to occasional use and the development of tolerance and physical dependence are poorly understood processes. Factors leading to increased use and habituation or addiction appear to include peer or group pressure and emotional distress that is symptomatically relieved by specific drug effects. Factors involved in the mechanisms leading to drug abuse include sadness, low self-esteem, social alienation, and environmental stress, particularly if accompanied by feelings of impotence to effect change or to accomplish goals. The medical profession may rarely contribute to harmful psychoactive drug use inadvertently through overzealous drug application to the problems of living and through failure to prevent the diversion of drugs by ruse. Advertising in mass media may contribute to social expectations that drugs can safely relieve distress or gratify needs.

Pharmacologic factors: Persons who become addicted or dependent have no known biochemical, drug dispositional, or physiologic responsiveness differences from those who do not, although many efforts have been made to find such differences. After 2 to 3 days of treatment with full doses of a narcotic analgesic, some physical dependence may exist. Such patients have a mild withdrawal syndrome, scarcely noted, or described as a case of influenza; they do not become addicted. Even patients with chronic pain problems requiring long-term administration usually are not addicts, although they may experience some problems with tolerance and physical dependence. Some substances have a high potential for physiologic dependence and are more prone to abuse even when used in a social or recreational setting. Pharmacologic effects are important, but not exclusive, factors in the development of drug dependence.

Personality factors: The "addictive personality" has been described variously by behavioral scientists, but there is little scientific evidence that characteristic personality factors exist. Some have concluded that addicts are basically escapists, persons who cannot face confronting realities and who run away. Others have described addicts as schizoid individuals who are fearful, withdrawn, and depressed, and who have a history of frequent suicide attempts and numerous self-inflicted injuries. Addicts have also been described as basically dependent and grasping in their relations and frequently exhibiting overt and unconscious rage and immature sexuality. These descriptions may have a genesis in the describer's attitudes. Clinicians, patients, and the culture are prone to highlight drug abuse in the matrix of a dysfunctional life or life episode and choose to place blame on the drug or drug use.

Abuse of prescription drugs and avoidance of illegal drugs may occur in person with an advanced education and professional status. Before developing the drug dependence, they did not demonstrate the pleasure-oriented, irresponsible behavior usu

ally prejudicially attributed to addicts. Sometimes the patient justifies the use of medication because of a crisis, job pressure, or family catastrophe that produces temporary anxiety or depression. Most of these patients abuse alcohol or another drug at the same time and may have repeated hospital admissions for overdose, adverse reactions, or withdrawal problems.

DEPENDENCE ON ALCOHOL

The development of characteristic deviant behaviors associated with prolonged consumption of excessive amounts of alcohol. Alcoholism is considered a chronic illness of undetermined etiology with an insidious onset, showing recognizable symptoms and signs proportionate to its severity.

The discussion of alcoholism needs 2 separate foci. Consumption of large amounts of ethyl alcohol is usually accompanied by significant clinical toxicity and tissue damage, the hazards of physical dependence, and a dangerous abstinence syndrome. Additionally, the term alcoholism is applied to the social impairment occurring in the lives of addicted individuals and their families. Usually, the 2 foci are recognized simultaneously, but occasionally one predominates to the apparent exclusion of the other.

An **alcoholic** is identified by severe dependence or addiction and a cumulative pattern of behaviors associated with drinking. (1) Frequent intoxication is obvious and destructive; it interferes with the individual's ability to socialize and to work. Drunkenness may lead to (2) marriage failure and eventually, after work absenteeism becomes intolerable, to (3) being fired. Alcoholics may (4) seek medical treatment for their drinking. They may (5) suffer physical injury, (6) be apprehended for driving while intoxicated, or (7) be arrested by the police for drunkenness. Eventually, they may (8) be hospitalized for delirium tremens or cirrhosis of the liver. Women alcoholics have been, in general, more likely to drink alone, and less likely to experience some of the social stigmata.

The frequency and severity of these 8 symptoms and the age at which they occur are accepted as defining the alcoholic. The earlier in life these behaviors are evident, the more crippling is the disorder.

Incidence of alcoholism among women, children, adolescents, and college students is increasing. The male:female ratio is now approximately 4:1. It is generally assumed that 75% of American adults drink alcoholic beverages, and 1 in 10 will experience some problem with alcoholism.

Etiology

The etiology is unknown. Psychologic hypotheses have noted the frequent incidence of certain personality traits, including (1) schizoid qualities (isolation, loneliness, shyness), (2) depression, (3) dependency, (4) hostile and self-destructive impulsivity, and (5) sexual immaturity. Families of alcoholics tend to have a higher incidence of alcoholism. Genetic or biochemical defects leading to alcoholism are suspected but have not been clearly demonstrated, although a higher incidence of alcoholism has been consistently reported in biologic children of alcoholics, as compared to adoptive children. Societal factors affect patterns of drinking and consequent behavior, the attitudes transmitted through the culture or child rearing. Alcoholics frequently have histories of broken homes and disturbed relationships with parents.

Physiology and Pathology (see also Ch. 73)

Alcohol is absorbed into the blood, principally from the small intestine. It accumulates in the blood because absorption is more rapid than oxidation and elimination. Depression of the CNS is a principal effect of alcohol: A blood alcohol level of 50 mg/dL produces sedation or tranquility; 50 to 150 mg/dL, lack of coordination; 150 to 200 mg/dL, intoxication (delirium); and 300 to 400 mg/dL, unconsciousness. (For

symptoms of unconsciousness due to acute alcoholism, see Ch. 118.) Blood levels > 500 mg/dL may be fatal. The legal driving level is 100 mg/dL or less in most states, and intoxication is often defined as present at this level. From 5 to 10% of ingested alcohol is excreted unchanged in urine, sweat, and expired air; the remainder is oxidized to CO_2 and water at a rate of 5 to 10 mL/h (of absolute alcohol), each mL furnishing about 7 kcal. Blood alcohol is seldom actually measured; it is estimated from the amount present in expired air.

The most common forms of specific organ damage seen in alcoholics are cirrhosis of the liver, peripheral neuropathy, brain damage, and cardiomyopathy, often accompanied by arrhythmias. Gastritis is common and pancreatitis may also develop. Alcohol seems to have a direct hepatotoxic effect, although inadequate nutrition secondary to heavy alcohol intake may exacerbate this effect. Irreversible impairment of liver function occurs in some alcoholics; this may prevent adequate glycogen storage and promote a tendency to hypoglycemia from inability to mobilize glucose. Symptomatic hypoglycemia may result from the absence of adequate food intake. (See also discussions of alcoholic ketoacidosis in DIABETES MELLITUS and HYPOGLYCEMIA in Ch. 94.) Both the direct action of alcohol and the accompanying nutritional deficiencies (particularly of thiamine) are considered responsible for the frequent peripheral nerve degeneration and brain changes. Alcoholic cardiomyopathy may develop after approximately 10 yr of heavy alcohol abuse and is attributed to a direct toxic effect of alcohol on the heart muscle, independent of nutritional deficiencies. It is manifested clinically as cardiomegaly and congestive heart failure and pathologically usually as diffuse myocardial fibrosis and hypertrophy with glycoprotein infiltration. In addition, thiamine deficiency associated with alcohol abuse can produce a cardiomyopathy ("beri-beri heart disease") in which high output failure is prominent, and cardiac conductive disturbances can occur related to electrolyte imbalance. The presence of ECG abnormalities and the occurrence of sudden death in youthful alcoholics raises the possibility that alcohol in excess may have a significant arrhythmic effect. Gastritis in alcoholics may be related to the effect of alcohol on gastric secretions, which are increased in volume and acidity while the pepsin content remains low.

Tolerance, Physical Dependence, and Abstinence Syndromes

Patients who drink large amounts of alcohol repetitively become somewhat **tolerant** to its effects, a phenomenon also noted with other CNS depressants (opioids, barbiturates, meprobamate, etc); later doses do not have the same intoxicating effect as earlier ones. This tolerance is not based primarily on changes in drug disposition or metabolism but is caused by adaptational changes of CNS cells (cellular or pharmacodynamic tolerance). Those tolerant to alcohol may have incredibly high blood alcohol concentrations; a few have survived concentrations of > 700 mg/dL. Even so, the tolerance is incomplete and individuals can always manifest some degree of intoxication and impairment with a high enough dose. In fact, in tolerant animals, the *lethal* dose increases minimally. The **physical dependence** accompanying tolerance is profound, and withdrawal produces a series of adverse effects that may lead to death. Individuals tolerant to alcohol are cross-tolerant to many other CNS depressants (barbiturates, nonbarbiturate hypnotics, and benzodiazepines).

Alcohol withdrawal syndrome: A continuum of symptoms and signs accompanies alcohol withdrawal, usually beginning 12 to 48 h after cessation of intake. The mild withdrawal syndrome includes tremor, weakness, sweating, hyperreflexia, and GI symptoms. Some patients may suffer generalized grand mal seizures, usually not more than 2 in short succession (**"alcoholic epilepsy"** or **"rum fits"**).

Alcoholic hallucinosis follows prolonged excessive use of alcohol. The symptoms are auditory illusions and hallucinations, frequently accusatory and threatening; the patient usually is apprehensive and may be terrified. The condition resembles schizophrenia, but there is generally no thought disorder and the history is not typical of

schizophrenia. The symptoms do not resemble the delirious state of an acute organic brain syndrome as much as do delirium tremens or the other pathologic reactions associated with withdrawal. Consciousness remains clear, and the signs of autonomic lability seen in delirium tremens usually are absent. When the syndrome occurs, it generally precedes delirium tremens, and frightening dreams may occur in this stage. The hallucinosis usually is transient and responds to treatment with moderately large doses of phenothiazines. Chlorpromazine or thioridazine 100 to 300 mg qid is recommended. Recovery usually occurs in 1 to 3 wk; recurrence is likely if the patient resumes drinking.

Delirium tremens (the severe withdrawal syndrome) begins with anxiety attacks, increasing confusion, poor sleep (accompanied by frightening dreams), marked sweating, and a profound depression. Autonomic lability, evidenced by diaphoresis and increased pulse rate and temperature, accompanies the delirium and parallels its progress. Mild delirium is usually accompanied by marked diaphoresis, a pulse rate of 100 to 120/min, and a temperature of 37.2 to 37.8 C (99 to 100 F). Marked delirium, with gross disorientation and cognitive disruption, is associated with significant restlessness, a pulse greater than 120/min, and temperature over 37.8 C (100 F).

Initially, fleeting hallucinations and nocturnal illusions that arouse fear and restlessness may occur. Typical of these delirious, confused, and disoriented states is a return to a habitual activity—eg, the patient frequently imagines that he is back at work and attempts to perform some related activity. Visual hallucinations are frequent and often incite terror. The patient is suggestible to all sensory stimuli and particularly to objects seen in dim light. Vestibular disturbances may cause him to believe that the floor is moving, walls are falling, or the room is rotating. As the delirium progresses, a persistent coarse tremor of the hand at rest develops, sometimes extending to the head and trunk. Marked ataxia is present; care must be taken to prevent self-injury. Symptoms vary among patients but are usually the same with each recurrence for a particular patient.

Temperature may be elevated during the withdrawal of any agent that has caused physical dependence, but elevated temperature in alcohol withdrawal is a poor prognostic sign. Although death may occur in delirium tremens, the course usually is self-limited, terminating in a long sleep. The acute period persists from 2 to 10 days but can be more prolonged in severe withdrawal syndromes. Delirium tremens should begin to clear within 12 to 24 h, and if improvement is not marked within this interval, other conditions such as subdural hematoma, a systemic disorder, or other disturbances of mentation should be suspected.

Patients with **cirrhosis and impending hepatic coma** become dull, lethargic, and stuporous and develop a "flapping" tremor of the extended arms **(asterixis).** The apprehension, panic, and restlessness seen in delirium tremens are absent. These patients are extremely ill and require immediate medical intervention. (See also PORTAL-SYSTEMIC ENCEPHALOPATHY, in Ch. 67.)

Korsakoff's syndrome (see also Chs. 118 and 120) is characterized by *a gross disturbance in recent memory, often compensated for by confabulation.* The syndrome usually is associated with excessive alcohol intake, chronic malnourishment, and a diet deficient in the B vitamins, particularly thiamine, but may occur with other organic brain diseases. Korsakoff's syndrome may begin insidiously, or suddenly follow bouts of delirium tremens. The prognosis is poor because the patient usually does not alter his previous pattern of excessive alcohol intake. The outcome is graver if **Wernicke's disease or encephalopathy** (ocular palsy, impaired mentation, ataxia, and polyneuropathy) also develops (see Ch. 120).

Pathologic intoxication is a rare syndrome characterized by repetitive and automatic movements and the occurrences of extreme excitement with aggressive, uncontrolled irrational behavior after ingesting a relatively small amount of alcohol. The episode

may last for minutes or hours and is followed by a prolonged sleep with amnesia for the event upon awakening.

Treatment

Medical evaluation is needed initially to detect any intercurrent illness that might complicate withdrawal and to rule out any CNS symptoms from injury that might mimic or be masked by the withdrawal syndrome. It is especially important to differentiate delirium tremens from the mental changes found in acute hepatic insufficiency, because of the difference in management.

Delirious patients are extremely suggestible and respond well to reassurance. They generally should not be restrained. Fluid balance must be maintained and large doses of vitamin C and B-complex vitamins, particularly thiamine, given promptly. A dehydrated alcoholic patient should be given 1000 mL of 5% dextrose in physiologic saline solution followed by 1000 mL of 10% dextrose in distilled water.

Some drugs frequently used to treat alcohol withdrawal are similar to alcohol in pharmacologic effects. In fact, the most useful agents are apparently those to which alcohol induces cross-tolerance. All patients entering withdrawal are candidates for CNS-depressant drugs, but not all need them. Nondrug "detoxification" can be utilized in many individuals if proper attention is paid to psychologic support, reassurance, and a nonthreatening approach and environment. Unfortunately, most of these are not readily available in a general hospital or emergency room venue.

Rapidly acting barbiturates (pentobarbital and secobarbital) are seldom used today, but phenobarbital is quite useful. However, benzodiazepines have become the mainstay of therapy. **Chlordiazepoxide** is recommended in most situations in initial 50- to 100-mg oral doses that may need repetition q 3 h. **Diazepam** is a useful alternative, given 5 mg IV or orally hourly until sedation occurs. (NOTE: Alcoholics may achieve intoxication and even physical dependence and withdrawal with diazepam or chlordiazepoxide.) Isolated seizures need no specific therapy, and repeated seizures will respond to 1- to 3-mg doses of IV diazepam. **Phenothiazines** are not recommended, since they may not control severe delirium tremens and they lower the seizure threshold. The routine administration of **phenytoin** is not necessary. Outpatient therapy with phenytoin is almost always a waste of time and drug, because these seizures only occur under the stress of alcohol withdrawal, and withdrawing (or heavily drinking) patients do not take their antiseizure medication.

The first treatment phase consists of complete withdrawal of alcohol. The delirious state that may accompany withdrawal and its management has been described above. After correction of any nutritional deficiencies associated with excessive alcohol intake (see in Ch. 120; and under THIAMINE [VITAMIN B_1] DEFICIENCY in Ch. 81), the patient's behavior must be changed to eliminate drunkenness. Maintaining sobriety once it has been established is difficult because the patient has fixed patterns of nonsobriety. The patient should be warned that after a few weeks, when he has recovered from his last bout, he is likely to find some excuse to take a drink. He should also be told that he may be able to drink in a controlled manner for a few days or, rarely, even for a few weeks, but with depressing regularity he will repeat the pattern and again drink without control.

Various types of psychotherapy have been recommended for alcoholism, but a general belief is that group processes are superior to one-on-one processes. Some feel that newer behavioral technics may hold promise.

Alcoholics Anonymous (AA): No other approach has benefited so many alcoholics as effectively as the help they have offered themselves through AA. The patient must find an AA group in which he is comfortable, preferably one where he has common interests with the other members in addition to his alcohol problem; eg, in some metropolitan areas there are AA groups of physicians and dentists. These groups provide the patient with nondrinking friends who are always available as well as an area in which

to socialize—away from the tavern. The patient also hears others, more expert than he, confess before the group every rationalization the patient has ever thought up privately to justify his own drinking. Finally, the help he gives to other alcoholics may afford him the self-esteem and confidence formerly found only in alcohol.

Disulfiram therapy: Disulfiram interferes with the metabolism of acetaldehyde (an intermediary product in the oxidation of alcohol) so that acetaldehyde accumulates, producing toxic symptoms and great discomfort. Drinking alcohol within 12 h after taking disulfiram produces facial flushing in 5 to 15 min, then intense vasodilation of the face and neck with suffusion of the conjunctivae, throbbing headache, tachycardia, hyperpnea, and sweating. Nausea and vomiting follow in 30 to 60 min and may be so intense as to lead to hypotension, dizziness, and sometimes fainting and collapse. The reaction lasts 1 to 3 h. Discomfort is so intense that few patients will risk taking alcohol as long as they are taking disulfiram. The patient should also avoid medications containing alcohol (eg, tinctures, elixirs, some OTC liquid cough/cold preparations, which contain as much as 40% ethanol).

Disulfiram may be given on an outpatient basis after the patient has been free of alcohol for 4 or 5 days. The initial dose is 0.5 gm orally once/day for 1 to 3 wk. The maintenance dose is adjusted individually; 0.25 to 0.5 gm once/day is usually adequate, but some patients may require more. Both patient and relatives should be warned that the effects of disulfiram may persist for 3 to 7 days following the last dose. The patient must want to be helped, must cooperate, and should be seen periodically by the physician to encourage his continuing to take disulfiram as part of an abstinence program.

Few studies convincingly indicate a general usefulness of the drug, and many patients are noncompliant. However, when patients succeed they are often users of disulfiram, and the lack of proof should not interfere with its availability to patients and therapists. Disulfiram therapy is **contraindicated** in pregnancy and in decompensated cardiac patients.

DEPENDENCE OF THE OPIOID TYPE

A strong psychic dependence manifested as an overpowering compulsion to continue taking the drug, the development of tolerance so that the dosage must be continually increased in order to obtain the initial effect, and physical dependence that increases in intensity with increased dosage and duration of use. The physical dependence necessitates continued administration of the same opioid or a related drug to prevent withdrawal. Withdrawal of the drug or administration of an antagonist precipitates a characteristic and self-limited abstinence syndrome.

Tolerance and **physical dependence** on the opioids and synthetic narcotics develop rapidly; therapeutic doses taken regularly over a 2- to 3-day period can lead to some tolerance and dependence, and the user may show symptoms of withdrawal when the drug is discontinued. Opioid drugs induce cross-tolerance. Abusers may substitute one for another. With increased use of methadone in detoxification and maintenance programs, illicitly obtained methadone has become an abused drug. People who have developed tolerance may show few signs of drug use and function normally in their usual activities. Tolerance to the various effects of these drugs frequently develops unevenly; for example, a meperidine user may tolerate large doses but show many of the stimulant and atropine-like side effects. Heroin users may become completely tolerant to the euphoric and lethal effects but will still have constricted pupils and constipation.

Symptoms and Signs

Acute intoxication with opioids is characterized by euphoria, flushing, itching of the skin, miosis, drowsiness, decreased respiratory rate and depth, hypotension, bradycardia, and decreased body temperature.

The **withdrawal syndrome** from an opioid generally includes symptoms and signs opposite to the drug's pharmacologic effects (eg, CNS hyperactivity). The severity of the withdrawal syndrome increases with the size of the opioid dose and the duration of dependence. Symptoms begin to appear as early as 4 to 6 h after withdrawal and reach a peak within 36 to 72 h for heroin. The initial anxiety and craving for the drug are followed by other symptoms increasing in severity and intensity. A reliable early sign of abstinence is an increased resting respiratory rate, > 16/min, usually accompanied by yawning, perspiration, lacrimation, and rhinorrhea. Other symptoms include mydriasis, piloerection ("gooseflesh"), tremors, muscle twitching, hot and cold flashes, aching muscles, and anorexia. The withdrawal syndrome in persons who have been taking methadone develops more slowly and is overtly less severe than heroin withdrawal, although users may perceive it as worse.

Complications

Many but not all complications of heroin addiction are related to unsanitary administration of the drug. The more frequent complications include pulmonary problems, hepatitis, arthritic conditions, immunologic alterations, and neurologic disorders. The effect of heroin addiction on pregnancy (see below and in DRUGS IN PREGNANCY in Ch. 176) merits special mention.

Pulmonary problems: Pulmonary conditions found in narcotic addicts include aspiration pneumonitis, pneumonia, lung abscess, septic pulmonary emboli, atelectasis, and pulmonary fibrosis from talc granulomatosis. Chronic heroin addiction results in a decreased vital capacity and a mildly to moderately decreased pulmonary diffusion capacity. These effects are distinct from the unusual pulmonary edema that may be associated with overdose. In addition, many addicts smoke one or more packages of cigarettes/day. As a result, the addict is particularly susceptible to a variety of pulmonary infections.

Liver disturbance: Heroin addicts have a higher incidence of viral hepatitis, both Type A and Type B. The combination of viral hepatitis and the frequently high alcohol intake may account for a high incidence of liver dysfunction.

Musculoskeletal conditions: The most common problem is osteomyelitis (particularly lumbar vertebral), probably due to hematogenous spread of organisms from unsterile injections. Infectious spondylitis and sacroileitis have been reported. **Myositis ossificans ("drug abuser's elbow")** is extraosseous metaplasia of muscle damaged by inept needle manipulation; injury to the brachialis muscle is followed by replacement of the muscle bundle by a calcific mass.

Immunologic abnormalities: Hypergammaglobulinemia, involving both IgG and IgM, may be detected in up to 90% of addicts. A number of serologic tests have been found to be positive in heroin addicts (see TABLE 138–2). The reason for the immunologic changes is unknown, but they may reflect repeated antigenic stimulation, either from infections or from the daily parenteral injection of foreign substances. This altered immune state in heroin addicts may lead to such problems as splenomegaly, arthritis and arthralgia, lymphadenopathy, nephritis, and false-positive VDRL (Venereal Disease Research Laboratory) test results. Recently added to this problematic list is evidence that IV drug users are at risk for AIDS (see in Ch. 19), presumably secondary to transmission of the HTLV-III/LAV virus type.

Neurologic disorders that occur in heroin addicts are usually noninfectious complications of coma and cerebral anoxia. They may suffer from toxic amblyopia (apparently due to quinine contamination of heroin), transverse myelitis, and a variety of mono- and polyneuropathies, as well as Guillain-Barré syndrome. Cerebral complications include those secondary to bacterial endocarditis (bacterial meningitis, mycotic aneurysm, brain abscess, and subdural and epidural abscesses), acute cerebral falciparum

TABLE 138–2. PERCENTAGE FREQUENCY OF POSITIVE SEROLOGIC TESTS IN HEROIN ADDICTS ENTERING TREATMENT

Serologic Tests	*Frequency* (%)
VDRL	15–30
Latex fixation	20
Tests for mononucleosis	10
C-reactive protein	20–30
Serum hepatitis	5–10
Lymphogranuloma venereum	20
Typhoid, O and H	15–25
Paratyphoid, A and B	10–30
Proteus OX-19	15–25
Q fever	5–15
Brucella	10–25
Coombs	5

malaria, and the cerebral complications of viral hepatitis and tetanus. Some neurologic complications are thought to be due to allergic responses to the heroin–adulterant mixture.

Other complications include superficial cutaneous abscesses, cellulitis, lymphangitis, lymphadenitis, and phlebitis from contaminated needles. Many heroin addicts begin with subcutaneous injections ("skin popping"). They may return to this mode when extensive scarring makes their veins no longer accessible. As addicts become more desperate, cutaneous ulcers in unlikely sites may be found. Contaminated needles and inoculum may also lead to bacterial endocarditis.

Pregnancy and opioid addiction: Problems of the heroin-addicted mother are transferred to the fetus; because heroin and methadone freely cross the placental barrier, the fetus readily becomes drug-dependent. Pregnant addicts seen early enough should be encouraged to enter a methadone maintenance program. Obviously, such plans should include the obstetrician and pediatrician who will treat the dependent infant. Pregnant women withdrawn from heroin or methadone late in the 3rd trimester of pregnancy risk the precipitation of labor. Pregnant women seen at or near term may best be stabilized on methadone. Abstinence would be better for the fetus but experience has indicated that withdrawn mothers often revert to heroin and withdraw from prenatal care. The methadone-maintained mother may nurse her newborn without apparent clinical problems in the child, and the minimal concentrations in breast milk have been confirmed. The infants of opioid-dependent mothers may present with tremors, a high-pitched cry, jitters, convulsions, and tachypnea. For a discussion of problems of the neonate, including **drug withdrawal** and **fetal alcohol syndromes,** see METABOLIC PROBLEMS IN THE NEWBORN in Ch. 186 and DRUGS IN LACTATING MOTHERS in Ch. 182. See also DRUGS IN PREGNANCY in Ch. 176.

Treatment

The clinical management of opioid addicts is extremely difficult. Physicians treating them must be fully aware of the federal, state, and local regulations concerning the treatment of addicts. Few physicians have had formal training or experience in dealing with opioid addicts and their companions and families, as well as the attitudes of society (including law enforcement officers, other physicians, and allied health personnel) toward the treatment of such individuals. The physician should be aware of locally available resources and usually should refer opioid addicts to specialized treatment centers rather than attempt to care for them in an office. If there are no specialized

centers, the physician can closely supervise the patient, with frequent contacts and close work with the patient's family and friends.

In order to legally use an opioid drug in treating an addict, the existence of a physiologic heroin dependence must be established. This is a difficult diagnosis, since many individuals seeking treatment have minimal physical opiate dependence; this high incidence of psychologic heroin dependence has occurred because at times only low-grade heroin has been available and most addicts may not maintain a high enough level of heroin use to produce physiologic dependence. The following are helpful in assessing physiologic dependence: (1) a history of 3 or more narcotic injections/day, (2) the presence of fresh needle marks, (3) observation of withdrawal symptoms and signs, and (4) the presence of morphine in a properly obtained urine specimen. Morphine (and its glucuronide metabolite) is the most abundant urinary opioid in heroin users.

Management of acute intoxication (overdose): Naloxone (0.4 to 0.8 mg) given IV is the drug of choice, since it possesses no respiratory depressant properties. If the patient's unconsciousness is due to an opioid, dramatic recovery occurs immediately following the administration of this antagonist. Since some patients become agitated, delirious, and combative as they recover from their comatose state, secure physical restraints may be required and should be applied before the antagonist is given. All patients treated for overdose should be hospitalized and observed for at least 24 h, since the action of the opioid antagonist is relatively short and respiratory depression may recur within several hours (especially with methadone). Pulmonary edema that may be severe enough to cause death from hypoxia is usually not responsive to naloxone and has an unclear relationship to overdosage.

The opioid withdrawal syndrome is self-limited, and although severely discomforting is not life-threatening. A patient admitted for withdrawal should be told that he will experience some unpleasant symptoms and should be reassured that they will not be allowed to progress to an odious level but that the medication he receives will be based on some objective physical signs of withdrawal. The patient's drug-seeking behavior usually begins with the first symptoms of withdrawal, and hospital personnel must always be alert to the possibility that he will try to obtain illicit supplies of drugs. Visitors may have to be restricted. Many patients with withdrawal symptoms have other medical problems that must be diagnosed and treated. Opioid users may have **mixed addictions,** and although providing appropriate withdrawal measures for each drug is theoretically feasible, for practical purposes this is not required.

Currently, **methadone substitution** is the preferred method of opioid withdrawal. Methadone is given orally in the smallest amount that will prevent severe signs of withdrawal but not necessarily all signs. Close observation of the patient is important, since his subjective symptoms are unreliable. Many of the symptoms of withdrawal can be mimicked by anxiety states. Generally, 20 mg/day of methadone will block the symptoms of severe withdrawal in most addicts. Higher doses should be given only on direct observations of the physical signs of withdrawal, since addicts are unreliable in reporting the size of their habits. Doses of 25 to 45 mg can produce unconsciousness if the person has not developed tolerance for heroin or methadone. Once a suppressing dose has been established, it should be reduced progressively *by not more than 20% each day*. Patients commonly become emotionally upset and frequently request additional medication. Chloral hydrate 500 to 1000 mg may be given orally for several nights to improve sleep. The acute manifestations of withdrawal usually subside within 7 to 10 days, but patients often complain of weakness, insomnia, and a severe pervasive anxiety for several months. Minor metabolic and physiologic effects of withdrawal may persist for up to 6 mo. It is appropriate to treat heroin withdrawal with oral

methadone, but the usual low-grade level of dependence can be treated with propoxyphene napsylate or even benzodiazepines, which are not cross-tolerant to opiates.

It is now well documented that the central α-adrenergic drug **clonidine** can halt essentially all signs of opioid withdrawal. This probably relates to diminution of central adrenergic outflow secondary to stimulation of central α receptors (the same mechanism by which clonidine lowers BP). This theory supports the importance of central adrenergic discharge in the evolution of the opioid withdrawal syndrome. Clonidine is not a benign drug. Besides causing hypotension and drowsiness, its withdrawal may precipitate restlessness, insomnia, irritability, tachycardia, and headache. It is now labeled by the FDA for use in opioid withdrawal and may be so used by the generalist. However, its overall contribution to therapy is minor. Withdrawal is not a difficult problem for patient or clinician. Abstinence, which clonidine does not aid, is.

Withdrawal from methadone: The abstinence syndrome induced by methadone is like that of heroin, but onset is more gradual and delayed, beginning 36 to 72 h after discontinuing the drug. Deep muscle aches and "bone pains" are frequent complaints. Because the abstinence syndrome begins gradually, methadone addicts may be initially observed on admission. A urine sample should be obtained to document the methadone habit, and methadone provided as symptoms develop. Methadone withdrawal for individuals coming from methadone maintenance programs may be particularly difficult, since the addict's dose of methadone may be as high as 100 mg/day. In general, ambulatory detoxification should be started by reducing the dose to 60 mg/day or less over several weeks before attempting complete detoxification. Clonidine may be particularly useful in aiding withdrawal from methadone.

Treatment of chronic opioid dependence: No consensus exists regarding long-term treatment of opioid-dependent users. Thousands of American opioid addicts are in methadone maintenance programs. It was hoped that large enough doses of oral methadone in treating addicts (chiefly heroin) would enable them to move to socially productive lives because their supply problems would be met. Additionally, the methadone would block any effects of injected heroin and alleviate user's "drug hunger." For some, the plan has worked. For others, methadone just adds another drug problem to their alcohol use, intermittent heroin use, and desperate lives. Additionally, the widespread availability of methadone has established its role as an important drug of abuse in the culture.

Experiments with **L-acetyl α-methadol (LAAM),** a longer-acting synthetic opioid, give hope of help to some addicts and of removing the problem of expensive daily client visits or take-home medication which insures some diversion. The culture's loss of faith in methadone maintenance or at least the lessening commitment of public money has diminished the number of treatment facilities and the amount of research given to LAAM.

Naltrexone, an orally bioavailable opioid antagonist, has been released for general use. It has little agonist effect, and many opioid addicts will not voluntarily consume it. Motivated patients may do well. There are reports of its usefulness in health professionals addicted to opioids. The usual dose is 50 mg/day or 350 mg/wk in 2 or 3 divided doses.

The therapeutic community concept emerged nearly 25 yr ago in response to the heroin problem. Synanon, Daytop Village, and Phoenix House pioneered this nondrug treatment in residential centers, and the movement has grown. The communal, relatively long-term (usually 15-mo) residential setting would, it was hoped, by training, education, and redirection help users achieve new lives. Like methadone maintenance, this mode has helped, indeed transformed, some. How well it works, how widely it may be applied, and how much funding society will give remain unanswered questions.

DEPENDENCE OF THE BARBITURATE TYPE

Psychic dependence that may lead to periodic, as often as continuous, abuse; and a physical dependence that can be detected only after consumption of amounts considerably above the usual therapeutic or socially acceptable levels. (Barbiturates and ethanol are strikingly similar in their syndromes of dependence, withdrawal, and chronic intoxication.) When barbiturate intake is reduced below a critical level, a self-limited abstinence syndrome ensues. Symptoms of withdrawal from barbiturates and other sedative-hypnotics can be suppressed completely with a barbiturate. **Tolerance** to barbiturates develops irregularly and incompletely so that considerable behavioral disturbances and psychotoxicity persist, depending on the drug's pharmacodynamic effects. Some mutual but incomplete cross-tolerance exists between alcohol and the barbiturates as well as the nonbarbiturate sedative-hypnotics, including benzodiazepines.

Symptoms and Signs

Drug effects: In general, those dependent on sedatives and hypnotics, including barbiturates and benzodiazepines, prefer the rapid-onset drugs (eg, secobarbital and pentobarbital). The signs of progressive sedative intoxication are depression of superficial skin reflexes, fine lateral-gaze nystagmus, slightly decreased alertness with coarser or rapid nystagmus, ataxia and slurred speech, and a positive Romberg's sign. With progression there is nystagmus on forward gaze, somnolence, marked ataxia with falling, confusion, deep sleep, small pupils, respiratory depression, and ultimately death. Patients on large doses of depressants frequently have difficulty thinking and show slowness of speech and comprehension with some dysarthria, poor memory, faulty judgment, narrowed attention span, and emotional lability. In general, the combination of slow thinking, slurred speech, and bruises on the extremities from falling may suggest dependence on depressants.

Withdrawal effects: In susceptible patients, psychologic dependence on the drug may develop rapidly; and, after only a few weeks, attempts to discontinue it exacerbate any initial insomnia and result in restlessness, disturbing dreams, frequent awakening, and feelings of tension in the early morning. The extent of physical dependence is related to the barbiturate dose and the length of time that it has been taken; for example, pentobarbital 200 mg/day may be ingested for many months without significant tolerance developing; 300 mg/day may induce an abstinence syndrome on terminating medication if ingested for more than 3 mo; and 500 to 600 mg/day may provoke an abstinence syndrome after 1 mo. Large doses of barbiturates (4 to 10 times the usual hypnotic dose) taken for 1 mo or more will probably induce some form of abstinence syndrome.

An abrupt withdrawal syndrome from large doses of barbiturates or tranquilizers produces a severe, frightening, and potentially life-threatening illness essentially similar to delirium tremens. Withdrawal from barbiturates carries a significant mortality rate and should always be undertaken in the hospital. Once the withdrawal syndrome has begun, reversing it is difficult, but with a careful schedule the symptoms can be minimized. The reestablishment of CNS stability requires about 30 days. Occasionally, after even properly managed withdrawal over 1 to 2 wk, a seizure may occur in the following 2 wk. Within the first 12 to 20 h after the withdrawal of a short-acting barbiturate, the patient becomes increasingly restless, tremulous, and weak. By the 2nd day, the tremulousness becomes more prominent, the deep tendon reflexes may be increased, and the patient becomes weaker. During the 2nd and 3rd days, convulsions occur in 75% of all patients taking 800 mg/day or more. The convulsions may progress to status epilepticus and death. From the 2nd to the 5th day, the untreated abstinence syndrome includes delirium, insomnia, confusion, and frightening visual and auditory hallucinations. Hyperpyrexia and dehydration often occur. With longer-acting barbi-

turates, symptoms may not begin for > 24 h, do not reach a peak for 5 to 7 days, and may last as long as 10 to 14 days.

A withdrawal syndrome similar to the barbiturate syndrome, although seldom as severe, may occur with benzodiazepines, particularly diazepam. Many patients so described have been heavy users of alcohol. The syndrome with these agents may be very long in developing because of continued presence of the drugs in the body. A withdrawal syndrome of varying severity may occur in individuals taking normal doses. Probably all patients taking benzodiazepines other than diazepam with some regularity for > 3 to 4 mo should be switched to diazepam and withdrawn over 2 to 4 wk.

Treatment

The procedure for treating dependence on depressants, particularly barbiturates, is to reintoxicate the patient and then withdraw the drug on a strict schedule, being alert for signs of marked withdrawal. Before beginning withdrawal from barbiturates, one can evaluate sedative tolerance with a test dose of pentobarbital 200 mg orally given to the nonintoxicated, fasting patient; 1 to 2 h later this test dose produces drowsiness or sleep with response to arousal in individuals with no tolerance to pentobarbital. Patients with intermediate levels of tolerance may show some impairment, while patients tolerant to 900 mg or more show no signs of intoxication. If the 200-mg dose has no effect, the tolerance level can be determined by repeating the test q 3 to 4 h with a larger dose. Severe anxiety or agitation may increase the patient's tolerance. Once the 24-h dose to which the patient is tolerant has been ascertained, that dose of pentobarbital is usually given qid for 2 or 3 days to stabilize the patient, and is then decreased by 10%/day.

Alternatively, phenobarbital can be used: it does not produce the "high" of the more rapidly acting drugs, its action is prolonged so that it provides smoother sedation, and it is the anticonvulsant of choice. Rapid-onset barbiturates or other sedative-hypnotics or minor tranquilizers can be replaced by a dose of phenobarbital equivalent to 1/3 the average daily dose of the drug on which the patient has become dependent (see TABLE 138–3). Phenobarbital is given orally qid, and the initial phenobarbital dose is reduced by 30 mg/day until the patient is drug-free; eg, if the patient has been taking secobar-

TABLE 138–3. DOSES OF SOME COMMON SEDATIVES AND TRANQUILIZERS THAT HAVE PRODUCED PHYSICAL DEPENDENCE

Drug	*Doses Producing Dependence (mg/day)*	*Time Necessary to Produce Dependence (days)*	*Dosage Equivalent to 30 mg Phenobarbital (mg)*
Secobarbital	500– 600	30	100
Pentobarbital ("yellow jackets")	500– 600	30	100
Amobarbital ("blues")	500– 600	30	100
Amobarbital-secobarbital combination ("rainbows")	500– 600	30	100
Glutethimide	1250–1500	60	500
Methyprylon	1200–1500	60	300
Ethchlorvynol	1500–2000	60	500
Meprobamate	2000–2400	60	400
Chlordiazepoxide	200– 300	60	25
Diazepam	60– 100*	40	10
Methaqualone	1800–2400	30	300
Chloral hydrate	2000–2500	30	500

* See also discussion of withdrawal effects, above.

bital 1000 mg/day, the stabilizing dose of phenobarbital is 300 mg/day or 75 mg q 6 h. Since the initial daily dose must be estimated from the patient's history, there is obviously a large margin of error, and the patient must be observed closely for the 1st 72 h. If he remains agitated or anxious, the dosage should be increased; if he is drowsy, dysarthric, or has nystagmus, the dosage should be decreased. While patients are being detoxified, other sedatives and psychotropic medications should be avoided. However, if the patient is also taking antidepressant medications, especially the tricyclics, the antidepressant should not be abruptly discontinued but should be reduced over 3 to 4 days. Methaqualone, a pervasively misused drug, has been moved to Federal Schedule I and is no longer available in the USA. Fake methaqualone (usually imitating Quaalude®) contains over-the-counter antihistamines or, rarely, large doses of diazepam.

DEPENDENCE OF THE CANNABIS (MARIJUANA) TYPE

Chronic or periodic administration of cannabis or cannabis substances producing some psychic dependence because of the desired subjective effects, but no physical dependence; there is no abstinence syndrome when the drug is discontinued. Cannabis can be used on an episodic but continuous basis without evidence of social or psychic dysfunction. In many users the term dependence with its obvious connotations probably is misapplied.

Use of the drug is widespread. In the USA it is commonly used in the form of cigarettes made from the dried plant, *Cannabis sativa*, or as hashish, the pressed resin of the plant. Recently, synthetic Δ-9 tetrahydrocannabinol **(THC)**, an active constituent of marijuana, has become available for research and limited clinical use; despite claims of dealers and users, it does not appear on the street.

Symptoms and signs: Cannabis produces a dreamy state of consciousness in which ideas seem disconnected, uncontrollable, and freely flowing. Time, color, and spatial perceptions are distorted and enhanced. In general, there is a feeling of well-being, exaltation, excitement, and inner joyousness that has been termed a "high." Many of the psychologic effects seem to be related to the setting in which the drug is taken. An occasional panic reaction has occurred, particularly in naive users, but these have become unusual as the culture has gained increasing familiarity with the drug. Communicative and motor abilities are decreased during the use of these drugs. Difficulty in depth perception and altered sense of timing, both of which are particularly hazardous during automobile driving, have been demonstrated. There are now several published reports of the exacerbation of schizophrenic symptoms by marijuana even in patients being treated with antipsychotic medication (eg, chlorpromazine).

Metabolic products of marijuana are retained in the tissues for a lengthy time. Lowered testosterone levels have been reported, although the biologic significance of this is uncertain.

In recent years, critics of marijuana use have become prominent and have enlisted much scientific data in support. A counter-reform movement opposed to decriminalization and the easy acceptance of the drug in American society has emerged. Many of the claims regarding severe biologic impact are still uncertain, but some other points are not. Despite the acceptance of the "new" dangers of marijuana, there is still little evidence of biologic damage even among relatively heavy users. This is true even in the areas intensively investigated, such as pulmonary, immunologic, and reproductive function. The surveys that continually showed an increased prevalence and increasing daily use by high school students have in recent years shown a diminution of use.

Marijuana used in the USA has a higher THC content than in the past. Many critics have incorporated this fact into warnings, but the chief opposition to the drug rests on a moral and political, and not a toxicologic, foundation.

DEPENDENCE OF THE COCAINE TYPE

Psychic dependence, sometimes leading to profound psychic addiction, produced by high doses of this stimulant drug that cause euphoric excitement and, occasionally, hallucinatory experiences, properties highly esteemed by experienced drug users. Neither tolerance nor physical dependence have been noted, and there is therefore no abstinence syndrome when the drug is withdrawn. The tendency to continue taking the drug is strong.

Symptoms and signs: Effects differ strikingly with different modes of use. When injected or inhaled, cocaine produces a condition of hyperstimulation, alertness, euphoria, and feelings of great power. The excitation and "high" are similar to that produced by injection of high doses of amphetamine. Since cocaine is a very short-acting drug, heavy users may resort to injecting it IV q 10 or 15 min. With this repetition, toxic effects such as tachycardia, hypertension, mydriasis, muscle-twitching, formication ("cocaine bugs"), miniaturized visual hallucinations, sleeplessness, and extreme nervousness appear. Hallucinations and paranoid delusions may develop, as well as violent behavior; the individual may be dangerous at this time. The action of the drug, however, is sufficiently brief to prevent sustained aggressive activity. The pupils are maximally dilated, and elevations of heart rate, BP, and respiration result from the drug's sympathomimetic effect. An **overdose** of cocaine produces tremors, convulsions with a temporal lobe seizure pattern, and delirium. Death may be due to a cardiovascular collapse or respiratory failure. Since the removal of cocaine from plasma requires intact serum esterase, there is speculation that subjects with extreme clinical toxicity may have genetically diminished (atypical) serum cholinesterase.

Severe toxic effects occur in the compulsive heavy user, who often also has a history of heroin use. Probably a majority of users are episodic recreational users who voluntarily curtail their use, or find that the drug's high cost mandates episodic use. However, cocaine use and the development of addictive behavior in some users has continued to increase in North America in recent years.

Two recent developments should be mentioned. The smoking of "free-base" cocaine (one version is now widely labeled as "crack") has become popular. This necessitates the conversion of the hydrochloride salt to the more combustible form. A flame is held to the converted material and the smoke inhaled. The speed of onset is shortened and the intensity of the high is magnified. Because the extraction utilizes flammable solvents, there have been serious explosions and burns.

Procaine when snorted produces local sensations not unlike cocaine and may even produce some "high." Powdered procaine is widely used to cut cocaine and is occasionally mixed with mannitol or lactose and sold as cocaine. It is widely sold by mail-order suppliers and is sometimes called "synthetic cocaine."

Treatment: Many nonspecific therapies including support and self-help groups have emerged, and cocaine "hotlines" have generated much publicity. Extremely expensive in-patient therapy is available to those whose wealth enabled them to purchase enormous amounts of cocaine initially.

Treatment of acute cocaine intoxication is generally unnecessary because of the extremely short action of the drug. If an overdose requires intervention, IV barbiturates or diazepam may be used. However, the respiratory depression that accompanies cocaine poisoning can be worsened with large doses of sedatives. Anticonvulsants do not effectively prevent convulsions in cocaine overdose. Discontinuing the chronic and sustained use of cocaine requires considerable assistance, and the depression that may occur requires close supervision and treatment.

DEPENDENCE OF THE AMPHETAMINE TYPE

Some psychic dependence produced by these widely used stimulants and anorexiants that cause elevated mood, increased wakefulness, alertness, concentration, and physical performance, and induce a feeling of well-being. There is significant sale of fake amphetamine, and many users now consume large amounts of caffeine along with **phenylpropanolamine, pseudoephedrine,** or **ephedrine.** This problem became so visible that the FDA has effectively outlawed the manufacture of the fakes by declaring that any combination of a stimulant phenethylamine with caffeine is a new drug that must be registered with the agency.

Symptoms and Signs

The **withdrawal** syndrome, if one exists, is not severe. Withdrawal is followed by a state of mental and physical depression and fatigue. Qualitatively, the psychologic effects are similar to those produced by cocaine; the psychologic dependence is variable. Unlike cocaine and most other CNS stimulants, amphetamine induces **tolerance.** Tolerance to amphetamine develops slowly, but a progressive increase in dosage can occur and permits the eventual ingestion or injection of amounts several hundredfold greater than the original therapeutic dose. The tolerance to various effects develops unequally, so that nervousness and sleeplessness persist and psychotoxic effects, such as hallucinations and delusions, may occur. However, even massive doses are rarely fatal. Chronic drug users have reportedly injected as much as 15,000 mg of amphetamine in 24 h without observable acute illness. For neophytes, however, rapid injection of 120 mg *may be fatal,* although some individuals have survived 400 to 500 mg.

Abusers of amphetamine are prone to accidents because of the excitation and grandiosity produced and the accompanying excessive fatigue of sleeplessness. IV administration may lead to serious antisocial behavior and can precipitate a schizophrenic episode. **Adverse reactions** to continued high doses of methamphetamine include (1) anxiety reactions during which the person is fearful and tremulous and concerned about his physical well-being; (2) an amphetamine psychosis in which the person misinterprets others' actions, hallucinates, and becomes unrealistically suspicious; (3) an exhaustion syndrome, involving an intense feeling of fatigue and need for sleep, after the stimulation phase; and (4) a prolonged depression during which suicide is a possibility.

A **paranoid psychosis** almost inevitably results from long-term use of high doses IV but also can result from large oral doses. This psychosis may rarely be precipitated either by a single large dose or by chronic moderate doses. Typical features of the amphetamine psychosis include delusions of persecution, ideas of reference, and feelings of omnipotence. Those who use high doses IV usually accept that they will sooner or later experience paranoia and are often able to cope with it. Nevertheless, when drug use becomes very intense, or toward the end of a long run, even well-practiced intellectual awareness may fail, and the user may respond to a delusional system. Recovery from even prolonged amphetamine psychosis is usual. The slow but complete recovery of users who have become thoroughly disorganized and paranoid is a striking phenomenon. The more florid symptoms fade within a few days or weeks, although some confusion and memory loss and some delusional ideas may commonly persist for months.

Treatment

Although there are no symptomatic withdrawal phenomena (other than general fatigue, sleepiness, and depression), EEG changes are seen that fulfill physiologic criteria for dependence. Abrupt discontinuance of amphetamine is not without complications; withdrawal can uncover an underlying depression, or it may precipitate a depressive reaction, often with a suicidal potential. In many persons whose amphetamine intake masks chronic fatigue, withdrawal is followed by 2 or 3 days of intense

tiredness or sleepiness. Patients recovering from an amphetamine psychosis may demonstrate severe anxiety and extreme restlessness. Therefore, withdrawal generally should be undertaken in a drug-free environment where hospital and nursing facilities are available.

The acute agitated psychotic state with paranoid delusions and auditory and visual hallucinations responds remarkably to phenothiazines; chlorpromazine 25 to 50 mg IM rapidly reverses the toxic psychotic conditions but may produce severe postural hypotension. Haloperidol 2.5 to 5 mg IM has been used effectively, since it rarely produces hypotension, but it greatly increases the risk of an alarming acute extrapyramidal motor reaction. Usually, reassurance and a quiet, nonthreatening environment will permit the patient to recover. Acidification of the urine with ammonium chloride 500 mg orally q 4 h aids amphetamine excretion.

DEPENDENCE OF THE HALLUCINOGEN TYPE

Hallucinogens include lysergic acid diethylamide (LSD), psilocybin, mescaline, peyote, 2,5-dimethoxy-4-methylamphetamine (DOM, "STP"), 3,4-methylenedioxymethamphetamine (MDMA), and other substituted amphetamines. Generally, other than LSD, the listed hallucinogen exotica are not available on the street, despite the beliefs of dealers and users, although in recent years a number of samples of a street product called "Ecstasy" have contained relatively pure methylene dioxyamphetamine (MDA) or its N-methyl congener, MDMA.

Symptoms and Signs

These substances induce a state of excitation of the CNS and central autonomic hyperactivity, manifested as changes in mood (usually euphoric, sometimes depressive) and perception. True hallucinations apparently rarely occur. Psychic dependence on hallucinogens varies greatly but usually is not intense. No evidence of physical dependence can be detected when the drugs are abruptly withdrawn. A high degree of **tolerance** to LSD develops and disappears rapidly. Individuals tolerant to any of these drugs are cross-tolerant to the others. Chief dangers to the individual are the psychologic effects and impairment of judgment, which can lead to dangerous decision-making or accidents.

Responses to the hallucinogens depend on several factors, including the individual's expectations, the setting, and his ability to cope with the perceptual distortions. Untoward reactions to LSD apparently have become rare. **Adverse reactions** to hallucinogens appear as anxiety attacks, extreme apprehensiveness, or panic states. Most often, these reactions quickly subside with appropriate management in a secure setting. However, some individuals (especially after using LSD) remain disturbed and may even show a **persistent psychotic state.** It is unclear whether the drug use has precipitated or uncovered a preexisting psychotic potential or whether this can occur in previously stable individuals.

Some persons, especially among those who are chronic or repeated users of hallucinogenic drugs and particularly with the use of LSD, may experience drug effects after they have discontinued use of the drug. Referred to as **"flashbacks,"** these episodes most commonly consist of visual illusions but can include distortions of virtually any sensation (including perceptions of time, space, or self-image) or hallucinations. Such episodes can be precipitated by use of marijuana, alcohol, or barbiturates, by stress or fatigue, or they may occur without apparent reason. The mechanisms that produce flashbacks are not known, but they tend to subside over a period of 6 mo to a year.

Treatment

Reassurance that the bizarre thoughts, visions, and sounds are due to the drug and not to a "nervous breakdown" usually suffices in acute adverse reactions to hallucinogens. **Phenothiazines must be used with extreme caution,** because of the danger of hypo-

tension, particularly if phencyclidine (see below) has been ingested. Short-acting barbiturates or minor tranquilizers such as chlordiazepoxide or diazepam may help reduce overwhelming anxiety.

For heavy users of hallucinogens, withdrawal of the drug is the simplest part of treatment; some may need psychiatric treatment for associated problems. Frequent contact and establishing a helpful relationship with a physician can be beneficial. Maintaining the patient's social functioning (eg, school or work performance) may be more realistic than aiming for complete abstinence.

Persistent psychotic states or other psychologic disorders require appropriate psychiatric care. Flashbacks may be transient and may not be unduly distressing to the patient, requiring no special treatment. However, they may be associated with anxiety and depression and may require therapy similar to that of the acute adverse reactions.

DEPENDENCE ON PHENCYCLIDINE (PCP)

PCP has emerged as an important drug of abuse. It is not easily classified and should be considered separately from the hallucinogenic drugs. It has a bewildering number of effects in the CNS, and its neuropharmacology is only poorly understood.

PCP was tested as an anesthetic agent in humans in the late 1950s because of an ability to isolate humans from noxious sensory input (dissociative anesthesia). It was withdrawn because individuals often experienced severe anxiety, delusional states, or frank psychosis postoperatively. Clinical testing stopped in 1962 and PCP appeared as a street drug in 1967. Initially sold deceptively as "THC," in recent years it has established its own market. Although once available as a veterinary anesthetic, essentially all street material results from illegal synthesis, not difficult to perform. Occasionally injected or ingested, it is most frequently sprinkled on smoking material (parsley, mint leaves, tobacco, marijuana), combusted, and inhaled. In recent years, much random violence and crime has been attributed to users of this drug, although as with past drug horror stories, this is not often well documented. Since the frequent reports of problems with PCP in 1978, the number of reports has declined significantly. Its current use and the attention directed to that use have declined.

Symptoms and signs: A giddy euphoria usually occurs with lower doses, often followed by bursts of anxiety or mood lability. Effects of higher doses include a withdrawn catatonic state, ataxia, dysarthria, muscular hypertonicity, and myoclonic jerks. Rotatory nystagmus is often present and helps in making the diagnosis. Cardiovascular status is usually unaffected. At very high doses, coma, convulsions, severe hypertension, and death may occur, although fatalities are unusual. Prolonged psychotic states have apparently followed use of this drug.

In treatment, diazepam often is helpful, and is mandatory when seizure activity is present. Some clinicians feel that haloperidol is useful. Hypotension may occur when chlorpromazine is used. Diazoxide may be used when severe hypertension is present. PCP is highly lipid-soluble and may have a prolonged biologic persistence. It or its metabolites may remain in the CNS for lengthy periods. The alkaline character of the drug leads to surprisingly high secretion into the stomach, and prolonged gastric lavage has recovered large amounts of PCP. Lavage must be accompanied by acidification with ammonium chloride (or other agents) because this maneuver results in dramatic ionic trapping in the stomach and urine. Anecdotally, street users may resort to cranberry juice to hasten urinary excretion.

DEPENDENCE ON VOLATILE SOLVENTS

A state of intoxication achieved by use of industrial solvents and aerosol sprays continues to be an endemic problem among juveniles. These volatile solvents (eg, aliphatic and aromatic hydrocarbons, chlorinated hydrocarbons, ketones, acetates) along with

ether, chloroform, and alcohol produce temporary stimulation before depression of the CNS occurs. Partial tolerance to the fumes develops with daily use, as does psychologic dependence, but an abstinence syndrome does not occur.

Acute **symptoms** of dizziness, drowsiness, slurred speech, and unsteady gait are seen early. Impulsiveness, excitement, and irritability may occur. As the CNS becomes more deeply affected, illusions, hallucinations, and delusions develop. The user experiences a euphoric dreamy "high," culminating in a short period of "sleep." Delirium with confusion, psychomotor clumsiness, emotional lability, and impairment of thinking are seen. The intoxicated state may last from minutes to an hour or more.

Complications may result from the effect of the solvent or from other toxic ingredients such as lead in gasoline. Carbon tetrachloride may cause a syndrome of hepatic and renal failure. Injuries to brain, liver, kidney, and bone marrow occur and may be the effects of heavy exposure or hypersensitivity. Death most often occurs from respiratory arrest, cardiac arrhythmias, or asphyxia due to occlusion of the airway.

Treatment of solvent-dependent children is difficult, and relapse is frequent. Intensive attempts to improve the patient's self-esteem and status in family, school, and society may be helpful.

DEPENDENCE ON VOLATILE NITRITES

Inhalation of amyl nitrite ("poppers") to alter consciousness and enhance sexual pleasure has emerged in recent years. This use has been particularly prominent in urban male homosexual society. When amyl nitrite was returned to the prescription drug category, entrepreneurs began to market other nitrites (butyl, isobutyl) under a variety of tradenames; eg, "Locker Room," "Rush," and others. At this time there is little evidence that the products have significant hazard, although they produce a predictable nitrite vasodilating effect with brief hypotension, dizziness, and flushing, followed by reflex tachycardia.

---

139. PSYCHOSEXUAL DISORDERS

Accepted norms of sexual behavior and attitudes vary greatly within and among different cultures. **Masturbation,** once widely regarded as a perversion and a cause of mental disease, is now recognized as a normal sexual activity throughout life and is considered a symptom only when it suggests an inhibition of partner-oriented behavior. Its cumulative incidence is approximately 97% in males and 80% in females. While masturbation per se is harmless, guilt created by disapproving and punitive attitudes may cause considerable distress and damage the capacity for sexual performance. Guilt and shame may also be induced by the discomfort of "forbidden" (eg, sadomasochistic or fetishistic) fantasies. Each year ± 1000 autoerotic fatalities occur, caused by asphyxia resulting from hanging or other methods of respiratory interference.

The Kinsey report revealed that about 5% of the population are preferentially **homosexual** for their entire lives. Several countries have passed laws permitting homosexual relationships between consenting adults. The American Psychiatric Association no longer considers homosexuality a psychiatric disease but suggests treatment for homosexuals whose desires create distress and who wish to reduce their homosexual arousal and increase their capacity for heterosexual arousal.

Frequent sexual activity with many partners, often one-time-only encounters, indicates diminished capacity for pair-bonding. **Extramarital sexuality** is discouraged by most cultures, but **premarital coitus** is accepted as normal by most. In the USA over 80% of both males and females have intercourse prior to marriage, in keeping with a recent shift in developed countries toward more freedom of sexual expression. **Dysfunction of**

desire, arousal, and orgasm in the male and female is discussed in Ch. 165. **Illegitimacy** (teenage unwed pregnancies are discussed in Ch. 202) arouses disapproval and causes social disadvantage in many countries, while in others a high proportion of children are born out of wedlock and are well tolerated. Illegitimate children reared by a single parent or by surrogates who may not form a close emotional bond with the child in the formative years may be less likely to mature normally and may be more susceptible to developing emotional disorders or frank mental illness. Data show a slight risk of increased mental illness in selected groups of children; eg, young children (not illegitimate) raised by a single, divorced parent. The prognosis is better when the single parent has a support system.

Individuals whose sexual practices include small amounts of **fetishism** and **sadomasochism** generally have normal love relationships. Such tendencies may excite anxiety and distress but call for reassurance rather than therapy. However, if sexual drives are absorbed almost entirely in submission to flagellation, are vented mostly on articles of clothing, or are expressed to a great extent in **exhibitionism** or **voyeurism,** the individual's capacity for establishing love relationships is stunted, and other aspects of his personal and emotional adjustment suffer.

Doctors can offer sensitive, disciplined advice on sexual matters and should not miss opportunities for helpful intervention, keeping in mind the influence of cultural diversity. The strength of the sexual drive, the needs of individuals, and the frequency of sexual contact are subject to great variation.

Etiology and Incidence

Etiology is complex and highly variable among individuals. Inherited or subtle constitutional factors probably play a part. The important role of fetal androgens in preparing the brain for later sexual activity suggests that interference with this process may render a person vulnerable to damaging environmental influences during childhood psychosexual development. Parental attitude toward sexual behavior is important. A forbidding puritanical rejection of physical sexuality engenders guilt and shame and inhibits the capacity for enjoying sex.

In forming a secure **sexual identity** (*sense of maleness or femaleness*) and **gender identity** (*sense of masculinity or femininity*—see below) the character of the parents' emotional bond and the relationship that each of them has with the child are important. The parent of the same sex must be a person with whom the child can identify. The opposite-sex parent must engender enough love and trust so that the child later feels comfortable with members of the opposite sex. Relations with parents may be damaged by excessive emotional distance, by punitive behaviors, or by seductiveness and exploitation. Children exposed to hostility, rejection, and cruelty are liable to sexual maladjustment. The child needs to feel accepted and lovable. (Establishing the individual's confidence that he is capable and worthy of being loved for himself is one of the goals of therapy.)

These potentially damaging parent-child relationships can lead to disorders of gender identity such as transsexualism, to one of the paraphilias, possibly to homosexuality (all discussed below), or to dysfunctions in sexual performance (see Ch. 165). For gender identity disorders in children, see Ch. 201. **Dissociation of sexual behavior** also may occur, in which emotional bonds can be formed with others from the individual's own social class or intellectual circle, but physical sexual relationships are possible only with those considered as inferiors, such as prostitutes, with whom the individual has no affinity and no emotional ties. In this type of maladjustment the sexual act with one's spouse is associated with guilt and anxiety, and sexual release is found in relationships or practices in which tender, caring feelings are not aroused.

Paraphilias are far more common among males than females, and this unequal distribution has been found in most cultures studied. Since reproductive competence in the

female is of decisive importance for the species, and less so in the male, biologic reasons for the unequal distribution may exist. Developmentally, males must transfer their infantile identification with their mothers to their fathers during the preschool or oedipal period, from about the age of 3 to about 6, whereas females need not pass through this process of changing identification. The need to "disidentify" during a critical period of psychosexual development creates greater vulnerabilities for the male, hence the enormous preponderance of males affected by the paraphilias.

The pattern of erotic arousal is fairly well developed before puberty; therefore, if something goes awry, the causes for gender or paraphiliac disorders should be sought in the prepubertal years. Three general factors are present: (1) anxiety interferes with normal psychosexual development; (2) a displacement to another pattern of arousal allows the person to avoid the standard pattern of erotic arousal while retaining the capacity for sexual pleasure; and (3) the pattern of sexual arousal often has both symbolic and conditioning facets (eg, the fetish "chosen" symbolizes the object of arousal but may have developed by an accidental association of the fetish with sexual curiosity, desire, and excitement). Whether *all* transsexual or paraphiliac development is created by these psychodynamic processes is still controversial; for many, it is true.

GENDER IDENTITY DISORDERS

DSM-III defines these as *disorders due to feelings of discomfort and inappropriateness about one's anatomic sex*. When sex labeling and rearing are confusing, children will become uncertain about their gender identity. However, even the presence of ambiguous genitalia usually will not affect the child's gender identity if sex labeling and rearing are unambiguous. Transsexuals (see below) often have had gender identity problems as children (see GENDER IDENTITY DISORDER OF CHILDHOOD in Ch. 201).

Transsexualism

A transsexual believes that he is the victim of a biologic accident, cruelly imprisoned within a body incompatible with his real sexual identity. The majority of transsexuals are males who consider themselves to have feminine gender identity and regard their genitalia and masculine features with repugnance. Their primary objective in seeking psychiatric help is not to obtain psychologic treatment but to secure surgery that will give them as close an approximation as possible to a female body. The diagnosis is made only if the disturbance has been continuous (not limited to periods of stress) for at least 2 yr and is not associated with genital ambiguity or genetic abnormality. Differential diagnosis must separate transsexuals from transvestites, cross-dressing homosexuals, and schizophrenics.

In true **male transsexuals** the condition begins in early childhood with indulgence in girls' games, fantasies of being female, avoidance of rough and tumble play and of competitive games, repugnance at the physical changes that attend puberty, and thereafter a quest for a feminine gender identity. Many transsexuals are adept at acquiring skills enabling them to adopt a feminine gender identity. Some patients are satisfied with achieving a more feminine appearance, together with employment and an identity card allowing them to work and live in society as women. Others are not content with changing their social identity but can be helped to achieve a more stable adjustment with small doses of feminizing hormones. Many transsexuals request feminizing operations in spite of the sacrifices entailed. The decision for surgery often raises grave social and ethical problems. Since some follow-up studies have provided evidence that *some* true transsexuals achieve more happy and productive lives with the aid of surgery, it is justified only in highly motivated true transsexuals with stable social and work records. After surgery, the patients need assistance with movement, gesture, and voice production. A few homosexual men, schizophrenics, or those with serious per-

sonality problems request reallocation surgery. The results in these patients are unsatisfactory from both a medical and social viewpoint.

Female transsexuals increasingly appear in medical and psychiatric practice. The patient asks for mastectomy, hysterectomy, and oophorectomy and also wants androgenic hormones to alter her voice and promote a more masculine appearance. She may ask for an artificial phallus to be fashioned by plastic surgery. Stable and effective personalities whose social adaptation in most spheres of their lives has been successful may sometimes be helped to achieve greater satisfaction through surgical help. Patients must be carefully selected, because anatomic results of heroic surgery are often less satisfactory than in the male-to-female procedure.

PARAPHILIAS

Gross impairment in the capacity for affectionate sexual activity between adult human partners (see also under Etiology, above). Many of the paraphilias are rare, and all occur mostly in males. Long-term psychotherapy usually is necessary but is not always successful. It is less useful when coercive, eg, by court order. **Group therapy** for some sex offenders is helpful, as is **anti-androgen treatment** for pedophiliacs, rapists, and lust murderers.

Fetishism

The use of nonliving objects as the preferred exclusive method of producing sexual excitement, usually beginning in adolescence. (The diagnosis of transvestism rather than fetishism should be made when a male is sexually stimulated and gratified by wearing, rather than simply fondling, some feminine garment, usually underclothing.) The fetish may replace sexual activity with a partner or may be integrated into sexual behavior with a partner. When the latter occurs, the fetish is required for erotic arousal. Commonly used fetishes are female undergarments, shoes, and boots—less commonly, parts of the human body such as hair or nails. Minor fetishistic behavior incorporated into heterosexual behavior is not aberrant. More intense fetishistic arousal patterns may generate serious problems in a relationship. When the fetish becomes the sole object of sexual desire, normal sexual relations are avoided.

Transvestism

Dressing by heterosexual males in female clothes, generally beginning in childhood or early adolescence. Transvestites usually achieve a certain amount of sexual excitement, and public display may give them much satisfaction. Despite their deviation, many transvestites have reasonably happy marriages. When their wives are cooperative, men have intercourse in feminine attire. When their wives are not cooperative, anxiety, depression, guilt, and shame associated with the desire to cross-dress are common. Few transvestites seek treatment unless there is marital conflict.

Zoophilia

Sexual excitement produced by the act or fantasy of engaging in sexual activity with animals as the preferred or exclusive method. DSM-III states that the animal may be the object of intercourse or may be trained to sexually excite the human partner by licking or rubbing. The animal is preferred even when other forms of sexual outlet are available. Zoophilia is extremely rare but the desire is intense and persistent; shame, guilt, and social isolation with depression, anxiety, and loneliness may result. This is the only paraphilia, other than sadomasochism, in which females come close to males in incidence.

Pedophilia (see also Ch. 190)

A preference for repetitive sexual activity with prepubertal children, usually beginning in middle age. Arbitrarily, the age difference between the adult with this disorder and the child victim is set at 10 yr or more. When the child is postpubertal, the disorder

frequently is labeled as child molestation rather than pedophilia, but the distinction often is arbitrary. Pedophiliacs prefer opposite-sex children to same-sex children 2:1. Heterosexually oriented males tend to prefer girls 8 to 10 yr; in most cases, the adult is known to the child. Looking or touching seems to be more prevalent than genital contact. With homosexually oriented males, the preferred partner's age is 10 to 13 yr, and acquaintanceship is more casual than in the heterosexually oriented group. Bisexual adult pedophiles choose children under the age of 8.

Sexual offenses against children constitute a significant proportion of reported criminal sexual acts. The recidivism rate for homosexual pedophilia is second only to exhibitionism, and ranges from 13 to 28% of those apprehended—roughly twice the rate of heterosexual pedophilia.

Exhibitionism

As described by DSM-III, *repetitive acts of genital exposure to an unsuspecting stranger for the purpose of producing sexual excitement.* Peak age at onset is in the mid 20s; rarely the first act occurs at either end of a spectrum ranging from preadolescence to middle age. Further sexual contact is almost never sought. About 30% of apprehended male sex offenders are exhibitionists. These persons have the highest recidivism rate of all sex offenders; about 20% get rearrested. The victim usually is a female adult or child. Most exhibitionists are married, but the marriage often is troubled by poor sexual adjustment, including frequent psychosexual dysfunction. A very few cases of exhibitionism in females have been reported—many females have exhibitionistic tendencies (usually not to strangers) sanctioned by society. Folklore has it that "women exhibit everything but the genitals; men, nothing but" (Romano).

Voyeurism

Sexual arousal by looking at unsuspecting females who are naked, disrobing, or engaging in sexual activity. Age at onset usually is early adulthood. Adolescent voyeurism generally is reported leniently; few are arrested. The essential feature is a repetitive seeking-out of these situations. Orgasm usually produced by masturbation may occur during the voyeuristic activity. The voyeur does not initiate further sexual contact. The disorder has to be differentiated from normal sexual curiosity occurring between people who know each other.

Sexual Masochism

Intentional participation in an activity in which the individual is physically harmed or the individual's life is threatened in order to produce sexual excitement, or if the preferred or exclusive mode of producing sexual excitement is to be humiliated, bound, beaten, or otherwise made to suffer. Age at onset commonly is early adulthood. Masochistic fantasy without masochistic behavior is an insufficient basis for the diagnosis of sexual masochism. Fantasies are fairly frequent, whereas masochistic behavior is relatively uncommon. A potentially dangerous form entails various types of physical self-constraint and partial asphyxiation by hanging, which can lead to accidental death. A few cases have been reported in women, but the vast majority are in men.

Sexual Sadism

The inflicting of physical or psychologic suffering on the sexual partner as a method of stimulating sexual excitement and orgasm. Age at onset commonly is early adulthood. Generally there are insistent and persistent fantasies in which sexual excitement is produced as a result of suffering inflicted on the partner, but the fantasies alone without behavior are an insufficient basis for the diagnosis. The diagnosis is warranted if bodily injury is extensive or mortal, whether the partner is consenting or not. Sadism is different from minor manifestations of aggression in normal sexual activity. At the extreme end of the spectrum of intensity for sexual sadism are individuals who require the partner to suffer in order for sexual excitement to occur; such individuals may

brutally rape or torture victims. Even more extreme are lust murderers, in whom sexual excitement is produced by the death of the victim.

The act of rape is essentially aggressive, not sexual, and most rapists are not motivated by sexually sadistic impulses. Approximately 1 rapist in 4 experiences enhanced sexual excitement by sadistic fantasies or behavior.

HOMOSEXUALITY

Homosexuality is no longer regarded as a mental disorder by the American Psychiatric Association. DSM-III lists **ego-dystonic homosexuality** as a special category (see Treatment and Prognosis, below). Society is slowly accepting homosexuality as a sexual variant, but great hostility and prejudice are still widely prevalent.

A transient stage of homosexual conduct in puberty and adolescence is common (1/3 of male adolescents), but almost all persons who experience this, even those who engage in some form of physical contact, later become exclusively heterosexual in their preferences. Approximately 5% of males are exclusively homosexual during their entire lives. A majority report some heterosexual contact that was soon abandoned after initial experiences. Perhaps 33% of male homosexuals and a larger percentage of female homosexuals **(lesbians)** are capable of heterosexual performance and even pleasure, although they are preferentially homosexual. About 20% of homosexual men and 33% of homosexual women marry, but their heterosexual marriages tend to be unstable.

Preferential or exclusive homosexuality has to be distinguished from **situational (facultative) homosexuality,** frequently exhibited by males and females confined for long periods with members of their own sex, as on board ship or in prison. Usual sexual behavior is resumed on release from such environments.

Sexual acts between homosexuals consist of expressions of tenderness, fondling, caressing, and kissing that usually culminate in orgasm—achieved through mutual masturbation, fellatio (taking the penis in the mouth), or anal intercourse. It is uncommon for one partner to adopt an exclusively active or passive role, and most homosexuals participate in the relationship in a variety of ways.

About 25% of male homosexuals are capable of long-lasting partnerships. Casual, shallow contacts with strangers are more frequent; 28% of male homosexuals report having more than 1000 partners. Because of this promiscuity, sexually transmitted diseases are frequent. AIDS (see Ch. 19) is found predominantly among male homosexuals. Only 5% of homosexuals posture effeminately; most are repelled by such behavior. Many homosexuals are emotionally stable, conducting normal lives and considering themselves happy, but the prevalence of depression, psychosomatic illness, and suicide seems higher among homosexuals than in the general population. Some indication exists that, unless they have formed "close-coupled" relationships, homosexuals suffer increasing isolation and rejection as they advance to middle or late life and are rejected by the homosexual culture, which seems to value highly youth and physical attractiveness.

The majority of female homosexuals are capable of "close-coupled" relationships, and engage in casual sexual contacts far less frequently than their male counterparts. Psychiatric illnesses are also less common among lesbians than among male homosexuals. This may be intrinsic or due to more favorable societal reactions, or both.

Etiology

Etiology is not known. Some psychiatrists ascribe the condition to failure of identification with the parent of the same sex and a close-binding seductive relationship with the parent of the opposite sex; however, many children raised in such environments do not exhibit homosexual behavior. Constitutional factors involving hormonal program-

ming of the brain during fetal life may be a significant factor. Some support for this hypothesis is to be found in the higher-than-expected prevalence of homosexual fantasies and behavior in men and women whose mothers received diethylstilbestrol (DES) during pregnancy.

Treatment and Prognosis

If a sustained pattern of homosexual arousal persistently causes distress, and the patient wishes to acquire or increase heterosexual arousal, **ego-dystonic homosexuality** is diagnosed, and treatment is warranted. Therapy is directed toward increasing heterosexual comfort, arousal, and behavior, or toward overcoming the patient's internal homophobia, making it possible for the patient to accept a homosexual orientation.

Unless there is a wish to change sexual orientation, treatment for homosexuality is not indicated. Some homosexuals enter treatment to alleviate distress due to problems with relationships or employment, and develop a motivation for change, but most have no wish to do so. Help in overcoming crises or mitigating emotional distress, and simple psychotherapy to assist individuals in achieving realistic, satisfying adjustment to their social predicament are all that is needed in most cases. For those homosexuals who are strongly motivated to change (and change is possible only if motivation is high), the best therapy draws on both behavioral technics and psychotherapy, including group therapy. Prognosis for change is better with a history of heterosexual behavior and fantasies. Otherwise, limited goals must be set. Endocrine treatments are valueless. The advice of specialists should be sought to plan treatment aimed at altering fundamental attitudes.

---

140. THE NEUROSES

Disorders in which specific, usually ego-alien, and distressing neurotic symptoms occur; ie, anxieties, phobias, obsessions, compulsions, hysterical conversion and dissociative phenomena, and certain symptoms relating to posttraumatic stress.

The neuroses comprise one of the 3 major categories of nonorganic psychiatric disorders, which also include the psychoses and personality (or character) disorders. Neurotic illness is not usually characterized by the major alterations in mental function and severe disturbances in cognitive and perceptual processes (eg, delusions, hallucinations) seen in the **psychoses**; also, the capacity to distinguish between fantasy and reality (reality testing) remains generally intact in neurotic illness, in contrast to its partial or complete absence in the psychoses. The significant aberrations in behavior patterns and personal relationships seen in the **personality disorders** also may occur in neurotic individuals.

Classification

In 1980, the American Psychiatric Association published the 3rd edition of its *Diagnostic and Statistical Manual of Mental Disorders* **(DSM-III)**, which revised the diagnostic classification of many of the mental illnesses. DSM-III omits the diagnostic class of Neuroses, placing anxiety neurosis, phobic neurosis, and obsessive-compulsive neurosis under the general heading of Anxiety Disorders (see TABLE 140–1); and splitting hysterical neurosis between the DSM-III category of Somatoform Disorder (which includes conversion hysteria, hypochondriasis, and somatization disorder), and Dissociative Disorder, which comprises dissociative hysteria (including psychogenic amnesia and fugue, and multiple personality) and depersonalization neurosis. The classification used here (which gives equal weighting to the various neuroses) generally follows that set forth in the latest (9th) edition of the *International Classification of Disease* (ICD-9).

TABLE 140–1. ANXIETY DISORDERS

Disorder	Subcategories
Phobic disorders (phobic neuroses)	Agoraphobia With panic attacks Without panic attacks Social phobia Simple phobia
Anxiety states (anxiety neuroses)	Panic disorder Generalized anxiety disorder Obsessive-compulsive disorder (Obsessive-compulsive neurosis)
Posttraumatic stress disorder	Acute Chronic or delayed
Atypical anxiety disorder	

ANXIETY NEUROSIS

(Generalized Anxiety Disorder; Anxiety Reaction)

A neurotic disorder characterized by chronic, unrealistic anxiety often punctuated by acute attacks of anxiety or panic. Anxiety neurosis afflicts 5% of the population, is characteristically a disorder of young adults, and affects women twice as often as men.

Etiology

Both psychologic and physiologic factors cause anxiety neurosis, and evidence of a genetic influence exists.

Psychologic factors: Emotional stress often precipitates anxiety (eg, threatened or actual changes in personal relationships). The precipitant is less obvious when inner emotional drives (sexual, aggressive, or dependency needs) cause conflict, because psychologic defenses keep them from the individual's conscious awareness. The drives are aroused by environmental events to which the person is especially sensitized, and anxiety represents the individual's fear of losing control of these drives and of his resulting actions.

Physiologically, the symptoms of anxiety (see below) are the direct manifestation of peripheral autonomic nervous system discharge (fight or flight reactions) set in motion by the arousal of frightening fantasies, impulses, and emotions. In the central nervous system, noradrenergic neurotransmitters play a prominent role in the production of anxiety, and recent studies point to the locus ceruleus, with its widespread connecting neural pathways to the rest of the brain, as an important mediating center.

Symptoms and Signs

Anxiety is a symptom in all psychiatric disorders, but it occurs alone or as the primary symptom in anxiety neurosis. **Acute anxiety attacks (panic disorders)** form the cardinal feature of anxiety neurosis and are among the most painful life experiences. They may occur repetitively over a period of time and are self-limited, generally lasting a few minutes to an hour or 2. The patient experiences a subjective sense of terror that arises for no evident reason, and a haunting dread of some nameless, imminent catastrophe, temporarily preventing rational thinking. Of the somatic symptoms integral to anxiety, the most common are cardiorespiratory, with tachycardia, palpitations, occasional premature beats, and precordial pain usually described as sharp or sticking in quality. Trembling, visible as a fine tremor of the outstretched hands, sweating, complaints of "butterflies in the stomach," and generalized motor weakness and dizziness

are common; nausea and occasionally diarrhea occur. The patient may notice a feeling of unreality and loss of contact with people and objects in his environment. A sense of air hunger leading to hyperventilation often is experienced. This can result in a secondary respiratory alkalosis, and varying degrees of muscular stiffness in the extremities and a feeling of pins and needles or numbness around the mouth and in the fingers and toes—**hyperventilation syndrome** (see RESPIRATORY ALKALOSIS in Ch. 84 and the discussion of psychogenic dyspnea in Ch. 31). These secondary symptoms compound the patient's anxiety and add to his frequent conviction that he is about to lose consciousness or die.

Chronic anxiety: Symptoms are similiar to those of acute anxiety attacks, but are less intense and of longer duration, lasting days, weeks, or months. The patient is aware of a generalized tension and apprehension, a tendency to startle easily, an uneasiness and nervousness at work or with people, a vague, nagging uncertainty about the future that may be accompanied by chronic fatigue, headaches, insomnia, and a variety of subacute autonomic symptoms. Although the syndrome is not completely disabling, the patient is chronically uncomfortable in his daily activities and personal relationships, and often finds his capacity for effective work compromised by chronic fatigue and difficulties in concentration.

Diagnosis

Because of the cardiac manifestations, anxiety attacks may be mistaken for myocardial infarction. Similarly, the autonomic symptoms secondary to a pheochromocytoma and the hyperarousal resulting from Graves' disease may imitate the clinical picture of anxiety neurosis. Appropriate physical and laboratory examinations usually establish the proper diagnosis.

Course and Prognosis

Mild anxiety tends to be chronic, punctuated by acute anxiety attacks of varying frequency and intensity. Roughly 1/3 of patients recover, with men having a better prognosis than women. Anxiety symptoms often become less severe and troublesome with middle age.

Treatment

Psychologic measures: Insight psychotherapy (in patients properly selected by the criterion of psychologic-mindedness), aimed at uncovering the unconscious conflicts, may bring about psychologic changes that lead to increased self-knowledge and tolerance of internal drives. **Supportive psychotherapy** may reduce symptoms through reassurance and the relationship with an understanding, sympathetic physician. **Relaxation technics** permit some voluntary control over autonomic functions that diminish hyperactivity. **Meditation** is a specific and often effective form of relaxation. In individuals with a capacity for entering hypnotic trance, **hypnosis** can potentiate the effects of the relaxation technics.

Pharmacologic measures: (See also ANTIANXIETY AGENTS in Ch. 281.) Medications that lower responsiveness to stress are helpful. Minor tranquilizers are often effective in controlling the symptoms of chronic or anticipatory anxiety. Panic attacks may be prevented with therapeutic doses of tricyclic antidepressant medication or monoamine oxidase **(MAO)** inhibitors. Clinical studies show a similar improvement in panic attacks following treatment with alprazolam. The use of β-blocking agents (propanolol, atenolol) has been suggested for the treatment of both panic and chronic anxiety, since in therapeutic doses they do not have the sedative property of the benzodiazepines or the unpleasant side effects of the antidepressant drugs. Clinical studies, however, have not shown any significant advantage of β-blockers over the benzodiazepines and antidepressants, and the latter 2 types of medication are currently generally accepted as the pharmacotherapeutic agents of choice.

Medications generally should be used along with, not as a substitute for, appropriate psychotherapy. (Since benzodiazepines are symptomatic treatment, care must be taken to avoid high dosage and prolonged continuous use that may result in physiologic dependence.)

PHOBIC NEUROSIS

(Phobic Disorders; Phobic Reactions)

A neurotic disorder characterized by the presence of irrational or exaggerated fears of objects, situations, or bodily functions not inherently dangerous or the appropriate source of the anxiety. Anxiety, both acute and chronic, is a prominent feature, but unlike the free-floating anxiety of anxiety neurosis, it is bound to and associated with exposure to specific environmental stimuli. Phobic disorders affect less than 1% of the population, comprise about 5% of neuroses found in patients > 18 yr, and occur more frequently in women.

Etiology

Etiology is in many respects similar to that of neurotic anxiety in general; ie, phobias appear to be associated with an increased family history of anxiety disorders, and the anxiety itself is a fearful reaction to the threatened emergence of forbidden, unconscious drives, a reaction that is expressed in excessive activity of the autonomic nervous system. However, further psychologic mechanisms **(projection, displacement)** focus the anxiety on specific external objects or situations, which then come to represent the underlying, original source of the anxiety. The shifting and binding of the anxiety to the external secondary symbol enable the individual to utilize the further defensive maneuver of **avoidance** of the object in order to control arousal of the painful anxiety. Choice of the phobic symbol is often determined by a chance exposure to the object at a time when the anxiety over a threatening inner impulse first appeared. The phobic object, in other words, becomes a conditioned stimulus, and the phobic neurosis is, in effect, a learned response.

Symptoms and Signs

The very thought of the phobic object is sufficient to induce anxiety, and as the patient comes closer in reality to the phobic stimulus, the anxiety mounts to an intensity reaching panic. As a result, the patient protects himself from experiencing the anxiety by avoiding the phobic stimulus, which often leads to a disabling constriction in his daily life and capacity for normal functioning. In some phobic individuals, **counterphobic behavior** develops (*the active seeking out of exposure to phobic, often dangerous situations*; eg, the individual with a fear of heights who becomes an alpine rock climber).

Agoraphobia (*a fear of open, public places or of situations where crowds are to be found*) is the most common (60%) of the phobic disorders. The individual's activities are severely restricted; in the extreme he cannot leave the security of his home. Agoraphobia often begins with the sudden onset of a panic attack in some public place; subsequently, anticipatory anxiety that the attack will recur causes the individual to remain at home to avoid a reemergence of the painful affect. Frequently, the agoraphobic patient can face the phobic situation without undue discomfort if in the company of someone with whom he has a close relationship—the so-called **obligatory companion.**

Phobias of objects (simple phobias) are *irrational fears of objects or situations other than those felt in agoraphobia or social phobias.* Simple phobias are commonly seen as transitory phenomena during early childhood (eg, fear of the darkness or of animals). Adults also may develop specific, localized neurotic fears (eg, dogs, insects; closed spaces—**claustrophobia;** or heights—**acrophobia).** If the objects are uncommon or easily avoided, no serious disability results. However, great inconvenience may occur; eg, in a businessman with a phobia of planes whose work requires frequent air travel.

Phobias of function (social phobias), in which *anxiety is aroused by the presence of others and by the irrational fear of embarrassing or humiliating oneself in public*, are less common than the other types. Most frequent manifestations are a fear of blushing, **erythrophobia** (the victim shuns social situations), and a fear of eating (public dining is avoided).

Diagnosis

The sudden outbreak of severe phobias may herald the onset of a schizophrenic psychosis or occasionally may be seen in patients with a chronic schizophrenic disorder. The course of the latter illness and the presence of thought disorder and other psychotic features (hallucinations, delusions) suggest a psychosis. Phobic patients sometimes become depressed because of their failure to overcome their phobic avoidance, but this is secondary to the phobic neurosis itself and disappears when the phobia is resolved.

Course and Prognosis

Phobic disorders usually begin in early adulthood and have chronic courses of exacerbations and remissions. Agoraphobia is not only severely disabling but is the least likely of the phobic disorders to manifest significant remissions. Spontaneous remission of phobic neurosis is less likely in patients steadily symptomatic for over a year.

Treatment

Psychotherapy: Insight psychotherapy may be effective. However, despite significant changes in the patient's psychologic functioning and structure, the phobic symptoms may persist and require more active technics focused specifically on bringing about their removal; eg, **behavior therapy.** These technics decondition the patient to the phobic stimulus by requiring him to confront the stimulus while using relaxation technics (including hypnosis) to combat the anxiety aroused by the stimulus (reciprocal inhibition). **Flooding** is an extreme behavioral procedure based on the experimental observation that the fear aroused in animals confronted by a frightening conditioned stimulus tends to dissipate if the animal is not allowed to escape. Clinical flooding technics require patients to imagine or actually confront the anxiety-provoking situation and to continue their exposure until the resulting intense anxiety abates. Since flooding is a highly painful procedure and, in clinical trials, generally produces no better therapeutic results than desensitization, it is not commonly used by behavior therapists.

Pharmacotherapy: (See also ANTIANXIETY AGENTS in Ch. 281.) Minor tranquilizers are helpful in reducing the intensity of the anticipatory anxiety, enabling the patient better to face the phobic stimulus and work toward complete desensitization. Panic attacks may be effectively controlled by tricyclic antidepressants, MAO inhibitors, and alprazolam. The use of β-blockers in the treatment of panic (see treatment of ANXIETY NEUROSIS, above) has not as yet been generally adopted in modern clinical practice.

OBSESSIVE-COMPULSIVE NEUROSIS

(Obsessive-Compulsive Disorder; Obsessional Neurosis)

A neurotic disorder characterized by the presence of recurrent ideas and fantasies ***(obsessions)*** *and repetitive impulses or actions* ***(compulsions)*** *that the patient recognizes as morbid and toward which he feels a strong inner resistance.*

Anxiety is a central feature, but in contrast to the phobias (where the patient is anxious in the face of external dangers of which he perceives himself to be the passive victim), the anxiety arises in response to internally derived thoughts and urges that the patient fears he may actively carry out despite his wishes not to. Obsessive-compulsive patients comprise less than 5% of those with neurotic disorders, and about 0.05% of the population at large. The neurosis affects men and women equally and tends to be found in individuals from upper socioeconomic levels and with higher intelligence.

Etiology

There is some evidence of a higher incidence in the families of obsessive-compulsive patients than in control populations.

Psychodynamic theory: The obsession is the ideational component of an underlying, forbidden impulse, most commonly aggressive in quality, that emerges into consciousness. Through the defense mechanism of **isolation,** the affective component of the drive is separated from the ideational content, so that the individual experiences only an insistent thought, unaccompanied by any awareness of a wish to realize the idea or that it stems from a hidden impulse. Despite the defense of isolation, the idea is too close to the forbidden drive. Therefore, the idea becomes the source of anxiety and motivates the further defensive maneuver of **undoing,** in the form of a secondary magical compulsive act.

Learning theory: An originally neutral thought becomes capable of arousing anxiety through its association with an unconditioned anxiety-provoking stimulus. When a subsequent action reduces that anxiety, the act becomes fixed as a compulsive ritual and a stable, but nonadaptive, learned psychologic structure is created.

Symptoms and Signs

Obsessions: Ideas, words, and images, usually disconnected and unrelated to what the individual is doing, force themselves on his attention with a power and insistence that he cannot resist. They are often colored by an aggressive, sexual, or scatologic quality that the individual perceives as totally alien to himself as a person. The patient frequently is convinced that he has done something harmful or antisocial, and feels considerable concern and anxiety. Despite this, he recognizes that the ideas are untrue and nonsensical, but at the same time spends considerable energy trying to resist them and banish them from his consciousness. His efforts may be momentarily successful; but inevitably the ideas return again moments later, and the struggle is renewed.

Compulsions and compulsive acts: A compulsion has the same autonomous characteristics as an obsession, but rather than being merely an idea or image, it is an overwhelming urge to do something aggressive, disgraceful, or obscene. As with the obsessions, the patient experiences anxiety, recognizes the absurdity of the impulse, and resists putting it into action. Not infrequently, however, he does in fact act on the compulsive urge and indulges in a repetitive behavioral pattern in the form of compulsive acts or rituals. These are often found to be secondary to a primary obsessional idea and serve the function of combating or neutralizing its harmful qualities. A young man, for example, had the insistent thought every time he turned off an electric light: "My father will die" (obsession). To quell the anxiety associated with that thought, he would feel compelled to touch the light switch again and say to himself, "I take back that thought" (compulsion). The quality of **magical thinking** characterizes both obsessions and compulsions. Neither has anything to do with the real, physical world of cause and effect—a fact of which the patient is aware.

Diagnosis

The often bizarre quality of obsessive-compulsive ideas and rituals may at times resemble the similar bizarreness of schizophrenic thinking, but in the obsessional patient reality testing is intact.

Course and Prognosis

Onset of symptoms occurs during early adolescence in 10 to 15% of patients. The disorder tends to run a chronic, remitting course, with symptomatic periods generally lasting < 1 yr before a remission brings relief. With treatment, about 25% of patients improve markedly; the rest are partially improved or unchanged. Prognosis is better for those patients who begin treatment early.

Treatment

Properly selected patients may respond to **insight psychotherapy** with disappearance of symptoms, but in many patients the symptoms are stubbornly resistant. **Supportive therapy,** with an emphasis on reassurance and encouragement to activity, may provide sufficient relief to enable patients to perform daily activities fairly comfortably. **Behavioral technics,** especially those aimed at **flooding** (see PHOBIC NEUROSIS, Treatment, above) the patient with anxiety by forcibly preventing him from carrying out compulsive rituals, have been reported to be successful, but are still experimental.

Pharmacotherapy: (See ANTIANXIETY AGENTS in Ch. 281.) The recent literature contains isolated reports of dramatic relief from obsessions and compulsive rituals following the administration of tricyclic antidepressants and MAO inhibitors, but the appraisal of the general usefulness of these drugs must await controlled clinical studies. When depression is significantly present, its successful treatment with antidepressant medication may also be accompanied by the disappearance of the obsessive-compulsive symptoms.

POSTTRAUMATIC STRESS DISORDER

A neurotic disorder produced by exposure to an overwhelming environmental stress and characterized by recurrent episodes of reexperiencing the traumatic event, numbing of emotional responsiveness, and a dysphoric general hyperarousal. The pathogenic effects of exposure to emotionally traumatic stress have long been recognized, but the severity and prevalence of such reactions in returning Vietnam war veterans has forced these reactions into prominence and has led to this DSM-III diagnostic category. The occurrence of the disorder is not accurately known, although figures as high as 80% have been reported in the survivors of some major civilian disasters.

Etiology

The etiologic *sine qua non* of the disorder is exposure to an overwhelming environmental stress. Since not every individual responds to such stress with a posttraumatic stress syndrome, it is evident that a variety of factors in clinical combination are required to produce the pathologic state. These include (1) the suddenness and unexpectedness of the stress, as in major fires, explosions, and airplane crashes, or in natural disasters like floods, earthquakes, and tornadoes; (2) the bloody brutality and horror of events associated with active armed combat or terrorist attacks; (3) the more prolonged and chronic stress of exposure to inhumane treatment such as occurs in POW and concentration camps, with the frequently associated torture and atrocities; (4) the psychologic and constitutional strengths and weaknesses of the victim; (5) concurrent bodily injury (especially of the head) suffered by the victim; and (6) the nature and availability of social supports.

Symptoms and Signs

A central feature is the reexperiencing of the trauma. This may occur in the form of intrusive, uncontrollable waking recollections of nightmares reproducing the stressful events, or of dissociated states of consciousness in which the patient appears vividly to relive the traumatic experience as if it were actually taking place. These more discrete episodes occur against a background of chronic anxiety, hyperalertness, and insomnia, often accompanied by difficulty in concentrating or impairment of memory. Some individuals develop phobic reactions to situations that recall memories of the events, and forced exposure to such situations may cause an exacerbation of acute symptoms and precipitate a dissociative, fugue-like reproduction of the experience itself. Not infrequently patients are emotionally labile, irritable, restless, and tremulous, and on occasion may manifest explosive outbursts of violent behavior. Many patients resort to

alcohol or drug abuse in an apparent attempt to diminish their painful inner state of hyperarousal. Most patients, furthermore, complain of a numbing of their responsiveness to people, objects, and events in the world around them. They lose interest in their usual pursuits, feel emotionally dead and unreal, and experience detachment and estrangement from others.

Diagnosis

Posttraumatic stress disorder is to be differentiated from depressive, anxiety, and phobic disorders. Although the posttraumatic syndrome may include anxious, depressive, and phobic symptoms, these do not dominate the clinical picture and are clearly secondary to the trauma. A careful neurologic examination should be part of the evaluation of every patient with suspected posttraumatic stress disorder in order to rule out the presence of brain lesions underlying the changes in memory and the difficulty in concentration.

Course and Prognosis

Many patients experience the outbreak of symptoms a few days to a few weeks after the trauma, but onset also may be delayed for many months. The rapidly appearing acute form is often self-limited, the symptoms disappearing spontaneously within 6 mo. In others the disorder runs a chronic course, lasting months or years and frequently causing significant disability. In patients with a delayed onset or chronic symptoms the prognosis is generally poor, and recovery may be compromised by the secondary gain associated with receiving compensation for their trauma.

Treatment

Treatment is largely aimed at relieving the prominent hyperarousal and anxiety symptoms. Behavioral desensitization and relaxation technics are particularly helpful, and where dissociative mechanisms underlie symptom formation, psychotherapy aimed at producing catharsis, abreaction, and insight may be useful. Antianxiety and antidepressant medications may be used adjunctively when necessary, but it should be remembered that this group of patients is particularly prone to develop dependency on drugs, so that prolonged pharmacotherapy generally is contraindicated.

HYSTERICAL NEUROSIS

(Conversion Reaction; Conversion Disorder; Dissociative Reaction; Dissociative Disorder)

A neurotic disorder characterized by a wide variety of somatic and mental symptoms resulting from dissociation, typically beginning during adolescence or early adulthood and occurring more commonly in women than men. Since the concept of hysteria as a disease is over 2000 yr old, its limits as a disorder have become blurred by a variety of definitions. This chapter restricts discussion to those phenomena classified as **conversion and dissociative disorders of consciousness,** which have a common basis in the mental phenomenon of dissociation.

Etiology

The concept of **dissociation,** *a process whereby specific internal mental contents (memories, ideas, feelings, perceptions) are lost to conscious awareness and become unavailable to voluntary recall,* is central to an understanding of the genesis of hysterical symptoms. Though unconscious, these mental contents can be recovered under special circumstances (eg, in dreams or a hypnotic trance). Furthermore, they are able to affect the individual's awareness and behavior in a variety of ways. For example, the dissociation and loss from consciousness of memories of motor patterns lead to paralysis; the emergence of a fragment of a dissociated visual memory may produce an ego-alien visual hallucination; the emergence of a complex of mental associations forming

a dissociated personality may effect a complete change in the individual's behavior. All phenomena of conversion and dissociative hysteria may be viewed as the effects of either the dissociation itself or of the eruption into consciousness of portions of the dissociated mental contents of varying degrees of complexity. Proneness to dissociation may in part be genetic.

Two factors concerning dissociation should be noted: (1) It is closely correlated with hypnotizability, and individuals prone to spontaneous dissociation rate high on hypnotizability scales. (2) It works as a psychologic defense; ie, it provides a mechanism for banishing anxiety-provoking, painful, unpleasant mental contents from consciousness. However, the individual becomes subject to the unconscious substitution of hysterical symptoms.

Symptoms and Signs

Conversion symptoms: Almost any organ disease symptom can be simulated on an hysterical basis; eg, symptoms mimicking the illness of a deceased relative. A variety of **sensorimotor symptoms** have been considered to be specific to and characteristic of hysterical neurosis. (Conversion symptoms are also commonly seen in nonpsychiatric practice in patients who do *not* have classical hysterical neurosis; see in PSYCHOSOMATIC MEDICINE, Ch. 135.) Weakness and paralysis of muscular groups are common; spasms and abnormal movements, less frequent. The motor disturbances are usually accompanied by altered sensibility, especially those involving touch, pain, temperature, and position sense. Especially characteristic are the "glove" and "stocking" distribution of the motor and sensory disturbances when these affect the limbs; ie, the distribution is determined by the body-image concept of a functional arm and leg rather than the dermatome innervation of the area affected. Another common distribution is complete hemianesthesia, which extends exactly to the midline of the body fore and aft. Less frequently, special senses and functions may be affected, such as in hysterical blindness, deafness, and aphonia; both visual and auditory hallucinations may occur.

Dissociative phenomena: A variety of altered states of consciousness may result from the dissociative process. In **somnambulism** (see also Ch. 122), the patient appears to be out of contact with his environment, is seemingly unresponsive to external stimuli, and in many cases appears to be living out a vivid, hallucinated drama, often the memory of some past emotionally traumatic event. In **amnesia,** the most common form of dissociative hysteria, the patient typically has a complete loss of memory for all past events covering a period of several hours to several weeks. **Anterograde amnesia** may occur, wherein the amnesia covers the memory of events as they are experienced, the patient forgetting continuously from moment to moment what he has just been thinking, feeling, and doing. For a discussion of amnesia as a functional syndrome in organic cerebral disease, see Ch. 118.

Far less common but more dramatic and eye-catching are the conditions of fugue states and multiple personalities. Central to both is a loss of personal identity. Typically, in a **fugue state** the individual suddenly loses all recollection of his past life and any awareness of who he is. He disappears from his usual haunts, leaving family and job, and traveling far from home, begins new work with a new identity, quite unaware of any change in his existence or life. Suddenly after a matter of days to weeks, he "comes to." Totally amnesic for the period of the fugue, he recaptures his former identity and, greatly distressed, wonders how he came to be in such strange surroundings. In the **multiple personality** a similar sudden change of identity occurs without, however, any wandering from home and with a frequent, unpredictable alternation between personalities. Most commonly 2 such personalities exist: the primary, or A personality, often afflicted with disabling neurotic symptoms and with no awareness of the existence of the B, or secondary personality. The latter, on the contrary, is fully

aware of all the thoughts and activities of A, and whereas A is chronically depressed and sick, B is healthy, vivacious, and scornful of the restricted life and personality that characterize A's existence.

Diagnosis

The sensorimotor symptoms of hysteria are distinguished from neurologic disease by the absence of pathologic neurologic signs, by recognition of precipitating psychosocial stress and conflict, and by the specific characteristics of the distribution of hysterical motor and sensory disturbances. Dissociative disorders of consciousness are differentiated from those caused by gross brain disease by the absence of positive indications of the latter (eg, EEG changes, abnormal CT scan, pathognomonic changes in tests of cognitive functions). When the hysterical symptoms imitate those of medical diseases, the diagnosis is often more difficult. It is best established by the absence of findings pointing to disorders in organ functions and by the positive stigmas of hysteria, such as high hypnotizability, a previous history of clear-cut conversion or dissociative symptoms, and evidence that the symptoms represent a symbolic expression and resolution of psychologic conflicts.

Course and Prognosis

The paucity of studies on the natural history of hysteria precludes definite statements about its course and prognosis. Clinical experience suggests that it is a chronic illness. While patients may recover from specific symptoms, these are frequently replaced by others, especially during periods of emotional tension and stress, as a result of the propensity for dissociation.

Treatment

Psychoanalytic treatment, once thought to be specific for hysterical symptoms, is effective in a small number of hysterical patients who are capable of using the insights gained by psychoanalytic exploration. For others, family therapy, environmental manipulation (eg, job changes, homemaking assistance), reassurance, and a supportive physician relationship may be helpful. Hypnosis can remove specific symptoms, but a substitute symptom often arises. However, in patients with amnesia, hypnosis can be an effective tool to bring repressed ideas and feelings into consciousness, enabling the patient to face and resolve them more directly as the first step in the therapeutic process. Continued psychotherapeutic work is necessary to help the patient come to a more healthy and adaptive resolution of his problem.

SOMATIZATION DISORDER
(Briquet's Syndrome)

A neurotic illness characterized by the presence of multiple somatic symptoms, including those seen in classical conversion hysteria. Patients usually consult a physician other than a psychiatrist. Formerly considered a form of hysteria and viewed by many as a hysterical personality disorder (see Narcissistic Personalities in Ch. 137), somatization disorder has been allocated a diagnosis of its own as a neurosis in DSM-III on the basis of phenomenologic clinical research. The disorder begins in adolescence or early adulthood, occurs predominantly in women (1 to 2% of the female population), and tends to be associated with sociopathy and alcoholism in male relatives.

Etiology

Etiology is not known, although the disorder often runs in families, and it is clear that the narcissistic personality structure of these patients (ie, their marked dependency needs and exaggerated rage when frustrated) is involved in their somatic complaints. The symptoms are a somatized message expressing a desperate plea for help and attention, and their intensity and persistence reflect the extreme degree of the wish to be cared for in every aspect of the patient's life.

Symptoms and Signs

Central to the disorder is the presence of multiple, vague somatic complaints that may be referable to any part of the body but most commonly take the form of headaches, nausea and vomiting, abdominal pain, bowel difficulties, dysmenorrhea, fatigue, syncope, dyspareunia, and sexual frigidity. Anxiety and depression are common accompaniments. The somatization appears to be part of a personality disorder, which has other characteristics. In their relationship with the doctor and others, patients are seen to be dramatic and emotional in presenting their complaints, and may be openly seductive and exhibitionistic. As the relationship develops, a marked, insatiable dependency emerges. Patients increasingly demand help and emotional support, may exhibit outbursts of rage when they feel that their needs are not gratified, and often attempt to manipulate others by threatening or attempting suicide. Often dissatisfied with their care, they go from doctor to doctor.

Diagnosis

Differentiation from hypochondriacal neurosis is discussed under that subchapter, below. Somatization disorder is distinguished from anxiety neurosis, hysterical neurosis, and depression by the predominance, multiplicity, and persistence of somatic complaints, the absence of the biologic signs and symptoms characterizing endogenous depression, and the gestural, manipulative nature of the suicidal behavior. The most difficult challenge lies in assessing the presence or absence of physical disease. Since such patients may develop concurrent physical illnesses, appropriate physical and laboratory examinations should be carried out during the initial clinical evaluation or whenever a significant shift occurs in the symptomatic picture.

Course and Prognosis

The disorder tends to run a fluctuating but chronic course. Complete relief of symptoms is rare, and unnecessary examinations and medical and surgical procedures may add to the patient's complaints or dysfunction. In some patients, depression becomes more prominent after many years, the frequent references and gestures relating to suicide become more ominous, and suicide may be carried out.

Treatment

Treatment usually is extraordinarily difficult, requiring tact and patience. The physician must walk a narrow clinical line between avoiding unnecessary diagnostic procedures and being alert to the possibility of developing physical disease. Medications do not help significantly, and attempts to provide insight with specific psychotherapeutic technics usually fail. The patient needs a calm, firm, supporting relationship with a physician who provides reassurance and sets effective, appropriate limits to the patient's histrionically exaggerated behavior and demands.

HYPOCHONDRIACAL NEUROSIS

(Hypochondriasis; Atypical Somatoform Disorder)

A neurotic disorder characterized by a preoccupation with bodily functions and a morbid fear that one is suffering from serious disease. The peak incidence of onset is in the 30s in men, the 40s in women.

Etiology

Etiology is unknown, but some clinical evidence suggests that hypochondriasis, like somatization disorder, is related to a narcissistic character organization marked by excessive concern with self and with the gratification of dependency needs.

Symptoms and Signs

The hypochondriacal patient complains of symptoms in a wide variety of body parts, most commonly in the abdominal viscera, chest, head, and neck. The specific

symptom may be based on a heightened awareness of bodily sensation (heartbeat, peristaltic action) or minor disorders of function such as mild, localized pain or discomfort. The complaints often are described in minute, specific detail with respect to location, quality, and duration, but follow no pattern recognizable as organic dysfunction, and are usually not associated with abnormal physical findings. Although the symptoms described by the patient may be odd or bizarre, in *hypochondriasis,* as contrasted with hypochondriacal symptoms seen in psychotic disorders, they are not delusional in quality, and the patient exhibits no other signs of psychosis.

Diagnosis

Although hypochondriasis shares with somatization disorder a central complaint of somatic symptoms, the disorders differ in that hypochondriacal neurosis begins at a later age and the somatic complaints of the hypochondriac are richly detailed and sharply localized. Hypochondriacal symptoms are frequently associated with endogenous depressions, are then usually delusional in quality, and disappear when the affective disorder is relieved.

Course, Prognosis, and Treatment

The course is chronic, fluctuating in some, steady in others. Only a very small proportion of patients (perhaps 5%) recover permanently. The presence of hypochondriacal complaints in association with depression presages a poor prognosis for recovery from the basic affective illness.

Hypochondriasis is notoriously resistant to all forms of treatment, and all such measures are only palliative. Patients may gain some relief from a sympathetic, supportive relationship with a physician, and it is often helpful to work with the patient's family, giving them an awareness of the nature and course of the disorder so that they can provide a supportive home environment.

---

141. MOOD DISORDERS

(Affective Disorders)

Psychopathologic states in which a disturbance of mood is either a primary determinant or constitutes the core manifestation. The term **affective disorder,** more commonly used in English-speaking countries, is being replaced by the internationally preferred and more accurate **mood disorder.** These conditions, especially the depressive forms, are heterogeneous and common in both psychiatry and general medicine.

Terminology and Classification

Moods are sustained emotions; **affects,** more short-lived expressions. Anxiety, anger, depression, and elation—the most commonly encountered emotions in clinical psychiatry—occur in many psychiatric disorders; depression and elation predominate in mood disorders.

Normal affects (sadness, grief, and joy) are part of the fabric of everyday life and should be differentiated from the more sustained morbid states of mood disorder. Sadness, or "normal" depression is a universal human response to defeat, disappointment, or other adverse situations; the response may be adaptive by permitting withdrawal to conserve inner resources. Transient depressive periods also occur as reactions to certain holidays or significant anniversaries, as well as during the premenstrual phase and the first week postpartum. Such **holiday blues, anniversary reactions, premenstrual depressions,** and **maternity blues** are not in themselves psychopathologic, but those predisposed to mood disorder may break down during these times.

Grief (*bereavement reaction*), the prototype of **reactive depression**, also manifests with anxiety symptoms such as initial insomnia, agitation, and autonomic nervous system hyperactivity. These reactions occur in response to significant separations and losses; eg, death, marital separation, romantic disappointment, leaving familiar environments, or forced emigration. Like other types of adversity, bereavement and loss seem not to cause clinical depression, except for those predisposed to mood disorder.

Elation, although not studied systematically, is popularly linked to success and achievement. However, "paradoxical depressions" also may follow such positive events, possibly because of the associated increased responsibilities. Elation is sometimes conceptualized psychodynamically as a defense against depression or as a denial of the pain of loss; eg, the rare form of bereavement reaction where elated hyperactivitiy may completely replace the expected grief. The concept of "flight into health" is invoked to explain the brief lucid and energetic periods encountered in dying patients or in those who need to take superhuman action in the face of unusual life duress. Whether such reactions form the prelude to clinical mania in predisposed individuals is speculative.

Morbid mood states (mood disorders) occur when sadness or elation is overly intense and continues beyond the expected impact of a stressful life event. The morbid mood may also arise "endogenously"; ie, without apparent life stress. Furthermore, in different subtypes of mood disorder signs and symptoms cluster into discrete full or major syndromal episodes sustained for at least 15 days—typically longer—or pursue a course of low-grade intermittent chronicity. Tendency for recurrence (especially on a periodic or seasonal basis) and familial affective loading are other characteristics that set apart morbid mood states from normal emotional reactions.

It is clinically useful to distinguish between **bipolar** (having depressive and elevated periods) and **unipolar** (depressions only) mood disorders. Bipolar disorder has younger age of onset and shorter **cycles** (*time from onset of one episode to that of the next*)—hence higher episode frequency and higher rates of disruption in developmental and social functioning. These prognostic features are particularly accentuated in **rapid-cycling** illness (*increased frequency of mood cycles of shorter duration, usually defined as ≥ 4 episodes/yr*).

Bipolar mood disorder *commonly begins with depression and is characterized by at least one elevated period sometime during the course of the illness.* In **Bipolar I disorder,** full-blown manic—and typically major depressive—episodes alternate with each other. In **Bipolar II disorder,** major depressive episodes alternate with hypomanic (ie, mild, non-psychotic, excited) periods of short duration. These hypomanic periods may be adaptive and sometimes associated with "supernormal" social functioning (typically, not leading to clinical referral) and often require expert evaluation for proper clinical diagnosis. Precise subtyping is crucial, because a mistaken diagnosis of unipolar illness and chronic treatment with tricyclic antidepressants may lead to rapid-cycling. In **cyclothymic disorder,** both elevated and depressive periods occur on a lower plane of severity, lasting from a few days to 2 wk, with an intermittently irregular course. Cyclothymia often is the precursor of bipolar I and II disorders, though it may continue as a lifelong trait without superimposed major episodes.

Unipolar mood disorder (major depressive disorder) occurs as *syndromal episodes of depression that are typically recurrent, but in 1/3 of cases occur once in a lifetime.* The term **melancholia** is reserved for *the most typical forms of major depressive disorder with such manifestations as marked agitation, weight loss, pathologic guilt, middle or early morning insomnia, diurnal variation in mood and activity with a nadir in the morning, and loss of the capacity to experience pleasure.* Melancholia requires somatic therapies; eg, showing dramatic response to tricyclic antidepressants **(TCAs)** and/or electroconvulsive therapy **(ECT).** Major unipolar illness is characteristically episodic with relatively

TABLE 141–1. PREDICTORS OF BIPOLAR OUTCOME IN DEPRESSION

Age <25	Psychotic depression
Acute onset	Hypomania upon antidepressant therapy
Postpartum onset	Family history of bipolar disorder
Severe psychomotor retardation and hypersomnia	Loaded affective pedigrees in 3 generations

asymptomatic phases between episodes; residual chronicity which occurs in 15 to 20% of cases is usually of late onset (ie, after age 50). **Atypical depressive disorder** is different in that *its course tends to fluctuate with significant mixtures of phobic anxious features and "reverse vegetative signs" such as hyperphagia, evening worsening, initial insomnia, and morning hypersomnolence.* Although atypical depression is not an established nosologic entity, it is believed by some authorities to predict good response to monoamine oxidase inhibitors **(MAOIs). Dysthymic disorder** is *intermittent or chronic low-grade depression of insidious early onset, typically < 21 yr*; superimposed major episodes commonly occur, but return to the low-grade baseline is generally the rule.

One out of 5 patients with first attacks of depression eventually become bipolar. TABLE 141–1 summarizes features that predict which depressive persons are at risk for bipolar transformation over time; 90% of all switches from unipolar to bipolar occur within a decade from the onset of clinically identifiable depressive manifestations.

Incidence and Epidemiology

Although about 1 of every 4 individuals experiences some form of affective disturbance, the lifetime risk for clinically significant mood disorders is probably ≤ 15% (12% in men and 18% in women). The rates are higher in women for the milder forms of depression, and nearly even in manic-depression. Bipolar disorders usually begin in the teens, 20s, and 30s. Unipolar conditions are more uniformly distributed throughout the life span and, on the average, begin a decade later than bipolar.

As the most prevalent psychiatric condition, depression varies from about 25% in public mental institutions to almost 40% in outpatient psychiatric clinics, reaching 50% in private psychiatric facilities, and up to 70% of all psychiatric diagnoses in nonpsychiatric medical practice. Although sadness and transient depressive affect are universal human experiences, clinical depression is limited to those individuals with a special vulnerability.

Culture, social class, and race have not been shown to make significant differential contributions to the overall rates of mood disorders. However, sociocultural factors modify the clinical manifestations; eg, somatic complaints, worry, tension, and irritability are more common in the lower socioeconomic classes; guilty ruminations and self-reproach are more characteristic of depressions in Anglo-Saxon cultures; and in some Mediterranean and African countries, as well as in American blacks, mania tends to manifest itself more floridly.

Etiology and Pathogenesis

The syndromes of depression and mania, like many medical conditions (eg, congestive heart failure) represent the final common pathways of various processes.

Secondary affective states are chronologically superimposed on preexisting nonaffective disorders and are often understandable developments from them—somatically (see TABLE 141–2), psychologically, or via both mechanisms. Some, such as myxedema depression, are largely attributable to physiochemical factors and are considered "symptomatic" depressions. Others, such as the chronic depressive states that accompany seriously debilitating cardiopulmonary diseases, are explained as depressive "re-

TABLE 141–2. COMMON CAUSES OF SYMPTOMATIC DEPRESSIONS AND ELATIONS

Type of Cause	*Depressions*	*Elations*
Pharmacologic	Steroidal contraceptives Reserpine; α-methyldopa Anticholine-esterase insecticides Amphetamine withdrawal Cimetidine; indomethacin Phenothiazines Thallium; mercury Cycloserine Vincristine; vinblastine	Corticosteroids Levodopa; bromocriptine Cocaine Amphetamines; methylphenidate Most heterocyclic antidepressants Monoamine oxidase inhibitors
Infectious	General paresis (tertiary syphilis) Influenza; viral pneumonia Viral hepatitis; infectious mononucleosis TB	General paresis (tertiary syphilis) Influenza St. Louis encephalitis
Endocrine	Hypo- and hyperthyroidism Hyperparathyroidism Cushing's disease Addison's disease	Hyperthyroidism
Collagen	SLE RA	SLE Rheumatic chorea
Neurologic	Multiple sclerosis Parkinson's disease Head trauma Complex partial seizures (temporal lobe) Cerebral tumors Stroke Dementing diseases in early stages Sleep apnea	Multiple sclerosis Huntington's chorea Head trauma Complex partial seizures (temporal lobe) Diencephalic and 3rd ventricle tumors Stroke
Nutritional	Pellagra Vitamin B_{12} deficiency	
Neoplastic	Cancer of the head of the pancreas Disseminated carcinomatosis	

action" to the limitations imposed by the underlying condition. More commonly both causes are operative; eg, in the schizophrenics' depression which could stem from high doses of depressant neuroleptics, as well as from the profound sense of demoralization imposed by a malignant mental disorder; or in the depressive psychosis of Cushing's disease, where the changes in body image in a female afflicted with acne, hirsutism, obesity, striae, etc are as relevant as the endocrine impact on the brain. Interestingly, excessive endogenous production of corticosteroids results in depression, while exogenous administration of corticosteroids is more likely to cause euphoria; fortunately, corticosteroids are often given to very sick individuals where some degree of flight into health is both expected and desirable.

Psychiatric conditions at high risk for depression include anxiety disorders, alcoholism and other substance use disorders, schizophrenic disorders, antisocial personality and somatization disorder, and ego-dystonic homosexuality. Bipolar disorder is virtually never seen as a complication of another psychiatric condition; if alcohol and

substance abuse chronologically precede a bipolar disorder, they are most likely prodromal manifestations of mood swings that the patient has attempted to self-treat with available substances.

In affective states associated with nonaffective disorders, incomplete syndromes of depression and mania are common, as well as admixtures with paranoia, anxiety, delirium, or dementia. When a full-blown affective syndrome develops in the setting of a medical condition, etiologic factors important in the primary mood disorders are probably operative. For instance, the so-called "reserpine depression" is most commonly a pseudodepression; it is partly attributable to the sedative side effects of the drug and is fully reversible upon its discontinuation. The less frequently occurring irreversible reserpine depressions are seen predominantly in predisposed individuals with family or personal history of mood disorder. This example highlights the arbitrary nature of the primary-secondary distinction and suggests a continuum of pathogenesis for all affective states. However, in clinical practice the dichotomy is useful to facilitate therapy aimed at reversible causes.

Primary mood disorders arise in the absence of factors leading to secondary affective states. The exact pathogenetic mechanisms are unclear, but an interaction between several contributory causes is most likely.

Heredity is an established predisposing factor, although sporadic (nonfamilial) forms occur. Unipolar depressions are hypothesized to be transmitted polygenically, and bipolar disorders by single dominant genes (either X-linked or autosomal). Alternatively, either disorders may lie on a polygenic continuum of severity. The metabolic end results appear to reflect some form of dysregulation in limbic-diencephalic neurotransmission, possibly at the level of postsynaptic receptors, but no direct evidence exists for neurotransmitter abnormality in mood disorders. However, indirect neurophysiologic, -pharmacologic, and -endocrine evidence implicates such abnormalities; eg, blunted growth hormone response to the α_2-agonist clonidine, shortened rapid eye movement (REM) latency, arecoline REM-induction, augmented melatonin suppression by light, abnormal dexamethasone suppression test **(DST)** results, and blunted thyroid-stimulating hormone **(TSH)** response to thyrotropin **(TRH).** Cumulatively, such findings support the notion of dysregulation in cholinergic and catecholaminergic neurotransmission. Indirect evidence also is emerging for serotonergic dysregulation as measured by decreased serotonin uptake by platelets in depression and decreased 5-hydroxy-indoleacetic acid **(5-HIAA)** in the CSF of patients—whether clinically depressed or not—who engage in violent suicidal acts.

Stressful life events (especially separations) commonly precede affective episodes, predominantly unipolar. However, such events may represent the prodromal manifestations of an affective episode rather than its cause; eg, affectively ill persons often alienate their loved ones. The role of psychologic precipitants is even less certain in bipolar conditions. The switch from depression to mania is often heralded by total insomnia for 1 to 3 days (and experimentally induced by total sleep or REM deprivation).

Any **personality type** can develop clinical depression, but the more recurrent unipolar forms are associated with introversion and passive-dependence. Such individuals lack the requisite social skills to adjust to significant departures from routine imposed by life events. The personality structure in bipolar illness tends to be more "normal"; ie, extroverted and compulsive.

Childhood loss of a parent does not place one at higher risk for a mood disorder, but such persons tend to have their first depressions at an earlier age, more often pursue an intermittently chronic course, and attempt suicide more often. Unsubstituted childhood loss may prevent the development of adult coping skills and thereby may contribute to the genesis of personality traits such as passive-dependent helplessness and related maladaptive attitudes of low self-esteem and lack of confidence.

The higher vulnerability of women to depression is customarily traced to their presumed greater passive-dependence and helplessness in controlling their destiny in male-oriented societies. However, biologic vulnerabilities are at least as relevant: women have two X chromosomes (important in bipolar illness, if dominant X-linkage is involved), have more precarious thyroid function, use depressant steroidal contraceptives, undergo premenstrual and postpartum endocrine changes, and compared to men, have higher levels of monoamine oxidase (the enzyme that degrades the neurotransmitters considered important for mood).

Symptoms, Signs, and Diagnosis

Diagnosis is made on clinical grounds: symptomatic picture, course, and family history, and sometimes on the basis of unequivocal response to somatic interventions. These approaches have recently been buttressed by laboratory findings believed to tap limbic-diencephalic dysfunction, especially the **dexamethasone suppression test (DST)** and sleep EEG (**R**apid **E**ye **M**ovement **[REM]** latency). DST is performed by giving 1 mg of dexamethasone at 11 PM and measuring serum cortisol the next day at 4 PM and 11 PM; 50% of melancholics fail to suppress cortisol, giving rise to levels $\geq 5\ \mu g/dL$ (with competitive-protein binding) or ≥ 4 mg/dL (with radioimmunoassay). False-positive results are obtained in pregnancy, high-dose estrogen usage, Cushing's disease, severe weight loss, uncontrolled diabetes mellitus; during alcohol withdrawal; and with phenytoin sodium, barbiturates, or carbamazepine. **REM latency,** *the time elapsed between onset of sleep and the first REM*, has a mean duration of 90 min in normal persons (range 70 to 110 min). In a drug-free patient, when narcolepsy is excluded, shortening of this latency to < 70 min on 2 consecutive nights is strongly suggestive of primary mood disorder.

Although there is no current consensus on the sensitivities and specificities of these tests, their judicious use can enhance conventional clinical wisdom in selected diagnostic and prognostic decisions discussed below. The tests are not useful for screening and routine use, nor can they substitute for clinical examination and judgment.

Unipolar illness: In the **depressive syndrome** (see TABLE 141–3), the mood typically is depressed, irritable, or anxious, or a combination thereof. However, in **masked depressions,** consciously experienced depression may be paradoxically absent. Instead, the patient complains of being somatically ill and may even wear a defensive mask of apparent cheerfulness **(smiling depression).** Others complain of various aches and pains, fears of calamity, and fears of becoming insane. Finally, in some the morbid affect is of such depth that tears dry up; here, a return of the ability to cry usually is a sign of improvement. In such depressions the patient complains of the inability to experience usual emotions—including grief, joy, and pleasure—and a feeling that the world has become colorless, lifeless, and dead.

The morbid mood is accompanied by preoccupation with guilt, self-denigrating ideas, decreased ability to concentrate, indecisiveness, diminished interest in usual activities, social withdrawal, helplessness and hopelessness, and recurrent thoughts of death and suicide.

Marked psychomotor and vegetative signs occur in full-blown depressive conditions in both uni- and bipolar illness. Psychomotor retardation or slowing of thinking, speech, and general activity may progress to **depressive stupor,** where all voluntary activities cease. Some patients have psychomotor agitation, with restlessness, wringing of the hands, and pressure of speech. Some patients, especially bipolar depressives, are hypersomnolent, while most major depressives typically complain of insomnia, with difficulty falling asleep, multiple arousals, or early morning awakening; subgroups of dysthymic and atypical depressives, however, may have hypersomnia. Anorexia and weight loss are sometimes serious enough to lead to emaciation and secondary disturbances in electrolyte balance; overeating and weight gain are less common and more

TABLE 141–3. CLINICAL MANIFESTATIONS OF DEPRESSIVE AND MANIC STATES

	Depressive Syndrome	*Manic Syndrome*
Mood	Depressed, irritable, or anxious (the patient may, however, smile or deny subjective mood change and instead complain of pain or other somatic distress)	Elated, irritable, or hostile
	Crying spells (the patient may, however, complain of inability to cry or to experience emotions)	Momentary tearfulness (as part of mixed state)
Associated psychologic manifestations	Lack of self-confidence; low self-esteem; self-reproach	Inflated self-esteem; boasting; grandiosity
	Poor concentration; indecisiveness	Racing thoughts; clang associations (new thoughts triggered by word sounds rather than meaning); distractibility
	Reduction in gratification; loss of interest in usual activities; loss of attachments; social withdrawal Negative expectations; hopelessness; helplessness; increased dependency	Heightened interest in new activities, people, creative pursuits; increased involvement with people (who are often alienated because of the patient's intrusive and meddlesome behavior); buying sprees; sexual indiscretions; foolish business investments
	Recurrent thoughts of death and suicide	
Somatic manifestations	Psychomotor retardation; fatigue Agitation	Psychomotor acceleration; eutonia (increased sense of physical well-being)
	Anorexia and weight loss, or weight gain	Possible weight loss from increased activity and inattention to proper dietary habits
	Insomnia, or hypersomnia	Decreased need for sleep
	Menstrual irregularities; amenorrhea	
	Anhedonia; loss of sexual desire	Increased sexual desire
Psychotic symptoms	Delusions of worthlessness and sinfulness	Gradiose delusions of exceptional talent
	Delusions of reference and persecution	Delusions of assistance; delusions of reference and persecution
	Delusions of ill health (nilhilistic, somatic, or hypochondriacal)	Delusions of exceptional mental and physical fitness
	Delusions of poverty	Delusions of wealth, aristocratic ancestry, or other grandiose identity
	Depressive hallucinations in the auditory, visual, and (rarely) olfactory spheres	Fleeting auditory or visual hallucinations

characteristic of milder depressions. There is often loss of sexual desire, with orgasmic difficulties; amenorrhea also can occur.

Psychotic manifestations are present in 15% of depressions, most commonly in melancholia. Patients have delusions of having committed unpardonable sins or crimes; hallucinatory voices accuse them of various misdeeds or condemn them to death. The uncommon hallucinations of vision take the form of coffins or deceased relatives. Feelings of insecurity and worthlessness may lead some patients to believe that they are being observed, watched, and persecuted. Others think they harbor incurable and "shameful" illnesses, like cancer and sexually transmitted disease; and that they are contaminating other people. Rarely a patient may kill family members to "save" them from future misfortune, and then commit suicide.

Diagnosis of a **melancholic episode** usually is not difficult; problems arise when the clinical picture is mild, atypical, or chronic. Patients with clinical depressions that represent the incomplete recovery phase of major unipolar illness show residual signs of vegetative irregularity and secondary interpersonal trouble in their conjugal life. **Early-onset dysthymia,** like its nosologic precursor "neurotic depression," is characterized by milder subsyndromal and nonpsychotic depressive manifestations with less prominent somatic signs but marked lowering of self-esteem and characterologic difficulties. However, not all dysthymias are unipolar. In some, the dysthymic pattern represents an attenuated, subaffective intermittent form of retarded bipolar illness, with hypomania manifest on pharmacologic challenge only. A positive diagnosis of dysthymia as a subaffective disorder is not easily made on clinical grounds if family history and pharmacologic response patterns are not documented. However, shortened REM latency and DST nonsuppression support the diagnosis. More commonly, however, dysthymia is related to the atypical depressions, with strong neurotic coloring of symptomatology; past or current history of panic attacks is probably the best clinical marker of such atypical cases.

Bipolar illness: In the full-blown **manic psychosis,** the mood typically is one of elation, but irritability and frank hostility with cantankerousness are not uncommon. The morbid mood colors patients' entire experience and behavior to such an extent that they believe they are in their best mental state. Their lack of insight and inordinate capacity for activity lead to a dangerously explosive psychotic state, in which the individual is impatient, intrusive, and meddlesome, and responds with aggressive irritability when crossed. Interpersonal friction results and may lead to secondary paranoid delusional interpretations of being persecuted. Psychomotor acceleration is experienced as racing thoughts and is manifested by flight of ideas, which in the extreme is difficult to distinguish from the loose associations of the schizophrenic. Attention is quite distractible, with the patient constantly shifting from one theme or endeavor to another. Thoughts and activities are expansive and may progress into frank delusional grandiosity; ie, false convictions of personal wealth, power, inventiveness, and genius, or temporary assumption of a grandiose identity. Patients may believe they are being assisted or persecuted by external agents. Fleeting auditory and visual hallucinations are sometimes present, occur at the height of mania, and are usually understandably linked with the morbid mood. The need for sleep is decreased. Manic persons are inexhaustibly, excessively, and impulsively involved in various activities without recognizing the social dangers involved. In the extreme, activity is so frenzied that any understandable link between mood and behavior is lost (a kind of senseless agitation known as **delirious mania**). This counterpart of depressive stupor, which is rare today, constitutes a medical emergency, as patients may die from sheer physical exhaustion.

Mixed states are *labile mixtures between depressive and manic manifestations or rapid alternation from one to the other*, and occur in 1/3 to 1/2 of manic-depressives at one time

or another. The most common examples include momentary switches into tearfulness and suicidal ideation, seen at the height of mania, or racing thoughts in the context of a depressive state. Less commonly, the entire affective episode is a mixed state, with dysphorically elevated mood, insomnia, psychomotor agitation, racing thoughts, suicidal ideation, grandiosity, persecutory delusions, auditory hallucinations, etc. Alcohol and sedative-hypnotic abuse often contribute to such full-fledged mixed states. Tricyclic antidepressants may also at times contribute to dysphoric-irritable mixed states that may be protracted beyond natural bipolar episodes (ie, > 3 to 4 mo).

An **alternation of major episodes of mania and depression in a cyclical pattern** is one of the most distinctive clinical pictures in medicine. Diagnostic difficulties arise when elated periods are of milder or hypomanic intensity. In diagnosing **bipolar II disorder,** emphasis should be placed on abrupt termination of episodes with brightening of mood, decreased need for sleep, and psychomotor acceleration beyond the patient's usual mode; often the switch into hypomania is caused by tricyclic antidepressants.

In **cyclothymia,** the clinical manifestations are similar to those described for manic-depressive illness, but are attenuated. Most typically, there are brief cycles (usually days) of alternating retarded depression and elevated periods or labile irritability. In another form, depressive features predominate; the bipolar tendency is shown by the ease with which elation or irritability is elicited by the administration of tricyclic antidepressants. In a form rarely seen clinically, and termed **hyperthymic disorder** or **hypomanic personality,** elevated periods predominate, with occasional periods of irritability. Although these milder forms of bipolar disorder tend to contribute to success in business, leadership, achievement, and artistic creativitiy in some individuals, it is important to recognize cyclothymic disorders because their affective nature is often masked by serious interpersonal and social problems, such as repeated marital failure or romantic breakups, episodic promiscuous behavior, uneven work and school record, geographic instability, and dilettantism, and an episodic pattern of alcohol and drug abuse. A family history for frank bipolar psychosis is a useful clue to diagnosis. In some cases, the only way to establish a definitive diagnosis is to give a therapeutic trial with lithium carbonate.

Differential Diagnosis

The most common diagnostic error equates affective psychosis with **schizophrenia** or **schizoaffective disorder** (see also Ch. 142). Differential diagnosis between affective and schizophrenic psychoses (TABLE 141–4) is important clinically because of the relative specificity of lithium for treating recurrent mood disorders (and the potential for neurotoxicity in schizophrenia), and because affectively ill individuals should be protected from the unnecessary risk of tardive dyskinesia. No pathognomonic differentiating features exist, and diagnosis must be based on the overall clinical picture, family history, course, and associated features. Not only mood-congruent psychotic features occur in mood disorders; mood-incongruent delusions or hallucinations are sometimes secondarily superimposed on the basic mood disorder because of the concomitant presence of alcoholic hallucinosis, sedative-hypnotic withdrawal, psychedelic-induced psychosis, or other systemic or brain disease producing psychotic symptoms. In a remitting illness with mixed affective and schizophrenic features, a schizoaffective diagnosis should not be made unless such complicating factors are excluded. When in doubt, because of the better prognosis of mood disorders, **therapeutic trial** with a thymoleptic drug (an antidepressant or lithium carbonate) is indicated. In making such clinical decisions, it helps to remember that the thyrotropin-releasing hormone **(TRH)** test is almost never blunted in nuclear schizophrenic conditions; and that thyroid-stimulating hormone **(TSH)** blunting and DST nonsuppression, even in the presence of schizophreniform features, tend to predict good response to thymoleptic drugs.

TABLE 141–4. DIFFERENTIATION OF AFFECTIVE AND SCHIZOPHRENIC PSYCHOSES

Validating Criteria	*Affective Psychosis*	*Schizophrenic Psychosis*
Age	Any	Rarely begins after 40 yr
Premorbid traits	Dysthymic, compulsive, cyclothymic, or extroverted	Often schizotypal
Onset	Usually abrupt	Usually insidious
Affect	Usually "infectious"	Rigid, blunted, or inappropriate
Thought processes	Usually intelligible: slowed down or accelerated	Typically difficult to follow (loose associations)
Delusions and hallucinations	Usually mood-congruent, but incidental Schneiderian symptoms can also occur	Typically idiosyncratic, bizarre, and involving multiple areas of the patient's life; commonly Schneiderian in form
Family history	Mood disorder; alcoholism	Schizophrenia
Course	Usually remitting or periodic; personality generally preserved	Usually nonremitting; social functioning often deteriorated
Biologic tests	Shortened REM latency; abnormal dexamethasone suppression test (DST); blunted thyroid-stimulating hormone (TSH) response to thyrotropin-releasing hormone (TRH)	Normal results with these tests (except in some schizophreniform psychoses)

(Adapted from H.S. Akiskal and V.R. Puzantian, *Psychiatric Clinics of North America* Vol. 2, No. 3, pp. 419–439, 1979. Copyright by W.B. Saunders Company. Used with permission.)

Therapeutic trial with thymoleptics also is justified in elderly individuals to clarify the differential diagnosis between **early dementia** (which often presents with affective change) and **pseudodemented depression.** (See also Ch. 118.) In the latter, psychomotor retardation, decreased concentration, and memory impairment contribute to the appearance of dementiform features. Because of the better prognosis of depressive illness, it should be preferentially diagnosed, especially when past episodes have occurred or when family history is suggestive. More traditional testing (eg, blood chemistry, CT scan, EEG) is more likely to aid differential diagnosis in these situations than DST, TRH, and sleep EEG findings.

The dual and related concepts of **masked depression** and **affective equivalents** are often invoked to explain certain disorders with prominent somatic symptoms or behavioral disturbance with minimal or absent mood change. These include antisocial acting out (especially in children and adolescents), substance use disorders, pain, hypochondriasis, anxiety states, and psychophysiologic disorders. In the absence of clear-cut affective symptoms, the diagnosis of a mood disorder is not recommended unless past episodes of mood disorders have occurred, the condition is periodic, and the family history is positive for affective illness. DST and REM latency findings may serve as corollary data in this type of differential diagnosis. Therapeutic trial with a thymoleptic drug also may be helpful in differential diagnosis if unequivocal response occurs.

Mood disorders are relatively uncommon before adolescence, at which time they often herald the onset of manic-depressive illness. The basic manifestations of **childhood depressive illness** (see also Ch. 201) are not radically different from adults; they are simply manifested in areas of typical concern to children and parents, such as

school work and play. In the presence of standard "adult" signs and symptoms of depression, the diagnosis of mood disorder should be made in preference to adjustment reactions or neurotic and behavior disorders; the latter often are given exaggerated prominence in child psychiatry. Conversely, when affective symptoms are lacking, hyperactivity and behavioral disturbances should not be considered affective equivalents unless validating criteria as outlined above are present. *Mood disorders, including bipolar psychoses, do occur in mentally retarded children (and adults),* in whom somatic symptoms and behavioral disturbances are especially likely to mask the basic mood disorder. Depressive manifestations in **adolescents,** especially those with stuporous or psychotic presentations, often herald the onset of bipolar illness; mania in adolescence often is confused with schizophrenia, but a cyclical pattern of retarded depression and an accelerated psychosis with good premorbid and intermorbid functioning strongly favors an affective diagnosis. The diagnostic status of laboratory tests is generally uncertain in juvenile affective disorders, though positive DST findings (with 1/2 of the adult 1-mg dose of dexamethasone) may corroborate the clinical impression of primary depressive disorder.

Unipolar depression is less often a cause of **alcoholism** and drug abuse than has been thought. Alcohol is more likely to be abused by the manic patient; while an attempt to treat the sleep disorder may be the motive in both, manics may sometimes seek enhanced excitement. Affective symptoms, especially depression, of a transient or intermittent nature (due to pharmacologic or social causes) that often accompany **substance use disorders** should not be confused with major mood disorders that most typically have a sustained duration of several months. Differentiation from intermittently chronic mood disorders such as cyclothymia and dysthymia is more problematic. Although primary alcoholism, other substance use disorders, and antisocial personality are the most likely diagnoses in individuals with flagrant alcohol and drug histories, polysubstance abuse in some teenagers may represent self-treatment for cyclothymic mood swings. Furthermore, episodic substance abuse (especially that of alcohol—**dipsomania**) or onset after age 30 favors the diagnosis of primary mood disorder with secondary substance abuse. When in doubt, a therapeutic trial with thymoleptic agents is indicated, because DST, TRH, and REM latency data are *unreliable* in the differential diagnosis of mood and substance use disorders.

Neurotic symptoms such as anxiety, phobias, and obsessions are common in primary depressive disorders; they disappear when the affective episode remits. In primary neurotic syndromes, on the other hand, there are usually irregular exacerbations and remissions of the neurotic symptoms beginning with early adulthood. Nevertheless, such conditions as periodic obsessional or anxiety states, especially if making their first appearance after age 40, are often due to primary mood disorder. Differentiating neurotic and mood disorders is more problematic when mild symptoms common to both groups of illnesses coexist. Such conditions, variously referred to as **mixed anxiety-depression, anxious depression,** or **atypical depression** usually have chronically intermittent courses. Some authorities consider them as the neurotic end of an affective spectrum. Despite symptomatologic overlap, however, primary mood (especially recurrent and bipolar) conditions and primary neurotic syndromes are biologically distinct, including genetic background (monozygotic twin data do not show a discordance pattern whereby one twin has primary depression, the other an anxiety state), DST and REM latency findings (generally negative in anxiety states), and lactate infusion. The latter procedure tends to elicit panic attacks in those with classic anxiety neurosis and is not characteristic of primary depressive illness.

Treatment of Unipolar and Bipolar Illness

The clinical pharmacology of thymoleptic agents: Psychopharmaceuticals effective in the treatment of mood disorders can be divided into 3 classes: the heterocyclic antidepressants **(HCAs),** monoamine oxidase inhibitors **(MAOIs),** and lithium salts.

TABLE 141–5. CLASSIFICATION OF SELECTED SIDE EFFECTS AND DOSAGE RANGE OF THE HETEROCYCLIC ANTIDEPRESSANTS (HCAs)

HCA	*Sedation*	*Anticholinergic*	*Dosage Range (Mg/day)*
III° and II° amine tricyclic antidepressants			
Amitriptyline	+++	+++	50–300
↓			
Nortriptyline*	++	++	50–150
Imipramine	++	++	50–300
↓			
Desipramine*	+	+	50–300
Other tricyclic antidepressants			
Doxepin	+++	++	50–300
Trimipramine	+++	++	50–400
Clomipramine†	++	++	50–300
Protriptyline	±	+++	10–60
Newer antidepressants			
Amoxapine	++	+	150–600
Maprotiline	++	+	50–300
Trazodone	+++	0	150–600
Alprazolam	++	0	0.5–4

* Arrows indicate biotransformed secondary amine tricyclic; such transformation is usually complete with imipramine and variable with amitriptyline.

† As THE MANUAL goes to press, clomipramine is not yet available for clinical use in the USA.

HCAs comprise the largest class of antidepressants (TABLE 141–5). Formerly known as tricyclic antidepressants **(TCAs)**, these agents are called heterocyclic because of the recent marketing of monocyclic, bicyclic, and tetracyclic drugs. Unlike amphetamine-type drugs, HCAs have no immediate euphoriant effects and hence no effect on normal sadness—probably why they pose no risk of abuse potential. Acutely, by blocking re-uptake, these agents or their metabolites increase the availability of the biogenic amines norepinephrine and serotonin (5-HT) in the synaptic cleft. Upon chronic administration they downregulate β_1 adrenoreceptors on the postsynaptic membrane; even an HCA like trazodone (which is presynaptically a 5-HT uptake blocker) and the benzodiazepine, alprazolam (which may have modest antidepressant action and which does not seem to act presynaptically), do produce such downregulation. In addition, all HCAs produce significant suppression of REM sleep, believed to be important in their mechanism of action (trimipramine seems to be the only exception), exert local anesthetic action, and increase cerebral capillary permeability.

Most HCA side effects derive from their α_1 adrenolytic and muscarinic-blocking actions (postural hypotension, quinidine-like cardiotoxicity and peripheral anticholinergic side effects). Sedation, depending on its desirability from the point of view of sleep induction and maintenance, may or may not be considered a side effect; it derives largely from histamine$_1$ and 5-HT$_2$ blockade. Of the "classical" agents, the secondary amine tricyclics (nortriptyline and desipramine) have the least amount of side effects with respect to the adrenolytic (α_1), anticholinergic, and antihistaminic mechanisms. Thus, nortriptyline, which has the virtue of producing negligible postural hypotension, has been safely used in depressed stroke patients. Of the new-generation

drugs, trazodone is virtually free of anticholinergic and cardiovascular side effects. Trazodone is also highly sedating and therefore useful in anxious melancholias; desipramine produces little if any sedation and therefore is useful in treating retarded depressives. Most HCAs tend to lower the seizure threshold, and this is particularly accentuated with maprotiline.

HCAs appear equally effective in about 70% of clinically depressed patients. The rate of response climbs to 90% in those with melancholic signs and symptoms. Other predictors of antidepressant response include previous response, family history of response, and experimentally, euphoric response to a 20- to 30-mg single dose of dextroamphetamine, and REM suppression with 2 nights of HCA use. HCAs tend to precipitate hypomania in bipolar depressives and should not be used on a chronic basis in such patients. However, in those without personal and familial history of bipolarity, these agents have been given safely for as long as 2 decades to prevent relapse in chronic unipolar patients.

Indications other than primary mood disorders include (1) prevention of school phobia and panic attacks (most studies have been conducted with imipramine); (2) childhood enuresis (imipramine); (3) palliation of peptic ulcer in depressed patients (doxepin, trimipramine, and amitriptyline); (4) symptomatic alleviation of idiopathic hypersomnia and sleep apnea (protriptyline given in the AM); (5) bulimia (imipramine and desipramine); (6) narcolepsy manifesting predominantly with cataplexy (imipramine); (7) pain syndromes even in the absence of a strong depressive component (sedating HCAs generally preferred); (8) attention deficit disorder (imipramine); (9) obsessive-compulsive disorder (clomipramine and others—see TABLE 141-5).

MAOIs inhibit the oxidative deamination of the 3 classes of biogenic amines—noradrenergic, dopaminergic, and 5-HT—as well as other phenylethamines (TABLE 141–6). Those marketed as antidepressants in the USA (eg, phenelzine, isocarboxazid, and tranylcypromine) are nonselective MAOIs which can cause hypertensive crises if tyramine- or dopamine-containing food or sympathomimetic agents are ingested concurrently (most common with tranylcypromine). More selective agents are under experimental trial as antidepressants and may offer relative freedom from such interaction. These agents are underused in the USA because of clinicians' "fear" of paradoxical hypertension due to dietary or drug interactions, described below under Treatment of Cyclothymic, Dysthymic, and Other Atypical Mood Disorders. Actually, postural hypotension—and consequent lightheadedness—is more of a problem with these agents. Erectile difficulties (least common with tranylcypromine) and insomnia are 2 other troublesome side effects. Potential for cardiotoxicity and anticholinergic side effects is minimal. Hepatotoxicity (the reason why the first MAOI, iproniazid, was withdrawn) is fortunately quite rare in the MAOIs in current use (least likely with tranylcypromine).

TABLE 141–6. CLASSIFICATION OF PROTOTYPIC MONOAMINE OXIDASE INHIBITORS (MAOIs)

Enzyme	*Substrate*	*Drugs*
MAO-A	Serotonin	Clorgyline†
MAO-B	Phenylethylamine Dopamine	Deprenyl† Pargyline*
Nonselective	Tyramine (plus others)	Phenelzine Isocarboxazid Tranylcypromine

* Marketed as an antihypertensive agent.
† Not available for clinical use in the USA.

The efficacy of phenelzine is now clearly established for panic disorder. Recent evidence for its efficacy in selected depressive nosologic types with anxious or atypical features has rekindled clinicians' motivation to prescribe it. However, even "typical" melancholias sometimes respond to this agent. Tranylcypromine is sometimes prescribed for hypersomnic-retarded bipolar patients experiencing a relapse under lithium prophylaxis. Again, some unipolar patients refractory to the HCAs may show dramatic response to tranylcypromine. Like the HCAs, and perhaps somewhat more consistently, MAOIs can precipitate euphoric or hypomanic responses, usually in those with bipolar diathesis. However, they have little or no effect on normal mood, and despite some direct amphetamine-like action possessed by tranylcypromine, MAOIs generaly are safe from an abuse standpoint.

Lithium is a naturally occurring alkali metal. By the early 1970s its efficacy had been demonstrated and methods of safe administration established. Its precise mechanism of stabilizing the unpredictable, often explosive, mood swings and behavior of bipolar patients is unknown. It may be any or all of the following: hyperpolarization of the neuronal membrane; increased presynaptic deamination of norepinephrine and decreased norepinephrine release; blocking β-adrenoreceptor-stimulated adenyl cyclase; decreased dopaminergic turnover; increased tryptophan uptake and consequent stabilization of 5-HT synaptic dynamics; inhibition of the synthesis of prostaglandin E_1; and slowing of biologic rhythms.

Lithium, usually given as a carbonate salt, is rapidly and completely absorbed via the GI tract and peaks in the serum in 1½ h. It is not biotransformed; 95% is excreted via the kidney, a process enhanced by a Na^+ load. Thus, any condition that leads to sodium loss—via disease or diuretics—poses a risk for toxicity. The elimination half-life is 24 h, which tends to increase with age and with the decreased glomerular filtration rate that accompanies kidney disease, dictating extreme caution and use of lower doses in such patients. Steady state is reached in 4 to 6 days—hence the latency in acute anti-manic action. During a manic episode, the patient retains lithium and excretes Na^+; oral dosage and the blood level need to be higher during acute treatment compared with maintenance prophylaxis. **Acute lithium side effects** (eg, fine tremor, stomach irritation, and diarrhea) are minimized when the dosage is divided throughout the day (eg, tid) or when slow-release forms are used. This is convenient during the first 6 to 12 mo of stabilization. However, once the dosage is established for a given patient (usually 600 to 1500 mg/day), it may be prudent in those at risk for kidney disease to give the entire dose following the evening meal—which may improve compliance despite possible peaking of side effects at night; the troughs in the blood level with single daily dose are believed to "protect" the kidneys.

Although lithium attenuates bipolar mood swings, it has no effect on normal mood. It also appears to have an anti-aggressive action, but it is unclear whether this occurs in patients without a bipolar diathesis. By its direct action, lithium produces no sedation nor, ordinarily, cognitive impairment; should the latter occur, it is often, though not always, due to lithium-induced hypothyroidism. Lithium does not produce dependence. Eighty-five percent of bipolar patients respond to it. Predictors of good response include a classic manic picture as part of primary mood disorder; episode frequency $< 2/\text{yr}$; and past and family history of lithium response. Promising uses of lithium include periodic alcoholism, polysubstance abuse, and episodic aggression—all of which might represent bipolar variants—and, experimentally, aplastic anemia (lithium regularly induces a modest leukocytosis).

Unipolar illness.

1. Medical or neurologic causes should be excluded, especially after age 40.

2. Hospitalization: Persistent suicidal ideation (particularly when family support is lacking), stupor, agitated-deluded depression, and physical debilitation require hospitalization and, often, electroconvulsive therapy **(ECT)**; the response to 4 to 8 treatments

in such cases usually is dramatic and may be lifesaving. A 2- to 4-wk course with maximal doses of sedating HCAs and, if necessary, buttressed with neuroleptics (eg, thioridazine up to 300 mg/day orally given in 2 to 3 divided doses, or thiothixene up to 30 mg/day orally or IM given in 2 to 3 divided doses) represents an alternative in agitated psychotic patients; to avert the risk of tardive dyskinesia, the neuroleptic should be discontinued as soon as possible. Continuation therapy for 6 to 9 mo (and up to 2 yr in patients > 50 yr) with an HCA usually prevents relapse in ECT- or drug-treated patients.

3. The outpatient setting is where most depressives are treated today. Pharmacotherapy is the treatment of choice for depressions of melancholic depth; nonmelancholic depressions are treated either with drugs or psychotherapy or, preferably, by combining the 2. Initially, the patient is seen on a weekly or biweekly basis to provide support and monitor progress. Since most patients are embarrassed and demoralized by the implications of having a mental disorder, especially one that seriously diminishes the capacity for work, it is extremely important to tell the patient, his family, and his employer (when appropriate) that depression is a self-limiting medical illness with a generally good prognosis; an explanation also may be given in terms of our current understanding of the biologic basis of depression.

4. Guidelines for drug therapy: The family history of response to a specific MAOI or HCA guides drug choice. Prominence of phobic anxiety suggests phenelzine. Otherwise, because of ease of administration, it is best to begin with an HCA. Although different HCAs are considered to be equally effective in the average case of depression, certain practical and pharmacodynamic considerations provide reasonable guidelines in their choice. First, it may be best to try one of the classical TCAs because we know more about their effectiveness and side effects. Furthermore, it is convenient to treat the agitated insomniac patient with a sedating HCA, the retarded insomniac patient with a less sedating HCA, and the hypersomnic retarded patient with an activating HCA. For patients with cardiac disease, or those who cannot tolerate anticholinergic side effects, or where such effects could lead to clinical catastrophes (eg, angle-closure glaucoma, prostatic hypertrophy), several of the new HCAs offer relative freedom from cardiotoxic and anticholinergic side effects. For many patients who should stay alert with the least amount of dry mouth, desipramine is preferred. Amitriptyline as well as other sedating HCAs help the depressed patient with concurrent pain and insomnia (not an uncommon combination) while decreasing the need for analgesic and spasmolytic medication in such conditions as GI disorders where the anticholinergic and antihistaminic properties of some HCAs may provide an advantage.

It is generally best to begin with the lowest unit dose marketed, and increase gradually over a period of 2 to 3 wk. Ordinarily, an average of 1/3 to 1/2 of the maximal allowable dose listed in TABLE 141–5 will suffice, but some may need doses higher than this maximum for remission; individual and population differences in the pharmacokinetic handling of the HCAs are the most likely explanation. It is also likely that the relatively high doses recommended by research clinicians, especially in the USA, are based on experiences with relatively refractory patients.

Giving the entire dose at bedtime usually renders hypnotics unnecessary, minimizes side effects during daytime, and improves compliance; however, some elderly patients may better tolerate daily divided doses. Therapeutic response is seen in approximately 2 to 3 wk (it can be as early as 4 days or as late as 4 to 5 wk). Within 1 to 2 mo following response, a downward adjustment of dosage is attempted, to be maintained at 2/3 of the effective therapeutic dose for the natural duration of an episode. Abrupt withdrawal should be *avoided* to prevent cholinergic rebound; eg, nightmares, nausea, colic, etc.

The indications and dosage range of the HCAs for preadolescent depressions are not established; in the rare melancholic child, conservative doses and increments are best, as is true with the elderly (about half the adult dose). Seizures and behavioral symp-

toms due to toxicity (excitement, confusion, hallucinations, or oversedation) are especially likely to occur in elderly individuals with organic brain disease, dictating lower initial and therapeutic doses.

The most troublesome, though generally benign, **side effects of the HCAs** include sedation, dry mouth, tremor, postural dizziness, blurred vision, sweating, constipation, and urinary hesitancy. During the first 10 to 15 days when the patient is largely reaping side effects and little therapeutic benefit, he should be informed that these are expected effects, that they are the prelude to therapeutic response, and that they will abate with time. The most serious but fortunately rare undesirable effects are precipitation of angle-closure glaucoma, prostatism, cardiac arrhythmias, myocardial infarction, and stroke. Patients with such potential should be excluded from therapy with traditional TCAs by appropriate ophthalmologic, urologic, and cardiologic consultation; the newer HCAs appear safer. TABLE 141–7 summarizes the most important and potentially serious interactions of the HCAs with medical conditions and other drugs.

Where anxiety is prominent, a benzodiazepine tranquilizer (eg, diazepam 2 to 5 mg orally bid or tid or lorazepam 1 to 2 mg orally bid or tid) can be added for 2 to 3 wk to the HCA regimen. Although neuroleptics alone, such as thioridazine 25 to 100 mg orally bid or tid, also are advocated for anxious depressions, it is best to reserve them for refractory cases in order not to expose the patient to unnecessary risk for tardive dyskinesia. There is recent suggestion that the new benzodiazepine alprazolam in doses of 0.5 to 2 mg bid might be singly effective in controlling both anxiety and depressive components. The MAOI phenelzine (up to 75 mg/day) is another alternative.

ECT or a potent MAOI such as tranylcypromine 10 to 30 mg orally bid may be given for those who are poor risks with HCAs, cannot tolerate them, or fail to improve on full courses of 2 different HCAs for 4 to 5 wk each (after dosage adjustment suggested by plasma drug levels). Plasma levels are most useful in determining causes of inadequate clinical response on standard oral doses, or when pronounced side effects occur on small doses, or when anticipated side effects might be dangerous because of heart disease or old age.

Especially when combined with a MAOI, the 5-HT precursor L-tryptophan given 6 to 8 gm/day orally has been advocated for **refractory depressions** on an experimental basis; L-tryptophan and a 5-HT HCA can be similarly combined. In 5 to 10% of depressions (usually women, detected by augmented TSH response to TRH stimulation) significant potentiation of tricyclic antidepressant activity may be provided by tri-iodothyronine 25 to 50 μg/day orally. A lithium-heterocyclic combination may also be beneficial in cases where an eventual bipolar course is suspected. After a 10-day period of a tertiary amine TCA such as amitriptyline 75 to 100 mg orally, the addition of gradually increasing doses of phenelzine 30 to 60 mg/day orally in divided doses appears to be safe, and might help selected refractory cases; but the addition, in reverse order, of a TCA on a MAOI may result in hypertensive crisis. The antiepileptic carbamazepine in doses 400 to 1200 mg/day has also been recently used in refractory cases, especially those where sleep-deprived EEG or nasopharyngeal leads reveal abnormal temporal spiking. Because of the risk of agranulocytosis, clinical vigilance and periodic CBC are prudent. All of these unorthodox approaches to refractory cases are best reserved for specialized mood disorder units or clinics.

5. Brief individual psychotherapy may improve coping skills once the acute melancholic phase is over. Couples' therapy may help resolve conjugal conflicts. Elaborate long-term psychotherapy is unnecessary except in the presence of significant personality disturbance.

Recurrent depressions occurring on an infrequent basis can be treated as outlined above for a single episode. However, unipolar illness recurring at intervals shorter than 2 yr is often treated with maintenance HCAs, the dosage periodically adjusted with

TABLE 141–7. CLINICALLY SIGNIFICANT INTERACTIONS BETWEEN HCAs AND SELECTED SOMATIC OR PSYCHIATRIC CONDITIONS AND DRUGS

Conditions/Drugs	*Interaction*	*Clinical Recommendation*
Cardiac disease	Arrythmias, heart failure	Coordinate treatment with cardiologist
Angle-closure glaucoma	Occular hypertension	Coordinate with ophthalmologist; consider trazodone or MAOI
Prostatic hypertrophy	Urinary retention	Give urecholine; consider trazodone or MAOI
Esophageal hiatus hernia	Increased reflux	Reduce dose; consider trazodone or MAOI
Debilitated physical state	Sluggish reflexes predispose to postural hypotension	Slow build-up of nortriptyline; consider ECT*
Pregnant, 1st trimester	Teratogenic	Treat depression with psychotherapy; reserve ECT* for severe cases
Organic mental disease	Hallucinations, disorientation, confusion	Use lower dose of HCA
Chronic schizophrenia	Exacerbation of hyperactive, aggressive psychotic state	Discontinue HCA; institute neuroleptic or raise its dose
Seizure disorder	Precipitation of seizure	Lower dose of HCA; consider concurrent use of antiepileptic medication
Neuroleptics	Increased blood levels of both drugs	Avoid combination unless absolutely necessary
Bipolar depression	Precipitation of hypomania or mania	Reduce dosage or discontinue; consider lithium carbonate
Ethanol	Potentiation of CNS depression	Do not prescribe HCAs to alcoholics unless depressive syndrome is sustained
Guanethidine	Decreased uptake by sympathetic neuron, thereby diminishing its hypotensive action	Trimipramine and trazodone have minimal effect on guanethidine pump
Clonidine	Inhibition of α_2-adrenergic receptors leads to abolition of antihypertensive action	Consider ECT* in severe cases
Advanced liver disease	Decreased degradation, increased blood level	Begin with very small doses; monitor plasma level of HCA
Heavy smoking, phenobarbital, and carbamazepine	Increased degradation, decreased blood level	Monitor plasma level; use higher HCA dose as needed
Cimetidine	Decreased degradation, increased blood level	Monitor plasma level; use lower HCA dose
Thyroid hormone	Potentiation of central effects	Adjust dosage as necessary

* ECT = Electroconvulsive therapy.

(Modified from Akiskal, H.S., "Clinical Overview of Depressive Disorders and Their Pharmacological Management," in *Neuropharmacology of Central and Behavioral Disorders*, edited by G. Palmer, 1981. Copyright by Academic Press. Used with permission.)

respect to mood level and side effects. Family history for bipolar illness is often positive in depressions with high episode frequency, and patients must be observed for hypomania. As expected, maintenance lithium carbonate (see below) is at least equally effective in such cases and may be the preferred treatment to avoid rapid-cycling. Relapses are not uncommon with maintenance chemotherapy; supportive psychotherapy may therefore assist in boosting morale, improving coping skills, and identifying early manifestations of relapse.

Bipolar illness. Many bipolar patients with recurrent depressions experience pleasant elevation of mood, usually at the end of a depression, but do not report it unless specifically questioned. In the absence of documented history for hypomanic or manic episodes, the **depressive phase** of bipolar illness may not be easily distinguishable from unipolar depression; predictors of bipolar outcome are summarized in TABLE 141–1. TCAs may sometimes overcorrect the mood in a hypomanic direction, giving a clue to the bipolar nature of the illness; such pharmacologic hypomania also is seen with ECT and MAOIs, and probably all centrally acting sympathomimetic drugs. Lithium has a modest acute antidepressant effect in the depressive phase of bipolar illness, and can be given alone or in conjunction with an HCA.

Manic psychosis often presents as a social emergency and is preferably managed on an inpatient basis; hypomania, usually on an outpatient basis. After preliminary laboratory evaluation (CBC, urinalysis, T_4, TSH, serum electrolytes, creatinine, and BUN), lithium carbonate is started 300 mg orally bid or tid and increased over a 7- to 10-day period until a serum level of 0.8 to 1.5 mEq/L is reached. Acutely manic patients have high tolerance for lithium and preferentially retain it during the first 10 days, while excreting sodium; regular diet is recommended. Teenagers, who enjoy excellent glomerular function, need higher doses of lithium to achieve the same level of equilibrium in the serum, while the reverse is true for elderly patients. Because lithium's onset of action has a 4- to 10-day latency period, it is sometimes initially necessary to also administer haloperidol 5 to 10 mg IM as needed (up to 60 mg/day) or another suitable neuroleptic until the manic psychosis is under control. In psychotic, extremely hyperactive patients with precarious food and fluid intake, it is preferable to give neuroleptics and supportive care for a week before initiating lithium. Mixed states of manic-depressive illness are also best treated with a neuroleptic-lithium combination. In all combination therapies, the neuroleptic can usually be discontinued in a few weeks. Carbamazepine up to 1200 mg/day is another alternative for extremely psychotic excitements and mixed states. Therapy for an isolated manic episode should continue for at least 6 mo; but most manias occur as part of recurrent bipolar illness.

Recurrent bipolar illness with frequent episodes is best treated with indefinite maintenance on lithium, with serum level of 0.4 to 0.8 mEq/L, usually achieved with two to five 300-mg capsules/day. Doses of HCA in the lower range (as given in TABLE 141–5) can be added when needed (preferably for a few weeks at a time), especially during the first 2 yr of maintenance therapy, to control moderate to severe depressive swings; and chlorpromazine or thioridazine (50 to 300 mg/day), again for a few days to a few weeks at a time, when hypomanic swings or mixed states supervene. There is growing concern that HCAs given to some bipolar patients even when protected by lithium carbonate, may induce rapid-cycling. Low doses of MAOIs (eg, 10 to 30 mg/day) might be preferable in such patients. Thus, in the approach to bipolar depressives, it is best to continue lithium, to avoid any antidepressants for mild relapses, to limit HCAs or MAOIs to the lowest possible dose for a few weeks in moderate relapses, and to treat severe cases with ECT.

Bipolar patients may complain of being overcontrolled, and of being less alert and creative; therefore, considerable psychotherapeutic skills are needed to assure compliance to maintenance doses of lithium, as well as interventions with the patient's spouse or family

to abate interpersonal crises secondary to mercurial moods. Actual decrease in creativity is relatively uncommon, as lithium generally offers the opportunity for more "even" periods devoted to interpersonal, scholastic, professional, and artistic pursuits. Individual psychotherapy may assist patients to cope better with their living problems and adjust to their new self-identities. In the noncompliant, cantankerous manic patient, a depot phenothiazine such as fluphenazine decanoate 12.5 to 25 mg IM every 3 to 4 wk is customarily given; because of the risks for tardive dyskinesia, lithium should be substituted as soon as feasible. In bipolar patients with mood-incongruent psychotic features beyond the usual boundaries of a "pure" mood disorder, intermittent courses of such neuroleptics often are necessary as well; recent clinical experience suggests that carbamazepine may be the drug of choice in such patients, especially when rapid-cycling.

Precautions in pregnancy: In females who wish to have a baby, it is best to wait for at least 2 yr of episode-free prophylaxis before prescribing a lithium holiday, which should come *before* giving up contraceptive measures. This is to avoid the risk of cardiovascular (Ebstein's) anomalies in the 1st trimester. For a serious relapse in the 1st trimester, ECT would be a safer alternative to thymoleptic medication. Such medication, if absolutely necessary, can be used at other times of pregnancy, but should be stopped 1 to 2 wk before delivery and resumed a few days postpartum. Such mothers should not nurse, as thymoleptic drugs pass through the milk.

The most common acute benign side effects of lithium consist of tremor, fasciculation, nausea, diarrhea, polyuria, polydipsia, and weight gain (partly attributed to high-calorie beverages). These usually are transient and often respond to a slight decrease in dosage (and use of diet soft drinks). Empirically, some clinicians advocate short courses of propranolol 10 mg orally tid or qid for incapacitating tremor.

Toxic effects are initially manifested by gross tremor, increased deep tendon reflexes, persistent headache, vomiting, and mental confusion, and may progress to stupor, seizures, and cardiac arrhythmias. Apart from overdose, lithium toxicity is more likely in patients with renal disease with decreased creatinine clearance and with sodium loss that may result from fever, excessive sweating, vomiting, diarrhea, or diuretics; nonsteroidal analgesics other than aspirin may also contribute to hyperlithemia. None of these represent absolute contraindications to lithium, but may dictate assessment of baseline renal function (eg, creatinine clearance), lower doses, dietary sodium supplementation, frequent serum lithium determinations, follow-up of renal function with 24-h urine volume, urine concentration, and creatinine clearance tests. It is likewise desirable to obtain TSH response to TRH challenge and other thyroid indexes when thyroid disease is suspected, and plan for frequent serum lithium determinations. Otherwise, in healthy subjects with relatively stable mood, quarterly serum checks and weight recording—together with biannual determination of creatinine and TSH—usually are sufficient.

The more common **chronic side effects** of lithium include mild leukocytosis (of no functional significance), exacerbation of acne and psoriasis (which may require dermatologic management), hypothyroidism (successfully managed with thyroid supplementation), and nephrogenic diabetes insipidus (may respond to reduction of dosage or temporary interruption of lithium therapy). Individuals with past history of parenchymal kidney disease may be at some risk for structural damage to the distal tubule; therefore, serum lithium levels generally should be maintained at the lowest level compatible with freedom from incapacitating mood swings. Some lithium experts believe that giving the entire therapeutic dose at bedtime may protect against kidney complications. For **lithium overdose,** see under Complications, below.

Treatment of Cyclothymic, Dysthymic, and Other Atypical Mood Disorders

Cyclothymia can be treated very much like recurrent bipolar illness, with considerable psychotherapeutic attention paid these persons' stormy interpersonal relations.

The decision to give a lithium trial depends on the functional impairment produced by the unpredictable mood swings.

For **dysthymia,** especially with bipolar family history, a vigorous trial of a catecholaminergic HCA such as desipramine (later buttressed with lithium carbonate) may help. The value of HCAs or lithium is not established in the other types of chronic depression. Thus, **secondary chronic dysphorias** that often accompany incapacitating nonaffective diseases are best handled with various combinations of supportive, group, and family therapies. However, where insomnia, anxiety, or pain (due to demonstrable organic pathology or psychologic factors, or both) is prominent, a sedating HCA such as trazodone in the 100- to 300-mg range can be adjunctively given. **Characterologic neurotic depressions,** although traditionally the domain of psychodynamically oriented psychotherapy, are being increasingly treated by behavioral and cognitive approaches. Sedating HCAs also can be given adjunctively for their tranquilizing or hypnotic properties; minor tranquilizers are generally best avoided. Trial with a MAOI is worthwhile if these approaches fail. The **atypical depressions** respond favorably to maintenance treatment with MAOIs, notably phenelzine, beginning with 15 mg bid or tid. The dose can be raised by 15 mg/wk until a ceiling of 60 to 75 mg/day is reached. Response may occur as early as a few days or as late as 8 wk. Treatment should continue for 12 mo or longer. Common side effects include insomnia, erectile difficulties, nausea, edema, weight gain, and postural hypotension. **To avert paradoxical hypertensive crises,** the patient should be instructed to avoid sympathomimetic drugs, reserpine, meperidine, and antihistamines, as well as tyramine– or L-dopa–containing beers and wine (including sherry), liqueurs such as Chartreuse and Drambuie, or foods with such content (overripe fruits, fava or broad beans, yeast extracts, canned figs, raisins, yogurt, cheese, sour cream, soy sauce, pickled herring, caviar, liver, and extensively tenderized meats). Patients receiving MAOIs—and who also may need anti-asthmatic, anti-allergic, local anesthetic, and general anesthetic medication—should be treated with the joint expertise of a pharmacologically oriented psychiatrist and an internist, dentist, or anesthesiologist with the requisite experience in neuropharmacology.

Complications

Social consequences. Frequent episodes of bipolar illness, often due to inadequate treatment or lack of compliance with maintenance chemotherapy, result in uneven productivity, dilettantism, bankruptcy, ruined careers, and repeated marital breakdown. Furthermore, all types of recurrent chronic mood disorders may poison family life and rob children of optimal parenting. Early recognition and comprehensive approaches (ie, psycho-, socio-, and pharmacotherapeutic) to the treatment of recurrent mood disorders tend to minimize such complications.

Secondary alcoholism and sedative-hypnotic abuse, the latter often iatrogenically facilitated, are common risks in inadequately treated or unrecognized recurrent mood disorders. Detection of mood disorders and their pharmacologic management is important for primary care physicians; minor tranquilizers and sedative-hypnotics are of little value as primary treatment.

Modest increase in mortality from cardiovascular causes occurs in bipolar illness, is not accounted for by cardiotoxicity from lithium and tricyclics, and tends to involve nonaffective first-degree biologic relatives as well. The reasons for this are obscure.

Suicide, the most serious risk, causes 15% of deaths in untreated mood disorders and tends to occur within 4 to 5 yr from the first clinical episode. The recovery phase from depression (when psychomotor activity is returning to normal but the mood is still dark) is a major risk period, as are the premenstrual phase and personally significant anniversaries. (See also Ch. 144).

Recent findings from mood and lithium clinics suggest that changes may be occurring in the epidemiology of suicide, in that lithium and ECT-treated patients are

under-represented in suicide statistics. This may be due to efficient follow-up strategies by such clinics, or the lithium correction of the serotonergic deficit that is correlated with suicidal mortality. Recent research (based on small sample size) has provided us with the provocative possibility of biochemical prediction in that those attempters with the lowest amount (< 15 mg/mL) of cerebrospinal 5-hydroxy-indoleaceticacid (5-HIAA) are at the highest risk for suicide. Central serotonergic deficiency appears to be correlated with impulsive acts of violence against the self and others. Other biologic risk factors include family history of suicide—even when the proband was raised away from the biologic relative—and continuous nonsuppression of the DST; these findings dictate close clinical vigilance in such cases, even when relatively asymptomatic.

Some skeptics have argued that the suggestive findings from mood clinics on prevention of suicide—by better control of the most common psychiatric disorder contributory to suicide—are deceptive. They believe that such a decline (if it can be demonstrated) is not due to primary prevention, but reflects secondary prevention through more rigorous treatment of suicidal overdoses, including more effective methods for treating barbiturate coma. Barbiturates are much less commonly used today, and all emergency physicians and those in primary care must be familiar with **TCA and lithium overdose,** the most likely medications to be ingested by suicidal patients; ethanol often is a complicating factor. TCA overdose presents as a hyperactive coma with atropinism, and the usual causes of death are cardiac arrhythmias and status epilepticus. Because of protein-binding, forced diuresis and hemodialysis are useless here; treatment effort centers on measures to stabilize cardiac and cerebral function. Similar effort also is vital with lithium overdose, but forced diuresis with sodium chloride or mannitol and alkalinization of urine and hemodialysis could prove lifesaving.

142. SCHIZOPHRENIC DISORDERS

(See also Ch. 201)

The schizophrenic disorders, as defined by **DSM-III** (the American Psychiatric Association's *Diagnostic and Statistical Manual,* Third Edition), are *mental disorders with a tendency toward chronicity which impairs functioning and which is characterized by psychotic symptoms involving disturbances of thinking, feeling, and behavior*. Six specific criteria for the diagnosis include (1) certain psychotic symptoms, delusions, hallucinations, formal thought disorder; (2) deterioration from a previous level of functioning; (3) continuous signs of the illness for at least 6 mo; (4) a tendency towards onset before age 45; (5) not due to mood (affective) disorders; and (6) not due to organic mental disorder or mental retardation.

The DSM-III definition eliminates several entities included in the DSM-II concept. Syndromes which look like schizophrenia but which last < 6 mo are called **schizophreniform.** Psychotic syndromes of < 2 wk duration which follow a significant psychosocial stressor are now called **brief reactive psychoses.** Borderline or latent schizophrenia and simple schizophrenia are now diagnosed **borderline** or **schizotypal personality disorders.** Late onset of schizophrenia-like syndromes (eg, the involutional paraphrenias) are diagnosed **paranoid disorder** or **atypical psychosis.** Organic mental disorder or mental retardation and affective disorder are specifically excluded.

The category of **schizoaffective disorder** (see below under Differential diagnosis) has been significantly narrowed. Most patients with mixtures of schizophrenic and affective symptoms are better diagnosed as schizophrenics or suffering from mood (affective) disorders (see also Ch. 141).

Subtypes of schizophrenia are **disorganized (hebephrenic), catatonic, paranoid, undifferentiated,** and **residual.** According to the course, they can be **subchronic** (< 2 yr),

chronic (> 2 yr), **subchronic with acute exacerbation, chronic with acute exacerbation,** and **in remission.**

Historical Background

Important differences exist among patients with schizophrenia's characteristic cluster of signs and symptoms, and providing a clear line between this behavior and other types of madness has proved difficult. Perceptive, seasoned clinicians from the 17th to the 19th century did their best to differentiate what today we call schizophrenia from melancholia, from mania due to fever and that due to wine, from the enfeeblement of the aged, and from those who suffered brain damage in war. (The notion of **paranoia** had emerged long before that, its first meaning being simply, "beyond understanding.") Although schizophrenia had many names (stupidity, foolishness, vesania, idiocy, insanity of puberty, monomania, paranoia, etc) the early clinicians described the characteristics of family origin, endogenous cause, early onset, remitting or progressive course, bizarre ideas, dissociation of thought and emotion, and social withdrawal, thus moving toward a useful psychiatric classification by using the criteria of symptomatology, course, and outcome.

The concept of dementia praecox was developed from 1896 on, based on the early onset of the tendency toward a deteriorating course. Soon the idea of underlying disturbances in certain psychologic processes, and the distinction between primary and secondary symptoms, were introduced, with attempts to interpret the latter according to freudian psychoanalytic theory. The name "schizophrenia" was coined in 1908, referring to the disconnection or splitting of the psychic functions, believed to be an outstanding symptom of the whole group. It was thought that the illness need not always begin early and could end in various ways, including a so-called social remission; but it was not certain that full recoveries occurred without leaving a scar. No definite pathologic anatomic or biologic abnormality was established. However, the unmistakable disturbances of thinking, perception, and feeling had been recognized.

Incidence

Schizophrenia occurs worldwide. Using a relatively narrow concept of the disorder, studies of European and Asian populations show the lifetime prevalence to be from 0.2% to almost 1%. Higher rates have been found in the USA and USSR, but the criteria used are much broader. Schizophrenia most commonly becomes manifest in late adolescence or early adult life, although paranoid schizophrenia typically has a later onset. Even with available forms of treatment, schizophrenic patients occupy about 1/2 the hospital beds of mentally ill and mentally retarded patients, and about 1/4 of all available hospital beds. The high prevalence in lower socioeconomic classes has been mainly attributed to social disorganization and consequent stresses, but there is evidence that this association arises partly because some patients in a prepsychotic phase drift down the social scale.

Etiology

Winston Churchill's description of the Soviet Union as being a riddle wrapped in mystery inside an enigma applies to schizophrenia. Most cases are now thought to be caused by a complex interaction between inherited and environmental factors. Several scientific models preempt the field: Those regarding schizophrenia as primarily biologic in origin (genetic, internal environment, or neurophysiologic model) with the environmental factors playing only a minor role; and those that consider the cause primarily environmental (ecologic, developmental, or learning model), with the biologic factors playing the minor role. Even in the most advanced biologic (the genetic) model, no direct evidence exists that the inherited genetic makeup of the person who develops one or more episodes of schizophrenia is in any way different from that of the individual who is not subject to such a hazard. It is only an inference based on the facts that an individual who has a consanguineous relative suffering with schizophrenia

has a higher risk of developing an episode, and that the risk varies with the degree of consanguinity. As none of the theories can be shown to be both necessary and sufficient, the vulnerability model, an elaboration of the diathesis stress model, is introduced to integrate the others and include the potential etiologic sources. A genetic predisposition is probably necessary if schizophrenia is to occur at all, but the overt manifestations of illness seem to be decided partly by stressful life experiences, such as faulty patterns of upbringing and disturbed relationships. Those who develop schizophrenia in middle age or later often are unmarried or widowed, or suffer from a serious physical handicap, such as being deaf.

Currently being investigated are attempts to identify the nature of the schizophrenic defect before its symptomatic manifestations—eg, the study of a schizophrenic patient's blood relatives who are not ill; and psychologic studies of eye tracking, reaction time crossover, and span of attention. Other technologies are being borrowed to learn more about how the brain processes information: from experimental psychology, masking and dichotic learning; from psychometrics, the development of interviewing technics; and from information processing, memory retrieval. Advanced technology in genetics may make it possible to identify certain traits in parallel with the presence of given mapping markers of genes. There are also new investigations in neuropathology, CT, MRI, positron emission tomography, and cerebral blood flow measures.

Premorbid personality: Although no specific personality type is seen in all cases, many patients who develop schizophrenia show such traits as hypersensitivity, shyness, unsociability, lack of affect, and paranoid attitudes. Difficulty in personal relationships and social isolation inevitably result. The term **schizoid personality** is used to denote persons with defective capacity to form social relationships; the term **schizotypal personality** describes those who, in addition to their deficiencies in social relations, show oddities of thinking, perception, communication, and behavior which are not severe enough to meet the criteria for schizophrenia. Schizoid and schizotypal personalities are discussed in Ch. 137.

Symptoms and Signs

Thought disorder: Clear, goal-directed thinking becomes increasingly difficult, as shown in a diffuseness or woolliness and circumstantiality of speech. Sudden and incomprehensible changes of subject and obvious flaws in reasoning occur because distraction by fringe associations and the patient's private symbolism determines his thinking as much as does normal logic. "I have always believed in the good of mankind but I know I am not a woman because I have an Adam's apple" seems nonsensical. However, the patient who said this suffered doubts about his sexual identity and believed that a battle for good and evil was raging within him; his implicit identification of women with evil, the switch from mankind to woman (presumably because of the syllable "man"), the search for reassurance by choosing a minor sexual difference because of its symbolism, and the condensation of the themes illustrate the schizophrenic disturbance of thinking. Some schizophrenics report a stoppage of thinking **(thought blocking)** or may claim that their thoughts are **broadcast** or shared with other people; delusional interpretations of these experiences (see below) lead to the belief that their minds are being controlled by external agencies. Thinking may be impoverished in many schizophrenic patients who have been ill for a long time.

Emotional (affective) changes: Blunting and inappropriateness (incongruity) of affect are the most characteristic emotional changes and are obvious and not easily overlooked in severe cases. Minor blunting and incongruity may be difficult to evaluate, since their assessment is subjective and therefore unreliable. Any mood disturbance—depression, excitement, anxiety, elation—may occur, and perplexity is not uncommon in acute schizophrenia.

Perceptual disorders: Auditory hallucinations are the most common, but hallucinations of sight, touch (including sexual sensations), smell, and taste may occur. The

auditory hallucinations range from whistling, humming, or machinery sounds to an indirect muttering of voices or clear, complex conversations. Auditory hallucinations can occur in many disorders, but certain types, especially hallucinations of a running commentary on the patient's actions or of voices talking about the patient, strongly suggest schizophrenia.

Delusions: Delusions of persecution are frequent, as well as those involving hypochondriacal or religious ideas, jealousy, and sexual identity (particularly homosexuality). Delusions of grandeur are common but also are often found in other disorders, such as in the manic phase of manic-depressive psychosis. Delusional interpretations of strange experiences such as thought blocking or broadcasting and depersonalization may lead the patient to believe that telepathy is occurring, that a mechanical device is recording his thoughts and conversation, or that he is under the control of an external agency. The patient suddenly may develop a delusional system that explains in a flash a whole succession of preceding puzzling events that he viewed with ill-defined suspicion, perplexity, or an inexplicable feeling of menace. This type of delusion, almost invariably diagnostic of schizophrenia, may convince the patient of his special significance—that he is the Messiah or the innocent victim in the center of a conspiracy—or provide immovably strong explanations for previous experiences. The delusional system may seem illuminating to the patient but is baffling and incomprehensible to others.

Catatonic signs: Disturbances of movement range from gross overactivity and excitement to marked retardation and even stupor with mutism. Posturing may occur, and the patient may take up a bizarre position (crucifix, or head raised several inches from the pillow) for prolonged periods. Extreme negativism or automatic obedience is sometimes seen. Mannerisms such as a mincing gait, grimaces, or overemphasis of normal movements are more common. Chemotherapy and improved individual management have made severe catatonic symptoms increasingly rare. Catatonic signs are also observed in patients with organic brain disease; eg, carbon monoxide intoxication, cerebral neoplasms.

Violent behavior: Although threats of violence and even minor aggressive outbursts are common in acute schizophrenic states and relapses, dangerous behavior occurring when the patient obeys commanding voices or attacks his persecutors is uncommon. Occasionally, grotesque violence, with self-mutilation (often of sexual organs) or murderous attacks, may occur. Matricide, the rarest form of murder, is most often perpetrated by schizophrenics, as is filicide. Petty crimes may be committed by a "down and out" chronic schizophrenic patient. The risk of suicide is increased in all stages of schizophrenic illness.

In addition to violent behavior associated with the psychotic state (including organic brain disease), there are individuals with personality disorders, including the schizoid or schizotypal types, who become severely isolated, depressed, and paranoid and who may seek resolution of their difficulties in an act of aggression (eg, physical attack, murder, assassination) against someone whom they perceive as a single source of their abject state. The victim is usually someone in authority (eg, a parent, teacher, popular idol, or prominent political leader), or a sweetheart, spouse, or child. In their tormented thinking, these patients appear to seek recognition, love, and honor for their "heroic" act, but at the same time they seem to expect and welcome death as punishment and escape.

Nonspecific symptoms: Withdrawal from external reality and failure to coordinate internal drives are frequent findings. There may be abnormalities of psychomotor activities; eg, rocking, pacing, peculiar motor responses, or immobility. The patient may often appear perplexed, eccentrically groomed or dressed, and disheveled. Poverty of speech is common and ritualistic behavior associated with magical thinking often occurs. The patient may be depressed and exhibit anxiety, anger, or a mixture of these.

There may be ideas of reference and hypochondriacal concerns. Rarely, during a period of excitement, a patient may be found to be confused or disoriented, but usually there is no significant disturbance in the sensorium.

Course and Diagnosis

Even in cases with **acute onset** (commonly of the catatonic or paranoid subtypes) and with an apparent relationship to stressful events in the environment, careful history taking often will reveal a prodromal period of weeks or months of increasing withdrawal and disorganization of the previous level of functioning. During the active phase, characteristic symptoms involve psychologic processes (content of thought, language, perception, affect), volition, motor behavior, sense of self, and relationship to the external world. A residual phase often follows the active phase and may be similar to the prodromal phase, but at times with persistent delusional beliefs and with emotional blunting.

In order to distinguish schizophrenic disorders from short-term reversible illnesses, DSM-III requires that schizophrenia be diagnosed only when continuous signs have lasted for at least 6 mo during the person's life, and that this period include an active phase of psychotic symptoms with or without a prodromal or residual phase. However, in many patients the deterioration is so **gradual** that it is difficult to trace back to a specific time when illness supervened in the schizoid personality. In the early stages of schizophrenia, the patient may become increasingly uneasily aware that his psychologic integrity is impaired. He may worry over his lack of concentration or fear that he is going insane. His personal identity may be threatened by doubts of his sexual gender. He may symbolize his awareness of illness in terms of an internal battle between good and evil or project his feeling of internal dissolution onto the environment as fantasies of the annihilation of the world by some holocaust.

DSM-III has classified the course as **subchronic** (< 2 yr), **chronic** (> 2 yr), **subchronic with acute exacerbation, chronic with acute exacerbation,** and **in remission.** In the past, schizophrenia was divided into 2 distinct patterns of onset. The first **(reactive)** is the development of illness in a person who has shown satisfactory social functioning but who often possesses an anxious and insecure temperament. This type of illness is frequently precipitated by a traumatic event and has a rapid onset. Patients with the second pattern **(process type)** have a history of poor social functioning, have few friends, and show occasional bizarre habits. They are described as isolated, shy, and withdrawn (schizoid). There is no distinct precipitating event; the illness begins with a gradual downhill course into withdrawal and isolation.

Certain symptoms commonly cluster together but no clear demarcation exists between **subtypes of schizophrenia,** and individual patients may shift from one to another in successive episodes or even in the same illness. The term **undifferentiated** is used when the episode is characterized by prominent psychotic symptoms not classifiable in any specific subtype, or meeting the criteria for more than one. Currently, those subtypes of schizophrenia without overt psychotic symptoms (ie, latent, borderline, or simple schizophrenia) are to be diagnosed as **borderline or schizotypal personality disorders.** The emphasis in **hebephrenia (disorganized type)** is on silliness and incongruity of affect and thought disorder with increasing autism. Delusions, hallucinations, and other minor catatonic symptoms (eg, mannerisms) are often present, and the personality is severely disorganized. In **catatonia,** movement disorders predominate, with increasing motor agitation or retardation and gross posturing. Autism is extreme. **Paranoid schizophrenia** includes delusions of persecution or grandeur, thought disorder, and hallucinations, but there is less personality disintegration than in other subtypes. In **chronic schizophrenia** all subtypes tend to a clinical picture where blunting of emotion and drive, and incoherence or poverty of thought are the dominant features. Delusions, hallucinations, passivity, and catatonic symptoms all may persist, usually

with diminished intensity. The diagnostic criteria for **residual type** include a history of at least one previous episode of schizophrenia with chronic psychotic symptoms, and a clinical picture without any prominent psychotic symptoms but continuing evidence of the illness (eg, blunted affect, social withdrawal, and poverty of thought).

Differential diagnosis: Altered states of consciousness are rare in schizophrenia. However, when this occurs accompanied by a clustering of schizophrenic symptoms, it may indicate an organic cerebral etiology caused by toxic (drug, metabolic, infection) or other organic factors. The organic delusional symptoms associated with amphetamines, cocaine, and phencyclidine should be considered particularly. Paranoid disorders are usually distinguished from schizophrenia by the absence of prominent hallucinations, incoherence, or bizarre delusions.

DSM-III asserts that affective symptoms are consistent with the diagnosis of schizophrenia and that schizophrenic symptoms are consistent with the diagnosis of affective disorders. The distinction for syndromes with both kinds of symptoms rests upon course. **Schizoaffective disorder** (see also Ch. 141) should be diagnosed whenever the clinician is unable to make a differential diagnosis between schizophrenia and affective disorders. The diagnosis of schizoaffective disorder is to be used when there is an episode of affective illness in which preoccupation with mood-incongruent delusions or hallucinations (persecutory delusions, bizarre delusions) dominates the clinical picture and when affective symptoms are no longer present. DSM-III's use of the diagnoses of **schizophreniform syndromes, brief reactive psychoses,** and **borderline** or **schizotypal personality disorders** are described in the introduction to this chapter.

Prognosis

Schizophrenia is not necessarily a chronic disorder. About 30% of patients recover completely, and most of the remainder show some improvement. The florid symptoms can nearly always be controlled, but blunting of emotion and drive may remain intractable. Although even minor defects may impair personal relationships and work efficiency, partial remission is compatible with a reasonable life adjustment. With treatment, an active psychosis commonly is controlled within 4 to 8 wk, but residual defects of varying severity may persist for weeks or months before further improvement. Relapse is common unless adequate follow-up and medication intake are maintained. Acute exacerbations requiring therapeutic intervention often occur; residual impairment usually increases between episodes. A favorable prognosis is associated with good premorbid personality with adequate social functioning, the presence of precipitating events, abrupt onset, onset late in life, a clinical picture that includes confusion or perplexity, and a family history of affective disorder.

Treatment

The mainstays of treatment are chemotherapy, the development of a therapeutic relationship with a skilled counselor, social support, and graded rehabilitation and retraining. For a first illness or an acute relapse, **hospitalization,** even if involuntary, is usually indicated to stabilize the patient on a suitable chemotherapeutic regimen; to ensure the physical safety of the patient or other persons; to prevent damage to finances, work prospects, or personal relationships; and to relieve the family. Although most states have enacted legal restrictions insisting that hospitalization take place only on the basis of the patient's being dangerous to himself or to others, the prevailing practice remains dependent on the psychiatrist's clinical judgment of the necessity for hospitalization. However, since schizophrenic patients are readily susceptible to institutionalism and since family ties are loosened by prolonged separation, hospitalization for more than a few months is harmful unless the severity of the illness makes it essential or it is part of an active rehabilitation program.

The onset of schizophrenic behavior in the **adolescent** period often makes it difficult to reach a clear diagnosis. Atypical depressions, anxiety states, identity confusion, and

most particularly drug abuse and alcohol, may mask, herald, or compound the onset of the psychosis. In the adolescent, when the illness is identified, it is most important to engage those involved in the patient's social network in order that they be properly informed and supported and become ready to cooperate in the care of the patient. These include not only the parent and siblings but teachers, counselors, employers, etc.

Chemotherapy: (See also ANTIPSYCHOTIC DRUGS in Ch. 281.) The rapid neuroleptization methods used for the management of **acute psychotic episodes** have not improved outcome. Currently, management has become more conservative. A highly disturbed or distressed patient can be given haloperidol 5 to 10 mg orally or IM q 4 to 6 h until the acute episode subsides. The various antipsychotic medications are equally effective in equivalent doses. Choice of drug must be based on side effects. Low potency drugs like chlorpromazine pose the risk of orthostasis and sedation; high potency drugs, such as haloperidol, may cause extrapyramidal syndromes. Oral chlorpromazine 200 to 500 mg/day or an equivalent dose of another antipsychotic drug is given initially or after the parenteral drugs. However, both high and low potency neuroleptics can cause extrapyramidal symptoms.

Antiparkinsonian drugs are prescribed now only when extrapyramidal symptoms become manifest or if the risk of extrapyramidal symptomatology is great. The prophylactic use of antiparkinsonian drugs is indicated when the medical risk of certain complications (eg, respiratory distress) is present, or when patients have reacted adversely to neuroleptic medication in the past. Usually, antiparkinsonian drugs are given for a short period of time, perhaps < 10 days, but in some instances with continuing parkinsonism, the use may be extended. Since antiparkinsonian agents are not without potential toxicity, periodic attempts to discontinue them are warranted.

The clinical efficiency and side effects of the butyrophenones, thioxanthenes, dihydroindolones, and dibenzoxazepines are the same as those of the phenothiazines. (For adverse effects of phenothiazine administration, including tardive dyskinesia and the neuroleptic malignant syndrome, see ANTIPSYCHOTIC DRUGS in Ch. 281.) The full dosages of antipsychotic medication given to younger patients are liable to cause marked side effects and are rarely required. Elderly patients (> 65 yr) are particularly prone to the full panoply of toxicities, including orthostasis, urinary retention, and parkinsonism. For this reason and because of altered kinetics in the elderly, caution should be used in arriving at the appropriate, generally lower, dosage.

Many schizophrenic patients will not continue to take oral antipsychotic medication. Long-acting depot injections of fluphenazine enanthate or decanoate or haloperidol decanoate are, therefore, often preferred for maintenance treatment, and they reduce the risk of relapse. Depot fluphenazine is given IM or s.c. in 25- to 37.5-mg doses every 2, 3, or 4 wk from the onset of treatment. Haloperidol decanoate is given 50 to 150 mg every 3 to 4 wk. Depot therapy requires backup facilities. Recently, special medication clinics have been established, and nurses have been trained to give defaulting patients their injections at home.

With rapid and complete recovery from an acute episode, drug treatment need not be continued for more than 3 to 6 mo after recovery. In more serious forms of illness, drugs should be continued for 2 to 3 yr, and some patients may require antipsychotic medication indefinitely. A general rule of thumb of maintenance medication is to continue the patient at 1/3 to 1/5 of the dosage he has required during the acute phase of his psychosis. The maintenance phase should be continued for 3 to 6 mo after discharge and tapered slowly for a trial period. Periods of stress (family discord, job difficulties, emotional losses, physical illness) may require reinstitution of medication. Depressive periods due to personal problems or a primary affective swing are not uncommon in otherwise well-controlled schizophrenics and require appropriate counseling and perhaps the prescribing of an antidepressant drug such as amitriptyline or imipramine.

Electroconvulsive therapy (ECT): In catatonic patients or those with severe depression, elation, or excitement, ECT accelerates the response to antipsychotic drugs; 4 to 10 treatments may be required. Controlled trials comparing ECT with neuroleptics show no advantage for ECT. In essence, ECT has limited usefulness.

Psychotherapy, counseling, and social management: Working with the patient and his family helps to alleviate distress and problems of work and personal relationships, to establish patterns of readjustment, and to uncover and work out stresses precipitating schizophrenic episodes. Depth or analytic psychotherapy is not indicated, but establishing a therapeutic relationship with frequent discussions and the therapist's patient concern and interest, is essential. In the initial stages (except rarely when there is no alternative) the therapist should not argue or flatly deny the reality of the patient's psychotic beliefs. Agreeing with the patient, on the other hand, risks compounding and reinforcing such beliefs. A neutral attitude may be achieved by focusing discussions on problems (including the patient's distress) to which the beliefs have given rise. With increasing insight, simple interpretation of certain ideas may be discussed.

Occupational therapy and graded social involvement should be arranged. For those who are more disabled, a comprehensive structured rehabilitation program including employment retraining may be planned. The needs of the family should be considered, and a trained social worker may be helpful.

Primary in the care of chronic schizophrenics is careful control of environmental pressure. Overstimulation (in the form of high expectancies, high emotional involvement with relatives, or excessive work loads) can cause either a florid exacerbation of symptoms or autistic withdrawal. Understimulation may occur in the home, particularly with overprotective parents, and in the hospital (institutionalism). In evaluating the handicaps of a chronic schizophrenic patient, it is good practice to assume, in order to avoid therapeutic nihilism, that secondary handicaps from over- or understimulation are present and outweigh the primary defects of the illness. Individual psychotherapy combined with appropriate family and milieu therapy helps foster direct, forthright, and less stressful communication between the patient and his world.

The number of self-help/mutual-aid groups of spouse, parents, and children has greatly increased, and these groups contribute to the reduction of shame, guilt, and fear through their concerted efforts to help members support each other, reduce myth and misinformation, and promote hope. The range of treatments that focus on practical help for patients and their families in managing everyday problems includes family management (the patient's family is encouraged to keep stress in the home minimal); hiring neighbors to look after schizophrenics; 24-h crisis teams; and the use of protected environments, in which sheltered jobs and living space for schizophrenics leaving hospitals are made available.

143. PARANOID DISORDERS

States of heightened self-awareness with a marked tendency to self-reference and projection of the patient's own ideas to others. In common usage "paranoid" implies persecutory ideas or attitudes held by the patient.

Paranoid states range imperceptibly from a circumscribed delusional system with no impairment of affect or associative processes, to the more complete disorganization seen in paranoid schizophrenia. This is reflected in inadequate affective responses, increasingly disorganized associations, and symbolization and projection of mental material as hallucinations.

Etiology, Symptoms, and Signs

The personality that spawns a paranoid illness reflects a need to shield sensitive portions of inner life, a hunger for recognition, and the fears and guilt feelings these

conflicts and strivings evoke. Sexual conflicts, often unconscious, may be operative, and homosexual tendencies are often noted. The paranoid patient characteristically has a tense and expectant affective state that stimulates his attention; he sees connections where none exist and at times rationalizes his concepts into an extensive delusional system.

Brief paranoid states: These states, which are often of a psychotic intensity, are reactive illnesses in persons whose personalities are characterized by extreme sensitivity, insecurity, inferiority, and suspiciousness. Isolation from social contact and physical problems (eg, deafness) often are exacerbating factors, and alcoholism is commonly involved. In acute and chronic brain syndromes, the impaired comprehension and dulling of consciousness favor paranoid interpretations and delusions.

Usually, these disorders are of < 6 mo duration. The onset generally is quite sudden, and the condition rarely becomes chronic.

Paranoid psychosis: Typically, a highly elaborated delusional system gradually develops without hallucinations, disorganization of thinking, or other characteristic schizophrenic symptoms. A few patients, however, eventually progress into frank schizophrenic illness. In one form of paranoid psychosis, core symptoms center on some minor real or imagined physical defect. The patient delusionally misinterprets facial expressions or overheard scraps of conversation as confirming his belief that he is discriminated against because of this defect. In other patients, a trivial or illusory asymmetry of face or enlargement of the nose is the focus for a paranoid system. Such patients may trail from specialist to specialist incessantly demanding plastic surgery. Real or imagined slights or injustices may lead to never-ending litigation, or religious fanaticism may insidiously progress to grandiose but encapsulated messianic beliefs.

In one dangerous form of paranoid psychosis, delusional sexual jealousy is the central theme. Jealousy has a complex psychopathology, and morbid jealousy **(Othello syndrome)** occurs in a variety of conditions, including paranoid states. A primary depression may underlie the illness. The patient's anguish over delusions of his spouse's infidelity is readily converted to rage. The patient may unceasingly make accusations, spy upon or follow his spouse, examine undergarments for seminal stains, and misinterpret simple actions, such as the way a curtain is drawn, as a message to the lover. He may demand confession constantly and assert that forgiveness will ensue. Physical assault is a real danger.

A persecutory delusional system may develop as a result of a close relationship with another person who already has a disorder with persecutory delusions. This type of induction psychosis is a result of sharing the delusions of the dominant person. In the past this disorder has been termed **"folie à deux."** In rare instances more than 2 persons may be involved. The prognosis for what is now called **shared paranoid disorder** is a function of the emotional strength of the person in whom the psychosis has been induced.

Symptoms and Signs

The history may show that, as a child, the patient needed special appreciation, was moody, resented school and parental discipline, could not form good play adjustments, and was suspicious. While growing up, the rigidity and tendency to pride may have increased, as well as the patient's sensitivity to others' attitudes toward him. Before the psychosis becomes manifest, prodromal symptoms may occur. The patient may have reacted to numerous situations with wounded and bitter pride. He overanalyzes his moods and sensations, may become hypochondriacal, is reserved, and withdraws in disdain from discussing his problems. Gradually, the idea may be born that his failures have been due to the enmity of others, and he sees new and hidden significance in commonplace events, leading to the belief that people deliberately slight him and that his situation is endangered. He experiences vague fears, becomes increasingly resentful, and defends his suspicions vigorously. Hallucinations may or may not occur.

Patients with classic paranoia or reactions closely approximating it probably never recover; however, they do not necessarily deteriorate and may not require hospitalization. If their conduct remains within bounds, society may view them as "cranks." However, some patients who at first appear to be suffering from circumscribed paranoid psychoses are later recognized to be schizophrenic.

Diagnosis

In contrast to mania, paranoid ideas are more sustained and are supported by a less changeable affect than manic vacillations. The mental operations are exaggerations of normal mechanisms, and differentiating patients with paranoid psychoses from nonpsychotic patients with extremely paranoid embittered personalities can be difficult. A patient is psychotic if the reaction is continuous, if his beliefs cannot be corrected, if they tend to spread, and if they are completely illogical and cause major functional impairment. These reactions can be classified as approximating either the paranoid or the schizophrenic pole by evaluating the degree of disturbance in the individual's contact with reality; the more the repressed material comes into consciousness as delusions and hallucinations and the more archaic the form of adjustment, the nearer the reaction approaches schizophrenia.

The rapid development of a paranoid illness, particularly in a previously well-adjusted personality, should lead to a very careful clinical assessment and investigations to exclude an underlying organic disorder due to systemic illness (eg, hypothyroidism), brain disease (eg, neurosyphilis), or drug toxicity (eg, amphetamines).

Treatment

Whether the patient should be hospitalized is determined by his potential danger to himself and to others. If delusions are directed against specific persons, confinement probably is necessary; the greater the expressed hatred, the more imperative is commitment. (See also the discussion of commitment under treatment of schizophrenia, above, and in Ch. 133.) Establishing a relationship with the patient is a vital step; psychotherapy then will alleviate distress and often modify behavior, even though essential delusional thinking is unaltered. In dealing with paranoid patients, honesty and truthfulness are necessary. The patient's concerns should be discussed, and the therapist should try to express an understanding of the patient's point of view, without agreeing with his delusions or belittling or strongly contradicting them. Often the patient will follow reasonable suggestions and greatly modify his behavior. The physician may become the patient's one confidant and can help him by being tolerant and combining a philosophic detachment with sympathetic humility, discretion, understanding, warmth, and a sense of humor about his own possible ineptness as well as the patient's peccadilloes. Thus, at least temporary serenity may be achieved by helping the paranoid patient to achieve a calmer environmental adjustment. The physician also can aid in unraveling family problems or irritating work situations.

Phenothiazines and other neuroleptic drugs, as described above for schizophrenia, are helpful and often minimize symptoms, though complete remission is uncommon even after prolonged drug treatment. In morbid jealousy, phenothiazines are most effective when onset was not insidious. However, it is difficult to persuade patients with this illness to undergo prolonged treatment.

---

144. SUICIDAL BEHAVIOR

(See also Chs. 141 and 201)

Suicidal behavior includes both completed and attempted suicide. An **attempted suicide** is a suicidal act that was not fatal, possibly because the self-destructive intention was slight, vague, or ambiguous. Most persons who attempt suicide are ambiva-

lent about their wish to die, and the attempt may result from a strong wish to live and a need to communicate a plea for help. When suicide plans and actions appear unlikely to succeed, they are often termed **suicide gestures** and are predominantly communicative in nature. However, a suicide gesture should not be dismissed lightly; it is an important cry for help and requires thorough evaluation and treatment aimed at relief of misery and prevention of further attempts, especially since 1 in 5 of those persons who attempt suicide repeats the attempt within a year, and 1 in 10 finally takes his or her life. **Completed suicides** differ in many respects from attempted suicides; the differences are discussed below. However, the distinction is not absolute, since attempted suicides also include acts by persons whose determination to die is thwarted only because they are discovered early and resuscitated effectively, and since a suicide attempt may be fatal by miscalculation.

The discussion in this chapter is based on the above categorization. However, a distinction also can be made between **direct destructive behavior** (which usually includes 3 distinctly different groups of phenomena: suicidal thoughts, suicide attempts, and completed suicides) and **indirect self-destructive behavior** (characterized by taking a life-threatening risk without an intention of dying, generally repeatedly, and often unconsciously in such a way that the consequences are ultimately likely to be destructive to the individual). This latter behavior covers a wide variety of phenomena; eg, excessive drinking and drug use, heavy smoking, overeating, neglect of one's health, self-mutilation, polysurgical addiction, hunger strikes, criminal behavior, and deviant traffic behavior.

Incidence

Statistics on suicidal behavior are based mainly on verdicts recorded on death certificates and at inquests, and they underestimate the true incidence. Even so, suicide ranks among the first 10 causes of death for adults in urban communities, and accounts for 10% of deaths between the ages of 25 and 34 and for 30% of deaths among university students. It is the third-ranking cause of death among adolescents (see also Ch. 201). Of the approximately 200,000 suicide attempts in the USA each year, 10% are successful. More than 70% of completed suicides are over 40 yr of age, and the incidence rises sharply above age 60, particularly for men. About 65% of attempted suicides are under the age of 40.

Attempted suicides account for about 20% of emergency medical admissions and for 10% of all medical admissions. Women make 2 to 3 times as many suicide attempts as men, but men are generally more successful in their attempts. Adolescent single girls are overrepresented among attempted suicides, and the incidence also is high among single men in their 30s. Several studies have found a higher incidence of suicides among the families of patients who have attempted suicide.

Marriage, for both sexes (particularly a secure relationship), is associated with a significantly low suicide rate; suicide attempts and completed suicide are higher among those alone because of separation, divorce, or death.

Among blacks, the suicide rate is lower than among whites, but suicide among black women has increased 80% in the last 20 yr. Among **American Indians** the rate has risen in recent years, and in some tribes it is 5 times the national average.

A number of suicides take place in **prisons,** particularly by young men who have not committed violent crimes. Hanging is the usual method, and the suicide is most likely to occur during the first week of incarceration. Hunger strikes accompanied by suicidal declarations, particularly among political prisoners, occur from time to time. Here, the intention to manipulate attitudes and behavior of others is at its most obvious. Self-injury and death are means to an end rather than goals. **Group suicides,** whether in large numbers or only involving two (as in lovers' or spouse suicides), represent extreme forms of identification with others. Suicides in large groups tend to occur in highly emotive settings that overcome the strong drive to self-preservation.

Professional persons, including lawyers, dentists, military men, and physicians, seem to have higher than average suicide rates. The physician rate is largely due to women physicians, whose annual rate of suicide is 4 times that of a matched general population. As for the suicide method, there is a high incidence of overdosage with drugs among both male and female physicians (as compared with the general population), possibly because of easy access and knowledge as to what constitutes a fatal dose. Of the medical specialties, the highest rate is among psychiatrists.

Suicide is less frequent among practicing members of most **religious groups** (particularly Roman Catholics), who are generally prohibited by their doctrines from taking their lives and are provided with close social bonds protecting against acts of self-destruction. The low rates that have been reported from Catholic countries are only in part due to a tendency of coroners to avoid verdicts of suicide; the rate appears to be actually reduced. However, religious affiliation and strong religious beliefs do not necessarily prevent impetuous, unpremeditated suicidal actions that occur in settings of frustration, anger, and despair.

Suicide notes are left by about 1 in 6 persons who complete suicide. The notes often refer to personal relationships and events that will follow the patient's death. In the elderly, they often express concern for those left behind, whereas in younger people they may be angry or even vindictive. In attempted suicides, a note indicates premeditation and a serious risk of repeated attempts and later, completed suicide.

Methods Used in Suicidal Acts

The choice of methods is determined both by cultural factors and the availability of the agent. The methods used also may reflect the seriousness of intention, since some (eg, jumping from heights) make survival virtually impossible, whereas others (eg, drug ingestion) provide a chance of being rescued. However, the use of a method that proves not to be fatal does not necessarily imply that the intention is less serious. A bizarre suicide method suggests an underlying psychosis.

Drug ingestion is the most frequent method used in suicide attempts. Barbiturates are used less often than before, while psychotropic drug use is increasing. Salicylate use has dropped from > 20% of cases to about 10%, with the more frequent prescribing of acetaminophen (a safer analgesic with regard to causing gastric irritation).

Two or more methods or a combination of drugs are used in about 20% of attempted suicides, increasing the risk of a fatal outcome, particularly when drugs with serious interactions are combined. Multiple drug ingestion makes it important to determine blood levels of all the possibilities when a patient is seen.

Violent methods such as shooting and hanging are uncommon among attempted suicides. Use of firearms has been the leading method of completed suicide in the USA for males, and the percentage has increased (from 58% in 1970 to 63% in 1980). For females the most frequent method in the past was poisoning, followed by firearms. However, as of 1980, the frequencies for females have reversed (firearms, 39%; poisoning, 27%).

Etiology

The psychologic mechanisms leading to suicidal behavior resemble those frequently implicated in other forms of self-destruction such as alcoholism, reckless driving, self-mutilation, and violent antisocial acts. Suicide is often the final act in a course of self-destructive behavior. Traumatic childhood experiences, particularly the distresses of a broken home or parental deprivation, are significantly more common among persons with a tendency to self-destructive behavior, perhaps because these persons are more likely to have serious difficulties establishing secure, meaningful relationships. Recent studies have shown an association between attempted suicide and the phenomena of battered wives and child abuse, reflecting a cycle of deprivation and violence within the family.

TABLE 144–1. HIGH SUICIDE RISK FACTORS

Personal and Social Factors	*Clinical Features and Symptoms*
Male sex	Depressive illness, especially at onset or toward end of illness
Age >55 yr	Marked motor agitation, reslessness, and anxiety
Recent separation, divorce, or widowhood	Marked feelings of guilt, inadequacy, and hopelessness; self-denigration or nihilistic delusion
Social isolation with real or imagined unsympathetic attitude of relatives or friends	Severe hypochondriacal preoccupations: delusion or near-delusional conviction of physical disease; eg, cancer, heart disease, or sexually transmitted disease
Impulsive, hostile personality	Command hallucinations
Personally significant anniversaries	Alcohol or drug abuse
History of suicide in family, or of affective disorder	Physical illness that is chronic, painful, or disabling, especially in patients who have previously enjoyed good health
Unemployment or financial difficulties, particularly if causing a drastic fall in economic status	Use of drugs (eg, reserpine) that can cause severe depression
Previous suicide attempt	
Detailed planning and taking precautions against being discovered	

Suicidal acts usually result from multiple and complex motivations. The principal causative factors (see also TABLE 144–1) include **mental disorders** (primarily depression), **social factors** (disappointment and loss), **personality abnormalities** (impulsivity and aggression), and **physical illnesses.** Often, one factor (commonly a disruption in important relationships) is the final straw. An aggressive component often is evident; when its distressing impact is considered, the act appears to be directed at other, significant persons. Homicide followed by suicide provides clear evidence of aggression, as does the high incidence of suicide among prisoners serving terms for violent crimes.

Depression causes over half of all attempted suicides, and although endogenous depression may be involved, in most cases the depression is reactive or neurotic. **Social factors** such as marital disharmony, broken and unhappy love affairs, disputes with parents among the young, and recent bereavements (particularly among the elderly) may precipitate the depression. Depression associated with **physical illness** may precipitate a suicide attempt, but physical disability, particularly if chronic or painful, is more commonly associated with completed suicide. Physical illness in the elderly, particularly serious, chronic, and painful illness, plays an important role in about 20% of suicides.

Among **schizophrenic** patients, suicide sometimes occurs, and in chronic schizophrenia may result from the phases of depression to which these patients are prone. The suicide method is usually bizarre and often violent. Attempted suicide is uncommon; i[illegible] may be the first gross sign of psychiatric disturbance, occurring in the early stages o[illegible] the illness, possibly when the patient becomes aware of the disorganization of hi[illegible] thought and volitional processes.

Alcohol predisposes to suicidal acts by aggravating the intensity of any depressiv[illegible] mood swing and by lowering self-control. About 30% of patients who attempt suicid[illegible] have consumed alcohol before the act, and about half of these were intoxicated at th[illegible] time. Since alcoholism itself, particularly "binge alcoholism," often causes deep fee[illegible] ings of remorse in the intervening periods, alcoholic patients are particularly suicide prone even when sober. In one follow-up study of alcoholics, 1 in 10 patients com

mitted suicide. Improved treatment facilities for alcoholics probably would reduce the suicide rate.

Organic brain disease in its acute form of **delirium** (which may be due to drugs, infection, heart failure, etc) or as **dementia** may be accompanied by emotional lability, when serious violent acts of self-injury may occur during a deep but transient depressive mood swing. Consciousness usually is impaired during the act, and the patient may have only a vague recollection of the event. **Epileptic** patients, especially those with temporal lobe epilepsy, frequently suffer brief but profound episodes of depression, which, together with the availability of drugs prescribed for their condition, put epileptic patients at a greater than normal risk of suicidal behavior.

Individuals with **personality disorders** are prone to attempted suicide, especially emotionally immature persons with a psychopathic personality, who tolerate frustration poorly and react to stress impetuously with violence and aggression. A history of excessive alcohol consumption, drug abuse, or criminal behavior is found sometimes. The large number of attempted suicides among separated or divorced persons may reflect an inability to form mature, lasting relationships as well as reflecting reduced social opportunity, loneliness, and depression. The precipitants in such cases are the stresses that inevitably result from the dissolution of even troubled relationships and the burdens of establishing new associations and life-styles. Another important aspect in attempted suicide is the element of "Russian roulette," in which the person decides to let fate determine the outcome. Some unstable persons find a source of excitement in this aspect of such perilous activities as reckless driving, dangerous sports, and other forms of toying with death.

Prevention of Suicide

Any suicide act or threat must be taken seriously. Although some attempted or completed suicides are a surprise and shock even to close relatives and associates, in most cases clear warnings are given, generally to relatives, friends, medical personnel, or volunteers in lay organizations offering a 24-h service to those in distress. Emergency suicide prevention centers attempt to identify the potentially suicidal person, maintain conversation, evaluate the risk, and offer help with immediate problems, usually calling upon others (family, physician, police) for urgent assistance in the crisis and trying to guide the suicidal person to appropriate facilities for follow-up assistance. Despite this logical approach to helping potentially suicidal individuals, no hard data indicate that it does reduce suicide incidence.

The average physician encounters 6 or more potential suicides in his office each year. More than half of suicides have consulted their physicians within the previous few months, and at least 20% have been under psychiatric care during the preceding year. Since depressive illness is a major cause of suicide, recognition and treatment of depression are the most important contributions a physician can make to suicide prevention. Each depressed patient should be questioned carefully about any thoughts of suicide. The fear is baseless that such inquiry, even in a tactful and sympathetic form, may implant the idea of self-destruction in the patient. The questioning aids the physician in obtaining a clearer picture of the depth of the depression, encourages constructive discussion, and conveys the physician's awareness of the patient's deep despair and hopelessness.

Features indicating a possibly high risk of suicide are shown in TABLE 144–1, above. Treatment of depression is outlined in Ch. 141. The risk of suicide is increased early in the treatment of depression, when retardation and indecisiveness are ameliorated but a depressed mood and feelings of gloom still persist. Early results of treatment may, therefore, enable the patient to set about self-destruction effectively in a state of only partially lifted depression. Psychotropic drugs must be prescribed carefully and in controlled amounts. Hypnotics used to treat insomnia in depressed patients are espe-

cially dangerous; insomnia may be a symptom of depression, and to treat it with drugs without treating the underlying depression is not only ineffective but highly dangerous.

For **dealing with an acute suicide threat** (eg, a patient who calls and declares that he is going to take a lethal dose of a drug or the person who threatens to jump from a height), only general advice can be given. In these situations the desire to die is ambivalent and often transient, and the physician or other person to whom the patient appeals for help must ally himself with the desire to live. The person threatening suicide is in an immediate crisis, and the physician should offer hope that it can be resolved. Emergency psychologic aid may be provided by (1) establishing a relationship and open communication with the patient; (2) reminding him of his identity (ie, using his name repeatedly) and helping him identify the problem that has brought on the crisis; (3) offering constructive help with the problem and encouraging the patient to constructive action; (4) involving the patient's family and friends, reminding the patient that others care for him and want to help.

If a patient calls to say that he has already committed a suicidal act (eg, taken a drug or turned on the gas) or is in the process, his address should be obtained, if possible, and someone else should contact the police at once to trace the call and rescue the patient. He should be kept talking on the telephone until the police arrive.

A comprehensive follow-up service providing adequate psychiatric and social aftercare is, at present, the best means of reducing further suicide attempts and completed suicide. Since many successful suicides have a previous history of suicidal attempts, a psychiatric assessment (see below) is important for *all* patients as soon as feasible after a suicide attempt. This defines the problems that contributed to the act and permits appropriate treatment to be planned.

Management of Attempted Suicide

Many attempted suicides are admitted to a hospital emergency ward in a comatose state. The usual management of a comatose patient is discussed in Ch. 118. When it is certain that the patient has ingested an overdose of a hypnotic, sedative, tranquilizer, or antidepressant, it is important to (1) remove the poison from the patient, attempting to prevent absorption and expedite excretion; (2) institute symptomatic treatment to keep the patient alive; and (3) administer any known antidote if the specific drug ingested can be firmly identified (see Ch. 289). Every case of life-threatening self-injury should be hospitalized both to treat the physical injury and for psychiatric assessment. Most patients are well enough to be discharged as soon as the physical injury is treated, but *all should be offered follow-up care* (see below; and under Prevention of Suicide, above).

Psychiatric assessment is made immediately after a suicide attempt, and at this time the patient may deny any problems. Not uncommonly, the severe depression that led to the suicidal act is followed by a short-lived mood elevation, a cathartic effect probably responsible for the finding that further suicide attempts are rare immediately after the initial attempt. Nevertheless, the risk of later, completed suicide is high unless the patient's problems are resolved. The patient needs a secure, strong source of help, which begins when the physician provides sympathetic attention and clear indications of his concern and commitment as well as his understanding of the patient's troubled feelings.

Steps in the psychiatric assessment: (1) establishment of rapport; (2) understanding the suicide attempt, its background, the events preceding it, and the circumstances in which it occurred; (3) appreciation of the current difficulties and problems; (4) thorough understanding of personal and family relationships, which often are pertinent to the suicide attempt; (5) full assessment of the patient's mental state, with particular emphasis on the recognition of depression, alcohol or drug abuse, and mental illness,

which require specific treatment in addition to crisis intervention; (6) an interview with the spouse, close relative, or friend, and contact with the family physician.

Involvement of nonmedical personnel trained in the management of suicidal behavior can provide an effective team to cope with most suicidal patients. Whether all attempted suicides must be seen by a psychiatrist, or could be satisfactorily dealt with by a trained nurse or social worker, remains a controversial issue.

Hospitalization: Duration of stay and the kind of treatment required vary. Patients with psychotic illness, organic brain disease, or epilepsy, and some with severe depression whose crisis situation has not resolved, should be admitted to a psychiatric unit for continued supervision until their underlying problems are resolved or they can cope with the problems. The role of the patient's family physician after a suicide attempt is central. If he is not in charge of the case, he should be kept fully informed and given specific suggestions for follow-up care.

Impact of Suicide on Others

Any suicidal act has a marked emotional impact on the associated persons. The completed suicide, especially, leaves physician, family, and friends with strong feelings, which include guilt, shame, and remorse at not having prevented the latest attempt, as well as anger, directed toward the suicide or others. However, the physician must realize that neither he nor the patient's family are omniscient or omnipotent and that the patient's eventual successful suicide was ultimately not preventable. The physician also should recognize that he has the remaining important task of helping the suicide's family and friends deal with their guilt feelings and sorrow.

The impact of attempted suicide on the associated persons is similar in nature to that produced by the completed suicide, but with the important difference that the opportunity remains to resolve these feelings by recognizing and responding appropriately to the "cry for help."

---

145. PSYCHIATRIC EMERGENCIES

An emergency may be created as much by circumstances as by an event. Behavior that excites comment and action in a public place may be tolerated in the home and regarded as hardly worthy of comment in a psychiatric ward. For the purposes of this chapter the circumstances are those of a general practitioner's office, an emergency ward, or a medical ward. Optimally, the setting should provide privacy, safety, and security for both patient and physician.

Obtaining a good history in an emergency may be impossible, and accounts given by excited relatives or bystanders can be biased or colored by personal involvement in the dramatic and unusual situation. At times, attention to the emotional concerns and needs of family is essential. In some emergencies diagnosis is critical to decision-making, but in others a symptom such as excitement or aggression constitutes the emergency, and diagnosis may have to await its control.

The term **acute psychosis** has been used to characterize certain disorders with impaired capacity to process information. Some cases involve organic abnormalities (eg, delirium—see below and in Ch. 118). Other cases, with unknown causes, are often called **acute functional psychosis** (eg, acute schizophrenia or acute mania)—for their management, see Chs. 141 or 142.

Panic; Anxiety Attacks (see also in Ch. 140)

In battle and in periods of civil catastrophe, anxiety is a normal state, but individuals who are subjected to particularly severe stress or who are perhaps especially

vulnerable can be incapacitated by terror. They may manifest tremors or dissociative symptoms and bizarre or dangerous behavior. Sedation is valuable, and a tactical withdrawal from the stressful situation for a few days is helpful. Prolonged withdrawal, however, is associated with a considerable risk of chronicity.

In less stressful situations, attacks of acute anxiety occur in susceptible patients; a phobic anxiety state commonly underlies those attacks. Many anxiety attacks are so brief that the acute phase is over before the patient can reach a doctor. In most cases the anxiety is generalized, but diagnostic problems can arise if various body systems are affected to different degrees, so that cardiovascular manifestations are prominent in one patient and GI symptoms in another. If **overbreathing (hyperventilation)** is the salient feature, the patient may complain of dizziness, lose consciousness, or show signs of tetany.

In everyday circumstances it may be difficult to determine what precipitated an anxiety attack, and advice to separate the patient from the anxiety-provoking situation often is gratuitous. Reassurance sometimes is sufficient to allay the patient's distress, and reassuring relatives and bystanders is helpful. If mild sedation is required, the benzodiazepines (eg, diazepam 5 to 10 mg or oxazepam 15 to 30 mg orally) usually are effective. In more disturbed patients diazepam 10 mg may be given IM or even IV. Major tranquilizers have no advantage over the benzodiazepines in these circumstances. It has been suggested that tricyclic or monoamine oxidase inhibitor (MAOI) antidepressants may prevent the occurrence of phobic anxiety states. Hyperventilation usually will stop if the patient's attention is drawn to it, and he is given quiet and supportive reassurance (see also RESPIRATORY ALKALOSIS in Ch. 84 and the discussion of psychogenic dyspnea in Ch. 31).

Delirium (see also Ch. 118)

Delirious patients are a common problem in medical and surgical wards. Acute delirium may be due to ingestion of drugs such as LSD or marijuana; overdose of prescribed medication; alcohol, barbiturate, or other drug withdrawal; electrolyte imbalance; metabolic disorders; infection; or seizures. Acute delirium also may occur as an idiosyncratic reaction to a normal dose of medicine, and is not uncommonly seen in situations of intense stress, such as cardiac care units.

Difficulties arise when a confused patient with impaired comprehension passively interferes with his medical treatment, or when a patient who becomes paranoid or delusional and begins to hallucinate becomes actively uncooperative and threatens or attacks the nursing staff or dismantles therapeutic equipment. Some patients are elated and overcheerful and disturb the ward by shouting and singing. Others are panic-stricken and may injure themselves in attempts to escape from imaginary persecutors.

Treatment of the cause of the delirium and good nursing care along with general measures to make the patient comfortable and keep him safe are needed. For example, keeping lights on during the night, and permitting someone known to the patient to stay with him are effective calming maneuvers. Often a major tranquilizer or diazepam orally or parenterally must be given urgently; the pharmacologic treatment is similar to that of an excited patient (see below).

Acute Memory Disturbances

Although disturbances of memory are most commonly organic (see Ch 118), memory loss that presents as an emergency usually is hysterical (see in Ch. 140). Patients with massive dissociation can no longer recall their identity or events of their past; language and knowledge of social customs generally survive. In hysterical pseudodementia, of which the Ganser syndrome is one example, cognitive functions are more profoundly dissociated, and regressive behavior results. In many of these patients a traumatic and often "shameful" event precedes the onset of the dissociation. The

patient's memory may return with quiet and persistent interviewing, but hypnosis or abreactive drugs such as amobarbital sodium IV (200 mg slowly infused usually is adequate) may be indicated. Other hysterical symptoms (eg, loss of vision, deafness, muteness, or paralysis) may require similar treatment.

Transient global amnesia (see in Ch. 118) creates similar difficulties and may be mistaken for hysterical amnesia. Remote memory is unaffected. There is no treatment for an attack of transient global amnesia; memory is recovered spontaneously in a few hours.

Dementia (see in Ch. 118) rarely presents as an emergency but may create one. A solitary patient who has been quietly deteriorating for months or years may be found in a state of indescribable squalor and neglect or may be brought to a doctor's office or emergency ward with no history and no informant.

Stupor (see also IMPAIRED CONSCIOUSNESS in Ch. 118)

Unconsciousness is always an emergency, and in some psychiatric disorders the degree of withdrawal is so substantial that a noncommunicative and unresponsive patient appears unconscious. The symptom of **catatonia** may be associated with organic brain disease such as carbon monoxide intoxication, encephalitis lethargica, and brain tumors. This condition may also occur in catatonic schizophrenia, severe depressive illness, and hysteria. If a history is available from a friend or relative, earlier characteristic symptoms may indicate the diagnosis, but great care must be taken to ensure that organic causes are not overlooked. Amobarbital sodium IV (200 mg slowly infused usually is adequate) is useful diagnostically in distinguishing hysterical, catatonic, and organic states; may relieve hysterical stupors; and often leads to a temporary remission in catatonic stupor. The technic should be used only by those with specific training and experience. Both catatonic and depressive stupor respond to ECT.

Excitement, Anger, and Aggression

Although excitement, anger, and their physical concomitant, aggression, occur in a wide range of psychiatric disorders (schizophrenia, mania, psychopathy, and, rarely, in temporal lobe lesions including epilepsy and delirium), the precise diagnosis may be academic if the patient is disturbed and violent. Calm words may not stem the patient's wrath, but meeting his anger with further anger will only aggravate the situation. Violent and potentially violent patients are secured as soon as the diagnosis is made or suspected.

An attempt to persuade the patient to take medication should be made; eg, diazepam 5 to 40 mg or haloperidol 5 to 10 mg orally. However, in most cases a parenteral route will be necessary, despite the patient's verbal and physical objections. This raises medico-legal questions, and physicians should be familiar with laws and regulations that apply in their locations to the management (including commitment) of acutely disturbed patients. Consultation with a psychiatrist or appropriate judicial authority will help protect the patient and the physician. Once the decision to give an injection has been made, adequate forces should be mustered; in all cases security personnel are required. Once the patient has been secured, a major neuroleptic, such as haloperidol 5 to 10 mg, should be injected in the properly restrained patient as carefully as it would be in any other individual. The injection may be repeated hourly or more frequently until there is a satisfactory reduction of symptoms, or oversedation or other serious side effects intervene. Total dosage varies greatly for different individuals, but failure to respond to 50 mg on the first day calls for reevaluation of the diagnosis. Six to 12 h after control is achieved, the patient may be given haloperidol orally, with the dosage based on the patient's individual needs. With this treatment, side effects (especially acute dystonic reactions) are common. They may be prevented by giving oral benztropine 1 to 2 mg bid.

Suicide (see Ch. 144, above)

§13. GENITOURINARY DISORDERS

146. CLINICAL EVALUATION OF GENITOURINARY DISORDERS

Symptoms of GU disorders may be nonspecific, but careful acquisition and analysis of data from the history, physical examination, and appropriate laboratory studies should provide accurate diagnosis.

A family history of renal disease in an adult may suggest polycystic disease or, if associated with ear and eye disorders, may indicate other hereditary nephropathy. A history of recent infectious diseases involving the skin, respiratory tract, or endocardium is helpful in evaluating possible causes of glomerulonephritis. A specific history of renal disease, trauma to the urinary system, stones, or prior urinary system surgery is important, as is a previous history of hypertension or a systemic disease known to affect the kidney (eg, diabetes mellitus, SLE). The clinical approach to such data is discussed here; specific disorders are discussed separately in the following chapters.

SYMPTOMS AND SIGNS

Fever, weight loss, and malaise are common. The presence of fever plus UTI symptoms helps evaluate the site of infection. Simple acute cystitis is afebrile; acute pyelonephritis or prostatitis usually produces high fever. Renal carcinoma occasionally is associated with fever. Weight loss is to be expected in the advanced stages of cancer but also may be noticed with renal insufficiency from any cause.

Changes in Micturition

Most people void about 4 to 6 times/day, mostly in the daytime. **Frequency** (*frequent micturition*), unassociated with an increase in urine volume, is a symptom of lessened bladder effective filling capacity. Infection, foreign bodies, stones, or tumor may injure the bladder mucosa or underlying structures, leading to inflammatory infiltration and edema. Mild stretching of the bladder and a loss of bladder elasticity results, producing a functional decrease, pain, and **urgency** (*a compelling need to urinate*). Involuntary urination may occur if voiding is not immediate. Voidings usually are small in volume

and the desire to urinate may be felt as almost constant **urinary tenesmus** (*painful straining*) until the irritative process resolves. **Dysuria** (*painful urination*) suggests irritation or inflammation in the bladder neck or urethra, usually due to bacterial infection. Persistent symptoms in the absence of such infection require careful evaluation of the bladder and urethra. **Nocturia** (*voiding during the night*) is an abnormal, but nonspecific, symptom, which may reflect early renal disease with a decrease in concentrating capacity but is commonly associated with cardiac and hepatic failure without evidence of intrinsic urinary system disease. Nocturia also may occur without disease; eg, as a result of excessive fluid intake in the late evening or from urine retention secondary to bladder neck obstruction (eg, prostatism). **Enuresis** (*bed-wetting at night*) is physiologic during the first 2 or 3 yr of life but becomes an increasing problem after that age. It may be produced by delayed neuromuscular maturation of the lower urinary tract, or it may indicate organic disease; eg, infection or distal urethral stenosis in girls, posterior urethral valves in boys, or neurogenic bladder. (See also Ch. 159 and BEHAVIORAL PROBLEMS in Ch. 188.)

Hesitancy, straining, decrease in force and caliber of the urinary stream, and terminal dribbling are common symptoms of obstructions distal to the bladder. In men, these are most commonly associated with prostatic obstruction, less often with urethral stricture. Similar symptoms in a male child suggest posterior urethral valves, congenital urethral stricture, or meatal stenosis. In women these symptoms suggest meatal stenosis.

Incontinence (*a loss of urine without warning*—see also Ch. 159) is associated with exstrophy of the bladder, epispadias, vesicovaginal fistula, ectopic ureteral orifices, congenital or acquired neurogenic (peripheral neuropathy, stroke, dementia) bladder dysfunction, as well as injuries sustained during prostatectomy or childbirth. In women, incontinence with mild physical stress such as coughing, laughing, running, or lifting is commonly associated with a cystocele as a result of aging or stretching of pelvic floor muscles following childbirth. Loss of urine due to bladder outlet obstruction or a flaccid bladder may produce **overflow incontinence** when the intravesicular pressure exceeds outlet resistance. Residual urine always is present with overflow incontinence.

Pneumaturia (*the passage of gas in the urine*), a rare symptom, usually indicates a fistula between the urinary tract and the bowel. This may be a complication of diverticulitis, with abscess formation, enterocolitis, carcinoma of the colon, or vesicovaginal fistula. Rarely, pneumaturia may be due to gas formation from bacteriuria alone. **Chyluria** is *lymph in urine* produced by rupture of a lymph vessel, chiefly due to obstruction from filariasis.

Changes in Urinary Output

Normally, adults void between 700 and 2000 mL daily. Impairment in renal concentrating capacity may occur with many forms of renal disease and may cause **polyuria** (*a daily urine volume > 2500 mL*—see also TABLE 88–3 in Ch. 88). **Oliguria** (*< 500 mL/day*) tends to be acute and may be due to decreased renal perfusion (prerenal factors), ureteral or bladder outlet obstruction (postrenal factors), or primary renal disease. **Persistent anuria** (*< 100 mL/day*) always is associated with uremia, and may signal acute renal failure or the end stage of chronic progressive renal insufficiency. Since anuria also can be due to urinary obstruction that may be reversible, this possibility must be ruled out when acute anuria occurs.

Changes in the Appearance of Urine

Urine may be clear during water diuresis or may be a deep yellow color due to the presence of chromogens (eg, urobilin) when maximally concentrated. If excretion of food pigments (usually red in color) or drugs (brown, black, blue, green, or red) can be excluded, colors other than yellow suggest the presence of disease such as hematuria,

hemoglobinuria, myoglobinuria, pyuria, porphyria, or melanoma. Urine frequently appears cloudy, suggesting pyuria due to a urinary tract inflammation, but this is more commonly due to precipitated amorphous phosphate salts in an alkaline urine. Microscopy of the urine sediment and chemical analysis of the urine usually identify the cause.

Hematuria (*blood in the urine*) can produce red to brown discoloration depending on the amount of blood present and the acidity of the urine. Slight hematuria may cause no discoloration and be detected only by chemical testing or microscopic examination. When hematuria is noted, the presence or absence of pain related to the urinary system is important. Hematuria without pain usually is due to renal, vesical, or prostatic disease. In the absence of RBC casts (which indicate glomerulonephritis), silent hematuria may be caused by bladder or kidney tumor. Such tumors usually bleed intermittently, and complacency must not occur if the bleeding stops spontaneously. Other causes of asymptomatic hematuria include stones, polycystic disease, renal cysts, sickle cell disease, hydronephrosis, and benign prostatic hyperplasia. When discomfort such as renal colic accompanies hematuria, a ureteral stone is suggested, although a clot from renal bleeding could cause the same type of pain. Hematuria with dysuria also is associated with bladder infections or lithiasis.

Milky urine may be caused by precipitated phosphates in an alkaline urine. **Brick dust urine** usually is produced by precipitated urates in an acid urine.

Pain (see also renal colic in Ch. 160)

Pain related to renal disease usually is in the flank or back between the 12th rib and the iliac crest, with occasional radiation to the epigastrium. Stretching of the pain-sensitive renal capsule is the probable cause and may occur in any condition producing parenchymatous swelling, such as acute glomerulonephritis, pyelonephritis, or acute ureteral obstruction. There is often marked tenderness over the kidney in the costovertebral angle formed by the 12th rib and the lumbar spine. Inflammation or distention of the renal pelvis or ureter causes pain in the flank and hypochondrium, with radiation into the ipsilateral iliac fossa and often into the upper thigh, testicle, or labium. The pain is intermittent but does not completely remit between waves of colic.

The most common cause of **bladder pain** is bacterial cystitis, and the discomfort is usually suprapubic and referred to the distal urethra during urination. Acute urinary retention causes agonizing pain in the suprapubic area, but chronic urinary retention due to bladder neck obstruction or neurogenic bladder usually causes little discomfort.

Prostatic disease generally is painless, but with prostatitis a vague discomfort or fullness in the perineal or rectal area may be noted. On the other hand, **testicular pain** due to trauma or infection usually is severe and felt locally.

Edema

Edema usually represents excessive water and sodium in the extracellular space due to abnormal renal excretion, but it may be caused by cardiac, hepatic, or renal disease. Initially, the problem is evident only by an increase in weight, but later, edema becomes overt. Edema associated with renal disease may be noted first as facial puffiness rather than swelling in dependent or lower parts of the body, but this characteristic is neither essential nor specific. If fluid retention continues, **anasarca** (*generalized edema*) with fluid transudates (effusions) in the pleural and peritoneal cavities may be seen; it is most frequently associated with continuous, heavy proteinuria (the nephrotic syndrome).

Hematospermia

Fewer than 2% of urologic referrals are due to bloody semen. Most patients have repeated episodes of hematospermia, although some experience it just once. It is usually idiopathic but may be associated with prolonged sexual abstinence, frequent coitus, interrupted coitus, and bleeding disorders. Many urologists ascribe the symptoms

to seminal vesiculopathy as a result of some unidentified infection or vascular congestion. The disorder is benign and rarely associated with malignancy or serious infection. It is always useful, however, to evaluate such patients for prostatic infection or urethral strictures. Because the etiology is unknown in most cases, treatment is largely empiric. Some urologists advocate a 5- to 7-day trial of tetracycline 250 mg qid followed by gentle massage. In the absence of overt urologic disease, patients should be reassured that the problem is not serious or progressive.

Nonspecific Symptoms and Signs

Most patients with progressive decompensation of the urinary system are asymptomatic early in the process. However, when sufficient renal function is lost (GFR < 10% of normal), disturbances of multiple organ systems occur producing symptoms ascribable to **uremia** (*toxic condition associated with excessive accumulation in the blood of protein metabolism byproducts*). Weight loss, weakness, fatigue, dyspnea, anorexia, nausea and vomiting, itching, failure to grow, tetany, peripheral neuropathy, pericarditis, and convulsions are the usual symptoms and signs. Most of these can be ameliorated or reversed by dialysis or renal transplantation and good nutrition.

Hypertension in childhood occasionally is secondary to renal disease (vascular anomalies or occlusion, glomerulonephritis); progressive renal failure in children and adults usually produces hypertension. However, not more than 5% of adult hypertension is due to renovascular causes (with major renal artery or segmental artery obstruction and demonstrable increased renin secretion from the obstructed side).

The skin may show pallor, suggesting anemia, commonly associated with renal disease; excoriations, suggesting pruritus; and infections (eg, carbuncles or cellulitis), which may be due to glomerulonephritis. Occasionally, skin lesions from vasculitis or endocarditis are present, suggesting a possible cause of renal disease.

Examination of the **optic fundi** helps to evaluate vascular disease and may reveal hemorrhages, exudates, and papilledema. The **mouth** may reveal stomatitis or an ammoniacal odor; the **face, abdomen,** or **extremities,** edema. The finding by palpation of **enlarged kidneys, bladder,** or **prostate** is important in diagnosing urinary system disease.

DIAGNOSTIC PROCEDURES

In an otherwise asymptomatic patient, hypoproliferative anemia may be a clue to renal failure; but many other causes (such as neoplasia and systemic inflammatory diseases) must be excluded. Likewise, polycythemia may occur in renal cell carcinoma or polycystic disease, but more common causes should be considered first.

Serum chemistries often are abnormal when renal dysfunction is present, but the changes are nonspecific and may be produced by variations in renal blood flow **(RBF)** as well as by parenchymatous renal disease. Hypernatremia, for instance, is most frequently due to lack of adequate water intake in an obtunded patient but also can be produced by excessive water loss from a renal concentrating defect due to tubulointerstitial disease (eg, nephrogenic diabetes insipidus; hypercalcemic or potassium depletion nephropathy). As another example, the serum bicarbonate may be reduced as a consequence of metabolic acidosis due to renal disease, but other causes such as lactic acidosis or ketoacidosis must be excluded. The most specific serum chemical determination for the diagnosis of renal dysfunction is the serum creatinine (see Measurement of Renal Function, below).

Urinalysis

The best guide to intrinsic GU disease, urinalysis includes a qualitative evaluation for the presence of protein, glucose, ketones, blood, and nitrites; determination of the urinary pH; and microscopic examination of the sediment. The solute concentration of urine should be measured by either refractometry (sp gr) or osmometry (osmolarity).

Proteinuria (see also in NEPHROTIC SYNDROME, Ch. 150): Commercially available

dipsticks permit simple and rapid testing. The dipstick technic is sensitive to as little as 5 to 20 mg/dL of albumin, the predominant protein in most renal diseases, but is less sensitive to globulins and mucoproteins and may be negative in the presence of Bence Jones proteins (found in multiple myeloma or a related lymphoproliferative disorder). Electrophoresis, immunoelectrophoresis, and radioimmunoassays also are available to separate or quantitate various urinary proteins.

The major mechanisms producing proteinuria are (1) elevated plasma concentrations of normal or abnormal proteins ("overflow" proteinuria such as lysozymuria in myelomonocytic leukemia or Bence Jones proteinuria in multiple myeloma); (2) increased tubular cell secretion (Tamm-Horsfall proteinuria); (3) decreased tubular resorption of normal filtered proteins; and (4) an increase of filtered proteins caused by altered glomerular capillary permeability.

In most adults with proteinuria, the abnormality is first observed as an "isolated" finding during a routine physical examination in an asymptomatic subject who appears healthy and exhibits no evidence of systemic or renal disease. Daily total protein excretion usually is < 1 gm (urine protein/creatinine ratio < 0.1). Different qualitative patterns of proteinuria have been described although the correlation of these patterns with long-term prognosis is not well established. Two types of classification have been used, the first based on body posture: (1) Repetitive tests identify proteinuria as **"constant"** if it is present during recumbency and quiet upright ambulation, and **"orthostatic"** when it is present only in the upright position. (2) The pattern is **"intermittent"** if proteinuria comes and goes, and **"persistent"** if proteinuria is found in all urine samples examined. The exact significance of intermittent or orthostatic proteinuria is not clear; most patients do not show any deterioration of renal function and in about 50% the proteinuria ceases after several years. The presence of constant or persistent proteinuria is more serious. Although the course is indolent in the absence of other indicators of renal disease, such as microscopic hematuria, most patients continue to demonstrate proteinuria over many years; many develop an abnormal urine sediment and hypertension, and a few progress to renal failure.

When proteinuria is constant or persistent, quantitative measurements of protein excretion are useful for diagnosis and to follow patients' clinical progress. These are accomplished by measuring the total protein voided in a timed interval, usually 24 h; normally, < 150 mg/day of protein are excreted. Alternatively, a random sample of urine is used to relate the amount of protein present to its creatinine content. Normally, the protein/creatinine ratio is < 0.1. Heavy proteinuria (> 2 gm/sq m/day or a protein/creatinine ratio ≥ 3) usually is found in patients with glomerulopathy producing the nephrotic syndrome. Proteinuria usually is minimal, intermittent, or absent in diseases primarily involving the tubulointerstitial area (eg, pyelonephritis, analgesic nephropathy, benign nephrosclerosis, and nephropathies of hypercalcemia and potassium depletion).

Exercise proteinuria sometimes is seen in joggers, marathon runners, and boxers. It is accompanied by elevation of catecholamines; and hemoglobinuria, hematuria, or even myoglobinuria may be associated.

Glucosuria: Testing by dipstick is both specific and very sensitive, detecting as little as 100 mg/dL of glucose. The most common cause of glucosuria is diabetic hyperglycemia with normal renal glucose transport. However, if glucosuria persists with normal blood glucose concentrations, renal tubular dysfunction should be considered.

Ketonuria: The dipstick reagent is much more sensitive to acetoacetic acid than to acetone. The reagent does not react with β-hydroxybutyric acid. In most instances ketonuria is nonspecific, and acetoacetic acid, acetone, and β-hydroxybutyric acid are all excreted in the urine. Consequently, a test that principally determines one of these 3 compounds generally is satisfactory for the diagnosis of ketonuria. Ketonuria offers clues to the causes of metabolic acidosis. It is present in starvation, uncontrolled

diabetes mellitus, and occasionally in ethanol intoxication. It is not specific for intrinsic urinary system disease.

Hematuria: The dipstick reagent is sensitive to free Hb and myoglobin. A positive test in the absence of RBCs on microscopic examination suggests the presence of hemoglobinuria or myoglobinuria—an important clue to etiology in the patient with acute renal failure.

Nitrituria is determined by a dipstick test that uses the conversion of nitrate (derived from dietary metabolites) to nitrite by the action of certain bacteria in the urine. If nitrite is present, a pink color forms. Normally no detectable nitrite is present. When there is significant bacteriuria, the test will be positive in 80% of cases where the urine has incubated for at least 4 h in the bladder. Thus, a positive test is a reliable index of significant bacteriuria. However, a negative test should never be interpreted as indicating the absence of bacteriuria. At least 4 reasons exist for a negative test when bacteriuria is present: (1) insufficient bladder incubation time for conversion of nitrate to nitrite; (2) low urinary excretion of nitrate; (3) absence in some urinary pathogens of the enzymes to convert nitrate to nitrite; and (4) reduction of nitrates all the way to nitrogen by bacterial enzymes.

Urine pH: The dipstick is impregnated with various dyes that respond with different color changes to a pH in the range of 5 to 9. Although this test is routinely done, it neither identifies nor excludes patients with urinary system disease. However, it is often useful to aid in identifying various crystals that may be found in urine on microscopy. Specific pH testing of urine with a pH meter is critical in the diagnosis of the "distal" type of renal tubular acidosis where the diagnosis is suggested by a urine pH greater than 5.5 following an acid load. Patients with other types of renal disease usually can vary urinary pH in a relatively normal manner even though the quantitative capacity to excrete titratable acid and ammonia may be reduced.

Urine solute concentration: Osmolarity (*the total concentration of solutes in urine, expressed as mM/L of urine water*) is best determined by an osmometer. However, for most clinical purposes, the measurement of urinary sp gr or its refractive index may suffice because of the correlation between these measures and urinary osmolarity. The customary hydrometer (urinometer) has been superseded by the more accurate refractometer, which is calibrated in terms of sp gr as well as refractive index. Readings are easy and rapid and only a few drops of urine are needed. Although the correlation is not a linear one, it is satisfactory for clinical applications except when large amounts of glucose or high mol wt solutes such as protein or organic iodides (radiographic contrast chemicals) are present. In these situations sp gr and refractometry give abnormally high values in contrast to the lower osmolarity values.

Normal urine osmolarity varies between 50 to 1200 mOsm/L depending on the circulating titer of ADH and the rate of urinary solute excretion. Although the loss of urinary concentrating capacity is a sensitive test of renal dysfunction, the measurement of urine osmolarity (or sp gr) in a randomly voided urine is only helpful when it is > 700 mOsm/L (sp gr 1.020), as it excludes significant tubulointerstitial disease. Osmolarity values less than this may be normal or abnormal depending on the prior state of hydration. Proper use of this test as a measure of renal function is described under Measurement of Renal Function, below.

Urinary sediment examination: Normal urine contains a small number of cells and other formed elements shed from the entire length of the urinary system. With disease, these cells are increased and may help to localize the site and type of injury. Particulate elements in urine can be separated and concentrated by forcing urine through a membrane filter; the residue on the filter requires special staining technics for proper microscopic visualization but provides a permanent record. More commonly, 10 to 15 mL of freshly voided urine is centrifuged for 5 min at a slow speed (1500 rpm), and the

supernatant decanted. The sediment residue at the bottom of the centrifuge tube is best visualized in a special glass chamber of fixed volume, but an ordinary glass slide and coverslip will suffice. Using reduced light with the low-power objective, several fields are scanned to detect casts and cells. Then the light is increased, and with the high-power objective, specific cells and casts are identified. A semiquantitative estimation of the numbers of these formed elements is made by a per-high- or low-power field count (eg, 10 to 15 WBCs/high-power field **[hpf]**).

A classification of urinary formed elements is listed in TABLE 146–1. Voided urine in women contains genital tract cells. It is uncommon to observe more than one leukocyte, erythrocyte, or epithelial cell/hpf (400X) in a normal male, or more than 4 leukocytes/hpf in a normal female. An increased number of cells suggests urinary system disease. Excessive numbers of RBCs may indicate infection, tumor, stones, or inflammation. Excessive leukocytes may indicate infection or other inflammatory diseases. The finding of occasional bacteria in a centrifuged urine sediment is not necessarily evidence of a significant UTI. However, the finding of bacteria in an uncentrifuged *fresh* urine sample commonly is associated with urine cultures of $> 10^5$ organisms/mL of voided urine and suggests UTI rather than contamination. Crystals of various salts (oxalate, phosphate, urate) or drugs (eg, sulfonamides) may also be found when their concentrations and urinary pH exceed the limits of their solubility.

The finding of **casts** (*cylindrical masses of mucoprotein in which cellular elements, protein, or fat droplets may be entrapped*) in urine sediment is most important in distinguishing primary renal disease from diseases of the lower tract. The types of casts possible and the diseases with which they are associated are noted in TABLE 146–2. **RBC casts are virtually pathognomonic of glomerulonephritis** (exceptions are rare). Although **WBC casts** suggest pyelonephritis, they are specific only for the presence of tubulointerstitial inflammation and also are common in certain stages of proliferative glomerulonephritis. On the other hand, the rare **bacterial cast** is pathognomonic of bacterial pyelonephritis. **Renal cells with fat inclusions** are common with various types of tubulointerstitial disease; however, a large number of such cells and fatty casts rarely are present, except when the nephrotic syndrome exists. Lastly, the finding of **waxy** and **broad casts,** which are formed in the most distal parts of the nephron, suggests diffuse, widespread nephron involvement with tubular dilatation of residual nephrons and thus is common in far-advanced renal failure.

Although a thorough examination of fresh, unstained, properly prepared urine sediment usually will reveal to the expert all of the important diagnostic elements present, a **stained urine sediment** may speed and enhance recognition of certain morphologically similar elements in urine such as renal tubular cells and leukocytes. Special stains such as Sudan III also will clarify the presence of free and cellular fat globules. TABLE 146–3 lists some of the commonly used supravital stains and their characteristics.

Urine cultures. Collection of specimens (see also LOWER URINARY TRACT AND MALE GENITAL TRACT INFECTIONS in Ch. 153): To diagnose UTI, one must obtain a sample

TABLE 146–1. URINARY FORMED ELEMENTS

Cells from Blood	*Cells from GU System*	*Foreign Cells*	*Crystals*
Erythrocyte	Epithelial	Bacterial	Oxalate
Leukocyte	Renal tubular	Fungal	Phosphate
Plasmacyte	Transitional	Parasitic	Urate
	Squamous	Neoplastic	Drug
	Sperm		

(Modified from W. H. Chapman et al, *The Urinary System,* p. 236. Copyright 1973 by W. B. Saunders Company. Used with permission.)

TABLE 146–2. URINARY CASTS

Type	*Description*	*Significance*
Plain cast		
Hyaline	Mucoprotein matrix secreted by tubules	Nonspecific; present in normal urine but increased numbers when urine flow is low
Waxy	Matrix contains serum proteins. Formed in distal nephron	Present in advanced renal failure
Casts with inclusions		
RBC	Protein matrix variably filled with red cells. Often have red-orange appearance	Present in proliferative glomerulonephritis. (Rarely, may also be found with cortical necrosis and occasionally with acute tubular injury.)
Epithelial cell	Protein matrix variably filled with tubular cells	Found with acute tubular injury, glomerulonephritis, and nephrotic syndrome
WBC	Protein matrix variably filled with leukocytes	Found with proliferative glomerulonephritis and interstitial nephritis
Granular	Tubular protein droplets in hyaline cast	Present with any form of nephritis causing tubular injury
Fatty	Free fat droplets or tubular cells with fat droplets in a protein matrix	Found with any form of nephritis but most abundant with nephrotic syndrome and Fabry's disease
Mixed	Hyaline cast with various cells such as red, white, and tubular	Usually found in proliferative glomerulonephritis
Miscellaneous	Crystals or bacteria	Bacterial cast pathognomonic of bacterial pyelonephritis
Pseudocasts	Composed of clumped urates, leukocytes, bacteria, artifacts	Important not to confuse with true cast

TABLE 146–3. URINARY SEDIMENT STAINS

Stain	*Characteristics*
Benzidine or orthotolidine	Used to identify hemoglobin; can distinguish yeast from RBC or pigmented casts from hemoglobin casts
Gram	Used to differentiate between gram-positive (purple) and gram-negative (red) bacteria
Papanicolaou	Useful in identifying malignant cells, cellular inclusion bodies in measles, and intranuclear inclusions in cytomegalic disease
Prescott-Brodie	Peroxidase stain plus eosin stains WBC blue-gray to black and other cells pink-red
Sternheimer-Malbin	A crystal violet and safranin stain that identifies white cells (granular motility or "glitter" cells)
Sudan III	A red, fat-soluble azo dye in 70% alcohol that stains fat pink-red
Wright	A mixture of eosin and methylene blue that is useful in identifying various types of leukocytes

that reflects bladder urine without undue contamination from other sources. This can be accomplished directly by a urethral catheter or suprapubic needle aspiration of the bladder. However, noninvasive technics using clean-voided urine collections and quantitative culture methods can give adequate information without the hazards of instrumentation in most patients. Culture of a clean-voided specimen in asymptomatic women is representative of bladder urine about 80% of the time; this increases to 90% when 2 consecutive specimens are positive, and to 100% when 3 consecutive specimens are positive and all demonstrate the same organism in a concentration of $\geq 10^5$ bacteria/mL of midstream urine. In the adult male who is circumcised or has retracted the foreskin and cleansed the glans, and in the dysuric woman, a urine colony count of $\geq 10^2$ bacteria/mL has high specificity.

Localization of infection (see also Ch. 153): Bacteriuria can occur from infection in any part of the urinary tract as well as certain parts of the reproductive system. Most patients, however, appear to have only bladder bacteriuria without evidence of tissue invasion. In the absence of urinary tract obstruction, such cases readily respond to appropriate antimicrobial treatment, and localization studies are not indicated. However, in the patient who has frequent relapsing infections, localization may help to uncover the cause and lead to different therapeutic management.

Localization studies may be divided into several types as shown in TABLE 146–4. **Ureteral catheterization** and **bladder washout technics** have become the standards for distinguishing lower from upper tract infections. These methods are based on the hypothesis that bacteria coming from the ureters suggest renal infection. Actually, such localization studies do not prove the existence of renal infection, since renal tissue is not sampled. The bladder washout method is probably the most benign localization procedure, since it avoids cystoscopy and ureteral catheterization.

For localization of lower UTIs **in men,** the voided urine and expressed prostatic secretions are partitioned into segments: the first voided 5 to 10 mL represents urethral fluid; the midstream portion, bladder; and the secretions expressed by prostatic massage and the first voided 5 to 10 mL immediately after prostatic massage indicate prostatic secretions.

In women, the presence of **antibody-coated bacteria** in the urine correlates closely with renal bacteriuria as determined by the bladder washout method. Apparently antibody-coated bacteria appear in the urine only when tissue invasion has occurred that elicits a local antibody response. These antibodies react with the surface antigens of the bacteria. The presence of antibody coating the bacteria can then be detected by fluorescein-conjugated immunoglobulins raised against human antibodies in an animal. Although these immunoglobulins are present in the urine of patients with cystitis, the immuno-

TABLE 146–4. USEFUL METHODS FOR LOCALIZING URINARY TRACT INFECTION

Methods	*Comments*
Clinical	Distinct features of pyelonephritis, perinephric abscess, cystitis, prostatitis, urethritis
Urinalysis	Bacterial cast pathognomonic of pyelonephritis; WBC cast suggests nonspecific tubulointerstitial inflammation; tissue may indicate papillary necrosis
Differential culture	Controlled voidings plus prostatic secretions or semen; bladder washout methods or ureteral catheterization to distinguish upper from lower tract infection
Antibody-coated bacteria	Indicate bacterial invasions of tissues (kidney, prostate)

globulins do not react with bacteria in urine. This further supports the hypothesis that antibody-coating of bacteria occurs only in infected tissue. As with all localization tests that depend on indirect evidence, the antibody-coated bacteria may not be specific. Nonspecific fluorescence may be observed with certain organisms (pseudomonas, staphylococci, and yeasts). **In men,** the test often is positive in bacterial prostatitis and pyelonephritis. However, uncertainty exists concerning the specificity and sensitivity of the test in both men and women, and it is not now recommended for clinical use.

Measurement of Renal Function

Renal function tests are useful in evaluating the severity of kidney disease and in following its progress. They can be divided into specific aspects of nephron function, such as glomerular filtration, blood flow, and tubular transport. TABLE 146–5 provides a summary of tests that have been found useful.

In clinical practice, the **GFR** is adequately estimated from the endogenous creatinine clearance. The normal value for men is between 140 to 200 L/day (70 ± 14 mL/min/sq m) and for women, 120 to 180 L/day (60 ± 10 mL/min/sq m). Serum concentration of creatinine varies inversely with the GFR and therefore is a useful index of the GFR if production (related to muscle mass, age) and metabolism (increased in uremia) are considered. The upper limit of serum creatinine concentration in men with normal GFR is 1.2 mg/dL; in women, 1 mg/dL. A formula useful for calculating the creatinine clearance, an estimation of the GFR, from the serum creatinine concentration in men is:

$$Cl_{creat} = \frac{(140 - \text{age [yr]})(\text{body wt [kg]})}{(72)(\text{serum creat [mg/dL]})}$$

In women, the calculated values are multiplied by 0.85.

Creatinine clearance is not useful for detecting early kidney damage due to hypertrophy of residual glomeruli. After loss of 50 to 75% of the normal glomerular filtration surface, a decrease in creatinine clearance is clearly detectable. Thus, a normal creatinine clearance cannot exclude the presence of mild renal disease. Because of clinical convenience, **serum creatinine** measurements are used as an index of renal function.

TABLE 146–5. RENAL FUNCTION TESTS

Nephron Function	*Specific Test*	*Clinical Test*
Glomerular filtration	Clearance of inulin ^{125}I-Iothalamate ^{169}Yb-DTPA ^{51}Cr-EDTA	Creatinine clearance Serum creatinine Serum urea
Renal plasma flow	Clearance of PAH ^{125}I-Hippuran	
Proximal tubular transport	T_m glucose (reabsorption) T_m PAH (secretion)	Serum phosphate, urate Urinary amino acids
Distal tubular transport	Maximal urine/plasma osmolarity Acidifying capacity (urine pH, TA, NH_4^+)	Maximal urinary osmolarity Acid and bicarbonate loading

DTPA = Diethylenetriaminepentoacetic acid; EDTA = Ethylenediaminetetraacetic acid; PAH = Para-aminohippurate; T_m = Transport maximum; TA = Titratable acid.

(Modified from W. H. Chapman et al, *The Urinary System,* p. 239. Copyright 1973 by W. B. Saunders Company. Used with permission.)

This is possible because creatinine production and excretion are reasonably constant in the absence of muscle disease. In contrast to the serum creatinine, the **blood urea nitrogen (BUN)** is unsuitable as a single measure of renal function (the blood concentration is influenced by variations in urine flow rate as well as the production and metabolism of urea). The BUN/creatinine ratio often is used to differentiate prerenal, renal, or postrenal (obstructive) azotemia. A ratio > 15 is abnormal and suggests prerenal or postrenal azotemia. The BUN/creatinine ratio also is elevated whenever urea production is increased by diet or glucocorticoid therapy, with some neoplasms and antibiotics, and with excessive protein catabolism as seen in infections and uncontrolled diabetes mellitus. The causes of prerenal azotemia include shock, dehydration, and massive GI hemorrhage. The BUN/creatinine ratio is normal in renal azotemia. A low ratio is found in pregnancy, overhydration, severe liver disease, and malnutrition.

Measurement of the **renal plasma flow** is no more useful clinically than the GFR and is considerably more difficult and costly. However, tests of **renal concentrating ability** are simple and diagnostically helpful. A loss of concentrating capacity in the presence of adequate ADH stimulation is associated with tubulointerstitial disease (edema, infiltrate, fibrosis) except when nephrogenic diabetes insipidus **(NDI)** is present. The loss of concentrating ability frequently is present long before a depression of GFR is measurable.

Renal concentration capacity is best tested by 2 procedures: (1) **water deprivation** for a period of 12 to 14 h; and (2) **the response to exogenous vasopressin**. After the patient has fasted for 12 to 14 h overnight, the osmolarity of the initial morning urine and subsequent hourly samples is measured. When there is < 0.001 sp gr or < 30 mOsm/L difference in consecutive hourly measurements, the maximum concentration capacity has been reached with water deprivation. Aqueous vasopressin 5 u. s.c. is given, and the urine osmolarity measured after another hour. The results of this type of testing are noted in FIG. 146–1. (CAUTION: *In persons with renal failure, water deprivation may be harmful and usually is not useful in diagnosis; the concentrating capacity is always abnormal when the GFR is significantly reduced.*) A lack of response either to water deprivation or exogenous vasopressin suggests an intrinsic renal concentrating defect that may be due to one or more of the following: **functional tubular impairment,** which may be congenital (eg, NDI or Fanconi's syndrome) or acquired (eg, osmotic diuresis, certain diuretics [furosemide, bumetanide, ethacrynic acid], potassium deficiency, or hypercalcemia). Otherwise, one considers **tubulointerstitial disease,** as seen in sickle cell disease, toxic nephritis, pyelonephritis, nephrosclerosis, or any renal disease severe enough to produce azotemia. For other responses to these tests, and their interpretations, see DIABETES INSIPIDUS in Ch. 88.

Additional special tests of renal tubular function usually require research laboratories and are reserved for patients with specific problems. However, tests that measure plasma phosphate and urate, urinary amino acids, and urine pH are readily available and may prove useful in screening specific clinical problems.

Imaging Procedures

Radionuclide procedures (see Ch. 266)

Radiographic procedures: A **plain x-ray of the abdomen** (kidney, ureter, bladder [KUB]) is performed first to demonstrate the size and location of the kidneys. Since GI and GU diseases tend to mimic each other, the x-ray may be helpful in differential diagnosis. However, the renal outline can be obscured by bowel content, lack of perinephric fat, or a perinephric hematoma or abscess. This difficulty may be overcome by tomography. Congenital absence of a kidney may be suggested. If both kidneys are unusually large, polycystic kidney disease, multiple myeloma, lymphoma, amyloid disease, or hydronephrosis may be present. If both are small, the end stage of a sclerosing

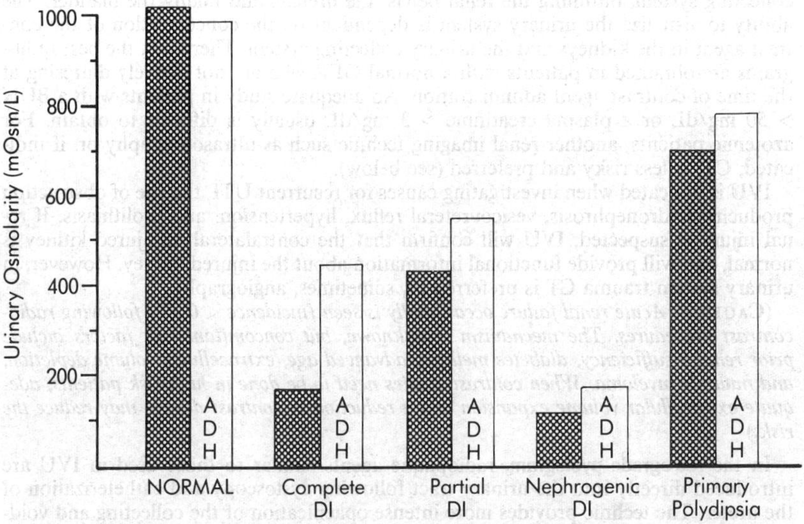

FIG. 146–1. Maximum urinary osmolarities after water deprivation (shaded bars) **vs. urinary osmolarity after administration of exogenous vasopressin** (open bars). DI = diabetes insipidus. (Data taken from "Recognition of partial defects in antidiuretic hormone secretion," by M. Miller et al, *Annals of Internal Medicine,* Vol. 73, No. 5, pp. 721–729, November 1970. Used with permission of The American College of Physicians and the author.)

disease such as glomerulonephritis, tubulointerstitial nephritis, or nephrosclerosis must be considered. Unilateral enlargement should suggest renal tumor, cyst, or hydronephrosis, whereas a small kidney on one side is compatible with congenital hypoplasia, atrophic pyelonephritis, or an ischemic kidney. Normally, the left kidney is 0.5 cm longer than its mate.

In 90% of cases, the right kidney is lower than the left because of displacement by the liver. The long axes of the kidneys are oblique to the spine and tend to parallel the borders of the psoas muscles. If both kidneys are parallel to the spine, the possibility of horseshoe kidneys should be considered. If only one kidney is displaced, a tumor or cyst may be present.

Because an x-ray film is 2-dimensional, a positive diagnosis of a stone in the urinary tract is practically impossible except in the instance of a staghorn calculus. However, suspicious opaque bodies may be noted in the region of the adrenal, kidney, ureter, bladder, or prostate. Oblique and lateral films, as well as visualization of the urinary tract with radiopaque fluids, are necessary in order to place the calcification specifically within these organs.

Intravenous urography (**IVU**; excretory urography; commonly but incorrectly referred to as intravenous pyelography—IVP) is used to visualize the kidney and lower urinary tract. Studies are done by an IV infusion of a triiodinated benzoic acid derivative. The iodine molecule provides radiopacity, while the benzoic acid molecule is rapidly filtered by the kidney. After IV injection of a contrast agent, the drug becomes concentrated in the renal tubules within the first 5 min, providing a nephrogram. Tomography of the kidney often is done routinely at this stage to show renal outlines that may otherwise be obscured by overlying gas or bowel content. In addition, cysts frequently can be differentiated from solid neoplasms. Later, the contrast agent appears in the

collecting system, outlining the renal pelvis, the ureters, and finally the bladder. The ability to visualize the urinary system is dependent on the concentration of the contrast agent in the kidneys and the urinary collecting system. Therefore, the best radiograms are obtained in patients with a normal GFR who are not actively diuresing at the time of contrast agent administration. An adequate study in patients with a BUN > 50 mg/dL or a plasma creatinine > 3 mg/dL usually is difficult to obtain. For azotemic patients, another renal imaging technic such as ultrasonography or, if indicated, CT, is less risky and preferred (see below).

IVU is indicated when investigating causes for recurrent UTI, the site of obstruction producing hydronephrosis, vesicoureteral reflux, hypertension, and urolithiasis. If renal injury is suspected, IVU will confirm that the contralateral uninjured kidney is normal, and will provide functional information about the injured kidney. However, in urinary system trauma CT is preferred or, sometimes, angiography.

(CAUTION: *Acute renal failure occasionally is seen [incidence < 0.5%] following radiocontrast procedures. The mechanism is unknown, but concomitant risk factors include prior renal insufficiency, diabetes mellitus, advanced age, extracellular volume depletion, and multiple myeloma. When contrast studies need to be done in high-risk patients, adequate extracellular volume expansion and a reduction in contrast dosage may reduce the risk.*)

In the **retrograde pyelogram,** radiopaque agents similar to those used in IVU are introduced directly into the urinary tract following cystoscopy and catheterization of the ureter. The technic provides more intense opacification of the collecting and voiding system when the IVU has been unsuccessful owing to poor renal function. Retrograde evaluation also may be indicated to assess the degree, type, cause, and length of ureteral obstruction or when the patient is allergic to IV radiopaque chemicals. Retrograde pyelography is useful for detailed examination of the pelvocalyceal collecting system, ureters, and urinary bladder. Disadvantages are (1) potential infection; (2) distortion of the calyces by overdistention; (3) backflow phenomena that obscure detail; (4) acute ureteral edema and secondary stricture formation; and (5) the need for anesthesia.

The cystogram is obtained as a part of the IVU but may be unsatisfactory owing to poor opacification or incomplete filling. Controlled bladder filling utilizing a catheter **(retrograde cystogram)** is then necessary for adequate visualization. Retrograde cystograms are advisable for study of neurogenic bladder, bladder rupture, or recurrent UTIs. Such causes as vesicoureteral reflux or vesical fistulas can be diagnosed by this technic or by radionuclide bladder scan. Films also are taken during and following voiding.

The male urethra may be examined during voiding following the cystogram **(voiding urethrocystography)**. If a urethral catheter cannot be inserted, retrograde injection of a contrast agent **(retrourethrocystography)** is used to delineate urethral pathology.

Ultrasound (US), a noninvasive, innocuous technic, is advantageous in that visualization does not depend on function. Nevertheless, some functional information can be inferred, especially in the fetus, in whom the kidneys can be identified with certainty after about 20 wk gestation, permitting measurement of urine production rate by serial estimations of the bladder volume. For neonates, US is a first-choice technic for investigating abdominal masses, UTI, and suspected anomalies of the urinary system, since the procedure is atraumatic and results are highly accurate.

The kidney can be effectively outlined and the pelvocaliceal echo pattern critically examined by scanning in multiple positions. US has proved particularly effective in diagnosing polycystic kidney disease, differentiating between renal cysts and tumors, detecting hydronephrosis and perirenal fluid collections or intrarenal hemorrhage, estimating renal size and parenchymal thickness, and locating the optimal site for percutaneous renal biopsy or nephrostomy. US is the preferred diagnostic method in a

uremic patient when uptake of contrast agent or isotope is impaired. US is effective in evaluating renal transplantation for sudden changes in kidney size; in detecting obstruction, lymphocele, or perirenal hemorrhage; and in detecting retroperitoneal pathology such as tumor, lymphadenopathy, or hemorrhage.

The urine-filled bladder is readily outlined by US. Normally, bladder wall contour changes depend on the amount of urine present. Absence of normal contour changes, distortion of bladder position, or abnormal wall thickness indicates pelvic or bladder wall pathology. Although bladder tumors may be observed with US, CT is a superior evaluation technic.

Computed tomography (CT) is more expensive than ultrasound and IVU but offers specific advantages. CT scans are most useful in evaluating the character and extent of renal mass lesions or determining the etiology of a retroperitoneal mass distorting the normal urinary tract (eg, an enlarged abdominal lymph node). Renal cysts are of low density on CT scanning, and following an IV injection of contrast material there is no enhancement—the cyst stands out as a prominent "lucency" against the contrast-containing parenchyma. Renal carcinoma, on the other hand, generally is isodense on the unenhanced scan and following administration of an IV contrast agent shows an increased density due to hypervascularity of the lesion. Contrast enhancement often helps demonstrate necrotic areas within the mass and areas of fat content that suggest angiomyolipoma. The extent of extrarenal involvement by a tumor often can be determined by CT scan.

When bladder carcinoma is suspected or known, CT after sequential intravesical air and contrast agent is another technic for evaluating the extent of these lesions.

Angiography is the most invasive of all renal imaging procedures and is reserved for special indications. Technics for introducing contrast agents include the retrograde method, in which a catheter is introduced through a peripheral artery (femoral, axillary) and extended to the desired area in the aortic lumen; and the translumbar method, now rarely used, in which percutaneous needle puncture of the aorta is performed. The retrograde method is safest and simplest and provides superior angiograms. In many institutions, conventional arteriography has been replaced by digital subtraction technics, which are safer because lower contrast loads and smaller catheters can be used.

Angiography is best reserved for investigating (1) possible vascular lesions, such as aneurysm; (2) an indeterminate CT examination for a mass lesion; (3) tumor embolization; and (4) inadequate CT visualization of renal veins or the inferior vena cava. Arteriography for a vascular map occasionally is desirable for bulky tumors.

Angiography also may be useful for (1) suspected renal hypertension; (2) congenital renal anomalies of structure, position, or vascular supply; (3) persistent unilateral renal bleeding in the presence of a normal IVU; (4) a poorly functioning kidney of relatively recent onset when the retrograde pyelogram is normal, or if retrograde ureteral catheterization is technically unsuccessful; and (5) cases in which accurate knowledge of blood supply is necessary before an operation; eg, for partial nephrectomy or transplant donors. **Complications** include injury to the cannulated vessels and neighboring organs, reactions to the contrast agent, and bleeding.

Venography: Visualization of the inferior vena cava for diagnostic purposes usually is done by percutaneous puncture of the femoral vein. Complications of this procedure have been few and are limited to those of extravasation of blood and the contrast agent in the area of injection. Renal vein catheterization provides samples for renal vein renin assays, for diagnosing renal vein thrombosis, and in evaluating the extent of malignant renal neoplasms when ultrasound or CT is indeterminate.

Magnetic resonance imaging (MRI) offers additional information about renal masses that cannot be determined by other imaging technics. MRI allows direct imaging in the transverse, coronal, and sagittal planes. Morphologic data is obtained from 3-

dimensional reconstruction of the tissue. MRI is the only imaging technic that can distinguish blurring of the corticomedullary junction secondary to edema, an early sign of transplant rejection. Solid and cystic renal lesions are as readily distinguished as with CT, but MRI provides information about the cyst fluid to help distinguish between hemorrhage or infection. In addition, MRI gives excellent definition of vascular and perirenal structures, permitting the diagnosis of thrombosis or neoplastic extension. In the pelvis, MRI shows tissue planes and can demonstrate the seminal vesicles and the extent of wall invasion of bladder cancer. MRI is limited by respiratory motion and peristalsis. Intrarenal calcifications are poorly defined because calcifications have few mobile protons.

Morphologic Procedures

Renal biopsy is performed for 4 reasons: (1) to help establish a histologic diagnosis; (2) to help estimate prognosis and the potential reversibility or progression of the renal lesion; (3) to estimate the value of therapeutic modalities; and (4) to determine the natural history of renal diseases. The only absolute contraindication to a biopsy is an uncontrollable bleeding disorder. The biopsy of a solitary kidney is a relative contraindication to be weighed against the need for information. Biopsies of a single, functioning, transplanted kidney are done frequently to diagnose and study possible graft rejections. Conditions associated with an increased morbidity following biopsy are deemed relative contraindications; these include renal tumors, large renal cysts, hydronephrosis, perinephric abscesses, severe reduction in blood or plasma volume, severe hypertension, and advanced renal failure with symptoms of uremia.

Of the 2 biopsy technics, **open** and **percutaneous,** the latter is most common. The open surgical method is rarely necessary—only when the percutaneous method has been unsuccessful or when direct visual control of the biopsy is critical. For the percutaneous technic the patient is sedated, and the kidney is visualized by radiographic or ultrasonic technics. With the patient in the prone position, and following local anesthesia of the overlying skin and muscles of the back, the biopsy needle is inserted and tissue is obtained for light, electron, and immunofluorescent microscopy.

Urine cytology is useful in screening for possible urinary tract neoplasia in high-risk populations such as workers with industrial dye; patients with painless hematuria from nonrenal causes, and in following patients after resection of bladder tumors. The 2nd voided morning urine sample is best, since the exfoliated cells in the initial morning specimen often show extensive deterioration. Abnormal cytology is seen in 70 to 85% of patients with known urinary tract epithelial neoplasia, but inflammatory or reactive hyperplastic lesions of the urinary tract may produce falsely positive results. Falsely negative examinations usually are associated with neoplasia having a low-grade histologic appearance. Diagnostic accuracy may be increased by vigorous bladder lavage with a small volume of 0.9% sodium chloride solution (50 mL pushed in and then aspirated by syringe through a catheter). The cells collected in the saline are concentrated and examined.

---

147. RENAL FAILURE

(See also Renal Disease and Diabetes Mellitus in Ch. 178; and the Hepatorenal Syndrome under Renal and Electrolyte Abnormalities in Ch. 67)

ACUTE RENAL FAILURE (ARF)

The clinical conditions associated with rapid, steadily increasing ***azotemia,*** *with or without oliguria (< 500 mL daily).*

Etiology and Classification

The causes of ARF can be grouped into 3 diagnostic categories: **prerenal** (inad-

equate renal perfusion), **postrenal** (obstruction), and **renal**. Major causes are noted in TABLE 147–1. Prerenal and postrenal causes are potentially reversible if diagnosed and treated early, and some of the causes of primary renal injury that result in acute vascular and tubulointerstitial nephropathy also are treatable, such as malignant hypertension, vasculitis, bacterial infections, drug reactions, and metabolic disorders (eg, hypercalcemia or hyperuricemia).

Pathophysiology

Prerenal azotemia is caused by inadequate renal perfusion due to extracellular volume depletion, cardiac or hepatic failure, or sepsis. Oliguria occurs as a result of reduced GFR and enhanced sodium and water resorption, normal responses to an inadequate circulating blood volume.

Intrinsic renal causes of ARF are multifactorial, with the most common being prolonged renal ischemia or a nephrotoxin. In experimental studies the factors that initiate and those that maintain ARF may differ. At least 3 mechanisms appear responsible for oligura: (1) a marked decrease in GFR due to renal cortical ischemia and/or a marked change in glomerular membrane permeability; (2) tubular obstruction from cellular and interstitial swelling and/or blockage from cellular debris; and (3) diffusion of glomerular filtrate across injured tubular epithelium. These factors are interdependent but all are not necessarily present in every patient; moreover, they vary in importance from patient to patient, and even in the same patient from time to time. The importance of all these factors in producing ARF points up the inadequacy of the previously popular term **"acute tubular necrosis"** as a description of the basic abnormality. The tubular lesions are variable, but edema and inflammation of the interstitial tissue are always present. While the general structural integrity of the vessels appears normal, the glomerular epithelial cells usually are swollen when viewed with scanning electron microscopy.

Postrenal azotemia usually is associated with glomerular and tubular dysfunction, and the urinary changes may mimic those in patients with primary renal injury.

Symptoms, Signs, and Diagnosis

Specific symptoms depend on the degree of renal dysfunction, the rate of renal failure, and the etiologic factors (see in CHRONIC RENAL FAILURE, below).

Initially, diagnostic focus rests on the exclusion of immediately reversible prerenal or postrenal factors. Extracellular volume depletion, cardiac and liver failure, and vasodilatation from sepsis may be the principal factors causing renal hypoperfusion and prerenal azotemia. Correction of the underlying hemodynamic abnormality with abatement of ARF is conclusive evidence.

In the absence of prerenal factors, obstructive causes are excluded. Bladder outlet

TABLE 147–1. MAJOR CAUSES OF ACUTE RENAL FAILURE

Prerenal	*Postrenal*	*Renal*
Fluid and electrolyte depletion Hemorrhage Septicemia Cardiac failure Liver failure Heatstroke (myoglobinuria ± fluid/elect depletion) Burns (fluid/elect depletion + myoglobinuria and hemoglobinuria)	Prostatism Bladder, pelvic, or retroperitoneal tumors Calculi	Acute tubular injury (ischemia, toxins, radiocontrast agents, hemoglobinuria, myoglobinuria) Acute glomerulonephritis Disseminated intravascular coagulopathy with cortical necrosis Arterial or venous obstruction Acute tubulointerstitial nephritis (drug reaction, pyelonephritis, papillary necrosis) Intrarenal precipitation (hypercalcemia, urates, myeloma protein)

obstruction probably is the most common cause of sudden, and often total, cessation of urinary output. A history of voiding difficulty or urinary stream reduction is particularly important in infants and older men. An enlarged kidney or palpable bladder is suggestive. Rectal and vaginal examinations are done when obstructive uropathy is suspected.

A history of intrinsic renal disease often is absent, but edema, the nephrotic syndrome, or signs of arteritis in the skin and retina may suggest glomerulonephritis. A history of hemoptysis may suggest Wegener's granulomatosis or Goodpasture's syndrome; a skin rash suggests polyarteritis or SLE. A history of drug ingestion and a maculopapular or purpuric skin rash may suggest drug allergy and tubulointerstitial nephritis. Primary vascular causes of ARF may be present without symptoms or signs. Bilateral renal artery occlusion may cause a bruit or flank pain but usually is asymptomatic. In infants, bilateral renal vein thrombosis usually results in enlarged, tender kidneys.

Oliguria or **anuria** suggests ARF or end-stage renal failure. However, a daily urine output of 1 to 2.5 L frequently is seen in ARF. Anuria suggests obstruction or intrinsic renal disease.

Laboratory findings: The **urinary sediment** may give valuable etiologic clues. In prerenal azotemia the sediment usually is unremarkable. This may also be true with obstructive uropathy, although white and red cells are not infrequently seen, as well as casts (granular and tubular cells). With primary renal injury, the sediment characteristically contains tubular cells, tubular cell casts, and many brown pigmented granular casts. Urinary eosinophils suggest an allergic tubulointerstitial nephritis; red cell casts suggest vasculitis or glomerulonephritis.

A progressive daily rise in the serum creatinine is diagnostic of ARF. However, urinary and serum chemical analyses permit the use of indexes early in the course of ARF, which may help to distinguish the various etiologies (see TABLE 147-2). Although the urine to plasma osmolarity ratio, urine sodium concentration, urine creatinine to serum creatinine ratio, and fractional excretion of sodium are discriminating in most patients, the most discriminating index is the "renal failure index," which is < 1 in prerenal azotemia or acute glomerulonephritis and > 2 in patients with postrenal or other renal causes of ARF.

Characteristic laboratory findings in ARF are those of progressive azotemia, acidosis, hyperkalemia, and hyponatremia. A modest daily rise in serum creatinine (1 to 2 mg/dL) and urea nitrogen (10 to 15 mg/dL) usually occurs. A rise of the serum creatinine > 2 mg/dL daily suggests that overproduction is occurring from rhabdomyolysis. Acidosis is ordinarily moderate, with a serum CO_2 content between 15 and 20 mEq/L. Serum potassium concentration increases slowly. However, when catabolism is markedly accelerated by trauma, sepsis, surgery, or steroids, or urea generation is accelerated by amino acid infusions, the serum urea nitrogen may rise at an excessive rate of 30 to 100 mg/dL/day and the serum potassium by 1 to 2 mEq/L/day. Hyponatremia usually is moderate (serum sodium 125 to 135 mEq/L) and is related to a surplus of water. The hematologic picture is that of a normochromic-normocytic anemia of moderate severity (see Ch. 96). Hct usually ranges from 25 to 30%.

In evaluating suspected postrenal azotemia, a postvoiding urethral catheterization helps assess bladder outlet obstruction. Urolithiasis as a cause of obstructive azotemia is not usually missed, as it is rarely silent, and simultaneous blockage of both ureters is unlikely. An x-ray of the abdomen can detect 90% of urinary tract calculi that are radiopaque. Ultrasound and radionuclide scans also are used in assessing possible upper tract obstruction and may obviate the need for retrograde ureteral catheterization. Intravenous urography should be cautiously used in this setting, as it occasionally may cause or worsen ARF.

ARF from acute tubular injury may have 3 typical phases: prodromal, oliguric, and

TABLE 147-2. DIAGNOSTIC INDEXES IN ACUTE RENAL FAILURE

	Prerenal	*Postrenal*	*Renal*	*AGN**
U/P osm†	> 1.5	1 to 1.5	1 to 1.5	1 to 1.5
Urine sodium, mEq/L	< 20	> 40	> 40	< 30
FE_{Na}‡	< 1	> 4	> 2	< 1
Renal failure index§	< 1	> 2	> 2	< 1

* Acute glomerulonephritis.
† Urine to plasma osmolarity ratio.
‡ Fractional excretion of sodium, U/P sodium ÷ U/P creatinine.
§ Urine sodium, mEq/L/urine to serum creatinine ratio.

(Adapted from T. R. Miller et al, "Urinary Diagnostic Indices in Acute Renal Failure," *Annals of Internal Medicine* Vol. 89, No. 1, pp. 47–50, July 1978. Used with permission of the American College of Physicians and the author.)

postoliguric. The **prodromal phase** varies in duration depending on causative factors such as the amount of toxin ingested or the duration and severity of hypotension. During the **oliguric phase,** urine output typically varies between 50 to 400 mL/day. However, a considerable number of patients are never oliguric and have a lower mortality, morbidity, and need for dialysis. Although the average oliguric period is about 10 to 14 days, the range varies from only 1 to 2 days to 6 to 8 wk. Serum creatinine typically increases by 1 to 2 mg/dL daily and the urea nitrogen by 10 to 20 mg/dL. However, serum urea nitrogen levels may be misleading as an early index of renal function because elevated values frequently are associated with increased protein catabolism due to surgery, trauma, burns, transfusion reactions, and GI or internal bleeding.

In the **postoliguric phase,** urine output gradually returns to normal levels; however, serum creatinine and urea levels may not fall until several days later. Tubular dysfunction may persist and is manifested by sodium wasting, polyuria (*which may be massive*) unresponsive to vasopressin, or hyperchloremic metabolic acidosis.

Prognosis

Renal failure and its immediate complications (eg, hyperkalemia, uremia, bleeding diathesis) are treatable, but the survival rate (about 50%) is not apparently improving, perhaps because more profoundly ill patients are now treated and because of the intrinsic mortality of associated conditions; eg, sepsis, pulmonary failure, major wounds, burns, surgical complications, and consumption coagulopathy.

Prophylaxis and Treatment

ARF often can be prevented by proper maintenance of normal fluid balance, blood volume, and BP during and after major surgery; by adequate infusions to maintain normal plasma volume in patients with severe burns; and by prompt transfusion in hemorrhagic hypotension. When a vasopressor agent is required, dopamine at an IV rate of 1 to 10 μg/kg/min may augment renal blood flow and urine output and prevent some cases of ARF. When intravascular hemolysis or rhabdomyolysis is detected, mannitol or furosemide should be given until pigment has disappeared from the urine. In incipient ARF, furosemide 2 to 3 mg/kg IV combined with mannitol 0.5 to 1 gm/kg IV or dopamine 0.5 to 3 μg/kg/min IV may reestablish normal urine flow or convert oliguric to nonoliguric ARF, but evidence of their beneficial effects otherwise is inconclusive except when they are given prophylactically in certain high-risk patients (eg, those undergoing aortic or open-heart surgery).

Dehydration and ECF depletion should be avoided in the patient requiring cholecystography or the patient with renal insufficiency requiring urography, particularly

those with multiple myeloma. Urography and angiography should be avoided whenever possible in any patient with renal insufficiency because of the high incidence of renal deterioration. The higher incidence in elderly patients correlates with the natural fall in GFR with aging. Severe hyperuricemia (> 10 mg/dL) should be treated with allopurinol before radiographic contrast studies. To prevent intrarenal tubular blockade with urates during cytolytic therapy in patients with neoplastic disease, prior treatment with allopurinol should be considered along with alkalinizing the urine (oral sodium bicarbonate and/or acetazolamide) and increasing urine flow with increased oral fluids.

Dialysis (see Ch. 148, below) should be started as soon as possible after the diagnosis is established, since patients with advanced azotemia may deteriorate in an unpredictable manner. The use of dialysis allows more aggressive nutrition and may improve prognosis.

The management of ARF without dialysis requires meticulous limitation of the intake of all substances requiring renal excretion, and is only advocated when dialysis is not available. Water intake should be restricted to a volume equal to urine output and measured extrarenal losses plus an allowance of about 500 mL/day for insensible loss. Daily weight determination serves as a check on fluid intake, since any weight gain must be attributed to excess fluid. Sodium and potassium intake are eliminated. Dosages of certain drugs that are principally eliminated by the kidney (eg, digoxin and some antibiotics) must be modified. To prevent negative nitrogen balance, oral or IV administration of essential amino acids in addition to glucose has been advocated; risks of such therapy include fluid overload, hyperosmolarity, and infection. An indwelling bladder catheter should be used with extreme caution and only when necessary.

In the postoliguric phase, careful attention to fluid and electrolyte balance is mandatory to prevent extracellular volume, osmolar, acid-base, and potassium disturbances that may be serious or even lethal.

CHRONIC RENAL FAILURE (CRF)

The clinical condition resulting from a multitude of pathologic processes that lead to derangement and insufficiency of renal excretory and regulatory function **(uremia)**.

Etiology and Classification

CRF may result from any cause of renal dysfunction of sufficient magnitude. The functional effects of CRF can be grouped into 3 stages: **diminished renal reserve, renal insufficiency (failure),** and **uremia.** The concept of renal functional adaptation explains the observation that a loss of 75% of renal tissue only produces a fall in GFR to 50% of normal. With diminished renal reserve there is a measurable loss of renal function, but homeostasis is preserved at the expense of some hormonal adaptations such as secondary hyperparathyroidism and intrarenal changes in glomerulotubular balance. At the stage of renal insufficiency, there is slight retention of nitrogenous compounds **(azotemia),** reflected in elevated plasma urea and creatinine. With further renal dysfunction, fluid and electrolyte balance is disturbed, azotemia increases, and systemic manifestations **(uremia)** occur. This is usually seen with a GFR < 6 mL/min/sq m.

Symptoms and Signs

Patients with mildly diminished renal reserve are asymptomatic, and renal dysfunction can only be detected by careful testing. A patient with mild to moderate renal insufficiency may have only vague symptoms despite the elevated BUN and creatinine; nocturia is noted at this stage, principally due to a failure to concentrate the urine during the night. Lassitude, fatigue, and decreased mental acuity often are the first manifestations of uremia. Neuromuscular features include coarse muscular twitches, peripheral neuropathies with sensory and motor phenomena, muscle cramps, and con-

vulsions (usually the result of hypertensive encephalopathy). GI manifestations (anorexia, nausea, vomiting, stomatitis, an unpleasant taste in the mouth) are almost uniformly present. In advanced disease, GI ulceration and bleeding are common. Malnutrition leading to generalized tissue wasting is a prominent feature of chronic uremia. The skin may develop a yellow-brown discoloration, and, occasionally, urea from sweat may crystallize on the skin as **uremic frost.** Pruritus is an especially uncomfortable feature of chronic uremia in some patients. Hypertension often is present in advanced renal insufficiency and usually is related to hypervolemia and, in an occasional case, to elevated serum angiotensin levels. Hypertension and renal retention of sodium and water may lead to congestive heart failure. Pericarditis, usually seen in chronic uremia, may occur in acute, potentially reversible, uremia.

Laboratory Findings

Characteristic findings are those of nitrogen retention, acidosis, and anemia. Urea and creatinine are elevated. Plasma sodium concentrations may be normal or reduced. Acidosis ordinarily is moderate, with the serum CO_2 content between 15 and 20 mEq/L. Hypocalcemia and hyperphosphatemia are found regularly. The serum potassium is normal or only moderately elevated (< 6.5 mEq/L). Urinary volume often is relatively fixed between 1 and 4 L/day and does not respond readily to variations in water intake. Urinary osmolarity is usually fixed close to that of plasma (300 to 320 mOsm/L). The findings on urinalysis depend on the nature of the underlying disease, but broad (especially waxy) casts often are prominent in advanced renal insufficiency of any cause. The hematologic picture (see also Ch. 96) is that of a normochromic-normocytic anemia of moderate severity. Hct usually ranges from 20 to 30% except in the patient with polycystic kidney disease, who may have a Hct of 35 to 50%.

Prognosis

The outcome depends on the nature of the underlying disorder and superimposed complications. The latter may cause acute reductions in renal function that are reversible with therapy. However, progression of underlying chronic renal disease generally is not susceptible to specific treatment. Reducing dietary protein early in CRF may reduce glomerular hyperfiltration and slow the rate of renal decompensation. When oliguria, progressive hyperkalemia, and pericarditis appear, they often indicate a preterminal state, but even in these situations, if no other major organ failure exists, dialysis or transplantation may improve the outlook.

Treatment

Factors aggravating or producing kidney failure (eg, salt and water depletion, nephrotoxins, congestive heart failure, infection, hypercalcemia, obstruction) must be treated specifically. If uremia is the result of a progressive and untreatable disorder, conservative management often will prolong useful, comfortable life until dialysis or transplantation is required. General principles of conservative management follow.

Meticulous attention to dietary management as renal failure progresses from moderate to end-stage disease is important. Anorexia is an early symptom of uremia, requiring evaluation of caloric intake. Increased caloric intake should be coupled with a reduction in the total content of dietary protein (see TABLE 147–3). Endogenous protein catabolism is minimized by providing sufficient carbohydrate and fat to meet energy requirements and prevent ketosis. An intake of 0.6 gm/kg of a mixed protein diet, which includes some low-quality protein to add variety, improves patient acceptance. To this basic protein allowance should be added the equivalent of daily urinary protein loss. Though life is not prolonged, many uremic symptoms (fatigue, nausea, vomiting, twitching, confusion) are markedly improved and the immediate need for dialysis or transplantation may be deferred for a short time.

Hypertriglyceridemia is commonly observed in uremia. Since reduction of carbohydrate intake and a proportional increase in protein is not possible in uremia, clofibrate

TABLE 147–3. SAMPLE MODIFIED GIOVANNETTI DIET (18–20 GM PROTEIN)*

Breakfast	*Lunch*	*Dinner*
1/2 cup cranberry juice 1/2 cup cream of rice, unsalted 2 slices toast, low-protein 4 tsp butter 2 tsp honey 1/4 cup milk 2 tsp sugar 1 cup tea	1 egg, soft-cooked 1/2 cup cooked carrots 1/2 cup rice 6 slices cucumber on 1 leaf lettuce 2 slices bread, low-protein 6 tsp butter 1 tbsp grape jelly 2 low-protein cookies 1 cup Kool-Aid®	Special fruit plate: 2 peach halves and 2 pineapple slices on lettuce 2 slices bread, low-protein 4 tsp butter 1 tbsp grape jelly 1/2 cup milk
Midmorning Nourishment	*Midafternoon Nourishment*	*Evening Nourishment*
2 slices low-protein rusk 4 tsp butter Cinnamon and 2 tsp sugar	6 pieces low-protein caramels 1 cup lemonade with sugar	2 low-protein cookies 6 oz 7-Up®

Approximate Composition:

Protein	20 gm	Sodium	1417 mg
Fat	95 gm	Potassium	888 mg
Carbohydrate	456 gm	Kilocalories	2760

* This diet provides 18 to 20 gm of high-quality protein primarily in the form of 1 egg and 6 oz of milk. Protein of low biologic value (vegetables, grains) can be added to give more variety and increase daily intake to 0.6 gm/kg. Caloric intake should be as high as possible. Foods are cooked without salt, and fluid is drained from the food when served.

(High-quality protein has a high proportion of essential amino acids; ie, those amino acids necessary for proper endogenous protein synthesis. Low-quality protein does not have a high proportion of essential amino acids.)

has been used successfully. Because this drug is eliminated in large part by the kidney, the customary dose must be reduced to 500 mg 3 times/wk. A reduction in **vitamin intake** often accompanies the dietary reductions in uremia; patients should take a multi-vitamin preparation containing water-soluble vitamins. There is no demonstrated need for administration of vitamins A or E.

Water intake may exceed limited renal concentrating and diluting capacities and should be controlled to maintain a serum sodium concentration of 135 to 145 mEq/L. **Sodium intake** should be unrestricted, unless contraindicated by edema or hypertension. **Potassium intake** is closely related to meat, vegetable, and fruit ingestion and does not usually require adjustments. Occasionally, supplementation may be required for the hypokalemia associated with renal tubular dysfunction or vigorous diuretic therapy. Except for hyporeninemic-hypoaldosteronism or potassium-sparing diuretic therapy, hyperkalemia is infrequent until end-stage renal failure, or in severe metabolic acidosis or with potassium loads (GI bleeding, excessive oral intake). Mild hyperkalemia (< 6 mEq/L) can be treated by reducing protein intake and correcting metabolic acidosis. Severe hyperkalemia (> 7 mEq/L) is an indication for dialysis, but a cation-exchange resin such as sodium polystyrene sulfonate 50 gm in a 10 or 20% glucose solution as a retention enema for 30 to 60 min, or 20 to 50 gm in 100 mL of a 20% sorbitol solution qid orally, may be useful if dialysis is not immediately contemplated. The benefits of cation-exchange resins are relatively slow—30 to 60 min when used rectally and 1 to 2 h when taken orally. **Activity** need not be restricted, as fatigue and lassitude usually keep it within acceptable limits.

Mild acidosis requires no therapy. However, when the plasma CO_2 content is < 15 mEq/L (mM/L), alkali therapy may help to reduce such symptoms as anorexia, lassitude, and dyspnea. Alkali therapy consists of sodium bicarbonate (initial dose is 1 gm tid) or sodium citrate (initial dose is a 10% solution, 1 tsp tid). Doses are increased gradually until the CO_2 is about 20 mEq/L (mM/L) and symptoms are relieved, or until evidence of sodium overloading prevents further therapy.

A chronic decline in renal function is associated with **abnormalities of calcium, phosphorus, parathyroid hormone (PTH), and vitamin D metabolism.** As the GFR falls, a rise in PTH and a decrease in serum 1,25-dihydrovitamin D_3 (calcitriol) concentration occurs. These changes probably are caused by an initial retention of phosphate as renal function decreases and a concomitant fall in the serum ionized calcium concentration. If left untreated, **hypocalcemia** and **hyperphosphatemia,** although asymptomatic, along with **osteodystrophy** (**osteitis fibrosa** or **osteomalacia**) develop. Treatment of these abnormalities usually prevents the development of symptomatic bone disease and also may reduce the rate of decline in renal function. Initial management includes control of hyperphosphatemia with careful dietary restriction of phosphorus plus administration of oral phosphate-binding compounds. Although aluminum hydroxide gels and aluminum carbonate are commonly used, the evidence of aluminum absorption and toxicity (encephalopathy, osteodystrophy, microcytic anemia) is considerable, and emphasis is now on oral calcium carbonate supplements (0.5 to 1.5 gm calcium tid with meals) to both reduce dietary phosphate absorption and improve calcium balance. Only if hyperphosphatemia is not adequately controlled or hypercalcemia occurs are aluminum salts in low doses considered. When hyperphosphatemia is controlled, eucalcemia usually occurs but frequently requires oral supplementation with calcitriol 0.25 to 1 μg/day to adequately raise the serum calcium high enough to suppress parathyroid hormone concentrations and heal osteodystophic lesions. The effect of therapy is monitored by frequent measurements of calcium, phosphate, and alkaline phosphatase. If rapid alkalinization produces hypocalcemic tetany, IV calcium gluconate may be useful.

The anemia of uremia (see in Ch. 96) responds only to transfusion, which should not be undertaken unless anemia is severe (Hct < 18%) or symptomatic. Transfusions should be given slowly, and packed RBCs should be used to avoid circulatory overloading. It is always appropriate to check for and treat other sources of anemia, particularly nutritional deficiencies such as iron, folate, and cyanocobalamin.

Congestive heart failure, most commonly due to fluid retention by the kidney, responds to sodium restriction. If myocardial damage is present, digitalis may be necessary, but it must be remembered that the distribution volume and excretion rate of digoxin are reduced in renal failure. Diuretics such as furosemide and bumetanide usually are effective even when renal function is markedly reduced. **Moderate or severe hypertension** should be treated by careful reduction of BP to avoid the deleterious effect of persistent hypertension on renal function. Patients who fail to respond to moderate reduction in sodium intake (100 mEq/day) need further dietary sodium restriction and diuretic therapy (furosemide 80 to 240 mg bid or bumetanide 1 to 5 mg bid). Adjunctive doses of hydrochlorothiazide 50 mg bid or metolazone 5 to 10 mg/day may be carefully added to high-dose furosemide or bumetanide therapy if hypertension or edema is not controlled. If careful reduction of the extracellular volume does not control BP, then conventional antihypertensive drugs are added.

When the limits of effectiveness of conventional therapy have been reached, long-term dialysis (see below) or transplantation (see Ch. 22) should be considered. When chronic dialysis is used to treat irreversible uremia, anemia and hypertension may still persist and require transfusions and restriction of fluid and salt intake, respectively. Occasionally, peripheral neuropathy may progress and become disabling despite fre-

quent dialysis. Fatigue and lassitude may be problems in the days just after each dialysis.

148. DIALYSIS AND FILTRATION PROCEDURES

In renal failure of any cause there are several physiologic derangements. Homeostatic balance of water, minerals (Na, K, Cl, Ca, P, Mg, SO_4), and excretion of the daily metabolic load of fixed hydrogen ions is no longer possible. Toxic end products of nitrogen metabolism (urea, creatinine, uric acid, and others) accumulate in blood and tissue. Finally, the kidney is no longer able to function as an endocrine organ in the production of erythropoietin and 1,25-dihydroxycholecalciferol.

Dialysis (hemodialysis and peritoneal dialysis) is *the process of separating elements in a solution by* ***diffusion*** *across a semipermeable membrane.* Diffusive solute transport depends on movement down a concentration gradient. **Hemofiltration** differs from dialysis in that it uses ***convective*** *transport of solute through ultrafiltration across the membrane* rather than diffusion. Convective solute transport depends on the movement of dissolved substances concomitant with fluid flow through a filtering membrane. Dialysis and filtration procedures can manage some of the derangements of renal failure, but not the endocrine deficits. Accumulated water and dissolved sodium chloride may be removed by ultrafiltration: hydraulic, in hemodialysis and hemofiltration; osmotic, in peritoneal dialysis. Homeostatic balance of minerals (K, P, Mg, SO_4) and removal of toxic end products of nitrogen metabolism may be accomplished by diffusive or convective transport. Correction of the metabolic acidosis is accomplished by diffusive transport of bicarbonate or bicarbonate precursors (acetate, lactate) in dialysis procedures and by infusion of these same materials in hemofiltration.

Indications

Absolute indications for dialysis and filtration procedures in **acute** or **chronic renal failure** (**ARF** or **CRF**) are similar and will be considered together: uremic encephalopathy, pericarditis, intractable metabolic acidosis, congestive heart failure, and life-threatening hyperkalemia. However, many physicians prefer to act prophylactically in oliguric ARF, using the procedure on a regular basis until the polyuric phase ensues. Strategy employed in CRF is empiric and varies. Some physicians begin dialysis when the residual creatinine clearance reaches the 5 to 10 mL/min range, others when the patient loses the stamina to maintain normal daily work and activity. Some authorities recommend for anephric individuals that the dialysis/filtration procedure produce a urea clearance of 1 to 1.5 L/wk/kg. Others arbitrarily begin 4-h thrice weekly hemodialysis (or a 56 L/wk continuous ambulatory peritoneal dialysis **[CAPD]** regime), adjusting the frequency and intensity of treatment to keep the predialysis (or steady-state) serum urea nitrogen concentration < 80 mg/dL. Still others use kinetic modeling to predict precisely the duration and frequency required to achieve this serum urea nitrogen concentration. This takes into account the patient's generation rate for urea, residual renal function, diet, and the expected clearance of the procedure. Definitions of the adequacy of depuration for renal failure vary, but most accept as adequate a treatment regime that permits the patient to be rehabilitated, eat a reasonable diet, make blood, and maintain a normal BP, and prevents progression of uremic neuropathy. Dialysis may be used solely as therapy for CRF, or to support renal transplantation.

Patients with **stable chronic renal failure** may not require dialysis. However, if an intercurrent illness such as gastroenteritis, congestive heart failure, sepsis, or lactic

acidosis produces acute metabolic or circulatory decompensation, the patient's condition may suddenly deteriorate. Congestive heart failure may be difficult to correct in these patients because response to diuretics is poor. Likewise, they may not tolerate the sodium load produced when metabolic acidosis is corrected with sodium bicarbonate. Dialysis corrects the metabolic acidosis without expanding the ECF volume, which it can actually reduce by ultrafiltration.

Acute drug intoxication can be survived by many patients if prompt and proper respiratory and cardiovascular support is given. However, dialysis can be effective in treating many specific drug poisonings (see Ch. 289). The decision to institute dialysis depends on the clinical and biochemical characteristics of the poisoning, including the severity of coma, whether a potentially lethal dose was ingested, whether an impaired route of excretion may make autodetoxification unlikely, and whether the poison can be metabolized to a more toxic form (eg, oxidation of ethylene glycol to oxalic acid). The hazards of prolonged coma and the relationship between toxicity and blood concentration are important factors in the clinical assessment. Furthermore, the risk of compromised ventilatory support during transit must be considered before moving a patient to a medical center which has an artificial kidney program.

PERITONEAL DIALYSIS

The peritoneum, consisting of visceral and parietal components, has a surface area approximating BSA (1 to 2 sq m in adults), and is permeable to solutes of mol wt up to 30,000 daltons. Total splanchnic blood flow is 1200 mL/min at rest, but only a small portion of that flow (70 mL/min) comes in contact with the peritoneum. Peritoneal dialysis is accomplished by instilling fluid into the peritoneal space and periodically draining and replenishing it in a tidal fashion. Solute concentrations in the peritoneal dialysate equilibrate slowly. Clearance of small molecules is a function of dialysate flow rate and contact time. Since larger molecules never reach equilibration, their clearance is a function primarily of peritoneal contact time.

Technic

Soft silicone rubber catheters are favored for both acute and chronic peritoneal dialysis; they have good flow characteristics and little tendency to perforate a viscus. These catheters may be implanted in the operating room under direct visualization or by insertion through a specially designed trocar, and should permit dialysate to fill or drain at 200 mL/min. Most such catheters incorporate a fabric collar—either polyester or expanded polytetrafluoroethylene **(PTFE)**—which allows tissue ingrowth at the skin and/or preperitoneal fascia, resulting in a watertight, bacteria-impervious seal.

A variety of schedules and devices are used. The simplest technic is **manual intermittent peritoneal dialysis (IPD),** using a Y-type infusion and drainage set. In adults, 1.5- to 3-L bottles or bags of dialysate are warmed to 37 C using dry heat, infused rapidly (over 10 min), allowed to dwell in the peritoneal cavity for 10 min, and drained in about 10 min. This rapid exchange technic achieves the highest solute clearance and is useful chiefly in the treatment of acute uremia. The treatment duration may be 12 to 48 h, depending on the needs of the patient. **Automated cycler IPD** was developed to permit these exchanges without the need for constant nursing attention; many patients can use automated cycler IPD on themselves at home. They usually set up the cycler at bedtime and allow the treatment to take place while they are sleeping; treatments are required 3 to 7 nights/week. **Continuous ambulatory peritoneal dialysis (CAPD)** is manual peritoneal dialysis using extremely long dwell times. A typical adult patient has 1.5 to 3 L of dialysate continuously present in the peritoneal cavity. This solution is drained and replenished tid or qid. Since the solutions come in collapsible polyvinyl chloride bags, the empty bag can be folded, tucked into a garment, and used for subsequent drainage, eliminating the need to disconnect and connect from a Y-type infusion-drainage system. Patients generally perform 3 of these exchanges (which take 30 to 45

min), spaced at intervals no shorter than 4 h, during the daytime and allow a longer 8- to 12-h exchange to take place at night while they are sleeping.

Continuous cycling peritoneal dialysis (CCPD) is similar to CAPD in concept, but differs in diurnal rhythm: long exchanges during the daytime; short exchanges while sleeping at night, using an automatic cycler. This allows daytime freedom from the necessity to perform exchanges but inhibits patient mobility because of cumbersome equipment.

Equilibrium peritoneal dialysis (EPD) was developed to permit continuous peritoneal dialysis for hospitalized (nonambulatory) patients, with efficient use of specialized personnel. A multiple-prong administration manifold and drainage bag is used to perform manual IPD with long dwell times. Sterile connections are established by specially trained nurses; routine staff nurses perform the exchanges by unclamping the bags sequentially without the need to use sterile technics.

Complications and Contraindications

Mechanical complications: hematoma in the peri-catheter tract, intra-abdominal bleeding, perforation of a viscus (early and late), dialysate leakage around the catheter, dissection of fluid into the abdominal wall, and obstruction of inflow and/or outflow by clots, fibrin, omentum, or fibrous encasement. **Infectious** complications include peritoneal infection (see also CHRONIC PERITONITIS in Ch. 55) at the skin interface with the peritoneal catheter, and abscess in the tract of the peritoneal catheter. **Cardiovascular** complications include hypotension, pulmonary edema, and cardiac arrhythmia. **Pulmonary** complications include atelectasis, pleural effusion, and pneumonia. **Metabolic** complications include hyperglycemia and hypoalbuminemia. **Miscellaneous** complications include peritoneal sclerosis (manifested by partial small bowel obstruction), hypothyroidism, seizures, and abdominal and inguinal hernias.

No **contraindications** are absolute, but several are relative: cellulitis of the abdominal wall, abnormal thoracoabdominal communication, fresh intra-abdominal vascular prosthesis, and fresh abdominal wound.

EXTRACORPOREAL PROCEDURES

Both hemodialysis and hemofiltration require extracorporeal circulation of the blood. **Long-term access** to the circulation is provided by subcutaneous arteriovenous fistulas. These avoid the recurrent infections and clotting associated with the formerly used external arteriovenous shunts. The radial artery is anastamosed to the cephalic vein in an end-to-end, end-to-side, or side-to-side fashion. The forearm veins dilate and eventually arterialize, and are suitable for repeated puncture. For those patients whose native vasculature is insufficient for a successful endogenous arteriovenous fistula, the autogenous saphenous vein graft, an exogenous prosthesis made from expanded polytetrafluoroethylene (PTFE), or a bovine carotid xenograft may be suitable. Recently developed implantable vascular valve systems allow one to tap into a vascular channel without skin puncture, but have the same complications of former arteriovenous shunts; ie, clotting and infections. Long-term results with these devices are pending. **Temporary access** to the circulation may be achieved by inserting single or double lumen catheters into the subclavian or femoral veins. Complications of vascular access include thrombosis, infection, and hemorrhage.

HEMODIALYSIS

In a hemodialysis system, blood is removed from the patient via a suitable access and pumped to the membrane unit. Dialyzed blood is returned to the patient through tubing that incorporates an air embolus protector. The dialysate delivery system mixes water (generally purified by reverse osmosis or deionization) with an electrolyte con-

centrate, warms it to body temperature, and checks the conductivity to ensure that it is isotonic to the patient's blood. Typical dialysate for hemodialysis is unsterile, but is prepared from water meeting rigid bacteriologic and chemical standards. The dialysate compartment of the membrane unit is under negative pressure relative to the blood compartment. This hydraulic pressure gradient permits ultrafiltration of excess fluid across the membrane.

Technic: To prevent clotting in the extracorporeal circuit, a loading dose of heparin (30 to 100 u./kg) is given to the patient to produce systemic anticoagulation (whole blood clotting time > 30 min), which is maintained with a sustaining infusion of heparin (about 7 to 15 u./kg/h). The level of anticoagulation is monitored, and the dosage of heparin is individualized. For patients with recent surgery or concomitant bleeding, lower doses of heparin are used (exposing the patient to greater risk of clotting the extracorporeal circuit); or regional heparinization (limited to the extracorporeal circuit) is accomplished by matched infusions of heparin (into the blood before it enters the dialyzer) and protamine (into the blood before it returns to the body).

Membrane units come in different sizes with differing surface areas, clearance characteristics, and hydraulic coefficients for ultrafiltration. Manufacturer's instructions generally give these specifications. A typical hemodialysis treatment takes 3 to 5 h. It reduces the serum urea nitrogen concentration by 50% and temporarily corrects metabolic acidosis and hyperkalemia. Most patients with CRF require thrice weekly hemodialysis to maintain a state of well-being.

Complications of hemodialysis include **fever**—due to bacteremia, pyrogens, or overheated dialysate; **anaphylaxis; cardiovascular problems**—hypotension (due to excessive ultrafiltration), cardiac arrhythmia, air embolus, pericardial tamponade; **hemorrhage**—GI, intracranial, retroperitoneal, or intraocular; **metabolic problems**—hyponatremia, hypernatremia, hypo- and hyperkalemia, hypercalcemia, hypermagnesemia; and **miscellaneous**—pruritus, seizures, muscle cramps, restlessness, insomnia, and dementia.

Contraindications for hemodialysis: There are only 2 relative ones, hypotension and active bleeding.

HEMOFILTRATION

In a typical hemofiltration circuit the blood circuit is similar to that used in hemodialysis. Ultrafiltration is accomplished by applying a vacuum to the outside of the membrane or partially occluding the blood outflow line, thereby increasing the pressure in the blood compartment of the membrane unit. Excess fluid removed by hemofiltration must be replaced by infusion of isotonic replacement fluid, downstream from the hemofilter. Occasionally the system employs predilution of this blood with replacement fluid to limit protein-caking on the filtration membrane. In addition to fluid removed in the hemofiltration process, dissolved solutes present in the blood will pass through to a greater or lesser extent depending on the particular membrane. Because of this *it is very important to replace excess crystalloid removed by hemofiltration procedures*. Hemofiltration is used in 3 different circumstances:

(1) As an adjunct to hemodialysis. Using conventional hemodialysis membranes, ultrafiltration is performed for a 1-h period prior to hemodialysis either by connecting the dialysate port to a vacuum source or by placing the dialysis machine in bypass mode under negative pressure. This technic is used in patients with chronic renal failure who are subject to intermittent excesses of fluid weight gain. It permits removal of large amounts of fluid without the osmotic shift of water into the intracellular compartment associated with hemodialysis, reducing the risks of muscle cramps and hypotension. The primary disadvantage (where duration of therapeutic session is a

limiting constraint) is that the subsequent hemodialysis treatment is shortened and therefore less effective in removing small solutes.

(2) Slow continuous ultrafiltration (SCUF) is used primarily in patients with oliguric acute renal failure who require large volumes of IV hyperalimentation. Blood from an arteriovenous fistula perfuses a special hemofiltration membrane (polysulfone or polyacrylonitrile) under its own arterial pressure. Ultrafiltration is regulated by applying a screw clamp to the ultrafiltrate line. Filtrate is continuously collected in a urine drainage bag. The chief advantage of this technic is the ability to remove large volumes of fluid on a daily basis (14 L/day). Disadvantages include the fact that the clearance of small solutes may be inadequate, requiring adjunctive hemodialysis, and intensive nursing care is required throughout this treatment, because the patient is anticoagulated and large fluid volumes are being removed.

(3) Maintenance hemofiltration differs from SCUF in that its purpose is the convection-based removal of uremic solutes. It has been employed on an experimental basis as a substitute for hemodialysis in the management of chronic renal failure. The extracorporeal circuit generally uses a blood pump. Ultrafiltration using special membranes (as in SCUF) is accomplished by application of a vacuum to the membrane or by partial occlusion of the blood outflow line. Excess ultrafiltrate (large volumes) is replaced by infusion of balanced electrolyte solutions after the hemofilter. Some devices have an elaborate control system to insure that volume balance of these solutions is maintained. The chief advantage reported for this technic is better control of BP. The theoretical benefit of enhanced clearance of "middle molecules" has not been clinically demonstrated. The disadvantages of maintenance hemofiltration are the need for large volumes of sterile IV solutions and for elaborate fluid control systems.

Complications of hemofiltration are the same as for hemodialysis.

NONDIALYTIC MANAGEMENT CONSIDERATIONS

Patients maintained on chronic dialysis programs have special needs that require a multidisciplinary approach involving cooperation between nephrologist, psychiatrist and/or social worker, specially trained nurses, nutritionist, and frequently the transplant surgical team. Ideally, assessment of the patient should begin when it is clear that progressive, irreversible renal disease is present, but before the actual need for dialysis or transplantation is present. Patients can then (1) have their psychosocial strengths and weaknesses assessed in a noncrisis atmosphere; (2) be informed so as to participate in the choice of therapy; and (3) have a vascular access created early, allowing time for maturation. The choice of therapeutic modality is individualized, considering the trade-offs inherent in each, the patient's psychosocial resources and desires, and the medical resources of the community.

Dialysis patients require special dietary care and medications and awareness and support regarding the psychosocial aspects of dialysis (see PSYCHOSOCIAL ASPECTS OF CHRONIC DIALYSIS, below).

Diet: Generally, patients eat a diet of defined protein content, 1 to 1.2 gm of protein/kg ideal body weight/day. This diet emphasizes high biologic value proteins, and is limited to 2 gm of Na and 2 gm of K. Limitation of phosphorus intake also may be required. Daily fluid intake is limited to 500 to 1000 mL plus measured urinary output, and must be monitored by weight gain. **Patients on peritoneal programs** require a more liberal intake of protein (1.25 to 1.5 gm/kg) to replace peritoneal losses (10 to 20 gm/day). Fluid, K (4 gm), and Na (3 to 4 gm) restrictions are not as severe as in hemodialysis programs.

Medications commonly prescribed for patients on chronic dialysis include multivitamin supplements (to replace estimated dialytic loss of the water-soluble vitamins, B-complex, folic acid, vitamin C); ferrous sulfate 500 to 900 mg/day (to replace iron lost in residual blood left in hemodialysis membranes); an anabolic steroid (eg, nandrolone

decanoate or testosterone enanthate, for its stimulating effect on erythropoiesis); and oral phosphate binders to maintain the predialysis serum phosphate within normal levels.

Some dialysis patients develop an **iron overload syndrome** because of multiple transfusions. In these patients ferrous sulfate supplementation should be avoided. Patients who develop **calcium oxalate urolithiasis** while on dialysis should not take dietary supplements of vitamin C because oxalic acid is a metabolic byproduct.

Management of the **hyperphosphatemia** of chronic renal failure is currently controversial. It is clear that patients who have a calcium × phosphorus product > 70 are at risk to develop extraosseous deposits of calcium. For this reason physicians have often prescribed aluminum hydroxide or aluminum carbonate gel preparations to bind dietary phosphate in the intestines. In recent years patients have been recognized who have **aluminum-related osteomalacia and/or dialysis dementia** (see below), in which the most likely source of aluminum was orally administered phosphate binders. For this reason some nephrologists use calcium carbonate as a phosphate binder instead, beginning at doses of 500 mg elemental calcium with each meal. Patients on calcium carbonate must be watched for the development of hypercalcemia. Whichever binder is chosen, it should be administered at meal time. Both types of phosphate binder can be constipating.

Aluminum-related osteomalacia may be diagnosed by needle biopsy of bone with special stains for aluminum. In addition, the magnitude of the body burden of aluminum may be estimated by administering a test dose of desferoxamine mesylate and measuring the increment of serum or plasma aluminum. Both aluminum-related osteomalacia and dialysis dementia have responded to intermittent IV or intraperitoneal doses of desferoxamine mesylate.

Hypertension is better controlled with continuous peritoneal dialysis technics than IPD dialysis or hemodialysis; patients on continuous technics seldom require antihypertensive medications. In approximately 80% of hemodialysis patients, hypertension can be controlled simply by achieving dry weight through ultrafiltration during dialysis. In the remaining 20%, antihypertensive drugs may be required. In resistant cases, a combination of agents is frequently used; eg, minoxidil in combination with a β-blocker because of reflex tachycardia. Antihypertensives which regularly produce orthostatic hypotension (methyldopa, guanethidine) usually are avoided in hemodialysis patients, but, if necessary, dosage may be omitted on days when hemodialysis is performed. Impaired renal excretion must be considered when any drug is given to these patients; eg, digoxin and aminoglycoside antibiotic doses are always reduced.

Certain peculiarities in the management of patients receiving peritoneal dialysis must be kept in mind; eg, constipation often interferes with catheter drainage. Many patients may require bulk laxatives (psyllium hydrocolloid) or stool softeners.

ALTERED NEUROLOGIC AND MENTAL STATES IN DIALYSIS PATIENTS

The symptoms and signs of **acute uremic encephalopathy** (see Ch. 147) are generally reversed rapidly by dialysis, although in rare cases restoration to the premorbid state may take 2 wk. However, sensitive psychologic tests can demonstrate differences in function before and after dialysis in otherwise stable patients. Furthermore, patients on chronic dialysis therapy may develop a variety of neurologic and psychiatric disorders which affect their mental functioning. Since hemodialysis patients are regularly anticoagulated, problems such as **subdural hematoma** and **intracerebral hemorrhage** may develop. Disequilibrium associated with osmotic shifts produced by hemodialysis may produce **seizures**. Because of enhanced atherosclerosis in renal failure, **thrombotic strokes** may occur.

A peculiar neurologic syndrome, **dialysis dementia,** is characterized by progressive dementia, dyspraxia, facial grimaces, myoclonic seizures, and characteristic EEG. This disorder may be associated with high brain aluminum concentrations. The exact source of the aluminum is controversial, but high concentrations in tap water have been found in areas where epidemics of this condition have occurred. Another source may be the aluminum-containing antacids prescribed to control phosphorus balance (see above). Secondary hyperparathyroidism also may be pathogenetic.

Besides organic brain syndromes, dialysis patients are also subject to a wide range of **functional disorders,** from schizophrenia and manic depression to maladaptive coping behavior (see PSYCHOSOCIAL ASPECTS OF CHRONIC DIALYSIS, below). The differential diagnostic approach used to separate these disorders is the same as that used for patients who do not have kidney failure. A careful neurologic and psychiatric evaluation is always warranted before assuming the disorder is functional or attempting symptomatic relief.

PSYCHOSOCIAL ASPECTS OF CHRONIC DIALYSIS

The chronic dialysis patient depends on his regular dialysis treatments for his life. Medical, social, and emotional complications make the patient and family constantly vulnerable to crises. How patients, families, and the treatment team cope with these pressures affects not only adjustment but also patient survival. In general, psychosocial problems are reduced by dialysis programs that encourage patient independence and resumption of former life interests as much as possible.

Psychosocial Stresses of Chronic Dialysis

Losses or threatened losses in every area of the patient's life abound; **loss of independence** is major among these. The patient is dependent on the treatment team to manage the illness and treatment; dialyses, often scheduled for the convenience of others, influence the patient's work and leisure activities. Regular employment may be precluded, and usual family roles and responsibilities are often modified, creating tension and feelings of guilt and inadequacy. Community help often is necessary for high treatment costs, medications, special diets, and transportation.

Also stressful are **losses and changes in body image and function**, including loss of urination and of physical energy; loss or change in sexual function; changed appearance due to access surgery, peritoneal catheter, needle marks, bone disease, or other signs of physical deterioration; and ultimately, the threat of loss of life.

Chronic dialysis has a major psychosocial **impact on the patient's family**, particularly in home dialysis when a family member is the treatment partner; but in any setting, patient dependence and reduced work capacity and physical abilities may cause role reversals in the family. The marital relationship is especially vulnerable.

Reactions of Patients and Families

Favorable prognostic indicators for long-term adjustment to dialysis include those premorbid personality factors and life adjustments that demonstrate the patient's adaptability, independence and self-control, tolerance to frustration, and optimistic perception of life. An emotionally stable and encouraging family also fosters adjustment. A consistently supportive approach from the treatment team towards patient and family and their inclusion as key participants are essential. Sex, educational status, and other socioeconomic factors seem to be less important. While age is not a critical indicator of long-term adjustment to dialysis, young adults and adolescents, who are coping with normal-age identity, independence, and body image issues, find these issues complicated by dialysis. Persons of many different personality types can adjust to dialysis.

Coping reactions among dialysis patients range from full rehabilitation to suicide. **Stages of adjustment** may include a "honeymoon" period at dialysis onset experienced by persons who are physically much improved, optimistic, and euphoric; a period of depression, disillusionment, and discouragement, when the long-term reality of the illness and treatment sets in; and finally, the beginning of long-term adaptation, characterized by the individual's premorbid personality and coping skills.

Specific coping reactions include **denial**, particularly useful in helping a patient to avoid the reality of his dependence on the treatment and his life-threatening situation. Thus, the patient is not overwhelmed and can resume life activities. However, if denial is excessive, the patient may reject the need for treatment and die. Lack of some denial may result in severe anxiety or depression and lead to psychosis or suicide.

Increased dependence or independence is a common coping reaction. Dependent personalities may more easily accept their circumstances, but excessive dependence can create extreme demands on others and impede rehabilitation. Some patients may accept the sick role too well and be unable to relinquish it. Independence as a coping reaction may create adjustment problems to the treatment and the sick role initially, and lead to rejection of advice and treatment. However, ultimately it can favor social rehabilitation and patient responsibility, reducing the burden on family members.

Depression, a normal response to loss, may be especially pronounced. **Guilt, hostility, and ambivalence** are seen in patients who view the treatment as both miracle and monster. They may feel both grateful and resentful toward those on whom they depend, and may be ambivalent about their very desire to live.

Some dialysis patients **act out** their feelings; eg, by noncompliance with diet and medication or arriving late or not at all for dialysis. The treatment team or the home dialysis partner may become the target for the patient's anger. However, many patients express their feelings and direct their energy in productive ways. They may return to work, resume former interests, or become "lay counselors" to fellow dialysis patients. Self-care and home dialysis help the patient regain a sense of control and independence by allowing him to be largely responsible for his own treatment, able to integrate it into his life more flexibly.

Coping reactions in patients' families are similar. Denial can be functional or can interfere with emotional support to the patient. Depression, resentment, guilt, ambivalence, and psychosomatic and behavioral problems are manifested by family members. However, families can provide very important support to their ill members and can also develop a network of mutual support with other dialysis families.

Impact of Treatment Alternatives

The development and more widespread use of several differing treatment modalities have facilitated patient-family adjustment. Hemodialysis, continuous ambulatory peritoneal dialysis, intermittent peritoneal dialysis, and continuous cycling peritoneal dialysis differ in method, time schedule, and complexity, and offer the option of partner-assisted or totally self-care dialysis. The potential for choice in treatment, patient involvement in selecting a modality, and recognition of the importance of psychosocial as well as medical factors in the choice of modality all influence compliance, adjustment, morbidity, and mortality.

Special Demands on the Treatment Team

The treatment team in dialysis programs generally consists of physicians, nurses, social workers, and dietitians. These professionals are intensely involved with patients, whom they see gradually deteriorate rather than get well. Strong emotional attachments are inevitable. Like patients, they sometimes cope by using denial, but it is generally an unsatisfactory reaction. Denying the seriousness of the patient's illness and his limitations may lead to unrealistic staff expectations. The resulting feelings of guilt in the patient and resentment in the staff impede meeting realistic rehabilitation

goals. Realistically appropriate staff attitudes promote the patient's desire to live, self-esteem, and rehabilitation.

149. IMMUNOLOGICALLY MEDIATED RENAL DISEASES

(Immune Renal Diseases; IRD)

Glomerular and tubulointerstitial renal diseases that are mediated by host immune mechanisms. IRD may result from "normal" sequelae of the host's immune responsiveness or from a variety of congenital or acquired immunologic derangements. In this chapter, we describe mechanisms by which renal immune injury occurs (see TABLE 149–1) and discuss methods of diagnosing and treating IRD. Related discussions of immune mechanisms are in Chs. 17 and 20.

An antigenic stimulus triggers nearly all immune responses, with resultant kidney inflammation. However, the precise antigen responsible for the majority of IRD is rarely known. In general (see TABLE 149–2) antigens involved in IRD may be categorized on the basis of whether their initial formation is within the kidney itself (renal antigen) or outside of the kidney (nonrenal antigen). Further, renal and nonrenal antigens may be either (1) endogenous (self) antigens which normally are constituents of the host; or (2) exogenous (nonself) antigens which normally are not constituents of the host. The nonrenal antigen (with or without antibody) ultimately finds its way to and localizes within the kidney.

Categorization of the histopathologic changes resulting from IRD are based on the type of immune response occurring in the kidney. These hypersensitivity reactions are discussed further below; and in Ch. 20.

Pathogenesis of IRD

The renal transplant as the prototypic IRD: The antigens of the graft may be identical to those of the host (transplantation in identical twins); in this case, no response occurs. However, in most renal transplants, the kidney provides antigens that are nonself and therefore trigger an immune response in the host, usually the **cellular** response. Renal antigens present on nucleated cells of the transplant are processed by the monocyte/macrophage system which releases interleukin-I and activates helper T cells. Activated helper T cells stimulate other T cells in the presence of interleukin-II, transforming them to cytotoxic T cells that attack the foreign antigens of the graft, resulting in cell-mediated immune inflammation.

The foreign renal antigens of the graft in a presensitized host also may trigger an **antibody-mediated** attack on renal capillary endothelium **(hyperacute rejection)** resulting in acute renal ischemia, infarction, and transplant loss.

Theoretically, histocompatibility antigens (β_2-microglobulins) released into the circulation may trigger an **immune complex (IC) reaction** resulting in IC deposition within the renal mesangium or glomerular basement membrane **(GBM)**. This type of immune renal injury is not common in renal transplants, but may be seen in extended-survival grafts. Rarely, the renal transplant may undergo **IgE-mediated** injury which causes vasospastic ischemia within the allograft. This vasospasm appears to be reversible if treated appropriately and promptly with antirejection medication.

IRD not involving transplantation may occur via any of the classical forms of immune response as described in Ch. 20. Since IC–mediated IRD is the most common form, it will be considered first.

Immune complex (IC, Type III) renal diseases *result from "planting" of endogenous or exogenous antigens along with specific antibody as antigen-antibody-complement com*

TABLE 149–1. PATTERNS OF IMMUNOLOGICALLY MEDIATED RENAL DISEASES

Type of Immune Reactivity	*Associated Renal Disease*	*Antigen or Cause*	*Pattern of Deposition of Immune Components*		
			Ig	*Complement*	*Fibrin*
IgE mediated (Anaphylactic, immediate, Type I)	1. Immune tubular interstitial disease	Various (eg, penicillin)	Interstitial	—	—
Cytotoxic (Antibody-mediated, Type II)	1. Anti-GBM disease	GBM	Linear along GBM	Linear along GBM (sometimes absent)	Extracapillary
	2. Anti-TBM disease	Tubular antigens	Linear along TBM	Linear along TBM	—
	3. Hyperacute rejection	Class I HLA antigens	Diffuse vascular	—	Diffuse cortical vascular
Immune complex (IC, Type III)	1. Immune complex GN, (eg, poststreptococcal, serum sickness, hepatitis B, SLE)	Variety of exogenous & endogenous	"Lumpy-bumpy" in capillary wall or interstitium	"Lumpy-bumpy" in capillary wall or interstitium	Minimal
Cell-mediated (Delayed, Type IV)	1. Chronic renal allograft rejection	Class II HLA antigens	Diffuse granular	Diffuse granular	Vascular
	2. Chronic GN	Renal antigens	Variable	Variable	Vascular
Direct complement activation (alternative pathway)	1. Membranoproliferative GN	IC, C_3 nephritic factor	Often none, occasional IgG in mesangium	C3, subendothelial or intramembranous	Rare
Acquired immuno-deficiency (AIDS)	1. Focal segmental GN	T cell virus	Focal and segmental IgM	Focal and segmental	—
Congenital complement component deficiency	1. Lupus-like syndrome	Complement deficiency	Focal mesangial	Focal mesangial	—
	2. Hemolytic-uremic syndrome	Factor H deficiency	Ischemic and coagulative necrosis	—	—

GBM = Glomerular basement membrane; TBM = Tubular basement membrane; HLA = Histocompatibility antigens; GN = Glomerulonephritis.
(Modified from J. A. Bellanti, *Immunology III*, p. 433, 1985. Copyright 1985 by W. B. Saunders Company. Used with permission.)

TABLE 149–2. PATHOGENESIS OF IRD CLASSIFIED BY TYPE OF ANTIGENIC STIMULUS

Antigen	*Endogenous (Self)*	*Exogenous (Non-Self)*
Renal (tissue fixed)	Anti-GBM disease Anti-GBM disease with pulmonary hemorrhage (Goodpasture's syndrome) Anti-TBM disease	Renal transplant rejection
Nonrenal ("planted")	Nuclear proteins (lupus nephritis) Tumor antigens	Antibiotics (methicillin-induced interstitial nephritis) Nonsteroidal anti-inflammatory drugs (NSAIDs)

GBM = Glomerular basement membrane; TBM = Tubular basement membrane.

plexes in the mesangium, interstitium, or glomerular capillary wall of the kidney. The type and location of antibody identified by immunofluorescence microscopy in renal biopsy sections is regarded as the "fingerprint" of the underlying immune mechanism. IC are classically planted in a **"lumpy-bumpy" pattern**. In IC renal diseases, circulating IC also may be demonstrated in the blood.

The underlying mechanisms of IC renal diseases have been determined by analogy to experimental IRD produced in laboratory animals by administration of foreign proteins. The foreign protein stimulates production of specific antibody, which combines with the antigen in one of 2 ways: within the kidney after the antigen has been planted, or in the circulation to form a circulating IC which subsequently becomes deposited. The former mechanism appears to be the more common process. The deposited antigen attracts its specific antibody as the antibody circulates through the kidney, and a local IC is formed. Alternatively, if the complexes are formed in the circulation, as antibody production increases, the size of the circulating IC increases, favoring localization in the mesangium or glomerular capillary wall. Small IC are not deposited and large complexes are preferentially removed by reticuloendothelial organs (spleen, liver, and lymphatics), minimizing localization in the kidney. As described above, a variety of endogenous and exogenous substances may function in the role of antigen in IC formation. For example, endogenous nuclear proteins may result in DNA–anti-DNA IC in lupus nephritis; or streptococcal cell wall antigens may form IC in poststreptococcal glomerulonephritis (**PSGN**—see TABLE 149–2).

Whatever the source of the antigen, deposition of IC in the glomerular capillary wall, predominantly in subepithelial sites, underlies the pathogenesis of IC immune glomerular diseases by activation of the complement system. On exposure to IC, the series of proteins known as complement **(C)** combine to form immune reactants capable of mediating injury. (See also THE COMPLEMENT SYSTEM in Ch. 17.) An example of one such immune reactant is chemotactic factor (C567), which causes polymorphonuclear leukocytes and other phagocytic cells to localize in the area of immune injury. These phagocytic cells release their intracellular enzymes (lysozymes) which are capable of causing tissue damage. Once completely activated through C9, C is capable of causing direct tissue destruction.

The precise mechanism whereby IC are planted remains unclear. Some antigens may have specific affinity for the GBM as described for single-stranded DNA to the mouse

GBM. Alternatively, planted antigens may actually be altered native antigens or viruses that gain access to renal tissues via the circulation. Regardless of the type or source of the antigen, a variety of factors appear to influence or favor such localization, including release of vasoactive substances to enhance vascular permeability, and the size, shape, and antigen:antibody ratio of the complexes. Nevertheless, none of these factors provides a complete explanation for the depositing of IC.

An additional explanation has been provided by demonstrating 2 forms of normally occurring binding sites for host immune reactants: one for activated complement (C3b) on the glomerular epithelial cell, and another for the Fc fragment of IgG in the renal interstitium. Hypothetically, IC containing antigen-antibody and C3 may attach to the subepithelial cells of the capillary wall. IC passage to the C3 binding site may be affected by release of vasoactive amines as well as the structure of the IC molecule. In tubulointerstitial IC IRD, localization of IgG-containing IC may result from attachment to interstitial Fc binding sites.

Cytotoxic (antibody-mediated or Type II) IRD results from *the fixation of cytotoxic antibody to kidney tissue, with subsequent activation of the C sequence and propagation of immune inflammatory injury*. Although not as common as IC IRD, the cytotoxic form is the more clearly understood. For example, **anti-GBM disease (Goodpasture's syndrome)** results from the fixation of the specific antibody to the GBM of the kidney. Often, the cytotoxic, GBM-fixing antibody can be detected in the serum as well. In contrast to the "lumpy-bumpy" pattern of antibody deposition in IC IRD, antibody in cytotoxic IRD is deposited in a smooth, linear fashion. The cytotoxic antibody is directed against kidney antigens resulting in tissue injury by local activation of C. As in IC IRD, the antigens within the kidney may be self (the GBM, as in Goodpasture's syndrome) or foreign (histocompatibility antigens, as in hyperacute renal graft rejection—see TABLE 149-2).

Cell-mediated (delayed—Type IV) IRD is characterized by *the infiltration of lymphocytes that have become sensitized to antigens within the kidney*. Sensitized lymphocytes may cause tissue injury either directly or by releasing soluble products (lymphokines) that have the capacity to support local inflammation with release of tissue-destructive intracellular enzymes. Although not completely proved, **chronic glomerulonephritis (GN)** may represent an example of cell-mediated sensitization to self-renal antigens, stimulated by exposure to cross-reactive streptococcal cell wall antigens. Sensitization to nonself renal antigens is exemplified by **chronic renal allograft rejection.**

IgE-mediated (immediate or Type I hypersensitivity) IRD *result from the action of IgE on basophils and mast cells after contact with specific antigen*. As one of their mechanisms of action, these vasoactive substances trigger platelet-mediated coagulation, thrombosis, and fibrin deposition. Participation of IgE-mediated mechanisms in IRD has not been definitively established; however, a number of renal diseases are associated with IgE deposition. It is likely that IgE-mediated hypersensitivity in part underlies the tubulointerstitial renal disease associated with the administration of penicillins, especially methicillin. This IRD is associated with eosinophilia, eosinophilic infiltration in the kidney, the deposition of IgE response to corticosteroids, and improvement on discontinuation of the drug.

Direct complement (C)-mediated IRD also may result from *direct activation of C through the alternative pathway* (see also TABLE 149-1, above; and THE COMPLEMENT SYSTEM in Ch. 17) *in the apparent absence of antigen or antibody*. The renal injury is characterized predominantly by the deposition of C3 and another serum protein **(properdin)** in the mesangium and glomerular capillary wall. Early components of complement and immunoglobulin are not demonstrable using immunofluorescence technics. Alternative pathway activation of the C system results when properdin cleaves C3, using as cofactors C3 proactivator, C3 proactivator convertase, and native C3 in the

presence of magnesium ions. While all these compounds are constituents of normal serum, activation normally proceeds at a controlled rate without resulting in renal deposition of activated C3. The exact mechanism whereby alternative pathway activation becomes disordered, with resultant renal C3 deposition, is not clear. About half the patients who develop IRD associated predominantly with C3 deposition have a serum protein capable of direct cleavage of C3 to active C3b. This molecule, called **C3 nephritic factor,** is a heat-stable 7S-globulin of 150,000 mol wt that is not an immunoglobulin. C3b may then deposit in the phagocytic mesangium of the kidney or in C3b binding sites within the capillary wall, which causes local immune inflammatory injury.

Direct C activation results in IRD characterized by proliferation of cellular elements within the renal corpuscle and increase in capillary wall thickness. These changes in renal biopsy sections are called **membranoproliferative GN** (see also in Ch. 150), of which 3 forms have been described: Types I, II and III (the latter seems to be characterized by features of both I and II). In IgE-mediated disease, deposited immune components are found mostly in the mesangium and subendothelial sites (Type I). In cytotoxic-type disease, the deposits are found intramembranously within the capillary wall (Type II). Although both forms appear to result from alternative pathway C3 activation, the subendothelial variety may be associated with IC activation of the alternative pathway, while cytotoxic disease is more commonly associated with the presence of C3 nephritic factor in the serum.

Renal disease in acquired immune deficiency syndrome: AIDS may be associated with a form of progressive renal disease characterized by focal segmental glomerulosclerosis and focal deposition of IgM and C3. Heroin addiction appears to be a significant risk factor; however, the disease also has been found in patients without antecedent heroin abuse. The pathogenesis is not yet clear, but the abnormal immunologic status of patients with AIDS may predispose to IRD; eg, via unbridled antibody-mediated immunity, since polyclonal hypergammaglobulinemia has been described in AIDS. An alternative explanation may be that renal damage proceeds via T cell-mediated immune injury.

Congenital C component deficiencies are associated with a number of renal diseases (see TABLE 149–1), including one manifested by an SLE-like syndrome, perhaps resulting from impaired handling of autologous proteins released into the circulation. Also, renal hemolytic-uremic syndrome has been described in patients with factor H deficiency. The exact mechanisms are not clear, but the perturbation of the normal immunologic environment of the host, whether in the direction of excess or deficiency, predisposes to the development of IRD.

Diagnosis

Renal biopsy: Although analyses of blood and urine usually are performed first, renal biopsy material ultimately provides the definitive data for the diagnosis of IRD, and possibly important indicators for prognosis and treatment. Consideration of the normal structure and the basic pathologic changes that are possible provides an understanding of IRD. The renal corpuscle consists of cells and extracellular material **(ECM)**. Possible cellular changes are an increase in number (hyperplasia), a decrease in number (atrophy), necrosis, and exudation (infiltration by neutrophils). The possible ECM changes are an increase in amount of material (sclerosis or scarring) or the accumulation of foreign protein deposits. All of every glomerulus **(diffuse change),** all of a few glomeruli **(focal change),** or part of a few glomeruli **(local change)** may be involved.

The **type and pattern of C deposition** help in diagnosing and distinguishing IRD. C deposition usually follows the pattern of immunoglobulin deposition. However, the

presence of C3 deposition in the absence of immunoglobulin, Clq, or C4 deposition suggests alternative pathway activation and membranoproliferative GN.

These histopathologic changes can be observed using light, immunofluorescence, and electron microscopy. **Light microscopic examinations** may reveal cellular proliferation, basement membrane thickening, sclerosis, hyalinization, alteration in vascular endothelial cells, and changes in the types of numbers of cells present in the renal tissue. Since various immune mechanisms may result in similar morphologic changes, **immunofluorescence microscopy** using fluorescein-labeled specific antibodies may be useful to characterize the type and location of immune components in the kidney. Recently, fluoresceinated monoclonal antibodies specific for types of lymphoid cell subsets have been used to identify the type and frequency of such subsets as T_4 (helper/inducer) or T_8 (suppressor/cytotoxic) lymphocytes. **Electron microscopy** provides a high degree of resolution to visualize submicroscopic changes in the thickness and composition of glomerular and tubular structures, and the presence of deposits which usually correlate with immunofluorescence findings.

Urine examination: In many instances, a precise diagnosis of IRD can be made by carefully examining the urine, which in IRD nearly always contains abundant protein and lipid-laden macrophages (the **Maltese crosses** seen by polarized light microscopy). Thus, the nephrotic syndrome (**NS**—see in Ch. 150) is present in virtually all forms of IRD. The excretion of excess protein into the urine appears to result from loss of ability by the glomerular capillary wall to retain large mol wt proteins or to repel negatively charged albumin molecules. The latter may be the consequence of immune injury altering the normal negative charges on the epithelial cell surface. While NS may be observed in nonimmune renal diseases such as diabetes mellitus, the presence of nephrotic-range proteinuria suggests an underlying immune mechanism.

RBCs, WBCs, and cellular casts also may be found in the urine. Injury resulting in necrosis, as in acute cytotoxic-type (Type II) injury of anti-GBM disease, causes significant hematuria. Forms of Type III (IC) injury (eg, postinfective glomerulonephritides) are associated with hematuria and RBC casts. SLE, with active renal disease, is associated with hematuria, lymphocyturia, RBC casts, and epithelial cell casts. This type of urine is called the **"telescopic urine"** of SLE nephritis and some other collagen vascular diseases. Membranous, membranoproliferative, focal sclerosing, and minimal-change glomerulonephritides are associated with NS but usually have otherwise benign urinary sediments.

Serologic analyses: In Type II IRD, cytotoxic antibodies may be present in the circulation (eg, anti-GBM or anti-kidney antibodies). Circulating antinuclear antibodies may be seen in SLE, or circulating IC in a variety of IC IRD.

Alterations in levels of C proteins often are useful in differentiating the types of IRD. When alternative pathway C activation predominates, early components of C (Clq and C4) are *not* depressed, since C consumption occurs via direct activation of C3 (eg, membranoproliferative GN **[MPGN]** and frequently in poststreptococcal GN **[PSGN]**). In classical pathway activation (as in SLE), early components of C are depressed. The presence of C3 nephritic factor with depressed C3 but normal Clq and C4 virtually establishes the diagnosis of MPGN with alternative pathway C activation.

Other helpful serologic analyses include rising titers of antibodies to streptococcal antigens in PSGN. Other postinfective glomerulonephritides can be diagnosed by serologic findings such as a positive test for syphilis, hepatitis-associated antigen, or rising antibody titers to certain other infective organisms.

Course and Prognosis

These are highly variable and depend on the underlying pathogenesis, the categories of which are discussed in Ch. 150.

Treatment

Although the immunologic mechanisms underlying many renal diseases are now understood, treatment in most instances is nonspecific or unavailable. Principles of therapy involve modulation of host immune mechanisms by removing antigen, antibody, or IC, inducing immunosuppression, and/or administering anti-inflammatory agents and in some cases platelet-inhibiting and anticoagulation agents (see TABLE 150–2 in Ch. 150, below). If the antigenic stimulus cannot be removed, the goal is to reduce the antigen load and create antibody excess to favor reticuloendothelial removal of IC. A few diseases are particularly responsive to corticosteroid therapy (eg, minimal change disease, SLE, and possibly membranous GN). Azathioprine may provide additional benefit in transplant rejection and SLE. Cyclophosphamide appears to be helpful in Wegener's granulomatosis. Cyclosporine is appropriate antirejection therapy in organ transplantation and may find application in other forms of IRD.

Results with dipyrimidole and acetylsalicylic acid in membranoproliferative glomerulonephritis **(MPGN)** Type I are promising enough that treatment with platelet inhibitors is recommended (no other treatment has proved effective). In MPGN Type II, depressing the level of cytotoxic antibodies is difficult, because the stimulating antigen remains. Therapeutic benefit has been achieved by plasmapheresis in anti-GBM disease, acute allograft rejection, and SLE. It is important that plasmapheresis be given only in combination with both corticosteroid and immunosuppressant maintenance medication (see also TABLE 150–4 in Ch. 150, below). Unfortunately, the majority of IRD remain resistant to therapy.

150. THE GLOMERULAR DISEASES

A group of diverse conditions including, but not limited to, glomerulonephritis **(GN)**, *in which the disease process appears mainly to affect the glomerulus.* Structural, functional, and clinical similarities exist within the group because of the limited number of ways that a tissue can respond to injury and that these injuries can be expressed as symptoms and signs. Clear-cut differentiation may be impossible. Furthermore, although pathologic differences may provide an understanding of the glomerular disease, correlations between morphologic changes and clinical features are not completely reliable in regard to prognosis and response to treatment.

Glomerular damage produces changes in glomerular capillary permeability, resulting in various degrees of proteinuria, hematuria, leukocyturia, and urinary casts. Microthrombosis, commonly accompanied by epithelial "crescents" formed from leaked fibrinogen and precipitated fibrin may occur, and if damage is severe, hemodynamic changes may produce oliguria. Commonly, tubular function is deranged by inflammatory changes in the interstitium. Measurable changes consist of reduction in the urinary concentrating capacity, acid excretion, and varying disturbances in nephron solute exchange. Because there is some inherent capacity for glomerular hypertrophy, such defects in tubular function usually occur before the GFR is much reduced. As glomerular derangement progresses, however, the total filtration surface is significantly reduced, the GFR falls, and azotemia occurs.

These varied glomerulopathies can be grouped into 5 major syndromes, based on their clinical presentation: (1) **acute nephritic syndrome**—acute onset and early resolution; (2) **rapidly progressive nephritic syndrome**—acute onset and rapid progression; (3) **idiopathic renal hematuric syndromes**—persistent, asymptomatic, minimal urinary abnormalities; (4) **nephrotic syndrome**; and (5) **chronic nephritic syndrome**. They may be either primary glomerulopathies or secondary to systemic disease.

ACUTE NEPHRITIC SYNDROME

(Acute Glomerulonephritis [AGN]; Postinfectious Glomerulonephritis [PIGN])

A disease most common in children, characterized pathologically by diffuse inflammatory changes in the glomeruli and clinically by the abrupt onset of hematuria with RBC casts and mild proteinuria, and in many cases hypertension, edema, and azotemia.

Etiology and Pathogenesis

The classic example of glomerular disease of acute onset is **poststreptococcal glomerulonephritis (PSGN).** In this immune complex **(IC)** disease, Group A β-hemolytic (nephritis strains 1, 4, 12, 29) streptococcal antigens provoke an antibody response, and the resulting circulating antigen-antibody complexes are deposited in the glomerular capillary walls. These complexes activate a cascade of events that are described in Ch. 149. PSGN may occur during epidemics of streptococcal infection or sporadically. The streptococcal infection is most often in the upper respiratory tract; however, infections at other sites (skin, middle ear) may precede nephritis, particularly in the first decade of life. Cultures of urine and renal tissue grow no streptococci. Antibiotics do not halt progression of the nephritis, unlike their effect in rheumatic fever. Clinically, AGN due to other infections (see TABLE 150–1) is indistinguishable from PSGN.

Other forms of PIGN thought to induce immunologic injury include the glomerulopathy associated with SBE, infected ventriculoatrial shunts (established to relieve hydrocephalus), varicella, infectious hepatitis (HBsAg-positive), syphilis, and malaria. The last three may cause a sclerosing lesion and severe proteinuria **(nephrotic syndrome)** rather than acute glomerular disease, possibly because of chronic but low-level antigenemia.

Pathology

The lesion is mainly confined to the glomeruli, which become enlarged and hypercellular, initially with numerous neutrophils and/or eosinophils and later with relatively large numbers of mononuclear cells. Epithelial cell hyperplasia is a common early, transient feature after onset of the clinical syndrome, and cellular crescents may be found in a few glomeruli. True synechiae (bridges of basement membrane between the capillary loops and Bowman's basement membrane) are rare. Endothelial cells increase in number and the usual fenestration of their cytoplasm may not be apparent. The mesangial regions often are greatly expanded by edema, and contain neutrophils, dead cells, cellular debris, and deposits of electron-dense material (ICs from the circulation or formed in situ).

The most notable feature of the glomerular basement membrane **(GBM)** is the large

TABLE 150–1. CAUSES OF ACUTE NEPHRITIC SYNDROME

Primary Renal Disease	*Secondary Disease*
Membranoproliferative glomerulonephritis (MPGN)	Poststreptococcal glomerulonenephritis (PSGN)
IgA nephropathy	Postinfectious glomerulonenephritis (PIGN)
Rapidly progressive glomerulonephritis (RPGN)	Polyarteritis nodosa
Focal glomerulonephritis (focal GN)	Goodpasture's syndrome
Acute interstitial nephritis	Systemic lupus erythematosus
	Henoch-Schönlein purpura
	Hemolytic-uremic syndrome
	Wegener's granulomatosis
	Thrombotic thrombocytopenic purpura
	Mixed IgG-IgM cryoglobulinemia
	Serum sickness

number of deposits in its epithelial side, chiefly near or in mesangial regions. Experimental evidence indicates that these are formed in situ. The foot processes of the epithelial cells are invariably effaced over the deposits. Fluorescence microscopy shows diffuse granular deposits of IgG and C3 distributed irregularly along the GBM and in the mesangium.

Symptoms, Signs, and Diagnosis

PSGN is most common in children > 3 yr of age and in young adults, but 5% of cases occur after age 50. There is a latent period of 1 to 6 wk (average, 2 wk) between the infection and the onset of nephritis. The presenting complaints are edema, oliguria, dark urine (blood content), and, if fluid retention is severe enough, hypervolemia. Headaches and visual disturbances may occur secondary to hypertension. A history of a sore throat, impetigo, or, better yet, a culture-proven streptococcal infection 1 to 6 wk before onset of these symptoms, and elevated serum titer of antistreptococcal antibodies, are clues to the diagnosis. The course is not stereotyped. About 50% of patients are symptom-free. In many cases, the first indicator is the incidental discovery of gross or microscopic hematuria. Transient renal insufficiency is common; in the majority of cases, the symptoms and signs abate gradually. In severe cases, complications include hypertension, with or without congestive heart failure, and hypertensive encephalopathy. The nephrotic syndrome (see below) develops in approximately 30% of patients. In an unfortunate few, onset of the disease is with anuria, severe hypervolemia, and hyperkalemia, and death may occur unless the patient is dialyzed.

Other forms of PIGN usually are easier to diagnose than PSGN, having a much shorter lag period or being present when the infection is apparent. However, the nephritis of **SBE** can pose a diagnostic enigma: A wide spectrum of renal involvement is possible, the systemic manifestations often mimic other diseases (eg, SLE or polyarteritis nodosa), and blood cultures may be sterile.

Laboratory Findings

The urine may be scanty and appears brown, smoky, or frankly bloody. From 0.5 to 2 gm of protein/sq m/day may be excreted. The urinary sediment contains RBCs, WBCs, and renal tubular cells; casts containing RBCs and Hb are characteristic, and WBC casts and granular (protein droplets) casts are common. **The RBC cast is pathognomonic of any form of glomerulitis,** but in association with the clinical picture just described is strongly indicative of glomerular disease of acute onset.

The antibody titer against the causal infectious agent usually rises within 1 to 2 wk. In particular, the increase in antibodies to streptococcal antigenic products can be measured: antistreptolysin-O **(ASO),** antistreptokinase **(ASKase),** antihyaluronidase **(AHase),** and antideoxyribonuclease B **(ADNase B).** ASO is the best indicator of upper respiratory infections; AHase and ADNase B, of pyoderma. Serum complement levels (C3, C4, CH_{50}) usually are diminished during the active phase of the disease. Complement levels return to normal within 6 to 8 wk in 80% of PSGN, but virtually never in Henoch-Schönlein purpura, hemolytic-uremic syndrome, IgA nephropathy, and Goodpasture's syndrome. Cryoglobulinemia usually persists for several months, whereas circulating ICs are detectable for only a few weeks. Ultrasound studies may help to distinguish acute disease (usually normal or slightly enlarged kidneys) from an exacerbation of chronic disease (small kidneys). Renal function (GFR) can be estimated from the serum creatinine concentration or urinary creatinine clearance. Although the GFR usually returns to normal over 1 to 3 mo, proteinuria may persist for 6 to 12 mo and microscopic hematuria for several years. Transient changes in urinary sediment may recur with minor respiratory infections.

Course and Prognosis

IC glomerular disease of acute onset such as **PSGN** usually carries a good prognosis if the initial renal damage is not severe and the source of antigenemia can be reduced

or removed. However, in some cases (1% in children, 10% in adults), the acute nephritic syndrome evolves into rapidly progressive glomerulonephritis **(RPGN)**. In patients with remittent disease, renal cellular proliferation disappears within weeks, but the severity of the inflammatory response varies widely and residual sclerosis is common. Most children (85 to 95%) retain or regain normal renal function but are at increased risk for hypertension. An abnormal urinalysis (proteinuria, hematuria) may continue for years; occasionally the condition may progress to chronic renal failure. A marked decline in GFR or the development of the nephrotic syndrome, together with extensive extracapillary proliferation (crescent formation) and necrosis, indicates rapid progression to end-stage renal failure. PSGN carries a poorer prognosis in adults. The urinary abnormalities persist in about 40% of cases and healing is characterized by scarring. Thus, the prognosis depends on the patient's age and the stage of the renal lesion when the inflammatory stimulus is removed.

PIGN secondary to an infected vascular prosthesis has a good prognosis if the infection (usually *Staphylococcus epidermidis [albus]*) can be eradicated; this often requires removal of the prosthesis, plus antibiotic therapy. **In SBE,** as in other forms of PIGN, removal of the source of the antigen usually (70 to 80%) is followed by resolution of the renal injury if extensive damage (crescents, necrosis) has not occurred before effective antimicrobial therapy.

Treatment

No specific treatment is available in most cases. Immunosuppressive agents and corticosteroids are ineffective—the latter may even worsen the condition. If a bacterial infection is still present when nephritis is discovered, it should be treated with antimicrobial drugs, and any other secondary causes (TABLE 150–1) should be treated (TABLE 150–2). If azotemia and metabolic acidosis are present, dietary protein is restricted. Sodium intake is restricted only when circulatory overload, edema, or severe hypertension is present; diuretics such as the thiazides and loop diuretics may help in the management of the expanded ECF volume. Hypertensive encephalopathy may require initial parenteral therapy with antihypertensive agents (hydralazine, diazoxide, labetalol, nitroprusside) when oral agents cannot be taken.

RAPIDLY PROGRESSIVE NEPHRITIC SYNDROME

(Rapidly Progressive Glomerulonephritis [RPGN]; Crescentic Glomerulonephritis)

A syndrome characterized pathologically by focal and segmental necrosis and epithelial cell proliferation (crescents) in most glomeruli and clinically by fulminant renal failure associated with proteinuria, hematuria, and RBC casts.

Etiology, Incidence, and Pathogenesis

Fortunately, RPGN is uncommon. The pathogenesis is unknown in most instances and the immediate causes are varied (see TABLE 150–3). RPGN may occur in most conditions that produce the acute nephritic syndrome (see above). The syndrome occurs as part of a multisystem disease in about 40% of cases. This chapter discusses the roughly 60% of RPGN cases that have primary renal involvement; of these, about half are idiopathic, a third appear to be caused by antibody directed against the GBM, and the rest are IC disease. The idiopathic cases also may be due to immunologic damage: Absence of deposits of immunoglobulins **(Ig)** or complement **(C)** in glomerular biopsy tissue may be due to a sampling error or represent a phase in the evolution of the disease that is free of residual immunologic factors.

The initiating events leading to autoimmunity directed against the GBM are unknown. Antibodies to the GBM are present in the blood and can be demonstrated by the immunofluorescence technic on the GBM. In certain patients, a circulating antibody is present that cross-reacts with pulmonary alveolar basement membrane, leading to a pulmonary–renal complex called Goodpasture's syndrome (see Ch. 44).

TABLE 150–2. THERAPY FOR GLOMERULONEPHRITIS INCLUDING IMMUNE RENAL DISEASE

Disease	Treatment
Poststreptococcal glomerulonephritis (PSGN)	No specific therapy available
Rapidly progressive glomerulonephritis (RPGN)	
Idiopathic	High-dose IV methylprednisolone; If fulminant disease, same as anti-GBM therapy
Immune complex (IC) disease	High-dose IV methylprednisolone
Anti-glomerular basement membrane (anti-GBM)	Plasmapheresis + maintenance prednisone + cyclophosphamide or chlorambucil
Focal glomerulonephritis (focal GN)	No specific therapy available
IgA nephropathy	Resistant to known therapeutic agents
Minimal-change disease (MCD)	Initial: prednisone. Maintenance: alternate-day predisone Corticosteroid-resistant or frequent relapses: prednisone on alternate days + daily cyclophosphamide; or cyclosporine
Focal glomerulosclerosis (FGS)	Usually corticosteroid-resistant. Give trial prednisone ± cyclophosphamide; or cyclosporine
Membranous glomerulonephritis (MGN)	High-dose alternate-day prednisone
Membranoproliferative glomerulonephritis (MPGN)	
Type 1	Platelet inhibitors: dipyridamole + acetylsalicylic acid
Type 2	No specific treatment available
Type 3	No specific treatment available
Mesangial proliferative glomerulonephritis	Mainly corticosteroid-resistant. Trial of oral prednisone
Goodpasture's syndrome	Plasmapheresis + maintenance predisone + cyclophosphamide or chlorambucil
Systemic lupus erythematosus	Intermittent IV cyclophosphamide + low-dose corticosteroids; plasmapheresis in resistant cases
Wegener's granulomatosis	Cyclophosphamide ± prednisone
Thrombotic thrombocytopenic purpura/hemolytic-uremic syndrome	Plasmapheresis + anti-platelet inhibitors (dipyridamole and acetylsalicylic acid)
Henoch-Schönlein purpura	No specific therapy available. Trial with plasmapheresis
Renal allograft rejection	
Acute	High-dose corticosteroids; ALG; ATG; irradiation; plasmapheresis
Chronic	Prednisone; cyclosporine; azathioprine; cyclophosphamide
Allergic interstitial nephritis	Trial with prednisone

ALG = antilymphocyte globulin.
ATG = antihymocyte globulin.

TABLE 150–3. CAUSES OF RAPIDLY PROGRESSIVE NEPHRITIC SYNDROME

Primary Renal Disease	*Secondary Extrarenal Disease*
Idiopathic	Henoch-Schönlein purpura
Immune complex	Polyarteritis nodosa
Anti-GBM* nephritis	Wegener's granulomatosis
	Systemic lupus erythematosus
	Goodpasture's syndrome
	Mixed IgG-IgM cryoglobulinemia
	Poststreptococcal glomerulonephritis (PSGN)
	Infective endocarditis
	Shunt nephritis
	Visceral sepsis
	Hepatitis

* GBM = Glomerular basement membrane.

Pathology

Focal proliferations of glomerular epithelial cells, in some cases interspersed with numerous neutrophils, form a crescentic cellular mass, filling Bowman's space. The glomerular tuft collapses, usually appearing hypocellular. Necrosis within the tuft or involving the crescent is not uncommon but may be the most prominent abnormality. In such patients, histologic evidence of vasculitis should be sought.

Interstitial edema often is a striking early finding. Most often it is diffuse and associated with infiltration of diverse types of inflammatory cells. Infiltration by mononuclear leukocytes between tubular cells is seen when interstitial infiltration is extensive. Later, the interstitium becomes diffusely fibrosed and the number of inflammatory cells decreases. Initial changes in the tubules include the formation of vacuoles and hyaline droplets and occasional RBC and hyaline casts in distal tubules. As the disease progresses, atrophy occurs and the GBM thickens.

Linear deposition of IgG (usually associated with C3 arranged segmentally) along the GBM is the most prominent abnormality seen on fluorescence microscopy, but this pattern is inconstant and nonspecific. In severe IC disease, there are diffuse irregular deposits of IgG and C3, commonly with proliferation of intraglomerular cells and crescent formation. In other cases, no Ig or C deposits are detected. However, fibrin occurs within the crescents, regardless of the fluorescence pattern.

Symptoms, Signs, and Diagnosis

The clinical presentation may be similar to that of acute nonprogressive disease, but most often the onset is more insidious, with weakness, fatigue, and fever as the most prominent symptoms; nausea, anorexia, vomiting, arthralgias, and abdominal pain also are common. A few patients have a history of proteinuria, hematuria, or hypertension. About 50% have edema and a history of an acute influenzalike illness within 4 wk of the onset of renal failure. This usually is followed by severe oliguria, and most patients are azotemic when first seen. Hypertension is uncommon and rarely severe.

Clinical findings and laboratory data usually indicate the diagnosis. Renal biopsy may help in differential diagnosis and in defining other potentially reversible lesions that may present similarly with RPGN.

Laboratory Findings

Azotemia of varying degree is typical. Hematuria, often macroscopic, always is present. RBC casts are invariable, and a "telescopic" sediment (RBC, WBC, granular,

waxy, and broad casts) is common. Anemia, sometimes severe, is a constant finding, and leukocytosis is common.

Serologic findings may help distinguish an anti-GBM antibody nephritis from severe IC disease. The latter is suggested by rising titers of antibodies to streptococci, circulating ICs, or cryoglobulinemia. Hypocomplementemia is uncommon in anti-GBM antibody nephritis but common in IC disease. A serum assay for circulating anti-GBM antibodies is helpful when positive. The kidneys may appear enlarged on ultrasound or radiographic imaging (done without contrast enhancement) initially, but they become progressively smaller.

Course and Prognosis

Although the course of the disease may take several months, it is common for many patients to present in the terminal stages of renal failure. Irreversible anuria is common, and without dialysis death occurs within a few weeks. The prognosis depends on preceding factors. If PSGN, SLE, or polyarteritis nodosa is the cause, renal function may improve with therapy. If the RPGN is idiopathic, however, spontaneous remission is rare. Patients who ultimately recover normal renal function have histologic changes, principally in the glomeruli, consisting chiefly of hypercellularity, with little or no sclerosis within the glomerular tuft or the epithelial cells and minimal fibrosis of the interstitium.

Treatment

A renal biopsy early in the course of suspected RPGN is essential to establish diagnosis, estimate prognosis, and plan management. Serologic tests and a check for infectious disease should be done. Where severe crescentic disease is found on biopsy (> 75% of glomeruli) without extensive glomerular obsolescence, tubulointerstitial lesions, multisystem or infectious disease, and the GFR exceeds 6 mL/min/sq m, drug therapy should be instituted (TABLE 150–2). Treatment should be started as early as possible, when the chance of best results is optimal. Treatment with anticoagulants, formerly advocated, has been abandoned. In general, corticosteroids given orally with or without cytotoxic drugs are ineffective.

For **idiopathic and IC RPGN,** however, high-dose parenteral methylprednisolone therapy is beneficial: 30 mg/kg (maximum, 3 gm) infused IV over 20 min, on days 1, 3, and 5; then, starting on day 8, 2 mg/kg orally on alternate days, tapering off in 3 to 6 mo. For **anti-GBM and fulminant IC RPGN,** a combination of plasmapheresis (see TABLE 150–4) and maintenance doses of prednisone (1 mg/kg/day) and cyclophosphamide or azathioprine (2 mg/kg/day) may be effective.

TABLE 150–4. PLASMAPHERESIS* IN RENAL DISEASE

Indications	*Complications*
Goodpasture's syndrome	Hypotension (volume depletion–inadvertent)
Anti-GBM nephritis	Hemorrhage (loss clotting factors)
Rapidly progressive glomerulonephritis (RPGN)	Arrhythmias
Polyarteritis nodosa and other vasculitides	Hypocalcemia
Systemic lupus erythematosus	Opportunistic infections
Thrombotic thrombocytopenic purpura	Hepatitis
Hemolytic-uremic syndrome	Hormone and/or enzyme depletion
Scleroderma	
Acute renal allograft rejection	

* Exchanges of between 2–4 L/day or 40 mL/kg sequentially for 5 days. Serum IgG may be a useful indicator of effectiveness.

Use concomitant immunosuppression for maintenance and to prevent rebound phenomena.

If the disease has progressed to a later stage, maintenance dialysis should be offered and therapy to treat the primary renal condition should be withheld. The alternative is renal transplantation, although this carries the risk of development of the original disease in the implanted kidney.

IDIOPATHIC RENAL HEMATURIC SYNDROMES

(IgA Nephropathy; Focal GN)

A group of disorders featuring recurrent episodes of macroscopic hematuria, mild proteinuria, glomerular changes, and slow or no progression to renal failure.

The idiopathic hematuric syndromes include a wide variety of primary disorders (IgA nephropathy, idiopathic focal GN), and may be the mode of presentation for several heredofamilial (Alport's syndrome, Fabry's disease, sickle cell), multisystem (SLE, Henoch-Schönlein purpura, vasculitis, Wegener's granulomatosis), and infectious (bacterial endocarditis, resolving PIGN) diseases. Histologically, the 2 main types are **mesangial IgA nephropathy (Berger's disease)** and **idiopathic focal GN**. IgA nephropathy affects up to 6 times as many males as females, is rare in blacks, and may be more common in orientals (25 to 40% of biopsies). No gender predilection is seen with focal GN.

Pathology

IgA nephropathy, one of the most common forms of primary GN, can be differentiated from other causes of idiopathic renal hematuria by immunofluorescence microscopy of renal biopsy tissue. The distinguishing (but nonspecific) feature is a granular deposition of IgA and C3 in the widened mesangium, with foci of segmental proliferative or necrotizing lesions. HLA-DR4 is detectable in about 50% of patients. Available evidence suggests that nephropathy occurs through mucosal immunization with polymeric IgA deposition in the kidney. The glomerular IgA deposits may occur in other diseases such as Henoch-Schönlein purpura, SLE nephritis, and chronic alcoholic hepatic cirrhosis.

Focal GN: Renal abnormalities range from minimal changes to mild diffuse proliferative GN. The most common lesion is focal, segmental, proliferative GN with various types of deposits.

Symptoms, Signs, and Diagnosis

About 50% of patients with recurrent renal hematuria have prominent mesangial IgA deposits in their renal tissue, and about half of these patients have increased serum IgA. Both IgA nephropathy and focal GN present initially during childhood or young adulthood. The syndrome is described most often as occurring 1 or 2 days after a febrile upper respiratory illness, thus mimicking PSGN, except that the onset of the hematuria is coincident with the febrile illness. There is no evidence of a systemic disease. Mild proteinuria (< 1 gm/day) is typical, but the nephrotic syndrome (see below) develops in up to 20% of patients who have IgA nephropathy. Microscopic hematuria always is present but RBC casts are noted infrequently, at least initially. The serum creatinine and complement levels usually are normal, but the IgA level commonly is increased in IgA nephropathy. Hypertension is unusual at the time of diagnosis. Loin pain may accompany the hematuria, more commonly in patients who have focal GN.

Patients with recurrent hematuria and a positive family history should be suspected of having hereditary nephritis (Alport's syndrome) and should have careful auditory and ocular examinations (see also Ch. 156).

Prognosis and Treatment

The long-term outlook for patients with **focal GN** appears benign. In most patients the hematuria remits spontaneously and renal function is well preserved. In **IgA ne-**

phropathy, however, the disease usually progresses, albeit slowly, with renal insufficiency and hypertension developing in 15 to 20% within 10 yr. Persistent heavy proteinuria, reduced GFR, and diffuse proliferative GN are unfavorable prognostic findings. Treatment of uremia is discussed under CHRONIC RENAL FAILURE in Ch. 147. Renal transplantation has been successful, although immunologic evidence of the disease in the implant has been recorded in some cases.

NEPHROTIC SYNDROME (NS)

A predictable complex that follows a severe, prolonged increase in glomerular permeability for protein. The main feature is proteinuria (> 2 gm/day/sq m), but hypoalbuminemia (< 3 gm/dL), generalized edema, and lipemia also are frequently present.

NS occurs at any age; in children, it is most common between ages 1.5 and 4 yr. There is a predilection for males in the young, and more equal sex distribution in older patients. New cases of NS in children average 2:100,000/yr in the USA and UK, and a survey of adults yielded 3 new cases/1,000,000/yr. The literature contains conflicting reports of the percentages of **minimal-change disease** (**MCD**—"lipoid nephrosis," "nil disease") in various age groups. The variations depend on selection of patients and referral patterns, local incidence of **focal glomerulosclerosis (FGS),** and geographic prevalence of predisposing diseases (eg, schistosomiasis in Egypt, malaria in Nigeria).

Etiology and Classification

NS may be due to primary glomerular disease (MCD, IC nephritides, focal segmental and mesangial diseases) or secondary causes. A simplified classification of causes of NS is in TABLE 150–5; the disorders touch almost every branch of medicine.

NS also is associated with a vast array of systemic diseases, neoplasms such as Hodgkin's and other lymphomas, as well as infections (TABLE 150–5). In North America, the most common of these causes is diabetes mellitus, followed by multiple myeloma, amyloid disease, and SLE; malignancy accounts for only 11% of cases in adults.

Familial nephrotic syndromes occur. Congenital NS (Finnish type) is hereditary (autosomal recessive), rapidly progressive, and usually requires dialysis within 1 yr.

Pathology

MCD is thought to be caused by secretion of a lymphokine, and an imbalance in T suppressor and T helper lymphocyte subpopulations, producing a disorder in cellular immunity. Morphologic change is apparent only on electron microscopy, which shows endothelial edema with diffuse swelling (effacement) of foot processes of the epithelial podocytes, proportionate to proteinuria. Vacuoles, lysozymes, and increased numbers of organelles may be detected; mesangial hypercellularity occurs in about 5%.

In **FGS,** segmental hyalinization, and IgM and C3, occur in a nodular and coarse granular pattern with diffuse loss of the foot processes. FGS begins in the juxtamedullary glomeruli and thus easily is missed on biopsy sampling. **Global sclerosis** may occur, leading to obsolete glomeruli.

In **membranous glomerulonephritis (MGN),** ICs are seen as dense deposits by electron microscopy. Subepithelial dense deposits occur with early disease, with spikes of lamina densa between the deposits. Later the deposits appear within the basement membrane, and marked thickening of the GBM occurs. There is a diffuse and granular pattern of IgG along the GBM, but no cellular proliferation, exudation, or necrosis. SLE glomerulonephritis is characterized by subendothelial, intramembranous, or subepithelial deposits. Wherever ICs are deposited, immunofluorescence staining is positive for complement **(C)** and for IgG, IgA, and IgM in varying proportions. A C receptor has been identified on the epithelial podocyte.

Based on differences in the glomerular ultrastructure, 3 forms of idiopathic **membra-**

TABLE 150–5. COMMON CAUSES OF THE NEPHROTIC SYNDROME

		Approximate Incidence	
		Children	Adults
Primary renal disease		**90%**	**75%**
Minimal-change disease (MCD)		65	15
Focal glomerulosclerosis (FGS)		10	15
Membranous glomerulonephritis (MGN)		5	30
Membranoproliferative glomerulonephritis (MPGN)		10	7
Others: mesangial proliferative glomerulonephritis, IgA nephropathy, rapidly progressive glomerulonephritis (RPGN), focal glomerulonephritis (focal GN)		10	3
Secondary disease		**10%**	**25%**
Metabolic	Diabetes mellitus, amyloidosis		
Immunogenic	Systemic lupus erythematosus, Henoch-Schönlein purpura, polyarteritis nodosa, Sjögren's syndrome, sarcoid, serum sickness, erythema multiforme		
Neoplasms	Leukemias, lymphomas, Hodgkin's lymphoma, multiple myeloma, carcinoma (bronchus, breast, colon, stomach, kidney), melanoma		
Nephrotoxins/drugs	Gold, penicillamine, mercury, street heroin		
Allergens	Insect stings, snake venoms, antitoxins, poison ivy, poison oak		
Infections	Bacterial —poststreptococcal glomerulonephritis (PSGN), shunt nephritis, infective endocarditis, leprosy, syphilis Viral —hepatitis B, infectious mononucleosis, varicella Protozoa —malaria Helminthic—schistosomiasis, filariasis		
Congenital nephrotic syndrome	Finnish type		
Heredofamilial	Alport's syndrome, Fabry's disease		
Miscellaneous	Toxemia of pregnancy, malignant hypertension		

noproliferative glomerulonephritis (MPGN) are recognized. In type I MPGN (mesangiocapillary GN), glomerular deposits, predominantly C3 and IgG, are subendothelial and the glomerular basement membrane is intact. In type II MPGN (intramembranous dense-deposit disease), deposits of C3 are present in a discontinuous linear pattern on either side of the capillary wall, in the tubular basement membrane, and in Bowman's capsule. Type III MPGN, probably a variant of type I, is characterized by both subendothelial and subepithalial deposits; basement-membrane–like material formed on the surface of these deposits eventually produces a glomerular basement membrane that has a fenestrated and duplicated appearance. The glomerular sclerosis that leads to renal failure in all 3 types appears to be caused by chronic deposition of ICs in the glomeruli. In **mesangial proliferative GN,** mesangial cells and matrix are increased and there are IgM and C3 deposits.

Proliferation may be focal or diffuse in the NS associated with acute PSGN, RPGN, Henoch-Schönlein purpura, Goodpasture's syndrome, and other glomerulonephritides. Most of the other etiologies of NS have distinctive lesions; eg, with diabetic nephropathy there is diffuse or nodular intercapillary glomerulosclerosis; amyloid has a fibrillar infiltrate that is diagnostic on electron microscopy and on polarizing microscopy with Congo red; and in sickle-cell nephropathy, a microangiopathy occurs.

In NS of any etiology, tubules may show granularity and contain vacuoles. Various clinical renal syndromes are associated with such changes in the tubulointerstitial compartment.

Symptoms and Signs

An early sign of NS, noted by patients, is "foamy" urine (bubbles on its surface). At presentation, proteinuria usually exceeds 2 gm/day/sq m or a random urine protein/creatinine concentration ratio > 3. Symptoms and signs include anorexia, malaise, puffy eyelids, retinal sheen, abdominal pain, wasting of muscles, and edema. Anasarca with ascites and pleural effusions is not uncommon.

Focal edema may be the reason for seeking help for such varied complaints as difficulty breathing (pleural effusion or laryngeal edema), substernal chest pain (pericardial effusion), scrotal swelling, swollen knees (hydroarthrosis), swollen abdomen (ascites), and (in children) abdominal pain from edema of the mesentery. Most often, the edema is mobile—detected in the eyelids in the morning and the ankles after standing. Fluid accumulates primarily by Starling forces (dependent on the relationship between hydraulic and oncotic pressure in capillaries and interstitium) and by systemic factors that increase fractional reabsorption of sodium such as the renin-angiotensin-aldosterone mechanism. Parallel white lines in fingernail beds are a clinical finding of uncertain etiology.

Orthostatic hypotension and even shock may develop in children. Adults may be hypo-, normo-, or hypertensive, depending on the degree of stimulation of their angiotensin production. It is important to be alert for muscle wasting, which may be masked by edema. Oliguria and even acute renal failure may develop because of hypovolemia and diminished perfusion; occasionally oliguric acute renal failure occurs.

Complications

Certain carrier proteins are lost in the urine in nephrosis, leading to low levels of 25-hydroxycholecalciferol (a precursor of active vitamin D), serum calcium, and adrenocortical and thyroid hormones.

A wide variety of clinical syndromes may develop in prolonged NS: nutritional deficiencies, including protein malnutrition resembling kwashiorkor; brittle hair and nails; alopecia; stunted growth; demineralization of bone; glucosuria; hyperaminoaciduria of various types; potassium-depletion syndromes; myopathy; decreased total calcium; tetany; and hypometabolism. Spontaneous peritonitis may occur and opportunistic infections are prevalent. The high incidence of infection is thought due to the loss of immunoglobulins **(Igs)**. Coagulation disorders, together with decreased fibrinolytic activity and episodic hypovolemia, are a serious thrombotic risk (notably, renal-vein thrombosis). Hypertension with cardiac and cerebral complications is most likely in diabetics and patients who have collagen vascular diseases.

Laboratory Findings

The initial urinalysis shows marked proteinuria with a daily excretion of > 20 gm. The urine sediment usually contains hyaline, granular, fatty, waxy, and epithelial-cell casts. Microscopic hematuria and RBC casts also may be present depending on the etiology of the glomerular disease. Leukocytes are prominent in exudative diseases and SLE. Amyloid fibrils may be seen on electron miscoscopy.

Hypoalbuminemia is detected by chemical measurement or quantitatiave electrophoresis. Albumin often is < 2.5 gm/dL, and in children it is sometimes < 1 gm/dL; values as low as 0.2 gm/dL have been recorded. Usually low are α- and γ-globulins, as well as ceruloplasmin, transferrin, ASO protein, C, and other Igs. By contrast, in SLE the IgG level usually is elevated; in FGS the IgG levels frequently are depressed; and in MGN the C3 level is normal. Serum urea nitrogen or creatinine concentrations vary according to the degree of renal impairment.

Urine sodium concentration often is < 1 mEq/L in the accumulation phase of ne-

phrotic edema. **Urine potassium** usually is high; the Na:K ratio exceeds 1. **Aldosterone** secretion and secretion rates are elevated during this stage, but may be normal at other times despite the continued presence of edema. Nephrotic patients excrete a salt load poorly, indicating a defect in the renal handling of sodium.

Lipemia may be detectable visually as lactescent sera. Such patients have lipoprotein-lipase deficiency (transiently correctable by heparin) or a problem in converting high- to low-density lipoprotein. In the laboratory, lipemia is documented by increased total cholesterol, triglycerides, free and esterified cholesterol, and phosphatides. Unesterified fatty acids are normal. Greatly increased lipid levels (up to, or even exceeding 10 times normal) are associated with severe hypoalbuminemia.

Lipiduria is determined by Sudan staining of casts containing lipid granules, identifying macrophages and renal tubular cells containing fatty droplets (oval fat bodies), and finding anisotropic crystals (doubly refractile fat bodies) with polarized light microscopy.

Microcytic anemia may be present because of the urinary loss of siderophyllin. **Coagulation disorders** are common, perhaps because of the loss of factors IX, XII, and thrombolytic factors (urokinase and antithrombin III) in the urine and increased serum levels of factor VIII, fibrinogen, and platelets.

Diagnosis

Diagnosis of NS is based on the clinical features and laboratory findings, but determination of the cause depends on renal histology. **Severe proteinuria** (> 2 gm/sq m/day) is the cardinal finding and essential to the diagnosis. The selection of a single value for the separation of nephrotic- and nonnephrotic-range proteinuria is arbitrary. However, it is useful because diseases that principally affect the extraglomerular vasculature and/or tubulointerstitial areas do not commonly evoke proteinuria of this magnitude. Other causes of proteinuria that are not in the nephrotic range are discussed in Ch. 146. Patients with primary NS have heavy proteinuria and its biochemical consequences as the main clinical problem; renal failure rarely is a presenting finding. However, renal insufficiency may occur in primary NS after a lengthy illness. Thus, heavy proteinuria in the nephritic patient often indicates that the disease is far advanced and is, therefore, an ominous sign. By contrast, patients with NS in association with a secondary cause of NS frequently have renal insufficiency at the time of onset or acquire it soon thereafter.

MCD occurs most commonly in children and is characterized by NS without hematuria, hypertension, or azotemia. By contrast, **MPGN,** also mainly a disease of children, presents with NS in 60 to 80%, with macroscopic hematuria in 50%, and with azotemia and hypertension in a smaller fraction. However, MPGN can be asymptomatic, with only hematuria and proteinuria. **FGS** commonly presents with hematuria, hypertension, and renal dysfunction in association with NS. In **MGN,** NS of insidious onset occurs, often with microscopic hematuria and sometimes associated with other conditions (eg, chronic IC disease, chronic infection, drug-induced states, neoplasm, and collagen vascular disease). With **mesangial proliferative GN,** NS occurs in > 75% of cases, microscopic hematuria in 20%, and hypertension in 35%.

Secondary causes of NS, including drugs, should be sought. Urinary and serum protein electrophoresis and immunoelectrophoresis differentiate glomerular from tubular proteinuria, and detect light chains (Bence Jones protein) or a monoclonal band (excludes multiple myeloma). Screening for commonly underlying systemic diseases, such as diabetes mellitus and SLE, should be done. If the histology confirms MGN, and particularly if the patient has lost weight or is elderly, a search for malignancy should be undertaken.

Prognosis

Prognosis varies with specific etiology. Complete remissions may occur if NS is secondary to treatable disorders (eg, infection, malignancy, drug-induced), which oc-

cur in about 50% of cases in childhood but at a lower rate in adulthood. The prognosis generally is favorable in the corticosteroid-responsive disorders and in the immunosuppressed frequent relapsers (see Treatment, below). Certain of these diseases, such as MGN, remit spontaneously even after 5 yr.

MCD has the best prognosis, with 90% of children and nearly as many adults responding to therapy. Relapses are common but progression to renal failure is rare. It has been suggested that after a year of remission a recurrence is unlikely during pregnancy.

MGN, a disease mainly of adults, runs an indolent course, progressing to renal failure in 50% of patients over 15 yr; 50% will be in remission or have persistent proteinuria or NS with adequate renal function. The majority of children will have complete spontaneous remission of proteinuria within 5 yr of diagnosis.

FGS and **MPGN** respond poorly to therapy and the prognosis is guarded. Over 50% of patients with FGS have renal failure by 10 yr; in 20% the course is more malignant, end-stage renal disease occurring within 2 yr; and the disease is more rapidly progressive in adults than in children. Similarly, 50% of patients with MPGN progress to renal failure within 10 yr, with remission in only a few (< 5%). Those with **mesangial proliferative GN** are virtually all nonresponders to corticosteroids. In **SLE, amyloidosis,** and **diabetic nephropathy,** treatment is chiefly palliative, although newer treatment protocols are improving the prognosis for SLE. In diabetic NS, renal failure usually develops within 3 to 5 yr.

In all cases of NS, the prognosis may be altered drastically by infection, hypertension, significant azotemia, or thromboses in cerebral, pulmonary, peripheral, or renal veins.

There is a high recurrence rate of NS in transplanted kidneys in patients who have FGS, SLE, IgA nephropathy, and especially type II MPGN, but less so in type I. Recurrence in transplants also occurs in some cases of MGN and mesangial proliferative GN.

Treatment

Treatment of NS is directed at the underlying pathogenetic process and is dependent on the renal pathology determined from biopsy tissue (TABLE 150–2).

In MCD, spontaneous remissions do occur, but several drug regimes have proved effective, and children especially experience a predictable, rapid recovery. Response to treatment is indicated by cessation of proteinuria and a diuresis if edema is present. Ninety percent of children respond to initial therapy (prednisone 60 mg/sq m or 2 mg/kg/day orally for 4 wk), most within the 4 wk; but 75% of these relapse. Adults are less responsive to corticosteroid therapy (prednisone 1.0 to 1.5 mg/kg/day orally for not more than 4 to 6 wk), and responders relapse at about the same rate as children. Adults are more prone to iatrogenic complications, particularly with increasing age and hypertension.

For all patients who respond, after continuing medication for another 2 wk, a change is made to a maintenance regime: prednisone 2 to 3 mg/kg on alternate days (to minimize toxicity) for 4 wk, tapering off during the next 4 mo. All patients should be carefully observed for signs of relapse. For both corticosteroid nonresponders and frequent relapsers, prolonged remission may be obtainable with the combination of prednisone on alternate days with a cytotoxic agent (usually, cyclophosphamide 2 to 3 mg/kg/day for 8 wk, or chlorambucil 0.2 mg/kg/day for 12 wk). An alternative approach is oral cyclosporine, 5 mg/kg/day in 2 divided doses, adjusted to obtain a whole blood trough concentration between 150 and 750 μg/L. Some initial responders may relapse when dosage is reduced.

Cytotoxic agents pose the hazards of gonadal suppression (most serious in prepubertal adolescence) and hemorrhagic cystitis. Dosage should be monitored by frequent blood counts, and cystitis excluded by urinalysis. In MCD, the risks of therapy should

be weighed against the advantages of reducing proteinuria, possibly without influencing the outcome of other manifestations of NS.

For FGS, treatment usually is ineffective, although in occasional patients the disorder remits spontaneously or responds to a course of corticosteroids. If it only improves slightly or relapses with this therapy, the addition of cyclophosphamide may induce remission. Therefore, a 4-wk course of corticosteroid therapy probably is acceptable to delineate the few responders. The usefulness of anticoagulants and antithrombotics has not been established. An improvement in GFR and a reduction in proteinuria may occur with cyclosporine dosage as described for MCD.

In MGN, patients significantly benefit from alternate-day corticosteroid therapy, starting before the onset of renal insufficiency (prednisone 100 to 150 mg every other day for 2 mo, then gradually reduced over the next 2 mo). Such treatment protects against deterioration in renal function rather than altering the rate of remission. Trials of large-dose therapy with methylprednisolone, or combined corticosteroid and immunosuppressive drugs, to obtain remission in MGN, have been encouraging but still are experimental. In adults with **type I MPGN,** a randomized prospective trial of the platelet inhibitors dipyridamole 225 mg/day and acetylsalicylic acid 975 mg/day stabilized renal function. In children with MPGN, alternate-day prednisone 2.5 mg/kg (maximum, 80 mg) as a single dose appears to prolong renal survival. In **mesangial proliferative GN,** spontaneous remissions are frequent but the condition is corticosteroid-resistant (5 to 20% response).

In the secondary causes of NS (eg, constrictive pericarditis, Hodgkin's lymphoma, and other neoplasms), remission of the renal manifestations can occur with specific therapy. Treatment of infectious antigens may cure NS (eg, staphylococcal and *Streptococcus viridans* endocarditis, "shunt" nephritis, malaria, syphilis, and schistosomiasis). Heroin addicts with NS due to FGS can experience complete remission of the NS if they cease taking heroin early in the disease. Colchicine produces favorable results in some cases of amyloid NS associated with familial Mediterranean fever (see in Ch. 15). Careful desensitization may reverse NS associated with nephroallergens such as poison oak or ivy and insect antigens. Removal of nephrotoxins such as gold, mercury, penicillamine, and trimethadione may be followed by remission.

Congenital nephrosis is rarely compatible with life beyond 1 yr, but a few patients have been supported nutritionally to the stage of renal failure and then managed with dialysis or transplantation.

Supportive therapy requires nutritional guidance to provide a diet normal in protein (about 1 gm/kg/day), high in biologic value, low in saturated fat, low in sodium (< 100 mEq/day), liberal in potassium, and with supplemental multivitamins, vitamin D, and iron. Graded exercise should be instituted.

If **hyponatremia** is present, fluid intake is restricted. If a brisk diuresis occurs and edema remits, sodium may need to be liberalized. If ascites is present, frequent small meals may be helpful. To **control symptomatic edema,** judicious use of thiazide or loop diuretics is recommended (CAUTION: *Diuretics, by reducing plasma volume further, may compromise renal function and predispose to thrombosis*). If **hypovolemia** is severe and life-threatening, an infusion of plasma or albumin may be justified. **Hypertension** should be treated, usually with diuretics; occasionally other agents may be necessary. **Infections** (especially bacteriuria, endocarditis, and peritonitis) are life-threatening; they should be watched for and treated promptly. **Thrombosis** is frequent and should be watched for (particularly deep-vein thrombosis and pulmonary emboli); anticoagulants may be helpful.

With alteration in serum protein levels, binding of many drugs may be changed, altering the degree of therapeutic efficacy. Sunlight, routine immunization, nephroallergens, insect bites, and potentially nephrotoxic drugs may have to be avoided in hypersensitive persons.

Children and their families should be counseled, to avoid the "deprived sibling" syndrome when a nephrotic child dominates parental energies, and to deal with other psychologic aspects such as cosmetic effects of the disease and corticosteroid therapy. Management of a child with chronic disability is discussed in Ch. 183.

151. TUBULOINTERSTITIAL DISEASE

Tubulointerstitial abnormalities occur in most renal diseases (see TABLE 151–1). Most are discussed in THE MANUAL in different chapters according to the etiology of the disorders (eg, bacterial pyelonephritis in Ch. 153; inherited tubular disorders in Ch. 155; malignancy-associated nephropathy in Ch. 163; toxic nephropathy in Ch. 152; transplant rejection in Ch. 22; and radiation nephropathy in Ch. 257). This chapter deals with selective circumstances in which tubulointerstitial nephritis **(TIN)** predominates, producing syndromes that may be due to diverse causes.

ACUTE NONINFECTIVE TUBULOINTERSTITIAL NEPHRITIS

*A syndrome of acute renal failure **(ARF)** most commonly due to drug hypersensitivity affecting tubules and interstitial tissue.*

Etiology

Drug-induced ARF is now common. Nephropathy is due either to direct toxicity (eg, amphotericin, aminoglycosides, radiocontrast agents) or a hypersensitivity reaction (eg, penicillins, sulfonamides, diuretics, nonsteroidal anti-inflammatory drugs).

Pathology

Glomeruli usually are normal. The earliest finding is interstitial edema typically followed by interstitial infiltration with lymphocytes, plasma cells, eosinophils, and small numbers of polymorphonuclear leukocytes. Tubular epithelium varies from necrotic to normal. The disorder is believed to be immunologic, but immunoglobulins and drug antigens have been found in the tubulointerstitial area in only a few cases. Histologic changes usually are reversible if the cause is recognized and removed; however, some severe cases progress to fibrosis and renal failure.

Symptoms and Signs

The initial presentation is varied. Some patients have UTI features such as fever, dysuria, pyuria, and flank pain. Others have few symptoms but present as ARF with or without oliguria. In others, renal function declines, in association with features of a hypersensitivity reaction (eg, fever, skin rash, eosinophilia). The urinary reaction may be minimal with only a trace of protein or pyuria, but often is striking with nephrotic-range proteinuria, hematuria (microscopic or gross), or marked pyuria including eosinophils. Although eosinophiluria is rare, it is pathognomonic for hypersensitivity TIN. Many patients develop **signs of tubular dysfunction** such as polyuria (concentration defect), volume depletion (defect in sodium conservation), hyperkalemia (defect in potassium excretion), and metabolic acidosis (defect in acid excretion). The kidneys usually are large because of interstitial edema, and avidly take up radioactive gallium or radionuclide labeled leukocytes. The interval between exposure to drugs and development of renal involvement varies between 5 days and 5 wk.

TABLE 151–1. DISORDERS ASSOCIATED WITH TUBULOINTERSTITIAL NEPHRITIS (TIN)

Acute TIN	*Chronic TIN*
Drug-induced hypersensitivity nephritis (see FIG. 152–1)	Obstructive uropathies (including reflux uropathy)
Pyelonephritis (bacterial, fungal, viral)	Pyelonephritis (bacterial, fungal, viral)
Immunologic reactions	Immunologic reactions
Acute transplant rejections	Transplant rejections
Acute glomerular disease association	Glomerulonephritis-associated
Metabolic diseases	Nephrotoxicity (see TABLE 152–1)
Hypercalcemia	Metabolic diseases
Hypokalemia	Nephrocalcinosis and/or nephrolithiasis
Hyperuricemia	Oxalosis
Nephrotoxicity (see TABLE 152–1)	Cystinosis
Obstructive uropathies	Gout (uric acid tophi)
Idiopathic	Inherited and multisystem disorders
	Polycystic disease
	Medullary cystic disease
	Hereditary nephritis
	Medullary sponge kidney
	Sickle cell disease
	Sjögren's syndrome
	Sarcoidosis
	Malignancy
	Radiation nephritis
	Balkan nephritis
	Idiopathic

Clinical Course, Prognosis, and Treatment

If severe prolonged oliguria is present, patients are treated for ARF. Patients usually recover renal function on withdrawal of the offending drug, although some residual scarring is common. Irreversible cases have been reported. Corticosteroid therapy (eg, prednisone 1 mg/kg once a day for 3 days followed by decreasing doses over the next 7 to 10 days) may be of value in accelerating recovery of function when TIN is caused by hypersensitivity or immunologic reactions.

CHRONIC TUBULOINTERSTITIAL NEPHRITIS

This term includes *all those chronic kidney disorders in which generalized or localized changes in the tubulointerstitial area predominate over glomerular or vascular lesions.* Since some tubulointerstitial changes are associated with all renal diseases, this distinction may be difficult. Furthermore, more than one condition associated with tubulointerstitial inflammation (eg, diabetes mellitus and UTI) may be present in a patient. Current data suggest that 1/3 to 1/2 of chronic renal failure cases develop as a result of chronic TIN.

The conditions commonly associated with chronic TIN are listed in TABLE 151–1. General features of TIN are discussed here; specific disorders are discussed separately in THE MANUAL.

Pathology

Although the causes and pathologic changes are variable, certain features are consistent. Grossly, the kidneys are small and atrophic. TIN due to toxins, metabolic diseases, and inherited disorders, and Balkan nephritis result in symmetric and bilateral

disease; with other causes, renal scarring may be unequal and involve only one kidney. The pelvic structures may not be affected except in pyelonephritis or obstructive uropathy. However, many disorders (eg, analgesic abuse, obstructive uropathy, diabetes mellitus) may be associated with renal papillary damage and calyceal dilation, with widening of the calyces and an overlying cortical scar. Histologically, glomeruli vary from normality to complete destruction. Tubules may be absent or atrophied. Tubular lumina vary considerably in diameter, but may show marked dilation, with homogeneous casts producing a thyroidlike appearance. The interstitium contains varying degrees of inflammatory cells and fibrosis. Nonscarred areas appear reasonably normal.

Symptoms, Signs, and Diagnosis

Certain clinical features are common to all types of TIN. Generally, symptoms indicating progression of renal disease are absent. Edema usually is not present, proteinuria is minimal, hematuria is uncommon, and the BP is normal or only mildly elevated in the early stages. When present, heavy proteinuria or marked hematuria suggests a complicating glomerular disease. Signs of tubular dysfunction similar to those described above for acute TIN may be present. Patients with chronic TIN due to oxalosis, hypercalcemia, hyperuricemia, or sarcoidosis may also have nephrolithiasis.

ENDEMIC TUBULOINTERSTITIAL NEPHRITIS OF THE BALKANS

In certain well-defined regions of the Balkans, a chronic nephropathy with the histologic characteristics of tubulointerstitial nephritis is endemic. The cause is unknown; an environmental fungal toxin is suspected. The disease is not familial and there are no associated hearing or ocular defects. Onset is never acute and occurs insidiously between ages 30 to 60 yr. The disease is rare in the young, and those who leave the endemic areas when young are spared.

The disease is discovered on routine examination by the presence of proteinuria or findings of chronic renal insufficiency. Special clinical features are the absence of edema, the rarity of hypertension, and the presence of severe anemia. The condition deteriorates slowly, with chronic end-stage disease appearing within 10 to 20 yr after the first signs. Malignant urinary system tumors are found in 30 to 40% of affected patients.

152. NEPHROTOXIC DISORDERS

(Toxic Nephropathy)

A poisonous substance, through its chemical actions, may kill, injure, or impair the function of an organism. Toxic nephropathy is *any functional or morphologic change in the kidney produced by a drug or a chemical or biologic agent that is ingested, injected, inhaled, or absorbed.* By extension, the concept applies to normal ions circulating in abnormal concentrations (eg, hypokalemic, hyperkalemic, hypomagnesemic, and hyperuricemic nephropathy).

The kidney has many unique features that render it susceptible to toxicity and its discovery. The various functions of the kidney can be measured quantitatively with accuracy, and subtle effects detected early. Its effluent (urine) can be measured by physical, chemical, microscopic, bacteriologic, and immunologic methods (see Ch. 146). Its affluent (blood) is the core of biochemistry. The kidney has the highest blood supply/gm of any tissue in the body (about 3.5 mL/gm/min vs. about 0.07

mL/gm/min for most organs except the lung). Circulating agents are thus delivered at 50 times the "usual" rate for tissues. The kidney has the largest endothelial surface area/gm, with 2 complete capillary beds in series. The first bed (glomerulus) has the highest hydrostatic pressure and greatest filtration fraction. Non-bound solutes leave the circulation via filtration at 100-plus mL/min, far above the mean of most organs. Thus the kidney gets a disproportionate sample of absorbed agents presented via arterial circulation.

Physiologic reduction of glomerular filtrate to form concentrated urine may expose the luminal surfaces of cells to as much as 300 times the plasma concentration of *filtered* molecules or 1000 or more times the plasma concentration of those agents undergoing *tubular secretion*. The surface area exposed is astronomical because of a fine brush border on proximal tubular cells. A countercurrent flow mechanism acts to increase concentration of both urine and the interstitial fluid of the medulla. No other tissue fluid in the body is exposed to such concentrations, which may range to 4 times plasma concentration. Tubular transport separates drugs from *protein binding*, a device commonly protective for other cells. Transcellular transport uniquely exposes the interior of the cell and its organelles to newly encountered chemicals. Binding sites (eg,

TABLE 152–1. COMMON NEPHROTOXIC AGENTS

Heavy metals	Inorganic mercury (chloride), organic mercury salts (methyl, ethyl, phenyl, sodium ethyl mercurithiosalicylate, mercurial diuretics), inorganic lead, organic lead (tetraethyl), cadmium, uranium, gold (especially sodium thiomalate), copper, arsenic, arsine (arsenic trihydride), iron, chromium (especially trioxide), thallium, selenium, vanadium, bismuth
Antibiotics	Aminoglycosides, sulphonamides, amphotericin B, polymyxin, neomycin, bacitracin, rifampin, trimethoprim, cephaloridine, methicillin/oxacillin, aminosalicylic acid, oxy- and chlorotetracyclines
Analgesics	Salicylates, acetaminophen, phenacetin, all nonsteroidal anti-inflammatory drugs, phenylbutazone, all prostaglandin synthetase inhibitors
Solvents	Methanol, amyl alcohol, ethylene glycol, diethylene glycol, cellosolves®, carbon tetrachloride, trichlorethylene, miscellaneous hydrocarbons
Oxalosis-inducing agents	Oxalic acid, methoxyflurane, ethylene glycol, antirust agents
Anticancer drugs	Cyclosporin, cisplatin, cyclophosphamide, streptozocin, methotrexate, nitrosoureas (CCNU, BCNU, methyl CCNU), doxorubicin, daunorubicin
Diagnostic agents	Sodium iodide, all organic iodide contrast agents
Herbicides and pesticides	Paraquat, cyanide, dioxin, diphenyl, cyclohexamides, and organochlorine insecticides: endrin, aldrin, endosulfan, dieldrin, lindane, benzene hexachloride (BHC), dichlorodiphenyl-trichloroethane (DDT), heptachlor, chlordecone, terpene polychlorinates, chlordane, dicofol (kelthane), chlorobenzilate, mirex, methoxychlor
Botanicals and biologicals	Mushrooms (eg, *Amanita phalloides*—severe muscarine poisoning), snake and spider venoms, insect bites, aflatoxins
Methemoglobin formers	See TABLE 152–3
Immune complex inducers	Penicillamine, captopril, levamisole, gold salts
Antiepileptics	Trimethadione, paramethadione, succinamide, carbamazepine
Unknown	(Balkan nephropathy)

TABLE 152–2. EXAMPLES OF AGENTS CAUSING NEPHROTOXICITY INDIRECTLY

Agent	*Mechanism*
Ethylene glycol, methoxyflurane	Via oxalic acid
Phencyclidine (PCP) and amphetamines	Via rhabdomyolysis
Methysergide	Via retroperitoneal fibrosis
Ergot alkaloids	Via severe arteriolar constriction
Heroin	Via lead, staphylococcus and fungal toxin, or other contaminants of illicit use
Chemotherapy of hematopoietic neoplasms and uricosuric drugs	Via obstruction with uric acid crystals—intra- or extra-renal
Vitamin D + milk + alkali + vitamin D analog	Nephrocalcinosis and lithiasis
Diphenyl and some pesticides	Via cysts and dysplasia
Mushroom and colchicine poisoning	Via diarrhea and fluid loss
Aniline, *p*-phenetidine, and a host of drugs, foods and industrial agents*	Via methemoglobin formation
Phenacetin and oxidant drugs	Only in G6PD-deficient patients

* See TABLE 152–3.

TABLE 152–3. AGENTS INDUCING METHEMOGLOBIN PRODUCTION

Medical Intoxications	*Industrial Intoxications*	*Food Intoxications*
Nitrates	Nitrites	Nitrites
Ammonium nitrate	Chlorides	Brines
Bismuth subnitrate	Potassium ferricyanide	Confusion between nitrite and sodium chloride
Nitrites	Aniline and derivatives	Nitrates
Potassium chloride	Trichlorocarbanilide	Contaminated water
Potassium permanganate	*p*-Nitroaniline	Spinach, carrots
Phenacetin	Phenylhydrazine	Sodium nitrate
Acetanilide	Toluidine and xylidine	Nitrobenzene (bakery goods)
Phenylhydrazine	Nitro- and dinitrobenzene	Essence of mirbane
Local anesthetics	Mono- and dinitrophenol	
Benzocaine	Dinitro-4,6-ortho-cresol	
Prilocaine	Nitrogenous derivatives of toluene	
Aminosalicylic acid	Nitroglycerin	
Dinitrophenol	Nitrocellulose	
Polyphenols	Naphthalene and derivatives	
Resorcinol	*p*-Dichlorobenzene	
Pyrogallol	Polyphenols	
Phenazopyridine		
Sulfones		
Sulfonamides*		
Primaquine*		
Methylene blue		

* Use caution in treatment with methylene blue (risk of hemolysis). This intoxication often reveals a latent red cell enzyme defect.

(From *Nephrology*, edited by J. Hamburger, J. Crosnier, and J. P. Grunfeld. Copyright 1979 by John Wiley & Sons. Used with permission of John Wiley & Sons, and also of the publisher of the French original, Flammarion, Paris, France.)

sulfhydryl [SH] groups) may facilitate *entry* but retard *exit* (eg, heavy metals). The kidney has the highest O_2 consumption/gm and glucose production/gm, and is, therefore, vulnerable to poisons affecting *cell energetics*. As the leading site of *immune complex deposition,* it is uniquely susceptible to *immunologic* injury.

Special mesangial cells have Ia receptors and can process antigen to stimulate appropriate T cells and recruit B cells for cellular immune reactions. The mesangium is a site for invasion of monocytes, phagocytes, and other biologically active cells migrating from the blood. The immunologic events in the mesangium also may control physiologic events in the vascular supply; eg, angiotensin receptors. The epithelial cell (podocyte) is the location of a complement (C_3) receptor in the human capillary.

Etiology

TABLE 152–1 lists most of the clinically important drugs and chemicals known to produce nephrotoxicity. Most of these are directly toxic to cells by known or unknown mechanisms. Other agents can produce renal injury by indirect mechanisms—often not apparent from a knowledge of the biochemistry of the agent. A partial list of such agents is presented in TABLE 152–2. Many agents are nephrotoxic via methemoglobin formation; a list is in TABLE 152–3. A diagrammatic mapping of the effects of some antibiotics on varied portions of the nephron is presented in FIG. 152–1.

In patients with pretreatment renal disease, one should be particularly alert to drugs that depend on the kidney as a major pathway for elimination. TABLE 152–4 provides a partial list. In renal failure there are significant changes in protein binding of acidic drugs. Protein binding not only is a major determinant of pharmacokinetics but also of cell toxicity in many organs. Renal failure also affects drug oxidation and reduction;

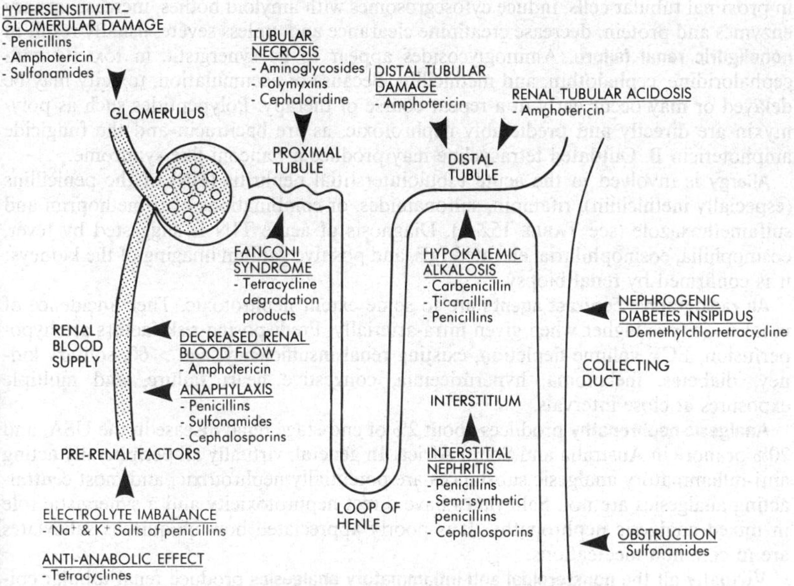

FIG. 152–1. Nephrotoxicity of antimicrobial agents. (Redrawn from Nephrotoxic Sites of Antimicrobial Agents, by G. B. Appel and H. C. Neu, in *The New England Journal of Medicine,* Vol. 296, No. 12, March 24, 1977, p. 665. Reprinted by permission of *The New England Journal of Medicine* and the author.)

TABLE 152–4. SOME DRUGS FOR WHICH THE KIDNEY IS A MAJOR PATHWAY OF ELIMINATION

Acetohexamide	Cimetidine	Nadolol
Amantadine	Clofibrate	Netilmicin
Amikacin	Cycloserine	Penicillins
Ampicillin	Digoxin	Procainamide
Atenolol	Ethambutol	Ranitidine
Carbenicillin	Flucytosine	Streptomycin
Cefamandole	Gentamicin	Sulfinpyrazone
Cefazolin	Kanamycin	Tetracycline
Cefoxitin	Lithium	Ticarcillin
Cephalexin	Methotrexate	Tobramycin
Cephalothin	Metoclopramide	Vancomycin

(Modified from M. Reidenberg and D. Drayer, "Drug Therapy in Renal Failure," *Annual Review of Pharmacology and Toxicology* Vol. 20, 1980. Copyright © 1980 by Annual Reviews Inc. Used with permission.)

glucuronide, sulfate, and glycine conjugation; acetylation; and hydrolysis. A list of such interactions is given in TABLE 152–5.

Only a few nephrotoxins can be discussed here in greater detail. In hospitals, by far the leading cause of nephrotoxic renal failure (about 25% of all acute renal failure) is **antibiotics,** with aminoglycosides leading the list. Streptomycin, kanamycin, neomycin, gentamicin, tobramycin, amikacin, and sisomicin all are nephrotoxic. They accumulate in proximal tubular cells, induce cytosegrosomes with amyloid bodies, increase urinary enzymes and protein, decrease creatinine clearance and, unless severe, usually result in **nonoliguric renal failure.** Aminoglycosides appear to be synergistic in toxicity with cephaloridine, cephalothin, and methicillin. Because of accumulation, toxicity may be delayed or may occur early in a repeat course of therapy. Polypeptides such as polymyxin are directly and predictably nephrotoxic, as are bacitracin and the fungicide amphotericin B. Outdated tetracycline may produce a Fanconi-like syndrome.

Allergy is involved in the acute tubulointerstitial nephritis **(TIN)** of the penicillins (especially methicillin), rifampin, sulfonamides, or combinations of trimethoprim and sulfamethoxazole (see TABLE 152–6). Diagnosis of acute TIN is suggested by fever, eosinophilia, eosinophiluria, elevated IgE, and positive gallium imaging of the kidneys; it is confirmed by renal biopsy.

All radiographic contrast agents are to some extent nephrotoxic. Their incidence of renal toxicity is higher when given intra-arterially. Predisposing risk factors are hypoperfusion, ECF volume depletion, existing renal insufficiency, age > 60, solitary kidney, diabetes, melanoma, hyperuricemia, congestive heart failure, and multiple exposures at close intervals.

Analgesic nephropathy produces about 2% of end-stage renal disease in the USA, and 20% or more in Australia and South Africa. In general, virtually all peripherally acting anti-inflammatory analgesic substances are potentially nephrotoxic, and most central-acting analgesics are not. Salicylates have direct nephrotoxicity and a synergistic role in mixed analgesic nephropathy. It is poorly appreciated how ubiquitous salicylates are in common medications.

Virtually all the **nonsteroidal anti-inflammatory analgesics** produce renal tubular epithelial damage and are, with varying potency, prostaglandin synthetase inhibitors and can produce hypoperfusion, papillary necrosis, and chronic TIN. Many of these agents are now available.

Most **heavy metals** accumulate in segments of the proximal nephron because of

TABLE 152–5. CLINICALLY SIGNIFICANT DRUG METABOLITES WHICH ACCUMULATE IN RENAL FAILURE

Drug	*Metabolite*
Acebutolol	N-acetyl analog
Acetohexamide	Hydroxyhexamide
Allopurinol	Oxypurinol
Azathioprine	6-Mercaptopurine
Cephalothin	Desacetylcephalothin
Chlorpropamide	2-Hydroxychlorpropamide
Clofibrate	Chlorophenoxyisobutyric acid
Daunorubicin	Daunorubicinol
Diazepam	Oxazepam
Digitoxin	Digoxin
Digoxin	Digoxigenin-bis-digitoxoside Digoxigenin-mono-digitoxoside
Doxorubicin	Adriamycinol
Meperidine*	Normeperidine
Methsuximide	N-desmethylmethsuximide
Methyldopa	*a*-Methyldopamine
Primidone	Phenobarbitone
Procainamide	N-acetylprocainamide
Propoxyphene	Norpropoxyphene
Rifampin	Desacetylrifampin
Sulfonamides	Acetylated metabolites

* Accumulation following high or prolonged dosing can produce neurotoxicity.

transport or binding sites such as sulfhydryl (SH) groups. Toxic effects of lead are seen from pica, industrial exposure, contaminated water, wine or alcohol, mining or inhalation of smoke, or leaded gasoline. Tetraethyl lead goes through intact skin and lungs. **Chronic lead syndrome** includes shrunken kidneys, uremia, hypertension, anemia with basophilic stippling, encephalopathy, peripheral neuropathy, and Fanconi syndrome. More acutely, lead colic may occur. Mercury, bismuth, and thallium nephrotoxicity seem to be decreasing, but cadmium, copper, gold, uranium, arsenic, and iron are still prevalent—the latter associated with proximal myopathy in hemochromatosis and in other forms of iron overload, such as dialysis patients with multiple transfusions.

TABLE 152–6. AGENTS ASSOCIATED WITH HYPERSENSITIVITY TIN

Semi-synthetic penicillins (especially methicillin; ampicillin, nafcillin, oxacillin, carbenicillin)	Allopurinol
Sulfonamides	Azathioprine
Rifampin	Antipyrine
Diuretics (especially thiazides, furosemide)	Anticonvulsants (especially phenytoin)
	Gold
	Phenylbutazone

Solvent nephrotoxicity occurs mainly from inhaled hydrocarbons (Goodpasture's syndrome), methanol, glycols, and halogenated compounds such as carbon tetrachloride and trichloroethylene. Halogenated anesthetics (eg, methoxyflurane) have also been implicated.

Drugs inducing immune complex disease in the kidney, proteinuria, and many features of nephrotic syndrome include D-penicillamine, captopril, levamisole, and gold salts used by injection for RA.

Diagnosis

Diagnosis of toxic nephropathy requires a detective's mentality. In addition to a broad knowledge of drugs and toxicology, the clinician must be alert to the psychologic profiles associated with possible suicide or homicide, and to the patient's possible exposures to toxic agents—at work, during recreation, and from his environment, hobbies, food, and water. Has he had radiation exposure > 2000 rads, or multiple doses of contrast materials, or does he have risk factors such as dehydration with a single dose of contrast material? Does he have contact with unusual hydrocarbons such as are found in pesticides, paint or stripping agents, solvents, cleaners, or fertilizers? Is he exposed to unregulated foods or alcohol (eg, lead in moonshine) or street drugs with their contaminants (eg, glue sniffing)? Does he self-medicate inordinately (analgesics, laxatives, diuretics, ointments)? Does he "borrow" prescription drugs from others? Does he live downstream from a pollution source or drink well water from a contaminated aquifer? (There are 400 industrial-waste, deep injection wells in 22 states.) What is his allergic history and his family history of immunologic disease?

Treatment

Treatment guides are found elsewhere in the discussions of syndromes produced by the particular toxic agent (eg, acute and chronic renal failure, nephrotic syndrome, tubular acidosis, interstitial nephritis, and in the section on poisoning).

General measures include withdrawal of the offending agent—induction of emesis, enhancing of excretion (eg, chelates, diuretics) while function remains, and by direct removal from the bloodstream via the most efficient method: usually, hemodialysis with large-surface dialyzer; hemoperfusion over charcoal or resins; plasmapheresis; or sorbapheresis.

Combination therapy may be indicated; eg, for methanol, dialysis plus infusion of ethanol to compete for alcohol dehydrogenase—thus decreasing any metabolism of methanol to more dangerous neuro- and ocular toxins. Bicarbonate infusions for acidosis due to the production of formic acid may be coindicated. Combination therapy can save both the life and sight in "fatal" levels of methanol poisoning and other solvents producing lactic acidosis.

---

153. INFECTIONS OF THE KIDNEY, URINARY TRACT, AND MALE GENITAL TRACT

(For urinary tract infections in children, see Ch. 191)

ACUTE BACTERIAL PYELONEPHRITIS

(Acute Infective Tubulointerstitial Nephritis)

An acute, patchy, often bilateral, pyogenic infection of the kidney. Clinically, renal pelvic infection cannot be distinguished from parenchymal infection, and both pelvis

and parenchyma usually are affected. Acute infective tubulointerstitial nephritis is a more descriptive term. (**Chronic bacterial pyelonephritis** is discussed separately below.)

Etiology

Infections usually occur by the ascending route after entering the urethral meatus. Obstruction (strictures, calculi, tumors, prostatic hypertrophy, neurogenic bladder) predisposes to infection. The role of obstruction, whether anatomic or physiologic (eg, neurogenic bladder), in predisposing to infection cannot be overemphasized; obstruction causes stasis, stasis abets growth of invading bacteria, and infection is established. Controversially, some believe that adults with diabetes mellitus may have a higher frequency of symptomatic bacteriuria than nondiabetics, perhaps due both to more frequent urinary instrumentation and a greater susceptibility to tissue invasion. Pyelonephritis is especially likely in females in their childhood or during pregnancy, and after urethral catheterization or instrumentation, but is uncommon in males free from urinary tract abnormalities. *Escherichia coli* is the most common bacterium and accounts for about 85% of uncomplicated infections, followed by *Klebsiella, Proteus,* and *Enterobacter*. *Pseudomonas,* staphylococci, and Group D streptococci account for 5 to 10% of the remainder. Hematogenous spread to the kidney may occur from any systemic infection but is most common with staphylococcal bacteremia that produces cortical and perinephric abscesses. Patients subjected to instrumentation or indwelling catheters, who become infected while in the hospital, who are on chronic antimicrobial therapy, or those being treated with corticosteroids or immunosuppressive drugs are particularly likely to colonize with unusual organisms, such as *Serratia, Acinetobacter,* and *Candida*.

Pathology

The kidney usually is enlarged. The parenchyma shows extensive destruction of tissue by the acute inflammatory process, particularly in the cortex. Arteries, arterioles, and glomeruli show considerable resistance to infection. Polymorphonuclear leukocytes are present in large numbers in the interstitial tissue and in the lumina of many tubules, particularly collecting ducts. Chronic inflammatory cells appear within a few days, and medullary abscesses and acute necrosis of papillary tissue may be found. The pelvic and calyceal epithelia show acute inflammation. An important feature of the kidney with acute pyelonephritis is the patchy nature of the disease. Discrete wedge-shaped areas of involvement with no spread of infection outside them are a striking feature.

Symptoms and Signs

Typically, the onset is rapid and characterized by chills, fever, flank pain, nausea, and vomiting. Bladder irritation from infected urine may result in frequency and urgency. Physical examination sometimes shows some abdominal rigidity, which must be distinguished from that produced by intraperitoneal disease. If rigidity is absent or slight, a tender, enlarged kidney may sometimes be palpable. Costovertebral tenderness is generally present on the infected side. In children, symptoms often are slight and less characteristic.

Diagnosis

Diagnosis is suggested by urinary symptoms (frequency and dysuria) associated with signs of sepsis and renal inflammation (chills, fever, costovertebral tenderness); the laboratory provides confirmation. Urine should be collected aseptically (a midstream voiding in the male, a "clean-catch" in the female) for culture and microscopic examination. On urinalysis, the pH may be alkaline because of urea-splitting organisms, proteinuria is minimal (< 1 gm/day), bacteria are found in fresh uncentrifuged urine, and RBCs and WBCs usually are seen. WBC casts, when seen, are pathognomonic of renal inflammation (also seen in glomerulonephritis or noninfective tubulointerstitial nephritis) but may be difficult to separate from renal tubular cell casts unless

special stains are used. Bacteria usually are evident on Gram stain of the unspun urine. Culture usually shows > 100,000 organisms/mL. Males, patients with renal colic, and those who do not respond promptly to treatment require further urologic investigation. Intravenous urography (**IVU**) may disclose calculi, anomalies, deformities, or obstructive lesions (see also DIAGNOSTIC PROCEDURES in Ch. 146).

Treatment

Antimicrobial therapy should be instituted as soon as the diagnosis has been established and urine has been sent to the laboratory for culture and sensitivity tests. The length of treatment is a debatable issue. Single-dose therapy should be reserved for those patients with acute urethral syndrome and acute cystitis if the diagnosis can be made with certainty. If renal infection cannot be excluded, treatment is continued for 5 to 10 days. In patients with frequent relapsing infections with the same organism and without evidence of urinary tract obstruction, 4 wk of treatment is warranted. Urine cultures are repeated during therapy only in patients who do not show resolution of symptoms within 3 days. Cultures following treatment are helpful in establishing early asymptomatic patients who have frequent recurrent infections. If obstruction is present, surgery may be required. (For specific treatment, see in LOWER URINARY TRACT AND MALE GENITAL TRACT INFECTIONS, below.)

CHRONIC BACTERIAL PYELONEPHRITIS

(Chronic Infective Tubulointerstitial Nephritis)

A chronic, patchy, often bilateral, pyogenic infection of the kidney that produces atrophy and calyceal deformity with overlying parenchymal scarring. The disorder causes end-stage renal failure in about 10 to 15% of patients who are treated by dialysis or transplantation. The term pyelonephritis should not be used to describe any tubulointerstitial nephropathy without documented urinary tract infection (**UTI**). Despite chronic renal bacteriuria, progressive renal failure is infrequent except when associated with obstructive uropathy.

Pathology

The histologic picture is nonspecific and similar to that seen with other diseases producing chronic tubulointerstitial nephropathy. The most specific change is a parenchymal scar associated with retraction of the adjacent papilla. Perhaps some initial insult (bacterial or other) produces papillary damage followed by focal tubulointerstitial atrophy, dilated calyces, and overlying cortical sclerosis.

Symptoms, Signs, and Diagnosis

Clinical clues, such as fever and flank or abdominal pain, are often vague and inconsistent. A history of UTI and recurrent acute pyelonephritis is helpful but infrequently obtained except in children with vesicoureteral reflux. A history of recurrent UTI and a typical pattern of renal dysfunction occasionally occurs and strongly suggests the diagnosis. An abnormal urogram showing a dilated calyceal system with an overlying scar is almost diagnostic alone, although a high degree of vesicoureteral reflux without bacteruria can produce similar findings. Frequently, obstructive uropathy (strictures, stones, reflux, myoneurogenic disease, etc) is present. In these patients, a positive urine culture does *not* distinguish the site of infection. Localization studies to differentiate upper from lower tract disease have been suggested; however, there is no conclusive evidence that they are of any clinical value in the management of patients with UTIs.

Proteinuria is absent, minimal, or intermittent until scarring of the kidneys is far advanced. Even then, proteinuria usually is < 1 gm/sq m/day. Urinary sediment tends to be scanty, but renal epithelial cells, granular casts, and, occasionally, WBC casts are found. Renal function studies may disclose defects in concentrating ability, and hyperchloremic acidosis before azotemia is found.

Clinical Course and Prognosis

The course is extremely variable, but typically the disease progresses extremely slowly, with patients having adequate renal function for 20 yr or more after the onset. Two important factors influence the outcome of the disorder: (1) recurrent pyelonephritis, and (2) the type of urinary obstruction. Frequent exacerbations of acute pyelonephritis, even though controlled, usually produce some further deterioration of renal structure and function. Continued obstruction acts both by predisposing to or perpetuating renal infection, and by increasing the pelvic pressure, which damages the kidney directly.

Treatment

The most important therapeutic measures are the elimination of obstruction and eradication of urinary bacteria. Where obstruction cannot be eliminated and recurrent infections are common, long-term antimicrobial therapy with drugs such as nitrofurantoin or trimethoprim/sulfamethoxazole (see LOWER URINARY TRACT AND MALE GENITAL TRACT INFECTIONS, below) are useful. The use of methenamine salts should be *avoided* because they are not effective in suppressing renal bacterial infections. In the absence of demonstrable obstruction or renal dysfunction, it has not been clearly established that covert renal bacteriuria is deleterious. Therefore, repeated courses of antimicrobials or suppressive therapy are probably not indicated. If uremia or hypertension develops, the principles of treatment are as outlined in the chapters dealing with these subjects.

LOWER URINARY TRACT AND MALE GENITAL TRACT INFECTIONS

Bacterial infections of the lower urinary tract are very common. They occur about 10 times more frequently in the female than in the male, except in the neonatal period when prevalence is about equal in both sexes. During infancy and adolescence in females, the prevalence of UTI is about 1%, rising to 2 to 3% between 20 and 60 yr of age, and then to 10 to 20% thereafter. In institutionalized elderly men and women, prevalence of covert bacteriuria is between 30 and 50%.

During infancy, organisms enter the GU system most often by hematogenous or lymphatic spread. In older children and in adults, the main route of infection is an ascending one (from the perineum-vagina-urethra-bladder). Antibacterial therapy and surgical procedures have markedly improved prognosis for most GU tract infections.

While urinary tract obstruction does not in itself cause UTI, its presence often predisposes to infection and makes infection much more difficult to clear with medical therapy. Urologic investigation is not routinely needed or useful in adult women with recurrent symptomatic or asymptomatic UTI, as it does not influence therapy. However, intravenous urography frequently is helpful in evaluating recurrent infections in children, adult women with a history of childhood infections, possible nephrolithiasis, relapsing infections or painless hematuria, and in symptomatic males of any age.

The majority of UTIs are caused by gram-negative bacteria. The most common gram-negative organisms are *Escherichia coli* (up to 85% of uncomplicated UTIs), followed by *Klebsiella* species, *Proteus* species, *Enterobacter (Aerobacter) aerogenes*, and *Pseudomonas aeruginosa*. Except for *Staphylococcus saprophyticus*, the 3rd most common cause of infection, gram-positive organisms such as *Staphylococcus epidermidis (albus)*, *S. aureus*, enterococci (*Streptococcus faecalis*), α-hemolytic streptococci, and β-hemolytic streptococci are much less frequently seen pathogens. Infection of the GU system by *Mycobacterium tuberculosis*, always a secondary manifestation of tuberculous disease in another site, is now uncommon. TB is discussed in Ch. 8.

SPECIFIC SITES OF LOWER URINARY TRACT INFECTION

Urethra

The urethra may be the site of acute and chronic infections. The bulbous and pendulous portions of the male urethra and the entire female urethra are richly invested with periurethral glands. Organisms gaining access to the urethra may colonize these glands and produce acute and chronic infection.

Women who have acute urethritis often have symptoms that are similar to those of acute bladder infections. Urethritis in men usually presents with a urethral discharge that is purulent (in cases due to *Neisseria gonorrhoeae*) or whitish-mucoid (in cases of nonspecific type). **Gonorrheal urethritis** is very common in men (see also in Ch. 14). Inadequately treated gonococcal urethritis can cause urethral strictures. Urethral stricture predisposes to proximal urethritis, occasionally with development of a periurethral abscess. Urethral diverticula may follow and serve as foci of continuing infection because of urinary stasis. Periurethral abscess may penetrate to and perforate the perineum or scrotum, and a urethral fistula may result. Although gonococcal urethritis may occur in women, the primary sites of infection are the vagina, cervix, and reproductive organs.

Nonspecific or nongonococcal urethritis may be due to infection with *Chlamydia trachomatis* or *Ureaplasma urealyticum*. Men usually experience burning on urination, urgency and frequency of urination, and inflammation of the urinary meatus. The scrotal contents may be involved (see EPIDIDYMITIS, below).

Bladder

Cystitis in women is usually due to ascending infection from the vagina through the urethra, and often occurs after sexual intercourse. Those women who develop recurrent UTIs differ from normal women in that they tend to carry large numbers of abnormal organisms for long periods of time on their vaginal vestibules. These pathogenic vaginal bacteria may find their way through the urethra and into the bladder and cause the next bladder infection. Thus the cause of recurrent UTI in women appears to be a lack of some form of local defense mechanism that allows the colonization of these bacteria on the vaginal vestibule. These women may also have decreased cervicovaginal antibody to enterobacteria.

Cystitis in men generally results from ascending infection of the urethra or prostate or occurs secondary to urethral instrumentation. The most common cause of relapsing bladder infection in men is chronic bacterial prostatitis. Although the bladder urine can readily be sterilized with an appropriate antibacterial agent, most antibacterial agents do not diffuse from plasma into prostatic fluid. Therefore, when drug therapy is stopped, the prostatic pathogen eventually reinfects the bladder urine.

Symptoms and signs: Acute cystitis classically presents with burning on urination or painful urination, urinary urgency and frequency, suprapubic and often low back pain, and nocturia. Gross hematuria also may occur, particularly in women. Many women with frequency and dysuria do not have bacteriuria, and symptoms usually resolve. Such symptoms may be caused by infections with gonococci, *Chlamydia*, *S. saprophyticus*, or viruses, or be secondary to vaginitis.

High back pain or loin pain, chills, fever, nausea and vomiting, and other signs of general toxicity usually imply a kidney infection, such as **acute pyelonephritis, renal abscess,** or **perirenal abscess.**

Recurrent cystitis in both men and women that is associated with passage of air in the urine, especially when changing or multiple organisms are involved, usually implies a vesicoenteric fistula. Recurrent cystitis in women is sometimes secondary to a small and otherwise essentially asymptomatic vesicovaginal fistula.

Hemorrhagic cystitis is an acute bacterial cystitis that presents with gross hematuria, frequency, urgency, and dysuria. **Cystitis cystica** and **vesicular cystitis** are usually sec-

ondary to chronic infections with mucosal and submucosal cystic changes similar to those seen in ureteritis cystica (see below). **Cystitis emphysematosa** is due to infection with gas-forming bacilli involving the submucosal layer of the bladder wall and is characterized by symptoms of infection plus pneumaturia. **Cystitis glandularis** is associated with chronic infections and exhibits characteristic histologic changes of encysted epithelialized spaces beneath the mucosal lining of the bladder. **Interstitial cystitis** is probably not an infectious disease and is discussed separately, below.

Prostate and Seminal Vesicles

Acute bacterial prostatitis is an acute infection of the prostate gland characterized by chills, high fever, urinary frequency and urgency, perineal and low back pain, varying degrees of symptoms of obstruction to voiding, dysuria or burning on urination, nocturia, and often arthralgia and myalgia. Gross hematuria sometimes accompanies acute prostatitis. The prostate gland is tender, focally or diffusely swollen and indurated, and usually warm to the palpating finger in the rectum. Culture of the expressed prostatic secretions usually yields large numbers of the bacterial pathogen. Enteric, gram-negative organisms are the most common cause of infection. However, because of the danger of bacteremia, the physician should *not* massage an acutely inflamed prostate gland until adequate blood levels of an appropriate antibacterial agent have been established. Since acute cystitis usually soon accompanies acute prostatitis, the bacterial pathogen usually can be identified by culture of the voided bladder urine.

Treatment: Hospitalization with bed rest, analgesics, and hydration generally is required. If sepsis is suspected, ampicillin or amoxicillin should be given for 7 to 10 days. To prevent the development of chronic bacterial prostatitis, trimethoprim/sulfamethoxazole therapy is recommended for 30 days. In patients allergic to penicillin, an alternative treatment until testing of antibacterial susceptibility of the pathogen is completed is an aminoglycoside. Should complete urinary retention occur, bladder drainage by punch suprapubic cystostomy is preferred over a urethral catheter (which may lead to bacteremia).

In **chronic bacterial prostatitis,** the spectrum of symptoms is variable. The hallmark of the disease is relapsing UTI due to the same pathogen as in the prostatic secretions. Some patients are essentially asymptomatic except for bacilluria that relapses between courses of antimicrobial therapy. Most patients, however, experience low back and perineal pain, urinary urgency and frequency, and painful urination. Prostate infections may involve the scrotal contents, producing intense localizing discomfort, swelling, erythema, and severe tenderness to palpation (see EPIDIDYMITIS, below). Rectal palpation of the prostate usually discloses no specific findings, but the prostate may be moderately tender and irregularly indurated or boggy. Secretions may be copious and numerous. WBCs, often in large clumps, may be identified, but the presence of large numbers of WBCs and lipid-laden macrophages (oval fat bodies) does not distinguish between bacterial prostatitis and nonbacterial prostatitis. The only accurate way of making the diagnosis of chronic bacterial prostatitis by laboratory means is with lower-tract localization cultures of the urethra, bladder, and prostatic secretions (see Diagnosis, below).

Chronic nonbacterial prostatitis is even more common than is bacterial prostatitis. Symptoms of this condition simulate those of chronic bacterial prostatitis; likewise, these patients usually show an increase in the number of WBCs and oval fat bodies in their expressed prostatic secretions. However, these patients rarely have a history of UTI, and lower-tract localization cultures fail to reveal a pathogenic organism.

The cause of nonbacterial prostatitis is unknown; thus, the condition is difficult to treat effectively. Antimicrobial agents do not relieve symptoms. Hot sitz baths and anticholinergic drugs provide some symptomatic relief. Some patients improve symptomatically with periodic prostatic massage, especially for congestive prostatitis.

Seminal vesiculitis, an infection of the seminal vesicles, is an uncommon condition and is impossible to prove by culture technics. It may be the cause of blood in the ejaculate.

Ureter

Ureteritis generally accompanies pyelonephritis and may accompany cystitis. Chronic ureteral infection may lead to decreased ureteral peristalsis and ureteral dilation with urinary stasis. One peculiar manifestation of chronic ureteritis is **ureteritis cystica,** the development of submucosal blebs that produce negative filling defects in the ureterogram.

DIAGNOSIS OF LOWER URINARY TRACT INFECTIONS

In normal men and women the bladder urine is sterile. The urethral flora normally is either sterile or contains small numbers of gram-postive organisms (*S. epidermidis [albus]*, *Streptococcus* species, diphtheroids, or lactobacilli). External vaginal cultures show a similar normal flora. The presence of gram-negative organisms in either the urethral culture of men or women or in vaginal cultures of women usually is abnormal, and may precede cystitis. (See also the discussion of urine cultures in Ch. 146.)

A clean-catch midstream urine specimen, the most commonly used specific diagnostic study, must be obtained scrupulously for culture and antimicrobial-sensitivity tests when an infection is suspected. **Quantitative urine cultures** are generally available and markedly reduce the need for specimens obtained by more complex procedures. The presence of > 100,000 organisms/mL in a carefully collected clean-voided urine specimen is presumptive evidence of a UTI. The presence of 3 or more species of bacteria in large numbers strongly suggests that the urine was contaminated during collection or was improperly stored (eg, kept at room temperature for an extended period) prior to culture, unless collected from a patient on chronic long-term catheter drainage.

The most accurate means of establishing the diagnosis of UTI is quantitative culture of the urine obtained by means of suprapubic needle aspiration of the bladder. A clean-voided midstream urine culture suffices in men to establish the diagnosis of UTI. In women the 2nd most accurate way to diagnose UTI is a urine culture obtained by bladder catheterization. Although urethral flora may be pushed into the bladder during catheterization, studies have shown that a bacterial colony count of > 1000 colonies/mL in a carefully collected catheterized specimen usually means that a bladder infection is present. Urinary infections rarely occur following bladder catheterization if careful, meticulous sterile technic is used.

In women, lower-tract localization cultures differentiate vaginal, urethral, and bladder infections. The patient is well hydrated to assure a full bladder. The lithotomy position is used. An external vaginal culture is obtained without preliminary skin preparation by swabbing the vaginal introitus with a sterile cotton-tipped applicator and then placing this cotton tip in 5 mL of saline or standard transport broth. With the nurse holding the patient's labia apart, the patient voids while on the table and the first 5 to 10 mL of urine are collected for a urethral culture. The patient then voids about 200 mL and a midstream sample is obtained by the nurse for a bladder culture. When the bacterial colony count of the vaginal culture significantly exceeds those of the urethral and midstream cultures, the diagnosis is vaginitis; when the urethral culture count exceeds the other cultures, the diagnosis is urethritis; when the midstream culture reveals a bacterial count of 100,000/mL, the diagnosis of a bladder or kidney infection is established.

In men, lower-tract localization cultures sort out urethral, bladder, and prostatic infections. The patient is well hydrated to assure a full bladder, and the foreskin is fully retracted to prevent washings from the prepuce from contaminating the specimen. The

glans penis is cleansed with an antiseptic solution. The patient voids, and the first voided 10 mL of urine are collected for a urethral culture. The patient next voids about 200 mL, and a midstream aliquot is obtained for a bladder specimen. The patient then bends forward and continues to retract the foreskin. The physician massages the prostate gland and collects drops of expressed prostatic fluid for prostatic culture. The patient voids again, and the physician collects the first voided 10 mL of urine immediately following prostatic massage (prostatic culture). The specimens are refrigerated immediately, cultured, and the quantitative bacterial colony counts of the 4 specimens are compared.

When the bacterial count of the urethral specimen significantly exceeds the other specimens, the diagnosis of bacterial urethritis is established. When the bacterial colony counts of the prostatic specimens significantly exceed those of the urethral and bladder specimens, the diagnosis of bacterial prostatitis is established. If the bacterial count of the midstream urine culture is 100,000/mL or greater, the diagnosis of a bladder or kidney infection is established. In the latter case the patient should be treated with a suitable antibacterial agent, and the localization cultures should be repeated in 4 to 5 days. If the patient has bacterial prostatitis, even though the urine will be sterilized by the antibacterial agent, the prostatic fluid cultures may still grow the pathogenic organism, and the diagnosis of bacterial prostatitis is established.

The normal centrifuged midstream or catheterized urine specimen should not contain > 5 WBCs/high-power field; more than this amount constitutes definite pyuria. Similarly, more than 2 RBCs/high-power field is considered abnormal and warrants further investigation. When the urine sample contains > 100,000 bacteria/mL, bacteria usually are readily seen on a wet-mount of the unspun sediment. A finding of > 20 bacteria/field of urine sediment, or a Gram stain of uncentrifuged urine demonstrating bacteria in every field, or > 8 WBCs/μL (cytologically determined in a hemacytometer chamber) has an 85% correlation with significant bacteriuria (> 100,000 organisms/mL) by quantitative culture. There is, however, no substitute for quantitative urine culture of carefully prepared samples in making the diagnosis of GU tract infection, and judging the sensitivity of the bacteria to specific antibiotics.

An **intravenous urogram (IVU) with a post-evacuation film** should be done in the evaluation of initial symptomatic UTI in men and relapsing infections in women, because congenital anomalies, obstructive uropathy, urolithiasis, or other abnormalities may complicate UTI. Repeated examinations are seldom warranted. IVU is of special value if pyelonephritis is suspected, and to determine residual urine volume without catheterization in the male. It is usually of little value for uncomplicated cystitis in the female. Retrograde pyelography is rarely indicated. **Voiding cystourethrograms** are important to evaluate the possibilities of vesicoureteral reflux, particularly in children, and may identify urethral strictures or valves as well. **Retrograde urethrography** is useful in both men and women to evaluate the possibilities of urethral strictures, diverticula, or fistulas. **Cystoscopy** may be helpful when a UTI fails to respond readily to therapy.

TREATMENT OF LOWER URINARY TRACT INFECTIONS

Obstructive uropathy, anatomic abnormalities, and neuropathic GU tract lesions may require correction by surgical means. Catheter drainage of an obstructed urinary tract aids in prompt control of UTI. On occasion, as with renal cortical abscess or perinephric abscess, surgical drainage is necessary. Instrumentation of the lower urinary tract in the presence of infected urine should be deferred, if possible, until the urine is sterilized with appropriate antimicrobial therapy to avoid bacteremia with septic shock, especially in the male.

Before antimicrobial treatment, uncomplicated and complicated (structural or neurologic abnormalities, foreign bodies) UTI should be distinguished. **For an initial course**

of therapy of uncomplicated infections, sulfonamides, tetracycline, ampicillin or amoxicillin, trimethoprim, or trimethoprim/sulfamethoxazole usually are adequate (see TABLE 153-1—dosages, where indicated, are for the average adult with normal renal function. Dosages of most agents must be altered in states of decreased renal function). Therapy for 7 to 10 days is customary, although 1 to 3 days may be adequate for most initial infections. Post-treatment follow-up is desirable to ascertain cure and rule out asymptomatic bacteriuria. Clinical symptoms of frequency, urgency, and dysuria are better guides to management than urine cultures in these patients.

The treatment of **recurrent uncomplicated infections** is slightly more complex. Recurrent infections can be relapses or reinfections. Sensitivity tests are highly desirable to guide antimicrobial selection. Most recurrences in girls and women are a reinfection with a new organism from the perineal-fecal reservoir and can be treated in the man-

TABLE 153–1. ANTIMICROBIAL DRUG DOSAGE FOR URINARY TRACT INFECTION IN ADULTS†

Drug	*Oral Daily Dose*	*Parenteral Daily Dose*	*Dosing Interval (hr)*
Amikacin		15 mg/kg	8–12
Amoxicillin	750–1500 mg		8
Amoxicillin with clavulanic acid	750 mg (amoxicillin)		8
Ampicillin	1–2 gm	1–2 gm	6
Carbenicillin	4–8 tablets*	6–12 gm	6
Cefaclor	750–1500 mg		8
Cefadroxil	1–2 gm		12–24
Cefamandole		1.5–6 gm	4–8
Cefazolin		1–2 gm	8
Cefoxitin		3–4 gm	6–8
Cephalexin	1–2 gm		6
Cephalothin		2–4 gm	4–6
Cephapirin		2–4 gm	6
Cephradine	2 gm		6
Demeclocycline	600 mg		6
Doxycycline	100–200 mg		12
Gentamicin		3–5 mg/kg	8–12
Methenamine hippurate	2 gm		12
Methenamine mandelate	4 gm		6
Nalidixic acid	2–4 gm		6
Netilmicin		4–6 mg/kg	8
Nitrofurantoin	200–400 mg		6
Norfloxacin	800 mg		12
Sulfonamides	2–4 gm		6
Tetracycline	1–2 gm		6
Ticarcillin		4–12 gm	6
Tobramycin		3–5 mg/kg	8–12
Trimethoprim	200 mg		12
Trimethoprim/sulfamethoxazole	320/1600 mg		12

* Each tablet provides 382 mg of carbenicillin.

† For dosages in children, see in Ch. 191.

ner of an initial acute uncomplicated infection. Recurrence within a few weeks of successful treatment may be caused by a relapse—reemergence of a partially suppressed organism. It is often caused by an inadequate course of therapy, urologic abnormalities, or renal infection. For relapses, tetracycline, ampicillin or amoxicillin, an oral cephalosporin, trimethoprim/sulfamethoxazole, or nitrofurantoin should be considered. The latter 2 agents are particularly useful for recurrences because the development of bacterial resistance is minimized. Therapy of relapses occasionally may require higher doses and 4 to 6 wk of treatment.

Long-term prophylaxis is appropriate for most patients who have > 2 infections a year. The annual cost of prophylaxis is also only 1/4 the cost of treating 3 to 4 infections each year. A prophylactic regimen of trimethoprim/sulfamethoxazole (1/2 tablet), nitrofurantoin (50 to 100 mg), or trimethoprim alone (100 mg) taken daily, thrice weekly, or after sexual intercourse is effective in reducing recurrent infections to near zero. Caution is indicated if nitrofurantoin is used for long-term use, as one study has shown serious adverse effects, including occasional fatal pulmonary reactions.

Complicated infections will respond to antimicrobial agents for only a few days unless the urologic abnormality can be corrected. Therefore, treatment should be reserved for acute episodes of tissue invasion in order to avoid the occurrence of highly resistant organisms. Aminoglycoside (gentamicin, tobramycin, amikacin) therapy of acute episodes of complicated infections is started after urine cultures because resistance to other antimicrobial agents is common. After initial treatment, sensitivity studies may indicate a less toxic agent can be substituted for the aminoglycoside for the 7- to 10-day course of treatment. When frequent septic recurrences occur, suppression of bacteriuria may be successful with nitrofurantoin, trimethoprim/sulfamethoxazole, or trimethoprim alone.

Symptomatic therapy: A variety of preparations are used for relief of UTI symptoms (especially frequency, urgency, and dysuria). These drugs include the anticholinergic agents (atropine, hyoscyamine, flavoxate, propantheline, or oxybutynin), which produce an antispasmodic effect on the smooth muscle of the urinary tract; and a topical urinary analgesic (phenazopyridine). Often alkalinization of the urine with oral sodium bicarbonate 0.5 tsp in 1/2 glass of water q 3 to 4 h may relieve symptoms. These drugs may be used *in conjunction with specific antibacterial drug therapy* for 1 or 2 days only in the early stages of treatment when symptomatic relief for the patient is highly desirable, or for treating symptoms when cultures are negative.

Chronic covert bacteriuria (*significant bacteriuria detected by the screening of apparently healthy populations*. The term is preferred to the older one, **asymptomatic bacteriuria**). Covert bacteriuria is rare in the male and should always prompt a thorough search for obstruction, prostatitis, or a hematogenous source. The prevalence of covert bacteriuria is about 1% in schoolgirls and increases with age and sexual activity. Except during pregnancy, when therapy is indicated to prevent acute bacterial pyelonephritis, the proper management of covert bacteriuria in the patient without obstruction is controversial. A common plan is to treat with a 7- to 10-day course of an appropriate oral antimicrobial for each recurrent infection. If recurrence occurs after 2 or 3 short courses of treatment, urologic studies should be done; if no correctable lesion is found, a 6-wk course can be tried. If covert bacteriuria again recurs, 2 choices are possible: treatment of symptomatic episodes only, or prophylaxis with nitrofurantoin or trimethoprim/sulfamethoxazole, or trimethoprim alone, for several months.

EPIDIDYMITIS

Acute bacterial epididymitis usually is a complication of bacterial urethritis or prostatitis and may be unilateral or bilateral. Torsion of the testis (see under RENAL AND GENITOURINARY DEFECTS in Ch. 187) must also be considered as an important differ-

ential diagnosis in patients under age 30 yr. Acute bacterial epididymitis is characterized by fever and pain in the scrotum. Physical examination reveals swelling, induration, and marked tenderness of a portion or all of the affected epididymis and at times, the adjacent testis. The infecting organism usually can be identified by urine culture or expressed prostatic secretions. In men < 35 yr, most cases are due to the sexually transmitted pathogens *Neisseria gonorrhoeae* or *Chlamydia trachomatis*. Most of these men have demonstrable urethritis.

Treatment consists of bed rest, scrotal elevation, scrotal ice packs, analgesics, and antimicrobial therapy. In men > 35 yr, most cases are due to coliform gram-negative bacilli. These men have pyuria, infected urine, and urologic abnormalities or recent urologic procedures. In addition to symptomatic therapy, ampicillin, amoxicillin, or trimethoprim/sulfamethoxazole can be given orally. If sepsis is suspected, a parenteral aminoglycoside or 3rd-generation cephalosporin may be useful until the infecting organism and its sensitivities are known. Posttreatment cultures are important to establish adequate treatment. Unless abscess formation occurs, surgical drainage usually is not required. When the inflammation involves the vas deferens, vasitis ensues; when the entire spermatic cord structures also are involved, the diagnosis is funiculitis. **Recurrent bacterial epididymitis** secondary to a chronic urethritis or prostatitis that cannot be cured usually can be prevented by means of vasoligation (vasectomy). Occasionally, **chronic epididymitis** requires an epididymectomy for relief of symptoms. Patients who must continuously wear an indwelling urethral catheter are prone to develop **recurrent epididymitis and epididymo-orchitis**. Prophylactic bilateral vasectomy should be considered, since most cases result from retrograde infection via the vasa. Placement of a suprapubic cystostomy or institution of a self-catheterization regimen may be useful adjuncts.

Nonbacterial epididymitis and epididymo-orchitis are of unknown etiology but are not rare. They may occur secondary to a retrograde extravasation. Urinalysis often is normal, and urine and prostatic fluid cultures are negative. The symptoms simulate those of bacterial epididymitis and treatment is similar, except that antimicrobial therapy may not be effective. Nerve block of the spermatic cord with a local anesthetic solution can provide marked symptomatic relief.

PARASITIC URINARY TRACT DISEASES

(See also Ch. 13)

Parasitic diseases such as schistosomiasis (bilharziasis), malaria, filariasis (*Wuchereria bancrofti*), *Trichomonas vaginalis*, *Entamoeba histolytica*, and *Echinococcus granulosus* affect large numbers of people and are frequent causes of renal and lower urinary tract disease. Parasitic infections often are chronic or recurrent, and it is not surprising that immunologic types of renal disease have been described. In Africa the most common type of childhood renal disease is the nephrotic syndrome associated with quartan malaria and a variety of glomerulopathic changes. Similarly, glomerulopathies are commonly associated with schistosomiasis, especially *Schistosoma mansoni* and *S. japonicum*. However, *S. haematobium* infestations are associated with obstructive uropathy, hydronephrosis, and pyelonephritis—a common cause of end-stage renal disease along the Nile river. Chronic cystitis is another frequent complication of schistosomiasis and frequently results in carcinoma of the bladder.

Filariasis involves the lymphatic system, with obstruction leading to chyluria and chronic elephantiasis that may involve the scrotum and legs. **Echinococcosis** is transmitted by the tapeworm ova and leads to hydatid cysts that most often involve the liver but also the kidney in a significant number of cases. ***Trichomonas vaginalis*** is a common cause of vaginitis in women but can lead to urethritis and prostatitis in men.

Amebiasis usually affects the GI tract, but may involve the kidney, bladder, and male or female genitalia, usually by blood-borne spread.

Treatment of trichomoniasis is discussed in Chs. 14 and 171. Treatment of the other infections is discussed in Ch. 13.

FUNGAL DISEASES
(See also Ch. 9)

A few mycotic diseases occasionally affect the GU system. *Candida* species are the most frequent fungal agents colonizing or infecting the urine. Multiple antibiotic therapy, antineoplastic drugs, corticosteroids, and chronic catheterization are predisposing factors. Urinary tract infections with *Candida* species may respond to flucytosine orally 150 mg/kg/day in divided doses q 6 h for 7 to 10 days, but emergence of resistant organisms is a frequent complication. Renal infections may require systemic therapy with amphotericin B (see General Therapeutic Principles in Ch. 9). Cystitis usually will respond to bladder instillations of amphotericin B over a 6- to 10-day period. **Blastomycosis,** a rare cause of prostatic, scrotal, and kidney infections, as well as hematospermia and bladder outlet obstruction, is presumptively diagnosed by the microscopic demonstration of round, budding, yeastlike cells, and is definitely established by culture. GU involvement may occur in 1/3 or more of male patients with this infection. Treatment is with amphotericin B (see General Therapeutic Principles in Ch. 9) or hydroxystilbamidine (see BLASTOMYCOSIS in Ch. 9). In **disseminated coccidioidomycosis** involvement of the GU tract, usually the kidney, and coccidioiduria are not uncommon. The inflammatory response is similar to TB, although there is less ureteral involvement. Amphotericin B is the mainstay of therapy. Rarely, a granulomatous reaction in the prostate occurs that resembles granulomatous prostatitis, although it is a vascular or allergic phenomenon, not an infection.

INTERSTITIAL CYSTITIS
(Hunner's Ulcer)

Interstitial cystitis is probably not an infectious disease, but is included here because of the clinical manifestations of bladder inflammation and irritation. This entity may be related to the collagen diseases, may be an autoimmune disease, may be an allergic manifestation, or may be secondary to an infectious agent not yet identified. It should not be confused with changes produced by radiation therapy and treatment with such drugs as cyclophosphamide, which also can cause severe cystitis. Carcinoma in situ of the urinary bladder often can mimic the symptoms of interstitial cystitis and must always be ruled out in such cases by means of repeated urinary cytology and bladder biopsy. Histologically, the bladder wall shows a unifocal or multifocal inflammatory infiltration with mucosal ulceration and scarring that ultimately results in contraction of the smooth muscle, diminished urinary capacity, and symptoms of frequent, painful urination and hematuria. Typically, middle-aged women are affected.

No single form of therapy is universally successful. Typical therapy has been repeated dilation and distention of the bladder under anesthesia and sometimes fulguration of the ulcerative lesions. Treatment with anticholinergic drugs such as propantheline bromide 15 mg qid or oxybutynin chloride 5 mg 2 to 3 times/day offers some relief. Bladder instillations of dimethyl sulfoxide (DMSO) also are being used with some success to relieve symptoms. Rarely, augmentation cystoplasty using ileum or sigmoid may be undertaken to increase bladder capacity, and occasionally the disease process may be so severe as to demand cystectomy with urinary diversion by ileal or colon conduit, ureterosigmoidostomy, or other methods.

154. VASCULAR DISEASE

VASCULAR DISEASES OF ACUTE ONSET

Excluding vasculitis (see in Ch. 110), 5 types of acute vascular disease produce renal syndromes: (1) malignant nephroangiosclerosis, (2) infarction from occlusion of major renal vessels, (3) atheromatous embolization, (4) renal cortical necrosis, and (5) renal vein thrombosis.

MALIGNANT NEPHROANGIOSCLEROSIS

(Malignant Nephrosclerosis; Malignant Hypertension)

Renal arteriolar necrosis associated with hypertension and rapidly progressive renal failure. Most cases of malignant nephroangiosclerosis appear as accelerated cardiovascular disease in the course of idiopathic hypertension, especially in untreated cases. Although 1% of patients with idiopathic hypertension have been reported to develop this complication, the incidence apparently is decreasing. However, about 20% of patients with this condition may have renovascular hypertension. The peak incidence in men occurs during their 40s and 50s; in women, about a decade earlier.

Pathology

The size of the kidneys varies greatly and presumably depends on the length of the clinical course and the presence of preexisting disease. The most striking glomerular change, the hallmark of malignant hypertension, is fibrinoid necrosis of arterioles. Proliferation of intraglomerular cells as well as epithelial crescents may be present. Interlobular arteries usually show considerable intimal thickening by a fine concentric layering of collagen, often causing a virtual obliteration of the vascular lumen.

Symptoms, Signs, and Diagnosis

Patients present with symptoms representing varying degrees of involvement of the brain, the heart, and the kidneys. On physical examination, neuroretinopathy (hemorrhages, exudates, and papilledema) is present. The heart is enlarged, with evidence of left ventricular hypertrophy. Congestive heart failure findings also may be present. Headaches, blurring of vision, and varying degrees of obtundation usually are present at some time during the disease. Coma may be present, due to cerebral hemorrhage.

Varying degrees of renal insufficiency are present. The urinary findings include proteinuria (occasionally in the nephrotic range) and microscopic hematuria. An occasional red cell cast may be found; but the numbers are small, except with those renal syndromes associated with proliferative glomerulonephritis. Granular casts are common, and if renal failure is far advanced, broad and waxy casts may be seen. Hematologic abnormalities are common and include coagulopathies as well as hemolysis. Extremely high levels of renin and aldosterone are typical.

Diagnosis is based on a persistent diastolic BP > 120 mm Hg and on neuroretinopathy, along with the other clinical features of cardiac and renal involvement described above.

Prognosis and Treatment

Untreated patients die in a relatively short period of time—about 50% by 6 mo, and most of the remainder within 1 yr. Death usually results from uremia (40%), cerebral atherothrombotic infarction (40%), or myocardial infarction (15%). Although some patients have spontaneous remissions, aggressive lowering of BP (see ARTERIAL HYPERTENSION in Ch. 26) and management of renal failure significantly reduce the mortality and morbidity. With therapy, fewer patients die, especially from renal failure and cerebrovascular disease, but the proportion developing myocardial infarction in-

creases. Patients with lesser degrees of renal failure improve most, and if hypertension can be reduced satisfactorily with dietary and drug therapy, most patients will be alive after 3 to 5 yr. Even patients with progressive renal insufficiency can be kept alive by dialysis and have occasionally shown improvement in renal function, permitting dialysis to be discontinued.

RENAL INFARCTION

A localized area of ischemic necrosis caused by either renal arterial or venous occlusion. Occlusion of the renal artery is rare and most frequently due to embolism, arteriosclerotic narrowing, and trauma. **Therapeutic infarction** via selective catheterization occasionally is used for renal tumors and massive proteinuria or severe uncontrollable hypertension in end-stage renal disease.

Symptoms and Signs

Small occlusions of the renal artery frequently occur without any urinary or systemic symptoms. Typically, however, a steady aching flank pain develops that is localized to the affected renal area. Fever, nausea, and vomiting may occur. When infarction is a result of arterial occlusion, the kidney is small and not palpable. However, with thrombosis of the renal veins, the kidney usually is tender and may be enlarged enough to be palpated. Hypertension occurs infrequently after infarction; if it occurs, it usually is transient. Leukocytosis, proteinuria, and microscopic hematuria typically are present. Gross hematuria is extremely rare. Serum and urine enzymes such as lactic dehydrogenase, alkaline phosphatase, and glutamic oxalacetic transaminase frequently are elevated early in the disease.

Diagnosis

When infarction is suspected, renal imaging is indicated. During the first 2 wk after a large renal infarction, excretion of contrast medium or radionuclide on the involved side is diminished or absent. Because impaired excretion also can be due to obstruction of the ureter, ultrasonography or retrograde urography is indicated to evaluate this possibility. A combination of history (atrial fibrillation, recent myocardial infarction or trauma, past embolic episodes), symptoms and signs, virtual absence of excretory function on the involved side, and a normal collecting system is strong evidence for renal infarction. Arteriography is definitive, but is done only if an attempt to relieve the obstruction is being considered. The extent of functional return may be evaluated by repeated intravenous urography **(IVU)** or radionuclide scanning at intervals of 1 mo.

Treatment

Surgical embolectomy may cause some reversal of renal dysfunction even up to 6 wk after embolization. However, conservative medical therapy with anticoagulants usually is indicated, especially in those with serious cardiac disease or unilateral infarction. Although reported experience is limited, percutaneous transluminal angioplasty or fibrinolytic (intraluminal or systemic) therapy may be more effective than previous procedures for arterial embolism. Anticoagulants remain the safest effective therapy for venous thrombosis. Although renal function may improve with treatment, a return to the premorbid state is unusual.

ATHEROEMBOLIC RENAL DISEASE

A clinical syndrome involving either rapid deterioration of renal function or a more slowly progressive renal failure. depending on the amount of atheromatous material obstructing the renal arteries. The syndrome may occur spontaneously or subsequent to vascular surgery or arteriography. In patients with severe erosive disease of the aorta,

the frequency of atheroembolic renal disease is approximately 15 to 30%; in patients with mild atherosclerosis, peripheral embolism has an incidence of only 1%. Embolization to the kidneys occurs most commonly in elderly patients and increases in incidence with age.

Symptoms, Signs, and Diagnosis

Atheroemboli to the kidney should be suspected in patients > 60 yr of age with renal failure of unknown etiology, especially if they have signs of advanced arteriosclerosis. The precise time of embolism is difficult to determine in patients with spontaneous atheroembolism, unlike in those with atheroembolism following arteriography. Most patients with spontaneous atheroembolism are azotemic when first seen, and progressive renal failure subsequently develops.

Patients with this disorder and renal failure usually are hypertensive. In those known to be previously normotensive, a substantial rise in BP occurs with the onset of atheroembolism. Embolisms of other abdominal organs such as the pancreas and the intestinal tract commonly occur. Signs of widespread peripheral embolism such as livedo reticularis, painful muscle nodules, or overt gangrene strongly suggest the diagnosis but are not often present. Furthermore, this syndrome may be confused with polyarteritis because of the multiple organ involvement. Embolization to the retina can cause sudden blindness, and bright yellow crystalline plaques can be seen lodged at bifurcations of arterioles on fundoscopic examination.

There are no distinctive laboratory or urinary sediment abnormalities. Diagnosis is confirmed only by renal biopsy.

Prognosis and Treatment

No treatment reverses advanced renal failure. The likelihood of atheroembolism of the renal arteries can be minimized during surgery involving an atheromatous aorta by careful technic.

RENAL CORTICAL NECROSIS

A rare form of arterial infarction characterized by necrosis of cortical tissues with sparing of the medulla.

Etiology and Incidence

Renal cortical necrosis can occur at any age; about 10% of cases occur in infancy and childhood. In neonates, over 50% are associated with abruptio placentae; the next most common association is bacterial sepsis. In children, infections, dehydration, shock, and hemolysis are associated. Other predisposing conditions are nephrotoxins, renal ischemia, intravascular coagulation, and hyperacute renal allograft rejection. Suggested mechanisms include vasospasm, activation of the clotting mechanism, endotoxin, immunologic injury, and direct endothelial cell injury. The lesion closely resembles the animal experimental forms of generalized Schwartzmann phenomenon.

Symptoms, Signs, and Diagnosis

Distinguishing this form of acute renal failure from many others may be difficult, but cortical necrosis should be considered when abrupt anuria occurs in any of the clinical settings noted above, and when gross hematuria and flank pain are present. Fever and leukocytosis are common even in the absence of sepsis. The urine contains much protein and RBCs; WBCs and casts (RBC, renal cell, and broad) frequently are seen. If measured early enough, serum LDH and AST (SGOT) levels are elevated. In the early stages, mild hypertension, or even hypotension, is common. However, in surviving patients who regain some residual renal function, accelerated or malignant hypertension is typical.

Although a biopsy showing patchy or diffuse cortical necrosis is the only means of confident diagnosis, renal x-rays also are useful. Serial x-rays initially show enlarged kidneys; renal size then diminishes and may be reduced to about 50% of normal in 6 to 8 wk. At this stage, calcification appears, often linear, and especially marked at the corticomedullary junction. The diagnosis is firmly established only from the typical histologic findings obtained by biopsy, which shows focal or patchy cortical necrosis.

Treatment

Management does not differ from other forms of acute renal failure, although more problems may be encountered because of the prolonged anuria and the precipitating causes. All appropriate means, including maintenance dialysis, are used to allow recovery of any residual function. A few patients may regain enough function to discontinue maintenance dialysis after several months. For the majority, however, chronic dialysis or renal transplantation is the usual solution.

RENAL VEIN THROMBOSIS

Etiology and Incidence

Primary renal vein thrombosis is the most common cause. This disease occurs as a **childhood variety** usually associated with volume depletion and hypercoagulability, or an **adult variety,** usually associated with the nephrotic syndrome **(NS)**. Various **secondary** causes also exist: (1) malignant renal tumors (usually renal cell carcinoma); (2) extrinsic compression of the renal vein (vascular abnormalities, tumor, retroperitoneal disease); (3) infection (pyelonephritis, perirenal abscess, TB, sepsis, osteomyelitis); (4) trauma; (5) thrombosis of the inferior vena cava (prolonged bed rest, external compression, hepatomegaly, retroperitoneal tumor, ligation of the inferior vena cava, pregnancy, oral contraceptives) with secondary renal involvement; and, rarely, (6) thrombophlebitis migrans, which may produce partial occlusion.

The incidence is difficult to determine because, aside from the acute forms, most cases induce only mild symptoms that often go unnoticed.

Symptoms, Signs, and Diagnosis

Clinically, 2 different pictures are seen: (1) With acute onset at any age, loin pain, fever, hematuria, oliguria, edema, leukocytosis, and renal failure are found. Acute thrombosis usually produces hemorrhagic infarction. (2) In adults, onset of the syndrome is most often gradual, with the appearance of proteinuria and a deterioration of GFR. Partially occlusive, slowly progressive thrombosis, more common in adults, is associated with nephrotic syndrome **(NS)** even with unilateral thrombosis. The diagnosis usually is considered only in the presence of the NS. (Whether the thrombosis is a primary cause of NS or is secondary to the hypercoagulable state associated with NS is still debated.)

If the disease is acute, ultrasonography may show an enlarged kidney; slowly progressive thrombosis produces an atrophic kidney. IVU shows poor or no excretion of the contrast agent. Cavography or selective renal phlebography may show thrombosis manifested by filling defects or a filling of collateral veins. In some patients, computed tomography, digital subtraction angiography, or renal arteriography may be preferred. Preliminary results with echo-Doppler duplex flowmeters and radionuclide-labeled platelets appear promising.

Prognosis and Treatment

Death due to renal vein thrombosis is rare and usually is related to the primary condition producing the thrombosis or to complications such as pulmonary embolism. The effect on renal function is variable, depending on whether one or both kidneys are

involved, on the development of collateral circulation or recanalization of the thrombus, and on the prior state of kidney function. These multiple factors influence the natural course of the disease and render evaluation of any treatment difficult. However, surgery is rarely used, and nephrectomy is performed only in certain cases of total infarction or for reasons related to the primary disease. Thrombolytic therapy with streptokinase or urokinase has been infrequently tried and is unproved. Anticoagulant therapy usually is associated with improvement of renal function, is particularly useful in preventing pulmonary embolism, and improves patient survival.

SLOWLY PROGRESSIVE VASCULAR DISEASE

Arteriosclerosis is a phenomenon of aging that is accentuated by hypertension. In the kidney, the lesion usually is described as **benign nephrosclerosis** although a more accurate term would be **nephroangiosclerosis**. The vascular lesions are quite distinct from those associated with malignant hypertension, where fibrinoid necrosis of the arteries is the hallmark of the vascular damage. Arteriosclerotic disease is discussed under ARTERIOSCLEROSIS; ATHEROSCLEROSIS in Ch. 26. See also HYPERTENSION in Ch. 26.

RENOVASCULAR HYPERTENSION

(See HYPERTENSION in Ch. 26)

155. RENAL DISEASE ASSOCIATED WITH SYSTEMIC AND METABOLIC SYNDROMES

Renal disease may be prominently involved in many systemic disorders. These include the collagen vascular diseases (eg, SLE, progressive systemic sclerosis, polyarteritis, Wegener's granulomatosis); hemorrhagic disorders (eg, the hemolytic-uremic syndrome, thrombotic thrombocytopenic purpura, Henoch-Schönlein purpura); plasma cell dyscrasias (eg, multiple myeloma); anemia (eg, sickle cell disease); liver disease (see Ch. 67); pregnancy (see Ch. 178); and endocrine and metabolic disorders (eg, diabetes mellitus and amyloidosis). Changes in the concentrations of various electrolytes and body fluids may have profound effects on renal function, especially seen in the presence of hypophosphatemia, hypercalcemia, potassium depletion, and gout. The renal abnormalities involved in the above disorders are included in their discussions elsewhere in THE MANUAL.

ANOMALIES IN KIDNEY TRANSPORT

RENAL TUBULAR ACIDOSIS (RTA)

Impaired ability to secrete hydrogen ions in the distal nephron or to resorb bicarbonate ions proximally, leading to chronic metabolic acidosis which, in the distal form, may be accompanied by potassium depletion and by rickets or osteomalacia.

Distal RTA (Type I) usually is a sporadic disorder, but familial cases occur either in association with another genetic disease or rarely as an isolated autosomal dominant disease. Sporadic cases may develop as a **primary** disease, nearly always in women, or **secondary** to a predisposing cause; eg, an autoimmune disease with hypergammaglobulinemia (especially Sjögren's syndrome), amphotericin B or lithium therapy, renal transplantation, nephrocalcinosis, renal medullary cystic disease, or chronic obstruction.

Proximal RTA (Type II) accompanies several inherited diseases, including Fanconi's syndrome, hereditary fructose intolerance, Wilson's disease, and Lowe's syndrome. It also occurs in multiple myeloma, vitamin D deficiency, and chronic hypocalcemia with secondary hyperparathyroidism; after renal transplantation; and following treatment with certain drugs, including acetazolamide, sulfonamides, outdated tetracycline, and streptozotocin.

Type IV RTA, in which the major defect is diminished renal ammonia production, occurs chiefly in association with selective hypoaldosteronism (hyporeninism).

Pathophysiology, Symptoms, and Signs

In distal (classic, Type I) RTA the ability to develop a high concentration of hydrogen ions in the distal tubule and collecting duct is impaired so that urine pH does not fall below about 6. In proximal (Type II) RTA, the capacity of the proximal tubule to resorb bicarbonate ion (**HCO_3^-**) is diminished so that at normal levels of plasma HCO_3^-, increased amounts of HCO_3^- reach the distal tubule and are excreted in the urine. At low levels of plasma HCO_3^-, the proximal tubule resorbs enough of the filtered HCO_3^- to allow urinary acidification to occur.

With either Type I or Type II, chronic metabolic acidosis develops. In the distal form this results in potassium wasting and decreased citrate excretion in the urine, and continued mobilization of bone calcium with hypercalciuria. Potassium depletion induced by chronic metabolic acidosis causes muscle weakness, hyporeflexia, and paralysis. The continued loss of bone calcium results in rickets and osteomalacia. In the presence of alkaline urine with reduced citrate, it also results in calcium precipitation; stone formation, which may be seen on x-ray, may cause renal colic and nephrocalcinosis. Renal parenchymal damage and chronic renal failure may develop eventually. In hereditary types, nephrocalcinosis has been seen by age 6.

Diagnosis

Low plasma HCO_3^- and low blood pH with a normal level of undetermined anions are present. Distal RTA is confirmed by an **acid load test**: Ammonium chloride 100 mg/kg orally normally reduces urine pH to < 5.2 within 3 to 6 h. In distal tubular acidosis, urine pH remains > 6.

A **bicarbonate titration test** helps to identify proximal RTA. Sodium bicarbonate is slowly infused in order to raise plasma HCO_3^-. In proximal tubular acidosis, HCO_3^- will appear in the urine before plasma HCO_3^- reaches the normal range.

Treatment

Bicarbonate administration relieves the symptoms and prevents or stabilizes renal failure and bone disease. In distal tubular acidosis, sodium bicarbonate 80 to 200 mg/kg/day (1 to 3 mEq/kg/day) orally in divided doses will eliminate the acidosis and reduce the occurrence of stones. In the proximal form, doses of 800 mg/kg/day or more may be necessary. **Shohl's solution** (140 gm citric acid and 90 gm sodium citrate dihydrate made up to 1 L with water), 50 to 100 mL/day in divided doses, can be substituted for sodium bicarbonate solution and may be better tolerated. Potassium supplements may be required in selected cases after alkalinization.

The acidosis accompanying the syndrome of hyporeninemia and hypoaldosteronism is usually mild. When necessary, it can be treated with sodium bicarbonate as described for distal RTA, above.

RENAL GLUCOSURIA

(Renal Glycosuria)

Excretion of glucose in the urine in the presence of normal or low blood glucose levels.

Renal glucosuria may be associated with many renal tubular defects involving aminoaciduria and renal tubular acidosis. When it occurs as an isolated finding with

otherwise normal renal function, it is usually inherited as an autosomal dominant trait; occasionally it is a recessive trait. The maximum rate at which glucose can be resorbed (normally 320 mg/min) is termed the **transport maximum (T_m)** for glucose. In Type A renal glucosuria, the T_m for glucose is reduced and sugar escapes in the urine. In Type B the T_m is normal, but the renal threshold is reduced so that glucose appears in the urine at a lower than normal plasma concentration. Combined forms of the disease occur. Intestinal glucose transport is normal except in the rare glucose-galactose malabsorption (see CARBOHYDRATE INTOLERANCE in Ch. 58).

Renal glucosuria is asymptomatic and without serious sequelae. A few patients eventually develop diabetes mellitus, which should be ruled out by establishing the diagnosis of glucosuria. **Diagnosis** is made by demonstrating glucose in the urine after an overnight fast in a patient having normal glucose tolerance. Glucosuria should be demonstrated by a specific test for glucose, such as the glucose oxidase test, to distinguish it from other abnormalities wherein reducing substances are found in the urine. No treatment is necessary.

NEPHROGENIC DIABETES INSIPIDUS (NDI)

(See also DIABETES INSIPIDUS in Ch. 88)

A disease in which renal function is normal except for an inability to concentrate the urine due to lack of response of the renal tubules to antidiuretic hormone.

NDI occurs as an X-linked, probably recessive, disease. Affected males are completely unresponsive to **antidiuretic hormone (ADH, vasopressin)**. Heterozygous females show normal or slightly impaired responsiveness to ADH.

Concentration of the urine in normal individuals is the consequence of secretion of ADH by the posterior pituitary in response to changes in the osmolality of the plasma and increased water resorption in response to ADH by the distal convoluted tubule and collecting duct. These parts of the nephron are normally impermeable to water in the absence of ADH, resulting in high flow rates of dilute urine. ADH increases the permeability of the distal tubule and collecting duct to water, allowing it to be passively resorbed along the medullary concentration gradient created by the countercurrent mechanism.

In NDI, the formation and secretion of ADH by the posterior pituitary are normal but the nephron is unresponsive to the hormone. The consequences are polydipsia, polyuria, and hypotonic urine, the same features as are seen in pituitary DI, from which the disease must be distinguished (see in Ch. 88). Usually the disease appears soon after birth. Since the infant cannot communicate its thirst, severe water depletion may result, with hypernatremia, fever, vomiting, and convulsions. *Brain damage with permanent mental retardation may occur if the cause of the symptoms is not recognized.* Urine osmolality is usually 50 to 100 mOsm/L but may rise to 280 mOsm/L during a solute diuresis. Other evidence of abnormal tubular function is lacking, and the GFR is normal. Physical growth is often retarded.

An **NDI syndrome** may be seen in disorders preferentially affecting the medulla or distal nephrons, resulting in impaired ability to concentrate the urine and apparent insensitivity to ADH: medullary and polycystic disease; sickle cell nephropathy; release of obstructing periureteral fibrosis; medullary pyelonephritis; hypokalemic, hypercalcemic, and hypomagnesemic nephropathies; the nephrotic syndrome; amyloidosis; Sjögren's syndrome; and myeloma. Certain nephrotoxins, especially aminoglycosides, lithium, and demeclocycline, also are causes.

Treatment of NDI consists of ensuring that the patient has an adequate free water intake. As long as the patient can increase his water intake in response to thirst, serious sequelae seldom occur, but polyuria and polydipsia may be nuisances. Sodium restriction, thiazide diuretics, and indomethacin or tolmetin may be helpful.

BARTTER'S SYNDROME

A combination of fluid, electrolyte, and hormonal abnormalities characterized by renal potassium and sodium wasting, hypokalemia, hyperaldosteronism, hyperreninemia, and normal BP. The syndrome usually appears in childhood, either as a sporadic or a familial, usually autosomal recessive, disorder.

Etiology, Pathophysiology, and Symptoms and Signs

Bartter's syndrome results from a complex disturbance of renal electrolyte handling. The underlying renal tubular disorder (or disorders) has not been defined. The proximal tubule, the ascending thick limb of the loop of Henle, and the distal nephron have all been suggested as possible sites of transport defects which might be etiologic. Potassium, sodium, and chloride wasting occur, each contributing to the stimulation of renin release, which is accompanied by hyperplasia of cells of the juxtaglomerular apparatus. Elevated levels of aldosterone are present. Potassium depletion is not eliminated by correction of the hyperaldosteronism. Sodium wasting results in a chronically low plasma volume, which is reflected by a normal BP despite high levels of renin and angiotensin, and by an impaired pressor response to angiotensin infusion. Metabolic alkalosis often develops. Inhibition of platelet aggregation is present. Hyperuricemia and hypomagnesemia may occur.

Excretion of prostaglandins and kallikrein in the urine is increased. Inhibition of prostaglandin synthesis results in correction of most of the abnormalities, but potassium depletion is only partially eliminated. Abnormalities in prostaglandin synthesis in fibroblasts and in sodium transport in erythrocytes are present in some cases.

Affected children have poor growth rates and appear malnourished. Muscle weakness, polydipsia, polyuria, and mental retardation may be present.

Diagnosis and Treatment

Bartter's syndrome is distinguished from other diseases associated with hyperaldosteronism by the absence of hypertension (as in primary hyperaldosteronism) and edema (as in secondary aldosteronism). When the features of the disease are first seen in adults, vomiting or surreptitious diuretic abuse must be explicitly eliminated as causes.

Potassium supplementation plus spironolactone, triamterene, propranolol, or indomethacin will correct most features, but no drug completely eliminates potassium wasting. Indomethacin 1 to 2 mg/kg/day usually maintains plasma potassium level close to the lower limit of normal.

LIDDLE'S SYNDROME

A rare disorder of renal epithelial transport which clinically resembles primary hyperaldosteronism (see Ch. 91) *with hypertension and hypokalemic metabolic alkalosis.* Accelerated sodium resorption and potassium secretion occur despite low aldosterone levels. The disorder is unresponsive to spironolactone. Treatment with triamterene or amiloride is effective.

---

156. INHERITED AND CONGENITAL DISORDERS

CYSTIC DISORDERS

The cystic disorders of the kidney represent types of dysplastic malformations, with single or multiple cysts varying in size from < 1 cm to > 10 cm in diameter. Some

disorders are congenital, some are acquired, and sometimes a distinction cannot be made. The major groups are (1) polycystic disease (adult and infantile types); (2) renal dysplasias (multicystic, focal and segmental, familial, secondary to lower urinary tract obstruction); (3) cortical cysts (simple [solitary and multiple], diffuse glomerular, and microcysts); (4) medullary cystic (medullary sponge kidney, medullary cystic disease complex); (5) cysts in hereditary disorders (Meckel's syndrome, Zellweger cerebrohepatorenal syndrome, Jeune's thoracic dystrophy, tuberous sclerosis complex, Lindau's disease); and (6) miscellaneous (inflammatory, neoplastic, extraparenchymal types).

POLYCYSTIC RENAL DISEASES

Inherited kidney disorders characterized by many bilateral cysts that cause enlargement of the kidney but reduce, by compression, the functioning renal tissue. The disease usually is classified by the inheritance pattern. Two types are recognized: the **adult form,** an autosomal dominant disorder that progresses to renal insufficiency in middle age; and an **infantile form,** a rare autosomal recessive disease that produces renal failure in childhood (see Ch. 187). The adult type usually develops clinical symptoms after the 2nd decade, although it has been described in a fetus from an affected patient and in several neonates. The incidence of the adult type is approximately 1:500 in autopsied series, but clinical recognition is only about 1:3000. The penetrance of the dominant type means 100% of carriers will manifest the disease by age 80 yr. About 5% of patients with end-stage renal disease have this disorder. Mechanisms for the development of polycystic disease and progressive enlargement of the cysts are not known. The cysts are dilated nephrons and collecting ducts. The cysts of glomerular origin may end blindly in the cortex, while those of tubular origin communicate proximally with the glomerulus and distally with the renal pelvis.

Symptoms and Signs

Since adult polycystic disease is slowly progressive over many years, it is often asymptomatic initially but may be discovered by ultrasonography in childhood. Clinical onset is in early or middle adult life, although occasionally the disease is not discovered until autopsy. Symptoms usually are related to effects of the cysts, such as lumbar discomfort or pain, hematuria, infection, and colic, or may be related to a loss of renal function with uremic symptoms. Chronic infection frequently is superimposed and contributes to the progressive loss of renal function. In about 33% of cases, cysts are present in the liver but are of no functional significance. About 10% of cases have associated intracranial aneurysms. Hypertension is common; about 75% of patients have this finding at the time of diagnosis.

Diagnosis

In advanced cases, when the kidneys are grossly enlarged and palpable, the diagnosis is obvious. The urine shows mild proteinuria and varying degrees of hematuria, but RBC casts are infrequent. Pyuria is common even in the absence of bacterial infection. Episodically, the urine is grossly bloody, apparently because of hemorrhage from a ruptured cyst or a dislodged calculus. The intravenous urogram (**IVU;** excretory urogram; IVP) is characteristic, with large kidneys showing irregular outlines because of the many cysts. The calyces, infundibula, and pelvis are compressed and elongated by cysts, giving what is referred to as a "spidery" appearance. Renal and hepatic sonograms and CT scans show a typical "moth-eaten" appearance due to the cysts that displace functional tissue; they may be diagnostic in early stages of the disease before typical changes are noted in the IVU. Polycystic kidney disease, with its progressive azotemia, is distinguished from solitary or multiple cysts of the kidney that do not distort a sufficient portion of the renal parenchyma to cause uremia. The distinction is made on clinical grounds and by ultrasound, IVU, or radionuclide scanning.

Prognosis and Treatment

Though over 50% of patients become uremic within 10 yr of onset of symptoms, the course is quite variable; for many, end-stage renal failure will not occur for > 20 yr. Without dialysis or transplantation, death usually is due to uremia or the complications of hypertensive cardiovascular disease, and occurs at an average age of 50. About 10% of patients die of intracranial hemorrhage from rupture of aneurysms.

Management of urinary infections and secondary hypertension may prolong life considerably. Genetic counseling is recommended. When uremia supervenes, its management is the same as in other renal diseases (see Ch. 147, above). With dialysis, patients with polycystic kidney disease have higher Hcts than any other group of patients. Transplantation is feasible, but the use of parental and sibling donors may be impractical in view of the familial characteristics of the disease.

MEDULLARY CYSTIC DISEASE

A diffuse nephropathy, either genetic or congenital in origin, usually seen in children or young adults and characterized by the insidious onset of uremia.

The commonly described variants and their incidence are juvenile nephronophthisis, 50%; adult-onset medullary cystic disease, 20%; and renal-retinal dysplasia, 15%. A family history is common and a recessive pattern of transmission is suggested, although cases with no family history comprise about 15%. In a few families the renal disease has been accompanied by pigmentary retinal degradation. The adult-onset variety is less common and shows a dominant pattern of transmission. The renal lesion is similar in all variants.

Symptoms, Signs, and Diagnosis

Symptoms usually begin in the first 2 decades of life, although the disease has been observed as late as the 60s. Polyuria due to a vasopressin-resistant renal concentrating defect often is the earliest symptom. Urinary sodium wastage frequently is present and commonly is severe enough to require a sodium intake of several hundred mEq/day to prevent extracellular volume depletion. Unexplained uremia is a good early clue in some cases. Retarded growth and evidence of bone disease are common in children. In many patients these problems develop slowly over a period of years and are so well compensated that they are not recognized as abnormal until significant uremic symptoms appear.

Serum chemistries are similar to those in patients with chronic renal failure. Proteinuria is minimal or absent and the urinary sediment is not remarkable. IVU demonstrates only small kidneys, but ultrasound and arteriography may reveal medullary cysts. Because cysts may be few and small, they can be overlooked or missed by any one or all of these imaging studies.

Prognosis and Treatment

Progression of the disease is variable and depends on the degree of renal dysfunction when the patient is first seen. As a rule, the disease progresses slowly but inexorably. When uremia supervenes, its management is the same as in other renal diseases (see Ch. 147, above). These patients may do very well with transplantation.

MEDULLARY SPONGE KIDNEY

Tubular ectasia or dysplasia resulting in congenital dilatation of the collecting tubules.

The disorder is unrelated to medullary cystic disease (see above). The true incidence is unknown but is probably about 1:5000. Sponge kidney leads to urinary stasis and nephrocalcinosis.

Symptoms, Signs, and Diagnosis

The condition usually is asymptomatic unless the complications of calculus colic (the most common presenting complaint), hematuria, or infections supervene. Nephrocalcinosis is found in > 50% of affected kidneys. Sonography usually is not helpful because the cysts are small and located deep in the medulla. The lesion must be differentiated from renal cystic disease, papillary necrosis, pyelonephritic cysts, TB, and other conditions causing nephrocalcinosis. Diagnosis is by urography, which shows pyramidal cavities filled with contrast material, giving the appearance of a bouquet of carnations. Medullary sponge kidney has been noted with increased frequency in Ehlers-Danlos syndrome and congenital hemihypertrophy.

Prognosis and Treatment

If uncomplicated, the condition has an excellent prognosis. Treatment is given only for complications. Usually, noncalcinotic forms are asymptomatic and need no therapy. Although nephrocalcinosis may be progressive, no specific medical treatment has been adequately assessed. However, thiazides (eg, hydrochlorothiazide 50 mg bid), high fluid intake, and a low calcium diet may inhibit stone formation and reduce obstructive complications. Infections are treated in the usual manner. Surgery is indicated only when obstruction occurs or if renal involvement is segmental. Extirpation of the affected tissue has proved beneficial.

HEREDITARY CHRONIC NEPHROPATHIES

Many of the genetically transmitted renal disorders produce functional or structural abnormalities, or both. Those involving mainly tubular transport defects (see Ch. 155) or metabolic defects with renal involvement as in Fabry's disease (see LIPIDOSES in Ch. 85) are discussed elsewhere. The hereditary, noncystic nephropathies discussed in this section are hereditary nephritis and the nail-patella syndrome.

HEREDITARY NEPHRITIS
(Alport's Syndrome)

A familial disorder characterized by hematuria, renal functional impairment, perceptive deafness, and, on occasion, ocular abnormalities.

Most evidence suggests an autosomal dominant inheritance with variable penetrance, although X linkage may be present in some families. There are no distinguishing histologic changes by light or immunofluorescence microscopy. Ultrastructural studies in some families show thickening and thinning of the glomerular and tubular basement membrane with multilamination of the lamina densa in a focal or local distribution. Dense deposits have not been found.

Symptoms, Signs, and Diagnosis

Onset of the disease may be similar to that of acute glomerulonephritis, but many patients are asymptomatic and the disease is detected by finding hematuria. The urine may contain small amounts of protein, WBCs, and casts of various types. The nephrotic syndrome occurs rarely. Afflicted females usually are asymptomatic and have little functional impairment, while most males with the disease develop evidence of renal insufficiency between ages 20 and 30. Perceptive deafness frequently is present, usually in the higher frequencies. Some individuals with a family history may have nerve deafness alone without renal disease; such persons are capable of transmitting the renal disease to a subsequent generation. Eye lesions occur less frequently than acoustic ones; cataracts are most common, but anterior lenticonus, spherophakia, nystagmus, retinitis pigmentosa, and blindness also have been noted. Other nonrenal manifestations include polyneuropathy and thrombocytopenia.

Treatment

Treatment is only indicated when uremia occurs; its management is the same as in other renal diseases. Successful transplants have been done using kidneys from cadavers or living, related adult females with hematuria but no sign of progression. Genetic counseling is indicated.

NAIL-PATELLA SYNDROME

(Osteo-onychodysplasia; Arthro-onychodysplasia; Onycho-osteodysplasia)

A rare familial disorder of mesenchymal tissue characterized by abnormalities of bone, joints, fingernails, and kidneys.

Inheritance occurs as an autosomal dominant trait linked to the ABO blood group locus. The most common skeletal dysplasia is unilateral or bilateral hypoplasia or absence of the patella, subluxation of the radial heads at the elbows, and bilateral accessory iliac horns. The fingernails are either absent or hypoplastic with pitting and ridges. Heterochromia of the irises may occur, but deafness is not found. The renal lesion is characterized by abnormal lamina production. Histologic changes by light microscopy are nonspecific with localized thickening of the capillary wall. Focal glomerular deposits of IgM and C3 may occur. The characteristic ultrastructural changes are localized areas of rarefaction of the glomerular basement membrane with intramembranous deposits having the appearance and periodicity of collagen.

Symptoms and Signs

Renal dysfunction occurs in about 50% of patients with this disorder and is manifested by proteinuria and, rarely, hematuria. Proteinuria usually is minimal but occasionally may reach nephrotic syndrome ranges. The disease is diagnosed by the typical clinical and radiographic findings and can be further confirmed by renal biopsy. About 30% of patients with renal involvement will slowly progress to renal failure.

Treatment

Genetic counseling is indicated. Management of progressive renal failure is the same as in other renal diseases. Successful transplants have been done without evidence of recurrence of the disease in the renal graft.

157. OBSTRUCTIVE UROPATHIES

Urine flow may be obstructed at any level from the glomerulus to the external urethral meatus and in some instances even beyond. The consequences include increased intraluminal pressure, urinary stasis, infection, stone formation, and loss of renal function. Presenting symptoms and signs depend on the nature, duration, and level of the obstruction.

HYDRONEPHROSIS

Dilatation of the renal pelvis and, usually, of the infundibula and calyces beyond the normal capacity of 3 to 10 mL.

Etiology

Primary hydronephrosis, without ureteral dilatation, results from obstruction at the ureteropelvic junction. This may be due to intrinsic stricture; high insertion of the ureter into the renal pelvis; a defect in continuity of smooth muscle at the ureteropelvic junction; kinking of the junction from nephroptosis; or extrinsic compression by fibrous bands or an aberrant artery or vein, or from a renal pelvis stone or tumor.

Secondary hydronephrosis results from obstruction distal to the ureteropelvic junction or occurs as a result of vesicoureteral reflux. Some causes are ureteral stones or tumors, extrinsic ureteral compression by primary or metastatic tumor, myoneurogenic disease of the ureter or bladder, fibrosis secondary to surgery or radiation, retroperitoneal fibrosis, ureterocele, congenital or acquired vesicoureteral reflux, malignancies of the bladder or other pelvic viscera, bladder outlet obstruction due to prostatic enlargement or carcinoma, or urethral obstruction such as stricture, congenital valves, or meatal stenosis. The hydronephrosis occasionally seen in pregnancy is due to mechanical factors and the effects of progestational hormones. It is usually transient, though some dilatation may persist following delivery. Occasionally, a severe UTI may induce temporary atony of the ureter, with hydronephrosis.

Pathology

Chronic dilatation of the renal pelvis causes muscular atony, fibrosis, and loss of peristaltic activity. Since urine is normally excreted at extremely low pressure, prolonged and severe hydronephrosis ultimately results in pressure atrophy of the renal parenchyma; this affects the collecting tubules and medullary interstitium initially, and then the proximal tubules, cortical interstitium, and glomeruli, with gradual loss of renal function.

Symptoms and Signs

When acute, hydronephrosis usually is manifested by colicky pain; when chronically progressive, it can be asymptomatic or attended by intercurrent attacks of dull, aching flank discomfort. A flank mass may be palpable, particularly in massive hydronephrosis of infancy and childhood. Intermittent hydronephrosis due to nephroptosis or acute overdistention of the renal pelvis **(Dietl's crisis)** generally produces excruciating pain. Hematuria is seen in about 10% of patients with hydronephrosis. Urinary infection with pyuria, fever, and localized discomfort is a fairly common finding. Calculi may result from stasis, and azotemia may occur when a solitary kidney is obstructed or both kidneys are involved. Unexplained, vague GI symptoms (eg, nausea, vomiting, and abdominal pain) may be due to hydronephrosis, and are often seen in children with congenital ureteropelvic obstruction.

Diagnosis

Urologic investigation (see also discussions of urinary system evaluation procedures in Ch. 146) includes abdominal ultrasound and/or an intravenous urogram (**IVU**; excretory urogram; IVP) performed by infusion, and may require tomography. Cystourethrograms may show lower tract obstruction, neurogenic disorders, or vesicoureteral reflux. Cystoscopy and retrograde urethrography or ureteropyelography may delineate the anatomic deformity. Following instillation of contrast material and removal of the ureteral catheter, the normal renal pelvis will empty contrast material in 5 to 10 min. Delayed emptying by a hydronephrotic kidney confirms a functional or anatomic abnormality, unless dehydration (which prolongs the emptying time) is a factor. Assessment of the degree of hydronephrosis as well as the comparative delay in emptying time, by either IVU, nuclear scan, or the retrograde technic, may be enhanced by establishing diuresis with a suitable diuretic before the contrast material or radioisotope is injected. A kidney that is nonfunctioning by delayed films on pyelography can be investigated by radioisotope scan to determine perfusion and identify functional renal parenchyma. Hydronephrosis usually is well documented by noninvasive ultrasound studies, which are particularly useful in children.

Treatment

Intensive UTI treatment and renal failure management are imperative. Prompt surgery for primary hydronephrosis is indicated if renal function is compromised, infection persists, or pain is significant. Temporary nephrostomy drainage may be needed

in severe obstruction, infection, or stones. The percutaneous technic can be used; eg, acute obstruction with sepsis is best managed initially by percutaneous nephrostomy drainage. Secondary hydronephrosis is corrected by attention to the cause; eg, relief of lower tract obstructive uropathies. Catheter drainage or urinary diversion is often helpful.

Prognosis

Surgical correction of primary hydronephrosis, either unilateral or bilateral, is successful in most cases when infection can be controlled, renal function has been preserved, and calculous disease has not supervened. The prognosis is more guarded in secondary hydronephrosis. Surgery must eliminate stasis or reflux, infection must be treated, and normal intraluminal pressure gradients must be preserved to ensure stabilization of renal function.

URETERAL OBSTRUCTION

Ureteral strictures can be congenital or due to trauma, infection, tumor, surgery, or external radiation. Ureteral segments lacking myoneural continuity cause proximal ureterectasis and hydronephrosis. Primary resection and reanastomosis of the ureter may adequately relieve obstruction and hydronephrosis due to strictures or atonic segments. **Retroperitoneal fibrosis** may be idiopathic or secondary to surgery or drugs, primarily methysergide. Management involves dissection and mobilization of the ureters with intraperitoneal transplantation and omental wrapping to avoid recurrence of obstruction. **Ureteral obstruction at the ureterovesical junction** may result from the trauma of stone passage or extraction, hypertrophy of the bladder wall in neurogenic diseases, defects in continuity of ureteral muscle, bladder outlet obstruction, or occasional congenital strictures. If more conservative management fails, vesicoureteral reimplantation is generally the surgical procedure of choice. **Ureteral obstruction by calculi** is very common and can cause chronic hydronephrosis. See Ch. 160 for treatment.

BENIGN PROSTATIC HYPERPLASIA (BPH)

(Benign Prostatic Hypertrophy)

Benign adenomatous hyperplasia of the periurethral prostate gland commonly seen in men over age 50, causing variable degrees of bladder outlet obstruction. The etiology is unknown but may involve alterations in hormonal balance associated with aging.

Pathology

Multiple fibroadenomatous nodules occur in the periurethral region of the prostate gland, probably originating within the periurethral glands themselves rather than in the true fibromuscular prostate **(surgical capsule),** which is displaced peripherally by progressive growth of the hyperplastic nodules. The hyperplastic process may involve the lateral walls of the prostate **(lateral lobe hyperplasia)** or may include tissue at the inferior margin of the vesical neck **(middle lobe hyperplasia)**. Histologically, the tissue is glandular with varying amounts of fibrous stroma interposed. Secondary infection may induce chronic prostatitis. As the lumen of the prostatic urethra is compromised, the outflow of urine is progressively obstructed, with hypertrophy of the bladder detrusor, trabeculation, cellule formation, and diverticula. Incomplete bladder emptying causes stasis and predisposes to infection with secondary inflammatory changes in the bladder and the upper urinary tract. Prolonged obstruction, even though incomplete, can produce hydronephrosis and compromise renal function. Urinary stasis also predisposes to calculus formation.

Symptoms and Signs

Bladder outlet obstruction symptoms include progressive urinary frequency, urgency, and nocturia due to incomplete emptying and rapid refilling of the bladder. Hesitancy and intermittency with decreased size and force of the urinary stream occur. Sensations of incomplete emptying, terminal dribbling, almost continuous overflow incontinence, or complete urinary retention may ensue. On rectal examination the prostate usually is enlarged, with a rubbery consistency and, frequently, loss of the median furrow. However, the size can be misleading. A prostate that is small by rectal examination may be sufficiently enlarged to cause urethral obstruction. Congestion of superficial veins of the prostatic urethra and trigone can cause hematuria secondary to rupture while the patient is straining to void. Burning on urination and chills and fever indicate urinary infection. Episodes of acute complete urinary retention may follow prolonged attempts to retain urine, immobilization, exposure to cold, anesthetic agents, anticholinergic and sympathomimetic drugs, or the ingestion of alcohol. The distended urinary bladder may be palpable or percussible on physical examination. Prolonged urinary retention, partial or complete, may cause progressive renal failure and azotemia.

Diagnosis

BPH with bladder outlet obstruction is suspected on the basis of the symptoms and signs. An indurated and tender prostate suggests prostatitis, while a stony, hard, nodular prostate usually indicates carcinoma or, occasionally, prostatic calculi. An IVU may disclose upward displacement of the terminal portions of the ureters **(fishhooking)** and a defect at the base of the bladder compatible with prostatic enlargement. With prolonged obstruction, dilatation of the ureters and hydronephrosis are noted. The postvoiding cystogram indicates the amount of residual urine. Catheterization after voiding measures residual urine and permits preliminary drainage, to stabilize renal function and adequately control urinary infection. Cystoscopy permits estimation of the gland size and the appropriate surgical approach, plus an opportunity to differentiate between vesical neck contracture, chronic prostatitis, and other obstructive phenomena. Instrumentation should be avoided until there is a commitment to definitive therapy, since manipulation may induce increased obstruction, trauma, and infection.

Treatment

When urinary infection or azotemia accompanies bladder outlet obstruction, initial therapy should be medical, directed toward stabilizing renal function, discontinuing anticholinergic and sympathomimetic drugs, and eradicating infection. Catheter drainage, either urethral or suprapubic, may be desirable in advanced bladder outlet obstruction. Slow decompression of the chronically obstructed, distended bladder is advised, and postobstructive diuresis may occur. Definitive therapy is surgical. Transurethral resection of the prostate **(TURP)** is the preferred operative procedure and has the advantage of patient acceptance, since no incision is required and TURP is associated with low morbidity and mortality. Larger benign prostates may be managed by open surgery using the suprapubic or retropubic approach that permits enucleation of the adenomatous tissue from within the surgical capsule. All surgical methods require postoperative catheter drainage for a few days. The prognosis is excellent and the patient usually maintains preoperative sexual potency, which usually is associated with retrograde ejaculation.

URETHRAL OBSTRUCTION

Obstruction **in the male** may result from BPH, prostatic carcinoma, chronic prostatitis with fibrosis, a foreign body, contracture of the vesical neck, or congenital urethral valves. Urethral strictures and meatal stenosis may be acquired or congenital. **In the**

female, urethral obstruction is rare but may occur secondary to tumor, radiation therapy, surgery, or instrumentation.

Diagnosis requires urologic investigation, which may include cystourethrography and cystourethroscopy. Treatment consists of elimination of the obstruction by medical (eg, hormone therapy for carcinoma of the prostate), surgical, or instrumentation technics.

---

158. MYONEUROGENIC DISORDERS

The urinary tract is subject to congenital and acquired disorders of smooth muscle and innervation that result in inadequate urinary storage or control, urinary stasis, infection, calculi, and renal damage. These complications of the underlying myoneurogenic disorders can be life-threatening and require careful evaluation and meticulous attention to management.

Urinary incontinence is discussed in Ch. 159; nocturnal enuresis in children, under BEHAVIORAL PROBLEMS in Ch. 188.

NEUROGENIC BLADDER

Vesical dysfunction resulting from congenital abnormality, injury, or disease process of the brain, spinal cord, or local nerve supply to the urinary bladder and its outlet.

Classification

Because of the complexity and variability of neurogenic bladder dysfunction, clinical classification is difficult. However, the distinction between the **hypotonic** (flaccid) and the **spastic** (contracted) neurogenic bladder is important in treatment. Congenital spinal cord defects generally result in a hypotonic neurogenic bladder, while acquired disease processes exhibit slowly progressive signs of either hypotonia or hypertonia. Neurogenic bladder dysfunction following acute spinal cord injury presents as a flaccid hypotonic bladder persisting for days, weeks, or months (shock phase) before permanent spasticity or flaccidity is established.

Etiology

Normal urinary control and voiding are the result of complex interactions of smooth muscle, voluntary muscle, cerebral inhibition, and the autonomic nervous system. Congenital neurogenic bladder may be due to myelomeningocele, filum terminale syndrome, or other lesions of the spinal cord, including the cauda equina. The most common acquired cause of severe neurogenic bladder dysfunction is spinal cord injury resulting in paraplegia or quadriplegia, the result of transverse myelitis or transection of the cord. Disease processes that result in neurogenic bladder dysfunction—either hypotonic or hypertonic—include syphilis, diabetes mellitus, brain or spinal cord tumors, cerebrovascular accidents, ruptured intervertebral disk, and the demyelinating or degenerative diseases such as multiple sclerosis and amyotrophic lateral sclerosis.

Symptoms and Signs

Neurogenic bladder dysfunction may manifest itself as partial or complete urinary retention, incontinence, or frequent urination. In the chronic phase, with inadequate emptying, urinary infection is common. Urinary calculi result from immobilization, with increased urinary calcium excretion, urinary stasis with crystallization, and superimposed urinary infection. In acute spinal cord injuries, the **"shock bladder"** is atonic and distended and may exhibit continuous overflow dribbling. With lower spinal cord (sacral and lumbar) lesions, the bladder becomes flaccid within a few weeks. Upper cord lesions (thoracic and cervical) produce an automatic or spastic reflex bladder that

may empty spontaneously or as the result of somatic stimuli; the effectiveness of emptying depends on urethral resistance. Contracture of the vesical neck is common, particularly in spastic neurogenic bladder, and vesicoureteral reflux with renal damage may follow any type of congenital or acquired neurogenic bladder. Associated sphincter dyssynergia may also be present.

Diagnostic Evaluation

Serial imaging studies such as intravenous urography (**IVU**; excretory urography; IVP), ultrasonography, cystography, and urethrography demonstrate urinary calculi and help to assess the anatomic patterns and progressions seen secondary to the neurogenic bladder. Cystourethroscopic evaluation determines the degree of bladder outlet obstruction. Serial cystometrograms during the recovery phase of flaccid paralysis provide an index of detrusor functional capacity and hence an indication of rehabilitation prospects. Also helpful are urodynamic assessment of voiding flow rates, sphincter electromyograms, and urethral pressure profile studies.

Treatment

In flaccid paralysis of the bladder following acute spinal cord injury, continuous catheter drainage or periodic intermittent catheterization should be established *immediately* to prevent overdistention with consequent infection and damage to the detrusor muscle.

Long-term management: Patients who develop an automatic or reflex bladder may be managed by condom catheter drainage. Persistent residual urine and contracture of the vesical neck may require transurethral resection on one or more occasions, or incision of the external sphincter (sphincterotomy) in the male, to minimize outlet resistance and to maximize emptying. Electrical stimulation of the bladder, the sacral nerves, or the spinal cord remains experimental.

Pharmacologic management may improve bladder storage, emptying, and control. Detrusor spasticity and involuntary contractions usually can be reduced or eliminated with medications producing an antispasmodic or anticholinergic effect on the bladder (eg, in adult dosages—oxybutynin chloride 5 mg 2 to 4 times/day; imipramine 50 mg 2 to 4 times/day; or propantheline bromide 15 mg 2 to 4 times/day. Side effects include dry mouth and constipation. Sphincter dyssynergia may respond to phenoxybenzamine hydrochloride 10 mg 1 to 2 times/day; postural hypotension is a possible side effect. The most commonly prescribed oral medication for detrusor hypotonia in the adult is bethanechol chloride 50 mg 2 to 4 times/day. This medication produces parasympathetic stimulation, and its possible related side effects. Improvement in sphincter control may result from such drugs as phenylpropanolamine hydrochloride and imipramine.

Continuous urethral catheter drainage may be required in some instances and is tolerated better in the female. In the male, the continuing presence of the catheter predisposes to urethritis, periurethritis, abscess formation, and urethral fistula. **Intermittent catheterization,** preferably done by the patient, is used when feasible rather than indwelling catheter drainage. **Permanent urinary diversion** is occasionally appropriate in some patients with congenital or acquired neurogenic bladder dysfunction, especially those in whom flaccidity persists and reflux occurs (increasing the risk of upper tract damage), or when spasticity or quadriplegia prevents the use of satisfactory continuous or intermittent drainage. **Permanent upper tract diversion** is best accomplished by ileal or colon conduit. **Permanent suprapubic cystostomy** affords adequate control in some patients, and **cutaneous vesicostomy** with an external appliance and no indwelling catheter may be a convenient method of urinary control in patients with no upper tract damage. **Not advised** are ureterosigmoidostomy (because most patients with neurogenic bladder dysfunction also lose rectal sphincter control) and cutaneous intubated ureterostomies and nephrostomies (since the inlying catheters increase the chances for stone formation and infection).

Continued monitoring of renal function, control of urinary infection, high fluid intake, early ambulation, frequent change of position, and dietary calcium restriction to inhibit stone formation are essential, with or without attendant urinary diversion or catheter drainage. Though total recovery in any form of neurogenic bladder is uncommon, rehabilitation may be excellent with vigorous and appropriate therapeutic measures. Artificial sphincter devices may be surgically inserted to control urinary continence in selected patients.

MEGACYSTIS SYNDROME

The syndrome of megacystis ("large bladder") is poorly understood. It is often seen in girls with large, thin-walled, smooth bladders without evidence of outlet obstruction. The presenting symptoms are related to UTIs. Vesicoureteral reflux is common. IVU with the bladder empty may disclose normal-appearing upper tracts, while cystourethrograms may exhibit reflux with massive upper tract dilatation. Rehabilitation by ureteral reimplantation and reduction cystoplasty may be effective, although some patients benefit from drug therapy or intermittent catheterization or require urinary diversion, generally by the ileal or colon conduit method.

URETERAL DYSFUNCTION

Abnormalities of ureteral smooth muscle or nerve supply may cause ureteral dilatation, segmental or total, with demonstrable obstruction. With **megaloureter** (*severe ureteral dilatation, unilateral or bilateral*), obstruction and reflux are not evident. Ureteral dilatation and relative atony may develop above a segmental defect in peristaltic transmission due to failure of smooth muscle continuity or of nerve impulse propagation (adynamic segment).

Treatment is surgical; prognosis depends on the neuromuscular integrity of the proximal ureter.

159. URINARY INCONTINENCE

Involuntary loss of urine during the day or night. (**Nocturnal enuresis** *or* **bed-wetting** is the *involuntary loss of urine during periods of sleep*—see also BEHAVIORAL PROBLEMS in Ch. 188).

Urge incontinence is characterized principally by *an urgent desire to void followed by involuntary loss of urine*. It may occur alone or with varying degrees of stress incontinence. In the absence of urinary tract infection, the most common causes are idiopathic; uninhibited neurogenic bladder dysfunction; multiple sclerosis; obstructive uropathy; bladder calculi, neoplasms, or TB; and interstitial cystitis. **Therapy** is directed toward correction of the underlying cause. Cases of the adult idiopathic variety are best treated with anticholinergic drugs, such as propantheline 15 mg, imipramine 50 mg, or oxybutynin 5 mg orally qid. The dosage should be adjusted to the individual patient's needs and tolerance.

Stress incontinence (partial incompetence of the urinary sphincter) is the *involuntary loss of urine on coughing, straining, sneezing, lifting, or any maneuver that suddenly increases intra-abdominal pressure*. **In men**, stress incontinence is seen occasionally following prostatectomy or trauma to the membranous urethra or bladder neck. **In women**, stress incontinence is the most common cause of involuntary loss of urine. It may be due to shortening of the urethra and loss of the normal posterior urethrovesical angle resulting from pelvic relaxation (cystocele) that characteristically occurs with

aging or multiparity. **Diagnosis** is established by history, pelvic examination, and demonstrating loss of urine with coughing or straining, which may be stopped by finger elevation of the paraurethral vaginal tissues at the bladder neck (the Marshall-Marchetti test). Mild cases may respond to a series of pubococcygeal muscle exercises (Kegel's exercises —see under SEXUAL DYSFUNCTION IN THE FEMALE in Ch. 165) or to sympathomimetic (α-adrenergic) drug therapy, which increases proximal urethral resistance. More severe cases require surgical correction by anterior vesicourethropexy, vaginal repair, or an endoscopic bladder neck suspension procedure.

Urinary retention with overflow incontinence (paradoxical incontinence) occurs when *the bladder becomes acutely or chronically overdistended and the intravesical pressure increases, eventually overcoming urinary sphincter resistance.* Urine then dribbles from the urethra, and the patient may be unable to initiate or maintain a good urinary stream. Examination of the abdomen reveals the distended bladder. The bladder's inability to empty may result from obstruction to urine outflow or from impaired detrusor contraction. **In children**, the most common causes of obstructive uropathy of the lower urinary tract include urethral meatal stenosis, urethral strictures, and urethral valves; rarely, the cause is bladder neck contracture. **In adults**, bladder outlet obstruction usually is due to vesical neck contracture, benign prostatic hyperplasia, carcinoma of the prostate, or urethral stricture. Myelomeningocele, spina bifida occulta, tumors, cerebrovascular accidents, chronic anticholinergic drug therapy, and injury to the sacral spinal cord may be associated with a bladder that lacks motor impulses, impairing voiding contraction.

Ectopic ureter in female patients characteristically presents a history of *lifelong, constant leakage of urine day and night despite voiding normal amounts of urine at regular intervals throughout the day.* The ectopic ureteral orifice may be located near the bladder neck, in the urethra, or within the vagina. Diagnosis is facilitated by careful inspection of the vagina and vaginal vestibule, cystoscopy, excretory urography, and voiding cystourethrography. Surgical correction is necessary for cure.

In the male, the ectopic ureter drains proximal to the external sphincter and does not produce urinary incontinence.

Total incompetence of the urinary sphincter is characterized by *a constant involuntary dripping of urine from the urethra day and night without bladder distention*, as determined by physical examination of the abdomen and measurement of residual urine. **In children**, congenital failure of the urethra to close properly (eg, epispadias) results in this form of incontinence. **In women,** it is usually due to trauma to the vesical neck and urethra. **In men,** the most common cause is surgical trauma to the vesical neck and prostatomembranous urethra. Postprostatectomy incontinence, particularly following radical prostatectomy for cancer, is due to damage to the urinary sphincter mechanism.

Various surgical procedures have been devised to treat this form of urinary incontinence, including the application of artificial sphincters.

Neurogenic bladder dysfunction: Various forms may underlie urinary incontinence (see Ch. 158, above).

Urinary fistulas in women cause *involuntary urine loss from the urethra or vagina*; the common symptom is loss from the vagina. Such fistulas usually are secondary to operative trauma, neoplasms, radiation therapy, automobile accidents, traumatic delivery, or gunshot wounds, where a tract becomes established and conducts urine from the ureter, bladder, or urethra into the vagina. The amount of urine lost varies with the fistula's size and location. Leaking may be constant or intermittent and may or may not be associated with voiding. **Diagnosis** usually can be established by excretory urography, voiding cystourethrography, and urethrocystoscopy. Inspection of the vagina

following filling of the bladder with indigo carmine solution helps identify whether the fistulous opening is from the urethra, bladder, or ureter. **Therapy** consists of surgical excision of the fistulous tract when feasible. Fistulas due to tumor or radiation therapy may require urinary diversion.

Psychogenic incontinence (see also BEHAVIORAL PROBLEMS in Ch. 188) occasionally is seen in **children** and even in **adults** who have underlying emotional disturbances. Diagnosis can be established only after all other causes of incontinence are ruled out. Treatment consists of α-adrenergic or anticholinergic drugs and psychotherapy.

Mixed types of incontinence are sometimes seen. **A child** may have incontinence secondary to both an uninhibited neurogenic bladder dysfunction and psychogenic factors; or an **adult male** may have both overflow incontinence due to prostatic obstruction and neurogenic bladder dysfunction secondary to diabetic neuropathy or cerebrovascular insufficiency. A complete urodynamic evaluation, including excretory urography, voiding cystourethrography, retrograde urethrography, cystoscopy, cystometrograms, and a careful neurologic examination may be required to detect these mixed forms. Therapy is directed toward identifying and treating the specific types of incontinence present.

---

160. URINARY CALCULI

(Nephrolithiasis; Urolithiasis)

Urinary calculi **(stones)** may occur anywhere in the urinary tract and are common causes of pain, obstruction, and secondary infection.

Incidence and Pathogenesis

Approximately 1 in every 1000 adults is hospitalized annually in the USA because of urinary stones. They are found in about 1% of all autopsies. The pathogenesis is related to (1) factors increasing the supersaturation of the urine with stone-forming salts, which include overexcretion states and conditions that lead to inadequate amounts of urine; (2) preformed nuclei, such as uric acid crystallites and other stones; and (3) abnormal crystal growth inhibitors.

Calculi vary in size from microscopic crystalline foci to stones several cm in diameter. A large stone, a so-called staghorn calculus, may be shaped by and virtually fill an entire renal calyceal system. About 80% of stones in the USA are composed of calcium, mainly calcium oxalate; 5% are uric acid; 2% cystine; and the remainder, magnesium ammonium phosphate, or "infection" stones. Stones may have characteristic colors or appearances, but crystallographic analysis should be used to determine the composition.

Symptoms and Signs

Many calculi are "silent." Back pain or **renal colic** may occur when calculi obstruct one or more calyces, the renal pelvis, or the ureter; stones in the bladder may cause suprapubic pain. Typical symptoms of renal colic include excruciating intermittent pain, usually originating in the flank or kidney area and radiating across the abdomen along the course of the ureter, frequently into the region of the genitalia and inner side of the thigh. GI symptoms (nausea, vomiting, abdominal distention, the clinical picture of ileus) may obscure the urinary origin. Chills, fever, hematuria, and frequency of urination are common, particularly as a calculus passes down the ureter. The affected kidney transiently may become nonfunctioning in acute renal colic due to ureteral calculus, even for some time after the stone has been spontaneously passed.

Diagnosis

The symptoms of colic, together with flank or costovertebral angle tenderness, increased sensitivity in the lumbar and groin areas, or complaints of pain in the genitalia with no obvious localized lesions suggest renal colic from stones. Diagnosis is supported by urinalysis and x-ray findings. Intravenous urography **(IVU)** should be done to evaluate extent of obstruction and to detect radiolucent stones. Differential diagnosis includes appendicitis, cholecystitis, peptic ulcer, and pancreatitis.

Urinalysis: The urine may be normal despite multiple calculi. Macroscopic or microscopic hematuria is common. Pyuria with or without bacteria may be seen. Various crystalline substances may be identified in the sediment, but the stone's composition should be determined by crystallography. The only exception is the presence of the typical benzene-ring crystals of cystine in a concentrated, acidified specimen, which strongly suggests cystinuria.

Roentgenography: Most urinary calculi are demonstrable on x-ray. Only pure uric acid calculi, rare xanthine calculi, and some "matrix stones" (composed largely of protein matrix) are radiolucent. Pyramidal calcium deposits within the renal parenchyma are diagnostic of **nephrocalcinosis** and suggest renal tubular acidosis, sarcoidosis, Cushing's disease, hyperparathyroidism, or the milk-alkali syndrome. Retrograde or intravenous urography may show opaque or nonopaque calculi, as well as the extent and degree of obstruction.

Treatment

Many small solitary calculi, uncomplicated by obstruction or infection, require no specific therapy. Eradication of infection should be attempted; if impossible, chronic suppressive therapy may be necessary. Symptoms of colic may be relieved by narcotics (morphine 10 to 15 mg or meperidine 100 mg IM q 3 to 4 h), but antispasmodics are unsatisfactory. Obstructing stones can be removed surgically if they do not pass spontaneously, but ultrasound disruption (**extracorporeal shock-wave lithotripsy**), where available, can spare most patients open surgery for impacted stones, provided the stones are in the renal pelvis or the uppermost ureter. Another alternative to open surgery is the use of percutaneous technics to remove renal calculi. Calculi impacted in the renal pelvis or ureter may require surgery, particularly when associated with infection. Calculi < 1 cm in diameter in the lower ureter may be approached endoscopically; cystoscopic basket extraction is successful when the calculus is not impacted in an edematous ureter. Uric acid calculi in the upper or lower urinary tract occasionally may be dissolved by prolonged alkalinization of the urine, but chemical dissolution of other calculi is not possible.

Prophylaxis

Identification of the type of stone is the first step in determining pathogenesis. Measurements of stone-forming substances in the urine and the clinical history are then needed to plan prophylaxis, beginning with recovery and analysis of the stone, preferably by crystallographic technics. A **cystine stone** is diagnostic of cystinuria, which is discussed under ANOMALIES IN KIDNEY TRANSPORT in Ch. 187.

Calcium stones: Approximately 5% of calcium stone formers have primary parathyroidism. Other rare causes of calcium stones are sarcoidosis, vitamin D intoxication, hyperthyroidism, renal tubular acidosis, multiple myeloma, metastatic cancer, and primary hyperoxaluria.

Idiopathic hypercalciuria, a hereditary condition, is present in 50% of men and 75% of women calcium stone formers, and is the main risk factor for calcium stones in the USA. Hypercalciuria is defined by an excretion rate of 300 mg/day (men), 250 mg/day

(women) or 4 mg/kg for either sex. Thiazide diuretics, such as trichlormethiazide 2 mg bid lowers urine calcium excretion and supersaturation with calcium oxalate. New stone production falls dramatically with the use of thiazides. Patients with stones are encouraged to increase their water intake to at least 1.3 L/day. Low calcium diet and sodium cellulose phosphate should be used cautiously, since there is a possibility of producing chronic negative calcium balance. Oral orthophosphate has not been thoroughly studied.

Hyperoxaluria: In addition to primary hyperoxaluria, hyperoxaluria is caused by enteric disease or excess ingestion of oxalate-containing foods (eg, rhubarb, spinach, cocoa, nuts, pepper, and tea). The amount of oxalate in the urine and clinical history will discriminate among the causes of hyperoxaluria. Patients with small-bowel disease can be treated with a combination of a low-oxalate, low-fat diet; calcium loading; or cholestyramine.

Hyperuricosuria is defined as > 750 mg (women) or 800 mg (men) per 24 h of uric acid in the urine. Uric acid crystals provide a nidus on which calcium oxalate crystals can orient themselves and grow. These patients can form what appear to be pure calcium stones, because the uric acid nidus is not measurable by commercial laboratories, or mixed calcium and uric acid stones. The pathogenesis of hyperuricosuria is virtually always excess consumption of purine, in the form of meat, fish, and poultry. If the diet cannot be changed, allopurinol 100 mg bid or 300 mg each morning can be used to lower the uric acid production.

There is a small group of **patients in whom no metabolic abnormality is found**. These people seemingly cannot tolerate normal amounts of stone-forming salts in their urine without crystallization. Thiazide diuretics and increased fluid intake reduce their stone production rate.

Uric acid stones occur because of increased urine acidity in which undissociated uric acid crystallizes. Increasing the urine pH to between 6 and 6.5 with alkali as sodium bicarbonate tablets 650 mg, 2 tid, or citrate (sodium or potassium salt) 0.5 to 1 mEq/kg/day in 2 or 3 divided doses; and if necessary, using allopurinol 100 mg bid or reduced purine intake, and increasing the water intake are treatment maneuvers that work in the majority of cases.

Magnesium ammonium phosphate stones (struvite): This crystal indicates the presence of UTI, with urea-splitting bacteria in the urinary system. The stones themselves are loci of infection and must be treated as infected foreign bodies. In contrast to the other types of stones, infection stones occur mostly in women. Fastidious attention to even small numbers of urea-splitting bacteria as well as treatment of any metabolic causes of stone may delay the need for surgery.

---

161. MALE GENITAL LESIONS

Abnormalities of the external male genitalia (penis, scrotum, and scrotal contents) are psychologically disturbing and sometimes life-threatening for the patient. A careful, gentle examination and correct diagnosis are mandatory.

Penile Lesions

Balanoposthitis (*generalized inflammation of the glans penis and foreskin*) is commonly caused by bacterial and yeast infections beneath the foreskin of the uncircumcised male. Such inflammation predisposes to meatal stricture, phimosis, paraphimosis, and cancer. Balanoposthitis is discussed in Ch. 14.

Erythroplasia of Queyrat, a premalignant lesion, is *a well-circumscribed area of reddish, velvety pigmentation, usually on the glans or at the corona.* Biopsy should be considered, and treatment consists of topical application of 5% fluorouracil cream. Careful follow-up is indicated.

Balanitis xerotica obliterans, the result of chronic inflammation, is *an indurated, blanched area near the tip of the glans, surrounding the meatus and often causing constriction.* Local antibacterial and anti-inflammatory agents may be used, and meatotomy may be required in some instances.

Bowen's and **Paget's diseases** (see Ch. 244) are rare skin cancers that may appear on the penis. For **carcinoma**, see Ch. 163. **Other rare penile lesions** include those due to TB, mycotic penile disease, and herpes zoster. **Herpes simplex** is more common. **Chancre,** the primary lesion of syphilis, and **genital warts (condylomata acuminata)** are discussed in Ch. 14.

Priapism

Painful, persistent, and abnormal penile erection, unaccompanied by sexual desire or excitation.

The mechanisms of priapism are poorly understood, but probably involve a complexity of vascular and neurologic abnormalities. Pelvic vascular thrombosis is most often incriminated. Priapism may be secondary to prolonged sexual activity; leukemia, sickle cell disease or trait, or other blood dyscrasias; pelvic hematoma or neoplasm; cerebrospinal disease such as syphilis or tumor; or infection and inflammation of the male genitalia such as prostatitis, urethritis, or cystitis, especially if complicated by a bladder calculus. Several drugs have been suspected of producing priapism (eg, trazodone, chlorpromazine, methaqualone, prazosin, tolbutamide, and certain antihypertensives, anticoagulants, and corticosteroids). The corpora cavernosa are rarely thrombosed completely, usually containing only thick, dark venous blood of motor oil consistency. The corpus spongiosum and glans penis are not involved.

Treatment is difficult and frequently unsuccessful. Neurogenic priapism may be alleviated by continuous caudal or spinal anesthesia. Estrogens are ineffective, and anticoagulants are effective only in the earliest stages. The corpora may be decompressed by introduction of large-bore needles (12- or 16-gauge) with evacuation and irrigation, though tumescence usually recurs. Creation of a fistula between the glans and corpus cavernosum has proved successful and can be done with a biopsy needle. Semipermanent diversion by means of a saphenous vein shunt from one or both corpora or a cavernoso-spongiosum shunt may result in detumescence for a period of time sufficient to permit reestablishment of pelvic circulation. Underlying causes should be treated. **Prognosis** for recovery of sexual function is poor unless treatment is prompt and effective.

Peyronie's Disease

Dysplasia of the cavernous sheaths consisting of a fibrous thickening and contracture of the investing fascia of the corpora not unlike Dupuytren's contracture. The cause is unknown. The disease occurs in adult males. The contracture usually results in deviation of the erect penis to the involved side, occasionally causes painful erections, and may prevent intromission. Later, the fibrotic process may extend into the corpus cavernosum, compromising tumescence distally.

Treatment is varied and results unpredictable. Resolution may occur spontaneously over many months. Surgical removal of the plaque and replacement with a patch graft may be successful or result in further scarring and exaggeration of the defect. An asymptomatic plaque does not warrant treatment. High-potency corticosteroid local injections may be effective; oral corticosteroids have not been. Local ultrasonic treatment has proved beneficial in relieving symptoms in some cases.

Scrotal Masses

Scrotal masses may be due to trauma, inflammatory conditions involving the scrotal wall or contents, neoplasms of the testis or testicular appendages, or mechanical abnormalities involving the scrotal contents or adjacent structures.

Epididymo-orchitis (*inflammation of the epididymis and testis*) may be a complication of urinary infection with prostatitis or urethritis, a sequel to gonorrhea, a complication of prostatic surgery, or a result of infection secondary to an indwelling catheter. Gram-negative bacteria and *Chlamydia trachomatis* are the organisms usually involved. Tuberculous epididymitis, syphilitic gummas, and the mycotic diseases (actinomycosis, blastomycosis) are rare today. Treatment consists of bed rest, scrotal support (adhesive bridge), ice bags, and systemic antibacterials. Scrotal abscesses tend to drain spontaneously and incision rarely is necessary. However, abscess formation and failure to respond to antibiotics may necessitate surgical intervention with possible epididymo-orchiectomy, especially in elderly, debilitated patients.

Acute **mumps orchitis** is discussed in Ch. 191.

Urethral stricture and **diverticulum** may be accompanied by abscess formation and extravasation of urine into the scrotum and perineum. Urinary diversion by suprapubic cystotomy, incision and drainage, and antibiotics are indicated. Persistent strictures are treated with open or endoscopic surgery.

Hydrocele is a common intrinsic scrotal mass. It results from excessive accumulation of sterile fluid within the tunica vaginalis due to overproduction (inflammation of the testis and its appendages) or diminished resorption (lymphatic or venous obstruction in the cord or retroperitoneal space). Congenital hydrocele is discussed in Ch. 187. Treatment of persistent, symptomatic hydrocele is surgical. Aspiration is only a temporary measure and may introduce secondary infection. **Hematocele** is usually secondary to trauma and is an accumulation of blood within the tunica vaginalis. Unlike hydrocele, it does not transilluminate. Treatment is surgical, if the hematocele is large and does not absorb with conservative management or is associated with laceration of the tunica albuginea of the testis. **Spermatocele (spermatic cyst)** occurs adjacent to the epididymis and usually contains sperm. When it is large, differentiating it from a hydrocele may be difficult, since each will transilluminate and is cystic and painless. Spermatocele, usually occurring at the upper pole of the testis adjacent to the epididymis, may suggest a "third testis." Surgical excision is indicated if the cyst becomes large and symptomatic.

Inguinal hernia, direct or indirect, may extend into the scrotal compartment. Hernia must be differentiated from hydrocele or hematocele. In the former, the examiner cannot palpate the cord above the mass, while with a hydrocele and hematocele, normal cord structures are usually palpable above the mass. Surgical repair of inguinal hernia is recommended because of the probability of progression and possibilities of incarceration and strangulation.

Testicular torsion: See Ch. 187, and MANAGEMENT OF THE NORMAL NEWBORN in Ch. 182.

Testis tumors: See Ch. 163.

Varicocele is a collection of large veins, usually occurring in the left scrotum and feeling like a "bag of worms." It is present in the upright position and should empty in the supine position. Surgical correction may be indicated in treating infertility, or if the varicocele is symptomatic (eg, producing pain or a feeling of scrotal fullness).

Lymphedema of the scrotum may result from abdominal venous compression, an intra-abdominal tumor, cirrhosis with ascites, filariasis, or Milroy's disease (idio-

pathic lymphedema). Treatment is with a scrotal suspensory, though resection and scrotoplasty may be necessary.

162. GENITOURINARY TRAUMA

Trauma to the GU tract may be caused by penetrating or perforating wounds, blunt crushing injuries, surgery, instrumentation, or irradiation. Hematuria, oliguria, pain, and anuria are the principal manifestations. Localized tenderness, swelling, and ecchymosis may be present; shock may develop. Prompt diagnosis and treatment can be lifesaving and are essential to preserve renal function and micturition.

Kidney

Blunt external force is the usual cause of traumatic injury to the kidneys. Penetrating or perforating injuries can result from gunshot or stab wounds. Damage varies widely: contusion may cause massive hematuria without anatomic defect; laceration may be capsular and/or parenchymal; fragmentation or "shattered kidney" may cause massive bleeding and extravasation of urine; laceration or complete disruption of the renal pedicle (artery or vein) may result in shock and sudden death. Intravenous urography **(IVU)** with tomography usually establishes a diagnosis, but computed tomography **(CT)** with IVU gives the most information and should be considered for more serious injuries. Retrograde pyelography is seldom required. Arteriography may be used when there is nonvisualization on IVU or when a major injury is suspected, which could require surgical intervention.

Therapy begins with whole blood or blood substitutes to prevent or control shock. Maintenance of BP and establishment of urinary flow also facilitate accurate radiographic diagnosis. Conservative management with bed rest will suffice in many cases. However, severe injuries resulting in uncontrolled bleeding or excessive urine extravasation can require surgical intervention or arterial embolization under radiologic control. **Prognosis** is good with prompt diagnosis and appropriate management. Renal hypertension may be a late consequence of renal injury with segmental ischemia or infarction and subsequent scarring, or may be due to perinephric fibrosis.

Ureter

Most ureteral injuries are due to pelvic surgery (radical urologic, gynecologic, or colonic procedures) and are frequently unrecognized until oliguria, pain, fever, anuria, or a fistula appears. Ureteral injury from external trauma is uncommon but may occur secondary to penetrating trauma. Blunt injuries, particularly with extreme hyperextension of the trunk, may rarely cause avulsion of the ureter at the renal pelvis or at the pelvic brim. Diagnostic measures should include IVU with tomography and, in some instances, retrograde pyelography. Percutaneous nephrostomy with antegrade pyelography can be valuable for diagnosis and therapy.

Treatment: Prompt recognition of injury caused by suture ligation of the ureter may result in satisfactory surgical correction. Postsurgical obstruction or urinary fistula may require temporary urinary diversion (nephrostomy, proximal ureterostomy) or primary repair (ureteroureterostomy, ureteroneocystostomy, or transureteroureterostomy). Ureteral catheterization and prolonged ureteral catheter stenting (3 to 6 wk) may dilate a stricture or allow a fistula to close. Penetrating knife or gunshot injuries usually require prompt surgical intervention.

Bladder

Rupture of the overdistended bladder is common with crushing external trauma as can occur in automobile accidents, and is usually associated with pelvic fracture. Rupture can be intra- or extraperitoneal. The principal presenting signs are oliguria, hema-

turia, or anuria. Diagnosis may be established by cystography with sterile contrast materials, which will also identify extravasation of urine. Displacement of the bladder as noted radiographically may or may not indicate rupture, since extravesical bleeding into the paravesical space may cause massive distortion (a "tear-drop bladder" configuration due to extrinsic compression).

Treatment for minor lacerations may only require catheter drainage for 7 to 10 days. With more severe injuries, treatment usually consists of prompt exploration, repair of lacerations, and establishment of urinary drainage, preferably with both suprapubic and urethral catheters.

Urethra

Common causes of urethral injury include pelvic fracture with shearing tears (usually at the prostatomembranous junction), perineal straddle injuries, and traumatic urethral instrumentation. Anuria with suprapubic, scrotal, or perineal extravasation of fluid may be presenting signs. Diagnosis is established by retrograde urethrogram. Cystourethrography defines the location and extent of injury.

Treatment: Minor urethral injuries require careful insertion of a catheter and stenting for a few days. More severe injuries require surgical repair. Suprapubic bladder catheter drainage should be established, and in many instances, urethral surgery may be deferred and done electively. Urethral stricture at the site of injury is a frequent long-term complication, demanding subsequent urethral dilation, endoscopic urethrotomy, or secondary surgical repair. Impotence is a possible complication of severe proximal urethral injury in males.

External Male Genitalia

While penetrating and perforating injuries of the penis or scrotum and its contents can occur, the severe injuries are from crushing blows and avulsion of the skin or genitalia. Avulsion injuries happen; eg, among industrial and farm workers when clothing is caught in machinery. Penile injuries occur secondary to a variety of devices such as penile rings and vacuum cleaner attachments, or to excessive trauma during intercourse, masturbation, or fellatio. Testicular trauma usually is secondary to physical combat such as a kick.

Treatment: Avulsed skin should be conserved, cooled, and reapplied as quickly as possible. Debridement should be conservative. Skin grafting may be necessary. When the entire scrotum is avulsed, the testes are buried, if possible, under the skin of the thigh or the lower abdomen, in hope of retaining spermatogenesis and hormonal function. Complete traumatic avulsion of the penis is uncommon. Gunshot wounds and other penetrating injuries require debridement and drainage. Hematomas and hematoceles may result from external trauma to the scrotum and are usually managed conservatively, while rupture of the tunica albuginea of the testis may require prompt surgical exploration and repair.

---

163. NEOPLASMS

(See also Ch. 105)

GU neoplasms occur at any age and in both sexes. They account for approximately 30% of cancer in the male and 4% in the female.

KIDNEY

TUBULOINTERSTITIAL DISEASE IN MALIGNANCY

Renal parenchyma may be invaded by proliferative malignant cells in leukemia and lymphosarcoma. The kidneys are enlarged, often asymmetrically. Intravenous urog-

raphy (**IVU**) reveals elongation and narrowing of the calyces due to this diffuse infiltration. Despite the extensive interstitial involvement, functional changes are minimal. Proteinuria is absent or insignificant and there is rarely a rise in the blood urea or creatinine levels unless some other complication occurs, such as uric acid nephropathy, hypercalcemia, or bacterial infection.

CARCINOMA OF THE KIDNEY
(Hypernephroma)

Adenocarcinoma of the kidney accounts for approximately 1 to 2% of adult cancers. The male-to-female ratio is estimated at 2:1. Most solid kidney tumors are malignant.

Symptoms, Signs, and Diagnosis

Hematuria, gross or microscopic, is the most common presenting sign, followed by flank pain, palpable mass, and FUO. Hypertension due to segmental ischemia or pedicle compression, and polycythemia secondary to increased erythropoietin activity also are seen in some cases.

Increasingly, renal cell carcinoma is being incidentally detected as a result of the increased use of abdominal ultrasound and CT scans. Occasionally, a kidney cancer is suspected in the interpretation of a radioisotope bone or renal perfusion scan. IVU confirms the presence of a mass, and CT scan offers information regarding the density of the mass, local extension, and nodal and venous involvement. Inferior venacavography offers more information regarding renal vein and vena cava extension and is especially valuable in staging right kidney lesions. Aortography and selective renal artery angiography may be required to define the nature of a kidney tumor as well as to provide a more accurate description of the number of renal arteries present and the vascular pattern in preparation for surgical intervention. A chest film is essential, since pulmonary metastases occur frequently. Preoperative staging is quite accurate, allowing for more definitive therapeutic planning.

Prognosis and Treatment

Transabdominal radical nephrectomy with removal of regional nodes offers a reasonable chance for cure in localized disease. Tumor involvement of the renal vein and even the vena cava, without distant metastases, still is a surgically curable stage of the disease. Metastatic renal carcinoma has a poor prognosis, since the tumor is radioresistant and chemotherapeutic agents, singly or in combination, are ineffective. Spontaneous regression of metastatic lesions following nephrectomy is rare. Treatment with progestational agents has not significantly improved survival. The role of immunotherapy is being investigated.

RENAL PELVIS AND URETER

Malignancies of the renal pelvis and calyces and ureter are histologically similar (usually transitional cell in character, but occasionally squamous cell). Hematuria is the principal presenting sign, and colicky pain may accompany obstruction. Diagnosis is established by finding a negative filling defect on IVU or retrograde pyelography. CT may aid in staging and can help in differentiating a nonopaque stone from a tumor or clot. Cytology may be helpful. **Treatment** usually is radical nephroureterectomy, including a cuff of bladder. Occasionally, local excision of a ureteral lesion is indicated (eg, decreased renal function, solitary kidney). **Prognosis** in operable, localized lesions is good. Periodic follow-up cystoscopies are indicated, since tumors tend to occur in the urinary bladder and may be treated by transurethral resection if detected in an early stage.

URINARY BLADDER

Etiology and Incidence

Known urinary carcinogens include β-naphthylamine, *p*-aminodiphenyl (aniline dyes), certain chemical intermediates in the manufacture of rubber, tryptophan metabolites, and, possibly, excretory products of tobacco tars. Chronic irritation as seen in schistosomiasis and with bladder calculi predisposes to bladder cancer. The incidence of bladder malignancies in men vs. women is about 3:1, and there are approximately 40,500 new cases/year (1986 estimate).

Pathology

Transitional cell carcinoma is the most common type. Squamous cell carcinoma is seen less frequently and usually is associated with parasitic infestation or chronic irritation of the mucosa. Adenocarcinoma also may occur as a primary tumor, but spread from a bowel carcinoma should be ruled out. Transitional cell carcinoma may present as a well-differentiated, superficial papillary tumor or as a highly invasive, poorly differentiated neoplasm with a spectrum between these characteristics. Squamous cell carcinoma of the bladder usually is highly infiltrative and has a poor prognosis.

Symptoms, Signs, and Diagnosis

Hematuria, pyuria, dysuria, burning, and frequency are the most common presenting symptoms. Pain occurs with invasion, infection, or fixation. A mass may be palpable on bimanual examination. Microhematuria may be the earliest sign of bladder carcinoma.

Filling defects of the bladder by cystogram or in the cystographic phase of the IVU suggest vesical neoplasm. Urinary cytologies are frequently positive for tumor cells. Diagnosis is by cystoscopy and transurethral resectional biopsy. Bimanual examination under anesthesia aids in staging the disease. Pelvic CT scan, ultrasound, and MRI may also be of value in staging.

Prognosis and Treatment

Malignancies that are superficial or invade only the most superficial portion of the bladder musculature respond to endoscopic therapy, but recurrence at the same or another site in the bladder is relatively common. Deeply invasive lesions of the bladder musculature respond poorly. Bladder malignancies that have metastasized are usually incurable, though cystectomy and urinary diversion may prolong life and be palliative.

Superficial and early lesions may be treated effectively by transurethral resection, but the incidence of recurrence is high. Tumors that invade the bladder wall in depth usually are treated by partial, total, or radical cystectomy, the latter methods necessitating concomitant urinary diversion. Preoperative irradiation may be effective in retarding tumor growth. Combined use of radiation therapy and surgery seems to yield the best results. Radiation therapy alone may be curative in some instances. Systemic chemotherapy is not effective. Certain selected superficial growths may be treated by repeated bladder instillations of chemotherapeutic agents such as thiotepa, mitomycin C, or doxorubicin. BCG instillation therapy has also proved to be effective in controlling superficial bladder carcinoma.

PROSTATE

Adenocarcinoma of the prostate accounts for a significant number of malignancies in men over age 50, and the incidence increases with each decade. There are approximately 90,000 new cases a year in the USA. The etiology is unknown, but appears to be hormone-related. Sarcoma of the prostate is rare, occurring primarily in children. Undifferentiated prostatic carcinoma, squamous cell carcinoma, and ductal transi-

tional carcinoma of the prostate also occur and are less responsive to the usual measures of control.

Pathology

The usual prostatic malignancy is glandular, not unlike the histologic configuration of normal prostate. Large nucleoli, mitoses, stromal invasion, and involvement of perineural lymphatics are the principal histologic criteria of diagnosis.

Symptoms and Signs

Prostatic carcinoma generally is slowly progressive, and may cause no symptoms. Late in the course of the disease, symptoms of bladder outlet obstruction, ureteral obstruction, hematuria, and pyuria may appear. Metastases to the pelvis, ribs, and vertebral bodies may cause bone pain. Stony hard induration or a nodule of the prostate palpated on rectal examination suggests prostatic malignancy and must be distinguished from granulomatous prostatitis, prostatic TB, prostatic calculi, and other more unusual prostatic diseases. The firm and nodular, irregular prostate is pathognomonic of prostatic carcinoma, and later exhibits extension of induration and fixation of the gland laterally and to the seminal vesicles.

Diagnosis

Prostatic carcinoma must be suspected on the basis of rectal findings. A solitary firm prostatic nodule or more extensive involvement may be diagnosed by transrectal or transperineal needle biopsy. Early incidental histologic diagnoses may occur when malignant changes are found in a specimen removed for benign prostatic hypertrophy. An **elevated serum acid phosphatase** indicates local extension or metastases. Other diseases causing elevation of this enzyme are benign prostatic hyperplasia (slight elevation following vigorous prostatic massage), multiple myeloma, Gaucher's disease, and hemolytic anemia. Radioimmunoassay methods for determination of prostatic acid phosphatase may give added information regarding the detection of localized prostatic carcinoma as well as later stages of the disease. The acid phosphatase level declines after successful treatment and rises again with recurrence.

Prostatic carcinoma frequently produces osteoblastic bony metastases. Their detection on bone scan or by radiographic imaging in the presence of a stony hard prostate is usually diagnostic.

Prognosis

Ten-year cure rates approaching 65% occur with localized prostatic carcinoma treated by radical prostatectomy or radiation therapy. Prostatic malignancies not amenable to radical surgery or radiation therapy may respond for several years to adequate hormonal control and/or orchiectomy. This is particularly true in older men and when the carcinoma is well differentiated. The presence of metastases at the time of initial diagnosis obviously worsens the prognosis, but therapy may yield significant long-term palliation without cure.

Treatment

Localized prostatic carcinoma may be cured by radical retropubic prostatectomy or radiation therapy. Extensive local disease, age or general health of the patient, or the presence of metastases may preclude cure by these modalities. In these situations, palliation may result from hormone control therapy, irradiation, or bilateral orchiectomy. Oral diethylstilbestrol 1 to 3 mg/day usually provides adequate control of disease for prolonged periods. Long-term high-dose oral estrogen therapy may result in thromboembolic complications. Short-term, high-dose IV diethylstilbestrol diphosphate may provide dramatic symptomatic relief in a few days. Other forms of treatment used to decrease testosterone levels and provide palliation include cyproterone acetate, flutamide, ketoconazole, aminoglutethimide, and analogs of luteinizing hormone-releasing hormone. Bilateral orchiectomy may be performed for advanced

disease when first recognized or after hormone therapy has been tried. Local radiation therapy may provide relief of pain due to bony metastases refractory to other treatment and also may be effective in controlling local disease in the prostatic area. Chemotherapy after hormone failure has not been effective.

URETHRA

Carcinoma of the urethra is rare. It occurs in both males and females and may be a squamous or transitional cell tumor, or occasionally adenocarcinoma. Hematuria and a local mass are the presenting symptoms. Obstructive symptoms may be present. Friable and bleeding masses presenting at the external urethral meatus in the female must be suspect. Differentiation between carcinoma of the urethra, urethral prolapse, and urethral caruncle may require biopsy. In the male, a history of urethral stricture is common. Irradiation and radical surgery are equally effective, although the prognosis remains guarded.

PENIS

Carcinoma of the penis is more common in uncircumcised males who practice poor local hygiene. The usual lesion, arising in the region of the corona or beneath the foreskin, is epidermoid, extending locally and metastasizing relatively late. Metastases are via the penile lymphatics to the superficial and deep inguinal nodes, often necessitating total or partial penectomy with associated inguinal lymphadenectomy. Penile carcinomas are usually refractory to radiation, and chemotherapy is rarely effective. Partial penectomy may be curative in early lesions, with a penile stump that is satisfactory for urination and sexual activity.

TESTIS

The origin and nature of scrotal masses must be accurately determined, since most growths arising within the testis are malignant, while extratesticular scrotal masses usually are benign.

Etiology and Incidence

Etiology is unknown. Testicular tumors account for the majority of solid malignancies in males < 30 yr. Cryptorchid testes have been variously reported to be affected by malignancy between 2.5 to 20 times as often as descended testes. This seems to be true even if the cryptorchid testis has been brought down surgically.

Pathology

Most malignant testicular tumors arise from the primordial germ cell and are classified as seminoma, teratoma, embryonal carcinoma, teratocarcinoma, and choriocarcinoma, in order of increasing malignancy. Functional interstitial cell carcinomas of the testis are rare. Tumors arising in the testicular appendages and the cord usually are benign fibromas, fibroadenomas, adenomatoid tumors, and lipomas, although sarcomas occasionally may occur.

Symptoms and Signs

The usual presenting sign in testicular tumor is a scrotal mass, progressively increasing in size and sometimes associated with pain. Many patients relate the mass to minor trauma, indicating the time when the mass was first discovered. Hemorrhage into a rapidly expanding tumor may produce exquisite local pain and tenderness. A firm mass arising from the testis is cause for immediate clinical suspicion of testicular tumor.

Diagnosis

Physical examination and ultrasound may localize the lesion to the testis. The diagnosis is established by exploration, exposing and clamping the cord through an inguinal incision before mobilization of the tumor. Diagnostic studies should include chest x-ray and IVU for direct or indirect evidence of metastases. Radioimmunoassays of α-fetoprotein and the β subunit of human chorionic gonadotropin are reliable markers indicating the presence of tumor and are valuable in follow-up of patients with proven testicular tumors, especially of the nonseminomatous types. Abdominal CT scans are important in the staging process, and pedal lymphangiography may offer additional information in staging of seminoma.

Prognosis

This depends on the histology and extent of the malignancy. Five-year survival rates > 80% are seen with seminomas localized to the testis or even metastatic to the retroperineum. The 5-yr survival rate with highly malignant rarer choriocarcinomas is very low. Other tumors range between these extremes.

Treatment

Inguinal orchiectomy must be performed. Transabdominal retroperitoneal lymph node dissection usually is recommended for terato- and embryonal carcinoma and adult teratoma. Irradiation may be effective in seminoma, using 3000 to 5000 R to the abdominal and mediastinal lymphatics as well as the left supraclavicular area, depending on staging. Chemotherapy with cisplatin in combination with other agents may cause regression and control of metastatic, nonseminomatous testicular tumors but is highly toxic. Cure is still possible in the presence of metastatic disease for both seminoma and nonseminomatous primaries (see also under ANTINEOPLASTIC CHEMOTHERAPY in Ch. 105).

§14. SEXUALLY RELATED DISORDERS

164. SEXUALLY TRANSMITTED DISEASES

(See Ch. 14)

165. DISORDERS OF SEXUAL FUNCTION

INTRODUCTION

Psychosexual disorders have been classified in Ch. 139, which discusses gender identity, the paraphilias, and homosexuality, although the latter is not considered a disorder per se. Sexual dysfunction, the most common of the psychosexual disorders encountered by the practicing physician, is discussed here.

Proper sexual functioning in men and women depends on an anticipatory mental "set" (the sexual motive state) or state of *desire,* effective vasocongestive *arousal* (erection in the male, lubrication in the female), and *orgasm*. Orgasm in the male includes emission and ejaculation. Emission produces a sensation of ejaculatory inevitability and is mediated by contractions of the prostate, seminal vesicles, and urethra. Orgasm in the female is accompanied by contractions, not always subjectively experienced as such, of the muscles that line the wall of the outer third of the vagina. In both sexes, generalized muscular tension, perineal contractions, and involuntary pelvic thrusting usually occur. Orgasm is followed by *resolution,* a sense of general relaxation, well-being, and muscular relaxation. During this phase men are physiologically refractory to further erection and orgasm for a period of time. In contrast, women may be able to respond to additional stimulation almost immediately.

The sexual response cycle is mediated by a delicate (or balanced) interplay between the sympathetic and parasympathetic nervous systems. Vasocongestion is largely mediated by parasympathetic outflow, whereas orgasm is predominantly sympathetic. Ejaculation is almost entirely sympathetic, whereas emission involves a much more

finely balanced combination of sympathetic and parasympathetic stimulation. All these reflex responses are easily inhibited by cortical influences or by impaired hormonal, neural, or vascular mechanisms. Alpha- and beta-adrenergic blocking agents may desynchronize emission, ejaculation, and the perineal muscle contractions occurring during orgasm.

The American Psychiatric Association's *Diagnostic and Statistical Manual of Mental Disorders*, Third Edition **(DSM-III)** states that **inhibitions in the response cycle** may occur at one or more of the sexual response phases, although inhibition in the resolution phase rarely is clinically significant. Generally, both the *subjective* dimensions of desire, arousal, and pleasure and the *objective* performance, vasocongestion, and orgasm are disturbed, although either component occasionally may occur alone.

All of the dysfunctions may be **primary** (lifelong, with effective performance never having been experienced in any situation, and generally due to intrapsychic conflicts) or **secondary** (acquired after a period of normal function); generalized, or limited to certain situations or with certain partners; and total or partial (degree or frequency of disturbance). Most patients complain of anxiety, guilt, shame, and frustration, and many develop somatic symptoms. Although dysfunction usually occurs during sexual activity with a partner, it is useful to inquire about function during masturbation.

Etiologic factors for both primary and secondary dysfunction can be similar. Poor communication is always present. **Psychologic factors** include *anger* directed toward the partner; *fear* of the partner's genitals, or of intimacy, losing control, dependency, or pregnancy; *guilt* following a pleasurable experience; *depression;* and *anxiety* created by marital discord, stressful life situations, aging, ignorance of behavioral norms (eg, frequency and duration of intercourse, oral-genital sex, or sexual practices), or sexual myths (eg, the assumed deleterious effects of masturbation, hysterectomy, or menopause). The so-called **"immediate" causes** of anxiety are the fear of failure, demand for performance, spectatoring (observing one's physical responses), an excessive wish to please the partner, and avoidance of sex and of talking about sexual concerns. These exacerbating factors additionally impair performance and satisfaction, and the consequent further avoidance of sexual activity with impaired communication creates a vicious circle.

Other related inhibitory factors include ignorance (often the consequence of inhibited learning, itself based on anxiety, shame, or guilt) of the sex organs and their function; traumatic events in childhood or adolescence (eg, incest or rape); feelings of inadequacy; religious training; excessive modesty; and puritanical aversion to intercourse.

Interpersonal and situational causes include marital discord and boredom in the relationship, and may be related to place, time, or a particular partner.

Physical factors are discussed under the individual disorders below. Even when these factors are identified, secondary psychogenic elements are almost always present and complicating.

INHIBITED SEXUAL DESIRE (ISD)

This disorder is defined by DSM-III as *persistent and pervasive inhibition of sexual desire in a woman or a man.*

Etiology

Sexual desire is a psychosomatic process based on brain activity (the "generator" or "motor" running in a rheostatic cyclic fashion) and cognitive scripting that includes sexual aspiration and motivation. Desynchronization of these components results in inhibited sexual desire **(ISD).** Acquired ISD is commonly caused by boredom in the relationship; depression (which leads more often to decreased interest in sex than it

does to impotence in the male or inhibited excitement in the female); psychoactive drugs; antihypertensive medication; and hormonal deficiencies. ISD also can be secondary to impaired sexual function. Lifelong generalized inhibitions of sexual desire are related to traumatic events in childhood or adolescence, the suppression of sexual fantasies, or, occasionally, low levels of androgens. Generally, testosterone levels < 300 ng/dL in the male and < 10 ng/dL in the female are considered potential causes.

Clinical Manifestations

The patient complains of a lack of interest in sex, even in ordinarily erotic situations. The disorder usually is associated with infrequent sexual activity, often causing serious marital conflict. Some patients, however, have sexual encounters fairly often to please their partners and may not show any difficulty with performance but continue to have sexual apathy. When boredom is the cause, frequency of sex with the usual partner decreases, but sexual desire may be normal or even intense with others (real or fantasized). A generalized anhedonia (see below) may be present.

SEXUAL DYSFUNCTION IN THE MALE

INHIBITED SEXUAL EXCITEMENT
(Erectile Dysfunction; Impotence)

Inability to attain or sustain an erection satisfactory for normal coitus. The dysfunction may be primary, which is rare and, if not organic, generally indicates severe psychopathology; or it may be secondary, in which erectile dysfunction prohibits completion of successful sexual intercourse in about 25% (or more) of opportunities.

Etiology

Primary erectile dysfunction is almost always due to intrapsychic factors. In rare cases, biogenic factors, usually associated with low testosterone levels and reflecting disorders of the hypothalamic-pituitary-gonadal axis, provide the major etiology. Occasionally, vascular abnormalities are found. Intrapsychic factors include an abnormal fear of the vagina, sexual guilt, fear of intimacy, or depression. Of the **secondary** cases, about 70% are caused by psychic factors. A transient episode of erectile dysfunction for any reason may be followed by secondary psychologic factors labeled "immediate" causes (see above).

Erectile dysfunction may be situational, involving place, time, a particular partner, some perceived competitive defeat, or damage to self-esteem.

Physical factors include systemic diseases (eg, diabetes mellitus [the most common], syphilis, alcoholism, drug dependency, hypopituitarism, and hypothyroidism); local disorders (eg, congenital abnormalities and inflammatory diseases of the genitalia); vascular disturbances such as aortic aneurysm and Leriche's syndrome; neurogenic disorders (eg, multiple sclerosis, spinal cord lesions, pituitary microadenoma with hyperprolactinemia, and cardiovascular accident); drugs such as hypertensives, sedatives, tranquilizers, and amphetamines; and surgical procedures such as sympathectomy. Prostatectomy and castration produce varying effects. Impotence is usually not produced after transurethral prostatectomy, whereas it almost always occurs after perineal prostatectomy. However, retrograde ejaculation is produced in the vast majority of men, irrespective of the type of prostatectomy.

Aging is not an inevitable cause of impotence, even into the 70s or 80s. While the amount and force of the ejaculate and thus sexual tension and the need to ejaculate are decreased, the capacity for erection often is retained.

Diagnosis

Psychic factors are implicated if the patient has situational impotence, has morning erections, or can achieve a firm erection with masturbation. Since a combination of

physical and psychic factors is possible, it must be determined whether the psychic factors are primary or secondary. Inability to have an erection under any circumstances requires a search for organic causes. Procedures include general medical evaluation, including history of drugs and alcohol, examination of the genitalia, neurologic evaluation, search for signs of vascular or endocrine dysfunction, and laboratory procedures including a glucose tolerance test and testosterone, luteinizing hormone **(LH)**, follicle-stimulating hormone, and prolactin levels (taken at 9 AM to avoid diurnal variations).

Particularly important in evaluating cases in which the etiology is uncertain is the examination for nocturnal penile tumescence **(NPT)**. Episodes of NPT accompany rapid-eye-movement **(REM)** sleep. Absence of erections during sleep strongly suggests, but does not prove, an organic basis. The patient can be monitored for nighttime erections in a special sleep laboratory. The number of erections, the duration of each erection, and the amount of penile vasocongestion during the course of a night's sleep can be evaluated to devise a quantitative estimate of erectile capacity. It is important to correct for artifacts by correlating erections with REM sleep and, usually, by direct observation.

Treatment

Psychic erectile dysfunction may respond to brief counseling to alleviate secondary factors. Every effort should be made to include the patient's partner. Reassurance following a careful physical examination and any necessary laboratory studies is a key first step. Education to dispel myths and misinformation and to help establish a nondemanding and mutually pleasurable situation may be sufficient. A specific technic is the 3-stage sensate focus method of Masters and Johnson, involving stepwise nongenital pleasuring, genital pleasuring, and nondemanding coitus. If about 6 counseling sessions do not bring results, referral to a sex therapist should be considered.

If physical abnormalities are found, therapy is directed toward alleviating the underlying disorder. If androgen levels are low (< 300 ng/dL), treatment with injectable testosterone 200 mg IM every 2 wk for 3 to 4 mo should be tried. (First, however, prolactin, FSH, and LH levels should be ascertained, since hyperprolactinemia can be successfully treated with bromocryptine.) Subcutaneous testosterone pellets are favored by some. There is often a short-lived positive placebo response to the administration of oral testosterone. Testosterone seems to increase sexual desire, especially spontaneous fantasies.

INHIBITION OF ORGASTIC CONTROL

(Premature Ejaculation)

The constant failure to maintain intromission of sufficient duration to satisfy a responsive partner. Because specific criteria vary, it may also be defined as *ejaculation occurring before the individual wishes.* Since normal biologic response is to ejaculate within 2 min after vaginal penetration and since few women are able to reach orgasm within 2 min, most men must learn how to retard emission and ejaculation.

Etiology and Diagnosis

In the adolescent, premature ejaculation is common. It may be aggravated by a feeling of sinfulness about sex or by a fear of discovery, of impregnating the girl, or of getting a sexually transmitted disease, as well as by anxiety over performance. In the adult similar concerns may persist, as well as interpersonal factors. Occult somatic factors are rare, although prostatitis or diseases affecting the neural pathways may be involved.

Treatment

Sometimes an explanation of the mechanism of premature ejaculation, reassurance, and simple advice are curative. Increasing the number of opportunities for ejaculation may decrease sexual tension. The "stop-and-start" technic involves stimulation of the penis either manually or during intercourse until the patient begins to recognize that he will soon ejaculate unless stimulation ceases. He signals his partner to cease stimulation, and stimulation is resumed after about 20 or 30 seconds. The partners rehearse this technic at first with manual stimulation, and later during coitus, stopping 3 times; with the 4th stimulation, they permit ejaculation to occur. With repetition, the patient learns ejaculatory control (for 5 or 10 min or even longer) in over 95% of the cases. Occasionally premature ejaculation masks deep-seated intrapsychic or interpersonal conflict and the patient may have to be referred for individual psychotherapy or marital therapy.

INHIBITED ORGASM
(Retarded Ejaculation)

A relatively rare phenomenon in which intravaginal ejaculation does not occur or, more rarely, there is *inability to masturbate to ejaculation.* The etiology usually is psychologic, but diabetes mellitus, thioridazine and mesoridazine (piperidyl variants of the phenothiazines), or some antihypertensive drugs may impair ejaculation. In some spinal cord diseases (eg, multiple sclerosis), erection but not ejaculation may be possible. Retarded ejaculation must be distinguished from the retrograde ejaculation that almost inevitably follows prostatectomy. Some drugs (amoxapine, desipramine, imipramine, and protriptyline) or neurologic disorders (eg, multiple sclerosis) can produce retrograde ejaculation or, rarely, emission without ejaculation.

Treatment: The partner stimulates the patient to ejaculation outside the vagina, then at the lips of the vagina, and finally inside the vagina. Psychotherapy is indicated if this behavioral technic fails.

SEXUAL ANHEDONIA

Rarely, a patient experiences *erection and ejaculation with no pleasure during orgasm.* The cause is psychogenic penile anesthesia in either a hysterical or obsessive person. Psychiatric consultation is indicated unless there is evidence of spinal cord damage or peripheral neuropathy. Loss of tactile sensation over the penis is unlikely to be neurogenic unless there are also anesthetic areas around the anus or scrotum.

SEXUAL DYSFUNCTION IN THE FEMALE

INHIBITED SEXUAL EXCITEMENT
("Frigidity")

DSM-III defines this disorder as *recurrent and persistent inhibition of sexual excitement during sexual activity, manifested by partial or complete failure to attain or maintain the lubrication–swelling response of sexual excitement until completion of the sexual act.* This inhibition occurs despite what the clinician judges to have been adequate sexual stimulation in focus, intensity, and duration. The disorder may be primary or, more frequently, secondary, and restricted to the partner.

Etiology

Psychic, acquired factors cause most cases; eg, inadequate sexual stimulation by the partner, marital discord (about 80% of cases), depression, and stressful life situations

(see also INTRODUCTON, above). Ignorance of genital anatomy and function is common, particularly of clitoral function and of effective arousal patterns and technics. Lifelong causes, in addition to ignorance, are related to the association of sex with sinfulness, and sexual pleasure with guilt. Fear of intimacy may also play a part.

The physical causes include localized diseases (endometriosis, cystitis, vaginitis), systemic diseases (hypothyroidism, diabetes mellitus—though its impact is greater on men), peripheral or CNS disorders (multiple sclerosis), muscular disorders (muscular dystrophy), drugs (oral contraceptives, antihypertensives, tranquilizers have variable effects), and ablative surgery (hysterectomy, mastectomy, which may have a negative impact on the woman's sexual self-image).

Aging: Although women can be orgasmic throughout their lives, sexual activity often decreases after age 60 because of the relative lack of partners, as well as untreated physiologic changes (eg, atrophy of the vaginal mucosa).

Diagnosis and Treatment

The history and physical examination help to establish (1) whether the origin of the condition is predominantly psychic, physical, or a combination of the 2; and (2) the degree of dysfunction. The physician should comfortably discuss sexual matters and elicit precise data, usually by asking questions that gradually move from the more general areas of concern to those of greater sensitivity. Organic factors are investigated by the physical examination and appropriate laboratory studies.

The patient's complaints are usually directed to the lack of orgasm, although it is not uncommon to hear women say, "I don't get turned on." The discussion of treatment appears in INHIBITED ORGASM, below, since inhibited sexual excitement almost invariably leads to inhibition of orgasm, and the treatment of both disorders is similar.

INHIBITED ORGASM

The essential feature of this disorder as indicated by DSM-III is *inhibition of orgasm following the normal sexual excitement phase during sexual activity that is assessed as adequate in focus, intensity, and duration.* Frequently the patient has both an inhibition of sexual excitement and of orgasm. The disorder may be primary, secondary, or situational. About 10% of women do not attain orgasm through any source of stimulation or in any situation. Most women can attain orgasm with clitoral stimulation, but probably > 50% of women are unable to regularly attain orgasm *during coitus*. When a woman responds to noncoital clitoral stimulation but cannot attain coital orgasm, a thorough sexual evaluation and even a trial of treatment is required to judge whether it represents a normal variation of response or if psychopathology is present.

The **etiology** is similar to that of inhibited sexual excitement. However, if lovemaking is consistently terminated before the aroused woman reaches climax (eg, due to inadequate foreplay, ignorance of clitoral/vaginal anatomy and function, or premature ejaculation), the frustration created may result in resentment or aversion, and dysfunction. Also, women who have no difficulty developing adequate vasocongestion may be fearful of "letting go," especially during intercourse. This may be due to guilt following a pleasurable experience or to the fear of abandoning oneself to a pleasurable situation requiring dependency on the partner. It may also represent a fear of losing control.

Treatment

Organic disorders should be treated. When psychic factors predominate (see in INTRODUCTION, above), counseling to remove the secondary causes is helpful; usually both partners should attend these sessions.

The Masters and Johnson 3-stage sensate focus exercises that involve the couple in stepwise nongenital pleasuring, genital pleasuring, and nondemanding coitus are generally beneficial to women with all levels of sexual inhibition. Less responsive to this

treatment format are those women accustomed to clitoral but not coital orgasms. Individual psychotherapy or group therapy sometimes is useful.

A woman's knowledge of the function of her sexual organs and of her responses is essential. This includes understanding of the best methods of stimulating her clitoris, and of the enhanced vaginal sensations possible by strengthening voluntary control of the **pubococcygeus muscle (PCG).** The PCG, which also controls urine flow, contains the nerve endings that provide pleasurable sensations in the outer third of the vagina. **Kegel's exercises** develop control of the PCG, which is contracted 10 to 15 times tid. In 2 to 3 mo perivaginal muscle tone improves, as does the woman's sense of control.

Women classified as having lifelong inhibition of orgasm (with or without inhibitions of sexual desire or excitement) should be referred to a psychiatrist. In any case, the nonspecialist should limit himself to about 6 counseling sessions, referring complex situations to a sex therapist or a psychiatrist.

DYSPAREUNIA

Painful or difficult coitus.

Etiology

Primary dyspareunia appears during initial attempts at sexual intercourse and is usually introital. The cause may be psychogenic or due to local trauma such as hymenal tears, laceration of the fourchet, or bruising of the urethral meatus. Subsequent to the injury, painful superficial ulcerations may develop. Forceful pressure against a sensitive urethra during coitus may be a factor. Other causes include inadequate lubrication, usually secondary to improper or insufficient loveplay; improper intromission; introital lesions due to inflammatory conditions such as skenitis; infections (eg, abscesses of Bartholin's glands or ducts); inflammation of labial sweat glands; irritation due to the use of improperly fitted or inadequately lubricated prophylactics; allergic reactions to contents of contraceptive foams, jellies, etc; and abnormalities of the female genital tract (eg, congenital septum or a rigid hymen).

Secondary dyspareunia is unrelated to first coitus and often develops years later. Causes include menopausal involution with dryness and thinning of the mucosa, tight perineorrhaphies following an episiotomy or plastic repairs of the vagina, marked retroflection of the uterus with ovaries prolapsed into the cul-de-sac, endometriosis, vaginitis, suburethral diverticulum, and pelvic inflammatory disease. Radiation therapy for treatment of malignancy or sterilization may precipitate an acute onset. For psychogenic causes and related factors, see INTRODUCTION, above.

Diagnosis

Pain during or following coitus is the chief complaint. The location and nature of the pain may be helpful guides to the diagnosis; ie, pain on deep thrusting indicating lesions of the uterus and/or broad ligament. A general and sexual history and a physical and pelvic examination usually uncover the etiology. Local introital lesions and uterine displacements or other pelvic pathology can be detected by examination, for which anesthesia is sometimes required (see VAGINISMUS, below). Inadequate stimulation or psychic inhibition of arousal may result in inadequate vaginal lubrication and cause coital pain.

Prophylaxis

Premarital examination of both partners and a frank explanation of the reproductive organs and their functions and of physiologic and psychologic factors involved in sexual intercourse, and guidance in its technics may prevent problems. Existing lesions or defects should be corrected, if possible. For example, a rigid hymen may be stretched as an office procedure. An anesthetic ointment (eg, 1% lidocaine) should be used before each treatment.

Treatment

Therapy of uncomplicated injuries is simple. Temporary avoidance of intercourse is important. A soothing ointment (eg, 1% dibucaine or 1% lidocaine) may be applied externally, in addition to sitz baths, for the relief of vulval distress. Pain and spasm can usually be prevented by liberal use of a lubricant just before coitus; sometimes a more posterior intromission that avoids pressure on a sensitive urethra may help. For treatment of more severe vaginismus, see below. A local estrogenic preparation is helpful in postmenopausal vaginitis, although to avoid risk of endometrial or breast cancer, oral estrogen in low doses for 20 days followed by a progestin for 8 to 10 days is preferred.

Cysts or abscesses should be excised; inflamed labia must be kept clean and dry; leukorrhea is treated in the usual manner. If the vulva is swollen and painful, a wet dressing of dilute aluminum acetate solution may be applied locally. At times, codeine 30 to 60 mg orally q 4 h and sedation (eg, phenobarbital 15 or 30 mg orally tid) may be indicated. Uterine retroflexion and prolapsed ovaries often can be corrected by a pessary. If trauma to sacrouterine ligaments is caused by an ill-fitting diaphragm, adjustment or elimination of the diaphragm is indicated.

Educational discussions may be needed for both partners (see Prophylaxis, above). However, longstanding cases of dyspareunia and cases in which the underlying psychic factors cannot be uncovered should be referred to a psychiatrist.

VAGINISMUS

Spasm of the vagina, a conditioned contraction of the lower vaginal muscles resulting from a woman's unconscious desire to prevent penetration. Since intromission is often impossible, vaginismus is frequently seen in cases of unconsummated marriage. Some women with vaginismus enjoy clitoral orgasms.

Etiologic factors are similar to those of dyspareunia (see above).

Diagnosis is confirmed by observation of an involuntary vaginal spasm during pelvic examination and, sometimes, by an avoidance reaction by the patient as the examiner approaches. The physical or psychogenic causes are established by history and physical examination. Anesthesia, local or general, may be required to overcome the spasm induced by even the gentlest vaginal inspection. The local injection of 1% xylocaine at the hymenal ring or a pudendal block may help some patients.

Treatment begins with correction of any painful physical disorders (see DYSPAREUNIA, above). If vaginismus then persists, technics to eliminate the vaginal muscle spasm, such as the **graduated dilation technic,** have been successful. With the patient in the lithotomy position, well-lubricated rubber or glass dilators in graduated sizes starting with a wire-thin one, are introduced into the vagina and allowed to remain in place for 10 min. A variation preferred by some is to use Young's rectal dilators because they are shorter than the vaginal ones and will cause less discomfort. A good practice, with usually less resistance on the patient's part, is to have the patient herself place the dilators in the vagina. It is helpful if the patient employs the Kegel exercises while the dilator is in place. By contracting her perivaginal muscles as long as she can and then relaxing them, while paying attention to the sensation when she lets go, she develops a sense of mastery over her vaginal muscles. It is also useful to have the patient place one hand on her inner thigh and ask her to contract and relax those muscles. That generally relaxes both thighs and, in the process, her perivaginal muscles. The procedure should be carried out by the physician at least 3 times/wk, and self-insertion with her fingers practiced by the patient at home bid.

Intercourse is attempted after the patient has tolerated insertion of the larger dilators without discomfort (with the rectal dilators, usually No. 5). This procedure must be accompanied by educational counseling (see Prophylaxis for DYSPAREUNIA, above). It is often helpful, prior to the institution of the technic of graduated dilation, to perform a sexologic examination. In the presence of the husband, the physician points

out the anatomic parts to the patient, letting her examine herself with the aid of a hand mirror. This often allays anxiety in both partners and encourages communication about sexual matters.

166. INFERTILITY

Failure to achieve conception by couples who have not used contraception for at least 1 yr.

Infertility affects about 15% of married couples in the USA. Although its etiology often is multiple, causes can be identified in 90% of cases. Of these, appropriate treatment produces pregnancy in about 40% of couples treated. Of 100 subfertile couples, about 40 will show a male factor etiology, 20 a female hormonal defect, 30 a female peritoneal factor, 5 a "hostile" cervical environment; and in about 5, the infertility remains unexplained after a full evaluation. About 30% of cases involve both male and female factors. Psychogenic influences in infertility are poorly understood, since some emotional stress is to be expected. Infertility can strongly affect the self-image, self-esteem, and sexuality of men and women. The impression that adoption increases fertility is unsubstantiated; there is no known somatic basis for psychologically induced infertility.

In counseling, even though one partner appears to have a specific disorder, it is important to remember that the problem is shared by 2 persons; both require support while each patient's ability to initiate or conceive a viable pregnancy is being evaluated and optimized. Because investigation of infertility in women is time-consuming and expensive, prompt evaluation of the male is essential (see also Ch. 203).

INFERTILITY IN MEN

Infertility: *Inability to fertilize the ovum.* **Sterility:** *Lack of sperm production.*

Etiology

Male fertility depends on adequate production of spermatozoa by the testes, unobstructed transit of sperm through the seminal tract, and satisfactory deposition within the vaginal vault. Causes of **impaired spermatogenesis** include certain environmental toxins (eg, radiation, some halogenated hydrocarbons, heat); undescended testis or testes; varicocele; traumatic or infection-related testicular atrophy; drug effects (eg, alcohol abuse, chronic marijuana use, exogenous testosterone); prolonged fever; and any endocrine disorders that affect the hypothalamic-pituitary-gonadal axis (see Chs. 87 and 88). **Antisperm antibodies** are a factor in certain couples with infertility, either in the male or female. **Obstruction of the seminal tract** may result from congenital anomalies, orchitis, epididymitis, vasitis, prostatitis, seminal vesiculitis, urethritis, urethral stricture, or surgical division of the vasa (vasectomy). **Defective delivery of sperm** into the vagina may result from surgery of the bladder neck, prostatectomy, hypospadias, premature ejaculation before intromission, functional or organic impotence, or structural abnormalities of the female genital tract.

Diagnosis

The **history** may suggest childhood cryptorchidism, mumps orchitis, or a sexual problem that precludes proper deposition of sperm. **Physical examination** may reveal structural abnormalities of the external genitalia. Particular attention should be given to the presence of a varicocele. This is best demonstrated by examining the patient in a standing position, using a Valsalva maneuver. Theories as to the pathophysiology of the varicocele include increased intrascrotal and testicular temperatures that may im-

pede sperm formation, or backflow of inhibiting adrenal or renal substances through the spermatic vein system. Testicular measurement and evaluation of testicular consistency are important. Normal testicular size should be 4 to 5 cm in its longest diameter or 20 to 25 cu cm; the consistency should be uniformly firm, not soft or nodular. Prostatitis may be diagnosed by palpation of the prostate gland and by examination of prostatic secretions, which should contain not > 10 WBCs/high-power field on microscopic examination of the smear. General evaluation of male secondary sex characteristics may provide clues to an underlying endocrine disorder.

Evaluation of the ejaculate is not only essential for fertility studies but is increasingly required to establish the effectiveness of vasectomies.

Collection of specimen: A minimum of 2 to 3 specimens should be analyzed before determining ejaculate adequacy. Analysis is best performed after 2 to 3 days of sexual continence, though this is not an absolute prerequisite. The specimen is collected by masturbation or interruption of intercourse, with ejaculation into a clean glass jar. Condoms are not suitable, since they contain chemicals that inactivate spermatozoa. Semen taken from the vagina may be altered by secretions and other vaginal contents. Decreased sperm survival in the cervical mucus may be corroborative evidence for a sperm viability defect as well as a sign of abnormality in the mucus itself. The specimen is analyzed within 2 h of collection and should be kept at room temperature until the motility analysis is completed. The time of the last previous ejaculation is recorded, as is the time of collection of the specimen.

Gross examination: Normally, semen is slightly viscous, opaque or opalescent, and yellowish-white or cream-colored. The usual volume of a specimen is 1 to 5 mL. Volume and sperm density often may be diminished following frequent ejaculations. The specimen should be examined microscopically for pus or blood.

Microscopic examination: For **direct examination,** a small amount of semen is placed on a slide and covered with a cover slip. Normally, > 60% of spermatozoa are motile and demonstrate purposeful forward movement. For **sperm count,** the semen is drawn to the 0.5 mark of a WBC pipette, which is then filled to the 11 mark with distilled water to immobilize the sperm. The pipette is shaken for 45 sec. A hemacytometer counting chamber is filled and the number of spermatozoa in 5 of the small squares is determined. The addition of 6 zeros gives the number of sperm/mL of semen.

Sperm morphology is analyzed by preparing 2 thin smears in the same manner as a thin blood smear. The smears are air-dried and stained with either hematoxylin and eosin or by the standard Papanicolaou technic. Using an oil-immersion objective, 100 sperm are counted and classified according to their shape as being either normal (oval), tapered, amorphous, duplicated, or immature. A count of > 40% abnormal sperm is pathologic.

Minimal requirements for the likelihood of fertilization are generally accepted as an **ejaculate volume** of 1 to 5 mL; a **sperm density** of > 20 million/mL; a sperm **motility** (ie, sperm that are "moving" at time of inspection) of > 60% when examined < 2 h after ejaculation; a qualitative determination of the **type of movement** exhibited by the *majority* of motile sperm, where a score of one equals movement in place only, and 4 equals fast, purposeful forward progression (an average score is > 2); and > 60% **normal morphologic forms.**

Results of semen analysis are recorded in 5 categories: (1) adequate, (2) aspermia, (3) azoospermia, (4) diffuse semen abnormality, or (5) isolated semen defects.

Aspermia, *absence of ejaculate,* is seen with an incompetent bladder neck following bladder neck surgery or with neurogenic dysfunction. Decreased seminal volume is less common and may indicate partial retrograde ejaculation or a hypoandrogenic state. **Azoospermia,** *absence of sperm in the semen,* is associated with primary testicular disorders, complete obstruction of the seminal tract, or an unstimulated hormonal state. Qualitative determination of seminal fructose indicates whether the ejaculatory ducts

are patent. Resorcinol is mixed with the semen and the mixture heated; an orange color indicates the presence of fructose. Cystourethrography and cystourethroscopy may demonstrate stricture, diverticulum, or evidence of inflammatory disease. Seminal vesiculograms and vasograms are accomplished by endoscopic catheterization of the ejaculatory ducts (rare) or by direct injection of contrast medium into the vasa using a microsurgical technic in an effort to define vasal obstruction. Ductile obstruction is confirmed by operative inspection when corrective microsurgery can be attempted. Testicular deficiency may be primary or secondary and these can be differentiated by endocrine, chromosome, and biopsy analyses as described below.

Oligospermia, *lowered sperm density*, often is idiopathic but may be associated with decreased spermatogenesis as seen with a varicocele. A sperm density of < 20 million/mL makes fertility statistically less likely. **Diminished motility and impaired sperm forward progression** are the commonest of the *isolated* abnormal seminal parameters and the earliest abnormality seen with varicoceles. They also may be impaired by a locally infectious process (prostatitis, seminal vesiculitis, urethritis), epididymal disease, or the presence of a sperm-immobilizing or sperm-agglutinating antibody. **Abnormal sperm morphology** as an isolated impairment is rare and most likely denotes a transient nonspecific insult; eg, a viremia.

Antisperm antibodies are best evaluated by antibody testing on either the seminal plasma or the serum. Several technics are used; a common one is the macroagglutination technic (Kibrick method). By using serial dilutions, the level of antisperm antibodies is quantitated.

Disorders to be ruled out include **hypothyroidism** (although rarely seen, it should be tested for when clinically suspected—see Ch. 89); **adrenogenitalism or other functional adrenal disorders** (see Ch. 91), which are excluded by such determinations as radioimmunoassay of cortisol, but are rarely if ever truly significant causes of male infertility; and **hypogonadism** (see Ch. 196), which is assessed by radioimmunoassay of serum gonadotropins (follicle-stimulating hormone; luteinizing hormone) and testosterone. In addition, special studies using the newer stimulatory agents (clomiphene, gonadotropin-releasing hormone) may demonstrate previously missed **abnormalities of the hypothalamic-pituitary-gonadal axis** (see also Chs. 87 and 88). Karyotyping may be of further value if one suspects a **genetic disorder** (suggested by unusual body habitus or severe gonadal dysgenesis—see also INTERSEX STATES in Chs. 187 and 203). Testicular biopsy is indicated in the azoospermic or severely oligospermic individual and may identify hyalinized seminiferous tubules (**Klinefelter's syndrome**—see under THE TESTES in Ch. 196) or inhibition of spermatogenesis. Karyotyping of testicular tissue may reveal a mosaic abnormality.

Treatment

Hypopituitarism and hypothyroidism respond to appropriate endocrine management. Secondary hypogonadism is discussed in THE TESTES in Ch. 196. Empirical treatment for endocrinopathy when a discrete abnormality is *not* found is rarely successful, although clomiphene citrate and human chorionic gonadotropin (HCG) have been suggested.

If poor sperm deposition, indicated by abnormal postcoital tests (see below), is due to hypospadias or penile deformity, corrective surgery or artificial insemination is indicated. Ligation of the internal spermatic vein may be curative in varicocele. Surgical treatment of inflammatory obstruction of the vasa and anastomosis of the proximal vas to the epididymis (epididymovasostomy) may improve passage of spermatozoa. Reconstruction of vasa previously divided by vasectomy, using a microsurgical technic, is technically successful in 80% of such patients.

If retrograde ejaculation is demonstrated, as seen following retroperitoneal procedures or surgery of the bladder neck, epinephrine-like drugs (pseudoephedrine 30 to 60 mg orally qid or imipramine hydrochloride 25 mg orally qid) may be useful.

The oligospermic patient and his wife should be instructed in appropriate technics of sexual activity to ensure optimum frequency of intercourse, timing in relation to the ovulatory cycle, and retention of spermatozoa following ejaculation. Kits are available for home use that can quite accurately determine the time of ovulation. Optimum frequency for the majority of patients is q 48 h; optimum timing is at the time of ovulation (just prior to or concomitant with the temperature elevation seen in women taking daily basal temperatures [see below], or roughly 14 to 15 days preceding the first day of menstruation); and optimum retention of spermatozoa is achieved by the woman's not douching but remaining in bed with the knees slightly bent to better place the cervix in the intravaginal seminal pool.

Artificial insemination: Since sperm and prostatic fluid are emitted before seminal fluid, the first portion of the ejaculate has the greatest density of sperm, and split-ejaculation collection can be useful for insemination when large-volume ejaculates are present. The patient collects the first portion of the ejaculate in a separate container, the physician using this for direct placement on the cervical os; or the couple themselves can mimic this by interrupting intercourse. Artifical insemination of **live** or **frozen donor semen** also can be used to initiate pregnancy in the normal female when other procedures have failed, or for men who are carriers of a genetic disorder.

In vitro fertilization has been used successfully for oligospermic men, men with autoantibodies to sperm, and in some cases where donor semen is used. An alternative procedure, **gamete intrafallopian transfer (GIFT),** can be attempted where sperm production is deficient and the fallopian tubes are patent. GIFT is described in treatment of infertility in women, below. Also see below for psychologic, ethical, and legal considerations in these procedures.

INFERTILITY IN WOMEN

Infertility: *Absence of conception after 1 yr of regular intercourse without use of contraceptives.* **Sterility:** *the inability to ovulate.* Either condition may or may not be reversible.

Etiology and Incidence

Causes of female infertility include disorders of the reproductive organs: ovaries (eg, dysgenesis, infection, polycystic ovary [Stein-Leventhal] syndrome, radiation damage); fallopian tubes (eg, absence, obstruction, salpingitis, endometriosis); uterus (eg, absence, anomalies, tumors, infection); cervix (displacement, cervicitis, stenosis). Vaginitis and sexually transmitted disease may be factors, as may endocrine disorders (eg, pituitary failure, thyroid disturbances, adrenal hyperplasia); systemic diseases (eg, diabetes mellitus); genetic disorders (eg, chromosomal abnormalities, testicular feminization syndrome); or immunologic causes (antisperm antibodies).

Age and race are factors: The risk of infertility among women 35 to 44 yr is double that of women 30 to 34 yr; the risk is 1½ times higher for black women than for white.

Diagnosis

Normal ovarian function first must be established. Ovarian physiology is discussed in Ch. 169; evaluation of abnormal ovarian function is found under AMENORRHEA in Ch. 170. (Conception and implantation are discussed in Ch. 175.) Once it is established that ovulation occurs regularly (by basal body temperature curves, appropriately timed examination of cervical mucus, ovarian ultrasonography, plasma progesterone level, and endometrial biopsy), the reproductive tract should be investigated for functional and anatomic competence to permit union of sperm and ovum in the fallopian tubes.

Basal body temperature curves: Normally, a rise in body temperature of 0.5 C (± 1.0 F) follows ovulation. Charts made by recording waking oral temperatures will show a biphasic curve, with temperatures rising about 14 days before the next menses

is due (suggesting ovulation) and then dropping just before menses. (Sustained elevation over 18 days suggests pregnancy.) If there is any question about ovulation time, **biopsy of the endometrium** can be obtained in the postovulatory secretory phase, usually on the 5th postovulatory day or just before menses. **Plasma progesterone** of 5 mg/mL or above is consistent with ovulation. An inadequate luteal phase, assumed to be due to inadequate progesterone production, may result in failure to maintain the endometrium sufficiently to support a fertilized ovum.

It may be important to use the various tests of ovulation in combination. The **luteinized unruptured follicle (LUF)** may be more common than previously anticipated. In this condition, the ovarian follicle matures and is functional endocrinologically, but may not release the ovum. While the temperature chart and plasma progesterone values may be suggestive of ovulation, it is only with the use of **serial ultrasound examinations (folliculograms)** in addition to basal body temperature charts and/or plasma progesterone that one will be able to ascertain that ovulation has, in fact, not occurred.

The postcoital test is performed on the expected date of ovulation, between 2 and 16 h after intercourse. A specimen of endocervical mucus is inspected for clarity, ferning, elasticity, and the number and activity of spermatozoa. In this way, the adequacy of coital position, intromission, and ejaculate content, as well as of the cervical environment, can be evaluated. Sperm survive in mucus that is abundant, clear, and elastic. The presence of this type of mucus indicates adequate local cervical and ovarian function. While the normalcy of this test as determined by the number of viable sperm seen remains somewhat controversial, certainly > 10 highly active sperm/high-power field should be visualized.

For evaluation of antibodies to sperm, see in INFERTILITY IN MEN, above.

Tubal patency can be readily evaluated by radiographic tests; eg, hysterosalpingography. However, direct visualization by laparoscopy or, occasionally, culdoscopy is extremely important, because this enables one to assess accurately not only tubal patency but also peritubal and peritoneal status. Furthermore, when conditions such as endometriosis or peritubal adhesions are encountered, these can be surgically treated at the time of a diagnostic laparoscopy. Laparoscopic treatments using the carbon dioxide laser and/or cauterization of lesions is becoming increasingly important in the management of female factor infertility.

Uterine factors: The multiple anatomic variations in uterine displacement from the usual anterior position are not considered significant, but congenital anomalies of the uterine cavity or submucous myomas may require treatment.

Treatment

When no identifiable abnormalities are found, reassurance and education of the patient are frequently helpful. Repeatedly poor results after postcoital examinations, despite documented ovulation, make investigation of male factors and coital habits imperative. Anatomic abnormalities of the cervix or hostile mucus resulting from erosions, infections, and other local disorders (eg, sperm antibody production) should be treated specifically. Abnormalities of the uterine cavity such as congenital anomalies and submucous myomas warrant surgery if associated with otherwise unexplained infertility. Tubal occlusion or endometriosis, diagnosed by laparoscopy, often requires surgical correction.

Ovulatory agents such as **clomiphene citrate** and **human menopausal gonadotropin (HMG)** are very useful therapeutic agents for specific causes of anovulation. Clomiphene appears to cause the hypothalamus to discharge the releasing factor, with a resulting increase in follicle-stimulating hormone **(FSH)** and luteinizing hormone **(LH)** and in turn stimulation of ovarian follicular growth. Estrogen from the ovary brings about a surge in LH, which induces ovulation. Repeated courses of the drug are given; beginning on the 5th day after spontaneous or induced bleeding, one 50-mg tablet is

given orally for 5 days. The occurrence of ovulation is determined by graphing the basal body temperature.

HMG, which is obtained from the urine of postmenopausal women and purified to contain approximately 75 IU each of FSH and LH, may be a very useful agent in managing certain ovulatory disorders. Responses to HMG are highly variable, and patients must be monitored closely to ensure that the correct dose be given and to avoid complications—the two most serious of which are multiple gestation and hyperstimulation. Monitoring of patients receiving HMG includes patient evaluations, serum estradiol, and ultrasound monitoring of the developing follicles. Pelvic examinations should be limited to avoid possible rupture of enlarged ovaries. The risk of multiple gestation is approximately 20 to 25%. The hyperstimulation syndrome should be *avoided*, since this is a life-threatening condition with massive accumulation of intraperitoneal and, occasionally, intrathoracic fluid with major fluid and electrolyte imbalances. This condition can be avoided if the ovulatory stimulus is withheld in potentially precarious situations. HMG should be used with caution and only by physicians experienced in its use.

Gonadorelin (synthetic gonadotropin-releasing hormone [GnRH]) is presently approved for diagnostic use only. Since its mode of action and method of administration have become more clearly understood, it is an extremely useful agent in certain ovulatory disorders—most notably, hypothalamic amenorrhea. In addition, it has been used to stimulate multiple follicular development in patients undergoing in vitro fertilization and GIFT (see below).

Artificial reproductive technics: For women with uncorrectable tubal abnormalities that do not permit ovum passage, the extraction of egg cells, their **in vitro fertilization** by the husband's sperm, and implantation in the uterus has been successful. Ultrasound has been used to guide the removal of the ovum. Another form of **embryo transfer** is used for women who are carriers of genetic disorders. A female ovum donor is inseminated with the husband's sperm and the fertilized egg is then transferred to the wife, who carries it to term.

Gamete intrafallopian transfer (GIFT) consists of the extraction of oocytes and their immediate mixing with approximately 100,000 sperm. The gametes are then inserted into the fallopian tube using a small tube, and fertilization occurs in the oviduct. In successful cases, the zygote continues into the uterus where implantation will occur. GIFT is a useful treatment in patients with unexplained infertility and in certain cases of male factor infertility. It is clearly not feasible in patients with surgically absent fallopian tubes.

The use of **frozen embryos** permits remaining embryos from some of the above technics to be saved for later attempts at gestation. Since the egg-retrieval process (and concomitant use of cycle-affecting drugs) need only be done once, this procedure has attractive aspects but is accompanied by ethical and legal questions (see below). Use of **frozen oocytes** is still experimental.

Surrogate motherhood (*the bearing of a child by another woman for an infertile couple*) is performed through artificial insemination or the frozen embryo technic (the embryo produced by in vitro fertilization of the couple's sperm and egg). This procedure is illegal in some states, in part because of state laws forbidding the "sale" of children.

Ethical and legal problems abound with some of these technics; eg, the disposition of stored frozen embryos (especially in cases of the death of the couple, or their separation or divorce); and determination of legal parentage in cases of semen or egg donation or of surrogate mothers. The current *presumption* is that the woman who carries the baby to birth is the legal mother, but clear legal determinations have not been universally established for these questions and others.

Psychologic impact: Since conception is so complex, for those couples attempting to correct their infertility, the remedial process can stretch over years and be not only an

extreme financial burden, but a cause of great emotional stress. There may be suppressed grief or guilt over past losses; eg, miscarriages, stillbirths, or abortions. A feeling of being defective is common and can extend to all areas of life, including sexuality and work performance. If one member of the couple has the greater infertility problem, feelings of guilt, anger, and resentment can arise in both partners. Many couples find the testing process intrusive and degrading, feeling exposed during this most intimate aspect of their lives. They may be left with increased sexual inhibition and decreased communication.

Irreversible infertility: Couples who have to deal with this verdict may undergo a mourning process for the child they cannot conceive. When denial, guilt, and anger are resolved, they can consider alternatives such as childlessness or adoption. A national support group, Resolve, exists for infertile couples.

167. THE MEDICAL EXAMINATION OF THE RAPE VICTIM

Rape is the *illegal sexual penetration of any body orifice.* Except when a child is seduced by offers of affection or bribes, rape is usually a sexual act committed by threat or use of force against an unwilling person. Reported cases of female victims in the USA total 75,000/yr; estimates of unreported rape range from 2 to 10 times that number. Approximately 90% of rapists attack victims of the same race; 50% are known to their victims and are often members of the extended family. This is particularly important for preteen and teenage victims and has implications for follow-up and child abuse prevention (see also Ch. 190). Most rapes are planned (not the result of sudden impulse), and over half the attacks involve a weapon, usually a knife. Approximately 50% of female rape victims show signs of physical trauma; over 10% require emergency treatment.

Although rape is usually thought of in the context of the female victim, a growing number of rape victims are males who are not necessarily part of a prison or homosexual community. The male victim is more likely to have physical trauma than the female, to have been victimized by several assailants, and to be more unwilling to report the crime. For both males and females, however, the assault is the sexual expression of aggression, anger, or need for power. It is a violent, even more than a sexual, act (see also Ch. 139). A few cases of female rapes of males have been reported in the last several years.

Evaluation Procedures

Although provision of medical care and psychologic support for the rape victim is the first concern, the patient is a victim of a crime, and forensic medicine requires certain special details of medical evaluation and record-keeping. TABLE 167–1 may serve as a guide for examination procedures and the medical record, to be adapted according to local requirements. Such a record is sometimes admissible in court and aids recall if testimony is required later. The record should never, unless subpoenaed, be released without written consent of the patient.

Wherever possible, the patient should be treated in a rape treatment center, which should be separate from routine emergency-room care and staffed by trained, concerned support personnel.

History and physical examination: A brief account of the attack by the patient will indicate areas for medical investigation and treatment. However, recounting the events is often frightening for the patient, and a complete history may have to be deferred until more immediate needs have been met. The reasons for the questions asked and for the examination procedure are not always clear to patients; eg, it may need to be

TABLE 167–1. EXAMINATION FOR ALLEGED RAPE

Name of patient: Date of examination:
Address: Time:
Phone: Location:
Age:
Sex:
Name of guardian, if patient is under age:
Address:
Phone:
Name of person accompanying patient to hospital:
Address:
Phone:
Name of police officer, badge number, and department:

HISTORY

Circumstances of attack
Date and time:
Location (familiar to patient?):
Assailant(s):
Number:
Name(s), if known:
Description(s):
Weapon:
Type of sexual contact (vaginal, oral, rectal):
Condom used?
Activities of patient after attack
Douche: Medication:
Bath: Other:
Clothing change:
Last menstrual period:
Date of previous coitus and time, if recent:
Contraceptive history (oral, IUD, etc):

PHYSICAL EXAMINATION

General trauma (extragenital)
Head: Chest: Arms:
Face: Abdomen: Legs:
Throat: Back: Other:
Genital trauma
Perineum: Vulva: Cervix:
Hymen: Vagina: Anus:
Foreign material on body (stains, hair, dirt, twigs, etc):
Evidence of alcohol or other drugs:
Evidence of existing pregnancy:

PSYCHOLOGIC ASSESSMENT

Patient's emotional or mental state:

(Continued)

explained to the female patient that knowledge of the last menstrual period, or the use of a contraceptive, will help determine the risk of pregnancy, or that information concerning the time of the last previous coitus is important in establishing validity of sperm testing.

Since the patient has been through an experience to which he or she did not consent, enlisting the patient's cooperation and requesting permission for the examination is important. Details of the pelvic examination should be described and explained as it proceeds, and the results should be reviewed with the patient. Rape victims may feel anxiety at being examined by a physician of the opposite sex. Therefore, and also for

TABLE 167–1. EXAMINATION FOR ALLEGED RAPE *(Cont'd)*

LABORATORY FINDINGS

Clothing:	Note condition (damaged, stained, foreign material adhering) Provide small samples, including unstained sample, or give clothing to police or laboratory		
Hair samples:	Loose hairs adhering to patient or clothing Semen-encrusted pubic hair Clipped pubic hair of victim—at least ten (for comparison)		
Other specimens, as indicated by the history or physical examination:			
	Tests	*From*	*To determine*
Semen	Papanicolaou Saline suspension* Acid phosphatase† Other (eg, bacterial cultures)	Vagina Cervix Rectum Mouth Thighs Other	Sperm motility, nonmotility Sperm morphology Presence of A, B, or H blood group substances‡ Gonorrhea
Baseline VDRL and gonorrhea cultures			
Blood (including dried samples on patient's body and clothing)			Blood group Presence of drugs, alcohol Pregnancy
Urine			Presence of drugs, alcohol Pregnancy

TREATMENT

REFERRAL

PHYSICIAN'S CLINICAL COMMENTS

Signed: MD State License No:

WITNESS TO EXAMINATION

Signed:

DISPOSITION OF EVIDENCE

Delivered by: Date: Time:

Received by: Date: Time:

* Should be performed by examining physician if time factor permits discovery of motile sperm.

† A useful test, since no sperm will be found if the assailant had a vasectomy, is oligospermic, or used a condom. If test cannot be performed immediately, specimen should be placed in a freezer.

‡ In 80% of cases, blood group substances are found in semen.

(Adapted from I. Root, W. Ogden, and W. Scott, "The Medical Investigation of Alleged Rape," *The Western Journal of Medicine* Vol. 120, No. 4, pp. 329–333, April 1974. Used with permission of *The Western Journal of Medicine* and the authors.)

the purpose of corroborating the procedures, if the physician is of the opposite sex, a nurse or volunteer of the victim's sex should be present during the examination.

The evidence collected during the examination, and all laboratory specimens, are placed in individual packages and carefully labeled, dated, and sealed. Receipts should be obtained upon delivery to the laboratory or police.

Psychologic assessment: Rape presents both psychologic and social problems for the victims, who must handle their own feelings as well as face the often negative reactions (eg, judgmental, derisive) of friends, family, and officials. Patients should be viewed as undergoing a **post-traumatic stress disorder** that typically has an *acute phase* lasting a few days to a few weeks, followed by a *long-term process* of reorganization and recovery.

Acute phase reactions are fear and anger, although patients' outward responses

range from talkativeness, tenseness, crying, and trembling to shock and disbelief, with dispassion, quiescence, and smiling. The latter responses are rarely an indication that the patient is unconcerned; they may be avoidance reactions or may occur in patients who have coping styles that require control of emotion or who are physically exhausted. Patients are usually severely frightened and embarrassed, and feel degraded. The anger felt by many victims may be displaced onto hospital personnel, who should be aware of this and not troubled by it.

Long-range effects of rape include reexperiencing the assault, aversion to sex, anxiety, phobias, suspiciousness, depression, nightmares and sleep disorders, somatic symptoms, and social withdrawal. Guilt feelings and shame occur when the patient feels, generally irrationally, that somehow he or she provoked or should have prevented the attack, or feels that the attack was a punishment for some wrongdoing.

The physician's report may include a brief account of the attack in the patient's words and a statement of the physician's clinical determination as to injuries and sexual activity. It is not necessary to state whether rape occurred, since that is a legal determination, but one should record a diagnosis including all probable or possible physical and psychologic problems.

Treatment

Most physical trauma is minor and treated conservatively, but severe injuries occur and may require surgical repair. Overall, the psychosocial aspects are the most potentially damaging and require sophisticated management. It is very important to treat patients with respect, to see that they are not left alone, to demonstrate understanding and empathy, to assure them that they are safe, and to explain in detail how the evaluation will proceed.

Psychologic trauma: An unhurried, nonjudgmental, listening attitude by the examiner is therapeutic. Since patients are in a traumatic state and many details may be embarrassing, they often omit important data. Therefore, specific details of the attacker's aggression, threats, violent behavior, and of the sex acts committed must be elicited with careful questioning. Empathy can be shown by acknowledging that the questions may be embarrassing or may exacerbate the patient's fears. Properly done, such a potentially distressing interview may begin the therapeutic process. *The full psychologic impact cannot be ascertained at the first examination, and follow-up visits must be scheduled.* At the first visit, the patient should be given an explanation of the possible psychologic and social sequelae and arrangements should be made for introduction to someone trained in rape crisis intervention. If the patient's acute stress reactions do not subside or if long-range psychologic problems seem likely, psychiatric referral is indicated. NOTE: Some patients appear to adjust quickly by unconsciously denying the rape and rapidly returning to normal activities, but later manifest the symptoms and signs of post-traumatic stress disorder.

Support network: The physician often has to deal with the intense reactions of family and friends, who can be sources of support or of additional stress. In the immediate situation, the physician has to try to decrease their strong feelings of anxiety, anger, or guilt, for these usually increase the intensity of the patient's emotional reactions. Instead, family and friends must be shown how to listen to the patient in a supportive fashion, and they can do this only if they can control their feelings when they are with the patient. A support network of health workers, friends, and family is a vital ingredient of long-term care.

Prophylaxis for sexually transmitted disease: If it is suspected that the assailant had gonorrhea or syphilis, the patient is immediately given probenecid 1 gm orally followed by procaine penicillin G/benzathine penicillin G 4.8 million u. IM in divided doses at 2 sites. Penicillin-allergic patients should be given (for gonorrhea) tetracycline

hydrochloride 0.5 gm orally qid for 5 days; for syphilis, the dosage is for 15 consecutive days.

Pregnancy: Factors determining the possibility of a pregnancy include the patient's menstrual cycle phase and whether or not contraceptives were used. HCG tests make such determinations easier. Although rape-induced pregnancy is very rare, if it seems possible, a birth control pill such as 0.5 mg norgestrel/0.05 mg ethinyl estradiol given 2 tablets orally immediately plus 2 tablets 12 h later, will induce menses (99% effective) if given within 72 h of rape. Antiemetic medication such as oral hydroxyzine will counter nausea and vomiting. If it is suspected that the patient was pregnant at the time of the rape, estrogens should not be given until this possibility is evaluated. The patient's attitude toward abortion should be explored.

Additional considerations include: (1) Provision of privacy for examination and consultation. (2) Provision of cleansing facilities and toilet. Many patients will want to wash (some will have been urinated on or have been raped out of doors); some will want to use a mouthwash. (3) Provision of money or transportation to get home. (4) If a rape crisis team operates in the area, referral can provide helpful medical, psychologic, and legal support to the victim.

Follow-up should include tests for gonorrhea, syphilis, and pregnancy within 6 wk. If pregnancy occurs, consideration should be given to its termination. A further test for syphilis should be done at 6 mo. (See also discussion of follow-up in Psychologic trauma, above.)

§15. GYNECOLOGY AND OBSTETRICS

168. GYNECOLOGIC PRACTICE AND APPROACH TO THE PATIENT

A patient's personal expectations, interpretations, and response to symptoms and therapy, as well as disease patterns, are influenced by her culture and socioeconomic status. Modesty may make the physical examination, particularly the pelvic examination, an ordeal. The patient may be ignorant of generative and sexual functions. Religious and cultural backgrounds influence attitudes about pregnancy, contraception, and abortion. Visual exploration of any portion of the genital tract may be proscribed. For some, an absolute requirement, or highly desirable one, may be virginity at marriage, frequently equated with the size of the hymenal orifice; thus, an appropriate examination may be limited or prevented. On the other hand, premarital sexual activity of young people with multiple partners is common and leads to infection, cervical neoplasia, and unplanned pregnancy. Taboos and attitudes toward menstruation vary markedly; eg, menses were traditionally associated with soiling, shame, and "sickness," or the menstrual flow was thought of as "cleansing," so that a heavy flow might be welcomed as feminine, and a light flow or longer interval interpreted as unhealthy.

Gynecologic and obstetric problems account for 20% of female office visits. Many women have physical examinations only because of need for contraception, pregnancy

detection and subsequent care, or sexual counseling. Many women postpone examinations until an urgent problem arises, and important symptoms considered too minor or embarrassing to mention (eg, annoying discharge, dyspareunia, urinary incontinence, or pelvic pressure) may be elicited only by careful interviewing and examination. Patients may or may not be aware of psychologic stress that may be augmenting or causing their symptoms. The patient may use minor symptoms as "tickets of admission" to explore other problems, such as fear of cancer or venereal disease, pregnancy, need for counseling in sexual or reproductive functions, or effects of menopause.

Increasingly, women are becoming better educated, working outside the home, having fewer children, changing residences, being divorced or separated, rearing children alone, and outliving their mates. The pressures of these changes may affect a woman's health, needs, and ability to handle problems. An affluent and better educated woman who has easy access to health care is more likely to practice preventive care and seek attention for early symptoms, although there is great variation and each patient's attitudes must be individually assessed.

About 40% of obstetric and gynecologic patients are adolescents, among whom venereal disease, pregnancy, and sexual dysfunction are occurring in epidemic proportions. Physicians have unique opportunities to establish continuing relationships, teach about body function and health care maintenance, and counsel. This contact must be nonjudgmental, as the developing woman will perceive insensitivity regarding her physical and emotional feelings. Her vulnerability accentuates the positive or negative effects of the physician's attitude on her own personality and on her attitudes toward future medical care. Confidentiality must be observed and affirmed to the adult or adolescent patient. The rights of minors who do not want parents informed of medical problems, especially regarding sexual activities, should be respected. Women now are less passive and expect to be involved in decisions affecting their health care. Therefore, the patient must have support and counsel, and sufficient information to understand the problem, the nature of therapy, and available alternatives.

The Gynecologic History

Rapport begins with the physician's courtesy, attention, and friendly, unhurried manner while compiling the medical record. A nonjudgmental approach in questions, gestures, and attitudes avoids moralizing or expressing dogmatic opinion and encourages an accurate history. Since physician and patient may have different attitudes about the role of women, care is necessary to avoid making the patient feel embarrassed, helpless, or dependent. A response appropriate to her needs is one that recognizes her unique worth and encourages realization of her independence.

The patient's **primary complaint** should be identified and then explored in detail. **Background data** reveal the patient as an individual. **Menstrual history** includes the age of menarche of the patient (and other family members), frequency, regularity, duration, amount of flow, pain or other symptoms with or before menses, abnormal bleeding, and dates of the last 2 menses. **Sexual activity,** orientation, and possible problems can influence further questioning. The possibility of pregnancy should be explored, along with attitudes, knowledge, and prior experience with contraceptives. **History of pregnancy** includes the number of pregnancies, their dates and outcomes, and problems in becoming pregnant. **Pain,** if present, should be described: when and where it occurs, its severity, its tendency to radiate, what exacerbates it or gives relief, and any relationship to GI or urinary functions. **Fever** is noted.

A **review of past illnesses** follows, including hospitalization and surgery, with details of abdominal or pelvic surgery. Any **history of radiation therapy** for benign disease—eg, mastitis, "enlarged thymus," menorrhagia, or skin disorders—should be elicited as well as reports of possible exposure to diethylstilbestrol **(DES)** by mothers who were pregnant or daughters born during the years (1947 to 1971) of its use. The patient's **general health** should be reviewed, including her **psychologic status,** with particular attention to

depression, anxiety, or drug abuse. **Drug intake** is noted with reference to allergies and especially drugs affecting the present condition, as they may conflict with proposed treatment or be contraindicated in pregnancy.

Since the **urinary tract** is frequently involved in gynecologic disease, questions are asked regarding frequency, nocturia, dysuria, involuntary loss of urine, and vaginal protrusion. Similarly, **GI symptoms** should be reviewed: change of bowel habit, stool color, anorexia, nausea, vomiting, abdominal pain, food intolerance, and past or present possible symptoms of liver disorder.

Breast problems, including pain or growths, should be noted. A review of general **endocrine status** includes abnormal hair growth, abnormal lactation, and symptoms of other endocrine dysfunction. A history of **bleeding abnormalities,** anemias, phlebitis, or other abnormal clotting may give clues to the cause of abnormal menses or preclude hormone medication. The **cardiac status** or history of cardiac disease, hypertension, smoking, or cholesterol or triglyceride abnormality may also influence therapy. A history of migraine headache or seizures may modify treatment; drugs used to control migraine may be detrimental in pregnancy. A **family history** may reveal hereditary disease; especially pertinent are ovarian, uterine, and breast cancer; diabetes; and genetic abnormalities.

The Gynecologic Examination

The bladder must be emptied before pelvic examination; the urine specimen is examined for sugar, albumin, and bacteria. Examination of blood for Hb or Hct is done as indicated (eg, heavy menses, tiredness, pallor, or previous anemia).

The **physical examination** includes height, weight, BP, and a check of heart, lungs, and lymph nodes. Abnormal body hair texture or distribution is noted. The thyroid gland may be enlarged, nodular, or tender.

A thorough **breast examination** (see Ch. 172) in both sitting and prone positions notes maturation, tenderness, symmetry, retraction of skin or nipples, or masses. Gentleness and warm hands are appreciated. The physician uses this occasion to instruct the patient in self-examination for early detection of malignancy.

Abdominal examination always begins away from an area of pain. Using a flat hand, probing, not poking, the physician systematically searches each quadrant of the abdomen for masses and tenderness. The following are noted: presence of a mass, its size, location, mobility, and tenderness; scars or distention; ascites or suggestion of other abdominal fluids; liver size and possible tenderness; whether or not the kidneys, liver, or spleen is palpable. Bowel sounds are checked if there is an abdominal complaint. If tenderness is present, its severity, location, and any accompanying rigidity of the abdominal wall are noted. Referral of tenderness elsewhere in the abdomen or rebound tenderness indicates peritoneal irritation.

The **pelvic examination** is usually deferred until last. With unhurried explanations and a sensitive and gentle, but matter-of-fact attitude, the physician helps the patient to relax; not only is she happier, but the examination is more thorough. Having emptied her bladder, the patient assumes the lithotomy position (in which the hips and knees are flexed with the buttocks at the edge of the table and the legs supported by heel or knee stirrups). **Inspection** of the genital area shows hair distribution, clitoral size, vulvar lesions, discoloration, discharge, inflammation, and degree of patency of the hymenal orifice. A gentle touch on the inner thigh just before touching the genitalia reduces the startle reflex.

To expose the cervix and avoid pressure on the urethra, a warmed, water-lubricated speculum is inserted into the upper vagina at a 45° angle, rotated, and then opened. (Lubricating jelly is avoided, since it may interfere with the Pap test.)

The **Papanicolaou (Pap) test** examines exfoliated cells to detect preinvasive lesions (eg, dysplasia, carcinoma-in-situ) as well as invasive lesions. The Pap test should detect 95% of cervical malignancies and premalignant states. The patient should have re-

frained from douching or using vaginal medication for 24 h. False negative results may result from inadequate sample or infection of a malignant lesion. Endometrial malignancies are detected in only 50%. Virus and other infections may be diagnosed, as well as the estrogen level.

An endocervical sample is taken with a saline-moistened cotton-tipped applicator that is rotated or rolled thinly on a slide and immediately fixed by immersion in equal volumes of ethyl ether and 95% ethyl alcohol (or 95% ethyl alcohol alone). The visible cervix is then firmly scraped circumflexually with an Ayre spatula; a sample from the posterior fornix ("vaginal pool") may be included. DES-exposed women should also have vaginal wall scrapings.

With the speculum in place, gross lesions are noted; specimens are taken if discharge or other symptoms warrant. The vaginal walls are inspected as the patient bears down and the speculum is gradually withdrawn.

Bimanual palpation of the uterus is attained with the index and middle finger of one hand in the vagina and the fingers of the other hand on the abdomen. The uterus is normally felt as a pear-shaped, smooth muscular organ; the fingers, shifting from anterior to posterior fornix, ascertain its position, size, consistency, surface contour, mobility, and tenderness. A retroflexed uterus is more difficult to outline and may seem larger than its actual size. **Enlargements** may be due to pregnancy, myoma, adenomyosis, simple hypertrophy, malignancy, or inflammation. **Softening** may be due to pregnancy, malignancy, degenerating myoma or sarcoma, or to low estrogen—as with immaturity or post-menopause. **Irregularities** may be due to myoma or myomas, varying in size from several millimeters to many centimeters; anomalies of the uterus, usually felt as an indentation of the fundus; malignancies; or adhesions of other pelvic structures, such as between ovary and uterus. **Adnexal structures** are carefully palpated by approximating the fingers of the 2 hands, the painful side last. The normal adult ovary, 3 by 2 by 2 cm, may be difficult to feel, especially if the abdominal wall is thick or tense; but this skill is important, because early diagnosis of malignant lesions depends upon early findings in an asymptomatic patient. Enlargements of ovary or adnexal mass, including tubes, should be noted, as well as signs mentioned above in palpating the uterus. On the right, the position of **the cecum** may be differentiated by its mobility and the presence of gas. The *cul-de-sac* area behind the uterus is palpated now, and then again with the rectal examination. The vagina is palpated, to search for vaginal cysts or nodules. **Pelvic support** may be evaluated with 2 fingers held gently against the posterior vaginal wall; the physician checks for descensus of the uterus and evidence of cystocele, rectocele, and enterocele by noting support both before and after the patient bears down. Protrusion of the anterior wall is termed **cystocele**. Posteriorly, the levator ani muscles offer support, with weakness and protrusion of the posterior wall termed **rectocele**. Herniation near the apex of the vagina between the major supporting uterosacral ligaments is an **enterocele**. This can also occur after a hysterectomy. The apex of the vagina may descend to varying degrees following hysterectomy.

Rectovaginal examination is done last, with the index finger in the vagina and the second finger in the rectum to confirm the findings. One palpates uterosacral ligaments, the back of the uterus and cervix, and the contents of the *cul-de-sac* (pouch of Douglas) and parametria to search for masses, tenderness, or induration. This part of the examination is especially important when the uterus is retroflexed. **Rectal lesions** within the range of the examining finger are noted (eg, hemorrhoids, fissures, polyps, masses); the presence of blood is noted.

The upper posterior vagina between the uterosacral ligaments, the thinnest layer of the abdominal wall, is a common site for needle aspiration of fluid contents of the peritoneum **(culdocentesis).**

The physician, using diagrams or pictures as indicated, should discuss the findings with the patient so that she understands her condition and the alternatives of therapy.

169. REPRODUCTIVE ENDOCRINOLOGY

Normal human reproductive function requires the complex interplay of endocrine and target organs (see FIG. 169–1). **Gonadotropin-releasing hormone (GnRH),** also known as luteinizing hormone-releasing factor or hormone **(LRF, LHRH, LRH),** is a small peptide (secreted by the hypothalamus) that regulates release of the pituitary gonadotropins **luteinizing hormone (LH)** and **follicle-stimulating hormone (FSH)** from the anterior pituitary gland (see Chs. 87 and 88). LH and FSH, termed "gonadotropins," are important in stimulating secretion of hormones by the gonads and also play an essential role in inducing maturation of germ cells. Androgens from the testes in men and estrogens from the ovaries in women in turn stimulate the target organs of the reproductive tract (ie, breasts, uterus, and vagina in women and accessory reproductive organs in men) and exert feedback effects on the CNS-hypothalamic-pituitary unit to influence its hormone secretion.

Steroids are polycyclic compounds derived from cholesterol with carbon atoms arranged in 4 rings. They circulate in the bloodstream bound almost entirely to various plasma proteins. Only free or unbound steroids appear to be biologically active. Steroid hormones can exert both **negative** and **positive feedback** effects on gonadotropin secretion. Negative feedback occurs when steroids *inhibit* release of LH and FSH; positive feedback occurs when steroids *stimulate* gonadotropin secretion.

Virtually all hormones are released in short bursts or pulses at intervals of 1 to 3 h. Constant levels are not observed in the circulation. The patterns described are therefore merely idealized representations on which the minute-to-minute fluctuations must be superimposed. Such factors must be considered in interpreting single hormonal values obtained for clinical purposes.

Infancy, Childhood, and Puberty

Both LH and FSH are elevated at birth but fall to low levels within a few months and remain low through the prepubertal years (see FIG. 169–2). Serum FSH levels are generally slightly higher than LH levels in children, when expressed in terms of milliinternational units **(mIU)**/mL. The hypothalamic-pituitary unit appears to be exquisitely sensitive to extremely low levels of circulating steroid, and negative feedback influences predominate. Early in puberty there is a decrease in the sensitivity of the hypothalamus to gonadal steroids, resulting in increased secretion of pituitary gonadotropins, stimulation of gonadal steroid production, and the development of secondary sexual characteristics. Increased secretion of both LH and FSH first occurs only during sleep and is associated with increased gonadal steroid secretion. Later, secretion of LH and FSH increases throughout the 24-h period. The patterns of increase in basal LH and FSH levels differ between boys and girls, but in both, basal LH levels exceed those of FSH.

The adrenal androgens, dehydroepiandrosterone **(DHEA)** and its sulfate **(DHEAS)** begin to increase several years prior to puberty in both sexes. It is possible that the increase in adrenal androgens may play a role in activation of other pubertal events and may be important in initiation of pubic and axillary hair growth (ie, adrenarche). Since ACTH and cortisol do not increase with these androgens, it has been suggested that another as yet unidentified pituitary peptide initiates adrenal androgen secretion (see Ch. 91).

The mechanisms responsible for initiating puberty are not understood. There must be some "CNS program" for initiating puberty. In addition to decreased sensitivity to the inhibitory feedback effects of circulating gonadal steroids, maturation of a positive

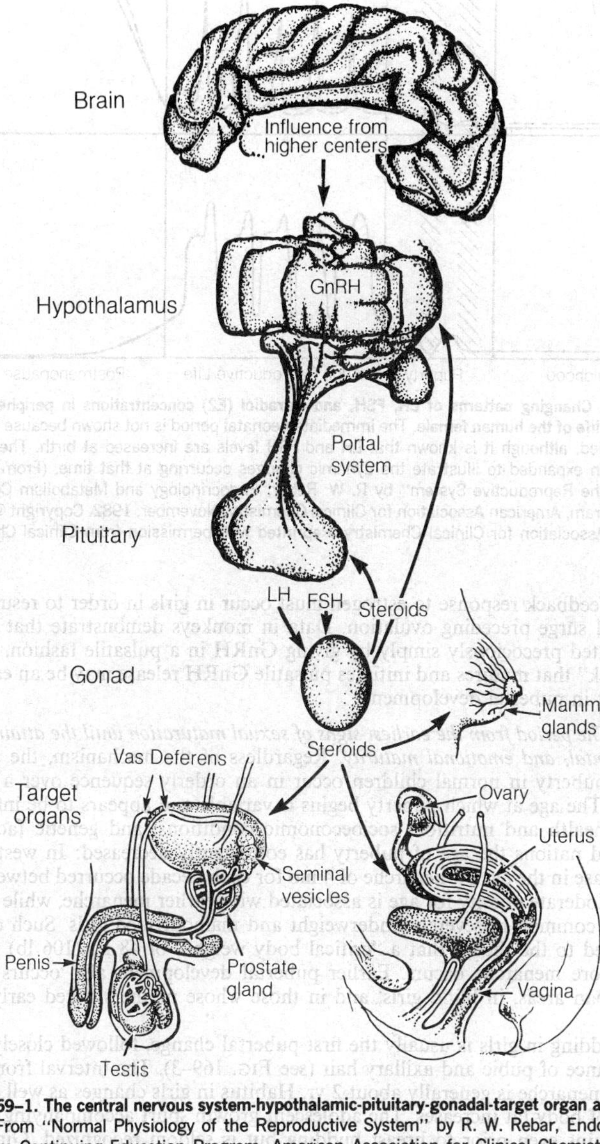

FIG. 169–1. The central nervous system-hypothalamic-pituitary-gonadal-target organ axis in men and women. (From "Normal Physiology of the Reproductive System" by R. W. Rebar, Endocrinology and Metabolism Continuing Education Program, American Association for Clinical Chemistry, November, 1982. Copyright © 1982 by the American Association for Clinical Chemistry. Reprinted with permission from Clinical Chemistry.)

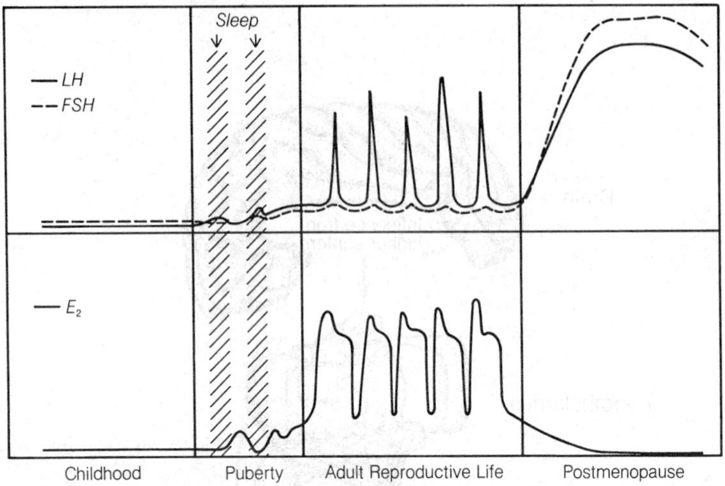

FIG. 169–2. Changing patterns of LH, FSH, and estradiol (E2) concentrations in peripheral blood throughout the life of the human female. The immediate neonatal period is not shown because it has not been well studied, although it is known that LH and FSH levels are increased at birth. The pubertal period has been expanded to illustrate the dynamic changes occurring at that time. (From "Normal Physiology of the Reproductive System" by R. W. Rebar, Endocrinology and Metabolism Continuing Education Program, American Association for Clinical Chemistry, November, 1982. Copyright © 1982 by the American Association for Clinical Chemistry. Reprinted with permission from Clinical Chemistry.)

stimulating feedback response to estrogen must occur in girls in order to result in the midcycle LH surge preceding ovulation. Data in monkeys demonstrate that puberty can be initiated precociously simply by giving GnRH in a pulsatile fashion. Thus, a central "clock" that matures and initiates pulsatile GnRH release may be an early and critical event in pubertal development.

Puberty: *The period from the earliest signs of sexual maturation until the attainment of physical, mental, and emotional maturity.* Regardless of the mechanism, the physical changes of puberty in normal children occur in an orderly sequence over a definite time frame. The age at which puberty begins is variable and appears to be influenced by general health and nutrition, socioeconomic conditions, and genetic factors. In industrialized nations the age of puberty has consistently decreased: In western Europe a decrease in the age of menarche of 4 mo for each decade occurred between 1850 and 1950. Moderate obesity for age is associated with earlier menarche, while delayed menarche is common in severely underweight and malnourished girls. Such observations have led to the theory that a "critical body weight" of 48 kg (106 lb) must be attained before menarche occurs. Earlier pubertal development also occurs in girls living in urban areas, in blind girls, and in those whose mothers noted early sexual maturation.

Breast budding in girls is usually the first pubertal change, followed closely by the first appearance of pubic and axillary hair (see FIG. 169–3). The interval from breast budding to menarche is generally about 2 yr. Habitus in girls changes as well, and the percentage of body fat increases. The adolescent growth spurt accompanying puberty typically begins even prior to breast budding but is seldom recognized. Girls reach peak height velocity early in puberty prior to menarche and have only limited growth potential following menarche.

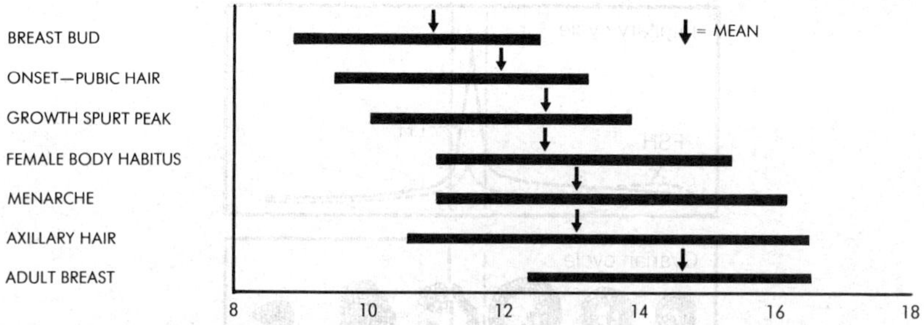

FIG. 169–3. Puberty—age of development of female sexual characteristics.

General Characteristics of the Menstrual Cycle

A **menstrual cycle** *begins with the first day of genital bleeding (day 1) and ends just prior to the next menstrual period.* **Menarche** refers to *the onset of menses*, **menopause** to *the cessation of menses*. Although the median menstrual cycle length is 28 days, only 10 to 15% of normal menstrual cycles are exactly 28 days in length; the range is about 18 to 40 days. Maximal variation with the longest intermenstrual intervals generally occurs in the years following menarche and those preceding menopause, when anovulatory cycles are more common.

Hormonal events during the menstrual cycle: On the basis of known endocrine events, the menstrual cycle can be divided into 3 distinct phases (see FIG. 169–4). The **preovulatory** or **follicular phase** varies in length, beginning with the first day of bleeding and extending to the day prior to the preovulatory LH surge. During the first half of the follicular phase, slightly increased FSH secretion from the anterior pituitary gland initiates growth and development of a cohort of 3 to 30 follicles, consisting of oocytes and their surrounding cells. One of these follicles is destined to ovulate; all the others will undergo degeneration **(atresia).** In the absence of appropriate increase in FSH, follicular development will not be normal. Circulating LH levels begin to rise slowly during this time, beginning 1 to 2 days after the FSH rise. Steroid hormone estrogen and progesterone secretion by the ovaries is relatively constant and remains low during this period.

In the **ovulatory phase**, a series of complex endocrine events culminates in the massive release (ie, preovulatory surge) of LH by the pituitary gland. The mechanism for the process of ovulation itself is unclear, but this LH surge is necessary to cause release of the ovum from the mature preovulatory (ie, graafian) follicle, generally 16 to 32 h after onset of the surge. (In discussing endocrine changes during the menstrual cycle, the day of maximal LH release is referred to as day 0. Hormonal events are centered around this surge, with days prior to the LH surge numbered negatively from 0 and days after the surge numbered positively.) Although ovulation may result, the subsequent luteal phase may be short and inadequate and preclude pregnancy.

About 7 to 8 days before the preovulatory surge, estrogen (particularly **estradiol, E_2**) secretion from the ovaries begins to increase slowly, but then accelerates and generally peaks during the day of or the day before the LH surge. This rise in estrogen is accompanied by a slow but steady increase in LH and a fall in FSH levels. This divergence in LH and FSH levels may be due to the preferential inhibitory action of estrogens on FSH, compared to LH release, and possible secretion of **inhibin**, also termed **folliculostatin,** a peptide hormone presumably secreted by the developing follicle that inhibits FSH secretion. Just prior to the LH surge **progesterone** levels also begin to increase significantly.

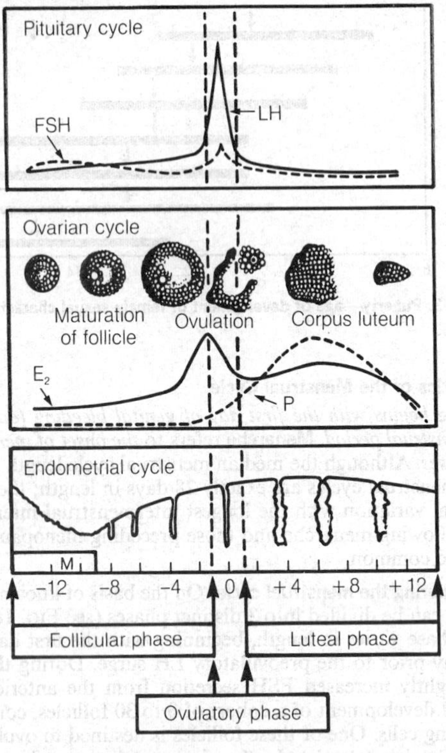

FIG. 169–4. The idealized cyclic changes observed in pituitary gonadotropins, estradiol (E2), progesterone (P), ovarian follicles, and uterine endometrium during the normal menstrual cycle. The data are centered about the day of the LH surge (day 0). Days of menstrual bleeding are indicated by M. (From "Normal Physiology of the Reproductive System" by R. W. Rebar, Endocrinology and Metabolism Continuing Education Program, American Association for Clinical Chemistry, November, 1982. Copyright © 1982 by the American Association for Clinical Chemistry. Reprinted with permission from Clinical Chemistry.)

During the ovulatory phase rapid release of LH occurs, partly as a result of positive estrogen feedback, and leads to final maturation of the follicle and ovulation. Although there is a smaller simultaneous increase in FSH secretion, its significance is not understood. With rising LH levels, estradiol levels fall but progesterone concentrations continue to increase. The LH surge typically lasts 36 to 48 h and is composed of several large bursts of LH release in a pulsatile fashion.

The **postovulatory** or **luteal phase** is the most constant half of the cycle, averaging 14 days in length in the absence of pregnancy and ending with the onset of menstruation. This phase's name and length come from the functional lifespan of the **corpus luteum** (ie, yellow body) of the ovary that supports the released ovum by secreting progesterone. After ovulation the granulosa and theca cells comprising the follicle reorganize to form the corpus luteum. The corpus luteum secretes increasing quantities of progesterone, peaking with secretion of about 25 mg during each 24-h period 6 to 8 days after the LH surge. Circulating LH and FSH levels decline and are low throughout most of the luteal phase but begin to increase again with menstruation.

Cyclic Changes in the Ovary

By the 6th wk of gestation, primordial germ cells, now called **oogonia**, have migrated by ameboid movement from their site of origin in the yolk sac to the genital ridges (ie, presumptive ovaries). Their number increases by mitosis markedly through the 20th wk of fetal age. The germ cells then undergo meiosis so that all germ cells are arrested in the diplotene stage of meiotic prophase by the 7th mo of gestation and can then be called **oocytes.** Between 7 and 9 mo of gestation the fetal ovary becomes organized and each oocyte becomes a part of a **primordial follicle,** consisting of a basement membrane, a single layer of squamous epithelial granulosa cells, and an oocyte arrested in meiosis. These primordial follicles represent the pool of nongrowing follicles from which all mature follicles develop. Thus, the human female is born with a limited number of germ cells (ova). These are eliminated from the ovary by atresia, which accounts for elimination of 99.9% of all germ cells, and by ovulation. The estimated number in the ovaries throughout life is cited in TABLE 169–1. Each viable oocyte remains arrested in meiotic prophase until following the midcycle LH surge of the cycle in which it is ovulated, making it one of the longest lived cells in the body (from embryo up to about 50 yr).

Follicle growth involves the transformation of a small primordial follicle 50 μm in diameter into a mature graafian follicle 1 to 2.5 cm in diameter (see FIG. 169–5). Follicle growth begins with the oocyte increasing in diameter from 15 to 150 μm. This larger oocyte becomes surrounded by a **zona pellucida**, a translucent "shell" of glycoproteins. The fully grown oocyte surrounded by a single layer of granulosa cells is termed a **primary follicle**. Development into a **secondary follicle** occurs with mitosis of granulosa cells so that the oocyte becomes surrounded by 2 or more cell layers. The initiation of oocyte and follicular growth is not controlled by gonadotropins and is not understood.

Although the oocyte itself fully differentiates early in follicular development, it cannot be extruded from the ovary until the follicular unit develops into a mature graafian follicle capable of responding to the midcycle LH surge. This phase of follicular maturation is completely dependent upon gonadotropin and steroid hormones and is controlled by changes in the type and number of hormone receptor sites on the granulosa and theca cells of the follicle.

FSH induces the appearance of FSH receptors on granulosa cells, necessary to stimulate the aromatase enzyme needed to convert androgens to estrogens. Specific steroid receptors for estradiol and testosterone appear in granulosa cells with the

TABLE 169–1. THE ESTIMATED POTENTIAL OF HUMAN OVARIES

Parameter	*Approximate Number*
Maximum number of oocytes in both fetal ovaries	7–20 million
Oocytes present at birth	2 million
Oocytes present at menarche	200–400,000
Oocytes undergoing some development during reproductive life	8000
Number of ovulatory menstrual cycles during reproductive life	300–400
Number of follicles beginning to develop each cycle	3–30
Number of ova normally shed at each ovulation	1 (rarely 2)

(Modified from "Normal Physiology of the Reproductive System" by R.W. Rebar, Endocrinology and Metabolism Continuing Education Program, American Association for Clinical Chemistry, November, 1982. Copyright 1982 by the American Association for Clinical Chemistry. Used with permission.)

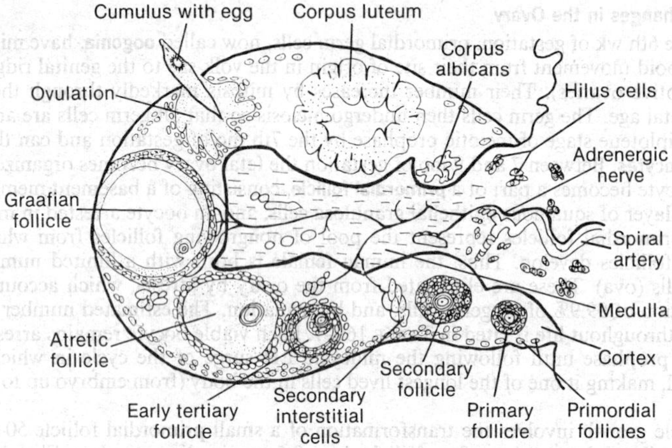

FIG. 169–5. Morphology and histology of a human ovary. The follicles, corpora lutea and secondary interstitial cells are embedded in the outer cortex, while the hilus cells, autonomic nerves, and spiral arteries are found in the medulla. (From G. F. Erickson in *Gynecology and Obstetrics,* edited by J. D. Sciarra, 1984. Harper and Row, publishers, Philadelphia. Used with permission.)

appearance of the FSH receptors. The estrogen-receptor interaction stimulates multiplication of granulosa cells and thus follicular growth, while androgen-receptor interaction has been implicated in follicular atresia.

Theca interstitial cells begin to develop around the basement membrane surrounding the granulosa cells shortly after the oocyte completes its growth. The theca develop specific receptors for LH but not FSH. LH stimulates the theca to synthesize androgens, mainly androstenedione and testosterone. The androgens produced in the theca diffuse across the basement membrane into the granulosa cells where they are converted into estradiol, which rises throughout the follicular phase and then diffuses into the systemic circulation to feed back on the hypothalamic-pituitary unit (see under Neuroendocrine Regulation of the Menstrual Cycle, below).

The mature tertiary, preovulatory, **graafian follicle** contains an antrum or fluid-filled cavity, created by proliferating granulosa cells, which secrete fluid and mucopolysaccharides. The tertiary follicle grows from 200 μm to 1 to 2.5 cm in diameter, primarily because of accumulation of follicular fluid under the control of FSH, which also induces the appearance of specific LH receptors on granulosa cells. These LH receptors are responsible for the stimulation of progesterone secretion prior to ovulation and for continued production of progesterone in the luteal phase. Granulosa cells also develop specific membrane receptors for prolactin in early tertiary follicles, but these decrease as the follicles mature and their physiologic role is unclear. About 2 wk are required for the presumptive preovulatory follicle to complete its growth and expel a mature oocyte. The mechanism of preovulatory selection from the cohort of developing follicles is unknown, but intraovarian factors must be important. This is also apparent because the fully grown oocyte is inhibited from resuming meiotic maturation by granulosa-oocyte interactions until after ovulation, even though it is able to do so.

Within 36 h of the LH/FSH surge, the oocyte completes the first meiotic division when each cell receives only 23 chromosomes of the original 46 and the first polar

body is extruded. The 2nd meiotic division, when each chromosome divides longitudinally with identical pairs, is not completed and the 2nd polar body extruded unless the egg is penetrated by a spermatozoan. During the LH surge, the preovulatory follicle swells and bulges above the ovarian epithelium. A **stigma** or avascular spot appears on the follicle surface. A small vesicle forms on the stigma, the vesicle breaks, and the oocyte and some granulosa cells surrounding the oocyte (forming the **cumulus** mass) are extruded. Lysozymes in the epithelial cells overlying the preovulatory follicle appear to play an important role in rupturing the follicle. Prostaglandin production by the follicle itself, perhaps under the regulation of LH and/or FSH, also appears essential for the ovulatory process.

The corpus luteum produces progesterone and estradiol for about 14 days and then degenerates unless fertilization occurs. Because progesterone is also thermogenic, basal body temperature increases by at least 0.33 C (0.6 F) in the luteal phase and remains elevated until menstruation. Prostaglandins and prolactin may play a role in regulating the life-span of the corpus luteum; however, this is as yet poorly understood. If fertilization occurs, **human chorionic gonadotropin (HCG)** from the fertilized ovum supports the corpus luteum until the fetoplacental unit can support itself endocrinologically. HCG is structurally and functionally similar to LH; however, pregnancy tests typically utilize antibodies specific to the β subunit of HCG and have little if any cross-reactivity with LH.

Cyclical Changes in the Other Target Organs of the Reproductive Tract

During the menstrual cycle, the **endometrium** undergoes remarkable histologic and cytologic changes that culminate with menstrual bleeding. The endometrium is composed of 3 layers: (1) the "nonfunctioning" **basal layer** that is not lost during menses and serves to regenerate the other 2 layers during the menstrual cycle, (2) the **superficial layer** of **compact** epithelial cells that line the uterine cavity, and (3) the intermediate **spongiosa layer**. These latter 2 layers are "functioning," show the greatest changes during the menstrual cycle, and are shed with menstruation. Following menstruation in the early follicular phase, the endometrium, which is composed of glands and stroma, is thin. The endometrial glands are narrow and straight with low columnar epithelium, and the endometrial stroma is dense. With rising levels of estradiol during the late follicular phase, the endometrium undergoes progressive proliferation and extensive mitoses (ie, regeneration from the basal layer), the mucosa thickens, and the tubular glands lengthen but remain straight. In the luteal phase, under the influence of progesterone, the glands become coiled, saw-toothed, and secretory with increased vascularity of the stroma. As both estradiol and progesterone decline in the late luteal phase, the stroma becomes increasingly edematous, endometrial and blood vessel necrosis occurs, and endometrial bleeding ensues. Because the histologic changes during the menstrual cycle are characteristic, endometrial biopsies may be used to accurately date the stage of the cycle and to assess the tissue response to gonadal steroids. Although the mechanism for the onset of menstruation is not understood, prostaglandins have been implicated in causing the initial vasoconstriction and subsequent tissue anoxia and necrosis. Since prostaglandin release may also explain the uterine contractions accompanying menstrual flow, the use of prostaglandin inhibitors to treat dysmenorrhea is logical and should be effective (see under PRIMARY DYSMENORRHEA in Ch. 171). The average duration of menstrual bleeding is 5 ± 2 days with a blood loss averaging 130 mL (range 13 to 300 mL). A saturated pad or tampon absorbs 20 to 30 mL. Menstrual blood does not usually clot (unless bleeding is very heavy) probably because fibrinolysin and other factors inhibiting clotting are present.

Cyclical changes in the diameter of the external cervical os, dimensions of the cervical canal, quantity and biophysical properties of cervical mucus, and tissue vascularity are also observed during the menstrual cycle. During the follicle phase, there is a progressive increase in cervical vascularity, congestion and edema, and in secretion of

cervical mucus. The external cervical os opens to a diameter of 3 mm at ovulation and then decreases to 1 mm. Under the influence of increasing levels of estrogen, there is a 10- to 30-fold increase in the quantity of cervical mucus. The elasticity or **spinnbarkeit** increases. "Palm leaf" arborization or **ferning** becomes prominent when cervical mucus obtained just prior to ovulation is allowed to dry on a glass slide and examined microscopically. This ferning is a result of increased NaCl in cervical mucus from estrogenic stimulation. Under the influence of progesterone in the luteal phase, cervical mucus thickens, becomes less watery, and loses its elasticity and ability to fern. The characteristics of cervical mucus are of use clinically in evaluating the stage of the cycle and the hormonal status of the individual.

Proliferation and maturation of the vaginal epithelium are also influenced by estrogen and progesterone. When ovarian estrogen secretion is low in the early follicular phase, vaginal epithelium is thin and pale. As estrogen levels increase in the follicular phase, the vaginal epithelium thickens and the squamous cells mature and become cornified. During the luteal phase, the number of precornified intermediate cells increases and there are increased numbers of leukocytes and debris as the mature squamous cells are shed. Changes in the vaginal epithelium can be quantitated histologically and are useful qualitative indices of estrogenic stimulation. The vagina and cervix are the most sensitive indicators of estrogenic stimulation in the body.

Neuroendocrine Regulation of the Menstrual Cycle

The release of both LH and FSH appears to be dependent on the secretion of GnRH from the hypothalamus as detailed in Ch. 87. No separate releasing hormone for FSH has been identified. Since strong evidence suggests that LH and FSH are sometimes found in the same cells, differential release of LH and FSH must be dependent upon interactions of various inputs such as GnRH and estradiol and the different disappearance rates of LH (half-life 20 to 30 min) and FSH (half-life 2 to 3 h) from the circulation. Like virtually all hormones, both LH and FSH are secreted in an episodic or pulsatile fashion. The frequency and amplitude of the pulses are modulated by ovarian steroids and vary throughout the menstrual cycle. GnRH also appears to be secreted in a pulsatile fashion and is responsible for the pulsatile gonadotropin secretion.

Of the ovarian steroids, 17β-estradiol is the most potent *inhibitor* of gonadotropin secretion, apparently acting on both the hypothalamus and the pituitary gland. Surgical removal of the ovaries leads to rapid increases in LH and FSH, and administration of estradiol to hypoestrogenic women leads to a prompt decline in circulating gonadotropin levels. For ovulation to occur, estradiol must also exert a *positive* effect on gonadotropin secretion. The feedback effects of estradiol appear to be both time and dose dependent. High physiologic concentrations of estrogen stimulate synthesis and storage of gonadotropin and also augment the effect of GnRH in stimulating gonadotropin release. In the normal menstrual cycle, the positive feedback action of estradiol leading to the midcycle LH/FSH surge is preceded by a period when lower estradiol levels are present with their negative feedback effects.

Thus, the secretion of LH and FSH is determined by the direct input of GnRH modulated by the feedback effects of gonadal steroids. Early in the follicular phase, the gonadotropes in the anterior pituitary gland have relatively small amounts of LH and FSH available for release. Increasing estradiol augments synthesis of LH and FSH but inhibits their secretion. As estradiol increases further to midcycle, it finally induces the midcycle release of LH and FSH, aided by the low but increasing quantities of circulating progesterone. Whether pulsatile release of GnRH is also increased at midcycle in women is unknown. The onset of the midcycle surge could represent merely a rapid increase in the number of GnRH receptors (stimulated by estrogen) present on the gonadotropes.

Menopause (see also MENOPAUSE in Ch. 171)

The time at which cyclic ovarian function as manifested by menstruation ceases. Menopause generally occurs at 51 yr of age, but may normally occur in women as young as 40 yr; typically there is a strong genetic factor affecting the age of onset. Symptoms and signs of the **menopause syndrome** are primarily related to decreased concentrations of circulating estrogen.

Symptoms include hot flushes, insomnia, paresthesias, palpitations, cold hands and feet, headache, vertigo, anxiety, irritability, nervousness, depression, fatigue, forgetfulness, inability to concentrate, and weight gain. The hot flush has been characterized most thoroughly. The woman feels warm or hot and may perspire, sometimes profusely; the hot flush or "flash" lasts from a few seconds to 3 to 5 min. The skin, especially of the head and neck, becomes red and warm. The flush may be followed by chills. These vasomotor symptoms of the hot flush occur coincident with the onset of LH pulses, but not every rise in LH is associated with a hot flush, suggesting that anterior hypothalamic centers independently control both flushes and pulsatile release of LH. Since hot flushes occur in women following pituitary ablation who do not secrete LH and FSH, the 2 events must be independent.

A number of other objective changes occur at menopause. Most apparent is the cessation of menstrual flow. Any genital bleeding in a woman who has not bled for 6 mo or more demands investigation. Gross osteoporosis of bone occurs in about 25% of menopausal women, especially among those who are thin and white. The vulvar skin and vaginal epithelium are thin, and the labia minora, clitoris, uterus, and ovaries decrease in size.

Many hormonal changes occur in the "perimenopausal" period (see FIG. 169–2). Regular menstrual cycles may continue up to the menopause. However, the cycles may become shorter, due to a shortened follicular phase, with increased FSH and decreased estradiol and progesterone levels in comparison to normal ovulatory cycles. Cycles may become quite variable in length, with some being ovulatory and other being anovulatory. Such changes must be due to decreasing ovarian follicular activity, but a few viable appearing oocytes have been observed in the ovaries of postmenopausal women.

Circulating LH and FSH levels are greatly increased in postmenopausal women, with the ratio of FSH to LH typically being > 1 (in terms of mIU/mL) because of decreased negative feedback by estradiol. Obviously, estrogen levels are markedly reduced. Androgen levels are also decreased, but only slightly, because the stroma of the postmenopausal ovary (as well as the adrenal) continues to secrete substantial amounts of androgen. These androgens are converted to estrogens in the periphery, especially in fat cells and skin. This peripheral conversion of androgens accounts for most circulating estrogen found in postmenopausal women (see also MENOPAUSE in Ch. 171).

170. AMENORRHEA AND ABNORMAL GENITAL BLEEDING

AMENORRHEA

Absence of menstruation, ie, either lack of menarche or cessation of menses.

Normal menstruation: By definition, the first day of menstrual flow is day 1 of the cycle. The interval is 28 ± 3 days for 65% of women, with a range of 18 to 40 days; once a menstrual pattern has been established the variation does not normally exceed 5 days. The average duration of menstrual flow is 5 ± 2 days with a blood loss averaging 130 mL (range 13 to 300 mL), usually heavier on the 2nd day. A saturated pad or tampon absorbs 20 to 30 mL.

Amenorrhea indicates failure of hypothalamic-pituitary-gonadal interaction to produce cyclic changes in the endometrium resulting in menses and thus may indicate an abnormality at any level of the reproductive tract. It is important to remember that amenorrhea is merely a sign, potentially of any of a large number of disorders involving several organ systems. Amenorrhea is **physiologic** *when it occurs in the prepubertal girl, during pregnancy and early lactation, and after the menopause.* At any other time it should be considered **pathologic**. It is traditional to categorize amenorrhea as **primary** (*the absence of menarche by age 16*) or **secondary** (*the absence of menstruation for 3 mo or more in women with past menses*) as noted above. However, such categorization may lead to diagnostic omissions and should not be considered in the evaluation of the amenorrheic woman.

Menarche may be delayed physiologically until the age of 18 yr. **Physiologic delay** must always be a diagnosis of exclusion. Evaluation is indicated in girls with no evidence of puberty by age 13 and in those in whom 5 or more years passes from the onset of pubertal development without menarche. Girls in whom evaluation as outlined below is normal should be reassured and followed at 3- to 6-mo intervals for pubertal progression. Although some physicians suggest use of exogenous progestins and/or estrogens to induce cyclic bleeding, this is unnecessary once normalcy of the outflow genital tract is established. Additionally, continued administration of sex steroids can obscure both initiation of menses and pathologic processes.

Clinical Evaluation

Even subtle hormonal alterations may be manifested by symptoms and signs. Central to the diagnostic evaluation is the history and physical examination with regard to the influence of altered hormonal secretion on the pubertal process and secondary sexual characteristics. Patients should be questioned for evidence of psychologic disturbances, dietary and exercise habits, lifestyle, environmental stresses, a family history of genetic anomalies, and abnormal growth and development. Patients should also be asked about the presence of any signs of increased androgen secretion **(hyperandrogenism)**, especially **hirsutism,** which may be defined as *an increase in sexually stimulated hair.* **Virilization** refers to *an increase in masculine secondary sexual characteristics* **(masculinization)**, including hirsutism, temporal balding, voice deepening, increased muscle mass, clitoromegaly, and increased libido, and to a decrease in feminine secondary sexual characteristics **(defeminization)**, including decreased breast size and vaginal atrophy. In addition, any history of **galactorrhea,** defined as *nonpuerperal secretion of milk or lactation*, should be sought.

Although the entire physical examination is important, special emphasis should be placed on evaluating (1) body dimensions and habitus, (2) the extent and distribution of body hair, (3) breast development and secretions, and (4) the genitalia. In normal individuals the arm span is similar to the height, while in hypogonadal individuals the span is typically > 2 in. (5 cm) greater than the height. The distribution and quantity of hair should be considered in light of the family history. **Hypertrichosis,** *the excessive growth of hair on the extremities, head, and back*, must not be mistaken for true hirsutism and virilization. Some hypertrichosis is not uncommon in women of Mediterranean descent, while any facial hair growth in the relatively hairless and androgen-insensitive Oriental woman may require thorough evaluation. The extent of hirsutism should be recorded, preferably by photographs. It is most practical only to grade facial hirsutism (since this is generally the reason the patient seeks aid) from 0 to 4+, giving 1+ each for excess chin, upper lip, or sideburn hair, and 4+ for a full beard.

The breasts should be inspected and development noted according to the method of Tanner (see FIG. 170–1). Any breast secretion should be elicited by applying pressure to all sections of the breast beginning at the base and working up toward the nipple while the patient is seated. Secretions should be examined microscopically for the

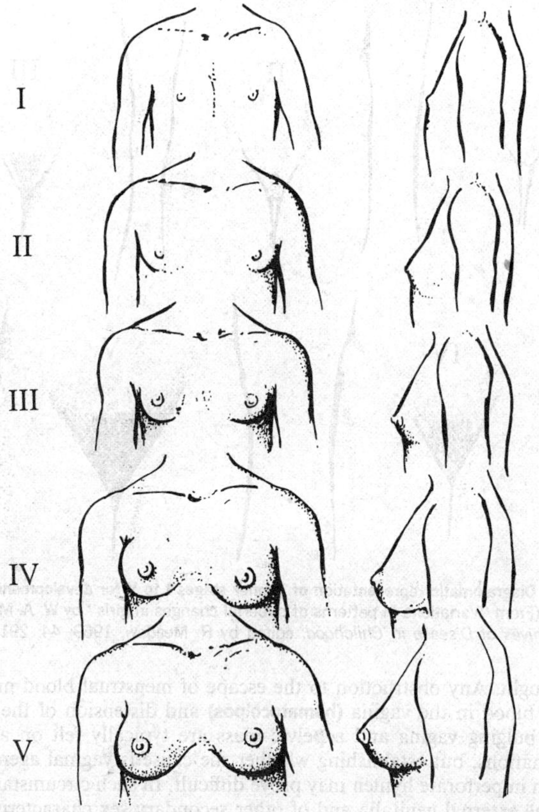

FIG. 170–1. Diagrammatic representation of Tanner stages I to V of human breast maturation. (From "Variations in patterns of pubertal changes in girls" by W. A. Marshall and J. M. Tanner, in *Archives of Disease in Childhood,* edited by R. Meadow, 1969; 44: 291–303. Used with permission.)

presence of thick-walled, perfectly round fat globules of varying sizes, proving the discharge is milk.

Lastly, the female genitalia should be examined carefully because they are sensitive indicators of hormonal milieu. The stage of pubic hair development should be noted (see FIG. 170–2). Since the sensitivity of the genitalia to androgens decreases in time from the early stages of fetal development to the adult individual, the extent of any virilization is important. The most marked changes, fusion of the labia and enlargement of the clitoris (with or without formation of a penile urethra) are observed in women exposed to androgens during the first 3 mo of their fetal development and in patients with congenital adrenal hyperplasia, hermaphroditism, and drug-induced virilization (see Ch. 91). Significant development of clitoromegaly postnatally requires marked hormonal stimulation and, in the absence of a history of intake of exogenous steroids, strongly implicates an androgen-secreting tumor. Estrogen-induced change becomes apparent with the development of the labia minora at puberty.

In the remainder of the pelvic examination, overt anomalies of müllerian duct derivatives, including imperforate hymen, vaginal and uterine aplasia, and vaginal septae

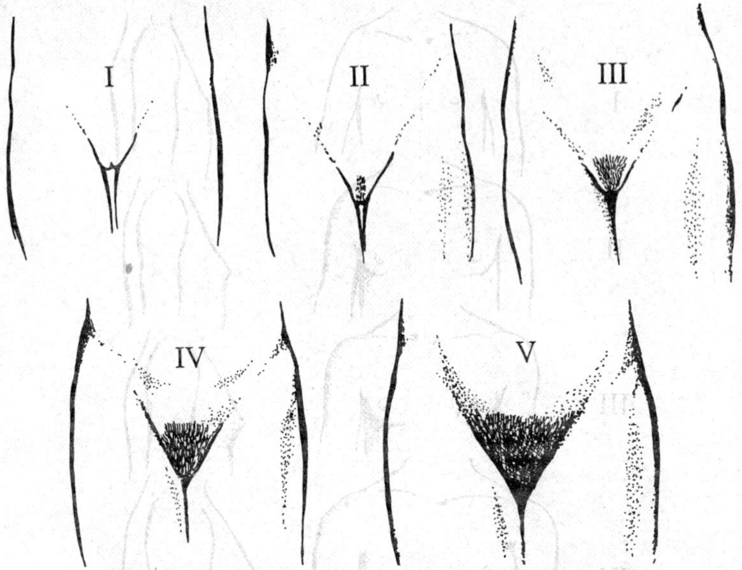

FIG. 170–2. Diagrammatic representation of Tanner stages I to V for development of human pubic hair in the girl. (From "Variations in patterns of pubertal changes in girls" by W. A. Marshall and J. M. Tanner, in *Archives of Disease in Childhood*, edited by R. Meadow, 1969; 44: 291–303. Used with permission.)

should be sought. Any obstruction to the escape of menstrual blood may lead to the collection of blood in the vagina **(hematocolpos)** and distension of the uterus **(hematometria)**. A bulging vagina and a pelvic mass are typically felt on abdominal and rectal examinations, but establishing whether the cause is vaginal agenesis, a vaginal septum, or an imperforate hymen may prove difficult. In such circumstances the development of the external genitalia and of other secondary sex characteristics is normal (because of normal ovarian function), but the presence of associated urinary tract and skeletal abnormalities is frequent (about 15 to 40%) in the first 2 instances. The external genitalia also appear normal in testicular feminization, but pubic and axillary hair is decreased, breast development is incomplete, and the vagina is of variable length with no identifiable cervix or uterus. Bimanual palpation can also document the existence of pelvic pathology, including tumors. Visual inspection of the quality of the vaginal mucosa and the cervical mucus is important because of their exquisite sensitivity to estrogen. Under the influence of estrogen, the vaginal mucosa progresses during sexual maturation from a tissue with a shiny, bright red appearance with sparse, thin secretions to a dull, gray-pink rugated surface with copious, thick secretions.

The history and physical examination should permit classification of the patients into the categories listed in TABLE 170–1. The various disorders of sexual differentiation and the physiologic and pathologic end-organ causes are often apparent on inspection. The stigma of **Turner's syndrome,** for example, including short stature of < 63 in., shield-like chest, webbed neck, short 4th metacarpals and metatarsals, hypoplastic nails, multiple pigmented nevi, and congenital heart disease generally make the diagnosis, which may be confirmed by karyotype (XO) (see GONADAL DYSGENESIS [TURNER'S SYNDROME] under SYNDROMES ASSOCIATED WITH SEX CHROMOSOME ABERRATIONS in Ch. 203). In male pseudohermaphrodites and in women with mülle-

TABLE 170–1. CLINICAL CATEGORIZATION OF AMENORRHEA

I. Physiologic causes
- A. Prepuberty
- B. Pregnancy
- C. Postmenopause

II. Chronic anovulation
- A. Due to CNS-hypothalamic-pituitary dysfunction
- B. Due to inappropriate feedback (ie, polycystic ovary syndrome)
- C. Due to thyroid and adrenal disorders

III. Ovarian failure

IV. Pathologic end-organ
- A. Gestational trophoblastic disease
- B. Asherman's syndrome

V. Disorders of sexual differentiation
- A. Müllerian agenesis and dysgenesis
- B. Gonadal dysgenesis
- C. Male pseudohermaphroditism

rian abnormalities, the abnormal genitalia should raise suspicions. Individuals with suspected intersex disorders should have a karyotype obtained (see INTERSEX STATES in Ch. 187). Likewise, pregnancy and gestational trophoblastic disease may be suspected and confirmed by measuring human chorionic gonadotropin. In women with amenorrhea developing following curettage or acute endometritis, the possibility of intrauterine adhesions or synechiae **(Asherman's syndrome)** must be entertained. Without laboratory studies it may be impossible to distinguish individuals with chronic anovulation from those with ovarian failure.

A **progestational challenge** can assess the competence of the outflow tract and the level of endogenous estrogens. Parenteral progesterone in oil (100 to 200 mg) is given or orally active medroxyprogesterone acetate (10 mg for 5 days). Within 10 days after conclusion of progestational medication, the patient will or will not bleed. Any bleeding excludes the possibility of Asherman's syndrome in most patients and suggests strongly, but does not confirm, the diagnosis of anovulation. If bleeding does not occur, orally active estrogen, such as conjugated estrogens 2.5 mg/day for 21 days, with the addition of 10 mg oral medroxyprogesterone acetate for the last 5 of those days will produce bleeding in the absence of a uterine abnormality. TB affecting the endometrium and Asherman's syndrome may preclude bleeding, although a hysterosalpingogram and hysteroscopy may be required for definitive diagnosis, since some patients continue to have cyclic bleeding.

Laboratory Studies

Basal levels of serum LH, FSH, and prolactin should be obtained in all women with amenorrhea. LH and FSH levels will show 1 of 4 patterns:

1. **A hypogonadotropic pattern** (LH and FSH both < 10 mIU/mL of the 2nd International Reference Preparation of human Menopausal Gonadotropin) is found in individuals with panhypopituitarism, isolated gonadotropin deficiency (who may also present with anosmia, color blindness, cleft lip or other midline defects as Kallman's syndrome), anorexia nervosa, amenorrhea-galactorrhea, and severe hypothalamic chronic anovulation.

2. **A normogonadotropic pattern** (LH and FSH both 7 to 20 mIU/mL with at least one ≥ 10 mIU/mL) includes women with hypothalamic chronic anovulation and, less frequently, inappropriate steroid feedback (ie, polycystic ovary syndrome).

3. **An inappropriate increase in the LH to FSH ratio** to > 2 with LH > 20 mIU/mL, includes women with chronic anovulation due to inappropriate feedback (a typical finding in polycystic ovary syndrome) and rarely testicular feminization. Such levels may also be seen at the time of the midcycle LH surge (in which case menses will occur 2 wk later), in pregnant women, and in those with trophoblastic disease (since immunoassay determinations of LH cross-react with those of HCG).

4. **A hypergonadotropic pattern** (LH > 20 and FSH > 40 mIU/mL) is suggestive of ovarian "failure." As discussed subsequently, ovarian "failure" may be reversible in some instances. The presence of elevated FSH levels in a young amenorrheic woman indicates the need for a karyotype.

Basal prolactin levels are elevated in perhaps 1/3 of women with amenorrhea. Because prolactin levels are increased by nonspecific stressful stimuli, sleep, and food ingestion, an elevated value (generally > 20 to 30 ng/mL, depending on the laboratory) should be repeated before more extensive testing. Prolactin is typically increased by a number of pharmacologic agents as well, including phenothiazines, L-dopa, reserpine, and oral contraceptive agents. If either galactorrhea or persistent hyperprolactinemia is present, or thyroid dysfunction is suspected, thyroid function studies are warranted to rule out primary hypothyroidism, with elevated TSH levels being diagnostic. In primary hypothyroidism, increased secretion of TRH stimulates increased prolactin as well as increased TSH release.

X-rays of the sella turcica are indicated in euthyroid women with hyperprolactinemia of < 100 ng/mL to rule out large pituitary tumors (see Ch. 88). Sellar x-rays should not be obtained in hypothyroid individuals with mild hyperprolactinemia and amenorrhea-galactorrhea because any enlargement of the sella turcica will return to normal following appropriate thyroid hormone replacement. Views of the sella turcica are also indicated whenever gonadotropin concentrations are low, regardless of the prolactin level, to rule out a pituitary neoplasm.

Pituitary testing, especially of adrenal and thyroid function, is warranted whenever panhypopituitarism is suspected or a large tumor is present. CT scanning of the sella will determine if the patient has any suprasellar extension of a pituitary neoplasm or if she suffers from the **empty sella syndrome,** in which the sella turcica is enlarged but has been largely replaced by CSF. Formal visual field testing is indicated whenever a pituitary neoplasm is ≥ 10 mm in diameter on x-ray or there is evidence of suprasellar extension (see Ch. 88).

In evaluating the anovulatory woman with masculinization (hyperandrogenic women), the aim of the evaluation is the exclusion of serious disorders. In most cases, this can be done easily at the bedside and confirmed with the aid of laboratory tests. Inappropriate gonadotropin secretion with elevated LH and low to normal FSH levels is commonly present, but both may be in the normal range. Total circulating androgen levels may be elevated but need not be because of altered metabolic clearance and decreased levels of sex hormone binding globulin **(SHBG),** which binds androgens in plasma. **Hirsutism** may also result because of increased sensitivity of the pilosebaceous unit (ie, hair follicle) to normal quantities of androgen. It is now recognized that so-called "idiopathic" hirsutism results from increased conversion of testosterone to dihydrotestosterone (DHT) within the hair follicle.

Initial laboratory evaluation of hirsute women should include measurement of serum testosterone (T) and dehydroepiandrosterone sulfate **(DHEA-S)** concentrations. T levels > 200 ng/dL should lead to investigation for an androgen-producing tumor, most commonly of ovarian origin. DHEA-S levels twice as high as the upper limit of the normal range for the laboratory should lead to evaluation for an adrenal neoplasm. There is no need for extensive testing if T or DHEA-S are not markedly elevated, because the possibility of a serious cause has been eliminated. Likewise, the presence of hirsutism obviates the need to measure biologically free T. The measurement of 3α-

androstanediol glucuronide has been suggested to determine if there is increased metabolic activity within the pilosebaceous unit in response to the circulating androgens. 3α-Androstanediol glucuronide has been shown to be elevated in all hirsute women. Consequently, its measurement adds little to the physical examination and is not recommended.

If T and DHEA-S measurements are obtainable, there is no need to measure urinary 17-KS and 17-hydroxycorticosteroid excretion. It is difficult to obtain complete 24-h urine collections, and results are inconclusive. 17-KS secretion is a poor indicator of testosterone secretion and of ovarian androgen production. Major sources of urinary 17-KS are secreted by the adrenal gland and, if 17-KS excretion is > 20 mg/24 h, the source of excess androgens is probably adrenal. Measurement of 17-hydroxycorticosteroid excretion is of no value in the diagnosis of androgen excess, although it is elevated in most cases of Cushing's syndrome (ie, adrenocortical hyperfunction). Likewise, the use of dexamethasone suppression and of stimulation with ACTH and HCG is not of consistent value in evaluating the hirsute woman. Individuals with suspected Cushing's syndrome should be screened for cortisol excess as discussed in Ch. 91.

Hirsute women with a history and examination suggestive of **congenital adrenal hyperplasia** (**CAH**; most commonly due to 21-hydroxylase deficiency) can have the diagnosis confirmed by the presence of elevated levels of 17-hydroxyprogesterone **(17-OHP)** in the serum or pregnanetriol in the urine. Patients with severe hirsutism beginning during adolescence, high levels of T and/or DHEA-S, a strong family history of hirsutism, or hypertension are candidates for the measurement of 17-OHP. (Individuals with mild 21-hydroxylase deficiency generally present with heterosexual precocity and short stature with a masculinized habitus and failure to develop female secondary sexual characteristics and menstrual periods—see Ch. 91.) Basal levels of 17-OHP > 3 ng/mL but < 8 ng/mL require ACTH stimulation testing to make a distinction between CAH and other disorders such as polycystic ovary syndrome **(PCO)**. Levels > 8 ng/mL are virtually diagnostic of CAH. Many protocols for ACTH testing have been utilized. A plasma level of 17-OHP > 3 ng/mL 15 min after IV administration of exogenous ACTH at a dose of 10 $\mu g/m^2$ body surface area in a patient suppressed with dexamethasone (2 mg orally at midnight before morning testing) is diagnostic of 21-hydroxylase deficiency.

Sonography, CT, and selective adrenal and ovarian vein angiography with androgen measurement are useful in attempting to localize any androgen-producing neoplasm prior to surgical excision. Selective adrenal and ovarian vein sampling should be performed only in specialized centers familiar with this procedure. The neoplasms should be inspected pathologically at the time of surgery to assess malignant potential.

CHRONIC ANOVULATORY DISORDERS

Chronic anovulation may be viewed as a steady state in which the monthly rhythm manifested by menses is no longer operational. The term chronic anovulation further implies that functional ovarian follicles remain and that cyclic ovulation can be induced or reinitiated with appropriate management. Chronic anovulation is the most frequent form of amenorrhea when there are no anatomic abnormalities of the target organs precluding menstruation (see Table 170–2). Selected syndromes are discussed in this chapter. Other disorders listed in Table 170–2 are discussed elsewhere in The Manual. Rational and appropriate management can be instituted only after the etiology of the anovulation has been determined. Unfortunately, until the mechanisms for the several forms of chronic anovulation are better understood, the anovulation can be interrupted only by transient and nonspecific ovulation induction in a large percentage of affected individuals.

TABLE 170–2. CLASSIFICATION OF CHRONIC ANOVULATION

I. Chronic anovulation of supra-pituitary origin
- A. Hypothalamic chronic anovulation (HCA)
  1. Psychogenic
  2. Exercise-associated
  3. Associated with malnutrition
  4. Of mixed or unknown etiology
- B. Anorexia nervosa
- C. Pseudocyesis (ie, false pregnancy)
- D. Forms of isolated gonadotropin deficiency

II. Chronic anovulation of pituitary origin
- A. Hypopituitarism
- B. Pituitary tumors
- C. Forms of isolated gonadotropin deficiency

III. Chronic anovulation due to inappropriate feedback (ie, polycystic ovary syndrome)
- A. Excessive extraglandular estrogen production (ie, obesity)
- B. Abnormal buffering involving sex hormone-binding globulin (including liver disease)
- C. Functional androgen excess (adrenal or ovarian)
- D. Neoplasms producing androgens or estrogens
- E. Neoplasms producing chorionic gonadotropin

IV. Chronic anovulation due to other endocrine or metabolic dysfunctions
- A. Adrenal hyperfunction
  1. Cushing's syndrome and disease
  2. Congenital adrenal hyperplasia (female pseudohermaphroditism)
- B. Thyroid dysfunction
  1. Hyperthyroidism
  2. Hypothyroidism
- C. Prolactin and/or growth hormone excess
  1. Hypothalamic dysfunction
  2. Pituitary dysfunction (micro- and macroadenomas)
  3. Drug-induced
- D. Malnutrition

(Modified from "The Reproductive Age: Chronic Anovulation" by R.W. Rebar in *The Ovary,* edited by G.B. Serra. Published by Raven Press, New York, 1983. Copyright 1983 by Raven Press. Used with permission.)

HYPOTHALAMIC CHRONIC ANOVULATION (HCA)

Evidence suggests that HCA is a heterogeneous group of disorders with similar manifestations. Emotional and physical stresses, diet, body composition, exercise, environment, and other unrecognized factors contribute in varying proportions to the anovulation. (Anorexia nervosa is a related but distinct entity discussed in EATING DISORDERS in Ch. 202.) These disorders are characterized by low to normal levels of gonadotropins and relative hypoestrogenism. Psychologic counseling and/or a change in the lifestyle of the individual is often effective in inducing ovulation. Ovulation may also be induced with clomiphene citrate. If these measures are ineffective, then treatment with human menopausal gonadotropin and human chorionic gonadotropin **(HMG-HCG)**, or with gonadotropin-releasing hormone **(GnRH)** given in a pulsatile fashion by a reproductive endocrinologist may be required. Hormonal treatment of patients not desiring pregnancy is controversial. Some authorities believe only periodic observation is indicated, but others advocate the use of exogenous estrogens supplemented cyclically with an oral progestin to prevent osteoporosis in those women with

low concentrations of circulating estrogen. An oral regimen of 0.625 to 1.25 mg conjugated estrogens, 20 μg ethinyl estradiol, or 0.5 to 1.0 mg micronized estradiol-17β for the first 25 days of each month with oral medroxyprogesterone acetate 5 to 10 mg added for days 16 to 25 can be used.

CHRONIC ANOVULATION DUE TO PITUITARY DYSFUNCTION

Hypopituitarism, pituitary tumors, and forms of isolated gonadotropin deficiency are discussed in Ch. 88. Following appropriate therapy for the pituitary dysfunction, ovulation can be induced if pregnancy is desired. Gonadal stimulation with HMG-HCG is required if the pituitary no longer produces gonadotropins.

CHRONIC ANOVULATION DUE TO INAPPROPRIATE FEEDBACK SIGNALS

A heterogeneous group of disorders with great clinical and biochemical variability in which chronic anovulation, because of inappropriate feedback signals to the hypothalamic-pituitary unit, appears to be the common denominator. The most prominent example is **polycystic ovary syndrome (PCO; Stein-Leventhal syndrome).** Included are such disorders as Cushing's syndrome, mild congenital adrenal hyperplasia, virilizing tumors of adrenal or ovarian origin, hyper- and hypothyroidism, and obesity, all of which are discussed in greater detail elsewhere in THE MANUAL.

Symptoms and Signs

Typically, patients present with amenorrhea, hirsutism, and obesity, but affected individuals may instead complain of irregular, profuse uterine bleeding (because of endometrial hyperplasia that results from unopposed estrogenic stimulation—see under ABNORMAL GENITAL BLEEDING, below), have no hirsutism, and be of normal height. Current evidence indicates that the hypothalamic-pituitary unit is intact, but that a functional derangement resulting in abnormal gonadotropin secretion is present. Excess androgen from any source or increased extraglandular conversion of androgens to estrogens can lead to the constellation of findings observed. In all these disorders, the ovaries may be enlarged with smooth and thickened capsules, or they may be normal in size. Typically, the ovaries contain many 2- to 6-mm follicular cysts, and thecal hyperplasia surrounding the granulosa cells is present. Large cysts containing atretic cells may be present.

Diagnosis

In PCO, the irregular menses, mild obesity, and hirsutism usually begin in the pubertal years and generally worsen with time. Although patients may present with either primary or secondary amenorrhea (as well as uterine bleeding), the common feature is that all patients are clinically well estrogenized with abundant cervical mucus on examination. LH levels are typically elevated with relatively low and constant FSH levels, but both may be in the normal range. Generally, levels of most circulating androgens tend to be mildly elevated. Hirsutism should be evaluated as described above. The aim of the diagnostic evaluation is to discover an etiology (eg, a neoplasm) that can be treated definitively. PCO itself is a benign disorder.

Treatment

No ideal therapy for either PCO or hirsutism exists. Patients may require therapy to induce ovulation if pregnancy is desired and to prevent estrogen-induced endometrial hyperplasia. The treatment selected must be individualized to the needs and desires of the patient.

In the anovulatory woman who is not hirsute and does not desire pregnancy, intermittent progestin (eg, medroxyprogesterone acetate 5 to 10 mg orally for 10 to 14 days q

1 to 2 mo) or oral contraceptives (if she is under age 35, does not smoke, and has no other significant risk factors [see ORAL CONTRACEPTIVES in Ch. 174]) should be given to reduce the increased risks of endometrial hyperplasia and carcinoma present in such a woman with unopposed estrogen. An endometrial biopsy should be obtained before initiating medical therapy in any woman with a prolonged history of anovulatory bleeding and in all affected women over age 35. Women using intermittent progestins should be cautioned about the need for contraception because of the possible (although unproven) association of these agents with birth defects if taken during early pregnancy.

In the anovulatory woman who is hirsute and does not desire pregnancy treatment differs, but is similar to, that offered to the ovulatory hirsute woman. The use of physical treatment modalities (including bleaching, electrolysis, plucking, waxing, and depilation) should be encouraged. No pharmacologic modality is ideal or completely effective, and the various pharmacologic agents have not been compared directly in controlled studies. **Oral contraceptive agents** are the first line of therapy for patients with mild hirsutism. These drugs suppress gonadotropin and steroid secretion and increase production of sex hormone binding globulin **(SHBG)**, thus reducing biologically active free testosterone levels. Unfortunately, several months are required to observe any effect, and that effect is often slight. All preparations seem to be equally efficacious. For the patient for whom oral contraceptives are undesired or contraindicated, continuous suppression with oral progestin (medroxyprogesterone acetate 5 to 20 mg/day) can be used. Side effects of progestin include mastodynia, bloating, and depression.

Cyproterone acetate, a potent progestational agent and an antiandrogen, appears to control hirsutism in 50 to 75% of affected women. It is used to treat hirsute women throughout the world except in the USA, where it has not been approved because of its propensity to cause breast cancer in beagle dogs and to cause fetal anomalies when given to pregnant rats. Cyproterone is generally used in a cyclic manner with ethinyl estradiol so that periodic withdrawal bleeding occurs. Contraception should be used. Significant side effects include decreased libido and mental depression.

Spironolactone, a mild diuretic which also inhibits the biosynthesis of androgen and competes with androgens for the androgen receptor in target tissues such as the hair follicle, has been used effectively to treat hirsutism at doses of 100 to 200 mg/day orally. Side effects have included initial diuresis and postural changes (including syncope and hypotension), mastodynia, and irregular uterine bleeding. This agent has not been approved for such use in the USA, and effects on a developing fetus are unknown. Thus, contraception should be used. Furthermore, the long-term effects of spironolactone remain unknown.

Glucocorticoids, used to achieve adrenal suppression, are not indicated in most hirsute women because no advantage of adrenal over ovarian suppression has been demonstrated and because the source of excess androgen in most hirsute women is largely ovarian. The potential hazards of adrenal steroids would seem to mitigate against their use except in patients with documented adrenal hyperfunction or enzyme defects in the steroidogenic pathway.

In the future, both GnRH agonists and antagonists may have potential in the treatment of hirsutism. These agents suppress gonadotropins and thus gonadal steroid secretion and produce what has been called a "medical oophorectomy." Effective topical antiandrogens also are being sought.

In women with PCO who desire pregnancy, clomiphene citrate 50 to 100 mg/day for 5 days remains the first choice with which to induce ovulation because of its simplicity and high success rate (75% ovulation rate; 35 to 40% pregnancy rate). Previous failure to induce ovulation with clomiphene should not contraindicate its use in the future. Other methods of ovulation induction used by endocrinologists include use of HMG-

HCG, human purified FSH (experimental), pulsatile administration of GnRH (experimental), and ovarian wedge resection. **Wedge resection** should be reserved for individuals in whom all other methods fail, there is a question of an ovarian tumor because of ovarian size or circulating androgen levels, and/or where fertility is not an issue (because pelvic adhesions can follow the surgery).

GALACTORRHEA

(See under ANTERIOR LOBE DISORDERS in Ch. 88)

PREMATURE OVARIAN FAILURE

(Premature Menopause)

Several disorders in which women under 40 yr of age present with symptoms and signs due to estrogen deficiency and have elevated circulating levels of gonadotropins (especially FSH) and low levels of estradiol. See TABLE 170–3 for the disorders presenting as ovarian failure.

Although the association between high levels of gonadotropin as observed in cas-

TABLE 170–3. CAUSES OF ELEVATED LEVELS OF GONADOTROPINS

I. Menopause

II. Physical causes
- A. Surgical extirpation of the gonads
- B. Irradiation of the gonads
- C. Viral agents
- D. Chemotherapeutic agents

III. Gonadotropin-producing neoplasms (rare)

IV. Chromosomal abnormalities
- A. Gonadal dysgenesis
  1. With stigmata of Turner's syndrome (45,XO)
  2. Pure (46,XX or 46,XY)
  3. Mixed
- B. Trisomy X with or without chromosomal mosaicism

V. Gonadotropin gonadal receptor and/or post-receptor defects (resistant ovary or savage syndrome)

VI. Defects in gonadotropin secretion
- A. Secretion of biologically inactive forms
- B. Defects in α or β subunits

VII. Enzymatic defects
- A. 17 α-Hydroxylase deficiency
- B. Galactosemia

VIII. Autoimmune disorders
- A. Polyglandular involving ovarian failure and any combination of thyroiditis, hypoadrenalism, hypoparathyroidism, diabetes mellitus, pernicious anemia, myasthenia gravis, vitiligo, and mucocutaneous candidiasis
- B. Isolated ovarian failure

IX. Congenital thymic aplasia

X. Idiopathic premature ovarian failure

trate and postmenopausal women with the absence of oocytes in the ovaries is very high, it is now clear that there are several rare circumstances in which high gonadotropin levels are found in women whose ovaries still contain viable follicles. Rare pregnancies have been reported in sexually active patients with hypergonadotropic hypogonadism during and following treatment with estrogens. Other patients have resumed regular menses and conceived after several years of hypergonadotropic amenorrhea.

All patients under age 35 in whom the diagnosis of ovarian failure has been made on the basis of elevated gonadotropins should have a karyotype determination. The presence of a Y chromosome requires laparotomy and excision of gonadal tissue to prevent the 25% incidence of malignant tumor formation occurring in such patients. Genetic evaluation is unnecessary in women presenting with elevated gonadotropin levels who are over age 35, because gonadal neoplasms have not been reported in these older women. They should be presumed to have premature menopause.

A number of cases of ovarian failure occur in association with other autoimmune disorders, including thyroiditis, hypoparathyroidism, hypoadrenalism, diabetes mellitus, rheumatoid arthritis, myasthenia gravis, and pernicious anemia. Some patients have been reported to have circulating antibodies to ovarian tissue (presumably to ovarian receptors for FSH). In view of these observations, in young women desiring pregnancy, blood tests to evaluate the possibility of an autoimmune disorder seem indicated. Such tests may also indicate which patients may develop other endocrine disorders with time. These tests should include measurement of serum calcium and phosphorus to rule out hypoparathyroidism, thyroid function tests and antibodies to rule out thyroiditis, and an AM cortisol to rule out hypoadrenalism. Also indicated are a CBC, sedimentation rate, total protein, albumin/globulin ratio, rheumatoid factor, and antinuclear antibody. Serum gonadotropin and estradiol levels can be determined weekly on 2 to 4 occasions. If LH levels are ever greater than FSH levels or if estradiol is ever > 50 pg/mL, then ovarian follicles should be present.

Ovulation induction with gonadotropins can be offered empirically, but any patients electing treatment must recognize that the possibility of pregnancy is very low.

ABNORMAL GENITAL BLEEDING

Abnormal uterine bleeding includes (1) excessive duration or amount of menstruation or both **(hypermenorrhea, menorrhagia)**, *(2) too frequent menstruation* **(polymenorrhea)**, *(3) nonmenstrual or intermenstrual bleeding* **(metrorrhagia)**, *and (4)* **postmenopausal bleeding**, *which denotes any bleeding occurring 6 mo or more following the last normal menstrual period at the menopause.*

Abnormal genital bleeding is due to organic causes in about 25% of patients; in the remainder there is a functional abnormality of the hypothalamic-pituitary-ovarian axis **(dysfunctional uterine bleeding)**. In considering the individual patient, age is the most important factor. Dysfunctional bleeding is much more common during the early reproductive years, while organic causes, including neoplasias of the genital tract, become more frequent with advancing age (see below).

Infancy and Childhood

Newborn girls may have some spotting for a few days because of stimulation of the endometrium in utero by estrogens produced by the placenta. Any other bleeding from the reproductive tract is rare in childhood and warrants investigation. Accidental traumatic lesions of the vulva and vagina are most common. Vaginitis (often as a result of a foreign body), prolapse of the urethral meatus, and tumors of the genital tract can

also present with bleeding. Ovarian tumors generally do not present with bleeding unless they are endocrinologically active.

Precocious puberty (see also Ch. 202) must always be considered in the differential diagnosis of bleeding in childhood and can be recognized in most cases by the development of secondary sexual characteristics. The cause for precocious development remains unknown in many cases but may be due to drug ingestion, CNS lesions, hypothyroidism, or adrenal or ovarian neoplasms.

Bleeding and vaginal discharge are the presenting symptoms in > 80% of cases of **vaginal adenosis** and **clear cell adenocarcinoma of the vagina and cervix**, lesions that have been linked to exposure to diethylstilbestrol **(DES)** in utero. These lesions are diagnosed by cytologic smear and colposcopically directed biopsy of suspicious areas. In the absence of malignancy, most lesions do not require treatment and the patients can be followed with periodic examinations.

Women of Reproductive Age

Hematologic disorders with abnormal clotting, whether primary (ie, idiopathic thrombocytopenia purpura, leukemia, bone marrow aplasia, hemolytic anemia) or secondary to systemic causes (ie, uremia, liver disease, anticoagulant therapy) can lead to abnormal bleeding throughout the reproductive years. Hematologic evaluation is indicated in adolescents and in others with a history suggestive of clotting disorders.

Complications of pregnancy are the most frequent organic causes of abnormal bleeding in women of reproductive age. Patients who present with symptoms of pregnancy or with a confirmed early pregnancy and uterine bleeding spontaneously abort the pregnancy in perhaps half the cases. Ectopic pregnancy and gestational trophoblastic disease are the most important entities to be considered in the differential diagnosis. These topics are discussed in Chs. 173 and 177. Endometritis and infected retained products of conception usually cause bleeding shortly after delivery or abortion but occasionally may present 2 wk or more later (see Ch. 180).

Endometriosis (see below) causes dysfunctional uterine bleeding in from 20 to 88% of affected women by unknown mechanisms.

Vulvar bleeding in the reproductive years is almost always due to trauma.

Vaginal lesions vary greatly and may cause bleeding during this time of life. Vaginitis causes bleeding more commonly in the child and in the postmenopausal woman because the vaginal mucosa is thinner then, but spotting may occur in severe cases during the reproductive years. Granulomatous tissue formed following surgery (especially hysterectomy) may also cause bleeding. Biopsy may be necessary to rule out malignancy. Although cauterization with silver nitrate or cryotherapy is sufficient to stop bleeding in most cases, surgical resection may be required for large lesions. Vaginal adenosis, which frequently presents with bleeding, was discussed above as a cause of bleeding in children. Malignant lesions of the vagina, which may also cause bleeding, are discussed in Ch. 173.

Cervical cancer (see Ch. 173) and several **benign cervical lesions** are associated with bleeding. Cervicitis only rarely causes bleeding, except in association with **ectropion of the cervix** (extension of columnar epithelium to the exposed portion of the cervix). Patients may complain of postcoital spotting, but the usual complaint is a vaginal discharge tinged with blood. Diagnosis and treatment are discussed in Ch. 171. Cervical polyps may present with intermenstrual or postcoital bleeding. Most are easily removed by merely twisting the polyp off at the pedicle. Endometrial polyps and submucosal myomas should be considered in the differential diagnosis. Condylomata accuminata of the cervix can cause bleeding and can be treated with cryotherapy, surgical resection, or laser therapy as discussed in Ch. 14.

Endometrial hyperplasia, a common cause of uterine bleeding, is discussed under Dysfunctional Uterine Bleeding, below.

Adenomyosis, *the benign invasion of endometrium into the myometrium*, is a common disorder that causes symptoms in only a small percentage of affected patients, most commonly late in the reproductive years. Menorrhagia and intermenstrual bleeding are the most common complaints, followed by nonspecific pelvic pain and bladder and rectal pressure. On pelvic examination, the uterus may feel enlarged, globular, and softer than normal; and there may be associated leiomyomas. Hysterectomy may be indicated for symptomatic relief in some patients.

Leiomyomas may be present in the uteri of as many as 40% of women by age 40, but in only a few women are they symptomatic. Any kind of bleeding abnormality can be caused by myomas. Hysterectomy is indicated for women in whom fertility is not an issue who are symptomatic, those with a uterus > 12 to 14 wk gestation in size, those in whom the uterus is increasing rapidly in size, and those with significant bleeding not controlled by medical methods.

Functional ovarian cysts are relatively common, and > 50% present with some form of menstrual irregularity, ranging from amenorrhea to menorrhagia. In young women cystic adnexal masses may disappear spontaneously. Adnexal masses of > 5 cm which persist for > 1 mo require surgical exploration to exclude a neoplasm. Although any ovarian tumor may cause abnormal uterine bleeding, bleeding is common only in endocrinologically active neoplasms. Treatment of these neoplasms is discussed in Ch. 173.

Contraceptives, including birth control pills, the IUD, and progestins may cause abnormal bleeding. It is unclear if tubal ligation is followed by an increased incidence of menstrual irregularities. These issues are discussed in Ch. 174.

Thyroid dysfunction may also be associated with menstrual irregularity. Although oligomenorrhea and amenorrhea are more common, menorrhagia can result.

Postmenopausal Bleeding

Gynecologic malignancies must be ruled out in any postmenopausal woman presenting with genital bleeding (see Ch. 173). Of the benign conditions associated with postmenopausal bleeding, the most frequent are atrophic vaginitis (see Ch. 171), an atrophic endometrium, endometrial polyps, and endometrial hyperplasia. Why a patient with atrophic endometrium bleeds is not clear. Endometrial polyps need no further treatment after diagnostic curettage but need to be observed for possible recurrence. Hyperplastic endometrial changes should generally be treated by hysterectomy in older women (see below).

DYSFUNCTIONAL UTERINE BLEEDING (DUB)

(Functional Uterine Bleeding)

Abnormal uterine bleeding not associated with tumor, inflammation, or pregnancy.

DUB, the most common cause for abnormal uterine bleeding, must be a diagnosis of exclusion. It occurs most commonly at the extremes of reproductive life; > 50% of the cases of DUB occur in women over age 45, and 20% are seen in adolescents. Although DUB may occur in association with either ovulatory or anovulatory cycles, > 70% of episodes are associated with anovulation. Thus, DUB is common in women with polycystic ovary syndrome **(PCO)**. The bleeding in anovulatory women is generally the result of stimulation of the endometrium with unopposed estrogen and may result in **endometrial hyperplasia**. The endometrium, thickened by the estrogen, then sloughs incompletely and irregularly, and bleeding becomes irregular, prolonged, and sometimes profuse. Abnormal bleeding may also occur in women taking some form of exogenous estrogen. In ovulatory cycles the abnormal bleeding is generally due to luteal phase abnormalities.

History and physical examination cannot distinguish patients with abnormal uterine

bleeding who have endometrial hyperplasia from those who do not. Individuals aged 35 or more, those with PCO and/or a prolonged history of anovulatory bleeding, and obese and nulliparous women should have an endometrial biopsy before initiation of medical therapy because such women are at increased risk for endometrial carcinoma (see Ch. 173). A Hct and Hb should be done on each patient presenting with abnormal bleeding to evaluate the chronicity and severity of the bleeding.

Treatment

Treatment varies with the age of the patient, the extent of the bleeding, pathologic assessment of the endometrium, and the patient's desires. Even acute episodes of profuse bleeding in anovulatory women can generally be treated by giving 1 combination oral contraceptive pill q 6 h for 5 to 7 days. Bleeding should stop in 12 to 24 h, but patients will have heavy bleeding, often with cramping, 2 to 4 days after stopping therapy. Recurrence is prevented by giving combination oral contraceptive agents cyclically for at least 3 mo. Should spontaneous cyclic menses not resume and pregnancy not be desired, the patient can be treated with cyclic progestin (medroxyprogesterone acetate 5 to 10 mg orally for 10 to 14 days each month). Uterine curettage is indicated in patients failing to respond to hormonal therapy (as indicated in a subsequent biopsy) and in those in whom irregular bleeding persists. If pregnancy is desired, then ovulation can be induced as discussed in treatment of PCO, above.

An alternative approach to the treatment of an acute episode of anovulatory bleeding is the administration of conjugated estrogens 25 mg IV q 4 h up to 3 doses until bleeding abates. Progestin therapy (medroxyprogesterone acetate 5 to 10 mg orally for 10 days) should be started simultaneously. Following cessation of therapy, withdrawal bleeding will result. The patient can then be treated with oral contraceptive agents for at least 3 cycles.

For individuals with anovulatory bleeding without a profuse bleeding episode, treatment with cyclic oral contraceptive agents or progestin can be offered if pregnancy is not desired. Ovulation induction with clomiphene citrate can be offered those desiring pregnancy. Similarly, clomiphene citrate can be used to treat luteal dysfunction. HCG 2500 to 5000 IU IM q 2nd or 3rd day beginning with the midcycle increase in basal body temperature and progesterone 12.5 mg/day IM in oil or 25 mg bid as rectal or vaginal suppositories have also been used to treat luteal dysfunction.

Treatment of women with endometrial hyperplasia must be individualized based on the pathologic findings, the age of the patient, and the patient's reproductive desires. Women with adenomatous and atypical adenomatous hyperplasia are most easily treated with hysterectomy regardless of age because of the risk of subsequent adenocarcinoma of the uterus. A fractional D & C should be performed prior to any therapy in any women with atypical hyperplasia on biopsy to rule out coexisting carcinoma. In women who are poor surgical risks and in those who desire to preserve future fertility, medroxyprogesterone acetate 20 to 40 mg/day orally can be given for 3 to 6 mo. Patients can then undergo repeat endometrial biopsy. If the biopsy indicates resolution of the hyperplasia, patients may be cycled with medroxyprogesterone acetate (5 to 10 mg/day orally for 10 to 14 days each month) or treated with clomiphene citrate to induce ovulation if pregnancy is desired. Women with more benign cystic hyperplasia can generally be treated with cyclic medroxyprogesterone acetate but again should undergo repeat biopsy in about 3 mo.

ENDOMETRIOSIS

The presence of endometrial tissue in abnormal locations, is common in women of reproductive age. Intra-abdominal endometriosis may be due to retrograde flow of menstrual tissue through the fallopian tubes, but the finding of endometriosis at dis-

tant sites (eg, nasal mucosa and lung) suggests vascular or lymphatic transport of endometrial fragments. Another possible cause is the transformation of coelomic epithelium into endometrial-like glands.

Symptoms, Signs, and Diagnosis

Since it is estimated that 25 to 50% of infertile women have endometriosis, it should be suspected in any woman with infertility. Dysmenorrhea, particularly beginning after several years of pain-free menses, and dyspareunia may occur. Suprapubic or rectal pain may be present, and abnormal bleeding is frequent, although the cause is unknown.

Examination may be normal or may reveal visible lesions on the vulva or cervix, in the vagina, in the umbilicus, and in surgical scars. There may be a retroverted and fixed uterus, enlarged ovaries, or uterosacral nodularity. In the absence of external visible lesions, the diagnosis can only be made by laparoscopy. Staging of the extent of the disease into mild, moderate, and severe forms is important in evaluating response to therapy and in communicating the seriousness of the disorder to other physicians.

Treatment

Treatment is controversial and must be individualized, depending on the patient's age, symptoms, desire for pregnancy, and extent of disease. In general, treatment consists of medically suppressing ovarian function to arrest the activity of the aberrant endometrial implants, surgical resection of as much of the tissue as possible, or a combination of the two. There is question as to whether the fertility rate is improved by treatment of mild or minimal endometriosis. For young women in whom mild endometriosis is accidentally discovered, suppression with danazol 400 to 800 mg/day, medroxyprogesterone acetate 10 to 20 mg/day, or continuous oral contraceptive pills for 4 to 6 mo followed by cyclic oral contraceptive pills may be helpful in preventing proliferation of the endometriosis. Experimental protocols are now evaluating the effectiveness of GnRH agonists in suppressing ovarian function.

Side effects of suppressive medical therapy are unpleasant. The most common side effects of danazol, some of which occur in > 80% of users, are weight gain, fluid retention, fatigue, decreased breast size, acne, oily skin, hot flushes, muscle cramps, and emotional lability. When oral contraceptives are given continuously, patients complain of bloating, weight gain, breast tenderness, chloasma, and irregular bleeding. Continuous progestin therapy may cause breast tenderness, bloating, depression, and irregular bleeding. With oral contraceptives and progestins, irregular bleeding can generally be controlled by the addition of oral 20 μg ethinyl estradiol during the episode of bleeding only.

Moderate to severe cases are most effectively treated by surgical removal of as many implants as possible while preserving reproductive potential (so-called "conservative surgery"). Great care must be taken to prevent adhesion formation following surgery. The success of surgery in relieving infertility is directly related to the severity of the endometriosis. Patients with moderate disease will achieve pregnancy about 60% of the time, while only 35% become pregnant following surgery for severe disease. There is growing support for use of danazol for 2 to 3 mo prior to conservative surgery. The use of suppressive medical therapy after surgery is also controversial but seems to be of benefit when used for 3 to 6 mo immediately following surgery for severe endometriosis. If pregnancy does not occur within 2 yr of surgery, the chances of it ever occurring are poor. Repeat surgery or surgery for recurrent endometriosis is very unlikely to be followed by pregnancy. If pregnancy is not an issue in the symptomatic patient, "radical" surgery consisting of hysterectomy and bilateral salpingo-oophorectomy can be performed. If all the endometriosis can be removed, consideration can be given to preserving one uninvolved ovary with the understanding there is a small risk for recurrent disease.

171. COMMON GYNECOLOGIC PROBLEMS

(See also Ch. 170)

PELVIC PAIN

Pelvic pain is a common complaint. Its nature and intensity may fluctuate, and its cause is often obscure. Pelvic pain may originate in genital or extragenital organs; in some cases no pathology can be demonstrated. Causes include intense muscular contractions or cramps, inflammation or direct irritation of nerves, and psychogenic factors. Both smooth and skeletal muscles can produce pain by strong or sustained contractions that result from overdistention or obstruction of a hollow viscus, ischemia, or tetany. Nerves can be irritated by acute or chronic trauma, fibrosis, pressure, or intraperitoneal irritation. Psychogenic factors can cause pain or aggravate minor aches. Often pelvic pain is due to multiple causes.

In evaluating acute lower abdominal pain, prompt decisions must be made about which conditions are surgical emergencies; ie, twisted ovarian cyst, ectopic gestation, ruptured tubo-ovarian abscess, appendicitis, and bowel perforation. A ruptured corpus luteum cyst and pelvic inflammation are usually treated medically.

The cause of pelvic pain can often be established by a careful history, with special attention to type of discomfort, distribution and radiation of the pain, time and suddenness of onset, circumstances at onset, duration of pain, associated symptoms, relation to various activities such as movement or defecation, frequency of recurrence, and relationship to the menstrual cycle, sleep, coitus, eating, and micturition. Physical and laboratory findings will aid the diagnosis.

Differential Diagnosis

Colicky pain is caused by contraction of an obstructed hollow viscus such as intestine, ureter, gallbladder, or appendix. **Sudden onset of pain** usually occurs from ischemia (eg, twisted ovarian cyst) or following sudden perforation and spillage into the peritoneal cavity. A more insidious onset over several hours occurs with inflammation or obstruction (eg, salpingitis, appendicitis, intestinal obstruction). **Localized pain** may represent a localized inflammation or problem with one adnexa or part of the uterus. **Pain involving the entire abdomen** suggests a generalized reaction (eg, flooding of the peritoneum with blood, pus, or intestinal contents). Pain from intraperitoneal irritation usually increases with movement of the abdomen, with general body movement, with bowel or bladder movement, or with examination. A **tender adnexal mass** suggests an ectopic gestation, ovarian cyst, or inflammatory mass. **Vomiting** occurs early with acute appendicitis or cholecystitis and may or may not accompany salpingitis or pyelonephritis; it occurs later in bowel obstruction.

Pain of genital origin: Sudden severe pelvic pain associated with a pelvic mass is usually not difficult to diagnose. When the pain is less severe and especially when it is chronic, the diagnosis is less obvious unless a mass is present. However, the mass may not be the cause of the pain. **Acute salpingitis** is usually bilateral and causes severe lower abdominal pain and tenderness, especially on movement of the cervix. The pain is usually accompanied by fever, leukocytosis, and a purulent discharge from the cervical canal. There are usually few findings related to the GI tract and no mass during the first few days of symptoms. If the salpingitis persists for several days, a pelvic abscess may develop, most often pointing toward the vagina or rectum. A sudden easing of symptoms may mean that the abscess has ruptured intra-abdominally and immediate laparotomy is required.

Ectopic gestation is most commonly signaled by pelvic pain, menstrual irregularity, and an adnexal mass (see Ch. 177). In pregnant women, sudden pelvic pain also may

be due to an associated torsion of an ovarian cyst, to acute degeneration of a uterine myoma, to placental abruption, to rupture of the uterus, or, if fever is present, to parametritis.

Ovarian cysts, including malignant tumors, are frequently asymptomatic; but the pressure of an abdominal mass may cause discomfort, aching, or heaviness. Sudden or sharp pain may indicate rupture, hemorrhage, or torsion; varying degrees of tenderness, fever, leukocytosis, or signs of shock may be present. Hemorrhage into a cyst is common and produces pain. Follicular or corpus luteum cysts that have thin walls usually result in little bleeding when ruptured and are treated conservatively. Cysts with thicker walls rarely rupture. Severe peritonitis can follow a catastrophic intra-abdominal event (eg, ruptured dermoid cyst, perforated endometrioma) and intra-abdominal hemorrhage may ensue. Twisted ovarian cysts produce intermittent colicky pain; the cyst should be removed without untwisting the pedicle, which might risk an embolism. **Malposition of the uterus** rarely causes pelvic pain unless it is retrodisplaced and fixed by adhesions or scar tissue. Pain may be due to an **invasive neoplasm,** a result of invasion of pelvic tissue or pelvic nerve roots.

Endometriosis may cause pain and tenderness by direct action on nerve endings locally or by interfering with function of involved or adjacent organs. Characteristically the pain is worse a few days before menstruation and during the early period of flow. Occasionally a patient experiences severe hypogastric pain for a few hours during midcycle **(mittelschmerz)** from ovary bleeding following ovulation; this pain may be mistakenly diagnosed as appendicitis.

Pelvic congestion, most commonly between ages 30 to 50, may cause discomfort 7 to 10 days before menses. Pelvic pain present on sitting or standing, but relieved by lying down, is frequently accompanied by low back and leg aches, increased vaginal discharge, and dyspareunia. The condition may worsen during stress or anxiety, when women often have additional premenstrual symptoms of fatigue, headache, and insomnia. The uterus is usually tender and may be retroverted. The condition may be due to chronic pelvic hyperemia and vascular congestion or to psychosomatic factors.

Pain with intercourse (dyspareunia) is discussed in Ch. 165.

Pain of extragenital origin: Most pelvic pain of extragenital origin is related to the urologic or GI systems, to skeletal and supporting tissues, or to psychologic factors. **Pain of urologic origin** is frequently associated with urinary symptoms such as frequency, dysuria, burning, fever, chills, hematuria, and ureteral colic. Occasionally, the only finding is suprapubic tenderness or tenderness in the area of the bladder trigone. Urinalysis, cystoscopy, and urodynamic and urographic studies are usually helpful in diagnosis.

Pain of musculoskeletal origin from the spine or pelvis may be at the site of the involvement or be referred. Pain that radiates down the legs or is aggravated by motion of the involved part rather than by vaginoabdominal or rectovaginal examination suggests a skeletal etiology, as does pain or hyperesthesia in other areas within the pelvis, such as the skin or abdominal wall. Various disturbances in the pelvic supporting tissues, such as cystocele, rectocele, and uterine descensus, can produce symptoms of pressure, pelvic heaviness, and insecurity ("as if organs will drop out"). Pelvic tumors and threatened abortion may produce a similar discomfort. The slow progression of the severity of symptoms may make the patient irritable, or she may have adapted and not even be aware of the symptoms until surgical correction relieves the anatomic displacements. **Backache** is common but seldom due to gynecologic disease except in cases of advanced tumors. Backache may be due to poor posture, lack of exercise, strain or other trauma, or primary disease of the skeletal system, eg, osteoporosis, herniated nucleus pulposus, osteoarthritis, or bone tumors. In some women during pregnancy, pelvic joints may be loosened so much that motion is painful, a

diagnosis that can be confirmed (and symptoms relieved) by tightening a belt around the pelvic girdle to stabilize the bony pelvis.

Pain originating from the GI tract or its appendages, especially appendicitis or diverticulitis, is often confused with pain of gynecologic origin. In GI disturbances, tenderness and accompanying muscle spasm usually are more intense away from the area of the uterus and adnexa, and nausea, vomiting, and disturbance of bowel motility (diarrhea or constipation) are more pronounced. Peritonitis from pelvic infection is difficult to differentiate from that arising from the bowel. During pregnancy, the pain of appendicitis tends to be less severe and more variable in intensity; after the first trimester it may occur higher in the abdomen. If pelvic pain is predominantly left-sided and recurrent, the possibility of diverticulitis should be considered. Functional disease of the bowel (irritable or spastic colon) is often diagnosed in patients complaining of pelvic pain. The pain is not directly related to eating. The colon may be palpable and tender, and rolling the examining fingers across the colon usually reproduces the pain. Whenever the diagnosis is not clear but the findings do not require immediate surgery and GI symptoms predominate, further search for the cause is indicated. Surgical emergencies must be ruled out, but usually radiologic studies of the gallbladder and bowel and endoscopy can be deferred until after the acute episode if the pain is not progressive and if fever and leukocytosis are not present. If there is doubt that acute surgical conditions can be ruled out, surgery is usually indicated without undue delay.

In **psychogenic pain,** extensive laboratory studies may be needed to rule out other disorders. WBC counts help to establish the presence or absence of infection, and other hematologic studies rule out porphyria and blood dyscrasias. Radiologic studies rule out disease of the gallbladder, GI tract, and urinary tract. Endoscopic examination and psychiatric or orthopedic evaluation may be indicated. Surgery, except for diagnostic endoscopy, is seldom indicated except with clear-cut evidence that it will correct the cause of the pain; exploratory laparotomy should rarely be needed for diagnosis. Diagnostic laparoscopy for examination of the pelvis may be useful, especially for early diagnosis of ectopic pregnancy, differential diagnosis of appendicitis vs. pelvic inflammation, and endometriosis.

Treatment

Treatment of pelvic pain should be directed at the specific cause, but may be only symptomatic. Specific treatments are discussed with each condition. Hypnosis by experienced persons has been useful in pelvic pain due to functional causes that are not amenable to surgery. Presacral and sacrouterine neurectomy are helpful in selected patients, especially those with endometriosis. Nerve block or transection may be helpful in inoperable malignancies, but usually the disease has spread beyond the area that can be included in the nerve block.

ENDOMETRIOSIS

(See in Ch. 170)

VULVOVAGINITIS

Infectious diseases and other inflammatory conditions affecting the vaginal mucosa and often secondarily involving the vulva; vaginal discharge is common.

Etiology

Most vulvovaginitis and symptomatic vaginal discharges are caused by bacteria, usually *Gardnerella vaginalis* in combination with various anaerobes. Protozoa (*Trichomonas vaginalis*) cause 1/3 of all cases; Candida infection is a frequent cause in pregnant women and diabetics, and occasionally oral contraceptives increase susceptibility. Less common causes are other bacteria (eg, *Neisseria gonorrhoeae*, chlamydiae, mycoplasmas, streptococci, *Escherichia coli*, and staphylococci), foreign bodies, viral infec-

tions (herpes and condyloma accuminata), pinworm (*Enterobius vermicularis*), fistulas, radiation, and tumors of the generative tract. Extensive vaginal and cervical adenosis, as found in some women exposed to diethylstilbestrol **(DES)**, may produce excessive discharge. Frequent douching, especially with chemicals, may disturb normal vaginal milieu. Deodorant sprays, laundry soaps and fabric softeners, and bath water additives may cause vulvar irritation. Tight, nonporous, nonabsorbent underclothing, as well as poor hygiene, may foster fungal and bacterial growth. Occasionally, sensitivity to spermicides, coital lubricants, or latex in a diaphragm or condom may cause irritation.

Etiology must also be considered by age groups because of differences in estrogen and sexual activity. In the **reproductive years**, when estrogen is present, vulvitis is usually secondary to vaginal infection, whereas **premenarchal and postmenopausal females** commonly have vulvitis alone.

Newborns may have a sterile mucoid discharge that is secondary to maternal estrogen effect and subsides in < 2 wk; a small amount of bleeding may occur from this "estrogen withdrawal" effect.

During **childhood**, *E. coli* are most commonly found with vulvitis; streptococci, staphylococci, and Candida are found less often. Occasionally, pinworms or *N. gonorrhoeae* cause infection. Bubble baths or soaps may cause irritation. When discharge is present, especially with blood, a foreign body must be considered as well as a DES-related tumor. The immature anatomy and poor hygiene contribute to infection. Premenarchal girls have small labia minora, thin vaginal mucosa, and little cervical secretion. They have scant discharge, and it is usually alkaline in pH, with few bacteria. The amount of discharge increases when estrogen production increases, up to a year or more before menarche.

In the **reproductive years**, a milky white, watery or mucoid discharge arises primarily from the cervix or desquamation of vaginal cells. The amount and type of discharge vary during the menstrual cycle and with sexual stimulation, from transudation of fluid from the vagina and Bartholin gland secretion. Normally, 4 or 5 kinds of bacteria are present, chiefly lactobacilli and corynebacteria, and small numbers of fungi. The vaginal pH is normally 3.5 to 4.5; acidity tends to be decreased by menstrual blood, infected cervical mucous, vaginal transudate, or semen. The glycogen content is high, the vaginal mucosa is thick, and the labia are well developed. Elevated hormonal levels, as in pregnancy and oral contraceptive use, can change the metabolism of the vagina. Vaginal discharges due to infections are discussed below.

In **postmenopausal women**, bacteria and fungi most commonly are the infecting agents, and Trichomonas is less common. Menopausal estrogen depletion due to aging, ovariectomy, or radiation of the pelvis, or temporary low estrogen states (similar to those during lactation) cause vulvar structures to regress and vaginal mucosa to thin. Discharge becomes scant and the pH rises to from 4.5 to 5.5. The atrophic vaginal and vulvar epithelium is more easily traumatized and infected. Dystrophies and tumors, symptomatic and asymptomatic, become increasingly common with aging. Folliculitis and other dermatological disorders can affect the skin of the vulva. Foreign bodies, especially forgotten pessaries, can be the cause.

Symptoms, Signs, and Diagnosis

The most common complaint is of vaginal discharge, with or without vulvar irritation. Vaginal discharge is abnormal when the odor is offensive; when pruritis, irritation, or pain occurs; or when the amount distresses the patient.

The initial visit should include a complete physical examination and history, with details on the discharge (color, consistency, presence of odor, duration, and symptoms; also, when it occurs in a cycle; whether it is recurrent; responses to previous therapy; whether vulvar itching, burning, pain, or lesion is present; and what aspect of the problem is most troublesome to the patient). The type of discharge may suggest the

cause or may be misleading. Questions should also concern sexual activity; contraceptive use; whether the consort has had urethral discharge, pruritis, penile lesions, postcoital irritation, or therapy for infection; use of chemicals on the vulva or vagina; recent change in laundry products; any venereal disease or parasitic infection, present or past; and if anyone in the household has pubic itching.

After the general physical examination, the vulva is examined for redness, edema, excoriation, and abnormal lesions. Biopsy of discrete vulvar lesions should be done; if much of the vulva is white and thickened (as in lichen sclerosis) or otherwise appears abnormal, a biopsy site may be selected with toluidine blue 1% staining, then decolorized with acetic acid 2 to 3% (vinegar diluted 1:1 with water). Parasites should be searched for, enlarged nodes palpated, ulcers cultured for viruses, and urethral and Bartholin gland discharge noted. In **children** a culture may be obtained from the vulva or fourchette; if discharge is present, a vaginal culture should be done. The child should be checked for a foreign body and for pinworms.

Physiologic discharge is annoying because of the feeling of wetness and soiled clothing, but it is not malodorous nor does it produce vulvitis.

Gardnerella infection tends to produce a white, gray, or yellowish turbid discharge with a foul or "fishy" odor that increases when the discharge becomes alkaline, such as after coitus or after washing with soap. Vulvar pruritus or irritation may be present, but redness or edema of the vulva is not usually marked.

Candida infection (see also GENITAL CANDIDIASIS in Ch. 14) is suggested by moderate to severe vulvar itching and burning, with redness and possibly excoriation. The thick, cheesy discharge that may be present tends to cling to the vaginal walls. Symptoms usually increase in the premenstrual week. Poorly controlled diabetics and patients on chronic use of tetracycline for acne are candidates for recurrence.

Trichomas infection is marked by a purulent, watery, sometimes greenish, frequently malodorous discharge that begins shortly after menses. The bubbles in the discharge as well as the odor are probably due to a coexisting, gas-producing, bacterial infection. Itching is severe. Acute inflammation of the vagina with small "strawberry spots" may be found.

A watery discharge, especially if bloody, suggests **malignancy** of the vagina or upper generative tract. **Cervical polyps** or **vaginal endometriosis** may also produce this type of discharge, with bleeding after coitus.

A discharge may be related to **atrophic vaginitis, radiation vaginitis**, or **foreign body**. The atrophic vagina is fragile, and bleeding sites may be identified. An acutely painful lesion of the vulva suggests **herpes infection** or **local abscess**. Chronic itching or discomfort of the vulva suggests **lichen sclerosis** or **carcinoma in situ**. In chronic vulvitis, atypical dystrophies and malignancy should be ruled out by biopsy.

Using a water-lubricated speculum, the physician inspects the vagina and, with a cotton-tipped applicator, obtains a specimen. It is diluted on 2 slides—one with normal saline, the other with 10% potassium hydroxide, at the same time checking the latter specimen for released odor. With microscopic examination, *T. vaginalis* can be seen as motile unicellular flagellated organisms. White cells, "clue cells" (granular-appearing epithelial cells), and many bacteria suggest Gardnerella infection. In potassium hydroxide, mycelia and/or spores of Candida are seen. A culture for *N. gonorrhoeae* is usually indicated; cultures for chlamydia may be done, but other cultures are not helpful.

The cervix is inspected, a Pap smear taken, and the remainder of the bimanual examination performed.

Treatment

Physiologic discharge requires only reassurance of normalcy and, if a discharge is

annoying, occasional douching with water to reduce the amount. Prepubertal girls should be instructed about perineal hygiene. Foreign bodies should be removed.

Specific causes of discharge require specific therapy. Topical anti-inflammatory agents such as hydrocortisone 0.5% tid can be used until specific therapy is instituted after culture results have been obtained. If labial adhesions have occurred secondary to previous inflammation of labia, applying 3 mm/day of estrogen cream for 7 to 10 days usually opens the labia. Povidone iodine douche 15 to 30 mL/L (2 tbsp/qt) of water may give relief until specific therapy is effective and may reduce recurrences of Candida.

Candida is treated topically with miconazole 2% or clotrimazole 1% cream or vaginal tablets or suppositories for 3 to 7 days. Ketoconazole may be indicated in recurrent disease. **Trichomonas** is treated with metronidazole 250 mg tid or 500 mg bid orally for 5 days; 2 gm in a single daily dose may be used. If infection recurs, the consort should also be treated. **Gardnerella or anerobic infections** are treated similarly to Trichomonas, with metronidazole. About 25% of patients have recurrences and require retreatment in 2 to 3 mo. Lowering vaginal pH with propionic acid jelly may help. **Chlamydial infections** are treated with tetracycline or erythromycin, 250 mg qid orally for 10 days. **Mycoplasma** is treated with doxycycline 100 mg bid orally for 10 days. For any of these infections, consorts should be treated simultaneously, if possible.

Acute vulvitis: The causal factor should be treated as discussed above, and measures should be taken to reduce acute inflammation; eg, wearing loose, absorbent clothing that allows air circulation, and keeping the vulva clean (soaps should be avoided). Intermittent use of ice packs reduces soreness and pruritis; sometimes warm sitz baths or compresses may help. Topical steroids are useful, and oral antihistamines may be helpful, especially at night when a sedative effect may be welcome. Acyclovir ointment applied to primary herpetic ulcers may reduce symptoms and shorten the course. Symptomatic treatment with pain relievers and bland coating ointments (petrolatum) or anesthetic ointments may be helpful.

Atrophic vaginitis is treated with estrogen replacement; many patients respond to oral estrogen (eg, conjugated estrogen, one 0.3-mg tablet qid for 1 wk, then 0.3 mg q 3 to 7 days) and do not require specific treatment of the infecting agent. Other patients do better with estrogen vaginal cream (1/2 applicator [2.0 gm] every night for 1 wk, then 1/2 applicator q 7 to 10 days).

Chronic vulvitis often leads to chronic inflammation. Occasionally it is due to poor hygiene, especially in elderly patients who are incontinent and bedridden, and responds to cleanliness. Conditions of the skin that can cause chronic vulvitis, such as psoriasis or tinea versicolor, need appropriate treatment, and infection is treated with specific antibiotics. All substances that may cause chronic irritation should be removed.

Vulvar dystrophies: Hyperkatotic or white lesions can occur at any age, but usually are postmenopausal. **Benign dystrophy** has been called lichen sclerosis et atrophicus. Testosterone propionate 2% in petrolatum applied in small amounts bid is often beneficial. Chronic use of topical steroid or estrogen cream may cause further drying and irritation. Surgical excision is not indicated. Follow-up examinations with constant search for progressive change and possible malignancy are essential. **Atypical dystrophies** should be removed.

SALPINGITIS

(Pelvic Inflammatory Disease [PID])

Infection of the fallopian tubes. The term **pelvic inflammatory disease (PID)** is used by some to include infection of the cervix (cervicitis), the uterus (endometritis), or the ovaries (oophoritis) as well, but the term should not be used as a catch-all for pelvic pain of unknown etiology.

Etiology and Pathogenesis

Salpingitis occurs predominantly in young women under age 25 who are sexually active and is the result of infection transmitted most commonly by intercourse, less often by childbirth (puerperal fever) or abortion. Patients with intrauterine devices (IUDs) are especially vulnerable, probably because the transcervical appendage assists pathogen transport. Salpingitis rarely occurs before the menarche, after the menopause, or during pregnancy. Infection may have a single organism or be polymicrobial. *Neisseria gonorrhoeae* is the responsible organism in 40 to 60% of acute nonpuerperal PID. Other organisms, primarily *Chlamydia trachomatis*, but also gram-negative bacilli and gram-positive cocci, mycoplasmas, and viruses, are being implicated with increasing frequency. Tuberculous salpingitis has become quite uncommon, especially in the absence of systemic TB (see Ch. 8). When salpingitis follows pregnancy or abortion, anaerobic streptococci or staphylococci are usually involved.

Salpingitis due to actinomycosis, schistosomiasis, leprosy, oxyuriasis, sarcoidosis, and foreign bodies (eg, x-ray contrast media) has been reported.

Infection begins intravaginally in most cases. The endocervical glands provide an optimum environment for organisms, especially *N. gonorrhoeae*, to flourish before spreading upward to produce a superficial endometritis and an endosalpingitis. Although symptoms and signs may predominate on one side, both tubes are probably affected. The tubal infection produces a profuse exudate and leads to agglutination of mucosal folds, adhesions, and tubal occlusion. Peritonitis, from spread of the exudate to the pelvic peritoneum, is common; the ovaries tend to resist infection, but may also be invaded.

Symptoms and Signs

Acute salpingitis: Onset is usually shortly after menses. Severe lower abdominal pain increases progressively with guarding, rebound tenderness, and discomfort that increases with cervical motion. Unless related to an IUD, involvement is usually bilateral. Vomiting may occur; bowel sounds are normal early, although paralytic ileus may ensue. High fever, leukocytosis, and copius purulent discharge from the cervix are common.

Chronic salpingitis may follow an acute attack with subsequent tubal and pelvic scarring and adhesions, chronic pain, menstrual irregularities, and, possibly, infertility. An obstructed tube may distend with fluid **(hydrosalpinx).** In **chronic interstitial salpingitis,** the tube is enlarged due to a thickened wall. Exacerbations may occur, commonly from organisms other than gonococcus.

Abscesses may develop in the tubes, ovaries, or pelvis during the acute or subacute stage. If a small perforation occurs, it may seal off but still respond to antibiotics; those that do not respond require surgical removal, usually with hysterectomy and bilateral salpingo-oophorectomy. Massive perforation of an adnexal abscess is a **surgical emergency,** rapidly progressing in a characteristic pattern of severe low abdominal pain, generalized peritonitis, nausea, vomiting, and shock secondary to peritonitis and endotoxemia (see SEPTIC SHOCK in Ch. 6). **Pyosalpinx,** in which one or both fallopian tubes are filled with pus, may be sterile but almost always is associated with symptoms of inflammation. The ovary, if involved, becomes incorporated into the tubal inflammatory mass, producing a **tubo-ovarian abscess. Hydrosalpinx** occurs with late or incomplete therapy, the result of closure of the fimbriated end of the fallopian tube. It may be present without symptoms for years. As a result of the mucosal destruction and tubal occlusion, **infertility** is a common sequel of salpingitis.

Diagnosis

The history may disclose recent coitus, insertion of an IUD, childbirth, or abortion. Temperature and WBC may be elevated. The sedimentation rate is usually elevated. On pelvic examination, the most striking finding is that moving the cervix or palpating

the adnexa produces severe pain. Peritoneal irritation frequently produces marked abdominal tenderness, and referred and rebound tenderness (therefore, gentle palpation is important if pelvic mass is to be identified). Surgical emergencies must be ruled out, especially appendicitis and ectopic gestation. Cultures and smear for Gram stain should be obtained from the cervical, urethral, and rectal areas and from the pharynx. Culdocentesis, with examination of the fluid, may help in differential diagnosis as well as in identifying organisms.

Treatment

Acute gonorrheal salpingitis requires immediate and vigorous treatment to stop the infection and prevent infertility. An STS should be performed and used as a baseline study for comparison with another such test in 5 to 6 wk. Antibiotics should be started as soon as specimens have been obtained for culture and sensitivity tests, without waiting for the results of these studies. Aqueous procaine penicillin or ampicillin is preferred for early stages of salpingitis. Probenecid 1 gm orally is followed by procaine penicillin G 4.8 million u. (3 gm), given in doses of 2.4 million u. (1.5 gm) IM in 2 separate sites, followed by ampicillin 4 to 6 gm orally or tetracycline 1.5 to 2 gm/day given orally for 7 to 10 days. Patients allergic to penicillin can be given spectinomycin 2 gm plus probenecid 1 gm orally. Severely ill patients having severe pain require hospitalization and larger antibiotic doses—crystalline penicillin 10 to 40 million u. (6.25 to 25 gm) IV over the first 24 h. The parenteral penicillin therapy should be continued until there is a favorable response, which should occur within 36 to 72 h. Oral penicillin (or ampicillin 500 mg qid) is then continued for at least 10 days. Patients hypersensitive to penicillin may be given tetracycline 500 mg IV qid for the first 24 to 48 h, then 500 mg orally qid to complete 10 days of therapy. (CAUTION: *Pregnant women and patients with renal failure should not be given tetracycline.*)

Current optimal inpatient therapy usually is combined antibiotic therapy, because infertility increases with degree of inflammation. One regimen is a triple therapy of ampicillin 1 gm q 6 h IV, tobramycin 2.9 mg/kg IV loading dose, then 1.5 mg/kg q 8 h IV, and clindamycin 600 to 1200 mg q 6 h IV. After clinical improvement, therapy can be changed to oral medication, ampicillin 500 mg with clindamycin 450 mg q 6 h.

Supportive treatment includes bed rest, and the patient may require IV fluids. If ileus is present, nasogastric suction may be necessary. Abscesses usually require drainage; intra-abdominal rupture of an abscess requires immediate exploration of the abdomen. Hydrosalpinx and tubal obstruction may require surgery. Repeated episodes of acute salpingitis tend to respond less readily to antibiotic therapy and may also require surgical management.

Adequate treatment of women with acute gonococcal salpingitis must include examination and treatment of sexual contacts, many of whom may be found to have nonsymptomatic urethral gonococcal infection. Failure to treat male sexual partners is a major cause of recurrent gonococcal salpingitis.

Post-treatment follow-up of patients with acute salpingitis is necessary and should include repeated pelvic examination and cultures for *N. gonorrhoeae.*

PREMENSTRUAL SYNDROME (PMS)

(Premenstrual Tension)

A condition characterized by nervousness, irritability, emotional instability, depression, and possibly headaches, edema, and mastalgia; it occurs during the 7 to 10 days before menstruation and disappears a few hours after onset of menstrual flow.

Etiology

The syndrome seems to be related to fluctuations in estrogen and progesterone. Estrogen exerts fluid-retaining action, and transitory increases in fluid in different body tissues seem to explain symptoms such as weight gain, edema, breast tenderness, and, possibly, bloating. However, many symptoms do not correlate in intensity with fluid retention and weight gain; eg, diuretics promote sodium and water excretion but do not relieve all of the symptoms and may have no effect on the symptom complex.

Estrogen-progesterone imbalance, excessive aldosterone or ADH, carbohydrate metabolism changes, hypoglycemia, hyperprolactinemia, allergy to progesterone, retention of sodium and water by the kidneys, and psychogenic factors have all been implicated.

Symptoms and Signs

Most women experience some symptoms referable to the menstrual cycle; in many women the symptoms are significant but of short duration and are not disabling. Other women have one or more of a broad range of symptoms that temporarily disturb normal functioning. Symptoms last from a few hours to 10 to 12 or more days and usually cease with onset of menses; however, in perimenopausal women, symptoms may persist through and after menses. Type and intensity of symptoms vary in the general population and may also vary in individuals.

With onset of menses, in many women PMS is replaced by **dysmenorrhea**. Significant dysmenorrhea is more common in the teens and tends to diminish as the woman matures. Conversely, PMS may begin in the twenties and increase with age.

The most common complaints are **mood alteration and psychological effects**: irritability, nervousness, lack of control, agitation, anger, insomnia, difficulty in concentrating, lethargy, depression, and severe fatigue. Symptoms related to **fluid retention** are edema, transient weight gain, oliguria, and breast fullness and pain. **Neurologic and vascular symptoms** include headache, vertigo, syncope, paresthesias of extremities, easy bruising, and cardiac palpitation. Epilepsy may be aggravated. **GI symptoms** include bloating, constipation, nausea, vomiting, and changes in appetite. **Pelvic heaviness or pressure** and **backache** may occur. **Skin problems** of acne, neurodermatitis, and aggravation of other skin disorders may also occur. **Respiratory problems** (allergies and infection) and **eye complaints** (visual disturbance and conjunctivitis) may be worse premenstrually.

Treatment

Treatment involves symptomatic relief and, when possible, correcting the cause. **Fluid retention** may be relieved by reducing sodium intake and using a diuretic (eg, hydrochlorothiazide 50 to 100 mg/day orally), starting just before the time when symptoms are usually noted. **Counseling** about the symptoms can increase self-understanding and lead to modification of activities for **stress reduction**. Because of the normal variation of the disorder, having the patient record symptoms and therapies helps to determine the effectiveness of the treatment. **Partner involvement**, directly or indirectly, may help both to cope with the PMS. **Hormonal manipulation** is effective for some women. Possible regimens include (1) natural progesterone by vaginal suppository (25 to 400 mg/day) or injection (progesterone in water, 100 mg/day IM) for 10 to 12 days premenstrually, (2) birth control pills, or (3) long-acting progestin (eg, medroxyprogesterone acetate 200 mg IM every 2 to 3 mo) to eliminate cyclic changes. **Tranquilizers** (eg, diazepam 2 to 5 mg tid orally) may be used in patients with irritability, nervousness, and lack of control, especially if they are unable to change their stressful environments. **Dietary changes**, increasing protein and decreasing sugars as well as supplementation with vitamin B complex (especially pyridoxine and/or magnesium), may be helpful for some women. Other regimens, using spironolactone, bromocriptine, or MAO inhibitors, do not show clear benefits.

PRIMARY DYSMENORRHEA

(Functional Dysmenorrhea)

Cyclic pain associated with menses during ovulatory cycles, but without demonstrable lesions affecting the reproductive cycle.

Etiology and Incidence

The pain is thought to result from uterine contractions and ischemia, probably mediated by the effect of prostaglandins produced in secretory endometrium; therefore, primary dysmenorrhea is almost always associated with ovulatory cycles. The passage of tissue through the cervix, a narrow cervical os, malposition of the uterus, lack of exercise, and anxiety about menses may be contributing factors. This common disability, which causes significant absence from school or work, usually appears during adolescence and tends to decrease with age and following pregnancy.

Symptoms and Signs

Low abdominal pain is usually crampy or colicky, but may be a dull constant ache and may radiate to the lower back or legs. It may start prior to or with menses, tends to peak after 24 h, and usually subsides after 2 days. Sometimes endometrial casts **(membranous dysmenorrhea)** or clots are expelled. Headache, nausea, constipation or diarrhea, and urinary frequency are often present; vomiting occurs occasionally. Premenstrual syndrome symptoms (see above) of irritability, nervousness, depression, and abdominal distention may persist during part or all of the menses.

Treatment

Assurance that her reproductive organs are normal will give a woman psychologic support. Local heat, supplied by a heating pad, may relieve discomfort. Conservative treatment also includes drugs with antiprostaglandin effects; aspirin, naproxen, ibuprofen, and mefenamic acid have been used; effectiveness may be increased if the drug is started 24 to 48 h before menses and continued through 1 or 2 days of the cycle. If an antiprostaglandin is ineffective, pain-relieving drugs such as codeine or pentazocine may be added. Occasionally, sympathomimetics can relieve spasm-type cramps. If pain continues to interfere with normal activity, suppression of ovulation with low-dose estrogen-progesterone birth control pills is advisable. The drug is given cyclically for 3 to 4 mo, then discontinued, and restarted as necessary. A sexually active woman without a medical contraindication can use the pills on a long-term basis for contraception in addition to pain relief. Although antiemetics may be used, nausea and vomiting usually disappear as cramps subside. The woman should get adequate rest and sleep, and regular exercise may be beneficial.

SECONDARY DYSMENORRHEA

(Acquired Dysmenorrhea)

Pain with menses caused by demonstrable pathology.

Etiology

One of the most common causes is endometriosis; adenomyosis also causes dysmenorrhea. A few women have an extremely tight cervical os, usually secondary to cauterization, that results in pain when the uterus attempts to expel tissue. Cramping pain occurs occasionally when a pedunculated submucosal fibroid or an endometrial polyp is being extruded from the uterus (although it may be painless).

Chronic pelvic inflammatory disease and adhesions may cause diffuse low abdominal pain that is vague and continuous. Patients with both acute and chronic pelvic inflammatory disease tend to have increased pain with menses. Acute pain may be associated with acute pelvic inflammation, fever, and diffuse abdominal symptoms during or just after menses.

Treatment

Counseling about the physiologic causes and the concerns, fears, and stresses related to this phase of life is important. When psychic factors dominate, psychotherapy is indicated and, if necessary, antidepressants, minor tranquilizers, and mild sedatives can be used as adjunctive therapy for, respectively, depression, anxiety and irritability, and insomnia.

Estrogen replacement is the only consistent and satisfactory therapy to sustain systems dependent on ovarian hormone secretion and to relieve **hot flushes**. Patient selection, determination of risk/benefit ratio, and observation during therapy are necessary. When hot flushes and fatigue and insomnia from night-awakening decrease, the feeling of well-being usually returns. When estrogens are contraindicated, treatments for reducing discomfort due to hot flushes include sedative-hypnotics (eg, barbiturates or benzodiazepines), progestin (medroxyprogesterone acetate 20 mg orally or 150 mg IM/mo), propanolol, or clonidine.

Symptomatic **vaginal atrophy and vaginitis** and **atrophic changes of the lower urinary tract** (especially of the urethra and trigone of the bladder) with urinary frequency, dysuria, and sometimes incontinence, are reversible with estrogen therapy.

Preventing **osteoporosis** (see also in Ch. 113) requires extended estrogen replacement. Adequate nutrition, including elemental calcium (1000 mg/day for premenopausal and estrogen-treated women, 1500 mg/day for untreated postmenopausal women), and weight-bearing exercise are also necessary. For those who have inadequate daily exposure to sunlight, vitamin D supplementation (600 u. bid) is indicated. The efficacy and safety of other modalities have not been established (eg, sodium fluoride, calcitriol, calcitonin, weak androgenic anabolic steroids, thiazides, diphosphonates, and 1–34 parathyroid hormone). To prevent falling, side effects of other drugs need to be considered and home hazards should be minimized.

The therapeutic effects of estrogen replacement on atherosclerosis, myocardial infarction, hypertension, and arthritis are not clear. Nor is there conclusive evidence that estrogen therapy prevents heart disease in menopausal women or that treated postmenopausal women are at increased risk of coronary disease.

Estrogen administration should be cyclic. If the patient has a uterus, a progestin is added to the cycle. Estrogen (conjugated estrogen 0.3 to 1.25 mg/day or ethinyl estradiol 0.02 to 0.05 mg/day) is taken orally once a day from the first through the 25th day each month. Progestins (eg, medroxyprogesterone acetate 10 mg or norethindrone acetate 2.5 to 5 mg orally) are given from the 16th through the 25th day each month. Bleeding, if it occurs, should happen only during the hormone withdrawal period; if bleeding occurs at other times, an endometrial biopsy should be done. Some physicians think that an endometrial biopsy should be obtained before therapy and at yearly intervals thereafter; others believe it need be done only if symptoms warrant, as it is an uncomfortable procedure, increases expense, and has a low yield in asymptomatic women. Estrogen can be increased or decreased according to the symptoms. If hot flushes occur during the end of the cycle, the days without estrogen can be decreased by 1 day each month until symptoms are relieved. Topical estrogen (eg, conjugated estrogen vaginal cream) may be used for atrophic vaginal changes and dyspareunia, 1 applicator/night for 5 nights, then 1/2 applicator/wk. The estrogen is readily absorbed systemically from the vaginal mucosa. Injectable estrogen (estradiol valerate 10 to 20 mg IM q 4 wk) is rarely indicated, except immediately following oophorectomy.

Contraindications to estrogen therapy include a history of estrogen-dependent neoplasia of the endometrium or breast, a history of thrombophlebitis or thromboembolism, and the presence or a history of severe liver disease. There are also relative contraindications.

Mammography should be routine in the postmenopausal age group and is particu-

Treatment

Secondary dysmenorrhea can be relieved symptomatically or by correction of the underlying abnormality as described elsewhere in THE MANUAL. Dilation of a narrow cervical canal may give 3 to 6 mo of relief and also permits diagnostic curettage. Interruption of uterine nerves by presacral neurectomy and division of the sacrouterine ligaments may help selected patients; hypnosis has also been useful.

MENOPAUSE

The physiologic cessation of menses as a result of decreasing ovarian function. It is usually a retrospective diagnosis, made when there have been no menses for a year. Menopause may be natural, artificial, or premature.

Etiology

Natural menopause occurs at an average age of 49 to 50 yr. As ovaries age, response to pituitary-produced gonadotropins (FSH and LH) decreases, initially with shorter follicular phases (hence, shorter cycles), fewer ovulations and decreased production of progesterone, and more cycle irregularity. Eventually, the follicle fails to respond and, without feedback of estrogen, the circulating gonadotropins rise substantially. Circulating levels of estrogens and progesterone are markedly reduced; androgen (androstenedione) is reduced by half, but testosterone decreases only slightly. This transitional phase beginning prior to menopause and continuing after it, during which a woman passes from her reproductive stage, is properly referred to as the **climacteric,** although most people refer to it also as menopause. **Premature menopause** refers to ovarian failure of unknown cause that occurs before age 40. Smoking is associated with early menopause. Menopause can also be hastened by radiation exposure, chemotherapeutic drugs, and surgery that impairs ovarian blood supply. **Artificial menopause** follows ovariectomy or radiation of the pelvis, including the ovaries.

Symptoms and Signs

Menopause may be asymptomatic, or symptoms may be severe. Hot flushes and sweating secondary to vasomotor instability affect 75% of women. Most have hot flushes for > 1 yr, and 25 to 50% for > 5 yr. Psychologic and emotional symptoms of fatigue, irritability, insomnia, and nervousness may be related to both estrogen deprivation and the stress of aging and changing roles. Lack of sleep due to disturbance by recurrent hot flushes contributes to fatigue and irritability. Intermittent dizziness, paresthesias, and cardiac symptoms of palpitations and tachycardia may occur; the incidence of heart disease increases. Dyspareunia, increasing pelvic relaxation, urinary incontinence, cystitis, and vaginitis tend to occur. Nausea, flatulence, constipation, diarrhea, arthralgia, and myalgia are common complaints.

Osteoporosis is the major health hazard. Those at highest risk are women who are slender, Caucasian, smokers, on steroids, or those who have little physical activity. Bone mass losses average 1%/yr after menopause and result in numerous fractures. Primary sites are the vertebrae, which show anterior collapse and lead to stooping and backache; hip fractures (200,000/yr in the USA); and wrist fractures. These fractures may occur with little trauma, and in the elderly, with no trauma.

Diagnosis

Menopause is usually obvious. In younger patients, elevated FSH substantiates the diagnosis. Endocrine disorders such as thyroid disease or diabetes should be ruled out. Patients with symptomatic osteoporosis should be investigated for causes other than menopause (eg, hyperparathyroidism).

larly pertinent as a screen and baseline in the estrogen-treated group. Most evidence indicates that estrogen therapy does not increase the risk of breast cancer.

---

172. BREAST DISORDERS

Etiology

Except in identifiable infections and certain varieties of trauma, little is known about the etiology of most breast lesions. However, certain major factors influence development of breast conditions and, therefore, presumably play a role in their etiology: (1) **Sex**: Certain neoplasms are at least 100 times more common in the female than in the male. (2) **Heredity**: Breast cancer and cysts develop more frequently in individuals with a family history of the disease. (3) **Endocrine influence**: In many women, breast discomfort occurs periodically before menstruation, and certain breast masses, especially cysts, enlarge transiently immediately before menstruation; in addition, the incidence of certain benign conditions (eg, fibrocystic disease) drops sharply after menopause, while the incidence of breast cancer rises. Pregnancy occurring before age 25 is somewhat protective against later development of breast cancer. The known effects of specific hormones on the course of breast cancer have been used in ablative procedures such as oophorectomy, adrenalectomy, and hypophysectomy and in administering exogenous estrogens, progesterones, androgens, corticosteroids, and the estrogen antagonist tamoxifen.

Symptoms and Signs

The history of a woman with a breast mass should include the family history; the patient's age; a description of the lesion—its duration, its relationship to hormone ingestion, pregnancy, lactation, menses, or menopause, any fluctuations in its size, its rate of growth; the presence or absence of nipple discharge; and history of trauma, discomfort, or pain.

Nipple discharge is always significant and may accompany a number of breast conditions. In addition to its physiologic occurrence during pregnancy and lactation, it may occur during infections of the breast as a purulent discharge; with certain types of carcinoma (especially malignant intraductal papillary carcinoma) as a bloody discharge; and with some benign conditions, notably fibrocystic disease, intraductal papilloma, and mammary duct ectasia (a rare form of fibrocystic mastitis in which the terminal ducts are dilated and filled with detritus). Occasionally, spontaneous galactorrhea (see also in Ch. 88) may be a sign of a prolactin-secreting pituitary adenoma. Since nipple discharge in the absence of lactation is uncommon, patients with this symptom should be referred to a surgeon.

Local pain or tenderness only rarely accompanies malignant breast diseases, even in advanced carcinoma. This lack of pain may be unfortunate, since patients usually seek medical advice promptly for a painful breast lesion.

Breast Examination

Various mammary gland disorders are readily detectable, because the breast can be inspected and palpated regularly by the patient. Unfortunately, so few periodic self-examinations are made that many breast masses are palpated only accidentally. Physicians should teach women proper technics and the importance of self-examination. FIG. 172–1 shows the usual positions for examining the breast.

Inspection: A good light is essential; otherwise, some of the most characteristic signs of breast cancer will be missed. The examiner should look for asymmetry (remembering that in women one breast is often slightly larger than the other), including elevation of one breast (FIG. 172–1, G), deviation or retraction of the nipple, and flattening

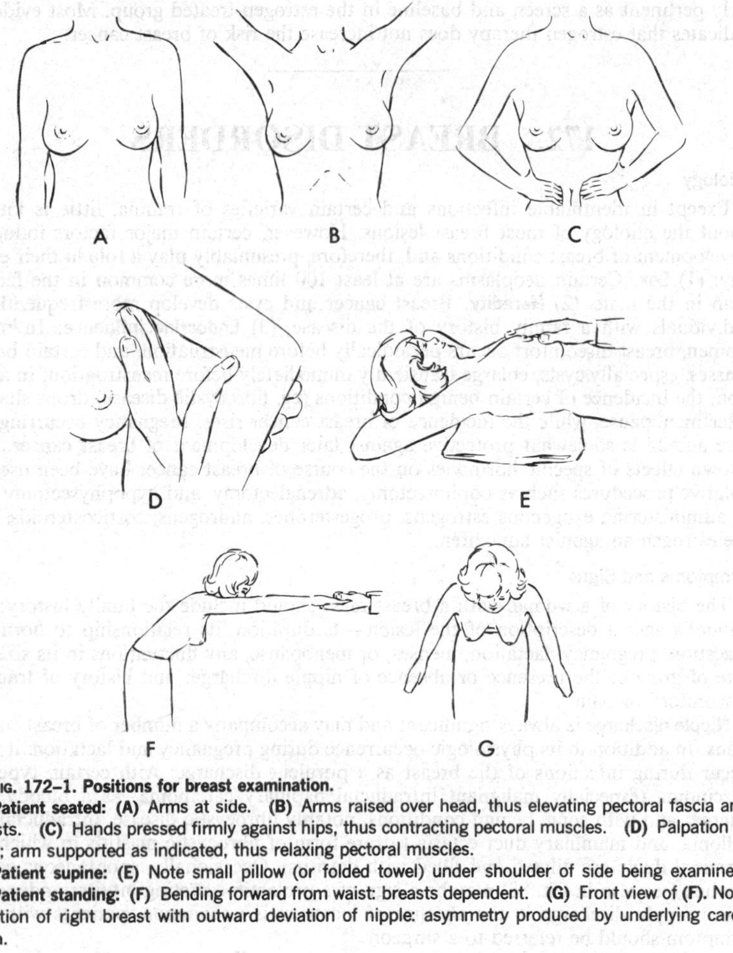

Fig. 172–1. Positions for breast examination.

Patient seated: **(A)** Arms at side. **(B)** Arms raised over head, thus elevating pectoral fascia and breasts. **(C)** Hands pressed firmly against hips, thus contracting pectoral muscles. **(D)** Palpation of axilla; arm supported as indicated, thus relaxing pectoral muscles.

Patient supine: **(E)** Note small pillow (or folded towel) under shoulder of side being examined.

Patient standing: **(F)** Bending forward from waist: breasts dependent. **(G)** Front view of **(F)**. Note elevation of right breast with outward deviation of nipple: asymmetry produced by underlying carcinoma.

or indentation of the normal breast contour. Also highly suggestive are redness or edema of the skin with peau d'orange appearance (pitted like an orange skin), nipple discharge with or without crusting, and localized retraction or dimpling of the skin, which the maneuvers shown in Fig. 172–1, B, C, and F may elicit.

Palpation is best carried out with the patient supine (Fig. 172–1, E). A small pillow is placed under the shoulder of the side to be examined, and the breast is gently palpated with the flat of the hand. The consistency of the breast tissue should be noted, and any tender areas, masses, or thickening of the parenchyma searched for. Large cysts may feel fluctuant, fibroadenomas are rubbery, and cancer is often firm or hard. Skin dimpling may be demonstrated by moving the integument over a subjacent mass or thickened area. This **retraction sign** involving either skin, nipple, or areola

always represents destruction of tissue within the breast. The destruction may be due to fat necrosis, accidental or iatrogenic trauma, infection (past or present), mammary duct ectasia, or malignancy. Carcinoma will be present in almost every instance in which the other causes can be eliminated.

Mobility of a mass is very significant. Well-circumscribed, freely mobile tumors are generally benign. Those that are fixed, ill-defined, or seem to blend with the surrounding parenchyma may be malignant. The axillas must be examined (FIG. 172–1, D) for possible lymph node involvement, and the terminal ducts should be gently milked toward the nipple to detect possible discharge.

Additional Diagnostic Technics

Aspiration of discrete breast masses with a 20-gauge needle is a useful diagnostic practice and, except for open incisional biopsy, is the most reliable method of diagnosing carcinoma. Recovery of greenish or straw-colored fluid indicates a cyst. (Following such aspiration, the mass should disappear.) However, this fluid recovery does not eliminate the possibility of a carcinoma lying adjacent to the cyst and this should be ruled out by mammography. Blood in a cyst aspirate is an indication for biopsy. Tissue fluid recovered from aspiration of solid breast masses should be smeared on a glass slide, sprayed with or placed in a fixative solution, and sent for cytological evaluation to a pathologist who is familiar with the range of cytological appearances seen in breast diseases.

Mammography or xeroradiography (soft-tissue x-ray) of the breast: A fine calcific stippling concentrated in the area of a mass is suspicious of carcinoma and may occasionally be seen even without a palpable mass. However, a negative mammogram does not rule out malignancy. In women younger than 35 yr, mammography is almost without value and should seldom be performed except as a baseline study. The American Cancer Society currently recommends: between ages 35 and 40, a baseline mammogram; between ages 40 and 49, mammography every 1 or 2 years, especially in "high-risk" women (those with a family history of breast cancer and women who have had cancer in one breast); and over age 50, a mammogram every year.

Ultrasonography is an imaging technic effective in differentiating cystic from solid breast masses. However, since this differentiation is easily made by simple aspiration, ultrasonography has only minimal value and is useless as a screening technic for detecting early, nonpalpable breast cancers.

Thermography, a technic for detecting and displaying the heat pattern given off by the skin, is not useful as a screening technic or for detecting small nonpalpable breast tumors, since it lacks sufficient sensitivity and specificity and false-positive results are common.

Biopsy of the lesion or suspected area is the only certain diagnostic procedure and should be performed whenever a dominant mass persists or does not disappear after aspiration (see above) of a cyst, or when the aspirate is bloody. Under such circumstances, a negative mammogram is *not* a reliable substitute for biopsy.

BENIGN BREAST CONDITIONS

INFECTIONS

Breast infections occur most frequently during lactation or shortly thereafter. **Recurrent subareolar abscesses,** low-grade chronic infections, may occur at other times. **TB of the breast** is rare and is generally associated with pulmonary or glandular TB. **Treatment** includes antibiotics and either excision or incision and drainage of abscesses.

TRAUMA

Aside from nipple fissures caused by nursing, the most common type of breast trauma is simple **contusion**. Contusions may be followed by **fat necrosis,** a benign condition that appears as a firm, irregular mass that may mimic carcinoma because it is often associated with skin retraction.

HYPERTROPHY

Uni- or bilateral hypertrophy may be seen in either sex, especially during early adolescence. Hypertrophy in men **(gynecomastia)** occurs as a discoid enlargement of breast tissue beneath the areola. In pubescent boys, the condition is ordinarily bilateral; in men over age 50, it is usually unilateral. In both age groups, the phenomenon is usually physiologic and tends to resolve spontaneously within 6 to 12 mo. Other causes of gynecomastia include testicular or pituitary tumors, some syndromes of male hypogonadism, cirrhosis of the liver (presumably because circulating estrogens are not inactivated), administration of estrogens for prostatic carcinoma, and therapy with steroidal compounds (eg, digitalis, spironolactone). Marked gynecomastia in a young man may require removal of breast tissue for psychologic reasons. In adults, biopsy is sometimes indicated to rule out carcinoma.

TUMORS AND CYSTS

FIBROEPITHELIAL TUMORS

Fibroadenomas are the most common benign breast tumors. As a pathologic entity they rank 3rd behind cystic disease and carcinoma, respectively. These tumors, seen most frequently in young women, are usually readily recognized because they feel encapsulated. They have a firm, rubbery consistency, are well circumscribed, and are easily "popped" about within the mammary tissue. The usual treatment is excision.

A rare form of fibroadenoma, **cystosarcoma phyllodes,** is characterized by its large size and rapid growth. Like a malignant tumor, it tends to recur locally if inadequately removed, but it only rarely metastasizes to regional lymph nodes or distant organs. Radical mastectomy is unwarranted; wide excision or simple mastectomy generally is the treatment of choice.

FIBROCYSTIC DISEASE OF THE BREAST
(Chronic Cystic Mastitis)

Fibrocystic disease, a benign condition and the most common disorder of the female breast, occurs in about 50% of premenopausal women. The fact that new cysts do not usually appear after menopause suggests that ovarian hormones are involved in the etiology of this disease. Pain or premenstrual breast discomfort is a frequent symptom, and the cysts may be tender; but the condition is more often asymptomatic and the patient generally seeks medical advice because of accidental palpation of one or more cysts.

The condition is usually bilateral. Solitary cysts often occur, but multiple cysts of many sizes are common. Characteristically, the breast has a nodular consistency. When the cysts are relatively large and near the surface, they may be moved about freely within the breast, though not so freely as a fibroadenoma. They are generally tense and may be tender. Aggregations of various-sized cysts deep within the breast are frequently indistinguishable from carcinoma, and surgical biopsy is mandatory in all dubious situations.

Evidence indicates that about 1/3 of women with biopsy-proven fibrocystic disease will show some degree of proliferative hyperplasia and have a 2 to 5 times higher risk

of developing breast cancer. The women in a small subset (4%) who have *atypical* hyperplasia combined with a family history of breast cancer have the highest risk (11%) of developing cancer. These patients should be examined at least every 6 mo, and annual mammography or xeroradiography, beginning at age 50, should be included in the follow-up.

Treatment of fibrocystic disease is rarely required. However, it has been shown that many women who complain of painful, lumpy breasts with recurrent cyst formation may be helped by eliminating methylxanthine-containing substances, such as coffee, tea, cola, and chocolate. These substances, by halting the actions of the catabolic enzyme phosphodiesterase, cause formation of fibrous tissue, increased cell growth, and cyst fluid. In addition, vitamin E in doses of 600 to 800 IU/day has been shown to relieve symptoms of fibrocystic disease in a majority of women and to cause regression in some. The mechanism is unknown, but may be related to alteration of blood levels of various hormones, including adrenal androgens and gonadotropins.

The clinical problem involves accurate differentiation of the numerous types of fibrocystic disease (single or multiple cysts, adenosis, fibrous mastopathy, duct ectasia, lobular neoplasia, or intraductal papillomatosis) from carcinoma. A dominant breast mass that does not completely disappear after cyst aspiration cannot be considered benign unless so proved by incisional or excisional biopsy and microscopic diagnosis. Aspiration biopsies, mammograms, xeroradiograms, and thermograms are too inaccurate for definitive diagnosis.

Intraductal Papillomas

Benign intraductal papillomas are relatively uncommon tumors occurring within the terminal nipple ducts of the breast. They are frequently too small to be palpated, and the symptom that brings the patient to the physician is generally a serous, serosanguineous, or frankly bloody **discharge from the nipple**. Treatment is careful excision of the affected ducts or the involved segment of the breast. With nipple discharge, especially if bloody, malignancy must be ruled out.

Lipomas

Lipomas of the breast are not uncommon. Though benign, they may be confused with malignant neoplasms if they are poorly encapsulated or unusually firm in consistency. Treatment is by excision.

CARCINOMA OF THE BREAST

(See also Ch. 105)

Breast carcinoma is the most common malignancy among women and shares with lung carcinoma the highest fatality rate of all cancers affecting females. One of every 11 women in the USA will develop breast cancer. For white women, the probability is about 1 in 10; for black women, the rate is close to 1 in 14. The annual mortality rate from 1930 to the present has remained fairly constant at about 27:100,000 females, and slightly higher for whites than for blacks. Breast cancer in men is rare and tends not to be recognized until late; thus, the results of treatment are poor. In women, breast carcinoma is rare before age 30, and the incidence rises rapidly after menopause. (For breast cancer in pregnancy, see under MALIGNANCY in Ch. 178.) Postmenopausal breast masses should be considered cancer until proved otherwise. Except for cystosarcoma phyllodes, other malignancies of the breast are rare enough to be considered pathologic curiosities.

Symptoms and Signs

Most breast cancers, including those frequently designated as **scirrhous, infiltrative, papillary, ductal, medullary,** and **lobular,** appear as a slowly growing, painless mass, though a vague discomfort may be present. Physical signs (see also under BREAST EXAMINATION, above) include a retracted nipple; bleeding from the nipple; distorted areola or breast contour; skin dimpling over the lesion; attachment of the mass to surrounding tissues, including the underlying fascia and overlying skin; edema of the skin of the breast with peau d'orange appearance; and enlarged axillary or supraclavicular lymph nodes. In far-advanced disease, skin nodules with ultimate breakdown and ulcer formation may be seen. Metastases should always be sought. The disease metastasizes by direct extension and via the lymphatics and the bloodstream. Among the most common sites are the lungs and pleura, the skeleton (especially skull, spine, and pelvis), and the liver. Whenever possible, distant spread of the disease should be confirmed by lymph node biopsy, by x-ray surveys of skeleton and chest, and, when appropriate, by liver and bone scans using radioactive isotopes.

Two atypical types of carcinoma are inflammatory carcinoma and Paget's disease. In **inflammatory carcinoma** the tumor grows very rapidly; the skin over it is edematous and becomes red, warm, indurated, and painful (ie, the symptoms resemble an infection). Diagnosis is established by biopsy. Any form of radical surgery is contraindicated because the disease tends to recur locally with great rapidity in the postoperative period. Treatment is palliative and includes radiotherapy (with or without simple mastectomy) followed by hormonal or chemotherapy as indicated.

In **Paget's disease** the nipple becomes crusted and has a chronic eczematoid appearance, because malignant cells (Paget cells) grow upward along the nipple ducts from an intraductal carcinoma originating deeper in the breast. These cells eventually invade the epidermis of the nipple. Sometimes the deeply situated tumor cannot be palpated and biopsy of the nipple is essential for accurate diagnosis. Treatment is the same as for any of the common breast carcinomas.

Diagnosis

While history, physical examination, and mammography may strongly suggest breast cancer, the diagnosis can be made only by microscopic examination of tissue removed by open or aspiration biopsy.

Treatment

Therapy depends mainly on the extent of the disease and the patient's age. If there is evidence of substantial involvement of axillary, supraclavicular, or internal mammary lymph nodes or of wider metastatic spread, treatment is palliative. When there is no evidence of peripheral spread (or, at most, signs of limited involvement of the axillary lymph nodes on the affected side), the treatment most often recommended is **total mastectomy and axillary dissection** (modified radical mastectomy). This procedure is now accepted as an equivalent alternative to conventional radical mastectomy for treating all primary operable breast cancers. The entire breast is removed together with virtually all of the axillary lymph nodes but, since the pectoral muscles are preserved and their function is left intact, the cosmetic result is far superior. In addition, the procedure lends itself far better to breast reconstruction with a plastic implant, which often can be inserted 6 to 12 mo after surgery. Cure rates for both operations appear identical. Even in the best circumstances, 10-yr survival rates > 50% have been unusual and some "clinical cures" may recur with fatal outcome as late as 20 yr after surgery. However, adjuvant chemotherapy programs are promising.

Over the past 10 yr increasing evidence has shown that many, if not most, primary operable Stage I and Stage II breast carcinomas can be conservatively managed by **partial mastectomy ("lumpectomy") plus a standard axillary node dissection followed in about 3 wk by irradiation of the remaining breast** with 5000 rads using 4 MeV and 6 MeV

photon beam linear accelerators or cobalt 60. This is followed by an additional boost of 1500 rads to the site of the excisional biopsy by external beam electrons or an interstitial implant of iridium 192. Results at 5 and 10 yr, in terms of disease-free survival and absolute survival, appear comparable to those for conventional modified radical mastectomy. The cosmetic results are for the most part outstanding. In the event of a late local recurrence in the ipsilateral breast (the reported incidence is between 5 and 10%), delayed mastectomy is still an option. If these results hold up for the next 5 or 10 yr, the mastectomy operation may become almost obsolete for Stage I and II breast cancers.

The relative value of mastectomy alone or in combination with postoperative radiotherapy, as compared to total mastectomy and axillary dissection in clinically negative and clinically positive axillary node groups, has been evaluated; the 10-yr survival data have failed to show an advantage for any particular treatment for either group. Finally, segmental mastectomy plus axillary dissection with and without postoperative irradiation has been compared to total dissection. To date, no advantage has been documented in any of the 3 treatment arms in absolute survival or distant disease-free survival. However, postoperative breast irradiation in the segmental mastectomy group did reduce the rate of reoccurrence of tumor in the ipsilateral breast from 22 to 5%.

Radiotherapy is sometimes used as an adjuvant to surgery. If axillary metastases are found after radical mastectomy or total mastectomy and axillary dissection, the ipsilateral internal mammary lymph node chain may be irradiated because of the high incidence of occult lymph node metastases in this area when the disease has already reached the axilla. Radiation should not be given to the already dissected axilla because the radiation greatly increases the possibility of postoperative lymphedema of the arm. For recurrent cancer, palliative radiotherapy can be valuable in controlling local chest wall or cervical lymph node recurrences and relieving pain from skeletal metastases. Radiation is of little value for visceral metastases.

Hormonal therapy, by addition or subtraction, is of greatest use in palliation of symptoms or in delaying advance of the disease. Hormonal therapy is often combined with radiotherapy when cancer recurs following mastectomy and when the tumor is so advanced that surgery is not indicated or is only palliative.

When disease recurs in *premenopausal* patients whose tumors are known to possess estrogen and progesterone receptor protein, castration may be tried first, preferably by bilateral oophorectomy rather than by radiotherapy. If there is no response or if the disease again becomes symptomatic after a beneficial response, androgens may be used; eg, testosterone propionate 100 mg IM 3 times/wk or, more conveniently, fluoxymesterone 20 mg/day orally. The masculinizing effects of these compounds can be avoided without sacrificing antineoplastic properties by substituting oral testolactone 300 mg/day. In general, androgens are most effective in controlling bone pain due to metastases. In a patient who is 10 or more years *postmenopausal* and has recurrent breast cancer, estrogens should be tried first, working up to 20 mg/day of diethylstilbestrol orally. If this fails, androgens may sometimes produce a remission. Megestrol acetate, a progesterone-like hormone, has also been useful in treating advanced breast cancer.

If neither androgens nor estrogens are effective or if they become ineffective after having produced a remission, corticosteroids (eg, prednisone 20 mg/day orally) may be tried either alone or in combination with various chemotherapeutic agents. Bilateral adrenalectomy or hypophysectomy may also temporarily retard recurrent disease, but selecting patients for such ablative procedures is difficult and is now rarely performed. Generally, if the tumor has not responded to previous hormonal manipulations, it will not respond to adrenalectomy or hypophysectomy. Even among tumors that have been shown to possess some estrogen dependence, only about 30% will respond further to such ablative procedures.

Presence or absence of estrogen- and progesterone-receptor protein in primary or metastatic tumor tissue is used to predict which patients may be expected to respond to additive or ablative endocrine therapy. In one study, primary and/or metastatic tumors of 1100 women were analyzed; of these, 70% were classified as estrogen-receptor negative **(ER–)** and 30% as estrogen-receptor positive **(ER+)**. Among the ER+ group, roughly 65% experienced an objective remission to hormonal manipulation, while only 5% of the ER– group responded.

Tamoxifen, a nonsteroidal estrogen antagonist, inhibits estrogen binding in breast cancers that are ER+ and PR+. Tamoxifen 20 mg/day orally should produce a partial or complete remission in about 50% of patients with recurrent ER+ and PR+ tumors, but is effective in < 10% of patients with ER– tumors.

In general, ER+, PR+ cancers have a better prognosis than ER–, PR– tumors and are more apt to be found in postmenopausal women. Tamoxifen as a single agent has been recommended for treating postmenopausal women with positive nodes and positive hormone receptor levels. Further studies are now comparing tamoxifen alone and in combination with cytotoxic agents.

Cytotoxic chemotherapy: Prophylactic chemotherapy may be useful in patients at high risk of developing recurrent cancer (ie, those with axillary lymph node metastases). Chemotherapy is also used in patients with recurrent breast cancer, sometimes in conjunction with hormonal manipulations and/or tamoxifen. A number of protocols using one or more chemotherapeutic agents in various combinations given at stated intervals for varying periods of time have been introduced and are being tested and evaluated. Sometimes these protocols add a corticosteroid (to suppress endogenous adrenal function) or the estrogen antagonist tamoxifen. The most commonly used and most effective chemotherapeutic agent is 5-fluorouracil. Others include cyclophosphamide, methotrexate, chlorambucil, vincristine, doxorubicin, and melphalan. Since all of these agents are to some degree immunosuppressive as well as cytotoxic and leukopenic, their use is not without risk and should be managed only by those experienced in cancer chemotherapy (see ANTINEOPLASTIC CHEMOTHERAPY in Ch. 105). These agents have demonstrated value in halting or delaying the appearance of metastases, especially in premenopausal patients, and in treating recurrences.

Biological response modifiers (eg, interferons, interleukins, LAK cells, anti-tumor monoclonal antibodies, tumor necrosis factor, adoptive immunotherapy) are agents or approaches that modify the host's biological response to tumor cells with resulting therapeutic benefit. They are a recent development in cancer research, and several are under study in clinical trials. These agents appear likely to provide new and better therapy.

---

173. GYNECOLOGIC NEOPLASMS

ENDOMETRIAL CARCINOMA

(Adenocarcinoma of the Uterus)

Of the malignancies affecting women, endometrial carcinoma ranks 3rd in frequency after breast and colorectal cancers. This adenocarcinoma of the uterus arises from the epithelial elements of the endometrium and is usually postmenopausal, with peak incidence between ages 50 and 60.

Etiology and Pathology

Endometrial carcinoma is more frequent in women with estrogen-producing ovarian tumors; with prolonged, and especially atypical, adenomatous endometrial hyperplasia; with delayed menopause; or with a disturbed menstrual history and infertility

Obesity, hypertension, diabetes mellitus, breast cancer, conditions that predispose to unopposed estrogen (ie, absence of ovulation and therefore no periodic progesterone), and a family history of breast or ovarian cancer possibly predispose to endometrial carcinoma.

Endometrial carcinoma spreads (1) down the surface of the uterine cavity into the cervical canal; (2) through the myometrium to the serosa and into the peritoneal cavity; (3) by transplantation via the lumen of the fallopian tube to the ovary, broad ligament, and peritoneal surfaces; (4) via the bloodstream, leading to distant metastases; or (5) via the lymphatics. Downward spread may lead to cervical stenosis and pyometra. Vaginal metastases may cause a mucosanguineous discharge, which leads to examination and diagnosis of the metastases in the more advanced stages.

Symptoms, Signs, and Diagnosis

The cardinal symptom is inappropriate uterine bleeding, such as any postmenopausal bleeding or recurrent metrorrhagia in the premenopausal patient; *as many as $^1/_3$ of all cases of postmenopausal bleeding are due to endometrial carcinoma.* The presence of myomas should not engender complacency regarding abnormal bleeding, especially in susceptible women (see Etiology, above). A mucoid or watery discharge may precede bleeding by several weeks or months.

In **diagnosis,** the **Papanicolaou test (Pap test**—see below under CERVICAL CARCINOMA) is helpful but undependable, since 30 to 40% of smears are false-negatives. Obtaining cellular material by aspiration of the endocervix may increase the rate of detection by Pap test to 70%. Vaginal douching should be avoided for at least 24 h prior to the examination. A good **endometrial biopsy** may give a positive finding of carcinoma 92% of the time. However, the diagnostic procedure of choice is **fractional curettage** (endocervical curettement, sounding of the uterus, dilation of the cervical canal, and curettement of the endometrium). This procedure permits histologic confirmation and grading of the tumor and staging of the extent of the tumor, including determining any extension of the lesion into the cervix, which is important in planning therapy. Caution should be exercised with biopsy, sounding of the uterus, or curettement, as perforation may occur with these procedures.

IVP, cystoscopy, proctosigmoidoscopy, barium enema, and chest x-ray should be performed prior to therapy. Other studies, such as mammography, bone scan, liver scan, arteriography, and lymphangiography, may be considered and performed when appropriate, but are not part of the routine staging procedure.

The international clinical staging system (FIGO) for endometrial carcinoma is outlined in TABLE 173–1.

Treatment and Prognosis

In the USA, the surgical approach includes extrafascial total abdominal hysterectomy with a wide vaginal cuff, combined with bilateral salpingo-oophorectomy and retroperitoneal lymph node sampling. Radical hysterectomy with retroperitoneal lymph node dissection is not warranted unless the cervix is clearly involved.

Progesterone therapy has been used for patients with advanced or recurrent disease, with regression occurring in 35 to 40% of cases. Continuous, large doses of nonestrogenic progesterone derivatives (hydroxyprogesterone caproate 1 gm/wk IM or medroxyprogesterone acetate 500 mg/wk IM) are given, or megestrol acetate 20 to 40 mg qid orally may be used. Treatment continues indefinitely if a favorable response is noted. It has produced regression of pulmonary, vaginal, and mediastinal metastases, and difficulties with sodium and water retention are rarely encountered. Remissions may last 2 to 3 yr or, occasionally, longer.

Recently, cytotoxic chemotherapy has been used with progestins for metastatic cancer. Monthly chemotherapy combining cyclophosphamide 500 mg/m², doxorubicin 50 mg/m², and cisplatin 50 mg/m², given IV, plus megestrol acetate 120 mg/day orally

TABLE 173–1. CLINICAL STAGING OF ENDOMETRIAL CARCINOMA AS A GUIDE TO TREATMENT AND PROGNOSIS*

Stage	Description
0	Carcinoma in situ, with histologic findings suspicious of malignancy
I†	Carcinoma confined to the corpus
IA	The length of the uterine cavity is 8 cm or less
IB	The length of the uterine cavity is > 8 cm
II	Carcinoma has involved the corpus and the cervix
III	Carcinoma has extended outside the uterus but not outside the true pelvis
IV	Carcinoma has extended outside the true pelvis or has obviously involved the mucosa of the bladder or rectum‡

* Staging as described by the International Federation of Gynecology and Obstetrics.

† Stage I subgroupings according to histologic type of adenocarcinoma are: G1—highly differentiated adenomatous carcinomas; G2—differentiated adenomatous carcinomas with partly solid areas; G3—predominantly solid or entirely undifferentiated carcinoma.

‡ A case should not be assigned to Stage IV only because of the presence of bullous edema (frequently but not always associated with submucosal extension).

has improved the overall objective response in 60% of patients. Frequent monitoring and complete knowledge of potential toxicity are essential with this regimen.

The **prognosis** is influenced by the histologic appearance and grading of the tumor, age of the patient (older women have a poorer prognosis), and tumor-spread before therapy. The overall 5-yr survival rates for endometrial carcinoma are encouraging. Almost 63% of patients will be alive without evidence of disease 5 yr or more after treatment; 28% will succumb within 5 yr of treatment; 9% will be alive with disease still present. In Stage I disease, the reported 5-yr survival rate is between 70 and 89%.

Rarely, malignancies originate from other histologic components of the uterus: sarcomas, carcinosarcomas, and mixed mesodermal tumors. Results of therapy in these cases are uniformly poor. Degenerating myomas rarely become sarcomatous, but when they do, if the lesion has remained within the myoma, cure rates with hysterectomy approach 80%.

CERVICAL CARCINOMA

Carcinoma of the uterine cervix, the 2nd most common malignancy of the female reproductive tract, most commonly affects women aged 40 to 55 yr. The incidence is higher among women from lower socioeconomic groups and among those with a history of early and frequent coitus and multiple sexual partners. Recently, venereal transmission of human papilloma virus **(HPV)** and herpesvirus type 2 **(HSV-2)** have been implicated as important in the etiology of cervical neoplasia.

Pathology

The earliest histologic change in what is considered a continuum from normal to invasive cancer (see also under DIAGNOSIS AND STAGING in Ch. 105) is **minimal cervical dysplasia,** in which abnormal cell proliferation occurs in the lower 1/3 of the epithelium. Most of the minimal dysplasias are self-limiting and regress to normal, but most **severe dysplasias** (2/3 of the epithelium showing abnormal proliferation) progress to **carcinoma in situ,** in which a full thickness of epithelium contains abnormal cells. When cancer cells penetrate the basement membrane and invade the stroma **("invasive carcinoma"),** they can spread by direct extension to adjacent pelvic organs or by lymphatic permeation and dissemination.

Of cervical carcinomas, 85 to 90% are squamous cell carcinomas. These vary from

well-differentiated cells with keratinization to highly anaplastic spindle cells. Of cervical tumors, 10 to 15% are adenocarcinomas. Sarcoma is rare.

Diagnosis

Early cervical neoplasia can be detected preclinically by cytologic examination of cervical smears obtained during routine annual pelvic examinations, as it is asymptomatic in this stage. The **Pap test** can detect 90% of early cervical neoplasias, and its use has reduced deaths from cervical cancer by > 50% through recognition and treatment of preinvasive neoplasia. Cervical cancer could be eliminated as a cause of death if all women had an annual Pap test; unfortunately, < 40% of women do so. (See directions for taking Pap test specimens in Ch. 168.)

Pap test results may be grouped into 4 categories: **Class I,** no abnormal cells seen; **Class II,** atypical cells seen, usually caused by inflammation; **Class III,** cells suspicious of carcinoma; **Classes IV and V,** carcinoma cells present. Most cytopathologists and many clinicians prefer to report findings descriptively (eg, smear is consistent with infection, dysplasia, etc.) rather than by class.

***Biopsy** is mandatory if a suspicious lesion (a friable mass or an ulcer) is seen.* Dysplasia or carcinoma detected on Pap smear can be investigated with the colposcope. If colposcopy is not available, the most abnormal areas may be identified for biopsy by staining the cervix with iodine solution, such as Lugol's (strong iodine) or Schiller's (potassium iodide 2 gm, iodine 1 gm, and water 300 mL). Nonstaining areas may be malignant, dysplastic, atypical, or glandular areas on the cervix. Outpatient **cervical punch biopsy and endocervical curettage** (to uncover lesions higher in the cervical canal) diagnose invasion in 90% of cases with abnormal cytology. **Colposcopy** may reveal the pathologic site for biopsy and avoid cone biopsy in 85% of cases. **Cold knife** (noncautery) **cone biopsy** or **laser cone biopsy** with fractional D & C performed under anesthesia is used only when simple biopsy fails to establish the presence or absence of invasion, or when colposcopic examination is inconclusive or unsatisfactory.

Clinical staging of cervical carcinoma by physical examination of the pelvis is the basis for estimating prognosis and planning therapy (see TABLE 173-2). In addition, a metastatic survey, including cytoscopy and sigmoidoscopy (with biopsies as needed in each), IVP, and chest x-rays are always done.

Treatment

Carcinoma in situ: Localized preinvasive lesions may be totally excised by cold knife conization with diligent follow-up or by total hysterectomy. The choice depends upon the patient's desire to remain reproductive and her reliability in follow-up. If conization is chosen, Pap tests should be repeated every 3 mo to ensure that all of the lesion has been removed and that it does not recur. Cryotherapy and occasionally laser therapy are currently being evaluated as outpatient methods of treatment in carefully selected patients when colposcopy and biopsy have clearly defined the lesion and invasive cancer has been ruled out.

Invasive squamous cell carcinoma remains well localized for a considerable length of time, with distant metastases occurring only late in its course. Since the tumor spreads by contiguity and via the lymphatics, effective treatment must include affected nodes as well as the primary tumor, but without excessively or irreversibly damaging surrounding normal body tissues. Radiotherapy and surgery used alone or together are effective. The cure rates are nearly identical.

Radiotherapy: A common and effective technic consists of 2 radium applications to the cervix (17,000 to 20,000 rads) for about 35 h each, followed by external radiation therapy encompassing the lymphatics along the pelvic sidewall. The radium applications are sufficient to destroy the primary tumor, and the external therapy raises irradiation to tumor-destroying levels in critical node regions. External therapy may precede radium applications in order to shrink bulky or very advanced disease. Major

TABLE 173–2. CLINICAL STAGING OF CERVICAL CARCINOMA AS A GUIDE TO TREATMENT AND PROGNOSIS*

Stage	Description
0	Carcinoma in situ, intraepithelial carcinoma
I	Carcinoma strictly confined to the cervix (extension to the corpus should be disregarded)
IA	Microinvasive carcinoma (early stromal invasion)
IB	All other cases of Stage I; occult cancer should be marked "occ"
II	Carcinoma extends beyond the cervix but not onto the pelvic wall; carcinoma involves the vagina, but not the lower third
IIA	No obvious parametrial involvement
IIB	Obvious parametrial involvement
III	Carcinoma extends onto the pelvic wall; on rectal examination there is no cancer-free space between the tumor and the pelvic wall; tumor involves the lower third of the vagina; includes all cases with hydronephrosis or nonfunctioning kidney
IIIA	No extension onto the pelvic wall
IIIB	Extension to the pelvic wall or hydronephrosis, or nonfunctioning kidney, or both
IV	Carcinoma has extended beyond the true pelvis or has clinically involved the mucosa of the bladder or rectum (bullous edema as such does not permit a case to be allotted to Stage IV)
IVA	Spread of the growth to adjacent organs
IVB	Spread to distant organs

* Staging as described by the International Federation of Gynecology and Obstetrics.

complications of radiotherapy include radiation proctitis and cystitis and occasionally recto- and vesicovaginal fistula formation. With primary radiotherapy for invasive squamous cell carcinoma, the overall 5-yr survival rate is about 55%. In Stages I and II, 5-yr cure rates are about 75 to 90%.

Surgical therapy: Primary surgical treatment is limited to patients whose ovarian function can be preserved, whose lesions display limited local spread, and in whom para-aortic lymph node biopsy is negative. Young women with Stage IB and IIA lesions are preferred candidates. Surgery involves radical hysterectomy, including all of the parametria, and bilateral retroperitoneal lymph node dissection ending at the bifurcation of the aorta. Five-year cure rates of 85 to 90% for women with Stage IB and IIA lesions have been reported following radical hysterectomy. The major complication of radical surgery is uretero- and vesicovaginal fistula formation, which occurs in about 1 to 2% of operations. If para-aortic node biopsy is positive or if the disease extends outside the pelvis, surgery is generally contraindicated.

If tumors are restricted to the pelvis but have involved the rectum or bladder, exenteration (excision of all pelvic organs) may be used to treat physically and psychologically appropriate patients. Exenteration usually is the treatment of choice for recurrent or persistent cancer confined to the central pelvis following conventional radiotherapy; occasionally it is used as primary therapy for advanced disease. It is successful in 25 to 45% of cases.

Chemotherapy: Systemic treatment provides only temporary pain relief in most instances. Distant metastases appear to respond better than the primary area in radiation failures. Many cytotoxic agents are being investigated, but only about 25 to 30% of tumors show objective regression.

Cervical carcinoma in pregnancy: About 1% of all cervical carcinomas are complicated by pregnancy or occur in recently pregnant women. With carcinoma in situ

treatment is delayed until after delivery, which may occur vaginally. Invasive disease is treated as in nonpregnant women: in the 1st trimester, radical hysterectomy or therapeutic irradiation will terminate the pregnancy; in the 2nd trimester, the uterus must be emptied by hysterotomy, followed by x-ray therapy or surgical excision for early lesions; in the 3rd trimester, a short delay to achieve fetal viability is encouraged. In invasive cervical disease vaginal delivery is contraindicated because it lowers the cure rate, whatever the treatment.

OVARIAN CARCINOMA

Of gynecologic neoplasms, 18% are ovarian carcinomas; the peak incidence occurs in women in their 50s. Since an ovarian neoplasm usually remains occult until it enlarges or extends enough to produce symptoms (see also under DIAGNOSIS AND STAGING in Ch. 105), early detection is difficult, and the disease has become extensive within or beyond the pelvis in 70 to 80% of patients before diagnosis. Thus, if routine pelvic examination reveals an ovary enlarged > 5 cm in diameter, careful follow-up is required. In the young woman, functional cysts are common; reexamination after 6 wk will show whether or not spontaneous resolution has occurred. The fact that size may be the only criterion for surgery indicates both the virulence of the disease and the inability to detect it. As a result, 1 in 4 ovarian tumors removed surgically is malignant. This ratio increases with the age of the patient. Ovaries in postmenopausal women are small and normally are not palpable. *Any enlargement of the ovary in a postmenopausal woman should signify a malignancy that requires prompt surgical excision.* Serous cystadenocarcinoma is the most common type (50% of cases) and occurs bilaterally in 30 to 50% of patients.

Pathology

Of malignant ovarian tumors, about 80% arise from the ovarian epithelium and have been classified histologically as (1) serous cystadenocarcinomas, (2) mucinous cystadenocarcinomas, (3) endometrioid tumors (similar to adenocarcinoma of the endometrium), (4) celioblastomas (Brenner tumors), (5) clear cell carcinomas, and (6) unclassified carcinomas. Tumors arising from germ cells or stroma not classified in this system include granulosa-theca cell tumors, Sertoli-Leydig cell tumors, dysgerminomas, and malignant teratomas.

Ovarian cancer tends to spread by both direct extension and lymphatics to regional nodes in the pelvis and para-aortic region. With lymphatic involvement, dissemination to the abdominal and pelvic peritoneum usually occurs. With abdominal involvement, hematogenous dissemination can lead to liver and pulmonary involvement.

Symptoms, Signs, and Diagnosis

An ovary may grow to considerable size before clinical symptoms appear. The earliest symptoms are vague lower abdominal discomfort and mild digestive complaints. Inappropriate endometrial bleeding is uncommon and presumably results from hormone secretion by the tumor. Abdominal swelling due to ovarian enlargement or accumulation of ascitic fluid, pelvic pain, anemia, and cachexia appear very late in the course. Additional physical signs include functional-tumor effects (hyperthyroidism, feminization, or virilization) or, more commonly, a lobulated fixed solid mass associated with nodular implants in the cul-de-sac. A Pap smear of the vaginal pool or pleural or peritoneal fluids may contain cells diagnostic of ovarian malignancy. X-rays show distant metastases to lung and bone.

Although usually a patient with a pelvic mass and ascites has a malignant ovarian tumor, a benign fibroma of the ovary may rarely be associated with ascites and right hydrothorax **(Meigs' syndrome).**

Clinical staging for ovarian carcinoma is outlined in TABLE 173–3.

TABLE 173–3. CLINICAL STAGING OF OVARIAN CARCINOMA AS A GUIDE TO TREATMENT AND PROGNOSIS*

Stage	Description
I	Growth limited to the ovaries
IA	Growth limited to one ovary; no ascites
IAi	No tumor on the external surface; capsule intact
IAii	Tumor present on the external surface, or capsule(s) ruptured, or both
IB	Growth limited to both ovaries; no ascites
IBi	No tumor on the external surface; capsule intact
IBii	Tumor present on the external surface, or capsule(s) ruptured, or both
IC	Tumor either stage IA or IB, but with ascites** present or with positive peritoneal washings
II	Growth involving one or both ovaries, with pelvic extension
IIA	Extension and/or metastases to the uterus and/or tubes
IIB	Extension to other pelvic tissues
IIC	Tumor either stage IIA or IIB, but with ascites** present or with positive peritoneal washings
III	Growth involving one or both ovaries with intraperitoneal metastases outside the pelvis, or positive retroperitoneal nodes, or both. Tumor limited to the true pelvis with histologically proved malignant extension to small bowel or omentum
IV	Growth involving one or both ovaries with distant metastases. If pleural effusion is present, there must be positive cytology to allot a case to stage IV. Parenchymal liver metastasis equals stage IV
Special Category	Unexplored cases that are thought to be ovarian carcinoma

* Staging as described by the International Federation of Gynecology and Obstetrics.

** Ascites is a peritoneal effusion that, in the opinion of the surgeon, is pathologic, or clearly exceeds normal amounts, or both.

Treatment and Prognosis

Standard therapeutic approaches are hindered by the variety of histologic types of tumors, by late discovery, and by the prevalence of widespread metastases, bilateral involvement, and extension to the uterus and contiguous structures. Not all lesions require extensive or radical therapy. In a young patient with a unilateral lesion of low histologic grade (such as a mucinous tumor), reproductive capability can be preserved by excising only the involved ovary and tube. In advanced disease, total abdominal hysterectomy and bilateral salpingo-oophorectomy with omentectomy are applied for excisable tumors, but there is considerable latitude in the treatment of each case. Radical surgery with node dissections or exenterations are ineffective, but radiotherapy and, more importantly, chemotherapy are becoming increasingly useful and are under continuous reevaluation. When tumor involvement precludes a realistic expectation of total excision, the initial laparotomy is performed for diagnosis and grading and to remove as much tumor as possible; chemotherapy or abdominal radiotherapy follows.

Widespread disease and Stage IV tumors must be treated with chemotherapy after adequate surgical excision. Most oncologists agree that combination therapy using 3 or more cytotoxic agents is preferable to single-agent treatment in patients with advanced Stages III and IV tumors. (See drugs and dosage recommendations listed above for cytotoxic chemotherapy with megestrol for treatment of endometrial cancer.)

The overall 5-yr survival rate without evidence of recurrence is 15 to 45% for the common epithelial tumors. Prognosis for the rare germ cell and stromal tumors varies considerably and depends upon the stage at diagnosis. For recurrent disease, the factor

most strongly correlated with survival is the time between diagnosis and start of multiagent therapy. With aggressive tumor reductive surgery and combination chemotherapy, the long-term survival rate for all ovarian cancers is improving (67% Stage III in one series). However, the death rate from ovarian cancer surpasses the combined rate for cervical and corpus cancer and ranks 5th in cancer fatalities in women.

CARCINOMA OF THE VULVA

Malignancy of the vulva accounts for about 3 to 4% of all gynecologic neoplasms and is most common after the menopause. Though patients can readily visualize and palpate these malignancies, they may not seek treatment for up to 3 yr because of embarrassment or fear. Also, the physician may cause delay by striving to provide symptomatic relief of the accompanying pruritus rather than obtaining an immediate biopsy.

Pathology

Squamous cell carcinoma comprises about 90% and basal cell carcinoma about 4% of cases; the remainder include intraepithelial carcinomas, such as Paget's disease, adenocarcinoma of Bartholin's gland, fibrosarcoma, and melanoma. The intraepithelial lesions are frequently of multifocal origin. Growth is initially superficial, but later the tumors extend into the vagina, the urethra, or the anus. The superficial inguinal and femoral nodes are involved in up to 50% of cases. Squamous cell carcinoma may be well differentiated or anaplastic.

Symptoms and Signs

Epithelial alterations, such as typical and atypical hyperplastic dystrophy, coexist in 40% of patients, and foci of lichen sclerosus may be seen in association with the cancer but are not necessarily considered to be precancerous. **Kraurosis vulvae**, a gross clinical diagnosis characterized by shrinkage and constriction of the vaginal outlet, is histopathologically identical to lichen sclerosus. Until the lesion reaches 1 to 2 cm or more in diameter, it is often asymptomatic, although carcinoma in situ tends to be pruritic. When the tumor becomes necrotic and infected, symptoms are those of an ulcer with bleeding and/or watery discharge.

Diagnosis

Diagnosis is made by simple biopsy in most instances. Biopsy sites can be delineated by staining the vulva with toluidine blue (1%) and then decolorizing with dilute (2 to 3%) acetic acid after allowing the dye to be absorbed for 3 to 5 min. Abnormal areas retain the blue dye. Differential diagnosis must include the various venereal diseases (granuloma inguinale, chancroid, lymphogranuloma venereum, and syphilis); basal cell carcinoma (rodent ulcer); intraepithelial (in situ) cancers characterized by small, red, white, or pigmented friable papules; Paget's disease, manifested by red, moist, elevated patches; and bowenoid papulosis, usually small elevated lesions considered a carcinoma in situ. Melanomas frequently appear as bluish-black, pigmented, or papillary lesions; they metastasize via the lymphatics and/or the bloodstream. The prognosis depends on the depth of involvement into the underlying epidermis.

Treatment

Since **squamous cell carcinoma** of the vulva spreads by local extension as well as by lymphatic embolization, all present and potential sites of tumor in this region should be removed. The tumors drain to the inguinal lymph nodes; however, those extending deep into the vagina drain into the retroperitoneal nodes. A correlation between tumor size and lymph node involvement has been noted.

The treatment of choice is radical vulvectomy and bilateral superficial inguinal and femoral node dissection. Recent reports demonstrate the importance of individualiza-

tion in specific instances, such as unilateral lesions with minimal invasion. Retroperitoneal lymph node dissection is warranted only if the superficial nodes are affected or if the tumor extends deeply into the vagina. Nevertheless, with deep pelvic nodal involvement there are few if any 5-yr survivors; thus irradiation should be considered in such cases. Up to 1/3 of the distal urethra may be excised without producing urinary incontinence. Lymphedema is a common problem for a year or so until collateral lymph channels have been established.

Preoperative external radiotherapy can be used to sterilize and/or decrease the size of large tumors. Radium needle implants may be used for inoperable tumors or for metastases.

The treatment of **basal cell carcinoma** is local excision. Paget's disease requires total vulvectomy, since the presence of an underlying malignancy must be ruled out. The treatment of **in situ carcinoma** should be individualized, since 40% or more of the cases are found in patients under age 40 yr, in whom vulvectomy is rarely indicated.

VAGINAL CARCINOMA

About 1% of gynecologic malignancies are vaginal carcinomas; the peak incidence is from age 45 to 65.

Etiology and Pathology

Except for clear cell carcinoma, where development of the tumor has been linked to intrauterine exposure to diethylstilbestrol **(DES)**, the etiology is unknown. Current evidence suggests that, as with cervical neoplasia, exposure to human papilloma virus **(HPV)** or herpesvirus type 2 **(HSV-2)** may be important.

Of malignancies arising primarily in the vagina, 95% are squamous cell carcinomas. The rest include primary and secondary adenocarcinomas, secondary squamous cell carcinomas in older women, clear cell adenocarcinoma in young women, and botryoid sarcoma (embryonal rhabdomyosarcoma) in infancy and childhood. Extension to the bladder and rectum is common.

Symptoms, Signs, and Diagnosis

Bleeding occurs after coitus or examination. Ulceration of the tumor may cause bleeding and infection. Watery discharge, dyspareunia, and, when the bladder or rectum is involved, urinary frequency or urgency or painful defecation occur. The tumor is most commonly found in the upper 1/3 of the vagina on the posterior wall.

In clinically unsuspected lesions, a Pap test may disclose carcinomatous cells, and a Schiller's test may outline the area to be biopsied. Extension is usually superficial toward the cervix, following the lymphatics. Every girl who has been or may have been exposed prenatally to DES should be examined at menarche, regardless of symptoms, and at regular intervals (at least yearly) thereafter.

Treatment and Prognosis

Treatment depends partly on the location and extent of the disease (it is complicated by extension to the bladder or rectum) and partly on the age and physical condition of the patient. A tumor localized in the upper 1/3 of the vagina is treated either by radical hysterectomy with upper vaginectomy and pelvic lymph node dissection or with radium and external radiotherapy. Treatment of secondary carcinomas and the primary carcinoma is usually combined and may be either radiotherapy or radical surgery. The 5-yr survival rate without recurrence is about 30%.

CARCINOMA OF THE FALLOPIAN TUBE

Primary carcinoma of the oviduct is rare, the peak incidence being from age 50 to 60. Chronic salpingitis or TB has been considered as a possible etiologic factor, but probably is unimportant. Infertility is not uncommon.

Pathology, Symptoms, Signs, and Diagnosis

These tumors spread either directly or by the lymphatics. Lymphatic spread is chiefly to the iliac, lumbar, and preaortic nodes. The tumors are usually unilateral and located in the distal 1/3 of the tube. As with any enlarging pelvic mass, symptoms are usually related to a vague feeling of discomfort due to pressure on the bladder or rectum. Occasionally a watery or blood-tinged vaginal discharge occurs. The diagnosis is rarely made preoperatively. Physical findings may include enlargement of the abdomen secondary to a large pelvic mass or to ascites, so the usual preoperative diagnosis is ovarian carcinoma. The tumor may close the fimbriated end of the tube, simulating the gross appearance of a hydrosalpinx.

Treatment

The 5-yr survival rate without evidence of recurrence varies from 5 to 48%. The treatment of choice is identical to that of the more common ovarian cancers: total abdominal hysterectomy and bilateral salpingo-oophorectomy with omentectomy followed by combination chemotherapy. Radiotherapy (confined to the pelvis) may be useful in the earlier disease.

TROPHOBLASTIC DISEASE

Neoplasms of trophoblastic origin that can follow intra- or extrauterine pregnancy.

A **hydatidiform mole** is the end stage of a degenerating pregnancy in which the villi have become hydropic and the trophoblastic elements have undergone variable amounts of proliferation. **Persistent trophoblastic disease (PTD, chorioadenoma destruens)** or locally invasive mole demonstrates local invasion of the myometrium by the villi of the hydatidiform mole. In contrast, **metastatic trophoblastic disease (MTD, choriocarcinoma,** chorioepithelioma) is an invasive—usually widely metastatic—tumor composed of syncytiotrophoblastic and cytotrophoblastic elements only.

A mole is more common in older patients. Molar pregnancies occur in about 1:2000 gestations in the USA; however, for unknown reasons, the incidence in Asiatic countries approaches 1:200. Over 80% of hydatid moles are benign. However, 15% lead to local invasion characteristic of PTD; 2 to 3% are followed by MTD. The locally invasive variant may cause uterine perforation, hemorrhage, and sepsis. A mole always precedes PTD, but precedes only 50% of MTDs. MTD occurs in about 1:25,000 to 1:45,000 pregnancies.

Symptoms, Signs, and Diagnosis

Hydatidiform mole often manifests itself shortly after conception by a rapid increase in the size of the uterus, which often is larger than it should be by dates. Vaginal bleeding, lack of fetal movement, lack of fetal heart tones at the appropriate time (12 wk with Doppler ultrasonography), and severe nausea and vomiting arouse clinical suspicion. Passage of typical grapelike molar tissue suggests the diagnosis, and histologic examination confirms it. Without such proof the diagnosis may be difficult to differentiate from other pregnancy complications involving a possibly normal fetus.

Ultrasound provides a sensitive diagnostic test that, while not infallible, usually demonstrates absence of an amniotic sac with a fetus in it. When ultrasound is not diagnostic, especially in cases of molar pregnancy, injection of contrast medium (eg, sodium diatrizoate) into the amniotic cavity should show a moth-eaten, honeycombed pattern on x-ray; however, this procedure is rarely required.

Human chorionic gonadotropin **(HCG)** is produced by the proliferating trophoblastic tissue, and high levels of HCG found on radioimmunoassay are valuable in evaluating treatment. Serum and urinary HCG levels are elevated during the first 100 days of gestation (higher with multiple pregnancy); therefore, the value of the test early in pregnancy is diminished. Radioimmunoassay for β subunit HCG, a more specific test for gonadotropin of chorionic origin, is very useful in evaluating treatment.

Complications of a mole include intrauterine infection and septicemia, hemorrhage, toxemia of pregnancy (the only condition in which true toxemia is seen in the first half of pregnancy), and development of MTD. PTD, because it is intramural, tends especially to cause bleeding; it may infiltrate adjacent tissue and occasionally metastasize to distant sites. MTD metastasizes early and widely via the venous and lymphatic systems and is highly malignant.

Treatment

Evacuation of **hydatidiform mole** is essential. The treatment of choice is suction curettage, followed by oxytocin stimulation and curettage of the uterus. Hysterotomy is no longer used for evacuation. Hysterectomy may be selected, based on the age, parity, and possible future pregnancy plans of the patient. For follow-up after evacuation, serial chest x-rays should be taken and determinations of urinary HCG titers or β subunit, preferably by radioimmunoassay, should be made. The titer should progressively fall to a normal level in 8 wk. If it fails to fall or rises after once falling, studies for malignant progression should be done. The patient should use contraception for a year, since detection of malignant change is compromised by pregnancy.

Patients with persistent or rising HCG levels may have either **PTD** (invasive mole) or **MTD** and should receive chemotherapy with methotrexate or dactinomycin. Chemotherapy has largely replaced hysterectomy in both conditions; results are good, reproductive capacity is preserved, and major surgery is avoided. Hysterectomy may be considered in patients >40 yr or those desiring sterilization and may be required for those with infection, uncontrolled bleeding, or invasion through the uterine wall. For patients with trophoblastic malignancy, the overall remission rate is 75 to 85%.

174. FAMILY PLANNING

One or both members of a couple can use **contraception** to avoid pregnancy temporarily or **sterilization** to prevent pregnancy permanently. **Induced abortion** can be used to correct failures of contraception. The couple's decision to begin, prevent, or interrupt a pregnancy may be influenced by **prenatal diagnosis** or **genetic counseling** (see Ch. 203). **Infertility** is discussed in Ch. 166.

CONTRACEPTION

Each contraceptive technic has advantages and disadvantages that should be explained so that the woman can choose the one most suitable for herself and her partner. The methods most used in the USA are—in order of popularity—oral steroid "pills," condom, intrauterine device **(IUD)**, spermicides, diaphragm, withdrawal, and rhythm. Many factors affect rates of contraceptive failure. Age, level of education, and degree of motivation are inversely related to contraceptive failure rates. In general, methods used at the time of coitus (eg, diaphragm, condom, foam, sponge, rhythm, withdrawal) are more effective in theory than in practice. Overall effectiveness is greater with methods unrelated to coitus (eg, oral contraceptives, IUD) because patient involvement is simpler. Over a period of several years, use/pregnancy rates are about 1%/yr for oral contraceptives and IUDs and are several times higher for coitus-related methods.

Diaphragm and Cervical Cap

The **diaphragm,** a dome-shaped rubber cup with a flexible rim that fits over the cervix, acts as a barrier to sperm. The diaphragm must be carefully fitted by the health provider, and the woman must know how to insert it so that the cervix is covered. Contraceptive cream or jelly should always be used with the diaphragm to improve

contraceptive effectiveness in case the diaphragm is displaced during coitus. The diaphragm should cause no discomfort, and neither partner should be aware of its presence. It should be inserted prior to coitus and remain in place for 8 h after the last coitus. Additional spermicide should be added prior to each coital act, to improve effectiveness. When the diaphragm is properly used, the pregnancy rate is about 3%; the overall failure rate is about 14%.

The **cervical cap** is similar to the diaphragm, comes in several sizes, and must be fitted by a clinician. It can be left in place for 72 h. It has not been approved for general, unrestricted use in the USA. Failure rates are similar to those with the diaphragm.

Vaginal Foams, Creams, Suppositories, and Sponges

These agents must be placed into the vagina before each coital act. They contain a spermicide, usually nonoxynol 9, that immobilizes or kills sperm on contact; they also provide a mechanical barrier to sperm. No type of foam or suppository seems to be more effective than another. As the woman's age increases, their efficacy increases greatly; in women > 30 yr, it is similar to that of the IUD. The contraceptive sponge contains the same spermicide but has the advantage of remaining effective for 24 h. Its failure rate is about the same as that of the diaphragm.

Rhythm

The rhythm method depends on abstinence during the fertile period. Ovulation most often occurs about 14 days before onset of the next menstrual period. Although the human ovum may be fertile for only about 24 h, motile sperm have been identified up to 7 days after coitus; fertilization has occurred following coitus 3 days before ovulation. For the rhythm method to be successful, the woman's menstrual cycles should be regular. To determine the period of abstention, 18 days should be subtracted from the length of the shortest of the previous 12 cycles and 11 days from the longest. Thus, if the woman's cycles vary between 26 and 29 days, the couple must abstain from coitus from day 8 through day 18 of each cycle. A more effective method is based on measuring the woman's basal body temperature each morning before arising. Basal body temperature rises about 0.6 F, from a relatively lower level before ovulation to a somewhat higher level, usually > 98 F (37 C), after ovulation. The couple abstains from intercourse until at least 48 to 72 h after the temperature rise. Noting an increased amount of cervical mucus (usually near the time of ovulation) has been used in an attempt to more accurately determine the "fertile time." The failure rate of the rhythm method is about 15 to 25%. Accurate use of temperature charts reduces the failure rate. Combining the cervical mucus changes with temperature changes, the "Sympto-Thermal" method has been advocated recently; however, even with these adjuvants, the failure ratio is about 10%.

Condom

Condom use, the 3rd most common contraceptive method in the USA (after male/female sterilization and oral contraceptives) is the only reversible effective male method other than coitus interruptus (withdrawal). If used properly, the condom also provides considerable protection against sexually transmitted diseases and may possibly prevent premalignant changes of the cervix. The condom should not be applied tightly (the tip should overlap about ½ in. to collect the ejaculate) and must be removed carefully so that none of the contents is spilled. The failure rate with careful use is 3 to 4%. Adding a spermicidal agent, either in the lubricant or by insertion into the vagina, may further lower this rate.

Oral Contraceptives (OCs)

There are 2 major categories of OCs: **combination** and **progestogen only**. Combination types contain both a synthetic estrogen and a synthetic progestogen and are given continuously for 3 wk. No medication is given in the 4th wk, to allow for withdrawal

bleeding. Using progestogen alone, a small dose of a synthetic progestogen is given every day; this regimen is associated with a relatively high incidence of irregular bleeding episodes and a pregnancy rate of 2 to 8%/yr and is recommended only when estrogen is contraindicated—eg, when breast-feeding.

Effectiveness does not differ significantly among the various combination formulations; if no tablets are omitted, the pregnancy rate is < 0.2% at the end of 1 yr. However, formulations with 50 μg or more of estrogen have a higher incidence of adverse effects and, in general, should not be prescribed. Low-dose formulations with 30 to 35 μg of ethinyl estradiol should generally be given to new users of OCs. These formulations are as effective as those with higher dose formulations, but the incidence of breakthrough bleeding **(BTB)** may be somewhat higher in the first few months of use.

The benefits of OCs must be weighed against risks for the individual patient. Not taking OCs may result in an unwanted pregnancy, and the risk of death associated with normal pregnancy as well as elective abortion is greater than that associated with OCs.

Starting OC treatment: All women receiving OCs should be examined initially, 3 mo later (to determine if BP has changed), and at least annually thereafter. When a personal or family history suggests increased risk of diabetes mellitus or arteriosclerotic cardiovascular disease, it is wise to obtain a 2-h postprandial blood glucose and a serum lipid profile that includes HDL-and LDL-cholesterol, total cholesterol, and triglycerides. If the glucose or lipids are abnormal, OCs should not be used. At each visit, breast and pelvic examinations should be performed and the liver carefully palpated. BP and weight should be determined. New users should be started on low-dose formulations, as mentioned above.

OC use following pregnancy: The woman who has had a term delivery differs from the postabortal woman in the interval between resumption of ovulation and recurrence of menstruation. The first episode of menstrual bleeding in the postabortal woman is usually preceded by ovulation, which generally occurs between 2 to 4 wk. Following a term delivery in a nonnursing mother, the first menstruation is usually anovulatory, but occasionally ovulation occurs 4 to 5 wk after delivery. Nursing mothers usually do not ovulate until 10 to 12 wk after delivery, but they may ovulate before the first menses. After spontaneous or induced abortion of a fetus < 12 wk gestation, OCs should be started immediately. Following termination of pregnancy between 12 and 28 wk, starting OCs should be delayed 1 wk. Since the risk of thromboembolism normally increases postpartum and may be enhanced by OCs, for patients who have a delivery after 28 wk gestation and are not nursing, OCs should be started 2 wk after delivery During lactation OCs diminish the amount of milk produced and reduce the concentrations of protein and fat in the milk; also, measurable amounts of the hormona compounds can be found in the milk. Therefore, combination OCs are *not* advised fo nursing mothers and progestogen-only formulations should be used. **Galactorrhea** is a uncommon side effect.

No benefits of intermittently stopping therapy have been documented. OCs nee not be stopped for any interval (unless the woman wishes to conceive), as long as sh does not develop adverse effects or other contraindications to their use. A health young woman can take OCs continuously until age 35. *Women* ***over age 35*** *who smok cigarettes or have other risk factors (eg, untreated hypertension or hypercholesterolemic have been reported to have an increased risk of death from circulatory diseases, includin stroke and myocardial infarction.* With advancing age, risks of such serious adver effects with OCs increase while risks associated with IUDs decline and with sterilization remain low. After age 35, use of OCs should be discouraged and alternative forn of contraception or sterilization should be recommended. Nonsmokers, however, ca safely take low-dose OCs until age 40 without increased risk of cardiovascular diseas

Physiology: The action of OCs results from a negative feedback on the hypothal

mus, inhibiting gonadotropin-releasing hormone; therefore, the pituitary does not secrete gonadotropins at midcycle to stimulate ovulation. The endometrium of the uterus becomes thin, and the cervical mucus becomes thick and impervious to sperm.

Side effects and contraindications: Women who develop BTB while taking OCs should receive an increased estrogen dose by increasing the amount given or by using a more estrogenic formulation. For women who develop amenorrhea, the progestogenic component should be decreased and the estrogen content may have to be increased. Many side effects, such as nausea, breast tenderness, fluid retention, higher BP, and depression, are related to the dose of estrogen. Progestogens produce anabolic effects, such as weight gain, acne, and a sensation perceived by some women as nervousness. Potency and weight of the progestogen in the formulation are important considerations with regard to adverse effects. Levonorgestrel is 10 to 20 times as potent as the other 3 progestogens used in OCs—norethindrone, norethindrone acetate, and ethynodiol diacetate, which are about equal in potency.

In addition to effects on the female genital tract, the metabolic activities of synthetic hormonal components of OCs affect nearly every other organ system. Serious complications, however, are relatively rare. **Absolute contraindications** to OCs include pregnancy, active liver disease, hyperlipidemia, uncontrolled hypertension, diabetes mellitus with vascular changes, and a history of thromboembolic phenomena, thrombophlebitis, coronary artery disease, stroke, sickle cell disease, estrogen-dependent cancer, liver adenoma, and cholestatic jaundice of pregnancy, as well as prolonged immobilization of a lower extremity. **Relative contraindications** include depression, migraine headache, oligomenorrhea, undiagnosed amenorrhea, and heavy cigarette smoking.

Inhibition of ovulation persists in a few women after they stop taking the tablets, but OCs do not cause permanent sterility or affect the outcome of pregnancies conceived any time after stopping OCs.

Most **serum protein changes** that occur during OC therapy do not represent medical hazards, but *results of some clinical laboratory tests are altered.* Serum copper and iron levels increase, while tests of thyroid function are altered to the same extent as in pregnancy; eg, thyroxin-binding globulin capacity increases, while free thyroxine remains normal. There is no evidence, however, that OCs alter thyroid function itself. However, increased levels of the globulins involved in the clotting process, particularly Factors VII and X, result in a hypercoagulable state.

The incidence of **deep vein thrombophlebitis** and **thromboembolism** in OC users is estimated to be 3 to 4 times higher than in nonusers, and mortality from thromboembolic disease associated with using hormonal contraceptives is estimated to be about 3:100,000 women/yr. Thrombus formation appears to be related to increases in blood-clotting factors and, possibly, increased platelet adhesion. These changes are produced by the estrogenic component, and the increased incidence of thromboembolism is related to the amount of estrogen given. The incidence of these disorders has steadily decreased as amounts of estrogen in the formulations have been lowered. There is no evidence that the incidence of thromboembolism is increased in women with varicosities of the leg veins. If a woman develops signs of deep vein thrombophlebitis or pulmonary embolism while receiving OCs, she should discontinue them and further diagnostic studies should be done. Because of the increased risk of thromboembolic disease, OCs should be discontinued 1 mo before elective surgery.

CNS effects of OCs include cerebrovascular accidents, as well as nausea and vomiting, headache, and depression. The risk of hemorrhagic stroke and possibly thrombotic stroke is estimated at 3 times greater in OC users than in nonusers. Women who have headaches more frequently or who develop any peripheral neurologic symptoms, fainting, or aphasia while taking OCs should discontinue them, since these symptoms may be prodromes of a cerebrovascular accident. Depression and sleep disturbances are noted in 1 to 2% of OC users.

Estrogen increases production of angiotensin, which causes some OC users to develop **increased BP.** With lower-dose estrogen formulations, there is a lessened incidence of increases in BP. BP should be monitored in all women before and during treatment with OCs. The steroids should be stopped if BP increases, as it will return to normal when OCs are discontinued.

Alterations in glucose metabolism, both impairment of glucose tolerance and increased plasma insulin levels, have been associated with OCs. However, this deterioration of glucose tolerance is usually reversible and occurs less frequently or not at all with low-dose formulations. OCs can be prescribed for patients who previously have had an elevated blood glucose test but are not currently diabetic. A 2-h postprandial blood glucose test should be performed annually in all women using OCs who are likely to develop diabetes mellitus; eg, those who have a family history of diabetes mellitus, whose infants were large at birth, or who have had a history of unexplained fetal deaths. If this test is abnormal, a glucose tolerance test should be performed and, if abnormal, the OCs should be stopped. It is best if insulin-dependent diabetics with vascular changes do not take OCs, as their use may increase the risk of cardiovascular disease.

Estrogens may cause **sodium retention;** some users develop **edema** and may gain 3 to 5 lb in weight. Progestogens are anabolic, and some women gain weight because of increased appetite. Thus, if a woman gains > 10 lb/yr, OCs should be discontinued or an OC containing a less potent progestogen should be used.

Serum levels of some vitamins, trace elements, and lipids may be altered by OCs. Levels of pyridoxine, folic acid, and most other B vitamins, as well as ascorbic acid, calcium, manganese, and zinc, are decreased, while vitamin A levels are increased. These changes have no known clinical significance, and women taking OCs do not need vitamin supplements. Serum lipid levels may be slightly altered in OC users. However, the slight decrease in high density lipoprotein cholesterol appears to be of no clinical significance.

Drug interactions: Although synthetic sex steroids can retard biotransformation of certain drugs such as phenazone and meperidine due to substrate competition, such interference is not important clinically. OC use has not been shown to inhibit the actions of other drugs. However, certain drugs (barbiturates, sulfonamides, cyclophosphamide, and rifampin) can interfere with the action of OCs by inducing liver enzymes that accelerate biotransformation of the steroids to more polar and less biologically active metabolites. A relatively high incidence of OC failure in women taking rifampin has been reported, and the 2 agents should not be given concurrently. Data concerning OC failure in users of other antibiotics (eg, penicillin, ampicillin, and sulfonamides) and other agents (eg, phenytoin and phenobarbital) are based on anecdotal reports and are less clear. Until controlled studies have been reported, it may be prudent to suggest use of a barrier method in addition to the OCs. Therapeutic doses of antibiotics are also prescribed. Epileptic patients who ingest phenobarbital daily should use a 50-μg estrogen formulation.

The incidence of **cholelithiasis** in OC users increases during the first few years of use, and then declines. Thus, OCs accelerate gallstone formation. Women who develop **idiopathic recurrent jaundice of pregnancy** (cholestasis of pregnancy) may also become jaundiced when treated with OCs and should not use them. **Active liver disease** is also a contraindication to hormonal contraceptive therapy, but hepatitis followed by complete recovery is not an absolute contraindication. Women with a history of liver disease should have normal liver function before taking OCs. Rarely, **benign liver adenomas** develop in OC users and may rupture spontaneously. The incidence is related to duration of use and is estimated to be about 1:30,000 to 500,000 users. The adenomas usually regress spontaneously after therapy is stopped. **Hepatic vein thrombosis** with Budd-Chiari syndrome has occurred in OC users, but a causal relationship has not been established.

Melasma, similar to that which develops in pregnancy, occurs in some patients receiving OCs. This change is accentuated by exposure to sunlight and disappears slowly after stopping the OCs. Since treatment is difficult (see HYPERPIGMENTATION in Ch. 241), it is best to stop OCs when melasma becomes apparent.

After 25 yr of use, there is no evidence that OCs increase the risk of any type of **cancer** in humans, including breast or liver cancer. Although cervical cancer is increased in OC users, its increase together with cervical dysplasia appears to be related to the sexual practices of OC users, not to the steroids. OC users therefore should have annual Pap smears. OCs have been shown to decrease the risk of the lethal endometrial and ovarian cancers by about 50%. Other documented noncontraceptive health benefits of OC use include decreased incidences of menorrhagia, dysmenorrhea, premenstrual tension, iron deficiency anemia, benign breast disease, and functional ovarian cysts; reduced incidences of ectopic pregnancy and salpingitis associated with their use should lessen infertility. These benefits result in an estimated reduction of 50,000 hospitalizations/year in the USA.

Intrauterine Devices (IUDs)

Only about 2 million women in the USA use IUDs for contraception, even though they are very effective. IUDs are not as effective as OCs but have some advantages: their effects are limited to the female genital tract and insertion requires only one decision by the patient. The various types of IUDs have little significant difference in effectiveness. Pregnancy rates at the end of 1 yr of use usually range from 1 to 3%. Differences in pregnancy rates among devices in various studies are due more to differences in insertion technics than differences in the devices themselves. A high fundal insertion must be obtained, especially with the copper devices. For any type of device, the pregnancy rate is greater in the first year than the second, and pregnancy rates are higher for smaller devices than for larger ones of the same design.

Discontinuation rates for IUDs are approximately the same for all devices, about 20 to 30% in the first year and about 10 to 15% in the second year. There is no need to change a plastic unmedicated IUD unless the patient develops increased bleeding after it has been in place for > 1 yr. The roughness of calcium salts deposited on the plastic over time, however, can cause ulceration and bleeding of the endometrium. If increased bleeding develops after 1 yr or more, the old IUD should be removed and a new one inserted.

The T- or 7-shaped devices wound with copper wire are very effective. These devices are no longer marketed in the USA, but they are approved for use by the FDA and do not need to be removed ahead of schedule from women wearing them. Because of the continuous dissolution of the copper, these devices should be replaced at 3- to 4-yr intervals. The plastic types may be left in situ for long intervals if no untoward symptoms develop. The T-shaped, progesterone-releasing IUD needs to be re-inserted annually. Despite its disadvantages, it is the only IUD currently marketed in the USA. Significantly less monthly blood loss occurs with the copper devices and progesterone device than with the larger plastic IUDs, such as the loop or double coil.

Physiology: A sterile tissue reaction in the endometrial cavity is generally accepted as the main cause of the contraceptive effect. There is bacterial contamination for 24 h after insertion of an IUD, and although the endometrial cavity rapidly becomes sterile, inflammation persists after the bacterial infection disappears. Breakdown products of intrauterine neutrophils are toxic to the sperm and blastocyst. The major mechanism of action of IUDs is prevention of fertilization because of this toxic effect on the sperm. The inflammatory foreign body reaction is transitory and ceases when the IUD is removed. The monthly incidence of conception in the first year after removal of an IUD is the same as after stopping usage of condoms or diaphragms; at the end of 1 yr, 90% of women who wish to conceive have done so.

Side effects and complications: Bleeding and pain are the major medical reasons for removing an IUD; these problems account for > 50% of all discontinuances and occur in about 15% of patients during the first year and 7% during the second year of use. Insertion during menses is usually less painful than at other times in the menstrual cycle.

The **expulsion rate** for most devices is about 10% during the first year. IUDs are expelled most frequently in the first few months after insertion and more frequently in the first year than the second year of use. Smaller devices are expelled more frequently than larger ones of the same design, and the expulsion rate is higher in younger women and in nulligravidas. If another IUD is inserted, there is a good chance it will be retained. *About 20% of expulsions are unnoticed and can be followed by an unwanted pregnancy*; therefore, a plastic string should be attached to the IUD so that the user can check periodically, especially after menses, to see that the device has not been expelled.

Perforation of the uterus is a potentially serious but uncommon problem. Its incidence varies among the different devices, but for all those in current use it is about 1:1000 insertions. Perforation most commonly occurs at the time of insertion and can usually be prevented by straightening the uterine axis with a tenaculum, determining the direction of the cavity with a probe, and inserting the IUD carefully. Sometimes only the distal portion of the IUD penetrates the uterine muscle at the time of insertion, and then uterine contractions during the next few months force the IUD into the peritoneal cavity. Perforation should always be suspected if a patient states she cannot feel the string but did not notice that the device was expelled. If the device or the tail is not visible after pelvic examination, the uterine cavity should be probed (unless pregnancy is suspected). If the device cannot be felt with a uterine sound or biopsy instrument, a sonogram or an x-ray should be obtained. A lateral x-ray with contrast medium inside the uterine cavity should be obtained, since an IUD located in the cul-de-sac can be missed on an ordinary anteroposterior film. All intraperitoneal IUDs should be removed, as they may cause bowel adhesions. Extrauterine IUDs containing copper can cause more severe intraperitoneal reactions and should be removed promptly. They can usually be removed via laparoscopy.

Bacterial contamination of the endometrial cavity occurs at the time of insertion and clears rapidly after 24 h. IUD appendages do not provide continuous access for bacteria to enter the endometrial cavity. However, an IUD should not be inserted in a patient with clinical evidence of salpingitis, since additional bacteria would be introduced. Most infections occurring after an IUD has been in place for 30 or more days are sexually transmitted and are not caused by the IUD; they can be treated without removing it, unless the infection is severe or the patient is pregnant. Although IUD users have a threefold greater incidence of clinical salpingitis than nonusers, the increased risk with the loop and copper IUDs occurs during only the first 4 mo after insertion and probably is related to bacteria introduced at the time of insertion. Prophylactic systemic antibiotic use following insertion is not cost effective. An IUD should not be inserted if there is clinical evidence of cervicitis. Since the shield type of IUD with its multifilament tail string has been associated with increased risk of salpingitis, all IUDs of this type should be removed. Individuals at high risk for developing salpingitis, including those with a prior history of pelvic inflammatory disease, nulliparous women under age 25 yr, and women with multiple sexual partners, should not use IUDs.

The incidence of congenital defects in babies born to mothers with an IUD in place is no greater than that of the general population; nor is the incidence of fetal death increased, but the incidence of **spontaneous abortion** is significantly higher (about 55%). If a woman who becomes pregnant with an IUD in place wishes to continue the pregnancy and the appendage is visible, the IUD should be removed, since the abortion rate is lower after removal of the device. The IUD will not be located in the

amniotic sac, since implantation does not occur immediately adjacent to the device. If the appendage is not visible, the uterus should not be probed in an attempt to remove the IUD. A number of serious and even fatal **systemic infections** have been reported in women who became pregnant with the IUDs (particularly the shield type with its multifilament tail) in place, and it is recommended that all IUDs be removed if pregnancy occurs and the string is visible. If the string is not visible, removal will result in abortion. *Therefore, if the patient refuses removal and wants to retain the pregnancy, she must be warned of the possibility of sepsis and should report symptoms of infection promptly.* If uterine infection during pregnancy occurs with an IUD in place, appropriate antibiotics should be given and the endometrial cavity should be evacuated.

Ectopic pregnancies are not effectively prevented by IUDs; a woman who becomes pregnant with an IUD in place has about a tenfold greater than normal (or 3 to 9%) chance of having an ectopic pregnancy. After an induced abortion for an IUD failure, the uterine contents should be examined histologically to ensure that the gestation was intrauterine.

Several long-term studies have shown no clinical evidence that IUDs cause adenocarcinoma of the endometrium or carcinoma of the cervix.

STERILIZATION

One partner is sterilized in about 1/3 of all married couples in the USA who use some method of family planning. Sterilization is the most popular contraceptive method for couples in whom the wife is over age 30. In contrast to the methods discussed above, *sterilization should always be considered permanent.* Reanastomosis following vasectomy or tubal ligation is possible, but the reconstructive operation is much more difficult following vasectomy; pregnancy rates following reanastomosis of the vas range from 45 to 60% and those following oviduct reanastomosis range from 50 to 80%. Both partners should be counseled regarding the risks and irreversibility of the procedures.

Sterilization in men is performed by vasectomy, an outpatient procedure that takes about 20 min and requires only local anesthesia. The vas deferens is isolated and cut, the ends of the vas are closed either by ligation or fulguration and then replaced in the scrotal sac, and the incision is closed. About 15 to 20 ejaculations are usually required after the operation before sterility is achieved. Semen analysis should be performed after the procedure, and *the man is not considered sterile until 2 sperm-free ejaculates have been produced.* Complications of vasectomy include hematoma (with an incidence up to 5%), sperm granulomas (inflammatory responses to sperm leakage), and spontaneous reanastomosis, which usually occurs shortly after the procedure.

Female sterilization is by tubal ligation, a more complicated procedure requiring an intraperitoneal incision and general anesthesia. Ligation can be performed through a small infraumbilical incision either directly after delivery in the operating room or the following day without prolonging the hospital stay. The same operative technics can be used for female sterilization at other times ("interval sterilization"). The oviducts can usually be easily and rapidly ligated through an abdominal incision or through a colpotomy incision. If a small, 2-cm suprapubic incision is made ("minilaparotomy"), the patient may be cared for in an ambulatory surgery setting, as with laparoscopy (see below). The "minilaparotomy" is usually performed under general anesthesia, but it can also be done under local anesthesia. The same technic as that used with laparoscopy can be used—eg, fulguration; occluding the tubes with bands or clips; or ligation/partial excision, such as the Pomeroy method.

Laparoscopy has become a popular gynecologic operative technic. Working through the laparoscope, the oviducts can be fulgurated and cut through 1 or 2 small intraperitoneal punctures. Although general anesthesia is usually used for laparoscopic sterilization, the patient does not have to be hospitalized overnight. The failure rate

following laparoscopic fulguration is reported to be only 1:1000 procedures. The incidence of complications following laparoscopic fulguration ranges from 1 to 6%; major complications, such as hemorrhage or puncture or burns of the bowel, occur at a rate of 0.6%. The rate of bowel injury is less with bipolar than with unipolar coagulation operations, and the former should always be used for fulguration.

Various mechanical devices (Silastic® bands and spring-loaded clips) are being used to occlude the tubes instead of fulgurating or cutting them, thereby avoiding problems associated with electric current. Because of less tissue damage, sterilization performed with these devices is potentially more reversible; but even with microsurgical technics, reversibility rates are only about 75%.

Elective vaginal hysterectomy is accepted for sterilization alone in some communities. If other chronic problems with the uterus exist (such as menorrhagia, cervical dysplasia, or severe dysmenorrhea), abdominal or vaginal hysterectomy may be the preferred method of sterilization. Although the morbidity, blood loss, and hospital stay are greater after hysterectomy than after tubal sterilization, there are long-term benefits, such as 100% effectiveness and the absence of menstrual disorders or the possibility of development of leiomyomas or cancer.

INDUCED ABORTION

Throughout history, women have used abortion to terminate unwanted pregnancies. Its legal status worldwide varies from complete prohibition to elective procedures on request. About 2/3 of the women in the world have legal abortion available; about 1/12 of all women are in countries with strictly enforced abortion prohibitions. In the USA, abortion is permitted on request in the first trimester; after 12 wk, each state may regulate abortion in ways reasonably related to maternal health.

The number of reported abortions in the USA has progressively increased, especially since 1974, when the laws were liberalized. In 1963, the *rate* of abortions was 0.13/1000 women in childbearing years (15 to 44); in 1980, the rate was 29.3/1000; therefore, ≅ 3% of women aged 15 to 44 have abortions in a year. The *ratio* of abortions to live births increased more markedly, from 13/1000 in 1963 to 362/1000 in 1980. Abortion is one of the most common surgical procedures in the USA; > 1.5 million abortions were reported in 1980. About 30% were done on women under age 20; 35% were 20 to 24, and the remaining 35% were 25 or older; 25% of the women were married. In 1980, > 90% of abortions were in the first trimester (12 wk or less), with > 50% of these at 8 wk or less. About 96% were performed by curettage, 2.2% by saline instillation, 0.5% by prostaglandin instillation, and < 1.5% by other methods, including major surgical procedures.

Abortion methods currently used are (1) instrumental evacuation through the vagina; (2) medical induction, with stimulation of uterine contractions; and (3) uterine surgery (hysterotomy or hysterectomy). The procedure varies with the length of gestation. "Weeks of gestation" are calculated from the *last menstrual period* with the assumption that ovulation occurred at about day 14 of the cycle. **Instrumental evacuation** is used in 96% of abortions. In pregnancies < 12 wk, curettage is virtually the only procedure used. **Suction curettage** at 4 to 6 wk of gestation (sometimes called "menstrual extraction," a term from earlier days when sensitive early pregnancy tests were not readily available), requires little or no dilatation of the cervix. The curet most commonly used is a small, flexible cannula (4, 5, or 6 mm in diameter); rigid, 6-mm plastic curets are also used, as well as metal endometrial aspiration biopsy curets. The cannula, attached to a vacuum source (usually a machine suction pump, but hand pumps and occasionally vacuum syringes are also used) is inserted through the cervix. The uterine cavity is gently and thoroughly curetted. Failure to terminate the pregnancy occurs more frequently in these early weeks than later.

After 7 wk, the cervix usually requires dilatation in order to use the larger-diameter suction curets needed to evacuate the larger amount of products of conception. The

cervix may be gently dilated by using tapered dilators of progressively increased sizes until the diameter of the desired cannula is reached. The size of the disposable cannula generally correlates with gestational age—eg, 8 mm for 8 wk of gestation, up to a maximum of 10 mm for 12 wk. To reduce potential injury to the cervix by mechanical dilatation, *Laminaria* (dried seaweed stems) are frequently used. After insertion into the cervical canal through the internal os, they are left for 4 to 5 h, usually overnight; the cervix dilates because of expansion of the *Laminaria* and/or stimulation of prostaglandin release.

In pregnancies > 12 wk, dilatation and evacuation **(D & E)** is the method most commonly used; it is progressively replacing medical methods of termination because its rate of serious complications is lower. Before 1979, patients with gestations of 13 to 15 wk had to wait to 16 wk, when medical induction could be effectively performed. **D & E** has replaced medical induction as the most common method used for termination at 13 to 15 wk and has replaced amniotic instillation as the method most commonly used at 16 to 20 wk. In this procedure (after 12 wk), the cervix is dilated (usually with one or multiple *Laminaria*), forceps are used to dismember and remove the fetus, and a 14- to 16-mm suction cannula is used to aspirate the amniotic fluid, placenta, and fetal debris. In more advanced pregnancies, multiple *Laminaria* may be used to gently dilate the cervix to 3 to 4 cm to make the evacuation easier and safer. D & E requires more skill than does suction curettage.

Although D & E has been shown to have lower rates of minor morbidity than medical induction through 20 wk, medical induction is still used—especially after 18 wk—because with D & E the risk of major morbidity (including bowel injury and uterine injury requiring hysterectomy) is greater.

First trimester abortion has been performed without **anesthesia**. However, the procedure usually produces considerable pain, and anesthesia should be used for humane reasons and also because the operator is more likely to remove all of the tissue if the patient is not in acute discomfort. In the first trimester, local anesthesia is more commonly used, with paracervical block the preferred method. Local anesthetic is injected into the paracervical tissue at 4 and 8 o'clock and into the anterior cervix; after a 5- to 10-min wait, good anesthesia is usually obtained. Local or general anesthesia is used for D & E.

Abortion may be initiated by **medical induction** of uterine contractions, especially in the 2nd trimester. In the USA, the most common procedure involves instilling hypertonic saline solution via a needle or small catheter through the abdominal wall and uterus into the amniotic sac. Commonly, 50 to 200 mL of amniotic fluid is removed and 200 mL of hypertonic (20%) saline is carefully injected into the sac. Labor usually starts within 24 h, and fetus and placenta are delivered about 36 h after instillation. Complications include hypernatremia, coagulopathy, hemorrhage, infection, cervical injuries, and water intoxication.

Prostaglandins stimulate uterine contractions. Without removing amniotic fluid, prostaglandin $F_{2\alpha}$, 40 mg, can be injected into the sac. This procedure produces a shorter instillation-to-abortion time but has an increased incidence of retained placenta and is more likely to result in abortion of a live fetus. Using intravenous oxytocins accelerates the process but increases the risk of lower uterine tears and hypernatremia. Prostaglandin E_2, injected extraamniotically or in suppositories, has also been used with considerable success. These suppositories are more commonly used to supplement other methods, especially when membranes rupture without active contractions occurring. Prostaglandins have also been used to soften the cervix prior to mechanical dilatation. Using *Laminaria* singly or multiply in the 2nd trimester prior to medical induction usually shortens labor and decreases the incidence of cervicovaginal lacerations. Side effects of prostaglandins include nausea, vomiting, diarrhea, hyperthermia, facial flushing, vasovagal symptoms, and bronchospasm. Prostaglandins may precipitate bronchial asthma in susceptible patients; patients with severe kidney and

liver disease may have decreased activation of the drug; patients with epilepsy may develop seizures. Intramuscular injection of 15 methylprostaglandin $F_{2\alpha}$ is also a method of terminating 2nd trimester pregnancy. The success rate is > 95%, and the treatment-to-abortion time is 8 to 12 h.

Injecting substances such as ethacridine, prostaglandin $F_{2\alpha}$, or saline via a catheter between fetal membranes and the uterine wall has been used between 13 and 16 wk. Urea has been used, but is generally considered less effective; it usually also requires the use of intravenous oxytocin or prostaglandin. Hypertonic glucose should *not* be used because it increases the risk of infection.

One major surgical procedure, **hysterotomy**, in essence a cesarean section, is rarely indicated. The uterine scar increases the risk of uterine rupture in a subsequent pregnancy. **Hysterectomy** should be reserved for women who have had a previous indication for hysterectomy and who recognize that permanent sterilization follows. The mortality of these procedures is 44 times that of a first-trimester curettage.

Complications

Complication rates are directly related to the gestational age of the pregnancy and to the method used. They double q 2 wk after 8 wk. If any doubt exists about the gestational age, an ultrasound examination should be done. Bleeding after conception may be misconstrued as the "last menstrual period"; the retroflexed uterus as well as the uterus of an obese patient may be difficult to assess. Serious early complications include perforation of the uterus (0.1%) by one of the instruments used for abortion (sometimes the intestine or other organs are also injured); major hemorrhage (0.06%) may occur secondary to trauma or atonic uterus; late hemorrhage may be due to retained placenta or infection. Laceration of the cervix (0.1 to 1%) ranges from superficial tenaculum tears to cervicovaginal fistula (associated with an instillation procedure in the 2nd trimester). Untoward effects of general or local anesthesia may occur. Additional complications of medical inductions have been noted previously.

The most frequent delayed complications include postabortion bleeding due to retention of fragments of placenta; infection (0.1 to 2%), ranging from mild endometritis to severe pelvic inflammation, peritonitis, and septicemia; and thrombophlebitis. Sterility may occur secondary to pelvic infection or from synechiae in the endometrial cavity. Rh sensitization may occur if Rh immune globulin is not used in susceptible Rh-negative women. The effect of elective abortion on subsequent pregnancies continues to be disputed. Recent extensive studies report no significantly increased risk. Forceful dilatation of the cervix in more advanced pregnancies may predispose to incompetent cervix. Complication rates, including mortality, have progressively decreased, especially since 1972. The safest method is suction curettage, followed by D & C, D & E, prostaglandin instillation, saline instillation, hysterotomy and hysterectomy.

In general, contraception has a much lower complication rate than abortion, especially for young women. Morbidity in permanent sterilization with tubal ligation is ≅ 5%; mortality is 10 to 20/100,000 cases. Maternal mortality in 1982 was 8.9/100,000 live births; the rate for nonwhite women was 3 times the rate for white women, and the rate for women > 35 was 3 times the rate for younger women. Therefore, contraception or sterilization should be used to *prevent* unwanted pregnancy, and abortion should be used for failure of safer technics.

Psychologic Aspects

For most women, abortion is not a threat to mental well-being and has no adverse psychological sequelae. Before abortions were easily and legally obtainable, psychological difficulties may have been related more to the problems and stress desperate women encountered in obtaining the procedure. The women more prone to psychologic sequelae are those who had psychiatric symptoms before pregnancy, who terminated a desired pregnancy for medical reasons (maternal or fetal), who have considerable ambivalence, or who are young adolescents or of late gestational age.

175. CONCEPTION, IMPLANTATION, PLACENTATION, AND EMBRYOLOGY

CONCEPTION

Ovulation and conception occur about 14 days before a menstrual period. If the periods are irregular, the time of conception and thus the due date of the pregnancy may be difficult to determine.

At the time of ovulation, the mucus of the cervix becomes less viscid, facilitating rapid transit of sperm from the vagina to the endometrial cavity. Under experimental conditions, sperm have migrated from the vagina to the fimbriated end of the uterine tube in 5 min. Before ovulation, sperm may be stored in the cervix for at least a few days.

Conception, or fertilization, occurs in the uterine tube, usually near the fimbriated end. The tubal epithelium must function properly for the sperm and ovum to unite and for continued division and development of the zygote during its transit down the tube to the endometrial cavity. The zygote moves from the fimbriated end of the tube to the endometrial cavity in 3 to 5 days and to the site of implantation in 1 to 2 more days. During this time the conceptus is dividing, and at the time of implantation it has formed a blastocyst, a single layer of cells surrounding a central cavity. On one wall of the blastocyst is a thickening 3 to 4 cell layers deep. This is the embryonic pole of the blastocyst; it will shortly be recognizable as an embryo.

IMPLANTATION

Implantation usually occurs in either the front or back wall of the endometrial cavity near the fundus. Trophoblast cells proliferate from the surface of the blastocyst and invade and penetrate the endometrium so that the blastocyst burrows into the central layer of endometrium. This process begins between day 5 and 8 and is completed by day 9 or 10.

By day 10 both syncytial and cytotrophoblast cells are identifiable. Beginning about day 10, fluorescent staining shows chorionic gonadotropin in syncytial cells. Presumably all the other trophic hormones made by the placenta appear in the syncytial cells relatively shortly thereafter. The blastocyst wall changes into the chorion and becomes the outer layer of the membranes surrounding the fetus and amniotic fluid.

The amniotic sac develops about day 10 to 12 as a split in the embryonic ectodermal layer; the sac fills with fluid and expands to cover the embryo and to line the inner wall of the future chorionic membrane. The old blastocyst cavity disappears.

The embryo continues to grow, but the pregnancy is confined within one wall of the uterine cavity until the 12th wk. At that time the endometrium or decidua overlying the pregnancy comes in such close contact with the decidua of the opposite wall of the uterus that they fuse and obliterate the endometrial cavity. After that time the only cavity in the uterus is the amniotic cavity, containing amniotic fluid and the fetus.

PLACENTATION

The first evidence of placental formation is development of the trophoblast cells at day 10. Invasion of these trophoblast cells into maternal blood vessels causes blood to leak into the space between cells, forming lakes or lacunae, which will become the intervillous space. Meanwhile, the fetus derives its nourishment from the lacunae. Initially the placenta surrounds the entire blastocyst and transmits nutrients and discharges wastes directly across cell membranes. Vessels appear within the placenta at day 19, and from that time the villar pattern of transfer from maternal blood to fetal

blood begins. Villi begin to form on the chorionic surface as early as day 11 to 12 and bud out around the entire surface of the pregnancy; they branch and rebranch in a complicated tree-like arrangement.

Beginning at about 12 wk and apparently influenced by the location of the major source of the maternal blood supply, the true, or discoid, placenta begins to demarcate at the old embryonic pole of the blastocyst; it is attached by anchoring villi to the decidua directly overlying maternal spiral arterioles. These spiral arterioles empty into the intervillous space so that the maternal blood circulates around and through the latticework of villi and drains out through 2 or 3 venous sinuses associated with each spiral arteriole. The villi are divided into groups called cotyledons, each supplied by 1 or 2 spiral arterioles. A placenta at term contains between 10 and 20 cotyledons. Nutrients are transferred from maternal blood in the intervillous space, across the trophoblast cells, through the fibrous core of the villus, and through the endothelial cells of the fetal capillaries to the fetal blood itself. Wastes move in the opposite direction. This arrangement is called a hemochorial placenta, since maternal blood is in apposition with fetal chorionic, or trophoblast, tissue.

The discoid placenta reaches its final form at 18 to 20 wk of pregnancy. At 12 wk the remaining villar structures covering the chorionic sac begin to atrophy, and they disappear entirely by 16 to 18 wk. The placenta grows throughout pregnancy until it reaches its final size of about 500 gm (1 lb) at delivery.

EMBRYOLOGY

The conceptus first becomes recognizable as an embryo about 10 days after fertilization, when the future ectoderm splits to form the amniotic sac. All 3 germ layers (ectoderm, mesoderm, endoderm) are present and can usually be distinguished. The primitive streak, or future neural tube, begins to develop thereafter, and around day 16 to 17 the mesoderm thickens near the cephalic end and forms a central channel ultimately to become the heart and great vessels. The heart begins to pump plasma through the vessels on day 20, and on day 21 fetal RBCs appear. At this time they are nucleated, since they are very premature forms; however, nucleated RBCs disappear shortly and reappear only in erythroblastosis. Fetal vessels develop throughout the body shortly thereafter. Some arise within the body stalk, which connects the allantoic sac to the fetal abdomen at the umbilicus and contains blood vessels and the extension of the urachus through which urine drains from the bladder into the allantoic sac.

The allantoic sac atrophies rapidly, and the body stalk becomes the umbilical cord connected to vessels within the placenta. Umbilical vessels carry blood to and from the placenta. Organ formation is complete by the 12th wk of pregnancy (70 days from conception) except in the CNS, which continues to develop throughout pregnancy. Most malformations occur during the first 12 wk, when outside teratogenic influences such as the rubella virus are most destructive. All medications or immunizations should be avoided until after the 12th wk of pregnancy, unless they are essential to protect the mother's health; great care should be taken to avoid a teratogenic drug.

---

176. NORMAL PREGNANCY, LABOR, AND DELIVERY

DIAGNOSIS OF PREGNANCY

The first sign of pregnancy and the first reason most pregnant women see a physician is absence of an expected menstrual period. If a patient's periods are usually regular, absence of menses for 1 wk or more is presumptive evidence of pregnancy.

Breast engorgement and nausea with occasional vomiting may also be noted. The engorgement is caused by increased levels of estrogen and progesterone, particularly estrogen, and is an extension of premenstrual breast engorgement. Nausea and vomiting may be caused by human chorionic gonadotropin **(HCG)** and estrogen, which the syncytial cells of the placenta begin to produce in increasing amounts 10 days after fertilization. HCG stimulates the corpus luteum in the ovary to continue to secrete high levels of estrogen and progesterone in order to maintain the integrity of the pregnancy. Many women become fatigued at this time, and an occasional patient notices abdominal enlargement (bloating) very early in her pregnancy.

Pregnancies are usually dated in weeks, starting from the first day of the last menstrual period. Thus, if the patient's menses were regular and if ovulation did occur on day 14 of the cycle, obstetric dates are about 2 wk longer than embryologic dates. If the patient's periods are irregular, the difference will be greater or less than 2 wk. Usually, 2 wk after missing a period the patient is considered to be 6 wk pregnant and the uterus is correspondingly enlarged.

By the time a patient whose periods were regular has missed a period for 2 wk, she is usually certain she is pregnant. Pelvic examination shows uterine enlargement compatible with pregnancy. The cervix is softer, and the uterus is irregularly softened and enlarged. The vagina and cervix usually become bluish to purple, apparently because they are engorged with blood.

A blood or urine test usually will be positive. Latex inhibition tests take only a few minutes to perform. The sensitivity for detecting HCG in urine ranges from 3500 mIU/mL (Gravindex®) to 1000 to 2000 mIU/mL (Pregnosticon Dri-Dot®); therefore, these tests are not reliable until at least 2 wk following missed menses. Urine tube tests using hemagglutination-inhibition reactions take longer but are more sensitive and accurate. Their sensitivity ranges from HCG levels of 1250 mIU/mL (e.p.t.®, in-home early-pregnancy test) to 700 to 750 (Pregnosticon® tube test). Radioimmunoassays **(RIAs)** and antibody tests of the beta subunit of HCG **(β-HCG)** can detect HCG at very low levels (10 to 15 mIU/mL) and can detect pregnancy 10 days after fertilization.

During the first 60 days of normal single gestation, HCG levels double about every 2 days, demonstrating an exponential rise. The concentration correlates closely with gestational age. Abnormal pregnancy, spontaneous embryonic abortion, blighted ovum abortion, and ectopic pregnancy have HCG levels that fall off the normal curve at some point.

The uterus at 6 wk of pregnancy sometimes can be easily flexed on the markedly softened isthmus. At 12 wk the uterus is larger than the cavity of the pelvis and rises out of the true pelvis into the abdomen; it can be palpated above the symphysis pubis. At 20 wk the upper pole of the uterus is at the level of the umbilicus (and about 20 cm from symphysis to top of uterus by tape measurement), and at 36 wk it is near the xiphoid process.

Positive proof of pregnancy is delivery of a fetus. Traditionally, 3 other signs have been accepted as positive: (1) fetal heart tones heard by a physician or recorded via phonocardiography or a Doppler detection instrument (fetal heart tones can ordinarily be detected with a stethoscope at 18 to 20 wk, and as early as 10 to 12 wk with a Doppler ultrasound device if the uterus is accessible abdominally); (2) fetal movements felt or heard by the examining physician; and (3) identification of a fetal skeleton on x-ray, usually after 16 wk. Today, however, positive proof can be obtained by noting a doubling of HCG levels and by ultrasound detection of an intrauterine sac and a fetus with cardiac motion. The presence within the uterus of a cavity compatible with pregnancy can be diagnosed at about 6 wk (4 wk after ovulation) using ultrasound scanning. Fetal cardiac motion may also be seen at this time with real-time ultrasound scanning and is detectable at 8 wk in > 95% of cases. The patient ordinarily begins to detect fetal motion between 16 and 20 wk.

Pregnancy is considered to last 266 days from the time of conception or 280 days from the first day of the last menstrual period if menses are regular at 28 days. **Nagele's rule** calculates the estimated date of confinement **(EDC)** by subtracting 3 mo from the first day of the last menstrual period and adding 7 days. This calculation is only approximate; 10% of patients or fewer will deliver on the calculated day, but 50% will deliver within 1 wk and 74 to 88% within 2 wk. Patients should be told that the EDC is ± 2 wk and that delivery 2 wk earlier or later is normal.

A pregnant woman is described as a "gravida." Each pregnancy (twins are one pregnancy) increases gravidity, so that a patient with 2 pregnancies is a gravida 2. Parity describes outcome and may be recorded in 2 fashions. Each delivery past 20 wk is recorded as para 1, 2, or 3 (twins are each 1 para). Each loss prior to 20 wk is recorded as abortus 1, 2, or 3. The sum of para and abortus equals gravidity. A newer, more widely used and more informative system records para in 4 numbers: The first indicates the number of deliveries past 20 wk; the 2nd, the number of abortuses; the 3rd, the number of premature deliveries, and the 4th, the number of living children. Thus, a woman pregnant for the 3rd time with 1 set of twins born at 32 wk and 1 abortion would be recorded as gravida 3, para 2–1–1–2.

PHYSIOLOGY

Pregnancy causes physiologic changes in all organ systems, most of which revert to normal after delivery.

Cardiovascular Physiology

Cardiac output (CO) rises 30 to 50%, beginning by 6 wk of pregnancy and peaking between 16 and 28 wk (usually at about 24 wk). CO remains elevated until after 30 wk, then may decrease slightly because the enlarging uterus obstructs the vena cava. During labor, CO increases another 30%. After delivery, the uterus contracts and CO drops markedly to about 15 to 25% above normal, then slowly declines over the next 3 to 4 wk until at about 6 wk postpartum it reaches the prepregnancy level. Increased CO is accompanied by an increase in heart rate from the normal 70 beats/min to 80 or 90 beats/min and by proportional stroke volume increases. BP usually drops (with a widening pulse pressure) as the uteroplacental circulation expands during the 2nd trimester, but may return to normal in the 3rd trimester.

The rise in CO is probably due to changes in uteroplacental circulation. As the placenta and fetus develop, the uterus requires greater blood flow. At term, blood flow to the uterus is about 1 L/min or 20% of normal CO. Since the volume of the uteroplacental circulation also increases markedly, more blood is needed. In addition, the circulation within the intervillous space acts partly as an arteriovenous shunt to further increase requirements for blood volume and CO.

Exercise causes greater increases in CO, heart rate, O_2 consumption, and respiratory volume/min during pregnancy than postpartum. The hyperdynamic circulation of pregnancy increases the frequency of functional murmurs and accentuates heart sounds. X-ray or ECG examination may show the heart displaced into a horizontal position, rotating to the left, with increased transverse diameter. Premature atrial and ventricular beats are common during pregnancy. All these changes should be recognized as normal, to avoid an erroneous diagnosis of heart disease, and usually can be managed with reassurance alone. However, paroxysms of atrial tachycardia occur more frequently in pregnant women and may require prophylactic digitalization.

Blood volume increases proportionally with CO, but the increase in plasma volume is greater (close to 50%) than the increase in RBC mass (about 25%), and the Hb may be lowered by dilution, from 13.3 gm to 12.1 gm.

The **WBC count** (from 5000 to 7000) increases slightly to 9,000 to 12,000. The total mass of WBCs must also increase to fill the increased blood volume. The reason for

this increase in WBCs is unknown. A marked leukocytosis (20,000 or more) occurs during labor and the first few days postpartum.

Iron requirements increase to about 1 gm during pregnancy. The fetus and placenta use about 300 mg of iron, and the increased maternal RBC mass requires an additional 500 mg. Excretion accounts for 200 mg. Supplemental iron therapy is needed, since the average woman has iron stores of only 0.3 to 0.5 gm. The amount absorbed from diet, with that absorbed from stores, is usually insufficient to meet the demands of pregnancy. Iron requirements become great during the 2nd half of pregnancy—6 to 7 mg/day. Supplemental iron is therefore valuable during pregnancy. Iron salts providing 30 mg of iron/day should be used, or 60 to 90 mg/day if anemia is present.

Renal Physiology

Changes in kidney function parallel those in cardiac function. GFR increases 30 to 50%, peaks between 16 and 24 wk of pregnancy, and remains at that level until nearly term, when it may decrease slightly because of positional stasis due to pressure on the vena cava. Renal plasma flow rises correspondingly. Back-up, due to pressure from the pregnant uterus on the ureters and hormonal influences (predominantly progesterone), markedly dilate the ureters. These increases in kidney function cause the BUN to drop, usually to < 10 mg/dL, and creatinine levels correspondingly drop to 0.7 mg/dL.

Kidney function, as well as cardiac function, is very responsive to posture during pregnancy. Normally, kidney function is increased in the supine position and decreased in upright positions; this difference is accentuated in pregnancy. In addition, kidney function and cardiac function are also markedly increased in the lateral position because in the supine position the heavy pregnant uterus resting on the great vessels causes stasis in the lower extremities. This increase is one reason a pregnant woman feels a need for frequent urination when trying to sleep.

Pulmonary Physiology

Changes in lung function during pregnancy are due partly to the hormonal stimulus of progesterone and partly to positional problems caused by the enlarging uterus. Tidal volume, respiratory rate, minute volume, and plasma pH and O_2 consumption increase, while inspiratory reserve, expiratory reserve, residual volume, residual capacity, and plasma P_{CO_2} decrease. Vital capacity and plasma P_{O_2} do not change. Thoracic circumference increases about 10 cm. Considerable hyperemia and edema of the respiratory tract, occasional symptomatic nasopharyngeal obstruction and nasal stuffiness, transient blockage of eustachian tubes, and changes in tone and quality of voice occur. Mild dyspnea on exertion is consistently noted, and frequency of deep respirations increases.

Gastrointestinal and Hepatobiliary Physiology

Constipation may occur as pregnancy progresses, due to the enlarging uterus pressing against the rectum and lower portion of the colon. In addition, GI motility decreases because elevated progesterone levels relax smooth muscle. Heartburn and belching are common, possibly because of the delay in gastric emptying time and relaxation of the sphincter at the junction of the esophagus and stomach, with reflux of gastric fluids; relaxation of the hiatus in the diaphragm adds to this complaint. Peptic ulcer disease, however, is uncommon in pregnancy, and preexisting ulcers often improve; HCl production decreases. The incidence of gallbladder disease is somewhat increased, and women who have been pregnant have more gallbladder problems than women who have not. Physiologic changes in the liver are discussed in Ch. 178.

Endocrine Physiology

Pregnancy alters the function of most endocrine glands, partly because most hormones are circulated in protein-bound forms and protein binding is increased in pregnancy. **Thyroid function** changes markedly; thyroid tests indicate an increase in

function that mimics hyperthyroidism, and the symptoms and signs of hyperthyroidism—tachycardia, palpitations, excessive perspiration, emotional instability, and an enlarged thyroid gland—are frequently present. However, true hyperthyroidism occurs in only 0.08% of pregnancies. **Adrenal hormone levels** increase, which probably causes the pink skin stria ("stretch marks") and may contribute to edema.

Increased levels of glucocorticoids, estrogens, and progesterone modify **glucose metabolism** and increase the need for insulin, as does the stress of pregnancy and possibly the increased level of human placental lactogen. Also, insulinase manufactured by the placenta may affect insulin requirements, so that patients with prediabetes frequently develop more overt forms of the disease. Diabetes mellitus and pregnancy are discussed in Ch. 178.

The **trophic hormones manufactured by the placenta** include HCG, which functions much like follicle-stimulating hormone and luteinizing hormone from the anterior pituitary gland in maintaining the corpus luteum and thereby prevents ovulation. The placenta also manufactures a hormone, similar to thyroid-stimulating hormone, that changes thyroid function, and a melanocyte-stimulating hormone that increases skin pigmentation. The placenta may also produce a variety of ACTH that increases adrenal gland function.

Skin

Melasma ("mask of pregnancy"), a blotchy brownish pigment, occurs over the forehead and malar eminences. Increased pigment of the mammary areolae and a dark line down the midabdomen commonly occur. There is increased incidence of spider angiomas (usually only above waist level) and thin-walled dilated capillaries (especially in the lower legs).

PRENATAL CARE

Ideally, all patients should be examined between 6 and 8 wk of pregnancy (ie, when a menstrual period is 2 to 4 wk late) so that duration of pregnancy can be estimated early and the EDC can be determined more accurately.

The **first examination** should include a **complete physical examination**, including weight, height, and BP; palpation of the neck and thyroid gland; auscultation of heart and lungs; examination of the breasts, abdomen, and extremities; and, ideally, a funduscopic examination of the eyes. **Laboratory tests** should include a CBC; STS; culture for gonorrhea; blood typing for the major blood groups, Rh factor, and antibody screening; a rubella antibody titer (unless a previous titer was positive); a complete urinalysis and screening test for bacteria in the urine, and a pap test of the cervix. Black patients should be tested for sickle cell trait or disease. Genetic studies should be offered to those in higher risk categories (see PREVENTION OF GENETIC DISORDERS in Ch. 203). Women from Asia or south of the US border should have skin tests for TB. A chest x-ray is needed only when there is a history of heart or lung disorder; otherwise, x-ray exposure should be avoided during pregnancy, especially during the first 3 mo. If an x-ray is required, the fetus should be shielded.

At 15 to 16 wk, an *a*-fetoprotein **(AFP)** test (see also in OTHER PROCEDURES under PREVENTION OF GENETIC DISORDERS in Ch. 203) should be offered. Elevated AFP may indicate neural tube defect **(NTD),** multiple pregnancy, or miscalculation of dates. An abnormally low AFP may be associated with chromosomal abnormalities.

Screening for abnormal carbohydrate metabolism should be done early in the 2nd trimester in women with a history of large infants or unexplained fetal losses, persistent glucosuria, or a strong family history of diabetes. At 28 wk, all women should be screened: glucose 50 gm in water or soda should be consumed by the patient at a random time (without fasting) and blood sugar determined 1 h later. Those with blood sugar ≥ 135 should be screened with a standard 100-gm, 3-h glucose tolerance test.

The first examination should also include a **full pelvic examination** with cytologic smear of the cervix and bimanual and rectovaginal examination to determine the size and configuration of the uterus and normality of adnexa. Pelvic capacity can be determined by attempting to touch the sacral promontory with the middle finger in the vagina; if the distance to the sacral promontory is > 11.5 cm from the under side of the symphysis, the pelvic inlet is almost certainly adequate. The distance between the ischial spines should also be estimated; 9 cm or more is considered normal. The length of the sacrospinous ligaments should be estimated to judge the depth of the pelvis; 4 to 5 cm or more is considered normal. The subpubic arch in a normal woman is 90° or wider. X-ray pelvimetry is rarely indicated. The combination of adequate pelvic examination for size and configuration, ultrasound examination for position and abnormality, and trial of labor for dilatation and descent will usually suffice for either vertex or breech presentation. Other presentations can also be determined.

Ultrasound is the imaging method of first choice in obstetrics. Many obstetricians believe each pregnancy should have at least one ultrasonic examination to ensure that progress is satisfactory. The equipment is portable, so the obstetrician can use it in the office or the labor room. The fluid-filled uterus improves ultrasonic visualization of the fetus and the placenta, while the rounded contour of the pregnant abdomen makes scanning more effective. Before examination, especially in early pregnancy, the patient is required to drink water, since a full bladder pushes the uterus out of the pelvis and improves visualization of its contents. The pregnancy can be visualized as early as the 4th or 5th wk, and fetal growth can be followed until delivery. By establishing a nomogram based on ultrasonic measurements of either fetal biparietal or chest diameters or both, fetal growth can be estimated in terms of weight. This makes it possible to detect sudden changes in fetal growth, check fetal size with predicted delivery dates, and determine fetal growth if early delivery is indicated for the mother's health. A "biophysical profile" of a fetus suspected of being in distress has been devised; it includes measurement of amniotic fluid, fetal tone, movement, and breathing pattern. Doppler monitoring of the fetal heart or monitoring of fetal respiratory movement has been advocated to detect a high-risk pregnancy. Ultrasound also is used to determine multiple pregnancy, hydatidiform mole, polyhydramnios, placenta previa, placental location, fetal position and size, ectopic pregnancy, needle guidance for amniocentesis or fetal transfusion, and the reason a uterus is too large or too small for given dates of gestation.

Technics for diagnosing in utero fetal structural abnormalities (eg, anencephaly, hydrocephaly, congenital heart defects, bowel obstruction, urinary tract obstruction, and polycystic kidney disease) are steadily improving. With real-time scanning, one can directly observe fetal and heart movements. In most hospitals, ultrasonography is used routinely for needle guidance during amniocentesis and fetal transfusion.

Follow-up visits should occur at 4-wk intervals until 32 wk of pregnancy, at 2-wk intervals until 36 wk, and then weekly until delivery. At each examination, the patient's weight and BP should be noted, and the size and shape of the uterus examined to determine whether growth and advancement are normal for gestational age. The urine should be tested for albumin and glucose. Fetal heart tones may be heard at 10 to 12 wk with Doppler ultrasound. Beginning at 18 wk, fetal heart tones should be listened for with a specially designed (DeLee-Hillis) stethoscope and recorded at each visit. The patient's ankles should be examined for edema. The Hct should be measured in each trimester. The patient at high risk for gonorrhea should have a culture for gonorrhea performed at the first visit and again at 36 wk. If the patient is Rh negative, an Rh antibody titer should be repeated at 26 to 27 wk; if Rh negative and the father of the baby is known *with certainty* not to be Rh negative, at 28 wk the patient should be given $Rh_o(D)$ immune globulin 300 μg (see also under PREPARATION OF DONOR AND RECIPIENT BLOOD AND ITS COMPONENTS in Ch. 97). A similar dose should also be

given if amniocentesis is performed or whenever there is significant bleeding. Titers should not be done thereafter. A weakly positive direct Coombs' test may be found in fetal cord blood, but it is not significant. If the infant is Rh_0(D) positive, the mother should receive more Rh_0(D) immune globulin.

These follow-up examinations can be performed by a physician's assistant or nurse and do not require the presence of a physician unless abnormalities are detected. If the EDC is uncertain, the pregnancy should be dated by ultrasound scanning. Dating is most accurate within the first 12 wk. Dating accuracy has a range of ± 4 days at 8 wk, ± 10 days at 13 wk, and ± 3 wk in the 3rd trimester. If normal uterine growth does not occur, fetal growth can be evaluated by ultrasound. This can be done as early as 18 wk and is most accurate between 28 and 32 wk. At each examination, some time should be spent answering questions and preparing the woman for labor and delivery, and she and her husband or other support person should be encouraged to attend childbirth education classes. The combination of early first-trimester pelvic examination, ultrasound in the first or early 2nd trimester, and heart tones by auscultation at 18 wk (weekly until heard) is accurate for dating in normal pregnancies and should be done in all pregnancies. Late in pregnancy, decisions concerning repeat cesarean section, premature rupture of membranes, or preterm labor can be made with certainty, based on these data.

Weight gain during pregnancy should be about 25 to 30 lb for an average-size woman, or 2 to 3 lb/mo of pregnancy. Weight gain beyond 30 to 35 lb is excessive and represents fat on both the fetus and the mother. The patient should be cautioned that it is more difficult to control weight gain late in pregnancy, and she should not gain most of the total weight during the first months; however, failure to gain weight is an ominous sign, especially if weight gain is < 10 lb. Fluid retention due to stasis in the legs may occasionally cause weight gain but may be relieved by having the patient lie on her side (preferably her left side) for 30 to 45 min tid or qid.

About 250 kcal should be added to the patient's daily **diet** to provide for fetal nutrition. Although protein should supply most of these calories, the diet should be well balanced, including fresh fruits and vegetables. High-fiber, sugar-free cereals should be encouraged. Salt (preferably iodized) may be used in moderation, but excessively salty foods and foods with added preservatives should be avoided. Dieting during pregnancy is not recommended, even for a grossly obese patient; some weight gain is essential for proper fetal development, and dieting reduces the supply of nutrients to the fetus. The fetus does have first choice of nutrients, but the choice must be of something worth having. The value of a nutritious and well-balanced diet should be emphasized throughout pregnancy.

Drugs, including vitamins and aspirin, should be discouraged. No drugs should be prescribed unless specifically indicated (see also DRUGS IN PREGNANCY below). An iron supplement is necessary for most women, and ferrous sulfate 300 mg orally bid will usually suffice. Ferrous gluconate 450 mg orally bid may be better tolerated. If the diet is adequate, no other vitamin or supplement is necessary.

For **nausea and vomiting,** dietary management should precede medication. The patient should be advised to drink or eat only small amounts frequently, avoiding hunger, and to limit herself to bland foods such as bouillon or consommé. Soda crackers and a soft drink will frequently relieve the nausea. Eating before rising may be helpful. No drugs for morning sickness have been approved by the FDA. If nausea and vomiting are so intense or persistent that the patient becomes dehydrated, develops ketosis, or loses weight, she may require hospitalization and IV fluids.

Edema, especially of the legs, is common. **Varicosities** of the legs and vulva are also common and may give discomfort. Clothing should be nonconstrictive at the waist and legs. Elastic support hose, increased rest with elevation of the legs, or preferably, lying on the side, usually decreases edema. **Hemorrhoids** are common; if symptomatic they

should be treated by using stool softeners, topically applied anesthetics, and warm soaks. **Backache** in variable degrees is common; eliminating excessive strain and wearing a light-weight maternity girdle may be helpful. **Symphysis pubis pain** occurs occasionally. **Heartburn** is common and usually is caused by reflux of gastric contents into the lower esophagus. Treatment includes eating smaller meals, avoiding bending or lying flat for several hours after eating, and using antacid preparations (except sodium bicarbonate). **Fatigue** is common, especially in the first trimester and again in late pregnancy. Pregnant women frequently develop increased **vaginal discharge,** which is usually nonpathologic. Trichomonas vaginalis and candidiasis are common, but probably should be treated only if symptomatic. **Pica,** a bizarre craving for strange foods or, at times, inedible materials (eg, starch or clay) may occur. Occasionally, profuse salivation, **ptyalism,** may cause distress.

Normal activities and **customary exercises** may be continued throughout pregnancy. Swimming and other mildly strenuous sports are permissible, and there is no reason a pregnant woman cannot ride horseback or engage in similar vigorous activity if she is accomplished at it and is cautious. Many women find that their sexual desire is changed (increased or decreased) during pregnancy. Sexual intercourse is permissible throughout pregnancy but should be prohibited if there is any vaginal bleeding, pain, or leakage of amniotic fluid. Several maternal deaths have been reported from blowing air into the vagina during cunnilingus.

Any of the following warning symptoms should be reported promptly: persistent headaches, persistent nausea and vomiting, dizziness, visual disturbances, pain or cramps in the lower abdomen, vaginal bleeding, rupture of membranes, swelling of hands or feet, diminished urinary output, or any illness or infection. The patient should also be encouraged to consult her physician about any problems that puzzle her.

Finally, the **signs of beginning labor** should be reviewed with the patient. The principal guideline is the onset of back pain or lower abdominal contractions that recur at regular intervals. A multipara with a history of rapid labors should notify the physician even earlier. Toward the end of pregnancy, after 36 wk, many doctors prefer to examine the patient vaginally to try to predict when labor will occur. This procedure is *contraindicated* if the head is floating above the inlet, because of the possibility of placenta previa, unless the placenta has been localized in normal position by a previous ultrasound.

FETAL MONITORING

Several methods for fetal monitoring are proving to be more reliable than auscultation with a fetoscope and observation of fundal height and apparent uterine growth.

Electronic fetal monitoring with external devices applied to the maternal abdomen detects and records fetal heart tones and uterine contractions. Internal leads may also be placed, with an electrode attached to the fetal scalp and a catheter through the cervix into the uterus to measure amniotic fluid pressure. The external devices are generally used for normal pregnancies and the internal methods are reserved for high risk or problem pregnancies.

External fetal monitoring can also be used as a non-stress test **(NST)** or as a contraction stress test **(CST)**, sometimes called the oxytocin challenge test **(OCT)**. In these tests, fetal heart rate is recorded and compared to fetal movement (NST) or to contractions induced by oxytocin (OCT) or those occurring spontaneously or secondary to breast stimulation. These tests are frequently used to monitor problem pregnancies.

External fetal monitoring is routinely used in all labors by many obstetricians. If a problem occurs or has been previously identified, internal monitoring is used to provide more reliable information about fetal heart rate patterns and uterine contraction patterns.

DRUGS IN PREGNANCY

Drug use in pregnancy is complicated by the changing biochemical dynamics of the mother and the fetus. Drug use by pregnant women appears to be high.

Drugs circulate between mother and fetus by the same pathway that provides the fetus with substances for growth and development and that removes waste products. The exchange takes place primarily in the placenta, where maternal arterial blood empties into sinuses (intervillous spaces) and then drains into the maternal uterine veins to be returned to the maternal systemic circulation. Maternal and fetal blood do not merge; exchange of solutes takes place across fetal capillaries contained in villi protruding into the intervillous spaces. Solutes must cross the epithelial cells of the villi and the endothelium of the fetal capillaries, from which they are carried to the fetus by the fetal placental veins, which converge into the umbilical vein.

Drugs given during pregnancy can affect the fetus by (1) direct effect on the embryo—lethal, toxic, or teratogenic; (2) effect on the placenta (constriction of vessels), affecting gas and nutrition exchange between fetus and mother; (3) effect on the myometrium (eg, oxytocin causing asphyxia or injuring the fetus); or (4) effect on biochemical dynamics of the mother, indirectly affecting the fetus.

The magnitude and seriousness of the effect of a drug on fetal development or reactivity is determined largely by **fetal age, potency,** and **dosage**. Drugs given during the embryo or zygote stage (before the 20th day after conception) act in an all-or-none fashion, either killing the embryo or not affecting it at all. The fetus is highly resistant to teratogenesis during this stage. The period of organogenesis (between the 3rd and 8th wk) is critical for the teratogenic effect of drugs. Drugs reaching the embryo at this stage may result in (1) no measurable effect, (2) abortion, (3) a sublethal gross anatomic defect (true teratogenic effect), or (4) a permanent subtle metabolic or functional defect that might manifest itself later in life (covert embryopathy). Drugs given after organogenesis (ie, in the 2nd and 3rd trimesters) are unlikely to be teratogenic, but they may alter the growth and the physiologic and biochemical functions of normally formed fetal organs and tissues.

The characteristics of drug diffusion across the placental barrier are similar to the passage across other epithelial barriers (see Drug Absorption in Ch. 270). After maternal administration, the concentration of a drug is higher in cord venous plasma than in cord arterial plasma and least in fetal plasma. Equilibration between maternal blood and fetal tissues takes at least 40 min. To avoid toxicity, drugs that pass through the placenta, such as those commonly used during labor (ie, local anesthetics, narcotics), should be given with great caution within the hour before delivery, since after the cord is cut the newborn (whose metabolizing enzymes and kidneys are still immature) must assume the task of clearing the transferred drug from its body. Some potential adverse effects of drugs on the fetus are discussed below.

Antineoplastic agents are foremost among the teratogens. Since embryonic tissues undergo rapid growth characterized by a high DNA turnover rate, they resemble neoplastic tissues and are very susceptible to antineoplastic agents. Aminopterin was the first drug shown to be teratogenic in man. Many antimetabolites and alkylating agents (including methotrexate, 6-mercaptopurine, cyclophosphamide, chlorambucil, and busulfan) can cause fetal abnormalities such as intrauterine growth retardation, mandibular hypoplasia, cleft palate, cranial dysostosis, ear defects, and club foot. Colchicine, vinblastine, vincristine, and actinomycin D are teratogenic in animals, but have not proved to be so in man. Colchicine has been shown to increase abnormal chromosomes in lymphocyte cultures; this raises concerns about increasing the risk of Down's syndrome in offspring.

Other potential teratogens: Cortisone, which is teratogenic in animals, causes abnormalities in humans when given in large doses. Congenital anomalies and limb defects have been reported to be associated with the use of sex hormones, including contracep-

tive pills, during pregnancy. Evidence indicates that triploidy and possibly polyploidy are more frequent in abortuses from women who become pregnant soon after ceasing oral contraceptives. It is wise to stop using oral contraceptive pills and use other forms of contraception for at least 3 mo when there is intent to conceive. **Androgenic hormones** and synthetic **progestins** given during the first 12 wk of gestation produce masculinization of the external genitalia in female fetuses. Correlation between adenocarcinoma of the vagina in adolescent girls and their mothers' using **diethylstilbestrol (DES)**, a synthetic nonsteroidal estrogen, has been reported. Besides the occurrence of clear adenocarcinoma in children exposed to DES, the following abnormalities were observed in females: poor preovulatory mucus, incompetent cervix, abnormal endometrial cavity, menstrual dysfunctions, spontaneous abortions, increased rate of ectopic pregnancy, and an increase in perinatal mortality. In males exposed to DES, meatal stenosis and hypospadias have been observed. Other human tumors have appeared many years after exposure to carcinogens (thymus radiation, aniline, etc), but this DES effect is the first implication of transplacental carcinogenesis in man. **Meclizine,** an agent frequently prescribed for motion sickness, nausea, and vomiting, is teratogenic in rodents, but this has not been documented in man. Increasing reports of cleft palate, cardiac abnormality, craniofacial anomalies, nail and digit hypoplasia, chromosomal aberrations, visceral defects, and mental subnormality in the offspring of epileptic mothers on **anticonvulsants** strengthen an association of anticonvulsant drugs and fetal abnormalities. However, risk factors for teratogenesis in epileptic mothers include not only the inherent teratogenicity of anticonvulsant drugs but also the frequency and severity of epileptic seizures, other complications of pregnancy, and socioeconomic class. The anticonvulsants trimethadione and valproic acid have been clearly shown to be strongly teratogenic and are contraindicated. The previous association of "fetal hydantoin syndrome" (a group of anomalies: craniofacial anomalies, deficient growth, mental retardation, and limb defects) with phenytoin is now disputed because studies have shown similar defects in babies born to untreated epileptic mothers. During the first day of life, newborns exposed to phenytoin and phenobarbital in vitro may develop bleeding tendencies that may be due to drug-induced vitamin K deficiency. This can be prevented by vitamin K injections for the mother before delivery and for the newborn after delivery. During pregnancy, epileptic symptoms must be treated with anticonvulsants, phenytoin, carbamazepine, or phenobarbital, with the smallest effective doses under careful monitoring. **Immunization with live virus** should be *avoided* when pregnancy is suspected; eg, giving rubella vaccine virus risks placental and fetal invasion.

Thyroid drugs: Radioactive iodine (^{131}I), when used to treat thyroid disease, can cross the placenta and completely destroy the thyroid gland of the fetus or produce severe hypothyroidism. Triiodothyronine, propylthiouracil, and methimazole also can cross the placenta and can cause fetal goiter.

Oral hypoglycemics given chronically to diabetic mothers can cause profound hypoglycemia in newborns.

Narcotics, sedatives, and analgesics (see also discussions on pregnancy and opioid addiction in Ch. 138 and medications for mood disorders in Ch. 141): Narcotics, barbiturates, and salicylates cross the placental barrier and attain significant levels in the fetus. A twofold increase in the incidence of spontaneous abortions has been seen among medical personnel chronically exposed to gaseous anesthesia. Neonates born to narcotics addicts may show withdrawal symptoms 6 h to 8 days after birth. Maternal phenobarbital administration alters the usual course of physiologic jaundice in the neonate, perhaps due to induction of the conjugating enzymes of the neonate. Babies born to epileptic mothers taking barbiturates and phenytoin may show blood coagulation abnormalities. Vitamin K given in the last month of pregnancy and during labor may counteract this. Salicylates compete with bilirubin for albumin binding sites and

may produce kernicterus. Large doses of aspirin reduce birth weight and increase the possibility of prepartal bleeding, necessitating cesarean section.

The **fetal alcohol syndrome** is seen in babies born to mothers who are heavy drinkers of alcohol. The syndrome consists of prenatal growth retardation, microcephaly, reduced palpebral fissures, borderline mental deficiency, and, less frequently, joint anomalies, cardiovascular defects, perinatal mortality, and postnatal failure to thrive. An absolutely safe level of alcohol consumption during pregnancy has not been established. Recent studies indicate that ingesting > 2.2 gm/kg/day of absolute alcohol increases the frequency of fetal alcohol syndrome; a daily intake of < 2 oz of wine probably would not produce fetal abnormalities.

Tranquilizers and antidepressants: Phenothiazines have been used during pregnancy as antiemetics and psychotropics. They readily pass the placental barrier and may produce retinopathy in the fetus.

A large follow-up study of antenatal exposure to meprobamate and chlordiazepoxide showed no evidence of increased malformations or fetal death rates. Mental and motor tests at age 8 mo and intelligence tests at 4 yr showed no evidence of brain damage. However, because of reports that some fetal abnormalities have been associated with intake of tranquilizers, the FDA requires that tranquilizer labels should warn about the increased risk of congenital malformation during administration in the first trimester of pregnancy. Tricyclic antidepressants have been associated with congenital malformations. Isolated cases of neonates born to mothers who received tricyclics just prior to delivery were observed to suffer from tachycardia, respiratory distress, and urinary retention.

Antibacterials: Tetracyclines pass the placenta and are concentrated and deposited in fetal bones and teeth, where they complex with calcium; the period of risk is from the middle to the end of pregnancy. Permanent yellowish discoloration of the teeth, enamel hypoplasia, and decreased resistance to caries have been observed in children of mothers given tetracyclines during pregnancy. Bone growth may be retarded. Tetracyclines have also been incriminated as a cause of congenital cataracts.

Streptomycin, gentamicin, kanamycin, and other ototoxic drugs should be avoided in pregnancy, since they cross the placenta and may damage the fetal labyrinth. Chloramphenicol, even when given to the mother in large doses, does not produce adverse effects in the fetus, except in the perinatal period. The neonate cannot adequately metabolize chloramphenicol, and the resulting high blood levels may lead to circulatory collapse **(the gray baby syndrome)**. Penicillins appear to be safe in pregnancy, but sensitization may occur in utero.

The long-acting sulfonamides also pass the placenta; being highly protein-bound, they can displace bilirubin from binding sites. If the sulfonamides are given well before the perinatal period, the placenta serves as an efficient excretor of the bilirubin and minimizes harm to the fetus. When sulfonamides are given near or at the perinatal period, severe jaundice and kernicterus may develop because the neonate is unable to clear the bilirubin, owing to the deficient conjugation system.

Anticoagulants: Coumarins given during pregnancy can pass to the fetus, which is highly sensitive to them. If a coumarin derivative is indicated, dosage should be kept strictly within the therapeutic range and the drug should be withdrawn 4 wk before delivery. Coumarin anticoagulants given early in pregnancy have been associated with fetal anomalies, but cause and effect have not been definitely established. High doses of salicylates given in late pregnancy may cause hypoprothrombinemia and fetal or neonatal hemorrhage. Heparin appears to be relatively harmless to the fetus.

Cardiovascular drugs: Cardiac glycosides cross the placenta, but neonates (and children) are relatively resistant to their toxicity. Of a dose of ^{14}C-digitoxin injected into the mother, only 1% appeared in the fetus as unchanged digitoxin and 3% as metabo-

lites. Higher concentrations of digitoxin have been observed in fetuses, mostly in the first trimester. Neonates born to mothers using digoxin have a plasma concentration approximating that of the mother, with no indication of ill effects on the fetus. Among mothers of children with congenital heart defects there is a high incidence of amphetamine use, which suggests a possible teratogenic association.

Antihypertensive drugs frequently used in mothers with preeclampsia or eclampsia also cross the placenta and can affect the neonate. Magnesium sulfate causes respiratory depression. Ganglionic blockers may produce autonomic effects such as hypotension and paralytic ileus. Reserpine given a few days before delivery can produce nasal stuffiness, with consequent respiratory distress and bradycardia. Propranolol passes the placental barrier and can cause bradycardia and hypoglycemia; respiration is depressed and the time to sustain respiration is prolonged. Thiazide diuretics should be avoided in pregnancy. Thiazide contracts the plasma volume of the mother and can compromise fetal oxygenation and nutrition. It can also cause hyponatremia, hypokalemia, and thrombocytopenia in the neonate.

Oxidant drugs such as primaquine, nitrofurantoin, naphthalene, vitamin K, sulfonamides, and chloramphenicol may cause hemolysis in fetuses with a genetic G6PD deficiency.

Drugs commonly used during labor and delivery: Placental transfer of local anesthetics (mepivacaine, lidocaine, prilocaine) from various sites of administration (epidermal, caudal, paracervical) have been associated with fetal CNS depression and bradycardia. Catecholamines and oxytocin given to mothers affect the fetus by their vasoconstricting action and myometrial effect, possibly causing anoxia, asphyxia, and trauma. Narcotics, scopolamine, barbiturates, ketamine, and analgesics all pass the placental barrier. Thiopental, which is commonly used during delivery, is concentrated in the fetal liver, shielding the CNS from high concentrations.

There have been reports of hypotonia, hypothermia, low Apgar scores, impaired metabolic response to cold stress, and neurological depression in babies born to mothers who received large doses of diazepam prior to delivery. These case reports of fetal impairment due to diazepam are not conclusive evidence that it is teratogenic.

Cigarette smoking: The mean birth weight of infants born to mothers who smoke during pregnancy is 6 oz less than that of infants born to nonsmoking mothers. The incidence of spontaneous abortion, stillbirth, and neonatal death may also be increased in pregnant women who smoke.

MANAGEMENT OF NORMAL LABOR

Labor consists of a series of rhythmic, progressive contractions of the uterus that cause effacement and dilation of the uterine cervix. The stimulus for labor is unknown. Circulating oxytocin secreted by the posterior pituitary gland may initiate labor, but no direct evidence supports this thesis. Labor usually begins within 2 wk (before or after) of the estimated date of confinement. In a first pregnancy, labor usually lasts a maximum of 12 to 14 h; succeeding labors are shorter, averaging 6 to 8 h.

The patient in labor has contractions that increase in duration, intensity, and frequency. The rhythmic contractions of actual labor are usually preceded by a latent phase, with irregular contractions of varying intensity that apparently ripen or soften the cervix. This latent phase may be intermittent over several days or may last only a few hours. Bloody show (a small amount of blood with mucous discharge) may precede the onset of labor by as much as 72 h.

Occasionally the amniotic and chorionic sac (the membranes) ruptures before labor begins, and amniotic fluid leaks through the cervix and vagina. A woman whose membranes rupture should contact her physician immediately. About 80 to 90% of these patients go into labor spontaneously within 24 h. If not and if the fetus is at term, labor is usually induced because of risk of infection.

Upon admission, the patient's BP, heart and respiratory rates, temperature, and weight should be recorded, and the presence or absence of edema noted. A urine specimen should be collected to be checked for protein and glucose, and blood should be drawn for a CBC and for blood type if not known. Physical examination should be done. Examination of the abdomen includes estimating the size, position, and presentation of the fetus, and noting the presence or absence of fetal heart tones. Preliminary estimates of the quality of contractions and their duration and frequency should also be recorded.

Vaginal examination should be performed with a clean glove after washing the patient's vulva carefully. Vaginal examination is *contraindicated* if there is any bleeding and may be *contraindicated* if the membranes are ruptured, unless they were ruptured by the physician. If membranes are ruptured, the presence of fetal meconium producing greenish discoloration should be noted, as it may be a sign of fetal distress. The amount of **dilation and effacement of the cervix** should be established, the degree of descent **(station)** of the fetus within the pelvic cavity should be recorded, and the presentation and position should be noted. **Presentation** describes the lowermost part, such as breech, vertex, or shoulder. **Position** describes the relationship of the presenting part to the pelvis, such as occiput left anterior **(OLA)** or sacrum right posterior **(SRP)**. Dilation is recorded in centimeters as the diameter of a circle. Effacement is estimated in percentages from zero effacement to 100% taking up of the cervix. Station is determined in centimeters above or below the level of the ischial spines. At this time it should be determined whether or not the membranes are intact.

The patient should be admitted to the labor suite for observation until delivery. An enema is not necessary; there is no evidence that it stimulates labor, and it contaminates the vulva and perineum throughout labor and delivery. Shaving (or clipping) vulvar hair is also not indicated; shaving is irritating and may lead to infection. An IV infusion of Ringer's solution may be started, using a large-bore indwelling catheter inserted in a vein in the hand or forearm. This infusion prevents the dehydration that may develop during labor and thus prevents hemoconcentration and provides an adequate circulating blood volume. During a normal labor of 6 to 10 h, the patient should receive 500 to 1000 mL of solution. The IV infusion also provides immediate access for drugs or blood in case of an emergency and for drugs to stimulate contraction of the uterus; fluid pre-loading is also of value if conduction anesthesia is to be used.

The patient should be observed carefully and frequently during labor. She should receive little by mouth, to prevent possible vomiting and aspiration during delivery. An antacid should be given orally on admission and q 3 h to neutralize gastric acidity. Maternal heart rate and BP and fetal heart rate should be checked every 15 to 30 min during the 1st stage of labor. In the 2nd stage, the patient should be attended constantly and fetal heart tones should be checked after every contraction or every 3 min, whichever is closer together. Many institutions electronically monitor the fetal heart rate and uterine contractions for all deliveries, since 30 to 50% of babies who develop fetal distress or die during delivery show no antecedent signs that would call for intense observation. Babies can frequently be saved and the quality of their lives improved by electronic monitoring (see also FETAL MONITORING under PRENATAL CARE, above).

Analgesia may be provided during labor as necessary, but as little drug as possible should be given because of effects on the fetus. With better preparation and education for childbirth, anxiety is lessened and need for an analgesic is markedly decreased. Meperidine and morphine sulfate are the narcotics most commonly used for analgesia. Small doses given IV—meperidine 25 to 50 mg or morphine sulfate 5 mg—q 60 to 90 min provide good analgesia with only a small total amount of drug. Although both narcotics cross the placenta and affect the fetus, naloxone (0.01 mg/kg) can be given IM, IV, or s.c. to the newborn as a specific antagonist, if necessary. "Synergistic" drugs (eg, promethazine) are popular but are not ideal, since there is no antidote if an

overdose is given or a problem arises. These drugs are more additive than synergistic; if more analgesia is needed, meperidine or morphine is better.

The 1st stage of labor, *from onset of labor to full dilation of the cervix* (about 10 cm) can be divided into several phases. In the **latent phase,** the contractions progressively become better coordinated, discomfort is minimal, and the cervix effaces but has minimal dilation. The duration of this phase varies, but averages 8½ h in nulliparas and 5 h in multiparas. The **active phase,** during which the cervix dilates from 2 to 3 cm to full dilation and the presenting part descends well into the midpelvis, lasts about 5 h in nulliparas and 2 h in multiparas. The patient may begin to feel the urge to bear down as the presenting part descends in the pelvis. However, she should be discouraged from pushing until the cervix is fully dilated, to avoid tearing the cervix and wasting her energy before it is useful.

The 2nd stage of labor, *the time from complete cervical dilation to delivery of the fetus,* lasts about 60 min in nulliparas and 15 min in multiparas. In addition to contractions of the uterus, expulsive bearing-down efforts are required of the mother for spontaneous delivery.

Various abnormalities of both 1st and 2nd stages of labor (problems of fetal distress, abnormal presentations, disproportions between fetus and maternal pelvis, bleeding disorders, infection, or premature labor) require special investigation, correction of the problems if possible, and possible use of forceps, vacuum extraction, or cesarean section delivery (see Ch. 179).

MANAGEMENT OF NORMAL DELIVERY

Ideally, when delivery is imminent the patient is taken to the delivery room with the IV infusion of Ringer's solution still running. The father or other support person should be offered the opportunity to accompany her. In the delivery room the patient is washed and draped and delivery accomplished.

Commonly used **anesthetics** for delivery are pudendal block, conduction anesthesia, and general anesthesia. In all cases training and experience are required for safe, effective anesthesia. **Pudendal block** involves injecting a local anesthetic through the wall of the vagina so that the pudendal nerve is flooded with anesthetic as it swings around the ischial spine. The nerve pathways are such that anesthesia is provided for the lower part of the vagina, the perineum, and the posterior portion of the vulva; the anterior vulva is enervated elsewhere and is not anesthetized. Pudendal block is useful for uncomplicated deliveries in which the mother wishes to push and there are no contraindications. **Paracervical block** is no longer recommended because of high incidence (> 15%) of fetal bradycardia. Infiltration of the perineum is also commonly used, although anesthesia is not as effective as well-administered pudendal block.

Several **types of conduction anesthetic** are available. The conduction anesthetic most frequently used for labor and delivery is lumbar epidural injection of local anesthesia. Caudal injection is rarely used today. Spinal anesthesia may be used for cesarean section, but is used less often because of the greater risk of spinal headache afterwards. Constant attendance and frequent (q 5 min) BP check must be done to detect and treat possible hypotension.

General anesthetics such as halothane and methoxyflurane can be very depressing to both mother and fetus, and, therefore, are not recommended for routine delivery. Greater interest in prepared childbirth has lessened their use, except for breech or twin delivery or cesarean section. Considerable experience is required to use them safely.

A vaginal examination is done to determine the position and station of the head. The patient is instructed to bear down and strain with each contraction, to move the head down through the pelvis, and to progressively dilate the vaginal introitus so that more and more of the head will appear. When about 3 or 4 in. of the head is visible in

a primipara during a contraction (somewhat earlier in a multipara), the following maneuvers can facilitate delivery and reduce the possibility of perineal laceration: The left palm is placed over the baby's head during a contraction to control and, if necessary, slightly retard its progress, while the curved fingers of the right hand are placed against the dilating perineum through which the baby's brow or chin is felt. Pressure against the brow or chin by the curved fingers helps to advance the head; its advancement or retardation is controlled by the physician to effect slow and controlled delivery. (These directions are for a right-handed physician.)

Use of forceps for delivery is often an arbitrary decision. If an epidural anesthetic that precludes vigorous straining is used, forceps are likely to be required and are safe. However, if a local anesthetic that allows bearing-down efforts is used, forceps usually are not necessary unless complications interfere. If the 2nd stage of labor is likely to be prolonged because the patient is having difficulty straining, forceps should be used.

An **episiotomy,** *surgical incision of the perineum,* substitutes a surgical incision for excessive stretching and possible tearing of the perineal tissues. The incision is easier to repair properly than a tear, and decreases anterior tears. Episiotomy should be performed for almost all patients having their first baby and for most patients who have had a previous episiotomy and have not had a subsequent delivery without episiotomy. The most common episiotomy is a midline incision made with scissors from the midpoint of the posterior fourchette directly backward toward the rectum. This type risks the complication of extension into the rectal sphincter or rectum itself; however, if recognized, the extension can be repaired successfully and will heal well. Episioproctotomy (intentionally cutting into the rectum) is not recommended because the incidence of rectovaginal fistula is unacceptably high. Tears or extensions into the rectum can usually be prevented by keeping the head well flexed until the occipital prominence passes beyond the subpubic arch. Another type of episiotomy is a mediolateral incision made with scissors from the midpoint of the posterior fourchette at a 45° angle laterally on either side. Although this type usually will not extend into the sphincter or rectum, postoperative pain and healing time are increased, and unless problems are expected, the midline episiotomy is recommended.

Following delivery of the head, the baby's body rotates so that the shoulders are in an anteroposterior position, and *gentle* downward pressure on the head delivers the anterior shoulder under the symphysis. The head is *gently* lifted, the posterior shoulder slides over the perineum, and the rest of the baby's body follows without difficulty. The baby's nose, mouth, and pharynx are aspirated with a bulb syringe to remove obstructions (mucus and fluids) and help establish respirations. The cord should be double-clamped, cut between the clamps, and tied. The baby is then placed into a warmed resuscitation bassinet. Care of the newborn is described in Ch. 182.

The 3rd stage of labor *begins after delivery of the infant and ends with delivery of the placenta.* After delivery, the operator's hand is placed gently on the uterine fundus to detect contractions; placental separation usually occurs during the 1st or 2nd contraction, often with a gush of blood from behind the separating placenta. The mother can usually push out the placenta. If not, and if significant bleeding occurs, the placenta can usually be expressed by firm, downward pressure on the uterus. If this is not effective, the umbilical cord is held taut while the uterus is pushed *upward,* away from the placenta. (Manual removal by inserting the entire hand into the uterine cavity, separating the placenta from its attachment, then extracting the placenta may be necessary.) The placenta should be examined for completeness, as fragments left in the uterus can cause delayed hemorrhage. If the placenta is incomplete, the uterine cavity should be explored manually. Many obstetricians routinely explore the uterus after each delivery. Immediately after delivery of the placenta, an oxytocic drug should be given (oxytocin 10 IU IM or, if the IV is running, in the IV fluid) to aid in firm contraction of the uterus. Oxytocin should *not* be given as a single large IV dose, since

cardiac arrhythmia may occur. Any laceration in the cervix or vagina should be repaired.

After inspection to rule out or repair lacerations and to make sure the uterus is contracting, and after repair of the episiotomy, the patient may be taken to the recovery room. If all is well, the infant can be presented to the mother so that they can be wheeled together to the recovery room. Many mothers wish to begin breast feeding soon after delivery, and this should be encouraged. Mother, infant, and father should remain together in a warm, private area for an hour or more, as this may increase parent-infant emotional attachment (bonding). The baby may then be taken to the nursery (see Ch. 182). The mother should be observed for about 1 h for bleeding, BP problems, and general well-being. The time from delivery of the placenta to 4 h postpartum is frequently called the **4th stage of labor;** most complications, especially hemorrhage, occur at this time, and frequent observation is mandatory.

PSYCHOLOGIC ASPECTS

For many women, the father's presence during labor is helpful and should be encouraged. His moral support, encouragement, and expressions of affection decrease the need for analgesia and make the process of labor less frightening and unpleasant. Childbirth education classes are available to prepare both the father and mother for a normal labor and delivery. Sharing the stresses of labor, the sight of their own child and the sound of its crying constitute a dramatic episode that tends to create strong bonds between parents and with the child. The couple should be fully informed regarding any complications.

HOME DELIVERY

Although home delivery has been advocated by some, it is not recommended because of the incidence of unexpected complications during labor and delivery, such as sudden abruption (premature separation) of the placenta, fetal distress during labor, unexpected multiple pregnancy, or unexpected postpartum complications, such as neonatal depression or abnormality or maternal hemorrhage. Hospitals are responding to patients' desires with homelike birthing room facilities and decreased formalities and rigid regulations, but with the availability of emergency equipment and personnel.

---

177. ABNORMALITIES AND COMPLICATIONS OF PREGNANCY

SPONTANEOUS ABORTION
(Miscarriage)

Physicians generally define abortion as *delivery or loss of the products of conception before the 20th wk of pregnancy*, but definitions may vary. For this discussion, 20 wk of gestation, which corresponds to a fetal weight of about 500 gm, will be used as the limit for abortion. *Delivery between 20 and 38 wk is considered* ***preterm birth.***

Incidence and Etiology

About 20 to 30% of women bleed or have cramping sometime during the first 20 wk of pregnancy; 10 to 15% actually spontaneously abort. Since in 60% of spontaneous abortions the fetus is either absent or grossly malformed, and in 25 to 60% it can be found to have chromosomal abnormalities incompatible with life, spontaneous abortion may be a natural rejection of a maldeveloping fetus.

About 85% of spontaneous abortions occur in the 1st trimester and tend to be

related to fetal causes; maternal factors more often cause 2nd trimester abortion. Maternal factors that have been suggested as causes of spontaneous abortion include an incompetent, amputated, or lacerated cervix; congenital or acquired anomalies of the uterine cavity; hypothyroidism; diabetes mellitus; chronic nephritis; acute infection; or severe emotional shock. Many viruses, most notably cytomegalo-, herpes-, and rubella viruses, have been implicated as causative. The importance of uterine fibroids, uterine retroversion, and impaired corpus luteum function appears to have been overestimated. A relationship to physical trauma has not been substantiated.

Classification

An abortion is termed either **early** (before 12 wk of pregnancy) or **late** (between 12 and 20 wk). This distinction is made because more difficulties are encountered in treating late abortions. After 12 wk of pregnancy, the cavity of the uterus is obliterated and instrumentation is more likely to cause perforation. Also, a definitive placenta has begun to form with a more organized and larger blood supply, so that bleeding is more likely. Fetal bones have also begun to form, and the long bones of the limbs may perforate the uterus during evacuation. Because of the size of a fetus at > 12 wk of pregnancy, it is also difficult to dilate the cervix enough to pass the fetus.

Abortions may be spontaneous or induced. **Spontaneous abortions** occur without any instrumentation. **Induced abortions** are those done for medical or elective reasons, and are discussed in Ch. 174. Abortions performed to save the mother's life or health are referred to as **therapeutic.**

Spontaneous abortions may be threatened, inevitable, incomplete, or complete. **Threatened abortion** is defined as any bleeding or cramping of the uterus in the first 20 wk of pregnancy. **Inevitable abortion** is intolerable pain or bleeding that threatens the mother's well-being. If part of the products of conception is passed or if the membranes are ruptured, the abortion is **incomplete.** If all of the products of conception are passed, the uterus has contracted toward normal size, and the cervix has closed, the abortion is **complete.**

If a patient has 3 or more consecutive spontaneous abortions, she is said to have **habitual abortion,** and extensive diagnostic investigation is required. Genetic and chromosomal studies should be done. Among the endocrinopathies and metabolic diseases to be ruled out are hypo- and hyperthyroidism, diabetes mellitus, and chronic renal disease. Defective corpus luteum function is always suspected. Anatomic uterine abnormalities (eg, polyps, fibroids, congenital defects) should be evaluated by hysterography, D & C, or hysteroscopy. Specific treatment, such as unification of a double uterus, excision of septum, and myomectomy, may be needed.

Missed abortion occurs when the fetus has died but has been retained in utero 4 wk or longer. After 6 wk in utero the **dead fetus syndrome** may develop with disseminated intravascular coagulation **(DIC)** and progressive hypofibrinogenemia and possible massive bleeding when delivery finally occurs. The dead fetus syndrome usually occurs only with 2nd trimester loss. Missed abortion should be suspected when the uterus fails to grow, when the fetal heart is not heard at the appropriate time with Doppler ultrasound, or when the fetal heart sound was present previously but is now absent. A serum or urine test for the β subunit of HCG will become negative earlier than expected. Ultrasound will fail to show cardiac activity. The diagnosis can be confirmed with ultrasound, and treatment can be started much earlier.

Septic abortion develops when the contents of the uterus become infected before, during, or after an abortion. The patient is acutely ill, with symptoms and signs of infection and threatened or incomplete abortion—chills, high temperature, septicemia, and peritonitis. Leukocytosis (WBC count 16,000 to 22,000) is present. Critically ill patients may evidence bacterial shock (**septic** or **endotoxin shock**) with vasomotor collapse, hypothermia, hypotension, oliguria or anuria, and respiratory distress. Causative organisms include *Escherichia coli*, *Enterobacter aerogenes*, *Proteus vulgaris*, hemolytic

streptococci, staphylococci, and some anaerobic organisms, such as *Clostridium perfringens*. If septicemia develops with the latter, anuria, anemia, jaundice, and thrombocytopenia with ecchymoses may result. In the USA prior to legalization of abortion, septic abortions were often associated with induced abortions done by untrained persons using nonsterile technics and were commonly called **criminal abortions**. The incidence of septic abortion in the USA has fallen dramatically.

Treatment

Treatment of **threatened abortion** is conservative; bed rest should be suggested, since it seems to lessen the amount of bleeding and cramping. The diagnosis should be confirmed with ultrasound. If an empty sac is found or if cardiac activity has disappeared, evacuation of the uterus is indicated. Intercourse should be avoided, although there is no evidence that it is harmful; however, guilt feelings associated with abortion immediately after intercourse may be great enough to warrant abstention. The patient should be encouraged not to work and to stay off her feet at home. There is no evidence that hormones save pregnancies except in very few instances, and they may cause fetal congenital anomalies, particularly transposition of the great vessels of the heart. Also, vaginal cancer or other genital abnormality in female offspring has been associated with the use of estrogen for threatened abortions. **Inevitable** and **incomplete abortions** must be completed, usually by D & C or suction. Many physicians feel that curettage is mandatory to prove that a spontaneous abortion is complete; others prefer to watch the patient for a few days and, if no further bleeding occurs, avoid the curettage.

In spontaneous abortions due to incompetence of the internal cervical os, the cervix seems unable to resist the progressive pressure of the enlarging pregnancy, and cervical dilation occurs. The cervical connective tissue may be weakened congenitally or secondary to deep cervical lacerations or previous overzealous operative dilation. Cervical cerclage may enable the pregnancy to continue to term.

Missed abortion should be completed by physician intervention as soon as the diagnosis is certain; with ultrasound examination, the death of a fetus in utero can be diagnosed earlier than was previously possible. Up to a gestational age of 28 wk, missed abortion or retained dead fetus is frequently managed by inserting a 20-mg dinoprostone (E_2 prostaglandin) suppository into the vagina q 3 or 4 h as necessary to achieve contractions. Pretreatment of the cervix with *Laminaria* decreases complications. This drug is not approved for use after the 28-wk gestational age limit. Vigorous antibiotic management and early emptying of the uterus are mandatory to save the mother's life in cases of **septic abortion**.

Late spontaneous abortion may be completed with a dilute IV infusion of oxytocin, which causes contraction of the uterus and delivery of the products of conception. After the uterus has contracted following delivery of the fetus, curettage may be needed to remove fragments of the placenta. Suction curettage is now used up to 18 wk of pregnancy.

Psychologic problems may develop in the woman who has a spontaneous abortion with her first pregnancy or who is having a second or third consecutive spontaneous abortion. Some psychologic upset probably occurs in every patient who has an abortion, whether it is spontaneous, therapeutic, or induced. Usually the couple can be reassured and their difficulties minimized with sympathetic discussion and support.

ECTOPIC PREGNANCY

Pregnancy in which implantation occurs outside the endometrium and endometrial cavity; ie, in the cervix, uterine tube, ovary, or the abdominal or pelvic cavity. The incidence, 1:100 to 1:200 diagnosed pregnancies, is rising and is higher in nonwhites. Its likelihood increases with previous tubal disease, ectopic pregnancy (10 to 25%), or induced abortion. Intrauterine devices do not prevent ectopic pregnancies.

The most common site of ectopic implantation is somewhere in a uterine tube. In many cases (50%) tubal implantation is caused by a previous tubal infection. Cervical, ovarian, and abdominal pregnancies are rare and will not be discussed.

The death rate for ectopic pregnancy has been falling, but much less rapidly than for maternal mortality in general. In the USA, it is estimated at 1:826. Untreated ectopic pregnancy is usually fatal.

Symptoms, Signs, and Diagnosis

In ectopic pregnancy, spotting and cramping pain usually begin shortly after the first missed menstrual period. The symptoms are similar to those of threatened abortion. Gradual hemorrhage from the tube causes pain and pressure, but rapid hemorrhage results in hypotension or shock. Often, uterine bleeding precedes these events as HCG levels decrease. Physical examination shows signs of hemorrhage, shock, and lower abdominal peritoneal irritation that may be lateralized. On pelvic examination, the uterus is enlarged (but smaller than anticipated from dates), the cervix is tender to motion, and a tender mass may be palpated in one fornix. The cul-de-sac may bulge. If the serum or urine test for the β subunit of HCG is positive and ectopic pregnancy is suspected, ultrasound should be performed. Serial titers of β subunit HCG are helpful in questionable cases. In normal pregnancy, the titer doubles about q 48 h; in ectopic pregnancy, the HCG titer may be lower than expected for the gestation time and frequently does not show normal doubling time. Also, when the HCG titer is 6500 mIU/mL, a gestational sac in the uterus is normally found on ultrasound. An empty uterus strongly suggests ectopic pregnancy. If, in addition, a mass is detected in the adnexa, the diagnosis is confirmed. Culdocentesis may be helpful; blood aspirated from the cul de sac does not usually clot. Laparoscopy can be very helpful. At about 6 to 8 wk of pregnancy, marked sudden lower abdominal pain may occur, followed by fainting. This usually indicates rupture of the tube with intra-abdominal hemorrhage.

Interstitial (cornual) pregnancies have a somewhat longer course, since the uterine wall provides support and delays rupture. In these patients the uterus is usually asymmetric and somewhat tender on examination. The usual signs include cramping and spotting. Cornual pregnancies rupture between 12 and 16 wk, and the rupture is catastrophic.

Treatment

Even if a tubal pregnancy is diagnosed before rupture, treatment is surgical. However, every effort should be made to conserve the tube by salpingotomy and evacuation of the pregnancy, with repair of the tube. If a damaged portion of the tube must be resected, as much tube as possible should be left behind. Future tubal reconstructive surgery may allow a subsequent pregnancy. After cornual pregnancy, the tube and ovary involved can usually be resected and the uterus repaired; rarely, repair is impossible and hysterectomy must be performed.

ANEMIA

Anemia during pregnancy is defined as a Hb concentration < 10 gm/dL, and may be found in as many as 80% of some gravid populations. Practically speaking, however, any patient with a Hb level < 11 to 11.5 gm/dL at onset of pregnancy must be treated as anemic, since the hemodilution that occurs as pregnancy advances will bring the Hb level into the anemic range.

Etiology

Most anemia during pregnancy is due to dietary iron deficiency (especially in teenage girls), to the normal loss of iron in blood with menses (which approximates the amount normally ingested each month, so iron stores are never built up), or to previous pregnancy. Rarely, anemia during pregnancy may be due to folic acid deficiency.

This condition is sometimes called megaloblastic anemia because in extreme cases early forms of RBCs are found in the peripheral circulation. Both types of anemia are discussed more fully in Ch. 96. In certain populations, both sickle cell trait and sickle cell anemia as well as thalassemia minor and major may be found. Other hemoglobinopathies are occasionally diagnosed. All are special problems in pregnancy and are discussed more fully in Ch. 96.

Diagnosis

Iron-deficiency anemia is diagnosed from the CBC and by finding characteristic hypochromic microcytic RBCs in the peripheral blood smear. It can be confirmed by RBC indices and serum iron and iron-binding capacity measurements. If the anemia does not respond to therapy for iron deficiency, folic acid deficiency should be suspected.

Treatment

Iron-deficiency anemia is treated with supplemental iron, preferably as ferrous sulfate 300 mg given not more often than bid. The side effects of the iron (gastric upset and constipation) are increased if > 2 tablets/day are given. Also, if > 2 tablets are taken daily, one dose blocks absorption of the succeeding doses and thereby reduces total intake. **Megaloblastic anemia** due to folic acid deficiency is treated with folic acid 1 mg bid. True megaloblastic anemia may require hospitalization for bone marrow examination and further treatment. These anemias can be profound enough (Hb 6 gm/dL or lower) to necessitate transfusion. Resistant iron-deficiency anemia or megaloblastic anemia warrants consultation for definitive treatment. Shotgun vitamin therapy or administration of iron by injection is occasionally warranted.

There is conflicting evidence that routine supplemental iron therapy is necessary in pregnancy. However, most pregnant patients should be given supplemental iron, ferrous sulfate 300 to 600 mg/day, even though the Hb level is normal at the beginning of the pregnancy. This prophylactic measure prevents depletion of reserves and the anemia that may ensue with any abnormal bleeding or with a subsequent pregnancy.

Treatment of **sickle cell anemia** is more controversial. Exchange transfusion for the mother is recommended by some but disputed by others. No evidence confirms any treatment other than supportive care.

HYPEREMESIS GRAVIDARUM

Malignant nausea and vomiting to the extent that the pregnant woman becomes dehydrated and acidotic. Ordinary "morning sickness" with nausea and vomiting is discussed under PRENATAL CARE in Ch. 176; the term *hyperemesis gravidarum* should be limited to women in whom starvation, dehydration, and acidosis are superimposed on the vomiting syndrome.

Pathology

Persistent hyperemesis gravidarum may be associated with serious liver damage. Necropsies in such cases usually show severe necrosis in the central portion of the lobules or widespread fatty degeneration similar to that seen in starvation. Hemorrhagic retinitis is a serious complication and indicates a grave prognosis: the mortality rate in such patients is 50%.

Symptoms, Signs, and Diagnosis

Patients with hyperemesis gravidarum do not gain weight and usually lose weight. Weight loss and dehydration confirm that the vomiting is extensive. Many pregnant women with morning sickness feel as though they are vomiting everything they ingest, but if they continue to gain weight and are not dehydrated, the condition is not hyperemesis gravidarum. Psychologic factors are prominent in this syndrome but do not lessen the danger. Investigation for unsuspected liver disease, kidney infection,

pancreatitis, intestinal obstruction, GI tract lesions, and intracranial lesions is required, since these conditions can cause vomiting.

Treatment

Hyperemesis gravidarum is treated by correcting the acidosis and dehydration with IV infusion of water, glucose, and electrolytes. The patient should be kept in bed in a hospital and given nothing by mouth for 24 h. Antiemetics and sedatives should be used as necessary. Occasionally IV vitamin therapy may also be required. After the dehydration and acute vomiting are corrected, bland oral feedings in small amounts at frequent intervals may be started and may progress as tolerated. Usually vomiting ceases within a few days, but sometimes the regimen of fasting, IV fluids, and small meals may have to be repeated once or twice.

Repeated ophthalmoscopic examinations are imperative, and if hemorrhagic retinitis appears, the pregnancy should be terminated at once. Even in the absence of a developing retinitis, termination of the pregnancy should be considered in the rare cases that do not respond to therapy (as evidenced by continued weight loss, jaundice, and increasing pulse rate).

PREECLAMPSIA AND ECLAMPSIA

Preeclampsia: *Development of hypertension, albuminuria, or edema between the 20th wk of pregnancy and the end of the first week postpartum.* **Eclampsia**: *Coma and/or convulsive seizures in the same time period, without other etiology*. The etiology of eclampsia and preeclampsia is unknown. Preeclampsia develops in 5% of pregnant women and characteristically occurs in primigravidas and women with preexisting hypertension or vascular disease. If untreated, preeclampsia characteristically smolders for a variable length of time and suddenly progresses to eclampsia. Eclampsia develops in 1:200 preeclamptic patients and is usually fatal if untreated. A major complication of preeclampsia is abruptio placentae (see below under THIRD TRIMESTER BLEEDING), apparently caused by the vascular disease.

Symptoms, Signs, and Diagnosis

Any pregnant woman who develops a BP of 140/90, edema of the face or hands, or albuminuria of 1+ or greater or whose BP rises by 30 mm Hg systolic or 15 mm Hg diastolic (even though it does not reach levels above 140/90) must be considered to have preeclampsia. Mild preeclampsia develops as borderline hypertension, unresponsive edema, or albuminuria. Patients with a BP of 150/110 or with marked edema or albuminuria are considered to have severe preeclampsia. All routine laboratory tests (CBC, urinalysis, electrolytes) should be obtained, and any abnormalities corrected. BUN and creatinine levels should also be obtained to rule out unsuspected kidney disease.

Treatment

Treatment is aimed at preserving the life and health of the mother; the fetus usually will also survive. A patient with **mild preeclampsia** may occasionally be treated as an outpatient who requires bed rest, but she should be seen by her physician every 2 days. If her condition does not immediately improve, she should be hospitalized. *The primary treatment of preeclampsia and eclampsia is delivery*. No data indicate that delay in delivery enhances neonatal survival, except in the patient with unusually mild and immediately responsive preeclampsia. Therefore any patient with preeclampsia that is nonresponsive or is more than very mild should be stabilized and delivered.

Diuretics have no place in the treatment of preeclampsia, since they further disturb the already deranged electrolyte balance and reduce both renal and uteroplacental perfusion. A low-salt diet is also of no value. The patient needs a normal salt intake and an increased intake of water. If she is kept in bed and encouraged to lie on her left side, her urinary output will promptly increase, and the intravascular dehydration and

hemoconcentration will lessen. Since the etiology of preeclampsia and eclampsia is unknown, the treatment prior to delivery is to lessen symptoms, and the principal drug agent is magnesium sulfate **($MgSO_4$)** as described below.

In **severe preeclampsia** more vigorous therapy is indicated. Upon admission, an IV infusion of a balanced salt solution (eg, Ringer's solution) is started through a large-bore catheter. Then 4 gm of $MgSO_4$ is given slowly IV over 15 min until the hyperreflexia that usually accompanies this disorder diminishes, thereby decreasing the risk of convulsions. Concomitant lowering of BP will usually occur. With infusion of 3 or 4 L of balanced salt solution in a 24-h period, a rise in urinary output and lessening in edema will also occur. $MgSO_4$ should be given continually via a pump through the IV infusion at about 1 to 2 gm/h with supplemental doses as necessary. Usually within 4 to 6 h, BP will stabilize at a lower level and hyperreflexia will be dampened. At that time delivery can be accomplished. If BP does not respond to $MgSO_4$ therapy, an IV infusion of hydralazine (40 mg/1000 mL) may be started with the rate of infusion titrated to BP levels. BP should never be lowered to < 130/80 in cases of severe preeclampsia or eclampsia, because perfusion of the uterus would be decreased so markedly that the fetus would be jeopardized. Calcium gluconate 1 gm IV is a specific antidote for excess $MgSO_4$. If urinary output does not increase, addition of furosemide 10 to 20 mg IV will produce diuresis; diuretics are not used otherwise. Sedatives should not be used because of effects on the fetus. Stabilization can be accomplished in 6 to 8 h, and delivery at that time is indicated. Once the decision to treat preeclampsia with other than bed rest has been made, delivery should be the objective.

The patient who is admitted with **established eclampsia** should be treated in the same fashion. Early administration of $MgSO_4$ usually controls the seizures. If not, IV diazepam in doses of 5 mg may be added until the seizures are controlled. Constant monitoring and attendance is required; BP, pulse, respirations, and reflexes should be recorded every 15 min, and urinary output and IV intake should be recorded hourly. Observation for complications such as blurring of vision, confusion, pain, vaginal bleeding, or loss of fetal heart tones must be made and recorded every 15 min. Again, the condition should be stabilized in 4 to 6 h, and delivery accomplished at that time.

Delivery should be accomplished by the most efficient method. If the cervix is ripe and vaginal delivery seems probable, amniotomy should be performed and a dilute infusion of oxytocin started, to induce labor. If the cervix is unfavorable and vaginal delivery is unlikely, cesarean section should be performed.

After delivery the patient must be monitored as carefully and frequently as during labor; 25% of eclampsia occurs in the postpartum period, usually in the first 2 to 4 days. As the patient gradually improves, a mild sedative such as phenobarbital 30 to 60 mg tid orally may be added and ambulation allowed. Hospitalization may be prolonged, and medication may be necessary after discharge. The patient should be seen every 2 wk or more often during the postpartum period. It is not unusual for her BP to remain elevated as long as 6 to 8 wk, but if it remains elevated beyond this time, a possible diagnosis of hypertension must be considered. Throughout this time CBC, urinalysis, BUN, and creatinine determinations must be obtained regularly.

THIRD TRIMESTER BLEEDING

ABRUPTIO PLACENTAE

Premature separation of a normally implanted placenta from the uterus. All degrees of placental separation, from a few millimeters to complete detachment, may occur. The etiology is unknown. Abruptio placentae occurs in 0.4 to 3.5% of all deliveries.

Symptoms, Signs, and Diagnosis

Retroplacental bleeding occurs, and the blood may pass behind the membranes and through the cervix **(external hemorrhage)** or may be retained behind the placenta **(con-**

cealed hemorrhage). Symptoms and signs depend on the degree of separation and blood loss. In severe cases, they include vaginal bleeding, a tender and tightly contracted uterus, evidence of fetal cardiac distress or death, and maternal shock. Abruptio placentae may be confused with placenta previa (see below). The diagnosis can usually be established by use of ultrasound. Serious complications, particularly with preexisting toxemia, include hypofibrinogenemia with disseminated intravascular coagulation **(DIC),** acute renal failure, and uteroplacental apoplexy **(Couvelaire uterus).**

Treatment

If the patient's bleeding is not life-threatening, if the fetal heart tones are normal, and if the pregnancy is not near term, bed rest is advisable in the hope that the bleeding will lessen. If the condition improves, ambulation may be allowed and the patient may even be discharged if there is no further bleeding and she has easy access to the hospital. If the bleeding continues or worsens, delivery is indicated in both fetal and maternal interests. Once the decision to deliver promptly has been made, vaginal examination is indicated. If the cervix is dilated, the membranes should be ruptured, as this seems to lessen the incidence of DIC. However, unless vaginal delivery is imminent, cesarean section is indicated in both maternal and fetal interests. With vigorous and active treatment, maternal and fetal or neonatal morbidity and mortality are markedly lessened.

PLACENTA PREVIA

Implantation of the placenta over or near the internal os of the cervix. The placenta may cover the internal os completely **(total previa)** or partially **(partial previa),** or it may encroach on the internal os (**low implantation** or **marginal previa**). Placenta previa occurs in 1:200 deliveries, usually in multiparas or in patients with abnormalities of the uterus, such as fibroids, that inhibit normal implantation.

Symptoms, Signs, and Diagnosis

The symptoms are sudden, painless vaginal bleeding beginning late in pregnancy when the lower uterine segment begins to thin and lengthen, followed by painless, massive, bright red bleeding. Placenta previa frequently cannot be distinguished from abruptio placentae (see above) by clinical findings. Vaginal examination is contraindicated until the diagnosis of abruptio placentae has been firmly established, since inadvertent vaginal examination in the presence of placenta previa will precipitate greater hemorrhage. The best way to differentiate the 2 diagnoses is with ultrasound examination.

Treatment

If bleeding is minor and the patient is not near term, bed rest is advised. If the bleeding stops, ambulation is allowed. The patient may be discharged from the hospital if the bleeding remains stopped, transportation is good, and distance to the hospital is short.

Once the decision for delivery has been reached, cesarean section almost always is preferable; very rarely, with a marginal or low-lying placenta previa on the anterior wall of the uterus, vaginal delivery may be allowed if the head effectively tamponades the placenta. Blood must be available for replacement as needed.

ERYTHROBLASTOSIS FETALIS

Hemolytic anemia of the fetus or neonate, caused by transplacental transmission of maternal antibody, usually evoked by maternal and fetal blood group incompatibility.

Etiology and Pathophysiology

Rh incompatibility may develop when an Rh-negative woman is impregnated by an Rh-positive man and an Rh-positive fetus is conceived. RBCs from the fetus cross the

placenta and enter the mother's circulation throughout pregnancy (the greatest transfer is at delivery) and stimulate maternal antibody production against the Rh factor. The antibodies reach the fetus via the placenta and cause lysis or destruction of the fetal RBCs. The resulting anemia may be so profound that the fetus may die in utero. To overcome the anemia, the fetal bone marrow releases immature RBCs, or erythroblasts, into the fetal peripheral circulation.

The Hb from the lysed RBCs breaks down to bilirubin, which is cleared from the fetus in utero by crossing the placenta into the mother's blood. After birth, however, bilirubin builds up in the newborn's circulation; high levels can be deposited in the basal ganglia of the brain and result in **kernicterus,** *a clinical syndrome of poor feeding, flaccidity, opisthotonus, seizures, apnea, and neonatal death.* Survivors may have choreoathetosis, mental retardation, and hearing loss.

Incidence

The incidence and severity of isoimmunization and the reaction are influenced by (1) the variable potencies of different antigens (producing variable antibody responses), (2) the distribution of the antigen in the population (affecting the probability of parents' having antigenically dissimilar RBCs), and (3) the zygosity of the father—if homozygous, all of his offspring will have the antigen; if heterozygous, 50% of his offspring will have the antigen. In the USA, 85% of whites are Rh-positive, and about 13% of marriages among whites result in pairing of an Rh-positive man and an Rh-negative woman. Only 1:27 children born to these couples will have erythroblastosis.

Unless the mother was previously sensitized by transfusion, a first pregnancy is rarely affected. The risks of sensitization increase with each subsequent pregnancy. In women who have developed Rh sensitization, the second pregnancy often produces a mildly affected infant, although 1/3 of infants who die do so in the first sensitized pregnancy. Succeeding pregnancies produce more seriously affected infants until, at the third, fourth, or fifth pregnancy, the fetus dies in utero.

Feto-maternal **incompatibilities of the ABO system** leading to neonatal erythroblastosis are less severe but more common. In these cases, production of maternal anti-A or anti-B antibodies is sensitized by fetal RBCs carrying these antigens. The most frequent pairing resulting in sensitivity is maternal blood group O and fetal blood group A. Neonatal jaundice rarely reaches serious levels, and a Coombs' test of the newborn's blood may be negative or only weakly positive.

Prevention and Treatment

Since antibody production does not usually begin in a previously unsensitized mother until after delivery, erythroblastosis can be prevented by injecting a high-titer anti-Rh γ-globulin preparation within 72 h after delivery. The preparation must be given after each pregnancy—whether it ends in delivery, ectopic pregnancy, or abortion. The anti-Rh antibody destroys fetal cells that crossed the placenta before they could stimulate the maternal immune system endogenous antibodies. If a massive fetal-maternal hemorrhage has occurred, additional injected anti-Rh antibody may be necessary. This technic has a failure rate of about 1 to 2%, apparently because of sensitization of the mother during pregnancy rather than at delivery. Therefore, all Rh negative mothers with no apparent sensitization (as indicated by amniotic fluid study—see below) should be treated with a standard 300-mg dose of anti-Rh antibody at about 28 wk of pregnancy. These exogenous antibodies are gradually destroyed over the next 3 to 6 mo, and the mother remains unsensitized.

At the first prenatal visit, all patients should be screened for blood and Rh type (see also in the discussion of immunohematology under PREPARATION OF DONOR AND RECIPIENT BLOOD AND ITS COMPONENTS in Ch. 97). If the patient is Rh-negative, the husband's blood type and zygosity should also be investigated. If he is Rh-positive and the mother's Rh antibody titer is negative, maternal Rh antibody titers should be

repeated antepartum at 26 to 27 wk. While titers are of limited value in patients who are already sensitized, they are very useful in patients at risk but not yet affected.

If the titers are > 1:32, **amniocentesis** and spectrophotometric determinations of bilirubin concentration in amniotic fluid should be done at 2-wk intervals beginning at 28 wk. Patients already sensitized to the Rh factor are candidates for amniocentesis at 26 to 30 wk, depending on the estimated severity of the disease. High-resolution spectrophotometric determination of the bilirubin level of amniotic fluid (see TABLE 177–1) is useful in the antepartum assessment of erythroblastosis fetalis.

If bilirubin levels in amniotic fluid remain normal, the pregnancy can be allowed to continue to term and spontaneous labor. If bilirubin levels are elevated, indicating impending intrauterine death, the fetus can be given **intrauterine transfusions** at 10-day to 2-wk intervals generally until 32 to 34 wk gestation, at which time delivery should be performed. Intrauterine transfusion is done by inserting a needle through the maternal abdominal and uterine walls and the fetal abdominal wall into the fetal abdominal cavity. RBCs from blood transfused into the fetal abdominal cavity are absorbed intact into the fetal circulation. This procedure must be performed in an institution equipped for care of high-risk pregnancies.

Delivery should be as nontraumatic as possible. The placenta should not be removed manually. An infant born with erythroblastosis should be attended immediately by a pediatrician who is prepared to do an immediate **exchange transfusion** if required (see HEMATOLOGIC PROBLEMS in Ch. 186).

HERPES GESTATIONIS

A polymorphous, vesiculobullous, nonviral-related eruption occurring during pregnancy or puerperium. The term herpes is a misnomer—the eruption is not associated with herpes or any other type of virus.

Etiology

Herpes gestationis, an uncommon disease, usually begins in the 2nd or 3rd trimester or immediately postpartum. It is thought to have an autoimmune etiology, since complement and immunoglobulins are localized to the skin basement membrane zone, the site of earliest histopathologic change, where the vesicle forms.

Symptoms and Signs

The eruption is very pruritic and may be polymorphic; vesicles and bullae are usually present. Lesions often start on the mother's abdomen and become widespread, and may be annular with vesicles on the outer border. In addition, the lesions may be grouped as in herpes zoster or simplex. Exacerbation of the eruption in the immediate postpartum period is common. The eruption usually remits within a few weeks to a few months postpartum, and may recur with subsequent pregnancies or with oral contraceptive usage. The infant may be born with erythematous plaques or vesicles that resolve in a few weeks without therapy.

TABLE 177–1. LEVEL OF BILIRUBIN IN AMNIOTIC FLUID

Clinical Interpretation	*Net Spectrophotometric Absorptivity*	*Total Bilirubin (mg/dL)*
Normal or possibly affected	< 0.20	<0.28
Affected but not in jeopardy	0.20–0.34	0.28–0.46
Distressed and probably in failure	0.35–0.70	0.47–0.95
Impending fetal death	> 0.70	>0.95

Diagnosis

Herpes gestationis may be confused clinically with several other pruritic eruptions of pregnancy, particularly with pruritic urticarial papules and plaques of pregnancy **(PUPPP)**, discussed below. Herpes gestationis can be diagnosed with certainty by direct immunofluorescence examination of perilesional skin: The third component of complement (C3) and occasionally IgG are deposited linearly at the epidermal basement membrane zone.

Treatment

Treatment aims at suppressing eruption of new lesions and relieving the intense pruritus. Some patients with mild disease require only frequent applications (5 to 6 times/day) of 0.1% triamcinolone acetonide cream. Others, with more widespread disease, require prednisone 10 mg qid for several days to control the eruption, then tapered to a level where only an occasional lesion erupts. At parturition the dosage may have to be increased because of severe exacerbations of itching and lesions.

PRURITIC URTICARIAL PAPULES AND PLAQUES OF PREGNANCY (PUPPP)

A common pruritic eruption of pregnancy of unknown etiology.

Symptoms and Signs

Intensely pruritic, erythematous, urticaria-like papules and plaques, at times with minute vesicles in the center, begin on the abdomen (frequently on the striae distensae) and spread to involve the thighs, buttocks, and occasionally the arms. Often halos of blanching surround the papular lesions. The eruption most frequently begins in the last 2 to 3 wk of pregnancy (occasionally in the last few days) but may begin at any time during the 3rd trimester. Most patients have hundreds of lesions. Although the eruption is itchy enough to keep the patient awake, excoriated lesions are rare. The eruption usually resolves promptly after delivery and does not usually recur in subsequent pregnancies.

Diagnosis

PUPPP must be differentiated from other pruritic eruptions of pregnancy. There is no specific diagnostic test for PUPPP as there is for herpes gestationis, from which it is, at times, difficult to differentiate.

Treatment

Symptoms and lesions usually resolve within 2 to 4 days with frequent (5 to 6 times/day) applications of 0.1% triamcinolone acetonide cream. At times, the intensity of symptoms and lack of response to topical corticosteroids necessitate use of oral prednisone, which should be given in divided daily doses totalling 30 to 40 mg. The dosage can be tapered by 5 mg q 3 to 4 days. Systemic corticosteroids, especially late in pregnancy, do not seem to harm the fetus.

---

178. PREGNANCY COMPLICATED BY DISEASE

CARDIAC DISEASE

Cardiac disease in pregnancy is becoming uncommon in the USA, mainly because of the marked decline in rheumatic heart disease (even though better diagnosis and treatment of other types of cardiac disease are allowing more of those patients to

achieve pregnancy and delivery). Cardiac disorders in pregnancy are predominantly congenital diseases that frequently have been corrected surgically.

The physiology of the cardiovascular system in pregnancy (discussed in Ch. 176) is the basis for the symptoms and treatment of heart disease in pregnancy, since pregnancy imposes predictable burdens on the cardiovascular system. Knowing that the patient has a history of heart disease is helpful, since primary diagnosis of cardiac lesions during pregnancy is complicated by frequent systolic functional murmurs, venous distention, tachycardia, and chest x-ray distortions that are related to pregnancy and not to disease. On the other hand, the unexpected finding of a diastolic or presystolic murmur during pregnancy demands investigation. Symptoms appear for the first time in about 25% of patients with mitral stenosis.

The functional status classification of the New York Heart Association is helpful in managing patients with heart disease and assessing their prognosis in pregnancy. Almost all deaths from congestive heart failure during pregnancy are in Class III and IV patients. Class I and II patients with mitral stenosis sometimes advance rapidly to higher-risk classifications. Class III patients need digitalis as well as bed rest beginning in the 20th wk of pregnancy. Class IV patients may be considered candidates for early therapeutic abortion.

In women with preexisting heart disease, pregnancy is associated with a maternal mortality of about 1%, but these deaths account for about 10% of all maternal mortality. Pregnancy, if successful, does not shorten life or permanently diminish the functional capacity of mothers with heart disease. Congenital heart disease is more common among the children of mothers with congenital heart disease. Patients in Class I or II have no increased risk of death during pregnancy, even when their predominant lesion is mitral stenosis. Patients who are symptomatic after limited activity or at rest (Class III or IV) have an increased risk of maternal and fetal death and should not conceive until they have been carefully evaluated and have had maximum improvement with medical and surgical therapy.

In patients with rheumatic heart disease (RHD), the murmurs of mitral and aortic stenosis are amplified, while murmurs associated with mitral and aortic insufficiency are diminished. Patients with **mitral or aortic insufficiency** who are asymptomatic or only mildly symptomatic usually tolerate pregnancy without difficulty; those with severe symptoms should be advised to have valve replacement before becoming pregnant. There is relatively little information about **aortic stenosis** and pregnancy, but reported maternal and fetal mortality rates are high, and patients with severe stenosis should be advised to have surgical correction before becoming pregnant. **Mitral stenosis** is especially dangerous because the tachycardia, increased blood volume, and increased cardiac output of pregnancy interact with this lesion to elevate pulmonary capillary pressure; atrial fibrillation also is common. Together, these factors increase the risk of pulmonary edema, the most lethal complication of mitral stenosis. Mitral stenosis often leads to pulmonary capillary hypertension before the menopause, but left ventricular failure secondary to mitral regurgitation or aortic valve disease is unusual during childbearing years. Mitral valvulotomy can be performed during pregnancy, but open-heart surgery increases the risks of abortion and fetal damage.

Maximum improvement of RHD should be achieved by surgical and medical means before conception. Prophylactic antibiotic therapy should be continued for pregnant women with RHD. Medical management is based on limitation of physical activity, fatigue, and anxiety; prevention or prompt treatment of anemia; and prompt treatment of infection. In all patients with mitral stenosis, digoxin 0.25 mg/day orally is used prophylactically if atrial fibrillation develops. Labor and delivery are best tolerated at full term, and careful attention to analgesia and relief of anxiety is essential. Occasionally, sudden postpartum episodes of pulmonary congestion occur, but generally the major hazard is at the time of peak cardiac output (20 to 34 wk). Antibiotics

should always be used in the immediate postpartum period as well as when risk of infection is increased—eg, with premature rupture of the membranes **(PROM)**.

Most asymptomatic patients with **congenital heart disease** are not under an increased hazard during pregnancy. Patients with **Eisenmenger's syndrome** and **primary pulmonary hypertension** (and perhaps isolated pulmonary stenosis) are liable to sudden collapse and death during labor or the postpartum period; this danger also exists following abortion later than the 20th wk of pregnancy. The cause of death in these patients is unclear, but the hazard is great enough to make pregnancy inadvisable. If pregnancy occurs, delivery should be accomplished under the best available conditions, with careful attention to anesthesia, availability of cardiac resuscitation, and prevention of right-to-left shunting by maintaining peripheral vascular resistance and minimizing pulmonary vascular resistance. Venous return must be maintained. Patients with **Marfan syndrome** are at increased risk of aortic dissection and rupture of aortic aneurysms during pregnancy; childbearing is not advised.

Occasionally cardiomyopathy begins near term or in the postpartum period. This syndrome, called **peripartal cardiomyopathy**, is especially apt to affect women over age 30, multiparas, those carrying twins, and those whose pregnancy is complicated by toxemia. The syndrome is associated with a 50% mortality within 5 yr and also with a high probability of recurrence in subsequent pregnancies, which are therefore contraindicated.

In pregnancy, the cardiac patient's status may deteriorate despite the precautions of frequent visits to her physician, ample rest, elimination of stress or anemia, prophylactic penicillin, and weight restriction. Abnormalities of cardiac rhythm or evidence of pulmonary congestion requires hospitalization and bed rest. Periods of special concern, when digitalization may be required, occur between 28 and 34 wk, during labor, and immediately postpartum, when the heart experiences maximum physiologic loads.

The fetus shares the increased risk from maternal cardiac disease. The fetus may die during an episode of maternal congestive failure, or the neonate may succumb due to prematurity.

Labor and delivery are threatening to a cardiac patient, since the work of labor, straining in the 2nd stage, and the increased amount of venous blood returning to the heart from the contracting uterus markedly alter cardiac hemodynamics. Cardiac output is raised about 20% during each uterine contraction. A skilled anesthesiologist should be in attendance during labor. Conduction anesthesia is preferred for patients with mitral valve disease, but patients with aortic valve disease cannot tolerate the stasis and occasional drops in BP that occur with conduction anesthesia and therefore should have local anesthesia, although general anesthesia may be necessary for these patients. No straining should be allowed in the 2nd stage of labor, since during this effort all oxygenation is stopped and the patient can become anoxic within seconds. Forceps delivery should be performed if feasible, or a cesarean section should be done if indicated (see Ch. 179). Forceps delivery is preferable, since the threat to the patient is less with an easy forceps delivery than with a cesarean section.

In the **postpartum period,** the patient should be monitored very carefully, because mobilization of fluid produces wide swings in cardiac function. Diuretic therapy must be administered carefully, and appropriate digitalis therapy should be continued. These patients are not out of danger for several weeks postpartum.

THROMBOPHLEBITIS

Thrombophlebitis rarely occurs in pregnancy and is slightly more common postpartum, although levels of circulating fibrinogen and other clotting agents rise during pregnancy but are markedly decreased after delivery. Stasis is greater during pregnancy than afterwards. Thrombophlebitis is discussed in Ch. 30.

HYPERTENSION

Hypertension is defined as a BP of 140/90 or greater before the onset of pregnancy or in the 1st trimester. Patients whose BPs were not measured as abnormal before pregnancy are difficult to diagnose as having hypertension during pregnancy. Because of hemodynamic adjustments within the uteroplacental circulation, BP usually drops to as low as 90/60 during the 2nd trimester, making diagnosis of hypertension difficult during that period.

About 75% of patients with hypertension have no difficulty with pregnancy; the other 25% have to be delivered early to avoid abruptio placentae or unexplained intrauterine death. Patients with **severe hypertension** should be managed similarly to those with renal disease (see below); they should be hospitalized at 28 to 30 wk, and renal function should be monitored by creatinine clearance as the key to timing of delivery. If the disease does not worsen and creatinine clearance remains stable, the pregnancy may be continued toward term. If it worsens or if clearance drops, delivery should be accomplished. Cesarean section is usually needed, and sterilization should be considered, since cure of the hypertension is unlikely.

In **mild hypertension**, patients should have a drop in BP in the 2nd trimester, just as in normal pregnancy. For patients who have mild hypertension and are on medication at the start of pregnancy, diuretics and other drugs should be stopped. If the BP remains level in the 2nd trimester, the incidence of superimposed preeclampsia rises from 4 to 16%. For those whose BP rises during pregnancy, the incidence of preeclampsia rises to 32%. Therefore, if BP fails to fall or rises in the 2nd trimester, or rises later in pregnancy, patients should be treated with methyldopa or hydralazine hydrochloride in usual dosages (see in HYPERTENSION in Ch. 26). *Diuretics should not be used*, since plasma volume expansion is delayed and is correlated with intrauterine growth retardation. If a rise in BP occurs late in pregnancy, preeclampsia must be considered (see Ch. 177). Patients with mild hypertension that does not worsen during pregnancy can be delivered at 38 to 40 wk, but they should not be allowed to go beyond term.

RENAL DISEASE

Occasional pregnancies are complicated by a significant decrease in renal function due to congenital renal anomalies or acquired renal disease. As a rule, a patient with significant dysfunction (serum creatinine > 3 mg/dL or BUN > 30 mg/dL) before pregnancy cannot carry to term. Nevertheless, some women with more severe renal disease have borne viable infants. Similar success has occasionally occurred in women on maintenance dialysis or following renal transplant. Pregnancy seems to have no significant effect on the occurrence of noninfectious renal disease as long as hypertension is absent or controlled.

Management requires close consultation with a nephrologist. Frequent office visits for monitoring of kidney function are needed. BUN and creatinine levels plus creatinine clearance should be measured at least monthly, and BP and weight should be recorded at 2-wk intervals. Sodium restriction is indicated and diuretics are given only to control BP or excessive edema; other drugs may be needed to control BP in some instances. The incidence of preeclampsia is high. Hospitalization after 28 wk of pregnancy should be considered, since delivery before term may be necessary to save the infant. Oxytocin challenge test **(OCT)** and nonstress test **(NST)** should be done (see in FETAL MONITORING under PRENATAL CARE in Ch. 176); as long as they are normal the pregnancy can continue. The lecithin/sphingomyelin **(L/S)** ratio should be determined. If it is > 2:1, especially with falling creatinine clearance or abnormal OCT, or NST, delivery should be accomplished. If the cervix is ripe and vaginal delivery appears easy, this route may be chosen, but cesarean section is usually necessary.

URINARY TRACT INFECTION

Urinary tract infection **(UTI)** is common in pregnancy, apparently because hormonal dilation and hypoperistalsis of the ureters and pressure of the pregnant uterus against the ureters cause stasis of urine. Asymptomatic bacteriuria occurs in about 15% of pregnancies and in some cases progresses to symptomatic cystitis or pyelonephritis. Frank UTI is not always preceded by asymptomatic bacteriuria. Diagnosis and management of UTI are similar to those processes in nonpregnant patients, except for avoidance of drugs that may harm the fetus, and are discussed in Ch. 153.

DIABETES MELLITUS

(See also DIABETES MELLITUS in Ch. 94)

Diabetes mellitus is a genetically and clinically heterogeneous group of disorders that share carbohydrate intolerance in common. In pregnant women it is important to define and classify the syndrome as accurately as possible because the complex metabolic alterations of normal gestation complicate diabetic control and may place the fetus in jeopardy. Thus, individualized management guidelines are recommended for women with different types of diabetes. In modern perinatal and neonatal centers, with preconception counseling and early prenatal care, the risks for diabetic mothers and their infants no longer exceed those of women without diabetes. A successful diabetic pregnancy requires (1) preconception counseling and optimal diabetic control before, during, and after the pregnancy and meticulous management by a diabetes team or by an obstetrician, internist, or family physician well-versed in diabetes in pregnancy, and a pediatrician; (2) prompt diagnosis and treatment of both trivial and serious complications of pregnancy; (3) careful timing and appropriate mode of delivery; (4) at delivery, attendance of a pediatrician who is knowledgeable in assessing and caring for infants of diabetic mothers; and (5) proximity of a neonatal intensive care nursery.

Classification

New nomenclature adopted by the National Diabetes Data Group is presented in TABLE 178–1. The former classification was based on age at outset, duration, and complications of the disease. **Gestational diabetes (GDM)**, a special category for pregnant women, is defined as carbohydrate intolerance of variable severity with onset or first recognition during the present pregnancy. *All pregnant women should be screened for GDM* because unrecognized or untreated gestational carbohydrate intolerance is associated with increased fetal and neonatal loss and higher neonatal and maternal morbidity (see also PRENATAL CARE in Ch. 176). GDM occurs in 1 to 3% of all pregnancies; the figure is much higher in selected populations. Pregnancy is a metabolic stress test for diabetes; women who fail the test and develop GDM may be obese, hyperinsulinemic, and insulin-resistant or thin and relatively insulin deficient. Thus, GDM is also a heterogeneous syndrome.

Management of Diabetic Pregnancies

Good diabetic control at conception and throughout gestation is important for an excellent maternal/infant outcome. Most diabetes centers use a team approach that combines the skills of physicians, nurses, nutritionists, and social workers. In addition, in regional perinatal centers, experts in ophthalmology, renal disease, neurology, cardiology, anesthesiology, perinatology, and neonatology are readily available.

Preconception counseling and diabetes control are important because congenital malformations in pregnancy complicated by diabetes may be linked to disturbances in maternal metabolism during the period of embryogenesis, and organogenesis is completed by the 6th or 7th wk of gestation.

TABLE 178–2 is a simple guide for managing pregnant women with Type I (IDDM), Type II (NIDDM, but always **insulin requiring** during gestation), and GDM. Details

TABLE 178–1. CLASSIFICATION OF GLUCOSE INTOLERANCE IN PREGNANT WOMEN

Nomenclature	*Former Names*	*Clinical Characteristics or Condition*
Type I, insulin-dependent diabetes mellitus (IDDM)	Juvenile diabetes (JD) Juvenile-onset diabetes (JOD) Ketosis-prone diabetes Brittle diabetes	Ketosis-prone. Insulin-deficient because of islet cell loss. Often associated with specific HLA types with predisposition to viral insulitis or autoimmune (*islet cell antibody*) phenomena. Occurs at any age. Common in youth. These women are usually of normal weight, but may be obese
Type II, non-insulin–dependent diabetes mellitus A. non-obese B. obese	Adult-onset diabetes (AOD) Maturity-onset diabetes (MOD) Ketosis-resistant diabetes Stable diabetes Maturity-onset diabetes of youth (MODY)	Ketosis-resistant. More frequent in adults but occurs at any age. Majority are overweight. May be seen in family aggregates as an autosomal dominant genetic trait. *Always require insulin for hypoglycemia during pregnancy.* Previous history of "borderline diabetes." Impaired glucose tolerance or treatment with oral hypoglycemic agents. $HbA_{1C} \geq 9\% \geq 20$ wk gestation
Type III, gestational diabetes (GDM)* A. non-obese B. obese	Gestational diabetes	Screening tests: All pregnant women. 50-gm oral glucose load given randomly (need not be fasting). A plasma glucose 1 h later ≥ 140 mg/dL or above is an indication for an oral glucose tolerance test (OGTT)**
Type IV, secondary diabetes	Conditions and syndromes associated with impaired glucose tolerance	Cystic fibrosis; endocrine disorders—eg, acromegaly, hyperprolactinemia, Cushing's syndrome, insulin receptor abnormalities, or aberrant forms of insulin; drugs or chemical agents; renal dialysis; organ transplantations; certain genetic syndromes

* All pregnant women at higher risk for gestational diabetes should be screened at the first prenatal visit. Risk factors are glycosuria, family history of diabetes in a first-degree relative, history of a stillbirth or spontaneous abortion, presence of fetal demise in a previous pregnancy, a previous heavy-for-date baby, obesity in the mother, a high maternal age, or parity of 5 or more.

** Diagnosis of gestational diabetes based on National Diabetes Data Group with a 100-gm glucose load that 2 or more of the following plasma glucose excursions be met or exceeded: Fasting 105 mg/dL (5.8 mmol/L); 1-h 190 mg/dL (10.5 mmol/L); 2-h 165 mg/dL (9.1 mmol/L); 3-h 145 mg/dL (8.0 mmol/L).

(Modified from "Maternal Metabolism in Normal Pregnancy and Pregnancy Complicated by Diabetes Mellitus," by D.R. Hollingsworth, in *Clinical Obstetrics and Gynecology* 28:1985. Copyright by J.B. Lippincott Company/Harper & Row, 1985. Used with permission.)

of treatment vary from one center to another and patient care must be carefully individualized.

In Type I patients, **overinsulinization** is a risk of tight metabolic control regardless of the route of administration. In some Type I patients hypoglycemia does not trigger the normal release of counterregulatory hormones (catecholamines, glucagon, cortisol, and growth hormone). These individuals may experience hypoglycemic coma *with no premonitory symptoms*. All such patients should have glucagon kits, and they and their families should be instructed about s.c. injection of glucagon for severe hypoglycemia

(unconsciousness, confusion, or plasma glucose levels < 40 mg/dL). In pregnancy, good diabetic control is defined by *absence* of wide glucose excursions with marked hyperglycemia or hypoglycemia, HbA_{1c} concentration of < 8%, quantitative urinary glucose loss of < 1 gm/day. During pregnancy, normal fasting blood glucose levels are 76 ± 1 SD 10 mg/dL and 2-h postprandial values are ≤ 120 mg/dL. Purified pork and human insulin (*as opposed to beef*) are recommended during pregnancy to minimize antibody formation. Insulin antibodies cross the placenta, but their effect (if any) in the fetus is unknown.

Complications of Diabetic Pregnancies

Medical and obstetric complications such as infection, diabetic ketoacidosis, premature labor, and pregnancy-induced hypertension are managed by current perinatal principles. No differences have been found in prevalence or severity of retinopathy, nephropathy, or neuropathy in women who have or have not experienced pregnancy. Diabetic retinopathy and nephropathy are not contraindications for conception or reasons for terminating pregnancy, but require preconception counseling and careful management during gestation. Initial and monthly ophthalmologic examinations are recommended. Patients with proliferative retinopathy noted at the first prenatal visit should receive photocoagulation treatment as early in pregnancy as possible to prevent progressive deterioration. Women who have background retinopathy are followed expectantly.

No evidence indicates that diabetic renal disease worsens because of pregnancy, and renal complications during pregnancy are quite rare. In women with chronic renal failure who are on hemodialysis, successful pregnancy is rare, but surviving infants have been reported. One of 50 women with functional renal transplants becomes pregnant. Pregnancy-induced hypertension occurs in 25% of such pregnancies and

TABLE 178–2. MANAGEMENT OF DIABETES MELLITUS IN PREGNANCY

Type	*Care Before Conception*	*Prenatal Care*	*Labor and Delivery*
I*	Regulate diabetes HbA_{1c} concentration should be ≤ 8% at conception	Start care after missed period Prenatal clinic visits each week Individualize diet following 1979 ADA† giuidelines and coordinate with insulin administration Recommend 3 meals and 3 snacks/day; emphasize consistent timing Individualize amount and type of insulin. In AM, 2/3 of total dosage (60% NPH, 40% regular); in PM, 1/3 (50% NPH, 50% regular)‡ Recommend moderate exercise after meals—with caution Instruct in home blood-glucose monitoring Check HbA_{1c} level every 4–6 wk Caution about dangers of hypoglycemia during exercise and at night Instruct patient and family in glucagon administration Fetal monitoring with non-stress tests from 35 wk to term	Induce labor after 37–38 wk when amniotic fluid lipid profile shows ≥ 3% phosphatidylglycerol (evidence of fetal lung maturity). A mature lecithin/sphingomyelin ratio (≥ 2.1) does not assure fetal lung maturity in diabetic pregnancies Deliver with constant low-dose insulin infusion or alternatively give usual PM NPH insulin dose and withhold insulin on AM of labor induction. Administer regular insulin s.c. as needed during labor and delivery

(Continued)

TABLE 178–2. MANAGEMENT OF DIABETES MELLITUS IN PREGNANCY *(Cont'd)*

Type	*Care Before Conception*	*Prenatal Care*	*Labor and Delivery*
II*	Encourage weight loss if patient is obese Control hyperglycemia§ HbA_{1c} concentration should be ≤ 8% at conception Recommend diet low in fat, relatively high in complex carbohydrates, high in dietary fiber Encourage exercise	Obese patients: prescribe regular insulin before each meal Normal-weight patients: In AM, 2/3 total dosage of insulin (60% NPH, 40% regular); in PM, 1/3 (50% NPH, 50% regular); for all, individualize amount and type. Use highly purified pork or human insulin Individualize daily caloric intake to void excessive weight gain (> 9.0 kg, or > 20 lb) No daytime snacks Recommend moderate exercise after meals Instruct in home glucose monitoring Monitor weekly at clinic visits: 2-h postbreakfast plasma glucose Check HbA_{1c} level every 4–6 wk	Same as for Type I
Gestational		Modify diet: eliminate concentrated sweets, monitor caloric intake to prevent excessive weight gain (> 9.0 kg, or > 20 lb) No daytime snacks Recommend moderate exercise after meals Prescribe small doses of purified pork or human short-acting insulin before meals if postprandial plasma glucose levels are > 120 mg/dL Monitor weekly at clinic visits: 2-h post-breakfast glucose level	Deliver at term; avoid prolonged gestation (> 42 wk)

* Suggested guidelines only. Marked individual variations require appropriate adjustments.

† ADA, American Diabetes Association

‡ Some hospital programs recommend up to 4 daily insulin injections. Continuous s.c. insulin infusion (CSII) given in medical research settings is a possible alternative. This is labor-intensive and should be employed only in special circumstances and at a diabetes center.

§ Women taking oral hypoglycemic drugs should stop this medication and control plasma glucose levels with insulin; possibility of an adverse effect on fetal development due to oral agents cannot be excluded.

other complications are common. The incidence of prematurity is related to maternal renal function and time interval from transplantation; the best prognosis for term deliveries of normal birth weight is 2 yr after transplantation.

The major cause of neonatal mortality is congenital malformation incompatible with life. Therefore, a maternal serum α fetoprotein determination is recommended at 16 to 18 wk gestation and a careful ultrasound examination at 18 to 22 wk (with measurement of amniotic fluid α-fetoprotein level if the maternal serum value was abnormal). Maternal serum and amniotic fluid tests or an abnormal ultrasound examination sug-

gest neural tube or other developmental defects. Congenital malformations of major organs have been positively correlated with elevated HbA_{1c} concentrations at conception and during embryogenesis (the first 8 wk).

Labor and Delivery

During the 3rd trimester, the 3 major aspects of care for diabetic women are control of maternal plasma glucose, assessment of fetal well-being, and determination of fetal pulmonary maturation.

Most women with **GDM** have spontaneous onset of labor at term and are delivered vaginally. When induction of labor is necessary, it is initiated with IV oxytocin and amniotomy. If these pregnancies are permitted to go beyond term (> 42 wk), the fetus is at risk for death in utero. Even when maternal glucose levels have been normal or nearly so throughout pregnancy, infants of mothers with GDM are at risk for macrosomia. Thus, cesarean section may be necessary if there is dysfunctional labor or cephalopelvic disproportion, or to avoid shoulder dystocia and injuries to the infant and the birth canal.

In diabetes Types I and II, the obstetrician should assess fetal well-being at 35 wk by external fetal heart rate monitoring (non-stress tests). In addition, the patient is instructed to count fetal movements for 30 min daily. A sudden decrease in fetal movement should be reported immediately to the obstetrician. Non-stress tests may begin earlier in women with complications such as hypertension, hydramnios, premature rupture of membranes, intrauterine growth retardation, premature labor, infection, or developmental defects.

Most diabetologists and perinatologists do not measure maternal serum or urinary estriol levels, since these expensive assays are no longer regarded as the most practical or useful tests to assess fetal well-being.

At 37 to 38 wk of gestation, patients should undergo ultrasonographic examination and amniocentesis. The amniotic fluid lipid profile is determined. In infants of diabetic women, a mature lecithin/sphingomyelin ratio ≥ 2 may not ensure normal neonatal respiratory function. When there is evidence of fetal lung maturity (3% or more phosphatidylglycerol), labor is induced with oxytocin. Vaginal delivery is planned unless labor fails to progress, there is marked fetal macrosomia, or the patient has had a previous cesarean section and a trial labor is considered undesirable.

Control of plasma glucose levels during labor and delivery is easier when insulin is administered as a continuous, low-dose infusion during the intrapartum period (TABLE 178–3). The patient is hospitalized one day before delivery and given her usual diet and insulin dose. Plasma glucose levels are obtained at bedtime and at 3 AM. The

TABLE 178–3. LOW-DOSE, CONSTANT INSULIN INFUSION FOR THE PERIPARTUM PERIOD*

Blood Glucose (mg/dL)	*Insulin (u./h)*	*Fluids (124 mL/h)*
< 100	0.5	Lactated Ringer's solution with 5% dextrose
100–140	1.0	Lactated Ringer's solution with 5% dextrose
141–180	1.5	0.9% sodium chloride
181–220	2.0	0.9% sodium chloride
> 200	2.5	0.9% sodium chloride

* Rough guideline. Each patient must be carefully monitored on an individual basis. Infection or insulin resistance alters insulin requirements.

(Modified from "Timing and Management of Labor and Delivery" in *Pregnancy, Diabetes and Birth* by D.R. Hollingsworth, 1984. Copyright© 1984 by The Williams and Wilkins Co., Baltimore. Used with permission.)

following morning, an IV cannula is inserted into a forearm vein and 1 L of lactated Ringer's solution with 5% dextrose is infused q 8 h. Insulin (usually 0.5 to 2.0 u./h) is infused from a syringe pump. Plasma glucose values are checked hourly and the insulin dose is carefully monitored to maintain normal glucose levels (70 to 120 mg/dL). A pediatrician should attend the delivery, to assess and care for the infant.

Postpartum Care

An immediate decrease in insulin requirement occurs following delivery and is related to the abrupt loss of the placenta, which has synthesized high levels of peptide and steroid hormones throughout pregnancy. Immediately postpartum, women with GDM and many of those with Type II require no insulin. In Type I patients, insulin requirements decline dramatically but gradually increase after about 72 h.

During the first 6 wk postpartum, women with Types I and II require careful readjustment of their insulin regimens to obtain close control. They should check blood glucose levels before meals and at bedtime. There are no contraindications for breast-feeding by diabetic mothers. In women with Type II diabetes, continuation of insulin therapy rather than oral hypoglycemic agents is recommended during lactation.

Women who have had GDM should have a 2-h oral glucose tolerance test with 75 gm of glucose at 6 to 12 wk postpartum to determine whether they are normal, clearly diabetic, or have impaired glucose tolerance.

Infants of diabetic mothers require careful neonatal assessment. These infants are at risk for respiratory distress, hypoglycemia, hypocalcemia, hyperbilirubinemia, polycythemia, and hyperviscosity.

THYROID DISEASE

Thyroid problems are common during pregnancy. Mild to moderate **hypothyroidism** may be associated with pregnancy, since affected women frequently have normal menstrual cycles. If the diagnosis was established before pregnancy, the usual replacement dose of L-thyroxine is continued. Modest increases or decreases in L-thyroxine may be necessary as pregnancy progresses. When hypothyroidism is first diagnosed during gestation, oral replacement therapy with L-thyroxine 0.1 to 0.15 mg/day is started as soon as the diagnosis is confirmed. Response to therapy is monitored by repeating serum T_4 and TSH determinations and free T_4 index calculations after several weeks and adjusting medication accordingly.

Treatment of **Graves' disease** during pregnancy varies in different medical centers. In general, the lowest possible dose of oral propylthiouracil (50 to 100 mg q 8 h) is recommended. *Caution is exercised*, as this drug crosses the placenta and may cause fetal goiter and hypothyroidism. The therapeutic response occurs gradually over 3 to 4 wk, and usually the dose does not need to be adjusted at shorter intervals. Simultaneous administration of L-thyroxine or L-triiodothyronine is *contraindicated*, since they may mask the effects on the mother of excessive doses of propylthiouracil and cause fetal hypothyroidism. Maternal thyroid status is monitored by physical examination and serum T_4, free T_4 index, and/or free T_4 determinations. In some centers with experienced thyroid surgeons, a 2nd-trimester thyroidectomy may be considered when the mother is euthyroid. If this treatment is selected, the mother should receive a full replacement dose of L-thyroxine (0.15 to 0.2 mg/day) beginning 24 h after surgery. Radioactive iodine (diagnostic or therapeutic) and iodide solutions are *contraindicated* during pregnancy because of adverse effects on the fetal thyroid. β-Blocking agents (eg, propranolol) are *not* recommended (unless drug reactions to propylthiouracil or the similar blocking agent methimazole are encountered) because of neonatal side effects such as bradycardia, floppiness, and severe hypoglycemia.

In Graves' disease, maternal thyroid status does *not* correlate with fetal thyroid function. Women with Graves' disease or a history of the disorder can be clinically

euthyroid, hyperthyroid, or hypothyroid. Regardless of which of these conditions prevails, their thyroid stimulatory immunoglobulins **(TSIs)** cross the placenta and may be associated with **fetal hyperthyroidism** in utero. Thyroid-blocking antibodies, if present, also cross the placenta; fetal thyroid status reflects the relative titers of the stimulatory or blocking immunoglobulins received. In infants at risk for in utero hyperthyroidism, fetal tachycardia (> 160/min) and intrauterine growth retardation documented by ultrasonography may indicate fetal hypermetabolism. In infants of women receiving propylthiouracil, congenital Graves' disease may not become apparent until 7 to 10 days after birth, as the effect of the drug subsides. Mothers and infants should be followed carefully postpartum to monitor their metabolic status.

Hashimoto's thyroiditis (see under THYROIDITIS in Ch. 89) is the most common cause of hypothyroidism. Maternal immune suppression associated with pregnancy often ameliorates the course of chronic thyroiditis. In some women, however, hypo- or hyperthyroidism occurs and may require treatment to maintain a maternal euthyroid status.

Acute (subacute) thyroiditis (see Ch. 89), a common problem during pregnancy, often is misdiagnosed as Graves' disease. A tender goiter is noted along with or following a respiratory infection. *Transient* symptoms of hyperthyroidism are associated with serum T_4 levels above normal pregnancy values. Usually, no treatment is necessary.

Postpartum maternal thyroid disease occurs in many women. Transient or, occasionally, persistent hypothyroidism may occur in women with goiter and high titers of microsomal antibody during pregnancy. In women with Graves' disease, a recurrence of hyperthyroidism after delivery may be either transient or persistent.

Painless thyroiditis with transient hyperthyroidism, a newly recognized postpartum entity, is probably an autoimmune disorder. It develops abruptly in the first few weeks after delivery, is associated with a low radioactive iodine uptake, and is characterized histologically by lymphocytic infiltration. In contrast to subacute thyroiditis, this disorder may be persistent or progressive, and recurrent transient episodes of hyperthyroidism are described.

HEPATIC DISORDERS

Normal pregnancy has subtle effects on hepatic function, especially bile transport, but routine function tests are normal. Alkaline phosphatase values progressively rise during the 3rd trimester and may reach 2 to 3 times normal at term; this is due to placental production rather than hepatic dysfunction. Jaundice may be due to the usual hepatic disorders or to conditions unique to pregnancy.

Not Unique to Pregnancy

Jaundice may be due to **drugs** (see Ch. 72), often from phenothiazines prescribed for morning sickness. Acute cholecystitis and biliary obstruction due to **gallstones** appear to be more common during pregnancy, probably due to increased lithogenicity of bile and impaired gallbladder contractility.

Viral hepatitis is the most common cause of jaundice during pregnancy. The course generally is unremarkable but may be unusually severe in patients in underdeveloped countries. The reason for this is unclear, but malnutrition may be responsible. There is no clear evidence that hepatitis is teratogenic in the first trimester. Hepatitis B surface antigen **(HBsAg)** may be transmitted to the infant at parturition or, less often, transplacentally. Transmission is particularly likely if the mother is e-antigen positive and is either a chronic HBsAg carrier or has contracted hepatitis during the 3rd trimester. Affected babies often become carriers of hepatitis B and have subclinical liver dysfunction, but only occasionally develop frank neonatal hepatitis. Prophylaxis prenatally and with immune globulin and vaccination for hepatitis-B exposed infants is discussed under NEONATAL INFECTIONS in Ch. 186.

Unique to Pregnancy

Minor hepatic dysfunction may develop in **hyperemesis gravidarum**. Jaundice may occur in **septic abortion** or severe **eclampsia;** the underlying illness is usually obvious, and the jaundice is unimportant. Occasionally women with preeclampsia develop a poorly understood syndrome of hepatic dysfunction accompanied by evidence of disseminated intravascular coagulation. **Spontaneous rupture of the liver** from subcapsular hematoma with intra-abdominal hemorrhage is a rare but life-threatening event associated with pregnancy; the pathogenesis is unknown, but it is usually associated with toxemia and may represent an extreme vascular complication of the disorder.

Cholestasis (pruritus) of pregnancy is a relatively common disorder, apparently caused by idiosyncratic exaggeration of hormonal effects on bile transport. Intense pruritus, the earliest manifestation of cholestasis, develops in the 2nd or 3rd trimester; dark urine and jaundice sometimes follow. Hepatic inflammation is not present and there are no systemic symptoms. The condition is benign and disappears after delivery; however, it tends to recur with each pregnancy, and affected women often develop the same syndrome if given oral contraceptives. When pruritus is severe, oral cholestyramine 8 to 12 gm daily in 2 or 3 divided doses usually relieves the itching. Bleeding from hypoprothrombinemia occasionally develops, but is readily reversed by vitamin K therapy (phytonadione 5 to 10 mg/day IM for 2 to 3 days).

Fatty liver of pregnancy ("obstetric yellow atrophy") is a rare and poorly understood grave illness that occurs near term and mimics fulminant viral hepatitis. The etiology is unknown. Mortality for both mother and fetus is high, although less severe cases are increasingly being recognized. It is debatable whether immediate termination of pregnancy alters the outcome, though this is usually advised. At autopsy, diffuse small droplets of fat in the hepatocytes and minimal apparent necrosis are seen. Recovery is complete if the patient survives, and the disorder does not recur in subsequent pregnancies. A seemingly identical illness may develop at any stage of pregnancy if tetracyclines are given IV in high doses.

Pregnancy in Women with Chronic Liver Disease

Women with chronic active hepatitis and especially cirrhosis often have decreased fertility; with severe liver disease, pregnancy is relatively uncommon. When it does occur, fetal losses are high because of spontaneous abortion and prematurity and successful pregnancy outcome is unpredictable. In contrast, prognosis for the mother is generally favorable, as maternal mortality is not substantially increased. Although pregnancy may temporarily worsen cholestasis in primary biliary cirrhosis and other cholestatic disorders, pregnancy per se is not detrimental to patients with underlying chronic liver disease. Increased plasma volume in the 3rd trimester enhances the risk of variceal hemorrhage in cirrhotic patients, a relatively uncommon event. Most patients can tolerate cesarean section.

Corticosteroids given for chronic active hepatitis need not be stopped during pregnancy, as there is no proven fetal hazard. Need for azathioprine and other immunosuppressive drugs must be balanced against potential hazards.

INFECTIOUS DISEASE

Infectious diseases other than urinary tract infections and common viral infections rarely complicate pregnancy and usually are not a problem. Bacterial infections can be treated specifically. However, certain viral diseases are important because they can have specific effects on the fetus. These diseases are discussed very briefly here in relation to pregnancy; more detailed discussions are elsewhere in The Manual.

Rubella is a major cause of congenital anomalies, particularly of the cardiovascular system and inner ear. **Cytomegalovirus** can cross the placenta and damage the fetal liver. Likewise, **toxoplasma** can affect the fetal brain. Patients should avoid cats during

pregnancy unless the cats are strictly confined to the house and are not exposed to street cats. **Infectious hepatitis** (see HEPATIC DISORDERS, above) follows a clinical course like that in the nonpregnant patient, but can be particularly devastating during pregnancy, especially in malnourished women. The fetus may be infected in the latter part of pregnancy, and the incidence of premature delivery is increased in patients with clinical infectious hepatitis. **Herpes** infection of the vulva can lead to serious and frequently fatal intrauterine or neonatal disease. Fetal infection can occur transplacentally during viremia in the mother, by ascent after rupture of the membranes, and by direct contact during vaginal delivery. If active vulvar herpes infection is present, cesarean section should be done to prevent fetal involvement, unless > 6 h has passed since premature rupture of membranes. The effects of other viral illnesses on the fetus are not well documented at this time.

MALIGNANCY

Malignancy of any kind is generally treated as if the patient were not pregnant. Malignancies of the upper abdomen, lung, or extremities are fortunately uncommon in pregnancy and should be treated as usual. (See also MALIGNANT MELANOMA in Ch. 244.) **Breast cancer** is a major problem because the breast engorgement that occurs during pregnancy makes recognizing a new lump difficult. Any solid or cystic breast mass should be investigated. This can usually be done by ultrasound guided needle aspiration or biopsy. Excisional biopsy may rarely be indicated. Delay may be fatal for the patient. **Malignancy of the lower abdomen,** excluding the genital tract, should be treated as in nonpregnant women. However, for **rectal cancers,** hysterectomy may be needed to remove the cancer adequately. Delay should not be allowed, and after 28 wk of pregnancy, cesarean section should be performed in an attempt to save the infant. Prior to that time the fetus should be sacrificed unless the patient refuses.

Malignancy of the genital tract is somewhat different. As soon as **ovarian cancer** is recognized, it should be treated by bilateral oophorectomy. Before the 12th wk of pregnancy the ovaries are usually easily palpable, but after that time they rise out of the pelvis with the uterus, and the cancer may be missed. Survival rates for these patients are very low. **Endometrial** and **tubal carcinomas** rarely occur during pregnancy.

Carcinoma of the cervix is becoming less common, since cytologic smears allow early diagnosis of the preinvasive form. However, cancer of the cervix can develop during pregnancy, and an abnormal Pap smear should not be attributed to pregnancy but must be followed up with colposcopically directed biopsies. Conization usually can be avoided. If biopsy shows **mild forms of dysplasia,** the patient can be allowed to deliver normally, and appropriate follow-up by cytologic smear and biopsy can start at the 6-wk checkup. **Severe dysplasia or carcinoma-in-situ (CIS)** warrants further investigation during pregnancy. A very superficial conization of the cervix may be necessary for complete diagnosis to rule out invasion, although colposcopy is usually accurate. If true severe dysplasia or CIS is found, hysterectomy may be offered at the time of delivery, but further investigation can be delayed until the 6-wk checkup and appropriate treatment instituted then. If **invasive cancer of the cervix** is diagnosed in the first 20 wk of pregnancy, either hysterotomy and radical hysterectomy with lymph node dissection or whole pelvis irradiation followed by intravaginal radium treatment is required. Evidence is accumulating that during pregnancy radical surgical therapy is more successful than irradiation. If the cancer is diagnosed after 20 wk, some patients prefer to wait for treatment until 32 wk, when there is some chance for survival of the infant; but if abortion is acceptable, treatment should be begun. Near term, cesarean section combined with radical hysterectomy and lymph node dissection is preferred.

Leukemia and **Hodgkin's disease** are uncommon in pregnancy. If they are diagnosed early in the pregnancy, they should be treated appropriately with assistance and guidance by a hematologist or oncologist. Many infants have developed normally while the

mothers were treated with antileukemic drugs, but use of such drugs also has been associated with loss of the pregnancy and fetal anomalies. Since leukemias are rapidly fatal, no attempt should be made to save the pregnancy, and the disease must be treated promptly. Hodgkin's disease is not so rapidly fatal, and cure is possible. If Hodgkin's disease is confined above the diaphragm, a pregnant patient may receive appropriate irradiation therapy with shielding of the abdomen. If the disease is below the diaphragm, abortion may be required for adequate treatment.

DISORDERS REQUIRING SURGERY

Most of these disorders in young women are confined to the abdomen and may cause problems during pregnancy, since pregnancy may obscure the diagnosis and affect necessary surgical procedures. When surgery must be performed, mother and fetus tolerate it well if the supportive care before and during surgery is good and if anesthesia is performed carefully so that hypotension and hypoxia do not occur. Certain conditions are particular diagnostic problems during pregnancy.

Appendicitis mimics the general cramping pain that patients may experience during pregnancy, and the WBC count of pregnant patients is normally somewhat elevated. In addition, since the appendix rises in the abdomen as pregnancy progresses, pain in the right lower quadrant does not reliably establish this diagnosis. If appendicitis is suspected, laparotomy should be performed *without delay* (the death rate from a ruptured appendix during pregnancy is high) or in the immediate puerperium (when appendicitis is more common).

Benign ovarian cysts can develop during pregnancy. Unless the cyst is obviously malignant, operative intervention should be delayed during the 1st trimester, since the cyst may be a corpus luteum. The operation should be delayed, if possible, until after 12 wk of pregnancy; however, if the cyst continues to enlarge or if there is tenderness, exploration is necessary. After 12 wk of pregnancy, ovarian tumors are difficult to diagnose because the ovaries rise out of the pelvis with the uterus and are difficult to find. Torsion or infarction can mimic appendicitis and will be discovered at laparotomy.

Gallbladder disease occurs occasionally and, if possible, should be treated expectantly; if the patient does not improve, immediate surgery is needed. **Bowel obstruction** can be devastating during pregnancy. Loss of pregnancy can occur if gangrene of the bowel with accompanying peritonitis develops. Prompt exploration is warranted in a patient with signs and symptoms of small or large bowel obstruction and a history of previous surgical intervention or intra-abdominal infection that might predispose to intestinal obstruction.

---

179. ABNORMALITIES AND COMPLICATIONS OF LABOR AND DELIVERY

INDUCTION OR STIMULATION OF LABOR

Elective induction of labor is rare and is usually used only when patients live long distances from the hospital, so that weather may make transportation difficult. Some of these patients should be hospitalized when they are near term. Dating must be accurate, and amniocentesis for lecithin/sphingomyelin **(L/S)** ratio is advisable.

When induction of labor is indicated in obstetrical or medical disease, the disease process should be under control and the reasons for the induction should be precise

and should be recorded. The most successful and safest method for induction is giving dilute intravenous oxytocin, using an infusion pump for precise control. Labor usually starts at a 2 to 5 mU/min flow; if contractions are inadequate, dosage increases are made at 30-min intervals. External fetal monitoring is essential. Internal monitoring should be performed as soon as the membranes can be safely ruptured. Ordinarily, a total of 40 mU/min should not be exceeded, since at that point water retention becomes a hazard.

Stimulation of labor with oxytocin (as above) is indicated when the patient has developed contractions with an unsatisfactory pattern; before stimulation is attempted, the diagnosis must be reasonably precise. If the patient is in the latent phase of labor—ie, has little effacement, minimal dilatation, and irregular contractions—then rest, walking, or support are better treatments than oxytocin. After true labor has begun (4-cm dilatation with nearly completed effacement), progress should be > 1-cm dilatation/h. If true labor does not occur, the patient is considered to have **hypotonic uterine dysfunction.** The best treatment is dilute oxytocin stimulation until a more normal pattern of contractions is achieved.

An occasional patient has **hypertonic dysfunctional labor**, in which contractions are too strong, too close together, or both. This contraction pattern is difficult to control. Administration of any oxytocic agent should be discontinued promptly. Repositioning the patient and administering analgesia may help. A tocolytic agent, such as ritodrine, may be effective.

PREMATURE LABOR

Onset of labor with effacement and dilation of the cervix before 37 wk of gestation.

Premature labor associated with vaginal bleeding or rupture of the membranes is difficult to stop. Bed rest helps occasionally, but if dilation and effacement of the cervix begin, labor usually progresses to delivery. Premature labor not associated with bleeding or leaking amniotic fluid can be stopped in 50% of patients by bed rest and hydration. Ethyl alcohol and barbiturates should not be used because of maternal and fetal side effects. **Ritodrine,** a β-adrenergic sympathomimetic agent and the best drug available, has a 70 to 80% success rate; however, side effects include maternal tachycardia and hypotension and fetal tachycardia. If ritodrine is not tolerated, $MgSO_4$ infusion (similar to that used for preeclampsia—see in Ch. 177) may also be effective. If premature labor is arrested, treating the mother with dexamethasone 5 mg q 12 h for 4 doses (betamethasone and hydrocortisone are also used) before delivery appears to accelerate maturation of the fetal lungs and decreases the incidence of neonatal respiratory distress syndrome (see under RESPIRATORY DISORDERS in Ch. 186). The problems to which premature infants are predisposed are discussed in GESTATIONAL AGE AND BIRTH WEIGHT in Ch. 186.

PREMATURE RUPTURE OF MEMBRANES (PROM)

Rupture of the membranes 1 or more hours before onset of labor. It was once felt that all these patients should be delivered promptly because of risk of neonatal infection. This no longer is the case. The patient with PROM should *not* have a digital examination of the cervix. Rather, examination with a clean speculum is done to verify rupture, estimate dilatation, and collect fluid for maturity studies. Firm diagnosis of rupture of membranes is made by seeing fluid escaping from the cervix or by the presence of fetal vernix or meconium; other less reliable tests are determination of pH with nitrazine paper (amniotic fluid is alkaline, giving blue color), and microscopic fern pattern of fluid dried on a glass slide. If the amniotic fluid indicates by L/S ratio or other tests that the fetal lungs are not mature, an attempt should be made to delay delivery until maturity. Bed rest will work in some patients. Ritodrine may be necessary in many. If

no digital or repeat speculum examination is performed, the risk of infection is minimal. The patient should be kept at bed rest and her temperature and pulse should be recorded at least twice daily. Delivery should be accomplished if infection is suspected or when amniotic fluid studies indicate maturity.

PROLAPSE OF THE UMBILICAL CORD

Prolapse of the umbilical cord is rare; it can be occult or overt. **Occult prolapse** occurs with intact membranes when the cord presents ahead of the presenting part or is trapped in front of a shoulder. A specific pattern on the electronic fetal monitoring tracing is generally diagnostic. **Treatment** is changing the patient's position to relieve pressure on the cord. Occasionally, cesarean section is necessary.

Overt prolapse occurs with ruptured membranes when the cord presents in front of the presenting part. This most commonly occurs spontaneously with breech presentation. It also occurs with vertex presentation, particularly when membranes are ruptured with the presenting part not engaged. The cause may be iatrogenic and is one of the reasons why membranes should not be artificially ruptured unless the head is well engaged in the pelvis. **Treatment** is immediate delivery, usually by cesarean section, to avoid fetal damage. An attendant or the obstetrician must hold the presenting part up off of the prolapsed cord in order to prevent further and prolonged compression of the cord.

AMNIOTIC FLUID EMBOLISM

Amniotic fluid embolism is extremely rare. It can occur at any gestational age, usually with tumultuous labor and ruptured membranes. Amniotic fluid is embolized into the pulmonary circulation and the patient responds as though a blood clot had embolized to the lungs, with collapse, shock, tachycardia, cardiac irregularity and arrest, and death. Autopsy will reveal fetal squamous cells and hair in the pulmonary circulation. If the patient survives, disseminated intravascular coagulation is a common complication (see in Ch. 99).

POSTDATISM AND POSTMATURITY

***Postdatism**: Pregnancy continuing after 42 wk. **Postmaturity**: An uncommon syndrome of failing placental function and fetal jeopardy that occurs after 42 wk.*

Since calculation of the expected date of confinement is subject to error, the diagnosis of **postdatism** may also be uncertain. If the mother's menstrual cycles were 35 days or longer, delivery may be late by definition although the infant is really only at term. The **signs of postmaturity** are lessening in uterine size and decrease in fetal motion in a pregnancy that is > 42 wk gestation by dates. Postmaturity can be confirmed by finding yellow coloring on amniocentesis, secondary to meconium staining of the amniotic fluid. Frequently, however, the amount of amniotic fluid is markedly decreased in postmature pregnancies, and amniocentesis may be difficult.

Postdatism can be treated expectantly, as long as no signs of postmaturity occur. Accurate dates should be established as early as possible in pregnancy. If dates cannot be established because of an irregular or unobtainable menstrual history, ultrasound examination should be performed early in pregnancy to determine the length of gestation. Later in pregnancy, prior to 32 wk, serial ultrasound examinations for biparietal diameter of the fetal head can confirm the date. If the pregnancy has continued past 42 wk, a nonstress test or an oxytocin challenge test should be performed to help to evaluate the condition of the fetus. If abnormal, delivery should be accomplished. If the cervix is not ripe, cesarean section should be done. Problems associated with postmaturity are discussed in GESTATIONAL AGE AND BIRTH WEIGHT in Ch. 186

PROBLEMS IN LABOR AND DELIVERY

FIRST AND SECOND STAGES OF LABOR

Most of the problems that occur during delivery can and should be anticipated beforehand. Signs of danger during the 1st stage of labor include **vaginal bleeding** (see THIRD TRIMESTER BLEEDING in Ch. 177) or **abnormal fetal heart rate**. Other problems include **abnormal fetal presentation and position**. All of these problems must be accurately diagnosed early in the first stage of labor so that appropriate therapy can be started at the proper time. Failure to diagnose potential problems at the initial examination threatens both mother and baby.

Occasionally for various reasons an infant is born apneic although no problems existed before delivery. Appropriate resuscitative measures must be started immediately (see ASPHYXIA AND RESUSCITATION in Ch. 186). There should always be some individuals besides the obstetrician in the delivery room who are trained in resuscitation and who can be freed from providing anesthesia or tending to maternal problems.

The primary event of the 2nd stage of labor is descent of the presenting part into the pelvis. In general, both cervical dilation and descent of the head into the pelvis should proceed by at least 1 cm/h; if they do not, **fetopelvic disproportion** is likely and appropriate treatment should be instituted. If disproportion is not present and labor does not progress normally with good descent of the infant, oxytocin infusion (see above) should be tried. If that is unsuccessful, a cesarean section should be done. Fetal heart tones must be monitored carefully; any significant abnormality of heart rate requires immediate delivery by forceps or cesarean section (see below).

In fetopelvic disproportion, forceps delivery or cesarean section is required. When an attempt at forceps delivery turns out to be too difficult, the obstetrician should realize that the pull is too hard to be safe and should perform a cesarean section.

Abnormal Presentations

When the fetal occiput is posterior in the pelvis rather than anterior (the most frequent abnormal presentation), the fetal neck is usually deflexed to some extent and a larger diameter of the head is presented for passage through the maternal pelvis. If there is any degree of disproportion, labor may be prolonged and delivery difficult. The obstetrician must evaluate this problem and decide between forceps delivery and cesarean section (see below). In **face presentation,** the head is hyperextended, and the chin presents; if the chin is posterior and remains so, vaginal delivery is not possible. **Brow presentation** rarely persists; vaginal delivery is not possible.

In breech presentation, the next most common abnormality, the fetal buttocks present rather than the head. The perinatal death rate is 4 times that of cephalic presentations; prematurity is a major factor contributing to this loss. In breech deliveries, complications can be prevented only by diagnosing the problem earlier. There are several varieties of breech presentation: In a **frank breech presentation** the fetal hips are flexed but the knees are extended. In a **complete breech presentation** the infant seems to be sitting with hips and knees flexed. Single or double **footling presentation** occurs when one or both legs are completely extended and present before the breech. *The primary problem with breech presentation is that the soft parts of the lower portion of the body and trunk can mold to fit through the pelvis, but the head has no chance to undergo molding.* Thus, disproportion is not discovered until the body has been delivered and the head is caught. These infants may die. The incidence of nerve damage due to stretching the extremities or spinal cord and brain damage due to anoxia is increased in breech presentation. Anoxia develops because, when the umbilicus of the infant is visible at the introitus, the cord is being compressed by the fetal head against the inlet of the pelvis so that little exchange of O_2 takes place. These problems are compounded

in primigravidas because the pelvic tissues have not been softened by previous deliveries. Many obstetricians feel that most breech presentations in primigravidas and all premature breech presentations should be delivered by cesarean section.

Other abnormalities occur. Occasionally an infant presents shoulder-first with a transverse lie in which the long axis is not parallel to the mother's long axis but is oblique or perpendicular to it; these infants, except second twins, should be delivered by cesarean section.

Twins occur in 1:70 to 1:80 deliveries and can be diagnosed before delivery by ultrasound, by x-ray, or by recording 2 distinct heart-rate patterns on the fetal ECG. **Complications of twin presentations**: Twins are usually small and premature because an overdistended uterus tends to go into labor before term. They present in various ways, and abnormal presentations may complicate delivery. The uterus contracts after delivery of the first twin and tends to shear away the placenta of the second twin, so that morbidity and mortality are higher for second twins. Finally, the overdistended uterus may not contract well after delivery and may cause maternal hemorrhage. The obstetrician should decide whether to deliver vaginally or by cesarean section.

Shoulder Dystocia

An uncommon occurrence in which the anterior shoulder in vertex presentation impinges on the symphysis pubis. The head, following delivery, appears to be pulled back tightly against the vulva. The crisis in this event is that the baby is unable to breathe because the chest is compressed by the vaginal canal and the mouth is kept shut by pressure against the vulva, so that the operator cannot insert any kind of tube. Oxygen deficit occurs within 4 to 5 min. This condition occurs most commonly with large infants, but the only consistent predictor is the need to perform mid-forceps delivery. Large babies cannot be accurately predicted and do not always have shoulder dystocia.

When this situation occurs, the first step is to dislodge the shoulder by suprapubic pressure combined with fundal pressure to disengage the shoulder and allow the baby to descend farther into the pelvis. Hyperflexing the mother's hips may be helpful by flattening the lower spine and causing the birth canal to be straighter. Failing this, a hand should be inserted into the posterior part of the vagina and pressure placed on either the anterior or posterior part of the posterior shoulder to rotate the baby in whichever direction it will go easily. With rotation, the anterior shoulder should disengage.

If neither attempt works, the posterior shoulder is pushed up into the hollow of the sacrum, the operator's hand is inserted to the fetal elbow, the fetal elbow is flexed, and the fetal hand is grasped and pulled outside to deliver the entire fetal arm. The arm is then used (like a crank for an old automobile) to turn the entire baby and disengage the anterior shoulder.

Forceps Delivery

Forceps delivery is **elective** when used to ease delivery or to provide greater control of the head. Forceps delivery is **indicated** in problems of fetal distress or fetal position, or to shorten the 2nd stage of labor when there are no complications but lengthy vaginal delivery is anticipated. The 2nd stage occasionally fails to progress when use of conduction anesthesia prevents the patient from adequate bearing-down effects. The decision to use forceps must be made by an obstetrician, since cesarean section may be a better alternative in each of these situations.

Contraindications to vaginal (forceps) delivery include cephalopelvic disproportion, incomplete dilatation of the cervix, failure of engagement, indeterminate presentation or position, and insufficient skill of the operator. An alternative to forceps delivery is vacuum extraction, but the operator must have had specific and sufficient training in the use of a vacuum extractor.

Major complications that occur with use of either forceps or vacuum extraction are

injury to the fetus and to the mother. Only specific training, skillful use, and experience will avoid these complications.

Cesarean Section

Cesarean section (*surgical delivery by incision in the body of the uterus*) should be performed whenever it is safer for the mother or baby than vaginal delivery. About 20% of deliveries are done by cesarean section. The decision and procedure require an obstetrician, and management of anesthesia and resuscitation of newborns require an anesthesiologist and neonatologist or someone skilled in neonatal resuscitation. Cesarean section is safe because of modern anesthesia, IV therapy, antibiotics, blood transfusions, and early ambulation.

Two types of uterine incision for cesarean section are used: classical and lower segment. A classical incision is longitudinal in the anterior wall of the uterus, starting at the top or fundus. This incision is usually reserved for patients with placenta previa or a transverse lie of the fetus. The uterine wall is more vascular in this area, blood loss is greater than with a lower segment incision, and the scar is not as strong in subsequent pregnancies. A lower segment incision is made in the thinned, elongated lower portion of the uterine body behind the bladder reflection; it may be either transverse or longitudinal. A longitudinal incision should be used for most abnormalities of presentation or for excessively large infants to avoid lateral extension of a transverse incision into the uterine arteries. Blood loss is lessened and, since the incision is covered by bladder and peritoneum, adhesions are reduced. Because scar tissue in the uterus is weaker than the myometrium, many obstetricians feel that any patient who has had a cesarean section must have a repeat cesarean section with each subsequent pregnancy. However, attempting vaginal delivery after cesarean section has recently become popular, with the success rate being > 50%. The best treatment for repeat cesarean section is correct management of the previous labor.

THIRD STAGE OF LABOR
(Delivery of the Placenta)

Maternal hemorrhage must be prevented during the 3rd stage. Ordinarily 400 to 500 mL of blood is lost during delivery; if any more is lost, the reasons must be sought. Possible sources of bleeding include uterine atony, vaginal or cervical lacerations, or retained portions of the placenta. If the uterus does not contract, hemorrhage will occur, since the primary mechanism for hemostasis within the uterus is contraction of myometrium. When the placenta has dropped into the lower uterine segment and presents at the cervix, the corpus may be depressed toward the pelvis to help push the placenta into the vagina. However, the uterus can be inverted if this procedure is done incorrectly, especially if traction is made on the cord before the placenta is completely separated. Exploration of the uterine cavity and birth canal for lacerations or retained placental fragments is discussed in Ch. 176. During this time a trained individual, preferably an anesthesiologist, must observe maternal well-being. The mother's BP, heart rate, respirations, and alertness must be monitored.

---

180. POSTPARTUM CARE

THE NORMAL PUERPERIUM

The clinical manifestations of the **puerperium**, *the 6-wk period following delivery*, are numerous and variable. They generally reflect reversal of the physiologic changes that occurred in pregnancy, and are mild and temporary and should not be confused with

more serious conditions. Within the first 24 h, the mother's pulse rate drops and her temperature may be slightly elevated. WBCs increase during labor, and in the first 24 h postpartum marked leukocytosis (to 20,000) occurs. Vaginal discharge is grossly bloody **(lochia rubra)** for 3 or 4 days, but over the next 10 to 12 days its color changes to pale brown **(lochia serosa)** and finally to yellowish white **(lochia alba)**. The total volume is about 250 mL; intravaginal tampons or external pads may be used to absorb it. Urine temporarily increases in volume and may contain protein and sugar. Loss of fluid elevates the Hct and ESR for a few days. The uterus involutes progressively; after 5 to 7 days it is firm and nontender and extends midway between symphysis and umbilicus. By 2 wk it is no longer palpable abdominally. Contractions of the involuting uterus are often painful and may require analgesics.

Management in the Hospital

The possibility of maternal infection, hemorrhage, and pain must be minimized. Observation, periodic uterine massage, and dilute oxytocin drip administration (or IM injection of 10 u. of oxytocin) are required for 1 h immediately after delivery of the placenta, to ensure that the uterus contracts and remains contracted to prevent excess bleeding. If general anesthesia was used during delivery, additional supervision (preferably in a recovery room equipped with facilities for suction), O_2 administration, a ready source of cross-matched or O-negative blood, and IV fluids must be available for 2 to 3 h after delivery.

After the first 24 h, postpartum recovery is rapid. Regular diet should be offered as soon as the patient requests food, sometimes shortly after delivery. Full ambulation is encouraged as rapidly as possible. Exercises to strengthen abdominal muscles may be started after 1 day. "Sit ups" done lying in bed with the knees elevated tighten only the abdominal muscles and will not cause a backache.

The perineum should be washed with warm water 2 or 3 times daily. Shower baths can be encouraged, but vaginal douching is prohibited during the early puerperium. Pain from an uncomfortable or painful episiotomy can be relieved with hot sitz baths several times daily as long as necessary; codeine 30 mg and aspirin 650 mg q 4 h may be required (if nursing, use acetaminophen 650 mg with codeine instead of aspirin).

Bladder care is important. Urine retention, bladder overdistention, and need for catheterization should be avoided if possible. Rapid diuresis may occur, especially when oxytocins are discontinued. Ambulation, encouragement to void, and surveillance to prevent asymptomatic bladder overfilling are essential.

The patient should be encouraged to defecate before leaving the hospital; laxatives may be needed if constipation exists. If a bowel movement has not occurred within 3 days, a mild cathartic can be given. Hemorrhoids can be prevented by maintaining good bowel function and can be treated with hot sitz baths.

A CBC should be done before discharge, to verify that the mother is not anemic. Seronegative women should be immunized against rubella on the day of discharge. If the mother is Rh negative, is not sensitized, and has an Rh-positive infant, she should be given 300 μg of γ-globulin with a high titer of anti-Rh within 72 h of delivery to prevent sensitization.

Breast engorgement may become very painful during early lactation, when the amount of milk is beginning to increase. Managing engorgement in the nursing mother is discussed under MANAGEMENT OF THE NORMAL NEWBORN in Ch. 182. If the mother is *not* going to breast feed, lactation can be suppressed by giving bromocriptine mesylate 2.5 mg bid with meals for 14 days. Firm support is needed, since drooping of the breasts stimulates the letdown reflex and encourages milk flow.

Postpartum depression ("blues") usually appears within 24 h of delivery, is usually limited to 72 h, and is common. If this depression lasts longer than 72 h or is associated with lack of interest in the infant, suicidal or homicidal thoughts, hallucinations, or psychotic behavior, it is pathologic. True psychosis is probably the emergence of

preexisting mental illness in response to the physical and psychic stress of pregnancy and delivery; psychotherapy is needed.

Management at Home

The mother and child can be discharged as early as the 2nd postpartum day if both are normal. Medication may be offered for sleep and pain as necessary, but should be limited in the nursing mother, since most drugs are secreted in breast milk. Normal activities may be resumed at will. Many family-centered obstetrical units discharge as early as 6 h postpartum if the patient did not have major anesthesia or complications. Major problems are rare, but a home visit or close follow-up regimen is necessary.

Intercourse may be resumed as soon as desired and comfortable; however, contraceptive measures are required, since pregnancy is possible. Contraceptive pills should be started after the first menstrual period, but only in women who are not breast feeding. Some authorities advocate starting birth control pills within the first postpartum week in non-nursing mothers. A diaphragm should be fitted only after complete involution of the uterus at 6 to 8 wk. In the meantime, foams, jellies, or condoms should be used. In non-lactating women, earliest ovulation is about 6 wk postpartum, usually following the first menses. However, conception has been reported as early as 2 wk postpartum, so ovulation can occur earlier. Nursing mothers tend to ovulate, *then* menstruate, usually at 10 to 12 wk postpartum. An occasional nursing mother will ovulate and menstruate (and become pregnant) as quickly as a nonlactating woman. It is better to avoid pregnancy for several months to allow complete recovery. *Rubella immunization mandates a delay of 3 mo before a woman should become pregnant.*

PUERPERAL INFECTION

Puerperal infection is presumed when the temperature rises to 38 C (100.4 F) or above on any 2 successive days after the first 24 h postpartum and other causes are not apparent. Infections directly related to delivery commonly involve the genital tract; they occur in the vagina, uterus, or parametria. Renal infections also commonly occur early after delivery. Other causes of fever, such as femoral thrombophlebitis and breast infection, tend to occur after the 3rd postpartum day.

Etiology

Febrile amnionitis during labor may be followed by a secondary endometritis, myometritis, parametritis, and puerperal pyrexia. Certain conditions predispose normal vaginal bacteria (such as anaerobic streptococci and staphylococci) to become pathologic in the puerperium; these include anemia, preeclampsia, prolonged rupture of the membranes, prolonged labor, traumatic deliveries, repeated examinations, retention of placental fragments within the uterus, and postpartum hemorrhage. The same factors enable exogenously introduced contaminants (*Escherichia coli*, β-hemolytic streptococcus, *Streptococcus faecalis*, anaerobic organisms, and even *Clostridium perfringens*) to multiply in the uterus and vagina.

Symptoms, Signs, and Diagnosis

Even in the first 12 h, a significant fever must be evaluated by examining the lungs and uterus and obtaining cultures of the urinary tract and lochia. After 2 or 3 days of low-grade fever, higher elevations occur. The most common cause of fever in early puerperium is dehydration, but puerperal infection begins typically with evidence of uterine infection.

Chills, headache, malaise, and anorexia are common. Pallor, tachycardia, and leukocytosis are the rule. The uterus is soft, large, and tender. Lochia may be diminished or profuse and malodorous; the prognosis is more ominous when uterine drainage is reduced. When the parametria are involved, pain and pyrexia are severe and the large,

tender uterus is fixed by hard, painful induration located at the base of the broad ligaments and extending to the pelvic walls.

Peritonitis and/or pelvic thrombophlebitis (with risk of pulmonary embolization) may complicate the illness. Endotoxemia, endotoxic shock, and renal tubular or cortical necrosis may follow virulent puerperal sepsis due to aerobic streptococci or other anaerobes and *E. coli*, and may be fatal.

Treatment

Preventing or decreasing the predisposing factors is primary. Although vaginal delivery cannot be made sterile, postpartum infections are uncommon today because of better aseptic technics. The most commonly occurring organism is *E. coli*; coagulase-negative staphylococci, enterococci, anaerobic cocci, and *Bacteroides* have been isolated frequently.

An initial antibiotic (eg, ampicillin 500 mg q 6 h or, if penicillin allergy exists, tetracycline 250 mg q 6 h) should be infused IV. With proper treatment, a puerperal infection responds readily and will not prolong hospital stay beyond a few days. After discharge, oral antibiotics and weekly office visits are required.

PYELONEPHRITIS

Pyelonephritis may occur postpartum if the kidneys become infected by bacteria ascending from the bladder. The infection may begin as asymptomatic bacteriuria during pregnancy and is sometimes associated with catheterizing the bladder to relieve urinary distention during and after labor. The symptoms include high fever, flank pain, general malaise, constipation, and, occasionally, painful urination. The causative organism is usually coliform, and **treatment** is as described above, with oral antibiotic therapy continuing for at least 10 days or preferably for 2 wk. High intake of liquids should be encouraged to maintain good kidney function. Many authorities feel that a urinary antimicrobial agent such as nitrofurantoin 100 mg orally q 8 h should be given for 6 to 8 wk. A repeat urine culture 6 to 8 wk after delivery is required to verify cure.

OTHER PUERPERAL INFECTIONS

A fever between days 4 and 10 postpartum may indicate a developing femoral thrombophlebitis; it should be treated by standard methods (see Ch. 30). Latent pulmonary TB may be activated by lowering the diaphragm following delivery and should also be treated by standard methods (see Ch. 8). Febrile reactions late in the puerperium are frequently due to mastitis, though cystitis is not uncommon. Breast abscesses are exceedingly rare and are treated with antibiotics aimed at streptococcal organisms, primarily ampicillin or erythromycin. Breast feeding need not be stopped if the infection improves.

POSTPARTUM HEMORRHAGE

Blood loss of > 500 mL during or after the 3rd stage of labor. Postpartum hemorrhage is the major cause of maternal mortality after infection. The causes vary, and most are avoidable. They include hemorrhage from the placental site (associated with an atonic uterus as a result of overdistention, prolonged or dysfunctional labor, grand multiparity, or relaxant anesthesia) and hemorrhage from lacerations, retained products of conception, or hypofibrinogenemia. Serious blood loss usually occurs early but may appear as late as 1 mo after delivery.

Treatment, as for infection, begins with prevention. Antepartum correction of anemia, recognition of hydramnios or multiple gestation, discovery of an unusual blood type, or history of puerperal hemorrhage are helpful. Careful, unhurried delivery, with a minimum of intervention, is always wise. After placental separation, oxytocin 10 IU

IM or dilute oxytocin drip (10 IU/1000 mL) generally ensures uterine contraction and reduces the inevitable blood loss. The placenta must be examined carefully for completeness. If it is incomplete, the uterus must be explored manually and missing fragments recovered. If the placenta does not separate spontaneously within 30 min after delivery, manual removal is advised. Rarely, curettage may be required to remove infected placental fragments and decidua. Uterine contraction and the amount of vaginal bleeding must be observed for 1 h after completion of the 3rd stage of labor.

If hemorrhage occurs, bimanual uterine massage and IV oxytocin drip are required. If bleeding persists, blood should be replaced and the uterus explored for lacerations or retained secundines. The cervix and the vagina are also examined. Injection of prostaglandin $F_{2\alpha}$ directly into the myometrium has been used with success; although the FDA has not yet approved use for this purpose, it should be tried before resorting to surgery. If contractions cannot be stimulated in a refractory atonic uterus, hypogastric ligation or hysterectomy may be required.

INVERTED UTERUS

A crisis that occurs when the corpus turns inside out, emerging through the cervix into the vagina or out beyond the introitus. It most commonly occurs with too much fundal pressure by an inexperienced operator or with too much traction on the cord of a placenta that is adherent.

The easiest and simplest way to reinvert the uterus is by pushing the corpus up into the vaginal canal, then passing a catheter into the vagina and occluding the introitus with the examiner's hand. Saline is flushed by hydraulic pressure (the saline is held 3 to 4 ft above the patient's abdomen) so that it inflates the vagina and reinverts the uterus.

Manual attempts to reinvert the uterus may result in its inadvertent puncture by the examiner's fingers. Rarely, surgical exploration is necessary. The constricting ring between the uterosacral ligaments is incised and the uterus is reinverted.

§16. PEDIATRICS AND GENETICS

---

181. INTRODUCTION

In recent years, pediatrics has enlarged its scope to include perinatology and adolescent medicine; has placed increasing emphasis on prevention and early recognition of disease; and has acknowledged the importance and interdependency of the behavioral, sociologic, economic, and political aspects of child health care.

Because in this section THE MANUAL discusses medical care of the newborn, infant, child, and adolescent, it is helpful to define those age groups as they are used here: ie, **the neonate (newborn)**—birth to 1 mo; the **infant**—1 mo to 1 yr; **early childhood**—1 yr through 5 yr; **late childhood**—6 yr through 12 yr; **adolescence**—13 yr through 17 yr. The term "child" may be used in a general way from birth on, as in discussions of the number of children in a family. Specifically, "child" refers to ages 1 through 12.

Prenatal diagnosis and genetic counseling are discussed in the last chapter of this section, Ch. 203. Diseases and disorders occurring in the pediatric age group that are also prevalent in adults are covered more fully elsewhere in THE MANUAL.

---

182. HEALTH MANAGEMENT IN NORMAL NEONATES, INFANTS, AND CHILDREN

INTRODUCTION

Most pediatricians in the developed countries, especially the USA and Canada, are primary care practitioners who direct their efforts to keeping neonates, infants, and children well. This is done through illness prevention, early detection and treatment of diseases, and provision of guidance and support to parents in their child-rearing practices. Health management as described below accounts for 35 to 50% of visits to pediatricians' offices and 55 to 60% of pediatricians' practice time. Except for the care of normal newborns, little of the primary care pediatrician's time is spent in hospital. Most childhood diseases do not require hospitalization and those that do most often are managed by pediatric subspecialists practicing in tertiary care hospitals.

MANAGEMENT OF THE NORMAL NEWBORN

PERINATAL PHYSIOLOGY

How does the transition from fetal to neonatal life occur? The successful transition of the term fetus, immersed in amniotic fluid and totally dependent on the placenta for gas exchange, nutrition, and excretion, to a squalling air-breathing neonate is a source of wonder. A number of neonatal disorders can now be seen as failures to successfully accomplish this transition. Several specific areas of "perinatal physiology" will be reviewed briefly.

Ventilation/Lungs

The placenta provides gas exchange for the fetus. Fetal lungs develop anatomically throughout gestation, and fairly well developed alveoli are present by the 25th wk. The fetal lungs continually produce fluid, a transudate from pulmonary capillaries plus some pulmonary surfactant secreted by type II pneumonocytes. Fetal breathing movements occur intermittently, usually during rapid eye movement (REM) sleep that is present about 1/3 of the time in the fetus. During these breathing movements, lung fluid moves up through the tracheobronchial tree and contributes to amniotic fluid. Fetal breathing movements appear to be essential for development of neuromuscular control of breathing that the neonate will require to survive.

Surface tension is not involved in fetal breathing movements, since fetal lung alveoli are fluid-filled. Following the first breath after delivery, however, the air spaces contain air, and air-fluid interfaces exist at an alveolar-surface–lining layer of water. Pulmonary surfactants must now be present in this layer of water; otherwise, excessively high surface tension would cause alveolar collapse **(atelectasis)**, greatly increasing the work of breathing. **Pulmonary surfactant** (a complex mixture of phospholipids, including phosphatidyl choline, phosphatidyl glycerol, phosphatidyl inositol, and lipoproteins) is largely stored in lipoprotein lamellar bodies or inclusions in the type II pneumonocytes or alveolar lining cells during fetal life. At the first breath, surfactant is secreted into the alveolar lining water layer. By 35 wk gestation there is usually sufficient surfactant present to prevent diffuse atelectasis, the primary defect in respiratory distress syndrome (RDS), which may complicate more premature birth (see in Ch. 186, below).

For normal respirations to occur, pulmonary interstitial and alveolar fluid must be cleared promptly at birth. There are 2 mechanisms to accomplish this. The 1st is

mechanical: During vaginal delivery the fetal thorax is compressed, expelling some lung fluid. As the thorax is delivered, elastic recoil of the ribs draws some air in the pulmonary tree. The 1st strong inspiratory efforts further fill the alveoli with air. Secondly, a great increase in pulmonary lymph flow at birth acts to resorb residual lung fluid. Fetal epinephrine and norepinephrine levels resulting from the stress of labor appear to induce this increased flow of lymph. Neonatal **wet lung syndrome (transient tachypnea of the newborn**—see RESPIRATORY DISORDERS in Ch. 186, below) is believed to be caused by delayed resorption of fetal lung fluid.

Changes in the Circulation at Birth

A profound change in the circulation coincides with the first breath of air. Pulmonary arteriolar resistance is very high in the fetal circulation; as a result, there is little blood flow to the fetal lungs (only 5 to 10% of cardiac output). In contrast, there is low resistance to blood flow in the systemic circulation, largely because of low resistance to blood flow through the placenta. Low fetal systemic arterial tension **(Pa_{O_2})**—about 25 mm Hg—along with locally produced prostaglandins keeps the fetal ductus arteriosus dilated. Blood ejected by the right ventricle preferentially flows right to left, from the pulmonary artery into the aorta, through the ductus arteriosus because of the high pulmonary resistance. Another right-to-left shunt occurs through the foramen ovale. Left atrial pressure is low in the fetus because little blood is returned from the lungs, while right atrial pressure is relatively high because of the large volume of blood returning from the placenta. The difference in atrial pressures keeps the flap of the foramen ovale open and permits blood to shunt from the right to left atrium.

The first breaths of air enhance pulmonary blood flow and closure of the foramen ovale. Pulmonary arteriolar resistance drops acutely, the result of vasodilation caused by expansion of the lungs, by increased Pa_{O_2}, and by reduction in arterial carbon dioxide tension **(Pa_{CO_2})**. Air breathing also creates alveolar air-fluid interfaces that exert force towards alveolar collapse, which is counteracted by the elastic forces of the ribs and chest wall. Pulmonary interstitial pressure therefore drops, reducing tissue pressure on the pulmonary capillaries, further enhancing pulmonary blood flow.

As pulmonary blood flow is established, venous return from the lungs increases and left atrial pressure is raised. When air breathing begins, the umbilical arteries contract in response to an increased Pa_{O_2}. Placental blood flow is reduced or ceases, and blood return to the right atrium is reduced. Right atrial pressure falls while left atrial pressure increases; the foramen ovale therefore closes as air breathing begins and pulmonary blood flow increases.

Soon after birth systemic resistance becomes higher than pulmonary resistance, a reversal of the relative resistances seen in the fetal state. Therefore, the direction of blood flow through the patent ductus arteriosus reverses, creating left-to-right shunting of blood. This state of circulation in which pulmonary blood flow has been established, placental circulation has been removed, and blood flows from left to right through the ductus arteriosus is called the **transitional circulation**. It lasts from moments after birth (when the pulmonary blood flow and functional closure of the foramen ovale occur) until about 24 h of age when the ductus arteriosus closes. Blood entering the ductus and its vasa vasorum from the aorta has a high oxygen tension **(P_{O_2})** which, along with alterations in prostaglandin metabolism, leads to constriction and closure of the ductus arteriosus. Once the ductus arteriosus has closed, an adult-type circulation exists. The 2 ventricles are now pumping in series, and there are no major shunts between the pulmonary and systemic circulations.

During the first days following delivery, a stressed newborn may revert to a fetal-type circulation. Asphyxia with hypoxia and hypercarbia cause the pulmonary arterioles to constrict and the ductus arteriosus to dilate, reversing the processes described above, resulting in right to left shunting through the now patent ductus arteriosus and the reopened foramen ovale. As a consequence, the newborn becomes severely hypoxe-

mic. This condition is called **persistent pulmonary hypertension** or **persistent fetal circulation** (of course, there is no umbilical circulation). The goal of treatment is to reverse the conditions which produced pulmonary vasoconstriction; ie, a ventilator is used to induce hyperventilation with 100% O_2.

Bilirubin Excretion (see also METABOLIC PROBLEMS IN THE NEWBORN in Ch. 186)

In the fetus, bilirubin is cleared from the circulation by transfer across the placenta into the mother's plasma following the concentration gradient. The maternal liver then conjugates and excretes the bilirubin of fetal origin.

At birth, the placenta is lost and the neonatal liver must then take up, conjugate, and excrete bilirubin into bile so it can be eliminated when the infant passes stools. These steps required for neonatal bilirubin elimination apparently function, at least in part, during fetal life. Fetal hepatocytes contain Y and Z binding proteins, which take up free bilirubin from blood in the hepatic sinusoids. The bilirubin is then diglucuronidated and secreted into bile, which makes its way into meconium but cannot be eliminated from the body, since the fetus does not normally pass stools. The enzyme β-glucuronidase, present in the fetus' small intestinal luminal brush border, is released into the intestinal lumen, where it breaks the bilirubin glucuronide bonds; free (unconjugated) bilirubin is then reabsorbed from the intestinal tract and reenters the circulation. The **fetal enterohepatic circulation of bilirubin** "anticipates" the steps in bilirubin metabolism and excretion that will be required in the newborn. However, fetal bilirubin is still cleared by the placenta. Following delivery, feedings produce the gastrocolic reflex and bilirubin is excreted in the stools before it can be deconjugated and reabsorbed.

Delay in initiating feedings and circumstances that prevent enteral feedings (eg, intestinal atresia) are often complicated by unconjugated hyperbilirubinemia. One reason appears to be that β-glucuronidase still present in the neonate's GI tract results in a continuing enterohepatic circulation of bilirubin when GI transit time is prolonged (see also HYPERBILIRUBINEMIA in METABOLIC PROBLEMS IN THE NEWBORN in Ch. 186).

Fetal Hb

Because of its high affinity for O_2, fetal Hb is especially suited to extract O_2 from maternal Hb across the placenta. This increased O_2 affinity is less useful following delivery, because fetal Hb less readily gives up O_2 to tissues; this may be deleterious if severe pulmonary or cardiac disease with hypoxemia exists. The transition from fetal to adult Hb begins prior to delivery.

The abrupt increase in Pa_{O_2} from about 25 to 30 mm Hg in the fetus to 90 to 95 mm Hg in the normal newborn results in a drop in serum erythropoietin, which accounts for a shutdown of erythrocyte production that normally occurs at birth and persists for 6 to 8 wk. This bone marrow shutdown results in **physiologic anemia,** particularly in premature newborns whose body mass and blood volume are now increasing rapidly. However, the falling Hb results in reduced tissue O_2 tension and an appropriate increase in erythropoietin release, which stimulates the bone marrow to produce new erythrocytes. (This anemia should not be confused with iron-deficiency anemia, which is not usually seen until age 4 to 6 mo.)

IMMUNOLOGIC STATUS OF THE FETUS AND NEWBORN

Individual host defense factors develop at different rates in the fetus. At the time of birth, the function of most immune mechanisms is proportional to gestational age, but, even in term infants, is lower than in adults. Thus the newborn and young infant (especially between ages 3 and 12 mo) have a significant transient immunodeficiency

involving all limbs of the immune system, causing the neonate to be at risk for overwhelming infection. The risk can be enhanced by prematurity, traumatic delivery, maternal illness, neonatal stress, and some medications. (Immunization procedures are discussed below in IMMUNIZATION PROCEDURES THROUGHOUT CHILDHOOD).

Phagocytic System

Phagocytic cells, first seen at the yolk sac stage of development, are critical for the inflammatory response that combats bacterial and fungal infection. Granulocytes and monocytes can be identified in the 2nd and 4th mo of gestation, respectively. In general, their level of function increases with gestational age, but is still low at term. The newborn's decreased inflammatory response contributes to increased susceptibility to infections and may help explain the absence of localized clinical signs (eg, fever or meningismus) that are seen in older children with infections.

Ultrastructure of newborn neutrophils is normal, but membrane deformability and adherence are decreased, possibly influencing cell functions such as chemotaxis and phagocytosis. In most neonates, neutrophil and monocyte **chemotaxis** is decreased because of an intrinsic abnormality of cellular locomotion and a decreased ability of newborn sera to generate chemotactic factors (substances that attract phagocytes to sites of microbial invasion). Decreased chemotaxis of newborn monocytes may contribute to their cutaneous anergy. Chemotaxis does not reach adult levels until several years of age. Neutrophil and monocyte **phagocytosis** and microbial killing usually are normal in healthy infants after 12 h of age, but are decreased in low-birth-weight or stressed term newborns.

Opsonization is necessary for efficient phagocytosis of many microorganisms. Serum opsonic factors include IgG and IgM antibody (heat-stable) and complement (heat-labile). IgM opsonizes gram-negative bacteria more efficiently than IgG, but complement is needed for optimal serum opsonic activity. Unlike IgG, IgM and complement components do not cross the placenta. Significant levels of IgM production begin only after birth unless stimulated by intrauterine infection. Synthesis of complement components begins as early as 5½ wk gestation, but levels of most classical and alternative pathway components are only 50 to 75% of adult levels at term. Therefore, normal newborns have very low serum levels of IgM and complement components. Newborn leukocytes have normal Fc and C3 receptors for both groups of opsonins. Serum opsonic activity varies with gestational age. Low-birth-weight infants have decreased opsonization of all organisms tested. Term infants usually have decreased opsonization of some organisms, particularly gram-negative bacteria.

The circulating monocyte is the precursor of the fixed tissue macrophage, which is capable of phagocytosis in utero and has low-to-normal microbicidal activity at term. Pulmonary alveolar macrophages migrate into position at or near the time of birth and help clear the alveoli of amniotic fluid debris as well as microorganisms. These and other tissue macrophages, including those in the spleen, have diminished phagocytic capacity. Decreased efficiency of the reticuloendothelial system of the newborn is, at least in part, due to decreased serum opsonic activity.

Cellular (T Cell) Immunity

In man, the thymus anlage is generated from the epithelium of the 3rd and 4th pharyngeal pouches at about the 6th wk of gestation; by the 12th wk it can participate in the immune response. The thymus is most active during fetal development and in early postnatal life. It increases in size rapidly in utero and is readily noted on chest x-ray in the normal neonate, and then involutes gradually over many years. The thymus is considered to be the mediator of the tolerance to "self" antigens during the fetal and perinatal periods and is essential to the development and maturation of peripheral lymphoid tissue. The epithelial elements in the thymus produce humoral substances that are important in T cell differentiation and maturation.

At birth, delayed hypersensitivity skin test responses are markedly diminished and skin graft rejection is impaired. These functions improve during the 1st few months of life. In contrast, T cell numbers, T cell subsets (helpers and suppressors), and T cell proliferative responses to mitogens and allogeneic cells are normal or increased. Some lymphokines (migration inhibitory factor, interferon-α), but not all (lymphotoxin, IFN-γ), are produced in near normal quantities by newborn lymphocytes. Cytotoxic activity, including natural killer, antibody-dependent, and cytotoxic T cell killing is considerably lower than in adult lymphocytes. Also, there is significant T cell suppression of B cell differentiation and antibody production. The net effect is a partial T cell immunodeficiency which may cause increased susceptibility to infection, and under rare circumstances, engraftment of transfused or maternal lymphocytes. A number of factors such as viral infections, hyperbilirubinemia, drugs taken by the mother late in pregnancy (eg, corticosteroids or antimetabolites) may depress T cell function in the neonate.

Antibody (B Cell) Immunity

B cells are found in fetal bone marrow, blood, liver, and spleen by 12 wk of gestation. Trace amounts of IgM and IgG synthesis occur by 20 wk and IgA synthesis by 30 wk. However, since the fetus normally is in an antigen-free environment, only small amounts of immunoglobulin (predominantly IgM) are produced in utero. Elevated levels of cord serum IgM (> 20 mg/dL) indicate in utero antigen challenge, usually congenital infection. Almost all IgG is acquired from the mother via the placenta. By the time of term birth, the term infant has IgG levels comparable to or greater than adult levels (110% of maternal level). IgG levels at the time of birth in premature infants are decreased in proportion to their gestational age. After birth, catabolism of the transplacental IgG with a half life of about 25 days results in a "physiologic hypogammaglobulinemia" by age 2 to 6 mo, which begins to resolve after 6 mo as the infant's rate of IgG synthesis begins to exceed catabolism of maternal antibody. By 1 yr of age the IgG level is about 70% of average adult values. IgA, IgM, IgD, and IgE do not cross the placenta. Their levels increase slowly from very low to about 30% of adult levels by 1 yr of age. Adult immunoglobulin levels are achieved approximately as follows: IgM, 1 yr; IgG, 8 yr; and IgA, 11 yr.

The newborn has deficient antibody responses to a number of antigens, including vaccine antigens. Antibody responses to polysaccharide antigens such as hemophilus and pneumococcal polysaccharides are particularly poor in the first 2 yr of life. When an antibody response occurs, usually there is a prolonged IgM response and a diminished IgG response. Immunization of an infant too early may result in the development of tolerance or a decreased antibody response to subsequent challenge with the same antigen.

Passive transfer of immunity from the mother in the form of transplacental IgG antibody and immune factors in breast milk helps compensate for the newborn's immature immune system. The maternal IgG antibody gives the neonate immunity to many serious bacterial (eg, pneumococcus, hemophilus, meningococcus) and viral pathogens (eg, measles, varicella). However, passively acquired maternal IgG antibody occasionally also can inhibit the newborn's response to immunization against agents such as as measles or rubella. Breast milk contains many antimicrobial factors, such as IgG, secretory IgA, leukocytes, complement proteins, lysozyme, and lactoferrin. These substances coat the GI and upper respiratory tracts and help prevent invasion of mucous membranes by respiratory and enteric pathogens. Breastfeeding is particularly important where the water supply may be contaminated.

The morbidity and mortality due to neonatal infections remain significant despite appropriate antibiotic therapy. Attempts have been made to augment the neonate's immature immune system in the prevention and treatment of infection. Animal studies suggest a possible role for fresh frozen plasma or immune or hyperimmune globulin in

some kinds of neonatal infection (eg, group B streptococcal disease). Data on the efficacy of exchange and leukocyte transfusions are conflicting and the advisability of their routine use awaits the results of controlled trials.

INITIAL CARE

At birth, the normal newborn breathes spontaneously once his airway is cleared of mucus and debris by gentle bulb suction. The cord is clamped and cut after the first breath; one vein and 2 arteries should be visible on the fresh-cut surface. The newborn is dried gently and placed on a sterile, dry receiving blanket on a warm table; maintaining body temperature is critical.

Initial delivery-room inspection is limited to identifying any life-threatening or major abnormalities, such as gross deformities (omphalocele, myelomeningocele, cleft lip and palate) and orthopedic anomalies (clubfoot, an abnormal number of digits on hands or feet). Other abnormalities to be noted include scaphoid abdomen, as seen in diaphragmatic hernia, and asymmetry or increased anteroposterior diameter of the chest, as seen in both diaphragmatic hernia and spontaneous pneumothorax. Color is noted using the Apgar score (see ASPHYXIA AND RESUSCITATION in Ch. 186). Generalized cyanosis indicates significant heart or lung disease; differential cyanosis indicates specific cardiac lesions. Many normal newborns have transient cyanosis that clears by the 5-min Apgar score. The heart and lungs are auscultated and the abdomen palpated. Gestational age is estimated (see method in FIG. 182–1) in order to plan special care for any neonate < 37 wk or > 42 wk gestation, or whose weight is inappropriate for his estimated gestational age (see GESTATIONAL AGE AND BIRTH WEIGHT in Ch. 186).

Except in resuscitation efforts, a tube should not be passed to check the esophagus and stomach until the newborn is stable (a minimum of 5 to 10 min after birth), since this maneuver may produce severe vaso-vagal reflex apnea in an otherwise normal infant. After 10 min of life, a tube is passed to check patency of the nares and esophagus in newborns born to mothers with polyhydramnios or diabetes, in those born in the breech position or by cesarean section delivery, and in *any* newborn with increased secretions, in order to rule out tracheoesophageal fistula and other anomalies of the esophagus and stomach. The stomach, if reached, is aspirated, and the volume of its contents measured. Neonates delivered in the vertex position may have little fluid left in the stomach, but this does not rule out obstruction. In premature newborns, the normal stomach volume is as follows:

Birth Weight	*Fluid Volume*
2.5 kg	12–15 mL
2.0 kg	10 mL
1.5 kg	7– 8 mL
1.0 kg	5 mL

As soon as possible the newborn is swaddled to maintain body temperature, being sure to cover the head, a large surface area capable of losing considerable heat. Two drops of 1% silver nitrate solution, or an antibiotic ointment such as erythromycin, are instilled in each eye. The newborn may now be held by the mother and put to breast if she wishes (see FEEDING, below). *Good hand-washing technic must be used by all personnel, since the newborn's defense mechanisms against infection are not fully developed.*

On arrival in the nursery, if the newborn's temperature is < 35.5 C (96 F), a heated crib is required. Normally, the crib is left flat and the newborn is placed on his side to

Physical Maturity

Score	0	1	2	3	4	5
Skin	edema gelatinous red, trans-parent	sl. edema smooth pink, vis-ible veins	no edema pink superficial peeling, and/or rash few veins	pale pink cracking pale area rare veins	pink hands feet parchment deep cracking no vessels	leathery cracked wrinkled
Lanugo	none	abundant	thinning	bald areas	mostly bald	
Plantar Creases	no crease	faint red marks	anterior transverse crease only	creases anterior 2/3	creases cover entire sole	
Breast	barely perceptible	flat areola no bud	stippled areola 1–2 mm bud	raised areola 3–4 mm bud	full areola 5–10 mm bud	
Ear	pinna flat, stays folded	sl. curved pinna soft with slow recoil	well-curved pinna, soft but ready recoil	formed & firm with instant recoil	thick cartilage ear stiff	
Genitals ♂	scrotum empty no rugae	at least one testis palpable	testes descend-ing, few rugae	testes down good rugae	testes pendulous deep rugae	
Genitals ♀	prominent clitoris & labia minora	labia majora visible	majora & minora equally prominent	majora large minora small	clitoris & minora completely covered	

Maturity Rating

Score	Weeks
5	26
10	28
15	30
20	32
25	34
30	36
35	38
40	40
45	42
50	44

Neuromuscular Maturity

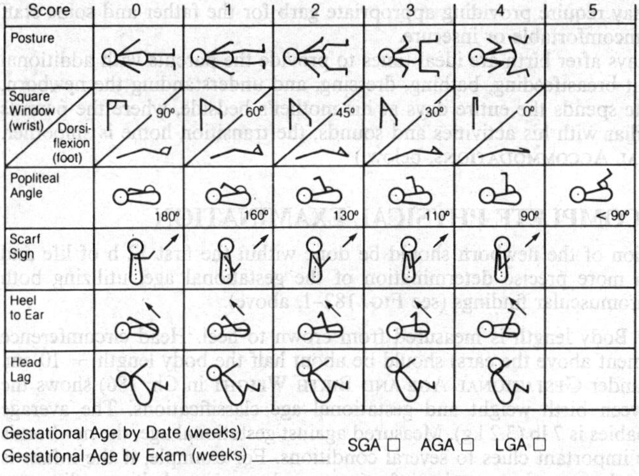

Score
0
1
2
3
4
5
Posture
Square Window (wrist)
Dorsi-flexion (foot)
90°
60°
45°
30°
0°
Popliteal Angle
180°
160°
130°
110°
90°
< 90°
Scarf Sign
Heel to Ear
Head Lag

Gestational Age by Date (weeks) ________ SGA ☐ AGA ☐ LGA ☐

Gestational Age by Exam (weeks) ________

FIG. 182–1. Assessment of gestational age. (Modified from "A simplified score for assessment of fetal maturation of newly born infants," by Jeanne L. Ballard et al., in *The Journal of Pediatrics*, Vol. 95, No. 5, Part I, pp. 769–774, Nov. 1979. Copyright 1979 by the C. V. Mosby Company.)

facilitate mucus drainage. Vitamin K_1 (phytonadione) 1 mg IM is given to prevent hypoprothrombinemia, which causes hemorrhagic disease of the newborn. Triple Dye® may be applied with a swab to the fresh-cut cord and periumbilical area to prevent infection; one application is sufficient.

The admission bath is not given for 6 h or until the temperature has been stabilized at 37 C (98.6 F) for 2 h. The bath should not remove all the **vernix caseosa** (*a whitish, greasy material that covers most of the body at birth*), as it provides some antibacterial protection. A mild soap such as castile may be used with thorough rinsing. Oils, powders, and ointments should not be routinely used.

Initial Parent-Infant Interactions

Although pregnancy gives a woman an opportunity to prepare herself psychologically for the new baby and to share that preparation with the father, there are important events that enhance parenting during and following birth. The physiologic aspects of birth include adaptations of the woman's body to the movement of the fetus from the uterus to the outside world. Participation in the birth by a prepared, knowledgeable woman and her spouse makes the new role of parenting go more smoothly. An optimal environment that helps the couple be secure and confident also helps the mother relax and work with her body during labor and delivery.

Parental feelings at the first moments of their newborn's life vary from ecstasy to disappointment; for some, these moments are totally forgotten because of concurrent events requiring priority such as resuscitation of the infant or obstetric complications in the mother. (Parent-infant bonding with the sick neonate is discussed in Ch. 183, below). It has been suggested that early physical contact with the infant, looking eye to eye, established an early bond essential to a lasting parental love and relationship. In humans, however, such a "critical period" may not exist. Unquestionably, mothers can relate well to their infants even when the first hours are not spent enraptured with each other.

Immediately following a normal birth, the mother should be helped to hold and cuddle her baby while warmth and stabilization are provided for the newborn. The mother should be offered opportunity to put the newborn to breast for the first suckling (see FEEDING, below), and the father should have the opportunity to share these moments. This may require providing appropriate garb for the father and some staff support if he is uncomfortable or insecure.

The first few days after birth are ideal times to provide the parents with additional information about breastfeeding, bathing, dressing, and understanding the newborn. When the neonate spends the entire days at his mother's bedside, where the parents can become familiar with his activities and sounds, the transition home is smoother. (See also HOSPITAL ACCOMMODATIONS, below.)

COMPLETE PHYSICAL EXAMINATION

This examination of the newborn should be done within the first 12 h of life and should include a more precise determination of the gestational age, utilizing both physical and neuromuscular findings (see FIG. 182–1, above).

Measurements: Body length is measured from crown to heel. Head circumference (largest measurement above the ears) should be about half the body length + 10 cm. FIG. 186–1 (see under GESTATIONAL AGE AND BIRTH WEIGHT in Ch. 186) shows the relationship between birth weight and gestational age classifications. The average weight for term babies is 7 lb (3.2 kg). Measured against gestational age, the newborn's size may provide important clues to several conditions. For example, if the infant is small for gestational age, an intrauterine infection or a chromosomal abnormality may be the cause; an infant may be large for gestational age because of maternal diabetes mellitus or hyperinsulinism, as in Beckwith's syndrome; cyanotic congenital heart

disease due to transposition of the great vessels; maternal obesity; or familial predisposition, as in Crow and Cheyenne Indians in Montana.

Skin: The skin is usually ruddy, and acrocyanosis is common in the first few hours. Dryness and peeling often occur in a few days, especially at foot and ankle creases. Petechiae may be seen over the scalp and face because of pressure exerted during delivery but are not normally present below the umbilicus. Vernix caseosa covers most of the body after 24 wk of gestation.

Head: In a vertex delivery the head will be molded, with overriding of the cranial bones at the sutures and some swelling and/or ecchymosis of the scalp **(caput succedaneum)**. In breech deliveries the head is usually unmolded, with swelling and ecchymosis occurring in the presenting part (ie, buttocks, genitalia, or feet). The fontanels may vary from a fingertip breadth to several centimeters in diameter. A **cephalhematoma** is an accumulation of blood between the periosteum and the bone, producing a swelling that does not cross suture lines. It may present over one or both parietal bones and occasionally over the occiput. Cephalhematomas gradually disappear over several months and should not be aspirated.

Asymmetry of the face may be present because of in utero positioning. Facial nerve palsy should be suspected when there is asymmetry of the nasolabial folds and the creases around the eyes when the baby cries. The **eyes** should open symmetrically. Pupils should be equal and react to light, and the fundi should be visualized. If a red reflex is obtained on ophthalmoscopic examination, opacities may be excluded. Scleral hemorrhages are common. The **ears** are inspected for gestational age determination and positioning; low-set ears often signal a renal or genetic abnormality. The ear canals should be patent and the tympanic membranes visible. Although inexpensive portable devices are available to test the newborn's hearing, their reliability and validity have not been demonstrated except for gross screening purposes. Auditory evoked response testing (see in Ch. 204) may be available for high-risk patients, who should be identified by careful history of family deafness, fetal rubella, neonatal jaundice, or maternal or neonatal treatment with aminoglycosides.

The **mouth** should be inspected for an intact palate and uvula, gum cysts, and a congenitally short frenulum **(tongue-tie)**. Small pearl-like elevations **(Epstein's pearls)** and small ulcerations **(Bednar's aphthae)** on the hard palate are normal. The infant's ability to suck should also be evaluated.

Cardiorespiratory system: Respirations are normally abdominal and range between 40 and 50/min. Breath sounds are harsh but should be heard equally throughout the chest. Heart sounds are audible by stethoscope, most prominently beneath the sternum. The heart rate is 100 to 150/min (average, 120). There may be marked sinus arrhythmia. Heart murmurs are frequently heard, but only about 10% are associated with congenital heart disease (see Ch. 187).

Severe congenital heart diseases, such as aortic atresia or hypoplasia of the right or left ventricle, may present with cyanosis or heart failure in the newborn period. Femoral pulses are palpable and their strength should be checked and compared; if the pulses are weak, aortic coarctation or left ventricular abnormalities may be present. Weak pulses should be confirmed with a flush or doptone BP taken in all extremities. **Flush BP** is a technic in which blood is removed from a limb by elevating it until the skin pales. A previously applied BP cuff is pumped up as in taking regular BP; then, with the limb at the patient's side, pressure is gradually dropped and a reading is taken when color returns to the limb. **Doptone BP** is a technic using a doppler tone to "bounce" off a vessel. A cuff is used with a sensor imbedded in it. Sound is intensified and audible.

Abdomen: The abdominal examination is very important, as 10% of all newborns have anomalies or findings that require careful monitoring during the first few days of

life, including abnormal shape, size, or position of the kidneys or other organs. (See also RENAL AND GENITOURINARY DEFECTS in Ch. 187.) Normally, the liver is felt 1 to 2 cm below the costal margin and the spleen tip is easily palpated. Both kidneys are ordinarily palpable, the left more easily than the right; if they cannot be palpated, agenesis or hypoplasia may be suspected. Large kidneys may be caused by obstruction, tumor, or cystic disease. Failure of the male infant to void may indicate posterior urethral valves. An umbilical hernia, due to a weakness of the umbilical ring musculature, is common, but rarely causes symptoms or needs therapy.

Genitalia: In the full-term male, the testes should be present in the scrotum. Hydroceles and inguinal hernias are encountered in the newborn. A firm, discolored scrotal mass may represent **testicular torsion,** particularly in breech deliveries. Although rare, and apparently not painful in the neonate, *torsion represents a surgical emergency*. Torsion can be distinguished from simple bruising by the distribution of the ecchymoses and the firmness of the testes if torsion is present. The mass will transilluminate if it is a hydrocele. In females, the labia are prominent. Mucoid and occasionally serosanguineous secretions (pseudomenses) may occur and are transient and nonirritating. A small tag of tissue at the posterior fourchette, believed to be due to maternal hormonal stimulation, will disappear over the first few weeks.

Neuromuscular system: The extremities should be symmetrically placed and actively mobile. Completely abducting the thighs to the surface of the examining table while the infant is supine with the hips and knees flexed should be possible; limited abduction and a palpable "clunk" as the femoral head slides into the hip socket are the cardinal signs of **congenital hip dislocation**. (See also MUSCULOSKELETAL DEFECTS in Ch. 187.) Female infants and those delivered in the breech position are particularly prone to have a dislocated hip. If hip mobility is in question, an x-ray should be obtained and an orthopedic specialist consulted. With minimal congenital dysplasia of the hip joint, using double or triple diapers may be adequate treatment. In more severe cases, an orthopedist should apply an abduction splint, but only after an x-ray is reviewed. If a specialist is not available immediately, triple diapers should be used 24 h/day until a splint can be applied. If **clubfoot** or any other significant orthopedic abnormality is present, therapy should begin immediately. (See MUSCULOSKELETAL DEFECTS in Ch. 187.)

The **neurologic examination** should include elicitation of the Moro, suck, and rooting reflexes. The deep tendon reflexes should be present and equal. (Neurologic congenital abnormalities are discussed in Ch. 187.)

THE FIRST FEW DAYS

Weight: Loss of 5 to 10% of birth weight in the first few days of life is considered normal and is common for most newborns. Passage of meconium, loss of vernix caseosa, and drying of the umbilical cord account for some weight loss, but most is due to urinary and insensible water losses. **Umbilical cord**: The plastic cord clamp should be removed in 24 h to avoid undue tension on the drying stump. Daily application of 70% alcohol to the stump hastens drying and reduces infection. The cord should be observed daily for redness or drainage, since it is an excellent portal of entry for infection. It is the first area to colonize with bacteria and usually is the site cultured in infection control programs (see also INITIAL CARE, above). **Circumcision,** if indicated, generally is performed within the first few days of life but should be delayed indefinitely if there is any displacement of the urethral meatus, hypospadias, or any other abnormality of the glans or penis, since the prepuce may be used later in plastic repair. Circumcision usually is requested by the parents and is rarely indicated medically. It should not be done if a family history of hemophilia or other bleeding disorders exists,

or if the mother is taking medication associated with coagulation disturbances, such as anticoagulants or aspirin.

Voiding: The first urine voided is concentrated and often contains urates, which turn the diaper pink. Failure to void within the first 24 h of life must be investigated thoroughly. Delayed voiding is more common in males and may be associated with a tight foreskin, or edema and swelling of the penis in the recently circumcised infant. **Defecating** (stooling): **Meconium** *is a sticky green-black substance that consists of lanugo and squamous epithelial cells from swallowed amniotic fluid and intestinal secretions.* **Every infant should pass meconium by age 24 h.** The infant who is meconium-stained at birth may delay defecating, but in this case it is evident that the anus is patent. Delayed defecation is most commonly the result of a plug of inspissated meconium (see GASTROINTESTINAL DEFECTS in Ch. 187).

Skin: Erythema toxicum, a benign self-limited rash, is the most common lesion and may occur at any time during the first week but most often on the second day. Usually found where clothing rubs the arms, legs, and back, and rarely on the face, the rash appears as a blotchy erythematous wheal with a central papule that may become quite prominent. A Wright-stained smear of the papule contents reveals eosinophils. A family history of allergy should be sought in severe cases; if found, use of lotions, powders, perfumed soaps, and plastic pants should be avoided. **Subcutaneous fat necrosis** may occur over any bony prominence subjected to trauma or pressure, especially the head, cheek, and neck where forceps are applied. Lesions are indurated, isolated, and well demarcated. A lesion may rupture through to the skin surface, releasing a clear yellow, sterile fluid that should disappear spontaneously or with use of a "pressure doughnut" dressing.

Jaundice may occur in normal newborns but is not **physiologic** if it appears before 24 h of age, and may not be physiologic if the serum bilirubin is > 10 mg/dL. (See under HYPERBILIRUBINEMIA in METABOLIC PROBLEMS in Ch. 186.)

Screening tests for metabolic and hematologic disorders should be undertaken. (See SCREENING PROCEDURES FOR INFANTS AND CHILDREN, below.)

FEEDING

(See also INFANT NUTRITION, below)

The normal newborn has active rooting and sucking reflexes and can receive oral feedings immediately. Ordinarily, these should not be delayed > 4 h.

Spitting and regurgitating mucus are common during the first day, but if they persist the stomach should be emptied by gentle aspiration through a feeding tube and washed out with 5% D/W until the returns are clear of mucus. If vomiting continues in a bottle-fed newborn, a hypoallergenic milk formula should be tried, and, if unsuccessful, a more comprehensive diagnostic assessment should be done. A breastfed newborn who continues to vomit should have a full diagnostic workup for obstruction, since babies are not allergic to human milk.

Bottle Feeding

The first offering tests whether or not the newborn can coordinate suck, swallow, and gag reflexes. Sterile distilled water is given, since even 5% D/W may irritate the newborn lung if aspirated. If this is not regurgitated, the next feeding can be a milk formula. Full-term newborns are usually fed on a 4-h schedule for the sake of hospital efficiency.

Prepackaged formulas are available in sterile 4-oz bottles providing 13 or 20 kcal/oz with adequate vitamins for the normal newborn. Full-term neonates can tolerate 20 kcal/oz immediately. The mother should be told not to overfeed the newborn simply

because 4 oz of formula are available. Feedings should be increased gradually during the first week of life from 1 or 2 oz to 3 or 4 oz given 6 times/day. This supplies 120 kcal/kg (55 kcal/lb).

The newborn should be offered water between feedings, particularly in hot weather or in a hot, dry environment. Newborns should retain at least 65 mL of fluid/kg the first 24 h, 75 mL/kg the second 24 h, and up to 100 mL/kg the third 24 h. Those who fall appreciably behind these amounts are given 5% glucose in 0.25% sodium chloride by IV drip to make up the deficit. A cause for the poor feeding pattern should be sought.

Breastfeeding

Over 50% of mothers breastfeed their infants today and the number is increasing, primarily in higher socioeconomic groups. Given adequate support and encouragement, most women can nurse their infants successfully. Physicians should discuss infant feeding with the mother, prenatally presenting the benefits of breastfeeding (nutritional, infection protection, immunologic, and psychologic—see also INFANT NUTRITION, below; and IMMUNOLOGIC STATUS OF THE FETUS AND NEWBORN, above) and other points to be aware of (see DRUGS IN LACTATING MOTHERS, below), so each mother can make an informed choice. The chief contraindication is the mother's lack of desire and interest.

When breastfeeding is planned, the technic should be familiar before delivery. Physicians who counsel nursing mothers should be conversant with the better literature on this subject before they recommend any reading to their patients. The physician should discuss the physiology of lactation with the mother and answer her questions. It is often helpful if the mother talks to a woman who has nursed successfully, even observes the process. Preparation of the nipple before delivery is not necessary, nor is manual expression of the breast, which at this time may lead to mastitis or early labor. Nature prepares the areola and nipple for the suckling by secreting a lubricant from the Montgomery glands to protect the surface. This lubricant should *not* be buffed away with a towel or elaborate nipple exercises.

At delivery, if the mother has had little medication and a normal delivery and the newborn is alert and active, he may be put to breast immediately for a few minutes on each side. He will receive a small amount of colostrum, a high-caloric, high-protein, thin yellow fluid present in the breast before birth and for the first few days thereafter, which contains antibodies, lymphocytes, and macrophages as well as nutrients. Colostrum also stimulates the passage of meconium.

Whether or not the newborn is nursed in the delivery room, he can be taken to the mother for nursing by 4 h of age. The mother should assume a comfortable, relaxed position, such as lying almost flat and turning from one side to the other to offer each breast. The newborn should be placed so he faces the mother, ventral surface to ventral surface. The mother should hold her breast with thumb on top and fingers below to support breast. This will assure that the breast is centered in the mouth, minimizing any soreness. The corner of the newborn's mouth should be stimulated with the nipple so that he will root and grasp the breast. Suction should be broken before removing the newborn from the breast. Feedings are started on alternate sides, initially at least 2 min at each breast. Although there should not be stop-watch timing, excessive suckling initially should be avoided, as sore nipples are easier to prevent than cure. On the other hand, milk production is dependent on adequate suckling time. Nursing times are gradually increased until the "milk is in." Ten minutes at the first breast and a time sufficient to satisfy the newborn at the second is usually appropriate. In primiparas, lactation is established in 72 to 96 h; less time is required in multiparas. If the mother is especially fatigued, the 2 AM feeding may be replaced with water until full milk secretion begins. Feeding should be on demand rather than by the clock, and feeding duration should also reflect infant needs.

Breast engorgement, which occurs during early lactation, may be prevented by early frequent feeding of the newborn. Engorgement can be alleviated if the mother wears a comfortable nursing brassiere 24 h/day for support. Manually expressing milk during a warm shower may provide considerable comfort. The mother may have to express her milk manually just before nursing to allow the newborn to get the swollen areola into his mouth, but excessive expression between feedings encourages continued engorgement and should be done only to relieve discomfort. Should sore nipples occur, positioning of the baby should be checked as above. Sometimes the newborn will draw in his lower lip and suck the lip, which is irritating to the nipple. The mother can ease the lip out with her thumb. Between feedings, she can use a hairdryer set on low to warm and dry her nipples for 15 min, letting the milk dry on the nipples. Plastic brassiere liners should be avoided.

Special dietary increases during lactation include 600 extra kcal, of which 20 gm are protein. The major nutrient a mother must add is 400 mg extra calcium (dairy products are an excellent source). If milk products are not tolerated, nuts and green vegetables should be increased, or calcium gluconate supplements by capsule may be used.

All newborns, but breastfeeding ones in particular, should be seen by the physician at 10 days to 2 wk of age to evaluate progress and answer any questions the mother may have before they become problems. This is especially urgent if the mother is a primipara. A normal newborn wets 6 to 8 diapers a day or more, stools daily, and has a vigorous cry, good skin turgor, and a good suck reflex. Weight gain is also a good test of adequate feeding. Although sleeping long periods of time between feedings may be a sign of a good milk supply, it can be associated with inadequate supply and starvation; thus all newborns should be checked early.

DRUGS IN LACTATING MOTHERS

Drugs pass into the breast milk of lactating mothers differentially, depending on the drug's lipid solubility, pK_a, and protein-binding capacity, and on the pH of the milk. The concentration gradient is the primary determinant of drug transfer between plasma and milk.

The pH of milk is slightly lower than plasma pH; hence weak bases tend to have a higher milk-to-plasma ratio than weak acids. Lincomycin, erythromycin, antihistamines, alkaloids, isoniazid, antipsychotics, antidepressants, lithium, quinine, thiouracil, and metronidazole—all weak bases—have concentrations in milk equal to or higher than in plasma. Barbiturates, phenytoins, sulfonamides, diuretics, and penicillins—weak acids—have concentrations in milk equal to or lower than in plasma.

Almost all drugs pass to some extent into breast milk, but the clinical significance of this depends on (1) the degree of drug passage into milk; (2) the amount of milk ingested by the infant at the feeding; (3) whether the amount ingested at each feeding is the same; (4) the frequency of feeding; (5) whether the drug is absorbed by the infant; and (6) whether the infant is affected by the drug.

There are problems in determining what drugs are contraindicated in lactating mothers because of very limited human studies. Data often are taken from case reports, human studies with very small numbers of subjects, or anecdotal reports of adverse effects in nursing infants associated with drug medication of the mother. Animal data are inappropriately projected to humans on a theoretical basis. The concentrations of drugs in milk are generally expressed relative to the mother's plasma concentration. A milk/plasma ratio of 1 or greater creates a false alarm for potential adverse effects in the nursing infants, not considering that milk concentration does not equate with plasma concentration in relation to target sites of action. A clear example is isoniazid. Given at therapeutic dose, the plasma concentration achieved is 6 μg/mL. Assuming that the milk/plasma ratio is 1, an infant consuming 8 oz of milk will ingest only 1.4 mg/feeding. The therapeutic dose of isoniazid for children is 10 to 20 mg/kg.

Considering absorption, distribution, metabolism, and excretion processes of the drug, one would expect an insignificant plasma concentration in the infant. Unless a drug is highly potent and toxic even in very low concentrations or has cumulative effects in infants because of the infant's immature drug metabolism and excretion, drug excretion in milk would not be a hazard to infants. As more studies are reported on drugs and lactation, fewer drugs are considered **absolute contraindications** to nursing infants. These are the anticancer drugs, radiopharmaceuticals, ergot and its derivatives (methysergide, etc), lithium, chloramphenicol, phenylbutazone, atropine, thiouracil, iodides, and mercurials.

Over-the-counter medications are increasingly important to consider because of their availability to consumers and the increasing trend in self-diagnosis and -treatment of self-limiting minor illnesses. The nonprescription drugs include (1) analgesics—aspirin and acetaminophen; (2) antihistamines in the cold, sinus, and cough remedies and antivertigo and sleeping aids; (3) sympathomimetics like ephedrine, pseudoephedrine, phenylephrine, and phenylpropanolamine, which are selectively utilized for anticongestant, anorexiant, and antiasthmatic medications; (4) antacids, laxatives, and cathartics; (5) topical medications (skin, rectal, and vaginal), which include corticosteroids, local anesthetics, astringents like zinc and bismuth, and antihistamines. In general, all the above medications *are safe* for nursing mothers, when taken for short-term and in doses prescribed on the labels. Over-the-counter drugs are formulated using the least toxic class of drugs at the lowest effective therapeutic doses.

Some controversies exist over the significance in breast milk of propylthiouracil, methimazole, warfarin, dicumarol, morphine, codeine, methadone, neuroleptics and antidepressants, sedatives and tranquilizers, isoniazid, contraceptives, alcohol, nicotine, and metronidazole. Although some studies have shown that these drugs have been given to nursing mothers without ill effects in their nursing infants, experts advise that these drugs should only be used when critically indicated. When they are prescribed, close observation of the infant is required because of potential toxicity with prolonged medication in specific conditions.

Analgesics: **Salicylates** are excreted into the breast milk in moderate amounts. With larger doses and chronic medication, nursing neonates may achieve plasma concentrations that can cause hyperbilirubinemia, hemorrhagic problems, and hemolysis in G6PD-deficient babies. **Acetaminophen** appears safe when taken in therapeutic doses. **Narcotic analgesics** (eg, codeine, morphine, meperidine, or methadone) in therapeutic doses are excreted in the milk at very low concentrations that minimally affect the nursing infants. However, in narcotic addicts using high doses of drugs, significant amounts are excreted in milk, affecting the nursing infant and causing withdrawal symptoms when feeding is missed (see above in this chapter; Ch. 138; and METABOLIC PROBLEMS IN THE NEWBORN in Ch. 186).

Antibiotics generally can be prescribed to nursing mothers without significant hazards to their infants. However, because almost all antibiotics are excreted in milk, infants may develop hypersensitivity, diarrhea, and candidiasis. Levels of **penicillin** are detectable in breast milk as early as 1 h and as long as 9 h after IM injection. **Tetracycline** is significantly excreted in milk, but because it is precipitated by calcium in the milk, absorption by nursing infants could be insignificant to cause adverse effects. However, the tetracyclines (eg, minocycline, which is 100% absorbed orally and not affected by food) should be avoided by nursing mothers. **Metronidazole**, a useful antiprotozoal and antibacterial for giardiasis, trichomoniasis, and hemophilus vaginitis, and a radiosensitizer in the treatment of various tumors, is significantly excreted in breast milk. The agent is carcinogenic in rodents and metagenic in bacteria. When metronidazole is inevitably indicated, breastfeeding should be suspended during the course of treatment and resumed 9 days after treatment. **Nalidixic acid, sulfonamides, and other oxidant drugs** can cause hemolysis in G6PD-deficient infants. The orally

nonabsorbable antibiotics like **streptomycin, kanamycin,** and **gentamicin** pose no systemic problems in infants, but their continuous ingestion may alter the infant's intestinal flora and consequently affect some immune mechanisms.

Antihypertensives, diuretic drugs, digoxin, and β-blockers can be continuously prescribed without significant adverse effects in nursing infants. **Hormones** that are orally absorbed, when given to nursing mothers in large doses, can attain high concentrations in milk. **Oral contraceptive pills** often are prescribed postpartum to prevent pregnancy. The hormones ethinyl estradiol and mestranol are excreted into breast milk; they can reduce milk production and also reduce pyridoxine (vitamin B_6) in the milk. Nursing infants can develop CNS symptoms (eg, irritability, shrill cries, seizures, or rigid opisthotonus). Breast enlargement may be observed in male infants. **Corticosteroids,** when given to the mother in large doses, can attain high concentrations in milk and pose the danger of suppressing growth and interfering with endogenous corticosteroid production in the infant. **Barbiturates** and **phenytoin** can induce microsomal oxidizing enzymes in infants, enhancing the degradation of endogenous steroids. **Diazepam** is excreted in breast milk and causes lethargy, drowsiness, and loss of weight in breastfed infants. Evidence indicates the metabolism of diazepam by nursing infants of mothers on moderate diazepam medication (30 mg/day or more). Since diazepam is metabolized by glucuronide conjugation, competition with bilirubin by diazepam for glucuronic acid may predispose neonates to kernicterus. The **antipsychotics** and **tricyclic antidepressants** pass into the milk but are not likely to produce any significant adverse reactions, since low plasma concentration is achieved in the infant because of poor absorption from the GI tract. **Warfarin and dicumarol** can be given cautiously to nursing mothers. **Heparin** does not pass to the milk.

Tetrahydrocannabinol (9-THC), the most psychoactive component of marijuana, is highly bound to lipoproteins after oral absorption, and the excretion to breast milk is very low in animals. Since the half-life of 9-THC in plasma in man may be as long as 2 days, it is wise for nursing mothers to avoid marijuana.

Drugs taken by nursing mothers that are not generally considered hazardous to the infant include insulin, epinephrine, alcohol, nicotine, and caffeine. However, *large doses of alcohol, caffeine, and theophylline can adversely affect the infant.* Nursing infants of mothers who are ingesting or taking large doses of caffeine and theophylline develop hyperirritability.

Drugs to be avoided in the absence of studies on their excretion in breast milk are those with long half-lives; those that are potent toxins to the bone marrow; those given in high doses chronically; insecticides, pollutants, and other toxins; and vaccines.

The following drugs can **suppress or inhibit lactation** in nursing mothers: bromocriptine, bendroflumethiazide, estradiol, oral contraceptives, levodopa, and the antidepressant, trazodone.

HOSPITAL ACCOMMODATIONS

Rooming-in is an arrangement that permits the infant to remain with the mother in her hospital room all or part of each day. Properly done, it facilitates establishing the critically important mother-child relationship. The primipara can learn about her baby with professional help available, while the experienced mother is reassured that her baby is being managed her way. The plan provides a flexible feeding and sleeping routine and may reduce the risk of cross-infection. This service is more an attitude than a physical facility and can be offered in any hospital with sympathetic medical and nursing personnel. Alternatively, **nursery care** generally allows the mother more rest and permits more direct continual supervision of the infant by nursery personnel when these considerations are paramount.

Early discharge from the hospital (under 48 h) should be accompanied by a plan to closely supervise home management with home or office visits.

HEALTH SUPERVISION OF THE WELL CHILD

Periodic health supervision visits intended to promote the optimal health of infants and children.

The objectives are (1) prevention of disease through routine immunizations (see IMMUNIZATION PROCEDURES THROUGHOUT CHILDHOOD, below) and through educational means (parental instruction on nutrition, accident prevention (see Ch. 189), sanitation, etc); (2) early detection of disease through interview, physical examination, and screening procedures (discussed separately below); (3) early treatment of disease; and (4) provision of guidance in child rearing to afford optimal conditions for normal emotional and intellectual development. To meet these objectives, child and parent are seen at regular intervals throughout the early years of life. The frequency and content of these visits are determined by the child's age, the population served, and the physician's opinion of their value.

Inquiries as to the child's intellectual and psychosocial development are essential in preventive health care. Personal adaptive development (social, language, gross motor, fine motor) can be estimated by using the Denver Developmental Screening Test (DDST). Routine testing should be started at age 4 to 6 mo, and can be repeated into early childhood.

Assessing the parents' perception of their child and the interactions between parents and child cannot be accomplished easily by any convenient, standardized method, but require skillful interviewing and observation, beginning with discussions at the first contact in the hospital. Some parents and physicians prefer to meet prior to the baby's delivery, usually during the early 3rd trimester, to discuss parental expectations for their newborn and plans for care during infancy and childhood. Subsequently, parental attitudes may be identified tactfully by determining how the parents feel they are being affected by caring for a new infant, how they handle difficult situations, and how easily they can obtain help when feeling tired or short-tempered. In helping to establish good parent–child interactions, the physician is performing an ongoing, integral responsibility that requires individualized attention.

The American Academy of Pediatrics has recommended preventive health care schedules (see FIG. 182–2) for children who have not manifested any important health problems and who are growing and developing satisfactorily. More frequent and sophisticated visits usually are required for children who do not meet these criteria. If a child comes under care for the first time at a late point on the schedule, or if any items are not accomplished at the suggested age, the schedule should be brought up to date as soon as possible.

SCREENING PROCEDURES FOR INFANTS AND CHILDREN

Screening procedures are a means of implementing the concept of preventive health care in infants and children, often before frank symptoms of disease exist. To be useful, screening must show that early detection of a disorder can improve an infant's health through therapeutic intervention or that genetic counseling may be provided to aid the family. The number of cases detected by screening tests varies greatly with each disorder but, in general, is low, and false positives may be anticipated. Some patients need retesting, reevaluation, or referral to an appropriate specialist before a clear, definitive diagnosis can be reached.

Testing in the Newborn Period

Screening of the neonate is important for identifying a number of physical anomalies and diseases, such as hip dislocation, renal masses, or cataracts. A complete phys-

ical examination should be performed (see MANAGEMENT OF THE NORMAL NEWBORN in Ch. 182), and each parent's family history and the mother's pregnancy history should be reviewed. Screening for metabolic and hematologic disorders also should be undertaken, especially for the following conditions.

Metabolic diseases (Recognition markers for certain diseases are discussed in PREVENTION OF GENETIC DISORDERS in Ch. 203): At the time of hospital discharge, the newborn should have capillary blood specimens taken to screen for a number of diseases (phenylketonuria **[PKU]**, hypothyroidism, tyrosinosis, homocystinuria, maple syrup urine disease, galactosemia). Many metabolic disorders (eg, PKU) are proving to be amenable to dietary management. **Galactosemia** (see GENETIC ABNORMALITIES OF CARBOHYDRATE METABOLISM in Ch. 196) may be reliably diagnosed and treated before affected infants must risk the consequences of high blood galactose levels (liver disease, cataracts, brain damage due to hypoglycemia, or death). **Hypothyroidism** diagnosed and treated before age 3 mo has a greatly improved prognosis. (Hypothyroidism in children is discussed in Ch. 196.)

Sickle cell screening: Newborn testing must be done by hemoglobin electrophoresis because Hb S levels are low. Because of cost and technical limitations, newborn testing is not done routinely in all USA states. However, the physician may want to do this test on an individual basis. When a neonatal test is positive, both parents should be tested for a sickle cell trait to investigate the potential of this disease in a subsequent pregnancy. (Prenatal testing for sickle cell disease is discussed under PREVENTION OF GENETIC DISORDERS in Ch. 203.)

Anemia: Blood loss during birth or in the neonatal observation period (when extensive studies may require multiple blood samples) may cause anemia. Determining the Hct or Hb level at the time of discharge provides a baseline value for tests taken later in infancy.

Babies of mothers whose blood type is O and/or Rh-negative should be typed and a Coombs' test performed. Those with a positive indirect Coombs' test should be watched for jaundice. Many recommend a total bilirubin determination on discharge as a routine procedure.

G6PD deficiency: About 10% of black American males suffer from a mild form of this disorder, and only occasionally have symptoms in early infancy; Orientals and some groups of Mediterranean origin develop a more severe form, with a hemolytic anemia and hyperbilirubinemia. Sensitivity of RBCs to various drugs occurs later. These selected groups should be screened during the neonatal period.

Procedures After the Newborn Period

Growth and development: Length (crown-heel), weight, and head circumference should be measured at each visit or health examination during the first year of life. Continued systematic plotting of the infant's measurements on a growth curve with percentiles facilitates growth-rate monitoring. The infant's developmental level and performance should be assessed at each visit. (See also FIG. 182-2 and the discussion below in GROWTH AND DEVELOPMENT FROM BIRTH THROUGH CHILDHOOD.)

Hips, legs, and feet: When unstable or dislocated hips are (occasionally) undetected in the newborn, later signs provide clues: unequal leg length or adductor tightness. Internal tibial torsion is common and may need orthopedic evaluation. Forefoot adduction usually is not apparent at birth and should be sought at each infant's examination. It is easily corrected at a young age. (See also COMMON FOOT AND LEG PROBLEMS IN CHILDREN AND ADOLESCENTS in Ch. 197.)

Cardiac auscultation should be performed to identify the presence of murmurs, and femoral pulses should be palpated at each health examination.

Abdominal palpation also should be repeated at every visit, since many masses, particularly Wilms' tumor and neuroblastoma, may be apparent only as the infant grows.

	Infancy						Early Childhood					Late Childhood					Adolescence			
Age[1]	By 1 mo	2 mo	4 mo	6 mo	9 mo	12 mo	15 mo	18 mo	24 mo	3 yr	4 yr	5 yr	6 yr	8 yr	10 yr	12 yr	14 yr	16 yr	18 yr	20+ yr
History																				
Initial/Interval	●	●	●	●	●	●	●	●	●	●	●	●	●	●	●	●	●	●	●	●
Measurements																				
Height and Weight	●	●	●	●	●	●	●	●	●	●	●	●	●	●	●	●	●	●	●	●
Head Circumference	●	●	●	●	●	●														
Blood Pressure										●	●	●	●	●	●	●	●	●	●	●
Sensory Screening																				
Vision	S	S	S	S	S	S	S	S	S	O	O	O	O	O	S	O	O	S	O	O
Hearing	S	S	S	S	S	S	S	S	S	S	O	O	S[2]	S[2]	S[2]	O	S	S	O	S
Development/Behavioral Assessment[3]	●	●	●	●	●	●	●	●	●	●	●	●	●	●	●	●	●	●	●	●
Physical Examination[4]	●	●	●	●	●	●	●	●	●	●	●	●	●	●	●	●	●	●	●	●
Procedures[5]																				
Hereditary/Metabolic Screening[6]	●																			
Immunization[7]		●	●	●			●	●				●					●			
Tuberculin Test						●	←	←	●[8]	→	→	←	←	●[8]	→	→	←	←	●[8]	→
Hematocrit or Hemoglobin[9]	←	←	←	←	●	→	←	←	●	→	→	←	←	●	→	→	←	←	●	→
Urinalysis[10]	←	←	←	●	→	→	←	←	●	→	→	←	←	●	→	→	←	←	●	→
Anticipatory Guidance[11]	●	●	●	●	●	●	●	●	●	●	●	●	●	●	●	●	●	●	●	●
Initial Dental Referral[12]										●										

● = to be performed; **S**= subjective, by history; **O**= objective, by a standard testing method.

Fig. 182–2. Guidelines for child health supervision. Recommendations approved by the Executive Board of the American Academy of Pediatrics in March 1982. (Modified from "Guidelines for Health Supervision," *News and Comment,* American Academy of Pediatrics, May 1982. Used with permission.)

1. If a child comes under care for the first time at any point on the schedule, or if any items are not accomplished at the suggested age, the schedule should be brought up to date at the earliest possible time.
2. At these points, history may suffice; if problem suggested, a standard testing method should be used.
3. By history and appropriate physical examination; if suspicious, by specific objective developmental testing.
4. At each visit, a complete physical examination is essential, with infant totally unclothed, older child undressed and suitably draped.
5. These may be modified, depending on entry point into schedule and individual need.
6. PKU and thyroid testing should be done at about 2 wk. Infants initially screened before 24 h of age should be rescreened.
7. Schedule(s) per Report of Committee on Infectious Disease, ed. 18, 1982.
8. The Committee on Infectious Diseases recommends tuberculin testing at 12 mo of age and every 1 to 2 yr thereafter. In some areas, tuberculosis is of exceedingly low occurrence and the physician may elect not to retest routinely or to use longer intervals.
9. Present medical evidence suggests the need for reevaluation of the frequency and timing of hemoglobin or hematocrit tests. One determination is therefore suggested during each time period. Performance of additional tests is left to the individual practice experience.
10. Present medical evidence suggests the need for reevaluation of the frequency and timing of urinalyses. One determination is therefore suggested during each time period. Performance of additional tests is left to the individual practice experience.
11. Appropriate discussion and counseling sould be an integral part of each visit for care.
12. Subsequent examinations as prescribed by dentist.

Note: Special chemical, immunologic, and endocrine testing are usually carried out upon specific indications. Testing other than newborn (eg, inborn errors of metabolism, sickle disease, lead) are discretionary with the physician.

Hearing (see also CLINICAL MEASUREMENT OF HEARING IN CHILDREN, below): About 1:1000 neonates has a significant hearing loss. Detecting this problem in infancy depends on understanding high-risk conditions as well as behaviors and responses that suggest a hearing loss. **High-risk factors** include birth weight < 1500 gm; Apgar score ≥ 5 at 5 min; serum bilirubin > 22 mg/dL in an infant whose birth weight is > 2000 gm, 17 mg/dL in a baby < 2000 gm; anoxia; neonatal sepsis or meningitis; neonatal hyperbilirubinemia; seizures or apneic spells; congenital intrauterine infection, such as rubella, cytomegalovirus, toxoplasmosis; drugs such as streptomycin; or a history of early hearing loss in a parent or close relative.

In about 1/3 of infants deaf from birth, a hereditary recessive etiology that is not present in either parent is assumed. These children must be identified by **observations that the parents can learn to make**. By age 3 mo an infant can be expected to startle to a nearby loud sound, stir or awaken from sleep when someone talks or makes a noise, and be soothed by the mother's voice. By age 6 mo an infant should look toward an interesting sound, turn when his name is called, make sounds such as "moo," "ma,", "da," and "di" to toys or objects, and coo when listening to music. By age 10 mo the infant should make sounds on his own, imitate some sounds made by others, and understand "no" and "bye-bye." By age 18 mo the appropriate use of a few single words, the understanding of many single words or commands, and babbling in sentence-like patterns is expected. Infants who do not pass these minimal performance standards should be referred for hearing testing.

Ear infections, serous fluid middle ear accumulations, or frequent respiratory infections may cause enough hearing loss in infants and children to seriously affect development of language skills. Prompt audiologic referral may be indicated.

Vision: While sight cannot at present be easily or very satisfactorily tested < 3 yr of age, attention to the infant's and young child's eyes should start early in life. **The premature infant** < 32 wk gestation must be repeatedly examined for evidence of **retinopathy of prematurity** (see under PREMATURE INFANT, below). This is best done by an ophthalmologist. Such infants also commonly develop refractive errors as they grow.

In the first 2 to 4 wk of life, an eye examination by the primary physician should note abnormalities of the globe (globe size in particular, since congenital glaucoma causes enlargement of the globe), color of the iris, pupillary size and asymmetry, character of the red reflex, and whether choroidal vessels can be visualized by direct ophthalmoscopy. A cataract may be seen, or merely suspected, when the red reflex is missing or distorted. Untreated cataracts may cause amblyopia (visual loss) if not detected early. **By age 6 wk,** the infant should begin to fix the parent with his eyes. Strabismus that persists after age 6 mo may cause loss of visual acuity, and an ophthalmologist should be consulted. Other conditions that obscure vision are ptosis and eyelid hemangioma.

In the growing child, alignment of the eyes should be examined repeatedly. Esotropia (inward deviation) accounts for much of childhood amblyopia. A cover test is of value in such testing. **By 3 or 4 yr of age,** vision testing by Snellen charts or newer testing machines can be done routinely. The E charts are better than pictures. Vision at < 20/30 performance should be checked by an ophthalmologist.

Further laboratory studies: (1) Newborn screening tests for phenylketonuria (PKU) are discussed in ANOMALIES IN AMINO ACID METABOLISM in Ch. 196. (2) Hct or Hb should be determined at age 8 to 9 mo on full-term infants and at age 5 to 6 mo on premature infants. (3) Sickledex® test for Hb S can be done at age 6 to 9 mo (diagnosis of sickle cell disease is discussed in Ch. 96). (4) Periodic blood testing for lead exposure should begin at age 1 yr in all children living in substandard or old housing, even if there is no history of paint chip consumption (see also Ch. 189).

After the age of 3, children should be routinely checked as follows. **Blood pressure** measured with a small 3-in. cuff should be done routinely (see FIG. 182–3). Larger

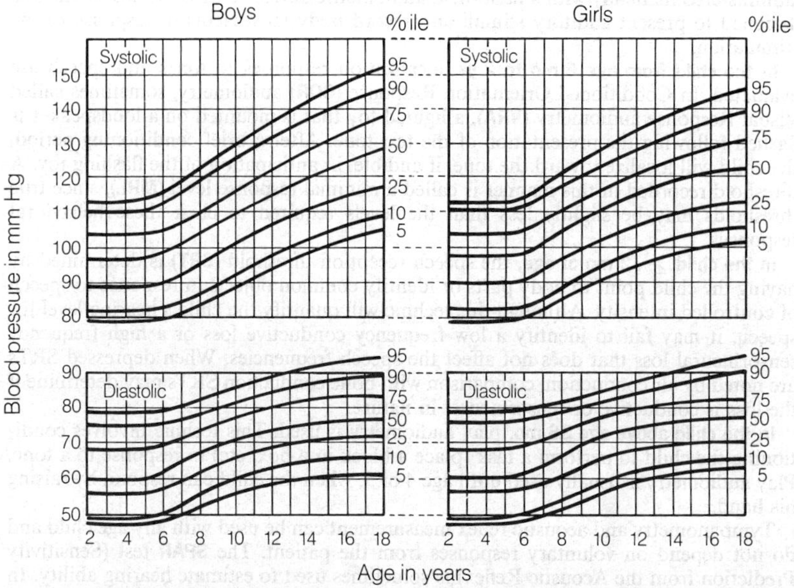

FIG. 182–3. Blood pressure measurements and percentiles for boys (left) and girls (right) measured in the right arm with the child seated. Since most children's pressures vary considerably, a single high value (eg, > 95th percentile) should not be considered an abnormal finding. Measurements should be repeated over time to indicate a trend. (From Task Force on Blood Pressure Control in Children in *Pediatrics* Vol. 59, No. 5 [Supplement], p. 803, May 1977. Copyright 1977 by *Pediatrics*. Used with permission of *Pediatrics*.)

cuffs can be used on older children, depending on arm sizes. **Scoliosis** can quickly be checked along with evaluation of posture. Shoulder tip and scapular symmetry, torso list, and spine position and rotation on forward bending are useful tests. **Urinalysis** should be done by dipstick testing on all regular visits. Repeated testing for **lead exposure** by erythrocyte protoporphyrin (EPP), zinc protoporphyrin (ZPP), as well as blood lead, should be done in all children whose lead studies are elevated.

CLINICAL MEASUREMENT OF HEARING IN CHILDREN

(See also CLINICAL MEASUREMENT OF HEARING in Ch. 204)

Early identification and correction of hearing loss is essential for normal development of communication skills. If history-taking identifies risk factors, infant audiometry should be done by age 3 mo. Profound hearing loss may be suspected by parents if their infant does not seem to respond to a spoken voice or ordinary household sounds. Parents' observations are very important, and questions they raise about a child's hearing should be investigated. Risk factors and simple tests of hearing are discussed in SCREENING PROCEDURES, above.

Special audiometric technics, usually performed by an audiologist, can assess hearing ability starting at birth. These tests use reflexive, behavioral, and physiologic auditory responses to stimuli of controlled intensity.

In the infant from birth to age 6 mo, evaluation involves eliciting reflexive responses **(auropalpebral, Moro, startle)** to relatively intense levels of sound. These tests may be

administered manually with a hand-held audiometric device or with automated devices designed to present auditory stimuli and record body movements in response to the stimulation.

In the child from age 6 mo to 2 yr, localization responses to tones and speech are evaluated. In Conditioned Orientation Response **(COR)** audiometry, sometimes called Visual Response audiometry **(VRA),** a lighted toy that is mounted on a loudspeaker is flashed following the presentation of the test tone. After a brief conditioning period, the child will localize toward the tone, if audible, in anticipation of the flashing toy. A threshold recorded in this manner is called a minimal response level **(MRL),** since true thresholds may be slightly less than the levels required to elicit these behavioral responses.

In the child ≥ 12 mo of age, the speech reception threshold **(SRT)** is determined by having the child point to body parts or identify common objects in response to speech of controlled intensity. Although this technic will quantify the child's hearing level for speech, it may fail to identify a low frequency conductive loss or a high frequency sensorineural loss that does not affect the speech frequencies. When depressed SRTs are noted by air conduction, comparison with bone conduction SRTs may determine if the loss is conductive or sensorineural in nature.

In the child above age 36 mo, play audiometry is used. This technic involves conditioning the child to perform a task (place a block in a box, etc) in response to a tone. Play audiometry is usually used until age 4 or 5, when the child can respond by raising his hand.

Tympanometry and acoustic reflex measurement can be used with any age child and do not depend on voluntary responses from the patient. The **SPAR** test (Sensitivity Prediction from the Acoustic Reflex) is sometimes used to estimate hearing ability. In the normal ear, the difference between acoustic reflex levels for broad band noise and pure tones is about 20 dB, but decreases in sensorineural losses. The determination of this difference can be used to predict hearing level in an uncooperative or unresponsive child. In addition to the SPAR, electrocochleography and brainstem-evoked response audiometry may be used.

GROWTH AND DEVELOPMENT FROM BIRTH THROUGH CHILDHOOD

PHYSICAL DEVELOPMENT

A multifaceted process involving genetic, nutritional, and environmental (physical and psychologic) factors. Disturbances in any of these may alter growth. Optimal growth requires optimal health.

Growth from birth to adolescence occurs in **2 distinct patterns.** The 1st (from birth to about age 2 yr) is one of rapid but decelerating growth. The 2nd (from about 2 yr to the onset of puberty) shows more consistent and steady annual increments. A child's position relative to his peers tends to remain the same. An exception may occur during the 1st yr of life, when a child grows faster or slower than his peers, before establishing his own pattern. This early growth restraint may be due to maternal factors (eg, due to uterine size). Boys and girls have little differences in sizes and growth rates during infancy and childhood.

Height (see also FIGS. 182–4 and 182–5): Linear growth is measured in length (child lying down) < 2 yr of age, and as height (child standing) after that. Typically, the infant increases his length approximately 30% by age 5 mo and > 50% by age 1 yr; subsequently, height doubles by age 5 yr. Height velocity continues to decrease until the onset of puberty. If puberty is delayed, growth in height may virtually cease.

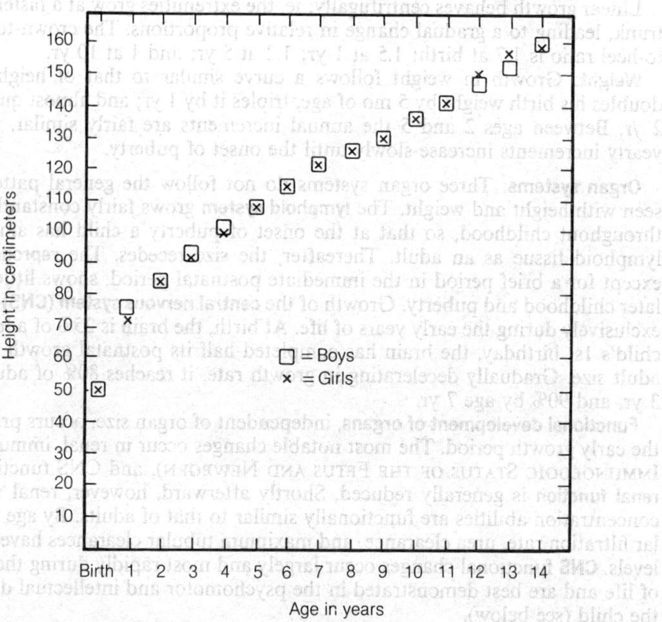

FIG. 182–4. Height and age equivalents in boys and girls.

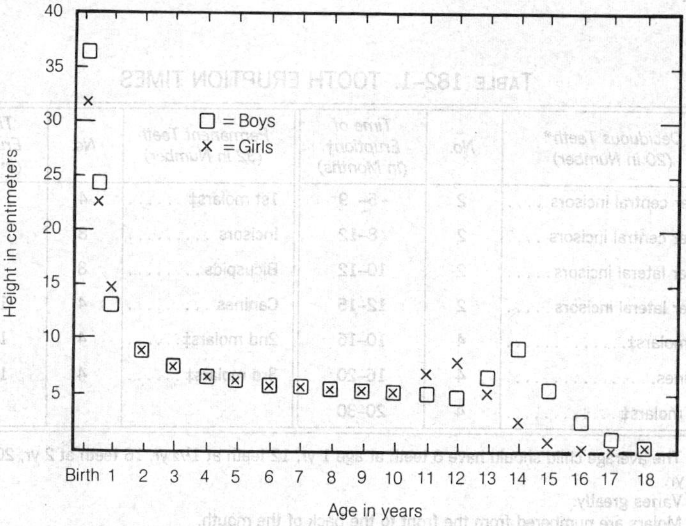

FIG. 182–5. Velocity of linear growth (height) in boys and girls in cm/yr.

Linear growth behaves centrifugally; ie, the extremities grow at a faster rate than the trunk, leading to a gradual change in relative proportions. The crown-to-pubis:pubis-to-heel ratio is 1.7 at birth; 1.5 at 1 yr; 1.2 at 5 yr; and 1 at 10 yr.

Weight: Growth in weight follows a curve similar to that of height. The infant doubles his birth weight by 5 mo of age, triples it by 1 yr; and almost quadruples it by 2 yr. Between ages 2 and 5 the annual increments are fairly similar. Subsequently, yearly increments increase slowly until the onset of puberty.

Organ systems: Three organ systems do not follow the general pattern of growth seen with height and weight. The **lymphoid system** grows fairly constantly and rapidly throughout childhood, so that at the onset of puberty a child has almost twice the lymphoid tissue as an adult. Thereafter, the size recedes. The **reproductive system,** except for a brief period in the immediate postnatal period, shows little growth until later childhood and puberty. Growth of the **central nervous system (CNS)** occurs almost exclusively during the early years of life. At birth, the brain is 25% of adult size. By the child's 1st birthday, the brain has completed half its postnatal growth and is 75% of adult size. Gradually decelerating in growth rate, it reaches 80% of adult size by age 3 yr, and 90% by age 7 yr.

Functional development of organs, independent of organ size, occurs primarily during the early growth period. The most notable changes occur in renal, immune (see above, IMMUNOLOGIC STATUS OF THE FETUS AND NEWBORN), and CNS functions. At birth, **renal function** is generally reduced. Shortly afterward, however, renal acidifying and concentration abilities are functionally similar to that of adults. By age 1 yr, glomerular filtration rate, urea clearance, and maximum tubular clearances have reached adult levels. **CNS** functional changes occur largely and most rapidly during the first 4 to 5 yr of life and are best demonstrated in the psychomotor and intellectual development of the child (see below).

Deciduous teeth: The timing of tooth eruption (see TABLE 182–1) is more variable than other developmental parameters, primarily because of familial factors. Infrequently, tooth eruption may be significantly retarded because of hypothyroidism. Eruption of deciduous teeth is similar in both sexes; permanent teeth tend to appear

TABLE 182–1. TOOTH ERUPTION TIMES

Deciduous Teeth (20 in Number)*	*No.*	*Time of Eruption† (in Months)*	*Permanent Teeth (32 in Number)*	*No.*	*Time of Eruption† (in Years)*
Lower central incisors	2	5–9	1st molars‡	4	5–7
Upper central incisors	2	8–12	Incisors	8	6–8
Upper lateral incisors	2	10–12	Bicuspids	8	9–12
Lower lateral incisors	2	12–15	Canines	4	10–13
1st molars‡	4	10–16	2nd molars‡	4	11–13
Canines	4	16–20	3rd molars‡	4	17–25
2nd molars‡	4	20–30			

* The average child should have 6 teeth at age 1 yr, 12 teeth at 1½ yr, 16 teeth at 2 yr, 20 teeth at 2½ yr.

† Varies greatly.

‡ Molars are numbered from the front to the back of the mouth.

earlier in girls. Deciduous teeth generally are smaller than their permanent counterparts. The presence of supernumerary teeth or their congenital absence is not uncommon.

Body composition: The most notable changes prior to puberty are the amounts of body fat and water. At birth, **body fat** is about 12% of body weight. Its proportion increases rapidly to 25% at 6 mo and then somewhat more slowly to 30% at 1 yr, accounting for the chubby appearance of the 1-yr-old infant. Subsequently there is a slow fall until age 5 to 6 yr, when body fat approximates that at the newborn period. Following this nadir, there is again a slow rise until the onset of puberty. The rise continues in girls at that time, while boys become somewhat thinner.

Body water measured as a percentage of body weight is 75% at birth, dropping to 60% at 1 yr (about equal to the adult percentage). This change is fundamentally due to a decrease in extracellular fluid from 45 to 28% of body weight. Intracellular fluid stays relatively constant. After age 1 yr, there is a slow and somewhat variable fall in the extracellular fluid and rise in the intracellular fluid to adult levels of approximately 16 and 47% respectively. The relatively large amount of body water, its high turnover rate, and the comparatively high surface losses (due to a proportionately large surface area) make the infant more susceptible to fluid deprivation than the older child and adult.

BEHAVIORAL AND INTELLECTUAL DEVELOPMENT

Behavioral and intellectual development is a continuous process that occurs in the same sequence in all children. The rate of development, however, varies from child to child; and even in a specific child, temporary pauses may occur in 1 or more spheres (eg, speech). This development proceeds from the head down (head and hand developmental function precede that of legs and feet), and from the universal or generalized response to the specific (gross motor function develops in advance of fine motor function). The process is primarily dependent on CNS maturation. It may be slowed somewhat with lack of sufficient practice (eg, in a child whose activity is limited by a prolonged illness); but conversely it cannot be significantly accelerated by increased practice or forced attempts at speeding the attainment of an as-yet-underdeveloped function.

The developmental process is affected by innate **intelligence** (in general, the higher the intelligence, the more rapid the development); **familial patterns** (eg, late walking, talking, or bladder control, all commonly seen); **environmental factors** (eg, a lack of appropriate stimulation can impede normal development); and **physical factors** (eg, hypotonia or deafness may alter normal development).

The major developmental events are summarized below.

Birth: The newborn sleeps most of the time. He can eat, clean his airway, and respond with crying to discomforts and intrusions. **Six weeks**: The infant regards objects in the line of vision, begins to smile when spoken to, lies flat on his abdomen, and has head lag when pulled to a sitting position. **Three months**: Smiles spontaneously, vocalizes, and follows a moving object with his eyes. His head is steady on sitting, and objects are grasped when placed in his hand. **Six months**: Sits with support and rolls over, supports himself in a standing position, transfers an object from hand to hand, and babbles to toys. **Nine months**: Sits well, crawls, and pulls himself to a standing position; says "mama" and "dada"; plays pat-a-cake; waves bye-bye; and holds his bottle. **One year**: The child walks with his hand held, speaks several words, and helps to dress himself. **Eighteen months**: Walks well, can climb stairs holding on, turns several book pages at a time, speaks about 10 words, pulls toys on strings, and partially feeds himself. **Two years**: Runs well, climbs up and down stairs alone, turns single book pages, puts on simple clothing, makes 2- or 3-word sentences, and verbal-

izes toilet needs. **Three years**: Rides a tricycle, dresses well except for buttons and laces, counts to 10 and uses plurals, questions constantly, and feeds himself well. **Four years**: Alternates feet going up and down stairs, throws a ball overhand, hops on one foot, copies a cross, knows at least one color, washes his hands and face, and takes care of toilet needs. **Five years**: Skips, catches a bounced ball, copies a triangle, knows 4 colors, and dresses and undresses without assistance.

IMMUNIZATION PROCEDURES THROUGHOUT CHILDHOOD

GENERAL CONSIDERATIONS

1. Basic immunization with killed or inactivated antigens (eg, pertussis vaccine, diphtheria or tetanus toxoid, or a combination of these agents) generally consists of either 2 or 3 **primary** injections (depending on the nature of the product and the age of the patient) and a **booster** dose about 7 to 12 mo later. The booster dose is essential for adequate long-term immunization.

2. Choice of product: Since alum-precipitated or alumina-adsorbed preparations are generally more effective than fluid preparations, they are frequently preferred for basic immunization as well as for subsequent boosters. Little if any evidence supports the belief that fluid preparations will induce a more rapid primary immune response.

3. Scheduling of injections: Schedules of recommended **routine** immunizations (diphtheria, tetanus, pertussis, poliomyelitis, measles, mumps, rubella), including booster inoculations where applicable, are presented in TABLES 182–2 to 182–4. The schedules recommended are reasonably flexible; longer intervals than those given in these tables will not impair the immune response. Therefore, basic immunization should not be repeated just because a scheduled injection was missed or delayed.

In neonates, the efficiency of the immune response improves rapidly in the first few months of life. Moreover, placentally transmitted antibodies, mainly in IgG, may interfere with the immune response of a young infant. For these reasons, routine immunization of infants is now generally scheduled to begin at 15 mo of age for live measles, live mumps, and live rubella virus vaccines; and at about age 2 to 3 mo for most other vaccines.

4. Dose per injection: Doses recommended by the manufacturer for basic immunization should generally be followed, but when the patient's condition or medical history indicates need for caution, individual doses may be reduced provided that the total dosage is given eventually. Booster doses may be reduced whenever indicated (eg, to avoid or minimize a reaction in a known hyperreactive patient), since the desired immunologic response to booster doses is less dependent on the amount of antigen injected.

5. Route of injection: Alum-precipitated or alumina-adsorbed preparations are best given IM, especially in children, to avoid nodules or "antigenic cysts." Fluid preparations should be given subcutaneously except for typhoid booster injections, which may be given (in doses of 0.1 mL or less) intradermally on the upper arm. (CAUTION: *IV injection of any active immunizing agent is* ***contraindicated***)

6. Combined immunization: The long-available combinations (eg, diphtheria-tetanus-pertussis, diphtheria-tetanus, tetanus-diphtheria [adult type]) are accepted widely and are more effective in some respects than the separate components. However, in certain situations (eg, risk of pertussis in a young infant), the physician may prefer to immunize with the antigen most urgently needed, then follow up with the others separately. Combinations of live viral vaccines—measles and mumps; rubella and mumps; and

TABLE 182–2. RECOMMENDED SCHEDULE FOR ACTIVE IMMUNIZATION OF NORMAL INFANTS AND CHILDREN

*Age**	*Vaccine(s)†*	*Comments*
2 mo	DTP-1‡; OPV-1§	Can be given earlier in areas of high endemicity
4 mo	DTP-2; OPV-2	Interval of 6 wk to 2 mo desired between OPV doses to avoid interference
6 mo	DTP-3	An additional dose of OPV at this time is optional for use in areas with a high risk of polio exposure
15 mo**	MMR††	
18 mo**	DTP-4; OPV-3	Completion of primary series
24 mo	Hib	*Hemophilus influenzae* b vaccine
4–6 yr‡‡	DTP-5; OPV-4	Preferably at or before school entry
14–16 yr	Td§§	Repeat every 10 yr throughout life

* These recommended ages should not be construed as absolute; ie, 2 mo can be 6 to 10 wk, etc.

† For all products used, consult manufacturer's package enclosure for instructions for storage, handling, and administration. Immunobiologics prepared by different manufacturers may vary, and those of the same manufacturer may change from time to time. The package insert should be followed for a specific product.

‡ DTP, diphtheria and tetanus toxoids and pertussis vaccine.

§ OPV, oral, attenuated poliovirus vaccine contains poliovirus types 1, 2, and 3.

** Simultaneous administration of MMR, DTP, and OPV is appropriate for patients whose compliance with medical care recommendations cannot be assured.

†† MMR, live measles, mumps, and rubella viruses in a combined vaccine.

‡‡ Up to 7th birthday.

§§ Td, adult tetanus toxoid and diphtheria toxoid in combination, contains the same dose of tetanus toxoid as DTP or pediatric diphtheria and tetanus toxoid (**DT**) and a reduced dose of diphtheria toxoid.

(Modified from *Morbidity and Mortality Weekly Report,* January, 14 1983, Vol. 32, No. 1, Centers for Disease Control, Atlanta, Georgia.)

measles, mumps, and rubella—are commercially available. There appears to be no interference with development of immune responses, as indicated by adequate elevations of antibodies to all viruses.

7. Booster immunization: Periodic booster immunization is indicated for many immunization procedures. The interval recommended will vary with the product; it can be as long as 5 to 10 yr for tetanus or diphtheria toxoid, but may be as short as 1 yr for influenza vaccine.

8. Reactions and contraindications: Mild local and febrile reactions are not uncommon after pertussis vaccine and, in older children or adults, diphtheria toxoid. Arthralgia is fairly common in adults after administration of rubella vaccine; occasionally arthritis also occurs. Antipyretics and analgesics usually control symptoms. Routine immunizations should be postponed in children with acute infections or neurologic disturbances. However, emergency indications for immunization override this precaution. During pregnancy there is a theoretical risk from live measles vaccine or bacterial vaccines that are apt to cause reactions. Thus, active immunization (except with influenza vaccine) should generally be **avoided** during pregnancy. *Persons with sensitivity to egg protein should not receive viral vaccines prepared in eggs.* (See also SPECIFIC IMMUNIZATIONS, below, for additional contraindications.)

9. Passive immunization is the only protective immunologic procedure currently available against certain infectious diseases; for example, acute viral hepatitis A (see also in Ch. 71).

TABLE 182–3. RECOMMENDED IMMUNIZATION SCHEDULE FOR INFANTS AND CHILDREN UP TO 7TH BIRTHDAY NOT IMMUNIZED AT THE RECOMMENDED TIME IN EARLY INFANCY*

Timing	*Vaccine(s)*	*Comments*
First visit	DTP-1†; OPV-1‡; (if child is ≥ 15 mo of age, MMR§)	DTP, OPV, and MMR can be administered simultaneously to children ≥ 15 mo of age
2 mo after first DTP, OPV	DTP-2; OPV-2	
2 mo after 2nd DTP	DTP-3	An additional dose of OPV at this time is optional for use in areas with a high risk of polio exposure
6–12 mo after 3rd DTP	DTP-4; OPV-3	
24 mo	Hib	*Hemophilus influenzae* b vaccine
Preschool** (4–6 yr)	DTP-5; OPV-4	Preferably at or before school entry
14–16 yr	Td††	Repeat every 10 yr throughout life

* If initiated in the first year of life, give DTP-1, 2, and 3 and OPV-1 and 2 according to this schedule, and give MMR when the child becomes 15 mo of age.

† DTP, diphtheria and tetanus toxoids with pertussis vaccine. DTP may be used up to the 7th birthday.

‡ OPV, oral attenuated poliovirus vaccine contains poliovirus types 1, 2, and 3.

§ MMR, live measles, mumps, and rubella viruses in a combined vaccine.

** The preschool dose is not necessary if the 4th dose of DTP and 3rd dose of OPV are administered after the 4th birthday.

†† Td, adult tetanus toxoid and diphtheria toxoid in combination, contains the same dose of tetanus toxoid as DTP or pediatric diphtheria and tetanus toxoid (**DT**) and a reduced dose of diphtheria toxoid.

(Modified from *Morbidity and Mortality Weekly Report,* January 14, 1983, Vol. 32, No. 1, Centers for Disease Control, Atlanta, Georgia.)

TABLE 182–4. RECOMMENDED IMMUNIZATION SCHEDULE FOR PERSONS 7 YR OF AGE OR OLDER

Timing	*Vaccine*	*Comments*
First visit	Td-1*; OPV-1†; MMR‡	OPV not routinely administered to those ≥ 18 yr of age
2 mo after first Td, OPV	Td-2; OPV-2	
6–12 mo after 2nd Td, OPV	Td-3; OPV-3	OPV-3 may be given as soon as 6 wk after OPV-2
10 yr after Td-3	Td	Repeat every 10 yr throughout life

* Td, tetanus and diphtheria toxoids (adult type) are used after the 7th birthday. The DTP doses given to children < 7 who remain incompletely immunized at age 7 or older should be counted as prior exposure to tetanus and diphtheria toxoids (eg, a child who previously received 2 doses of DTP needs only 1 dose of Td to complete a primary series).

† OPV, oral, attenuated poliovirus vaccine, contains poliovirus types 1, 2, and 3. When polio vaccine is to be given to individuals ≥ 18 yr, inactivated polio vaccine (**IPV**) is preferred.

‡ MMR, live measles, mumps, and rubella viruses in a combined vaccine. Persons born before 1957 can generally be considered immune to measles and mumps and need not be immunized. Rubella vaccine may be given to persons of any age, particularly to women of childbearing age. MMR may be used, since administration of vaccine to persons already immune is not deleterious.

(Modified from *Morbidity and Mortality Weekly Report,* January 14, 1983, Vol. 32, No. 1, Centers for Disease Control, Atlanta, Georgia.)

10. "Health Information for International Travel," a pamphlet containing immunization requirements and recommendations for foreign travel, is published annually by the U.S. Public Health Service. The latest edition, sold by the Superintendent of Documents, U.S. Government Printing Office, Washington, D. C. 20402, should be used.

SPECIFIC IMMUNIZATIONS

Diphtheria immunization: All children should receive active immunization with diphtheria toxoid, the type of toxoid or combination used depending on the age of the child. Schick tests generally are unnecessary; instead of a follow-up Schick test, a booster dose of toxoid is given at the recommended time. For those > 12 yr, the best procedure is to immunize or boost with tetanus-diphtheria toxoid, adult type.

Pertussis immunization: Active immunization may be started at age 1 to 3 mo, either with separate injections of pertussis vaccine or through the use of DTP vaccine. In either case, the manufacturer's recommendations should be followed, since the dose may vary from preparation to preparation. For those > 6 yr, routine use of pertussis vaccine, either separately or in combination, is not recommended.

If any of the following adverse events occurs after DTP or single-antigen pertussis vaccination, further vaccination with a vaccine containing pertussis antigen is *contraindicated*: (1) Allergic hypersensitivity. (2) Fever of 40.5 C (105 F) or greater within 48 h. (3) Collapse or shocklike state (hypotonic-hyporesponsive episode) within 48 h. (4) Inconsolable crying persisting ≥ 3 h or an unusual, high-pitched cry occurring within 48 h. (5) Convulsions, with or without fever, occurring within 3 days. All children with convulsions, especially those with convulsions occurring within 7 days of receipt of DTP, should be fully evaluated to clarify their medical and neurologic status before deciding to initiate or continue vaccination with DTP. (6) Encephalopathy occurring within 7 days. This includes severe alterations in consciousness, with generalized or focal neurologic signs. (A small but significantly increased risk of encephalopathy has been shown only within the 3-day period following DTP receipt. However, most authorities believe that an encephalopathy occurring within 7 days of DTP should be a contraindication to further doses of DTP.)

Tetanus immunization: The initial DTP immunization series is followed by a DTP booster at age 18 mo and another when the child reaches school age. Subsequent routine tetanus boosters (indicated for all children and adults) every 10 yr should maintain protection. More frequent boosters are unwarranted, since untoward reactions to toxoid may occur. At any interval after basic immunization, immunity can be reestablished by a single booster dose; however, after an interval of > 10 yr since the last injection of toxoid, the rate of the booster response may be somewhat slower. (For procedure in handling injuries when tetanus is a potential threat, see TETANUS under CLOSTRIDIAL INFECTIONS in Ch. 8.)

***Hemophilus influenzae* type b immunization**: The purified capsular polysaccharide *H. influenzae* type b **(Hib)** vaccine is recommended for all infants at 24 mo of age. Need for a booster dose has not been determined. Infants who attend day-care facilities and those at high risk because of chronic disease should be immunized at 18 mo of age.

Poliomyelitis immunization: Primary immunization of infants with trivalent oral (live) vaccine should begin at about age 2 mo, integrating the schedule with other routine immunization procedures, as shown in TABLE 182–2. For primary immunization of children up to age 6, 2 doses are given at approximately 8-wk intervals, followed by a 3rd dose given about 1 yr later. Inactivated poliovirus is recommended for children with immunodeficiency diseases.

Revaccination is not presently considered necessary for the child who has completed a primary course. However, a single dose of trivalent vaccine on entering school has

been recommended to fill in any possible antibody gaps resulting from failure of a "take." Adults should be immunized only when a risk of infection exists (eg, foreign travel or a local epidemic).

Measles immunization is recommended as a routine procedure for all susceptible infants or children. Live attenuated vaccine is the agent of choice in healthy children and is given at about 15 mo of age, when about 95% of children will have an antibody response. If exposure to measles is likely before that age, the vaccine should not be withheld; reimmunization at an older age may be necessary. Vaccine may be given at any later age to those not vaccinated earlier. Reimmunization is recommended for patients (1) who received killed vaccine alone or who received killed vaccine followed within a year by live vaccine; (2) who received live attenuated measles vaccine alone or with gamma globulin before 1 yr of age; or (3) with an unclear immunization history.

Live attenuated measles vaccine is *not* recommended for (1) children with leukemia or other generalized malignancies, (2) those under treatment with irradiation, corticosteroids, or antimetabolites, or (3) those suffering from other severe or debilitating illness. Instead, one should depend on protective doses of immune serum globulin immediately following exposure (see MEASLES under VIRAL INFECTIONS in Ch. 191).

Mumps immunization is recommended as a routine procedure for all susceptible infants or children. Live attenuated vaccine is the agent of choice for infants or children aged not less than 12 mo and should be given in accordance with the manufacturer's directions. (See also MUMPS under VIRAL INFECTIONS in Ch. 191.)

Rubella immunization: See RUBELLA under VIRAL INFECTIONS in Ch. 191, and CONGENITAL RUBELLA under NEONATAL INFECTIONS in Ch. 186.

Other immunizations—eg, for smallpox, influenza, hepatitis B, pneumococcal pneumonia, rabies, cholera, typhoid, plague, yellow fever—are discussed under the specific disorder.

INFANT NUTRITION

Measurement of diet adequacy cannot be precise. Increases in the infant's weight and length only grossly reflect nutritional progress. The daily requirements for adequate nutrition are especially significant for the growing child compared to the adult (see TABLES 79–2 and 79–3 in Ch. 79; and TABLE 182–5 in this chapter). Protein is one constituent of the diet that varies with the rate of growth as well as the state of health. Because of a deceleration in growth rate as compared to body weight, the caloric needs of the child calculated as a function of body weight gradually decrease as the child grows older so that < 6 mo the requirement is 50 to 55 kcal/lb/day (110 to 120 kcal/kg); at 1 yr, 45 kcal/lb/day (95 to 100 kcal/kg); and at age 15 yr, 20 kcal/lb/day (50 kcal/kg). When protein and calories are provided by human milk, the requirements between 3 and 9 mo of age may actually be lower than those stated. The relative need for protein, vitamins, and minerals remains constant and is greater than that of adults. Requirements for various vitamins depend on the intake of calories, protein, fat, carbohydrate, and specific amino acids.

Nutritional deficiency diseases are unusual in our culture today, unless associated with another disease that alters intake, absorption, or metabolism; therefore, personal opinion regarding nutrition often is applied more than scientific data. Since the stomach is not very discriminating, babies may be satisfied on nearly any diet, but the retention of a formula does not necessarily make it adequate for optimal growth and development.

For the infant, drinking and eating are intense experiences, comprise most of his socializing, and are integral parts of his developmental progress. Thus, the act of feeding provides emotional and psychologic benefits, as well as an opportunity to

TABLE 182–5. RANGE OF AVERAGE WATER REQUIREMENTS OF CHILDREN AT DIFFERENT AGES UNDER ORDINARY CONDITIONS

Age	*Average Body Wt in Kg*	*Total Water in 24 h, mL*	*Water/Kg Body Wt in 24 h, mL*
3 days	3.0	250–300	80–100
10 days	3.2	400–500	125–150
3 mo	5.4	750–850	140–160
6 mo	7.3	950–1100	130–155
9 mo	8.6	1100–1250	125–145
1 yr	9.5	1150–1300	120–135
2 yr	11.8	1350–1500	115–125
4 yr	16.2	1600–1800	100–110
6 yr	20.0	1800–2000	90–100
10 yr	28.7	2000–2500	70–85
14 yr	45.0	2200–2700	50–60
18 yr	54.0	2200–2700	40–50

(From "Nutrition and Nutritional Disorders" by L. A. Barness, p. 138, in *Nelson Textbook of Pediatrics*, ed. 12, 1983, edited by R. E. Behrman and V. C. Vaughan, III; W. E. Nelson, Senior Editor. Copyright 1983 by W. B. Saunders Company. Used with permission.)

gratify both sucking and nutritional needs. Problems caused by failure to satisfy these needs are discussed in COMMON FEEDING AND GASTROINTESTINAL PROBLEMS, below.

Breastfeeding

Management of breastfeeding in the hospital is discussed under FEEDING in MANAGEMENT OF THE NORMAL NEWBORN, above. Once the mother and baby are discharged, nursing usually settles into a routine pattern. A modified ad lib schedule that allows the infant to sleep as long as possible at night is usually best. Infants generally should not be put to breast more often than q 2 h. Some infants, however, have a regular fussy period daily, and more frequent feeding may temporarily be necessary.

The mother's diet should be well balanced, and she should avoid foods that may cause colic, such as garlic, onions, legumes, cabbage, chocolate, and excessive amounts of exotic or seasonal fruits (melons, rhubarb, peaches), unless trial shows that they are tolerated. Maternal fatigue and emotional stress result in failure to satisfy the infant more often than any other factors. **Breast engorgement,** which occurs during early lactation, is discussed under FEEDING in MANAGEMENT OF THE NORMAL NEWBORN, above.

Human milk contains nutritional substances ideal in quantity and quality for optimal growth and development of the human infant. For example, breast milk contains a predominance of monounsaturated fatty acids, which are easily absorbed and do not combine with calcium to make unabsorbable soaps; it also contains lipase, which facilitates the digestion of fat; it has the highest lactose content of the mammalian milks, providing a readily available energy source compatible with neonatal enzymes; it contains large amounts of vitamin E, which may be related to preventing anemia and is an important antioxidant in fat metabolism; and it has a calcium:phosphorus ratio of 2:1, preventing calcium-deficiency tetany (the ratio in cow's milk is almost reversed). In addition to its nutritional value, breast milk favorably changes the pH of stools and the intestinal flora, thus protecting against bacterial diarrheas. Because of the protective quality of these factors, all infectious diseases are less frequent in breastfed than in bottle-fed infants.

If the mother's diet is adequate, the only supplement that the breastfed infant may require is fluoride (in drops) 0.25 mg/day orally for the first 6 mo, since this passes into

breast milk poorly. In areas with little sunshine, infants, especially those with dark skins, may require 400 u. of vitamin D daily.

Drugs in lactating mothers are discussed under FEEDING in MANAGEMENT OF THE NORMAL NEWBORN.

Weaning should be related to the individualized needs and desires of both mother and baby. Nursing at least 6 mo, until solid foods are added to the diet, is considered by many as an ideal minimum. Gradual weaning over weeks or months is easiest. One breastfeeding/day should be replaced by a bottle or cup of fruit juice, modified formula, or fresh cow's milk when the infant is about 7 mo old. Weaning to a cup can be completed by age 10 mo; some infants will cling to 1 or 2 nursings daily, often until age 18 to 24 mo. Some infants are nursed even longer but should also receive solid foods and fluids by cup.

Bottle Feeding

By the time the infant leaves the hospital, he has adapted to the bottle and usually takes 2 to 3 oz/feeding, approximately q 4 h. A modified ad lib schedule is satisfactory for most infants. If more volume is needed, water may suffice, especially in warm weather. A baby should be held and cuddled for all feedings; *the bottle should never be propped.*

Nutritional requirements: Commercial infant formulas have made formula-making at home rare. They are generally available as powder, concentrated liquid, and prediluted liquid, and are generally preferable to cow's milk. Preparing 20 kcal/oz of prepared formula requires 1 tbsp powder to 2 oz water, 1 oz liquid concentrate to 1 oz water, and no adjustment in the prediluted form. Each type contains the minimum daily requirement of vitamins and is available with iron 10 to 12 mg/qt, a maintenance dose. Special hypoallergenic or carbohydrate-free formulas are available, as are predigested formulas with triglycerides, amino acids, and monosaccharides, and simulated breast milk; each has a different vitamin content and preparation procedure. If a **nonproprietary formula** is desired, the most reliable, easily made, and flexible formula is made from 13 oz evaporated milk, 1 to 3 tbsp sugar (for additional calories), and 19 oz water. This will provide 21 kcal/oz of formula. Each infant should receive 50 to 55 kcal/lb/day (120 kcal/kg) and 2 to 2½ oz of fluid/lb/day (150 mL/kg).

Nutritionally, milk is a well-balanced food for an infant except that it lacks iron. An infant not receiving a proprietary formula with iron may require an iron supplement, such as ferrous sulfate drops 75 mg/day, after neonatal stores begin to deplete, at age 4½ to 6 mo. When an evaporated, skim, or whole milk formula is used, the infant should also receive supplemental vitamins A, C, and D daily for the first year of life and the second winter in cold climates. Fluoride is provided by using fluoridated water to prepare the formula or by giving fluoride drops (0.25 mg/day orally) when fluoridated water is not available or when prediluted liquid formula is used.

Initiating Solid Foods

The time to start solid foods depends on the infant's needs and readiness, but infants do not need solids before age 6 mo. The infant must develop a new movement for tongue and mouth. Neurologic development has progressed sufficiently for this to occur at about 3 to 4 mo in full-term infants. Infants can swallow solids at a younger age if the food is placed on the back of the tongue, but refusal is normal. Some parents coax the infant to take large amounts of solid food in an effort to get the baby to sleep through the night; no sound evidence supports this practice. Some infants who are force-fed early rebel and develop feeding problems later.

Many infants take solids *after* being bottle-fed, which satisfies the need to suck and more rapidly appeases hunger. Solids should be offered by spoon and should be introduced individually to determine tolerance. Many commercial baby foods, especially desserts and soup mixtures, are high in starch, which has no vitamins or minerals and

is high in calories, and cellulose, which is poorly digested by infants. Some commercial baby foods have a high sodium content (over 200 mg/jar); they can be identified by reading labels carefully and should be avoided. (The daily infant sodium requirement is 17.6 mg/kg.) Pureed home foods are adequate. Meat should be introduced in preference to foods that are high in carbohydrates; but, since many infants tend to reject meat, it should be introduced with care and attention, so that it is accepted well. Wheat, eggs, and chocolate should be avoided until the child is 1 yr of age to prevent unnecessary food sensitivities.

COMMON FEEDING AND GASTROINTESTINAL PROBLEMS

Most common feeding and GI problems are not serious medically, and many can be handled by explanation and reassurance with a minimum of medication and formula manipulation. However, such problems may be of major concern to parents, and careful appraisal of the infant always is indicated to determine the problem's significance and severity. The evaluation of parental complaints should include observing the parent–child interaction in the office and checking the infant's length and weight. If the infant's growth rate is normal when plotted on a standard growth chart, and the parent's complaints appear out of proportion to the findings, this over-concern may be a clue to deeper anxieties or problems in the parent–child relationship requiring further exploration.

A number of disorders mentioned in this chapter are further detailed elsewhere in THE MANUAL. In addition, eating problems of older children are discussed in BEHAVIORAL PROBLEMS in Ch. 188.

Regurgitation and Vomiting

Infants commonly bring up small amounts (seldom > 5 to 10 mL) of milk during or soon after feedings, often as the baby is burped. Feeding too fast and swallowing air may be related to this; using bottles with firmer nipples and smaller holes, and burping the baby more often may help. Study of this problem is seldom indicated and a formula change usually is valueless. Excessive regurgitation may be due to overfeeding (see below). However, **vomiting** may signal a more serious condition. Repeated projectile vomiting of increasing amounts may indicate **pyloric stenosis** or **gastroesophageal reflux. Upper small bowel obstruction** from duodenal bands, duodenal stenosis, or volvulus causes bile-stained vomitus. **Metabolic disorders** (eg, adrenogenital syndrome and galactosemia) may present with vomiting. Vomiting with fever and/or lethargy may signal **infection;** eg, sepsis or meningitis.

Underfeeding

Adequately fed infants usually become quiet or sleep soon after a feeding. The underfed infant often remains restless, almost seems to look around for more to eat, and awakens 1 to 2 h after being fed, appearing to be hungry. Such clear signs of underfeeding are not always present or may not be fully appreciated by a parent. Weight gain < 200 to 250 gm/wk (6 to 8 oz) in infants under age 4 mo is inadequate. A detailed feeding history must be taken to determine whether the difficulty is underfeeding or a more serious metabolic or systemic problem. Constituents and proportions of the formula should be reviewed. Underfeeding also may be a sign of parental inadequacy; eg, lack of concern or neglect of the baby are factors to be considered seriously. Breastfed infants who do not show adequate weight gain may be weighed before and after several feedings to determine their milk intake more accurately. The breastfed infant's diet may be supplemented with an appropriate milk formula and cereal; treatment of the formula-fed infant may include a change of the formula constituents and an increase in total quantity of formula offered.

Overfeeding

Monitoring the infant's weight by serial recording on a standard growth chart readily shows when an infant is gaining too rapidly. Other signs of overfeeding include crying and excessive regurgitation. Since problems of obesity may begin with excessive eating in infancy, attempts to control the infant's rate of weight gain may be of value, particularly if the infant has 2 obese parents and, therefore, an 80% chance of becoming obese. The overweight infant's daily intake should be reviewed, and the parents should be encouraged to reduce the amounts offered.

Diarrhea

Frequent loose bowel movements (4 to 6 a day) may occur in the normal infant; they are of no concern unless anorexia, vomiting, weight loss, failure to gain weight, or passage of blood also occurs. Breastfed infants tend to have frequent, frothy bowel movements, especially if they are not receiving solid baby foods.

Sudden onset of diarrhea with vomiting, bloody stools, fever, anorexia, or listlessness may be due to **infection**. A low-grade diarrhea persisting for weeks or months may result from several conditions, such as (1) **gluten-induced enteropathy (celiac disease)**: The gluten fraction of wheat protein causes a malabsorption of dietary fats, resulting in malnutrition, anorexia, and bulky, foul-smelling stools. Removing gluten from the diet by excluding all wheat products corrects the condition. (2) **cystic fibrosis**: Pancreatic insufficiency results in trypsin and lipase deficits, causing high fecal losses of protein and fats with consequent malnutrition and growth retardation. The stool is large in quantity and often foul-smelling. Pancreatic extract may be given orally to improve this problem. (3) **sugar malabsorption**: Intestinal mucosal enzymes, such as lactase, which splits lactose to galactose and glucose, may be congenitally absent or temporarily deficient secondary to GI infection. Improvement after eliminating carbohydrates from the diet or after substituting a lactose-free formula strongly suggests such a malabsorption state. (4) **allergic gastroenteropathy**: Milk protein may cause some cases of diarrhea, especially those associated with vomiting and the presence of blood in the stools, but intolerance to the carbohydrate fraction of the ingested food should be suspected also. Symptoms often abate promptly on substitution with a soybean formula and return with a challenge feeding of cow's milk. Those infants intolerant of cow milk commonly are soy-intolerant, so there may be a need to use one of several special elemental noncarbohydrate-based formulas available. Spontaneous improvement usually occurs toward the end of the first year of life, regardless of alterations in the content of the formula offered to the infant.

Constipation

The infant's bowel movements vary so much in frequency that it is difficult to define constipation. The same infant who has a bowel movement 4 times a day may, at other times, have one every 2 days. Most infants pass a hard, large stool with minimal discomfort, while some cry when passing a soft one. Infants < 2 to 3 mo commonly have a minor degree of anal stenosis that causes persistent straining and passage of small-caliber stools. A gentle digital examination of the anus easily identifies this condition, revealing a tight band-like circum-anal constriction. Anal dilation once or twice provides relief of symptoms. A large bowel movement may cause an **anal fissure,** which presents with pain on defecation and the occasional passage of a small amount of bright red blood. The fissure can be identified by inspecting the anal canal with an anuscope or an otoscope, using a large speculum. In infants, most fissures clear quickly without intervention, but a mild stool softener, such as dioctyl sodium sulfosuccinate 3 to 5 mg/kg/day divided into 2 to 3 doses, may be used for 7 to 10 days to allow the fissure to heal; the value of locally applied corticosteroid cream has not been proved. Persistent constipation, particularly if it begins before age 1 mo, may be a symptom of **congenital megacolon** (see under Distal Small Bowel and Large Bowel Obstruction under Gastrointestinal Defects in Ch. 187).

COLIC

A symptom complex of early infancy that is characterized by paroxysms of crying, apparent abdominal pain, and irritability.

Etiology, Symptoms, and Signs

Colic may begin shortly after a baby comes home from the hospital, but often begins some weeks later, and may persist until age 3 or 4 mo. The term "colic" is descriptive, suggesting a cause of intestinal origin, but the specific mechanisms of infantile colic are unknown. Typically, the colicky infant eats and gains weight well, may seem excessively hungry, and often will suck vigorously on almost anything available, but paroxysms of crying may transform a peaceful home into chaos and strain family tempers. Colic often occurs at a predictable time of day or night, but a few infants cry almost incessantly. Excessive crying causes aerophagia, which results in flatulence and abdominal distention. Such crying *may* be an early manifestation of an insistent, impatient personality style, which may have counterpart behavior patterns in the older child. Parents are apt to assume that the infant is irritable because of the way they handle him; some explanation of the infant's individuality is justified to overcome any such guilt feelings.

Diagnosis

Before colic is diagnosed, other reasons for similar behavior must be ruled out. A hungry baby may cry incessantly, but shows an inadequate weight gain. An over-attended infant may not get sufficient sleep. Sickness, such as a fever, a cold, or an ear infection, may cause irritability. A physical examination may reassure both physician and parents; a blood count, urinalysis, or other study may be indicated. Careful questioning may reveal that crying is not the chief concern, but a symptom that the parents have used to justify their visiting the doctor to present another problem—eg, concern over the death of a previous child or over their feelings of inability to cope with a new infant.

Treatment

The infant who cries for short periods of time may respond to being held, rocked, or patted gently. An infant with a strong sucking urge who fusses soon after a feeding may need more sucking stimulus. If a bottle feeding takes < 20 min, new nipples with smaller holes should be tried; a pacifier also may quiet the infant. A very active, restless infant may respond, paradoxically, to being swaddled rather tightly with a small sheet and placed on his stomach. A short trial of a milk substitute formula is useful to ascertain whether a form of milk intolerance may exist. In exceptional circumstances, the judicious use of a sedative such as phenobarbital (in liquid form) 2 mg/kg/day orally in 2 divided doses may help when given 1 h before the anticipated fussy period. Parents should be assured that the colicky infant is basically healthy, that this behavior will cease in a few weeks, and that too much crying is not harmful.

---

183. SPECIAL CONSIDERATIONS IN CARING FOR SICK CHILDREN AND THEIR FAMILIES

PARENT-INFANT BONDING: THE SICK NEONATE

Strong psychologic attachments between parents and their newborn that begin to develop in the first hours and days following birth. The process is influenced by the parents' own experiences as they were reared by their parents, by their cultural and social

attitudes toward childrearing, by their personality development, by their desire to have a child, and by the psychologic planning for the arrival of the newborn, which progresses through the pregnancy. Parent–infant bonding establishes the intense emotional ties that normally exist between parents and their children. It ensures the necessary parental support of the child during his developmental years, and supports the development of the child's personality (see also INITIAL CARE in Ch. 182).

When the neonate is sick or premature, the situation is much more difficult and special care must be taken to be realistically encouraging to the parents and to help them understand the newborn's problems. Parents should be encouraged to visit their newborn early and frequently and to participate in his care as much as possible. Supportive attention to the parents helps minimize their anxiety and promotes the bonding process.

Particular difficulties arise when a critically ill newborn must be transferred to an **intensive care nursery**. The parents may be separated from their infant for many days or weeks, and the development of normal attachments may not be possible. In the past, parental visiting and contact with premature or very ill neonates were either impossible or extremely limited, and in many such cases parental neglect or abuse of these children developed. In the modern intensive care nursery, parents and close relatives are encouraged to visit the newborn frequently and as soon after birth as possible. After appropriate hand washing and gowning, they should be helped to touch or hold the newborn as his condition allows. *No newborn, even if on a respirator, can be considered too ill for the parents to see and touch*. Parent–newborn bonds are strengthened if the parents can feed, bathe, and change their newborn, and if the mother can give her breast milk to her sick neonate, even if he must initially be fed by tube. (See also MANAGEMENT OF CHRONIC DISABILITY, below.)

Malformed newborns: When a newborn has a birth defect, the parents should see him together as soon after birth as possible, regardless of his medical condition. Parents sometimes are strongly discouraged from seeing their malformed or critically sick newborn, but this often leads them to imagine his appearance and condition to be much worse than is actually the case. Intensive parental support is essential, with as many counseling sessions as are needed for questions and concerns to be answered and to achieve understanding and then acceptance of their newborn's condition. It is important to emphasize what is normal about the child and what potential he has, and not to dwell totally on the abnormalities.

When an infant dies, parents who have never seen or touched him may feel as though they had never had a baby. Such parents have reported exaggerated feelings of emptiness; prolonged pathologic depression may result because the parents could not grieve for the loss of a "real infant." The process of mourning will then be incomplete. In most situations, parents who have not been able to see or hold their infant will be helped if allowed to do so after the infant has died. In all cases, follow-up visits with the physician and a social worker are helpful to review the circumstances of the infant's illness and death, to answer questions that often arise later, and to assess and alleviate inappropriate guilt feelings. This also gives the physician an opportunity to recommend genetic counseling and/or counseling with a perinatologist regarding possible future pregnancies. The physician can evaluate the parents' grieving process, and if it is pathologic, he can provide appropriate guidance or make a referral for more extensive support.

MANAGEMENT OF CHRONIC DISABILITY

The term chronic disability comprises a range of disorders, from ***chronic illness*** *(illness lasting at least 3 mo, and usually persisting for several years or an indefinite period)* to ***physical*** and ***mental handicaps*** *(permanent incapacitations that make normal*

achievement difficult). Children with chronic disability generally have more pronounced physical–adaptive needs than normal children. Their educational, psychologic, and social requirements are similar to those of all children, but meeting these needs often requires specialized programs.

When chronic disability is apparent at birth, improving the newborn's health receives the emphasis of care; however, the family's need for support should not be ignored. If a newborn is severely disabled or has limiting congenital defects, his physical problems are complicated by the possibility of initial negative parental reactions, such as shock, dismay, grief, and guilt. Parents should nevertheless be promptly informed if chronic disability exists or is suspected, even though extensive discussions may be deferred until consultations are held with appropriate specialists. As soon as a factual, realistic, honest appraisal of the severity of the condition, the medical care available, and the prognosis is known, it should be shared with the parents. The parents must be encouraged to express their feelings and to work through them. They must be helped to establish a supportive, close relationship with their child (see also PARENT–INFANT BONDING: THE SICK NEONATE, above), and they should participate in care plans. Community acceptance of the handicapped youngster, and community commitment to providing early nonmedical services and opportunities (eg, preschool programs) that meet his or her special needs are very important.

Establishment of Specific Goals

A set of management goals and **a treatment plan** must be established, understood, and accepted by the physicians and other health professionals involved. The child's parents should participate in the planning, which should take into account their values, priorities, and limitations. However, to prevent later guilt feelings, final determinations regarding care should not be solely the parents'. The objectives should be realistic; should be based on the physical, emotional, intellectual, and social needs of the child; and should include maximal development of his assets. A balance must be set between overprotection and too much pressure; frequently, however, the scholastic and behavioral expectations are set too low. Children who are obviously different are often viewed as incapable of coping with ordinary lifestyles. Whining, biting, crying, hitting, "giving up," and other inappropriate behavior should not be tolerated in them any more than in other children.

Each person involved in the child's care (including his parents) should have a *written statement* of the short- and long-term goals that have been agreed upon and of the services that will be needed to accomplish these goals in a specific period of time. Goals should be reviewed, updated, and redefined at regular intervals. Attainment of physical objectives can be assessed through the use of goal-oriented medical records and by parental diary-keeping. Appraisal of psychologic goals is made by clinical observation, evaluation of behavioral symptoms, and investigation into family and peer relationships, and may require psychologic testing and developmental evaluation. Assessment of scholastic achievement commensurate with the child's abilities and of the services needed to accomplish it requires close contact with school personnel, who must be adequately informed about the child's disabilities and must agree with the established educational goals.

Goal-setting may involve balancing the benefits of a treatment against its potential harm; achieving one treatment objective may therefore sacrifice the degree to which another is accomplished. For example, the timing of hospitalization or surgery may not always be optimal with regard to psychologic or social considerations.

The physician may be able to influence community acceptance of chronically disabled children and may wish to exercise leadership in this area. Programs are needed to teach these children the skills necessary for participation in social interaction, and providing such programs may require reassessing how, where, and why public money is spent.

Involvement of the Family

The physician must understand the strains that will be placed on the parents, affecting such areas as marital relations, social life, the amount of attention other children receive, and financial resources. This requires knowledge of the family structure, the strengths of the marriage, the relationships that exist between the siblings, and the presence of other health problems. Knowledge of the family situation will help the physician to recognize and understand the parents' phases of adaptation (their progression from disorganization and reintegration to mature adaptation); and the reasons for their frequent use of denial, their feelings of guilt, and their tendency to project their feelings or to become dependent on the doctor. Parents must be helped to recognize and interpret these reactions, permitted to ventilate their anxieties and other feelings, and helped to identify their strengths and weaknesses—all without becoming overly dependent on the doctor.

Recognition of Physician Problems

Because the prevalence of very complex specific disorders (eg, cystic fibrosis, rheumatoid arthritis, congenital amputations) tends to be low in an average pediatric practice, primary-care physicians may understandably be concerned about their ability to handle some of the more difficult technical aspects of treatment. The resultant sharing of responsibilities with specialists provides optimum care to a patient, but presents the primary-care physician with a variety of potential problems requiring great maturity, patience, and the ability to communicate well and to prevent or resolve conflicts. In some circumstances the family physician cannot realistically assume the major responsibility for the comprehensive management of the patient and his family. In these situations specialists should be clearly informed that they will be expected to accept broader and more comprehensive responsibilities.

Physicians' understanding of *their own* feelings and attitudes toward chronically ill and handicapped patients and their families is an important factor in successful management. They risk rejecting these patients or according them a low priority because the patients so rarely show dramatic improvement directly related to the physicians' actions; or they may identify with patients or parents, becoming anxious, overzealous, and, later, disappointed and resentful. Self-evaluation and discussion with others will help them to recognize these normal, but adverse, reactions.

---

184. SPECIAL CONSIDERATIONS OF DRUG TREATMENT IN NEONATES, INFANTS, AND CHILDREN

(See also appropriate chapters in §23; and DRUGS IN LACTATING MOTHERS, above)

Effective and safe drug therapy in neonates, infants, and children requires understanding maturational changes in drug action, metabolism, and disposition during growth and development. Virtually all pharmacokinetic parameters change with age. Pediatric drug dosage regimens must be adjusted for age (the major determinant), disease states, sex, and individual needs. Failure to make such adjustments may lead to ineffective treatment or to toxicity.

Drug absorption: GI absorption of drugs may proceed for longer than in adults, especially in the newborn with prolonged gastric emptying time and in children with celiac disease. Absorption of some drugs given IM (digoxin, kanamycin) may be erratic in neonates. Dermal and percutaneous absorption of drugs is remarkably enhanced in newborns and young infants; eg, topically administered epinephrine may cause systemic hypertension, and dermal absorption of dyes and antibacterials (hexa-

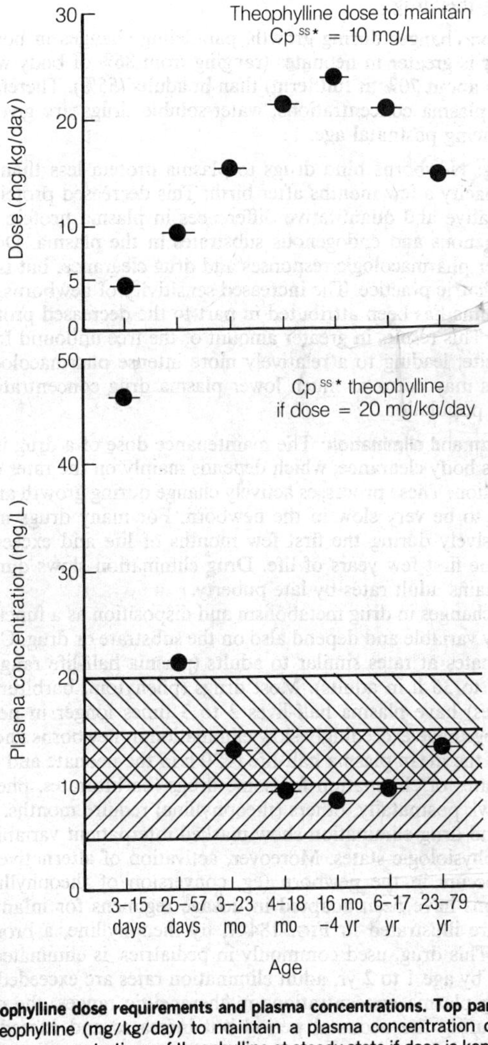

FIG. 184–1. Theophylline dose requirements and plasma concentrations. Top panel: Estimated dose requirements of theophylline (mg/kg/day) to maintain a plasma concentration of 10 mg/L. **Lower panel:** Estimated plasma concentrations of theophylline at steady state if dose is kept at 20 mg/kg/day. Shaded areas indicate tentative therapeutic level for bronchodilatation and anti-apneic activity.

*Cp^{ss} = Plasma concentration at steady state.

(From "Maturational Changes in Theophylline and Caffeine Metabolism and Disposition: Clinical Implications" by J. V. Aranda, in *Proceedings of the Second World Conference on Clinical Pharmacology and Therapeutics,* July 31-August 5, 1983, p. 870, edited by L. Lemberger and M. M. Reidenberg. Copyright by the American Society for Pharmacology and Experimental Therapeutics, Bethesda, 1984. Used with permission.)

chlorophene) may result in poisoning. Theophylline administered percutaneously to premature newborns with apnea is well absorbed and maintains plasma therapeutic concentrations of this drug.

Drug distribution changes during growth, paralleling changes in body composition. Total body water is greater in neonates (ranging from 86% of body weight in premature newborns to about 70% at full term) than in adults (55%). Therefore, to maintain equivalent drug plasma concentrations, water-soluble drugs are given in decreasing doses with advancing postnatal age.

Protein binding: Newborns bind drugs to plasma protein less than adults, but approach adult capacity a few months after birth. This decreased protein binding could be due to qualitative and quantitative differences in plasma protein and also to the presence of exogenous and endogenous substrates in the plasma. Decreased protein binding may alter pharmacologic responses and drug clearance, but is seldom considered in older pediatric practice. The increased sensitivity of newborns to certain drugs such as theophylline has been attributed in part to the decreased protein-bound fraction of the drug. This results in greater amount of the free unbound fraction available at the receptor site, leading to a relatively more intense pharmacologic effect. Thus, adverse reactions may occur at much lower plasma drug concentrations, considered safe in the adult population.

Drug metabolism and elimination: The maintenance dose of a drug is largely a function of the drug's body clearance, which depends mainly on the rates of drug metabolism and elimination. These processes actively change during growth and development. Their rates tend to be very slow in the newborn. For many drugs metabolism rates increase progressively during the first few months of life and exceed adult rates of elimination by the first few years of life. Drug elimination slows during adolescence and probably attains adult rates by late puberty.

Maturational changes in drug metabolism and disposition as a function of postnatal age are extremely variable and depend also on the substrate or drug. Carbamazepine is excreted by neonates at rates similar to adults (plasma half-life ranges: 8 to 28 h in neonates and 21 to 36 h in adults). Most drugs (phenytoin, barbiturates, analgesics, cardiac glycosides) have plasma half-lives 2 to 3 times longer in newborns than in adults. Other drugs have exceedingly slow elimination in newborns and young infants; eg, theophylline: the mean plasma half-life is 30 h in the neonate and 6 h in the adult. Whereas adult rates of elimination for some drugs (barbiturates, phenytoin) may be achieved 2 to 4 wk postnatally, others (theophylline) require months.

Metabolism and drug elimination show marked interpatient variability and vulnerability to pathophysiologic states. Moreover, activation of alternative biotransformation pathways occurs in the newborn (eg, conversion of theophylline to caffeine). These observations have been adapted in dosage regimens for infants and children. The principles are illustrated in FIG. 184–1, by theophylline, a bronchodilator and CNS stimulant. This drug, used commonly in pediatrics, is eliminated very slowly in the neonate; but by age 1 to 2 yr, adult elimination rates are exceeded. Thus, in order to maintain drug plasma concentrations in therapeutic ranges, the dose/body wt is extremely low during the neonatal period but increases and exceeds adult dosages within 6 mo to 4 yr of age.

Renal drug elimination is the primary route for antimicrobial agents, which are the most commonly used drugs in newborns and young children. Renal elimination reflects and is dependent on glomerular filtration and secretion. Both functions are deficient in the newborn and undergo active maturational changes during the first 2 yr of life. Neonatal glomerular filtration rate is about 30% of adults and is greatly influenced by gestational age at birth. Effective renal blood flow **(RBF)** affects the rate at which drugs are presented to and eliminated by the kidneys. The effective RBF is low

during the first 2 days of life (34 to 99 mL/min/1.75 sq m), increasing to 54 to 166 mL/min/sq m by 14 to 21 days and further increasing to adult values of about 600 mL/min/sq m by age 1 to 2 yr. Plasma clearances of drugs are significantly increased in early childhood beyond the 1st yr of life. This is partly due to increased renal and hepatic elimination of drugs in early childhood relative to adults, especially the elderly. Dose regimens of aminoglycosides and other antimicrobials are adjusted to account for these maturational changes.

Pediatric Drug Dosages

No rules are adequate to guarantee efficacy and safety of drugs in the pediatric patient, especially for the newborn. Dosages based on pharmacokinetic data for a given age group adjusted to the patient's desired response and individual drug handling capability are the most rational approach to pediatric drug dosage calculations.

Many drugs currently used in pediatric practice have not been studied adequately or at all in a pediatric population. Many formulas have been suggested for calculating the dose for the child from the adult dose (eg, Clark's, Dilling's, and Young's rules), assuming incorrectly that the adult dose is always right and that the child is a miniature adult. As shown in FIG. 184–1, dosage requirements constantly change as a function of age. Dosage based on body weight is practical but not ideal. Infants receive an underdosage if given doses in mg/kg satisfactory for adults. The **body surface area (BSA)** method of calculating drug dosages (BSA [sq m] divided by 1.7 and multiplied by adult dose equals approximate pediatric dose) gives a more consistent dosage requirement throughout all the age groups, *but this method does not apply to the premature and full-term newborn.*

Pharmacokinetic considerations and therapeutic monitoring: Knowledge of a drug's kinetic profile allows manipulation of the dose to achieve and maintain a given plasma concentration. Many drugs exhibit a biexponential plasma disappearance curve in the neonate and older pediatric patient; ie, the log of the plasma drug concentration decreases linearly as a function of time with a brief but fast distributive (alpha) phase and a slower elimination (beta) phase. This exemplifies a 2-compartment model and first-order kinetics, where a certain percentage or fraction (not amount) of the drug remaining in the body is eliminated with time; and after the distribution phase, the plasma concentration reflects or is proportional to the concentration of drug in other portions of the body. This model is applicable to a wide variety of drugs used in newborns and older pediatric patients, although some drugs (eg, gentamicin, diazepam, digoxin) may fit a multicompartmental model; others (eg, salicylates) exhibit saturation kinetics (ie, a certain amount—not a percentage or fraction—of the drug is eliminated per unit time). In the young toddler and prepubertal child the alpha phase may be very short relative to the beta phase, and its contribution to overall elimination and to dosage computations may not be significant. Similarly, drugs given to the newborn usually have an extremely prolonged elimination phase relative to the distributive phase. Thus, the entire body during the newborn period could be considered as if it were a single compartment for purposes of dose calculations.

Administering a loading dose (mg/kg) may be useful to achieve a given plasma concentration quickly when rapid onset of drug action is required. For many drugs, loading doses are generally greater in neonates and young infants than in older children or adults. However, the prolonged elimination of drugs in the first few weeks of postnatal life warrants substantially lower maintenance doses given at longer intervals to prevent toxicity or overdosage. Rapid changes in drug elimination with increasing age require adjustment of maintenance doses with advancing postnatal age. This adjustment also depends on the drug being used.

Monitoring drug concentrations from serum or other biologic fluids (saliva, urine, CSF, etc) is useful if the desired pharmacologic effect is not attained or if adverse reactions occur. Monitoring is also useful in making dose adjustments to individualize therapy and to monitor a patient's compliance.

Routes of drug administration are dictated by the clinical needs and circumstances in a given patient. In the sick premature newborn, almost all medications are administered IV, since GI function and therefore drug absorption is impaired and the IM route is precluded because these neonates have very poor muscle mass. In older preterm neonates, full-term newborns, and older pediatric patients, the oral route is predominant. Drug absorption through the skin is currently being evaluated for the neonate, in whom the thin dermal layers allow drug absorption. For the acutely ill child and those with vomiting, diarrhea, and impaired GI function, the parenteral route is recommended.

Adverse drug reactions and toxicity: Beside the usual desired routes, there are unintentional portals of drug entry in fetal and pediatric patients; eg, transplacentally, or via breast milk; by inadvertent direct fetal injection; and pulmonary, skin, or conjunctival entry. Underestimation of the degree of drug entry through these routes, and lack of awareness of the altered drug disposition and metabolism have led to therapeutic tragedies. Maturation of metabolic factors is also important; eg, failure to recognize the deficient glucuronyl transferase activities in the newborn led to the **gray baby or toddler syndrome** characterized by acute cardiovascular collapse due to chloramphenicol toxicity (for a discussion of chloramphenicol, see in Ch. 3). Displacement of bilirubin from the albumin binding sites by sulfa drugs led to **kernicterus** or **bilirubin encephalopathy** in neonates. Dermal absorption of hexachlorophene produced **cystic brain lesions** and **neuropathologic abnormalities** in young infants. Boric acid and aniline dye poisoning also occurred from unexpected absorption of these agents from the diapers.

Drug toxicities usually are exaggerations of the known pharmacologic effects of a drug as observed with overdosage (eg, cardiac arrhythmias with overdosage of cardiac glycosides). However, host factors such as **hypersensitivity** or **genetic abnormalities** (eg, G6PD deficiency) may predispose the patient to adverse drug reactions (see Ch. 277). Withdrawal of the offending drug generally results in disappearance of the adverse drug reaction. Management of persistent toxic reactions depends on the specific drug involved.

COMPLIANCE

Research has documented disturbingly low levels of compliance; eg, among children put on a 10-day course of penicillin for streptococcal infections, 56% were found not to be receiving the medicine by the 3rd day; 71% were noncompliant by the 6th day; only 18% were receiving the medicine by the 9th day. Noncompliance in pediatric settings ranges between 50 to 75%, with even higher levels in the case of chronic conditions (eg, juvenile diabetes, asthma) requiring complex regimens of long duration, and that alter existing behavior patterns.

The probability of poor compliance cannot be assessed on the basis of general characteristics or sociodemographic data, but requires specific efforts by the physician to assess levels of adherence. Each situation is unique and *every* parent must be viewed as a *potential* noncomplier. Some major factors contributing to noncompliance, and strategies that are helpful in improving compliance will be discussed (see also Ch. 278).

1. Uncertainty concerning physician instructions. Some parents do not clearly understand what is expected of them, partly because of poor recall of information. Patient recall decreases rapidly: 15 min after meeting with the physician, about 1/2 the infor

mation is forgotten. Also, patients recall best what occurred during the first 1/3 of the discussion, and more is remembered about the diagnosis than about the details of the prescribed therapy.

Strategies: The physician describes the regimen details orally, writes them down, and reviews the written instructions again. The importance and details of the regimen are emphasized. Technical information about the disease, action of the medication, etc are avoided (such information usually does *not* increase compliance). These instructions are given early in the discussion, and common medical terms not generally understood are avoided (eg, void, incubation period, workup, prn).

2. Complicated regimens. Compliance levels decrease when the regimen is complex, inconvenient, expensive, or of long duration, or requires alterations in life style.

Strategies: The regimen is kept as simple as possible, by reducing the number of different medications, the number of doses, and variations in scheduling. If clinically appropriate, larger, less frequent doses, and preparations that combine several drugs or provide more sustained action are used; doses are synchronized when more than one medication is required. Routine prescribing of additional nonessential medications (eg, OTC cough and cold preparations, decongestants, vitamins) is avoided and critical aspects of the treatment plan are emphasized (eg, giving the antibiotic regularly for the full course of the regimen). In unavoidably complex regimens, the treatment plan might be divided into less complex stages to be implemented sequentially (eg, gradually increasing urine-testing frequency for diabetes patients). Matching the regimen schedule to the parent's/patient's regular daily activities minimizes both inconvenience and forgetfulness.

Scheduling follow-up visits or phone calls in quick succession (eg, 3 to 4 days) can demonstrate progress or identify problems, offers an illusion of short-term therapy, and provides motivation for adherence and opportunity for suggestions to overcome difficulties or concerns about the therapy. If lifestyle must be modified (eg, changes in diet or exercise), changes should be introduced one at a time over the course of several visits. Realistic goals should be set (eg, if the child should lose 30 lb, a target is set to lose 2 lb by a 2-wk follow-up visit). Good compliance should be reinforced with praise, and only then should the next objective be added. The cost of the regimen may be reduced by prescribing generically, and by avoiding unnecessary and OTC prescribing.

3. Obstructive health beliefs. Parental health beliefs and attitudes, often based on prior incorrect knowledge about, or experience with, the illness or regimen, lead the parent to decide not to follow some or all of the physician's recommendations.

Strategies: The patient's or parents' beliefs must be elicited by specific questions and often can be altered. The physician should ask if the parent (a) agrees with the diagnosis; (b) perceives the condition (or its sequelae) as serious; (c) feels the recommended treatment will work; (d) fears regimen side effects; and (e) believes the regimen will be difficult to follow.

The parent may possess powerful, well-defined (although scientifically erroneous) health beliefs that conflict with the assessment and diagnosis ("My child can't have the flu because he's had it before and you don't get that twice—it's like measles"). Such beliefs have multiple origins, including cultural standards, handed-down family beliefs, prior illness experience, misinterpretation of factual information, and acceptance of erroneous information from nonmedical sources.

The physician should encourage parents to discuss concerns about the diagnosis or the treatment plan. If it is determined that certain beliefs may contribute to noncompliance, corrective factual information is provided. Effective persuasion may require appeals to feelings of responsibility or support from what the parent perceives to be a more credible source (eg, other parents whose children were successfully treated with the same regimen).

4. Troubled physician-parent interaction. Parental dissatisfaction with the amount of information and emotional support obtained from the physician, inability to express concerns, difficulty in understanding responses to their questions, and unfulfilled expectations for the visit are associated with negative outcomes for children (eg, failure to keep follow-up appointments, lack of problem resolution, and noncompliance). **Strategies:** Correcting these problems requires that the physician recognize their existence. This means that privacy and adequate time must be provided for discussion and that the physician be secure and sensitive enough to encourage parents to express their expectations, concerns, misconceptions, and complaints. Compliance will improve when the parent perceives that sincere concern and sympathy have been shown and when *responsive* information about the condition and progress is provided.

Other strategies: Although physicians are becoming aware that noncompliance is a significant problem, surprisingly little **monitoring of regimen adherence** is performed. Poor adherence should always be considered as a possible explanation for inability to achieve the desired therapeutic goal, and should be ruled out before starting other diagnostic/treatment efforts. **Utilizing other health care providers** can be beneficial. **Nurses** and **pharmacists** can execute most of the strategies described above. They can provide verbal and written reinforcement of regimen information; send telephone or mailed reminders at the time the patient's supply of the medication would be running out; issue written instructions concerning special precautions to be taken with various types of drugs; and maintain a patient medication profile, to aid in preventing overdose, allergic reactions, and adverse drug interactions, and also serve as a mechanism to monitor compliance.

185. FLUID AND ELECTROLYTE DISORDERS IN INFANTS AND CHILDREN

Dehydration, usually due to diarrhea, remains a major cause of morbidity and mortality in infants and children worldwide. Too much fluid and electrolyte may be as devastating as too little in seriously ill pediatric patients with cerebral edema, with impairment of renal or circulatory function, or with immature organ systems (eg, premature infants). In general, the younger the child, the more careful the calculations of fluid and electrolyte requirements must be.

The young infant is compromised by being unable to communicate thirst or seek fluid. In addition, the infant has a relatively large obligatory evaporative loss of fluid; this is in part due to the high ratio of BSA to volume. The infant's metabolic rate is 2 to 3 times that of the adult when expressed per unit of body weight; heat generated by metabolic activity must be dissipated (largely through evaporation), and solute products must be excreted (largely in the urine). The net result is a more rapid turnover of body fluids in the infant than in the adult and less margin for error in calculating fluid and electrolyte needs.

In the clinical management of infants and children with fluid and electrolyte disorders, complete precision is impossible; nevertheless, sufficient accuracy can usually be attained to restore and maintain normal balance and to avoid serious complications. Attention to basic principles, a commitment to monitor progress carefully, and experience are required. Situations that demand particular attention to detail are those in which organ function (especially skin, heart, brain, or kidney) is critically compromised.

Fluid and electrolyte problems are most easily approached by considering separately the **deficit, maintenance,** and **ongoing losses** and by calculating first the **amount** of fluid required, then its **composition** (electrolytes)—see TABLE 185-1—and, finally,

TABLE 185–1. APPROACH TO FLUID AND ELECTROLYTE PROBLEMS

Problem	*Amount (Fluid)*	*Composition (Electrolyte)*
Deficit	Short-term weight change Clinical estimate (TABLE 185–2)	TABLE 185–3
Maintenance	Calculate by either surface area method OR caloric methods	TABLE 185–6
Ongoing loss	Measure	TABLE 185–7 or Measure

the **rate of replacement**. In this way, even complex problems can be dissected and are not as overwhelming as they first may appear.

Deficit

Deficit refers to *the losses incurred prior to beginning corrective measures.*

The **amount** can best be determined directly from changes in body weight when such information is available. An acceptable presumption is that a short-term weight loss in excess of 1% body weight/day represents a fluid deficit. When the child's prior weight is unknown, a clinical estimate of fluid loss must be used, although there are shortcomings and pitfalls in this method (see TABLE 185–2).

The **composition** of fluid required to replace a deficit depends on (1) the duration of the loss, (2) the nature of fluid lost, and (3) present serum electrolyte concentrations. If the loss is hyperacute, ie, minutes to a few hours, the composition is essentially that of serum. In the usual situation, however, dehydration develops over 2 to 3 days, and there is more time for equilibration between extracellular fluid **(ECF)** and intracellular

TABLE 185–2. CLINICAL ESTIMATE OF THE SEVERITY OF DEHYDRATION

*Infant EWL**	*Infant mL/Kg*	*Adolescent EWL**	*Adolescent mL/Kg*	*Severity of Dehydration*	*Clinical Data*	*Problems in Assessment*
5%	50	3%	30	Mild	Dry mucous membranes	Oral mucosa may be dry in chronic mouth-breathers
					Oliguria	Frequency of urination may be unknown in infantile diarrhea, especially in girls
10%	100	5%	50	Moderate	Marked oliguria	As for oliguria, above
					Poor skin turgor	Affected by serum Na concentration ([Na])**
					Sunken fontanel	Infants only
					Tachycardia	Affected by fever, [Na],** underlying disease
15%	150	7%	70	Severe	Hypotension	Affected by [Na],** underlying disease
					Poor perfusion	Affected by [Na],** underlying disease

* EWL = Estimated Weight Loss.
** [Na] > 150 mEq/L gives falsely low estimate of severity; [Na] < 130 mEq/L exaggerates clinical estimate of severity.

TABLE 185–3. USUAL DEFICITS OF ELECTROLYTES BY CAUSE OF DEHYDRATION (mEq/L)

Cause	*Sodium*	*Potassium*
Fasting and thirsting	50	10
Diarrhea		
Isotonic dehydration	80	80
Hypotonic dehydration	100	80
Hypertonic dehydration	20	10
Pyloric stenosis	80	100
Diabetic ketoacidosis	80	50

fluid **(ICF)**; thus, less sodium and more potassium are required. TABLE 185–3 presents approximate concentrations of electrolytes to replace deficit losses in the most frequently encountered clinical situations leading to dehydration.

The patient's current serum electrolyte concentrations (and in particular the **sodium** concentration) guide the selection of fluid composition after initial "resuscitation" of the circulation (see also HYPO- and HYPERNATREMIA under REGULATION OF WATER AND SODIUM HOMEOSTASIS in Ch. 84). Abnormalities of serum sodium concentration also affect the clinical estimation of the severity of dehydration (see TABLE 185–2).

The rate at which the deficit is replaced depends on the severity of dehydration and the rate of fluid loss. In general, when signs of circulatory compromise exist, 20 mL/kg of ECF-like fluid (eg, Ringer's lactate, isotonic saline) is infused IV over 30 to 60 min to restore adequate perfusion—the "resuscitative phase." If the circulation does not improve satisfactorily, more ECF-like fluid or 10 mL/kg of a colloid (eg, plasma; plasma protein fraction, human; blood) is infused rapidly; the need for this additional resuscitative measure must alert the physician to anticipate the many possible complications and sequelae of acute shock (see Ch. 26). The remainder of the deficit can be replaced over 8, 12, 24, or 48 h, depending on the patient's apparent need for volume and on practical considerations. If serum electrolyte concentrations were abnormal initially, the post-resuscitative phase of the deficit replacement must be tailored accordingly.

Maintenance

Fluids are required to maintain homeostasis, to dissipate the heat generated by metabolic activity, and to excrete the solute products of cellular metabolism. Evaporative losses from the skin and respiratory tract (in a ratio of 2:1) account for about 50% of maintenance fluid needs. The other 50% is provided for urine formation, to permit excretion of solute in urine that is neither concentrated nor dilute (ie, 300 mOsm/L, sp gr about 1.010).

The **amount** of maintenance fluid required depends on metabolic rate and thus bears a complex relationship to weight: the younger the child, the greater the metabolic activity/kg body wt (50 kcal/kg for newborn, 26 to 28 cal/kg for adult). Thus, the amount of fluid for maintenance needs cannot be determined directly from body weight with the same ease as deficit needs can be.

Three systems for estimating the amount of maintenance fluid required are currently in wide use: one is based on body surface area, the others on caloric expenditure. Surface area, like metabolic rate, is not a linear function of weight and requires the use of a table or nomogram (see FIG. 185–1). The advantage of this system is the convenience of a single number to remember: maintenance needs for individuals of all ages are about 1500 to 2000 mL/sq m/day.

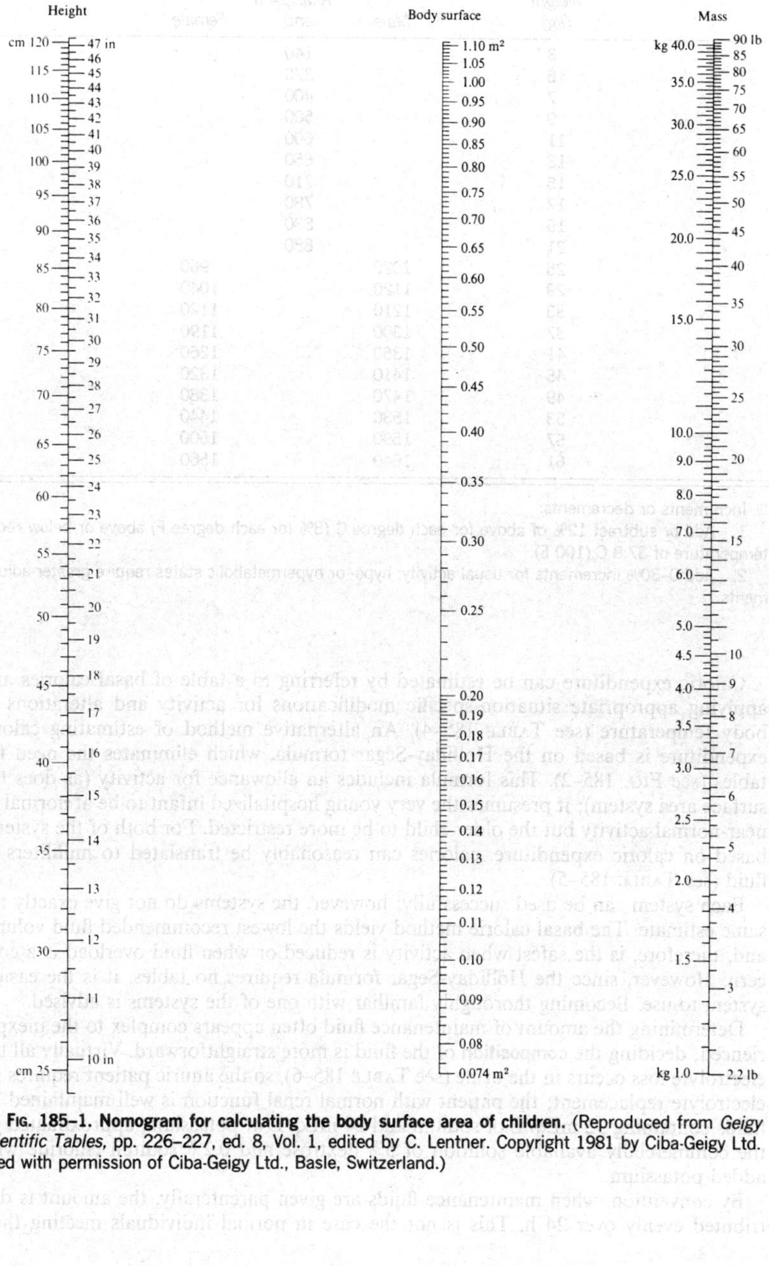

FIG. 185–1. Nomogram for calculating the body surface area of children. (Reproduced from *Geigy Scientific Tables*, pp. 226–227, ed. 8, Vol. 1, edited by C. Lentner. Copyright 1981 by Ciba-Geigy Ltd. Used with permission of Ciba-Geigy Ltd., Basle, Switzerland.)

TABLE 185–4. STANDARD BASAL METABOLIC RATES

Weight (kg)	Male	Kcal/24 h and	Female
3		140	
5		270	
7		400	
9		500	
11		600	
13		650	
15		710	
17		780	
19		830	
21		880	
25	1020		960
29	1120		1040
33	1210		1120
37	1300		1190
41	1350		1260
45	1410		1320
49	1470		1380
53	1530		1440
57	1590		1500
61	1640		1560

Increments or decrements:

1. Add or subtract 12% of above for each degree C (8% for each degree F) above or below rectal temperature of 37.8 C (100 F).
2. Add 0–30% increments for usual activity; hypo- or hypermetabolic states require greater adjustments.

Caloric expenditure can be estimated by referring to a table of basal calories and applying appropriate situation-specific modifications for activity and alterations in body temperature (see TABLE 185–4). An alternative method of estimating caloric expenditure is based on the Holliday-Segar formula, which eliminates the need for tables (see FIG. 185–2). This formula includes an allowance for activity (as does the surface area system); it presumes the very young hospitalized infant to be at normal or near-normal activity but the older child to be more restricted. For both of the systems based on caloric expenditure, calories can reasonably be translated to milliliters of fluid (see TABLE 185–5).

Each system can be used successfully; however, the systems do not give exactly the same estimate. The basal calorie method yields the lowest recommended fluid volume and, therefore, is the safest when activity is reduced or when fluid overload is a concern. However, since the Holliday-Segar formula requires no tables, it is the easiest system to use. Becoming thoroughly familiar with one of the systems is advised.

Determining the amount of maintenance fluid often appears complex to the inexperienced; deciding the **composition** of the fluid is more straightforward. Virtually all the electrolyte loss occurs in the urine (see TABLE 185–6), so the anuric patient requires no electrolyte replacement; the patient with normal renal function is well maintained by fluids containing 32 mEq/L of sodium and 24 mEq/L of potassium, approximated by the commercially available solution of 5% dextrose and 0.2% sodium chloride with added potassium.

By convention, when maintenance fluids are given parenterally, the amount is distributed evenly over 24 h. This is not the case in normal individuals meeting their

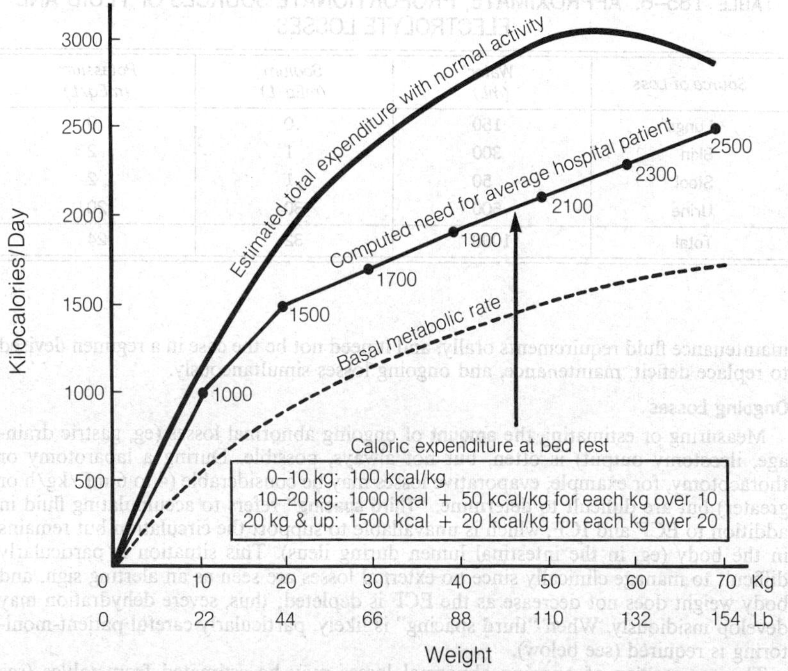

Fig. 185–2. Estimated caloric expenditures under basal conditions ***(bottom curve),*** **under conditions of bed rest** *(middle curve),* **and under conditions of full activity** *(top curve).* The middle curve can be divided into 3 segments according to slope: from 0 to 10 kg = 100 kcal/kg; from 10 to 20 kg = 50 kcal/kg; > 20 kg = 20 kcal/kg. These slopes can be used to formulate reasonable estimates of caloric expenditure for maintenance fluid therapy without use of a graph. Thus, estimated caloric expenditure for a 23-kg child = (100 kcal/kg × first 10 kg) + (50 kcal/kg × next 10 kg) + 20 kcal/kg × last 3 kg) = 1560 kcal. (From "The Maintenance Need for Water in Parenteral Fluid Therapy" by M. A. Holliday and W. E. Segar, in *Pediatrics,* 19:823, 1957. Copyright American Academy of Pediatrics 1957. Used with permission of *Pediatrics.*)

Table 185–5. THE RELATIONSHIP BETWEEN CALORIC EXPENDITURE AND MAINTENANCE FLUID REQUIREMENTS

Source of Water Loss	*Usual Losses (mL H_2O/100 kcal metabolized)*
Lungs	15–20
Skin	30–40
Stool	5
Urine	55–65
Total	115
Water generated Metabolism ($CH_2O + O_2 \rightarrow H_2O + CO_2$)	−15
Net	100

TABLE 185–6. APPROXIMATE, PROPORTIONATE SOURCES OF FLUID AND ELECTROLYTE LOSSES

Source of Loss	*Water (mL)*	*Sodium (mEq/L)*	*Potassium (mEq/L)*
Lungs	150	0	0
Skin	300	1	2
Stool	50	1	2
Urine	500	30	20
Total	1000	32	24

maintenance fluid requirements orally, and it need not be the case in a regimen devised to replace deficit, maintenance, and ongoing losses simultaneously.

Ongoing Losses

Measuring or estimating the **amount** of ongoing abnormal losses (eg, gastric drainage, ileostomy output) is often, but not always, possible. During a laparotomy or thoracotomy, for example, evaporative losses may be considerable (4 to 6 mL/kg/h or greater) but are difficult to determine. **"Third spacing"** refers to accumulating fluid in addition to ECF and ICF, which is unavailable to support the circulation but remains in the body (eg, in the intestinal lumen during ileus). This situation is particularly difficult to manage clinically since no external losses are seen as an alerting sign, and body weight does not decrease as the ECF is depleted; thus, severe dehydration may develop insidiously. When "third spacing" is likely, particularly careful patient-monitoring is required (see below).

The **composition** of ongoing abnormal losses may be estimated from tables (see TABLE 185–7), but it is wise to chemically analyze the fluid if the amount is large or the loss is expected to continue for several days.

The easiest method for delivering fluid and electrolytes to replace ongoing losses is by adding them to the already instituted infusion of maintenance and/or deficit fluids ("piggy-back"); this obviates the need for mixing special solutions and permits flexibility in the replacement schedule.

TABLE 185–7. APPROXIMATE COMPOSITION OF EXTERNAL ABNORMAL LOSSES (mEq/L)

Fluid	*Sodium*	*Potassium*	*Chloride*
Gastric	20–80	5–20	100–150
Pancreatic	120–140	5–15	40–80
Small intestine	100–140	5–15	90–130
Bile	120–140	5–15	80–120
Ileostomy	45–135	3–15	20–115
Diarrheal	10–90	10–80	10–110
Sweat			
Normal	10–30	3–10	10–35
Cystic fibrosis	50–130	5–25	50–110
Burns	140	5	110

Gains

Not all fluid and electrolyte problems are those of deficits and losses; some result from **overhydration** (particularly when there is disordered renal or cardiac function), or excessive electrolyte administration, or both. It is important to be alert to additional sources of fluid and electrolytes, such as the diluent used to reconstitute medications, eg, Sterile Water for Injection or Sodium Chloride Injection.

The principles used for restoring homeostasis in dehydration can, with some modification, be applied to problems of excess: fluid amounts and compositions are estimated, and the appropriate restrictions on intake are applied.

Monitoring

All of the guidelines discussed are approximations and in no way obviate the need for careful monitoring of the patient. Unfortunately, there is no single, simple sign or test that infallibly reflects fluid and electrolyte balance; 10 measures are listed in TABLE 185–8 in rough order of practical value, considering degree of ease, availability, invasiveness, time to perform, and cost. Frequency of monitoring must be individualized, depending on the present severity of the disorder and the potential rate of change. Once daily is rarely sufficient.

Practical Example

An infant has diarrhea for 3 days with weight loss of 1 kg (from 10 kg to 9 kg). Clinical findings support the estimate of 10% fluid deficit—dry mucous membranes, poor skin turgor, markedly decreased urine output, and tachycardia, but BP is normal and adequate peripheral perfusion is shown by compression-release of the nail beds. Serum sodium is 136 mEq/L; potassium, 4 mEq/L; chloride, 104 mEq/L; and bicarbonate, 20 mEq/L.

TABLE 185–8. SIGNS AND TESTS TO MONITOR STATE OF HYDRATION

Sign or Test	*Problem*
1. Physical signs of dehydration (see TABLE 185–2)	May be deceiving if [Na] abnormal; may be influenced by fever (esp. pulse); etc. (see TABLE 185–2)
2. Body weight	Can be fooled by "third spacing"
3. Urine volume	Low output may represent the syndrome of inappropriate antidiuretic hormone (SIADH), dehydration, or renal failure
4. Urine specific gravity	Concentrating ability of infant kidney limited; high sp gr may indicate dehydration, SIADH, or renal failure; low sp gr may indicate good hydration, pyelonephritis, or acute tubular necrosis
5. Intake and output with direct measure of all losses (and gains)	Must estimate maintenance; cannot measure "third space" loss
6. Urea nitrogen (SUN, BUN)	GFR severely reduced before urea nitrogen rises; elevated by blood in GI tract; infant normally lower than adult; need creatinine to differentiate dehydration from renal disease
7. Hematocrit	Useful serially, but not as single value; much less helpful if patient is actively bleeding
8. TSS (total serum solids) or TSP (total serum protein)	Good serially in same patient but not as single value
9. Concurrent serum & urine osmolalities	Good for detecting SIADH problem
10. Serum electrolyte concentrations	By themselves, say little about state of hydration

Calculations

Deficit

Amount (from TABLE 185–2): 1 L

Composition (Electrolyte losses from TABLE 185–3: Diarrhea-isotonic): 80 mEq of sodium, 80 mEq of potassium

Maintenance

Amount:

Surface area method: 0.47 sq m × 1500 to 2000 mL/sq m/day = 705 to 940 mL/day

Basal calorie method: 550 basal kilocalories + 20% for activity = 660 kcal ∼ 660 mL/day

Holliday-Segar formula: 100 kcal/kg × 10 kg = 1000 kcal ∼ 1000 mL/day

Composition: 5% dextrose and 0.2% sodium chloride + 20 mEq/L of potassium acetate

Ongoing losses

Amount: to be determined as course progresses

Procedure

Resuscitative portion of deficit

Ringer's lactate at 20 mL/kg × 1 h

Amount: 20 mL/kg × 10 kg = 200 mL

Composition: 130 mEq/L of sodium; 4 mEq/L of potassium

Remainder of deficit

Amount: 1000 mL (total deficit) − 200 mL (already given) = 800 mL

Composition of sodium: 80 mEq (deficit) − 26 mEq (given in the Ringer's lactate) = 54 mEq. The 54 mEq in 800 mL is a concentration of 68 mEq/L and approximates the sodium content of commercially available 5% dextrose and 0.45% sodium chloride (77 mEq/L).

Rate: arbitrary; let us choose 100 mL/h × 8 h

Maintenance

Amount: 660 to 1000 mL

Composition of sodium: 5% dextrose and 0.2% sodium chloride

Rate: If begun after deficit replacement, then the first day requirements must be given over 15 rather than 24 h

$$\left(\text{so rate} = \frac{660 \text{ to } 1000}{15} \cong 50 \text{ to } 60 \text{ mL/h}\right).$$

After the first day, the maintenance fluids can be distributed evenly over the full 24-h period

$$\left(\text{rate} = \frac{660 \text{ to } 1000}{24} \cong 30 \text{ to } 40 \text{ mL/h}\right).$$

Ongoing losses

As occur

Summary:

Ringer's lactate, 200 mL/h × 1 h

5% dextrose and 0.45% sodium chloride, 100 mL/h × 8 h

5% dextrose and 0.2% sodium chloride, 50 to 60 mL/h × 15 h

5% dextrose and 0.2% sodium chloride, 30 to 40 mL/h thereafter

Notes

1. Only sodium needs are calculated in this example: the amount and rate of potassium administered is governed by safety, and full replacement is not achieved acutely. Once urine output is assured and it is thus considered safe to administer potassium, 20 to 40 mEq/L is added to the replacement solutions.

2. Sequential replacement of deficit and maintenance fluids is demonstrated in the example; the method is convenient and illustrates the approach presented in the text. Many clinicians prefer to combine deficit and maintenance replacement and to proceed more slowly; that method is equally acceptable and is preferred in hypernatremic dehydration (see below).

HYPERNATREMIA IN INFANTS AND CHILDREN

A serum sodium (Na) concentration > 150 mEq/L. Hypernatremia results from water loss in excess of solute loss **(Hypernatremic dehydration)**, solute overload **(salt poisoning)**, or both. Water loss in excess of solute loss occurs commonly in disorders such as diarrhea, but hypernatremic dehydration only develops when fluid intake is insufficient to offset the loss. Clinical situations of particular concern include those in which intake is compromised and/or the fluid loss is underestimated or overlooked.

Salt poisoning most commonly results from an error in the preparation of infant formula or from the administration of hyperosmolar solutions, and appears less frequently nowadays, presumably due to the introduction of partially and fully preprepared formulas.

As hypernatremia develops, the "extra" sodium does not diffuse into the cell but remains an obligatory extracellular ion; water then leaves the cell and enters the extracellular space in an attempt to reduce the osmolarity of the extracellular fluid. This serves to bolster the intravascular volume—but at the expense of cellular size and function. Intracranial hemorrhage and acute renal tubular necrosis are the major complications.

Because the intravascular volume is preserved, the physical examination provides an underestimate of the degree of dehydration. The presence of doughy skin and subcutaneous tissue (when present) is a suggestive physical sign, as is a dissociation between the severe degree of dehydration (as judged by weight loss and by the state of the mucous membranes) and the relatively mild degree of circulatory compromise. **Diagnosis** is established by measurement of the serum sodium concentration. Additional laboratory findings may include an increase in the BUN, a modest increase in blood glucose, and, if serum potassium is low, a depression in the level of serum calcium.

Treatment is designed to avoid a rapid fall in serum osmolality, since the osmotic gradient favoring movement of water into cells may cause cerebral edema. Correction of hypernatremia should be extended over 2 to 3 days (48 to 72 h). The fluid *volume* administered is the sum of the estimated deficit and 2 to 3 days of maintenance requirements; this total amount is divided by 48 to 72 to determine the hourly volume and is given at a constant *rate* over the 48 to 72 h of correction. The *composition* of the fluid is 5% dextrose with approximately 70 mEq/L of cation. Initially the cation is sodium; once evidence of adequate urine output is demonstrated, the cation should be sodium and potassium in approximately equal amounts. Extreme hypernatremia (sodium > 200 mEq/L) caused by salt poisoning should be treated by peritoneal dialysis.

Prophylaxis requires attention to the volume and composition of unusual fluid losses and of solutions used to maintain homeostasis. In newborns and young infants, who are unable to signal thirst effectively and to replace losses voluntarily, the opportunity

for dehydration is greatest; factors which increase radiant heat loss (including warmers and phototherapy lights) raise the risk of hypernatremia. The composition of feedings whenever mixing is involved (eg, some infant formulas, concentrated preparations for tube feeding) requires particular attention, especially when the potential for developing dehydration is high, such as during episodes of diarrhea, poor fluid intake, vomiting, or high fever.

---

186. DISTURBANCES IN NEWBORNS AND INFANTS

GESTATIONAL AGE AND BIRTH WEIGHT

CLASSIFICATION

Each newborn is classified as premature, full-term, or postmature. This permits anticipation of clinical problems, since the level of organ system maturation is primarily determined by gestational age. The neonate is also classified as large, appropriate, or small for gestational age. The fetal growth rate may be altered by genetic factors and by abnormal intrauterine states, which can also predispose the infant to perinatal problems. Each infant's intrauterine growth status should be determined at birth by plotting his weight for gestational age (see FIG. 186–1). FIG. 182–1 in INITIAL CARE also deals with gestational age assessment.

PREMATURE INFANT

Any infant born before 37 wk gestation. Previously, any infant weighing < 2.5 kg (5.5 lb) was termed premature; this definition was inappropriate, since many newborns weighing < 2.5 kg are actually mature or postmature but small for gestational age **(SGA)** and have a different appearance and different problems than do premature infants.

Etiology

In most cases, the cause of premature labor or premature rupture of the membranes followed by premature labor is unknown. However, the histories of women having premature deliveries commonly show low socioeconomic status, lack of prenatal medical care, poor nutrition, poor education, unwed state, and intercurrent, untreated illness or infection. There has often been inadequate prenatal care. Since premature birth and its related problems are the greatest causes of neonatal morbidity and mortality, the underlying etiologies and methods of prevention must be found. The use of drugs to arrest premature labor and to hasten maturation of the fetal lungs if premature delivery is likely is discussed in Ch. 179.

Signs

The premature infant is small, usually weighs < 2.5 kg, and tends to have thin, shiny, pink skin through which the underlying veins are easily seen. Little subcutaneous fat, hair, or external ear cartilage exists. Spontaneous activity and tone are less in premature infants, and their extremities are not held in a flexed position. In males the scrotum may have few rugae and the testes may be undescended. In females the labia majora do not yet cover the labia minora.

Problems

Most problems of premature infants relate to the immature functioning of organ systems.

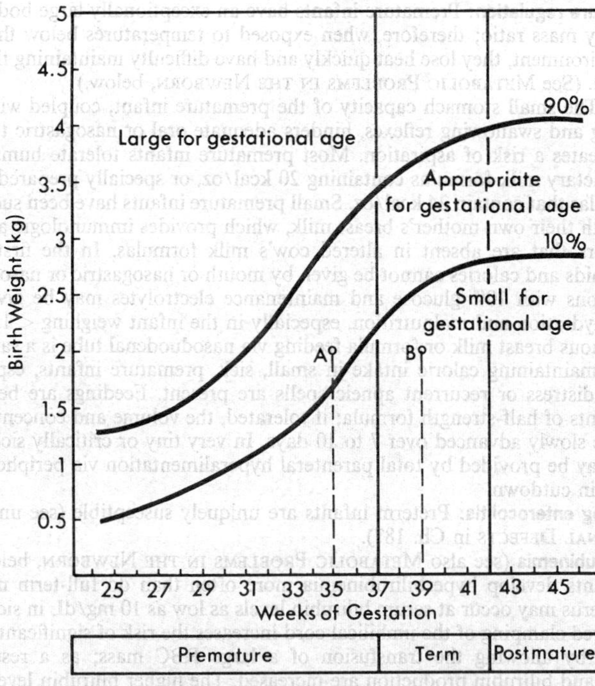

Fig. 186–1. Level of intrauterine growth based on birth weight and gestational age of liveborn, single, white infants. Point A represents a premature infant, while point B indicates an infant of similar birth weight, who is mature but small for gestational age; the growth curves are representative of the 10th and 90th percentiles for all of the newborns in the sampling. (Adapted from "Classification of the Low-Birth-Weight Infant" by A. Y. Sweet, in *Care of the High-Risk Neonate,* ed. 2, 1979, by M. H. Klaus and A. A. Fanaroff. Copyright 1979 by W. B. Saunders Company. Used with permission.)

Lungs: In many premature infants, surfactant production is not adequate to prevent alveolar collapse and atelectasis, which results in the respiratory distress syndrome (**RDS**—see under Respiratory Disorders, below).

CNS: Inadequate sucking and swallowing reflexes in the infant born before 34 wk gestation may require that the infant be fed IV or by gavage. Immaturity of the respiratory center in the brainstem results in periodic breathing and apneic spells (see Premature Apnea under Respiratory Disorders, below). Apnea may also result from nasopharyngeal and soft palate obstruction ("obstructive apnea"). The periventricular germinal matrix (see Birth Trauma, below) is prone to hemorrhage in preterm infants, and this hemorrhage may extend into the cerebral ventricles **(intraventricular hemorrhage)**. Hemorrhagic infarction of the periventricular white matter may also occur in premature infants, but the reasons for this are not understood. Hypotension, inadequate or erratic brain perfusion, and BP peaks (as when fluid or colloid is given rapidly IV) may all contribute to cerebral injury or hemorrhage.

Infection: The risk of developing sepsis or meningitis is about 4 times greater in the premature infant than in the full-term newborn. (See Neonatal Infections in Ch. 186; and Immunologic Status in Ch. 182.)

Temperature regulation: Premature infants have an exceptionally large body surface area to body mass ratio; therefore, when exposed to temperatures below the neutral thermal environment, they lose heat quickly and have difficulty maintaining their body temperature. (See METABOLIC PROBLEMS IN THE NEWBORN, below.)

GI tract: The small stomach capacity of the premature infant, coupled with immature sucking and swallowing reflexes, hinders adequate oral or nasogastric tube feedings and creates a risk of aspiration. Most premature infants tolerate human breast milk, proprietary milk formulas containing 20 kcal/oz, or specially prepared "premature" formulas that contain 24 kcal/oz. Small premature infants have been successfully tube-fed with their own mother's breast milk, which provides immunologic and nutritional factors that are absent in altered cow's milk formulas. In the first days, if adequate fluids and calories cannot be given by mouth or nasogastric or nasoduodenal tube, solutions with 10% glucose and maintenance electrolytes may be given IV to prevent dehydration and malnutrition, especially in the infant weighing < 1.5 kg (3.3 lb). Continuous breast milk or formula feeding via nasoduodenal tube is a satisfactory method of maintaining caloric intake in small, sick, premature infants, especially if respiratory distress or recurrent apneic spells are present. Feedings are begun with small amounts of half-strength formula; if tolerated, the volume and concentration of feedings are slowly advanced over 7 to 10 days. In very tiny or critically sick infants, nutrition may be provided by total parenteral hyperalimentation via peripheral IV or a central vein cutdown.

Necrotizing enterocolitis: Preterm infants are uniquely susceptible (see under GASTROINTESTINAL DEFECTS in Ch. 187).

Hyperbilirubinemia (see also METABOLIC PROBLEMS IN THE NEWBORN, below): Premature infants develop hyperbilirubinemia more often than do full-term newborns, and kernicterus may occur at serum bilirubin levels as low as 10 mg/dL in sick prematures. Delayed clamping of the umbilical cord increases the risk of significant hyperbilirubinemia by allowing the transfusion of a large RBC mass; as a result, RBC breakdown and bilirubin production are increased. The higher bilirubin levels in premature infants may be partially due to inadequately developed hepatic mechanisms for excreting bilirubin, including deficiencies in the uptake of bilirubin from the serum, in its conjugation to bilirubin diglucuronide in the liver, and in its excretion into the biliary tree. In addition, decreased bowel motility enables more bilirubin diglucuronide to be deconjugated within the intestinal lumen by the enzyme β-glucuronidase before excretion, permitting increased reabsorption of free bilirubin (enterohepatic circulation of bilirubin). Early feedings can significantly decrease the incidence and severity of physiologic jaundice by increasing bowel motility, thus interrupting the enterohepatic circulation of bilirubin as the bilirubin is excreted in the stools.

Hypo- and hyperglycemia: See METABOLIC PROBLEMS IN THE NEWBORN, below.

Kidney: Renal function is immature, so that concentration or dilution of urine is less effective than in the full-term infant. The inability of the immature kidney to excrete fixed acids, which accumulate with high-protein formula feedings and as a result of bone growth, may cause metabolic acidosis (late metabolic acidosis of the premature) and resultant growth retardation. Late metabolic acidosis is easily treated with oral sodium bicarbonate; and although the amount given depends on the severity of acidosis, 1 to 2 mEq/kg/day in 4 to 6 divided doses is often adequate and may need to be continued for several days. Reduction of the protein content of the formula may also be necessary.

RETINOPATHY OF PREMATURITY
(Retrolental Fibroplasia)

A bilateral disorder characterized by abnormal peripheral retinal vessels that occurs mainly in premature infants in whom the immature retinal vascular bed was exposed to

high postnatal incubator O_2 concentrations. Rarely, the condition has also been noted in premature infants not exposed to excess O_2. Immature retinal vessels are especially sensitive to O_2, but the exact level or duration of arterial PO_2 that results in injury is unknown. Considerable individual variation in susceptibility is likely. Affected infants usually weigh < 1500 gm at birth. Controversy exists about the exact pathogenetic mechanism for the condition; however, the insult affects primarily the temporal retina and its developing retinal vascular bed. An abnormal ridge of vascular tissue forms between the vascularized and nonvascularized temporal retina. If severe, the neovascularization invades the vitreous and may cause retinal detachment. If mild, the abnormal vessels may regress spontaneously. Delayed cicatricial changes occur in some during the lst yr of life, resulting in dragging of the retinal vessels and macula into a temporal retinal fold. Myopia is a common finding. Other associated problems include glaucoma, retinal detachment (which can occur even in later life), and mental retardation.

Prevention and Treatment

Careful monitoring of incubator O_2 is needed. The lowest concentration necessary to prevent hypoxic brain injury should be used. The ocular danger increases with $O_2 > 30\%$. Vitamin E administration is said to reduce the incidence of retinopathy of prematurity, but is experimental at this time. Recent data suggest that the bright lighting of neonatal intensive care nurseries, which is usually maintained around the clock, may be detrimental and that efforts be made to reduce the intensity of such lighting. Once retinopathy has developed, cryosurgical therapy to the retina may be useful. Patients should be closely monitored by an ophthalmologist.

POSTMATURE INFANT

Any infant born after 42 wk gestation.

Etiology

The cause of postmature delivery generally is unknown. Very rarely, abnormalities of the fetal pituitary–adrenal axis (eg, anencephaly or adrenal agenesis) can result in postmaturity.

Signs

Postmature infants are alert and appear mature, but there is a decreased amount of soft tissue mass, particularly subcutaneous fat; the skin may hang loosely on the extremities and is often dry and peeling. The finger- and toenails are long. The nails and umbilical cord may be meconium-stained if meconium has been passed in utero.

Problems

The main clinical problem encountered is that past term the placenta involutes, and multiple infarcts and villous degeneration produce the **placental insufficiency syndrome**. The fetus may receive inadequate nutrients from the mother, resulting in fetal soft tissue wasting. **Asphyxia** during labor may occur secondary to placental insufficiency (see ASPHYXIA AND RESUSCITATION, below). Postmature infants also are prone to develop the **meconium aspiration syndrome** (see under RESPIRATORY DISORDERS, below), which may be unusually severe since, past term, amniotic fluid volume is decreased and the aspirated meconium is less diluted. Postmature infants are also predisposed to neonatal **hypoglycemia** because of insufficient glycogen stores at birth. This condition is exaggerated if perinatal asphyxia has occurred, during which anaerobic metabolism rapidly utilizes the last of the glycogen stores. Neonatal hypoglycemia is discussed in METABOLIC PROBLEMS IN THE NEWBORN, below.

SMALL-FOR-GESTATIONAL-AGE (SGA) INFANT

(Dysmaturity; Intrauterine Growth Retardation)

Any infant whose weight is below the 10th percentile for gestational age, whether premature, full-term, or postmature. Despite his size, a full-term SGA infant does not have the problems related to organ system immaturity that the premature infant has.

Causes

An infant may be small at birth because of genetic factors (short parents or a genetic disorder associated with short stature) or from other factors that can retard intrauterine growth. These usually are not operative before 32 to 34 wk gestation, and include fetal malnutrition, generally from placental insufficiency that often results from maternal disease involving the small blood vessels (as in preeclampsia, primary hypertension, renal disease, or longstanding diabetes); placental involution accompanying postmaturity; or infectious agents such as cytomegalovirus, rubella virus, or *Toxoplasma gondii*. An infant may be SGA if the mother is a narcotic addict or a heavy user of alcohol and, to a lesser degree, if she smokes cigarettes during pregnancy.

Signs

Despite their small size, SGA infants have physical characteristics and behavior similar to normal-sized infants of like gestational age. Thus, a 1.4-kg infant born between 37 and 42 wk gestation may have the skin, external ear cartilage, sole creases, and genital development of a full-term infant, as well as the neurologic development, alertness, spontaneous activity, and zest for feeding. If the intrauterine growth retardation has been caused by chronic malnutrition, SGA infants may demonstrate "catch-up" growth following delivery if they maintain an adequate caloric intake.

Problems

Birth asphyxia: If intrauterine growth retardation is due to placental insufficiency, the infant will be at risk of asphyxia during labor, since each uterine contraction slows or stops maternal placental perfusion via the spiral arteries. Therefore, when placental insufficiency is suspected, the fetal state should be assessed prior to labor and the fetal heart rate should be monitored during labor. If fetal asphyxia is imminent, rapid delivery, often by cesarean section, is indicated. The SGA infant with asphyxia is likely to have low Apgar scores and mixed acidosis at birth (see ASPHYXIA AND RESUSCITATION, below). Perinatal asphyxia is the greatest problem for these infants, and if it can be avoided, their neurologic prognosis appears to be quite good. Infants who are SGA because of genetic factors, congenital infection, or maternal drug use may not have such a good prognosis.

Meconium aspiration: During birth asphyxia, SGA infants, especially those who are post-term, may pass meconium into the amniotic sac and begin deep gasping movements. The consequent aspiration of meconium is likely to result in meconium aspiration syndrome after delivery (see under RESPIRATORY DISORDERS, below).

Hypoglycemia: The SGA infant is very prone to hypoglycemia in the first hours and days of life because of lack of adequate glycogen stores (see also METABOLIC PROBLEMS IN THE NEWBORN, below.)

LARGE-FOR-GESTATIONAL-AGE (LGA) INFANT

Any infant whose weight is above the 90th percentile for gestational age, whether premature, full-term, or postmature.

Etiology

Other than genetically determined size, the major cause of an infant's being large for gestational age is **maternal diabetes mellitus**.

Signs

The infant of a diabetic mother is generally large, obese, and plethoric; is often listless and limp; and may feed poorly.

Problems

Delivery: Because of the infant's large size, vaginal delivery is often difficult and may be traumatic. Shoulder dystocia, fractures of the clavicles or limbs, and birth asphyxia may occur. Therefore, cesarean section delivery should always be considered when the fetus is thought to be LGA, especially if the mother's pelvic measurements are not adequate.

Hypoglycemia: The infant of a diabetic mother is very likely to become hypoglycemic in the first 1 to 2 h following delivery because of his state of hyperinsulinism and the sudden termination of a glucose infusion from the mother when the umbilical cord is cut. This can be prevented by close prenatal control of the mother's diabetes and by prophylactic use of 10% glucose in water IV in the infant until early frequent feedings can be instituted to provide calories and glucose. The blood glucose should be closely monitored during the transition period. (See also METABOLIC PROBLEMS IN THE NEWBORN, below.)

Hyperbilirubinemia (see also METABOLIC PROBLEMS IN THE NEWBORN): Infants of diabetic mothers frequently develop hyperbilirubinemia because of their intolerance for oral feedings in the first days of life (increased enterohepatic circulation of bilirubin), because of their relatively high Hct (one manifestation of macrosomia; ie, RBC mass), and probably because of other, unknown factors.

Lungs: In infants of diabetic women, pulmonary maturation with production of surfactant may be delayed until late in gestation; therefore, these infants may develop respiratory distress syndrome even if delivered only a few weeks prematurely. Following amniocentesis, the lecithin/sphingomyelin ratio and the presence of phosphatidylglycerol (PG) in the amniotic fluid can be determined to evaluate fetal lung maturity. As a result, the optimal time for safe delivery may be determined.

ASPHYXIA AND RESUSCITATION

(Asphyxia Neonatorum)

A newborn who does not breathe spontaneously or is in shock requires immediate resuscitation to sustain life and minimize the possibility of brain damage. Although instituting ventilation usually is the main concern, rapid correction of hypovolemia to support circulation may be equally critical.

Etiology and Pathophysiology

High-risk pregnancies can be anticipated in about 70% of cases. Newborns are likely to require resuscitation in situations such as premature labor, multiple births, prolapsed umbilical cord, severe maternal bleeding, maternal hypotension, toxemia, or intrauterine growth retardation. During an otherwise apparently uncomplicated labor, the appearance of meconium in amniotic fluid, abnormalities of the fetal heart rate pattern, or a drop in the fetal scalp blood pH to below 7.25 may indicate fetal distress, especially when more than one finding is present.

Perinatal asphyxia may be due to placental or neonatal pulmonary dysfunction. The infant may become asphyxiated before or during labor and may be in a critical state at the moment of delivery, or may become asphyxiated after delivery when effective spontaneous breathing does not begin. Asphyxia in utero may result from severe uteroplacental insufficiency, abruptio placentae, umbilical cord compression, uterine tetany, maternal hypotension, or fetal exsanguination. The newborn may not breathe spontaneously because of prior asphyxiation, because of placental passage of maternal analgesics and anesthetics, or because of malformations (eg, choanal atresia, diaphragmatic

hernia, or hypoplastic lungs). A premature infant with immature lungs and surfactant deficiency may not be able to establish adequate respirations at birth because of low lung compliance.

Asphyxia produces both hypoxemia and hypercapnia. Respiratory acidosis results from CO_2 retention; superimposed metabolic acidosis occurs as tissues are deprived of adequate O_2 and lactic acid accumulates. Secondary effects include a fall in cardiac output **(CO)** with a drop in pulse rate and BP, hypovolemia from pooling of blood in central veins or escape of fluid from the capillary bed damaged by hypoxemia, and CNS depression. Anaerobic glycolysis causes increased use of glycogen stores; therefore, asphyxiated infants, particularly those small for gestational age, are prone to early hypoglycemia.

Clinical Evaluation

The Apgar scoring system (see TABLE 186–1) estimates the severity of respiratory and neurologic depression at birth by rating certain physical signs. Every baby should be rated at exactly 1 and 5 min after birth, and both scores should be recorded. The maximum score of 10 is rare; the lower the score, the more severely depressed is the infant (≤ 5 indicates severe depression). Low scores, particularly at 5 min, are more likely to predict residual neurologic damage or neonatal death, although most infants with low 5 min Apgar scores survive and are normal.

The low Apgar score may be caused by either perinatal asphyxia or respiratory and neurologic depression from transplacental passage of anesthetics given to the mother. An infant with low Apgar scores due to perinatal asphyxia will appear cyanotic or pale and have a slow heart rate and low BP, while a baby depressed by anesthetics is likely to have normal color, heart rate, and BP at birth. A cord-blood pH < 7.20 is a more direct measure of perinatal asphyxia.

Preparations for Effective Resuscitation

Delivery room personnel must be skilled in initiating resuscitation, as the apneic infant cannot wait for a consultant. In high-risk situations, preparations should be made in advance, and trained personnel should be present at the delivery. Personnel must be familiar with the following equipment, which should be simple, dependable, and in working order: sources of O_2 and suction, suction catheters of various sizes, infant airways, an infant resuscitation bag and mask, a laryngoscope with newborn- and premature-size blades (sizes 1 and 0), endotracheal tubes (sizes 2.5, 3, and 3.5 mm), an endotracheal tube stylet, and umbilical catheters (sizes 5 and 8 French). Fluids (eg, 5 or 10% D/W and 5% human serum albumin) should be on hand, as

TABLE 186–1. THE APGAR SCORE

Criteria	Score 0	Score 1	Score 2
Color	Blue; pale	Body pink; extremities blue	All pink
Heart rate	Absent	< 100	> 100
Respiration	Absent	Irregular; slow	Good, crying
Reflex response to nose catheter	None	Grimace	Sneeze, cough
Muscle tone	Limp	Some flexion of extremities	Active

should sodium bicarbonate (see Step 4, below). Basic equipment and drugs (in common doses and dilutions) may be displayed clearly on a pegboard in the delivery room. To maintain the infant's body temperature during evaluation and resuscitation, a radiant heater is essential.

Treatment

Step 1. Airway: The airway must be quickly cleared of secretions, fluid, or blood by gently suctioning the pharynx and nostrils with a soft catheter. Suctioning is limited to 5 to 10 sec, since prolonged vigorous suctioning of the posterior pharynx may cause apnea or bradycardia (by stimulating the vagal reflex).

The well-oxygenated infant who is depressed by anesthetic agents may be stimulated repeatedly (eg, by gently slapping the feet) before other efforts at resuscitation are begun. However, if central cyanosis or bradycardia develops, positive pressure ventilation (see Step 2, below) must begin immediately.

For a neonate who is covered with meconium and depressed, it is essential to intubate the trachea at once; endotracheal suctioning is repeated until the airway is clear of aspirated meconium. An endotracheal tube with the largest possible diameter should be used (a 3.5-mm tube can usually be used for full-term infants, a 3-mm tube for infants < 1.5 kg, and a 2.5-mm tube for infants ≤ 1 kg), so that the largest possible size suction catheter can be inserted. The trachea can then be suctioned further by the mouth-to-endotracheal tube technic (with intervening face mask). To prevent severe anoxia, these procedures must be performed quickly and followed by positive pressure ventilation with O_2, using a bag and an endotracheal tube.

Step 2. Ventilation: Positive pressure ventilation (with 60 to 80% O_2) can usually be effectively and safely provided with bag and mask resuscitation, by placing the infant's head in the neutral position and raising the jaw slightly to ensure an unobstructed airway. So that valuable time is not lost or errors made, only experienced personnel should perform endotracheal intubation. Ventilation rate should be started at about 40/min; its effectiveness is judged by watching chest wall movement (since hearing transmitted breath sounds is not always a reliable indicator of adequate ventilation).

Step 3. Circulation: If the infant does not rapidly become pink with effective positive pressure ventilation, the circulation may be inadequate. If the pulses are thready and capillary refill is poor (> 2 sec), cardiac massage is begun by placing the thumbs over the midsternum with both hands encircling the chest or placing 1 or 2 fingers over the midsternum in the midline and compressing the chest about 100 to 120 times/min about ⅔ the distance to the anterior vertebral column. After 3 or 4 chest compressions, one positive pressure ventilation is given to maintain a respiratory rate of about 40/min. This sequence is repeated smoothly and requires 2 experienced persons. If the heart rate is < 100/min and pulses are thready with low BP and poor skin perfusion, give epinephrine 0.1 to 0.2 mL/kg of a 1:10,000 solution IV. In emergency situations, if IV access is not available, 0.2 mL of a 1:20,000 dilution of epinephrine can be given endotracheally. Following severe asphyxia, dopamine or dobutamine may be required as a continuous IV infusion to maintain CO and perfusion.

Step 4. Fluid and glucose: For the severely asphyxiated infant with a poor CO, rapid infusion of fluid using a plasma expander (eg, 10 mL/kg of either 5% human serum albumin or fresh frozen plasma) will improve circulation and facilitate the distribution and buffering of fixed acids. In emergencies, infusions and sampling of blood are most quickly accomplished through an umbilical vein catheter. Sodium bicarbonate may be needed to correct metabolic acidosis. Whenever possible, the acid-base status should be determined first; otherwise, the infant may be given sodium bicarbonate 2 mEq/kg IV. Sodium bicarbonate comes as a hypertonic solution (44.5 mEq/50 mL) and should be diluted three- to fourfold with sterile water and then infused over 5 to 10 min while

positive pressure ventilation is continued. Since asphyxiated infants are prone to hypoglycemia, the blood glucose levels should be monitored and 10% D/W should be given IV, starting shortly after delivery.

Step 5. Depression secondary to narcotics: If the infant's respiratory depression may be due to narcotics given to the mother, naloxone (a narcotic antagonist) 0.01 mg/kg IV is given. This may need to be repeated several times at 5- to 20-min intervals if the initial response is good, since naloxone has a short half-life compared to narcotics. Naloxone is not indicated for any other type of drug or anesthetic depression in the neonate, as it is an antidote only for narcotics.

Step 6. Temperature: Maintaining the infant's temperature during resuscitation is essential. Cooling may double or triple the infant's basal metabolic rate, thus increasing O_2 requirements. In the face of O_2 lack, severe O_2 debt can ensue rapidly and result in neurologic damage or death. After the infant is dried thoroughly, radiant heating (rather than blankets) is recommended to permit continuous observation of the infant's color and activity.

Sequelae

Infants with significant asphyxia at birth require close observation for evidence of sequelae. Cerebral hypoxia may produce **hypotonia** and **lethargy** or **coma** initially, as well as **convulsions** that may not occur for 1 or 2 days. The premature infant with cerebral hypoxia is more likely to develop **germinal matrix hemorrhages** that can rupture into the lateral ventricles, resulting in **intraventricular hemorrhage** of varying severity. (See also BIRTH TRAUMA, below.) Following asphyxia, fluid intake should be restricted initially (eg, 10% D/W 60 mL/kg/day IV) and q 12 h weight, urine output, and serum electrolytes should be monitored, since **inappropriate ADH secretion** may develop. Also, severe renal hypoxia and hypoperfusion can result in **acute tubular necrosis,** also resulting in fluid retention and hyponatremia. **Ischemia of the bowel wall,** particularly in premature infants, may damage the mucosa and its ability to secrete mucus, which protects against enteric bacterial invasion. Several days later, after milk feedings are begun, **necrotizing enterocolitis,** possibly associated with peritonitis or sepsis, may occur. For this reason, feedings may be delayed for 5 to 7 days in such infants, and nutrition provided as total parenteral nutrition given IV. Meconium-stained, asphyxiated infants may develop **meconium aspiration syndrome** with respiratory distress, pneumomediastinum, and tension pneumothorax.

All organ systems, except the CNS, usually will recover from hypoxic insults. The infant with asphyxia at birth is at risk for long-term residual CNS damage including mental retardation, cerebral palsy, and seizure disorders. Unless damage is proved, being reasonably optimistic and supportive, but honest, will help parents relate positively to their infant. Most infants who have sustained perinatal asphyxia will be normal. Parental attachment is essential for developing the warm, loving, and stimulating home environment that will in large measure ultimately determine the child's mental development.

RESPIRATORY DISORDERS

RESPIRATORY DISTRESS SYNDROME (RDS)
(Hyaline Membrane Disease)

A disorder primarily of prematurity, manifested clinically by respiratory distress and pathologically by pulmonary hyaline membranes and atelectasis.

Etiology

RDS is due to diffuse lung atelectasis that develops when pulmonary surfactants are deficient at birth. The air-fluid interfaces of the water film lining the alveoli exerts large

forces causing the alveoli to collapse if surfactants are lacking. Pulmonary surfactant is manufactured in the Type II alveolar cells and is a mixture of phospholipids and a surfactant apoprotein. (For a discussion, see PERINATAL PHYSIOLOGY in Ch. 182.)

RDS almost always occurs in infants born before 37 wk gestation; the more premature the infant, the greater the chance of developing RDS. RDS is also more likely to develop in infants of diabetic mothers, but is less likely to develop in infants whose mothers have toxemia or hypertension and in infants with signs of fetal growth retardation. Prolonged rupture of the membranes also seems to afford some protection against RDS.

Fetal lung maturity with regard to surfactant production may be assessed before delivery by measuring surfactants in amniotic fluid obtained by amniocentesis or collected from the vagina (if the membranes have ruptured). Fetal lung maturity is shown if the lecithin/sphinogomyelin ratio (L:S ratio) is > 2 and phosphotidyl glycerol is present. Use of this information to choose the optimal time for delivery in a variety of maternal disorders as well as for repeat cesarean section has reduced the incidence of RDS (see Chs. 177 to 179). Also systemic administration of β-methasone to the woman who must be delivered when the fetal lung profile is immature may induce fetal surfactant within 24 h, reducing the risk of RDS (see Chs. 177 to 179).

Symptoms and Signs

The infant with RDS has almost always been born prematurely. A diagnosis of RDS in an infant of ≥ 37 wk gestational age is unusual and should make one suspect that the mother may have had unrecognized diabetes mellitus or that the diagnosis is incorrect (eg, early onset Group B streptococcal pneumonia and sepsis can mimic RDS clinically and radiographically).

The infant will usually develop rapid, labored respirations immediately or within a few hours after delivery. There will be supra- and substernal retractions, nasal alae flaring, and "grunting" retractions. Both the amount of atelectasis and the severity of respiratory failure will increase with time. The lack of surfactant causes lung compliance to be very low and the work of inflating the "stiff" lungs is increased. The premature infant is further handicapped because his ribs are cartilagenous and easily deformed; respiratory effort is wasted in deforming the ribs (substernal retractions). In severe disease, the diaphragms and intercostal muscles fatigue and CO_2 retention and respiratory acidosis develop. Additionally, there is shunting of blood through the atelectatic portions of lung and the infant becomes hypoxemic. Unless adequate O_2 is delivered, metabolic acidosis will supervene. Ultimately, if untreated, severe hypoxemia will result in multiple organ failure and death.

Not all infants with RDS will present with signs of respiratory distress; tiny, very low birth weight infants (eg, < 1000 gm) may be unable to initiate respirations at birth because their lungs are so stiff, and will present with primary apnea in the delivery room. All such infants must be immediately intubated and given positive pressure ventilation.

Premature infants with RDS are at greater risk of intraventricular hemorrhage **(IVH)** and neonatal death. Intracranial pathology (from ischemia and IVH) has been associated with hypoxemia, hypercarbia, hypotension, and swings in arterial BP and cerebral perfusion. Tension pneumothorax, which may occur as a complication of RDS, produces sudden circulatory changes and also may result in reduced cerebral blood flow (see NEONATAL NEUROLOGY under BIRTH TRAUMA and HEMORRHAGIC SHOCK AND ENCEPHALOPATHY in Ch. 186).

Diagnosis

The diagnosis is based on the history (eg, premature labor, maternal diabetes, immature fetal lung profile done on an amniotic fluid sample), physical examination (eg, respiratory distress, cyanosis), and laboratory assessment. Arterial blood gases **(ABG)**

show variable degrees of hypoxemia and hypercarbia. Chest x-ray shows diffuse atelectasis and roughly correlates with the clinical severity of the RDS: **Grade I RDS**: Reticulogranular pattern of the lung parenchyma with aerated areas (black dots) exceeding atelectatic areas (white dots); **Grade II RDS**: Reticulogranular areas of lung parenchyma with white dots (airless, atelectatic lung) in excess of aerated lung; **Grade III RDS**: Same as Grade II plus prominent air bronchograms; and **Grade IV RDS**: Almost total loss of heart borders because of severe diffuse atelectasis.

Once the infant is placed on a respirator, positive pressure inflation of the lung may reduce the extent of the atelectasis. Early onset Group B streptococcal pneumonia and sepsis can masquerade as RDS radiologically as well as clinically.

Treatment and Prognosis

Monitoring: Treatment is proportional to the clinical severity of the disease, and it is important to monitor respiratory and circulatory status closely, so that appropriate support can be provided. An umbilical artery catheter **(UAC)** is usually placed in infants with moderate-to-severe respiratory disease; ie, those who require the percent of inspired O_2 (FIO_2) $\geq$ 40%. If a UAC cannot be inserted, a percutaneous radial artery catheter can be used for continuous BP monitoring and for sampling ABGs.

Transcutaneous monitors that can continuously and noninvasively monitor both transcutaneous O_2 and CO_2 tension (**$TcPO_2$** and **$TcPCO_2$**) make a major contribution to care by reducing the need for blood samples. After transcutaneous monitor values have been correlated with simultaneously obtained arterial samples, they can be used to follow trends in ABGs and ABG responses to changes in ventilator settings. Intermittent blood gas sampling (eg, radial artery punctures or heel sticks) has the disadvantage of causing pain, and may yield results that are different (usually worse) than the infant's true ABG values at rest.

Acceptable PaO_2 in preterm infants is 50 to 70 mm Hg, because these infants have fetal Hb, which is almost fully saturated at these values. Higher PaO_2 may increase the risk of **retinopathy of prematurity,** while delivering very little additional O_2 to tissues.

Normal $PaCO_2$ is 35 to 45 mm Hg. We prefer to maintain the $PaCO_2$ in the low end of this range during the first few days of ventilator therapy. This reduces the infant's gasping and respiratory efforts as the respirator performs the work of breathing. Some data suggest that the variations in systemic BP and cerebral blood flow associated with gasping respirations may increase the risk of intracranial hemorrhage.

Specific treatment is individualized. Infants with mild RDS may do well with supplemental O_2 administered by hood; more severe RDS will respond to administration of continuous positive airway pressure (CPAP) with the infant breathing spontaneously; the sickest infants will require ventilator support. As RDS resolves, usually in 4 to 5 days, the type of support is reduced proportionally: The infant may be weaned from a ventilator, to CPAP, to an O_2 hood.

O_2 hood: O_2 must be mixed with air using a blender and the percent O_2 being delivered must be measured and recorded using an O_2 analyzer. O_2 delivery should never be measured as L/min, since the flow rate tells nothing about how much O_2 the infant is actually inspiring. The O_2 should be warmed (36 to 37 C) and humidified to prevent cooling.

Continuous positive airway pressure (CPAP) is indicated for an infant who requires a $FIO_2 \geq 40\%$ to maintain a normal PaO_2 (50 to 70 mm Hg). It may be started earlier in an infant whose RDS is worsening rapidly. CPAP can be delivered via nasal prongs, nasopharyngeal tube, or an endotracheal tube. It delivers an O_2 mixture to the airway of a spontaneously breathing infant under positive pressure, usually 5 to 8 cm H_2O pressure. The positive pressure holds alveoli open throughout the respiratory cycle and improves oxygenation by reducing the amount of shunting of blood through airle

portions of lung (see PERINATAL PHYSIOLOGY in Ch. 182). As the Pa_{O_2} improves, it is usually possible to reduce the FI_{O_2}.

Ventilator support is required if the infant has respiratory failure with a $Pa_{CO_2} > 60$ mm Hg, apnea, or cannot be oxygenated with CPAP. Clinical judgment plays a large role: Infants who are at risk of severe RDS and IVH (eg, infants weighing < 1500 gm at birth) and infants whose RDS is worsening rapidly may do better if started on a ventilator without waiting for respiratory failure or hypoxemia to develop.

The infant is intubated with an appropriate-size endotracheal tube (the smallest is a 2.5-mm diameter tube for infants < 1250 gm; a 3-mm tube is usually appropriate for infants of 1250 to 2500 gm; and a 3.5-mm tube is used for those > 2500 gm). Intubation is safer if O_2 is insufflated into the airways during the procedure; special laryngoscopic blades have been designed for this.

Ventilators may be designed to deliver gas at either a predetermined pressure or volume. Both types have advantages and indications. Many neonatal intensive care units find the pressure-limited, time-cycled continuous flow ventilators easy to use in tiny infants. The inspired O_2 concentration, inspiratory time (IT), expiratory time (ET), peak inspiratory pressure (PIP), and positive end expiratory pressure (PEEP) are each set independently.

It is beyond the scope of this text to describe all the details of ventilator therapy in the neonate. Initial settings are estimates based upon past experience and judgment of the severity of the lung disease. Typical settings for an infant with moderate RDS would be: $FI_{O_2} = 40\%$; IT = 0.75 sec; ET = 0.75 sec, (rate = 40 breaths/min), PIP = 25 cm H_2O, PEEP = 5 cm H_2O. The infant's color, chest wall movements, breath sounds, and respiratory efforts should be observed; the first ventilator settings are often adjusted, depending on the clinical response. Readjustments are based on arterial or transcutaneous gas monitoring. Pa_{CO_2} is lowered by increasing the minute ventilation by the following maneuvers: Increase tidal volume (increase PIP or decrease PEEP) or increase rate (decreasing ET). The Pa_{O_2} will be increased by either increasing the FI_{O_2} or increasing the mean airway pressure (increase PIP, increase PEEP, or prolong IT).

Any sudden change in the infant's condition, including changes in oxygenation, blood gases, BP, or perfusion should lead one to check the endotracheal tube immediately for its position and patency. The tip of the tube is in proper position when it is palpated through the tracheal wall just at the jugular notch. If there is any doubt, the tube should be removed and the infant supported by bag and mask ventilation until a new tube is inserted.

Tension pneumothorax, *an emergency that must be treated at once*, is another cause of sudden clinical deterioration. It may be detected by clinical signs (loss of breath sounds and shift of the heart away from the affected side, positive transillumination, and by x-ray). The free air may be drained with a scalp vein needle or angiography catheter and syringe until a chest tube can be inserted. The chest tube should be attached to water seal with 10 to 15 cm of continuous suction.

As the infant's respiratory status improves, he can be weaned from intermittent mandatory ventilation **(IMV)** by lowering the FI_{O_2}, inspiratory pressure, and rate (by prolonging the expiratory time). Continuous flow positive pressure ventilators permit the infant to breathe spontaneously against a positive expiratory pressure (PEEP) while the ventilator rate is progressively slowed. This permits a gradual transition; when the ventilator rate is turned to zero, the infant will be on endotracheal CPAP. The final steps involve extubation and support with nasal (or nasopharyngeal) CPAP, and then use of a hood to provide humidified O_2 or air. Some very low birth weight infants may be weaned earlier if they are begun on aminophylline (6 mg/kg IV loading dose, and maintenance of 1.5 mg/kg IV q 8 h, adjusted as needed to maintain a blood level of 7 to 14 mg/mL). Alternatively theophylline may be given orally or by gastric

tube at the same dose. Xanthines are respiratory stimulants that increase ventilatory efforts and may prevent apneic and bradycardic episodes that may interfere with successful weaning.

TRANSIENT TACHYPNEA OF THE NEWBORN (TTNB)

(Neonatal Wet Lung Syndrome)

Respiratory distress with rapid respirations and hypoxemia requiring O_2 supplementation, a condition caused by delayed resorption of fetal lung fluid.

Infants with TTNB are usually born at or close to term. They are more likely to have been delivered by cesarean section, and to have had perinatal distress. Although tachypneic, these newborns may not show signs of respiratory distress (eg, grunting and retractions), but they may be cyanotic. Chest x-ray shows hyperinfiltrated lungs with heavy perihilar markings, giving the appearance of a shaggy heart border. Fluid is often present in the fissures. The lung periphery remains clear. The mechanism for resorption of fetal lung fluid is described in PERINATAL PHYSIOLOGY in Ch. 182.

Treatment involves administering O_2 by hood and monitoring blood gases by arterial sampling or by transcutaneous monitoring. Some infants may require support with CPAP, and rarely may require IMV. Recovery within 2 to 3 days is the rule.

APNEA OF PREMATURITY

Many infants of ≤ 34 wk gestation will have apnea spells, usually beginning after the first 2 to 3 days. The incidence is greatest at the lowest gestational ages. These infants often have **periodic breathing** (*rapid respirations with brief pauses*), which is attributed to immaturity of the medullary respiratory center control. If the respiratory pauses las > 10 sec they may be associated with hypoxemia and bradycardia, and active interven- tion may be required to initiate respirations. Hypoxemia briefly stimulates respirator efforts in the newborn, but, after a few seconds, acts to *suppress* respirations.

Central apnea may occur and is due to a lack of sufficient neural impulses from th respiratory center in the medulla to the respiratory muscles; the infant is flaccid an makes no respiratory efforts. Other apnea spells are due to upper airways obstructio **(obstructive apnea)** in which apposition of the posterior pharyngeal wall with th tongue occludes the nasopharynx; the infant makes respiratory efforts, but cann inhale air into the lungs and becomes hypoxemic and bradycardic. Obstructive apne will not be detected by an apnea monitor, because chest wall movements are presen Therefore, low-birth-weight infants at risk for apnea should be on a heart rate monito and they must be observed closely to detect color change and to confirm the presen of apnea or bradycardia.

Treatment

While it is common for well low-birth-weight infants to have spells of apnea, apn is a common sign of neonatal disorders (eg, hypoglycemia, sepsis, and intracrani hemorrhage). Therefore, it is important to evaluate each premature infant who dev ops apnea to avoid missing these underlying, treatable conditions.

The infant should lie with the neck in the neutral position or slightly extended prevent upper airways obstruction (obstructive apnea). Slightly lowering the enviro mental temperature (eg, to lower the skin temperature from 36.5 C [97.7 F] to 36.2 [97.1 F]) may reduce the frequency of apnea in some infants. If apnea spells contin especially if they are associated with cyanosis or bradycardia, the infant can be trea with aminophylline, a central-acting respiratory stimulant. A loading dose of 6 mg/ IV is given, followed by maintenance doses of 1.5 mg/kg q 8 h. If the infant is tak enteral feedings, theophylline may be given orally or into the gastric tube at the sa dose. The aminophylline or theophylline blood level should be maintained at 7 to μg/mL.

If apnea continues despite treatment with a xanthine, the infant may be treated with continuous positive airway pressure **(CPAP)**; it can be started at 5 cm H_2O pressure and be administered by nasal prongs or nasopharyngeal tube. Intractable apneic spells require ventilator support (see RESPIRATORY DISTRESS SYNDROME, above).

Aminophylline treatment is stopped after the infant has been apnea-free about 7 days and the infant may be sent home after another 10 days if there is no recurrence of apnea after theophylline treatment has been discontinued. Most premature infants will stop having apneic spells by the time they reach about 37 wk gestational age. Those who continue to experience apnea or bradycardia, including those who have intracranial hemorrhage or porencephaly, may be considered possible candidates for home monitoring to avoid sudden infant death syndrome (see in Ch. 186). A 24-h pneumogram may help with this evaluation.

PERSISTENT PULMONARY HYPERTENSION (PPH)

(Persistent Fetal Circulation)

A life-threatening disorder in which there is a return to the fetal condition with the pulmonary arterioles vasoconstricted and the effective pulmonary blood flow reduced to a fraction of normal. As in the fetus, blood is shunted from right to left, either through the foramen ovale or through a persistent patent ductus arteriosus. (For a description of the perinatal circulation and the development of PPH, see PERINATAL PHYSIOLOGY in Ch. 182). The right-to-left shunting leads to profound hypoxemia, even when the infant is breathing 100% O_2.

Etiology, Symptoms, and Signs

In many infants who have died with PPH, pathologic examination of the lungs has shown abnormal muscular hypertrophy of the walls of the small pulmonary arterioles, which may have been the result of chronic hypoxemia in utero. PPH occurs most commonly in term or post-term infants and in infants with fetal growth retardation secondary to placental insufficiency (eg, preeclampsia, maternal hypertension). Commonly, an episode of perinatal or postdelivery asphyxia seems to trigger the persistence or recurrence of pulmonary hypertension. If postmature, these infants are also very prone to meconium aspiration syndrome (see below). PPH has also been observed following maternal treatment with large doses of prostaglandin synthetase inhibitors (eg, aspirin or indomethacin), presumably because these drugs may have produced constriction of the fetal ductus arteriosus in utero leading to an abnormally high pulmonary blood flow with a secondary "protective" hypertrophy of the pulmonary arteriolar walls. Congenital diaphragmatic hernia **(CDH)** is also often associated with muscular hypertrophy of the pulmonary arterioles in both lungs, also presumed secondary to an abnormally high pulmonary blood flow in utero (the left lung is usually severely hypoplastic and all the pulmonary blood flow must go through the right lung). PPH often complicates the course of infants with CDH, and accounts for the high mortality rate in that condition.

Diagnosis

The diagnosis usually is clear on the basis of history, physical findings, and x-ray and laboratory data. The infant with PPH will be near term or post term, and will be and will remain hypoxemic even when breathing or being ventilated with 100% O_2. The lungs may be entirely clear on chest x-ray, but parenchymal lung disease (eg, meconium aspiration syndrome or neonatal pneumonia) or congenital diaphragmatic hernia may be present. Occasionally, it may be difficult to exclude the possibility of cyanotic congenital heart disease. A cardiac workup with ECG and echocardiogram will resolve most of these questions. In PPH the echocardiogram may show a prolonged right ventricular pre-ejection phase reflecting pulmonary hypertension. Occasionally cardiac catheterization may be needed to rule out congenital heart disease.

The increased pulmonary vascular resistance that leads to pulmonary hypertension and right-to-left shunting is worsened by hypoxemia and hypercarbia. Therefore, PPH should be suspected in any near-term infant with arterial desaturation, as it is important to begin treatment as quickly as possible to prevent progression of the pulmonary hypertension.

Treatment

Treatment involves hyperventilation with 100% O_2 to produce a marked respiratory alkalosis. The goal is to lower the Pa_{CO_2} to 15 to 20 mm Hg and to raise the pH to 7.5 to 7.6. A low Pa_{CO_2}, high pH, and high Pa_{O_2} all act to decrease the pulmonary vascular resistance. Extreme hyperventilation may be required to achieve pulmonary vasodilation with an increase in Pa_{O_2}. Giving sodium bicarbonate to produce metabolic alkalosis may also help to dilate the pulmonary arterioles. Some infants do better if muscle paralysis is induced (eg, pancuronium bromide 0.1 mg/kg IV repeated as needed to prevent voluntary movements). Rapid bag and mask ventilation with 100% O_2 for 10 to 20 min may help to establish hyperventilation. The ventilator settings used to maintain hyperventilation will vary widely depending on the nature of any underlying parenchymal lung disease (eg, meconium aspiration, pneumonia, pulmonary hypoplasia).

If hyperventilation does not lead to improved arterial oxygenation, treatment with an α-adrenergic blocker to induce pulmonary vasodilation may be tried. Tolazoline is given in a loading dose of 1 to 2 mg/kg IV over 5 to 10 min, then 1 to 2 mg/kg/h IV. Since tolazoline may also induce systemic vasodilation and hypotension, it should be given by a route that will provide maximum delivery of the drug to the pulmonary circuit; in PPH with a right-to-left shunt at the atrial level this is done by giving it into a vein in the upper part of the body (upper extremity or scalp vein) or directly into a catheter in the pulmonary artery. Systemic hypotension should be treated immediately, because it will increase the right-to-left shunting. Initially, a volume expander can be used (eg, 5% human albumin 10 mL/kg over 10 min). If BP or perfusion remain decreased after 2 to 3 doses of albumin, treatment should be begun with dopamine 2 to 20 mg/kg/min IV (*maximum dose 40 mg/kg/min; never given through an arterial line*) or dobutamine 2.5 to 7.5 mg/kg/min IV (*never given through an arterial line*). Tolazoline causes histamine release, and upper GI bleeding has been associated with its use; antacids may be given prophylactically.

Since these infants may have a right-to-left shunt at the ductal level, it is useful to monitor Pa_{O_2} above and below the level of the ductus by simultaneously measuring blood gases from arterial catheters in both the right radial artery and the abdominal aorta, or with transcutaneous monitors placed on the right side of the chest and on the abdomen or thigh.

Careful attention also must be paid to maintenance of fluid, electrolyte, glucose, and Ca homeostasis. Infants should be kept at the neutral thermal environment, and treated with antibiotics for possible sepsis. Once Pa_{O_2} has been stabilized in the range of 80 to 100 mm Hg, weaning is begun, first by reducing the F_{IO_2} in very small decrements of 2 to 3% O_2. Later F_{IO_2} and ventilator pressures can be reduced alternately. The goal is to avoid any large changes, since a sudden drop in the Pa_{O_2} can lead to a recurrence of pulmonary vasoconstriction.

NEONATAL PNEUMONIA

(See NEONATAL INFECTIONS, below)

MECONIUM ASPIRATION SYNDROME (MAS)

Aspiration of meconium that has entered the amniotic sac, leading to a chemical pneumonitis and mechanical obstruction of bronchi. Complete bronchial obstruction result

in atelectasis, while partial blockage leads to hyperinflation of the lungs and pulmonary air leaks (eg, pneumomediastinum or pneumothorax).

This occurs in the setting of fetal distress that may be associated with placental insufficiency (eg, in maternal preeclampsia, hypertension, or postmaturity). The fetus passes meconium stools in response to stress and also gasps forcefully, aspirating meconium mixed with amniotic fluid into the tracheobronchial tree. MAS is often most severe in post-term infants who have a reduced amniotic fluid volume, because the meconium is less dilute and the thicker particulate meconium is more likely to cause airways obstruction.

Diagnosis

The infant with MAS will have mild to extremely severe respiratory distress. Air-trapping caused by partial bronchial obstruction with meconium, or a secondary tension pneumothorax may cause an increased anteroposterior chest diameter, giving a barrel-chested appearance. The infant may appear dysmature or postmature, and there may be meconium staining of the skin and nails.

Chest x-rays show patchy atelectasis and intervening areas of emphysematous hyperinflation. Progressive air-trapping may lead to pulmonary interstitial emphysema or cysts, pneumomediastinum, or pneumothorax. Occasionally, fluid is seen in the major fissures or in the pleural spaces.

Treatment

Treatment should begin in the delivery room. Immediate suctioning of the upper airways, including the trachea, will remove much of the meconium. This should be accomplished before beginning positive pressure resuscitation (if needed), and optimally before the first spontaneous breaths have been taken.

When meconium is noted in the amniotic fluid, the delivering physician can suction the infant's nasopharynx and pharynx with a DeLee trap and catheter. Personnel trained to perform endotracheal suctioning should be present in the delivery room. Endotracheal intubation with a 3.5- or 4.0-mm endotracheal tube is performed at once if thick meconium is present or if there is thin meconium and the infant has not begun spontaneous, vigorous respirations (neonatal respiratory depression). The endotracheal tube is first suctioned with the largest possible catheter. Since large clumps of meconium may not come up through a suction catheter, mouth to endotracheal tube suction is then applied (with an intervening face mask) and continued while the tube is removed. If large amounts of meconium are recovered, this procedure may need to be repeated several times.

Next, the infant is reintubated and given positive pressure respirations with O_2. If the infant is severely depressed (cyanosis, slow heart rate), it may be necessary to proceed rapidly to positive pressure resuscitation.

After admission to the nursery, intermittent chest physiotherapy and airways suctioning and the administration of humidified air or O_2 may help to loosen meconium and secretions.

Respiratory support is provided according to the severity of the pneumonitis and varies from supportive care and chest physiotherapy to providing supplemental O_2 by hood, or to administering positive pressure ventilation. Infants with MAS, especially those who are post-term, are susceptible to developing persistent pulmonary hypertension **(PPH)** and it is essential to anticipate this life-threatening complication and to initiate treatment for it at once (see PPH, above). If the infant's blood gases are only marginally satisfactory in an O_2 hood, or are worsening over time, it may be safest to initiate positive pressure ventilation to avoid hypoxemia or hypercarbia, which may trigger the chain of events leading to PPH.

Infants with MAS trap air beyond bronchi that are partially blocked with aspirated meconium. During the first few days they are prone to develop air leak syndromes

(pneumomediastinum and pneumothorax). Regular evaluations by auscultation of breath sounds, transillumination of the chest, and chest x-rays are important to detect these complications. Evaluation and treatment for tension pneumothorax or for an endotracheal tube plugged by meconium should be instituted at once if the infant's BP, perfusion, or ABG values suddenly worsen (see PULMONARY AIR-BLOCK SYNDROME, below).

Since meconium may enhance bacterial growth and it is difficult to rule out bacterial pneumonia on the radiographs, it is customary to obtain cultures of blood and tracheal aspirate and begin these infants on antibiotics (ampicillin and gentamicin or tobramycin).

ASPIRATION OF OTHER SUBSTANCES

During delivery infants may also aspirate vernix caseosa, amniotic fluid, and maternal or fetal blood. Then they may exhibit respiratory distress and show signs of aspiration pneumonia on chest x-ray. As in meconium aspiration, treatment is supportive; if bacterial infection is suspected, cultures are taken and antibiotics are begun.

PULMONARY AIR-BLOCK SYNDROME

(Pulmonary Interstitial Emphysema [PIE]; Pneumomediastinum; Pneumothorax; Pneumopericardium)

Dissection of air (air-leaks) out of the normal pulmonary air spaces.

Air leak has been described following delivery in 1 to 2% of normal infants, probably as a result of the large negative intrathoracic forces of the first breaths of air. Many of these infants are asymptomatic or have only tachypnea.

Usually, however, pulmonary air leaks occur in infants with serious lung diseases (eg, RDS or MAS—see above) who are predisposed because of poor lung compliance and the need for high distending pressures (eg, RDS infant on a respirator) or because of increased airways resistance (eg, meconium partially obstructing bronchi in MAS).

Pulmonary Interstitial Emphysema (PIE)

PIE occurs if *air dissects from the alveoli into the pulmonary interstitium, lymphatics, or subpleural space.* This often occurs in infants with poor lung compliance being treated with positive pressure ventilation, but may occur spontaneously. The location of PIE is highly variable: it may involve one or both lungs, and may be focal or generalized within each lung. The infant's respiratory status may become much worse (raised Pa_{CO_2}, lowered pH, lowered Pa_{O_2}) if there is diffuse dissection of air, as lung compliance is suddenly reduced.

Chest x-ray shows several or many cystic or linear lucencies in the lung fields that are too large or too peripheral to represent bronchi. Some lucencies are elongated, while others appear as enlarged subpleural cysts and may be several cm in diameter.

The course of PIE is highly variable. It may resolve dramatically over 1 or 2 days or persist on x-ray for weeks or months. Some infants develop bronchopulmonary dysplasia **(BPD)** and the cystic changes of PIE then merge into the x-ray picture of BPD.

Treatment: The goal is to lower the ventilator inspiratory pressure as much as possible to allow the lung to heal. It would be reasonable to achieve adequate oxygenation in the presence of PIE by increasing the F_{IO_2} in order to lower the inspiratory pressure but this may be difficult or impossible if the lungs with diffuse PIE become very noncompliant.

If PIE is very severe in one lung, and mild or absent in the other lung, differential bronchial intubation may be attempted. An endotracheal tube is advanced into the mainstem bronchus on the less involved side; this may be facilitated by turning the

head and neck to the side opposite the bronchus to be intubated. If lung auscultation is performed during this maneuver, breath sounds will be lost over the lung with PIE when differential bronchial intubation has been achieved. Position is confirmed on x-ray, which will soon show total atelectasis of the lung with PIE. Since only one lung is now being ventilated, ventilator settings and FIO_2 may need to be increased at once. After 24 to 48 h, the endotracheal tube is pulled back into the trachea, in hopes that the PIE has resolved. There have also been reports of the successful treatment of severe PIE using very high frequency jet ventilators, but this approach is still experimental.

Pneumomediastinum (PM)

PM results *if pulmonary interstitial emphysema dissects into the loose connective tissue of the mediastinum.* Usually, the infant will not develop additional signs of respiratory distress, but the chest may transilluminate positively, and, on x-ray, air in the mediastinum will be seen lifting the lobes of the thymus away from the cardiac silhouette. Air may dissect further into the subcutaneous tissues of the neck and scalp; subcutaneous air is asymptomatic and will resolve spontaneously.

Specific treatment is not needed. However, since PM indicates that an air leak has occurred, it may be advantageous to try to lower ventilator pressures.

Pneumothorax

Pneumothorax develops *when air dissects into the pleural space from a pneumomediastinum or from the rupture of a subpleural bleb (PIE).* Although sometimes asymptomatic, pneumothorax is often a life-threatening complication, especially in an infant with severe parenchymal lung disease (eg, RDS, MAS) on positive pressure ventilation.

Clinical signs of a **tension pneumothorax** may include a sudden increase or fall in BP, poor skin perfusion, poor pulses, and reduced or absent breath sounds on the affected side. Heart sounds may be muffled if the pneumothorax is on the left side. Positive transillumination with a fiberoptic light source strongly suggests that there is free air in the thorax. If the infant's condition permits, a chest x-ray will confirm the diagnosis.

Treatment: Immediate evacuation of a pneumothorax with a syringe and needle is required in the infant with lung disease or on positive pressure ventilation. Definitive treatment is by insertion of a 5 or 8 French chest tube. Chest tubes should be inserted with a curved hemostat after a small incision is made in the skin (NOTE: Insertion of a chest tube with a trocar is more likely to result in lung laceration). The tube should be positioned with the tip anteriorly in the chest, since free air will collect in the most superior space (anteriorly when the infant is supine). The chest tube should be connected to a trap and 10 to 15 cm of H_2O suction. Follow-up auscultation, transillumination, and x-ray will confirm that the tube is functioning properly.

In an infant free of underlying lung disease, a pneumothorax may produce only mild tachypnea or even be asymptomatic. In this situation, it is possible simply to wait for spontaneous resolution while the infant is closely observed.

Other Air Leaks

In an infant on positive pressure ventilation, air may dissect into the pericardial sac causing **cardiac tamponade** with reduced cardiac output and BP. X-ray will show air within the pericardial sac entirely surrounding the heart. Rapid evacuation of the air using a scalp vein needle, followed by surgical insertion of a pericardial tube may be lifesaving.

Occasionally a pulmonary air leak may result in free air dissecting retroperitoneally and then into the peritoneal cavity producing a **pneumoperitoneum**. This will resolve spontaneously, but it needs to be distinguished from pneumoperitoneum due to a ruptured abdominal viscus, which is a surgical emergency.

BRONCHOPULMONARY DYSPLASIA (BPD)

A chronic lung disorder that may occur in infants who require ventilator support.

Etiology

Injury to the lung may be associated with barotrauma from positive pressure ventilation, high inspired O_2 concentrations, and endotracheal intubation; it is more common among infants of low gestational age. It is often a sequel of RDS and its treatment, and is more likely to develop during the occurrence of pulmonary interstitial emphysema (see PIE, above). The transition from RDS to BPD is gradual; often the infant simply fails to wean from intermittent mandatory ventilation **(IMV)** at the age of 5 to 6 days (when RDS should have resolved).

Since BPD is at least in part caused by ventilator use, it is important to wean infants from ventilator support as soon as possible. In an infant with RDS who fails to wean from IMV at an appropriate time, possible underlying problems (eg, PDA and nursery-acquired pneumonia) should be sought and treated if present. Early use of aminophylline as a respiratory stimulant may help to wean preterm infants from IMV.

Symptoms and Signs

In the early stages of BPD there is inflammation and exudate. The alveolar epithelium may slough, and macrophages may be found in the tracheal aspirate. At this time the chest x-ray may show only a diffuse haziness of the lung fields. Later, scarring and breakdown of alveolar walls occur. Alternating areas of emphysema with hyperaeration and pulmonary scarring lead to a "hobnail appearance" pathologically, and a multicystic appearance with many course streaks and hyperinflation on chest x-ray. There may be muscular hypertrophy of the peribronchial and arteriolar smooth muscle, and squamous metaplasia of the bronchial epithelium.

Prognosis and Treatment

BPD may require weeks or months of additional ventilator support and/or supplemental O_2. Ventilator pressures and F_{IO_2} should be reduced as tolerated, but the infant should not be allowed to remain hypoxemic, mainly because low Pa_{O_2} will cause pulmonary vascular constriction and may result in pulmonary hypertension, cor pulmonale, and right heart failure. This can be evaluated by echocardiography, as pulmonary hypertension will be manifested by a prolonged right ventricular pre-ejection time. Arterial oxygenation may be continuously monitored with a transcutaneous monitor or a pulse oximeter.

Infants with chronic lung disease may have a compensated respiratory acidosis while breathing spontaneously. It is therefore appropriate to let the P_{CO_2} rise above normal while weaning from the ventilator as long as the pH remains normal (pH > 7.30) and the infant's respiratory distress is not too great.

Good nutrition is necessary in these chronically ill infants who often have increased caloric needs because of the increased work of breathing. Nutrition may be provided by venous alimentation, or nasoduodenal or orogastric tube feedings, depending on the infant's condition. Infants with BPD may be very susceptible to developing pulmonary congestion or edema if challenged with excessive fluids. It is often necessary to restrict the daily fluid intake to 100 to 120 mL/kg/day; this may present a challenge to provide adequate calories (eg, by adding glucose polymers or medium chain triglyceride oil to supplement enteral feedings).

Chronic diuretic therapy is customarily used to treat these infants, because of their tendency to develop pulmonary congestion with decreased lung compliance. Furosemide 1 mg/kg IV, IM, or orally given once daily to tid may be used for short periods, but prolonged use causes hypercalciuria with resultant osteopenia, fractures, and renal stones. Chronic diuretic therapy can be more safely provided with the combination o

chlorothiazide 10 to 20 mg/kg/day and spironolactone 1 to 2 mg/kg/day both given orally bid. The state of hydration and serum electrolytes should be closely monitored.

After the infant with BPD is weaned from a ventilator, supplemental O_2 may be required for an additional period of weeks. This may be given by nasal cannula with gradual reduction in the O_2 flow rate. Oxygenation can be monitored with a transcutaneous monitor or pulse oximetry.

The parents will require a great deal of emotional support, because the course of resolution of BPD may be both slow and unpredictable, and some infants may die after many months of care. Surviving infants' respiratory distress gradually resolves, although reduced lung compliance and increased airways resistance may persist for several years. These infants are at increased risk of lower respiratory tract infection, especially viral infections, in the first years, and may quickly develop respiratory decompensation if pulmonary infection supervenes. The infant will likely require rehospitalization if signs of a respiratory infection develop or there is increased respiratory distress.

RESPIRATORY DISORDERS DUE TO ALTERED RBC MASS AND BLOOD VOLUME

(See Hematologic Problems in this chapter, below)

BIRTH TRAUMA

The incidence of neonatal injury from a difficult or traumatic delivery is decreasing. Improved prenatal diagnosis and monitoring during the course of labor have helped to prevent neurologic injury. In addition, cesarean section, which now presents fewer risks to the mother than in the past, often replaces attempts at difficult versions, vacuum extractions, or mid- or high-forceps deliveries.

A traumatic delivery is anticipated when the mother has small pelvic measurements, when the infant seems large for gestational age (often the case with the infants of diabetic mothers), or when there is a breech or other abnormal presentation, especially in a primipara. In such situations, both the labor and the fetal condition should be monitored. If fetal distress is detected, the mother should be positioned on her side and given O_2. If fetal distress persists, an immediate cesarean section should be performed.

INJURIES TO THE CENTRAL AND PERIPHERAL NERVOUS SYSTEMS

(See also Cerebral Palsy Syndromes in Ch. 198)

The mechanics of labor and delivery are such that physical injury to the infant can easily occur. The strength of these forces is apparent from the head molding that follows vertex deliveries, but even severe molding usually does not cause problems or require treatment.

Head trauma varies in degrees: **Caput succedaneum,** edema of the presenting portion of the scalp, results from mild trauma as this area is forced against the uterine cervix. **Subgaleal hemorrhage** results from greater trauma and is characterized by a boggy feeling over the entire scalp, including the temporal regions. **Cephalhematoma,** or hemorrhage beneath the periosteum, can be differentiated from more superficial bleeding because it is sharply limited to the area of a single bone, the periosteum being adherent at the sutures. Cephalhematomas are commonly unilateral and parietal in location. A small percent have an associated **linear fracture** in the bone underlying them. Cephalhematomas do not require treatment, but anemia or hyperbilirubinemia may rarely

result from bleeding associated with them. **Depressed skull fractures** are uncommon. Most result from forceps pressure; rarely, they are caused by the head resting against a bony prominence in utero. They can be seen and felt as depressions, and must be differentiated from the depressions secondary to an elevated periosteal rim seen with cephalhematomas. X-rays will confirm the diagnosis. Depressed fractures may require neurosurgical elevation. Depressed skull fractures or other head trauma may be associated with subdural bleeding, subarachnoid hemorrhage, or even contusion or laceration of the brain itself (see INTRACRANIAL HEMORRHAGE, below).

Trauma to cranial nerves primarily involves the **facial nerve**. Involvement of other cranial nerves is uncommon and not usually due to birth injuries. Although frequently attributed to forceps pressure, most such injuries probably occur from pressure on the nerve in utero. This may be due to fetal positioning (eg, from the head lying against the shoulder) or to pressure against the nerve by the sacral promontory or a uterine fibroid.

Facial nerve injury is usually peripheral, and the face appears asymmetric. In complete peripheral 7th nerve injuries, movement of facial muscles on the entire involved side is absent. Injury also occurs in individual branches of the 7th nerve, most frequently the mandibular. Intrauterine pressure on the mandible can also lead to facial asymmetry, but the muscle innervation is intact. Comparison of the maxillary and mandibular occlusal surfaces, which should be parallel, differentiates this from a true 7th nerve injury. No test or treatment is needed for peripheral facial nerve injuries, which usually resolve by age 2 to 3 mo.

Injuries to nerve roots and peripheral nerves may result from difficult deliveries and are usually seen in the upper extremities. **Brachial plexus injuries** follow stretching caused by shoulder dystocia, breech extraction, or hyperabduction of the neck in cephalic presentations. The injury can be due to simple stretching, hemorrhage within a nerve, tearing of the nerve or root, or avulsion of the roots with associated cervical cord injury.

The site and type of injury determine the prognosis. Injuries of the upper brachial plexus (C5, 6) affect muscles about the shoulder and elbow, while lesions of the lower plexus (C7, 8; and T1) primarily affect muscles of the forearm and hand. **Erb's palsy** is an upper brachial plexus injury causing adduction and internal rotation of the shoulder with pronation of the forearm; ipsilateral paralysis of the diaphragm is common. Treatment consists of passive range of motion to maintain joint mobility, and pinning the arm above the head to place the muscles opposing those paralyzed at rest. **Klumpke's palsy** is a lower plexus injury resulting in paralysis of the hand and wrist, often with an associated ipsilateral Horner's syndrome (miosis, ptosis, anhidrosis). Passive range of motion is the only treatment indicated. Neither of these brachial plexus injuries is usually associated with demonstrable sensory loss. Improvement in both is usually rapid. If a significant deficit persists over 3 mo, then surgical exploration and repair should be considered.

When the entire brachial plexus is injured, there is no movement of the involved upper extremity, and sensory loss is often present. Ipsilateral pyramidal signs should be sought, since their presence indicates associated spinal cord trauma. Passive range of motion is used to prevent contractures, and surgical exploration should be considered. The prognosis for recovery is poor. Subsequent growth of the involved extremity may be impaired.

Injuries to other peripheral nerves, such as the radial, sciatic, and obturator, are rare in the newborn and are not ordinarily related to the birth process. They are usually secondary to a local traumatic event; eg, an injection in or near the sciatic nerve or fat necrosis over the radial nerve. The muscles antagonistic to those paralyzed should be placed at rest until recovery occurs. In most peripheral nerve injuries recovery is complete. Neurosurgical exploration of the nerve is seldom indicated.

Trauma to the spinal cord is rare. It is usually seen in breech deliveries and follows excess longitudinal traction to the spine. Sometimes a click or snap is heard at delivery. It can also follow hyperextension of the fetal neck in utero (the "flying fetus"). The trauma usually occurs in the lower cervical region (C5, 6, 7), since higher lesions generally are fatal. The injury may consist of hemorrhage into the spinal cord or varying degrees of spinal cord disruption. Initially there is spinal shock with total flaccidity below the level of injury. Spasticity usually develops within days or weeks. Breathing is diaphragmatic, since the phrenic nerve arises higher (C3, 4, 5). There is paralysis of intercostal and abdominal muscles, and voluntary control of rectal and bladder sphincters cannot develop. Sensation and sweating are lost below the involved level, and can result in fluctuations of body temperature with environmental changes. The CSF usually is bloody. X-rays of the neck are normal. The usual causes of death are progressive loss of renal function, making evaluation of the urinary tract essential, and recurring pneumonia. Some infants survive for many years. Treatment of spinal cord injury consists of nursing care to prevent skin ulcerations, prompt treatment of urinary and respiratory infections, and regular evaluations to identify obstructive uropathy early (see Ch. 157).

INTRACRANIAL HEMORRHAGE

Hemorrhage in or around the brain is a major problem in the newborn infant, especially when premature. Hypoxia, pressures exerted on the infant's head during labor, and the presence of the germinal matrix in prematures are 3 major reasons. Small hemorrhages frequently are found at autopsy in the subarachnoid space, falx, and tentorium. Larger hemorrhages are less common but usually more serious. About 40% of premature infants < 1500 gm have intracranial hemorrhage. Cranial ultrasound and CT studies can detect blood and are useful in diagnosis. Hemorrhage can occur into several spaces related to the CNS. **Bleeding into the subarachnoid space** probably is the most common in full-term infants and may account for the RBCs so often seen in the newborn's CSF. The diagnosis, made by examining the CSF and performing a CT scan, should be suspected in any infant with apnea, seizures, lethargy, or an abnormal neurologic examination. The associated meningeal inflammation may lead to a communicating hydrocephalus as the baby grows. **Bleeding into the subdural space,** which occurs less often as obstetric technics have improved, results from tears in the falx, the tentorium, or the bridging veins. Such tears are most common in infants of primiparas, in large infants, or after difficult deliveries. All these conditions can produce unusual pressures on the skull. The presenting finding may be seizures, a rapidly enlarging head, or an abnormal neurologic examination with hypotonia, a poor Moro response, retinal hemorrhages, or a positive transillumination of the skull.

Hemorrhages within the ventricles or parenchyma are the most serious type of intracranial bleeding. They occur mostly in premature infants, generally during the first 3 days of life. Some are asymptomatic, but there can be apnea, cyanosis, or even a sudden collapse. Hemorrhage in premature infants is frequently bilateral and usually arises in the **germinal matrix** (*a mass of embryonic cells lying over the caudate nucleus, and present only in the fetus*) on the lateral wall of the lateral ventricles. Most bleeding episodes are subependymal or have a small amount of blood in the ventricles. In severe ones, there may be casts of the ventricular system and large amounts of blood in the cisterna magna and basal cisterns. Hypoxia, particularly in premature infants, often precedes intraventricular and subarachnoid bleeding. Hypoxia damages the capillary endothelium, impairs cranial vascular autoregulation, and increases cerebral blood flow and venous pressure, all of which make hemorrhage more likely.

Suspected intracranial hemorrhage requires careful evaluation for skin petechiae or hemorrhage from other sites, which suggest a systemic hematologic or vascular disorder; eg, vitamin K deficiency, hemophilia, or disseminated intravascular coagulation.

Laboratory evaluation of an infant with suspected intracranial hemorrhage should begin with a lumbar puncture. The CSF should be examined for RBCs, and usually contains gross blood. A CBC (especially Hct and platelet count) and metabolic studies to identify other causes of neurologic dysfunction (hypoglycemia, hypocalcemia, electrolyte imbalance) should be done. Clotting studies may also be needed. Cranial ultrasound or CT scan can readily identify blood within the ventricles or brain substance, but thin layers of subarachnoid or subdural blood lying over the hemispheres may be missed. An EEG may be helpful in establishing the prognosis if the infant survives the acute bleeding episode.

Treatment of most intracranial hemorrhages is supportive unless a hematologic abnormality has contributed to the bleeding. The infant should receive vitamin K if it was not previously given. Platelets should be given if they are deficient. Treatment of subdural hematomas consists of daily bilateral subdural taps until the spaces are dry. *Only 10 to 15 mL of subdural fluid should be removed from each side initially, as removing larger amounts may precipitate shock.* If 2 wk of daily drainage fails to prevent reaccumulation of subdural fluid, a craniotomy with membrane stripping or a subdural shunting procedure should be considered.

The **prognosis** for infants with large intraventricular hemorrhages is poor, especially if they extend into the parenchyma. Most infants with smaller hemorrhages survive the acute bleeding episode and do well. A few may be left with variable degrees of neurologic deficit. The prognosis is much better if the hemorrhage is subarachnoid. The outlook for infants with subdural hematomas is guarded, but some do well.

FRACTURES

Midclavicular fracture, the most common fracture during birth, usually occurs with shoulder dystocia or when the obstetrician must fracture the clavicle to facilitate a difficult breech delivery. The infant is first noted to be irritable and does not move the arm on the involved side either spontaneously or when the Moro reflex is elicited. Most clavicular fractures are greenstick and heal rapidly and uneventfully. A large callus forms at the fracture site within a week, and remodeling is completed within a month. The major significance of clavicular fractures is their association with brachial plexus injury and with pneumothorax from perforation of the apical pleura.

The **humerus** and the **femur** may be fractured in difficult deliveries. Most of these are greenstick, mid-shaft fractures, and excellent remodeling of the bone usually follows, even if there is an initial moderate degree of angulation. A long bone may be fractured through its epiphysis, but even here the prognosis for newborns is excellent.

SOFT TISSUE INJURIES

Any of the soft tissues are susceptible to injury with subsequent edema and hemorrhage if they have been the presenting part or the fulcrum for the forces of uterine contraction. Edema and ecchymosis of the periorbital and facial tissues commonly occur in face presentations, while the scrotum or labia are traumatized during breech deliveries. Breakdown of blood within the tissues and conversion of heme to bilirubin result whenever a hematoma develops in any injury. This added burden of bilirubin in borderline cases may produce sufficient neonatal jaundice to require exchange transfusion (see Hyperbilirubinemia under Metabolic Problems in the Newborn, below). No other treatment is needed.

HEMATOLOGIC PROBLEMS

To evaluate anemias in the newborn during the first week of life, blood should be obtained by venipuncture; Hcts obtained by heel prick may be as much as 15% too high due to sludging of blood in skin capillaries.

ACUTE BLOOD-LOSS ANEMIA

Massive perinatal blood loss may result from abnormal placental separation, as in abruptio placentae or placenta previa; from a traumatic tear of the umbilical cord or of a vessel if there is velamentous insertion of the cord into the placenta; or from incision into an anterior-lying placenta during cesarean section delivery. If the umbilical cord is wrapped tightly around the infant's neck or body, arterial blood from the infant may be pumped into the placenta, while compression of the cord prevents blood from returning via the umbilical vein to the infant; clamping the cord immediately upon delivery may then result in significant acute blood loss (into the placenta).

In such cases, shock and severe asphyxia may occur before delivery or at birth. The infant is hypotensive and extremely pale, has weak or absent pulses, makes poor respiratory efforts, and does not respond to the usual steps in CPR. The Hct and Hb should be determined; a normal Hct does not rule out acute massive blood loss, however, because it may not have had time to equilibrate downward.

Acute blood loss with hypovolemic shock should be corrected by immediate transfusion of whole blood via an umbilical vein catheter. Start by giving 10 mL/kg over 5 to 10 min and give repeat doses until an adequate circulation has been restored. If blood is not immediately available, circulation may be supported by infusing colloid (5% human albumin or fresh frozen plasma). If shock persists, more blood or colloid should be given. Central venous pressure may be monitored via an umbilical vein catheter (after the catheter tip is radiologically confirmed as being above the diaphragm), to help determine when the blood deficit has been replaced.

A **twin-to-twin transfusion** may occur in identical twins who have an anastomotic vessel between their portions of one placenta. A chronic transfusion of blood from one twin into the other results. The donor is usually small for gestational age and anemic; the recipient is significantly larger and plethoric. The donor may need exchange or simple blood transfusion to raise the Hct rapidly to a safe level, while the recipient, who may suffer from polycythemia (see below), may require partial exchange transfusion with plasma to lower the Hct to a safe level (< 65%).

HEMOLYTIC ANEMIAS OF THE NEWBORN

(See also ERYTHROBLASTOSIS FETALIS in Ch. 177)

RHESUS (RH) INCOMPATIBILITY

Rh incompatibility may occur when an Rh-negative woman carries an Rh-positive fetus. Isoimmunization of the mother occurs after some (incompatible) fetal RBCs cross the placenta and induce an immunologic response of maternal antibodies that subsequently cross the placenta into the fetus and lead to hemolysis. The severity of the hemolytic process can be evaluated by doing sequential amniocenteses to measure the amount of bilirubin present in the amniotic fluid. These are measured as the optical density at 450 mμ (OD 450) and are corrected for gestational age (see TABLE 177–1).

The first immunization may occur with a miscarriage or in a pregnancy with an Rh-positive fetus. The severity of isoimmunization increases in subsequent pregnancies, and each subsequent infant is more likely to be affected. Rh incompatibility usually indicates that group D RBC surface antigen is present, although C and E factor incompatibilities of the Rh system may also occur. Rh isoimmunization can usually be prevented by proper administration of Rh_o(D) immune globulin to the unsensitized Rh-negative woman at 20 wk gestation and again following delivery or at the time of miscarriage. (See also ERYTHROBLASTOSIS FETALIS in Ch. 177.)

Symptoms and Signs

The most severely affected fetuses develop profound anemia in utero and are delivered with **hydrops fetalis,** which may be diagnosed before delivery on fetal ultrasound examination, which shows scalp edema, cardiomegaly, hepatomegaly, or ascites. Polyhydramnios may also be present. These newborns are extremely pale and may have severe generalized edema, including pleural effusions and ascites. The liver and spleen are enlarged because of extramedullary hematopoiesis. Heart failure may occur. Because of anemia and prematurity, asphyxia is more likely during labor and delivery, and cesarean section may be indicated. Prematurity and asphyxia, along with hypoproteinemia, predispose these infants to respiratory distress syndrome **(RDS),** the signs of which may be difficult to distinguish from those of heart failure. Less severely affected neonates may be anemic, but do not have edema or other signs of hydrops; others may have little or no anemia at birth. Affected infants usually develop severe hyperbilirubinemia soon after delivery because of the continuing hemolytic effect of Rh antibodies that have crossed the placenta; **kernicterus** may develop if this is not treated (see HYPERBILIRUBINEMIA, below).

Treatment

An infant with hydrops fetalis or severe erythroblastosis fetalis without hydrops is critically ill and should be delivered at a perinatal intensive care facility. Fetal heart rate should be monitored during labor; and if signs of asphyxia occur or if the infant is severely affected, cesarean section delivery is indicated.

The mainstay of treatment is exchange transfusion using Rh-negative erythrocytes. An exchange blood transfusion using twice the infant's calculated blood volume (a 2-volume transfusion) removes 85% of the infant's blood, including circulating antibodies, sensitized RBCs, and accumulated bilirubin.

In hydrops fetalis, profound anemia should be treated at once by doing a partial (1-volume) exchange transfusion using packed Rh-negative RBCs (Hct 70%). After the infant's condition stabilizes, a 2-volume exchange transfusion with Rh-negative blood should be performed. In addition, digoxin and diuretics for heart failure, alkali therapy for metabolic acidosis, and supportive treatment for RDS may be required.

When an Rh-negative, sensitized woman delivers, the cord blood should be examined immediately to determine the infant's blood type, and the direct Coombs' test should be performed. If the infant is Rh-positive and the direct Coombs' test is positive, the infant's Hct and reticulocyte count should be determined, and a blood smear should be obtained to check for reticulocytes and nucleated RBCs. The bilirubin level in cord blood should be determined also. A cord-blood Hct < 40% or a cord bilirubin > 5 mg/dL are indications of severe hemolysis.

Laboratory and clinical evaluations of some infants suggest such a severe rate of hemolysis that exchange transfusion will almost certainly be required in the future. If the infant's condition is stable, an early exchange transfusion will remove sensitized RBCs and antibodies before hemolysis produces large amounts of bilirubin, and may avert the need for multiple exchange transfusions at a later time. **Criteria suggesting the need for an early, but not emergency, exchange transfusion include** a Hct < 40%, reticulocytes > 15%, and a bilirubin concentration > 5 mg/100 mL at birth; the most useful information is obtained by observing the rate at which serum bilirubin rises over a period of several hours. If the bilirubin level rises at ≥ 1 mg/dL/h, the infant will likely come to exchange transfusion.

If an exchange transfusion is not indicated immediately, the infant can be followed by clinical evaluation and by serial determinations of both serum bilirubin and Hct. Should bilirubin levels become dangerously elevated (see HYPERBILIRUBINEMIA in PREMATURE INFANT AND POSTMATURE INFANT and METABOLIC PROBLEMS IN THE NEWBORN in Ch. 186), or significant anemia develop, exchange transfusion is indicated.

Many affected Rh-positive infants will not require an exchange transfusion in the newborn period; however, the Hct must be followed serially *for several weeks or months,* as severe anemia may develop because of slow, ongoing hemolysis. Such infants will require a simple transfusion with packed Rh-negative RBCs.

ABO Blood Group Incompatibility

In almost all cases of ABO incompatibility, the mother's blood type is O and the infant's is either A or B. (See also Erythroblastosis Fetalis in Ch. 177.) Anti-A sensitization is more common, but anti-B sensitization is likely to produce more severe hemolytic disease when it occurs. Although the infant may develop anemia in utero, it is almost never severe enough to cause hydrops fetalis or intrauterine death. The major clinical problem is the development of significant hyperbilirubinemia following birth.

The required laboratory studies are similar to those for Rh disease. The direct Coombs' test is usually weakly positive, but may occasionally be negative; this does not rule out ABO incompatibility if other criteria for diagnosis are met. Usually anti-A or anti-B antibodies can be found in the infant's serum (positive indirect Coombs' test) or following elution from the infant's RBCs. Also, numerous microspherocytes in the infant's blood and reticulocytosis suggest ABO incompatibility. Principles of surveillance and treatment of these infants are identical to those for Rh incompatibility.

Rare Blood Group Incompatibilities

Many rare blood group incompatibilities have been documented (eg, Kell, Duffy). Although infrequent, they may be severe; and because hemolysis is involved, they produce anemia and hyperbilirubinemia as does Rh or ABO incompatibility. Treatment is similar to that for Rh incompatibility; blood used for exchange transfusion must lack the sensitizing antigen.

Anemia Due to Congenital Spherocytosis

(See also Anemias Due to Excessive Red Cell Destruction—Hemolytic Anemias in Ch. 96)

Hemolysis in infants born with congenital spherocytosis often causes significant hyperbilirubinemia. Anemia may develop as well. Significant splenomegaly usually does not occur in neonates. Spherocytes are seen on the blood smear, and the RBCs have increased osmotic fragility. This disorder may be inherited as a dominant trait, so a family history of one parent with hemolytic anemia or splenectomy may help in making the diagnosis. However, in many cases the family history is negative for spherocytosis. Early hyperbilirubinemia, if severe, is treated by exchange transfusion. Splenectomy may be required at a later age to control chronic hemolytic anemia.

Nonspherocytic Hemolytic Anemias

Occasionally neonates develop hemolytic anemia secondary to RBC enzymatic defects, such as **pyruvate kinase deficiency** or **G6PD deficiency** (see Anemias Due to Excessive Hemolysis in Ch. 96). If a Heinz body preparation is positive in an infant with hemolytic anemia, these disorders are suspected and specific tests for enzyme activity can be performed. A definitive diagnosis may be difficult to make in the neonate, and the course of the hemolytic anemia should be observed over time. If the hemolytic process continues, amounts of blood large enough to diagnose specific RBC enzymatic defects can more easily be obtained when the infant is older.

Hemolytic Anemia Due to Infections

Hemolysis is found in many congenital infections (eg, toxoplasmosis, rubella, cytomegalovirus disease, herpes simplex, and syphilis) and in infections due to hemolytic bacteria (eg, *Escherichia coli* or β-hemolytic streptococci). Jaundice, which is often present also, should suggest the possibility of an infectious process, particularly if the direct serum bilirubin is elevated (> 1.5 mg/dL).

HEMOGLOBINOPATHIES

(See also Anemias Due to Defective Hemoblogin Synthesis in Ch. 96)

Most clinical hemoglobinopathies involve abnormalities of the β-chain of Hb (sickle cell disease, β-thalassemia). Since the newborn has a large amount of fetal Hb (α-2, γ-2), these disorders are *not* clinically evident at birth, but most are gradually manifested later, in the first 6 mo of life. However, the rare disorder α-thalassemia results in **hydrops fetalis** with either fetal or early neonatal death due to profound intractable anemia. Methods that are available to screen for various hemoglobinopathies in the newborn period are being done routinely in some states.

POLYCYTHEMIA AND HYPERVISCOSITY

Increased viscosity due to a high Hct (usually 70% or more), which may result in stasis of blood within vessels, pulmonary congestion, cardiomegaly, and, possibly, vascular thrombosis. The affected newborn may appear plethoric, or can present with neurologic signs (eg, seizures, lethargy, poor feeding), or cardiorespiratory distress (tachypnea, tachycardia, cyanosis). Symptomatic newborns with a central venous Hct > 65% should receive a partial exchange transfusion in which aliquots of blood are removed and replaced by equal volumes of plasma to reduce the Hct to safe levels; *simple phlebotomy alone should not be used,* because hypovolemia results and the symptoms may worsen. A possible association between neonatal polycythemia and subsequent developmental delay has been suggested, but remains unproven.

METABOLIC PROBLEMS IN THE NEWBORN

HYPOTHERMIA

An abnormally low body temperature. Newborn infants are prone to becoming hypothermic on exposure to a cool environment. Hypothermia is a serious hazard that can result in hypoglycemia, metabolic acidosis, and death. Since the infant's O_2 requirement (metabolic rate) increases with cold stress, hypothermia may also result in tissue hypoxia and neurologic damage in infants with respiratory insufficiency (eg, the preterm infant with respiratory distress syndrome). Prolonged unrecognized cold stress may divert calories to heat production and impair growth.

Newborns respond to cooling by a discharge of norepinephrine by the sympathetic nerves to the "brown fat." This specialized organ of the newborn, located in the nape of the neck, between the scapulas, and around the kidneys and adrenals, responds by lipolysis followed by oxidation or reesterification of the fatty acids that are released. These reactions produce heat locally, and a rich blood supply to the brown fat helps to transfer the heat produced to the rest of the infant's body. This reaction may increase the infant's metabolic rate and O_2 utilization two- to threefold.

Despite this response, the low-birth-weight infant may become hypothermic because he has a large surface area to body weight ratio and rapidly loses heat by radiation. Evaporative heat loss (eg, an infant wet with amniotic fluid in the delivery room), and conductive and convenctive heat losses can also be significant.

Hypothermia can be prevented by rapidly drying the infant in the delivery room (to avoid evaporative heat loss) and then swaddling him (including his head) in a warm blanket. If the infant is exposed for resuscitation or closer observation, or to provide skin-to-skin contact with the mother, he should be warmed under a radiant warmer. Use of a warmer with a servo-control mechanism and careful observation will prevent hypothermia or hyperthermia.

The infant's thermal environment is determined by factors such a relative humidity, air flow, and the proximity of cold surfaces (to which heat is lost by radiation) as well as by the ambient air temperature.

Sick newborns should be maintained at the **neutral thermal environment** —the environmental conditions under which the metabolic rate is minimal while maintaining a normal core temperature (37 C or 98.6 F). This can be approximated by setting the isolette temperature indicated in Table 186–2 according to the infant's birthweight and postnatal age. An alternative approach is to use an isolette or radiant warmer with a servo-control mechanism set to maintain the infant's skin temperature at 36.5 C (97.7 F).

HYPOGLYCEMIA

(See also Ch. 94)

A blood glucose < 40 mg/dL in the full-term infant, or < 30 mg/dL in the premature infant. The correlation between symptoms and low blood glucose levels is inexact, as is the correlation between hypoglycemia and subsequent neurological damage. Some infants with low blood glucose will suffer neurologic damage, so it is important to prevent neonatal hypoglycemia, or to treat it promptly when it develops.

Etiology

Hypoglycemia usually occurs because of deficient glycogen stores at birth or secondary to hyperinsulinism. Glycogen stores may be deifcient in very low birth weight infants who are therefore prone to hypoglycemia unless they receive a sustained input of exogenous glycose. Glycogen stores are also depleted in infants who experience intrauterine malnutrition because of placental insufficiency (small-for-gestational-age infants). If they also sustained perinatal asphyxia with hypoxia, any glucose stores (as glycogen) will have been rapidly consumed during anerobic glycolysis. Infants with deficient glycogen stores may become hypoglycemic at any time in the first few days, especially if there is a prolonged interval between feedings or if oral intake is poor.

Hyperinsulinism is seen in infants of diabetic mothers (inversely to the degree of diabetic control), in severe erythroblastosis fetalis, and in **Beckwith-Wiedmann syndrome.** Elevated insulin levels characteristically result in a rapid fall in the blood glucose in the first 1 to 2 h after birth when the continuous supply of glucose from the placenta is interrupted. Hypoglycemia may also occur if an IV infusion of glucose in water is abruptly interrupted.

Symptoms and Signs

Although many infants remain asymptomatic, listlessness, poor feeding, hypotonia, jitteriness, apneic spells, tachypnea, and seizures may occur.

Prophylaxis and Treatment

Infants in the following categories are at risk for developing hypoglycemia: infants of diabetic mothers, premature infants, small-for-gestational-age infants, infants with severe isoimmune hemolytic disease, infants with Beckwith-Weidemann syndrome, and infants who have experienced perinatal asphyxia. Those at risk infants who are sick, extremely premature, or have respiratory distress should receive their maintenance fluids as 10% glucose IV. Because they frequently develop early hypoglycemia and often feed poorly, infants of insulin dependent diabetic women should also be

TABLE 186–2. NEUTRAL THERMAL ENVIRONMENTAL TEMPERATURES*

Age and Weight	*Starting Temperature (C)*	*Range of Temperature (C)*
0–6 h		
Under 1200 gm	35.0	34.0–35.4
1200–1500 gm	34.1	33.9–34.4
1501–2500 gm	33.4	32.8–33.8
Over 2500 gm (and > 36 wk)	32.9	32.0–33.8
6–12 h		
Under 1200 gm	35.0	34.0–35.4
1200–1500 gm	34.0	33.5–34.4
1501–2500 gm	33.1	32.2–33.8
Over 2500 gm (and > 36 wk)	32.8	31.4–33.8
12–24 h		
Under 1200 gm	34.0	34.0–35.4
1200–1500 gm	33.8	33.3–34.3
1501–2500 gm	32.8	31.8–33.8
Over 2500 gm (and > 36 wk)	32.4	31.0–33.7
24–36 h		
Under 1200 gm	34.0	34.0–35.0
1200–1500 gm	33.6	33.1–34.2
1501–2500 gm	32.6	31.6–33.6
Over 2500 gm (and > 36 wk)	32.1	30.7–33.5
36–48 h		
Under 1200 gm	34.0	34.0–35.0
1200–1500 gm	33.5	33.0–34.1
1501–2500 gm	32.5	31.4–33.5
Over 2500 gm (and > 36 wk)	31.9	30.5–33.3
48–72 h		
Under 1200 gm	34.0	34.0–35.0
1200–1500 gm	33.5	33.0–34.0
1501–2500 gm	32.3	31.2–33.4
Over 2500 gm (and > 36 wk)	31.7	30.1–33.2
72–96 h		
Under 1200 gm	34.0	34.0–35.0
1200–1500 gm	33.5	33.0–34.0
1501–2500 gm	32.2	31.1–33.2
Over 2500 gm (and > 36 wk)	31.3	29.8–32.8
4–12 Days		
Under 1500 gm	33.5	33.0–34.0
1501–2500 gm	32.1	31.0–33.2
Over 2500 gm (and > 36 wk)		
4–5 days	31.0	29.5–32.6
5–6 days	30.9	29.4–32.3
6–8 days	30.6	29.0–32.2
8–10 days	30.3	29.0–31.8
10–12 days	30.1	29.0–31.4

(*Continued*)

* These are appropriate isolette temperatures if the room is warm and the isolette wall temperature is within a degree of the air temperature in the isolette. In a cool room, add 1 C to the isolette temperature given in the table for every 7 C that the room is below the isolette temperature.

(Modified from "The Physical Environment" by A. A. Fanaroff, in *Care of the High-Risk Neonate*, ed. 2, by M. H. Klaus and A. A. Fanaroff. Copyright 1979 by W. B. Saunders Company. Used with permission.)

TABLE 186–2. NEUTRAL THERMAL ENVIRONMENTAL TEMPERATURES* *(Cont'd)*

Age and Weight	*Starting Temperature (C)*	*Range of Temperature (C)*
12–14 Days		
Under 1500 gm	33.5	32.6–34.0
1501–2500 gm	32.1	31.0–33.2
Over 2500 gm (and > 36 wk)	29.8	29.0–30.8
2–3 Wk		
Under 1500 gm	33.1	32.2–34.0
1501–2500 gm	31.7	30.5–33.0
3–4 Wk		
Under 1500 gm	32.6	31.6–33.6
1501–2500 gm	31.4	30.0–32.7
4–5 Wk		
Under 1500 gm	32.0	31.2–33.0
1501–2500 gm	30.9	29.5–32.2
5–6 Wk		
Under 1500 gm	31.4	30.6–32.3
1501–2500 gm	30.4	29.0–31.8

started on an IV glucose infusion at birth. At risk infants who are not "sick" should be started on early, frequent formula feedings to provide a source of carbohydrate and other nutrients. In addition, all infants who are at risk for hypoglycemia should have their blood glucose checked at frequent intervals. This can be screened at the bedside using diagnostic glucose test strips (eg, Chemstrip bG®); low values should be confirmed by blood glucose tests in the hospital laboratory.

If the infant develops hypoglycemia, it should be treated at once by IV infusion of 10% glucose in water, 5 to 10 mL/kg over 10 min. The infusion of 10% glucose should then be continued at a rate that provides adequate maintenance fluids; about 4 to 8 mg/kg/min of glucose. Blood glucose values must be monitored so that further adjustments in the infusion rate or additional therapy can be provided. Once the infant's condition has improved, enteral feedings can gradually replace the IV infusion while the blood glucose is monitored. The IV infusion of glucose should always be tapered, as sudden discontinuation may result in hypoglycemia.

If there is difficulty in starting an IV infusion promptly in a hypoglycemic infant, the administration of glucagon 300 μg/kg IM will usually rapidly raise the blood glucose, an effect lasting 2 to 3 h. However, glucagon often will not raise the blood glucose in infants whose glycogen stores are depleted. Hypoglycemia that is refractory to high rates of glucose infusion may be treated with hydrocortisone 5 mg/kg/day IM in 2 divided doses. If hypoglycemia is refractory to treatment, an endocrine evaluation and search for other etiologies (eg. sepsis) should be considered.

HYPERGLYCEMIA

An abnormal increase of the blood glucose above 120 mg/dL in newborns. This condition occurs less frequently than hypoglycemia. However, very low birth weight infants (< 1.5 kg) may not tolerate rapid IV infusions of glucose during the first few days and may become significantly hyperglycemic. Very severely stressed or septic newborns may also develop hyperglycemia. **Transient neonatal diabetes mellitus** is a rate entity

that usually occurs in small-for-gestational-age infants; until this resolves spontaneously, usually within a few weeks, glucose homeostasis and hydration should be carefully maintained.

Severe hyperglycemia with serum hyperosmolarity may cause neurologic damage. Another risk is that hyperglycemia may cause glycosuria with osmotic diuresis and dehydration.

Treatment includes reducing the glucose infusion rate (either by changing the concentration from 10% glucose to 5% glucose, or by slowing the rate). Fluid and electrolyte losses resulting from diuresis are replaced IV. If hyperglycemia persists at low glucose infusion rates (eg, 4 mg/kg/min) it may be an indication of relative insulin deficiency or of insulin resistance. Human insulin may be added to the IV 10% glucose infusion at a ratio of 1 to 2 u./40 gm glucose (or 2 to 6 u./kg/day). The hypoglycemic response to insulin therapy is unpredictable in the newborn, and it is extremely important to monitor the blood glucose frequently.

HYPOCALCEMIA

(See also Ch. 84)

A serum calcium (Ca) concentration < 8 mg/dL. Neonatal hypocalcemia occurs fairly frequently among infants in the intensive care nursery. High-risk groups include premature infants, infants of diabetic mothers, small-for-gestational-age infants, and infants who have experienced perinatal asphyxia.

Etiology

The etiology of **early-onset hypocalcemia** is not well understood. Some preterm or sick newborns appear to have a transient period of relative hypoparathyroidism following birth; when the constant infusion of ionized Ca from the placenta is interrupted their serum Ca falls. This may be exaggerated in infants of diabetic mothers, as these women have higher than normal ionized Ca levels during pregnancy and at birth the neonatal parathyroid glands therefore do not function as well to maintain a normal serum Ca level. Hypocalcemia may also be seen in infants of women with hyperparathyroidism for the same reason. In other infants there appears to be a lack of the normal phosphaturic renal response to parathyroid hormone. Perinatal asphyxia may cause increased serum calcitonin, which inhibits Ca release from bone and leads to hypocalcemia.

After 3 days of age, **late hypocalcemia** may present with tetany of seizures. It is usually due to feedings of cow's milk or formula preparations with too high a phosphate **(PO_4)** load and elevated serum PO_4 leads to hyocalcemia.

Symptoms and Signs

Infants with hypocalcemia are often asymptomatic, but may present with hypotonia, apnea, poor feeding, jitteriness, or seizures. A prolonged QTc interval on the ECG is suggestive of hyocalcemia. Signs of hypocalcemia rarely occur unless the total serum calcium is < 7 mg/dL.

Treatment

Early onset hypocalcemia ordinarily resolves in a few days and treatment usually is not required if the infant is asymptomatic. Infants with serum Ca levels > 7 mg/dL rarely require treatment. Those with levels < 7 mg/dL, should be treated with 10% calcium gluconate solution, 200 mg/kg of calcium gluconate (2 mL/kg) by slow IV infusion over 5 to 10 min. Ten percent calcium gluconate solution contains 100 mg calcium gluconate/mL, and 9 mg elemental calcium/mL. Too rapid an infusion can cause bradycardia, and the heart rate should be monitored during the infusion. The IV site should also be watched closely as tissue infiltration by Ca solution is very irritating and may cause local tissue damage.

After acute correction of hypocalcemia, calcium gluconate may be mixed in the IV fluids and given continuously. Starting with 400 mg/kg/day of calcium gluconate, the dose may be increased gradually to 800 mg/kg/day if needed to prevent recurrence of hypocalcemia. When oral feedings are begun they may be supplemental with the same daily dose of calcium gluconate.

The goal of treatment in late onset hypocalcemia is to add sufficient Ca to the formula to provide a 4:1 molar ratio of Ca to PO_4. This will precipitate calcium phosphate in the GI tract, prevent PO_4 absorption from the GI tract, and enhance Ca absorption.

HYPERNATREMIA

(See also Chs. 84 and 185)

Serum sodium **(Na)** *> 150 mEq/L.* An increase in serum Na concentration may be caused by excessive body loss of free water (hypertonic dehydration), or administration of Na in excess of renal losses. Extreme hypernatremia has been associated with seizures, intracranial hemorrhage, and later neurologic impairment.

Excessive losses of free water frequently occur in association with dehydration in very low birth weight infants **(VLBW)** via cutaneous evaporation of water (insensible water losses) and immature renal function with reduced ability to produce a concentrated urine. The skin of VLBW infants of 24 to 28 wk gestation lacks a stratum corneum and is extremely permeable to water. Skin blood flow and insensible water loss are much increased if the infant is nursed under a radiant warmer or is under bililites. These infants may require up to 150 to 200 mL/kg/day of water given IV in the first few days, after which insensible water loss decreases. Body weight, serum electrolytes, urine volume, and sp gr must be checked at least every 6 to 12 h in these tiny infants, so fluid administration can be adjusted appropriately. Hypernatremia due to excessive water losses is treated by water replacement as 5 or 10% glucose in water IV.

Hypernatremia may also occur if Na in isotonic or hypertonic fluids is administered in excess of renal losses. Daily Na maintenance for low-birth-weight infants is 3 to 4 mEq/kg/day. It is important to remember that fresh frozen plasma and human serum albumin are isotonic Na solutions. Even catheter flushes of isotonic saline may provide a significant amount of Na to VLBW infants. Sodium bicarbonate is a hypertonic solution and should be diluted 1:3 with water before administration. The infant with hypernatremia secondary to excess Na administration will often be edematous and will have high urine Na excretion unless there is cardiac or renal insufficiency. **Treatment** is by stopping the administration of Na and maintaining the administration of water as 5 or 10% glucose IV until the serum Na concentration returns to normal.

In the past, errors in preparing evaporated milk formulas by adding excess sodium chloride resulted in neurologic damage or death of some infants. Infants formulas should not be prepared at home and it is also inadvisable to alter proprietary formulas at home by the addition of salt.

HYPERBILIRUBINEMIA

(See also Ch. 67)

With the breakdown of each gram of Hb, 34 mg of bilirubin are produced. Hyperbilirubinemia will result if bilirubin is overproduced, undersecreted, or both; therefore, the appearance of jaundice can signal a variety of disorders. Known causes of neonatal hyperbilirubinemia are listed in Table 186–3.

Significantly great bilirubin accumulation may result in brain damage due to deposition of bilirubin in the basal ganglia and brainstem nuclei **(kernicterus)**. Early symptoms of kernicterus in term infants are lethargy, poor feeding, and vomiting; opisthotonos, oculogyric crisis, seizures, and death may follow. Kernicterus may not

TABLE 186–3. CAUSES OF NEONATAL HYPERBILIRUBINEMIA

Overproduction	*Undersecretion*	*Mixed*
Fetal–maternal blood group incompatibility—Rh, ABO, others	Metabolic–endocrine	Sepsis
Hereditary spherocytosis (eliprocytosis, somatocytosis)	Familial nonhemolytic jaundice Types 1 and 2 (Crigler-Najjar syndrome)	Intrauterine infections
Nonspherocytic hemolytic anemias	Gilbert's disease	Toxoplasmosis
G6PD deficiency and drugs	Hypothyroidism	Rubella
Pyruvate kinase deficiency	Tyrosinosis	Cytomegalovirus inclusion disease
Other red-cell enzyme deficiency	Hypermethioninemia	Herpes simplex
α Thalassemia	Drugs and hormones	Syphilis
β-δ Thalassemia	Novobiocin	Hepatitis
Acquired hemolysis due to vitamin K_3, nitrofurantoin, sulfonamides, antimalarials, penicillin, oxytocin?, bupivacaine, or infection	Pregnanediol	Respiratory distress syndrome
Extravascular blood—petechiae; hematomas; pulmonary, cerebral, or occult hemorrhage	Lucey-Driscoll syndrome	Asphyxia
Polycythemia	Diabetic mother	Infant of diabetic mother
Maternal–fetal or feto–fetal transfusion	Prematurity	Severe erythroblastosis fetalis
Delayed umbilical cord clamping	Hypopituitarism and anencephaly	
Increased enterohepatic circulation	Obstructive disorders	
Pyloric stenosis*	Biliary atresia*	
Intestinal atresia or stenosis, including annular pancreas	Dubin-Johnson and Rotor's syndromes*	
Hirschsprung's disease	Choledochal cyst*	
Meconium ileus or meconium plug syndrome	Cystic fibrosis* (inspissated bile)	
Fasting or other cause for hypoperistalsis	Tumor or band* (extrinsic obstruction)	
Drug-induced paralytic ileus (hexamethonium)	α_1 Antitrypsin deficiency*	
Swallowed blood	Parenteral nutrition	

* Jaundice may not be seen in neonatal period.

(Adapted from "Neonatal Hyperbilirubinemia," by R. L. Poland and E. M. Ostrea, Jr., in *Care of the High-Risk Neonate,* by M. H. Klaus and A. A. Fanaroff, ed. 2. Copyright 1979 by W. B. Saunders Company. Used with permission.)

be associated with recognizable clinical signs in preterm infants. Later in childhood, late signs of kernicterus may be manifested as mental retardation, choreoathetotic cerebral palsy, sensorineural hearing loss, and paralysis of upward gaze. It is not known if minor degrees of bilirubin encephalopathy can result in less severe neurologic impairment (eg, perceptual-motor handicaps and learning disorders in school).

Normal Route of Bilirubin Excretion

Old or damaged RBCs are removed from the circulation by reticuloendothelial cells, which then metabolize the heme to bilirubin. The bilirubin (unconjugated), attached to serum albumin, is carried to the liver and transferred to binding proteins (Y and Z proteins) in the hepatocytes. Glucuronyl transferase then conjugates the bilirubin with uridinediphosphoglucuronic acid (UDPGA) to bilirubin diglucuronide (conjugated,

direct-reacting bilirubin), which is actively secreted into the bile ducts and enters the GI tract. The newborn lacks proper intestinal bacteria for oxidizing bilirubin in the gut; consequently, unaltered bilirubin is excreted in the stools, giving them a typical bright yellow color. However, the newborn's (and fetus') GI tract contains β-glucuronidase, which deconjugates bilirubin so that unconjugated bilirubin can be rebsorbed and returned to the circulation from the intestinal lumen. The **enterohepatic circulation of bilirubin** allows reabsorption of bilirubin from the fetus' GI tract so that it can be excreted by the placenta, but it may contribute to **physiologic jaundice** because it persists in the newborn.

The exact cause of physiologic hyperbilirubinemia is not known; limiting rates in the binding of bilirubin in the hepatocytes, in the conjugation of bilirubin with glucuronic acid, and in bile secretion have all be implicated, as well as the enterohepatic circulation of bilirubin. Physiologic jaundice appears after 24 h in about 50% of full-term infants and in a higher percentage of premature infants. It usually is not accompanied by constitutional symptoms or signs and disappears within 1 wk. However, excess bilirubin accumulation from any cause (see TABLE 186–3) can produce kernicterus, especially in the preterm or sick neonate.

Etiology

An increased production of bilirubin (eg, from elevated Hb from hypertransfusion, hemolytic diseases, hematomas), a decreased ability to excrete bilirubin (eg, from decreased glucyronyl transferase in the preterm infant, hepatitis, biliary atresia), or both will result in neonatal hyperbilirubinemia (see TABLE 186–3). Neonatal hyperbilirubinemia is most often of the unconjugated (indirect reacting) type. Conjugated hyperbilirubinemia is now seen fairly often due to cholestasis as a complication of parenteral alimentation. Other causes of direct hyperbilirubinemia are listed in TABLE 186–3. The specific etiology must always be sought and treated. For instance, extrahepatic biliary atresia may progress to irreversible cirrhosis if it is not diagnosed and surgically corrected in the first 4 to 6 wk.

Evaluation of Neonatal Hyperbilirubinemia

Jaundice appearing on the first day in any newborn, and a bilirubin concentration > 10 mg/dL in premature infants or > 15 mg/dL in full-term infants, warrants investigation. The blood level of bilirubin is about 4 to 5 mg/dL when jaundice becomes visible. With increasing bilirubin levels, visible jaundice advances in a head-to-foot direction.

In addition to a complete history and physical examination, evaluation of neonatal hyperbilirubinemia should include determination of both total and direct serum bilirubin concentration, direct Coombs' test, Hct, blood smear, reticulocyte count, and the determination of blood type and Rh group of both infant and mother. Other studies, such as blood, urine, and spinal fluid cultures, or determination of RBC enzyme levels, may be indicated by the history, physical examination, or initial laboratory findings (see TABLE 186–3).

Breast milk jaundice: The mechanism of breast milk jaundice is not understood. Occasional term infants who are breast fed will develop progressive unconjugated hyperbilirubinemia during the first week; the problem tends to recur in subsequent pregnancies. If the bilirubin level continues to increase to 17 or 18 mg/dL it may be necessary to change from breast milk to formula feedings and phototherapy may also be indicated. It will only be necessary for the infant to be off of breast milk for one or two days and the mother should be encouraged to continue to express breast milk regularly so that she will be able to commence nursing as soon as the infant's bilirubin level is < 15 mg/dL. She should also be assured that the hyperbilirubinemia has not caused any harm and that she may safely return to breast feeding. Since breast milk jaundice is diagnosed by exclusion, it is important for the physician to evaluate the

infant for other possible causes of the hyperbilirubinemia that may require specific treatment (see also PREMATURE INFANT under GESTATIONAL AGE AND BIRTH WEIGHT in Ch. 186).

Pathogenesis of Kernicterus

There is no clinically proven test available that indicates the risk of kernicterus in a particular infant. Bilirubin is firmly bound to serum albumin and is not free to cross the blood brain barrier and cause kernicterus as long as there are free bilirubin binding sites on serum albumin. The risk of kernicterus is therefore greater in infants who have a low albumin concentration or who have substances present in their serum that compete for bilirubin binding sites on albumin. Such substances include free fatty acids, hydrogen ion, and certain drugs such as sulfisoxazole and aspirin. Serum albumin concentrations are lower in preterm infants putting them at greater risk. Competing molecules (eg, free fatty acids and hydrogen ion) are likely to be elevated in the serum of infants who undergo fasting, are septic, or have respiratory or metabolic acidosis. These clinical conditions would therefore place an infant at increased risk of kernicterus.

Since there is no exact test to determine the risk of kernicterus and hence the level at which exchange transfusion is necessary, the following rule of thumb has proved useful as rough guide. The "exchange transfusion" is set as 0.1 times the weight in kilograms. A 1000 gm infant would receive an exchange transfusion at a bilirubin level of 10 mg/dL, and a 2000 gm infant at 20 mg/dL. It is rarely necessary to do an exchange transfusion if the total serum bilirubin is < 10 mg/dL. Traditionally in term infants exchange transfusion has been done if the toal serum bilirubin reaches 20 mg/dL. Although clinical correlations are not available, in the absence of hemolytic disease the bilirubin may safely be allowed to rise slightly above 20 mg/dL if the infant is not sick. In addition to the determination of exchange transfusion level based upon weight, it it customary to lower the exchange transfusion level by 1 to 2 mg/dL if the infant has clinical factors that would increase the risk of kernicterus (eg, fasting, sepsis, acidosis, etc). Only unconjugated hyperbilirubinemia can cause kernicterus; if the conjugated bilirubin is significantly elevated, only the level of unconjugated bilirubin is used to calculate the need for exchange transfusion.

Treatment

Early frequent feedings of newborns will reduce the incidence and severity of hyperbilirubinemia by increasing GI motility and frequency of stools, thereby minimizing the enterohepatic circulation of bilirubin. The type of feedings does not appear important in increasing bilirubin excretion.

Phototherapy: Exchange transfusion remains the definitive treatment for hyperbilirubinemia that has reached the level where kernicterus may occur. However, phototherapy has proved to be an apparently safe and effective method to prevent or treat hyperbilirubinemia and it has greatly reduced the need for exchange transfusion. Since there are many biological effects of exposure of the neonate to bright light, phototherapy should be used for specific indications.

It is important to carefully consider all possible etiologies for hyperbilirubinemia before starting phototherapy, otherwise the symptom of "jaundice" may be treated without making the correct diagnosis. Phototherapy can be started when the serum bilirubin reaches within 3 or 4 mg/dL of the serum concentration at which exchange transfusion would be performed (see Pathogenesis of Kernicterus, above). Phototherapy produces configurational photoisomers of bilirubin in the skin and subcutaneous tissues; these more water soluble configurations can be rapidly excreted by the liver without the need for prior glucuronidation. Temporary intestinal lactose intolerance occurs during phototherapy, but the resultant diarrhea is not usually a significant problem.

Exposing newborns with hyperbilirubinemia, particularly premature infants, to visible light in the blue range is most effective for reducing hyperbilirubinemia. However, if blue lights are used, cyanosis cannot be detected; therefore, phototherapy using broad-spectrum white light is preferred by many.

A Plexiglas® shield should be placed between the phototherapy lights and the infant to screen out ultraviolet radiation, and the infant should be blindfolded during phototherapy to prevent eye damage. Care must be taken to avoid nasal obstruction by the blindfold, and skin color should not be trusted to evaluate the severity of jaundice, since visible jaundice may disappear during phototherapy while the serum bilirubin remains elevated. The light should be turned off and the blindfold removed during feedings, and also when blood is taken for bilirubin determinations, since bilirubin in the collection tubes may photo-oxidize rapidly. Phototherapy is not indicated if there is biliary or intestinal obstruction since the photoisomers then cannot be excreted. Brownish discoloration of the serum and skin has occurred in such circumstances **(bronze baby syndrome),** but it is not known if this condition is hazardous to the infant.

Exchange transfusion: Traditionally, dangerous levels of bilirubin are treated by exchange blood transfusion via an umbilical vein catheter. Overall mortality is < 1% for this procedure when done by experienced personnel, and should be much less when the procedure is done on otherwise healthy full-term newborns. The level of hyperbilirubinemia at which exchange transfusion is indicated (ie, risk of kernicterus exists if not treated) is given above in Pathogenesis of Kernicterus.

INBORN ERRORS OF METABOLISM

Many inherited biochemical disorders may be detected at or soon after birth. In many states newborns are routinely screened for the more common inborn errors of metabolism including congenital hypothyroidism, galactosemia, hemoglobinopathies, and phenylketonuria. Inborn errors of metabolism are discussed elsewhere in THE MANUAL.

FETAL ALCOHOL SYNDROME (FAS)

Maternal alcohol abuse during pregnancy is the most important cause of drug-induced teratogenesis. The most serious consequence is severe mental retardation, due to impaired brain development. Affected infants have growth retardation and are microcephalic. Multiple malformations may occur—microphthalmia, short palpebral fissures, midfacial hypoplasia, abnormal palmar creases, cardiac defects, and joint contractures; no single finding is pathognomonic. The mental retardation is felt to be part of ethanol teratogenesis since infants of alcoholic women are often retarded even if raised in foster homes.

FAS has been diagnosed in infants born to chronic alcoholics who drank heavily throughout pregnancy. Lesser degrees of alcohol abuse result in less severe manifestations of FAS. Because it is not known when during pregnancy ethanol is most likely to harm the fetus, or whether there is a lower limit of ethanol use that can be considered safe, pregnant women should be advised to avoid all alcohol intake. When a child is affected, the mother's other children should be examined carefully for subtle manifestations of FAS.

DRUG WITHDRAWAL SYNDROMES

The infant of a woman addicted to **narcotics** (eg, heroin, morphine, or methadone) should be observed for the development of withdrawal symptoms within 72 h after delivery. Characteristic signs include irritability, jitteriness, hypertonicity, vomiting, diarrhea, sweating, convulsions, and hyperventilation that produces respiratory alkalo-

sis. Mild withdrawal symptoms are treated by swaddling and frequent feedings to reduce restlessness. Severe symptoms can be controlled by diluting tincture of opium, which contains 10 mg morphine/mL, 25-fold with water and giving 3 to 6 drops q 4 to 6 h as needed. Phenobarbital 5 to 7 mg/kg/day given in 3 divided doses may also control withdrawal symptoms. Treatment is tapered and stopped over several days or weeks as symptoms subside.

Prolonged maternal use of **barbiturates** may cause neonatal drug withdrawal with jitteriness, irritability, and fussing that often does not develop until 7 to 10 days postpartum when the infant has been discharged from the nursery. Sedation with phenobarbital 5 to 7 mg/kg/day given in 3 divided doses may be required and then tapered over a few days or weeks, depending upon the duration of symptoms.

Newborn infants rarely die from drug withdrawal, but long-term effects have not been studied. *Most crucial in the management of infants of mothers addicted to narcotics is evaluation of the home situation to determine if the infant will be safely cared for following hospital discharge.* The supportive help of relatives, friends, and visiting nurses may enable the mother to care for her infant. Otherwise, foster home care or an alternative care plan may be in the best interests of the child. The incidence of **sudden infant death syndrome** is greater in infants born to narcotic addicts, even in those placed in foster homes, and evaluation for cardiorespiratory monitoring at home should be considered.

SEIZURE DISORDERS IN THE NEWBORN

(See also Ch. 121)

General Considerations

Seizures are a frequent and serious neonatal problem and require immediate evaluation to determine their etiology and treatment. They are usually focal and may be difficult to recognize; migratory clonic jerks of extremities, alternating hemiseizures, or primitive subcortical seizures (respiratory arrest, chewing movements, persistent deviations of the eyes, episodic changes in tone) are common. A typical grand mal seizure is infrequent. The focal nature of neonatal seizures may be due to the lack of myelination, the primarily inhibitory nature of the newborn cortex, or incomplete formation of dendrites and synapses in the brain at this age.

Seizures can only arise from an abnormal CNS discharge, but this may be from a primary intracranial process (meningitis, tumor, encephalitis, intracranial hemorrhage) or secondary to a systemic or metabolic problem (anoxia, hypoglycemia, hypocalcemia, hyponatremia, etc). The type of seizure seen in the newborn is not helpful in distinguishing focal CNS lesions from metabolic problems. It is important to separate the clonic activity seen with hypertonicity and jitteriness from true seizure activity. Jitteriness produces clonus only with stimulation, and holding the extremity will stop it. Seizures occur spontaneously, and their motor activity can be felt to continue when the limb is held.

Etiology

Since specific treatment for many causes of neonatal seizures is known, the etiology must be pursued. **Hypoglycemia** is common in infants born to diabetic mothers, infants small for gestational age, and those with a hypoxic insult or other stress. In full-term infants, blood sugar levels < 30 mg/dL are considered hypoglycemic; in low-birth-weight infants, < 20 mg/dL. Not all infants have symptoms at hypoglycemic levels. Whether asymptomatic hypoglycemia leads to neurologic damage is unknown, but the possibility exists. **Hypocalcemia,** defined as a serum calcium level < 7.5 mg/dL, is usually accompanied by a serum phosphorus level of > 3 mg/dL and, like hypoglycemia, can be asymptomatic. It is often associated with prematurity or difficult births. **Hypomagnesemia** is uncommon, but can produce seizures when the serum magnesium

level is < 1.4 mEq/L. Hypomagnesemia is often associated with hypocalcemia and should be considered in a hypocalcemic infant when the seizures continue after adequate calcium therapy. Either **hyper-** or **hyponatremia** may cause seizures. Hypernatremia can result from accidental sodium chloride overloading. Hyponatremia can be dilutional or may follow sodium loss in stool or urine.

Seizures are frequent with **meningitis**. They also occur in **sepsis**, but generally are not a presenting sign. Intracranial and systemic infections are often caused by gram-negative organisms. Cytomegalovirus, herpes simplex virus, rubella virus, *Treponema pallidum*, and *Toxoplasma gondii* should also be considered. **Pyridoxine deficiency** or dependency is a rare but readily treated cause of seizures. Other causes in newborns are more difficult to diagnose and to treat. They include the sequelae of **hypoxia, intraventricular hemorrhage, birth trauma, malformations of the CNS,** and **drug withdrawal.**

Diagnosis

The evaluation of neonatal seizures should begin with blood sugar, calcium, magnesium, and electrolyte determinations. Commercially available test strips provide a rapid blood sugar determination, but a concomitant true blood glucose should also be obtained. Next, infection is sought through cultures from peripheral sites, blood, and CSF. The CSF should also be examined for abnormal numbers of RBCs or WBCs, and for the sugar and protein content. The need for further metabolic tests, such as arterial pH, blood gases, serum bilirubin, or urine amino acids, depends on the clinical situation. X-rays of the skull may reveal intracranial calcifications, and long-bone films may show changes due to congenital infectious diseases such as rubella and syphilis. An EEG is useful in documenting and following the seizures; it is especially helpful if there is difficulty in deciding whether or not the infant is having seizures. The presence of a normal or focal EEG during a seizure has been shown clinically to be a good prognostic sign, while a diffusely abnormal EEG is a poor one. Cranial ultrasonography can document intracranial hemorrhage. If other etiologies have been excluded or maternal addiction is suspected, the mother should be studied as a help in diagnosing neonatal drug withdrawal seizures.

Prognosis and Treatment

Although conditions causing neonatal seizures have a high mortality and are often associated with permanent neurologic damage, nearly 50% of neonates who have seizures and survive will be normal at age 5 yr.

Therapy should be directed primarily at the underlying pathology and secondarily at the seizure. Except for seizures presenting as apnea, it is usually not necessary to stop a seizure in progress, since they generally are self-limited and rarely compromise vital function in a newborn. If blood glucose is low, 50% dextrose 1 to 2 mL/kg IV is given. If hypocalcemia is present, 10% calcium gluconate can be given IV in a dose up to 10 mL in term infants and 6 mL in premature infants. *Calcium gluconate should be given no faster than 1 mL/min and with continuous cardiac monitoring.* Extravasation should be avoided, since sloughing of the skin can result. If magnesium deficiency is diagnosed, 1 mL of a 50% magnesium sulfate solution is given IM. Infections should be treated with the appropriate antibiotics.

Symptomatic treatment of the seizure itself should begin immediately after completing the initial efforts to identify its cause. Phenobarbital is the drug of choice and should be given in a loading dose of 15 to 20 mg/kg. Maintenance therapy, consisting of 5 to 8 mg/kg/day in 2 divided doses, should be started 12 h later. Phenobarbital should be given IV, especially if seizures are frequent or prolonged. When the seizures are controlled, the oral route can be used. Phenytoin in similar doses can also be used, if necessary, or added, if 2 drugs are needed to control seizures. It is only effective IV in neonates, and should be given slowly to avoid hypotension or arrhythmias. Signs of

phenytoin toxicity may be difficult to detect in newborns, and prolonged high levels may be harmful. If blood levels can be monitored, the risk is smaller. Therapeutic blood levels for phenobarbital are 15 to 40 μg/mL; for phenytoin, 10 to 20 μg/mL. Infants taking anticonvulsant medication need close observation, since overmedication with resulting respiratory depression and even arrest may at times be more dangerous to them than the seizures themselves.

CONGENITAL SENSORINEURAL HEARING LOSS

In the past, epidemics of rubella resulted in the birth of large numbers of children with congenital deafness. Particularly during the first trimester of pregnancy, the rubella virus may invade the developing inner ear **(viral endolymphatic labyrinthitis)** and produce much destruction and a profound sensorineural hearing loss. Other causes of profound congenital sensorineural hearing loss are anoxia during birth, bleeding into the inner ear from trauma to the base of the skull during delivery (particularly in premature infants), ototoxic drugs given to the mother, erythroblastosis fetalis, and numerous hereditary conditions including Waardenburg's syndrome, albinism, and Hurler's syndrome.

Diagnosis and Treatment

If a child does not develop speech normally, a differential diagnosis of deafness, mental retardation, aphasia, and autism must be considered.

Since children must hear language to learn it, deaf children do not develop language without special training. They require special education, beginning as soon as the hearing loss is identified. Because there is an optimum time for acquisition of language, early diagnosis of deafness in infants is essential.

Amplification with a **hearing aid** should be started as early as possible after diagnosis (even as early as 6 mo of age). In bilateral sensorineural hearing loss, binaural amplification using postauricular or in-the-ear aids is indicated to maximize hearing and permit development of auditory localization. For information on various types of hearing aids, see Ch. 207.

NEONATAL INFECTIONS

ANTIMICROBIAL THERAPY FOR NEWBORNS

Rapid physiologic changes during the neonatal period significantly affect the pharmacokinetic and toxicologic properties of antimicrobial agents. Absorption, distribution, metabolism, and excretion of drugs vary in neonates according to body weight, surface area, and gestational and chronologic ages (see below and the appropriate chapters in Rx). These changes necessitate complex dosing and frequency interval selections based on cmpiric data derived from studies of antimicrobials in newborns (see TABLE 186–4).

Pharmacologic Principles

Antibiotic distribution: The extracellular fluid compartment comprises up to 40% of total body weight in neonates. This increases the volume of distribution of certain drugs (eg, aminoglycosides) and requires larger doses relative to weight than those used in adults. Lower serum albumin concentrations in premature infants may affect antibiotic protein binding. Drugs that displace bilirubin from albumin (eg, sulfonamides) may increase the risk of kernicterus.

Antibiotic metabolism and excretion: Absence or deficiency of certain enzymes during early neonatal life may prolong the half-life of certain drugs and increase the risk of toxicity. For example, immaturity of hepatic glucuronyl transferase activity in neo-

nates diminishes conjugation of chloramphenicol to the inactive form. This can cause cardiovascular collapse and death, the **"gray baby syndrome,"** in infants treated with excessive dosages of chloramphenicol. Diminished GFR and renal tubular secretion in neonates increases the half-life values of penicillins and aminoglycosides. With changing renal function during the first month of life, dosage and frequency of administration of these antibiotics must be readjusted.

When using antibiotics that have unpredictable pharmacokinetics or a narrow therapeutic index (eg, chloramphenicol and aminoglycosides), plasma drug levels should be measured at appropriate intervals to assure sufficient but not excessive levels. Chloramphenicol levels should be measured, especially when the infant is given concurrent treatment with rifampin, phenobarbital, or acetaminophen, because of interference with hepatic metabolism. The measurement can usually be done in the USA in reference or university laboratories.

Route of administration: Vasomotor instability of infants with serious bacterial infection results in unpredictable drug absorption when drugs are given s.c. or IM. Therefore, antibiotics for severe infections should preferentially be given IV. Oral antibiotics can be used for outpatients who are not seriously ill (see TABLE 186–5).

Antibiotic therapy in pregnant or lactating women: Most commonly used antimicrobial agents cross the placenta and are excreted in human breast milk. Sulfonamides, chloramphenicol, and tetracyclines should particularly be avoided in pregnant and nursing mothers (see DRUGS IN PREGNANCY under PRENATAL CARE in Ch. 176).

Choice of antimicrobial regimen: Specific therapy should be tailored according to the results of cultures and antimicrobial susceptibility testings. Empiric treatment, usually a combination of ampicillin and an aminoglycoside, is often started pending these results (see also in NEONATAL SEPSIS in this chapter, below). Knowing the prevalence of antibiotic-resistant gram-negative bacilli in a particular nursery is helpful in choosing the first-line antibiotic regimens. If skin lesions are present or catheter-associated infections are suspected, additional antistaphylococcal coverage is recommended.

Physicians should be cautious when using potent broad-spectrum antimicrobial agents such as the newer cephalosporins; these agents can induce drastic changes in bowel flora, bleeding disorders, emergence of resistant organisms, and superinfections with yeasts or enterococci.

TABLES 186–4 and 186–5 recommend dosages for selected antimicrobial agents for newborns. Pharmacologic data and safety and efficacy data are limited for many drugs; however, as new, safer agents become available, those older drugs with known toxic effects and unpredictable pharmacokinetics will no longer be used routinely. Other drugs, although less commonly used in the newborn, that do have specific therapeutic values are vancomycin for infections caused by methicillin-resistant staphylococci; metronidazole for anaerobic infections; ceftazidine for *Pseudomonas aeruginosa*; trimethoprim-sulfamethoxazole for shigellosis, salmonellosis, *Pneumocystic carinii*, and rare cases of gram-negative bacillary meningitis refractory to other regimens; and rifampin for TB and prophylaxis for meningococcal and *Hemophilus influenzae* diseases.

NOSOCOMIAL INFECTION IN THE NEWBORN

Infections contracted while in the hospital or from organisms acquired in the hospital. By definition, infant infections caused by organisms acquired during or after birth in a hospital are considered nosocomial even when they are acquired from the mother. Obviously, not all nosocomial infections are preventable.

About 1% of *term* newborns develop infection while in the hospital; in others the infection becomes apparent shortly after going home. The incidence of sepsis, however, is low—about 1:1000 live births. By contrast, about 15% of *premature* and *sick*

TABLE 186–4. DOSAGE RECOMMENDATIONS FOR SELECTED PARENTERAL ANTIMICROBIAL AGENTS FOR NEWBORNS

Antimicrobial Agent	*Route of Adm.*	*Individual Dose*	*Interval of Administration* Infant Weight < 2000 gm, Age 0–7 days	Infant Weight < 2000 gm, Age ≥ 8 days	Infant Weight ≥ 2000 gm, Age 0–7 days	Infant Weight ≥ 2000 gm, Age ≥ 8 days	*Comments*
Aqueous penicillin G	IV						
Meningitis		100,000 u./kg	q 12 h	q 8 h	q 8 h	q 6 h	Maximum for group B streptococcal meningitis, 400,000 u./kg/day
Other diseases		50,000 u./kg	q 12 h	q 8 h	q 8 h	q 6 h	
Penicillin G	IM						
Benzathine		50,000 u./kg	q 24 h	q 24 h	q 24 h	q 24 h	
Procaine		50,000 u./kg	q 24 h	q 24 h	q 24 h	q 24 h	
Ampicillin	IM, IV						
Meningitis		50 mg/kg	q 12 h	q 8 h	q 8 h	q 6 h	
Other diseases		25 mg/kg	q 12 h	q 8 h	q 8 h	q 6 h	
Ticarcillin	IM, IV	75 mg/kg	q 12 h	q 8 h	q 8 h	q 6 h	No primary indication. Use in combination with aminoglycoside against *P. aeroginosa.* Potential bleeding with renal failure
Carbenicillin	IM, IV	100 mg/kg	q 8 h	q 8 h	q 8 h	q 6 h	
Mezlocillin	IM, IV	75 mg/kg	q 12 h	q 8 h	q 8 h	q 6 h	Limited data
Methicillin	IM, IV						
Meningitis		50 mg/kg	q 12 h	q 8 h	q 8 h	q 6 h	Monitor renal functioning
Other diseases		25 mg/kg	q 12 h	q 8 h	q 8 h	q 6 h	
Nafcillin, oxacillin	IV						
Meningitis		50 mg/kg	q 12 h	q 8 h	q 12 h	q 8 h	Limited data
Other diseases		25 mg/kg	q 12 h	q 8 h	q 12 h	q 8 h	
Cephalothin*	IV	20 mg/kg	q 12 h	q 8 h	q 8 h	q 6 h	No primary indication. Limited data. Do not use for initial therapy of sepsis or meningitis
Cefazolin*	IM, IV	20 mg/kg	q 12 h	q 12 h	q 12 h	q 8 h	
Cefotaxime	IM, IV	50 mg/kg	q 12 h	q 8 h	q 12 h	q 8 h	Limited data
Ceftazidime	IV, IM	50 mg/kg	q 12 h	q 8 h	q 12 h	q 8 h	

Moxalactam	IM, IV	50 mg/kg	q 12 h	q 8 h	q 12 h	q 8 h	Loading dose of 100 mg/kg in meningitis. Not active against group B streptococci or *Listeria monocytogenes*. Potential bleeding
Cefamandole	IM, IV	30 mg/kg	q 8 h	q 6 h	q 6 h	q 6 h	Limited data. No primary indication
Ceftriaxone	IM, IV						
Meningitis		50 mg/kg	q 12 h	q 12 h	q 12 h	q 12 h	Limited data.
Other diseases		50 mg/kg	q 24 h	q 24 h	q 24 h	q 24 h	
Kanamycin† and	IM, IV	10 mg/kg	—	q 8 h	q 12 h	q 8 h	Monitor serum peak drug levels (kanamycin or amikacin = 15–25 μg/mL; gentamicin or tobramycin = 5–10 μg/mL). Reduce dose for impaired renal function. Reduce frequency in very small premature infants (q 18 h)
Amikacin†		7.5 mg/kg	q 12 h	—	—	—	
Gentamicin†	IM, IV	2.5 mg/kg	q 12 h	q 8 h	q 12 h	q 8 h	
Tobramycin†	IM, IV	2 mg/kg	q 12 h	q 8 h	q 12 h	q 8 h	
Chloramphenicol	IV, IM	25 mg/kg	q 24 h	q 24 h	q 24 h	q 12 h	Adjust doses by monitoring serum drug levels and hematologic parameters
Vancomycin	IV	15 mg/kg loading dose, then 10–15 mg/kg	q 12 h	q 8 h	q 12 h	q 8 h	Limited data. Give by slow IV infusion, no less than 60 min. Monitor serum levels, adjust doses in renal failure
Metronidazole	IV	7.5 mg/kg	q 12 h	—	q 12 h	—	Give loading dose of 15 mg/kg. Limited data
		15 mg/kg	—	q 12 h	—	q 12 h	
Trimethoprim/ sulfamethoxazole‡	IV	3.5 mg/kg TMP, 12.5–25 mg/kg SMX	q 12 h	q 12 h	q 12 h	q 12 h	Limited data. Monitor bilirubin and hematologic and renal parameters
Amphotericin B	IV	0.25 – 1 mg/kg	Dilute in D5W (do not use saline solution) Limited data. Start at 0.25 mg/kg single daily dose over 4–h infusion. After patient improves, give dose every other day. Increase by 0.25 mg/kg every other day, up to 1 mg/kg/day. Total dose over a 4– to 6–wk period, about 30–35 mg/kg. Monitor hematologic and renal functions				

* Does not cross the blood-brain barrier.

† Sample to be obtained after end of IV infusion or 60 min after IM injection.

‡ In shigellosis, 2 mg/kg TMP and 10 mg/kg SMX loading dose followed by 0.6 mg/kg TMP and 3 mg/kg SMX q 12 h. In gram-negative meningitis and *P. carinii* pneumonitis, use higher doses. Measure TMP levels on the 3rd day of therapy (desirable peak of TMP is 5 to 6 μg/mL.

TABLE 186–5. DOSAGE RECOMMENDATIONS FOR SELECTED ORAL ANTIMICROBIAL AGENTS FOR NEWBORNS

Antimicrobial Agent	*Dosage (mg/kg/dose)*	*Interval*	*Comments*
Amoxicillin Cefaclor	15	q 8 h	Limited data
Erythromycin estolate	10	q 8–12 h	For chlamydia or pertussis
Erythromycin ethyl succinate	10	q 6 h	
Neomycin Colistin	3–4	q 6 h	For gastroenteritis caused by enteropathogenic strains of *E. Coli,* and for prophylaxis of neonates at high risk for necrotizing enterocolitis. May be systemically absorbed in the presence of significant diarrhea. Unproven efficacy and safety
Rifampin	10	q 24 h	For tuberculosis
	5	q 12 h	For meningococcus prophylaxis for 2 days
	10	q 24 h	For *H. influenzae* prophylaxis for 4 days
Flucytosine	25	q 6 h	Limited data. Use only in combination with amphotericin, to retard emergence of resistance

infants in some studies have developed one or more nosocomial infections, with a high risk of death.

Most infants are born from a sterile environment to a world teeming with microorganisms. Colonization with bacteria and other organisms is inevitable, but exposure to more virulent organisms before a balanced and inhibitory normal flora is established can result in illness. Premature or ill infants may not have fully functional defenses (see IMMUNOLOGIC STATUS OF THE FETUS AND NEWBORN under MANAGEMENT OF THE NORMAL NEWBORN in Ch. 182) and are likely to undergo multiple invasive diagnostic, therapeutic, and monitoring procedures that further breach barriers to infection.

Term nurseries: Skin infection with *Staphylococcus aureus* acquired in the nursery is the most frequent nosocomial infection in term infants. Other types of infection include meningitis or sepsis with group B β-hemolytic *Streptococcus, Citrobacter,* or *Listeria monocytogenes*; diarrhea caused by enterotoxigenic or enteropathogenic *Escherichia coli,* salmonella, or rotaviruses; disease with herpes simplex, enteroviruses, or respiratory syncytial virus; ophthalmitis or complicated infection with *Neisseria gonorrhea*; or conjunctivitis or pneumonitis with *Chlamydia trachomatis.* The majority of these infections are transmitted from mother to infant during the perinatal period, although transmission among infants in the nursery is possible if appropriate control measures are not followed. Sepsis with *E. coli* or other gram-negative pathogens is uncommon in healthy term infants, but clusters of infection caused by virulent strains occur. Except for group A streptococcal infection, most postpartum maternal genital infections are not likely to be transmitted to the newborn. Consequently, a febrile postpartum woman who feels well enough and has no infection that endangers her

infant may be allowed to handle and feed her newborn if she washes her hands thoroughly, wears a clean hospital gown, and prevents the baby from contacting any contaminated items.

***Staphylococcus aureus* disease and skin care regimens**: Pustular skin lesions in the periumbilical or diaper area are the most frequent manifestations, although complicated and disseminated infections including osteomyelitis, pneumonia, and meningitis occur. Staphylococcal **scalded skin syndrome,** ranging in severity from scarlatiniform erythema to bullous lesions to generalized exfoliative disease **(Ritter's disease)** is caused by *S. aureus* producing exfoliative toxin. Clinical onset of *S. aureus* infection varies from a few days to several months of age, but usually occurs at 2 to 3 wk. *S. aureus* pathogens resistant to methicillin, gentamicin, and other antibiotics are becoming more common in nurseries.

Colonization of infants in the nursery with *S. aureus* ranges from < 10 to 70% or more. Since different strains vary markedly in virulence, the probability of disease in colonized infants also varies greatly, and a high colonization rate per se is not an indication for instituting specific control measures. In fact, colonization with a noninvasive strain may "interfere" with colonization by disease-producing strains. Therefore, culturing of infants for surveillance should be undertaken only if the nursery is experiencing **disease** due to *S. aureus*. Since most such infections appear after the infant has left the nursery, a surveillance system to assess infections occurring within the first month of life should be established with the community's infant health care providers.

Although nursery personnel who are *S. aureus* nasal carriers and disseminators are potential sources of infection for infants, colonized infants in the nursery are most frequently the reservoir; transmission is from infant to infant on the transiently colonized hands of personnel. The umbilical stump and groin are the most frequently colonized sites during the first few days of life, while the nares are more frequently colonized later.

Skin care for newborns may affect colonization patterns. Bathing infants with 3% hexachlorophene decreases frequency of *S. aureus* colonization, but *routine* use of this product is inadvisable because of its potential neurotoxicity, particularly in low birth weight infants. The American Academy of Pediatrics recommends dry skin care for infants, but in some hospitals this has resulted in high rates of colonization with *S. aureus* and epidemics of disease. During disease outbreaks, applying triple dye to the cord area or bacitracin ointment to the cord and/or nares and circumcision site helps reduce colonization, and hospitals troubled with *S. aureus* disease may temporarily institute daily bathing of the diaper area of each term infant with 3% hexachlorophene emulsion, which should then be rinsed off.

Special-care nurseries: The bacterial floras colonizing premature and sick infants in special-care nurseries tend to be the predominantly gram-negative organisms prevalent there (eg, *Klebsiella*, *Enterobacter*, *Pseudomonas*, and *Proteus*), which frequently are resistant to multiple antibiotics.

Organisms are transmitted via the hands of personnel and the multiple invasive procedures used for these infants: long-term arterial and venous catheterization for intravascular pressure monitoring, parenteral nutrition, or access for fluids, medicine, or blood sampling; endotracheal intubation with ventilatory assistance or continuous airway pressure; and nasogastric or nasojejunal feeding tubes for alimentation. All these procedures have been implicated as causes of epidemic or endemic nosocomial infections. Prevention of colonization and infection requires providing sufficient space (80 to 100 sq ft/infant in intensive care; 50 sq ft/infant in intermediate care; 6 ft between incubators or warmers, edge-to-edge in each direction) and personnel (nurse to patient ratio 1:1 to 2 in intensive care, 1:3 to 4 in intermediate care); knowledge of

recommended methods for patient-care (including technics for placement and care of invasive devices); and meticulously cleaning and disinfecting or sterilizing equipment between use on successive infants. Active surveillance for infections (not colonization) and monitoring of procedure methodology are essential.

Establishing a strict cohort of infected or colonized babies is impractical in most special-care nurseries. However, many infected infants can be cared for in these units if personnel follow appropriate isolation technic, including the use of gowns (to prevent contamination of uniforms and forearms) and gloves (when touching lesions or handling items potentially contaminated with infectious secretions or excretions). Forced-air incubators provide limited protective isolation but should not be relied upon to prevent transmission from an infected infant; the exteriors and interiors of the units rapidly become heavily contaminated, and personnel are likely to contaminate their hands and forearms while working with the infants in the units.

Prophylaxis: Although frequently used, nonspecific antibiotic prophylactic therapy is *not* effective, hastens development of resistant bacteria in the unit, alters the balance of normal flora in the infant, and predisposes the infant to colonization with more resistant strains. Routine prophylactic antimicrobial therapy is recommended only for prevention of gonorrheal ophthalmia neonatorum (see NEONATAL CONJUNCTIVITIS, below) or complicated gonococcal infection in exposed infants. Antibiotics against specific pathogens may be considered under special circumstances; eg, penicillin G for prophylaxis against group A streptococcal infection or oral colistin or neomycin for prophylaxis against enterotoxigenic or enteropathogenic *E. coli* during a confirmed nursery epidemic. Prophylaxis for neonatal hepatitis B virus is discussed below, under NEONATAL HEPATITIS B VIRUS INFECTION.

An infant who remains in the hospital > 2 mo should be immunized against diphtheria, tetanus, and pertussis **(DTP)** according to the routine schedule for age (see IMMUNIZATION PROCEDURES THROUGHOUT CHILDHOOD in Ch. 182). To avoid cross-infection with other infants in the nursery, oral (live virus) polio vaccine should not be given in the hospital.

Screening blood prior to transfusions is now routinely done to detect units that may be contaminated with human T-lymphotropic virus, type III (HTLV-III). Infants born to cytomegalovirus (CMV) seronegative mothers are at risk of serious infection or death if transfused with CMV-contaminated blood; every effort should be made to transfuse infants with only blood or components screened for CMV. (See Ch. 19 and CONGENITAL AND PERINATAL CYTOMEGALOVIRUS INFECTION, below.)

Routine practices for nursery personnel include active surveillance for infections; knowledge of disease transmission; providing sufficient room (in the term nursery, 30 sq ft of floor space/bassinet, and 40 sq ft in the admission-observation nursery; a minimum of 3 ft between bassinets, edge-to-edge in each direction) and personnel (1 nurse/6 to 8 term infants requiring routine care); and emphasis on handwashing between infant contacts. Providing each infant with his own supplies and equipment in a separate bassinet reduces the risk for cross-contamination. Since airborne transmission of disease in a nursery is relatively uncommon, infants with various infections may be cared for in a general nursery if personnel are meticulous in technics to avoid transmission between infants, as described above. The environs of infants with diarrhea or draining skin lesions may be heavily contaminated; a separate room for these infants is desirable. Similarly, a separate room or strict cohort is desirable for infants with many types of congenital infection (CMV, rubella, syphilis) or those with potentially serious viral infections (herpes simplex, respiratory syncytial virus, coxsackievirus).

Nursery personnel should wear short-sleeved scrub clothes provided and laundered by the hospital, but long-sleeved gowns are recommended for handling infants outside incubators and bassinets. Caps, beard bags, and masks are recommended and sterile gloves are essential only during invasive procedures, such as inserting an umbilical

catheter. *Handwashing is the keystone to infection control in the nursery*. At the start of a shift, personnel should scrub hands and forearms to the elbows. Between handling infants, a vigorous 15-second wash with an antiseptic agent is recommended (vigorous washing is more important than the antiseptic agent chosen). Disposable gloves may limit hand contamination when working with infected infants or contaminated items. Personnel should not wear jewelry while on duty.

Personnel with respiratory tract infections (including pharyngitis), furuncles, draining skin lesions, diarrhea, or fever should not work with infants. Those with *active* nasolabial herpes preferably should not work with infants, but the risks of compromising patient care by excluding essential personnel must be weighed against the risk of infecting an infant. Personnel with chronic dermatitis on their hands should be individually evaluated. Serology for rubella should be performed on all personnel; susceptible women should be counseled about the risk of infection and offered rubella vaccine or the option of working in another area during pregnancy.

Encouraging mothers to room-in with their infants and establishing alternate birth centers as part of the delivery facility can enhance the birth experience without increasing the risk of infection to mother or infant when instituted with care. Having sufficient personnel is important (1 nurse/3 mother-infant pairs for rooming-in). The presence of siblings at the birth and liberal visiting policies with the mother (eg, in a family lounge or private room) should be encouraged; only visitors with active infectious illness should be excluded.

In an epidemic, establishing cohorts of diseased or colonized infants is useful; unexposed infants may be discharged early or may room with their mothers rather than be admitted to the nursery. Continuing surveillance of infants for 1 mo post-discharge is necessary for assessing the adequacy of controls instituted to abort an epidemic.

NEONATAL CONJUNCTIVITIS

(Ophthalmia Neonatorum)

Purulent ocular drainage is common during the neonatal period. The major causes are, in decreasing order, chemical, chlamydial, and bacterial. Chemical conjunctivitis is generally secondary to the instillation of silver nitrate drops for ocular prophylaxis. *Chlamydia trachomatis*, the most frequent infectious cause of neonatal conjunctivitis, occurs in 2 to 4% of live births. Chlamydial inclusion conjunctivitis (inclusion blennorrhea), acquired by the infant during parturition, may account for 1/3 to 1/2 of all cases of conjunctivitis seen in infants < 4 wk of age. The prevalence of maternal chlamydial infection ranges from 2 to 20%; about 33% of infants born to affected women will develop conjunctivitis and 10% will develop pneumonia. Other bacteria, including *Streptococcus pneumoniae* and *Hemophilus influenzae*, account for another 15% of all cases of neonatal conjunctivitis. The frequency of ophthalmia neonatorum in the USA due to *Neisseria gonorrhoeae* is 2 to 3/10,000 live births. Aside from *H. influenzae* and *N. gonorrhoeae*, isolation of other bacteria, including *Staphylococcus aureus*, may represent colonization and not infection. The major viral agent that causes neonatal conjunctivitis is herpes simplex virus **(HSV),** types 1 and 2.

Clinical Presentation

The different causes of neonatal conjunctivitis are difficult to distinguish on clinical grounds alone because they overlap in both presentation and onset. **Chemical conjunctivitis** secondary to silver nitrate usually appears within 6 to 8 h after instillation and disappears spontaneously within 24 to 48 h. **Gonococcal ophthalmia** produces an acute purulent conjunctivitis that appears 2 to 5 days after birth, or earlier if there has been premature rupture of membranes. The infant has severe eyelid edema followed by chemosis and a profuse purulent exudate that may spurt out of the lids when they are separated. If treatment is delayed, corneal ulcerations may occur. **Inclusion conjunctivi-**

tis due to *C. trachomatis* usually occurs 5 to 14 days after birth. It may range from mild conjunctivitis with minimum mucopurulent discharge to severe edema of the eyelids with copious drainage and pseudomembrane formation. Unlike in older children and adults, follicles are not present in the conjunctiva in neonates with this infection. The onset and presentation of conjunctivitis due to other bacteria are extremely variable, ranging from 4 days to 3 wk. **Keratoconjunctivitis** due to HSV can occur as an isolated infection or in conjunction with disseminated or CNS infection. Herpetic conjunctivitis can be mistaken for bacterial or chemical conjunctivitis, but the presence of dendritic keratitis is pathognomonic.

Diagnosis

The first diagnostic procedure should be a culture and Gram stain of the conjunctiva. *Gonococcal infection must be ruled out.* The presence of intracellular gram-negative, coffee-bean–shaped diplococci suggests gonococcal infection. Cultures should be placed on appropriate media (eg, Thayer-Martin) for isolating *N. gonorrhoeae*. Examining the Gram stain also helps to suggest other bacterial pathogens. In chlamydial infection, a smear of the conjunctiva should show a predominantly mononuclear reaction with no organisms.

The most sensitive means of diagnosing chlamydial ophthalmia is a direct culture of the conjunctiva. Since *C. trachomatis* is an intracellular parasite, it must be grown in cell culture. Cultures of the conjunctiva can be obtained by firmly stroking the everted lower eyelid with a calcium alginate swab. The results of examining Giemsa-stained *epithelial* scrapings for cells containing characteristic basophilic cytoplasmic inclusions correlate well with culture results. However, in order to obtain an adequate sample of epithelial cells (not just exudate), a blunt spatula should be used. Two rapid, nonculture diagnostic methods are now commercially available: a monoclonal antibody test that detects chlamydiae in smears, and an enzyme-linked immunoassay. Both appear to be very sensitive and specific for detecting chlamydiae in conjunctival specimens.

The diagnosis of herpetic conjunctivitis can best be confirmed by isolating the virus, detecting specific HSV-1 or HSV-2 antigen by immunofluorescence in conjunctival scrapings, or identifying HSV particles by electron microscopic evaluation.

Prophylaxis

Routine use of 1% silver nitrate, erythromycin, or tetracycline ophthalmic ointments or drops instilled into each eye after delivery is recommended by the CDC for prevention of neonatal **gonococcal conjunctivitis**. Erythromycin and, possibly, tetracycline will also prevent **chlamydial conjunctivitis.** Since infants born to mothers with untreated gonorrhea are at increased risk of infections at other sites, full-term exposed infants should be treated prophylactically with a single injection of aqueous crystalline penicillamine G, 50,000 u. IM or IV and low-birth-weight infants should receive 20,000 u. IM or IV.

Treatment

For **gonococcal ophthalmia,** the infant should be hospitalized and given aqueous penicillin G 100,000 u./kg/day IM in 4 divided doses for 5 to 7 days. Frequent irrigation of the eye with saline will prevent secretions from adhering. Topical antimicrobial preparations alone are not sufficient and are not required if appropriate systemic antibiotic therapy is given. For infections due to penicillinase-producing *N. gonorrhoeae*, neonates can be treated with either cefotaxime 100 mg/kg/day IV in 3 divided doses for 7 days or ceftriaxone 125 mg IM as a single dose. Conjunctivitis due to other bacteria usually responds to topical ointments containing polymixin plus bacitracin, erythromycin, or tetracycline. Since at least 1/2 of the infants with **chlamydial conjunctivitis** also have nasopharyngeal infection and some develop chlamydial pneumonia, systemic therapy is preferable to topical therapy. Erythromycin ethylsuccinate 50 mg/kg/day orally q 6 or 12 h for 10 days to 2 wk is recommended. **HSV conjunctivitis**

should be treated (*in association with an ophthalmologist*) with trifluorothymidine ophthalmic drops or ointment q 2 to 3 h while the infant is awake and in combination with idoxuridine ointment at bedtime, until 3 to 5 days after healing appears to be complete. If there is no response within 7 to 8 days, therapy with systemic acyclovir should be considered. Specific diagnosis is important, since ointments containing steroids may seriously exacerbate eye infections due to *C. trachomatis* and HSV.

ACUTE INFECTIOUS NEONATAL DIARRHEA

A syndrome caused by pathogenic bacteria and viruses, characterized by passage of formless stool and often associated with an abnormal increase in stool frequency and vomiting. It must be differentiated from the normal stool patterns of breast-fed infants as well as from other noninfectious causes of diarrhea (see TABLE 186–6). Acute infectious gastroenteritis in older infants and children is discussed in Ch. 191.

Etiology and Epidemiology

Infectious agents can be acquired during the first month by several routes: (1) maternal organisms ingested during passage through the contaminated birth canal; (2) bacteria from other infants or toddlers with gastroenteritis, usually transmitted on the hands of nursery personnel or parents; (3) organisms acquired directly from the con-

TABLE 186–6. NONINFECTIOUS CAUSES OF NEONATAL DIARRHEA

Anatomic Disorders	**Metabolic and Enzymatic Disorders**
Hirschsprung's disease	Congenital disaccharidase deficiency (lactase, sucrase-isomaltase deficiency)
Massive intestinal resection (short-bowel syndrome)	Congenital glucose-galactose malabsorption
Intestinal lymphangiectasia	Secondary disaccharide, monosaccharide malabsorption
Inflammatory Disorders	1. After GI surgery
Cow-milk protein intolerance	2. After infection
Soy protein intolerance	3. With milk-soy protein sensitivity
Regional enteritis	Cystic fibrosis
Ulcerative colitis	Syndrome of pancreatic insufficiency and bone marrow dysfunction (Schwachman syndrome)
Primary Immunodeficiency Disorders	Physiologic deficiency of pancreatic amylase
Wiskott-Aldrich syndrome	Intestinal enterokinase deficiency
Thymic dysplasia	Congenital bile-acid deficiency syndrome
Miscellaneous	Abetalipoproteinemia
Irritable colon of childhood (chronic nonspecific diarrhea)	Acrodermatitis enteropathica
Phototherapy for hyperbilirubinemia	Congenital chloride diarrhea
Familial dysautonomia (Riley-Day syndrome)	Primary hypomagnesemia
Familial enteropathies	Congenital adrenal hyperplasia
High sulfates in water	Intestinal hormone hypersecretion
Phenolphthalein poisoning/child abuse	1. Non-β islet cell hyperplasia (vasoactive intestinal peptide—**VIP**)
Narcotic withdrawal	2. Neural crest tumors
Necrotizing enterocolitis	Wolman's disease
	Transcobalamin II deficiency
	Hereditary tyrosinemia (hepatorenal type)
	Methionine malabsorption (oasthouse disease)
	Hartnup disease

(Modified from "Microorganisms Responsible for Neonatal Diarrhea" by S. M. Marcy and R. L. Guerrant, in *Infectious Diseases of the Fetus and Newborn Infants,* ed. 2, 1983, edited by J. Remington and J. O. Klein. Copyright 1983 by W. B. Saunders Company. Used with permission of W. B. Saunders Company and the author.)

taminated hands of symptomatic or asymptomatic contacts; (4) airborne or droplet infection; (5) fomites; (6) contaminated formula or solid food supplements; and (7) household pets. Routes 1 and 2 are probably most common.

There are few longitudinal studies on the etiology of sporadic community-acquired diarrhea in neonates. Most reports are based on observations during outbreaks in newborn nurseries or infant wards. The apparent etiology has varied according to season, geography, and diagnostic technics available. Major bacterial pathogens that have been implicated in industrialized nations include *E. coli*, *Salmonella* spp., and *Campylobacter* spp. At present, 3 different diarrheagenic types of *E. coli* are recognized: enteropathogenic *E. coli* **(EPEC)**, enterotoxigenic *E. coli* **(ETEC)**, and invasive *E. coli* **(IEC)**. The mechanism of action of EPEC is uncertain but may be partly due to close destructive adherence to the intestinal brush border or to a cytotoxin; ETEC secrete a heat-labile and/or heat-stable enterotoxin. IEC produce an invasive shigella-like enterocolitis (see also Ch. 57).

Nursery outbreaks have been attributed to ECHO viruses 5, 11, 14, 17, and 18, coxsackie viruses A and B, and enteric adenoviruses. Rotavirus, the agent responsible for most cases of enteritis in older infants, is occasionally implicated in neonatal illness, although asymptomatic carriage is more frequent. The possible role of other agents such as a Norwalk-like agent, astrovirus, calicivirus, and coronavirus in neonatal illness is still under investigation.

Rare cases of infantile diarrhea in nurseries have been associated with the isolation of enterotoxigenic strains of *Klebsiella*, *Pseudomonas*, *Citrobacter*, *Proteus*, and *Providencia*. The development of selective media is permitting evaluation of the role of *Campylobacter jejuni* and *Yersinia enterocolitica* in neonatal disease. *Staphylococcus aureus*, *Candida albicans*, amoeba, and giardia may be responsible for GI disease on rare occasions.

Symptoms and Signs

Dehydration and electrolyte imbalance can develop rapidly in newborns with diarrhea, particularly if accompanied by vomiting. Documented weight loss, poor feeding, and irritability are important early findings. Dry oral mucous membranes, diminished skin elasticity, sunken eyes and fontanels, and listlessness are late signs and usually reflect fluid losses of 10% or more. Oliguria in the first weeks of life, before renal concentrating mechanisms are fully matured, is also a late sign of dehydration.

Mucoid, slimy, bloody stools indicate colitis, usually due to *Shigella*, *Salmonella*, or *Campylobacter*. Passage of watery, yellow or green, voluminous, relatively odorless, nonbloody stools, abrupt in onset, is associated with enteritis caused by rotavirus, ETEC, or EPEC.

Bacteremia due to *Salmonella* and *Campylobacter*, or "secondary" sepsis caused by normal enteric organisms that enter the bloodstream through areas of necrosis or ulceration in the colon, may accompany diarrheal disease. Infants with prolonged or severe symptoms should be carefully examined for metastatic foci of infection. Fever is often absent, even in seriously infected neonates.

Laboratory Diagnosis

Two stool cultures with antibiotic susceptibility studies should be obtained. Technics appropriate for isolating more fastidious organisms, such as *C. jejuni* or *Y. enterocolitica*, should be used whenever possible. Stool cultures should also be taken from close contacts with enteric disease (eg, family members or nursery staff). Seriously ill neonates must be evaluated for systemic infection by examination and culture of the CSF, urine, and blood, and by chest x-ray.

Examining a freshly passed stool may help in making an etiologic diagnosis. Large numbers of fecal polymorphonuclear leukocytes, often accompanied by RBCs, indicate an invasive colitis due to *Shigella*, *Salmonella*, *Campylobacter*, *Yersinia* or IEC. If

the diarrhea is unusually persistent or relapsing, secondary sugar-malabsorption due to villous brush-border damage should be suspected. Testing watery stools promptly (within 30 min) for pH (< 6) and reducing substance (> 0.5%) helps to confirm the diagnosis. (In interpreting the test results, it should be borne in mind that altered intestinal flora due to antibiotic therapy, breast-feeding, or use of an elemental formula may normally result in acid pH and reducing substances in the stool.)

Additional helpful technics include dark-field or phase-contrast microscopy (*Campylobacter*); enzyme-linked immunosorbent assay **(ELISA)** (rotavirus); fluorescent antibody stains (*Shigella sonnei*, EPEC); electron-microscopy (viruses). Serotyping to identify EPEC can be accomplished through agglutination tests with commercially available typing sera; confirmation of toxigenic properties of *E. coli* requires special laboratory facilities.

The WBC count and differential are of little value in determining the etiology or severity of gastroenteritis but can be useful in suspected bacteremia or focal infection. Serum electrolytes and BUN or creatinine are important aids in guiding fluid and electrolyte therapy in hospitalized patients.

Treatment

Primary attention must be directed to restoring and maintaining fluid and electrolyte balance. Excessive diarrhea or weight loss, vomiting, fever, unreliable caretakers, or an impression that the infant looks "sick" indicates need for hospitalization.

Infants with cardiovascular instability, those with persistent vomiting of small-volume oral feedings, and those who refuse to drink require parenteral IV fluid therapy. Infants in shock with collapsed peripheral veins can be given emergency fluids via tibial bone marrow or intraperitoneal routes.

Following an initial evaluation to establish baseline weight and clinical appearance, most infants—whether in hospital or at home—can be treated with *carefully monitored* oral fluid therapy. Infants who are breast-feeding may continue to do so ad libidum, but should be offered supplementary fluids such as those described below. Others should be started on small, frequent feedings of oral rehydrating fluids such as proprietary sugar-electrolyte solutions (Pedialyte®, Lytren®, Infalyte®). Avoid fluids containing red dyes that may color the stool and lead to an erroneous diagnosis of hematochezia.

World Health Organization oral rehydration solution (WHO-ORS) may also be used—each liter contains 90 mEq sodium, 80 mEq chloride, 20 mEq potassium, 30 mEq bicarbonate, and 110 mmoles of sucrose (40 gm/L) or glucose (20 gm/L). Alternatively, a satisfactory WHO-ORS can be made by mixing the following ingredients: isotonic saline 450 mL, 5% glucose 500 mL, potassium chloride injection USP 10 mL, and 8.4% sodium bicarbonate 30 mL. Whichever solution is used, *one volume of water or breast milk should follow every 2 volumes of solution, or serious hypernatremia may result.*

After initial rehydration and stabilization with sugar-electrolyte solutions, lactose-free soy-based formula may be offered to non-breast-fed infants. Milk or formula feedings can be resumed cautiously a few days later. If diarrhea recurs because of temporary lactose malabsorption, soy formula should be restarted and continued for 2 or 3 wk. Occasionally, elemental or casein-hydrolysate formulas or even IV hyperalimentation will be required to control diarrhea and prevent protein–calorie malnutrition. Prolonged diarrhea with continued weight loss despite these measures mandates hospital observation and a search for alternate etiologies.

Optimal antimicrobial therapy for **bacterial enteritis** varies from one geographic area to another and even at different hospitals within the same city. Thus, although the drugs recommended below are generally adequate, the clinician should keep informed of changing patterns of antibiotic resistance among organisms isolated from his patient population.

***Shigella* infections** should be treated with ampicillin 50 to 75 mg/kg/day parenterally for 5 to 7 days. If an ampicillin-resistant strain is isolated, 10 mg trimethoprim/50 mg sulfamethoxazole/kg/day orally or IV in 2 divided doses may be used. Sulfa drugs are contraindicated in jaundiced infants, and their use in neonates requires informed consent. Chloramphenicol is a less desirable alternative. In very ill infants, consideration of possible "secondary" sepsis would indicate need for an aminoglycoside in addition to the primary anti-shigella therapy.

Antibiotic therapy does not benefit a neonate with mild ***Salmonella* gastroenteritis.** Newborns with fever, moderate to severe diarrhea, suspected concurrent septicemia, or localized infection should, however, receive treatment. Parenteral chloramphenicol 25 to 50 mg/kg/day (depending on weight, age, and serum levels when possible) for 5 to 7 days is sufficient in most cases. Ampicillin 50 to 75 mg/kg/day (depending on weight and age) can be used to treat infection caused by susceptible strains. Focal complications require more prolonged therapy. Occasionally, a protracted mild colitis with failure to thrive may respond to antibiotic therapy. The asymptomatic carrier state should not be treated.

If an **EPEC or ETEC infection** is identified, epidemic spread in a nursery and the duration of illness may be reduced by treating for 3 to 5 days with colistin 15 mg/kg/day orally in 3 divided doses. Resolution of ***Campylobacter* enteritis,** if still symptomatic at the time the agent is identified, may be hastened through the use of oral erythromycin estolate 30 mg/kg/day in 3 divided doses. When bacteremia is suspected or proven, addition of parenteral gentamicin 5 to 7.5 mg/kg/day (monitoring plasma levels) is indicated. There are no clinical data upon which to base recommendations for antimicrobial therapy for *Yersinia* or IEC enterocolitis in newborns; both organisms are usually susceptible to aminoglycosides and chloramphenicol.

Any attempt to alter the course of neonatal gastroenteritis with antiperistaltics or antidiarrheal agents is contraindicated. Impairment of bowel motility not only potentiates persistent colonization of the host with enteropathogens, but also permits significant sequestration of fluid in the bowel, masking the seriousness of dehydration by decreasing the number of stools and preventing weight loss.

Persons responsible for the care of a neonate with diarrhea must be instructed in simple enteric precautions—particularly handwashing. Up to 50% of neonates may continue to excrete *Salmonella* organisms for 3 mo, 10% for 1 yr. A carrier state may also follow *Shigella* and *Campylobacter* enterocolitis. Follow-up stool cultures should be taken when infection with these organisms is present. Epidemiologic investigation must be initiated in the event of a nursery outbreak.

NEONATAL SEPSIS
(Sepsis Neonatorum)

Invasive bacterial infection that occurs in the first 4 wk of life. Bacterial infections, the primary cause in 10 to 20% of neonatal deaths, occur 5 times more often in low-birth-weight **(LBW)** newborns than in full-term newborns.

Neonatal sepsis occurs in from 1:500 to 1:1600 live births; the highest rates occur in lower socioeconomic groups. The risk is greater in males (2:1) and in neonates with congenital malformations, particularly those of the GU tract.

The newborn may be predisposed to neonatal sepsis by obstetric complications, eg, premature rupture of the membranes **(PROM)** occurring 24 or more hours before birth (or as little as 6 h before, if accompanied by active labor), maternal bleeding (placenta previa, abruptio placentae), toxemia, precipitous delivery, maternal infection (particularly of the urinary tract or endometrium), and newborn resuscitation procedures. Neonatal sepsis is usually diagnosed in the first 7 days of life when the newborn's history includes a perinatal complication. By contrast, sepsis most commonly develops

after 7 days of age without known predisposing factors; this group includes those who acquire nosocomial infections.

Advances in antimicrobial therapy and supportive care for neonatal sepsis have not significantly decreased the mortality rate (25 to 70%). The fatality rate occurring within 72 h after birth is higher than when sepsis occurs later without predisposing factors, and it is twice as high in LBW as in full-term neonates.

Etiology

Before 1940 Group A β-hemolytic streptococcus was the major cause of neonatal sepsis, but was replaced by gram-negative enteric bacilli. Coagulase-positive staphylococci caused the nursery epidemics of the late 1950s. During the 1960s, coliforms returned to prominence (perhaps in part because of the introduction of routine hexachlorophene bathing) with *Escherichia coli* (predominantly those containing the K_1 polysaccharide capsule) being the most common cause of neontal sepsis. In the 1970s, the Group B streptococcus (*Streptococcus agalactiae*) emerged to equal or exceed them.

It is helpful to distinguish whether the infection most likely was derived from the maternal vaginal vault or from the environment. Pathogenic organisms acquired before, during, or immediately after birth are likely to cause sepsis identified within the first 7 days of life **(early-onset sepsis)**, while those acquired from the environment (the mother, nursery personnel, or inanimate objects used for infant support) generally appear after the first week of life **(late-onset sepsis)**. Group B streptococci or *E. coli* cause approximately 70% of early-onset neonatal sepsis; other gram-negative enteric bacilli—*Listeria monocytogenes*, Group D streptococci (enterococcus and *Streptococcus bovis*) and occasionally *Streptococcus pneumoniae, Hemophilus influenzae* type b, and *Neisseria meningiditis*—cause the remaining 30%. *Staphylococcus epidermidis* is emerging as a major pathogen in intensive care nurseries in infants after the first 48 h of life.

Gonococcal infection should be considered in evaluating a septic neonate, since asymptomatic gonorrhea occurs in 5 to 10% of pregnancies. Because an infected newborn is at risk for both ophthalmia and disseminated gonococcal disease, endocervical cultures should be performed routinely during pregnancy and at delivery.

The role of anaerobes (particularly *Bacteroides fragilis*, which requires special culture media for identification) in neonatal sepsis is unclear, although neonatal deaths have been attributed to *Bacteroides* bacteremia. Anaerobes may account for some culture-negative cases in which autopsy findings indicate sepsis, and should be suspected in the presence of foul-smelling amniotic fluid at birth.

These comments on etiology pertain to the predominant pathogens in North American nurseries, but in other areas different pathogens (eg, *L. monocytogenes* in Spain and gram-negative enteric bacilli—particularly *Salmonella* spp—in Latin America) may predominate.

Group B streptococcal disease may present as a fulminating, primarily bacteremic and pulmonic form that may be caused by serotypes I, II, or III. In this form there is a high incidence of associated obstetrical complications and of desperately ill newborns who rapidly develop respiratory distress and shock, with a mortality rate of 50 to 80%; meningitis is frequently absent. The late-onset, meningitic form occurs at 1 to 12 wk and is caused almost exclusively by serotype III. This form is not always associated with demonstrable maternal cervical colonization—a fact which suggests that postnatal acquisition of the organism may occur.

L. monocytogenes also may occur in an early form—respiratory distress and shock with a fulminant course within the first several days of life and primarily involving the lungs (granulomatosis infantiseptica)—or in a later, predominantly meningitic form with a better prognosis.

E. coli is the predominant pathogen in early-onset neonatal sepsis; 40% of *E. coli* causing septicemia and 80% of those causing meningitis possess the K_1 capsular antigen, a virulence factor for *E. coli*.

A distinct bacteriologic profile exists for those organisms derived from the environment that cause **late-onset sepsis.** The nosocomial infection rate for newborns hospitalized for > 48 h in a regional newborn intensive care unit may be as high as 25%. *Staphylococcus aureus* and gram-negative enteric bacilli (particularly *Klebsiella* spp, *E. coli*, *Proteus* spp, *Pseudomonas aeruginosa*, as well as enterococcus and Candida) are the predominant pathogens. Most commonly, nosocomially acquired cases occur sporadically but epidemics occur and may be due to single, usually multiply-resistant organisms (eg, *Klebsiella pneumoniae*, *Enterobacter cloacae*, and *S. aureus*). More recently, *Staphylococcus epidermidis* has emerged as a common nosocomial pathogen, most frequently associated with indwelling intravascular devices.

Pathogenesis

The clustering of neonatal bacterial infections in the perinatal period suggests that pathogens usually are acquired during labor and delivery. Hematogenous and transplacental dissemination of maternal infection occurs in the transmission of viral (eg, rubella, cytomegalovirus), protozoal (eg, *Toxoplasma gondii*), and treponemal (eg, *Treponema pallidum*) agents. A few bacterial pathogens (eg, *L. monocytogenes*, *Mycobacterium tuberculosis*) reach the fetus transplacentally, but most are acquired by the ascending route in utero (as in PROM) or as the fetus passes through the birth canal. Organisms may invade the fetal circulation by contaminating superficial chorionic vessels, but more commonly by fetal aspiration or swallowing of contaminated amniotic fluid and subsequent invasion of the bloodstream. The ascending route of infection helps to explain the high incidence of PROM in neonatal infections, the significance of adnexal inflammation (amnionitis being more commonly associated with neonatal sepsis than is central placentitis), the increased risk of infection to the twin closer to the birth canal, and the bacteriology of sepsis, which reflects the flora of the maternal vaginal vault.

Foci of infection become established in the paranasal sinuses, middle ear, lungs, or GI tract, and may be disseminated to meninges, kidneys, bones, joints, peritoneum, and skin. Pneumonia is the most common invasive bacterial infection in the neonate.

Newborns (particularly those of LBW) are immunologically immature and ill-suited to defend against the polymicrobial flora to which they are exposed during and after parturition. The role of passively acquired IgG antibody in protecting the fetus is vividly demonstrated by serotype-III Group B streptococcal infections. Mothers without significant antibodies against this organism give birth to newborns with significantly higher risk of developing the disease than those born to mothers with the antibodies. Similar protection by maternal antibodies against other bacteria causing early-onset neonatal sepsis (eg, *E. coli*) has not been convincingly demonstrated.

Certain bacterial "virulence" factors (eg, Group B streptococcus serotype-III polysaccharide and the K_1 antigen in *E. coli*) seem to play a role, particularly in meningitis.

Most important, perhaps, are certain deficiencies in the newborn that are related to birth weight and the host. They include low levels of complement (and consequent opsonization deficiency), chemotactic and cytotoxic monocyte dysfunction, and certain polymorphonuclear leukocyte abnormalities (including deformability, altered chemotaxis, phagocytosis and bacterial killing, and depressed oxidative responses). (See IMMUNOLOGIC STATUS OF THE FETUS AND NEWBORN under MANAGEMENT OF THE NORMAL NEWBORN in Ch. 182.)

Risk factors for nosocomial infection include associated illness (eg, respiratory distress syndrome—which may only be a marker for increased use of invasive supportive technics), exposure to antimicrobial agents, prolonged hospitalization, contaminated laboratory support equipment, and intravenous or enteral solutions. The gram-positive organisms (eg, *S. aureus*) may be introduced by nursery personnel; gram-negative enteric bacteria are almost always derived from the patient's endogenous flora, which frequently has been altered by antecedent antibiotic therapy. Once colonized, however,

all of these organisms spread via the hands of nursery personnel. Therefore, situations (chiefly, crowding, high nurse-to-newborn ratios, and poor handwashing) that increase exposure of the neonate to these bacteria result in a higher nosocomial infection rate in the newborn nursery.

Symptoms and Signs

Because the newborn can respond to perinatal insults in only a few ways, the early signs of neonatal sepsis are frequently nonspecific and subtle. Diminished spontaneous activity or less vigorous sucking, temperature instability (hypo- or hyperthermia), respiratory distress, apnea, neurologic signs (eg, seizures, jitteriness), jaundice (especially occurring within the first 24 h of life without Rh or ABO incompatibility), vomiting, diarrhea, and abdominal distention all occur with varying frequency, but none of these signs is specific for sepsis.

Specific signs of an infected organ may pinpoint the primary source or a metastatic site. Examination of the ears, preferably with pneumatic otoscopy, may identify otitis media. Periumbilical erythema, discharge, or bleeding in a neonate without a hemorrhagic diathesis (infection prevents obliteration of the umbilical vessels) suggests omphalitis. Coma, seizures, opisthotonos, or a bulging fontanel signals severe CNS dysfunction and suggests meningitis or brain abscess. Decreased spontaneous movement of one extremity and/or swelling, warmth, erythema, and tenderness over a joint indicate pyogenic arthritis and/or an underlying osteomyelitis. Unexplained abdominal distention may indicate peritonitis or necrotizing enterocolitis (particularly when accompanied by bloody diarrhea with fecal leukocytes).

Diagnosis

Early diagnosis requires awareness of risk factors (particularly in LBW newborns) and a high index of suspicion when any newborn deviates from the norm in the first few weeks of life. Remarks by parents or nurses that the neonate is "not doing well" or any signs of sepsis require prompt investigation. The following laboratory tests include those likely to produce helpful diagnostic information and should be performed as part of the routine workup of a newborn for suspected sepsis.

WBC count, differential, and smear: The "normal" WBC in the newborn varies, but values < 4,000 or > 25,000 are abnormal. An absolute band count > 1500 is highly predictive of neonatal sepsis, as is an immature:total ratio of > 0.14. Examination of the peripheral blood smear for toxic granulation, vacuolization, and Döhle bodies may be a valuable index of bacteremia.

Buffy coat: Gram stain of the buffy coat may reveal organisms in 35% or more of the neonates with a positive blood culture, probably reflecting relatively large numbers of bacteria that circulate in the newborn in sepsis.

Lumbar puncture should be performed in any neonate suspected of sepsis. A needle with a trocar is used, to avoid introduction of epithelial tissue and subsequent development of epitheliomas. The CSF, even if bloody or acellular, should be cultured.

Blood cultures: Umbilical vessels are frequently contaminated by organisms on the umbilical stump and yield unreliable cultures. Blood for culture should be obtained by venipuncture, preferably at 2 peripheral sites, each carefully prepared first with an iodine-containing liquid, followed by 95% alcohol. Blood should be cultured for both aerobic and anaerobic organisms.

Urinalysis and culture: Urine should be obtained by suprapubic aspiration, not by urine collection bags. Finding ≥ 5 WBC/high-power field **(hpf)** in the spun urine or any organisms in a fresh unspun gram-stained sample (regardless of collection method) is presumptive evidence of a UTI, which in the newborn suggests antecedent bacteremia. Absence of pyuria does not rule out UTI.

Counterimmunoelectrophoresis (CIE) and latex agglutination (LA) tests, using high-titered, type-specific antiserum, detect antigen in body fluids (eg, CSF, concentrated

urine) with great reliability in the newborn. They can contribute additional information by detecting capsular polysaccharide antigen of Group B streptococcus, *E. coli* K_1, *S. pneumoniae*, *H. influenzae* type B, and *N. meningiditis*.

External ear canal fluid: Gram-stain examination and culture of this fluid may indicate the infecting organism. The presence of 3 or more polymorphonuclear leukocytes **(PMNs)**/hpf frequently predicts a positive blood culture, with the same organism being cultured from the otic fluid.

Gastric fluid: Only one in 30 neonates having 5 or more PMNs/hpf in the gastric aspirate will develop sepsis within 72 h of birth, but missing that one infant is rare when using this criterion for predicting positive blood-culture results.

Treatment

Newborns with **early-onset sepsis** should receive ampicillin or penicilin G plus an aminoglycoside. Sepsis recognized or suspected after the 1st wk of life should be treated initially with methicillin plus an aminoglycoside or a 3rd generation cephalosporin (see NEONATAL MENINGITIS below). Once an organism is identified, antibiotic therapy is adjusted according to sensitivities and the site of infection. If foul-smelling amniotic fluid is present at birth, therapy for anaerobes (chloramphenicol) should be considered in the initial antibiotic coverage. Chloramphenicol should be given only if serum levels of the drug can be closely monitored. There are insufficient pharmacokinetic data to provide guidelines for the use of clindamycin in newborns.

The choice of an aminoglycoside for early-type sepsis is dictated by the antibiotic sensitivity pattern for the nursery of each hospital. When 10% of isolated *E. coli* strains are resistant to a particular aminoglycoside, it should not be used for at least 6 mo. Subsequently, if resistance drops to < 10%, that aminoglycoside may be returned to use with continued surveillance of resistance rates.

Initial therapy of patients with **late onset sepsis** should include methicillin plus an aminoglycoside (or a 3rd-generation cephalosporin). Newborns previously treated with an aminoglycoside who need retreatment should receive a different aminoglycoside.

If *S. epidermidis* is isolated from blood or other normally sterile fluid and is considered to be a pathogen, initial therapy with vancomycin is recommended, since about 35% of *S. epidermidis* isolates are resistant to semisynthetic penicillins (eg, methicillin). However, if the organism is found to be sensitive to this class of antibiotics, then vancomycin should be discontinued and replaced by methicillin. Removal of the source of this organism (usually an indwelling intravascular catheter) is essential.

Vaginal or rectal cultures of women at term may show colonization rates of up to 30% by Group B streptococcus; at least 50% of their newborns will also become colonized. Only 1 in 100 of those colonized will develop invasive disease due to Group B streptococcus. At present, there is insufficient data to recommend routine culture and treatment of mothers at term or routine culture and treatment of newborns who are colonized at only superficial sites (eg, umbilicus, perineum, throat).

Humoral deficiencies (including decreased amounts of maternally-derived specific antibody and low complement levels) may be corrected by administering fresh plasma or fresh-frozen plasma **(FFP)**. (NOTE: These materials should be used only if they can be demonstrated to be CMV-antibody negative, HBsAg negative, and negative for antibody against HTLV-III, the agent of AIDS. If HTLV-III antibody testing is not available, only blood products obtained from individuals with no known risk factors for AIDS should be used). Fifteen mL/kg of either preparation should be given IV over 3 h daily for as long as the patient remains clinically ill.

Newborns with absolute granulocyte counts ≤ 1500/µL are at excess risk of death from neonatal sepsis and may benefit from granulocyte transfusion. PMNs are obtained from normal adult donors with red cell antigens compatible with their neonatal recipient. To prevent graft vs. host disease, each granulocyte pack must be treated with 1500 rads before transfusion. Granulocyte transfusions of 15 mL/kg of a suspension

containing 0.5 to 1 × 10^9 granulocytes/15 mL with < 10% lymphocytes should be used. Infusions are administered once or twice daily for 5 days.

Patients with disseminated intravascular coagulation or shock may benefit by exchange transfusion using 160 mL/kg of citrated blood < 48 h old, repeated q 8 to 12 h up to 4 times until clinical stabilization occurs. After the first exchange transfusion, most infants who will survive demonstrate increased mean arterial pressure and pH, and improved tissue perfusion.

These newer measures (FFP, granulocyte, and exchange transfusions) may represent significant gains over other, routinely employed supportive measures for sick newborns and should be viewed as promising additions to be used judiciously in attempting to diminish the still-high mortality rate due to bacterial sepsis of the newborn.

NEONATAL PNEUMONIA

Neonatal pneumonia, like sepsis, may be of early or late onset.

EARLY-ONSET PNEUMONIA

Pneumonia as part of generalized sepsis and present at or within hours of birth.

Etiology

Early-onset pneumonia often occurs following prolonged rupture of the amniotic membranes or amnionitis. The fetus is surrounded by infected amniotic fluid, and respiratory efforts result in aspirating into the lungs organisms that cause pneumonia and sepsis. These organisms may also gain entry by being swallowed by the fetus, or through the conjunctiva or the scalp after it has been broken by electrode insertion. Neonatal pneumonia has also been associated with low Apgar scores and perinatal complications; eg, premature labor, placental abruption, and difficult forceps delivery.

Group B streptococcus is the most common cause of early-onset sepsis and pneumonia, but occasionally *Listeria monocytogenes, Hemophilus influenzae, Escherichia coli, Klebsiella*, and other gram-positive and gram-negative organisms are responsible.

Symptoms, Signs, Diagnosis, and Treatment

The infant's appearance depends on the severity of the sepsis and pneumonia, ranging from infants who simply have transient tachypnea of the newborn **(TTNB)** or labored respirations to those with respiratory failure and septic shock from the time of birth. The delivery history (eg, amnionitis) may suggest the diagnosis, but bacterial pneumonia cannot be distinguished clinically from other causes of neonatal respiratory distress, such as respiratory distress syndrome **(RDS)**, TTNB, meconium aspiration, or persistent pulmonary hypertension. Chest x-rays also may not distinguish between causes of respiratory disease. X-rays of neonatal pneumonia may show patchy infiltrates, interstitial fluid, or, rarely, lobar consolidations; or the x-rays may look like those of RDS, TTNB, or meconium aspiration.

Evaluation for suspected pneumonia is the same as for sepsis (see NEONATAL SEPSIS, above). Cultures of blood, tracheal aspirate, and CSF are most important. A CBC with platelet count and a urine test for latex agglutination for Group B streptococcus are useful.

Treatment of both early- and late-onset pneumonia is the same as that for NEONATAL SEPSIS, above.

LATE-ONSET PNEUMONIA

Pneumonia usually seen after 7 days of age and most common in neonatal intensive care units in infants who require prolonged endotracheal intubation because of chronic lung disease or who have long-term vascular catheters that provide another site for bacterial invasion.

Symptoms, Signs, and Diagnosis

Onset of nursery-acquired pneumonia may be gradual, with increased secretions being suctioned from the endotracheal tube and need for increased ventilator settings. Other infants may be acutely ill and have temperature instability and neutropenia. Chest x-ray may show new infiltrates, but these may be difficult to recognize if the infant has severe bronchopulmonary dysplasia.

Evaluation includes cultures of blood and tracheal aspirate. Coagulase-negative staphylococcus, resistant to oxacillin, in recent years has been a common cause of nursery-acquired sepsis and pneumonia. Vancomycin is the drug of choice, but a less nephrotoxic antibiotic may be substituted when the sensitivity reports are available. In infants likely to have been on a variety of broad-spectrum antibiotics, a wide spectrum of pathogens may be found, including coagulase-positive staphylococcus, *E. coli*, *Klebsiella*, *Pseudomonas*, *Proteus*, and *Serratia*, as well as *Candida albicans* and other fungi (see NEONATAL SEPSIS, above).

For **treatment**, see NEONATAL SEPSIS, above.

NEONATAL MENINGITIS

Inflammation of the meninges due to bacterial invasion in the first 4 wk of life. It occurs in 2:10,000 full-term and 2:1,000 LBW infants; there is a male predominance. It is a frequent concomitant to neonatal sepsis (see above).

E. coli containing the K_1 polysaccharide and Group B streptococcus (predominantly Type III) account for 70% of meningitis in the newborn. Meningitis due to Group B streptococcus may be present in the first week of life, when it accompanies early-type pneumonic illness. Usually, however, it occurs after this period (and up to 3 mo of age) as an isolated illness characterized by absence of antecedent obstetric or perinatal complications, predominance of serotype III, presence of more specific signs of meningitis (eg, fever, lethargy, seizures), and a mortality rate (15 to 20%) that is significantly lower than that with the earlier-onset type.

Other enteric gram-negative bacilli, *Listeria monocytogenes*, and enterococcus are less common—but significant—causes of neonatal meningitis.

Most affected infants have a history of LBW and one or more of the obstetric or perinatal complications that predispose to neonatal sepsis. Usually the meninges are seeded by bacteremia from another focus (70% of cases have a positive blood culture), but direct extension to the CNS from a contiguous focus may occur (eg, otitis media, emphasizing the importance of the middle ear examination).

Signs and Diagnosis

CNS signs usually are subtle and nonspecific (eg, jitteriness, apnea, vomiting, diarrhea, jaundice). A high index of suspicion is required. Definitive diagnosis can be made only by examining the CSF; lumbar puncture should be performed in any infant suspected of sepsis. The CSF should be examined by Gram stain and cultured, and cell count and protein and glucose determinations made. The CSF of normal newborns during the first several days of life contains up to 32 WBCs/mm³ (mean = 8), which declines to 10 by 1 mo of age. As many as 60% of those cells may be polymorphonuclear neutrophil leukocytes. Similarly, the CSF protein may be as high as 170 mg/dL in the first week of life. Since a normal newborn blood glucose may be as low as 40 to 60 mg/dL, it is important to obtain a peripheral blood glucose for comparison with the CSF glucose. The normal CSF/blood glucose ratio is ≥ 50%.

Ventriculitis is a frequent concomitant of neonatal meningitis, particularly when caused by gram-negative enteric bacilli. A poor prognosis is correlated with the presence of ventriculitis, persistence of positive CSF cultures, a CSF WBC count ≥ 10,000, and a CSF protein ≥ 500 mg/dL. Brain abscess (frequently caused by *Citrobacter diversus*) or subdural empyema may occur. The mortality rate in neonatal meningitis is 15 to 60% (the better prognosis is for those due to Group B streptococcus), and 3/4 of

the survivors suffer severe CNS dysfunction (eg, hydrocephalus, deafness, psychomotor retardation), particularly when caused by gram-negative enteric bacilli.

Treatment

Treatment of gram-negative meningitis is constantly being reevaluated because the mortality rate remains unacceptably high. Aminoglycosides penetrate variably or poorly into the CSF. They do not reach the ventricles in therapeutic concentrations, even when given intrathecally in the lumbar space, and no clinical advantage has been demonstrated for intrathecal administration over parenteral administration. Since ventriculitis is common in gram-negative enteric meningitis, after it is diagnosed by ventricular tap aminoglycosides (eg, gentamicin 2 to 3 mg q 18 to 24 h) may be administered into the ventricles by placement of an Ommaya or a Salmon-Rickham reservoir. However, this mode of therapy has not demonstrably improved the outcome and is controversial.

Third-generation cephalosporins (eg, moxalactam, cefotaxime, ceftizoxime, ceftazidime, and ceftriaxone) are being evaluated; their excellent broad-spectrum in vitro activity and achievable high bactericidal concentrations in the CSF make them look promising for the treatment of suspected or proven gram-negative meningitis in newborns. All of them except moxalactam have good activity against the group B streptococcus, but none is satisfactory in treating the enterococcus or *L. monocytogenes*. Therefore, when these antibiotics are used to treat neonatal meningitis in which the pathogen has not yet been identified, they should be supplemented with ampicillin.

In treating Group B streptococcus, initial dosages of up to 300,000 u./kg/day of penicillin G are recommended until the individual organism's sensitivity can be determined, because some strains are relatively penicillin-resistant. In vitro synergy of penicillin G plus gentamicin has been demonstrated, but its clinical significance is unknown. Third-generation cephalosporins, with the exception of moxalactam, show excellent activity against this organism, but penicillin G is still the antibiotic of choice.

Therapy for enterococcal meningitis is penicillin G or ampicillin plus gentamicin, and for *L. monocytogenes*, ampicillin and gentamicin.

Parenteral therapy for gram-positive meningitis is continued for 1 wk after CSF sterilization (minimum duration of therapy is 2 wk); for gram-negative meningitis, therapy is continued for 2 wk after CSF sterilization (minimum, 3 wk).

Specific clinical situations in which the meningitis has occurred may alter selection of initial antibiotics; eg, a newborn who received ampicillin and gentamicin for suspected neonatal sepsis in the first week of life and several weeks later in an intensive care nursery develops sepsis and meningitis should be considered to have a multiply-resistant gram-negative organism or *Staphylococcus aureus*. This newborn should receive a combination of an aminoglycoside different from the one previously used (eg, amikacin) or a 3rd-generation cephalosporin (eg, cefotaxime) plus methicillin. The initial drug of choice for *Staphylococcus epidermidis* is vancomycin until the isolate can be demonstrated to be sensitive to a semisynthetic penicillin (eg, methicillin). Once a pathogen is isolated, antibiotic regimens are tailored to in vitro sensitivities.

The roles of fresh frozen plasma, granulocyte transfusions, and exchange transfusion in treating neonatal meningitis are unknown but should be considered in treating neonatal meningitis.

Close follow-up for neurologic complications during the first 2 yr of life should be undertaken.

NEONATAL LISTERIOSIS

(See also Listeriosis under Bacterial Diseases Caused by Aerobic Bacilli in Ch. 8)

Transplacental infection with *Listeria monocytogenes* can result in fetal dissemination with granuloma formation in many organs (eg, liver, adrenals, lymphatic tissue,

lungs, and brain)—**"granulomatosis infantiseptica."** Aspiration or swallowing of amniotic fluid or vaginal secretions can lead to perinatal infection. *L. monocytogenes* is the 3rd most common cause of neonatal meningitis.

Symptoms and Signs

Infections in pregnant women are characterized by a primary bacteremia, presenting as a nonspecific "flu-like" illness. In the fetus and newborn, clinical presentation depends on the timing and route of infection. Abortion, premature delivery with amnionitis (with a characteristic murky amniotic fluid), stillbirth, or neonatal sepsis commonly occurs. In the newborn, infection may be apparent within hours or a few days, or it may be delayed up to several weeks. Infants with early-onset disease frequently are of LBW, have associated obstetric complications, and show evidence of sepsis with circulatory and/or respiratory insufficiency. The delayed-onset form presents as meningitis or sepsis in a term, previously well infant. Neonatal mortality varies from 10 to 50%, being higher in those infants with early-onset disease.

Diagnosis

In neonatal listeriosis, specimens should be taken from cord blood, the infant's CSF and meconium, the mother's lochia and cervical and vaginal exudates, and grossly diseased parts of the placenta.

Cultures of blood and cervix should be obtained from any pregnant woman with a febrile disease. The laboratory should be asked to look for *L. monocytogenes*. Evaluation for sepsis (see above) should be performed in a sick neonate or infant born to a mother with listeriosis during pregnancy. CSF examination may show a predominance of mononuclear cells. Gram-stained smears are frequently negative or may show pleomorphic, gram-variable coccobacillary forms. The clinician should be careful not to disregard them as "diphtheroid" or streptococcal contaminants.

Prophylaxis

Avoidance of food products contaminated by *L. monocytogenes* is important, since they cause maternal (and fetal) infection. Pregnant women who have previously given birth to infected infants should have a cervical culture done during the 3rd trimester to identify a carrier state of *L. monocytogenes*. Such recognition may allow prophylactic treatment prior to delivery or intrapartum, to prevent vertical transmission to the newborn.

Treatment

Ampicillin is the treatment of choice and should be given parenterally for a minimum of 2 wk. Synergy of ampicillin or penicillin with an aminoglycoside or rifampin has been demonstrated, and trimethoprin-sulfamethoxazole and imipenem are active antibiotics against *L. monocytogenes*, but these regimens have not been well evaluated in the newborn. Other adjuncts to the newborn with bacterial sepsis should be given (see NEONATAL SEPSIS, above).

CONGENITAL RUBELLA

Etiology and Epidemiology

Infection of the fetus results from primary maternal infection during pregnancy or up to 3 mo prior to conception. The frequency of congenital rubella thus depends upon the proportion of women of childbearing age who are susceptible and the frequency of rubella infection in the community. Before rubella virus vaccine was developed, epidemics of rubella and congenital rubella occurred about every 6 to 9 yr. During epidemic years congenital rubella infection was found (using serologic tests to identify subclinical cases) in as many as 2% of newborns. The incidence has dropped dramatically in the USA; only 20 cases were reported in 1983.

Pathogenesis

Both the rate of in utero transmission of rubella and the consequences of fetal infection are related to the stage of gestation at the time of maternal infection. Infection during the first 8 wk of pregnancy results in a fetal infection rate of about 50%; subsequently, the rate of in utero transmission drops sharply to < 10% by the 16th wk. The proportion of infected fetuses with damage due to rubella follows a similar pattern; with maternal rubella at 8, 12, 13 to 20, and > 20 wk, approximately 85, 50, 15, and 0%, respectively, of infected live-born infants have defects apparent at birth or during early childhood. These gestational influences probably are due to a number of factors, including timing in relation to organogenesis, maturation of fetal host mechanisms, and maturation of the placental barrier.

Developing fetal organs are damaged by infection of cells in blood vessels in both the placenta and fetus. These vascular lesions are characterized by endothelial necrosis and are often accompanied by petechiae and hemosiderin-laden macrophages in fetal organs. In addition, rubella can produce cytolytic infection of host cells; cellular damage due to virus has been identified in a number of tissues, including myocardium, CNS, skeletal muscle, and epithelial cells of the developing inner ear, lens, and teeth.

Symptoms and Signs

As many as ⅔ of infants with congenital rubella will be free of any abnormality at birth. The **classic rubella syndrome** has been characterized by the combination of cardiac, ocular, and hearing defects, although infection and damage can occur in every organ system. Of the abnormalities likely to be present at birth, cardiovascular (pulmonary artery hypoplasia, patent ductus arteriosus), low birth weight for gestational age, osteitis, hepatosplenomegaly, retinopathy, and cataracts are the most common; encephalitis, microcephaly, adenopathy, pneumonitis, jaundice, thrombocytopenia, petechiae or purpura, and anemia may also be seen.

Congenital rubella should be viewed as a chronic infection capable of producing progressive damage. Clinical follow-up and testing have shown that ultimately CNS damage (hearing loss, intellectual and motor deficiencies) is the most frequent and significant clinical problem associated with congenital rubella. Most patients who are symptomatic at birth and many of those who lack signs of infections eventually will have some degree of hearing loss or psychomotor damage.

Diagnosis

The diagnosis should be suspected when maternal seroconversion or a compatible illness occurs during pregnancy, when a neonate has clinical signs of congenital rubella, and in any infant with hearing loss, retinitis, or encephalopathy of unknown etiology. Even with a high index of suspicion, many cases will be missed, since many mothers and infected newborns also lack clinical signs of rubella.

Virologic and serologic laboratory technics can confirm the diagnosis; both methods are best when applied very early in life. Children with congenital rubella usually shed virus for about 6 mo. Virus may be present in the pharynx, urine, WBCs, conjunctiva, feces, and CSF; a pharyngeal swab is probably the best source. If eye or CNS disease is present, then conjunctiva and CSF also yield good material for isolation. Since the rate of viral shedding declines steadily, viral isolation attempts should be made as early as possible, preferably within the first 3 mo. Antibody to rubella can be measured by various technics; hemagglutination inhibition **(HAI)** is the most widely used. IgM antibodies can be measured by indirect fluorescence and other methods. Although the presence of IgM antibody to rubella in a newborn is strong evidence of congenital infection, one must be careful to check for RF, which will produce false positives and is frequently present in congenital cytomegalovirus infection and in syphilis. When rubella-specific IgM antibody is present, the diagnosis of congenital rubella should be confirmed by viral isolation or serial antibody determination.

Passively acquired maternal IgG antibodies decline gradually and are usually undetectable after age 6 mo; thus, serial determinations of IgG antibody levels are required. Antibody that increases or persists distinguishes infected infants from those with passively acquired maternal antibody. *Because of the prognostic implications for CNS damage, a diagnosis should not be presented to the family until it is secure.* Subtle, perhaps progressive, damage to the CNS (including organs of perception) is likely to accompany congenital rubella; therefore, appropriate examinations of vision, hearing, and psychomotor development should be performed throughout childhood.

Prevention

There is no treatment for maternal or congenital rubella infection; *prevention therefore assumes paramount importance.* The major thrust in the USA has been to reduce the chances for susceptible women to acquire rubella during pregnancy by immunizing young children with the goal of preventing epidemics. It is currently recommended that children receive rubella immunization at age 15 mo (along with mumps and measles in a combined vaccine). In many areas immunization is required for children entering school. Antibody to rubella persists in > 95% of vaccinees for at least 10 yr.

The American Committee on Immunization Practices has emphasized the importance of immunizing adolescents and adults who have no evidence of rubella immunity. Evidence is a documented history of rubella immunization or serologic proof of immunity; a clinical history of rubella infection is not sufficient. Immunization of all susceptibles among women of childbearing age and adult males in populations at high risk for rubella outbreaks, such as college students, military recruits, and hospital personnel, has been recommended. Although follow-up studies of women who received rubella vaccine during pregnancy indicate little if any risk of congenital rubella syndrome, pregnant women should not receive this vaccine and women who are immunized should be cautioned not to become pregnant for 3 mo.

NEONATAL HERPES SIMPLEX VIRUS (HSV) INFECTION

Neonatal HSV infection results in serious disease with high mortality and significant morbidity. The incidence is estimated to be between 1:5,000 and 1:10,000 live deliveries. HSV type 2 causes about 80% of cases; the remainder are caused by HSV type 1. HSV-2 is usually transmitted to the newborn during delivery by passage through an infected maternal genital tract (see also INFECTIOUS DISEASE in Ch. 178). Infrequently, transplacental transmission of virus and nosocomial spread from one neonate to another by hospital personnel or family have also been implicated as sources of infection. Mothers of newborns with HSV infection tend to be young and without a past history or symptoms of genital infection at the time of delivery.

Clinical Manifestations

Rapid and specific diagnosis of neonatal HSV infection is essential if therapy is to be efficacious. Disease manifestations generally occur between the first and 2nd wk of life; however, symptoms may not appear until as late as age 4 wk. The hallmark of infection is skin vesicles, which frequently lead to progressive or more serious forms of disease over a period of 7 to 10 days if therapy is not instituted. Importantly, as many as 15% of babies will have no skin vesicles; usually, these babies have brain infection. Other signs of infection, which can be present singly or in combination, include temperature instability, lethargy, hypotonia, respiratory difficulty (apnea or pneumonia) convulsions, hepatitis, and/or disseminated intravascular coagulopathy. They provide the basis for classifying the disease into 2 major categories. Newborns considered to have **disseminated disease** with visceral organ involvement have hepatitis, pneumonitis and/or disseminated intravascular coagulopathy with or without encephalitis or skin disease. The mortality rate is 85%. The 2nd major group, those with **localized disease** can be further subdivided into 2 groups. The first group has encephalitis manifested b

neurologic findings and CSF pleocytosis and elevated protein, with or without concomitant involvement of the skin, eyes, and mouth. In the absence of therapy, encephalitis in the newborn has a mortality rate of about 50% and at least 95% of the survivors have sequelae. The other form of localized disease includes babies having only skin, eye, and mouth involvement and no evidence of CNS or organ disease. Death is uncommon in this group, except as the result of concomitant medical problems, but approximately 30% develop neurologic impairment, which may not become manifest until 2 to 3 yr of age.

The morbidity associated with each form parallels its mortality and is directly proportional to the extent of the disease. About 90% of infants with viscerally disseminated neonatal HSV infection have subsequent sequelae. Only 5% of those with CNS infection return to normal. Neonatal herpes is, therefore, a rapacious viral infection in the newborn period.

Diagnosis

Neonatal HSV infection can be confirmed by isolation of virus in tissue culture. The most common site for virus retrieval is skin vesicles; the mouth, eye, and CSF are also high-yield sites. In some newborns presenting with encephalitis, virus is found only in the brain. Isolation of virus can be accomplished in various cell lines of human or nonhuman origin. Cytopathologic effects can usually be demonstrated within 24 to 48 h after inoculation of the specimens. The diagnosis can also be confirmed by neutralization with appropriate high-titer antiserum monoclonal antibodies or by direct immunofluorescence. If no diagnostic virology facilities are available, a Pap smear of the lesion base can be obtained for characteristic histopathology (multinucleated giant cells and intranuclear inclusions). Other studies include electron microscopy and immunofluorescence of lesion scrapings, particularly using monoclonal antibodies.

Treatment

Vidarabine, the only available therapy (acyclovir is under evaluation), halves the mortality rate and increases from 10% to 35% the number of newborns who will develop normally. Vidarabine 30 mg/kg/day in standard IV fluid should be given over a period of 12 h. This dosage is repeated each day for 10 to 14 days. Treatment also requires vigorous supportive therapy, including appropriate IV fluids, alimentation, respiratory support, correction of clotting abnormalities, and control of seizure disorders. The appearance of herpes keratoconjunctivitis requires topical therapy with an agent such as trifluridine (see also NEONATAL CONJUNCTIVITIS in this chapter, above).

NEONATAL HEPATITIS B VIRUS INFECTION

(See also Ch. 71)

Of the recognized forms of viral hepatitis (hepatitis A, hepatitis B, and non-A, non-B hepatitis), the neonatal disease produced by the hepatitis B virus **(HBV)** is the only form that has been studied, primarily because of the absence, until recently, of a marker to identify hepatitis A or non-A, non-B infections. This discussion, therefore, focuses on neonatal infections caused by HBV—a broad spectrum of disease, with most neonates developing chronic subclinical hepatitis.

Etiology and Epidemiology

Hepatitis B is caused by the HBV, a 42-nm, double-shelled DNA virus. The surface antigen (HBsAg) is found on the surface of the virus and on accompanying 22-nm spherical and tubular forms that represent excess virus-coat material.

In the USA, the major source of neonatal HBV infection is infected mothers. Another source, exposure to contaminated blood products, has been virtually eliminated by screening blood donors for HBsAg. Neonates may also acquire HBV through horizontal acquisition; however, this is not a significant route in countries such as the USA, where the HBsAg carrier rate in the general population is quite low (about

0.1%). Maternal acute hepatitis B during the 3rd trimester of pregnancy or within 2 mo of delivery is associated with a 70% risk of maternal–infant transmission of HBV; in contrast, only 5% of infants born to mothers with acute hepatitis B during the 1st or 2nd trimester develop the disease. There also is a high risk of maternal–infant transmission of HBV from asymptomatic HBsAg-positive carriers who possess the e antigen. Carriers who lack the e antigen or possess anti-HBe may still (although are less likely to) transmit the disease.

Maternal–infant transmission of HBV occurs primarily as a result of either micro maternal-fetal transfusions during labor and/or infant contact with infectious maternal secretions in the birth canal. Transplacental transmission is unusual. Postpartum transmission occurs rarely, through neonatal exposure to infectious maternal blood, saliva, stool, urine, or breast milk. Neonatal HBV infection may be an important reservoir of this virus in certain communities.

Symptoms, Signs, and Course

Most neonates infected with HBV develop chronic, subclinical hepatitis characterized by persistent hepatitis B antigenemia and variably elevated transaminase activity. Histologically, this disease resembles the **"chronic persistent hepatitis"** seen in adults (see in Ch. 71). Long-term prognosis for these neonates is not known, although there is evidence that chronic HBsAg carriage, especially when acquired early in life, increases the risk of subsequent liver disease (eg, chronic-active hepatitis, cirrhosis, and primary hepatocellular carcinoma). Infrequently, newborns infected with HBV may develop acute hepatitis B, which is usually mild and self-limited, with jaundice, lethargy, failure to thrive, abdominal distention, and clay-colored stools. Occasionally, infants may be severely affected with hepatomegaly, ascites, and hyperbilirubinemia (primarily conjugated); on rare occasions the disease may be fulminant and even fatal. Fulminant hepatitis B is seen more frequently in infants born to chronic carriers rather than to mothers with acute hepatitis B. Many children born to women with acute hepatitis B during pregnancy are of low birth weight, regardless of whether or not they are infected with HBV.

Diagnosis and Differential Diagnosis (see in Ch. 71)

Prophylaxis

Treatment to prevent hepatitis B should be given to infants born to all HBsAg-positive mothers. Mothers belonging to groups known to be at high risk of HBV infection should be routinely tested for HBsAg during a prenatal visit. Such groups include women of Asian, Pacific Island or Alaskan Eskimo descent (whether immigrants or born in the USA); born in Haiti or Sub-Saharan Africa; with histories of acute or chronic liver disease or multiple episodes of venereal disease; working or being treated in a hemodialysis unit; working or residing in an institution for the mentally retarded; ineligible as blood donors; receiving blood transfusions on repeated occasions; having frequent occupational exposure to blood in medicodental settings; having household or sexual contact with known HBsAg carriers; or known to use illicit injectable drugs.

While the optimal prophylactic treatment regimen has yet to be determined, the following approach is effective: hepatitis B immune globulin **(HBIG)** at a total dose of 0.5 mL IM within 12 h of birth; then 3 doses of inactivated hepatitis B virus vaccine 0.5-mL IM. The first dose should be given concurrently with HBIG but at a different site; however, this first dose may be given within 7 days of birth. The 2nd and 3rd doses should be given at 1 mo and 6 mo, respectively, after the first. Testing for HBsAg and anti-HBs at 12 to 15 mo is recommended.

Separating an infant from an HBsAg-positive mother is not recommended and breast feeding does not appear to increase the risk of postpartum transmission of HBV, particularly if HBIG and hepatitis B virus vaccine have been given. However, if

a mother has cracked nipples, abscesses, or other breast pathology, breast feeding could potentially transmit HBV to her infant.

Treatment

Neonates with acute hepatitis B should receive symptomatic care and adequate nutrition. Neither steroids nor HBIG have been shown to be of value in this situation. There is no specific treatment for neonates with chronic, subclinical hepatitis, but periodic liver function tests are necessary because of the potential risk of developing significant disease.

CONGENITAL AND PERINATAL CYTOMEGALOVIRUS INFECTION

(See also CYTOMEGALOVIRUS INFECTION under HERPES VIRUSES in Ch. 12)

Etiology and Epidemiology

Cytomegalovirus **(CMV)**, the leading cause of congenital viral infection, occurs in 0.4 to 2.2% of all live births in most populations. CMV can occur in the mother as an endogenous reactivation of latent virus **(recurrent infection)** or as an exogenous **primary gestational infection;** in either case, she can transmit CMV to the fetus. The former type is probably more frequent, since in many populations almost all women of childbearing age are seropositive. In some developing nations nearly 100% of the people are infected during childhood; in upper-middle income groups in the USA and Great Britain, about 50% of young adults are susceptible.

In addition to in utero transmission, infants can acquire CMV from their mothers by exposure to genital tract secretions during birth **(perinatal infection)** and from breast milk. Although infants who acquire CMV through these routes shed virus for years, as do those with congenital infection, there is no evidence that either perinatally acquired or breast-milk–acquired infections produce any damage to the CNS, vision, or hearing. However, transfusing premature newborns (≤ 1500 gm) of seronegative women with multiple units of blood from seropositive donors can lead to CMV infection in 10 to 18% of cases. Infection results in clinically significant disease in about 50 to 60% of cases, with mortality reaching 20% of the more seriously affected infants.

Pathogenesis

The mechanisms through which CMV produces damage at the cellular level are poorly understood. Lytic infection with host cell death occurs, but it is not clear that this accounts for all of the disturbances that may result from congenital CMV infection. The outcome of the infection (abortion, fatal neonatal illnesses, sick newborn with survival, normal newborn with or without late sequelae) most likely depends upon such factors as type of maternal infection (primary or recurrent), fetal age at time of infection, genetic factors controlling host immune response, and even viral strain virulence. The contrast between the lack of morbidity associated with perinatal acquisition and the serious illness that often accompanies transfusion-acquired CMV infection in premature newborns of seronegative women suggests that the presence of antibody reduces virulence in these early postnatal infections.

Symptoms and Signs

No clinical disease is evident in > 90% of newborns with congenital CMV infection. CMV in most of the infants who are symptomatic at birth or who develop sequelae probably is due to primary maternal infection. The abnormalities of those symptomatic at birth vary widely in type and severity. The most frequent manifestations are microcephaly, hepatosplenomegaly, petechiae, jaundice, and growth retardation. Laboratory tests are likely to show thrombocytopenia, increased total IgM, conjugated hyperbilirubinemia, elevated AST (SGOT), and atypical lymphocytosis. Ten to 30% of infants with *symptomatic* congenital CMV infection die within a few months of birth.

Although CNS involvement is not usually evident at birth, its signs appear within a few years in > 90% of children with symptoms at birth and include microcephaly (70%), intellectual impairment (60%), neuromuscular disorders (35%), hearing loss (30%), and chorioretinitis or optic atrophy (22%). Sequelae also occur in about 10% of children who are *asymptomatic* at birth. In this group, hearing loss is by far the most frequent handicap; overt neurologic signs do not appear, but retinochoroiditis, intellectual deficits, and behavioral problems have been associated with asymptomatic congenital CMV infection.

Diagnosis

Congenital CMV infection should be considered in any newborn with signs of congenital infection (eg, hepatosplenomegaly, jaundice, petechiae), a maternal seroconversion or mononucleosis-like illness during pregnancy, or an abnormal result on screening tests for congenital infection. The most sensitive and specific means of proving congenital CMV infection is isolation of virus from urine or other body fluid within the first 2 wk of life. Since CMV is stable in urine at refrigerator temperature for weeks, specimens can be shipped to a reference laboratory for viral isolation. Demonstration of virus by electron microscopy or immunologic methods is less sensitive and often less available than viral isolation. Since CMV acquired during or shortly after birth can result in viral shedding by 1 mo of age, congenital infection can be proven only if virus is recovered during the first 2 wk of life. The presence in cord blood of RF, an IgM level > 20 mg/dL, or a specific IgM antibody to CMV has been used to screen for congenital CMV infection. Each of the 3 lacks either sensitivity or specificity and cannot be recommended for general use; confirmation must be by viral isolation.

Treatment and Prevention

There is no treatment for congenital CMV infection. Vidarabine has been used in a small number of patients; viral shedding was reduced during treatment but returned afterward. Prevention of primary maternal infection during pregnancy is not possible, since the major sources of virus have not been identified. An attenuated live virus vaccine is under investigation, but cannot be recommended for general use in susceptible women until it is clear that primary maternal infection is more likely to produce fetal damage than recurrent infection.

Transfusion-acquired CMV infection in newborns can be prevented by screening the patient and potential donors for antibody to CMV. *Seronegative newborns ≤ 1500 gm should receive blood products from only seronegative donors or blood products rendered noninfectious* by other means (eg, frozen deglycerolized RBCs).

To enhance developmental potential and provide appropriate therapy, all children with congenital CMV infection should receive audiologic, ophthalmologic, and psychomotor evaluations at yearly intervals during childhood.

CONGENITAL TOXOPLASMOSIS

An infection caused by transplacental acquisition of the ubiquitous protozoan Toxoplasma gondii. The disease occurs throughout the world with an estimated incidence of 1:1000 to 1:3000 live births.

Etiology and Pathogenesis

T. gondii, a small, banana-shaped parasite, exists in 3 forms: the trophozoite or proliferative form invades and multiplies asexually within nucleated host cells of any warm-blooded animal; the tissue cyst or latent form occurs in the extraintestinal tissues of cats and other mammalian or avian hosts; and the oocyst or resistant form multiplies sexually by gametogony in the lining epithelium of the intestinal tract of cats. Toxoplasmosis is transmitted by ingestion of raw or poorly cooked meat contain-

ing tissue cysts or by direct or indirect exposure to oocysts shed in cat feces. Infectivity of the oocyst in soil may be preserved for several months, and certain invertebrate vectors, such as flies and cockroaches, have been implicated in transmission.

It is generally agreed that congenital transmission occurs only when the infection is acquired during gestation. Nearly 35% of women who acquire toxoplasmosis during pregnancy give birth to congenitally infected infants. The rate of transmission is directly related to the gestational age at the time of infection (17, 25, and 65% for the 1st, 2nd, and 3rd trimesters of pregnancy, respectively); however, the degree of fetal damage has an inverse relationship. This phenomenon explains why the majority of infants with congenital toxoplasmosis appear normal or only moderately sick at birth.

Symptoms and Signs

At birth about 70% of infected infants are asymptomatic, 10% are born with ocular involvement only (retinochoroiditis, optic nerve atrophy, blindness), and the remaining 20% suffer from symptomatic infection that manifests itself as either an acute generalized form of illness (hepatosplenomegaly, jaundice, abnormal CSF, anemia, fever, pneumonitis, maculopapular rash, thrombocytopenia) or as neurologic sequelae (micro- or hydrocephalus, intracranial calcifications, convulsions, mental retardation, ocular involvement). The disease may run a fulminating course leading to death in a matter of days or a few months. Most survivors of severe symptomatic infection have severe neurologic and ocular sequelae. Despite standard therapy, even infants with inapparent infection at birth may develop in later years a wide range of intellectual deficits and retinochoroiditis, which can lead to blindness.

Diagnosis

Maternal infection is seldom symptomatic and requires serologic confirmation. Indirect fluorescent antibody **(IFA)** and Sabin-Feldman **(SF)** dye tests are the most widely accepted serologic tests. Because toxoplasma antibodies are commonly present in women of childbearing age, serologic diagnosis of a primary infection (recent, acute) can be convincingly demonstrated only by the de novo appearance of antibody between acute and convalescent sera. Four-fold rises or high, stable, antibody titers are only suggestive of a recent infection. The most important diagnostic aid is determination of IgM-specific antibodies. An IgM-IFA titer of > 1:256 strongly suggests recent infection. The parasite has been isolated from amniotic fluid in a few cases.

When congenital toxoplasmosis is suspected clinically, eye examination, skull x-rays, and CSF analyses must be obtained. The diagnosis can be confirmed by demonstrating persisting or rising levels of specific IgG antibodies (antibodies of maternal origin decline and eventually disappear between 6 and 9 mo), presence of IgM antibodies in cord or neonatal sera, or isolation of *T. gondii* from placenta, cord blood, or CSF. Determination of IgG antibodies is the only method available to most clinicians. Its main drawback is the 4 to 6 mo required to confirm the diagnosis (by a persistently high or rising titer). Screening for asymptomatic congenital toxoplasmosis is not yet practical because of the low sensitivity and poor specificity of available procedures. **Differential diagnosis** includes other viral (rubella, herpes simplex virus **[HSV]**, cytomegalovirus **[CMV]**), bacterial (bacterial sepsis), protozoan (trypanosomiasis), and treponemal (syphilis) infections.

Treatment

The combination of pyrimethamine with sulfadiazine or triple sulfonamides (but not sulfisoxazole) is the only effective regimen available in the USA. Because of its potential teratogenic effects, pyrimethamine should not be used in the 1st trimester of pregnancy. A therapeutic abortion may be considered, but only after an irrefutable diagnosis of recently acquired toxoplasmosis has been made. All infants with proven infection should receive at least a 1-mo course of therapy with pyrimethamine 2 mg/kg/day the first day, followed by 1 mg/kg/day on the following 29 days, and

sulfadiazine or triple sulfonamides 150 mg/kg/day. To prevent bone marrow depression, leucovorin calcium 5 mg/day should be given. If there is evidence of active eye involvement, treatment should be supplemented with prednisone 2 mg/kg/day for 20 days. *Prednisone must never be given alone.* Exacerbations of retinochoroiditis should be similarly treated. During therapy, bone marrow depression should be monitored at weekly intervals with a CBC, including platelet and reticulocyte counts. Although the efficacy remains unproven, it has been recommended that this course of therapy be given every other month for at least the first year of life. There is no known treatment for the late sequelae of congenital toxoplasmosis.

CONGENITAL SYPHILIS

Infectious disease caused by Treponema pallidum *and transmitted from mother to fetus via the placenta.* Risk of transplacental infection of the fetus is related to the stage of the mother's infection; ie, untreated early syphilis is almost invariably transmitted, while the frequency is much less with the latent and tertiary stages. In untreated mothers with late syphilis, a healthy child may be born between 2 others who have congenital syphilis. Congenital syphilis is preventable and occurs only in untreated pregnant women. If routine prenatal serologic tests for syphilis **(STS)** (see in Ch. 14) are carried out on all pregnant women, the incidence of congenital syphilis can be greatly reduced.

Symptoms and Signs

In **early congenital syphilis,** skin lesions are found on the infant. Bullous eruptions or a macular copper-colored rash on the palms and soles, and papular lesions around the nose and mouth and in the diaper area are the most characteristic. Generalized lymphadenopathy is also present. The infant may fail to thrive, have a characteristic "old man" look, develop fissured lesions around the mouth (rhagades), have a mucopurulent or blood-stained nasal discharge causing snuffles, and have an enlarged liver and spleen. A few infants may develop meningitis, choroiditis, hydrocephalus, or convulsions, and others may be mentally retarded. Within the first 3 mo of life, osteochondritis (chondroepiphysitis) may result in pseudoparalysis of the limbs with characteristic radiologic changes in the bones.

Many patients with congenital syphilis remain in the **latent stage** of the disease throughout their lives and never present any active manifestations. In others, late stigmas appear: gummatous ulcers tend to involve the nose, septum, and hard palate, while periosteal lesions result in "saber shins" and bossing of the frontal and parietal bones. Neurosyphilis may be meningovascular in type, but juvenile paresis and tabes may develop. Optic atrophy, sometimes leading to blindness, may occur. Interstitial keratitis is the most common eye lesion and frequently relapses, often resulting in scarring of the cornea. Sensorineural deafness, which is often progressive, may appear at any age. **Hutchinson's incisors, Moon's molars,** and maldevelopment of the maxilla resulting in "bulldog" facies are frequently present.

Diagnosis

Clinical suspicion of **early congenital syphilis** is confirmed by demonstrating *Treponema pallidum* in scrapings from the skin or mucosal lesions.

Since most neonates will not have signs of disease during their nursery stay, the newborn born to a mother with a history of any sexually transmitted disease before and especially during pregnancy should be investigated. Positive STS may be due to passive transfer of maternal antibody across the placenta. Therefore, a positive STS in an otherwise asymptomatic infant should be interpreted with caution. A positive **fluorescent treponemal antibody-immunoglobin M (FTA-ABS-IgM)** test and a rising titer in a Venereal Disease Research Laboratory (**VDRL**—see in Ch. 14) test on the infant's serum are strong evidence that the infant is infected.

Late congenital syphilis is diagnosed by the clinical history, distinctive physical signs, and positive serologic tests (see also the discussion on screening tests for syphilis in Ch. 14). **Hutchinson's triad** of interstitial keratitis, Hutchinson's incisors, and 8th nerve deafness is diagnostic. Sometimes the standard STS are negative, and the *T. pallidum* immobilization **(TPI)** test may also be negative, but the fluorescent treponemal antibody-absorption **(FTA-ABS)** test is usually positive. The diagnosis should be considered in cases of unexplained deafness.

Prophylaxis

Adequate treatment given to the mother during pregnancy usually cures both mother and fetus. However, in some cases, treatment late in the pregnancy, while eliminating the infection, may have been given too late to prevent development in the fetus of some stigmas that will be apparent after birth.

When a diagnosis of congenital syphilis is made, the other members of the family should be examined. Both infant and mother should be examined at regular intervals. Re-treatment of the mother in subsequent pregnancies is necessary only if the titer of the serologic tests remains high.

Treatment

For **pregnant women with syphilis,** benzathine penicillin G 2.4 million u. IM as a single injection (1.2 million u. may be given in each buttock) or, alternatively, aqueous procaine penicillin G 600,000 u./day IM for 10 days is recommended. Those allergic to penicillin may be treated with penicillin after desensitization or with erythromycin 500 mg q 6 h for 15 days. Neonates of those treated with erythromycin should be treated with penicillin, since transfer of erythromycin to the fetus is poor. Tetracycline is *contraindicated.*

For **early congenital syphilis,** the Centers for Disease Control recommend that infants with CSF abnormalities be given aqueous procaine penicillin G 50,000 u./kg IM daily for 10 days; infants with normal CSF may be given benzathine penicillin G 50,000 u./kg IM as a single or divided dose at one session. Occasionally a severe Jarisch-Herxheimer reaction occurs after such therapy. Prolonged surveillance well into adult life is advisable. Usually the prognosis is favorable if serious damage has not already been done. The mother and other infected members of the family should also be treated.

In **late congenital syphilis,** the CSF should be examined before treatment is started. If the CSF is nonreactive, treatment should be as for primary and secondary syphilis; if reactive, as for latent syphilis (see in Ch. 14). Interstitial keratitis is usually treated with corticosteroids and atropine drops; an ophthalmologist should be consulted. Patients with nerve deafness may benefit from combining penicillin therapy with a corticosteroid such as prednisone 0.5 mg/kg/day orally in divided doses for 1 wk, followed by 0.3 mg/kg/day for 4 wk, after which the dose is gradually reduced over a period of 2 to 3 mo. (Steroids have not been critically evaluated in either of these conditions.) Family contacts should be traced and patients should be kept under long-term surveillance.

PERINATAL TUBERCULOSIS

Infants may acquire TB (1) by transplacental spread through the umbilical vein to the fetal liver, (2) by aspiration or ingestion of infected amniotic fluid, or (3) by postnatal exposure to active TB in a close contact (family or nursery personnel) via airborne inoculation. About 50% of children born to mothers with active pulmonary TB develop the disease during the first year of life if chemoprophylaxis or BCG vaccination is not given. Routine neonatal BCG vaccination is not indicated in developed countries, but may curb the incidence of childhood TB or decrease its severity in selected populations.

Symptoms and Signs

The clinical presentation of neonatal TB is nonspecific, but multiple organ involvement is usually present. The infant may look acutely or chronically ill. Fever, lethargy, respiratory distress, hepatosplenomegaly, or failure to thrive should alert the physician to the possibility of TB in an infant with a history of TB exposure.

Diagnosis

Screening for TB by detailed history and skin testing is an essential part of prenatal evaluation. A pregnant woman with a positive tuberculin reaction should have a chest x-ray (with precautions against exposure of the fetus to radiation) and her close contacts should also be screened for TB.

The result of skin testing may be difficult to interpret in the newborn infant: it may be negative in the neonate with active TB. Conversely, a false-positive test may result from transference of tuberculin-sensitized lymphocytes to the fetus by maternal–fetal transfusion or to the neonate via ingested breast milk. Examination and culture of tracheal aspirates, urine, gastric washings, and CSF for acid-fast bacteria can be helpful. Chest x-ray usually shows miliary infiltrates. Biopsy of the liver, lymph nodes, or lung and pleura may be necessary to confirm the diagnosis.

Prophylaxis and Treatment

1. Chemoprophylaxis during pregnancy: Use of isoniazid **(INH)** by the woman without acute TB can be deferred until the 3rd trimester or after delivery because of the potential hepatotoxicity of INH in pregnancy. Increased risk of TB to the newborn of a mother with a positive PPD occurs primarily during the postpartum period rather than during pregnancy. Newborns whose mothers have a positive PPD but are without clinical or radiologic evidence of infection do not need prophylaxis but should be skin-tested every 3 mo for 1 yr. If the reaction becomes positive, the infant should receive INH 5 to 10 mg/kg/day orally in 1 or 2 divided doses for 1 yr and should be carefully followed.

2. Pregnant women with active TB: Limited clinical experience suggests that INH, ethambutol, and rifampin used in recommended doses during pregnancy are not teratogenic to the human fetus. If the disease is not extensive, pregnant women can be treated with a combination of INH (300 mg), pyridoxine (50 mg), and ethambutol (15 to 25 mg/kg). If a 3rd antituberculous drug is warranted, rifampin (600 mg) should be added. All these drugs can be given in single daily doses. Streptomycin is potentially ototoxic to the developing fetus and should not be used early in pregnancy unless rifampin is contraindicated. Other antituberculous agents should be avoided because of teratogenicity (eg, ethionamide) or lack of clinical experience during pregnancy. Breast feeding is not contraindicated for mothers on therapy who are not infective.

3. Asymptomatic infant of a woman with active TB: The infant usually should be separated from the mother until she is under effective treatment and acid-fast stains of her sputum become negative (usually 2 to 12 wk). Family contacts should be investigated to detect undiagnosed TB before sending the infant home. If compliance can be reasonably assured and the familial environment is nontuberculous, the infant should be treated with INH and may be sent home at the usual time and then skin-tested at ages 6 wk and 3 mo. If the infant remains tuberculin negative after that period, INH may be discontinued and the infant followed with skin tests every 3 mo for the first year of life.

If, on the other hand, good compliance in a nontuberculous environment *cannot* be assured, within the first week of life the infant should receive BCG vaccine and INH should be started. (Although INH inhibits the multiplication of BCG organisms, clinical trials and anecdotal reports support such combined use.) This infant is separated from the mother until she has received antituberculous therapy and her sputa for acid-fast bacilli are negative. The infant may then be sent home and tuberculin skin-tested

at age 6 wk. A positive test is then indicative of a successful BCG "take," and the INH may be discontinued at that point. BCG vaccination does not insure against development of tuberculous disease but offers the infant significant protection against serious and widespread invasion (eg, tuberculous meningitis). Therefore, these infants should be closely followed for development of tuberculous illness, particularly in the first year of life.

4. Newborn with active TB: Treatment with INH 10 to 15 mg/kg/day and rifampin 15 mg/kg/day, both given orally in 2 divided doses, is recommended. However, little is known about the pharmacology and safety of these drugs in the newborn. Streptomycin 20 mg/kg/day divided into 2 doses IM can be used as a 3rd drug in severe cases. **When the CNS is involved,** the initial therapy should include corticosteroids (prednisone 1 mg/kg/day for 4 to 8 wk, then gradually tapered), INH 20 to 30 mg/kg/day, rifampin 15 mg/kg/day, and streptomycin 20 mg/kg/day, and should be continued until all signs of meningitis have disappeared and cultures are negative on 2 successive lumbar punctures at least 1 wk apart. At this point, INH and rifampin at lower dosages (10 to 15 mg/kg/day) should be given for 1 to 2 yr. Monitoring for drug toxicity (hematologic, hepatic, and otologic) should be frequent.

SUDDEN INFANT DEATH SYNDROME (SIDS)

The sudden death of any infant or young child which is unexpected by history and in which a thorough postmortem examination fails to demonstrate an adequate cause for death. SIDS is the most common cause of death between 2 wk and 1 yr of age, accounting for 30% of all deaths in this age group. Distribution of SIDS is worldwide, occurring in 1.5/1000 live births in the USA. Peak incidence is between the 2nd and 4th mo of life. Incidence is increased in the cold months, in lower socioeconomic groups, in prematurely born infants, in subsequent siblings of SIDS victims, and in infants born to mothers who are narcotic-addicted or who smoke during pregnancy. Many risk factors for SIDS apply to nonSIDS infant deaths as well. Almost all SIDS deaths occur when the infant is thought to be sleeping.

Etiology and Diagnosis

The cause is unknown, although it is most likely due to dysfunction of neural cardiorespiratory control mechanisms. The dysfunction which causes the death may be only intermittent or transient, and it is likely that multiple mechanisms are involved. Less than 5% of SIDS victims have been noted to have episodes of prolonged apnea prior to their death, so the overlap between the SIDS population and infants with recurrent prolonged apnea is very small.

The diagnosis, while largely one of exclusion, cannot be made without an adequate autopsy to rule out other causes of sudden, unexpected death, such as intracranial hemorrhage, meningitis, and myocarditis.

Management

Parents who have lost a child from SIDS are grief-stricken, are not prepared for the tragedy, and, because no definitive cause can be found for their baby's death, usually have excessive guilt feelings. These may be aggravated by the nature of investigations conducted by police, social workers, or others who become involved because of the sudden unexpected death. Family members require support not only during the days immediately following the infant's death, but for several months thereafter to help them deal with their grief and dispel their guilt reactions. This includes, whenever possible, an immediate home visit to (1) help the parents deal with their initial panic and prevent them from rushing carelessly to the hospital, endangering themselves and others; (2) observe the circumstances in which SIDS occurred; and (3) begin to inform and counsel the parents concerning the cause of death.

Autopsy should be performed quickly. As soon as the preliminary autopsy results are known (usually within 8 to 12 h), a 2nd home visit should be made to continue the earlier discussions with the family concerning SIDS. A 3rd meeting with the parents 2 to 3 days later reinforces the earlier discussions and answers many new questions raised. In a month or so a 4th meeting should be held, to give the family the final (microscopic) autopsy results and to discuss their adjustment to their loss, especially their attitude toward having other children. Much of the counseling and support can be complemented by specially trained nurses or by lay persons who have themselves experienced the tragedy of, and adjustment to, SIDS (eg, a member of a local chapter of the National Foundation for Sudden Infant Death Syndrome or of the International Guild for Infant Survival).

HEMORRHAGIC SHOCK AND ENCEPHALOPATHY

(Newcastle Syndrome)

Acute onset of severe shock, encephalopathy, hyperthermia, and other symptoms in previously healthy infants, often leading to severe neurologic sequelae and death. The syndrome was first described in 1979 in 5 patients thought to be suffering from heatstroke. Since then, many more patients have been reported in England and the USA.

Etiology and Pathology

The cause is unknown. Postmortem examinations have not revealed an etiology. Diffuse cerebral edema with herniation and focal hemorrhages in the cerebral cortex, jejunum, ileum, and other organs are consistently noted. Multiple nonspecific changes are described, including patchy swelling and degeneration of hepatocytes; but no panlobular fatty degeneration consistent with Reye's syndrome is seen. Viral and bacterial cultures, both pre- and postmortem, reveal only normal flora. Hematologic abnormalities are consistent only with severe disseminated intravascular coagulation **(DIC)**. Serum chemical analysis usually reveals a marked acidosis, moderate abnormalities in liver function, mild hyponatremia, and normal glucose and ammonia. Elevations in trypsin and below normal α_1-antitrypsin levels have been observed. Urine and blood toxic screens are universally negative. Septicemia, overwhelming viremia, Reye's syndrome, toxic shock, heatstroke, and toxin-induced disease have failed as significant explanations when evaluated in light of the clinical course and laboratory findings.

Symptoms and Signs

Characteristic manifestations are (1) acute onset with no (or only mild) prodromal illness in a child 3 to 8 mo old (one child was 26 mo old); (2) hyperpyrexia (fevers up to 42.1 C [107.78 F] rectally); (3) encephalopathy marked by generalized convulsions (often unresponsive to anticonvulsants), coma, and hypotonia; (4) profound shock resistant to fluid therapy and pressor support; (5) eventual death or severe neurologic impairment. Associated symptoms include watery diarrhea immediately preceding or during the acute episode, severe DIC, renal failure, acidosis, and hepatic dysfunction. Respiratory and cardiac functions are minimally impaired.

Treatment

There is no specific treatment other than rapid and aggressive support. Large fluid infusions (up to 300 mL/kg) as well as multiple pressors usually are required to maintain adequate perfusion. Elective intubation and hyperventilation may be of some help in decreasing cerebral edema, and multiple IV anticonvulsants may be needed. DIC that progresses in the face of fresh frozen plasma administration has responded to exchange transfusion in a few cases.

187. CONGENITAL ABNORMALITIES

Structural defects present at birth.

GENERAL CONSIDERATIONS

Congenital malformations may be isolated or multiple, inherited or sporadic, apparent or hidden, or gross or microscopic. They cause about 10% of neonatal deaths. A major anomaly is apparent at birth in 3 to 4% of newborns; by age 5 yr, up to 7.5% of all children manifest a congenital defect. The incidence of specific congenital anomalies varies with (1) the individual defect (common malformations such as cleft lip and cleft palate occur in 1:1000 births); (2) the geographic area, because of factors such as differences in the genetic pool or the environment (the occurrence of spina bifida is 3 to 4:1000 births in areas of Ireland; under 2:1000 in the USA); (3) cultural practices (where marriages between relatives are frequent, the incidence of certain defects increases); and (4) certain ante- and perinatal problems (see Etiology, below).

Etiology

Several factors associated with pregnancy and delivery signal the increased likelihood of congenital malformation: (1) a primipara over age 35 yr (Down's syndrome is a particular risk); (2) breech presentation, which is also often accompanied by birth asphyxia; and (3) poly- or oligohydramnios. Excess amniotic fluid is present when the fetus has difficulty swallowing (eg, severe CNS disorders such as anencephaly) or the fluid cannot reach the GI tract to be absorbed (eg, esophgeal atresia); decreased fluid is associated with GU anomalies that lower fetal urine output.

The specific etiology of many congenital malformations is unknown. A variety of insults to the developing fetus may produce the same defect if they occur at similar times during embryogenesis when an organ system is most susceptible.

Genetic factors are responsible for many single malformations as well as syndromes. These can follow simple mendelian laws and be autosomal dominant, autosomal recessive, or sex-linked. Where the inheritance is more complex, as in spina bifida, multiple factors are probably involved. These may include a genetic predisposition or an increased susceptibility to certain environmental factors. Some syndromes result from chromosomal abnormalities and can be identified by chromosomal study; eg, Down's syndrome (trisomy 21). (See also Ch. 203.)

Teratogenic agents include (1) drugs taken by the mother during pregnancy (see in Ch. 176)—eg, thalidomide, which produced defects of the extremities; and, recently, valproic acid, which has been associated with spina bifida; (2) maternal illness such as diabetes mellitus and hypothyroidism; (3) various infectious agents—eg, rubella virus, cytomegalovirus, and *Toxoplasma gondii* (microcephaly, with subsequent motor and intellectual retardation, is one serious consequence); and (4) irradiation. Although irradiation can produce congenital malformations experimentally, its teratogenicity in man is less clear.

Treatment

Prenatal evaluation using ultrasound, amniocentesis, and chorionic villus biopsy (see in Ch. 203) permits diagnosis of some defects during pregnancy. When a serious defect is identified, parents can then decide if they wish to continue the pregnancy or, alternatively, both physician and parents can make realistic plans for the labor and delivery of a child with defects. Prenatal therapy also becomes possible. In utero treatment has been tried for obstructive uropathy and hydrocephalus, but is not presently successful.

If a congenital malformation is identified or suspected, the parents should be informed promptly, even though extensive discussion may be deferred until specialists

are consulted. The family should be given a realistic, honest appraisal of the severity of the condition, the medical care available, and the prognosis. Parents should participate in decision making; however, to prevent later guilt feelings, the final determinations regarding care should not be theirs alone. (See also PARENT–INFANT BONDING: THE SICK NEONATE, and MANAGEMENT OF CHRONIC DISABILITY in Ch. 183.) When genetic factors are suspected, the parents should receive genetic counseling (see Ch. 203); if the condition is not inherited, they should be given that reassurance.

Discussions of some specific congenital defects follow.

CONGENITAL HEART DISEASE (CHD)

Defects of the heart and major great vessels produced by abnormalities at various stages of fetal development and present at birth, but which may not be diagnosed until later. The incidence of such anomalies is 1:120 live births. In some instances, a specific etiology may be identified. Chromosomal defects (eg, Trisomy 13, Trisomy 18) usually have severe congenital cardiac anomalies. Other chromosomal or genetic diseases (eg, Trisomy 21, Turner's syndrome [XO], Holt-Oram) are frequently associated with congenital cardiac anomalies. Maternal illness (eg, diabetes mellitus, SLE), environmental exposure (eg, thalidomide), and combinations of the above may be implicated. The risk of CHD with an affected first degree relative is generally considered to be 2 to 3%, with a higher risk from children of affected individuals.

Identification and diagnosis of CHD depends on the recognition of affected cardiac function—heart murmurs, representing turbulent flow, altered systemic and pulmonary blood flow, shunting in either direction, and evidences of altered workload of the cardiac chambers. Routine history, physical examination, ECG, and chest x-ray are usually adequate for specific anatomic diagnosis, with supportive and confirmatory data from echocardiography, cardiac catheterization, angiocardiography, and other laboratory data.

Cardiovascular Adaptation at Birth (see PERINATAL PHYSIOLOGY under MANAGEMENT OF THE NORMAL NEWBORN in Ch. 182)

Normal Circulation (see FIG. 187–1)

In the presence of a normal heart (after the neonatal period of cardiovascular adaptation with closing of the foramen ovale and ductus arteriosus and a decrease in pulmonary vascular resistance to normal adult levels), there is complete separation of the systemic and pulmonary circuits and all right heart pressures are lower than their left heart counterparts. The consequences of congenital heart disease are dependent on those differences.

Pathophysiology

Many congenital cardiac defects, while clearly a result of abnormal cardiac development, produce no significant hemodynamic alteration. Defects with more significant effects on hemodynamics will show the results of ventricular volume load, ventricular pressure load, atrial emptying abnormalities, admixture of unoxygenated and oxygenated blood, or inadequate systemic CO. Defects characterized by obstruction to blood flow (eg, pulmonic or aortic stenosis) are not dependent on a drop in pulmonary vascular resistance and are therefore usually audible at birth, producing ejection murmurs, which have a crescendo/decrescendo quality as pressure within the ventricle rises in systole to overcome the obstruction. Ventricular hypertrophy on the ECG reflects this increased pressure workload on the heart, but because hypertrophy of ventricular muscle at moderate levels does not produce ventricular enlargement, the changes are not well seen on x-ray.

Since left-to-right shunts are dependent on decreasing pulmonary resistance for shunting to occur, they are not generally apparent until some time after birth—several

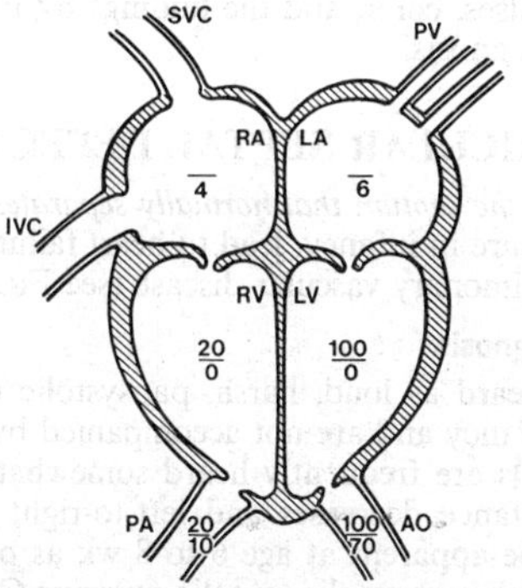

Fig. 187–1. Normal circulation with representative right and left heart pressures. Representative right heart saturation = 75%. Representative left heart saturation = 95%. **AO** = aorta; **IVC** = inferior vena cava; **LA** = left atrium; **LV** = left ventricle; **PA** = pulmonary artery; **PV** = pulmonary veins; **RA** = right atrium; **RV** = right ventricle; **SVC** = superior vena cava.

days to a few weeks for high-pressure shunts (ie, ventricular or great vessel level), and considerably later for low-pressure atrial level shunts. Ventricular dilation, the result of left-to-right shunting, is well demonstrated by cardiomegaly on x-ray, but produces a less obvious ECG pattern.

Heart murmurs and thrills are the result of turbulent flow within the heart or great vessels and are transmitted to the surface at the point where they are generated, making careful localization of murmurs of great diagnostic help. Increased flow across the pulmonic valve produces a soft murmur with characteristics similar to an ejection murmur. Regurgitant flow from an atrioventricular valve or flow across the ventricular septum produces a pansystolic murmur, possibly obscuring the heart sounds as its intensity increases. Flow in the great vessels is continuous and a murmur arising from aortic-pulmonary flow is continuous and uninterrupted by the heart sounds when pulmonary artery pressure is not high. The quality of the heart sounds reflects adequacy of ventricular function and arterial closing pressures. An ejection sound may be heard easily after the first sound when valve opening is restricted.

Increased pulmonary blood flow with increased pulmonary venous pressure may lead to signs of respiratory distress with tachypnea and dyspnea. Tachycardia and hepatomegaly are other consequences of heart failure. Increases in pulmonary blood flow are easily seen by chest x-ray. Cyanosis, as a presenting symptom of CHD, is seen in the neonate, but a careful search for noncardiac causes is required. Many neonatal respiratory problems are accompanied by cyanosis when there is obstruction to air flow within the bronchial tree, when large masses occupy space otherwise occupied by lung, or when alveolar disease prevents adequate gas exchange. Recognition of cyanosis is dependent on the absolute amount of unsaturated Hb and may therefore be masked by anemia. Clubbing and polycythemia are the result of longstanding arterial unsaturation. Harlequinism, mimicking cyanosis, is not rare in the neonate or young infant. Hypothermia, hypoglycemia, hypocalcemia, sepsis, and CNS dysfunction also commonly present with cyanosis in the newborn.

Inadequate systemic perfusion presents as diminished or impalpable pulses, cold extremities, poor capillary refill and, if prolonged, evidences of organ dysfunction (eg, decreased urine output and renal failure). Assessment of the characteristics of heart

murmurs, adequacy of pulses, color, and the findings by ECG and x-ray will usually allow a precise cardiac diagnosis.

VENTRICULAR SEPTAL DEFECT (VSD)

Opening or openings in the septum that normally separates the ventricles, which may undergo spontaneous closure in infancy, lead to heart failure, require surgical closure, or be accompanied by pulmonary vascular disease (see FIG. 187–2).

Symptoms, Signs, and Diagnosis

VSDs are frequently heard as loud, harsh, pansystolic murmurs at the lower left sternal border in early infancy and are not accompanied by hemodynamic abnormality. More significant VSDs are frequently heard somewhat later at age 2 to 3 wk as pulmonary vascular resistance decreases and left-to-right shunting increases. Heart failure (see below) may be apparent at age 6 to 8 wk as pulmonary flooding occurs. There is a long, loud, harsh pansystolic systolic murmur Grade 3 to 4/6 at the lower left sternal border, a mid-diastolic apical murmur of mitral flow if there is a large shunt, accentuation of the pulmonic closure sound when pulmonary artery pressure is elevated, and signs of heart failure when present. X-ray findings include cardiomegaly, left atrial and left ventricular enlargement, and increased pulmonary arterial flow. ECG findings are initially those of left ventricular volume load, but may include increasing right ventricular hypertrophy as right ventricular and pulmonary artery pressures increase. Cardiac catheterization and angiocardiography to determine VSD location, pulmonary vascular resistance, and the presence of associated, and sometimes masked, anomalies (eg, ductus or coarctation) is usually done before surgery.

Prognosis and Treatment

Anticongestive measures (eg, digitalis, diuresis, salt restriction) and treatment of respiratory infections may control heart failure and allow the child to maintain normal growth and development. In children who respond well to these measures, the heart failure usually disappears in the first or second year and the defect becomes less significant and may not require surgery.

In infants who respond poorly or not at all to anticongestive measures, it may be necessary to consider VSD closure in the first year of life. Infants with large shunts or heart failure who have not been well stabilized are at considerably higher risk for viral

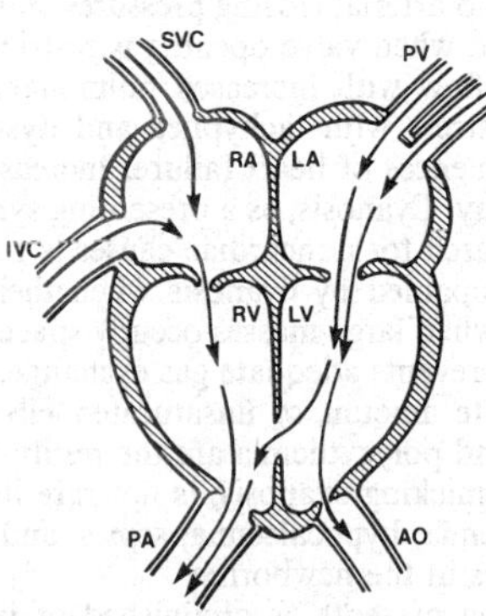

FIG. 187–2. Ventricular septal defect: Increased pulmonary blood flow, increased left atrial volume, and increased left ventricular volume. (For abbreviations, see FIG. 187–1.)

pneumonias (eg, respiratory syncytial virus) than are infants with smaller shunts and deserve consideration of early repair. VSDs that remain significant with cardiomegaly, growth failure, or symptoms, but without heart failure, may require closure later in childhood. All children with VSD should receive adequate protection against infective endocarditis (see ENDOCARDITIS in Ch. 27).

ATRIAL SEPTAL DEFECT
(Ostium Secundum; Sinus Venosus)

Opening in the septum, which normally separates the atria (see FIG. 187–3).

Symptoms, Signs, and Diagnosis

The typical murmur of atrial septal defect is usually present after age 1 yr when pulmonary blood flow has increased significantly and a Grade 2 to 3/6 flow murmur is audible at the upper left sternal border in association with splitting of the second sounds throughout all phases of respiration. In the presence of a large left-to-right shunt (in which the pulmonary to systemic blood flow ratio ≥ 2:1), there may be a low-pitched diastolic murmur of tricuspid flow. By x-ray, there is dilation of the right atrium and right ventricle and an increase in pulmonary arterial flow. The ECG shows a moderate right axis, a moderate right ventricular volume load, normal left ventricular forces and, in some patients, a slightly prolonged PR and/or P wave abnormalities. Partial anomalous pulmonary venous flow is common with a sinus venosus atrial defect, and persistence of the left superior vena cava is not uncommon. The diagnosis is usually apparent on clinical grounds and the defect is usually seen by 2-D echocardiogram. However, catheterization is often done preoperatively, not only to assess the size of the shunt and to determine the presence of anomalous systemic or pulmonary veins, but also to evaluate left ventricular function.

Treatment

Surgical repair is recommended electively at age 4 to 6 yr in children in whom the pulmonary to systemic flow ratio is > 1.5:1, although most patients undergoing atrial defect closure have a 2.5 to 3:1 ratio. Surgery may be done earlier if very large shunts are present or if atrial dysrhythmias appear. Continued medical observation is justified in children with lesser shunts, if they have no cardiomegaly or symptoms and if continued medical care can be assured. Prediction of which children will develop pulmonary hypertension in adulthood is not yet possible.

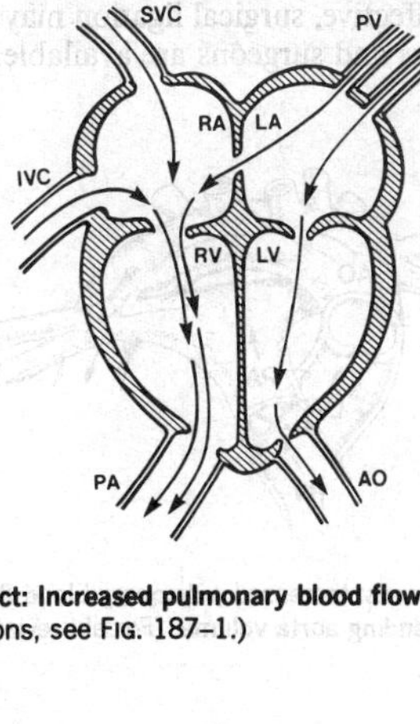

FIG. 187–3. Atrial-septal defect: Increased pulmonary blood flow, and increased right atrial and ventricular volumes. (For abbreviations, see FIG. 187–1.)

PATENT DUCTUS ARTERIOSUS (PDA)

Failure to close of the fetal communication between the pulmonary artery and the aorta (see FIG. 187–4).

Symptoms, Signs, and Diagnosis

PDA in the premature infant is a frequent occurrence with increased pulmonary blood flow and further compromise of gas exchange, particularly in the infant with respiratory distress syndrome. The infant will have bounding pulses, a hyperdynamic precordium, increased pulmonary closure sound, and a pulmonic area murmur that may be continuous, systolic with a short diastolic component, or systolic alone. In some infants, there is no murmur, but the other findings are present. These infants will usually have normal ECGs for the degree of prematurity (ie, left ventricular prominence), but may show a left ventricular volume load. By x-ray, they will have cardiomegaly and, if the pulmonary findings of respiratory distress syndrome are not severe, an increase in pulmonary arterial flow. Echocardiogram may be helpful with demonstration of left atrial size exceeding the aortic root diameter.

Persistent PDA in full-term infants is usually identified after age 6 to 8 wk by a continuous murmur at the upper left sternal border. The peripheral pulses are full with a widened pulse pressure and the ECG may reflect left ventricular volume load. The x-ray will show prominence of left atrium, left ventricle, ascending aorta, and an increase in pulmonary blood flow if the ductus has significant flow. Care must be taken to be sure that the ductus is not compensating for pulmonary atresia and that the murmur does not represent a systemic arteriovenous fistula, branch pulmonary stenosis, or aortic-pulmonary window. Evaluation of femoral pulses and leg BP is necessary to rule out a hidden coarctation.

Prognosis and Treatment

If the respiratory status of **the premature infant** is compromised by ductal patency, attempts at closure are indicated. These include fluid restriction (90 to 100 mL/kg/day), diuresis, and consideration of pharmacologic closure with indomethacin or surgical ligation. Indomethacin is a prostaglandin inhibitor and, in the absence of excessive jaundice (indirect bilirubin > 10 mg/dL), renal failure (creatinine > 1.4 mg/dL, BUN > 35 mg/dL), or thrombocytopenia (platelet count < 100,000/μL) usually will produce prompt ductal closure after one dose of 0.2 mg/kg IV or 0.2 mg/kg orally 3 times. Moderate fluid restriction should be maintained for 2 to 3 days with subsequent gradual and steady fluid increase. If contraindications to indomethacin exist or if indomethacin is ineffective, surgical ligation may be undertaken at little risk, if experienced anesthesiologists and surgeons are available. While less significant duc-

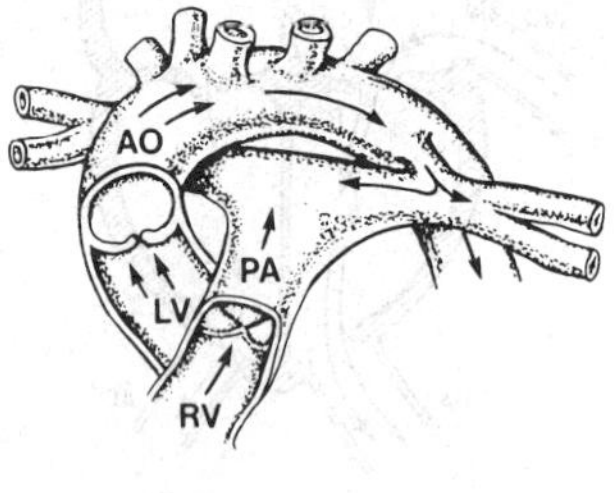

FIG. 187–4. Patent ductus arteriosus: Increased pulmonary blood flow, increased left atrial and ventricular volumes, and increased ascending aorta volume. (For abbreviations, see FIG. 187–1.)

tuses in premature infants will frequently undergo spontaneous closure or will close with fluid restriction alone, some will remain patent and require surgical closure at age 1½ to 2½ yr. **In full-term infants** with persistent PDA, surgical repair by ligation or transection is indicated if heart failure occurs or electively at age 6 mo to 3 yr to remove the risk of infective endarteritis.

ATRIOVENTRICULAR (AV) CANAL DEFECTS

(Ostium Primum Atrial Septal Defect; Complete AV Canal Defect [or Endocardial Cushion Defect])

AV canal defects are openings in the atrial and/or ventricular septa at the level of the AV valves and are usually accompanied by mitral and/or tricuspid valve abnormalities (see FIG. 187–5).

Symptoms, Signs, and Diagnosis

Complete AV canal defects, frequently seen in infants with Down's syndrome, may present with cyanosis at birth, the result of right-to-left shunting at either atrial or ventricular level, and may have systolic regurgitant murmurs of mitral and/or tricuspid insufficiency. Heart failure may be present early as the result of large volume shunts or AV valve insufficiency or both. The diagnosis may be made from the typical ECG pattern of a superior, left axis deviation and counterclockwise loop due to congenital absence of the anterior division of the left bundle, frequent prolongation of the PR interval, and the presence of left ventricular hypertrophy and/or right ventricular hypertrophy, depending on the specific hemodynamic changes in the individual infant. The x-ray will show cardiomegaly with a typical bulge of the upper right atrial shadow, right and left ventricular dilation, prominent main pulmonary artery segment, and increased pulmonary artery flow. The diagnosis may be confirmed by 2-D echocardiography. Cardiac catheterization and left ventricular angiography usually are done before surgery, although the echocardiographic delineation of ventricular chamber size and chordal attachments provides the major information needed preoperatively.

Treatment

Surgical repair of complete AV canal defects should be done early to prevent fixed pulmonary vascular disease, clearly under age 2 yr, and possibly in the second half of the first year. The indication for surgical repair should be taken in the context of the patient's overall medical state, since many are severely retarded.

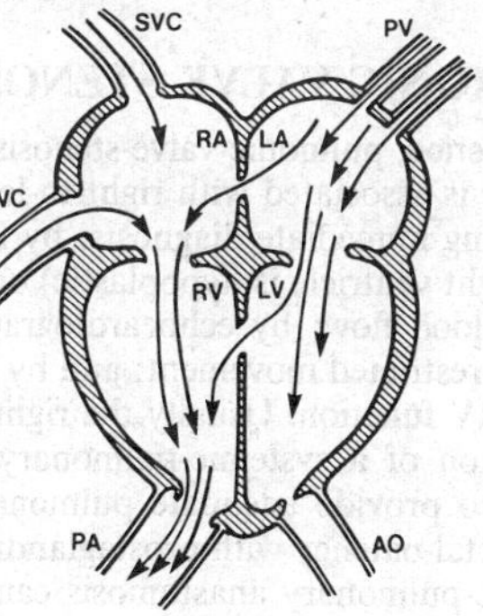

FIG. 187–5. Atrio-ventricular canal defect: Increased pulmonary blood flow, increased volumes of all chambers; increased pulmonary vascular resistance frequent. (For abbreviations, see FIG. 187–1.)

CONGENITAL AORTIC VALVE STENOSIS

Congenital aortic valve abnormalities, usually a bicuspid valve, may produce severe left ventricular **(LV)** outflow tract obstruction in infancy with severe LV dysfunction, heart failure, evidence of ischemic changes by ECG, and poor systemic output. This is uncommon but requires an immediate attempt at aortic valvotomy to prevent death. Surgical results are not uniformly good and residual aortic valve insufficiency may result. Valve replacement is usually required at a later age when the child has grown.

More commonly, bicuspid aortic valve with stenosis and sometimes with insufficiency is found later in childhood. There are usually no symptoms and there is an ejection systolic murmur heard loudest at the upper right sternal border, usually with a prominent systolic ejection click, and an accentuated aortic closure sound. There may be a soft, early diastolic murmur of aortic insufficiency. The ECG shows increasing evidence of LV hypertrophy and ischemia as severity of LV dysfunction increases, but it is not well correlated with the degree of obstruction. The x-ray may reflect poststenotic dilation of the ascending aorta and, in longstanding obstruction, may show LV hypertrophy. Complete evaluation by echocardiography, cardiac catheterization, and angiocardiography may be necessary at any age if there is evidence of severe obstruction or if symptoms occur (eg, exercise-induced chest pain or syncope), but this is usually delayed until adolescence.

A decision as to surgical palliation by aortic valvotomy is based not only on a significant LV-aortic gradient ($\geq$ 50 mm Hg) but on evidence of LV dysfunction and symptoms as well. Aortic valvotomy must be considered palliative rather than curative and restenosis requiring aortic valve replacement is frequent. Significant aortic insufficiency following surgery may require valve replacement as well.

LV outflow tract obstruction **at the subaortic level** by a fibrous ridge or by muscular hypertrophy will have essentially the same findings except that the ejection click will not be heard, the murmur may be most intense over the mid-sternum, and there will be no poststenotic dilation. **Supravalvar aortic obstruction** is not common, but is frequently seen in hypercalcemia syndrome (Williams syndrome). Surgical repair, while possible, is difficult.

Congenitally bicuspid aortic valves occasionally produce severe obstruction in childhood and commonly become obstructive in adult life, at that time requiring valve replacement. Appropriate antibiotic prophylaxis against infective endocarditis/endarteritis is indicated in any patient in whom the diagnosis of bicuspid aortic valve is made.

PULMONIC VALVE STENOSIS

In the immediate neonatal period, pulmonic valve stenosis with severe obstruction to right ventricular **(RV)** outflow is associated with right-to-left atrial shunting and presents as an emergency, requiring immediate diagnosis: by ECG showing either diminished RV forces (when the right ventricle is hypoplastic) or RV hypertrophy; by x-ray with decreased pulmonary blood flow; by echocardiography, which may identify a severely narrowed valve with restricted movement; and by catheterization and angiography to evaluate potential RV function. Usually the right ventricle is severely hypoplastic and immediate creation of a systemic-pulmonary anastomosis (eg, Blalock-Taussig shunt) is indicated to provide adequate pulmonary blood flow. Temporary palliation by maintaining ductal patency with prostaglandin E_1 (0.05 μg/kg/min) may be lifesaving until a systemic-pulmonary anastomosis can be performed. Pulmonary valvulotomy may also be indicated. These are palliative procedures; further surgery may be necessary in later childhood to provide further relief of RV outflow obstruction.

In older children, there is no cyanosis, although somewhat poor peripheral color may be the result of a prolonged circulation time and a wide atrioventricular O_2 difference. There is an ejection murmur, usually with a prominent ejection click, at the upper left sternal border with an increasingly late peak with increasing degrees of obstruction. The pulmonic component of the second sound is progressively delayed and diminished. RV hypertrophy of increasing degrees of severity is seen on the ECG. The x-ray shows a normal heart size and prominence of the main pulmonary artery segment with increasing RV hypertrophy. Cardiac catheterization to evaluate the degree of obstruction, the nature of the pulmonic valve, and RV function is indicated before surgery, which is usually performed electively in the immediate preschool period in children in whom RV pressure is greater than about 60 mm Hg.

PERIPHERAL PULMONIC STENOSIS

Many neonates have soft systolic flow murmurs in the distribution of the branch pulmonary arteries without evidence of significant elevation of right heart pressures. These murmurs usually disappear by the end of the first year as growth occurs. However, in certain conditions (eg, congenital rubella, hypercalcemia syndrome [Williams syndrome], and in some otherwise normal children), anatomic obstruction to flow to the branch pulmonary arteries occurs and may produce a continuous murmur. This is rarely amenable to surgical repair because there are multiple areas of obstruction within the lung itself and because there is usually an associated hypoplasia of the pulmonary arterial tree distal to the obstruction.

COARCTATION OF THE AORTA

Infants with coarctation of the aorta may have very sudden onset of heart failure, cardiovascular collapse, and severe metabolic acidosis as the ductus closes and distal perfusion is compromised. They require immediate treatment with supportive medications, intubation and ventilatory support if necessary, and may benefit from an infusion of prostaglandin **(PG)** E_1 at 0.05 μg/kg/min to reopen the ductus arteriosus. The response to PGE_1 infusion will be gradual, usually over a period of hours, but most infants will stabilize with increased distal perfusion and improved renal blood flow and allow surgical repair of the coarctation and closure of the patent ductus.

Older children with coarctation of the aorta have upper extremity hypertension relative to the lower extremities and may have an absolute hypertension. A soft bruit, louder in the back, is often heard over the coarctation site. The femoral pulses, while frequently palpable, are clearly diminished and delayed when compared with the brachial pulses. The ECG is usually normal but may show left ventricular hypertrophy, and the x-ray shows a normal heart size with coarctation visible in a slight left anterior oblique view. Rib notching may be seen in older children. Catheterization and angiography are not necessary unless significant associated defects (eg, aortic stenosis, aortic insufficiency, mitral valve disease, ventricular septal defect) are present or there is evidence that the narrow segment is not in the usual location just distal to the left subclavian artery or if of greater length than usual. Dilated collateral arterial vessels are usually palpable at the scapular margin. Surgical repair by resection and direct anastomosis, left subclavian artery "roofing" technics, or, if needed, grafting is recommended at age 4 to 6 yr, or earlier with persistent upper extremity hypertension, heart failure, or other complications. Prophylaxis against endocarditis is needed.

TETRALOGY OF FALLOT

An anatomic abnormality with severe or total right ventricular outflow tract obstruction and a ventricular septal defect allowing right ventricular unoxygenated blood to bypass the pulmonary artery and enter the aorta directly (see FIG. 187–6).

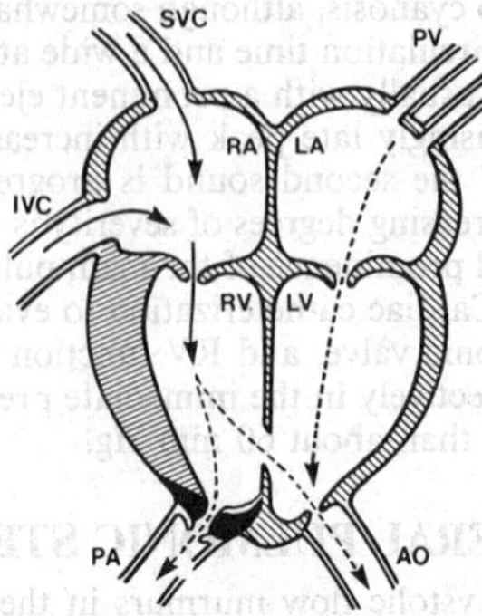

FIG. 187–6. Tetralogy of Fallot: Decreased pulmonary blood flow; right ventricular hypertrophy, unoxygenated blood enters aorta. (For abbreviations, see FIG. 187–1.)

In most instances, the upper left sternal border ejection murmur of right ventricular (RV) outflow tract obstruction is heard at or shortly after birth with the gradual development of cyanosis thereafter. Infants with tetralogy of Fallot with pulmonary valve atresia and ductus-dependent pulmonary blood flow, however, will present with severe cyanosis and a continuous murmur of ductal flow. Prostaglandin E_1 infusion at 0.05 µg/kg/min will usually maintain ductal flow until surgical palliation by a systemic-pulmonary anastomosis can be performed. Prostaglandin infusion may lead to respiratory arrest and equipment for mechanical ventilation should be available. Prompt tapering of the infusion to the lowest effective dose should be done as quickly as possible.

Older infants will have an ejection murmur, right axis deviation, and RV hypertrophy by ECG; x-ray shows a small heart, and concave main pulmonary artery segment with diminished pulmonary blood flow. Right aortic arch is common. Assessment of the intracardiac anatomy should be performed in infancy to determine the possibility of complete intracardiac repair or the need for palliative increases in pulmonary blood flow by systemic-pulmonary anastomoses.

In some infants, tetralogy hypercyanotic "spells" with anxiety, air hunger, respiratory distress, increasing cyanosis, and altered level of consciousness may occur, usually precipitated by activity. Treatment of "spells" consists of supplemental O_2, knee-chest position, and morphine 0.1 to 0.2 mg/kg IM. Propranolol 0.25 mg/kg or more orally q 6 h is useful to prevent further spells, but catheterization, angiography, and surgical palliation or repair are urgent.

TRANSPOSITION OF THE GREAT ARTERIES

An anatomic abnormality where the aorta arises directly from the right ventricle and the pulmonary artery arises from the left ventricle, producing severe systemic hypoxemia (see FIG. 187–7).

Infants with transposition of the great arteries present with severe cyanosis immediately after birth with rapid progression to metabolic acidosis, secondary to poor tissue oxygenation and a compensatory respiratory alkalosis. They are usually otherwise healthy. Examination findings may be limited to cyanosis alone. Chest x-ray shows a narrow base as the great vessels are superimposed rather than side-by-side; there is absence of the main pulmonary artery segment in its usual location, and the overall

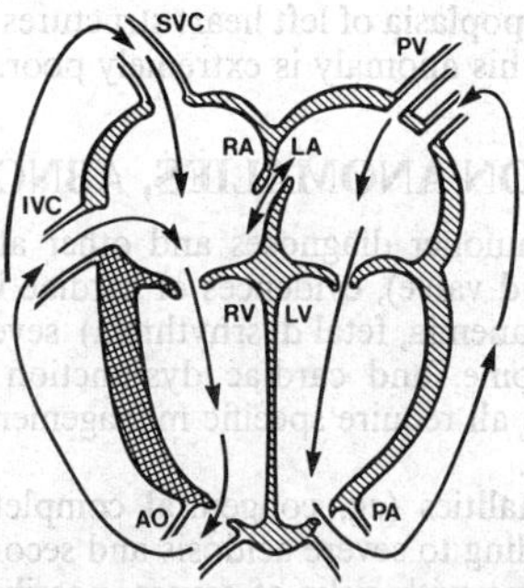

FIG. 187–7. Transposition of the great arteries: Unoxygenated blood enters aorta; right ventricular hypertrophy; foramen ovale permits minimal mixing. (For abbreviations, see FIG. 187–1.)

picture is "an egg on side." Pulmonary venous congestion may develop rapidly. The ECG is normal for the newborn.

Immediate confirmation of the diagnosis by echocardiography or cardiac catheterization is indicated, and palliation by balloon atrial septostomy to improve atrial mixing and decompress the left atrium is necessary. In those infants in whom life-threatening hypoxemia exists, temporary palliation by administration of prostaglandin E_1 will produce ductal opening, leading to an increase in pulmonary blood flow and temporary improvement in systemic oxygenation. This does not negate the need for immediate atrial septostomy. Surgical repair by redirection of systemic and pulmonary venous return (Mustard or Senning technic) or, in some infants, by arterial switching technic is performed in early infancy.

COMPLEX CYANOTIC CONGENITAL HEART DISEASE

More complex anomalies (eg, single ventricle with or without pulmonary stenosis, tricuspid atresia with normally-related or transposed great vessels, tricuspid and pulmonic atresia, mitral atresia, and truncus arteriosus) are less common. Specific anatomic diagnosis is usually possible by the usual methods of evaluation, but management is assisted by confirmatory testing (eg, angiography). The initial management of most of these infants consists of assuring adequate pulmonary blood flow by systemic-pulmonary anastomosis or by protection of the pulmonary vascular bed and control of increased pulmonary blood flow by pulmonary artery banding. Restoration of normal blood flow patterns and separation of oxygenated and unoxygenated blood in some of these infants is possible by the modified Fontan technic in which blood flow is directed from the right atrium to the pulmonary artery, excluding the ventricle from the right-sided circulation. Conduit repair of truncus arteriosus is also possible for some infants.

UNDERDEVELOPED LEFT VENTRICLE SYNDROME

The abrupt appearance of severe heart failure with loss of peripheral pulses and evidence of a severe decrease in systemic perfusion in a 2- or 3-day-old infant who has been considered healthy strongly suggests the presence of aortic and/or mitral valve atresia with ductus-dependent systemic blood flow and cardiovascular collapse occurring as the ductus closes. Cardiomegaly, pulmonary venous congestion, and an ECG

with no evidence of left ventricular forces are strongly suggestive and echocardiography demonstrating severe hypoplasia of left heart structures is confirmatory. The prognosis for most infants with this anomaly is extremely poor.

LESS COMMON ANOMALIES, ABNORMALITIES

Combinations of the commoner diagnoses and other abnormalities (eg, Ebstein's malformation of the tricuspid valve), evidences of cardiac involvement with fetal disease (eg, prolonged in utero anemia, fetal dysrhythmia), severe cardiac anomalies associated with asplenia syndrome, and cardiac dysfunction secondary to noncardiac disease (eg, hypothyroidism) all require specific management guided by their manifestations in the specific infant.

Many other rare abnormalities (eg, congenital complete heart block, congenital metabolic errors usually leading to severe acidosis and secondary myocardial dysfunction, prolonged QT syndrome with risks of severe, possibly fatal dysrhythmia), and rare defects (eg, cor triatriatum) require skilled diagnostic and therapeutic intervention.

Pulmonary vascular disease **(Eisenmenger reaction)** may be a limiting factor in the care of infants and children with such congenital defects as VSD, AVC, truncus where high-pressured (ventricular, aortic-pulmonary) shunts occur, and may exist alone as primary pulmonary hypertension. In these situations, pulmonary vascular resistance is maintained at a high level with medial muscular hypertrophy of the pulmonary arterioles and occlusion of the many smaller branches. As pulmonary vascular resistance approaches and equals systemic vascular resistance, left-to-right shunting is decreased and right-to-left shunting occurs, leading to systemic desaturation and visible cyanosis. Surgical repair is usually contraindicated when calculated pulmonary vascular resistance is > ½ the calculated systemic vascular resistance. Persistent and increasing right-to-left shunting leads to increasing peripheral hypoxemia and increasing polycythemia. Increased O_2-carrying capacity is provided by a Hct of up to 65% but, at higher levels, increased viscosity leads to decreasing O_2 delivery to the tissues. Cautious phlebotomy with maintenance of total blood volume may be beneficial, reducing Hct levels to about 60% when they exceed 65% and when the patient is symptomatic (eg, slurred speech, visual problems, and increased fatigue).

HEART FAILURE (HF)

(See also CONGENITAL HEART DISEASE, above)

A clinical syndrome that occurs when the heart, acting as a pump, is unable to maintain CO sufficiently to satisfy the metabolic demands of the body. A recognizable constellation of clinical and laboratory abnormalities reflect acute and chronic pulmonary and/or systemic congestion, as well as the findings of the underlying cardiac abnormality; eg, pulmonic stenosis can produce heart failure *without* pulmonary congestion.

Etiology

TABLE 187–1 gives an average age of onset of HF in infancy and childhood related to specific etiologies. In utero, HF is uncommon and is the result of compromise of the pump function of the heart and its inability to maintain forward flow, rather than to shunts or obstruction. HF in utero may be produced by sustained intrauterine tachycardia, chronic anemia with a subsequent volume load, myocardial dysfunction secondary to myocarditis, etc. Some of these may be treated by managing the underlying abnormality; eg, maternal digitalization and diuresis may treat fetal tachycardia.

HF occurring immediately after birth may be the result of the above and also perinatal asphyxia with myocardial damage, severe tricuspid and/or pulmonic insufficiency related to hypoxia or to structural valve defects. Metabolic defects (eg, hypo-

TABLE 187–1. AGE OF ONSET OF HEART FAILURE WITH COMMON CAUSES

Birth to first few hours of life
Severe chronic (intrauterine) anemia
Intrauterine or neonatal paroxysmal supraventricular tachycardia
Perinatal asphyxia
Severe tricuspid and/or pulmonic insufficiency
Underdeveloped left ventricle syndrome
Metabolic abnormalities (ie, hypoglycemia)
Critical pulmonic or aortic stenosis
Systemic or placental arteriovenous malformations
First month of life
All of above
Transposition of great vessels
Coarctation of aorta, with or without associated abnormalities
Anomalous pulmonary vein drainage, particularly with pulmonary vein obstruction
Infancy
Ventricular septal defect, single ventricle
Truncus arteriosus
Patent ductus arteriosus
Atrioventricular canal defects
Rare metabolic diseases (ie, glycogen storage disease)
Childhood
Acute rheumatic fever with carditis
Rheumatic heart disease
Viral myocarditis
Bacterial endocarditis
Volume overload in course of a noncardiac disease

thermia, hypoglycemia, or severe metabolic acidosis from whatever cause) may also lead to HF immediately after birth. Critical aortic or pulmonic stenosis may be associated with early neonatal HF. Underdeveloped left ventricle syndrome is usually manifested at 48 to 72 h by abrupt HF and metabolic acidosis secondary to poor systemic perfusion.

HF occurring in the 1st wk of life is the result of any of the above, complicated coarctation, various transpositions, systemic arteriovenous fistulas, or left-to-right shunts in premature infants (eg, ductus arteriosus). Cardiac abnormalities with high-pressured left-to-right shunts (eg, ventricular septal defect, patent ductus arteriosus, truncus arteriosus) usually show HF by age 6 to 8 wk as pulmonary vascular resistance decreases. More complex lesions (eg, anomalous pulmonary venous return, atrioventricular canal defects, single ventricle) may cause HF, depending on the degree of pulmonary artery flooding and pulmonary venous obstruction.

Symptoms and Signs

The onset of HF in infants may be gradual, but is usually rapid and occasionally is extremely rapid. Tachycardia, with heart rates > 120 to 140/min and up to 200/min, is usually present. Signs of left and right heart failure usually occur together in infants. **Left ventricular failure** is manifested by respiratory difficulties. Dyspnea and tachypnea, with a respiratory rate of 60 to 100/min or more in the absence of primary lung disease, are frequently found and are due to pulmonary venous congestion, increased pulmonary capillary pressure, and transudation of fluid into alveolar, interstitial, and bronchiolar spaces. Superimposed infection may accentuate these problems. Rales and

rhonchi are variable but not uncommon, while frank pulmonary edema with frothy, blood-stained sputum is rare. Coughing and wheezing are common. Fatigue from increased respiratory rate and work, as well as the increased metabolic demands to sustain the increase in respiration, lead to poor feeding, inadequate intake, and failure to thrive, although head circumference and growth in length are not usually compromised. Growth failure may be partially masked by fluid retention, decreased urine volume, and inappropriate weight gain. Other symptoms include restlessness, irritability, and excessive sweating.

Cardiomegaly is seen, except with constrictive pericarditis and severe pulmonary venous obstruction. Poor myocardial function is reflected in poor heart sounds, gallop rhythm, and signs of poor peripheral perfusion with cool extremities and decreased pulse volume and capillary filling, as well as a grayish rather than blue color. Cyanosis, an indicator of right-to-left intracardiac shunting, may also reflect inadequate alveolar gas exchange secondary to pulmonary venous congestion or a low output state with an increase in arterial-venous O_2 difference.

In **right ventricular failure,** hepatomegaly is a common and reliable sign of HF in infancy, and is a sensitive guide to the effectiveness of therapy. Pain and tenderness secondary to hepatic engorgement and abnormalities of the jugular venous pulse, while useful signs in older children, are not reliable in infants. Peripheral edema occasionally is seen, particularly on the backs of hands and feet and in the periorbital area.

There are few specific laboratory findings in HF. Dilutional anemia and hyponatremia may be seen. A decrease in urine volume and albuminuria may be present. Hypoglycemia secondary to depletion of and inadequate stores of glycogen, as well as hypermetabolic state, is frequent, particularly in neonates. The WBC count may reflect associated infection, and prolonged systemic arterial desaturation usually results in polycythemia and later iron deficiency.

Diagnosis

HF is identified by the symptoms and signs described above. Evaluation of the infant or child in HF includes an attempt at a specific anatomic diagnosis by evaluating the history, physical examination, and basic laboratory and x-ray findings.

The precordium should be palpated for thrills, heaves, location of the maximal impulse, and sounds. Heart sounds are evaluated by listening for quality, intensity, 2 semilunar valve closures and their relative timing, and extra sounds. Heart murmurs are identified by their location, timing, duration, intensity, and quality. Examination of the lungs for evidence of congestion or infection is required. Assessment of peripheral pulse quality and BP in all extremities is necessary. The degree of peripheral O_2 desaturation and of anemia can be determined by an examination of conjunctivae, mucous membranes, lips, and nailbeds. Liver size and fullness, as well as peripheral edema, should be noted. Fluid retention can best be determined by recording serial, carefully measured, weight increments. Frequent reevaluation of these physical findings serves as a guide to effectiveness of therapy and, as they change, as an aid to specific diagnosis.

ECG changes are of little benefit in diagnosing HF, but are of major value in making a specific anatomic diagnosis. Echocardiography, phonocardiography, vector cardiography, cardiac catheterization, and angiocardiography are required for complete anatomic diagnosis in some instances, but are unnecessary in diagnosing HF. They are rarely performed before the HF and other acute problems (eg, electrolyte abnormality and infection) are controlled.

Prognosis and Treatment

Treatment is initially aimed at relieving the HF, but the prognosis is primarily influenced by the underlying disease and its treatment.

TABLE 187–2. PEDIATRIC DIGOXIN DOSES

Age	*Digitalizing Dose (μg/kg)*	*Maintenance Dose (μg/kg/day)*
Premature	20	5–8
Term, 0–1 wk	30	8–10
0–2 yr	30–50	10–12
2–5 yr	30	10–12
5+ yr	30	5–10

Digoxin is the most widely used drug for HF (see TABLE 187–2 for doses). The initial digitalizing dose may be given IV or orally, either in 3 divided doses, with a larger initial portion, or on a schedule of q 4, 6, or 8 h, depending on urgency. IM digoxin is rarely indicated. Digoxin maintenance divided into 2 doses daily usually provides a smoother response than does 1 daily dose. *Caution* in digoxin prescribing is important. Digoxin concentration in the elixir for oral use is 50 μg/mL (0.05 mg), while in digoxin for IV use it is 250 μg/mL (0.25 mg). Digoxin levels in neonates and infants are not very helpful or reliable.

In very severe HF with inability to improve CO by other means, dopamine and/or dobutamine may be beneficial, beginning with 5 μg/kg/min and increasing to 15 μg/kg/min if needed. Higher doses should be *avoided* because of an adverse effect on renal blood flow. Afterload reduction with nitroprusside 0.5 to 3.0 μg/kg/min IV, hydralazine 0.5 to 5.0 mg/kg/day orally (in 3 divided doses), and captopril 0.5 to 6.0 mg/kg/day orally (in 2 to 4 divided doses) are rarely needed in children, but are available, if used with appropriate caution.

Diuresis with a rapid-acting drug (eg, furosemide or ethacrynic acid 1 mg/kg IV or 2 mg/kg orally) produces an immediate response. Either drug may be repeated in 4 to 6 h, and the dose may be doubled if an adequate response is not obtained. Chlorothiazide 20 to 40 mg/kg/day orally in 2 divided doses may be given in long-term diuretic management of infants and children. Interrupting therapy (eg, for 3 or 4 days/wk) helps to prevent electrolyte imbalance, but K supplements may be necessary. Caution must be used in prescribing diuretics if acute or chronic renal disease is present.

Therapy that may be beneficial during initial management includes humidified O_2 given by croupette, mask, or nasal prongs with adequate inspired O_2 (< 40% to prevent pulmonary epithelial damage) to prevent cyanosis and alleviate respiratory distress; sedation with morphine sulfate 0.2 mg/kg s.c. q 4 to 6 h as needed; and head elevation. Limiting Na and, to a lesser extent, fluid intake to daily maintenance levels helps to maintain a favorable response to treatment, although care should be taken to avoid serum Na levels < 130 mEq/L. Rotating tourniquets, phlebotomy, and mechanical respiratory assistance are less commonly needed. Other general support measures (eg, attempts to increase caloric intake by formulas of increased caloric density, rigorous fever control, treatment of anemia) are of value.

GASTROINTESTINAL DEFECTS

Many GI anomalies with intestinal obstruction in the newborn present as acute surgical emergencies. Immediate medical management includes decompression of the bowel by continuous nasogastric suction to prevent aspiration pneumonia or further abdominal distention with respiratory embarrassment, and rapid referral to a center where neonatal surgery can be performed. Maintaining the infant's body temperature, preventing hypoglycemia with 10% D/W IV, and preventing or treating acidosis and

infections so that the infant is in good condition for surgery are also vital. Since an infant with one anomaly is likely to have others, any neonate with a GI abnormality should be evaluated for malformations of other organ systems.

HIGH ALIMENTARY TRACT OBSTRUCTION

Maternal hydramnios should suggest the possibility of a high (esophageal, gastric, duodenal, jejunal) obstruction, since this disorder prevents the fetus from swallowing and absorbing amniotic fluid. When a high obstruction is suspected, a nasogastric tube should be passed into the stomach immediately following delivery. In esophageal atresia, the tube will not pass into the stomach. The finding of a large volume (> 20 mL) of fluid in the stomach at birth, especially if bile-stained, supports the diagnosis of upper GI obstruction.

Esophageal atresia is usually associated with **tracheoesophageal fistula**, most commonly a fistula from near the carina of the trachea to the lower esophageal segment (Type III B in FIG. 187–8).

In the neonate, characteristic symptoms of esophageal atresia with a tracheoesophageal fistula are excessive secretions, coughing and cyanosis after attempts at swallowing, and aspiration pneumonia. With a Type III B lesion, abdominal distention develops rapidly because, as the infant cries, air from the trachea is forced through the fistula into the lower esophagus and stomach. Diagnosis of atresia can be established by inability to pass a nasogastric tube into the stomach; if a radiopaque catheter is used, its final location can be determined by x-ray. Rarely, a small amount of water-soluble radiopaque dye must be put into the upper pouch through the tube under fluoroscopy to document discontinuity of the esophagus, and then the dye should be carefully aspirated, since its entry into the infant's lungs can cause a chemical pneumonitis. This procedure should be done only at a referral center.

The aim of preoperative management is to prevent aspiration pneumonia, which makes surgical correction more hazardous. Oral feedings are withheld. A suction catheter is inserted into the upper esophageal pouch and attached to continuous suction to prevent aspiration of swallowed saliva. The infant may be positioned with the right side down to facilitate gastric emptying and to minimize the risk of aspirating gastric acid through the fistula. If definitive repair must be deferred because of extreme prematurity, aspiration pneumonia, or associated congenital malformations, gastrostomy is performed to decompress the stomach. Once the gastrostomy tube is placed to suction, gastric contents are not likely to reflux through the fistula into the tracheobronchial tree. When the infant's condition is stable, a thoracotomy can be performed to repair the esophageal atresia and close the tracheoesophageal fistula. Occasionally,

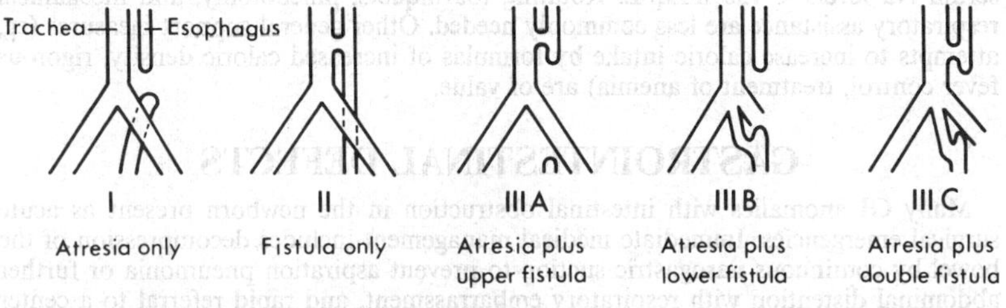

FIG. 187–8. Types of tracheoesophageal fistula. (From A. J. Schaffer and M. E. Avery, *Diseases of the Newborn*, ed. 4, 1977, p. 110. Copyright 1977 by W. B. Saunders Company. Used with permission of W. B. Saunders Company and the authors.)

the gap between the esophageal segments is too great to perform a primary repair, and technics to stretch the esophageal segments gently prior to later anastomosis may be beneficial, or repair by interposing a segment of colon between the esophageal segments may be required. Prognosis is good once the hazards of preoperative management and surgery are passed, but in some infants the lower esophageal sphincter may be incompetent, causing difficulties due to gastroesophageal reflux.

Diaphragmatic hernia (*protrusion of abdominal contents into the thorax through a defect in the diaphragm*) usually occurs on the left side and in the posterolateral portion of the diaphragm (foramen of Bochdalek hernia). Loops of bowel, even most of the abdominal contents, may protrude through the defect into the hemithorax on the involved side. If there is a large congenital diaphragmatic hernia, the lung on the affected left side is always hypoplastic. After delivery, as the newborn cries and swallows air, the loops of bowel quickly fill with air, and this rapidly enlarging mass can cause further acute respiratory embarrassment as the heart and mediastinal structures are pushed to the right, compressing the normal lung. In severe cases following delivery, respiratory distress is immediate and the infant is desperately ill; in others, mild respiratory difficulty develops a few days later as abdominal contents progressively herniate through the diaphragmatic defect. When very small, the abnormality may appear only as a small diaphragmatic defect found on a routine chest x-ray.

X-ray reveals numerous air-filled loops of bowel in the involved hemithorax, and contralateral displacement of the heart and mediastinal structures. If the x-ray is taken immediately at birth before the infant has swallowed air, the diaphragmatic hernia may present as an opaque mass. As soon as diaphragmatic hernia is diagnosed, a large nasogastric tube should be passed into the stomach and continuous suction begun to prevent swallowed air from entering the GI tract and causing further lung compression. If any respiratory distress occurs, the infant must be immediately intubated and ventilated. Paralysis with pancuronium may facilitate ventilation and prevent the swallowing of air. Bag and mask ventilation should *not* be used, as it further distends the bowel loops and worsens the infant's condition. Surgery is required to place the bowel in the abdomen and to close the diaphragmatic defect. The combination of one hypoplastic and one atelectatic lung often makes ventilator management extremely challenging. In infants with a hypoplastic left lung, the right lung may contain abnormal, small pulmonary arteries with smooth muscle hyperplasia; this leads to increased pulmonary vascular resistance with decreased pulmonary blood flow (persistent pulmonary hypertension), right-to-left shunting, and severe hypoxemia. Pulmonary vessel constriction may be relieved by hyperventilation with a respirator (see Persistent Pulmonary Hypertension in Ch. 186). Tolazoline can also help to reduce the increased pulmonary vascular resistance. *It is important that the empty hemithorax not be put to water-sealed drainage, as excessive negative pressure and mediastinal shift may result.* Recently, some infants with diaphragmatic hernia, pulmonary insufficiency, and persistent pulmonary hypertension unresponsive to respirator support have been saved by the use of extracorporeal membrane oxygenation.

Hypertrophic pyloric stenosis *(obstruction of the pyloric lumen due to pyloric muscular hypertrophy)* may almost completely block the GI tract.

The muscular hypertrophy is rarely present at birth but develops over the first 4 to 6 wk of life, and symptoms of obstruction do not commonly appear until then. Forceful projectile vomiting of feedings without bile usually begins late in the first month of life. Visible gastric peristaltic waves may be present, crossing the epigastrium from left to right. Delay in diagnosis may lead to repeated vomiting, dehydration, failure to gain weight, and hypochloremic metabolic alkalosis. Diagnosis can be made by palpation of a discrete, 2- to 3-cm, firm, movable pyloric "olive" deep in the right side of the epigastrium. If the diagnosis is uncertain, a barium-swallow x-ray will show delayed gastric emptying and the typical "string sign" of a markedly narrowed, elongated

pyloric lumen. The treatment of choice is a pyloromyotomy, which leaves the mucosa intact and separates the incised muscle fibers. Postoperatively, the infant usually tolerates feedings well within a few days.

Duodenal obstruction has several possible etiologies, including atresia or stenosis. After the ileum, the duodenum is the most common site of primary intestinal atresia. Obstruction at this site is quite often found in infants with Down's syndrome. Newborns with anomalies of bowel position (see Malrotation, below) may have peritoneal bands that stretch across the duodenum and cause partial or complete occlusion. Choledochal cyst or annular pancreas may also cause duodenal blockage by extrinsic pressure.

Since the obstruction is high, there usually is a history of hydramnios, and the infant develops forceful vomiting *of bile* after the first feedings. Infants with choledochal cysts may also present with variable degrees of obstructive jaundice. In contrast to the single large, air-filled stomach seen in pyloric obstruction, plain x-rays show the characteristic "double bubble" sign, with one large, air-filled bubble representing the stomach and a second bubble representing air in the dilated duodenum proximal to the point of blockage. A barium swallow may identify the point of obstruction as well as extrinsic pressure from a choledochal cyst, while a barium enema will detect GI malrotation.

When duodenal obstruction is suspected, the infant should not be fed. Continuous suction via a nasogastric tube is begun to decompress the stomach and to prevent vomiting and aspiration of vomitus. Surgical exploration is indicated to define and correct the obstruction. The type of repair required will depend on the findings at surgery.

DISTAL SMALL BOWEL AND LARGE BOWEL OBSTRUCTION

In most cases of distal small-bowel or large-intestine obstruction, no history of maternal hydramnios exists, since much of the swallowed amniotic fluid can be absorbed from the fetal bowel proximal to the obstruction. The first few feedings are usually tolerated, but late in the first day or on the second day abdominal distention appears, often accompanied by bilious or fecal vomiting. The infant may pass a small amount of meconium at first, but thereafter does not pass stools. If intestinal obstruction is suspected, a small specimen of meconium may be examined microscopically for squamous cells and lanugo hair. Since these are normally present (from swallowed amniotic fluid), they provide evidence against a complete intestinal obstruction **(Farber test)**. However, obstruction of a previously patent bowel may occur during gestation, so this finding does not absolutely rule out intestinal atresia.

The general diagnostic approach and preoperative management of distal small bowel and large bowel obstruction include discontinuing feedings, placing a nasogastric tube for suction to prevent further intestinal distention or possible aspiration of vomitus, correcting any fluid and electrolyte disturbances, and performing appropriate x-ray studies beginning with plain films and a barium enema.

In **meconium plug syndrome**, thick, inspissated, rubbery meconium forms a cast of the colon and even part of the terminal ileum, and can cause complete intestinal obstruction, with distention and vomiting. A contrast enema with dilute meglumine diatrizoate will demonstrate the plug, and the contrast enema or subsequent gentle enemas with 0.45% sodium chloride solution (10 to 20 mL) will usually separate the plug from the bowel wall and expel it, relieving the obstruction. Although most infants with meconium plug syndrome will thereafter be normal, diagnostic studies may be indicated to identify the small number with underlying Hirschsprung's disease (see below) or cystic fibrosis (see also meconium ileus below). Meconium plug is more common in infants of diabetic mothers and of toxemic mothers treated with magnesium sulfate.

Meconium ileus is almost always an early manifestation of cystic fibrosis (see also Ch. 193). The abnormal meconium is thick, extremely tenacious, and stringy, adhering to the bowel walls and causing obstruction at the level of the ileum. Distal to the ileal obstruction, the colon is narrowed in diameter and contains dessicated meconium pellets. The tenacious meconium of meconium ileus is easily distinguished from the rubbery meconium plug described above. In meconium ileus, loops of intestine can often be palpated through the abdominal wall, and may have a characteristic doughy feel. Diagnosis is supported by the presence of undigested albumin in the meconium. (After a meconium-and-water mixture [1:1] has been shaken and then centrifuged, 10% trichloroacetic acid is added to the supernatant. A heavy, white precipitate indicates undigested albumin.) The luminal contents may appear granular on plain films because small air bubbles are trapped in the abnormal meconium.

The loops of small bowel, distended with thick, tenacious meconium, may twist around each other to form a volvulus in utero. The bowel may then lose its vascular supply and may infarct, producing a sterile meconium peritonitis seen on x-ray as calcified meconium flecks on the peritoneal surfaces and even in the scrotum. The infarcted loop may be resorbed, leaving an area or areas of bowel atresia, or it may be walled off as a large cyst.

If meconium ileus is diagnosed or strongly suspected, the obstruction in uncomplicated cases (eg, no perforation, volvulus, or atresia) may be relieved by giving one or more enemas with a contrast medium (eg, a diluted solution of meglumine diatrizoate and sodium diatrizoate) under fluoroscopy. The large GI water losses that result from hypertonic enemas must be replaced concurrently by vein in order to prevent dehydration. If the enema does not relieve the obstruction, laparotomy is required. A "double-barreled" ileostomy with repeated N-acetylcysteine lavage of both loops is usually required to remove the abnormal meconium and relieve the obstruction.

Surviving infants who develop cystic fibrosis (almost 100%) have the same prognosis as others with that disease. Children with cystic fibrosis and meconium ileus have no worse pulmonary disease than the group as a whole. A positive sweat test is needed to make a definitive diagnosis of cystic fibrosis.

Bowel atresia occurs most frequently in the ileum, followed in order by the duodenum (see discussion of duodenal obstruction, above), jejunum, and colon. Ileal atresia usually presents late on the first or second day. Abdominal distention progressively increases, the infant fails to pass stools, and finally feedings are regurgitated. The general diagnostic approach and preoperative management are similar to those for the other types of distal small bowel or large bowel obstruction (see above). At surgery, the entire bowel should be inspected for additional areas of atresia. The atretic portion of bowel is resected and a primary anastomosis is usually performed. However, at times the proximal portion of the ileum is markedly dilated, while the distal, unused part is hypoplastic. In such cases, the surgeon may perform a "double-barreled" ileostomy and defer anastomosis until the distended proximal bowel has diminished in size. Prognosis is excellent following surgery.

Anomalies of bowel position (malrotation) may cause intestinal obstruction. During embryonic development, the primitive bowel protrudes from the abdominal cavity. As it returns to the abdomen, the large bowel normally rotates counterclockwise, with the cecum finally coming to rest in the right lower quadrant. If rotation is incomplete or abnormal so that the cecum ends up elsewhere (usually in the right upper quadrant or midepigastrium), bowel obstruction may result, either from **retroperitoneal bands** that stretch across the duodenum, or from a **volvulus** of the small bowel that, lacking its normal peritoneal attachment, twists on its narrow stalk-like mesentery. The clinical presentation initially is the same as with other forms of bowel obstruction. A barium

enema will show that the cecum does not lie in the right lower quadrant. *Volvulus is an acute surgical emergency, since the involved bowel may become gangrenous if the obstruction is not immediately relieved.* Upper GI series of a patient with volvulus will show obstruction at the level of the ligament of Treitz with typical radiologic findings.

Hirschsprung's disease (congenital megacolon) is caused by congenital absence of Meissner's and Auerbach's autonomic plexuses in the bowel wall, usually limited to the colon. Peristaltic activity in the involved segment is absent or abnormal, resulting in continuous spasm and partial or complete obstruction with accumulation of intestinal contents and massive dilation of the more proximal normally innervated bowel. Most commonly anal, the obstruction may extend proximally to involve varying portions of the colon, occasionally the entire colon, or even the terminal ileum, and very rarely the entire GI tract. "Skip" lesions almost never occur. The infant presents with obstipation, distention, and finally vomiting. Occasionally, infants have only mild or intermittent constipation, often with intervening bouts of mild diarrhea, and Hirschsprung's disease may not be diagnosed until later in infancy. However, it is important to make the correct diagnosis as early in infancy as possible, because the longer the disease goes untreated, the greater is the chance of toxic enterocolitis, which may be fatal. In older infants, symptoms and signs may include anorexia, lack of a physiologic urge to defecate, empty rectum on examination, palpable colon, and visible peristalsis. The child also may fail to thrive.

A barium enema shows the colon dilated proximal to the site of obstruction, and the narrow, distal segment, which lacks normal innervation. However, a barium enema in the newborn period may not be diagnostic of congenital megacolon. **Rectal biopsy,** disclosing the absence of nerve ganglia, makes the definitive diagnosis. Neonatal Hirschsprung's disease should be treated with a colostomy at a site in the colon proximal to the aganglionic segment. Resection of the entire aganglionic portion of the colon and definitive repair with a "pull-through" procedure can then be deferred until the infant is larger.

The obstipation of Hirschsprung's disease may lead to superimposed **toxic enterocolitis** with small intestinal overgrowth of bacteria and production of bacterial toxins. The consequent *fulminant, catastrophic diarrhea* results in massive fluid loss and may rapidly result in dehydration and death. Fluid replacement and antibiotics are important, but unlikely to be successful unless the obstruction can be quickly relieved by colostomy. Saline lavage of the colon using a rectal tube may be helpful in the initial stages of stabilization before performing a colostomy.

Following surgical repair of Hirschsprung's disease by a pull-through procedure, the prognosis is good; most of these infants eventually achieve good bowel control.

Anal atresia is obvious on examination, since the anus is not patent. Should the diagnosis be missed on routine examination and the infant be fed, all the signs of distal bowel obstruction will, of course, soon develop. Male infants with anal atresia often have a **fistula** from the anal pouch to either the urethra or the perineum. If a fistula is present in females, it extends from the anal pouch to the vagina or, rarely, the bladder. The space between the blind anus and the skin of the perineum may be several centimeters long, or as narrow as a thin membrane of skin covering the anal opening. A cutaneous fistula generally indicates low atresia, and definitive repair via a perineal approach is usually possible. If no perineal fistula exists, a high lesion is likely and will probably require a colostomy, with definitive repair deferred until the infant is older (and larger). The urine should be examined for the presence of meconium or bacteria. By using the lateral prone position for x-rays and fistulograms, a skilled radiologist can define the level and type of lesion. The surgical approach will depend on the findings, especially the length of the atresia.

DEFECTS IN ABDOMINAL WALL CLOSURE

An **omphalocele** is *a protrusion of variable amounts of abdominal viscera from a midline defect at the base of the umbilicus.* The herniation is covered by a thin membrane and may be small, including only a few loops of bowel, or may contain most of the abdominal viscera, including all the intestines, the stomach, and the liver. The immediate dangers are drying of the viscera, hypothermia due to heat loss through evaporation of water from the exposed viscera, and infection of the peritoneal surfaces. Immediately after delivery, the exposed viscera should be covered with sponges wet with sterile saline, and covered with an occlusive dressing to prevent evaporation, to avoid hypothermia, and to maintain sterility. Another useful technic to maintain sterility and prevent evaporative water and heat loss is to place the infant's body up to the level of the axillae in a sterile "bowel bag" containing warm sterile saline. *Surgical repair of the defect is indicated as quickly as possible.*

Primary closure is performed as soon as feasible. With a large omphalocele, the abdominal cavity may be too small to contain the viscera. In this case, the viscera are covered by a pouch or chimney of Silastic® sheeting, which is progressively reduced in size over several days as the abdominal capacity slowly increases until all of the viscera can be returned to the abdominal cavity.

In **gastroschisis,** the abdominal viscera protrude through an abdominal wall defect, usually on the right side of the umbilical cord insertion. There is no membranous covering and the intestines are markedly edematous and appear shortened from being bathed in amniotic fluid containing fetal urine (ie, chemical peritonitis). It often takes several weeks before intestinal function recovers and oral feedings can be given.

Associated bowel anomalies (eg, atresia) must be looked for in infants with omphalocele or gastroschisis. Anomalies of other organ systems may accompany omphalocele, but are rarely seen in infants with gastroschisis.

MISCELLANEOUS SURGICAL EMERGENCIES

Inguinal hernias develop most often in the male newborn and particularly in premature infants. Since hernias can become incarcerated, repair should be early, usually when the infant weighs about 2.27 kg (5 lb). (In contrast, **umbilical hernias** rarely become incarcerated, close spontaneously after several years, and should not ordinarily be operated on.) **Intussusception,** *prolapse of one portion of the bowel into another,* although rare in neonates, is an extreme emergency because of the danger of intestinal gangrene, as is **volvulus,** discussed under anomalies of bowel position, above. Extensive **bowel infarction** may rarely occur from occlusion of the mesenteric arteries due to mural thrombi or emboli following high placement of an umbilical artery catheter. **Perforation** of the stomach or bowel wall from a rigid nasogastric or nasojejunal feeding tube may cause peritonitis. Most gastric perforations in newborns are spontaneous and may occur because of a congenital defect in the stomach wall.

BILIARY ATRESIA; NEONATAL HEPATITIS

The **neonatal hepatitis** ("giant cell hepatitis") syndrome is usually of unknown etiology, though infection with cytomegalovirus or hepatitis B virus or α_1-antitrypsin deficiency are rarely responsible. **Biliary atresia** reflects total or partial agenesis of the biliary tree, and usually affects extrahepatic, rather than intrahepatic, bile ducts. Recent evidence indicates that biliary atresia and neonatal hepatitis probably represent a spectrum of overlapping disorders rather than distinct entities. In most cases biliary atresia develops several weeks after birth, probably following inflammation and scar-

ring of the bile ducts, and is rarely found in stillborns or in the immediate neonatal period. The etiology for the inflammatory response is not known.

In both conditions, cholestatic jaundice with mixed hyperbilirubinemia, progressively dark urine (conjugated bilirubin), acholic stools, and hepatomegaly are usually first noted about 2 wk after birth. By age 2 to 3 mo, retarded growth, irritability from pruritus, and signs of portal hypertension may be present. Liver function tests reflect both cholestasis and hepatocellular necrosis. Appropriate investigations can usually exclude other specific causes of neonatal obstructive jaundice (eg, specific infectious etiologies, α_1-antitrypsin deficiency, galactosemia, and cystic fibrosis), but differentiation between neonatal hepatitis and biliary atresia may be difficult. Direct and total bilirubin values, AST (SGOT), ALT (SGPT), alkaline phosphatase, and serum levels of bile acids often will not clearly distinguish biliary atresia from neonatal hepatitis with severe cholestasis. Ultrasound **(US)** examination of the gallbladder and extrahepatic bile ducts may be helpful. The absence of a recognizable gallbladder and of extrahepatic bile ducts on US examination is strongly suggestive of biliary atresia. Placement of a nasoduodenal tube and collection of a 24-h sample of duodenal fluid by gravity drainage may reveal the presence of bile (bilirubin can be measured biochemically); bile excretion is strong evidence against a diagnosis of complete bile-duct atresia. Fecal excretion of ^{131}I rose bengal 72 h after the dye is given IV usually exceeds 10% in hepatitis, but is less in atresia. Overlap occurs, however, and despite recent changes, this test is not infallible. Recently, liver scan using Tc99m-Tc-PIPIDA has proven useful in identifying extrahepatic bile flow. Percutaneous liver biopsy is often very useful in questionable cases (see Ch. 68), and if interpreted by an experienced pathologist, it is probably the most accurate diagnostic test available.

If the diagnosis is still uncertain, laparotomy must be done before 2 mo of age because infants with biliary atresia will develop irreversible biliary cirrhosis if operation is deferred. At laparotomy, an intraoperative cholangiogram to delineate the state of the biliary tree and an open liver biopsy for frozen section morphology are obtained. Atretic ducts can be successfully reanastamosed in only 5 to 10% of cases. However, a modification of the Kasai procedure, a hepatoportoenterostomy, is performed in the others. The majority will reestablish bile flow, but unfortunately many will continue to have significant chronic medical problems, including cholestasis, recurrent ascending cholangitis, and failure to thrive with late mortality occurring in a significant number. Cholestasis due to neonatal hepatitis usually resolves slowly, but permanent hepatic damage may ensue. Supportive therapy is discussed in Ch. 67. In recent years liver transplantation has saved the lives of some infants with liver failure from biliary atresia and cirrhosis.

NECROTIZING ENTEROCOLITIS (NEC)

An acquired disease, primarily of preterm or sick neonates. There is mucosal or deeper intestinal necrosis and the commonest site is the terminal ileum, with the colon and the proximal small bowel involved less frequently. The necrosis begins in the mucosa, and may progress to involve full thickness of the bowel wall, resulting in perforation. There is associated sepsis in 1/3 of infants.

Etiology and Pathogenesis

In infants who develop NEC, 3 factors are usually present: a preceding ischemic insult to the intestine; bacterial colonization of the intestine; and intraluminal substrate in the bowel, ie, enteral feedings.

The etiology of NEC is not known, but it is believed that an ischemic insult damages the bowel so that the mucosa does not produce normal protective mucus; abnormal peristalsis also may permit bacterial overgrowth. Once feedings are begun, ample substrate is provided for proliferation of luminal bacteria. These organisms can penetrate

into the bowel wall; there they produce hydrogen gas that collects, producing the characteristic appearance of "pneumatosis intestinalis" on x-ray. Gas may also enter the portal veins, and intraportal gas may be seen on plain films of the abdomen or by US examination of the liver. Progression of the disease may lead to full-thickness bowel necrosis, peritonitis, sepsis, and death.

The ischemic insult may result from vasospasm of the mesenteric arteries, which may be produced by an anoxic insult triggering a primitive "diving reflex" that markedly diminishes intestinal blood flow. The increased incidence of NEC reported with the use of umbilical artery **(UA)** catheters may be secondary to vasospasm due to the presence of the catheter or to the fluids infused, to thromboemboli from the catheter tip, and/or to the anoxia inherent in the respiratory distress for which UA catheterization is used. Ischemic intestinal insult may result as well from low blood flow states encountered during an exchange transfusion or in sepsis, or from the use of hyperosmolar formulas. Similarly, congenital heart disease with reduced systemic blood flow or arterial O_2 desaturation may lead to bowel hypoxia/ischemia and predispose to NEC. The suggestion that feeding breast milk may offer protection from NEC has not been proven.

NEC may occur as clusters of cases or "outbreaks" in neonatal units. Epidemiologic studies in some "outbreaks" have found infection and/or colonization of affected infants by specific organisms (eg, *Klebsiella* or *E. coli*), but often no common organism can be identified. However, because of concern that at least some outbreaks may have an infectious etiology, it is recommended that isolation of infants with NEC and cohorting of possibly exposed infants be considered if several cases of NEC occur in a short time span within a neonatal unit.

Epidemiology and Clinical Findings

Certain neonates are at particular risk of developing NEC; 75% of NEC occurs in prematures, particularly if there has been prolonged rupture of the membranes with amnionitis or asphyxia at birth. There may also be a higher incidence in infants fed hypertonic formulas, or who have undergone exchange transfusion. The ileus may be manifested by abdominal distention, bilious gastric residuals following feedings that may progress to vomiting, and/or gross or microscopic GI bleeding. Screening the stools of premature infants who are being fed for occult blood or reducing substances may help to diagnose NEC at an early stage. Sepsis may be manifested by lethargy, temperature instability, increased apneic spells, and metabolic acidosis.

Early x-rays may be nonspecific and reveal only ileus. However, a fixed, dilated bowel loop that does not change on repeated x-rays indicates NEC. Specific x-ray signs of NEC are pneumatosis intestinalis and portal venous gas. Pneumoperitoneum indicates bowel perforation.

Treatment

The treatment of NEC is nonoperative in about 70% of cases. Feedings must be discontinued at once if NEC is suspected and the bowel should be decompressed with a nasogastric tube attached to suction. Appropriate colloid and crystalloid parenteral fluids must be given to support the circulation, as extensive bowel inflammation and/or peritonitis may lead to considerable third-space fluid losses. Total parenteral nutrition will be needed for 14 to 21 days while the bowel heals. Systemic antibiotics should be started at once with ticarcillin or mezlocillin and amikacin or gentamycin, and treatment continued for 10 days. (For dosage, see TABLE 187-3.) Most important, the infant with NEC requires frequent clinical re-evaluation (eg, at 6-h intervals), with sequential abdominal x-rays, CBCs, platelet counts, and blood gases.

Operative therapy will be necessary in up to 1/3 of neonates with NEC. Absolute indications for operative intervention are intestinal perforation (pneumoperitoneum),

TABLE 187–3. DOSAGE OF SYSTEMIC ANTIBIOTICS FOR INFANTS

Drug and Route		Age < 1 to 7 days	Age > 7 days
Ticarcillin	IV, IM	15 mg/kg/day q 12 h*	15–22.5 mg/kg/day q 8–12 h*
Mezlocillin	IV, IM	150–225 mg/kg/day q 8–12 h*	225–300 mg/kg/day q 6–8 h*
Amikacin	IM, IV	15 mg/kg/day q 12 h*	15–22.5 mg/kg/day q 8–12 h*
Gentamicin	IM, IV	5 mg/kg/day q 12 h*	7.5 mg/kg/day q 8 h*

* Given in divided doses.

signs of peritonitis (absent bowel sounds and diffuse guarding and tenderness or erythema of the abdominal wall), or aspiration of purulent material from the peritoneal cavity by paracentesis. Erythema and edema of the abdominal wall is a sign of peritonitis in the newborn and is an indication for surgery. Serious consideration for surgery should be given in an infant with NEC whose clinical and laboratory condition worsens over time despite support with antibiotics, colloid, etc. At surgery, gangrenous bowel is resected, and ostomies created. With resolution of sepsis and peritonitis, bowel continuity can be re-established several weeks or months later. Rarely, infants treated nonoperatively will develop an intestinal stricture over the following weeks or months, usually at the splenic flexure of the colon. These infants will then require resection of the stricture to relieve intestinal obstruction. About ⅔ of infants with NEC will survive; the outcome has been improved by aggressive supportive measures and judicious timing of surgical intervention.

MUSCULOSKELETAL DEFECTS

This chapter discusses some important and common disorders of the newborn musculoskeletal system; others are found elsewhere in THE MANUAL.

Various **craniofacial abnormalities** arise from maldevelopment of the 1st and 2nd visceral arches, which form the facial bones and ears at about the 7th wk of embryonic development. These malformations include cleft lip and cleft palate, Treacher Collins syndrome (mandibulofacial dysostosis), Pierre Robin and Waardenburg syndromes, hypertelorism, and deformities of the external and middle ear. Most infants with craniofacial abnormalities have normal intelligence.

Cleft lips and **cleft palates** are the most common 1st arch defects and may involve either or both the hard and soft palates. They occur once in 700 to 800 births. The cleft may vary from involvement of the soft palate only, to a complete cleft of the soft and hard palates, the alveolar process of the maxilla, and the lip. Cleft lips cause no disability but are cosmetically distressing, while a cleft palate interferes with feeding and with speech development. Use of a feeder with which formula can be delivered with mild pressure (such as a plastic bottle) often is helpful. There are special cleft palate nipples and devices to occlude the cleft that rarely need to be used. Plastic surgery can significantly improve either disorder. Dental, orthodontic, psychiatric, and speech therapy may be required.

Infants with defects associated with small mandibles **(Pierre Robin** and **Treacher Collins syndromes)** cannot be fed easily and may have bouts of cyanosis because the tongue tends to fall backwards, obstructing the pharynx. Feeding problems can be avoided by gavage. If cyanosis or respiratory problems persist, tracheostomy or surgery to fix the tongue in a forward position may be required. An otologic evaluation is indicated, since these syndromes may involve the ear.

Congenital torticollis (*head tilt present at birth*): Fractures, dislocations, or subluxations of the cervical spine (especially C-1 and C-2), or odontoid abnormalities are rare but serious causes, since permanent neurologic damage may result. Cervical x-rays can help exclude these conditions, but traumatic injury may occur before or during delivery. The most common etiology for torticollis is neck trauma during delivery, with hematoma, fibrosis, and contracture of the sternocleidomastoid **(SCM)** muscle. The torticollis is not present at birth; it appears in the first few days or weeks of life, and a nontender mass is noted in the SCM in the segment nearest the occiput. Passive stretching of the involved muscle is indicated (achieved by rotating the head and flexing the neck laterally to the opposite side). Other causes include abnormalities of the bony spine, such as **Klippel-Feil syndrome** (*fusion of the cervical vertebrae*), or of the atlas to the occipital bone **(atlanto-occipital fusion)**. CNS tumors, bulbar palsies, and ocular dysfunction are prominent neurologic causes but rarely are present at birth.

Congenital scoliosis is rare, but **vertebral anomalies** such as hemi-, wedge, or butterfly vertebrae are more common. Bony spinal defects should be suspected when there are posterior midline cutaneous abnormalities, bony torticollis, or congenital anomalies of the lower extremities. Since growth can lead to serious deformity, treatment with braces or body jackets should begin early. Surgery may be needed if the curvature progresses. Associated renal anomalies are common, and intravenous urography (IVU; IVP) is indicated.

Congenital dislocation of the hip, more common in breech presentations and female infants, has an uncertain etiology but seems to be secondary to laxity of the ligaments about the joint or to in utero positioning. The dislocation can be uni- or bilateral. If unilateral, the involved leg is shorter and there may be asymmetric skin creases in the thigh. The major sign of subluxation or dislocation is inability to completely abduct the thigh to the surface of the examining table when the hip and knee are flexed. This adductor spasm is often present even if the hip is not actually dislocated at the time of the examination. If the hip is dislocated, abduction and external rotation of the femur may produce an audible or palpable "clunk" as the femoral head reenters the acetabulum. Minor "clicks" are more commonly found, are less significant, and should disappear within a month or two. Since partial or complete dislocation may be difficult to detect at birth and can appear during the first year of life, periodic testing for limitation of abduction is advised. X-rays of the hip may be difficult to interpret early and are helpful only if they confirm the clinical impression. Early treatment is critical, since the hip usually can be reduced immediately after birth, and with growth the acetabulum will then form almost normally. If therapy is delayed, the outcome is progressively less satisfactory, since the potential for correction with growth declines steadily. Medical treatment consists of devices (eg, splint, slings, harnesses, or large padded diapers) that hold the affected hips abducted and laterally rotated, thus encouraging the acetabulum to form properly as growth occurs.

Femoral torsion or twisting, either internal (anteversion—knees pointing toward each other) or external (retroversion—knees pointing in opposite directions), is typical of newborns, in whom either condition may be striking. Spontaneous correction of even dramatic femoral torsion generally occurs when the infant stands and walks. Sleeping prone can prolong retroversion. Hip x-rays for dislocation should be considered. Positioning and passive exercises may be helpful.

Knee dislocation anteriorly with hyperextension at birth is rare, but requires emergency treatment. The dislocation may be related to muscle imbalance (if myelodysplasia or arthrogryposis is present) or intrauterine positioning, and is often associated with ipsilateral hip dislocation. Immediate treatment with daily passive flexion movements and splinting in flexion frequently results in a functional knee, if the infant is otherwise normal.

Bowing and twisting (torsion) of the tibia are common at birth and seldom pathologic. Bowing with x-ray changes of a narrow sclerotic intramedullary canal is an exception, with a high risk of fracture and pseudarthrosis; a protective orthosis is needed.

Abnormalities of the feet are common. Of the **clubfoot (talipes) deformities,** the most frequently seen is **equinovarus;** the foot is plantar flexed, inverted, and markedly adducted. Deformities from in utero positioning can mimic clubfoot, but they can be passively corrected while pathologic changes cannot. Orthopedic care beginning in the nursery with repeated cast applications to normalize the foot's position is optimal. In severe cases, surgery may be required if casting is not successful. In the **calcaneovalgus** position, the foot is flat or convex, dorsiflexed, and can easily be approximated against the lower tibia. Early treatment with a cast to place the foot in the equinovarus position or with use of corrective shoes usually is successful. **Metatarsus adductus** (adduction of the forward part of the foot) does not require treatment. However, if the foot is also inverted and cannot be passively straightened with ease **(metatarsus varus),** serial casts usually are required.

Congenital absence of individual muscles or groups of muscles may occur. Partial or complete agenesis of the pectoralis major is one of the most common of these defects, and can be an isolated phenomenon or can be associated with ipsilateral hand abnormalities **(Poland's anomaly)**. One or more layers of the abdominal musculature may also be absent at birth (eg, **prune-belly syndrome**). This deficiency often is associated with severe GU abnormalities, particularly hydronephrosis. Incidence is highest in male infants, who often also have undescended testes. The prognosis is poor, even with early relief of the urinary tract obstruction. Malformations involving the feet and rectum often accompany agenesis of the abdominal musculature.

The **chondrodystrophies** are *diseases affecting the manner in which cartilage is converted to bone*. Of these, **achondroplasia** is the best known. All are characterized by dwarfism (usually with a trunk of normal size, but with short extremities) and are often associated with abnormalities elsewhere. The osteochondrodysplasias, osteopetroses, and osteochondroses are discussed in Ch. 197. In most of the chondrodystrophies, x-rays of the long bones are needed for accurate diagnosis. Mental development usually is normal. Hypothyroidism should be ruled out. Treatment is supportive.

The **mucopolysaccharidoses (MPS**—see under INHERITED DISORDERS OF CONNECTIVE TISSUE in Ch. 197) have similarities with the chondrodystrophies, but some types also have visceral and CNS involvement with mental deficiency; and truncal shortening and limb contractures are more common. The MPS are not usually apparent in newborns.

Osteogenesis imperfecta, *abnormal fragility of bone*, is a serious newborn disease that diffusely affects bone. Several forms have been described, but the newborn type **(congenita)** is the most severe. Infants are born with multiple fractures, which lead to shortening of the extremities. The skull is soft, has many wormian bones, and feels like a "bag of bones" when palpated. The sclerae are abnormally thin and translucent and may appear blue because a deficiency in connective tissue allows the color of the underlying vessels to show through. (Blue sclerae do not, however, always indicate osteogenesis imperfecta.) Some infants also have a hearing loss, presumably from otosclerosis due to abnormal connective tissue around the ossicles of the middle ear. Delivery trauma may lead to intracranial hemorrhage and stillbirth because of the soft skull. Infants born alive may often die suddenly during the first few days or weeks of life, but some survive as deformed dwarfs. Mental development is normal unless head trauma with CNS injury occurs. There is no effective treatment.

Congenital hypophosphatasia is due to absence of alkaline phosphatase in the serum and results in a diffuse lack of calcium deposition in the bones. Vomiting, failure to gain weight, and enlargement of the epiphyses like that seen in rickets usually occur.

Bony deformities and dwarfism, but normal mental development, are present in patients who survive infancy. There is no effective treatment.

Congenital amputations are *transverse or longitudinal limb deficiencies due to primary intrauterine growth inhibition or secondary intrauterine destruction of normal embryonic tissues*. The etiology often is unclear, but teratogenic agents (eg, thalidomide) and amniotic bands are 2 known causes. In transverse deficiencies, all elements beyond a certain level are absent, and the limb resembles an amputation stump. In longitudinal deficiencies, specific maldevelopments occur; eg, complete or partial absence of the radius, fibula, or tibia. Infants with either transverse or longitudinal limb deficiencies may also have hypoplastic or bifid bones, synostoses, duplications, dislocations, or other bony defects. One or more limbs may be affected, and defects may be of a different type in each limb. X-rays are essential in determining which bones are involved. CNS abnormalities are rare.

Treatment consists mainly of providing a prosthesis, and is highly individualized. Prosthetic devices are most valuable in lower extremity deficiencies or when there is complete or nearly complete absence of an upper limb. If any activity in an arm or hand exists, no matter how great the malformation, functioning capacity must be carefully assessed before a prosthesis or operation is recommended. Therapeutic amputation of any limb or portion of a limb should be **avoided** unless essential for fitting of a prosthetic device, and should be considered only after evaluating the functional and psychologic implications of the loss.

An upper limb prosthesis should be designed to serve as many needs as possible so that the number of devices is kept to a minimum. A child uses a prosthesis most successfully when it is fitted early and becomes an integral part of his body during the developmental years. With effective orthopedic and ancillary support, most children with congenital amputations lead normal lives.

ARTHROGRYPOSIS MULTIPLEX CONGENITA (AMC)

The presence at birth of fibrous ankylosis of multiple joints. AMC is heterogenous and consists of several disease entities. However, the AMC label often is loosely and incorrectly placed on some well-defined disorders in which limited joint movement is only one of several abnormalities present, or in which a primary cause of joint rigidity is evident.

Etiology and Pathology

The cause is unknown. AMC is nongenetic in most instances. Affected individuals have normal chromosomes. Impaired intrauterine fetal movement may be the pathogenic mechanism.

AMC can be neurogenic, with histologic and electromyographic evidence of nervous system involvement, or myopathic, with muscle fiber changes shown by electromyography. Neurogenic and myopathic AMC may correspond to typical and atypical clinical forms, but this is unproved.

Symptoms and Signs

In typical AMC, the joints of all limbs are fixed. The shoulders generally are adducted and internally rotated, the elbows are extended, and the wrists and digits are flexed. The hips may be dislocated and usually are slightly flexed. The knees are extended and the feet are often in equinovarus.

The muscles are hypoplastic and the limbs tend to be tubular and featureless. Soft tissue webbing often is present over the ventral aspects of the flexed joints. The spine usually is uninvolved, and apart from slenderness of the long bones, the skeleton is radiographically normal. Occasional associated abnormalities include cleft palate,

cryptorchidism, cardiac lesions, and urinary tract malformations. Physical handicap may be severe, but intelligence usually is unimpaired.

A relatively common, atypical form of AMC is characterized by limited joint involvement and absence of muscle wasting and associated abnormalities.

Differential Diagnosis

Congenital joint contractures may be secondary to many conditions, including spinal defects (spina bifida, sacral agenesis) and spasticity due to cerebral cortical damage. Joint rigidity also may be present in acquired disorders (juvenile RA) and several genetic conditions. Since AMC usually is not inherited, recognition of inheritance patterns is diagnostically important.

Prognosis and Treatment

The deformities are at their worst at birth. AMC is not progressive; any change that occurs will be an improvement. Considerable handicap may be present, and orthopedic correction usually is required. The angle of joint ankylosis can be surgically altered, but enhanced mobility is difficult to attain. Active physiotherapy and manipulation during the first few months of life may produce considerable improvement.

NEUROLOGIC DEFECTS

Some of the most serious congenital abnormalities of the nervous system, such as anencephaly, encephalocele, and spina bifida, develop in the first 2 mo of gestation and represent defects in neural tube formation **(dysraphia)**. Others, such as hydranencephaly and porencephaly, occur later and appear to be secondary to destructive processes of the brain after it has formed. Some defects are relatively benign; eg, meningocele.

Accurate in utero detection of many CNS malformations is now possible using amniocentesis and ultrasound (see PREVENTION OF GENETIC DISORDERS in Ch. 203). Genetic counseling for parents of a child with a major neurologic abnormality is important, since the risk of a subsequent child having such a defect is high. These parents also need psychologic help and support.

Some of the more serious neurologic disorders are discussed below.

Anencephaly, *absence of the cerebral hemispheres*, is incompatible with life. The absent brain is sometimes replaced with malformed cystic neural tissue, which may either be exposed or covered with skin. Varying portions of the brainstem and spinal cord may be missing or malformed. No diagnostic or therapeutic efforts are helpful, and these infants either are stillborn or die within a few days.

Other malformations of the cerebral hemispheres may occur: the hemispheres may be large or small; the gyri may be absent, unusually large (and mushroom-shaped on cross section), or multiple and small; microscopic sections of a normal-appearing brain sometimes show disorganization of the normal laminar neuronal arrangement; a decreased head size **(microcephaly)** is often present. These defects are usually associated with severe motor and mental retardation. Therapy is that of general support, and anticonvulsants if needed to control seizures.

Encephalocele, *a protrusion of brain or heterotopic nervous tissue along with meninges through a skull defect*, is associated with incomplete closure of the cranial vault or **cranium bifidum**. Encephalocele usually occurs in the midline and is nasal or occipital but can be asymmetrically frontal or parietal. Small encephaloceles may resemble cephalhematomas, but x-rays show a bony skull defect at their base. Most encephaloceles should be repaired, since even large ones may contain mostly heterotopic nerve tissue which can be removed without leaving major functional disability. When other serious malformations coexist, the decision to repair may be more difficult. The hydro-

cephalus (see below) often associated with encephalocele requires definition by CT scan or ultrasonography and, if it is progressive, surgical treatment with a shunt. About ½ of affected infants have other congenital defects. The prognosis is good for many of these patients.

Porencephaly, *a cyst or cavity in a cerebral hemisphere that communicates with a ventricle*, may occur pre- or postnatally. The defect may be caused by a developmental anomaly, inflammatory disease, or a vascular accident such as intraventricular hemorrhage with parenchymal extension. The neurologic examination is usually abnormal. Cranial transillumination may be positive. Diagnosis is confirmed by CT scan or ultrasonography. Progressive hydrocephalus may require a shunt procedure. Prognosis is variable; a few patients develop only minor neurologic signs and have normal intelligence.

Hydranencephaly is *an extreme form of porencephaly in which the cerebral hemispheres are almost totally absent*. Usually, the cerebellum and brainstem are formed normally and the basal ganglia are intact. The meninges, bones, and skin over the cranial vault are normal. Results of neurologic examination in the newborn period may be normal or abnormal, but the infant fails to develop normally. Externally, the head appears to be normal, but when transilluminated, light shines completely through. A CT scan or ultrasonography confirms the diagnosis. Treatment is supportive.

Dandy-Walker cysts and the Arnold-Chiari malformation are major malformations of the posterior fossa that often lead to hydrocephalus.

Dandy-Walker cysts are *developmental malformations in which the 4th ventricle is cystic*; hydrocephalus usually results. Diagnosis is made by observing superior displacement of the lateral sinus groove on x-ray, or by transillumination of the posterior fossa, and is confirmed by a CT scan or ultrasonography. The hydrocephalus usually requires a shunt.

The **Arnold-Chiari malformation** is a defect in the formation of the brainstem. It consists of *elongation of the cerebellar tonsils, which protrude through the foramen magnum; beaking of the colliculi; and thickening of the upper cervical spinal cord.* Diagnosis is made by CT scan or ventriculography. Hydrocephalus may result from blockage of the 4th ventricular outlets or an associated aqueductal stenosis. Either may require a shunt procedure to relieve the obstruction. The Arnold-Chiari malformation may occur alone, but is frequently associated with spina bifida (see below) and syringomyelia (see Ch. 130).

Spina bifida, *defective closure of the vertebral column*, is one of the most serious neural tube defects compatible with prolonged life. Its severity varies from the occult type with no findings to a completely open spine **(rachischisis)** with severe neurologic disability and death. In spina bifida cystica, the protruding sac can contain meninges **(meningocele),** spinal cord **(myelocele),** or both **(myelomeningocele)**. The open types can be diagnosed in utero using amniocentesis for elevated α-fetoprotein, and ultrasonography. Spina bifida is commonly seen in the lumbar, low thoracic, or sacral region, and usually extends for 3 to 6 vertebral segments. The sac in myelomeningocele usually consists of meninges with a central neural plaque. If not well covered with skin, the sac can easily rupture, increasing the risk of meningitis.

When the spinal cord or lumbosacral nerve roots are involved in the spina bifida, as is usual, varying degrees of paralysis occur below the involved level. Since this paralysis is present in the fetus, there can be orthopedic problems, such as clubfoot, arthrogryposis, or dislocated hip (see under MUSCULOSKELETAL DEFECTS, above) present at birth. The paralysis usually affects the sphincters of the bladder and rectum, and the resulting GU disorder can eventually lead to severely damaged kidneys. Kyphosis, sometimes associated with spina bifida, can hinder surgical closure and preclude the patient from lying supine. Hydrocephalus occurs frequently and may be related to

aqueductal stenosis or an Arnold-Chiari malformation (see above). Other congenital anomalies may be present.

Laboratory evaluation begins with x-rays of the spine, skull, hips, and, if malformed, the lower extremities. Urinary evaluation is essential and includes urinalysis, urine culture, BUN and creatinine determination, and intravenous urography. Further testing depends on the associated defects and may include intracranial studies (CT scan or ultrasonography) and CSF evaluation.

Prognosis is determined by the number and severity of abnormalities, and is poorest for those patients who have total paralysis below the lesion, kyphosis, hydrocephalus, early hydronephrosis, and associated congenital defects. With proper care, however, many children do well.

Treatment requires a united effort by specialists from several disciplines. Initially essential are neurosurgical, urologic, orthopedic, pediatric, and social service evaluations. The decision of how aggressively to treat should be made before neurosurgery is undertaken, since closure of the defect assures at least temporary survival. Thorough evaluation of the infant and counseling of the family should precede intervention. The decision depends on the type, level, and extent of the lesion; the associated defects and the infant's health status in general; the treatment resources, including availability of ongoing care; the family's desires and strengths; and the estimated potential for the patient's habilitation.

If the defect is leaking CSF, urgent neurosurgical evaluation and repair will reduce the risk of meningeal or ventricular infection. Hydrocephalus may require a shunt procedure. Kidney function must be carefully followed, and urinary tract infections should be treated promptly. Obstructive uropathy either at the bladder outlet or ureteral level must be treated vigorously, especially when infection is present. Loss of renal function or shunt complications are the usual causes of death in older patients with spina bifida. Orthopedic care should begin early with application of a cast for clubfoot, if present, and close observation of the hip joints, since dislocation is frequent. Other continuing orthopedic concerns are scoliosis, pathologic fractures, development of pressure sores, and muscle weakness and spasm, which may cause further deformities.

Hydrocephalus, *excessive accumulation of CSF within the ventricles*, is the most common cause of abnormally large heads in neonates. Obstruction is most frequently seen in the aqueduct of Sylvius but can also occur at the outlets of the 4th ventricle (foramina of Luschka and Magendie) or in the subarachnoid spaces around the brainstem or over the hemispheres. **Communicating hydrocephalus** is present when CSF flows freely into the subarachnoid space; **noncommunicating hydrocephalus** indicates blockage at a site within the ventricular system or between it and the subarachnoid space. Communicating hydrocephalus usually results from meningeal inflammation, either secondary to infection or to blood in the subarachnoid space.

Laboratory evaluation of the infant with hydrocephalus begins with skull x-rays or a CT scan. Either may show separation of sutures, areas of thinning of the bones, or intracranial calcifications (associated with congenital infections). Plain skull films may show a "beaten metal" appearance of the bones (common in infants with myelomeningoceles and hydrocephalus), indicating a prolonged increase in intracranial pressure. A CT scan will show the ventricular size and can also indicate the site of obstruction. Ultrasonography can define the degree of ventricular dilatation, and serial studies can document progression of the hydrocephalus. Ultrasound is especially valuable following intraventricular hemorrhage, since ventricular dilatation may be transient and require either no specific treatment or only medical treatment. When congenital infection is suspected, serologic studies for *Toxoplasma gondii*, rubella virus, *Treponema pallidum*, and herpes- and cytomegalovirus are indicated, and evidence of liver involve-

ment is sought. If seizures are present, an EEG may be helpful. Further evaluation may consist of subdural taps, CSF evaluation, or a CT scan.

Differential diagnosis includes intracranial space-occupying lesions such as subdural hematomas, porencephalic cysts, and tumors. These can be identified by CT scan. An abnormally large, usually malfunctioning brain **(megalencephaly)** can also occur.

Treatment depends on etiology. Medical treatment with acetazolamide and glycerol or lumbar punctures (if the hydrocephalus is communicating) can sometimes be helpful temporarily. However, progressive hydrocephalus, especially if the head circumference is growing too rapidly, requires a shunt procedure to reduce the pressure. It is important to ascertain prior to operation that the hydrocephalus is progressive, since some hydrocephalics arrest spontaneously. The type of shunt performed depends on the neurosurgeon's experience and preference. Ventriculo-peritoneal shunts are generally preferred, since complications are fewer. After placement of the shunt, the infant's progress should be followed with attention to occipitofrontal head circumference, development, and the increased risk of infections related to the shunt. Periodic, partial CT scans or ultrasound (if the anterior fontanel is open) can be used to monitor ventricular size. Some children cease to need the shunt as they become older, but it is difficult to determine when this occurs, and shunts are rarely removed. Fetal surgery to treat congenital hydrocephalus before birth has been attempted, but has been unsuccessful and is presently experimental.

CONGENITAL EYE DEFECTS

CONGENITAL GLAUCOMA

(Infantile Glaucoma; Buphthalmos; Hydrophthalmos)

A rare condition due to a congenital defect in the region of the iridocorneal angle of the anterior chamber that obstructs the outflow of aqueous, causing a chronic increase in the intraocular pressure. The disorder is usually bilateral and is seen in infants and children. The eyeball becomes considerably enlarged; the cornea thinned, milky, and bulging; the pupil large and fixed; the anterior chamber deep. If the disease is permitted to progress, the optic nerve becomes damaged and blindness ensues. **Treatment** by early surgical intervention offers the only real hope of preserving useful vision.

CONGENITAL CATARACT

Developmental or congenital cataracts are present at birth, and can be the result of chromosomal abnormalities, intrauterine infection (eg, rubella), metabolic disease (galactosemia), or other maternal disease during pregnancy. The cataracts may be nuclear or cortical, and may not be noticed unless fundoscopy is performed at birth. If the cataracts are sufficiently dense to obscure the view of the optic disk and vessels, an ophthalmologist should be asked to estimate the possible effect on the infant's vision. Early surgery (within a few months of birth) is now advocated to permit development of appropriate retinal fixation and cortical visual responses. While the surgery is technically straightforward, postoperative visual correction with spectacles or contact lenses is difficult but must be done to achieve good vision.

Juvenile or adult cataract is discussed in Ch. 221.

RENAL AND GENITOURINARY DEFECTS

Congenital anomalies of the GU tract are more common than those of any other organ system. The kidneys and ureters, bladder and bladder outlet, and gonads are involved most frequently. Complications include urinary obstruction and stasis with infection and stone formation, impairment of renal function, and sexual disability or infertility. Treatment of significant anatomic anomalies is usually surgical.

KIDNEY

Fusion anomalies: The most common is **horseshoe kidney** (*the 2 kidneys are joined at their corresponding [usually the lower] poles, generally with an isthmus of renal parenchyma across the midline at the joined poles*). Since the ureters course medially and anteriorly over this isthmus, secondary obstruction may develop. About 1/3 of patients with horseshoe kidney have no difficulty, 1/3 may develop hydronephrosis that requires surgery, and 1/3 may suffer abdominal pain accentuated by hyperextension. Surgical resection of the isthmus occasionally is required, and may be indicated to facilitate resection of the abdominal aorta, which lies behind the isthmus.

Other fusion anomalies include **fused pelvic kidney (pancake kidney),** in which *a single pelvic renal mass is served by 2 collecting systems and ureters* that frequently become obstructed because of anomalous position and drainage. **Crossed fused renal ectopia** also occurs, with both kidneys on one side, and usually requires no treatment unless obstruction is present.

Renal ectopia and malrotation (*displacement or failure of ascent or rotation of either or both kidneys*) may be evident on abdominal ultrasound, CT scan, or urography even though the patient has been asymptomatic. **Pelvic kidney,** usually lying over the sacral promontory, may complicate pregnancy because of outflow obstruction. **Malrotation** of a normally positioned kidney may compromise urinary drainage and cause hydronephrosis that requires surgical correction.

Agenesis: Bilateral renal agenesis (*congenital absence of both kidneys*—Potter's syndrome) is incompatible with life. **Unilateral renal agenesis** is not uncommon and usually is accompanied by ureteral agenesis with absence of the ipsilateral trigone and ureteral orifice. The congenitally solitary kidney usually is both hyperplastic and hypertrophic, maintaining normal renal function.

Duplication anomalies: *Supernumerary collecting systems*—**accessory renal pelvis, double pelvis and ureter,** or **"duplex kidney"** —may be unilateral or bilateral and may involve the renal pelvis, calyces, the ureter, and/or one or both ureteral orifices. **"Double kidney"** is a misnomer, since the single renal mass has more than one collecting system. Surgical correction is unnecessary unless renal function is compromised or complications such as hydronephrosis, infection, reflux, urinary incontinence, or obstruction develop.

Renal dysplasias (*developmental abnormalities*) with consequent compromise of renal function may result from abnormal development of the renal vasculature, the renal tubules, the collecting system, or the drainage apparatus.

Cystic hydronephrosis (*ureteral agenesis and atresia resulting in renal cystic degeneration resembling a cluster of grapes*) is due to formation of urine in the lobular segments of the fetal kidney, progressive hydrostatic atrophy, and ultimate cessation of renal function.

Renal hypoplasia (*underdevelopment of a kidney*) usually is associated with incomplete development of the main renal artery or its branches. The kidney is small, with histologically normal nephrons. Complications include ureteral abnormalities, hydronephrosis, and infection.

Polycystic kidney disease in children is discussed below; in adults, in Ch. 156. **Medullary sponge kidney** also is discussed in Ch. 156.

CHILDHOOD POLYCYSTIC DISEASE

A rare (1/10,000 births) autosomal recessive cystic disease of both kidneys and liver producing renal failure in childhood. It is the most common genetically determined childhood cystic disease of the kidneys. Adult renal polycystic disease is discussed in Ch. 156.

Symptoms, Signs, and Diagnosis

Affected neonates have a protuberant abdomen with huge, firm, smooth-surfaced, symmetric kidneys. The enlarged liver is abnormal with periportal fibrosis, bile duct proliferation, and rare cysts; the remainder of the hepatic parenchyma is normal. These pathologic findings are responsible for perisinusoidal portal hypertension with minimal or absent hepatic dysfunction. Ultrasonography is the best diagnostic tool. The diagnosis can be suspected in utero in most cases where ultrasonography of the fetus is done late in pregnancy. Based on the severity of liver involvement and on the degree of renal failure, 4 subcategories have been defined: perinatal, neonatal, infantile, and juvenile.

Perinatal disease is severe, with > 90% of the renal tubules showing cystic deformity. Although the liver is abnormal, death occurs from renal failure within 6 to 8 wk after birth. In the **neonatal** form, about 60% of the renal tubules are involved and hepatic enlargement is pronounced but clinically silent. If the perinatal respiratory problems are survived, death from renal failure is common within the first year of life. In the **infantile** variety, hepatomegaly is the most common feature with less frequent evidence of nephromegaly or splenomegaly. Either portal hypertension or renal failure dominates the clinical findings. Survival into adolescence is not uncommon. In the **juvenile** form, portal hypertension predominates and fewer than 10% of the renal tubules are cystic. Patients often survive into the 3rd decade.

If the disease is not diagnosed at birth, the physical findings are less specific. Nephromegaly is less marked, and slowly progressive renal insufficiency, anemia, and mild hypertension become the major problems. Diagnosis in early childhood may be difficult in the absence of a positive family history. Between ages 5 and 10 yr, subtle signs of portal hypertension appear, such as esophageal and gastric varices, and hypersplenism (leukopenia, thrombocytopenia). Urographic studies are helpful, but biopsies of kidney and liver may be necessary to establish the diagnosis.

Prognosis and Treatment

The prognosis is limited, whether hepatic or renal dysfunction predominates. In most patients death occurs soon after birth from uremia or other associated complications. Infants who survive the first few years show progressive renal failure. For those with less renal involvement, progressive portal hypertension ensues. Portacaval or splenorenal shunts have been successful in reducing morbidity but not mortality. Control of hypersplenism is important, to obviate difficulty with immunosuppression if renal transplantation is attempted, although transplant experience is limited. Dialysis is performed on the same basis as for other children with chronic renal insufficiency.

URETER

Congenital ureteral anomalies are frequently associated with renal anomalies, but may occur independently. Complications include obstruction, infection, and stone formation, as well as problems of urinary control.

Duplication anomalies (*partial or complete duplication of one or both ureters, together with duplication of the ipsilateral renal pelvis*) may occur. Duplication of only the lower ureter is rare. When complete duplication of the ureters exists, the ureter from the uppermost portion of the kidney opens at a more distal point than the orifice of the lower pole ureter. Ectopia of one or both orifices, vesicoureteral reflux into the lower or both ureters, ureterocele, or stenosis of one or both ureteral orifices is common. Surgery is unnecessary unless vesicoureteral reflux, obstruction, infection, incontinence, or compromised renal function develops. (See also Ectopic orifices, below.)

Ectopia. Retrocaval ureter (*anomalous development of the ureter, usually behind a persistent right cardinal vein*) can cause obstruction. A retrocaval ureter on the left is seen

only with persistence of the left cardinal vein system or complete situs inversus. Surgical treatment consisting of division of the ureter with uretero-uretero anastomosis anterior to the vena cava or iliac vessel is indicated if significant obstruction is present.

Ectopic orifices: *Displaced openings of single or duplicated ureters* may occur on the lateral bladder wall (predisposing to vesicoureteral reflux), distally along the trigone, in the bladder neck, in the female urethra distal to the sphincter (leading to incontinence), in the genital system (prostate and seminal vesicle in the male, uterus or vagina in the female), or externally. Ectopic orifices frequently lead to reflux, obstruction, incontinence, and infection. Surgical correction may be indicated.

Stricture and stenosis: Congenital stricture may occur at any portion of the ureter, and frequently at the ureterovesical junction, where it is managed by surgical reimplantation of the ureter into the bladder. Defects in the continuity of ureteral smooth muscle may result in dysfunctional segments, disposing to proximal ureterectasis. **Megaloureter** (*congenital ureteral dilatation with no evident cause*) may be the result of such localized segmental muscular abnormality or neurogenic deficit.

Ureterocele (*bulging of the lower end of the ureter into the bladder*) may produce progressive and self-obstructing cystic dilatation leading to ureterectasis, hydronephrosis, calculus formation, and potential loss of renal function. Diagnosis is established urographically and cystoscopically. Treatment, when indicated, is surgical. The prognosis is good if the condition is recognized before significant renal dysfunction occurs.

VESICOURETERAL REFLUX

Reflux of urine from the bladder into the ureter is abnormal and may result in damage to the upper urinary tract by bacterial infection and by increased hydrostatic pressure.

Etiology

Vesicoureteral reflux most often is due to congenital anomalous development of the ureterovesical junction. Incomplete development of the intramural ureteral tunnel causes a failure of the valvelike action at the ureterovesical junction and permits the reflux of bladder urine into the ureter and renal pelvis, often under the increased intravesical pressures of voiding. Other causes of vesicoureteral reflux include bladder outlet obstruction with increased intravesical pressures, lower urinary tract infection with edema and distortion of the ureteral orifice, neurogenic dysfunction of the detrusor and vesical neck mechanism, and iatrogenic reflux secondary to surgical or instrumental manipulation of the ureteral orifice.

Pathology

Intraureteral pressures rarely are greater than 10 or 12 cm of water pressure; voiding pressures may reach levels of 50 to 200 cm. Such increased pressures may be followed by progressive hydrostatic damage to the kidney when they are transmitted into the ureter and renal pelvis. Bacteria in the lower urinary tract are transmitted by reflux to the upper tract, causing persistent urinary infection with potential loss of renal function.

Symptoms, Signs, and Diagnosis

Abdominal or flank pain, persistent or recurrent urinary infection, dysuria or flank pain with voiding, frequency and urgency, or the uremic syndrome may be secondary to vesicoureteral reflux. Pyuria, hematuria, proteinuria, and bacteriuria may be present.

Intravenous urography **(IVU)** may show calicectasis, ureteral "ribboning," and ureterectasis with dilatation of the upper collecting system. Filling and voiding cystourethrograms demonstrate vesicoureteral reflux. Cystoscopy may confirm ureteral

malimplantation, with ectopia and distortion of the ureteral orifice, or bladder outlet obstruction. Reflux may also be demonstrated by isotope cystogram scan.

Prognosis and Treatment

Conservative medical management usually is adequate for mild reflux of the "high pressure" (voiding) type with no renal damage and normal orifices, and easily controlled infection. Reflux may disappear in many such cases. Severe "low pressure" (filling) reflux secondary to malimplantation or ectopia of the ureteral orifice is best treated by vesicoureteral reimplantation. This is usually successful in eliminating reflux and may preserve renal function. Vesicoureteral reflux in association with massive hydroureteral nephrosis or myoneurogenic disorders may require primary urinary diversion (cutaneous ureterostomies, vesicostomy, ileal or colon segment urinary diversion). Medical management of associated urinary infection and azotemia, renal rickets, hypoproteinemia, and anemia is imperative.

BLADDER

Congenital anomalies of the urinary bladder include exstrophy, agenesis, duplication, persistent urachus, and the megacystis syndrome, which may be a primary myoneural defect.

Exstrophy of the urinary bladder is an easily detectable and serious major anomaly. The open (unroofed) bladder is seen in the suprapubic region with urine dripping from the ureteral orifices. The bladder mucosa is continuous with the abdominal skin, and the pubic bones are separated. Attempts at primary closure have been successful. Ureterosigmoidostomy, with or without proximal colostomy, and ileal or colon loop urinary diversion are the most common procedures when primary closure is not feasible or fails. Reconstruction of the genitalia is required. The prognosis for maintenance of normal renal function is relatively good.

Congenital bladder diverticula occur and predispose to urinary infection. Diagnosis is made by cystography and cystoscopy. Surgical removal of diverticula and reconstruction of the bladder wall may be indicated.

Contracture of the vesical outlet may occur in association with neurogenic diseases or as a primary congenital entity. Abdominal pain, weak and dribbling stream, distended urinary bladder, and persistent pyuria should suggest bladder outlet obstruction. Vesicoureteral reflux may occur. Cystography and cystoscopy establish the diagnosis. Endoscopic resection or open plastic surgical revision of the vesical orifice usually provides relief. **Congenital bladder neck obstruction** is a rare entity and an overworked diagnosis.

PENIS AND URETHRA

The penis in the male and the urethra in both male and female may be congenitally absent. Other anomalies include double penis, congenital penile curvature or malrotation, microphallus, and urethral stricture, stenosis, and duplication.

Hypospadias (*displaced urethral opening*): In the female, the urethra opens into the vagina. In the male, the urethral opening may be on the underside of the penile shaft, at the penoscrotal junction, between the scrotal folds, or in the perineum. **Chordee** (*ventral curvature of the penis, most apparent on erection*), usually is associated with hypospadias and is caused by a fibrous band along the usual course of the corpus spongiosum. Also present is a "dorsal hood" formed by incomplete foreskin development. The principal complications are meatal stenosis, the patient's inability to direct the urinary stream, and sexual disability in later life. Early surgical correction consists

of an initial procedure to release the chordee and straighten the shaft, followed by plastic reconstruction of the urethra. One-stage surgical repairs often are performed. Prognosis is good.

Epispadias: *A dorsal fusion defect of the urethra, partial or complete, the ultimate representing exstrophy of the urinary bladder*. Epispadias occurs in both males and females, but more commonly in males. Urinary control can be satisfactory with incomplete epispadias. Reconstruction may be effective, but is often difficult and associated with persistent incontinence.

Urethral valves: *Congenital folds of the urethra acting as valves* occur in both sexes, but are much more common in the prostatic urethra of the male. Complications are due to obstruction, which may be severe and lead to massive upper tract damage. Symptoms and signs include weak and dribbling urinary stream, overflow incontinence, and urinary infection. Diagnosis is established by urography and endoscopy. Prompt surgical intervention may obviate the need for urinary diversion.

Stenosis: The most common form of congenital urethral stenosis is **meatal stricture**. Urethral meatotomy usually is successful.

Phimosis (*congenital or acquired [inflammatory] constriction of the foreskin, which cannot be retracted*) and **paraphimosis** (*inability of the retracted constricting foreskin to be reduced over the glans*). Surgical treatment by circumcision is indicated. A preliminary dorsal slit may be required. The prognosis is excellent.

TESTES AND SCROTUM

The scrotum may fail to develop unilaterally **(hemiscrotum)** or bilaterally, often associated with cryptorchidism. Congenital **hemangiomas** of the scrotum may require surgical removal, since bleeding or progressive enlargement can be anticipated. **Penile-scrotal transposition** is a striking anomaly amenable to surgery.

UNDESCENDED TESTES
(Cryptorchidism)

Incomplete or improper prenatal descent of one or both testes is common. Hormonal function generally is normal. However, the undescended testis may show progressive failure of spermatogenesis if untreated. The cryptorchid testis has a higher incidence of carcinoma, which may manifest itself many years later.

In true **cryptorchidism,** the testis remains within the abdominal cavity or retroperitoneally, the result of hormonal or mechanical abnormalities. In **incomplete descent** or **maldescent of the testis,** or **arrested testis,** the testis lies within the inguinal canal but has been obstructed in its passage by mechanical factors. The **ectopic testis** lies outside the usual course of descent, suprapubically, within the perineum, or along the inner aspect of the thigh. **Hypermobile or retractile testes** may lie within the scrotum at times (eg, during a hot tub bath) but then retract into the inguinal canal.

Treatment

Chorionic gonadotropin (HCG) 500 to 1000 IU given IM 2 or 3 times/wk for periods up to 6 wk may promote bilateral testicular descent. The usual surgical treatment is orchiopexy before 2 yr of age. Delay in surgery beyond age 5 yr may impair spermatogenesis, a critical factor when bilateral cryptorchidism occurs. Surgery generally is unnecessary for hypermobile (retractile) testes, since normal descent occurs at puberty. Orchiectomy usually is the treatment of choice when unilateral cryptorchidism is discovered in the postpubertal patient.

TESTICULAR TORSION

Twisting of the testis on its cord, spontaneously or following strenuous activity, may result from anomalous development of the tunica vaginalis and spermatic cord. Immediate **symptoms** of torsion are severe local pain, nausea, and vomiting, followed by scrotal edema and fever. Torsion must be differentiated from inflammatory conditions within the scrotum, trauma, and testicular tumor. Radioisotope scrotal scan may aid in diagnosis. **Immediate surgical intervention** is advised when torsion is suspected, since exploration within a few hours offers the only hope of testicular salvage. Fixation of the contralateral testis is performed to prevent torsion on that side. (See also under COMPLETE PHYSICAL EXAMINATION in MANAGEMENT OF THE NORMAL NEWBORN in Ch. 182.)

ANOMALIES IN KIDNEY TRANSPORT

CYSTINURIA

An inherited defect of the renal tubules in which resorption of the amino acid cystine is impaired, urinary excretion is increased, and cystine calculi often form in the urinary tract.

Cystinuria is inherited as an autosomal recessive trait. Heterozygotes may excrete increased quantities of cystine in the urine, but seldom enough to result in stone formation.

Pathophysiology

The diminished renal tubular resorption of cystine increases its concentration in the urine. Cystine is poorly soluble in acid urine; when its concentration exceeds its solubility, precipitation in the urinary tract results, both as crystals and stones.

Renal tubular resorption of dibasic amino acids (lysine, ornithine, and arginine) is also impaired, although these amino acids have an alternative transport system separate from that shared with cystine. Since the dibasic amino acids are more soluble in urine than is cystine, their increased excretion does not result in precipitation. Absorption of cystine and the dibasic amino acids is decreased in the small intestine as well as in the renal tubule. Several patterns of impaired intestinal absorption of these amino acids have been described.

Symptoms, Signs, and Diagnosis

Radiopaque cystine stones form in the renal pelvis or bladder. Staghorn calculi are common. Symptoms usually appear between ages 10 and 30, and renal colic is the most common presenting complaint. UTI and renal failure due to obstruction may develop. In longtime survivors, end-stage renal disease is the rule.

Cystine may occur in the urine as yellow-brown hexagonal crystals. The presence of excessive cystine in the urine may be detected by the nitroprusside cyanide test. The diagnosis is confirmed by chromatography or electrophoresis.

Treatment

The concentration of cystine in the urine can be reduced by increasing urine volume. Fluid intake must be sufficient to provide a urine flow rate of 2 mL/min, especially at night when the pH of the urine drops. Alkalinization of the urine to pH > 7.5 with sodium bicarbonate 15 to 30 gm/day orally in divided doses, and acetazolamide 250 mg orally at bedtime, will increase the solubility of cystine significantly. D-Penicillamine 250 mg/day orally initially and gradually increased to 1 to 2 gm/day may be effective when high fluid intake and alkalinization do not reduce stone formation. D-

Penicillamine reduces cystine excretion by forming the more soluble disulfide, cysteine-penicillamine. *Toxicity of penicillamine limits its usefulness.* About half of all patients treated develop some toxic manifestation, including fever, rash, arthralgias, and, less commonly, nephrotic syndrome, pancytopenia, or an SLE-like reaction.

FANCONI'S SYNDROME

An acquired or inherited disorder, often associated with cystinosis, with characteristic abnormalities of renal proximal tubular function including glucosuria, phosphaturia, aminoaciduria, and bicarbonate wasting.

Occurrence and Genetics

As an inherited trait, Fanconi's syndrome usually accompanies another genetic disorder, particularly cystinosis. (See TABLE 196–4 in ANOMALIES IN AMINO ACID METABOLISM in Ch. 196.) When associated with cystinosis, it is an autosomal recessive disease. Heterozygotes may show cystine accumulation in cells but lack other clinical and laboratory manifestations. Fanconi's syndrome may also accompany Wilson's disease, hereditary fructose intolerance, galactosemia, glycogen storage disease, Lowe's syndrome, and tyrosinemia.

Acquired Fanconi's syndrome may be caused by 6-mercaptopurine or outdated tetracycline, renal transplantation, multiple myeloma, amyloidosis, intoxication with heavy metals or other chemical agents, and vitamin D deficiency.

Pathophysiology, Symptoms, and Signs

A variety of defects of proximal tubular function occur, including impaired resorption of glucose, phosphate, amino acids, bicarbonate, uric acid, water, potassium, and sodium. The aminoaciduria is generalized and, unlike the case in cystinuria, increased cystine excretion is only a minor component. The basic abnormality underlying these diverse changes is unknown. The chief clinical features (proximal tubular acidosis, hypophosphatemic rickets, hypokalemia, polyuria, and polydipsia) usually appear in infancy in hereditary Fanconi's syndrome.

In the **nephropathic form associated with cystinosis,** failure to thrive and growth retardation are common. The retinas show patchy depigmentation. Interstitial nephritis develops, leading to progressive renal failure that may be fatal before adolescence.

Diagnosis and Treatment

Diagnosis is made by demonstrating the abnormalities of renal function, particularly glucosuria, phosphaturia, and aminoaciduria. In cystinosis, slit-lamp examination may show cystine crystals in the cornea.

There is no specific treatment. Acidosis may be improved by giving sodium bicarbonate. **Shohl's solution** (140 gm citric acid and 90 gm sodium citrate dihydrate made up to 1 L with water) given 50 to 100 mL/day in divided doses can be substituted for sodium bicarbonate solution and may be better tolerated. For treatment of hypophosphatemic rickets, see below. Potassium depletion may require replacement therapy. Renal transplantation has been successful in renal failure; however, when cystinosis is the underlying disease, progressive damage may continue in other organs and eventually end in death.

HYPOPHOSPHATEMIC RICKETS

(Vitamin D-Resistant Rickets)

A familial or, rarely, acquired disorder characterized by impaired resorption of phosphate in the proximal renal tubules with consequent hypophosphatemia, defective intestinal absorption of calcium, and rickets or osteomalacia that is unresponsive to vitamin D.

Familial hypophosphatemic rickets is inherited as an X-linked dominant trait. Affected females have less severe bone disease than males and may show only hypophosphatemia. Sporadic acquired cases sometimes are associated with benign mesenchymal tumors **(oncogenic rickets).**

Pathophysiology, Symptoms, and Signs

The major physiologic abnormality is decreased proximal tubular resorption of phosphate; decreased intestinal calcium and phosphate absorption also occurs. Parathyroid hormone and vitamin D levels are normal. Two types of hypophosphatemic rickets occur. In Type I, impaired renal synthesis leads to a subnormal plasma level of 1,25-dihydroxy vitamin D_3. In Type II, 1,25-dihydroxy vitamin D_3 in plasma is normal or elevated and the disease is due to an impaired cellular response to this substance.

The disease is manifested as a spectrum of abnormalities from hypophosphatemia alone, to severe rickets or osteomalacia with bowing of the legs and other bone deformities, pseudofractures, bone pain, and short stature. Blood phosphate levels are depressed, calcium is normal, and alkaline phosphatase often is elevated. Bony outgrowth at muscle attachments may limit motion. The rickets of the spine or pelvis seen in vitamin D deficiency is rarely found. Craniostenosis and convulsions may be present in children. The age of onset is usually < 1 yr.

Hypophosphatemic rickets must be distinguished from **vitamin D-dependent rickets,** an autosomal recessive disorder with similar clinical features except that hypocalcemia is present, hypophosphatemia is mild or absent, tetany and convulsions are common, and rickets of spine and pelvis are frequent (see also Ch. 81).

Treatment

Treatment of Type I hypophosphatemic rickets consists of oral phosphate 1 to 3 gm/day in divided doses, as neutral phosphate solution, plus calcitriol 0.5 to 3 μg/day (15 to 50 ng/kg/day). Increase in plasma phosphate concentration, decrease in alkaline phosphatase, healing of rickets, and improvement of growth rate occur. Hypercalciuria or secondary hyperparathyroidism may complicate the treatment. Type II hypophosphatemic rickets responds poorly to treatment. In adults with oncogenic rickets, dramatic improvement has followed removal of the tumor.

HARTNUP DISEASE

A rare disease due to abnormal absorption and excretion of tryptophan and other amino acids, characterized clinically by rash and CNS abnormalities.

Hartnup disease is inherited as an autosomal recessive trait. Consanguinity is common. Heterozygotes are normal. Small intestine absorption of tryptophan, phenylalanine, methionine, and other monoaminomonocarboxylic amino acids is abnormal. Accumulation of unabsorbed amino acids in the GI tract increases their metabolism by bacterial flora. Some tryptophan degradation products including indoles, kynurenine, and serotonin are absorbed by the bowel and appear in the urine. Renal amino acid resorption is also defective, causing a generalized aminoaciduria involving all neutral amino acids except proline and hydroxyproline. Conversion of tryptophan to niacinamide is also defective.

Symptoms and signs are due to niacinamide deficiency and resemble those of pellagra, particularly the rash on parts of the body exposed to the sun. Neurologic manifestations include cerebellar ataxia and psychologic abnormalities. Mental retardation, short stature, headache, and collapsing or fainting are common. Symptoms may be precipitated by sunlight, fever, drugs, or other stresses. Poor nutritional intake nearly always precedes appearance of symptoms. The eventual prognosis is good and the frequency of attacks usually diminishes with age.

Diagnosis is made by demonstrating the characteristic amino acid excretion pattern in the urine. Presence of indoles and other tryptophan degradation products in the urine provides supplementary evidence of the disease. **Treatment**: Attacks can be prevented by maintaining good nutrition and supplementing the diet with niacinamide or niacin.

FAMILIAL IMINOGLYCINURIA

An autosomal recessive benign defect in the renal tubular resorption of imino acids and glycine. Homozygotes excrete abnormal amounts of imino acids (proline and hydroxyproline) and glycine; heterozygotes have glycinuria only. Plasma levels of amino acids are normal. Intestinal absorption of proline may be impaired. Iminoaciduria is normal in the newborn.

INTERSEX STATES

(See also Ch. 203 and Congenital Adrenal Hyperplasia in Ch. 196)

Conditions in which the appearance of the external genitalia is either ambiguous or at variance with the chromosomal, gonadal, or genetic sex of the individual.

Etiology and Classification

The genitalia develop during the first trimester of intrauterine life under the influence of the sex steroids. Abnormalities of sexual development may arise as a consequence of endocrine or morphologic derangements, the latter often associated with karyotypic abnormalities. **Female pseudohermaphrodites** are normal females exposed to excessive amounts of androgenic steroids in utero. They have 46,XX karyotypes and normal internal genitalia, but ambiguous external genitalia. The offending androgen may be derived from external sources, as is the case when the mother is given progesterone to prevent miscarriage; but more often the ambiguity is due to an internal accumulation of androgen caused by an enzymatic block in steroidogenesis **(adrenogenital syndrome). True hermaphrodites** have both ovarian and testicular tissue, and mixed masculine and feminine genital structures; a rare individual may be fully masculinized externally. The majority of true hermaphrodites have had 46,XX karyotypes, but the pattern can be quite variable.

Male pseudohermaphrodites have testicular tissue only, and usually a 46,XY karyotype. Etiologically they are complex; in general, however, the disorder arises from (1) failure to generate adequate amounts of androgen or (2) failure to metabolically respond to the androgens produced. The former group includes some rare forms of disordered steroidogenesis as well as certain types of gonadal dysgenesis (the only type of male pseudohermaphrodite likely to have a karyotype other than 46,XY). Male pseudohermaphroditism due to an altered response to androgen includes the **testicular feminization syndrome** (a key androgen receptor is absent); **pseudovaginal perineoscrotal hypospadias** (the enzyme responsible for the conversion of testosterone to dihydrotestosterone is lacking in the tissues); and **receptor-positive defects** (nuclear binding seems to be at fault). Patients with **simple hypospadias** may have a variety of poorly defined and sometimes transient endocrinologic disturbances. In the above disorders, as with most intersex patients, the external genitals are ambiguous. These variants are present at birth.

Patients with **mixed gonadal dysgenesis** have both testicular tissue and primitive gonadal tissue called "streaks." They usually have a 46,XY/45,XO karyotype, and tend to be short of stature as adults. **Pure gonadal dysgenesis** is the name given to those with gonadal "streaks" bilaterally. Unlike the other intersex states in which the external genitalia are likely to exhibit some degree of ambiguity, these patients appear phenotypically to be normal females; diagnosis often is delayed until they reach puberty and fail to feminize.

Diagnosis

Patients with genital ambiguity, phenotypic females with palpable gonads, and phenotypic males with impalpable gonads should be evaluated for intersexuality. Males with hypospadias usually do not require such an evaluation if both testes are descended and appear palpably normal, but hypospadias associated with one or both testes undescended should be investigated.

Assessment of intersex patients is urgent, not only because of pressures to establish a correct sex assignment, but also because of the need to identify a patient with the **adrenogenital syndrome** (see in Ch. 91) so that treatment can be started before life-threatening hyponatremia develops. **Buccal smears** for nuclear membrane chromatin, **vaginograms** to demonstrate a cervix or uterine canal, and **sonography** to show a uterus behind the bladder are studies that can be done quickly but are somewhat nonspecific. When positive, they are suggestive but not diagnostic of the adrenogenital syndrome. **Hormonal assays** are more definitive. Patients with the adrenogenital syndrome characteristically show elevations of urinary 17-ketosteroids, 17-hydroxysteroids, and pregnanetriol. Even more specific is an elevated serum 17-hydroxyprogesterone. Elevated serum renin levels indicate the impending hyponatremia that ultimately will be reflected in declining serum sodium and rising serum potassium levels. **Karyotyping** establishes the definitive diagnosis in most intersex patients although it may be redundant in the adrenogenital syndrome, where the diagnosis rests primarily on the biochemical data.

Patients in whom the adrenogenital syndrome can be ruled out, either because they have palpable gonads externally, or because they do not exhibit the necessary biochemical abnormalities, usually require early surgical exploration and gonadal biopsy for definitive diagnosis. Sex assignment in these individuals should not be delayed beyond the 1st wk of life, if this can be avoided.

Treatment

Assignment of sex appropriate to the individual is the most important element. Generally, **female pseudohermaphrodites** are sex-assigned as females. **True hermaphrodites** are best sex-assigned according to the ease with which their genital construction can be carried out along one sexual line or another, but most have been reconstructed as males. This may be a particularly attractive option if the individual has a normally descended testis to provide hormonal function at puberty. **Male pseudohermaphrodites** are sex-assigned according to their potential as determined by genital development and hormonal activity. Those with the full-blown **testicular feminization syndrome** must be sex-assigned as females, but for many of the other male pseudohermaphrodites, male sex assignment is reasonable and appropriate. When uncertainty exists in smarginal cases, 1 or 2 courses of testosterone (in oil) 25 mg IM help determine the ability of the genitalia to respond to androgen—an essential requirement in male sex assignment.

Patients with **mixed gonadal dysgenesis** are best sex-assigned as females, not only because of short stature, but also because of the propensity of these testes to develop tumors. Those with **pure gonadal dysgenesis** appear phenotypically as females, and should be raised as such.

Timing of the surgical reconstruction of the genitalia is variable. Sex-assigned females other than those with the adrenogenital syndrome should have a clitoral resection as early as possible to facilitate familial acceptance in their assigned role. Those with the adrenogenital syndrome have to be deferred some months until they have been rendered endocrinologically stable by steroid therapy. Vaginal reconstruction in all of these patients is best deferred until puberty because of the high incidence of stenosis when it is done early in life. Correction of hypospadias in males usually is done at about 2 to 3 yr of age.

188. DEVELOPMENTAL PROBLEMS

FAILURE TO THRIVE

Failure of growth and development to meet realistic expectations because of genetic, physical, or psychosocial factors. Growth and development in infants, children, and adolescents are sensitive indicators of their health. Failure to thrive most often presents in an infant as insufficient weight gain, in a child as shortness, and in the early teenager as a combination of shortness and lack of sexual development. Presented with a patient who is failing to thrive, the physician must first determine whether the child is reaching his or her realistic potential. The expectations of parents or others may be realistic and pathologic causes are involved, or they may be unrealistic, which can lead to psychologic problems.

Etiology

Any pathologic process severe enough to interfere with normal metabolism will inhibit body growth. When deranged metabolism is related to acute illness, as is usually the case, the duration is brief and has little or no long-range effect on growth or development. With prolonged or frequent abnormalities, however, growth is likely to be impeded and possibly permanently affected. Whatever the etiology, malnutrition often is a mediating influence, particularly in the infant. Failure to thrive may be only one of many manifestations of a complex disease process and may even go unnoticed, overshadowed by the severity of other symptoms. A categorization of possible etiologies follows, most of which are discussed in more detail elsewhere in THE MANUAL.

Genetic factors. Tall parents as a rule have tall children; short parents, short children. However, children inherit not only this potential for ultimate development but also the pattern for obtaining it. Parents who were small as children, with a late onset of puberty and a late cessation of growth (eventually falling within the normal range), may have offspring who follow the same pattern, which is a form of **constitutional delay** (see also discussion below, in Unknown causes). These parents may seek help in hurrying along their children's growth so that the youngsters will not suffer the indignities the parents did.

Children with **chromosomal abnormalities** (eg, Turner's syndrome, the trisomies) characteristically do not grow well and have low birth weights for gestational age. These children also have multiple congenital anomalies.

Defects in function of major organ systems. Endocrine system: Deficiency of thyroid hormone or somatomedin (the compound that mediates the effect of growth hormone on cartilage), or of their respective pituitary trophic hormones, thyroid-stimulating hormone (TSH) and growth hormone (GH), leads to profound growth retardation and, in the case of thyroid deficiency, also to developmental delay. Lack of the sex hormones or their pituitary trophic hormones causes failure of secondary sexual development and its accompanying growth spurt. **Pituitary dwarfism** is discussed in Ch. 196. Excesses of adrenocortical hormones, endogenous or therapeutic, interfere with growth, a point often helpful in differentiating simple obesity from Cushing's syndrome. **CNS**: Damage to the brain may lead to feeding difficulties or to changes in endocrine function that affect growth and development. **Cardiovascular and respiratory systems**: Metabolic processes will be disturbed and tissues will not grow if there is a breakdown of the physiologic mechanisms for delivering nutrients and O_2 to the tissues and removing waste products and CO_2. **Hematopoietic system**: Since optimal cell metabolism and normal growth require O_2, children with moderate to severe anemia will have tissue hypoxia and growth failure.

GU system: Because the kidneys eliminate the toxic waste products of metabolism and help to maintain a normal extracellular electrolyte concentration and pH, chronic

renal failure with uremia leads to growth failure. Renal tubular defects, congenital or acquired (eg, renal tubular acidosis), may also disturb the cellular environment to the extent that normal growth cannot take place. **GI system**: Structural lesions such as pyloric stenosis, with its concomitant vomiting, or mucosal malfunction or absence of digestive enzymes (as in malabsorption syndromes) may reduce the amount of nutrients reaching the tissues. **Skeletal system**: In abnormalities of bone formation (eg, achondroplasia) normal lengthening of the skeleton cannot be achieved. **Systemic disease processes**, particularly noninfectious diseases that affect multiple systems (eg, collagen vascular diseases and the "storage" diseases [the mucopolysaccharidoses, cystinosis, etc]) retard growth.

Malnutrition is interwoven with the complex etiology of failure to thrive and may be caused by inadequate food intake, malabsorption, or faulty metabolism. Specific deficiencies of essential nutrients, as well as general malnutrition, may cause profound growth retardation, as in marasmus, kwashiorkor, or rickets.

Psychosocial and environmental influences: A supportive, loving parent–child interaction is important. If physically or emotionally deprived, infants and young children may stop growing. Parental withdrawal, rejection, or hostility produces emotional deprivation and can result from a number of causes; eg, an unwanted pregnancy, the death of another child, parental jealousy or insecurity, or disappointment over the sex, appearance, or growth of the child. The socioeconomic status of the family may be an important factor in a child's growth; it can affect nutrition, living conditions, and parental attitudes. Environmental factors that may interfere with growth include ex posure to infections, parasitic infestations, and intoxication by a variety of foreign substances.

Unknown causes: A form of **constitutional delay** is seen in some children whose growth inexplicably appears to stand still for a period of time. Occasionally, this can be related to some stressful event such as a family move, a hospitalization, or some intercurrent illness. As inexplicably as it stopped, growth starts again. The lost growth may not be regained, but an approximately normal rate of development is maintained from that point on. As in the hereditary form of constitutional delay, pubescence and final cessation of growth are delayed, but these children ultimately achieve a reasonably normal adult stature. **Primordial dwarfism** is a type of growth failure frequently associated with a variety of congenital abnormalities, many of which appear as minor structural defects (see below, Physical examination, under Diagnosis). These children are frequently small at birth despite normal gestational age, and manifest no obvious cause for their lack of growth. It has been assumed that their cells do not respond to environmental and controlling mechanisms as do normal cells.

Diagnosis

The history, including prenatal, birth, neonatal, psychosocial, and family information, is of particular importance because often the physical examination is not unusual except for the smaller-than-normal height and weight measurements.

Information from the antepartal and neonatal periods provides important diagnostic clues: Was the pregnancy complicated by such factors as inadequate prenatal care, toxemia, maternal diseases (eg, diabetes mellitus or thyroid disease), intrauterine infection? Was there birth trauma? Was the infant premature or small for gestational age? Family history should include age-related heights of relatives in order to give an indication of genetic potential; developmental patterns such as the time of the mother's menarche and the age when the father stopped growing; any stressful events affecting attitudes toward the child, such as a sibling's death; the kind of relationship that exists between the mother and child; the emotional climate in the home. Observing the parent–child interaction can be especially illuminating.

All obtainable previously recorded heights, weights, and head circumferences are plotted on any of the standard growth charts (keeping in mind the potential variability if the figures are obtained from different sources). This data, along with the parents' heights, will show how far below his expected growth the child is. (The child's growth, although within the normal range on the standard chart, may be abnormal based on his own growth potential.) The data also may indicate when growth stopped, and will give values for annual growth increments. If a standstill period is found, the physical and psychosocial events of that time are investigated. If the child is small but annual height and weight increments are appropriate for age, constitutional delay is likely. In general, children who fail to thrive because of a pathologic process grow at less than the normal rate and tend to fall progressively behind their peers.

Psychomotor development also should be assessed, searching for possible CNS lesions. Finally, each major organ system should be thoroughly reviewed and evaluated.

Physical examination: Height, weight, and body proportion measurements are obtained (eg, upper to lower body segment ratios, arm span vs. height). From height and weight, a height age and weight age (that age at which each measurement matches the median on standard growth charts) can be determined. A weight age considerably below height age suggests a nutritional disorder. The maintenance of infantile body proportions suggests developmental delay as well as growth failure, as seen in hypothyroidism.

Minor structural abnormalities, such as a high-arched palate, low-set ears, hypoplastic nails, shortened metacarpals, or inability to fully extend joints, should be sought. Their presence suggests Turner's syndrome in a female or primordial dwarfism in the male or female.

In the older child, pubertal development is assessed (see also Chs. 169 and 170). The earliest manifestation of puberty in a girl usually will be budding of the breasts; in the male, testicular enlargement. In general, a testis longer than 2.5 cm is a stimulated testis.

The physician should be alert for signs of neglect or abuse (see Ch. 190). If there are serious questions about the child's growth rate, a period of simple observation may be indicated prior to an extensive laboratory investigation.

Laboratory studies: A **CBC** may reveal anemia or suggest infection. An **ESR** is helpful to eliminate infection or inflammatory disease. **Urinalysis** should include sp gr to assure optimal concentrating power (> 1.020), pH to determine adequate acidifying ability (< 6), and other screening tests for renal tubular disease, diabetes mellitus, nephritis, or renal infection. A **BUN** or **serum creatinine** should be obtained to rule out a silent uremic state. **Thyroid function** should also be determined. Hypothyroidism can be very subtle in its presentation, but is easily checked and treated. An **x-ray for bone age** should be obtained. In a child ≥ 3 yr old, this may be done with a wrist film. Below age 3, films of multiple areas lead to greater accuracy. Hypothyroidism is characterized by a bone age that falls below the height age; constitutional short stature, by a bone age that is essentially identical to the height age; and other organic and primordial conditions, by a bone age that is more advanced than the height age. In conjunction with current height, bone age may be useful in predicting ultimate height. If the bone age is behind the chronologic age, growth potential is greater than that expected for the chronologic, which may be reassuring to parents and child.

Special studies: Special studies may be indicated to evaluate more completely the function of various organ systems or to detect other etiologies. In a short girl, especially if she is sexually underdeveloped and beyond the normal age for puberty, Turner's syndrome is possible. Either a buccal smear for sex chromatin or chromosomal analysis of peripheral blood would be diagnostic. If emotional deprivation or any other disturbed parent–child relationship is suspected, removing the child from the

environment, generally to a hospital for observation, may be helpful for both diagnosis and therapy. Hypothalamic–pituitary function (see PITUITARY DWARFISM in Ch. 196; and HYPOPITUITARISM IN THE ADULT in Ch. 88) should be evaluated in children whose growth rate is less than optimal, who do not have multiple abnormalities (as in primordial dwarfism), and in whom no abnormality is identified by the above procedures.

Treatment

Treatment depends on the etiology—it may be as simple as providing a proper diet or as complex as doing a renal transplant. In malnutrition, nutritional rehabilitation is essential and often must be implemented while diagnostic studies are being made. When psychosocial factors are involved, treatment must include management of the family and living conditions. If the period of failure to thrive has been relatively short and its cause is corrected, one can generally anticipate a period of catch-up growth followed by return to a normal pattern. If the failure has been prolonged, its effect may be long-lasting, and return to normal height and weight for age may never be achieved. There is at present no known therapy for primordial dwarfism.

Those children with constitutional delay are, in general, best reassured that they will reach a normal height without treatment. Anabolic steroids or sex hormones have been used, with controversial results. They may increase bone development relatively faster than height, in effect potentially *reducing* the growing period and thus the ultimate height. Their use therefore should be restricted to those children who are having severe psychologic problems because of their small size and who thoroughly understand and accept the possible risks.

BEHAVIORAL PROBLEMS

Many behaviors that can lead to significant problems are typical of a certain stage of development (eg, the oppositional behavior of a 2-yr-old) or of a common temperamental pattern (eg, the "difficult" child who has irregular biologic functions, intense reactions, predominantly negative mood, and slowness in adapting to changes). Differentiation between difficult but normal behaviors and significant behavioral problems often is unclear. A significant problem is more likely when the behavior is frequent and chronic, when more than one problem behavior is involved, and particularly when the behavior interferes with social and cognitive functioning. A parent's or teacher's perception that a problem is significant warrants attention. Looking beyond the chief complaint often uncovers information essential for understanding a significant problem.

Prevalence figures vary according to how "behavioral problems" are defined and measured, but several population studies cite a rate of at least 10% for significant behavioral problems in all pediatric age groups. National surveys of office-based pediatric practice, however, show the diagnosis of behavioral problems to be < 2%.

General Principles of Dealing with Behavioral Problems

The context in which the problem evolved must be understood, including interactions between the child and caregivers, and the social environment surrounding those interactions. Contributing factors include characteristics of the child; eg, health (past and current), developmental status, and temperament (difficult, or slow-to-warm-up). Parental factors include misinterpretations of typical stage-related behaviors, dissonance between parental expectations and child characteristics, and parental characteristics such as depression, disinterest, rejection, and overprotectiveness (to the point of stifling steps toward independence). Social environmental factors include stresses like marital discord, unemployment, and significant personal losses, particularly in the context of weak social supports.

A broad-based history is required, which at least briefly surveys the child and parental and environmental factors that may be contributory. Prescribing technics to modify

behavior without some understanding of the etiology merely treats symptoms. The specific behavior may be successfully modified, but if a significant underlying problem exists it is likely to manifest itself as a new symptom.

A complete, chronologic description of the child's **activities in a typical day** provides precise details about the problem behavior. Focus should be on the immediate context in which the problem behavior occurs and the parental response to the behavior. **Direct observation** of parent-child interaction during the office visit provides valuable clues. These observations and the parent's history should be supplemented whenever possible by the observations of other relatives, teachers, nurses, etc.

Feelings of guilt and incompetence, almost universal in parents of children with behavioral problems, are difficult for parents to express. Identifying with parental frustrations and pointing out the prevalence of such problems often can allay some of the guilt and facilitate a constructive approach.

Early intervention is preferable because the longer maladaptive behaviors exist, the more difficult they are to change.

Changing behavior is a learning process for the child. **Consistency** in rules and **limit-setting** across time and among caregivers facilitate this process. Parents should try to **minimize expressions of anger** when enforcing rules. Highly charged emotions may interfere with or distort the learning process.

Increasing the amount of **positive contact** between the parent and child is crucial to successful change of unacceptable behavior in the child. Mutually enjoyable interactions build the self-esteem of the parent and the child and help break vicious circle patterns (see below) that have developed.

For simple problems, parental education, reassurance, and a few specific suggestions often are sufficient; but follow-up is important to be certain that the problem is not more complex than initially assumed.

For complex or chronic problems, a more comprehensive assessment is indicated, possibly requiring multiple visits. An initially confusing history may be clarified if a detailed parental diary is kept of the timing and frequency of the problem behavior, including preceding activities and parental responses. Depending on the nature of the problem and the expertise of the clinician, referral to a psychologist, psychiatrist, neurologist, or other specialist may be indicated.

Interactional Problems in Early Infancy

The first few months of life can be a difficult adjustment period for the infant and new parents. The infant's feeding and sleeping schedules usually are unpredictable, and most infants do not sleep through the night until 2 to 3 mo of age. Many infants have periods of frequent, prolonged, intense crying in the first 3 mo (see COLIC under COMMON FEEDING AND GASTROINTESTINAL PROBLEMS in Ch. 182). Periods of alertness in the infant are still brief, providing relatively little positive feedback to the parents for their exhausting new job. A mother's ability to cope during this period may be further diminished by a difficult pregnancy or delivery, postpartum depression, or lack of adequate support from a spouse, relatives, or friends.

The quality of mother–infant interactions in the early months is related to later cognitive and social development of the infant. In extreme cases interactional failure may result in failure to thrive. Other manifestations include persistent, excessive crying or irregularity of schedules, or failure to develop positive interactive games with the infant by 3 to 4 mo. Since a variety of factors (child, parental, or environmental) can contribute to the interactional problem, a careful history and assessment of the infant and the parent–infant interaction are indicated (see above). **Treatment** includes parental education about infant development and the temperamental characteristics of their infant in particular; reassurance if appropriate; and attempts to improve the support available to the parents (eg, emotional support, help with housework and childcare, and other resources as needed).

Discipline

The noun "discipline" has several meanings, including instruction and self-control, in addition to punishment. **Positive reinforcement** for appropriate behavior as a disciplinary tool for molding a child's behavior is a powerful one, with no adverse side effects. Efforts to control a child's behavior through scolding or physical punishment may work briefly, if used sparingly, but are ineffective when frequently used and may be detrimental to the child's sense of security and self-esteem. Threats to leave or send the child away are damaging.

A good approach to altering unacceptable behavior is the use of a **"time-out" procedure**. This requires a small, portable kitchen timer, a chair in a dull place (no TV or toys, not in the bedroom, and not dark or scary), and agreement among caregivers about the specific behavior(s) that will result in time-out. Since time-outs are a learning process for the child, they are best used for one specific type of inappropriate behavior, or at most a small number of behaviors at one time. Before using time-out, the rules are explained clearly to the child, including the targeted behavior, and the procedure demonstrated. The steps are as follows:

1. After an inappropriate behavior, it is briefly described to the child, who is calmly told to go to the time-out chair or is led there if necessary.
2. When the child is sitting in the chair, the timer is set to last 1 min for each year of age up to a maximum of 5 min.
3. If the child gets up from the chair before the bell rings, he is replaced and the timer reset. If the child gets up repeatedly, it may be necessary to hold him in the chair (not in one's lap), avoiding talking and eye contact. If it is necessary to hold him down for the entire period until the bell rings, the timer is set again.
4. If the child stays in the chair but does not quiet down before the bell rings, the timer is reset.
5. When it is time for the child to get up, he is asked the reason for the time-out; anger and nagging are avoided. If he does not recall the correct reason, he is briefly reminded.
6. Within a short period of time, praiseworthy behavior should be sought. This may be easier to achieve if the child is started in a new activity away from the scene of the inappropriate behavior.

Since most children prefer the attention they get for inappropriate behavior to no attention at all, special times for pleasant interactions with the child must occur each day. The pleasant interactions also provide an opportunity for reinforcing positive behavior.

Common Vicious Circle Patterns

Parental reaction to a child's behavior causing an adverse response from the youngster which in turn leads to continued detrimental parental response.

In the most common vicious circle, the **aggressive-resistant child** is responded to with scolding, yelling, and spanking. This pattern may arise from parental reactions to the stage-related negativism of the 2-yr-old or back talk of the 4-yr-old, or it may evolve from parental attempts to cope with a child who has had a "difficult" temperament since birth. These children often react to stress and emotional discomfort with stubbornness, back talk, aggressiveness, and temper outbursts rather than crying.

The circular pattern may be interrupted if parents ignore behavior that does not encroach on the rights of others (tantrums, refusals to eat) and use distraction or temporary isolation to limit behavior that cannot be ignored. Friction also can be reduced and appropriate behavior reinforced by judicious use of praise. In addition, the parents and child should spend at least 15 to 20 min/day involved in a mutually pleasurable activity. If the mother is at home all day, she should be encouraged to spend some time away from the child on a regular basis.

Another circle evolves when parents react to a **fearful, clinging, or manipulating child** with overprotection and overpermissiveness. Initial complaints to the physician often are medical, but the description of a typical day reveals conflicts at mealtime, difficulties with separation, parental inability to limit behavior that encroaches on the rights of others, and a parental tendency to perform tasks for the child that he can do himself (eg, dressing, feeding).

Frequently, the history includes complications during the pregnancy or a serious familial illness that is believed to increase the child's vulnerability. The parents need reassurance that the child is physically well, and encouragement to set reasonable limits on dependency-seeking and manipulating behavior in order to reestablish a balance of mutual respect.

When any conflicting parent–child interaction develops, the physician must provide empathetic support while the parents try to modify their response pattern. If there is no change in 3 to 4 mo, reevaluation of the problem or psychiatric consultation is indicated.

Problems Related to Eating

Not eating enough and eating the wrong foods are common complaints of parents with 2- to 8-yr-olds. At mealtime while the parents coax and threaten, the child may sit with food in his mouth or may respond to attempts at force-feeding by vomiting. The decrease in appetite usually is related to the slowing in growth rate that is normal at this time. The parents should be educated about the growth patterns of young children, reassured about the child's current height and weight status, and instructed to reduce emotions at mealtime by putting the food in front of the child and removing it in 15 or 20 min without comment about what is or is not eaten. This, along with restricting between-meal snacks, generally will restore the relationship between appetite, the amount eaten, and the child's nutritional needs. If the feeding problem is part of a pattern of overcoercion or overconcern about the child's health, a more detailed history is needed in order to determine appropriate management (see General Principles of Dealing with Behavioral Problems, above).

Sleep Problems (see also Ch. 122)

Normal sleep consists of cycles of **REM** sleep (rapid-eye-movement, light sleep) and **NREM** sleep (non-rapid-eye-movement, deep sleep). NREM sleep can be divided into four EEG stages, with stages 3 and 4 representing the deepest sleep. From age 2 to 3 through adulthood, individuals cycle through the stages of NREM and REM sleep about every 90 min, beginning with a sustained NREM period. About 80% of the total sleep time is spent in NREM sleep. Newborns have less well defined stages, enter sleep through active REM, and spend about half their sleep time in REM. The mature pattern gradually develops over the first 2 to 3 yr.

Nightmares are frightening dreams that occur during REM sleep. The child usually becomes fully awake and can vividly recall the details of the dream. Frightening experiences, including scary stories or television violence, can precipitate a nightmare, particularly in 3- to 4-yr-olds who cannot readily distinguish fantasy from reality. An occasional nightmare is normal, and comfort from the parent may be all that is required. Persistent or frequent nightmares, however, suggest an environmental problem that warrants evaluation.

Somnambulism (*persistent sleepwalking*) and **night terrors** are disorders of arousal that share many clinical features. They occur during arousal from deep sleep (stage 3 or 4 NREM sleep), usually in the first 1 to 3 h of sleep. Episodes last from seconds to many minutes and are characterized by sudden awakening, blank or confused stares, incomplete arousal with poor responsiveness to people, and amnesia for the episode.

Night terrors are dramatic because of the screaming and inconsolable panic of the child during the episode. They are most common between ages 3 and 8 yr. Somnambu-

lism involves clumsy walks during which objects usually are avoided. The child appears confused but not frightened. At least one episode of sleepwalking is estimated to occur in 15% of children between 5 and 12 yr of age. Persistent sleepwalking occurs in 1 to 6% of the population, most commonly in school-aged boys. Stressful events sometimes may trigger an episode. Both disorders are almost always self-limited, though sporadic episodes may occur for years. When these disorders persist to adolescence and adulthood an underlying psychologic disorder should be considered. A **differential diagnostic consideration** is temporal lobe epilepsy that may occur at night manifested by hallucinations, incomplete arousal, fear, and automatic behavior. Suspicions of seizure activity when awake, a large degree of autonomic activation, and enuresis during the episode warrant an EEG.

Treatment consists of education and assurance. Diazepam (2 to 5 mg before sleep) may be given for very frequent episodes.

Resistance to going to bed is a common problem, which generally peaks between 1 and 2 yr of age. The child cries when left alone in the crib or climbs out and seeks his parents. This behavior is related to separation anxiety (see below) and to increasing attempts by the child to control his environment, both of which are common at this age. Long naps late in the afternoon; rough, overstimulating play before bedtime; a disturbance in the parent–child relationship; or tension in the home also may cause the problem.

Letting the child get up, staying in the room and comforting him at length, or spanking and scolding all are ineffective. Settling the child with a brief story, offering a favorite doll or blanket, and using a night light are helpful, but sitting quietly in the hallway in sight of the child and making sure that he stays in bed may be needed to control the problem. Once the child learns that he will not be allowed out of bed or cannot entice the parent into the room for more stories or play, he will settle down and go to sleep.

Night awakening occurs in about 50% of infants between 6 and 12 mo of age, and is related to the development of separation anxiety (see below). In older children, episodes often follow a move, illness, or other stressful event. Allowing the child to sleep with the parents, playing, feeding, or spanking and scolding usually prolong the problem. Returning the child to his bed with simple reassurance or sitting outside the open bedroom door until he settles down usually is more effective. Some 3-yr-olds wander around the house without waking the parents; installing a hook-and-eye lock on the outside of the child's bedroom door will solve the problem, but this procedure must be used judiciously and should not be indiscriminately employed to isolate or control the child.

Problems of Toilet Training

Most children are consistently trained for bowel control between ages 2 and 3 yr and for urinary control between 3 and 4. By age 5 the average child can go to the toilet alone, managing all aspects of dressing, undressing, and wiping. However, wide individual variations occur; eg, about 30% of normal 4-yr-olds and 10% of 6-yr-olds have not achieved regular nighttime continence.

The key to avoiding problems lies in recognizing the child's readiness to train, which is signaled when the child has dry periods lasting several hours, shows interest in sitting on a potty chair or wanting to be changed when wet, and can carry out simple verbal commands. This generally occurs between ages 18 and 24 mo.

The most common approach to toilet training is the **timing method**. After demonstrating readiness, the child is introduced to the potty chair and gradually required to briefly sit on it fully clothed and then to practice taking his pants down, sitting on the potty chair for no more than 5 or 10 min, and redressing. Simple explanations of the purpose for the exercise are given repeatedly and emphasized by placing wet or dirty

diapers in the pot. The crux of this method involves the parent's anticipation of the child's need to eliminate, and then positive reinforcement for successful elimination with praise or rewards. Anger or punishment for lack of success or accidents may be counterproductive. This method works well for children with predictable elimination schedules. For the child with unpredictable schedules, however, it is difficult to provide the contingent reinforcement, and training must await the ability of the child to anticipate elimination himself.

A second training method involves **modeling** with a doll. After readiness is demonstrated, the child is taught the steps of the toileting process as the parent gives positive reinforcement to the doll for dry pants and for successful completion of each step of the process. Then the child imitates this process with the doll repeatedly, assuming the parent's role as reinforcer. Lastly the child performs the steps himself as the parent provides praise and rewards.

If the child resists sitting on the toilet, allowing him to get up and trying again after a meal is recommended. If resistance continues for days, postponing the training for several weeks is the best strategy. Behavior modification, with a reward for sitting on the toilet and producing results, has succeeded with both normal and retarded children. Once the pattern is established, rewards are given for every other success and then gradually withdrawn. In any case, *power struggles must be avoided*, since they are detrimental and may result in a strained parent-child relationship. If a repetitive pattern of pressure and resistance occurs, it should be managed as discussed under Common Vicious Circle Patterns, above.

Nocturnal Enuresis (see also Ch. 159)

Involuntary and repeated passage of urine while asleep occurring at an age when voluntary control could be expected. Nocturnal enuresis is present in 30% of children at age 4 yr, 10% at age 6, 3% at age 12, and 1% at age 18. It is more common in boys than girls, appears to be familial, and is sometimes associated with sleep disorders (eg, sleepwalking and night terrors). An **organic etiology** is found in only 1 to 2% of cases, and they usually involve a UTI. Although rare, other diagnoses to consider include congenital anomalies, sacral nerve disorders, diabetes mellitus or insipidus, or a pelvic mass. These can be excluded by a careful history, physical examination, urinalysis, and urine culture. Positive findings may indicate the need for an intravenous urogram and cystourethrogram, a urologic consultation, or other evaluations. Bedwetting occasionally is associated with moderate to severe individual or family psychopathology, indicating psychiatric referral. Bedwetting usually represents only a delay in maturation that resolves with time. **Secondary enuresis,** in which previous bedtime control is lost, usually is due to a psychologically stressful event or condition. There is, however, a greater chance of an organic etiology (eg, UTI or diabetes mellitus) than in primary nocturnal enuresis.

Treatment: Four different modalities are commonly used, each claiming a cure rate higher than the spontaneous cure rate of 15%/yr after age 6. Even higher spontaneous cure rates before age 6 argue against imposing a treatment regimen before that age. Other factors, like embarrassment preventing camp or overnight experiences during the school years, favor treatment after age 6.

Motivational counseling has been the most common approach, involving the following recommendations: (1) The child assumes an active role by keeping a calendar to record wet and dry nights, by talking to the physician himself, by urinating before going to bed, and by changing his clothing and bedding when wet. (2) Fluids are not consumed for 2 to 3 h before bed. (3) Punishments are discontinued and angry parental responses are avoided. (4) Positive reinforcement is given for dry nights (a star calendar or other rewards depending on the age). (5) Reassurance is given about the etiology and prognosis of enuresis, with the aim to remove blame and guilt.

Bladder exercises are proposed when the etiology is believed to be the inability of a small bladder to hold a whole night's volume of urine. The child is encouraged to increase fluid intake early in the day, and then to delay urination after the urge to urinate (for seconds initially, gradually increasing to minutes). In addition, the child is instructed to interrupt the urinary stream midway through bladder emptying for a similar period of time before completing urination. One study found a cure rate of 35%.

Enuresis alarms have proved to be by far the most effective treatment currently available. Two studies, involving 5- to 15-yr-olds, reported a 70% cure rate with only a 10 to 15% relapse rate. These alarms are easy to set up, cost about 40 dollars, and are triggered by a few drops of urine. The disadvantage is the time required for complete success. In the first few weeks of use the child awakens after full voiding; in the next few weeks partial inhibition of urination is achieved. Eventually, the child awakens with a conditioned response to bladder contractions before urination occurs. The alarm should be used for 3 wk beyond the last wetting episode before discontinuation.

Imipramine is falling out of favor in the treatment of enuresis because of the greater long-term success rate of alarms, side effects of the drug, and the potential for life-threatening accidental ingestions. If other modalities fail and the family strongly favors treatment, imipramine may be used (50 mg 1 h before bed in 8- to 12-yr-olds, and 75 mg over age 12). If imipramine is likely to succeed, a response usually occurs in the first week of treatment. This is the one real advantage of the drug, particularly if it is very important to the family and child to achieve a rapid response. After 1 mo without enuresis, the drug should be tapered over 2 to 4 wk and then discontinued. Relapses are very common after discontinuation of the drug, reducing the long-term cure rate to only 25%. If relapse occurs, a 3-mo course may be tried. Blood counts should be done every 2 to 4 wk while on imipramine to detect the rare occurrence of agranulocytosis.

Encopresis and Constipation

Encopresis (*fecal incontinence in the absence of organic defect or illness*) occurs in about 17% of 3-yr-olds and 1% of 4-yr-olds. Most of this soiling is from resistance to toilet training (see above), but sometimes overflow fecal incontinence associated with chronic constipation is the cause. The latter may result from stool withholding due to a painful anal fissure, from resistance to coercive attempts at toilet training, or from Hirschsprung's disease (see under DISTAL SMALL BOWEL AND LARGE BOWEL OBSTRUCTION in GASTROINTESTINAL DEFECTS in Ch. 187).

Treatment depends on the diagnosis. Onset of symptoms in the first year of life, absence of stool in the rectum, and a lack of a physiologic urge to defecate are more characteristic of Hirschsprung's disease, but lack of response to a medical regimen of phosphate enemas followed by either daily mineral oil (the Davidson regimen, see below) or milk of magnesia more reliably identifies children who need further diagnostic study. Soiling also may accompany severe psychopathology in the child, particularly those 5 yr of age and older; taking a careful family history and noting other behavioral symptoms may suggest the need for psychiatric evaluation along with physical management.

The **Davidson regimen** can be used to treat constipation and to identify those children requiring further study. Fecal impactions are removed by 2 hypertonic phosphate enemas given about 1 h apart (about 30 mL/10 kg body wt [1 oz/20 lb] up to a maximum of 120 mL [4 oz]/enema). This is done once or twice/day until clear returns indicate that the impaction has been removed.

The child is then started on mineral oil, 1 tbsp morning and night. This is increased by 1 tbsp/day until 4 or 5 loose bowel movements occur daily, which usually requires about 5 tbsp bid (the maximum dose is 10 tbsp bid). Children under age 2 yr may need supplemental fat-soluble vitamins given at midday between doses of mineral oil. If 2 or 3 wk of this treatment do not correct the constipation, further diagnostic studies, such

as a barium enema, sigmoidoscopy, and rectal biopsy, are indicated to rule out Hirschsprung's disease or other organic obstruction.

For the next phase, the child (if over age 3) is placed on a potty seat at a regular time each day for 5 to 15 min, with his feet on a firm surface against which he can push while performing Valsalva's maneuver. When this training procedure has developed regular bowel habits, the mineral oil can be gradually withdrawn over a 6- to 8-wk period. Follow-up is required to detect recurrences of constipation, which are treated similarly.

Some physicians prefer to use milk of magnesia rather than mineral oil. The initial dose is 1 tbsp every morning, with increases of 1 to 2 *tsp* every few days until a daily bowel movement is maintained. Giving the dose with chocolate syrup may make it more palatable. Bowel training is then undertaken as above. The whole sequence may take 3 to 6 mo with either agent.

Acquired megacolon, resulting from prolonged stool retention, usually is seen in mentally retarded or psychotic children who refuse to try to defecate. The rectum is distended and full of feces, causing inadequate anal control. The colon also gradually becomes distended. Fecal soiling is a prominent symptom. Treatment of acquired megacolon in children is principally psychiatric; however, laxatives and enemas also are necessary until the child can be persuaded to undertake bowel training.

Separation Anxiety, Fears, and Phobias

Separation anxiety: Crying when the mother leaves the room or when a stranger approaches is a normal developmental stage, beginning around age 8 mo and persisting until 18 to 24 mo. The intensity of this behavior varies with each child.

Some parents, especially those with their first child, suspect an emotional problem and respond by becoming protective and avoiding separations or new situations. Fathers often interpret the behavior as a sign of a spoiled child and may criticize the mother or try to modify the child's behavior by scolding and punishment. Discussing the expected appearance of this behavior at the 6-mo well-baby visit often can prevent parental concerns. The parents' response to the behavior should be reviewed at later visits so that the physician can recognize and stop unwise methods of handling the problem. If the parents' response only reinforces the child's distress (ie, leads to a vicious circle), a more extensive evaluation will be needed before a management plan can be devised.

In cases where separating the mother and child is necessary but can be planned, such as in elective surgery, the physician should recommend separation during a less threatening age—before 6 mo or after 3 yr.

Fears of the dark, monsters, bugs, and spiders are common in 3- and 4-yr-olds; fears of injury and death are more common in older children. Frightening stories, movies, or television shows are often upsetting and intensify fears. Statements made by the parents in anger or jest may be taken literally by preschool children and can be disturbing. A shy child may initially react to new situations with fear or withdrawal; repeated exposure and reassurance, without pressure, help him adapt.

Phobias: Normal developmental stage-related fears must be differentiated from those caused by tension in the home or by internalized conflicts (phobias). The screening outlined under General Principles of Dealing with Behavioral Problems, above, usually helps to identify the child or family with more serious problems. If the phobia is intense, is out of proportion to the potential danger involved, and interferes with the child's activity, and if the child does not respond to simple reassurance, a psychiatrist should be consulted.

School phobia: Children 6 and 7 yr old may show separation anxiety by refusing to go to school. The child may frankly refuse to go or complain of stomachaches, nausea, or other symptoms that justify his staying home. He may be reacting from fear of a

teacher's strictness or reproofs, which can frighten a sensitive child, or fear of harassment by peers. More often, the mother has become overprotective of a dependent-manipulating child. With older children (ages 10 to 14) school phobia may indicate more serious psychopathology requiring psychiatric evaluation and therapy. If the physician recognizes that complaints such as chronic abdominal pain or headaches may be due to separation anxiety or other emotional problems, he can avoid giving a series of tests in search of organic diseases. Such tests can be costly, time-consuming, and painful, and can complicate the real problem.

For the younger child, immediate return to school is necessary to minimize disability from falling behind in school work. The physician should then explore the family situation in more detail and decide whether some form of brief intervention therapy is appropriate or whether referral to a mental health professional is indicated. Relapses may occur after a bona fide illness or a vacation period. With the pre- or early adolescent, immediate return to school is not so urgent and management depends on the results of a detailed psychiatric evaluation.

Overactivity

Parents of 2-yr-olds generally indicate that their child is active and seldom still, and in 4-yr-olds a high activity and noise level is common. In both age groups such behavior is stage-related, but frequently leads to parent–child conflicts and causes parental concern.

Hyperactivity is not easily defined, since claims that a child is hyperactive often reflect the tolerance level of the annoyed person. Some children are clearly more active and have shorter attention spans than average, and they create management problems for many people encountering them.

This syndrome may arise from a variety of etiologies, such as an emotional disorder, CNS dysfunction, or a genetic component, or it may simply be an exaggeration of a normal temperament trait.

Adults most frequently try to suppress overactivity by scolding and punishment, but these responses usually increase the activity level. Not requiring the child to sit still for a long time or finding a teacher who is skilled in coping with an overactive child may help.

When hyperactive behavior is extreme and is associated with signs of perceptual, motor, or psychologic disorders, the condition is clearly pathologic, and further evaluation is indicated. Children with such problems are discussed in ATTENTION DEFICIT DISORDER, below.

LEARNING DISORDERS

Inability to acquire, retain, or generalize specific skills or sets of information because of deficiencies or defects in attention, memory, or reasoning, or deficiencies in producing responses associated with desired and skilled behavior. The term **learning disorder** encompasses learning problems along the entire continuum of cognitive abilities with difficulties noted in the learning of adaptive, perceptual-motor, social, language (communication), and academic skills. The term **learning disability** is more limited; it assumes normal cognitive abilities and refers specifically to problems in reading, arithmetic, spelling, and written expression.

Descriptions of learning disorders are diverse, and numerous syndromes have been identified. Educationally, the terms **learning disability, mental retardation,** and **autism** refer to learning disorders. Other labels, such as **neurologically impaired, minimal brain dysfunction, perceptual deficit disorder, dyslexia,** and **attention deficit disorder** or **hyperkinesis** have been associated with learning disorders and are used to describe behavior perceived as independent and constituting specific syndromes.

Etiology and Incidence

Learning disorders are multidimensional and affected children are heterogenous. No single cause or set of core symptoms has been defined. Genetic influences may be obvious, as in Down's syndrome, or subtle, as in developmental reading disabilities. About 3 to 15% of the school population in the USA has been cited as having learning disorders. Males tend to outnumber females by 5 to 1, suggesting familial and biologic influences.

Symptoms and Signs

Since learning disorders occur in young children who cannot express their feelings, difficulties, and symptoms well or at all, defining the characteristics of these disorders is limited to physical and behavioral signs observed by others. Although signs are manifested at early ages, most are not recognized until the child reaches school age and encounters the rigors of symbolic and figurative learning. Most students with learning disorders have positive neurologic findings or demonstrate lags in neurodevelopmental integrity. The neurologic factors frequently are interrelated with cognitive and behavioral liabilities, but no single sign or set of signs predicts later difficulties. Problems with visual-motor coordination, gross motor movement, and delay in paired associative learning (eg, color-naming, labeling, counting, and letter-naming) are predominant indicators of early problems with formal learning. Disturbances or delays in receptive and expressive vocabulary and comprehension of language are better predictors of academic problems beyond the preschool years. Other warning signs that are often overlooked are short attention span and distractibility, limited verbal fluency, restricted memory span, and signs related to fine motor problems (eg, poor printing and copying).

Behaviorally, difficulties with impulse control, non–goal-directed behavior and overactivity, discipline problems, withdrawal and avoidance behavior, and aggressiveness may be early indications of cognitive and communication disorders and impending school difficulties.

Cognitive disturbances: Although basic cognitive processes and learning strategies appear to be age-dependent and vary with cognitive ability (IQ), most learning disorders are related intrinsically to deficiencies in brain functions and the relationships between different functions. Problems may exist in (1) **perceptual functions**, exhibiting difficulties in personal and extrapersonal orientation, visual-spatial abilities, selective attention, pattern recognition, sound discrimination and analysis, and visual-motor integration; (2) **memory functions**, including short- and long-term information retention, memory (rehearsal) strategies, and verbal retrieval and production; and (3) **reasoning abilities**, such as concept formation, abstracting, generalizing, and organizing and planning information for problem solving. A number of subgroups of children with specific reading–learning disorders have been identified, ranging from basic language dysfunctions, dysnomia, and poor comprehension of spoken language, to visual–spatial disorders and problems in pattern recognition. Other subtypes have been noted in arithmetic disorders; eg, **anarithmia** (*disturbances in basic concept formation, and failure to acquire computation skills*); and **ageometria** (*arithmetic problems due to disturbances in spatial reasoning*). Other subtypes may exist; however, most learning disorders are complex or mixed, with problems emanating from deficiencies in more than one system.

Diagnosis

Since signs of learning disorders vary and disorders share similar and overlapping characteristics, diagnostic criteria must be comprehensive and precise. A **multidisciplinary evaluation** consisting of medical, psychologic, social, educational, speech and language, and emotional–behavioral factors is essential to establish functioning levels and skill indexes, to plan treatment, and to monitor a child's progress.

The **medical evaluation** should include detailed family history, the child's medical, developmental, and school history, a general physical examination, and a traditional and adaptive neurologic examination. Young children should be evaluated for developmental level using standardized criteria. Although causal relationships have not been firmly established, use of ototoxic drugs, maternal illnesses, and all complications during pregnancy and delivery should be noted (eg, spotting, toxemia, prolonged labor, precipitous delivery), as well as neonatal problems (eg, prematurity, low birth weight, jaundice, perinatal asphyxia, postmaturity, respiratory distress, and minor physical anomalies). Children with learning problems often have several cumulative minor physical abnormalities. Chronic and acute ear infections and insidious hearing loss, allergies, and repeated illnesses associated with autoimmune deficiencies also have been implicated.

Verbal and nonverbal intelligence testing should be done. Significant differences within and between verbal and nonverbal systems often indicate differences in ability to process information, learning preference, and learning disorders. Children with reading and generalized learning disabilities tend to have more difficulties with functions controlled by the left hemisphere than the right. Comprehensive assessment of neuropsychologic functions often is needed to test anterior and posterior brain functions of left and right hemispheres and the preferred manner in which a child processes information; eg, holistically or analytically, and visually or auditorially. These methods allow for qualitative as well as quantitative assessment and encourage comparisons of each child's development relative to his ability.

Intellectual, educational, psychologic, and language assessments are essential and must be integrated to determine the degree of discrepancy in skills, deficiencies in subskills and prerequisite skills, deficiencies in use of effective learning strategies (eg, rehearsal), and the degree of intactness of memory and reasoning. An **educational evaluation** identifies reading, writing, arithmetic, and spelling skills and deficits. **Reading evaluations** measure abilities in word decoding and recognition, passage comprehension, and passage fluency. **Arithmetic levels** should be established for computation skills, knowledge of operations, and understanding of mathematical concepts. Functional assessment to determine if the child applies all 3 of these processes to everyday experiences should be conducted. **Writing samples** should be obtained to evaluate spelling, syntax, and fluency of ideas. Dyspraxia and developmental maladroitness also should be investigated if writing problems exist.

Psychologic evaluation defines conduct disorders, poor self-esteem, and early childhood depression that frequently accompany learning disorders. Attitudes toward school, motivation, peer relationships, and self-confidence should be assessed.

Treatment

Treatment centers on effective *educational* management of the child's problem and, when necessary, the use of medical, behavioral, and psychologic therapy. No single educational program, technic, or procedure has resolved basic learning problems in children with either diverse or pervasive learning disorders or specific learning disabilities. **Direct instruction** adapted to meet a child's learning differences is advocated. Diagnostic tests, as suggested above, should be used to help determine the most effective teaching program, which may take a remedial, compensatory, or strategic (teaching the child) approach. Testing also is used for classification and educational placement decisions. When a child's learning preference and learning problem is mismatched with the instructional method implemented, the learning disorder may be aggravated.

Many children will need supplementary specialized instruction in one area only while continuing to attend regular education programs. Others will need separate and intense educational programs to accommodate their learning needs. Optimally, chil-

dren with learning disorders should attend programs in the least restrictive environment compatible with the severity and extent of their learning difficulties.

Most medical, neurologic, or biochemical therapies popularly recommended for children with learning disorders are *unsubstantiated* by clinical and applied research; eg, eliminating food additives, prescribing large doses of vitamins, and analyzing the system for trace minerals. Similarly, medication has minimal impact on academic achievement, intelligence, and general learning ability, although certain medications (eg, psychostimulants) may be effective in enhancing attention and concentration, allowing the child to respond more efficiently to instruction (see ATTENTION DEFICIT DISORDER, below). Therapies such as patterning by sensory stimulation and passive movement, sensory integrative therapy through postural exercises, and optometric training to remedy visual perceptual and sensory-motor coordination processes are controversial and there is little positive data to encourage their use. The effectiveness of treatments such as visual and auditory perceptual and perceptual-motor training also has been difficult to substantiate through controlled investigations. Although many learning-disordered children have deficits in these processes, specific interventions designed to promote perceptual competence have not been conclusively demonstrated to improve reading and language comprehension.

ATTENTION DEFICIT DISORDER (ADD)

(Hyperactivity; Hyperkinesis; Minimal Brain Dysfunction)

Developmentally inappropriate inattention and impulsivity, with or without hyperactivity. This definition conforms to the American Psychiatric Association's *Diagnostic and Statistical Manual* (DSM-III), shifting the focus of the disorder from excessive physical activity. Although the use of the term ADD (and others indicated in the synonyms above) as an independent diagnosis of a specific syndrome has been challenged, no study or critique has been able to discount the constellation of signs used to describe the disorder. ADD is implicated in learning disorders, and except for severe and profound mental retardation can influence the behavior of children at any cognitive level. ADD is estimated to affect 5 to 10% of school-aged children, precipitating half of the childhood referrals to diagnostic clinics. ADD is seen 10 times more frequently in boys than girls. **Etiology** is unknown. Several theories advocating biochemical, sensory and motor, physiologic, and behavioral correlates and manifestations have been proposed.

Symptoms and Signs

The **primary signs** of ADD with or without hyperactivity are a child's display of inattention and impulsivity. ADD with hyperactivity is diagnosed when the signs of overactivity are obvious. Although children with ADD and without hyperactivity may not manifest high activity levels, most exhibit restlessness or jitteriness, short attention span, and poor impulse control. These are qualitatively different from those seen in conduct and anxiety disorders. **Inattention** is described as *a failure to finish tasks started, easy distractibility, seeming lack of attention, and difficulty concentrating on tasks requiring sustained attention.* **Impulsivity** is described as *acting before thinking, difficulty taking turns, problems organizing work, and constant shifting from one activity to another.* Impulsive responses are especially likely when involved with uncertainty and the need to attend carefully. **Hyperactivity** is featured as *difficulty staying seated and sitting still, and running or climbing on things excessively.* In general, children with hyperactivity are described as "always on the go."

Primary signs tend to appear when the ADD child is involved in vigilance and reaction-time tasks, and tasks requiring visual and perceptual search, paired associate learning, systematic listening, and directed attention. These signs tend to restrict devel-

opment of academic skills and concepts, thinking and reasoning strategies, motivation for school, and adjustment to social demands. Behavior often is more resistant to treatment than that of children with other behavioral disorders.

Associated or secondary signs are frequently noted: motor incoordination, nonlocalized "soft" neurologic findings, perceptual–motor dysfunctions, EEG abnormalities, emotional lability, opposition, anxiety, aggressiveness, low frustration tolerance, and poor peer relationships.

Onset of ADD occurs typically before age 3 yr and invariably before age 7 yr. The peak age for referral has been between 8 and 10 yr. Early indicators vary, but most children diagnosed as ADD with or without hyperactivity at school age exhibited delays in their motor development, tended to have brief attention spans (eg, did not play with toys or did so in brief intervals), and usually had higher activity levels than normal during their preschool years. Children with hyperactivity often were described as hyperexcitable and were difficult to manage as toddlers and preschoolers. In school these signs persist, and difficulty with visual motor tasks such as copying and printing may become apparent. Right–left confusion and immature coordination after age 7 yr is prevalent in both types of ADD. Some children with ADD signs also have been less responsive to positive and negative reinforcement. They often seem to lack intrinsic motivation and do not consider long-term consequences of their behavior. In general, children with ADD during the school years are a more homogeneous group than those referred before age 6 yr. Many ADD signs expressed during the preschool years indicate communication disorders, anxiety, and conduct disorders, whereas ADD signs during later childhood usually are specific and qualitatively distinct; eg, such children often exhibit continuous movement of the lower extremities, motor impersistence such as the purposeless movement and fidgeting of hands, impulsive talking, and a seeming lack of awareness of their environment. Most are not aggressive or oppositional. Some studies have found that approximately 25% of children with ADD exhibit depression, but it is uncertain if depression is secondary to or independent of the symptoms.

Adolescents and adults may display residual symptoms of inattention and impulsivity such as fidgetiness, restlessness, difficulty completing assigned tasks (eg, homework), and difficulty focusing attention for extended periods of time. Although hyperactivity tends to diminish with age, residual symptoms and signs can extend well into adulthood.

Diagnosis

Diagnosis often is difficult. No particular organic signs or set of neurologic indicators are specific. Although organic factors may have a role in diagnosis, the primary signs are behavioral, varying with situation and time. Rating scales and checklists, the predominant mode of identification, often are unable to distinguish ADD from other behavioral disorders. Such data often are based on subjective observations made by untrained personnel. In a clinical setting most behavior is not obvious and, unless the child is excessively overactive or impulsive, diagnosis is impossible without the use of specific tasks; eg, vigilance and reaction-time tasks, tasks sampling paired associate learning, and tasks increasing response uncertainty, and without the use of behavioral recording technics that allow the observer to document objectively the type of overactivity, inattention, and impulsivity associated with ADD. Social and medical histories and school reports are essential for diagnosis.

Treatment and Prognosis

No single treatment has been completely effective with all children; however, psychostimulant medications combined with behavioral and cognitive therapies (eg, self-recording, self-monitoring, modeling, and role-playing) have the greatest controlling influence on symptom expression. Used alone, medication has been effective predomi-

nantly with less aggressive ADD children coming from stable home environments. Elimination diets, megavitamin treatments, psychotherapy, and biochemical interventions (eg, the administration of neurochemicals) have had the least effect, and most studies have found minimal change in behavior and no sustained, positive long-term outcomes when such treatments have been implemented.

Methylphenidate is the drug of choice. Its use has proved more effective than tricyclic antidepressants (eg, imipramine), caffeine, and other psychostimulants (eg, pemoline and deanol) and has fewer side effects than dextroamphetamine. Common side effects of methylphenidate are sleep disturbances (eg, insomnia), depression or sadness, headache, stomachache, suppression of appetite, elevated BP, and, with use of large continuous doses, a reduction of growth. Behavior changes with methylphenidate are related to dosage; learning often is enhanced at lower doses (0.3 mg/kg/administration) and decreased with higher doses. Improvements in social behavior occur most often when medication levels exceed 1.0 mg/kg/administration. Dosage often is titrated, beginning at low doses and increasing to optimal levels (decrease in symptoms, improvement in task performance, and no side effects). Response to medication often is individual and dosage is prescribed depending on the severity of the behavior and the child's ability to tolerate the substance. Medication often is prescribed to help the child only in school. Drug holidays are recommended; eg, the medication is not given on weekends, school holidays, or during summer vacations. Placebo conditions or periods when no medication is administered are recommended to investigate and challenge the need for medication. Challenge conditions should occur for 5 to 10 school days to insure reliability of observations. Long-term benefits of medication have not been conclusively demonstrated. However, some research indicates that use of medication permits participation in activities previously inaccessible because of poor attention and impulsivity. Medication often interrupts the cycle of inappropriate behavior, enhancing behavioral and academic interventions.

The use of cognitive–behavior modification, self-monitoring technics, environmental control of noise and visual stimulation, appropriate task length, and teacher proximity often have positive effects on classroom behavior. Parents should be referred for parent training and behavior management technics when difficulties persist at home. Children with ADD with hyperactivity and poor impulse control are often helped at home when structure, consistent parenting technics, and well-defined limits are established. The use of behavior management technics and contingencies such as token economies and self-monitoring with reinforcement often is effective. Parents should be encouraged to seek professional assistance.

Follow-up studies have found that children identified as ADD do not grow out of their difficulties. Later problems in adolescence and adulthood occur predominantly as academic failure, low self-esteem, and difficulty learning appropriate social behavior. Some studies have found that adolescents and adults with histories of ADD have a high incidence of personality trait disorders and antisocial behavior; most continue to display impulsivity, restlessness, and poor social skills.

DYSLEXIA

(Congenital Word Blindness; Primary Reading Disability)

Disparity between apparent intellectual potential and achievement in reading and, often, spelling. Educationally, the term dyslexia is applied when a child, usually of normal or better intelligence, is ≥ 2 yr behind his expected grade level in reading. The inability to read is inconsistent with achievement in other school subjects, such as arithmetic. A family history of language disorders is common, and boys are affected more often than girls. All socioeconomic levels are involved.

Etiology is unknown. Dyslexic children do not have an increased incidence of eye problems over the normal population. A brain defect in perception has been postu-

lated; ie, the processing (developing the connotation) of the visual image. Evidence exists of a problem in translating perceptions from one sensory system to another (inability to match seeing, feeling, and hearing). One type of dyslexia may be caused by a defect in the cerebellum. Sensory deficits and neurologic impairment are absent.

Alexia (*loss of the ability to comprehend written language*) is a similar condition that develops later in life because of a neurologic lesion.

Symptoms and Signs

The child almost never reads for pleasure. Spelling and handwriting ability often are impaired. Confusion in orientation of letters is manifested in several ways: reading from right to left, failure to see (and sometimes to hear) similarities or differences in letters or words, or inability to work out the pronunciation of unfamiliar words. Attempts to read or write are characterized by letter and word reversals (eg, "p" for "g," "saw" for "was") that are typical of normal first- and second-graders, but persist in the dyslexic child. Other reading errors include omitting words or losing the place on the page. A better-than-normal facility at mirror-reading or -writing is common. In some dyslexic children images seem to blur at a relatively low speed. The dyslexic child often is left-handed, but may be right-handed or ambidextrous or have mixed dominance.

In attempting to satisfy demands that he read, the child may make up a story if the text contains a picture or may substitute words for those he cannot read. He may be able to vocalize words; ie, to read aloud but without comprehension.

Symptoms of frustration are inevitable. The reading disability and its effects on learning and school performance may lead to behavioral problems, delinquency, aggression, withdrawal, and alienation from other children, parents, and teachers.

Diagnosis

Before dyslexia is diagnosed, the child with a reading problem must have thorough ophthalmic, auditory, psychologic, and neurologic examinations to verify that his poor reading is not due to some other disorder. Early diagnosis is important, since the prognosis is much better if the defect can be identified and treated before a pattern of frustration and failure is established. When the cause is cerebellar, an optokinetic tape or visual presentation, available to most ophthalmologists, will detect the defect.

A battery of psychologic tests is required to provide a profile of the child's abilities and deficits. The child should be referred to a consultant who is experienced in evaluating the complex and often subtle deficits found in dyslexia.

Treatment

Treatment is multidimensional, by remedial, corrective, and compensatory education, since there is no known way to correct perceptual deficits. The psychologic test results help to identify the child's areas of strengths and weaknesses so that a suitable teaching program can be designed. Remedial steps are aimed at teaching around the problem, using the child's abilities and unimpaired capabilities to compensate for his areas of weakness. Thus, auditory perception may be emphasized for a child who has difficulty in comprehending purely visual symbols; eg, by having him name and pronounce letters aloud as he traces them and, later, by having him read aloud instead of silently. Curricula such as bookless teaching through audio cassettes may be one treatment in certain specific dyslexias.

Reading skills, the child's progress in other areas, and the treatment program should be reviewed regularly. The importance of balancing the child's academic difficulties with enjoyable, successful activities should never be forgotten.

In many children, by the age of 7 or 8, cognitive abilities take over; and these children may overcome or cope with their problem. With others, dyslexia remains a lifelong problem, preventing them from achieving their intellectual potential.

MENTAL RETARDATION (MR)

(Mental Handicap; Mental Subnormality)

Subaverage intellectual ability present from birth or early infancy, manifested by abnormal development and associated with difficulties in learning and social adaptation. Traditionally, 3% of the total population are reported to be mentally retarded, but only about 1 to 1.5% are actually identified. The birth rate of children with IQs < 50 is 3.6:1000 live births.

Etiology

Intelligence is polygenetically and environmentally determined. The genetic and environmentally caused predispositions to MR may be indistinguishable. The incidence of familial retardation in the offspring of 2 retarded persons is 40%; for one, it is 20%. In 80% of cases, the cause of MR is unknown. The etiology is more likely to be identified in the more severely retarded child. Factors causing MR may occur in the prenatal, perinatal, and postnatal periods.

Prenatal abnormalities causing MR may be due to chromosomal defects or genetic factors (see Ch. 203), congenital infections, drugs, radiation, or unknown conditions affecting implantation and embryogenesis.

Chromosomal abnormalities comprise the largest number of known genetic causes (see also Ch. 203). Most common are the trisomies, which involve an additional chromosome (47 instead of the normal 46), such as Trisomy 18 (Edwards' syndrome) and Trisomy 13 (Patau's syndrome). The cri du chat syndrome results from a partial deletion of chromosome 5. Down's syndrome is a form of Trisomy 21 or (less often) a translocation from the 13–15 group to chromosome 21. Trisomy 21 is the most common trisomy, occurring in 1:600 live births. Abnormalities in sex chromosomes, such as Klinefelter's syndrome (XXY), Turner's syndrome (XO), and various mosaics, may also be associated with MR. A recently described chromosomal defect associated with MR is the **fragile X syndrome** (see X-LINKED MENTAL RETARDATION under CHROMOSOME ABERRATIONS in Ch. 203). Males are affected more frequently than females. Associated physical features include normal to increased head size, macro-orchidism, a prominent jaw, and protruding ears.

Genetic metabolic disorders: The oculocerebrorenal (Lowe's), Lesch-Nyhan (hyperuricemia), and Hunter's (a mucopolysaccharidosis variant) syndromes are sex-linked recessive defects that cause MR. Other metabolic disorders, such as phenylketonuria, galactosemia, maple syrup urine disease, and other aminoacidurias and acidemias, are autosomal recessive disorders. Tay-Sachs disease, Niemann-Pick disease, Gaucher's disease, and Hurler's syndrome (mucopolysaccharidosis) are autosomal recessive lysozymal defects.

Genetic neurologic disorders: Primary microcephaly may be caused by an autosomal recessive gene. Tuberous sclerosis, neurofibromatosis, and myotonic dystrophy are all autosomal dominant disorders.

Congenital infections are a major cause of MR and have been due to rubella virus, cytomegalovirus (a common cause—1:600 to 1:1000 live births), *Toxoplasma gondii*, and *Treponema pallidum*. Other viruses infecting the pregnant woman have been causally implicated but not proved.

Drugs: Children born to chronic alcoholic mothers may have the **fetal alcohol syndrome,** which includes anomalies such as microcephaly, micrognathia, blepharophimosis, cardiac defects, intrauterine growth retardation, and MR (see also under METABOLIC PROBLEMS in Ch. 186). **Fetal hydantoin** (phenytoin) **syndrome** develops in about 11% of children whose mothers receive hydantoin during pregnancy. This syndrome may include mental deficiency, prenatal and postnatal growth failure, microcephaly, cranial facial abnormalities, nail or distal phalangeal hypoplasia, and associated cardiac defects.

Perinatal complications related to prematurity, CNS bleeding, breech or high forceps delivery, multiple births, placenta previa, preeclampsia, and asphyxia neonatorum may increase the risk of MR. Small-for-gestational-age infants have an increased incidence of MR; the intellectual impairment often is related to the cause of decreased weight. Premature infants < 32 wk gestation who weigh < 1.5 kg have a 10 to 50% chance of being retarded, depending on their weight, perinatal events, and the quality of care provided. Infants at risk of being mentally retarded require close developmental observation during the first several years of life. The outcome of mild untoward perinatal events is often directly related to the socioeconomic status of the parents.

Postnatal factors may include viral and bacterial encephalitides and meningitides, poisoning by such substances as lead and mercury, and accidents that result in severe head injuries or asphyxia.

Prenatal, fetal, or postnatal malnutrition in the mother or infant may affect brain development, resulting in MR. This is a major concern in developing countries where famine and hunger are commonplace. Malnutrition, coupled with environmental deprivation (lack of the physical, emotional, and cognitive support required for developmental growth and social adaptation), may be the most common cause of MR worldwide.

Diagnosis and Prognosis

Accurate diagnosis provides prognosis, suggests an educational and training program, forms the foundation of genetic counseling, and relieves guilt. FIG. 188–1 provides a general diagnostic approach to use when MR is suspected. Skull x-rays should be obtained when one suspects premature closure of the sutures. The CT scan is very helpful in diagnosing cerebral malformations, cerebral atrophy, CNS hemorrhage, hydrocephalus, tumor, and intracranial calcifications associated with toxoplasmosis, cytomegalovirus infection, or tuberous sclerosis. An EEG should be performed when a seizure disorder is suspected. Urine and blood amino acid and enzyme studies are indicated when inborn errors of metabolism are suspected. The major clinical manifestations of these metabolic errors may be associated with failure to thrive, lethargy, vomiting, seizures, hepatosplenomegaly, coarse facial features, abnormal urinary odor, or macroglossia.

Subaverage intellectual ability can be identified and measured by **standardized intelligence tests.** Such tests have a middle-class bias, but in general they reasonably appraise a child's intellectual ability, particularly in a child aged 9 to 10 yr. Psychologic tests, such as the Bayley Scale of Infant Development, for children under age 2 yr; the Stanford-Binet, for ages 2 to 4 yr; the Wechsler Preschool and Primary Scale of Intelligence, for ages 3 yr 10 mo to 6 yr 7 mo; and the Wechsler Intelligence Scale for Children, for ages 4 yr to 15 yr 11 mo, should be given by qualified psychologists. The Denver Developmental Screening Test provides a gross assessment of developmental achievement for children up to age 5 yr and can be given by the physician or his assistant. It should be used as a screening test only. Isolated delays in sitting or walking **(gross motor skills)** and in pincer grasp, drawing, or writing **(fine motor skills)** may be due to a neuromuscular disorder, while deficits in language and personal–social skills may be caused by emotional problems, environmental deprivation, learning disorders, or sensory defects without MR. Intelligence tests are subject to error and should be questioned when they do not support clinical findings. Illness, language barriers, or cultural differences may hamper a youngster's test performance.

Mentally retarded children function at various levels. The child who has **borderline intelligence** or is a slow learner (IQ 84 to 71) is rarely identified before he begins school. At this time educational and behavioral problems become evident. About 14% of children tested in school have IQs identified as borderline retardation; however, after leaving school these children are likely to blend into the general population without attracting attention to their lower intellectual skills. They can support themselves

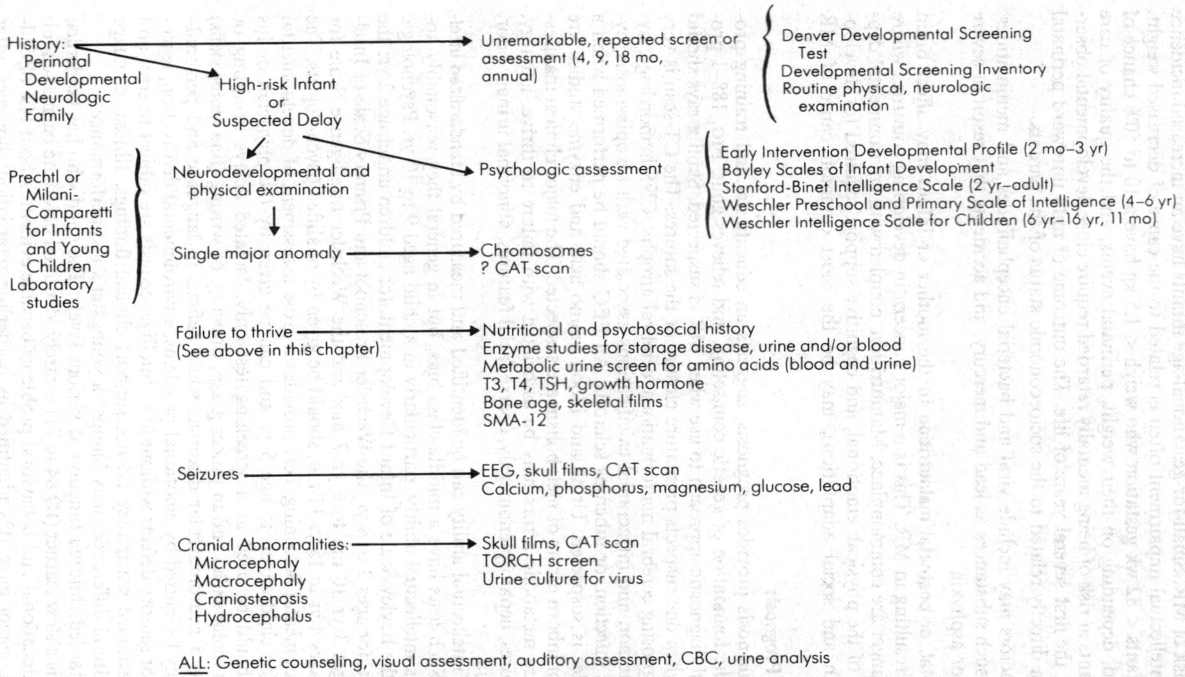

Fig. 188–1. The diagnostic process. This is meant to be a general guide. The laboratory studies should be determined by careful history and physical examination. References for the Prechtl and Milani-Comparetti examinations are as follows: Prechtl, H. F. R., Beintema, D., Neurological examination of full-term new born infants. Clinics of Developmental Medicine, No. 12. London: Spastic International Publications, J. B. Lippincott Co., 1964; and Milani-Comparetti, G., Routine developmental examination in normal and retarded children. Developmental Medicine and Child Neurology, 9:631–638, 1967. (From "The child with mental retardation," p. 210, by A. P. Scheiner and N. A. McNabb, in *The Practical Management of the Developmentally Disabled Child*, by A. P. Scheiner and I. F. Abroms. Published by C. V. Mosby Co., St. Louis, 1980. Used with permission.)

as long as job opportunities exist that require only basic skills or manual performance.

Children with **mild retardation** (IQ 70 to 50) are educable. Those at the upper level may attain 4th- to 6th-grade reading skills. These individuals can provide for their basic self-help needs and depending on their level of function have varying degrees of educational achievement and social and occupational skills. They require some supervision and support, special educational and training facilities, and, frequently, a sheltered living and work situation. They usually are free from gross physical defects but may have a higher-than-normal incidence of epilepsy. Although they have difficulty reading, most mildly retarded individuals can learn the basic educational skills needed for everyday life. Socially they are often immature and unsophisticated, with a poorly developed capacity for social interaction. Because their thinking is concrete and they are often unable to generalize, adjusting to new situations is difficult, and their poor judgment, lack of foresight, and gullibility make them susceptible to delinquency. Serious offenses are uncommon, but the mildly retarded may commit impulsive crimes, often as a member of a group and sometimes in order to achieve peer group status. Those children at the lower mild retardation level and the **moderately retarded,** trainable child (IQ 49 to 35) have obvious language and motor delays.

Given adequate training and support, mildly and moderately retarded adults can live with varying degrees of independence within the community. Some can cope with minimal support in halfway houses, while others need greater supervision, and most will need a sheltered workshop.

The **severely retarded** child (IQ 34 to 20) is trainable, but to a lesser degree. The **profoundly retarded** child (IQ 19 and below) usually cannot learn to walk and has minimal language skills.

The life expectancy of retarded individuals may be shortened, depending on the etiology and severity of MR. In general, the more severely impaired a child is, the higher the mortality; but with modern medical technology, this tends to vary widely.

Mental illness can occur in mentally handicapped persons of all ability levels, as it can in people with normal intelligence. It may cause sudden behavior changes. Language deficits may make it difficult to identify thought disorders and delusions, but the relatively sudden development of a flat affect and hallucinations may suggest **schizophrenia. Depression** may occur when an adolescent retarded person is socially rejected by the normal peer group at school, or when he realizes others see him as different and deficient. Appropriate neuroleptic and antidepressive medication (in dosages similar to those used in the nonretarded) may be used in treatment. Psychotherapy and active care and training aimed at alleviating the person's sense of worthlessness or modifying unrealistic goals may also be helpful. The use of psychotropic drugs in the absence of psychotherapy and environmental changes is *rarely* effective.

Behavior disorders are the most common reason for psychiatric referral and the most common psychiatric condition in institutionalized populations. Explosive outbursts, temper tantrums, and physically aggressive behavior usually are excessive responses to normal stresses; they are often situational, and precipitating factors usually can be found. Lack of training in socially responsible behavior, inconsistent discipline, and the reinforcement of faulty behavior are the major underlying causes of unacceptable behavior; brain damage and impaired ability to communicate are important predisposing factors. In institutional settings, overcrowding, understaffing, and lack of occupation are important aggravating factors, and the incidence of behavioral difficulties falls dramatically when living conditions are improved and proper training and occupation introduced.

Prevention

Genetic counseling provides parents with knowledge and understanding of the cause of retardation and the risk of recurrence. Siblings can learn of their own risk for having

a retarded child. Amniocentesis may detect inherited metabolic disorders, carrier states, and the presence or absence of CNS defects such as myelodysplasia and anencephaly. (Ultrasound also can identify these CNS defects.) Prenatal diagnoses permit the option of abortion and subsequent family planning. Amniocentesis is indicated in all pregnant women over age 35 yr because of their increased risk for having a child with Down's syndrome, as well as in women with a family history of mucopolysaccharidosis, galactosemia, Tay-Sachs disease, and maple syrup urine disease. (See also PREVENTION OF GENETIC DISORDERS in Ch. 203.)

The use of rubella vaccine has all but eliminated congenital rubella as a cause of MR. A vaccine is being sought for cytomegalovirus infection. Continuing improvements in obstetric and neonatal care, such as the use of exchange transfusion and Rho immunoglobulin to prevent hemolytic disease of the newborn (erythroblastosis fetalis), the regionalization of neonatal intensive care units, and improved knowledge and technology have further reduced the incidence of MR.

Treatment

Environmental factors can make a significant difference to the infant or child who is at high risk for developmental disabilities. Infants developmentally vulnerable because of a perinatal insult may overcome their vulnerability in a facilitating environment. Referral to an early intervention program during infancy may prevent MR.

As soon as retardation is confirmed or strongly suspected, the parents should be informed; whenever possible, they should be informed together. The findings of the various consultants must be coordinated and interpreted, and many hours spent discussing causes, impact, prognosis, and education and training with the parents. If the family physician cannot do this, the family should be referred to a center with a multidisciplinary team that evaluates and serves children with developmental disabilities; but the physician should plan to provide continuing medical care and advice.

A comprehensive, individualized program is developed with the help of appropriate specialists. Formal psychologic assessment may be deferred until age 3 yr unless the diagnosis is uncertain or the physician cannot assess the child's development himself. A neurologist should investigate all cases of moderate to severe retardation, progressive disability, neuromuscular deterioration, or suspected seizure disorders. Orthopedists, physical therapists, and occupational therapists should be included in evaluating and managing retarded children who have cerebral palsy or other major motor deficits. Speech pathologists and audiologists are helpful with major language delays or with a suspected hearing loss. Nutritionists, social workers, educators, ophthalmologists, psychiatrists, and dentists all can be helpful.

Family support and counseling are of major importance; however, realistic methods of caring for the child are paramount. Whenever possible the retarded child should attend a normal day-care center or a regular public school. Level of social competence is more important than IQ when evaluating an individual's handicap due to retardation. IQ and social competence are highly correlated at the lower end of the IQ scale, but with higher scores other factors such as the presence of physical handicaps, personality defects, other mental illness, and social factors are increasingly important in determining effective functioning and the need for care.

Every effort should be made to have the child live at home or in a community-based residence. Institutionalization should not be considered without extensive family discussion—the presence of a mentally retarded child in the home can be disruptive, but is rarely the primary cause of family discord. However, the family must have psychologic support and may need help with the burdens of daily care. This can be provided by such services as day-care centers, homemakers (trained nonprofessionals who come to the home to help with household chores and child care), and temporary foster homes. The retarded adult should be provided with long-term residence in apartment clusters, hostels, and nursing homes.

189. ACCIDENTS AND POISONINGS

ACCIDENTS

Accidents are the most common cause of death in childhood, killing more children than cancer, poliomyelitis, meningitis, congenital malformations, and heart disease combined. Even the infant under age 1 yr is at risk, with > 3000 deaths in this age group each year from falls, burns, drowning, and suffocation. Accidents are also the leading cause of child disability. For every accidental death, 100 children are seriously injured.

Accidents are due to a sequence of events, most of them preventable, and the child's curiosity is usually the catalyst. Accidents are more common when the child is hungry or tired (as before meals or naps); is being cared for by a mother substitute; is in new surroundings (a recent family move or vacation); or is hyperactive. Accidents are likely to occur when parents are ill or the mother is pregnant; when the marital relationship is poor; when parents are rushed and busy; or when parents do not anticipate the risks associated with each new level of development in their child.

Safety education for parent and child is the key preventive measure. Passive protection is not enough. The child must be protected from some hazards and taught to deal with those that are unavoidable. Parents need to be taught to avoid situations known to precipitate accidents. Preventive care includes safe storage of inedible materials; use of safety caps and containers; and using safety belts and safe car seats for children in automobiles (see below). Parents must set good safety examples (eg, wearing seat belts), since children mimic their parents' actions.

The physician aids accident prevention by educating parents, distributing safety information in his office, setting a good example himself, and anticipating potentially high-risk situations (suggesting that a mother who is occupied with the care of a sick child obtain appropriate help with her other children).

Prevention of Injury in Auto Accidents

Injury in auto accidents is a major cause of death among all age groups claiming 12/100,000 infants at 2 mo of age, 3/100,000 children aged 6 to 11 yr, and increasing even more during the adolescent years. Untethered children may be the only casualty of a sudden stop that causes no property damage or other personal injury.

To reduce the incidence and severity of human impact in a crash, all occupants should be restrained. State laws vary but most states now have child restraint laws. *A child held by a restrained adult is not safe as the adult cannot hold the child who will be thrown by tremendous force even at minimal speed* (10-lb child, traveling 30 miles/hour, would require the strength to lift 300 lb 1 ft off the ground). The unrestrained adult may also be thrown forward and crush the child against the interior of the car with a force equal to the adult weight × $(\text{speed})^2/2$.

Child restraints must be properly used to be effective. The child must be strapped into the restraint, which should be designed for his size and development. The entire restraint must be secured to the car according to manufacturer's instructions or it will only serve to facilitate the trajectory path of the child in a crash. Older children should be secured by seat belts in both front and back seats. The evidence of the effectiveness of car restraints at reducing trauma is undeniable.

There are a number of USDA-approved seats. Restraints that meet Federal Crash Standards are appropriately marked. A current list of approved models is available from Academy of Pediatrics or the National Safety Council. The infant seat, which is used facing the rear, is appropriate up to 15 lb wt. Restraints for children from 16 to 40 lb face forward and are equipped with shoulder restraints and lap guards and provide stability for the head as well.

Head Injury

A high percentage of deaths from trauma in childhood are due to craniocerebral trauma and its complications. Serious side effects on the developing nervous system often result in residual impairment, both physical and mental.

Head injury is the most common form of trauma for which children are admitted to the hospital. The greatest number of head injuries occur in children < 1 yr of age. Boys exceed girls as victims and injuries are predominantly due to falls in and around the home, although the single greatest cause is bicycle accidents. Falls from a height are a major cause of accidental death in urban children. A major campaign to prevent falls from windows in New York City produced a 96% decrease in these accidents in 1 yr.

The **clinical syndrome** will depend on the location and extent of the injury. The most frequent manifestations are minor trauma without unconsciousness, concussion, contusion, and fractures. Far more serious but infrequent are subdural and epidural hematomas. The history of the event and the time that follows is extremely important and the details should be meticulously gathered from family and witnesses. Time, type of injury, and patient's immediate response in terms of consciousness is critical to management. Minor head trauma without loss of consciousness and without neurologic signs may be associated with vomiting, pallor, irritability, or lethargy.

Concussion is *a transient and rapidly reversible state of neuronal dysfunction associated with a loss of consciousness immediately following the head injury*. Victims often have amnesia for the event and the time just prior to the event but have no neurologic signs.

Contusion is *the focal bruising or tearing of cerebral tissue accompanied by parenchymatous hemorrhage and local edema*. The neurologic signs depend on the focus, but the ventral surface of the frontal lobe and inferolateral aspects of the temporal lobes are the most common sites. There may be disturbances of strength and sensation and even an increase in intracranial pressure.

Linear skull fractures are important because they indicate the intensity of the trauma, but their significance for possible complications depends on their location and extent. Fractures across the middle meningeal artery, the sagittal sinus, the orbit, the sinuses, or the foramen magnum may be associated with neurologic signs. Leakage of spinal fluid or blood from the auditory or nasal passages or postauricular ecchymosis indicates a basilar fracture that is usually not visible on x-ray.

Depressed skull fractures require immediate intervention. Subdural hematoma, the collection of blood between the dura and the brain, may be either acute or chronic with symptoms and signs evolving over hours or days. Altered level of consciousness, symptoms and signs of intracranial hypertension, or a focal deficit are characteristic and require immediate surgical intervention. Chronic subdural hematoma develops slowly and treatment is controversial.

Treatment: Most children with mild head trauma can be observed at home by competent parents. Children with altered consciousness at time of examination, or with a history of unconsciousness for a period of time, those with a fracture, and those with focal or diffused neurologic findings should be observed in the hospital. If circumstances suggest possible child abuse, these children should also be observed (see Ch. 190).

Hospitalized children must be closely observed for level of consciousness, vital signs, and changing neurologic status, especially with focalization or lateralization of signs or pupillary changes. Most diagnostic studies are of little help in children although a CT scan is safest and provides the most information. It should be done if the status worsens.

Although nothing can be done to alter the primary damage, secondary brain dysfunction may lead to respiratory and circulatory failure. Brain swelling and intercranial hypertension with elevated intracranial pressure requires immediate

appropriate management to prevent further interference with O_2 delivery and cellular metabolism.

Special precautions are necessary to avoid cerebral edema as the immature brain of the infant and child are especially susceptible. Water intoxication due to overhydration may precipitate cerebral edema. Fluids therefore should be restricted to 75% of maintenance and should be given at a uniform rate over the 24-h period.

Change in level of consciousness is always important. When the patient has been unconscious throughout the observation period, vital signs become doubly important along with pupillary signs and deep tendon reflexes. In multiple trauma, it is important to remember that restless agitation may be due to a problem elsewhere (eg, hypoxia, pain elsewhere, or a full bladder). The possibility of cerebral hypoxia or shock from other causes in auto accidents, falls from great heights, or other multiple trauma should not be overlooked. Careful monitoring for hypoxia includes maintenance of a good airway and obtaining blood gases. When cyanosis or air hunger appear, the child is in serious trouble. Hypoxia also predisposes to cerebral edema.

If the child has normal blood gases and no evidence of an expanding lesion (epidural or subdural) and continues to deteriorate, hypertonic agents (eg, mannitol) may be indicated. Mannitol in a 20% solution, with a dose range of 1 to 3 mg/kg may be infused over 1 h. Glycerol, given in a 10% solution 1 to 1.5 gm/24 h orally is an alternative treatment when oral therapy is possible. It can be used in renal failure. Its effect on cerebral edema lasts 24 to 48 h and there is no apparent rebound. Although not universally effective for all causes of increased intracranial pressure, dexamethasone is usually effective in focal trauma. The effect is rarely evidenced before 12 h. In a child, 0.25 to 2 mg of dexamethasone or 1 to 10 mg methylprednisolone can be given IM q 6 h.

The belief that fixed dilated pupils, loss of oculovestibular reflexes, and decerebrate posturing are irreversible and untreatable led to suboptimal care. Early management directed toward maintaining adequate pulmonary gas exchange and brain perfusion will reduce risk of increased intracranial pressure and secondary complications.

Seizures occur in about 5% of children > 5 and 10% of those < 5 yr old during the first week post trauma. Early seizures have a more benign prognosis than those which occur later. Recovery depends on the age, duration of coma, and site of maximal trauma. Common problems during recovery include retrograde amnesia, behavior changes, sleep disturbances, and decreased intellectual ability. Functional recovery in most children is remarkably good. Of the nearly 5 million children who sustain a head injury each year, 4000 die and 15,000 require prolonged hospitalization. Of those with severe injury whose coma exceeds 24 h, 50% suffer major neurologic sequelae. Between 2 and 5% remain severely handicapped. (See also HEAD INJURY in Ch. 124.)

POISONING

Poisoning is still the most common cause of nonfatal accidents in the home, despite the many educational programs aimed at its prevention. In a case of ingestion where additional information is needed as to the contents of a trade name product or of the appropriate therapy indicated, the nearest Poison Control Center should be consulted.

The most common serious poisonings in children (acetaminophen, aspirin, caustics, lead, and hydrocarbons) are discussed here. (See also Ch. 289.)

ACETAMINOPHEN POISONING

Acetaminophen is *not* a "harmless" alternative to aspirin. Its toxicity has been well documented in the British literature since 1960. There are > 100 products sold OTC that contain acetaminophen. There are many childrens' preparations in liquid, tablet,

and capsule form. The measurement of toxicity is very different from aspirin and therefore, the treatment of overdose is different. Symptoms are usually mild until 48 h or later post ingestion.

The Cytochrome P 450 dependent enzyme system produces a potentially toxic metabolite of acetaminophen that is cleared by the hepatic glutathione stores under normal circumstances. In an acute overdose, excessive levels of the metabolite deplete the glutathione stores in the liver and hepatic necrosis results (see Ch. 72).

Acetaminophen in young children is rarely fatal, even when AST (SGOT) levels reach 20,000 IU/L. The reason for this age-related difference continues to be under investigation. Children > 12 yr appear to respond as adults to the hepatic challenge of acetaminophen. An increase in symptoms and a prolongation of abnormal liver functions have been observed in adolescents.

Acetaminophen overdose can be described in 4 stages:

Stage I (first few hours): No symptoms or symptoms of GI irritability occur within 12 to 24 h in 100% of patients with large ingestions.

Stage II (after 24 h): GI symptoms may diminish, but liver function tests become abnormal. AST (SGOT) and ALT (SGPT), bilirubin, and prothrombin time are elevated in that order.

Stage III (3 to 5 days): Levels of AST (SGOT), ALT (SGPT), bilirubin, and prothrombin time peak. Symptoms of hepatic failure appear.

Stage IV (after 5 days): Hepatic toxic reaction resolves or death from hepatic failure occurs.

A dose of ≥ 140 mg/kg in a child or > 10 gm in an adult is toxic.

Plasma half-life is 2½ h in normal dosage. A half-life > 4 h correlates with severe hepatocellular injury.

Treatment

The stomach is immediately emptied by emesis or lavage. Apomorphine 0.07 mg/kg or 0.03 mg/lb s.c. or IM may be used for emesis since its effect can be reversed with naloxone 0.4 to 2 mg s.c. or IM in adults or 0.01 mg/kg in children if vomiting persists and oral N-acetylcysteine cannot be retained. If the patient has ingested > 140 mg/kg of acetaminophen, acetylcysteine will be necessary. Activated charcoal should *not* be used, as it will impede the treatment.

At 4 h or later, post-ingestion, a plasma assay for acetaminophen should be obtained and compared to the Rumack-Mathew Nomogram (see FIG. 189–1). If the plasma level is below the possible risk zone and no toxic symptoms have developed, no medication is necessary. If the plasma level is above the possible risk zone (≥ 15 µg/mL plasma), a loading dose of acetylcysteine 140 mg/kg should be given *orally or by stomach tube* and the medication should be continued using 17 additional doses of 70 mg/kg at 4-h intervals; any doses vomited within 1 h should be repeated (some centers employ less than the total dosage).

Acetylcysteine is available as a 20% solution (200 mg/mL) in vials of 4, 10, and 30 mL and should be diluted 1:4 in a carbonated beverage or fruit juice before use. A 20-kg child would need a loading dose of 140 mg/kg = 2800 mg or 14 mL of 20% solution. This would require 56 mL of the 1:4 diluted solution. If 24 h have lapsed since ingestion, acetylcysteine is generally not to be used and supportive measures instituted appropriate to the magnitude of liver failure. If prothrombin time is 3 times normal, phytonadione 1 to 10 mg IM is given. Fresh plasma or clotting factor may be necessary. IV dextrose solution is given to maintain hydration. Forced diuresis may be harmful. Peritoneal or hemodialysis is ineffective beyond 10 h post ingestion.

Since antihistaminics, steroids, phenobarbital, and ethacrynic acid stimulate hepatic Cytochrome P 450 system activity, they should be avoided during the management of an acute acetaminophen overdose.

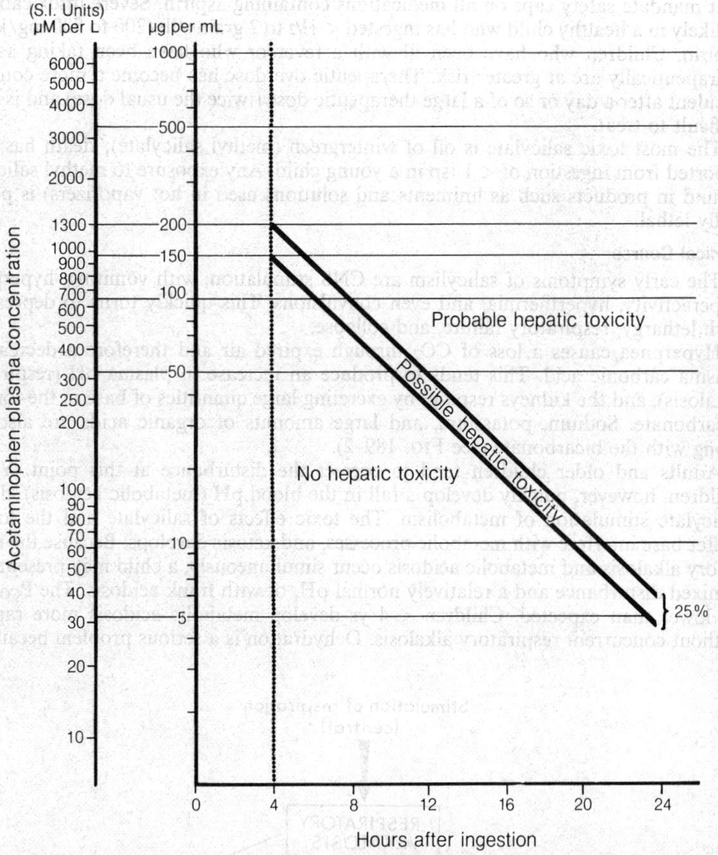

Fig. 189–1. Rumack-Matthew nomogram for acetaminophen poisoning. Semi-logarithmic plot of plasma acetaminophen levels vs. time. *Cautions for use of this chart:* (1) The time coordinates refer to time of ingestion. (2) Serum levels drawn before 4 h may not represent peak levels. (3) The graph should be used only in relation to a single acute ingestion. (4) The lower solid line 25% below the standard nomogram is included to allow for possible errors in acetaminophen plasma assays and estimated time from ingestion of an overdose. (Adapted from *Pediatrics* Vol. 55, No. 6, June 1975. Used with permission of *Pediatrics.*)

Residual structural and functional hepatic abnormalities do not occur following recovery from acute acetaminophen overdose in previously healthy individuals. The effects of chronic excessive use or repeated overdoses are still under study.

ASPIRIN AND OTHER SALICYLATE POISONING
(Salicylism)

One of the most common accidental poisoning is from ingestion of aspirin (acetylsalicylic acid). This is true even for children under age 5 yr despite safety packaging laws that limit the size of a bottle of infant aspirin to thirty-six 1¼-grain tablets, and

that mandate safety caps on all medications containing aspirin. Severe intoxication is unlikely in a healthy child who has ingested < 1½ to 2 grains/lb (200 to 300 mg/kg) of aspirin. Children who have been ill with a fever or who have been taking aspirin therapeutically are at greater risk. Therapeutic overdose has become a more common accident after a day or so of a large therapeutic dose (twice the usual dose) and is more difficult to treat.

The most toxic salicylate is oil of wintergreen (methyl salicylate); death has been reported from ingestion of < 1 tsp in a young child. Any exposure to methyl salicylate (found in products such as liniments and solutions used in hot vaporizers) is potentially lethal.

Clinical Course

The early symptoms of salicylism are CNS stimulation, with vomiting, hyperpnea, hyperactivity, hyperthermia, and even convulsions. This quickly turns to depression, with lethargy, respiratory failure, and collapse.

Hyperpnea causes a loss of CO_2 through expired air and therefore a decrease in plasma carbonic acid. This tends to produce an increase in plasma pH (respiratory alkalosis), and the kidneys respond by excreting large quantities of base in the form of bicarbonate. Sodium, potassium, and large amounts of organic acids are also lost along with the bicarbonate (see FIG. 189–2).

Adults and older children tend to correct the disturbance at this point. Young children, however, quickly develop a fall in the blood pH (metabolic acidosis), due to salicylate stimulation of metabolism. The toxic effects of salicylate and the loss of buffer base interfere with metabolic processes, and ketosis develops. Because the respiratory alkalosis and metabolic acidosis occur simultaneously, a child may present with a mixed disturbance and a relatively normal pH, or with frank acidosis. The P_{CO_2} will be lower than expected. Children < 4 yr develop metabolic acidosis more rapidly, without concurrent respiratory alkalosis. Dehydration is a serious problem because of

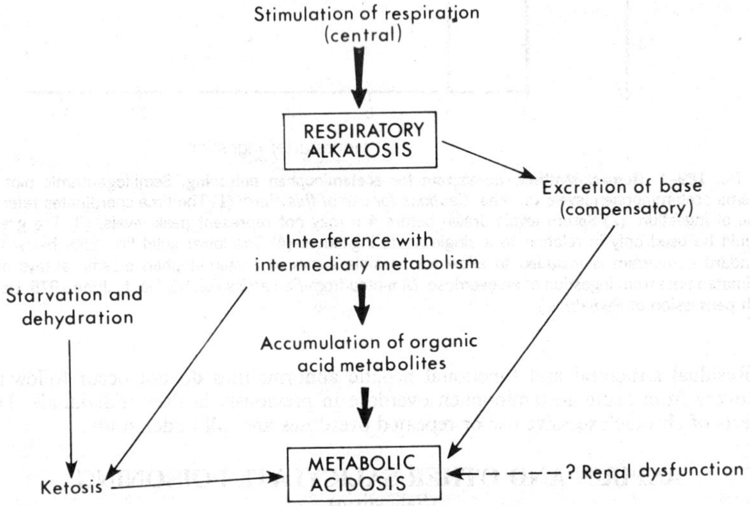

FIG. 189–2. Pathogenesis of acid-base disturbance in salicylate poisoning. (From "Drug Intoxication" by A. K. Done, in *The Pediatric Clinics of North America*, Vol. 7, No. 2, pp. 235–255, May 1960. Copyright W. B. Saunders Company, 1960. Used with permission.)

insensible water loss and increased renal water loss (from an increased urine solute load). Severe losses of sodium and potassium are not uncommon.

Laboratory Findings and Diagnosis

A useful qualitative screening test for salicylic acid is performed by adding a few drops of glacial acetic acid or 0.1 N hydrochloric acid to 1 mL of urine, followed by 3 drops of 10% ferric chloride solution. A burgundy red color appears and persists if salicylic acid is present (color may turn reddish brown in the presence of phenothiazines). A serum salicylate level can be obtained in most laboratories. Commercially available test strips may be used with urine as well as serum or plasma to determine the presence of salicylic acid. These tests react only with salicylic acid and therefore do *not* work on stomach contents or pills, but any salicylate is hydrolyzed in the body to salicylic acid and would be present as such in blood or urine.

Other laboratory tests to assist in assessment and treatment include blood pH, serum CO_2, or P_{CO_2} (any 2); serum sodium; serum potassium; BUN; blood glucose; and urine pH and sp gr. These determinations and the serum salicylate level should be followed serially during therapy.

The manifestations of salicylate toxicity are related to the peak level rather than the level of a given moment. For single-dose ingestions of salicylate, an estimate of the relative severity of the illness can be determined by use of a nomogram, provided the approximate time of ingestion and a single serum salicylate level are known (see FIG. 189–3).

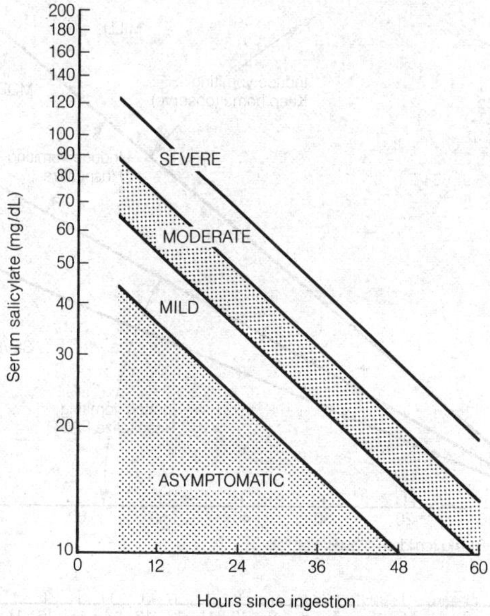

FIG. 189–3. Nomogram for estimating severity of salicylate poisoning at varying intervals in time, after ingestion of a single dose. (From "Salicylate Intoxication; Significance of Measurement of Salicylate in Blood in Cases of Acute Ingestion" by A. K. Done, in *Pediatrics,* Vol. 26, pp. 800–807, November 1960. Copyright American Academy of Pediatrics 1960. Used with permission of *Pediatrics.*)

Treatment

Early emptying of the stomach is critical and is best accomplished by giving ipecac syrup (see GENERAL PRINCIPLES OF TREATMENT in Ch. 289), unless the patient is comatose. The stomach should, however, be emptied even 6 to 8 h after ingestion. A cathartic such as sodium sulfate 5 to 10 gm orally is given to hasten the salicylate through the intestinal tract. A cathartic is not necessary in small children who have received ipecac, because ipecac has a cathartic effect on infants. A dose of activated charcoal (15 gm in 4 oz of water) should be given orally or by stomach tube. Oral administration of sodium bicarbonate is contraindicated, as it enhances the absorption of salicylate.

A general plan of treatment can be made by relating the patient's size to the dose taken and the serum salicylate level (see FIG. 189–4). Mild cases are treated with oral fluids alone; eg, milk or fruit juice hourly, up to 100 mL/kg in the first 24 h. Potentially severe cases are treated with IV fluids immediately. A hypotonic, polyionic solution containing 1 part 0.9% sodium chloride solution and 2 parts 10% D/W can be used before the serum salicylate level is known. The initial rate of administration is rapid (400 mL/sq m BSA or 15 mL/kg in the first hour) to restore hydration and establish renal blood flow. When shock is present, plasma or whole blood is also given (10 to 15 mL/kg in 1 h). After urinary output has been established, and if severe

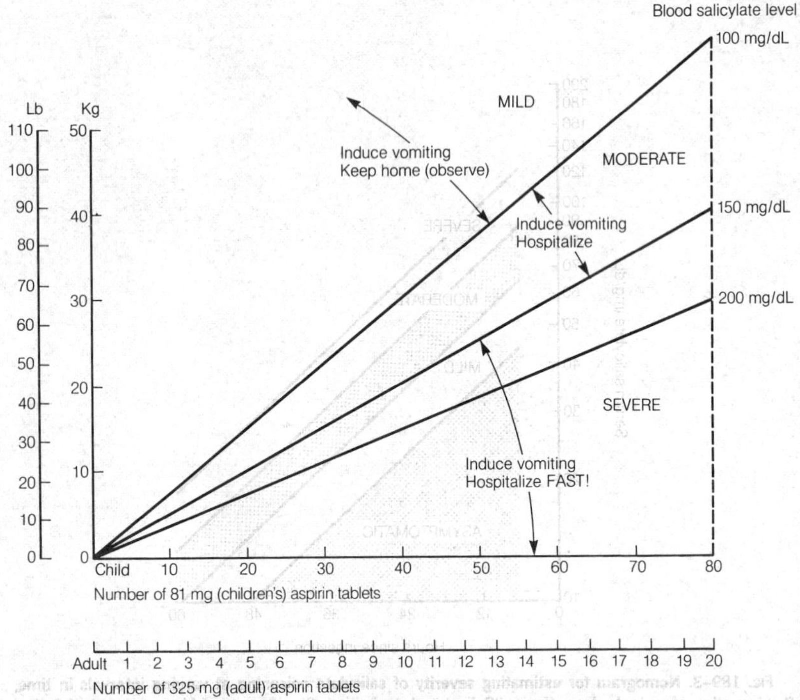

FIG. 189–4. Aspirin ingestion graph, relating severity of intoxication to the patient's size and the amount ingested. (Courtesy of University of Rochester School of Medicine, Department of Pediatrics.)

TABLE 189–1. SCHEDULE OF INTRAVENOUS FLUID ADMINISTRATION FOR SALICYLATE INTOXICATION

Condition	*Fluid*	*Rate*
Initial hydration	A	400 mL/sq m BSA in 1 h
If shock present	plasma or blood	10–15 mL/kg in 1 h, then fluid as for initial hydration
After urine flow established		
Mild or no acidosis	B	2.5–3.5 L/sq m BSA/24 h
Severe acidosis	C	3–5 L/sq m BSA/24 h
Additional urgent buffering of profound acidosis	sodium bicarbonate	3–5 mEq/kg in 2–4 h
	or, if acidosis unresponsive or Na restriction desired	
	Tromethamine	3–5 mL of 0.3 M soln in 1 h
	Determine further needs by blood pH measurement (< 7.18)	

Composition (mEq/L) and preparation of fluids

Fluid	*Na*	*K*	*Cl*	*HCO_3 or lactate*	*Preparation*
A	75	0	50	25	330 mL 10% D/W 170 mL 0.9% sodium chloride 14 mL 7.5% sodium bicarbonate (44.6 mEq/mL)
B	40	35	40	20	Electrolyte 75, Electrolyte 75 with 5% dextrose, Ionosol T with 5% dextrose
C	55	35	40	35	500 mL Fluid B 8.5 mL 7.5% sodium bicarbonate

Sodium bicarbonate should not be added until the pH is known, especially in children.

(Modified from "Treatment of Salicylate Poisoning," by A. K. Done and A. R. Temple, in *Modern Treatment,* Vol. 8, pp. 528–551, Aug. 1971. Used with permission of Lippincott/Harper & Row.)

acidosis is present, sodium bicarbonate can be given (3 to 5 mEq/kg IV in 2 to 4 h). However, children may not be severely acidotic (some adults become alkalotic). Thus, sodium bicarbonate may have a minimal effect on excretion. Potassium restoration is essential for successful alkalinization of the urine and excretion of salicylate (35 mEq/L potassium chloride solution is given IV at a rate of 2500 mL/sq m BSA/24 h or 100 mL/kg/24 h). See TABLE 189–1 for a summary of IV fluid administration.

Fever is controlled by tepid water (not alcohol) sponging. Vitamin K_1 (phytonadione) 25 mg/day IM or IV (CAUTION: *For IV administration, see Ch. 81*) in a single dose is given for bleeding due to hypoprothrombinemia, which is seen only rarely. Renal failure is rare; if it occurs, hemodialysis is indicated.

INGESTION OF CAUSTICS

Ingestion of strong acids and alkalies, causing burns and direct tissue damage, is not unusual. The most common sources of caustics are drain and toilet bowl cleaners and electric dishwasher detergents. Formerly sold as solids, these products are now also available in the more damaging liquid form, containing sodium hydroxide or sulfuric acid. With the solid products, the burning sensation of a particle sticking to a moist surface keeps the child from consuming much. Since the liquid preparations do not stick, more is easily consumed and the entire esophagus can be destroyed.

Clinical Course

Pain is immediate. The burned areas become edematous and swollen, dysphagia ensues, and secretions accumulate. Edema may obstruct the airway. The pulse is often rapid and weak. Respirations are shallow, and shock is common.

Patients who survive the initial insult may succumb to secondary infections, or the esophagus or stomach may be perforated after a week or more. Perforation into the mediastinum occurs acutely, with severe chest pain. Even with a benign early course, stricture can develop weeks later if the acute episode is untreated. Death can result from such complications as circulatory shock, asphyxia due to pharyngeal edema, perforation of the esophagus, or pulmonary irritation.

Treatment

All patients should be seen by a physician; most will require hospitalization.

Dilution of the chemical by drinking water is required immediately. A mild neutralizing solution of acid or alkali is *not* indicated, as it generates a heat-producing reaction. Milk, a demulcent, is preferred for children. It has the advantage of coating and soothing the mucous membranes and replacing tissue protein as the target of the destruction. However, milk can confuse the interpretation of findings at esophagoscopy performed within 30 min of giving milk. Contaminated clothing is removed and the contaminated skin is washed. Emptying the stomach by emesis or lavage is *contraindicated.*

The presence or absence of mouth burns is not an indication of whether or not the esophagus is burned. Endoscopy is indicated whenever caustics are ingested to be sure the esophagus is intact. In the presence of esophageal lesions, corticosteroid therapy is started (prednisone 60 mg/day, orally if possible, in 4 divided doses for 4 days, gradually decreasing the total dose over 2 to 3 wk and discontinuing when inflammation has cleared). A broad-spectrum antibiotic is given if there is fever or evidence of perforation. In mild cases, oral fluids are started early; otherwise, IV therapy is instituted until oral fluids can be tolerated. A tracheostomy may be indicated to provide an airway. If strictures are not prevented, subsequent dilation therapy will be required for months or years.

LEAD POISONING

Lead poisoning (plumbism) is a chronic disorder, sometimes punctuated by recurrent acute symptomatic episodes, that may result in chronic irreversible effects (eg, cognitive deficits in the child and progressive renal disease in adults). "High-dose" lead sources include repetitive ingestion of chips of lead pigment paint; retention of a metallic lead object (shot, curtain weight, fishing weight, bauble, etc.) in the stomach, where lead is slowly dissolved; contamination of acidic foods and beverages (fruits, fruit juices, cola drinks, tomatoes, tomato juice, wine, cider) by storage in improperly lead-glazed ceramic ware; burning of lead-painted wood in home fireplaces or stoves or of battery casings; folk medicines containing lead compounds; cottage industry manufactured items (lead-glazed ceramic ware, leaded glass, etc); illicit lead-contaminated whiskey, wine; inhalation of fumes of leaded gasoline; and occupational exposures without protection (respirator, ventilation, dust suppression). "Low-dose" lead sources, mainly lead-contaminated dust and soil, have been associated with asymptomatic increased lead absorption in children (see TABLE 189–2 for a classification of lead poisoning).

Symptoms, Signs, and Diagnosis

The risk of symptomatic plumbism increases with blood lead concentration **(PbB)** > 60 to 70 μg Pb/dL whole blood. When PbB is > 100 μg/dL whole blood, the risk of encephalopathy is great but unpredictable. In children, sustained PbB > 40 to 50

TABLE 189–2. LEAD POISONING CLASSIFICATION

Class	*Risk*	*Laboratory Findings (Whole Blood)*
I	Normal	PbB 5–29 μg/dL FEP < 49 μg/dL
II	Moderate	PbB 30–49 μg/dL FEP 50–109 μg/dL
III	High	PbB 50–69 μg/dL FEP 110–249 μg/dL
IV	Urgent	Asymptomatic PbB 70–100 μg/dL and/or FEP 250 μg/dL
V	Encephalopathy or impending encephalopathy: any symptomatic patient, or any patient with PbB > 100 μg/dL	

PbB = Whole blood lead concentration.
FEP = "Free" erythrocyte protoporphyrin.

μg/dL whole blood increases the risk of long-term cognitive deficits; these adverse effects may begin at PbB > 30 μg/dL whole blood.

In the adult, a characteristic sequence of symptoms may develop over several weeks or longer: personality changes, headache, metallic taste, anorexia, vague abdominal discomfort culminating in vomiting, constipation, and colicky abdominal pain. Encephalopathy is rare in adults. **In young children,** onset of clinical symptoms usually is abrupt with the appearance over 1 to 5 days of persistent and forceful vomiting, ataxic gait, seizures, alterations in consciousness, and, finally, intractable seizures and coma. These manifestations of acute encephalopathy are due primarily to cerebral edema and may be preceded by several weeks of irritability and decreased play activity. Brain abscess, brain tumor, acute encephalitis, and meningitis should be included in the differential diagnosis. In children, chronic plumbism should be included in the differential diagnosis of mental retardation, seizure disorders, aggressive behavior disorders, developmental regression, and persistent pica. Symptoms may abate spontaneously if excessive exposure is interrupted, only to recur with renewed exposure. A hypochromic, microcytic anemia may be present in both children and adults due to lead, concurrent iron deficiency, or both. Inhalation of tetraethyl- or tetramethyl-lead produces a different picture, with manifestations primarily of a toxic psychosis.

Definitive diagnosis requires measuring PbB. Another useful test that reflects lead exposure is the measurement of "free" erythrocyte protoporphyrin **(FEP)**; see Laboratory Findings in TABLE 189–2. FEP is a more sensitive indicator of metabolically active lead found in soft tissue and loosely found in bone. FEP is a direct measurement of the toxic effects of lead on heme synthesis. It is a good screening test for routine checks of at-risk children. Measurement of the total lead output in urine during the first day of chelation therapy is also highly useful. Diagnosis is confirmed if the ratio (μg Pb excreted/mg CaEDTA administered) exceeds 1. Blood and urine samples *must* be collected with "lead-free" equipment. To get reliable results, tests should be done by laboratories experienced in lead analysis. In acutely symptomatic cases chelation therapy usually must be begun before blood and urine lead data are available. Presumptive diagnosis can be made on the basis of bone marrow aspirates showing basophilic stippling in > 60% of normoblasts, urinary tests for coproporphyrin and δ-aminolevulinic acid, and, in the child, positive abdominal and long-bone x-ray films. Moderate glycosuria is suggestive.

Treatment

In acute lead encephalopathy (Class IV and V), combination treatment with dimercaprol **(BAL)** and edetate calcium disodium **(CaEDTA)**, according to the dosage schedule in TABLE 189–3, is recommended and should be started as soon as urine flow is established. This is maximum dosage and should not be continued beyond 5 days, to avoid depleting body stores of essential metals, particularly zinc. Dosages are preferably calculated in terms of BSA rather than body weight. In asymptomatic, or very mildly symptomatic, patients with confirmed PbB in excess of 70 to 100 μg/dL whole blood (Class IV), the regimen is modified as follows: Stop BAL after 48 h, but continue CaEDTA for an additional 48 to 72 h in reduced dosage of 1000 mg/sq m/day divided into 2 or 3 IM doses given at 8- to 12-h intervals. Patients receiving BAL should be given maintenance parenteral fluids or clear liquids orally to avoid the vomiting that BAL often causes. When PbB is 50 to 69 μg/dL whole blood (Class III), CaEDTA only is sufficient (TABLE 189–3). Brief courses of chelation therapy are usually associated with rebound in PbB, presumably due to internal redistribution of lead. This rebound often can be suppressed with oral D-penicillamine **(PCA)** instituted after a 2-day rest period following CaEDTA treatment. Prophylactic amounts of iron, zinc, and copper probably should be given to minimize depletion of these metals during long-term treatment with PCA.

TABLE 189–3. DOSAGE SCHEDULE FOR CHELATING AGENTS

	Combined BAL-CaEDTA*
Dosage:	BAL† 83 mg/sq m of BSA/dose (IM); CaEDTA‡ 250 mg/sq m of BSA/dose (IM)
Administration:	For the first dose, inject BAL (IM) only; beginning 4 h later and q 4 h thereafter for 5 to 7 days, inject BAL and CaEDTA simultaneously at separate and deep IM sites; rotate injection sites.
	CaEDTA Only
Dosage:	500 mg/sq m of BSA/dose q 12 h (IM).
Administration:	IM injection simpler in children, but if IV route preferred as in adults, infuse each dose over a 6-h period; allow 2 to 3 wk between each 3 to 5 day course of therapy.
	D-Penicillamine§
Dosage:	Up to 500 mg/sq m of BSA/day for long-term oral therapy.
Administration:	Give entire daily dose on empty stomach 2 h before breakfast; contents of capsule may be mixed in a small amount of chilled fruit or fruit juice immediately prior to administration.

* See text for critical aspects of supportive care and precautions with chelating agents.

† BAL (dimercaprol). The dosage recommended for adults by the FDA is 2.5 mg/kg body wt/dose q 4 h, which is equivalent to approximately 100 mg/sq m of BSA/dose, or about 20% higher than the dose recommended here for children.

‡ CaEDTA. Edetate calcium disodium, available in 20% solution. For IM use, add sufficient procaine to yield a final concentration of 0.5% procaine. IM injection is more convenient in children and permits better control of IV fluids, a vital consideration in cases of encephalopathy. If given IV in combination with IM BAL, infuse the total daily dose (1500 mg/sq m of BSA) over 24-h period and monitor ECG continuously.

§ D-Penicillamine (PCA), available in 250- and 125-mg capsules. Classified as an investigational drug by the FDA when used to treat lead poisoning; see recommendation of AMA Council on Drugs.

(Adapted from "Increased lead absorption and acute lead poisoning" by J. J. Chisholm, Jr., in Gellis and Kagan, *Current Pediatric Therapy* Vol. 9, 1980. Copyright 1980 by W. B. Saunders Company. Used with permission.)

CaEDTA followed by PCA may be of some benefit in children with confirmed PbB ≥ 50 μg/dL whole blood by reducing the time that the developing brain is exposed to excess lead; at lower PbB, treatment is mainly reduction in exposure and dietary improvement.

The use of combined BAL-CaEDTA treatment in acute lead encephalopathy is described in detail in the literature. CaEDTA is given IV or IM but is most effective as a continuous IV infusion over 6 h in a concentration < 0.5% in dextrose and water or 0.9% sodium chloride injection. The dose in severe cases is up to 1500 $mg/m^2/24$ h. The important points are: (1) Careful supportive therapy is just as vital to survival as chelation therapy. (2) BAL-CaEDTA treatment must be instituted promptly with the first dose of BAL preceding the first dose of EDTA by at least 4 h. BAL 75 mg/m^2 is given by deep IM injection and repeated q 4 h (maximum 450 $mg/m^2/24$ h). (3) Parenteral fluids are restricted to basal fluid requirements and a minimal estimate of replacement of deficits due to dehydration, protracted vomiting, or concurrent renal injury due to lead. (4) Adequate, but not excessive, urine flow must be established before CaEDTA can be given; mannitol may be necessary to accomplish this quickly. (5) Diazepam is used for initial control of seizures, and further control of convulsive activity is maintained with paraldehyde until the patient is improved. After this, long-term treatment with phenytoin may be instituted. Hypertonic solutions and surgical decompression to relieve intracranial pressure and reduce cerebral edema are *contraindicated.* (6) Attempts to evacuate residual lead from the lower bowel by enema are futile and the attendant delay can jeopardize a child's life. (7) It is judicious to hospitalize patients without clinical evidence of increased intracranial pressure (vomiting, altered state of consciousness) as incipient cases of encephalopathy; monitor parenteral fluids and urine output, and restrict oral intake during the initial 24 to 48 h of treatment. (8) Lumbar puncture is *contraindicated unless absolutely necessary for differential diagnosis.* Even then, only a few drops of CSF should be withdrawn *dropwise.*

Precautions in the use of chelating agents: EDTA is not metabolized; it is excreted unchanged exclusively by renal glomerular filtration. CaEDTA must be withheld in anuric patients. In the combined BAL-CaEDTA regimen, CaEDTA at the dosage level in TABLE 189–3 should not exceed 5 successive days; however, in very severe, slowly responsive cases of encephalopathy it may be given cautiously for no more than 2 additional days. The lower daily dosage of CaEDTA (1000 mg/sq m/day) advised for mildly symptomatic or asymptomatic cases is safer, but should not be used for more than 5 successive days with a rest period of 1 wk or more between courses. While the diagnostic CaEDTA test (1000 mg/sq m over 1 day only) is safe in asymptomatic persons, CaEDTA probably should not be given therapeutically in non–life-threatening situations when acute renal disease is present.

Serious reactions to CaEDTA include rising BUN, proteinuria, microscopic hematuria, shedding of renal tubular epithelial cells in urine, hypercalcemia, fever, and diarrhea. Renal toxicity, which is dose-related, is usually reversible. Side effects to CaEDTA are probably due to depletion of zinc. **PCA** is *contraindicated* in renal disease and penicillin sensitivity. Patients on PCA must be monitored weekly for side reactions (eg, diffuse erythematous rashes, angioneurotic edema, neutropenia, and proteinuria), which are reversible if the drug is stopped promptly. **BAL** should not be given in the presence of severe hepatocellular injury, but may be given cautiously early in oliguric, encephalopathic patients. BAL can induce moderate to severe acute intravascular hemolysis in patients with G6PD deficiency. Unlike CaEDTA and D-penicillamine, BAL may *not* be given concurrently with medicinal iron. Contraindications to the use of *any* chelating agent in asymptomatic persons include the concurrent presence of liver or kidney disease. In severely symptomatic cases the risks of chelation therapy must be carefully weighed. None of these drugs should be given for prophylactic purposes to lead work-

ers or when any patient is concurrently overexposed to lead, as they can cause a net increase in the absorption of lead present in the GI tract. *Long-term treatment requires reducing exposure to lead.*

IRON POISONING

Because of the wide distribution of iron **(Fe)** preparations, ingestion of Fe-containing products is a common potentially lethal pediatric problem. Elemental Fe has a toxic effect on the GI, cardiovascular, and central nervous systems. The oral lethal dose of elemental Fe ranges from 200 to 250 mg/kg but as little as 130 mg of elemental Fe has been fatal in children. There are > 100 commercial Fe preparations on the market; however, ferrous sulfate (20% elemental Fe), ferrous fumarate (33% elemental iron), and ferrous gluconate (12% elemental iron) are most widely prescribed. In general, up to 10 tablets in a child is associated with mild poisoning, up to 20 tablets with moderate toxicity, and > 20 tablets with severe poisoning. On the basis of body weight, 20 to 60 mg elemental iron/kg is mild-to-moderate toxicity, 200 to 250 mg/kg is life-threatening.

Establishing whether Fe has been ingested may be facilitated by abdominal x-ray, since Fe tablets are radiopaque. Gastric fluid, when tested with a solution of 30% hydrogen peroxide and distilled water, will produce color if Fe is present, ranging from light orange to dark red depending upon the amount of Fe.

Diarrhea, vomiting, leukocytosis, hyperglycemia and a positive abdominal radiograph are associated with serum Fe concentrations > 300 mg/dL. If any one of these findings are positive, the level will likely exceed 300. If no symptoms develop in the first 6 h, the patient is at minimal risk.

There are 4 characteristic stages of iron toxicity. In **stage I**, which occurs within 6 h, vomiting, explosive diarrhea, irritability, abdominal pain, seizures, lethargy, and coma may be present. Irritation of GI mucosa may lead to hemorrhagic gastritis. Tachypnea, tachycardia, hypotension, and metabolic acidosis may also occur when serum Fe levels are high. Shock or coma in the first 6 h is a grave prognostic sign. During **stage II** (within 10 to 14 h of ingestion), there is a latent period of up to 24 h of deceptive improvement. In **stage III** (12 to 48 h post ingestion), shock, hypoperfusion, and hypoglycemia may be present. Serum Fe levels may be normal. Elevated ALT (SGPT) due to liver damage, fever, leukocytosis, bleeding disorders, inverted T waves on the ECG, disorientation, restlessness, lethargy, convulsions, coma, shock, acidosis, and death may occur. There may be a **stage IV** 2 to 5 wk later if late complications due to pyloric, antral, or intestinal obstruction, hepatic cirrhosis, or CNS damage occur.

When possible, a serum Fe and an Fe-binding capacity should be determined promptly. If the serum Fe exceeds the Fe-binding capacity, there is a potential for systemic toxicity. If the serum Fe exceeds normal (110 μg/dL) but is < 350 μg/dL, it is highly unlikely that any free Fe exists, and the patient need not be hospitalized unless symptoms are present. If the serum Fe is > 350 μg/dL, or if symptoms are present, hospitalization is necessary.

The provocative chelation test can be performed to determine if any free Fe exists in the patient's blood. Deferoxamine 25 mg/kg (not > 1 gm) is given IM. Free Fe will be chelated by the deferoxamine and eliminated in the urine producing a reddish color, if the Fe level exceeds the Fe-binding capacity. A lack of reddish color in a symptomatic child is a false-negative reaction. Whenever the serum Fe is > 500 μg/dL, deferoxamine therapy should be started immediately.

Treatment

Initially, a vigorous effort to remove the Fe from the stomach should be initiated. If the patient is awake and alert, emesis should be induced with ipecac syrup; in the hospital, apomorphine can be used IM or s.c. Gastric lavage with a large bore tube can

be carried out with 5% sodium bicarbonate as the wash solution. The use of sodium dihydrogen phosphate solution (Fleet® enema diluted 1:4) has been recommended but has the risk of also producing hyperphosphatemia and hypocalcemia unless volumes are closely controlled and not > 100 mL used. If an x-ray still shows radiopaque tablets following emptying the stomach, the process should be repeated. Activated charcoal does not absorb Fe and should not be used.

Deferoxamine therapy should be instituted in (1) any patient with a serum Fe level ≥ 350 μg/dL and evidence of free Fe, (2) all patients with a serum Fe level ≥ 500 mg/dL, and (3) any patient with symptoms when blood Fe levels are not available. In a normotensive patient, the dose of deferoxamine is 1 gm IM regardless of the patient's age, followed by 1 gm q 4 to 12 h up to 6 gm/day depending on clinical signs and laboratory response to treatment. If the patient is hypotensive, the drug should be given IV not to exceed 15 mg/kg/h. In massive overdose this may not be adequate as 1 gm deferoxamine chelates only 85 mg of Fe. Peritoneal dialysis, hemodialysis, or exchange transfusion should be considered. Exchange transfusion is particularly effective and is important if renal shutdown develops. Follow-up for potential sequelae should be carefully planned at 2 to 6 wk post ingestion. There may be the paradox of Fe deficiency anemia due to GI blood losses and chelation of Fe stores. The corrosive effects on the GI tract are predominantly gastric and pyloric stenosis or stricture. Radiographs at 6 wk post ingestion including an upper GI series should be done.

Prognosis is good. Mortality is about 10% when shock and coma develop; overall it is about 2 to 3%.

HYDROCARBON POISONING

Every year the ingestion of petroleum distillates (eg, gasoline, kerosene, paint thinners) and halogenated hydrocarbons (eg, carbon tetrachloride, ethylene dichloride) is responsible for > 25,000 poisonings in children under age 5 yr. One fourth of all the deaths from accidental poisonings fall in this group. Viscosity and surface tension are the most important physical properties of these hydrocarbon derivatives, as they determine the degree of hazard of their aspiration—small quantities can spread rapidly over large surface areas of the lung. The lower the viscosity, the higher the risk of pulmonary aspiration, with certain additives contributing to other toxic effects. Mineral seal oil (used in products such as furniture polish) is the most dangerous of the more viscous of these liquids.

Clinical Course

Symptoms and signs relate chiefly to the respiratory system, GI tract, and CNS. Initially, the victim coughs and chokes, even with only one small taste. Cyanosis, breath-holding, and persistent coughing may then occur. Older children may complain of a burning sensation in the stomach, and vomit spontaneously. CNS symptoms include lethargy, coma, and convulsions. These effects are usually dose-related and are most severe with lighter fluid and mineral seal oil ingestions.

In animal experiments, hydrocarbon in the respiratory tract is 140 times more toxic than hydrocarbon in the GI tract. If this finding were applied to humans, death could occur with 350 mL in the stomach of a child or with only 2.5 mL in the lungs. In severe cases, cardiac dilation, atrial fibrillation, and fatal ventricular fibrillation may occur. Damage to kidneys and bone marrow has been described. When death occurs from pneumonitis, it usually does so within 24 h. Resolution of uncomplicated pneumonia takes about 1 wk, except when due to mineral seal oil ingestion, when it usually takes 5 to 6 wk.

Laboratory Findings

A chest x-ray is the single most important diagnostic test, and is obtained in all cases involving children under age 10 yr regardless of symptoms. The most severe cases have

visible x-ray evidence of hydrocarbon aspiration pneumonia within 2 h; 90% of all cases with pneumonia have positive films by 18 h; however, no new cases develop after 24 h. A WBC count, WBC differential, and urinalysis may help to identify secondary infection and renal involvement. Blood hydrocarbon levels have no practical value. If there are no signs (WBC, fever) or symptoms (tachypnea, tachycardia, cough or rales) within 8 h and chest film is negative, the patient may be discharged. When there is evidence of pulmonary involvement, determining arterial blood gas levels will aid both diagnosis and treatment.

Treatment

All children who ingest hydrocarbons should be seen by a physician at a hospital, since x-rays are needed and admission is frequently required.

Immediately, at home, any contaminated clothing is removed, and the child's skin is washed. A glass of milk (*never with mineral oil*) is given to dilute the ingested material and reduce stomach irritation. Water is immiscible with hydrocarbons.

Where the risk of CNS effects is high because of the type or volume of hydrocarbon ingested, gastric lavage may be performed *with extreme care to avoid aspiration*, using copious amounts of water. Following lavage, 30 to 60 mL of olive oil and a saline cathartic should be left in the stomach.

Early pneumonitis is chemical in nature and does not respond to antibiotics.

Supportive therapy with IV fluids and O_2 is appropriate. Corticosteroids generally are not effective. However, controlled studies have not been done with a large series of life-threatening cases, and corticosteroids may be appropriate in severe cases with a rapid onset of symptoms and x-ray findings of pneumonia.

When a hydrocarbon containing another poisonous substance is ingested, treatment must be directed at both poisons.

190. CHILD ABUSE AND NEGLECT

The physical or mental injury, sexual abuse, negligent treatment, or maltreatment of a child under the age of 18 by a person who is responsible for the child's welfare, under circumstances which indicate the child's health or welfare is harmed or threatened thereby. Physicians are required by law to report incidents wherein child abuse or neglect may be suspected in any child whom they examine or treat and are granted immunity from suit or liability for so reporting. The reports usually are made to a specifically designated agency of child protection.

Abuse and neglect of children are complicated problems of parent–child interactions that often coexist and may not be easily differentiated. Neglect probably occurs 10 to 15 times more frequently than abuse. All social classes and races contribute to these incidents. About 25% of cases occur in children under age 2 yr. Sexes are affected equally. The incidence is difficult to determine accurately, but more than a million children are involved annually. As many as 20% of physically abused children are permanently injured, and about 4000 deaths from abuse and neglect occur annually in the USA. Sexual abuse or molestation reporting has increased greatly, and presently is thought to involve 200,000 children yearly.

Etiology

Abuse generally is caused by the breakdown of impulse control in the parent or guardian. Four contributing factors are recognized: **(1) Parental personality features**: The childhood experience of the parent lacked affection and warmth, often included abuse, and was not conducive to the development of adequate self-esteem or emotional maturity. Lacking an early loving environment, abusive parents may look toward their

children as a source of the affection and support they never received. As a result, they may have unrealistic expectations of what their child can supply for them; they are frustrated easily and lose control, unable to give what they never experienced. Parents' use of drugs or alcohol may provoke them to impulsive and uncontrolled behaviors toward their children. Less commonly a parent may be frankly psychotic. **(2) A "different" child**: Irritable, demanding, or hyperactive children may provoke parents' tempers. Handicapped children, often more dependent and needing care, are susceptible. Premature or sick infants separated from parents early in infancy, and stepchildren or those biologically unrelated may not form adequately strong ties with their parents or guardians. Parents may have unrealistic expectations of what a child's performance should be and may punish him severely with little justification. **(3) Inadequate support**: Parents may be isolated, unprotected, and vulnerable in the absence of relatives, friends, neighbors, or peers who normally can provide physical and psychologic support in times of stress. **(4) A crisis**: Situational stress often may precipitate abuse, particularly at a moment when support is not at hand.

Neglect often is seen among multiproblem families with poorly organized lifestyles. Acute or chronic depression, especially maternal, is often present. Desertion by the father, himself inadequate or unable or unwilling to assert a controlling influence in the family, often may precipitate neglect. Drug or alcohol abuse by one or both parents frequently results in chronic impoverishment and a distortion of priorities in family life. Chronic medical problems of a parent may contribute.

Manifestations of Abuse

History: Features that are suggestive of abuse are (1) parental reluctance to give a history of injury; (2) an inconsistent history that may be at variance with the apparent stage of resolution of the injury and may vary dependent on the source of the injury; (3) history of injury that is incompatible with the developmental capability of the child; (4) an inappropriate response by the parents to the severity of the injury; and (5) delay in reporting the injury.

Physical: Skin lesions, such as ecchymoses, hematomas, burns, welts, and abrasions in various stages of development, are common (eg, round cigarette burns, arcuate bruises from extension cord whipping, symmetric scald burns of upper or lower extremities). Serious traumatic injury to the mouth, eye, internal abdominal organs, and CNS may produce permanent damage. Fractures may be single or multiple, and a skeletal survey may show bony injuries in varied stages of resolution. Metaphyseal fractures and subperiosteal elevations in long bones occur in infancy. Major diagnostic considerations in the examination are (1) multiple injuries at different stages of resolution or development; (2) cutaneous lesions specific for particular sources of injury; and (3) *repeated* injury, which is suggestive of abuse (or inadequate supervision).

Emotional: Emotional manifestations of abuse are less easily defined than are the physical signs. In infants failure to thrive (see above) is a common early observation. Inadequate parental stimulation and interaction with a small child often causes delays in development of social and language skills. Small children may be distrustful, superficial in interpersonal relationships, passive, and overly concerned with pleasing adults. The emotional impact on children usually becomes obvious at school age, when difficulties develop in forming relationships with teachers and peers. Often, emotional effects can be documented only when they improve after the child is placed in another environment.

Sexual abuse or molestation: Acts of adults upon children include exposure, genital manipulation, sodomy, fellatio, and coitus. The perpetrating adult may be unknown or unrelated, in which case the abuse is considered **rape** if vaginal penetration occurred. More often, the adult is biologically related or within the close circle of family, in which case the offense is termed **incest**. Where young children are involved the offense most often is nonviolent and repetitive, and may be covered over by collusive collabo-

ration within the family. Physical signs may include difficulty in walking or sitting, vaginal discharge or pruritus, recurrent UTIs, or a sexually transmitted infection. However, there may be no physical indications of injury, and the behavior of the child (irritability, fearfulness, insomnia, or other behavior problems) may be the only clue. Careful interviewing of the child may be the only means of adding necessary details. Older children may be threatened with physical injury by the offender if they "tell," and thus may conceal repeated assaults. Sexually transmitted disease of any sort in any child < 12 to 13 yr must be viewed as the result of sexual molestation until this is ruled out.

Manifestations of Neglect

Failure to meet basic physical needs: Inadequate provision of food, clothing, or shelter, despite available supportive community resources, is common (eg, malnutrition, fatigue, lack of hygiene or appropriate clothing). Desertion or death by starvation may occur in extreme cases. As many as ½ of infantile failure-to-thrive cases may be due to neglect.

Emotional deprivation: In early infancy, retardation of emotional growth may occur with blunting of affect and lack of interest in the environment. This commonly accompanies failure to thrive and is often misdiagnosed as mental retardation or physical illness. Signs in older children include poor school attendance and excessive home responsibilities.

Failure to meet health needs: Failure to seek preventive medical attention, such as immunizations and routine health supervision, and delay in seeking care for illness may be clues to inadequate family functioning.

Treatment of Abuse and Neglect

Providing care to involved families must be seen in long-range perspective, because the disturbed patterns of personal interaction are usually longstanding. In both abuse and neglect settings, *families should be approached in a helping rather than a punitive manner.*

A careful review of the family setting and of the parents' deficiencies and needs is essential diagnostically and is the first step in treatment. Hospitalization of the child (emergency temporary removal from the home) may be indicated, but usually is not required, and depends on how well rapport can be established with the parents. When hospitalization occurs, parents should be told that the studies to be undertaken will include discussions with them as well as the diagnostic tests on their child.

Social work consultation: Adequate understanding of the parents' backgrounds usually requires considerable review of medical records and of prior contacts with various community service agencies. If available, a social work consultant can provide valuable assistance in conducting such reviews and may help with interviews and family counseling.

Reporting to a social service or welfare department: When abuse or neglect cases are reported, a face-to-face conference should be held with a child protective services representative to assure clear understanding and help in planning management. The parents should be told beforehand by the physician that such a report is being made pursuant to the law.

Care planning: Many communities have a multidisciplinary team consisting of a social worker, psychiatrist, pediatrician, and others to provide diagnostic assistance and guidance in designing a treatment program. A source of primary medical care is fundamental and should be acceptable to both the family and the reporting physician. Periodic or ongoing social work contact usually is needed. Psychiatric assistance in understanding personality disorders and in dealing with specific conditions, such as depression, often is indicated.

Management of sexual molestation: Sex offenses of children may have lasting psychologic effects on the child's development and future sexual adaptations. Effects are more lasting and intense on older and teenage children. Counseling or psychotherapy of both the child and the adults concerned may prevent these effects.

Community care programs: Day-care centers for small children can relieve a mother under stress, allowing her a few hours each day for herself. Homemaker services can be arranged to give assistance. Parent aide programs, utilizing trained nonprofessional people to relate closely to abusing and neglecting parents, are being developed in some communities. "Parents Anonymous" groups also have been successful.

Temporary removal from the home: If the home setting carries a high risk to the child's health or if work with the family has not progressed, temporary removal may be indicated. Temporary removal on an acute basis should be strongly considered in cases of physical or sexual abuse when, after disclosure by the child, the child will be returning to a situation in which there will be contact with the suspected perpetrator(s), and other caretakers do not support the allegations of the child. Removal requires a court petition, presented by the legal counsel of the appropriate welfare department. The procedure varies from state to state, but usually entails family court testimony by a physician. When the court decides in favor of removing the child from the home, a disposition is arranged. The family's physician should participate in this disposition planning. If not, his agreement and consent to the disposition should be sought. While the child is in temporary placement, the physician should maintain contact with the parents and be assured that adequate efforts are being made to help them. He should also participate when the decision is made to reunite child and parents. As the dynamics of the family setting improves, it may be possible for the child to remain in the parents' care.

Follow-up: The families of abused and neglected children frequently relocate, making continuity of care very difficult. Broken appointments are common; outreach and home visiting by welfare workers or a public health nurse may be needed to keep all who are concerned aware of the patient's progress.

Prevention

Knowing which settings may cause abuse and neglect of children helps to identify certain at-risk families. Parents having their first baby and teenage mothers who may be rebelling against their parents are in the high-risk group. In addition, events during pregnancy, delivery, or early infancy that increase the risk of infant morbidity can weaken the parents' emotional ties to the infant (see also PARENT–INFANT BONDING: THE SICK NEONATE in Ch. 183). Therefore, throughout pregnancy, the neonatal period in the hospital, and early infancy, inquiries may elicit the parents' feelings about their own and each other's adequacies and about the baby's well-being. How well can they tolerate a small baby in the house? Does the father provide moral and physical support to the mother? Do they have relatives or friends who can help in times of need? If not, can help be arranged? The physician who is alert to the possibility of child abuse and neglect often can provide the guidance and support necessary to prevent these tragic health problems.

---

191. CHILDHOOD INFECTIONS

BACTERIAL INFECTIONS

DIPHTHERIA

An acute contagious disease caused by Corynebacterium diphtheriae, *characterized by the formation of a fibrinous pseudomembrane, usually on the respiratory mucosa, and by*

myocardial and neural tissue damage, secondary to an exotoxin. **Cutaneous diphtheria** lesions are also common.

Epidemiology

Three biotypes (*mitis, intermedius,* and *gravis*) of *C. diphtheriae* exist. Only toxigenic isolates produce exotoxin. Nontoxigenic organisms may produce symptomatic diphtheria, but the clinical course is usually milder than that caused by toxigenic isolates. Spread is chiefly by the secretions of infected persons, directly or via contaminated fomites. Sporadic cases usually result from exposure to carriers who may never have had apparent disease; cases occurring during an epidemic can usually be traced.

Cutaneous diphtheria can occur when any disruption of the integument is colonized by *C. diphtheriae*. Indigent adults living in an endemic area are particularly at risk, since poor personal and community hygiene contribute to the spread of cutaneous diphtheria. Skin diphtheria is not restricted to tropical zones. Large outbreaks have occurred in temperate climates.

Pathology

Ordinarily, the organisms lodge in the tonsil or nasopharynx and, as they multiply, toxigenic *C. diphtheriae* may produce exotoxins lethal to the adjacent host cells. Occasionally the primary site is the skin or mucosa elsewhere. The exotoxin also damages cells in distant organs, to which it is carried by the blood. Pathologic lesions are found in the respiratory passages, oropharynx, myocardium, nervous system, and kidneys.

The diphtheria bacillus first destroys a layer of superficial epithelium, usually in patches, and the resulting exudate coagulates to form a grayish pseudomembrane containing bacteria, fibrin, leukocytes, and necrotic epithelial cells. The membrane is formed in the wake of the spreading infection, and the areas of bacterial multiplication and toxin absorption are wider and deeper than indicated by the size of the membrane.

The myocardium may show fatty degeneration or fibrosis. Degenerative changes in the cranial or peripheral nerves occur chiefly in the motor fibers. Anterior horn cells and anterior and posterior nerve roots may show damage in severe cases, in direct proportion to the duration of infection before antitoxin has been given. The kidneys may show a reversible interstitial nephritis with extensive cellular infiltration.

Symptoms and Signs

The incubation period (1 to 4 days) and prodromal period (12 to 24 h) are among the shortest in bacterial diseases. Initially, the patient with tonsillar or faucial diphtheria has only a mild sore throat, dysphagia, a low-grade fever with an increased heart rate, and a rising polymorphonuclear leukocytosis. Nausea, emesis, chills, headache, and fever are more common in children.

The characteristic membrane is usually tonsillar, but may be found in other areas (eg, the nasopharynx); it is dirty gray, tough, and fibrinous, and may be firmly adherent so that removal causes bleeding. Depending on the duration of infection, the membrane may be punctate or extensive and yellow-gray or creamy. In small children, who may show no signs of illness until the disease is well established, a membrane is often present at the first examination. In older children and adults, complaints of sore throat and fatigue may antedate appearance of the membrane. Some patients never develop a membrane.

The disease may remain mild. When it progresses, dysphagia, signs of toxemia, and prostration become prominent. Edema of the pharynx and larynx obstructs breathing. If the membrane involves the larynx or the trachea and bronchi, it may partially obstruct the air passage or become detached and suddenly cause complete obstruction. The cervical lymph glands are enlarged. In severe cases, diffusion of exotoxin into the neck tissue may produce such edema that the patient appears "bull-necked." A serosanguineous nasal discharge, often unilateral, may appear if the nasopharynx is affected.

The lesions of **cutaneous diphtheria** are not morphologically specific. Any break in the skin can be secondarily infected with *C. diphtheriae*; lacerations, abrasions, ulcers, burns, and other wounds are potential reservoirs of the organism. The lesions occur most commonly on the extremities and if left untreated may become anesthetic due to local infiltration of the exotoxin. Cutaneous diphtheritic lesions usually also harbor Group A β-hemolytic streptococci, *Staphylococcus aureus*, or both. A pseudomembrane is uncommon. Concomitant nasopharyngeal infection with the same biotype occurs in 20 to 40% of the cases. Ocular infection with *C. diphtheriae* is rare and may be seen regardless of other cutaneous lesions.

Complications

Severe complications are especially likely when antitoxin is not given promptly. Myocarditis is usually manifest by the 10th to 14th day but can appear during the 1st to the 6th wk. Heart failure may follow; sudden death may occur. Insignificant ECG changes occur in 20 to 30% of patients. However, A-V dissociation, complete heart block, and ventricular arrhythmias are associated with a high mortality. Dysphagia and nasal regurgitation, from bulbar paralysis, may be seen in the 1st wk of illness; peripheral nerve palsies appear from the 3rd to the 6th wk. Spontaneous reversal is slow over many weeks. Myocarditis and palsies are not modified by corticosteroids or delayed administration of antitoxin.

Diagnosis

This is based on the clinical appearance of the membrane, pending confirmation by culture. Gram stain of the membrane may reveal gram-positive rods with metachromatic (beaded) staining in a typical Chinese-character configuration. Löffler's or tellurite medium is preferred for primary isolation of the organism, but it grows well on other artificial media. The laboratory should be notified that this now rare organism is suspected. Cutaneous diphtheria should be considered when a patient develops skin lesions during an outbreak of respiratory diphtheria.

Immunization

Active immunization should be given routinely to all children and all susceptible contacts (see IMMUNIZATION PROCEDURES THROUGHOUT CHILDHOOD in Ch. 182). For previously immunized contacts, a booster dose, adult type (Td), is sufficient.

Treatment

Symptomatic patients should be hospitalized in intensive care units. **Diphtheria antitoxin must be given early,** since the antitoxin neutralizes only toxin not yet bound to cells. In suspected cases, antitoxin must be given immediately upon clinical diagnosis, without waiting for culture confirmation. CAUTION: *Diphtheria antitoxin is derived from horses; hence, a skin test to rule out sensitivity should always precede administration* (see SERUM SICKNESS in Ch. 21). If, after 30 min, no erythema or a flat erythema < 0.5 cm in diameter appears about the site of the skin-test injection, administration of antitoxin may proceed. The dose ranges from 20,000 to 100,000 u. The amount given is decided empirically. Moderately symptomatic diphtheritic pharyngitis would require 20,000 to 40,000 u., while patients presenting with more severe symptoms or with complications would require larger doses.

Antitoxin may be given IM or IV. Doses above 20,000 u. may be added to 200 mL isotonic saline and given slowly IV over 30 to 45 min to facilitate delivery of the large volume.

An urticarial wheal in response to the skin test indicates sensitivity and mandates **extreme caution** in giving the antitoxin. The patient must first be desensitized with dilute antitoxin, given in graduated doses, as described in SERUM SICKNESS in Ch. 21. Epinephrine 1:1000 should be available for immediate injection of 0.3 to 1 mL s.c., IM, or slowly IV if untoward symptoms appear. In the highly sensitive patient, IV administration of antitoxin is **contraindicated.**

Supportive treatment is important, particularly with the complications of diphtheria. Bed rest is necessary, as are careful nursing with emphasis on nutrition, fluid intake, proper oxygenation, constant observation for signs that endotracheal intubation or a tracheostomy is needed, continuous monitoring for cardiac problems, and frequent examination for CNS complications. Since the membrane can easily be dislodged, tracheostomy is the preferred emergency airway. Eradication of the organism with antibiotics is important. Adults may be given procaine penicillin G 600,000 u. IM q 12 h for 10 days or enteric-coated erythromycin 250 to 500 mg or erythromycin ethylsuccinate 400 mg orally q 6 h for 7 days. Children weighing < 25 kg should receive procaine penicillin G 300,000 u. IM q 12 h or erythromycin 40 mg/kg/day (maximum 1 gm/day) orally or IV in 4 divided doses. Ampicillin is also effective—75 mg/kg/day in 4 divided doses for children or 250 to 500 mg orally q 6 h for adults. Clindamycin and rifampin have also been used.

Recovery from severe diphtheria is slow, and patients must be prevented from resuming activities too soon. Even normal physical exertion may harm the patient recovering from myocarditis.

Management of an Outbreak

1. Isolate and treat all **symptomatic patients** as described above until 2 throat (or skin, if appropriate) cultures are negative for *C. diphtheriae*. The cultures should be taken 24 and 48 h after cessation of antibiotics. If positive cultures persist after clinical recovery, re-treat for 10 days with erythromycin (2 gm/day orally in 4 divided doses for adults, 50 mg/kg/day for children). To avoid impaired absorption from food, use the enteric coated base or ethylsuccinate forms of erythromycin. With current antibiotic regimens, tonsillectomy is no longer indicated for eradication of persistent foci.

2. Submit all isolates of *C. diphtheriae* to the local health department for biotyping and toxigenicity determination. Nontoxigenic and toxigenic biotypes may coexist in a community.

3. For all **close contacts** of known diphtheria patients, obtain nasopharyngeal and throat cultures for *C. diphtheriae*. Examine the throat and integument; hospitalize *symptomatic* patients and treat as described above, pending culture reports. Confine *asymptomatic* contacts with positive throat cultures for *C. diphtheriae* **(carriers)** at home, without visitors, for the duration of therapy, and give erythromycin orally, 250 to 500 mg q 6 h for adults; 50 mg/kg/day in 4 divided doses for children. Do *not* give antitoxin to carriers. After 3 days of treatment, the "breadwinner" may resume work while taking antibiotics. *Recheck cultures after therapy*. Erythromycin treatment failures are usually due to failure to take the medicine rather than to drug resistance of the organism. Occasional resistance of *C. diphtheriae* to erythromycin has been recognized within the USA. Isolates from treatment failures should have antimicrobial sensitivities performed.

4. Update diphtheria immunization of **all contacts**, including hospital personnel; use adult type (Td) immunization.

5. Persons with negative cultures and full immunization may be presumed safe from both personal and public health standpoints.

PERTUSSIS
(Whooping Cough)

An acute, highly communicable bacterial disease, characterized by a paroxysmal or spasmodic cough that usually ends in a prolonged, high-pitched, crowing inspiration (the whoop).

Etiology and Epidemiology

The causative agent is *Bordetella pertussis*, a small, nonmotile, gram-negative coccobacillus. *B. parapertussis* closely resembles this organism; it causes **parapertussis,** which

may be clinically indistinguishable from pertussis, but is usually milder and less often fatal.

Transmission is by aspiration of *B. pertussis* sprayed into the air by a patient, particularly in the catarrhal and early paroxysmal stages. Transmission by contact with contaminated articles is rare. Patients usually are not infectious after the 3rd wk of the paroxysmal phase.

Pertussis is endemic throughout the world. In a given locality it becomes epidemic every 2 to 4 yr. It occurs at all ages, but about ½ of all cases occur before age 2, since infants usually have no protective antibodies. One attack does not confer natural immunity for life, but second attacks, if they occur, are usually mild and often unrecognized.

Symptoms and Signs

The incubation period averages 7 to 14 days (maximum, 3 wk). *B. pertussis* invades the mucosa of the nasopharynx, trachea, bronchi, and bronchioles, causing increased secretion of mucus, initially thin and later viscid and tenacious. The disease lasts about 6 wk and is divided into 3 stages: catarrhal, paroxysmal, and convalescent. The **catarrhal stage** begins insidiously, generally with sneezing, lacrimation, or other signs of coryza; anorexia; listlessness; and a troublesome, hacking nocturnal cough that gradually becomes diurnal. Fever is rare.

The cough becomes **paroxysmal** after 10 to 14 days. There are 5 to > 15 rapidly consecutive coughs followed by the whoop, a hurried, deep inspiration. After a few normal breaths another paroxysm may begin. Copious amounts of viscid mucus may be expelled (usually swallowed by infants and children but also occurring as large bubbles via the nares) during or following the paroxysms. Vomiting subsequent to paroxysms, or due to gagging on the tenacious mucus, is characteristic. In infants, choking spells (with or without cyanosis) may be more common than whoops.

The **convalescent stage** usually begins within 4 wk; paroxysms are not so frequent or severe, vomiting decreases, and the patient looks and feels better. The average duration of illness is 51 days (range, 3 wk to 3 mo). Paroxysmal coughing may be reinduced for months, usually by irritation from a URI.

The WBC count is usually between 15,000 and 20,000, but may be normal or as high as 60,000; there are usually 60 to 80% small lymphocytes.

Diagnosis

The catarrhal stage is often difficult to distinguish from bronchitis or influenza. Adenoviral infections and TB should also be considered in the differential diagnosis, since either can mimic the pertussis syndrome. Lymphocytosis of 70% or more in an afebrile or slightly febrile child over age 3 with a suspicious cough often suggests pertussis but does not distinguish from adenoviral pertussis-like syndrome. Cultures of nasopharyngeal specimens are positive for *B. pertussis* in 80 to 90% of cases in the catarrhal and early paroxysmal stages. Best results are obtained with small sterile cotton swabs on 28-gauge, zinc-coated wire passed through the nostril to the nasopharynx. Freshly prepared Bordet-Gengou or charcoal-agar medium, containing penicillin or cephalexin to inhibit overgrowth by other flora, should be used. Specific fluorescent antibody testing of nasopharyngeal smears is an accurate means of early diagnosis, but is not as sensitive as culture. Parapertussis is differentiated only by culture or by the fluorescent antibody technic.

Prognosis and Complications

Pertussis is serious in children under age 2; mortality is about 1 to 2% before age 1. The disease is troublesome but rarely serious in older children and adults, except in the aged.

The most frequent complications are respiratory, including asphyxia in infants. Bronchopneumonia and cerebral complications cause the majority of fatalities in in-

fants and young children. Bronchopneumonia is also a frequent complication in the aged, and may be fatal at any age. Interstitial emphysema, subcutaneous emphysema, and pneumothorax are infrequent consequences of the increased intrathoracic pressure during paroxysms. Bronchiectasis, particularly in debilitated children, and residual emphysema can result. Atelectasis may result when a mucus plug occludes a bronchiole. A primary tuberculous lesion may be extended by simultaneous occurrence of pertussis. Convulsions are common in infants but rare in older children. Hemorrhage into the brain, eyes, skin, and mucous membranes can result from severe paroxysms and consequent anoxia. Cerebral hemorrhage, cerebral edema, or toxic encephalitis may result in spastic paralysis, mental retardation, or other neurologic disorders. An ulcer of the frenum of the tongue may develop from lower incisor trauma during paroxysms. Umbilical hernia and rectal prolapse occasionally occur. Otitis media is frequent.

Prophylaxis

Active immunization: See IMMUNIZATION PROCEDURES THROUGHOUT CHILDHOOD in Ch. 182. **Passive immunization** is unreliable and is not recommended.

Oral erythromycin therapy (12.5 mg/kg qid) commencing during the incubation period and continuing for 14 days may abort the infection in contacts, but efficacy is not yet fully established.

Patients should particularly be quarantined from susceptible infants for at least 4 wk from onset of disease or until symptoms have subsided. If quarantine is uncertain or difficult, erythromycin estolate therapy (12.5 mg/kg orally qid) for 14 days usually eradicates nasopharyngeal carriage of the organism, thus diminishing infectivity to others; however, there is no recognized therapeutic benefit to the patient after the paroxysms have begun.

Treatment

Hospitalization is recommended for seriously ill infants because expert nursing care is important. Bed rest is unnecessary for older children with mild disease. Small, frequent meals are advisable. Parenteral fluid therapy may be required to replace salt and water losses if vomiting is severe. In infants, careful suction to remove excess mucus from the throat may be lifesaving, and tracheostomy or nasotracheal intubation is occasionally needed. O_2 should be given if cyanosis persists after removal of mucus. Seriously ill infants should be housed in a darkened, quiet room and disturbed as little as possible, since any disturbance can precipitate serious paroxysmal spells with anoxia. Close attention should be paid to the nutritional needs of the infant, since preexisting or developing malnutrition can contribute significantly to an adverse outcome.

Expectorant cough mixtures, cough suppressants, and mild sedation are of questionable value, and should be used cautiously or not at all. Adrenergic drugs such as theophylline or salbutamol, and corticosteroids have also been suggested for the treatment of severely ill patients; however, further controlled studies are needed to assess their effectiveness and potential hazards. Antibiotics should be used only for bacterial complications such as bronchopneumonia and otitis media.

OCCULT BACTEREMIA

Pathogenic bacteria in the bloodstream of young febrile children who have no apparent foci of infection and look well enough to be managed as outpatients. This disorder should be distinguished from sepsis, neonatal sepsis, and septic shock. (For children > 2 yr of age, see Ch. 6 and for neonates, see NEONATAL SEPSIS and NEONATAL MENINGITIS under NEONATAL INFECTIONS in Ch. 186.)

Etiology and Epidemiology

Occult bacteremia is caused by *Streptococcus pneumoniae* in 65 to 75% of cases and by *Hemophilus influenzae* type b in 15 to 25%; a variety of bacteria, including *Neisseria meningitidis* and *Salmonella* spp, cause the remainder.

Occult bacteremia is detected in about 3 to 4% of febrile infants between 1 and 24 mo of age. In most instances the children who look well enough to be managed as outpatients but who later are found to be bacteremic are < 2 yr of age; most cases occur in infants between 6 and 24 mo of age. Incidence does not vary with sex or race.

Symptoms and Signs

Occult bacteremia is most often associated with URIs, pharyngitis, or fever alone; however, the percentage of bacteremic infants with one of these complaints is very small. It is unlikely that a child with a temperature of < 38.5 C (101.3 F) is bacteremic. The risk of bacteremia increases with higher temperatures.

Diagnosis

Diagnosis depends on isolating bacteria from the blood. Cultures usually take 24 to 48 h to become positive and often are contaminated with microorganisms from the skin, but more rapid technics are not sensitive enough (latex particle agglutination tests and enzyme-linked immunoassays deserve further evaluation).

Nonspecific tests may help to determine the risk of a particular child's being bacteremic. In most bacteremic children the WBC is elevated and thus is sensitive; however, only about 10% of children with WBC counts of > 20,000/μL are bacteremic. Acute-phase reactants add little to the WBC count. Combining risk factors—eg, 1 to 24 mo of age, fever > 38.5 C (101.3 F) and high WBC count—helps, but at best identifies only 10 to 25% of infants with bacteremia.

Prognosis

Of the children who receive antibiotics before it is known that they are bacteremic, > 75% will be clinically improved and < 10% will have persistent bacteremia. In contrast, < 33% of children who do not receive antibiotics will be clinically improved and nearly 33% of those with *S. pneumoniae* bacteremia and 50% of those with *H. influenzae* bacteremia will still be bacteremic at the 2nd visit. The incidence of meningitis, however, is essentially the same in children who receive oral antibiotics as in those who do not.

Treatment

By the time it is determined that ambulatory patients are bacteremic, about 50% are already receiving oral antibiotics because about 50% of those in whom bacteremia is suspected have treatable foci of infection—usually otitis media or pneumonia.

Some authorities advocate treatment of infants between the ages of 6 and 24 mo with temperatures > 40 C (104 F) and WBC counts > 15,000 while awaiting the results of outpatient blood cultures. Others feel it is not necessary to start treatment if close observation can be guaranteed. In either case, careful observation and follow-up are essential.

URINARY TRACT INFECTION (UTI) IN CHILDREN

Significant bacteriuria in a child, either asymptomatic or with the manifestations of cystitis, pyelonephritis, or septicemia.

The urinary tract from the kidneys to the bladder is normally sterile, in spite of probable frequent contamination with colonic bacteria via the urethra. Mechanisms that maintain the tract's sterility include urine acidity and free flow, a normal empty-

ing mechanism, intact ureteral and urethral valves, and immunologic and mucosal barriers. Abnormality in any of these mechanisms and urinary stasis are major predisposing factors to UTI.

Etiology and Incidence

In abnormal urinary tracts many different organisms can cause infection, but in relatively normal tracts, the organisms usually are strains of *Escherichia coli* with specific attachment factors for transitional epithelium of the bladder and ureters. *E. coli* causes > 75% of UTI in all pediatric age groups. The remaining cases are due to other gram-negative enterobacteria such as *Klebsiella*, *Proteus mirabalis*, and *Pseudomonas aeruginosa*. Enterococci (group D streptococci) and coagulase-negative staphylococci such as *S. saprophyticus* are the most frequently implicated gram-positive organisms. Fungi and mycobacteria are unusual causes of UTI. Adenoviruses are implicated in a syndrome of hemorrhagic cystitis.

One to 2% of **newborns** develop UTI, and the male:female ratio is 5:1. The infections in males often are bacteremic. Predisposing factors include malformations and obstructions of the urinary tract, prematurity, indwelling catheters, and lack of circumcision; major renal abnormalities are present in 20 to 40% of newborns with UTI.

UTIs occur in 2% of **young children beyond the newborn period,** and in 5% of **school age children**. The female-to-male ratio rises with age and is > 10:1 beyond age 4 yr. Infections in females usually are ascending and not associated with bacteremia. The marked female preponderance is attributed to the shorter female urethra. Other predisposing factors in this age group include indwelling catheters, constipation, Hirschsprung's disease, and anatomic abnormalities of the urinary tract such as obstructions, neurogenic bladder, and ureteral duplications. Other associated risk factors include pinworms, IgA deficiency, diabetes, trauma, and, in **adolescents,** sexual intercourse. Five to 15% of school age children with UTI have renal anomalies that will require surgery; 30 to 40% have vesicoureteral reflux that will require antibiotic prophylaxis. The incidence of reflux varies inversely with age.

Symptoms and Signs

In **newborns,** symptoms and signs are nonspecific and often mimic those of neonatal sepsis. Poor feeding, diarrhea, failure to thrive, vomiting, mild jaundice, lethargy, fever, or hypothermia can suggest UTI.

Infants and toddlers also present with poorly localizing signs. Some children are asymptomatic and diagnosed on routine screening; others have symptoms referable to the GI tract (eg, vomiting, diarrhea, or abdominal pain). In **children > 2 yr,** the more classical picture of cystitis or pyelonephritis can be seen although, again, as many as 40% of UTIs may be asymptomatic. Symptoms of cystitis include dysuria, frequency, hematuria, urinary retention, suprapubic pain, urgency, pruritus, incontinence, foul-smelling urine, and enuresis. Symptoms of pyelonephritis include those of cystitis plus high fever, chills, costovertebral pain, and tenderness.

Diagnosis

Bladder urine is normally sterile but usually acquires some colonic and skin bacteria during passage through the urethra. The diagnosis of UTI requires demonstration of significant bacteriuria in a culture of properly collected urine.

Newborns and young children: Urine is best obtained by suprapubic aspiration or direct catheterization of the urinary bladder. Bagged specimens are reliable if negative, but a positive culture always should be confirmed with a repeat specimen, preferably suprapubic or catheterized. In **older children,** clean-voided urine specimens are acceptable, but the culture should be repeated prior to initiating antimicrobial therapy unless the signs are so obvious that immediate therapy is warranted. If the urine is obtained by suprapubic aspiration of the bladder, the presence of any gram-negative bacteria is significant, as is the presence of > 1000 coagulase-negative staphylococci/mL of urine.

In a catheterized specimen, > 10^3 colonies/mL usually are significant. Clean-voided specimens from males are significant with colony counts > 10^4; from females, with colony counts > 10^5. Repeating the culture improves the diagnostic accuracy of a positive result. Occasionally UTI may be present in spite of low colony counts, possibly due to prior antibiotic therapy, very dilute urine (sp gr < 1.003), or obstruction to the flow of grossly infected urine.

Urine should be cultured as soon as possible or stored at 4 C if a delay of > 10 to 20 min is anticipated. Urine is best cultured in blood agar plates and incubated 24 to 48 h at 37 C. The urine is streaked on the plates using quantitative bacteriologic loops. When urine is from a suprapubic aspirate or is catheterized, 0.001 mL *and* 0.1 mL should be cultured. Specimens from a bag, or clean-voided, are sufficiently cultured at 0.001 mL. For office bacteriology, culturing on blood agar plates is the procedure of choice, although kit methods such as the dipslide or filter paper are sensitive. Chemical tests for the presence of bacteria, such as the nitrite test, are useful for screening.

Microscopic examination of the urine is useful but not definitive. Pyuria (> 5 WBCs/high-power field in the spun urine sediment) usually indicates UTI, but is absent in 60% of culture-proven UTIs. The urine Gram stain can be a sensitive procedure for identifying UTI. The presence of one bacterium/oil immersion (1000x) field in an unspun urine, or > 100 bacteria in a spun urine sediment, correlates with the presence of > 10^5 bacteria/mL of urine.

Distinguishing upper from lower tract disease is not always clear-cut. When the child presents with high fever, costovertebral angle tenderness, and gross pyuria with casts, there is little doubt the child has pyelonephritis. However, when sensitive distinguishing technics (eg, bladder washout, concentrating ability, or the presence of antibody-coated bacteria) have been applied in research settings, many children with asymptomatic UTIs or with only symptoms of cystitis had upper tract disease. These specialized tests are not indicated in the usual clinical settings, but the physician should be aware that any child with UTI may have upper tract disease.

Treatment and Prognosis

The major goal is to preserve renal parenchymal function and to minimize acute morbidity. **All children with suspected UTI** should be examined for abdominal masses, enlarged kidneys, urethral abnormalities, costovertebral angle tenderness, and signs of lower spinal malformations. Force of the urinary stream may be the only clue to obstruction or neurogenic bladder. BP, height, and weight should be recorded. Hct, BUN, and creatinine should be checked in children with documented UTI.

In the newborn, blood and urine cultures should be obtained and treatment begun parenterally with ampicillin and an aminoglycoside in dosage appropriate for neonatal sepsis (see TABLE 186–4 in ANTIMICROBIAL THERAPY FOR NEWBORNS in Ch. 186). If blood cultures are negative, clinical response is good, and repeat urine culture 48 to 72 h into therapy is negative, an appropriate oral antibiotic such as ampicillin, amoxicillin, or a cephalosporin can be used to complete a 10-day course. Another urine culture should be obtained 7 to 10 days after the end of therapy. A poor response suggests either a resistant organism or an obstructive lesion, and warrants urgent evaluation.

Beyond the newborn period, children with UTI can be treated with oral antibiotics unless they have high fever, prominent signs of toxicity, or are vomiting, in which case parenteral treatment is indicated. The initial antibiotics of choice are ampicillin, amoxicillin, sulfisoxazole, trimetroprim/sulfamethoxazole **(TMP/SMZ)**, or a cephalosporin (see TABLE 191–1). These agents provide adequate coverage for *E. coli*. Children hospitalized with acute pyelonephritis and signs of sepsis should receive ampicillin and an aminoglycoside parenterally. Length of treatment for UTI is 10 to 14 days, although many children can be successfully treated with a short course of antibiotics; eg, amikacin 7.5 mg/kg IM in a single dose may achieve a cure rate and a recurrence rate

TABLE 191–1. ANTIMICROBIAL DRUG DOSAGES FOR URINARY TRACT INFECTION IN CHILDREN

Drug	*Daily Dose, Oral (mg/kg/day)*	*Daily Dose, Parenteral (mg/kg/day)*	*Dosing Interval (hr)*
Amikacin		15	8–12
Amoxicillin	30		8
Ampicillin	50	100	6
Carbenicillin		50–200	6
Cefadroxil	30		12
Cefamandole		50–100	6
Cefazolin		25–50	8
Cefotaxime		100	6
Cefoxitin		80–160	6
Ceftriaxone		50	12
Cefuroxime		75	8
Cephalexin	25–50		6
Cephalothin		40–80	6
Cephapirin		40–80	6
Gentamicin		3–5	8
Kanamycin		15	8
Methenamine hippurate	75		12
Methenamine mandelate	75		6
Nitrofurantoin	5–7		6
Sulfonamides	150		6
Tetracyclines*	25–50		6
Ticarcillin		100–200	6
Tobramycin		3–5	8–12
Trimethoprim/ sulfamethoxazole	6 TMP/ 30 SMX	6 TMP/ 30 SMX	12

* Tetracyclines should be avoided in children < 8 yr of age.

similar to 10 days of oral sulfisoxazole. Ampicillin, amoxicillin, TMP/SMZ, or cefadroxil for 1 to 3 days achieves similar results in uncomplicated cystitis. This approach appears promising but presently should not be used for treatment of recurrences.

In all children with UTI, urine should be recultured 2 to 3 days after start of therapy and again 7 to 10 days after stopping antibiotics to document efficacy of treatment. Failure to sterilize the urine after 48 h of antibiotics may be due to a resistant organism, an obstructive lesion, or poor compliance.

All children with diagnosed UTI should undergo evaluation of their urinary tract with an intravenous urogram **(IVU)** to search for major malformations, and a voiding cystourethrogram **(VCUG)** to detect significant reflux. Reflux of infected urine into the renal pelvis, or the presence of infected urine behind an obstruction, can lead to chronic pyelonephritis, renal scarring, poor kidney growth, and renal failure. The IVU can be performed at any time, but is recommended earlier in younger infants. The VCUG is best postponed 3 to 6 wk to allow the transient reflux usually associated with cystitis to resolve and thus obtain a more accurate evaluation of the competence of the ureterovesical valves. Some physicians postpone radiologic evaluation in girls > 3 yr old until after the 2nd UTI. Significant experience is accumulating with ultrasound and renal scans for evaluation of the upper tract.

Management of vesicoureteral reflux **(VUR)** should be based on the **grade** as defined by the International Reflux Study Committee. In grade I, the ureters only are involved; in grade II, the reflux reaches the calyces; in grade III, there is dilatation of the ureter and renal pelvis; in grade IV, the dilatation is increased and there is obliteration

of the sharp angle of the fornices; in grade V, there is gross dilatation of ureter, pelvis and calyces, with frequent absence of papillary impressions. Children with a normal radiologic evaluation or mild, grade I vesicoureteral reflux can be followed with periodic urine cultures. Those infants with grade II or III reflux are candidates for antibiotic prophylaxis. If grade IV or V reflux or a major renal anomaly is detected, formal urologic referral is indicated and surgery may be necessary (see Ch. 158).

Symptomatic or asymptomatic UTIs recur in about 50% of cases. The risk is increased in those with urologic abnormalities. Repeat urine cultures should be done 3 to 4 times during the 1st yr after diagnosis, and at least twice a year during the next 2 or 3 yr (or any time the child develops UTI symptoms).

Prophylactic antibiotics are indicated for children with Grade II or higher reflux to reduce recurrences and prevent kidney damage. Nitrofurantoin 2 mg/kg/day or TMP/SMZ (1 mg/kg/day of the TMP) is administered once daily, usually at night.

The overall prognosis for children with UTI is good. It is unusual for properly managed patients to progress to renal failure unless they have uncorrectable renal abnormalities.

ACUTE INFECTIOUS GASTROENTERITIS

(See also Ch. 57)

A syndrome of vomiting and diarrhea, caused by pathogenic microorganisms, that may lead to dehydration and electrolyte imbalance. Infants and children are more apt than adults to have gastroenteritis and its complications; 500 million cases occur annually in children worldwide. Incidence in the developed countries has decrease 100-fold since 1900, but acute infectious gastroenteritis is the leading cause of death in children < 4 yr old in underdeveloped and developing countries. Infectious diarrhea in neonates is discussed under NEONATAL INFECTIONS in Ch. 186.

Etiology

The causative agent usually is not identified in most clinical situations. However, **bacterial pathogens** can be identified by stool culture and those isolated most often are a variety of strains of *Escherichia coli*, *Shigella*, *Salmonella* (almost exclusively non-*S. typhi*), *Campylobacter jejuni*, and *Yersinia enterocolitica* in North America and *Vibrio cholera* in Asia. **Viral agents** implicated include enterovirus strains (echo-, polio-, coxsackie-), astroviruses, paroviruses, adenoviruses, and picornoviruses. The most common agent is human rotavirus, causing 40 to 50% of acute diarrhea in children requiring hospitalization (usually those < 36 mo old). Parvovirus-like particles have been isolated in epidemics of diarrhea in several communities.

Symptoms, Signs, and Diagnosis

The epidemiology and the duration, character, and frequency of vomiting and diarrhea in relation to the child's age may indicate the etiology and severity of the illness. More often than not, one or more members of the patient's family or close contacts have had symptoms recently of gastroenteritis or of a respiratory infection. Infants < 3 mo old may develop dehydration and electrolyte imbalance as early as 24 h after onset; those between 3 and 6 mo by 36 h; and those > 6 mo by 48 h. However, severe dehydration and metabolic acidosis may develop within 24 h of onset at any age if vomiting is intractable, diarrhea explosive, or fluid intake drastically reduced. Physical examination should exclude any extra-intestinal cause and determine the state of hydration. Lethargy, anorexia, fever, oliguria, and substantiated weight loss are signs of dehydration.

In older infants and overweight young children and when hypernatremia is present, some signs may not appear until dehydration is critical. These include warm, dry skin with poor tissue turgor, a sunken anterior fontanel, sunken eyes with absent tearing

(softened eyeballs are a late sign in severe dehydration), dry oral mucous membranes, weak or absent sucking, and lethargy. Five percent dehydration is usually accompanied by dry oral mucous membranes and the absence of tears, while 10% dehydration is characterized by sunken eyes, a sunken anterior fontanelle, and poor tissue turgor.

The Hct and serum electrolytes may reflect the state of hydration and electrolyte balance. Urinary sp gr helps assess the state of hydration, and microscopic examination of urine for bacteria determines whether or not a UTI (a common cause of symptoms similar to those of gastroenteritis) may be present. The WBC count does not usually help in the differential diagnosis or to assess the severity of the condition particularly when dehydration is present and the total WBC count rises due to hemoconcentration. A shift to the left in the differential WBC count, even under these circumstances, may indicate the presence of accompanying sepsis. Stool cultures may be useful to differentiate bacterial from viral gastroenteritis, and sensitivity studies may suggest specific antibiotic therapy in the severely ill. A Wright-, Gram-, or methylene blue-stained smear of a watery stool specimen usually shows abundant polymorphonuclear leukocytes when bacterial infection is present.

Treatment

Treatment of acute gastroenteritis has 3 purposes: (1) to replace and maintain fluids and electrolytes; (2) to control vomiting, diarrhea, and abdominal pain; and (3) to eliminate the infectious agent, if possible.

For the ambulatory patient, fluid and electrolyte balance is maintained by offering frequent small amounts of hypotonic fluids such as plain or sugar water; half-strength flavored gelatin products (red-dye–colored gelatins should be avoided because they may resemble blood when passed in diarrheal stools); apple or grape juice; decarbonated ginger ale, cola, or other soda beverages; and hypotonic electrolyte solutions ordinarily used for parenteral administration (eg, a solution of 5% dextrose and 0.2% sodium chloride solution [2 gm sodium chloride/L] or 34 mEq/L each of Na^+ and Cl^-, and containing potassium [20 mEq/L] and lactate, citrate, or bicarbonate [30 mEq/L]). Unboiled skim milk or dilute formula can be added to the diet as the symptoms subside. Gradual return to a full diet in 3 or 4 days usually is possible.

Most hospitalized patients require IV fluid therapy; oral fluids are usually withheld to place the GI tract at rest. In enterotoxigenic diarrhea due to *V. cholera* and some strains of *E. coli*, an oral glucose–electrolyte solution (sodium chloride 2.5 gm, sodium bicarbonate 2.5 gm, potassium chloride 1.25 gm, glucose 25 gm, and water to make 1 L) should be given ad lib.

Antiemetics and preparations designed to absorb water, give bulk to the stool, and diminish diarrhea are not particularly effective. Anticholinergics, diphenoxylate, and paregoric are *contraindicated* for most infants and young children because of their side effects. In children > 5 yr old paregoric 0.1 to 0.25 mL/kg orally q 3 to 4 h will reduce cramping and the frequency of bowel movements.

Antibiotics should be reserved for *E. coli* epidemics in the hospital (neomycin 100 mg/kg/day orally in 3 divided doses for 3 to 5 days) or for severe cases of shigellosis when it is known that local strains are frequent invaders and susceptible to ampicillin (50 mg/kg/day orally in 4 divided doses for 4 to 5 days). Amoxicillin should not be used as an alternative to ampicillin. Trimethoprim/sulfamethoxazole (10/50 mg/kg/day orally in 2 or 3 divided doses for 4 to 5 days) can be used in ampicillin-resistant shigellosis. *Salmonella* gastroenteritis should *not* be treated with antibiotics, since the course of the disease is not affected, fecal excretion of the organism is prolonged, and the emergence of resistant strains is enhanced. However, when salmonella invade the bloodstream or become localized in extra-intestinal sites, ampicillin (100 to 300 mg/kg/day) or chloramphenicol (25 mg/kg/day for infants and 50 to 100 mg/kg/day for children) is given in divided doses q 6 h IV dependent upon in vitro

susceptibility tests. Infants < 6 mo old and T-cell deficient children should be treated in this way even without evidence of sepsis or extra-GI localization. *Yersinia* gastroenteritis usually subsides without antibiotic therapy. *V. cholera* gastroenteritis should be treated with tetracycline (50 mg/kg/day orally in 4 divided doses for 3 days). *Campylobacter jejuni* enterocolitis severe enough to require hospitalization should be treated with erythromycin (30 to 50 mg/kg/day orally in 3 divided doses for 7 days).

For discussion of infant botulism, see Ch. 57.

PERIORBITAL AND ORBITAL CELLULITIS

Infections that primarily affect children, cause acute swelling and redness of the eyelid and surrounding skin **(periorbital cellulitis)** *or of the eyelid and orbital contents* **(orbital cellulitis)**, *progress rapidly, and can result in serious systemic and ocular complications.*

Etiology and Incidence

Periorbital and orbital cellulitis can result from an external focus of infection (eg, a wound or insect bite), an internal source of infection (eg, sinusitis), or seeding from bacteremia. *Hemophilus influenzae* type b can be isolated from the blood of about 33% of patients who have no evidence of trauma or another external focus of infection. The most common pathogens associated with external foci are *Staphylococcus aureus* and *Streptococcus pyogenes*, but these are seldom isolated from the blood. In general, a bacterial pathogen is isolated from < 50% of the patients with periorbital cellulitis.

Periorbital cellulitis occurs much more frequently (85 to 90% of patients) than orbital cellulitis (10 to 15%). Periorbital cellulitis occurs commonly in children < 5 yr of age, while orbital cellulitis is more frequent in children > 5 yr.

Anatomy and Pathophysiology

The orbit is a conical cavity bounded by the paranasal sinuses. The floor of the frontal sinuses forms the roof of the orbit, the lateral walls of the ethmoid sinuses form the medial wall, and the roof of the maxillary sinus lies just below the floor of the orbit. The orbital contents are separated from the eyelids and protected anteriorly by the orbital septum. The orbital septum or palpebral fascia is a membranous extension of the periosteum, which is attached to the entire margin of the orbit and extends to the levator palpebra superior in the upper lid and to the tarsal plate in the lower lid. The orbital septum helps prevent infection from spreading from the eyelids to the orbit.

Periorbital and orbital cellulitis most often result from direct extension from infected ethmoid sinuses or local cutaneous infections. Extension of the infection is aided by the extensive venous network around the eye. These veins do not have valves, so infection can spread in either direction. Local inflammation can also result in venous or lymphatic obstruction that gives rise to swelling distant from the site of actual infection.

Symptoms and Signs

Swelling and redness of the eyelids are usually the first signs of periorbital or orbital cellulitis. Involvement is unilateral > 90% of the time, and signs of trauma or local infection can be found in about 33% of patients. Most children have fever; about 20% have nasal discharge and another 20% have conjunctivitis. Chemosis can be seen with only preseptal involvement, but ophthalmoplegia, proptosis, eye pain, or decreased visual acuity indicate orbital disease.

Complications: The most common complications of orbital cellulitis are central retinal artery or retinal vein thrombosis, and retinal damage secondary to ischemia caused by increased intraocular pressure. Intracranial complications, which occur when the infection is not contained within the orbit, include epidural, subdural, or cerebral abscesses, cavernous sinus or cortical vein thrombosis, or bacterial meningitis.

Diagnosis

The eye must be examined, to evaluate the position of the globe, eye movement, and visual acuity. Since lid swelling frequently makes it necessary to use lid retractors in order to evaluate the globe, it is best to consult an ophthalmologist whenever possible. TABLE 191–2 summarizes the findings in patients with periorbital cellulitis and varying degrees of orbital involvement. The direction of proptosis may be a clue to the location of the infection; eg, extension from the frontal sinus pushes the globe down and out, and extension from the ethmoid sinus pushes the globe laterally and out. If examination of the eye fails to demonstrate proptosis, ophthalmoplegia, or decreased visual acuity, the major question becomes whether an external focus of infection can be found. If there is no evidence of local injury or infection, an infection of the sinuses should be sought. Blood cultures yield pathogens in 20% of patients, but other laboratory tests are not particularly helpful. Roentgenographs of the sinuses are useful for diagnosing sinusitis in children > 1 yr of age, but generally do not differentiate preseptal from postseptal involvement. When orbital involvement is suspected, CT scanning can best assess sinus involvement, subperiosteral elevation, and intraorbital abscess formation, and should be done as soon as specimens for culture have been taken and antibiotics begun.

Differential diagnosis of swelling and erythema of the eyelid includes trauma, insect bites, allergy, and tumor. Other inflammatory diseases (eg, hordeolum, dacrocystitis, dacroadenitis, and conjunctivitis) can usually be distinguished by location and appearance.

Treatment

Children with periorbital or orbital cellulitis should be hospitalized and treated promptly. An ophthalmologist and otolaryngologist should be consulted early, in case surgical drainage is necessary. With an obvious external focus of infection, gram stain and cultures of exudate or subcutaneous aspirate should be obtained and an antibiotic begun that treats both *S. aureus* and *S. pyogenes*. With no obvious external focus of infection, blood cultures should be obtained and therapy for *H. influenzae* type b and *Streptococcus pneumoniae* begun. In an infant < 1 yr of age with no external focus of infection, a lumbar puncture should be performed. Aspirates of cellulitis should be obtained if this can be done without violating the orbital septum. Since usually it is difficult to be sure there is no external focus of infection, it is best to obtain specimens for culture and begin antibiotics (chloramphenicol with nafcillin or cefuroxime alone) that effectively treat *H. influenzae* type b as well as gram-positive aerobes. When CNS involvement is suspected, chloramphenicol with nafcillin will provide adequate antibacterial coverage until culture results are known.

TABLE 191–2. FINDINGS IN PERIORBITAL AND ORBITAL INFECTIONS

Infections	*Lid Swelling and Erythema*	*Ophthalmoplegia*	*Proptosis*	*Visual Acuity*
Periorbital cellulitis	+	–	–	Normal
Orbital cellulitis	+	+	+	±
Subperiosteal abscess	+	+	+	Abnormal
Orbital abscess	+	+	+	Abnormal
Cavernous sinus thrombosis	+	+	+	Abnormal

+ = present; – = absent.

(Modified from "Management of the child with a red and swollen eye" by D. W. Teele, in *Pediatric Infectious Diseases* 2:258–262, 1983. Copyright © by The Williams and Wilkins Company, 1983. Used with permission.)

IMPETIGO; ECTHYMA

Impetigo (impetigo contagiosa): *A superficial vesiculopustular skin infection.* **Ecthyma:** *An ulcerative form of impetigo.*

Etiology, Symptoms, Signs, and Diagnosis

A Group A β-hemolytic streptococcus **(GABHS)** has been the most frequent cause of pyodermas (superficial skin infections), but there has been a marked shift, with *Staphylococcus aureus* now much more common than GABHS as the initial cause. A staphylococcus is the primary pathogen in bullous impetigo wherever it may occur on the body and crusted impetigo of the face; its role in ecthyma varies in different parts of the world. An upsurge of furuncles and several more serious staphylococcal infections have also been recognized. Purulent infections of the ears or nostrils may be the source of staphylococci, but cutaneous staphylococci seldom come from the nose or throat. Spread of untreated infection to others is often suspected, but deliberate experimental infections are difficult to induce.

The arms, legs, and face are more susceptible to impetigo and ecthyma than are unexposed areas. Both impetigo and ecthyma may follow superficial trauma with a break in the skin; or the infection may be secondary to pediculosis, scabies, fungal infections, other causes of dermatides, or insect bites. Impetigo may occur on normal skin, especially on the legs in children. Lesions vary from a pea-sized vesicopustule to large, bizarre, circinate ringwormlike lesions. In impetigo, the lesions caused by *S. aureus* progress rapidly from maculopapules to vesicopustules or bullae to exudative and then honey-colored, crusted, circinate lesions. Ecthyma is characterized by small, purulent, shallow, punched-out ulcers with thick, brown-black crusts and surrounding erythema. Itching is common, and scratching may spread the infection. **Diagnosis** is usually based on clinical findings.

Prognosis

Neglected infection in adults can result in cellulitis, lymphangitis, or furunculosis. In children, untreated erythematous lesions may persist for months. Pigmentary changes with or without scarring may result.

Prompt recovery usually follows appropriate treatment. Acute glomerulonephritis in children, but not acute rheumatic fever, may follow cutaneous infection with a GABHS (however, nephritis is less common because strains of streptococci that are nephrogenic are now less prevalent). Ecthyma penetrates more deeply than impetigo and therefore results in ulceration with subsequent scarring.

Treatment

Systemic antibiotics are clearly superior to the present topical antibacterials. Local treatment is usually unnecessary, but tap-water compresses can be used for debridement. Because most cases are now caused by penicillinase-producing staphylococci, cloxacillin or a first-generation cephalosporin is the drug of choice. Penicillin-sensitive patients should receive cephalexin for 10 days—125 mg qid for children, 250 mg qid for adults—because erythromycin-resistant staphylococci are becoming more frequent (10 to 40%) and erythromycin is less effective in treating these staphylococcal infections. Most streptococci are sensitive to erythromycin but rarely to tetracycline. In pure staphylococcal pyoderma a penicillinase-resistant penicillin (eg, cloxacillin 125 mg qid for children or 250 mg qid for adults) should be given for 10 days.

In secondary impetigo, the underlying condition must also be treated.

INFECTIOUS MYRINGITIS

(See Ch. 206)

OTITIS MEDIA

(See Ch. 206)

ACUTE MASTOIDITIS

(See Ch. 206)

ACUTE EPIGLOTTITIS

(Supraglottitis)

A severe, rapidly progressive infection of the epiglottis and surrounding tissues that may be quickly fatal because of sudden respiratory obstruction by the inflamed structures.

Etiology and Incidence

Hemophilus influenzae type b is almost always the pathogen; very rarely, streptococci may be responsible. The incidence of *H. influenzae* type b epiglottitis is highest in children aged 2 to 5 yr; the disease is uncommon in children < 2 yr, but it may occur at any age.

Pathophysiology

Infection, acquired through the respiratory tract, may produce initial nasopharyngitis. Subsequent downward extension produces a supraglottic cellulitis with marked inflammation of the epiglottis as well as the vallecula, the aryepiglottic folds, the arytenoids, and the ventricular bands. Bacteremia is common. The inflamed epiglottis mechanically obstructs the airway; the work of breathing increases and CO_2 retention and hypoxia may result. Clearance of inflammatory secretions is also impaired. These combined factors may result in fatal asphyxia within a few hours.

Symptoms and Signs

Onset frequently is acute and fulminating. Sore throat, hoarseness, and, usually, high fever develop abruptly in a previously well child. Dysphagia and respiratory distress characterized by drooling, dyspnea, tachypnea, and inspiratory stridor develop rapidly and cause the child to lean forward and hyperextend the neck. On physical examination the child may appear moribund or restless and in severe respiratory distress. There are deep suprasternal, supraclavicular, intercostal, and subcostal inspiratory retractions. Breath sounds may be diminished bilaterally and rhonchi may be heard. The pharynx is usually inflamed.

H. influenzae type b pneumonia, occasionally with empyema, may occur concurrently with epiglottitis. Metastatic infection to the joints, meninges, pericardium, or subcutaneous tissues that results in an abscess or cellulitis may occur, though infrequently.

Diagnosis

The patient should be hospitalized immediately whenever the diagnosis is ***suspected*** *clinically*. Direct visualization of the epiglottis is diagnostic, but manipulation may initiate sudden, fatal airway obstruction. Visualization should be attempted *only* by designated trained personnel with equipment to establish an airway if necessary. If direct laryngoscopy confirms the diagnosis by revealing a "beefy" red, stiff, and edematous epiglottis, an artificial airway should be placed immediately. The type of airway may depend on the expertise of the staff, but endotracheal tubes are generally associated with fewer complications. *H. influenzae* type b may then be cultured from the upper respiratory tract and, usually, the blood.

The major differential diagnostic concern is acute **viral croup** (laryngotracheobronchitis). Croup is usually less fulminant in onset, and its characteristic barking cough is uncommon in epiglottitis. The epiglottis in croup may be erythematous, but is not markedly edematous and crimson as in epiglottitis. **Lateral and anteroposterior neck x-**

rays will differentiate the two, showing subepiglottic narrowing and a normal-sized epiglottis in croup and, in epiglottitis, an enlarged epiglottis and distention of the hypopharynx. **Bacterial tracheitis** (pseudomembranous croup) may also cause acute onset of dyspnea, fever, and stridor. It is characterized by a thick, exudative membrane that covers the larynx and that may be observed on x-ray or seen directly. **Diphtheria** (see in this chapter, above) should be considered in an unimmunized patient.

Treatment

Speed is vital. A continually adequate airway must be assured, and specific parenteral antibiotics given. Sudden complete airway obstruction occurs so unpredictably that an airway must be secured immediately, preferably by nasotracheal intubation. Alternatively, tracheostomy may be performed. Each institution should have a predetermined protocol for the emergent care of such children that involves the pediatrician, otolaryngologist, and anesthesiologist. Careful and skilled nursing care is required, since secretions can cause obstruction even after intubation or tracheostomy. The nasotracheal tube is usually required only until the patient has been stable for 24 to 48 h (usually a total intubation time < 60 h). The inflammation is effectively controlled with parenteral antibiotics. Chloramphenicol 75 to 100 mg/kg/day IV in 4 divided doses should be used initially, since ampicillin-resistant *H. influenzae* type b organisms are common. Rarely, *H. influenzae* type b strains resistant to chloramphenicol have been isolated. Where this has occurred, both chloramphenicol and ampicillin therapy should be started. If the organism is isolated and proves to be ampicillin-sensitive, ampicillin 200 mg/kg/day IV in 4 divided doses can be given. Some strains are resistant to both ampicillin and chloramphenicol; in this case, a 3rd-generation cephalosporin or cefuroxime may be used. Sedatives should be *avoided.*

ADENOID HYPERTROPHY

Enlargement of adenoidal tissue due to lymphoid hyperplasia.

Adenoidal lymphoid hyperplasia occurs in children and may be physiologic or secondary to infection or allergy. Consequent obstruction of the eustachian tubes may result in recurrent acute, chronic, or secretory (serous) otitis media; obstruction of the choanae may cause chronic sinusitis, mouth breathing, a hyponasal voice, and purulent rhinorrhea. Chronic adenoiditis is common.

Treatment

Adenoidectomy is frequently indicated in persistent serous and chronic otitis media to reduce exacerbations of chronic otitis media and improve the results of tympanoplasty. Adenoidectomy for recurrent acute otitis media depends on the duration of the earache after antibiotic is initiated, the presence of spontaneous perforation, the frequency with which myringotomy is required, and the severity of systemic symptoms. Adenoidectomy for nasal obstruction depends on the severity of the obstruction and the patient's age, since lymphoid hyperplasia reaches its maximum at puberty. Purulent rhinorrhea or sinusitis that recurs or persists despite adequate antibiotic treatment in otherwise normal children may be corrected by adenoidectomy.

RETROPHARYNGEAL ABSCESS

Retropharyngeal abscesses usually occur in infants or young children as complications of suppurative retropharyngeal lymph nodes to which infection has spread from the pharynx, sinuses, adenoids, nose, or middle ear. These abscesses are unusual in adults because the retropharyngeal lymph nodes diminish or disappear after childhood. Occasional causes in adults or children are TB or perforation of the posterior pharyngeal wall by foreign bodies or instrumentation.

The major manifestations are painful swallowing, fever, cervical lymphadenopathy, and, if airway obstruction occurs, stridor, dyspnea, and hyperextension of the neck. The cervical vertebrae cannot be palpated through the posterior pharyngeal wall, which is boggy and fluctuant, with a definite, usually unilateral, bulging. Widening of the prevertebral space can be demonstrated on lateral radiographs of the neck. **Complications** include hemorrhage; rupture of the abscess into the airway, causing asphyxia or pulmonary aspiration; laryngeal spasm; mediastinitis; and suppurative thrombophlebitis of the internal jugular veins.

Treatment includes draining the abscess through an incision in the posterior pharyngeal wall and giving penicillin G 150,000 u./kg/day IV in 4 equal doses for 3 to 4 days; then orally for a total of 14 days, unless culture and sensitivity studies of the drained abscess material indicate use of an alternate antimicrobial agent.

VIRAL INFECTIONS

(For a condensed review of differential diagnoses of the more common exanthems, see TABLE 191–3)

MEASLES

(Rubeola; Morbilli; Nine-Day Measles)

A highly contagious acute disease characterized by fever, cough, coryza, conjunctivitis, eruption **(Koplik's spots)** *on the buccal or labial mucosa, and a spreading maculopapular cutaneous rash.*

Etiology and Epidemiology

Measles is caused by a paramyxovirus and is spread largely by droplets from the nose, throat, and mouth of a person in the prodromal or an early eruptive stage of the disease, or by airborne droplet nuclei. Indirect spread by uninfected persons or by objects is unusual. The communicable period of the disease begins 2 to 4 days before the rash appears and continues during the acute stages. The virus disappears from nose and throat secretions by the time the rash clears. Persons who develop mild desquamation following the rash are no longer infectious.

Measles and chickenpox appear to be among the most readily transmitted of all infectious diseases. Before widespread immunization programs began, measles epidemics occurred every 2 or 3 yr, with small localized outbreaks during intervening years. In recent years in the USA, age-specific attack rates have shifted; outbreaks now occur frequently in teenagers and young adults, with sporadic cases in infants and young children. An infant whose mother has had measles receives transplacental passive immunity lasting most of the first year of life; thereafter, susceptibility is high. One attack of measles confers lifelong immunity.

Symptoms and Signs

After a 7- to 14-day incubation period, typical measles begins with prodromal fever, coryza, hacking cough, and conjunctivitis. The pathognomonic **Koplik's spots** appear 2 to 4 days later, usually on the buccal mucosa opposite the lst and 2nd upper molars. These spots resemble tiny grains of white sand surrounded by an inflammatory areola. If they are numerous, the entire background may be a mottled erythema. Pharyngitis and inflammation of the laryngeal and tracheobronchial mucosa develop. Characteristic multinucleated giant cells appear in nasal secretions, pharyngeal and buccal mucosa, and, often, urinary sediment.

The characteristic rash appears 3 to 5 days after onset of symptoms, usually 1 to 2 days after the Koplik's spots appear. It begins in front of and below the ears and on the side of the neck as irregular macules that soon become maculopapular and spread rapidly (within 24 to 48 h) to the trunk and extremities, at which time they begin to

fade on the face. Petechiae or ecchymoses may be present with particularly severe rashes.

At the peak of the illness, the temperature may exceed 40 C (104 F), and periorbital edema, conjunctivitis, photophobia, a hacking cough, extensive rash, and mild itching are present. Leukopenia with a relative lymphocytosis is usual. The constitutional symptoms and signs parallel the severity of the eruption and vary with the epidemic. In 3 to 5 days, the fever falls by lysis, the patient feels more comfortable, and the rash begins to fade rapidly, leaving a coppery-brown discoloration followed by desquamation.

Atypical measles syndrome (AMS) is commonest in adolescents and young adults and is usually associated with prior immunization using the original killed measles vaccines, which are no longer available. However, live, attenuated measles vaccine administration has also been known to precede development of AMS, perhaps as a result of inadvertent inactivation due to improper storage. Presumably, inactivated measles virus vaccines do not prevent wild virus infection and can sensitize patients so that disease expression is altered significantly. AMS may begin abruptly, with high fever, toxicity, headache, abdominal pain, and cough. The rash may appear 1 to 2 days later, often beginning on the extremities, and may be maculopapular, vesicular, urticarial, or purpuric. Edema of the hands and feet may occur; pneumonia and hilar adenopathy are common, and nodular densities in the lungs may persist for 12 wk or longer. Moderate to severe abnormalities in the ventilation/perfusion ratio in the lungs may result in significant hypoxemia.

Prognosis and Complications

Measles has a low mortality rate and is usually benign unless complications ensue. Pneumonia (especially in infants), otitis media, and other bacterial infections are common. Patients with measles are highly susceptible to streptococcal infection. Measles causes transient suppression of delayed hypersensitivity, leading to a transient reversal of previously positive tuberculin and histoplasmin skin tests, and sometimes to worsening of active TB or reactivation of latent mycobacterial infection. An exacerbation of fever, change in blood count from leukopenia to leukocytosis, and development of malaise, pain, or prostration suggest a complicating bacterial infection.

Acute thrombocytopenic purpura, at times with severe hemorrhagic manifestations, may complicate the acute phase of measles.

Encephalitis occurs about once in 600 to 1000 cases. It usually occurs 2 days to 3 wk after onset of the exanthem, often beginning with high fever, convulsions, and coma. Although in most instances the CSF lymphocyte count is between 50 and 500/μL and the protein level is increased, a normal CSF at the time of initial symptoms does not rule out encephalitis. The course may be brief, with recovery in about a week, or may be prolonged and terminate in serious CNS impairment or death.

Measles virus is also associated with **subacute sclerosing panencephalitis (SSPE)**, which is discussed in this chapter, below. SSPE is a previously unexplained chronic brain disease of children and adolescents that occurs months to years (usually years) after an attack of measles, causes intellectual deterioration, convulsive seizures, and motor abnormalities, and is usually fatal. Measles virus has been identified in brain tissue by electron microscopy, demonstration of measles antigen through fluorescent antibody technics, and isolation of the agent from brain biopsies.

Diagnosis

Typical measles may be suspected in a patient with coryza, photophobia, and evidence of bronchitis, but before the rash appears a definite diagnosis can be made only by identifying Koplik's spots. These, followed by high fever, malaise, and the rash with its characteristic cephalocaudal progression, establish the diagnosis in most cases. The virus can be grown in tissue culture, and serologic tests are available.

TABLE 191–3. DIFFERENTIAL DIAGNOSIS OF

Condition	Incubation (days)	Period of Communicability	Symptoms and Signs
Measles (Rubeola)	7–14	From 2 to 4 days before appearance of rash until 2 to 5 days after onset	Koplik's spots; fever, coryza, cough, conjunctivitis, photophobia, usually mild pruritus
Rubella (German measles)	14–21	Shortly before onset of symptoms until rash disappears; infected newborns are usually infective for many months	Malaise, fever, headache, rhinitis; postauricular & suboccipital lymphadenopathy, with tender nodes
Roseola infantum (Exanthem subitum)	Probably 5–15	Unknown	Infants & preschool children affected. Characteristic disappearance of high fever & simultaneous appearance of rash
Erythema infectiosum (Fifth disease)	Probably 5–10	Undetermined	Low-grade fever, occasional arthalgias
Chickenpox (Varicella)	14–21	From a few days before onset of symptoms until all crops of vesicles have crusted over	Moderate fever, headache, malaise, occasional sore throat
Infectious mononucleosis	10–50	Undetermined	Malaise, headache, fever, sore throat, splenomegaly, generalized lymphadenopathy
Scarlet fever (Scarlatina)	3–5 (Occasionally slightly shorter or longer)	Usually from 24 h before onset of symptoms until 2 to 3 wk thereafter, or even longer if complications occur (eg, sinusitis, otitis media)	Sore throat, chills, fever, headache, vomiting; strawberry tongue; cervical lymphadenopathy; circumoral pallor, rapid pulse
Drug rash	History of use of drug	None	Variable, including fever, malaise, arthralgia, nausea, photophobia, pruritus

THE MORE COMMON EXANTHEMS

Eruption			*Laboratory Findings*
Site	Character	Onset; Duration	
Starts around ears, on face, neck, spreading over trunk & limbs. Limbs escape in mild cases	Maculopapular; brownish-pink in color & irregularly confluent in severe cases or even petechial. Discrete in mild cases	3 to 5 days after onset of symptoms; lasts 4 to 7 days	Granulocytic leukopenia. Virus in blood & nasopharynx
Face, neck, & spreading to trunk & limbs	Fine pinkish macules which become confluent & often scarlatiniform or pinpoint on 2nd day	1 or 2 days after onset of symptoms; lasts 1 to 3 days	WBC count usually normal or slightly reduced. Virus in blood and nasopharynx
Chest & abdomen, with moderate involvement of face & extremities	Either diffuse macular or maculopapular	On about 4th day; rash appears as temperature drops suddenly to normal; lasts 1 to 2 days	Granulocytic leukopenia
Starts on cheeks, spreads to arms, legs, trunk	Maculopapular; often blotchy or reticular	Shortly after onset of symptoms; lasts 5 to 10 days; may recur for several weeks	Mild lymphocytosis & eosinophilia
Usually 1st on trunk, later on face, neck, extremities; infrequently on palms & soles	Lesions discrete; progress from macule to papule to vesicle to crusting; appear in crops, hence these various stages of development are present simultaneously	Shortly after onset of symptoms; lasts a few days to 2 wk	Presence of virus in vesicle fluid
Most prominent over trunk	Occurs in about 15% of cases, as a morbilliform, scarlatiniform, or vesicular rash	Appears 5 to 14 days after onset of illness; lasts 3 to 7 days	Positive heterophil antibody test; leukocytosis with atypical enlarged lymphocytes ("mononucleosis"); appearance of antibodies to Epstein-Barr virus
Face, neck, chest, abdomen, spreading to extremities. Entire body surface may be involved	Diffuse pinkish-red flush of skin, blanching on pressure & with Schultz-Charlton blanching reaction	On 2nd day; lasts 4 to 10 days	Granulocytosis; throat culture positive for β-hemolytic streptococcus, erythrogenic-toxin producing
Generalized; sometimes restricted to exposed surfaces	May be morbilliform, scarlatiniform, erythematous, acneform, vesicular, bullous, purpuric, or exfoliating	Variable	Agranulocytosis may be present; test urine for drug

Differential diagnosis of typical measles includes rubella, scarlet fever, drug rashes, serum sickness, roseola infantum, infectious mononucleosis, adenovirus, and echo- and coxsackievirus infections. Distinguishing features of rubella include its mild course with few or no constitutional symptoms, enlarged (and usually tender) postauricular and suboccipital lymph nodes, low fever, normal blood count, usual absence of a recognizable prodrome, and short duration. Scarlet fever may be suggested at first by the pharyngitis and fever, but the leukocytosis of scarlet fever is absent. Koplik's spots, the severe cough, and the characteristic rash of measles clarify what might be a difficult diagnosis. Drug rashes (eg, from phenobarbital or sulfonamides) resemble the measles eruption, but the typical prodrome, cough, and cephalocaudal progression of the rash are absent and the palms and soles are more likely to be prominently involved. Here, even more than usual, the history is important. Roseola infantum produces a skin rash similar to that of measles, but is seldom seen in children over age 3. It can usually be differentiated by its high initial temperature, absence of Koplik's spots and malaise, and appearance of the rash simultaneously with defervescence.

The differential diagnosis of AMS is similar to that of typical measles; however, the pleomorphism of the rash and the severe constitutional signs sometimes observed may suggest Rocky Mountain spotted fever, leptospirosis, hemorrhagic varicella, or meningococcal infection; other differential diagnoses include certain bacterial or viral pneumonias, appendicitis, collagen-vascular diseases such as juvenile RA, and Kawasaki syndrome (mucocutaneous lymph node syndrome). A history of measles exposure and prior receipt of killed vaccine suggest the diagnosis, but virus isolation and/or serologic studies may be necessary to confirm it.

Prophylaxis

A live attenuated virus vaccine is available that provides the same permanent immunity as natural measles. The vaccine produces mild, or inapparent, noncommunicable infection and an antibody response near that of natural measles. Fever over 38 C (101 F) occurs 5 to 12 days after inoculation in < 5% of vaccinees and is often followed by a rash. CNS reactions are exceedingly rare, and simultaneous administration of measles immune globulin **(MIG)** or immune serum globulin with the vaccine is unnecessary and contraindicated.

Contraindications to the use of any live measles virus vaccine include generalized malignancies (eg, leukemia, lymphoma), immunologic deficiency diseases, and therapy with corticosteroids, irradiation, alkylating agents, or antimetabolites. Reasons to defer vaccination include pregnancy, any acute febrile illness, active untreated TB, or administration of antibody (as whole blood, plasma, or any immune globulin) within the past 8 wk.

For **routine immunization,** see IMMUNIZATION PROCEDURES THROUGHOUT CHILDHOOD in Ch. 182.

Exposed susceptibles may be protected if the live vaccine is given within 2 days of exposure. Alternatively (eg, in pregnant patients, children < 3 yr of age, or patients with TB or an acute febrile illness), MIG or immune serum globulin 0.25 mL/kg IM is given immediately, followed by a live vaccine 8 wk later or as soon after that as health permits. An exposed susceptible patient with a condition that contraindicates use of *any* live measles virus vaccine (leukemia, immunosuppression, combined immunodeficiency, etc) is given MIG or immune serum globulin 0.5 mL/kg IM (maximum, 15 mL). If such an immunocompromised patient also has a bleeding disorder—eg, thrombocytopenia, IV gamma globulin should be considered.

Treatment

Treatment is symptomatic. Patients should be protected from exposure to streptococcal infections. Secondary bacterial complications require appropriate antimicrobial drugs. Immune serum globulin is ineffective in encephalitis; symptomatic care is the only available treatment.

RUBELLA
(German Measles; Three-Day Measles)

A contagious exanthematous disease, usually with mild constitutional symptoms that may result in abortion, stillbirth, or congenital defects in infants born to mothers infected during the early months of pregnancy. Congenital rubella is discussed under NEONATAL INFECTIONS in Ch. 186.

Etiology and Epidemiology

The disease is caused by an RNA virus spread by airborne droplet nuclei or by close contact. A patient can transmit the disease from 1 wk before onset of the rash until 1 wk after it fades. (Congenitally infected infants are potentially infectious for many months after birth.) Rubella is apparently less contagious than measles, and many persons are not infected during childhood; as a result, 10 to 15% of young adult women are susceptible. Many cases are misdiagnosed or are mild and go unnoticed. Epidemics occur at irregular intervals during the spring; major epidemics occur at about 6- to 9-yr intervals. Immunity appears to be lifelong following natural infection.

Symptoms and Signs

After a 14- to 21-day incubation period, a 1- to 5-day prodrome, usually consisting of malaise and lymphadenopathy, occurs in children but may be minimal or absent in adolescents and adults. Tender swelling of the suboccipital, postauricular, and postcervical glands is characteristic, and, with the typical rash, suggests the diagnosis.

The rash is similar to that of measles but is less extensive and more evanescent. It begins on the face and neck and quickly spreads to the trunk and extremities. At the onset of the eruption, a flush simulating that of scarlet fever may appear, particularly on the face. A mild enanthem of discrete rose-colored spots is present on the palate, later coalescing into a red blush and extending over the fauces. There is a reddening of the pharynx at the onset, but no complaint of sore throat. The rash usually lasts about 3 days. On the 2nd day, it often becomes more scarlatiniform (pinpoint) with a reddish flush. The slight skin discoloration that remains as the rash fades may disappear in a day.

Constitutional symptoms in children are mild—slight malaise and occasional arthralgias. Adults characteristically complain of few or no constitutional symptoms, although fever, malaise, headache, stiff joints (occasionally with overt, transient arthritis), a slight feeling of lassitude, and mild rhinitis may be noted. They may become aware of the disease by noting the rash on the chest, arms, or forehead, or by discovering the characteristic postauricular lymphadenopathy while washing or on combing the hair. Encephalitis is a rare but occasionally fatal complication that has occurred during extensive outbreaks of rubella among young adults in the armed services. Transient testicular pain is also a frequent complaint in affected adult males.

Diagnosis

Measles, scarlet fever, secondary syphilis, drug rashes, erythema infectiosum, infectious mononucleosis, and echo-, coxsackie-, and adenovirus infections must be considered. Rubella is clinically differentiated from measles by the milder, more evanescent rash, and by the absence of Koplik's spots, coryza, photophobia, and cough. The typical patient with measles is much sicker, and the illness lasts longer. With even mild scarlet fever, there are usually more constitutional symptoms than in rubella, including a severely red, sore throat. The WBC count is elevated in scarlet fever but normal in rubella. Observation for a day usually establishes the diagnosis in scarlet fever.

The eruption and adenopathy of rubella can be simulated by secondary syphilis, but the adenopathy of syphilis is not tender and the skin eruption usually becomes prominent on the palms and soles. If there is doubt, a qualitative STS should be done and follow-up quantitative testing may be necessary. Infectious mononucleosis may also

cause a rubella-like adenopathy and skin rash but can be differentiated by the initial leukopenia followed by leukocytosis, the many atypical mononuclear cells in the blood smear, the appearance of antibodies to the Epstein-Barr virus, and, in many cases, an increase in the heterophil antibody titer. In addition, the pharyngeal angina of infectious mononucleosis is usually prominent, and malaise is greater and lasts much longer than in rubella.

A clinical diagnosis of rubella is subject to error without laboratory confirmation, especially since enteroviral exanthems closely mimic rubella. Therefore, a history of "German measles" is an unreliable guarantor of infection and immunity. Acute and convalescent sera should be obtained, if possible, for serologic testing; a four-fold or greater rise in specific antibodies is confirmatory.

Prophylaxis (see also IMMUNIZATION PROCEDURES THROUGHOUT CHILDHOOD in Ch. 182)

Rubella immunization programs prevent some of the catastrophes associated with congenital rubella, but the most successful policy for immunization is not yet known. Routine use of live rubella vaccine in all susceptible mothers immediately following delivery has been suggested, but routine vaccination of children between the ages of 15 mo and puberty is recommended. The hope is that the latter procedure will eradicate the reservoir of infection in the early age group that is presumed responsible for most adult exposures. This strategy has been largely successful in the USA. Another suggested procedure is to screen women of childbearing age for rubella antibodies (the history, whether positive or negative, being too unreliable a criterion of immunity) and immunize those who are seronegative. Such immunization, however, should not be undertaken unless conception is prevented for at least 3 mo afterward.

Live virus vaccine now prepared in human diploid fibroblast cell cultures has been shown to be effective, with antibody production in > 95% of recipients. Transmission of vaccine virus from vaccinees to susceptible contacts rarely, if ever, occurs and is not a contraindication to immunization. Vaccine virus is transmissible to the fetus but has not been causally implicated in producing congenital rubella. In children vaccinated with live virus vaccines, solid immunity lasts 15 yr or more.

Fever, rash, lymphadenopathy, polyneuropathy, arthralgia, or overt arthritis are rare with vaccination in children; joint pain and swelling occasionally follow vaccination in adult women.

Vaccine should not be given to any person with a defective or altered immune mechanism (eg, with leukemia, lymphoma, other malignancy, or a febrile illness, or during prolonged corticosteroid or x-ray treatment). Data suggest that vaccine can infect a fetus during early pregnancy and, although the risk of fetal damage is considered to be extremely low (estimated to be ≤ 3%), its use is **contraindicated** throughout pregnancy.

Treatment

Rubella requires little or no treatment. Otitis media, a rare complication, requires appropriate treatment. There is no specific therapy for encephalitis.

ROSEOLA INFANTUM

(Exanthem Subitum; Pseudorubella)

An acute disease of infants or very young children characterized by high fever, absence of localizing symptoms or signs, and appearance of a rubelliform eruption simultaneously with, or following, defervescence.

Etiology and Epidemiology

The cause and mode of spread are not known, but the disease is probably communicable and caused by a neurodermotropic virus. It occurs most often in the spring and fall. Minor local epidemics have been reported.

Symptoms and Signs

The incubation period is probably 5 to 15 days. Fever of 39.5 to 40.5 C (103 to 105 F) begins abruptly and persists for 3 to 5 days without any evident cause. Convulsions are common during the early phase, particularly as the temperature rises. Leukopenia with relative lymphocytosis is present, usually by the 3rd day. Lymphadenopathy in cervical and posterior auricular regions is often noted, and the spleen may be slightly enlarged.

The fever usually falls by crisis on the 4th day, and the macular or maculopapular eruption appears; it is profuse on the chest and abdomen and mild on the face and extremities, and may last for a few hours to 2 days. The temperature is normal at this stage, and the child feels and acts well. The evanescent rash may be unnoticed in mild cases.

Diagnosis and Treatment

If roseola is known to be in the community, it should be suspected when a child aged 6 mo to 3 yr develops a persistently high temperature without apparent cause. A presumptive diagnosis usually can be made, to the relief of the parents, if pyelonephritis, otitis media, meningitis, sepsis, and bacterial pneumonia can be ruled out.

Treatment is symptomatic and includes careful antipyretic measures to keep the child comfortable. For treatment of convulsions, see Ch. 121. When the temperature falls to normal and the eruption appears, the patient is so nearly well that further treatment is unnecessary.

ERYTHEMA INFECTIOSUM
(Fifth Disease)

An acute viral disease characterized by mild constitutional symptoms and a blotchy or maculopapular rash beginning on the cheeks and spreading primarily to the exposed areas of the extremities.

Etiology and Epidemiology

The disease is caused by the recently discovered human parvovirus B19 agent. It occurs most often during spring months, and localized outbreaks among children and adolescents are common. Parvovirus B19 is now also recognized as the primary cause of aplastic crises in patients with chronic hemolytic disorders, such as sickle-cell disease. Spread is thought to be usually by the respiratory route, and inapparent infection can occur.

Symptoms and Signs

The incubation period is 4 to 12 days. Signs and symptoms can vary among different individuals. In "classical" cases, manifestations are low-grade fever, slight malaise, and an indurated, confluent erythema over the cheeks ("slapped face" appearance). Within 1 to 2 days a symmetric eruption appears that is most prominent on the arms, legs, and trunk, usually sparing the palms and soles. The rash is maculopapular, tending toward confluence; it forms slightly raised blotchy areas and reticular or lacy patterns, usually most prominent on the exposed areas of the arms. The duration of illness is usually 5 to 10 days, but the eruption may recur for several weeks afterward, exacerbated by sunlight, exercise, heat, fever, or emotional stress. Mild joint pain and swelling are sometimes observed in adults with this disease.

Diagnosis and Treatment

The appearance and pattern of spread of the rash are the only diagnostic features; however, such a diagnosis must be made with caution, since rubella and some enteroviruses have been known to mimic this disease. If there is any doubt, rubella infection should be ruled out by serologic testing.

Only symptomatic treatment is necessary.

CHICKENPOX
(Varicella)

An acute viral disease, usually ushered in by mild constitutional symptoms that are followed shortly by an eruption appearing in crops and characterized by macules, papules, vesicles, and crusting.

Etiology and Epidemiology

Chickenpox and herpes zoster are caused by the varicella-zoster virus, chickenpox being the acute invasive phase of the virus, and zoster (shingles) being the reactivation of the latent phase.

Chickenpox, like measles, is highly communicable. Epidemics occur in winter and early spring in 3- to 4-yr cycles (the period required to develop a new group of susceptibles). Susceptibility is high from birth until the disease is contracted, but some infants may have partial immunity, probably acquired transplacentally, until age 6 mo.

Chickenpox is believed to be spread by infected droplets from the nose and throat and is most communicable during the short prodrome and early stages of the eruption. The usual incubation period is 14 to 16 days, and communicability to others is considered possible from 10 to 21 days after exposure. When the final lesions have crusted, the patient can no longer transmit the disease. Isolation for 6 days after the first vesicles appear is usually sufficient to control cross-infection. Indirect transmission (by immune third persons) probably does not occur.

Symptoms and Signs

Mild headache, moderate fever, and malaise may be present 11 to 15 days after exposure, about 24 to 36 h before the first series of lesions appears. The prodrome is usually unrecognized in young children, is more likely to be present in children over age 10, and is usually severe in adults.

The initial rash, a macular eruption, may be accompanied by an evanescent flush. This rash evolves within a few hours to characteristic itchy monolocular "teardrop" vesicles, containing clear fluid and standing out from their red areolas; at this time diagnosis can usually be made. The typical individual chickenpox lesions progress from macule to papule to vesicle and begin crusting within 6 to 8 h. Lesions erupt in successive crops, some macules just appearing as earlier crops are beginning to crust. The eruption may be generalized in severe cases; otherwise, the face and extremities are partially spared. When only a few lesions are present, the upper trunk is the most frequent site. Lesions may also be present on the mucous membranes, including the upper respiratory tract, palpebral conjunctiva, rectal, and vaginal mucosa. In the mouth the vesicles rupture immediately, are indistinguishable from those of herpetic stomatitis, and often cause pain on swallowing. Laryngeal or tracheal vesicles may cause severe dyspnea. Lesions are frequently present on the scalp and result in tender, enlarged suboccipital and posterior cervical lymph nodes. The acute phase of illness usually lasts 4 to 7 days. New lesions usually cease to appear by the 5th day, the majority are crusted by the 6th day, and most crusts disappear in < 20 days after onset.

Chickenpox in childhood is usually benign. However, it may be severe or fatal in patients with leukemia or those receiving corticosteroids.

Complications

Secondary streptococcal infection of the vesicles may lead to erysipelas, sepsis, acute hemorrhagic nephritis, or, rarely, gangrene of the skin. Staphylococci may also infect the vesicles and cause bullous impetigo. Pneumonia as a complication of severe chickenpox is encountered in adults and newborns, but is unusual in young children. Myocarditis, transient arthritis, and hemorrhagic complications have also been re-

ported. Hemorrhagic varicella should raise suspicion of varicella-associated thrombocytopenic purpura or secondary meningococcal sepsis.

Post-chickenpox encephalitis is unusual; it occurs in < 1 in 1000 cases. Like that following measles, it tends to occur toward the end of the disease or 1 to 2 wk after its termination. One of the most common neurologic complications is acute cerebellar ataxia. Transverse myelitis, cranial nerve palsies, and multiple-sclerosis–like clinical manifestations have also occurred. Encephalitis may be fatal, but the prognosis for complete recovery from CNS complications is generally good and is far better than in measles encephalitis. Reye's syndrome, an unusual, but severe, complication, may begin 3 to 8 days after onset of the rash (see REYE'S SYNDROME in MISCELLANEOUS INFECTIONS, below).

Diagnosis

Secondary syphilis, impetigo, infected eczema, insect bites and stings, drug rashes, contact dermatitis, erythropoietic porphyria (hydroa aestivale), and, occasionally, coxsackievirus and disseminated herpes simplex virus infections must be considered in the differential diagnosis.

Prophylaxis

Chickenpox can be prevented or modified by administering IM zoster immune globulin **(ZIG),** derived from the sera of patients recovering from herpes zoster, or varicella-zoster immune globulin **(VZIG)** prepared from pooled plasma containing high titers of specific antibody. The recommended dose in 125 u. (approximately 1.25 mL/10 kg, with a maximum dose not to exceed 625 u. Such preparations should be given within 96 h after exposure to be effective; their use is primarily for exposed susceptibles with leukemia, immune deficiency syndromes, or other severe debilitating illness. Also, newborns whose mothers developed chickenpox within 5 days prior to delivery or 2 days after delivery are candidates for prophylaxis. Inquiries regarding availability of these globulins may be directed to local American Red Cross Blood Services centers. Large doses of pooled human γ-globulin have also been shown to modify the disease if given shortly after exposure, but the quantity required is so great (0.6 to 1.2 mL/kg IM) that this is not generally recommended. Limited studies suggest that zoster immune plasma **(ZIP)** at doses ranging from 3 to 14 mL/kg IV or pooled γ-globulin at doses of 4 to 6 mL/kg IV may also be useful prophylactically if given within 6 days after exposure. These preparations have no therapeutic value after the illness has begun. Live, attenuated vaccines are currently under study and appear to be very effective, but are not now available for routine use.

Treatment

Mild cases require only symptomatic treatment. Wet compresses may be applied to control itching, which may be extreme, and to prevent scratching, which may lead to widespread infection and disfigurement. Systemic antihistamines may be used in severe cases. Because of the frequency of staphylococcal or streptococcal superinfection of the vesicles, patients should be bathed often with soap and water and kept in clean underclothing; hands should be kept clean and nails clipped. Antiseptics should not be applied to individual lesions unless they become secondarily infected. Staphylococcal or β-hemolytic streptococcal infection is treated with appropriate systemic antibiotics. **In severe cases** with existing widespread disease or known immunocompromise, vidarabine or acyclovir may be given IV.

RESPIRATORY SYNCYTIAL VIRUS (RSV)

RSV is one of the most important causes of lower respiratory illness (including bronchiolitis and pneumonia) in infants and young children and can be fatal. The

sudden death of a baby with respiratory disease is often believed to be due to RSV infection. In normal adults and older children, RSV causes milder respiratory illness, but it is also an important cause of the influenza syndrome, bronchopneumonia, and exacerbations of chronic bronchitis. Elderly people and those with underlying pulmonary diseases may be quite susceptible to infection with RSV.

Etiology

RSV is an RNA virus, classified as a paramyxovirus. Only one serotype has been recognized to have clinical importance. Biologically and behaviorally it resembles influenza and parainfluenza viruses more than other taxonomic virus groups, but is serologically and, in other ways (eg, by its failure to grow in eggs or produce hemagglutinin), biologically distinct from them.

Epidemiology

RSV is associated with a sharp annual outbreak of acute respiratory disease occurring in late autumn or in winter. Like influenza, it increases morbidity and mortality from bronchitis and pneumonia. The annual recurrence of a single RSV serotype indicates that reinfection, with illness, occurs. Although about 70% of persons have serum antibody against RSV by age 5, infections continue to occur in persons of all ages. The poorly protective effect of serum antibody against infection, and, perhaps, its immunologic enhancement of disease are indicated by the increased severity of infection seen in some infants < 6 mo old, who have maternal antibody but develop severe lower respiratory tract disease that causes an appreciable number of deaths.

Symptoms and Signs

The clinical manifestations of RSV infection are variable and, in general, differ with age and host factors. The syndrome is of little help in identifying the specific cause of the infection. Dyspnea, cough, and wheezing are the most prominent symptoms; fever and bronchiolitis are the most frequent findings. Crepitant rales are characteristic; bronchopneumonia is often apparent in chest x-rays. The leukocyte count is normal, but granulocytes may be moderately elevated. In adults and older children, infection may be inapparent or only an afebrile URI (the common cold), but RSV infections can mimic influenza and they also account for 15% of hospital admissions for acute exacerbations of chronic bronchitis. Secondary bacterial pneumonia (most commonly pneumococcal) may signify a preceding infection with RSV.

Diagnosis

RSV can be isolated from respiratory secretions on susceptible tissue cultures. Since the virus poorly tolerates freezing and thawing unless protected by special media, it may be difficult to store or ship specimens. RSV infection is usually confirmed serologically. A rise in serum antibody can be detected by CF with a standard antigen. However, serologic findings may be difficult to evaluate. Very young infants often have maternal antibody, children may show acquired antibody in the early-phase serum, an antibody rise may not be demonstrable in young children, and mild disease in adults causes no increase in titer. An enzyme-linked immunosorbent assay **(ELISA)** is now commercially available. It is a more sensitive and convenient technic for detecting RSV antigens in secretions and for titration of antibody.

Treatment

Mild and inapparent infections are probably quite frequent and resolve without special attention. Severe disease in infants and children requires hospitalization and careful observation to ensure adequate respiration. In studies done in infants with bronchiolitis or pneumonia caused by RSV, ribavirin, a newly licensed antiviral drug, reduced virus shedding and accelerated recovery from illness in patients with severe

disease. Ribavirin 10 mg/kg was administered as a small-particle aerosol for 12 h for 3 to 5 days. Adults with bronchopneumonia and acute bronchitis also may require respiratory support.

ENTEROVIRAL DISEASES

(See also TABLE 191–4)

A group of diseases caused by enteroviruses ***(polio-, coxsackie-, or echoviruses).***

Etiology and Epidemiology

Because of similar biologic, chemical, and physical properties, the **enteroviruses** and the rhinoviruses are placed together taxonomically as subgroups of the family **picorna-**

TABLE 191–4. SYNDROMES CAUSED BY ENTEROVIRUSES

Disease	*Serotypes Most Often Implicated*	*Comments*
Herpangina	Coxsackievirus A 2, 4–6, 8, 10; probably 3 and others	Most common in infants and children; characteristic pharyngeal lesions
Hand-foot-and-mouth disease	Coxsackievirus A 16 Enterovirus 71	Most common in young children; vesicular exanthem usually brief and benign
Epidemic pleurodynia (Bornholm disease)	Coxsackievirus B 1–6	Most common in children, but any age group may be affected
Aseptic meningitis	Coxsackievirus A 2, 4, 7, 9, 23 and others, B 1–6 Poliovirus 1–3 Echovirus 4, 6; others less commonly	Most common in infants and children; course usually benign
Paralytic disease	Poliovirus 1–3 Coxsackievirus A 7 and others Echovirus 4, 6, and others Enterovirus 71	See POLIOMYELITIS
Myocarditis Pericarditis	Coxsackievirus B 2–5 Coxsackievirus A 23, B 1–5 Echovirus 1, 6, 8, 16	May occur at any age; myocarditis neonatorum has high mortality
Exanthems: With fever alone	Coxsackievirus A 23, B 2, 3, 5; A 4–6, 9, 16 also implicated Echovirus 4; 2, 6, 11, 14, 16, 18, 30 also implicated	Course generally benign
With aseptic meningitis	Coxsackievirus A 16, 23; B 4 Echovirus 4, 16	Course generally benign
Respiratory disease	Echovirus 4, 8, 20, and others Coxsackievirus A 21, B 1, 3, 4, 5 Poliovirus 1–3	Most common in infants and children; course generally mild
Gastroenteritis	Echovirus 6, 14, and 18 proved cause in newborns; many other enteroviruses suspected in all age groups	Probably most important in newborn or premature nursery
Conjunctivitis	Enterovirus 70 Coxsackievirus A27 Echovirus 7	Outbreaks of hemorrhagic conjunctivitis most common with enterovirus 70

viruses (*pico*, small; *rna*, their characteristic nucleic acid component). For a discussion of the polioviruses, see POLIOMYELITIS, below. For rhinoviruses, see THE COMMON COLD in Ch. 12.

The **coxsackieviruses** are an antigenically heterogeneous group divided into Groups A (23 types) and B (6 types). They resemble the polioviruses in size, resistance to physical and chemical agents, prevalence during summer and fall, and largely person-to-person spread. They have been isolated from oral secretions, stools, blood, and CSF.

The **echoviruses** (**e**nteric **c**ytopathogenic **h**uman **o**rphan), like the coxsackieviruses, are small, heterogeneous, most prevalent in summer and fall, and widely distributed geographically; 31 serotypes are recognized. These viruses have been isolated from the pharynx, feces, blood, CSF, and CNS tissues.

More recently identified enteroviruses have growth and host characteristics that variably overlap with coxsackieviruses and echoviruses. These are simply classified as higher-numbered enteroviruses (types 68 to 72).

RECOGNIZED DISEASE ENTITIES

Herpangina

Numerous Group A coxsackieviruses and, occasionally, other enteroviruses may cause herpangina. It tends to occur in epidemics, most commonly in infants and children, and is characterized by sudden onset of fever with sore throat, headache, anorexia, and, frequently, pains in the neck, abdomen, and extremities. Vomiting and convulsions may occur in infants. Within 2 days after onset, a few (rarely > 12) small (1 to 2 mm in diameter), grayish, papulovesicular lesions with erythematous areolas appear, most frequently on the tonsillar pillars, but also on the soft palate, tonsils, uvula, or tongue. During the next 24 h, the lesions become shallow ulcers, seldom > 5 mm in diameter, that heal in 1 to 5 days. Complications are unusual, and the patient is generally asymptomatic by the 7th day. Permanent immunity to the infecting strain follows infection, but repeated episodes, caused by other Group A viruses, are possible. Coxsackievirus A10 has been shown to cause a similar disease, but oral and pharyngeal lesions are raised, whitish to yellowish nodules. This entity is called **lymphonodular pharyngitis.**

Diagnosis is based on the symptoms and characteristic oral lesions. It is best confirmed by isolating the virus from the lesions or by demonstrating a rise in specific antibody titer. Differential diagnosis includes herpetic stomatitis (which occurs during any season and shows larger, more persistent ulcers) and recurrent aphthae and Bednar's aphthae (which rarely occur in the pharynx and generally are not associated with systemic symptoms). **Treatment** is symptomatic.

Hand-Foot-and-Mouth Disease

This is usually associated with coxsackievirus A 16 and occurs particularly among young children. The course is similar to that of herpangina, but a vesicular exanthem is distributed over the buccal mucosa and palate and similar lesions appear on the hands and feet and occasionally in the diaper area. **Treatment** is symptomatic.

Epidemic Pleurodynia (Bornholm Disease)

This disease may occur at any age, but it is most common in children. It may be caused by any of the 6 Group B coxsackieviruses and is characterized by sudden onset of severe, frequently intermittent, pain in the epigastrium or lower anterior chest, with fever and often headache, sore throat, and malaise. Local tenderness, hyperesthesia, muscle swelling, and myalgias of the trunk and extremities may occur. The disease usually subsides in 2 to 4 days, but relapse may develop within a few days and symp-

oms may recur for several weeks. In some cases, symptoms continue for a few weeks. Complications include orchitis, fibrinous pleuritis, pericarditis, and, rarely, aseptic meningitis.

Diagnosis is obvious during an epidemic. However, in sporadic cases or in the early tages of an epidemic, the disease may be mistaken for poliomyelitis, myocardial in-arction, spontaneous pneumothorax, acute appendicitis, pancreatitis, costochondritis, a perforated viscus, or an influenza-like respiratory infection. Laboratory diagnosis consists of isolating the virus from the throat or stool, or demonstrating a rise in pecific neutralizing antibody titers.

Prognosis is good in uncomplicated cases, although a few deaths have been reported. Repeated infections with other Group B coxsackieviruses are possible.

Treatment is entirely symptomatic.

Aseptic Meningitis

Aseptic meningitis in infants and young children is frequently caused by a Group A or B coxsackievirus, or an echovirus; viruses other than enteroviruses are often respon-sible in older children and adults (see ARBOVIRUS ENCEPHALITIDES in Ch. 12, and ACUTE VIRAL ENCEPHALITIS AND ASEPTIC MENINGITIS in Ch. 125). Headache, pain and stiffness in the neck and back, and muscular aches may be abrupt in onset or preceded by prodromal fever, malaise, anorexia, and vomiting. Kernig's and Brudzin-ski's signs usually are positive. Symptoms generally subside by the end of a week, but fatigue and irritability may persist for months. CSF findings consist of a normal or slightly elevated protein level, a normal glucose level, and a cell count usually < 500/cu mm; neutrophils may predominate in the early stages, but lymphocytes are more common later. Encephalitic signs occasionally develop and may be severe.

Meningitis due to coxsackie- or echovirus is usually impossible to differentiate clini-cally from other viral meningitides during the acute stages. Occasionally a patient presents with CSF hypoglycorrhachia in addition to a neutrophile predominance, sug-gesting meningitis. If there is also an associated petechial rash, further confusion can result. **Diagnosis** is made by isolating the virus from the throat, stool specimens, or occasionally the CSF, or by demonstrating a rise in neutralizing antibody titer.

Prognosis is generally good, but death may occur in the newborn. **Treatment** should follow that for nonparalytic poliomyelitis (see POLIOMYELITIS, below), since the two diseases are clinically indistinguishable in the acute stages.

Paralytic Disease

Certain Group A and B coxsackieviruses (especially A 7), several echoviruses, and enterovirus type 71 may produce muscle weakness or paralysis that is clinically indis-tinguishable from paralytic poliomyelitis. The causative virus can be identified by laboratory technics; **treatment** is the same as for paralytic poliomyelitis.

Myocarditis; Pericarditis

Myocarditis neonatorum, caused by Group B coxsackieviruses and some echovi-ruses, occurs in newborns infected after birth (rarely in utero). Usually, several days of well-being are followed by sudden onset of fever, feeding difficulties, pharyngitis, tachycardia, cyanosis, and tachypnea; frequently there are associated cardiac murmurs and hepatomegaly. The ECG may show signs of myocarditis. CNS, hepatic, pancre-atic, or adrenal lesions may be present concomitantly. Recovery may occur within a few weeks, but death due to circulatory collapse is not unusual.

Myocarditis or pericarditis in older children or adults also may be due to a Group B coxsackievirus, and, in a few instances, to a Group A coxsackievirus or an echovirus. Symptoms and signs are usually localized only to the myocardium or pericardium, and complete recovery is usual.

Diagnosis is made, as in other coxsackievirus infections, by virus isolation or anti-body titer studies. **Treatment** is symptomatic, including strict bed rest and control of

heart failure and arrhythmias. The value of corticosteroids has not been established; their use is best reserved for severe cases of myocarditis with associated cardiac failure.

Exanthems With or Without Aseptic Meningitis

Certain echo- and coxsackieviruses may cause a rubelliform rash that is generally discrete, nonpruritic, nondesquamative, and usually confined to the face, neck, and chest. The rash is sometimes maculopapular or morbilliform, occasionally hemorrhagic or vesicular. Fever is common. Aseptic meningitis may develop. The disease is usually epidemic, with exanthems predominating among infants and children, but sporadic cases occur. The course is generally benign.

Respiratory Disease

Enteroviruses have been implicated in some infants' and children's respiratory illnesses characterized by fever, coryza, and pharyngitis, sometimes with diarrhea and vomiting. Bronchitis and interstitial pneumonia have occasionally occurred in infants. **Treatment** is symptomatic (see THE COMMON COLD in Ch. 12).

Diarrhea; Gastroenteritis

Enteroviruses, particularly echoviruses 6, 14, and 18, have occasionally been isolated from the stools of newborn infants with acute diarrheal disease. A large variety of enteroviruses and a few adenoviruses have been isolated from the stools of older infants and young children with acute gastroenteritis, but their importance in the etiology of this disease is questionable. Other enteric viruses, called "epidemic gastroenteritis viruses," have been demonstrated by oral inoculation of volunteers with stool filtrates, and by electron microscopy of the feces in acute cases, particularly in specimens from infants and young children. Not all of these viruses have been clearly identified, but most do not appear to be enteroviruses. **Treatment** of enteric infections is symptomatic (see ACUTE INFECTIOUS GASTROENTERITIS under BACTERIAL INFECTIONS in this chapter, above).

Conjunctivitis

Acute hemorrhagic conjunctivitis has occurred rarely in epidemics in the USA, but importation from Africa and Asia, where outbreaks have occurred, is considered to be more likely in the future. The disease, associated with infection by enterovirus type 70, is characterized by rapid onset of swelling of the eyelids, with congestion, pain, and increased lacrimation. Some patients also develop subconjunctival hemorrhages and epithelial keratitis. Systemic illness is unusual, although a few cases of transient lumbosacral radiculomyelopathy or poliomyelitis-like illness have been recorded. Recovery is usually complete within 1 to 2 wk of onset. Other enteroviruses associated with conjunctivitis include some strains of coxsackievirus A24 and echovirus 7; these are usually not associated with hemorrhagic manifestations.

Treatment is symptomatic.

POLIOMYELITIS

(Infantile Paralysis; Acute Anterior Poliomyelitis)

An acute viral infection with a wide range of manifestations, including nonspecific minor illness, aseptic meningitis (nonparalytic poliomyelitis), and flaccid weakness of various muscle groups (paralytic poliomyelitis).

Etiology and Epidemiology

Poliovirus is an enterovirus belonging to the picornoviridae, whose major properties include a single-stranded RNA genome, small size (22 to 30 nm), lack of an envelope, and insensitivity to ether and other lipid solvents. Of the 3 immunologically distinct poliovirus serotypes, type I is the most paralytogenic and the most common cause of epidemics.

Man is the only natural host for polioviruses. The infection occurs through direct contact and is highly contagious. Inapparent infections (the main source of spread) are common in unimmunized populations, but overt disease is rare; even in epidemics, the ratio of inapparent infections to clinical cases exceeds 100:1. The paralytic disease had been thought to be uncommon in developing (mainly tropical) countries, but recent surveys of lameness indicate an incidence as high as in the peak years in the USA before introduction of vaccines. In such areas, where sanitation and hygiene are poor, virus circulation is extensive and occurs year round, infection and immunity are acquired in the first few years of life, there are no epidemics, and > 90% of paralytic cases are confined to children < 5 yr. In contrast, as sanitation and hygiene improved in economically developed countries, infection was delayed, many older children and young adults remained susceptible, and summer epidemics involving increasingly older age groups occurred. Extensive use of vaccines has almost eliminated the disease in the industrialized world.

Pathology and Pathogenesis

Virus enters the mouth and primary multiplication occurs in lymphoid tissues in the oropharynx and intestinal tract, mainly the ileum. Small amounts of virus reach the blood and are carried to other sites in the reticuloendothelial system, where extensive multiplication occurs. Secondary viremia is followed by invasion of the CNS. Under certain circumstances, the virus may also reach the CNS via autonomic nerve fiber endings in the alimentary tract. The agent is present in blood, throat, and feces during the incubation period, and after onset persists in throat washings for 1 to 2 wk and in feces for 3 to 6 wk or longer. Viremia lasts several days but disappears by the time of onset, when antibodies have already developed.

The spinal cord and brain are the only sites of significant virus-induced pathology. The motor neurons of the anterior horn of the spinal cord, the medulla, and certain other parts of the brain, including the cerebellum and the motor cortex, are involved. Damage to neurons by the virus, the primary event, excites an intense inflammatory reaction and eventually neuronophagia. The site and severity of paralysis is determined by the distribution of the neuronal lesions. Factors predisposing to serious neurologic damage include increasing age, recent tonsillectomy, inoculations (most often DTP), pregnancy, and physical exertion concurrent with onset of the CNS phase.

Symptoms and Signs

Clinical forms vary, but the 2 basic patterns are the "minor illness" (abortive type) and the "major illness" (which may be paralytic or nonparalytic). The **minor illness,** accounting for 80% to 90% of clinical infections, occurs chiefly in young children, is mild, and does not involve the CNS. Symptoms are slight fever, malaise, headache, sore throat, and vomiting, which develop 3 to 5 days after exposure. Recovery occurs within 24 to 72 h.

Symptoms of the **major illness** may follow several days of well-being, but more commonly appear without a previous minor illness, particularly in older children and adults. Incubation is usually 7 to 14 days, but may be as long as 35 days. Fever, severe headache, stiff neck and back, deep muscle pain, and sometimes hyperesthesias and paresthesias may be present. There may be no further progression from this picture of aseptic meningitis or the disease may go on, with loss of tendon reflexes and asymmetric weakness or paralysis of muscle groups, depending on the location of lesions in the spinal cord or medulla. Dysphagia, nasal regurgitation, and nasal voice are early signs of bulbar involvement. Encephalitic signs occasionally predominate. The CSF sugar is normal, the protein is slightly elevated, and the cell count commonly ranges from 20 to 300 cells/μL (predominantly lymphocytes). The peripheral WBC counts may be normal or moderately increased.

Diagnosis and Differential Diagnosis

Asymmetric flaccid limb paralyses or bulbar palsies without sensory loss during an acute febrile illness in a child or young adult almost always indicate poliomyelitis, though rarely certain coxsackieviruses and echoviruses may produce the same clinical picture (see above in this chapter in the general discussion of enteroviral diseases). In the Guillain-Barré syndrome, often confused with paralytic poliomyelitis, there is usually no fever, muscle weakness is symmetric, sensory findings are characteristically present, and CSF protein is markedly elevated in the presence of a normal cell count. CNS involvement due to mumps or herpes viruses, tuberculous meningitis, or brain abscess should also be considered, and, in certain geographic areas, meningoencephalitis due to arborviruses. Nonparalytic poliomyelitis cannot be distinguished clinically from aseptic meningitis due to other agents; virus isolation from throat and/or feces or demonstration of a rise in specific antibody is required to confirm the diagnosis.

Prognosis

In the abortive and nonparalytic forms, recovery is complete. In paralytic poliomyelitis, fewer than 25% of patients suffer severe permanent disability, about 25% have mild disabilities, and over 50% recover with no residual paralyses. The greatest return of muscle function occurs in the first 6 mo, but improvement may continue for 2 yr. Mortality is 1 to 4% but may increase to 10% in adults or those with bulbar disease. **Recently, a new syndrome has been described**: progressive paralysis and atrophy occurring years after acute paralytic poliomyelitis. The syndrome is thought to be due to physiologic changes and aging, with further loss of anterior horn cells in a population of neurons depleted by earlier poliovirus infection.

Prophylaxis

Active immunization is recommended for all infants and children (see IMMUNIZATION PROCEDURES THROUGHOUT CHILDHOOD in Ch. 182). Two vaccines have been used: **inactivated Salk vaccine (IPV),** given in a series of injections with periodic booster doses, and **oral Sabin live attenuated virus vaccine (OPV).** Both vaccines induce circulating antibodies, but OPV also induces alimentary tract resistance associated with local secretory (IgA) antibody production that blocks virus implantation. Because of its immunologic superiority and logistic simplicity, trivalent OPV is recommended for routine childhood immunization in the USA. Very rarely OPV has been associated with paralytic poliomyelitis. OPV is contraindicated in immunodeficient persons, who should receive IPV. Nor should OPV be used in families with an immunodeficient member because of the possibility of contact infection from recipients who excrete the virus. Because poliomyelitis incidence in the USA is extremely low, primary vaccination of adults (> 18 yr) is not recommended. Adults who have never been immunized and are travelling to endemic or epidemic areas should be given a course of IPV; if the time is too short to permit at least 2 doses of IPV, a single dose of trivalent OPV is indicated.

Treatment

Therapy is nonspecific. Patients with abortive or mild nonparalytic poliomyelitis need only bed rest for several days. Symptomatic treatment with analgesics and antipyretics may be useful. **During active myelitis,** rest on a firm bed (with footboards, to help prevent footdrop) is indicated. Muscle spasm and pain may be relieved by several 20-min applications/day of hot, moist packs. Urinary retention, a frequent complication in patients with leg paralysis, may respond to a parasympathomimetic such as bethanechol 5 to 30 mg orally or 2.5 to 5 mg s.c. 3 or 4 times/day, but catheterization is frequently necessary. All patients who require catheterization should be on an intermittent catheterization program to decrease the possibility of developing urinary tract infection. If infection occurs, treatment with an appropriate antibiotic and a high fluid intake to prevent formation of urinary calcium phosphate stones is indicated. Physical

therapy is the most important part of management of paralytic poliomyelitis during convalescence.

Respiratory failure may be due to spinal cord involvement causing paralysis of the muscles of respiration, or to damage by the virus to the respiratory centers in the medulla and paralysis of muscles innervated by the cranial nerves. Artificial respiration is the treatment for both types. In patients with pharyngeal muscle weakness, difficulty in swallowing, inability to cough, and pooling of bronchotracheal secretions, postural drainage and suction should be instituted. Tracheostomy is frequently required to keep the airway clear. Pulmonary atelectasis is common in respiratory failure, and bronchoscopy and aspiration are often necessary. Further details regarding respiratory intensive care can be found in Ch. 34. Antimicrobial agents are not recommended unless infection occurs.

MUMPS
(Epidemic Parotitis)

An acute, contagious, generalized viral disease, usually causing painful enlargement of the salivary glands, most commonly the parotids.

Etiology and Incidence

The causative agent, a paramyxovirus, is spread by droplet infection or direct contact with materials contaminated with infected saliva. The virus probably enters through the mouth. It may be found in the saliva for 1 to 6 days before the salivary glands swell and for the duration of glandular enlargement (usually 5 to 9 days). It has been isolated from patients' blood and urine, and from the CSF in patients with CNS involvement.

Mumps is endemic in heavily populated areas, but may occur in epidemics when many susceptible individuals are crowded together. Communicability is less than in measles and chickenpox. Incidence peaks in late winter and early spring. Although the disease may occur at any age, most cases are in children aged 5 to 15; the disease is unusual in children < 2 yr, and infants up to 1 yr ordinarily are immune. One attack usually confers permanent immunity even though only one parotid has been enlarged. About 25 to 30% of cases are clinically inapparent.

Symptoms, Signs, and Course

After a 14- to 24-day incubation period, onset occurs with chilly sensations, headache, anorexia, malaise, and a low to moderate fever that may last 12 to 24 h before salivary gland involvement is noted. These prodromal symptoms may be absent in mild cases. Pain on chewing or swallowing, especially on swallowing acidic liquids such as vinegar or lemon juice, is the earliest symptom of parotitis. There is marked sensitivity to pressure over the angle of the jaw. With development of parotitis, the temperature frequently rises to 39.5 or 40 C (103 or 104 F). Swelling of the gland reaches maximum about the 2nd day and is associated with tissue edema extending beyond the parotid in front of and below the ear.

Both parotid glands are involved in most cases. Occasionally, the submaxillary and sublingual glands also swell; more rarely, these are the only glands affected. Swelling of the neck beneath the jaw occurs in such cases, or, with submaxillary gland involvement, suprasternal edema may develop. The oral duct openings of the involved glands are "pouting" and slightly inflamed. The skin over the glands may become tense and shiny. Involved glands are acutely tender during the 24- to 72-h febrile period. The WBC count may be normal, though a slight leukopenia with a reduction in granulocytes is usual.

Prognosis is excellent in uncomplicated mumps, although rarely a relapse occurs after about 2 wk.

Complications

Particularly in postpuberal patients, the disease may involve organs other than the salivary glands. Symptoms may precede, accompany, or follow salivary gland involvement, and may also occur without primary sialadenitis.

Orchitis occurs in about 20% of postpuberal male patients and is usually unilateral. Some testicular atrophy may ensue, but sterility is exceedingly rare; hormonal function is not lost. Gonadal involvement in females **(oophoritis)** is less commonly recognized, is far less painful, and has not been associated with subsequent infertility.

Meningoencephalitis: Headache, stiff neck, and CSF pleocytosis is common in mumps; CSF glucose levels are usually normal but occasionally are low, between 20 and 40 mg/dL, mimicking bacterial meningitis. More severe encephalitic signs occur in about 5 to 10%, with drowsiness or even coma or convulsions that may be abrupt in onset. About 30% of CNS mumps infections occur without associated parotitis. The prognosis is favorable in most cases with CNS involvement, and considerably better than in measles encephalitis, although permanent sequelae, such as unilateral (rarely bilateral) nerve deafness or facial paralysis, may result. As in other viral diseases, a para- or post-infectious form of encephalitis may occur, but is rare. Other unusual manifestations include acute cerebellar ataxia, transverse myelitis, and polyneuritis.

Pancreatitis: Toward the end of the first week, a few patients may have sudden severe nausea and vomiting, with abdominal pain that is most severe in the epigastrium and suggests pancreatitis. These symptoms disappear in about a week and the patient completely recovers.

Miscellaneous: Prostatitis, nephritis, myocarditis, mastitis, polyarthritis, and lacrimal gland involvement are seen occasionally. Inflammation of the thyroid and thymus glands may cause edema and swelling over the sternum, but this is more common secondary to submaxillary gland involvement.

Diagnosis

Diagnosis of typical cases during an epidemic is easy, but sporadic cases are more difficult to detect. Swelling of the parotid or other salivary glands due to mumps virus must be distinguished from (1) bacterial parotid involvement in streptococcal throat infections, diphtheria, or debilitated patients with poor oral hygiene, typhoid, or typhus fever; (2) Mikulicz's syndrome, a chronic, usually painless parotid and lacrimal gland swelling of unknown etiology that occurs with TB, sarcoidosis, SLE, leukemia, and lymphosarcoma; (3) malignant and benign salivary gland tumors; (4) drug-related parotid enlargement (eg, from iodides or guanethidine); and (5) obstruction produced by a calculus in Stensen's duct. Enlarged lymph nodes along the mandible may be mistaken for swollen salivary glands. Mumps meningoencephalitis, sometimes the only clinical manifestation, must be differentiated from other viral meningitides.

Paired acute and convalescent sera permit diagnosis by means of the CF test, preferably with both soluble **(S)** and viral **(V)** antigens. S antibodies increase in the first week of infection and drop rather rapidly, often disappearing after 6 to 8 mo; V antibodies usually rise later than S antibodies but drop slowly to a plateau. A single serum specimen may occasionally be diagnostic if both CF antigens are used. Other serologic tests are also available. An elevated serum amylase level may also suggest the diagnosis. If virological diagnostic services are available, the virus can be readily isolated from the throat, CSF, and, occasionally, the urine.

Prophylaxis

The patient should remain in isolation until glandular swelling subsides. Susceptible contacts should be followed closely from the 14th to the 28th day after exposure. Mumps immune globulin and immune serum globulin are not helpful.

Live mumps virus vaccine is the agent of choice for active immunization (see IMMUNIZATION PROCEDURES THROUGHOUT CHILDHOOD in Ch. 182). A mumps neutralization antibody titer of 1:2 or greater is protective. This vaccine produces no significant local or systemic reaction and requires only one injection. It is not yet clear whether revaccination is required to maintain lifelong immunity. Postexposure vaccination does not protect against mumps from that exposure.

Treatment

Treatment is symptomatic. A soft diet reduces pain caused by chewing. Analgesics may be used for headache and general malaise.

Complications are also treated symptomatically. Patients with orchitis require bed rest. Supporting the scrotum in cotton on an adhesive-tape bridge between the thighs to minimize tension, or applying ice packs, often helps to relieve pain.

If nausea and vomiting of pancreatitis are severe, oral feedings should be withheld and fluid balance restored by IV dextrose and saline solutions.

Corticosteroids are not usually necessary, although they may diminish pain and swelling in acute orchitis.

SUBACUTE SCLEROSING PANENCEPHALITIS (SSPE)

A progressive, usually fatal, neurologic (brain) disorder occurring months to years (usually years) after an attack of measles and characterized by mental deterioration, myoclonic jerks, and seizures.

Etiology and Epidemiology

The mode of spread is not known. An altered measles virus, acquired naturally or by vaccination, is the probable cause. Measles virus has been demonstrated in brain tissue and isolated from brain biopsies. Males are affected more frequently than females. The incidence has been declining in the USA and Western Europe.

Symptoms and Signs

Onset is usually before age 20. Often the first signs are diminished performance in schoolwork, forgetfulness, temper outbursts, distractibility, sleeplessness, and hallucinations. Seizures follow the mental changes and initially are myoclonic jerks—sudden flexion movements of the extremities, head, and trunk; grand mal seizures may occur. Patients show further intellectual decline; changes in speech; and abnormal involuntary movements, including athetosis, chorea, and ballistic or throwing movements. Dystonic movements and transient periods of opisthotonos are seen. Later, rigidity of the body musculature, difficulty in swallowing, cortical blindness, and optic atrophy may be noted. Focal chorioretinitis and other funduscopic abnormalities are seen in a number of patients. In the final phases, the patient becomes increasingly rigid, with intermittent signs of hypothalamic involvement (eg, hyperthermia, diaphoresis, and disturbances of pulse and BP).

The disease, almost invariably fatal within 1 to 3 yr and often as the result of terminal bronchial pneumonia, sometimes has a more protracted course, with pronounced neurologic deficits. A few patients have remissions and exacerbations.

SSPE patients have a typical EEG: paroxysmal bursts of 2 to 3 cycles/sec, high-voltage, diphasic waves occurring synchronously throughout the recording. The CT scan may show cortical atrophy or low-density lesions of the white matter. The CSF usually is under normal pressure and has a normal cell count and protein content. The CSF γ-globulin is almost always markedly elevated and may comprise as much as 20 to 60% of the total spinal fluid protein. The patient's serum and CSF contain elevated levels of measles virus antibodies. Antimeasles IgG appears to increase as the disease progresses. Despite vigorous serologic responses to measles virus, SSPE patients do not develop antibodies to the M protein of the measles virion.

Diagnosis

SSPE should be considered in a child or adolescent who shows progressive mental deterioration and myoclonic jerks or seizures. The diagnosis is confirmed by the characteristic EEG, an elevated CSF γ-globulin, and an excessive quantity of measles virus antibody in the serum and spinal fluid.

Treatment

A number of antiviral agents have not proved helpful, but isoprinosine has been reported to retard the disease. Generally, only symptomatic treatment with anticonvulsants and supportive measures can be offered.

PROGRESSIVE RUBELLA PANENCEPHALITIS

A progressive neurologic disorder occurring in a child with the stigmata of congenital rubella, and presumably due to reactivation of the rubella virus infection.

Symptoms and Signs

Children with congenital defects due to rubella virus (eg, deafness, cataracts, microencephaly, and mental retardation) develop this disease in their early teens. They show progressive spasticity, ataxia, mental deterioration, and seizures. The condition can be confused with measles-virus–related subacute sclerosing panencephalitis **(SSPE)**, described above, but myoclonic seizure activity is more frequent in SSPE.

Diagnosis and Treatment

The diagnosis is considered when a patient with congenital rubella develops progressive neurologic deficit associated with elevated CSF cell count, total protein, and γ-globulin; elevated rubella virus antibody titers in CSF and serum; and recovery of rubella virus from brain tissue. Unlike SSPE, measles antibody titers are normal and the EEG does not show the "burst suppression" pattern typical of SSPE. CT scan may show ventricular enlargement, particularly of the 4th ventricle, due to cerebellar atrophy.

There is no specific treatment for the disorder.

CROUP
(Acute Laryngotracheobronchitis)

An acute viral inflammation of the upper and lower respiratory tracts, characterized by inspiratory stridor, subglottic swelling, and respiratory distress that is most pronounced on inspiration.

Etiology, Epidemiology, and Pathophysiology

The parainfluenza viruses, especially Type 1, are the major pathogens. Less common causes are respiratory syncytial virus **(RSV)** and influenza A and B viruses, followed by adeno-, entero-, rhino-, and measles viruses and *Mycoplasma pneumoniae*. Croup caused by influenza may be particularly severe and may occur in a broader age range of children. Seasonal outbreaks are common; cases due to parainfluenza viruses tend to occur in the fall, and those due to RSV and influenza viruses are likely to occur in the winter and spring. Spread is most likely to be by the airborne route or by contact with infected secretions. Croup is primarily a disease of children aged 6 mo to 3 yr, though it may occasionally occur earlier or later.

The infection produces inflammation of the larynx, trachea, bronchi, bronchioles, and lung parenchyma. However, obstruction, caused by swelling and inflammatory exudate, is most pronounced in the subglottic region. Obstruction increases the work of breathing and, as the child tires, results in hypercapnia. Hypoxemia without hyper-

capnia commonly occurs due to parenchymal pulmonary infection. Atelectasis may occur concurrently if the bronchioles become obstructed.

Symptoms and Signs

Croup is usually preceded by a URI. A "barking," often spasmodic cough, and hoarseness may mark the acute onset of inspiratory stridor, commonly at night. The child may awaken during the night with respiratory distress, tachypnea, and supraclavicular, suprasternal, substernal, and intercostal inspiratory retractions. In severe cases, cyanosis with increasingly shallow respirations may develop as the child tires. The obvious respiratory distress and the harsh inspiratory stridor are the most dramatic physical findings. Auscultation reveals prolonged inspiration and stridor, often with some expiratory rhonchi and wheezes. Rales also may be present. Breath sounds may be diminished with atelectasis. Fever is present in about ½ the children. Leukocytosis with increased polymorphonuclear cells may be present initially, with a subsequent shift to leukopenia and lymphocytosis. With involvement of the lung parenchyma, arterial blood gas analysis reveals hypoxemia with or without hypercapnia. In hospitalized cases, hypoxemia has been shown to be present in about 80% of patients. Subepiglottic narrowing may be seen on anteroposterior neck x-ray. The child's condition may appear improved in the morning but may worsen again at night. The illness usually lasts 3 to 4 days. Croup occurring in children who are subject to recurrent episodes is often called **"spasmodic croup."** Allergy or airway reactivity may play a role in spasmodic croup, but the clinical manifestations of an episode cannot be differentiated from the usual case of viral croup, and spasmodic croup is also usually initiated by a viral infection.

Differential Diagnosis

Croup must be differentiated from **epiglottitis**. Distinguishing features are given in the discussion of epiglottitis, above. **Bacterial tracheitis** is a separate and unusual entity and is most likely to be confused with epiglottitis because of its rapid onset and severe, progressive course. It is characterized by the acute onset of fever, dyspnea, and stridor in young and older children. Although it may rarely follow viral croup, it should be differentiated from viral croup by the greater degree of toxicity and respiratory distress, the left shift of the WBC, the thick secretions, and the laryngeal shaggy, exudative membrane, which may be visualized on x-ray or directly. Cultures of the membrane or deep tracheal secretions obtained by suctioning are most likely to grow a pure culture of *Staphylococcus aureus* or β-hemolytic Group A streptococcus. Pneumococci and *Hemophilus influenzae* type b are less-frequent causes. A **foreign body** may cause respiratory distress and a typical croupy cough, but fever and a preceding URI are absent. X-rays of the neck may show a foreign body, but indirect and direct laryngoscopy may be required to confirm the diagnosis. **Diphtheria** is excluded by a history of adequate immunization, or confirmed by identification of the organism in special cultures of scrapings from the typical grayish diphtheritic pharyngeal or laryngeal membrane. Rarely, **retropharyngeal abscess** may present with stridor. It may be diagnosed by finger palpation of the mass or by lateral x-ray of the neck.

Bacterial tracheitis, a recently described and uncommon infection affecting children of any age, needs to be differentiated from viral croup because of its severe and rapidly progressive course. The pathogens most frequently involved are *Staphylococcus aureus*, Group A β-hemolytic streptococci, and *Hemophilus influenzae* type b. The disease is acute in onset and produces respiratory stridor, high fever, and often copious purulent secretions. The child may appear to have epiglottitis with marked toxicity and respiratory distress that may progress rapidly and may require intubation. The **diagnosis** is indicated on direct laryngoscopy by evidence of purulent secretions and inflammation in the subglottic area, or by a lateral neck roentgenogram showing an area of subglottic narrowing with a shaggy, purulent membrane.

Treatment

Home therapy: The mildly ill child may be cared for at home with supportive measures. The child should be made comfortable and should be kept well hydrated. Rest is important, as fatigue and crying can aggravate the condition. Home humidification devices (eg, "cold-steam" vaporizers or humidifiers, or steam from a hot shower in an enclosed bathroom) may ameliorate upper airway drying, but the water droplets produced are too large to help in mobilizing secretions in the lower respiratory tract. Increasing or persistent respiratory distress, tachycardia, fatigue, cyanosis, or dehydration indicates need for hospitalization.

Hospital therapy: Since moderate hypoxemia may exist without cyanosis, arterial blood gas analysis is indicated initially in all hospitalized croup patients. If the Pa_{O_2} is initially < 60 mm Hg, humidified O_2 should be administered. A 30 to 40% inspired O_2 concentration is usually adequate. CO_2 retention (Pa_{CO_2} > 45 mm Hg) generally indicates fatigue and necessitates close surveillance of the patient. *The need for intubation should be anticipated, and equipment and personnel should be ready*. The need for airway intervention is indicated by (1) increasing CO_2 retention despite adequate oxygenation, nebulized mist therapy, and hydration; (2) hypoxemia that is unresponsive to O_2 administration; and (3) secretions that cannot be mobilized by coughing. Nasotracheal intubation, if performed early by skilled personnel, causes fewer complications than does tracheostomy.

The viscosity of tracheobronchial secretions may be reduced and their clearance enhanced by mist therapy. Standard jet-type nebulizers improve laryngeal humidification, but bronchiolar humidification requires use of an ultrasonic nebulizer fitted to a mask or an oxygen tent.

The viruses that most commonly cause croup do not usually predispose to secondary bacterial infection, and antibiotics are rarely indicated. Nebulized racemic epinephrine has been successful in producing symptomatic improvement and relieving fatigue. However, it should only be used with the understanding that the effects are transient, and that the course of the illness, the Pa_{O_2}, and the prognosis are not altered, and tachycardia and other side effects may occur. The use of corticosteroids remains controversial, but many physicians use steroids early in the course of severe, hospitalized cases of viral croup.

BRONCHIOLITIS

An acute viral infection of the lower respiratory tract affecting infants and young children and characterized by respiratory distress, expiratory obstruction, wheezing, and crackles.

Bronchiolitis often occurs in epidemics and mostly in children < 18 mo of age, with a peak incidence in infants < 6 mo—the ages of predilection for respiratory syncytial virus **(RSV)** and parainfluenza 3 virus. Annually, 10 to 15/1000 children of this age require medical attention for bronchiolitis, but the actual incidence is estimated to be much greater.

Etiology and Pathophysiology

The major pathogens of bronchiolitis are RSV and parainfluenza 3 virus; influenza A and B, parainfluenza 1 and 2, and adenoviruses are less frequent causes. *Mycoplasma pneumoniae*, rhinoviruses, enteroviruses, and measles virus are uncommon etiologic agents.

The infecting virus spreads from the upper respiratory tract to the medium and small bronchi and bronchioles and causes epithelial necrosis. The developing edema and exudate result in partial obstruction, which is most pronounced on expiration and

leads to air trapping within the alveoli. With complete obstruction and absorption of the trapped air, multiple areas of atelectasis may follow.

Symptoms and Signs

Typically, an affected infant has had a preceding URI, followed by rapid onset of respiratory distress with tachypnea, tachycardia, and a hacking cough. Increasing distress is evidenced by circumoral cyanosis; deepening retractions of the subcostal, intercostal, and suprasternal areas; and audible wheezing. The child often appears markedly lethargic, but fever is not always present. Dehydration may develop from vomiting and decreased oral intake. With fatigue, respirations may become more shallow and ineffective, leading to respiratory acidosis. The chest is hyperresonant on percussion, and auscultation reveals wheezing, prolonged expiration, and, often, fine moist crackles. X-ray usually shows hyperinflated lungs, depressed diaphragm, and prominent hilar markings. Infiltrates may be present from atelectasis as well as RSV pneumonia, which is relatively common with RSV bronchiolitis.

Diagnosis

Initial laboratory findings are *not* diagnostic. About ⅔ of the children have WBC counts of 10,000 to 15,000. Most have 50 to 75% lymphocytes. In severe cases, serum electrolytes reveal the degree and type of dehydration, and blood gases are apt to show hypoxemia. Specific etiologic diagnosis is made by viral isolation or rapid diagnostic technics, such as immunofluorescence.

Asthma is the major consideration in the differential diagnosis and is the more likely diagnosis in a child > 18 mo of age, especially if previous episodes of wheezing and a family history of allergy have been documented. Gastric reflux may also produce the clinical picture of bronchiolitis; multiple episodes in an infant may be a clue to this diagnosis. Foreign body aspiration may occasionally cause wheezing and should be considered if the history or epidemiologic setting is suggestive and if the onset is sudden and not associated with prior upper respiratory tract signs (eg, nasal congestion).

Prognosis and Treatment

Most children can be treated at home and recover in 3 to 5 days without sequelae. The mortality rate is < 1% when medical care is adequate. Increasing respiratory distress, cyanosis, fatigue, and dehydration are indications for hospitalization.

Oxygenation: Recognizing and treating hypoxemia is most important. In the hospital, arterial blood gas determinations are performed, since the degree of hypoxemia cannot be accurately defined clinically. Adequate levels of oxygenation ($Pa_{O_2} > 60$ mm Hg) are usually attained with a 30 to 40% O_2 mixture delivered by tent or face mask. Endotracheal intubation is indicated if progressive CO_2 retention occurs, if the child cannot clear bronchial secretions, or if hypoxemia is unresponsive to O_2 administration. Following intubation, one should continue giving O_2 and attend to clearing secretions (by postural drainage and tracheal suctioning) and humidifying the lower tracheobronchial tree with ultrasonic nebulization.

Fluids: At home, hydration is maintained with frequent small feedings of clear liquids. In the hospital, fluids should be given IV initially and the level of hydration monitored by urine output and sp gr, and serum electrolyte determinations.

Pharmacologic agents: Corticosteroids are valueless, and sedatives are contraindicated. Antibiotics should be withheld unless a secondary bacterial infection, a rare sequela, occurs. Bronchodilators are usually ineffective, and repeated administration may harm the young infant. A new antiviral agent, ribavirin, is now available for hospitalized patients with bronchiolitis from respiratory syncytial virus. The drug is administered as a small-particle aerosol with equipment employing a generator run by compressed air. Usually ribavirin is given for 12 to 18 h/day for 3 to 5 days.

MISCELLANEOUS INFECTIONS

FEVER OF UNKNOWN ORIGIN (FUO) IN CHILDREN

A rectal temperature (or its equivalent) of 38.5 C (101.3 F) or higher measured on at least 4 occasions over a minimum period of 2 wk. This definition excludes most of the brief, self-limited, febrile illnesses that account for about 30% of outpatient pediatric visits in the USA. Because of a paucity of data, FUO in the pediatric age group is not as well delineated as in adults, but certain differences are apparent.

Etiology

As with adults, the etiology depends partly on locale; the data presented here are derived from children in the temperate climate of the USA.

Infection is the cause in about 50% of FUO in children; in almost 50% of these cases, viruses are the presumptive etiology. The type of infection varies with age: upper respiratory tract and viral infections are most common in children < 2 yr, while endocarditis and infectious mononucleosis occur predominantly in children > 6 yr. Of all children with an infectious etiology for FUO, 65% are ≤ 6 yr old. Children tend to have more viral and common bacterial diseases than adults, in whom TB, occult abscesses, and less common organisms are found.

Collagen vascular diseases (CVD) account for about 20% of FUO in childhood. Again, age helps in differential diagnosis. Of the children in this group who present with FUO, including almost all of the patients with inflammatory bowel disease (Crohn's disease of the small or large intestine, ulcerative colitis), 80% are > 6 yr. Juvenile RA is a common childhood CVD cause of FUO.

Neoplasia causes 10% of FUO in pediatric patients, with leukemia the most common disease entity. In adults, neoplasia accounts for 20% of FUO, with a predominance of solid tumors (eg, lymphoma, disseminated carcinomatosis). Neoplasia as a cause of FUO in childhood has no age predilection.

Miscellaneous causes (eg, milk allergy, Behçet's syndrome, diencephalic syndrome, thyroiditis) account for about 10% of children with FUO. The cause of FUO is **unknown** in about 15% of children (7% of adults), despite exhaustive diagnostic investigation.

Symptoms, Signs, Diagnosis, and Prognosis

Nonspecific symptoms (eg, anorexia, weight loss, fatigue, chills, sweats) are common and have little differential diagnostic or prognostic value. In contrast, patients with cutaneous symptoms and signs (eg, pruritus, rash, pigmentary changes) are more likely to have a serious illness (malignancy or CVD) with a poor prognosis. Chest pain, dyspnea, significant heart murmur, arthropathy, and cyanosis are similarly associated with serious underlying diseases (eg, bacterial endocarditis, SLE). Localizing findings are present in only 60% of patients with FUO but in nearly all patients with a fatal outcome.

Rare diseases are uncommon causes of FUO in children; > 85% of FUO in children can be assigned an etiology, usually a disease entity commonly seen in pediatrics. Hospitalization to perform sophisticated, often invasive, and usually expensive diagnostic procedures is less often needed in evaluating the child than the adult with FUO.

Routine CBC, urinalysis, and chest x-ray are not often helpful in detecting a serious illness or identifying a specific etiology. On the other hand, the ESR is elevated and the albumin/globulin ratio is reversed in about 75% of patients with CVD or malignancy, while only 10% of patients with FUO due to viral or benign illnesses exhibit these abnormalities.

The physician's skills in obtaining a history, performing a physical examination, selecting screening laboratory tests, and synthesizing available clinical information are especially important in evaluating the child with FUO; the data obtained suggest further diagnostic evaluation. Bone marrow examination may be particularly helpful: It may diagnose infection (by culture, particularly in *Salmonella* infections) or certain malignancies and may suggest CVD (by revealing plasma cell predominance) or infection (by an increase in the myeloid/erythroid ratio). Tissue biopsies (eg, lymph node, skin lesions) are diagnostic in about 40% of children in whom they are obtained. Laparotomy and selective angiographic and radioisotopic technics are less frequently needed as diagnostic tools (although they may be helpful in selected patients), primarily because of the different causes of FUO in children. Ultrasound, CT, and ^{67}Ga scanning help to define lesions usually already suspected on clinical grounds and should be used selectively to elucidate suspected pathology, not to screen patients in diagnostic evaluations of FUO.

At some time during the illness, 80% of children with FUO receive antibiotics and nearly 100% receive antipyretics. These therapies are not generally helpful in diagnosis, as they may mask the underlying process.

Prognosis is related to the underlying cause. Complete recovery can be expected by etiologic group: infection, 90%; CVD, 10%; undiagnosed, 33%. In malignancy, the outcome depends on the type and stage of the tumor.

REYE'S SYNDROME

The syndrome of acute encephalopathy and fatty degeneration of the viscera **(AEFDV)** *that tends to follow some acute viral infections.*

Reye's syndrome was first characterized as a distinct clinical and pathologic entity in 1963. The etiology is unknown, but viral agents (eg, influenza A or B, varicella virus), exogenous toxins (eg, *Aspergillus flavus* aflatoxin), salicylates, and intrinsic metabolic defects in urea-cycle enzymes such as ornithine transcarbamylase have been implicated as associated or interrelated factors.

Epidemiology

The syndrome usually is seen in children under age 18 yr. In the USA, most cases occur in late fall and winter. Both geographic and temporal clusters, as well as sporadic cases, have been described. Widespread outbreaks have occurred in association with regional influenza epidemics. Varicella virus, the enteroviruses, Epstein-Barr virus, and the myxoviruses have been associated with sporadic cases. In Thailand, AEFDV has been associated with aflatoxin ingestion. An increased incidence among siblings has been noted, but whether environmental factors (eg, common exposure to exogenous toxins or viruses) or genetic predispositions (eg, an inherited enzyme deficiency) account for the familial clustering is unknown.

Pathology

With light microscopy, uniform intracytoplasmic panlobular microvesicular fatty infiltration of the liver is seen, which stains with oil red O (a Sudan dye) on frozen section. Fatty accumulation in the pancreas, heart, kidney, spleen, and lymph nodes, and pulmonary histiocytes have also been described. Fatty infiltration is thought to be neutral lipid (probably triglyceride) and hepatic inflammation is generally absent or slight. An occasional patient, especially one who has had significant hypotension, may show zonal hepatic necrosis that is typically central in the hepatic lobule. Electron microscopic sections of liver show mitochondrial injury that varies with the severity of the disease but includes glycogen depletion, smooth endoplasmic reticulum prolifera-

tion, peroxisome damage, and swelling of the mitochondrial matrix. Histologic abnormalities of the liver usually return to normal by 8 to 12 wk after onset of the disease.

CNS findings are generally nonspecific and include cerebral edema, gyral flattening, swollen white matter, and ventricular compression. On microscopy, perineuronal and perivascular clear spaces with swollen astrocytes are seen.

Symptoms and Signs

Severity of the disease varies greatly, but the syndrome is characterized by a biphasic illness: initially a viral infection, usually a URI (occasionally exanthematous) is followed on about day 6 by the onset of *pernicious* nausea and vomiting and by a sudden change in mental status. When associated with varicella, the encephalopathy usually develops on the 4th to 5th day of the rash. The changes in mental status may vary from a mild amnesia and noticeable lethargy to intermittent episodes of disorientation and agitation that often progress rapidly to deepening stages of coma manifested by progressive unresponsiveness, decorticate and decerebrate posturing, seizures, flaccidity, fixed dilated pupils, and respiratory arrest. Focal neurologic findings are usually not present. Hepatomegaly occurs in about 40% of cases, but jaundice is rare.

Complications include electrolyte and fluid disturbances, diabetes insipidus, inappropriate ADH syndrome, hypotension, cardiac arrhythmias, bleeding diatheses (especially GI), pancreatitis, respiratory insufficiency, and aspiration pneumonia. In fatal cases, the mean time from hospitalization to death is 4 days.

Diagnosis and Laboratory Findings

Reye's syndrome should be suspected in any child exhibiting the acute onset of an encephalopathy (without known heavy metal or toxin exposure) *associated with hepatic dysfunction.* Liver biopsy provides the definitive diagnosis and is especially useful in sporadic cases and in young children. The diagnosis may also be made when the typical clinical findings and the history are associated with a constellation of laboratory findings: increased liver transaminases (AST [SGOT], ALT [SGPT] > 3 times normal), usually normal bilirubin, increased blood ammonia level, and prolonged prothrombin time. CSF examination usually shows increased pressure, < 8 to 10 WBC/L, and normal protein; the glutamine level may be elevated. Hypoglycemia and hypoglycorrachia are seen in 15% of cases, especially in children under age 4 yr.

Signs of widespread metabolic derangements also may be present and include elevated serum levels of the amino acids glutamine, alanine, lysine, and α-amino-N-butyrate, and of the medium-chain free fatty acids; acid-base disturbances, usually hyperventilation with mixed respiratory alkalosis and metabolic acidosis; and other electrolyte abnormalities such as hyper- and hypo-osmolality, hypernatremia, hypokalemia, and hypophosphatemia.

Differential diagnosis includes other causes of coma and hepatic dysfunction, such as sepsis or hyperthermia (especially in infants); potentially treatable inborn abnormalities of urea synthesis or of fatty acid oxidation—eg, systemic carnitine deficiency or medium chain acyl-CoA dehydrogenase **(MCAD)** deficiency with episodic hypoglycemia and hyperammonemia; inborn errors of urea synthesis with episodic hyperammonemia (also especially in infants); phosphorus or carbon tetrachloride intoxication; acute encephalopathy caused by salicylism or other drugs or poisons; viral encephalitis or meningoencephalitis; and acute hepatitis. Similar light-microscopy findings on liver biopsy may be seen with idiopathic steatosis of pregnancy and tetracycline liver toxicity.

Prognosis

Outcome is related to the severity and rate of progression of coma, severity of the increased intracranial pressure, and degree of blood ammonia elevation. A recom-

TABLE 191–5. STAGING OF REYE'S SYNDROME

Signs	*Stages*				
	I	II	III	IV	V
Level of consciousness	Lethargy, follows verbal commands	Combative or stuporous	Coma	Coma	Coma
Posture	Normal	Normal	Decorticate	Decerebrate	Flaccid
Response to painful stimuli	Purposeful	Purposeful or nonpurposeful	Decorticate	Decerebrate	None
Pupillary reaction	Brisk	Sluggish	Sluggish	Sluggish	None
Doll's eyes (oculocephalic reflex)	Normal	Conjugate deviation	Conjugate deviation	Inconsistent or absent	None

(From NIH Consensus Development Conference, Diagnosis and Treatment of Reye's Syndrome, in JAMA 246:2441–2444, November 27, 1981.)

mended staging system for evaluating Reye's syndrome patients is shown in TABLE 191–5. Progression from Stage I to higher stages can be anticipated when the initial blood ammonia level exceeds 100 μg/dL (60 μmol/L) and the prothrombin time is 3 sec or longer than that of the control. Fatality rates average 21%, but range from < 2% among patients in Stage I to > 80% in patients in stages IV or V. Fortunately, most patients are diagnosed while in Stage I, and it is believed that early intervention may ameliorate or prevent progression. Fatality rates average 21% but may be > 80% in patients who have seizures, flaccidity, and respiratory arrest. Prognosis for survivors usually is good. Recurrences are uncommon. The incidence of neurologic sequelae (mental retardation, cranial nerve palsies, motor dysfunction) is unknown but may be related to the severity of coma.

Treatment

Since the cause of the syndrome is uncertain and widespread metabolic derangements are present, no universally accepted therapy exists. Early diagnosis and prompt institution of intensive supportive care are the mainstays of treatment. Meticulous and constant attention to the neurologic, electrolyte, metabolic, cardiovascular, respiratory, and fluid status is essential to cope with rapid changes. Treatment includes IV fluid and electrolyte solutions containing glucose, usually 5 to 10% but occasionally up to 50%; judicious use of cathartics and nonabsorbable antibiotics (eg, neomycin 100 mg/kg/day orally in divided doses q 6 h); and vitamin K_1 5 mg/day IV or IM. Increased intracranial pressure must be controlled with such agents as mannitol 0.5 to 1.0 gm/kg given IV over 45 min, dexamethasone 0.5 mg/kg/day IV, or glycerol 3 to 6 gm/kg/day by gastric tube; close monitoring of intracranial pressure may help to guide this therapy. Common procedures include monitoring blood gases, blood pH, and blood pressure by arterial catheters; inserting an endotracheal tube; and controlling ventilation. Other treatment modalities, eg, exchange transfusion, hemodialysis, and induction of deep coma with the use of barbiturates (to reduce intracranial pressure), have not been proved to be effective. Attempts to reduce the hyperammonemia by using agents such as sodium benzoate are being evaluated.

KAWASAKI SYNDROME

(Mucocutaneous Lymph Node Syndrome [MLNS])

A syndrome usually occurring in infants and children < 5 yr of age, consisting of a characteristic exanthem, enanthem, fever, lymphadenopathy, and polyarteritis of variable severity.

Etiology, Epidemiology, and Pathology

The etiology is unknown. First described in Japan in the 1960s, thousands of cases have been reported worldwide in diverse racial and ethnic groups, but children of Japanese descent have a higher prevalence. Most patients have been 2 mo to 5 yr of age, but Kawasaki syndrome has been reported in individuals up to 34 yr. The male:female ratio is about 1.8:1. No clear-cut seasonal or geographic pattern has been observed. In Japan, it has been suggested that genetic factors affect susceptibility to the syndrome; the histocompatibility antigen HLA-Bw22 was found in these patients about twice as often as in the general population (25% vs. 12%), but no single HLA antigen is common to all cases.

The pathology is nearly identical to infantile periarteritis nodosa, with vasculitis primarily affecting large- and medium-sized arteries. There is a particular predilection for the coronary vessels. An immunologic basis for the pathological findings is generally suspected.

Symptoms and Signs

The illness tends to progress through stages, beginning with fever, usually remittent and > 39 C (102.2 F), associated with irritability, often lethargy, and occasional intermittent, colicky abdominal pain. Usually within a day of fever onset, a polymorphous, erythematous macular rash appears, primarily over the trunk, especially in the perineal region. The rash varies and may, for example, be urticarial and pruritic. This is followed within several days by mucous membrane changes, including injected pharynx; reddened, dry, fissured lips; bilateral conjunctival injection; and a red "strawberry" tongue.

The most characteristic changes occur in the distal parts of the extremities. During the first week of illness, pallor of the proximal portion of the fingernails or toenails (leukonychia partialis) may be apparent. Erythema or a purple-red discoloration and variable edema of the palms and soles usually appear on about the 3rd to 5th day of illness. While edema may be slight, it is often tense, hard, and not subject to pitting with pressure. Periungual, palmar, and plantar desquamation begin on about the 10th day after onset. The superficial layer of the skin sometimes comes off in large casts, revealing new, normal skin. Cervical lymphadenopathy is often present throughout the course. The illness may last from 2 to 12 wk or longer. Relapses may occur.

The most feared additional expressions of the disease include those related to the heart and usually begin about the 10th day, as the rash, fever, and other early acute manifestations begin to subside; ie, in a subacute phase of the syndrome. Inflammation of the coronary arteries occurs in 5 to 20% of all cases and sometimes leads to acute myocarditis with congestive heart failure, arrhythmias, pericarditis, cardiac tamponade, thrombosis, infarction, or development of coronary artery aneurysms.

Other findings indicate involvement of many systems. Arthritis or arthralgias occur in about 1/3 of patients (mainly involving large joints). Other findings may include pneumonia, aseptic meningitis, diarrhea, and tympanitis. Less common manifestations are hepatitis, hydrops of the gallbladder, anterior uveitis, encephalopathy, pleural effusions, tonsillar exudate, and unusual exanthems—petechial, vesicular, or pruritic.

Laboratory Findings

Leukocytosis, frequently with a marked increase in immature ("band") forms, is common in the acute phase of the illness. Other hematologic findings include a mild anemia, thrombocytosis (500,000/μL or greater) in the 2nd or 3rd wk of illness, and

elevated ESR. Serum immunoglobulins are characteristically increased, particularly IgE. Serum complement and transaminase values are often mildly elevated.

Other laboratory abnormalities may be observed, depending on the organ systems involved, and include pyuria, proteinuria, CSF pleocytosis, and ECG changes (arrhythmias, decreased voltage, or left ventricular hypertrophy). Echocardiography, a very good means of detecting coronary artery aneurysms, probably should be performed in all patients in about the 5th wk. Coronary arteriography is useful in selected cases.

Cultures for bacteria and viruses, as well as serologic tests for evidence of infection, have been unrevealing. Some patients have shown positive antibody responses to proteus OX-19 or OX-K antigens, but specific rickettsial serologies have been negative.

Diagnosis

This is based on the clinical findings and reasonable exclusion of other diseases. The diagnosis is accepted only if 5 of the following 6 criteria are noted: (1) fever of 5 or more days; (2) bilateral conjunctival injection; (3) lip, tongue, and oral mucosa changes (injection, drying, fissuring, "strawberry tongue"); (4) changes of the peripheral extremities (edema, erythema, desquamation); (5) polymorphous truncal exanthem; (6) cervical lymphadenopathy.

The **differential diagnosis** includes bacterial diseases (especially scarlet fever, staphylococcal exfoliative syndromes, and leptospirosis), viral exanthems (eg, measles), rickettsial disease (eg, Rocky Mountain spotted fever), toxoplasmosis, acrodynia, Stevens-Johnson syndrome, juvenile RA, and infantile periarteritis nodosa.

Prognosis

The overall case–fatality ratio is estimated at 1 to 2% and is most commonly related to cardiac complications. Unfortunately, the fatalities are unpredictable; > 50% occur during the first month after onset, 75% within 2 mo, and 95% within 6 mo. Death has also been reported to occur as long as 10 yr later, and can be sudden and unexpected at any time. However, if no coronary artery disease can be demonstrated, the prognosis for complete recovery is excellent. Aneurysms tend to regress within 1 yr, although it is not known whether residual coronary lesions remain.

Treatment

There is no specific therapy. During the acute, febrile phase, aspirin at doses of 80 to 150 mg/kg, divided at 6-h intervals, is thought to reduce the risk of coronary artery involvement. Doses are adjusted to achieve serum levels of 20 to 25 mg/dL. Following the febrile phase, aspirin 5 to 10 mg/kg once daily has been recommended, primarily for its antithrombotic effect. ECGs should be checked frequently, and some authorities recommend close follow-up with two-dimensional echocardiography and consideration of coronary angiography whenever a coronary aneurysm is suspected. The duration of aspirin therapy is guided by the clinical course and is usually continued for several months. If coronary aneurysms develop, treatment should be continued indefinitely until they disappear.

In Japan, a multicenter controlled trial comparing treatment with aspirin alone and treatment with aspirin and a 5-day course of IV γ-globulin **(IVGG)** demonstrated significantly fewer coronary artery lesions in the group that received IVGG.

Corticosteroids are not recommended as routine therapy in this syndrome; in fact, there is some evidence that they may increase the risk of development of coronary aneurysms.

PINWORM INFESTATION

(Enterobiasis; Oxyuriasis)

An intestinal infestation by Enterobius vermicularis *characterized by perianal itching.* The pinworm is the most common parasite infesting children in temperate climates.

The prevalence of *Enterobius* in the general childhood population is at least 20%; for institutionalized children it is as high as 90%.

Etiology

Infestation usually results from finger transfer of eggs from the perianal area to fomites (clothing, bedding, toys), from which the ova are picked up by the new host, transmitted to the mouth, and swallowed. Airborne eggs may be inhaled and then swallowed. Reinfestation (or autoinfestation) easily occurs through finger transfer of eggs from the perianal area to the mouth.

The parasites reach maturity in the lower GI tract within 2 to 6 wk. The female worm migrates to the perianal region (usually at night) to deposit her eggs within the skin folds. The sticky gelatinous substance in which the ova are deposited and the movements of the female worm cause pruritus. The ova normally survive for as long as 3 wk. In that time the larvae may hatch and migrate back within the rectum and lower intestine (retroinfestation).

Symptoms and Signs

Most who harbor pinworms have no symptoms or signs. Some will, however, experience perianal itching and develop excoriations in this area from persistent scratching. Abdominal pain, toxic synovitis, insomnia, convulsions, and many other conditions have been attributed to pinworm infestation, but a causal relationship has not been demonstrated. Appendicitis due to obstruction of the appendiceal lumen by pinworms may occur but is rare.

Diagnosis

Pinworm infestation can be diagnosed by finding the female worm, which is about 10 mm long (males average 3 mm), in the perianal region 1 or 2 h after the child has been put to bed for the night, or by low-power microscopic identification of the ova. The ova are obtained in the early morning before the child arises, by patting the perianal skin folds with a strip of transparent adhesive tape, placed sticky side out over the end of a tongue depressor. The tape is then put sticky side down on a glass slide. A drop of toluene between tape and slide will dissolve the mucilage and eliminate the air bubbles in the tape that can hamper identification of the ova.

Treatment and Prognosis

Since the parasitic relationship is seldom harmful, prevalence is high, and reinfestation is probable, treatment is usually not indicated. However, most parents are shocked by the concept of infestation and actively seek treatment even when their children have had pinworms many times. Pyrantel pamoate in 1 dose of 11 mg/kg (maximum 1 gm) given orally and repeated after 2 wk will eradicate pinworms in about 90% of cases. Retro- and reinfestation are likely, since ova may be deposited for as long as 1 wk following therapy, and the ova deposited in the environment prior to therapy will survive for as long as 3 wk. Treatment of only one family member is useless, since multiple infestations within the household are the rule. Meticulous hand washing and housekeeping have little effect on the control or treatment of pinworm infestation.

Carbolated petrolatum or other antipruritic creams or ointments used topically in the perianal region 2 to 3 times daily may relieve the itching.

When infestation recurs, complete eradication of pinworms for a single family would be possible in most instances under the following extreme regimen: (1) all family members receive the therapeutic dose of pyrantel pamoate; (2) the family move out of their home for 3 wk, preferably taking a vacation, during which time they stay at a different place each night; and (3) pyrantel pamoate is given to all again at the end of 2 wk.

Since only 20% of the childhood population harbor pinworms, and a large percentage of those who encounter this parasite never receive treatment, there must be unknown means by which an individual rids himself of enterobius or the enterobius gives up its parasitic relationship with humans.

192. NEOPLASMS

Childhood neoplasms are also discussed elsewhere in THE MANUAL (eg, Chs. 101, 105, and 126).

WILMS' TUMOR
(Nephroblastoma)

An embryonal adenomyosarcoma of the kidneys with heterogeneous carcinomatous elements that occurs fetally and may not manifest itself clinically for years. A genetic defect has been associated in some cases (see under GENETICS OF MALIGNANT DISEASE in Ch. 203).

Symptoms, Signs, and Diagnosis

The diagnosis usually is made in children < 5 yr of age, but the tumor occasionally can be detected in adults. The most frequent presenting finding is a palpable abdominal mass; other findings include abdominal pain, hematuria, fever, anorexia, nausea, and vomiting. Hematuria (15 to 20% of cases) indicates invasion of the collecting system. Hypertension may occur secondary to ischemia from renal pedicle or parenchymal compression.

The intrarenal tumor usually distorts the functioning parenchyma. Abdominal ultrasound defines the cystic or solid nature of the mass, and excretory urography usually is diagnostic. Renal arteriography, vena cavography, or retrograde pyelography seldom is required. CT scan of the abdomen is helpful in staging the tumor but may be difficult to perform in small children. Chest films are indicated, since metastatic pulmonary involvement is fairly common at the time of initial diagnosis. Bilateral synchronous Wilms' tumors occur in about 4% of cases. Congenital anomalies, such as aniridia and hemi-hypertrophy, are associated with an increased incidence of Wilms' tumor.

Prognosis and Treatment

Prognosis depends on the histologic appearance of the tumor, the stage at the time of diagnosis, and the age of the patient. However, when treated with surgery alone or in combination with radiation and chemotherapy, the disorder has a high cure rate.

Prompt surgical exploration of potentially resectable lesions is indicated, with examination of the contralateral kidney. Chemotherapy with actinomycin D and vincristine, and radiation therapy are used depending on the stage of the disease. (For further discussion of treatment, see under ANTINEOPLASTIC CHEMOTHERAPY in Ch. 105.) The National Wilms' Tumor Study Group has established staging criteria and suggestions for treatment.

NEUROBLASTOMA

A common solid tumor of childhood arising mainly in the adrenal gland, but also from any portion of the extra-adrenal sympathetic chain, including in the retroperitoneum or chest. A familial incidence of neuroblastoma is observed (see under GENETICS OF MALIGNANT DISEASE in Ch. 203). Many neuroblastomas are functional, producing

elevated levels of serum or urinary catecholamines. **Ganglioneuroma** is a benign neoplasm that occasionally represents maturation of neuroblastoma; ganglioneuroma usually occurs in adults.

Symptoms, Signs, and Diagnosis

Approximately 75% of these tumors are diagnosed in children < 5 yr of age. About 50% begin in the abdomen; 15 to 20%, in the thorax. Presenting symptoms and signs depend on the site of origin and disease stage. A palpable abdominal mass or evidence of a metastatic lesion to liver, lung, or bone, especially to the skull in the orbital region, may be the initial presentation. If bones are involved, bone pain may be present. Bone marrow involvement may cause pallor (anemia), petechiae (thrombocytopenia), and leukopenia. Other tumor sites are not uncommon, including the skin and brain. Hemorrhage and necrosis into the tumor occur, and abdominal tumors may cross the midline. Differential diagnosis includes Wilms' tumor; renal masses; rhabdomyosarcoma, hepatomas, and other tumors; and tumors of GI and genital origins. Diagnostic tests include ultrasound, bone marrow examination, intravenous urography, and bone and CT scans. Elevated urinary vanillylmandelic acid (VMA) is diagnostic (a 24-h urine collection).

Prognosis and Treatment

Surgical excision of localized primary lesions provides the best chance for cure. For more advanced disease, a staging procedure is necessary. However, most patients (especially if > 1 yr of age) present with metastatic disease to liver, lung, or bone. Chemotherapeutic agents such as vincristine, cyclophosphamide, doxorubicin, and cisplatin are used, as well as radiation therapy for advanced disease. Spontaneous regression of neuroblastomas has been reported with hemorrhage and necrosis. The younger the child at the time of diagnosis (< 2 yr) the better the prognosis for cure, partly because younger children tend to have less disseminated disease.

RETINOBLASTOMA

A malignant tumor that arises from the immature retina. It occurs in 1:15,000 to 1:30,000 live births and represents about 2% of childhood malignancies. The disease may be inherited or the result of a new germinal mutation. About 10% of patients have a family history of retinoblastoma and another 30% have bilateral disease; all of these (ie, 40% of the patients) will pass the trait to their children as an autosomal dominant. The remaining 60% of patients have unilateral and nonheritable disease. A small proportion of cases have a deletion involving chromosome 13*q*14, but all heritable cases carry a mutant gene, "the retinoblastoma gene" at locus 13*q*14 (see also under GENETICS OF MALIGNANT DISEASE in Ch. 203).

Diagnosis is usually made before age 2 yr when a white reflex from the pupil ("cat's eye") or strabismus is investigated. Both fundi must be carefully examined by indirect ophthalmoscopy with the pupils widely dilated and the child under anesthesia. The tumors appear as single or multiple gray-white elevations in the retina; tumor "seeds" may be visible in the vitreous. In almost all tumors, calcification can be detected by CT scan.

Treatment: If diagnosed when the tumor is intraocular, > 90% can be cured. Unilateral retinoblastoma is usually managed by enucleation with removal of as much optic nerve as possible. In asymmetric bilateral cases, the more involved eye often is enucleated and the other eye treated by photocoagulation, cryotherapy, radiation, and systemic antimetabolites—often in combination. Ophthalmologic reexamination of both eyes and retreatment, if necessary, are required at 2- to 4-mo intervals. Studies of spinal fluid and bone marrow for malignant cells are conducted concomitantly. Other

malignancies frequently develop in later life in retinoblastoma patients. Siblings and other family members should be examined, and should be informed about the genetic implications and risks.

---

193. PULMONARY DISORDERS

CYSTIC FIBROSIS (CF)

(Mucoviscidosis; Fibrocystic Disease of the Pancreas; Pancreatic Cystic Fibrosis)

An inherited disease of the exocrine glands, primarily affecting the GI and respiratory systems, and usually characterized by the triad of chronic obstructive pulmonary disease, exocrine pancreatic insufficiency, and abnormally high sweat electrolytes.

Etiology and Incidence

CF, the most common lethal genetic disease in the white population, occurs in the USA in about 1:2000 white and 1:17,000 black live births; it is rare in Orientals. Twenty percent of patients in the USA are adults. It is inherited as an autosomal recessive trait (carried by about 5% of the white population). Heterozygotes are clinically unaffected. The basic defect remains unknown.

Pathology and Pathophysiology

Nearly all exocrine glands are affected but in varying distribution and degree of severity. Involved glands fall into 3 types: (1) those that become obstructed by viscid or solid eosinophilic material in the lumen (pancreas, intestinal glands, intrahepatic bile ducts, gallbladder, submaxillary glands); (2) those that produce an excess of histologically normal secretions (tracheobronchial and Brunner's glands); and (3) those that are normal histologically but secrete excessive Na and Cl (sweat, parotid, and small salivary glands). Duodenal secretions are viscid and contain an abnormal mucopolysaccharide. Aspermia and infertility are seen in 98% of adult men secondary to maldevelopment of the vas deferens. In women fertility is decreased secondary to viscid cervical secretions, but many women with CF have carried pregnancies to term. However, there is a high incidence of maternal complications and fetal wastage.

Evidence suggests that the lungs are normal at birth. The pulmonary lesion is probably initiated by diffuse obstruction of the small airways by abnormally thick mucus secretions. Secondary to obstruction, there is bronchiolitis and mucopurulent plugging of the airways. Bronchial changes are more common than parenchymal changes. Emphysema is not a prominent feature. Early in the course, *Staphylococcus aureus* is the pathogen most often isolated from respiratory tract secretions, but as the disease progresses *Pseudomonas aeruginosa* becomes the most frequent sputum isolate. A mucoid variant of pseudomonas is uniquely associated with CF. As the pulmonary process progresses, bronchial walls thicken, the airways remain filled with purulent and viscid secretions, areas of atelectasis develop, and hilar lymph nodes enlarge. Chronic hypoxemia results in muscular hypertrophy of the pulmonary arteries, pulmonary hypertension, and right ventricular hypertrophy. Death usually results from a combination of respiratory failure and cor pulmonale.

Symptoms and Signs

Meconium ileus due to obstruction of the ileum by viscid meconium is the earliest possible sign (see in GASTROINTESTINAL DEFECTS in Ch. 187), which is present at birth in 7% to 10% of affected infants. It is often associated with volvulus, perforation, or atresia, and, with rare exceptions, is always followed by the other signs of CF. In the newborn period CF may also be associated with the **meconium plug syndrome**, a tran-

sient form of distal intestinal obstruction secondary to 1 or more plugs of inspissated meconium in the anus or colon.

In infants without meconium ileus, onset is frequently heralded by a delay in regaining birthweight and inadequate weight gain at 4 to 6 wk of age. Pancreatic insufficiency is clinically apparent in 85 to 90% of patients. Manifestations include the passage of frequent, bulky, foul-smelling, oily stools; abdominal protuberance; and poor growth pattern with decreased subcutaneous tissue and muscle mass, despite a normal or even voracious appetite. Rectal prolapse occurs in 20% of untreated infants and toddlers. Clinical signs may be related to deficiency of the fat-soluble vitamins; CF should be considered in every infant with hypoprothrombinemia. Infants with CF who have been on soy protein formula or breast milk may develop hypoproteinemia with edema and anemia secondary to protein malabsorption. Excessive sweating (as in hot weather or with fever) may lead to episodes of hypotonic dehydration and circulatory failure. In arid climates infants may present with chronic metabolic alkalosis. Findings of salt crystal formation on the skin and a salty taste on the skin are highly suggestive of CF.

Fifty percent of all patients present with **pulmonary manifestations** usually consisting of chronic cough and wheezing associated with recurrent or chronic pulmonary infections. Cough is the most troublesome complaint, often accompanied by gagging, vomiting, and disturbed sleep. With progression of disease, there are intercostal retractions, use of accessory muscles of respiration, a barrel-chest deformity, digital clubbing, and cyanosis. Upper respiratory tract involvement includes nasal polyposis and opacification of the paranasal sinuses. Teenagers may have retarded growth, delayed onset of puberty, and a declining tolerance for exercise. Pulmonary complications in adolescents and adults include pneumothorax, hemoptysis, and right heart failure secondary to pulmonary hypertension. Insulin-requiring diabetes develops in 2 to 3% of patients, and multinodular biliary cirrhosis with varices and portal hypertension develops in 4 to 5% of adolescents and adults. Chronic and/or recurrent abdominal pain may be related to intussusception, pancreatitis, gastroesophageal reflux, gallbladder disease, or episodes of partial intestinal obstruction secondary to abnormally viscid fecal contents.

Laboratory Findings

Since meconium in most neonates with CF contains large amounts of serum proteins (especially albumin), meconium examination has been used as the basis of a newborn screening test. However, since such testing does not detect the 10 to 15% of patients with normal or near-normal pancreatic enzymes, it is not recommended for mass screening. Pancreatic insufficiency is present in about 85% of patients with CF. The duodenal fluid is abnormally viscid and shows absence or diminution of enzyme activity and decreased HCO_3^- concentration; stool trypsin and chymotrypsin are absent or diminished. Tests of fat absorption, including 72-h fecal fat excretion, provide an indirect assessment of pancreatic exocrine function. Patients with normal exocrine pancreatic function fail to produce HCO_3^- following IV secretin stimulation. About 40% of patients show a diabetic oral glucose tolerance curve secondary to a reduced and delayed insulin response. Fasting blood levels of carotenoids, vitamins A and E, essential fatty acids, and cholesterol are reduced in patients with steatorrhea. Total serum protein is initially normal, but with advanced disease, the α_1-, α_2-, and γ-globulin fractions are elevated and albumin is decreased.

The serum concentration of immunoreactive trypsin has been reported to be elevated in newborns with CF and is being evaluated as a means of newborn screening; a radioimmunoassay has been developed for use with dried blood spots routinely collected for newborn metabolic screening.

Chest x-ray findings may be helpful in suggesting the diagnosis of CF. Hyperinflation and bronchial wall thickening are the earliest findings. Subsequent changes include areas of infiltrate, atelectasis, and hilar adenopathy. With advanced disease

segmental or lobar atelectasis, cyst formation, bronchiectasis, and pulmonary artery and right ventricular enlargement are seen. Branching, finger-like opacifications, representing mucoid impaction of dilated bronchi, are characteristic. Pulmonary function tests reveal hypoxemia, reduction in forced vital capacity, forced expiratory volume in 1 sec and $FEV_1/FVC\%$, and an increase in residual volume and the ratio of residual volume: total lung capacity.

Diagnosis

There is no reliable test for prenatal diagnosis or for heterozygote (carrier) detection. In the general population, however, the recent discovery of linkage markers for the CF gene on chromosome 7 allows for prenatal diagnosis and heterozygote detection in families with a previously affected child. The diagnosis is usually confirmed in infancy or early childhood, but 10% of patients escape detection until adolescence or early adulthood.

Diagnosis of CF is suggested by the clinical and laboratory features described above and then confirmed by demonstrating an elevation of Na and/or Cl concentrations in sweat. The only reliable test is the **quantitative pilocarpine iontophoresis sweat test**: localized sweating is stimulated pharmacologically, the amount of sweat collected is measured, and the electrolyte concentration determined. In patients with a suggestive clinical picture or a positive family history, a Na or Cl concentration > 60 mEq/L confirms the diagnosis of CF. It is estimated that < 1:1000 patients with CF will have a sweat chloride < 50 mEq/L. False-negative results are rare, but may occur in the presence of edema and hypoproteinemia or with inadequate quantities of sweat. False-positive results are usually related to technical errors or use of inappropriate equipment. Although results of the sweat test are valid after the first 24 h of life, it may be difficult to obtain an adequate sweat sample (> 50 mg) before 3 to 4 wk of age. Concentrations of electrolytes in sweat normally increase slightly with age; nevertheless, the sweat test is valid in adults.

A small subset of patients, labeled as **CF variants,** have chronic pseudomonas bronchitis, normal pancreatic function, and intermediate sweat Cl concentrations in the range of 40 to 60 mEq/L.

Prognosis

The course of CF, largely determined by the degree of pulmonary involvement, varies greatly from patient to patient. However, deterioration is inevitable, leading to debilitation and eventual death. The prognosis has steadily improved over the past four decades, mainly due to institution of aggressive treatment before the onset of irreversible pulmonary changes. Median survival is to 20 yr of age. Long-term survival is somewhat better for males than for females. Over the course of the illness, caregivers, including physicians, nurses, physical therapists, counselors, and social workers have opportunity to form the kind of supportive environment for these patients and their families that will make their condition more tolerable. With appropriate support, most patients can make an age-appropriate adjustment at both home and school. Despite myriad problems, the occupational and marital successes of these patients are impressive. Most patients work or attend school until shortly before death.

Genetic counseling can be useful for at-risk families to explain the inheritance pattern of CF and empiric risk figures and to outline the possibilities for prenatal diagnosis and carrier detection.

Treatment

A comprehensive and intensive therapy program is essential, directed by an experienced, available physician in conjunction with the services of personnel in nursing, nutrition, physical and respiratory therapy, and counseling. The goals of therapy include maintenance of adequate nutritional status, prevention or aggressive therapy of

pulmonary complications, encouragement of physical activity, and provision of adequate psychosocial support.

Obstruction in uncomplicated meconium ileus can sometimes be relieved with enemas containing a hyperosmolar radiopaque contrast material, with surgical intervention if needed. After the newborn period, episodes of partial intestinal obstruction (**"meconium ileus equivalent"**) can be treated with enemas containing a hyperosmolar radiopaque contrast material or N-acetylcysteine. Oral administration of dioctyl sodium succinate or N-acetylcysteine may be helpful in preventing such episodes. When **pancreatic insufficiency** is present, pancreatic enzyme replacement in the form of powder, tablets, or capsules should be given with each meal, the dosage varying with the size of the meal, potency of the preparation, and stool pattern. The most effective enzyme preparations consist of pancrelipase in pH-sensitive, enteric-coated microspheres.

Diet therapy includes (1) sufficient calories and protein to promote normal growth—exceeding usual Recommended Dietary Allowance requirements (of the Food and Nutrition Board of the National Research Council) by 50%, (2) a normal-to-high total fat intake to increase the caloric density of the diet, (3) multivitamins in double the recommended daily allowance, (4) supplemental vitamin E in water miscible form, and (5) salt supplementation during periods of thermal stress and increased sweating. Infants on broad-spectrum antibiotics and patients with liver disease and hemoptysis should be given vitamin K supplements. Formulas containing protein hydrolysates and medium-chain triglycerides may be used instead of modified whole milk for infants with severe pancreatic insufficiency. Glucose polymers and medium-chain triglyceride supplements can be used to increase caloric intake. Long-term benefit has not been demonstrated for parenteral nutritional support.

Prophylaxis against respiratory infections consists of maintenance of pertussis and measles immunity, and annual influenza vaccination. There has been no demonstrated increase in susceptibility to or morbidity from pneumococcal infections and routine use of pneumococcal vaccine is *not* advocated.

Treatment of pulmonary manifestations includes prevention of airway obstruction and control of infection. Chest physical therapy consisting of postural drainage, percussion, vibration, and assisted coughing is recommended at the first indication of pulmonary involvement (see Ch. 33). If there is evidence of reversible airway obstruction, bronchodilators may be given orally and/or by aerosol. O_2 therapy is indicated in patients with severe pulmonary insufficiency and hypoxemia. In general, assisted ventilation is not indicated for CF patients with chronic respiratory failure. Its occasional use should be restricted to the patient with good baseline status in whom acute respiratory failure develops, or in association with pulmonary surgery.

Pneumothorax can be treated by closed chest tube thoracostomy in combination with the intrapleural installation of a sclerosing agent, eg, quinacrine 2% (100 mg in 50 mL isotonic saline) instilled daily for 3 days or by open thoracotomy with resection of blebs and pleural abrasion.

Aerosolized mucolytics and oral expectorants are widely used, but few data support their efficacy. The use of home mist tents is no longer recommended as studies of aerosol deposition, pulmonary function, chest x-ray changes, and sputum viscosity have failed to demonstrate any benefit. Tracheobronchial lavage provides temporary improvement in some patients, but results have not been shown to be superior to those obtained with an intensive course of chest physical therapy and IV antibiotics. The use of IPPB devices is not recommended because of the possibility of causing a pneumothorax.

Antibiotics: In symptomatic outpatients, bacterial pathogens in the respiratory tract should be treated with effective doses of appropriate drugs as determined by culture and sensitivity testing. Penicillinase-resistant penicillins, eg, cloxacillin or dicloxacillin,

or a cephalosporin are the agents of choice for *Staphylococci*. Erythromycin, ampicillin, trimethoprim/sulfamethoxazole, tetracycline, or occasionally chloramphenicol may be used individually or in combination for protracted ambulatory therapy of pulmonary infection due to a variety of organisms. For severe pulmonary exacerbations, especially in patients colonized with *Pseudomonas*, admission to the hospital for parenteral antibiotic therapy is advised. Combinations of an aminoglycoside with an anti-*pseudomonas* penicillin are frequently used by the IV route. Some of the newer cephalosporins with anti-*pseudomonas* activity may be useful. Serum aminoglycoside concentrations should be monitored and dosage adjusted to achieve a peak level of 8 to 10 μg/mL and a trough value of 1 μg/mL. Patients with CF may require high doses of aminoglycosides to achieve acceptable serum concentrations. They also show enhanced renal clearance of some penicillins and may require large doses to achieve adequate serum levels. The goal of treating pulmonary infections should be to improve the clinical picture sufficiently so that continuous use of antibiotics is unnecessary. However, in some ambulatory patients with recurrent pulmonary exacerbations, long-term use of appropriate antibiotics may be indicated. In selected patients chronic anti-*pseudomonas* therapy delivered by aerosol may be effective.

Massive or recurrent hemoptyses are treated by embolization of the involved bronchial arteries. Patients with symptomatic **right heart failure** should be treated with diuretics, salt restriction, and O_2.

Surgery may be indicated for the following: localized bronchiectasis or atelectasis that cannot be effectively treated medically; nasal polyps; bleeding from esophageal varices secondary to portal hypertension; gallbladder disease; and intestinal obstruction due to a volvulus or an intussusception that cannot be medically reduced.

---

194. GASTROINTESTINAL DISORDERS

RECURRENT ABDOMINAL PAIN (RAP)

(See also Abdominal Pain in Ch. 55)

Three or more episodes of pain over at least 3 mo. The persistence, recurrence, and chronicity of RAP distinguish it from the presentation of children with an "acute" abdomen. Incidence in the general population is slightly > 10%; the ratio of girls to boys is 4:3. RAP is rare in children < 4 to 5 yr old and most common between ages 8 to 10 yr, with a second peak noted among early adolescent girls.

There are 3 distinct types of RAP depending upon whether it arises secondary to organic disease, a dysfunctional state, or stress that results in psychogenic pain.

RAP OF ORGANIC ORIGIN

An organic cause for symptoms is found in only 5 to 10% of children with RAP. Table 194–1 lists the most commonly occurring organic diseases that should be considered in the differential diagnosis. Of these conditions, inflammatory bowel disease, chronic appendicitis, peptic ulcer disease, parasitism (especially in endemic areas), urinary tract disease, and sickle cell disease are found most frequently. In adolescent girls, pelvic inflammatory disease and ovarian cyst should be considered.

Symptoms, Signs, and Diagnosis

Pain from organic disease has certain distinctive characteristics. It is commonly described as constant or cyclical (associated with certain activities or related to diet) and is well localized, especially to areas other than the periumbilical region, and may penetrate to the back. It frequently may wake the child from sleep. Associated find-

TABLE 194–1. ORGANIC ETIOLOGIES OF RECURRENT ABDOMINAL PAIN

Etiology	Diagnostic Approach
GU Disorders	
Congenital abnormalities	IV urogram
UTI	Urine culture
Pelvic inflammatory disease	Pelvic examination
Ovarian cyst, endometriosis	Gynecologic consultation
GI Disorders	
Hiatus hernia	Barium swallow, fluoroscopy
Hepatitis	Liver function tests
Cholecystitis	Cholangiogram, ultrasound
Pancreatitis	Serum amylase level
Peptic ulcer disease	Upper GI series, endoscopy, stool for occult blood
Parasitic infestation (eg, Giardiasis)	Stool examination for ova, parasites
Meckel's diverticulum	Technetium scan
Granulomatous enterocolitis	ESR, barium enema
Intestinal TB	Tuberculin test
Ulcerative colitis	Sigmoidoscopy, rectal biopsy
(Postoperative) adhesive bands	Upper GI series
Pancreatic pseudocyst	Ultrasound
Chronic appendicitis	Abdominal x-ray, ultrasound
Systemic Disorders	
Lead intoxication	Blood lead, free erythrocyte protoporphyrin levels
Henoch-Schönlein purpura	History, urinalysis
Sickle cell disease	Sickle preparation, Hb electrophoresis
Food allergy	Elimination diet
Abdominal epilepsy	EEG
Porphyria	Urine uroporphyrin level
Familial Mediterranean anemia, familial angioneurotic edema, migraine equivalent	Family history

(Adapted from "Recurrent Abdominal Pain" by G. J. Barbero, in *Pediatrics in Review* Vol. 4, p. 30, 1982. Copyright 1982 by *Pediatrics.* Used with permission of *Pediatrics.)*

ings, which vary according to the underlying disease, include recurrent or persistent fever; jaundice; changes in bowel consistency, color, or elimination pattern; blood in the stools; vomiting; hematemesis; abdominal distention; joint symptoms; change in appetite; and weight loss.

Two entities deserve particular attention in pediatric patients because their presentation can be confusing: **(1) Peptic ulcer disease** is often missed because the typical relationship of food intake to pain sensation and the usual epigastric location of the pain, as seen in adults, are seen infrequently in children. **(2) UTI**, in which the pain may be described by the child as abdominal or pelvic in origin with no referral to the flank or the urethra, will be missed unless tested for specifically.

Treatment

When an underlying organic disorder is suspected, appropriate testing (see TABLE 194–1) should be done immediately and specific therapy instituted accordingly.

RAP ARISING FROM A DYSFUNCTIONAL STATE

Pain arising from a non-diseased organ as a result of interaction between constitutional and environmental factors. This classification is relatively new and its exact incidence in

RAP has not been quantified, but it probably occurs as frequently as organic disease. It is important because it contains a number of entities, each with a clearcut pathophysiologic basis for the pain that usually responds well to specific therapy; eg, diet change or drugs.

Etiology

Why some individuals with dysfunctional states develop abdominal pain and others do not is unknown. Perhaps anxiety alters autonomic and intestinal function, which then becomes expressed as pain in individuals with a constitutionally defined temperament prone to experience pain when stressed.

Diagnosis

Differential diagnosis of RAP arising from a dysfunctional state includes conditions such as constipation or fecal retention and incontinence secondary to inappropriate diet, ineffective toilet training, or improper toilet facilities for the child's size; dysmenorrhea; mittelschmerz (see Ch. 171); and lactose intolerance (see in Ch. 58) secondary to the normal physiologic decline in lactase activity seen in many population groups after the age of 4 to 5 yr. Because pain may not occur for up to 2 h after ingestion of milk or a milk product, the etiology of pain due to lactose intolerance may not be suspected initially.

A careful history defining associated symptoms or precipitating factors (eg, a 24-h diet recall to investigate food allergy or dietary indiscretion as the source of pain; menstrual history, etc) is the most important diagnostic tool. Once the underlying dysfunctional state has been identified, therapeutic efforts should be directed toward habit or diet change or appropriate analgesic therapy and patient/family education.

RAP OF PSYCHOGENIC ORIGIN

In 80 to 90% of all cases, RAP is of psychogenic origin. Its pathophysiology is unknown, but it appears to be linked to stress and anxiety, depression, or tension.

Symptoms and Signs

Pain may occur daily or several times a week or month. Occasionally, the child is symptom-free for weeks or months. Rarely sharp, the pain is generally vague and ill-defined, but sometimes is reported as crampy or colicky. Awakening during the night with pain is unusual, although some patients awake early because of discomfort.

Pain in psychogenic RAP is most often periumbilical, and it has been suggested that the farther the pain is from the umbilicus, the greater the likelihood of an organic disorder. However, this tendency is not diagnostic, and psychogenic pain can mimic any symptom complex. Thus, frequency, nature, and localization of pain are not reliable discriminators between the different types of RAP. Any change in the location or pattern of pain deserves immediate evaluation, because acute abdominal conditions of organic etiology can occur in patients with chronic psychogenic pain just as in any other population group.

Diagnosis and Differential Diagnosis

Distinguishing children with underlying organic conditions from children with dysfunctional or psychogenic abdominal pain can be difficult. Psychogenic pain, not a diagnosis of exclusion, must be documented by historical, personality, and family characteristics, findings on physical examination, and laboratory results consistent with the diagnosis.

The history: A most significant finding is that symptoms progress little or not at all; the child gets no worse with time. It is important to begin with the first attack of pain, documenting its frequency, nature, location; relationship to meals, defecation and voiding; and results of using any treatment including position change, home remedies, and OTC and prescription drugs. Important characteristics that suggest, but are not

pathognomonic of psychogenic pain, include *lack* of consistent bowel symptoms, fever, weight loss, or growth failure. Associated symptoms are common and can include headache, dizziness (not vertigo), facial pallor, and diaphoresis. Fatigue, anorexia, nausea, vomiting, diarrhea, constipation, and limb pains occur occasionally but are less common in psychogenic pain than with RAP of organic or dysfunctional etiology.

Psychosocial characteristics include evidence of immaturity, unusual dependence on parents, anxiety or depression, apprehension, tension, and perfectionism. Often parents see these children as special, either because of their position in the family (only child, youngest sibling, or only male or female child in a large sibship) or because of an early problem (colic or eating difficulty) or a minor unrelated medical condition. Parents are often described as anxious, overprotective, authoritarian, and preoccupied with the child. Data should be obtained regarding the occurrence of any possible precipitating factor such as illness, family discord, separation and loss, or school-related stress; evidence of primary gain (what the child avoided because of pain) or secondary gain (what psychosocial benefits may be derived from being sick); and the child's personality.

The family history frequently is positive for chronic somatic complaints or pain, peptic ulcer disease, headaches, "nerves," or depression. The history should include questions about similar or related illnesses in other family members, especially the parents at a similar age.

What constitutes a **"stressful situation"** is relative; these patients appear to be stressed easily. The physician can usually detect specific precipitating events at home (recent illness, financial problems, separation or loss) or at school (concern about performance or interpersonal relationships with teachers or peers). The illness itself also may compound any preexisting problems; eg, it may result in significant school absenteeism, isolation from peers, and increased sibling rivalry.

Physical examination: Most children are seen initially when they are symptom-free. Therefore, before making a final diagnosis, an evaluation should be performed during an episode of pain to observe for bowel distention and to be reassured that no signs of an organic disorder are overlooked. Except for evidence of periumbilical discomfort on palpation of the abdomen, findings on examination are typically negative. Once the physician is certain of the findings, frequently repeated examinations are to be avoided lest they focus on or magnify the physical complaints or instill or perpetuate the idea that the physician lacks confidence in the diagnosis.

Laboratory studies should be ordered promptly to allay patient and parent anxiety. Initial laboratory investigation, however, should be limited to a search for the most likely organic or dysfunctional causes of RAP. Appropriate tests to consider include Hb, Hct, blood smear, WBC count, and ESR; urinalysis and urine culture; examinations of the stool for ova, parasites, blood, pH, and reducing substances; a tuberculin test; liver function studies; serum amylase levels; and a plain x-ray of the abdomen. A test for sickle cell disease might be appropriate in selected at-risk patients. Specific, well-documented food intolerances, eg, lactose, should be evaluated appropriately (eg, by a trial of a lactose-free diet). Further evaluation, including contrast studies of the GI or urinary tract, EEG, or endoscopy, should be reserved for patients with specific indications.

Treatment

At least 2 extended visits will be necessary. Management begins with the initial evaluation, when the tone of the relationship between physician and family is established. Parents and child should be interviewed separately, and then together; all should be asked what they think (or fear) might be causing the problem. Parental

reaction to the pain and perceptions of their child's reactions to pain should be elicited.

The physical examination should be complete and performed in the presence of the parent(s), if appropriate, to impress upon them the care and thoroughness with which it was done. A list of laboratory studies desired and the reason why each has been selected should be shared with the family.

During the initial visit, it is premature to suggest specific treatment for the pain, even if the physician is fairly certain that the primary problem is psychogenic. Most parents are concerned about an underlying organic cause; unless this concern is adequately addressed through appropriate investigation, they are unlikely to react favorably or consistently to a behavioral management plan. Rather, between the initial evaluation and the follow-up visit, it is helpful to have the child and family keep a diary to record fully any episode of pain: its nature, intensity, and duration; precipitating factors; diet; defecation; and any remedies applied and the results obtained. By use of this diary method, inappropriate patterns of behavior and exaggerated responses to pain sometimes become obvious to the patient and family, facilitating cooperation in a behaviorally-oriented management strategy.

The follow-up appointment should be scheduled as soon as possible after results of the laboratory tests are available, so that findings can be shared and put into perspective, and a management plan outlined. Each parent's and child's specific concerns about cause or prognosis should be addressed and appropriate reassurance that the child is not in physical danger provided. The physician must redefine the problem for the family by reviewing the data that established the diagnosis, followed by demonstration of a clear understanding of the nature of the problem, and clarification of the mechanism of pain generation and its perception in the child.

In describing how the symptoms appear to be related to stress and tension, the difficulty should not be ascribed to an "emotional problem," which families erroneously interpret as meaning that the child is imagining pain or is "crazy"—fears and defensiveness about this issue may lead to resistance to further advice or therapy. Instead, by using the analogy of a stress or tension-related headache (experienced by most people at one time or another) the explanation is more likely to be understood and accepted.

The next step is to engage the family's cooperation in removing as many sources of excessive stress and tension as possible and helping the child to cope with unavoidable stress in a different, more effective, way. The goal is to avoid perpetuating the negative psychosocial aspects of chronic pain (eg, prolonged absences from school or withdrawal from peer activities).

The treatment plan should promote age-appropriate activities and increase independence and self-reliance, fostering the attitude that the child can either control or learn to live with the symptoms while participating fully in everyday activities. It is important to point out that as the parents change their attitude and stop treating the child as special or ill, *the symptoms may become worse for a period of time before they abate.*

Follow-up visits for support should be scheduled periodically (weekly, monthly, or bimonthly, depending upon the family's needs) until the problem has resolved *and* for some months afterward. Psychiatric referral may be required (up to 50% of families in some reports) when the symptom persists despite appropriate supportive counseling, especially when there is evidence of depression in the child or chronic marital conflict or serious psychologic difficulties in the parents.

Medications are not recommended; no drug has proved effective, and drugs can reinforce hypochondriasis or may lead to dependency.

Hospitalization is usually reserved for patients whose families have difficulty accepting a non-organic diagnosis or in whom further studies (including psychologic evalu-

ation and family interaction observation) are necessary. The hospitalization should be brief and goal-directed, to avoid reinforcing symptoms or unduly magnifying any aspect of the problem.

Prognosis

Long-term prognosis is guarded, and no single treatment regimen is universally successful. Some children later develop a variety of other somatic complaints or emotional difficulties.

CHILDHOOD PEPTIC ULCER

The diagnosis of peptic ulcer is not commonly made in infants and children. One reason may be that a satisfactory clinical history cannot be obtained in infants and young children. In the neonatal period, perforation and hemorrhage may be the first recognized manifestation. Hemorrhage may continue to be a first recognized symptom in later infancy and early childhood, although repeated vomiting or evidence of abdominal pain may be a clue to the diagnosis. After reaching school age, the child may be better able to localize the pain, describe it, and relate it to time of day and eating. Relationship to eating and occurrence at night suggest an ulcer. A barium x-ray study should be done first to establish the diagnosis. If it is negative and ulcer is still suspected, 2 options are open. The first option and the best way of making a definitive diagnosis would be to perform fiberoptic endoscopy, which, under the age of 7 or 8 yr, requires general or narcoleptic anesthesia. For definitive treatment, either ranitidine (10 to 20 mg/kg/day) or cimetidine (20 to 40 mg/kg/day) may be used orally, though neither has been tested formally in children for efficacy or safety. The second option, if endoscopy is not feasible and after excluding other possible causes of ulcerlike pain (see RECURRENT ABDOMINAL PAIN, above), is to treat the child for a presumptive diagnosis of ulcer with antacids or histamine H_2 antagonists as above. It is prudent to limit the duration of therapy to 6 to 8 wk. Recurrences and complications may occur as in adults, but obstruction is rare and the possibility of a gastric ulcer's being malignant is remote. Treatment follows the principles of adult care (see PEPTIC ULCER in Ch. 54).

MECKEL'S DIVERTICULUM

A congenital sacculation following incomplete obliteration of the vitello-intestinal duct. It may be found 30 to 150 cm (1 to 5 ft) proximal to the ileocecal valve in 1 to 2% of the population. Islands of gastric epithelium, occasionally found in a Meckel's diverticulum, can be identified by technetium scan. Peptic ulceration may develop in the adjacent tissue with pain, perforation, or massive hemorrhage as complications of the ulcer. A Meckel's diverticulum may precipitate intussusception, particularly during childhood. The diverticulum may resemble the appendix with similar potential for obstruction or infection; thus, it may mimic appendicitis with similar complications and treatment (see APPENDICITIS in Ch. 55). A chronic inflammatory process may lead to adhesions and obstruction of the small intestine or to ileal stricture and the signs and symptoms of lower obstruction (see BOWEL OBSTRUCTION in Ch. 55). **Treatment** is surgical excision.

---

195. NUTRITIONAL DISORDERS

NUTRITIONAL STATUS OF CHILDREN

Although frank deficiency states are rare in children of advanced western societies, marginal undernutrition is not uncommon in families living in poverty or consuming

restricted dietaries for alleged health reasons. Under such circumstances growth is primarily affected, usually resulting in a greater falling off in gain in weight than in height. Deviations can be detected by measurements at regular intervals and the use of standard growth charts. Single observations are insignificant, as individual children vary in their growth potential. Additionally, blood levels of vitamins A and C, thiamine, riboflavin, iron, and transferrin saturation are low in a significant proportion of these children. Zinc deficiency may be responsible for retarded growth and hypogeusia (see Ch. 82).

Any child suspected of having impaired nutritional status should have a careful history of dietary intake taken, including any suspected intolerance to certain foods (see FOOD ALLERGY AND INTOLERANCE in Ch. 21). A general physical examination should be made and systemic disease that causes undernutrition and impaired growth (eg, intestinal, liver, hormonal, renal, and heart disease) should be excluded. Specific tests for vitamin or trace element deficiencies are only necessary if the history or physical examination suggests their presence. In the absence of any evident cause for poor growth, reassurance should be given, but growth should be observed at regular intervals and dietary intake monitored.

ESSENTIAL FATTY ACIDS (EFA)

EFAs are unsaturated fatty acids that cannot be synthesized in the body and therefore must be provided by the diet. They are essential for many physiologic processes including growth, the integrity of cell membranes, and the synthesis of prostaglandins (see Ch. 284). The 3 most important EFAs are linoleic, linolenic, and arachidonic acids (see in NUTRITION in Ch. 79).

In infants, EFA deficiency has been observed following prolonged administration of fat-free diets or total parenteral nutrition and may result in a scaly dermatitis, thrombocytopenia, failure to thrive, poor wound healing, and increased susceptibility to infection. Low plasma levels of linoleic and arachidonic acids are diagnostic of early EFA deficiency.

For the maintenance of proper health, 2 to 3% of the total calories in the diet should be in the form of EFAs. Common vegetable oils (eg, corn, cottonseed, and soybean oil) are excellent sources of linoleic and linolenic acids. Arachidonic acid can be synthesized in the body from linoleic acid. In deficiency states up to 10 gm/day of EFA may be required.

INFANTILE SCURVY

(See also VITAMIN C DEFICIENCY in Ch. 81)

Scurvy: *An acute or chronic disease characterized by hemorrhagic manifestations and abnormal osteoid and dentin formation and caused by a deficiency of ascorbic acid.* Primary deficiency in infants is due to lack of supplementary vitamin C.

Symptoms and Signs

Infantile scurvy usually occurs between the 6th and 12th mo of life. Early symptoms include irritability, anorexia, and failure to gain weight. The child screams when moved and may keep his legs motionless because of pain from subperiosteal hemorrhage. Advanced cases show angular enlargements of the costochondral junctions (scorbutic rosary), swelling over the ends of the long bones (especially at the lower end of the femur), and a tendency to hemorrhage, as shown by swollen hemorrhagic gums surrounding erupting teeth. Skin hemorrhages at this age are rare, and gingivitis does not develop until teeth have erupted. Fever, anemia, and increased pulse and respiration rates are common. The anemia is usually normocytic and normochromic; however, macrocytosis and a megaloblastic bone marrow may be seen due either to a

combined deficiency of vitamin C and folic acid, or to oxidation of tetrahydrofolates to 10-formylfolic acid in the absence of vitamin C.

X-ray findings are characteristic. The ends of the long bones show a transverse thickening and increased density—the **white line.** Immediately shaftward of the white line is a localized area of rarefaction, first evident at the lateral margins and appearing in the x-ray as a small fracture. The trabecular markings of the shaft become indistinct, giving it a ground-glass appearance. After 7 to 10 days of therapy, some calcification results; x-ray shows a club-like swelling extending from the white line to the middle of the shaft (never into the joint). The blood is resorbed, and the bone resumes its normal shape as treatment proceeds.

Diagnosis

Infantile scurvy must be differentiated from rickets, poliomyelitis, osteomyelitis, rheumatic fever, and from hemorrhagic disorders (eg, blood diseases, severe anemias, allergic purpuras). Rickets often occurs before the 5th mo, scurvy almost never before the 6th. The diseases may rarely occur simultaneously. Hemorrhagic manifestations are absent in rickets. The costochondral junctions are enlarged in either condition, but in scurvy the swellings are angular while in rickets they tend to be rounded. Poliomyelitis is often considered because the baby does not move his legs and cries when moved; in scurvy, the absence of neurologic changes, the presence of bleeding, and bone changes permit differentiation. Joint involvement may suggest rheumatic fever, but this disease is uncommon before age 2. The bone swellings in scurvy never extend into the joint. Other diseases that cause bleeding can usually be excluded by their characteristic tests (see Ch. 99). In doubtful cases, a therapeutic trial of ascorbic acid 300 to 500 mg orally will stop the pain of infantile scurvy within 24 to 48 h and will decrease gingival swelling and bleeding within 72 h.

Prophylaxis

In industrialized countries proprietary infant formulas are fortified with vitamin C and liquid multivitamin preparations are readily available. Alternatively, unboiled orange juice, beginning with 1 tsp daily in the 2nd to 4th wk of life, with progressive increases until at 5 mo the intake is 2 to 3 oz, may be given. Tomato juice at 3 times these doses may be used.

Treatment

Ascorbic acid 50 mg qid should be given orally for 1 wk in **infantile scurvy,** then 50 mg tid for 1 mo, with prophylactic doses thereafter. In vomiting or diarrhea, one half the recommended oral dose may be given IM or IV as sodium ascorbate.

196. ENDOCRINE AND METABOLIC DISORDERS

CONGENITAL GOITERS

An enlarged thyroid gland present at birth occurring with or without hypothyroidism. Four types of congenital goiters have been described. *Type 1* involves a defect in iodide transport, probably secondary to an alteration in synthesis of cell surface proteins necessary for transport. *Type 2* is associated with several defects in iodination mechanisms within the thyroid. One involves the absence of the enzyme peroxidase, necessary for the organification of iodine, which can result in goitrous cretinism. Another defect, which is inherited as an autosomal recessive, appears to involve hydrogen peroxide generation and is associated with deaf mutism, a complex known as **Pen-**

dred's syndrome. These patients are usually euthyroid; therefore, the deafness is not secondary to hypothyroidism. A third defect, associated with abnormal peroxidase, allows sufficient compensation for maintenance of a euthyroid state. *Type 3* congenital goiters are found in patients with dehalogenase defects. Although the precise biochemical abnormality is unclear, patients have complete or partial deiodination defects of monoiodotyrosine and diiodotyrosine within thyroglobulin. *Type 4* congenital goiters are associated with defects in the synthesis of thyroglobulin. **Athyreotic cretinism** is found in children born without a thyroid gland.

HYPOTHYROIDISM

A deficiency of thyroid activity. **Hypothyroidism in the young** produces symptoms and signs that differ from adult hypothyroidism (see HYPOTHYROIDISM in Ch. 89). **Neonatal hypothyroidism (cretinism)** is characterized by respiratory distress, cyanosis, jaundice, poor feeding, hoarse cry, umbilical hernia, and retardation of bone growth. Diagnosis requires a high index of suspicion and is greatly aided by routine determination of serum T_4 and TSH in umbilical cord blood, or filter paper blood spots taken at 2 to 5 days of age. Prompt treatment with exogenous thyroid (no later than the first week to 10 days of the postnatal period) prevents or markedly reduces abnormalities in mental development. Appropriate doses of thyroid hormone in the 1st yr of life range from 25 to 90 μg sodium L-thyroxine orally/day. Treatment is monitored by measuring serum T_4 and TSH and changes in the symptoms and signs associated with hypothyroidism such as macroglossia and slow growth rate, which may take many months to normalize. Caution must be taken not to overtreat and produce hyperthyroidism. **Childhood (juvenile) hypothyroidism** is characterized by growth retardation, delayed dentition, and mental deficiency. The symptoms and signs of **adolescent hypothyroidism** are similar to those of adults; additionally there may be short stature and precocious puberty with an enlarged sella turcica.

HYPERTHYROIDISM

Neonatal Graves' disease is a serious and potentially life-threatening occurrence in infants born of mothers who have or have had Graves' disease. Frequently the mothers are under treatment for Graves' disease during the pregnancy and almost invariably have high titers of thyroid-stimulating antibodies **(TSAb)** in their blood, which presumably cross the placenta and stimulate the infant's thyroid gland. Clinical manifestations of neonatal Graves' disease may occur as early as several days after birth and differ in several respects from those observed in juvenile or adult hyperthyroidism. Feeding problems, vomiting, and diarrhea can result in significant electrolyte imbalance; the thyroid goiters may cause respiratory difficulty, and tachycardia may result in heart failure. Ophthalmopathy is rare.

Affected infants generally recover within 3 or 4 mo, although occasionally the course is prolonged—6 mo to 1 yr or more. The duration of the disease appears to be a function of the concentration of TSAb in the infant's blood after birth and the rate the TSAb are metabolized. Since the half life of the TSAb is about 2 wk, disease persisting > 3 or 4 mo after birth is difficult to explain on the basis of passive transfer of TSAb. Therefore, infants with neonatal Graves' disease are probably a heterogeneous group with different pathogenetic mechanisms for hyperthyroidism.

Morbidity and mortality are significant. Persistent elevations of thyroid hormone may result in premature fusion of cranial sutures, impaired intellect (as determined by IQ), hyperactivity later in childhood, and growth retardation. The mortality may be as high as 15 to 20%. Intrauterine Graves' disease also may result in either death of the fetus in utero, stillbirth, or premature birth. Thus, the possibility of neonatal Graves' disease must be considered in advance in any pregnant woman having active Graves'

disease or a history of Graves' disease, and titers of TSAb should be determined during pregnancy (see also SCREENING PROCEDURES FOR INFANTS AND CHILDREN in Ch. 182).

Treatment: During the hyperthyroid phase the cornerstone of therapy is oral propylthiouracil 5 mg/kg/day in 3 divided doses. Iodine solution (Lugol's) may be given in a dose of 6 to 12 mg/day (1 or 2 drops). Infants with severe cardiovascular manifestations may require digitalis and/or a β-adrenergic blocking drug such as propranolol. Severe cases, with high titers of TSAb, may require exchange transfusion.

PITUITARY DWARFISM

Abnormally short stature due to hypofunction of the anterior pituitary. Height is less than the 3rd percentile, growth velocity is ≤ 4 cm/yr, and bone age is ≥ 2 yr behind chronologic age.

Etiology

The potential etiology of pituitary dwarfism is varied, as detailed in TABLE 196–1, and most children with short stature will not have an identifiable pituitary disorder. Although endocrine disorders constitute a minority of all causes of growth retardation, it is important to identify them because they are treatable.

Children with hypopituitarism most commonly have either a **pituitary tumor** (generally a **craniopharyngioma**)or no demonstrable etiology **(idiopathic hypopituitarism)**. In some patients, the combination of lytic lesions of bone in the skull and diabetes

TABLE 196–1. MAJOR ENDOCRINE CAUSES OF SHORT STATURE

I. Decreased GH Secretion
- A. Hypothalamic causes
  - 1. Decreased secretion of GRH
  - 2. Organic lesions
- B. Pituitary causes
  - 1. Decreased secretion of GH alone or with other pituitary hormones
  - 2. Organic lesions
- C. Functional GH deficiency (emotional deprivation)

II. Defective GH Action
- A. Defective GH receptors (Laron dwarfism)
- B. Secretion of abnormal forms of GH
- C. Nutritional impairment of GH-induced somatomedin formation (kwashiorkor)

III. Impaired Skeletal Response to Somatomedin (or GH)
- A. Constitutional short stature
- B. Gonadal dysgenesis (Turner's syndrome)
- C. Primary cartilagenous or bone disease
- D. Chronic renal disease
- E. Chronic inflammatory disease
- F. Corticosteroid excess
  - 1. Pituitary and adrenal disorders
  - 2. Treatment with pharmacologic doses of corticosteroids

IV. Hypothyroidism (Primary or Secondary)

V. Precocious Puberty
- A. Organic
  - 1. Central (CNS) ("true precocious puberty" with early epiphiseal closure)
  - 2. Pseudoprecocious puberty
- B. Idiopathic ("true precocious puberty")

VI. Diabetes Mellitus

VII. Adrenocortical Insufficiency

insipidus will suggest **Hand-Schüller-Christian** disease (see HISTIOCYTOSIS X in Ch. 45). **Isolated growth hormone (GH) deficiency** may occur in association with midline defects, such as cleft palate, absence of the septum pellucidum, optic nerve hypoplasia, and nystagmus. GH deficiency, either alone or in association with other abnormalities, is hereditary in 10% of cases. (See also FAILURE TO THRIVE in Ch. 188.)

Symptoms and Signs

Growth retardation with normal proportions is the hallmark of hypopituitarism in childhood. Individuals with hypopituitarism will also fail to begin pubertal development. Those with isolated GH deficiency have normal body proportions as well, will undergo normal (although sometimes delayed) pubertal development, and have normal reproductive potential.

Determination of bone age from hand x-rays is important in evaluating growth problems, as is the careful recording of height and weight over time on any of several available growth charts. In pituitary dwarfism, epiphyseal maturation is usually retarded to the same extent as height. Obviously, radiologic evaluation of the sella turcica is also indicated to rule out calcification and neoplasms. In addition, the sella is abnormally small in 10 to 20% of children with pituitary GH deficiency.

Diagnosis

Diagnosis of GH deficiency must be made on the basis of reduced responses to provocative stimuli to GH release, even though interpretation of results of such testing is often difficult (see HYPOPITUITARISM IN THE ADULT in Ch. 88). Should GH responses be normal, then levels of somatomedin-C (identical to insulin-like growth factor I, IGF-I) can be measured. Normal somatomedin-C levels in children > 6 yr of age rules out severe GH deficiency. In younger children, the difference between normal and low somatomedin-C levels is too small to permit reliable screening. Since somatomedin-C levels are low in conditions other than GH deficiency (eg, protein malnutrition), the diagnosis must be confirmed with provocative tests of GH secretion. If GH responses indicate GH deficiency, then the other pituitary hormones must also be evaluated. Prolactin levels may be increased in children with craniopharyngiomas.

The great majority of children below the 3rd percentile for stature have normal levels of GH and somatomedin-C. Both the bone and height ages are generally somewhat retarded. A family history of short stature or delayed puberty is common. Such children are generally diagnosed as having either **hereditary (familial) short stature** or **constitutional (physiologic) delayed puberty**. As diagnostic tests improve, some of these children may prove to have somatomedin receptor and postreceptor defects. The short stature of certain racial groups, as exemplified by the African pygmy, also may be due to a similar abnormality.

Children with normal levels of GH and very low levels of somatomedin-C have also been described. Since such children do show increases in somatomedin-C and growth velocity when given exogenous GH, it is suspected that these individuals secrete biologically inactive GH.

Emotional deprivation may also retard growth, apparently by hypothalamic inhibition of GRH release. Characteristically the family environment is poor. Resumption of normal growth occurs rapidly after removing the child from the oppressive environment.

Patients with **Laron dwarfism** have severe proportionate growth retardation, elevated GH levels, and low somatomedin-C levels. After administration of exogenous GH, somatomedin-C levels and growth velocity do not increase, implying a defect in the GH receptor.

In **hypothyroidism**, growth retardation is not proportionate; the extremities are particularly short in comparison to the rest of the body.

In **Turner's syndrome,** the short stature is often confused with pituitary dwarfism. Turner's syndrome may be strongly suspected in short girls with primary amenorrhea,

webbed neck, a low nuchal hairline, short fourth metarcarpal or metatarsal bones, a shield-like chest with widely spaced nipples, and cardiac abnormalities, especially coarctation of the aorta. Rarely, individuals with short stature and gonadal dysgenesis have none of the stigmata usually associated with Turner's syndrome. Patients with these disorders have abnormalities involving the X chromosome as discussed in GONADAL DYSGENESIS under SYNDROMES ASSOCIATED WITH SEX CHROMOSOME ABERRATIONS in Ch. 203. Thus, chromosomal evaluation should be a part of the workup of short girls who have no obvious cause of growth retardation.

The possibility of an occult **chronic inflammatory disease** also should be considered. Children with juvenile rheumatoid arthritis, rheumatic fever, and inflammatory bowel disease often present with growth failure. A thorough evaluation will usually suggest the cause. **Corticosteroids** should be used to treat affected children when indicated, but it must be remembered that excess glucocorticoids from any source also inhibit skeletal growth.

A number of **congenital and hereditary diseases of the skeleton** must be considered, but disproportionate growth is generally easily recognized (see MUSCULOSKELETAL DEFECTS in Ch. 187, and Ch. 197).

Many **renal diseases**, including chronic renal insufficiency, renal tubular acidosis, and Bartter's syndrome, are also associated with growth retardation. Since clinical abnormalities may be absent in many such patients, all individuals in whom growth failure is unexplained should undergo tests to screen for renal disease.

Children with severe congenital **heart disease** and mentally retarded children with **CNS disease** may also suffer from retarded growth.

Treatment

Replacement therapy with exogenous human GH is indicated for all children with short stature who have documented GH deficiency. Semi-purified GH, prepared from both cold acetone-preserved and freshly collected human pituitary glands, has been used for this purpose for several years. However, the recent demonstration of fatal Creutzfeldt-Jakob disease in 4 young adults who had been treated with human GH has resulted in a ban in the USA on the use of GH prepared from human pituitaries. It is now apparent that GH purification procedures did not include steps known to exclude and inactivate agents causing the subacute spongiform viral encephalopathies. (The potential for transmission of infectious diseases with other purified hormones derived from human sources must always be remembered.)

Human GH that is *genetically engineered in bacteria* has been released to replace the natural product, and intensive work is in progress to develop a fully synthetic duplicate of the human hormone. In preliminary studies, results with bacterially synthesized methionyl human GH appear to be identical to those obtained with GH purified from human pituitaries. Although many dosage regimens have been examined, no ideal treatment schedule has been developed. The usual therapeutic dosage of biosynthetic GH (somatrem) in the USA has been about 0.1 mg/kg (0.2 IU/kg) given IM 3 times each week. Such dosages have been used because of limited GH availability and not because of experimental evidence that such regimens induce optimal growth. Larger doses may lead to more rapid growth, and it has been suggested that the growth response is directly related to the logarithm of the dose between 30 and 100 mIU/kg. Increases in height of 10 to 15 cm frequently occur in the first year of treatment, but growth may slow thereafter, due sometimes to the development of antibodies to the impure preparations. Allergic and acute reactions to GH injections are uncommon. Withholding GH therapy for several months may restore responsiveness in refractory individuals. Other therapeutic agents are of little value in the treatment of GH deficiency.

As GH preparations become more available, the question arises whether children with short stature and normal GH secretion should be treated. Preliminary studies

suggest that children with "constitutional short stature" demonstrate accelerated growth velocity with GH treatment. No controlled studies have been conducted to determine if the accelerated growth initiated in such individuals will be sustained nor whether there are any untoward side effects from such treatment. The use of GH in children with short stature from other causes has not been investigated.

Replacement of cortisol (see Chs. 91 and 283) and thyroid hormone (see Ch. 89) should be provided whenever indicated. Overtreatment of thyroid and adrenal deficiencies must be avoided or will impair the response to GH. Replacement with gonadal steroids is not indicated until normal puberty occurs, treatment with exogenous GH is completed, or pubertal development needs to be induced with gonadal steroids because of hypogonadism. Steroids in high doses initiate epiphyseal closure, thereby *limiting* ultimate height.

CONGENITAL ADRENAL HYPERPLASIA

The term congenital adrenal hyperplasia covers a group of disorders caused by defects in hydroxylation of cortisol precursors (see TABLE 196–2). The resulting low levels of cortisol induce increased secretion of corticotropin (ACTH), causing adrenal hyperplasia. In the most common forms, 21-hydroxylase and 11-hydroxylase defects, the net effect is an increased secretion from the adrenal gland of cortisol precursors and androgens. Hypersecretion of adrenal androgens during intrauterine life causes masculinization of the female external genitalia **(pseudohermaphroditism)**. See INTERSEX STATES in Ch. 187. Differentiation of ovaries, tubes, and uterus remains normal. If hypersecretion occurs before 12 wk gestation, there may be a persistent genitourinary sinus, a single opening for vagina and urethra, and even labioscrotal fusion. After 12 wk, only clitoral hypertrophy is produced. (Synthetic progestational agents or andro-

TABLE 196–2. TYPES OF METABOLIC BLOCKS IN CONGENITAL ADRENAL HYPERPLASIA

Missing Enzyme	*Deficient*	*Excess*	*Phenotype*
Desmolase	All steroid hormones	Lipid in adrenal	Adrenal insufficiency
3β-OL Dehydrogenase	Corticoids Aldosterone	Dehydroepiandrosterone	Sodium loss, adrenal insufficiency Male: hypospadias Female: mild virilism
17-Hydroxylase	Androgens Estrogens Cortisol Aldosterone	Corticosterone 11-Deoxycorticosterone	Immature female; ambiguous genitalia in males Hypertension Low potassium Alkalosis
21-Hydroxylase	Aldosterone Corticoids	Androgens	Masculinization Sometimes sodium loss, adrenal insufficiency
11-Hydroxylase	Corticoids Aldosterone	Androgens 11-Deoxycorticosterone	Masculinization Hypertension
18-Hydroxylase	Aldosterone	Corticosterone	Salt loss

(Modified from *Metabolic Control and Disease* [formerly *Duncan's Diseases of Metabolism*], ed. 8, 1980, edited by P. K. Bondy and L. E. Rosenberg. Copyright 1980 by W. B. Saunders Company. Used with permission.)

gens taken during the first trimester of pregnancy may also cause masculinization of the external genitalia.) The phallus is enlarged in boys **(macrogenitosomia)**, but the testes and prostate remain small at puberty because of suppression of luteinizing or interstitial-cell–stimulating hormone **(LH or ICSH)** and follicle-stimulating hormone **(FSH)** by excessive androgens. These children grow at an accelerated rate when young, but show advanced skeletal maturation. Because of premature closing of the epiphyses, their ultimate height is below average. If the defect in cortisol production is sufficiently severe, and especially if aldosterone production is also blocked, the neonate may develop life-threatening adrenal failure immediately after birth, which requires *immediate* treatment with cortisol and mineralocorticoid as well as appropriate fluid and electrolyte therapy. In patients with 11-hydroxylase block, an excess of the mineralocorticoid, deoxycorticosterone is produced, which causes hypertension but protects against early adrenal failure.

Other defects, especially of 17-hydroxylase, cause phenotypic feminization of genetically male infants, in association with other characteristics of excessive mineralocorticoid activity.

Elevated urinary 17-KS with normal or decreased 17-OHCS suggests the diagnosis of 11-hydroxylase or 21-hydroxylase defect. Raised serum 17-OH progesterone is found in patients with the 21-hydroxylase defect. The presence of excessive pregnanetriol excretion gives strong support to the diagnosis of 21-hydroxylase defect, whereas in 11-hydroxylase block, excessive amounts of tetrahydro S and tetrahydro deoxycorticosterone are excreted and serum deoxycorticosterone and deoxycortisol levels are elevated. Plasma testosterone levels are elevated in both defects.

The female genotype in pseudohermaphrodite girls can be confirmed by leukocyte karyotyping. In boys with macrogenitosomia, true precocious puberty (see in DEVELOPMENTAL CONDITIONS in Ch. 202) must be ruled out.

Treatment

Therapy with hydrocortisone arrests the disorder. Administration of hydrocortisone 0.3 mg/kg/day or 10 to 20 mg/m²/day in divided doses s.c. in infants for 3 days reduces 17-KS by more than 50%. In patients old enough to take pills, hydrocortisone may be given orally, starting at 25 mg bid or 20 to 25 mg/m²/day. Prednisolone 5 mg bid can be substituted. Patients with sodium-losing syndromes may require deoxycorticosterone or fludrocortisone as in adrenocortical insufficiency (see ADRENAL HYPOFUNCTION in Ch. 91). Dosage should be titrated to maintain normal plasma 17-OH progesterone levels (< 50 ng/dL in childhood) or excretion levels of 17-KS (< 0.5 mg/24 h for each year of age until puberty). Serum electrolyte levels and BP should be followed closely, especially if the patient has the salt-losing form of the disease (11-hydroxylase defect). The rate of growth should be monitored frequently, and bone age should be checked every few years. Ordinarily, these will be within normal limits if steroid suppression has been maintained. Surgical reconstruction of the external genitalia is often necessary in girls. Hydrocortisone therapy permits feminization of girls; menstruation occurs and treated patients have had normal pregnancies. Hydrocortisone suppresses androgen secretion in boys and permits secretion of luteinizing hormone and follicle-stimulating hormone at puberty so that testicular development and spermatogenesis may take place.

THE TESTES

MALE HYPOGONADISM

Decreased functional activity of the testes (either endocrine, gametogenic, or both).

The testes serve 2 functions—synthesis and secretion of testosterone by the interstitial (Leydig) cells, and production of sperm within the seminiferous tubules. Hypogo-

nadism can refer to hypofunction of either component, but this section will deal mainly with hormonal disorders due to testosterone deficiency. For syndromes of androgen resistance see INTERSEX STATES in Ch. 187; for congenital disorders of the testes and scrotum, see RENAL AND GU DEFECTS in Ch. 187.

Testicular Development and Function

The embryonic gonad has the potential for becoming either testis or ovary. The H-Y antigen, a product of the Y chromosome, interacts with plasma membrane receptors to induce differentiation of the Sertoli cells that then direct the distribution of the germ cells in the developing testis. The Sertoli cell secretes a peptide that causes regression of the primordial müllerian duct. Under the influence of the Y chromosome, fetal Leydig cells mature and, in response to pituitary luteinizing hormone **(LH)**, secrete **testosterone.** This steroid causes differentiation of the vas deferens and seminal vesicles, whereas its 5α-reduced metabolite, **dihydrotestosterone,** induces differentiation of the prostate and the external genitalia.

Following birth, the Leydig cells regress and, except for a poorly understood, brief period of function during the first 6 mo, remain quiescent until puberty. The bulk of the testis is composed of the tubules that grow slowly prepubertally. As plasma follicle-stimulating hormone **(FSH)** levels begin to rise, at about age 9, there is rapid tubular growth and an increase in testicular volume. A volume > 5 mL or a diameter longer than 2.5 cm is thus the first indication of beginning pubescence. Generally within a year or 2 of this time, evidences of androgen effect appear. It is known that some FSH is necessary to *initiate* spermatogenesis, and it is probable that at least small amounts of testosterone must also be present. In the experimental animal and in man, spermatogenesis can be *maintained* at almost normal levels by human chorionic gonatropin **(HCG)** alone.

The regulation of testicular function follows, in general outline, that of other glands responding to peptide hormones. LH stimulates the Leydig cell via the mediator—cyclic AMP. FSH binds only to the Sertoli cell, generates cAMP, and activates spermatogenesis by as yet unknown mechanisms. FSH synergizes with LH to increase testosterone secretion and both growth hormone and prolactin have also been shown to synergize with LH.

The Leydig cell secretes testosterone and small amounts of dihydrotestosterone and estradiol. Testosterone and its metabolites, estradiol and dihydrotestosterone, act at pituitary and hypothalamic sites in the negative feed-back loop modulating the secretion of LH. These same steroids and a tubular secretory protein, **inhibin,** will suppress FSH secretion. Thus, destruction of the tubules will increase FSH, whereas loss of Leydig cell function will cause an increase of LH and FSH. The synthesis and secretion of the gonadotropins are regulated by the pulsatile secretion of the hypothalamic peptide hormone, **gonadotropin-releasing hormone (GnRH).**

Symptoms and Signs

Testosterone has a role in the developing fetus (see above), and its absence will result in a female phenotype. If dihydrotestosterone synthesis is inadequate because of a deficiency of 5α-reductase, there will be ambiguous external genitalia. A lack of testosterone at the expected time of pubescence is manifest by delayed closure of epiphyses and eunuchoidal skeletal proportions (span > height by 2 in., heel to pubic symphysis length greater than pubic symphysis to crown by 2 in.); no deepening of the voice; delayed and scanty growth of pubic and axillary hair; absence of beard and mustache growth; small prostate; small penis and a nonpigmented, nonrugated scrotum; low testicular volume with absent spermatogenesis; poor muscular development; and, usually, psychosocial immaturity. The patients are usually brought to the physician by their parents, who are worried about poor growth and development.

When Leydig cell function is severely impaired after puberty, libido and potentia decrease, ejaculate volume diminishes, there may be hot flashes, and there is a partial regression of the coarse sexual hair to a thinner hair requiring less frequent shaving.

In the adult male, cessation or diminution of testosterone secretion is difficult to appreciate clinically. The symptoms of loss of libido and impotence are not specific for androgen lack and most often occur in men with normal Leydig cell function. A decrease in frequency of shaving, early soft wrinkling of the face, and a softening of the testis may be present.

Laboratory Assessment of Leydig Cell Function

1. **Serum testosterone levels**: The normal range is wide (0.3 to 1.0 μg/dL). There is no correlation between testosterone concentrations > 0.3 μg/dL and libido or potency.

2. **Serum gonadotropins**: Bioassay of *urinary* gonadotropins for the diagnosis of gonadal disorders is no longer acceptable. Elevated *serum* gonadotropins indicate testicular disease, and an elevated FSH is a reliable index of severe, irreversible tubular disease. It is difficult to distinguish low from normal serum gonadotropins. Evaluation of gonadotropins that are inappropriately low in the presence of low plasma testosterone concentrations requires either clomiphene or GnRH tests.

3. **Clomiphene stimulation test**: The nonsteroid weak estrogen agonist clomiphene stimulates the release of gonadotropins. Since it acts as an anti-estrogen, it is only effective when testosterone/estradiol levels are above those of anorchid males. In men with borderline low levels of testosterone and gonadotropins, failure of clomiphene (100 mg daily for 7 days) to cause a 50% increase in LH indicates hypothalamic pituitary insufficiency. This test is not consistently normal until stage III of puberty and is of little use in differentiating between hypogonadotropic hypogonadism and delayed puberty (see in DEVELOPMENTAL CONDITIONS in Ch. 202).

4. **GnRH stimulation**: A standard test consists of administering 100 μg GnRH IV and obtaining a peak rise of LH at about 20 min to levels 3 times control. In hypothalamic disease, repeated injections over a period of several days to 2 wk may be necessary to elicit a normal response. An exaggerated response indicates a relatively low level of feedback inhibition (testosterone/estradiol for LH; tubular factor(s) for FSH). As with the clomiphene test, the response of LH to GnRH only becomes normal at stage III of puberty; thus it too does not clearly distinguish hypogonadotropic hypogonadism from delayed puberty.

5. **Karyotype**: A buccal smear will often be sufficient to indicate the extra X chromosome in Klinefelter's syndrome (although it is usually normal in mosaicism). Karyotyping is rarely necessary in male hypogonadism when there is no ambiguity of the male phenotype. It should be noted that hypospadias may be the only indication of an abnormal genotype.

6. **HCG stimulation**: When there is a testis present, a testosterone response can almost always be obtained with repeated HCG stimulation. A satisfactory test for Leydig cell function is a 50% increase in plasma testosterone 24 to 72 h after a single injection of 5000 IU of HCG. This test is rarely indicated but may be used in boys with cryptorchidism and delayed puberty.

Classification of Hypogonadism

Hypogonadism may be due to Leydig cell dysfunction **(primary hypogonadism)** or to disorders of the hypothalamic-pituitary unit **(secondary hypogonadism)**. Secondary hypogonadism may be differentiated into pituitary and hypothalamic hypogonadism by testing with GnRH. In primary hypogonadism, the gonadotropins in serum or urine are elevated because of decreased feedback at the pituitary-hypothalamic unit.

PRIMARY HYPOGONADISM

Leydig cell function is depressed in malnutrition, in renal failure, myotonic dystrophy, in chronic disease, to a variable extent with aging, and by certain toxins such as lead and alcohol.

Klinefelter's syndrome: This most frequent cause of primary hypogonadism is defined as *the presence of one or more extra X chromosomes in at least one tissue*. Almost invariably, the testes are small, containing sclerosed tubules with only rare Sertoli cells, and there is usually azoospermia. Gynecomastia occurs with high frequency. More variable clinical features of the syndrome include eunuchoid habitus, mental retardation, increased frequency of diabetes mellitus, poor wound healing, and rare skeletal deformities. When there is **mosaicism** (in which some cells contain the normal 46 chromosomes, while others contain one or more extra X chromosomes) with the XXY genotype occurring in only a few cell lines, many of these clinical findings may be absent and the disease manifests itself only by infertility or decreased fertility.

XX males: This syndrome closely resembles Klinefelter's syndrome but is rare and probably not associated with mental retardation. In recent studies, the H-Y antigen has been identified in all such patients, accounting for the presence of the testis and the similarity to seminiferous tubule dysgenesis.

Testicular agenesis (vanishing testis syndrome): These patients are normal phenotypic males having no testes. The male phenotype implies normal fetal testosterone secretion so that testicular destruction must have occurred after fetal organogenesis was completed.

Sertoli-cell-only syndrome (germinal aplasia): These patients present as essentially normal men with slightly reduced testicular volume, and infertility. There is an absence of germinal cells in the tubules. Although plasma testosterone is normal, an exaggerated LH response to GnRH indicates that there is compensated Leydig cell dysfunction.

Noonan's syndrome (male Turner's): These boys have a normal XY karoytype, some of the features of Turner's syndrome (such as hypertelorism, short stature, epicanthal folds, and right-sided congenital heart disease), and various skeletal malformations. In contrast to Turner's syndrome, mental retardation is often present. Leydig cell function may be normal or decreased and some patients may have cryptorchidism.

Enzymatic defects: Since all congenital interruptions of testosterone biosynthesis and action lead to a female phenotype or ambiguous genitalia, these do not enter into a discussion of Leydig cell hypofunction in the normal male.

SECONDARY HYPOGONADISM

Delayed pubescence: The prepubertal male is hypogonadotropic. FSH stimulation of tubular development (stage II-III of puberty) is the first evidence of pubescence. At present, there is no reliable test to distinguish between delayed puberty and hypogonadotropic hypogonadism unless there are signs suggesting Kallmann's syndrome.

Hypogonadotropic hypogonadism: Kallmann's syndrome is the most frequent cause of secondary hypogonadism. It is inherited as an autosomal dominant with variable penetrance and is characterized by low FSH and LH levels, anosmia or hyposmia, and the variable occurrence of short fourth metacarpals, syndactyly, midline skeletal defects, and mental retardation. Inadequate secretion of FSH and LH may occur as an isolated defect as well. In both cases the disease can be shown to be hypothalamic in origin, since repeated injections of GnRH will eventually elicit a normal gonadotropin response. Boys remain sexually prepubescent until either testosterone secretion is induced by HCG or androgen is given.

Isolated LH deficiency (fertile eunuch syndrome): This is a rare syndrome in which boys have pubertal testicular size and some spermatogenesis in the absence of signs of androgen effect. The deficiency of LH is not complete and HCG will produce virilization and increased sperm counts.

Panhypopituitarism: Destruction of the pituitary gland or interruption of hypothalamic transmission of GnRH may be due to tumors, granulomatous or infectious disease, trauma, and metastatic disease. When panhypopituitarism occurs before puberty, sexual infantilism persists. Small tumors, secreting prolactin, have also been shown to suppress gonadotropin secretion, presumably by direct effect at the pituitary-hypothalamic level rather than by destruction of the pituitary gland. (See also HYPOFUNCTION OF THE ANTERIOR PITUITARY under ANTERIOR LOBE DISORDERS in Ch. 88.)

Several congenital diseases, such as Laurence-Moon-Biedl syndrome, Prader-Willi syndrome, cerebellar ataxia, Alstrom syndrome, congenital icthyosis, and others that are associated with hypogonadotropic hypogonadism, will not be discussed here.

Treatment

Patients with **primary hypogonadism** can be virilized with exogenous androgens. Doses of testosterone enanthate or cypionate 200 to 300 mg IM every 2 to 3 wk will provide satisfactory replacement. Patients with primary hypogonadism cannot become fertile and gonadotropin treatment need not be considered.

Treatment of patients with **secondary hypogonadism** depends on goals. In boys or young men, virilization can be attained using testosterone enanthate or cypionate at doses of 200 to 300 mg IM every 2 to 3 wk. In adults, the dose can be titrated by measuring plasma testosterone levels or assessing sexual responses. The IM injection of HCG 2000 IU 3 times/wk is also satisfactory. Neither treatment compromises the capacity for tubular development and spermatogenesis, but the administration of long-acting testosterone every 2 wk is convenient. If fertility is the goal, then FSH at doses of 25 to 75 u. 3 times/wk with HCG as above will induce spermatogenesis after one to 2 mo of treatment. Once spermatogenesis has been induced, it can be maintained with HCG alone, providing that treatment is started before regression of spermatogenesis begins.

Boys with delayed puberty may encounter difficult psychosocial adjustment and may therefore need to be virilized. The use of testosterone enanthate or cypionate is appropriate and has not been shown to preclude normal development. At intervals of about 6 mo, treatment should be stopped to see if pubescence is beginning. Increased testicular size is indicative of effective therapy.

Clomiphene is rarely useful in hypogonadotropic hypogonadism, since testosterone levels are very low. Pulsatile injection of GnRH agonists may be used therapeutically to stimulate pituitary secretion of gonadotropins.

Infertility due to oligospermia is a poorly defined condition. Since hypogonadotropic males given FSH and HCG can impregnate their wives with sperm counts between 1 and 5 million/mL, the number of sperm cannot be the decisive factor. Attempts to use clomiphene citrate or androgen rebound therapy have generally been unsuccessful.

GENETIC ABNORMALITIES OF CARBOHYDRATE METABOLISM

GALACTOSEMIA

A metabolic abnormality, inherited as an autosomal recessive trait, involving conversion of galactose to glucose, caused by absence of the enzyme galactose-1-phosphate uridyl transferase. The gene for this enzyme is located on the short arm of chromosome 9. In

this disorder galactose and galactose-1-phosphate accumulate in many tissues, damaging them by interfering with their normal metabolic processes. The incidence in Great Britain is about 1 in 80,000 births, giving a gene frequency of 1 in 150 of the population.

The infant appears normal at birth, but within a few days or weeks of being fed with milk, which contains galactose and lactose (a disaccharide which on hydrolysis yields glucose and galactose), the child becomes anorexic, vomits, ceases to grow, and becomes jaundiced. The liver enlarges, there is proteinuria and aminoaciduria, and ultimately ascites, and edema. If treatment is delayed, the child remains physically stunted and mentally retarded, and many have cataracts; however, mild cases may occur without serious impairment. The **diagnosis** may be suspected from the presence of non–glucose-reducing substances (galactose and galactose-1-phosphate) in the urine and confirmed by the absence of the transferase enzyme in erythrocytes. If there is reason to suspect the diagnosis antenatally, it can be made at birth using the erythrocytes from a few drops of cord-blood. Prenatal diagnosis by amniocentesis is also possible but is not ethically justified.

Treatment

If the mother has high blood galactose levels, the fetus may be damaged (including permanent mental impairment), whether or not it is deficient in galactose-1-P-uridyl transferase. Amniocentesis will not reveal whether the fetus' brain development has been impaired.

Milk and milk containing foods should be eliminated from the diet at once, preferably during pregnancy in women who are known carriers of the trait. Synthetic galactose- and lactose-free milk substitutes and foods are available. Strict dietary restriction should be maintained for as long as possible, certainly up to school age. Prognosis for physical development is good if galactose has been eliminated from the diet, but although their I.Q. is within the normal range, children with galactosemia tend to remain underachievers. Prevention is through genetic counseling.

GALACTOKINASE DEFICIENCY

An inability to metabolize galactose due to a deficiency of the enzyme galactokinase, inherited as an autosomal recessive defect. The gene for this enzyme is located on the long arm of chromosome 17. As in the more common galactosemia, plasma and urinary galactose concentrations are elevated, but no GI or brain disturbances occur. Unless galactose is removed from the diet, cataracts develop rapidly because of the accumulation of galactitol in the lens. Enzyme tests for galactose-1-phosphate uridyl transferase are normal, but galactokinase activity is absent in the erythrocytes. **Treatment** is as for galactosemia.

GALACTOSE EPIMERASE DEFICIENCY

A rare inherited metabolic disorder in which there is a deficiency of uridyl diphosphate galactose 4-empiridase and in which galactose-1-phosphate accumulates in erythrocytes and leukocytes, but without causing significant dysfunction. It may be detected during screening for galactosemia. No treatment is required.

GLYCOGEN STORAGE DISEASES
(Glycogenoses)

A group of hereditary disorders caused by lack of one or more of the many enzymes involved in glycogen synthesis or breakdown, and characterized by the deposition of abnormal amounts or types of glycogen in the tissues (see TABLE 196–3 for classification and characteristics). Symptoms and signs arise either through accumulation of glycogen or

TABLE 196–3. CHARACTERISTICS OF THE GLYCOGENOSES

Type	Enzyme System Affected	Organs Involved	Clinical Symptoms	Eponym
0	UDPG-glycogen transferase	Liver, muscle	Large fatty liver, fasting hypoglycemia	------
Ia	Glucose-6-phosphatase	Liver, kidney	Large liver and kidney; growth retardation; severe hypoglycemia; acidosis; hyperlipemia; hyperuricemia	von Gierke
Ib	Glucose-6-phosphatase translocase	Liver, leucocytes	As above but less severe; neutropenia, recurrent GI infections	------
II	Lysosomal glucosidase (various types)	All organs	Large liver and heart; no abnormal blood chemistry	Pompe
III	Debrancher enzyme system	Liver, muscle, heart, leukocytes	Enlarged liver, fasting hypoglycemia, variable muscle involvement	Forbes
IV	Brancher enzyme system	Liver, muscle, and most tissues	Progressive cirrhosis in juvenile type; myopathy and heart failure in late-onset type	Andersen
V	Muscle phosphorylase	Skeletal muscle	Cramps on exercise with no rise in blood lactate	McArdle
VI	Liver phosphorylase	Liver	Enlarged liver, fasting hypoglycemia but often no symptoms at all	Hers
VII	Phosphofructokinase	Skeletal muscle erythrocytes	Cramps on exercise but no rise in blood lactate, hemolysis	Tarui

VIII, IX, X: Rare disorders involving various components of the liver phosphorylase activating–deactivating cascade

other intermediate metabolites, or through lack of an end product of glycogen breakdown, particularly glucose. Glycogen and some of the intermediate metabolites can be detected noninvasively by nuclear magnetic resonance. The incidence of all forms of glycogen storage diseases is 1 in 40,000, but this may well be a considerable underestimate because some forms of glycogenosis cause only minimal disturbances and may therefore remain undiagnosed. Variations in severity and age of onset of clinical manifestations are due to involvement of different isoenzymes or other components of the affected enzyme systems. Inheritance is autosomal recessive, except in Type IX, which is X-linked. Types O, I, IV, and VI mainly affect the liver. Types II and III involve most tissues. Types V and VII are restricted to skeletal muscle (see Glycogen Storage Diseases of Muscle in Ch. 132); Type II also affects the myocardium.

Diagnosis is by demonstrating absence of the specific enzyme in a biopsy of the affected tissue. **Treatment** in Types O, I, and III is directed toward preventing hypoglycemia and lactic acidosis by frequent small carbohydrate feeding: raw (not boiled) cornstarch, 2 gm/kg given q 4 or 6 h day and night has proved particularly helpful in

maintaining a steady blood glucose level. With it, catch-up growth and reduction of lactic acidemia, hyperuricemia, and hyperlipidemia can be achieved. Alternatively, continuous overnight feeding of a high dextrin preparation (eg, Vivonex®) through a nasogastric tube may be attempted, but this method carries with it the risk of accidental aspiration of the feed. Limiting anaerobic (ischemic) exercise reduces the muscle symptoms of types V and VII. No effective treatment is known for the other types.

HEREDITARY FRUCTOSE INTOLERANCE

A metabolic inability to utilize fructose caused by absence of the enzyme phosphofructoaldolase and inherited as an autosomal recessive trait. The incidence of this disorder is 1 in 20,000 in Switzerland where it was first described. Fructose-1-phosphate accumulates in the body inhibiting glycogenolysis and gluconeogenesis. Ingestion of more than very small amounts of fructose or sucrose (which on hydrolysis yields glucose and fructose) induces hypoglycemia, with sweating, tremor, confusion, nausea, vomiting, and possibly convulsions and coma. With prolonged ingestion of fructose, proximal renal tubular acidosis may occur with urinary loss of phosphate and glucose; cirrhosis of the liver and mental deterioration may also develop. Patients protect themselves by developing a strong dislike for sugar-containing sweets and fruit; their teeth are usually completely free of caries.

Diagnosis is suggested by the onset of symptoms in infancy and finding fructose in the urine. It is confirmed by demonstrating the absence of the enzyme in a liver biopsy or by demonstrating a fall in blood glucose 5 to 40 min after giving fructose 250 mg/kg IV, followed by the administration of IV glucose as soon as the fall in blood glucose has been documented.

Treatment is to exclude fructose (found chiefly in sweet fruits), sucrose, and sorbitol from the diet. Attacks of fructose-induced hypoglycemia are treated with glucose.

FRUCTOSURIA

A harmless excretion of fructose in the urine, caused by an autosomal recessive lack of the enzyme fructokinase. The incidence in the general population is about 1 in 130,000. This benign asymptomatic defect prevents normal utilization of ingested fructose, resulting in abnormal levels in the blood and urine. Fructosuria may lead to an incorrect diagnosis of diabetes mellitus (fructose will reduce copper sulfate, but will not react with glucose oxidase). No treatment is required.

FRUCTOSE-1,6-DIPHOSPHATASE DEFICIENCY

A rare metabolic disorder caused by a deficiency of fructose-1,6-diphosphatase, a key enzyme of gluconeogenesis. This results in hypoglycemia and acidosis owing to the accumulation of gluconeogenic precursors—certain amino acids, lactic acid, and keto acids. The symptoms can be relieved by giving glucose orally, or IV if hypoglycemia is severe.

PENTOSURIA

A harmless autosomal recessive metabolic derangement characterized by the excretion of L-xylulose in the urine due to absence of the enzyme L-xylulose dehydrogenase. It occurs almost exclusively in Jews, with an incidence of 1 in 2500 in American Jews. As with fructosuria, its only importance is the danger that the presence of xylulose in the urine may lead to an erroneous diagnosis of diabetes mellitus. Treatment is not required.

INHERITED ABNORMALITIES OF PYRUVATE METABOLISM

Pyruvate appears in the metabolic pathway of carbohydrates, fats, and amino acids. Inborn errors of pyruvate metabolism can therefore cause a wide variety of disturbances.

Deficiency of the pyruvate dehydrogenase complex: Deficiency of one of the proteins in this multi-enzyme complex results in inadequate production of acetyl CoA and subsequently of acetylcholine, which is essential in the normal development of the nervous system. Clinical manifestations are predominantly ataxia and psychomotor retardation. This deficiency may be one of the causes of Reye's syndrome. There is no known treatment for this disorder.

Pyruvate carboxylase deficiency: The absence of this enzyme results in inadequate production of oxaloacetate; gluconeogenesis is therefore reduced and causes fasting hypoglycemia and lactic and ketoacidosis. Amino acid synthesis is also impaired and results in reduced formation of amino acid neurotransmitters with a variety of neurologic symptoms. Hypoglycemia and acidemia may be relieved by frequent feeding with carbohydrate-containing foods, but there are no reports of specific replacement with neurotransmitter (eg, dopamine, tyrosine) for treatment of the neurologic symptoms.

DIABETES MELLITUS IN CHILDREN

Diabetes mellitus **(DM)** is the most common endocrine disorder of childhood. In the USA the prevalence of DM is about 0.9/1000 children. Its frequency, however, has been found to increase with age—about 1 case/1430 children at 5 yr of age to about 1 case/360 children at 16 yr of age. The peak ages of onset are between 5 to 7 yr of age and puberty; both sexes are equally affected. A seasonal variation has been noted with new cases being recognized more in autumn and winter. No apparent correlation with socioeconomic status has been found. The incidence is much higher in Israel, Great Britain, Sweden, and USA as compared to France, Germany, Spain, and Italy.

The major forms of diabetes and carbohydrate intolerance are presented in TABLE 94–1 in Ch. 94 and in TABLE 178–1 in Ch. 178. Most children have **Type I, insulin-dependent diabetes mellitus (IDDM),** formerly known as juvenile-onset diabetes mellitus, which is characterized by insulinopenia and dependence on exogenous insulin. These patients frequently develop ketoacidosis in the absence of exogenous insulin. **Type II, noninsulin-dependent diabetes mellitus (NIDDM),** formerly known as adult- or maturity-onset diabetes, is discussed in DIABETES MELLITUS in Ch. 94.

Etiology

The etiology of DM is incompletely understood, but may be related to various factors: (1) **Virus infections**—Data suggest that mumps and Coxsackie B are possible diabetogenic agents, but irrefutable evidence is lacking. (2) **Autoimmune destruction of pancreatic islet cells**—IDDM may occur in some predisposed individuals. It is more prevalent among individuals with Hashimoto's thyroiditis, Addison's disease, pernicious anemia, and in other autoimmune disorders. Several of these diseases are also associated with certain HLA surface antigens. Islet cell antibodies have been found in about 75% of patients with IDDM studied at the time of diagnosis and prior to insulin therapy. (3) **Inheritance**—IDDM may be associated with genetic factors but not to the same extent as NIDDM. Twin concordance is found to be < 50% in IDDM. The inheritance of HLA B8 or BW15 antigens appears to increase the risk of acquiring IDDM 2 to 3 fold. When both of these antigens are present in an individual, the risk of developing IDDM increases seven- to tenfold.

Symptoms and Signs

Most diabetic children present with a history of polydipsia and polyuria secondary to an osmotic diuresis, with renal losses of water, minerals, and calories. Anorexia is

far more common than polyphagia and, together with polyuria, accounts for reduction in body weight. Other complaints include lethargy, weakness, and sometimes the onset of enuresis in a previously continent child. Glycosuria also predisposes the child to vaginal monilial infections. Other infections are not common presenting problems.

In < 10% of children early symptoms may be overlooked or ignored until **diabetic ketoacidosis (DKA)** develops. DKA is a problem in IDDM patients in poor control, or it may be precipitated by infection or fever. Mortality in DKA ranges from 5 to 15%. Early manifestations of DKA include anorexia, excessive thirst, nausea, vomiting; if untreated, air hunger with Kussmaul breathing, confusion and coma may occur. An acetone odor may be detected in the breath. In the early phases polyuria is preeminent but, as dehydration progresses and glomerular filtration rate declines, urinary output gradually decreases. Visual disturbances and severe abdominal pain may predominate during this period. DKA initially may be confused with viral gastroenteritis and abdominal pain may be confused with acute appendicitis, especially since the WBC count is frequently elevated. However, there is marked increase in blood glucose and the hepatic generation of β-hydroxybutarate and acetoacetate secondary to insulin deficiency, leading to metabolic acidosis, hyperosmolarity, and dehydration.

Diagnosis

Diabetes is diagnosed by elevated fasting blood glucose values and glucosuria (ketonuria may also be present), together with a history (in about 80% of children > 2 yr of age) of polyuria, polydipsia, and weight loss. The usual interval between onset of symptoms and diagnosis is 2 to 4 wk. Polyuria and polydipsia, *without* glycosuria, are the primary features in diabetes insipidus, either central or renal (see DIABETES INSIPIDUS under POSTERIOR LOBE DISORDERS in Ch. 88).

A urine test alone is not adequate to establish a diagnosis of diabetes. Renal glycosuria without elevated blood sugar may occur in several diseases associated with a renal proximal tubular defect (eg, Fanconi's syndrome, heavy metal poisoning, Wilson's disease, cystinosis, and inborn errors of intermediary carbohydrate metabolism). Isolated renal glycosuria, detected often on routine urine screening of asymptomatic individuals, is an innocuous renal tubular defect requiring no further attention.

If the fasting blood glucose level is > 120 mg/dL or a 2-h postprandial level is > 140 mg/dL, DM should be considered. In a small subgroup of patients, a definite diagnosis may be difficult to make, and provocative tests are indicated; eg, an oral glucose tolerance test **(OGTT)**. Severe stress due to infection or trauma may occasionally cause transient hyperglycemia and glucosuria and, infrequently, patients may require short-term insulin therapy. Following recovery, it is advisable to do an OGTT, since the stress may have uncovered a prediabetic condition. For a detailed discussion of the OGTT, see under Diagnosis in DIABETES MELLITUS in Ch. 94.

An **intravenous glucose tolerance test** is usually done in patients with GI diseases such as malabsorption. The **intravenous sodium tolbutamide test** is rarely used in diagnosing IDDM because of the high risk of severe hypoglycemia.

Complications of Diabetes Mellitus

The complications of DM (eg, nephropathy, retinopathy, neuropathy) are discussed below and elsewhere in THE MANUAL. Diabetic arteriosclerotic disease is discussed in Ch. 26.

In IDDM, the younger the age of onset and longer the duration, and the more frequent the episodes of ketoacidosis, the more likely the patient is to have **diabetic nephropathy**. Almost all diabetics with IDDM have histologic evidence of glomerulosclerosis, but only about 35% develop clinical nephropathy, usually about 15 to 20 yr after diagnosis. Renal failure secondary to obliterative lesions in glomerular capillaries accounts for 48% of all deaths in diabetics who acquire the disease before age 20.

Diagnosis of nephropathy is based on the presence of marked proteinuria, decreased creatinine clearance, and hypertension. Hypertension is a harbinger of significant un-

derlying renal involvement. Microalbuminuria is a good predictor of nephropathy, even in the asymptomatic, seemingly healthy diabetic.

Treatment of diabetic nephropathy consists mainly of dietary restriction of protein, potassium, and phosphorus if creatinine clearance is decreased to < 20 mL/min. Microalbuminuria is potentially reversible by good glycemic control. With chronic hemodialysis survival is 40 to 75% at 2 yr; chronic peritoneal dialysis is preferable if there is chance of renal transplant, but hyperglycemia and peritonitis are major complications.

Diabetic retinopathy (see under VASCULAR RETINOPATHIES in Ch. 223).

Symptomatic neuropathy is uncommon in childhood; however, impaired nerve conduction can be detected early. **Growth failure** is commonly seen in poorly controlled diabetics. Low serum somatomedin-C levels, in the face of a paradoxical growth hormone elevation, increased protein wasting and urinary nitrogen loss may be contributing factors. **Necrobiosis lipoidica diabeticorum** is an uncommon but characteristic lesion located in the pretibial area of diabetic patients. **Vitiligo** is another skin condition that may be present. **Infections** are more common in diabetic patients in poor control, primarily as a consequence of impaired WBC function and attenuated tissue perfusion. Phagocytosis by inflammatory cells in the diabetic is abnormal. **Hyperglycemic hyperosmolar nonketotic coma** and **lactic acidosis** are discussed under Diagnosis of Ketoacidosis and Hyperosmolar Coma in DIABETES MELLITUS in Ch. 94.

Treatment

The main goals of therapy are to (1) maintain normal physical growth and adequate nutrition, (2) control symptoms, (3) prevent ketoacidosis as well as long-term complications, and (4) provide psychological support of the patient with this chronic disease requiring life long care.

Diet: The goal is to maintain blood sugar as close to normal as possible without compromising growth and nutrition. Diet is chosen according to individual needs, taking into account the dosage of insulin, physical activity, growth, and body habitus. This is achieved by avoiding concentrated sweets (eg, candy, cakes) and maintaining the day-to-day temporal regularity of food intake to avoid hypoglycemia—usually 3 well balanced meals and a snack in the afternoon and before bed. Unless the patient is overweight, caloric restriction is usually undesirable in a young growing diabetic. Patients are encouraged to use the food exchange system prepared by the American Diabetes Association to regulate the proportions of protein, fat, and carbohydrate in the diet. If the patient has hypertriglyceridemia, the diet is adjusted accordingly.

Exercise and activity: Exercise must be assessed when reviewing the overall blood glucose control. Diabetic children are encouraged to participate in sports and activities like their nondiabetic peers but are advised not to swim or take long bicycle rides alone. The blood glucose level declines after strenuous exercise. It is important to keep a readily absorbable carbohydrate (eg, honey or candy) on hand during athletic events should hypoglycemia occur. Exercise may also increase the rate of absorption of insulin from the injection site, especially if administered where blood flow may be enhanced. This increased insulin uptake may suppress hepatic glucose production and with increased blood glucose utilization by muscle may lead to symptomatic hypoglycemia. To avoid hypoglycemia patients are advised to (1) increase carbohydrate intake before exercise, (2) inject insulin in a nonexercised area of the body, and (3) decrease insulin dose if necessary.

Initiation of Insulin Therapy

For a discussion of various insulins, insulin therapy, and complications of and resistance to insulin therapy, see under Treatment of DIABETES MELLITUS in Ch. 94.

Most children with IDDM are hospitalized at the initiation of therapy, to establish insulin dosages and for comprehensive instructions concerning diabetic management. The precise dose of insulin cannot be predicted, since this usually changes as the disease evolves. Commonly, the patient is started on 0.6 u./kg/day of total insulin dose, of which ⅔ is given in the morning before breakfast and ⅓ before supper in the evening. Of the ⅔ in the A.M., ⅓ is given as regular rapid-acting insulin and the remainder as intermediate-acting NPH. Before the evening main meal, the insulin dose is divided almost equally between intermediate-acting and rapid-acting. After reviewing the daily blood sugar records, the dose and combination of the 2 insulins is adjusted. Because of the variability of the renal threshold and hydration status of each patient, and the inability to detect hypoglycemia, adjustment of insulin doses based on urine sugar levels is unreliable. Insulin dosage is increased by 10% increments of the total daily dose and is adjusted to keep the blood glucose level as close to normal as possible, the target level being 80 to 120 mg/dL. In very young children, who are incapable of recognizing and communicating the symptoms of hypoglycemia, it is desirable to keep the blood glucose level slightly above normal.

Some diabetics wake up with high blood glucose levels and require more insulin in the early morning than expected. This is known as the "dawn phenomena" and is presumed to be due to increased clearance of insulin or nocturnal growth hormone surges. This rise in blood sugar is difficult to manage by increasing the evening insulin dose (given the associated risk of precipitating nocturnal hypoglycemia). A long-acting insulin (such as ultralente) is sometimes used with the intermediate variety in patients who develop recurrent hypoglycemia and where a peak action is not desired.

Insulin therapy alone is inadequate without patient education. The family is taught to monitor the child's diabetes on a day-to-day basis with blood glucose reagent strips. Ideally, with home glucose monitoring, patients analyze the relationship between activity and diet on their blood glucose level and appropriately change their insulin dosage, food intake, or exercise. Various types of reagent strips are available for home blood glucose monitoring. Patients are advised to monitor their blood glucose at least bid to qid, usually preprandially, and at bedtime (for details, see Ch. 94).

Glucosylated Hb (Hb A_1C), the nonenzymatic glucosylation of the B chain, is helpful in assessing the mean blood glucose level over the previous 2 to 3 mo and is especially useful in assessing patients with wide day to day variations of blood sugar.

In some patients there are unexplained swings of blood glucose varying from severe hyperglycemia to hypoglycemia despite seemingly valid insulin adjustments. Such patients are termed **"brittle diabetics."** Management of these patients is more complex (see Ch. 94).

ANOMALIES IN AMINO ACID METABOLISM

Anomalies of amino acid metabolism may be categorized as those of transport and those of catabolism. Both are genetically determined. Although the latter are usually considered the only true metabolic anomalies, defects in amino acid transport in the renal tubule or GI mucosa are also metabolic, since they are caused by enzyme defects. Abnormalities in plasma levels of various metabolites occur in the catabolic group, but are absent in the transport group. Newly discovered entities and recognition of variations in many of the original or classic types are leading to the definition of increasing numbers of catabolic disorders.

The salient features of catabolic amino acid metabolic diseases are listed in TABLE 196–4. Phenylketonuria as a prototype is discussed in greater detail below, since it was the first of the group to be described and is the most common.

TABLE 196–4. ANOMALIES IN AMINO ACID METABOLISM

Disease	*Amino Acid Affected*	*Enzyme Defect*	*Clinical Features*	*Treatment*
Phenylketonuria	Phenylalanine	Phenylalanine hydroxylase	Neurologic symptoms; mental retardation	Controlled phenylalanine intake
Tyrosinosis (Medes)	Tyrosine	Tyrosine α-ketoglutarate aminotransferase (?)	One reported case, probably benign	
Tyrosinemia	Tyrosine	Tyrosine aminotransferase (?)	Mental retardation, keratitis, dermatitis	Controlled phenylalanine and tyrosine intake
Tyrosinemia	Tyrosine and methionine	Fumarylacetoacetate fumarylhydrolase	Fanconi's syndrome, hepatic cirrhosis, fulminating hepatic failure	Controlled phenylalanine, tyrosine, and methionine intake
Albinism	Tyrosine	Tyrosinase	Absent pigment in skin, hair, eyes	Protection of skin & eyes from actinic radiation
Alkaptonuria	Tyrosine	Homogentisic oxidase	Arthritis, dark urine	
Histidinemia Classic	Histidine	L-Histidine ammonia lyase (liver and skin)	Retardation, neurologic manifestations; frequently benign	Low-protein diet, controlled histidine intake
Variant	Histidine	L-Histidine ammonia lyase (liver only)	As above	As above
Maple syrup urine disease (branched chain ketoaciduria) Classic	Leucine Isoleucine Valine Alloisoleucine	Branched chain keto-acid decarboxylase	Reflex changes, hypertonicity, odor of urine and perspiration, convulsions, coma, death	Controlled intake of branched chain amino acids, exchange transfusion and peritoneal dialysis for acute episodes
Intermittent	Same	Same, but some activity	Symptoms only with stress (fever, infection)	Same for acute episodes, none necessary between episodes
Intermediate	Same	Degree of activity between classic and intermittent	Retardation, neurologic symptoms; full-blown picture develops with stress	Protein intake limited to requirement
Thiamine-responsive	Same	Same, presumably cofactor deficiency	Similar to mild picture of intermediate	Thiamine—large doses

Valinemia	Valine	Valine aminotransferase	Retardation	Controlled valine intake
Homocystinemia	Methionine	Cystathionine synthetase (1) Pyridoxine-responsive (2) Non–pyridoxine-responsive	Skeletal abnormalities, ectopia lentis, retardation, thromboembolic disease	(1) Massive doses of pyridoxine (2) Controlled intake of methionine and cystine supplementation, also folic acid supplementation
Cystinosis	Cystine	Unknown	Cystine accumulation throughout RE system, WBC, cornea; Fanconi's syndrome, renal failure	Symptomatic for Fanconi's syndrome; renal transplant for failure Cysteamine
Cystathioninemia	Methionine	Cystathionase	Retardation (?), large number of individuals have no clinical symptoms—benign trait	Large doses of pyridoxine
Glycinemia (non-ketotic)	Glycine	Glycine cleavage enzyme system	Convulsions, retardation	Low-protein diet, strychnine (?)
β-Alaninemia	β-Alanine	β-Alanine-α-ketoglutarate amino transferase	Seizures, somnolence, death	Pyridoxine (?)
Prolinemia, Type I	Proline	Proline oxidase	Hereditary nephritis, nerve deafness (?)	May be benign trait
Prolinemia, Type II	Proline	Δ^1Pyrroline-5-carboxylate dehydrogenase	Convulsions, mental retardation	Low-protein diet, low proline & glutamic acid
Hydroxyprolinemia	Hydroxyproline	Hydroxyproline oxidase	Mental retardation, CNS symptoms	Low-protein diet (?) Benign (?)
Lysinemia	Lysine	Lysine-ketoglutarate reductase	Muscle weakness, retardation, benign in some instances	Controlled lysine intake (?)
Lysine intolerance	Lysine Arginine	Lysine: NAD oxidoreductase (deaminating)	Vomiting, coma	Low-protein diet, controlled lysine intake
Saccharopinuria	Lysine	Aminoadipic semialdehyde–glutamate reductase	Retardation	Controlled lysine intake
Pipecolicacidemia	Lysine	Pipecolate oxidase	Retardation	Controlled lysine intake
AGA deficiency	Ammonia	*N*-Acetylglutamate synthetase deficiency	Lethargy, coma, vomiting	Low protein diet, arginine, sodium benzoate

(*Continued*)

TABLE 196–4. ANOMALIES IN AMINO ACID METABOLISM *(Cont'd)*

Disease	*Amino Acid Affected*	*Enzyme Defect*	*Clinical Features*	*Treatment*
Carbamyl phosphate synthetase deficiency	Ammonia	Carbamylphosphate synthetase	Vomiting, lethargy, acidosis, death, coma	Low-protein diet; essential amino acid mixture, ketoacid analogs of amino acids; arginine; sodium benzoate
Ornithine transcarbamylase deficiency	Ammonia	Ornithine transcarbamylase	Recurrent vomiting, irritability, lethargy, coma, seizures, X-linked, lethal in the male	Low-protein diet; essential amino acid mixture, ketoacid analogs of amino acids; arginine; sodium benzoate
Citrullinemia	Citrulline	Argininosuccinic acid synthetase	Vomiting, coma, convulsions	Low-protein diet; essential amino acid mixture, ketoacid analogs of amino acids; arginine; sodium benzoate
Argininosuccinic-acidemia	Argininosuccinic acid	Argininosuccinase	Seizures, retardation, coma, vomiting	Low-protein diet; essential amino acid mixture, ketoacid analogs of amino acids; arginine; sodium benzoate
Argininemia	Arginine	Arginase	Retardation, seizures, spasticity	Essential amino acid mixture, ketoacid analogs of amino acids
Ornithinemia	Ornithine	Ornithine keto-acid transaminase	Gyrate atrophy of choroid & retina	Low-protein diet, low arginine; proline supplement
Syndrome of hyperornithinemia, hyperammonemia, & homocitrullinemia	Ornithine Ammonia Homocitrulline	Transport defect into mitochondria (?)	Seizures, retardation	Low-protein diet
Sarcosinemia	Sarcosine	Sarcosine dehydrogenase	Mental retardation (?), no symptoms	May be benign trait, no treatment indicated
Glutamicacidemia	Glutamic acid	?	Mental and physical retardation, seizures, trichorrhexis nodosa	?

Pyroglutamic acidemia	Pyroglutamic acid	?	Episodic vomiting, retardation	?
Isovaleric acidemia	Leucine	Isovaleryl CoA dehydrogenase	Vomiting, lethargy, acidosis, retardation, odor of sweaty feet, neonatal death	Controlled leucine intake; glycine
β-Hydroxyisovaleric aciduria	Leucine	β-Methylcrotonyl-CoA carboxylase	Retardation, muscle atrophy, unpleasant urine odor	Controlled leucine intake
HMG CoA lyase deficiency	Leucine	3-Hydroxy-3-methyl-glutaryl coenzyme A lyase	Acidosis, hypoglycemia, hypotonia, lethargy	Low protein diet Controlled leucine intake Control of hypoglycemia
α-Methylacetoacetate accumulation	Isoleucine	Acetyl-CoA thiolase	Episodes of acidosis, coma; retardation	Low-protein diet, controlled isoleucine intake
Propionicacidemia (form of ketotic glycinemia)	Threonine Isoleucine Methionine	Propionyl-CoA carboxylase (1) Apoenzyme deficiency (2) Coenzyme deficiency	Acidosis, lethargy, coma, mental and physical retardation	(1) Low-protein diet, controlled intake of threonine, isoleucine, and methionine (2) Large doses of biotin
Multiple carboxylase deficiency	Leucine Isoleucine Valine	Holocarboxylase synthetase; biotinidase	Acidosis, skin rash, alopecia, hypotonia, defective T- and B-cell immunity	Biotin 5–10 mg/day
Methylmalonic acidemia (form of ketotic glycinemia)	Isoleucine Valine Threonine Methionine	Methylmalonyl-CoA mutase (1) Apoenzyme deficiency (2) Vitamin B_{12} cofactor deficiency	Acidosis, lethargy, coma, mental and physical retardation	(1) Low-protein diet, controlled isoleucine, valine, threonine intake (2) Massive doses of vitamin B_{12}
	Same	Methylmalonyl-CoA racemase (?)	Same	Same as (1) above
Methylmalonic acidemia-homocystinuria	Isoleucine Valine Threonine Methionine	Methylmalonyl-CoA mutase and homocysteine: methyl tetrahydrofolate methyl transferase	Retardation, failure to thrive, seizures, megaloblastic anemia	Hydroxocobalamin

PHENYLKETONURIA

(PKU; Phenylalaninemia; Phenylpyruvic Oligophrenia)

An inborn error of metabolism, characterized by a virtual absence of phenylalanine hydroxylase activity and an elevation of plasma phenylalanine, that frequently results in mental retardation.

Etiology and Incidence

Excess phenylalanine, an essential amino acid, is normally eliminated from the body by hydroxylation to tyrosine. The enzyme phenylalanine hydroxylase is essential for this reaction. If it is inactive, phenylalanine accumulates in the blood and is excreted in excess in the urine; some is transaminated to phenylpyruvic acid, which may be further metabolized to phenylacetic, phenyllactic, and *o*-hydroxyphenylacetic acids; all are excreted in the urine. The exact etiology of the mental retardation is not known, but it is the consequence of the biochemical defect. This enzyme defect, transmitted as an autosomal recessive trait, is found in most population groups but is rare in Ashkenazi Jews and in blacks. Incidence in the USA of the typical variety is approximately 1:16,000 live births.

Clinical Features

Clinical symptoms of PKU are usually absent in the newborn period, hence *laboratory screening tests are mandatory for its detection.* Rarely an infant may be lethargic or may feed poorly. Mental retardation is the most important symptom; the majority of untreated patients manifest some degree of mental retardation, usually severe. They tend to have lighter colored skin, hair, and eyes than unaffected family members. Some infants may have a rash similar to infantile eczema.

Many neurologic symptoms and signs, especially affecting reflexes, occur. Both petit and grand mal seizures are common in older children, and the incidence of abnormal EEGs is 75 to 90%. Children manifest extreme hyperactivity and psychotic states, and often exhibit an unpleasant "mousy" body odor that is caused by phenylacetic acid in the urine and sweat.

Diagnosis

Early diagnosis depends on detecting a high plasma phenylalanine level together with a normal or low plasma tyrosine. The exact plasma level that serves as a cut-off point between classic PKU and the variants of this disease cannot be fixed, although 20 mg/dL (1.2 mM/L) has been proposed. Better methods of differentiation are required. Prenatal diagnosis is now possible in the majority of PKU families. DNA is isolated from cultured amniotic cells or chorionic villus samples, analyzed by restriction fragment length polymorphism, and the profiles compared with those of the parents and the proband.

After the newborn has consumed a moderate amount of milk (the source of phenylalanine) for at least 48 h, he should be screened for PKU. The **Guthrie inhibition assay test** is usually used. A strain of phenylalanine-dependent *Bacillus subtilis* is cultured in a medium on which is placed a filter paper disc impregnated with several drops of capillary blood and other discs containing varying amounts of phenylalanine (controls). The zone of growth around the disc containing the blood sample is proportional to the phenylalanine content. After 4 to 6 wk of age, abnormal levels of phenylalanine metabolites may appear in the urine, including phenylpyruvic acid, phenyllactic acid, phenylacetic acid, and *o*-hydroxyphenylacetic acid. **Another screening test** involves the addition of a few drops of 10% ferric chloride solution to a urine sample or wet diaper (a paper test strip is commercially available). A deep bluish green color indicates the presence of phenylpyruvic acid in the urine. Urine testing is done *after* the neonatal period and should be repeated at regular intervals for 1 yr if the

infant has a family history of PKU. The results of all screening must be confirmed by more exact tests using fluorimetric methods or ion exchange column chromatography.

Variants

Screening programs have detected a number of infants with abnormally high phenylalanine levels. In many, the finding is secondary to neonatal (developmental) tyrosinemia, which can be distinguished by abnormal plasma tyrosine levels. The remaining cases can be divided into classic PKU and mild and severe forms of "**hyperphenylalaninemia.**" Mild forms usually exhibit plasma levels of below 8 to 10 mg/dL while on a normal diet; the severe forms are associated with greater elevations. The distinction between severe hyperphenylalaninemia and classic PKU cannot be made by plasma phenylalanine measurements alone. Exact differentiation requires assay of liver phenylalanine hydroxylase activity, which is virtually absent in classic PKU and present in amounts varying from 5 to 15% of normal in the hyperphenylalaninemias. The liver is normally the only place where measurable quantities of phenylalanine hydroxylase may be found.

No sequelae to the mild variants are expected. The consequences of the more severe forms are not known and these patients should be treated the same as those with classic PKU until more information is available.

Elevated plasma phenylalanine levels may also occur as a result of **tetrahydrobiopterin deficiency.** Dietary therapy can correct the abnormal plasma phenylalanine level but severe neurologic deterioration continues. This occurs because tetrahydrobiopterin is a cofactor in the synthesis of dopamine, norepinephrine, and serotonin; deficiency of these neurotransmitters may account for the neurologic symptoms. Tetrahydrobiopterin deficiency may occur either as a result of a defect in the synthesis of biopterin or a deficiency of dihydropteridine reductase, which reduces biopterin to its active form, tetrahydrobiopterin. Substitution therapy with levodopa, carbidopa, 5-OH tryptophan, and tetrahydrobiopterin, in addition to dietary treatment, may have a beneficial effect on these variants if started early in life.

Maternal phenylketonuria, if left untreated, has a profound effect on the fetus. Over 90% of such pregnancies result in an infant with mental and physical retardation, and there is a high incidence of microcephaly. Control of the maternal blood phenylalanine level before pregnancy may prevent these sequelae, but experience is too limited to be certain of the efficacy of early treatment.

Treatment

Treatment consists in limiting the phenylalanine intake of the child so that his essential amino acid requirement is met but not exceeded. This allows normal growth and development but prevents accumulation in the body of phenylalanine and its abnormal end products. Monitoring of the child and his plasma phenylalanine levels is required. Since all natural protein contains about 4% phenylalanine, it is impossible to satisfy the protein requirement without exceeding the phenylalanine requirement. Hence, casein hydrolysates (treated to remove the phenylalanine) or mixtures of amino acids should constitute the protein moiety of the diet. Lofenalac®, a widely used product in the USA, is a complete food (except for its phenylalanine content) and is used in place of the usual milk in the diet. Low-protein natural foods, such as fruits, vegetables, certain cereals, etc, are allowed. The phenylalanine requirement is supplied by measured quantities of natural protein and the residual phenylalanine content of Lofenalac® (80 mg/100 gm of dry powder). The requirement in terms of body wt decreases with age; it varies from 60 to 90 mg/kg/day during the first months of life and decreases to 20 to 30 mg/kg/day by the end of the first year. Dietary products completely free of phenylalanine are now available. They facilitate control of the blood phenylalanine level and allow a little more leeway in the use of natural foods. Phenyl-

free (Mead Johnson) is a complete food except for phenylalanine, PKU-1, PKU-2 (Milupa) and Maxamaid (Scientific Hospital Supplies) do not contain fat, and hence provide fewer calories than the other preparations.

Treatment must be initiated during the first days of life to prevent mental retardation. Treatment started after 2 to 3 yr of age may be effective only in controlling the extreme hyperactivity and intractable seizures. The length of time that treatment must be continued is unknown. Some clinicians believe that it must be continued for life; others think that it may be terminated when myelinization of the brain is virtually complete, at about 5 yr of age. However, there are a number of reports of a drop in IQ and the development of behavior problems and learning difficulties when therapy is terminated at this age. This has resulted in an increasing number of patients who are being maintained on therapy indefinitely.

Prognosis

The prognosis in untreated PKU, while not life-threatening, is poor for intellectual development. Early and well-maintained treatment makes normal development possible and prevents CNS involvement.

---

197. MUSCULOSKELETAL AND CONNECTIVE TISSUE DISORDERS

RHEUMATIC FEVER

A nonsuppurative acute inflammatory complication of Group A streptococcal infections, characterized mainly by arthritis, chorea, or carditis appearing alone or in combination, with residual heart disease as a possible sequel of the carditis. Subcutaneous tissues (nodules) and the skin (erythema marginatum) also can be involved.

Etiology and Incidence

Group A streptococcus is the precursor, but the role of the host's constitutional and environmental susceptibility has not yet been clarified. Environmentally, malnutrition and overcrowding seem to predispose to the infections and subsequent rheumatic episodes. The attack rates of rheumatic fever range from 0.1% in untreated people with mild or asymptomatic streptococcal infections to as high as 3% in those with febrile exudative pharyngitis. Rheumatic fever occurs most often during school age, with first attacks rare before age 4 and uncommon after 18. Familial susceptibility is of significant but not paramount importance. For unknown reasons, rheumatic fever is now a rare disease in the USA, even when streptococcal pharyngitis is not treated.

Exact incidence rates of acute rheumatic fever are difficult to determine because the physician does not see many episodes, particularly those with only mild asymptomatic carditis. Though incidence rates have declined in recent years in developed countries, rheumatic fever still flourishes in underdeveloped countries. The contribution of antibiotics is difficult to separate from a reduction due to the use of more specific diagnostic criteria. The prevalence of rheumatic heart disease is also difficult to determine because diagnostic criteria are not standardized for the living, and necropsy is not performed routinely. According to recent surveys, rheumatic heart disease is the most common cardiac abnormality of school children, found in about 1 to 2%. It is responsible for about half of the rejections from military service for cardiovascular reasons and in 1975 caused 12,930 deaths in the USA, compared with 5615 deaths during the same interval attributed to syphilis, TB, and infectious enteritis.

Pathology

The histopathology of acute rheumatic fever is difficult to assess because few patients die during the acute attack. Aschoff lesions are often, but not consistently, found in the myocardium and other parts of the heart of the patient with carditis. Biopsy of subcutaneous nodules shows certain features resembling Aschoff lesions, but no characteristics distinguish the nodules from those of RA. Biopsy of inflamed synovial membrane shows nonspecific edema and hyperemia; erythema marginatum has no specific histopathologic lesions. Only hyperemia has been found in the brains of patients who died during an acute episode of chorea or in those who died years later.

The most characteristic and potentially dangerous anatomic lesion of rheumatic inflammation is the gross effect on cardiac valves. The mitral valve is involved most commonly; the aortic valve, often; the tricuspid valve, infrequently; and the pulmonic valve, rarely. An acute interstitial valvulitis may cause edema, thickening, fusion, and retraction or other destruction of leaflets and cusps, leading to stenotic or regurgitant functional changes. Similar involvement can shorten, thicken, or fuse chordae tendineae, adding to the regurgitation of damaged valves or producing regurgitation for a valve that is itself unaffected. Dilation of valve rings may be a 3rd mechanism causing regurgitation. Regurgitation and stenosis are the usual effects on the leaflets of mitral and tricuspid valves; the aortic valve generally becomes regurgitant initially and stenotic only later.

Fibrinous nonspecific pericarditis, sometimes with effusion, is seen only in the presence of endocardial inflammation and almost always subsides without permanent damage.

Symptoms and Signs

Because the 5 major manifestations of rheumatic fever (carditis, migratory polyarthritis, chorea, erythema marginatum, and subcutaneous nodules) can appear alone or in combinations, rheumatic fever has many clinical patterns. Cutaneous and subcutaneous features are uncommon and almost never occur alone, usually developing in a patient who already has arthritis, chorea, or carditis. Fever is a prominent symptom, but is not specific.

1. **Arthritis** is the most common clinical manifestation. Joints become painful and tender, and may also be red, hot, and swollen, sometimes with effusion. Involved joints usually are the ankles, knees, elbows, or wrists. The shoulders, hips, and small joints of hands and feet also may be involved, but almost never alone. If vertebral joints are affected, other disease should be suspected. Rheumatic arthropathy can be mono- or polyarticular, and the typical pattern of migratory polyarthritis is now seen mainly when bed rest and anti-inflammatory therapy have not been started promptly. Tenosynovitis may develop at the site of muscle insertions.

2. **Chorea** can occur alone or in association with other rheumatic manifestations (see SYDENHAM'S CHOREA in Ch. 198).

3. **Carditis** has its own spectrum of manifestations, with the appearance, alone or in various combinations, of pericardial rub, murmurs, cardiac enlargement, or heart failure. In first attacks of rheumatic fever, carditis is present in about 50% of patients with arthritis. In the absence of arthritis (or chorea), a patient with carditis will seek medical attention only if sufficiently febrile, if pericarditis is present and painful, or if cardiac decompensation produces respiratory, peripheral, or abdominal manifestations. In the absence of these provocations, the cardiac damage may not be discovered until much later, when the patient is found to have "rheumatic heart disease without a history of rheumatic fever." In about 50% of adults, the carditis develops in this insidious manner, with the ailment initially undetected.

Since murmurs are the most frequent manifestation of carditis, careful auscultatory technics and rigorous interpretative criteria are required to avoid errors. The soft diastolic blow of aortic regurgitation (heard best along the lower left sternal border) and the presystolic murmur of mitral stenosis (heard focally above or medial to the apex) may be undetected when present.

Cardiac decompensation in acutely ill children may be undiagnosed because its manifestations may be different from those expected in adults. Children's symptoms may be dyspnea without rales, nausea and vomiting (due to gastric hyperemia), a right upper quadrant or epigastric ache (due to distention of the hepatic capsule), and a hacking nonproductive cough (due to pulmonary congestion).

4. **Subcutaneous nodules,** which occur most frequently on the extensor surfaces of large joints, usually coexist with evidence of carditis. Ordinarily, the nodules are painless, transitory, and responsive to whatever agent is used for the associated joint or heart inflammation.

5. **Erythema marginatum,** a serpiginous, flat, painless rash, is transient, sometimes lasting less than a day. Its appearance is often delayed after the inciting streptococcal infection; if it appears as (or even after) other aspects of rheumatic inflammation subside, it should not be mistaken for a new attack.

Other manifestations: Abdominal pain and **anorexia** can occur in rheumatic fever either via the hepatic mechanism described under cardiac decompensation, above, or via a concomitant mesenteric adenitis. Because of the elevated WBC count and abdominal guarding, the situation may resemble acute appendicitis, particularly when other rheumatic manifestations are absent. A prompt response to diuretic or anti-inflammatory agents may confirm the diagnosis.

The arthralgias **("growing pains")** often attributed to rheumatic fever are due to nonspecific myalgia or tenodynia in the para-articular zone and can be distinguished from rheumatic arthropathy by the absence of tenderness during passive movement of the allegedly involved joint. Isometric contraction of the neighboring muscles or tendons often reproduces the pain.

The lethargy, malaise, or fatigue often ascribed to rheumatic fever can be caused by heart failure. "Rheumatic" pneumonia or pleurisy is no longer regarded as specific to rheumatic fever. The manifestations may be caused by other diseases (such as RA or SLE), or by conventional types of pulmonary infection or infarction, occurring in association with decompensated rheumatic heart disease.

Laboratory Findings

The clinical pathology of rheumatic fever is manifested in systemic and local indexes of acute inflammation. Systemically, the ESR is elevated, often to levels > 120 mm/h in the Westergren method and > 50 in the uncorrected Wintrobe test. The WBC count reaches values of 12,000 to 20,000 and may go higher with corticosteroid therapy. Serum C-reactive protein is abnormally high; since it rises and falls faster than the ESR, a negative test is useful to confirm the absence of inflammation in a patient whose ESR remains elevated for some time after an acute rheumatic episode has subsided clinically.

Local indexes of inflammation are found in synovial fluid, although aspiration is seldom necessary for diagnosis or therapy. The fluid is usually clear and sterile, with normal mucin concentration, an elevated WBC count, and a ropy acetic acid precipitate.

Prolongation of the P-R interval is the most common abnormality in the ECG. This finding has *not* correlated well with prognosis or with other evidence of carditis, and it is now regarded as due to a nonspecific abnormality, unrelated to cardiac inflammation, that chemically causes delayed A-V electrical conductivity in about 30% of patients with poststreptococcal complications. Other ECG abnormalities, when present, are due to pericarditis, enlargement of ventricles or atria, or cardiac arrhythmias.

Diagnosis

No single test or other evidence is pathognomonic of rheumatic fever. Diagnosis usually is based on fulfillment of the modified Jones criteria, which require the presence of at least 1, and preferably 2, of the 5 major manifestations cited earlier, together with evidence not only of recent Group A streptococcal infection (scarlet fever, positive throat culture, or elevated ASO or other streptococcal antibody titers), but also of such "minor" manifestations of acute inflammation as fever and an elevated ESR or WBC count.

Gout, sickle cell anemia, leukemia, SLE, embolic bacterial endocarditis, serum sickness, drug reactions, traumatic arthritis, or gonococcal arthritis usually can be distinguished by history or specific laboratory tests. The main diagnostic source of confusion is juvenile RA (see below), which sometimes begins with a relatively abrupt onset, occasionally with rheumatoid cardiac involvement, and often without positive serologic tests for rheumatoid factor. The absence of an antecedent streptococcal infection and the long clinical course of an arthropathic episode usually distinguishes rheumatoid from rheumatic arthritis.

Congenital heart disease with murmurs, cardiomegaly, or congestive heart failure in children and adolescents is distinguished by characteristic murmurs and by cyanosis, when present; echocardiography, cardiac catheterization, or angiography can be used to verify difficult diagnoses. Subendocardial fibroelastosis has been increasingly recognized as an uncommon mimic of rheumatic cardiac abnormalities; it can be suspected when there is no convincing evidence of rheumatic or congenital lesions.

Clinical Course and Prognosis

Except for carditis, all manifestations of rheumatic fever subside without residual effects. Joint pain and fever usually subside within 2 wk, often more rapidly, and seldom last longer than a month; the ESR usually returns to normal within 3 mo in the absence of carditis. Patients with carditis generally have overt acoustic evidence of it when first encountered; if no worsening occurs during the next 2 to 3 wk, new manifestations of carditis seldom occur thereafter. Since murmurs often do not disappear and new cardiac phenomena are uncommon, inflammatory rather than cardiac manifestations are the best indexes of therapeutic response. The evidence of acute inflammation, including ESR, usually subsides within 5 mo in uncomplicated carditis.

About 5% of rheumatic patients have **prolonged attacks** (8 mo or longer) with clinical and laboratory manifestations of inflammation appearing in **spontaneously recurrent episodes** unrelated to intervening streptococcal infection or to cessation of anti-inflammatory therapy. Such recurrent attacks are more likely to be associated with carditis.

Rheumatic fever does not seem to produce chronic "smoldering" cardiac inflammation. Scars left by acute valvular damage may contract and change, and secondary hemodynamic difficulties may develop in the myocardium without the persistence of acute inflammation.

The long-term outcome depends on the severity of the initial carditis. Patients without carditis seldom develop valvular damage, are less likely to have rheumatic recurrences, and are unlikely to develop carditis during recurrences. Those with severe carditis during the acute episode are usually left with residual heart disease that is often worsened by the rheumatic recurrences to which they are particularly susceptible. Murmurs eventually disappear in about half of the patients whose acute episodes were manifested by mild carditis without major cardiac enlargement or decompensation. Susceptibility to recurrences in this group is intermediate between the low risk of the "no carditis" and the high risk of the "severe carditis" patients, but the recurrences may create permanent or further cardiac damage.

Treatment

In patients with **arthritis** only, therapy is directed toward relief of pain. In mild cases, codeine, other analgesics, or relatively small doses of aspirin are adequate. In

more severe situations, complete **salicylization** is necessary. Aspirin is given in an escalating pattern, resembling that of digitalization, until clinical effectiveness has been attained or toxicity supervenes. Measurements of blood or urinary levels of salicylate are only necessary to help deal with signs of toxicity. The starting dose of aspirin for children and adolescents is 60 mg/kg (about 30 mg/lb), divided into 4 daily doses. If not effective overnight, the dose is increased to 90 mg/kg the next day, 120 mg/kg on the following day, and 180 mg/kg on the day after. High doses can be divided into 5 or 6 doses/day. Aspirin should be abandoned in favor of a corticosteroid if a therapeutic effect has not been produced after the 4th day.

Enteric-coated, buffered, or complex salicylate molecules appear to have no advantages over ordinary aspirin. Local gastric reactions can be avoided (or treated, when they occur) by giving milk or antacids 1/2 h after ingestion of the aspirin. Systemic toxicity of salicylate is manifested by tinnitus, headache, or tachypnea and may not appear until after a week or more of fixed dosage. Toxicity is managed by reducing the dosage if the drug appears therapeutically effective, or by abandoning the drug.

Carditis: The goal is to suppress inflammation while avoiding a posttherapeutic rebound. **Salicylate** is the first choice, because an 8-wk course is seldom followed by a rebound, and adverse effects are less serious than those of high-dosage corticosteroid therapy. However, with severe carditis, particularly when heart failure is present, salicylates may not be effective. A **corticosteroid program** then should be started promptly. One useful regimen consists of prednisone 40 to 80 mg/day, depending on the size of the patient. If inflammation is not suppressed after 2 days at this dosage, a total daily amount of 120 to 160 mg may be needed. The fully suppressive dose should be maintained until the ESR has remained normal for at least 1 wk; the dose is then halved for the next week. To prevent poststeroid rebounds, an overlap of full-scale salicylate therapy is begun simultaneously, maintained throughout the tapering of the corticosteroid, which may proceed at the rate of 5 mg every 2 days, and continued until 2 wk after the corticosteroid has been stopped.

Cardiac arrhythmias or decompensation should be treated with appropriate agents. A posttherapeutic rebound manifested only by fever or joint pain often subsides spontaneously, but heart failure in a rebound, if uncontrollable by cardiotonic agents, requires resumption of anti-inflammatory therapy. In patients with prolonged, spontaneously recurrent attacks with carditis, treatment with immunosuppressive agents may be effective.

Other therapeutic procedures: The acutely ill patient's choice of **physical activities** is usually as wise as arbitrary medical decisions. Patients generally limit themselves appropriately if symptomatic with arthritis, chorea, or heart failure. In the absence of carditis, no restrictions are needed after the acute episode subsides. Advice about physical restrictions is most difficult for asymptomatic patients with carditis; strict bed rest has no proved value, and its enforcement may create undesirable psychologic reactions. **Physical restrictions** seem advisable only in patients with symptomatic heart failure to reduce or remove the symptoms.

Though poststreptococcal inflammation is well developed by the time a rheumatic patient is detected, an eradicating course of **antibiotics** is useful to remove any lingering organisms. Appropriate regimens are described under Course and Treatment of streptococcal infections in Ch. 8.

Antistreptococcal prophylaxis should be maintained continuously after an attack of acute rheumatic fever (or chorea) to prevent recurrent attacks. The most effective method is benzathine penicillin G in a monthly IM injection of 1.2 million u., but the injections are painful and require monthly medical attention. Sulfadiazine, in a single oral dose of 1 gm/day (500 mg/day in patients < 27 kg [60 lb]), is as effective as other oral regimens. The daily prophylactic dose of oral penicillin G or V is 200,000 to 250,000 u. bid.

The optimum duration of antistreptococcal prophylaxis is uncertain. Some authorities believe it should be maintained for life in every patient who has had rheumatic fever or chorea, or as long as they have close contact with children, who have higher rates of carriage of Group A streptococci. Others recommend prophylaxis only for the first few years after an acute attack, in all patients under age 18, and for life only in patients with severe cardiac damage. In patients with mild cardiac damage (ie, murmurs but no cardiomegaly or decompensation), prophylaxis can be maintained or discontinued in favor of early treatment of future streptococcal infections.

In patients with known or suspected rheumatic valvular disease, prophylaxis against bacterial endocarditis should be instituted for **dental or oral surgical procedures** likely to cause gingival bleeding, for **surgery on the upper respiratory tract**, and for **surgery or instrumentation of the GU and lower GI tracts**. Patients undergoing dental procedures and surgical procedures on the upper respiratory tract should be given 2 gm of oral penicillin V 1 h before the procedure and 1 gm 6 h later; or a single oral dose of amoxicillin 3 gm 1 h before the procedure, with this dose repeated 6 h later for high-risk procedures. Patients allergic to penicillin should be treated with erythromycin 1 gm orally at the time of the procedure and 500 mg orally 6 h later. Another alternative is vancomycin 1 gm IV, slowly over 1 h, starting 1 h before the procedure.

For GI and GU tract surgery or instrumentation, patients should receive ampicillin 2 gm IM or IV plus gentamicin 1.5 mg/kg IM or IV given 30 min to 1 h before the procedure. A similar dose of both drugs is given 8 h later. Alternatively, amoxicillin 3 gm can be given orally 1 h before minor or low-risk procedures, followed 6 h later by 1.5 gm. Patients allergic to penicillin should be given vancomycin 1 gm IV over 1 h plus gentamicin 1.5 mg/kg IM or IV. The antibiotics should be begun 1 h before the procedure, and may be repeated once 8 to 12 h later.

Note that recently approved regimens of amoxicillin 3 gm orally can be used as standard prophylaxis for oral, GU, and GI procedures.

JUVENILE RHEUMATOID ARTHRITIS

Rheumatoid arthritis ***(RA)*** *beginning before 16 yr of age, similar in many respects to adult RA, but which can be divided into 3 subtypes (systemic, pauciarticular, polyarticular), each presenting with different clinical features.* The disease tends to affect the larger joints that may result in interference with growth and development. Micrognathia (receded chin) due to impaired mandible growth may be seen.

About 20% of children have a **systemic onset** (often called **Still's disease**). High fever, rash, splenomegaly, generalized adenopathy, serositis, and a striking neutrophilic leukocytosis frequently are present. At times these systemic features precede appearance of the arthritis. Rheumatoid factor **(RF)** usually is absent. **Pauciarticular onset** affects about 40% of children. Girls, especially, with this type of onset often have antinuclear antibodies and a high incidence of chronic iridocyclitis. Iridocyclitis often is asymptomatic and is detected only with periodic slit-lamp examinations. A subgroup of boys with pauciarticular onset includes many who have HLA-B27 antigen; most of them subsequently develop classic clinical features of one of the seronegative spondyloarthropathies. The remaining 40% of children with RA have a **polyarticular onset** that often is similar to adult RA. However, RF usually is negative except with teenage onset, mostly in girls. In this group RF implies a poor prognosis. Otherwise, the outlook in general is more favorable than in adults. In fact, complete remissions occur in up to 75% of patients.

Treatment

Therapy is somewhat similar to that for adults. Aspirin is well tolerated and effective, provided large and anti-inflammatory doses (80 to 130 mg/kg/day) are prescribed; serum salicylate levels should be checked for therapeutic levels (20 to 30 mg/dL) with the higher doses. Elevated AST (SGOT) levels may occur, but they return

to normal once aspirin is stopped. In children under age 15, only aspirin and tolmetin are approved for use in the USA, but if these drugs prove to be toxic or ineffective, other nonsteroidal anti-inflammatory drugs **(NSAIDs)** may be tried. Systemic corticosteroids usually can be avoided except for treatment of severe systemic disease. Growth retardation is the major hazard of using prolonged corticosteroids in children. Intra-articular corticosteroids can be given, the dosage being adjusted to the smaller size of affected joints. IM gold salts are administered to children who do not respond to aspirin or other NSAIDs. Dosage is built up gradually with precautions, as in adults, being adjusted to the body weight: 1 mg/kg weekly initially, then slowly weaned to 1 mg/kg/mo. (A discussion of use of gold in RA is in RHEUMATOID ARTHRITIS in Ch. 108.) Although penicillamine and hydroxychloroquine are not approved for use in children, they may be effective in patients in whom gold salts are ineffective or not tolerated.

Active exercises, splints, and other supportive measures help to prevent flexion contractures. Adaptive devices can help children live as normal lives as possible. Ophthalmologic examinations should be given semiannually to detect asymptomatic iridocyclitis (anterior uveitis—see Ch. 222), thereby facilitating early treatment with ophthalmic corticosteroid drops (and mydriatics).

COMMON FOOT AND LEG PROBLEMS IN CHILDREN AND ADOLESCENTS

As children develop, the musculoskeletal system changes dramatically, with varying angulations, rotations, and longitudinal growth. Many lower extremity problems relate to these variations and either improve or worsen as growth occurs. For example, in infancy, external rotation of the hip (femoral retroversion), medial rotation of the tibia (tibial torsion), and metatarsus adductus are common. With time and conservative treatment, improvement generally occurs.

Evaluation for foot and leg problems in children requires cooperation and sequential individual analysis of each part of the extremity. Asymmetric findings or progressive deformity are *not* typical of normal variation, and a neurologic cause should be sought (myelodysplasia, cerebral palsy, etc). The range of mobility at each joint should be tested, and angulation or rotation of femur, knees, and feet checked with the patient standing. To assess tibial torsion, seat the patient with knees flexed 90° and the legs hanging free. Next align the longitudinal tibial axis and tibial tubercle with the 2nd metacarpal. Now imagine a line between the 2 malleoli. The angle at which these 2 lines intersect, as seen looking along the tibia, will approximate the degree of internal or external tibial torsion. Gait also should be observed.

Hips and femurs: Internal torsion of the femur is common in children, since femoral anteversion decreases from 40° to 15° between birth and teen age. Marked **femoral anteversion** results in "kissing knees," toeing-in, and clumsiness. Sitting in the "W" position or sleeping prone with the legs extended or flexed (knee-chest) and internally rotated may contribute and should be avoided. If marked findings persist after age 8 yr, orthopedic referral is needed. **External femoral torsion** is commonly seen before children walk and apparently is due to an abduction/external rotation soft-tissue contracture following in utero positioning. Sleeping prone with the legs externally rotated can prolong the condition. Internally rotating the lower extremities with diaper changes may be helpful, but most cases begin to correct spontaneously when the child walks. A careful check for hip dislocation is indicated (see MUSCULOSKELETAL DEFECTS in Ch. 187).

Hip pain and limp are characteristic of a slipped femoral capital epiphysis in adolescents, or Legg-Calvé-Perthes disease in younger children. The pain sometimes is referred to the knee or anterior thigh. Early diagnosis of a **slipped epiphysis** dramatically

improves the outcome. Slippage generally is slow and occurs most commonly in obese teenage boys. It is bilateral in 20% of patients. The cause is unknown, but hormonal factors are suspected. X-rays confirm the diagnosis and exclude acetabular dysplasia or arthritic changes. Treatment is surgical. **Legg-Calvé-Perthes disease** is discussed below under THE OSTEOCHONDROSES.

Knee or femoral-tibial angular deformities are of 2 major types: (1) bowlegs (genu varus); and (2) knock-knees (genu valgus). Both variations can result in adult osteoarthritis of the knee if untreated. **Bowlegs** are common in toddlers and usually correct spontaneously by age 18 mo. If bowlegs persist or increase in severity, then **Blount's disease** (tibial osteochondrosis) should be suspected. Early diagnosis of Blount's disease is difficult, since x-rays may be normal. Rickets should be ruled out. Treatment using the Danish night splint is effective if started early; otherwise, surgery may be needed. **Knock-knees** are less common, and even severe degrees usually correct spontaneously by age 9 yr. Skeletal dysplasia or hypophosphatasia should be excluded. Treatment is surgical stapling of the medial distal femoral epiphysis if marked deformity persists after age 10 yr.

Knee pain with swelling over the tibial tubercle in adolescence usually is **Osgood-Schlatter disease** (see below in THE OSTEOCHONDROSES). Adolescents also are prone to develop **chondromalacia patellae** (*softening of the patellar articular cartilage*). Angular or rotational changes in the leg apparently produce this by unbalancing elements of the quadriceps with patellar misalignment during movement. Knee pain occurs when climbing, especially up or down stairs. Treatment consists of isometric quadriceps strengthening, aspirin, and avoiding pain-producing activities.

Tibial twisting or torsion occurs with growth, going from 0° of lateral external rotation at birth to 20° by adult life. External tibial torsion rarely is a problem. Internal or medial tibial torsion is common at birth, but improves with growth. It is associated with toeing-in and bowlegs. Rickets or a neuromuscular problem should be excluded. Occasionally, passive exercises (external rotation of the foot) or corrective shoes (wedges on inner heel and outer sole, Thomas or torque heel) may be useful. Torsion persisting after age 7 yr needs orthopedic care.

Forefoot abnormalities occur in 1 out of every 100 births. Fortunately most are functional, such as metatarsus adductus, rather than structural, such as partial clubfoot (talipes varus) or metatarsus varus. In **metatarsus adductus,** the forefoot can be passively abducted and everted beyond neutral and lacks inversion, and when the sole is stimulated lateral movement of the forefoot is seen. Resolution without treatment usually occurs in the first year of life. **Metatarsus varus** may require treatment with corrective casting by an orthopedist. **Pronation, flatfoot,** and **pes planovalgus** are recognized by a flattened medial longitudinal arch with outward rolling of the foot. There is eversion of the hindfoot and eversion and abduction of the forefoot. Most children have some pronation when they begin to walk because of ligament laxity and a wide-based gait, but the pronation corrects without treatment by age 2½ yr. Infants often appear falsely flatfooted because of a fat pad below the medial longitudinal arch. The arch usually is restored when standing on tiptoe if the deformity is functional. If there are pains or cramps in the feet, then treatment with corrective shoes is indicated (arch support or shoes with a long medial counter and a Thomas heel).

INHERITED DISORDERS OF CONNECTIVE TISSUE

EHLERS-DANLOS SYNDROME

An inherited connective tissue disorder characterized by articular hypermobility, dermal hyperelasticity, and widespread tissue fragility. Though usually inherited as an autoso-

mal dominant condition, Ehlers-Danlos syndrome is heterogeneous based on different gene mutations affecting the structure or assembly of different collagens, and at least 10 varieties have been described including uncommon X-linked and recessive forms. In the usual dominant form, no specific biochemical or histologic changes have been demonstrated, though cross-linking of the collagen fibrils is thought to be defective. In a recessive type, the enzyme lysyl hydroxylase is deficient.

Symptoms, Signs, and Diagnosis

Clinical findings vary widely, depending on the specific gene mutation and resultant type of Ehlers-Danlos syndrome. This discussion covers the range of possibilities that appear to varying degrees in individual patients.

The skin can be stretched several cm but returns to its normal position on release. Wide papyraceous scars are often present over bony prominences, particularly the elbows, knees, and shins. The extent of joint hypermobility varies but may be marked. Affected individuals have become the "elastic ladies" or "India rubber men" of circus side shows. A bleeding tendency may be present but is troublesome in only a minority of patients (see in VASCULAR DISORDERS in Ch. 99). Fleshy outgrowths (molluscoid pseudotumors) frequently form on top of scars or at pressure points. Subcutaneous calcified spherules may be palpated or demonstrated radiologically.

Minor trauma may cause wide gaping wounds but little bleeding; wound closure may be difficult, since sutures tend to tear out of the fragile tissue. Surgical complications arise because of deep tissue fragility. Synovial effusions, sprains, and dislocations occur frequently. Talipes equinovarus is present in 5% of patients, congenital dislocation of the hip in 1%, spinal kyphoscoliosis in 25%, and thoracic deformity in 20%. Pes planus is present in 90% of adult patients. GI hernias and diverticula are common. Spontaneous hemorrhage and perforation of portions of the GI tract occur rarely, as do dissecting aneurysm of the aorta and spontaneous rupture of large arteries. Medullary sponge kidney has been reported in a very small proportion of Ehlers-Danlos patients. Tissue extensibility in an affected mother may cause premature birth; fetal membrane fragility and consequent early rupture may occur if the fetus is affected. Maternal tissue fragility may complicate episiotomy or cesarean section. Ante-, peri-, and postnatal bleeding may occur. Epicanthus is common in children; myopia in adults. Scleral fragility and perforation of the globe of the eye have been described in a rare autosomal recessive form of the disease.

Prognosis and Treatment

Although numerous and varied complications may occur, the life span usually is normal. The prevalence of lethal complications may be very high in a minority of kindreds.

There is no specific treatment. Trauma should be minimized. Protective clothing and padding may be helpful. If an operation is performed, hemostasis must be meticulous. Wounds should be carefully sutured and tissue tension avoided. Obstetric supervision during pregnancy and delivery is mandatory. Genetic counseling should be provided.

MARFAN SYNDROME

An inherited disorder of connective tissue transmitted as an autosomal dominant trait, resulting in ocular, skeletal, and cardiovascular abnormalities. The marfanoid hypermobility syndrome and congenital contractual arachnodactyly are uncommon but distinct variants. An abnormality of the aortic media is the principal structural defect in the great vessels, the histologic changes resembling those of Erdheim cystic medial necrosis.

Symptoms and Signs

The severity of the syndrome varies greatly. Marfan syndrome patients are taller than average for age and family, with arm span exceeding height. The digits are dispro-

portionately long and thin (arachnodactyly). Deformity of the sternum—outward displacement (pectus carinatum) or inward displacement (pectus excavatum)—is frequent. Hyperextensibility of joints, backward curvature of the legs at the knees (genu recurvatum), flat feet, and kyphoscoliosis occur often. Hernias are common. Subcutaneous fat usually is sparse. The palate is often high-arched.

Ocular findings include subluxation or dislocation of the lens (ectopia lentis) and iridodonesis (tremulousness of the iris). The margin of the dislocated lens often can be seen through the undilated pupil. High-grade myopia may be present, and spontaneous detachment of the retina sometimes occurs.

Cardiovascular changes are associated with weakness of the aortic media in areas subject to greatest hemodynamic stress. The ascending aorta undergoes progressive dilation or acute dissection beginning in the coronary sinuses as early as the first or as late as the fifth decade of life. Aortic regurgitation may precede x-ray evidence of aortic dilation. Bacterial endocarditis may develop. Mitral valve prolapse or regurgitation due to redundant cusps and chordae tendinae may occur, producing systolic clicks and a late systolic murmur. Cystic disease of the lungs and recurrent spontaneous pneumothorax have occurred.

Diagnosis

This is made by recognition of the cardiovascular, ocular, and skeletal manifestations, especially with a positive family history. Diagnosis can be difficult because many patients have few major features, specific histologic or biochemical changes are lacking, and there are no objective tests for diagnostic confirmation. Homocystinuria may be confused with Marfan syndrome because of similar clinical features, but can be differentiated by demonstrating homocystine in the urine.

Appropriate genetic counseling is indicated. At present, antenatal diagnosis is not feasible.

Prognosis and Treatment

In very general terms, the liability to serious complications is proportional to the severity of the manifestations.

For girls who are very tall, induction of precocious puberty by age 10 with estrogens and progesterone may reduce ultimate height. Anabolic steroids may help children and adults with aortic dilation, but masculinizing effects limit their use in females. Reserpine or propranolol reduces the abruptness of ventricular ejection and has been prescribed in an attempt to prevent aortic dilation and dissection. The results have not been consistent. The ascending aorta has been replaced successfully in some patients.

PSEUDOXANTHOMA ELASTICUM (PXE)

(Grönblad-Strandberg Syndrome)

A generalized connective tissue disorder characterized by premature dermal infiltration and laxity in the flexural creases of skin, angioid streaks in the ocular fundi, and hemorrhagic arterial degeneration. PXE is heterogeneous, but the common form is inherited as autosomal recessive.

The earliest histologic changes occur in the elastic fibers. Elastin fibers in the skin, the media of intermediate- and small-sized arteries, and occasionally the endo- and pericardium are basophilic and calcified, and may be rodlike or granular. Basophilia and subsequent cracking of Bruch's membrane cause the retinal angioid streaks.

Symptoms, Signs, and Diagnosis

The skin of the neck, axillas, and inguinal and periumbilical areas is thickened, grooved, inelastic, lax, and redundant, with yellowish pebbly nodules in the later stages. The skin changes resemble those in actinic (senile) elastosis, but only exposed areas are involved in the latter. Brownish or gray angioid streaks, wider than retinal

veins but similarly coursing over the fundus, are characteristically present in the retina. Retinal hemorrhage and severe vision loss may occur. Weak or absent pulses, intermittent claudication, and easy fatigability occur in the extremities. Arterial calcification may be radiographically apparent at an early age. Brachial arteriography shows radial and ulnar artery occlusion with dilated interosseous arteries supplying blood to the hands. Angina pectoris and hypertension are common. Uterine, GU tract, nasal, and subarachnoid hemorrhage may occur.

Prognosis and Treatment

The clinical course varies with the severity and location of vascular involvement. Deaths from the disease or its complications have been reported in patients aged 30 to 70. Treatment is conservative and symptomatic.

CUTIS LAXA

A rare disorder characterized by lax skin hanging in loose folds. A comparatively benign form of cutis laxa is inherited as an autosomal dominant condition; a potentially lethal form with cardiorespiratory complications, as an autosomal recessive condition. Acquired cutis laxa occurs rarely.

In all forms of cutis laxa, histologic examination of the skin shows fragmented elastin. The underlying defect is unknown.

Symptoms and Signs

Inherited forms: Dermal laxity may be present at birth or may develop later, occurring wherever the skin is normally loose and hanging but most obvious on the face. Affected children have a mournful or "Churchillian" facies because of the lax skin folds. Hernias and diverticula of the GI tract are common. Progressive pulmonary emphysema may precipitate cor pulmonale in severely affected patients.

Acquired cutis laxa is clinically distinct from the genetic forms. It may develop insidiously during adulthood and sometimes leads to death from aortic rupture and pulmonary complications. It also may develop following a severe illness involving fever, polyserositis, and erythema multiforme, usually in children or adolescents.

Differential Diagnosis

The dermal fragility and articular hypermobility of **Ehlers-Danlos syndrome** are absent in cutis laxa. Localized areas of loose skin are sometimes found in other disorders; eg, **Turner's syndrome** (see also Ch. 203), in which the affected newborn female's folds of lax skin at the base of the neck tighten and resemble webbing as the child grows older; and **neurofibromatosis** (see also Ch. 131), in which pendular plexiform neuromata occasionally develop that are unilateral and have a configuration and texture distinguishing them from cutis laxa.

Treatment

There is no specific therapy. Plastic surgery considerably improves appearance in inherited cutis laxa; healing usually is uncomplicated, but dermal laxity may recur. Plastic surgery is less successful in acquired cutis laxa. Cardiorespiratory complications should be treated appropriately.

THE MUCOPOLYSACCHARIDOSES (MPS)

Genetic conditions characterized by increased urinary mucopolysaccharide excretion and variable systemic manifestations, including a typical facies, skeletal dysplasia, mental deficiency, corneal opacity, and hepatosplenomegaly. Each MPS has distinct clinical features, a specific genetic biochemical defect, and a predictable prognosis (see TABLE 197–1). The disorders are designated MPS I through MPS VII (with specific eponyms)

TABLE 197–1. GENETIC MUCOPOLYSACCHARIDOSES

	Designation	Clinical Features	Excessive Urinary Mucopolysaccharide	Substance Deficient
MPS I H	Hurler syndrome*	Early clouding of cornea; grave manifestations; death usual before age 10	Dermatan sulfate Heparan sulfate	α-L-Iduronidase (formerly called Hurler corrective factor)
MPS I S	Scheie syndrome	Stiff joints; cloudy cornea; aortic regurgitation; normal intelligence; ?normal lifespan	Dermatan sulfate Heparan sulfate	α-L-Iduronidase
MPS I H/S	Hurler-Scheie compound	Phenotype intermediate between Hurler and Scheie	Dermatan sulfate Heparan sulfate	α-L-Iduronidase
MPS II	Hunter syndrome (severe and mild forms)	No clouding of cornea; milder course than in MPS I H but death usual before age 15 In the mild form, survival to age 30 to 50; fair intelligence	Dermatan sulfate Heparan sulfate	L-Iduronosulphate sulphatase
MPS III	Sanfilippo syndrome (several forms)	Identical phenotype: Mild somatic and severe central nervous system effects	Heparan sulfate	Heparan sulfate sulfatase N-Acetyl-α-D-glucosaminidase in some forms
MPS IV	Morquio syndrome	Severe bone changes of distinctive type; cloudy cornea; aortic regurgitation	Keratan sulfate	N-Acetylhexos-aminidase-6-SO_4 sulphatase
MPS V	Vacant			
MPS VI	Maroteaux-Lamy syndrome	Severe osseous and corneal change; normal intellect	Dermatan sulfate	Arylsulphatase B
MPS VII	β-Glucuronidase deficiency (more than 1 allelic form?)	Hepatosplenomegaly; dysostosis multiplex; WBC inclusions; mental retardation	Dermatan sulfate	β-Glucuronidase

* Other rare metabolic disorders such as the mucolipidoses bear a clinical resemblance to Hurler syndrome, but they may be differentiated biochemically.

(Modified from *Heritable Disorders of Connective Tissue*, ed. 4, by V. A. McKusick. Copyright 1972 by the C. V. Mosby Co., St. Louis. Used with permission of The C. V. Mosby Co. and the author.)

by identifying the excess urinary mucopolysaccharide. The primary enzyme defect has been identified in some instances.

Diagnosis

The clinical features of MPS are not usually apparent at birth. During infancy and childhood, short stature, bony dysplasia, hirsutism, and abnormal development become apparent; diagnosis is further suspected in the presence of the characteristic coarse facies, with thick lips, an open mouth, and a flattened nasal bridge. Family history can be helpful. With the exception of MPS II, which is X-linked, all forms of MPS are inherited as autosomal recessives.

The MPS group of conditions can be diagnosed antenatally by estimation of enzymatic activity in cultured amniotic fluid cells. Postnatal urine screening tests must be interpreted cautiously, since false-negative and false-positive results are common. Even in severely affected individuals, tests may be negative in early infancy. The diagnosis is confirmed by estimation of specific enzymatic activity in leukocytes, cultured fibroblasts, or, in some conditions, serum. Cultured dermal fibroblasts also stain with a characteristic metachromasia. Radiologic skeletal changes are typical of dysostosis multiplex; they vary in severity with the form of MPS and may be sufficiently specific to allow a precise diagnosis. However, these radiologic features vary considerably throughout childhood and must be interpreted cautiously.

Prognosis and Treatment

For prognosis, see TABLE 197–1.

At present, no worthwhile therapy is available. Attempts at replacement of the deficient enzyme by plasma infusion or skin grafting have had only limited and temporary success. Bone marrow transplantation has produced a biochemical remission in some instances, but impairment of intellectual function has persisted. A high rate of morbidity and mortality accompanies bone marrow transplantation, and the procedure's value in these disorders is questionable.

THE OSTEOCHONDRODYSPLASIAS

A group of inherited disorders in which growth abnormalities of bone or cartilage lead to skeletal maldevelopment and dwarfism. **Achondroplasia** is the most common and best known, but many other distinct forms of short-limbed dwarfism have been described. These differ widely in genetic background, course, and prognosis, and diagnostic precision is essential. Genetic counseling can be effective, since the pattern of inheritance in most of the osteochondrodysplasias is known. Antenatal diagnosis is possible in some cases by fetoscopy or ultrasonography. Conditions in which fetal limb shortening are severe can be recognized by ultrasonography. New radiographic and molecular technics have future promise. Features of the most important disorders in this group are summarized in TABLE 197–2.

Management: Surgical intervention (eg, prosthetic joint replacement of the hip) is proving to be of value. Hypoplasia of the odontoid process is an inconsistent feature which predisposes to subluxation of 1st and 2nd cervical vertebrae and compression of the spinal cord. For this reason, the status of the odontoid should be evaluated preoperatively by x-ray studies, and the patient's head should be carefully supported if it is hyperextended for endotracheal intubation during anesthesia.

Organizations such as the Little People of America provide social contact for affected individuals and act as a pressure group on their behalf. Similar societies have been founded in Australia and Great Britain.

LETHAL SHORT-LIMBED DWARFISM

Osteochondrodystrophies that present as lethal or potentially lethal short-limbed dwarfism in the newborn. Characteristic x-ray changes are diagnostic, and a whole-baby x-ray study should be obtained in every newborn short-limbed dwarf. This is important even if the infant is stillborn, as diagnostic precision is essential for genetic prognostication. These conditions are summarized in TABLE 197–3.

TABLE 197–2. FORMS OF DISPROPORTIONATE DWARFISM

Disorder	*Additional Clinical Manifestations*	*Usual Mode of Inheritance*	*Reported Cases*
Achondroplasia	Bulky forehead, saddle nose, lumbar lordosis, bow legs	AD	Common
Hypochondroplasia	Resembles achondroplasia in mild degree. Heterogeneous ?	AD	100
Pseudoachondroplasia	Normal facies. Dwarfism and kyphoscoliosis vary in degree. At least 4 forms	AD/AR	200
Diastrophic dysplasia	Severe dwarfing with rigid hitchhiker thumb and fixed talipes equinovarus	AR	200
Multiple epiphyseal dysplasia	Mild dwarfism. Spine and face normal. Digits sometimes stubby. Often presents with hip dysplasia. Very heterogeneous	AD	Common
Spondyloepiphyseal dysplasia	Kyphoscoliosis is a major feature. Myopia and a "flat" facies are sometimes present. Heterogeneous	AD/AR/XL	100
Metaphyseal chondrodysplasia	Many different eponymous types (eg, Jansen, Schmid, McKusick). Associated features in some include malabsorption, neutropenia, and thymolymphopenia	AR/AD	200
Mesomelic dysplasia	Shortening of the forearms and shanks predominates. The face and spine are normal. Several eponymous forms (eg, Nievergelt, Langer)	AD/AR	50
Chondrodysplasia punctata	All forms have pug nose, icthyotic skin lesions, and radiographic epiphyseal stippling		
a) Rhizomelic form	Marked proximal limb shortening. Lethal in infancy	AR	30
b) Conradi-Hunermann form	Mild asymmetric limb shortening. Benign	AD/XL dominant	100
Chondroectodermal dysplasia (Ellis-van Creveld syndrome)	Distal limb shortening. Postaxial polydactyly. Structural cardiac defects	AR	100

TABLE 197–3. FORMS OF LETHAL SHORT-LIMBED DWARFISM

Disorder	*Additional Features*	*Mode of Inheritance*	*Reported Cases*
Achondrogenesis	Gross limb shortening. Hydropic head and trunk. Heterogeneous	AR	50
Thanatophoric dysplasia	On AP* x-rays, vertebrae are "H-shaped" and femora have a "telephone receiver" configuration	Polygenic	Common
Asphyxiating thoracic dysplasia (Jeune's syndrome)	Constriction of upper thorax. Polydactyly sometimes present. Prognosis variable	AR	50
Short rib–polydactyly syndromes	Thoracic constriction. Polydactyly. Invariably lethal. Heterogeneous	AR	50
Chondrodysplasia punctata (severe rhizomelic form)	Severe proximal limb shortening, saddle nose, icthyosis	AR	30
Campomelic dysplasia	Marked bowing of lower limbs. Heterogeneous	AR	30
Osteogenesis imperfecta congenita	Limb deformity due to multiple fractures (see also MUSCULOSKELETAL DEFECTS in Ch. 187)	AR/AD	100

* Anteroposterior

Specific histologic abnormalities have been recognized in some osteochondrodysplasias, and further subdivision and delineation are anticipated on the basis of these findings.

THE OSTEOPETROSES
(Albers-Schönberg Disease; Marble Bones)

Increased bone density and abnormalities of skeletal modeling characterize these genetic disorders of unknown pathogenesis. Formerly loosely grouped together under the above synonyms, the disorders can now be separated into categories on a basis of predominance of bone sclerosis or defective skeletal modeling: **osteoscleroses, craniotubular dysplasias,** and **craniotubular hyperostoses**. Since some of these conditions are comparatively benign and others progressive and fatal, diagnostic accuracy is crucial. There is no specific therapy for the majority of these disorders. Surgical decompression may be required for elevation of intracranial pressure and for entrapment of the facial and auditory nerves. Malocclusion of the teeth may necessitate specialized orthodontic measures. Facial distortion due to bone overgrowth is sometimes severe and may cause psychologic problems.

The most important of the disorders are summarized below.

Osteoscleroses

Increased skeletal density with little disturbance of modeling.

Osteopetrosis with delayed manifestations (in childhood, adolescence, or young adulthood): The designation **Albers-Schönberg disease,** in the strict sense, pertains to *the autosomal dominant **(AD)** delayed, tarda, or benign form of osteopetrosis*, which is relatively common with wide geographic and ethnic distribution. Affected individuals may be totally asymptomatic, the diagnosis often reached by chance when x-ray studies are

taken for some unrelated purpose. The facies, physique, mentality, and life span are normal, and general health is unimpaired. Occasionally the presenting feature is facial palsy or deafness resulting from cranial nerve compression by bone overgrowth. A mild anemia is an infrequent complication.

The skeleton usually is radiologically normal at birth, bone sclerosis becoming increasingly apparent as childhood progresses. Bony involvement is widespread but patchy, and the extremities are sometimes spared. The calvaria is dense and the sinuses may be obliterated. In the spine, sclerosis of the vertebral endplates gives rise to the characteristic "rugger jersey" appearance.

Osteopetrosis with precocious manifestations *(the autosomal recessive [AR] precocious, malignant, or congenita form of osteopetrosis presenting in infancy)* is an uncommon, potentially lethal disorder clinically and genetically distinct from the benign AD type. Bone overgrowth is associated with marrow dysfunction, and presenting symptoms include failure to thrive, spontaneous bruising, abnormal bleeding, and anemia. Hepatosplenomegaly develops, and palsies of the optic, oculomotor, and facial nerves occur in later stages. Death from anemia, overwhelming infection, or hemorrhage usually occurs in the 1st yr of life.

Generalized bone density is the predominant radiologic feature. Penetrated films of long bones reveal transverse bands in the metaphyseal regions and longitudinal striations in the shafts. As the condition progresses, the ends of the long bones, particularly the proximal humerus and distal femur, develop a flask-shaped configuration. Endobones form in the vertebrae, pelvis, and tubular bones; the skull becomes thickened; and the spine shows the "rugger jersey" appearance.

Bone marrow transplantation has produced excellent initial results in a few infants, but the long-term outcome is unknown.

Pyknodysostosis (AR inheritance): Short stature becomes evident in early childhood; adult height does not exceed 150 cm (5 ft). Other manifestations of disorder (enlarged skull, short and broad hands and feet, dystrophic nails, and blue sclerae) usually are recognized in infancy. Affected individuals resemble each other closely, having small faces, receding chins, and carious, misplaced teeth. The cranium bulges and the anterior fontanelle remains patent. The terminal phalanges are short and fingernails dysplastic. Pathologic fractures are an important complication.

On x-ray, bone sclerosis appears during childhood, but neither bone striations nor endobones are seen. The calvaria is not particularly dense but fontanelles are patent and multiple wormian bones are present. Facial bones and paranasal sinuses are hypoplastic, and the mandibular angle is obtuse. Clavicles may be gracile, with underdevelopment of their lateral portions; the distal phalanges are rudimentary.

Craniotubular Dysplasias

Abnormal skeletal modeling, with minor bone sclerosis.

Metaphyseal dysplasia (Pyle disease) is a rare AR disorder often confused semantically with craniometaphyseal dysplasia (see below). Individuals with metaphyseal dysplasia are clinically normal, apart from valgus knee deformities, although scoliosis and bone fragility are occasional complications. Diagnosis usually is reached by chance following x-ray studies for an unrelated purpose.

In contrast to the mild clinical signs, x-ray changes are striking. The long bones are undermodeled and bony cortices generally thin. Tubular bones of the legs have gross "Erlenmeyer flask" flaring, particularly in the distal portions of the femora. The skull is virtually spared, apart from a supraorbital prominence; the mandibular angle is obtuse; and the bones of the pelvis and thoracic cage are expanded.

Craniometaphyseal dysplasia (AD inheritance) is relatively common compared to the other conditions in this group. Paranasal bossing develops during infancy, and progressive expansion and thickening of the skull and mandible distort the jaw and face.

Bone encroachment leads to entrapment and dysfunction of the cranial nerves, particularly the 7th and 8th. Malocclusion of the jaws may be troublesome, while partial obliteration of the sinuses predisposes to recurrent nasorespiratory infection. Height and general health are normal, but progressive elevation of intracranial pressure is an infrequent and serious complication.

X-ray changes are age-related, usually evident by age 5. The main feature in the skull is sclerosis, which is maximal in the base although the cranium is always involved to some degree. Long bones have widened metaphyses with a club-shaped configuration, particularly at the lower end of the femur. However, these changes are much less severe than in Pyle disease. The spine and pelvis are uninvolved.

Frontometaphyseal dysplasia: Distinct AD and X-linked forms may exist. The disorder becomes evident in early childhood. The supraorbital ridge is prominent, resembling a knight's visor. The mandible is hypoplastic, with anterior constriction. Dental anomalies are common, and deafness develops in adulthood because of sclerotic narrowing of the internal acoustic foramina and the middle ear. Long bones of the legs are moderately bowed. Progressive contractures in the digits may simulate RA. General health is good and height is normal.

On x-ray, bone overgrowth of the frontal region is obvious; patchy sclerosis is present in the cranial vault. The vertebral bodies are dysplastic but not sclerotic. The iliac crests are abruptly flared and the pelvic inlet distorted. Femoral capital epiphyses are flattened, with expansion of the femoral heads and coxa valga deformity. Finger bones are undermodeled, with erosions and loss of joint space.

Craniotubular Hyperostoses

Overgrowth of bone, causing both alteration of contour and increase in skeletal density.

Endosteal hyperostosis (van Buchem's disease): The classical form is inherited as AR. A mild AD variety has also been reported. Overgrowth and distortion of the mandible and brow become evident in mid childhood. Subsequently, entrapment of the cranial nerves leads to facial palsy and deafness. The life span is not compromised, stature is normal, and the bones are not fragile. Major x-ray features are widening and sclerosis of the calvaria, cranial base, and mandible. Endosteal thickening is present in the diaphyses of the tubular bones.

Sclerosteosis (AR inheritance) is most prevalent in the Afrikaner population of South Africa. Overgrowth and sclerosis of the skeleton, particularly the skull, develop in early childhood. Height and weight are often excessive, and deafness and facial palsy due to cranial nerve entrapment may be a presenting feature. Distortion of the facies, apparent by age 10, eventually becomes severe. In adults, elevation of intracranial pressure may cause headache, and several sudden deaths have occurred from impaction of the brainstem in the foramen magnum. Cutaneous or bony syndactyly of the 2nd and 3rd fingers distinguishes sclerosteosis from the other disorders in this group.

Predominant x-ray features are gross widening and sclerosis of the calvaria and mandible. The vertebral bodies are spared, although their pedicles are dense. Pelvic bones are sclerotic but with normal contours. Cortices of the long bones are sclerosed and hyperostotic, and their shafts undermodeled.

Diaphyseal dysplasia (Camurati-Engelmann disease) is a comparatively well known AD disorder that presents in mid childhood with muscular pain, weakness, and wasting, typically in the legs. These symptoms usually resolve by age 30. Cranial nerve compression and raised intracranial pressure are occasional complications. The manifestations are variable; some patients are severely handicapped whereas others are virtually asymptomatic.

The predominant x-ray feature is marked thickening of the periosteal and medullary surfaces of the long bones' diaphyseal cortices. The medullary canals and external

bone contours are irregular. The extremities and the axial skeleton usually are spared. Infrequently, the skull is involved, with calvarial widening and basal sclerosis. As with the clinical features, the x-ray changes are quite variable. Corticosteroid therapy may be effective in relieving bone pain and improving muscle power.

THE OSTEOCHONDROSES

A group of disorders affecting the epiphyses during childhood characterized by noninflammatory, noninfectious derangements of the normal process of bony growth occurring at various ossification centers at the time of their greatest developmental activity. Etiology is unknown. The osteochondroses do *not* have a simple genetic basis. They differ in their anatomic distribution, course, and prognosis; their importance lies in their orthopedic implications. Rare osteochondroses include Freiberg's disease (head of 2nd metatarsal), Panner's disease (capitulum), Sever's disease (calcaneus), and Johansson-Larsen syndrome (patella).

Legg-Calvé-Perthes Disease

Idiopathic aseptic necrosis of the femoral capital epiphysis. The disease is by far the most common of the osteochondroses. It has a maximum incidence between the ages of 5 and 10 yr, with a predilection for males. It usually is unilateral.

Symptoms, signs, and diagnosis: Major symptoms are pain in the hip joint and disturbance of gait, usually of gradual onset and slow progression. Joint movements are limited and the thigh muscles may become wasted. X-rays initially reveal flattening and, later, fragmentation of the femoral head, which contains areas of lucency and sclerosis.

The inherited skeletal disorders, notably multiple epiphyseal dysplasia, frequently are misdiagnosed as Legg-Calvé-Perthes disease. In any atypical bilateral or familial case, a skeletal survey to exclude conditions of this type is *mandatory*, as the prognosis and optimal form of management differ in these various disorders. Hypothyroidism, sickle cell anemia, and trauma also must be excluded.

Management is orthopedic, and includes prolonged bed rest, mobile traction, and slings, and containment of the femoral head by abduction plaster casts and splints. Some authorities advocate subtrochanteric osteotomy with internal fixation and early ambulation.

The untreated case usually follows a prolonged but self-limiting course (2 to 3 yr). When the condition eventually becomes quiescent, residual distortion of the femoral head and acetabulum predispose to secondary degenerative OA. For the treated case, these sequelae are less severe.

Osgood-Schlatter Disease

Osteochondritis of the tibial tubercle occurs between ages 10 and 15 yr and is more common in boys than girls. The etiology is thought to be trauma from excessive traction by the patella tendon on its immature epiphyseal insertion. The disorder usually is unilateral.

Symptoms, signs, and diagnosis: Major features are pain, swelling, and tenderness over the tibial tubercle at the site of patellar tendon insertion. There is no systemic disturbance. Lateral radiographs of the knee show fragmentation of the tibial tubercle.

Management: The condition usually resolves spontaneously after a course lasting weeks or months. Relief of pain and avoidance of sport and excessive exercise, especially deep knee bending, are the only necessary measures. Immobilization in plaster, injection of hydrocortisone, and surgical removal of loose bodies, drilling, and grafting are procedures required infrequently.

Scheuermann's Disease

A relatively common condition in which backache and kyphosis are associated with localized changes in the vertebral bodies. The condition presents in adolescence, and

boys are more frequently affected than girls. Scheuermann's disease probably is heterogeneous (ie, not a single entity but a group of conditions sharing similar features), but the etiology and pathogenesis are a matter of debate. Osteochondritis of the upper and lower cartilaginous vertebral endplates has been incriminated, but trauma sometimes is a causative factor. Some affected persons have disproportionate limb lengths; others show a familial tendency.

Symptoms, signs, and diagnosis: A "round-shouldered" posture and persistent low-grade backache are the usual presenting features. Mild cases often are recognized during routine screening of school children for spinal deformity. The major clinical finding is an increase of the normal thoracic kyphosis, which may be diffuse or localized. Scheuermann's disease course is long (very variable—often several years) but mild; trivial spinal malalignment often persists when the disorder has become quiescent.

Lateral x-rays of the spine show anterior wedging of the vertebral bodies, usually in the lower thoracic and upper lumbar region. The endplates become irregular and sclerotic in later stages. Spinal malalignment is predominantly kyphotic, but an element of scoliosis sometimes is present. The x-ray changes often are inconsistent, possibly reflecting underlying heterogeneity. In atypical cases, a generalized skeletal dysplasia and spinal tuberculosis must be excluded.

Management: Mild nonprogressive cases can be treated by reduction of weight-bearing stress and by avoidance of strenuous activity. Occasionally, when the kyphosis is more severe, a spinal brace or rest and recumbency on a rigid bed are indicated. Surgical stabilization and correction of malalignment are infrequently required for progressive cases.

Köhler's Disease

A rare form of osteochondritis of the navicular bone of the tarsus. The disease affects children between ages 3 and 5 yr and has an increased incidence in boys.

Symptoms, signs, and diagnosis: The foot becomes swollen and painful, with tenderness maximal over the medial longitudinal arch. Weight-bearing and walking increase the discomfort, and the gait is disturbed. The condition has a chronic course but rarely persists for > 2 yr.

On x-ray, the navicular bone initially is flattened and sclerotic and later becomes fragmented, prior to reossification. The condition is unilateral, and comparative x-rays of the unaffected side are valuable for assessment of progression.

Management is symptomatic, requiring rest, pain relief, and avoidance of excessive weight-bearing. In the acute case, a few weeks in a below-knee walking plaster, well molded under the longitudinal arch, may be helpful in early stages.

198. NEUROLOGIC DISORDERS

SYDENHAM'S CHOREA

(Chorea Minor; Rheumatic Chorea; St. Vitus' Dance)

A CNS disease, often of insidious onset but of finite duration, characterized by involuntary, purposeless, nonrepetitive movements, and subsiding without neurologic residua.

Etiology

Sydenham's chorea is generally regarded as an inflammatory complication of Group A β-hemolytic streptococcal infections. After the infection, the time interval before onset of chorea (sometimes up to 6 mo) is longer than that of other rheumatic manifes-

tations, and the chorea may begin as, or after, other clinical and laboratory features have returned to normal. If it is a sole clinical feature of poststreptococcal inflammation, Sydenham's chorea may thus appear to be an isolated, unrelated event.

The disease is more common in girls than boys; in childhood; and (for temperate climates) in the summer and early fall, after the spring and early summer peak incidence of rheumatic fever. Chorea occurs in up to 10% of rheumatic attacks.

Symptoms and Signs

The patient develops rapid, purposeless, nonrepetitive movements that may involve all muscles except the eyes. Voluntary movements are abrupt, with impaired coordination. Facial grimacing is common. The patient may appear clumsy in mild cases, and may have slight difficulties in dressing and feeding. In extreme cases, the patient may need vigorous sedation and protection to avoid self-injury from flailing arms or legs. The neurologic examination shows no defect in muscle strength or sensory perception except for an occasionally pendulous knee jerk.

The course of chorea is variable and difficult to measure because of its insidious onset and gradual cessation. A month or more may elapse before the movements become intense enough to make the patient or his parents seek medical attention. The episode may end within another 3 mo but, occasionally, may last 6 to 8 mo.

Diagnosis

The athetoid movements of chorea are pathognomonic. They resemble those of cerebral palsy, from which they can be distinguished by the history of recent onset. Other conditions that must be differentiated are habit spasms, which are repetitive; and the movements of hyperkinetic children, which are purposeful. Huntington's chorea is usually associated with a family history and appears in adulthood. The Parkinson-like side effects of tranquilizers, given to control the apparently "hyperactive" child, may confuse the diagnosis of chorea until the drugs are discontinued and the unaltered choreic movements can be noted.

Aside from occasional lingering evidence of previous streptococcal infection, chorea has no characteristic laboratory features. The CSF is usually unremarkable, and the EEG shows no more than nonspecific dysrhythmias.

Treatment

No medication is consistently effective. Sedation with a barbiturate may be attempted when the movements are severe, in dosage adequate to make the patient barely drowsy. A tranquilizer—such as diazepam 5 mg 4 to 6 times/day—may be effective if barbiturates fail. If both of these agents fail, a salicylate or a corticosteroid may be given in the dosage described for rheumatic fever (see in Ch. 197, above).

Chorea is best regarded and treated as a transitory, reversible form of cerebral palsy. It is important to reassure patients and those who deal with them—family, friends, nurses, teachers, classmates—that the ailment is self-limited, that it will ultimately subside without residual damage, and that the temporary impairment of motor functions will not affect intellectual capacity. Patients should miss school only if movements are uncontrollably severe and should return to school as soon as they can manage the necessary locomotion, even if some residual dysfunction is still present. Many of the so-called psychologic effects ascribed to chorea in the past were due not to the disease itself, but to the associated scholastic deprivation and to the patients' anxiety and dismay at the bizarre movements and at the reactions they invoke in people who do not understand.

Severe cardiac involvement is seldom present in patients with active chorea, but, if present, can be managed as described for rheumatic fever (see in Ch. 197, above). After completion of an attack, antistreptococcal prophylaxis against recurrences of chorea (or rheumatic fever) should be maintained as described for rheumatic fever.

CEREBRAL PALSY (CP) SYNDROMES

A loose descriptive term applied to a number of nonprogressive motor disorders resulting from gestational or perinatal CNS damage and characterized by an impairment of voluntary movement. The term is not a diagnosis, but provides a useful therapeutic classification for children with static spastic paresis, incoordination, or involuntary movements who will require complex training and therapy to attain their optimum potential.

Etiology and Incidence

Between 0.1% and 0.2% of children (about 0.5% of pediatric hospital admissions) have CP syndromes; up to 1% of premature babies or those small for gestational age are afflicted. The etiology often is hard to establish, but in utero disorders, birth trauma, neonatal asphyxia, and neonatal jaundice play important roles. Spastic paraplegia is especially common after premature birth, spastic quadriparesis after perinatal asphyxia, and athetoid and dystonic forms after perinatal asphyxia or kernicterus. Severe systemic disease during early infancy (eg, meningitis or other infections; water or salt depletion) may also cause a CP syndrome.

Symptoms and Signs

A number of syndromes have been described, grouped into 4 main categories: spastic, athetoid, ataxic, and mixed forms.

Spastic syndromes are the most common, representing about 70% of cases. The spasticity is due to upper motor neuron involvement and may mildly or severely affect motor function. **Hemiplegia** connotes involvement of both limbs on one side; the arm usually is affected more severely. **Paraplegia** connotes involvement of both legs, with relative or complete sparing of the arms. **Quadriplegia** or **tetraplegia** connotes involvement of all limbs to a similar degree. **Diplegia** refers to a form intermediate between para- and quadriplegia, with predominant involvement of the legs.

The affected limbs usually are underdeveloped, and show increased deep tendon reflexes and muscular hypertonicity, weakness, and a tendency to contractures. A "scissors gait" and toe-walking are characteristic. In mildly affected children, symptoms may be seen only during certain activities such as running. With quadriplegia, an associated corticobulbar impairment of oral, lingual, and palatal movement, with consequent dysarthria, is common.

Athetoid or **dyskinetic syndromes** occur in about 20% of cases and result from basal ganglia involvement. The resultant slow, writhing, involuntary movements may affect the extremities (athetoid), or the proximal parts of the limbs and the trunk (dystonic); abrupt, jerky distal movements (choreiform) also may occur. The movements increase with emotional tension and disappear during sleep. Dysarthria is present and often severe.

Ataxic syndromes are uncommon (about 10% of cases) and result from involvement of the cerebellum or its pathways. Weakness, incoordination, and intention tremor produce unsteadiness, a wide-based gait, and difficulty with rapid or fine movements.

Mixed forms are common: most often, spasticity and athetosis; less often, ataxia and athetosis.

Associated disorders: Convulsive seizures occur in about 25% of patients, most often in those with hemiplegia. Strabismus and other visual defects may be seen. Children with athetosis due to kernicterus commonly display nerve deafness and paralysis of upward gaze.

Children with spastic hemiplegia or paraplegia frequently have normal intelligence

and a good prognosis for social independence; spastic quadriplegia and mixed forms often are associated with disabling mental retardation.

Diagnosis

It is only rarely possible during early infancy to establish that a child is suffering from CP. Nevertheless, early diagnosis and therapy are highly desirable, and children known to be unusually at risk (those with evidence of birth trauma, asphyxia, jaundice, or meningitis, or with a neonatal history of seizures, hypotonia, or reflex suppression) should have close follow-up surveillance.

Specific forms of CP often cannot be characterized until the 2nd yr. Before the specific motor syndrome develops, the child will show lagging motor development and, often, persistent infantile reflex patterns, hyperreflexia, and altered muscle tone. It is important to distinguish the specific CP syndromes from progressive hereditary neurologic disorders or those requiring surgical or other specific forms of neurologic treatment. The relatively uncommon ataxic forms are particularly hard to distinguish, and many ataxic children ultimately are found to have progressive cerebellar degenerative disease.

Laboratory tests are useful in excluding certain progressive biochemical disorders that involve the motor system, such as Tay-Sachs disease, metachromatic leukodystrophy, and the mucopolysaccharidoses. Other progressive disorders, such as infantile neuroaxonal dystrophy, cannot be excluded by laboratory tests and must be diagnosed by clinical or pathologic criteria. Children with pronounced mental retardation and symmetric motor abnormalities should be evaluated for amino acid and other metabolic abnormalities.

Athetosis, self-mutilation, and hyperuricemia in boys identify the **Lesch-Nyhan syndrome**. Cutaneous or ocular abnormalities may indicate **tuberous sclerosis, neurofibromatosis, ataxia telangiectasia, von Hippel-Lindau disease,** or **Sturge-Weber syndrome;** these disorders are usually, but not always, progressive. Infantile spinal muscular atrophy, spinocerebellar degenerations, and the muscular dystrophies generally lack signs of cerebral disease. **Adrenoleukodystrophy** has an onset later in childhood.

Treatment

The treatment goal is development of maximal independence within the limits of the patient's motor and associated handicaps. Many patients, especially those with spastic paraplegia or hemiplegia, can lead near-normal lives with proper management of the motor handicap. Seizures require the use of anticonvulsants for control (see Ch. 121). Physical therapy, occupational therapy, bracing, orthopedic surgery, and speech training may all be required. Attendance in a regular school class is desirable when intellectual and physical handicaps are not severe.

Complete social independence is not a realistic goal for many CP patients, who will require varying degrees of supervision and assistance throughout their lives. For these children, special schooling is highly desirable. Even the severely affected can profit from training in simple daily functions that increase independence in self-care activities such as washing, dressing, and feeding, and that greatly reduce the burden for families or chronic-care facilities.

As with all chronically handicapped children, the parents need continuing assistance and guidance in understanding the child's status and future potential, and in relieving their own feelings (see MANAGEMENT OF CHRONIC DISABILITY in Ch. 183). These children will reach their maximal potential only with the help of stable and sensible parental care combined with the assistance of public and private agencies (eg, community health agencies, vocational rehabilitation organizations, and lay health organizations such as the United Cerebral Palsy Association).

199. NOSE AND THROAT DISORDERS

(See also §17)

FOREIGN BODIES

Common in young children, foreign bodies in the nose result in a foul-smelling, bloody, unilateral discharge. Mineral salts are deposited on a long-retained foreign body, producing a rhinolith. **Treatment**: Removal usually requires general anesthesia in a child. Vasoconstriction with a topically applied sympathomimetic amine (eg, 10 drops of phenylephrine 0.25%) may facilitate removal. A blunt hook is placed behind the foreign body and then drawn forward. Attempts at grasping smooth, firm foreign bodies with forceps tend to push them farther posteriorly. Rhinoliths are difficult to remove because their shape tends to conform to the contour of the nasal passage.

JUVENILE ANGIOFIBROMA

A benign tumor arising from the connective tissue in the nasopharyngeal vault and occurring almost exclusively in males at puberty. The angiofibroma is red and firm and is composed of fibrous tissue and numerous thin-walled vessels without contractile elements. Epistaxis is the major symptom. The angiofibroma may obstruct the nasal cavity, encroach upon the paranasal sinuses, and invade the orbit and the cranial cavity. The pterygomaxillary fissure is frequently widened by extension of the tumor into the infratemporal fossa. The widening of the fissure may be determined radiographically; the extent of the tumor may be determined with CT. The source of the blood supply and the presence of intracranial extension are determined with bilateral selective internal and external carotid angiography.

Although angiofibromas usually involute with maturity, **treatment** is usually necessary. To control recurrent massive bleeding, estrogen therapy with diethylstilbesterol (5 mg orally tid for 6 wk prior to excision) reduces the size and vascularity of the tumor. Angiographic embolization followed by excision is the more definitive method of treatment, but radiation therapy is the treatment of choice for patients with intracranial or orbital extension.

JUVENILE PAPILLOMAS

Benign tumors of the larynx that may grow so exuberantly at multiple sites that tracheotomy is required to maintain an adequate airway. They are thought to be of viral etiology, and they may appear as early as 1 yr of age and occur in epidemics. **Treatment** is by periodic excision or laser vaporization. Recurrence is common. Regression usually occurs spontaneously at puberty.

---

200. OPHTHALMOLOGIC DISORDERS

Disorders of the eye are also discussed in §18; under CONGENITAL EYE DEFECTS in Ch. 187; and under VISION AND EYE MOVEMENT DISORDERS in Ch. 119.

STRABISMUS

(Squint; Cross-Eyes; Heterotropia)

Deviation of one eye from parallelism with the other. **Paralytic (nonconcomitant) strabismus** results from paralysis of one or more ocular muscles and may be caused by a

specific oculomotor nerve lesion. It is characterized by limitation of eye motion and increasing diplopia in the fields of action of the paralyzed muscles (see also VISION AND EYE MOVEMENT DISORDERS in Ch. 119). Diplopia is not present if the paralysis is congenital, since vision in the deviated eye is suppressed. **Nonparalytic (concomitant) strabismus** usually results from unequal ocular muscle tone caused by a supranuclear defect within the CNS. A concomitant strabismus may be convergent **(esotropia)**, divergent **(exotropia)**, or vertical **(hyper-** or **hypotropia)**. The deviation from parallelism does not vary with ocular movements and the function of individual muscles is usually intact, unless secondary contraction occurs. **Latent strabismus (phoria)** is concomitant and may occur as **esophoria, exophoria,** or **hypo-** or **hyperphoria**. In phorias, the muscle imbalance is overcome by the neurologic (central) tendency to fuse the images from each eye. Phorias, unless large, rarely cause symptoms and are apparent only when fusion is suppressed artificially.

Examination for strabismus can be initiated by having the patient fix on a pencil or flashlight held in front of the examiner. By alternately covering and uncovering an eye, the examiner can detect a shift in the eye that is being uncovered as that eye picks up fixation on the object. In the presence of exotropia, the eye that was covered will have to turn *in* to achieve fixation; esotropia requires the eye to rotate *out* to fixate. The amount of tropia can be estimated by using prisms oriented in a fashion that makes it unnecessary for the deviating eye to move to fixate. The power of the prism (in diopters) used to prevent deviation also quantitates the tropia.

Amblyopia (reduced visual acuity) usually results from suppressing the image from the deviating eye to avoid the confusion of diplopia. Disuse of an eye, as in cases of severe refractive error or impaired vision due to disease, may also result in strabismus.

Treatment

Since strabismus may be the result of serious ocular or neurologic disease, complete evaluation of the eyes (corneas, lenses, retinas, and optic nerves) and neurologic status of the patient, regardless of age, is mandatory. Ocular deviation, if constant, should be investigated shortly after birth; if intermittent, by age 6 mo. It should never be merely observed, assuming that it will be outgrown, since serious disease may be overlooked. If muscle imbalance alone is responsible, strabismus should be treated early with corrective glasses or contact lenses, miotics (eg, 0.03% echothiophate iodide bid), orthoptic training (eg, eye exercises, patching the normal eye), or surgical restoration of the muscle balance. Early treatment may prevent amblyopia and allow a better prognosis for development of binocular vision. Permanent visual loss can occur if strabismus and its attendant amblyopia are not treated before age 4 to 6 yr, and intermittent follow-up examinations are required at least until the child is 10 yr old.

201. PSYCHIATRIC CONDITIONS IN CHILDHOOD AND ADOLESCENCE

CHILDHOOD PSYCHOSIS

Psychoses are manifested by pathology in all areas of mental function: behavior, cognition, and affect. They are relatively rare (4 to 5 cases/10,000 children), but they pose significant problems for medical care. They can be differentiated into 3 major categories, each differing in age of onset, course, and prognosis: infantile autism, and childhood-onset pervasive developmental disorder; disintegrative psychosis; and childhood schizophrenia.

INFANTILE AUTISM

(Kanner's Syndrome)

A syndrome of early childhood characterized by (1) abnormal social relationships; (2) language disorder with impaired understanding, echolalia, and pronominal reversal; (3) rituals and compulsive phenomena (an insistence on the preservation of sameness); and (4) uneven intellectual development, in most cases.

The ratio of male to female cases is 4:1. An epidemiologic study of all cases in England in which autism was known to have occurred in at least one of a pair of twins revealed that the concordance rate in monozygotic twins was significantly greater than that in dizygotic pairs; this points to an important role for genetic factors. When the syndrome was originally identified, its differentiation from mental deficiency and from manifest brain injury was emphasized; however, it is now defined by its behavioral manifestations, and the level of intellectual function and the presence or absence of neurologic damage are recorded separately using a multiaxial diagnostic system.

Symptoms, Signs, and Diagnosis

Infantile autism usually is manifest in the first year of life; *its onset is not later than age 30 mo.* The syndrome is characterized by extreme aloneness (lack of attachment, failure to cuddle, avoidance of eye gaze); insistence on sameness (resistance to change, rituals, morbid attachment to familiar objects, repetitive acts); speech and language disorder (which varies from total muteness through delayed onset of speech to markedly idiosyncratic use of language); and markedly uneven intellectual performance. Autistic children are difficult to test; they usually do better on performance than on verbal items in standard IQ tests and may show islets of age-appropriate performance despite retardation in most areas. Nonetheless, in the hands of an experienced examiner, an IQ test provides a useful predictor of outcome. Those children with IQ < 50 have an almost uniformly poor prognosis; about half those who test higher can do moderately well. The disorder tends to maintain a consistent symptomatic picture throughout development, with some individuals acquiring symptoms of schizophrenia (delusions and hallucinations) in adolescence or young adulthood.

Neurologic examination commonly yields nonfocal findings, although about 20 to 50% of the children (particularly those with IQ < 50) develop seizures before adolescence. EEG examination usually is uninformative. CT scans have isolated a subgroup of autistic children with enlarged ventricles. Individual cases of autism have been associated with the congenital rubella syndrome and cytomegalic inclusion disease.

Treatment

For the most severely impaired children, the systematic application of behavior therapy, a technic that can be taught to parents, helps to manage the child in the home and at school. These benefits are considerable for autistic children who try the patience of the most loving parents and the most devoted teachers. Butyrophenones provide limited benefit, mainly in controlling the most severe forms of aggressive and self-destructive behavior; they do not abort the psychosis. The use of electric shock, tried in the past, is to be condemned. Speech therapy should begin early. For mute children, the value of learning sign language is not yet established.

For those children in the near normal or higher IQ range, psychotherapy and special schooling often are very helpful.

CHILDHOOD-ONSET PERVASIVE DEVELOPMENTAL DISORDER

A new nosologic entity aimed at distinguishing a syndrome similar to infantile autism but with a later age of onset (30 mo to 12 yr). It is characterized by abnormal social relations (eg, aloofness, inappropriate affect, and a lack of skill in making friendships),

and bizarre mannerisms, which commonly include oddities of motor movement, bizarre gestures, and unusual speech patterns. The disorder is not fully expressed until after age 30 mo, although some features may appear earlier. As with autism, delusions and hallucinations are characteristically absent.

Except for a later age of onset, the syndrome appears to be a variant of autism. The disorder often coexists and tends to become blurred with symptoms of Tourette's disorder, obsessive-compulsive disorder, and hyperactivity. **Treatment and prognosis** are similar to that described for autism, above.

DISINTEGRATIVE PSYCHOSIS

A heterogeneous collection of syndromes with onset after age 3 yr and a history of prior normal development. The typical history is that of a child with normal development to age 3 or 4 (including the acquisition of speech, toilet training, and adequate social behavior). Following a period of vague illness and mood change in which the child is irritable and complaining, he undergoes marked regression with loss of the developmental landmarks previously acquired. The child deteriorates to a grossly defective level. Disintegrative psychosis includes some cases that later may be identifiable as specific neurodegenerative syndromes (eg, slow virus diseases [see CENTRAL NERVOUS SYSTEM VIRAL DISEASES in Ch. 12], juvenile cerebromacular degeneration) as well as those in which no cause can be identified. The course is inexorably grave, and the child will require lifelong care as a severe mental defective; longevity may not be impaired in the nonspecific cases. At present, there are no specific treatments for any of the disorders within this category.

CHILDHOOD SCHIZOPHRENIA

(See also Ch. 142)

Psychotic states with onset after age 7 yr and with behavioral similarities to adult schizophrenia. Evidence concerning cause suggests that environmental stress precipitates manifest illness in individuals with a genetic predisposition. Although biochemical hypotheses implicating abnormalities of dopamine metabolism have been tested, results have not been conclusive.

The prevalence of this disorder increases with age. Whereas infantile autism and childhood-onset pervasive developmental disorder are distinctly different from the adult schizophrenias, childhood schizophrenia forms a continuum with the adolescent and adult forms of the disorder. It is characterized by withdrawal of interest, flat affect, thought disorder (blocking and perseveration), ideas of reference, hallucinations and delusions, and complaints of thought control. **Diagnosis** is based on descriptive clinical phenomena.

Treatment

Combined psychotropic and psychotherapeutic treatment is required. Phenothiazines (eg, thiothixene 0.10 to 0.40 mg/kg/day) and butyrophenones (haloperidol 0.15 to 0.30 mg/kg/day) may be effective in controlling acute psychotic symptoms, but relapse is common. (*Because children are susceptible to extrapyramidal side effects with those drugs, they must be used with caution.*) Hospitalization is useful in the management of acute exacerbations; some children require continuing inpatient psychiatric care.

AFFECTIVE DISORDERS (DEPRESSION AND MANIA)

(See also Ch. 141)

Severe affective (mood) disorders, comparable to those seen in adults, are relatively rare among children. However, in recent years, attention has been drawn to the recog-

nition of depression in school-age children. When severe symptoms are present, association with a family history of depressive disorder is likely. Studies of adults support the belief that there is a major genetic component in affective disease, with a higher incidence in the pedigree than in the general population.

Symptoms, Signs, and Diagnosis

The symptoms of **depression** include a sad and unhappy appearance, apathy and withdrawal, reduced capacity for pleasure, feeling rejected and unloved, difficulty in sleeping, somatic complaints (headaches, abdominal pain, insomnia), episodes of clowning or foolish behavior, and persistent self-blame. Chronic depressive reactions are associated with anorexia, weight loss, and despondency. Some contend that depression may be "masked" by overactivity and aggressive and antisocial behavior.

Bipolar affective disorder (manic-depressive psychosis) is exceedingly rare before puberty and unknown in early childhood. Some children do manifest marked mood swings (cyclothymic temperament), but these do not reach psychotic proportions, except when the result of exposure to toxins and drugs.

Treatment

Evaluation of the family and social setting is required to identify stresses that may have precipitated these disorders. Appropriate measures directed at the family and school must accompany direct treatment of the child, focusing on enhancing his self-esteem. Brief hospitalization may be necessary in acute crises. Although controlled studies remain to be done, most clinicians believe that tricyclic antidepressant drugs (eg, imipramine 1 to 2.5 mg/kg/day) are useful adjuncts to treatment. Whether lithium is useful in preventing recurrence has yet to be established; its use in children remains experimental because there are no data on possible toxic effects on the developing organism, particularly on the kidney, thyroid, and brain. Given individual variation in pharmacokinetics of tricyclic antidepressants, monitoring plasma concentration is useful in determining optimal dosage levels. A plasma level of 125 to 200 ng/mL is considered the range of therapeutic effectiveness, although an upper level in children has not been firmly established.

GENDER IDENTITY DISORDER OF CHILDHOOD

DSM-III (*Diagnostic and Statistical Manual of Mental Disorders* of the American Psychiatric Association, Third Edition) describes the essential features of this disorder as a persistent feeling of discomfort and inappropriateness in a prepubertal child about his or her anatomic sex and a desire to be, or a conviction that he or she is, of the opposite sex. Apparently rare, the disorder must be differentiated from the much more frequent rejection of stereotypical sex-role behavior (eg, tomboyishness in girls or sissyish behavior in boys). Children with a gender identity disorder have a profound disturbance of the normal sense of maleness or femaleness, and will strongly and persistently state a desire to be of the other sex, or will insist that they are. (Individuals who develop **transsexualism** [see in Ch. 139] have evidenced gender identity problems as children.)

Girls regularly have male peer groups and are avidly interested in sports and rough-and-tumble play; they are not interested in playing with female-type dolls or in playing house. They insist on wearing stereotypical masculine clothing. Boys invariably are preoccupied with female stereotypical activities such as dressing in girls' or women's clothes, or have a compelling desire to participate in the girls' games. They choose toys and games that are most usually favored by girls, and frequently demonstrate gestures and actions usually regarded as feminine. They encounter considerable male peer-group teasing and rejection.

Of the boys who cross-dress, 75% begin prior to their 4th birthday. Doll-playing begins during the same period. Social ostracism and conflict become significant at

about age 7 or 8. The age of onset in females is also early, but a majority give up this pattern in late childhood or adolescence. A minority of the girls remain identified as males, and some of these develop a homosexual arousal pattern. A smaller number from each sex may later develop transsexualism. The condition may be reversible with long-term psychotherapy and family therapy; the data are not yet conclusive.

Intersexuality

Confusion over gender identity may arise if the child is born with ambiguous genitalia. These children are sometimes called **hermaphrodites,** although most are **pseudohermaphrodites.** Male pseudohermaphrodites have testicular tissue; females have ovarian tissue. In true hermaphrodites, both testicular and ovarian tissues coexist.

The sex of rearing should be determined by the probable course of development at adolescence. If corrective surgery is recommended, it should be carried out very early, whenever possible prior to 18 mo of age. Intersex states are discussed in more detail in Chs. 187 and 203.

ADOLESCENT PSYCHIATRIC CONDITIONS

The adolescent population is no more psychiatrically ill than any other age group. The mistaken assumption that psychopathology is typical in adolescence leads to both over- and under-diagnosis (if all teenagers are "disturbed," disturbance is normal). Follow-up studies suggest that those adolescents seen in clinics and emergency departments for behavioral problems are in fact different from the great majority of their peers and are likely to remain so without adequate intervention.

Some problems typical of adolescence are discussed here, but detailed information on psychiatric conditions occurring in all groups can be found in §12. Suicide in adolescents is discussed separately, below.

Adjustment Disorder

An acute response to environmental stress by an adolescent with a basically good adaptive capacity; symptoms abate as stress diminishes. This diagnosis often is misapplied to chronic difficulties of adjustment and to more serious psychopathology because of a reluctance to give an unfavorable label and prognosis to adolescents. However, it is appropriate when there is strong doubt about the presence of such an underlying disorder and when the environmental stress is impressive.

Occasionally, a generally stable adolescent who is coping with major stresses suffers a **catastrophic reaction** with extreme and even bizarre symptoms and behavior. Resolving the stressful situation, frequently a school or family problem, is the first goal in treatment even when more profound disturbance is suspected. Crisis intervention is worthwhile, since the essentially normal adolescent has a great capacity for responding to help. Recognition of this syndrome and prompt display of empathy, support, and guidance may lead to rapid remission.

Conferences with parents or family group therapy may help, but with some older adolescents or in instances of insoluble family pathology, the teenager should be treated alone. Referral to a social agency, with arrangements for reporting to the physician, may be used. Psychiatric referral may be necessary.

Substance Use Disorders (see also Ch. 138)

Patterns of adolescent substance abuse change. Daily use of marijuana and experimentation with a variety of compounds have diminished since the late 1970s, while alcohol use is unchanged and cocaine and other stimulants may be used more frequently. Reported rates are unreliable and probably underestimated. Although substances change in favor, the susceptible adolescent is the same: less able in school, more invested in recreation, more likely to have a job and money. There is apparently a predictable sequence from alcohol through marijuana to other compounds; a rise in

alcohol use on departure for college; and a relatively stable pattern of use thereafter. Most persons begin serious abuse before age 20 yr, but adolescent preventive programs have not been as effective as hoped. However, the gradual diminution in male adolescent tobacco use suggests that favorable changes can occur. At the individual level, if substance abuse is self-medication for depression or dysphoria, therapeutic intervention—group or individual therapy, antidepressant medication—can be helpful. Detailed information on alcohol and substance abuse should be sought in confidence during the course of routine examination, particularly when academic and behavioral problems are reported.

Conduct Disorders

These disorders are more frequent and more difficult to treat than adjustment disorder. They usually are complained of by someone other than the patient. Persons with **undersocialized** conduct disorders show selfishness, a failure of normal bonds with others, and a lack of appropriate guilt. **Socialized** types have group loyalties—often, however, at the expense of outsiders. Those with **aggressive** conduct disorders engage in repetitive antisocial violence; **nonaggressive** types avoid such acts but may violate familial and social norms by repeated lying, running away, truancy, or substance abuse. Adolescents with conduct disorders tend to have higher-than-expected incidences of medical pathology and psychotic illness at follow-up. Treating medical, neurologic, and psychiatric conditions may improve the patient's self-esteem and -control. Moralizing or dire admonitions are ineffective and should be avoided. Often, only separation from a damaging environment and external discipline offer hope of success.

Attention Deficit Disorder (see under LEARNING DISORDERS in Ch. 188)

Conversion and Somatization Disorders

These disorders are discussed in Ch. 140 and PSYCHOSOMATIC MEDICINE in Ch. 135. However, they deserve mention here because they often begin at early adolescence, often occur together, are underdiagnosed, and may be inadvertently reinforced by vigorous medical intervention. **Conversion disorder** occurs when unacceptable psychic conflict is expressed as a somatic symptom, often as a neurologic disease. Incidence in children is equal in both sexes but more common in girls by midadolescence. The diagnosis in **somatization disorder** requires a multitude of symptoms in patients—nearly all female—who make illness a way of life. Both conditions occur more frequently where parents and other family members are symptomatic, providing models for a youth's symptomatology. Each disorder may afford both "primary gain" (by keeping the basic conflict unconscious) and "secondary gain" (by avoiding an undesired situation or by affording extra attraction). Although once synonymous with hysteria, both conditions actually occur in a wide range of psychopathology: depression, particularly, but schizophrenia, retardation, and many personality disorders as well.

When these disorders are suspected, the physician should avoid extensive laboratory evaluations, which indicate diagnostic uncertainty and may tend to be interpreted by the patient as confirmation of a physical problem. A psychiatric examination often will be unacceptable, since it threatens the patient's symptomatic solution. However, relatively short visits, with reassurance and inquiries into nonmedical areas, may gradually wean the patient away from the condition. Reassurance and support of family members help to minimize somatic symptoms as the "ticket" for continued medical attention.

SUICIDE IN CHILDREN AND ADOLESCENTS

(See also Ch. 144)

Suicide has increased in childhood, at least in boys, and has particularly increased in adolescents (the 3rd leading cause of adolescent death). In the 15- to 24-yr age group

male suicide has increased 50% since 1970; female suicide, only slightly. For all adolescents 15 to 24 yr, the 1981 suicide rates were 12.3/100,000 (the male:female ratio was 4:1). Suicide rates for all children between ages 5 and 14 were 0.5/100,000 in 1981. These rates represent minimum incidence figures because official designation of a death as suicide requires proof of intention.

Identifying the suicidal patient: Suicidal incidents often are preceded by medical visits, when recent changes in behavior may be revealed (eg, despondent mood, low self-esteem, sleep and appetite disturbances, inability to concentrate, truancy from school, somatic complaints, and suicidal preoccupation). Statements such as "I wish I had never been born" or "I'd like to go to sleep and never wake up" should be taken seriously as possible indications of suicidal intent. Directly questioning pediatric patients about suicide diminishes the risk. **Predisposing factors** include a history of suicide in family members or close friends; deaths in the family; alcoholism; and conduct disorders (see above under ADOLESCENT PSYCHIATRIC CONDITIONS), because of the associated potential for action. **Precipitating factors** often are **losses**: eg, of self-esteem, as in family arguments, a humiliating disciplinary episode, pregnancy, or school failure; of a boy- or girlfriend; of familiar surroundings (school, neighborhood, friends) due to a geographical move. Other factors may be a lack of structure and boundaries, leading to an overwhelming feeling of lack of direction, or the intense pressure to succeed in certain families, and the belief by the child or adolescent that he is falling short of expectations. A frequent motive for a suicide attempt is the effort to manipulate or punish others with the fantasy "You'll be sorry after I'm dead." Publicity around dramatic suicides often is followed by similar episodes. A rise in suicides among self-identified populations (eg, a single high school, a college dormitory) also indicates the importance of suggestion. Fortunately these trends usually are self-limiting.

Responding to suicidal behavior: *A suicidal threat or attempt represents an important communication about the intensity of experienced despair.*

When somatic complaints bring a child or adolescent to the physician's office, early recognition of the risk factors mentioned above may help prevent a suicide attempt. In responding to these early cues, or when confronted with threatened or attempted suicide, a vigorous intervention is appropriate and patients should be directly questioned about their unhappy or self-destructive feelings. The physician should not provide reassurance without full understanding of the circumstances, since to do so can undermine his credibility.

Every suicide attempt is a medical emergency. Once the immediate threat to life has been removed, a decision must be made on the necessity for hospitalization. This rests on weighing the balance between the degree of risk and the family's capacity to provide support. Lethality of intent can be assessed by the degree of forethought, the suicidal method, and the circumstances. A negative or unsupportive parental response is ominous. If the family response shows love and concern, a positive outcome is possible. Hospitalization is the surest form of protection and usually is indicated if severe depression and/or psychosis is suspected. Psychiatric referral is most successful if continuity with the primary caretaker is assured. Essential in the follow-up treatment process is the rebuilding of morale and the restoration of emotional equilibrium within the family.

---

202. PHYSICAL CONDITIONS IN ADOLESCENCE

The most common health problems of adolescence relate to growth and development, appearance, increased socialization, and certain metabolic and infectious disor-

ders that are prevalent during this time. Periodic medical evaluations are important to document and evaluate growth and development and maintain a favorable doctor–patient relationship. For immunization procedures in adolescents, see Ch. 182.

Accidents are the leading cause of death during adolescence, and many such fatalities are due to motor vehicle mishaps. Nonfatal accidents, such as burns (see in Ch. 254) and multiple fractures, are responsible for many teenage hospitalizations. A detailed, comprehensive history should be obtained if an accident occurs, because premorbid behavioral problems are common in adolescents who experience serious injuries. Any teenager with a significant history of behavioral problems, such as running away, depression, or truancy, requires further psychologic evaluation (see ADOLESCENT PSYCHIATRIC CONDITIONS, above).

DEVELOPMENTAL CONDITIONS

NORMAL GROWTH AND DEVELOPMENT

Adolescent physical growth includes both somatic and sexual maturation. The age of onset and rapidity of development vary with each individual and are influenced by genetic and environmental factors. Girls begin maturation and complete their growth about 2 yr before boys. Maturity begins at an earlier age today than a century ago, probably because of improvements in nutrition, general health, and living conditions. For example, the age at menarche in the USA has decreased 3 to 4 mo/decade during that time.

Somatic growth of both males and females includes attainment of adult height and weight, musculoskeletal growth, and increased size of all organs, except the lymphatics, which decrease in size, and the brain, which plateaus during adolescence. The growth spurt in boys occurs between ages 13 and 15½ yr; a gain of 4 in. can be expected in the year of peak velocity. For girls, the growth spurt begins at about age 12 yr, may reach 3½ in. in the year of peak velocity, and is almost completed by 13½ yr. In general, boys are heavier and taller than girls because they have a longer growth period. At age 18, growth is 99% complete; about 2 cm of growth remain for boys, slightly less for girls. One adolescent may develop early, another late, but both may reach the same height. Factors that control bone age progression also exert a considerable influence over menarche and, to a lesser extent, over pubic hair development.

Once **sexual changes** begin, they proceed in an established sequence in both boys and girls. **In the male**, sexual changes begin with growth of the scrotum and the testes, followed by the appearance of pubic hair and growth of the seminal vesicles and the prostate. The height spurt usually begins a year after the testes start growing. Axillary and facial hair appear about 2 yr after pubic hair. The median age for first ejaculation (between 12½ and 14 yr in the USA) is affected by psychologic and cultural, as well as biologic, factors. First ejaculation takes place about 1 yr after the accelerated penis growth. Mature spermatozoa appear between ages 14 and 16 yr, but maximum fertility is not reached until the late teens or early 20s. Uni- or bilateral gynecomastia is common in teenage boys and usually resolves within 1 yr.

In the female, sexual changes chronologically are bony pelvis growth; breast development; uterine, vaginal, labial, and clitoral growth; secondary sexual hair appearance; and menarche. Menarche occurs about 2 to 2½ yr after breast development begins and when deceleration of the height spurt is greatest; the onset of menstruation is met with varying degrees of joy, shame, disgust, and fear. The stages of breast growth and pubic hair development can be detailed using Tanner's criteria (see in AMENORRHEA in Ch. 170). If the order of sexual changes is disturbed, growth is abnormal and the physician should suspect pathologic reasons.

See below for discussions of delayed sexual maturation and precocious puberty

IDIOPATHIC SCOLIOSIS

A structural lateral curvature of the spine. Sixty to 80% of cases occur in girls. Scoliosis may first be suspected when one of the teenager's shoulders is noticed to be higher than the other or when clothes do not hang straight. An initial complaint may be fatigue in the lumbar region after sitting or standing for a long period. This may be followed by muscular backaches in areas of strain, such as the lumbosacral angle. Pain, a late manifestation, may become more persistent as irritation of the ligaments increases. New estimates indicate that of the 4% of children age 10 to 14 yr who have a detectable variation from normal spinal alignment, ½ will necessitate treatment or continuing medical observation; ½ can be screened in school for progression.

The teenager should bend forward for examination, because the spinal curve is more pronounced in that position. Most curves are convex to the right in the thoracic area and to the left in the lumbar area, so that the right shoulder is higher than the left. One hip may be more prominent than the other. X-ray examination should include anteroposterior and lateral views of the spine with the patient standing.

The prognosis depends on the site and severity of the curve and the age of onset of symptoms. The type of curve is related to the complications. The greater the curve, the greater the likelihood of progression after skeletal maturity. Prompt referral to an orthopedist is indicated, so that the means of preventing further deformity (a cast or Milwaukee brace) or correcting the deformity (surgery or electrospinal stimulation) can be instituted. Scoliosis and its treatment threaten the teenager's self-image. Wearing a brace or a cast can cause concern about being different from peers, and hospitalization and surgery challenge the youngster's independence, but the alternative is a significant deformity. Counseling and support are the major components of the family doctor's care of teenagers with scoliosis.

SLIPPED FEMORAL EPIPHYSIS

Etiology is not known, but may be related to the effects of growth hormone and estrogen on the thickness of the epiphyseal plate. The disorder is often seen in overweight teenagers. The onset is usually insidious, and symptoms are associated with the stage of slippage. Initially there may be hip stiffness that improves with rest. This is followed by a limp, and then by hip pain that radiates down the anteromedial thigh to the knee. Examination of the hip in the early stages may reveal no pain or limitation of movement. In more advanced stages, there may be pain on motion of the affected hip, with limited flexion, abduction, and medial rotation; knee pain, without specific knee findings; and a limp. The affected leg is externally rotated. If the blood supply to the area is compromised, avascular necrosis and collapse of the epiphysis may occur.

Early diagnosis is vital, as treatment becomes more difficult in the more advanced stages. Anteroposterior and lateral x-rays of both hips should be obtained. X-rays of the affected hip show widening of the epiphyseal line or displacement posteriorly and inferiorly of the femoral head. Orthopedic referral is important to confirm the diagnosis and evaluate the need for corrective surgery. Surgical treatment requires immobility, which limits the adolescent's independence.

OSGOOD-SCHLATTER DISEASE

(See in The Osteochondroses in Ch. 197)

DELAYED SEXUAL MATURATION

(See also Pituitary Dwarfism in Ch. 196)

Delayed sexual maturation is present in boys if there is no testicular enlargement by age 13½ or if there are > 5 yr between the initial and complete growth of the genitalia.

For girls, no breast development by age 13 or a period of > 5 yr between the beginning of breast growth and menarche indicates delayed sexual maturation. Short stature signals delayed maturation in both boys and girls.

The major causes of delayed puberty are (1) **Constitutional delay**, occurring in the teenager whose family has a history of late growth. The youngster's prepubertal growth rate is normal and his skeletal growth and adolescent growth spurt are delayed. He experiences late, but normal, sexual maturation. (2) **Genetic disorders**, including Turner's syndrome (gonadal dysgenesis) in the female and Klinefelter's syndrome (primary testicular dysfunction) in the male. (3) **CNS conditions**, such as a destructive tumor of the pituitary, which results in decreased gonadotropin secretion. (4) **Chronic illnesses**, such as diabetes mellitus, chronic renal disease, and cystic fibrosis.

PRECOCIOUS PUBERTY

The onset of sexual maturation before age 8 in a girl and age 10 in a boy.

True precocious puberty is activation of the hypothalamic-pituitary axis with consequent enlargement and maturation of the gonads, and the development of secondary sexual characteristics, adult serum gonadal steroid levels, and spermatogenesis or oogenesis. In **pseudoprecocious puberty,** by contrast, secondary sexual characteristics develop because of high circulating levels of androgens or estrogens, usually secreted from a gonadal or adrenal tumor, but the gonads remain immature and spermatogenesis or oogenesis does not occur. Other causes of pseudoprecocious puberty are HCG-secreting tumors, such as hepatoblastomas and rare pineal tumors.

The incidence of true precocious puberty is 2 to 5 times greater in females, and about 80% of female cases have no identifiable abnormality. In contrast, 60% of male cases have underlying organic disease. Organic causes in either sex include lesions of the hypothalamus (hamartomas, rarely craniopharyngiomas), intracranial tumors (pinealomas), and a few rare diseases.

In a recently recognized syndrome, a small group of boys has been identified with apparently autonomous, **gonadotropin-independent, Leydig-cell function**. In this syndrome, both gametogenesis and steroidogenesis are stimulated in the absence of any increase in gonadotropin secretion.

Precocious pubarche refers to the appearance of pubic hair alone prior to age 8 in a girl and age 10 in a boy; **precocious adrenarche** refers to the appearance of axillary and pubic hair alone prior to age 8 in a girl and age 10 in a boy; and **precocious thelarche** refers to the onset of breast development prior to age 8 in a girl. These conditions may herald the onset of precocious puberty, but precocious pubarche and thelarche may occur independently of any further development. When these latter 2 conditions do occur alone and there is no pubertal progression, they are generally benign. Careful follow-up of affected children is warranted.

Symptoms, Signs, and Diagnostic Evaluation

In both true and pseudoprecocious puberty, boys exhibit facial, axillary, and pubic hair; penile growth; and increased masculinity. Girls develop breasts and pubic and axillary hair. In true precocious puberty, girls also begin to menstruate. Linear growth is initially rapid in both sexes, but the adult height is shortened by premature closure of the epiphyses. Testicular or ovarian enlargement, which occurs in true precocious puberty, is absent in pseudoprecocious puberty.

Laboratory evaluation should include bone age, skull x-rays, and serum testosterone, dehydroepiandrosterone sulfate, 17-hydroxyprogesterone, estrogen, luteinizing hormone **(LH),** follicle-stimulating hormone **(FSH),** and prolactin levels. CT scanning of the brain is indicated in all children with true precocious puberty. Gonadotropin-independent precocious puberty can be documented by establishing prepubertal gona-

dotropin responses to exogenous gonadotropin-releasing hormone **(GnRH)** in boys with no neoplasm or other obvious cause for early development.

Treatment

A GnRH agonist, an analog of luteinizing hormone-releasing hormone **(LHRH)**—such as His6, Pro9, NEt, or D-Trp6-Pro9-Net-LHRH at a dose of 4 to 8 μg/kg s.c. daily, or 6 D Ser-(TBU)-GnRH (1–9) ethylamide 400 to 800 μg/day in 2 to 4 divided intranasal doses—can be given until the time of normal puberty and will desensitize the pituitary gland for secretion of LH and FSH, thereby halting precocious puberty. Treatment has been successful in all cases of true precocious puberty in boys and girls.

For gonadotropin-independent precocious puberty, androgen antagonists (eg, spironolactone 1.5 mg/kg/day in 3 divided oral doses or cyproterone acetate 75 to 100 mg/sq m in 3 divided oral doses) ameliorate the effects of the excess androgen.

TEENAGE PREGNANCY AND CONTRACEPTION

In 1982, 523,531 infants were born to teenagers in the USA (an estimated 14% of all births). Of these, 51% were born out of wedlock. Approximately 9773 babies were born to mothers under age 15. About 433,900 abortions were performed on teenagers in 1978. The divorce rate for teenage marriages is 50% within 2 yr, 80% by 5 yr. Many teenage mothers have histories of school failure and psychologic problems and are likely to have repeated pregnancies.

Prenatal management should include rigorous medical and psychosocial care, while planning with the adolescent about her future. Teenagers who are pregnant, particularly the very young, may have a higher incidence of anemia and toxemia than do women in their 20s; but, if they receive prepartum care, they should not experience greater obstetric morbidity than adult women of similar background. Infants of young mothers have an increased incidence of prematurity, respiratory distress syndrome, and low birth weight (especially with mothers under age 15).

Teenagers are in a developmental transition, and pregnancy or marriage usually adds emotional strains. Pregnant girls and their partners tend to drop out of school or vocational training, thus increasing their economic problems, loss of self-esteem, and strained interpersonal relationships. Easy access to abortion does not remove the psychologic problems of the unwanted pregnancy for the girl or the boy. Emotional crises occur when pregnancy is diagnosed, when the decision to have an abortion is made, during the postabortal period (similar to the postpartum period of depression), the date when the baby would have been born, and on anniversaries of that date. Follow-up care is imperative and should include family counseling and psychosocial planning for both the boy and the girl and contraceptive education and treatment.

Despite sexual activity, many adolescents are ignorant of anatomic details and of how they may become pregnant. Non-pregnant, sexually active adolescents who seek information regarding pregnancy should be counseled and given contraceptives, if indicated.

The medical issues of contraception (see Ch. 174) are similar during adolescence and adulthood, but are more complicated in teenagers because of their potentially lesser knowledge and experience and their developmental stresses. Areas of concern include irregularity in pill taking (adolescents often fail to take medication regularly); the romantic wish to think of intercourse as unplanned and spontaneous, which complicates the use of contraceptives; the tendency for "accidents" to occur; concerns about the pill, often because of misinformation acquired from others; and limited options for birth control methods, since the diaphragm, in particular, requires preplanning and must be in place prior to intercourse in order to be effective. Despite these difficulties, even young teenagers can effectively manage contraceptive technics with adequate professional guidance.

EATING DISORDERS

ANOREXIA NERVOSA AND BULIMIA

Disorders characterized by a disturbed sense of body image and morbid fear of obesity, manifested by abnormal patterns of handling food, self-induced marked weight loss, and amenorrhea in women. Females are affected predominantly; about 5 to 10% of cases are male. Onset is usually in adolescence, occasionally prepubertal, and much less commonly in adulthood. A high percentage of patients are reported to be found in middle and upper socioeconomic families. The incidence is increasing in Western society.

Anorexia nervosa may be mild, but can be severe and life-threatening; mortality rates have often been reported between 2 to 5% and, in some follow-up studies, as high as 15 to 21%. However, since most mild cases are probably not specifically diagnosed, the true prevalence of the disorder and its mortality rate are not really known.

Etiology

The etiology is unknown, but anorexia nervosa is rare where there is a genuine shortage of food. Social factors appear to play an important role. Emphasis on the desirability of being thin pervades our society, and obesity is associated with a wide variety of undesirable traits. Recent surveys reveal that 80 to 90% of prepubertal children are aware of these attitudes and > 50% of these girls attempt diets and other measures to control their weight. Since only a small percentage develops anorexia nervosa, other factors must be important. Some are probably predisposed because of as-yet-undefined intrinsic psychologic and, possibly, genetic and metabolic vulnerability.

Symptoms and Signs

Even before the onset of illness, many patients are described as being very meticulous, compulsive, intelligent, and oriented to high achievement and success. The first specific indication of the impending disorder is a concern about obesity (even if the patient is lean—only about 30% of patients are obese at onset), and the start of restricting food intake. Preoccupation and anxiety about weight persist even as emaciation develops, and denial of the illness is a prominent feature. Patients do not complain of anorexia or weight loss, usually resist treatment, and are brought to the physician's attention by their families, by intercurrent illness, or by complaints about other symptoms; eg, bloating, abdominal distress, constipation.

Anorexia is a misnomer, as appetite remains unless the patient becomes cachexic. Patients are preoccupied with food: they study diets and calories; hoard, conceal, and waste food; collect recipes; and prepare elaborate meals for others. Binge eating **(bulimia)** followed by induced vomiting and the use of laxatives and diuretics **(binge-purge behavior)** occurs in 50% of anorectics. Amenorrhea is universal in women anorectics and often appears before appreciable weight loss. In men and women, there is usually a loss of interest in sex. Other common findings include bradycardia, low BP, hypothermia, the development of lanugo hair or frank hirsutism, and edema. Parotitis is common, and together with dental erosion (as a result of induced vomiting) is a useful physical sign in patients who are also bulimic. Remarkably, even patients who appear cachexic tend to remain very active (including pursuing vigorous exercise programs) and free of symptoms of nutritional deficiencies or unusual susceptibility to infections. Depression is commonly present, and patients tend to be very manipulative. They often lie about food intake and conceal behavior such as induced vomiting.

Many endocrine changes have been reported, including pre- or early pubertal patterns of luteinizing hormone secretion and low levels of thyroxine and triiodothyronine. Dysfunction may be found in virtually every major organ system in the severely malnourished patient, but the most dangerous are cardiac and fluid and electrolyte

disorders. There is decreased cardiac muscle mass, chamber size, and output. Dehydration, metabolic acidosis, and low serum K may be present; all are aggravated when the patient induces vomiting and uses laxatives and/or diuretics. Sudden death is not rare, most likely due to ventricular tachyarrhythmias. Some patients have been found to have prolonged Q-T intervals (corrected for heart rate), which, in addition to the risks imposed by hypokalemia, may predispose to such arrhythmias.

Bulimia is now considered a separate disorder (which may coexist with anorexia nervosa); and a malignant form, **bulimia nervosa,** is now recognized as a discrete diagnostic entity in the new Diagnostic and Statistical Manual III-R of the American Psychiatric Association. It is characterized by recurrent episodes of binge eating during which the patient experiences a feeling of loss of control over eating and regularly engages in either self-induced vomiting, use of laxatives and/or diuretics, or rigorous dieting or fasting to overcome the effects of the binges. A frequency of 2 binge-eating episodes a week for at least 3 mo is required for the DSM III-R diagnosis. Typically, a binge involves rapid consumption of food (especially of high caloric value); ≥ 15,000 calories may be eaten in a few hours. Binges tend to be episodic, are often triggered by psychosocial stress, and may occur as often as several times a day; they are carried out in secret. Although bulimic patients are anxious about becoming obese, unlike patients with overt anorexia nervosa, they tend not to become emaciated. They may even become obese, but more often tend to fluctuate 10 to 15% below or above ideal body weight.

Binge eating can cause acute gastric dilatation and even rupture. Induced vomiting is associated with erosion of dental enamel, parotitis, esophagitis, and esophageal rupture. Aspiration pneumonia occurs when induced vomiting is associated with reduced consciousness (during drug or alcohol use). Hypokalemia can result from vomiting and purging, and death has been reported from abuse of ipecac taken to induce vomiting.

People with bulimia tend to be more aware of and remorseful or guilty about their behavior than those with anorexia and are more likely to admit their concerns when questioned by a sympathetic physician. They appear to be less introverted than patients with anorexia nervosa and more prone to impulsive behavior and overt depression.

Diagnosis

Anorexia nervosa usually is apparent from the constellation of symptoms described above, particularly the association of loss of ≥ 25% of body weight in a young person who fears obesity, becomes amenorrheic, denies illness, and otherwise appears well. The key to diagnosis is eliciting the central fear of obesity, which is not diminished by weight loss. In severe cases, marked depression or symptoms suggesting another disorder such as schizophrenia may require differentiation or may be additional diagnostic entities.

Bulimia may be suspected in patients expressing marked concern about weight gain and manifesting wide fluctuations in weight, especially if there is evidence of excessive use of laxatives or unexplained hypokalemia. Suspicion is also aroused by swollen parotid glands, scars on the knuckles of the hand (from induced vomiting), and dental erosion. However, the diagnosis depends on the patient's description of binge or binge-purge behavior.

Treatment

Treatment of **anorexia nervosa** can be divided into 2 distinct phases—short-term intervention to restore body weight and save life, and long-term therapy to ameliorate longstanding personality and family problems.

When weight loss has been severe or rapid, or when weight has fallen below some arbitrary level (eg, 80% of ideal), prompt restoration of weight becomes the overriding

consideration, and hospitalization is imperative. When in doubt, hospitalize. Simply removing the patient from her home sometimes reverses a downhill course, but more energetic psychiatric treatment is often required. Tube feeding or parenteral alimentation is sometimes necessary, and patients who are depressed may benefit from antidepressant medication.

Once the patient's nutritional and water and electrolyte status has stabilized, there begins a difficult treatment, complicated by the patient's abhorrence of weight gain, denial of illness, and manipulative behavior. The physician should attempt to provide a calm, concerned, stable relationship, while encouraging a reasonable caloric intake. Combined management by a family doctor and psychiatrist may be useful. Family therapy is often helpful, as is individual psychotherapy—behavioral, cognitive, and psychodynamic.

Approaches to the treatment of **bulimia** and **bulimia nervosa** are relatively new, and there is no current consensus as to which is the most effective. More severe cases have generally been treated by psychiatrists with antidepressant medication and less severe cases by psychologists with behavior therapy. Each approach has achieved successes and, unfortunately, all-too-frequent failures. As with anorexia nervosa, consultation with a specialist in the disorder can be helpful.

OBESITY

(See also Ch. 83)

Arbitrarily, body weight 20% over standard height-weight tables. **Morbid obesity**: *> 100% overweight.*

Obesity in adolescence is as difficult and discouraging to treat as at any other age, and is one of the most common presenting complaints in adolescent clinics in the USA. Primary endocrine or metabolic disorders are uncommon, but some of the secondary medical problems seen in overweight adults may be evident; eg, hypertension, and knee and back problems. Not infrequently, a mildly obese adolescent rapidly gains weight during the teenage years and becomes significantly obese. Untreated, the likelihood of continuing obesity throughout adulthood is markedly increased. The obese adolescent is likely to have a poor self-image, and to become more sedentary and socially isolated. Parents often are overprotective and may subtly encourage overeating behavior.

Treatment approaches are numerous but success rates are low. School is an appropriate place for specialized education in nutrition and physical activity; however, there are few programs designed for overweight adolescents. Presently available drugs should be avoided because they are not helpful in the long run. Surgical approaches such as operations to reduce stomach size may be used in morbid obesity. Behavioral approaches are best because they encourage the factors essential to long-term success: reduction and control of caloric intake with well-balanced choices of ordinary foods, permanent changes in eating habits, and increased physical activity (walking, hiking, swimming, and dancing are excellent).

INFECTIOUS MONONUCLEOSIS

An acute disease characterized clinically by high fever, sore throat, and generalized lymphadenopathy; pathologically by diffuse hyperplasia of lymphatic tissue; hematologically by an increase in lymphocytes, many of which are atypical; and serologically by development of transient heterophil antibodies to sheep, horse, and beef erythrocytes, and of persistent antibodies to the Epstein-Barr virus.

Etiology

Infectious mononucleosis is caused by the Epstein-Barr virus **(EBV)**, a member of the herpes group. The disease occurs only in persons who previously had no antibodies to

the virus. EBV-specific antibodies emerge during the late incubation period, reach peak titers in the acute phase, and then decline to lower levels where they persist indefinitely and serve as reliable indicators of immunity to the disease. The virus is regularly present in oropharyngeal secretions during the acute phase and often also the convalescent phase, and intermittently thereafter for life. EBV is detected by its ability to transform cord-blood lymphocytes in vitro into continuously growing lymphoblasts that harbor EB viral DNA and express the EBV-determined nuclear antigen **(EBNA)**. The transforming activity is a biologic property of the virus and restricted to B-lymphocytes. Permanently growing, EBV-genome-carrying B-lymphoblast cultures can be established regularly also from peripheral blood lymphocytes of patients with infectious mononucleosis. There is evidence now that EBV can replicate in some epithelial cells of the oro- and nasopharynx. As with other herpesviruses, a persistent EBV carrier state uniformly follows primary EBV infections. This is evident from the lifelong maintenance of EBV-specific antibodies, the establishment of continuous, EBNA-positive lymphoblast cultures from peripheral leukocytes or lymph nodes of seropositive (but not seronegative) donors; and intermittent oropharyngeal excretion of the virus.

Epidemiology

Despite the regular oropharyngeal shedding of EBV, infectious mononucleosis is not very contagious. The annual incidence among susceptible college students of ≤ 15% is not increased in roommates of patients. The disease is mainly transmitted by healthy viral carriers through close salivary contact. Under conditions of poor hygiene or crowding, most primary EBV infections occur in early childhood and remain silent or are too mild to be specifically diagnosed. In affluent population segments, primary exposure to EBV is often delayed until adolescence or later, when it leads in about 50% of individuals to typical infectious mononucleosis. Characteristic cases are observed occasionally, however, in infants and children < 2 yr if one searches for them. They occur also in adults well > 40 yr, when failure to include infectious mononucleosis in the differential diagnosis can lead to unnecessary invasive diagnostic procedures; eg, bone marrow aspiration or lymph node biopsy.

The EBV-transformed B-lymphocytes have a permanent growth potential (one of the attributes of malignant cells) but are controlled by cellular immune defenses in immunocompetent persons. When this control does not develop or is abolished in severely immunocompromised patients, unrestrained polyclonal proliferation of EBV-transformed, EBNA-positive B-lymphocytes occurs. This has been observed in genetic immunodeficiencies (eg, ataxia-telangiectasia); in renal, cardiac, or marrow allograft recipients; and in patients with AIDS. EBV is intimately associated with > 95% of the cases of endemic African Burkitt's lymphoma (see also BURKITT'S LYMPHOMA in Ch. 102), a monoclonal B-cell tumor with a characteristic translocation between chromosomes 8 and 14, or less frequently between 8 and 2 or 22. With this translocation, the MYC oncogene is moved from chromosome 8 to the vicinity of immunoglobulin gene regions of chromosome 14, 2 or 22 and derepressed. The tumor cells contain EB viral DNA and express EBNA. Of sporadic cases of Burkitt's lymphoma in the USA and Europe, < 20% are EBV-associated. EB viral DNA is regularly present also in undifferentiated nasopharyngeal carcinoma and the carcinoma cells are EBNA-positive. This tumor has its highest incidence among Southern Chinese but occurs at low frequency everywhere. Like Burkitt's lymphoma, nasopharyngeal carcinoma is a monoclonal tumor, which denotes that EBV genomes were present in the very first malignantly transformed cell. It is certain, however, that development of these 2 tumors requires additional, but as yet, unidentified factors.

Symptoms, Signs, and Complications

After a 4- to 7-wk incubation period, vague grippe-like malaise, fatigue, headache, and chilliness develop, typically followed by high fever, sore throat, and generalized

lymphadenopathy. Symptoms and signs may be confusing, since almost any organ may be affected. EBV does not replicate in cells of the affected organs; rather, EBV-transformed B-lymphocytes become widely disseminated and proliferate until attacked by activated T-lymphocytes. This interaction or products (lymphokines?) released by it are thought to be responsible for most of the signs and symptoms. Splenomegaly is present in 50% of the patients; rarely, the spleen may rupture spontaneously or following trauma, including overly vigorous palpation. Liver function tests are abnormal in almost all patients; hepatomegaly is noted in about 20%, jaundice in < 5%. Eyelid and orbital edema is often noted. A transient maculopapular rash is seen in about 10% of the patients and is often precipitated by ampicillin therapy. Punctate petechiae may be found on the border between the soft and hard palates. Pericarditis and myocarditis occur occasionally. Chest pain, dyspnea, and cough indicate pneumonitis. CNS involvement in the form of meningoencephalitis, Guillain-Barré syndrome, transverse myelitis, Bell's palsy, or cerebellar ataxia may emerge during or after the acute phase and may occasionally be the only clinical manifestation. Reye's syndrome has been observed in association with primary EBV infections. Renal involvement is rare and due, most likely, to antigen-antibody complexes. Hemolytic anemia, thrombocytopenic purpura, agranulocytosis, and pancytopenia are infrequent but severe complications.

The typhoidal form, characterized by minimal or no sore throat and by delayed development of hematologic and serologic changes, occurs in < 10% of the cases.

Patients usually recover fully in < 4 wk, but as many as 10% complain for many months or even several years of persistent fatigue, intermittent fever, and recurrent lymphadenopathy, at times to the extent of being unable to work. In some of these **chronic active** cases, EBV-specific antibody titers are persistently elevated or occasionally extraordinarily high; but in many the antibody titers do not differ significantly from those of patients who recover rapidly.

Diagnosis

Blood-smear examination and serologic tests are the cornerstones of diagnosis. Demonstrating EBV in oropharyngeal secretions is not diagnostic, since virus carriers also excrete the virus intermittently.

Hemogram: By the 2nd or 3rd wk, the total WBC count is usually elevated to 10,000 to 15,000 with a relative and absolute lymphocytosis. Soon after onset, a transient increase in B cells occurs, followed by a transient increase in T cells. Both B and T cells contribute to an increase (> 10%) in the number of atypical lymphocytes, which frequently show cytoplasmic vacuolation; oval, kidney-shaped, or slightly lobulated nuclei; and great cell-to-cell variation in size and staining characteristics. An increased number of atypical lymphocytes is also found in cytomegalovirus infections, viral hepatitis, measles, rubella, and serum sickness.

Heterophil antibody test: Agglutinins for sheep and horse RBCs arise in infectious mononucleosis and are absorbed by beef RBCs but not by guinea pig kidney suspension (Forssman antigen). Beef RBCs are lyzed in the presence of complement. Rapid slide agglutination test kits with all reagents are available commercially. The following guidelines are helpful: (1) A positive slide reaction with a serum from an acutely ill patient whose blood smears show numerous atypical lymphocytes justifies a diagnosis of infectious mononucleosis; an antibody titer is not needed, since it reflects neither severity nor prognosis of the illness. (2) If the reaction is positive but the blood smears do not indicate infectious mononucleosis, the serum should be titrated in the differential absorption tube test with sheep RBCs **(Paul-Bunnell-Davidsohn test)** or, preferably, with more sensitive horse RBCs **(Lee-Davidsohn test).** If the beef cell absorbed titer equals or exceeds the guinea pig kidney absorbed titer, the slide test was falsely positive. If the pattern specific for infectious mononucleosis is noted (the guinea pig kidney

absorbed titer exceeds the beef cell absorbed titer), the patient should be asked whether he experienced an infectious-mononucleosis-like illness within the past 18 mo, because heterophil antibodies may remain detectable for many months at gradually declining titers. In such cases, EBV-specific serologic tests should be performed. (3) If the rapid test is negative but the blood smears are clearly compatible with infectious mononucleosis, the serum should be titrated by the differential absorption tube test, to determine whether the patient has a heterophil antibody titer too low (≤1:112) to register in the slide test, or whether heterophil antibodies are truly absent. A 2nd serum specimen should be examined after 7 to 10 days, to exclude a delayed heterophil antibody response. In such cases, EBV-specific and other serodiagnostic tests differentiate between heterophil negative infectious mononucleosis that is caused by EBV and infectious-mononucleosis-like illnesses induced by other agents (see Differential Diagnosis).

In adolescents and adults, heterophil antibodies are usually detectable within the first 2 wk of illness, but may occasionally arise later. They generally disappear 3 to 6 mo after onset; at times they persist longer. Heterophil antibody tests are consistently negative in < 10% of adult patients and in a somewhat greater percentage of infants and children. Because heterophil antibody titers are generally lower in early childhood than at an older age, false-negative slide agglutination tests are encountered more frequently in children than in adolescents and adult patients.

The heterophil antibodies are of the IgM class. Other (mostly IgM) antibodies may arise transiently in infectious mononucleosis; ie, potentially hemolytic cold agglutinins specific for red cell antigen i, rheumatoid factor, antinuclear antibodies, smooth muscle antibodies, Wassermann reagin and others. Total serum IgM levels may increase, therefore, by as much as 100% (IgG levels by 50%). Why primary EBV infections evoke these heterophil antibody responses is unknown.

Liver function tests should be performed, since hepatic involvement is common. Most indicative are tests for elevated alkaline phosphatase, SGPT (ALT), and SGOT (AST).

EBV-specific serodiagnostic tests are needed for accurate diagnosis when characteristic clinical, hematologic, or heterophil antibody responses fail to develop in a patient clinically suspected of having infectious mononucleosis or when unusual clinical manifestations are observed. They are based at present on titration of sera by immunofluorescence technics and use of cell smears prepared from selected EBV-transformed lymphoblast cultures that intrinsically (or after certain manipulations) express EBV-encoded antigens in some or all of the cells.

The key antigens are the EB viral capsid antigens **(VCA)**, the diffuse **(D)** and restricted **(R)** antigens of the EBV-induced early antigen **(EA)** complex, and the EBV-associated nuclear antigen **(EBNA)**. Antibodies to VCA, D, and R are titrated by indirect immunofluorescence, which permits determination of the immunoglobulin class of the antibodies by using fluorescein-labeled heavy-chain-specific antibodies. Antibodies to EBNA are measurable only by the highly sensitive anticomplement immunofluorescence technic. Applying this set of tests to a single serum specimen permits differentiation between current, recent, past, or, when negative, no preceding EBV infection.

A **current primary EBV infection** is characterized by high titers of IgM and IgG antibodies to VCA, transient antibodies to D in about 80% of cases, and, as yet, no antibodies to EBNA (these antibodies arise 3 wk to 3 mo after onset of illness). A **recent primary EBV infection** is identified by low or no longer detectable levels of IgM antibodies but high titers of IgG antibodies to VCA and no, or as yet barely detectable, titers of antibodies to EBNA. Absence of antibodies to EBNA is observed in certain immunodeficiencies and therefore does not always reflect a recent primary EBV infection. Antibodies to D may still be detectable or may have been replaced by

low transient titers of antibodies to R. After a **long-past primary EBV infection,** usually only moderate titers of IgG antibodies to VCA and EBNA are found. Antibodies to R, rarely to D, may be detected if the antibody titers to VCA are on the high side. This pattern may be noted in many cases of chronic infectious mononucleosis, but in a rare case extraordinarily high IgG antibody titers to VCA and D may persist for years. Immunosuppressive conditions may upset the equilibrium between EBV and host defenses and activate the persistent infection with increases in IgG antibody titers to VCA and D or R, but IgM antibodies to VCA do not reemerge. For **EBV-associated Burkitt's lymphoma,** high antibody titers to VCA and R are characteristic; and for **undifferentiated nasopharyngeal carcinoma,** both IgG and IgA antibody titers to VCA and to D.

Examining CSF in cases with CNS complication is unnecessary because EBV does not replicate in nervous tissue and thus does not evoke a local antibody response.

Differential Diagnosis

Infectious mononucleosis must be differentiated from other acute infections associated with fever, sore throat, and lymphadenopathy due to bacteria (streptococcus, diphtheria, Vincent's angina), other viruses (cytomegalovirus, rubella, adenoviruses, hepatitis A and B), and other agents (*Toxoplasma gondii*). Cytomegalovirus **(CMV)** causes a mononucleosis-like disease, but patients are usually adults; moreover, while splenomegaly, hepatomegaly, and atypical lymphocytes are commonly present, sore throat and cervical lymphadenopathy are usually absent, and heterophil antibody responses are always absent. The post-perfusion syndrome following open-heart surgery is usually caused by CMV (see CYTOMEGALOVIRUS INFECTION, under HERPES VIRUSES in Ch. 12), only rarely by EBV. In cases with CNS involvement, various other causative agents must be considered. On occasion, lymphoproliferative disorders (leukemia, Hodgkin's disease, lymphomas) must also be excluded, but their differentiation from infectious mononucleosis by EBV-specific serology is at times difficult because these diseases or their therapies have immunosuppressive effects with consequent activation of the persistent EBV infection. An acute syndrome in patients infected with the virus that causes acquired immunodeficiency syndrome **(AIDS)** may resemble infectious mononucleosis (see Ch. 19).

Prognosis

Infectious mononucleosis usually spends itself in 1 to 4 wk, but may linger for many months or years. Sequelae are unusual and the ultimate outlook is excellent. Rarely, death may follow splenic rupture, airway obstruction, acute pericarditis or myocarditis, CNS complications, agranulocytosis, or pancytopenia. In the severely immunosuppressed patient a primary EBV infection or activation of the persistent infection may lead to fatal, polyclonal B-cell proliferation.

Treatment

Therapy is usually symptomatic. Bed rest should be enforced during the acute phase of fever and malaise and prolonged in cases with hepatic involvement. Strenuous exercise must be avoided while the spleen is enlarged. Acetaminophen, rather than aspirin, should be used to control headache because of the rare association of EBV with Reye's syndrome. The analgesics and saline gargles relieve sore throat and other oropharyngeal symptoms. Antibiotics are of no value unless secondary bacterial infection is present. Corticosteroids should be given *only* to patients with severe complications such as airway obstruction, neurologic involvement, hemolytic anemia, thrombocytopenic purpura, myocarditis, or pericarditis. Rupture of the spleen requires immediate surgery and blood transfusions. Treatment by intravenous acyclovir **(ACV)** has shown a trend toward shorter duration of tonsillitis and pharyngitis and faster return to pre-illness weight as compared to untreated controls. Oral ACV is being

explored. (Acyclovir therapy is not presently recommended for uncomplicated cases.) Polyclonal proliferation of EBV-transformed B-lymphocytes in renal or cardiac allograft recipients is apparently brought to remission by the drug.

203. GENERAL PRINCIPLES OF MEDICAL GENETICS

(A glossary is provided at the end of the chapter.)

The development of an individual depends on 2 interacting influences—genetic factors and environment. The genetic composition, or **genome**, of an individual is established at conception; thereafter, a complex interaction of genes and environment (both internal and external) shapes his development. Though the genes remain largely unaltered, environmental experiences are constantly changing and may even alter the genome through **mutation**, or inheritable alteration of a gene.

Some genetic component probably exists in almost all diseases, but the extent of this component varies. For example, bacterial diseases are considered purely environmental, yet the human male is slightly more susceptible to most of them than the female. There is little doubt that genetic factors play a role here, though the precise role is not known. Conversely, diseases such as Down's syndrome (mongolism) and phenylketonuria **(PKU)** are due to specific genetic defects and the environment plays a relatively small role. Between the extremes is a host of conditions wherein genetic and environmental factors interact to produce birth defects, metabolic disorders, and other disease conditions.

The **genes**—the basic units of heredity—are molecules of DNA. The capacity of DNA to replicate itself constitutes the basis of hereditary transmission. DNA also provides the **genetic code**, which determines the development and metabolism of cells by controlling the synthesis of RNA. The sequential order of the components that make up RNA determines the amino acid composition of proteins, which in turn determines the functions of proteins and thereby the functions of cells.

The many thousands of genes are carried by the **chromosomes** (rod-like structures in the nuclei of cells). In man, each somatic or non-germ cell normally has 46 chromosomes, arranged in 23 pairs. One pair, the **sex chromosomes**, determines the sex of the individual. The female has two X chromosomes in every cell nucleus; the male has one X and one Y. The male sex chromosomes are **heterologous**, since the 2 members of the pair are not identical: the X chromosome is larger and carries genes responsible for many hereditary traits as well as for determination of sex; the Y chromosome is small, is shaped differently, and carries primarily, if not exclusively, genes concerned only with male sex determination. The remaining 22 pairs of chromosomes, the **autosomes**, are **homologous**, since both members of a pair are usually identical in size, shape, and genetic loci.

The genes are arranged along the chromosomes in linear order, and each gene has its own specific **locus**. The number and arrangement of the loci on homologous chromosomes are identical, and genes that occupy homologous loci are called **alleles**. Every individual has 2 alleles for each kind of gene, one on each chromosome of a pair. A person possessing a pair of identical alleles for a particular gene is a **homozygote**; one who possesses a dissimilar pair of alleles is a **heterozygote**. If a gene exerts its effect when it is present on only one chromosome, the gene is **dominant**. A **recessive** gene is expressed only when present in both members of a chromosome pair (or in the single X of a normal male or a 45,X female). The gene, or its corresponding trait, is **X-linked** if it is located on the X chromosome; otherwise it is **autosomal**.

Three types of genetically determined disorders are (1) **mendelian** or **single-gene mutations,** which are inherited in recognizable patterns; (2) **polygenic** or **multifactorial conditions,** in which genetic mutations involving more than one gene and nongenetic factors interact in ways that are not always clearly recognizable; and (3) **chromosomal aberrations** or **abnormalities,** which include both structural defects and deviations from the normal number.

INHERITED DISORDERS

CONSTRUCTION OF THE PEDIGREE

In man, the chief method of genetic study is the observation of family trees or **pedigrees,** which show the distribution of genetic traits in kindreds. A careful family history must be taken and a pedigree constructed in order to determine the pattern of inheritance. Some familial disorders with identical **phenotypes,** or observable features, are inherited in different patterns. For example, cleft palate may be due to an autosomal dominant, an autosomal recessive, or an X-linked recessive gene, or it may be a multifactorial condition (ie, familial, but with no precisely predictable pattern of inheritance).

FIG. 203–1 shows the symbols used in constructing a pedigree chart. As illustrated in the various pedigrees (FIGS. 203–2 to 203–5), the generations are numbered with Roman numerals, with the earliest at the top and the most recent at the bottom. Within each generation, individuals are numbered from left to right with Arabic numerals. Thus, each individual in the pedigree can be specifically identified by 2 numbers (eg, II, 4). A spouse who is included in the pedigree chart is also assigned an identifying number (eg, II, 6 in FIG. 203–2). Siblings are usually arranged in sequence by age, with the oldest on the left.

The study of a trait or a disease in a particular family begins with an affected person (the **proband, propositus,** or **index case**). When taking a family history, the pedigree must be drawn as the various relatives are being described. The inquiry begins with the siblings of the proband and proceeds to the parents; then to relatives of the parents, including brothers and sisters and their children; then to the grandparents; and so on. The number of relatives included in the pedigree is determined by the pattern of inheritance of the condition and by the extent of the informant's memory or knowledge.

SINGLE-GENE DEFECTS IN MAN

Genetic disorders determined by a single gene are the easiest to analyze and therefore have been the ones most fully studied. Single-gene defects may be autosomal or X-linked, and dominant or recessive.

AUTOSOMAL DOMINANT INHERITANCE

A typical pedigree is shown in FIG. 203–2. In general, the following rules apply: (1) Every affected person has at least one affected parent. (2) An affected person marrying a normal individual has, on the average, an equal number of affected and normal children. (3) Normal children of an affected parent have normal children and grandchildren. (4) Males and females are equally likely to be affected. (5) The trait can appear in every generation. (6) Heterozygotes are affected.

Variations in the above rules are as follows:

1. Expressivity and penetrance: The effects of a single gene may be influenced both by the individual's environment and by the thousands of other genes that may alter the

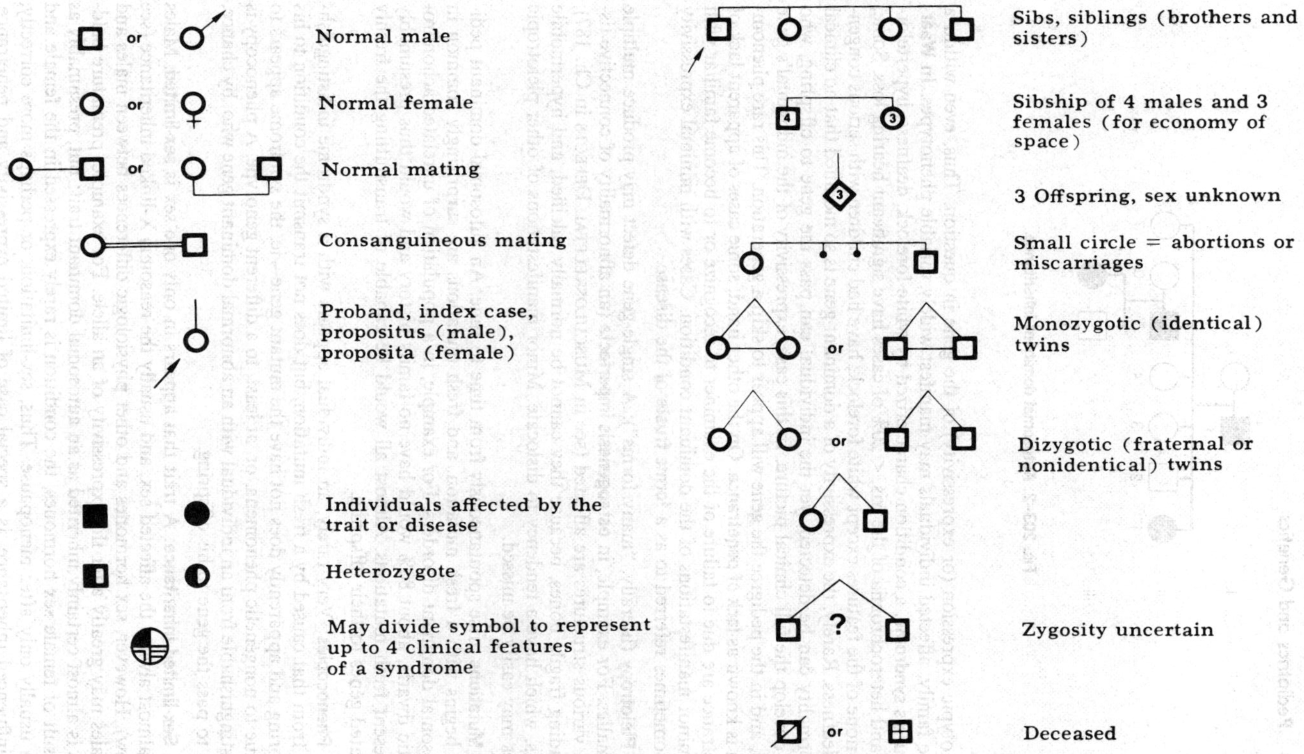

FIG. 203–1. Symbols used in constructing a pedigree chart.

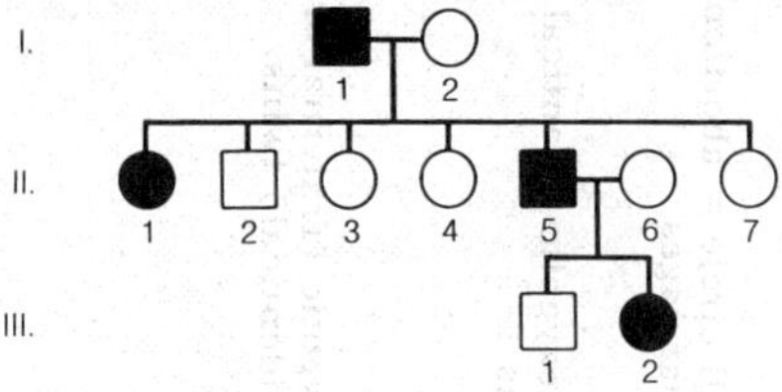

FIG. 203–2. Autosomal dominant inheritance.

phenotypic expression (or expressivity) of the gene in question. Thus, even within a single family, affected individuals may manifest widely variable phenotypes. In **Waardenburg's syndrome,** a condition characterized by white forelock, deafness, hypertelorism, and heterochromia of the iris, < 20% of cases have significant hearing loss. Some, with none of the features except white forelock, have had children with serious congenital deafness. Rarely, the expressivity of a dominant gene is so modified that no clinical abnormality can be detected, yet the individual can pass the gene to offspring, who may develop the full clinical picture. In this case, expressivity of the individual's gene is nil, and in the pedigree the gene will appear to skip a generation. This rare phenomenon is known as **lack of penetrance**. On the other hand, some cases of apparent lack of penetrance are due to failure of the examiner to recognize or to become familiar with the minor manifestations of the dominant condition. Cases with minimal expressivity are sometimes referred to as a **forme fruste** of the disease.

2. Pleiotropy (literally, "many forms"): A single-gene defect may produce multiple anomalies. For example, in **osteogenesis imperfecta** (an abnormality of connective tissue), various structures are affected (see in MUSCULOSKELETAL DEFECTS in Ch. 187), including fragile bones, because they cannot be normally calcified, and hypermobile joints, which have a tendency to dislocate. Minor manifestations of other pleiotropic genes may easily be missed.

3. Mutations arise spontaneously from time to time. An autosomal dominant pedigree begins with a fresh mutation, and fresh mutations are surprisingly common in autosomal dominant disorders. For example, in a population of unrelated achondroplastic dwarfs, about 80% would have no family history and would thus presumably represent fresh mutations. Almost all would be capable of transmitting the freshly mutated genes to their offspring.

4. Phenocopies: Very rarely, an individual appears with a syndrome indistinguishable from that caused by a fresh mutation, but does not transmit the condition to his offspring and apparently does not have the mutant gene—ie, the syndrome appears to be due to nongenetic phenomena, or, at least, to a different genotype. A phenocopy is indistinguishable from an individual with an abnormal dominant gene who, by chance, fails to pass the gene to his offspring.

5. Sex-limited inheritance: A trait that appears in only one sex is **sex-limited**. Males are almost always the affected sex, and usually the reason is X-linked inheritance (see below). However, sex hormones and other physiologic differences between males and females may greatly alter the expressivity of an allele. For example, premature baldness is almost certainly inherited as an autosomal dominant trait; but, presumably as a result of female sex hormones, the condition is rarely expressed in the female and then usually only after menopause. Thus, sex-limitation, or perhaps more correctly, sex-influenced inheritance, is a special case of limited expressivity and penetrance.

6. Homozygous dominant genotype: This can occur in the offspring of 2 individuals who are heterozygous (or homozygous) for the same dominant gene; eg, the offspring of 2 achondroplastic dwarfs. In theory, the homozygote for the dominant gene is phenotypically indistinguishable from the heterozygote. However, in the few known marriages between persons with the same autosomal dominant abnormality, some offspring have had much more severe anomalies than either parent, suggesting that a pair of dominant alleles may have a worse effect than one. Also, in some of these matings, an increased number of spontaneous abortions and stillborn infants with multiple malformations have occurred, suggesting that the presence of 2 dominant alleles may at times be lethal.

AUTOSOMAL RECESSIVE INHERITANCE

A typical pedigree is shown in FIG. 203–3. In general, the following rules apply: (1) If an affected person is born to normal parents, both parents are heterozygotes, and, on the average, 1/4 of their offspring will be affected, 1/2 will be heterozygotes, and 1/4 will be normal. (2) If affected siblings come from a consanguineous marriage, there is strong evidence of recessive inheritance. (3) If an affected person and a genotypically normal person marry, all of their children will be phenotypically normal heterozygotes. (4) If an affected person and a heterozygote marry, on the average 1/2 of their children will be affected and 1/2 will be heterozygotes. (5) If 2 affected people marry, all of their children will be affected. (6) Males and females are equally likely to be affected. (7) Heterozygotes are phenotypically normal but are carriers of the trait. Where a defect of a specific protein (eg, an enzyme) is recognized as the cause of the disease, the carrier usually has a reduced amount of that protein.

Most diseases due to homozygosity for autosomal recessive mutant genes are rare. Most of the inborn errors of metabolism are inherited in this pattern. Affected individuals are homozygous, and each parent is a heterozygote or carrier.

Consanguinity becomes an important factor in autosomal recessive diseases, since related individuals are much more likely to share the same mutant allele. A detailed family history taken from both parents may disclose an unknown or forgotten consanguinity.

X-LINKED RECESSIVE INHERITANCE

A typical pedigree is shown in FIG. 203–4. In general, the following rules apply: (1) Nearly all affected persons are males. (2) The trait is always transmitted through the heterozygous mother, who is phenotypically normal. (3) An affected male never transmits the trait to his sons. (4) The carrier female transmits the trait to 1/2 of her sons. None of her daughters will show the trait, but 1/2 will be carriers. (5) All daughters of an affected male will be carriers.

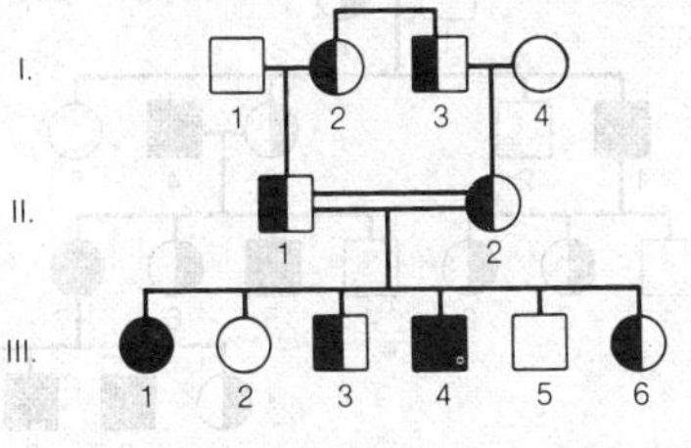

FIG. 203–3. Autosomal recessive inheritance.

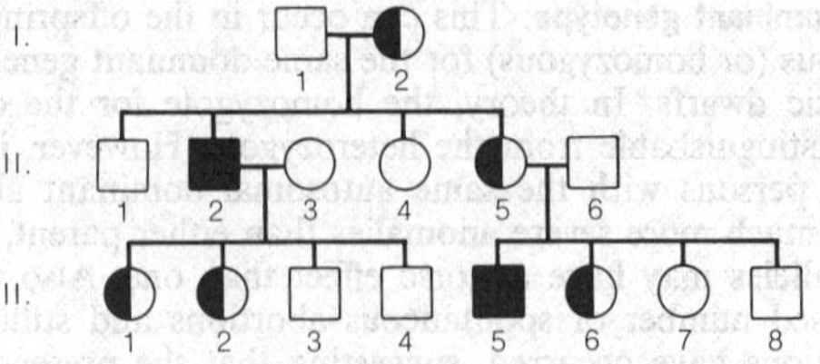

FIG. 203–4. X-linked recessive inheritance.

More than 150 traits, most of which are diseases (eg, inborn errors of metabolism), are a result of mutant genes on the X chromosome. Since the human male has only one X chromosome, the term **hemizygous** is applied. In males, all genes on the X chromosome, whether recessive or dominant, are expressed; this explains the predominance of males in X-linked recessive conditions. An affected female must be, with only rare exceptions, homozygous for the mutant allele; ie, it must be present in both of her X chromosomes. This can happen only if her father is affected and her mother is either heterozygous or else homozygous for the mutant allele. Since most X-linked mutants are rare, affected females are very rare (the incidence in females is the square of that in males). In addition, on the average, ½ of the maternal uncles of the proband will be affected, and since ½ of the maternal aunts will be carriers, some of the proband's male maternal first cousins will also be affected.

On occasion, females known to be heterozygous for X-linked mutations show varying degrees of expression, but rarely as severely as the affected (hemizygous) male (see The Lyon Hypothesis under SYNDROMES ASSOCIATED WITH SEX CHROMOSOME ABERRATIONS, below). In addition, a structural chromosomal rearrangement, such as an X-autosome translocation, can result in an affected female even though she is a heterozygote.

X-LINKED DOMINANT INHERITANCE

A typical pedigree is shown in FIG. 203–5. In general, the following rules apply: (1) Affected males transmit the trait to all of their daughters but none of their sons. (2) Affected heterozygous females transmit the condition to ½ of their children regardless of sex. (3) Affected homozygous females transmit the trait to all of their children.

X-linked dominant mutants are very rare, and females are usually more mildly affected than males. For example, in nephrogenic diabetes insipidus, females show

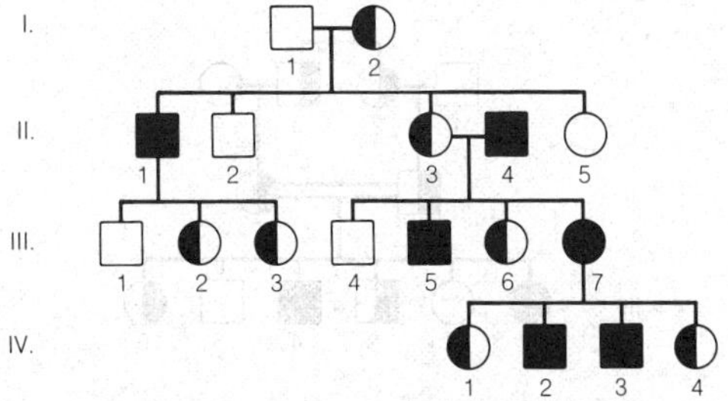

FIG. 203–5. X-linked dominant inheritance.

mild degrees of polydipsia and polyuria. In incontinentia pigmenti, the X-linked gene appears to be lethal in males and causes a peculiar swirling pattern of melanin pigmentation and other anomalies in affected females.

Since it is difficult to distinguish X-linked dominant from autosomal dominant inheritance, large pedigrees are required with particular attention given to the offspring of affected males, since male-to-male transmission rules out X-linkage.

Codominant Inheritance

Only a *trait* or *disease* can be dominant or recessive, not the *gene* itself, since presumably both alleles at a genetic locus produce some product. Codominance can only be observed if the phenotypes are qualitatively different, as with the blood group antigens (AB, MN), the leukocyte antigens, and serum proteins differing in electrophoretic mobility (albumin, haptoglobin, etc). Confusion occurs where heterozygotes are clinically normal and the condition is usually considered recessive, as in sickle cell disease. However, if the basis for the phenotype is taken to be the sickle cell preparation, which is positive in heterozygotes as well as homozygotes, the disorder could be considered dominant. Or, the condition can be thought of as codominant if one looks at the Hb electrophoresis, since the ratio of sickle Hb to normal Hb in the heterozygote is roughly 40:60.

MULTIFACTORIAL INHERITANCE

Close relatives tend to resemble each other with respect to a number of quantitative or measurable characteristics, such as height, weight, size and shape of nose and other facial features, BP, and "intelligence." Many of these traits have a distribution that fits the familiar bell-shaped curve known as the normal curve, a phenomenon that is compatible with determination of the trait by a number of genes. Each gene adds to or subtracts from the trait, and each acts in an additive manner independently of the others with no dominance. There are few individuals at the extremes of the distribution and many in the middle, since an individual is unlikely to inherit a large number of factors all acting in the same direction. In addition, a number of environmental factors, each adding to or subtracting from the final result, will also produce a normal distribution. Most of the time, the variation in the population results from a number of genes and environmental factors acting together to determine the final result. This is termed **multifactorial inheritance.**

A large number of relatively common congenital anomalies and diseases that are clearly familial do not fit the expectations for mendelian inheritance. More likely these conditions result from multifactorial inheritance of a continuously distributed variable, with a threshold separating the affected individual from the normal. Thus, the affected patient has a liability or predisposition to the condition representing the sum of genetic and environmental influences.

This concept explains the relatively high risk of the trait in first-degree relatives (siblings and children), who share 50% of their genes, and the much lower risk to the more distant relatives, who are likely to inherit only a few of the high-liability genes.

The **neural tube defects** (anencephaly, encephalocele, myelomeningocele), often referred to collectively as **spina bifida**, are a common example. In the North American white population they occur with a combined incidence of about 1.5:1000 live births. The parents of an affected infant, now identified as carrying a relatively large number of high-liability genes, have about a 1:30 chance of producing a 2nd affected offspring (this 3% risk has been calculated mathematically and confirmed by empiric data from population studies). Similarly, the patient with a neural tube defect, if able to have children, has a 3 to 4% chance of having an affected child. In the relatively rare instance where a couple has had 2 affected children, the risk for a 3rd rises further (7

to 8%). For the neural tube defects, environmental factors unquestionably play a role. For example, the incidence approaches 1:100 in areas in the western part of the United Kingdom, and clusters of cases have appeared in some neighborhoods. When people from these high-risk areas emigrate to North America, their risk falls but remains higher than that of the American population. The environmental agent(s) has never been identified, although recent data have implicated vitamin deficiency.

Other examples of multifactorial inheritance, with similar risks for siblings and offspring of affected individuals, are congenital anomalies of the heart (see in Ch. 187), idiopathic epilepsy (petit mal or grand mal), congenital megacolon (Hirschsprung's disease), most cases of cleft lip with or without cleft palate, and many forms of cancer (see below). Congenital pyloric stenosis provides an interesting variation on the multifactorial theme. There is a striking sex ratio of 5 males:1 female, suggesting that the threshold for girls is higher. Thus, the female apparently requires more potent liability genes in order to develop the condition, and ought to have more affected sibs and a greater risk of producing affected offspring than a male with pyloric stenosis. Family studies have confirmed this.

Currently, attention is being focused on a group of common disorders with multifactorial etiology; eg, arteriosclerotic heart disease, diabetes mellitus, cancer, and arthritis. Genetically determined predisposing factors, including positive family history and biochemical parameters, are being used to identify individuals at increased risk who would be most likely to benefit from preventive measures, such as drugs, special diets, changes in lifestyle, and changes in occupation (see PREVENTION OF GENETIC DISORDERS, below).

GENETIC HETEROGENEITY

The tremendous capacity of the human organism to vary, both phenotypically and genotypically, should be emphasized. Heterogeneity occurs in almost all inborn errors of metabolism, resulting from different alleles or mutations at different loci; eg, > 12 mutations are now known to produce the phenotype of Hurler syndrome (see TABLE 197–1 in INHERITED DISORDERS OF CONNECTIVE TISSUE, Ch. 197). Over 60 specific causes of congenital deafness have been identified; some are genetic, others result from rubella virus and other environmental agents. There is growing concern about the teratogenic effects of drugs taken during pregnancy. Women who consume large quantities of alcohol during pregnancy have a high risk of producing infants with severe intrauterine growth and mental retardation, as well as congenital malformations (the fetal alcohol syndrome—see METABOLIC PROBLEMS in Ch. 186).

Thus, phenotypically similar conditions may be due to different mutations, nongenetic factors, or combinations of both. In order to establish the cause of the patient's problem and to determine the risk for future offspring as accurately as possible, the physician must take a thorough family history, including an inquiry into possible environmental teratogens, keeping heterogeneity in mind.

GENETICS OF MALIGNANT DISEASE

Little is known of the genetics of most types of cancer, but the pieces of the puzzle are slowly falling into place. The new technics of molecular genetics have confirmed the existence of **"oncogenes"** —literally, tumor genes—which at least in some instances are normal genes that were responsible for control of embryonic or fetal development and are present in everyone. Normally they are inactivated and remain so. It is now clear, however, that the human genome is not as stable as once was thought and when some of these "regulatory" genes are relocated or rearranged as a result of a chromosomal translocation, inversion, or even simple breaking, they may act as the initiator of

a malignancy. The rearrangements may be induced by a variety of environmental agents or by genetically determined events that are as yet poorly understood.

In some families there seem to be many instances of various and apparently unrelated malignancies, while few cases of cancer appear in other families from similar environments. Most malignancies seem to occur in genetically predisposed individuals who are at some time exposed to environmental carcinogens (many of them as yet unknown). However, some malignancies clearly show mendelian or multifactorial inheritance.

Familial polyposis of the colon: See Ch. 63.

Neurofibromatosis (von Recklinghausen's disease): See Ch. 131.

Retinoblastoma, a relatively common tumor, accounts for 2% of childhood malignancies. Its multiple occurrence in about 40% of families indicates that some cases are due to an autosomal dominant gene, especially when the tumor is bilateral. Recent studies have demonstrated a deletion of a segment of the long arm of chromosome 13 in some retinoblastoma patients, and the gene was subsequently mapped to the 13q14 band. Gene probes have already been found for identification of potentially affected newborns, but until they are widely available, careful and repeated eye examinations of subsequent offspring are mandatory. With early diagnosis and treatment, survival and preservation of sight (even in the affected eye) can be anticipated. The closely related and more common childhood malignancy, **neuroblastoma,** is beginning to show a similar but less frequent familial incidence as more patients survive and have children. Urinary catecholamine levels should be determined in siblings and offspring at ages 6 and 12 mo. Similarly, a small fraction of **Wilms' tumors** is due to an inherited mutation, and the aniridia-Wilms' tumor syndrome invariably occurs in individuals with a specific chromosomal deletion in the short arm of number 11 (11p13).

Xeroderma pigmentosum is a rare, disfiguring syndrome, which is inherited as an autosomal recessive trait. Areas of depigmentation, hyperpigmentation, telangiectasia, and epidermal scarring occur, and epidermal carcinomas frequently develop (particularly on exposure to sunlight).

Immunologic deficiency diseases (the inherited agamma- and dysgammaglobulinemias) carry an increased risk of malignancies of the lymphoid system, particularly lymphomas and leukemias.

In patients with Down's syndrome (mongolism), **leukemia** develops about 15 times more often than in the normal population. Similarly, a group of **"chromosome instability" syndromes** (eg, Fanconi's anemia, Bloom's syndrome, ataxia telangiectasia) exists that are characterized by increased chromosome breakage and a high risk of leukemia or lymphoma; each is inherited as an autosomal recessive trait.

Carcinoma of the breast occurs significantly more often in daughters of similarly affected women than in the general population. Presumably, this is an example of multifactorial inheritance. Females at risk should be apprised of this, and regular self-examination of the breasts should be emphasized.

Carcinoma of the lung: First-degree relatives of individuals with lung cancer appear to be significantly more at risk, especially if they smoke cigarettes.

POPULATION GENETICS

Knowing the incidence of various mutations in different populations is important. For example, when a case of phenylketonuria (PKU) occurs, family members who are carriers of the abnormal gene will want to know their risk of marrying another carrier. This risk depends on the frequency with which that particular gene occurs in the

population. Furthermore, many genes that cause serious human disease occur with a different frequency in different racial and ethnic groups. For instance, Tay-Sachs disease is nearly 100 times more frequent among Ashkenazi Jews than among non-Jews, and the incidence of heterozygotes in Ashkenazis is 1:30 (see Screening Programs under PREVENTION OF GENETIC DISORDERS, below).

In the study of human genetics, representative samples of populations are surveyed in order to calculate gene frequencies. With autosomal dominant genes, the frequency in a given population can be calculated merely by identifying cases of the disease. The gene frequency for X-linked recessive genes can be simply calculated by determining the frequency of affected males in a male population. In autosomal recessive conditions, usually only the homozygote or affected individual can be detected with certainty; the asymptomatic carrier is seldom positively identifiable. However, the frequency of the carrier for autosomal recessive conditions can be determined from the frequency of the homozygote by using the following mathematical procedure. For any 2 alleles, A and a, there are 3 possible genotypes: AA, Aa, and aa. If the proportion of "A" genes in the population is represented as p and the proportion of "a" genes as q, then p plus q must equal 100%. Since gene frequencies are expressed as a fraction of unity, the equation is written $p + q = 1$. With random mating, the various combinations of gametes can be represented as a simple binomial expansion, and the frequencies of the various offspring will be in the proportion p^2 (AA), 2 pq (Aa), and q^2 (aa). This distribution of genotypes remains essentially the same from generation to generation (the **Hardy-Weinberg law**).

The analysis is more than an exercise in algebra because, by knowing the ratio of the various genotypes (p^2, 2 pq, q^2), their frequency can be determined if the frequency of the affected homozygote is known. For example, cystic fibrosis (aa) has a frequency, among Caucasians, of about 1:2500 live births. Thus:

$$\begin{aligned} & q^2 = 1/2500 \\ \text{therefore } & q = 1/50 \\ \text{but } & p = 1 - q \\ \text{therefore } & p = 1 - 1/50 \\ & = 49/50 \\ & \cong 1 \end{aligned}$$

$$\begin{aligned} \text{The frequency of carriers (Aa)} &= 2\,pq \\ &= 2 \times 1 \times 1/50 \\ &= 1/25 \end{aligned}$$

This simple example shows that *carriers of a recessive condition are much more common than affected individuals*. Since most recessively inherited diseases are rare, p can be considered as 1, and the carrier frequency can be quickly estimated by calculating q and multiplying by 2.

When **cystic fibrosis** has occurred in one or more siblings in a family, each normal sibling has a 2:3 chance of being a heterozygote (no accurate biochemical test yet exists for heterozygote detection). These normal siblings should know their risk of having affected children. If a normal sibling marries an unrelated individual, that individual has a 1:25 chance of being a carrier. If 2 heterozygous individuals marry, their chance of having an affected child is 1:4. Therefore, the risk of having an affected child is 2:3 × 1:25 × 1:4, or about 1:150.

Consanguinity is a common indication for genetic counseling; autosomal recessive conditions are the major concern. Every human being is heterozygous for 6 to 8 alleles

that would, in the homozygous state, lead to one of the several hundred known recessive diseases. Among incestuous unions, such as parent–child or brother–sister, where 50% of the genome is shared, abnormal offspring are common. Yet for the more often encountered first cousin unions, where 1:8 genes are shared, the risk of genetically determined disease is 3 to 5%, as compared to a risk of about 2% for nonconsanguineous parents. Some studies have suggested an increased incidence of spontaneous abortions, stillbirths, prematurity, cerebral palsy, multifactorial conditions (eg, congenital dislocation of the hip), and infertility for first cousin marriages, but the increases have been small and usually not statistically significant. For couples less closely related than first cousins, data are sparse, but the risks seem little if any increased over those for the nonconsanguineous population. Thus, there is little reason to discourage first cousin marriages and no reason to discourage unions between less closely related couples, unless dealing with highly inbred groups, such as the Amish or Mennonites, where heterozygosity for deleterious genes is often greatly increased.

GENETIC COUNSELING IN HEREDITARY DISORDERS

Physicians must recognize the hereditary nature of many human illnesses, and must impart this information to the patient or the family. Genetic counseling should be no different from counseling by a physician for any other illness. The facts should be clearly presented to all concerned family members so that they can make a rational decision about further pregnancies. Patients often misunderstand and misinterpret genetic information during the counseling session. Follow-up visits and written communications are usually very helpful.

Genetic counseling centers have been established at all medical schools in the USA and Canada, and private genetics programs are also appearing. Patients and families can be referred for diagnosis, counseling, and management, and the staff will provide physicians with up-to-date information should the referring physician wish to undertake the counseling himself. A working relationship with a genetics center has become essential for the practicing physician, in large part because of the rapidly developing applications of molecular genetics to patient care, particularly in early diagnosis, carrier detection, and prevention (see PREVENTION OF GENETIC DISORDERS, below).

SINGLE-GENE DEFECTS

More than 3000 conditions have been identified as single-gene defects for which the risk of producing affected offspring can be predicted mathematically.

Autosomal Dominant Conditions

The statistical risk of recurrence is 50%, regardless of the outcome of previous pregnancies; usually there is no sex predilection. If the family history is negative and the case is presumed to be a fresh mutation, the risk to siblings is nearly zero, but the affected individual risks transmitting the dominant mutant to ½ of his offspring. (This is not true of phenocopies.)

Huntington's disease (HD) exemplifies a major problem posed by some autosomal dominant diseases. Though the abnormal gene is present at conception, the disease is undetectable before symptoms occur, which is usually not until the mid 30s or later. By this time, the unsuspecting victim has already produced offspring, ½ of whom have inherited the HD gene and will eventually develop the disease. Most physicians feel, therefore, that all individuals at risk—all children and all siblings of an affected individual—should consider not having children. These are individual decisions, however, and the physician must not allow personal biases to interfere. Recent developments in molecular genetics have provided new options for HD families (see PREVENTION OF GENETIC DISORDERS, below).

Autosomal Recessive Conditions

The risk to siblings of an affected individual is 25%, and, again, families must realize that the same risk applies to *each* pregnancy. The analogy with drawing cards from a deck is useful: the chance of drawing a heart, club, spade, or diamond is 1:4, but it is not uncommon to draw 2 or even 3 cards of the same suit in a row.

Since consanguinity increases the risk, a family pedigree should be constructed before counseling, and the patient should be advised of the hazard of marrying a close relative. Heterozygote detection (see below) is also an important factor in autosomal recessive conditions.

X-Linked Recessive Conditions

A heterozygous female has a 25% chance of having an affected child, since the chance of having a male child is 50%, and 50% of male offspring are affected. Since heterozygous females have normal girls, prenatal detection of fetal sex by amniocentesis (see PREVENTION OF GENETIC DISORDERS, below) is a possible means of prevention. However, the rapidly increasing availability of X-linked gene probes will soon make detection of the affected male fetus a reality (see PREVENTION OF GENETIC DISORDERS, below).

X-Linked Dominant Conditions

Of the children of affected females, 1/2 will be affected regardless of sex; ie, the risk for offspring of affected females is the same as for autosomal dominant traits. *All* of the daughters and *none* of the sons of an affected male will be affected.

MULTIFACTORIAL CONDITIONS

Many congenital anomalies and syndromes are of multifactorial origin. The low recurrence risk is discussed above, and the possibility of prevention through prenatal diagnosis and selective abortion must be presented to couples at risk (see PREVENTION OF GENETIC DISORDERS, below).

HETEROZYGOTE DETECTION

This is a neglected, but extremely important, aspect of genetic counseling, especially in X-linked recessive conditions. In such families, female siblings of affected boys, as well as maternal aunts, run a high risk of being heterozygotes, and thus may themselves have affected children. It is the physician's responsibility to point this out to families and to keep up with the molecular genetic approaches to carrier detection.

Heterozygotes for X-Linked Conditions

Muscular dystrophy (Duchenne or pseudohypertrophic type—see also Ch. 132): In affected males, the diagnosis is made from the clinical picture, muscle biopsy, and high serum concentrations of enzymes released from damaged muscle. The most useful is the serum creatine kinase **(CK)**. In heterozygotes, CK levels lie between those of affected males and normal individuals. Unfortunately, CK values in normal and heterozygous females overlap considerably, so that only about 70% of heterozygous females can be positively identified. Nevertheless, because of the severity of the disease and the lack of therapy, prevention by contraception or by selective abortion of males should be discussed with the family. Fortunately this is one of the diseases for which a DNA probe will soon be available. This will provide the long-awaited means for accurate carrier detection and prenatal diagnosis of affected male fetuses (see PREVENTION OF GENETIC DISORDERS, below).

Hemophilia: Affected males have very low levels of serum antihemophilic globulin **(AHG)**. Heterozygous females have, on the average, 50% of normal amounts of AHG, and tests combining AHG activity with immunologic quantitation of AHG protein

appear to detect over 90% of the heterozygotes. New methods of therapy using self-administered AHG concentrates, and in the very near future, pure AHG produced by recombinant DNA technology, are changing the prognosis in hemophilia, and prevention by selective abortion of males is becoming questionable ethically.

Hunter syndrome (X-linked mucopolysaccharidosis): The affected hemizygous male and heterozygous female can both be detected biochemically with close to 100% accuracy, and the affected male is detectable prenatally through enzyme assay in cultured amniotic fluid cells (see Amniocentesis under PREVENTION OF GENETIC DISORDERS, below).

Lesch-Nyhan syndrome (hereditary hyperuricemia): Usually, affected males are severely mentally and physically retarded, have marked hyperuricemia, and exhibit a peculiar propensity to self-mutilation by chewing their lips and fingertips, which leads to tissue loss and scarring. The basic enzymatic defect is known, and cases and carriers are detectable with almost 100% accuracy through biochemical studies on cultured cells. Affected males can be detected prenatally, as with Hunter syndrome.

Autosomal Recessive Conditions

Heterozygote detection in autosomal recessive conditions is less vital than in X-linked conditions. Most autosomal recessive mutant genes that cause disease are rare, and thus, even though 2:3 of the phenotypically normal siblings of an affected person are heterozygotes, their chance of marrying a carrier of the same mutant is remote, and their chance of having affected offspring is even more remote. However, a consanguineous marriage greatly increases the risk of affected offspring. The actual risk for these situations can be calculated by using the formula given in POPULATION GENETICS, above. Heterozygote detection is important when the gene frequency is high, as occurs among certain ethnic and racial groups (see Screening Programs, below).

CHROMOSOME ABERRATIONS

Today it is relatively simple to culture cells and obtain chromosome preparations from many human cells and tissues, including circulating blood lymphocytes. Physicians in any location can mail a few milliliters of heparinized venous blood to a cytogenetics laboratory. Specimens should not be refrigerated, but must be packaged in a well-insulated container to avoid freezing or breakage. In the laboratory the RBCs are sedimented out and the leukocytes are incubated in culture medium for 2 to 3 days. A bean extract, phytohemagglutinin, both accelerates the precipitation of RBCs and stimulates the division of lymphocytes. Then colchicine, a drug that arrests mitosis during metaphase, is added to the culture. Thus a large number of cells accumulate in metaphase, the time during the cell cycle when chromosomes are best visualized. Each chromosome has replicated (made a copy of itself) and appears as 2 chromatids attached at the centromere or central constriction. A variety of chromosome staining technics is available, and after the treated cells are spread onto microscope slides, the chromosomes from single cells are photographed. Individual chromosomes can be cut out of the print and pasted onto a piece of paper. This chromosome picture is called a **karyotype**. Chromosomes can be stained using the Giemsa or G banding technic. The banding pattern produced by this procedure and a related technic using quinacrine mustard as the stain (the Q banding technic, yielding fluorescent bands) permits identification of each chromosome in the human complement and has greatly increased the precision of cytogenetic diagnosis (see FIG. 203–6 for a diagrammatic illustration of the chromosome bands).

The nomenclature for describing the human karyotype requires a brief explanation. The normal male and female are designated as 46,XY and 46,XX, respectively. In Down's syndrome, where there is an extra chromosome 21 (trisomy 21), the notation is 47,XX,21+ for a female and 47,XY,21+ for a male. When a chromosome has a

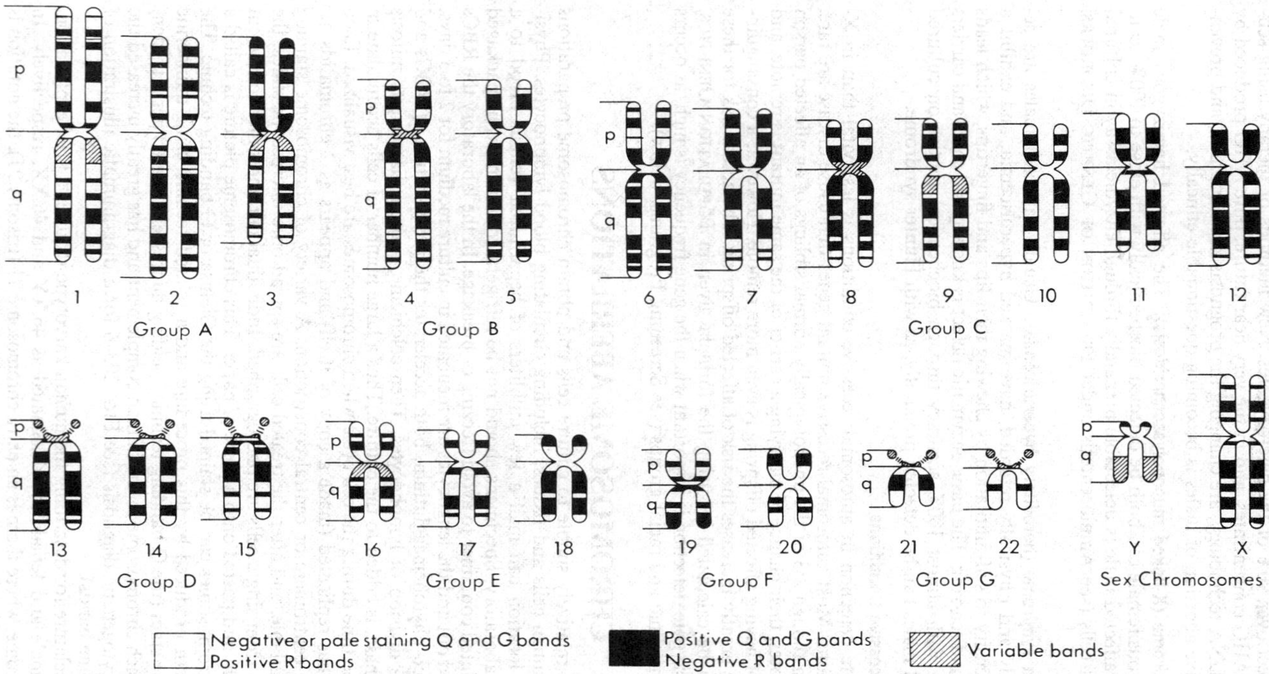

FIG. 203–6. A diagrammatic representation of chromosome bands as observed with the Q-, G-, and R-staining methods; centromere representative of Q-staining method only. Each chromosome appears as 2 chromatids joined at the centromere or central construction. The 23 pairs of chromosomes are sorted by size, position of centromere, and specific banding pattern, and the autosomes are numbered from 1 to 22. The sex chromosomes retain the classic X and Y designations. The older groupings of the chromosomes by letter, as done prior to the banding technics, are also shown. (Adapted from ISCN [1978]: An International System for Human Cytogenetic Nomenclature [1978]. Birth Defects: Original Article Series, Vol. XIV, No. 8 [The National Foundation, New York, 1978].)

structural abnormality, it is necessary to specify whether the long or short arm is affected; the letter "*p*" represents the short arm and "*q*" the long arm. Thus, for a deletion of the short arm of chromosome 5, as found in the cat-cry syndrome, the female karyotype is 46,XX,5*p*–. The typical 14/21 "balanced translocation carrier" parent (mother, in this example) of a translocation Down's syndrome patient is written as 45,XX,t(14*q*21*q*): The translocation chromosome is formed from the long arms of 14 and 21; the short arms are lost.

Not shown in the diagram is the numbering system: Each arm of the chromosomes is divided into one to 4 major regions, depending on length; and each band, positively or negatively staining, is given a number. The numbers rise as the distance from the centromere increases. For example, 1q23 refers to chromosome one, the long arm (q), the 2nd region distal to the centromere, and the 3rd band in that region.

SYNDROMES ASSOCIATED WITH AUTOSOMAL ABERRATIONS

Some syndromes associated with autosomal aberrations have clear-cut and well-established clinical findings and are described below. Additionally, the technics for banding human chromosomes precisely identify patients with specific chromosome defects even though clinical findings are few or relatively nondiscriminatory. New syndromes associated with trisomies, partial trisomies (due to translocations of portions of either short or long arms), and deletions of most of the chromosomes have been described; only the better established and more common clinical entities are included here.

DOWN'S SYNDROME

(Trisomy 21; Trisomy G; Mongolism)

In about 95% of cases of Down's syndrome, there is an extra chromosome 21. The overall incidence is about 1:700 live births, but there is a marked variability depending on maternal age—in the early childbearing years, the incidence is about 1:2000 live births; for mothers over age 40, it rises to about 1:40 live births. Just over 20% of infants with Down's syndrome are born to mothers > 35 yr, yet these older mothers have only 6 to 7% of the children. However, the number of women having babies after age 35 has been rising quite rapidly in the last few years. The extra chromosome 21 comes from the father in 1/4 to 1/3 of the cases.

Symptoms and Signs

Infants tend to be placid, rarely cry, and demonstrate muscular hypotonicity. Physical and mental development are retarded; the mean IQ is about 50.

Microcephaly, brachycephaly, and a flattened occiput are characteristic. The eyes are slanted, and epicanthal folds usually are present. **Brushfield's spots** (*gray to white spots resembling grains of salt around the periphery of the iris*) usually are visible in the neonatal period and disappear during the first 12 mo of life. The bridge of the nose is flattened, and the mouth is often held open because of a large, protruding tongue that is furrowed and lacks the central fissure. The hands are short and broad, with a single palmar crease **("simian crease")**; the fingers are short, with clinodactyly (incurvature) of the 5th finger, which often has only 2 phalanges. The feet have a wide gap between the 1st and 2nd toes, and a plantar furrow extends backward. Hands and feet show characteristic dermal prints (dermatoglyphics). Congenital heart disease is found in about 35% of patients; atrioventricular canal defects and ventricular septal defects are most common.

Prognosis

The life expectancy of the mongoloid child is decreased by heart disease and by susceptibility to acute leukemia. Today, most patients without a major heart defect survive to adulthood, but the aging process seems to be accelerated, with death occurring in the 4th or 5th decade.

Chromosomal Variants

1. Translocations: Some mongoloid children have 46 chromosomes. However, these children actually have the genetic material of 47 chromosomes—the additional chromosome 21 has been translocated. Most commonly, a 14/21 translocation occurs; that is, the additional chromosome 21 is transferred and attached to a chromosome 14. In about half the cases, both parents will have normal karyotypes, indicating a **de novo** translocation in the child. Among the remaining couples, one parent (almost always the mother), although phenotypically normal, has only 45 chromosomes, one of which is the 14/21 translocation chromosome. Theoretically, the chance is 1:3 that a mother with a 14/21 translocation will have a mongoloid child, but for unknown reasons the actual risk is lower (about 1:10). If the father carries the 14/21 translocation, the chance of having a mongoloid offspring is only 1:20; the reason for this is not known.

The next most common translocation is 21/22. In this case, the chance that the carrier will have a Down's syndrome child is also about 1:10, but the risk for carrier fathers is about the same as for mothers. In extremely rare instances, a parent may have a 21/21 translocation. In this case, 100% of surviving offspring will have Down's syndrome.

2. Mosaics: Presumably as a result of nondisjunction in the fertilized zygote, some cases of Down's syndrome have 2 cell lines, one normal and one with 47 chromosomes. The relative proportion of each cell line is highly variable, both from individual to individual and within different tissues and organs in the same individual. The prognosis, as far as intelligence is concerned, becomes difficult and presumably depends on the proportion of trisomy 21 cells in the brain. A few mosaic Down's syndrome patients have been found with barely recognizable clinical signs and normal intelligence, and thus the incidence of this variant is unknown. Curiously, in some cases both the physical stigmata and the intellectual deficit lessen as the affected child ages. The risk of having trisomy 21 offspring when either parent is a mosaic is increased by an incalculable factor depending on the degree of mosaicism in the gonads.

A complete cytogenetic investigation of the patient with trisomy 21 includes chromosome analysis of both parents to rule out mosaicism and permit a discussion of the availability, indications, and risks of amniocentesis in future pregnancies (see Prevention of Genetic Disorders, below).

Trisomy 18
(Edwards' Syndrome)

An additional chromosome 18 occurs in 1:3000 live births with little, if any, maternal age effect. There is a peculiar sex ratio—3 females:1 male.

The newborn infant is premature or small for gestational age, with marked hypoplasia of skeletal muscle and subcutaneous fat and hypotonia. The cry is weak, and response to sound is decreased. There is often a history of feeble fetal activity, polyhydramnios, a small placenta, and a single umbilical artery.

The occiput is prominent, and there is a narrow bifrontal diameter with hypoplasia of the orbital ridges, short palpebral fissures, small mouth, and micrognathia, all of which give the face a pinched appearance. Microcephaly, epicanthal folds, low-set malformed ears, and cleft lip and/or palate are common. The peculiar clenched fist with the index finger overlapping the 3rd and 4th fingers is almost pathognomonic. Absence of the distal crease on the 5th finger is common, as is a low-arch dermal ridge pattern on the fingertips. The nails are hypoplastic, and the big toe is shortened and

frequently dorsiflexed. Hypoplastic or absent thumbs, clubfeet, rocker-bottom feet, and syndactyly are also seen.

Ventricular septal defect, patent ductus arteriosus, atrial septal defect, anomalous pulmonary and/or aortic valves, and congenital anomalies of lung, diaphragm, kidneys, and ureters are frequent. Hernias and/or diastasis recti, cryptorchidism in the male, and redundant skin folds (particularly over the posterior aspect of the neck) also are common.

Survival for more than a few months is rare, and mental retardation is severe in those who do survive.

TRISOMY 13
(Patau's Syndrome)

This syndrome, caused by trisomy of chromosome 13, occurs in about 1:5000 births and is characterized by midline anomalies. Infants tend to be small at birth. Apneic spells in early infancy are frequent, and mental retardation is severe. Many appear to be deaf. Moderate microcephaly with sloping forehead, wide sagittal sutures, and widely patent fontanels are present. Gross anatomic defects of the brain, especially **holoprosencephaly** (*failure of the forebrain to divide properly*), are common. Myelomeningocele is found in almost 50% of cases. Microphthalmia, colobomas (fissures) of the iris, and retinal dysplasia occur frequently. The supraorbital ridges are shallow and the palpebral fissures usually are slanted. Cleft lip, cleft palate, or both are present in most cases. The ears are abnormally shaped and usually low-set.

Simian crease, polydactyly, and hyperconvex narrow fingernails are common. The fingers tend to be flexed, but not in the characteristic manner seen in trisomy 18. The feet show posterior prominence of the heel, and there may be a rocker-bottom foot. About 80% of cases show the congenital cardiovascular anomalies described under TRISOMY 18, above. Dextrocardia is common as well.

Capillary hemangiomas, especially on the forehead in the midline, are common. Other midline defects include dermal sinuses of the scalp and loose folds of skin over the posterior aspect of the neck. The genitalia are frequently abnormal in both sexes; cryptorchidism and abnormal scrotum occur in the male, and bicornuate uterus is found in the female. Hematologically, there is an increased frequency of nuclear projections in polymorphonuclear leukocytes and a persistence of fetal Hb. Most patients (70%) are so severely affected that they die before age 6 mo; < 20% survive beyond age 1 yr.

PARTIAL TRISOMY 22
(The Cat-Eye Syndrome)

The association between coloboma of the iris (cat eye) or anal atresia, or both, with an extra small chromosome 22 (22*q*+) has been confirmed. In addition, anomalies such as severe psychomotor retardation, hypertelorism, eyes with an antimongoloid slant, abnormal ears with preauricular tags or fistulas, and congenital heart disease occur. Full trisomy 22 has been reported in a few patients with a similar phenotype, but frequently microcephaly, micrognathia, and hypotonia occur as well.

DELETION SYNDROMES

In the rare **cat-cry syndrome (cri du chat syndrome, 5*p*– syndrome),** there is a deletion of the short arm of chromosome 5. The syndrome is characterized by a high-pitched, mewing cry, closely resembling the cry of a kitten, which is heard in the immediate newborn period, lasts several weeks, and then disappears. Affected infants show low birth weight, microcephaly, and a peculiar round or moon face with wide-set eyes, antimongoloid or downward-sloping palpebral fissures with or without epicanthal

folds, strabismus, and a broad-based nose. The ears are low-set and abnormally shaped, and frequently have narrow external canals and preauricular tags. Micrognathia, a short neck, and varying degrees of syndactyly are present; heart defects are frequent and the infants are hypotonic. Mental and physical development are markedly retarded. A significant number survive to adulthood, when facial asymmetry and malocclusion often lead to a grotesque appearance.

The **4*p*– deletion syndrome** is extremely rare. The short arm of chromosome 4 is deleted, and the syndrome shares most of the features of the cat-cry syndrome but lacks the cat-like cry. Mental retardation is profound. In addition, there are midline scalp defects, ptosis and colobomas, beaked nose, cleft palate, delayed bone age, and, in males, hypospadias and undescended testes.

LEUKEMIA
(See Ch. 101)

SYNDROMES ASSOCIATED WITH SEX CHROMOSOME ABERRATIONS

The Lyon Hypothesis (X-Inactivation Theory)

Sex determination in man is controlled by a unique pair of chromosomes, the X and the Y. The female has two X chromosomes, and the male has one X plus one Y. The Y chromosome is usually the smallest of the 46 chromosomes, and geneticists have been able to detect, at most, only one non–sex-related gene in it. On the other hand, the X is one of the largest chromosomes in group C and contains hundreds of genes, most of which have nothing to do with sex.

This situation would seem to create a genetic "dosage" problem, since the normal female has 2 loci for every X-linked gene as compared to the male's single locus. However, according to the **Lyon hypothesis,** *one of the two X chromosomes in each somatic cell of the female is genetically inactivated.* It is evident that the **Barr body,** or **sex chromatin mass,** seen within the nuclei of female somatic cells represents all (or at least most) of the 2nd X chromosome. In fact, no matter how many X chromosomes are present in the genome, all but one seem to be inactivated. Thus, the number of sex chromatin masses is one less than the total number of X chromosomes.

X-inactivation has interesting implications in clinical medicine. For example, X chromosome anomalies are relatively benign, compared to analogous autosomal anomalies. Females with three X chromosomes are usually normal physically and mentally, and are apparently fertile. In contrast, all of the known autosomal trisomies, such as Down's syndrome and trisomies 18 and 13, have devastating effects. The relatively benign nature of additional X chromosomes presumably results from inactivation of most of the extra chromosomal material. Similarly, the total absence of an autosome is lethal, whereas the total absence of one X chromosome, though it leads to a specific syndrome (Turner's syndrome), is relatively benign.

The symptomatic heterozygote for an X-linked recessive disorder may also be explained on the basis of this theory. Females who are heterozygous for hemophilia or muscular dystrophy occasionally show bleeding tendencies or muscle weakness, respectively. The Lyon hypothesis also suggests that X-inactivation is a random event and, in each individual, therefore, 50% maternal and 50% paternal X-inactivation should occur. However, a random process follows the normal distribution curve, and nearly all of the maternal X may be inactivated in some females, and the paternal X in other females. If, by chance, nearly all cells containing the normal allele were inactivated in a given tissue of a heterozygote, the disease in that individual and in the hemizygous affected male might be similar.

GONADAL DYSGENESIS
(Turner's Syndrome; Bonnevie-Ullrich Syndrome)

This syndrome is due, in general, to the complete or partial absence of one of the two X chromosomes in the female. Its incidence is about 1:3000 live female births. Many affected newborns present with marked dorsal lymphedema of the hands and feet, and with lymphedema or loose folds of skin over the posterior aspect of the neck. This appearance is almost pathognomonic.

The full picture in the older child or adult consists of short stature, webbing of the neck, low hairline on the back of the neck, ptosis, a wide chest with broad-spaced nipples, multiple pigmented nevi, short 4th metacarpals and hypoplasia of the nails, coarctation of the aorta, amenorrhea, failure of breast development, and juvenile external genitalia. The ovaries are replaced by bilateral streaks of fibrous stroma that are usually devoid of developing ova.

Renal anomalies and hemangiomas are frequent. Occasionally, telangiectasis occurs in the GI tract, with resultant intestinal bleeding. Mental deficiency is rare, but many patients suffer from spatial disorientation and thus score poorly in performance tests and in mathematics, even though they score average or above in verbal IQ.

Variants: (1) **Mosaics**: A number of patients with Turner's syndrome are mosaics (eg, 45,X/46,XX or 45,X/47,XXX). (2) **Ring chromosomes**: Occasionally, affected individuals have one normal X and one abnormal X that form a ring chromosome. (3) **Long arm isochromosomes**: Some patients have one normal X and one long arm isochromosome formed by the loss of short arms and development of a chromosome consisting of just the long arms. These individuals tend to have the complete syndrome, so that deletion of the short arm of the X chromosome appears to be the most important factor in the syndrome. (4) **Turner phenotype with normal sex chromosomes (Noonan's syndrome)**: In several families, both females and males have many characteristics of Turner's syndrome, though their chromosomes are 46,XX or 46,XY. This is apparently due to homozygosity for an autosomal recessive mutant in some cases, and to autosomal dominant inheritance in others. There are phenotypic differences, primarily a more normal stature, normal sexual development and fertility, pectus excavatum, and more frequent involvement of the right side of the heart (pulmonic stenosis) rather than coarctation of the aorta. Mental retardation occurs frequently but usually is not severe.

A cytogenetic analysis must be obtained on all patients with gonadal dysgenesis in order to rule out mosaicism with a Y-bearing cell line; eg, 46,XY/45,X. These patients are usually phenotypic females who have variable features of Turner's syndrome, although some are intersexes. They are at high risk of developing gonadal malignancy, especially gonadoblastoma, and should have the gonads removed prophylactically during early childhood.

THE TRIPLE X SYNDROME (47,XXX)

These individuals have three X chromosomes and two Barr bodies or sex chromatin masses. This condition, found initially in hospitals for the mentally retarded, has also been discovered in about 1:1000 apparently normal females during routine surveys of newborn populations. Though sterility sometimes occurs, several normal XXX females have had offspring who have been both chromosomally and phenotypically normal. Follow-up studies of the unselected infants ascertained in newborn surveys have revealed impaired intellect with IQ scores averaging < 90 and associated school problems in all subjects when compared with siblings. Most have moderate to severe deficits in language areas, reflecting their difficulties with visual-motor and sensory perceptual integration.

Rare Anomalies of the X Chromosome

Although rare, 48,XXXX or 49,XXXXX females have been found. There is no consistent phenotype, though the risk of mental retardation and congenital abnormalities increases markedly with an increase in number of X chromosomes, especially when there are > 3. The genetic imbalance early in embryonic life prior to X-inactivation may cause anomalous development.

Klinefelter's Syndrome (47,XXY)

This relatively common chromosome anomaly occurs in about 1:700 live male births. In the past, 47,XXY individuals were thought to be mentally retarded, and surveys of mental institutions have disclosed an incidence of about 1:50 mentally retarded male patients. The typical affected individual is tall and eunuchoid, with small, firm testes and gynecomastia. However, clinical variation is great, and we now know that most 47,XXY males are normal in appearance and intellect, and are found in the course of an infertility work-up (probably all are sterile) or in cytogenetic surveys of normal populations. Boys from the latter group have been followed developmentally. There has been no mental retardation but many have specific deficits in verbal IQ and reading. They are inefficient in their use of language and slow in auditory processing; speech and language therapy have been beneficial and they eventually do well in school. Testicular development varies from hyalinized nonfunctional tubules to some production of spermatozoa, and urinary excretion of follicle-stimulating hormone **(FSH)** is frequently increased.

Variants: Some patients with Klinefelter's syndrome have three, four, and even five X chromosomes along with the Y. In general, as the number of X's increases, the severity of mental retardation and of malformations also increases. Again, genetic imbalance prior to X-inactivation may be significant. A few individuals appear to be 46,XX; these cases probably result from a translocation of a minute, and therefore undetectable, fragment of a Y chromosome to one of the X's or to another chromosome. There are also rare mosaic individuals with Klinefelter's syndrome.

The 47,XYY Syndrome

This chromosome anomaly was first described in 1961 in a 6-ft white male with no particular problems. A number of males with this syndrome, particularly those who are aggressive or violent, are found in institutions for criminals with subnormal IQ, and it has been suggested that extra Y chromosomal material predisposes males to criminal aggressive tendencies. However, 47,XYY individuals are also found in normal populations with about the same high frequency as 47,XXY, and the role of the extra Y chromosome in criminal tendencies is questionable. Early test results on the boys identified by newborn screening show increased language dysfunction similar to that of the 47,XXY males.

X-Linked Mental Retardation

(Fragile-X Syndrome)

(See also Mental Retardation in Ch. 188)

Among persons institutionalized because of mental retardation, a 30 to 50% excess of males has been well documented. Family studies frequently revealed affected male sibs and maternal uncles, leaving no doubt that there is a group of X-linked mutant genes that cause mental retardation without major congenital anomalies. This at least in part accounts for the excess of retarded males. Some of these males have an X chromosome with a constriction near the end of the long arm, resulting in what looks like a small knob separated from the main portion of the chromosome by a thin stalk.

The stalk, often broken in preparing the karyotype, is referred to as a fragile site and its presence can be detected by using special cell culture technics. The clinical features include large testes, especially after puberty, large protuberant ears, and prominent chin and forehead. When affected males have this fragile-X chromosome, frequently, but not always, the fragile-X can be demonstrated in the carrier female. Some carriers are also mentally retarded; and, curiously, some of the males are mentally normal. Because the fragile-X cannot be reliably detected in cultured fibroblasts or amniotic fluid cells, prenatal diagnosis is not yet sufficiently accurate for general use. This fragile-X syndrome is of major importance because, next to Down's syndrome, it is the most common cause of mental retardation that can be specifically diagnosed.

INTERSEX STATES

(See also in Ch. 187)

Genetic disorders may be responsible for intersex states in a variety of ways. A useful approach to the diagnosis in cases of ambiguous genitalia is based on the results of chromosome analysis, and many patients can be placed into 1 of 3 categories:

1. Chromosome abnormalities. Sex chromosome abnormalities include a variety of mosaics with or without a Y chromosome, the gonadal dysgenesis syndromes (may be 46,XX or 46,XY) and true hermaphrodites (often 46,XX in lymphocytes but mosaic in the ovotestis). Ambiguous genitalia may also occur in trisomies 13 and 18 and in other autosomal chromosome disorders.

2. Masculinization of 46,XX females (female pseudohermaphrodites). The most common problem is congenital virilizing adrenal hyperplasia **(adrenogenital syndrome),** a group of disorders due to enzyme deficiencies in the adrenal cortical biosynthetic pathways, each of which is inherited as an autosomal recessive trait. Exogenous androgen from maternal ingestion or maternal tumors may also masculinize a fetus.

3. Undermasculinization of 46,XY males (male pseudohermaphrodites). Some of the enzyme deficiencies in congenital adrenal hyperplasia lead to production of abnormal androgens that fail to fully masculinize the male fetus. In addition, there is a group of **"androgen resistance syndromes"** due to deficiencies of cell membrane androgen receptors (total resistance causes the testicular feminization syndrome), most of which are X-linked.

It is important to note that most cases of ambiguous genitalia occur as components of multiple malformation syndromes or as development defects, often associated with anomalies of the genitourinary tract and/or lower intestinal tract. If the adrenogenital syndrome is suspected, the infant must be carefully monitored for sodium depletion or hypertension while awaiting results of assays for urinary steroid metabolites.

INDICATIONS FOR CHROMOSOME ANALYSIS

1. Congenital malformations. Infants with multiple congenital anomalies of unknown etiology often have chromosomal anomalies (see above). Single malformations, even when severe (eg, congenital heart defects, neural tube defects), are rarely associated with chromosome aberrations, but minor defects that are easily overlooked must be carefully sought. Frequently the radiologist will find unsuspected skeletal anomalies, and therefore x-rays are part of the work-up of any patient who may have a syndrome. Similarly, patients with **nonspecific mental retardation,** infants who **fail to thrive,** and **small-for-gestational age** newborns provide a low yield of abnormal karyotypes but may still constitute indications for analysis; the discovery of the chromosome anomaly may prompt a more detailed search for malformations, some of which may be correctable (eg, early diagnosis of a urinary tract obstruction or abnormal vertebrae could greatly benefit the patient).

2. Ambiguous external genitalia (see above, and in INTERSEX STATES in Ch. 187). Because of the wide variety of chromosomal variation that may lead to ambiguity, the buccal smear is no longer acceptable for even a presumptive diagnosis of either sex. In the rare event where the biologic sex must be obtained quickly (eg, to avoid serious psychologic problems for parents), a bone marrow aspirate may be used for immediate preparation of karyotypes.

3. Habitual abortion. Although a major chromosome anomaly is found in no more than 3% of couples who have had 2 or more spontaneous abortions, karyotyping both parents is part of the work-up.

4. Infertility. After anatomic defects are excluded as the cause, the couple should be karyotyped. Again, the buccal smear is inadequate. Both 47,XXY males and females with a variety of X chromosome anomalies may appear perfectly normal, but may be sterile.

5. Sperm donors. Males participating in artificial insemination by donor programs should be karyotyped in order to rule out a translocation or other heritable chromosome anomaly.

6. X-linked mental retardation. Special chromosome studies for the fragile X are indicated.

7. Cancer cytogenetics. Data from chromosome analyses are being used in the diagnosis and management of an increasing number of malignancies, especially leukemias and lymphomas.

GENETIC COUNSELING IN CHROMOSOME ANOMALIES

Fortunately, most syndromes associated with chromosome anomalies occur only once in a family, and an optimistic prognosis for future offspring can usually be given after appropriate studies are completed. Parental karyotypes are essential for all patients with a translocation or deletion syndrome to be sure that the rearrangement was not inherited. When either parent is found to be a balanced carrier of any chromosome rearrangement, the siblings of both the patient and the affected parent are at risk and additional chromosome studies are indicated. The availability of prenatal diagnosis and prevention through selective abortion must be presented to those at risk (see below).

Patients with **Down's syndrome** due to trisomy 21 present unique problems. Surprisingly, the majority of familial cases are trisomy 21 rather than translocations, and only a few result from parental mosaicism (mosaicism may lead to multiple cases but only within one sibship). Thus, regardless of maternal age, the parents of any child with Down's syndrome are at high risk (at least 1%) of having another affected child and should be made aware of amniocentesis. The siblings of these parents, however, are *not* at increased risk as long as there are no other close relatives with trisomy 21.

PREVENTION OF GENETIC DISORDERS

The goal of the medical geneticist is to identify individuals who, because of their particular hereditary background, conditioned by their lifetime of special experiences, are unsuited for the environment in which they find themselves. Neither genes nor environment cause disease, and when individuals at high risk are identified, methods are becoming increasingly available to mitigate the effects of both the genome and the uniquely offensive components of the environment. For conditions not yet treatable or detectable prenatally, prevention by contraception may be necessary, with adoption or artificial insemination as options (the latter is becoming more acceptable and should be discussed when appropriate).

THE IMPACT OF ADVANCES IN MOLECULAR GENETICS

The speed with which the new DNA technology is being moved from the laboratory bench to the care of patients is without precedent in the history of medicine. A few of the main acts in this rapidly developing drama are highlighted below.

The isolation of human genes: Technics for purification of DNA and RNA, separation of the 2 polynucleotide strands of the double helix, and understanding the triplet code for translating the sequence of bases in the genetic material to the corresponding sequence of amino acids in polypeptide chains were crucial. For example, the gene for human insulin was synthesized by first purifying the 2 polypeptide chains of the hormone itself. The sequence of amino acids yielded the sequence of bases that coded them, and the appropriate bases were chemically linked together in the correct order in vitro. The genes for the α- and β-hemoglobin polypeptide chains were synthesized from purified messenger RNA (mRNA). The specific RNA was relatively easy to purify from human erythroid precursor cells because about half of their total mRNA is for Hb production. Transcription from an RNA template to DNA occurs thanks to the enzyme, reverse transcriptase. Several additional methods for purifying and analyzing human genes have been developed, and it turns out that a gene is not simply a segment of DNA coding for the amino acid sequence of a polypeptide chain. Instead, it consists of coding sequences called **exons** that are interspersed by non-coding intervening sequences known as **introns.** The introns are transcribed initially but are spliced out of the messenger RNA before it leaves the cell nucleus. The function of the introns is unknown but many of the mutations that cause β-thalassemia, for example, lie within them. In addition, there are flanking sequences on both sides of structural genes that regulate their activity and provide start and stop signals for their transcription.

Restriction endonucleases are bacterial enzymes that break the genetic material into thousands of pieces, but each specific endonuclease breaks the DNA or RNA only when there is a very specific sequence of bases. For example, one endonuclease might recognize the sequence G-C-C-T-A-A and break the chain between the T and the A (the 4 bases that make up the DNA are *C*ytosine, *G*uanine, *T*hymidine, and *A*denine). This sequence will occur by chance over and over again in the human genome and thus the many fragments of varying lengths, as shown in FIG. 203–7.

Cloning the genes is the vital step whereby a piece, eg, of human DNA, be it a purified gene or not, is inserted into a cloning vehicle, usually a bacterial **plasmid** (*a circular bit of DNA present naturally in bacteria*), and then the bacterium is cultured. Each newly produced plasmid contains the human DNA, and literally billions of copies of the human gene or DNA segment can be produced in this bacterial factory. The circular plasmids can be opened for insertion of foreign DNA using restriction endonucleases. The combination of bacterial plasmid and a human DNA segment is one example of recombinant DNA.

The gene probe: Any segment of DNA or RNA will bind to its complementary sequence. That is how the **double helix** is formed from a single strand in the first place—G always binds to C, and A to T. Thus, if one takes the many copies of one of the cloned genes described above and adds a radioactive label to each copy, one has a labeled probe. The probe will seek out its complementary segment of DNA and can then be found by autoradiography. A probe added to a chromosome spread can actually locate a gene in a specific chromosome or use it to identify a piece of DNA in a "Southern blot," as illustrated in FIG. 203–7.

The Southern blot, a procedure named after the investigator who devised it, is the cornerstone of the applications of recombinant DNA to prevention of genetically determined disease. The technic is outlined in FIG. 203–7. Briefly, DNA is extracted

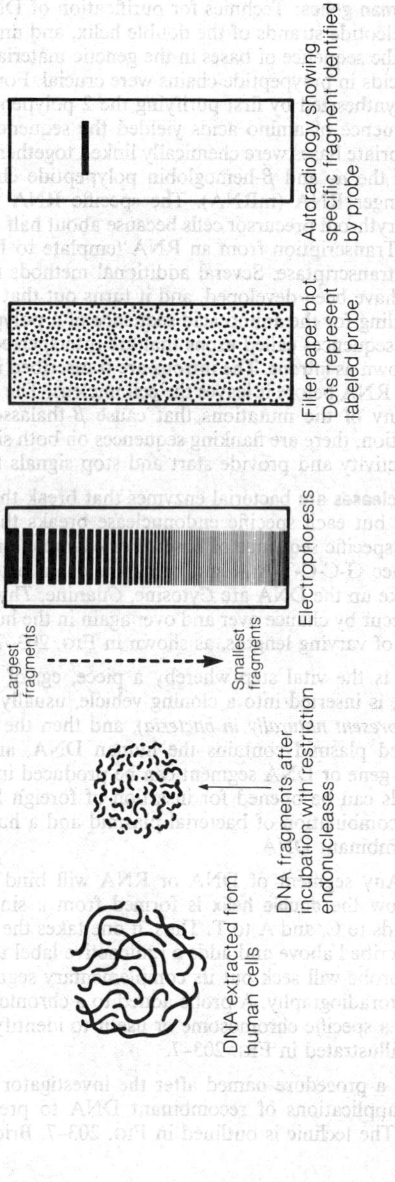

FIG. 203–7. The Southern blot technic.

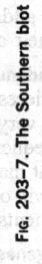

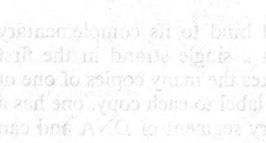

from cells of the patient and fragmented by one of the restriction endonucleases. The fragments are electrophoresed, which separates them primarily by size, the smaller ones moving more rapidly through the pores of the gel. The fragments are then blotted onto nitrocellulose filter paper and overlaid with a labeled probe. The probe will bind only to its complementary sequence and thus identify the gene of interest as a band or bands on the paper.

Restriction fragment length polymorphisms (RFLPs): The various available restriction endonucleases have revealed a remarkable amount of variability in the human genome. If just one base substitution occurs in the sequence recognized by the endonuclease, the DNA will not break at that site and instead of 2 small fragments, there will be one big one. The different-sized fragments will move to different places in the Southern blot procedure and the probe will identify the different-sized fragments, as shown in FIG. 203–8. Since these variants are so common, they have provided us with an almost unending series of markers known as RFLPs. If the base substitution occurs within the gene in question, and coincidentally at the site of the mutation that causes the disease,

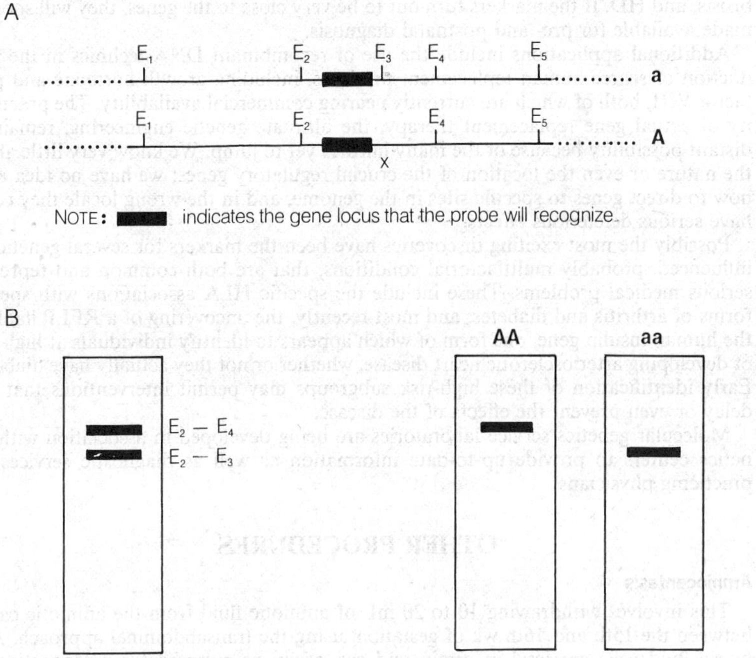

FIG. 203–8. Detection of restriction fragment length polymorphism (RFLP).

A. Depicted are small sections of 2 homologous chromosomes, **a** and **A**. E_1, E_2 . . . E_5 are the breakpoints caused by a restriction endonuclease, E.

In chromosome **A**, a base substitution is present at the site marked x; thus, the site is not recognized by E. No break occurs and a large fragment results. The probe will bind to both the E_2-E_3 fragment of chromosome **a** and the E_2-E_4 fragment of chromosome **A**, the latter being the larger. After Southern blotting and autoradiography, the probe will identify both fragments (see Figure B).

B. Some people will be homozygous **AA** and others **aa**. **AA** individuals will have only the large E_2-E_4 fragment; **aa** individuals, the E_2-E_3.

as is the case for sickle cell anemia, the marker will identify an individual's genotype without family studies. If the variant flanks the gene in question but is very close to it, as in Huntington's disease **(HD)**, family studies are required to determine which sized fragment is associated with the HD gene in a given family.

Medical applications: The technics above have already led to extraordinary advances in mapping the human genome, and it is just a matter of time for the development of probes for most of the human diseases resulting from single gene mutations even though the nature of the genetic defect is unknown. This will permit precise identification of genotype, including heterozygotes and homozygotes, and provide the means for diagnosis before birth and before the development of detectable clinical signs in such conditions as HD. Genes whose function is unknown, such as the HD and Duchenne muscular dystrophy genes, will soon be isolated and sequenced and their products deduced, which could lead to understanding of the basic defect and eventually to treatment approaches. Already reported are probes for the X-linked genes causing the hemophilias, Lesch-Nyhan syndrome, and Duchenne muscular dystrophy. Probes available for other medically important conditions due to autosomal mutant genes include the hemoglobinopathies, phenylketonuria, α_1-antitrypsin deficiency, cystic fibrosis, and HD. If the markers turn out to be very close to the genes, they will soon be made available for pre- and postnatal diagnosis.

Additional applications include the use of recombinant DNA technics in the production of scarce human replacement products, including growth hormone and pure factor VIII, both of which are currently nearing commercial availability. The practicality of actual gene replacement therapy, the ultimate genetic engineering, remains a distant possibility because of the many hurdles yet to jump. We know very little about the nature or even the location of the crucial regulatory genes; we have no idea as to how to direct genes to specific sites in the genome, and in the wrong locale they could have serious deleterious effects.

Possibly the most exciting discoveries have been the markers for several genetically influenced, probably multifactorial conditions, that are both common and represent serious medical problems. These include the specific HLA associations with specific forms of arthritis and diabetes, and most recently, the uncovering of a RFLP flanking the human insulin gene, one form of which appears to identify individuals at high risk of developing arteriosclerotic heart disease, whether or not they actually have diabetes. Early identification of these high-risk subgroups may permit interventions that will delay or even prevent the effects of the disease.

Molecular genetics service laboratories are being developed in association with genetics centers to provide up-to-date information as well as diagnostic services for practicing physicians.

OTHER PROCEDURES

Amniocentesis

This involves withdrawing 10 to 20 mL of amniotic fluid from the amniotic cavity between the 15th and 16th wk of gestation, using the transabdominal approach. Amniotic fluid cells are fetal in origin and can easily be cultured for cytogenetic and biochemical studies. The indications for amniocentesis are:

1. Advanced maternal age. The risk of producing a child with a trisomy, especially trisomy 21, begins to rise rapidly in the mid 30s. Discrepancies between liveborn and amniocentesis-based surveys exist, but from the latter, the incidence of Down's syndrome due to trisomy 21 ranges from 1:200 to 1:50 for ages 35 to 39, while in ages 40 to 45, the risks are between 2 to 6:100. Most physicians feel that women who will be over age 35 at the time of delivery should be told of the risk and offered amniocentesis. There is a minor paternal age effect but it is of little practical importance: For exam-

ple, the husband of a 34-yr-old woman would have to be 70 to increase her risk to that of a 35-yr-old woman.

2. Previous trisomic offspring. When a couple has produced a still- or liveborn child with any trisomy, the risk in a subsequent pregnancy is increased.

3. Translocation carriers. When one parent carries a chromosome translocation, 5 to 100% of the offspring may be aborted or liveborn with multiple malformations, depending on which parent and which chromosomes are involved. In general, in nonhomologous translocations the risk is greater when the mother is the carrier.

4. Sex determination. The karyotype constructed from cultured fetal cells permits determination of fetal sex before birth. Where the mother has been identified as a carrier of an X-linked mutant and a specific test for the affected fetus is not available, fetal sex determination may be carried out with the option to abort males, although half of them will be normal. The availability of specific X chromosome DNA probes will soon permit identification of the affected male (see above). Prenatal sex determination should not be offered to couples who wish to have a child of a specific sex for nongenetic reasons.

5. Metabolic diseases: If both parents have been identified as carriers of the same abnormal autosomal recessive gene (ie, they have already had a child with an inborn error of metabolism or participated in a heterozygote screening program) and the disease can be detected prenatally, amniocentesis should be offered. More than 100 conditions can now be diagnosed prenatally, including glycogen storage diseases, mucopolysaccharidoses, aminoacidurias, diseases of lipid metabolism, and miscellaneous conditions such as the adrenogenital syndrome. A few X-linked diseases (eg, Hunter and Lesch-Nyhan syndromes) are also detectable by enzyme assay of cultured amniotic fluid cells.

6. Previous neural tube anomaly: Couples who have produced a baby with a neural tube defect, such as anencephaly, myelomeningocele, or encephalocele, have a 2 to 5% risk of such a defect recurring in a subsequent pregnancy, as compared to the population incidence in North American whites of about 1:700 births. The incidence among blacks is $< 1:3000$. The same increased risk applies to the children of an affected parent. Second-degree relatives of an affected individual (nieces, nephews) have about a 1:100 risk; for first cousins, the risk is about 1:200. There is little if any increased risk for other family members. α-Fetoprotein is elevated in $> 90\%$ of the amniotic fluids of fetuses with open neural tube defects, and this test is used to screen pregnancies at high risk. Today most geneticists suggest amniocentesis and detailed ultrasound for first-degree relatives, and maternal serum α-fetoprotein with ultrasound for second- and third-degree relatives. Other conditions (eg, presence of fetal blood, threatened abortion, twins, omphalocele, exstrophy of the bladder, fetal death, Turner's syndrome, congenital nephrosis, duodenal atresia) also result in elevated α-fetoprotein, necessitating confirmation of diagnosis by ultrasonography and assay of amniotic fluid for acetylcholinesterase activity of neurologic origin. Neither spina bifida occulta nor isolated congenital hydrocephalus is considered to be a neural tube defect.

7. Other congenital defects: The technics for prenatal diagnosis of kidney anomalies such as renal agenesis (Potter's syndrome) and polycystic disease, lethal forms of short-limbed dwarfism (thanatophoric dwarf, achondrogenesis), anomalies of the gut (diaphragmatic hernia, obstruction), and micro- and hydrocephalus are being provided by rapidly advancing technology using ultrasonography and fetoscopy.

8. Maternal insulin-dependent diabetes: There is up to a tenfold increase in the risk of a neural tube defect, which brings the incidence to between 1 and 2%. In addition, the risk of other congenital anomalies, particularly those involving the sacrum and lower limbs, is increased. However, it is now clear that careful control of blood glucose, particularly prior to conception through embryogenesis, will significantly lower the risk of fetal malformations. Detailed ultrasound examinations of the fetus at 16 and 18 wk along with maternal serum α-fetoprotein should be offered.

Complications of amniocentesis at 16 wk are uncommon. Fetal loss due to the procedure occurs in about 1:200 amniocenteses, but other serious injury to the fetus has not been reported. Infection is rare. Although amniotic fluid leak, hemorrhage (fetal or maternal), or both occur in 1 to 2% of cases, they usually cease after a short period of bed rest. Cell culture failures and incorrect cytogenetic diagnosis are very rare in experienced laboratories.

Chorionic Villus Sampling (CVS)

This is a new prenatal diagnostic procedure that is being studied in several multicenter research projects, while already being offered as a service in some genetics centers. A sample of chorionic villi is obtained by inserting a flexible catheter through the vagina and cervix, and advancing it to the site of fetal implantation under direct ultrasound guidance. About 10 to 30 mg of villi are then aspirated into a syringe; any contaminating maternal tissue is removed under a dissecting microscope; and karyotypes can be prepared directly from the villi, which contain many dividing cells. Alternatively, short-term cell culture (3 days) may be carried out. Most, if not all, of the enzymes present in cultured amniotic fluid cells are also measurable in extracts of chorionic villi or cultured villus cells, and DNA can be extracted from these fetal cells for molecular genetic studies.

Important advantages of CVS are these: It is done at 8 to 10 wk of gestation, which is 2 mo earlier than amniocentesis, and results are available within hours or days rather than weeks. Thus, if a couple elects termination of pregnancy because of an abnormal result, a 1st trimester abortion is easier and safer than one at 20 wk.

The main problem with CVS is the risk—its magnitude is unknown. Data currently indicate a miscarriage rate of between 2 to 6% as a direct result of the procedure. In addition, data are insufficient on the chance of causing harm to the fetus that goes on to term after CVS.

If this procedure proves to be safe, relatively inexpensive, and acceptable to pregnant women, it will lead to at least one major ethical problem: Should it be offered to all, regardless of maternal age, for prenatal diagnosis of chromosome anomalies, 80% of which occur in the offspring of women *under* age 35?

Screening Programs

Newborn: Screening of newborn infants for **PKU** to detect the condition before significant CNS damage occurs is almost worldwide. When the diagnosis is confirmed, dietary treatment is started, so that mental retardation is prevented. Screening tests using dried blood spots on filter paper have been automated and expanded to permit early detection of other inborn errors of metabolism amenable to treatment, such as galactosemia, maple syrup urine disease, and some forms of homocystinuria. The same patient specimens have been adapted to detect congenital hypothyroidism, a relatively common cause of mental retardation (1:3000 births) in which early institution of therapy is crucial. Screening programs are under way throughout North America.

Screening for heterozygotes: Tay-Sachs disease, the model for this approach to prevention of genetic disease, is inherited as an autosomal recessive condition and is found primarily among the Ashkenazi (Eastern European) Jews. The disease can be diagnosed with precision, both pre- and postnatally, and the carrier or heterozygote can also be accurately detected. Screening programs in several urban centers determined the carrier frequency to be between 1:20 and 1:30 Ashkenazi Jews. Many couples at risk have been identified, and several affected fetuses have been detected prenatally by amniocentesis and have been aborted. Since only a fraction of the Jewish community has been screened, the physician should apprise every Ashkenazi Jewish couple of the risk of Tay-Sachs disease, preferably before any pregnancy occurs. The couple should then have the opportunity to be tested if they wish. Information for both

doctor and patient is available from the Tay-Sachs Foundation. This approach has resulted in the near disappearance of Tay-Sachs disease in the Jewish population.

Sickle cell disease, thalassemia, and other hemoglobinopathies are now preventable. The populations at risk have been identified (Southern Italians, Greeks, and other Mediterranean peoples for β-thalassemia; orientals for α-thalassemia variants; and blacks for both sickle cell disease and thalassemias), and carrier detection is readily available, accurate, and relatively inexpensive. Tests for accurate determination of affected fetuses using microliter amounts of fetal RBCs have been perfected, but reliable and safe methods of obtaining fetal blood specimens have yet to be established. Aspiration of placental blood using ultrasound guidance for placement of the needle and puncture of a placental vessel under direct vision with a fetoscope are being used, but fetal loss as a result of the procedure is about 5% even in the most experienced hands. However, new molecular technics using restriction endonucleases can identify the specific gene defect in amniotic fluid cells and chorionic villi (see above); fetal blood specimens are only rarely necessary for prenatal diagnosis of most hemoglobinopathies.

Screening for neural tube defects: Since 9:10 infants with such defects are born to couples with no prior history of an affected baby, amniocentesis for high-risk couples can have little effect on the incidence. However, in > 80% of cases, α-fetoprotein is significantly elevated in maternal serum at 16 to 18 wk gestation. Several pilot research projects in Canada, the USA, and the United Kingdom have shown that maternal serum α-fetoprotein screening for all pregnant women who wish to participate is feasible, sufficiently accurate, cost-effective, and acceptable to a large proportion of the population. The FDA has removed the restrictions on the reagents used in the serum test, and serum screening is now available in most of the USA. However, the physician must exercise great care in the choice of laboratory or center that he uses. Interpretation of serum and amniotic fluid α-fetoprotein levels requires experience and the collaboration of a skilled ultrasonographer, both for the confirmation of gestational age and for the detailed sonography required when the serum α-fetoproteins are consistently elevated.

Screening for Down's syndrome: Recently obtained data indicate that in most pregnancies where the fetus has Down's syndrome, the maternal serum α-fetoprotein is below the median. Cutoff points, below which amniocentesis for fetal karyotyping would be indicated, are in the process of being determined for various maternal ages.

GENETIC SCREENING IN THE WORKPLACE

This new concept is causing considerable conflict between labor and management. The issue is the employee or potential employee who, because of some genetically determined trait, is less suited to some specific job than an individual who does not have that trait. Many feel that such screening interferes with the individual's freedom of choice, could be considered an unfair labor practice, and would insist that the workplace be made safe for everyone, regardless of his or her genetic makeup.

On the other hand, this genetic approach may be reasonable for individuals making career or lifestyle decisions. First, however, unequivocal associations must be established between "deleterious genes" and specific environmental factors, and then interventions proved to be effective must be developed.

TERATOLOGY

Exposures to potentially teratogenic drugs (see also DRUGS IN PREGNANCY in Ch. 176), various forms of radiation, and industrial pollutants have become a major problem for physicians managing pregnancies. Up-to-date information pertaining to

humans is difficult to find and to interpret, and much of the available data has not been critically appraised. However, most genetics centers in North America now have access to well-designed, computerized teratogen information services that provide the latest information on both animal and human studies. Physicians would be well advised to find out about the availability of such a service in their areas and to use it whenever the questions arise.

GLOSSARY OF GENETIC TERMS

Allele (allelomorph): Alternative forms of a gene. There may be many alleles for a given gene, but each person possesses only 2 alleles for each gene, receiving one of each pair of alleles from each parent. A person with a pair of similar alleles is a homozygote; one with a dissimilar pair is a heterozygote.

Amniography: Opacification of amniotic fluid by injecting radiopaque material in order to visualize the fetal skeleton and soft tissues more clearly.

Aneuploidy: An irregular number of chromosomes (eg, 45, 47, or 48 chromosomes in man), caused by the loss or addition of one or more chromosomes or parts of chromosomes.

Autoradiography: The process by which a radioactive label is used to identify a specific biologic process or material by overlaying with x-ray film and observing exposed areas that usually appear as dots or bands.

Autosomal: Located on, or transmitted by, an autosome.

Autosomes: Those chromosomes that are not sex chromosomes. Man has 22 pairs of autosomes.

Barr body: The sex chromatin mass in somatic cells of the female (see Sex chromatin).

Carrier: An individual who carries a recessive gene, either autosomal or sex-linked, together with its normal allele, but who does not himself show any clinically detectable effects of the gene; ie, a heterozygote for a recessive gene.

Centromere: The constricted portion of the chromosome, which is the point of attachment to the equatorial plane of the mitotic or meiotic spindle.

Chromatid: A chromosome at prophase and metaphase consists of 2 strands attached to the centromere. Each strand is a chromatid (see Mitosis).

Chromatin: The substance in cell nuclei and chromosomes that stains intensely with basic dyes, composed of DNA combined with proteins. In the fixed intermitotic nucleus, it usually takes the form of an irregular network of long coiled threads, which are gradually condensed into individual chromosomes as the cell undergoes division.

Chromatin-negative: Refers to nuclei that lack the sex chromatin mass, or Barr body. Characteristic of the normal human male.

Chromatin-positive: Refers to nuclei containing the distinctive sex chromatin mass. Characteristic of the normal human female.

Chromosomal aberration (or **abnormality**): A deviation from the normal morphology of chromosomes.

Chromosome: One of a number of small bodies, occurring in pairs, into which the chromatin material of a cell nucleus resolves itself prior to cell division. Chromosomes are visible only during cell division. Homologous chromosomes are the 2 members of one pair, one of maternal and one of paternal origin. Chromosomes bear the vehicles of hereditary traits, the genes. The morphologic characteristics of the individual chro-

mosomes and their total number are constant for all the somatic cells of a given species. Major chemical components are DNA, RNA, histones, and nonhistone proteins.

Chromosome number: The number of chromosomes found in the somatic cells of an individual or of a species; normally, 46 in man.

Clone: A colony of cells that originated from a single cell.

Congenital: Present at birth; not necessarily genetic.

Consanguinity: Relationship by descent from a common ancestor.

Crossing-over: The exchange of corresponding segments between maternal and paternal homologous chromosomes, occurring when maternal and paternal homologous chromosomes are paired during prophase of the first meiotic division.

Cytogenetics: A branch of genetics dealing with the cytologic basis of heredity; ie, with the study of the chromosomes.

Diploid: The normal complement of chromosomes (in humans, 22 pairs of homologous chromosomes and the sex chromosomes).

Dizygotic (or **dizygous**) **twins**: Twins resulting from the simultaneous fertilization of 2 ova by 2 spermatozoa. Recurrence in families is common. (*Synonym*: Fraternal twins.)

Dominant gene: A gene that expresses its effect even when it is present on only one chromosome.

Empiric risk: The prediction of the probability that a genetic or congenital abnormality will occur in a family.

Exon: A segment of a gene that is represented in the mature messenger RNA and which codes for a portion of the structure of a protein.

Expressivity: The extent to which a trait is manifested. The kind or degree of phenotypic expression may be slight or pronounced.

Gamete: A male or female reproductive cell; a spermatozoon or ovum.

Gene frequency: Refers to the relative proportion of each of 2 or more alleles of a particular gene in a given population. The gene frequency may be expressed as a percentage (0 to 100%) or as a probability (0 to 1).

Genetic code: The sequential order of the bases of DNA, which carry the genetic information.

Genome: All the genes found in a diploid set of chromosomes.

Genotype: The full set of genes carried by an individual. The term is sometimes used in a more limited way to refer to the alleles present at one or more loci.

Haploid: The number of chromosomes in a normal gamete, which contains only one member of each chromosome pair; in man, the haploid number is 23.

Hemizygous: Since males have only one X chromosome, they are said to be hemizygous with respect to X-linked genes.

Hermaphrodite: An individual with both male and female gonadal tissue (not necessarily functional).

Heterologous: Chromosomes or chromosomal segments that are nonhomologous (see Homologous) or nonidentical.

Heterozygote: An individual possessing differing alleles at a given locus on a pair of homologous chromosomes. (*Adjective*: Heterozygous.)

Homologous: Chromosomes or chromosomal segments that are identical with respect to genetic loci and visible structure; eg, 2 normal chromosome 15s. (*Noun*: Homologues.)

Homozygote: An individual possessing a pair of identical alleles at a given locus on a pair of homologous chromosomes. (*Adjective*: Homozygous.)

Inborn error of metabolism: A genetically determined biochemical disorder in which a specific enzyme defect produces a metabolic block that may have pathologic consequences.

Incidence: The number of infants born with a condition/number of live births in a given population. (Compare with Prevalence.)

Intron: A segment of a gene that is initially transcribed but then spliced out of the messenger RNA: It is an intervening segment of DNA between 2 exons.

Isochromosome: A chromosome in which the arms on either side of the centromere are identical.

Karyotype: The full complement of chromosomes; the term covers the number, relative sizes, and morphology of the chromosomes.

Linkage: Genes that have their loci on the same chromosome are said to be linked. Also used to describe traits transmitted by a gene of known locus on a specific chromosome (eg, see X-linkage).

Locus: The precise location of a gene on a chromosome. Different forms of the gene (alleles) are always found at the same locus on the chromosome.

Meiosis: Nuclear division that occurs during the formation of gametes. Two consecutive cell divisions (the 1st and 2nd meiotic divisions) occur, but only one division of the chromosomes occurs. Thus, the number of chromosomes is reduced from the diploid (46) to the haploid (23) number. During meiosis, pairing of homologous chromosomes takes place, followed by chromosomal breakage and crossing-over. The end result of meiosis is 4 cells, each with 1/2 the number of chromosomes possessed by the original cell.

Metaphase: That stage of cell division (mitosis or meiosis) during which the chromosomes line up on the spindle equatorial plate.

Mitosis: A form of nuclear division in which each chromosome splits lengthwise (**replicates** itself), one chromatid of each chromosome passing to one daughter cell and the other chromatid to the 2nd daughter cell. Thus, each daughter cell receives the full complement of 46 chromosomes. This type of cell division is characteristic of somatic cells, and of germ cells before the onset of meiosis.

Monozygotic (or **monozygous**) **twins**: Twins resulting from the division into 2 embryos of a single zygote, following fertilization of a single ovum by a single spermatozoon. Recurrence within families is rare. (*Synonym*: Identical or one-egg twins.)

Mosaic: An individual with 2 or more cell lines differing in genotype.

Multifactorial inheritance: Inheritance of a trait governed by many genes or **multiple factors**. Each gene may act independently with cumulative total effect. Height, weight, and other body dimensions are determined by multifactorial inheritance.

Mutation: A permanent heritable change in the genetic material. Mutations are an important source of hereditary diversity.

Mutation rate: The frequency of detectable mutations/genic locus/generation.

Oncogene: A gene that can cause a tumor.

Penetrance: The frequency of phenotypic expression of a dominant gene or a homozygous recessive gene. When a dominant gene produces no detectable phenotypic expression, it shows **lack of penetrance.**

Phenocopy: An individual with all the hallmarks of a particular genetic disorder but with no hereditary cause apparent in his pedigree.

Phenotype: The total of all observable features of an individual (including his anatomic, physiologic, biochemical, and psychologic makeup, and his disease reactions, potential or actual). The phenotype is the result of interaction between the genotype and the environment. The term may also apply to the trait produced by a single gene or several genes.

Population genetics: The study of mutant genes in populations rather than in individuals.

Prevalence: The number of individuals with a specific condition in a given population.

Proband: The individual with an abnormality whose relatives are studied to determine the hereditary or genetic aspects of the trait. (*Synonyms*: Propositus [male]; proposita [female]; index case.)

Probe: A radioactive DNA or RNA sequence used to detect the presence of a complementary sequence by molecular hybridization.

Prophase: The first stage of cell division, during which the chromosomes become visible as discrete structures.

Recessive: A **trait** is recessive if it is expressed only in individuals who are homozygous (or hemizygous) for the gene concerned; a **gene** is recessive if it is expressed only in homozygous (or hemizygous) individuals.

Restriction endonucleases: A family of bacterial enzymes, each of which breaks DNA or RNA at specific base sequences. In bacteria, these enzymes "restrict" the entry of foreign genetic material (eg, viruses) that would be harmful.

Restriction fragment length polymorphism (RFLP): Different-length fragments of DNA present at the same site or locus in a chromosome and uncovered by restriction endonucleases.

Ring chromosome: A circular chromosome resulting from breakage in both arms of a chromatid followed by fusion of the broken ends to form a ring. Varying amounts of chromosomal material are lost or deleted from both arms.

Segregation: The separation of the 2 alleles of a pair of allelic genes during meiosis, so that they pass to different gametes.

Sex chromatin: A chromatin mass in the nucleus of interphase cells of females. It represents a single X chromosome, which is inactive in the metabolism of the cell. Normal females have sex chromatin, thus are **chromatin-positive;** normal males lack it, hence are **chromatin-negative**. (*Synonym*: Barr body.)

Sex chromosomes: Chromosomes responsible for sex determination (XX in females; XY in males).

Sex-limited: Affecting one sex only.

Sex-linkage: Inheritance by genes on the sex chromosomes, especially on the X chromosomes.

Somatic cell: Soma refers to body, and the term is used for all of the body's nonreproductive cells. Somatic cells are diploid; germ cells are haploid.

Southern blot: A technic for transferring DNA fragments separated by gel electrophoresis to nitrocellulose paper for molecular hybridization to labeled probes.

Teratogen: Any agent that causes a physical defect or defects in a developing embryo or fetus.

Translocation: A change in location of genetic material, either within a chromosome or from one chromosome to another.

Trisomy: The presence of 3, rather than 2, chromosomes in a particular set; eg, individuals with 3 sex chromosomes, XXX, XXY, or XYY, are trisomic for the sex chromosomes.

X chromosome: A sex chromosome that occurs singly in the normal male, in duplicate in the normal female.

X-linkage: Transmission of a trait by a gene on the X chromosome.

Y chromosome: A sex chromosome that occurs singly in the normal male, but is absent in the normal female.

§17. OTOLARYNGOLOGY

204. CLINICAL EVALUATION OF COMPLAINTS REFERABLE TO THE EARS

Hearing loss, tinnitus, vertigo, earache, and otorrhea are the principal symptoms attributed to the ears. A thorough history should be taken and a physical examination performed with emphasis on the ears, nose, nasopharynx, and paranasal sinuses to evaluate complaints referable to the ears. In addition, the teeth, tongue, tonsils, hypopharynx, larynx, salivary glands, and temporomandibular joints should be examined, since pain and discomfort may be referred from them to the ears. Radiography or CT of the temporal bones is usually indicated in trauma to the ear, possible basal skull fracture, perforation of the tympanic membrane, hearing loss, vertigo, facial paralysis, and otalgia of obscure origin. Measurements of auditory and vestibular functions are of great diagnostic importance in patients with complaints referable to the ears.

HEARING LOSS

Hearing loss caused by a lesion in the external auditory canal or the middle ear is called **conductive,** while hearing loss due to a lesion in the inner ear or the 8th nerve is called **sensorineural.** Conductive and sensorineural hearing loss can be differentiated by comparing the threshold of hearing by air conduction with that by bone conduction

(see also DIFFERENTIATION OF SENSORY [COCHLEAR] AND NEURAL [8TH NERVE] HEARING LOSSES, below).

CLINICAL MEASUREMENT OF HEARING

Hearing by air conduction is tested by presenting an acoustic stimulus, in air, to the ear. A hearing loss or elevation of the threshold demonstrated in this way can be caused by a defect in any part of the hearing apparatus—external auditory canal, middle ear, inner ear, 8th nerve, or central auditory pathways.

Hearing by bone conduction is tested by placing a sounding source (eg, the oscillator of an audiometer or the stem of a tuning fork) in contact with the head. This causes vibration throughout the skull, including the walls of the bony cochlea, and stimulates the inner ear directly. Hearing by bone conduction bypasses the external and middle ear and tests the integrity of the inner ear, 8th nerve, and central pathways.

If the air conduction threshold is elevated and the bone conduction threshold is normal, the hearing loss is *conductive*. If both air and bone conduction thresholds are elevated equally, the hearing loss is *sensorineural*. Occasionally, a **composite** or **mixed** loss of hearing occurs, with both conductive and sensorineural components. Under these circumstances, both bone and air conduction thresholds are elevated, the air conduction more than the bone.

The Weber and Rinne tuning fork tests are used to differentiate a conductive from a sensorineural hearing loss. For these tests, tuning forks with frequencies of 256, 512, 1024, and 2048 Hz are used. The **Weber tuning fork test** is performed by placing the stem of a vibrating tuning fork on the midline of the head and having the patient indicate in which ear the tone is heard. The patient with a unilateral *conductive* hearing loss hears the tone louder in the affected ear, for reasons that are unclear. By contrast, the patient with a unilateral *sensorineural* loss hears the tone in the unaffected ear, because the tuning fork stimulates both inner ears equally and the patient perceives the stimulus with the more sensitive, unaffected end organ and nerve.

The **Rinne tuning fork test** compares hearing ability by air conduction with that by bone conduction. The tines of a vibrating tuning fork are held near the pinna (air conduction) and then the stem of the vibrating tuning fork is placed in contact with the mastoid process (bone conduction) and the patient is asked to indicate which stimulus is louder. Normally the stimulus is heard longer and louder by air conduction than by bone conduction; eg, 40 sec by air conduction and 20 sec by bone conduction (AC>BC). With a conductive hearing loss, this ratio is reversed; the bone conduction stimulus will be perceived longer and louder than the air conduction stimulus (BC>AC). With a sensorineural hearing loss, both air and bone conduction perception are reduced, but the ratio remains the same (AC>BC).

The **audiometer** is used to quantitate hearing loss. With this electronic device, acoustic stimuli of specific frequencies (pure tones) are delivered at specific intensities in order to determine the patient's hearing threshold for each frequency. The hearing for each ear is measured from 125 or 250 to 8000 Hz by air conduction (using earphones) and by bone conduction (using an oscillator in contact with the head). Hearing loss is measured in decibels **(dB)**, which equal 10 times the logarithm of the ratio of the acoustic power of a stimulus required to achieve hearing threshold in a patient to the acoustic power required to achieve threshold in a normal individual. Test results are plotted on graphs called audiograms (FIG. 204–1). If intense tones are presented to one ear, they may be heard in the other ear. The Rinne tuning fork test and audiometry require the use of masking for accurate results. **Masking** is presentation of sound (usually noise) to the ear not being tested so that responses are based on hearing in the ear being tested.

Speech audiometry: The **spondee threshold (ST)**, the intensity at which speech is recognized as a meaningful symbol, is determined by presenting a list of spondee

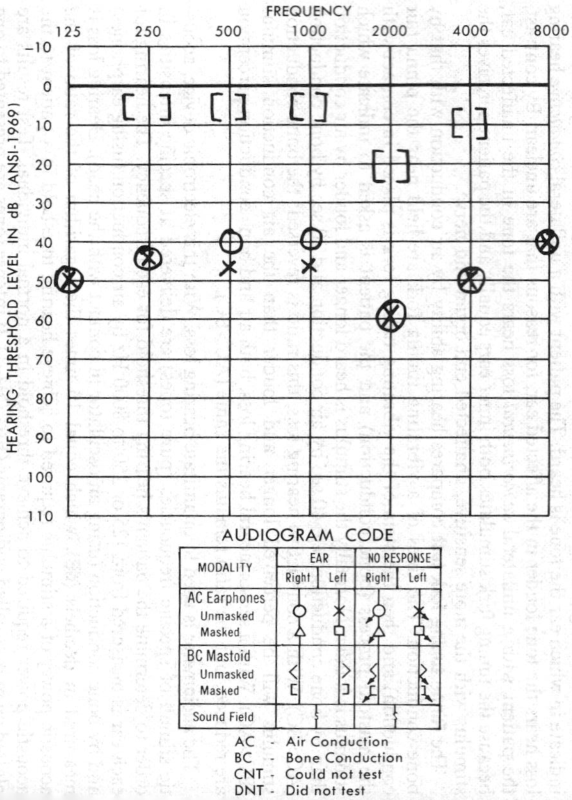

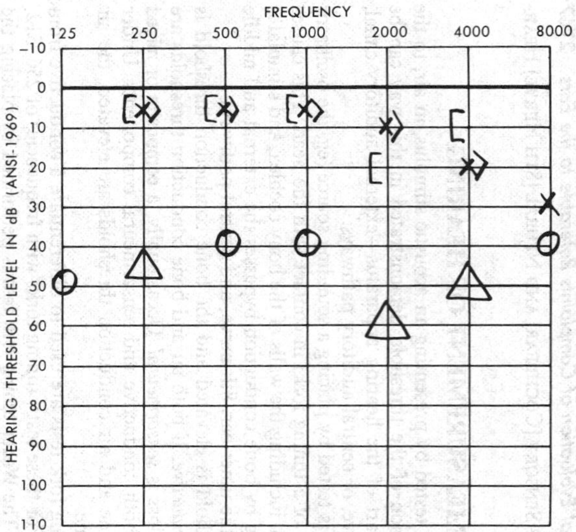

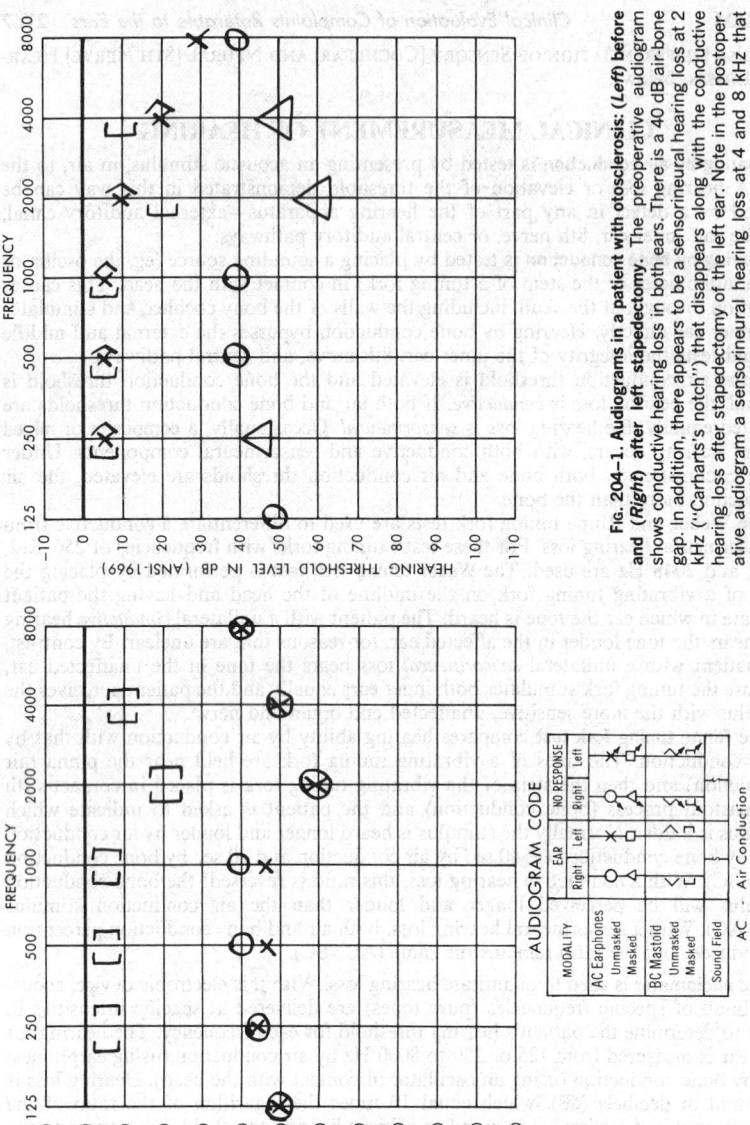

Fig. 204–1. Audiograms in a patient with otosclerosis: (*Left*) before and (*Right*) after left stapedectomy. The preoperative audiogram shows conductive hearing loss in both ears. There is a 40 dB air-bone gap. In addition, there appears to be a sensorineural hearing loss at 2 kHz ("Carhart's notch") that disappears along with the conductive hearing loss after stapedectomy of the left ear. Note in the postoperative audiogram a sensorineural hearing loss at 4 and 8 kHz that often develops following a stapedectomy.

AUDIOGRAM CODE

MODALITY	EAR		NO RESPONSE	
	Right	Left	Right	Left
AC Earphones				
Unmasked	○	✕		
Masked	△	□		
BC Mastoid				
Unmasked				
Masked	[	]		
Sound Field				

AC - Air Conduction
BC - Bone Conduction
CNT - Could not test
DNT - Did not test

words (2 syllables equally accented, such as *railroad, staircase, baseball*) at specific intensities, noting the intensity at which the patient repeats 50% of the words correctly. The ST usually approximates the average hearing levels at speech frequencies of 500, 1000, and 2000 Hz.

Ability to discriminate the various speech sounds or phonemes is determined by presenting 50 phonetically balanced one-syllable words, containing the phonemes in the same relative frequency as in conversational English, at an intensity of 25 to 40 dB above the ST. The percentage of words correctly repeated by the patient is the **discrimination score,** normally 90 to 100%. The discrimination score remains in the normal range in conductive hearing losses, but is reduced in sensorineural hearing losses because analysis of the speech sounds by the inner ear and 8th nerve is impaired. Discrimination tends to be poorer in neural than in sensory hearing losses.

Tympanometry measures the impedance of the middle ear to acoustical energy without voluntary participation by the patient and requires only that the patient remain quiet during the test; a sounding source and microphone sealed in the external auditory canal can measure the acoustical energy absorbed (passing through) or reflected by the middle ear. In conductive hearing loss, the middle ear absorbs relatively less sound and reflects relatively more sound. Normally the greatest compliance of the middle ear occurs with a pressure in the external auditory canal equal to atmospheric pressure. Increasing or decreasing the pressure in the external auditory canal demonstrates various patterns of compliance. With a relatively negative pressure in the middle ear, as in eustachian tube obstruction and middle ear effusion, maximal compliance occurs with a negative pressure in the external auditory canal. With discontinuity of the ossicular chain, as in necrosis or dislocation of the long process of the incus, no point of maximal compliance can be obtained. With fixation of the ossicular chain, as in stapedial footplate ankylosis in otosclerosis, compliance may remain normal or may be reduced. Tympanometry has been used to screen children for middle ear effusions (serous or secretory otitis media), to provide diagnostic clues, and to confirm the type of lesion in patients with conductive hearing losses.

This technic can detect changes in compliance produced by reflex contraction of the stapedius muscle; the acoustic reflex is initiated by presenting to the same or opposite ear a tone approximately 80 dB above the hearing threshold. The presence or absence of this reflex is important in the topographical diagnosis of facial nerve paralysis. The reflex adapts or decays in neural hearing losses, and presence or absence of acoustic reflex adaptation or decay, especially below 2000 Hz, aids in differential diagnosis of sensory and neural hearing losses. The acoustic reflex can also confirm voluntary threshold responses.

The minimum comprehensive audiologic assessment requires measuring pure-tone air and bone conduction thresholds, STs, and discrimination, performance intensity function for phonetically balanced words, tympanometry, and acoustic reflex testing, including reflex decay testing. Information gained from these procedures helps one decide if more definitive differentiation of a sensory from a neural hearing loss as described below is indicated.

When the patient cannot or will not respond voluntarily to acoustic stimuli, measuring the cochlear microphonic response and action potentials of the 8th nerve **(electrocochleography)** and evoked responses from the brainstem and auditory cortex **(brainstem response audiometry)** (see also under DIFFERENTIATION OF SENSORY [COCHLEAR] AND NEURAL [EIGHTH NERVE] HEARING LOSSES, below) to acoustic stimuli has been useful in evaluating infants and children suspected of having profound hearing loss (see also CLINICAL MEASUREMENT OF HEARING IN CHILDREN under SCREENING PROCEDURES FOR INFANTS AND CHILDREN in Ch. 182), individuals suspected of feigning or exaggerating a hearing loss (psychogenic hypacusis), and patients with sensori-

neural hearing loss of obscure etiology. Seven sequential wave forms have been identified that occur in the 8th nerve and central auditory pathways in response to acoustic stimuli. Lesions of the 8th nerve and brainstem auditory pathways result in changes in the amplitude and latency of the wave forms; these changes in latency of the wave forms are often of diagnostic value. Brainstem-response audiometry is used in coma to determine the functional integrity of the brainstem.

Clinical Measurement of Hearing in Children

(See under Screening Procedures for Infants and Children in Ch. 182)

DIFFERENTIATION OF SENSORY (COCHLEAR) AND NEURAL (8TH NERVE) HEARING LOSSES

The term *sensorineural* indicates that it is not certain whether the loss of hearing is due to a lesion in the inner ear or in the 8th nerve. The differentiation between sensory (cochlear) and neural (8th nerve) hearing loss is clinically important. **Sensory hearing losses** result from end-organ lesions (acoustic trauma, viral endolymphatic labyrinthitis, ototoxic drugs, Meniere's disease) that usually represent no threat to life. On the other hand, **neural hearing losses** are frequently due to potentially fatal cerebellopontine angle tumors and a wide variety of other neurologic disorders (see Hearing Loss in Ch. 119).

Sensory and neural hearing losses may be differentiated on the basis of tests for discrimination, performance intensity function for phonetically balanced words **(PI-PB)**, recruitment, acoustic reflex decay, sensitivity to small increments in intensity, pathologic adaptation, and auditory brainstem responses (see also Table 204–1).

Sensory hearing losses due to cochlear lesions are characterized by mild to moderate loss of discrimination for speech, improved discrimination with increasing intensity, presence of recruitment, absence of acoustic reflex decay, high sensitivity for small increments in intensity, mild tone decay, and well-formed waves with normal latencies in brainstem response audiometry.

Neural hearing losses are characterized by severe loss of discrimination for speech, deteriorating discrimination with increasing intensity, absence of recruitment, presence of acoustic reflex decay, poor sensitivity for small increments in intensity, marked tone decay, and abnormally long latencies of wave forms or absence of wave forms in brainstem response audiometry.

Table 204–1. DIFFERENCES BETWEEN SENSORY AND NEURAL HEARING LOSSES

Test Applied	*Type of Hearing Loss*	
	Sensory	Neural
Discrimination for speech	Moderate decrement	Severe decrement
Discrimination with increasing intensity	Improves	Deteriorates
Recruitment	Present	Absent
Acoustic reflex decay	Absent	Present
Sensitivity to small increments in intensity	Good	Poor
Tone decay	Mild	Marked
Waves in brainstem response audiometry	Well-formed, with normal latencies	Absent or with abnormally long latencies

The following diagnostic studies are used to differentiate sensory from neural hearing losses:

Discrimination for phonetically balanced words is described above.

Performance intensity function for phonetically balanced words (PI-PB), as mentioned above, is tested at 25 to 40 dB above the ST. Once the discrimination score is determined, discrimination may be determined at higher intensities. With sensory hearing losses, discrimination usually improves at higher intensities. With neural hearing losses, discrimination characteristically deteriorates at higher intensities. If an articulation function (discrimination as a function of intensity) is plotted, a "rollover" or decrement in discrimination is seen with increasing intensity in patients with an 8th nerve lesion.

Recruitment (abnormal increase in the perception of loudness or the ability to hear loud sounds normally despite a hearing loss) can be demonstrated by having the patient compare the loudness of sounds in the affected ear with the loudness of sounds in the normal ear. In sensory hearing losses, the sensation of loudness in the affected ear increases more with each increment in intensity than it does in the normal ear. In neural hearing losses, the sensation of loudness in the affected ear increases no more with each increment in intensity than it does in the normal ear (no recruitment) or increases less with each increment in intensity than it does in the normal ear (decruitment).

Acoustic reflex decay: As mentioned above, this reflex response adapts or decays with continuous presentation of a tone, particularly below 2000 Hz, over time mildly in sensory hearing losses and severely in neural hearing losses.

Sensitivity to small increments in intensity can be demonstrated by presenting a continuous tone at a hearing level (dB level above audiometric zero) of 75 dB and increasing the intensity by 1 dB briefly at irregular intervals. The percentage of small increments that the patient can detect yields the **short increment sensitivity index (SISI).** A high SISI (60 to 100%) is characteristic of sensory hearing losses, while a patient with an 8th nerve lesion can detect < 30% of the small changes in intensity.

Pathologic adaptation is demonstrated when a patient cannot continue to perceive a constant tone above the threshold of hearing **(tone decay).** The tone decay is mild in sensory lesions and severe in neural lesions.

Several of these phenomena may be demonstrated with the **Békésy automatic audiometer,** in which the intensity of the stimulus can be controlled by the patient. The patient is instructed to depress a button when he hears the stimulus, which causes the intensity of the stimulus to decrease. When the stimulus is no longer audible, the patient releases the button, and the intensity begins to increase. In this way the patient traces back and forth across his threshold of hearing. Over the course of a 6½-min period, the frequency of the test tone may be gradually increased from 100 to 10,000 Hz. If pathologic adaptation is present, it can be demonstrated by decay of the response to a continuous presentation of the test stimulus. Decay of the response can be reduced or eliminated by interrupting the tone for 0.5 second every second. Testing with continuous and interrupted tone presentations yields 5 patterns of tracings. In the Type I pattern, the continuous and interrupted tracings are superimposed. This pattern is found in normal hearing and in conductive hearing losses. In the Type II pattern, the 2 tracings are superimposed up to 1000 Hz. Above this frequency, the threshold for the continuous tones increases by about 20 dB from that of the interrupted tones, and in the higher frequencies the excursions of the continuous tracings become smaller. This pattern is characteristic of sensory hearing losses, as in Meniere's disease, and indicates mild pathologic adaptation. In the Type III pattern, the continuous tracing separates sharply from the interrupted tracing at a lower frequency, and excursions of the continuous tracing do not become smaller. This pattern is characteristic of neural lesions, such as acoustic neurinomas, and indicates severe pathologic adaptation. In the Type IV pattern, the continuous tracing separates from the inter-

rupted tracing at all frequencies, and excursions of the continuous tracing may or may not become smaller. This pattern indicates active cochlear lesions (such as a recent attack of Meniere's disease) or early neural lesions. In the Type V pattern, the apparent thresholds of the continuous and interrupted tones are separated but the apparent thresholds of the interrupted tones are greater than those of the continuous tones. This pattern occurs in psychogenic or feigned hearing loss.

Brainstem response audiometry (BRA) is the most powerful technic available to differentiate sensory from neural hearing losses. Five distinct electric waves, generated in the 8th nerve and brainstem in response to acoustic stimulation and categorized by Jewett as I, II, III, IV, and V, can be recorded from the head by computer averaging the responses to many stimuli. Each wave probably emanates from a distinct structure in the auditory pathway such as the 8th nerve, cochlear nuclei, superior olivary complex, lateral lemniscus, and inferior colliculus. With lesions of the 8th nerve, one or more wave forms may be lost, the latency of the wave forms from the onset of the acoustic stimuli may be increased, and the interwave latencies may be prolonged. With cochlear lesions, the wave forms are easily recognized and the latency relationships remain normal.

Patients with complaints referable to one cranial nerve, such as the 8th cranial nerve, deserve thorough neurologic evaluation. Emphasis has been placed in this discussion on thorough evaluation of the auditory division of the 8th nerve and its end organ. Further evaluation of the patient should include vestibular testing (see below) and may require CT of the head with enhancement (paying special attention to the internal auditory canals) and air-contrast, computed cisternography.

CENTRAL AUDITORY IMPERCEPTION

Lesions of the central auditory pathways (cochlear nuclei, brainstem pathways crossing the midline [trapezoid body, dorsal stria of Held, and stria of von Monakow], superior olivary complex, lateral lemniscus, inferior colliculus, medial geniculate body, auditory radiation, and auditory cortex) characteristically do not result in elevation of pure-tone and STs and decreased discrimination for single words. Special tests are required to bring out the deficit in auditory function with lesions of the central auditory pathways. These tests (1) measure discrimination of degraded or distorted connected speech, (2) measure discrimination in the presence of a competing message in the other ear, (3) evaluate the ability to fuse into a meaningful message incomplete or partial messages to each ear, and (4) localize sound in space (median plane localization) when the acoustic stimuli are delivered simultaneously to each ear.

Speech may be degraded or distorted with low frequency or high frequency filters, periodic interruptions, or time compression. There is a loss of discrimination of degraded or distorted connected speech in the ear contralateral to a cortical lesion. Likewise, presenting a competing message in the ipsilateral ear results in a loss of discrimination in the ear contralateral to a cortical lesion. Brainstem lesions produce a loss of ability to fuse incomplete messages presented to each ear into a meaningful message and impair the ability to make accurate localizations of sound in space.

TINNITUS

Perception of sound in the absence of an acoustic stimulus. Tinnitus, a subjective experience of the patient, is distinguished from **bruit,** noise that may be heard by the examiner and often by the patient as well.

Tinnitus may be of a buzzing, ringing, roaring, whistling, or hissing quality or may involve more complex sounds that vary over time. Tinnitus may be intermittent, continuous, or pulsatile (synchronous with the heart beat). An associated hearing loss is usually present.

The mechanism involved in tinnitus remains obscure. Tinnitus may occur as a symptom of nearly all ear disorders, including obstruction of the external auditory canal due to cerumen and foreign bodies, infectious processes (external otitis, myringitis, otitis media, labyrinthitis, petrositis, syphilis, meningitis), eustachian tube obstruction, otosclerosis, middle ear neoplasms such as the glomus tympanicum and glomus jugulare tumors, Meniere's disease, arachnoiditis, cerebellopontine angle tumors, ototoxicity (due to salicylates, quinine and its synthetic analogs, aminoglycoside antibiotics, certain diuretics, carbon monoxide, heavy metals, alcohol, etc), cardiovascular diseases (hypertension, arteriosclerosis, aneurysms, etc), anemia, hypothyroidism, hereditary sensorineural hearing loss, noise-induced hearing loss, acoustic trauma (blast injury), and head trauma.

Evaluation of the patient with tinnitus requires the minimum comprehensive audiologic assessment described above as well as CT of the temporal bone. Finding a sensorineural hearing loss indicates the testing described above for differentiating sensory and neural hearing losses. Pulsatile tinnitus requires investigation of the vascular system with carotid and vertebral arteriograms to exclude arterial obstruction, aneurysms, and vascular neoplasms.

Treatment

The patient's ability to tolerate the tinnitus varies. Treatment should be directed toward the underlying disease, since its amelioration may produce improvement in the tinnitus. Correction of the associated hearing loss usually results in relief of the tinnitus. Although there is no specific medical or surgical therapy for tinnitus, many patients find relief by playing background music to mask the tinnitus and even go to sleep with the radio playing. A hearing aid for the associated hearing loss often results in suppression of the tinnitus. Some patients benefit from use of a tinnitus masker, a device that is worn like a hearing aid and that presents a noise more pleasant than the tinnitus. Electrical stimulation of the inner ear, as with a cochlear implant, often reduces the tinnitus but is appropriate only for the profoundly deaf.

CLINICAL EVALUATION OF THE VESTIBULAR APPARATUS

Patients with vertigo, difficulty with balance, or a sensorineural hearing loss of unknown etiology should have vestibular function tested. Evaluation of vestibular function includes rapidly alternating movement, finger-to-nose, heel-to-shin, and Romberg tests; gait testing; and electronystagmography **(ENG)** with caloric testing. Since the results in each ear can be compared, caloric tests are more useful clinically than stimulation with acceleration or deceleration in rotational, torsion swing, and lateral swing tests.

Artificial stimulation of the vestibular apparatus produces nystagmus, past-pointing, falling, and autonomic responses such as sweating, vomiting, hypotension, and bradycardia. **Nystagmus** (see also in Ch. 119), the most useful response, can be monitored visually or, more reliably, by recording changes in the corneoretinal potential (electronystagmography). Vestibular nystagmus is a rhythmic movement of the eyes. It has a quick and a slow component and may be rotary, vertical, or horizontal. The direction of the nystagmus is determined by the direction of the quick component because it is easier to see. However, the slow component is the more fundamental response to vestibular stimulation, while the quick component is compensatory. The slow component moves in the direction of the movement of the endolymph. Past-pointing and falling are also in the direction of movement of the endolymph. The hallucination of the movement of the environment is in the direction of endolymphatic flow, and the hallucination of the movement of the subject is in the direction opposite to that of endolymphatic flow.

ENG electronically detects spontaneous gaze, or positional nystagmus that might

not be visually detectable. Eye tracking of a moving target and the response to optokinetic stimulation with a rotating striped drum are conveniently recorded electronically at the time of caloric testing.

Caloric stimulation produces convection currents within the endolymph. These currents cause movement of the cupula in the ampulla of the horizontal semicircular canal; the movement is in one direction during cooling and in the opposite direction during warming.

The **Hallpike caloric test,** an accurate and reproducible measure of vestibular sensitivity, is performed with the patient supine and the head elevated 30 degrees to bring the horizontal semicircular canal into a vertical position. Each ear is irrigated with 240 mL of water delivered in 40 sec, first at 30 C (86 F) and then at 44 C (110 F). The resulting nystagmus is monitored with the patient gazing straight ahead. Irrigation of the ear with cool water produces nystagmus to the opposite side; warm water produces nystagmus to the same side. A mnemonic device is COWS (cold to the opposite and warm to the same).

The duration of the nystagmus, the velocity of the slow component, or the frequency of the nystagmus may be measured. **Canal paresis,** a unilateral reduction or absence of sensitivity, and **directional preponderance,** a relative exaggeration of the nystagmic response in one direction, can be demonstrated. Various combinations of canal paresis and directional preponderance may coexist. The presence of canal paresis, directional preponderance, or combinations of the two signals an organic lesion—end organ, 8th nerve, brainstem, or cerebellar—but does not necessarily indicate on which side the lesion is. Occasionally, an important differential point rests on the caloric examination. Acoustic neurinomas frequently show canal paresis or complete lack of response on the side of the neoplasm.

Patients with vertigo should have a minimum comprehensive audiologic assessment and CT of the head with enhancement as well as the vestibular evaluation described above.

EARACHE

Pain occurs with infections and neoplasms in the external ear and middle ear, or is referred to the ear from remote disease processes. Even mild inflammation in the external auditory canal produces severe pain. Perichondritis of the pinna produces severe pain and tenderness. With eustachian tube obstruction, abrupt changes in middle-ear pressure relative to atmospheric pressure may result in painful retraction of the tympanic membrane. Infection in the middle ear results in painful inflammation of the middle-ear mucous membrane and pain due to increased pressure in the middle ear with bulging of the tympanic membrane. The commonest cause of earache in children, acute otitis media, requires prompt examination by a physician and antibiotic therapy to prevent serious sequelae. In the absence of disease in the ear, the source of referred otalgia should be sought in those areas receiving sensory supply from the cranial nerves that subserve sensation in the external ear and middle ear—ie, the trigeminal, glossopharyngeal, and vagus nerves. Specifically, the cause of obscure otalgia should be sought in the nose, paranasal sinuses, nasopharynx, teeth, gingiva, temporomandibular joints, mandible, tongue, palatine tonsils, pharynx, hypopharynx, larynx, trachea, and esophagus. Occult neoplasms in these locations often first make their presence known by pain referred to the ear.

Treatment depends on identifying the cause of the pain and providing the therapy appropriate for that disease.

VERTIGO

An abnormal sensation of rotary movement associated with difficulty with balance, gait, and navigation in the environment. The sensation may be subjective: the patient feels he

is moving relative to his environment; or it may be objective: he feels the environment is moving relative to him. Vertigo results from lesions or disturbances in the inner ear, 8th nerve, or vestibular nuclei and their pathways in the brainstem and cerebellum.

205. EXTERNAL EAR

OBSTRUCTIONS

Cerumen may obstruct the ear canal and cause itching, pain, and a temporary conductive hearing loss. It may be removed by irrigation, but rolling the cerumen out of the ear canal with a blunt curet or loop is quicker, less messy, and more comfortable for the patient. Irrigation is contraindicated if there is a history of otorrhea, perforation of the tympanic membrane, or recurrent external otitis. Allowing water into the middle ear through a perforation may exacerbate chronic otitis media. Cerumen solvents are not recommended because they often do not solve the problem and frequently cause maceration of the skin of the canal and allergic reactions.

Children insert all types of objects into their ear canals, such as beads, erasers, or beans. A **foreign body** in the ear canal is best removed by raking it out with a blunt hook. Forceps tend to push smooth objects deeper. A foreign body lying medial to the isthmus is difficult to remove without injuring the tympanic membrane and ossicular chain. Metal and glass beads may sometimes be removed by irrigation, but with a hygroscopic foreign body (eg, a bean) adding water causes it to swell and complicates its removal. A general anesthetic is needed for an uncooperative child or when there is a difficult mechanical problem.

Insects in the ear canal are most annoying while alive. Filling the ear canal with mineral oil will kill the insect and give immediate relief, and will facilitate its removal with forceps.

EXTERNAL OTITIS

Infection in the ear canal may be localized **(furuncle)** or diffuse, involving the entire canal **(generalized or diffuse external otitis)**. External otitis is more common during the summer swimming season. It is often called **swimmer's ear**.

Etiology

Generalized external otitis may be caused by a gram-negative rod such as *Escherichia coli*, *Pseudomonas aeruginosa*, or *Proteus vulgaris*; by *Staphylococcus aureus*; or, rarely, by a fungus. Furuncles are usually due to *S. aureus*. Certain persons (eg, individuals with allergies, psoriasis, eczema, and seborrhea dermatitis) are particularly prone to develop external otitis. Predisposing factors include getting water or various irritants such as hair spray or hair dye in the ear canal, and trauma from cleaning the canal. The ear canal is self-cleansing by the movement of desquamated epithelium, like a conveyor belt, from the tympanic membrane outward. The patient's attempts to clean the canal with cotton applicators interrupt the self-cleansing mechanism and promote accumulation of debris by pushing it in the direction opposite to the movement of the desquamated epithelium. Debris and cerumen tend to trap water allowed into the canal; the resulting skin maceration sets the stage for invasion of pathogenic bacteria.

Symptoms and Signs

Patients with diffuse external otitis complain of itching, pain, a foul-smelling discharge, and loss of hearing if the canal becomes swollen or filled with purulent debris. Tenderness on traction of the pinna and on pressure over the tragus tends to distin-

guish it from otitis media. The skin of the external auditory canal appears red, swollen, and littered with moist, purulent debris.

Furuncles cause severe pain and, when a furuncle drains, brief sanguineous purulent otorrhea.

Treatment

Systemic antibiotics are seldom necessary unless there is a spreading cellulitis. In **diffuse external otitis,** topical antibiotics and corticosteroids are effective. The infected debris is first gently removed from the canal with suction or dry wipes of cotton. A solution containing neomycin sulfate 0.5% and polymyxin B sulfate 10,000 u./mL is effective against the usual gram-negative rods, while adding a topical corticosteroid such as 1% hydrocortisone reduces the swelling and allows antibiotic penetration into the depth of the canal; 5 drops are instilled tid for 7 days. External otitis also responds to alteration of the pH of the canal with topical 2% acetic acid 5 drops tid for 7 days. An analgesic such as codeine 30 mg orally q 4 h is usually necessary for the first 24 to 48 h. If there is cellulitis extending beyond the ear canal, penicillin G 250 mg orally q 6 h for 7 days is indicated.

Furuncles should be allowed to drain spontaneously, since incision may lead to a spreading perichondritis of the pinna. Topical antibiotics are *ineffective*. Analgesics such as codeine 30 mg orally q 4 h are necessary to relieve the pain. Dry heat is also helpful in relieving the pain and hastens resolution.

PERICHONDRITIS

Trauma, insect bites, and incision of superficial infections of the pinna may initiate perichondritis, which causes an accumulation of pus between the cartilage and the perichondrium. The blood supply to the cartilage is provided by the perichondrium. If the perichondrium is separated from both sides of the cartilage, the resulting avascular necrosis leads to a deformed pinna. Septic necrosis also plays a role. The infection tends to be indolent, long-lasting, and destructive. Perichondritis is usually caused by a gram-negative rod. **Treatment:** Wide incision and suction drainage is used to reapproximate the blood supply to the cartilage. Systemic antibiotic therapy is indicated and should be guided by culture and sensitivity studies; often IV therapy with an aminoglycoside antibiotic and a synthetic penicillin is required.

AURAL ECZEMATOID DERMATITIS

Eczema, characterized by itching, redness, discharge, desquamation, and even fissuring leading to secondary infection, frequently involves the pinna and ear canal. Recurrences are common. **Treatment:** Dilute aluminum acetate solution (Burow's solution) is applied as often as required. Itching and inflammation can be reduced with topical corticosteroids. Topical antibiotic therapy as described above for diffuse external otitis may be needed occasionally.

MALIGNANT EXTERNAL OTITIS

Pseudomonas osteomyelitis *of the temporal bone.*

Malignant external otitis occurs mainly in elderly diabetics, beginning as an external otitis caused by *Pseudomonas aeruginosa* and becoming a pseudomonas osteomyelitis of the temporal bone. It is characterized by persistent and severe earache, foul-smelling purulent otorrhea, and granulation tissue in the external auditory canal. There may be varying degrees of conductive hearing loss. Frequently, facial nerve paralysis occurs. Increased radiodensity throughout the air-cell system in the temporal bone and middle ear and radiolucency of the temporal bone develop. Biopsy of the tissue in the ear canal is necessary to differentiate the condition from a malignant neoplasm. The osteomyelitis spreads along the base of the skull and may cross the midline. Surgical

therapy is usually not helpful or necessary. Careful control of the diabetes and prolonged (6 wk) IV therapy with an aminoglycoside antibiotic and a synthetic penicillin result in complete resolution in most cases.

TRAUMA

Hematoma

A subperichondrial hematoma may result from blunt trauma to the pinna. The external ear becomes a shapeless, reddish-purple mass when blood collects between the perichondrium and the cartilage. Since the perichondrium carries the blood supply to the cartilage, avascular necrosis of the cartilage may occur. The "cauliflower ear" characteristic of wrestlers and boxers is the consequence of an organized and calcified hematoma. **Treatment:** The clot must be evacuated through an incision, and the skin and perichondrium are reapproximated to the cartilage with suction drainage to keep the cartilage and its blood supply in close approximation.

Lacerations

For lacerations of the external ear that penetrate the cartilage and the skin on both sides, the skin margins are sutured, the cartilage is splinted externally with benzoin-impregnated cotton, and a protective dressing is applied. Sutures should not extend into the cartilage.

Fractures

Forceful blows to the mandible may be transmitted to the anterior wall of the ear canal (posterior wall of the glenoid fossa). Displaced fragments from fractures of the anterior wall of the canal may cause stenosis of the canal and must be reduced or removed under general anesthesia.

TUMORS

Sebaceous cysts, osteomas, and **keloids** may arise in and occlude the ear canal and cause retention of cerumen and a conductive hearing loss. Excision is the treatment of choice.

Ceruminomas arise in the outer third of the external auditory canal. Although these neoplasms appear benign histologically, *they behave in a malignant manner and should be excised widely.*

Basal cell and squamous cell carcinomas frequently develop on the external ear following regular exposure to the sun. Early lesions can be successfully treated with cautery and curettage or irradiation. More advanced lesions involving the cartilage require surgical excision of V-shaped wedges or larger amounts of the external ear. Invasion of cartilage makes irradiation therapy less effective and surgery the preferred treatment. Basal cell and squamous cell carcinomas may also arise in or secondarily invade the external auditory canal. Persistent inflammation in chronic otitis media may predispose to development of squamous cell carcinoma. Extensive resection is indicated, followed by radiation therapy. En bloc resection of the external auditory canal with sparing of the facial nerve is performed when lesions are limited to the canal and have not invaded the middle ear.

---

206. TYMPANIC MEMBRANE AND MIDDLE EAR

The patient with a middle ear disorder may present with one or more of the following complaints: a feeling of fullness or pressure in the ear; constant or intermittent,

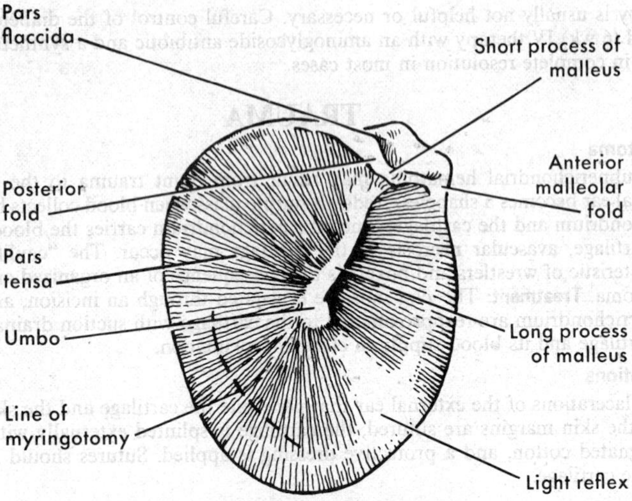

FIG. 206–1. The tympanic membrane (right ear).

mild to excruciating pain; otorrhea; diminished hearing; tinnitus; and vertigo. In acute otitis media, systemic symptoms (eg, fever) are commonly present in addition. The symptoms may begin with a feeling of fullness and progress serially in additive fashion. Infants and children, especially, may be febrile and present with other prominent systemic manifestations (anorexia, vomiting, diarrhea, lethargy, etc).

The symptoms may result from infection, trauma, and disturbed pressure relationships secondary to eustachian tube obstruction. In determining the cause, the physician should elicit information about antecedent and associated symptoms (eg, rhinorrhea, nasal obstruction, sore throat, upper respiratory infection, allergic manifestations; headache or other evidence of meningeal involvement; systemic symptoms). The appearance of the external auditory canal and tympanic membrane (see FIG. 206–1, above) often yields diagnostic clues; the nose, nasopharynx, and oropharynx should also be examined for signs of infection and allergy and for evidence of an underlying disorder—eg, a neoplasm of the nasopharynx.

The function of the middle ear should be evaluated with pneumatic otoscopy, the Weber and Rinne tuning fork tests, tympanometry, and audiometry.

TRAUMA

The tympanic membrane may be punctured and the tympanum penetrated by objects placed in the ear canal (eg, cotton applicators) or entering the canal accidentally (eg, twigs on a tree or missiles such as pencils or hot slag). A sudden overpressure, as in an explosion (acoustic trauma), a slap, or swimming and diving accidents, or a sudden negative pressure, as in a kiss over the ear, also can perforate the tympanic membrane. Penetration of the eardrum may cause dislocations of the ossicular chain, fracture of the footplate of the stapes, displacement of fragments of the ossicles or missile into the inner ear, a perilymph fistula from the oval or round window, or facial nerve paralysis.

Symptoms and Signs

Traumatic perforation of the tympanic membrane results in sudden severe pain followed by bleeding from the ear. A loss of hearing and tinnitus occur. The loss of

hearing is more severe if there has been a disruption of the ossicular chain or trauma to the inner ear. Vertigo suggests an associated injury to the inner ear, as occasionally a portion of the stapes or a missile is driven into the inner ear. Purulent otorrhea may begin in 24 to 48 h, particularly if water gets into the middle ear.

Treatment

Following perforation, oral penicillin G or V 250 mg q 6 h should be given for 7 days to prevent infection. Aseptic technic is used in examining the ear. If necessary, under local anesthesia and microscopic control, the displaced flaps of tympanic membrane may be laid in their original positions to facilitate healing. The ear is kept dry, and topical medication with 2% acetic acid, 5 drops tid, though not used prophylactically, may be employed if the ear becomes infected. Spontaneous closure of the perforation is usual; a tympanoplasty is indicated if the perforation does not heal spontaneously within 2 mo. A persistent conductive hearing loss suggests discontinuity of the ossicular chain, and the middle ear should be explored surgically and repaired. A sensorineural hearing loss or vertigo that persists for hours or longer following the injury indicates penetration of the inner ear and requires an exploratory tympanotomy to repair the damage as soon as possible.

BAROTITIS MEDIA

(Aerotitis)

Damage to the middle ear due to ambient pressure changes. During a sudden increase in ambient pressure, as in descent of an airplane or in deep sea diving (see appropriate chapters in §21), gas must move from the nasopharynx into the middle ear to maintain equal pressure on both sides of the tympanic membrane. If the eustachian tube is not functioning properly, as in URI or allergy, the pressure in the middle ear will be less than the ambient pressure and the relative negative pressure in the middle ear will result in retraction of the tympanic membrane, and a transudate of blood from the vessels in the lamina propria of the mucous membrane will form in the middle ear. If the difference in pressure becomes great, ecchymosis and subepithelial hematoma may develop in the mucous membrane of the middle ear and in the tympanic membrane. Very severe pressure differentials cause bleeding into the middle ear and rupture of the tympanic membrane. A perilymph fistula through the oval or round windows may occur. Pressure differentials between the middle ear and the ambient pressures usually produce severe pain and a conductive hearing loss. A sensorineural hearing loss or vertigo during descent suggests the possibility of a perilymph fistula while the same symptoms during ascent from an aquatic dive suggest bubble formation in the inner ear.

An individual with an acute URI or allergic reaction should be advised not to fly or dive, but if these activities are undertaken, a nasal vasoconstrictor such as phenylephrine 0.25% applied topically 30 min before descent is of prophylactic value.

INFECTIOUS MYRINGITIS

(Bullous Myringitis)

Inflammation of the tympanic membrane secondary to viral or bacterial infections. Vesicles develop in the tympanic membrane in viral infections and in acute bacterial (particularly *Streptococcus [Diplococcus] pneumoniae*) and mycoplasmal otitis media. Pain is sudden in onset and persists for 24 to 48 h. Hearing loss and fever, when they occur, suggest bacterial otitis media. **Treatment:** Since it is difficult to differentiate a viral from a bacterial or mycoplasmal otitis, antibiotic therapy as for acute otitis media is indicated. Pain may be relieved by rupture of the vesicles with a myringotomy knife or by analgesia with a narcotic such as codeine orally q 4 h as necessary.

ACUTE OTITIS MEDIA

A bacterial or viral infection in the middle ear, usually secondary to a URI. While it can occur at any age, it is most common in young children, particularly from age 3 mo to 3 yr. Microorganisms may migrate from the nasopharynx to the middle ear over the surface of the eustachian tube mucous membrane or by propagating in the lamina propria of the mucous membrane as a spreading cellulitis or thrombophlebitis.

Etiology

In newborn infants, gram-negative enteric bacilli, particularly *Escherichia coli*, and *Staphylococcus aureus* cause suppurative otitis media. In older infants and young children (< 8 yr of age), *Streptococcus [Diplococcus] pneumoniae, Hemophilus influenzae*, Group A β-hemolytic streptococci, and *S. aureus* are the causative microorganisms in suppurative acute otitis media. Viral otitis media usually becomes secondarily invaded by one of these microorganisms. In those > 8 yr of age, *H. influenzae* is a less frequent causative microorganism and *S. pneumoniae*, Group A β-hemolytic streptococci, and *S. aureus* are the causative organisms. The relative frequency of the microorganisms causing acute otitis media varies according to which microorganisms are epidemic in the community at any given time. After the neonatal period, *E. coli* rarely causes acute otitis media. Likewise, *Klebsiella pneumoniae* and *Bacteroides* species rarely cause acute otitis media.

Symptoms and Signs

The first complaint usually is of persistent, severe earache. Hearing loss may occur. Fever (up to 40.5 C [105 F]), nausea, vomiting, and diarrhea may occur in young children. The tympanic membrane is erythematous and may bulge; landmarks become indistinct, and the light reflex is displaced. Bloody, then serosanguineous and finally purulent, otorrhea may follow spontaneous perforation of the tympanic membrane.

Complications

Serious complications include acute mastoiditis, petrositis, labyrinthitis, facial paralysis, conductive and sensorineural hearing loss, epidural abscess, meningitis (the most common intracranial complication), brain abscess, lateral sinus thrombosis, subdural empyema, and otitic hydrocephalus. Symptoms of an impending complication include headache, sudden profound hearing loss, vertigo, and chills and fever.

Diagnosis

Diagnosis is usually made on clinical grounds. The exudate obtained at myringotomy should be cultured, as should spontaneous otorrhea. Nasopharyngeal cultures may be helpful but do not correlate well with the causative agent.

Treatment

Antibiotic therapy is indicated for acute otitis media to relieve the symptoms, hasten resolution of the infection, and reduce the chance of labyrinthine and intracranial infectious complications and of residual damage to the hearing mechanism of the middle ear.

Penicillin G or V 250 mg orally q 6 h for 10 days is the drug of choice in patients over age 8 yr. Amoxicillin 35 to 70 mg/kg/day orally in 3 equal doses q 8 h for 10 days is preferred for those < 8 yr because of the frequency of *H. influenzae* infections. Treatment is continued for 10 to 14 days to ensure resolution and to prevent sequelae. Subsequent therapy depends on cultures, sensitivities, and the clinical course. In penicillin allergy, erythromycin 250 mg orally q 6 h for older children and adults, and a combination of erythromycin 30 to 50 mg/kg/day orally in equally divided doses q 6 h and sulfisoxazole 150 mg/kg/day orally in equally divided doses q 6 h for children < 8 yr may be given for 10 to 14 days.

To improve eustachian tube function, topical vasoconstrictors such as phenylephrine 0.25% 3 drops q 3 h may be instilled into each nasal cavity while the patient is

supine and his neck is extended. Such therapy should not exceed 5 to 7 days. Systemic sympathomimetic amines such as ephedrine sulfate, pseudoephedrine, or phenylpropanolamine, 30 mg orally (for adults) q 4 to 6 h for 7 to 10 days, may also be helpful. Antihistamines, such as chlorpheniramine 4 mg (for adults) orally q 4 to 6 h for 7 to 10 days, may improve eustachian tube function in allergic patients but are not indicated for nonallergic individuals.

Myringotomy should be considered if the tympanic membrane is bulging or if pain, fever, vomiting, and diarrhea are severe or persistent. The patient's hearing, tympanometry, and the appearance and movement of the tympanic membrane should be followed until there is complete resolution.

SECRETORY OTITIS MEDIA

(Serous Otitis Media)

An effusion in the middle ear resulting from incomplete resolution of acute otitis media or obstruction of the eustachian tube. The effusion is often sterile but may contain pathogenic bacteria. Secretory otitis media is common in children. The eustachian tube obstruction may be due to inflammatory processes in the nasopharynx, allergic manifestations, hypertrophic adenoids, or benign or malignant neoplasms. The middle ear is normally ventilated 3 to 4 times/min as the eustachian tube opens during swallowing. O_2 is absorbed by the blood in the vessels of the middle ear mucous membrane, and if the patency of the eustachian tube is impaired, a relative negative pressure develops within the middle ear.

Symptoms and Signs

At first there is mild retraction of the tympanic membrane, with displacement of the light reflex and accentuation of the landmarks; then in the middle ear a transudate from the blood vessels in the mucous membrane develops, recognizable by the amber or gray color that it gives the eardrum and the immobility of the tympanic membrane. An air-fluid level or bubbles of air may be seen through the tympanic membrane; conductive hearing loss occurs. Tympanometry demonstrates maximal compliance with negative pressures in the external auditory canal.

Treatment

In view of the role of pathogenic bacteria in middle ear effusions, a trial of antibiotic therapy as described under acute otitis media is often beneficial and is the first step to be considered in therapy. It is effective in relieving eustachian tube obstruction due to bacterial infection and in sterilizing the middle ear.

Systemic sympathomimetic amines such as ephedrine sulfate, pseudoephedrine, or phenylpropanolamine, 30 mg orally tid (for adults), may improve eustachian tube function by their vasoconstrictive effect. Antihistamines such as chlorpheniramine 4 mg (for adults) orally q 4 to 6 h may relieve eustachian tube obstruction in allergic individuals. Myringotomy may be necessary for aspiration of the fluid and for insertion of a tympanostomy tube, which allows ventilation of the middle ear and ameliorates the eustachian tube obstruction regardless of the cause. The middle ear may be ventilated on a temporary basis with Valsalva's maneuver or politzerization.

Correction of any underlying condition in the nasopharynx is required. Children may require adenoidectomy, removing lymphoid aggregations on the torus of the eustachian tube and in Rosenmüller's fossa as well as the central adenoid tissue mass, to eradicate persistent and recurrent serous otitis media. Antibiotic therapy should be given to resolve bacterial rhinitis, sinusitis, and nasopharyngitis. Immunologic investigation (see Chs. 18, 20, and 21) is occasionally helpful. Any demonstrated allergen should be eliminated from the patient's environment, or immunotherapy should be tried (see Ch. 21).

ACUTE MASTOIDITIS

Infection in the mastoid process resulting in coalescence of the mastoid air cells due to bacterial infection. In acute purulent otitis media, the infection always extends into the mastoid antrum and cells, but progression and destruction of the bony portions of the mastoid process are aborted by suitable antibiotic therapy. The responsible bacteria are the same as those causing acute otitis media. Characteristically, **streptococcal mastoiditis** is preceded by early perforation of the tympanic membrane and profuse otorrhea; **pneumococcal mastoiditis** is likely to be less symptomatic but just as destructive, and advanced coalescence of the mastoid air cells may precede perforation of the tympanic membrane.

Symptoms and Signs

Acute mastoiditis becomes clinically apparent 2 wk or more after the onset of untreated acute otitis media, as one of the cortices of the mastoid process is destroyed. A postauricular subperiosteal abscess may develop as the lateral mastoid cortex is destroyed. Redness, swelling, tenderness, and fluctuation develop over the mastoid process and the pinna is displaced laterally and inferiorly. An exacerbation of the aural pain, fever, and otorrhea usually occurs. The pain tends to be persistent and throbbing, and a creamy, profuse discharge is common. Increasing hearing loss is characteristic.

In acute otitis media, radiographic density of mastoid air cells is increased due to swollen mucous membrane and purulent fluid in the air cells. In coalescent mastoiditis, cell partitions become indistinct and radio-opacity decreases. The individual septa can no longer be seen as the air cells coalesce.

Treatment

The initial antibiotic of choice is penicillin. After a sample of the otorrhea is taken for culture and determination of antibiotic sensitivities, penicillin G 1 million u. IV q 6 h is given. Subsequent IV therapy depends on cultures, sensitivities, and the clinical course. Antibiotic therapy should be continued for at least 2 wk.

A subperiosteal abscess calls for complete exenteration of mastoid air cells (mastoidectomy).

CHRONIC OTITIS MEDIA

A permanent perforation of the tympanic membrane.

Chronic otitis media can result from acute otitis media, eustachian tube obstruction, mechanical trauma, thermal or chemical burns, or blast injuries. Chronic otitis media can be divided into 2 major categories, depending on the type of perforation: (1) the benign central perforation of the pars tensa and (2) the dangerous attic perforations of the pars flaccida and marginal perforations of the pars tensa.

Some substance of the tympanic membrane remains between the rim of the perforation and the bony sulcus tympanicus in **central perforations** (see FIG. 206–2a). These perforations result in a conductive hearing loss. Exacerbations of chronic otitis media may follow URIs or occur when water gains access to the middle ear in bathing and swimming. They are often caused by gram-negative rods and *Staphylococcus aureus*, and result in painless, purulent otorrhea, which may be foul-smelling. Persistent exacerbations may produce **aural polyps** (granulation tissue that prolapses from the middle ear through the perforation into the external auditory canal) and destructive changes in the middle ear such as necrosis of the long process of the incus.

Pars flaccida (attic) perforations lead into the epitympanum (see FIG. 206–2b). **Marginal perforations** usually occur in the posterior-superior portion of the pars tensa and there is no substance of tympanic membrane between the edge of the perforation and

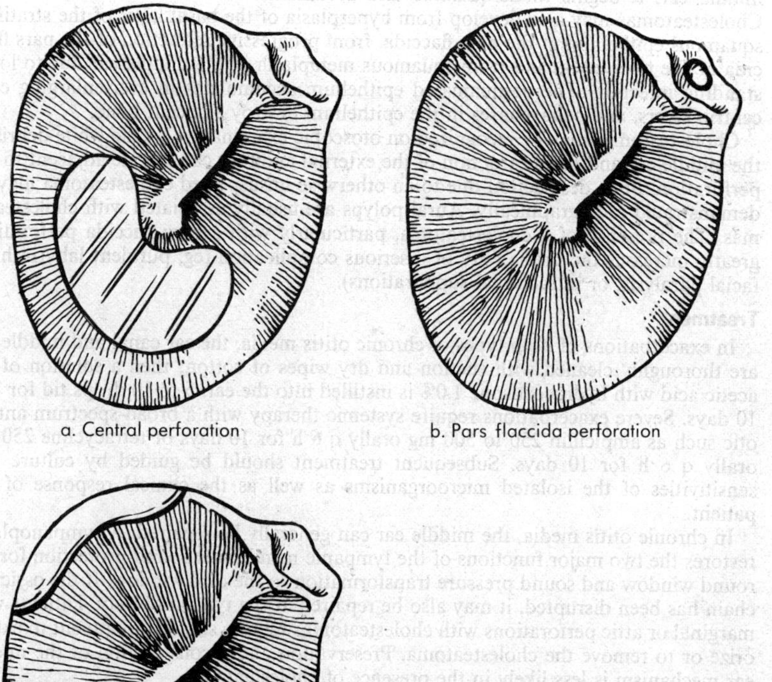

FIG. 206–2. Perforations of the tympanic membrane (right ear).

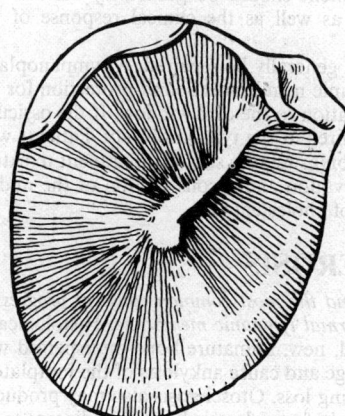

the bony sulcus tympanicus (see FIG. 206–2c). Marginal perforations result from an acute necrotizing otitis media that destroys large areas of the tympanic membrane, including the anulus tympanicus and the mucous membrane of the middle ear. These perforations may be associated with a conductive hearing loss, and exacerbations of otorrhea occur as with the central perforations. Complications such as labyrinthitis, facial paralysis, and intracranial suppuration are more likely to occur than with central perforations. Pars flaccida and marginal perforations are frequently associated with **cholesteatomas.**

During the healing of acute necrotizing otitis media, the remaining epithelium of the mucous membrane and the stratified squamous epithelium of the ear canal migrate to

cover the denuded areas. Once the stratified squamous epithelium is established in the middle ear, it begins to desquamate and accumulate and a cholesteatoma results. Cholesteatomas may also develop from hyperplasia of the basal layer of the stratified squamous epithelium of the pars flaccida, from progressive retraction of the pars flaccida or the pars tensa, and from squamous metaplasia in the middle ear due to longstanding infection. The desquamated epithelium accumulates in ever-enlarging concentric layers, and collagenases in the epithelium destroy adjacent bone.

Cholesteatomas may be recognized on otoscopic examination by the white debris in the middle ear and the destruction of the external auditory canal bone adjacent to the perforation. Bone destruction due to an otherwise unsuspected cholesteatoma may be demonstrated radiographically. Aural polyps are usually associated with cholesteatomas. The presence of a cholesteatoma, particularly with a pars flaccida perforation, greatly increases the probability of a serious complication (eg, purulent labyrinthitis, facial paralysis, or intracranial suppurations).

Treatment

In exacerbations of both types of chronic otitis media, the ear canal and middle ear are thoroughly cleaned with suction and dry wipes of cotton; then a solution of 2% acetic acid with hydrocortisone 1.0% is instilled into the ear, 5 to 10 drops tid for 7 to 10 days. Severe exacerbations require systemic therapy with a broad-spectrum antibiotic such as ampicillin 250 to 500 mg orally q 6 h for 10 days or tetracycline 250 mg orally q 6 h for 10 days. Subsequent treatment should be guided by culture and sensitivities of the isolated microorganisms as well as the clinical response of the patient.

In chronic otitis media, the middle ear can generally be repaired. A tympanoplasty restores the two major functions of the tympanic membrane: sound protection for the round window and sound pressure transformation to the oval window. If the ossicular chain has been disrupted, it may also be repaired at the tympanoplasty. Patients with marginal or attic perforations with cholesteatomas require surgical treatment to exteriorize or to remove the cholesteatoma. Preservation and reconstruction of the middle ear mechanism is less likely in the presence of cholesteatoma.

OTOSCLEROSIS

A disease of the bone of the otic capsule and the most common cause of progressive conductive hearing loss in the adult with a normal tympanic membrane. Histologically, foci of otosclerosis show irregularly arranged, new, immature bone interspersed with numerous vascular channels. These foci enlarge and cause ankylosis of the footplate of the stapes and a consequent conductive hearing loss. Otosclerosis also may produce a sensory hearing loss, particularly when the foci of otosclerotic bone are adjacent to the scala media.

The tendency to otosclerosis is familial. About 10% of adult white populations have foci of otosclerosis, but only about 10% of affected persons develop conductive hearing loss. It becomes clinically evident in the late teenage and early adult years. The fixation of the stapes may progress rapidly during pregnancy.

Treatment is with microsurgical technics: The stapes is removed and replaced by a prosthesis; the hearing loss is corrected in most cases. A hearing aid may also improve the hearing of the patient with otosclerosis.

TUMORS

Rarely, the middle ear is the site of origin of squamous cell carcinoma. The persistent otorrhea of chronic otitis media may be a predisposing factor. Radiation therapy and resection of the temporal bone are necessary.

Nonchromaffin paragangliomas (chemodectomas), known as glomus jugulare or glo-

mus tympanicum tumors, arise in the temporal bone from glomus bodies in the jugular bulb or the medial wall of the middle ear. They produce a pulsatile red mass in the middle ear. The first symptom is often a tinnitus that is synchronous with the pulse. Hearing loss and, later, vertigo develop. Excision is the treatment of choice. Palliation is achieved with radiation therapy for tumors too large to resect.

207. INNER EAR

For a discussion of the etiology, diagnosis, and treatment of **vertigo,** see also Chs. 119 and 204.

MENIERE'S DISEASE

A disorder characterized by recurrent prostrating vertigo, sensory hearing loss, and tinnitus, associated with generalized dilation of the membranous labyrinth **(endolymphatic hydrops).**

The etiology of Meniere's disease is unknown, and the pathophysiology is poorly understood. The attacks of vertigo appear suddenly, last from a few to 24 h, and subside gradually. The attacks are associated with nausea and vomiting. The patient may have a recurrent feeling of fullness or pressure in the affected ear. The hearing in the affected ear tends to fluctuate, but over the years the hearing progressively worsens. The tinnitus may be constant or intermittent, and may be worse before, after, or during an attack of vertigo. Although only one ear is usually affected, both ears are involved in 10 to 15% of patients.

In **Lermoyez's variant** of Meniere's disease, hearing loss and tinnitus precede the first attack of vertigo by months or years and the hearing may improve with the onset of the vertigo.

Treatment

Treatment is empirical. A number of operations, including sacculotomy, placement of a stainless steel tack through the footplate of the stapes, ultrasonic irradiation, endolymphatic-subarachnoid shunt, and cryosurgery have been advocated for patients who are disabled by the frequency of vertiginous attacks. Vestibular neurectomy relieves the vertigo and usually the hearing is preserved. A labyrinthectomy can be performed if the vertigo is sufficiently disabling and the hearing has degenerated to a useless level.

Symptomatic relief of the vertigo may be obtained with anticholinergic agents (eg, atropine 1 to 2 mg orally or scopolamine 0.6 mg orally or IM q 4 to 6 h or by transdermal patch) to minimize vagal-mediated GI symptoms, antihistamines (eg, diphenhydramine, meclizine, or cyclizine 50 mg orally or IM q 6 h) to sedate the vestibular system, or barbiturates (eg, pentobarbital 100 mg orally or IM q 8 h) for general sedation. Diazepam 2 to 5 mg orally q 6 to 8 h is particularly effective in relieving the distress of severe vertigo by sedating the vestibular system.

VESTIBULAR NEURONITIS

A benign disorder characterized by sudden onset of severe vertigo that is persistent at first and then becomes paroxysmal. The disease is thought to be a neuronitis involving the vestibular division of the 8th nerve, and to be viral in origin because of its frequent epidemic occurrence, particularly among adolescents and young adults.

The first attack of vertigo is severe, is associated with nausea and vomiting, and lasts for 7 to 10 days. There is persistent nystagmus toward the affected side. The condition is self-limited and may occur as only a single episode, or several subsequent attacks

may occur over the next 12 to 18 mo; each subsequent attack is less severe and of shorter duration. There is no associated hearing loss or tinnitus.

The diagnostic evaluation should include an audiologic assessment, electronystagmography with caloric testing, and CT of the head with enhancement with particular attention to the internal auditory canals to exclude other diagnostic possibilities, such as cerebellopontine angle tumor and brainstem hemorrhage or infarction.

Treatment: Acute attacks of vertigo may be suppressed symptomatically as in Meniere's disease (see above). With prolonged vomiting, IV fluids and electrolytes may be required for replacement and maintenance.

BENIGN PAROXYSMAL POSITIONAL VERTIGO

(Postural or Positional Vertigo; Cupulolithiasis)

Violent vertigo, lasting < 30 sec and induced by certain head positions. The vertigo occurs when the patient lies on one ear or the other. It also occurs when the patient tips his head backward to look up over his head. The vertigo is accompanied by nystagmus. There is no associated hearing loss or tinnitus. Benign paroxysmal positional vertigo usually subsides in several weeks or months but may recur after months or years.

Etiology

Granular basophilic masses in the cupula of the posterior semicircular canal have been demonstrated. It has been suggested that the cupular deposits represent calcium carbonate derived from the otoliths. Etiologic factors appear to be spontaneous degeneration of the utricular otolithic membranes, labyrinthine concussion, otitis media, ear surgery, and occlusion of the anterior vestibular artery.

Diagnosis

A **provocative test for positional nystagmus** may be performed. The patient is first seated on an examining table, then assumes the supine position with his head dependent over the end of the table and turned so that one ear is undermost. After the position has been assumed, a latent period of several seconds will be followed by vertigo, which is severe, is likely to last for 15 to 20 sec, and is accompanied by rotary nystagmus. If the left ear is affected, when it is put undermost the nystagmus will be clockwise; if the right ear, the nystagmus is counterclockwise. When the patient sits up, the response recurs, but the nystagmus is rotary in the reverse direction and is milder. The response fatigues, so that with immediate repetition of the test the response will be less strong.

Positional nystagmus may occur with end-organ or CNS lesions. The latency of the response, the severe subjective sensation, the fatigability of the response, the limited duration, and the direction of the rotary nystagmus distinguish benign paroxysmal positional vertigo from a CNS lesion. The positional nystagmus of CNS lesions lacks latency, fatigability, and the severe subjective sensation. The nystagmus may continue as long as the position is maintained. The positional nystagmus of CNS lesions may be vertical or changing in direction and, if rotary, is likely to be perverted (ie, not in the anticipated direction).

The diagnostic evaluation should include an audiologic assessment, electrostagmography with caloric testing, and CT of the head with enhancement with particular attention to the internal auditory canals, to exclude other diagnostic possibilities.

Treatment

The patient is instructed to avoid the provocative positions. If benign positional paroxysmal vertigo lasts for as long as a year it can be relieved in most cases by dividing the nerve to the posterior semicircular canal of the affected ear at tympanotomy.

HERPES ZOSTER OTICUS

(Ramsay Hunt Syndrome; Viral Neuronitis and Ganglionitis; Geniculate Herpes)

Invasion of the 8th nerve ganglia and the geniculate ganglion of the facial nerve by the herpes zoster virus, producing severe ear pain, hearing loss, vertigo, and paralysis of the facial nerve.

Vesicles can be seen on the pinna and in the external auditory canal in the distribution of the sensory branch of the facial nerve. Other cranial nerves are often involved, and some degree of meningeal inflammation is common. Lymphocytes may be present in the CSF, and the protein content is often increased. Evidence of a mild generalized encephalitis can be found in many patients. The hearing loss may be permanent or there may be partial or complete recovery. The vertigo lasts for days to several weeks. The facial paralysis may be transient or permanent.

Treatment

Corticosteroid therapy is the treatment of choice; eg, prednisone 40 mg/day orally for 2 days, then 30 mg/day orally for 7 to 10 days, followed by gradual tapering of the dose. Pain is relieved with codeine 30 to 60 mg orally q 3 to 4 h as necessary, while the vertigo is effectively suppressed with diazepam 2 to 5 mg orally q 4 to 6 h. Decompression of the fallopian canal, indicated when the nerve excitability declines or electroneurography demonstrates a 90% decrement, occasionally relieves the facial paralysis.

PURULENT LABYRINTHITIS

(Suppurative Labyrinthitis)

Invasion of the inner ear by a bacterium. Purulent labyrinthitis may occur secondary to acute otitis media or purulent meningitis. In acute otitis media, the microorganisms may gain access to the inner ear through the oval and round windows; in purulent meningitis, through the cochlear aqueduct. Purulent labyrinthitis is also frequently followed by meningitis as the microorganisms gain access to the subarachnoid space through the cochlear aqueduct.

Purulent labyrinthitis is characterized by severe vertigo and nystagmus. It invariably results in complete hearing loss and, in chronic otitis media and cholesteatoma, is often followed by facial paralysis. **Treatment** includes labyrinthectomy for drainage of the inner ear, radical mastoidectomy, and IV antibiotic therapy appropriate for meningitis.

SUDDEN DEAFNESS

Severe sensorineural hearing loss that usually occurs in only one ear and develops over a period of a few hours or less.

Sudden deafness occurs in about 1:5000 persons every year. Although the sudden onset suggests a vascular etiology (embolism, thrombosis, or hemorrhage) by analogy with vascular accidents in the CNS, the evidence supports a viral etiology in most cases. Sudden deafness tends to occur in children and young and middle-aged adults who have no evidence of vascular disease. The histopathologic findings in the temporal bone in sudden deafness are unlike those seen in the inner ear of animals with experimental vascular occlusion or embolization, but are similar to those seen in human viral infections of the inner ear that result in sudden deafness—eg, mumps and measles **(viral endolymphatic labyrinthitis).** The viruses of influenza, chickenpox, mononucleosis, the adenoviruses, and others also produce sudden deafness.

The pathologic findings in individuals with persistent hearing loss due to viral endolymphatic labyrinthitis are similar regardless of the causative virus. The organ of Corti is missing in the basal turn. Individual hair cells tend to be missing. Ganglion cell

populations are reduced in the basal turn. The stria vascularis becomes atrophic. The tectorial membrane is often rolled up and ensheathed in a syncytium. Reissner's membrane may be collapsed and adherent to the basilar membrane.

Perilymph fistulas between the inner and middle ears occasionally occur with severe ambient pressure changes and with strenuous activities like weight lifting. Fistulas in the oval or round windows result in a sudden or fluctuating sensory hearing loss and vertigo. The patient may experience an explosive sound in the affected ear when the fistula occurs.

Symptoms and Signs

The hearing loss is usually profound, but hearing returns to normal in most patients and partial recovery occurs in others. Tinnitus and vertigo may be present initially. The vertigo usually subsides in several days. If hearing is going to return, it is likely to do so in 10 to 14 days.

Treatment

Although vasodilators, anticoagulants, low mol wt dextran, corticosteroids, and vitamins have all been advocated, no form of treatment is of proven value. In view of the frequent micropetechiae and extravasation of blood that are characteristic of virus-induced inflammatory reactions, vasodilation and anticoagulation may not be indicated. Furthermore, in an inflammatory reaction the cochlear blood flow is already increased as much as is beneficial. Although corticosteroids are not of proven value, their use appears rational—eg, prednisone 40 mg/day orally for 2 days, then 20 mg/day orally for 5 to 7 days followed by a tapering of dosage. Bed rest also seems advisable.

Surgical exploration of the middle ear should be carried out for a suspected perilymph fistula, and the fistula should be repaired with an autogenous soft tissue graft of fat or fascia.

CONGENITAL SENSORINEURAL HEARING LOSS

(See in Ch. 186)

NOISE-INDUCED HEARING LOSS

Any source of intense noise, such as woodworking equipment, chain saws, internal combustion engines, heavy machinery, gunfire, or aircraft, may damage the inner ear. Exposure to intense noise results in loss of hair cells in the organ of Corti. Individuals vary greatly in susceptibility to noise-induced hearing loss, but nearly everyone will lose some hearing if exposed to sufficiently intense noise for a sufficient time. Any noise > 85 dB is damaging. Usually a high-frequency tinnitus accompanies the hearing loss. Loss occurs first at 4 kHz and gradually moves into the lower frequencies with further exposure. In contrast to most sensorineural hearing losses, damage is less at 8 kHz than at 4 kHz. Blast injury, termed acoustic trauma, produces the same kind of sensory hearing loss.

Prevention depends on limiting the length of exposure, reducing the noise at its source, and isolating the person from the sound source. As the intensity of the noise increases, the duration of exposure must be reduced to prevent damage to the inner ear. Noise may be attenuated by wearing ear protectors, eg, plastic plugs in the ear canals or glycerine-filled cups over the ears. With severe noise-induced hearing loss, a hearing aid is usually helpful.

PRESBYCUSIS

The sensorineural hearing loss that occurs as a part of normal aging. It begins after age 20, first affecting the highest frequencies (18 to 20 kHz) and gradually moving into the lower frequencies; it usually begins to affect the 4- to 8-kHz range by age 55 to 65,

although there is considerable variation. Some individuals are severely handicapped by age 60 and some are essentially untouched at 90. Men are affected more often and more severely than women. Stiffening of the basilar membrane and deterioration of the hair cells, stria vascularis, ganglion cells, and cochlear nuclei may play a role in pathogenesis, and presbycusis appears to be related in part to noise exposure.

Speech reading (lip reading); auditory training, making maximum use of nonauditory clues; and amplification with a hearing aid are helpful.

OTOTOXIC DRUGS

The aminoglycoside antibiotics, salicylates, quinine and its synthetic substitutes, and the diuretics ethacrynic acid and furosemide can be ototoxic. Though affecting both the auditory and vestibular portions of the inner ear, these drugs are particularly toxic to the organ of Corti (cortitoxic). Nearly all ototoxic drugs are eliminated through the kidneys, and renal impairment predisposes to the accumulation of toxic levels. Ototoxic drugs should be avoided in topical medication for the ear in the presence of a perforated tympanic membrane, since they can be absorbed into the inner ear fluids through the secondary tympanic membrane at the oval window.

Streptomycin damages the vestibular portion of the inner ear more readily than the auditory portion. Although vertigo and difficulty with maintaining balance tend to be temporary and eventually completely compensated, severe and permanent loss of vestibular sensitivity may persist, causing difficulty when walking in the dark and Dandy's syndrome (bouncing of the environment with each step). From 4 to 15% of patients receiving 1 gm/day for > 1 wk develop a measurable hearing loss, which usually appears after a short latent period (7 to 10 days) and slowly becomes worse if treatment is continued. Complete, permanent deafness may follow.

Neomycin has the greatest cortitoxic effect of any antibiotic. With large doses given orally or by colonic irrigation for intestinal sterilization, enough may be absorbed to affect hearing, particularly if GI ulceration or other mucosal lesions are present. Neomycin should *not* be used for irrigating wounds or for intrapleural or intraperitoneal irrigation because massive amounts of neomycin may be retained and absorbed and cause deafness. **Kanamycin** and **amikacin** are close to neomycin in cortitoxic potential. **Viomycin** shows both cochlear and vestibular toxicity. **Vancomycin** causes hearing loss, especially in the presence of renal insufficiency. **Gentamicin** and **tobramycin** have vestibular toxic properties in man and both vestibular and cochlear toxicity in laboratory animals.

Ethacrynic acid IV has caused profound and permanent hearing loss in gravely ill patients with renal failure who are given concomitant aminoglycoside antibiotic therapy. Transient hearing loss from **furosemide** has been reported.

Salicylates produce hearing loss and tinnitus that is usually reversible. **Quinine** and its synthetic substitutes produce a permanent loss of hearing.

Precautions

Ototoxic antibiotics should be **avoided** in pregnancy. Elderly persons and those with a preexisting hearing loss should not be treated with ototoxic drugs if other effective drugs are available. If possible, before treatment is begun with an ototoxic drug (especially an ototoxic antibiotic), the hearing should be measured in order to document a preexisting hearing loss. Hearing should be monitored audiometrically as often as daily while treatment is continued. The highest frequencies are usually affected first, and high-pitched tinnitus or vertigo may develop—though they are not reliable warning symptoms. If renal function is impaired, the dosage of renally eliminated ototoxic drugs should be adjusted so that the blood levels do not exceed those required therapeutically. Serum levels of the agent should be monitored to insure that adequate therapeutic levels have been achieved but not exceeded. Although there is some indi-

vidual variation in susceptibility, not exceeding the recommended blood level will usually conserve the hearing.

FRACTURES OF THE TEMPORAL BONE

Ecchymosis in the postauricular skin (Battle's sign) suggests a fracture of the temporal bone. Bleeding from the ear following a skull injury is pathognomonic of a temporal bone fracture. The bleeding may be medial to an intact tympanic membrane, may come from the middle ear through a ruptured tympanic membrane, or may come from a fracture line in the ear canal. A hemotympanum gives the eardrum a blue-black color. CSF otorrhea signifies a communication between the middle ear and the subarachnoid space. Fractures longitudinal to the petrous pyramid (80%) extend through the middle ear and rupture the tympanic membrane; they produce facial paralysis in 15% of cases and a profound sensorineural hearing loss in 35%. The middle ear damage may include disruption of the ossicular chain. Transverse fractures (20%) cross the fallopian canal and the cochlea and nearly always produce facial paralysis and a permanent hearing loss. The hearing can be assessed initially with the Weber and Rinne tuning fork tests and subsequently with audiometry. With CT of the head with special attention to the temporal bone, the fracture can usually be demonstrated.

Treatment

IV penicillin G 1 gm q 6 h should be given for 7 to 10 days to prevent meningitis. Persistent facial paralysis requires decompression of the nerve. Tympanoplasty with repair of the ossicular chain is carried out weeks or months later.

ACOUSTIC NEURINOMA

(Vestibular Schwannoma; Acoustic Neuroma; Eighth Nerve Tumor)

Acoustic neurinomas are derived from Schwann cells. They arise twice as often from the vestibular division of the 8th nerve as from the auditory division and account for approximately 7% of all intracranial tumors.

As the tumor increases in size, it projects from the internal auditory meatus into the cerebellopontine angle and begins to compress the cerebellum and brainstem. The 5th and later the 7th cranial nerves become involved.

Symptoms, Signs, and Diagnosis

A hearing loss and tinnitus are early symptoms. Although the patient complains of dizziness and unsteadiness, true vertigo is not usually present. The sensorineural hearing loss (see Ch. 204) is characterized by greater impairment of speech discrimination than would be expected with a cochlear lesion. Recruitment is absent, and the short increment sensitivity index **(SISI)** is low. Tone decay is marked. Usually Békésy audiometry shows a Type III or IV pattern. Acoustic reflex decay and absence of wave forms and increase in the latency of the 5th wave in the brainstem response audiometry provide further evidence of a neural lesion. As a rule, caloric testing demonstrates marked vestibular hypoactivity (canal paresis). Early diagnosis is based on the audiologic assessment, particularly brainstem response audiometry, and air contrast computed cisternography.

Treatment

Small tumors may be removed with microsurgical technics that allow preservation of the facial nerve, using a middle cranial fossa route to preserve the remaining hearing or a translabyrinthine route if no useful hearing remains. Large tumors are removed by a combined translabyrinthine and suboccipital approach.

HEARING AIDS

Amplification of sound with hearing aids is helpful for patients with conductive or sensorineural hearing losses that are > 30 dB in the speech frequencies. Hearing aids are also helpful to individuals with predominantly high-frequency sensorineural hearing losses and to individuals with unilateral hearing losses.

Air conduction hearing aids, usually coupled to the ear canal with an airtight seal or open tube, are generally superior to bone conduction hearing aids and are used except when there is some contraindication to using an ear mold or tube, as in atresia of the external auditory canal or persistent otorrhea. The **body aid** type, appropriate for profound hearing losses, is the most powerful; it is worn in the shirt pocket or in a body harness and connected by a wire to the earpiece, or receiver, which is coupled to the ear canal by a plastic insert, or earmold. In infants and young children with profound hearing loss in which it is not possible to determine which ear hears better, the amplification from the body aid is delivered to both ears by using a Y-cord. For moderate to severe hearing losses, a **postauricular** or **ear-level aid,** which fits behind the pinna and is coupled to the ear mold with flexible tubing, is appropriate. **Eyeglass aids,** which are built into the temple bar of eyeglasses, with tubing leading to the earmolds, are usually restricted to individuals who wear eyeglasses continually. The less powerful **in-the-ear aid** is contained entirely within the earmold and fits less conspicuously into the concha and the ear canal; it is appropriate for mild to moderate hearing losses. **Canal aids** are contained entirely within the ear canal and are cosmetically acceptable to many users who would otherwise refuse amplification. The **CROS aid** (for Contralateral Routing of Signals) is used for individuals with monaural hearing; a hearing-aid microphone is placed on the nonfunctioning ear and sound is routed to the functioning ear (either through a wire or miniature radio transmitter), allowing the patient to hear sounds from the nonfunctioning side and to develop a limited ability to localize sound. If the better ear also has a loss of hearing, the sound from the poorer side can be amplified and the sound coming to the better side can be amplified, the so-called **BiCROS aid.**

A **bone conduction aid** is sometimes used in hearing losses in which an earmold or tube cannot be used, as in atresia of the ear canal or persistent otorrhea. The oscillator is placed in contact with the head, usually over the mastoid, with a spring band over the head, and sound is conducted through the bone of the skull to the cochlea. Bone conduction hearing aids require more power and introduce more distortion than air conduction hearing aids and are less comfortable to wear.

In evaluating a patient for a hearing aid, professional advice is required. Selecting the proper hearing aid requires matching the electroacoustic characteristics of the hearing aid with the type of hearing loss on the basis of gain, saturation level, and frequency response. **Gain,** or amplification, refers to the difference between the input and the output of the hearing aid. The more severe the hearing loss, the more gain is generally required. **Saturation level,** the maximum output of the hearing aid regardless of input, is an important consideration for patients with reduced tolerance to sound (as in recruitment). In severe tolerance problems, special circuitry (automatic gain control, or AGC) is available that keeps the output of the aid at tolerable levels. **Frequency response** refers to the gain of the aid as a function of frequency. As a general rule, the frequency response should be selected to provide gain consistent with the patient's audiometric configuration. High frequency accentuation can also be achieved by venting the earmold, which benefits many individuals with a sensorineural hearing loss who have a greater loss in the high frequencies than in the low frequencies.

COCHLEAR IMPLANTS

Profoundly deaf individuals to whom hearing aids are of no help in speech reading (lip reading) or in hearing environmental sounds (doorbells, ringing of the telephone,

alarms, etc) may benefit from a cochlear implant. This electronic device consists of a battery-powered processor that converts sound into modulations of an electric current, an internal and external induction coil system that transmits the electrical impulses through the skin, and an electrode (some implants have more than one electrode) connected to the internal induction coil that stimulates the remaining fibers of the auditory division of the 8th cranial nerve. At mastoid surgery, the electrode is inserted into the scala tympani of the basal turn of the inner ear. The internal induction coil is implanted into the bone of the skull posterior and superior to the ear; the external conduction coil is held in place on the skin over the induction coil by magnets in the two coils.

Cochlear implants help with speech reading by allowing the profoundly deaf to distinguish when a word begins and ends, the intonation of the word, the rhythm of the speech, and some speech percepts. Some cochlear implants even allow minimal discrimination of words *without* visual clues. Cochlear implants allow deaf persons to hear and distinguish environmental sounds and warning signals. They also help deaf persons modulate their voices to make their speech more intelligible to hearing persons.

---

208. NOSE AND PARANASAL SINUSES

FRACTURES OF THE NOSE

The nasal bones are fractured more frequently than are other facial bones. The fracture usually includes the ascending processes of the maxilla and often the septum. The torn mucous membrane results in nosebleed. Soft tissue swelling develops promptly and may obscure the break. Septal hematomas may occur between the perichondrium and the quadrilateral cartilage and may become infected; abscess formation leads to avascular and septic necrosis of the cartilage, with a saddle deformity of the nose.

Diagnosis

A fracture should be suspected if blunt injury causes bleeding from the nose. Diagnosis can ordinarily be established by gently palpating the dorsum (bridge) of the nose for deformity, instability, crepitus, and point tenderness, and is confirmed by x-ray. The most common deformity is deviation of the dorsum of the nose in one direction and depression of the nasal bone and ascending process of the maxilla on the other side.

Treatment

Nasal fractures in adults may be reduced under local anesthesia; children require general anesthesia. The fracture is manipulated into a good position by internal and external traction. A blunt elevator is placed under the depressed nasal bone and the depressed bone is lifted anteriorly and laterally while pressure is applied to the other side of the nose, in order to bring the nasal dorsum to the midline. The position of the nose may be stabilized by internal packing and external splinting. Septal hematomas must be immediately incised and drained. Septal fractures are difficult to hold in position and often require nasal septal surgery later.

FOREIGN BODIES

(See Ch. 199)

SEPTAL DEVIATION AND PERFORATION

Deviations of the nasal septum from developmental abnormalities or trauma are common but often are asymptomatic and require no treatment. Septal deviation may cause

varying degrees of nasal obstruction and predispose the patient to sinusitis (particularly if the deviation obstructs an ostium of a paranasal sinus) and to epistaxis as a result of drying air currents. **Treatment** of symptomatic deviation of the nasal septum is by septoplasty or submucous resection of the septum.

Septal **ulcers** and **perforations** may follow nasal surgery, repeated trauma such as picking the nose, and granulomatous infections such as TB and syphilis. Crusting about the margins and repeated epistaxis may result. Small perforations may whistle. Topically applied bacitracin 500 u./gm in a petrolatum base reduces the crusting. Although perforations of the nasal septum may be repaired by using buccal or septal mucous membrane flaps, the problem can be more reliably controlled by closing the perforation with a silastic septal button.

EPISTAXIS

(Nosebleed)

Bleeding from the nose occurs secondary to local infections such as vestibulitis, rhinitis, and sinusitis; systemic infections such as scarlet fever, malaria, and typhoid fever; drying of the nasal mucous membrane; trauma (digital, as in picking the nose, and blunt, as in nasal fractures); arteriosclerosis; hypertension; and bleeding tendencies associated with aplastic anemia, leukemia, thrombocytopenia, liver disease, the hereditary coagulopathies, and Osler-Weber-Rendu syndrome (hereditary hemorrhagic telangiectasia—see in Ch. 99).

Treatment

Most nasal bleeding occurs from a plexus of vessels in the anteroinferior septum (Kiesselbach's area). **Bleeding may be controlled by pinching the nasal alae together for 5 to 10 min.** If this fails, the bleeding site must be found. The bleeding point may be cauterized; bleeding can be controlled temporarily by applying pressure over a cotton pledget impregnated with a vasoconstrictor such as phenylephrine 0.25% and a topical anesthetic such as tetracaine 1% until the site is anesthetized. Although electrocautery may be used, silver nitrate in a 75% applicator bead may be used to control bleeding without producing too deep a burn of the mucous membrane.

In epistaxis due to a hemorrhagic disorder, petrolatum gauze is used to apply pressure as atraumatically as possible to the bleeding point; cautery is not used, since the periphery of a cauterized area may begin to bleed. Attention is directed to identifying and correcting the bleeding disorder.

In arteriosclerosis and hypertension, bleeding is likely to be far posterior in the inferior meatus and may be difficult to control. Control requires ligating the internal maxillary artery and its branches or packing the posterior part of the nasal cavity. The arteries may be ligated under microscopic control with a surgical approach through the maxillary sinus. In order to pack the posterior part of the nasal cavity, the choana is obstructed with a postnasal pack made by folding and rolling 4-in. gauze squares into a tight bundle and tying the bundle with 2 strands of heavy silk suture. The ends of one suture are tied to a catheter that has been introduced through the nasal cavity on the side of the bleeding and brought out through the mouth. The catheter is withdrawn from the nose as the pack is placed behind the soft palate into the nasopharynx. The 2nd suture is trimmed below the level of the soft palate so that it can be used to remove the pack. (Alternatively, the balloon of a Foley catheter may be inflated in the nasopharynx to obstruct the choana.) The nasal cavity, particularly the posterior part of the inferior meatus, is firmly packed with petrolatum gauze and the first suture is tied over a roll of gauze at the anterior nares to secure the postnasal pack. The packing remains in place for 4 days. An antibiotic such as ampicillin 250 mg orally q 6 h is given to prevent sinusitis and otitis media. Postnasal packing lowers the arterial P_{O_2}, and supplementary O_2 should be given while the packing is in place.

In Osler-Weber-Rendu syndrome, multiple severe nosebleeds may occur from arteriovenous aneurysms in the mucous membrane and result in profound and persistent anemia that is not easily corrected with administration of iron. A split-thickness skin graft (septal dermoplasty) reduces the episodes of epistaxis and allows the anemia to be corrected.

Severe epistaxis is often associated with liver disease. Blood may have been swallowed in large amounts. It should be eliminated as promptly as possible with enemas and cathartics, and the GI tract sterilized with nonabsorbable antibiotics (eg, neomycin 1 gm orally qid) to prevent the breakdown of blood and absorption of ammonia.

Need for blood replacement is determined by the Hb level, vital signs, and the central venous pressure.

NASAL VESTIBULITIS

Infection of the nasal vestibule. **Low-grade infections** and **folliculitis** produce annoying crusts, and bleeding occurs as the crusts come away. Bacitracin ointment 500 u./gm applied topically bid for 14 days is effective.

Furuncles of the nasal vestibule are usually staphylococcal; they may develop into a spreading cellulitis of the tip of the nose. Systemic antibiotics should be employed along with hot soaks; penicillin G or V is the drug of choice. Furuncles of the central portion of the face should be allowed to drain spontaneously. Incision and drainage increase the risk of retrograde thrombophlebitis and subsequent cavernous sinus thrombosis, and are **contraindicated.**

RHINITIS

The most frequent of the acute upper respiratory infections, characterized by edema and vasodilatation of the nasal mucous membrane, nasal discharge, and obstruction.

Acute rhinitis is the usual manifestation of a common cold (see under RESPIRATORY VIRAL DISEASES in Ch. 12); it may also be caused by streptococcal, pneumococcal, or staphylococcal infections. **Chronic rhinitis** may occur in syphilis, TB, rhinosclerosis, rhinosporidiosis, leishmaniasis, blastomycosis, histoplasmosis, and leprosy, all conditions characterized by granuloma formation and destruction of soft tissue, cartilage, and bone. Rhinosclerosis also causes progressive nasal obstruction from indurated inflammatory tissue in the lamina propria. These conditions produce nasal obstruction, purulent rhinorrhea, and frequent bleeding. Rhinosporidiosis is characterized by bleeding polyps.

Diagnosis and Treatment

Diagnosis and treatment of **acute bacterial rhinitis** are based on pathogen identification and antibiotic sensitivities. Topical vasoconstriction with a sympathomimetic amine (eg, phenylephrine 0.25%), given q 3 to 4 h for not more than 7 days, provides symptomatic relief. Systemic sympathomimetic amines, such as pseudoephedrine 30 mg orally q 4 to 6 h, may be given for vasoconstriction of the nasal mucous membrane.

Diagnosis in **chronic rhinitis** is based on demonstrating the causative microorganism by culture or biopsy. Treatment consists of chemotherapy appropriate to the causative agent.

ATROPHIC RHINITIS

A chronic rhinitis characterized by an atrophic and sclerotic mucous membrane, abnormal patency of the nasal cavities, crust formation, and foul odor. The mucous membrane changes from ciliated pseudostratified columnar epithelium to stratified squamous epithelium, and the lamina propria is reduced in amount and vascularity. Anosmia results, and epistaxis may be recurrent and severe. The etiology is unknown, although bacterial infection plays a role.

Treatment is directed toward reducing the crusting and eliminating the odor. Topical antibiotics, such as bacitracin 500 u./gm in a petrolatum base and estrogens and vitamins A and D topically or systemically, may be effective. Occluding or reducing the patency of the nasal cavities, surgically or with a pledget of lamb's wool, decreases the crusting caused by the drying effect of air flowing over the atrophic mucous membrane.

VASOMOTOR RHINITIS

A chronic rhinitis characterized by intermittent vascular engorgement of the nasal mucous membrane, sneezing, and watery rhinorrhea. The turgescent mucous membrane varies from bright red to a purplish hue. The condition is marked by periods of remission and exacerbation. It appears to be aggravated by a dry atmosphere. The etiology is uncertain, and no allergy can be identified.

Treatment is empirical and not always satisfactory. Patients benefit from humidified air; eg, from a humidified central heating system or a vaporizer in the workroom and bedroom. Systemic sympathomimetic amines—eg, pseudoephedrine 30 mg orally (adult) q 4 to 6 h as necessary—give symptomatic relief but are not recommended for regular long-term use. Topical vasoconstrictors should be **avoided** because the vasculature of the nasal mucous membrane loses its sensitivity to stimuli—eg, the humidity and temperature of the inspired air—that result in vasoconstriction. Vasodilatation results, except after application of a strong stimulus, such as a topical sympathomimetic amine.

ALLERGIC RHINITIS

(See Atopic Diseases in Ch. 21)

POLYPS

Allergic rhinitis predisposes to polyp formation; polyps may also occur in acute and chronic infections. Nasal polyps form at the site of massive dependent edema in the lamina propria of the mucous membrane, usually around the ostia of the maxillary sinuses. As a polyp develops, it becomes teardrop-shaped; when mature, it resembles a peeled seedless grape. In acute infections, polyps may regress after the infection resolves. Bleeding polyps occur in rhinosporidiosis. Unilateral polyps occasionally occur in association with benign or malignant neoplasms of the nose or paranasal sinuses.

Treatment: Corticosteroids, such as beclomethasone dipropionate (42 mcg/spray) or flunisolide (25 mcg/spray) aerosols, 1 or 2 sprays in each nasal cavity bid, have reduced or eliminated polyps, although surgical removal is often still required. Polyps should be removed if they obstruct the airway or promote sinusitis, or if they are unilateral polyps that may be obscuring benign or malignant neoplasms. Polyps tend to recur unless the underlying allergy or infection is controlled. Following removal of nasal polyps, topical beclomethasone or flunisolide therapy tends to retard their recurrence. In severe and recurrent cases, maxillary sinusotomy or ethmoidectomy may be indicated.

WEGENER'S GRANULOMATOSIS

Wegener's granulomatosis, a vasculitis of unknown etiology characterized by granulomas of the nose and lung and glomerulitis of the kidney, is discussed fully in Ch. 110. Most destructive lesions of bone, cartilage, and soft tissue of the nose and paranasal sinuses are ultimately found on thorough biopsy to be malignant neoplasms such as a lymphoma or carcinoma.

ANOSMIA

Loss of the sense of smell. Anosmia requires careful evaluation for intranasal and intracranial diseases. Anosmia occurs when (1) intranasal swelling or other obstruction prevents odors from gaining access to the olfactory area; (2) the olfactory neuroepithelium is destroyed, as in viral infections, atrophic rhinitis, or the chronic rhinitis of granulomatous diseases and neoplasms; or (3) the olfactory nerve fila, olfactory bulbs and tracts, or their central connections are destroyed, as by head trauma, intracranial surgery, infections, or neoplasms. Head trauma is a major cause of anosmia in young adults; viral infections are a major cause in older adults. Anosmia occurs congenitally in male hypogonadism (Kallmann's syndrome). Most patients with anosmia have normal perception of salty, sweet, sour, and bitter substances, but they lack flavor discrimination, which is largely dependent on olfaction, and therefore often complain of loss of the sense of taste.

Diagnostic evaluation requires examination of the cranial nerves and upper respiratory tract (particularly the nose and nasopharynx), psychophysical measuring of odor and taste identification and threshold detection, and enhanced CT of the head to rule out neoplasms and unsuspected fractures of the floor of the anterior cranial fossa.

Treatment for allergic rhinitis and removal of nasal polyps and benign neoplasms often result in recovery of the sense of smell. Conditions causing destruction of the olfactory neuroepithelium or its central pathways do not lend themselves to effective therapeutic intervention, although spontaneous recovery frequently follows regeneration of the olfactory neuroepithelium and its central pathways.

SINUSITIS

An inflammatory process in the paranasal sinuses due to viral, bacterial, and fungal infections or allergic reactions.

Etiology and Pathogenesis

Acute sinusitis is caused by streptococci, pneumococci, *Hemophilus influenzae,* and staphylococci, and is usually precipitated by an acute viral respiratory tract infection. Exacerbations of chronic sinusitis may be caused by a gram-negative rod or anaerobic microorganisms. In about 25% of cases, chronic maxillary sinusitis is secondary to dental infection.

With a URI, the swollen nasal mucous membrane obstructs the ostium of the paranasal sinus, and the O_2 in the sinus is absorbed into the blood vessels in the mucous membrane. The resulting relative negative pressure in the sinus **(vacuum sinusitis)** is painful. If the vacuum is maintained, a transudate from the mucous membrane develops and fills the sinus, where it serves as a medium for bacteria that enter through the ostium or through a spreading cellulitis or thrombophlebitis in the lamina propria of the mucous membrane. An outpouring of serum and leukocytes to combat the infection results, and painful positive pressure develops in the obstructed sinus. The mucous membrane becomes hyperemic and edematous.

Symptoms, Signs, and Diagnosis

The symptoms and signs of acute and chronic sinusitis are similar. The area over the involved sinus may be tender and swollen. Maxillary sinusitis causes pain in the maxillary area, toothache, and frontal headache. Frontal sinusitis produces pain in the frontal area and frontal headache. Ethmoid sinusitis causes pain behind and between the eyes, and a frontal headache that is often described as "splitting." Pain from sphenoid sinusitis is less well localized and is referred to the frontal or occipital area.

There may be malaise. Fever and chills suggest an extension of the infection beyond the sinuses.

The nasal mucous membrane is red and turgescent; yellow or green purulent rhinorrhea may be present. The seropurulent or mucopurulent exudate may be seen in the middle meatus in maxillary, anterior ethmoid, and frontal sinusitis, and in the area medial to the middle turbinate in posterior ethmoid and sphenoid sinusitis.

The frontal and maxillary sinuses may be opaque to transillumination, but radiography of the paranasal sinuses more reliably defines the sites and the degree of involvement. Radio-opacity in acute sinusitis may be due to the swollen mucous membrane or a retained exudate. X-rays of the apices of the teeth are required in chronic maxillary sinusitis to exclude a periapical abscess.

Treatment

Improved drainage and control of infection are the aims of therapy in acute sinusitis. Steam inhalation effectively produces nasal vasoconstriction and promotes drainage. Topical vasoconstrictors such as phenylephrine 0.25% spray q 3 h are effective but should be used for a maximum of 7 days; systemic vasoconstrictors such as pseudoephedrine 30 mg orally (adult) q 4 to 6 h are less reliably effective.

In both acute and chronic sinusitis, antibiotics should be given for at least 10 to 12 days. In acute sinusitis, penicillin G or V 250 mg orally q 6 h is the initial antibiotic of choice, and erythromycin 250 mg orally q 6 h is the second choice. In exacerbations of chronic sinusitis, a broad-spectrum antibiotic such as ampicillin 250 or 500 mg or tetracycline 250 mg orally q 6 h is better. In chronic sinusitis, prolonged antibiotic therapy for 4 to 6 wk often results in complete resolution. The sensitivities of pathogens isolated from the sinus exudate and the patient's response guide subsequent therapy. Sinusitis not responsive to antibiotic therapy may require operative intervention (Caldwell-Luc operation for the maxillary sinuses, ethmoidectomy for the ethmoid sinuses, and sphenoid sinusotomy for the sphenoid sinuses) to improve ventilation and drainage and to remove inspiccated mucopurulent material, epithelial debris, and hypertrophic mucous membrane. Chronic frontal sinusitis is managed with an osteoplastic obliteration of the frontal sinuses.

NEOPLASMS

Unilateral bloody nasal discharge and obstruction, and facial swelling and numbness indicate cancer of the nose or paranasal sinuses until proven otherwise. **Exophytic papillomas** are squamous cell papillomas with a branching, vascular connective tissue stalk with finger-like projections on the surface. In the nasal cavity they often require repeated excision, but have a benign course. **Inverted papillomas** are squamous cell papillomas in which the epithelium is invaginated into the vascular connective tissue stroma. They are invasive and behave in a locally malignant manner; excision must include a large margin of normal tissue, including the bone of the lateral wall of the nasal cavity in a procedure called a lateral rhinotomy.

Other benign tumors that occur in the nasal cavity are fibromas, hemangiomas, and neurofibromas. Fibromas, neurolemmomas, and ossifying fibromas occur in the paranasal sinuses.

Squamous cell carcinoma is the most common malignant tumor in the nose and paranasal sinuses; others are adenoid cystic and mucoepidermoid carcinomas, malignant mixed tumors, adenocarcinomas, lymphomas, fibrosarcomas, osteosarcomas, chondrosarcomas, and melanomas. Hypernephroma is the most common metastatic tumor in the paranasal sinuses. Combined irradiation and radical resection give the best survival rates for the primary neoplasms.

209. NASOPHARYNX

ADENOID HYPERTROPHY

(See ADENOID HYPERTROPHY under BACTERIAL INFECTIONS in Ch. 191 and JUVENILE ANGIOFIBROMA in Ch. 199)

TORNWALDT'S CYST

(Nasopharyngeal Cyst)

A frequently infected cyst found in the midline of the nasopharynx. The cyst lies superficial to the superior constrictor muscle of the pharynx and is covered by the mucous membrane of the nasopharynx. If infected, it may cause persistent purulent drainage with a foul taste and odor, eustachian tube obstruction, and sore throat. Purulent exudate may be seen coming from the opening of the cyst. **Treatment** consists of marsupialization or excision.

NASOPHARYNGEAL CARCINOMA

Squamous cell carcinoma of the nasopharynx occurs in children and young adults. Rare in North America, it is one of the most common cancers in the Orient. The first symptom is often nasal or eustachian tube obstruction; the latter may result in middle ear effusion. Purulent bloody rhinorrhea, frank epistaxis, cranial nerve paralysis due to invasion of the parapharyngeal space and cranial cavity by the tumor, and cervical lymphadenopathy due to metastasis are common presenting complaints. **Diagnosis** is by biopsy of the primary nasopharyngeal tumor. Biopsy of the neck metastasis should be avoided until the nasopharynx has been inspected and palpated and any suspicious lesion there has been biopsied. The **treatment** of choice is supervoltage irradiation. The overall 5-yr survival rate is 35%.

---

210. OROPHARYNX

PHARYNGITIS

Acute inflammation of the pharynx. Usually viral in origin, it may be due to a Group A β-hemolytic streptococcus or occasionally to a pneumococcus or coagulase-positive staphylococcus. It is characterized by sore throat and pain on swallowing. Differentiating viral from bacterial pharyngitis on the basis of physical examination alone is difficult. In both, the pharyngeal mucous membrane may be mildly injected or severely inflamed and may be covered by a membrane and a purulent exudate. Fever, cervical adenopathy, and leukocytosis are present in both viral and streptococcal pharyngitis but may be more marked in the latter. (For pharyngitis in gonorrhea and in other sexually transmitted diseases, see in Ch. 14.)

Treatment includes aspirin, to relieve discomfort, and rest. Antibiotic therapy should usually be withheld pending positive cultures for bacteria. Penicillin G or V 250 mg orally q 6 h for 10 days is indicated for streptococcal pharyngitis and may be given for pneumococcal and staphylococcal pharyngitis if the symptoms and course warrant therapeutic intervention.

TONSILLITIS

Acute inflammation of the palatine tonsils, usually due to streptococcal or, less commonly, viral infection. Epidemics of viral tonsillitis occur among military recruits. Ton-

sillitis is characterized by sore throat and pain, most marked on swallowing and often referred to the ears. Very young children may not complain of sore throat but will refuse to eat. High fever, malaise, headache, and vomiting are common.

Diagnosis

The tonsils are edematous and hyperemic. There may be a purulent exudate from the crypts and a membrane—white, thin, nonconfluent, and confined to the tonsil—that peels away without bleeding. The **differential diagnosis** includes diphtheria, Vincent's angina (trench mouth), and infectious mononucleosis. In diphtheria, the membrane is dirty gray, thick, and tough, and bleeds if peeled away; it shows *Corynebacterium diphtheriae* on smear and culture. Vincent's angina, characterized by superficial, painful ulcers with erythematous borders, is caused by a fusiform bacillus and a spirochete that are demonstrable on smear. Infectious mononucleosis tonsillitis characteristically is associated with micropetechiae of the soft palate; atypical lymphocytes on smear and a positive heterophil agglutination test confirm the diagnosis of mononucleosis.

Treatment

In viral tonsillitis, symptomatic therapy is as for pharyngitis (above). Penicillin G or V 250 mg orally q 6 h is the treatment of choice in streptococcal tonsillitis and should be continued for 10 days. When possible, the throat should be recultured 5 to 6 days later. Family members' throats should also be cultured initially so that carriers may be treated at the same time. Tonsillectomy should be considered if, despite these precautions, acute tonsillitis repeatedly develops after adequate treatment, or if chronic tonsillitis and sore throat persist or are relieved only briefly by antibiotic therapy.

PERITONSILLAR CELLULITIS AND ABSCESS
(Quinsy)

An acute infection located between the tonsil and the superior pharyngeal constrictor muscle. Peritonsillar abscesses are rare in children but common in young adults. Although usually due to a Group A β-hemolytic streptococcus, anaerobic microorganisms such as bacteroides also cause peritonsillar infection. There is severe pain on swallowing; the patient is febrile and toxic, holds his head tilted toward the side of the abscess, and shows marked trismus. The tonsil is displaced medially by the peritonsillar cellulitis and abscess, the soft palate is erythematous and swollen, and the uvula is edematous and displaced to the opposite side.

Treatment

Cellulitis without pus formation will respond to penicillin in 24 to 48 h. Initially, penicillin G 1 million u. IV q 4 h is given. If pus is present and does not drain spontaneously, incision and drainage are required. Antibiotic therapy should be continued orally with penicillin G or V 250 mg q 6 h for 12 days. Peritonsillar abscesses tend to recur and tonsillectomy is indicated (usually performed 6 wk after the acute infection has subsided). With antibiotic therapy, the tonsillectomy can be performed at the time of the acute peritonsillar infection.

PARAPHARYNGEAL ABSCESS

Suppuration of a parapharyngeal lymph node with consequent abscess formation is usually secondary to pharyngitis or tonsillitis and may occur at any age. The abscess is lateral to the superior pharyngeal constrictor muscle and close to the carotid sheath. Pharyngeal inflammation may not be apparent. The anterior cervical triangle is markedly swollen. Penicillin G 150,000 u./kg/day IV in 4 equal doses (for a child) should be given initially and the abscess drained though a cervical, not pharyngeal, incision.

Subsequently, penicillin G or V 250 mg orally q 6 h is given to complete 12 days of therapy.

RETROPHARYNGEAL ABSCESS

(See under BACTERIAL INFECTIONS in Ch. 191)

VELOPHARYNGEAL INSUFFICIENCY

Incomplete closure of the velopharyngeal sphincter between the oropharynx and the nasopharynx, resulting in impaired speech and deglutition. The speech is characterized by nasal emission of air and weak oral plosive and fricative articulation.

Normal closure, achieved by the sphincteric action of the soft palate and the superior constrictor muscle, is impaired in patients with cleft palates, repaired cleft palates, congenitally short palates, submucous cleft palates, unusually large nasopharynges, and palatal paralysis.

Diagnosis and Treatment

Regurgitation of solid foods and fluids through the nose denotes gross velopharyngeal insufficiency, but normal speech is a more exacting criterion of competency. Inspection of the palate during phonation may reveal palatal paralysis. Palpation of the midline of the soft palate and transillumination with a nasopharyngoscope may demonstrate a submucous cleft. A lateral x-ray may demonstrate the congenitally short palate or an unusually large nasopharynx and, if taken during phonation, will indicate the degree of insufficiency; cinefluoroscopy during connected speech verifies an inability to maintain velopharyngeal valve closure.

Treatment requires speech therapy and surgical correction by a palatal push-back procedure, pharyngeal flap, pharyngoplasty, or Teflon paste injection of the posterior pharyngeal wall.

CARCINOMA OF THE TONSIL

Squamous cell carcinoma of the tonsil, second in frequency only to carcinoma of the larynx among malignancies of the upper respiratory tract, occurs predominantly in males and is associated with tobacco smoking and ethanol ingestion. Sore throat is the most common presenting complaint, and pain often radiates to the ear on the same side. A metastatic mass in the neck may be the first symptom. **Diagnosis** is made by biopsy. Direct laryngoscopy, bronchoscopy, and esophagoscopy are carried out to exclude a synchronous 2nd primary neoplasm. **Treatment** combines irradiation and surgery, consisting of radical resection of the tonsillar fossa, hemimandibulectomy, and radical neck dissection. The 5-yr survival rate approximates 50%.

ZENKER'S (PHARYNGOESOPHAGEAL) DIVERTICULUM

(See in Ch. 51)

211. LARYNX

VOCAL CORD POLYPS

Vocal cord polyps develop from voice abuse, chronic laryngeal allergic reactions, and chronic inhalation of irritants such as industrial fumes and cigarette smoke. They consist of chronic edema in the lamina propria of the true vocal cord and result in

hoarseness and a breathy voice quality. Biopsy of discrete lesions should be done to exclude carcinoma. **Treatment** involves surgical removal of the polyp at direct laryngoscopy to restore the voice, and attention to the underlying cause to prevent recurrence, including voice therapy if voice abuse is the cause.

VOCAL CORD NODULES

(Singer's Nodules)

Vocal cord nodules are caused by chronic voice abuse, such as yelling or shouting, or using an unnaturally low fundamental frequency. The nodules are condensations of hyaline connective tissue in the lamina propria at the junction of the anterior 1/3 and the posterior 2/3 of the free edges of the true vocal cords. Hoarseness and a breathy voice quality result. Carcinoma should be excluded by biopsy. **Treatment** involves surgical removal of the nodules at direct laryngoscopy and correction of the underlying voice abuse. Vocal nodules in children usually regress with voice therapy alone.

CONTACT ULCERS

Unilateral or bilateral ulcers of the mucous membrane over the vocal process of the arytenoid cartilage. Contact ulcers are usually due to voice abuse in the form of a sharp glottal attack (abrupt rise in intensity at the onset of phonation). Reflux of gastric contents may also be an etiologic factor. Mild pain on phonation and swallowing and varying degrees of hoarseness result. Biopsy to exclude carcinoma is important. Prolonged ulceration leads to nonspecific granulomas that produce varying degrees of hoarseness.

Treatment consists of prolonged voice rest (6 wk minimum) for healing of the ulcers. Patients must recognize the limitations of their voices and learn to adjust their vocal activities to avoid recurrent ulcers. Granulomas tend to recur after surgical removal but respond to voice therapy. Antacids, avoiding eating within 2 h of retiring, and elevation of the head of the bed should be employed if gastroesophageal reflux is demonstrated on an upper GI series.

LARYNGITIS

Inflammation of the larynx.

Etiology

Viral and bacterial URIs are the most frequent causes of acute laryngitis. Although viral laryngitis is commoner, β-hemolytic streptococcus and *Streptococcus pneumoniae* are causative microorganisms. It may also occur in the course of bronchitis, pneumonia, influenza, pertussis, measles, and diphtheria. Excessive use of the voice, allergic reactions, and inhalation of irritating substances can cause acute or chronic laryngitis.

Symptoms and Signs

Unnatural change of voice is usually the most prominent symptom. Hoarseness and even aphonia, together with a sensation of tickling, rawness, and a constant urge to clear the throat, may occur. Symptoms vary with the severity of the inflammation. Fever, malaise, dysphagia, and throat pain may occur in the more severe infections; dyspnea may be apparent if laryngeal edema is present. Indirect laryngoscopic examination discloses a mild to marked erythema of the mucous membrane that may also be edematous. If a membrane is present, diphtheria must be suspected (see DIPHTHERIA under BACTERIAL INFECTIONS in Ch. 191).

Treatment

There is no specific treatment for viral laryngitis. Penicillin G 250 mg orally q 6 h for 10 to 12 days is the drug of choice for streptococcal or pneumococcal laryngitis. Treatment of acute or chronic bronchitis may improve the laryngitis. Treatment of chronic bronchitis may require a broader spectrum antibiotic, such as ampicillin 250 or 500 mg or tetracycline 250 mg orally q 6 h for 10 to 14 days. Voice rest and steam inhalations give symptomatic relief and promote resolution of acute laryngitis.

ACUTE LARYNGOTRACHEOBRONCHITIS

(See ACUTE EPIGLOTTITIS under BACTERIAL INFECTIONS and CROUP under VIRAL INFECTIONS in Ch. 191)

VOCAL CORD PARALYSIS

Etiology

Vocal cord paralysis may result from lesions at the nucleus ambiguus, its supranuclear tracts, the main trunk of the vagus, or the recurrent laryngeal nerves. Intracranial neoplasms, vascular accidents, and demyelinating diseases cause nucleus ambiguus paralysis. Neoplasms at the base of the skull and trauma of the neck cause vagus paralysis. Recurrent laryngeal paralysis is caused by neck or thoracic lesions, eg, aortic aneurysm, mitral stenosis, neoplasms of the thyroid gland, esophagus, lung, and mediastinal structures, or trauma, thyroidectomy, neurotoxins (lead), neurotoxic infections (diphtheria), and viral illness. Viral neuronitis probably accounts for most cases of idiopathic vocal cord paralysis.

Symptoms and Signs

Vocal cord paralysis results in loss of vocal cord abduction, or adduction and abduction; may affect phonation, respiration, and deglutition; and may result in aspiration of food and fluids into the trachea. The paralyzed cord generally lies 2 to 3 mm lateral to the midline, and in recurrent laryngeal nerve paralysis may move with phonation but not on inspiration. In **unilateral vocal cord paralysis,** the voice is hoarse and breathy. There is usually no airway obstruction because the normal cord abducts sufficiently. In **bilateral vocal cord paralysis,** the cords are within 2 to 3 mm of the midline and the voice is of limited intensity but good quality. The airway, however, is inadequate, resulting in stridor and dyspnea on moderate exertion.

Diagnosis

The cause must always be sought. The evaluation may include laryngoscopy, bronchoscopy, and esophagoscopy. Neurologic examination; enhanced CT of the head, neck, and chest; thyroid gland scan; and upper GI series are also indicated. Cricoarytenoid arthritis may cause fixation of the cricoarytenoid joint and must be differentiated.

Treatment

In unilateral paralysis, augmenting the paralyzed cord by injecting a Teflon suspension may allow approximation of the cords for voice improvement and prevention of aspiration. Maintenance of an adequate airway is the problem in bilateral paralysis. Tracheotomy may be needed permanently or during URIs. An arytenoidectomy with lateralization of the true vocal cord will open the glottis and improve the airway but may adversely affect voice quality.

LARYNGOCELES

Evaginations of the mucous membrane of the laryngeal ventricle. Internal laryngoceles displace and enlarge the false vocal cord and result in hoarseness and airway obstruc-

tion. External laryngoceles extend through the thyrohyoid membrane, producing a mass in the neck. Laryngoceles are filled with air and can be expanded by Valsalva's maneuver. They tend to occur in musicians who play wind instruments. They appear on CT as smooth, ovoid, low-density masses. Laryngoceles may become infected (laryngopyocele) or filled with mucoid fluid. **Treatment** is excision.

NEOPLASMS

BENIGN

Juvenile papillomas are discussed in Ch. 199. Other benign laryngeal tumors include hemangiomas, fibromas, chondromas, myxomas, and neurofibromas. They may involve any part of the larynx. Removal restores the voice, the functional integrity of the laryngeal sphincter, and the airway.

MALIGNANT

Squamous cell carcinoma, the most common malignant neoplasm of the larynx, is also the most common malignancy of the head and neck. The incidence is higher in males. It is associated with cigarette smoking and ethanol consumption. The true vocal cords (particularly the anterior portion), epiglottis, pyriform sinus, and postcricoid area are common sites of origin. Cordal or glottic carcinoma produces hoarseness early, and all patients with hoarseness lasting > 2 wk should have indirect laryngoscopy. A discrete lesion of the laryngeal mucous membrane should be biopsied at direct laryngoscopy. Carcinoma of the supraglottic larynx (epiglottis), hypopharyngeal carcinoma (pyriform sinus), and postcricoid carcinoma cause pain and difficulty on swallowing. In the first 2 forms, a metastatic mass in the neck may be the first symptom.

Verrucous carcinoma is a rare variant of squamous cell carcinoma and usually arises in the glottic area. The diagnosis may require multiple biopsies.

Treatment

For **early glottic carcinoma,** radiation therapy or cordectomy results in a 5-yr survival rate of 85 to 95%. For **early cordal carcinoma,** radiation is preferred, since it usually results in a normal voice. For **advanced carcinoma** with anterior commissure involvement, impaired vocal cord mobility, thyroid cartilage invasion, or subglottic extension, surgery is necessary. A hemilaryngectomy, preserving laryngeal phonation and sphincteric functions, is often possible. More advanced glottic carcinoma requires total laryngectomy. **Early supraglottic carcinoma** can be effectively treated with radiation therapy. For more **advanced supraglottic carcinoma** that does not involve the true vocal cords, a supraglottic partial laryngectomy can be performed to preserve the voice and glottic sphincter. If there is true vocal cord involvement, a total laryngectomy is required. **Early hypopharyngeal carcinoma** may be managed by an extended partial laryngectomy; more advanced lesions require a total laryngectomy. **Postcricoid carcinoma** requires a total laryngopharyngectomy and replacement of the hypopharynx and cervical esophagus with a free jejunal graft with microvascular anastomoses. For **metastasis to the cervical lymph nodes,** laryngeal surgery is combined with radical or modified radical neck dissection. In **advanced supraglottic and hypopharyngeal carcinoma,** a combination of radiation therapy and operation is more successful than surgery alone. **Verrucous carcinoma** is treated surgically.

Rehabilitation after total laryngectomy requires developing a new voice by using esophageal speech or creating a tracheoesophageal fistula. **Esophageal speech** involves taking air into the esophagus during the negative intrathoracic pressure of inspiration and gradually eructating the air through the pharyngoesophageal junction to produce a sound that is articulated into speech by the pharynx, palate, tongue, teeth, and lips.

A **tracheoesophageal fistula,** created by inserting a one-way valve between the trachea and the esophagus, forces air into the esophagus during expiration to produce a sound that is converted into speech. With this technic, fluids and food may be aspirated into the tracheobronchial tree if the tracheoesophageal valve misfunctions.

An alternative method, using an **electrolarynx** as a sounding source, requires holding the device in place while it produces the sound that is articulated into speech.

212. NEOPLASMS OF THE HEAD AND NECK

Neoplasms of specific organs are discussed elsewhere in THE MANUAL. This discussion deals with important general principles of head and neck neoplasms and with the situation in which cervical metastasis is present and the primary neoplasm cannot be determined.

Etiology and Pathogenesis

A history of alcohol and tobacco consumption is present in 85% of patients with cancer of the head or neck. The most common cancer of the upper respiratory and alimentary tracts is squamous cell carcinoma of the larynx, followed by squamous cell carcinoma of the palatine tonsil and hypopharynx. People who practice poor oral hygiene, have ill-fitting dentures, dip snuff, or chew tobacco tend to develop oral cavity cancers.

The Epstein-Barr virus plays a role in pathogenesis of nasopharyngeal cancer. Patients who received small doses of radiation therapy 20 or more years ago (for acne, facial hair, enlarged thymus, hypertrophic tonsils, and adenoids) are predisposed to developing thyroid and salivary gland cancer.

Head and neck cancer usually spreads in an orderly fashion and remains localized to the head and neck for long periods. Local tissue invasion is followed by regional metastasis and then by distant metastasis. Hematogenous metastases are usually associated with large or recurrent tumors and with concurrent disease in immunosuppressed patients.

Epidemiology

In the head and neck, 90% of cancers are squamous cell (epidermoid) carcinoma; melanomas, lymphomas, and sarcomas make up another 5%. Patients with cancers of the salivary glands, thyroid, paranasal sinuses, and sarcomas are usually under age 59 yr, whereas those with squamous cell carcinoma of the oral cavity, pharynx, and larynx are generally over age 59 yr, the average age for all patients with head and neck cancers. Cancer of the nasopharynx is extremely prevalent in native-born and first-generation Chinese. Caucasians are more frequently afflicted with head and neck cancer than blacks.

Staging and Prognosis

Head and neck cancers are classified according to size and site of involvement of the primary neoplasm **(T)**, number and size of metastases to the cervical lymph nodes **(N)**, and evidence of distant metastases **(M)**. **Stage I:** The primary neoplasm is < 2 cm in diameter or localized to one anatomic site without regional or distant metastasis ($T_1N_0M_0$). **Stage II:** The primary neoplasm measures 2 to 4 cm in diameter or involves 2 areas within a specific site (eg, larynx) without regional or distant metastasis ($T_2N_0M_0$). **Stage III:** The primary neoplasm is > 4 cm or involves 3 adjacent areas in a specific head and neck site and/or has an isolated neck metastasis < 3 cm in diameter

(T_3N_0 or any $T_{1-3}N_1M_0$). **Stage IV:** The cancer is massive, invades bone and cartilage and/or extends outside of its site of origin into another site (eg, oral cavity into oropharynx); neck metastasis measures > 3 cm, involves multiple nodes or is fixed to surrounding tissue, and/or evidence exists of distant metastases ($T_4N_{1-3}M_{0-1}$).

With appropriate treatment, Stage I survival generally approaches 90%; Stage II, 75%; Stage III, 45 to 75%; and Stage IV, < 35%. Overall 5-yr survival is 65% for all patients with local Stage I and II squamous cell cancer of the head and neck. The rate drops to 30% for patients with metastasis to lymph nodes (Stage III). Patients over age 70 yr have longer disease-free intervals and better survival rates than younger patients.

Exophytic or verrucous-appearing tumors respond to treatment better than infiltrative, ulcerative, or indurated lesions. Cervical or distant metastasis is associated with limited survival. The more poorly differentiated the cancer, the greater the chance of regional and distant metastasis. Invasion of muscle, bone, or cartilage reduces cure rates. Perineural spread as evidenced by pain, paralysis, or numbness indicates a highly aggressive neoplasm with a high propensity for recurrence.

Treatment

Small soft-tissue lesions < 2 cm in diameter, regardless of location within the upper respiratory or alimentary tracts, respond equally to surgery or radiation. A 5-yr cure rate of 90% can be expected. With radiation therapy, some surgical procedures may be needed in order to achieve the 90% cure rate. Lesions > 2 cm or with bone or cartilage invasion (with or without regional neck metastasis) require surgery. If lymph node metastases are found, postoperative radiation is necessary. Alternatively, fair survival rates can be attained with radiation with or without chemotherapy. If the cancer recurs, the patient has recourse to surgery. In advanced (most stage II and all stages III and IV) squamous cell carcinoma, combining surgery and radiation offers a better chance of cure than treatment with either modality alone. Radiation therapy may be given preoperatively or postoperatively. Postoperative radiation is usually preferred.

Surgery is more effective than radiation and/or chemotherapy in controlling large primary cancers, while radiation is effective in controlling microscopic or nonpalpable metastases. Chemotherapy kills tumor cells at the local site, regional lymph nodes, and distant metastases. It is not clear whether adjuvant chemotherapy (in combination with surgery or radiation therapy) increases the cure rate; however, combined therapy does prolong the interval between cancer disappearance and recurrence. Several agents—cisplatin, fluorouracil, bleomycin, and methotrexate—provide useful palliation for pain and reduce neoplasm size in patients in whom surgery or radiation therapy cannot be used. A disadvantage of surgery is the need for rehabilitation for swallowing and speaking. Radiation produces skin changes, fibrosis, ageusia, xerostomia, and, rarely, osteoradionecrosis. Toxicities of chemotherapy include severe nausea and vomiting, transient hair loss, gastroenteritis, and hematopoietic and immune depression. In cancer excision after chemotherapy or irradiation, the surgeon must remove what was originally involved with the neoplasm before the anticancer therapy was started.

Recurring or persisting cancer: *A palpable mass or ulcerated lesion with edema or pain at the primary site after therapy*. Detecting recurrence after chemotherapy or radiation therapy is more difficult than after surgery alone; however, recurrence after surgery alone is usually more difficult to eradicate than recurrence after radiation and/or chemotherapy.

For adequate local control following surgical failure, all scar planes as well as reconstructive flaps must be excised in addition to the cancer. Radiation and/or chemotherapy following surgical failure is much less effective than when used before or with surgery. Gallium scan can in some cases detect recurrences or tumors that are ≥ 2 cm.

UNKNOWN PRIMARY AND CERVICAL METASTASES

After detection of cancerous cervical adenopathy, 80% of primary carcinoma will be found in the upper respiratory or alimentary tracts. If adenopathy occurs in the supraclavicular area, only 40% of patients will have the primary site of origin in the head and neck. Evaluation of a neck mass may require endoscopy and biopsy of all suspicious areas. Random biopsies of the tonsils, base of tongue, and nasopharynx are indicated if no lesions are found. Open biopsy of a neck mass suspicious for carcinoma is contraindicated unless definitive radical neck surgery is simultaneously undertaken; otherwise, open biopsy severely affects patient prognosis. In contradistinction, fine needle (20 to 22 gauge) aspiration biopsy of a cervical mass can be complementary to the workup of an unknown primary, without spreading cancer or affecting patient prognosis.

Treatment: Palpable cancerous cervical adenopathy requires surgical removal and radiation therapy to the nasopharynx, palatine tonsils, base of the tongue, and both sides of the neck. Nonpalpable cervical metastases with a squamous cell cancer primary in the head and neck respond equally to surgery or radiation.

PREMALIGNANT LESIONS

(See in Ch. 251)

§18. OPHTHALMOLOGIC DISORDERS

213. CLINICAL EXAMINATION

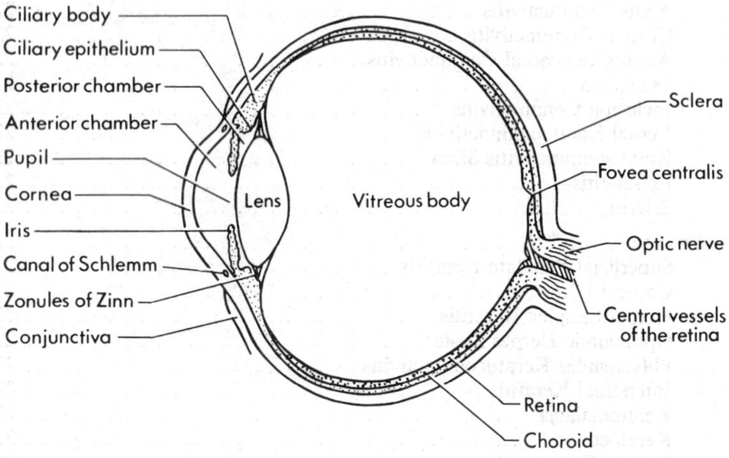

FIG. 213–1. **The eye—cross section.** The **zonules of Zinn** keep the lens suspended, while the muscles of the **ciliary body** serve to focus the lens. The **ciliary epithelium** secretes **aqueous humor,** which fills the **anterior and posterior chambers** and drains primarily via the **canal of Schlemm.** The **iris** regulates the light entering the eye by adjusting the size of its central opening, the **pupil.** The visual image is focused on the **retina,** the **fovea centralis** being the area of sharpest visual acuity. Note that the conjunctiva ends abruptly at the limbus. The cornea is covered with an epithelium that differs in many respects from the conjunctival epithelium.

Some ocular complaints are nonspecific, so that a complete history and examination of all parts of the eye and its adnexa are necessary to identify the source of the complaint. The patient should be asked about the location and duration of the symptom; the presence and nature of any pain, discharge, or redness; and any change in visual acuity.

Unless chemicals requiring immediate irrigation have splashed into the eye, the first step in ocular evaluation is to record the visual acuity. Vision is tested by having the patient wear his glasses and look at an eye chart 20 ft away. Covering each eye alternately, the acuity in each can be determined. In the usual Snellen notation, 20/40 indicates that the patient sees at 20 ft what the average person sees at 40 ft. Gross inspection of the glasses will provide an approximation of the degree of ametropia (eg, nearsightedness, farsightedness, astigmatism). Visual fields and ocular motility may also be determined at this time. The fields can be checked by confrontation examination, as described under assessment of visual fields under VISION AND EYE MOVEMENT DISORDERS in Ch. 119.

Under a focal light and magnification (eg, provided by a headband loupe), systematic examination of the eye should proceed. The eyelids are examined for lesions of the margins and subcutaneous tissues. The area of the lacrimal sacs is palpated and an attempt made to express any contents up through the canaliculi and puncta. The lids are then everted, and the palpebral and bulbar conjunctiva and the fornices are inspected for foreign bodies, signs of inflammation (eg, follicular hypertrophy, exudate, injection), or other abnormalities.

The cornea should be inspected closely. If pain and photophobia make it difficult for the patient to open his eye, topical anesthesia can be accomplished before examination by instilling 1 drop of 1% proparacaine or tetracaine. Fluorescein staining with sterile, individually packaged fluorescein strips will make corneal abrasions or ulcers more apparent. The strip is moistened with 1 drop of sterile saline and, with the patient's eye turned upward, is touched to the inside of the lower lid for several seconds. The eye is closed for 5 seconds, then examined under good magnification and illumination. Denuded areas will stain green.

The size and shape of the pupils and their reaction to light and accommodation should be noted. Ocular tension and anterior chamber depth should be estimated before dilation, as mydriasis can precipitate an attack of acute glaucoma if the anterior chamber is shallow.

Ophthalmoscopy is aided by dilating the pupil with 1 drop of 0.5% tropicamide or 2.5 or 5% phenylephrine (repeated in 5 to 15 min if necessary); for longer action, 0.5% cyclopentolate or 10% phenylephrine may be used. Care must be taken not to dilate the pupils in patients who have had head trauma or who may be suspected of having acute disease of the CNS. Atropine is not recommended because of its prolonged action. Ophthalmoscopy will disclose lesions of the cornea, lens, and retina, as well as vitreous opacities and optic nerve lesions. The strength of the ophthalmoscope lens required to bring the retina into focus will give an approximate measure of refractive error. The fundus may show changes due to systemic disease (eg, diabetes mellitus, hypertension).

Other instruments (eg, slit lamp, gonioscope, tangent screen, perimeter) may be needed for precise diagnosis; their use requires special training. The slit-lamp examination is especially helpful in distinguishing corneal lesions. Though other physicians can care for many diseases of the eye, when in doubt an ophthalmologist should be consulted, especially when the cause of pain or diminished vision is not apparent or when symptoms persist.

Ultrasonography delineates retinal tumors, detachments, and vitreous hemorrhages, even in the presence of opacities of the cornea and lens. Use of ultrasound in ophthalmology started early, with both A and B mode technics. A hand-held B scanner has

simplified ultrasonic examination of the eye and made it possible to do such studies in the ophthalmologist's office. Definition in the orbit is improved by using higher frequencies (7 to 10 MHz). Ultrasonography has also been useful in locating metallic and nonmetallic foreign bodies, and in the refraction prior to implantation of plastic lenses. The most successful application of ultrasonic tissue characterization has been in differentiating between melanoma and metastatic carcinoma of the orbit. By using a biologic standard, an accuracy of > 90% has been claimed.

214. OCULAR SYMPTOMS AND SIGNS

Some of the more common ocular symptoms and signs are discussed here and others are elsewhere in THE MANUAL: Exophthalmos is discussed in Ch. 216; strabismus, in Ch. 200; and nystagmus and extraocular muscle movements, under VISION AND EYE MOVEMENT DISORDERS in Ch. 119.

Hemorrhage

Subconjunctival hemorrhages may develop at any age, usually following minor trauma, straining, sneezing, or coughing; rarely, they occur spontaneously. They alarm the patient but are of no pathologic significance, with the rare exception of when they are associated with blood dyscrasias. They occur as gross extravasations of blood beneath the conjunctiva and are absorbed spontaneously within 2 wk. Topical corticosteroids, antibiotics, vasoconstrictors, and compresses are of little value in speeding reabsorption; reassurance is adequate therapy.

Vitreous hemorrhages are extravasations of blood into the vitreous and produce a black reflex on ophthalmoscopy. They may occur in such conditions as diabetic retinopathy or hypertension or result from trauma, retinal neovascularization, or retinal tears. In the 3 latter conditions, retinal detachment may ensue. Vitreous hemorrhages tend to absorb slowly, but they may become loosely organized and subsequently form proliferating bands that obscure vision and later contract and detach the retina. Localized bleeding from retinal vessels can sometimes be controlled by photocoagulation with light or laser beams. Periodic evaluation of vascular retinopathies by an ophthalmologist is important, particularly in diabetes mellitus.

Retinal hemorrhages may be flame-shaped in the superficial nerve fiber layer, as in hypertension or venous occlusion, or more localized ("dot and blot") in the deeper layers, as in diabetes mellitus or septic infarctions. Retinal hemorrhages are always significant, reflecting vascular disease that usually is systemic.

Spots

Seeing spots (floaters) before one or both eyes is a frequent adult complaint. The spots usually are most noticeable against a white background and seem to move slowly; they usually are without significance, and are due to vitreous debris derived from the membranous attachment of the vitreous body to the optic nerve and retina. They are more prevalent in highly myopic and older persons and tend to become less noticeable with time. A minute **vitreous hemorrhage** appears as a brown or red spot. **Retinal detachments** may be preceded by a shower of "sparks" or lightning flashes, and also may be accompanied by spots. Only after the retina actually separates from its underlying structure does a "curtain" of visual loss move across the visual field. Spots may be serious; they warrant meticulous examination of the fundus and media after dilation with a short-acting mydriatic or cycloplegic (eg, 1% cyclopentolate, 1 drop, repeated in 5 to 15 min). Examination is done best by indirect ophthalmoscopy, a technic used by most ophthalmologists. Vitreous floaters can be seen with a high plus

lens by looking into the red reflex at a distance of 6 to 12 inches. Repeated examinations are warranted if the complaint continues or worsens, if vision is affected, or if apprehension persists. Spots of recent origin or those accompanied by flashes of light should be evaluated by an ophthalmologist. Disturbance of vision always demands an explanation.

Photophobia

Abnormal visual intolerance of light is common in lightly pigmented persons. Usually it is without significance and may be relieved by wearing dark glasses. It is an important, but nondiagnostic, symptom in keratoconjunctivitis, intraocular inflammation, acute glaucoma, and traumatic corneal epithelial abrasions.

Pain

Ocular pain usually is important and, unless due to an obvious local cause such as a foreign body, acute lid infection, or injury, demands investigation (eg, for uveitis, especially iridocyclitis, or glaucoma). Sinusitis occasionally causes referred eye pain.

Scotomas

A blind spot in the field of vision is a **negative scotoma.** Frequently it goes unnoticed by the patient unless it involves central vision and interferes significantly with visual acuity. Negative scotomas noticed by the patient usually are due to hemorrhage or choroiditis. A scotoma found in the same visual field area in each eye is usually a quadrantic or hemianopic defect due to a lesion in the optic pathways. A **positive scotoma,** perceived as a light spot or scintillating flashes, represents a response to abnormal stimulation of some portion of the visual system; eg, as in the migraine syndrome.

Examination of the eyes, including the visual fields, always is mandatory to determine the cause of any scotoma. A bilateral scotoma, if not caused by bilateral retinal lesions, demands perimetric examination and neurologic evaluation.

Errors of Refraction

In **emmetropia** no optical defect exists and parallel light rays entering the eye focus clearly on the retina. In **ametropia,** an optical defect exists that may be of several varieties: In **hyperopia** (farsightedness), the most common refractive error, the point of focus lies behind the retina, either because the eyeball axis is too short or because the refractive power of the eye is too weak. A convex (plus) lens is used in corrective glasses. In **myopia** (nearsightedness), the image is focused in front of the retina because the axis of the eyeball is too long or the refractive power of the eye is too strong; a concave (minus) corrective lens is used. In **astigmatism,** the refraction is unequal in the different meridians of the eyeball. A cylindric corrective lens (a segment cut from a cylinder) is used that has no refractive power along the vertical axis and is concave or convex along the opposite axis.

Anisometropia, a significant difference between the refractive errors of the two eyes (usually > 2 diopters), is seen occasionally. When the refractive errors are corrected with lenses, image size differences **(aniseikonia)** are produced and can lead to difficulties in fusion and even to suppression of one of the images.

Presbyopia, a hyperopia for near vision that develops with advancing age, results from a physiologic change in the accommodative mechanism by which the focus of the eye is adjusted for objects at different distances. Beginning in the teens, the lens substance gradually grows less pliable and eventually cannot change shape (accommodate) in response to the action of the ciliary muscles. As a result, the individual becomes unable to focus well for near vision, but usually does not need corrective glasses until he reaches the early to mid-40s.

215. INJURIES

Trauma to the eye or adjacent structures requires meticulous examination to determine the extent of injury. Vision, range of extraocular motion, location of lid and conjunctival lacerations and of foreign bodies, and clarity of the ocular media should be carefully determined and recorded in detail for protection of patient, physician, and, in industrial cases, employer.

FOREIGN BODIES

1. **Conjunctival and corneal injuries** by foreign bodies are the most frequent eye injuries. Seemingly minor trauma can be serious if ocular penetration is unrecognized or if secondary infection follows a corneal abrasion.

Treatment: Adequate light, good anesthesia, and proper instruments are essential to ensure minimal trauma when removing embedded foreign bodies. Fluorescein staining (see Ch. 213) renders foreign bodies and abrasions more apparent. An anesthetic (eg, 2 drops of proparacaine 0.5%) is instilled onto the conjunctiva. Both lids are everted and the entire conjunctiva and cornea inspected with a binocular lens (loupe). Conjunctival foreign bodies are lifted out with a moist sterile cotton applicator. A corneal foreign body that cannot be dislodged by irrigation may be lifted out carefully on the point of a sterile spud or hypodermic needle, under loupe magnification. Unless steel or iron foreign bodies are removed immediately, they leave a "rust ring" on the cornea that also requires removal, under the light and magnification of the slit lamp.

If the foreign body was tiny, only an antibiotic ointment (eg, erythromycin 0.5% or bacitracin 500 u./gm) should be instilled. If larger, however, treatment is that for any **corneal abrasion:** dilating the pupil with a short-acting cycloplegic (eg, 1 drop of 1% cyclopentolate); instilling an antibiotic, usually erythromycin or bacitracin; and applying a patch firmly enough to keep the eye closed overnight. Ophthalmic corticosteroid preparations tend to promote the growth of fungi and are **contraindicated.** The corneal epithelium regenerates rapidly; under a patch, large areas heal within 1 to 3 days. Follow-up examination by an ophthalmologist 1 or 2 days after injury is wise, especially if the foreign body was removed with a needle or spud.

2. **Intraocular foreign bodies:** A foreign body that has penetrated the eye must be removed by an ophthalmic surgeon, but certain **emergency treatment** should be instituted immediately. The pupil is dilated with 2 drops of 1 to 4% atropine solution. Antimicrobials are indicated, both systemic and topical; eg, gentamicin 2 mg/kg/day (if kidney function is adequate) in combination with methicillin 1 gm IV q 6 h, and gentamicin 0.3% ophthalmic solution 1 drop hourly. Ointment should be avoided if the globe is lacerated. A patch and a metal shield are placed over the eye to avoid inadvertent pressure that could extrude ocular contents through the penetration site.

LACERATIONS AND CONTUSIONS

During the first 24 h, **lid contusions ("black eye")** should be treated with ice packs to inhibit swelling. The next day, hot compresses may aid absorption of the hematoma. Minor **lid lacerations** may be repaired with fine silk sutures. Lid-margin lacerations are best repaired by an ophthalmic surgeon, since particular care is needed to ensure apposition and avoid a notch in the contour. Major lacerations, especially those involving the lacrimal apparatus, should be repaired by an ophthalmic surgeon.

Trauma to the globe may severely damage internal structures. Hemorrhage into the anterior chamber, laceration of the iris, cataract, dislocated lens, glaucoma, vitreous hemorrhage, orbital-floor fractures, retinal hemorrhage or detachment, and rupture of the eyeball may result. **Emergency treatment** may be needed before care by a specialist.

It consists of alleviating pain (eg, with meperidine 50 mg IM q 3 h), keeping the pupil dilated with 2 drops of 1 to 4% atropine, applying protective dressings (including a metal shield), and combating possible infection with local and systemic antimicrobials as for an intraocular foreign body (see above). One should never forcibly open traumatized lids, as the injury may be aggravated. When a globe laceration is present, topical antibiotics should be given in the form of drops only, to avoid penetration of ointment into the globe. Because of the danger of fungal contamination, corticosteroids are **contraindicated** before open wounds are closed surgically.

Anterior chamber hemorrhage (traumatic hyphema) following blunt injuries is potentially serious and requires attention by an ophthalmologist. It may be followed by recurrent bleeding, glaucoma, and blood-staining of the cornea. The **immediate treatment** is complete bed rest, binocular bandaging, sedation, and, if intraocular pressure rises, a carbonic anhydrase inhibitor (eg, acetazolamide 250 mg to 1 gm/day orally in divided doses). The non-ophthalmologist should *not* use miotics or mydriatics in these cases. Rarely, recurrent bleeding with secondary glaucoma may require evacuation of the blood by an ophthalmologist.

BURNS

Eyelid burns should be cleansed thoroughly with sterile isotonic saline solution, followed by petrolatum gauze or an antimicrobial ointment (eg, bacitracin). Sterile pressure dressings are then applied and held by an elastic bandage or stockinet around the head until the surface has healed.

Chemical burns of the **cornea** and **conjunctiva** can be serious and should be treated immediately by copious irrigation with water or other bland fluids. The eye may be anesthetized with 1 drop of 1% proparacaine, if it is available, but irrigation should never be delayed and should be carried out for 5 to 30 min, depending on the estimate of chemical contact. Irrigation until the pH is neutral (as measured with paper indicators) is a reasonable end point. Pain results from loss of corneal epithelium and chemical iritis, which should be treated by instilling a long-acting cycloplegic (eg, 1% atropine solution), applying an antibiotic ointment, and patching. Prolonged use of topical anesthetics should be avoided. Initially, pain may require codeine 30 to 60 mg orally or meperidine 50 mg IM q 4 h. Severe burns require specialized treatment by an ophthalmologist to save vision and prevent major complications such as iridocyclitis, perforation of the globe, and lid deformities. All patients with significant redness of the eye or loss of normal epithelium should be seen by an ophthalmologist within 24 h.

---

216. ORBIT

ORBITAL CELLULITIS

(See also PERIORBITAL AND ORBITAL CELLULITIS under BACTERIAL INFECTIONS in Ch. 191)

Inflammation of the orbital tissues caused by infection that extends from the nasal sinuses or teeth, by metastatic spread from infections elsewhere, or by bacteria introduced via orbital trauma. Symptoms include extreme orbital pain, exophthalmos, impaired mobility of the eye, lid swelling, chemosis, fever, and malaise. Possible complications are loss of vision from optic neuritis, thrombophlebitis of the orbital veins resulting in cavernous sinus thrombosis, panophthalmitis, and spread of the infection to the meninges and brain.

Treatment with appropriate systemic antimicrobials is supplemented by general supportive therapy (including hot applications to localize the infection, bed rest, and

fluids). Meperidine 50 mg, or codeine 60 mg with aspirin or acetaminophen, orally q 4 h should be given for pain. Incision and drainage are indicated if suppuration is suspected or if the infection does not respond to antibiotic therapy.

CAVERNOUS SINUS THROMBOSIS

Thrombosis of the cavernous sinus usually results from direct spread of infection along the venous channels draining the orbit and face. It is often secondary to orbital cellulitis or a pyogenic skin infection in the central region of the face; rarely, it is due to metastatic spread from other pyogenic foci. Exophthalmos, papilledema, severe cerebral symptoms (headache, convulsions), and a septic temperature curve are present. The prognosis is grave.

Prompt intensive **treatment** with systemic antibiotics appropriate to the causative organism, IV fluids, and bed rest is imperative.

EXOPHTHALMOS

(Proptosis)

Protrusion of one or both eyeballs that results from orbital inflammation, edema, tumors, or injuries; cavernous sinus thrombosis; or enlargement of the eyeball (as in congenital glaucoma and unilateral high myopia). In hyperthyroidism, edema and lymphoid infiltration of the orbital tissues may cause unilateral or bilateral exophthalmos. Sudden unilateral onset is usually due to hemorrhage or inflammation of the orbit or accessory sinuses. A 2- to 3-wk onset suggests chronic inflammation or orbital pseudotumor (a non-neoplastic cellular infiltration and proliferation); slower onset suggests neoplasm.

An arteriovenous aneurysm involving the internal carotid artery and the cavernous sinus may produce a pulsating exophthalmos with bruit. Post-traumatic onset is probably due to carotid-cavernous fistula, confirmable by auscultation of the globe. Trauma or infection (especially facial) may cause cavernous sinus thrombosis with unilateral exophthalmos and fever. Unilateral high myopia or meningioma may cause unilateral exophthalmos. Thyroid studies should be performed when the cause is not apparent; if thyroid function is normal, the cause must be sought within the orbit by x-ray (including pneumograms, if necessary). The degree of exophthalmos can be followed with the exophthalmometer; if it is progressive, exposure of the globe can lead to corneal drying, ulceration, and infection.

Treatment

Etiology determines therapy. Ligation of the involved common carotid is necessary in arteriovenous aneurysm. The exophthalmos of hyperthyroidism may subside when the hyperthyroidism is controlled, but occasionally it follows a relentless course and requires surgical orbital decompression. Systemic corticosteroids are often beneficial in controlling edema and pseudotumor (eg, 60 to 80 mg prednisone orally, given daily for 1 wk, then on alternate days for 5 wk, then gradually reduced to the minimal amount needed to control the proptosis). Tumors must be removed.

---

217. LACRIMAL APPARATUS

DACRYOSTENOSIS

Stricture of the nasolacrimal duct, often resulting from a congenital abnormality or an infection. Congenital obstruction usually appears between ages 3 and 12 wk as a persistent tearing, **(epiphora)** of one eye or, rarely, of both. Epiphora is chronic overflow of

tears over the lid margin, onto the cheek. Adult patients may complain of tearing, but in fact do not have epiphora unless they or their family members notice the overflow of tears. The later onset and lack of purulent exudate in congenital obstruction differentiate it from neonatal conjunctivitis due to either silver nitrate instillation or bacterial infection. Pressure on the nasolacrimal sac frequently causes a copious reflux of mucus or pus from the punctum. In adults, dacryostenosis with epiphora may result from inflammatory obstruction of the duct due to chronic nasal infection, or from severe or chronic conjunctivitis. Fracture of the nose and facial bones may cause mechanical obstruction. Prolonged blockage usually leads to infection of the lacrimal sac (see DACRYOCYSTITIS below).

Treatment

Congenital dacryostenosis usually resolves spontaneously by age 6 mo. Milking the contents of the lacrimal sac through the nasolacrimal duct with fingertip massage bid may speed resolution; antibiotic drops may prevent infection. If resolution is not spontaneous, the punctum should be dilated and the nasolacrimal canal probed. Brief general anesthesia usually is necessary in infants. **In adults,** a local anesthetic such as 0.5% proparacaine is instilled and the punctum is dilated. Isotonic saline is irrigated gently through the nasolacrimal system with a fine, blunt canaliculus needle while the upper punctum is occluded with a punctum dilator. (A drop of fluorescein in the saline makes obstruction in the nose easily detectable.) If this fails, lacrimal probing may establish patency. Using probes of increasing size followed by irrigation with sterile isotonic saline may be successful in incomplete obstruction. Complete obstruction requires a surgical opening from the tear sac into the nasal passages.

DACRYOCYSTITIS

Infection of the lacrimal sac.

Etiology

Dacryocystitis is usually secondary to obstruction of the nasolacrimal duct. In infants, it is a complication of congenital dacryostenosis; in others, the duct obstruction results from nasal trauma, deviated septum, hypertrophic rhinitis, mucosal polyps, hypertrophied inferior turbinate, or residual congenital dacryostenosis.

Symptoms and Signs

Pain, redness and edema about the lacrimal sac, epiphora, conjunctivitis, blepharitis, fever, and leukocytosis are associated with **acute dacryocystitis;** in **chronic dacryocystitis,** slight swelling of the sac may be the only symptom. On pressure, pus may regurgitate through the punctum. The sac may become distended from retained secretions and form a large mucocele. Recurrent acute inflammations may result in a red, brawny, indurated area over the sac. An abscess, if present, may rupture and form a draining fistula.

Treatment

Acute dacryocystitis is treated by frequent application of hot compresses; incision and drainage if an abscess has formed; and procaine penicillin G 1.2 million u. IM, followed by penicillin V 250 to 500 mg orally q 6 h and topical antibiotic ophthalmic preparations to prevent secondary corneal infection. The systemic antibiotic can be changed after results of culture are available. **Chronic dacryocystitis** may be relieved by dilating the nasolacrimal duct with a probe after using a local anesthetic such as 0.5% proparacaine or tetracaine, or 4% cocaine. Contributory nasal or sinus abnormalities should be treated. If conservative treatment fails, removal of the sac, nasolacrimal intubation, or anastomosis may be necessary.

218. EYELIDS

LID EDEMA

Allergies (see OTHER ALLERGIC EYE DISEASES in Ch. 21) usually produce marked crinkly lid edema of one or both eyes and may be due to topical agents, such as eyedrops (eg, atropine or epinephrine), other drugs, or cosmetics. Plant allergens can cause lid edema in atopic individuals. **Trichinosis** produces lid edema that is usually bilateral and resembles the allergic type; the associated fever and other systemic symptoms may not be present initially. An eosinophilia > 10% is characteristic.

In allergic lid edema, removal of the offending cause is often the only treatment needed. Cold compresses over the closed lids may speed resolution; topical corticosteroid creams (eg, 0.1% triamcinolone) may be needed if swelling persists > 24 h.

BLEPHARITIS

Inflammation of the lid margins with redness, thickening, and often the formation of scales and crusts or shallow marginal ulcers.

Etiology

Ulcerative blepharitis is caused by bacterial infection (usually staphylococcal) of the lash follicles and the meibomian glands. The cause of nonulcerative (squamous or seborrheic) blepharitis is often obscure; it may be allergic in origin or associated with seborrhea of the face and scalp.

Symptoms and Signs

A foreign-body sensation is common. Itching, burning, and redness of the lid margins, lid edema, loss of lashes, and conjunctival irritation with lacrimation and photophobia may be present. In ulcerative blepharitis, tenacious adherent crusts appear and leave a bleeding surface when removed. Small pustules develop in the lash follicles and eventually break down to form shallow ulcers. During sleep, the lids become glued together by dried secretions. A history of repeated sties and chalazions is common. In the nonulcerative type, greasy, easily removable scales develop on the lid margins.

Prognosis

Patients should be warned that both types are indolent, recurrent, and stubbornly resistant to treatment. Exacerbations of the nonulcerative type are inconvenient and unsightly, but not destructive. Repeated attacks of the ulcerative type result in loss of eyelashes, scarring of the lids, and occasionally corneal ulceration.

Treatment

Erythromycin or bacitracin ophthalmic ointment should be applied tid to the lash margins, following 10-min application of warm compresses. Instilling sulfacetamide-corticosteroid drops is useful in treating secondary conjunctival and corneal irritation or bacterial invasion. Drops may be used 5 times/day during the day, and ointment at night and on arising; treatment is for 1 to 2 wk. Tonometry is indicated during long-term corticosteroid therapy. Neomycin can be used, but prolonged local treatment should be avoided because it risks local allergic reactions.

Nonulcerative seborrheic blepharitis also requires attention to the face and scalp (see SEBORRHEIC DERMATITIS in Ch. 230).

HORDEOLUM

(Sty)

An acute localized pyogenic infection of one or more of the glands of Zeis or Moll ***(external hordeolum)*** *or of the meibomian glands* ***(internal hordeolum, meibomian sty).***

Etiology

Staphylococci usually are responsible. Sties often are associated with and secondary to blepharitis. Recurrence is common.

Symptoms and Signs

External hordeolum usually begins with pain, redness, and tenderness of the lid margin followed by a small, round, tender area of induration. Lacrimation, photophobia, and a foreign-body sensation may be present. Though usually localized, edema may be diffuse. A small yellowish spot, indicative of suppuration, appears in the center of the induration ("pointing"). The abscess soon ruptures, with discharge of pus and relief of pain.

Internal hordeolum involving one of the meibomian glands is more severe. Pain, redness, and edema are more localized. Inspection of the conjunctival side of the lid shows a small elevation or yellow area at the site of the affected gland. Later, an abscess forms, pointing on the conjunctival side of the lid; it seldom points through the skin. Spontaneous rupture is rare, and recurrence is common.

Diagnosis

External sties are superficial and well localized, and appear to lie at the base of an eyelash. An internal sty is deeper and can be seen through the conjunctiva. If the hordeolum lies near the inner canthus of the lower lid, it must be differentiated from acute dacryocystitis (see in Ch. 217). Successful lacrimal irrigation rules out dacryocystitis.

Treatment

Suppuration may be aborted in the early stages by topical antimicrobials (eg, 0.5% erythromycin or 500 u./gm bacitracin ointment tid). Pointing is hastened by hot compresses applied for 10 min tid or qid. As soon as suppuration is evidenced by the formation of a central yellow area, the sty should be incised with a sharp, fine-tipped blade and its contents expressed. Antibiotic ophthalmic solutions or ointments (eg, 10 to 30% sulfacetamide), applied for several days, prevent spread of infection to neighboring structures. Systemic antibiotics are rarely needed.

CHALAZION

Chronic granulomatous enlargement of a meibomian gland from occlusion of its duct, often following inflammation of the gland.

Symptoms and Signs

At onset, a chalazion may be indistinguishable from a sty, with lid edema, swelling, and irritation. After a few days, however, it resolves, leaving a painless, slowly growing, round mass in the lid. The skin can be moved loosely over the swelling, which may be seen in the tarsus of the lid, generally presenting subconjunctivally as a red or gray mass. When the mass is in the lower lid near the inner canthus, chronic dacryocystitis must be ruled out.

Treatment

Most chalazions disappear after a few months, although incision and curettage may be indicated if there is no resolution after 6 wk. Hot compresses and topical antibiotic ointments (eg, 0.5% erythromycin or bacitracin 500 u./gm) are indicated initially. Systemic antibiotics rarely are necessary.

ENTROPION AND ECTROPION

Inversion of the eyelid **(entropion)** and *eversion* **(ectropion)** can result from aging or from scar formation. Entropion causes irritation as the lashes rub against the globe,

and may lead to corneal ulceration and scarring. Ectropion is generally the result of tissue relaxation with aging, and leads to poor drainage of tears through the nasolacrimal system. Symptoms may include redness, irritation, and epiphora. Both conditions, if persistent, are best treated surgically.

TUMORS

The skin of the eyelids can have both benign and neoplastic growths. **Xanthelasma** is a frequent, benign type, with yellow-white, flat plaques of lipid material that occur subcutaneously on the upper and lower lids. Except for cosmetic reasons, they need not be removed.

Basal cell carcinoma is frequently seen at the lid margins, at the inner canthus, and on the upper cheek. Biopsy establishes the diagnosis. **Treatment** is surgical excision or cryotherapy.

Other malignant tumors are less common; they include meibomian gland carcinoma and melanomas of several types.

---

219. CONJUNCTIVA

The conjunctiva lines the back of the lid, extends into the space between the lid and the globe and extends up over the sclera to the cornea. This tissue can respond to various stimuli with chemosis, hemorrhage, or inflammation. In addition, there are 2 common benign neoplasms of the conjunctiva: (1) A **pinguecula** is an accumulation of subepithelial lipid material just adjacent to the cornea at either the 3 or 9 o'clock position. It may be unsightly, but it has no tendency to grow onto the cornea and need not be removed. (2) A **pterygium** is a fleshy growth of conjunctiva onto the cornea and is more often found in hot, dry climates. This growth may distort the cornea, induce astigmatism, and change the refractive power of the eye. In some cases removal is indicated, to reduce irritation and to prevent changes in vision.

ACUTE CONJUNCTIVITIS

An acute conjunctival inflammation, usually caused by viruses, allergy, or bacteria.

Etiology

Viruses, especially adenoviruses (see under RESPIRATORY VIRAL DISEASES in Ch. 12) and allergies (see ALLERGIC CONJUNCTIVITIS in Ch. 21) are the most common causes in populations with good hygiene. Mixed or unidentifiable pathogens may be present. Conjunctival irritation from wind, dust, smoke, and other types of air pollution often is associated; conjunctivitis may also accompany the common cold, exanthems (especially measles), and corneal irritation due to the intense light of electric arcs, sunlamps, and reflection from snow. Acute hemorrhagic conjunctivitis, associated with infection by enterovirus type 70 (see under ENTEROVIRAL DISEASES in Ch. 191), has occurred in outbreaks in Africa and Asia.

Symptoms, Signs, and Diagnosis

TABLE 219–1 indicates prominent symptoms and signs found in acute conjunctivitis. The discharge should be cultured, particularly if it is purulent. Smears should be examined microscopically, stained with Gram's stain to identify bacteria and with Wright's stain to determine the leukocytic response. While cultures can be taken for viral disease, special tissue culture facilities are necessary for growth of the virus.

TABLE 219–1. DIFFERENTIATING FEATURES IN CONJUNCTIVITIS

Etiology	*Discharge; Cell Type*	*Lid Swelling*	*Node Involvement*	*Itching*
Bacterial	purulent; polymorphonuclear leukocytes	moderate	no	no
Viral	clear; mononuclear	minimal	yes	no
Allergic	clear, mucoid, ropy; eosinophils	moderate to severe	no	intense

Lymphoid follicles are present on the undersurface of the lid in viral infection; velvety papillary projections, in allergic disease. The preauricular node should be palpated in all cases; it tends to be enlarged and painful in viral conjunctivitis.

Examination of conjunctival scrapings will rule out inclusion conjunctivitis, trachoma, and vernal conjunctivitis: in the former two, inclusion bodies are present; in the last, eosinophils are present. Retained corneal or conjunctival foreign bodies and corneal abrasion or ulcer may be ruled out by staining the eye with fluorescein (see Ch. 213) and examining it, under magnification, with a good focal light.

The deep ciliary injection of iritis and of acute glaucoma is readily differentiated, since it is due to fine, straight, deep vessels that radiate from the limbus and are immobile when the conjunctiva is moved. The brick-red conjunctival injection of conjunctivitis is composed of coarse, tortuous superficial vessels that move with the conjunctiva; moreover, the conjunctiva blanches when a decongestant (eg, a drop of phenylephrine 0.125%) is instilled. Other features that distinguish conjunctivitis from acute iritis and acute glaucoma are given in TABLE 219–2.

TABLE 219–2. DIFFERENTIAL DIAGNOSIS OF CERTAIN ACUTE EYE DISORDERS

	Acute Iritis	*Acute Glaucoma*	*Acute Conjunctivitis*
Pain	Moderately severe	Very severe	Burning, but not severe
Vision	Moderately decreased	Considerably decreased	Normal
Eyeball tension	Usually normal or soft	Increased	Unchanged
Lacrimation or discharge	Lacrimation	Lacrimation	Mucous or mucopurulent discharge
Injection	Circumcorneal	Circumcorneal and episcleral	Superficial conjunctival
Cornea	Transparent precipitates may be present on posterior surface	Appears steamy	Normal
Anterior chamber	Normal depth	Very shallow	Normal depth
Iris	Dull and swollen	Congested and bulging	Normal
Pupil	Small, irregular	Mid-dilated	Normal

Treatment

After examining the patient, the physician must wash his hands thoroughly and sterilize his instruments to avoid transmitting infection. The patient should be told to use only his own towels. The eyes should be kept free of discharge and not patched. If bacterial infection is suspected, 10% sulfonamide drops and an antibiotic ointment (eg, 0.5% erythromycin) are applied tid. This treatment can be used for all forms of conjunctivitis; a poor clinical response after 2 or 3 days indicates that an insensitive bacterium is present, or that the cause is viral or allergic. Antibiotic therapy may be modified if necessary when the results of culture and sensitivity studies become available. Corticosteroids should not be used, either separately or with antibiotics, until a causative pathogen is identified or excluded, since herpes simplex virus may be present and may be spread from the conjunctiva to the cornea, with subsequent ulceration and perforation. If allergy is likely on the basis of history and lack of response to antibiotic therapy, topical corticosteroid therapy (eg, 0.12% prednisolone acetate drops tid) can be initiated. With long-term use of corticosteroids, intraocular pressure should be monitored and the lens examined periodically for cataracts.

CHRONIC CONJUNCTIVITIS

A chronic inflammation of the conjunctiva characterized by exacerbations and remissions that occur over months or years. The causal agents, when identifiable, are similar to those of acute conjunctivitis; ectropion, entropion, blepharitis, chronic dacryocystitis, and chronic exposure to irritants are also etiologically associated.

Symptoms and Signs

Symptoms are similar to those of acute conjunctivitis but less severe, and include itching, smarting, and a foreign-body sensation; a scant mucoid secretion may be present. The palpebral conjunctiva is reddened, thickened, and velvety. The bulbar conjunctiva may be slightly involved.

Treatment

Irritating factors must be eliminated. Overtreatment may produce drug sensitivity and should be avoided. Prophylactic expression of the meibomian glands with 2 glass rods, after topical anesthesia (eg, 1 or 2 drops of 0.5% proparacaine), may help. A short course of topical corticosteroid-antibiotic therapy may be soothing and beneficial.

CONJUNCTIVITIS NEONATORUM

(Ophthalmia Neonatorum)

(See NEONATAL CONJUNCTIVITIS under NEONATAL INFECTIONS in Ch. 186)

ADULT GONOCOCCAL CONJUNCTIVITIS

A rare, severe, purulent conjunctivitis that occurs in adults as a result of self-inoculation from a gonorrheal genital infection or is acquired from a gonorrheal contact. Usually only one eye is involved. Symptoms similar to those of conjunctivitis neonatorum, but more severe, develop 12 to 48 h after exposure; complications, including corneal ulceration, abscess, perforation, panophthalmitis, and blindness, are common. Treatment involves parenteral antimicrobial therapy and 10 to 30% sulfacetamide drops instilled into the affected eye q 2 h.

TRACHOMA

(Granular Conjunctivitis; Egyptian Ophthalmia)

A chronic conjunctivitis caused by Chlamydia trachomatis *and characterized by progressive exacerbations and remissions, with follicular subconjunctival hyperplasia, corneal vascularization, and cicatrization of the conjunctiva, cornea, and lids.*

Epidemiology

The disease is still endemic in poverty-stricken parts of the dry, hot Mediterranean countries and Far East. It occurs sporadically among American Indians and in mountainous areas of the southern USA. It is most contagious in its early stages and is transmitted by direct contact or, possibly, by handling contaminated articles (eg, towels, handkerchiefs). The causative organism, a **TRIC** agent (**TR**achoma and **I**nclusion **C**onjunctivitis), is a strain of *Chlamydia trachomatis* and is related to psittacosis and lymphogranuloma venereum (see Ch. 11).

Symptoms and Signs

After an incubation period of about 7 days, conjunctival congestion, eyelid edema, photophobia, and lacrimation gradually appear, usually bilaterally. Small follicles develop in the conjunctiva of the upper lids 7 to 10 days later and gradually increase in size and number for 3 or 4 wk, forming yellow-gray semitransparent "sago-grain" granulations surrounded by inflammatory papillae. Pannus formation begins during this stage, with invasion of the upper half of the cornea by loops of vessels from the limbus. The stage of follicular hypertrophy and pannus formation may last from several months to > 1 yr, depending on response to therapy. The entire cornea may ultimately be involved, reducing vision. Rarely, the pannus retrogresses completely and corneal transparency is restored without treatment.

Unless adequate treatment is given, the cicatricial stage follows. The follicles and papillae gradually shrink and are replaced by scar tissue that often causes entropion and lacrimal duct obstruction. The corneal epithelium becomes dull and thickened, and lacrimation is decreased. Ulcers form in ischemic areas of the pannus. On healing, the conjunctiva is smooth and grayish-white; the extent of residual corneal opacity and vision loss varies. Secondary bacterial infection is common and contributes to scarring and the chronicity of the disease.

Diagnosis

C. trachomatis can be isolated in culture. In the early stage, the presence of minute granular cytoplasmic inclusion bodies in Giemsa-stained epithelial conjunctival scrapings differentiates trachoma from acute conjunctivitis. Inclusion bodies are also found in inclusion conjunctivitis but the developing clinical picture distinguishes this from trachoma. Palpebral vernal conjunctivitis is similar to trachoma in its follicular hypertrophic stage, but eosinophilia and milky flat-topped papillae are present and inclusion bodies are not found in the scrapings.

Treatment

Tetracycline (or erythromycin) eye ointments, applied bid or qid for 4 to 6 wk, are usually effective. A concomitant oral tetracycline is helpful. Lid deformities should be treated surgically.

INCLUSION CONJUNCTIVITIS

(Inclusion Blennorrhea; Swimming Pool Conjunctivitis)

An acute conjunctivitis, known as ***inclusion blennorrhea*** *in the newborn and* ***adult inclusion conjunctivitis*** *or* ***swimming pool conjunctivitis*** *in the adult, caused by* Chlamydia trachomatis, *a TRIC agent* (see TRACHOMA, above). This organism can persist asymptomatically in the cervix for prolonged periods. As a form of ophthalmia neonatorum, inclusion conjunctivitis results from passage through an infected birth canal and occurs in 40 to 50% of the newborns exposed to it. Although most instances of acute inclusion conjunctivitis in adults result from exposure to infected genital secretions, adenovirus acquired in swimming pools has been implicated occasionally.

Symptoms, Signs, and Diagnosis

Intense papillary conjunctivitis, lid swelling, chemosis, and mucopurulent discharge develop, usually bilaterally, after a 5- to 14-day incubation period. Epithelial-cell inclusion bodies are present in conjunctival scrapings. Hypertrophied papillae may develop in both conjunctival folds and persist for several months. No corneal damage occurs. In adults, the conjunctivitis is less severe than in neonates (see in NEONATAL CONJUNCTIVITIS under NEONATAL INFECTIONS in Ch. 186) and usually unilateral; the secretion is less profuse but the papillae are larger. Preauricular lymph nodes may be swollen on the side of the involved eye.

Treatment

Tetracycline 1% ophthalmic ointment qid is specific and should be applied to both eyes in order to prevent bilateral infection. In adults, oral tetracycline 500 mg qid for 10 days is also given to cure concomitant genital infection.

VERNAL KERATOCONJUNCTIVITIS

A bilateral, recurrent conjunctivitis with concurrent corneal epithelial changes, usually allergic in origin, with recurrences in the spring and fall. It is most common in males aged 5 to 20. (See also ALLERGIC CONJUNCTIVITIS in Ch. 21).

Symptoms and Signs

Intense itching, lacrimation, photophobia, conjunctival injection, and a tenacious mucoid discharge containing numerous eosinophils are characteristic. Either the palpebral or the bulbar conjunctiva may be affected. In the **palpebral form**, square, hard, flattened, closely packed, pale pink to grayish "cobblestone" granulations are present, chiefly in the upper lids. The uninvolved tarsal conjunctiva is milky white. In the **bulbar (limbic) form**, the circumcorneal conjunctiva becomes hypertrophied and grayish. Occasionally, a small, circumscribed loss of corneal epithelium occurs, causing pain and increased photophobia.

Symptoms usually disappear during the cold months and become milder over the years, but the granulations often persist for life.

Treatment

Frequent applications of a topical corticosteroid are beneficial (eg, 0.1% dexamethasone drops q 2 h), supplemented if necessary by small oral doses. Dosage should be reduced as soon as possible, with long-term maintenance therapy of 0.25% prednisolone acetate applied once or twice/day the goal. If topical steroids are used for more than a few weeks, intraocular pressure must be checked routinely.

KERATOCONJUNCTIVITIS SICCA

(Keratitis Sicca; Dry Eyes)

A chronic, bilateral dryness of the conjunctiva and sclera leading to dessication of the ocular surface.

Symptoms and Signs

As an isolated phenomenon or in association with systemic diseases such as rheumatoid arthritis or lupus erythematosus (when it is termed **Sjögren's syndrome**), dryness of the eyes occurs more commonly in adult women. Initial reduction of tear production leads to burning and irritation. This proceeds to photophobia and blepharospasm as the corneal epithelium develops scattered cellular loss, termed superficial keratitis. In its advanced stages, keratinization of the ocular surface occurs, frequently associated with loss of the normal configuration of the conjunctival fornices. In advanced kerato-

conjunctivitis sicca, ulceration, vascularization, and scarring of the cornea may lead to severe visual disability.

Diagnosis

Diagnosis depends upon the history and examination. If the patient complains of dryness and irritation, particular attention should be paid to the adequacy of the tear meniscus as seen through the slit lamp, as well as the presence or absence of punctate erosion of the conjunctiva and cornea. A **Schirmer's test** is done by using standardized strips of filter paper placed, without anesthesia, at the junction between the middle and lateral third of the lower lid. Wetting of the paper of 2 mm or less in 5 min on 2 successive occasions confirms the diagnosis of dry eye.

Treatment

Frequent use of artificial tears containing methylcellulose or polyvinyl alcohol can be effective. Most cases are treated adequately throughout the patient's life with such supplementation. Intractable cases may respond to use of soft contact lenses, kept hydrated with frequent applications of saline drops. Occlusion of the nasolacrimal punctum can be tried before eyelid surgery, but in severe cases partial tarsorrhaphy can reduce loss of tears through evaporation.

EPISCLERITIS

Inflammation of the episcleral tissues, usually localized. A red to purplish tender patch is present just under the conjunctiva; a yellow nodule may also be present. The condition usually is self-limited and not associated with systemic disease. **Treatment** usually need not be extensive. However, frequent applications of topical corticosteroid, eg, 0.125% prednisolone acetate drops q 2 h for 5 days and gradually reduced over 3 wk, is usually effective in shortening the attack.

SCLERITIS

A deep, usually localized, inflammation of the scleral tissues, more purple in appearance than episcleritis. It may be associated with rheumatic disorders. If severe, perforation of the globe and loss of the eye may ensue.

Treatment

Some cases respond to a topical corticosteroid, but careful observation is necessary to forestall increased loss of scleral substance. Systemic corticosteroids may be tried when involvement is quite deep and response to topical therapy is poor, but the prognosis is guarded.

When the process is associated with rheumatoid disease, systemic immunosuppression with agents such as azathioprine or cyclophosphamide may be warranted. Such treatment requires careful monitoring of the hematopoietic, renal, and other organ systems, and should be undertaken only in conjunction with a specialist experienced in using these drugs.

---

220. CORNEA

SUPERFICIAL PUNCTATE KERATITIS

Scattered, fine, punctate loss of epithelium from the corneal surface of one or both eyes. It is often associated with trachoma, staphylococcal blepharitis, conjunctivitis, or a respiratory tract infection. It may be due to a viral infection or may be a reaction to local medication and is commonly the cause of intense pain after exposure to ultravio-

let rays (eg, from welding arcs, sun lamps). Symptoms include photophobia, pain, lacrimation, conjunctival injection, and diminution of vision. An enlarged preauricular node may be present in viral cases. Lesions due to ultraviolet ray exposure do not appear until several hours after the exposure; they last 24 to 48 h, while those secondary to viral or bacterial agents may last for months. Healing is spontaneous and residual vision impairment is rare, regardless of etiology.

Treatment

Topical antimicrobial therapy should be given promptly, particularly if a causative organism can be cultured and identified. For gram-positive organisms, 10 to 30% sulfacetamide drops q 2 h and 0.5% erythromycin or 500 u./gm bacitracin ointment tid can be used. Gram-negative organisms can be treated with 0.3% gentamicin or 0.3% tobramycin drops q 2 h, and bacitracin ointment tid. Dark glasses are useful for photophobia. A systemic analgesic may be needed for control of pain; *topical anesthetics may delay healing and should not be used.* Ultraviolet burns are treated with short-acting cycloplegics, antibiotic ointment, and patching for 24 h. Corticosteroids are not indicated.

CORNEAL ULCER

Local necrosis of corneal tissue due to invasion by microorganisms.

Etiology

A pneumococcal, streptococcal, or staphylococcal infection following trauma or complicating a corneal foreign body is the usual primary cause. Corneal ulcers also occur as complications of herpes simplex keratitis, chronic blepharitis, conjunctivitis (especially bacterial), trachoma, dacryocystitis, gonorrhea, and acute infectious diseases. **Indolent ulcers** are considered to be fungal until proved otherwise. Corneal ulcers may also result from disturbances in corneal nutrition secondary to vitamin A or protein malnutrition, or corneal exposure due to eyelid injuries or defective closure of the lids **(lagophthalmos).**

Symptoms and Signs

Pain, photophobia, blepharospasm, and lacrimation are present, but may be minimal. The lesion begins as a dull, grayish, circumscribed superficial infiltration and subsequently necroses and suppurates to form an ulcer. This stains green with fluorescein (see Ch. 213 for method) and is readily evident. Considerable ciliary injection is usual, and in long-standing cases blood vessels may grow in from the limbus **(pannus).** The ulcer may spread to involve the width of the cornea or may penetrate deeply; pus may appear in the anterior chamber **(hypopyon).**

Ulceration without extensive infiltration may occur in herpes simplex. Fungal ulcerations are densely infiltrated and show occasional discrete islands of infiltrate (satellite lesions) at the periphery.

Complications

The deeper the ulcer, the more severe the symptoms and complications. Ulcers of the cornea heal with fibrous tissue replacement, causing opaque scarring of the cornea and decreased vision. Iritis, iridocyclitis, corneal perforation with iris prolapse, hypopyon, panophthalmitis, and destruction of the eye may occur with or without treatment. Ulcers caused by fungi are indolent but serious; those caused by *P. aeruginosa* are especially virulent, and those associated with dendritic herpes simplex keratitis may be particularly refractory.

Treatment

Corneal ulcers should be treated only by an ophthalmologist.

HERPES SIMPLEX KERATITIS

Corneal herpes simplex virus infection, with a spectrum of clinical appearances, commonly leading to chronic inflammation, vascularization, scarring, and loss of vision. The initial infection is usually an undistinguished self-limiting conjunctivitis, which may be accompanied by a vesicular blepharitis. Recurrences usually take the form of **dendritic keratitis,** with a characteristic branched lesion of the cornea resembling the veins of a leaf, with knoblike terminals. A foreign-body sensation, lacrimation, photophobia, and conjunctival injection are early symptoms, followed rapidly by corneal hypoesthesia or anesthesia, an important diagnostic sign. Ulceration and permanent scarring of the cornea may result. **Disciform keratitis,** a deep, disc-shaped corneal inflammation with accompanying iritis, frequently follows dendritic keratitis and probably represents an immunologic response to the virus. Rarely, direct invasion of the corneal stroma by herpes simplex virus is seen, and occasionally a recurrent loss of corneal epithelium is seen in patients with herpes simplex virus but without active viral eruption.

Treatment

Idoxuridine **(IDU),** vidarabine, and trifluridine are specific, though not always effective. The agent, whether an ointment or solution, should be used several times daily. If the epithelium surrounding the dendrite is loose and edematous, debridement by gentle swabbing with a cotton-tipped applicator before beginning drug therapy may speed healing. If healing fails to occur after 3 to 5 days, debridement by gentle swabbing with a cotton-tipped applicator is indicated. Topical corticosteroids are **contraindicated** in the early stages of dendritic keratitis, but may be effective when used with an antiviral agent in the later stromal or uveitic involvement. Atropine 1% instilled tid is useful in cases with more than epithelial involvement. Cases that fail to heal after 1 wk and those with stromal or uveal involvement require referral to an ophthalmologist.

OPHTHALMIC HERPES ZOSTER

(See also HERPES ZOSTER under EXANTHEMATOUS VIRAL DISEASES in Ch. 12)

Involvement of the eyelid or palpebral conjunctiva by herpes zoster is not threatening to the globe. However, when the nasociliary nerve is affected, as indicated by a lesion on the tip of the nose, the cornea invariably becomes involved. Marked lid edema, ciliary and conjunctival injection, corneal infiltration, and pain are all present. Keratitis accompanied by uveitis may be severe, and is followed by scarring. Glaucoma, a common sequel, often develops much later.

Treatment

Unlike herpes simplex, herpes zoster *is* an indication for corticosteroids when the cornea and uveal tract are involved. Topical therapy (eg, 0.1% dexamethasone, instilled q 2 h initially) is usually adequate. The pupil should be kept dilated with 1% atropine or 0.5 to 1% cyclopentolate solution, 1 drop tid. Intraocular pressure must be monitored.

If the patient is in good general health, a brief course of high-dose steroids (eg, prednisone 60 mg/day for 3 days, then 45 mg for 3 days, and then 30 mg for 3 days) may prevent severe postherpetic neuralgia. Recently, experimental use of cimetadine 300 mg qid for 3 wk has been advocated to prevent postherpetic neuralgia.

PHLYCTENULAR KERATOCONJUNCTIVITIS

(Phlyctenular or Eczematous Conjunctivitis)

A conjunctivitis, usually occurring in children, characterized by discrete nodular areas of inflammation ***(phlyctenules)*** *and resulting from the atopic reaction of a hypersensitive*

conjunctiva or cornea to an unknown allergen. Proteins of staphylococcal, tuberculous, or other bacterial origin have been implicated. The disease is rare in the USA.

Phlyctenules appear as crops of small yellow-gray nodules at the limbus or on the cornea and bulbar conjunctiva and persist from several days to 1 to 2 wk. They ulcerate, but heal without a scar. When the cornea is affected, blepharospasm, severe tearing, photophobia, and pain may be prominent. Frequent recurrence, especially with secondary infection, may lead to corneal opacity with loss of vision. **Treatment** with a topical corticosteroid-antibiotic combination is valuable in combating the condition and any secondary infection.

INTERSTITIAL KERATITIS

(Parenchymatous Keratitis)

A chronic nonulcerative infiltration of the deep layers of the cornea, with uveal inflammation. It is rare in the USA. Most cases occur in children as a late complication of congenital syphilis. Ultimately, both eyes may be involved. Rarely, acquired syphilis or TB may cause a unilateral form in adults.

Photophobia, pain, lacrimation, and gradual loss of vision are common. The lesion begins in the deep corneal layers; soon the entire cornea develops a ground-glass appearance, obscuring the iris. New blood vessels grow in from the limbus and produce orange-red areas ("salmon patches"). Iritis, iridocyclitis, and choroiditis are common. The inflammation and neovascularization usually begin to subside after 1 to 2 mo. Some corneal opacity may remain, but vision may be impaired even when the cornea clears completely. An ophthalmologist should be consulted for treatment.

KERATOMALACIA

(Xerotic Keratitis; Xerophthalmia)

A condition associated with vitamin A deficiency and protein-calorie malnutrition, characterized by a hazy, dry cornea that becomes denuded. Corneal ulceration with secondary infection is common. The lacrimal glands and conjunctiva are also affected. Lack of tears causes extreme dryness of the eyes, and foamy Bitot's spots appear on the bulbar conjunctiva. Night blindness may be associated. Further details, including specific therapy, can be found under VITAMIN A DEFICIENCY in Ch. 81. Antibiotic ointments or sulfonamides (eg, sulfacetamide ophthalmic solution 30% or ointment 10%) are required if secondary infection exists.

KERATOCONUS

A slowly progressive ectasia of the cornea, usually bilateral, beginning between ages 10 and 20. The cone shape that the cornea assumes causes major changes in the refractive power of the eye and necessitates frequent change of spectacles. Contact lenses may provide better visual correction, and should always be tried when eyeglasses are not satisfactory. Surgery may be necessary if the cornea becomes thin or if scarring follows rents in the posterior corneal surface.

BULLOUS KERATOPATHY

A condition caused by excessive fluid accumulation in the cornea, most frequently the result of aging and failure of the corneal endothelium. It is seen occasionally after intraocular operations (eg, for cataract) where the mechanical stresses further interfere with the process of corneal detumescence.

The fluid-filled bullae on the corneal surface rupture, causing pain and decreased vision. The bullae and swelling of the corneal stroma can be seen on examination.

Treatment, including the use of dehydrating agents, soft contact lenses, and corneal transplantation, is best carried out by an ophthalmologist.

221. CATARACT

Developmental or degenerative opacity of the lens. (**Developmental or congenital cataracts** are discussed under CONGENITAL EYE DEFECTS in Ch. 187).

Juvenile or adult cataract is characterized by progressive, painless loss of vision. The cause may be senile degeneration, x-rays, heat from infrared exposure, systemic disease (eg, diabetes), uveitis, or systemic medications (eg, corticosteroids).

Symptoms and Signs

The cardinal symptom is a progressive, painless loss of vision. The degree of loss depends on the location and extent of the opacity. When the opacity is in the central lens nucleus (**nuclear cataract**), myopia develops in the early stages, so that a presbyopic patient may discover that he can read without his glasses ("second sight"). Pain occurs if the cataract swells and produces secondary glaucoma.

Opacity beneath the posterior lens capsule (**posterior subcapsular cataract**) affects vision out of proportion to the degree of cloudiness because the opacity is located at the crossing point of the rays of light from the viewed object. Such cataracts are particularly troublesome in bright light.

Diagnosis

Gradual loss of vision beginning in middle age or later is characteristic of glaucoma as well as cataract. Before dilation of the pupils for an ophthalmoscopic examination, increased intraocular tension and a shallow anterior chamber must be ruled out.

Well-developed cataracts appear as gray opacities in the lens. Ophthalmoscopic examination of the dilated pupil (see Ch. 213) with the instrument held about 1 ft away will usually disclose subtle opacities. Small cataracts stand out as dark defects in the red reflex. A large cataract may obliterate the red reflex. Slit-lamp examination provides more details about the character, location, and extent of the opacity.

Treatment

Frequent refractions and eyeglass prescription changes help maintain useful vision during cataract development. Occasionally, chronic pupillary dilation (2.5 to 10% phenylephrine) is helpful for small lenticular opacities. When useful vision is lost, lens extraction is necessary; it can be accomplished by removal of the lens intact, or by emulsification followed by irrigation and aspiration. Age is no contraindication to surgery. Corticosteroids must be given topically and systemically when surgery is needed in the presence of uveitis. Refractive correction postoperatively is accomplished by cataract spectacles, contact lenses, or intraoperative implantation of an intraocular prosthetic lens.

222. UVEAL TRACT

UVEITIS

Inflammation of the uveal tract (iris, ciliary body, and choroid). Inflammation of the contiguous retina (retinitis), by tradition, is included in the category of uveitis. Uveitis may be anatomically classified as **anterior (iritis and iridocyclitis), intermediate (cyclitis, peripheral uveitis), posterior (choroiditis and retinitis),** and **diffuse (iritis plus intermediate uveitis plus chorioretinitis).** Some of the uveitic diseases are associated with systemic

disease (see below) and others represent strictly ocular syndromes (eg, Fuchs' heterochromic iridocyclitis, pars planitis, birdshot retinochoroidopathy, etc).

Symptoms and Signs

The symptoms and signs generally are subtle: mainly diminished or hazy vision, black floating spots, or symptoms related to complications of uveitis (glaucoma, cataract, and retinal detachment). Severe pain, redness, and photophobia are classically described, but occur only in cases of acute iritis and iridocyclitis. The major signs of **anterior uveitis** include pupillary miosis and perilimbal flush (injection adjacent to the limbus). Cells and flare and keratic precipitates on the corneal endothelium are signs seen only by means of the biomicroscope (slit lamp). Signs of **intermediate uveitis** include cells in the vitreous, cellular aggregates in the inferior anterior vitreous humor, and exudation and membrane formation overlying the inferior pars plana of the ciliary body. While the vitreal cells and cellular aggregates may be seen with the direct ophthalmoscope, the membrane over the pars plana usually requires using the indirect ophthalmoscope (usually used only by ophthalmologists). Signs of **posterior uveitis** often include vitreal inflammatory cells and strands, white fuzzy fundus lesions, and inflammatory sheathing of retinal blood vessels.

The direct damage as well as secondary complications of uveitis are often severe and may develop with alarming rapidity; therefore, when uveitis is suspected, the patient should be referred as rapidly as possible for ophthalmologic evaluation.

Common Systemic Diseases Associated with Uveitis

Fuller discussions of these diseases are elsewhere in THE MANUAL. Although therapeutic suggestions are included here, it should be understood that treatment should never be attempted by anyone but an ophthalmologist.

Ankylosing spondylitis, a common cause of acute iridocyclitis, is more frequent in males and may be associated with attacks of pain, redness, and photophobia in one or both eyes. HLA-B27 and x-rays of the sacroiliac joint are usually positive. Treatment includes intensive local use of corticosteroid drops as well as mydriatic/cycloplegic drops.

Reiter's syndrome, another common cause of acute iridocyclitis, is seen mainly in males and is associated with HLA-B27 positivity. Treatment is the same as that for the uveitis associated with ankylosing spondylitis.

Juvenile rheumatoid arthritis (JRA) is characteristically associated with a bilateral chronic iridocyclitis. Symptoms are minimal—mainly blurred or diminished vision. This disease occurs primarily in girls with pauciarticular joint disease; 80% demonstrate a positive ANA. Inflammatory exacerbations require treatment with local steroids and mydriatic/cycloplegic therapy.

Toxoplasmosis is the most common cause of posterior uveitis. While toxoplasmosis may infect the individual by either the acquired or congenital route, the ocular disease almost always results from congenital transmission. The recurrent attacks of acute focal necrotizing retinitis produce diminished and hazy vision. Since there may be associated acute secondary iridocyclitis, some patients present with pain, redness, and photophobia. Laboratory testing for anti-toxoplasma antibodies by enzyme-linked immunoabsorbent assay **(ELISA)** or indirect fluorescent antibody is positive, but usually only in low titers. Systemic treatment with antitoxoplasmic agents such as pyrimethamine and sulfonamides combined with systemic corticosteroids is often recommended for retinal lesions that threaten the macula.

Cytomegalovirus (CMV) infection, like ocular toxoplasmosis, produces acute necrotizing retinitis secondary to congenitally acquired infection. Symptoms are usually only visual, since secondary iridocyclitis is rare. In adults, CMV retinitis is rare except in patients immunosuppressed for organ transplants, by anti-cancer treatment, or by AIDS. Laboratory testing is for CF antibodies to CMV and for examination of urinary

sediment for CMV inclusions. Available treatment is poor, but recently attempts have been made to use antiviral agents (eg, acyclovir).

Toxocariasis is most common in childhood and usually produces a single, unilateral, peripheral or posterior, retinal granuloma or, occasionally, generalized inflammation of the entire inner eye (endophthalmitis). Uveitis rarely occurs in generalized visceral larval migrans; more often it occurs after only minimal systemic infection with few larvae. The ELISA for Toxocara on serum, aqueous, or vitreous samples is usually positive. Treatment is limited to systemic steroids. Antihelminthic agents are not recommended.

Histoplasmosis may be associated with a multifocal choroiditis, especially in patients who have lived in the Ohio, Missouri, and Mississippi River valleys. The uveitis is always noted months to years after acutely acquired systemic histoplasmosis, when the complement fixation test has usually returned to negative. Skin testing with histoplasmin is positive in 80% of cases, and most patients who have macular disease demonstrate presence of the HLA-B7 antigen. Chest x-ray often is useful in showing pulmonary calcifications typical of pulmonary histoplasmosis. Treatment includes systemic and/or periocular corticosteroid injections. Laser photocoagulation may be the best way to halt the progress of macular disease.

Tuberculosis (TB), although now considered to be a rare cause of uveitis, may result in almost any type of uveitis, including a diffuse generalized inflammation of all of the intraocular tissues. Laboratory tests include PPD and chest x-ray. Treatment with antituberculous medication and systemic steroids is often necessary.

Syphilis, (secondary, tertiary, or latent), like TB, is relatively rare in association with any type of uveitis. Laboratory testing on serum includes the nonspecific Venereal Disease Research Laboratory **(VDRL)** test as well as the specific fluorescent treponemal antibody-absorption **(FTA-ABS)** test, and hemagglutination and microhemagglutination tests for *Treponema pallidum* antibodies. Examining the spinal fluid for reagin antibodies is often useful. After the diagnosis has been established, treatment includes systemic penicillin or synthetic or semisynthetic penicillins and corticosteroids.

Behçet's syndrome is rare in the USA. Acute recurrent bilateral iridocyclitis, with pain, redness, photophobia, and severe retinal vasculitis and papillitis, is common. The ocular findings often occur in association with oral and genital aphthae, dermatitis, thrombophlebitis, or other systemic symptoms related to a widely disseminated systemic occlusive vasculitis. Laboratory testing includes biopsy of suspected skin or mucous membrane lesions, and search for the HLA-B51 antigen. Treatment using local and systemic corticosteroids may quiet the acute inflammatory episode, but is usually ineffective in arresting the relentless progressive damage of the disease. Therefore many authorities recommend immunosuppressive drugs or cyclosporin for this condition.

Vogt-Koyanagi-Haradas (VKH) syndrome: VKH, or uveoencephalitis, is much more common in Orientals than in Caucasians. It often begins with bilateral attacks of acute iridocyclitis with pain, redness, and photophobia. Later, severe diffuse choroiditis may result in serous (inflammatory) detachment of the macular areas, with profound loss of vision. Associated systemic signs include alopecia arreata, poliosis, vitaligo, dysacusis, and meningeal headaches. The headaches may be fleeting. Lumbar puncture taken when the patient has a headache usually reveals pleocytosis of the spinal fluid—a valuable aid in diagnosis. Treatment using local and systemic corticosteroids or immunosuppressive drugs is often necessary.

Sarcoidosis, one of the more commonly associated diseases, may be accompanied by any type of anterior, posterior, or diffuse uveitis. The ocular inflammation often occurs independently of any systemic inflammation, thereby making diagnosis difficult. Laboratory tests of value include biopsy of conjunctival or lacrimal granulomas; serum

testing for angiotensin converting enzyme and lysozyme; testing for elevation of the ESR; chest x-ray for hialar adenopathy; and gallium scan of the head, neck, and chest.

Treatment is limited to local, periocular, and systemic corticosteroids.

ENDOPHTHALMITIS

Suppurative inflammation involving all the inner layers of the eye, the vitreous, and sclera may result from infection with bacterial or fungal agents. The infection may have been introduced exogenously (by a perforating wound of the eye or intraocular surgery) or endogenously via the bloodstream (from an infective focus elsewhere in the body or from the contaminated needle of an intravenous drug abuser).

The symptoms and signs of inflammation are often dramatic: severe pain, redness, photophobia, and profound loss of vision. Often the fundus cannot be visualized due to inflammation of the vitreous. Early testing of aqueous and especially vitreous aliquots for culture and microscopic examination is recommended.

Treatment *should be as in an emergency*, since delay of a few hours may result in blindness, and consists of systemic, periocular, and intraocular broad-spectrum antibiotics (eg, cefazolin or gentamicin). Supplemental steroids usually are needed. Often surgical vitrectomy is necessary.

MALIGNANT MELANOMA OF THE CHOROID

This is the most common primary ocular malignancy. It is rare in the black race. Malignant melanoma usually can be seen ophthalmoscopically (through a dilated pupil) and appears as a single, round or oval, slightly elevated, gray or nonpigmented lesion. Early detection is important, since the prognosis is related to the size of the lesion. When the lesion is small, treatment with laser or radioemitting plaques may result in regression of the tumor and save the eye. Larger tumors require enucleation. If the lesion is ignored, it may exit from the eye via scleral canals and involve the orbit or spread hematogenously to distant organs, especially the liver.

---

223. RETINA

VASCULAR RETINOPATHIES

Retinal hemorrhage, exudates, edema, ischemia, or infarction due to ocular or systemic vascular disorders.

Arteriosclerotic retinopathy is found in generalized arteriosclerosis and is often secondary to hypertension. The walls of the retinal arterioles become thickened, and the changes are reflected on ophthalmoscopy as a widened arteriolar light reflex. As the sclerosis progresses, one sees indentation of the veins at arteriovenous crossings and an increased difference between the sizes of the venous and arteriolar blood columns. The fine arterioles and veins may become tortuous, and the arteries may appear sheathed. Advanced sclerosis at arteriovenous crossings can cause branch retinal vein occlusion.

Hypertensive retinopathy occurs in chronic essential hypertension, malignant hypertension, and toxemia of pregnancy. The fundi show generalized or focal retinal arteriolar constriction in the early stages. As the disease progresses, superficial flame-shaped hemorrhages and small white or gray superficial foci of retinal ischemia ("cotton-wool spots") develop. Yellow "hard" exudates (drusen), due to lipid deposition deep in the retina and arising from leaking retinal vessels, are seen later and often produce a star-shaped figure around the macula. (See also HYPERTENSION in Ch. 26.) The optic disk

becomes congested and edematous in severe hypertension and resembles the choked disk caused by brain tumor (**papilledema**; see in Ch. 225).

Treatment

Arteriosclerotic and hypertensive retinopathies can be managed only by medical control of the primary systemic disorder.

CENTRAL RETINAL ARTERY OCCLUSION

Central retinal artery occlusion produces a painless, sudden, unilateral blindness. The occlusion may be due to embolism (disseminated atherosclerotic plaques, endocarditis, fat emboli [Purtscher's retinopathy], atrial myxoma) or to thrombosis in a sclerotic central artery. Another important cause is cranial arteritis (temporal arteritis; see in Ch. 30). The pupil is semidilated and responds poorly to direct light but constricts briskly when the other eye is illuminated. Ophthalmoscopy discloses a pale, opaque fundus with a bright red fovea ("cherry red spot"). The arteries are attenuated and may appear bloodless; the veins are narrow, with less blood than normal. An embolic obstruction is sometimes visible; if it is not relieved quickly, retinal infarction occurs and blindness is permanent. If a major branch is occluded rather than the entire artery, fundus abnormalities are limited to that sector of the retina and a permanent subtotal visual field loss follows unless the occlusion is relieved.

Branch retinal artery occlusion is almost always embolic.

Treatment

Immediate treatment is imperative. Reduction of intraocular tension by intermittent digital massage over the closed eyelids or anterior chamber paracentesis may dislodge an embolus and allow it to enter a smaller branch of the artery, thus reducing the area of retinal ischemia. Inhalation of 5 to 10% CO_2 in O_2 may relieve retinal arterial spasm.

CENTRAL RETINAL VEIN OCCLUSION

Central retinal vein occlusion usually appears in elderly arteriosclerotic patients. Glaucoma, covert diabetes mellitus, hypertension, increased blood viscosity, or an elevated Hct can be predisposing factors. Occlusion in a young person is uncommon; it may be idiopathic or result from retinal phlebitis. Painless visual loss occurs less abruptly than in arterial obstruction. The retinal veins appear distended and tortuous, the fundus is congested and edematous, and numerous retinal hemorrhages appear. These changes are limited to one quadrant if the obstruction involves only a branch of the vein. Neovascularization of the retina or of the iris **(rubeosis iridis)** with secondary (neovascular) glaucoma can occur weeks to months after the occlusion. Fluorescein angiography is essential to determine the state of the circulation. Patients with normal retinal vessel perfusion usually do well; those with poor perfusion are more likely to develop complications.

Treatment

There is no generally accepted medical therapy. Tonometry to detect predisposing glaucoma, a blood-clotting survey, and a glucose tolerance test are worthwhile. Destruction of secondary retinal neovascular overgrowth by photocoagulation may decrease vitreous hemorrhages. Secondary neovascular glaucoma requires panretinal photocoagulation.

DIABETIC RETINOPATHY

This major cause of blindness can be particularly severe in juvenile diabetics with insulin-dependent diabetes mellitus **(IDDM)** but is also frequent in chronic noninsulin-

dependent diabetes mellitus **(NIDDM).** Although the severity of the metabolic derangement is important, the degree of retinopathy seems more related to the duration of the diabetes than to its stability; retinopathy generally occurs after 10 yr. Hypertension has a further deleterious effect. Two types of diabetic retinopathy are recognized—nonproliferative and proliferative. **Nonproliferative retinopathy** (also known as **background** or **simple retinopathy**) is characterized by increased capillary permeability, microaneurysms, hemorrhages, exudates, and edema. The first signs are often venous dilation and small red dots seen ophthalmoscopically in the posterior retinal pole. The dots are caused by single or clustered **capillary microaneurysms** that can be demonstrated by fluorescein angiography. Visual symptoms are not encountered until an advanced state (macular edema or proliferative retinopathy) is reached. Dot and blot retinal hemorrhages and deep-lying edema and edema residues may impair macular function. Macular edema is a common cause of visual impairment in diabetics and may best be detected or confirmed by fluorescein angiography. The exudates of retinopathy may be soft (cotton-wool spots), which are microinfarcts caused by anoxia (acute vascular deficiency), and hard yellow exudates usually caused by chronic edema (damaged capillaries). Both types of exudates may impair normal vision.

Proliferative retinopathy is characterized by new vessel formation (neovascularization within the retina and extending into the vitreous) and scarring, resulting in **retinitis proliferans** in the posterior pole in advanced disease. The new vessels may extend into the vitreous cavity with subsequent vitreous hemorrhages, fibrous tissue formation, and secondary retinal detachment.

Treatment

Control of the diabetes and blood pressure is important; good control may retard the onset of diabetic retinopathy, but does not usually reverse it. Diabetics with IDDM should have careful annual retinal examinations (generally by an ophthalmologist), beginning 5 yr after diabetes has been diagnosed. Those with NIDDM should have annual examinations beginning at the time of diagnosis. Visual symptoms, including blurred vision for > 2 days not associated with a significant change in blood glucose, sudden loss of vision in one or both eyes, or black spots, cobwebs, or flashing lights in the field of vision, are indications for ophthalmologic referral at any time. Hypertension also should be controlled.

Panretinal photocoagulation (by xenon arc or argon laser) may diminish or eliminate proliferative retinopathy and iris neovascularization. Pituitary ablation is reserved for patients whose retinopathy has progressed beyond where photocoagulation can be used; the procedure produces major long-term endocrine deficiencies and candidates must be carefully selected. Vitrectomy is useful in many cases of longstanding vitreous hemorrhage.

MACULAR DEGENERATION OF THE AGED

(Senile Macular Degeneration [SMD])

Atrophy or degeneration of the macular disk. SMD is a leading cause of visual diminution in the elderly. The condition is without sex predilection, but is much more common in white than in black people. No predisposing systemic condition is known, and possibly the condition is hereditary. Two different forms of SMD can be defined: In the first, the **atrophic form,** there is pigmentary disturbance in the macular region but no elevated macular scar and little or no hemorrhage or exudation in the region of the macula; the second, called **disciform macular degeneration,** is characterized by formation of an exudative mound often surrounded by subretinal and intraretinal hemorrhage. Eventually this mound contracts and leaves a distinct elevated scar at the posterior pole. Both forms of SMD are generally bilateral and are often preceded by multiple drusen in the macular region.

Symptoms, Signs, and Diagnosis

A slow or sudden, painless loss of central visual acuity may occur. Occasionally the first symptom is visual distortion from one eye; this can easily be tested with an Amsler Grid. Funduscopy reveals pigmentary or hemorrhagic disturbance in the macular region of the involved eye; the contralateral eye almost always shows some pigmentary disturbance and the presence of drusen in the macula. Fluorescein angiography often demonstrates neovascular membranes beneath the retina, particularly in the disciform variety.

Treatment

No medical therapy is effective. Smoking probably should be eliminated. If fluorescein angiography shows a neovascular net, it should be treated by appropriate laser photocoagulation. The krypton or green argon laser may be used to treat choroidal new vessels lying in the juxtafoveal or subfoveal areas. For patients who have lost central vision, low vision devices are available and low vision service counseling is advised. Patients with SMD, though often "legally blind" (less than 20/200 vision), usually have good peripheral vision and useful color vision, and they should be advised that they will not lose all sight.

RETINAL DETACHMENT

Separation of the neural retina from the underlying retinal pigment epithelium.

Although detachment may be localized initially, without treatment the entire retina may detach. **Rhegmatogenous detachment** implies a through and through break in the retina and is seen most often in myopia, after cataract surgery, or following ocular trauma. In these cases fluid percolates through the hole from the vitreous into the subretinal space. **Nonrhegmatogenous detachments** can be produced by vitreoretinal traction (eg, proliferative retinopathy of diabetes or sickle cell disease) or by transudation of fluid into the subretinal space (eg, severe uveitis, especially in Vogt-Koyanagi-Harada disease, or primary or metastatic choroidal tumors).

Symptoms, Signs, and Diagnosis

Retinal detachment is painless. Premonitory symptoms include dark or irregular vitreous floaters, flashes of light, or blurred vision. As the detachment progresses, the patient notices a curtain or veil in the field of vision. If the macula is involved, central visual acuity fails drastically.

Any patient with a suspected or established retinal detachment should be seen, on an emergency basis, by an ophthalmologist. Prognosis is best if the condition is treated before macular involvement occurs. Visual acuity can be measured with the Snellen chart or any reading material. Each eye is tested separately (with glasses, if the patient wears them). Visual fields can be estimated by confrontation testing. Direct ophthalmoscopy may show retinal irregularities and a bullous retinal elevation with darkened blood vessels. Indirect ophthalmoscopy, including scleral depression, is necessary to detect peripheral breaks and detachment.

If a vitreous hemorrhage obscures the fundus, especially in a myopic, aphakic (post-cataract extraction), or injured eye, retinal detachment should be suspected and ultrasonography performed. The patient should be hospitalized, sedated, and kept in bed with his head elevated. Binocular patching and pupillary dilatation are used until an adequate examination can be carried out.

Treatment

Rhegmatogenous detachment is treated by finding the retinal holes and sealing them by diathermy or cryotherapy. The eye may be shortened by scleral "buckling" and by implanting silicone rubber sponges. Fluid may be drained from the subretinal space.

Anterior retinal breaks without detachment can be sealed by transconjunctival cryopexy; posterior breaks, by photocoagulation. More than 90% of rhegmatogenous detachments can be reattached surgically.

Nonrhegmatogenous detachments due to vitreoretinal traction may be treatable by intravitreal surgery; transudative detachments due to uveitis may respond to systemic corticosteroid therapy, but occasionally may require antimetabolite therapy. Primary choroidal neoplasms (malignant melanomas) may require enucleation, though radiation and local resection are used occasionally; choroidal hemangiomas respond to localized photocoagulation. Metastatic choroidal neoplasms (the usual primary sites are breast, lung, and GI tract) respond well to radiotherapy, and the eyes should *not* be enucleated.

RETINITIS PIGMENTOSA

A slowly progressive, bilateral, tapeto-retinal degeneration. A hereditary pattern is often difficult to establish, but in most cases it appears to be autosomal recessive. It may also be autosomal dominant or, infrequently, X-linked. It may occur as part of a syndrome complex (Bassen-Kornzweig, Laurence-Moon-Biedl).

The retinal rods are affected most, producing defective night vision that may become symptomatic in early childhood. A midperipheral ring scotoma (detectable by visual field testing) widens gradually, so that central vision frequently is also reduced by middle age. Total blindness may eventually ensue.

Ophthalmoscopic abnormalities usually are evident by age 10 yr. The most conspicuous finding is dark pigmentation in "bone-spicule" configuration in the equatorial retina. The retinal arteries and veins often appear narrowed and the disk, in some, may have a waxy yellow color. Other, later, manifestations can include macular degeneration, degenerative vitreous opacities, and cataract. Associated defects include myopia and deafness.

Diagnosis is aided by specialized testing (eg, dark adaptation, electroretinography **[ERG]**, electro-oculography **[EOG]**). Other retinopathies that can simulate retinitis pigmentosa (eg, congenital syphilis, congenital rubella, chloroquine toxicity) must be ruled out. Family members should be examined and tested to detect subclinical cases and to establish the hereditary mode if possible.

No **treatment** is effective except perhaps in Bassen-Kornzweig disease, where large doses of vitamin A have been advocated; genetic and career counseling are all that can be offered.

---

224. GLAUCOMA

A disorder characterized by increased intraocular pressure that may cause impaired vision, ranging from slight loss to absolute blindness. **Primary glaucoma** in adults may be of two types: (1) **chronic open-angle** (wide-angle) or (2) **acute or chronic angle-closure** (closed-angle, narrow-angle, congestive, acute glaucoma attack). **Congenital (infantile) glaucoma** is also primary (see also under CONGENITAL EYE DEFECTS in Ch. 187). **Secondary glaucoma** results from preexisting ocular disease, usually uveitis, intraocular tumor, or an enlarged cataract. Prolonged corticosteroid therapy, especially with topical ophthalmic preparations, can produce an increased pressure, particularly in patients with a predisposition, so-called steroid responders. It may be present after 1 wk, but usually occurs by the 6th to 8th wk of therapy. The increased pressure usually, but not always, subsides with cessation of therapy. Periodic tonometry is advisable during long-term corticosteroid use, to discover early elevated pressure and preclude damage

from a severe or prolonged intraocular pressure rise. **Absolute glaucoma** is the last stage of any form of uncontrolled glaucoma. The eye is blind from progressive atrophy of the optic nerve head. The pupil usually is widely dilated and fixed, the iris atrophied, and the disk deeply excavated. Pain is no longer prominent but may recur. The eyeball subsequently degenerates.

A competent gonioscopy of the anterior chamber angle is essential for proper diagnosis and classification of the glaucomas.

TABLE 224–1 lists the salient findings and usual treatment for the most common forms of glaucoma. Rarer forms may occur with associated congenital anomalies (eg, Sturge-Weber and Marfan syndromes) or with vascular or degenerative disorders.

PRIMARY GLAUCOMA

Etiology and Pathogenesis

The causes are unknown. Vasomotor and emotional instability, hyperopia, and especially heredity are among the predisposing factors. The increased intraocular tension is related to an imbalance between production and outflow of the aqueous humor. Obstruction to outflow appears to be mainly responsible for this imbalance. In **chronic open-angle glaucoma,** the anterior chamber and its anatomic structures appear normal, but drainage of the aqueous humor is impeded. In **acute and chronic angle-closure (congestive) glaucoma,** the anterior chamber is shallow, the filtration angle is narrowed, and the iris may obstruct the trabecular meshwork at the entrance of the canal of Schlemm. Dilation of the pupil may push the root of the iris forward against the angle, which may produce angle closure and thus precipitate an acute attack. Eyes with narrow anterior chamber angles are predisposed to acute angle-closure glaucoma attacks of varying degrees of severity.

CHRONIC OPEN-ANGLE GLAUCOMA (COAG)

A disorder characterized by a gradual rise in intraocular pressure, causing slowly progressive loss of peripheral vision and, when uncontrolled, late loss of central vision and ultimate blindness. The most prevalent form of glaucoma, it is common after age 30 but may occur in early childhood. It is usually familial. Rarely, it is unilateral.

Those at higher risk of developing COAG are those > 35 yr or those with diabetes (also those with positive glucose tolerance tests), myopia, pigment dispersion syndrome (Krukenberg's spindle), or a family history of glaucoma.

Diagnosis

Glaucoma should be suspected in any patient, especially if > 35 yr, who requires frequent spectacle lens changes, has mild headaches or vague visual disturbances, sees halos around electric lights, or has impaired dark adaptation. Since glaucoma can be asymptomatic until irreversible damage has occurred, every routine eye examination (and, optimally, every physical examination) in all adult patients should include examination with a tonometer. A single normal reading does not rule out glaucoma, since physiologic pressure shows diurnal variations of about 3 to 4 mm Hg (and even greater). The pressure rise in early glaucoma may be intermittent. A high-normal pressure reading is an indication for frequent follow-up examinations. In suspected cases, a complete glaucoma work-up by a glaucoma subspecialist is indicated.

Cupping of the optic disk is characteristic but a normal optic disk does not rule out glaucoma, since optic nerve damage develops insidiously and, in some cases, late in the disease. Visual field changes may be subtle, with normal-appearing disks. The earliest changes in the central visual field are a baring of the blind spot and small scotomata above or below fixation, with small and dim visual field targets. Subtle nasal peripheral field defects appear early. The external eye usually appears normal.

TABLE 224–1. CHARACTERISTICS OF

Type of Glaucoma	*Age*	*Iridocorneal Angle*	*Cornea*	*Pupil; Iris*
Chronic open-angle glaucoma	Rare in children and young adults; incidence rises from age 30 on	Wide open; may show pigment deposits	Not remarkable	Pupil not dilated. Iris may be atrophic late in the course
Angle-closure: acute; glaucoma attack	Any age, but more frequent after age 30	Closed during acute attack; narrow in interim	Cloudy. Microcystic edema of epithelium frequent	Pupil mid-dilated, fixed. Iris appears muddy
Glaucomato-cyclitic crisis (Posner-Schlossman syndrome)	Any age from young adulthood on	Narrow (not closed) or wide open	May be clear with keratic precipitates. Edema may be present	Pupil not dilated or only slightly dilated
Angle-closure: chronic; recurrent glaucoma attack	Any age	Narrow; closable with peripheral anterior synechiae	Usually cloudy during attack, clear between attacks	Pupil usually dilated during attack, normal between attacks
Congenital (infantile) glaucoma	Birth to 1st few mo of life (usually discovered before age 6 mo)	Closed by membrane	Large in diameter, cloudy	Pupil dilated. Iris may show atrophy
Secondary glaucoma	Any age (usually accompanying or following anterior uveitis)	Angle may be blocked by inflammatory debris or pigment	May be cloudy. Microcystic edema may be present	Pupil may be narrow. Iris may appear muddy
Corticosteroid-induced glaucoma	Any age in susceptible individuals ("steroid responders") after prolonged ophthalmic use	Wide open or narrow (not closed)	Usually clear	Pupil reacts; not constricted or dilated

THE COMMON FORMS OF GLAUCOMA

Optic Nerve Head & Visual Field	*Intraocular Pressure*	*Subjective Symptoms*	*Treatment of Choice*
May appear normal or show cupping. Progressive visual field defect if untreated	Elevated slightly (22 to 30 mm Hg) or markedly (30 to 45 mm Hg). Usually bilateral	Blurring of vision, frequent change of glasses. Occasional headaches, often ascribed by patient to "nervous tension" or "sinus problems"	*Topical:* Pilocarpine, timolol maleate, betataxolol HCl, epinephrine, dipivefrin, demecarium bromide, echothiophate iodide *Systemic:* Carbonic anhydrase inhibitors *Surgery:* Laser trabeculoplasty; subscleral filtering procedure if medication fails
Optic nerve head obscured during attack; may be normal. May show cupping after several attacks. Typical glaucomatous field defects may develop	40 to 70 mm Hg or even higher. Usually unilateral	Severe head & eye ache, blurred vision, halos around lights, general malaise, nausea, sometimes vomiting (GI symptoms may be misleading, delaying proper diagnosis)	*Topical:* Pilocarpine, timolol maleate *Systemic:* Osmotic agents, carbonic anhydrase inhibitors *Surgery:* Laser iridotomy or peripheral iridectomy when eye is quiet
Usually no cupping. *No* visual field loss!	May be 50 mm Hg or higher. Usually unilateral	Blurred vision, halos around lights, headache. Nausea rare	*Topical:* Corticosteroid drops *Systemic:* Carbonic anhydrase inhibitors *Surgery: Strictly contraindicated*
As for acute angle-closure glaucoma	Up to 70 or higher during attack. Between attacks normal. Usually unilateral	Severe headaches during attacks, blurred vision, halos around lights. Nausea rare.	*Surgery:* Laser iridotomy or iridectomy; filtering surgery if > 1/2 of iridocorneal angle is permanently closed
Usually hard to evaluate. Later atrophic and may show cupping	Markedly elevated (50 to 70 mm Hg). Usually bilateral	Not assessable	*Surgery:* goniotomy, goniopuncture, trabeculotomy
Initially may appear normal; if condition persists, may be cupped or atrophic. Glaucomatous field defect may develop	May be 50 mm Hg or higher. Usually unilateral	Blurred vision, halos, headache. Nausea rare	*Topical:* Anti-inflammatory management *Systemic:* Anti-inflammatory management, carbonic anhydrase inhibitors
Initially no cupping; if not treated, cupping may develop. Glaucomatous field defect develops	May be 50 mm Hg or higher. Frequently unilateral	Blurred vision and halos initially rare; headaches may be present. Blurred vision common in later stages	*Stop corticosteroids* *Topical:* Pilocarpine 1 to 4%, timolol maleate 0.25 or 0.5%, betataxolol HCl, demecarium bromide 0.125 or 0.25%, echothiophate iodide *Systemic:* Carbonic anhydrase inhibitors

Treatment

Most cases can be controlled with eyedrops. Beginning with the weakest available preparations (eg, 0.5% pilocarpine), the most effective concentration and frequency of administration are determined by trial. Preparations of choice are pilocarpine, timolol maleate, carbachol (only in patients who are not controlled by or react adversely to pilocarpine), and, in aphakic eyes only, potent cholinesterase inhibitors such as echothiophate iodide (CAUTION: *Patients treated with powerful miotics like demecarium, echothiophate, and isoflurophate may develop cataracts or retinal detachment, which must be looked for periodically during treatment).* Rarely, 2% pilocarpine ointment (must be individually prepared) is used at night to supplement other medication. Carbonic anhydrase inhibitors (eg, dichlorphenamide 50 to 200 mg/day or acetazolamide 125 to 250 mg qid orally) are of value when miotics alone do not control abnormal tension but should be used with great caution. Epinephrine 0.5 to 2%, 1 drop 1 to 2 times/day, may aid control by reducing aqueous production; recently it has been recommended that for more effective management dipivefrin hydrochloride 0.1% solution used once or twice a day may be substituted for epinephrine. The patient should avoid fatigue, emotional upsets, use of tobacco, and drinking large quantities of fluids. Tonometry and charting of visual fields should be performed semi-annually or more often when indicated. When medication fails to control intraocular tension or visual fields show increasing defects, laser trabeculoplasty or filtering surgery to improve aqueous drainage should be considered.

ACUTE ANGLE-CLOSURE GLAUCOMA

A disorder characterized by attacks of suddenly increased intraocular pressure, usually unilateral, with severe pain and loss of vision, caused by acute obstruction of aqueous drainage within the eye.

Symptoms and Signs

Prodromal symptoms occur as transitory episodes of diminished visual acuity, colored halos around lights, and pain in the eye and head. At such times, examination shows a somewhat dilated, poorly reacting pupil and shallow anterior chamber in the affected eye. These episodes may last only a few hours and recur at intervals before a typical prolonged attack of acute angle-closure glaucoma. The acute attack is characterized by rapid loss of sight and sudden onset of severe throbbing pain in the eye; the pain radiates over the sensory distribution of the 5th nerve. *Nausea and vomiting are common and may be mistaken for acute GI disease.* Upper lid edema, lacrimation, circumcorneal injection, chemosis, and a somewhat dilated, fixed pupil may be present. The cornea is steamy, the anterior chamber shallow, and the aqueous humor turbid enough to obscure the fundus. Intraocular pressure is increased considerably. (TABLE 219–1 in Ch. 219 lists findings that distinguish acute glaucoma, iritis, and conjunctivitis.) Symptoms usually subside after medical treatment, but may recur. Each acute attack progressively diminishes vision and contracts the visual field. The condition may be bilateral.

Glaucomatocyclitic crisis (Posner-Schlossman syndrome), a recurrent monocular rise in pressure, simulates acute angle-closure glaucoma but is associated with normal anterior chamber depth, keratic precipitates, and other signs of uveitis.

Treatment

Oral glycerin 1 to 2 gm/kg, mixed with an equal amount of water (cooled and preferably flavored with lemon), will often abort acute attacks, and is excellent initial therapy to reduce elevated intraocular pressure rapidly. Oral carbonic anhydrase inhibitors (eg, acetazolamide 500 mg), if given immediately, will generally abort an attack. If not, acetazolamide 500 mg IV and frequent instillation of miotics (eg, pilo-

carpine 4% q 15 min) for 1 to 2 h are indicated. Once the tension is normal, an oral carbonic anhydrase inhibitor q 6 h can be continued for several doses, together with miotics. If the initial therapy does not reduce the tension, 20% mannitol 500 mL by slow IV drip can be given (unless otherwise contraindicated), to be followed by miotics and a carbonic anhydrase inhibitor. Surgery, peripheral iridectomy or laser iridotomy, prevents further attacks and is often performed prophylactically on the unaffected fellow eye as well, if by gonioscopy the angle appears to be narrow.

Glaucomatocyclic crisis responds to systemic and topical corticosteroids and carbonic anhydrase inhibitors such as dichlorphenamide or acetazolamide; *surgery is strictly contraindicated.*

CHRONIC ANGLE-CLOSURE GLAUCOMA

A disorder characterized by recurrent attacks—usually unilateral, of increased intraocular pressure, pain, and impaired vision—similar to those of acute angle-closure glaucoma but less severe. The causes are similar, but the anterior angle is obstructed gradually, not suddenly. Factors that promote dilation of the pupil may be precipitating causes. The fellow eye frequently becomes involved later. A provocative test for this condition is the **darkroom test** after tonometry, exposing the patient (who must be awake) to 60 min of darkness with the head bent forward in a prone position (best performed leaning on a Mayo table), then promptly measuring the intraocular pressure again. A rise in the pressure of 6 mm Hg during the test is considered positive.

Treatment

One or two drops of pilocarpine 1 or 2% instilled 3 to 6 times/day is the treatment of choice for temporary management. Timolol maleate 1 drop 0.25 or 0.5% solution used 1 or 2 times/day can be *added,* to aid temporary management; it should not be used without pilocarpine because timolol maleate does not contract the pupil and therefore does not promote removal of the iris from the iridocorneal angle. Oral glycerin or mannitol by IV drip (see ACUTE ANGLE-CLOSURE GLAUCOMA, above) is useful in aborting attacks. Carbonic anhydrase inhibitors are used only during attacks in narrow-angle glaucoma, and are **contraindicated** in long-term therapy. Early laser iridotomy or peripheral iridectomy usually prevents further attacks. Permanent damage to the iridocorneal angle may necessitate management of the elevated intraocular pressure, even after successful laser iridotomy or iridectomy.

SECONDARY GLAUCOMA

Glaucoma secondary to an intraocular disorder, usually anterior uveitis.

Etiology and Pathogenesis

Secondary glaucoma is caused by any interference with the flow of aqueous humor from the posterior chamber through the pupil into the anterior chamber to the canal of Schlemm. Inflammatory disease of the anterior segment may prevent aqueous escape by causing complete posterior synechia and iris bombé, and may plug the drainage channel with exudates. Other common causes are intraocular tumors, intumescent cataracts, central retinal vein occlusion, trauma to the eye, operative procedures, and intraocular hemorrhage.

Treatment

Secondary glaucoma is best treated by an ophthalmologist; intensive therapy and probably mydriasis are indicated. The underlying cause, usually uveitis, must be treated. Treatment is begun with systemic corticosteroids, and the effect of a mild mydriatic (eg, 5% homatropine, 1% cyclopentolate, or 10% phenylephrine) is tested in the office; 1% atropine bid or tid is given if the mydriasis is successful. If this fails, use

of pilocarpine and/or timolol maleate should be considered. A carbonic anhydrase inhibitor or oral glycerin as for acute angle-closure glaucoma may be useful temporarily during the acute phase. Surgical intervention is indicated in iris bombé, tumor, and swollen cataract.

---

225. OPTIC NERVE; VISUAL PATHWAYS

PAPILLEDEMA

(Choked Disk)

Swelling of the optic nerve head due to increased intracranial pressure. It is almost always bilateral and occurs with brain tumor or abscess, cerebral trauma or hemorrhage, meningitis, arachnoidal adhesions, pseudotumor cerebri, cavernous sinus thrombosis, dural sinus thrombosis, encephalitis, space-occupying brain lesions, severe hypertensive disease, and pulmonary emphysema.

Vision is not affected initially, but the blind spot is enlarged. The degree of disk elevation is determined by comparing the highest plus lens necessary to bring the most elevated portion of the disk into sharp focus with that used to see an unaffected portion of the retina clearly. Engorged and tortuous retinal veins, a hyperemic disk, and retinal hemorrhages about the disk are usually observed. The absence of changes in the arterioles and a normal blood pressure help to differentiate the papilledema of brain tumor from that of hypertension. If the intracranial pressure is not reduced, secondary optic atrophy and loss of vision eventually occur.

PAPILLITIS

(Optic Neuritis)

Inflammation of that portion of the optic nerve visible ophthalmoscopically. It occurs with foci of inflammation in and about the optic nerve, as part of demyelinating conditions, following a viral illness, or with multiple sclerosis, as a result of infarction of a part or all of the optic nerve head in temporal arteritis or other occlusive disease of the ciliary vessels, from tumorous metastasis to the optic nerve head, from certain chemicals (eg, lead, methanol), after bee stings, during meningitis, and from syphilis. It is usually unilateral, though this depends on the etiology. In many cases the etiology remains obscure despite thorough evaluation.

Vision loss, varying from a small central scotoma to complete blindness and frequently maximal within 1 or 2 days, is the only symptom. Ophthalmoscopy discloses hyperemia and edema of the disk with fine vitreous opacities in the early stages, and more noticeable changes in advanced cases. The retina becomes edematous around the nerve head and its vessels become engorged; a few exudates and hemorrhages near or on the optic nerve head may be present.

A particularly important cause of papillitis in patients over age 60 is **cranial giant cell arteritis (temporal arteritis)** (see also TEMPORAL ARTERITIS in Ch. 30). It may present with papillitis in one eye associated with malaise and an elevated ESR. It can rapidly spread to the other eye and result in bilateral blindness. The diagnosis is confirmed by temporal artery biopsy.

With spontaneous remission or successful removal of the cause early in the course, vision is usually restored; otherwise, postneuritic optic atrophy develops, with varying degrees of vision loss depending on the etiology. **Treatment** with corticosteroids, either systemic (eg, prednisone 60 mg/day orally) or retrobulbar (eg, methylprednisolone acetate 20 mg), may be helpful. Treatment of cranial giant cell arteritis with systemic corticosteroids is highly effective; see also in Ch. 30.

RETROBULBAR NEURITIS

Inflammation of the orbital portion of the optic nerve, usually unilateral. Multiple sclerosis is responsible for many of the cases; some of the remainder are due to the same factors that cause papillitis, but idiopathic cases are even more common with retrobulbar neuritis than with papillitis. Rapid loss of vision and pain on moving the eye are the principal symptoms. In contrast to papillitis, the fundus usually appears normal, though some mild disk hyperemia is seen occasionally. Spontaneous remission, with normal vision restored, often occurs in 2 to 8 wk. In some cases a central scotoma and pallor of the temporal portion of the disk may remain. Relapses may occur, especially in multiple sclerosis. Each relapse increases the residual visual damage and temporal pallor; optic atrophy and permanent total visual loss may result. **Treatment** is the same as for optic neuritis.

TOXIC AMBLYOPIA

A reduction in visual acuity believed to be due to a toxic reaction in the orbital portion of the optic nerve. Toxic amblyopia overlaps with retrobulbar neuritis. It is usually bilateral and usually seen in patients who use excessive alcohol or tobacco. In the former case, malnutrition may be the true underlying etiology. Cases of true tobacco amblyopia are rare. Lead, methanol, chloramphenicol, digitalis, ethambutol, and many other chemicals have also been implicated.

An initially small central or pericentral scotoma slowly enlarges and progressively interferes with vision. It may become absolute and lead to blindness. Abnormalities are not usually seen, but later in the course a temporal disk pallor may develop.

Treatment

Vision may improve if the cause is removed immediately, unless the optic nerve has atrophied. Chelation is indicated in lead poisoning.

OPTIC ATROPHY

Atrophy of the optic nerve, commonly divided into primary and secondary. In **primary optic atrophy,** the disk is white or grayish with sharp edges and a saucer-shaped excavation. The lamina cribrosa is clearly visible and the retina is usually normal. In **secondary optic atrophy,** the disk is dirty white with irregular, indistinct margins and is covered by glial tissue that conceals the lamina cribrosa. Evidence of previous inflammation (such as sheathed vessels) may be seen in the retina.

Visual loss is roughly proportional to the degree of nerve atrophy. Total blindness with a pupil that is unreactive to direct light can be seen.

Optic atrophy is a sign of chronic optic nerve disease and not a diagnosis in itself; it demands search for an etiology. Dramatic return of vision can accompany reversal of certain pathologic processes (eg, return of central vision and visual field following decompression of a tumor).

HIGHER VISUAL PATHWAY LESIONS

The site of damage along the optic pathway determines the nature of visual field changes (see FIG. 225–1). Optic nerve lesions result in visual disturbances restricted to the affected eye. Lesions about the chiasm usually affect vision bilaterally. Lesions above or below the chiasm (eg, a pituitary tumor) destroy nerve fibers supplying the inner (nasal) half of both retinas with consequent defects in the temporal visual fields **(bitemporal hemianopia).** Lesions in the optic tract, optic radiations, or cerebral cortex produce **homonymous hemianopia,** with loss of function in the right or left halves of

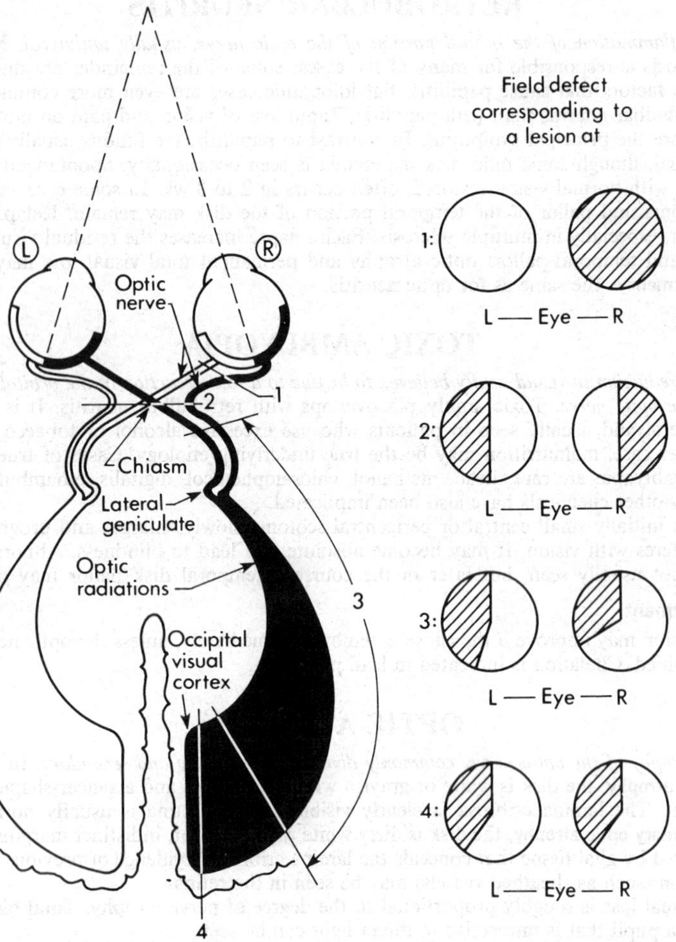

FIG. 225–1. Higher visual pathways—lesion sites and corresponding visual field defects.

both visual fields opposite to the side affected. This, the most common type of hemianopia, is usually caused by a brain tumor or CVA.

Treatment is that of the primary lesion.

---

226. CONTACT LENSES

Hard corneal contact lenses are thin, saucer-shaped disks made of a hard plastic, polymethyl methacrylate **(PMMA)**, that float on the tear layer overlying the cornea. They are 7 to 10 mm in diameter and cover part of the cornea. **Soft hydrophilic contact**

lenses are about 13 to 15 mm in diameter and cover the entire cornea. Made of poly-2-hydroxyethyl methacrylate **(HEMA)** and other soft plastics, they mold to the eye. **Flexible nonhydrophilic lenses** (eg, made of silicone) as well as gas-permeable lenses (hard) of pure silicone and of silicone PMMA admixtures are available. They permit increased O_2 transmission to the wearer's cornea.

Contact lenses often provide better visual acuity and peripheral vision than do eyeglasses and are prescribed to correct refractive errors (eg, nearsightedness and far-sightedness, astigmatism, presbyopia, anisometropia, aniseikonia, and aphakia after cataract removal) and for keratoconus. Either soft or hard lenses may be prescribed. Toric hard and soft contact lenses (similar to cylindrical lenses in spectacles) are used to correct astigmatism; they are very satisfactory in many cases.

Soft contact lenses are prescribed, by an ophthalmologist only, for treatment of bullous keratopathy and other corneal disorders ("bandage lenses"). These lenses are also well-tolerated occluders in children when occlusion therapy is needed (eg, for amblyopia). Prophylactic antibiotic eyedrops (eg, 0.5% chloramphenicol ophthalmic solution 1 drop bid or tid) may be advisable with a bandage-type soft contact lens. The soft lens as a vehicle for delivering topical medications to the eyes is being studied, but is not very promising. Extended wearing of contact lenses, especially for use in aphakia after cataract surgery, is practical but must be strictly monitored by the practitioner. The patient should see the practitioner at least twice a year and should clean the lenses once a week.

Hard contact lenses require an adaptation period sometimes as long as a week for complete wearing comfort; during this time the wearer gradually increases the daily number of hours the lenses are worn. Wearers usually experience temporary blurring of vision ("spectacle blur"), which should not exceed 2 h, when wearing eyeglasses after removing their contact lenses.

No pain should be present at any time; pain is a sign of an ill-fitting contact lens.

Hard and soft contact lenses may occasionally cause superficial corneal changes (which may be painless) or abrasions accompanied by severe pain, photophobia, and anxiety. Ill effect may be caused by poor fit of the lens or change in the lens parameters (especially with soft lenses); by the lenses being worn in a harmful (eg, oxygen-poor, smoky, windy) environment; by their being improperly inserted or removed; or by small foreign particles (eg, soot, dust) being trapped between the contact lens and the cornea. Discomfort may also occur after removing the lenses, especially after prolonged use ("overwearing syndrome"). Spontaneous healing may occur in a day or so if the lenses are not worn, or treatment may be required—dilation of the pupil with a mydriatic to prevent posterior synechiae of the iris, topical antibiotic eye drops or ointments, a firm eye patch, bed rest, and sedation may be necessary. Recovery usually is rapid, complete, and without vision impairment. An ophthalmologist should be consulted before the lenses are worn again.

Because of their size, soft lenses are easier for elderly persons to handle. Since soft contact lenses mold to the eye, they are not apt to eject spontaneously (as hard lenses may) and foreign bodies are less likely to lodge underneath them. Wearing comfort usually is immediate and little or no adaptation period is necessary. Soft lenses apparently do not damage the eye even when the eye is closed for short periods and may thus be better for patients who may become unconscious (eg, epileptics, diabetics). Such patients should carry an emergency card that identifies them as contact lens wearers. Soft lenses are brittle when dry and break easily. Hard lenses are usually somewhat simpler and less time-consuming to care for than are soft lenses, which require special care and handling.

Because most soft lenses are hydrophilic, conventional solutions for hard contact lenses should not be used with soft lenses. Most therapeutic eyedrops can be used in conjunction with soft lenses, though originally there was fear of concentrating the preservative of the eyedrops in the soft lens.

The manufacturer's instructions for hygiene and handling of either type of lens must be strictly observed by the user. Persons susceptible to eye infections, those with a hand tremor or arthritis that interferes with lens insertion or removal, and those who are insufficiently motivated to tolerate the temporary discomfort that may occur while adapting to lenses are unlikely to wear either type of lens successfully. Lenses should not be worn if the eyes are inflamed or infected, during sleep, or when swimming.

Presbyopia can be corrected with contact lenses. In one approach, the non-dominant eye is corrected for reading and the dominant eye for distant vision ("monovision"). Hard and soft bifocal and multifocal contact lenses are also successful, but are not popular with practitioners because the fitting procedure is often time consuming.

§19. DERMATOLOGIC DISORDERS

227. DIAGNOSIS OF SKIN DISEASES

Many skin diseases can be diagnosed by physical examination alone if one is familiar with the primary and secondary lesions and their arrangement and usual distribution. Except for obviously circumscribed diseases, such as a plantar wart, the patient

should undress and be examined completely, since he may not notice or report lesions on clothed areas of the body. The oral mucosa, anogenital area, scalp, and nails also will frequently provide clues to the diagnosis. A good light—preferably daylight—is essential. The history may be invaluable in assessing physical findings.

PRINCIPAL TYPES OF LESIONS

Primary Lesions

These, the earliest changes to appear, are the most important to recognize and, if necessary, to biopsy.

Macule: *A flat, discolored spot of varied size (< 10 mm) and shape.* **Patch:** *A similar spot > 10 mm.* Examples of macules are freckles, flat moles, tattoos, port-wine marks, and the rashes of rickettsial infections, rubella, and rubeola.

Papule: *A solid, elevated lesion usually < 10 mm in diameter.* **Plaque:** *A plateau-like lesion > 10 mm in diameter or a group of confluent papules.* Many cutaneous diseases begin with papules—warts, psoriasis, syphilis, lichen planus, drug eruptions, pigmented moles, seborrheic and actinic keratoses, some phases of acne, epitheliomas.

Nodule: *A palpable, solid lesion, > 5 or 10 mm in diameter, that may or may not be elevated.* Examples are keratinous cysts, small lipomas, fibromas, some types of lymphoma, erythema nodosum, and a variety of neoplasms. Larger nodules (20 mm or greater) are classified as **tumors,** benign or malignant.

Vesicle: *A circumscribed, elevated lesion < 5 mm in diameter containing serous fluid.* **Bulla (blister):** *A vesicle > 5 mm in diameter.* Vesicles or bullae are commonly caused by primary irritants, allergic contact dermatitis, physical trauma, sunburn, insect bites, or viral infections (herpes simplex, varicella, herpes zoster); other causes include drug eruptions, pemphigus, dermatitis herpetiformis, erythema multiforme, epidermolysis bullosa, and pemphigoid.

Pustule: *A superficial, elevated lesion containing pus.* Pustules may result from infection or a seropurulent evolution of vesicles or bullae. Possibilities include impetigo, acne, furuncles, carbuncles, certain deep fungus infections, acne, hidradenitis suppurativa, kerion, pustular miliaria, and pustular psoriasis of the palms and soles.

Wheal: *A transient, elevated lesion caused by local edema.* Wheals are a common allergic reaction; eg, from drug eruptions, insect stings or bites, or sensitivity to cold, heat, pressure, or sunlight.

Telangiectasia: *Dilated superficial blood vessels.* Telangiectasias may be seen in rosacea or certain systemic diseases (ataxia telangiectasia, scleroderma) and may result from long-term therapy with topical fluorinated corticosteroids, but most are of unknown etiology.

Secondary Lesions

These result either from the natural evolution of primary lesions (eg, a vesicle bursts, leaving an eroded area) or from the patient's manipulation of the primary lesion (eg, scratching a vesicle, leaving an eroded or ulcerated area).

Scales: *Heaped-up particles of horny epithelium* (may be a primary or secondary change). The most common scaling rashes are psoriasis, seborrheic dermatitis, superficial fungus infections, tinea versicolor, pityriasis rosea, and chronic dermatitis of any type.

Crust (scab): *Dried serum, blood, or pus.* Crusting is encountered in a wide variety of inflammatory and infectious diseases.

Erosion: *Loss of part or all of the epidermis.* Erosion is often seen in herpes-group virus infections and in pemphigus.

Ulcer: *Loss of epidermis and at least part of the dermis.* When ulcers result from physical trauma or acute bacterial infection, the etiology usually is apparent. Less obvious causes include chronic bacterial and fungus infections, self-inflicted ulcers, various peripheral vascular diseases and neuropathies, systemic scleroderma, and neoplastic tumors.

Excoriation: *A linear or hollowed-out crusted area, caused by scratching, rubbing, or picking.*

Lichenification: *Thickened skin with accentuated skin markings.* Atopic dermatitis and lichen simplex chronicus (localized scratch dermatitis) are typically associated with lichenification.

Atrophy: *Thinned and wrinkled skin, resembling cigarette paper.* Atrophy is seen in the aged, and in discoid LE with long-term use of topical fluorinated corticosteroids.

Scar: *The result of healing after destruction of some of the dermis.* Scars, like ulcers, may have easily recognized origins. Others are evolutionary changes, as in discoid LE.

ARRANGEMENT OF LESIONS

The lesions of certain skin diseases form distinctive patterns. The **grouping** of tense vesicles in herpes simplex and zoster, and their linear configuration in the latter, point to the diagnosis. **Annularity** (a tendency to form rings) is typical in granuloma annulare, erythema multiforme, dermatophyte infections, and secondary syphilis. **Linearity** of lesions is sometimes seen with epidermal nevi, linear scleroderma, and contact dermatitis. Lesions in psoriasis, lichen planus, and flat warts may mimic the shape of trauma to the skin **(the Koebner phenomenon, isomorphic reaction).**

DISTRIBUTION OF LESIONS

Much can be learned from lesion distribution. Occasionally, however, a disease does not follow its common pattern of distribution. Psoriasis, for example, appears most commonly on extensor surfaces, but may appear on flexor surfaces or even on the tip of the penis or on the palms.

Some common patterns of skin involvement are as follows:

Acne: Face, neck, chest, upper back. In "tropical acne" the entire trunk may be involved.

Atopic dermatitis: Characteristically involves the antecubital and popliteal spaces, face, neck, and hands. In infants its distribution is not characteristic.

Erythema multiforme: Primarily on palms, soles, and mucous membranes, but may be widespread.

Erythema nodosum: Lower legs, principally on pretibial surfaces.

Lichen planus: Oral mucosa, flexor surface of wrists, trunk, genitalia. Lesions may be widespread.

Chronic discoid LE: Principally on the face, scalp, ears, neck.

Photosensitivity reactions: Areas exposed to natural or artificial light; eg, the V of the neck, the arms below the sleeves, and the face (especially the cheeks and nose). This characteristic distribution frequently is not recognized and may be confused with contact dermatitis.

Pityriasis rosea: Trunk and proximal extremities in most cases, with the long axis of oval lesions running parallel to the lines of cleavage. Occasionally pityriasis rosea may affect only the extremities and spare the trunk.

Psoriasis: Elbows, knees, scalp, back, anogenital region, nails.

SPECIAL DIAGNOSTIC METHODS

Biopsy is essential for diagnosing any obscure dermatosis, particularly a chronic one, and is imperative if there is any suggestion of neoplasm. A fully developed typical lesion should usually be chosen for biopsy, but early lesions are best in vesicular, bullous, or pustular eruptions. The simplest biopsy procedure is to insert a sharp circular punch, 3 mm or more in diameter, well through the dermis, and snip off the base of the plug. An adequate biopsy of some relatively friable lesions (eg, seborrheic keratoses) may be obtained with a sharp curet. For a larger tissue sample, and for deep dermal or subcutaneous lesions, a wedge is removed and the incision sutured. For most small tumors, excision allows microscopic diagnosis and cure with one procedure. All pigmented lesions, including nevi, should be excised deeply enough so that the depth of the lesion can be evaluated histologically. Superficial biopsies are often inadequate for histologic diagnosis. A deep part of the biopsy specimen should be cultured when a mycobacterial or a deep fungal infection is suspected.

Examination of scrapings for fungi: In any suspected superficial fungal infection, the organisms can be demonstrated by microscopic examination of scales that have been taken from the lesion, covered with 10% potassium hydroxide, and warmed gently; hairs from a lesion must be examined in tinea capitis. In dermatophyte infections, only hyphae are seen, while in tinea versicolor and candidal infections both yeast and hyphae are seen; the distinction may be important in selecting specific chemotherapy.

Bacterial and fungal cultures: In acute bacterial infections of the skin, culture and antibacterial sensitivity testing are advisable, although treatment should be started promptly. Adequate sampling is essential. With frankly pustular lesions, a swab sample is sufficient; the swab should be placed immediately in broth culture and not allowed to dry out. In chronic infections (eg, TB or deep fungi), where the flora may be mixed and relatively sparse, more ample specimens (including even deep biopsy specimens) must be obtained and special culture media may be needed. Culture of superficial fungal infections will occasionally be positive when the scraping is negative.

Wood's light examination: When the skin is viewed in a darkened room under ultraviolet light filtered through Wood's glass ("black light"), tinea versicolor may fluoresce golden and erythrasma orange-red; scalp hairs in tinea capitis caused by *Microsporum canis* and *Microsporum audouini* are a light bright green. The earliest clue to a *Pseudomonas* infection, especially in burns, may be a green fluorescence under a Wood's light. The depigmentation of vitiligo can be differentiated from hypopigmented lesions by its ivory-white color on Wood's light examination.

Cytologic examination: The **Tzanck test** is rapid and reliable in diagnosing vesicular eruptions. A smear of cellular material scraped from the base of a vesicle and stained with Wright's or Giemsa stain shows multinucleated giant cells in herpes simplex, herpes zoster, and varicella, but not in vaccinia and smallpox. **Virus cultures** are more sensitive and are becoming very rapid—an improvement over the more difficult cytologic Tzanck test. If a virus or chlamydial infection is suspected early, vesicle fluid or cervical or urethral material can be put into special "transport media" for culture in most medical centers. Pemphigus can be diagnosed by finding typical acantholytic

cells, which have very large nuclei and scant cytoplasm and have lost attachment to each other.

Immunofluorescent (IF) tests: Fluorescent microscopy (see TYPE II HYPERSENSITIVITY REACTIONS in Ch. 20) is an important aid in diagnosing and managing certain skin diseases. The indirect IF test demonstrates that the serum of a patient with pemphigus or bullous pemphigoid contains specific antibodies that bind to different areas of the epithelium. In pemphigus, the antibody titer may correlate with the severity of the disease. In the direct IF test, biopsied skin of patients with pemphigus, pemphigoid, dermatitis herpetiformis, herpes gestationis, SLE, and discoid LE shows specific, diagnostic patterns.

Other special diagnostic methods include patch tests used for allergic contact dermatitis (see TYPE IV HYPERSENSITIVITY REACTIONS in Ch. 20) and darkfield examination for syphilis (see Ch. 14).

---

228. GENERAL PRINCIPLES OF TOPICAL DERMATOLOGIC THERAPY

Many substances are applied for topical treatment, including absorbents, anti-infectives, anti-inflammatory agents, astringents (drying agents that precipitate protein and shrink and contract the skin), cleansing agents, emollients (skin softeners), and keratolytics (agents that soften, loosen, and facilitate exfoliation of the squamous cells of the epidermis). These locally acting agents are used to (1) cleanse, debride, and protect the skin; (2) destroy causative agents (bacteria, fungi, or protozoa); (3) relieve symptoms such as pruritus, burning, and pain; and (4) reduce inflammation and promote healing.

The **vehicle** (base or carrier) for topical medication must be selected carefully, since it may alter the effectiveness of the active ingredient. Allergic and irritating reactions (eg, contact dermatitis) may be caused by ingredients of the vehicle as well as by the active agent.

Ointments are oleaginous and contain little if any water; they feel greasy, but are generally well tolerated. They are best used to lubricate, especially if applied over hydrated skin; they protect lesions with thick crusts, lichenification, or heaped-up scales, and may be less irritating than a cream on some eroded or open lesions such as stasis ulcers.

Creams, semisolid emulsions of oil in water or water in oil, are the mainstay of dermatologic therapy. They are easy to apply and "vanish" when rubbed into the skin.

Lotions originally were suspensions or dispersions of finely powdered material (eg, calamine) in a water or alcohol base; however, most modern "lotions" (eg, some corticosteroid lotions) are really oily emulsions. Convenient to apply, lotions cool and dry acute inflammatory and exudative lesions. The powder suspensions, however, may be irritating if they dry the skin too much. Lotions usually must be shaken before use.

Solutions, homogenous mixtures of 2 or more substances, are convenient to apply, especially in the scalp. Like lotions, solutions are drying. The most commonly used solvents are ethyl alcohol, propylene glycol, polyethylene glycol, and water.

CLEANSING AGENTS AND PROTECTANTS

The principal **cleansing agents** are detergents and solvents. Soap is the most popular detergent, but synthetic detergents are also used. "Baby type" shampoos are usually well tolerated not only in the eyes but also in cleaning wounds and abrasions and are useful in psoriasis, eczema, and other forms of dermatitis for removal of crusts and

scales. Badly irritated, weeping, or oozing lesions, however, should be cleaned only with water.

Various ingredients often are added to detergents and other dermatologic preparations to enhance or add certain properties. For antidandruff action, dipyrithione or selenium sulfide or tar extracts may be added to a shampoo.

Water is the principal solvent used for cleansing. Using plain **tap-water soaks, baths,** or **compresses** (made from gauze or old sheets) for 48 to 72 h (changing them at 1- or 2-h intervals) will generally soothe and cool acute weeping or oozing lesions, dry them, and often debride them as well. Wet dressings containing aluminum acetate, magnesium sulfate, etc, are seldom better than plain tap water. Ethyl alcohol, the most commonly used organic solvent for topical use, is usually well diluted with water.

Topical **protectants** cover and protect the skin against a deleterious influence. **Powders** are often used as protectants in intertriginous areas; ie, between the toes and in the intergluteal cleft, axillas, groin, and inframammary areas. Powders dry macerated skin and reduce friction by absorbing moisture, thereby providing comfort. However, some tend to "ball up" and can be irritating when they become moist. Powders may be incorporated into protective creams, lotions, and ointments. Collodion and other films are **mechanical protectants** that provide a flexible or semirigid continuous film or coating over the skin. Modern moist dressings (hydrophilic polymers) such as Vigilon® can be applied with a gauze cover. Zinc gelatin (Unna's boot) protects the skin by forming an occlusive dressing. **Sunscreens,** preparations that screen the skin from ultraviolet light, are also protectants (see Ch. 253).

ERADICATION OF CAUSATIVE AGENTS AND RELIEF OF SYMPTOMS

Eradication of specific agents causing skin infections is discussed in the appropriate chapters in SKN. In general, topical antibiotics are ineffective and in many instances are contraindicated. However, topical fungicides, scabicides, and pediculicides are commonly used in skin disorders, as are systemic antibiotics.

Relief of symptoms such as pruritus and pain is discussed elsewhere in THE MANUAL. In addition to analgesics for relief of pain, camphor 0.5 to 3% or menthol 0.1 to 0.2% may be used singly or together in topical creams or ointments. Local anesthetics such as lidocaine and dibucaine are generally not used on the skin because they are ineffective; they are sometimes useful on mucosal surfaces.

TOPICAL ANTI-INFLAMMATORY AGENTS

Corticosteroids, the most effective topical agents, are remarkably devoid of major side effects. Itchy and inflammatory dermatoses usually respond favorably to properly used corticosteroids. However, they may worsen a pilosebaceous condition such as acne or rosacea. Topical corticosteroids and other skin preparations are usually made up as creams, lotions, ointments, or solutions, and less commonly as aerosols and tapes.

TABLE 228-1 lists many of the topical corticosteroid preparations currently available. Since hydrocortisone 1%, a nonfluorinated preparation, does not induce facial telangiectasia, perioral dermatitis, atrophy, or striae, it may be preferable to a synthetic corticosteroid for treating facial dermatoses. Although some preparations are available in higher or lower concentrations, a full-strength preparation should usually be prescribed first. The preparations should be applied sparingly tid, or more frequently for some dermatoses. For maximum effectiveness, creams should be rubbed in gently until they vanish. The corticosteroid may be diluted with a bland base if large areas of skin are involved. Several hydrocortisone 0.5% preparations are now available without prescription.

TABLE 228–1. REPRESENTATIVE TOPICAL CORTICOSTEROID PREPARATIONS

Hydrocortisone Preparations*

Creams	0.125%–2.5%
Ointments	0.5%–2.5%
Lotions	0.125%–2.5%
Aerosol	0.5%, 1%

Synthetic Corticosteroid Preparations†

	Lowest Strength	*Low Strength*	*Full Strength*	*High Strength*
Creams	Dexamethasone 0.1%	Hydrocortisone valerate 0.2% Fluocinolone acetonide 0.01% Betamethasone valerate 0.01% Flurandrenolide 0.025% Triamcinolone acetonide 0.025%	Halcinonide 0.025% Betamethasone benzoate 0.025% Betamethasone valerate 0.1% Clocortolone 0.1% Desonide 0.05% Fluocinolone acetonide 0.025% Amcinonide 0.1% Flurandrenolide 0.05% Triamcinolone acetonide 0.1%	Fluocinolone acetonide 0.2% Fluocinonide 0.05% Halcinonide 0.1% Triamcinolone acetonide 0.5% Betamethasone dipropionate 0.05% Desoximetasone 0.25% Diflorasone diacetate 0.05%
Ointments	Methylpredniso-lone acetate 0.25%	Triamcinolone acetonide 0.025% Flurandrenolide 0.025% Methylpredniso-lone acetate 1.0%	Triamcinolone acetonide 0.1% Betamethasone valerate 0.1% Betamethasone benzoate 0.025% Halcinonide 0.025% Desonide 0.05% Flurandrenolide 0.05% Fluocinolone acetonide 0.025%	Triamcinolone acetonide 0.5% Betamethasone diproprionate 0.05% Halcinonide 0.1% Diflorasone diacetate 0.05% Fluocinonide 0.05%
Lotions		Triamcinolone acetonide 0.025%	Betamethasone benzoate 0.025% Betamethasone valerate 0.1% Flurandrenolide 0.05% Triamcinolone acetonide 0.1%	Betamethasone diproprionate 0.05%
Gels‡	Dexamethasone 0.1%		Betamethasone benzoate 0.025%	Fluocinonide 0.05%
Solutions		Fluocinolone acetonide 0.01%		Halcinonide 0.1%
Medicated adhesive tape				Flurandrenolide 4 μg/sq cm (7.5 cm wide roll × 60 cm/nm)

(Continued)

* More than 30 companies now provide generic- or brand-labeled hydrocortisone creams, ointments, and lotions. Concentrations of 0.5% are commonly available without prescriptions.

† Preparations within each group are therapeutically equivalent.

‡ Approximately equivalent to full-strength creams.

TABLE 228–1. REPRESENTATIVE TOPICAL CORTICOSTEROID PREPARATIONS (*Cont'd*)

Synthetic Corticosteroid Preparations† (*Cont'd*)

	Lowest Strength	*Low Strength*	*Full Strength*	*High Strength*
Aerosols	Dexamethasone 0.01%		Betamethasone diproprionate 0.1% Triamcinolone acetonide 0.2%	

Corticosteroid Suspensions for Intralesional Injection

Suspension	*Potency (Concentration)—mg/mL*
Triamcinolone acetonide	10, 40
Triamcinolone diacetate	25, 40
Triamcinolone hexacetonide	5, 20
Betamethasone sodium phosphate	4
Betamethasone acetate + betamethasone sodium phosphate	6 (3 mg/mL each of sodium phosphate and acetone esters)

A useful method for delivering a high concentration of corticosteroid to a chronic lesion or to one resistant to topical corticosteroids is direct **intralesional injection** of a corticosteroid suspension. The major problem with intralesional corticosteroids is dermal atrophy, which is usually reversible. In black skin, hypopigmentation may follow injection. Several corticosteroid suspensions for intralesional injection are listed in TABLE 228–1. These suspensions are usually diluted 2 to 4 times with sterile saline containing a preservative to minimize risk of local atrophy and hypopigmentation. The more insoluble preparations are more persistent and long-acting.

Absorption and effectiveness of topical corticosteroids are increased by covering the treated area with a nonporous occlusive dressing. This **occlusive therapy** is used in such conditions as psoriasis, atopic dermatitis, LE, and chronic hand dermatitis. Usually, a polyethylene film (eg, a common plastic household wrap) is applied overnight over a cream or ointment preparation, since these tend to be less irritating than lotions for occlusive therapy. A plastic tape impregnated with flurandrenolide is especially convenient for treating isolated or recalcitrant lesions. Miliaria, atrophic striae, and bacterial infections may follow occlusive therapy; children and, less often, adults, may suffer some pituitary and cortisol suppression after prolonged occlusive treatment of large areas.

The use of topical antibiotics, alone or in combination with topical corticosteroids, is seldom warranted, except in the treatment of acne, where topical antibiotics alone are beneficial (see Ch. 235). The combinations are no more effective than a corticosteroid alone, and allergic contact dermatitis from topical antibiotics, especially neomycin, may complicate the primary problem.

229. PRURITUS

(Itching)

A sensation that the patient instinctively attempts to relieve by scratching.

Etiology, Symptoms, and Signs

Itching may accompany a primary skin disease or may be a symptom of systemic disease—sometimes the only symptom.

Skin diseases in which itching is most severe include scabies, pediculosis, insect bites, urticaria, atopic dermatitis, contact dermatitis, lichen planus, miliaria, and dermatitis herpetiformis. Dry skin (especially in the elderly) often causes severe generalized itching.

Systemic conditions clearly associated with generalized itching include obstructive biliary disease, uremia (frequently associated with hyperparathyroidism), lymphomas, leukemias, and polycythemia rubra vera. During the latter months of pregnancy, itching may occur unaccompanied by primary skin lesions. Many drugs (especially barbiturates and salicylanilides) can cause pruritus. Other diseases believed to cause generalized itching, even though an association has not been proved, include hyperthyroidism, diabetes mellitus, and internal cancers of many types. One should be cautious in attributing a psychogenic etiology to the generalized pruritus, although this is a common problem.

Persistent scratching may produce redness, urticarial papules, excoriated papules, fissures, and elongated crusts along scratch lines. Lichenification and pigmentation may also result from prolonged scratching and rubbing. Frequently, however, the patient who complains of severe generalized itching has no signs of scratching or rubbing the skin.

Treatment

First and foremost, the cause of generalized pruritus should be sought and corrected. If no skin disease is readily apparent, an underlying systemic disorder or drug-related cause should be sought.

If feasible, all medications should be stopped or chemically unrelated drugs substituted. Irritating clothing, such as woolens, should be avoided. Bathing should be minimized, as it may aggravate generalized itching, whatever the cause. Emollients, such as white petrolatum or hydrogenated vegetable oil (eg, a cooking oil) containing 0.125 to 0.25% menthol, are good "moisturizers" if applied while the skin is still wet. The skin should then be blotted dry to remove water and excess oil. Proprietary anesthetics should be avoided. Ultraviolet B to the skin and oral cholestyramine can be helpful in uremia, cholestasis, and at times even when no underlying abnormalities are found. Topical corticosteroids seldom alleviate generalized itching (without dermatitis), but may uncommonly be useful in essential pruritus of the elderly.

If a drug has been adequately ruled out as the cause of the itching, one may prescribe a tranquilizer such as hydroxyzine or, for more severe cases, minimal and gradually increasing doses of chlorpromazine or doxepin. Antihistamines, if at all helpful, may be so mainly because of their sedative effect.

---

230. DERMATITIS
(Eczema)

Superficial inflammation of the skin, characterized by vesicles (when acute), redness, edema, oozing, crusting, scaling, and usually itching. Scratching or rubbing may lead to lichenification.

The terms *dermatitis* and *eczema* are used synonymously in this chapter. There is no general agreement among authorities as to the distinction between them. The term *eczematous dermatitis* is often used to mean a vesicular dermatitis, and some authorities still restrict the term *eczema* to chronic vesicular dermatitides.

For diagnostic purposes, the dermatitides are divided into those with exogenous causes and those with presumably endogenous causes (see TABLE 230–1). Many conditions (eg, hand dermatitis, exfoliative dermatitis) may be either exogenous or endogenous. Dermatitis may also accompany various immune deficiency diseases (eg,

TABLE 230–1. CLASSIFICATION OF DERMATITIDES

Endogenous	*Contact or Exogenous*
Atopic	Direct irritant
Seborrheic	Non–light-dependent
Nummular	Phototoxic
Chronic dermatitis of hands and feet	
Exfoliative	Allergic
Stasis	Non–light-dependent
Localized scratch dermatitis	Photoallergic
Pruritus ani or vulvae	
Drug eruptions	

Wiskott-Aldrich syndrome, X-linked agammaglobulinemia), inborn errors of metabolism (eg, phenylketonuria, ahistidinemia), or nutritional deficiency diseases (eg, pellagra).

CONTACT DERMATITIS

An acute or chronic inflammation, often sharply demarcated, produced by substances in contact with the skin.

Etiology

Contact dermatitis may be caused by a primary chemical irritant or may be a Type IV delayed hypersensitivity reaction (see Ch. 20).

Direct irritants may damage normal skin or irritate an existing dermatitis. Weak or marginal irritants, such as soap, acetone, or even water, may take several days of exposure to cause clinically recognizable changes. Strong irritants, such as acids, alkalis, or phenol, cause observable changes within a few minutes.

Allergic contact dermatitis is due to delayed hypersensitivity and requires a latent period ranging from 5 or 6 days (in the case of strong sensitizers such as poison ivy) to years between the time of first exposure and the reexposure that precipitates the dermatitis. Recent studies indicate that Langerhans' cells (a minor subpopulation of epidermal cells) are critical for presentation of allergens to T lymphocytes, which thereby become sensitized. Chemical mediators released from keratinocytes and Langerhans' cells may also contribute to sensitivity induction. Patients often find it difficult to believe that they have become allergic to substances they have used for years or to medications used to treat their dermatitis, but the **ingredients in topical medications** constitute a major cause of allergic contact dermatitis: antibiotics (penicillin, sulfonamides, neomycin), antihistamines (diphenhydramine, promethazine), anesthetics (benzocaine), antiseptics (thimerosal, hexachlorophene), and stabilizers (ethylenediamine and derivatives). Other commonly implicated substances include **plants** (poison ivy, oak, and sumac; ragweed, primrose); many potential **sensitizers used in the manufacture of shoes and clothing** (tanning agents in shoes; free formaldehyde in durable-press finishes; rubber accelerators and antioxidants in gloves, shoes, underpants, bras, and other wearing apparel); **metal compounds** (nickel, chromates, mercury); *p*-phenylenediamine and other **dyes;** and **cosmetics** (depilatories, nail polish, deodorants). **Industrial agents** capable of producing occupational dermatoses are almost innumerable.

Photoallergic and **phototoxic contact dermatitis** require exposure to light following topical application of certain chemicals. They are manifested as an exaggerated response to sunlight (polymorphous light eruptions—see in Ch. 253). Agents commonly

responsible for photoallergic contact dermatitis include aftershave lotions, sunscreening agents, and topical sulfonamides. Phototoxic contact dermatitis is commonly caused by certain perfumes, coal tar, psoralens, and cutting oils. Photoallergic and phototoxic contact dermatitis must be differentiated from photosensitivity reactions to systemically administered drugs.

Symptoms and Signs

Contact dermatitis ranges from transient redness to severe swelling with bulla formation; itching and vesiculation are common. Any part of the skin that comes in contact with a sensitizing or irritating substance may be involved. Thus, dermatitis on exposed skin surfaces may be due to an air-borne substance (eg, ragweed pollen, insecticide spray). Characteristically, the dermatitis at first is sharply limited to the site of contact; later it may spread to other areas.

The course varies. If the cause is removed, simple erythema disappears within a few days and blisters dry up. Vesicles and bullae may rupture, ooze, and crust. As the inflammation subsides, scaling and some temporary thickening of the skin occur. Continuing exposure to the causative agent or complications such as irritation from or allergy to a topical medication, excoriation, or infection may perpetuate the dermatitis.

Diagnosis

Since contact dermatitis may resemble other types of dermatitis, an allergen or irritant should be suspected as the cause or aggravating factor in any puzzling dermatitis. Characteristic skin changes and a history of exposure facilitate the diagnosis, but identifying the responsible agent may require exhaustive questioning and extensive patch testing. The patient's occupation, hobbies, household duties, vacations, wearing apparel, topical medications, cosmetics, and spouse's activities must all be considered. Knowing the characteristics of topical allergens or irritants, including the typical distribution of lesions, is helpful. The site of the initial lesion is often an important clue to the cause.

Patch testing (see TYPE IV HYPERSENSITIVITY REACTIONS in Ch. 20) with a standard group of contact allergens may be helpful if questioning is fruitless. A specialist should select the test concentrations (particularly for industrial agents or cosmetics, in which case an industrial specialist should be consulted). Patch testing is sometimes withheld during the acute phase of the dermatitis because the allergen may worsen the eruption in a very sensitive patient. A positive patch test reaction does not necessarily identify the agent causing the contact dermatitis. There must be a history of exposure to the test agent in the areas where the dermatitis originally occurred before a definite diagnosis can be made. Moreover, a negative patch test does not rule out contact dermatitis: it may only mean that the offending agent was not included in the tests.

Treatment

Treatment may be ineffective or the dermatitis may promptly recur unless the offending agent is removed. Patients with photoallergic or phototoxic contact dermatitis should avoid exposure to light as well. In the acute phase of dermatitis, such as that caused by poison ivy, gauze or thin cloths dipped in water and applied to the lesions are soothing and cooling; they should be applied for 30 min, 4 to 6 times/day. Blisters may be drained 3 times/day, but the tops should not be removed. An oral corticosteroid (eg, prednisone 40 to 60 mg/day) should be given for 12 to 16 days in severe or extensive cases or even in limited cases when there is severe facial inflammation. The prednisone dose can be decreased by 10 to 20 mg every 3 to 4 days. Topical corticosteroids are not helpful in the blistering phase, but once the dermatitis is less acute, a topical corticosteroid gel or, if the dermatitis is very dry, an ointment (see TOPICAL ANTI-INFLAMMATORY AGENTS in Ch. 228) should be rubbed in gently tid. Antihista-

mines (except for their sedative effect) and desensitization are ineffective in contact dermatitis.

ATOPIC DERMATITIS

A chronic, itching, superficial inflammation of the skin, usually occurring in individuals with a personal or family history of allergic disorders (eg, hay fever, asthma).

Etiology

The cause is unknown. Although the relationship to the dermatitis is not clear, these patients have high levels of cyclic AMP phosphodiesterase in their WBCs. Frequently, numerous inhalants and foods produce wheal-and-flare reactions on scratch or intradermal tests, but these reactions are usually nonspecific. Recent studies suggest that certain foods induce erythema and itching in young individuals. Patients with atopic dermatitis usually have high serum levels of reaginic (IgE) antibodies and peripheral eosinophilia, but the etiologic significance of these findings is unknown. Several studies have reported a defect of T cell regulation that may be associated with increased IgE responses.

Symptoms, Signs, and Course

Atopic dermatitis may begin in the first few months of life, with red, weeping, crusted lesions on the face, scalp, and extremities. In older children or adults, it may take a more localized chronic form. The course is unpredictable. Although the dermatitis usually subsides by age 3 or 4 yr, exacerbations and remissions frequently recur during childhood, adolescence, or adulthood.

Itching is a constant feature. The consequent scratching and rubbing lead to an itch-scratch-rash-itch cycle. In older children and adults, atopic dermatitis typically appears as erythema and lichenification in the antecubital and popliteal fossae and on the eyelids, neck, and wrists. The dermatitis may become generalized. Secondary bacterial infections and regional lymhadenitis are common. Frequent use of medications, proprietary or prescribed, exposes the atopic patient to many topical allergens, and contact dermatitis may aggravate and complicate the atopic dermatitis, as may the generally dry skin that is common in these patients. Intolerance to primary irritants is common, and emotional stress, environmental temperature or humidity changes, bacterial skin infections, and wool garments commonly cause exacerbations.

Complications

Patients with longstanding atopic dermatitis may develop cataracts while in their 20s or 30s. Herpes simplex or vaccinia may induce a grave febrile illness **(Kaposi's varicelliform eruption)** in atopic patients. Therefore, the patient with atopic dermatitis must not be vaccinated against smallpox or be exposed to patients with clinically active herpes simplex or to recently vaccinated persons.

Diagnosis

Diagnosis is entirely clinical and is based on the distribution of lesions, the long duration, and, often, a family history of atopic allergy. Because atopic dermatitis is often hard to differentiate from seborrheic dermatitis in infancy or from primary irritant dermatitis at any age, the patient should be seen several times before a definitive diagnosis is made. The physician must be careful not to attribute all subsequent skin problems to an atopic diathesis.

Treatment

The following general measures are advisable:

1. Patients should avoid as many offending agents as possible and should be advised against using complex topical medications.

2. Corticosteroid creams or ointments applied tid are the most effective medications. Because they are expensive, supplemental use of white petrolatum, hydrogenated vegetable oil (as for cooking), or hydrophilic petrolatum (if the patient is not allergic to lanolin) and water may be advisable. These emollients are applied between applications of the corticosteroid and help to hydrate the skin, an important objective in treatment. Prolonged, widespread use of high potency corticosteroid creams or ointments should be avoided in infants, as adrenal suppression (reversible) may ensue. Ineffectiveness after continuous use of topical steroids can be avoided by using simple emollients for a week or more, after which the steroids may again be effective.

3. Bathing should be minimized if the patient notices a deleterious effect, and use of soap on the area of dermatitis should be avoided, since soap and water may be drying and irritating. Oils help to lubricate the skin, and the above-mentioned corticosteroid or emollient ointments should be applied within 3 min after a bath, before the skin is dried, to enhance their emollient effects. The skin can then be patted dry.

4. For children, an antihistamine (eg, diphenhydramine elixir 25 to 50 mg) at bedtime may be a useful sedative when itching is worst. Doxepin, a dibenzoxepin tricyclic compound, is a very active antihistamine and also has a useful psychotherapeutic effect in itching patients. This agent may be tried, beginning with 10-mg capsules or 5 mg in a calibrated dropper, and increasing the dose slowly as needed and tolerated. Hydroxyzine hydrochloride 25 mg tid or qid (children, 50 mg/day in divided doses) may also be useful.

5. Fingernails should be kept short to minimize excoriations and secondary infections.

6. For secondary infections, oral cloxacillin or a cephalosporin 250 mg qid for adults and 25 to 50 mg/kg/day in divided doses for children is advised.

7. If the dermatitis resists home treatment, hospitalization, with its closer psychologic and dermatologic attention and the change in environment, often accelerates improvement.

8. Oral corticosteroids should be considered a last resort. Stunting of growth, osteoporosis, and the other side effects of prolonged systemic corticosteroids are serious hazards when atopic patients take the drug for years, and rebound exacerbations on stopping therapy are frequent. Alternate-day use of corticosteroids may be helpful (eg, for adults, prednisone 20 to 40 mg every other morning). The initial dose should be continued for several weeks, then slowly decreased while the patient is encouraged to use topical medications.

9. Older adults may benefit from psoralen plus UVA **(PUVA)**, described under PSORIASIS in Ch. 236. PUVA is available in most dermatologic centers. Because of its potential long-term side effects, it is rarely indicated for children or young adults.

SEBORRHEIC DERMATITIS

An inflammatory scaling disease of the scalp, face, and, occasionally, other areas of the body. Despite the name, the composition and flow of sebum are usually normal.

Symptoms and Signs

Onset in adults is gradual, and the dermatitis usually is apparent only as dry or greasy diffuse scaling of the scalp **(dandruff)** with variable itching. In severe disease, yellow-red, scaling papules appear along the hairline, behind the ears, in the external auditory canals, on the eyebrows, on the bridge of the nose, in the nasolabial folds, and over the sternum. Marginal blepharitis with dry yellow crusts and conjunctival irritation may be present. Seborrheic dermatitis does not cause hair loss.

Infants within the first month of life may develop seborrheic dermatitis, with a thick, yellow, crusted scalp lesion **("cradle cap")**, fissuring and yellow scaling behind the ears, and red facial papules. The infant may also have an associated stubborn diaper rash.

Older children may develop thick, tenacious, asbestos-like, scaly plaques in the scalp that may measure 1 to 2 cm in diameter.

Genetic and climatic factors seem to affect the incidence and severity of the disease; it is usually worse in winter. The prognosis is better than in atopic dermatitis. Very rarely, in infants or adults, the condition may become generalized.

Treatment

This depends on the location and severity of the seborrheic dermatitis. **In adults,** pyrithione zinc, selenium sulfide, sulfur and salicylic acid, or tar shampoo should be used daily or every other day until the dandruff is controlled and twice/wk thereafter. A corticosteroid lotion (eg, 0.01% fluocinolone acetonide solution or 0.025% triamcinolone acetonide lotion) should be rubbed into the scalp or other hairy areas bid until scaling and redness are controlled. Hydrocortisone 1% cream rubbed in bid or tid will rapidly improve seborrheic dermatitis of the postauricular areas, nasolabial folds, eyelid margins, and bridge of the nose; the cream is then used once daily if needed. Hydrocortisone cream is best for facial seborrheic dermatitis, as the fluorinated corticosteroids may produce such side effects as telangiectasia, atrophy, and perioral dermatitis. **For infantile seborrheic eczema,** a mild baby shampoo is used daily and a hydrocortisone cream is rubbed in bid. For the thick asbestos-like lesions seen in the scalps of young children, 10% salicylic acid in mineral oil or a corticosteroid gel is applied at bedtime to affected areas and rubbed in with a toothbrush. The scalp is shampooed daily until the thick scale is gone.

Studies have suggested that topical imidazoles (anti-yeast compounds) may be effective in some patients with seborrheic dermatitis and have focused attention on the possible role of *Pityrosporum ovale* (a common lipophilic yeast normally present in follicles) as a cause for this disease.

NUMMULAR DERMATITIS

Chronic dermatitis characterized by inflamed, coin-shaped, vesicular, crusted, scaling, and usually pruritic lesions.

The etiology of nummular dermatitis is unknown. It is seen most commonly in middle-aged patients under emotional stress and is frequently associated with dry skin, especially during the winter. Exacerbations and remissions may occur.

Symptoms and Signs

The discoid lesions start as pruritic patches of confluent vesicles and papules that later ooze serum and then form crusts. The lesions are widespread; they are frequently more prominent on the extensor aspects of the extremities and on the buttocks, but they also appear on the trunk.

Treatment

No treatment is uniformly effective. Oral antibiotics may be given empirically, since many types of bacteria can be cultured and the therapy has been found to decrease the severity of the lesions. Oral cloxacillin or a cephalosporin 250 mg qid and tap-water compresses are helpful when there is much weeping and pus. Less infected lesions may also improve with tetracycline 250 mg orally qid, which has a beneficial (although not necessarily antibacterial) effect. After the lesions have dried, a corticosteroid cream or ointment should be rubbed in tid and occlusion with a corticosteroid cream under polyethylene film or with flurandrenolide-impregnated tape should be applied at bedtime. Occasionally oral corticosteroids are required; a reasonable starting dose is 40 mg of prednisone given every other day to lessen side effects. Long-term systemic corticosteroid therapy should be avoided.

CHRONIC DERMATITIS OF HANDS AND FEET

The hands and feet are frequent sites of inflammatory eruptions—the hands because they are subjected to mechanical and chemical trauma; the feet because of the warm, moist conditions in shoes. The eruption commonly becomes chronic and can be crippling at home or at work.

The following primary dermatoses may involve the hands and feet:

1. Contact dermatitis (see above) is common. Many allergens or irritants—caustics, strong soaps, detergents, organic solvents, vacuum cleaner dust, topical medications—may cause or perpetuate the dermatitis. In any dermatitis of the feet, every effort should be made to obtain patch-test evidence of sensitivity to a component of shoes, since this sensitivity limits the choice of footwear.

2. "Housewives' eczema," a hand dermatitis frequently seen in housewives, has many causes. It is undoubtedly worsened by washing dishes, clothes, and babies, since repeated exposure to even mild detergents and water or prolonged sweating under rubber gloves may irritate dermatitic skin or may even cause a marginal irritant dermatitis. Occasionally, contact dermatitis that appears urticarial occurs in 10 to 20 min as a reaction to fresh foods.

3. Pompholyx is a chronic condition characterized by deep-seated itchy vesicles on the palms, sides of the fingers, and soles. Scaling, redness, and oozing often follow the vesiculation. The condition is also known as **dyshidrosis** —a misnomer, since sweating may be decreased, normal, or excessive. Though no cause is known in most cases, a primary cause, such as a fungus or a contact allergen, should always be sought.

4. Psoriasis localized to the hands presents on the dorsum as the typical thick, silvery, scaling papules or plaques, but palmar lesions are not always characteristic. Though pitted grooves in the nails often indicate psoriasis, they can occur with any dermatitis of the fingers.

5. Recalcitrant pustular eruptions of the palms and soles are characteristically crops of deep-seated sterile pustules of unknown etiology that resist treatment. They may be associated with psoriasis elsewhere.

6. Fungal infection of the feet is common; of the hands, uncommon. Patients with a hand dermatitis should be examined for a fungal infection of the feet, since the latter can produce a nonspecific dermatitis on the hands (**dermatophytid;** see Ch. 232).

Treatment

Treatment should be directed to removing the cause wherever possible. The following general principles are useful if no specific cause is found: (1) A topical corticosteroid cream or ointment applied tid may decrease the itching, but clearing the dermatitis may require overnight occlusive therapy with polyethylene gloves (or nonpermeable plastic bags on the feet), sealed at the wrists or ankles with cellophane tape, after a 4th application of the cream. (2) Oral cloxacillin or cephalosporin 250 mg qid, should be given if there is any evidence of secondary infection. (3) Wet chores should be limited to short periods, and white cotton gloves should be worn under rubber gloves. (4) A 14-day course of oral prednisone is needed occasionally, starting with 40 mg/day and slowly decreasing the dose while the patient is taught and encouraged to follow the above routines in order to decrease the exacerbation that may ensue when the oral corticosteroid is stopped. (5) If the dermatitis is longstanding and disabling or if benefit from oral corticosteroids is not lasting, 10 to 14 days of hospitalization may be helpful. This removes the patient from his environment, provides intensive therapy, and gives an opportunity for detailed patch testing, cultures, and other diagnostic studies. (6) PUVA delivered to just the hands and feet is often very effective, whatever the cause. (7) Oral retinoids (isotretinoin) 40 mg/day may be a last resort for severe psoriasis or idiopathic pustular eruptions of the hands and, if used with proper precautions, may greatly help these "dermatologic cripples."

GENERALIZED EXFOLIATIVE DERMATITIS

A severe, widespread erythema and scaling of the skin.

Etiology

No cause can be determined in most cases. In some patients, the disorder is secondary to certain dermatitides (eg, atopic, psoriatic, pityriasis rubra pilaris, contact); or it may be induced by a systemic drug (eg, penicillin, sulfonamides, isoniazid, phenytoin, or barbiturates) or an irritating topical agent. Exfoliative dermatitis may also be associated with mycosis fungoides or lymphoma.

Symptoms and Signs

The onset may be insidious or rapid. The entire skin surface becomes red, scaly, thickened, and, occasionally, crusted. Itching may be severe or absent. The characteristic appearance of any primary dermatitis is usually lost. Localized areas of normal skin may be seen when the exfoliative dermatitis is caused by psoriasis, mycosis fungoides, or pityriasis rubra pilaris. Generalized superficial lymphadenopathy is frequently present, and biopsy usually shows benign lymphadenitis.

The patient's temperature may be elevated, or he may feel cold from excessive heat loss, because of the increased blood flow to the skin and exfoliation. These may also cause weight loss, hypoproteinemia, iron deficiency, or even (in patients with borderline cardiac compensation) high-output congestive heart failure.

Diagnosis and Treatment

The disease may be life-threatening, and every attempt must be made to determine the cause. A history or signs of a primary dermatitis may be helpful. Biopsy is usually not helpful, but pemphigus foliaceus or mycosis fungoides may be diagnosed by skin biopsy, or lymphoma by a lymph node biopsy. Sézary syndrome may be diagnosed by a blood smear.

Hospitalization is often necessary. Because drug eruptions and contact dermatitis cannot be ruled out by history alone, all possible medications, systemic and topical, should be stopped. Essential systemic medicines should, if possible, be changed to chemically dissimilar ones. Petrolatum applied after tap-water baths will give temporary relief. Subsequent local treatment is the same as for contact dermatitis (see above).

Oral corticosteroids should be used only when topical measures are unsuccessful. Prednisone 40 to 60 mg is given every day; then, after about 10 days, every other day. Usually the dose can be further decreased, but prednisone will be required for long periods if an underlying cause is not found and eliminated.

STASIS DERMATITIS

Persistent inflammation of the skin of the lower legs with a tendency toward brown pigmentation, commonly associated with venous incompetency. (See also under VENOUS DISEASES in Ch. 30.)

Symptoms and Signs

The eruption is usually localized to the ankle, where erythema, mild scaling, and a brown discoloration are seen. Edema and varicose veins are common but by no means always present. Because of the relative lack of symptoms, the condition is often neglected. The usual consequences are increasing edema, secondary bacterial infection, and eventually ulceration. Recent studies have shown perivascular fibrin deposition and abnormal small-vessel vasoconstrictive reflexes that may be the real cause—not stasis per se.

Treatment

Both leg-elevation above the heart, to increase venous return and prevent tissue edema, and topical therapy are necessary. Topical therapy depends on the stage of the process. For acute dermatitis, tap-water compresses or the new "wet" hydrocolloid dressings should be applied, continuously at first and then intermittently. If the lesion is purulent, a more absorbent hydrocolloid dressing may be the best treatment. When the dermatitis becomes less acute, a corticosteroid cream or ointment should be applied tid or incorporated into zinc oxide paste. Ulcerative lesions are best treated with compresses and bland dressings such as zinc oxide paste. Recent studies have shown the superior efficacy of various new dressings, such as DuoDerm.® Oral antibiotics are useful when cellulitis is present; topical antibiotics are useless and often cause contact dermatitis. When the edema and inflammation subside, split-thickness skin grafts may be useful.

In selected instances, ulcers on ambulatory patients may be healed with an **Unna's paste boot** (zinc gelatin), the less messy **zinc gelatin bandage,** or one of the newer **"colloid" dressings,** which are all available commercially. The Unna's paste boot is being replaced by the more expensive but more effective new, absorptive, colloid-type dressings used under elastic support. At first it may be necessary to change the dressing q 2 or 3 days, but, as edema recedes and the ulcer heals, once or twice/wk is sufficient. Following healing, ambulation should always be with elastic support applied before getting out of bed in the morning.

Complex or multiple topical medications or nonprescription remedies should not be used, since the skin in stasis dermatitis is vulnerable to direct irritants and to potentially sensitizing topical agents (antibiotics; anesthetics; and vehicles of topical medications, particularly lanolin or wool alcohols).

LOCALIZED SCRATCH DERMATITIS

(Lichen Simplex; Neurodermatitis)

A chronic, superficial, pruritic inflammation of the skin, characterized by dry, scaling, well-demarcated, hyperpigmented, lichenified plaques of oval, irregular, or angular shape.

Etiology, Symptoms, and Signs

The disease may have a strong psychogenic component. Allergy appears to play no part. Women are affected more often than men, with onset usually between ages 20 and 50. An area of skin begins to itch recurrently, as a result of prior irritation or without apparent reason. The principal site is the occipital region, but arms or legs, especially ankles, are frequently involved. Vigorous scratching gives transient relief, but the itching recurs. Stress and tension increase the pruritus, and scratching may become an unconscious habit. The usual course is chronic.

A fully developed plaque has an outer zone of brownish discrete papules and a central zone of confluent papules covered with scales.

Pruritus ani and **pruritus vulvae** are often instances of circumscribed scratch dermatitis. The involved skin may only be red, moist, and hyperpigmented, or may even appear normal.

Diagnosis

Diagnosis can usually be made by inspection, but possible underlying causes should be excluded. The skin lesions are common in Asiatics and American Indians. Generalized itching without apparent skin lesions may occur in patients with a variety of systemic disorders (see Ch. 229). Most anal and vulvar pruritus is idiopathic, but may be due to pinworms, trichomoniasis, hemorrhoids, local discharges or fissures, candidiasis, warts, contact dermatitis, or occasionally psoriasis. Unusual but important

causes of anal or vulvar dermatitis are extramammary Paget's disease, Bowen's disease, and lichen sclerosis et atrophicus.

Treatment

It is important for the patient to realize that scratching and rubbing produce the skin changes. The pruritus may be controlled with medication; topical corticosteroids are the most effective. A cream may be rubbed in, but surgical tape impregnated with flurandrenolide (applied in the morning and replaced in the evening) may be best, since it simultaneously prevents scratching. Small areas may be locally infiltrated with a long-acting corticosteroid such as triamcinolone acetonide 2.5 mg/mL (achieved by diluting with saline), 0.3 mL/sq cm of lesion; this can be repeated every 3 to 4 wk. Oral 10-mg doses of chlorpromazine or doxepin at bedtime, increased to 25 to 50 mg/day if tolerated, may be useful.

Pruritus ani or vulvae is best treated with a hydrocortisone cream tid. Zinc oxide paste can be applied over the cream for protection; it may be removed with mineral oil. Patients should be cautioned not to rub hard with toilet paper after a bowel movement. Pinworms should be eradicated and warts treated. Hemorrhoids or hypertrophic "tags" should be removed and discharges or fissures corrected surgically if the course is chronic, but this will not always cure the pruritus ani because the itching is frequently of unknown etiology.

231. BACTERIAL INFECTIONS OF THE SKIN

The specific bacterial cause of a skin infection should be identified (see Bacterial and Fungal Cultures in Ch. 227). Knowledge of the normal skin flora helps in interpreting culture reports, since large numbers of bacteria, including micrococci, diphtheroids, and *Corynebacterium acnes*, normally inhabit the skin.

Infection may be the primary cause of a skin lesion or may be superimposed on another skin disease. Primary infections such as impetigo and erysipelas almost always respond promptly to *systemic* antibiotics, but secondary infections may clear more slowly. *Topical* antibiotics are ineffective in most bacterial skin infections and may cause allergic contact dermatitis. Recurrent infections should alert the physician to a possible underlying systemic disorder (eg, diabetes mellitus).

STAPHYLOCOCCAL DISEASES OF THE SKIN

(For IMPETIGO; ECTHYMA, see under BACTERIAL INFECTIONS in Ch. 191)

In the following syndromes, which must be differentiated because some are life-threatening, strains of *Staphylococcus aureus* either cause the syndromes or may be important in their development: **toxic shock syndrome (TSS)**, discussed under STAPHYLOCOCCAL INFECTIONS in Ch. 8; deep staphylococcal infections such as **cellulitis** (see Ch. 4) or **necrotizing fasciitis** (see Ch. 4); *Staphylococcus epidermitis* **septicemia** (caused by a usually nonpathogenic staphylococcus other than *aureus*); and **scalded skin syndrome (SSSS)**, described below, which must be distinguished from **toxic epidermal necrolysis (TEN)**, described in Ch. 237.

STAPHYLOCOCCAL SCALDED SKIN SYNDROME (SSSS)

(Ritter-Lyell Syndrome)

An acute, widespread erythematous process in which the epidermis peels off. It usually occurs in infants, young children, or immunosuppressed patients.

Etiology

Group II coagulase-positive staphylococci, usually phage Type 71 and often resist-

ant to penicillin, elaborate an epidermolytic toxin that splits off the upper part of the epidermis just beneath the granular cell layer. The toxin enters the circulation and affects the skin systemically, as in scarlet fever. SSSS may occur in epidemics in nurseries, with transmission from infant to infant on the hands of personnel. Most frequently, colonized infants are the source, although nursery personnel may be nasal carriers of *S. aureus*. The disease is also seen sporadically in children, usually < 6 yr of age, and in immunosuppressed adults.

Symptoms and Signs

Illness begins with a localized crusted infection (often impetigo-like), most often at the umbilical stump or in the diaper area during the first few days of life. When it occurs sporadically in children aged 1 to 6 yr, it starts with a superficial crusted lesion, frequently around the nose or ear. Within 24 h, tender bright red areas appear around the crusted area. The red areas may become painful and generalized and may progress rapidly to large, flaccid blisters that are easily broken to produce erosions. The epidermis peels off easily, often in large sheets, when the red areas are touched inadvertently or pushed by the examiner's finger. The disease progresses rapidly to widespread desquamation of the skin within 36 to 72 h and patients may become very ill with systemic manifestations, such as malaise, chills, and fever. Loss of the protective skin barrier exposes the patient to sepsis and to fluid and electrolyte imbalance. With prompt diagnosis and appropriate therapy (see below), mortality rarely occurs.

Diagnosis

Rapid and accurate differential diagnosis is essential, since proper therapy differs drastically in SSSS and toxic epidermal necrolysis (TEN). Age and milieu of the patient help in differential diagnosis; eg, SSSS almost invariably occurs only in infants, young children, and immunocompromised adults and starts with a staphylococcal infection (although the latter may not have been noted). Cultures should be obtained from the skin and nasopharynx. When TEN occurs in older individuals, it is usually due to drugs but may be a staphylococcal infection, as in children. Acute onset of a symmetrical erythematous skin eruption associated with systemic signs may suggest a drug hypersensitivity rash, viral exanthem, or scarlet fever, but none of these causes a *painful* rash. Bullae, erosions, and easily loosened epidermis occur in a number of disorders in which the epidermis is severely damaged, such as thermal burns, genetic bullous diseases (eg, some types of epidermolysis bullosa), and acquired bullous diseases (eg, pemphigus vulgaris and bullous pemphigoid [see Ch. 238]).

Defining the level of epidermal cleavage is crucial in differentiating SSSS and TEN (see Ch. 237). A scraping of the skin (Tzanck test, see Ch. 227) will often reveal the level. Biopsy shows cleavage and blister formation within the granular cell (outermost) layer of the epidermis in SSSS, but in TEN biopsy shows blister formation subepidermally (between epidermis and dermis) or at the level of the basal cell.

Treatment

Treatment with systemic penicillinase-resistant antistaphylococcal antibiotics (eg, cloxacillin or cephalexin) must be started as soon as the clinical diagnosis has been made and specimens for cultures have been taken, without waiting for culture reports. In early stages, oral cloxacillin 125 mg qid (in children) may be given, but in severe cases methicillin 25 to 50 mg/kg IV or IM should be given q 6 h until improvement is noted; oral cloxacillin 25 mg/kg qid should then be given for at least 10 days. Corticosteroids are *contraindicated* and topical therapy and patient handling must be minimized. If the disease is widespread and the lesions are weeping, the skin should be treated as if it were burned. Hydrolized polymer gel dressings may be very useful and reduce the number of dressing changes. Since the split is high in the epidermis, the stratum corneum is quickly replaced and healing is usually rapid—5 to 7 days after treatment

is started. Steps to detect carriers and prevent or deal with nursery epidemics are described in NOSOCOMIAL INFECTION IN THE NEWBORN under NEONATAL INFECTIONS in Ch. 186.

ERYSIPELAS

A superficial cellulitis caused by Group A β-hemolytic streptococci. The face (often bilaterally), an arm, or a leg is most often involved. The lesion is well demarcated, shiny, red, edematous, and tender; vesicles and bullae often develop. Patches of peripheral redness and regional lymphadenopathy are seen occasionally; high fever, chills, and malaise are common. Erysipelas may be recurrent and may result in chronic lymphedema. A nidus of infection may be an interdigital fungal infection of the foot that may require long-term griseofulvin therapy to prevent recurrent erysipelas.

Diagnosis from the characteristic appearance is usually easy. The causative organism is difficult to culture from the lesion, but it may occasionally be cultured from the blood. Erysipelas of the face must be differentiated from herpes zoster; of the arm or hand, from the rare erysipeloid (see in BACTERIAL DISEASES CAUSED BY GRAM-POSITIVE BACILLI in Ch. 8). Contact dermatitis and angioneurotic edema may be mistaken for erysipelas.

Treatment

Penicillin V or erythromycin 250 mg orally qid should be given for at least 2 wk. In acute cases, penicillin G 1.2 million u. IV q 6 h gives a rapid response and should be replaced by oral therapy after 36 to 48 h. In recent cases showing resistance to these antibiotics, cloxacillin or keflex has been used. Local discomfort may be relieved by cold packs; aspirin 600 mg, with codeine 30 mg if required, may be given orally for pain.

FOLLICULITIS; FURUNCLES; CARBUNCLES

Folliculitis: *A superficial or deep bacterial infection and irritation of the hair follicles.* It is usually caused by *Staphylococcus aureus*. The acute lesion consists of a superficial pustule or inflammatory nodule surrounding the hair. The condition may follow or accompany other pyodermas. Infected hairs are easily removed, but new papules tend to develop. Folliculitis may become chronic where the hair follicles are deep in the skin, as in the bearded area **(sycosis barbae).** Stiff hairs in the bearded region may emerge from the follicle, curve, and reenter the skin, producing a chronic low-grade irritation without significant infection (**pseudofolliculitis barbae**; see Ch. 235).

Furuncles (boils): *Acute, tender, perifollicular inflammatory nodules resulting from infection by staphylococci.* They occur most frequently on the neck, breasts, face, and buttocks, but are most painful when they occur in skin that is closely attached to underlying structures (eg, on the nose, ear, or fingers). The initial nodule becomes a pustule 5 to 30 mm in diameter, with central necrosis, which discharges a core of necrotic tissue and sanguineous purulent exudate. The condition may be recurrent and troublesome **(furunculosis)**, and often occurs in healthy young individuals. Miniature epidemics or clusters have been recorded among teenagers living in crowded quarters with relatively poor hygiene.

Carbuncles: *A cluster of furuncles with spread of infection subcutaneously, resulting in deep suppuration, often extensive local sloughing, slow healing, and a large scar.* Carbuncles develop more slowly than single furuncles and may be accompanied by fever and prostration. They occur most frequently in males and most commonly on the nape of the neck. Diabetes mellitus, debilitating diseases, and old age are predisposing factors, though carbuncles do occur in otherwise healthy persons.

Treatment

The treatment of acute folliculitis is similar to that of impetigo. Prompt treatment may prevent development of a chronic infection.

A single furuncle is treated with intermittent moist heat to allow the lesion to point and drain spontaneously, since extensive incision may spread the infection. A furuncle in the nose or central facial area should be treated with systemic antibiotics, the selection depending on the results of culture and sensitivity tests. Multiple furuncles and carbuncles require culture and sensitivity studies. Usually a penicillinase-resistant penicillin is required, such as cloxacillin 250 mg orally qid, or a cephalosporin in the same dosage. For recurrent boils, oral antibiotic therapy continuously for 1 to 2 mo may be advisable.

Clusters of cases are increasing—emphasizing the importance of finding and treating family and friends who may be sources of reinfection for the patients. Immunization with staphylococcal vaccines is ineffective. For all bathing, liquid soap containing either chlorhexidine gluconate with isopropyl alcohol or 2 to 3% chloroxylenol may be prophylactic but is not therapeutic.

HIDRADENITIS SUPPURATIVA

An inflammation of the apocrine glands resulting in obstruction and rupture of the ducts with painful local inflammation. Most lesions occur in the axilla or groin, but they may also be found around the nipples or anus. The lesions may be confused with furuncles but tend to be more persistent and are diagnosed primarily by their location and clinical course. Pain, fluctuation, discharge, and sinus tract formation are characteristic. In chronic cases, coalescence of inflamed nodules may cause palpable cordlike bands in the axilla. The condition may become extensive and disabling; if the pubic and genital areas are severely involved, walking may be difficult.

Treatment

Susceptible patients should avoid antiperspirants or other irritants. Early simple cases are treated with rest, moist heat, and prolonged systemic antibiotic therapy as for furunculosis. Surgical excision and plastic repair of the affected areas may be necessary if the disease persists. Isotretinoin orally has been effective in some patients. A rather large dosage is required—2 mg/kg/day—and recurrences are much more common than in acne. Etretinate in a slightly lower dose may also be effective. These drugs must be used with caution (see treatment of acne in Ch. 235).

CHRONIC GRANULOMATOUS DISEASE

(See under SPECIFIC IMMUNODEFICIENCIES in Ch. 18)

PARONYCHIAL INFECTIONS

Acute or chronic inflammation of the periungual tissues.

In acute paronychia, the causative organisms—usually micrococci, *Pseudomonas*, or *Proteus*, but sometimes *Candida* (see Ch. 232)—enter through a break in the epidermis resulting from a hangnail, trauma (eg, from manicuring), or chronic irritation (eg, from excessive exposure to water and detergents). The infection may follow the nail margin ("run-around"), or may extend beneath the nail and suppurate. Rarely, the infection penetrates more deeply into the finger; necrosis of the tendons and further extension of the infection along the tendon sheaths may result. Eventually the chronically infected nail becomes distorted.

Treatment

An acute infection is treated with hot compresses or soaks and, if bacterial, with an appropriate systemic antibiotic. The accumulated debris is painful and should be

drained. A purulent pocket should be opened cautiously with the point of a scalpel. Infection extending along the tendon sheaths requires prompt surgical incision and drainage.

In chronic recurrent inflammation, it is important to keep the hands dry. The subungual debris should be cultured. If *Candida* is not present on several cultures, cutting back the nail to the point of its detachment from the underlying skin and applying dilute tincture of iodine, 2 drops bid, will help to keep the subungual and paronychial areas dry and free of infection. If *Candida* is present, an antifungal lotion (eg, ciclopirox, miconazole, or tioconazole) should be applied tid to the paronychial and subungual areas after the nail is cut back. As the GI tract is a likely source of contamination with *Candida*, oral nystatin 500,000 u. qid may also be advisable. Women should be examined for an accompanying candidal vaginitis, which should also be treated. Grossly distorted nail plates may have to be removed.

ERYTHRASMA

A superficial skin infection caused by Corynebacterium minutissimum, *found most commonly in adults*. The incidence is higher in the tropics.

Erythrasma resembles a chronic fungus infection or intertrigo. In the toe webs, scaling, fissuring, and slight maceration occur, usually confined to the 3rd and 4th interspaces. In the genitocrural region, principally where the thighs contact the scrotum, patches are irregular and pink, later becoming brown with a fine scale. Erythrasma may widely involve the axillas, trunk, and perineum, particularly in obese middle-aged women or in patients with diabetes mellitus.

Differentiation from ringworm is essential. Diagnosis is established readily with a Wood's light, under which erythrasma shows a characteristic coral-red fluorescence.

Prompt clearing follows oral erythromycin or tetracycline 250 mg qid for 14 days, but recurrences 6 to 12 mo later are usual. Antibacterial soaps may also control the infection.

ERYSIPELOID

(See in BACTERIAL DISEASES CAUSED BY GRAM-POSITIVE BACILLI in Ch. 8)

232. SUPERFICIAL FUNGAL INFECTIONS

DERMATOPHYTE INFECTIONS
(Ringworm)

Superficial infections caused by dermatophytes—fungi that invade only "dead" tissues of the skin or its appendages (stratum corneum, nails, hair). Microsporum, Trichophyton, and *Epidermophyton* are the genera most commonly involved. Fomites are probably not responsible for transmission of infection. Some dermatophytes produce only mild or no inflammation; in such cases, the organism may persist indefinitely, causing intermittent remissions and exacerbations of a gradually extending lesion with a scaling, slightly raised border. In other cases an acute infection may occur, typically causing a sudden vesicular and bullous disease of the feet; or an inflamed boggy lesion of the scalp **(kerion)** may occur, which is due to a strong immunologic reaction to the fungus and is usually followed by remission or cure.

Clinical Types and Diagnosis

Since clinical differentiation of the related dermatophytes is difficult, these infections are conveniently discussed according to the sites involved. Diagnosis is con-

firmed by demonstrating the pathogenic fungus in scrapings of lesions, either by direct microscopic examination or by culture (see also SPECIAL DIAGNOSTIC METHODS in Ch. 227).

Tinea corporis (ringworm of the body) is usually caused by a *Trichophyton*. The characteristic papulosquamous annular lesions have raised borders, expand peripherally, and tend to clear centrally. Differential diagnosis includes pityriasis rosea, drug eruptions, nummular dermatitis, erythema multiforme, tinea versicolor, erythrasma, psoriasis, and secondary syphilis.

Tinea pedis (ringworm of the feet, athlete's foot) is particularly common. *Trichophyton mentagrophytes* infections begin in the 3rd and 4th interdigital spaces and later involve the plantar surface of the arch. The lesions often are macerated and have scaling borders; they may be vesicular. Acute flare-ups, with many vesicles and bullae, are common during warm weather. Infected toenails become thickened and distorted. *T. rubrum* produces scaling and thickening of the soles, often extending just beyond the plantar surface in a "moccasin" distribution. Inflammation or vesiculation may be slight or severe. Tinea pedis may be confused with maceration (from hyperhidrosis and occlusive footgear), with contact dermatitis (from sensitivity to various materials in shoes, particularly adhesive cement), with eczema, or with psoriasis.

Tinea unguium (ringworm of the nails), a form of onychomycosis, is usually caused by a *Trichophyton* species. Toenail involvement is common in longstanding tinea pedis; infections of the fingernails are less common. The nails become thickened and lusterless, and debris accumulates under the free edge. The nail plate becomes separated, and the nail may be destroyed. Differentiating a *Trichophyton* infection from *Candida* infection and psoriasis is particularly important because chemotherapy is specific and prolonged treatment is required.

Tinea capitis (ringworm of the scalp) mainly affects children. It is contagious and may become epidemic. *Trichophyton tonsurans* infection has become the common cause in the USA; other *Trichophyton* species, such as *T. violaceum*, are common in other parts of the world. *T. tonsurans* infection of the scalp is subtle in onset and characteristics. Inflammation is low-grade and persistent; the lesions are not annular or sharply marginated; and the hairs do not fluoresce under Wood's light. Affected areas of the scalp show characteristic black dots resulting from broken hairs. The fungus, an endothrix, produces within the hair chains of arthrospores that can be seen microscopically.

Trichophyton species may persist in adults. *Microsporum audouini* and *M. canis*, once predominant, are much less common. *M. audouini* lesions are small, scaly, semi-bald grayish patches with broken, lusterless hairs. Infection may be limited to a small area or extend and coalesce until the entire scalp is involved, sometimes with ringed patches extending beyond the scalp margin. *M. canis* and *M. gypseum* usually cause a more inflammatory reaction, with shedding of the infected hairs. A raised, inflamed, boggy granuloma **(kerion)** may also occur; it is followed shortly by healing. Diagnosis of a *Microsporum* infection is facilitated by examining the scalp under a Wood's light; infected hairs may fluoresce a light bright green. The organism is an ectothrix, producing spores to form a sheath around the hair. The sheath can be seen on microscopy. Culture of the fungus is also important in establishing the diagnosis.

Tinea cruris (jock itch) may be caused by various dermatophyte or yeast organisms. Typically, a ringed lesion extends from the crural fold over the adjacent upper inner thigh. Both sides may be affected. Scratch dermatitis and lichenification are often seen. Lesions may be complicated by maceration, miliaria, secondary bacterial or candidal infection, and reactions to treatment. Recurrence is common, since fungi may persist indefinitely on the skin or may repeatedly infect susceptible individuals. Flare-ups occur more often during the summer. Tight clothing or obesity tends to favor growth

of the organisms. The infection may be confused with contact dermatitis, psoriasis, erythrasma, or candidiasis. The scrotum is often acutely inflamed in candidal intertrigo, whereas in dermatophyte infections scrotal involvement is usually absent or slight.

Tinea barbae, a mycotic infection of the beard area, is rare. Infections in this area are more commonly bacterial (see FOLLICULITIS in Ch. 231), but may be fungal, especially in agricultural workers. The causative agent is established by microbiologic study.

Dermatophytids or "id" eruptions are fungus-free skin lesions that occur elsewhere on the body during an acute vesicular or inflammatory ringworm infection; they are thought to result from hypersensitivity to the fungus. Vesicular dermatitis of the hands is most commonly due to some other cause (see CHRONIC DERMATITIS OF HANDS AND FEET in Ch. 230).

Treatment

Griseofulvin is effective in treating tinea capitis, corporis, pedis, and unguium (onychomycosis) caused by *Trichophyton rubrum*, *T. schoenleini*, *T. mentagrophytes*, *T. sulfureum*, *T. verrucosum*, *T. interdigitalis*, *Epidermophyton floccosum*, *Microsporum audouini*, *M. canis*, or *M. gypseum*; but it is worthless in candidiasis or tinea versicolor and deep-seated mycoses (eg, histoplasmosis, coccidioidomycosis). The adult dosage is microsize griseofulvin 250 mg orally bid to qid and the drug is best given with a high-fat meal. The micronized form is better absorbed than the nonmicronized form. Some infections, especially those involving the nails, may require > 7 mo of therapy. The drug occasionally causes GI distress, skin rashes, or leukopenia. Angioedema has been reported. Headaches, vertigo, and, rarely, transient hearing reduction may occur. Topical imidazoles with oral griseofulvin increases the cure rate. A number of related imidazoles (miconazole, clotrimazole, ticonazole, econazole, bifonazole) as well as ciclopirox olamine cream have recently been marketed. The latter has been found to be the first effective topical cream for many (but not all) cases of onychomycosis. All of the imidazoles are about equal in efficacy and are very effective topical medications for the treatment of certain types of dermatophyte infections of the skin (but not tinea capitis or onychomycosis). **Ketoconazole,** an oral imidazole derivative, is an effective broad-spectrum agent for systemic therapy of candidiasis and some deep fungal infections. Although it is also effective orally for dermatophyte infections, occasional liver toxicity that can be severe or even fatal limits its use for superficial infections unless safer measures fail (see also General Therapeutic Principles in Ch. 9).

Tinea corporis: For small to moderately sized lesions, one of the imidazole or ciclopirox creams or lotions should be rubbed in bid until at least 7 to 10 days after lesions disappear. For extensive or resistant tinea corporis, the most effective therapy is oral griseofulvin. Tinea corporis usually responds readily to specific antifungal medication, but may be extensive and resistant to treatment in persons with debilitating systemic diseases.

Tinea pedis: Griseofulvin, the most effective treatment for mycologically proven tinea pedis, should be started even though it may have little immediate effect on the acute inflammatory infection. It is useful in chronic infections and in preventing acute exacerbations, but cure may require therapy for many months and is especially difficult if the toenails are involved. Concomitant topical imidazole or ciclopirox may reduce recurrences.

Good foot hygiene is essential. Interdigital spaces must be dried after bathing, macerated skin rubbed away, and a bland, drying dusting powder applied. Light permeable footwear is recommended, especially during warm weather; many patients benefit from going barefoot. During acute vesicular flare-ups, bullae may be drained at the margin, but the keratinous tops should not be removed. Tap-water soaks bid are drying.

Whitfield's tincture (3% salicylic acid and 6% benzoic acid in 70% alcohol solution) or Whitfield's ointment or any of the topical medications used for tinea corporis may be useful in the subacute or chronic phases. Cure with topical treatment is difficult but control may be obtained with long-term therapy.

Tinea cruris: Topical therapy with a cream or lotion, as in tinea corporis, is often effective. In some cases, griseofulvin orally for 3 to 4 wk may be needed.

Tinea unguium may respond to griseofulvin if treatment is continued until the nail has regrown completely and all infected material has been cast away. For fingernails, this may require 6 to 12 mo. Treatment of toenails should be discouraged, since 1 to 2 yr may be required, recurrence is usual, and complete cure is unlikely. Preliminary studies suggest that topical ciclopirox (which is uniquely water soluble) may be effective, with many months of only topical treatment in 1/2 or more of patients with chronic tinea unguium.

Tinea capitis: Children with *Trichophyton* infection should be given microsize griseofulvin 125 to 250 mg orally bid with meals or milk for at least 4 wk or until all signs of infection are gone. Until the tinea capitis is cured, an imidazole or ciclopirox cream should be applied to the affected child's scalp to prevent spread to other children.

Tinea barbae: Griseofulvin is the best treatment. If the lesions are severely inflamed, a short course of prednisone should be given in addition, starting with 40 mg/day orally (for adults) and tapering the dose over a 2-wk period.

YEAST INFECTIONS

CANDIDIASIS

(Candidosis; Moniliasis)

Candidiasis is usually limited to the skin and mucous membranes; uncommonly, the infection may become systemic and cause life-threatening visceral lesions. Systemic candidiasis (candidosis) is discussed in Ch. 9.

Etiology

Candida albicans is a ubiquitous, usually saprophytic, yeast that can become pathogenic if the organisms proliferate because of a favorable environment and if the host's defenses are weakened. The interrelation of these factors and the mechanisms that increase susceptibility to infection are discussed in Ch. 7. Specifically, intertriginous and mucocutaneous areas, where heat and maceration provide a fertile environment, are the sites most susceptible to candidiasis; and systemic antibacterial, corticosteroid, or antimetabolic therapy, pregnancy, obesity, diabetes mellitus or other endocrinopathies, debilitating diseases, blood dyscrasias, and immunologic defects increase susceptibility to candidiasis.

Symptoms and Signs

Symptoms vary with the site of the infection. **Intertriginous infections,** the most common, appear as well-demarcated, erythematous, sometimes itchy, exudative patches of varying size and shape. The lesions are usually rimmed with small, red-based pustules and occur in the axillas, inframammary areas, umbilicus, groin and gluteal folds (eg, diaper rash), between the toes, and on the finger-webs. **Perianal candidiasis** produces white macerative pruritus ani.

Vulvovaginitis is relatively common, especially in pregnancy or diabetes mellitus, and appears as a white or yellow discharge with inflammation of the vaginal wall and vulva. **Infection of the glans penis** and the underside of the preputium is less common but may be seen in men whose sexual partners have candidal vulvovaginitis and in

men with diabetes mellitus. This infection of the glans may be manifested by slightly scaling lesions and/or burning of the glans after coitus.

Oral candidiasis (thrush) appears as creamy white patches of exudate that can be scraped off an inflamed tongue or buccal mucosa (see also under STOMATITIS in Ch. 247). Although oral candidiasis is common in children and is benign, in young adults it may be the first sign of AIDS. **Perlèche,** which appears at the corners of the mouth and is characterized by inflammation with erosion and fissures, may be due to ill-fitting dentures and persistent moisture or to candida, or both.

Candidal paronychia begins around the nail as a painful red swelling that later develops pus. **Subungual infections** are characterized by distal separation of one or several fingernails **(onycholysis)** with white or yellow discoloration of the subungual area.

Defects in cell-mediated immune responses (which, in children, are sometimes genetic) may lead to **chronic mucocutaneous candidiasis (candida granuloma**—see also in Ch. 18), which is characterized by red, pustular, crusted and thickened lesions, especially on the nose and forehead. In patients with an immune deficiency, other, more typical, candidal lesions or systemic candidiasis is also seen.

Diagnosis

Candida can be demonstrated by finding both yeast and hyphae in gram-stained specimens or in potassium hydroxide mounts of scrapings from a lesion. Because *Candida* is a commensal of man, the culture of a species from the skin, mouth, vagina, urine, sputum, or stool should be interpreted cautiously. To confirm the diagnosis, a characteristic clinical lesion, exclusion of other causes, and, at times, histologic evidence of tissue invasion are needed.

Treatment

Topical nystatin, the imidazoles, and ciclopirox are all effective against skin and vaginal infections (for genital infections, see also GENITAL CANDIDIASIS in Ch. 14). A vehicle appropriate to the site of infection must be chosen and frequency of administration should be tid or qid. When anti-inflammatory and antipruritic actions are desired, equal amounts of the antifungal cream and a low-strength corticosteroid (eg, hydrocortisone) cream can be mixed. Recalcitrant or recurrent cases, especially of oral or anogenital candidiasis, benefit from nystatin oral suspension or tablets, 500,000 u. qid. When one sexual partner has recurrent candidiasis, both partners should be given topical and oral nystatin. For candidal diaper rash, the skin should be kept dry by changing diapers frequently and by generously applying talcum powder containing nystatin; in severe cases, rubber pants and plastic disposable diaper coverings should be avoided. Oral ketoconazole is effective for many forms (including vaginal) of acute as well as chronic mucocutaneous candidiasis. If an immune deficiency is present, ketoconazole followed by cimetidine may delay a relapse. The hepatic toxicity of oral ketoconazole must be considered and monitored. Treatment of paronychial infections is discussed in Ch. 231.

TINEA VERSICOLOR

An infection characterized by multiple, usually asymptomatic, patches of lesions varying in color from white to brown, and caused by Pityrosporon orbiculare (*formerly* Malassezia furfur). It is common in young adults. Tan, brown, or white, very slightly scaling lesions, which tend to coalesce, are seen on the chest, neck, and abdomen and occasionally on the face. The scaling may not be apparent unless the lesion is scratched. The patient may notice the condition only in the summer because the lesions do not tan; instead they appear as variously sized white "sun spots." Itching is rare and usually occurs only when the patient gets overheated. The condition is diagnosed from the clinical appearance and by finding groups of yeast and short plump hyphae on microscopic examination of scrapings from the lesions. The extent of involvement can

be determined by the golden fluorescence or pigment changes under a Wood's light. Culture of the organism is difficult without special media and is not needed for diagnosis.

Treatment

Selenium sulfide in shampoo form (CAUTION: *Keep out of reach of children*) is applied undiluted and widely to all involved areas, including the scalp, for 3 or 4 days at bedtime and washed off in the morning; the scrotum should be avoided. If irritation occurs, the selenium sulfide should be washed off after 20 to 60 min or treatment should be stopped for a few days. If irritation is too severe, 2% micropulverized sulfur and 2% salicylic acid in a shampoo base may be applied at bedtime for 2 wk. Oral ketoconazole is also effective, but long-term treatment for this usually trivial disease rarely seems warranted because of the potential toxicity; however, in preliminary studies one or two 200-mg tablets were effective in eliminating tinea versicolor for several months. The lesions may not become repigmented until the fungus is clear and the patient is exposed again to some sun. Eventual recurrence is almost universal after any treatment. The scalp may be the reservoir.

---

233. PARASITIC INFECTIONS OF THE SKIN

SCABIES

(The Itch)

A transmissible parasitic skin infection, characterized by superficial burrows, intense pruritus, and secondary infection.

Etiology and Incidence

Scabies is caused by the itch mite *Sarcoptes scabiei*. The impregnated female mite tunnels into the stratum corneum and deposits her eggs along the burrow. The larvae hatch within a few days and congregate around the hair follicles. Lesions are thought to result from hypersensitivity to the parasites.

Scabies is transmitted readily, often through an entire household, by skin-to-skin contact with an infected individual; eg, when people sleep together. It is sometimes spread by clothing or bedding. However, extensive cleaning or fumigating is not warranted, since the mite does not live long off the human body. Simply machine-laundering an infested person's clothing, bed linens, and towels should suffice.

Symptoms, Signs, and Diagnosis

Pruritus is marked and is most intense when the patient is in bed. The characteristic initial lesions are the burrows, seen as fine wavy dark lines a few millimeters to 1 cm long with a minute papule at the open end. The inflammatory lesions occur predominantly on the finger-webs, the flexor surface of the wrists, about the elbows and axillary folds, about the areola of the breasts in females and on the genitals in males, along the belt-line, and on the lower buttocks. The face is not involved in adults but may be in infants. Patients who have neurological disorders or various forms of immunodeficiency may have nonpruritic scaling due to infection with myriad mites (particularly on the palms and soles).

Burrows may be difficult to find (particularly when the disease has persisted for several weeks) because they are soon obscured by scratching or by secondary lesions—eg, urticaria, scratch dermatitis, eczema, or superimposed bacterial infection. Diagnosis can be confirmed by demonstrating the parasite in scrapings taken from a burrow, then mixed with any clear solution (eg, mineral oil, potassium hydroxide, or even water), and examined microscopically.

Treatment

Treatment is curative and may serve as a "therapeutic test" in doubtful cases. The patient may apply 1% lindane (gamma benzene hexachloride) or 25% benzyl benzoate cream or lotion (sometimes irritating) over the entire skin surface from the neck down. For infants < 2 yr, 5 or 10% sulfur ointment is preferred because of a potential neurotoxicity from absorption of gamma benzene hexachloride. (Permethrin 5% cream seems safer and more effective, but has not yet been approved by the FDA for use in scabies.) Warm bathing before application is no longer recommended. The application should be repeated the next morning but not again, because persistent inflammation and itching may be due to scratching, contact dermatitis, or secondary infection rather than to the mite, and further applications may cause irritant dermatitis. Contacts, both adults and children (eg, a whole family), should be treated simultaneously.

Retreatment is rarely needed, unless infection is reacquired. A 0.1% fluorinated corticosteroid ointment (see Ch. 228) bid may be used for persistent itching, which may take 1 to 2 wk to subside. Concomitant bacterial infections may require systemic antibiotics but often clear spontaneously when the scabies is cured.

PEDICULOSIS

Infestation by lice may involve the **head** (by *Pediculus humanus capitis*), the **body** (*P. humanus corporis*), or the **genital area** (*Phthirus pubis*). The head louse and pubic (crab) louse live directly on the host; the body louse, in the undergarments. Infestation is widespread where overcrowding or inadequate facilities for personal hygiene or clean clothing exist. The body louse is an important vector of the organisms that cause epidemic typhus, trench fever, and relapsing fever.

Symptoms, Signs, and Diagnosis

Pediculosis capitis is transmitted by personal contact and by such objects as combs and hats. It is common among school children, without regard to social status, and is less common in blacks. Infestation is localized predominantly on the scalp, though it sometimes involves the eyebrows, eyelashes, and beard. Itching is severe, and excoriation of the scalp, sometimes with secondary bacterial infection, may be seen. Moderate discrete posterior cervical adenopathy is frequent. In children, a generalized, nonspecific dermatitis is occasionally caused by lice infesting only the scalp. Diagnosis is simple if infestation is considered and the scalp is inspected, preferably with a magnifying lens. Small, ovoid, greyish-white nits (ova) are seen fixed to the hair shafts, sometimes in great numbers; unlike scales, they cannot be dislodged. The nits mature in 3 to 14 days. Lice may be found, less frequently than the nits, around the occiput and behind the ears.

Pediculosis corporis is uncommon under good hygienic conditions. Nits may be found on the body hairs, but both parasites and ova are easily found in underclothing, since the body louse primarily inhabits the seams of clothing worn next to the skin. Itching is invariable. Lesions are especially common on the shoulders, buttocks, and abdomen. Inspection may show small red puncta due to bites, usually associated with linear scratch marks, urticaria, or superficial bacterial infection. Furunculosis is an occasional complication.

Pediculosis pubis is usually transmitted venereally. The crab louse ordinarily infests the anogenital hairs but may involve other areas, especially in hairy individuals. In all itching dermatoses of the anogenital region, careful inspection for the parasites should be made; they may be few in number. The lice are large but not easily seen without a diligent search; they resemble the small crusts of scratch dermatitis. Sometimes the lice may be seen as small bluish spots on the skin, ordinarily on the trunk. The ova are commonly attached to the skin at the base of the hairs. A sign of infestation is a

scattering of minute dark brown specks (louse excreta) on undergarments where they come in contact with the anogenital region. Excoriation and secondary dermatitis, the latter often from self-medication, may develop early.

Treatment and Prevention

Cure is usually rapid with 1% lindane (gamma benzene hexachloride), applied once/day for 2 days in shampoo, cream, or lotion form or as a combination of shampoo followed by the cream or lotion; pyrethrin preparations or 0.5% malathione lotions can be effective, but lindane has neurotoxicity, and all may be irritating or inflammable. Application may be repeated in 10 days to destroy any nits that survived, but prolonged application of parasiticides should be **avoided.** A safer, more effective, and more pleasant product, 1% permethrin cream rinse, has been approved recently by the FDA. Infestation of eyelids and eyelashes may be more difficult to manage; the parasites usually must be removed with forceps. Plain petrolatum applications may kill or weaken the lice on eyelashes. Sources of infestation, such as combs, hats, clothing, or bedding, should be decontaminated by vacuuming, thorough laundering and steam pressing, or dry cleaning. Recurrence is common.

CREEPING ERUPTION
(Cutaneous Larva Migrans)

This disease is caused chiefly by *Ancylostoma braziliense*, the hookworm of the dog or cat. The ova of the parasites are deposited on the ground in dog or cat feces. The larva persists in warm moist ground or sand and penetrates unprotected skin where it contacts the soil. The feet, legs, buttocks, or back are most commonly involved. The haphazard progress of the parasite as it burrows in the epidermis produces a winding, threadlike trail of inflammation. Itching is marked, and scratch dermatitis and bacterial infection with a bizarre pattern are common.

Treatment

Applying the oral 10% suspension of thiabendazole topically to all affected areas qid for 7 to 10 days is promptly effective. Topical mebendazole incorporated into cream is said to be effective also, but fewer studies have been done.

234. VIRAL INFECTIONS OF THE SKIN

Herpes simplex and herpes zoster, though they may be considered viral skin infections, are discussed elsewhere in THE MANUAL.

WARTS
(Verrucae)
(See also GENITAL WARTS in Ch. 14)

Common, contagious, epithelial tumors caused by at least 35 types of human papilloma virus (HPV), some of which can become malignant. (See TABLE 234–1.) Viral warts may appear at any age, but are most frequent in older children and uncommon in the aged. Appearance and size depend on their location and on the degree of irritation and trauma to which they are subjected. The course may be erratic. Infection may persist as single or multiple lesions, and lesions may develop by autoinoculation. Complete regression after several months is usual with or without treatment, but warts may persist for years and may recur at the same or different sites.

The importance of serologic or cell-mediated immunity is not yet clear. Some feel that, because wart virus particles are seen only in the outer epithelium (granular layer

TABLE 234–1. TYPES OF WART VIRUS AND CLINICAL CORRELATIONS

Clinical Form	*Types*	*Clinical Correlations*
Common (including palmar, plantar, & periungual)	1, 2, 4, 7	Rarely malignant
Flat	3, 10	Usually benign
Genital (See Ch. 14), also found in mouth, perianal area, bladder, and lung	6, 11	In women, 28% have associated cervical dysplasia with koilocytic cells
	16, 18, 33	Found in >50% of tumors in women with invasive carcinoma of cervix; type 16 found in 80% of men and women with Bowenoid papulosis of external genitals. Lesions usually disappear spontaneously but future cancers may appear
	6a, b, c, d, e	Bushke Loewenstein giant condyloma often malignant; also in cervical dysplasia and laryngeal tumors
Butcher's (meat handler's)	7, 10	Common warts, usually benign
Malignant epidermodysplasia verruciformis	5a, b, 8	Often malignant; sunlight or x-ray therapy cofactors, especially with type 5
Epidermodysplasia verruciformis	1, 2, 3, 4, 7, 9, 10, 12, 14, 17, 18, 19, 20, 23, 24, 25	Most seem benign, except possibly 14, 17, 20
Cutaneous warts in immunosuppressed and transplant patients	8 or others	Often malignant; sunlight a cofactor
Laryngeal papillomas	6, 11, 16, 30	Both types may become malignant; either type may occur in infants on passage through the vaginal canal and in adults as a consequence of oral-genital sex. May spread to lungs as cancer.
Oral papillomatosis (Heck's disease)	13	Usually benign

and beyond), they have little chance to get deep enough to serve as good antigens. On the other hand, patients with epidermodysplasia verruciformis or immunosuppression from organ transplants lack immunity to the virus and get generalized cutaneous infections with many types of virus. This suggests that some types of immune mechanisms are significant. In addition, spontaneous cure of many warts in normal people and subsequent apparent lifelong immunity need further explanation.

Differential Diagnosis

The wart viruses are circular, double-stranded DNA, with about 8000 base pairs. To qualify as a separate type there must be < 50% of DNA cross-hybridization; subtypes, > 50%. Each type is indicated by a number and, in general, causes certain clinical lesions. Although each DNA is distinctive, most papillomas, including those of bovine origin, also have a common protein antigen that can be demonstrated histologically on fixed tissue with a test that is positive for all types of papillomas and is very useful in

diagnosis. When the papillomas become malignant, however, they no longer give a positive stain nor can recognizable papilloma particles be seen with the electron microscope. Oncogenic papilloma DNA can then be found in the cancers by modern molecular hybridization DNA technics. DNA typing is now available in only a few special research laboratories but is important for prognosis of genital warts and their consequences.

Common warts (verrucae vulgaris) are almost universal in the population and most do not become malignant. They are sharply demarcated, rough-surfaced, round or irregular, firm, light gray, yellow, brown, or grayish-black tumors 2 to 10 mm in diameter. They appear most frequently on sites subject to trauma (eg, fingers, elbows, knees, face, scalp) but may spread elsewhere. **Periungual warts** are common warts occurring around the nail plate.

Plantar warts are common warts on the sole of the foot; they are flattened by pressure and surrounded by cornified epithelium. They may be exquisitely tender and can be distinguished from corns and calluses by their tendency to pinpoint bleeding when the surface is pared away. **Mosaic warts** are plaques of myriad small, closely set plantar warts.

Filiform warts are long, narrow, small growths usually seen on the eyelids, face, neck, or lips. **Flat warts** are smooth, flat, yellow-brown lesions and occur more commonly in children and young adults, most often on the face and along scratch marks through autoinoculation. **Warts of unusual shape**—eg, pedunculated, or resembling a cauliflower—are most frequent on the head and neck, especially on the scalp and bearded region.

Moist or "venereal" warts (condylomata acuminata) are discussed in Ch. 14.

Treatment

Most **common warts** disappear spontaneously or with simple nonscarring treatment such as a flexible collodion solution containing 16% salicyclic acid and 16% lactic acid applied daily, after gentle peeling, by the patient or parent. Or the physician may freeze the wart (avoiding the surrounding skin) for 15 to 30 sec with liquid nitrogen. This procedure is often curative, but may need to be repeated in 2 to 3 wk. Electrodesiccation with curettage is satisfactory for a solitary lesion or a few lesions. Laser surgery may also be useful. Recurrence or appearance of new warts close by occurs in about 35% of patients within a year after any treatment, so that scarring methods should be avoided as much as possible.

Plantar warts may require more vigorous maceration with a 40% salicyclic acid tape kept in place for several days. The physician then removes the wart by debridement while it is still damp and soft; removal is followed by destruction by freezing or by caustics such as 30% trichloracetic acid.

In **common** or even **periungual warts,** cantharidin 0.7% in flexible collodion is also useful. The physician, using a tiny-tipped applicator and being careful to avoid normal skin, applies the preparation 2 to 3 times (after drying) at one visit and covers the wart with occlusive tape that is left in place for 7 h. The procedure can be repeated in 1 or 2 wk, if necessary. (Cantharidin should not be given to patients for treatment at home.)

Other destructive treatments, such as a CO_2 laser or various acids, will work in many cases; or even snipping off **filiform (long single) warts** may be sufficient.

X-ray therapy has no place in treating warts because of its potential to make them malignant; even in squamous cell carcinomas, which occur in patients with the rare epidermodysplasia verruciformis **(EDV),** x-ray therapy causes warts to become much more invasive. Ultraviolet exposure is also a potent cocarcinogen in patients with EDV immunosuppression for any reason.

Flat warts can often be treated successfully with daily application of tretinoin (retinoic acid 0.05%), as used in acne. If sufficient peeling does not occur for wart removal, another irritant such as 5% benzoyl peroxide or a 5% salicylic acid cream can be applied sequentially with tretinoin to remove lesions. Spontaneous resolution may follow unprovoked inflammation of the lesions.

Several new methods, whose long-term value and risks are not fully known, are available. One of these, intralesional injection of small amounts of 0.1% solution of bleomycin in saline, often produces necrosis and cures even stubborn plantar warts. However, reports of scleroderma of fingers where warts have been injected with bleomycin suggest caution in spite of its popularity and effectiveness.

Extensive warts, even in hitherto untreatable epidermodysplasia verruciformis, have improved or cleared with *oral isotretinoin, or etretinate,* which *must be used by physicians familiar with these drugs and their possible side effects, especially fetal abnormalities if used during pregnancy.*

Interferon, especially α-interferon, intralesionally or IM, has also cleared intractable lesions of skin and genitals. Its optimal administration and long-term results are under study in several countries.

MOLLUSCUM CONTAGIOSUM

A poxvirus infection characterized by skin-colored, smooth, waxy, umbilicated papules 2 to 10 mm in diameter. A "giant" single molluscum may grow 2 or 3 times as large.

Transmission is by direct contact, often venereal. Its contagiousness to others varies. The papules may appear anywhere on the skin and often occur as numerous small papules in the genital and pubic area. The lesions are usually asymptomatic, unless secondarily infected, and may be discovered only when the patient is examined for another sexually transmitted disease. They can be diagnosed easily by the characteristic central umbilication or dell, filled with a semisolid white material that, if expressed and Giemsa-stained, shows many large cells containing inclusion bodies. Inclusion bodies alone may be seen. The disease can spread by autoinoculation, but after months may disappear spontaneously. Areas of eczematous dermatitis may surround several mollusca, especially in young children; the cause of the dermatitis is not known.

Treatment, to be successful, usually requires destroying each lesion by cantharidin (as for common warts, above), by freezing, or by removing the central core of the papule with a needle or a comedo extractor.

235. DISORDERS OF HAIR FOLLICLES AND SEBACEOUS GLANDS

ACNE

A common inflammatory pilosebaceous disease characterized by comedones, papules, pustules, inflamed nodules, superficial pus-filled cysts, and, in extreme cases, canalizing and deep, inflamed, sometimes purulent, sacs.

Pathogenesis

The pathogenesis is complex. An interaction between hormones, keratinization, sebum, and bacteria somehow determines the course and severity of the disease. Acne begins at puberty, when the increase in androgens causes an increase in the size and activity of the pilosebaceous glands. It is thought that the earliest microscopic change is intrafollicular hyperkeratosis, which leads to blockage of the pilosebaceous follicle with consequent formation of the comedo, composed of sebum, keratin, and microor-

ganisms, particularly *Propionibacterium (Corynebacterium) acnes*. Lipases from *P. acnes* break down triglycerides in the sebum to form free fatty acids **(FFA)**, which irritate the follicular wall. Retention of sebaceous secretions and dilation of the follicle may lead to cyst formation. Rupture of the follicle, with release of FFA, bacterial products, and keratin constituents into the tissues, induces an inflammatory reaction that heals with scarring in severe cases.

Symptoms and Signs

For therapy and prognosis, acne is best classified as superficial or deep according to the severity of the predominating lesions. Spontaneous remission is the rule, but when this will occur cannot be predicted.

Superficial acne is characterized by comedones, either open (blackheads) or closed (whiteheads); inflamed papules; superficial cysts; and pustules. Large cysts occur occasionally, sometimes after manipulation or trauma to an otherwise uninflamed blackhead. In **deep acne,** deep inflamed nodules and pus-filled cysts are also present; some of them open on the skin surface and discharge their contents. Scarring is frequent in deep acne. The lesions are commonest on the face, but the neck, chest, upper back, and shoulders may also be affected. The prognosis for healing without scars is good in superficial acne, but clumsy attempts to extrude blackheads or superficial cysts and scratching of ruptured lesions may increase scarring.

Acne is often exacerbated during the winter and improved during the summer, probably because of the beneficial effect of the sun. Diet has little, if any, effect, but if a food is suspected it should be omitted for several weeks and then eaten in substantial quantities to see if eating it makes any difference. Most such trials prove that the acne is unrelated to food. Acne may cycle with the menses, and may clear or become worse during pregnancy. In many of those women who first develop acne in their 20s and 30s it seems to result from applying cosmetics (especially "moisturizers") that contain comedogenic oils.

Diagnosis

Diagnosis of acne is usually simple. Comedones are almost always present, and lesions at various stages of development are seen simultaneously. Rosacea may resemble acne, but there are no comedones. Corticosteroid-induced acneiform lesions are usually follicular pustules all in the same stage of development; comedones are absent.

Treatment

Disfiguring or even mild acne may embarrass adolescents, even though the disease is almost universal, and some may become withdrawn, using the acne as an excuse to avoid difficult personal adjustments. Supportive counseling for both patient and parents is helpful. Misconceptions about a relationship between acne and diet, athletics, or sex are common and need correcting. Some cosmetics aggravate acne (especially those with comedogenic ingredients such as isopropyl myristate), and most greasy products should be avoided.

Other treatment depends on the severity of the lesions:

Superficial acne: If the face is oily, it should be washed several times/day (although this has little effect on lesions). Any good toilet soap may be used. Antibacterial soaps are of no benefit, and abrasive soaps are irritating, which will make it difficult to use the more specific follicular medications, tretinoin or benzoyl peroxide (see below).

Large comedones may be removed carefully once or twice/wk, preferably with a Schamberg loop extractor after hot water compresses. The proper technic may be taught to a responsible member of the family. Many dermatologists doubt the lasting value of such manipulation. Inflammatory lesions should not be opened until they have pointed in a pustule. Picking the crust covering an opened lesion may delay healing for several weeks and produce a pitted scar.

Sunlight and irritating topical medications aid superficial lesions. Sunlight causes mild dryness and slight scaling; it is usually effective, but not always available, and the benefit may be difficult to duplicate with a sunlamp. Topical tretinoin (vitamin A acid; retinoic acid) 0.05% cream or liquid, or 0.01 or 0.025% gel, is often effective. It must be applied cautiously; the liquid should be applied with a cotton-tipped applicator. Tretinoin should be applied nightly (every other night if irritation is excessive), going over the entire affected area *only once*. The eyes, nasolabial folds, and creases of the mouth should be avoided. Exposure to sunlight and use of other medications often are restricted to prevent severe irritation. Improvement usually requires 3 to 4 wk, and the condition may appear worse at first. Blackheads can be removed easily after a month of treatment. Other topical medicines include 5 to 10% benzoyl peroxide, the best nonprescription topical medication, and various sulfur-resorcinol combinations; they are usually applied bid or one preparation at night and another in the morning. Oral tetracycline (see below) may also be helpful in superficial pustular acne.

Topical antibiotics (tetracycline, clindamycin, and erythromycin) in liquid vehicles are being used with some benefit.

Deep acne: Vigorous management is required to reduce residual scarring. Topical treatment is unsatisfactory for severe, deep lesions. Treatment of patients with a few deep lesions is usually a broad-spectrum oral antibiotic: the effect is probably due to reduction of bacterial organisms. Tetracycline is the most effective and produces the fewest side effects. A dose of 250 mg qid (between meals and at bedtime) should be continued for 4 wk and then decreased to the lowest amount that gives a good response. Because relapse ordinarily follows short periods of treatment, therapy must be continued for months to years, though as little as 250 or 500 mg/day is often sufficient. If the patient is pregnant, erythromycin in similar dosage may be used. The commonest side effect with prolonged antibiotic use is a candidal vaginitis. If local and systemic therapy (see CANDIDIASIS in Ch. 232) do not eradicate this problem, antibiotic therapy for the acne must be stopped. Long-term use of antibiotics may also produce a gram-negative pustular folliculitis, seen around the nose and in the center of the face. This uncommon superinfection is often difficult to clear; treatment should be based on culture and sensitivity of the responsible organism.

Oral isotretinoin is the best treatment in patients in whom treatment with antibiotics is not successful or in patients with very severe deep acne. This medication has revolutionized the treatment of acne, *but should be used only by physicians who are thoroughly familiar with its adverse effects*. Since isotretinoin is teratogenic, women taking the drug must use strict contraceptive measures while taking it and for at least 1 mo after stopping it. Pregnancy tests before beginning and at monthly intervals are important. Warnings against pregnancy should be put on every bottle dispensed. If pregnancy occurs while the woman is taking the drug, counseling about terminating the pregnancy is indicated because severe fetal abnormalities are likely to occur. The dosage of isotretinoin is usually 1 to 1.5 mg/kg/day for 20 wk. If the patient cannot tolerate this dosage because of side effects, the dose may be reduced to 0.5 mg/kg/day. The commonest side effect, seen in about 90% of patients, is dryness of conjunctivae and mucosae of the genitalia, and chapped lips. Petrolatum is usually beneficial in alleviating some of the symptoms associated with the dryness. Musculoskeletal symptoms, pain or stiffness of large joints or the lower back, may also occur in about 15% of patients. Symptoms often resolve with reduced dosage. Occasionally the drug must be discontinued. CBC, liver function, and triglyceride and cholesterol levels should be determined before treatment. Each, except for the CBC, should be reassessed at 2 wk and then monthly during treatment. Triglyceride levels may increase to a level where the drug should be discontinued. Liver function is only occasionally affected. Following the 20 wk of therapy, improvement of the acne may continue. Most patients do not require a 2nd course of treatment; when needed, it should be resumed only after the

drug has been stopped for 4 mo. Retreatment is required more often if the initial dosage is low (0.5 mg/kg/day).

For isolated lesions, incision and drainage is often beneficial when the lesion is fluctuant. For firm lesions, or after incision and drainage, injection of 0.5 mL triamcinolone acetonide suspension 2.5 mg/mL (the 10-mg/mL suspension must be diluted) into a cyst is helpful; local atrophy (due to the corticosteroid or to destruction of tissue by the cyst) is usually transient.

Dermabrasion for small scars is sometimes useful, but its permanent effect is controversial.

X-ray therapy is not justified. Topical corticosteroids, especially the fluorinated ones, may worsen acne. When other measures fail and acne seems related to the menses, an oral estrogen-progesterone in the usual contraceptive dosage may be tried; therapy for at least 6 mo is needed to evaluate the effect.

ROSACEA

A chronic inflammatory disorder, usually beginning in middle age or later, and characterized by telangiectasia, erythema, papules, and pustules appearing especially in the central areas of the face. Tissue hypertrophy, particularly of the nose **(rhinophyma),** may result. Occasionally, rosacea occurs on the trunk and extremities.

The cause is unknown, but the disease is most common in persons with a fair complexion. Diet probably plays no role in the pathogenesis. Rosacea may resemble acne, but comedones are never present; differential diagnosis also includes drug eruptions (particularly from iodides and bromides), granulomas of the skin, cutaneous LE, and perioral dermatitis.

Treatment

Topical metronidazole cream or broad-spectrum oral antibiotics are usually effective. Tetracycline is preferred because side effects with long-term use are few. A starting dose of 250 mg qid (between meals) should be reduced once a beneficial response is achieved. Often only 250 mg/day or every other day will control the disease. Recalcitrant cases often respond to oral isotretinoin as in acne (see above). Topical fluorinated corticosteroids aggravate rosacea and are contraindicated. Surgical correction may be required for rhinophyma, a bulbous red nose resulting from neglected rosacea.

PERIORAL DERMATITIS

A red papular eruption of unknown etiology occurring around the mouth and on the chin. The condition occurs predominantly in women aged 20 to 60. It may superficially resemble acne or rosacea. A zone of normal skin lies between the lesions and the vermilion border of the mouth. Some oily cosmetics, especially "moisturizers," may worsen the disorder, as do fluorinated steroids.

Treatment with tetracycline 250 mg qid (between meals) is often effective. The dose should be reduced gradually after 1 mo to the smallest amount that controls the disease. Recalcitrant, disfiguring cases may clear with oral isotretinoin as in acne (see above).

HYPERTRICHOSIS

(Hirsutism)

Excessive hair growth in areas usually not hairy. A familial tendency is common and occurrence is more frequent in people from the Mediterranean area. An endocrine disorder may be implicated in women and children—most frequently, adrenal virilism, basophilic adenoma of the pituitary, masculinizing ovarian tumors, and the Stein-

Leventhal syndrome. Hirsutism is seen frequently at menopause, with systemic androgenic steroid or corticosteroid therapy, and with some antihypertensive medications. It also may occur in porphyria cutanea tarda. (See also in ADRENAL VIRILISM under ADRENAL CORTICAL HYPERFUNCTION in Ch. 91, and in Ch. 170.)

Treatment

Any underlying disorder should be treated. The only safe permanent local treatment is destruction of individual hair follicles by electrolysis, a tedious process. Widely used temporary measures include plucking, shaving, and use of epilating wax. Chemical depilatories are acceptable if the directions are followed, but may irritate the skin. A hair bleach may mask the condition if the hair is fine. Women with endocrine abnormalities improve with spironolactone, but this drug must be considered experimental for such use because it is a tumorigen when given for long periods.

ALOPECIA

(Baldness)

Partial or complete loss of hair. It may result from genetic factors, aging, or local or systemic disease. (Seborrheic dermatitis and psoriasis, the two dermatoses that affect the scalp most commonly, do not produce alopecia.) **Nonscarring (noncicatricial) alopecia** occurs without scarring or gross atrophic changes; **scarring (cicatricial) alopecia** follows scar tissue formation resulting from inflammation and tissue destruction.

Nonscarring Alopecia

Male-pattern baldness is extremely common. It is familial and requires the presence of androgens, but other etiologic factors are unknown. The hair loss begins in the lateral frontal areas or over the vertex. If onset is in the mid-teens, subsequent baldness is commonly extensive. **Female-pattern alopecia** is not infrequent in women. It is confined ordinarily to thinning of the hair in the frontal and the parietal regions; complete baldness in any area is rare.

Toxic alopecia is usually temporary and may follow, by as long as 3 to 4 mo, a severe, often febrile, illness (eg, scarlet fever). It may also be seen in myxedema, hypopituitarism, or early syphilis, following pregnancy, and with some drugs—particularly cytotoxic agents, thallium compounds, and overdoses of vitamin A or retinoids.

In **alopecia areata,** sudden hair loss in circumscribed areas occurs in individuals who have no obvious skin disorder or systemic disease. Any hairy area may be involved, the scalp and beard most frequently. Rarely, all the body hair may be lost **(alopecia universalis).** The prognosis is poor if alopecia is extensive or begins in childhood, but alopecia first appearing in adult life and confined to a few areas is often reversed in a few months, though recurrences may occur. Serum antibodies to thyroglobulin, gastric parietal cells, adrenal cells, and thyroid may be present.

Hair pulling (trichotillomania) is a neurotic habit that usually appears in children; it may remain undiagnosed for a long time. The hairs may be broken off or pulled out. Some stubby regrowth may be visible, but the condition is often hard to differentiate from alopecia areata. Biopsy is sometimes helpful.

Scarring Alopecia

If hair loss is due to atrophy or scarring, little regrowth can be expected. In injuries (eg, burns, physical trauma, x-ray atrophy), the cause of the scarring will usually be apparent; if it is not obvious, it should be sought. Cutaneous LE, chronic deep bacterial or fungal infections; deep factitial ulcers; granulomas such as sarcoidosis, syphilitic gummas, or TB; or inflamed tinea capitis (kerion or favus) may produce scarring

alopecia. Certain slow-growing tumors may gradually extend in the scalp with resultant scarring. Some rare scarring alopecias are of unknown cause.

Examination should include the entire skin surface and mucous membranes, because related lesions will often be found. Biopsy should be done at an area of active inflammatory change, usually at the border of a bald patch. Cultures for bacteria and fungi may be indicated.

Diagnosis

Microscopic examination of plucked hair may differentiate some forms of nonscarring alopecia. Normally 80 to 90% of hairs are in a growing (anagen) phase; the rest are in a resting (telogen) phase. *All* of the hair (approximately 40 to 60 hairs) from a defined area of the scalp should be plucked, using a strong instrument, and an anagen/telogen count performed. Anagen hairs have sheaths attached to their roots, whereas telogen hairs have no sheaths and have tiny bulbs at their roots. Postpartum and post-illness alopecias are characterized by an increased percentage of telogen hairs, whereas alopecias due to thallium or antimitotic drugs are characterized by a normal percentage of telogen hairs. The anagen hair in the latter conditions may break easily because the hair shaft narrows. Alopecia areata is characterized by hairs that look like exclamation points.

Biopsy of the scalp may differentiate various forms of scarring alopecias. Either histologic or immunofluorescent examination may delineate LE, lichen planopilaris (lichen planus of the scalp), and scleroderma. Metastatic lesions, which may also produce localized scarring alopecia, are diagnosed by biopsy.

Treatment

No therapy is known for idiopathic male-pattern baldness, though transplants from hairy to bald areas are effective. Minoxidil, an antihypertensive medication, is being used topically in solutions of about 3%. Results vary, and the drug can be detected in the blood. When the drug is stopped, the new hair falls out. The long-term value of minoxidil and its dangers are unknown.

In alopecia areata, triamcinolone acetonide suspension can be injected intradermally if the lesions are small, but the results may not be lasting. Experimental induction of a mild allergic contact dermatitis has shown some benefit, as have other topical irritants.

In scarring alopecia, treatment is directed at eliminating the cause.

PSEUDOFOLLICULITIS BARBAE

Pseudofolliculitis of the beard **(ingrown hairs)** is seen most frequently in black men. The stiff hair tips penetrate the skin before leaving the follicle, or else leave the follicle, curve, and reenter nearby skin, provoking small pustules that are more a foreign-body reaction than an infection. The only consistently effective **treatment** is to have the patient grow a beard. Special razors have been used with varying results. A thioglycolate depilatory may be used every 2 to 3 days but is often irritating. Application of tretinoin (vitamin A acid; retinoic acid) 0.05% liquid or cream or 10% benzoyl peroxide cream daily or every other day may be effective in mild or moderate cases; they may be irritating and should be used every other day at first, then daily.

KERATINOUS CYST

(Wen; Sebaceous Cyst; Steatoma)

A slow-growing benign cystic tumor of the skin containing follicular, keratinous, and sebaceous material and frequently found on the scalp, ears, face, back, or scrotum. On palpation, the cystic mass is firm, globular, movable, and nontender; it seldom causes

discomfort unless infected. Puncture of the cyst produces characteristic cheesy, often fetid, contents formed of epithelial debris and greasy material; soft keratin often predominates, and at times calcium deposits may be found. Secondary bacterial infection with abscess formation occurs. A **milium** is a minute superficial keratinous cyst, usually found on the face or scrotum.

Treatment

For milia, expression of the contents through a tiny stab incision is curative. For larger lesions, a small incision is made and the contents are evacuated; then the cyst wall is removed through the incision with a curette or hemostat. Surgical excision is also effective. Any large cyst may recur after treatment if the cyst wall is not completely removed. Infected cysts can be incised and drained; a gauze drain is inserted and gradually removed over 7 to 10 days. Oral antibiotics such as cloxacillin or erythromycin may be required.

---

236. SCALING PAPULAR DISEASES

PSORIASIS

A common chronic and recurrent disease characterized by dry, well-circumscribed, silvery, scaling papules and plaques of various sizes.

Psoriasis varies in severity from 1 or 2 lesions to a widespread dermatosis with disabling arthritis or exfoliation. The cause is unknown, but the thick scaling is probably due to increased epidermal cell proliferation. About 2 to 4% of the white population, and far fewer blacks, are affected. Onset is usually between ages 10 and 40, but no age is exempt. A family history of psoriasis is common and usually reflects an autosomal dominant inheritance. General health is not affected, except for the psychologic stigma of an unsightly skin disease, unless severe arthritis or intractable exfoliation develops.

Symptoms and Signs

Onset is usually gradual. The typical course is one of chronic remissions and recurrences (or occasionally acute exacerbations) that vary in frequency and duration. Factors precipitating psoriatic eruptions include local trauma (which causes the **Koebner phenomenon**, with lesions appearing at the trauma site) and, occasionally, severe sunburn, irritation, topical medications, chloroquine antimalarial therapy, and withdrawal of systemic corticosteroids. Some patients (especially children) may have explosive psoriatic eruptions after an acute URI.

Psoriasis characteristically involves the scalp (including the postauricular regions), the extensor surface of the extremities (particularly at elbows and knees), the back, and the buttocks. The nails, eyebrows, axillas, umbilicus, or anogenital region may also be affected. Occasionally the disease is generalized.

The lesions are sharply demarcated, usually nonpruritic, erythematous papules or plaques covered with overlapping, silvery or slightly opalescent, shiny scales. The lesions heal without scarring, and hair growth is not altered. Papules sometimes extend and coalesce, producing large plaques in bizarre annular and gyrate patterns. Nail involvement may resemble a fungal infection, with stippling, pitting, fraying or separation of the distal margin, thickening, discoloration, and debris under the nail plate.

Psoriatic arthritis (see in Ch. 108) often closely resembles RA and may be equally crippling, but the patient's serum contains no rheumatoid factor. In **exfoliative psoriatic**

dermatitis, which may be intractable and may lead to general debility, the entire skin is red and covered with fine scales; typical psoriatic lesions may be obscured at first. **Pustular psoriasis** is characterized by sterile pustules that may be localized to the palms and soles or may be generalized; typical psoriatic lesions are not always present.

Diagnosis

Diagnosis by inspection is rarely difficult. In psoriasis of the scalp, as elsewhere, the well-defined, dry, heaped-up, lesions with large silvery scales are usually not hard to distinguish from the diffuse, greasy, yellowish scaling of seborrheic dermatitis. However, psoriasis may be confused with seborrheic dermatitis, squamous cell carcinoma in situ (when on the trunk), secondary syphilis, fungal infections, cutaneous LE, eczema, lichen planus, or localized scratch dermatitis. In psoriasis, removal of the superficial scale typically shows tiny bleeding points (Auspitz sign).

Biopsy findings may be typical, but many other skin diseases may have psoriasis-like histologic features that make them difficult to distinguish.

Prognosis and Treatment

The prognosis depends on the extent and severity of the initial involvement, and usually the earlier in life it begins, the greater the severity. Acute attacks usually clear up, but complete permanent remission is rare. No therapeutic method assures a cure, but most cases can be well controlled.

The simplest forms of treatment—lubricants, keratolytics, and topical corticosteroids—should be tried first for a limited number of lesions because effective remedies are not numerous. Exposure to sunlight is recommended, though occasionally sunburn may induce exacerbations. Systemic antimetabolites such as methotrexate (see below) should be used only in severe skin or joint involvement. Systemic corticosteroids should *not* be used because of the side effects, which include severe exacerbations or pustular lesions that may occur during treatment (even with increasing doses) or after therapy has been stopped.

Lubricating creams, hydrogenated vegetable (cooking) oils, or white petrolatum are applied—alone or with added corticosteroids, salicylic acid, crude coal tar, or anthralin (dithranol)—bid while the skin is still damp after bathing. Alternatively, crude coal tar ointment or cream may be applied at night and washed off in the morning, followed by exposure to natural or artificial (280 to 320 nm) ultraviolet **(UV)** light in slowly increasing increments sufficient to produce mild erythema.

Anthralin can be effective as a cream or an ointment, beginning with 0.1% and increasing to 1% if tolerated. Anthralin may be irritating and should not be used in intertriginous areas. Anthralin stains sheets and clothing as well as the skin. A new "short contact" treatment with anthralin avoids many of its disadvantages: 20 to 30 min after it has been applied, the patient washes it off by bathing well.

Topical corticosteroids may be used as an alternative or adjunct to anthralin or coal tar treatment. As an adjunct they are used bid or tid during the day and anthralin or coal tar is used at bedtime. Corticosteroids are most effective when used under occlusive polyethylene coverings or incorporated in adhesive tape. This may be done overnight and a corticosteroid cream rubbed in without occlusion bid or tid during the day. The initial choice of concentration usually depends on the extent of involvement. As the lesions improve, the corticosteroid should be applied less frequently or in lower concentration in order to prevent local side effects (atrophy, telangiectasias). After about 3 wk, a bland ointment should be substituted for 1 to 2 wk to prevent loss of steroid effectiveness (tachyphylaxis). Triamcinolone acetonide 0.1% (or equivalent—see Ch. 228) is most effective, but is expensive; 1 oz (30 gm) of cream is usually needed to cover the entire body. The commercial preparation may be diluted in an appropriate vehicle: ointment in petrolatum, or cream in a vanishing cream base; commercial preparations of lower strength are also available. If potent fluorinated topical cortico-

steroids are applied to large areas of the body, especially under occlusion, systemic effects can be observed and psoriasis may be aggravated, as with systemic corticosteroids. For small, localized lesions, flurandrenolide-impregnated tape left on overnight and changed in the morning is effective. Relapse after topical corticosteroids is often faster than with other agents. Rest periods, as suggested above, may prevent relapses and unresponsiveness.

Thick scalp plaques may be difficult to treat. A suspension of 10% salicylic acid in mineral oil or, if available, plain soft soap (sapo mollis, not tincture of green soap) may be rubbed in at bedtime with a toothbrush and washed out the next morning with a cosmetically acceptable tar shampoo. A shower cap can be worn in bed to enhance penetration and to avoid messiness. Nonresidual corticosteroid alcoholic solutions can be applied during the day.

Resistant skin or scalp patches may respond to *local* superficial injection of triamcinolone acetonide suspension diluted with saline to 2.5 mg/mL, the amount depending on the size of the lesion. Injections should not be repeated more often than every 3 wk, and may cause local atrophy. Systemic corticosteroids are usually contraindicated.

Methotrexate taken orally is the most effective treatment in severe disabling psoriasis, especially severe psoriatic arthritis or widespread pustular or exfoliative psoriasis, that is unresponsive to topical agents or psoralens and high intensity ultraviolet A **(PUVA)** therapy (see below). Methotrexate seems to act by interfering with the rapid proliferation of epidermal cells. Because the potential toxicity requires monitoring hematologic, renal, and hepatic function and because dosage regimens vary, *methotrexate therapy should be undertaken only by physicians experienced in its use for psoriasis.*

PUVA is usually highly effective in treating extensive psoriasis. Oral methoxsalen (average dose 40 mg) is followed, at a specific interval, by exposure of the skin to long-wave UV light (330 to 360 nm). The dosage of both the methoxsalen and the UV exposure must be tailored to each patient. Although the treatment is clean and may produce remissions for several months, repeated treatments with intensive light may increase UV-induced skin cancer (especially in those with either prior arsenic or x-ray therapy or a history of skin cancers). With appropriate precautions, adverse effects on eyes and blood seem minimal. Using oral retinoids along with PUVA decreases the dosage of UV light required to induce remissions.

Etretinate or isotretinoin can be particularly effective for pustular psoriasis. Patients should be warned about getting pregnant while taking retinoids and for at least 2 yr after etretinate because of its teratogenic potential and long-term retention in the body. Other drugs, such as cyclosporine and other retinoids, are under investigation.

PITYRIASIS ROSEA

A self-limited, mild, inflammatory skin disease characterized by scaly lesions, possibly due to an unidentified infectious agent. It may occur at any age but is seen most frequently in young adults. In temperate climates, incidence is highest during spring and autumn.

Symptoms and Signs

A "herald" or "mother" patch, found most commonly on the trunk, usually precedes the generalized eruption by 5 to 10 days. It is slightly erythematous, rose- or fawn-colored, and circinate or oval; it has a scaly, slightly raised border and resembles a superficial ringworm infection. Many similar lesions 0.5 to 2 cm in diameter follow the herald patch and sometimes continue to appear for weeks. The lesions usually appear on the trunk. On the back, their long axes parallel the lines of cleavage, typically radiating from the spinal column in a "Christmas tree" pattern. In blacks the eruption may be primarily papular, with little scaling.

At times, lesions principally affect the arms, with relative sparing of the trunk. The face is involved occasionally. Rarely, lesions become generalized, sometimes giving a scarlatiniform appearance. Systemic symptoms are usually absent, but slight malaise and headache occur rarely, and itching is sometimes troublesome. Spontaneous remission within 4 or 5 wk is usual, though the eruption may persist for 2 mo or longer. Recurrences are rare.

Differential Diagnosis

Pityriasis rosea must be differentiated from tinea corporis, tinea versicolor, drug eruptions, psoriasis, and, most importantly, secondary syphilis. A serologic test for syphilis should be done routinely.

Treatment

There is no specific treatment, and usually no treatment is needed. The patient should be reassured that the lesions will clear. Artificial or natural sunlight may hasten involution. Inflamed, itching lesions may be relieved by 0.25% menthol in a vanishing cream base. Prednisone—10 mg orally qid until the itching subsides, then decreased over a 14-day period—should be used only when itching is severe.

LICHEN PLANUS

A recurrent, pruritic, inflammatory eruption characterized by small discrete angular papules that may coalesce into rough scaly patches, often accompanied by oral lesions. Children are affected infrequently.

Etiology

The cause is unknown. Some drugs (eg, arsenic, bismuth, gold) or exposure to certain color-photography developers may cause an eruption indistinguishable from lichen planus. Quinacrine taken for long periods may produce hypertrophic lichen planus of the lower legs as well as other dermatologic and systemic disturbances.

Symptoms and Signs

Onset may be abrupt or gradual. The initial attack persists for weeks or months, and intermittent recurrences may be noted for years.

The primary papules are 2 to 4 mm in diameter, with angular borders, a violaceous color, and a distinct sheen in cross-lighting. Rarely, bullae may develop. Moderate to severe, often refractory, itching may be present. The lesions are usually distributed symmetrically, most commonly on the flexor surfaces of the wrists and on the legs, trunk, glans penis, and oral and vaginal mucosa. Lesions are occasionally generalized, but the face is rarely involved. Particularly on the lower legs, the lesions may become large, scaly, and verrucous **(hypertrophic lichen planus).** During the acute phase, new papules may appear along a site of minor skin injury such as a superficial scratch (the **Koebner phenomenon**). Hyperpigmentation (and sometimes atrophy) may develop as lesions persist. Rarely, a patchy scarring alopecia of the scalp appears.

The oral mucosa is involved in about 50% of patients, often before cutaneous lesions develop. The cheek mucosa, tongue margins, and mucosa in edentulous areas show asymptomatic ill-defined, bluish-white linear lesions that may be reticulated at first and increase in size in an angular configuration. An erosive form may occur in which the patient complains of shallow, often painful, recurrent oral ulcerations. Longstanding ulcers may result in mouth cancers. Chronic exacerbations and remissions are common.

Diagnosis

Lichen planus is histologically distinctive. Persistent oral or vaginal lichen planus, with thickening and coalescence of the lesions, may sometimes be difficult to differen-

tiate clinically from leukoplakia. Though always indicated, biopsy may not yield specific findings in old lesions.

Widespread erosive oral lesions must be differentiated from those of candidiasis, leukoplakia, carcinoma, aphthous ulcers, herpetic stomatitis, and erythema multiforme. The peripheries of the lesions should be examined for short dendritic extensions and characteristic delicate bluish-white lacy lesions.

Treatment

Asymptomatic lichen planus does not require treatment. If a drug or chemical is suspected as the cause, its use should be discontinued. An antihistamine (eg, hydroxazine 25 mg or chlorpheniramine 4 mg orally qid) may decrease moderate itching through a sedative effect. Localized pruritic or hypertrophic areas may be treated with triamcinolone acetonide suspension diluted with saline to 2.5 to 5 mg/mL and superficially injected into the lesion, using enough to elevate the lesion slightly (not to be repeated more often than every 3 wk); or with occlusive corticosteroid therapy (eg, triamcinolone acetonide 0.1% cream or equivalent under polyethylene wrapping at bedtime, or flurandrenolide-impregnated tape). Tretinoin 0.1% solution with corticosteroids can also be beneficial in treating lichen planus on glabrous skin. It should be applied with a cotton-tipped applicator at night, followed by tid application of a full-strength corticosteroid cream (see Ch. 228). For erosive oral lesions, viscous lidocaine mouthwashes before meals should be tried.

Erosive oral lesions and widespread severely pruritic skin lesions often require a systemic corticosteroid; eg, oral prednisone 40 to 60 mg every morning initially, with the dose decreased by about one third each week. Unfortunately, itching may return after systemic prednisone has been stopped; in this case, a systemic corticosteroid in continued low dosage given every other morning may be tried. Retinoids (*see precautions above, under* P*SORIASIS*) have also been reported to be effective.

The disease tends to be self-limiting but may recur after years.

---

237. INFLAMMATORY REACTIONS OF THE SKIN

DRUG ERUPTIONS

(Dermatitis Medicamentosa)

An eruption of the skin or mucous membranes following oral or parenteral administration of a drug. (See also DRUG HYPERSENSITIVITY in Ch. 21 and ADVERSE DRUG REACTIONS in Ch. 277.)

Etiology

Many drug eruptions are due to allergic mechanisms: specific antibodies to the drug or specifically sensitized lymphocytes may develop during a sensitization period that may be as short as 4 or 5 days after initial drug exposure. A later exposure to the drug results in an eruption, which may appear within minutes or not for hours or days. Other reactions are of unknown mechanisms or are caused by accumulation of a drug (eg, pigmentation from silver), pharmacologic action of a drug (eg, striae or acne from systemic corticosteroids; purpura from excessive anticoagulation) or interaction with genetic factors (eg, porphyria cutanea tarda from estrogens, which induce an enzyme involved in porphyrin metabolism).

Symptoms and Signs

Drug eruptions vary in severity from a mild rash to toxic epidermal necrolysis. Onset may be sudden (eg, urticaria or angioedema after penicillin) or delayed for

hours or days (morbilliform or maculopapular eruptions following penicillin or sulfonamides) or even years (exfoliation or pigmentation from arsenic). The lesions may be localized (fixed drug eruptions, oral ulcerations, or dermatitis in light-exposed areas), but many are generalized.

Some drugs produce characteristic eruptions, but reactions may imitate features of practically any dermatosis. The most frequently seen patterns with some typical causative agents are listed below. The drugs added most recently are most likely to be the cause, but drugs that have been taken for long periods must also be suspected.

Urticaria (penicillin, aspirin, tartrazine [the dye FD&C yellow No. 5]) is easily recognized by the typical well-defined edematous wheals.

Morbilliform or maculopapular eruptions (almost any drug, especially barbiturates, sulfonamides, and antibiotics) range in appearance from measleslike to an eruption resembling pityriasis rosea.

Mucocutaneous eruptions (penicillin; barbiturates; sulfonamides, including derivatives used in hypertension and diabetes mellitus) vary from a few small oral vesicles or urticaria-like skin lesions to painful oral ulcerations with widespread bullous skin lesions (see ERYTHEMA MULTIFORME and the Stevens-Johnson syndrome, below).

Acneiform eruptions (corticosteroids, iodides, bromides) resemble acne but lack comedones and usually begin suddenly.

Toxic epidermal necrolysis (barbiturates, hydantoins, penicillin, sulfonamides) is characterized by large areas of loosened, easily detached epidermis that give the skin a scalded appearance (see TOXIC EPIDERMAL NECROLYSIS, below). It is often fatal. A similar condition in infants, young children, and immunosuppressed patients is caused by a specific staphylococcal infection (scalded skin syndrome; see Ch. 231).

Exfoliative dermatitis (penicillin, sulfonamides) is characterized by redness, scaling, and thickening of the entire skin surface; it, too, may be fatal (see in Ch. 230).

Photosensitivity eruptions (phenothiazines, tetracyclines, sulfonamides, chlorothiazide, artificial sweeteners) appear as areas of dermatitis or gray-blue hyperpigmentation (phenothiazines and minocycline) on skin exposed to the sun.

Fixed drug eruptions (phenolphthalein, tetracycline) are well-circumscribed, frequently isolated, dusky red or purple lesions on the skin or mucous membranes (especially of the genitals) that reappear at the same sites each time the drug is taken.

Lichenoid or lichen-planus-like eruptions (antimalarials, gold, chlorpromazine) are angular papules that coalesce into scaly patches (see LICHEN PLANUS in Ch. 236).

Purpuric eruptions (chlorothiazide, carbromal, meprobamate, anticoagulants, apronalide) are nonblanching purple macules that vary in size but are usually tiny. They are most common on the lower extremities but may occur anywhere and may indicate a more serious purpuric vasculitis.

Erythema nodosum (sulfonamides, oral contraceptives, iodides, bromides) is described in this chapter, below.

Diagnosis and Treatment

Identification of the causative agent is essential. A detailed history is often required, with persistent inquiry about *all* medications, including nonprescription drugs used for sleep, pain, colds, constipation, and headache, and the use of eyedrops, nosedrops, and suppositories. It is important to remember that some drug eruptions start *after* the drug has been stopped (eg, ampicillin), some continue for weeks or months after the drug is stopped, and minute amounts of some drugs may produce a reaction.

Most drug reactions resolve when the offending drug is stopped and require no further therapy. Often, and especially in hospitalized patients who take many drugs, all but life-sustaining medicines must be discontinued, and each reinstituted in order of importance at weekly intervals. A physician well versed in the incidence and types of

drug eruptions can frequently withhold the most likely offender and continue the other drugs. When medicines are necessary to the patient's health, chemically unrelated compounds should be substituted when possible.

No laboratory tests are yet available to aid diagnosis, although lymphocyte transformation and penicillin skin tests are under study. Sensitivity can be confirmed only by readministration of the drug, which may be hazardous.

A lubricant (eg, white petrolatum) may be used for a dry, itching maculopapular eruption. A topical fluorinated corticosteroid ointment (see Ch. 228) should also be applied in one small area qid and, if effective, applied to the entire eruption. Disabling acute urticaria may require aqueous epinephrine (1:1000) 0.2 mL s.c. or IM, or the slower-acting but more persistent soluble hydrocortisone 100 mg IV, which may be followed by oral corticosteroid for a short period. For treatment of some serious drug reactions, such as severe erythema multiforme or the Stevens-Johnson syndrome, see below.

TOXIC EPIDERMAL NECROLYSIS (TEN)

A life-threatening skin disease in which the epidermis peels off in sheets, leaving widespread denuded areas. It most often occurs in adults and usually represents a drug reaction or is idiopathic.

Etiology

In about 1/3 of cases, the etiology is a drug; sulfonamides, barbiturates, nonsteroidal anti-inflammatory agents, phenytoin, allopurinol, and penicillin have been associated with many cases, while numerous other drugs have been implicated in single cases. In about 1/3 of cases, the cause is unclear because of concomitant serious disease (eg, graft-versus-host disease) and treatment with drugs. In most of the remaining cases, the etiology is unknown.

Symptoms and Signs

TEN typically begins with painful localized erythema that disseminates rapidly. At the sites of erythema, flaccid blisters occur or the epidermis peels off. It may peel off in large sheets with gentle touching or pulling. Malaise, chills, myalgias, and fever accompany the denudation. Widespread areas of erosion, including all mucous membranes (eyes, mouth, genitalia) occur within 24 to 72 h and the patient may become gravely ill. Affected areas of skin often look like second-degree burns. Mortality is caused by fluid and electrolyte imbalance, multiorgan sequelae (eg, pneumonia, GI bleeding), and infection.

Diagnosis

Rapid diagnosis is important so that a possibly offending drug can be stopped. Before widespread erythema and epidermal denudation occur it may be difficult to distinguish TEN from other morbilliform drug eruptions or erythema multiforme and Stevens-Johnson syndrome. TEN is often thought to be a continuum of the latter two diseases. Although TEN closely resembles staphylococcal scalded skin syndrome (**SSSS**), differentiation from SSSS is facilitated by the patient's age, by the clinical setting, and by defining the level of the epidermal split by biopsy, as described under SSSS in Ch. 231.

Treatment

Patients should be hospitalized; excellent nursing care and close observation are essential. *Potentially responsible or suspected drugs should be stopped immediately.* Patients should be isolated to minimize exogenous infection and managed as those with severe burns (see also Ch. 254), by protecting the skin and denuded areas from trauma and infection and replacing fluid and electrolyte losses.

Though their use is controversial, systemic corticosteroids have been tried in stop-

ping "allergic" drug reactions. Some severe cases require from 0.5 to 1.0 gm of methylprednisolone IV for several days to reverse the process. This type of steroid therapy has been associated with many adverse effects and should be administered under well-controlled conditions. Corticosteroids often seem to enhance gram-negative or other sepsis (without improving the skin) and increase the mortality rate. Septicemia, which often occurs with pulmonary infections, must be recognized and treated promptly, for it is the most common cause of death. Ophthalmologic consultation is often required, as there may be considerable crusting of the conjunctiva. Urologic consultation may also be necessary in order to prevent phimosis.

ERYTHEMA MULTIFORME

(Erythema Multiforme Exudativum or Bullosum)

An inflammatory eruption characterized by symmetric erythematous, edematous, or bullous lesions of the skin or mucous membranes.

Etiology

No cause can be found in > 50% of cases. In the remainder, drugs and x-ray therapy are usually implicated in adults and infectious causes in children and young adults, including herpes simplex (probably the most commonly found etiologic agent), coxsackie- and echoviruses, *Mycoplasma pneumoniae*, psittacosis, and histoplasmosis. Vaccinia, BCG, and poliomyelitis vaccines have also induced erythema multiforme. Almost any drug can cause erythema multiforme; penicillin, sulfonamides, and barbiturates are the most common causes. The mechanism by which infectious agents or drugs cause the condition is unknown, but it apparently is a hypersensitivity reaction.

Symptoms, Signs, and Diagnosis

Onset is usually sudden, with erythematous macules or papules, or wheals, vesicles, and sometimes bullae, appearing mainly on the distal portion of the extremities, including the palms and soles, and on the face; hemorrhagic lesions of the lips and oral mucosa can also occur (see under ORAL ERYTHEMA MULTIFORME in Ch. 247). The skin lesions (target or iris lesions) are symmetric in distribution and often annular, with concentric rings and a central purpura—a grayish discoloration of the epidermis—or vesicle. Itching is variable. Systemic symptoms vary; malaise, arthralgia, and fever are frequent. Attacks that last 2 to 4 wk and recur in the fall and spring for several years are sometimes seen.

Stevens-Johnson syndrome is *a severe form of erythema multiforme characterized by bullae on the oral mucosa, pharynx, anogenital region, and conjunctiva.* Typical erythema multiforme lesions may or may not be present elsewhere on the skin. The patient may be unable to eat or close his mouth properly and drools continually. The eyes may become very painful, and conjunctivitis with swelling and pus may make it impossible for the patient to open them. The conjunctival lesions may leave residual corneal scarring. The condition is occasionally fatal.

The skin lesions of erythema multiforme must be distinguished from bullous pemphigoid and dermatitis herpetiformis; the oral lesions, from allergic stomatitis, pemphigus, and herpetic stomatitis.

Treatment

When a cause can be found, it should be treated, eliminated, or avoided. Some cases of erythema multiforme are associated with mycoplasmal pneumonia and should be treated with a tetracycline. Local treatment depends on the type of lesion. Simple erythema often needs no treatment. Vesicles and bullous or erosive lesions can be treated with intermittent tap-water compresses. Cheilitis and stomatitis of erythema multiforme may require special care (see ORAL ERYTHEMA MULTIFORME under STOMA-

TITIS in Ch. 247). Systemic corticosteroids (see DRUG ERUPTIONS, above, and Treatment, in ORAL ERYTHEMA MULTIFORME in Ch. 247) are not routinely used; however, they have been beneficial in severe and in chronic erythema multiforme. Their use is controversial. Some patients, especially those with severe mouth and throat lesions, seem to succumb more readily to fatal respiratory infections if treated with systemic corticosteroids. Intensive systemic antibiotics (as indicated by culture and sensitivity), fluids, and electrolytes may be life-saving in patients with extensive mucous membrane lesions. If frequent or severe erythema multiforme is preceded by herpes simplex, acyclovir 200 mg orally 3 or 5 times daily is effective in preventing most attacks, but its long-term effects are unknown.

PRURITIC URTICARIAL PAPULES AND PLAQUES OF PREGNANCY (PUPPP)

(See Ch. 177)

ERYTHEMA NODOSUM

An inflammatory disease of the skin and subcutaneous tissue characterized by tender red nodules, predominantly in the pretibial region but occasionally involving the arms or other areas.

The nodules gradually change from pink to bluish to brown, resembling a bruise. Fever and arthralgia are frequent, hilar adenopathy less frequent. The condition is most common in young adults and may recur for months or years.

Erythema nodosum in children is most commonly caused by URIs, especially from streptococci; in adults, streptococcal infections and sarcoidosis are the most common causes. Less common causes (except in locales where the underlying disease is endemic) include leprosy, coccidioidomycosis, histoplasmosis, primary tuberculosis, psittacosis, lymphogranuloma venereum, and ulcerative colitis. The condition can also be a reaction to drugs (sulfonamides, iodides, bromides, oral contraceptives). A prolonged search for systemic infection or causative drug may be required, and in many cases no cause can be determined. An elevated erythrocyte sedimentation rate is the most common laboratory finding.

Treatment

Bed rest is helpful for relief of painful nodules. Appropriate antibiotic therapy—eg, long-term (at least 1 yr) penicillin, if an underlying streptococcal infection is suspected—is beneficial. If symptoms are severe and there is no evidence of underlying infection or drug etiology, aspirin may be helpful, although the lesions often recur. Systemic corticosteroids, often the only means of controlling the lesions, reduce the lesions but may mask an underlying systemic disease.

GRANULOMA ANNULARE

A benign, chronic dermatosis of unknown etiology characterized by papules or nodules that spread peripherally to form a ring with normal or slightly depressed skin in the center. The lesions are yellowish or the color of the surrounding skin, and one or more may be present. They are usually asymptomatic and are usually present on the feet, legs, hands, or fingers. The condition may be seen in children or adults. It is not associated with systemic diseases, except that among adults with many lesions there is a statistically increased incidence of diabetes mellitus. In about 10% of cases, exposure to sunlight has brought out showers of lesions. Spontaneous resolution is common. In addition to reassurance and explanation of the benign nature of the disease, high-

strength topical corticosteroids under occlusion every night, corticosteroid-containing tape, or intralesional corticosteroids (see Ch. 228) may hasten involution of the disease.

238. BULLOUS DISEASES

PEMPHIGUS

An uncommon, potentially fatal skin disorder characterized by intraepidermal bullae on apparently healthy skin and mucous membranes.

Etiology and Incidence

Pemphigus usually occurs in middle-aged or older persons and is rare in children. It is an autoimmune disease; the serum and skin of patients in the active stage contain readily demonstrable IgG antibodies that bind at the site of epidermal damage. These antibodies can induce the same pathologic process in vivo and in vitro. Foci of high incidence of pemphigus occur in South America, especially Brazil.

Symptoms and Signs

Tense or flaccid bullae of varying sizes are the primary lesions. They frequently occur first in the mouth, where they soon rupture and remain as chronic, often painful, erosions for variable periods of time before the skin is affected. On the skin, the bullae characteristically arise from normal-appearing skin and leave a raw, denuded, and, later, crusted area when they rupture. The extent of both skin and mucosal involvement varies (eg, lesions may occur in the oropharynx and upper esophagus). Itching is usually absent.

In some superficial varieties of pemphigus (eg, pemphigus foliaceus), bullae may not be prominent and usually are not present in the mouth, and the process may resemble exfoliative dermatitis, psoriasis, a drug eruption, or many other forms of dermatitis. The lesions may be localized to the face and may suggest a combination of seborrheic dermatitis and cutaneous LE.

Diagnosis

Pemphigus should be suspected in any bullous disorder or chronic mucosal ulceration. It must be differentiated from all other chronic ulcerative oral lesions and from other bullous dermatoses such as bullous pemphigoid, benign mucosal pemphigoid, drug eruptions, toxic epidermal necrolysis, erythema multiforme, dermatitis herpetiformis, and bullous contact dermatitis. In pemphigus the epidermis is easily detached from the underlying skin **(Nikolsky's sign)** and biopsy usually shows typical suprabasal epidermal cell separation. In pemphigus foliaceus, the separation occurs within the superficial part of the epidermis. A Tzanck test (see SPECIAL DIAGNOSTIC METHODS in Ch. 227) is frequently diagnostic when one does a Wright's or Giemsa stain on a smear of cells obtained by scraping the base of a lesion. The acantholytic cells typically seen in pemphigus are unattached and basal-cell-like, with large centrally placed nuclei and condensed cytoplasm. Direct immunofluorescence **(IF)** tests of perilesional skin or mucous membranes are most reliable and invariably show I_gG on the epidermal or epithelial cell surfaces. Indirect IF tests usually show pemphigus antibodies in the patient's serum, even when the lesions are localized in the mouth. The antibody titer may correlate with the severity of the disease.

Treatment

Treatment depends upon the extent and severity of disease. The mainstay of therapy is systemic corticosteroids. Some patients with few lesions may respond to low doses of

prednisone (eg, 20 to 30 mg/day), but most patients ultimately require higher doses. Patients who do not have extensive disease may be treated as outpatients with a starting dose of 60 to 80 mg/day orally.

Hospitalization and large doses of corticosteroids are indicated for patients with widespread disease because the condition is potentially fatal if inadequately treated. The aim of treatment, both immediate and subsequent, is to stop the eruption of new lesions. The initial dosage of prednisone, 30 to 40 mg bid (or equivalent) orally, should be doubled if new lesions continue to appear after 5 to 7 days. Skin infections should be treated with systemic antibiotics. Reverse isolation procedures (see BARRIERS in Ch. 2) may be required. Generous use of talc on patient and sheets may prevent oozing skin from adhering to the sheets, or the new hydrocolloid dressings may be useful. Silver sulfadiazine cream can be used on erosions to prevent secondary infection.

Corticosteroid dosage should be decreased gradually when no new lesions have appeared for 7 to 10 days, with the total daily dose given every morning at first, then every other morning. The maintenance dose should be as low as possible. It may be possible, usually after months or years, to discontinue maintenance therapy if no new lesions appear during a trial period of several weeks without treatment. Methotrexate, cyclophosphamide, azathioprine, and IM gold have each been used successfully, either alone or with corticosteroids, to avoid the undesirable effects of long-term use of corticosteroids, but these drugs carry their own serious risks. Some authorities advocate using one of the above therapies at the same time that corticosteroids are started because they are thought to be "steroid sparing." Plasmapheresis combined with immunosuppressives, a therapy directed at reducing antibody titers, is under investigation.

BULLOUS PEMPHIGOID

A chronic, benign bullous eruption seen chiefly in the elderly. It is considered an autoimmune disease because antibodies directed against the basement membrane zone of the epidermis (the site of histologic damage) are usually found in the serum and skin.

Symptoms and Signs

Characteristic tense bullae develop on normal-appearing or reddened skin, sometimes accompanied by annular, dusky red, edematous lesions with or without tiny peripheral vesicles. Occasionally, rapidly healing oral lesions are seen. Itching is common, but there are usually no other symptoms. As in many other bullous diseases, subepidermal blisters may be found on biopsy.

Diagnosis

The disease must be differentiated from pemphigus, erythema multiforme, drug eruptions, benign mucosal pemphigoid, dermatitis herpetiformis, and acquired epidermolysis bullosa. Finding serum antibodies to the basement membrane zone on an *indirect* immunofluorescence **(IF)** test is diagnostic. Antibodies or complement, or both, are bound to the basement membrane zone of perilesional skin in the *direct* IF test.

Treatment

The eruption usually improves with prednisone 40 to 60 mg orally every morning. The dose can be tapered slowly to a maintenance level after several weeks. Occasional new lesions in the elderly should be disregarded (rather than increasing the prednisone dosage, as in pemphigus) because of the burden of side effects. In trials, the corticosteroid dosage has been reduced by giving azathioprine adjunctively.

DERMATITIS HERPETIFORMIS

A chronic eruption characterized by clusters of intensely pruritic vesicles, papules, and urticaria-like lesions.

This disease occurs mainly in patients 15 to 60 yr old, and rarely in blacks and Orientals. Several immunologic abnormalities have been demonstrated, including IgA deposits in almost all normal-appearing and perilesional skin. Asymptomatic gluten-sensitive enteropathy is found in 75 to 90% of patients and in some of their relatives.

Symptoms, Signs, and Diagnosis

Onset is usually gradual. Tiny vesicles, papules, and urticaria-like lesions appear, usually distributed symmetrically on extensor aspects (elbows, knees, sacrum, buttocks, occiput). Vesicles and papules are not uncommon on the face and neck. Itching and burning are severe, and scratching often obscures the lesions.

The typical histopathologic picture is seen only in early lesions and is characterized by microvesicle formation in the dermal papillary tips, which are infiltrated with neutrophils. Direct IF tests for IgA deposition in the dermal papillary tips in normal-appearing and perilesional skin are always positive and provide an important diagnostic aid.

Treatment

Dapsone 50 mg orally tid or qid usually relieves symptoms within 1 or 2 days and improves the rash; dramatic relief in itching is seen in 1 to 3 days. Up to 100 mg qid can be given by increasing the dose at weekly intervals if there is no improvement. Most patients can be maintained eventually on 50 to 150 mg/day. Although less effective, sulfapyridine may be used as an alternative; initial dosage is 2 to 4 gm/day orally and maintenance dosage is 1 to 2 gm/day. Strict adherence to a gluten-free diet for prolonged periods may be very effective in controlling the disease in some patients, obviating or reducing the patient's requirement for drug therapy.

Patients receiving dapsone or sulfapyridine should have a CBC weekly for 4 wk, then every 2 to 3 wk for 8 wk, and every 10 to 12 wk thereafter, since hematologic changes are the most common side effects. CNS or liver toxicity occurs rarely. If considerable hemolysis occurs or if the patient has significant cardiopulmonary problems due to dapsone therapy, sulfapyridine should be used, as usually it does not induce significant hemolysis.

HERPES GESTATIONIS

(See in Ch. 177)

239. DISORDERS OF CORNIFICATION

ICHTHYOSIS

(Dry Skin; Xeroderma)

Skin texture is genetically determined, and several ichthyotic skin diseases are inherited. Ichthyosis also is a symptom in several rare hereditary syndromes and occurs in several systemic disorders.

1. **Xeroderma,** the mildest form, is neither congenital nor associated with systemic abnormalities. It usually occurs on the lower legs of middle-aged or older patients, most often in cold weather and in patients who bathe frequently. There may be mild to moderate itching and an associated dermatitis due to detergents or other irritants.

2. The **inherited ichthyoses,** all characterized by excessive accumulation of scale on the skin surface, are classified according to clinical, genetic, and histologic criteria (see TABLE 239–1).

TABLE 239–1. CLINICAL AND GENETIC FEATURES OF SOME OF THE INHERITED ICHTHYOSES

Disorder	*Inheritance Pattern*	*Age at Onset*	*Type of Scale*	*Distribution*	*Associated Clinical Findings*	*Histology*
Ichthyosis vulgaris	Autosomal dominant	Childhood	Fine	Usually back and extensor surfaces; spares flexors; usually many markings on palms and soles	Atopy; keratosis pilaris	May be diagnostic*
X-linked ichthyosis	X-linked	Birth or infancy	Large, dark (may be fine)	Prominent on neck and trunk; normal palms and soles	Corneal opacities	May be diagnostic*
Lamellar ichthyosis (nonbullous congenital ichthyosiform erythroderma; "collodion baby")	Autosomal recessive	Birth	Large, coarse	Most of body; thick palms and soles	Ectropion	Diagnostic
Epidermolytic hyperkeratosis (bullous congenital ichthyosiform erythroderma)	Autosomal dominant	Birth	Thick, warty	Most of body; especially warty in flexural creases	Blisters	Diagnostic

* These patients have been shown to have a steroid sulfatase enzyme deficiency.

3. Ichthyosis is a characteristic of **Refsum's syndrome** (a hereditary ataxia with polyneuritic changes and deafness), and of **Sjögren-Larsson syndrome** (hereditary mental deficiency and spastic paralysis); both syndromes are autosomal recessive.

4. Asymptomatic ichthyosis occurs in some systemic diseases (eg, leprosy, hypothyroidism, lymphoma, AIDS) and may be an early manifestation. The dry scaling may be fine and localized to the trunk and legs, or it may be thick and widespread. In sarcoidosis, a thick scaling may appear on the legs and biopsy usually shows the typical granulomas. In other systemic diseases, biopsy of ichthyotic skin is not diagnostic.

Treatment

In any ichthyosis, an emollient—preferably plain petrolatum or mineral oil—should be applied bid and especially after bathing (for 10 min to hydrate the stratum corneum), while the skin is still wet. Blotting dry with a towel will then remove undesirable excess oil. An agent particularly effective in removing the scale in ichthyosis vulgaris, lamellar ichthyosis, and sex-linked ichthyosis contains 6% salicylic acid in a gel composed of propylene glycol, ethyl alcohol, hydroxypropylene cellulose, and water. It should be applied after hydration of the skin, bid plus at bedtime, and should be covered overnight with an occlusive dressing (eg, thin plastic film or bags). In children, it should be applied only bid and should not be occluded. After the scaling has decreased, only occasional application is required. Other useful agents include 50% propylene glycol in water, hydrophilic petrolatum and water (in equal parts), and cold cream and the α-hydroxy acids (eg, lactic and pyruvic) in various bases. In lamellar ichthyosis, 0.1% tretinoin (vitamin A acid; retinoic acid) cream is effective.

Soaps should be used only in intertriginous areas. Hexachlorophene products should not be used because absorption and toxicity are increased.

Patients with epidermolytic hyperkeratosis (bullous ichthyosis) may need long-term cloxacillin 250 mg orally tid or qid or oral erythromycin (same dosage), for as long as the thick intertriginous scaling is present, to prevent formation of painful and foul-smelling pustules. Regular use of soaps containing chlorhexidine may also reduce the bacteria. Lubrication may slightly improve ichthyosis due to an underlying systemic disease, but remarkable improvement follows if the primary disease can be corrected. The most effective therapies for most of the ichthyoses are the synthetic retinoids, given orally. Etretinate (see precautions under PSORIASIS in Ch. 236) is effective in epidermolytic hyperkeratosis, ichthyosis vulgaris, and X-linked ichthyosis. Isotretinoin is more effective than etretinate in lamellar ichthyosis. Long-term (1 yr or more) treatment with isotretinoin has resulted in bony exostoses in some patients, and other long-term side effects may arise. The lowest doses possible should be used. Newer derivatives that may be safer are being studied. (CAUTION: *Oral retinoids are absolutely contraindicated in pregnancy*.)

KERATOSIS PILARIS

A common disorder of keratinization in which the orifices of the hair follicles are filled with horny plugs. Multiple small, pointed keratotic papules appear mainly on the lateral aspects of the upper arms, thighs, and buttocks. They are most prominent in cold weather. The cause is unknown, the problem is chiefly cosmetic, and **treatment** is usually unnecessary, but hydrophilic petrolatum and water (in equal parts), cold cream, or petrolatum may be beneficial and, with 3% salicylic acid added, may help to flatten the lesions. The 6% salicylic acid gel described for the treatment of ichthyosis or the buffered lactic acid lotions may be very effective.

CALLUS; CORN

(Tyloma; Heloma)

Callus: *A superficial circumscribed area of hyperkeratosis at a site of repeated trauma.*
Corn: *A painful conical hyperkeratosis, found principally over toe joints and between toes.*

Calluses and corns are caused by pressure or friction, usually over a bony prominence. **Calluses** are usually found on the hands or feet but may occur elsewhere, especially in a person whose occupation entails repeated trauma to a particular area (eg, the mandible and clavicle in a violinist). **Corns** are pea-sized or slightly larger and occur on the feet. "Hard" corns occur over prominent protuberances, especially on the toes; "soft" corns occur between the toes. Corns may ache spontaneously or be tender on pressure.

Diagnosis

Calluses may be differentiated from plantar warts by trimming away the horny skin. A wart (see also in Ch. 234) will appear sharply circumscribed, sometimes with soft macerated tissue or with central black dots resulting from thrombosed capillaries, and paring it will cause pinpoint bleeding. A callus shows only heaped-up keratin, and skin markings are preserved. A corn, when pared, shows a sharply outlined translucent core that interrupts the normal papillary line.

Treatment

Prophylaxis is important. Completely eliminating undue pressure on the affected site may not be practicable, but pressure should be reduced and redistributed when possible. For foot lesions, soft, well-fitting shoes are important, and pads or rings of suitable shapes and sizes, moleskin or foam-rubber protective bandages, arch inserts, or metatarsal plates or bars may help to redistribute the pressure.

The hyperkeratotic tissue may be removed with keratolytic agents such as 20% salicylic acid in collodion or 40% salicylic acid plasters (taking care to avoid applying the agent to normal skin), or with a nail file. A pumice stone, used while the patient is in a bath, is often most practical. Salicylic acid plasters can be used on calluses anywhere.

Patients with a tendency to calluses and corns need the regular services of a podiatrist, and those with impaired peripheral circulation, especially if associated with diabetes mellitus, require special care (see under PERIPHERAL ATHEROSCLEROTIC DISEASE in Ch. 30).

---

240. DECUBITUS ULCER

(Bedsore; Pressure Sore; Trophic Ulcer)

Ischemic necrosis and ulceration of tissues overlying a bony prominence that has been subjected to prolonged pressure against an external object (eg, bed, wheelchair, cast, splint). It is seen most frequently in patients who have diminished or absent sensation, or are debilitated, emaciated, paralyzed (eg, from spinal cord injuries or degenerative neurologic diseases), or are otherwise long bedridden. Tissues over the sacrum, ischia, greater trochanters, external malleoli, and heels are especially susceptible but other sites may be involved, depending on the patient's position. Decubitus ulcers can affect not only superficial tissues, but also muscle and bone.

Etiology

Both intrinsic and extrinsic factors precipitate decubitus ulcers. **Intrinsic factors** include loss of pain and pressure sensations that ordinarily prompt the patient to shift position and relieve the pressure, and the thinness of fat and muscle padding between bony weight-bearing prominences and the skin. Disuse atrophy, malnutrition, anemia, and infection play contributory roles. In a paralyzed extremity, loss of vasomotor control leads to a lowering of tone in the vascular bed and a lowered circulatory rate. Spasticity, especially in patients with spinal cord injuries, can place a shearing force on the blood vessels to further compromise circulation.

The most important of the **extrinsic factors** is pressure. Its force and duration directly determine the extent of the ulcer. Pressure severe enough to impair local circulation can occur within hours in an immobilized patient, causing local tissue anoxia that progresses, if unrelieved, to necrosis of the skin and subcutaneous tissues. The pressure is due to infrequent shifting of the patient's position; friction and irritation from ill-adjusted supports or wrinkled bedding or clothing may be contributory. Moisture, which leads to tissue maceration, predisposes to decubitus. It may result from perspiration or from urinary or fecal incontinence.

Symptoms, Signs, and Course

The stages of decubitus ulcer formation correspond to tissue layers. The **1st stage** consists of skin redness that disappears on pressure; the skin and underlying tissues are still soft. The **2nd stage** shows redness, edema, and induration, at times with epidermal blistering or desquamation. In the **3rd stage,** the skin becomes necrotic, with exposure of fat. In the **4th stage,** necrosis extends through the skin and fat to muscle; further fat and muscle necrosis characterizes the **5th stage.** In the **6th stage,** bone destruction begins, with periostitis and osteitis, progressing finally to osteomyelitis, with the possibility of septic arthritis, pathologic fracture, and septicemia.

Prophylaxis

The best treatment for pressure sores is prevention. *Pressure on sensitive areas must be relieved.* Unless a full-flotation bed (water bed) is used, providing even distribution of the patient's weight through hydrostatic buoyancy, the bedridden patient's position must be changed at least q 2 h until tolerance for longer periods can be demonstrated (by the absence of redness). Air-filled alternating-pressure mattresses, sponge-rubber "egg-crate" mattresses, and silicone gel or water mattresses decrease pressure on sensitive areas but do not negate the need for position changes q 2 h. An operative turning (Stryker) frame facilitates turning patients with cord injuries. Protective padding (eg, sheepskin or a synthetic equivalent) at bony prominences should be used under braces or plaster casts, and at potential pressure sites a window should be cut out of the cast. A wheelchair patient must be able to shift his position every 10 to 15 min even if he is using a pressure-relieving pillow.

Skin inspection is important. Pressure points should be checked for erythema or trauma at least once/day in an adequate light. Able patients, mobile or immobile, and their families must be taught a routine of daily visual inspection and palpation of sites for potential ulcer formation. Exquisite skin care for neurologically damaged parts is necessary to prevent maceration and secondary infection. Lying on a sheepskin helps to keep the patient's skin in good condition and minimize decubiti. Protective padding, pillows, or a sheepskin can be used to keep body surfaces separated.

Maintaining **cleanliness and dryness** helps to prevent maceration. Bedclothes should be changed frequently, using sheets that are soft, clean, and free from wrinkles and particulate matter. Essential hygienic measures include sponging the skin in hot weather and thorough drying after baths.

Oversedation should be avoided and activity encouraged. Physiotherapy, when practicable, may be carried out by means of passive and active exercises. Hydrotherapy is

also valuable. The special activated mattresses mentioned above or ones filled with fluids or tiny spheres seem very useful but are expensive.

Treatment

A well-balanced diet, high in protein, is important. Blood transfusions may be needed for anemia.

Threatened decubitus (lst and 2nd stages) requires energetic use of all the above prophylactic measures to prevent tissue necrosis. The area should be kept exposed, free from pressure, and dry. Stimulating the circulation by gentle massage can accelerate healing. The major problem in treating decubitus ulcer is that the ulcer is like an iceberg, a small visible surface with an extensive unknown base, and there is no good method of determining the extent of tissue damage. Ulcers that have not advanced beyond the 3rd stage may heal spontaneously if the pressure is removed and the area is small. New hydrophilic gels and dressings speed healing.

Fourth stage ulcers require debridement; some may also require deeper surgery. When the ulcers are filled with pus and necrotic debris, application of dextranomer beads or other and newer hydrophilic polymers may hasten debridement without surgery. Conservative debridement of necrotic tissue with forceps and scissors should be instituted. Some debridement may be done by cleansing the wound with 1.5% hydrogen peroxide. Wet dressings of water (especially whirlpool baths) will assist in debriding. The granulation that follows removal of necrotic tissue may be satisfactory for skin grafts to cover small areas.

More advanced ulcers with fat and muscle involvement require surgical debridement and closure. Affected bone tissue requires surgical removal; disarticulation of a joint may be needed. A sliding full-thickness skin flap graft is the closure of choice, especially over large bony prominences such as the trochanters, ischia, and sacrum, since scar tissue cannot develop the tolerance to pressure that is needed.

For spreading cellulitis, a penicillinase-resistant penicillin or a cephalosporin is necessary.

Many new dressings and topical agents are being tested and made available for use. No one powder, gel, or dressing is universally superior. The subject is complex; ie, some are wet and lead to Pseudomonas infection if used too long, others are painful, all are expensive, and some are of little value. The doctor treating skin ulcers will need to be cautious and learn the specific properties and precise method of use of such agents.

241. PIGMENTARY DISORDERS

HYPOPIGMENTATION

A congenital or acquired decrease in melanin production.

Albinism: *A rare autosomal recessive inherited disorder in which melanocytes are present but do not form melanin.* The hair is white, the skin pale, and the eyes pink; nystagmus and errors of refraction are common. Albinos sunburn easily and frequently develop skin cancers. They should avoid sunlight, use sunglasses, and during daylight hours apply on uncovered skin a sunscreen with a sun protection factor of 15 **(SPF 15).**

Vitiligo: *An absence of melanocytes, causing hypopigmented areas, usually sharply demarcated and often symmetric, and varying from 1 or 2 spots to near universality.* The hair in vitiliginous areas is usually white, and the lesions are white under a Wood's light. Lesions are prone to sunburn. The cause is unknown; although vitiligo usually is acquired, it is sometimes familial (autosomal dominant, with incomplete penetrance

and variable expression) or may follow unusual physical trauma, especially of the head. The association of vitiligo with Addison's disease, diabetes mellitus, pernicious anemia, and thyroid dysfunction, as well as a high incidence of serum antibodies to thyroglobulin, adrenal cells, and parietal cells, has led to a postulated immunologic and neurochemical basis. Antibodies to melanin have been demonstrated in some patients. **Treatment** is for the cosmetic disfigurement. Small lesions may be camouflaged with cosmetic creams or the newly developed tanning solutions that do not wipe off on clothing as other cosmetics do and that may last for several days (Dy-O-Derm® is widely accepted). Sunscreens with SPF 15 protect against sunburn. Oral and topical psoralens with ultraviolet A **(UV-A)** have been used, but the treatment is protracted and results vary. Cover-up cosmetics are much more satisfactory for most patients where cure is doubtful.

Postinflammatory hypopigmentation follows healing of certain inflammatory disorders (especially bullous dermatoses), burns, and skin infections, and appears in scars and atrophic skin. The skin may not be ivory white as in vitiligo, and spontaneous repigmentation may eventually occur. Cover-up cosmetics or solutions are again most satisfactory.

HYPERPIGMENTATION

Hyperpigmentation due to deposition of melanin may be a manifestation of hormonal changes as in Addison's disease, pregnancy, or use of anovulatory pills. Darkening may also result from increased melanogenesis, as is seen in hemochromatosis, or from silver deposits, as are seen in argyria.

Melasma (chloasma), dark brown, sharply marginated, roughly symmetric patches of pigmentation on the face (usually on the forehead, temples, and malar prominences) occurs mainly during pregnancy **(melasma gravidarum, the "mask of pregnancy")** and in women taking anovulatory hormones. It may, rarely, occur idiopathically in dark-skinned men. Exposure to sunlight accentuates the pigmentation. In women, the darkening fades somewhat after childbirth, on cessation of the hormone, and with time. **Treatment** with 2% hydroquinone in an alcoholic glycol base applied bid may decrease the pigmentation. Hydroquinone should be tested behind one ear for a week before it is used on the face, since it may cause dermatitis or may lighten the skin too much. Sequential use of topical 0.1% tretinoin will enhance the effect of hydroquinone. The patient must use an SPF 15 sunscreen over the hyperpigmented areas when outdoors and should avoid excessive exposure to the sun if the bleaching is to work. Only melanosis can be lightened. Hemosiderin (dermal) pigmentation is unaffected. Long-term application (years) of hydroquinone has, rarely, caused local ochronosis.

---

242. DISORDERS OF SWEATING

MILIARIA
(Prickly Heat)

An acute inflammatory pruritic eruption due to retained extravasated sweat. Because of duct obstruction and inflammation, sweat fails to reach the surface, is trapped in the epidermis or dermis, and causes irritation (prickling) and, frequently, severe itching. The characteristic minute lesions are vesicular if obstruction is superficial **(miliaria crystallina)** or red if inflammation is deeper **(miliaria rubra).** Miliaria is usually seen in warm humid weather, but it may occur in cool weather if the patient is overdressed. Treatment is symptomatic and prophylactic, and includes cooling and drying the involved areas and avoiding conditions that may induce sweating. Air conditioning is

ideal. Corticosteroid lotions, sometimes with 0.25% menthol added, are often used, but any topical treatment is less effective than changing the environment and the clothing.

HYPERHIDROSIS

Excessive perspiration due to overactivity of the sweat glands. It may be general or confined to the palms, soles, axillas, inframammary regions, or groin. The skin in affected areas is often pink or bluish white. In severe cases, the skin, especially on the feet, may be macerated, fissured, and scaling. The exudate may be malodorous **(bromhidrosis);** the fetid odor is caused by decomposition of the sweat and cellular debris by bacteria and yeasts.

Increased hydration of the skin may be a contributing factor in various skin diseases (fungal or pyogenic infections; contact dermatitis). Generalized hyperhidrosis frequently accompanies fever. An endocrine dysfunction (eg, hyperthyroidism) or, occasionally, a CNS disorder may also cause generalized sweating. The cause of localized hyperhidrosis is unknown; it usually occurs in otherwise normal individuals. Excessive sweating of the palms and soles may be psychogenic.

Treatment

For generalized hyperhidrosis, the underlying systemic disease must be treated. The hyperhidrosis may be refractory. Side effects make parasympatholytic agents impractical, and sympathectomy usually has only a temporary effect.

For localized hyperhidrosis, aluminum chloride as a 20% solution of aluminum chloride hexahydrate in absolute ethyl alcohol, applied at night to the dried axilla, palms, or soles and covered tightly with a thin polyethylene film, is usually effective. In the morning, the polyethylene film is removed and the area is washed free of salt. Two applications usually protect the area for 1 wk. A 5% solution of methenamine (available in some countries) in water may also be effective.

Bromhidrosis often responds readily to treatment. Scrupulous cleanliness is essential. Daily bathing with a liquid soap containing chlorhexidine and application of an aluminum chlorhydroxy complex preparation is usually adequate. Shaving the axillary hair may be necessary. Extreme axillary hyperhidrosis, especially when accompanied by bromhidrosis, may be relieved by excising the concentrated group of glands in the axillary vault if the anhydrous aluminum chloride treatment fails.

---

243. BENIGN TUMORS

WARTS

(See in Chs. 14 and 234)

KERATINOUS (SEBACEOUS) CYSTS

(See in Ch. 235)

MOLES

(Pigmented, Nevocytic, or Nevus-Cell Nevi)

Circumscribed pigmented macules, papules, or nodules composed of clusters of melanocytes or nevus cells.

Moles may be small or large; flesh-colored, yellow-brown, or black; flat or raised; smooth, hairy, or warty; and broad-based or pedunculated. Practically every human has a few moles. Most appear in childhood or adolescence. During adolescence and pregnancy, more moles may appear and existing ones may enlarge and darken.

About 40 to 50% of malignant melanomas (see also MALIGNANT MELANOMA in Ch. 244) arise from melanocytes in moles; the rest arise from melanocytes in normal skin. The very rare malignant melanomas of childhood arise from large, pigmented moles that are present at birth. Halo nevi usually resolve spontaneously but very rarely are melanomas.

Classification

A **lentigo** is a flat, uniformly pigmented, brown to black spot that is due to an increased number of melanocytes at the epidermodermal junction. Lentigines are darker, sparser, and more scattered than freckles, and do not darken or multiply with sun exposure.

Junctional nevi are usually flat but may be slightly elevated. Light brown to nearly black and from 1 mm to 1 cm in size, they result from clustering of melanocytes at the epidermodermal junction. Moles on the palms, soles, and genitalia are usually junctional.

Compound nevi are usually dark and may be slightly or considerably elevated. Nests of melanocytes occur at the epidermodermal junction and within the dermis.

Intradermal nevi are elevated, flesh-colored to black, and may be smooth, hairy, or warty. Both melanocytes and nevus cells are found, almost entirely confined to the dermis.

Halo nevi are pigmented moles, usually compound or intradermal nevi, surrounded by a ring of depigmented skin.

Dysplastic nevi (see also below) are irregular, pigmented lesions, ranging from tan to dark brown on a pink background.

Treatment

Since moles are extremely common and melanomas uncommon, it is not justifiable to remove moles prophylactically. However, a mole should be excised and examined histologically if it enlarges suddenly (especially with an irregular border), becomes darker or inflamed, shows spotty color changes, begins to bleed, ulcerates, or becomes painful or pruritic. If the mole is too large for simple complete excision, it should be biopsied deeply enough to make an accurate microscopic diagnosis. Extensive surgery—eg, wide primary excision—is inappropriate before an accurate microscopic diagnosis, since many lesions are misdiagnosed clinically as melanomas. Simple excision or biopsy does not increase the likelihood of metastasis should the lesion prove malignant, and it avoids unnecessary destructive procedures for benign lesions.

Moles can be removed for cosmetic purposes without fear of subsequent malignant changes, but all moles removed should be examined histologically. A hairy mole should be excised completely to prevent hair regrowth.

DYSPLASTIC NEVI

Acquired pigmented lesions that are irregular and ill-defined, with both macular and papular components.

Etiology

Dysplastic nevi can be **inherited** as an autosomal dominant trait or may be **sporadic** (ie, occurring with no dysplastic nevi detected in family members). The presence of multiple dysplastic nevi in 2 or more family members has been termed **dysplastic nevus syndrome.**

Symptoms and Signs

Dysplastic nevi, first recognized because of their unusual appearance and increased frequency in certain families, typically measure 5 to 12 mm in diameter and are larger than common moles (see above). Their color is variegated, ranging from tan to dark

brown on a pink background. Although they may appear anywhere on the body, their relatively more frequent occurrence on covered areas, such as buttocks, breast, and scalp, differs from the distribution of common moles. Most individuals have about 10 common moles, but individuals with dysplastic nevi may have > 100 lesions. Common nevi usually have appeared by early adult life, but dysplastic nevi continue to appear even after age 35.

Diagnosis

The entire skin, including the scalp, of the patient suspected of having one or more dysplastic nevi should be examined, and one or more atypical-appearing lesions should be biopsied. A family history should be obtained with special reference to moles and melanomas or other skin cancer. If this history suggests melanoma, first-degree relatives should also be examined for melanoma and dysplastic nevi. Persons with dysplastic nevi who are from melanoma-prone families—ie, families with 2 or more first-degree relatives having cutaneous melanomas—have a high lifetime risk of developing melanomas that arise within dysplastic nevi (evidence suggests that melanomas can arise directly from dysplastic nevi) or de novo in presumably normal skin. It is not known whether the risk of melanoma is increased in individuals who have dysplastic nevi and no family history of melanoma.

Accurate diagnosis of dysplastic nevus depends upon histologic confirmation of a biopsy deep enough to reveal the depth of the lesion.

Treatment

Lesions suggesting dysplastic nevi or early melanoma should be excised. The decision to excise such lesions is influenced by their color and progression (see MOLES, above). Patients with dysplastic nevi should avoid excessive sun exposure and use sun screens with an SPF of 15 (see in Ch. 241); they should be taught self-examination, to detect changes in existing nevi. Excellent color photographs of most of the patient's body should be taken for use in regular, complete follow-up examinations, to determine changes in individual lesions. Using photographs in this manner has been reported to reduce the mortality from melanomas.

SKIN TAGS

(Acrochordons)

Common soft, small, flesh-colored or hyperpigmented pedunculated lesions, usually multiple and occurring mainly on the neck, axilla, and groin. They are usually asymptomatic but may become irritated. **Treatment** by freezing with liquid nitrogen or cutting with a scalpel or scissors may be performed if the tags are irritating or for cosmetic reasons.

LIPOMAS

Soft, movable, subcutaneous nodules with normal overlying skin. Patients may have one or many lesions. They occur much more frequently in women than in men, and appear most commonly on the trunk, back of the neck, and forearms. They are rarely symptomatic, but pain may occur. **Diagnosis** is usually made clinically, but a biopsy should be performed if there is rapid growth of a lesion. Rarely, lipomas become malignant. **Treatment** is not usually required, but lesions may be surgically excised or removed by "liposuction" if they are bothersome.

ANGIOMAS

(Hemangioma; Vascular Nevus; Lymphangioma)

Localized vascular lesions of the skin and subcutaneous tissues, rarely of the CNS, that result from hyperplasia of blood or lymph vessels.

Angiomas are usually either congenital or appear shortly after birth and occur in

about a third of newborn infants. Most disappear spontaneously **(immature hemangiomas)**, but some persist and create cosmetic problems. Complications may follow overtreatment, post-traumatic ulceration, or localized tissue hypertrophy from a persistent angioma of the CNS (see ARTERIOVENOUS MALFORMATIONS under VASCULAR DISORDERS in Ch. 130), the face, or an extremity.

Classification and Treatment

Congenital hemangiomas may be classified as follows:

1. Nevus flammeus (portwine stain) is a flat, pink, red, or purplish lesion present at birth and due to vascular ectasia. These lesions are very commonly present in the nuchal area. Nevus flammeus of the trigeminal area may be a component of the **Sturge-Weber syndrome** (leptomeningeal angiomatosis with intracranial calcification). A nevus flammeus usually will not fade, though splotchy small red macular lesions in the area above the nose and on the eyelids may disappear in a few months. For **treatment,** carbon dioxide, argon, and other lasers and infrared beams are being used with fairly good results in some cases. A nevus flammeus can usually be hidden with an opaque cosmetic cream prepared by a cosmetician to match the patient's skin color.

2. Capillary hemangioma (strawberry mark) is a raised, bright red lesion that develops shortly after birth and consists of proliferations of endothelial cells. It tends to enlarge slowly during the first several months of life and usually involutes spontaneously within 2 to 5 yr. Regression is usually complete, but at times a brownish pigmentation and scarring or wrinkling of the skin remains. Since spontaneous regression is the usual course, **treatment** is not indicated, except when a lesion on or near the eye or a body orifice (eg, urethra, anus) might interfere with function. When treatment is required, prednisone 10 mg orally bid or tid should be given as soon as possible and for at least 2 wk. If resolution starts, the prednisone should be decreased slowly; if not, it should be stopped. Surgical excision, laser excision, electrocoagulation, injection of sclerosing solutions, or application of dry ice is used, but often leaves more scarring than would spontaneous resolution.

3. Cavernous hemangioma is a raised red or purplish lesion composed of large vascular spaces. The blood vessels and frequently the lymphatics are often mature, in which case the lesion may contain numerous arteriovenous shunts and vascular malformations. Cavernous hemangiomas rarely involute spontaneously. Partial involution may follow ulceration, trauma, or hemorrhage. **Treatment** must suit the type of lesion. Occasionally, in children, systemic prednisone (as for a capillary hemangioma) may induce spontaneous resolution. Surgical excision may be considered, especially if it is causing increased growth of an extremity. Small surface nodules may be excised individually or destroyed by electrocoagulation.

Spider angioma (vascular spider) is a bright red, faintly pulsatile lesion consisting of a central arteriole with slender branches that extend outward like spider legs. Compression of the central vessel temporarily obliterates the lesion. Vascular spiders are not congenital. Single or small numbers of these lesions may be seen in children or adults and are unrelated to internal disease. Most patients with hepatic cirrhosis also develop many vascular spiders that may become quite prominent. Many women develop lesions during pregnancy or while taking oral contraceptives. As they are asymptomatic and usually resolve spontaneously about 6 to 9 mo postpartum or after discontinuing oral contraceptives, treatment is not usually required. If the lesions do not resolve spontaneously or **treatment** is required for cosmetic purposes, the central arteriole can be destroyed with fine needle electrodesiccation. Lasers are also being used, but the superiority of the cosmetic results with this method has not been established.

Lymphangiomas are elevated lesions composed of dilated and cystic lymphatic ves-

sels, usually yellowish tan but occasionally reddish if small blood vessels are intermingled. Puncture of the lesion yields a colorless fluid. **Treatment** consists of deep excision.

PYOGENIC GRANULOMA

(Granuloma Telangiectaticum)

A bright red, brown, or blue-black vascular nodule composed of proliferating capillaries in an edematous stroma. The term "pyogenic granuloma" is a misnomer because the lesion is neither of bacterial origin nor a true granuloma, but, rather, granulation tissue. The lesion develops rapidly, often at the site of recent injury, and probably represents a vascular and fibrous response to injury. It must be differentiated from a melanoma or other malignant tumor, which it often resembles. There is no sex or age predilection. The overlying epidermis is thin, and the lesion tends to be friable, bleeds easily, and does not blanch on pressure. The base may be pedunculated and surrounded by a collarette of epidermis. During pregnancy, pyogenic granulomas may become large and exuberant—eg, gingival pregnancy tumors **(telangiectatic epulis).** Pyogenic granulomas sometimes involute spontaneously; if not, a biopsy should be done. **Treatment** consists of removal by excision or electrodesiccation. The lesions may recur.

SEBORRHEIC KERATOSES

(Seborrheic Warts; Senile Warts)

Pigmented superficial epithelial lesions that are usually warty but may occur as smooth papules. The cause is unknown. They occur commonly in middle-aged or older patients and most often on the trunk or temples, though in blacks, especially women, they frequently occur on the malar part of the face **(dermatosis papulosa nigra).** Seborrheic keratoses vary in size and grow slowly. Round or oval and flesh-colored, brown, or black, they usually appear "stuck on" and may have a waxy, scaling, or crusted surface. They are not premalignant, and need no **treatment** unless they are irritated, itchy, or cosmetically bothersome. Curettage with or without electrodesiccation after local injection of lidocaine 1%, or freezing with liquid nitrogen or CO_2 snow, removes the lesions with little or no scarring.

DERMATOFIBROMA

(Fibrous Histiocytoma)

A firm, red to brown, small papule or nodule composed of fibroblastic tissue and usually found on the lower legs. Dermatofibromas are common and are usually solitary and asymptomatic, but may be multiple and may or may not itch. Their cause is unknown. **Treatment,** by excision under local anesthesia, is unnecessary unless there are symptoms—irritation, erosion, sudden enlargement, or other change in surface characteristics.

KERATOACANTHOMA

A round, firm, usually flesh-colored lesion with a characteristic central crater containing keratinous material. Onset is rapid, and within 1 or 2 mo the lesion reaches its full size, which may exceed 5 cm. Common sites are the face, forearm, and dorsum of the hand. Spontaneous involution usually starts within a few months, but may result in scarring. This lesion is sometimes difficult to differentiate clinically and histologically from squamous cell carcinoma. If the diagnosis is certain and the patient can be observed frequently, no **treatment** may be necessary; but if there is any doubt, a lengthwise through-and-through midline biopsy should be done. Because the lesion involutes with scarring, surgical treatment may yield better cosmetic results.

KELOID

A smooth overgrowth of fibroblastic tissue that arises in an area of injury or, occasionally, spontaneously. Keloids are shiny, smooth, often dome-shaped, and slightly pink. They tend to appear on the upper back and chest and on the deltoid area, and may be seen as a consequence of severe acne in these sites. Keloids are more frequent in blacks. **Treatment** with a corticosteroid (eg, triamcinolone acetonide 40 mg/mL, in amounts up to 20 mg/lesion) injected into the base of the lesion monthly via a Luer-Lok syringe or by jet injection may flatten the keloid but is often ineffective. Surgical or laser excision followed by intralesional injection of the wound with a corticosteroid can also be tried.

244. MALIGNANT TUMORS

Skin cancers such as basal cell and squamous cell carcinoma are among the most common malignancies and are usually curable. Most of these tumors arise in sun-exposed areas of skin. The incidence is highest in outdoor workers, sportsmen, and sunbathers, and is related to the amount of melanin pigment in the skin; light-skinned persons are most susceptible. Such tumors may also develop years after x-ray or radium burns or arsenic ingestion.

Less common malignancies include malignant melanoma, Paget's disease of the nipple or extramammary Paget's (usually near the anus), Kaposi's hemorrhagic sarcoma, and cutaneous T cell lymphoma (mycosis fungoides—see in Ch. 102). For different reasons, some of these malignancies are increasing at alarming rates.

BASAL CELL CARCINOMA
(Rodent Ulcer)

Basal cell carcinomas may appear as small, shiny, firm nodules; ulcerated, crusted lesions; flat, scar-like indurated plaques; or lesions difficult to differentiate from psoriasis or localized dermatitis. Most commonly the carcinoma begins as a small shiny papule, enlarges slowly, and, after a few months, shows a shiny, pearly border with telangiectasias, and a central dell or ulcer. Recurrent crusting or bleeding is not unusual, and the lesion continues to enlarge slowly. Basal cell carcinomas rarely metastasize, but may cause trouble and, rarely, death by invading or impinging on underlying vital structures or orifices (eyes, ears, mouth, bone, dura mater).

Treatment should be by a specialist after the mandatory biopsy and histologic examination. The clinical appearance, size, site, and histologic findings determine choice of treatment—electrodesiccation and curettage, surgical excision, or occasionally x-ray therapy. Recurrences (about 5%) are treated with Moh's chemosurgery (microscopically controlled excision of the tissue). Topical fluorouracil is now known to be associated with extensive dermal spread under a healed epidermis and should *not* be used for local treatment of cancer.

SQUAMOUS CELL CARCINOMA

Squamous cell carcinomas arise from the malpighian cells of the epithelium. Most appear on sun-exposed areas, but they may occur anywhere on the body. A squamous cell carcinoma may develop in normal tissue or in a preexisting **actinic keratosis** or patch of leukoplakia. The tumor begins as a red papule or plaque with a scaly or crusted surface. It may then become nodular, sometimes with a warty surface. In some, the bulk of the lesion may lie below the level of the surrounding skin. Eventually it

ulcerates and invades the underlying tissue. About 1/3 of lingual or mucosal lesions have metastasized before they have been diagnosed.

A biopsy is essential. **Treatment** is as for basal cell carcinoma. Squamous cell carcinoma on the lip or other mucocutaneous junction should be excised; at times it is difficult to cure, but in general the prognosis for small lesions removed early and adequately is excellent. Recurrences should be treated with Moh's chemosurgery as with basal cell carcinoma.

Bowen's disease (intraepidermal squamous cell carcinoma) is a superficial squamous cell carcinoma in situ. The lesion is solitary or multiple and resembles a localized patch of psoriasis, dermatitis, or dermatophyte infection. It is red-brown and scaly or crusted, with little induration. **Treatment** is as for basal cell carcinoma. Topical therapy with fluorouracil is not curative except for mucosal superficial penile lesions.

Bowen's disease of the genitals may be associated with human papilloma virus and is thus infectious. It may lead to cervical or other urogenital infections and subsequent cancers (see GENITAL WARTS in Ch. 14).

MALIGNANT MELANOMA

(Melanoma)

A malignant tumor of melanocyte origin. Melanomas are increasing in frequency. Malignant melanomas arise in areas of the skin, mucous membranes, eye, and CNS where pigment cells occur. They appear in different sizes, shapes, and colors (most commonly pigmented), and vary in propensity for invasion and metastasis. Thus, malignant melanoma may be a highly malignant tumor that spreads so rapidly it is fatal within months of its recognition, while in some forms the 5-yr cure rate is nearly 100%. Early suspicion by inspection and an adequate biopsy for histologic determination of tumor thickness are the only means of effective management and an optimum prognosis.

Because the incidence of melanoma is increasing rapidly and early diagnosis and cure depend upon the patient's consulting a physician early, vigorous campaigns to alert the public are underway in Australia and several of the "Sun-Belt" states in the USA.

Most malignant melanomas arise from melanocytes in normal skin; about 40 to 50% develop from pigmented moles (see also MOLES and DYSPLASTIC NEVI in Ch. 243). Danger signals that suggest malignant transformation of pigmented nevi include changes in size; color, especially spread of pigmentation to surrounding normal skin and red, white, and blue colors; surface characteristics; consistency; shape; or surrounding skin, especially with signs of inflammation. Although melanomas are more common in pregnant than in nonpregnant women, pregnancy does not increase the likelihood that a mole will become a melanoma. Metastasis to the fetus is rare. Malignant melanomas are very rare in children, but can arise from very large pigmented moles (giant congenital nevi) that have been present from birth.

Types, Symptoms, and Signs

Four major types of melanoma have been described. There is, however, little clinical significance as far as prognosis is concerned, since prognosis largely depends upon the histologically determined thickness of the melanoma.

1. Lentigo-maligna melanoma arises from lentigo maligna (Hutchinson's freckle), which appears on the face or other sun-exposed areas in elderly patients as an asymptomatic, large (2 to 6 cm), flat, tan or brown macule with darker brown or black spots scattered irregularly on its surface. In lentigo maligna (malignant melanoma-in-situ), both the normal and malignant melanocytes are confined to the epidermis, whereas in lentigo-malignant melanoma, the malignant melanocytes invade the dermis. After vari-

able periods, about 1/3 of lentigo malignas develop a progressive malignant focus with cells invading the dermis; therefore, early excision—before the lesion is very large—is recommended. Most other treatment methods usually do not include the depths of the follicles that are involved and must be removed.

2. Superficial spreading melanoma accounts for 2/3 of all melanomas. It is initially much smaller than the lentigo-maligna melanoma, is usually asymptomatic, and occurs most commonly on the legs in women and on the torso in men. Consultation is sought because the patient notes enlargement or irregular coloration of the lesion. It usually appears as a plaque with raised, indurated edges, and often shows red, white, and blue spots or small, sometimes protuberant, blue-black nodules. Small indentations may be noted on the surface. Histologically the lesion is characterized by atypical melanocytes invading the dermis and epidermis.

3. Nodular melanoma comprises 10 to 15% of all melanomas. It may occur anywhere on the body and is seen in patients in their 20s to 60s. It also is asymptomatic, unless it ulcerates. Consultation is usually sought because dark, protuberant papules or a plaque rapidly enlarges, often with little radial growth. Colors vary from pearl to gray to black. Occasionally, a nodular melanoma contains little if any pigment.

4. Acrolentiginous melanoma is uncommon. It arises on palmar, plantar, and subungual skin and has a characteristic histologic picture similar to lentigo-maligna melanoma.

Differential Diagnosis

Many lesions colored by melanin pigment or blood can be mistaken for malignant melanomas. Pigmented basal cell carcinoma, seborrheic keratosis, dysplastic nevus (see DYSPLASTIC NEVI in Ch. 243), blue nevus, dermatofibroma, all types of moles, hematomas (especially on the hands or feet), venous lakes, pyogenic granulomas, and warts are among the most common lesions confused with melanomas. If doubt exists, an excisional biopsy (or, if impossible because of the size or site of the lesion, incisional biopsy) should be performed. The biopsy should include the full depth of the dermis and extend slightly beyond the edges of the lesion. This enables the pathologist, by doing step sections, to determine the maximal thickness of the melanoma. Definitive radical surgery should not be performed before obtaining a histologic diagnosis.

Diagnostic Criteria

Guidelines for selecting those pigmented lesions that need to be excised or biopsied include recent enlargement, darkening, bleeding, or ulceration. These features, however, usually indicate that the melanoma has already invaded the skin deeply. Earlier diagnosis is possible if biopsies can be obtained from lesions having (1) variegated colors—eg, brown or black with shades of red, white, or blue, (2) irregular elevations that are either visible or palpable, and (3) irregular borders with angular indentations or notches.

Histologic assessment: Therapy and prognosis largely depend on histologic criteria that define the maximum thickness of the melanoma measured histologically with an optical micrometer. Adequate biopsy specimens are necessary for histologic grading—biopsy should be excisional for small lesions and incisional for larger lesions. Melanomas arising in the CNS and subungual melanomas are not classifiable by these systems.

The degree of lymphocytic infiltration, which represents the patient's immunologic defense system, may correlate with the level of invasion. Lymphocytic infiltration is maximal in the most superficial lesions; it decreases with deeper levels of tumor cell invasion.

Prognosis and Treatment

The clinical type of tumor is less important to the survival rate than the thickness of the tumor at the time of diagnosis. Thickness is determined by measuring the depth of invasion of melanoma cells from the granular cell layer. Thus, for example, as indicated in TABLE 244–1, no metastases or recurrences have been found with tumors < 0.76 mm thick that show no signs of histologic regression.

Metastasis of malignant melanoma occurs via both lymphatics and blood vessels. Local metastasis results in the formation of satellite papules or nodules that may or may not be pigmented. Direct metastasis to skin or internal organs may occur, and occasionally metastatic nodules are discovered before the primary lesion is identified. Melanomas arising from mucous membranes have a poor prognosis even though they seem quite limited when first discovered.

Treatment of malignant melanoma is not yet standardized, but is becoming more rational as new data on grading of lesions accumulates. **Lentigo-maligna melanoma** and its premalignant precursor, lentigo maligna, are usually treated with wide local excision and, if necessary, with skin grafting. Intensive x-ray therapy is much less effective than surgery. **Nodular** or **spreading melanomas** are usually treated by wide local excision extending down to the fascia. Lymph node dissection is usually recommended only when there is node enlargement.

Patients with thick melanomas and those with regional (Stage II) or distant (Stage III) metastasis may benefit from consultation with experts in newer forms of therapy. Chemotherapy with dacarbazine (DTIC) or the nitrosoureas (BCNU, CCNU) are being used with limited success. Cis-platinum and others are currently under study. Results using BCG vaccine to alter the patient's immune response have been discouraging, but newer forms of immunotherapy are promising. Vaccines using melanoma antigen are being studied to measure the patient's antibody response and for possible therapy.

PAGET'S DISEASE OF THE NIPPLE AND EXTRAMAMMARY PAGET'S DISEASE

A rare type of carcinoma that appears as a unilateral dermatitis of the nipple and represents extension to the epidermis of an underlying mammary duct carcinoma. The redness, oozing, and crusting closely resemble dermatitis, but the physician should suspect carcinoma because the lesion is unilateral. Biopsy of the lesion shows typical histologic changes. Paget's disease also occurs at other sites, most often in the groin or perianal area (extramammary Paget's disease). An underlying carcinoma should be sought in all cases. Most cases of extramammary Paget's disease are now thought to arise from apocrine glands. **Treatment** is determined by the surgeon; mastectomy is usual for lesions of the nipple.

TABLE 244–1. MALIGNANT MELANOMA—RATE OF METASTASIS AS A FUNCTION OF THICKNESS

Depth of Invasion	*Metastasis*
<0.76 mm	0%
0.76–1.5 mm	33%
1.51–2.25 mm	32%
2.26–3.0 mm	69%
>3.0 mm	84%

MYCOSIS FUNGOIDES

(See in Ch. 102)

KAPOSI'S HEMORRHAGIC SARCOMA (KS)

(Multiple Idiopathic Hemorrhagic Sarcoma)

A neoplasm characterized by vascular skin tumors that may appear in 3 distinctive forms. KS lesions originate from multifocal sites in the mid-dermis and extend to the epidermis. Histopathology shows spindle cells and vascular structures admixed to various degrees. The cell of origin in many cases is the endothelial cell shown by specific staining for factor VIII; the tumor cells resemble smooth muscle cells, fibroblasts, and myofibroblasts. An **indolent form** of KS manifests nodular or plaquelike dermal lesions. A **lymphoadenopathic form** of KS is disseminated and aggressive, involving lymph nodes, viscera, and occasionally the GI tract. In a form associated with **acquired immunodeficiency syndrome (AIDS**—see in Ch. 19), the lesions are widely disseminated in the skin, mucous membrane, lymph nodes, and viscera.

Incidence

KS, although uncommon, once was most frequent in eastern Europe, Italy, and the USA and occurred mainly in the indolent form in men of Italian or Jewish ancestry > 60 yr of age. However, KS is endemic in equatorial Africa; there it is more aggressive, is seen commonly in children and young men, and comprises nearly 10% of all malignancies in Zaire and Uganda. In the past few years, the aggressive form of KS has occurred in at least ⅓ of patients with AIDS and has assumed epidemic proportions in the USA and many other countries (see in Ch. 19).

Clinical Manifestations

In older men, KS generally appears first on the toes or legs as purple or dark brown plaques or nodules that may fungate or penetrate soft tissue and invade bone; disseminated lymph node and visceral involvement follow in 5 to 10%. The KS lesions associated with AIDS may be the first notable manifestation of AIDS. They appear first primarily on the upper body or mucosa as barely elevated pink or red papules or plaques, but become widely disseminated on the skin and are associated with visceral lesions and disseminated lymph node involvement.

Treatment and Prognosis

For indolent superficial lesions, electrocoagulation or electron beam radiotherapy is used for lesions, while deeper or unresponsive dermal disease with lymphedema is treated by 1000 to 2000 rads of x-ray therapy, which, if needed, may be repeated after a few years. Vinblastine, an active, but weak, agent in treating AIDS-related sarcoma, further lowers immunity.

In the more aggressive and disseminated form, various treatments to manage the underlying immunodeficiency and its complications have been tried. In the indolent form, patients tend to live for 10 yr or more.

§20. DENTAL AND ORAL DISORDERS

245. DENTISTRY IN MEDICINE

MEDICAL-DENTAL CONSULTATION

A dentist should consult a physician when he suspects systemic disease, when he needs to evaluate a person's ability to withstand general anesthesia or extensive oral surgery, or when an emergency occurs in a dental office.

A physician should consult a dentist on behalf of a child with abnormal growth manifested by peculiar facies, delayed tooth eruption, or gross malformation or malalignment of teeth; or for a patient with cleft lip or palate, jaw fracture, oral neoplasm, or newly discovered lump in the neck. Dental consultation is also indicated for obscure facial pain, for unexplained swelling or cellulitis of the neck that might have originated in an infected tooth, or for infection of the parapharyngeal space that might have followed an abscess of a lower posterior tooth. Physicians should be familiar with dental procedures and the amount of trauma and risk involved to patients with systemic disease. Dentists who search for oral cancer and who refuse to extract teeth unless valid dental reasons exist are consultants to be prized.

Clarification of the cause of face, head, and neck symptoms often necessitates the pooled knowledge of both physician and dentist. Obscure causes of **face, head, and neck pain** include malocclusion, poorly fitting dental prostheses, disease of the temporomandibular joints, unilateral mastication, spasm of the muscles of mastication, and occult cavities in the jawbones. Referred pain may make diagnosis difficult; for example, pain referred to the ear may arise from an inflammation of the gingival flap about a partly erupted mandibular 3rd molar, or from the back of the tongue in glossopharyngeal neuralgia. Paresthesias of the lower lip may follow damage to the inferior alveolar nerve during extraction of a mandibular molar, but may also be a rare sign of an oral neoplasm compressing that nerve. Conversely, percussion tenderness in several maxillary teeth may indicate nasal or antral disease adjacent to the root tips.

Patients undergoing oral surgery warrant the same preoperative medical workups and postoperative care as those undergoing procedures of comparable scope and severity elsewhere in the body. Oral surgical procedures include simple extractions; removal of impacted teeth; alveoloplasty (cartilage grafts or resection of mucosa with reattachment to deepen the mucobuccal fold so that dentures can be retained better); repair of jaw fractures; correction of protruding mandibles or retruded or small jaws; orthognathic surgery (repositioning an area of alveolar bone and its contained teeth) for severe malocclusion; excision of soft tissues, bone cysts, and neoplasms; and surgery on the temporomandibular joint to remedy arthritis, developmental anomalies, or the results of trauma.

DENTAL CARE OF PATIENTS WITH SYSTEMIC DISORDERS

Dental care is occasionally hazardous. Its risks can be minimized by (1) doing elective dental procedures when the medical patient is best able to withstand the inherent trauma and (2) encouraging healthy individuals to practice oral hygiene so that, should systemic disease develop, massive dental treatment in a belated attempt to remedy prolonged neglect is unnecessary and will not delay medical therapy or cause additional complications.

Routine oral surgery or periodontal treatment puts medical patients at risk when the normal inflammation required for healing is inhibited by such drugs as corticosteroids, immunosuppressive agents used in organ transplantation, and cytotoxic drugs given for cancer. Hemorrhage, delayed healing, local infection, and even septicemia may occur. Dental care should be carried out and time for healing allowed before using such systemic drugs.

People with **bleeding disorders** should have teeth filled to avoid subsequent extractions. Filling a tooth is almost always a bloodless procedure. Exceptions occur: (1) Deep decay that has entered or has almost entered the pulp mandates completely removing the decayed tooth structure, to prevent recurrent caries; the minimal bleeding from the pulp that follows the removal is easily controlled by pressure. (2) Minimal gingival lacerations may occur from instrumentation during preparations for treating

interproximal caries. Cavity preparation involving the occlusal surface of a tooth that is not deeply decayed should be completely bloodless.

Suspected **bleeding or coagulation disorders** should be assessed prior to oral surgery. In patients with acute forms of **leukemia, thrombocytopenia,** or **hepatitis,** extractions should be delayed until the condition improves or stabilizes. Prolonged bleeding following extraction or periodontal procedures may occur in patients with **polycythemia vera** or **macroglobulinemia, disorders of platelet number and function,** and severe **liver disease** with diminished vitamin K-associated plasma coagulation factors or increased fibrinolytic activity. In coagulation disorders, extractions and regional block anesthesia often require pretreatment with the appropriate coagulation factor and perhaps aminocaproic acid immediately before, during, and after the oral surgical procedure.

In **leukemia,** oral hygiene is vital because periodontal disease favors occurrence of gingival bleeding and probably local tissue infiltration. Infection often follows extraction in disorders with **granulocytopenia.**

Cardiovascular patients may be adversely affected by dental procedures. Following a myocardial infarction, dental procedures should be delayed for 3 mo, if possible, and anticoagulant dosage may need temporary reduction (prothrombin time to about 1½ times the control value) to avoid undue postextraction bleeding. Individuals with pulmonary or cardiac disease who require inhalation anesthesia for dental procedures should be treated in a hospital. Tooth extraction, scaling (removal of calculus), or other periodontal procedures are followed by bacteremia; patients with mitral valve prolapse, congenital or rheumatic heart disease, or a prosthetic cardiac valve are predisposed to bacterial endocarditis and should receive antibiotics before and after such dental procedures. It is particularly important for them, as for patients with coagulation disorders, that teeth be filled to avoid extractions and that preventive oral hygiene be practiced to minimize tooth decay and gingivitis.

Epinephrine, used as a vasoconstrictor to potentiate the duration of local anesthetics, may cause arrhythmias or exacerbate hypertension as the exogenous hormone adds to the anxiety or fear-induced endogenous level; cardiac ischemia may result. Sedation or tranquilization is advantageous in fearful cardiovascular patients and facilitates treatment. Electrical equipment such as a cautery, a pulp tester, and even the dental handpiece (drill) can interfere with pacemakers. Such patients and their dentists should be forewarned so that appropriate measures may be taken. The horizontal position of a dental chair may be intolerable to patients with congestive heart failure, and those on antihypertensive drugs may develop orthostatic hypotension on arising.

Infections may follow dental procedures such as tooth extraction, particularly of abscessed or periodontally involved teeth. **Bacteremia** may result in endocarditis, mediastinitis, thrombophlebitis of the jugular veins, pneumonia, empyema, meningitis, brain abscess, and cavernous sinus thrombophlebitis. Mediastinitis, thrombophlebitis, a parapharyngeal abscess, or a cellulitis of the floor of the mouth may develop from contiguity with an abscessed tooth, whether or not endodontic treatment (root canal) was performed. Infectious material, such as fragments of teeth or fillings or pus from periodontal infection, may be aspirated and cause a lung abscess.

Chemotherapy for neoplasms includes drugs (eg, doxorubicin, 5-fluorouracil, bleomycin, dactinomycin, and methotrexate) that cause stomatitis; the severity is often related to the degree of periodontal disease present. Before instituting such drugs, it is advisable to remove calculus (tartar) and improve the health of periodontal tissue to minimize gingival hemorrhage, tissue sloughing, oral pain, and consequent poor food intake. Subsequent proper use of the toothbrush and dental floss will minimize the likelihood of stomatitis.

Prior to radiotherapy of the oral region, patients should have required oral surgery, periodontal treatment, restoration of salvageable teeth, and fluoride treatment (to minimize caries following xerostomia secondary to irradiation and destruction of the

salivary glands). Dental work should be completed and healing permitted before radiotherapy begins. *Extraction of teeth from previously irradiated tissues is commonly followed by* ***osteoradionecrosis*** *of the jaws, a catastrophic complication* (see OSTEORADIONECROSIS in Ch. 267). It is best to avoid extraction, if possible, by using dental restorations, dental splints, or endodontic treatment (root canal). Careful lifelong attention to oral hygiene is necessary to avoid oral or periodontal surgery. Frequent fluoride applications are also indicated for an indefinite period following radiotherapy. Tissue breakdown and persistent ulceration is likely beneath a partial or a complete denture because of scarring and inelasticity of irradiated tissue. The prostheses should be checked and adjusted whenever discomfort is noted.

Extraction of a tooth adjacent to a carcinoma of the gingiva, palate, or antrum favors invasion of the alveolus (tooth socket) by the neoplasm. Extraction should be done only in the course of definitive treatment.

Subcutaneous and mediastinal emphysema may rarely follow use of a high-speed air turbine dental drill or compressed air during a root-canal procedure, or to section a tooth or the alveolar bone during an extraction, as air is forced into the alveolus of the bone and then dissects along fascial planes. Acute onset of jaw and cervical swelling with characteristic crepitus on palpation of the swollen skin is diagnostic.

In **endocrine disorders,** tooth extraction is never routine. Dental treatment should usually be postponed until the systemic disease is well controlled. For example, tachycardia may occur in hyperthyroid individuals, accompanying the anxiety often present in dental patients. One exception to postponement is that poorly controlled diabetics may be more easily managed after they receive necessary dental care to improve poor oral hygiene. **Diabetics** are prone to periodontal disease and following periodontal surgery or extractions may require adjustment of insulin dosage and parenteral fluids or diet during the time when food intake is limited because of postoperative pain. Poorly controlled diabetics, often dehydrated, also have a decreased salivary flow that contributes to caries. To avoid undue interference with food intake, extensive extractions, restorative dentistry, or periodontal surgery should not be done in one visit. Patients with **adrenocortical insufficiency** may require supplemental corticosteroids during the stress of major dental procedures. Individuals who have **Cushing's syndrome** or are receiving corticosteroids for a systemic disease may have delayed wound healing and increased capillary fragility.

An **allergic** individual might, despite previous interrogation, receive an offending antibiotic, local anesthetic, or other medication given in conjunction with dental treatment.

In **Bell's palsy** the natural cleansing action of the lip and cheek on the tooth surfaces of the involved side is lost; without scrupulous oral hygiene and repeated fluoride treatments, unilateral decay will increase.

People with **convulsive disorders** should have fixed (not removable) small dental appliances, to prevent swallowing or aspirating them and causing airways obstruction or possibly esophagitis or enteritis due to the foreign body. Tracheoesophageal or enterocolonic fistulas may develop subsequently. **Quadriplegics** and individuals with severe upper extremity incoordination or tremor cannot have good oral hygiene unless those who care for them are very conscientious. Unexplained fever in them may have an oral basis that should be sought.

Hepatitis B virus rarely may be transmitted by dentists with antigenemia who are carriers of the disease to patients via open lesions on the dentist's fingers into the alveolus of an extracted tooth or into the patient's mouth and therefore the GI tract. The hazard is diminished if dentists with digital lesions, particularly with a history of hepatitis, wear rubber gloves. Unfortunately, autoclaving is not the usual means of sterilizing dental instruments, so the use of dental instruments or the probably rare reuse of hypodermic needles may infect a subsequent patient. If a patient with viral

hepatitis visits a dentist during the incubation period, additional individuals may be placed at risk.

DENTAL RESTORATIONS AND APPLIANCES

Fillings are inserted after removal of decay. A temporary filling is kept in place for weeks in the hope that the tooth will retain its vitality and deposit secondary dentin to seal a pulp exposure. Silicate, a type of porcelain cement, is used to fill cavities in anterior teeth because it resembles enamel. Recently, plastic resins have been used for the same purpose. The occlusal surfaces of posterior teeth, which bear the brunt of mastication, require stronger materials. The commonest ones used, amalgam and gold inlay, can be identified by color. A small, less common filling is gold foil.

If decay is extensive, placing several fillings in one tooth might undermine its structure. To avoid fracture of the natural crown, the dentist removes the decay and fills the sites with cement. He grinds and tapers the outer surfaces so that an artificial **crown,** usually of gold, may be placed. A porcelain jacket crown is used on anterior teeth for its natural appearance. During laryngoscopy, care must be exercised not to dislodge any artificial crowns fixed on anterior teeth.

When teeth are missing, a bridge or partial denture can be made. A **bridge** is usually smaller than a partial denture, but it is possible to make 1 or 2 bridges to cover an entire maxillary or mandibular dental arch. Stress in a bridge is largely borne by abutment teeth (usually on either side of the missing tooth or teeth). Abutment teeth have crowns cemented to them; thus, the bridge is a fixed appliance that is not easily removed. False teeth are soldered to the crowns and to each other. A **partial denture,** typically a removable appliance with clasps that snap over the abutment teeth, may be removed for cleaning. Part of the load of occlusion is borne by the soft tissues underlying artificial teeth, which often are on both sides of the jaw. This appliance is often used when there are no more natural teeth beyond the tooth or teeth to be replaced.

Complete dentures are removable appliances that help a patient chew solid foods and improve his speech and appearance, but they cannot achieve the efficiency or tactile sensations of natural dentition.

All **removable dental appliances** are generally removed before throat surgery, general anesthesia, or convulsive shock therapy to avoid loss, breakage, aspiration, or swallowing during the procedure. They should be stored in water to prevent dimensional changes that may occur with drying. However, some anesthesiologists believe that an appliance aids the passage of an airway tube, keeps the face in a more normal shape so the mask fits better, does not interfere with laryngoscopy, and prevents natural teeth from injuring the opposing gingiva of a completely edentulous jaw.

---

246. EXAMINATION OF THE ORAL REGION

Knowing the details and frequency of dental visits may alert the physician to a particular dental problem or to a lack of attention to dental care. **Inability to chew food well** suggests insufficient teeth for proper mastication, poorly fitting dental appliances, loose or painful teeth, or disorders affecting the temporomandibular joint **(TMJ)** or the muscles of mastication. **Slight, occasional bleeding** after brushing suggests bristle damage or mild gingivitis; **frequent, spontaneous, or profuse bleeding** may indicate severe gingivitis or a blood dyscrasia. A history of a **single, mild infection** after oral surgery does not necessarily have systemic implications; but **recurring oral and other infections** may indicate agranulocytosis, neutropenia, leukemia, immunoglobulin defects, or disorders of leukocyte function. **Root canal treatment**—a common dental procedure when

decay has reached the pulp or for devitalization after trauma—occasionally is associated with osteitis at the tip of the root. **Sores, lumps, or pain** may originate from both teeth and soft tissues. **Medication history** may reveal incompatibilites and duplications. **Abnormal taste sensations** may be due to psychiatric disorders. However, a search for local causes should always be made. A bitter taste may indicate pus originating from a periodontal or alveolar abscess. A salty taste may indicate bleeding or seepage of tissue fluid from beneath poorly fitting dentures or from inflamed periodontal tissues into the normally sodium-poor oral environment. Correction of such underlying dental problems results in disappearance of the symptom.

The Face

The face and mouth are inspected for marked asymmetry, lesions, or disproportions. An **unusual facial appearance** characterizes many head and neck syndromes of genetic or developmental origin and often occurs with atypical positioning or malformations of the pinnae or an unusual skull shape, with or without dental abnormalities. An underweight patient may lack teeth or have severe periodontal disease, caries, or poorly fitting dental appliances that interfere with chewing. Not all involuntary weight loss indicates systemic disease in such individuals.

Slight facial asymmetry is universal. It may be due to preferential chewing on one side causing unilateral enlargement of the masticatory muscles, differences in the contour of the dental arches, angulation of the teeth on one side compared to the other, or combinations of these. However, **marked facial asymmetry** occurs in individuals with lipodystrophy, hemiatrophy, hemihypertrophy of the face, or congenital absence of the condyle of the mandible. Awareness of the psychologic trauma of facial malformation should lead to referral for possible facial surgery.

Cheek **contours** depend mainly on the posterior teeth. **Swellings** of the face may be cutaneous (eg, neurofibromas or sebaceous cysts) or may arise from deeper tissues. If one or both cheeks appear swollen, the distension may be in the skin, in the parotid glands (which may be enlarged because of mumps, Sjögren's syndrome, or a tumor), or inside the mouth. An excessively thick denture flange gives the wearer a puffy appearance that disappears on removing the denture and can be remedied by a dentist's grinding down its outer thickness. An abscessed tooth may cause soft-tissue swelling as pus drains from the tooth toward the outer surface of the face or neck. Endodontic (root canal) treatment or extraction promotes drainage and mitigates against further spread of infection. Salivary gland and lymph node enlargement is evident on inspection of the preauricular and submandibular regions.

Fistulas may represent malformations of the embryologic branchial pouches or draining sinuses from abscessed teeth. An abscessed lower molar may drain below the angle of the mandible and eventually leave a depressed scar.

Breath Odor (see also Halitosis, Real and Imagined in Ch. 52)

The physician should wonder why a patient who is reeking from mouthwash is self-conscious about his breath. Is it only recent ingestion of alcohol, onions, or garlic, or use of tobacco, or is it for another reason? Extensive dental caries, periodontal disease, or tonsillitis causes a fetid odor often accompanied by a bad taste. Rhinitis, ozena, or sinusitis also causes halitosis. There are **systemic causes** of bad breath: in liver failure, a mousy odor is present; in uremia, a uriniferous smell; and in a lung abscess or bronchiectasis, a putrid odor. In diabetic ketosis, acetone is present in the expired air.

Lips

Lip movements normally betray emotion as the patient speaks; in scleroderma or Parkinson's disease, the lips are rigid. With a facial nerve paralysis (Bell's palsy), marked asymmetry occurs when the patient talks or smiles. The **vermilion border** (between the mucosa of the lips and the skin of the face) is the site of recurrent infections

(cold sores) and carcinoma. **Generalized thickening** of the lips occurs in myxedema, cretinism, and acromegaly. **Localized swellings** may indicate a lymphangioma or hemangioma, the latter causing purplish discoloration as well. Besides cosmetics to camouflage the deformity, more definitive treatment is available (see Ch. 243). In the absence of anterior teeth, the lips become shorter and more concave. They are attached to the jaws by prominent midline and smaller lateral frena. Other abnormalities are discussed in Ch. 251.

Temporomandibular Joint

The TMJ is palpated laterally and intrameatally for tenderness, range, smoothness of motion, and condylar deformity. As the patient opens his mouth, one notes any limitation or **deviation of jaw movement** indicating abnormality of the 5th cranial nerve or weakness of jaw muscles. Congenital malformation or absence of the TMJ can cause similar signs, and characteristic abnormalities appear on x-ray. Normally the jaw should move symmetrically, and with mouth open, 3 fingers should fit comfortably between the upper and lower incisors (40 to 50 mm). If less space exists, both articular and nonarticular conditions should be considered in the differential diagnosis, since they can produce similar types of dysfunction. The patient may have scleroderma, parotitis, malformation or arthritis of the TMJ, a peritonsillar abscess, or pericoronitis (infection of the gingiva about a partially erupted 3rd molar). Tetanus or a depressed fracture of the zygomatic arch impinging on the coronoid process of the mandible can also impair opening the mouth. Muscular problems (trismus, myofascial pain-dysfunction [MPD] syndrome) for which the cervical muscles and muscles of mastication should be palpated are more common causes of limited jaw movement than are joint problems (ankylosis, disk derangement). An unusually wide opening may indicate a subluxation of the mandible.

By placing his or her little fingers deeply into the patient's auditory canals, the physician can test the range and smoothness of mandibular condylar motion as the mouth opens and closes.

For complaints of ear or facial pain on chewing, the examiner can use a stethoscope in front of each ear as the patient opens and closes his mouth. Clicking or popping sounds indicate an internal disk derangement. A grating noise or crepitus suggests degenerative joint disease.

Teeth (see also under GROWTH AND DEVELOPMENT FROM BIRTH THROUGH CHILDHOOD in Ch. 182)

A useful shorthand representation for recording observations is shown in TABLES 246–1 and 246–2. The horizontal line represents the space between the jaws and the vertical line denotes the midline of the face. Another method of identifying teeth is using the letters A to T for the deciduous and numbers 1 to 32 for the permanent teeth; eg, in the permanent dentition, numbering begins with the 3rd maxillary right molar and goes to the left across the maxillary arch, then to the right across the mandibular arch to the 3rd mandibular right molar.

Oral hygiene reflects the patient's general attitude toward himself or his physical, psychologic, or economic ability to care for himself. Are teeth decayed or missing? Pain experienced when teeth are tapped with a tongue depressor suggests extensive dental caries or periodontal disease. Severe periodontal disease causes most instances of visible mobility of teeth, but rarely, erosion of the alveolar bone by an underlying tumor (eg, ameloblastoma) will loosen them. A deeply carious tooth may have an infected or necrotic pulp. A dentist can test the patient's reaction of pain to a weak electrical stimulus to determine whether a tooth is alive. A tooth with decay involving the pulp is a potential source of infection into surrounding alveolar bone. **Calculus (tartar),** if present, is deposited particularly near the orifices of the salivary ducts on the buccal surfaces of the maxillary molars and the lingual surfaces of the mandibular anterior teeth.

TABLE 246–1. RELATIONSHIP BETWEEN DECIDUOUS AND PERMANENT TEETH*

20 Deciduous		*32 Permanent*	
Symbol	**Name**	**Symbol**	**Name**
A	Central incisor	1	Central incisor
B	Lateral incisor	2	Lateral incisor
C	Canine (cuspid)	3	Canine (cuspid)
D	1st molar	4	1st premolar (bicuspid)
E	2nd molar	5	2nd premolar (bicuspid)
		6	1st molar
		7	2nd molar
		8	3rd molar

* Each quadrant (left or right half of each jaw) contains the teeth listed.

The commonest motor abnormality of the oral region is probably not Bell's palsy (see Ch. 131) but **bruxism** —the clenching or grinding of teeth that erodes and eventually diminishes the height of dental crowns. Such attrition is common with advancing years; in youth, it often indicates bruxism. The teeth may loosen. Although the patient may be oblivious of his habit, other family members are aware. The treatment requires that the patient consciously try to overcome the habit, perhaps with the help of sedatives or tranquilizers and abstinence from alcohol. Alcohol often aggravates bruxism. A dentist can make a splint to be worn over the teeth to prevent the grinding movements. Biofeedback may be tried.

Maxillary incisor **fractures** are common in children with neurologic disorders who fall often. Malocclusion can result in a front tooth contacting its opponent at an angle so that a corner of an incisor may be chipped.

Defects in tooth form: Once formed, teeth are never remodeled by systemic influences, only by local ones. Thus, the examiner may find evidence of developmental disorders or endocrinopathies. In **congenital syphilis** the contours of the incisors and 1st molars undergo characteristic changes: The incisors show a constriction at the incisal 3rd, which produces a pegged or screwdriver shape, and a characteristic notch

TABLE 246–2. SHORTHAND REPRESENTATION OF TEETH

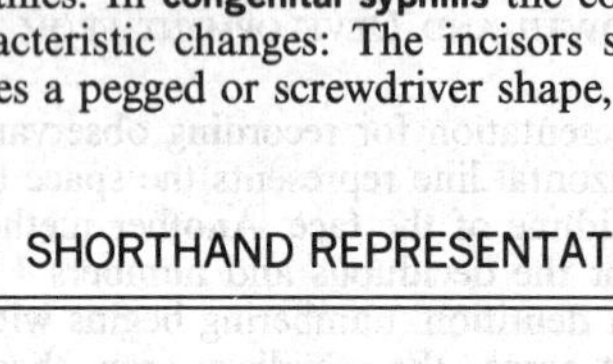

Using the symbol for the tooth from TABLE 246–1,

|D represents the mandibular left deciduous 1st molar;

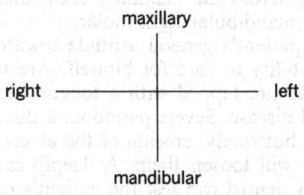

6| represents the maxillary right permanent 1st molar.

in the central portion of the incisal edge. The 1st molar is dwarfed, with constriction of the occlusal surface and roughening and hypoplasia of the enamel. With hereditary opalescent dentin **(dentinogenesis imperfecta),** an autosomal dominant trait, the dentin is abnormally formed and teeth are a dull bluish-brown. Such teeth cannot withstand occlusal stresses and rapidly become worn. **"Peg" lateral incisors** are congenitally narrow but are unassociated with systemic disease.

Defects in enamel or tooth color: A **dead tooth** appears gray. Darkening of the teeth and enamel hypoplasia follow **chronic administration of tetracyclines** during the second half of pregnancy or during tooth development in the child; the affected teeth, rather than fluorescing white in ultraviolet light, have a colored fluorescence characteristic of the type of tetracycline given. A dark band may be visible in ordinary light after only 5 days of therapy. The abnormal calcium metabolism associated with **rickets** results in enamel hypoplasia. A rough irregular band appears around each tooth. The location of the band indicates the area being calcified at the time of abnormal calcification, and thus provides an estimate of the age when the disease occurred and its duration. Such teeth are not unduly susceptible to dental caries. A **high fever** during odontogenesis can also interfere with enamel formation, and a narrow zone of chalky pitted enamel is visible after the tooth erupts. **Amelogenesis imperfecta,** an autosomal dominant hereditary disease, causes severe enamel hypoplasia. Children who drink water containing > 1 ppm of fluoride during the period of tooth development are likely to develop mottled enamel **(fluorosis).** The enamel changes can range, depending on the amount of fluoride ingested, from irregular whitish opaque areas to severe brown discoloration of the entire crown, with a roughened surface. Such teeth have a high resistance to dental caries. In **congenital porphyria,** teeth fluoresce a reddish color due to deposition of pigment in the dentin. Periapical x-rays show that hypopituitary dwarfs have small dental roots and people with gigantism have large roots. In acromegaly, one sees not only enlargement of the jaws but also hypercementosis of the roots.

The patient should be asked to remove dentures so that the underlying soft tissues may be seen. The likelihood of dropping or distorting a dental appliance is greater if the physician attempts to remove it.

With age, teeth darken and biting surfaces become worn **(attrition)** so that chewing is less effective. **Gingivae** may **recede** and thus expose more of the crowns and often even part of the roots. Since a small zone of exposed dentin is sensitive to touch or temperature alterations, noncarious teeth can become painful when enamel and cementum do not quite contact each other. The dentist can desensitize such teeth. Proper keratinization of the oral mucosa requires sex hormones. Hormonal therapy can ameliorate the poorly keratinized, inflamed mucosa commonly found after menopause.

In edentulous jaws of the aged, **atrophy of the alveolar process (senile atrophy)** is common. This diminishes the stability of artificial full dentures, particularly the lower one. Oral surgical procedures can improve the situation.

Normal Occlusion

Occlusion should be checked on both sides of the mouth; this can be done by retracting each cheek with a tongue depressor while the patient bites normally. In normal occlusion, the maxillary anterior teeth overlie the mandibular anterior teeth. The outer (buccal) cusps of the maxillary posteriors are external to the corresponding cusps of the mandibular posterior teeth. Since the outer parts of all the maxillary teeth are superficial to the mandibular teeth, the lips and cheeks are displaced from between the teeth so they are not bitten. Furthermore, the lingual (inner) surfaces of the lower teeth are in a smaller arc than that of the upper teeth, confining the tongue and minimizing the likelihood of its being bitten as the teeth occlude. All the teeth should contact their opponents, so that the powerful masticatory forces (which may be > 100 lb in the molar region) will be widely distributed. If these forces are applied to only a few teeth, the latter are likely to loosen.

Malocclusion

The commonest **classification** of deviation from the normal contact of the maxillary and mandibular teeth identifies 3 major forms of malocclusion. **Class I:** The upper and lower molars occlude normally, but the anterior teeth are crowded or malpositioned. **Class II:** The lower jaw is retruded and the facial profile is convex. **Class III:** The mandible protrudes.

Etiology: Malocclusion often reflects a disproportion between jaw and tooth size—ie, a jaw so small or teeth so large that the jaw cannot accommodate them all in proper alignment. Other causes are supernumerary, malformed, or missing teeth; delayed eruption or impaction of permanent teeth; ankylosis of the mandible; cleft lip or palate; and rarely, cleidocranial dysostosis or Hurler's syndrome. A frequent cause of acquired malocclusion is loss of teeth with shifting of adjacent teeth and extrusion of opposing teeth unless a bridge or partial denture is made. Premature loss of deciduous teeth in children often results in approximation of adjacent teeth causing insufficient space for eruption of the permanent successors. This shift can be prevented by a dental appliance termed a space maintainer. Less frequently, malocclusion is from habits like thumb- and finger-sucking or tongue-thrusting. Iatrogenic malocclusions can occur from improper dental restorations and appliances, improper fixation of jaw fractures, or a Milwaukee orthopedic back brace, which places constant pressure on the mandible. Rarely, teeth are displaced by an underlying jaw tumor.

Diagnosis and Treatment: Malocclusions are corrected primarily for oral health reasons, although the patient often needs help for cosmetic or psychologic reasons. Because early interceptive **orthodontics** usually eliminates a later need for more expensive and difficult technics, a child should have a dental consultation as soon as malocclusion is suspected. The evaluation includes x-rays of the skull, facial bones, and teeth, and study casts of the teeth. Malocclusion following facial trauma may suggest tooth displacement, often accompanied by a jaw fracture.

Therapy increases resistance to dental decay, anterior tooth-edge fracture, and periodontal disease, and it improves speaking and mastication. Occlusion can be improved by selective grinding where teeth or restorations contact prematurely, by aligning teeth properly, or by inserting crowns or onlays to build up teeth that are below the plane of occlusion. Applying a continuous mild force to the teeth by means of orthodontic appliances (braces) moves the teeth by gradually remodeling the alveolar bone. Some patients initially require extraction of 1 or more permanent teeth to obtain enough space for stable alignment. When the final relationship has been achieved, the patient wears a plastic retainer at night until the teeth stabilize in new positions. Where it is anticipated that orthodontic treatment may not suffice, surgical correction of jaw abnormalities contributing to malocclusion (orthognathic surgery) is often indicated. Orthodontic treatment of adults is now commonplace.

Oral Mucosa

With a finger cot for protection against infectious lesions, the cheek is palpated bimanually (with one finger inside and one outside) to delimit lesions. Most people have yellowish pinhead-size macules in the buccal mucosa. These are harmless **ectopic sebaceous glands** (Fordyce granules). Many persons have a thin white line (linea alba) on the buccal mucosa along the occlusal plane. It represents surface keratinization due to accidental, repeated cheek biting over the years.

The **color** of soft tissues can reflect anemia, polycythemia, cyanosis, or jaundice. One looks for generalized inflammation (stomatitis) as well as localized areas of inflammation, ulceration, petechiae, or thickening. Darkly pigmented areas may indicate a racial characteristic, Addison's disease, or, very rarely, melanoma.

Dryness of the mouth may be from dehydration, mouth breathing, or use of diuretics, or may reflect salivary gland dysfunction or disease (see Ch. 247). The orifices of

the parotid ducts open in the cheek beside the maxillary molars. The sublingual and submandibular salivary gland ducts open on the floor of the mouth behind the lower incisors. In case of pain or swelling in those regions, if saliva does not emanate from the appropriate duct, it may be obstructed by a calculus (sialolith).

The **distribution of keratinized and nonkeratinized oral mucosa** can be significant. Keratinized epithelium is on the facial aspect of the lips, the dorsum of the tongue, the gingiva around the base of the dental crowns and adjacent part of the roots of the teeth, and on the hard palate. It is less likely to be damaged by hard food particles than nonkeratinized mucosa that is mobile, as in the cheek, sides of the tongue, soft palate, and floor of the mouth. Keratinized mucosa in these areas is abnormal and a definite diagnosis must be made. White areas may be seen in the mucobuccal fold in adolescents or others who retain snuff or chewing tobacco there. Such leukoplakias are often precancerous (see Ch. 251).

Gingiva

The gum should be firm and nicely contoured about and adapted to the crowns of the teeth. Pink, stippled tissue should fill the entire interdental space. Keratinized gingiva is present near the crowns. More distant gingiva is nonkeratinized, highly vascular, and continuous with the buccal mucosa. A tongue depressor should express no blood or pus from the gingiva. At the gingival margin, a dark line suggests exposure to lead or a heavy metal. Gingivitis (see in Ch. 249) is common.

The Palate

The anterior portion of the hard palate is the site of the incisive papilla adjacent to the central incisors. Behind it are the rugae, firm ridges that keep food from slipping as the tongue crushes the food against them. A person with a cleft palate (see also under MUSCULOSKELETAL DEFECTS in Ch. 187) has a very nasal voice. Normal vocal resonance and articulation involve the anterior teeth, lips, tongue, and palate, as well as the lungs, vocal cords, and pharynx. A very **high palatal vault** is seen in Marfan syndrome (see under INHERITED DISORDERS OF CONNECTIVE TISSUE in Ch. 197). Punctate areas of inflammation about the ducts of the numerous minor salivary glands of the palate are common, especially in pipe smokers. The boneless soft palate should rise symmetrically when the patient says "ah." The uvula at the far end of the soft palate's midline varies greatly in length among individuals.

Tongue and Floor of the Mouth

As the patient touches the tip of his tongue to his soft palate, one can examine the floor of the mouth and the under surface of the tongue, where cancer often starts. The tongue, having a wide range of **movement,** should be able to twist its tip around the sides of the molar teeth. Normal tongue movement indicates good hypoglossal nerve function, but neuromuscular weakness may prevent its holding a midline position or moving rapidly. For a neurologic evaluation of taste, it is possible to use 0.1 M solutions of NaCl, HCl, sucrose, and urea. The tongue may be **enlarged** in myxedema, amyloidosis, or acromegaly, or if a rhabdomyoma is present. In edentulous individuals without complete dentures, the tongue tends to broaden.

The **papillae** may be normal or atrophied. The tongue is smooth and pale in pernicious anemia or smooth and fiery red in deficiencies of niacin or riboflavin (see GLOSSITIS in Ch. 247). Oral cancer often occurs on the lateral surface of the tongue (see NEOPLASMS in Ch. 251).

Salivary Glands

Saliva promotes retention of artificial dentures because of its mucin content. Thus, conditions characterized by diminished saliva flow often adversely affect the ease with which dentures may be worn. If natural teeth are present, salivary flow washes away bacteria and food debris and favors oral cleanliness. A reduction in flow facilitates

development of tooth decay. This may be caused by an abnormality of the salivary glands (see in Ch. 247).

247. DISORDERS OF THE LIPS, MOUTH, AND TONGUE

Most diseases affecting the mucous membrane can occur anywhere in the oral mucosa, but they will be mentioned under the most frequent sites. Also see Chs. 246 and 251.

LIPS

An acute swelling of the lip may be **angioedema** (see URTICARIA; ANGIOEDEMA in Ch. 21). Brownish-black melanin pigmentation spots in association with GI polyposis occur in the **Peutz-Jeghers syndrome. Exfoliative cheilitis** is a chronic desquamation of the superficial mucosal cells; if it persists despite abstention from very hot or irritating foods and alcoholic beverages and despite changes of lipstick or dentifrices, triamcinolone acetonide ointment should be tried. A **chancre** has a serosanguineous crust (see SYPHILIS in Ch. 14).

Mucocele (mucous retention cyst), most commonly found on the lower lip, is due to trauma severing the excretory ducts of the accessory salivary glands and permitting the mucin-containing saliva to escape into the tissues. A soft nodule forms. If the nodule is superficial, the overlying epithelium is thinned and assumes a bluish tinge. Treatment is excision.

Tiny painful vesicles characterize two common disorders: herpes labialis **("cold sore")**, found on the vermilion border, and recurrent aphthous ulcers **("canker sores")**, on the inner aspects of the lips (see also RECURRENT APHTHOUS STOMATITIS and ORAL HERPETIC MANIFESTATIONS in this chapter, below).

Cheilosis (angular cheilitis) is characterized by fissuring and dry scaling of the skin and vermilion surface of the lips and angles of the mouth. The condition is associated with deficiency of some of the B vitamins, particularly riboflavin and pyridoxine, and frequently accompanies other clinical signs of avitaminosis. One must also consider herpetic involvement, the split papule of syphilis, and the pseudocheilosis or wrinkling at the corners of the mouth accompanying loss of vertical dimension of the face (the distance between the jaws). In edentulous patients, wrinkling can be diminished by inserting dentures that separate the jaws. Loss of skin elasticity with aging normally results in overlapping of the skin at the corners of the mouth, so that saliva pools there and contributes to angular inflammation. Persistent lesions should be cultured to rule out a mycotic infection, particularly candidiasis **(Perlèche).** Mixed infections respond best to a combination of antifungal, antibacterial, and anti-inflammatory agents. High doses of vitamin B complex are beneficial if blood tests indicate a deficiency.

BUCCAL MUCOSA
(See also STOMATITIS, below)

Mucosal lesions may cause dentures to hurt or fit poorly. **Koplik's spots** are tiny, grayish-white macules with red margins occurring during the late prodromal and early eruptive stages of measles. **Aspirin burn** is a painful white area of coagulated tissue caused by the local caustic action of aspirin placed against the mucosa to relieve a toothache. Wiping off the white film reveals a reddened area. **Irritation "fibroma,"** composed of fibrous tissue, is not a true neoplasm because its growth is limited. It is

usually present opposite the occlusal plane where the patient chronically bites or sucks his cheek. Treatment is excision and breaking the habit or reducing the cusps of offending teeth. **Hereditary hemorrhagic telangiectasia** (see in Ch. 99) is characterized by localized dilated blood vessels in the oral cavity, nasal mucosa, and elsewhere. Should bleeding occur, applying local pressure and an absorbable gelatin sponge ordinarily suffices. If not, a cautery may be used. **Lichen planus** often occurs with cutaneous lesions (see Ch. 236). The mucosa is characteristically netlike and hardened, with papules or erosive areas. Violet atrophic or white hyperkeratotic variations may appear on the dorsum of the tongue. **Bullae** of short duration occur in various mucocutaneous disorders (eg, pemphigus and erythema multiforme), including the severe Stevens-Johnson syndrome. Behçet's syndrome has oral as well as ocular and genital mucosal ulcers. Herpangina, characterized by vesicles in the posterior part of the mouth, and hand-foot-and-mouth disease, with small ulcerated vesicles, are both due to coxsackieviruses (see in ENTEROVIRAL DISEASES under CHILDHOOD INFECTIONS in Ch. 191).

FLOOR OF THE MOUTH

This area may be the site of a **cellulitis** following extraction of, or root canal treatment on, an abscessed mandibular tooth. Incision, drainage, and aggressive antibiotic therapy (eg, two 500-mg tablets penicillin V, then 1 tablet q 6 h to a total of 40 tablets) are indicated. An extensive sublingual infection, termed **Ludwig's angina,** is very hard to palpation (see SUBMANDIBULAR SPACE INFECTION in Ch. 5).

An **epidermoid cyst** is an inclusion cyst in the floor of the mouth (usually in the midline) or the mucobuccal fold, which is the junction of the buccal mucosa and the alveolar mucosa. The midline of the floor of the mouth is the most common location for a **dermoid cyst,** which has a doughy feel. All cysts should be excised and carefully examined for evidence of malignancy.

SALIVARY GLANDS

Painless swelling of the parotid glands is often noted in hepatic cirrhosis, in sarcoidosis, in mumps, following abdominal surgery, or associated with neoplasms or infections. The common factors may be dehydration and inattention to oral hygiene. The latter promotes the growth of large numbers of bacteria that, in the absence of sufficient salivary flow, ascend from the mouth into the duct of a gland. Another cause of a painful salivary gland is **sialolithiasis** (salivary duct stone). The submandibular glands are most commonly affected. Pain and swelling associated with eating are characteristic. Calcium phosphate stones tend to form because of the high pH and viscosity of the submandibular gland saliva, which has a high mucin content. Stones are removed by manipulation or excision.

Autoimmune sialosis is the Mikulicz-Sjögren syndrome, a unilateral or bilateral enlargement of the parotid and/or submandibular glands, and often the lacrimal glands. Occasionally painful, it is associated with xerostomia (dry mouth) due to impaired saliva formation, which is most common in older women. (See SJÖGREN'S SYNDROME in Ch. 108).

THE PALATE

Torus palatinus is a common benign overgrowth of bone (osteoma) in the midline of the hard palate where the maxillae fuse. No treatment except reassurance is required unless a dentist wishes to cover the hard palate completely with a denture. If so, surgery is required.

A hole in the palate may be a **congenital cleft** involving either or both the hard and soft palates. Clefts of the palate or lip occur once in 700 to 800 births. The cleft may

vary from involvement of the soft palate only to a complete cleft of the soft and hard palates, the alveolar process of the maxilla, and the lip. The infant should be referred to a cleft palate team (pediatrician, orthodontist, speech pathologist, plastic surgeon, and psychologist). There are several etiologies of **perforating lesions** other than the congenital cleft; these include salivary gland tumors, the gumma of tertiary syphilis, carcinoma of the palate, and rarely, TB.

In infectious mononucleosis, **petechiae** may occur at the junction of the hard and soft palate. In neutropenia or agranulocytosis, there may be **ulcerations** with little inflammation. Clumps of asymptomatic red **papules** are seen in inflammatory hyperplasia of the palate (pseudopapillomatosis). A denture may irritate such lesions.

The palate may be the site of **Wegener's granulomatosis** (lethal midline granuloma—see in Ch. 110) in which there is destruction of bone with sequestration.

STOMATITIS

An inflammation of the mouth, often a symptom of systemic disease. Fetid breath odor and blood-tinged saliva may accompany any ulcerative lesions of the oral mucosa.

Etiology

Stomatitis may be caused by infection, trauma, dryness, irritants and toxic agents, hypersensitivity, or autoimmune conditions. Infectious agents include streptococci, gonococci, fusospirochetes, *Candida albicans*, *Corynebacterium diphtheriae*, *Treponema pallidum*, *Mycobacterium tuberculosis*, and the viruses of herpes simplex, coxsackie, measles, and infectious mononucleosis. Stomatitis may also result from avitaminosis, particularly lack of the B vitamins or vitamin C (as in pellagra, sprue, pernicious anemia, or scurvy); or from iron deficiency anemia with dysphagia **(Plummer-Vinson syndrome),** agranulocytosis, or leukemia. Lichen planus, erythema multiforme, SLE, Behçet's syndrome, and pemphigus vulgaris frequently present oral mucosa signs. Mechanical trauma from cheek biting, mouth breathing, jagged teeth, orthodontic appliances, ill-fitting dentures, or nursing bottles with hard or too-long nipples may produce characteristic lesions. Xerostomia resulting from drugs, the aging process, or radiation therapy predisposes the mouth to sensitivity and infection. Generalized stomatitis may follow excessive use of alcohol, tobacco, hot foods, or spices; or sensitization to toothpaste, mouthwash, candy dyes, lipstick, and, rarely, acrylic dentures. Phenytoin, iodides, bismuth, mercury, barbiturates, lead, and many other drugs may produce stomatitis. Chemical stomatitis of occupational origin may be due to dyes, heavy metals, acid fumes, or metal or mineral dust. The latter 3 may also cause abrasion of the hard tissues. Mercury causes marked salivation.

Symptoms and Signs

Clinical signs vary widely according to the type of stomatitis present. **Allergic stomatitis** is characterized by an intense, shiny erythema with slight swelling. Itching, dryness, or burning, often present, may be due to sensitivity to foods or to lipstick.

Vincent's infection (necrotizing ulcerative gingivitis—see VINCENT'S INFECTION in Ch. 249) causes ulceronecrotic lesions of the interdental papillae that may extend to the marginal gingivae or produce painful ulcers of the mucous membranes.

Thrush (candidiasis), caused by *C. albicans*, is characterized by white, slightly raised patches resembling milk curds that, when removed, expose a hyperemic area that may bleed slightly. The infection usually begins on the tongue and buccal mucosa and may spread to the palate, gums, tonsils, pharynx, larynx, GI tract, respiratory system, and skin. The mouth usually appears dry. Thrush is common in infants; the debilitated; the immunosuppressed; individuals on long-term antibiotic, corticosteroid, and antineoplastic therapy; and those with xerostomia. (See also SYSTEMIC CANDIDIASIS in Ch. 9.)

Pseudomembranous (or **membranous**) **stomatitis,** an inflammatory reaction that produces a membrane-like exudate, may be caused by chemical irritants (eg, gold, iodides)

as well as bacteria (streptococci, staphylococci, gonococci, *C. diphtheriae*). Fever, lymphadenopathy, and malaise may occur or the infection may be localized.

Mucosal lesions accompanying systemic disease include the mucous patches of syphilis; the strawberry, then raspberry, tongue of scarlet fever; Koplik's spots of measles; the ulcers of erythema multiforme; and the smooth, fiery red tongue and painful mouth of pellagra. Hemorrhagic lesions may occur in scurvy and disorders of platelet number and function. Unprovoked bleeding, decreased salivation, and an ammonia odor accompany uremic stomatitis.

The **mucocutaneous lymph node syndrome (Kawasaki syndrome)** affects children, causing erythema of the lips and oral mucosa. See KAWASAKI SYNDROME in Ch. 191.

Acrodynia occurs in children and is characterized by oral ulcerations, profuse salivation, and bruxism (see in Ch. 246) with loss of teeth. It is caused by a mercurial toxicity reaction.

Diagnosis

Establishing the etiology may be difficult. The history may disclose a systemic disease, a dietary deficiency, or contact with irritants or allergens. Physical examination is obligatory, since it may reveal lesions of other mucous membranes, as in erythema multiforme, candidiasis, or syphilis; lesions of the skin, as in pellagra, pemphigus, lichen planus, or SLE; signs of pulmonary TB, sprue, anemia, or another contributory disease; or a general decrease in exocrine secretions.

Direct smears and cultures from the lesions may disclose a pathogen. Any diphtheria-like membrane should be so examined *promptly*. Vincent's infection usually limits itself to the gingival tissue, differentiating it from primary herpetic gingivostomatitis. Darkfield examination of scrapings from the lesions and STS are indicated in an attempt to rule out syphilis before penicillin is given. In thrush, a history of recent antibiotic therapy is common. To identify *C. albicans*, scrapings from suspect lesions should be cultured and examined microscopically in 10% potassium hydroxide hanging drop preparations or methylene blue stained smears. Blood count, bone marrow examination, gastric analysis, or other laboratory procedures may be indicated.

A solitary, undiagnosed oral lesion of > 1 wk duration that does not respond to treatment must be considered malignant until biopsy proves otherwise.

Treatment

Underlying systemic disorders should be treated specifically. Oral hygiene is always necessary. Candidiasis usually responds to nystatin oral suspension 400,000 u. (4 mL) qid for 10 days as an oral rinse and then swallowed. Clotrimazole 10-mg oral lozenges 5 times a day for 14 days are effective in persistent overgrowths. When compliance is a problem, ketoconazole, one 200-mg tablet (for children, 1/4 tablet) orally once a day is effective. All antifungals should be continued for at least 3 days after signs and symptoms disappear. For oral bacterial infections, oral penicillin V is the drug of choice (see under PENICILLINS in ANTIMICROBIAL CHEMOTHERAPY in Ch. 3). Large, painful ulcers that prevent eating may be relieved temporarily by rinsing the mouth with 2% lidocaine viscous, 15 mL (1 tbsp) before each meal and q 3 h as needed for relief. A mouthwash of 1/2 tsp sodium bicarbonate in 250 mL (8 oz) warm water qid is soothing and cleansing. Rinsing (and spitting out) after each meal with elixir of dexamethasone 0.5 mg/5 mL (1 tsp) relieves discomfort and promotes healing of nonviral and nonbacterial oral lesions.

RECURRENT APHTHOUS STOMATITIS

Acute painful ulcers on the movable oral mucosa, occurring singly or in groups ***("canker sores")****.* Minor ulcers, the most common form, are < 1 cm in diameter, last 10 to 14 days, and heal without scarring; major ulcers, > 1 cm in diameter, last weeks to

months and heal with scarring. Recurrent attacks are common, with 2 or 3 ulcers during each attack; however, 10 to 15 ulcers are common in some individuals. Women are affected more often than men.

Etiology is unknown, but several factors point toward a localized immune reaction. Deficiencies of iron, vitamin B_{12}, and folic acid increase susceptibility. Stress and local trauma are usually the predominant precipitating factors.

Symptoms and Signs

Beginning as a shallow, ovoid erosion with a slightly raised, yellowish border surrounded by a narrow, red, hyperemic zone, the ulcer is covered within 5 to 7 days with a yellowish opaque material composed of coagulated tissue fluids, oral bacteria, and WBCs. The acutely painful phase lasts 3 or 4 days; symptoms then diminish until the lesion heals spontaneously, usually without scarring, in 7 to 10 days. Malaise, fever, and lymphadenopathy may accompany severe attacks. Recurrent attacks vary from one lesion 2 to 3 times/yr to an uninterrupted succession of multiple lesions.

Diagnosis

The mucosal lesion looks distinctive enough to differentiate aphthous stomatitis from primary or recurrent herpetic oral lesions (which may appear concurrently) and from the lesions of erythema multiforme, oral pemphigus, or benign mucosal pemphigoid. Aphthae rarely appear on the immovable mucosa (hard palate, attached gingiva), the prime areas for recurrent intraoral herpetic ulcers. The history and clinical examination exclude herpangina.

Treatment

A topical anesthetic such as 2% lidocaine viscous, 15 mL (1 tbsp) as an oral rinse q 3 h or before meals, provides short-term relief and facilitates eating. A dental protective paste (Orabase®) applied qid prevents irritation of the ulcers by the teeth, dental appliances, and oral fluids. An application of triamcinolone acetonide in emollient dental paste reduces discomfort and promotes healing.

For multiple lesions, tetracycline oral suspension (250 mg qid for 10 days) is held in the mouth for 2 to 5 min before swallowing, to coat the ulcers. If treatment is started early after onset, symptomatic relief occurs within a day and new lesions are aborted. Treatment must be repeated for each new attack. Occasionally this therapy results in oral (and vaginal) candidiasis. For severe episodes of minor aphthae or for major aphthae, corticosteroid therapy is indicated, both topical and systemic (elixir of dexamethasone 0.5 mg/5 mL [1 tsp] to rinse with [and spit out] after meals and at bedtime for 5 days).

ORAL ERYTHEMA MULTIFORME

(See also Erythema Multiforme in Ch. 237)

Acutely painful stomatitis characterized by diffuse hemorrhagic lesions of the lips and oral mucosa and usually associated with constitutional symptoms. Oral, ocular, genital, and dermal lesions can occur concurrently.

Symptoms, Signs, and Diagnosis

Prodromal symptoms may include rhinitis and sinusitis. Multiple vesicles form in the earliest stage. Typical lesions consist of diffuse hemorrhagic eroded areas throughout the mouth; the lips are commonly bloody and crusted, but the gingivae are rarely involved. Extensive oral, conjunctival, and genital lesions may be present, even without dermal eruption.

The patient may have fever as high as 40 to 40.6 C (104 or 105 F) during the early stages. Severe constitutional symptoms (fever, malaise, arthralgia) usually persist for 4 or 5 days; as they regress, the typical lesions develop. The constitutional symptoms

may be similar to those in allergic stomatitis, pemphigus, and herpetic stomatitis, which must be differentiated. The lesions are a deeper red than the mucous patches of secondary syphilis.

Treatment

Oral lesions in the acute phase may be treated with systemic corticosteroids (prednisone 10 mg orally tid for 5 days) or elixir of dexamethasone 0.5 mg/5 mL (1 tsp) to rinse with and swallow qid for 5 days. Without corticosteroids, the lesions may persist from 3 to 8 wk or longer. When intraoral lesions cause difficulty in eating, a liquid diet is helpful. Dehydration may necessitate IV fluid therapy. A warm mouthwash of 10% sodium bicarbonate solution and anesthetic troches, ointments, or solutions (eg, 2% lidocaine viscous) can be used 5 or 6 times/day. Petrolatum ointment may soothe lip lesions. With treatment, improvement is rapid and lesions usually heal without scarring. Recurrence is not usual.

ORAL HERPETIC MANIFESTATIONS

(See also HERPES SIMPLEX under RESPIRATORY VIRAL DISEASES in Ch. 12)

Acute, painful vesicular eruptions of the oral mucosa or vermilion borders, caused by the herpes simplex virus. Primary acute herpetic infection is common in infants and young children, and may occur in teenagers and young adults (see also HERPES SIMPLEX in Ch. 12). A history of recent contact with an adult having a herpes simplex eruption is frequent.

In childhood, the initial viral infection usually goes unrecognized unless the stomatitis causes feeding difficulties. After infection, antibody titer remains high throughout life and limits future response to the virus to an occasional recurrent lesion intraorally on the hard palate, or extraorally on the vermilion border, often extending to the skin surfaces of the lips. The latter are often called **fever blisters** or **cold sores.** Mild trauma such as that associated with dental treatment, abrasion of the vermilion border, sunburn, food allergy, anxiety, onset of menstruation, or any disease that produces a fever or an increased metabolic rate may precipitate lesions.

Symptoms and Signs

In **primary acute herpetic gingivostomatitis,** multiple shallow ulcers of varying size occur throughout the mouth. The oral ulcerations are preceded by inflamed gingivae resembling acute necrotizing ulcerative gingivitis and a 2- to 3-day prodromal period of malaise, fever, and cervical lymphadenopathy. During the first 4 or 5 days, pain may be severe enough to discourage a child from eating and drinking. Although the disease is usually self-limited and symptoms subside in 7 to 10 days, extensive systemic involvement and fatal viremia have occurred in infants and occasionally in older children.

In **recurrent herpes labialis,** patients usually experience a sensation of fullness, burning, and itching before the typical vesicle develops on slightly elevated, erythematous tissue at or near the junction of the vermilion and skin. The greatest extension of the lesion is usually toward the skin. A vesicular lesion may exist for hours before the vesicle breaks and a yellowish, crusted lesion forms. Underlying tissues are not indurated, though varying degrees of edema may be present. Lesions seldom last > 10 days.

Recurrent intraoral herpetic palatal and gingival lesions begin with multiple small vesicles that rupture quickly and unite to form large, superficial ulcerations with irregular margins. A large zone of erythema usually surrounds the ulcers.

Diagnosis

Primary acute herpetic stomatitis must be differentiated from drug eruptions and erythema multiforme, and, more rarely in adults, from pemphigus. Allergic forms of stomatitis can usually be suspected from the history. In both erythema multiforme and

pemphigus, accompanying skin lesions are common. **Erythema multiforme** (see in Ch. 237) may be discerned by more marked constitutional symptoms and widespread hemorrhagic lesions. In **pemphigus** (see also in Ch. 238), constitutional symptoms usually persist for several weeks, and the patient often recalls a prior episode of large painless bullae without accompanying prodromal symptoms.

Diagnosing the solitary lesion of **herpes labialis** is usually not difficult because of its characteristic appearance and location.

Treatment

In **primary herpetic stomatitis,** a topical analgesic relieves temporary pain; 2% lidocaine viscous, 5 mL (1 tsp) as an oral rinse q 3 h, or diphenhydramine elixir, 5 mL (1 tsp) as an oral rinse q 2 h is used as needed. A sodium bicarbonate mouthwash of 2.5 mL (0.5 tsp) in 250 mL (8 oz) warm water qid soothes and cleanses. Since children tend to decrease fluid intake, they must be watched for dehydration. Supportive therapy consists of increasing fluids and giving diet supplements (see TABLE 79–5 in Ch. 79). Systemic antibiotics may be used to guard against secondary infection.

Recurrent herpetic labialis (lip lesions) can be reduced in frequency by using a sunscreen containing amino benzoic acid during sun exposure. *All proposed treatment is more effective if started in the prodromal stage*, ie, at the first symptoms of local change in sensations.

Topically, antiviral agents such as vidarabine or acyclovir ointments will discourage spreading and act as lubricants. Applying ice locally will reduce swelling. Petrolatum will tend to prevent cracking, bleeding, and self-inoculation from manual spread.

Systemic treatment is directed toward improving resistance to the virus. A combination of equal parts of citrus bioflavanoids and ascorbic acid tablets 400 mg tid for 3 days may abort or greatly reduce the duration of the lesions. Where frequent recurrences interfere with daily function or nutrition, acyclovir 200-mg capsules 5 times/day will give relief.

Desiccating agents such as alcohol, ether, and chloroform are thought to fractionate the virus, thereby inviting resistant and mutagenic strains. Corticosteroids can spread the virus, especially on mucosal tissue.

There is no cure for herpes simplex.

TONGUE

Infants may have **mucocutaneous lymph node syndrome (Kawasaki syndrome**—see in Ch. 191) in which there is a bright red tongue and face, edema of the extremities, and thrombocytosis. **Ankyloglossia** (tongue-tie) may be diagnosed if the tip of the tongue cannot contact the alveolar ridge or the tips of the teeth or sweep from one corner of the mouth to the other. To increase mobility of the tongue, the lingual frenum may need cutting. Untreated tongue-tie may affect speech and interfere with mastication and passive cleansing of the teeth. A **burning sensation** is a frequent postmenopausal symptom in association with poor keratinization, or may be a symptom of diabetic neuropathy; both require treatment of the underlying endocrine disorder. In the absence of physiologic or anatomic abnormalities, depression or an anxiety state should be considered. Amitriptyline 25 mg at bedtime with a weekly increase of dosage is usually effective in 3 to 4 wk.

GLOSSITIS

An acute or chronic inflammation of the tongue.

Etiology

Glossitis may be either a primary disease or a symptom of disease elsewhere. The many and varied causes include the following:

Local: Infectious agents commonly found in the mouth; mechanical trauma (jagged teeth, ill-fitting dentures, oral habits, repeated biting during convulsive seizures); primary irritants (excessive use of alcohol, tobacco, hot foods, spices); or sensitization (by toothpaste, mouthwashes, breath fresheners, candy dyes, and, rarely, plastic dentures or restorative materials).

Systemic: Avitaminosis (particularly of the B group, as in pellagra), anemia (pernicious anemia, iron deficiency anemia), certain generalized skin diseases (lichen planus, erythema multiforme, aphthous lesions, Behçet's syndrome, pemphigus vulgaris, syphilis).

Symptoms, Signs, and Diagnosis

Clinical manifestations vary widely without strong correlation between the appearance of lesions and the severity of symptoms. Reddened tip and edges of the tongue may indicate incipient pellagra, pernicious anemia, irritation from excessive smoking, or a tooth with a rough surface. In later stages of pellagra, the entire tongue is fiery red, swollen, and often ulcerated. In iron deficiency and particularly in pernicious anemia, the tongue is pale and smooth. Painful ulcers may indicate primary herpetic or aphthous lesions, pulmonary TB with positive sputum, streptococcal infection, erythema multiforme, or pemphigus vulgaris. Whitish patches suggest candidiasis, the mucous patch of syphilis, lichen planus, leukoplakia, or mouth breathing. Denuded smooth areas, if not painful, may indicate **geographic tongue** (benign migratory glossitis), or if moderately painful, anemia or pellagra; if they are very distressing and persistent, they may be the lesions of **atrophic lichen planus** (slick, glossy, or glazed tongue). **Median rhomboid glossitis,** a developmental lesion, consists of a rhomboid-shaped smooth, reddish, nodular area on the dorsal surface of the back portion of the middle third of the tongue. **Hairy tongue,** due to a profuse overgrowth of the filiform papillae, is usually asymptomatic and often follows antibiotic therapy, fever, excessive use of O_2-liberating mouthwashes, or a reduction in salivary flow. Brown papillae are usually from tobacco staining or the overgrowth of chromogenic bacteria. Treatment is rectifying the underlying cause and brushing the tongue with a toothbrush.

Severe acute glossitis occasionally results from local infection, burns, or trauma. It may develop rapidly, producing marked tenderness or pain with swelling sufficient to cause protrusion of the tongue and the danger of airway obstruction and suffocation. Mastication, swallowing, and speaking are painful and sometimes impossible. Cervical and submandibular adenitis with evidence of systemic toxicity may be present. Immediate treatment with steroids may be indicated to reduce the edema.

Patients may complain of a painful burning tongue **(glossodynia** and **glossopyrosis)** without obvious clinical evidence of inflammation. Many patients are postmenopausal. Incipient candidiasis, anemias, diabetes mellitus, latent nutritional deficiencies, or malignancies should be excluded.

Each case of glossitis deserves study, since the tongue often mirrors disease. History may disclose an irritant, contact allergen, sensitizing drug, deficient diet, or other symptoms of disease. Other mucosal surfaces and the skin should be inspected for evidence of pellagra, erythema multiforme, syphilis, or lichen planus. Studies for an anemia, mild diabetes mellitus, sprue, and syphilis should be performed.

Prognosis

When the cause can be determined and corrected, response is usually prompt, but may be delayed in nonspecific or chronic involvement. The patient should be reassured that persistent lesions such as median rhomboid glossitis and geographic tongue are innocuous. Aphthous lesions, erythema multiforme, and hairy tongue often recur periodically. Solitary ulcerations that do not respond to treatment after 1 wk should be biopsied.

Treatment

General: Specific causative disorders are treated as indicated. Irritants and sensitizing agents are to be *avoided.* A bland or liquid diet, preferably cooled, is given. Meticulous oral hygiene is imperative.

Local: Oral infections call for specific therapy (see STOMATITIS, above). The pain of large lesions that interfere with eating may be relieved temporarily by rinsing with an obtundent mouthwash before each meal; topical anesthetics (lidocaine 5% ointment or 10% spray; benzocaine 2% ointment; dyclonine 0.5% liquid) applied to discrete lesions also give relief and encourage eating. Occasionally, systemic analgesics (aspirin or acetaminophen 650 mg q 4 h) are required. Topical application of triamcinolone acetonide 0.1% in emollient dental paste to specific lesions (except those of viral etiology) tid or qid will relieve symptoms and may promote healing.

The patient with symptoms of painful burning but a clinically normal tongue requires special management. Tests for vitamin B_{12} deficiency should be conducted, especially after menopause. For therapy of B_{12} deficiency, see Ch. 96. After systemic causes (anemia, diabetes mellitus) have been ruled out, an emotional basis may be presumed. Reassurance (especially regarding neoplasm) and encouragement are important.

248. DENTAL CARIES AND ITS COMPLICATIONS

TOOTH DECAY

A gradual pathologic disintegration and dissolution of tooth enamel and dentin, with eventual involvement of the pulp. Except for the common cold, this is the most prevalent human disorder.

Etiology

The interaction of 3 factors results in dental caries: a susceptible tooth surface, the proper microflora, and a suitable substrate for the microflora. Although several oral acidogenic microorganisms can initiate the carious lesion, laboratory and clinical evidence points to *Streptococcus mutans* as the primary pathogen. Its virulence stems from its ability to synthesize extracellular polysaccharide. Lactic acid, a by-product of this synthesis, contributes to tooth demineralization. Mono- and disaccharide sugars serve as the principal substrates for the process. The gummy extracellular polysaccharides increase the bulk of dental plaque and favor bacterial proliferation and attachment to the tooth surface. **Dental plaque**—a combination of these polysaccharides, salivary glycoproteins, and desquamated mucosal cells—serves as a localized site of acid production.

Dietary carbohydrates play a significant role. The types of carbohydrates and frequency of their ingestion are more important than the amounts consumed. Frequent between-meal snacks, especially of sucrose-containing foods, enhance the carious process; sticky foods that linger are potentially more harmful than nonsticky foods.

Pathogenesis

Dental caries begins on the external crown or exposed root surface of the tooth. Bacterial plaque, not food debris, causes caries. Plaque is not flushed away by the action of oral musculature or saliva. The role of saliva in preventing caries is in its buffering capacity and remineralization effect. Acid action first demineralizes enamel with its high inorganic content; proteolysis of its organic matrix follows. When the carious process reaches the dentin or begins on the root surface, the tooth becomes

sensitive to temperature or osmotic changes engendered by foods or by touch. Caries spreads rapidly because of the lower mineral content of dentin and cementum. As demineralization and necrosis of the dentin progress, microorganisms may invade the dentinal tubules. Microbial products preceding the organisms in the dentinal tubules may cause inflammation of the dental pulp before destruction of the surrounding dentin is evident.

Symptoms and Signs

The patient is often unaware of the presence of caries until the lesion is well advanced. Common early symptoms are sensitivity to heat and cold and discomfort after eating sugar-containing foods. A darkened area between anterior teeth or cavitation when the carious process has progressed sufficiently may be noticed. Caries is clinically diagnosed by the dentist when softened enamel or dentin is detected with a sharp instrument. Radiographically, caries appears as a radiolucent area, as do most resin filling materials and bases under metallic restorations. Consequently, radiographic diagnosis must be coupled with a visual examination.

Prophylaxis

Teeth are less susceptible to caries if optimum amounts of fluoride (approximately 1 mg/day) are ingested while the teeth are developing. Fluoride combines with some of the apatite crystals in the tooth structure to form the less soluble fluorapatite. Maximum benefit accrues when water containing 1 ppm of fluoride is consumed from birth until the permanent dentition completes eruption (age 11 to 13.) Nearly 1/2 the US population still does not have access to optimally fluoridated water. There is no proof that ingesting fluoridated water or fluoride supplements during pregnancy will significantly protect a child's deciduous teeth and permanent lst molars, although these calcify in utero.

Ingesting excessive fluoride before eruption, while the enamel is forming, may cause permanent mottling of the enamel. Once erupted, teeth cannot develop mottling when exposed to excessive fluoride. During pregnancy, the placenta acts as a barrier against marked increases in fluoride concentration and thus protects the calcifying fetal teeth against mottling.

If the water supply contains less than the optimum amount of fluoride for the local mean maximum air temperature (as prescribed by the Public Health Service Drinking Water Standards), children should take daily supplements during their tooth-forming years, by using bottled fluoridated water for drinking and cooking, or by taking a sodium fluoride tablet.

Applying fluoride compounds to erupted teeth enhances benefits from systemic fluorides in both children and adults; it is not a substitute, since the modes of action differ. Periodic applications should be supplemented by daily use of a fluoride-containing dentifrice. Daily use of a mouth rinse containing low fluoride concentrations is also effective for children as prophylaxis against caries. For highly caries-prone patients, custom trays for self-application of fluoride gel for 5 min/day are recommended.

Food particles and dental plaque should be removed from all accessible tooth surfaces at least once daily. Mechanical removal is the only effective method currently available. Proper use of a soft-bristled toothbrush removes plaque adequately from all areas except interproximal tooth surfaces and deep pits and fissures of the enamel. Interproximal surfaces, highly susceptible to dental caries, should be cleaned daily with dental floss or tape. Plaque-disclosing tablets or liquids composed of food coloring may be used to check the efficacy of plaque removal. Since fluorides are relatively less effective for preventing pit and fissure caries, sealing enamel pits and fissures with a BIS-GMA-type resin is highly effective in preventing caries and is performed increasingly by dentists. The sealed teeth should be checked annually and the sealant replaced when lost.

Treatment

Although caries may be arrested, destroyed tooth structure cannot regenerate. All affected tooth structure should be removed and replaced with a restorative material. For details of filling teeth, see DENTAL RESTORATIONS AND APPLIANCES in Ch. 245.

PULPITIS

Inflammation of the dental pulp (containing vascular, connective, and nervous tissue) and of the adjacent periodontal tissues, resulting in **toothache.**

Etiology and Pathology

Pulpitis may result from thermal, chemical, traumatic, or bacterial irritation of the pulp. Pulpal inflammation and infection secondary to caries is the most frequent cause. Since hard dentinal walls surround the pulp, an inflammatory reaction usually results in necrosis. The inflammation extends through the apex of the tooth and involves the periapical tissues (connective tissue of the periodontal membrane and bone).

Diagnosis

In acute suppurative pulpitis, a sharp, throbbing, shooting pain may be intermittent; it is less intense in pulpitis secondary to mechanical debridement of a cavity. A distinction must be made between caries-induced pulpitis and pulpitis secondary to traumatic occlusion. Intense pain may be difficult to localize. It may be referred to the opposite mandible or maxilla or to areas supplied by common branches of the 5th nerve. Radiographs, pulp testers, percussion, thermal tests, and palpation aid in diagnosis.

Treatment

In early pulpitis, cleansing the cavity to remove food debris and softened dentin, followed by packing the cavity with zinc oxide-eugenol cement (clove oil mixed with zinc oxide powder to form a thick paste), usually affords relief and prevents food debris from accumulating. Infected pulpal tissue should be removed and root canal therapy instituted, or the tooth should be extracted.

PERIAPICAL ABSCESS

(Dentoalveolar Abscess)

An acute or chronic suppurative process of the periapical region.

Etiology and Pathogenesis

The abscess is secondary to an infection of the dental pulp usually due to caries. However, it may occur after trauma to the teeth or from periapical localization of organisms, usually α-hemolytic streptococci or staphylococci.

Symptoms and Signs

Pain is gnawing and continuous. The involved tooth is painful when percussed, and often the teeth cannot close without added discomfort. Hot or cold foods may increase the pain. If treatment is delayed, the infection may spread through adjacent tissues, causing **cellulitis,** varying degrees of facial edema, and fever. The infection may extend into osseous tissues or into the soft tissues of the floor of the mouth. Local swelling and **gingival fistulas** may develop opposite the apex of the tooth, especially with deciduous teeth. Drainage into the mouth causes a bitter taste. **Abscesses** from lower molars may drain at the angle of the jaw.

A *chronic* periapical abscess usually presents few clinical signs, since it is essentially a circumscribed area of mild infection that spreads slowly. In time, the infection may become granulomatous. As the granuloma enlarges, the lesion may progress to an epithelium-lined cavity and a **periapical cyst** results. Persistent periapical cysts and granulomas may become infected. All are radiolucent on x-ray examination. Bacteria

may spread via the blood and by contiguity to involve the brain, cervical, and thoracic structures (see Ch. 245).

Treatment

Extraction or root canal therapy is usually indicated. If high fever persists, antibiotics (eg, penicillin G or V 250 to 500 mg q 6 h, or erythromycin or a tetracycline 250 mg q 6 h) should be given. Hot saline mouth rinses may encourage pointing. If the swelling becomes fluctuant, it should be drained, usually by intraoral incision. An analgesic (eg, aspirin or acetaminophen 650 mg alone or with codeine 30 to 60 mg orally q 3 to 4 h) is usually needed. Bed rest, a soft diet, and forced fluids may be necessary.

---

249. PERIODONTAL DISEASE

(Pyorrhea)

Inflammation or degeneration of tissues that surround and support the teeth: gingiva, alveolar bone, periodontal ligament, and cementum. Periodontal disease most commonly begins as gingivitis and progresses to periodontitis. If the severity of the disease is disproportionate to the amount of plaque and calculus, **systemic disease** may be present; however, in widespread periodontal disease, local factors are also present. For example, diabetes mellitus, scurvy, leukemia and other disorders of leukocyte number or function, hyperparathyroidism, and osteoporosis aggravate local factors.

GINGIVITIS

Inflammation of the gingivae, characterized by swelling, redness, change of normal contours, watery exudate, and bleeding. Swelling deepens the crevice between the gingiva and the teeth, and gingival pockets form. Gingivitis is common, and may be acute, chronic, or recurrent.

Etiology

The greatest single cause is poor hygiene, characterized by bacterial plaque (microbial colonies growing in carbohydrate residues tenaciously attached to the tooth surfaces). Other local factors such as malocclusion, dental calculus (calcified plaque, called tartar), food impaction, faulty dental restorations, and mouth breathing play important secondary roles.

Gingivitis is commonly noted at puberty and during pregnancy and is presumably due to endocrine factors. Gingivitis may be the first sign of a systemic disorder with lowered tissue resistance, eg, hypovitaminosis, leukopenic disorders, allergic reaction, endocrine disturbance (eg, diabetes mellitus), or a debilitating disease. Prolonged ingestion of phenytoin may cause enlargement of the gingiva; the use of birth control pills may increase inflammatory changes; heavy metals (eg, lead and bismuth) may also cause gingivitis. Correcting the factors causing the gingivitis would prevent most periodontal disease.

Symptoms, Signs, and Diagnosis

Simple gingivitis: The outstanding signs are a band of red, inflamed gum tissue surrounding the necks of teeth, edematous swelling of the interdental papillae, and bleeding on minimal injury. Pain is usually absent. The inflammation, sometimes acute in onset, may subside or persist.

Gingivitis of diabetes mellitus: Uncontrolled diabetics have an exaggerated response to gingival irritants; secondary infections and acute gingival abscesses are common. Rapid, progressive periodontal bone loss is a common radiographic finding.

Gingivitis of pregnancy: Mild inflammation of the gingiva may develop in pregnancy; hyperplasia, especially of the interdental papillae, is likely to occur. Pedunculated gingival growths **(pregnancy tumors)** often arise from the papillae in the first trimester, may persist throughout pregnancy, and may or may not subside after delivery. These growths tend to recur if excised before term and may or may not regress following delivery. A similar lesion, **pyogenic granuloma,** is a soft, reddish mass in the interdental gingiva that develops rapidly and then remains static. Treatment is excision. A similar gingivitis may accompany dysmenorrhea.

Desquamative gingivitis is characterized by deep red, painful, easily bleeding gingival tissue. Vesicles may precede the stage of desquamation. Desquamative gingivitis often occurs during menopause. The gingivae are soft because the cornified cells that would resist masticatory trauma are absent. Sequential administration of estrogens and progestins is often beneficial. A similar gingival lesion may be associated with bullous pemphigoid or benign mucosal pemphigoid, which responds to corticosteroid therapy (see Ch. 238).

Gingivitis in leukemia: Engorged, edematous, painful, enlarged, livid gums that bleed readily suggest leukemia. They result from reduced tissue resistance, the presence of leukemic infiltrates in the periodontal tissues, and characteristic bleeding abnormalities. The gingiva may become secondarily infected with fusospirochetal organisms, resulting in necrotizing ulcerative gingivitis (see VINCENT'S INFECTION, below).

Phenytoin gingivitis: Prolonged intake of phenytoin may cause fibrotic gingival hyperplasia. The interdental papillae enlarge initially. The process may progress until the gums are entirely involved and the teeth partially obscured. The hyperplastic tissue is firm and less prone to bleed than in other forms of gingivitis. Excision may afford temporary benefit. A folic acid supplement (3 mg/day) helps to control the hyperplasia. The drugs nifedipine and cyclosporine can produce a similar hyperplasia of the gingiva.

Gingivitis in hypovitaminosis: The gingiva in **scurvy** is inflamed, hyperplastic, engorged with blood, and bleeds easily. It may appear as "bags of blood." Petechial and ecchymotic areas may be on the gums and elsewhere in the mouth. Destruction of periosteum and periodontal tissue, resulting in loosened teeth, is common. Gum changes are not seen in edentulous patients. In **pellagra,** the gingiva is inflamed, bleeds easily, and is subject to secondary infection. The lips are reddened and cracked, the mouth feels scalded, the tongue is smooth and bright red, and tongue and mucosa may show ulcerations.

Pericoronitis: Recurrent episodes of acute inflammation of the gingival flap overlying a partially erupted tooth are common—most often around the 3rd molar; extraction may be considered after the acute process subsides. The gingival flap disappears when the tooth is fully erupted. Treatment is local aqueous irrigation. If the infection is severe, antibiotics may be required; eg, penicillin V 500 mg orally q 6 h for 10 days.

Gingival abscess (parulis) develops from a periapical abscess at the tip of the root of a nonvital tooth. Pus escapes from a sinus that opens on the mucosal surface. A periodontal abscess may drain similarly.

Prophylaxis

Daily removal of plaque with dental floss and a toothbrush, and routine cleaning by a dentist every 4 to 6 mo are essential preventive procedures, especially when systemic conditions predispose to gingivitis.

Treatment

The treatment is to control or correct both plaque and local and systemic factors. Some cases require extensive treatment such as scaling, selective grinding of teeth to eliminate traumatic occlusion, and replacement of overhanging fillings and poorly contoured restorations. Otherwise, food trapped against the gingiva may become im-

pacted into the gingival margin. Excision of excess gingiva is required in specific situations as noted above.

VINCENT'S INFECTION

(Trench Mouth; Necrotizing Ulcerative Gingivitis; Fusospirochetosis)

A noncontagious infection, associated with a fusiform bacillus and a spirochete, that begins on the interdental papillae and can affect the marginal and attached gingiva by direct extension. Lack of oral hygiene, physical or emotional stress, nutritional deficiencies, blood dyscrasias, debilitating diseases, insufficient rest, and heavy smoking predispose to this disease, which is seen most frequently in young adults.

Symptoms and Signs

Onset, usually abrupt, may be accompanied by malaise. Without a secondary infection, there is usually no fever. The chief symptoms are acutely painful bleeding gums, salivation, and fetid breath. The ulcerations, usually limited to the marginal gingivae and interdental papillae, have a characteristic punched-out appearance, are covered by a grayish membrane, and bleed on slight pressure or irritation. Swallowing and talking may be painful. Regional lymphadenopathy is often present. Lesions on the buccal mucosa are rare but may appear as diffuse ulcerations covered with an easily removed pseudomembrane. Rarely, lesions may occur on the tonsils, pharynx, bronchi, rectum, or vagina.

Diagnosis

The punched-out appearance of the interdental papillae, the interdental grayish membrane, spontaneous bleeding, and pain are pathognomonic. The presence of overwhelming numbers of fusospirochetal forms in stained smears from the lesions confirms the diagnosis. Early differentiation from diphtheria or agranulocytosis is essential when tonsillar or pharyngeal tissues are involved. The differential diagnosis must consider streptococcal or staphylococcal pharyngitis and primary herpetic stomatitis.

Treatment

Gentle but thorough local debridement, oral hygiene, adequate nutrition, high fluid intake, and rest are essential. Using a soft brush and irrigating under low pressure or rinsing the mouth with warm normal saline or 1.5% peroxide solution may be helpful for the first few days. Analgesics may be required during the first 24 h after initial debridement. The patient should avoid irritation (eg, from smoking or from hot or spicy foods) and should have appropriate rest, good nutrition, and high fluid intake. Marked improvement usually occurs within 24 h, and then debridement can be completed. Although the acute stage responds quickly to antibiotic therapy (eg, penicillin G or V, erythromycin, or a tetracycline, 250 mg q 6 h), antibiotics are seldom necessary and should be avoided unless high fever is present. Poor tissue topography, often produced during the acute phase, may need surgical correction to reduce the possibility of recurrence.

OTHER GINGIVAL DISORDERS

Enlargement of the gingivae occurs frequently during hormonal changes, ie, pregnancy and puberty, particularly where local irritation exists, as with malocclusion or calculus. **Idiopathic fibromatosis** is characterized by diffuse enlargement of the gingivae, either smooth or nodular (see also Phenytoin Gingivitis, above). The hypertrophied tissue is often removed after the etiologic factors have been controlled.

Gingival **fibromas** often occur near sites of chronic irritation. A **giant cell epulis,** which looks similar, may arise from the periodontal ligament. If the tissue contains

such cells, blood chemistry should be investigated for the possibility of hyperparathyroidism.

Denture sore mouth is chronic inflammation due to frictional trauma of the mucosa under a poorly fitting denture. Treatment is replacement with a proper fit. Frequently this condition is accompanied by an oral candidiasis that requires concomitant treatment with nystatin oral rinses or ointment applied to the tissue surface of the denture or clotrimazole troches, 10 mg, 5 times/day. Ketoconazole, one 200-mg tablet/day, may be required.

In thrombocytopenic purpura or disorders of platelet function, gingival petechiae and **hemorrhage** may occur. Localization is predominantly at sites of periodontal disease.

PERIODONTITIS

Progression of gingivitis to the point that loss of supporting bone has begun. It is the primary cause of tooth loss in adults.

Etiology

Periodontitis results from the same local and systemic factors that cause gingivitis. The duration and severity of these factors as well as the resistance and repair potential of the patient influence the rate of osseous resorption. Faulty occlusion causing an excessive functional load on the teeth may contribute to the progress of the disease.

Symptoms, Signs, and Diagnosis

The early symptoms and signs of periodontitis are similar to those of gingivitis. The gingival pockets between the gingivae and the teeth deepen, calculus deposits often enlarge, the gums lose their attachment to the teeth, and bone loss begins. The pockets collect debris and allow microbes to proliferate, thus promoting the disease. Destruction of the supporting osseous tissue in varying degree is the earliest evidence seen on x-ray. Loosening of teeth and possible recession of the gums follow progressive bone loss; tooth migration is common in later stages. Pain is usually absent unless an acute infection (eg, abscess formation in one or more periodontal pockets) is superimposed on the chronic process.

Treatment (see also GINGIVITIS, above)

Systemic disorders require correction. Astringent agents, mouthwashes, and antibiotics are of little value in long-term treatment. Dental referral is indicated to correct or eliminate local irritative factors and to instruct in home care that will limit further destruction. If abnormal gum shape and pockets go uncorrected, surgery will be required. Advanced periodontitis with deep pocket formation and tooth mobility is likely to require extensive periodontal surgery. Selective grinding of tooth surfaces to eliminate traumatic occlusion, and splinting of loose teeth may be necessary. Extractions are often imperative in advanced disease.

JUVENILE PERIODONTITIS

(Periodontosis)

An uncommon widespread degeneration of the periodontal tissues with loss of alveolar bone so that teeth may be lost at an early age. It differs from periodontitis in its lack of associated inflammation and pus formation. Typically, there is significant bone loss localized to the first molars and incisors during late childhood or the early teens. Specific microorganisms and a hereditary predisposition may be linked to the disease. By early adulthood, typical chronic inflammatory periodontitis may be superimposed on the original juvenile condition. While its cause and treatment are unknown, im-

proving the occlusion and splinting the teeth may be of value. Periodontal surgery may stabilize the condition.

---

250. TEMPOROMANDIBULAR JOINT (TMJ) DISORDERS

The TMJ is susceptible to common congenital and developmental anomalies, fractures, dislocations, ankylosis, arthritis, and neoplastic diseases. There may also be internal derangements of the intra-articular disc. Nonarticular disorders that affect the area and can mimic true TMJ disease and the muscular disorder known as **myofascial pain-dysfunction (MPD) syndrome** (see below), which may secondarily involve the TMJ, must be considered in differential diagnosis. (See also TEMPOROMANDIULAR JOINT in Ch. 246.)

CONGENITAL AND DEVELOPMENTAL ANOMALIES

Agenesis: Congenital absence of the condyloid process results in severe facial deformity. The coronoid process, the ramus, and parts of the mandibular body may also be absent. Abnormalities of the external, middle, and inner ear, the temporal bone, the parotid gland, the muscles of mastication, and the facial nerve are often associated. Without the condyle, the mandible deviates to the affected side, and the unaffected side is elongated and flattened. Mandibular skewing results in severe malocclusion. X-rays of the mandible and TMJ show the degree of agenesis and distinguish this condition from others that affect the growing condyle and produce similar facial deformities but are *not* associated with severe structural loss.

Treatment: Jaw reconstruction by autogenous bone grafting should be initiated as soon as possible to limit progression of the facial deformity. Mentoplasty and onlay grafts of bone, cartilage, or soft tissue are also frequently used to improve facial symmetry. Orthodontic treatment helps correct malocclusion.

Condylar hypoplasia may be developmental in origin but usually results from local injury by trauma, infection, or irradiation during the growth period. Hypoplasia produces facial deformity characterized on the affected side by a short mandibular body, fullness of the face, and deviation of the chin. On the unaffected side, the body of the mandible is elongated and the face appears flat. Malocclusion results from the mandibular deviation. Diagnosis is based on a history of progressive facial asymmetry during the growth period, x-ray evidence of condylar deformity and antegonial notching, and, frequently, a history of trauma. **Treatment** by surgically shortening the normal side of the mandible or lengthening the affected side is usually functionally and esthetically corrective. Presurgical orthodontic therapy helps to achieve an optimal result.

Condylar hyperplasia, a disorder of unknown etiology, is characterized by persistent or accelerated growth at a time when growth should be diminishing or ended. Slowly progressive unilateral enlargement of the mandible causes cross-bite malocclusion, facial asymmetry, and shifting of the midpoint of the chin to the unaffected side. The patient may appear prognathic. The lower border of the mandible is often convex on the affected side. On x-ray, the TMJ may appear normal or the condyle may be symmetrically enlarged and the mandibular neck elongated. The condition is self-limiting. Since chondroma and osteochondroma may produce similar symptoms and signs, they must be ruled out. These grow more rapidly and usually cause asymmetric condylar enlargement.

Treatment: Condylectomy is recommended during the period of active growth, as determined by serial cephalometric x-rays and bone scan. If growth has already stopped, orthodontics and surgical mandibular repositioning are indicated. If the height of the mandibular body is greatly increased, facial symmetry can be further improved by reducing the inferior border.

TRAUMA AND DISLOCATION

(See Ch. 252)

ANKYLOSIS

Ankylosis of the TMJ is most often a sequel to trauma or infection, though it may accompany RA or be congenital. Chronic, painless limitation of movement occurs. When associated with condylar growth arrest or tissue loss, facial asymmetry is usual (see **condylar hypoplasia**, above). True (intra-articular) ankylosis must be distinguished from false (extra-articular) ankylosis. The latter may be caused by such things as enlargement of the coronoid process, depressed fracture of the zygomatic arch, or scarring from surgery or irradiation. In most cases of true ankylosis, x-rays of the TMJ show loss of normal bony architecture.

Treatment: Forced opening of the jaws is generally ineffective because of bony fusion. Condylectomy can be used if the ankylosis is intra-articular. An ostectomy in the ramus may be needed if the coronoid process and zygomatic arch are also involved. Prolonged use of jaw-opening exercises is essential to maintain the surgical correction.

INTERNAL DISK DERANGEMENT

Internal derangement of the articular disk can be caused by chronic spasm of the lateral pterygoid muscle, trauma, or arthritic changes in the articulating surfaces. Such derangements take 2 forms: anterior disk displacement with reduction during function, which is accompanied by clicking or popping sounds on opening the mouth, and anterior disk displacement without reduction, which is characterized by painful limitation of jaw movement. This clinical distinction is confirmed by arthrography or CT scan.

Treatment

Nonsurgical treatment is effective in approximately 25% of the patients who have anterior disk displacement with reduction. It employs jaw repositioning appliances, nonsteroidal anti-inflammatory drugs, and, when there is lateral pterygoid spasm, muscle relaxants. For patients with persistent pain and clicking unresponsive to such modalities, the disk can be repositioned surgically.

For anterior displacement of the disk that is not self-reducing, surgical correction is indicated. If the disk is in satisfactory condition, it is merely repositioned. Otherwise, it is removed (meniscectomy) and replaced with an alloplastic implant.

ARTHRITIS

(See also Ch. 108)

Most forms of arthritis can involve the TMJ; the most common ones are infectious, traumatic, rheumatoid, and degenerative (osteoarthritis).

Infectious arthritis may be part of a generalized systemic disease, may arise from direct extension of adjacent infection, or may result from localization of blood-borne organisms from a distant infection. Inflammation and limited jaw movement are present. Early x-rays are negative but bone destruction becomes evident later. Local signs

of inflammation, associated with evidence of a systemic disease or an adjacent infection, suggest the diagnosis. In suppurative arthritis, joint aspiration may confirm the diagnosis and identify the causative organism.

Treatment includes antibiotics, proper hydration, control of pain, and restriction of motion. Suppurative infections should be aspirated or incised. Once the infection is controlled, jaw-opening exercises are important to prevent scarring and limitation of function.

Traumatic arthritis may be caused by acute injury or excessive opening—eg, during yawning, tooth extraction, or endotracheal intubation. Pain, tenderness, and limitation of motion occur. X-rays are negative except for occasional widening of the joint space due to intra-articular edema or hemorrhage. The diagnosis includes a history of trauma and x-rays negative for fracture. **Treatment** includes analgesics, heat application, a soft diet, and restriction of jaw movement.

In **RA,** the TMJ is involved in > 50% of cases, in both adults and children. Pain, swelling, and limited movement are the most common findings. In children, destruction of the condyle results in growth disturbance and facial deformity. Ankylosis may follow in all patients. X-rays of the TMJ are usually negative in early stages, but bone destruction is seen later and may result in an anterior open-bite deformity. The **diagnosis** is suggested by TMJ inflammation associated with polyarthritis and is confirmed by positive laboratory findings.

Treatment is similar to that for RA of other joints. In the acute stage, anti-inflammatory drugs are given and jaw function should be limited. When symptoms subside, mild jaw exercises help prevent excessive loss of motion. Surgical correction is necessary if ankylosis develops, but should not be undertaken until the condition is quiescent.

Primary degenerative arthritis (osteoarthritis) may involve the TMJ as well as other joints and usually occurs in persons over age 50. Relatively asymptomatic, patients complain only occasionally of stiffness, crepitation, or mild pain. Joint involvement is generally bilateral. X-rays may show flattening and lipping of the condyle. **Treatment** is symptomatic.

Secondary degenerative arthritis usually occurs in persons aged 20 to 40 after trauma or persistent MPD syndrome (see below), and is characterized by limitation of opening and unilateral pain on motion, joint tenderness, and crepitation. When associated with MPD syndrome, the symptoms intermittently become more severe and some muscles of mastication are tender. X-rays generally show condylar flattening, lipping, spurring, or erosion. The unilateral joint involvement helps to distinguish secondary from primary degenerative arthritis. **Treatment** is conservative, as for MPD syndrome, though arthroplasty or high condylectomy may be necessary. Intra-articular injection of corticosteroids or of 2% lidocaine may bring symptomatic relief but may harm the joint if repeated often.

NONARTICULAR CONDITIONS MIMICKING TEMPOROMANDIBULAR JOINT DISORDERS

Conditions unrelated to the TMJ that can produce preauricular pain, limitation of jaw movement, or a combination of both include pulpitis, pericoronitis, otitis, parotitis, trigeminal neuralgia, atypical (vascular) neuralgia, temporal arteritis, nasopharyngeal carcinoma, myositis and myositis ossificans, tetanus, scleroderma, depressed fracture of the zygomatic arch, and osteochondroma of the coronoid process. Pain due to these, unlike intrinsic TMJ disorders, is usually not exacerbated by finger pressure on the TMJ as the patient opens the mouth.

MYOFASCIAL PAIN-DYSFUNCTION (MPD) SYNDROME

The most common disorder involving the TMJ area, MPD syndrome occurs in women more frequently than in men. Most cases are psychophysiologic in origin and result from tension-relieving jaw-clenching or tooth-grinding habits, or a centrally generated increase in masticatory muscle tonus in response to stress. The ensuing muscle fatigue in turn induces spasm of the masticatory muscles, the immediate cause of MPD. Poorly aligned teeth or ill-fitting dentures occasionally contribute to the condition. Secondary degenerative arthritis may involve the joint in the late stages.

Diagnosis is based on clinical findings. Characteristically, the patient complains of unilateral, dull, aching preauricular pain that radiates to the temporal region, the angle of the jaw, and the occiput; tenderness in one or more of the muscles of mastication; jaw limitation; and occasional "clicking" or "popping" sounds in the joint (see INTERNAL DISK DERANGEMENT, above). Joint pain on awakening may indicate bruxism during sleep. X-rays are usually normal, although secondary degenerative changes are seen occasionally in very late stages. Degenerative arthritis, which causes similar symptoms, must be excluded. Primary degenerative arthritis is usually bilateral. Both primary and secondary degenerative arthritis usually produce x-ray changes in the joint, and secondary degenerative arthritis causes tenderness of the TMJ on lateral or intrameatal palpation; these findings help to distinguish the arthritides from MPD syndrome. However, secondary degenerative arthritis can be a sequel to MPD syndrome and therefore both conditions can be present simultaneously.

Treatment includes a soft, non-chewy diet; limited use of the jaw; hot, moist applications or diathermy; diazepam 2 to 5 mg qid (the last dose taken at bedtime) as a muscle relaxant and tranquilizer; analgesics (eg, aspirin 650 mg qid) for pain; and use of a biteplate. Clenching or grinding the teeth should be avoided. Possible causative life stresses should be discussed with the patient. Psychologic counseling may be helpful in persistent cases.

---

251. PRENEOPLASTIC AND NEOPLASTIC LESIONS

ORAL PRENEOPLASTIC AND EARLY LESIONS

Approximately 20,000 new cases of oral cancer (mainly squamous) are reported each year in the USA and account for about 5% of cancers in men and 2% in women. More than any other factor, the stage of these cancers determines the prognosis (see STAGING AND PROGNOSIS in Ch. 212). While oral cancers < 1 cm in diameter are easily cured, most lesions are *not* diagnosed before stage III or IV and ≥ 50% have metastasized to lymph nodes. Therefore, 5-yr survival rates remain at 30 to 40%. This unfortunate situation appears to result from inadequate knowledge of appropriate screening procedures and strongly entrenched misconceptions.

Persons at risk: While screening is easy enough to include all patients, careful attention to patients with clearly defined **risk factors** is mandatory; ie, individuals ≥ 40 yr old, those who smoke ≥ 1 pack of cigarettes/day, those who use smokeless ("chewing") tobacco, and those who drink alcoholic beverages regularly. Screening these individuals has been reported to increase discovery rates of early cancer in these high risk populations to 1/200 to 1/250.

Sites at risk: Next, it should be recognized that 90% of oral cancers are detected in only a few "high risk" sites: the floor of the mouth, the ventrolateral aspect of the tongue, and the soft palate complex (uvula, soft palate proper, anterior pillar, and

lingual aspects of the retromolar trigone). Buccal carcinoma should be considered in people who smoke cigars or pipes or use smokeless tobacco.

Misconceptions: Most physicians and dentists have been taught that **leukoplakia** (white lesions) are the most common precancerous lesions in the mouth and that early cancers are white lesions. In fact, < 5% of such lesions ultimately prove to be cancerous. Early, asymptomatic oral cancer appears most often as a **red (erythroplastic) lesion.** These lesions are not *pre*cancerous; they are early carcinomas. These areas look like an inflammation, probably as the result of a submucosal round-cell infiltrate that has arisen below the malignant squamous cells in response to the developing neoplasm. When dry, these red lesions appear more granular or slightly abraded. Therefore, they should be dried gently with a piece of gauze and examined carefully under good light. Two distinct types of erythroplastic lesions have been identified: (1) a red, granular lesion (appearing like worn velvet) speckled with islands of keratin (white) or normal mucosa within or peripheral to the red component, and (2) a smooth, nongranular, red lesion with minimal associated keratin, similar to a nonspecific inflammation. Both types may have irregular, ill-defined borders; generally, palpation is not helpful diagnostically, as few are indurated or raised. *Any erythroplastic lesion that does not respond to treatment and persists > 14 days should be considered carcinoma in situ or invasive carcinoma and requires biopsy.* Unfortunately, **squamous cell carcinoma** is not usually diagnosed in its earliest stages and later appears as a deep ulcer, with smooth, indurated, rolled margins, fixed to deeper tissues.

Other malignancies of the oral cavity are epidermoid carcinoma of the lip, cheek, and tongue; lymphoepithelioma; melanoma; and myelocytic and lymphocytic leukemias. **Benign lesions that may be confused with oral cancer include** irritation, fibroma, papilloma, granuloma (including pregnancy tumor), the glossitis of avitaminosis, geographic tongue, median rhomboid glossitis, hemangioma and lymphangioma, fibrous hypertrophy of the gingiva, melanosis, myoblastoma, retention cysts (including ranula), xanthomatosis, torus palatinus, submandibular duct calculus, hypertrophy of the foliate papillae, radiculodental cysts, and ameloblastoma. Syphilis, erosive lichen planus, benign ulcer, TB, leukoplakia, and dental abscess should also be considered. Exfoliative cytology is useful in screening, but biopsy is essential to establish the diagnosis.

Multiple carcinomas: *Patients with an oral cancer are at high risk (up to 33%) of developing a second primary neoplasm in the mouth, pharynx, larynx, esophagus, or lung.* Therefore, patients identified as having an oral cancer should be screened for cancer in all these sites and reexamined at yearly intervals (eg, examination of mouth and throat, indirect laryngoscopy, chest x-ray).

Treatment

Any recognizable irritation (eg, faulty restorations and prosthetic devices) should be corrected or removed. Tobacco in any form should be eliminated. Mucosal drying agents such as alcoholic beverages and mouth rinses with alcoholic vehicles should be discontinued.

Treatment of oral neoplasms generally consists of wide local excision for small lesions and en bloc excision of larger lesions in continuity with radical neck dissection if lymph nodes are involved. Radiotherapy alone may be appropriate for certain small or large lesions or may be combined with surgery. Chemotherapy may be used as palliation or as an adjunct to surgery and radiotherapy.

NEOPLASMS OF SPECIFIC TISSUES

Lips, gingiva, and tongue: Smoker's patch is a firm, brownish, keratotic plaque on the vermilion border of the lower lip and is most common in smokers who hold a cigarette or pipe in one location. *Only a biopsy can rule out squamous cell carcinoma.* Cessation

of smoking and careful observation are recommended even if the lesion is not malignant. **Actinic cheilosis** occurs in adults, especially redheads with fair skin, who spend much time out of doors. The lips are dry with many erosive areas. A person with this *precancerous* lesion should be seen every 3 to 6 mo, avoid prolonged exposure to sunlight, wear a broad-brimmed hat or cap, and use an antiactinic cream. **Squamous cell carcinoma** usually appears on the vermilion border of the lower lip as a nonhealing ulcer with a convex, indurated margin, or less commonly, as a keratotic patch. It may be fixed to the underlying tissues. If treated early, prognosis is excellent. In **leukemia,** the gingival tissue may be infiltrated and prone to bleed. **Rhabdomyoma** of the tongue causes a palpable interior mass. It is much rarer than squamous cell carcinoma, which arises in the mucosa.

Cheek: Irritation of the mucosa is commonly seen in the mucobuccal fold, where chewing tobacco or snuff may be habitually retained. The irritation may progress to erythroplakia or leukoplakia and squamous cell carcinoma. A firm, nodular, nonpainful swelling in the cheek covered by normal-appearing mucosa is rather common. It is usually the result of a cheek bite and is an **"irritation fibroma."** This is considered benign.

Palate: Accessory salivary gland tumor is usually a mixed tumor with both epithelial and mesenchymal components, an adenoid cystic carcinoma, or a mucoepidermoid carcinoma. Typically, it appears as a firm, smooth, painless mass lateral to the midline. Any such swelling that is not bony hard should be considered a salivary gland tumor until a biopsy proves otherwise. A **fullness of the palate** can represent extension of a malignant tumor of the lining of the nose or the antrum rather than a primary lesion of the palate. The soft palate may become immobile if a cancer is in the nasopharynx.

Jaws: If not initially detected on x-ray, jaw tumors are diagnosed clinically because their growth causes **swelling** of the face, palate, or alveolar process (the area of the jaw surrounding the teeth). They cause bone tenderness and severe pain originating in the involved bone. **Ameloblastoma,** the most common odontogenic neoplasm, most frequently arises in the posterior mandible and is slowly invasive, but rarely metastatic. On x-ray, it typically appears as a multiloculated or soap-bubble radiolucency. **Odontomas** are tumors of the dental follicle or the dental tissues that usually appear in the mandibles of young people; several types include fibrous odontomas and cementomas. An absent molar tooth suggests a composite odontoma. **Other neoplasms** include osteogenic sarcoma, giant cell tumor, Ewing's tumor, multiple myeloma, and metastatic tumors.

Salivary glands: The two main types of tumors are the **mixed tumor (pleomorphic adenoma),** 60% of which occur in the parotid glands, and **mucoepidermoid carcinoma.** These tumors occur not only in major salivary glands but about 20% are found in accessory salivary glands located mainly in the palate and the buccal mucosa (see above). One of 6 tumors in the parotid gland, 1/3 of those in the submandibular gland, almost 1/2 of all palatal tumors, and nearly all sublingual gland tumors are malignant.

Slowly developing parotid swellings may be painless and the patient complains of a change in appearance; but acute swelling of the parotid gland is painful because of dense fascia surrounding it. A parotid tumor causes facial paralysis if it compresses or infiltrates the facial nerve, which may also be damaged inadvertently during surgery to remove the tumor. Tumors of the submandibular salivary glands are often painful because of close association with the lingual branch of the trigeminal nerve.

252. DENTAL EMERGENCIES

Emergency dental treatment by a physician is sometimes required when dentists are unavailable, but dental consultation is desirable as soon as possible.

TOOTHACHE AND INFECTION

Pain localized to a particular tooth and provoked by sweets or cold is usually caused by **caries** that do not yet involve the dental pulp (nerve). Because this type of pain is usually fleeting, the patient should avoid provoking stimuli, use mild analgesics, and seek prompt treatment.

Localized pain that is usually intensified by heat most commonly denotes caries that has reached the dental pulp (see PULPITIS in Ch. 248). Associated **periapical inflammation,** often present, may be diagnosed by tenderness to percussion. (If all maxillary posterior teeth on one side are sensitive to percussion, maxillary sinusitis should be suspected.) Initial treatment with an analgesic (eg, acetaminophen 325 mg with codeine 30 mg orally q 4 h) and an antibiotic (eg, erythromycin, penicillin V, or a cephalosporin, 250 mg q 6 h) may be indicated until dental therapy can be initiated.

Periapical infection, often accompanied by swelling of contiguous soft tissues, will usually develop from untreated pulpitis. Emergency treatment consists of analgesics and antibiotics, as described above in periapical inflammation. A **periapical abscess** that has spread beyond the alveolar bone and is causing swelling and fluctuation in adjacent soft tissue requires incision and drainage; antibiotics alone are inadequate. An intraoral incision is usually appropriate, but a percutaneous incision may be necessary for dependent drainage. To aid in selecting the appropriate antibiotic, a specimen should be cultured. (See also PERIAPICAL ABSCESS in Ch. 248.) **Erupting or impacted molar teeth,** particularly 3rd molars, can be painful and may cause adjacent soft tissue inflammation that can progress to serious infection; erythromycin, penicillin V, or a cephalosporin, 250 to 500 mg orally qid, should be started. **Less common causes of acute perioral swelling** include periodontal abscess, infected cysts, antritis, allergy, salivary gland obstruction or infection, peritonsillar infection, or skin infection.

POSTEXTRACTION PROBLEMS

Swelling is normal after intraoral surgical procedures and is somewhat proportional to the degree of manipulation and trauma. If it does not begin to subside by the 3rd postoperative day, infection is likely and an antibiotic (eg, erythromycin, penicillin V, or a cephalosporin, 250 to 500 mg orally qid) should be started.

Postoperative pain, usually moderate, can be controlled with acetaminophen or aspirin 325 mg with codeine 30 mg orally q 4 h.

Postextraction alveolitis (dry socket) is usually peculiar to the removal of mandibular posterior teeth. Typically, the pain begins on the 2nd or 3rd postoperative day, is referred to the ear, and lasts from a few days to many weeks. Alveolitis is best treated with topical analgesic medication; ¼-in. gauze saturated in eugenol and/or guaiacol, placed in the socket and changed daily, usually reduces the need for prolonged systemic analgesics. Infection is uncommon. Rarely, **osteomyelitis** may be confused with alveolitis, but osteomyelitis is characterized by fever, local swelling, and later x-ray changes. If osteomyelitis is suspected, an antibiotic such as a cephalosporin or erythromycin should be instituted and the patient referred for definitive care.

Postextraction bleeding usually oozes from small vessels. After removing any superfluous clot with gauze, a pressure dressing (cotton wrapped in gauze, or a tea bag) is applied directly and continuously to the extraction site for 20 to 30 min. This is repeated 2 or 3 times. If the bleeding continues, the site may be anesthetized with 2% lidocaine with 1:100,000 epinephrine by nerve block or infiltration as appropriate, and the socket area sutured under tension, allowing space between the sutures for packing if necessary. Local hemostatic agents such as oxidized cellulose or topical thrombin on a gelatin sponge or microfibrillar collagen may be placed in the socket. If these measures fail, a systemic cause should be sought. Rarely, blood loss may require transfusion.

FRACTURED AND AVULSED TEETH

If a small portion of a crown is fractured and the dental pulp is not exposed, analgesic medication (eg, acetaminophen 650 mg q 4 h) and a topical covering with zinc-eugenol or similar cement are appropriate. If the pulp is exposed or the tooth is mobile, erythromycin, penicillin V, or a cephalosporin, 250 mg q 6 h should also be given. Partially avulsed teeth should be repositioned and stabilized. With any partially or completely avulsed tooth, antibiotic therapy should be prescribed for several days.

Permanent retention of a completely avulsed tooth may be possible *if it is immediately replaced into the socket without washing and with minimal handling.* If replacement is delayed a few minutes or if the tooth is washed or handled excessively, it may be retained for a few months to a few years, but the prognosis for indefinite retention is poor. Root resorption usually occurs after delayed replacement. Thus, the patient should be instructed to replace the avulsed tooth immediately and seek professional care to stabilize it. If this is not possible, the tooth should be kept moist in saline or in milk and then, if indicated, replaced and stabilized.

FRACTURES OF THE JAW AND CONTIGUOUS STRUCTURES

Fractures of the jaws and contiguous structures are diagnosed primarily by physical examination and x-ray. Fracture should be suspected if there is malocclusion, mobility of the maxillae, discrepancy in the smooth contour of the orbital rims, diplopia, infraorbital anesthesia, tenderness to palpation (particularly over the condyle or condylar neck of the mandible), and restriction or deviation when opening the mouth. A facial fracture is an emergency if there is airway obstruction, uncontrollable hemorrhage, or trauma to the eye or CNS. Routine x-rays usually confirm the diagnosis for fractures of the mandible, but CT scanning may be helpful for midface fractures. *Fracture of a cervical vertebra should be considered when a blow has been sufficient to fracture facial bones.* An oral-maxillofacial surgeon should be consulted for a fractured jaw; otherwise, unrecognized malocclusions may result.

Treatment: Manually holding the mandible in a protruded position or inserting an orotracheal or oropharyngeal airway may be necessary temporarily to maintain an airway (see Ch. 33). If there is hemorrhage into the oropharynx, an orotracheal airway should be placed or the patient positioned to allow the oropharynx to drain dependently. Until definitive care is available, the jaws usually can be temporarily stabilized and hemorrhage minimized by use of a Barton bandage. If a jaw fracture can be treated within the first few hours after injury, closure of lip lacerations is best delayed until the fracture has been reduced.

Fractures through a tooth socket are compound fractures, usually requiring antibiotic prophylaxis (eg, with penicillin V, erythromycin, or a cephalosporin, 250 to 500 mg orally in liquid form q 6 h).

Fractures of the mandibular condyle are usually characterized by preauricular pain, swelling, and limitation of opening. With a unilateral fracture, the jaw deviates to the affected side on attempted opening. Bilateral fracture can produce an anteriorly opened bite. Posterior-anterior and Towne's views of the mandible usually show the fracture on x-ray. **Treatment** is usually intermaxillary fixation for varying periods, though severely displaced, bilaterally fractured condyles may require open reduction and fixation. Jaw opening exercises are usually used to aid function after fixation is discontinued. In children, some abnormal growth may ensue.

DISLOCATED MANDIBLE

A dislocated mandible will be fixed in a markedly open position with only the most posterior teeth contacting. If the midline is deviated, the dislocation is unilateral rather

than bilateral. Injecting a local anesthetic agent (eg, 1% lidocaine 2 to 5 mL) in the joint area and in the area of insertion of the lateral pterygoid muscle may allow the mandible to reduce spontaneously.

Alternatively, or in addition, manual reduction may be necessary. Premedication with diazepam (5 mg IV) and a narcotic (eg, for the average healthy adult, meperidine 25 mg IV or 50 mg IM) is desirable. The patient should be well below the operator and the patient's head should be stabilized to obtain leverage; the operator places his thumbs on the external oblique line of the mandible (lateral to the 3rd molar area) and his fingers under the tip of the chin. A rotary motion is used, with the thumbs pressing inferiorly and anteriorly and the fingers pressing superiorly, until the mandible is reseated.

The jaw should be stabilized with a Barton bandage to maintain the mandible in the reduced position. The patient should avoid wide opening of the mouth for at least 6 wk. When the patient feels a yawn coming, he should place his fist under his chin to prevent wide opening of the mouth. If this is not the first such dislocation, an oral-maxillofacial surgeon should be consulted.

§21. DISORDERS DUE TO PHYSICAL AGENTS

253. REACTIONS TO SUNLIGHT

The skin responds to excessive sunlight with an acute reaction (sunburn); a chronic reaction that may lead to skin cancer after many years; or an unusual photosensitivity that may be due to the ingestion or application of certain drugs or chemicals, which may be indicative of systemic disease, or may be idiopathic.

Etiology and Predisposing Factors

Solar radiation that reaches the earth's surface ranges in wavelength from 290 to 1850 nanometers **(nm)** or 2900 to 18,500 angstroms **(Å)**. The character and amount of such radiation varies greatly with the seasons and with changing atmospheric conditions. Sunburn-producing rays—those below 320 nm (3200 Å)—are filtered out completely by ordinary window glass and to a great extent by smoke and smog; most are filtered out during the winter months in northern temperate zones, especially in urban areas. Large amounts of sunburn-producing rays may pass through light clouds, fog, or 1 ft of clear water and many persons unwittingly sustain severe reactions under such conditions or while swimming. Snow, sand, and bright sky enhance exposure by reflecting the rays.

Following exposure to sunlight, the epidermis thickens and the melanocytes produce melanin at an increased rate, providing some natural protection against further expo-

sure. Persons differ greatly in their reactivity to sunlight. Uneven melanin deposition occurs in many fairhaired individuals and results in freckling. Pigmentation does not occur in the skin of albinos because of a defect in melanin metabolism, nor in areas of vitiligo because of the absence of melanocytes. Blondes and redheads are especially susceptible and should avoid overexposure. Blacks and other nonwhites are not immune to the effects of the sun and can become sunburned with prolonged exposure. In recent years "tanning parlors" that utilize artificial light sources to induce tanning without sunburn have become popular. As all such light sources contain some UVB (see below), some long-term deleterious effects should be expected.

ACUTE SUNBURN

Ordinary sunburn results from overexposure of the skin to ultraviolet rays of 280 to 320 nm, UVB (2800 to 3200 Å). **Symptoms and signs** appear in 1 to 24 h and, except in severe reactions, pass their peak in 72 h. Skin changes range from mild erythema with subsequent evanescent scaling, to pain, swelling, skin tenderness, and blisters from more prolonged exposure. Sunburn affecting the lower legs, particularly the pretibial surfaces, is especially uncomfortable and often slow to heal. Constitutional symptoms (fever, chills, weakness, shock), similar to a thermal burn, may appear if a large portion of the body surface is affected; these may be due to heatstroke or heat exhaustion (see Ch. 255).

Secondary infection and miliaria-like eruptions (see in Ch. 242) are the most common late complications. Following exfoliation, the skin may be hypervulnerable to sunlight for one to several weeks.

Prophylaxis

Simple precautions will prevent most cases of severe sunburn. Initial summer exposure to bright midday sun should not be > 30 min, even in persons with dark brunette skin. In temperate zones, exposure is less hazardous before 10:00 AM and after 4:00 PM because sunburn-producing wavelengths are usually filtered out. In winter, the greatest danger of sunburn (and snow blindness) comes during foggy days that may be deceptive and have almost as much UVB as clear days on fresh snow; the danger is increased at high altitude.

Formulations of 5% aminobenzoic acid **(PABA)** as its esters in ethyl alcohol in a gel or in a cream are very effective in preventing sunburn. They take about 30 min to bind strongly to the skin, and therefore should be applied about 30 to 60 min before sun exposure so that wash off from perspiration or swimming will be minimized. PABA products rarely cause allergic or photoallergic contact dermatitis. Those who cannot tolerate PABA or its esters may use a benzophenone sunscreen. Opaque formulations containing zinc oxide or titanium dioxide physically block and prevent radiation from reaching the skin. When suitably colored with agents such as iron salts, they are cosmetically acceptable. Newer, highly effective, nonopaque lotions containing both a PABA ester and benzophenone are now available. **Sunscreens** are now rated in the USA by the FDA's SPF (sun protection factor) numbers: 15 is the most protective and 1 the least. In some other countries 10 is maximum and equal to US 15. Patients with photodrug reactions are rarely protected with these products.

Treatment

Further exposure should be *avoided* until the acute reaction has subsided. Topical corticosteroids are no more effective than cold tap-water compresses in relieving symptoms. Ointments or lotions containing local anesthetics such as benzocaine and other sensitizing agents should be *avoided.*

Early treatment of extensive and severe sunburn with a systemic corticosteroid (eg, prednisone 10 mg orally qid for 4 to 6 days for adults or teenagers) will decrease the

discomfort considerably. (For treatment of heatstroke and heat exhaustion, see Ch. 255.)

CHRONIC EFFECTS OF SUNLIGHT

Chronic exposure to sunlight ages the skin. Wrinkling and elastosis (yellow discoloration with small yellow nodules) and pigment alterations are the most common troubling consequences of long-term exposure, especially for women. The atrophic effects in some persons may resemble those seen after x-ray therapy. Precancerous keratotic lesions **(actinic keratoses)** are a frequent, disturbing consequence of many years' overexposure. Blondes and redheads are particularly susceptible; blacks are rarely affected. The keratoses are usually hard and sharp on palpation, and gray to dark in color. They should be differentiated from warty brown *seborrheic* keratoses, which increase in number and size with age but occur on covered as well as uncovered areas of the body and are not premalignant.

The incidence of squamous and basal cell carcinoma of the skin in fair, white-skinned persons is directly related to the amount of yearly sunlight in the area. Such lesions are especially common in those who were exposed as children and teenagers and in sportsmen, farmers, ranchers, sailors, and sunworshipers. Malignant melanomas may also increase in incidence with increasing sun exposure.

Treatment

If there are only a few lesions, cryotherapy, eg, freezing with liquid nitrogen, is the most rapid and satisfactory treatment for actinic keratosis. If there are too many lesions to freeze, actinic keratoses usually respond dramatically to small amounts of 5-fluorouracil **(5-FU)**, applied to the affected area nightly. For face lesions, 1% 5-FU in propylene glycol is best; elsewhere (eg, on the arm), 2 or 5% 5-FU cream can be used; if no response is seen within 10 days, 0.1% tretinoin solution should be applied a few hours before the 2 or 5% 5-FU application. Treatment is continued for at least 2 wk or until a brisk reaction with redness, scaling, and slight burning is seen, often including patches with no previously detected gross changes. If the reaction is too brisk, application should be suspended for 2 or 3 days. Masking cosmetics can make the treatment more acceptable. Topical 5-FU therapy is free of significant adverse effects but is so disfiguring and painful during treatment that freezing of individual lesions is returning to popularity. 5-FU treatment is no more lasting than individual destruction and has concealed serious underlying basal cell cancers. It should not be used to treat basal cell cancers.

PHOTOSENSITIVITY REACTIONS

In addition to the acute and chronic effects of sunlight, a variety of unusual reactions may occur after only a few minutes' exposure: eg, areas of erythema or frank dermatitis; urticarial and erythema multiforme-like lesions; bullae; and chronic, thickened, scaling patches.

Numerous factors (many unknown) may contribute to increased photosensitivity: (1) SLE or cutaneous LE—unless the cause is obvious, every patient with pronounced photosensitivity should be studied for these conditions; (2) ingestion of a variety of drugs (eg, sulfonamides, tetracyclines, thiazides, griseofulvin), though sensitivity appears in only a small percentage of patients taking such compounds; (3) external application of or contact with various substances (see also Ch. 230), including toilet waters and bergamot containing perfumes, sulfonamides, coal tar, soaps containing halogenated salicylanilides, and certain plants (eg, meadow grass, parsley); (4) xeroderma pigmentosum and certain porphyrias are less common but serious diseases also associated with photosensitivity.

Polymorphous light eruptions are unusual reactions to light that are not associated with systemic disease or drugs, as far as can be determined. Eruptions may be papular or plaque-like, dermatitic, urticarial, or erythema multiforme-like, and appear on sun-exposed areas. They are more common in people from northern climates when first exposed to spring or summer sun than in those who get sun year round. Direct immunofluorescence of a biopsied lesion and of normal-appearing skin is negative, as opposed to LE, where the result is usually positive. Diagnosis is by exclusion or by reproduction of the lesions with artificial or natural sunlight when the patient is not using any medication (systemic *or* topical).

Prophylaxis and Treatment

Avoidance of sunlight is important, and the patient should wear protective clothing (eg, hats and long-sleeved shirts) when outdoors on sunny days. Sunscreening preparations (see ACUTE SUNBURN, above) are sometimes helpful. Other treatment is directed to the underlying cause, where possible. Polymorphous eruptions manifested as papules, plaques, or dermatitis may respond to topical corticosteroids. In patients with polymorphous photosensitivity or cutaneous LE, prolonged (2 to 4 mo) administration of hydroxychloroquine 200 to 400 mg/day orally often reduces or completely suppresses photosensitivity and may be tried if treatment is required and sunscreens are not effective. Potential eye toxicity should be watched for by an ophthalmologist particularly by examining visual fields. PUVA (psoralens plus UVA) is also effective in preventing some cases of polymorphous light eruptions if used before sun exposure but should not be used in LE.

---

254. BURNS

Tissue injury caused by thermal, chemical, or electrical contact results in protein denaturation, burn wound edema, and loss of intravascular fluid volume due to increased vascular permeability. Systemic effects, such as hypovolemic shock, infection, or respiratory tract injury pose a greater threat to life than do local effects.

In spontaneous burn wound healing, dead tissue sloughs off as new epithelium begins to cover the injured area. In **superficial burns**, regeneration occurs rapidly from uninjured epidermal elements, hair follicles, and sweat glands; little scarring results unless infection occurs. With **deep burns** (destruction of the epidermis and much of the dermis), reepithelialization starts from the edges of the wound or from the scattered remains of integument. The process is slow, and excessive granulation tissue forms before being covered by epithelium. Such wounds generally contract and develop into disfiguring or disabling scars unless treated promptly by skin grafting.

Symptoms, Signs, and Assessment of Burn Injury

The **severity** of the burn is judged by the quantity of tissue involved. This quantity is represented by the percentage of the **body surface area (% BSA)** burned and by the **depth** of the burn. A reasonable classification of burns by severity is: small, or < 15% BSA; moderate, or 15 to 49% BSA; large, or 50 to 69% BSA; and massive, 70% or greater BSA.

The depth of the burn may be described as first, second, and third degrees. **First degree** burns are red, very sensitive to the touch, and usually moist. There are no blisters and the surface markedly and widely blanches to light pressure. **Second degree** burns may or may not have blisters. The bases of the blisters may be erythematous or whitish with a fibrinous exudate. The wound base is sensitive to touch and may blanch to pressure. **Third degree** burns may but generally do not present with blisters. The surface may be white and pliable when pressure is applied or it may be black, charred,

and leathery. Third degree burns may be pale in color and mistaken for normal skin, but the subdermal vessels do not blanch to pressure. The wound may be bright red due to fixed hemoglobin in the subdermal region. The third degree burn is generally anesthetic or hypoesthetic. Hair may be pulled from their follicles easily. Often, the distinction between deep second and third degree burns can be made only after 3 to 5 days of observation.

Respiratory tract ventilation injury accompanying thermal burns is due to inhalation of the incomplete products of combustion, which are potent chemical irritants to the respiratory mucosa. Only steam inhalation causes actual thermal damage to the respiratory tract. Inhalation of hot gases can cause immediate upper airway obstruction; airway edema can produce a slower developing upper airway obstruction; and small airway alveolar capillary injury can cause delayed progressive respiratory failure. Symptoms and signs of respiratory tract injuries are described under Initial Treatment, below.

In **electrical burns,** injury results from the generation of heat up to 5000 C. Since most of the resistance to electric current is at the point of skin contact with the conductor, electrical burns usually involve the skin and subjacent tissues and may be of almost any size and depth. Progressive necrosis and sloughing are usually greater than the original lesion would indicate. Electrical injury, particularly from alternating current, may cause immediate respiratory paralysis, ventricular fibrillation, or both (see CARDIAC ARREST AND CARDIOPULMONARY RESUSCITATION in Ch. 27).

Chemical burns may be due to strong acids and alkalies, phenols, cresols, mustard gas, or phosphorus. All produce necrosis that may extend slowly for several hours.

About 85% of burns are small and can be treated in outpatient facilities. Criteria establishing when to treat a burn victim as an outpatient are given below, following a description of the evaluation and treatment of the more extensively burned patient (> 15% BSA burns in adults, > 10% BSA in small children).

Initial Treatment of the Burn Victim

Immediate care requires establishment of an adequate airway for ventilation and oxygenation, stopping the burning process, replacement of acute plasma volume loss, recognition and management of any associated life-threatening major trauma, diagnosis of metabolic abnormalities, and protection from bacterial contamination.

Ventilation injuries, if severe, can be treated with tracheal intubation (the nasotracheal route is preferred) and mechanical ventilation. **Absolute indications for intubation** include rapid and shallow ventilation with tachypnea of 30 to 40 breaths/min; inadequate ventilation indicated by a respiratory rate of < 8 to 10 breaths/min; mechanical airway obstruction from trauma, edema, or laryngospasm; or signs of respiratory failure with arterial blood determinations of pH < 7.2, P_{O_2} < 60 mm Hg, or P_{CO_2} > 50 mm Hg. **Relative indications for intubation** may include history of an enclosed space explosion or fire; singed nasal hairs or oral mucosa, erythema of the palate, or soot in the mouth, larynx, or in the sputum; edema associated with a burn of the face or neck; and signs of respiratory distress such as nasal flaring, respiratory crowing or stridor, anxiety, agitation, or combativeness. If ventilation mechanics seem adequate, then O_2 may be administered by face mask or nasal cannula.

Stopping the burning process involves removing all clothing, especially any smoldering material such as melted synthetic shirts or hot tar-laden material. All chemical agents should first be flushed off the skin with copious amounts of water. **Acid and alkali burns** and burns caused by organic compounds such as **phenols or cresols** should be diluted with copious amounts of water. **Phosphorus burns** should be immersed immediately in water to avoid contact with air. Phosphorus particles are removed gently under water and the wound is washed with 1% copper sulfate solution to coat any residual particles with a protective film of copper phosphide; these fluoresce and

can be readily removed in a darkened room. Care must be taken to avoid excess absorption of copper. Following initial treatment, chemical burns should be treated as thermal burns of comparable size and extent.

Immediate volume replacement: Shock should be *anticipated* in third degree and extensive second degree burns involving > 25% BSA of adults or > 30% BSA of children. When hypovolemic shock is present, **volume replacement** should begin immediately with the establishment of a 14- to 16-gauge venous cannula in 1 or 2 veins. Although central lines may not be necessary initially, their later placement may be difficult. Therefore, if the need for central access is anticipated for fluid or K replacement or for hyperalimentation, a subclavian or internal jugular line should be placed early. If necessary, central or peripheral lines may be placed through burn eschar. A "cutdown" is avoided, since it more likely destroys the vein and precludes its future use, but more importantly, it carries a high risk of infection. Blood should be obtained for determination of Hb, Hct, blood type, and cross-match.

The immediate resuscitation fluid is Ringers lactate. A rapid estimate of the extent of burn injury to determine the initial flow rate can be obtained by the **rule of fourths,** in which the number of fourths of the body that are burned is determined. The area of the body burned is estimated as 1, 2, 3, or 4 fourths and multiplied by the flow rate of 1 L/h. For example, if the face and anterior chest are burned, then 1/4 of the body is burned. The fluid delivery rate is 1 × 1 L/h, or 1 L/h. This infusion rate can be used for the first 1 to 2 h, when a more detailed physical examination and accurate calculation of the fluid requirements can be done (see below). Proper fluid replacement is determined by careful monitoring of the patient and should be modified to optimize BP, pulse, and urinary output.

Pain from minor burns can usually be relieved by codeine 30 to 60 mg orally or s.c. and aspirin 650 mg orally q 4 to 6 h. In severe burns with peripheral vasoconstriction, morphine 0.1 mg/kg or meperidine 1.0 mg/kg should be given IV q 3 h.

A **tetanus toxoid booster,** 0.5 to 1 ml s.c. or IM, may be given to patients immunized within 4 to 5 yr; otherwise, tetanus immune globulin (human) 250 u. IM should be given (and repeated every 6 wk as necessary), and concomitant active immunization should be started.

Bacterial invasion occurs whenever the epidermis is broken. Dead tissue, warmth, and moisture provide ideal conditions for bacterial growth. Streptococci and staphylococci usually predominate shortly after a burn, and gram-negative bacteria after 5 to 7 days, but mixed flora are always found.

Penicillin G 5 million u. IM is given daily for 3 days as prophylaxis against streptococcal cellulitis.

Long Range Burn Treatment

Problems and therapeutic solutions should be identified after initial resuscitation. This requires a detailed history and physical examination with a careful evaluation of the injury, calculation of fluids required, monitoring vital signs and urinary flow to adjust the resuscitative fluids given, consideration of escharotomies, detection and treatment of metabolic abnormalities, and topical wound care.

History and physical examination: Accurate data about the burn episode usually comes from sources such as the ambulance driver, accompanying family member, coworker, police, or firefighter. The following details are important: (1) Where was the patient when the burn occurred? Was he in a closed space? (2) What exactly was the patient doing when the burn occurred? Was there an explosion? (3) What was the burn source (i.e., thermal, electrical, or chemical)? (4) How long was the patient exposed? (5) What exactly was done to eliminate the burn mechanism? (6) Did anything happen to the patient that would suggest the presence of any associated injuries?

Further medical history seeks information about allergies, medications, the presence

of heart, pulmonary, or renal disease, diabetes, or any other medical or psychiatric disorders. Smoking and drinking habits should also be noted.

A **complete physical examination** is performed to detect any pulmonary, cardiac, hepatic, neurologic, or renal disease and to determine the extent and severity of injury. This must be done before maturation of burn injuries, when physical findings may be more difficult to discern. A best estimate for height and weight is recorded to allow calculation of the patient's BSA. Often the height can be measured immediately and preburn weight estimated by a family member. Details of the body surface burned and the estimated depth are recorded on a burn diagram. The area involved is outlined, and the depth of the burn indicated by the type or style of the markings. **In adults,** the extent of the burn (% BSA) is estimated by comparing the burn diagram with the **rule of nines:** head and neck, 9% of BSA; each hand and arm (including deltoid), 9%; each foot and leg as far up as the inferior gluteal fold, 18%; anterior and posterior trunk including buttocks, 18% each; perineum, 1%. **In children,** a more accurate estimate for the % BSA involved may be obtained using the Lund-Browder chart (see FIG. 254–1).

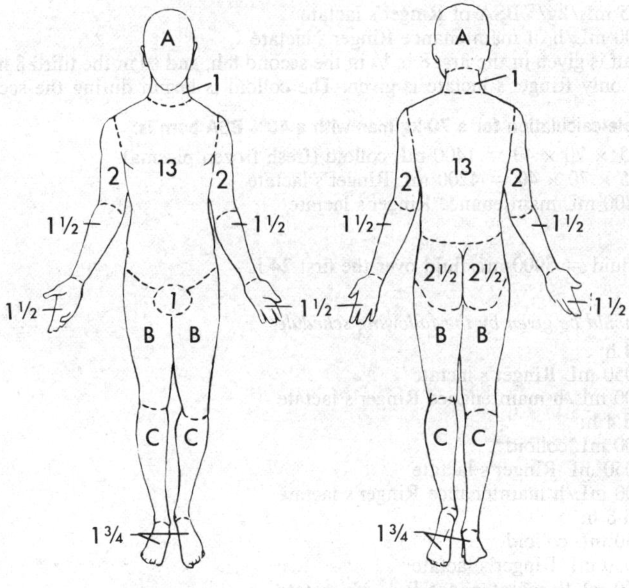

Relative percentage of areas affected by growth

	Age in years					
	0	1	5	10	15	*Adult*
A—1/2 of head	9 1/2	8 1/2	6 1/2	5 1/2	4 1/2	3 1/2
B—1/2 of 1 thigh	2 3/4	3 1/4	4	4 1/4	4 1/2	4 3/4
C—1/2 of lower leg	2 1/2	2 1/2	2 3/4	3	3 1/4	3 1/2

FIG. 254–1. Lund and Browder chart for estimating extent pf burns. (Redrawn from *The Treatment of Burns* by C. P. Artz and J. A. Moncrief, ed. 2, 1969. Copyright 1969 by W. B. Saunders Company. Used with permission of W. B. Saunders Company.)

Calculation of volume replacement: The object is to maintain normal physiology as reflected by urine, vital signs, and mental status. The fluid volume needed is related to the extent of the burn. Most formulas suggest 2 to 4 mL/kg/%BSA for the first 24 h. The colloid requirement (plasma, albumin, etc) is a matter of judgment. Whether to use colloid and when to start depends on the size of the burn, the patient's age, and concomitant diseases. Patients with small burns seldom require colloid. Patients with large or massive injuries, young children, elderly patients, and those with cardiac disease will require colloid in the first few hours. The exact volume and rate of crystalloid and colloid administration depends on each patient's response to the fluid delivery. Patients who have inadequate urine output despite administration of a high volume of crystalloid often respond to colloid. The object is to maintain normal physiology as reflected by urine volume, vital signs, mental status, and ventilatory function. Precalculated figures are seldom correct for the total period of resuscitation; formulas are used *only as a guide.*

A general formula that may be used as a guide for the first 24 h is:

0.5 mL/kg/%BSA of colloid
1.5 mL/kg/%BSA of Ringer's lactate
100 mL/h of maintenance Ringer's lactate

One half is given in the first 8 h, ¼ in the second 8 h, and ¼ in the third 8 h. For the first 4 h, only Ringer's lactate is given. The colloid is begun during the second 4 h.

A sample calculation for a 70-kg man with a 40% BSA burn is:

$0.5 \times 70 \times 40 = 1400$ mL colloid (fresh frozen plasma)
$1.5 \times 70 \times 40 = 4200$ mL Ringer's lactate
2400 mL maintenance Ringer's lactate

Total fluid = 8000 mL fluid over the first 24 h

This should be given by the following schedule:

First 4 h:
1050 mL Ringer's lactate
100 mL/h maintenance Ringer's lactate

Second 4 h:
700 mL colloid
1050 mL Ringer's lactate
100 mL/h maintenance Ringer's lactate

Second 8 h:
350 mL colloid
1050 mL Ringer's lactate
100 mL/h maintenance Ringer's lactate

Third 8 h:
350 mL colloid
1050 mL Ringer's lactate
100 mL/h maintenance Ringer's lactate

Rounding off the calculations, the sample orders would read:

Please administer the following IV solutions:

For the first 4 h:
Ringer's lactate at 360 mL/h

For the second 4 h:
Fresh frozen plasma at 180 mL/h
Ringer's lactate at 360 mL/h

For the second 8 h:
Fresh frozen plasma at 45 mL/h
Ringer's lactate at 220 mL/h
For the third 8 h:
Fresh frozen plasma at 45 mL/h
Ringer's lactate at 220 mL/h

Monitoring: Many parameters must be followed closely to prevent or recognize incipient problems as early as possible. Therefore, it is good procedure to establish a flow chart listing the items discussed here. The goal of fluid replacement is to maintain an adequate BP and a urine output of > 50 to 100 ml/h in an adult or 1 ml/kg/h in a child while avoiding overloading the circulation. An indwelling Foley catheter should be placed to monitor the urine output. Insufficient therapy can be recognized by a decline in urine volume, an increase in hemoconcentration, and symptoms of shock. Pulmonary edema and congestive failure should be prevented by monitoring the pulse, respiration, BP, and neck vein distention or the central venous pressure. The lung bases should be auscultated frequently for rales.

Patients with preexisting cardiovascular-renal disease present a special problem. Fluid, electrolyte, and colloid administration should be limited to amounts sufficient to produce minimal adequate urinary output (25 ml/h) and the patient watched for signs of circulatory overload.

Pulse, BP, temperature, ECG, and arterial blood gases should be monitored in severe burns, in the elderly, or in patients with preexisting disease. Most cardiac arrhythmias are caused by hypovolemia, hypoxia, acidosis, or hyperkalemia. These metabolic disorders should be evaluated and corrected before cardiac drugs are used. Ventricular tachycardia and fibrillation are exceptions, which should be treated immediately while underlying metabolic abnormalities are evaluated. If 0.5% silver nitrate is used as a topical antibacterial agent, it is well to remember that such a solution is hypotonic and leeches Na and Cl and some K from the tissues into the wet dressing. Losses may result in severe **hyponatremia, hypochloremia,** and **hypochloremic alkalosis.**

Serum K is aggressively maintained above 4 mEq/L. **Hypokalemia** is common in the early resuscitation period for 3 reasons: (1) Many patients present with depleted K stores secondary to prior diuretic therapy. (2) K is not generally included in the early vigorous fluid replacement. (3) Some K is lost into the hypotonic 0.5% silver nitrate dressings.

Hypoalbuminemia results from the combination of dilutional effects of crystalloid replacement therapy and enhanced loss of protein into the subeschar edema fluid. Colloid solution is continued throughout the resuscitation period at the rates previously described in order to maintain albumin levels at about 3 gm/dL and a total protein > 5 gm/dL. Most Ca in the serum is reversibly bound to albumin. **Hypocalcemia** may therefore be a result of hypoalbuminemia. The ionized fraction of serum Ca is usually normal but should be measured periodically. Replacement quantities of Ca, phosphate, and magnesium are given daily.

Generalized poor tissue perfusion, a result of hypovolemia or cardiac failure, results in **metabolic acidosis.** Blood pH < 7.2 should be treated with sodium bicarbonate IV (see METABOLIC ACIDOSIS in Ch. 84). Focal poor tissue perfusion can result from a constricting eschar or fascia that should be treated with escharotomy and fasciotomy (see Operative Management below).

Myoglobinuria can result from ischemic constrictions of muscle and from deep thermal or electrical burns of muscle, and should be treated by alkalinization of the urine with 50 mEq sodium bicarbonate q 4 to 8 h with frequent monitoring of both serum and urine pH. The goal is a urinary pH > 8. In severe myoglobinuria, mannitol 12.5 gm is given IV q 4 to 8 h for osmotic diuresis until the myoglobinuria clears. **Hemoglobinuria** may result from erythrocyte destruction following burns and is treated identi-

cally as myoglobinuria. Both myoglobinuria and hemoglobinuria may result in renal tubular necrosis if not promptly and accurately managed.

Hb is determined q 3 to 4 h for the first 72 h, and therapy is regulated so that the Hb does not rise above 16 or fall below 11 gm/100 mL. Hct should be maintained at about 40%.

Body temperature should be closely followed because hypothermia occurs frequently in the extensively burned patient. Those with rectal temperatures < 97 F (36 C) are treated by warming the resuscitation fluids. Rewarming patients from temperatures < 91 F (33 C) may be associated with fatal arrhythmias. These patients should be warmed slowly and monitored continuously (see Ch. 256).

Escharotomies: Indications for escharotomies are liberal in circumferential third-degree burns. The loss of a previously palpable pulse, or a nonpalpable pulse in a single extremity with easily palpable pulses in the remaining extremities, are indications for escharotomies. Peripheral ischemia is suspected when a single extremity is cooler than the others and has a poor capillary refilling time. A tense eschar is released even in the presence of Doppler pulses if peripheral ischemia is suspected. With injuries to the skin that do not involve deeper tissue, the depth of the escharotomy incision extends only through the dermis, excluding the hypodermis or fat. The incision should extend well beyond the tense region of eschar to assure complete release. Some full thickness eschars retain pain sensation, making the releasing incision painful. Anesthesia may be obtained with 1% lidocaine.

Topical wound care: Under aseptic conditions, the burned surface is washed with soap and water, cultured, treated with the appropriate topical agent, and covered with sterile dressings. Some of the common topical agents used are 0.5% silver nitrate solution, mafenide acetate, and 1% silver sulfadiazine. To use silver nitrate, the wounds are covered with as many as 8 layers of cotton roll bandages and the silver nitrate is poured over the dressing at 2-h intervals. This keeps the dressing moist and the concentration of the silver nitrate at the skin at about 0.5%. A lower concentration probably is not bactericidal. A higher concentration, which is a result of evaporation, can further burn the skin. Both the mafenide and silver sulfadiazine are directly applied to the wound as a cream and then may be covered with a few layers of cotton rolls. It is important to completely remove the old topical agents before the new application each day. Following topical applications of silver nitrate, patients may develop excessive Na losses, hypokalemia, hypochloremia, alkalosis, and methemoglobinuria. Mafenide acetate cream applied topically inhibits carbonic anhydrase activity and may produce compensated metabolic acidosis and, occasionally, proximal renal tubular acidosis.

Operative management: Excision or removal of the burn eschar creates a clean wound bed that can be covered with grafting material. Naturally, deep second- or third-degree burns separate and slough wound eschar over a period of time leaving a raw wound bed. Excision is best done during the first 1 to 4 days after the burn **(early excision).** This removes devitalized tissue, avoids subeschar sepsis, and allows early wound closure, which shortens hospitalization and improves the functional result of the burn wound.

In early excision, it is first determined whether a burned region is a deep second- or third-degree burn and thus requires grafting; then which part of the body should be excised first. The largest area of involvement is removed first, in order to remove the largest eschar possible, but no more than 20% BSA is excised at a single sitting. The back, chest, and abdomen are excised first and in that order. These are the most successful areas for graft acceptance. The neck and upper chest should be excised early to provide skin coverage for future central line placement. The upper extremities including the hands are excised before the lower extremities. The face is rarely excised.

Excision results in a burn wound bed that requires closure with graft material. Currently available graft materials are (1) autografts, the patient's own skin; (2) allografts, viable skin usually from cadaver donors; and (3) xenografts, skin from porcine sources. In the future, artificial skin will provide early wound closure, elimination of the inflammatory response in the burn wound bed, and subsequent wound bed contraction. Autografts can be transplanted as either sheet or meshed grafts. A sheet graft is a solid piece of skin. Mesh grafts are used when donor skin is scarce. To obtain mesh grafts, small incisions are made at regular intervals in the sheet of donor skin with a skin meshing instrument that permits the graft to cover a larger area. Meshed grafts heal with an uneven gridlike appearance. Autografts are histocompatible and therefore are not rejected. Sufficient autograft material is not available in burns > 50% BSA. However, autograft may be taken from the same donor site region repeatedly at 14-day intervals, which expands the autograft supply in time. Both allografts and xenografts are temporary and will be rejected at 10 to 14 days. They must be replaced with autograft, but their use is lifesaving in massive burns.

Physical and occupational therapy: Positioning, exercising, splints, and pressure garments help preserve function and appearance as burn wounds heal. Body surfaces with high skin tension and movement such as the face, joints, upper legs, and chest are most susceptible to formation of scars and contractures.

Splints to prevent contractures and keep specific joints in the position of function should be applied as soon as possible after admission. They must be fitted properly and constantly assessed in the early stages of treatment to avoid constriction of the extremity that may result in increasing edema. Later, as edema subsides, the splints often need to be remodeled for a closer fit. In extensive burns, splints are worn continuously until the area is grafted and shows substantial healing. Joints are also maintained in functional position throughout convalescence with dressings and blanket rolls.

With extensive burns, the total body position is considered. The **neck** is extended using soft foam pads fashioned to conform to the skull. The **axilla** is flexed about 30 to 60° with arm troughs and should be abducted. The **elbow** is positioned and splinted at extension or slight flexion. The **wrist** is slightly extended 20 to 30°. The **metacarpophalangeal joints** are flexed at 90°. The **proximal and distal interphalangeal joints** are extended completely to decrease the stretch of the dorsal skin over them and the possibility of ischemic necrosis. The **thumb** is in slight apposition to the palm. The **hips** should be abducted and are prevented from external rotation by lateral extensions of the ankle splints. The **ankle** is splinted at 90° dorsiflexion to stretch the achilles tendon.

Joints are put through active and passive range of motion exercises once or twice a day before grafting to preserve function. Both exercise and positioning become easier as the initial edema subsides. After skin grafting, the grafted part is usually kept immobile for 5 to 10 days awaiting stability of the graft before starting postoperative exercises.

Nutrition: Aggressive metabolic support is indicated in patients with > 20% BSA burn, preinjury malnutrition, complications such as sepsis or associated injury, and a weight loss in excess of 10% of the premorbid weight. This support begins 3 to 4 days after the fluid resuscitation phase of the burn therapy.

Oral feeding is preferred because of fewer complications and lower cost, but anorexia, facial burns, or dysphagia may make it difficult or impossible. If oral feeding is inadequate, but GI motility and absorption are normal, then **tube feedings** are used as a supplemental or total caloric source. **Parenteral nutrition** is indicated in those patients with prolonged gastric and colonic ileus related either to the burn wound, repeated operations, or sepsis. Complications are more likely in parenteral nutrition than with the enteral route. For further details of providing adequate nutrition, the use of elemental or defined formula diets, and parenteral nutrition, see Ch. 79.

Outpatient Burn Treatment

Superficial burns that involve a small body surface area and no inhalation injury may be treated in outpatient facilities. The general criteria are (1) first and superficial second-degree burns of < 15 to 20% BSA (adults) or < 10% BSA (small children), (2) moderate to deep second-degree burns involving < 10% BSA, and (3) third-degree burns of < 1% BSA. An estimate is made of time required for wound closure. The patient is admitted if a wound is not expected to heal spontaneously in 3 wk or less. Admission is planned either at the first encounter with the patient or at follow-up a few days later. Patients are more likely to be admitted if (1) the face, hand, perineum, or feet are involved with the deeper aspects of the burn, (2) if poor compliance with elevation and dressing changes is anticipated, or (3) the patient is < 2 yr of age or > 70 yr of age.

Outpatient treatment of burns requires a history and physical examination as described above (including estimates and recording of both the depth and the extent of the burn in terms of % BSA); cleansing and debriding the wound; topical therapy; splinting and positioning the wound; administration of medications; explanation of home care instructions; and arrangement for outpatient follow-up visits.

Wound cleaning, removing the burning agent, and debridement: Small burns should immediately be immersed in cold water, if possible. Chemical wounds should be copiously irrigated with water. The burn wound should be cleaned with soap and water.

The blisters of the burn wound should be sharply debrided away if they are already broken or are likely to be broken. If the depth of the burn wound is in question, blisters should be removed and the wound base examined for full thickness injury. All debris should be carefully removed from the wound. For deeply embedded dirt the wound may be anesthetized with a local infiltration of 1 to 2% lidocaine and scrubbed with a stiff brush and soap.

Topical therapy: Once the wound is clean, a topical agent may be applied. Silver sulfadiazine cream is commonly used. One layer of the cream is applied with sterile technic, using a sterile tongue blade as an applicator and the wound is covered with gauze roll bandages.

Splinting and positioning: If the burn involves a joint and is at least of second-degree depth, splinting is required (see also above). The hand is splinted by wrapping each finger individually with cotton roll gauze over the hand and wrist in a "figure 8" pattern. The palm should receive extra padding to maintain the metacarpophalangeal and interphalangeal joints in slight flexion. The wrist or elbow may be splinted by using an arm sling. The lower extremities are not usually splinted in outpatient care. *The most important therapeutic maneuver is elevation of the extremity*, especially in patients with a lower extremity or hand burn. The extremity should be placed above heart level at all times except for brief periods of ≤ 20 min during the day.

Medications: Patients with burns of second-degree or more are often given penicillin V 1 to 2 gm/day orally in 4 divided doses as prophylaxis for streptococcal cellulitis over the first few days. Erythromycin 1 to 2 gm/day orally in 4 divided doses may be used in patients with a penicillin allergy. Active immunization against tetanus is given as described above. Analgesic is prescribed as necessary.

Home care instructions: The patient should be advised to: (1) keep the wound clean and dry; (2) keep the wound elevated; (3) change the dressing twice daily as directed; (4) take the antibiotics as directed; and (5) the patient should know when and where to return for follow-up. The patient should especially understand to clean the wound completely with water to remove all the residual topical medication before applying a new layer.

Outpatient follow-up visits are required to: (1) monitor compliance with wound care; (2) debride the wound; (3) examine for cellulitis; (4) further assess the burn depth; (5

evaluate and arrange for ambulatory, occupational, and physical therapy; and (6) consider excisional therapy. The first follow-up visit is usually within 24 to 48 h after the burn or immediately if signs of sepsis occur. Subsequent outpatient visits are q 24 to 72 h as necessary, depending upon the severity of the burn depth and the ability of the patient to care for the wound.

255. HEAT DISORDERS

HEAT STROKE AND HEAT EXHAUSTION

Mild to grave reactions to high temperature due to inadequate or inappropriate responses of heat-regulating mechanisms.

Etiology

Prolonged exposure to high ambient temperatures may lead either to excessive fluid loss and hypovolemic shock (heat exhaustion) or to failure of heat loss mechanisms and dangerous hyperpyrexia (heat stroke). Dehydration, excessive sweating, vomiting, diarrhea, age, and debility predispose to either; high humidity, strenuous exertion, poor ventilation, and heavy clothing contribute. Many drugs (eg, antihistamines, anticholinergics, phenothiazines, numerous psychotropic drugs, and cocaine) increase susceptibility to heat illness, particularly heat stroke. Though stemming from the same cause, heat stroke and heat exhaustion are sharply different (see TABLE 255–1).

Prophylaxis

Common sense is the best preventive; strenuous exertion in a very hot environment, inadequately ventilated space, or heavy, insulating clothing should be avoided; loss of fluid and electrolytes (often imperceptible in very hot, very dry air) should be replaced by continuous oral fluids slightly salty to taste (ie, near isotonic). Sometimes exertion in a hot environment cannot be avoided; every effort should then be made to replace lost fluid and salt and to keep the skin temperature cool by evaporation. Salt tablets occasionally cause gastric distress and are less desirable than lightly salted beverages and foods.

TABLE 255–1. DIFFERENTIATION BETWEEN HEAT STROKE AND HEAT EXHAUSTION

	Heat Stroke	*Heat Exhaustion*
Cause	Inadequate or failure of heat loss	Excessive fluid loss—hypovolemic shock
Warnings	Headache, weakness, sudden loss of consciousness	Gradual weakness, nausea, anxiety, excess sweating, syncope
Appearance and Signs	Hot, red, dry skin; little sweating; hard rapid pulse; very high temperature	Pale, grayish, clammy skin; weak, slow pulse; low BP; faintness
Management	Emergency cooling by wrapping or immersion in cold water or ice; immediate hospitalization	As for simple syncope: head down; replace lost salt and water (usually orally, rarely IV)

HEAT STROKE

(Sunstroke; Hyperpyrexia; Thermic Fever; Siriasis)

Symptoms and Signs

An abrupt onset is sometimes preceded by prodromal headache, vertigo, and fatigue. Sweating is usually but not always decreased, and the skin is hot, flushed, and usually dry. The pulse rate increases rapidly and may reach 160 to 180; respirations usually increase, but BP is seldom affected. Disorientation may briefly precede unconsciousness or convulsions. The temperature climbs rapidly to 40 or 41 C (104 or 106 F) and the patient feels as if burning up. Circulatory collapse may precede death; after hours of extreme hyperpyrexia, survivors may have permanent brain damage.

Diagnosis and Prognosis

Hot, dry, flushed skin, high body temperature, and rapid pulse in a person exposed to a hot environment are usually enough to distinguish heat stroke from food, chemical, or drug poisoning. Heat stroke is a *serious emergency* and unless promptly and energetically treated, results in convulsions and death or permanent brain damage. Core temperature of 41 C (106 F) is a grave prognostic sign; temperature a degree higher is often fatal. Old age, debility, or alcoholism worsen the prognosis.

Treatment

Heroic measures should be instituted immediately. If distant from a hospital, the patient should be wrapped in wet bedding or clothing, immersed in a lake or stream, or even cooled with snow or ice while waiting for transportation. WARNING: *The temperature should be taken every 10 min and not allowed to fall below 38.3 C (101 F) to avoid converting hyperpyrexia to hypothermia.* Once in hospital, more exact control measures are instituted and the core temperature is monitored continuously to avoid hypothermia. Stimulants and sedatives including morphine are avoided; diazepam or a barbiturate may be given IV if convulsions are not otherwise controllable. Electrolyte determinations should guide IV therapy. Bed rest is desirable for a few days after severe heat stroke, and temperature lability may be expected for weeks.

HEAT EXHAUSTION

(Heat Prostration, Collapse, or Syncope)

Symptoms and Signs

Because of excessive fluid loss, this disorder gives adequate warning by increasing fatigue, weakness, anxiety, and drenching sweats, leading to circulatory collapse with slow thready pulse, low or imperceptible BP, cold, pale, clammy skin, and disordered mentation followed by a shock-like unconsciousness. Temperature is usually *below* normal and the picture is that of simple syncope.

Diagnosis and Prognosis

Heat exhaustion causing vasomotor collapse is more difficult to differentiate from insulin shock, poisoning, hemorrhage, or traumatic shock than is heat stroke. Usually the history of heat exposure, failure of hydration, absence of other apparent cause, and response to treatment are sufficient for diagnosis. The condition is usually transient and the prognosis is good unless circulatory failure is prolonged.

Treatment

Heat exhaustion requires restoration of normal blood volume and assurance of adequate brain perfusion. The patient should be placed flat or with head down. Small amounts of cool, slightly salty fluids should be given orally every few minutes to restore normovolemia. Isotonic saline IV, cardiac stimulants, or plasma volume ex-

panders (albumin, dextran) are seldom needed, and should be given cautiously to avoid overloading an embarrassed circulatory system.

HEAT CRAMPS

Severe cramps of striated muscle resulting from excessive sweating due to exertion and/or high ambient temperatures.

Etiology

Heat cramps are due to excessive loss of sodium chloride by profuse sweating during strenuous activity at high atmospheric temperatures (> 38 C [100 F]). It is common in manual laborers (eg, engine room personnel, steel workers, and miners), in mountaineers or skiers overdressed against the cold, and in those not acclimatized to hot, dry climates where excessive sweating is almost undetected because of rapid evaporation.

Symptoms and Signs

Onset is often abrupt, with muscles of the extremities affected first. Severe pain and carpopedal spasm may incapacitate the hands and feet. Often episodic, the cramping makes the muscles feel like hard knots. When the cramps affect only the abdominal muscles, the pain may simulate an acute abdomen. Vital signs are usually normal. The skin may be either hot and dry or clammy and cool, depending on the humidity.

Prophylaxis and Treatment

In most instances, heat cramp is prevented and also rapidly relieved by drinking fluids or eating foods containing sodium chloride. If the patient cannot take food or drink orally, 0.9% sodium chloride IV may be necessary. Sodium chloride tablets are often used for prophylaxis, but can cause stomach irritation, and overdose may lead to edema. Awareness of the problem is usually sufficient to prevent it.

---

256. COLD INJURY

(Frostnip; Frostbite; Accidental Hypothermia; Exposure; Immersion or Trench Foot; Chilblains; Pernio)

Injury by cold causing structural and functional disturbances of small blood vessels, cells, nerves, and skin; or generalized lowering of body temperature.

Etiology

Exposure to damp cold (temperatures around freezing) causes **frostnip** and **immersion (trench) foot.** Exposure to dry cold (temperatures well below freezing) causes **frostbite** and **accidental hypothermia.** Loss of body heat is by conduction (wet clothing, contact with metal), convection (windchill), and radiation (flow of heat from warm to cold object). Susceptibility to cold injury is increased by dehydration; drug or alcohol excess; impaired consciousness; exhaustion; hunger; anemia; impaired circulation due to cardiovascular disease, constricted vessels or polycythemia; and in very young or old age.

Hypothermia occurs when the body cannot sustain normal temperature. Wind chill, wet or inadequate clothing, substance abuse, or debility may cause dangerous hypothermia even though ambient temperature is no lower than 17 to 20 C (50 to 60 F). As shivering ceases, the body becomes unable to warm itself and the core temperature falls (see also ACCIDENTAL HYPOTHERMIA in Ch. 264).

Pathology

Ice crystals may form within or between cells, interfering with the sodium pump, thus rupturing cell walls; RBCs clump, and platelet micro-emboli form to cause

thromboses; neurovascular impulses shunt blood, often sacrificing an injured part to save the whole. Any or all of these events may produce from mild to severe injuries. **Dry cold injury** is usually superficial: the hard carapace of dry gangrene is often only a few mm thick over healthy tissue. **Wet gangrene** is often complicated by infection and tends to be deeper. **Immersion** or **trench foot** causes physiologic aberrations such as edema, blotchy cyanosis, increased sweating and paresthesias, rather than tissue loss. The pathology of long-lasting symptoms from cold injury **(chilblains)** is unknown.

Symptoms, Signs, and Diagnosis

Frostnip manifests as firm, cold, white areas on face, ears or extremities. Peeling or blistering (as from sunburn) may occur in 24 to 72 h, and occasionally mild hypersensitivity to cold persists. In **immersion** or **trench foot,** the extremity is pale, edematous, clammy, cold, and numb; tissue maceration and infection are likely. Increased sweating, pain, and hypersensitivity to temperature change may persist for years due to autonomic disturbance. In **frostbite,** the area is cold, hard, white, and anesthetic; on warming it becomes blotchy red, swollen and painful. Depending on the extent of injury, the area may recover normally or deteriorate to soft wet gangrene or to the black carapace of dry gangrene. **In hypothermia,** the falling core temperature leads to lethargy, clumsiness, mental confusion, irritability, hallucinations, slowed or arrested respiration, and slowed, irregular, and finally arrested heartbeat. Rectal temperature below 34 C (93 F) will help to differentiate hypothermia from cardiac disease, diabetic coma or hyperinsulinism, CVA, or substance abuse that may also be present.

Prophylaxis

Preventive measures, though obvious, are often ignored. Several layers of warm clothing, and protection against wetting and wind are important, even though weather may not seem to threaten cold injury. Gloves and socks should be kept as dry as possible, and insulated boots that do not impede circulation are essential in very cold weather. Warm head covering is particularly important, since 30% of heat loss is from the head. Ample fluid and food should be taken. Being alert for and warming cold numb parts may prevent damage. As the body cools, shivering, exertion, warm clothing, and hot drinks may prevent hypothermia.

Treatment

Frostnip is treated by warming with an unaffected hand or a warm object. **Frostbitten** extremities should be warmed rapidly in warm water, being careful not to burn the anesthetic tissues. Frozen feet should not be warmed if the victim must walk some distance to care, because trauma to thawed tissue increases the damage; refreezing after thawing is also dangerous. Warm drinks, snuggling with a warm companion, or warming hands or feet against a warm abdomen or axilla may be all that is possible in the field.

In the hospital, extremities should be warmed in large containers of water kept at 38 to 43 C (100 to 110 F) while overall assessment is made. Reserpine (0.5 mg) may be given into the brachial or femoral artery of the affected extremity to dilate vessels and decrease sludging; pit viper venom is preferred by European doctors. Tetanus toxoid should be given if damage is extensive and antibiotics if infection is apparent. After warming, extremities should be kept dry, open to air, and as sterile as practicable. Phenoxybenzamine 10 mg/day orally, increasing by 10 mg/day at 4- to 6-day intervals may decrease tissue loss. Heparin and dextran appear less effective. Oxygen is helpful only at altitude. Chemical or surgical sympathectomy is rarely needed. Nutrition and morale require special attention. Surgery should be delayed as long as possible, since the ominous black carapace often will be shed leaving viable tissue; "Freeze in January, operate in July" remains a valid adage. Whirlpool baths followed by gentle drying, rest, and time are the best long-term management. No treatment for the prolonged symptoms following immersion foot or frostbite is known.

In hypothermia, when shivering stops and lethargy and other symptoms increase, *a major emergency is imminent.* The victim is often found unconscious some distance from shelter. At the scene, further heat loss should be prevented and rapid assessment made. If the patient is conscious, warming by any means available may proceed while evacuation is planned. If unconscious, many factors must be considered, and there is debate whether warming should precede or follow removal to hospital. If a pulse is detectable, however faint, transport is preferred, preventing further heat loss and taking extreme care to avoid jarring or sudden motion which may trigger ventricular arrhythmia to which the cold heart is prone. If no pulse is detectable, cardiopulmonary resuscitation takes priority, but it may be difficult to restore sinus rhythm. Ventricular tachycardia or fibrillation may occur. Some authorities prefer to control fluids, pH, and oxygenation before resuscitation, providing this can be accomplished rapidly. Unconscious hypothermic victims cannot generate enough heat to warm spontaneously and must be warmed externally.

In the hospital rapid warming by total immersion in a tub of water kept at 45 to 48 C (113 to 118 F) is preferred. Inhalation of warm moist air or oxygen, heating pads, or thermal blankets should be used while the bath is prepared. In desperate cases, peritoneal dialysis with large volumes of warm saline may be lifesaving. Acidosis can be expected during warming, and pH, K, and Na levels should be monitored q 2 h until consciousness and rectal temperature of at least 35 C (95 F) are present. The ECG should be monitored to detect arrhythmia.

257. RADIATION REACTIONS AND INJURIES

The harmful effects—acute, delayed, or chronic—produced in body tissues by exposure to ionizing radiations.

Etiology

Harmful sources of ionizing radiation once were limited primarily to high-energy x-rays used for diagnosis and therapy and to radium and other naturally occurring radioactive materials. Present sources of potential radiation injury include nuclear reactors, cyclotrons, linear accelerators, alternating gradient synchrotrons, and sealed cobalt and cesium sources for cancer therapy. In addition, numerous radioactive materials have been produced artificially for use in medicine and industry.

Accidental escape of large amounts of radiation from reactors has occurred several times. The most publicized event in the USA was the accident involving the nuclear power plant at Three Mile Island in Pennsylvania on March 28, 1979. More recently, on April 26, 1986, a major accident occurred in the nuclear power complex at Chernobyl in the Ukraine, USSR. This accident resulted in several deaths due to radiation and a large number of injuries. In addition, significant radiation from the accident was detected in most of eastern Europe and parts of western Europe, Asia, and the USA. This event may have been unique because of the differences in design of Russian reactors and the lack of a containment vessel. Radiation exposure from such accidents during the first 40 yr of nuclear energy use up to 1985 (not including Chernobyl) resulted in 35 serious exposures (whole body irradiation $\geq$ 100 rems) with 10 deaths; none were associated with power plants. The Three Mile Island accident did not result in any major radiation exposure. Estimated doses received ranged from 73 mrem at 0 to 1 mile from the plant to 0 to 2 mrem at 10 to 20 miles. Doses received by the population in the immediate area of the Chernobyl plant were considerably higher. TABLE 257–1 puts these doses in perspective. Nuclear power generators in the USA must meet stringent federal standards that limit effluent radioactivity to extremely low

TABLE 257-1. ANNUAL WHOLE-BODY RADIATION DOSE-EQUIVALENT RATES IN THE U.S.A.

Source	Average (mrem/year)	Percent of Total
Natural background (cosmic, terrestrial, internal)	82	44.6
Medical radiation		
X-rays	77	41.8
Radiopharmaceuticals	14	7.6
Fallout (weapons testing)	4–5	2.4
Nuclear industry	<1	<0.5
Research	≪1	≪0.5
Consumer products	3–4	1.9
Airlines		
Travel	0.5	0.3
Transport of radiopharmaceuticals	0.01	0.005
	184	100%

(Reprinted from "The Effects on Populations to Low Levels of Ionizing Radiation," 1980, with permission of the National Academy Press, Washington, D.C.)

levels. Although background radioactivity in the earth and in its atmosphere increased after the years of atmospheric nuclear weapons testing, it appears to have stabilized at present levels.

Ionizing radiation—whether in the form of x-rays, neutrons, protons, α or β particles, or γ-rays—acts either directly or by secondary reactions to produce biochemical lesions that initiate a series of histologic changes and physiologic symptoms and signs that vary with the radiation dose and time.

The biologic effect of a given dose of radioactivity is also dependent on the rate at which it is administered. A single rapid dose of radioactivity may be fatal, while the administration of the same dose over a period of weeks or months may be tolerated with little measurable acute effect. Relationships between the degree of damage caused and the healing or death of a cell are quite complex. In addition to the early somatic effects of large doses (observable within days), changes in the DNA of rapidly proliferating cells may become manifest as a disease or as a genetic effect in offspring many years later.

Radiation usually is characterized in the lay press as low level or high level, with doses in the range of 20 to 30 rads often referred to as low level radiation. Medical doses are usually < 5 rads and frequently < 1 rad.

Total dose and dose rate determine somatic or genetic effects. The units of measurement commonly used in determining radiation exposure or dose are the roentgen, the rad, and the rem. The **roentgen (R)** is a measure of quantity of x or γ ionizing radiation in air. The **radiation absorbed dose (rad)** is the amount of energy absorbed in any tissue or substance from exposure and applies to all types of radiation. The R and the rad are nearly equivalent for practical purposes. The **rem** is used in describing the observation that some types of radiation, such as neutrons, may produce more biological effect for an equivalent amount of absorbed energy; thus the rem is equal to the rad times a constant called the "quality factor." For x and γ radiation, the rem is equal to the rad. The rad and the rem are currently being replaced in the scientific nomenclature by 2 units that are comparable with the International System of Units, namely, the **gray (Gy)**, equal to 100 rads, and the **Sievert (Sv)**, equal to 100 rem.

The **dose rate** is the radiation dose/unit of time. From the very low dose rates of unavoidable background radiation (about 0.1 rad/yr), where no effect can be detected, the probability of measurable effects increases as the dose rate and/or total dose increases. An observable effect becomes quite certain after a single dose of several hundred rads, but may require higher doses if given at a low dose rate or intermittently. Large doses are of concern because of their immediate somatic effects, while low doses are of concern because of their potential for late somatic and long-term genetic effects. The effects of radiation exposure on an individual are cumulative.

The **body area** exposed is also an important factor. The entire human body can probably absorb up to 200 rads without fatality; however, as the whole-body dose approaches 450 rads the death rate will approximate 50% (ie, LD_{50}), and a total wholebody dose of > 600 rads received in a very short time will almost certainly be fatal. By contrast, thousands of rads delivered over a long period of time (eg, for cancer treatment) can be tolerated by the body when small volumes of tissue are irradiated. **Distribution of the dose** within the body is also important. For example, protection of bowel or bone marrow by appropriate shielding permits survival of the exposed individual from what would otherwise be a fatal whole-body dose.

Pathophysiology

Tissues vary in response to immediate radiation injury according to the following descending order of sensitivity: (1) lymphoid cells, (2) gonads, (3) proliferating cells of the bone marrow, (4) epithelial cells of the bowel, (5) epidermis, (6) hepatic cells, (7) epithelium of the lung alveoli and biliary passages, (8) kidney epithelial cells, (9) endothelial cells (pleura and peritoneum), (10) nerve cells, (11) bone cells, (12) muscle and connective tissue. Generally, the more rapid the turnover of the cell, the greater the radiation sensitivity.

If the absorbed dose of radiation is sufficiently high, necrosis of any living cell will occur. Large but sublethal doses of radiation may produce disturbances in cell proliferation: (a) the rate of mitosis is decreased and (b) DNA synthesis is impaired in 2 ways—first, the rate of synthesis is slowed; second, cells may continue DNA synthesis and become polypoid. These and other ill-defined effects of radiation are reasonably certain to occur after significant doses in tissue categories 1 to 4, above, are received.

Diminished production of new cells in tissues that normally undergo continual renewal (eg, enteric mucosa, marrow, gonads) results in progressive hypoplasia, atrophy, and eventually fibrosis, depending on the dose. Some cells, injured but still capable of mitosis, may be so damaged that they will pass through 1 or 2 generative cycles, producing abnormal progeny such as giant metamyelocytes and hypersegmented neutrophils before they die.

Most of our estimates of the effects of very low levels of radiation exposure (< 10 rads) are obtained by extrapolation from studies of higher doses. These extrapolations usually are based on a linear relationship. Some workers believe there may be a threshold effect, citing experiments in which animals subjected to extremely low levels of increased radiation actually had *prolonged* survival compared to animals receiving radiation from background sources only. Regardless, there are very few objective data documenting the somatic and genetic effects of doses of radiation below 10 rads.

Symptoms and Signs

The disruption of cell renewal systems and direct injury of other tissues produce clearly defined clinical syndromes:

1. Acute radiation syndromes can be divided into cerebral, GI, and hematopoietic categories, depending on dose, dose rate, area of the body, and time after exposure.

The **cerebral syndrome,** produced by extremely high total body doses of radiation (> 3000 rads), is always fatal, and consists of 3 phases: a prodromal period of nausea and vomiting; then listlessness and drowsiness ranging from apathy to prostration

(possibly due to nonbacterial inflammatory foci in the brain or to radiation-induced toxic products); and, finally, a more generalized component characterized by tremors, convulsions, ataxia, and death within a few hours.

The **gastrointestinal syndrome** (400 or more rads) occurs when the total body dose of radiation is smaller but still high. It is characterized by intractable nausea, vomiting, and diarrhea that lead to severe dehydration, diminished plasma volume, vascular collapse, and death. The GI syndrome results from the initial "toxemia" due to necrosis of tissue and is perpetuated by progressive atrophy of the GI mucosa. Ultimately, the intestinal villi are denuded, with massive loss of plasma into the intestine. Regeneration of intestinal epithelial cells may be possible after large doses of radiation. Massive plasma replacement and antibiotics during the first 4 to 6 days will keep patients alive until the epithelium regenerates. However, even if the patient does survive, the respite is temporary, since hematopoietic failure will ensue within 2 or 3 wk.

The **hematopoietic syndrome** (200 to 1000 rads), characterized by anorexia, apathy, nausea, and vomiting, may be maximal within 6 to 12 h. Symptoms then subside, and within 24 to 36 h after exposure the subject is asymptomatic. During this period of relative well-being, lymph nodes, spleen, and bone marrow begin to atrophy, leading to pancytopenia. This atrophy is the result of 2 distinct processes—direct killing of radiosensitive cells and inhibition of new cell production. In the peripheral blood, lymphopenia commences immediately, becoming maximal within 24 to 36 h. Neutropenia develops more slowly. Thrombocytopenia may be prominent within 3 or 4 wk.

Increased susceptibility to infection develops due to (1) a dose-dependent decrease in circulating granulocytes and lymphocytes, (2) a dose-dependent impairment of antibody production, (3) impairment of granulocyte migration and phagocytosis, (4) decreased ability of the reticuloendothelial system to kill phagocytized bacteria, (5) diminished resistance to diffusion in subcutaneous tissues, and (6) hemorrhagic areas of the skin and bowel that encourage entrance and growth of bacteria. Susceptibility to infection by both saprophytic and pathogenic organisms is present. Hemorrhage is mainly due to the thrombocytopenia.

With acute total body radiation doses of > 600 rads, hematopoietic or GI malfunction will be fatal; with doses < 600 rads, the probability of survival is inversely related to the total dose.

2. Acute "radiation sickness" following therapeutic irradiation (particularly of the abdomen) is characterized by nausea, vomiting, diarrhea, anorexia, headache, malaise, and tachycardia of varying severity. The discomfort subsides within a few hours or days; its cause is not understood.

3. Delayed effects: (a) *Intermediate effects*: Prolonged or repeated exposure to low dose rates from internally deposited or external sources of radiation may produce amenorrhea, decreased fertility in both sexes, decreased libido only in the female, anemia, leukopenia, thrombocytopenia, and cataracts. More severe or highly localized exposure causes loss of hair, skin atrophy and ulceration, keratosis, and telangiectasia, and ultimately may cause squamous cell carcinomas. Osteosarcomas may appear years after ingestion of radioactive bone-seeking nuclides such as radium salts.

Serious injury to exposed organs may occur occasionally after extensive radiotherapy for cancer. Renal functional changes include a decrease in GFR and tubular function. Clinical manifestations may occur acutely after extremely high doses (after a latent period of 6 mo to 1 yr) and may include proteinuria, renal insufficiency of varying degree, anemia, and hypertension. When cumulative kidney exposure is > 2000 rads in less than 5 wk, radiation fibrosis and oliguric renal failure will occur in about 37% of cases. The remainder will develop variable changes over a prolonged time. Large accumulated doses to muscles may result in painful myopathy with atrophy and calcification. Very rarely, these changes may be followed by a neoplastic change, usually a sarcoma. Radiation pneumonitis and subsequent pulmonary fibrosis

may be severe when lung metastases are irradiated, and can be fatal after a cumulative dose of > 3000 rads if treatment is not spread over a sufficient period. Radiation pericarditis and myocarditis have been produced by extensive mediastinal radiotherapy. Catastrophic myelopathy may develop after a segment of the spinal cord has received cumulative doses > 4000 rads. Following vigorous therapy of abdominal lymph nodes for seminoma, lymphoma, or ovarian carcinoma, chronic ulceration, fibrosis, and perforation of the bowel may develop. Skin erythema and ulceration were observed fairly often during the era of orthovoltage x-ray therapy, but the high-energy photons produced by modern cobalt-60 units and linear accelerators penetrate deeply into tissues and have virtually eliminated these complications.

(b) *Late somatic and genetic effects*: Radiation alters the "information system" of proliferating somatic and germ cells. With somatic cells this may be manifested ultimately as somatic disease— eg, cancer (leukemia, thyroid, skin, bone) or cataracts—or, as suggested in animal models, by nonspecific shortening of life. Leukemia from substantial radiation in humans has been observed. It is asserted, but not proved, that there is no "threshold" dose for leukemia, and that the incidence increases with dose. Thyroid carcinoma has been observed 20 to 30 yr after x-ray therapy for adenoid and tonsillar hypertrophy, and x-ray treatment for nonmalignant conditions is now considered inappropriate except in highly unusual situations. However, several large studies have failed to show increased thyroid cancer in persons receiving up to 8 rads to the thyroid delivered by radioisotopes.

With germ cell exposure, mutations are increased. When mutations are perpetuated by procreation, animal studies indicate that an increasing number of genetic defectives will be expressed in the course of generations. Although this has not been observed in man as a direct result of germ cell irradiation, the possibility presents serious medical, ethical, and philosophic problems with respect to unborn generations. It imposes a moral obligation to limit radiation exposure to that which is absolutely necessary for valid diagnostic or therapeutic purposes, and to strictly control occupational exposure. The potential harm, however, should be kept in perspective. Some investigators believe that no measurable effects will occur below a certain threshold, while others insist that any radiation is potentially harmful. The long-term probability of a measurable genetic or somatic effect appearing in a given individual is estimated to be 10^{-4}/rad.

Diagnosis and Prognosis

When a person is receiving therapeutic radiation or has been exposed during a radiation accident, the etiology is obvious. Prognosis depends on the dose, the rate at which it was received, and its distribution within the body. Review of the data and serial hematologic and bone marrow studies to gauge the severity of marrow injury are necessary to accurately determine the prognosis.

When the cerebral or GI syndromes are present, the diagnosis is simple but the prognosis grave. Death occurs with the cerebral syndrome within hours to a few days; with GI symptoms within 3 to 10 days; and with hematopoietic symptoms in 8 to 50 days. In the latter, death may occur from a supervening infection in 2 to 4 wk or from massive hemorrhage between 3 and 6 wk.

In **chronic** cases, where external exposure is either unknown or overlooked, a diagnosis may be difficult or impossible. A search for possible occupational exposure is required. In institutions licensed by federal or state governments, records of exposure to radiation are maintained. Serial chromosome studies can be performed to watch for types and frequency of chromosomal abnormalities that are likely to occur after significant radiation exposure, but such abnormalities may have preexisted or been induced by nonradiation sources. Periodic examination for early cataracts is appropriate in chronic radiation exposure of the eye, especially from neutrons.

Cases of alleged exposure to radiation are difficult to evaluate since emotional or psychologic factors tend to predominate. Unless the individual has received a docu-

mented external or internal dose, exact diagnosis is probably impossible. Normal hematologic values and the absence of objective clinical illness would permit reassurance of the patient and others concerned.

Prophylaxis

Many drugs and chemicals increase the survival rate in animals if given prior to irradiation; eg, sulfhydryl compounds. However, none are currently of practical value in man. The only certain way to avoid fatal or serious overexposure is the rigorous enforcement of protective measures and adherence to the maximum permissible dose (MPD) levels. These values are listed in *Basic Radiation Protection Criteria*, NCRP Report No. 39, published by the National Council on Radiation Protection and Measurements (P.O. Box 30175, Washington, DC 20014).

Treatment

Contamination of the skin by radioactive materials should be immediately removed by copious water irrigation and special chelating solutions containing EDTA when available (Radiac Wash®). Small puncture wounds must be treated vigorously to remove contamination. Irrigation and debridement are indicated until the wound is free of radioactivity. Ingested material should be removed promptly by induced vomiting or lavage if exposure is recent. If radioiodine is inhaled or ingested in large quantities, the patient should be given Lugol's solution or saturated solution of potassium iodide to block thyroid uptake for days to weeks, and diuresis should be promoted. Monitoring of exposed patients is mandatory, using hand-type rate-meter probes or sophisticated whole-body counting. Urine should be analyzed for nongamma-emitting radionuclides if exposure to these agents is suspected. Radon breath analysis can be done in cases of suspected radium ingestion.

Since the **acute cerebral syndrome** is uniformly fatal, treatment is palliative and directed toward combating shock and anoxia, relieving pain and anxiety, and sedation for control of convulsions.

Symptoms of **radiation sickness due to therapeutic irradiation of the abdomen** can be diminished by an antiemetic (eg, prochlorperazine 5 to 10 mg orally or IM qid) and may be prevented by administering the drug beforehand. Attention to nutrition and fluid balance through close cooperation between radiotherapist and referring physician is mandatory. Most difficulties can be avoided or minimized by careful planning of the overall management (eg, dose, time interval between treatments, supportive therapy).

If the **gastrointestinal syndrome** develops after external whole-body irradiation, the type and degree of therapy will depend on the severity of the symptoms. After modest exposure, antiemetics and sedation may suffice. If oral feeding can be started, a bland diet is tolerated best. Fluid, electrolytes, and plasma, by appropriate routes, may be required in large volumes. The amount and type will be dictated by blood chemical studies (especially electrolytes and proteins), blood pressure, pulse, fluid exchange, and skin turgor.

Management of the **hematopoietic syndrome,** with its obvious potentially lethal factors of infection, hemorrhage, and anemia, is similar to therapy of marrow hypoplasia and pancytopenia from any cause (see HYPOPLASTIC [APLASTIC] ANEMIA under NORMOCHROMIC NORMOCYTIC ANEMIAS in Ch. 96). Antibiotics, fresh blood, and platelet transfusions are the main therapeutic aids. Rigid asepsis during all skin-puncturing procedures is mandatory as is strict isolation to prevent exposure to pathogens.

Concurrent antineoplastic chemotherapy or use of other marrow-suppressing drugs, unless strongly indicated because of some preexisting clinical condition or sudden complication, should be *avoided* because of the potential for further suppression of blood-forming elements in bone marrow.

Bone marrow transplants have proved helpful in genetically identical animals. If a

dose > 200 rads is suspected, tissue typing and search for a compatible bone marrow should be made. If an identical twin is available, a marrow transplant will increase the probability of survival. If granulocytes and platelets continue to decrease at a constant rate and fall to < 500 and 20,000/μL, respectively, homotransplantation of marrow should be considered, though the likelihood of success is small and the transplant may be followed by a potentially fatal immunologic graft-vs.-host reaction. (See BONE MARROW TRANSPLANTATION in Ch. 22.)

In dealing with **late somatic effects due to serious chronic exposure,** removal of the patient from the radiation source is the first step. With radium, thorium, or radiostrontium deposition in the body, prompt administration of oral and parenteral chelating agents (EDTA) will increase the excretion rate. However, in the late stages these agents are useless. Radiation ulcers and cancers require surgical removal and plastic repair. Radiation-induced leukemia is treated like any similar spontaneous leukemia. Anemia is corrected by whole-blood transfusion. Thrombocytopenic bleeding may be reduced by platelet transfusions. However, these measures are of only temporary value since the probability is slight that an extensively damaged bone marrow will regenerate. No effective treatment for sterility, or for ovarian and testicular dysfunction, except for hormonal supplementation, has been devised.

258. ELECTRIC SHOCK

Injury caused by an electric current passing through the body. The electricity may be atmospheric (lightning) or man-made; ie, high-voltage transmission and low-voltage lines. Potential injuries include physiologic aberrations and burns.

Pathogenesis

Factors that determine the form and severity of injury (which may range from a small minor burn to death) include (1) the type and magnitude of current, (2) the resistance of the body at the point of contact, (3) the current pathway, and (4) the duration of current flow.

The **type and magnitude of current** have a profound influence upon the injury sustained. In general, **direct current (DC),** which has zero frequency (although it may be intermittent or pulsating), is less dangerous than **alternating current (AC),** the type generally used in the USA. AC, particularly of the common 50-60 **Hz** (cycles/second) variety, is 3 to 5 times more dangerous than DC of the same voltage and amperage. DC tends to cause a convulsive contraction, often forcing the victim away from further current exposure. The effects of AC on the body depend to a great extent on the frequency—low-frequency currents, 50 to 60 Hz, usually being more dangerous than high-frequency currents. AC, 60 Hz, causes muscle tetany, often "freezing" the hand to the circuit as the fist clenches the current source resulting in prolonged exposure with severe burns. *Generally, the higher the voltage and the amperage, the greater the damage from either type of current.* Both AC and DC may affect the body by either altering physiologic functions (involuntary muscular contractions and seizures, ventricular fibrillation, respiratory arrest due to CNS injury or muscle paralysis, etc) or by producing thermal, electrochemical, or other damage (burns, necrosis of muscle and other tissue, hemolysis, coagulation, dehydration, vertebral and other skeletal fractures, muscle and tendon avulsion, etc). Electric shock often causes a combination of these effects.

The **threshold of perception** for DC entering the hand is about 5 to 10 milliamperes **(mA);** for AC, 60 Hz, about 1 to 10 mA. The maximum current that can cause contraction of the flexor musculature of the arm but still permit the subject to release his hand

from the current source is termed the **"let-go" current.** For DC this value is about 75 mA; for AC, about 15 mA and varies with muscle mass. A low-voltage (110 to 220 volts) 60-Hz AC traveling through an intact skin and a transthoracic pathway for a fraction of a second can induce **ventricular fibrillation** at currents as low as 60 to 100 mA; about 300 to 500 mA of DC are required. If the current has a direct pathway to the heart (eg, via a cardiac catheter or pacemaker electrodes), much smaller currents (< 1 mA, AC or DC) can produce fibrillation.

Body resistance (measured in $ohms/cm^2$) is concentrated primarily in the skin, and varies directly with the skin's condition. Dry, well-keratinized, intact skin has an average resistance of 20,000 to 30,000 $ohms/cm^2$, whereas the resistance of moist, thin skin is about 500 $ohms/cm^2$. If the skin is punctured (eg, from a cut or abrasion, or by a needle), or if current is applied to moist mucous membranes (eg, mouth, rectum, vagina), the resistance may be as low as 200 to 300 $ohms/cm^2$. A calloused palm or sole may have a resistance of 2 to 3 million $ohms/cm^2$. As current passes through the skin, much energy may be dissipated at the surface if the skin resistance is high, and large surface burns can result at both the entry and exit points with charring of tissues in between (heat = $amperage^2 \times resistance$). Tissues are also burned internally, depending on their resistance; nerves, blood vessels, and muscles conduct electricity far better than the denser tissues of fat, tendon, and bone. If the skin resistance is low, the patient may have few if any extensive burns but may still suffer cardiac arrest from the current reaching the heart.

The **pathway of current** through the body can be crucial in determining human injury. Conduction from arm to arm or between an arm and a foot at ground potential is much more dangerous than contact between a leg and ground since the current may traverse the heart. Electrical injuries to the head may cause seizures, intraventricular hemorrhage, respiratory arrest, ventricular fibrillation or asystole, and cataracts. The most common entry point for electricity is the hand followed by the head. The most common exit is the foot. Lightning rarely, if ever, has entry and exit wounds.

The **duration of current flow** through the body is important. While the heart is vulnerable to small currents at relatively low voltages, in general, the amount of injury to the body is directly proportional to the duration of exposure because tissue breakdown occurs with longer durations allowing internal current flow. Heat is produced by current flow through tissues, causing severe burns, protein coagulation, vascular thrombosis, and tissue necrosis.

When a victim freezes to a circuit (see "let-go" current above) he may suffer severe burns. Conversely, a lightning victim rarely suffers external or internal burns, despite the higher voltage, because the short duration of current is not enough to cause skin breakdown. It "flashes over" the victim, producing little internal damage other than electrical short-circuiting of systems (heart-asystole, brain-confusion and loss of consciousness).

Symptoms and Signs

The effects and clinical manifestations of electrical injuries depend on the complex interaction of the factors discussed above. Electricity can startle a person and cause him to fall down or to drop objects. It may cause severe, spastic stimulation and contraction of the muscles with accompanying fractures, dislocations, and loss of consciousness. Both respiratory paralysis (apnea) and cardiac arrhythmias or arrest may occur. Sharply demarcated electrical burns may be present on the skin and extend well into the subjacent tissues.

High voltage may cause coagulation necrosis of the internal tissues between the entry and exit points of the current. Massive edema may supervene as the veins coagulate and the muscles swell. Fluid and electrolyte disturbances as well as severe myoglo-

binuria may cause acute renal failure. Dislocations, fractures, and blunt injuries may be present from powerful muscle contractions or falls secondary to the electric shock.

"Bathtub" accident victims, where a wet (grounded) individual contacts a 110 v circuit, may show no burns but suffer cardiac arrest.

Lightning, because of its short duration, rarely leaves entry or exit wounds and seldom causes muscle damage or myoglobulinuria. Coma and other neurologic sequela may be present, but usually resolve within hours or days. Death is most frequently due to cardiopulmonary arrest or severe brain damage.

Prevention

Prevention of electrical injuries entails proper design, installation, and maintenance of all electric devices. Education and compliance, as well as common sense and respect in dealing with electricity, are essential. Any electric device that touches or may be touched by the body and has life-threatening potential should be properly grounded and incorporated in circuits containing fail-safe equipment. **Ground-fault circuit breakers,** which trip at current leakage to ground levels of as low as 5 mA, are excellent safety devices and are readily available.

Treatment

Treatment consists of (1) separating the patient from the current source, (2) reestablishing vital functions immediately, and (3) supportive care as required.

Breaking contact between the victim and the current source can be done either by **shutting off the current** or by **removing the person from contact with it.** The best method is to cut off the source, if it can be done rapidly (eg, throwing a circuit breaker or switch, disconnecting the device from its electrical outlet, or cutting the wires, using insulated tools); otherwise, the victim must be removed from the source. *For low voltage*, the rescuer should first ensure that he himself is well insulated from ground, and then should use an insulating material (eg, cloth, dry wood, rubber, leather belt) to pull the person free. *If it is suspected that high voltage lines are involved (> 1000 v), it is best to leave the victim alone until the power can be shut off*, since high and low voltage lines are not always easily differentiated.

Once it has been established that it is safe to touch the victim, **a rapid examination for vital functions should be performed** (eg, radial, brachial, or carotid pulses; respiratory function; level of consciousness). Airway stabilization is the first priority. If spontaneous respiration is not observed or cardiac arrest has occurred, immediate resuscitation is required. Heart-lung resuscitation technics are detailed in CARDIAC ARREST AND CARDIOPULMONARY RESUSCITATION, in Ch. 27. The treatment of shock and other manifestations of massive burns are discussed in Ch. 254.

Once vital functions have been reestablished, the full nature and extent of the injury must be evaluated (see Pathogenesis, above) and treated. A search for dislocations, fractures, cervical-spine and blunt injuries should be made. If myoglobinuria is present, fluid loading is essential and mannitol or furosemide may be indicated.

Lightning injuries are usually superficial, but victims may require cardiac resuscitation, monitoring, and supportive care. Fluid restriction is the rule due to potential brain edema. After being struck by lightning, patients without vital signs for 15 min or even longer have been revived by CPR, although this is unusual.

Tetanus prophylaxis is required for any burn. An ECG, cardiac enzymes, CBC, and a urinalysis especially for myoglobin are baseline determinations for all electrical injuries. Other tests may be indicated as necessary. Any suggestion of cardiac damage, arrhythmias, or chest pain requires monitoring for at least 24 h. Any deterioration in the level of consciousness mandates a CT scan to rule out intracranial hemorrhage.

259. MOTION SICKNESS

A disorder caused by repetitive angular and linear acceleration and deceleration and characterized primarily by nausea and vomiting. Sea-, air-, car-, train-, swing-, and space-sickness are specific forms. Prevention is easier than treatment.

Etiology

Excessive stimulation of the vestibular apparatus by motion is the primary cause. There is great individual variation in susceptibility. The pathways of the afferent impulses from the labyrinth to the vomiting center in the medulla are undefined, but motion sickness only occurs when the 8th nerve and cerebellar vestibular tracts are intact. Visual stimuli (eg, a moving horizon), poor ventilation (fumes, smoke, and carbon monoxide), and emotional factors (eg, fear, anxiety) commonly act in concert with motion to precipitate an attack. Motion sickness in space travel is referred to as the **space adaptation syndrome;** weightlessness or zero gravity is an etiologic factor. This syndrome is a major problem in the efficiency of astronauts in the first few days of space flight, but adaptation occurs over several days.

Symptoms and Signs

Cyclic nausea and vomiting are characteristic. They may be preceded by yawning, hyperventilation, salivation, pallor, profuse cold sweating, and somnolence. Aerophagia, dizziness, headache, general discomfort, and fatigue may also occur. Once nausea and vomiting develop, the patient is weak and unable to concentrate. With prolonged exposure to motion, individuals may adapt and gradually return to well-being. However, symptoms may be reinitiated by more severe motion or by recurrence of motion after a short respite.

Prolonged motion sickness with vomiting may lead to arterial hypotension, dehydration, inanition, and depression. Motion sickness can be a serious complication in patients who are already ill.

Prophylaxis and Treatment

Susceptible individuals should minimize exposure by positioning themselves where there is the least motion (eg, amidships or, in airplanes, over the wings). A supine or semirecumbent position with the head braced is best. Reading should be avoided. Keeping the axis of vision at an angle of 45° above the horizon will reduce the susceptibility. Avoiding visual fixation on waves or other moving objects is helpful to some. A well-ventilated cabin is important and going out on deck for a breath of fresh air is helpful. Alcoholic or dietary excesses before or during travel increase the likelihood of motion sickness. Small amounts of fluids and simple food should be taken frequently during extended periods of exposure; if the exposure is short, as in air travel, food and fluids should be avoided. In the space adaptation syndrome, movement aggravates the symptoms.

Prophylactic drugs should be given before nausea and vomiting occur. One hour before departure, susceptible individuals may be given diphenhydramine, meclizine, or cyclizine 50 mg orally; promethazine 25 mg or diazepam 5 to 10 mg orally; or scopolamine HBr 0.6 mg orally to minimize the vagal mediated GI symptoms. A smaller dose of scopolamine can be delivered via a dermal patch from which 0.5 mg is released over 3 days. If emotional factors are significant, phenobarbital 15 to 30 mg may be given orally 1 h prior to departure. Sedation with pentobarbital 100 mg orally to induce light sleep may be helpful if alertness is not required. However, sedation should be mild enough to allow mental clarity when the passenger arrives at the destination. All dosages should be appropriately modified for prolonged exposure. After vomiting be-

gins, medication must be given rectally or parenterally to be effective. With prolonged vomiting IV fluids and electrolytes may be required for replacement and maintenance.

260. MEDICAL ASPECTS OF AIR TRAVEL

Commercial aviation safely transports millions of passengers each year but imposes a variety of potential medical stresses. While absolute prohibitions on flying exist for very few medical conditions, planning and precautions are necessary for some patients who travel by air. Commercial pilots undergo rigorous screening and physical examinations and accidents due to their illness or to substance abuse are extremely rare.

General aviation, a rapidly growing area for business and recreational flying, also presents a number of potential health hazards. The FAA requires periodic medical examination of private pilots by specially designated physicians, but most of these approximately 1 million pilots licensed in the USA receive their medical care from private practitioners. Of the more than 4000 accidents that occur each year in general aviation, most happen in recreational aircraft and are often related to the injudicious use of alcohol or drugs. The physician may counsel his pilot patient in these matters, caution about side effects of medications (eg, antihistamines), and provide current tetanus immunization.

Aircraft of all types present increasing **environmental health hazards** in terms of urban noise and air pollution, occasional large scale disasters, and toxic contamination in agricultural areas. For patients living near large airports, continuous high level noise and air pollution can aggravate a wide variety of medical conditions. Local disaster facilities near airports should be prepared to provide initial management of major trauma and burns of air crash survivors. Physicians in agricultural communities should know the toxic manifestations of the chemicals used in aerial spraying that may accidentally contaminate farm workers or nearby populated areas (see Ch. 289).

Clinical Manifestations

Major problems imposed on the air traveler relate to (1) changes in barometric pressure, (2) decreased O_2 tension, (3) turbulence, (4) circadian dysrhythmia, and (5) psychologic stress.

Changes in barometric pressure: Modern jet aircraft, including the supersonics, maintain cabin pressure equivalent to between 5000 and 8000 ft. At such altitudes free air in body cavities tends to expand by about 25% and may aggravate certain medical conditions. The occasional accidental loss of cabin pressure and the fact that some airplanes are unpressurized must be kept in mind. Upper respiratory inflammation or allergy may obstruct eustachian tubes or sinus ostia, resulting in **barotitis media** (see Ch. 206) or **barosinusitis** (see also Ch. 208). Frequent yawning or closed-nose swallowing during descent, decongestant nasal sprays, and antihistamines taken before or during flight often prevent or relieve these conditions. Children are particularly susceptible to barotitis media and should be given oral fluids or feedings during descent to encourage swallowing (chewing gum or hard candy is more effective than eating). Facial pain of dental origin may occur with air pressure changes. Air travel is *contraindicated* in the following: patients with pneumothorax or potential for its development (eg, large pulmonary blebs or cavities); and where air or gas is trapped and even modest expansion may cause pain or stress tissue (eg, incarcerated bowel or recent [< 10 days] laparotomy). Patients with a colostomy should wear a large bag and expect frequent filling.

Decreased O_2 tension: Cabin pressure at a 7500-ft altitude-equivalent results in a Pa_{O_2} of about 70 mm, which is well tolerated by healthy travelers. Problems may arise,

however, in a number of conditions, including moderate or severe **pulmonary disease** (eg, asthma, emphysema, cystic fibrosis, etc), **congestive heart failure, anemia** with a Hb < 8.5 gm/dL, severe **angina pectoris, sickle-cell disease** (but not trait, see Ch. 96), and some **congenital heart diseases.** Patients with these conditions can usually fly safely with continuous O_2, available from most airlines if arranged for in advance (all commercial aircraft carry O_2 for use during an in-flight emergency). Patients recovering from **myocardial infarction** may fly when stable, often within 10 to 14 days. Ankle edema is common on long flights and should not be confused with increased congestive heart failure. **Hypertension** is affected by psychologic stress of flight and may be controlled by a mild pre-flight tranquilizer. Smoking can aggravate mild hypoxia and should be avoided. The impact of alcohol may be increased by fatigue and hypoxia. In general, anyone able to walk 100 yd or climb one flight of stairs and whose disease is stable should tolerate normal cabin conditions without additional O_2.

Turbulence may cause air sickness (see Ch. 259) or injury and can occur at any time. Passengers should keep their seat belts fastened at all times while seated.

Circadian dysrhythmia ("jet lag"): Rapid travel across multiple time zones creates many biologic and psychologic stresses; after long trips, travelers should plan on 24- to 48-h rest upon arrival and avoid major commitments or decisions during this adjustment period. A gradual shift in sleeping and eating patterns (a high protein, low calorie intake is recommended) before departure may partly alleviate the problem. Some therapeutic regimens require alteration to compensate for circadian dysrhythm, eg, diabetics using long-acting insulin may need to change to regular insulin until they have accommodated to the destination time, available food, and activity. Other medication schedules may require adjustment based on elapsed rather than local time.

Psychologic stress: Fear of flying and claustrophia are psychologic and not influenced by logic or reason; hypnosis and behavioral modification psychotherapy have reduced the fear of flying in some. Fearful passengers may benefit from mild sedation before and during flight. Hyperventilation may provoke unconsciousness, tetany-like convulsions, or simulate cardiovascular disease; physician-passengers may be asked to volunteer Good Samaritan services in such inflight situations. Psychotic tendencies may become more acute and troublesome in flight, and patients with violent or unpredictable tendencies must be accompanied by an attendant and be appropriately sedated.

Other Considerations: (1) Thrombophlebitis is a possibility for anyone sitting for long periods, especially during pregnancy and for patients with venous disease; frequent (q 1 to 2 h) walks around the cabin and short-movement exercises should be practiced while seated. **(2) Dehydration** may develop because of very low cabin humidity, but can be avoided by adequate intake of fluids and avoidance of alcohol. **(3) Wired jaw:** Maxillofacial injury immobilized by fixed wires, unless fitted with a special quick-release device, is a *contraindication* to air travel since air sickness may result in aspiration of vomitus. **(4) Pacemakers and metal prostheses:** Newer models of pacemakers are effectively shielded from interference from security devices; older units may be affected. Battery life sufficient for the length of travel should be assured. The metal content of pacemakers and of metal prostheses may trigger a security alarm; a physician's letter should be carried to avoid security difficulties. **(5) Communicable disease:** Patients with any communicable disease that may endanger others in a crowded aircraft are not acceptable as passengers. International immunization requirements change frequently; current information may be obtained from local or state health departments. **(6) Contact lens** wearers should instill artificial tears frequently to avoid corneal irritation resulting from low cabin humidity. **(7) Medications and records:** The experienced traveler carries on his person essential medications sufficient to assure continued therapy in the event of lost baggage, theft in hotels, delayed arrival, or local unavailability.

Patients who must carry narcotics should have a verifying letter from their physician to avoid possible security complications. A summary of a patient's medical record (including ECG) may be invaluable should a patient become ill away from home. Patients subject to disabling illness (eg, epilepsy) or who are at high risk should wear a medical identification bracelet or necklace (eg, as provided by Medic-Alert Foundation, Turlock, CA 95380). A recent dental checkup and carrying extra glasses are wise precautions. **(8) Uncomplicated pregnancy** through the 8th mo is acceptable; high-risk patients must be individually evaluated if travel is planned. Acceptance during the 9th mo usually requires a physician's written approval dated within 72 h of departure and indicating delivery date. Seat belts should be worn across the thighs. Thrombophlebitis is a specific risk when sitting for long periods (see above). **(9) Children:** Infants under 7 days of age are not accepted for travel. For children with chronic disease (eg, congenital heart disease, chronic lung disease, anemia), the same precautions apply as for adults. **(10) Elderly and the handicapped:** There is no upper age limit and airlines make all reasonable efforts to accommodate patients with handicaps. Wheel chair and litter patients can often be accommodated on commercial aircraft; otherwise, air ambulance service is necessary. Some airlines will accept patients requiring special equipment (IV fluids, respirators, etc) provided appropriate personnel accompany the patient and arrangements have been made in advance. **(11) Special foods,** including low-sodium, low-fat, and diabetic diets are usually available upon advance request.

Further advice regarding air travel may be obtained from the medical department of major airlines or from the FAA Regional Flight Surgeon. Special arrangements (eg, O_2, wheelchair, etc) can be made through regular reservations clerks, but at least 72 h advance notice is usually required.

Foreign travel may involve significant difficulties in case of illness. Millions travel abroad yearly; about 1 in 30 requires emergency care. Many insurance plans, including Medicare, are not valid in foreign countries; overseas hospitals often require a substantial cash deposit regardless of insurance. Special insurance programs, including some that will arrange for emergency evacuation (eg, NEAR, 1900 N. MacArthur, Oklahoma City, OK 73127) are available. Directories listing English-speaking physicians in foreign countries are available from several organizations (eg, InterMedic, 777 Third Avenue, New York, NY 10017, and International Association for Medical Assistance to Travelers, 736 Center Street, Lewiston, NY 14092); US Consulates may also assist in obtaining emergency medical services. *The Traveler's Medical Manual*, by Scotti and Moore, Berkley Books, 1985, contains valuable information for persons traveling abroad, including those with special health needs.

261. NEAR-DROWNING

Pathophysiology

Near-drowning victims, because of aspiration or laryngospasm, usually sustain significant hypoxemia, with the consequent danger of respiratory failure and hypercapnea. Acute reflex laryngospasm may result in asphyxia without aspiration of water. Aspiration of fluid and particulate matter may cause chemical pneumonitis, damaging cells lining the alveoli, and may impair alveolar secretion of surfactant, resulting in patchy atelectasis.

The perfusion of nonaerated, atelectatic areas of the lungs leads to intrapulmonary shunting of blood and aggravates hypoxemia. The more fluid aspirated, the greater the surfactant loss, atelectasis, and hypoxemia. Aspiration of large quantities of water may cause sizable areas of atelectasis resulting in stiff noncompliant lungs and respiratory failure (see Ch. 35). Respiratory acidosis with hypercapnea and hypoxemia can occur. A concomitant metabolic acidosis may also result from tissue hypoxia. Hypoxemia

and tissue hypoxia often result in pulmonary edema and even cerebral edema. On x-ray, pulmonary edema may simulate atelectasis and the 2 conditions may coexist.

The mammalian **diving reflex** in cold water allows survival after long periods of submersion. The diving reflex, first identified in seagoing mammals, slows the heartbeat and constricts the peripheral arteries, shunting oxygenated blood away from the extremities and the gut to the heart and brain. In cold water the O_2 needs of the tissues are reduced, extending the possible time of survival.

Respiratory insufficiency is more critical than changes in electrolytes and blood volume, which vary in magnitude depending on the type and volume of aspirated fluid. Sea water may cause a mild elevation of Na and Cl, but the levels are rarely life-threatening. By contrast, aspirating large quantities of fresh water can cause a sudden increase in blood volume, profound electrolyte imbalance, and hemolysis. Victims may succumb to the effects of these changes, asphyxia, and, possibly, ventricular fibrillation, at the scene of the tragedy. Cardiac arrest, usually preceded by fibrillation, causes many of the deaths attributed to drowning. However, current belief is that the pulmonary edema following near-drowning is a direct result of hypoxemia and analogous to pulmonary edema of high altitude, ie, noncardiogenic pulmonary edema.

Prevention

Eating and drinking shortly before swimming should be avoided. Children require proper supervision at beaches and near pools or ponds. All swimmers should be accompanied by an experienced swimmer or swim only in guarded areas. Nonswimmers and small children should wear flotation jackets when in boats or playing near bodies of water. Children should be taught to swim as early as possible, and adults and children over 12 should be familiar with the basics of resuscitation. Infants, children, the debilitated, and the elderly should not be left unattended in bathtubs.

Treatment

The key factors for surviving submersion without permanent injury appear to be duration of submersion, water temperature, age of the individual (the diving reflex is more active in children), and speed of resuscitation efforts. Survival depends more on the prompt correction of hypoxemia and acidosis (ventilatory insufficiency) than correction of electrolyte imbalance, the goal being to prevent pulmonary and cerebral edema due to tissue hypoxia.

If near-drowning takes place in very cold water, the victim *may be hypothermic*. Because of the diving reflex and the reduced metabolic needs associated with hypothermia, vigorous attempts should be made to resuscitate victims (especially children) even though they have been submerged for periods up to 1 h or longer. The management of hypothermia is discussed in Ch. 256.

Emergency mouth-to-mouth resuscitation should begin immediately if the victim is apneic—in the water, if necessary. If heart beat and carotid pulse cannot be detected, closed chest cardiac massage (see CARDIAC ARREST AND CARDIOPULMONARY RESUSCITATION in Ch. 27) is initiated as soon as artificial ventilation is started. Mechanical ventilators, which supply higher inspired O_2 concentrations, should be used if available. Electrical defibrillation may be necessary.

Time should not be wasted in attempts to drain water from the lungs in a fresh-water victim, because the hypotonic fluid passes rapidly into the circulation. Sea water, being hypertonic, draws plasma into the lung, and the Trendelenburg position may promote drainage.

Hospitalization is mandatory for all victims. Resuscitation should continue during transport, regardless of the patient's condition. Consciousness is not synonymous with recovery, since *delayed death from hypoxia can occur*.

Initial emphasis in the hospital continues to be intensive pulmonary care to achieve adequate arterial blood-gas and acid-base levels. Required measures range from simple

O_2 administration for a spontaneously breathing patient to continuous ventilatory support of an apneic patient by tracheal intubation with a cuffed tube connected to a mechanical ventilator. Sodium bicarbonate IV is usually indicated, since metabolic acidosis almost invariably accompanies the tissue and cellular hypoxia. Further bicarbonate administration, ventilatory support, and proper inspired O_2 concentrations are determined by monitoring blood gases. High supplemental levels of O_2 inhalation must be continued until the arterial blood-gas studies indicate that lesser O_2 concentrations are adequate.

Frequent manual hyperinflation of the lungs is indicated to re-expand atelectatic alveoli. β_2-Agonists by inhalation or injection help to reduce bronchospasm. Since near-drowning with fluid aspiration is a form of aspiration pneumonitis, corticosteroids and antibiotics may be considered depending on the individual case.

Fluid and electrolyte solutions are required to correct significant electrolyte imbalance. A large quantity of fluid may be extravasated into the lungs, producing a reduced blood volume that may be reflected by lowered central venous pressure; infusion of volume expanders may be indicated. Fluid restriction is usually not advisable, since the pulmonary and cerebral edema caused by hypoxia are related to direct pulmonary epithelial damage or osmotic gradients rather than to circulatory overload as in congestive heart failure. RBC replacement to increase the O_2-carrying capacity of the blood, and forced diuresis to facilitate excretion of the free plasma Hb may be necessary if there is significant hemolysis.

The patient who develops acute respiratory distress syndrome requires mechanical ventilation. Positive end-expiratory pressure (PEEP) may help to maintain patency of alveoli, prevent alveolar collapse, and expand collapsed alveoli (see Ch. 35). Pulmonary care may be necessary for hours or days, depending on the arterial blood-gas and pH analyses. Permanent brain damage from hypoxemia and tissue hypoxia may be a residual problem in some cases. Cerebral resuscitation measures and the role of neurologic classification for brain injury require further study. The following measures may be beneficial, but carry intrinsic risks: hyperventilation, hyperoxygenation with hyperbaric chambers, hypothermia, barbiturate coma, and steroids. Acetazolamide IV has been effective in relieving cerebral edema due to hypoxia.

---

262. MEDICAL ASPECTS OF DIVING AND WORK IN COMPRESSED AIR

Serious errors in diagnosis and treatment may occur when illness arises from diving or other activitives involving **increased environmental pressure.** Diving with **scuba** (**s**elf-**c**ontained **u**nderwater **b**reathing **a**pparatus) has grown enormously as a popular sport and in commercial and scientific applications. As a result, many individuals are now potential victims of conditions that were once confined to deep sea divers and construction workers in tunnels or caissons.

A patient with almost any disorder that develops during, or especially following, exposure to increased pressure could have decompression sickness or gas embolism and urgently need recompression. Physicians who see such patients must have a high index of suspicion and be ready to seek advice. This chapter provides basic information, and the **Divers Alert Network (DAN),** coordinated by the Duke University Medical Center, Durham, NC, provides consultation at any hour **(919–684–8111).**

DEPTHS AND PRESSURES

Increased pressure at depth results from the weight of water, just as barometric pressure on land reflects the weight of the atmosphere above. Pressures in diving are

often expressed in units of depth or atmospheres absolute **(atm abs; ATA).** A diver at 33 ft (10 m) in sea water is exposed to a pressure of 14.7 psi, 760 mm Hg, or one atmosphere **(atm)** greater than the barometric pressure at the surface. The **total pressure** at 33 ft, 2 atm abs, includes both the weight of the water and the barometric pressure at the surface. Every additional 33 ft of descent adds one atm of pressure. In a caisson or tunnel, compressed air is used to exclude water from the worksite and the interior pressure reflects the head of water outside.

Pathophysiologic Effects of Increased Pressure

Medical problems caused by exposure to increased pressure involve one or more of the following mechanisms:

1. Local differences in pressure ("squeeze"). When external pressure on the body increases with depth, the pressure of gas in the lungs and airways increases accordingly. If the eustachian tubes can be opened normally (eg, by swallowing or yawning), pressure in the middle ear can be kept equal to the increasing external pressure. If a structural anomaly, allergic or vasomotor rhinitis, or URI prevents such equalization, the excess external pressure is exerted directly on the eardrum. The external pressure is also fully transmitted to all blood vessels of the body including those in the mucosa of the middle ear, where if the pressure remains lower than the external pressure, the capillaries may dilate, leak, and rupture. If edema fluid and extravasated blood do not occupy enough space to equalize the pressure, the eardrum may rupture. Middle ear infection often follows such **barotitis media** (see also Ch. 206).

Barotrauma by the same mechanism may also occur in the paranasal sinuses. It is signaled by local pain or, in sphenoid sinus "squeeze," by pain referred to the occiput, vertex, or frontal area. Mucosal congestion causing inability to equalize pressure in the ears or sinuses may respond to local or systemic decongestants, but persistent efforts to dive without free equalization of pressure will usually produce some injury.

Any rigid or semi-rigid airspace attached to the body can also become the site of local "squeeze." Face masks are equalized by air from the nose, but goggles and some diving suits can cause discomfort, local hemorrhage, and tissue damage. Ear plugs form a closed space in the auditory canal and must *not* be used in diving.

2. Compression and expansion of gas. Boyle's Law indicates that the volume of a given mass of gas changes inversely with the absolute pressure; eg, 1 L of air at the surface (1 atm abs) is compressed to ½ L at 33 ft of depth (2 atm abs). Equalization of pressure in body airspaces during descent must compensate for such compression. Compression of lung gas limits the safe depth of a "breath-hold" dive, but breathing from a diving helmet or scuba regulator compensates for compression of gas in the respiratory system.

Changes in pressure and gas volume in the middle ear can produce **vertigo** by at least 3 different mechanisms. (1) If the eardrum ruptures when a diver is bareheaded in cold water, the effect is like that of a **caloric test** (see in Ch. 204) and can produce severe and potentially disastrous vertigo, disorientation, nausea, and vomiting. (2) Unequalized pressure differences in the middle ear may affect the inner ear via the round window and produce **alternobaric vertigo,** a possible cause of the dysequilibrium sometimes experienced by divers upon starting ascent. (3) **Perilymph fistula,** an uncommon but serious cause of vestibular disorder, requires prompt surgery. It can be confused with inner-ear decompression sickness when it becomes evident following a dive.

Compression of gas at depth produces **increased gas density** proportional to the pressure in atm abs. Since a scuba diver breathes at about the same rate and tidal volume at depth as during comparable work at the surface, the number of gas molecules respired per minute at depth increases in proportion to the pressure. Thus at 2 atm abs it is twice that at the surface. Not only does the diver's air supply duration decrease proportionately, but breathing becomes difficult at greater depths because of the gas-flow limitations of the diver's airways and of his breathing apparatus. Respira-

tory limitation can accentuate overexertion, respiratory exhaustion, and general fatigue—potentially significant problems of diving even under ideal conditions.

Life-threatening complications can arise from the expansion of pulmonary gas on ascent. If a diver breathes compressed gas at depth and then fails to let it escape freely on ascent, the expanding gas may overinflate the lungs. Possible consequences include **pneumothorax, mediastinal and subcutaneous emphysema,** and **gas (air) embolism;** the latter is an extreme emergency and a leading cause of death among scuba divers (see below and TABLE 262–1).

TABLE 262–1. CONDITIONS REQUIRING RECOMPRESSION

	Decompression Sickness	*Gas Embolism*
Symptoms and Signs	**Extremely variable.** Three main types (singly or in combination): 1. **"Bends"**—pain, most often in or near a joint 2. **Neurologic** involvement of almost any type or degree 3. **"Chokes"**—respiratory distress followed by circulatory collapse **(extreme emergency)**	Common: **unconsciousness,** often with convulsion Less common: milder cerebral manifestations (Mediastinal and subcutaneous emphysema and/or pneumothorax may also be present) **Assume that any unconscious diver has gas embolism and seek recompression promptly**
Onset and immediate course	Gradual or sudden onset during decompression or as long as 24 h after dive(s)* deeper than 30 ft (or hyperbaric exposures beyond 2 atm abs) (Also possible in exposure to low pressure, as at altitude) ***Repetitive dives** are frequently involved	Sudden onset during or very shortly after . . . 1. Ascent, even from a few feet of depth 2. Decompression from any increased pressure 3. Any accident or procedure that could permit gas to enter circulation
Proximate cause	**Usual:** Diving or hyperbaric exposure beyond no decompression limits and without proper decompression stops **Occasional:** 1. Dive or pressure exposure within "no decompression limits" or with appropriate decompression stops 2. Low-pressure exposure, as in loss of cabin pressure in aircraft at altitude	Usual: **Breath holding** or airway obstruction during ascent or reduction of pressure Other: Entry of free gas into cardiovascular system during heart surgery or other medical/surgical procedure
Mechanism	**Excess dissolved gas** forms bubbles in blood or tissues upon reduction of external pressure. Bubbles produce local mechanical effects or circulatory impairment	Usual: **Overinflation of lungs** causes entry of free gas into pulmonary vessels followed by embolization of the brain Other: Pulmonary, cardiac, or systemic circulatory obstruction by free gas from any source
Immediate management	**Essential emergency care as required (CPR, etc.)** 100% oxygen by close-fitting mask Trendelenburg position if feasible (*especially for suspected gas embolism*) **Transportation to nearest suitable chamber** Fluids orally, if conscious; otherwise IV	

3. Partial-pressure effects. The partial pressure of a gas is proportional to the number of molecules of that gas present in a given volume of gas. The concentration of O_2 in air is about 21%, and the partial pressure of O_2 in air at surface (1 atm abs) is about 0.21 atm. The concentration of O_2 in air remains the same at depth, but the partial pressure reflects the increasing pressure and compression of the gas. At 2 atm abs, the number of O_2 molecules per unit volume is twice what it is at the surface, and the partial pressure is double.

The physiologic effects of gases are related to their partial pressure and change according to depth. Toxic effects appear as the partial pressure of O_2 increases. **Pulmonary oxygen toxicity** can cause lung damage with extended exposure to a P_{O_2} much above 0.6 atm (equivalent to 60% O_2 at surface or 30% O_2 at 33 ft). **Oxygen convulsions** may occur, especially in working dives, as the P_{O_2} approaches or exceeds 2 atm (100% O_2 at 33 ft or 50% O_2 at 99 ft).

Increased partial pressures of N_2 produce **nitrogen narcosis,** a condition resembling alcohol intoxication. In divers breathing air, this becomes noticeable at 100 ft or less. It is generally incapacitating at about 10 atm abs (300 ft), where it produces an anesthetic effect resembling that of 30% nitrous oxide at sea level. Helium lacks this anesthetic property and is used in place of N_2 as the diluent for O_2 in deep diving.

Partial pressure of O_2 and CO_2 in alveolar gas are modified by the pressure of depth in **breath-hold diving** and in underwater swimming without breathing apparatus. The impulse to return to the surface and resume breathing depends largely upon CO_2 buildup in the body. When a breath-holding diver hyperventilates beforehand to extend his time underwater, he blows off CO_2 but adds little to his stores of O_2. He may then become **unconscious from hypoxia** without warning before his P_{CO_2} rises enough to become an effective stimulus.

Diving to a significant depth during the breath-hold complicates the situation by elevating the P_{O_2} and permitting extended O_2 uptake at depth. A diver who has "pushed his limits" under those circumstances may lose consciousness when his alveolar P_{O_2} falls to a low level on ascent. This phenomenon is probably responsible for many unexplained drownings among spearfishing competitors and others who do extensive breath-hold diving. The term **shallow-water blackout** is sometimes applied, but it is best reserved for its original meaning in connection with **CO_2 excess** in rebreathing types of scuba. **Hypoxia** is also a potential problem in rebreathing units.

Carbon dioxide poisoning. In normal individuals on land, hyperpnea and breathlessness usually provides ample warning of increased CO_2 in inspired gas. Such a response may be more the exception than the rule underwater, especially where a high P_{O_2} and exertion are also factors. Some individuals develop spontaneous **CO_2 retention** through an inadequate increase in pulmonary ventilation during exertion. Whatever the source, abnormally high P_{CO_2} per se can cause **loss** or **impairment of consciousness** at depth and can also increase the likelihood of **O_2 convulsions** and augment the severity of **nitrogen narcosis.** The tendency to retain CO_2 may be suspected in divers who frequently experience post-dive headaches or pride themselves on low air-use rates.

Inert-gas uptake in the blood and tissues occurs whenever the partial pressure of gases such as N_2 is increased. When the pressure is subsequently reduced by ascent, bubbles may form with various consequences (see TABLE 262–1, and DECOMPRESSION SICKNESS, below).

4. Pressure per se. Certain neuromuscular and cerebral abnormalities comprise the **high pressure neurologic syndrome (HPNS),** which is seen in deep diving and may appear at about 600 ft on descent. HPNS is attributed to hydrostatic pressure without reference to gas compression or partial pressures. It has no evident medical importance at shallower depths.

5. Complicating factors in diving include poor visibility, currents requiring excessive effort, and cold. **Hypothermia** can develop rapidly in water, and early effects may

include crucial loss of judgment and dexterity. Cold water can trigger fatal **cardiac arrhythmias** in susceptible individuals. **Hypoglycemia** is a serious hazard in insulin-dependent diabetics and in those who indulge in alcohol while neglecting adequate food intake. **Drugs,** including medications as well as **alcohol** and other drugs of abuse, may have unanticipated effects at depth.

CONDITIONS REQUIRING RECOMPRESSION

GAS EMBOLISM

(Air Embolism)

A disorder resulting from overinflation of the lungs by expanding pulmonary gas during reduction of surrounding pressure (eg, ascent from depth in diving), generally characterized by abrupt loss of consciousness and/or other CNS manifestations, and attributed to cerebral gas emboli originating in the lungs. (See TABLE 262–1.)

Etiology

Overinflation of the lungs is the usual cause of **arterial gas embolism.** The victim is most commonly a scuba diver who holds his breath during ascent from a dive. Running out of air at depth is a common precipitating event. Even swimming-pool depths are sufficient to cause gas embolism if the individual has access to a source of gas and takes even a single breath underwater. Gas inspired at any depth expands on ascent and, if not allowed to escape freely, overinflates the lungs and elevates alveolar pressure resulting in escape of gas into pulmonary veins returning blood to the heart. If this gas reaches the carotid arteries, embolization of the cerebral vessels is almost inevitable.

Symptoms, Signs, and Diagnosis

Immediate **loss of consciousness,** with or without convulsions or other cerebral manifestations, is the typical consequence of gas embolism. A diver who loses consciousness during or very shortly after ascent *must be assumed to have gas embolism and should be promptly recompressed* (see RECOMPRESSION TREATMENT, below). Milder symptoms and signs, ranging from behavioral changes to hemiparesis, may also be seen.

Overinflation of the lungs also can produce mediastinal and subcutaneous emphysema, alone or with gas embolism. Pneumothorax is less frequent but more consequential. Hemoptysis or bloody froth suggests pulmonary injury. Iatrogenic arterial gas embolism is not unknown. It may be suspected, eg, when a patient fails to regain consciousness after heart surgery.

Emergency Treatment

The patient must be transported to a suitable chamber for recompression without any delay for nonessential procedures. Transport by air may may be justified if it will save a significant amount of time, but exposure to reduced pressure at altitude must be minimized. Most authorities recommend the Trendelenburg position when gas embolism is suspected. Life-saving emergency measures take precedence where indicated (eg, CPR, control of bleeding, attention to the airway), but these, together with administration of a maximal concentration of O_2 and fluid therapy, can usually be carried out during transport. Recompression treatment is discussed below.

DECOMPRESSION SICKNESS

(Caisson Disease; The Bends)

A disorder resulting from reduction of surrounding pressure (as in ascent from a dive, exit from a caisson or hyperbaric chamber, or ascent to altitude), attributed to formation

of bubbles from dissolved gas in blood or tissues, and usually characterized by pain and/or neurological manifestations. (See TABLE 262–1.)

Pathophysiology

A diver or compressed-air worker breathing air under increased ambient pressure takes up additional quantities of O_2 and N_2 in solution in the blood and tissues. O_2 is utilized continuously, but N_2 (or any other "inert" gas present) leaves the body only via the reverse of its entry through the lungs and circulation. Gradients of partial pressure govern uptake and elimination of the gas, but the degree of **supersaturation** (excess of tissue gas pressure over ambient pressure) is crucial in determining whether symptomatic bubbles will form in the body during or after ascent.

The consequences of bubble formation from dissolved gas are known as **decompression sickness, caisson disease, or "the bends"** (see TABLE 262–1). Although "the bends" strictly refers to painful manifestations, it is often used as a synonym for decompression sickness.

Consequential bubble formation can usually be avoided by (1) restricting the uptake of gas, as by limiting the depth and duration of dives to a range that does not require decompression stops on ascent ("no-decompression limits"; see TABLE 262–2), or (2) using a standard air **decompression table,** as found in the *US Navy Diving Manual* (obtainable from the Superintendent of Documents, US Government Printing Office, Washington, DC 20402). The table provides a pattern of ascent that normally allows excess inert gas to escape harmlessly. Decompression sickness rarely occurs after dives within the limits given in TABLE 262–2 or when US Navy decompression tables are followed; but the diver's account of depth, duration, and decompression procedure is not necessarily reliable. Many divers incorrectly believe that large "safety factors" are built into US Navy diving tables and do not follow them accurately.

Repetitive dives are a major source of difficulty. Some divers are unaware that an excess of inert gas remains in the body after every dive and increases with each subsequent exposure. If the interval between dives is < 12 h, special repetitive dive tables (as provided by the *US Navy Diving Manual*) must be used.

US Navy decompression tables have not been tested for adequacy in females or in older divers; such persons should use them with caution. Dives conducted at **altitude** and **flying after diving** require special procedures or precautions.

Symptoms and Signs

Local pain ("the bends") is present in a large proportion of cases of decompression sickness, but it is often accompanied by neurologic abnormalities. In divers, pain is

TABLE 262–2. U.S. NAVY NO-DECOMPRESSION LIMITS

(Single dives not requiring decompression stops on ascent)

Depth in Feet	*Time in Minutes*	*Depth in Feet*	*Time in Minutes*
30	(no limit)	90	30
35	310	100	25
40	200	110	20
50	100	120	15
60	60	130–140	10
70	50	150–190	5
80	40		

Notes:
1. Times are from leaving surface to starting ascent.
2. This table *must not* be used for **repetitive dives** (see text).
3. Diver's impression of depth and time is often incorrect.

most commonly reported in or near an arm joint. In compressed-air workers, joints of the leg are more often affected. The pain is unusual, hard to describe, and often poorly localized. "Deep" and "like something boring into the bone" are expressions sometimes used. At first, pain may be mild or intermittent, but it is apt to increase steadily and may become very severe. Local inflammation and tenderness are usually absent and the pain may not be affected by motion.

Neurologic manifestations may accompany pain or be present independently. They are much more common following dives with scuba than in "hard-hat" diving or caisson work. Currently, the proportion of neurologic problems among cases of decompression sickness probably exceeds 50%. The spinal cord is especially vulnerable, and many divers are unaware of the dire significance of seemingly minor manifestations such as weakness or numbness in the extremities.

Neurologic symptoms and signs are exceedingly variable. They range from mild paresthesia to major cerebral problems. Vestibular involvement may produce severe vertigo and may be difficult to differentiate from **perilymph fistula.** Spinal cord lesions leading to paraplegia are a particular hazard, and delay in treatment may render the condition irreversible.

The condition known as **the chokes,** or **respiratory decompression sickness,** is rare in occurrence but grave in significance. It arises from massive bubble-embolization of the pulmonary vascular tree. Some cases resolve spontaneously, but rapid progression to circulatory collapse and death is not uncommon without prompt recompression. Substernal discomfort and coughing on deep inspiration or inhalation of tobacco smoke are often early manifestations of chokes. In animal studies, chokes are strongly associated with exposure to altitude soon after diving. Chokes and other serious manifestations appearing at **altitude** are not necessarily cured by return to ground level and may require prompt chamber recompression.

Other manifestations of decompression sickness include **itching,** skin **rash,** and exceptional **fatigue.** These have not customarily been treated by recompression, but they are sometimes forerunners of much more serious problems. Divers complaining of them should at least be kept under observation. One hundred percent O_2 by mask may relieve such symptoms. **Cutaneous edema** is a rare occurrence and probably reflects obstruction of lymphatic channels by bubbles. It deserves recompression if progressive or persistent. **Mottling** ("marbling") of the skin is uncommon but may precede or accompany conditions that require recompression. **Abdominal pain** may reflect bubble formation at the site; but, especially in the form of **girdle pain,** *it can be an important signal of spinal cord involvement.*

Late manifestations of decompression sickness include **aseptic bone necrosis** (dysbaric osteonecrosis). This is much more common in compressed-air workers than in divers, but divers are not immune. Bone necrosis is presumably a consequence of bone infarction by bubbles, as in inadequate or delayed treatment of bends. Lesions adjacent to articular surfaces are most common in the shoulder and hip and can cause great damage to the joint with chronic pain and severe disability. Bone necrosis is an insidious hazard because it becomes symptomatic or is detected by x-ray months or years after the responsible insult, which may be a single improper decompression.

Permanent neurologic defects, eg, **paraplegia,** are frequently attributable to delayed or inappropriate treatment of early signs of spinal cord involvement. In some instances, the initial damage may be too severe to remedy even with prompt and well-chosen treatment. However, repeated treatments with **hyperbaric oxygen** (see in Ch. 267) assist in recovery. The prognosis appears to be considerably more favorable in spinal cord injury from decompression sickness than from other forms of trauma.

Emergency Treatment

Decompression sickness requires recompression. *Transport to a suitable recompression facility takes precedence over any procedure that can be conducted during transport*

or postponed without serious risk to life. Transport should not be delayed even in cases that appear mild, since more serious manifestations may develop. O_2 in maximal concentration should be administered by mask. Shock may develop, especially in severe cases with delayed treatment. Adequate fluid intake should be ensured and both intake and output recorded along with the vital signs.

RECOMPRESSION TREATMENT

(See also Ch. 267)

Recompression is imperative in both decompression sickness and gas embolism and should be accomplished as soon as possible to avoid serious and lasting injury. Its objective is to compress bubbles to asymptomatic size, redissolve them, and restore adequate O_2 to affected tissues. Regardless of the distance to a chamber or how long the delay, it is likely to be beneficial. Unnecessary recompression involves far less risk than palliative treatment prescribed in the hope that the problem will subside without recompression.

Recompression in the water *must not* be attempted. Divers themselves, and medical facilities and rescue and police units in popular diving areas, should know the location of the nearest suitable chamber, the means of reaching it rapidly, and the most appropriate source of consultation by telephone. In the absence of such local forethought, the DAN number **(919–684–8111)** is invaluable.

When a physician recommends recompression but cannot be sure that the patient will receive proper treatment in a suitable chamber, he should obtain signed and witnessed acknowledgement of his recommendation. What constitutes a "suitable" chamber is currently being debated. Many cases can be treated successfully in one-man hyperbaric chambers available in many areas; however, the need for "hands-on" access to the patient or for greater pressure capability often cannot be foreseen and may be vital.

The need for recompression is determined by the fact that the individual has been exposed to increased pressure and has symptoms or signs suggestive of decompression sickness or gas embolism. Details of the history, physical examination, and laboratory findings usually add little of value. Sometimes, a conclusive diagnosis cannot be made without a "test of pressure." At some point, at least before leaving maximum treatment pressure, a careful **neurologic examination** is important to identify any defect that might require modifying the course of treatment.

Failure to provide prompt and appropriate treatment of decompression sickness or gas embolism entails entirely unacceptable risk of serious and lasting injury.

Tables for treatment and guidelines for their selection and use are found in the *US Navy Diving Manual.* The main difference in treatment between gas embolism and decompression sickness is that tables specifically designed for the former include an excursion to 6 atm abs with the aim of rapid compression of cerebral bubbles. Otherwise, treatment of both conditions normally relies upon breathing O_2 at pressures < 3 atm abs.

The US Navy treatment tables achieve a high percentage of success in cases of decompression sickness that follow ordinary diving with air as the breathing medium. Dives involving unusual gas mixtures or extraordinary depths or durations may require special therapeutic procedures.

Medical adjuncts to recompression: Patients will sometimes need medical or surgical procedures in addition to recompression. If it is impossible to provide both simultaneously, recompression takes precedence over any measure that can be postponed without serious risk to life. Intensive care, when required, can be provided in a well-equipped chamber.

Adequate fluid intake with monitoring is important. If IV fluids are required, 0.9% sodium chloride is generally preferred. The possibility of bladder paralysis and need

for catheterization should be kept in mind. Periodic measurement of Hct is desirable, and measurement of central venous pressure and circulating blood volume may be necessary in severely ill patients.

Corticosteroids (eg, dexamethasone sodium phosphate 20 to 40 mg IV, then 4 mg IM q 6 h) may be useful in curbing inflammation from decompression sickness and in controlling CNS edema. Additional measures for reducing brain/cord swelling are indicated when CNS manifestations are present, especially if the response to recompression is not prompt.

Sedatives and narcotics may obscure symptoms and cause respiratory insufficiency. They should be avoided before and during treatment or used in minimum effective dosage when urgently needed.

EVALUATION OF FITNESS FOR DIVING

Although asked to judge the fitness of individuals for diving or related pursuits, physicians usually cannot bar anyone from diving and function largely as advisors. It is advisable not only to explain unwelcome findings and their implications but to make them a matter of record with signed acknowledgement by the individual concerned.

In the absence of uniform standards, a few self-evident considerations can be cited:

(1) A diver must be able to take care of himself over a wide range of conditions. Diving can involve unusually **heavy exertion** even for individuals who do not plan to participate in any arduous underwater activities. Air cylinders are heavy, currents can necessitate strenuous swimming, etc. Divers should be free of any significant cardiac or pulmonary disease and possess normal to superior **aerobic capacity.** Gross **obesity** is often associated with poor exercise tolerance and increased susceptibility to decompression sickness. **Physical handicaps** must be assessed in terms of the individual's ability to aid a "diving buddy" as well as to function as a diver with minimal assistance himself.

Rigid **age limits** are inappropriate, but older aspirants deserve special scrutiny especially in **cardiopulmonary fitness.** Family history and coronary risk factors should be considered. Certain **cardiac arrhythmias,** including some that are acceptable in other sports, are contraindicated in diving even in younger people.

(2) **Divers must be able to equalize pressure uneventfully in all body air spaces.** Pulmonary conditions that involve air trapping may cause gas embolism on ascent. *Absolute contraindications* include lung cysts, asthma, emphysema, and a history of spontaneous pneumothorax. Chronic nasal congestion, perforated eardrum, and certain otologic operations are *contraindications*. Diving should be avoided during respiratory infections and exacerbations of vasomotor or allergic rhinitis. Habitual air-swallowing and a tendency toward regurgitation have unfavorable implications.

(3) **Divers must not be subject to impairment of consciousness, alertness, or judgment.** Such lapses, even if momentary, can lead to underwater mishaps endangering the diver and his companions. Epilepsy, syncope, insulin-dependent diabetes, and alcohol or drug abuse are incompatible with diving. Medications that cause drowsiness or reduce alertness are undesirable and may potentiate N_2 narcosis. Lack of emotional stability is perilous for a diver and his associates. It is suspected when motivation seems inappropriate or when the history suggests accident-proneness or impulsive behavior.

Women have taken up scuba diving in large and increasing numbers, and present knowledge suggests that, with only a few exceptions, fit and healthy women can dive as safely as men. One probable exception concerns susceptibility to decompression sickness; women should be even more conservative about **decompression** than men. Another exception concerns **pregnancy,** with the likelihood that diving increases the incidence of birth defects and fetal death. Safe limits of exposure cannot be specified with confidence, so diving is best avoided by women who are, or may be, pregnant.

Evaluation of professional divers and others at unusual risk warrants special procedures including pulmonary function testing, stress electrocardiography, audiometry, and bone x-rays.

Adequate training is an absolute necessity for safe diving, and the physician should emphasize its importance. Courses under the auspices of national organizations are widely available.

263. HIGH-ALTITUDE ILLNESS

(Acute Mountain Sickness [AMS]; High-Altitude Pulmonary Edema [HAPE]; High Altitude Cerebral Edema [HACE]; Soroche; Puna; Mareo)

Syndromes due to decreased O_2 at high altitudes.

Etiology, Pathology, and Pathophysiology

Atmospheric pressure decreases as altitude increases but the percentage of O_2 in air remains constant; as a result the partial pressure of O_2 decreases with altitude and at 18,000 ft (5500 m) is about 1/2 that at sea level. About 15% of persons ascending above 9000 ft (2700 m) in less than a day will develop symptoms and signs of altitude illness in which the dominant form may vary. Persons who have had one attack are slightly more susceptible to another under similar conditions, but there is great variation between individuals and even in the same person at different times. Children under six and women in the premenstrual phase are especially vulnerable. Very rapid ascent (as in unpressurized aircraft, balloons, or a decompression chamber) causes a different form of hypoxic illness.

Hypoxia stimulates breathing, which increases tissue oxygenation but also causes respiratory alkalosis, which contributes to the symptomatology until it is partially compensated by loss of HCO_3 in urine. Hypoxia impairs the O_2 dependent "sodium pump," resulting in the accumulation of Na and water within, and the movement of K out of cells; it is thought that the resultant swelling of cells is the basic pathophysiology of altitude illnesses. ADH secretion may be increased by hypoxia in some individuals causing further water retention.

No specific pathology has been demonstrated in AMS. Pulmonary artery pressure is invariably elevated by hypoxia, but systemic pressure may or may not increase. Interstitial edema precedes frank alveolar edema in HAPE; the edema fluid resembles plasma, which presumably seeps through lung capillary walls. Edema and petechial hemorrhages are found in the brains of patients dying from HACE and HAPE. Platelet and fibrin microemboli or gross thromboembolism are common in severe cases. Retinal hemorrhages, and splinter hemorrhage beneath nailbeds are often seen above 16,000 ft (5000 m), but nosebleed is rare. Endocrine glands are normal, though their function is often altered. Liver, kidneys, and heart are normal and passive congestion is not seen.

Symptoms, Signs, and Diagnosis

Various forms of altitude illness may occur separately or in combinations. **Acute mountain sickness (AMS)** is the most common and may appear at altitudes as low as 6500 ft (2000 m). It is characterized by headache, fatigue, nausea, dyspnea, sleep disturbance, and rapid, forceful heartbeat. Exertion aggravates the symptoms. Unless dehydration is severe or hyperventilation is excessive, AMS usually subsides within a few days. Laboratory studies are nonspecific and rarely required for diagnosis.

High-altitude pulmonary edema (HAPE) is less common but more serious, usually developing 24 to 72 h after rapid ascent above 9000 ft (2700 m). Long time high-altitude residents, returning after a brief stay at low altitude appear to be at a slightly greater risk. Children under six are much more susceptible than adults. HAPE is

characterized by increasing dyspnea; irritative cough that becomes productive of frothy, often bloody sputum; weakness; ataxia; and later coma. Cyanosis, tachycardia, and low grade fever are common, and together with fine and coarse rales (often audible without a stethoscope) may lead to a misdiagnosis of pneumonia. Chest x-ray shows Kerley lines and a patchy distribution of edema quite different from that seen in congestive heart failure. Atrial pressure is normal, but pulmonary artery pressure is even greater than that found in normal subjects during hypoxia. HAPE may worsen rapidly, and coma and death may occur within hours.

The absence of one pulmonary artery is a rare congenital anomaly that greatly increases the risk of HAPE even as low as 5000 ft (1500 m), probably because of the resulting mismatch between perfusion and ventilation. Persons who develop HAPE repeatedly or at unusually low altitude, should be studied for unsuspected pulmonary artery pathology.

High-altitude cerebral edema (HACE) is probably present to some degree in all altitude illness, but occasionally is seen in severe form with headache, mental confusion, gait ataxia, clumsy hand movements, and diplopia. Occasionally, coma develops rapidly after few symptoms or signs, but ususally ataxia and hallucinations give warning. Stiff neck is not seen and papilledema is not necessary for diagnosis. HACE must be differentiated from other causes of coma (such as infection, vascular accident, ketoacidosis) by history, absence of significant fever or paralysis, and by normal blood and spinal fluid studies.

High altitude retinal hemorrhages (HARH) are common above 17,000 ft (5200 m) but if seen at lower altitudes should be considered due to other illness. HARH may occur in the absence of any other altitude illness but are more common with HAPE and HACE. They are asymptomatic unless in the macular region and are absorbed without sequelae. "Cotton wool spots" occur rarely.

Prophylaxis

Altitude illness is best prevented by slow ascent, no faster than 1000 ft (300 m) a day from 5000 to 10,000 ft (1500 to 3000 m) and more slowly above this. Physical fitness and climbing experience, though they enable greater exertion for less O_2 consumption, do not protect against any form of altitude illness. Strenuous effort should be avoided for several days, but bed rest is less beneficial than mild exercise. Because of great individual variation, those going to altitude should learn how fast they can ascend without symptoms; a climbing party should be paced at the rate of its slowest member. Young children, and altitude residents returning from a sojurn at low altitude should be especially alert for symptoms.

Water loss is greatly increased by overbreathing the dry air at altitude, and dehydration with some degree of hypovolemia aggravates symptoms. Drinking much more water than usual is important, but additional salt should be avoided. Alcohol seems to worsen AMS. A light diet, high in easily digested carbohydrates (fruits, jams, starches) improves altitude tolerance and is recommended for the first few days.

Acetazolamide is an effective prophylactic for AMS. Dosage recommended is 250 mg orally q 8 h the day before, during, and a day after ascent; sustained release capsules may be used. Acetazolamide inhibits carbonic anhydrase and allows increased ventilation and better O_2 transport with less alkalosis; it halts periodic breathing (almost universal during sleep at altitude) thus preventing sharp falls in blood O_2. Low flow O_2 during sleep accomplishes the same but is inconvenient. Aspirin may relieve headache and possibly decrease the risk of HAPE by preventing platelet emboli. Prochlorperazine 10 mg orally q 6 h, a popular preventive in Europe, has not been widely used in the USA. Antacids are worthless. Phenytoin is currently being reevaluated because of its value as a membrane stabilizer. Dexamethasone 4 mg orally q 6 h may also prevent AMS.

Acclimatization: Persons exposed to altitude gradually develop an integrated series of responses that restore tissue oxygenation toward normal. Full acclimatization takes more time the higher the altitude, and above 18,000 ft (5500 m) deterioration is more rapid and there are no permanent residents. Major features of acclimatization include moderate sustained hyperventilation with slight alkalosis and decreased alkaline reserve, normal or low cardiac output, increased hemoglobin and myoglobin, increased tissue capillaries, and changes in cell enzyme activity. After many generations at altitude, different populations have acquired slightly different strategies of acclimatization. Although acetazolamide has been used to enhance acclimatization, its value is not proven.

Treatment

AMS seldom requires treatment other than fluid, analgesics, light diet, mild activity, and (rarely) descent. Acetazolamide 250 mg orally q 4 h is helpful in AMS and HAPE, but more controlled studies are needed. When **HAPE** is suspected, bed rest and O_2 may be tried, but if the condition worsens, *immediate descent is essential.* O_2 is less effective than descent. Although morphine may be effective, respiratory depression may outweigh its value. Digitalis, phlebotomy, and limb tourniquets are of no value since congestive heart failure is not at fault. Furosemide (20 to 40 mg orally q 2 h or 20 mg slowly IV) has been effective. (CAUTION: *Brisk diuresis may cause hypovolemic shock, since the patient is often already dehydrated; oral fluid replacement is essential.*) In hospital, treatment is based on ruling out other causes of pulmonary disease; adequate oxygenation, perhaps by intubation and Positive End Expiratory Pressure (PEEP); bedrest; judicious diuresis; postural drainage; and antibiotics, if superimposed infecton is suspected. Recovery is usual within 24 to 72 h. Persons who experience one episode of HAPE are likely to have another and should be warned. In severe **HACE,** dexamethasone (8 mg IV q 4 h) has been used and IV acetazolamide has been dramatically effective. **HARH** require no treatment, generally resolving during stay at altitude.

Chronic mountain sickness (CMS or Monge's disease), is an uncommon condition which affects longtime altitude residents; it is characterized by fatigue, dyspnea, aches and pains, excessive polycythemia, thromboembolism, and ultimately cardiac failure. CMS resembles **alveolar hypoventilation** (formerly called pickwickian syndrome) and both are thought caused by an inadequately sensitive respiratory center. The victim should descend to sea level; recovery is slow and return to altitude may cause recurrence. Repeated phlebotomy has been helpful but may not be the most desirable management.

§22. SPECIAL SUBJECTS

264. GERIATRIC MEDICINE

Geriatric medicine or geriatrics is an interdisciplinary approach to management of sickness and disability in the elderly. Gerontology includes the sciences describing the changes of normal aging as distinguished from disease effects. Most age-related biologic changes appear to show physiologic functions peaking before age 30 with subsequent gradual linear decline. Most changes have no practical implications for daily activity, but can become critical in periods of great stress. Thus, disease, rather than normal aging, is the prime decompensating factor in old age. Physiologic processes that decline with age include renal blood flow and creatinine clearance; in many individuals, maximum heart rate and thus cardiac output with exercise; glucose tolerance; vital capacity of the lung; lean body mass; and cellular immunity. But liver function and total lung capacity remain the same across the age spectrum, and secretion of ADH in response to osmolar stimuli actually increases with age. (See also Nutritional Disorders in the Elderly and Chronically Ill in Ch. 80.)

Studies on aging are difficult because as people age, healthy subjects become harder to find. Cross-sectional studies, which compare individuals of different ages, are relatively easy to do, but may be less useful than longitudinal studies in which long-term monitoring compares the same persons to their younger selves. Such studies are difficult because of the time factor and drop-out rate.

Caring for an elderly person with multiple interacting diseases—and often difficult socioeconomic circumstances—demands the highest expression of the diagnostic, analytic, and synthetic and interpersonal skills of the physician. The last is of major importance, for often it is the physician's familiarity with patient behavior, history, satisfaction, fears, and aspirations that underlies early recognition of disease and the preparation and acceptance of suitable interventions that may involve lifestyle adjustments. The value of knowing the patient through a thorough life history and mental status test cannot be emphasized enough. First signs of physical illness, often reversible, commonly are mental or emotional, tending to confirm the stereotype of "senility" and thereby deterring proper diagnosis and treatment if casually accepted.

DEMOGRAPHY AND HEALTH CARE DELIVERY

Maximum human life span (about 100 yr, but with an estimated potential of reaching 110 to 120 yr) has changed little compared with major increase in average life expectancy. The old-old population is mostly female, because women outlive men. Although they are an increasingly healthy and active group, many problems emerge, especially after age 75. Burdens of multiple diseases are complicated by social disadvantage, emotional vulnerability, and poverty (as individuals outlive their resources and supportive age peers). One hundred years ago, 2% of Americans were over age 65. At the turn of the century, 4% were over age 65. Currently, > 11% of our citizens (27 million) are over age 65, and there is a net daily gain of > 1000 people into the ranks of elders. A full picture suggests that more recent cohorts of elderly persons are reaching age 65 in better health than their predecessors. Old age in its conventional but erroneous image as severe debilitation after age 65 is more aptly applied to the post-75 population.

Today a 65-yr-old man has a 13-yr life expectancy; if he lives to 75, he has 9 more years ahead of him. A 65-yr-old woman will live 18 yr on the average, and at age 75 she can expect to live 12 more years. It is estimated that in 2030, when the peak of the post-World War II baby boom will reach age 65, there will be > 55 million Americans (1:5) over age 65. The "over 85s" are expected to experience the highest percentage increase of all. Women live about 8 yr longer than men, probably the result of genetic, biologic, and environmental factors. Survival differences may narrow some since women are smoking more and moving into traditionally male job markets. Despite increased smoking and stress-related morbidity, women will probably always outlive men.

Caring for increasing numbers of old and infirm citizens makes extraordinary demands on traditional systems of health care delivery; the strains increase disproportionately, since the elderly, having more illness and complicating psychosocial sequelae, use more medical and socially supportive services. Though only 11% of our population, the elderly occupy > 33% of our acute hospital beds, buy 25% of all prescription drugs, and spend 30% of our > 300 billion dollar health budget (> 50% of the federal health budget). Nursing home care cost 21 billion dollars in 1980 and is projected to reach 70 billion by 1990. As early as 1972, nursing home beds began to outnumber acute hospital beds. Of the 1.4 million nursing home beds in America, 90% are occupied by people over age 65, but < 5% of Americans over age 65 live in nursing homes or other institutions.

Other ways of looking at the same data give a different perspective. Among the "over 65s," nearly 1/4 will spend time in a nursing home before death, and of those surviving beyond 80, > 50% will die in a nursing home. Nursing home beds in America outnumber acute hospital beds, but twice as many immobilized elderly live in the community as in nursing homes, and 25% of the community-dwelling elderly have no living relatives. A segment of our "over 65" population can be identified as being institutionalized or at high risk for future institutionalization (especially in the absence of community services). These approximately 6 million older Americans consume a disproportionate share of health resources. Special attention to their needs and their function within our health care system could add quality and years to their lives while restraining cost increases.

Studies, done in the early 1950s in Scotland, examined the response of older people to illness; they illustrate *qualitatively* different demands on traditional health care delivery systems. Each patient had a doctor responsible for continuing outpatient care, the doctor's office was conveniently located, and care was free to the patient. Although this system appeared adequate, startling numbers of people were identified with multiple medical problems that were *unknown to the responsible physician*. The problems

unearthed by screening with history, physical examination, laboratory tests, and a questionnaire given in the home were not esoteric. Common treatable conditions, such as B_{12} or iron deficiency anemia, congestive heart failure, GI bleeding, uncontrolled diabetes mellitus, active TB, foot disease interfering with mobility, oral disorders interfering with eating, correctable hearing and vision defects, and a high incidence of dementia and depression often go undiagnosed in the elderly. Important characteristics of disease in old age include the following:

(1) Elderly patients tend to conceal legitimate complaints pointing to serious treatable diseases. Many elderly as well as young people, believe that old age is a time of sickness and disability, and that not feeling well is a natural part of aging. Elderly persons with symptoms tend to report them only to family members, who at least half the time do not pursue the symptoms further. The prevalence of depression, combined with the cumulative losses of old age and the discomfort of illness, reduces interest in regaining health. Impaired cognition impedes the patient's complaining and reduces the physician's diagnostic searching. Today's old people grew up when hospitals were places for dying, and are reluctant to seek care.

(2) The phenomenon of multiple disorders in the elderly complicates and interferes with diagnosis and treatment of the presenting illness. In one study an average of 6 diseases was found among several thousand people, and the primary physician was unaware of 1/2 of the disorders present. Disease in one organ system stresses another weakened system that begins an irreversible concatenation of deteriorations, passing multiple points of no return, leading to infirmity, dependence, and, if uninterrupted, death. Active case-finding surveillance mechanisms for the aging must be added to our current passive health care system. Alert early intervention may prevent compounding and improve the quality of life through relatively minor maneuvers.

(3) Disorders often present atypically (see below for further discussion).

(4) "Predeath," *a period of dependency due to immobility, incontinence, or impaired cognition* (frequently in combination) precedes nearly 3/4 of deaths in old age. This period, usually spent in hospitals or nursing homes, is strongly age-related and approaches 3 mo in the group > 85 yr old. The cost, in human suffering and in money, is substantial. Immobility, incontinence, and cognitive impairment are clarions of serious underlying disease that demand prompt evaluation and specific treatment to avoid prolonged dependency.

BASIC PRINCIPLES IN CARING FOR THE ELDERLY

Predictable hazards for aged hospitalized patients include (1) nighttime confusion or "sundowning," (2) falls, (3) fractures with no identifiable trauma, (4) sudden appearance of decubiti, (5) fecal impaction and urinary retention, (6) falling victim to diagnostic and therapeutic endeavors, (7) prolonged convalescence, and (8) loss of the home while the patient is hospitalized.

There is special need to **identify multiple concomitant pathologic processes.** Treating one disorder without considering simultaneous associated ones may accelerate decline rather than result in improvement. Common conditions coexist in the elderly (eg, congestive heart failure, chronic renal failure, angina pectoris, osteoporosis, osteoarthritis, frail gait, chronic constipation, urinary precipitancy, venous and arterial insufficiency in the legs, diabetes mellitus, chronic pain, sleep disturbance, depression, cognitive impairment, and multiple drug regimens with poor compliance). When multiple problems coincide in one elderly patient, bed rest, surgery, drugs, and other treatments may be disastrous if not scrupulously monitored and well integrated.

Disorders in old age can be divided into 2 broad groups—those seen commonly *only* in the elderly and those which, though occurring also in other age groups, present *unusual features* or present *without usual features* in the elderly.

DISORDERS COMMON ONLY IN THE ELDERLY

Problems usually restricted to the elderly include normal pressure hydrocephalus, accidental hypothermia, and urinary incontinence (these are discussed below). Other disorders common only in the elderly are diabetic hyperosmolar nonketotic coma; stroke; polymyalgia rheumatica—giant cell arteritis; decubitus ulcers; metabolic bone disease; degenerative osteoarthritis; hip fracture and its rehabilitation; dementia syndrome; falling; prostatic carcinoma; gammopathies, including multiple myeloma; chronic lymphatic leukemia; angioimmunoblastic lymphadenopathy with dysproteinemia (lymphoma); TB (especially miliary); herpes zoster; basal cell carcinoma; and parkinsonism. Separate discussions elsewhere in THE MANUAL are listed in the index.

NORMAL PRESSURE HYDROCEPHALUS (NPH)

Cerebral ventricular dilation with normal lumbar CSF pressure, presenting with a characteristic clinical syndrome of dementia, apraxia of gait, and urinary incontinence. Etiology may be attributed to previous surface inflammation of the brain, usually from subarachnoid hemorrhage or diffuse meningitis, presumed to result in scarring of the arachnoid villi over the brain convexities where CSF absorption usually occurs. Supporting data are meager, however, and many elderly NPH patients have no history of predisposing disease.

Clinical Manifestations

The syndrome consists of dementia, incontinence, and a distinctive apraxia of gait, associated with ventricular dilation and normal CSF pressure. There is neither motor weakness nor staggering, but rather what has been described as the "slipping clutch" phenomenon in which initiation of gait is hesitant, but eventually walking occurs. NPH has also been described in association with various psychiatric manifestations that are not distinctive, and it should be considered in the differential diagnosis of any new psychiatric illness in old age.

Treatment

Shunting CSF from the dilated ventricles sometimes results in clinical improvement, but the longer the disease has been present, the less likely shunting will be curative. Radiographic or pressure measurements in patients with the syndrome do not predict the clinical outcome of shunting.

ACCIDENTAL HYPOTHERMIA
(AH; Hypothermia)

Unexpected fall of body temperature to < 35 C (95 F). The sudden appearance of low body temperature in the elderly as a common winter event was noted 20 yr ago. The afflicted are at high risk for a potentially fatal clinical syndrome mimicking stroke or metabolic derangement. British investigations speculate that thousands of elderly people die each year in Great Britain from AH, but one American study could not find lowered temperature among high-risk community dwelling elders in Maine during the winter. The wide range of estimates can be explained by the lack of definitive pathologic evidence of hypothermia death. Stated simply, most dead people are cold; therefore, death cannot confidently be attributed to AH postmortem. Temperatures of elderly patients entering hospitals in Britain during winter months were accurately recorded using a low-reading thermometer, disclosing that > 3.5% of patients over age 65 had body temperatures below 35 C. Lack of central heating or indoor plumbing was not a risk factor for these patients. If these data can be extrapolated, nearly 50,000 elderly Americans may be entering hospitals each winter with occult hypothermia.

Etiology and Pathogenesis

Elderly people with borderline low temperatures have age-related autonomic defects producing low peripheral resting blood flow, a nonconstrictor vasomotor response to cold, and easily provoked orthostatic hypotension. These defects are exacerbated by phenothiazines, especially chlorpromazine, and correlate with hypothermia risk.

The provocative cold stress is not prolonged exposure to severe cold conditions; rather, these aged patients may become hypothermic while in their mildly cool homes (as warm as 18.3 C [65 F]), though most episodes are initiated by temperatures < 18.3 C. Besides inadequate environmental heating in the winter, contributory factors include diminished perception of cold and poor heat conservation mechanisms. AH takes many hours to several days to develop. Body temperature, once falling below 35 C, continues to fall slowly and insidiously, terminating in death if the environment is unaltered. The overall mortality rate is about 50% but survival is largely determined by the presence and severity of complicating disease.

A variety of drugs (including neuroleptics, sedatives and hypnotics, tranquilizers, alcohol); congestive heart failure; hypothyroidism; hypopituitarism; uremia; Addison's disease; starvation; ketoacidosis; pulmonary infection; sepsis; brain injury; and any immobilizing illness predispose to hypothermia.

Symptoms and Signs

As body temperature drops, the patient proceeds from fatigue, weakness, incoordination, apathy, and drowsiness to an acute confusional state that, when body temperature falls below 32.2 C (90 F), progresses to stupor and coma. Hallucinations, combativeness, and resistance to aid may be seen. While hands and feet of many people are cold to the touch in winter, these patients have cold abdomens as well. Shivering and pallor are strikingly absent, respirations are shallow and infrequent, slow pulse and low BP with a host of atrial and ventricular arrhythmias are common, and the face may be puffy and pink. The ECG may show a characteristic J wave early—a small positive deflection following the QRS complex in the left ventricular leads—which is found in no other condition. Unfortunately, it appears in slightly < 50% of hypothermic patients. More commonly, the ECG shows baseline oscillation produced by a fine rapid muscle tremor that is often mistaken for electrical interference or voluntary motion. This fine trembling is usually not apparent grossly but probably is the elderly hypothermic patient's physiologic equivalent of shivering. Neurologic signs of tremor, ataxia, pathologic and depressed reflexes, coma, seizures, and a marked increase in muscle tone resembling acute parkinsonism may all occur. If temperature fall is uninterrupted, death usually occurs between 23.9 C (75 F) and 29.4 C (85 F) from cardiac standstill or ventricular fibrillation.

General metabolic effects of hypoxia and tissue necrosis are the rule, though if the patient survives, low temperature may delay the onset of many complications. The commonest complications are pancreatitis, pulmonary edema, pneumonia, metabolic acidosis, renal failure, and gangrene of the extremities.

Diagnosis

Knowledge of the disorder, a high index of suspicion, and a low-reading thermometer are required. The standard clinical thermometer reads from 34.4 C (94 F) to 42.2 C (108 F) and is rarely shaken down below 35.6 C (96 F). A low-reading thermometer, registering 28.9 C (84 F) to 42.2 C (108 F), is available. Health personnel caring for the elderly must be oriented to look for low body temperature, since the usual custom is to document only normal or elevated temperatures when evaluating a patient.

Treatment

Slow spontaneous rewarming, which allows body temperature to return to normal gradually (not faster than 0.6 C [1 F]/h) by conserving heat still being produced by the

hypothermic patient, is recommended. *More rapid rewarming has often resulted in irreversible hypotension.* Heat conservation is achieved with blankets or more sophisticated insulating materials in a warm room. Careful monitoring and anticipation of common complications are essential to successful treatment (see also Treatment in Ch. 256).

URINARY INCONTINENCE

The involuntary loss of urine while awake or asleep is a malodorous social stigma, commonly concealed by its embarrassed victim with a mountain of absorbent pads. The prevalence ranges from 5 to 15% in people over age 65 at home, as high as 50% in those hospitalized, and is even higher in the chronic institutionalized elderly. As much as 25% of nursing time in geriatric hospitals is consumed dealing with incontinence. Such patients require a 200% increase in alloted nursing time to deal with bedpans and urinals, and nearly 600% more time to be bathed satisfactorily, compared with the nursing required by continent peers.

The causes of urinary incontinence may be temporary or fixed. Specific types and their management are discussed in Ch. 159.

DISORDERS WITH UNUSUAL PRESENTATIONS IN THE ELDERLY

The characteristic symptoms and signs of many disorders are frequently absent in old age, and are often replaced with one or more nonspecific manifestations, such as refusal to eat or drink, falling, incontinence, dizziness, acute confusion, increasing dementia, weight loss, and failure to thrive. Depression is probably the most common psychiatric disorder in the "over 65" population. Organic psychoses, other affective disorders, paranoid states, hypochondriasis, and suicide become more common with age; all may present atypically.

Diseases that are especially likely to be diagnostic enigmas in the elderly are drug intoxication, alcoholism, myxedema, myocardial infarction, pulmonary embolism, pneumonia, malignant disease (especially colon, lung, and breast), acute abdomen, and thyrotoxicosis, which is discussed illustratively below.

OCCULT HYPERTHYROIDISM

Apathetic and masked hyperthyroidism are 2 variant thyrotoxic syndromes lacking the readily recognizable symptoms and signs (see Ch. 89). Although > 50% of thyrotoxic patients are 40 to 60 yr of age, 15% are over age 65. Occult hyperthyroidism is found in 1 to 2% of newly hospitalized patients over age 65 in Great Britain. These patients show no goiter 40% of the time and no eye signs or tachycardia in > 50%. The constellation of diffuse goiter, eye signs, and thyroid bruit occurs in only 20% of older thyrotoxic patients. One explanation of the paucity of classic findings in the elderly is that their diminished physiologic reserve is depleted quickly by hypermetabolic stress. T_3 toxicosis is uncommon in the elderly.

Symptoms and Signs

Masked hyperthyroidism is the more common of the 2 syndromes. The usual features of multisystem involvement in thyrotoxicosis are absent, and symptoms and signs referrable to a single organ system, most often the heart, dominate the clinical picture. Congestive heart failure poorly responsive to digitalis, atrial fibrillation with slow ventricular response, other fixed or paroxysmal arrhythmias, cardiomegaly, and palpitations are common. GI involvement can include constipation, weight loss with anorexia, and hepatomegaly. Psychiatric manifestations include confusion, psychomotor retardation, chronic depression, and apparent "senile" dementia. Increased bone cal-

cium turnover is reflected in elevated serum calcium, bone pain, osteoporosis, and frequent fracture.

Apathetic hyperthyroidism, the less common occult presentation of thyrotoxicosis in the elderly, occurs in 10 to 15% of aged thyrotoxics. Apathy and inactivity replace the usual hyperkinesis and dominate the clinical picture even though there may be associated cardiac or other organ system findings. These patients look extremely old and wizened, but with treatment rapidly lose wrinkling and become more youthful-looking. They have been described as having a "characteristic senile appearance" of mild chronic illness, but when afflicted with an acute illness or stress, they "quietly and peacefully sink into coma and die an absolutely relaxed death without activation."

Laboratory values are generally the same for older and younger adults, but T_3 levels decline 10 to 20% in euthyroid elderly. **Treatment** is usually effective with radioactive iodine, but up to 50% of the patients need temporary prior and subsequent pharmacologic thyroid suppression (see also HYPERTHYROIDISM in Ch. 89).

DRUG THERAPY IN THE ELDERLY

Elderly patients, in or out of the hospital, are twice as susceptible to adverse drug reactions as younger patients. These reactions are likely to be more serious and extend hospitalization longer than for a younger patient. Old people at home take nearly 3 times as many drugs as the general population, with women taking twice as many as men. The average older person receives 13 prescriptions annually and spends 20% of personal funds on drugs. When the prevalence of intellectual and visual impairment in the elderly is juxtaposed to the similar size, shape, and color of many medicines, errors in administration occur. More than 50% of elderly patients do not take their drugs as prescribed and about 25% of them make errors likely to result in drug-induced illness.

Elderly patients are more susceptible to the adverse and toxic effects of most drugs, and the aged often bear the brunt of reflexive prescribing for uninvestigated symptoms. Changes with aging in body composition, and in drug distribution, metabolism, excretion, and response make the elderly more vulnerable to adverse reactions. Since most clinical trials and pharmacologic studies are performed in younger people, drug treatment standards thus developed and applied to the elderly are often hazardous.

Physiologic data demand that extreme care be used in selecting drugs and dosages to treat old people. An indicated drug should not be withheld because of a patient's age, but extra care is required in prescribing for and supervising the elderly.

Drug absorption can be influenced by numerous changes in the aging GI tract. Decline of gastric acid secretion, decreased mesenteric blood flow, shrinkage of total surface area of the gut, and decline of active transport mechanisms tend to decrease absorption and result in a lower serum level of an orally administered drug. Decreasing motility, largely due to higher pH of gastric contents, makes absorption more complete and thus elevates serum levels. The net effect of these factors is small, so that blood levels for most drugs in the elderly are not predictably influenced by differences in absorption.

Body composition changes occurring with age collaborate to make blood levels of drugs higher after standard doses. Weight declines, but body fat increases modestly (5 to 20%) in men and women. Lean body mass relative to total weight and total body water both decline, resulting in more drug/wt of metabolically active tissue, and generally a smaller volume of distribution with standard doses of drug. Serum albumin falls, so that the many drugs that bind substantially to protein circulate less bound and are more active. Such changes in body composition add up to make toxic accumulation of drugs more likely in the elderly.

Metabolism, largely by liver enzymes, accounts for inactivation of many drugs. The scanty available data suggest a decline in the maximum clearance rates of some hepatic enzyme systems, but currently there are insufficient data to make any general state-

ments about drug inactivation with age. Smoking and alcohol consumption have more influence on hepatic metabolism of drugs than does aging.

Decline in kidney function is a major factor in producing elevated blood levels of drugs in the elderly. Renal blood flow falls nearly 1%/yr after age 30, resulting in about a 30 to 40% decrease in most elderly. Diminished renal blood flow is reflected by a similar fall in GFR, and urea and creatinine clearance. However, serum creatinine, the commonly used measure of renal function, rises little or not at all, largely because of decreased muscle mass and creatinine production in the elderly. Similarly, BUN rises far less than expected because of diminished protein intake in old age. Therefore, creatinine clearance is a far more reliable indicator of drug-clearing capacity of the aging kidney, and is generally predictable by an age-creatinine clearance nomogram for individuals free of renal disease. A small subset of elderly individuals showed little or no change in renal function with age.

Changes in the aging brain reduce reserve capacity and make cognitive decline a particularly high-risk early event when elderly patients accumulate high blood levels of many drugs. Tissue sensitivity to some drugs increases, producing greater effects using standard doses.

---

265. AIDS FOR THE DISABLED PATIENT

The family that must provide long-term home care for a bedridden or partially disabled patient requires guidance in routine nursing care as well as instruction in more complicated procedures. Personnel from the Visiting Nurse Association or the local Board of Health can provide invaluable instruction and assistance.

The **ambulatory, partially disabled patient** and his family must learn together, at the beginning of treatment, the new methods of ambulation, the needed safety measures, and any ongoing treatments. The patient optimally should be able to direct and be responsible for any measures that he cannot manage for himself. Family members should be helped to acquire a proficiency that makes them relatively secure and they should feel free to ask questions.

Equipment

A **wheelchair** must have brakes and be chosen with consideration of the patient's disability, size, weight, and activity, so that a stable sitting position without contractures is maintained. Guidelines for selecting a wheelchair are available from manufacturers, distributors, and physical therapy departments. **Crutches** are measured and adjusted with the patient standing against a wall or supported by a chair. In use, the top bar should be 2 in. below the anterior axillary fold and the tips 6 to 8 in. ahead of and to each side of the toes, so that the crutches and legs form a supporting tripod. The patient's weight is borne on the hand pieces, which should be adjusted to allow a 15° angle at the elbow.

A **cane** should provide 25° of elbow flexion. To walk correctly with a cane, the patient stands in a normal walking position with the cane held on the side opposite to his weak leg. With his weight on the cane and the weak leg, he moves his good leg forward. Then he puts his weight on his good leg and moves the cane and the weak leg forward. An alternative method is to place the cane a step ahead of his feet, move his weak leg forward, shift his weight to the cane and his weak leg, and then move his good leg forward.

Building Modifications

Stairs should have a 10 in. deep tread, a maximum of 7 in. high, preferably snub nose, and have at least one **railing,** which should be 32 in. high and extend 18 in.

beyond the top and bottom steps. **Wheelchair access** requires 32-in. doorways; a space 60 × 60 in. for turns; and **ramps** with a nonskid surface, a grade of 1 in./ft (8.33%), and railings 48 in. apart, 32 in. high, and extending 1 ft beyond the ramp at top and bottom. A small wheelchair elevator is useful for outside accessibility when space prohibits a ramp. A seat-type elevator may be installed on an inside stairway.

Toilet bars should be 1½ in. in diameter, 33 in. above and parallel to the floor, and 1½ in. from the wall. Bars that can be attached to the toilet are available commercially. An elevated toilet seat may aid in wheelchair transfers. Two **tub grab bars** are needed: one parallel to the tub and 4 in. above the tub surface, and the other vertical to the tub starting 9 in. from the tub surface. Both should be 1½ in. from the wall. **Shower grab bars** should reach from the floor to head height (minimally knees to head) and be 1½ in. from the wall. A number of tub seats or shower seats are available, including shower chairs. Roll in shower chairs are available, and a "telephone" shower head allows greater independence for the severely disabled.

Kitchen requirements include counters 26¼ in. (or 26½ in.) from the floor or waist high; a stove with controls at the front, an oven at chair-arm height; and a sink that is open below and with the pipes flush to the wall to allow a chair to roll under.

---

266. NUCLEAR MEDICINE

The branch of medicine that deals with the use of unsealed radioactive materials for diagnosis and therapy. The most useful property of a radionuclide for imaging is its emission of electromagnetic radiation in the form of gamma rays (photons). These are easily detectable with modern instrumentation and can be both quantitated and localized within the body accurately and noninvasively. Radionuclides may be administered orally, parenterally, or through intracavitary routes and usually are associated with significantly lower doses of radiation than alternative radiographic technics.

Radionuclides decay at unique and characteristic rates (half-life). In the process of decay from unstable to more stable states, isotopes may emit gamma rays that are specific for a given radionuclide. The measurement of the energy spectrum of radiation emitted by a radioactive element and of the half-life of that element permit its accurate identification in microgram quantities (tracer dose), without exposing the patient to any pharmacologic toxicity. For example, a tracer dose of ^{131}I may be given safely to a patient with known iodine sensitivity. Patients with a history of contrast media sensitivity can be studied safely with alternative nuclear medicine technics.

Many nuclides emit beta particles as well as gamma rays. Negatively charged beta particles (negatrons) are emitted from the nucleus and may be useful in certain forms of in vitro analysis such as radioimmunoassay. However, beta particles cannot be used within the body for diagnosis because they are not measurable externally and they yield significant radiation to the patient (their entire energy is absorbed by the tissue in which they localize). Other forms of radiation include alpha particles, which are helium nuclei ejected from the nucleus and which, because of their relatively heavy mass and energy, are associated with the highest radiation dose and lowest penetrability.

Another form of emission of particulate matter is the positron. This is a positively charged particle that is emitted from the nucleus and on encountering an electron is annihilated, with the resultant production of 2 gamma rays of characteristic energy (511 KeV) that are emitted 180° from each other, permitting very accurate localization of the site of origin of the positron, as well as its quantitation. Many of the naturally occurring elements that are vital constituents of organic matter, including carbon, oxygen, and nitrogen, can be made radioactive and capable of positron emission. This attribute makes **positron emission tomography** a valuable method for evaluating normal

biochemical processes. Since most positron emitters have very short half-lives requiring on site production, positron emission tomography is mainly a research technic. **Single photon emission tomography** is a related technic that uses a tomographic principle for imaging conventional radionuclides. Much progress has been made in the use of emission tomographic technics and their clinical use is increasing; eg, by imaging a tomographic slice of activity, diagnosis may be improved by eliminating interference from parts of an organ overlying a suspected lesion.

Radioactive isotopes may be utilized as simple salts of an element, such as sodium radioiodine, or they may be chemically bound to another molecule to produce a "labeled" compound (radiopharmaceutical). Regardless of the mode of labeling of an element or compound, the substances generally behave physiologically and biochemically identical to the stable nonradioactive form. For example, radioactive ^{131}I behaves the same in the body as nonradioactive or stable ^{127}I. This property makes the use of Lugol's solution beneficial in people who have been exposed accidentally to radioiodine. By saturating the thyroid with a large amount of nonradioactive iodine, thyroid uptake of the radioactive form is reduced. Alternatively, small amounts of radioiodine (^{123}I, ^{131}I) may be used to measure thyroid function in the radioactive iodine uptake test. If radioiodine is attached to a molecule such as albumin, the molecule continues to behave as albumin, but its fate and location in the body may be traced easily by external detection of gamma rays from the radioiodine. Depending on the size of the molecule, the use of a radioactive label added to a compound in which it is not a normal constituent may or may not affect its physiologic and biochemical handling.

Therapy has not been a prominent part of nuclear medicine practice, with the major exception of radioiodine treatment of benign and malignant thyroid disease. Radiophosphorus is used in some hematologic disorders and colloidal gold has been of help in ascites secondary to malignancy. Problems relate to the difficulty of delivering an adequate amount of radioactive material to the target organ without excessive radiation exposure to the rest of the body. In nuclear medicine, the use of some radioactive materials in therapy overlaps to a small extent with the practice of radiotherapy where radioactive materials may also be used in the form of sealed sources.

RADIATION DETECTION

The growth of nuclear medicine is dependent on both improved methods for radiation detection and the synthesis and utilization of radiopharmaceuticals for studying specific organs. The earliest practical clinical radiation detector was the radiation probe. A probe consists of a carefully prepared crystalline block of sodium iodide doped with minute traces of thallium that make it highly sensitive to gamma radiation. The gamma radiation interacts in the crystal and the electromagnetic energy is absorbed resulting in the emission of an equivalent amount of energy from the crystal in the form of visible light. Another component of the probe is a light-sensitive photocathode placed behind the crystal to enable light to be detected and converted to an electrical current, which can then be amplified and finally used to quantitate the amount and energy of the original incident gamma rays.

The scintillation camera, a device with imaging capabilities, is essentially a combination of a number of photomultiplier tubes behind a very large crystal. It utilizes a sophisticated electronic system to analyze not only the number of gamma ray events in the crystal and their energy, but also the location of the events within the crystal. Lead collimators allow radioactivity to reach the crystal only at 90° to its surface. Each site in the body corresponds, therefore, to only one site on the crystal. This makes it possible to depict on a cathode ray oscilloscope the corresponding location beneath the crystal from which a gamma ray must have originated. If a radiopharmaceutical is concentrated in a specific organ, the radioactivity will cluster in the area of the organ and provide an image that can be interpreted both morphologically, based upon its

appearance, and physiologically, based upon the time activity relationships of the accumulation and disappearance of the tracer and its mechanism of uptake and metabolism or excretion.

The computer has become an intrinsic part of nuclear medicine, with rapidly increasing applications since the major impetus given by the development of methods for cardiovascular nuclear medicine studies. Routinely obtained gamma camera studies appear as rather simple images, but inherently they contain a large amount of potentially useful quantifiable data. The computer can quantitate the data, localize the information, and display it in a variety of forms including time activity curves. It can be used to evaluate portions of the image and to modify the images. Such additional analysis permits considerable enhancement of the information supplied by nuclear medicine studies and the acquisition of important physiologic data.

RADIATION DOSIMETRY

Nuclear medicine depends upon the administration of a radiopharmaceutical or radionuclide to a patient. Virtually all procedures used are dependent on internally distributed radioactive material, following either IV or oral administration. Units commonly in use today are the microcurie **(µCi)** and millicurie **(mCi),** which quantitate the amount of radioactivity present in the dose. These units will ultimately be replaced by the Becqueral **(Bq).** One millicurie equals 37 MBq and one microcurie equals 37 KBq. The dose of radioactivity given that relates to the amount of radionuclide used should be differentiated from the **radiation dose** that refers to *the radiation energy imparted to the exposed tissues.* The implications of radiation dosimetry, along with a table to illustrate relative commonly encountered doses, is given in Ch. 257. TABLE 266–1 may be used to gain a perspective of the radiation dosimetry involved in common nuclear medicine procedures.

With an IV urogram the skin may receive 3300 mrads; with an IV cholangiogram 29,000 mrads. Skin doses are of concern in radiographic procedures but are usually negligible in isotope procedures.

RADIOPHARMACEUTICALS

The key to the future of nuclear medicine lies more in the development of new pharmaceuticals than in improvements in instrumentation. The number and variety of procedures that can be performed is limited only by the ingenuity of the chemist in obtaining compounds that localize in specific organs and labeling the compounds with

TABLE 266-1. RADIATION DOSE TO THE PATIENT IN RADIONUCLIDE STUDIES*

Radiopharmaceutical	*Target Organ*	*Millirads*
^{57}Co-Vit B_{12} (Schilling Test)	Total Body	80
^{99m}Tc-Pertechnetate (Thyroid Scan)	Thyroid	150
^{99m}Tc-Diphosphonate (Bone Scan)	Bone	450
^{99m}Tc-Colloid (Liver Scan)	Liver	1000
^{99m}Tc-Microspheres (Lung Scan)	Lung	400
^{99m}Tc-DTPA (Kidney Scan)	Kidneys	150
^{131}I-Iodide (RAI)	Thyroid	4200
^{131}I-Hippuran (Kidney Scan)	Kidneys	300

*Calculated from the usually administered dose, 100 rads (100,000 mrads) equal 1 gray (Gy)

an appropriate radionuclide. There are a wide variety of mechanisms by which pharmaceuticals can be delivered to the organ of interest. They may depend upon active transport, in which the compound in question is actively removed from the blood and transported to the target organ. Key examples of this type of organ localization are the thyroid with its trapping of radioiodine, and the kidneys, which selectively concentrate ^{131}I-labeled orthoiodohippurate. Phagocytosis is relied upon for imaging of the liver and spleen, where the capability of the reticuloendothelial system to remove particulate matter such as technetium 99m sulphur colloid is used to gain excellent localization of these organs. Cell sequestration can be used to image the spleen by treating technetium 99m-labeled RBCs with heat, thereby damaging them and making them susceptible to removal from the bloodstream by the spleen. Capillary blockade provides the physiologic basis for lung scanning by trapping the radioactive particles within the capillaries of the lung.

Simpler, less specific approaches to radionuclide localization include exchange diffusion, in which a radioactive element such as xenon-133 gas is inhaled and an image of the ventilation of the lungs is obtained by the diffusion of the gas throughout the inspired air. Physicochemical adsorption represents a more complex process and is the probable basis for skeletal imaging, in which technetium 99m phosphonates are trapped in bone through exchange with normal bone constituents in the hydration shell. Compartmental localization takes advantage of normal barriers within the body, such as the vascular system, to restrict the diffusion of substances such as technetium 99m-labeled albumin and thereby provide an image of its route throughout the vascular system. Newer approaches to localization of radiopharmaceuticals include the use of compounds such as radioiodinated estrogens that are taken up by specific receptor sites and provide an index of the quantity of receptor sites and receptor activity in a given area. The development of monoclonal antibodies promises to further improve radiopharmaceutical localization by directing specific monoclonal antibodies labeled with radionuclides at targets of interest.

The major physical characteristics of many of the commonly used radionuclides are shown in TABLE 266–2.

SPECIFIC ORGAN IMAGING PROCEDURES

Although the diagnoses of specific diseases and disorders are discussed in their appropriate sections of THE MANUAL, an overview of nuclear medicine procedures follows:

Thyroid: The best known and understood test in nuclear medicine is the **thyroid uptake,** based on the concentration of radioiodine by the thyroid for incorporation into thyroid hormone. Several important points bear on this test. Radioiodine thyroid tests

TABLE 266–2. SOME COMMONLY USED RADIONUCLIDES

Substance	*Half-Life*	*Photon Energy (KeV)**	*Beta Emission*
^{99m}Tc	6 h	140	No
^{131}I	8.05 d	364	Yes
^{123}I	13 h	159	No
^{67}Ga	78 h	90–390	Yes
^{133}Xe	5.3 d	80	Yes
^{81m}Kr	13 s	190	No
^{111}In	2.8 d	170, 250	No
^{201}Tl	73 h	70, 135, 167	No

*Kiloelectron-volts

should not be ordered for in vivo evaluation of thyroid function prior to in vitro testing that yields accurate information without exposing the patient to radiation (see also Laboratory Testing of Thyroid Function under THYROID HORMONES in Ch. 89). When morphologic information in addition to functional information is required (eg, to evaluate thyroid nodules and other forms of neoplastic disease), a **thyroid scan** is necessary. However, thyroid scanning carries a significantly larger radiation burden than the thyroid uptake alone; therefore, the combination of an uptake and scan should not be ordered routinely.

Liver and spleen: Unfortunately, due to the great variety of space-occupying diseases that may affect the liver, no single test is uniformly successful in identifying disease. A scan of the liver with technetium 99m sulphur colloid provides morphologic and functional information about the state of the reticuloendothelial system. For instance, in patients with severe liver disease, a so-called "colloid shift" may be seen where more than the normal amount of colloid is taken up by the bone marrow and spleen due to reduced liver function. Similarly, uptake of colloid by the spleen provides information about the functional integrity of that organ. No simple guidelines exist for deciding between ultrasound, CT scanning, and nuclear medicine technics for liver and spleen studies. These tests are useful in a variety of overlapping conditions and consultation with specialists should be sought in choosing a first line of investigation.

Biliary scanning has been improved by the introduction of iminodiacetic acid derivatives that are easily labeled with technetium 99m. These compounds are actively concentrated and secreted by the liver providing morphologic and physiologic information about the integrity of the biliary tract and the gallbladder. They are particularly valuable in the diagnosis of acute cholecystitis, because visualization of the gallbladder with these agents does *not* occur in acute cholecystitis, providing evidence of the functional deficit. In addition, these agents provide information about bile production and flow, gallbladder emptying, and postoperative leaks or obstructions.

Stomach: Agents in which technetium 99m is incorporated into food are increasingly being used to evaluate gastric motility and emptying and as an adjunct to other evaluations of hiatal hernia. The test can be used to evaluate therapeutic interventions as well (eg, the administration of bethanacol in gastroesophageal reflux).

Intestines: GI bleeding can be diagnosed and localized very precisely with technetium 99m sulphur colloid or with technetium-labeled RBCs. The information is a valuable guide to the angiographer in precisely defining the bleeding site.

Lung perfusion scanning with technetium 99m-labeled microspheres to visualize the distribution of pulmonary arteriolar blood flow, and **ventilation scanning** using radioactive gases or aerosols to evaluate ventilation are very useful to detect pulmonary embolism (see Ch. 39). Lung scanning also can be used to evaluate pulmonary function and agents that improve pulmonary function, but these applications have not achieved widespread use.

Cardiovascular system: Several procedures are available to evaluate the possibility of myocardial infarction, including ^{99m}Tc phosphate scanning, in which active uptake of phosphate occurs in the presence of an infarct; thallium-201 imaging, in which an infarct causes a lack of uptake; and gated blood pool studies, in which radioactive-labeled RBCs can be observed in their course through the cardiac chambers permitting observation of abnormal wall motion associated with myocardial infarction. In addition, cardiac output and cardiac ejection fraction can be measured easily. Radioactive tracers can provide a wide range of information about myocardial perfusion and function, previously obtainable only through cardiac catheterization (see RADIONUCLIDE IMAGING OF THE HEART and CARDIAC CATHETERIZATION in Ch. 25).

Urogenital: Radiopharmaceuticals can be used to measure GFR (technetium 99m DTPA), renal plasma flow (^{131}I orthoiodohippurate), renal perfusion (technetium 99m pertechnetate), and renal morphology (technetium 99m DMSA, technetium 99m glucoheptonate). These nuclear medicine tests are safe and reliable and are useful in patients who have known contrast media sensitivity or underlying renal insufficiency. The tests offer morphologic and functional information, whereas IV urography or arteriography offer mainly morphologic information. Radionuclide renography coupled with diuretics is especially valuable in distinguishing nonobstructive from obstructive dilation of the urinary tract. Tracer technics can provide images of the kidneys in severe renal failure and can be used to evaluate the presence or absence of ureteral reflux and to differentiate torsion of the testicle from epididymitis.

Adrenal gland: ^{131}I-labeled 19-iodocholesterol can be used for adrenal cortex imaging in diseases such as primary hyperaldosteronism. ^{131}I-labeled benzylguanidine permits adrenal medulla imaging for diseases such as pheochromocytoma. These technics have a restricted application but offer potential for therapeutic as well as diagnostic use in adrenal diseases.

Bone and joint diseases are major subjects for applications of radionuclide technics. Technetium 99m-labeled phosphonates are highly sensitive to changes in bone turnover, and therefore are very useful in the early detection of bone and joint abnormalities. X-ray and other procedures for evaluating bone morphology depend on relatively extensive changes in bone composition before they become apparent. When bone disease is suspected and radiographs are normal, radionuclide technics offer a more sensitive form of diagnosis. Bone surveys should be carried out only with radionuclides, since they expose the patient to much less radiation and have a higher sensitivity than x-rays.

Brain: Although cisternography still is of use in selected patients with dementia, hydrocephalus, or suspected CSF leak, the role of nuclear medicine in brain and other neurologic diseases has been replaced largely by CT scanning and MRI. Newer agents that specifically measure brain receptors or are related to cerebral blood flow may provide applications in the future.

Vascular: Peripheral blood flow can be measured with radioactive xenon or sodium and can be estimated by muscle uptake of thallium. In addition, images of the aorta can be obtained to evaluate renal perfusion, aortic aneurysm, superior vena caval syndrome, and related conditions. These are simple screening tests that often may obviate the need for angiography.

Total body scanning is useful in a few situations; one is the possibility of bone disease, another is in the detection of an unknown infection site. Gallium 67 uniquely localizes in infection sites. Alternatively, indium 111-labeled WBCs can be used in whole body scanning to seek infection. Gallium-67 can also be used in suspected cases of interstitial nephritis, where its uptake is intense, and in diagnosing sarcoidosis where abnormal pulmonary uptake occurs.

Transplantation: Radioisotopes have been used in managing liver, lung, pancreas, and kidney transplantation. Their greatest use is in providing a very sensitive method for detecting renal transplant rejection, which is visually characterized by severely decreased perfusion and function, often in spite of continued urine production. Acute tubular necrosis in transplant recipients is characterized by modest perfusion reduction, better uptake of iodohippurate than in rejection, and virtual anuria. Kidney transplants also may concentrate technetium 99m sulphur colloid during rejection.

267. HYPERBARIC OXYGEN THERAPY

(HBO Therapy)

A medical treatment in which the patient is entirely enclosed in a pressure chamber breathing 100% oxygen **(O_2)** *at greater than one atmosphere* **(atm)** *pressure.* Either a monoplace chamber pressurized with pure O_2 or a larger multiplace chamber pressurized with compressed air where the patient receives pure O_2 by mask, head tent, or endotracheal tube may be used.

To locate hyperbaric facilities in the USA, Canada, and the Carribean area in an emergency, call the Divers Alert Network (DAN) at Duke University (919) 684–8111.

Contraindications and indications approved by the Committee on Hyperbaric Oxygenation of the Undersea Medical Society are presented below.

Contraindications

An **absolute contraindication** to HBO therapy is untreated pneumothorax, because with decompression the intrapleural air may double or triple in volume as normal atm pressure is approached. If pneumothorax occurs in the multi-place chamber under pressure, it must be relieved surgically before decompression. In the monoplace chamber, a McSwain dart or other chest tube is made ready, the chamber is decompressed not taking longer than 1 min, and the chest tube inserted as the patient emerges. **Premature infants** *are susceptible to retrolental fibroplasia and, therefore, HBO is contraindicated.* Full-term babies may be safely treated with HBO. Babies may require papoose restraints, and young children may need mild sedation. Concerns that HBO treatment of **pregnant women** might stimulate premature closure of the patent ductus in the fetus have been mitigated by research in the Soviet Union in which women in all stages of pregnancy, when treated with HBO, produced normal children. The chamber is used if there is an overriding need to treat a pregnant patient; eg, in CO poisoning (where the fetus suffers much more than the mother) or gas gangrene.

Relative contraindications: A history of spontaneous pneumothorax requires readiness to manage complications, as noted above. **Previous thoracic surgery** is a concern, as air trapping that could cause ruptured lung and air embolism are possibilities. Any pulmonary lesion may increase the possibility of air trapping, but patients with pneumonia and severe inhalation pneumonitis have been treated. In severe **emphysema with CO_2 intoxication,** removal of the hypoxic drive may cause respiratory arrest. **Upper respiratory infections** may make it difficult for the patient to equalize pressure in the ears and sinuses. Decongestants are indicated. If the patient has a **history of middle ear surgery** for the treatment of otosclerosis, a wire or plastic strut might be displaced by the application of pressure if the patient cannot equalize pressure in his ears. Tympanostomy tubes may be needed. **Seizure disorders** may increase susceptibility to O_2 seizures, and additional premedication (eg, with diazepam) may be advisable. **Uncontrolled high fever** may predispose to O_2 seizures and should be reduced before placing the patient in the chamber. **Respiratory viral infections** may tend to worsen with HBO. Such an infection is a reason to temporarily interrupt daily treatment of some chronic illnesses. In **congenital spherocytosis,** RBCs are fragile and high O_2 partial pressures may cause severe hemolysis. A **history of optic neuritis,** even if not active, has sometimes been associated with blindness following HBO treatment. Although rare, treatment should be halted immediately if the patient complains of a sudden change in vision.

Side Effects

O_2 seizures may occur, particularly when therapy is given at pressures > 2.4 atmospheres absolute **(ATA).** Some patients are idiosyncratically susceptible to high O_2 partial pressures. O_2 seizures cease when the O_2 is withdrawn; there are no known

sequelae. **Pulmonary O_2 toxicity,** consisting of substernal chest pain, cough, and patchy atelectasis, may occur but can be avoided if treatment protocols are adhered to.

After 20 or 30 treatments in the chamber, some patients complain of **numb fingers,** usually in the ulnar distribution; but this sensation disappears within 4 to 6 wk after therapy.

Serous otitis may result from breathing hyperbaric O_2 on a daily basis but usually is a minor problem; treatment is with decongestants.

A change in the refractive power of the lens is one of the most common side effects. Myopia, particularly in the elderly, tends to become worse, but presbyopes report an improvement in visual acuity, especially when reading. The original refractive state usually returns within 4 to 6 wk after therapy. The only cases in which visual acuity has not returned to pretreatment status are those with pre-existing lenticular opacities. It has been suggested, but not proved, that pre-existing cataracts mature more rapidly with HBO.

INDICATIONS

Carbon Monoxide Poisoning

Automotive exhaust gas, home heating, and industrial exposure are the most common sources. Fumes from paint strippers containing methylene chloride are metabolized to CO in the body and can cause severe symptoms. The diagnosis cannot be made unless one suspects exposure, especially in any afebrile individual or family group exhibiting flu-like symptoms. Headache, nausea, vomiting, weakness, and collapse often are followed by coma and death. "Cherry red" coloration of the skin is rare and an unreliable diagnostic sign. The percentage of carboxyhemoglobin in the blood likewise does *not* correlate with the prognosis and very often does not correspond to the patient's clinical condition, which is caused by tissue toxicity (inhibition of cytochrome A_3 oxidase).

Criteria for hyperbaric treatment: Unconsciousness, neurologic symptoms or signs, depression of the ST segment on the ECG, or a carboxyhemoglobin level > 40% are indications for HBO therapy. Evaluation of mental status is much more important than the carboxyhemoglobin level, and severity of acidosis is a good indication of the severity of the poisoning. Long exposures have a worse prognosis. If a hyperbaric chamber is located in the patient's hospital, treatment may be started at a lower carboxyhemoglobin level (25%) in the absence of other symptoms and signs. In the obtunded patient, treatment is indicated even if the CO level is zero if it is certain that CO poisoning caused the problem. The patient should be transferred to an HBO facility in the community (if available) or to the nearest facility available via rapid aircraft transport if practical. Although the mechanism is not completely understood, treatment may be effective even several days after the acute exposure.

Treatment: One hundred percent O_2 is given by tight-fitting mask (eg, aviator masks, anesthesia masks) or an endotracheal tube. Plastic "rebreather" masks commonly used in emergency rooms rarely deliver > 50 to 60% O_2 and *should not routinely be used in the treatment of CO poisoning.* Acidosis and arterial pH are corrected to ≥ 7.15, and it is important to supplement potassium **(K)** if needed. Low K is frequently seen, and arrhythmias can result from the vigorous administration of HCO_3 in hypokalemia.

In a monoplace chamber, the patient is treated for 90 min. If residual symptoms persist, retreatment can be carried out in 6 to 12 h. **In the multi-place chamber,** the patient is taken to 3 ATA and treated with two to three 23-min periods of 100% O_2 by mask with 5-min "air-breaks" in between. This is accomplished by removing the mask in the multiplace chamber or decompressing to the surface in the monoplace chamber

for this brief period. Treatment can then be continued at 1.9 ATA. In severe cases, US Navy Decompression Sickness Treatment Table 6 may be used from the onset. This provides at least 4 h of O_2 breathing at pressures starting at 2.8 ATA. In a conscious patient who cannot equalize his middle ear, myringotomy is indicated; it is optional in the unconscious patient but should not delay definitive treatment. Patients with a markedly impaired sensorium should be restrained, as they may awaken combative. Diazepam IV may be used to manage the combative patient.

Decompression Sickness and Gas (Air) Embolism (see CONDITIONS REQUIRING RECOMPRESSION in Ch. 262)

Air embolism also is seen in the hospital setting secondary to surgery, IV therapy, lung biopsy, ventilator accidents, renal dialysis, arterial catheterization, oral inflation of the vagina with air during pregnancy, and in victims escaping from submerged vehicles.

Gas Gangrene

Gas gangrene myonecrosis is discussed in HISTOTOXIC CLOSTRIDIAL DISEASE under CLOSTRIDIAL INFECTIONS in Ch. 8. *Clostridium perfringens* is the most common cause, although another organism or organisms are usually present. Pathogenesis is primarily mediated by alpha-toxin, a lecithinase, which dissolves RBCs (producing hemolysis and hematuria) and severely damages muscle, cell membranes, and renal tubules. Gas gangrene myonecrosis can produce profound shock that responds only to whole blood or packed cells. Death may ensue within 6 h of the diagnosis unless immediate corrective action is taken. HBO therapy, if available, must be carried out early in the course of the disease. If the patient with truncal gangrene is first treated in the chamber > 24 h after the diagnosis is made, the mortality is 75%; if treated within 24 h, the mortality falls to < 20%. When a limb is involved, mortality may be > 9% if HBO treatment is delayed > 24 h, but it approaches zero if instituted within 24 h, regardless of the type or time of surgery. If the syndrome progresses despite HBO therapy, amputation or major debridement must be carried out. The prognosis is especially grave in the elderly compromised host with gangrene of the abdomen or trunk. After the patient is no longer toxic, all necrotic material should be immediately removed surgically.

Surgery requiring general anesthesia should be deferred until after the first HBO treatment is given because: (1) Surgery prior to HBO treatment entails delay while the alpha-toxin damages all the organs of the body. (2) A general anesthetic given to a patient in septic shock vastly increases the morbidity and mortality. (3) A cleaner line of demarcation between the viable and necrotic tissue appears after 2 or more HBO treatments, often making possible less disfiguring surgery and even the salvage of entire limbs. (4) Large open debrided areas that constantly ooze blood and serum complicate fluid balance and subsequent chamber treatment.

HBO given at a pressure of 3 ATA in the multiplace chamber or 2.5 ATA in the monoplace chamber halts production of alpha-toxin when the tissue P_{O_2} rises to ≥ 300 mm Hg. Circulating alpha-toxin is fixed and deactivated in the tissues within about 30 min. Treatment is for 90 min.

In severely ill, febrile patients, the risk of convulsion can be diminished if an "air-break" (see Treatment of CO poisoning, above) of 5 min is provided in the middle of the 90-min treatment. Usually, 3 treatments are given in the first 24 h followed by 2 treatments in the ensuing two 24-h periods, making a total of 7 treatments. Fewer treatments may be given if the patient's signs of toxicity disappear, but up to 10 treatments may be necessary.

Crush Injury and Compartment Syndrome

Crush or degloving injuries (stripping of the skin and flesh from the bones, usually of the hands or feet as seen in wringer or industrial roller injuries) can interrupt both large vessels and the continuity of capillary beds. Large vessels must be repaired

surgically, but the ischemic anoxia associated with decreased capillary flow requires HBO treatment. Edema soon forms increasing the distance O_2 must diffuse from functioning capillaries. This often creates a vicious cycle and causes complications such as compartment syndrome and frank sloughing of compromised tissue.

Treatment: With a globally hypoxic limb, edema formation can be reduced by 50% if HBO treatment is initiated within about 8 h, assuming that damaged large vessels have been surgically repaired. HBO treatment reduces blood flow in muscle about 20%, reduces edema, and increases the amount of O_2 in physical solution in the plasma. Tissues receive abundant O_2, even though functioning capillaries may be sparse, thereby reducing tissue necrosis by about 50% in severely compromised compartments. Thus, HBO is most valuable in impending compartment syndrome but remains an adjunct to fasciotomy in established compartment compromise. Treatments are usually continued for 3 to 5 days.

Compromised Skin Grafts and Flaps

Most skin grafts and flaps will take without the adjunctive use of HBO therapy, but there is a 28% improvement in take in HBO-treated groups. Failing full-thickness flaps must be treated early, at the first signs of cyanosis or failure to take; treatment is continued bid for 3 to 7 days, depending on the appearance of the graft. In the compromised host where previous split thickness grafts have failed, graft take can often be achieved using HBO therapy to produce granulation tissue adequate for grafting and for 3 days bid following grafting.

Mixed Soft Tissue Infections

Most infections respond to adequate debridement and antibiotics, but in patients with peripheral ischemia (tissue $P_{O_2} < 30$ mm Hg), leukocyte killing cannot take place and HBO plays a role. Treatment daily or bid establishes granulation tissue to aid control of infection. If *Bacteroides* is the causative organism, initial HBO therapy should follow a gas gangrene protocol (see above). However, in treating the diabetic foot, an ankle arterial pressure (measured by Doppler) > 75 mm Hg is necessary or HBO will not be of value. Additionally, transcutaneous P_{O_2} measurements may be helpful. If $TcPO_2$ readings are > 40 mm Hg, healing with closure of the wound can probably be achieved using HBO therapy. If readings < 40 mm Hg rise to levels of ≥ 1000 when the patient is placed in the chamber at 2.4 ATA, healing will most likely occur. Otherwise, amputation is probably indicated.

Burns

Deep second-degree burns may deteriorate to full thickness loss, and HBO may be considered to reduce hypoxia and edema formation. HBO therapy reduces edema secondary to vasoconstriction and results in a 35% reduction in fluid requirement within the first 24 h. *To be effective, HBO therapy must be started within 24 h of the burn, preferably sooner.* HBO therapy will aid in the treatment of concomitant smoke inhalation and CO or cyanide poisoning (see Smoke Inhalation, below). Additionally, Curling's ulcer rarely appears, hypertrophic scarring and contracture are reduced, and burn encephalopathy is rare in patients treated with HBO.

Mafenide must be carefully removed before starting HBO therapy as it produces a peripheral vasodilation that, when coupled with the central vasoconstriction caused by HBO, produces worse results than when either HBO or mafenide is used alone. Silver sulfadiazine may be used. HBO is administered for 90 min q 8 h for the first 24 h, and then bid until all wounds are covered with epithelium or securely grafted. Burn therapy otherwise is as described in Ch. 254, but the necessity of controlling acidosis when HBO is used is especially important using 10 mEq bicarbonate/L of Ringer's solution. In order to avoid pulmonary O_2 toxicity, HBO is discontinued if the patient requires supplemental O_2 of 40% or greater outside the chamber. Tangential excision is used

with HBO and grafting is carried out as soon as there is uniformly healthy granulation tissue. HBO should be used only in established burn centers in accordance with rigid protocols.

Smoke Inhalation (see also Ch. 254)

Smoke inhalation usually consists of CO and/or cyanide poisoning combined with a severe chemical pneumonitis. (Modern building construction materials yield significant amounts of cyanide.) Bronchospasm and pulmonary edema typically worsen over the first 24 to 36 h, mandating that smoke inhalation patients be observed and have blood gases monitored for at least 24 h prior to discharge. HBO rapidly clears carboxyhemoglobin from blood and provides O_2 dissolved in plasma, while counteracting the tissue toxic effects of both CO and cyanide.

Initial therapy should be as for Carbon Monoxide Poisoning, above. Ventilatory support may be necessary, but early HBO treatment can reduce the need for intubation.

Soft Tissue Radiation Necrosis

Six to 18 mo following local radiation of tissue, medium-sized blood vessels begin to progressively sclerose, sharply limiting blood supply and causing profound tissue ischemia. Induration and fibrosis ensue and, if a break develops in the integument, infection usually supervenes and prevents healing. Wounds typically tend to enlarge when WBCs can no longer kill bacteria because of a fall in the tissue P_{O_2} to < 30 mm Hg. This problem is most common following radiation of head and neck tumors but also can be a serious problem in the abdomen and other areas.

Treatment: Prior to HBO therapy, surgery was the only treatment. Extirpation of the irradiated area and use of vascularized soft tissue grafts to close the defect are often successful. When this is not possible, due to the presence of critical structures (eg, the carotid artery), surgery should *not* be attempted until there has been adequate pretreatment with HBO to establish the necessary granulation tissue to support a graft.

In the hyperbaric chamber tissue P_{O_2} will rise to 75 to 80% of normal after 18 to 30 treatments, as vascular granulation tissue develops. Skin grafts then may be applied and HBO therapy is performed bid for at least 3 days following surgery and then once a day as necessary. Using pretreatment HBO, spontaneous closure of orocutaneous fistulas has been reported, and infections can be controlled when the P_{O_2} rises sufficiently. Wounds tend to be stable and do not exhibit long-term deterioration following adequate HBO treatment.

Osteoradionecrosis

Necrosis of bone caused by irradiation.

This condition most commonly involves the mandible secondary to radiation for head and neck tumors. Supervoltage x-ray results in aseptic degeneration, due to loss of viable osteoblasts and osteoclasts. Most cases of osteoradionecrosis of the jaw originate from tooth extraction, required because radiation caries develop with subsequent infection. The trauma of tooth removal causes a breakdown of gum tissue and subsequent progressive infection. Exposed bone is often visible and there is evidence of infection with pus formation, but the disorder is not a form of osteomyelitis. The infection is invariably periosseous in origin. Granulation tissue cannot form to bridge over dead bone, and the infection continues despite meticulous wound care and antibiotics; the resolution rate is only about 8%.

Prevention: When tooth extraction is necessary, it is best to give 20 preoperative HBO exposures on a once-a-day basis 5 or 6 days a week. Postoperatively, the patient is treated daily 10 more times with HBO. Perioperative antibiotics are used as appropriate. Even in patients who have received > 6000 rads to the jaw area, osteoradionecrosis is prevented in about 92%.

Treatment: If only a small patch of bone is exposed and x-ray reveals that radiation damage has not extended throughout the corpus of the mandible (a Stage I lesion), the patient is treated with HBO 30 times on a once-a-day basis while meticulous wound care is given. If the mucosa closes over the bone within 30 treatments, HBO is continued for 60 treatments total. Should the lesion not heal within 30 treatments, the lesion is classified as a Stage II and an alveolar sequestrectomy is performed with a watertight closure of the mucosa. Thirty more treatments are given.

X-ray evidence of total involvement of the mandible, an orocutaneous fistula, an extensive area of denuded bone, a pathologic fracture or dehiscence of a Stage II lesion is classified as a Stage III lesion. Thirty daily treatments are given, followed by resection of the mandible back to bleeding bone; the mandibular nerve is preserved and any orocutaneous fistulas are closed. Following operation, the position of the jaw is maintained with an external acrylic arch bar. Ten weeks later, 20 additional HBO treatments are given, followed by transcutaneous insertion of a bone graft, which is followed by at least 10 additional HBO treatments to assure take of the graft. About 94% of the cases will achieve freedom from pain, reestablishment of an intact mucosa, and normal shape and function with sufficient alveolar height to support dentures.

Chronic Refractory Osteomyelitis (see also Ch. 114)

When osteomyelitis does not resolve with surgery and antibiotics, there is often generalized host compromise due to another underlying disorder or local ischemic compromise of the wound. In the center of osteomyelitic wounds, P_{O_2} is often < 20 mm Hg, preventing leukocytes from killing bacteria, and fibroblast activity from producing collagen and scar formation. HBO treatment aims to produce O_2 levels in the infected area ≥ 30 mm Hg. Normally, only refractory osteomyelitis that fails to respond to surgery and antibiotics is considered for HBO therapy, but osteomyelitis of the skull or the sternum are exceptions. The skull because of the close proximity of the brain with the possible spread of the infection, and to avoid disfigurement if ablative surgery becomes necessary. With osteomyelitis of the sternum (a common complication of the sternum splitting approach used for cardiac surgery), HBO may be considered, if locally available, at the first indication of infection, as movement of the sternum caused by breathing can render irradication of persistent infections extremely difficult.

Treatment: HBO therapy is adjunctive to adequate saucerization, sequestrectomy, and IV antibiotic therapy. If the wound has been refractory for ≤ 2 yr, arrest of about 85% of the infections can be anticipated; later, the arrest rate may fall to 50%.

Treatment is given once a day and continued for 10 days after all drainage ceases and there is no further evidence of infection. After 30 treatments, if the wound continues to drain, it is wise to re-x-ray to see if a sequestrum has become evident. Occasionally, 40 to 60 treatments may be necessary.

Exceptional Blood Loss Anemia

In certain instances of blood loss (eg, in Jehovah's Witnesses who refuse blood products for religious reasons) and in cases of severe hemolysis or a rare blood type for which no adequate cross-match may be obtained, blood transfusions may not be possible. Patients with as little as 1 gm of Hb have been salvaged when HBO has been used. Enough O_2 can be physically dissolved in plasma at 3 ATA to support life, and there appears to be no inhibition of erythropoiesis when HBO is used intermittently. However, platelet loss is a major problem and continued bleeding is often difficult to control.

HBO may be required as often as every other hour with 1 h spent at pressures up to 2.5 ATA. More commonly, 1 or 2 h spent at 2 ATA suffices with a surface interval of from 2 to 6 h. Initial treatment frequencies are determined by signs of ischemia, eg, substernal pain or ischemic bowel. Later, the best indicator is the ECG; inverted T

waves indicate hypoxemia. Treatment is continued for up to 10 days with gradually lengthening intervals between treatments to bid or tid.

Actinomycosis

Most *Actinomycosis israeli* infections respond to surgery and antibiotics (see ACTINOMYCOSIS in Ch. 8). However, in rare refractory cases or where ablative surgery to irradicate the infection involves critical structures (eg, the middle ear) HBO may be indicated; O_2 has a direct effect on this organism. The patient is treated on a gas gangrene protocol (see Gas Gangrene, above).

268. LABORATORY MEDICINE

Introduction

Almost all known physical and chemical principles have been incorporated into instruments and systems to make clinical laboratory measurements. Among these are atomic absorption spectrophotometry; chromatography; colorimetry; potentiometry; coulometry; electrophoresis; flame photometry; fluorometry; immunodiffusion; isotopic technics; mass spectrometry; protein binding; immunoassays using radioisotopes, enzymes, or fluorescence to amplify readings; turbidimetry; nephelometry; osmometry; and ultracentrifugation.

The rates of speed with which measurements can be made and the variety of tests available vary considerably. The size of equipment varies, with the trend toward miniaturization. Current technology incorporates better quality control mechanisms, permitting operation by fewer and perhaps less highly trained people.

Laboratory utilization: A number of vectors affecting laboratory utilization are at play. In spite of significant efforts to curtail the utilization of medical resources, the overall number of laboratory tests has continued to climb, although at a slower rate, in response to their value as diagnostic tools and therapeutic monitors. In the USA, hospital admissions have declined, effecting a shift in testing to ambulatory patients. Broad survey studies on blood specimens are still found useful by practicing physicians as screening mechanisms, but the availability of instruments that permit random access and test selection make it possible to select more organ-specific panels to help detect abnormalities or state of health.

Economic considerations in response to mandates to curtail health care expenditures are becoming prominent. Capital and operating costs have come under careful scrutiny as cost efficiency is stressed. Clinical laboratories in hospitals, under prospective payment programs, are now considered cost centers rather than profit centers and must compete with commercial laboratories. All are offering more cost-effective services. Government regulations and third party payors (eg, insurance programs, industry) affect utilization, perhaps mostly by decreasing the number and length of stay of hospital admissions. Some offset occurs in the enhanced use of ambulatory services and the constant threat of lawsuits that encourage physicians to practice defensive medicine.

Miniaturization and simplification of technics and incentives to do more ambulatory procedures have made office and self-testing more attractive. The more commonly ordered tests (eg, glucose, urea nitrogen, potassium, hematocrit, urinalysis, and pregnancy tests) done in office settings provide rapid answers that may be used in the decision-making process while the patient is present. There also is an economic incentive for practitioners to do office testing under regulatory reimbursement schedules. Blood glucose is increasingly being self-determined from fingerprick specimens to set dosage in insulin-dependent diabetics. The availability of monoclonal antibodies for diagnostic purposes has made possible self-testing for pregnancy. Additional simple

tests will be available in the near future. More complex tests are still sent to clinical laboratories, many of which provide either pickup or mail service of specimens on a regional basis.

Interpretation of Tests

Standard methods of specimen collection, transportation, storage, and preparation are extremely important in assuring reliable results. The addition of appropriate anticoagulant, prevention of hemolysis, and timely separation of clot from serum are among the important considerations in specimen preparation.

Since the same test may be done by varying technics in different laboratories, it is necessary to know the normal ranges for each specific method and laboratory. The units may differ, giving divergent numerical values. The usually reported "normal range" encompasses the 95% confidence level for a *population* (± 2 standard deviations from the mean). Thus, 1:20 values may fall outside of the normal range, but still be normal for a specific patient; ie, a false positive result. Obviously, the more tests done on an individual the more likely such values will be obtained. Further study of these outlying tests can be anxiety-provoking and time- and resource-consuming with a very low yield of useful information.

Interpretation of results must not only be made in light of the total clinical picture, but also with knowledge of interfering substances that may occur either in vivo (eg, medications) or in vitro (eg, enzyme inhibitors or activators). To determine the usefulness of a test in the diagnosis of disease, 3 variables are important and must be considered: (1) its specificity (incidence of false positives), (2) sensitivity (incidence of false negatives), and (3) the disease prevalence in the population being tested.

Variations From normal-clinical conditions: TABLE 268–1 lists some of the more common tests ordered and the conditions in which variations from normal may occur. It is not meant to be all-inclusive. Many frequently used tests are described in THE MANUAL under the organ systems or diseases they are associated with.

TABLE 268–1. CONDITIONS IN WHICH VARIATIONS FROM SELECTED NORMAL CHEMISTRY VALUES MAY OCCUR

Analyte	*Increase*	*Decrease*
Alanine aminotransferase (ALT or SGPT)	Hepatitis, cirrhosis, liver metastases, obstructive jaundice, infectious mono, hepatic congestion	Pyridoxine (vitamin B_6) deficiency
Albumin	Dehydration, diabetes inspidus	Overhydration, malnutrition, malabsorption, nephrosis, hepatic failure, burns, multiple myeloma, metastatic carcinomas
Alkaline phosphatase	Bone Growth, bone metastases, Paget's disease, rickets, healing fracture, hyperparathyroidism, hepatic disease, obstructive jaundice, hepatic metastases, pulmonary infarction, heart failure, pregnancy	Pernicious anemia, hypoparathyroidism, hypophosphatasia
Aspartate aminotransferase (AST or SGOT)	Myocardial infarction, heart failure, myocarditis, pericarditis, myositis, muscular dystrophy, trauma, hepatic disease, pancreatitis, renal infarct, eclampsia, neoplasia, cerebral damage, seizures, hemolysis, alcohol	Pyridoxine (vitamin B_6) deficiency, terminal stages of liver disease

(Continued)

TABLE 268–1. CONDITIONS IN WHICH VARIATIONS FROM SELECTED NORMAL CHEMISTRY VALUES MAY OCCUR *(Cont'd)*

Analyte	*Increase*	*Decrease*
Bilirubin	Hepatic disease, obstructive jaundice, hemolytic anemia, pulmonary infarct, Gilbert's disease, Dubin-Johnson syndrome, neonatal jaundice	
Calcium	Hyperparathyroidism, bone metastases, myeloma, sarcoid, hyperthyroidism, hypervitaminosis D	Hypoparathyroidism, renal failure, malabsorption, pancreatitis, hypoalbuminemia, vitamin D deficiency, overhydration
Cholesterol	Hypothyroidism, obstructive jaundice, nephrosis, diabetes mellitus, familial, pancreatitis	Hyperthyroidism, infection, malnutrition, heart failure, malignancies
Creatinine	Renal failure, urinary obstruction, dehydration, hyperthyroidism	
Glucose	Diabetes mellitus, IV glucose, thiazides, corticosteroids, pheochromocytoma, hyperthyroidism, Cushing's syndrome, acromegaly, brain damage, hepatic disease, nephrosis	Excess insulin, insulinoma, Addison's disease, myxedema, hepatic failure, malabsorption
Lactate dehydrogenase (LDH)	Myocardial infarction, pulmonary infarction, hemolytic anemia, pernicious anemia, leukemia, lymphoma, malignancies, hepatic disease, renal infarction, seizures, cerebral damage, trauma, sprue	
Phosphorus	Renal failure, hypoparathyroidism, diabetic acidosis, acromegaly	Hyperparathyroidism, osteomalacia, rickets, Fanconi syndrome, cirrhosis, hypokalemia, excess IV glucose
Potassium	Hyperkalemic acidosis, cardiac arrhythmia, diabetic acidosis, hypoadrenalism, hereditary hyperkalemia	Cirrhosis, malnutrition, vomiting, metabolic alkalosis, diarrhea, nephrosis, diuretics, hyperadrenalism, familial periodic paralysis
Sodium	Dehydration, diabetes insipidus, excessive salt ingestion	Excess antidiuretic hormone, nephrosis, hypoadrenalism, myxedema, congestive heart failure, diarrhea, vomiting, diabetic acidosis, diuretics
Total protein	Multiple myeloma, myxedema, lupus, sarcoidosis, diabetes insipidus, dehydration, collagen disease	Burns, cirrhosis, malnutrition, nephrosis, malabsorption, overhydration
Triglyceride	Hereditary, nephrosis, cholestasis, pancreatitis, cirrhosis, diabetes mellitus, hepatitis, dietary	Malnutrition

(Continued)

TABLE 268–1. CONDITIONS IN WHICH VARIATIONS FROM SELECTED NORMAL CHEMISTRY VALUES MAY OCCUR *(Cont'd)*

Analyte	*Increase*	*Decrease*
Uric acid	Gout, renal failure, diuretic therapy, leukemia, lymphoma, polycythemia, acidosis, psoriasis, hypothyroidism, eclampsia, multiple myeloma, pernicious anemia, tissue necrosis, inflammation	Uricosuric drugs, allopurinol, Wilson's Disease, large doses of vitamin C
Urea nitrogen	Renal disease, dehydration, G.I. bleeding, leukemia, heart failure	Hepatic failure, overhydration, pregnancy

NORMAL VALUES

TABLE 268–2 lists reference values for selected clinical laboratory tests. Many important laboratory reference values (eg, steroid hormones, polypeptide hormones, thyroid hormones, vitamins, hematologic data [CBC, coagulation and platelet factors, hemoglobin], enzymes, and immunologic factors) are elsewhere in THE MANUAL—see the Index.

Note that SI units are given in addition to conventional units. These International System units have been used in the European literature for many years. An attempt is again underway for the American literature to do the same. Conversion factors can be worked out and are readily available. The benefits consist in scientific standardization in reporting and the use of molar concentration units of SI that are more meaningful because they represent relative combining power of chemical species.

TABLE 268–2. SELECTED CLINICAL LABORATORY TESTS—REFERENCE VALUES

Reference Values for Blood (B), Plasma (P), and Serum (S)

Test	*Normal Adult Range*	
	Conventional Units	*SI Units*
Acetoacetate plus acetone (B)	Negative	
Aldolase (S)	1.0–8.0 u./L	16.6–135 nkat/L*
Aminotransferase (S)		
Alanine (ALT, SGPT)	5–30 u./L	83–500 nkat/L*
Aspartate (AST, SGOT)	5–25 u./L	83–415 nkat/L*
Ammonia (B)	11–35 μmol/L	11–35 μmol/L
Amylase (S)	60–160 u./dL	111–296 u./L
Ascorbic acid (B)	0.4–1.5 mg/dL	23–85 μmol/L

(Continued)

* One katal **(kat, K)** is defined as the amount of enzyme that catalyzes a reaction rate of one mole per second in an assay system, regardless of reaction conditions (1 nanokat/L = 0.06 IU/L).

TABLE 268–2. SELECTED CLINICAL LABORATORY TESTS—REFERENCE VALUES *(Cont'd)*

Reference Values for Blood (B), Plasma (P), and Serum (S)

Test	Normal Adult Range	
	Conventional Units	*SI Units*
Bilirubin (S)		
Direct (Conjugated)	0.1–0.4 mg/dL	1.7–6.8 μmol/L
Total	0.3–1.1 mg/dL	5.1–19.0 μmol/L
Blood volume	8.5–9.0% of body weight (kg)	80–85mL/kg
Calcium (S)		
Ionized	2.1–2.6 mEq/L 4.25–5.25 mg/dL	1.05–1.30 mmol/L
Total	4.6-5.5 mEq/L 9.2–11.0 mg/dL	2.3–2.75 mmol/L
Carbamazepine (P)	3–12 μg/mL	12.75–51.0 μmol/L
CO_2 content (S)	24–30 mEq/L	24–30 mmol/L
CO (B)	<5% of total Hb	
Carotenoids (S)	0.5–3.0 μg/mL	0.9–5.6 μmol/L
Ceruloplasmin (S)	27–37 mg/dL	1.8–2.5 μmol/L
Chloride (S)	96–106 mEq/L	96–106 mmol/L
Cholesterol (S)	120–220 mg/dL	3.1–5.68 mmol/L
CK (S)		
Female	10–70 u./L	166–1167 nkat/L*
Male	25–90 u./L	416–1500 nkat/L*
CK isoenyzmes (S)	5% MB or less	
Copper (S)	70–155 μg/dL	11–24 μmol/L
Creatinine (S)	<1.5 mg/dL	<133 μmol/L
Digoxin (S)		
Therapeutic	0.8–2.0 ng/mL	1.0–2.6 nmol/L
Toxic	>2.5 ng/mL	>3.2 nmol/L
Ethanol (B)	Negative	
Glucose, fasting (P)	75–105 mg/dL	4.2–5.8 mmol/L
Iron (S)		
Total	50–150 μg/dL	9–27 μmol/L
Binding capacity	250–410 μg/dL	45–73 μmol/L
Lactate (B)		
Venous	4.5–20 mg/dL	0.5–2.2 mmol/L
Arterial	4.5–14.4 mg/dL	0.5–1.6 mmol/L
Lactic dehydrogenase (S)	50–115 u./L	833–1917 nkat/L*
Lead (B)	0–50 μg/dL	0–2.4 μmol/L
Lipase (S)	0–1.5 u. (Cherry-Crandall)	0–1.5 u. (Cherry-Crandall)
Lithium (S)		
Therapeutic	0.5–1.4 mEq/L	0.5–1.4 mmol/L
Toxic	2.0 mEq/L	>2.0 mmol/L
Magnesium (S)	1.3–2.1 mEq/L 1.8–3.0 mg/dL	0.7–1.1 mmol/L
5′-Nucleotidase (S)	1–12 u./L	16.6–200 nkat/L*
Osmolality (S)	280–295 mOsm/kg serum water	280–295 mmol/kg serum water
Oxygen saturation (B)		
Arterial	96–100%	0.96–1.00

(Continued)

TABLE 268–2. SELECTED CLINICAL LABORATORY TESTS—REFERENCE VALUES *(Cont'd)*

Reference Values for Blood (B), Plasma (P), and Serum (S)

Test	Normal Adult Range	
	Conventional Units	*SI Units*
P_{CO_2} (B)	35–45 mm Hg	4.7–6.0 kPa
pH (B)	7.35–7.45	7.35–7.45
P_{O_2} (B)	75–100 mm Hg	10.0–13.3 kPa
Phenobarbital (S)		
Therapeutic	15–50 μg/mL	65–215 μmol/L
Toxic	>50 μg/mL	>215 μmol/L
Phenytoin (S)		
Therapeutic	5–20 μg/mL	20–79 μmol/L
Toxic	>20 μg/mL	>79 μmol/L
Phosphatase, acid (S)	0.2–1.8 IU/L	3.3–30 nkat/L*
Phosphatase, alkaline (S)	23–71 IU/L	383–1185 nkat/L*
Phosphorus, inorganic (S)	3–4.5 mg/dL 1–1.5 mEq/L	1.0–1.5 mmol/L
Potassium (S)	3.5–5.0 mEq/L	3.5–5.0 mmol/L
Primidone (S)		
Therapeutic	5–12 μg/mL	23–55 μmol/L
Toxic	>15 μg/mL	>69 μmol/L
Procainamide (S)		
Therapeutic	4–10 μg/mL	17–42 μmol/L
Toxic	>16 μg/mL	>68 μmol/L
Protein (S)		
Total	6.0–8.0 gm/dL	60–80 gm/L
Albumin	3.5–5.5 gm/dL	35–55 gm/L
Globulin	2.0–3.5 gm/dL	20–35 gm/L
Electrophoresis		
Globulin		
α_1	0.1–0.4 gm/dL	1–4 gm/L
α_2	0.4–1.1 gm/dL	4–11 gm/L
β	0.5–1.6 gm/dL	5–16 gm/L
γ	0.5–1.4 gm/dL	5–14 gm/L
Pyruvic acid (B)	0.3–0.9 mg/dL	0.03–0.10 mmol/L
Quinidine (S)		
Therapeutic	1.2–4.0 μg/mL	3.7–12.3 μmol/L
Toxic	>10 μg/mL	>30 μmol/L
Salicylate (P)		
Analgesic	20–100 μg/mL	145–724 μmol/L
Anti-inflammatory	150–300 μg/mL	1086–2172 μmol/L
Toxic	>300 μg/mL	>2172 μmol/L
Sodium (S)	135–145 mEq/L	135–145 mmol/L
Sulfate (S)	2.9–3.5 mg/dL	0.3–0.36 μmol/L
Triglycerides (S)	35–160 mg/dL	0.40–1.81 mmol/L
Urea nitrogen (S)	8–23 mg/dL	2.9–8.2 mmol/L
Uric acid (S)	3–7 mg/dL	0.18–0.42 mmol/L
Vitamin A (S)	20–60 μg/dL	0.7–2.1 μmol/L
Vitamin D derivatives (S)		
1,25-dihydroxy	20–45 pg/mL	48–108 pmol/L
25-hydroxy	25–40 ng/mL	62.5–100 nmol/L

(Continued)

Reference Values for Urine

Test	*Normal Adult Range*	
	Conventional Units	*SI Units*
Acetone plus acetoacetate	Negative	
Amylase	1–17 u./h	1–17 u./h
Calcium	<300 mg./day	<7.5 mmol/day
Catecholamines		
Epinephrine	<10 µg/day	<55 nmol/day
Norepinephrine	<100 µg/day	<590 nmol/day
Chorionic gonadotropin	Negative	
Copper	0–50 µg/day	0–0.8 µmol/day
Coproporphyrin	30–250 µg/day	46–380 nmol/day
Creatine		
Females	<100 mg/day	<0.76 mmol/day
Males	<40 mg/day	<0.30 mmol/day
Creatinine	14–26 mg/kg/day	0.12–0.23 mmol/kg/day
Cystine or cysteine	Negative	
Hemoglobin and myoglobin	Negative	
17-Hydroxycorticosteroids	2–9 mg/day	5.5–25 µmol/day
5-Hydroxyindoleacetic acid	2–9 mg/day	10–47 µmol/day
17-Ketosteroids	4–18 mg/day	14–62 µmol/day
Lead	<0.08 µg/mL or <120 µg/day	<0.39 µmol/L
Phosphorus, inorganic	0.4–1.3 gm/day	13–42 mmol/day
Porphobilinogen	Negative	
Protein	<150 mg/day	<150 mg/day
Sugar, quantitative glucose	Negative	
Urobilinogen	0.1-0.8 EU/2h 0.5–4.0 EU/day	0.1–0.8 EU/2h 0.5–4.0 EU/day
Uroporphyrin	<50 µg/day	<60 nmol/day
Vanillylmandelic acid (VMA)	1–9 mg/day	5–45 µmol/day

269. READY REFERENCE GUIDES

CALCULATION OF DOSAGES FOR INFANTS AND CHILDREN

(See also Ch. 184)

Drug dosages for children can be calculated by using Young's, Cowling's, or Clark's rules. To use **Young's rule,** the child's age should be divided by the age plus 12; the result is the fraction of the adult dose recommended for the child. (For example, a child aged 3 yr will require $\frac{3}{3 + 12} = 1/5$ of the adult dose.) **Cowling's rule** divides the age at the next birthday by 24. (Thus, for a child aged 5 yr, the dose is 6/24 or 1/4 of the adult dose.) **Clark's rule** divides the weight (in lb) by 150 to give the appropriate fraction of the adult dose.

(Thus, for a 50-lb child, the dose is $\frac{50}{150}$ or 1/3 of the adult dose.)

Body surface area (BSA) can also be used to calculate pediatric drug dosages or fluid and electrolyte requirements. A nomogram for estimating the BSA is given in Fig. 185–1. The dosage is determined as follows:

$$\frac{\text{BSA (sq m)}}{1.7} \times \text{Adult Dose} = \text{Approximate Dose}$$

It should be emphasized that these calculations give only approximate values, that individual requirements vary widely, and that young children may be unduly susceptible to certain drugs (eg, opioids) or relatively insusceptible to others (eg, belladonna). Individual drug characteristics and idiosyncrasies make it prudent to review the manufacturer's instructions on the drug package insert.

WEIGHTS, MEASURES, AND EQUIVALENTS

TABLE 269–1. METRIC SYSTEM

Weight:		
1 kilogram (kg)	=	1000 grams (10^3 gm)
1 gram (g, gm)	=	1000 milligrams (10^3 mg)
1 milligram (mg)	=	1000 micrograms (10^{-3} gm)
1 microgram (μg, mcg)	=	1000 millimicrograms (10^{-6} gm)
	=	1000 nanograms (ng) (10^{-6} gm)
1 millimicrogram (mμg)	=	1000 micromicrograms (μμg) (10^{-9} gm)
	=	1000 picograms (pg) (10^{-9} gm)
Volume:		
1 liter (L)	=	1000 milliliters (mL)
	=	1000 cubic centimeters (cc)

TABLE 269–2. EQUIVALENTS
(all approximate)

Liquid:			
Metric		*Apothecaries'*	
30 mL	=	1 fluid ounce	
250 mL	=	8+ fluid ounces	
500 mL	=	1+ pint	
1000 mL (1 liter)	=	1+ quart	

Weight:				
65	mg	=	1	grain (gr)
28.35	gm	=	1	ounce (oz)
1	kg	=	2.2	pounds (lb)

Linear:				
1	millimeter (mm)	=	0.04	inch (in.)
1	centimeter (cm)	=	0.4	inch
2.5	centimeters	=	1	inch
1	meter (m)	=	39.37	inches

TABLE 269–3. HOUSEHOLD MEASURES
(with approximate equivalents)

1 teaspoon (tsp)	=	4 mL		
1 teaspoon, medical	=	5 mL		
1 dessert spoon	=	8 mL		
1 tablespoon (tbsp)	=	15 mL	=	1/2 fluid ounce
1 teacup	=	120 mL	=	4 fluid ounces

TABLE 269–4. ATOMIC WEIGHTS (APPROXIMATE) OF SOME COMMON ELEMENTS

Hydrogen (H)	= 1	Magnesium (Mg)	= 24
Carbon (C)	= 12	Phosphorus (P)	= 31
Nitrogen (N)	= 14	Chlorine (Cl)	= 35.5
Oxygen (O)	= 16	Potassium (K)	= 39
Sodium (Na)	= 23	Calcium (Ca)	= 40

MILLIGRAM-MILLIEQUIVALENT CONVERSIONS

The unit of measure of electrolytes is the milliequivalent (mEq), which expresses the chemical activity, or combining power, of a substance relative to the activity of 1 mg of hydrogen. Thus, 1 mEq is represented by 1 mg of hydrogen, 23 mg of sodium, 39 mg of potassium, 20 mg of calcium, and 35 mg of chlorine. Conversion equations are as follows:

$$\text{mEq/L} = \frac{(\text{mg/L}) \times \text{Valence}}{\text{Formula Wt}}$$

$$\text{mg/L} = \frac{(\text{mEq/L}) \times \text{Formula Wt}}{\text{Valence}}$$

(NOTE: Formula Wt = Atomic or Molecular Wt)

Milliosmol

The mEq is roughly equivalent to the milliosmol (mOsm), the unit of measure of osmolality or tonicity. Normally, the body fluid compartments each contain about 280 mOsm of solute/L.

TABLE 269–5. CENTIGRADE–FAHRENHEIT EQUIVALENTS

Centigrade°	*Fahrenheit°*	*Centigrade°*	*Fahrenheit°*
Freezing (water at sea level):		Pasteurization (holding), 30 min at:	
0	32	61.6	143.0
Clinical range:		Pasteurization (flash), 15 sec at:	
36.0	96.8	71.1	160.0
36.5	97.7	Boiling (water at sea level):	
37.0	98.6		
37.5	99.5	100.0	212.0
38.0	100.4		
38.5	101.3	Conversion	
39.0	102.2	To convert degrees F to degrees C, subtract 32, then multiply by 5/9 or 0.555	
39.5	103.1		
40.0	104.0		
40.5	104.9	To convert degrees C to degrees F, multiply by 9/5 or 1.8, then add 32	
41.0	105.8		
41.5	106.7		
42.0	107.6		

§23. CLINICAL PHARMACOLOGY

270. DRUG ABSORPTION AND BIOAVAILABILITY

Absorption: *The process of drug movement from the site of application toward the systemic circulation.*

Bioavailability: *The rate at which and the extent to which the active moiety (drug or metabolite) enters the general circulation, thereby permitting access to the site of action.*

Drug product: *The actual dosage form of a drug, consisting of the drug itself plus other ingredients formulated into a usable medicine; eg, as a tablet, capsule, or solution.*

In the present context, absorption describes drug movement, while bioavailability refers to a specific net result. Whereas the physicochemical properties of a drug govern its absorptive potential, the properties of the dosage form, or both, can be major determinants of its bioavailability. Hence, the concept of equivalence among drug products is important in clinical decisions. However, there is often confusion about different types of equivalence. **Chemical (pharmaceutical) equivalence** refers to *drug products that contain the same compound in the same amount in two or more dosage forms and meet present official standards*; however, inactive ingredients in the drug products may differ. **Bioequivalence** refers to *chemical equivalents that, when administered to the same individual in the same dosage regimen, result in equivalent concentrations of drug in blood and tissues.* **Therapeutic equivalence** refers to *two drug products that, when administered to the same individual in the same dosage regimen, provide essentially the same therapeutic effect or toxicity; they may or may not be bioequivalent.*

DRUG ABSORPTION

Drug products are formulated for administration by a variety of routes, including oral, buccal, sublingual, rectal, parenteral, topical, and inhalation. The physicochemical properties of drugs, their formulations, and the routes of administration are important in absorption. A prerequisite to absorption of any drug is that it be able to enter into a solution. The solid drug product (eg, tablet) must undergo disintegration and deaggregation, and the active ingredients must undergo dissolution before the drug can be absorbed.

Except when a drug is given IV, it must traverse several semipermeable cell membranes before it reaches the general circulation. These membranes act as biologic barriers that selectively permit the passage of certain solutes or drug molecules and are

remarkably similar in chemical composition and spatial arrangement throughout the body. Cell membranes are composed primarily of a bimolecular lipid matrix, containing mostly cholesterol and phospholipids, in which are embedded globular protein macromolecules of random size and composition. The membrane proteins may be involved in transport processes and may also function as receptors for cellular regulatory mechanisms. Membrane lipid confers both hydrophilic and hydrophobic properties, providing stability to the membrane and determining its permeability characteristics. Drugs are transported across this biologic barrier primarily by passive diffusion; however, facilitated diffusion, active transport, and pinocytosis may play a minor role.

Passive diffusion: *Transport across the cell membrane in which the driving force for movement is the concentration gradient of the solute.* Most drug molecules are transported across a membrane by simple diffusion from a high concentration area (eg, GI fluids) to a low concentration area (eg, blood) without expenditure of energy by the biologic system. Diffusion rate is directly proportional to this gradient and depends upon lipid solubility, degree of ionization, molecular size, and the area of the absorptive surface. Since the drug is transported away by the systemic circulation and distributed into a large volume, the concentration of drug in the blood is initially low compared to that at the site of administration, and the large concentration gradient serves as the driving force for absorption. However, since the cell membrane is lipoid in nature, drugs that are highly lipid-soluble diffuse more rapidly than drugs that are relatively lipid-insoluble. Small molecules tend to penetrate membranes more rapidly than do large molecules.

Most drugs exist as weak organic acids or bases in both undissociated and dissociated form in an aqueous environment. The undissociated or nonionized fraction is usually lipid-soluble and diffuses readily across the cell membrane. The dissociated or ionized form cannot penetrate the cell membrane easily because of its low lipid solubility. The importance of lipid solubility in transport can be illustrated by the absorption of three barbiturates as shown in TABLE 270–1. At pH 1, all are essentially nonionized, yet absorption rates vary because of their different lipid solubilities. The charged groups on the protein surfaces of the cell membrane may also impede passage of the ionized fraction. Thus, the combination of low lipid solubility and greater electrical resistance make penetration of the ionized form so slow that the penetration rate may be attributed mainly to the undissociated fraction.

The distribution of a weak electrolyte across a membrane will be determined by its pK_a and the pH gradient. If a pH gradient exists, the extent of ionization of a weak electrolyte on the two sides of a membrane will differ—for a weak acid, the higher the

TABLE 270–1. INFLUENCE OF LIPID SOLUBILITY ON RATE OF ABSORPTION

Barbiturate	*pK_a*	*Partition Coefficient* $CHCl_3/H_2O$	*% Absorbed from Stomach in 1 h at pH 1*
Barbital	7.8	1	4
Secobarbital	7.8	52	30
Thiopental	7.6	580	46

(Modified from L. S. Schanker et al: "Absorption of Drugs from the Stomach; I. The Rat," *Journal of Pharmacology and Experimental Therapeutics* Vol. 120, pp. 528–539, 1957. Copyright 1957 by The Williams and Wilkins Co., Baltimore. Used with permission of The Williams and Wilkins Co. and the author.)

pH, the lower the ratio of nonionized to ionized fractions. Consider the partitioning of a weak acid (eg, pK_a 4.4) between plasma and gastric juice. In plasma (pH 7.4) the ratio of nonionized to ionized forms is 1:1000; in gastric juice (pH 1.4) the ratio is reversed, ie, 1000:1. When the weak acid is given orally, a large concentration gradient is established between the stomach and the plasma, a condition favorable to diffusion through the gastric mucosa. At equilibrium, the concentration of nonionized drug will be equal in the stomach and in the plasma because it is the only moiety that can penetrate membranes. However, the concentration of ionized fraction in the plasma will be approximately 1000 times greater than that in the gastric lumen. For a weak base with a pK_a of 4.4, the situation is reversed. Thus, weakly acidic drugs (eg, aspirin) theoretically should be more readily absorbed from an acid medium (gastric lumen) than weak bases (eg, quinidine). However, regardless of pH, most drug absorption occurs in the small intestine because of its large surface area.

Facilitated diffusion: For certain molecules driven across the cell membrane by the concentration gradient, the rate of penetration is greater than would be expected on the basis of their low lipid solubility (eg, glucose). It is postulated that a "carrier component" combines reversibly with the substrate molecule at the cell membrane exterior and that the carrier-substrate complex diffuses rapidly across the membrane with release of the substrate at the interior surface. This carrier-mediated diffusion process is characterized by **selectivity** and **saturability.** The carrier mechanism accepts for transport only those substrates having a relatively specific molecular configuration and the process is further determined by the availability of carrier. No expenditure of energy is required by this process; substrate is not transported against a concentration gradient.

Active transport: In addition to the same selectivity and saturability described for facilitated diffusion, active transport *requires energy expenditure by the cell, and substrates may be accumulated intracellularly against a concentration gradient.* Active transport processes appear to be limited to agents with close structural similarities to normal body constituents. These agents are usually absorbed from specific sites in the small intestine. Active transport processes have been identified for various ions, vitamins, sugars, and amino acids.

Pinocytosis refers to *the engulfing of particles or fluid by a cell.* The cell membrane invaginates, encloses the particle or solute, and then fuses again, forming a vesicle which later buds off within the interior of the cell. This mechanism also requires the expenditure of energy. Pinocytosis probably plays a minor role in drug transport.

Absorption of Oral Solutions

The GI mucosa acts as a semipermeable barrier. Oral solutions may be absorbed along the entire alimentary canal and must pass through various fluids and tissues and survive encounters with several enzyme systems. The epithelial lining, its organization, and physiologic factors affecting acid secretion, stomach emptying, intestinal transit, and bile and mucus flow can affect drug absorption and bioavailability. Thus some segments favor the absorption process. The **oral mucosa** has a thin epithelium and a rich vascularity that favors drug absorption, but solutions are in contact too briefly for any appreciable absorption.

The **stomach** has a rich blood supply and a large epithelial surface, but the rate at which it empties determines how long a substance remains in the stomach and is influenced by many factors. For some drugs, physiologic processes that delay gastric emptying increase the degradation of the drug in the stomach and profoundly decrease systemic absorption. Penicillin G is an example of a drug that is acid-labile. The acidic environment of the stomach favors the absorption of weak acids that are largely lipid-soluble and nonionized. Under normal conditions, absorption from the stomach is highly variable and minor compared to absorption from the small intestine.

The **small intestine** presents the largest GI surface area for absorption; however, its environment varies. In the duodenum the pH is 4 to 5, but the intraluminal pH becomes progressively more alkaline farther along the alimentary canal (eg, the pH of the lower ileum is about 8). The GI flora may inactivate certain drugs, reducing their absorption and bioavailability. Compared to passage through the stomach, drug transit through the small intestine is usually slow, but other factors, including blood flow, metabolism in the intestinal wall, and permeability characteristics, influence the passage of intact drug across the intestinal mucosa. Decreased blood flow (eg, in shock) may lower the concentration gradient across the intestinal mucosa and decrease absorption by passive diffusion. (Decreased peripheral blood flow also alters drug distribution and metabolism.)

Certain physiologic factors and diseases can influence bioavailability after a drug has penetrated the intestinal wall but before it has reached the systemic circulation. For certain drugs (eg, propranolol) only a fraction of the drug absorbed from the intestine reaches the systemic circulation because of first-pass hepatic metabolism. Such metabolism can also occur during passage through the gut wall during absorption. Individual variations in age, sex, activity, genetic phenotype, stress, disease (eg, achlorhydria, malabsorption syndromes), and previous GI surgery can alter or impair drug bioavailability.

In contrast to the small intestine, the **large intestine** has no villi and its main function is not one of absorption. Nevertheless, molecules that escape absorption in the small intestine may be absorbed, albeit less efficiently, in the colon.

Absorption of Solid Dosage Forms

Most drugs administered orally are in the form of tablets or capsules primarily for convenience, economy, stability, and patient acceptance. They must disintegrate and dissolve before absorption can occur. **Disintegration** greatly increases the surface area of the drug, brings it into contact with the GI fluids, and promotes dissolution. Disintegrants and other excipients (eg, diluents, lubricants, surfactants, binders, and dispersants) are often added during manufacturing to facilitate these processes. Factors capable of causing variable or retarded disintegration of solid drug products include excessive pressure applied during the tableting procedure and special coatings applied to protect the tablet from the digestive processes of the gut. Hydrophobic lubricants (eg, magnesium stearate) may bind to the active drug and reduce its bioavailablility. Surfactants may influence the wettability, solubility, and dispersibility of the active drug and thereby alter its dissolution rate.

The **dissolution rate** determines the availability of the drug for absorption. When slower than the absorption rate, dissolution will be the rate-limiting step and can be altered by manipulating the drug or the dosage formulation. Some factors that may alter the dissolution rate are salt form, particle size, crystal form, and hydrates. For example, the Na salts of weak acids (eg, barbiturates and salicylates) dissolve faster than their corresponding free acids regardless of the pH of the medium. Reduction of particle size is frequently used to increase the surface area of a drug and is effective in increasing the rate and extent of GI absorption of a drug that is rate-limited by slow dissolution. Certain drugs exhibit polymorphism, existing in amorphous or various crystalline forms. Chloramphenicol palmitate exists as 2 polymorphs, A and B, but only the latter has sufficient dissolution, absorption, and bioavailability to be of clinical value. A hydrate is formed when one or more water molecules combine with a drug molecule in crystal formation. The solubility of such a solvate may be markedly different from the nonsolvate form of a drug. For example, anhydrous ampicillin has a greater rate of dissolution and in vivo absorption than its corresponding trihydrate.

The presence of food in the stomach can delay its emptying and the entry of drug particles into the intestine. Giving drugs with food may reduce bioavailability (eg,

increased degradation of penicillin by stomach acid), enhance absorption (eg, the poorly soluble drug griseofulvin given after a high fat meal), or have little or no effect.

Absorption from Parenteral Sites

Direct placement of a drug into the bloodstream (usually IV) ensures bioavailability of all the drug administered. However, administration by a route that requires drug transfer through one or more biologic membranes to reach the bloodstream precludes a guarantee that all of the drug will eventually be absorbed. IM or subcutaneous injection of drugs bypasses the skin barrier, but the drug must penetrate into the capillaries. The rate of entry into capillaries is usually determined for lipid-soluble drugs by their oil/water partition coefficients and for lipid-insoluble drugs by their molecular size. The rate of capillary blood flow is also a major factor in the rate of absorption. Thus, the injection site and the blood flow to it can markedly influence a drug's absorption rate. For example, the absorption rate of diazepam injected IM into a site with poor blood flow can be much slower than that following an oral dose.

Absorption may be delayed or erratic when salts of poorly soluble acids and bases are injected IM. For example, the parenteral form of phenytoin is the Na salt, which has a pH of about 12. When it is injected IM, tissue fluids act as buffers and the pH decreases, causing a shift in the equilibrium between the ionized and free acid form of the drug, forming more of the poorly soluble free acid, which precipitates and is absorbed very slowly.

Absorption via the lymphatic system contributes little to the total absorption of drug molecules because the flow of lymph is slow compared to that of blood. However, lymphatic absorption may be significant in the case of larger molecules (eg, insulin) or highly lipid-soluble drugs.

Prolonged-Release Dosage Forms

Prolonged- (controlled-) release dosage forms are designed to reduce the frequency of dosing and to maintain more uniform plasma drug concentrations, thus providing a more uniform pharmacologic effect. Additionally, greater patient convenience may improve compliance with the therapeutic regimen. Ideally, suitable drugs for such dosage forms are those that require frequent dosing because of a short biologic half-life and a short duration of effect. Drugs with a narrow therapeutic index (eg, anticoagulants) usually are not suitable candidates because of the larger doses required and variable absorption may lead to poor control of therapy or unwanted side effects.

Oral prolonged-release dosage forms are often designed to maintain therapeutic concentrations of drug for up to 12 h. They generally release a normal therapeutic dose of drug initially, and subsequently release sustaining amounts more slowly. Reduction of the absorption rate can be achieved in various ways: by coating the drug particles with wax or related water-insoluble material, by embedding the drug in a matrix from which it is released slowly during transit through the GI tract, or by complexing the drug with ion-exchange resins.

Topical prolonged-release dosage forms have been designed to provide drug release for extended periods. For example, nitroglycerin-impregnated polymer bonded to an adhesive bandage provides controlled drug delivery over a period of 24 h. Drugs for transdermal delivery must have suitable skin penetration characteristics and high potency.

Many nonintravenous parenteral preparations have been formulated to provide sustained blood levels. In some cases, insoluble salts (eg, fluphenazine enanthate) injected IM may provide activity for several weeks or a month. For other drugs, suspensions or solutions in nonaqueous vehicles are formulated; eg, insulin may be injected in crystalline suspensions for prolonged action. Amorphous insulin, with a high surface area for dissolution, has an intermediate onset and duration. The procaine salt of penicillin is poorly soluble and slowly absorbed when injected IM.

BIOAVAILABILITY OF DRUGS

The concept of bioavailability relates to the efficiency of the dosage formulation as an extravascular drug delivery system and permits comparison of drug products for relative availability or bioequivalence. It includes consideration of both the amount and rate of absorption into the systemic circulation following extravascular administration. Bioavailability depends upon a number of factors, including how a drug product is designed and manufactured, its physicochemical properties, and other factors that relate to the patient or the disease.

Absorption of a drug may be incomplete due to its physicochemical properties (eg, solubility), its pharmaceutical formulation (see DRUG ABSORPTION, above), the presence of food or other drugs in the GI tract, gastric emptying and intestinal transit times, pH of the GI tract, metabolizing bacteria in the gut, biliary flow, and GI disease. Although a drug may be absorbed completely, its rate of absorption may also be important. It may be too slow to maintain a therapeutic blood level or be too rapid, resulting in toxicity from high drug levels. The amount of drug reaching the systemic circulation from the GI tract is affected by first-pass hepatic metabolism and by the metabolism during passage through the intestinal wall.

Bioavailability is considered most commonly in orally administered drugs and is determined either by measuring the concentration of drug in body fluids or by the magnitude of the pharmacologic or therapeutic response produced.

Differences in the bioavailability of various pharmaceutical formulations of a given drug have clinical significance, since bioequivalence of therapeutic or toxic effects depends upon plasma drug levels. Differences in bioavailability between individuals and even in the same individual at different times make its determination difficult to assess. Such assessment is further complicated because bioavailability of a preparation in man does not always correlate with laboratory tests (eg, tablet dissolution rate) or with studies in animals.

Poor bioavailability is most commonly seen with oral dosage forms of poorly water soluble, slowly absorbed drugs. Slow or incomplete absorption may give capricious results, since more factors affect bioavailability in this situation than when drugs are rapidly and completely absorbed. Problems are encountered most frequently during long-term therapy when the patient who is stabilized on one pharmaceutical formulation receives a nonequivalent substitute. Clinically important examples of ineffective therapy or toxicity have been noted for digoxin and phenytoin, as well as other drugs.

Sometimes therapeutic equivalence may be achieved despite differences in bioavailability. For example, the margin between an effective concentration of penicillin and its toxic level is so wide that the prescribed dosage usually achieves a blood concentration far above the minimum effective level. Moderate blood concentration differences due to bioavailability differences in penicillin products might therefore not affect therapeutic effect or safety. In contrast, bioavailability differences would be important for a drug with a relatively narrow range between therapeutic and toxic levels.

Qualitative analysis of the serum concentration-time curve allows assessment of bioavailability, which usually involves three parameters: the maximum (or peak) serum drug concentration, the time of occurrence of maximum serum drug concentration, and the area under the serum concentration-time curve (FIG. 270–1). The serum drug concentration increases with the rate and extent of absorption; the peak is reached when the rate of drug removal equals the rate of absorption.

Bioavailability determinations based on maximum serum concentration alone can be misleading, since drug removal begins immediately upon entry into the bloodstream. The peak serum concentration time is related to the absorption rate and is the most widely used index of this parameter, but absorption is not complete when the serum concentration has peaked, except in the case of a rapid IV injection.

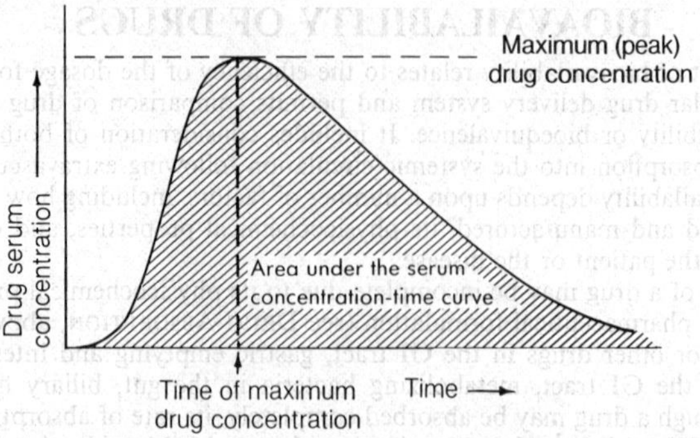

FIG. 270–1. Representation of serum concentration-time relationship after a single dose of a hypothetical drug.

The **area under the concentration curve (AUC)** is the most important measurement of bioavailability based on serum concentration determinations. It is directly proportional to the total amount of unchanged drug in the body. To describe the serum concentration curve accurately it is necessary to sample blood at frequent intervals; the extent of absorption is determined by taking samples for a sufficient time. Drug products may be considered bioequivalent if their serum level curves are essentially superimposable. Two drug products which have similar AUC's but different shapes of serum level-time profiles are equivalent in *extent* of availability but are absorbed at different *rates*.

Multiple dosing also permits evaluation of bioavailability, and this procedure has several advantages. In some cases, it more closely represents the usual clinical situation (eg, use of most antibiotics). Higher serum levels are usually achieved than following a single dose that facilitates drug analyses. After 5 to 10 consecutive doses of a drug are administered at an equal dosing interval, the blood concentration should reach an approximate steady state, provided the dosing interval is about equal to the elimination half-life of the drug. The extent of absorption can be analyzed by measuring the AUC during one dosing interval after reaching the steady-state.

For drugs that are primarily excreted unchanged in the urine, availability may be estimated by measuring the total amount of drug excreted. Ideally, urine collection should be made over a period of 7 to 10 elimination half-lives for complete recovery of the drug and to evaluate the extent of absorption. Comprehensive bioavailability studies utilize both serum and urinary excretion data.

271. DRUG DISTRIBUTION

After a drug enters the general circulation, it distributes throughout the body and partitions in various tissues. Distribution through various fluid compartments and tissues is generally unequal and is affected by the extent of protein binding, regional variations in pH, and the permeability of various membranes.

The rate of entry of a drug into a tissue depends upon the rate of blood flow to the tissue, the tissue mass, and the partition characteristics of the drug between blood and tissue. Richly vascular areas achieve equilibrium more rapidly than poorly perfused areas, if the drug readily crosses the vascular membrane barriers. After **distribution equilibrium** is attained, the concentrations of drug in tissues and extracellular fluids reflect changes in the plasma concentration. Metabolism and excretion occur simulta-

neously with distribution, making the process dynamic and complex. The means for measuring the rate and extent of drug distribution are described in Ch. 272, while factors affecting drug distribution are discussed below.

Magnitude of Distribution

If one assumes that the body acts as a single fluid compartment, the amount of fluid into which a drug appears to be distributed is called the **apparent volume of distribution** (see Ch. 272). Every drug is distributed in the body in a characteristic manner. It is useful and customary to describe the extent of distribution in terms of the water content of compartments that are anatomically and functionally distinct. For instance, a drug whose volume of distribution is approximately 3 L can be conceptualized as being contained almost completely within the plasma water. A volume of distribution of 12 L corresponds to that of extravascular interstitial fluid plus plasma water, and about 40 L is equal to the total water content of the body. To assume that a drug is contained within a particular compartment is an oversimplification; however, it does allow some valid generalizations about the extent of drug distribution. *The greater the volume of distribution of a drug, the smaller the fraction likely to reach the receptor site to produce the desired pharmacologic effect.*

Most drugs have a volume of distribution of < 500 L/70 kg; some typical values are shown in TABLE 271–1. Many acids (eg, warfarin and salicylic acid derivatives) are highly protein bound and too water soluble to enter the cellular water, and thus have a low volume of distribution. Many bases (eg, amphetamine and meperidine) are avidly taken up by the tissues and thus have a very large volume of distribution, which can be larger than the volume of the entire body. This paradox is the result of the mathematical method for calculating the "apparent" volume of distribution.

Drug Reservoirs

Drugs can accumulate in various tissues or body compartments and serve as drug depots in equilibrium with the drug in plasma. As the plasma level declines, stored drug is released into the circulation prolonging the drug action. The anesthetic thiopental is an example of a drug in which storage in tissue reservoirs prolongs drug action. It is highly lipid-soluble and rapidly distributed to the brain following a single-dose IV injection. Once plasma levels start declining, the concentration of drug in the brain follows that in plasma and the termination of anesthesia ends rapidly as the drug distributes in the body to a larger fraction of the body in a second phase. Thus, following a single dose, anesthesia is terminated rapidly because of a redistribution of

TABLE 271–1. SOME EXAMPLES OF THE VOLUME OF DISTRIBUTION

Drug	*Liters/70 kg*
Warfarin	8
Acetylsalicylic acid	12
Gentamicin	18
Theophylline	35
Phenytoin	45
Acetaminophen	66
Lidocaine	77
Procainamide	133
Quinidine	189
Propranolol	273
Amitriptyline	581

the drug. However, if drug levels are followed long enough, a third phase of distribution can be distinguished, which represents slow uptake of drug by fat. With continued administration of thiopental, large amounts can accumulate and be stored in fatty tissue; these tissues can act as a reservoir for thiopental and prolong its anesthetic action.

Protein binding: Drugs are transported in the bloodstream partly in solution (as free drug) and partly bound to various blood components (eg, plasma protein). The major determinant of the ratio of bound to free drug is the reversible interaction between a drug molecule and a molecule of protein, an interaction governed by the Law of Mass Action. Although many plasma proteins can interact with drugs, albumin is the most important and can interact with anions or cations. The extent to which a drug binds with an albumin molecule depends upon the molecular structure of the drug. Acidic drugs are generally bound more extensively than basic drugs. TABLE 271–2 gives some values for drug binding to serum albumin.

The α- and β-lipoproteins of the plasma are an important group of proteins with a high binding affinity, but a relatively low binding capacity, for many endogenous (eg, corticosteroids) and foreign compounds. Plasma γ-globulins do not interact significantly with drugs except where they occur as specific antibodies to protein hormones (eg, insulin). Such antibodies may lessen the hormone's therapeutic effects.

Since only unbound drug is available for passive diffusion to the extravascular or tissue sites where pharmacologic effects occur, plasma protein binding influences the distribution and pharmacologic activity of drugs. As free drug leaves the circulation, the remaining protein-drug complex begins to dissociate, releasing more free drug for diffusion. Some highly protein-bound drugs (eg, sulfonamides) may be confined largely to the plasma compartment, serving as depots and releasing more drug as it is removed from the circulation by metabolism and excretion. As the dose of a drug increases, the available protein-binding sites decrease, and the relative amount of free drug increases. If the dose exceeds protein-binding capacity, the addition of more drug will increase only the free drug concentration. In practice, saturation of protein-binding sites by drugs with high association constants (eg, sulfonamides) occurs only when such drugs are given in large (ie, gm) doses.

TABLE 271–2. SOME VALUES OF DRUG BINDING IN HUMAN SERUM

Drug	*Percent Bound*
Warfarin	99
Diazepam	99
Furosemide	96
Dicloxacillin	94
Propranolol	93
Tolbutamide	93
Sulfisoxazole*	88–92
Phenytoin	89
Quinidine**	71
Lidocaine	51
Digoxin	25

* Function of drug blood level, see text.
** Significant binding to serum protein other than albumin.

Generally, only unbound drug is available for metabolism; however, some highly bound drugs (eg, propranolol) are rapidly metabolized. Only free drug is available for glomerular filtration, but active processes such as secretion by the renal tubules and carrier-mediated transport across other cell membranes are not restricted to free drug.

Intracellular drug reservoirs: Some drugs accumulate in cells in higher concentration than they do in extracellular fluid. Such accumulation most commonly involves binding of drugs with protein, phospholipids, or nucleoprotein. The antimalarial agents such as chloroquine are notorious for intracellular binding and can reach intracellular concentrations in eye and liver tissue that are thousands of times higher than that of plasma. These stored drugs are in equilibrium with those in the plasma and are released into the plasma as the drugs are eliminated from the body, but their rate of release is usually too slow to produce pharmacologic effects. Consequently, this type of storage represents a site of loss (and possible local toxicity) rather than a depot for continued drug action.

Fat and other tissues can serve as reservoirs for lipid-soluble drugs. Changes in body composition (and circulation) may occur with age and affect the distribution and equilibration rate of drugs. For example, the ratio of fat to lean tissue is greater in the elderly. The enlarged fat compartment may affect the distribution and accumulation of lipid-soluble drugs such as diazepam. This may necessitate dosage adjustments for such drugs during chronic administration to prevent exaggerated or prolonged drug action.

Tetracycline may be stored in bone and teeth. In the fetus and the young, tetracycline can cause local toxicity that can persist long after therapy has ceased.

Passage of Drugs into the Central Nervous System

Drugs enter the CNS by 2 routes: the capillary circulation and the CSF. Although the brain receives a large proportion of the cardiac output (about 1/6), rapid distribution of drugs to brain tissue is restricted. While some lipid-soluble drugs (eg, thiopental) do enter and exert their pharmacologic effects very rapidly, many drugs, particularly the more water-soluble agents, enter the brain very slowly. The endothelial cells of the brain capillaries, which appear to be more tightly joined to one another than are those of other capillary beds, contribute to the slow diffusion of water-soluble substances. Another important barrier to water-soluble substances is the close approximation of the glial connective tissue cells (astrocytes) to the basement membrane of the capillary endothelium. The capillary endothelium and the astrocytic sheath together are referred to as the **blood-brain barrier.** They confer permeability characteristics on the brain different from those of other tissues and constitute a relative obstacle to drug penetration.

Drugs may enter the ventricular CSF directly via the choroid plexus, gaining access to brain tissue by passive diffusion from the CSF. The choroid plexus is also a site of active transport of organic acids (eg, penicillin) from CSF to blood.

The major factors that determine the rate of drug penetration into the CSF include the extent of protein binding, the ionization state, and especially the lipid-water partition coefficient of the compound. The penetration rate into the brain is slow for highly protein-bound drugs, and for the ionized form of weak acids and bases is so slow as to be virtually nonexistent. Differences in pH between the plasma and brain compartments may appreciably influence the distribution ratio of drugs between the compartments through an ion-trapping effect. Under normal conditions there is a small pH difference between plasma (pH 7.4) and CSF (pH 7.3), which particularly affects weak electrolytes with pK's near these pH values. Lipid-soluble substances diffuse across brain capillaries and capillary barriers elsewhere at similar rates.

272. PHARMACOKINETICS AND DRUG ADMINISTRATION

Pharmacokinetics is the study of the time course of a drug and its metabolites in the body following drug administration.

Drugs are administered to achieve a therapeutic objective, which requires the attainment and maintenance of a pharmacologic response. To accomplish this, an appropriate concentration of drug is required at the site of action. What is appropriate and the dosage needed to achieve it depend upon the patient's clinical state, the severity of the condition being treated, the presence of other drugs and concurrent disease, and other factors.

The pharmacologic response observed relative to the concentration at the active site depends upon the **pharmacodynamics** of the drug, while the attainment and maintenance of the appropriate concentration depends upon the **pharmacokinetics** of the drug. The former is concerned with how a drug acts on the body; the latter, which is emphasized in this chapter, deals with how the body acts on a drug.

Because of individual differences, successful therapy requires planning drug administration according to each patient's needs. Traditionally, this has been accomplished by empirically adjusting dosage until the therapeutic objective is met. This method is frequently inadequate because of delays or because of undue toxicity. An alternative approach is to initiate drug administration according to the expected absorption and disposition (distribution and elimination) of the drug in a patient and to adjust dosage by monitoring the plasma drug concentration, a reflector of drug at the active site, in addition to drug effects. This approach requires knowledge of the drug's pharmacokinetics as a function of age and weight, and of the presence and kinetic consequences of renal, hepatic, cardiovascular, or other disease.

To identify and quantitate the variables in pharmacokinetics, isolation of the input and disposition processes is helpful. Absorption, distribution, and elimination and the factors affecting them are described in Chs. 270, 271, and 273. The quantitative aspects of these processes and the application of pharmacokinetic principles to drug administration are discussed in this chapter.

BASIC PHARMACOKINETIC PARAMETERS

The pharmacokinetic behavior of most drugs may be summarized by parameters that relate variables to each other (see TABLE 272–1). The parameters are constants, although their values may differ from patient to patient and in the same patient under different conditions.

Bioavailability and Absorption Rate Constant

The extent of drug absorption into the general circulation is expressed by the **bioavailability,** the fraction of a dose reaching the plasma site of measurement. The rapidity of absorption is often expressed by the **absorption rate constant,** provided absorption follows Relationship 2 in TABLE 272–1. Changes in these two parameters influence the maximum (or peak) concentration, the time at which the maximum concentration occurs, and the area under the concentration-time curve after a single oral dose. In chronic drug therapy bioavailability is the more important measurement because it relates to the average level obtained, whereas only the degree of fluctuation is related to the absorption rate constant.

Volume of Distribution and Unbound Fraction

The **apparent volume of distribution** and the **fraction unbound** in plasma are the two most widely-used parameters for drug distribution. The volume of distribution is use-

TABLE 272–1. BASIC PHARMACOKINETIC PARAMETERS AND THEIR DEFINING RELATIONSHIPS

	Relationship		*Parameter*		
Absorption					
1.	Rate of absorption	=	Absorption Rate Constant	×	Amount remaining to be absorbed
2.	Amount absorbed	=	Bioavailability	×	Dose
Distribution					
3.	Amount in body	=	Volume of Distribution	×	Plasma drug concentration
4.	Unbound drug concentration in plasma	=	Fraction Unbound	×	Plasma drug concentration
Elimination					
5.	Rate of elimination	=	Clearance	×	Plasma drug concentration
6.	Rate of renal excretion	=	Renal Clearance	×	Plasma drug concentration
7.	Rate of metabolism	=	Metabolic Clearance	×	Plasma drug concentration
8.	Rate of renal excretion	=	Fraction Excreted Unchanged	×	Rate of elimination
9.	Rate of elimination	=	Elimination* Rate Constant	×	Amount in body

* Another conceptually useful parameter is biologic half-life. Its relationship to the elimination rate constant is: Half-life = 0.693/(Elimination Rate Constant).

ful because it allows estimation of the dose required to achieve a given concentration and, conversely, the concentration achieved on administering a given dose. The unbound fraction is useful because it relates the measured total concentration to the unbound concentration, which is presumably more closely associated with drug effects. It is a particularly useful parameter when plasma protein binding is altered, eg, in hypoalbuminemia, renal disease, hepatic disease, and displacement interactions.

Clearance, Renal Clearance, and Fraction Excreted Unchanged

The rate at which a drug is eliminated from the body is proportional to the plasma concentration, Relationship 5, TABLE 272–1; the parameter relating the two is clearance. The parameters relating rate of renal excretion of unchanged drug and rate of metabolism to the plasma concentration are **renal clearance,** Relationship 6, and **metabolic clearance,** Relationship 7, respectively. Because the rate of elimination is the sum of the rates of renal excretion and extrarenal elimination, usually metabolism, it follows that

Total clearance = Renal clearance + Extrarenal (metabolic) clearance

The ratio of the rate of renal excretion to the rate of total elimination, also the ratio of renal clearance to (total) clearance, is the **fraction excreted unchanged,** Relationship 8. This parameter is useful in assessing the potential effect of renal and hepatic diseases on drug elimination.

The rate of extraction of a drug from the blood in an eliminating organ, such as the liver, cannot exceed the rate of its presentation to the organ. Thus, clearance has a

limiting value. When high extraction exists, elimination is limited by drug delivery and hence by blood flow to the organ. Furthermore, when the eliminating organ is the liver and a drug is given orally, a portion of the dose administered may be lost on its requisite passage through the liver to the general circulation. This is called the **first-pass effect**; it applies to metabolism in the gut wall as well as in the liver. Thus, whenever a drug is highly extracted (high clearance) in either of these locations, the bioavailability is low, sometimes precluding oral administration or resulting in an oral dose much larger than the equivalent parenteral dose. A large first-pass effect is shown by a number of drugs, such as alprenolol, hydralazine, isoproterenol, lidocaine, meperidine, morphine, nifedipine, nitroglycerin, propranolol, and verapamil.

Elimination Rate Constant and Half-life

The **elimination rate constant** relates the rate of elimination to the amount of drug in the body. As the rate of elimination equals clearance times plasma drug concentration (Relationship 5, TABLE 272–1) and the amount of drug in the body equals volume of distribution times plasma drug concentration (Relationship 3), it follows that

$$\text{Elimination rate constant} = \frac{\text{Clearance}}{\text{Volume of distribution}}$$

Expressed in these terms, the elimination rate constant is a function of how a drug is cleared from the blood by the eliminating organs and how the drug distributes throughout the body.

Half-life (biologic) is a convenient parameter. It is the time required for the plasma drug concentration or the amount in the body to decrease by 50%. For most drugs, the half-life remains constant regardless of how much drug is in the body. It is related to the elimination rate constant by

$$\text{Half-life} = \frac{0.693}{\text{Elimination rate constant}}$$

VARIABILITY IN PARAMETER VALUES

Many of the variables affecting pharmacokinetic parameters have been recognized and can be taken into account to adjust drug administration to an individual patient's needs, although even after dosage adjustment sufficient variability usually remains to require careful monitoring of drug response and, in many cases, of plasma drug concentration.

Age and Weight

For some drugs, changes in pharmacokinetics with age and weight are well-established. In children (6 mo to 20 yr), renal function appears to correlate well with body surface area. Thus, for drugs primarily eliminated unchanged by renal excretion, clearance varies with age according to the change in surface area. In persons over age 20, renal function decreases about 1%/yr. Taking these changes into account permits dosage adjustment of these drugs with age. Body surface area also has been found to correlate with metabolic clearance in children, although exceptions are common. For neonates and young infants, both renal and hepatic functions are not fully developed and no generalization, except for the occurrence of rapid change, can be made.

Disease

Renal function impairment causes several pharmacokinetic changes. The renal clearance of most drugs appears to vary directly with creatinine clearance, regardless of the renal disease present. The change in (total) clearance depends upon the contribution of the kidneys to total elimination. Thus, (total) clearance is expected to be proportional

to renal function (creatinine clearance) for drugs solely excreted unchanged and not to change at all for drugs eliminated by metabolism.

Sometimes volume of distribution changes in renal failure. For digoxin, a decreased volume of distribution is observed because of decreased tissue binding. For phenytoin, salicylic acid, and many other drugs, volume of distribution increases because of decreased binding to plasma proteins.

In physiologic stress (eg, myocardial infarction, surgery, ulcerative colitis, and Crohn's disease) the concentration of the acute phase protein, α_1-acid glycoprotein, is increased. Consequently, the binding of several basic drugs, such as propranolol, quinidine, and disopyramide, to this protein is increased. The volume of distribution of these drugs is decreased accordingly.

Hepatic disease produces changes in metabolic clearance, but good correlates or predictors of the changes are unavailable. Dramatically reduced drug metabolism has been associated with hepatic cirrhosis. Reduced plasma protein binding is often observed in this disease because of lowered plasma albumin. Acute hepatitis, with elevated serum enzymes, is usually not associated with altered drug metabolism. Congestive heart failure, pneumonia, hyperthyroidism, and many other diseases also alter the pharmacokinetics of drugs.

Drug Interactions

Drug interactions can cause changes in pharmacokinetic parameter values and, therefore, in drug response. Interactions are known that affect each of the parameters in TABLE 272–1. Most of these interactions are graded, and the extent of the interaction depends upon the concentration of both of the interacting drugs. For these reasons, predicting and adjusting drug administration in these situations are difficult. The prevention and management of drug interactions are discussed in DRUG INTERACTIONS in Ch. 276.

Dose and Time Dependence

In some instances, the values of the pharmacokinetic parameters change with dose administered, concentration in plasma, or time; eg, a decreased bioavailability of griseofulvin as the dose is increased, a disproportionate increase in the steady-state plasma phenytoin concentration on increasing its dosing rate, and a decrease in plasma carbamazepine concentration during its chronic administration. The decreased bioavailability of griseofulvin is due to the drug's low solubility in the GI tract. Phenytoin shows a concentration (dose) dependency because the metabolizing enzymes have a limited capacity to eliminate the drug, and the usual rate of administration approaches the maximum rate of metabolism. Carbamazepine shows time dependence because it induces its own metabolism.

Although relatively uncommon, dose and time dependencies introduce variability into the kinetics and response to several drugs. Other causes of dose- and time-dependent kinetics are saturable plasma protein and tissue binding (phenylbutazone), saturable secretion in the kidney (high dose penicillin therapy), and saturable metabolism during the first pass through the liver (propranolol).

DRUG ADMINISTRATION

Pharmacokinetic parameter values are obtained experimentally. When these values are known, the kinetics of a drug can be predicted. The kinetic consequences of administering a drug as a single IV dose, by constant-rate infusion, as an oral dose, and in multiple doses are described below using the drug aminophylline as an example. The metabolism of this drug shows concentration dependence in some individuals, especially children; however, for illustrative purposes, consider a 70-kg individual (Patient A) whose metabolism is concentration independent. The patient's parameter values are

bioavailability, 1.0; absorption rate constant, 1.0 h^{-1}; volume of distribution, 0.5 L/kg; clearance, 43 mL/kg/h; and half-life, 8 h.

Single Intravenous Dose

The expected time course of theophylline in plasma following the IV administration of a single 320-mg dose of aminophylline (hydrous form is 80% theophylline) to Patient A is shown in FIG. 272–1 with both linear and semilogarithmic plots. The predicted initial plasma concentration is 7.3 mg/L (Dose of theophylline [256 mg]/Volume of distribution [L/kg × 70 kg]). The subsequent decline is estimated from the half-life; q 8 h the concentration decreases by a factor of 2.

The discrepancy between the observed (solid line) and the predicted (dashed line) concentration-time profiles is explained by the time required to distribute drug throughout the body. This is often called the **distribution phase** and explains why single doses of many drugs, including aminophylline, must be administered by a short-term infusion over 5 to 10 min or more.

Constant Rate Intravenous Infusion

The expected plasma concentration of theophylline on IV infusion of aminophylline to Patient A at a constant rate of 45 mg/h is shown in Curve A of FIG. 272–2.

Plateau concentration: The plasma concentration of theophylline and the amount of drug in the body rise until the rate of elimination equals the rate of infusion. The plasma concentration and amount of drug in the body are then at steady state—having reached a plateau level. From Relationships 5 and 9, TABLE 272–1, it follows that

Rate of infusion = Clearance × Plateau plasma drug concentration

and

Rate of infusion = Elimination rate constant × Plateau amount of drug in body

Thus, the plateau plasma concentration is controlled only by the clearance value and the rate of infusion; the plateau amount of drug in the body is determined only by the elimination rate constant and the rate of infusion.

Time to reach plateau: The time required to accumulate theophylline in the body depends on the half-life of the drug. This is demonstrated in FIG. 272–2 by the admin-

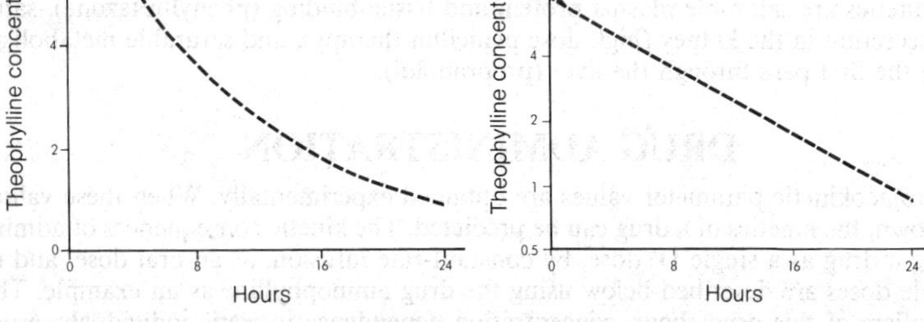

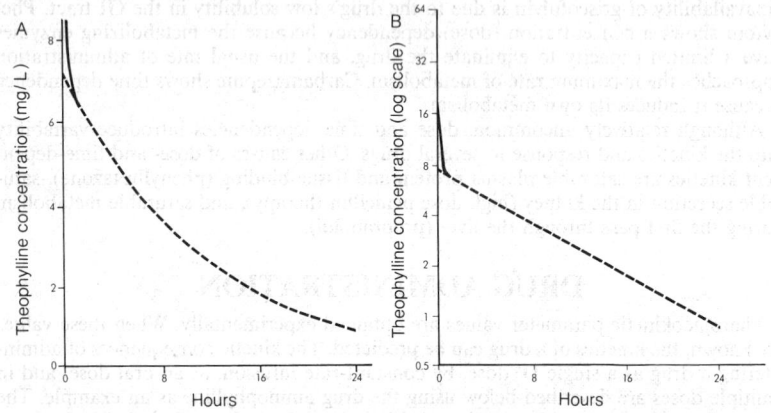

FIG. 272–1. Decline of the plasma theophylline concentration in Patient A following the IV administration of a single 320 mg dose of aminophylline. Shown on linear (A) and semilogarithmic (B) plots. Key: observation (—); prediction from parameter values given (-----).

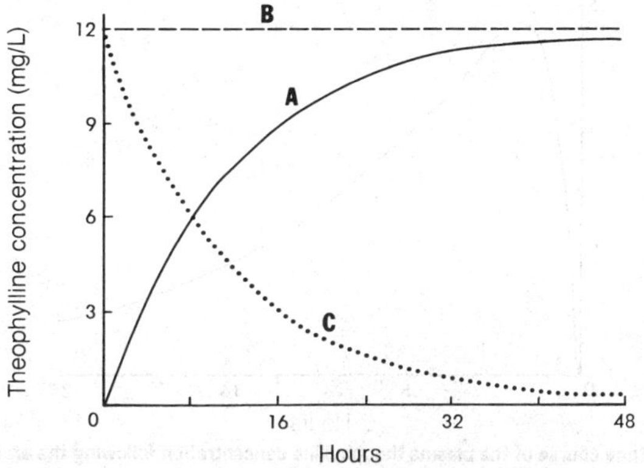

FIG. 272–2. Time course of the plasma theophylline concentration following the constant-rate IV infusion of 45 mg/h of aminophylline without (___, Curve A) and with (-----, Curve B) the administration of an IV loading dose of 530 mg. of aminophylline to Patient A. Curve C shows drug remaining from the loading dose.

istration of a single dose (530 mg) of aminophylline to attain a concentration of 12 mg/L followed immediately by an infusion of 45 mg/h of aminophylline to maintain the level, Curve B of FIG. 272–2. Drug from the loading dose disappears as shown in Curve C, with 1/2 remaining at one half-life, 1/4 at 2 half-lives, and so on. The amount of drug in the body from the infusion, therefore, increases (Curve A) so that 1/2 of the plateau amount is present at one half-life, 3/4 at 2 half-lives, etc.

If the infusion were stopped at 48 h, the postinfusion curve would resemble Curve C, but would be displaced in time. The important principle is that the time frame for both accumulation and disappearance of drug is determined by the half-life. In Patient A, without a loading dose, aminophylline must be infused for at least 32 h (4 half-lives in the patient) for the concentration to approach the plateau value. Measuring a plasma concentration after this time would then provide an accurate estimate of theophylline clearance.

Single Oral Dose

The predicted concentration of theophylline in this patient after orally administering a single 300-mg dose of aminophylline (anhydrous form is often used orally; it is 85% theophylline) is shown in FIG. 272–3. Several points are pertinent: (1) The time course is different from that of a single IV dose (FIG. 272–1), because time is required to absorb the drug; however, the area under the curve is the same because this drug is virtually totally available. (2) The more rapid the absorption, the closer the curve is to that of the IV dose. (3) At the peak concentration, absorption is not complete; here, the rate of absorption is simply equal to the rate of elimination.

Multiple Dosing, Drug Accumulation, and Dosage Regimens

On repetitively administering 300 mg of aminophylline orally q 6 h to Patient A, the theophylline concentration increases as shown in Curve A of FIG. 272–4. As with IV infusion, the average concentration at plateau depends upon the clearance, and the time required to accumulate the drug is a function of the half-life. Here, however, the levels fluctuate because of intermittent dosing. The kinetic consequence of an altered clearance of theophylline is demonstrated by Curves B and C. Curve B is the time course of plasma theophylline concentration in Patient B, who has congestive heart failure and whose clearance is only 21.5 mL/kg/h (about half that of Patient A). On administering 300 mg of aminophylline q 6 h to Patient B, the drug accumulates to

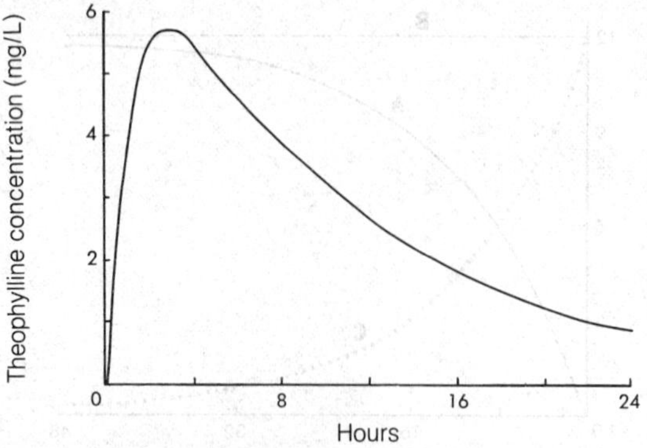

FIG. 272–3. Time course of the plasma theophylline concentration following the oral administration of a single 300 mg dose of aminophylline to Patient A.

levels about double those of Patient A. Furthermore, the time to reach the plateau levels is twice as long, a result of a 16-h half-life in Patient B.

Plasma concentrations of 10 to 20 mg/L are usually associated with optimal theophylline therapy. Above 20 mg/L the probability of toxicity increases. Thus, Patient B is at risk of developing toxicity (nausea, vomiting, CNS stimulation, seizures) that could have been averted, with prior knowledge of decreased metabolism in congestive heart failure, by decreasing the dosage. The slow metabolism also might have been detected by plasma concentration monitoring.

The requirement of Patient B for theophylline would probably be met with 200 mg aminophylline q 8 h (25 mg/h). However, because of the long half-life and the slow accumulation in this individual, rapid attainment of a therapeutic concentration (and

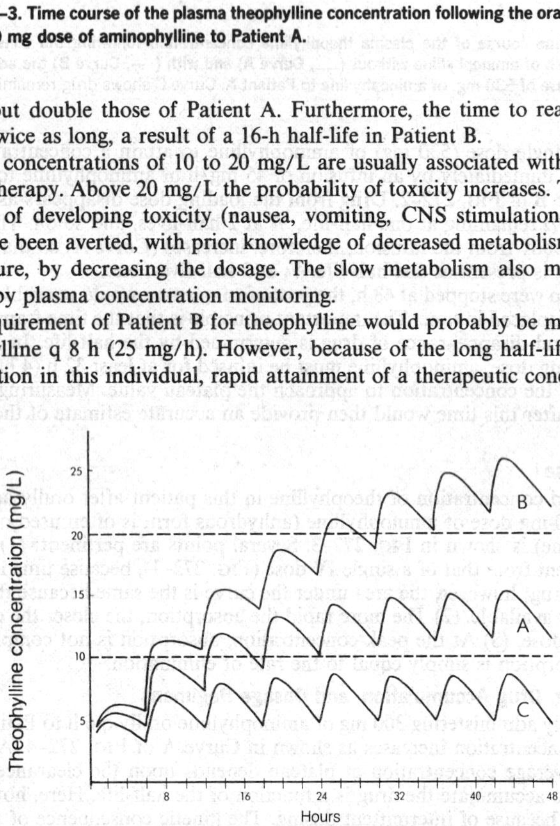

FIG. 272–4. Accumulation of theophylline on orally administering 300 mg. of aminophylline every 6 h. Curve A: in Patient A. Curve B: in Patient B, whose clearance is one-half that of Patient A. Curve C: in Patient C, whose clearance is twice that of Patient A. The dashed lines are the usual therapeutic limits and represent the *therapeutic window.*

response) cannot be achieved without administering a loading dose. The loading dose of aminophylline required (volume of distribution × desired theophylline concentration × factor to convert theophylline into aminophylline) is about 500 mg:

$$\left(35\text{ L} \times \frac{12\text{ mg}}{\text{L}} \times \frac{100\text{ mg aminophylline}}{85\text{ mg theophylline}}\right)$$

Curve C of FIG. 272–4 shows the time course of theophylline in a young, otherwise healthy, asthmatic adult (a heavy smoker). The clearance in this patient is 86 mL/kg/h and the half-life is 4 h. Administration of 300 mg aminophylline q 6 h (50 mg/h) would probably be ineffective. The need for more drug could have been anticipated. Measurement of a plasma concentration, just before the next dose, would support this need. However, administration of aminophylline to this patient would be difficult because of the short half-life, high clearance, and large dosage requirements (100 mg/h). This is an example of a patient for whom the use of prolonged-release type of dosage form may be indicated. Because absorption is more or less sustained, 600 mg q 6 h is reasonable, since widely fluctuating levels would be avoided.

In summary, pharmacokinetic principles can be helpful in initiating and monitoring drug therapy and in making adjustments to provide the optimum dosage requirements for each patient. The most useful pharmacokinetic parameters are bioavailability, clearance, volume of distribution, half-life, and fraction excreted unchanged.

273. DRUG ELIMINATION

The sum of the processes of loss of drug from the body. Removal of active drugs from the body depends on **metabolism** and **excretion.** Although these are separate and distinct processes, their functions in eliminating drugs are similar.

METABOLISM
(Biotransformation)

The process of chemical alteration of drugs in the body. The liver is the principal site of drug metabolism. Some metabolites are pharmacologically active (see TABLE 273–1). When the substance administered is inactive and an active metabolite is produced, the administered compound is called a **prodrug.** Metabolic reactions may be classified as nonsynthetic and synthetic.

In **nonsynthetic reactions,** the drug is chemically altered by either (1) oxidation, (2) reduction, (3) hydrolysis, or (4) a combination of these processes. These reactions usually represent only the first stage of biotransformation; metabolic products formed may subsequently undergo a synthetic reaction prior to elimination. Unlike the conjugated products of synthetic reactions, the metabolites of nonsynthetic processes may be pharmacologically active. Most oxidation and reduction reactions are catalyzed by the microsomal enzyme systems in the endoplasmic reticulum of the liver. Hydrolysis reactions and a few oxidative and reductive reactions are mediated by nonmicrosomal enzyme systems.

Examples of drugs metabolized by nonsynthetic reactions include amphetamine, chlorpromazine, imipramine, meprobamate, phenacetin, phenobarbital, phenytoin, procainamide, quinidine, and warfarin.

In **synthetic reactions** (or **conjugations**) the parent drug, or intermediate formed by nonsynthetic reactions, combines with an endogenous substrate, such as an amino acid

TABLE 273–1. EXAMPLES OF DRUGS FORMING THERAPEUTICALLY IMPORTANT METABOLITES

Drug	*Metabolite*
Acetohexamide	Hydroxyhexamide
Acetylsalicylic acid*	Salicylic acid
Amitriptyline	Nortriptyline
Chloral hydrate*	Trichloroethanol
Chlordiazepoxide	Desmethylchlordiazepoxide
Codeine	Morphine
Diazepam	Desmethyldiazepam
Flurazepam	Desethylflurazepam
Glutethimide	4-Hydroxyglutethimide
Imipramine	Desipramine
Lidocaine	Desethyllidocaine
Meperidine	Normeperidine
Phenacetin*	Acetaminophen
Phenylbutazone	Oxyphenbutazone
Prednisone*	Prednisolone
Primidone*	Phenobarbital
Procainamide	N-Acetylprocainamide
Propranolol	4-Hydroxypropranolol

* Prodrugs. Metabolites are primarily responsible for their therapeutic effects.

or glucuronic acid, to yield an addition or conjugation product. Metabolites formed from synthetic reactions are usually biologically inactive and, because they are more polar, are more readily excreted by the kidney (in urine) and the liver (in bile) than those derived from nonsynthetic reactions.

Several synthetic reactions are frequently encountered. **Glucuronidation,** the most common synthetic reaction, is the only one that takes place in the liver microsomal enzyme system. Glucuronides are eliminated in the urine and are also secreted in the bile. Examples of drugs metabolized this way are salicylic acid, morphine, meprobamate, and chloramphenicol. **Amino acid conjugation** with glutamine and glycine produces conjugates that are readily excreted in the urine but are not secreted via bile. **Acetylation** is the primary metabolic pathway for sulfonamides. Other drugs that are acetylated include hydralazine, isoniazid, and procainamide. **Sulfoconjugation** is the reaction between phenolic or alcoholic groups and inorganic sulfate, which is partially derived from sulfur-containing amino acids such as cysteine. The sulfate esters formed are polar and readily excreted in the urine. **Methylation** is a major metabolic pathway for inactivation of some catecholamines. Other compounds that are methylated are niacinamide and thiouracil.

Effects of age on drug metabolism: Neonates have partially developed liver microsomal enzyme systems and, consequently, have difficulty with the metabolism of many drugs, such as hexobarbital, phenacetin, amphetamine, and chlorpromazine. The experience with chloramphenicol in neonates highlights the serious consequences that may occur because of slower conversion to the glucuronide. Equivalent mg/kg doses of chloramphenicol that are well tolerated by older subjects can result in serious toxicity in neonates **(the gray baby syndrome)** and are associated with prolonged and elevated

blood levels of chloramphenicol. Elderly patients often show a reduced ability to metabolize drugs. The reduction varies depending on the drug and is not as severe as that in neonates. (See DRUG THERAPY IN THE ELDERLY in Ch. 264.)

Individual variation in the rate of drug metabolism (see also Ch. 276) makes it difficult to predict an individual's clinical response to a given dose of a drug. Some patients may metabolize a drug so rapidly that therapeutically effective blood and tissue levels are not achieved; in others, metabolism may be so slow that toxic effects result with usual doses. For example, phenytoin blood levels vary from 2.5 to > 40 mg/L in different persons given the same dose. Some of this variability is due to differences in the amount of the key enzyme, cytochrome P_{450}, available in the liver, and to differences in the affinity of the enzyme for the drug. Genetic factors play a major role in determining these differences. Concurrent disease states, particularly chronic liver disease, drug interactions, especially those involving induction or inhibition of metabolism, and other factors also contribute.

EXCRETION

The process by which a drug or metabolite is eliminated unchanged from the body. The kidney is the major organ of excretion and is responsible for eliminating water-soluble substances. The biliary system also excretes certain drugs and metabolites. Although drugs may also be eliminated via other pathways (eg, intestine, saliva, sweat, breast milk, and lungs), the overall contribution of these routes is generally small. An exception is the excretion of volatile anesthetics via the lung in expired air.

RENAL EXCRETION OF DRUGS

Glomerular filtration and tubular reabsorption: About 1/5 of the plasma reaching the glomerulus is filtered through pores in the glomerular endothelium; the remainder passes along the efferent arterioles to the renal tubules. Drugs bound to plasma proteins are not filtered; only unbound drug appears in the filtrate. The principles that govern renal tubular reabsorption of drugs are those of any transmembrane passage (see DRUG ABSORPTION in Ch. 270). Polar compounds and ions are unable to diffuse back into the circulation and are excreted unless a specific transport mechanism for their reabsorption exists, as there is, for example, for glucose, ascorbic acid, and the B vitamins.

Effects of pH on the reabsorption and excretion of drugs: Although the glomerular filtrate that enters the proximal tubule has the same pH as plasma, the pH of voided urine varies from 4.5 to 8.0, and this may markedly affect the rate of drug excretion. Since the nonionized forms of nonpolar weak bases and weak acids tend to be reabsorbed readily from the tubular urine, acidification of the urine increases the reabsorption (ie, decreases the elimination) of weak acids and decreases the reabsorption of weak bases (excreted more rapidly). The opposite is true for alkalinization of the urine.

These principles may be applied in some cases of overdosage to enhance the elimination of weakly basic or acidic drugs. With the weak acids phenobarbital or aspirin, for example, alkalinization of the urine increases their excretion. Conversely, urinary acidification may accelerate the urinary elimination of certain bases, such as methamphetamine. The overall extent to which changes in urinary pH alter the rate of drug elimination depends upon the contribution of the renal route to total elimination.

Tubular secretion: Mechanisms for active tubular secretion exist in the proximal tubule and are important in the elimination of many drugs; eg, penicillin, mecamylamine, and salicylic acid. This process is energy-dependent and may be blocked by metabolic inhibitors. The secretory transport capacity can be saturated at high concentrations and each substance has its own characteristic maximum secretion rate, termed

transport maximum (Tm). Anions and cations are handled by separate transport mechanisms. Normally, the anion secretory system eliminates metabolites that have been conjugated with glycine, sulfate, or glucuronic acid. The various anionic compounds compete with one another for secretion. This tendency can be used therapeutically; eg, probenecid blocks the normally rapid tubular secretion of penicillin resulting in higher plasma penicillin concentrations for a longer time. Organic cations also compete with each other but not with anions.

BILIARY EXCRETION OF DRUGS

Drugs and their metabolites that are extensively excreted in the bile are transported across the biliary epithelium against a concentration gradient, requiring an active secretory process. This transport mechanism may become saturated by high plasma concentrations of a drug (transport maximum), and substances with similar physicochemical properties may compete for excretion via the same mechanism.

Biliary elimination is enhanced by a mol wt over 300 (smaller molecules are generally secreted only in negligible amounts); the presence of both polar and lipophilic groups; and conjugation, particularly with glucuronic acid. Biliary excretion is only occasionally a major route of drug elimination.

When a drug undergoes biliary secretion and reabsorption from the intestine, it completes an **enterohepatic cycle.** Drug conjugates that are secreted into and hydrolyzed in the GI tract, where the drug is reabsorbed, also undergo enterohepatic cycling. Biliary excretion is a route of elimination from the body only when the enterohepatic cycling is incomplete, ie, when all the secreted drug is not reabsorbed.

274. PLASMA CONCENTRATION MONITORING

Once a therapeutic objective is defined and a drug and dosage regimen are chosen for a patient, drug therapy is conventionally managed by monitoring the incidence and intensity of both therapeutic and undesirable effects. Although preferable, the use of a direct measure of the therapeutic effect is not always possible. For a number of drugs alternative endpoints are used, eg, prothrombin time for oral anticoagulants, rosette inhibition test for immunosuppressive agents, blood or urine glucose for hypoglycemic drugs, and serum uric acid for uricosurics. Signs of toxicity are also used, eg, tinnitus and nystagmus in therapy with salicylate and phenytoin, respectively. Because minor toxicities do not always occur before more severe toxicities and because of the inherent undesirability of toxic reactions, this procedure clearly has limitations. An alternative procedure is **plasma concentration monitoring,** which can provide a more facile and rapid estimation of dosage requirements than by observing drug effects alone. For some drugs it is routinely useful; for others it can be helpful in certain situations.

MONITORING DRUG IN PLASMA

A plasma drug concentration may be useful in the initiation as well as in the maintenance of drug therapy. The basic idea is to achieve and maintain a target concentration or range of concentrations. Such monitoring is of value, for example, in reducing toxicity when the probability and severity of toxicity are closely related to the plasma concentration. Plasma concentration then serves as an intermediate therapeutic endpoint to help prevent toxicity.

A strategy for drug administration may be entirely developed based on the plasma drug concentration, but this approach must be placed in perspective with all methods of monitoring. Certain criteria have been established, some related to the drug and others to the circumstances of its use. A few of the criteria are absolutely necessary; others are only relatively important. However, most of them must be met for the strategy to be effective.

Criteria Related to the Drug

Direct effect-concentration relationship: The intensity and probability of therapeutic or toxic effects must quantitatively correlate with the plasma level.

Nature of the therapeutic regimen: The objective of the regimen must be to attain and maintain a therapeutic effect. This usually requires maintenance of plasma concentration within a limited range. Drugs for which only acute or intermittent effects are desired are therefore excluded. Tolerance also diminishes the potential for applying the method.

Lack of other dosing guides: When readily assessed therapeutic endpoints are lacking, plasma concentration monitoring becomes particularly attractive; eg, in antiepileptic therapy, for which the therapeutic endpoint is the absence of seizures.

Low therapeutic index: The probability of a therapeutic problem is greater for a drug with a narrow range between those concentrations giving the desired response and those producing toxicity; ie, a drug with a low margin of safety or a low therapeutic index.

Current state of information: Prior knowledge of the therapeutic concentrations and the pharmacokinetic parameters of a drug is essential for plasma concentration monitoring to be effective. Furthermore, knowledge of the conditions in which these concentrations and parameters are likely to be altered is also important. However, this requirement is relative; by monitoring the concentration, adjustments in dosage can be made.

Analytical procedure: A sensitive, accurate, and specific assay for the drug must be available; the results must be available quickly enough to permit prudent therapeutic decisions. The half-life of the drug is an index of this "turn-around" time, as it is the time frame of accumulation on multiple dosing and of disappearance on discontinuing the drug.

Variability in pharmacokinetics: Interindividual differences and, in certain conditions, intraindividual differences in the pharmacokinetics of drugs are principal reasons for monitoring plasma concentrations. Drugs with poor and erratic absorption and those that are primarily metabolized, in contrast to those mostly excreted unchanged, are often candidates for monitoring. The larger the variability in the absorption and disposition of the drug, the greater is the need for monitoring it.

TABLE 274–1 lists drugs for which plasma level monitoring is now commonly used as well as the respective plasma concentrations usually associated with optimal therapy—**the therapeutic window** (see below).

Criteria Related to the Situation

For some drugs, plasma level monitoring is not *routinely* suggested, but it may be helpful in certain situations.

Anticipation of a therapeutic problem: When there is a high probability of encountering a therapeutic failure because of the patient's clinical status, a plasma concentration measurement can be helpful. For a patient with GI disease or with a gastric resection, an orally administered drug known to have poor bioavailability may be a candidate for monitoring. Similarly, the presence of renal, hepatic, thyroid, or cardiovascular disease may also suggest monitoring. For drugs that are primarily excreted unchanged, the presence of renal disease requires special attention, particularly if renal function is severely impaired or is variable with time.

TABLE 274–1. COMMONLY MONITORED DRUGS AND THEIR THERAPEUTIC PLASMA CONCENTRATIONS

Drug	*Plasma Concentration Usually Associated with Optimal Therapy (mg/L)*
Digitoxin	0.01–0.03*
Digoxin	0.0006–0.002*
Phenobarbital †	10–30
Phenytoin	7–20
Procainamide ‡	4–8
Quinidine	1–4
Theophylline	10–20

* Often expressed in units of ng/mL: digitoxin, 10–30 ng/mL; digoxin, 0.6–2.0 ng/mL.
† When used as an anticonvulsant.
‡ Concentration of active metabolite, N-acetylprocainamide, is also monitored.

The concurrent administration of several drugs, especially those known to interact pharmacokinetically, is also a situation in which plasma monitoring should be considered (see DRUG INTERACTIONS in Ch. 276). Finally, plasma concentration monitoring may be useful where noncompliance is likely to occur (see Ch. 278).

Presence of a therapeutic problem: The lack of a response at usual or even higher dosages or a toxic reaction at customary or lower dosages are therapeutic problems. Appropriately planned plasma levels may help explain whether noncompliance, poor absorption, altered metabolism, or an unusual pharmacodynamic resistance or sensitivity to the drug is the cause of the problem.

TABLE 274–2 is an illustrative list of additional drugs for which situations may arise in which monitoring may be useful. As more clinical pharmacokinetic information becomes available the status of these drugs and those in TABLE 274–1 will undoubtedly change.

Complicating Factors

The occurrence of active metabolites is one of the major limitations. The antiarrhythmic agent, procainamide, for example, forms an active acetylated metabolite, N-acetylprocainamide, by a hepatic enzyme that shows genetic differences. Procainamide is partially excreted unchanged, while the metabolite is almost entirely handled by the kidneys. Thus, in patients who are rapid acetylators and who have compromised renal function, the correlation between response and procainamide concentration is expected to differ from that observed in patients who are slow acetylators and have normal renal function. The concentration of both the drug and its metabolite should be monitored, especially in the presence of renal disease.

Delay in the response to a given drug concentration: The effects of digoxin on the heart exemplify a delay caused by the time required to distribute drug to the active site. Therefore, digoxin concentrations should not be measured within 6 h of a dose, even after IV administration, as the plasma concentration will not reflect the concentration at the active site. An observed response that is an indirect measure of the actual drug effect may be another cause of delay. The measurement of serum uric acid concentrations following the administration of a uricosuric agent and the determination of the one-stage prothrombin time following use of an oral anticoagulant are examples.

TABLE 274–2. SITUATIONS AND ADDITIONAL DRUGS FOR WHICH PLASMA CONCENTRATION MONITORING MAY BE USEFUL*

Drug	*Plasma Concentration Usually Associated with Optimal Therapy (mg/L)†*	*Situation(s) Suggesting Monitoring of Drug Concentration*
Amikacin	12–25**	Patient with impaired or changing renal function
Ethosuximide	25–75	Question of compliance or when coadministered with other anticonvulsants & source of toxicity is desired
Gentamicin	4–12**	Patient with impaired or changing renal function
Kanamycin	12–25**	Patient with impaired or changing renal function
Lidocaine	1.4–6.0	Patient with chronic hepatic disease or when infusion of drug is prolonged
Lithium	0.7–2.0 (mEq/L)	Patient with partially impaired renal function or on a low sodium diet
Methotrexate		In high dose therapy, concentration is used as a measure of potential toxicity & of a requirement for citrovorum factor rescue
Nortriptyline	0.05–0.15 (50–150 ng/mL)	Inadequate patient response. Plasma concentrations above 0.15 are less effective
Propranolol	0.02–0.2 (20–200 ng/mL)	Question of compliance or low availability. Patient with chronic hepatitis
Primidone ‡	8–12	Question of compliance. Also when coadministered with other anticonvulsants & source of toxicity is desired
Salicylates §	100–300 (10–30 mg/100 mL)	Patient with impaired hearing or patient on high-dose antacid therapy that increases urine pH
Tobramycin	4–12**	Patient with impaired or changing renal function

* Selected examples of situations are given.

† For each drug the therapeutic window is defined in terms of the concentration at the time of sampling. Usually a trough concentration is measured. When concentration units other than mg/L are commonly used, they are so noted.

‡ Metabolized to phenobarbital. The concentration of phenobarbital should also be monitored.

§ Metabolism and protein binding are dose dependent. Serum albumin must be considered in the interpretation of a salicylate concentration. Therapeutic window refers to the anti-inflammatory use of the drug.

** Usually obtained 30 min after the end of a 30 min constant-rate infusion.

THE THERAPEUTIC WINDOW

The range of plasma concentrations with the greatest probability of therapeutic success. However, concentrations of a typical population may be inappropriate for an individual patient. Higher than usual values may be appropriate if the condition is severe and the converse if the condition is mild. Individual exceptions are not uncommon.

For drugs that are bound to plasma proteins and in situations in which an alteration in binding is anticipated, the total concentration (bound + unbound) must be adjusted to give the desired unbound concentration. Conditions which reduce binding to albumin (a protein to which many acidic drugs bind) include end-stage renal disease, cirrhosis, hypoalbuminemia, severe burns, and pregnancy. Binding to α_1-acid glycoprotein and lipoproteins (proteins to which many basic drugs bind) has been observed to be increased during stress and decreased in chronic hepatic disease. In these cases,

adjustment of the therapeutic window is accomplished by estimating the fraction unbound in plasma in the patient and comparing it to the usual fraction unbound. Thus,

$$\text{Adjusted concentration} = \frac{\text{Usual fraction unbound}}{\text{Anticipated fraction unbound}} \times \text{Usual concentration}$$

For example, the fraction unbound for phenytoin is increased from 0.1 to about 0.25 in severe renal disease. Therefore, the usual therapeutic window, 7 to 20 mg/L, becomes 3 to 8 mg/L after adjustment.

EVALUATION OF A MEASURED CONCENTRATION

In contrast to usual clinical laboratory tests, the interpretation of plasma drug concentrations requires the application of pharmacokinetic principles. The subsequent presentation is illustrative.

Collection of Data

The history of drug administration, the clinical status of the patient, and a firm knowledge of the clinical pharmacokinetics of the drug are required (see TABLE 274–3). The drug administration history, including doses, times of dosing, and times of sampling, is mandatory, as are the age and weight of the patient.

The need for other information (eg, renal, hepatic, and cardiovascular functions; serum proteins; active metabolites; assay methods) varies with the drug and the situation. This information must be known by the individual who evaluates the concentra-

TABLE 274–3. DATA COLLECTION

History of Drug Administration
Drug, dosage, dosage forms, routes of administration, times of administration, compliance, inpatient or outpatient
Time of Sampling (Relative to Dose)
Present and Previous (If Any) Plasma Drug Concentrations
Clinical Status of Patient
Weight, age, sex, condition being treated, concurrent disease states (especially cardiovascular, hepatic, and renal diseases)
Laboratory Data
Renal function (serum creatinine, creatinine clearance, blood urea nitrogen)
Hepatic function (prothrombin time, serum albumin, serum bilirubin, hepatic enzymes in blood)
Protein binding (plasma proteins and albumin)
Concurrent Drug Therapy
Drug interactions
Assay interferences
Active Metabolites
Assay Method (Accuracy, Sensitivity, and Specificity)
Usual Pharmacokinetic Parameters Associated with Type of Patient in Question
Bioavailability, absorption rate constant, volume of distribution, unbound fraction in plasma, renal clearance, hepatic clearance

tion. An ability to estimate renal function from a serum creatinine is also important (see Ch. 146).

Interpretation of Data

After collecting the information needed, including the present and any previous plasma concentrations, two approaches may be taken. One is to compare the observed value with that predicted from known information. This approach is helpful in identifying problems such as noncompliance, low or high bioavailability, or unusually slow or rapid elimination. The other approach is to determine the pharmacokinetic parameters of the drug in the individual, a particularly useful analysis in determining an individual patient's dosage requirements. Whether the measured value is a good estimate of the minimum, average, or maximum concentration at steady state on a fixed-dose, fixed-dosing-interval regimen, or a nonsteady-state value obtained shortly after starting the drug or following an unequal dosage schedule, must be immediately established from the dosing history and the time of sampling.

Steady state: A value that represents an estimate of the average steady-state concentration on a fixed-dose, fixed-dosing-interval regimen is most readily handled. For a concentration to approximate such a value, a plasma sample must be obtained after dosing for at least 3 half-lives (in the patient). Furthermore, the fluctuation of the concentration within a dosing interval must be small, especially if the sample is obtained just before the next dose. This condition is essentially satisfied if the dosing interval is < 1 half-life. For example, this occurs for the daily administration of digoxin (half-life of 2 days or more). The observed concentration can then be evaluated by comparing it with the expected concentration.

The predicted average concentration, C_{av}, is a function of the expected values of bioavailability, F, clearance, Cl, and the rate of administration, (D/τ, dose/dosing interval), that is,

$$C_{av}\,(\text{expected}) = \frac{F}{Cl}\,(\text{expected}) \cdot \frac{D}{\tau} \qquad (1)$$

If the ratio of concentrations, observed to predicted, is > 1, either the input is greater or the elimination is slower than expected, or both. The converse is true for a ratio < 1. Thus, there is a set of explanations consistent with either observation.

Causes of either an altered input or an altered elimination are summarized in TABLE 274–4. Perhaps the most common cause is the difference between how the patient takes the drug and how he is supposed to or is believed to take it—a compliance problem. Bioavailability is a factor that only needs to be considered for drugs in which its value is low or variable or where malabsorption is suspected. Renal and hepatic clearances may explain altered elimination depending on the major route of drug elimination. Plasma protein binding is a concern for highly bound drugs because of the dependence of clearance upon it.

Fluctuation: The dosage regimens of many drugs are such that there is considerable fluctuation in the plasma concentration. The dosing interval may be comparable to or greater than the half-life, or the regimen may be similar to a 9–1–5–9 regimen in which the drug is taken q 4 h for 4 doses followed by a 12-h interval. In either case, if there is much fluctuation it must be considered.

For drugs in which the regimen involves considerable fluctuation, the preferred time of sampling is usually just before the next dose. The concentration, C, expected at the

TABLE 274–4. CAUSES OF AN UNEXPECTED STEADY-STATE PLASMA CONCENTRATION

Factor Involved	Concentration Ratio > 1*	Comment	Concentration Ratio < 1	Comment
Compliance	Noncompliance—taking more than directed	Probably less frequently a cause than taking less than directed	Noncompliance—taking less than directed	A very frequent problem
Bioavailability	Higher than usual	Only an explanation if bioavailability is usually low	Lower than usual	A more frequent problem for drugs that are usually poorly absorbed
Renal Clearance	Lower than usual	A valid explanation for drugs whose major route of elimination is renal excretion. May be altered pH, inhibition of secretion, or simply decreased renal function	Greater than usual	Not a frequent explanation. May occur because of altered urine pH or flow. The renal route must usually be or become the major route of elimination
Hepatic Clearance	Lower than usual	An explanation for drugs whose major route of elimination is metabolism or biliary secretion. May be competitive inhibition by another drug, decreased blood flow, hepatic disease, or genetic in origin	Greater than usual	An explanation if hepatic elimination is or becomes the major route of elimination. May be enzyme induction, or activation, or genetic in origin
Plasma Protein Binding	Greater than usual	Not usually an explanation	Less than usual	May be a result of displacement, hypoalbuminemia, hepatic and/or renal disease

* Observed concentration divided by expected concentration

end of a fixed dosing interval, τ, following the administration of a fixed dose, D, under steady-state conditions, is

$$C = \frac{F \cdot D \cdot e^{-\frac{Cl}{V} \cdot \tau}}{V\left(1 - e^{-\frac{Cl}{V} \cdot \tau}\right)} \qquad (2)$$

where Cl is total clearance, V is the apparent volume of distribution, and F is the bioavailability. Again, the observed concentration may be compared to the value predicted from the expected values of the parameters.

A maximum concentration, from a sample obtained soon after an IV dose or at the peak time after an oral dose, is often unreliable. Either absorption or distribution, or both, may take time to be essentially complete; they also often vary with time and among patients.

When absorption and distribution are rapid, eg, after the IM administration of the aminoglycosides, measurement of plasma concentration soon after the dose and close to the peak has been found to be useful. Under these conditions, the peak concentration can be estimated from

$$C_{peak} = \frac{F \cdot D}{V\left[1 - e^{-\frac{Cl}{V} \cdot \tau}\right]} \qquad (3)$$

or from the relationship

$$C_{peak} = C + F \cdot D/V \qquad (4)$$

where F • D/V is the increment of change in the concentration on adding F • D to the body.

Nonsteady state: A plasma sample may be obtained at a time when the drug has not fully accumulated or following an erratic pattern of previous doses and dosing intervals. Steady-state principles cannot be applied in these circumstances; however, other methods may be used.

Estimation of Parameter Values

For adjusting dosage in an individual patient, the most useful procedure is to estimate the value of clearance and sometimes the values of the volume of distribution and half-life from the monitored concentration(s). Clearance is the most valuable parameter, because it is needed to predict the dosage required to achieve a given concentration and the converse.

From a steady-state value: When a concentration is a good estimate of an average steady-state concentration, bioavailability is not variable, compliance is assured, and the patient is on a fixed-dose fixed-interval dosage regimen, clearance is readily estimated from

$$Cl = \frac{F \cdot D/\tau}{C_{av}} \tag{5}$$

a rearrangement of equation 1. For example, if a digoxin concentration of 1.2 μg/L were obtained on chronically administering 0.125 mg IV (F = 1.0) per day to a patient, the clearance would be 104 L/day. From equation 1, then, a concentration of 1.4 μg/L, a value near the middle of the usual therapeutic window, would be expected on orally administering 0.25 mg/day of a dosage form with F = 0.60.

Clearance may be calculated from the relationship:

$$Cl = \frac{V}{\tau} \cdot \ln\left[\frac{F \cdot D}{V \cdot C} + 1\right] \tag{6}$$

when a trough concentration is obtained under steady-state conditions, large fluctuations are anticipated (dosing interval ≫ half-life), and the drug is given IV or absorption is rapid. For example, gentamicin is a drug whose concentrations fluctuate extensively because the usual half-life and dosing interval are 2 and 8 h, respectively. If a steady-state trough gentamicin concentration of 3 mg/L were obtained in a 70-kg patient on an IV regimen of 80 mg q 8 h, the clearance would be 2.0 L/h (F = 1, V = 0.25 L/kg). One's confidence in the estimate depends on several factors, including variability in the values of V and F, assay errors, and the assumptions above.

The dosage required to achieve a given average concentration can then be computed from the clearance and bioavailability estimates as follows:

$$D/\tau = \frac{Cl}{F} \cdot C_{av} \tag{7}$$

In the example of digoxin above, the daily oral dose required to achieve a concentration of 1.4 μg/L is 0.25 mg. For gentamicin, the 12-h IV dose required to maintain an average concentration of 3 mg/L, from equation 5, is then 72 mg. The peak, equations 3 or 4, and trough, equation 2, are then 5.5 and 1.4 mg/L, respectively.

From a nonsteady-state value: Clearance may also be estimated from a nonsteady-state concentration. As an example, consider the interpretations that would be given to theophylline concentrations obtained in 3 different 70-kg patients 12 h after starting an IV infusion of 42.5 mg/h (aminophylline, 53 mg/h). Clearance is highly variable for theophylline, whereas the volume of distribution is relatively constant (0.5 L/kg). On infusing the drug in patients A, B, and C who have clearances of 20, 40, and 80 mL/h/kg respectively, the plasma concentrations rise as shown in FIG. 274–1. The plasma concentration in patient A reaches toxic levels, but it takes > 24 h of infusion. The concentration in patient B approaches a steady-state value within the therapeutic window. The values for patient C remain subtherapeutic.

For a plasma sample obtained 12 h after starting an infusion, the concentration in patient C is close to a steady-state value and clearance is reasonably estimated using the steady-state approach. The concentrations in patients A and B are not near the steady-state, but the levels do provide some information. The concentration expected at this point in time may be calculated from the values of clearance, Cl, and volume, V, using the relationship

$$C = \frac{R}{Cl} \cdot \left(1 - e^{-\frac{Cl}{V}t}\right) \tag{8}$$

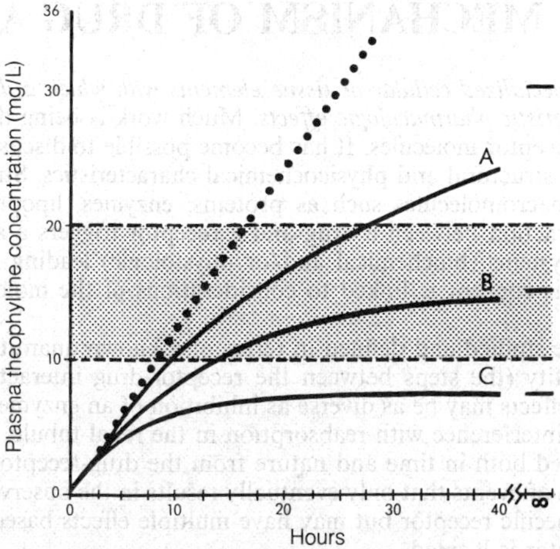

Fig. 274–1. Plasma theophylline concentration.

where R is the rate of infusion and t is the duration of the infusion. The steady-state concentration is R/Cl.

The observed concentration in patient B is identical to that calculated, indicating that a steady-state concentration of about 15 mg/L will be approached. For patient A, however, the observed value of 12 mg/L is above that expected at this time. A steady-state concentration in the potentially toxic range is possible, but one has little confidence in estimating what the value will be. The reason for the lack of confidence is seen by the dotted line in Fig. 274–1. This line represents the increase in the plasma concentration in a patient who is totally unable to eliminate the drug. The concentration at 12 h in patient A, about 12 mg/L, is close to that, 15 mg/L, which would be observed if no elimination occurs and, as a consequence of analytical and other sources of error, the only valid conclusions to be drawn are that the patient may approach potentially toxic levels, a decrease in dosing rate should be considered, and that a subsequent sample should be obtained.

Concentration Dependent Kinetics

For a drug, like phenytoin, whose clearance is concentration dependent, the principles above cannot be applied. Yet, because of its kinetic behavior, monitoring is particularly useful. Michaelis-Menten enzyme kinetic concepts apply here, but they are beyond the scope of this chapter.

FREQUENCY OF MONITORING

How frequently the concentration should be monitored depends on the drug, the confidence one has in estimates from previous measurements, and the presumed change in those factors that influence drug response. For example, digoxin may need to be monitored only occasionally in patients with congestive heart failure whose state of health and drug therapy remain stable; but if their health deteriorates or drugs known to interact with digoxin (eg, quinidine) are added, more frequent monitoring is indicated. For theophylline, daily or even more frequent monitoring may be required for a patient in an intensive care unit, especially if congestive heart failure, pulmonary edema, or severe constrictive airway disease is present. These conditions decrease theophylline metabolism; consequently, dosage requirements are likely to be less than normal.

275. MECHANISM OF DRUG ACTION

Receptors: *Specialized cellular or tissue elements with which a drug interacts to produce its characteristic pharmacologic effects.* Much work is being devoted to the isolation of actual receptor molecules. It has become possible to discuss receptors in terms of their specific structural and physicochemical characteristics. Structurally, receptors appear to be macromolecules such as proteins, enzymes, lipoproteins, and nucleic acids. The interaction between a drug and a receptor triggers a series of events that alter biologic systems (biochemical and/or physiologic) leading to a pharmacologic effect. Thus, this concept is linked to considerations of the molecular basis of drug action.

Receptors are studied and defined in terms of a known quantity (the drug) and an unknown quantity (the steps between the receptor-drug interaction and observable effects). These effects may be as diverse as inhibition of an enzyme, release of a neurotransmitter, or interference with reabsorption in the renal tubule. However, the effect may be separated both in time and nature from the drug-receptor interaction, which initiates a series of events that only eventually results in the observed response. A drug reacts with a specific receptor but may have multiple effects based upon the organ in which the receptor is located.

A variety of physicochemical forces attract the drug to the receptor site, bind it to the receptor, and trigger the characteristic response. Ionic forces (those between oppositely charged atoms) seem most important in the approach of a drug molecule to the receptor site. These are gross forces, however, and may not be as critical as hydrogen bonding and Van der Waals forces in properly aligning and stabilizing the drug-receptor complex. Covalent binding of drugs to receptors usually results in stable long-lasting complexes; such as the case with alkylating agents used in chemotherapy of neoplastic diseases.

The pharmacologic actions of certain drugs apparently are *not* mediated by receptor interaction. For example, neutralization of gastric acid by an antacid is a direct chemical reaction between an acid and a base. Osmotic diuresis is an example of drug action based on the physical properties of solutes. Chelation of heavy metals by some drugs is also not a classic receptor-drug interaction. The lack of reactivity of certain volatile general anesthetics and their varied chemical structures suggest that this action is not mediated by formation of a specific complex with endogenous macromolecules or receptors.

Several theories of drug-receptor interaction have been proposed, but most experimental observations are best explained by a combination of current hypotheses. The Law of Mass Action and the reversibility of drug-receptor interaction served as the basis for the receptor occupation theories, which postulate that the magnitude of the drug-induced effect is proportional to the concentration of the drug-receptor complex. Inherent in this theory are the concepts of **affinity** (the propensity of a drug to bind with a given receptor) and **intrinsic activity** or **efficacy** (the biologic effectiveness per unit of drug-receptor complex). A plot of the drug effect (in terms of **percent of maximum response**) vs. the logarithm of the dose results in a typical sigmoid curve (FIG. 275–1). The increase in response depicted by Curve A represents a graded, continuous process whose magnitude is directly proportional to the combination with, or occupancy of, receptors by the drug molecules.

Curves A and B in FIG. 275–1 illustrate the principles of intrinsic activity and maximal response, which are also called **potency** and **ceiling effect** in clinical terminology. Examination of the log dose-effect relationships for various doses of Drug A and Drug B reveals that more Drug B than Drug A is needed to confer the same degree of clinical response. Thus, Drug A has greater biologic activity per unit weight and is more potent than Drug B. In addition, no matter how much Drug B is given, there is

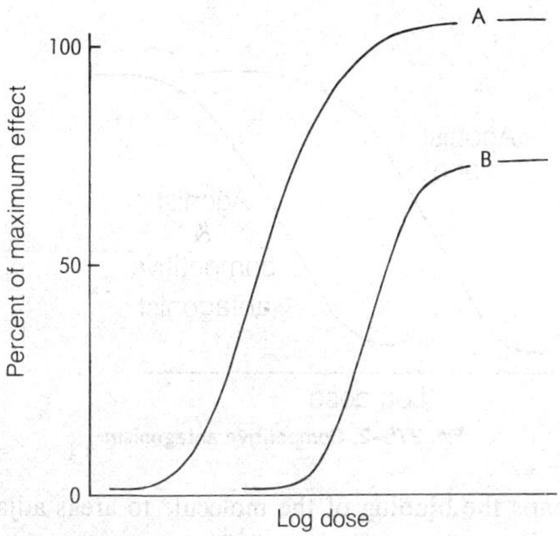

Fig. 275–1. Log dose-effect curves for drug A and drug B.

a point beyond which no further effect will occur. This is also true of Drug A, but the plateau occurs at a much greater degree of effect. Thus, Drug A is not only more potent than Drug B but it also has a higher maximum or ceiling of activity.

Dose-effect curves and the concepts of affinity and intrinsic activity are useful in defining the interaction of 2 drugs acting on the same receptors. Such interactions include competitive antagonism, noncompetitive antagonism, potentiation, and partial agonist (ie, dual agonist-antagonist) activity.

In some cases, the chemical structure or steric configuration of 2 different drugs is sufficiently similar that both molecules possess an affinity for the same receptor sites. **Agonists** are drugs whose interaction with a receptor initiates a biologic response that modifies cellular activity, increasing or decreasing it. Agonists possess both receptor affinity and intrinsic activity (efficacy). Drugs that interact with a receptor but do not initiate the sequence of events leading to an effect are referred to as **antagonists;** such drugs have affinity but lack intrinsic activity. There are 2 types of antagonists—competitive and noncompetitive. When both agonist and **competitive antagonist** are present in the same biologic system, they compete for the same receptor sites. A larger dose of agonist will then be required to induce the biologic effect at every response level. The dose-effect curve is shifted to the right but is parallel to the curve obtained with the agonist alone (Fig. 275–2). For example, naloxone (N-allyl noroxymorphone), which is structurally similar to morphine, has little or no morphine-like activity, but blocks the expected effects when given before or after morphine. More morphine is needed to overcome the competition, resulting in the characteristic shift to the right of the dose-response curve. Thus, in the presence of a competitive antagonist, the agonist's maximal effect may be achieved, but only at very high concentrations of agonist. Antagonist congeners (ie, modifications of molecular configuration resulting in altered structure-activity relationships) may block agonists to a greater or lesser degree.

One explanation for the phenomenon of competitive antagonism relates to the **stereospecificity** of the drug-receptor interaction. In some instances, only one of several stereoisomers of the same drug exhibits full agonist activity. Others may be partial agonists or even antagonists. The *d* and *l* isomers of epinephrine are structurally identical except for the spatial arrangement of the substitutions on one carbon atom, a seemingly minor difference that results in profound biologic differences. The spatial arrangement may affect the ease with which the drug can approach the crucial area of

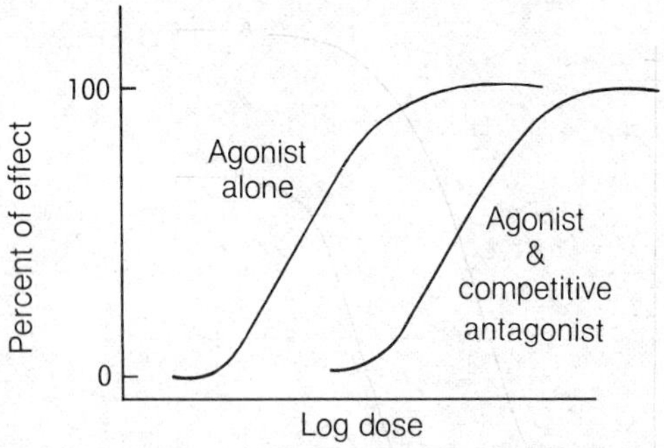

FIG. 275–2. Competitive antagonism.

the receptor or perhaps the binding of the molecule to areas adjacent to the specific receptor site.

Drugs are also **selective,** reacting only with **specific** receptors; selectivity and specificity are hallmarks of the receptor theory of drug action.

The term **noncompetitive antagonism** describes the effect of an antagonist that somehow alters the receptor or otherwise prevents an agonist from exerting any effect; eg, a noncompetitive antagonist may form a covalent bond with a receptor thus preventing the agonist attachment to or interaction with the receptor area. Noncompetitive antagonist effects may occur at distant sites that prevent the result of the receptor-agonist interaction. The efficacy of one drug is reduced as the concentration of the 2nd drug increases. In the distant effect form of noncompetitive antagonism, the affinity of the agonist for the its receptor remains unchanged. In noncompetitive antagonism, the log dose response (effect) curves begin at a similar point but shift to the right and have a depressed maximum effect as shown in FIG. 275–3. This is in contrast to the parallel shift of the dose response curve seen with a competitive antagonist.

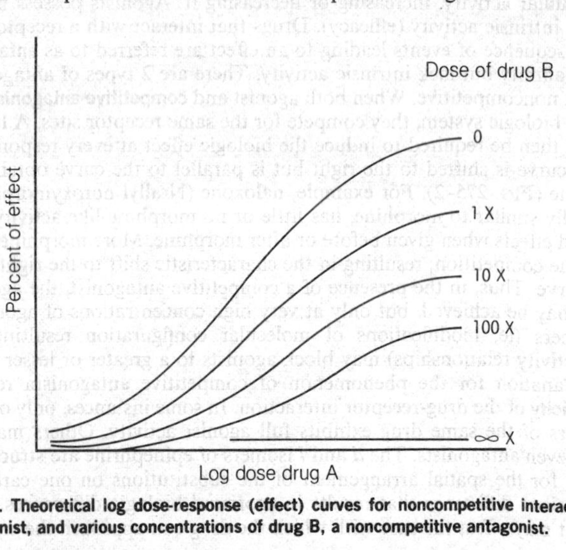

FIG. 275–3. Theoretical log dose-response (effect) curves for noncompetitive interaction between drug A, an agonist, and various concentrations of drug B, a noncompetitive antagonist.

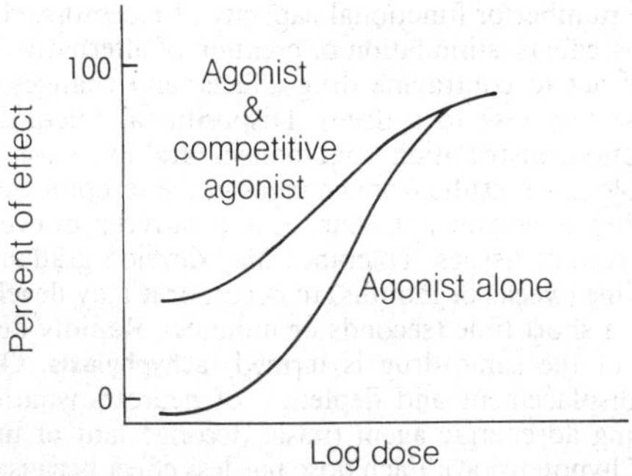

FIG. 275–4. Potentiation. Both agonist and competitive agonist react with the same receptor.

Two agonists that react with the same receptor, when administered together, may produce an additive or supra-additive effect at low concentrations. The maximum attainable response, however, is no greater than that elicited by the more active member of the drug pair because the tissues cannot respond to a greater degree (FIG. 275–4). The term **potentiation** describes the effect obtained by a drug combination that is greater than the algebraic sum of the effects of each component. However, the term is also used to describe the ability of one drug to increase the action of another by interfering with its inactivation or elimination.

Certain structural analogs of agonist molecules may exhibit a complex mixture of both agonist and antagonist activities; such dual-acting drugs are referred to as **partial agonists** (FIG. 275–5). Receptor activation is usually predominant at low concentrations, whereas receptor blockade is dominant at higher concentrations. Dichloroisoproterenol is a typical partial agonist; at low doses it produces adrenergic β-receptor-mediated effects similar to those of isoproterenol; at higher doses it acts similar to propranolol, blocking interaction of isoproterenol at β-receptor sites.

Tolerance is defined pharmacologically as *reduction in responsiveness to a medication following repeated administration. The concept of tolerance includes the lack of injury, relative impunity from undesired drug action, or of not being affected in any manner by a drug or poison.* Current medical usage looks at the practical aspects of tolerance—the need to increase the size of subsequent drug doses in order to achieve the same effect obtained previously. Tolerance may be present as a constitutional attribute or it may

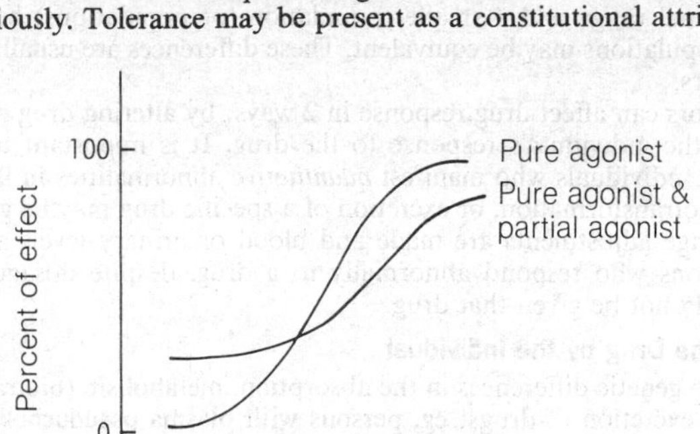

FIG. 275–5. Partial agonist activity.

be acquired. The complex causes for this phenomenon include preexisting genetic, physiologic, or pathophysiologic factors (eg, reduction in drug concentration at its site of action, changes in the number or functional capacity of receptors, changes in cellular responsiveness to drug effects, stimulation or creation of alternative biochemical or metabolic pathways that act to contravine drug effects, and changes in behavior or psychology that decrease response to a drug). Dispositional tolerance results from alterations in the absorption, distribution, metabolism, and excretion of the medication. So-called cellular tolerance results from changes in the receptor (perhaps through autoregulation as following beta agonists), changes in post-receptor events, or in other aspects of these cells or distant tissues. Tolerance may develop gradually and require many doses and a long time (weeks or months) to occur, or it may develop acutely and require a few doses over a short time (seconds or minutes). Rapidly developing tolerance to repeated doses of the same drug is termed **tachyphylaxis.** One example of tachyphylaxis involves displacement and depletion of neurotransmitter by repeated doses of an indirect-acting adrenergic agent (nasal decongestant or indirectly acting agonists for treatment of hypotension). Each dose has less effect because it releases less transmitter, since the pool of available transmitter has not been replenished.

276. MODIFICATION OF DRUG RESPONSE

PHARMACOGENETICS

Pharmacogenetics deals with *genetic factors responsible for variations in drug response among individuals*. The original definition was limited to genetic disorders initially revealed by the administration of a drug. Now, the scope includes all of the applications of formal genetic analysis to pharmacology and therapeutics (eg, therapy of genetic disorders). This discussion, however, is limited to conditions covered by the original definition. Many unexpected and peculiar adverse reactions occurring in a small percentage of individuals exposed to a drug, commonly referred to as **"idiosyncrasies,"** can be explained as genetically determined abnormal reactivity to a drug.

Just as normal ranges exist for physiologic parameters, a random population of individuals given the same dosage of a drug usually will show a quantitative range of responses. This variation is due to both environmental and hereditary factors and in most instances follows a unimodal normal distribution pattern. Occasionally, drug responses follow a more complex distribution pattern and there may be 2 or more recognizable populations (bimodal distribution). There may be a large population showing a normal range and a smaller population (or populations) behaving differently, or the populations may be equivalent. These differences are usually due to single inherited factors.

Genetic factors can affect drug response in 2 ways: by altering drug metabolism, or by modifying the individual's response to the drug. It is important to differentiate between them. Individuals who manifest *quantitative* abnormalities in the absorption, distribution, biotransformation, or excretion of a specific drug may be given that drug if suitable dosage adjustments are made and blood or urinary levels are monitored. However, persons who respond abnormally to a drug, despite dosage adjustments, should generally not be given that drug.

Alteration of the Drug by the Individual

This refers to genetic differences in the absorption, metabolism (biotransformation), transport, and excretion of drugs; eg, persons with plasma **pseudocholinesterase deficiency** (frequency, about 1:2500) have a decreased ability to inactivate succinylcholine, resulting in prolonged paralysis of the respiratory muscles when conventional dosages are used. Prolonged apnea may occur, requiring extended artificial ventilation.

About 50% of the population of the USA have a **defect in isoniazid acetylase** in the liver that results in slow inactivation of isoniazid and other drugs metabolized by the same enzyme system (eg, hydralazine, sulfamethazine, phenelzine). Slow acetylators tend to be more susceptible to adverse effects when given conventional dosages of these drugs; eg, peripheral neuritis with isoniazid and hydralazine-induced lupus erythematosus. **Deficient parahydroxylation of phenytoin** is a rare genetic biotransformation defect. In all these conditions, the dosage of the drug should be reduced or the dosage interval increased.

Normally, chemicals introduced into the body are metabolically detoxified, mainly in the liver. However, in the case of some drugs and chemical agents the metabolites are more toxic (eg, acetaminophen, methanol, glutethimide, and organophosphorus insecticides), a process that may be referred to as **metabolic toxification.** Agents that have an inducing effect on hepatic enzymes (see DRUG INTERACTIONS below) may lead to increased production of such metabolites. This is clinically relevant, for example, when a patient taking acetaminophen also consumes alcohol or phenobarbital. Inhibiting agents that block the appropriate metabolic pathway may be used to advantage in treatment; eg, giving N-acetylcysteine for acetaminophen overdose or ethanol for methanol overdose.

Alteration of the Individual's Response to the Drug

Persons with **glucose-6-phosphate dehydrogenase (G6PD) deficiency** may develop hemolytic anemia when given oxidant drugs such as antimalarials, sulfonamides, and certain analgesics. As G6PD is a key enzyme in RBC reduction reactions and these reactions appear to be essential for maintenance of cellular integrity, a deficiency of this enzyme results in an exaggerated sensitivity to the hemolytic effect of certain oxidant drugs. The condition is inherited as a sex-linked recessive trait. Many varieties of drug-induced hemolytic anemia have been described, but the two most important are the African and Mediterranean types. In the former (occurring in about 10% of U.S. blacks), the deficiency is manifested only in the older RBCs, the younger cells being normal. The G6PD levels in these persons are usually 8 to 20% of normal. In the Mediterranean type, levels are lower and the deficiency involves the entire RBC population. (See also ANEMIAS DUE TO EXCESSIVE HEMOLYSIS in Ch. 96.)

Malignant hyperthermia occurs in 1:20,000 surgical procedures involving muscle relaxants and general inhalation anesthetics (most often succinylcholine and halothane). Muscular rigidity is often the first sign of the disorder; other symptoms include tachycardia, arrhythmias, rapidly rising temperature, acidosis, and shock. This rapidly progressive reaction, which is inherited as an autosomal dominant trait, is often fatal (70% in untreated cases); *therapy should be initiated immediately*. All anesthetic agents should be discontinued at once and dantrolene administered by rapid IV push, starting with 1 mg/kg and continuing until symptoms begin to subside, or up to a total dose of 10 mg/kg. Corrective therapy should also include management of metabolic acidosis and core and surface cooling. Susceptible family members can be identified by elevated CK levels and muscle biopsy for histochemistry, electronmicroscopy, and in vitro exposure to halothane. If a susceptible person needs an operation, it should be done under local anesthesia or neuroleptic analgesia.

Approximately 5% of the U.S. population respond abnormally to **corticosteroids** by marked increases in intraocular pressure; glaucoma may develop. The condition is inherited as an autosomal recessive trait.

Genetic warfarin resistance is inherited as an autosomal dominant trait. The exact mechanism is unclear, but it probably operates at a receptor or enzymatic level in the liver. **Genetic warfarin sensitivity** also occurs.

In patients with certain types of **porphyria** (see ANOMALIES IN PIGMENT METABOLISM in Ch. 85), acute attacks can be precipitated by barbiturates and other drugs (eg, sulfonamides, phenylbutazone). The mechanism involves induction of the enzyme δ-

aminolevulinic acid synthetase (ALA synthetase), which results in increased porphyrin production.

INDIVIDUAL VARIATION DUE TO ENVIRONMENTAL FACTORS

Apart from the genetically determined differences in drug response mentioned above, individuals may differ widely in their response to drugs because of both internal and external environmental factors. Even within the same individual, for example, age, diurnal and circadian variations, changes in temperature, diet, disease, menstruation, drugs, and posture may influence response to a particular drug, mainly by altering its pharmacokinetics (eg, decreased renal function in elderly patients on conventional dosages of digitalis may lead to retention and an increased incidence of toxicity), and also by altering the response of the body to the drug (eg, hypokalemia, hypomagnesemia, or hypercalcemia may potentiate certain effects of digitalis).

DRUG INTERACTIONS

Alteration of the effects of one drug by the prior or concurrent administration of another. The usual result is an increase or decrease of the effects of one of the drugs. Desired interactions are usually considered in the context of combination therapy (eg, in the treatment of hypertension, asthma, certain infections, and malignancy), in which 2 or more drugs are used to increase therapeutic effects or reduce toxicity. Unwanted interactions can cause adverse drug reactions **(ADRs)** or produce therapeutic failure.

Since few of the known or suggested drug interactions have been sufficiently analyzed to determine their clinical significance, the possibility of problems developing must be viewed in perspective. If an interaction appears likely, therapeutic alternatives should be considered; but a patient should not be denied needed therapy because of the possibility of an interaction.

The mechanisms of drug interactions are usually pharmacodynamic or pharmacokinetic. Although the majority of drug interactions are of the pharmacodynamic type, most of the literature deals with the pharmacokinetic type.

PHARMACODYNAMIC INTERACTIONS

Pharmacodynamic interactions include the concurrent administration of drugs having the same (or opposing) pharmacologic actions and alteration of the sensitivity or the responsiveness of the tissues to one drug by another. Many of these interactions can be predicted from a knowledge of the pharmacology of each drug. By monitoring the patient clinically, deviations from the expected effect can often be quickly detected and the dosage adjusted accordingly.

Drugs With Opposing Pharmacologic Effects

Interactions resulting from the use of 2 drugs with opposing pharmacologic effects should be among the easiest to detect, but various factors may preclude early identification of such antagonism. For example, an ophthalmologist may prescribe a cholinergic drug (eg, pilocarpine) for a patient who is also taking an anticholinergic preparation (eg, propantheline) prescribed by his family physician for a GI condition. Although the anticholinergic drug may not alter intraocular pressure in many patients, some may experience difficulty.

Drugs With Similar Pharmacologic Effects

An example of this type of interaction is the increased CNS-depressant effect that often occurs when persons taking sedatives, tranquilizers, antihistamines, or other

drugs having depressant effects consume alcoholic beverages. Many individuals risk this combination and experience no difficulty, but it can be lethal.

An excessive anticholinergic effect can develop with the concurrent use of drugs that all produce such effects; for example, an antipsychotic agent (eg, chlorpromazine), an antiparkinson drug (eg, trihexyphenidyl), and a tricylic antidepressant (eg, amitriptyline). In some individuals, particularly geriatric patients, this additive effect may result in an atropine-like delirium that could be mistakenly interpreted as a worsening of the psychiatric symptoms. Distinguishing between the symptoms of the conditions being treated and the effects of the drugs being employed as therapy may be difficult, but is essential.

Interactions Involving the Adrenergic System

The enzyme monoamine oxidase **(MAO)** metabolizes catecholamines such as norepinephrine. Increased levels of norepinephrine accumulate within the adrenergic neurons when MAO is inhibited. Any drug that releases greater than usual amounts of norepinephrine can bring about exaggerated responses, including severe headache, hypertension (possibly a hypertensive crisis), and cardiac arrhythmias. Such an interaction may occur between MAO inhibitors (eg, isocarboxazid, phenelzine, tranylcypromine, and pargyline) and indirectly-acting sympathomimetic amines. Although most sympathomimetic amines (eg, amphetamine) are available only by prescription, others (eg, ephedrine, phenylephrine, and phenylpropanolamine), known to interact with MAO inhibitors, are present in many popular nonprescription cold and allergy remedies. Patients taking MAO inhibitors should *avoid* using such products.

Serious reactions (hypertensive crises) have occurred in patients being treated with MAO inhibitors following the ingestion of foods and beverages having a high tyramine content, including certain cheeses, beer and wines, chocolate, and pickled herring. Tyramine is metabolized by MAO, which is present in the intestinal wall and the liver; this enzyme protects against the pressor actions of amines in foods. When the enzyme is inhibited, unmetabolized tyramine can accumulate, releasing norepinephrine from adrenergic neurons.

The antineoplastic drug procarbazine and the anti-infective drug furazolidone (or probably its metabolite) can also inhibit MAO and the same warnings apply to these drugs as to other MAO inhibitors. With furazolidone, however, the enzyme inhibition usually does not occur within the first 5 days of therapy and the course of treatment is often completed within that time.

The antihypertensive agent guanethidine is transported to its site of action within adrenergic neurons by a system that is also responsible for the uptake of norepinephrine and several indirectly-acting sympathomimetic amines such as ephedrine and the amphetamines. Concentration of guanethidine in these neurons is necessary for its hypotensive effect. Tricyclic antidepressants can inhibit the uptake of guanethidine into the neuron terminal, thereby preventing its concentration at these sites and antagonizing the hypotensive effect. The effect of guanethidine is also antagonized by amphetamine, ephedrine, methylphenidate, chlorpromazine, and most other antipsychotic agents. Guanadrel is a newer analog of guanethidine, and it is likely that it will interact with other drugs in a similar manner.

Alteration of Electrolyte Levels (see Ch. 286)

PHARMACOKINETIC INTERACTIONS

Pharmacokinetic interactions are more complicated and difficult to predict because the interacting drugs often have unrelated actions and the interactions are mainly due to alteration of absorption, distribution, metabolism, or excretion, which changes the amount and duration of a drug's availability at receptor sites. The *type* of response expected from the component drugs is *not* changed, only the *magnitude* and *duration*.

Thus, a pharmacokinetic interaction is confined to an altered effect of one, or possibly both, of the participating drugs and is predictable from a knowledge of what the individual drugs can do. Such interactions may be detected by patient-monitoring procedures. A change in blood drug levels usually occurs and useful information may be obtained by measuring these levels.

Alteration of Gastrointestinal Absorption

Interactions that involve a change in drug absorption from the GI tract are of variable importance. Overall drug absorption may be reduced and its therapeutic activity compromised, or absorption may be delayed though the same amount of drug is eventually absorbed. A delay in drug absorption is undesirable when a rapid effect is needed to relieve acute symptoms, such as pain, or when the effects of a drug may be unduly prolonged (eg, the patient may have excessive residual sedation in the morning after taking a hypnotic drug at bedtime).

Alteration of pH: Many drugs are weak acids or weak bases, and the pH of the GI contents can influence absorption. Since the nonionized (more lipid-soluble) form of a drug is more readily absorbed than the ionized form, acidic drugs are usually more readily absorbed from the upper regions of the GI tract, where they are primarily in a nonionized form. By raising the pH of the GI contents, antacids may delay the absorption of pentobarbital, an acidic substance, and decrease, or delay, its hypnotic effect. Although changes in absorption might be predicted for many acidic and basic drugs, clinically important interactions are likely to occur in only a few situations.

Complexation and adsorption: Tetracyclines can combine with metal ions (eg, Ca, Mg, Al, and Fe) in the GI tract to form poorly absorbed complexes. Thus, certain foods (eg, milk) or drugs (eg, antacids, products containing Mg, Al, and Ca salts, or Fe preparations) can significantly decrease the amount of tetracycline absorbed. Absorption of doxycycline and minocycline is apparently not markedly influenced by food or milk and either drug might be preferred when gastric irritation occurs or appears likely. Aluminum-containing antacids will, however, decrease the absorption of these tetracyclines; it is likely that the increase in pH of the GI contents also contributes to the reduction of absorption of the tetracyclines.

Complexation can be expected with cholestyramine and colestipol. In addition to binding with and preventing reabsorption of bile acids, these agents can bind with drugs in the GI tract, having the greatest affinity for acidic drugs, eg, thyroid hormone or warfarin. To minimize the possibility of such an interaction, the interval between the administration of cholestyramine or colestipol and another drug should be as long as possible (preferably, at least 4 h).

The absorption of digoxin may be significantly reduced by the simultaneous use of kaolin-pectin mixtures or antacids. Physical adsorption of digoxin to these agents is the most likely reason, although other mechanisms also may be involved.

Alteration of motility: By *increasing* GI motility, metoclopramide or a cathartic may hasten the passage of drugs through the GI tract, resulting in decreased absorption, particularly of drugs that require prolonged contact with the absorbing surface and those that are absorbed only at a particular site along the GI tract. Similar problems can occur with enteric-coated and sustained-release formulations.

By *decreasing* GI motility, anticholinergics may either reduce absorption by retarding dissolution and slowing gastric emptying, or increase absorption by keeping a drug for a longer period of time in the area of optimal absorption.

Alteration of Distribution

Displacement of drugs from protein-binding sites may occur when 2 drugs capable of protein-binding are given concurrently, especially when they are capable of binding to the same sites on the protein molecule **(competitive displacement).** Since the number of

plasma or tissue protein-binding sites is limited, drugs can displace one another. Although the protein-bound fraction of a drug is not pharmacologically active, an equilibrium exists between the bound and unbound fractions. As the unbound or free drug is metabolized and excreted, the bound drug is gradually released to maintain the equilibrium and pharmacologic response. The risk of interactions from protein displacement is significant primarily with drugs that are highly protein-bound (> 90%) and have a small apparent volume of distribution, especially during the first few days of concurrent therapy.

Both phenylbutazone and warfarin are extensively bound to plasma proteins, especially albumin, but phenylbutazone has a greater affinity for the binding sites. When the 2 drugs are taken concurrently, fewer binding sites are available for warfarin, thus increasing the amount of free anticoagulant and the risk of hemorrhage. Phenylbutazone also inhibits the metabolism of warfarin, resulting in continued enhancement of anticoagulant effect.

The binding of acidic drugs to serum albumin has been most extensively studied; however, more recently, the importance of the binding of basic drugs to α_1-acid glycoprotein has been recognized.

Alteration of Metabolism

Stimulation of metabolism: Many drug interactions result from the ability of one drug to stimulate the metabolism of another by increasing the activity of hepatic microsomal enzymes involved in their metabolism **(enzyme induction).** In this manner, phenobarbital increases the rate of metabolism of coumarin anticoagulants such as warfarin, resulting in a *decreased* anticoagulant response. The dose of the anticoagulant must be increased to compensate for this effect, but this is potentially dangerous if the patient discontinues the phenobarbital without appropriately reducing the anticoagulant dose. The use of alternative sedatives (eg, the benzodiazepines) eliminates this risk. Phenobarbital also accelerates the metabolism of other drugs, such as digitalis and steroid hormones. Enzyme induction is also caused by other barbiturates and by various therapeutic agents (eg, rifampin) and chemicals (eg, insecticides).

Disturbed calcium metabolism and osteomalacia is associated with the use of anticonvulsants such as phenobarbital and phenytoin. Reduced serum calcium levels are caused by vitamin D deficiency, resulting from enzyme induction by the anticonvulsants. The risk of deficiency is greatest when the patient's dietary intake of vitamin D is borderline.

Pyridoxine can antagonize the activity of the antiparkinson drug levodopa by accelerating the conversion of the levodopa to its active metabolite, dopamine, in the peripheral tissues. In contrast to levodopa, dopamine cannot cross the blood-brain barrier, where it is required for the antiparkinson effect. In patients receiving both levodopa and carbidopa (a decarboxylase inhibitor), the addition of pyridoxine does not reduce the action of levodopa.

Studies show that the efficacy of certain drugs (eg, chlorpromazine, diazepam, propoxyphene, and theophylline) may be decreased in individuals who smoke heavily, because of increased hepatic enzyme activity from the action of polycyclic hydrocarbons found in cigarette smoke.

Inhibition of metabolism: One drug may inhibit the metabolism of another, causing its prolonged and intensified activity. For example, disulfiram, used in the treatment of alcoholism, inhibits the activity of aldehyde dehydrogenase, thus inhibiting the oxidation of acetaldehyde, an oxidation product of alcohol. This results in the accumulation of excessive acetaldehyde and causes the characteristic disulfiram effect (see under Treatment in DEPENDENCE ON ALCOHOL in Ch. 138). Disulfiram exhibits several other inhibitory actions. It enhances the activity of warfarin, phenytoin, and isoniazid, presumably by inhibiting their metabolism.

Allopurinol reduces the production of uric acid by inhibiting the enzyme xanthine

oxidase. However, xanthine oxidase is involved in the metabolism of such potentially toxic drugs as mercaptopurine and azathioprine; when the enzyme is inhibited, the effect of these 2 agents can be markedly increased. Therefore, when allopurinol is given concurrently, a *reduction* to about 1/3 to 1/4 the usual dose of mercaptopurine or azathioprine is advised. Thioguanine, which is closely related chemically and pharmacologically to mercaptopurine and azathioprine, is apparently not influenced by allopurinol.

Cimetidine inhibits oxidative metabolic pathways and is likely to increase the action of other drugs that are metabolized via this mechanism (eg, carbamazepine, phenytoin, theophylline, warfarin, and the benzodiazepines). Most benzodiazepines (eg, diazepam) are metabolized via oxidative mechanisms; however, lorazepam, oxazepam, and temazepam undergo glucuronide conjugation and their action is not affected by cimetidine. Unlike cimetidine, ranitidine does not significantly inhibit oxidative enzyme systems and is not likely to cause clinically significant interactions via this mechanism.

Increased bioavailability of propranolol and metoprolol in the presence of food has been reported. These drugs undergo considerable first-pass metabolism in the liver after oral administration, and it is suggested that the transient increase in hepatic blood flow associated with eating may reduce hepatic extraction of the drugs and first-pass metabolism. The increased bioavailability appears to be related to the protein content of the meal.

Alteration of Urinary Excretion

Alteration of urinary pH: Urinary pH influences the ionization of weak acids and bases and thus affects their reabsorption and excretion. A drug in its nonionized form more readily diffuses from the glomerular filtrate into the blood. More of an acidic drug is in the nonionized form in an acid urine than in an alkaline urine, where it primarily exists as an ionized salt. Thus, more of an acidic drug (eg, a salicylate) diffuses back into the blood from an acid urine, resulting in prolonged and perhaps intensified activity. Opposite effects are seen for a basic drug like dextroamphetamine. When the urinary pH was maintained at about 5 in one investigation, 54.5% of a dose of dextroamphetamine was excreted within 16 h, compared to a 2.9% excretion when the pH value was maintained at about 8.

Interference with urinary excretion: Probenecid increases the serum levels and prolongs the activity of penicillin derivatives, primarily by blocking their tubular secretion. Such combinations have been used to therapeutic advantage. For example, probenecid improves the effectiveness of penicillin and its analogs when used in single-dose regimens in the treatment of gonorrhea.

Significantly greater serum digoxin levels are found when quinidine is administered concurrently than when digoxin is given alone. Quinidine appears to reduce the renal clearance of digoxin, although other nonrenal mechanisms are probably also involved in this interaction.

Verapamil and nifedipine may increase serum digoxin levels by inhibiting both its renal and nonrenal elimination, and it is often necessary to reduce the dose of digoxin in their presence.

PRINCIPLES OF MANAGEMENT

The following general points concerning drug interactions warrant emphasis:

1. The drugs for which interactions are most significant clinically are those with potent effects, low safety margins, and a steep dose-response curve; eg, warfarin, digoxin, cytotoxics, hypotensives, and hypoglycemic agents.

2. It may be difficult to distinguish a drug interaction from other pathophysiologic factors affecting the response to therapy.

3. Not all patients develop reactions, even when it is known that interactions may

occur. Individual factors, such as dose and metabolism, determine whether the phenomenon occurs.

4. When the effects of drugs are being closely monitored, an interaction usually requires a change of dosage or therapy and does not result in significant problems for the patient.

5. In the displacement-from-protein-binding types of interaction, one fact is often overlooked. Any displacement alters the relationship between total and unbound drug and thus complicates the clinical interpretation of total drug levels in the blood. Total plasma concentrations of highly bound and displaceable drugs do not have the same meaning in the presence of displacing drugs as in their absence. Awareness of this becomes more important as blood levels are increasingly used to aid in the therapeutic control of patients on a variety of drugs. It would be desirable, and in some cases it may be necessary, to use ultrafiltrates of plasma samples rather than whole plasma for determining drug concentrations.

To minimize the incidence and clinical consequences of drug interactions, the prescriber should (1) know the patient's total drug intake, including agents prescribed by others and all OTC medications; (2) prescribe as few drugs in as low doses for as short a time as needed; (3) know the effects, both wanted and unwanted, of all the drugs used (since the spectrum of drug interactions is usually contained within these effects) and know the slope of dose-response curves (ie, the drug should be one for which the dosage range permits a considerable margin of error); (4) observe and monitor the patient for the drugs' effects, particularly after any alteration in therapy (some interactions, eg, metabolic effects depending on enzyme induction, may take a week or more to appear); and (5) consider drug interactions as possible causes of any unanticipated troubles. If unexpected clinical responses do occur, blood levels of drugs being taken should be measured, if possible; the literature or someone with specific knowledge of drug interactions should be consulted; and, most importantly, the dose of the drug should be altered until the desired effect is obtained. If this fails, the drug should be changed to one that will not interact with other drugs being taken.

---

277. DRUG TOXICITY

(For Drugs in Pregnancy, see PRENATAL CARE in Ch. 176; for Drugs in Lactating Mothers, see FEEDING under MANAGEMENT OF THE NORMAL NEWBORN in Ch. 182)

PRECLINICAL AND CLINICAL EVALUATION OF TOXICITY

Before a drug is approved for general clinical use by the FDA, preclinical and clinical data showing substantial evidence of safety and efficacy are required by law. Drug studies proceed through various phases, as follows.

Preclinical Investigation (Animal Studies)

Animal toxicity studies must precede human drug exposure. Two main principles are involved in all animal toxicity testing. First, the effects of chemicals in laboratory animals, when properly qualified, are applicable to man. Second, the use of high doses in experimental animals is a necessary and valid method to discover possible toxicity in man. Because the number of animals used in toxicity studies is relatively small and interest is in detecting the low incidence toxic response, larger doses must be given in order to validate the extrapolation to man.

Animal studies used to determine or define the safety of a drug include studies of acute, subchronic, and chronic toxicity in several animal species. **The initial acute toxicity studies** are to determine the **median lethal dose (LD50),** the toxic symptoms devel-

oped by the animals, and the time that they appear. At least 3 species of animals, one not a rodent, are usually used, and acute toxicity is usually determined by more than one route of administration. These initial studies give an indication of species differences, nature of the toxic effects, time periods, and dosages at which they will be elicited. The LD50 alone, however, has little predictive value unless accompanied by longer-term studies using measures of toxicity other than death.

Subchronic toxicity studies are conducted in at least 2 animal species and usually consist of daily administration of the test drug for up to 90 days. In each species, at least 3 dose levels are used, varying from the expected therapeutic doses to levels high enough to produce toxicity. Ideally, drug administration is by the route to be used in human trials. Physical and laboratory examinations are performed throughout the observation period. At the termination of the study, the animals are sacrificed and pathologic examinations conducted to determine the target organs of toxicity.

Chronic toxicity studies are carried out in at least 2 species, one of which is not a rodent. These studies usually last for up to the lifetime of the animal (ie, 2 yr in a rodent or longer in a nonrodent), but their length will depend on the intended duration of administration of the drug to humans. Three dose levels are again used, varying from low level or nontoxic to a greater than therapeutic dose level, high enough to produce a toxic response on chronic administration. Again, laboratory tests and observations are made at intervals throughout the period of drug administration. Some animals may be sacrificed periodically for gross and histologic postmortem examination when results of these chronic toxicity tests are to determine if the chemical is a potential carcinogen and is capable of inducing tumors.

Additionally, extensive **reproduction experiments** are carried out in rats and rabbits to detect any alterations in the reproductive cycle or any teratogenic effects on the unborn. These more specialized animal tests and the longer chronic toxicity studies may be conducted concurrently with the initial studies in human subjects, particularly when the drug is intended only for short-term human use.

The data from these studies are used to plot drug effects against the log dosage, providing dose-response curves for wanted and unwanted effects; the relationship between these indicates the safety margin. The dose ratio between toxic and therapeutic effects is the **therapeutic index** (see FIG. 277–1). In animals it can be expressed as the ratio LD50/ED50, where LD50 is the dose lethal to 50% of a population and the ED50 is the dose therapeutically effective in 50% of a comparable population. The greater the therapeutic index, the greater the safety margin for a particular drug. This concept becomes less important in clinical situations dealing with individuals, where the concern is usually related to nonlethal events and the smallest dose that will be associated

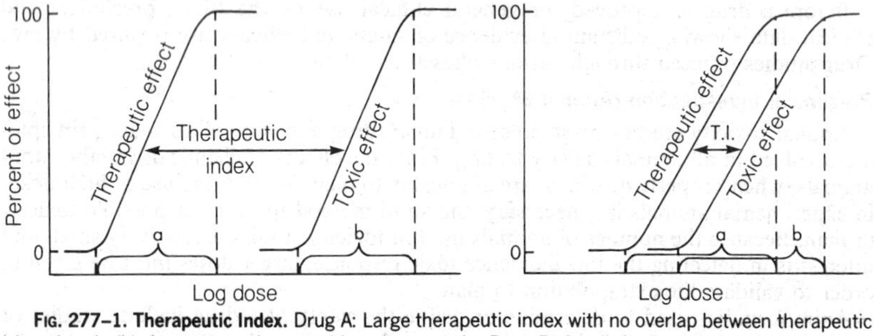

FIG. 277–1. Therapeutic Index. Drug A: Large therapeutic index with no overlap between therapeutic (a) and toxic (b) dose range; thus, a wide safety margin. Drug B: Small therapeutic index with overlap between therapeutic (a) and toxic (b) dose range; thus, a small safety margin.

with a serious toxic reaction. The concept is also more difficult to apply in clinical practice because of the multiplicity of toxic effects, each of which may have its own dose-response curve, and because the toxic and therapeutic curves may not be parallel.

Clinical Investigation (Human Studies)

Clinical studies of new drugs, prior to approval by the FDA for marketing, are conducted in 3 phases. The widespread general use of the drug and postmarketing surveillance of drug use can be regarded as a 4th phase. Some adverse effects of drugs cannot be discerned in animals; eg, symptoms such as dizziness, nausea, headaches, ringing in the ears, heartburn, and depression. It has been estimated that ≥ 50% of undesirable drug effects seen most frequently can be ascertained only during human trials.

Phase 1 represents the first administration of a new drug to man. Informed consent is a prerequisite, as are certain legal requirements; eg, submitting the results of animal studies, information about product composition and manufacture, the intended clinical study protocol, approval from the local Institutional Review Board **(IRB),** and information about the training and experience of the investigators to the FDA, whose permission is required to initiate the study. These investigational drug studies are performed under a permit from the FDA known as an **investigational new drug exemption permit (IND).** A small number of closely monitored subjects, mainly healthy volunteers, are usually involved. Initially, each receives a single dose of the drug to determine a safe dose range and assess pharmacokinetic data. The primary objective of this necessarily cautious phase of the investigation is to determine a safe and tolerated dosage in humans; however, observation of toxicity, if it occurs, and of absorption, metabolism, and excretion may also be made during Phase 1.

Phase 2 can begin after satisfactory preliminary evidence regarding safety has been obtained. It involves the supervised administration of the drug to patients for treatment of, or prophylaxis against, the disease or symptoms for which the drug is intended. These studies usually are conducted in randomized clinical trials comparing the new drug with the prototype drug, if any, for the particular indication. This is also often the first opportunity to observe the effect of long-term administration of the drug to humans. These are the most crucial tests in the development and evaluation of a new drug, since the decision to proceed with extensive trials in large populations must be made on the basis of the data obtained in a relatively small number of patients.

Phase 3 begins after the initial phases have provided reasonable evidence of safety and efficacy. It consists of more widespread clinical trials that may move from the realm of clinical investigators to practicing physicians. Phase 3 extends up to the time of release of the drug for general use. The studies in this phase are intended to yield data on which the sponsor and the FDA can base a decision that the drug is safe and effective for its intended use. As many as 150 clinicians may participate in these studies and the patients under their supervision usually number > 1500 and may even exceed 3000.

There are no definitive rules on what constitutes safety and efficacy. These quantities must be judged in relation to the specific clinical conditions for which the drug is to be used and to alternative therapeutic modalities. When sufficient data have been collected to justify continued use of the drug, a **New Drug Application (NDA)** is submitted. Usually at least 4 yr or more have elapsed between the time the drug was selected on the basis of the original pharmacologic screen and the date of completion and filing of the NDA.

Phase 4 is the study of the actual use of the drug in medical practice and, though often not recognized as a phase of clinical investigation, is a most important one from a clinical standpoint. This postmarketing surveillance that occurs after approval of the NDA is necessary to provide feedback from large-scale use of the drug. New therapeu-

tic or toxic effects may be discovered, including rare or long-term effects that were not discernible in small numbers of patients. The sponsor's claims of drug efficacy and safety that are to appear in brochures and advertising are reviewed and approved by the FDA. Reports concerning current clinical studies must be sent to the FDA periodically during this phase of clinical investigation; specifically, reports are due q 3 mo during the 1st yr, q 6 mo during the 2nd yr, and annually thereafter. These reports must also include information about the quantity of drug distributed and copies of mailing pieces, labeling, and advertising. Also, the manufacturer must transmit to the FDA any unexpected side effects, injury, and toxic or allergic reactions that have been made known to the manufacturer. Thus, the FDA is responsible for assuring that drugs are safe and effective before being marketed, and for continued surveillance of drugs after their introduction into clinical use.

ADVERSE DRUG REACTIONS

Adverse drug reactions (ADRs) embody *a wide variety of toxic drug reactions, dose- or non-dose-related, that occur in therapeutic situations.* The term usually excludes nontherapeutic overdosage (eg, accidental exposure or attempted suicide) or failure of the drug to have its intended effect (ie, excludes lack of efficacy).

Severity of ADRs is usually classified as **mild** (no antidote, therapy, or prolongation of hospitalization necessary); **moderate** (requires a change in drug therapy, although not necessarily cessation of the drug, and may prolong hospitalization or require special treatment); **severe** (potentially life-threatening, requires discontinuation of the drug and specific treatment of the adverse reaction); and **lethal** (directly or indirectly contributes to the death of the patient).

The incidence of ADRs varies widely, from about 1 to 30%. Admission to a hospital because of an ADR has been shown to account for between 3 and 7% of all admissions. Most prospective studies in hospitalized patients (excluding the mildly ill) show ADRs of 10 to 20%. About 10 to 20% of these are severe. The incidence of deaths due to ADRs is unknown; rates of about 0.5 to 0.9% of medical patients have been suggested, but these include many patients with serious and complex diseases.

The incidence and severity of drug toxicity can also be influenced by patient variables such as age, sex, disease, genetic factors, geographic factors, and by drug-related factors such as type of drug, route of administration, duration of therapy, dosage, and bioavailability. The extent to which misprescribing and patient compliance errors contribute to the incidence of ADRs is not clear.

The most commonly reported causes of drug-related deaths are (1) **gastrointestinal hemorrhage and peptic ulceration** (corticosteroids, aspirin, other anti-inflammatory drugs, anticoagulants); (2) **other hemorrhages** (anticoagulants, cytostatic agents); (3) **aplastic anemia** (chloramphenicol, phenylbutazone, gold salts, cytostatic agents; (4) **hepatic damage** (chlorpromazine, isoniazid); (5) **renal failure** (analgesics); (6) **infection** (corticosteroids, cytostatic drugs); and (7) **anaphylaxis** (penicillin, antisera). Allergy is an important factor in nonfatal drug reactions, but is less important as a cause of death.

Dose-Related, Predictable Drug Reactions

Although individuals vary considerably in their responsiveness to a particular drug effect, most drug toxicity is related to the amount of drug taken; the nature of the toxic manifestations is determined by the properties of the drug molecule. Previous contact with the drug is not necessary for the development of toxic reactions. Dose-related reactions can occur as side effects or overdosage toxicity, as defined below.

Side effects are *predictable pharmacologic effects that occur within therapeutic dose ranges and are undesired in the given therapeutic situation.* Side effects may be useful under certain circumstances. For example, the drowsiness produced by an antihista-

mine may be considered a "side effect" in the treatment of an allergy during the day, whereas the sedative-hypnotic effect may contribute to the desired overall therapy in the treatment of the allergy and associated insomnia at bedtime.

Overdosage toxicity is *the predictable toxic effect that occurs with dosages in excess of the therapeutic range for a particular patient.* It overlaps with side-effect toxicity to some extent, especially in drugs with a small therapeutic index. The severity of the reaction is usually dose-related (eg, hemorrhage with oral anticoagulants or convulsions due to local anesthetic agents). Some overdosage toxicity may occur because of drug accumulation caused by ineffective renal elimination or hepatic metabolism of the offending drug.

Non-Dose-Related, Unpredictable Effects

Drug allergy: Allergic reactions depend on altered reactivity of the patient as a result of prior contact with a drug that functions as an antigen or allergen. They are not dose-related; the symptoms and signs that develop are determined by antigen-antibody interactions and are largely independent of the pharmacologic properties of the drug molecule. Allergic reactions are not completely unpredictable; a careful clinical history and appropriate skin tests may suggest those at risk. This subject is discussed in greater detail under DRUG HYPERSENSITIVITY in Ch. 21 (see also DRUG ERUPTIONS in Ch. 237).

Idiosyncrasy is an imprecise term that has been used as a classification for unexpected and peculiar adverse reactions occurring in a small percentage of individuals exposed to a drug. Idiosyncratic reactions are not related to a drug's known pharmacologic effects and are not obviously allergic in nature. The aplastic anemia occurring with chloramphenicol might be considered as an example. Idiosyncrasy has been recently defined by some as *a genetically determined abnormal reactivity to a drug*, but not all idiosyncratic reactions have a pharmacogenetic cause. The term "idiosyncrasy" may become obsolete as specific mechanisms of adverse drug reactions become elucidated (see PHARMACOGENETICS in Ch. 276). For example, hemolysis occurring in individuals taking certain drugs (eg, antimalarials) can no longer be considered idiosyncratic, because a genetic predisposition (G6PD deficiency) can be detected in the laboratory and hemolysis is therefore predictable and dose-related.

Management and Prevention

Prevention requires a familiarity with the drug used and an awareness of the potential reactions to it. Mild ADRs can often be recognized before serious effects develop. If an ADR occurs, the type and any precipitating factors (eg, digitalis toxicity occurring from hypokalemia due to concurrent diuretic therapy) must be determined if possible. With dose-related ADRs, dose modification or attention to precipitating factors may suffice; increasing the rate of drug elimination is rarely necessary. With non-dose-related ADRs, the drug should usually be withdrawn and re-exposure avoided.

CARCINOGENESIS

(See also Ch. 105)

A carcinogen is a *chemical or physical agent that has the potential of producing neoplasia.* Chemical carcinogens are defined by their ability to produce tumors as measured by (1) development of types of tumors not seen in the controls (ie, unique); (2) an increased incidence of tumor types occurring in the treated animals compared to controls; (3) an occurrence of tumors earlier than in the controls; and (4) an increased multiplicity of tumors in individual animals. It is generally accepted that environmental or nutritional factors account for as much as 90% of human cancers. The factors include smoking, dietary habits, and chemical and drug exposure. Genetic, viral, and

radiation factors are estimated to cause the remaining 10%. Most carcinogenic effects of chemicals have a long latency period; 20 to 30 yr is not unusual prior to the development of tumors. Such delayed effects are rarely detected in early clinical trials of new drugs. Chemicals capable of producing cancer in laboratory animals have diverse structures, suggesting a high likelihood that numerous mechanisms are involved in the induction of cancer. Carcinogenesis is believed to be a multistep process with most carcinogens being unreactive compounds (procarcinogens or secondary carcinogens) that are converted in the body to primary carcinogens.

It has been proposed that carcinogens be divided into those that are **genotoxic** and **epigenetic.** The term genotoxic is applied to those agents that function as electrophilic reactants and interact directly with DNA to produce an altered DNA, thus producing or initiating an abnormal cell. Genotoxic compounds include all of the direct acting and primary carcinogens as well as many procarcinogens or secondary carcinogens. The epigenetic agents include those carcinogens for which there is no evidence of genotoxicity. To date, identified drug-carcinogens primarily fall into the epigenetic classification. This category includes some solid state carcinogens, many hormones and immunosuppressants, and the group of compounds called cocarcinogens and promoters (which are not carcinogens per se but potentiate the effects of a carcinogen). Promotion involves increased growth and development of dormant or latent tumor cells, and the time from initiation to the development of the tumor probably depends on the presence of such promoters.

Detection of low incidence of carcinogenic potential is a serious problem during the evaluation phase of new drugs. For example, it is normal for 100 animals to be used in any given dose or study and the incidence of tumor development would have to exceed 4% to be statistically significant. A 4% incidence of tumors would be extremely high for most drug categories.

Drugs with a high carcinogenic potential should be avoided but therapeutic decisions depend upon benefit-risk assessments. For example, though alkylating chemotherapeutic agents are potent carcinogens in a variety of animals, it would be illogical to withhold them from a patient with a potentially lethal disease. (The situation is analogous to exposure to x-rays, which also have carcinogenic potential.)

Very few drugs are in use for which there is good evidence of carcinogenesis in humans. Oral contraceptives appear rarely to cause hepatic adenomas, which are benign in terms of their own growth, but they are extremely vascular and can cause fatal hemorrhage. An association between reserpine and carcinoma of the breast has been claimed by some workers on the basis of case-control studies, but has not been confirmed by others in cohort studies. There is convincing evidence that some nondrug chemicals are carcinogens. This evidence includes the associations between aflatoxins and hepatoma, vinyl chloride and liver hemangiosarcoma, coal tars and skin cancer, cigarette smoke and lung carcinoma, and aniline dyes and bladder tumors.

Short-term mutagenicity testing is developing into a reasonably accurate method of detecting potential carcinogens prior to large-scale human exposure and holds promise of becoming an even better predictor of human carcinogenicity.

BENEFIT-TO-RISK RATIO

In every therapeutic endeavor, risks must be weighed against benefits for each particular clinical situation and patient. Drug therapy is justified only if the possible benefits outweigh the possible risks after considering the qualitative and quantitative impact of the use of a drug and the likely outcome if drug therapy is withheld. This decision depends on adequate clinical knowledge of the patient, knowledge of the disease and its natural history, and knowledge of the drugs and their potential adverse effects.

Although the term benefit-to-risk "ratio" is convenient and often used, for individual patients numerical predictions of benefit or risk do not exist, and the mathematical division (to obtain a ratio) is never performed. A more accurate term is benefit-to-risk "analysis." The following factors must be taken into account:

Patient factors: Age, sex, presence or capability of pregnancy, occupation, social circumstances, genetic traits, etc., may change the magnitude of risks and benefits by influencing the course and severity of the disease or the response to medication. Examples include the poor prognosis of very young or old patients with pneumonia that requires aggressive therapy, the sensitivity of the fetus to drugs that may be relatively safe for a nonpregnant woman, and industrial exposure to organophosphates or genetic cholinesterase deficiency resulting in increased sensitivity to depolarizing muscle relaxants. A 60-yr-old patient with atherosclerosis, a poor cerebral blood flow, and a BP of 200/120 requires different therapy than would an otherwise healthy young patient with the same blood pressure.

Disease factors such as the course, duration, mortality, and morbidity influence risks and benefits of treatment. It makes little sense to treat a self-limiting disease causing little debility, such as herpes labialis with a potent systemic drug such as cytarabine, whereas such therapy may be justified in herpetic encephalitis, which is otherwise usually fatal.

Drug factors include the frequency, severity, and predictability of adverse reactions, the relationship of such reactions to dosage, the means by which they can be prevented or treated, and the availability of alternative drugs or therapies. For example, penicillin anaphylaxis is rare, but it is potentially fatal and may sometimes be avoided by taking an adequate history and doing appropriate skin tests. If anaphylaxis occurs when one is prepared for it, successful treatment is possible. Penicillin, therefore, should not ordinarily be withheld in streptococcal pharyngitis for fear of anaphylaxis. On the other hand, aplastic anemia due to chloramphenicol is also fatal and relatively rare, but it is unpredictable and often irreversible. Therefore, although chloramphenicol is also effective against streptococcal pharyngitis, safer alternatives exist, and its use is not justified. However, for a serious disease such as *Haemophilus influenzae* meningitis, few alternative drugs exist and chloramphenicol therapy may be justified.

A drug's efficacy should also be known, including the predictability of a favorable response, whether the effect is symptomatic or curative, the relationship to dosage, and the duration of the beneficial effect. Acute myeloid leukemia in children responds to aggressive combination chemotherapy and is justified. However, use of aggressive chemotherapy is debatable in such malignancies as gastric carcinoma, where the response to chemotherapy is poor and therapy may increase morbidity.

Judicious use of drug combinations may increase benefits and reduce risks; eg, the use of adrenergic blocking agents with a thiazide diuretic and potassium supplements in the treatment of hypertension.

---

278. PATIENT COMPLIANCE

The degree to which patients adhere to a treatment plan.

Even the most thorough and well-designed therapeutic regimen will fail without patient compliance. Depending on the variable studied and the strictness of definition, from 15% to 95% of patients studied have been found to be noncompliant. Overall, probably a third to a half of patients make some error with their medications—incorrect dose, errors in timing, adding unprescribed medications, or not taking medication. Capricious or irregular dosing exposes a patient to the risks of medication without

concomitant therapeutic benefit. While most patients occasionally default or make errors, some never stray and others continually fail to comply.

It is difficult to identify patients who do not take their medications as prescribed. The same patient may act differently depending on the treatment, disease, adverse effects, or other factors in his life. In dealing with noncompliance, *the prescriber must discuss it with the patient and ascertain why the patient is not following the prescribed treatment*. The cause for noncompliance may be remediable with such a discussion, or the therapeutic regimen may need to be modified.

Patient factors in noncompliance: Age, sex, race, and educational level are not predictors of compliance. "Forgetfulness" is the most frequently cited reason, but it is not really an explanation. It may be a rationalization to cover unconscious or partly conscious concerns about the patient's health status, his diagnosis, and the taking of medication. Commonly, there is fear of adverse effects, of addiction, of the disease state that treatment implies, and of loss of independence. For example, patients with hypertension have an asymptomatic disease and must cope with medical advice from physicians, public health advertisements, and well-intentioned friends regarding their risks of stroke, heart attack, and renal disease. Many deal with the resultant anxiety by attempts at denial of illness, a prominent sign of which is neglecting to take medication. In other cases, medications may be stopped because symptoms and signs decrease or disappear. Although medications comprise a small fraction of total personal health expenditures, some patients decrease the dose or the duration of treatment to save money. More rarely, a patient may not fill the prescription at all for financial or other reasons.

Medication factors in noncompliance: Complex regimens with frequent dosing or many medications increase errors in dosage times, scheduling with meals, etc. If preparations look alike, patients may confuse medications and inadvertently repeat or omit doses. Other factors include adverse effects (real or imagined), unpleasant tastes or smells, and precautions imposed by therapeutic regimens (eg, no alcohol or cheese).

Disease factors in noncompliance: Certain types of illness, such as chronic diseases with day-to-day fluctuation in symptoms (or without symptoms), seem to be important in predisposing to compliance problems. When prophylactic medication is prescribed or when the medication causes more symptoms than the disease under therapy (eg, hypertension), noncompliance or defaulting is more likely.

The physician's role in improving patient compliance: Making a correct diagnosis and designing a simple, effective therapeutic regimen starts the therapeutic process. Good communication between the physician and the patient is essential. Directions must be clear, precise, and tailored to the vagaries and necessities of the patient's life and the disease process. Adverse effects should be discussed in a general way and the patient urged to mention the appearance of undesired or unexpected effects to a physician prior to stopping medication. Inappropriate termination of the therapeutic regimen may be prevented if the physician explains the delay associated with the onset of apparent benefit characteristic of some drugs, eg, antidepressants. Inquiring about adherence to the regimen and the reasons for any problems may help to correct noncompliance and is necessary, since patients often do not volunteer such information. The belief that education promotes rational choices and improves compliance is not supported by hard evidence. Dealing specifically with patient factors that underlie noncompliance is far more effective. Trust—in the personal physician, in the prescribed therapy, or perhaps in medical science in general—appears most crucial to patient compliance. Explaining the purpose of the components in the regimen and the beneficial and adverse effects of a medication, as well as its shape, color, and dosage schedule, are educational; but, more important, they may help create a relationship of trust.

The pharmacist's and nurse's role in improving compliance: Nurses or pharmacists may detect compliance problems. Information that patients do not discuss with physicians may be transmitted to less threatening figures and can be relayed to the physician; eg, by the pharmacist who notes that the patient cannot pay for a full prescription or does not obtain refills. Illogical or incorrect prescriptions, which may decrease compliance, may be noted by a pharmacist and corrected in consultation with the prescriber. Nurses and pharmacists may instruct patients on their medications, especially prior to discharge from the hospital. By reviewing the physical characteristics of medications, directions, side effects, drug interactions, precautions, specific patient concerns, and the necessity for each medication with the patient, they can uncover misunderstandings and fears and can enhance the patient's knowledge. Some institutions have experimented with programs of inpatient self-medication under supervision with promising results.

The role of the pharmaceutical industry and pharmacologists in improving compliance: The pharmaceutical industry and pharmacologists can help by discovering effective medications with few adverse effects and convenient dosage schedules. Making medications taste better and varying the shape and color of tablets also help. Better sustained-release and rational combination products may help improve compliance by reducing the number of doses needed per day and the number of medications ingested. New formulations and routes of administration (transcutaneous, sustained release, etc) have diminished some of the nuisance aspects of chronic medication ingestion.

Pharmacologists contribute to compliance by studying ways in which medications can be administered to take advantage of their pharmacokinetic properties with the goal of reducing missed doses and errors. For example, many psychotropic drugs have long half-lives and can be given once a day in a large dose (eg, at bedtime) instead of in 3 or 4 smaller doses throughout the day. Better definition of the patients who will respond to a medication and of those at risk for adverse effects should help the physician to assess pharmacologic response, maximize benefit, and design an optimum dosage schedule of the logical agent.

Misuse of medication, such as taking outdated prescription drugs or those prescribed for other apparently similar illnesses, also forms part of a broadened definition of compliance to therapy. Following the spirit but not the sense of prescription directions is another type of noncompliance. Examples include inappropriate ingestion of certain medications with food, and taking medications with interacting over-the-counter preparations. In addition, taking excessive doses or taking doses at inappropriate times of day that may result in adverse effects (eg, diuretics prior to bedtime) are another form of noncompliance that health professionals must watch for.

Patients may not take medications for valid and important reasons. In fact, "intelligent non-compliance" (where the patient discontinues or decreases the dose of medication based on a correct interpretation of the clinical situation) may decrease adverse effects and improve the therapeutic outcome. Too often, however, the therapist does not know of these efficacious maneuvers. If the patient can act as a therapeutic monitor, noting desirable and detrimental effects, then communicating these observations to the physician, both will benefit. The physician can better adjust therapy, exploring the dose-effect relationship or discontinuing unneeded drugs. Patients are more likely to have a satisfactory outcome through adherence to the *cooperatively* designed program. Finally, physicians can gain valuable knowledge about responses to medication and the course of a disease which may be valuable in treating other patients. Such cooperative compliance demands patient and physician education about therapeutic monitoring and involves time, money, and sharing responsibility. Nevertheless, it would seem beneficial to expend the time and effort to achieve cooperative compliance.

279. PLACEBOS

Inactive substances used in controlled studies for comparison with presumed active drugs or prescribed with the intent to relieve symptoms or meet a patient's demands. A placebo may be any type of therapeutic maneuver, including surgical and psychologic technics or medication in any form (eg, oral, parenteral, topical), but this discussion is limited to drug formulations.

The term placebo harks back to the 116th Psalm in the Hebrew Bible. Through a number of translating errors, the Vulgate Latin version came to contain the word "placebo" (I shall please). Over the centuries, the term placebo was applied to the Vespers for the Dead, derisively to servile flatterers and toadies, and to laments sung at funerals by professional mourners.

In 1785, the word placebo appeared in a medical dictionary for the first time as "a commonplace method or medicine." Two editions later, the placebo had become a "make-believe medicine," allegedly inert and harmless. We now know that administration of placebos may have profound effects, both good and bad.

The Binary Nature of Placebo Effects

The medical literature is replete with reports on the power of the placebo to help patients with anxiety, tension, melancholia, schizophrenia, pain of all sorts, headaches, cough, insomnia, seasickness, chronic bronchitis, the common cold, arthritis, peptic ulcer, hypertension, nausea, and senile dementia, among others. But the placebo is not only able to help; it has also been associated with "side effects." These have included nausea, headache, dizziness, sleepiness, insomnia, fatigue, depression, numbness, hallucinations, itching, vomiting, tremor, tachycardia, diarrhea, pallor, rashes, hives, ataxia, and edema, to name only a partial list.

This remarkable list of *subjective and objective* changes, both desirable and unwanted, becomes more understandable and is put into perspective once one recognizes that there are 2 components of the placebo response. One is the anticipation (usually optimistic) of effects because of the expectations associated with medication. One can call this "suggestibility," "faith," "hope," or whatever.

The 2nd component, however, is at times even more important— spontaneous change. If a placebo has been taken before spontaneous improvement, it may be given credit, just as a placebo may be blamed if someone spontaneously develops a headache or a rash after taking an inert capsule or tablet.

The "Placebo Reactor"

Studies to determine whether or not certain personality characteristics correlate with responses to placebos have disagreed extravagantly with one another. This is not surprising, since some investigators have called a "placebo reactor" one who gets benefit from placebos, and others have used the term for people who report side effects after placebos. It seems unlikely that the same personality traits would predispose to such different types of responses.

It is probably more correct to talk about a spectrum of "placebo reactivity" than about placebo reactors, since virtually anyone is suggestible under some circumstances. However, some people seem more prone to influence than others. We can only speculate, but these differences at times may relate to the recipient's personality; eg, dependent personalities, who tend to want to please their physicians, may be more likely to report beneficial effects, and histrionic personalities may be more likely to note some sort of effect, good or bad. Probably the most important factors are those that relate to specific attitudes toward the illness, medications, and physician. For example, when a patient with acute pain has a favorable attitude toward medicines and is given the placebo by a concerned and confident physician, a better response

may occur than when a patient has chronic pain, views drugs as dangerous chemicals, and is given the placebo by a gruff physician who appears uncertain.

Placebo addicts: At least 2 patients have been reported who were addicted to placebos. One consumed 10,000 placebos in 1 yr. The other showed many of the characteristics of a true drug addict: a tendency to increase the dose; inability to stop the "medicine" without psychiatric help; a compulsive desire to take the tablets; and an abstinence syndrome when deprived of the tablets.

Use in Research

Difficulty in sorting out the 2 components of the placebo response does not detract from the utility of the placebo as a standard in clinical trials, where it serves in much the same way as a "blank" serves the chemist to assay "background noise" that must be subtracted from the overall treatment effect. Whatever the relative importance of suggestibility and spontaneous change, the drug must perform better than placebo to justify its being marketed. In some studies, eg, comparison with a new drug to relieve angina pectoris, relief with placebo commonly exceeds 50%, presenting quite a challenge to demonstrate effectiveness with an active agent.

Use in Therapy

There is a placebo element in every therapeutic maneuver; therefore, the effects of a drug will vary from patient to patient and doctor to doctor, depending on placebo reactivity. People with a "positive" orientation to drugs, doctors, nurses, hospitals, etc. are more likely to respond favorably to placebos than are people with a "negative" orientation. The latter may deny benefit or complain of untoward effects. Thus, as with any other prescribed agent, giving a placebo has potential benefits and risks that must be evaluated. A positive placebo effect is more likely when both patient and doctor believe that therapeutic benefit will result from a drug. Thus, an active agent with no pharmacologic effect on the process being treated (eg, vitamin B_{12} in a patient with arthritis) may provide a favorable response, or a mildly active agent may have an enhanced effect (eg, a vasodilator in a patient with intermittent claudication).

With deliberate placebo use (which is extraordinarily rare in clinical practice, as opposed to research trials), in addition to the adverse effects described above, there are several major **hazards:** (1) Since the doctor is deceiving the patient, there may be an adverse alteration in the doctor-patient relationship. At the very least, the doctor must be more guarded, lest his deception be discovered. Should it be discovered, the patient will lose face, feel betrayed, and his confidence in the physician will be impaired. (2) The doctor may misinterpret the patient's response; particularly pernicious is the unwarranted conclusion that a positive response means that the patient's symptoms are psychogenic or neurotically exaggerated. (3) Where other doctors or nurses are involved in the deception (as in a group practice or hospital setting), the potential for adversely modifying the attitudes and behaviors of any or all of the others toward the patient and the potential for discovery are greatly increased. Considering the availability of a host of drugs that have at least the potential to alleviate most of the complaints seen in practice and the danger of destroying a patient-doctor relationship with placebo use, placebos qua placebos are rarely indicated.

Today, doctors may prescribe vitamin "tonics" or B_{12} injections that are often tantamount to placebos, although they rarely prescribe lactose tablets or "sterile hypos." For example, most young physicians pick up patients from another doctor who has left practice. Often, a physician acquires patients who have taken B_{12} or other vitamins as a "tonic" with great faith and perceived benefit for many years; denied their "medicine," such patients often feel ill and can become seriously upset. Based on cultural or psychologic sets, some patients genuinely seem to require and obtain benefit from either an unrequired medication or a particular dosage form (eg, by injection when an oral agent should suffice). Denying them may result in their turning to unscrupulous

charlatans and sometimes hazardous practices. In dealing with incurable chronic or malignant disease, placebos may also offer needed hope.

---

280. NEUROTRANSMISSION

Introduction

A **neurotransmitter (NT)** *is defined as a chemical that is selectively released from a nerve terminal by an action potential, interacts with a specific receptor on an adjacent structure, and produces a specific physiologic response.* The following criteria must be satisfied before a chemical can qualify as a NT: (1) The chemical must be present in the nerve terminal; (2) The chemical must be released from the nerve terminal by an action potential; (3) The chemical when applied experimentally to the receptor must produce the identical effect as would stimulation of the presynaptic neuron. Although evidence exists from in vitro and animal studies that certain chemicals function as NTs, little such evidence is available for human nerve tissue. Thus, all the NTs discussed below should be understood as being putative NTs in humans.

A nerve cell or neuron has 2 major distinguishing functions—propagation of the action potential along the axon, and transmission of the signal from the nerve to another nerve or cell structure (receptor) to elicit a response (eg, nerve impulse, muscle contraction). While impulses conducted along an axon are electrical in nature, the transmission of impulses from one neuron to another neuron or to a non-neuronal cell is chemical and depends upon specific NTs. All NTs derive from amino acids (or related compounds such as choline). Certain neurons synthesize only one, neuron-specific NT; others have been shown to synthesize 2 or more NTs. Some neurons modify amino acids to form the "amine" transmitters (eg, norepinephrine, serotonin, acetylcholine); others combine amino acids to form "polypeptide" transmitters (eg, endorphins, enkephalins), and still other neurons use amino acids unchanged or synthesized as transmitters.

A particular neuron generates the same action potential all the time and conducts it at a fixed speed along the axon. Thus, nerve propagation is basically an "all or none" response that is not subject to modulation. Drugs either do not affect propagation or abolish it completely (eg, local anesthetics). Only a few diseases alter the structure of the nerve (eg, multiple sclerosis) and interfere with propagation.

In contrast, transmission via NTs is a highly sensitive process that can be increased or decreased to accommodate any given physiologic situation. Many drugs modulate this process and many neurologic and psychiatric diseases are caused by an over-or-underactivity of neuronal transmission (see below).

Basic Principles of Neurotransmission

Neurotransmission involves (1) synthesis and storage of the NT in the prejunctional nerve structure; (2) release of the NT from the nerve terminal; (3) interaction of the NT with the postjunctional structure (receptor); and (4) rapid termination of the NT-receptor interaction (see FIG. 280–1).

The cell body, which contains the nucleus and DNA, forms the enzymes that are involved in the **synthesis** of most NTs. These enzymes act on precursor molecules that are taken up by the neuron to form the NT.

Storage of the NT occurs at the nerve terminal in distinct vesicles. These NT molecules are usually bound to specific proteins in the presence of ATP and certain cations. The amount of NT in one vesicle (usually several thousand) is termed a quantum.

Some NT molecules are constantly leaving the terminal, but the amounts are insufficient to elicit a significant physiologic response. However, an action potential arriving

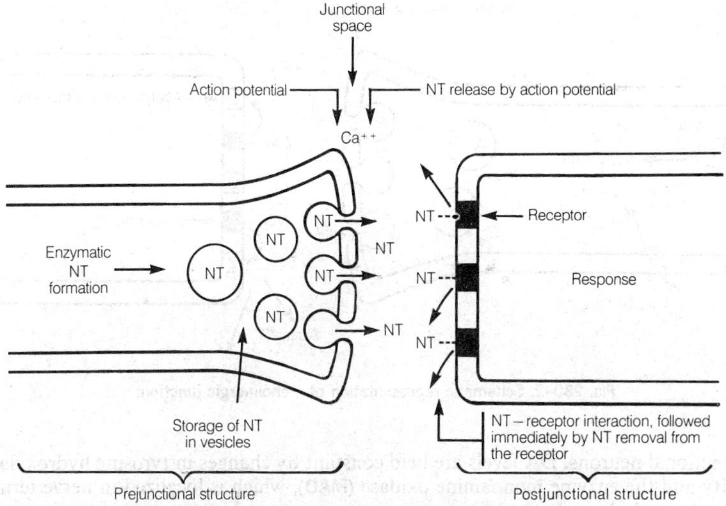

FIG. 280–1. Schematic representation of neurotransmission.

at the terminal (aided by a flux of Ca^{++}) causes the simultaneous **release** of NT molecules from many vesicles by fusing the walls of these vesicles to that of the nerve terminal and causing formation of an opening through which the NT molecules are expelled into the synaptic cleft (exocytosis).

The quanta released from these vesicles diffuse across the cleft and bind briefly to **receptors,** causing their activation and a physiologic response. NTs can be *excitatory* (initiation of a new action potential) or *inhibitory* (inhibition of the development of a new action potential). The response of non-neuronal structures (eg, skeletal, smooth or cardiac muscle cells, and glands) may also be stimulatory or inhibitory.

To assure rapid, consecutive activation of the same receptors ("morse code"), the NT-receptor interaction is followed by **termination.** The NT is quickly "pumped" back by active processes (reuptake) into the nerve terminals, destroyed by enzymes located near the receptors, or diffused into the surroundings.

Major Neurotransmitters (NTs)

Acetylcholine (Ach), the major NT of the motoneurons, autonomic preganglionic fibers, postganglionic cholinergic (parasympathetic) fibers, and many neurons in the CNS (basal ganglia, motor cortex) is synthesized from choline and mitochondrially derived acetyl-coenzyme A by the enzyme choline acetyltransferase **(CAT).** Upon release, Ach stimulates cholinergic receptors of adjacent structures. This interaction is rapidly terminated by hydrolysis of Ach to choline and acetate by the enzyme acetylcholinesterase **(ACE)** that is found on neurons and neuromuscular junctions. The levels of acetylcholine are regulated by the activity of choline acetyltransferase and by choline uptake (see FIG. 280–2).

Dopamine (DA) is the NT of some peripheral nerve fibers and of many central neurons (eg, substantia nigra, midbrain, hypothalamus). The amino acid tyrosine is taken up by dopaminergic neurons, converted by the enzyme tyrosine hydroxylase to 3,4-dihydroxyphenylalanine **(DOPA),** decarboxylated by the enzyme aromatic L-amino acid decarboxylase to DA, and stored in vesicles. After release, DA interacts with dopaminergic receptors and is then "pumped" back by active processes (reuptake) into the

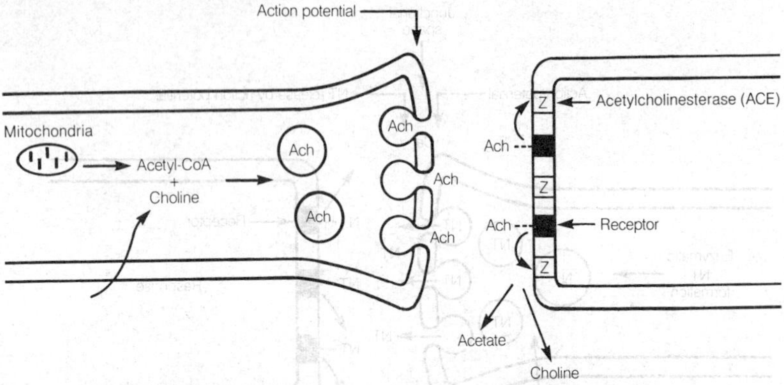

Fig. 280–2. Schematic representation of a cholinergic junction.

prejunctional neurons. DA levels are held constant by changes in tyrosine hydroxylase activity and the enzyme monoamine oxidase **(MAO)**, which is localized in nerve terminals and metabolizes dopamine.

Norepinephrine (NE) is the NT of most postganglionic sympathetic fibers and many central neurons (eg, locus ceruleus, hypothalamus). NE synthesis, like that of DA, also starts with the precursor tyrosine but continues as the DA is hydroxylated by dopamine-β-hydroxylase to form NE, which is stored in vesicles. Upon release, NE interacts with adrenergic receptors. This action is terminated largely by the re-uptake of NE back into the prejunctional neurons (see Fig. 280–3). Tyrosine hydroxylase and MAO regulate intraneuronal NE levels. Metabolism of NE occurs via MAO and catechol-O-methyltransferase (COMT) to inactive metabolites (eg, normetanephrine, 3-methoxy-4-hydroxyphenylethylene glycol [MHPG], 3-methoxy-4-hydroxymandelic acid [VMA]).

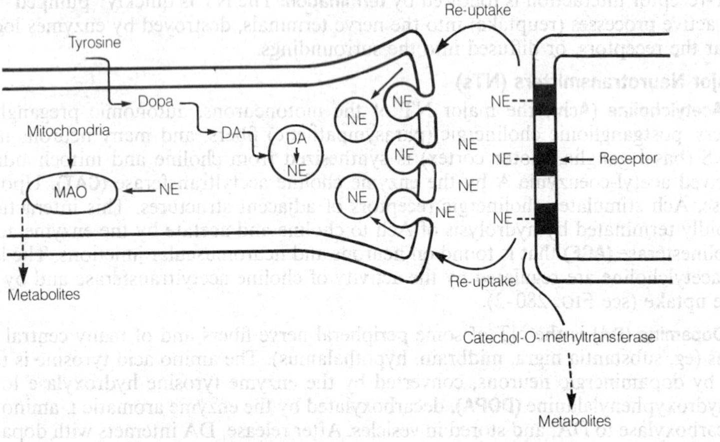

Fig. 280–3. Schematic representation of an adrenergic junction.

Serotonin (5-HT) is the NT of many central neurons (eg, raphe nucleus). Its synthesis begins with the uptake of tryptophan into serotonergic neurons. Tryptophan is hydroxylated by the enzyme tryptophan hydroxylase to 5-hydroxytryptophan, and then decarboxylated to serotonin (5-hydroxytryptamine) by the enzyme aromatic L-amino acid decarboxylase. Levels of 5-HT are controlled by the uptake of tryptophan and intraneuronal MAO. Metabolism occurs mainly via MAO to 5-hydroxyindoleacetic acid.

γ-Aminobutyric acid (GABA) is a major inhibitory NT in the CNS and is found in many central neurons (eg, basal ganglia, cerebellum). GABA is derived from glutamate, which is decarboxylated by glutamic acid decarboxylase. After interaction with receptors, GABA is actively "pumped" back into the prejunctional neurons. Regulation of intraneuronal GABA levels is not well understood.

β-Endorphin (β-End) is a polypeptide and is the transmitter of many central neurons (eg, hypothalamus, amygdala, periventricular thalamus, locus ceruleus). In the cell body, amino acids are assembled by several enzymes into a large polypeptide, called pro-opiocortin. This polypeptide is transported down the axon and is cleaved by specific peptidases into fragments, one of which is β-End containing 31 amino acids. After interaction with peptidergic (opioid) receptors, it is hydrolyzed by peptidases into smaller, inactive peptides and amino acids. Regulation of intraneuronal β-End levels is incompletely understood.

Methionine-enkephalin and leucine-enkephalin are the NTs of many central neurons (eg, globus pallidus, thalamus, caudate, central gray). Their synthesis is similar to that of endorphin in that larger precursor peptides are formed in the cell body (proenkephalin A and B) and split by specific peptidases in the axon into smaller peptides. Two of the fragments are the enkephalins having 5 amino acids and either methionine or leucine as the terminal amino acid. After interaction with peptidergic (opioid) receptors, the enkephalins are hydrolyzed by other peptidases into smaller, inactive peptides and amino acids. Regulation of intraneuronal enkephalin levels is not well understood.

Substance P is a peptide and is the transmitter of many central neurons (eg, dorsal root ganglia, basal ganglia, hypothalamus). Its synthesis and fate are similar to those of the endorphins and enkephalins.

Glycine, glutamate, and aspartate are NTs used directly by certain neurons without change (although glycine might also be synthesized from serine). Aspartate is mainly present in the cortex, glutamate in the cerebellum and spinal cord, and glycine in the interneurons of the spinal cord.

Other neurotransmitters, whose roles in neurotransmission have not been firmly established, include **epinephrine, histamine, vasopressin, vasoactive intestinal peptide, carnosine, bradykinin,** and others.

Major Receptors

A receptor is a small binding or recognition site (possessing a specific molecular configuration) on a cell surface that causes a physiologic response upon stimulation by a NT or other chemical, such as a drug or toxin. Some receptors cause inhibitory (eg, relaxation of a muscle) or excitatory (eg, contraction of a muscle) physiologic responses.

Receptors are protein complexes that are continuously synthesized and degraded. Their half-lives range from days to weeks. The number of receptors and their affinity for specific NT molecules is not constant but will vary. Receptors that are continuously stimulated by NTs or drugs (agonists) become hyposensitive **("down-regulation"),** whereas receptors that are not stimulated by their NT or are blocked by drugs (antago-

nist) become hypersensitive **("up-regulation")**. The result is a decreased or increased physiologic response of the effector cell.

Most NTs interact primarily with the **postsynaptic receptor (R-1)** to produce a physiologic response in the adjacent structure (see FIG. 280–4). However, receptors are also located on presynaptic neurons that control the release of a specific NT. These receptors can be divided into different classes. The **autoreceptors (R-2)** respond only to released NT and are of 2 types: (R-2,+) that increase the release of NT, and (R-2,) that inhibit the release of NT. These autoreceptors cause a brief, intense release of the NT as shown in FIG. 280–4. **Presynaptic receptors (R-3)** opposite impinging neurons can also increase or inhibit the release of a NT. In addition, **receptors for neuromodulators (R-4)** or substances that are not released from nerve terminals (eg, steroids, prostaglandins) can modulate the release of the NT. However, the following discussion will center mostly on postsynaptic receptors.

Receptors always interact physiologically with their respective NT. For instance, Ach released from cholinergic neurons interacts with all cholinergic receptors to produce a response. However, not all cholinergic receptors are identical and subclasses exist. Such subclasses reveal themselves by the action of chemicals or drugs. For example, muscarine preferentially stimulates only cholinergic receptors located on effector cells innervated by postganglionic cholinergic (parasympathetic) fibers, whereas nicotine preferentially stimulates only those cholinergic receptors located on skeletal muscle cells, autonomic ganglia, and the adrenal medulla. For this reason, the first receptors are called muscarinic and the latter, nicotinic receptors. This allows for the more selective action of drugs; ie, drugs can be developed that will not stimulate all cholinergic receptors, but only those of the muscarinic *or* nicotinic type.

Cholinergic receptors can be divided into nicotinic N_1 (adrenal medulla, autonomic ganglia) and N_2 (skeletal muscle) receptors as well as muscarinic M_1 (autonomic system, corpus striatum) and M_2 (autonomic system, hindbrain, cerebellum) receptors.

Adrenergic receptors can be divided into α_1 (postsynaptic in the sympathetic system) and α_2 (presynaptic in the sympathetic system and postsynaptic in the brain) receptors as well as β_1 (heart) and β_2 (other sympathetically innervated structures) receptors.

Dopamine receptors (cortex, limbic system, basal ganglia) can be categorized into D_1 receptors linked to a dopamine sensitive adenylate cyclase system, and D_2 receptors not linked to this enzyme.

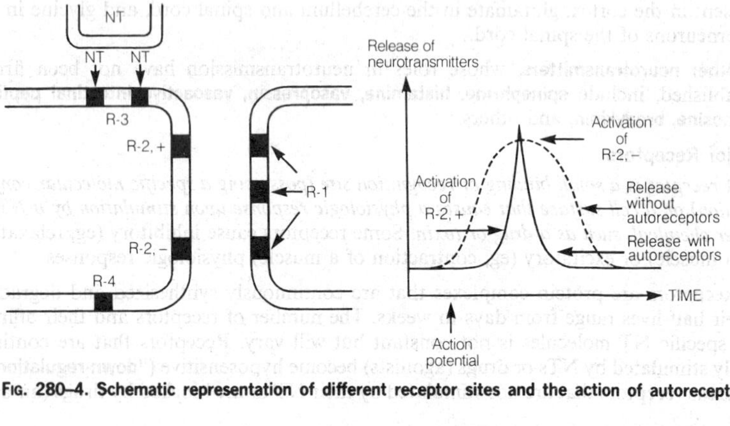

FIG. 280–4. Schematic representation of different receptor sites and the action of autoreceptors.

Serotonin (5-HT) receptors can be divided into serotonin 5-HT_1 and 5-HT_2 receptors whose exact locations are unclear.

Endorphin-enkephalin or opioid receptors are divided into mu (central pain regions), delta (limbic region), kappa (cerebral cortex), and sigma (hippocampus) receptors.

Specific receptors also exist for the other NTs but the existence of subclasses is still uncertain.

Second messenger system: Stimulation of some receptors by a NT causes a direct response of the cell (eg, opening of a Na^+ channel to cause an excitatory response or opening of Cl^- and K^+ channels to cause an inhibitory response); however, stimulation of other receptors by a NT ("first messenger") first activates a specific system causing formation of specific molecules (**"second" messenger**), which then produce the final cellular response.

Adenosine 3′,5′-monophosphate (**c-AMP**), guanosine 3′,5′-monophosphate (**c-GMP**), and inositol triphosphate (**IP3**) are "second" messengers and are synthesized by a complex series of reactions in the cell wall. A simplified version for the formation and action of c-AMP is shown in FIG. 280–5.

Pathology of Neurotransmission

Defects in the process of NT storage, release, synthesis, degradation, and changes in receptor sensitivity may occur that can lead to faulty transmission resulting in clinical disorders.

Defects in the synthesis, storage and/or release of a specific NT can lead to increased or decreased concentrations of NT in the synaptic cleft, resulting in improperly stimulated receptors. For example, it has been postulated that depression is associated with decreased synthesis and release of norepinephrine and/or serotonin in the brain, Parkinson's disease with reduced levels of presynaptic dopamine, Huntington's chorea with decreased levels of GABA, and mania with an excessive release of norepinephrine.

Increases or decreases in the affinity and/or number of receptors caused indirectly by changes in NT stimulation ("up or down regulation") or directly by pathologic changes of the receptor structure can alter the resulting physiologic response. For example, it has been postulated that destruction of neuromuscular acetylcholine receptors by antibodies leads to myasthenia gravis, hypersensitive dopamine receptors to schizophrenia and tardive dyskinesia, and hypersensitive β receptors (secondary to NE changes) to depression.

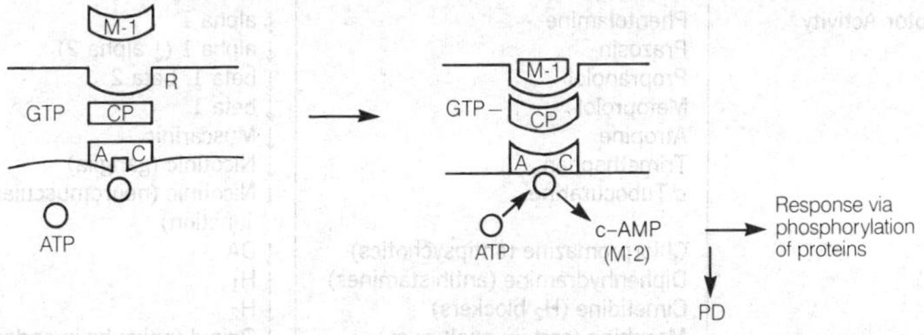

FIG. 280–5. Schematic representation of the formation of c-AMP. M-1 = Neurotransmitter ("first" messenger); R = Receptor; CP = Coupling protein (guanine nucleotide-binding regulatory protein); GTP-CP = Guanosine triphosphate complex protein, which activates AC; M-2 = c-AMP ("second" messenger); AC = Adenylate cyclase, which forms c-AMP; PD = Phosphodiesterase, which destroys c-AMP.

Pharmacology of Neurotransmission

Most drugs that affect the nervous system modulate the neurotransmission process. Correction of the neurotransmission defect that causes the disease therefore constitutes the mechanism underlying the therapeutic effect of such drugs. Interference with other, normal NT processes constitutes the mode of action of the side effects.

Drugs can increase or decrease the synthesis, storage, release, or degradation of a specific NT. This will usually occur in all neurons in the body and brain and these drugs are not very selective in their action on a specific organ. For instance, ephedrine increases the release of norepinephrine from all norepinephrine containing neurons and the released NE will stimulate all norepinephrine or adrenergic receptors in the body.

Drugs can more selectively stimulate (agonists) or block (antagonists) certain recep-

TABLE 280–1. EXAMPLES OF DRUG ACTION ON NEUROTRANSMISSION AND THE RESULTING EFFECTS

Process	*Drug*	*Result (Response)*
↑ NT Synthesis	L-DOPA	↑ DA
	Tryptophan	↑ 5-HT
↓ NT Synthesis	α-Methyl-DOPA (?)	↓ NE
↓ NT Storage	Reserpine	↓ NE, ↓ 5-HT
↑ NT Release	Ephedrine	↑ NE
↓ NT Release	Lithium	↓ NE, ↓ DA
↓ NT Uptake	Cocaine	↑ NE*
	Imipramine (antidepressant tricyclics)	↑ NE*
↓ NT Metabolism	Phenelzine (MAO-inhibitors)	↑ NE, ↑ 5-HT
	Neostigmine (anticholinesterases)	↑ Ach*
↑ Receptor Activity	Phenylephrine	↑ alpha 1
	Clonidine	↑ alpha 2†
	Epinephrine	↑ beta 1, beta 2 (plus alpha)
	Metaproterenol	↑ beta 2
	Neostigmine (certain anticholinesterases)	↑ Nicotinic
	Pilocarpine	↑ Muscarinic
	Diazepam‡ (anxiolytics)	↑ GABA
↓ Receptor Activity	Phentolamine	↓ alpha 1
	Prazosin	↓ alpha 1 (↓ alpha 2)
	Propranolol	↓ beta 1, beta 2
	Metoprolol	↓ beta 1
	Atropine	↓ Muscarinic
	Trimethaphan	↓ Nicotinic (ganglia)
	d-Tubocurarine	↓ Nicotinic (neuromuscular junction)
	Chlorpromazine (antipsychotics)	↓ DA
	Diphenhydramine (antihistamines)	↓ H_1
	Cimetidine (H_2 blockers)	↓ H_2
	Morphine (certain analgesics)	↓ Opioid (enkephalin-endorphin)

* In the synaptic or junctional space.
† Dose and time dependent.
‡ Acts on a regular or modular component of the GABA receptor and increases GABA binding and activity.

tors. Due to the presence of specific subsets of receptors on certain tissues, such drugs are often more selective (concentration dependent) in their effects; for instance, the sympathomimetic drug phenylephrine will activate only α-adrenergic receptors (see TABLE 280–1).

281. DRUGS ACTING ON THE CENTRAL NERVOUS SYSTEM

OPIOID ANALGESICS AND ANTAGONISTS
(Narcotic Analgesics and Antagonists)

Narcotic: *A drug derived from opium or an opium-like substance, that relieves pain, alters mood and behavior, and possesses the potential for dependence and tolerance.* **Opioid:** *A generic term describing substances, natural or synthetic, that bind to opiate receptors and produce an agonist action.* **Opioid antagonist:** *Opioid-like substances that bind to opiate receptors but produce little or no agonist activity.* The emergence of the concept of specific opiate receptors in the brain and the discovery of the endogenous endorphins and enkephalins has greatly enhanced our understanding of the mechanism of pain relief or analgesia. Consequently, the term "narcotic," while still important in medical-legal parlance, is becoming obsolete in pharmacology. While some authors designate the semisynthetic derivatives of opium as "opiates" and the synthetic compounds as "opioids," we prefer the term "opioid" for all such substances, natural, semisynthetic, or synthetic that activate opiate receptors.

Opioid analgesics and antagonists are among the most effective and valuable medications for treatment of serious pain. They are most often useful in acute short-term painful states such as the postoperative period. Patients with visceral pain seem to respond better to opioid analgesics although they are effective in any serious pain syndrome. They should be used judiciously, but not withheld for fear of adverse effects in patients with severe pain. The underlying cause of the pain should be sought and removed if possible. Therapeutic goals vary with the etiology, nature, and expected duration of the pain, and with the location of the treatment facility (home or hospital). A reasonable goal is to decrease pain to a level that allows the patient to eat, sleep, and convalesce with minimal disturbance. Since each patient is his own bioassay system, dosage should be modified after assessing the patient's response.

Drugs that exert their effect peripherally at the locus of pain (eg, local anesthetics, certain anti-inflammatory analgesics) usually relieve pain without disrupting the patient's ability to function. In contrast, centrally acting drugs alter the patient's perception of pain, tend to sedate, and may decrease his ability to function and limit him to bedrest. Patients with severe pain can often tolerate higher analgesic doses without untoward CNS depression, but such resistance disappears once the pain has been controlled. The patient's respiratory function and ability to clear tracheobronchial secretions must be maintained.

Opioid analgesics are often underused, resulting in needless suffering. The required dose is often underestimated and the duration of action overestimated. Physician and nurse's concerns about development of addiction are often excessive. Hospitalized patients given even large doses of opioids for 10 days or longer very rarely develop addiction. Adequate pain relief produced early during therapy may decrease the total amount of medication needed and increase the patient's comfort. This may be accomplished in the hospital by giving the drug **at the request of the patient** but no more often

than q 1 h for the first two doses. After that, it should be given no more often than q 3 h. The patient should be asked q 4 h if medication is needed. It is often helpful to analyze the 24 h pattern of a patient's pain. An increased or supplemental dose of analgesic at a particular time (eg, prior to a bath or procedure) may lessen discomfort dramatically and diminish the overall need for pain medication. Another approach is to administer the analgesic on a **fixed schedule.** This usually results in less total drug administered as steady-state levels provide continual relief of pain, permitting the patient to rest or sleep without constant anxiety over requesting medication, etc.

Opioid effects apparently are mediated via specific receptors in the CNS and other peripheral organs. Endogenous opioids (enkephalins, endorphins) are the primary ligands for these receptors, but these have not yet become clinically useful materials. Strong, opioid-like analgesics acting at these sites with fewer undesirable effects may be developed. Possible therapeutic interventions include a blockade of enzymes that degrade endogenous opioids, alteration of receptor site sensitivity, or other methods for increasing endogenous opioid stores.

Opioid Analgesics

Morphine, an opium alkaloid, is the prototype of the opioid analgesics. It provides analgesia at a dose (about 10 mg IM) that does not result in severe alterations in consciousness. Although its exact mechanism and locus of action are not known, morphine affects both the initial perception of pain and the emotional response to it. Total pain relief is difficult to achieve, but reduction in the level of distress or suffering is an achievable goal. Patients with severe pain rarely obtain pleasant, euphoric sensations after morphine administration, but may become drowsy and relaxed, partly because of decreased distress. Paradoxically, in people without pain morphine may produce unpleasant psychologic and physical sensations (dysphoria).

Many chemical variations of the morphine molecule have been developed to increase potency and oral effectiveness and to reduce undesired side effects; however, both beneficial and adverse effects are intertwined. Though the possibility of psychologic and physical dependence is a constraint on the use of morphine and related opioid analgesics, addiction from clinical prescribing rarely occurs (see DEPENDENCE OF THE OPIOID TYPE in Ch. 138).

Traditionally, morphine has not been considered to be effective when taken orally. It is rapidly transformed principally in the liver to inactive metabolites and excreted in the urine. However, several new developments, which compensate for first-pass degradation, may make oral morphine more effective. A slow-release tablet containing 30 mg released over 8 h, a concentrated oral solution, and a buccal tablet have all been developed recently in an attempt to make oral morphine more effective. These latter routes may provide long lasting pain relief with very low doses. Additionally, respiratory depression and sedation may be diminished, although such adverse effects are still possible. **Morphine sulfate** is the most commonly used water-soluble salt, and a reasonable starting dose for a 70 kg patient is 8 to 10 mg IM or s.c. If administered IV (2 to 10 mg), it must be given slowly (over 4 to 5 min) to prevent serious hypotension. Pain relief generally begins within 15 to 20 min (sooner after IV administration) and lasts 3 to 4 h. Higher doses provide greater analgesic effect and longer duration of action. The ceiling of morphine's analgesic effect is very high and, in large doses, it may be used as a surgical anesthetic. However, adverse effects limit the maximum tolerated dose. Elderly patients get more long-lasting analgesia from standard doses of morphine. Epidural and intrathecal morphine administration continue to be studied—these routes provide long-lasting (up to 24 h) effective pain relief with very low doses (as low as 1 mg). However, some patients find the sedative and relaxing effects of morphine beneficial, effects which may be absent with epidural or intrathecal administration.

Elderly patients seem to be more sensitive to morphine's analgesic effect. With increasing age, morphine's duration of action increases. Thus, the possibility of accu-

mulation of drug effect may occur in some elderly patients who receive frequent doses of morphine. Clinical observation and discussions with the patient remain the best methods for titration and dose adjustment in the elderly, as in all other patients.

Adverse effects of morphine are dose-related and include CNS depression, with decreased respiratory responsiveness to CO_2, decreased cough reflex, nausea, and vomiting. Morphine also produces miosis and stimulates release of ADH from the hypothalamus. Peripheral smooth muscle effects decrease propulsive movements in the GI tract, causing constipation (a useful effect in the treatment of diarrhea with opioids but a significant problem in patients with chronic pain, eg, cancer). The venules (capacitance vessels) dilate following morphine administration, and hypotension may occur in hypovolemic patients or those who suddenly assume an upright position. Depression of central vasomotor centers and histamine release may be involved in causing hypotension. The hypotensive effect of opioids is intensified by concomitant administration of phenothiazines.

Morphine and other opioids should be used with great caution (if at all) in patients with chronic obstructive pulmonary disease. Since morphine increases CSF pressure, patients with suspected CNS disease should probably not receive opioids. In patients with liver disease, smaller starting doses and careful titration are advisable. Patients with markedly decreased renal function may have unusually prolonged CNS depressant effects from opioids, so that repeated doses of opioid antagonists (perhaps for several days following the last opioid dose) may be needed to reverse respiratory depression in anuric patients. Neonates, especially premature babies, lack adequate metabolic pathways to eliminate morphine and other opioids and are unusually sensitive to them.

The development of tolerance to morphine varies from one physiologic system to another; eg, the pupillary and GI effects of morphine exhibit little tolerance. However, during chronic therapy it may become necessary to increase the dose to achieve the same degree of pain relief, since the duration of action shortens and the peak analgesic effect decreases. CNS stimulants such as amphetamines potentiate the analgesic effect of morphine.

Codeine, also derived from opium, has analgesic activity when given orally; 65 mg is equianalgesic to about 600 mg of aspirin. However, since codeine acts centrally, it complements aspirin, acetaminophen, and other peripherally acting analgesics. It is also useful in treating cough and diarrhea and has lower abuse potential than some other opiods. Unwanted effects of codeine (respiratory depression, nausea, vomiting, and constipation) are similar to those of other opioids.

Meperidine is a synthetic opioid analgesic. Between 75 and 100 mg parenterally is equianalgesic to 10 mg of morphine sulfate, but its duration of action (about 3 h) is shorter than that of morphine. The adverse effects of these drugs are similar, but meperidine has less smooth muscle effect and seems to have less depressant effect on the newborn, probably because it less readily crosses the placental barrier. Meperidine has a relatively high abuse potential and serious hypotension may occur when it is given concomitantly with monoamine oxidase inhibitors. Meperidine is not useful for cough or diarrhea.

Methadone is a synthetic analgesic with excellent activity when given orally. The usual dose for pain relief is 5 to 10 mg orally q 6 to 8 h. Methadone is used extensively in the USA for short-term treatment of heroin withdrawal (see DEPENDENCE OF THE OPIOID TYPE in Ch. 138), for long-term maintenance therapy of opioid addiction, and for analgesia in cancer patients. These uses are made possible by methadone's long duration of action, oral effectiveness, ability at high dosage to block heroin-induced euphoria, and less prominent sedation. Adverse effects of methadone resemble those of morphine and are reversible by opioid antagonists. Both the duration of analgesia and

the CNS (ie, respiratory) effects provided by methadone persist for a longer time than those of morphine. Therefore, unless tolerance has developed, the patient should be closely monitored after increasing the methadone dose or frequency of its administration, as serious respiratory depression may result. Methadone is easily differentiated from morphine by a urine test. Some opioid addicts treated with methadone function better socially than when taking heroin, although controversy surrounds such maintenance therapy. Another new development in the treatment of opioid addicts includes the use of orally active opioid antagonists such as naltrexone (see below).

Propoxyphene is related chemically to methadone and other opioids, but has less addiction liability. Propoxyphene 65 to 130 mg has central-type analgesic activity, but does not cause significant respiratory depression, GI upset, or clotting difficulties. It is clinically useful alone or in combination with aspirin or acetaminophen. The drug's toxicity resembles that of opioid analgesics. Sedation, nausea, and dizziness may occur. CNS depression caused by overdosage may be reversed by naloxone, an opioid antagonist. True physical dependence is rare with propoxyphene. Opioid restrictions are not presently necessary with propoxyphene, but deaths have occurred with overdosage and it should be prescribed with discretion. Its hazards are increased if the drug is combined with alcohol or other CNS depressants.

In analgesic activity, 100 mg of propoxyphene napsylate is equivalent to 65 mg of propoxyphene hydrochloride. Because of its physical characteristics, it is possible to make suspension and tablet formulations of the napsylate salt, allowing more flexibility in dosage and administration. Propoxyphene napsylate may be useful in "detoxifying" opioid addicts.

Combinations: Opioid analgesia may be potentiated by CNS stimulants such as amphetamine or cocaine. A liquid analgesic-stimulant-alcohol combination may be useful in selected patients with pain. However, many patients improve simply if the dose of opioid analgesic is adjusted appropriately.

Opioid Adjuvants

Phenothiazines, eg, chlorpromazine, fluphenazine, perphenazine, while having little direct analgesic activity, may be useful as analgesic adjuvants. Although the data are contradictory, phenothiazines may potentiate opioid analgesia and decrease associated nausea and vomiting; however, hypotension may also be potentiated. In some clinical syndromes (eg, postherpetic neuralgia and atypical facial pain), combinations of a phenothiazine and a tricyclic antidepressant or a tricyclic antidepressant alone are often effective.

Methotrimeprazine, a phenothiazine analgesic, does not induce tolerance or psychologic or physical dependence and thus has no abuse or addiction potential. In analgesic activity, methotrimeprazine 15 to 20 mg IM is equivalent to about 10 mg of morphine. This drug should *not* be given IV or s.c. Therapeutic doses do not produce respiratory depression, pupillary changes, or constipation, but orthostatic hypotension and sedation are common adverse effects.

Opioid Antagonists and Agonist-Antagonists

The N-allyl analogs of morphine and levorphanol (**nalorphine** and **levallorphan,** respectively) diminish or abolish the effects of opioids and methadone and precipitate an acute withdrawal syndrome in physically dependent addicts. However, they also have partial agonist activity and elicit opioid effects when given alone. CNS depression can be exacerbated if these antagonists are given to patients with respiratory depression caused by nonopioid drugs such as barbiturates or other sedative-hypnotics. **Nalorphine** is an effective analgesic, but its use is limited by a significant incidence of hallucinations.

Pentazocine, a weak opioid antagonist with considerable analgesic activity, is less

subject to abuse than pure opioid agonists. However, it has some abuse potential, especially if given parenterally. The analgesic activity of pentazocine 40 to 50 mg IM is comparable to 10 mg of morphine. The drug may also be given orally. Pentazocine can cause unpleasant hallucinations. There may be greater risk in giving pentazocine to patients during an acute myocardial infarction. If given to someone dependent on opioids, it can precipitate withdrawal symptoms. Pentazocine overdosage is reversible by naloxone, but not by other opioid antagonists.

Combinations of low doses of pentazocine and peripherally acting analgesics such as acetaminophen have been marketed. An oral preparation of pentazocine containing a low dose of naloxone is also available. In theory, parenteral abuse of pentazocine should be diminished by this preparation with maintained efficacy. Orally given naloxone will not block pentazocine analgesia. However, if anyone injects the dissolved tablet material, the parenteral naloxone will block the effects of the pentazocine.

Naloxone is almost a pure opioid antagonist without significant agonist action and is virtually free of the undesirable effects of the opioid agonist-antagonists. It does not cause respiratory depression nor psychotomimetic effects when given alone, and it can reverse the effects of pentazocine, propoxyphene, and all other opioid analgesics. Onset of action is extremely rapid (within minutes) when given IV and slightly less rapid when given IM. However, the duration of antagonism is usually not as long as the duration of opioid-induced respiratory depression, so that clinical vigilance and repeated doses of naloxone may be necessary. A common starting dose is 0.4 mg IV every 2 to 3 min as needed.

Naltrexone, an orally active opioid antagonist, has recently been approved by the FDA for use as an adjunct in opioid dependence. It has a long duration of action and is generally well tolerated. Naltrexone may have other potentially important applications that remain to be studied.

Newer opioid agonist-antagonist analgesics include **butorphanol, nalbuphine,** and **buprenorphine.** Each is derived from a different narcotic class. They have different ratios of antagonist to agonist properties and are all effective analgesics. Only buprenorphine is currently available in an orally administered form. The abuse potential of these drugs, while less than morphine or meperidine, has not yet been established. However, these compounds have the potential to precipitate withdrawal in patients dependent on narcotics.

ANTIANXIETY AGENTS

(Anxiolytics; "Minor" Tranquilizers; Sedatives)

Using drugs to relieve anxiety is common, although their precise efficacy is uncertain. Their utility is affected by patient and physician acceptance, placebo effect, and the episodic nature of most anxiety (see ANXIETY NEUROSES in Ch. 140).

The benzodiazepines have largely supplanted other antianxiety drugs, including the barbiturates, meprobamate, and hydroxyzine. The phenothiazines (eg, thioridazine) are occasionally used as antianxiety agents; however, their side effects make them ill-advised in ambulatory patients without *marked* anxiety or who do not respond to or tend to become dependent upon benzodiazepines. The degree of CNS depression produced by most anxiolytics is dose-dependent and can be severe. They continue to be the most common agents of drug suicide attempts (see Ch. 144).

Clinical Principles

Since most antianxiety drugs have a long half-life, once-a-day dosage is often sufficient. The benzodiazepines (particularly diazepam) may persist in the serum for over 24 h after a single dose. Since many patients with anxiety complain of insomnia, the

largest portion of the dosage may be given at bedtime, thus promoting sleep and providing some tranquilizing effect the next day. Smaller doses can be taken during the day as needed.

Dosage requirements vary widely and must be tailored to the individual and the degree of anxiety. Successful treatment does not imply a continuing need; some patients may need treatment only once or intermittently. Counseling and supportive maneuvers are always indicated and may preclude the need for constant drug therapy.

In pregnancy, the use of antianxiety drugs is not advised, especially during the first trimester, because of increased risk of congenital abnormalities, notably cleft lip and palate (0.2 to 0.4% incidence) and intrauterine growth retardation. They are sometimes used during labor and delivery to relieve anxiety and potentiate analgesia. However, such use can adversely affect the newborn; sedation, respiratory depression, poor sucking, hypotonia, hypothermia, and hyperbilirubinemia have been observed.

In the elderly, antianxiety drugs have been associated with oversedation, ataxia, confusion, reduced energy levels, and paradoxical excitement and delirium. The benzodiazepines are considered the safest antianxiety agents and are also the most commonly used sedative hypnotics. Unusual responses of the elderly may be explained by age-dependent changes in drug pharmacokinetics and increased target organ sensitivity. The elderly have diminished water and lean body mass with increased body fat, low plasma albumin, and diminished hepatic drug-metabolizing enzymes and drug elimination capacity. These factors can result in high serum concentrations of unbound active drug that distribute preferentially to lipid tissues, primarily the brain. Caution should be exercised in cases of dementia or depression, because benzodiazepines can worsen these conditions and occasionally induce florid delirium. Antianxiety drugs should be used primarily for short-term treatment in the elderly.

Diazepam, chlordiazepoxide, and flurazepam are very slowly eliminated and their half-lives increase considerably with age (4 to 6 fold at age 80); thus, the risk of toxic cumulation is high in the elderly. In contrast, the elimination of lorazepam, oxazepam, and alprezolam (which have shorter half-lives) is not significantly changed with age. In general, the benzodiazepines should be given in much lower doses (30 to 50% of the young adult dose), and at longer intervals for drugs with long half-lives. No change in the dose intervals is necessary for drugs with short half-lives.

Choice of an Antianxiety Drug

Since the antianxiety effects of the above drugs are nonspecific, the choice of agent depends on an evaluation of its potential toxicity. Individual drugs and their average adult daily dosages for anxiety are given in TABLE 281–1.

Phenobarbital is inexpensive and effective, but unwanted sedation is common. Meprobamate is occasionally useful and costs less than the benzodiazepines, but is generally regarded as less effective. Both meprobamate and the barbiturates have much greater abuse potential including tolerance, physical dependence, addiction, and a withdrawal syndrome than benzodiazepines and they present a greater hazard of CNS depression and death following overdose. However, barbiturates are still useful as an effective sedative, hypnotic, and anticonvulsant for certain conditions (see SEDATIVES AND HYPNOTICS in Ch. 122; see also Ch. 121).

β-Adrenergic blockers, such as propranolol, have recently been used to decrease some manifestations of anxiety (eg, tremor, palpitations). They block anxiety-induced tachycardia, decrease tremor, and also appear to have a central anxiolytic effect. They may be used alone or in combination with other anxiolytic drugs in short-term situational anxiety and acute panic symptoms. Propranolol is *not* effective in chronic anxiety or in anxiety where somatic symptoms are not prominent.

Benzodiazepines are highly effective in nonpsychotic anxiety, but they offer no benefits for thought disorder of schizophrenics and may even exacerbate it. These drugs

TABLE 281–1. COMMONLY USED ANTIANXIETY AGENTS

Drug	*Daily Dose Range (mg) Often Divided into 2–4 Daily Doses*
Barbiturates	
Phenobarbital	30–100
Butabarbital	25–120
Benzodiazepines	
Alprazolam	0.75–4.0
Clorazepate	15–60
Chlordiazepoxide	15–300
Diazepam	5–60
Halazepam	60–160
Oxazepam	10–120
Prazepam	20–60
Lorazepam	2–6
Other antianxiety agents	
Hydroxyzine	100–400
Meprobamate	800–2400
Tybamate	750–3000

have no mood elevating or antidepressant effect, but reduce anxiety in anxious depressed patients. Their use in depression can increase suicidal tendency. Benzodiazepines are useful in treating anxiety associated with allergies, dermatologic lesions, and GI and cardiovascular disorders. These drugs also control anticipatory anxiety in panic attacks and it has been suggested that alprazolam has specific antipanic activity. With therapeutic doses used for anxiety and other conditions, benzodiazepines are not likely to cause significant cardiovascular or respiratory depression, but they do potentiate the effects of other CNS depressants.

Diazepam relieves muscle spasm in neurologic and musculoskeletal disorders and is a good anticonvulsant. Benzodiazepines, especially chlordiazepoxide and diazepam, are the mainstay for the treatment of acute alcohol withdrawal syndrome because of their effectiveness and low incidence of respiratory and cardiovascular toxicity (see Treatment under DEPENDENCE ON ALCOHOL in Ch. 138). Benzodiazepines are also the preferred drugs for preanesthetic medication and for induction of anesthesia. The use of benzodiazepines as hypnotics is discussed under INSOMNIA in Ch. 122.

The **mechanism of action** of benzodiazepines is not completely established. Specific benzodiazepine receptors have been found in the brain and the affinity of benzodiazepines for such receptors is related to their pharmacologic potency. It has been hypothesized that binding a benzodiazepine to its receptor triggers the complex sequential events that enhance the inhibitory neuronal activity of γ-aminobutyric acid **(GABA).**

Pharmacokinetics, rather than inherent neuropharmacologic effects, appear responsible for differences in the clinical performances of the various benzodiazepines. Diazepam is rapidly absorbed after oral administration, reaching peak plasma concentrations in 1 h; chlordiazepoxide is slowly absorbed, reaching peak plasma concentrations in several hours. The plasma half-life of diazepam is 20 to 50 h; of chlordiazepoxide, 7 to 28 h. Benzodiazepines are highly protein bound, especially in plasma and in tissues of the GI tract and brain. Diazepam distributes rapidly to the adipose tissues after administration, explaining the initial rapid plasma decline in a few hours, followed by a slow decline and, in about 6 h, a resurgence of blood levels that is associated with another phase of drowsiness. Certain benzodiazepines such as chlordiazepoxide, chlorazepate, diazepam, halazepam, and prazepam are metabolized to active metabolites that concentrate in the brain and stay longer than the parent

compound. Because of the long plasma half-life of many of these metabolites, significant accumulation can occur. In contrast, alprazolam, oxazepam, and lorazepam (short-acting benzodiazepines) are biotransformed to inactive glucuronide metabolites that are readily eliminated by the kidney. Excretion of benzodiazepines and their metabolites is mainly renal and a small portion by hepatobiliary excretion and the feces.

Toxicity of benzodiazepines is low; skin rash, nausea, headache, impairment of sexual function, vertigo and lightheadedness occasionally occur. Unwanted effects, such as drowsiness and ataxia, may be extensions of the pharmacologic effects. Paradoxical responses of increased anxiety, psychosis, and sudden suicidal impulses have been reported. Changes in the pharmacokinetics of benzodiazepines by factors such as liver disease, renal failure, age (elderly), sex, and concomitant drug administration can enhance toxicity.

A **benzodiazepine withdrawal syndrome** may occur in patients who have been taking benzodiazepines for several months to years, even with dosages as low as 30 mg/day. Symptoms range from mild insomnia, dizziness, headache, and anorexia to severe signs like hypotension, hyperthermia, psychosis, seizures, muscle cramps, sweating, and coma. The severity of the syndrome appears to be related more to the duration of use than to dosage. Symptoms begin to appear on the 2nd or 3rd day after withdrawal of the long-acting benzodiazepines, such as chlordiazepoxide or diazepam, and abruptly and more severely after sudden withdrawal of the short-acting agents, such as oxazepam or lorazepam.

Meprobamate is rapidly absorbed from the GI tract, metabolized by the liver, and excreted by the kidneys. The usual adult dose for anxiety is 400 mg orally tid. Beneficial effects appear within a few days. The drug is relatively safe at normal doses. Drowsiness is the most common side effect. Adverse effects include allergic reactions, nausea and vomiting, hypotension, muscular weakness, and, rarely, blood dyscrasias. Tolerance and dependence may occur and chronic intoxication with confusion and ataxia can occur. In patients taking high doses (> 3 gm/day) for long periods, abrupt cessation of therapy produces a withdrawal syndrome that can present with convulsions or resemble delirium tremens.

ANTIPSYCHOTIC DRUGS

(Neuroleptics; "Major" Tranquilizers)

Introduction

Over the past 35 yr psychotropic drugs have produced major changes in the management of psychiatric illness (see Chs. 142, 143, and 201). Fewer patients need hospital care; family physicians offer more effective treatment in the office; and psychiatrists are consulted more selectively for diagnosis and treatment of difficult cases. As with many physical disorders, the realistic objective of psychiatric treatment may not be complete remission, but rather the restoration of an adequate level of basic functions necessary for a satisfying and productive life. When this goal is attained, medication must not be discontinued abruptly; maintenance therapy may be necessary. In schizophrenia, the more florid the symptoms and the more acute the onset, the more likely is a good response. Little change can be expected in chronic schizophrenics.

The antipsychotic drugs include phenothiazines, butyrophenones, thioxanthenes, dihydroindolone, dibenzoxazepine, and diphenylbutylpiperidine. TABLE 281–2 lists the antipsychotic drugs commonly used in the treatment of acute and chronic schizophrenia and the range of doses for various ages. The drugs listed are also useful in agitated depression, manic-depressive psychosis, other psychotic conditions, and confusion, delirium, and agitation commonly observed in the elderly. Haloperidol and pimozide are also indicated in Tourette's syndrome. Other medical uses of the antipsychotic drugs include control of nausea and vomiting, intractable hiccup, and Huntington's

TABLE 281–2. COMMONLY USED ANTIPSYCHOTIC DRUGS

Drug	*Daily Oral Dose (mg)*		
	Adult (15–65 yrs)	*Elderly (> 65 yrs)*	*Children (2–14 yrs)*
Phenothiazine (aliphatic)			
Chlorpromazine	50–2000	30–75	10–200
Triflupromazine	25–150		
Phenothiazine (piperidine)			
Mesoridazine	50–400		
Thioridazine	100–800	30–75	
Phenothiazine (piperazine)			
Fluphenazine	4–100	0.5–2	0.75–12.5
Perphenazine	16–80		
Prochlorperazine	25–150		
Trifluoperazine	5–60		5–20
Butyrophenones			
Haloperidol	4–150	0.5–2	0.75–12
Thioxanthenes			
Chlorprothixine	30–400		
Thiothixine	5–120	2–3	1–30
Dihydroindolone			
Molindone	20–200		1–2.5
Dibenzoxazepines			
Loxapine	20–160		15–50
Diphenylbutylpiperidine			
Pimozide	2–10		

chorea. These drugs are contraindicated in withdrawal syndrome from alcohol, barbiturates, and other sedatives because they may cause seizures by lowering the seizure threshold.

The suggested initiation of daily neuroleptic doses is in divided doses, tid or bid, starting with the low dose and increasing gradually to a maximum tolerated dose. Eventually, dosing can be changed to once a day to increase and insure compliance.

Selection of an Antipsychotic Drug

Paranoid schizophrenics do better on neuroleptics than do nonparanoid schizophrenics. Haloperidol (a butyrophenone) is preferred over the phenothiazines in nonparanoid patients. Among the phenothiazines, the more sedative ones such as chlorpromazine or thioridazine are preferable for agitated patients. Less sedative drugs such as trifluoperazine and perphenazine are best for patients with symptoms of withdrawal and retardation. *The notion that different antipsychotic drugs affect target symptoms selectively does not have convincing experimental support.* Currently available antipsychotic drugs do not differ appreciably among themselves with respect to clinical effectiveness. However, individual response to each drug varies, and may reflect pharmacokinetic differences more than inherent pharmacologic differences among them.

Often the choice of an antipsychotic drug depends on avoiding side effects detrimental to a particular patient. Haloperidol and the piperazine phenothiazines are preferred where sedation is undesirable and there is risk of CVS symptoms; eg, arrhythmias and

hypotension. Haloperidol is also preferred for patients with suspected liver abnormalities. If there is a risk of developing extrapyramidal symptoms (eg, in the aged, or in those with neurologic problems), thioridazine is the drug of choice. *Avoid* thioridazine in patients with heart disease and with ejaculation problems. Children and young adults are susceptible to extrapyramidal side effects; therefore, haloperidol and piperazine phenothiazines are best *avoided.* Chlorpromazine appears to be safest to use in children and young adults when doses are properly titrated.

The neuroleptics used commonly for the elderly are chlorpromazine, thioridazine, thiothixine, haloperidol, and fluphenazine. The elderly are more prone to extrapyramidal side effects, tardive dyskinesias, and hypotension. Occurrences of rare side effects (eg, skin pigmentation, leukopenia) are also increased in the elderly.

PHENOTHIAZINES

The clinically important subgroups of phenothiazines are the **aliphatics** (the most widely known is **chlorpromazine [CPZ]);** the **piperazines** (eg, fluphenazine, trifluoperazine, perphenazine); and the **piperidines** (eg, thioridazine). The pharmacologic properties of the various phenothiazines are qualitatively similar, but the relative potency and toxicity depend on the chemical structure. Clinically, the aliphatics are the least potent drugs. Piperidines have intermediate potency, and piperazines are generally the most potent.

Side effects also vary. Thioridazine (a piperidine derivative), for example, causes less hypotension and fewer extrapyramidal side effects than CPZ (an aliphatic derivative). Pigmentary retinopathy and ECG changes have been particularly observed with high doses (> 1000 mg) of thioridazine. The recommended ceiling dose is 800 mg/day. In contrast, the piperazine derivatives (fluphenazine, trifluoperazine, perphenazine, etc.) produce less drowsiness, hypotension, and tachycardia, but more extrapyramidal reactions than CPZ.

Plasma levels of CPZ vary widely in different patients with a given dose, due to differences in absorption, distribution, metabolism, and excretion of the drug. After absorption, CPZ is rapidly distributed and bound by most tissues, resulting in a high tissue/plasma concentration. There is extensive hepatic and extrahepatic metabolism of CPZ with more than 150 potential metabolites, some of which are pharmacologically active. The plasma half-life of CPZ is about 9 to 12 h and it takes 7 to 10 days of oral intake to achieve a steady state. CPZ and its metabolites are excreted in both urine and feces, where they can be detected in trace amounts for 6 to 18 mo after cessation of therapy. Psychotic patients with plasma levels < 50 ng/mL generally show no improvement. Those with 50 to 300 ng/mL show clinical improvement, and when plasma levels reach 700 to 1000 ng/mL, toxicity often appears (eg, convulsions or extrapyramidal symptoms). The optimum therapeutic plasma concentration in children is lower than that of adults (40 to 80 ng/mL). Unfortunately, CPZ plasma levels do not usually correlate with dosage, but are affected by such factors as (1) dosage form; (2) age (children are rapid metabolizers and, despite moderate doses of 3 to 10 mg/kg, they achieve low plasma concentrations); and (3) duration of therapy (institutionalized patients on long-term therapy achieve very low plasma levels—17 to 50% of values seen in patients on short-term therapy—despite moderately high [600 to 1000 mg/day] CPZ doses).

Clinical Effects

The phenothiazines are effective in acute and chronic schizophrenia and do not produce drug dependence. They have a marked effect on thought disturbances associated with paranoid ideation, delusions, anxiety, and agitation. CPZ, the prototype phenothiazine, produces psychomotor slowing, emotional quieting, and an affective indifference that is described as a neuroleptic action. CPZ also produces considerable

drowsiness and hypotension, to which tolerance develops quite rapidly, and has a central antiemetic and hypothermic effect. CPZ also has antihistaminic, anticholinergic, and muscle relaxant activity. Important biochemical effects are blockade of catecholamines (norepinephrine and dopamine), of serotonin uptake in the brain, and inhibition of dopamine-sensitive adenylate cyclase activity in the limbic system.

In acute psychosis, a starting dose of 300 to 400 mg/day of CPZ is increased rapidly to as much as 1000 to 2000 mg/day in 1 to 2 wk. Thereafter it is lowered to a maintenance dose of 300 to 400 mg/day, depending on the clinical picture. Young adults in their 20s should be given relatively lower doses in a therapeutic trial of not less than 3 to 6 wk. Single daily maintenance doses can be tried in order to improve patient compliance. Rapid neuroleptization, for the prompt treatment of acutely ill psychotic patients who are assaultive, aggressive, and combative, involves the IM injection of neuroleptics like chlorpromazine (50 to 100 mg), haloperidol (5 mg), or fluphenazine (5 mg) q 30 or 60 min for about 6 doses, until the patient improves or becomes sedated. This regimen, although effective, results in increased extrapyramidal effects and on rare occasions carries the risk of cardiovascular side effects, seizures, and neuroleptic malignant syndrome (see below).

Antipsychotic drugs do not cure schizophrenics. Regardless of which drug is prescribed, patients usually achieve maximal benefit in the first 3 to 6 mo of treatment. This initial improvement can be sustained with maintenance therapy in most patients. Some clinicians have proposed as a rule of thumb that after the first episode a schizophrenic patient should be maintained on medication for at least 1 yr, and after the second episode, for at least 2 yr; in the event of further relapse, the patient should be kept on drug therapy indefinitely. Early cessation of therapy has led to relapse in 25% of patients within 4 wk, in 50% within 8 wk, and in 75% within 12 wk.

Adverse effects of phenothiazines include drowsiness, sedation, hypotension, extrapyramidal symptoms (eg, akathisia, dystonia, tremors, and rigidity), reduction of convulsive seizure threshold, ocular and skin pigmentation, photosensitization, tardive dyskinesia, hepatotoxicity, and blood dyscrasias. Phenothiazines may produce abnormalities in myocardial repolarization and phenothiazine-induced arrhythmias are common. Endocrine effects include suppression of ovulation, induction of lactation, increased release of ADH, and inhibition of oxytocin release.

The phenothiazines may cause drug-induced **acute dystonia** with vigorous chorea and athetosis, muscular facial spasms, and torticollis. These appear to be idiosyncratic phenomena that begin within 48 h of initiation of treatment and are not dose-related. Treatment of severe reactions with diphenhydramine 50 mg IV or benztropine 2 mg IM is usually effective but may need to be repeated as the offending drugs have long half-lives. Small oral doses of benztropine, biperiden, trihexyphenidyl, or diphenhydramine usually suffice for mild reactions.

The **neuroleptic malignant syndrome** is *an uncommon life-threatening idiosyncratic reaction to neuroleptic therapy*. The pathophysiology of the neuroleptic malignant syndrome is not as clear as the pathophysiology of malignant hyperthermia (see under PHARMACOGENETICS in Ch. 276) due to inhalation anesthetics. The proposed theories are central dopaminergic blockade or catecholamine depletion resulting in derangement of central thermoregulation, vs. the peripheral hypermetabolic state of the skeletal muscle.

A review of 53 cases of neuroleptic malignant syndrome revealed the following: (1) Most of the patients had been on a wide variety of neuroleptics without previous history of neuroleptic malignant syndrome. (2) The drugs most commonly involved were the potent neuroleptics (haloperidol and the piperazine phenothiazines), although some of the cases involved less potent neuroleptics. (3) Of the 47 patients where sex was reported, 68% were men and 32% were women. The clinical signs observed were

very high temperature (102 to 104 F), tachycardia, tachypnea, profuse diaphoresis, rigidity, altered consciousness, autonomic dysfunction, hyper- or hypotension, seizures, tremors, leukocytosis, and marked elevation of serum CK. Rhabdomyolysis can also be a serious complication, producing extemely high CK, hyperkalemia, myoglobinuria, and acute renal insufficiency. Other complications include respiratory failure (due to aspiration, infection, shock, or pulmonary emboli), myocardial infarction, hepatic failure, and intravascular coagulation. The mortality rate is 15 to 20%.

Treatment consists of immediate withdrawal of neuroleptics, prompt institution of intensive supportive care with adequate hydration and nutrition, and measures to lower temperature. Dantrolene, oral or IV, has been tried with unequivocal benefit. It can be given IV at 60 mg q 6 h. Oral dantrolene can be given starting at 25 mg/day, increasing up to 25 mg tid and then by increments of 25 mg to as high as 100 mg bid to qid; this method has been shown to benefit some patients. Bromocriptine 5 mg tid and amantidine 50 mg tid can also be tried, as well as congentin and diazepam. Secondary complications such as hypoxia, acidosis, and renal failure must be treated vigorously. Patients who recovered from haloperidol-induced neuroleptic malignant syndrome have been slowly and cautiously reintroduced to other neuroleptics such as thioridazine, molindone, or fluphenazine when the psychiatric illness deteriorated. The use of these other agents was effective and did not result in any precipitation of the neuroleptic malignant syndrome.

Tardive dyskinesia is characterized by choreiform movements of the buccal-lingual-fascial muscles, less commonly the extremities. Rarely, focal or even generalized dystonia may be seen. Tardive dyskinesia may be caused by high doses of phenothiazines given over a long time, a common practice in young schizophrenics. Older patients, particularly women and those with brain injury, have a higher incidence of tardive dyskinesia. The problem does not disappear when the drug is discontinued and resists standard treatments for movement disorders. Anticholinergics can exacerbate tardive dyskinesia. The incidence has increased with the common and prolonged use of phenothiazines. Reintroduction or increase in dosage of piperazine phenothiazines or haloperidol may aggravate or, paradoxically, may suppress the dyskinesia. Reserpine 0.1 to 1.0 mg/day or clonazepam 1 to 3 mg/day is sometimes helpful. Deanol acetamidobenzoate and choline chloride, precursors for acetylcholine, are also sometimes helpful. Lithium, tricyclic antidepressants, and baclofen have also been useful in some patients. A recent theory is that receptor sensitivity modulation with dopamine agonists, like L-dopa and bromocriptine, may be useful in the treatment of tardive dyskinesia. The dopamine agonist, by stimulating dopamine autoreceptors, can inhibit dopamine synthesis and release.

Skin and eye complications, drowsiness, and hypotension appear to be dose-related. Extrapyramidal symptoms (eg, persistent dyskinesia) and hepatotoxicity are influenced by other factors such as age, sex, duration of drug administration, and individual hypersensitivity. Hepatotoxicity and blood dyscrasias appear to be hypersensitivity reactions. Altered immune reactions have been observed in patients treated with CPZ for 2-½ yr. In a study of 75 schizophrenic patients treated with CPZ, 50% showed positive antinuclear antibodies, 75% developed increased serum IgM and prolongation of partial thromboplastin time, and 50% had splenomegaly. These findings appear to be specific for chlorpromazine, since they were not observed with other neuroleptics.

Antipsychotic drugs taken by women during pregnancy, especially during the 3rd trimester, produce neurologic and behavioral changes in neonates, despite the absence of structural teratogenic effects. Neuroleptics, especially haloperidol, are excreted in breast milk.

Interaction of CPZ with other drugs includes the following: (1) CPZ potentiates the action of CNS depressants, eg, alcohol, narcotics, hypnotics, and sedatives; (2) CPZ plasma levels are lowered by trihexyphenidyl and possibly by other anticholinergics;

(3) CPZ absorption is impaired by insoluble antacids; (4) CPZ potentiates the hypotensive effect of antihypertensives; (5) the use of L-dopa in phenothiazine-induced parkinsonism in psychiatric patients aggravates schizophrenia and does not control the extrapyramidal symptoms; and (6) lithium lowers plasma CPZ levels.

Long-acting parenteral preparations of fluphenazine decanoate or enanthate may be used to manage problems of compliance, absorption, and erratic plasma levels, particularly in patients on long-term therapy. These dosage forms are given IM (25 to 50 mg) every 1 to 3 wk and are usually well tolerated. Recent studies showed that fluphenazine decanoate given at low doses of 1.25 to 5 mg IM q 2 wk was sufficient to prevent relapse in schizophrenic outpatients. Side effects generally consist of minor autonomic disturbances, infrequent hypotension, and dermatologic disorders. Drowsiness and lethargy may occur in some individuals after the initial injection, but are generally mild and abate spontaneously within 1 wk; when pronounced, they can be counteracted by methylphenidate 10 to 20 mg orally once or twice daily for a few days. Extrapyramidal symptoms occur within 4 to 5 days of treatment, in contrast to the greater delay often seen after oral therapy. With oral neuroleptics, 90% of dyskinesias, parkinsonism, and akathisias occur in 4 to 5, 72, and 73 days, respectively. With parenteral fluphenazine, dyskinesia may occur in some patients in 12 to 24 h, akathisia in 1 to 4 days, and parkinsonism in 2 to 5 days post-injection. Symptoms of parkinsonism are well controlled by anticholinergic antiparkinsonian agents such as benztropine mesylate. Akathisia responds to the same drugs and also to small doses of barbiturates or antihistamines. Dystonic reactions are readily relieved by diazepam IV or benztropine mesylate 1 to 2 mg IM. Convulsions, jaundice, agranulocytosis, and major skin and eye changes are rare complications of therapy. Interaction of fluphenazine decanoate with other drugs appears to be of minor significance.

BUTYROPHENONES

Haloperidol and droperidol are the only butyrophenones available in the USA at present; however, droperidol is used primarily as an adjunct to anesthesia rather than as a neuroleptic. Haloperidol blocks dopamine receptors in the CNS. It is effective against aggressive behavior in disturbed children, organic psychosis, alcoholic delirium, and assaultive behavior. It is also useful in managing confused, negativistic geriatric patients, senile psychosis, mania and paranoid reactions, and other behavior disorders of the elderly. Neurologic disorders such as Gilles de la Tourette's syndrome, Huntington's chorea, spasmodic torticollis, hemiballismus and hyperkinesia of organic origin, and intractable hiccups are also benefited by haloperidol. It is a potent antiemetic. Compared with the phenothiazines, it causes less hypotension, anticholinergic effects, cardiac complications, and sedation. The risk of drug-induced liver disease with haloperidol appears minimal. However, haloperidol-induced chronic cholestatic liver disease has been reported.

Haloperidol induces more extrapyramidal side effects than the aliphatic and piperidine phenothiazines; these effects may be minimized by using low doses. Young patients (children and adolescents) are most likely to develop dystonic reactions, middle-aged patients usually develop akathisia, and elderly individuals tend to develop parkinsonism.

Overdosage of haloperidol usually involves an exaggeration of the pharmacologic effects and adverse reactions. Gastric lavage or induction of emesis should be followed by administration of activated charcoal. Treatment is primarily supportive. Haloperidol should be used in pregnancy only if the benefits clearly justify a potential risk to the fetus.

The usual initial dosage of haloperidol for moderate symptoms is 0.5 to 2.0 mg orally bid or tid; for severe symptoms, 3 to 5 mg orally bid or tid. Daily dosages up to 100 mg for a limited time may be necessary in some cases. Infrequently, doses above

100 mg have been used in severely resistant patients. For maintenance, dosage is reduced to the smallest effective amount. Haloperidol is readily absorbed orally. Peak plasma concentration occurs 2 to 6 h after ingestion and may plateau for as long as 72 h; plasma levels may be detectable for weeks. In acute cases, haloperidol 2 to 5 mg IM may be given.

Haloperidol potentiates the effect of CNS depressants and anticoagulants. It diminishes the effect of L-dopa. It can diminish dyskinesia but aggravates parkinsonism in patients on L-dopa therapy. Since prolonged neuroleptic therapy is associated with development of tardive dyskinesias, haloperidol is not recommended for the treatment of tardive dyskinesias or L-dopa dyskinesias because it can mask the worsening of neuroleptic-related tardive dyskinesias.

THIOXANTHENES

Of the 4 thioxanthenes marketed in various countries, only **chlorprothixene** and **thiothixene** are available in the USA for clinical use. The thioxanthenes resemble the phenothiazines in chemical structure, absorption, metabolism, excretion, and clinical effects. Chlorprothixene and thiothixene have been used in the treatment of schizophrenia and depression. The average oral daily adult dosage is 75 to 200 mg for chlorprothixene and 10 to 30 mg for thiothixene; however, individual patient requirements vary.

Like other neuroleptics, the thioxanthenes interfere with conditioned reflex activity without affecting unconditioned reflex activity. They increase limbic system activity and inhibit proprioceptive arousal reactions. Psychoactive thioxanthenes share some of the properties of tricyclic antidepressants. Thiothixene is comparable to chlorpromazine in therapeutic impact and is particularly effective against affective symptoms. It is especially useful for patients who are socially withdrawn, and is also effective in the management of psychotic depression, tension-agitation, and anxiety.

Fever, fatigue, and drowsiness are the most frequent adverse effects. The sensitivity to sunlight seen with phenothiazines is usually not observed. The relative frequency of adverse effects with thiothixene is lower than with the corresponding phenothiazine analogs. The lower incidence of extrapyramidal effects in long-term maintenance therapy is especially advantageous. Thiothixene has fewer adverse effects on the myocardium than does thioridazine.

OTHER ANTIPSYCHOTIC DRUGS

Loxapine, a tricyclic dibenzoxazepine derivative, is chemically distinct from thioxanthenes, butyrophenones, and phenothiazines. Its pharmacologic and toxicologic properties are similar to those of the piperazine group of phenothiazines. Therapeutic efficacy is comparable with that of other neuroleptics in schizophrenia. Side effects include involuntary movements, hypotension, and somnolence. Oral doses range from 60 to 100 mg/day, although some patients may require up to 250 mg/day.

Molindone, a dihydroindolone derivative, is structurally different from the phenothiazines, butyrophenones, and thioxanthenes, but is also pharmacologically similar to the phenothiazines. The daily oral dose range is 20 to 200 mg.

GENERAL CENTRAL NERVOUS SYSTEM STIMULANTS AND ANOREXIANTS

CNS stimulants are used to increase alertness, inhibit fatigue, suppress the appetite, manage certain children with minimal brain dysfunction or hyperkinesis, and treat narcolepsy. Many of these drugs are related to amphetamine and share the phenethylamine structure. Their activity as psychostimulants is primarily due to an ability to act

indirectly by displacing endogenous catecholamines from storage sites in neural tissues, but may also be partly related to direct catecholamine-like adrenergic receptor activation in the CNS. Their use in clinical medicine continues to decline because of criticism of any use to induce brief mood elevation or to suppress fatigue and a fear that nonchalant prescribing may have contributed to abuse (see also Ch. 138).

The failure of most obese patients to lose weight satisfactorily by attempting to decrease food intake alone has led to widespread use of anorexiants. Though these drugs may be of value in beginning a weight reduction program, their long-term utility has been questioned. Amphetamine and related compounds such as diethylpropion, phentermine, and phendimetrazine are most effective for the first 3 to 6 wk. The suggestion that they might be useful intermittently over a long period to aid in weight control has been made. The dosage usually is divided and given before meals, but some agents have a long duration of action and may be given less frequently. Most anorexiants may disturb sleep if given late in the day. The use of agents less subject to abuse than amphetamine or phenmetrazine is recommended whenever feasible.

Amphetamine is the prototype CNS stimulant. There are a variety of amphetamine salts and mixtures in various formulations. Amphetamine produces mood elevation with increased wakefulness, alertness, concentration, and physical performance. Systolic and diastolic blood pressures are raised, the respiratory center is stimulated, and appetite is suppressed through a central effect. It is rapidly absorbed from the GI tract, reaches high concentrations in the CNS, and is largely metabolized. Its prolonged duration of sympathomimetic action relates to its resistance to metabolic degradation by enzymes that metabolize catecholamines. Amphetamine and related compounds, when taken repeatedly, induce tolerance to some degree, but this is partially dependent on dosage.

Insomnia, dizziness, excessive sweating, tremors, and euphoria may occur, and feelings of depression and fatigue often accompany withdrawal. Anxiety and panic states are seen, particularly at the high dosage levels associated with amphetamine abuse. Lethal overdose is uncommon because of the large difference between an effective and fatal dose and because tolerance has often occurred. For a detailed discussion of amphetamine abuse and its management, see Ch. 138.

Methylphenidate is a CNS stimulant with effects similar to that of amphetamine. It is used to treat hyperkinesis in children (see LEARNING DISORDERS in Ch. 188) and for narcolepsy (see Ch. 122).

Fenfluramine, a newer anorexiant, appears to have minimal abuse potential. Although a phenethylamine, it has sedation as its principal side effect and may be given late in the day without disturbing sleep. It should be *avoided* in patients with a history of mental depression and migraine. Some feel that a low night-time dose of fenfluramine may be combined with a daytime dose of phentermine or diethylproprion for effective and minimally symptom-inducing anorexia.

ANTIEMETICS

Drugs that prevent or relieve nausea and vomiting. Nausea and vomiting may be symptoms of disease processes, eg, metabolic or microbial toxins, or responses to stimuli such as drugs, radiation, or motion. The underlying cause should be sought and corrected if possible, as the etiology suggests which antiemetic is optimal for symptomatic treatment. Nausea and vomiting induced by noncytotoxic drugs such as digitalis, estrogens, and iron preparations should be treated by reducing the dose, changing the route of administration, or switching to another drug.

Stimulation of the vomiting center in the medulla can arise in the chemoreceptor trigger zone **(CTZ),** cerebral cortex, or vestibular apparatus, or can be relayed directly from peripheral areas (eg, gastric mucosa). Though the mechanism of action of the

antiemetics is not well understood, they appear to act on the CTZ, cerebral cortex, vestibular apparatus, or vomiting center.

Some nausea and vomiting is mild, self-limited (eg, usually that occurring during the first trimester of pregnancy), and does not require drug therapy. Drugs should be avoided if possible during the first 3 mo of pregnancy, but certain antihistamines may be tried if drug therapy is absolutely necessary. In other settings, untreated vomiting may delay or interrupt wound healing after surgery or may cause fluid and electrolyte loss perpetuating the symptoms of nausea and vomiting. Persistent vomiting precludes oral administration. Generally, drug therapy is more successful for prophylaxis than for treatment of vomiting, especially that caused by motion sickness, radiation, or cancer chemotherapy.

Most of the drugs mentioned in this chapter (See also TABLE 281-3) are discussed in more detail elsewhere in THE MANUAL; the primary focus here is on their antiemetic effect.

Antidopaminergics

Antidopaminergics include many of the phenothiazines (eg, prochlorperazine, fluphenazine) and the butyrophenones—haloperidol and droperidol. The phenothiazines and butyrophenones appear to act by selectively depressing the CTZ, and to a lesser extent, by acting on the vomiting center. They are useful in treating nausea and vomiting that is postoperative, radiation- or drug-induced, or associated with gastroenteritis, pregnancy, carcinoma, or uremia. Except for promethazine, phenothiazines are not useful in treating motion sickness. Since most phenothiazines (except thioridazine and mesoridazine) appear to be equally effective antiemetics, if given in sufficient dosage, the choice of drug may depend upon consideration of side effects (see PHENOTHIAZINES under ANTIPSYCHOTIC DRUGS, above).

Haloperidol is comparable in efficacy to the phenothiazines. It has been used to treat nausea and vomiting associated with anesthesia and surgery, radiation therapy, cytotoxic drugs, narcotics, and GI disorders. **Droperidol** is a sedative that is used parenterally as a preanesthetic medication and occasionally for intractable nausea and vomiting associated with cancer chemotherapy.

Metoclopramide stimulates the motility of the upper GI tract without stimulating gastric, biliary, or pancreatic secretions. Metoclopramide increases the tone and amplitude of gastric contractions, relaxes the pyloric sphincter and the duodenal bulb, and increases peristalsis of the duodenum and jejunum. The result is accelerated gastric emptying and intestinal transit. Metoclopramide, given orally or parenterally, relieves the symptoms associated with acute and recurrent diabetic gastroparesis or gastroparesis related to delayed gastric emptying (eg, nausea, vomiting, anorexia, and fullness after meals).

Metoclopramide is used for nausea and vomiting of various etiologies (emetogenic cancer chemotherapeutic agents, radiation therapy, surgery, pregnancy, and gastric ulcers). Its antiemetic activity is probably related to both its gastrokinetic effects and its dopamine antagonist actions. The drug inhibits the central and peripheral effects of the emetic substance, apomorphine. For prevention of chemotherapy-induced emesis, the initial 2 doses should be 2 mg/kg if highly emetogenic drugs such as cisplatin or dacarbazine are used. One mg/kg may be adequate for less emetogenic regimens. The dose should be diluted in 50 mL of a parenteral solution and infused slowly 30 min before chemotherapy; repeat q 2 h for 2 doses, then q 3 h for 3 doses. Side effects are primarily CNS (restlessness, lassitude, drowsiness, and fatigue) or GI (nausea and diarrhea). Extrapyramidal symptoms occur in about 0.2 to 1% of patients treated and are more common in children and young adults and at the higher doses used in prophylaxis of vomiting due to cancer chemotherapy. The drug is contraindicated when stimulation of GI motility might be dangerous (mechanical obstruction or perfo-

TABLE 281–3. SOME ANTIEMETIC DRUGS

Agent	*Usual Adult Dosage (mg)*	*Route of Administration*	*Frequency*
Antidopaminergics			
Chlorpromazine	10–25	oral	q 4–6 h
	50–100	rectal	q 6–8 h
	25	IM	q 3–4 h
Droperidol	2.5–10	IM	once, for premedication
	1.25–5	IV	once
Fluphenazine	1.25	oral	q 6–8 h
	1.25	IM	q 6–8 h
Haloperidol	1–5	oral	bid
	1–5	IM	bid
Metoclopramide	10	oral	qid 1/2 h before meals and at bed time
	10	IV	once
Perphenazine	8–16	oral	daily in divided doses
	5	IM or IV	only as necessary
Prochlorperazine	5–10	oral	tid or qid
	25	rectal	bid
	5–10	IM	q 3–4 h
Thiethylperazine	10	oral	once daily to tid
	10	rectal	once daily to tid
	10	IM	once daily to tid
Triflupromazine	20–30	oral	daily
	5–15	IM	q 4 h
	1–3	IV	daily
Antihistamines			
Buclizine	50	oral	bid
Cyclizine	50	oral	qid
	50	IM	q 4–6 h
Dimenhydrinate	50	oral	q 4 h
	50	IM or IV	q 4 h
Hydroxyzine	25–100	oral	tid or qid
	25–100	IM	q 4–6 h
Meclizine	25–50	oral	once daily
Promethazine	10–25	oral	bid
	12.5–50	rectal	bid
	12.5–25	IM	q 4–8 h
Anticholinergics			
Scopolamine	0.3–1.0	oral	prior to travel
	1 adhesive unit	topical	prior to travel
Miscellaneous			
Benzquinamide	50	IM	q 3–4 h
	25	IV	1st dose only
Dronabinol	5–15 mg/m²	oral	q 2–4 h beginning 1–12 h before chemotherapy and continuing 8–24 h after therapy
Diphenidol	25–50	oral	q 4 h
Timethobenzamide	250	oral	tid or qid
	200	rectal	tid or qid
	200	IM	tid or qid

ration), in pheochromocytoma, and in epileptics or in patients receiving drugs likely to cause extrapyramidal reactions.

Domperidone, like haloperidol and metoclopramide, is a dopamine antagonist. However, it has peripheral action because it does not cross the blood brain barrier and thus, does not produce CNS effects. Antiemetic action is presumedly due to a direct blocking effect of dopamine receptors in the CTZ. The drug appears to be effective in the treatment of nausea and vomiting associated with surgery and certain cancer chemotherapeutic agents. Facial flushing, headache, slight somnolence, and dry mouth are side effects reported with doses of 40 mg IV or 100 mg orally. Domperidone is an *investigational* agent in the USA; it is available in Europe. Optimal antiemetic dosage regimens are not yet established.

Antihistamines

These appear to act on the neural pathways originating in the labyrinth. Certain antihistamines (eg, promethazine, diphenhydramine, buclizine, cyclizine, meclizine) are effective in treating motion sickness and the vertigo of Meniere's disease. They are useful, but less effective, in treating postoperative nausea and vomiting and that associated with pregnancy.

The piperazine derivatives—buclizine, cyclizine, hydroxyzine, and meclizine have been demonstrated to be teratogenic in preclinical studies. Although the FDA has concluded that the data support neither a restriction on the use of cyclizine or meclizine nor a pregnancy warning, these drugs should be used with caution in pregnancy; the dose and duration of treatment should be kept to a minimum. (See also Prenatal Care in Ch. 176.)

Anticholinergics

Scopolamine is more effective than antihistamines for preventing motion sickness, but its clinical use is limited by a short duration of action and by side effects, including blurred vision, dry mouth, drowsiness, fatigue, and the possibility of increased intraocular pressure in patients with glaucoma. An adhesive film containing scopolamine is available and designed to be placed in an area of intact skin on the head behind the ear. It delivers the drug at a constant rate that is sufficient to combat motion sickness, yet is slow enough to avoid or minimize most side effects and prolong drug action for several days; nevertheless, dryness of the mouth and drowsiness may occur. Transdermal scopolamine is contraindicated in glaucoma and hypersensitivity to the drug or adhesive material.

Miscellaneous Agents

Benzquinamide appears to be as effective an antiemetic as the phenothiazines. The drug increases cardiac output and BP and may be useful in patients with CNS depression (eg, postoperative patients and those treated with sedatives or analgesics). Drowsiness is the most common side effect; shivering and chills, and reactions similar to those of phenothiazines have also been reported. Benzquinamide is administered IM or IV; no oral dosage form is available in the USA.

Dronabinol, Δ-9-tetrahydrocannabinol **(THC)** is approved for the treatment of nausea and vomiting caused by cancer chemotherapy in patients who have failed to respond to conventional antiemetic treatment. THC is the principal psychoactive component of marijuana. Its mechanism of antiemetic action is unknown, but cannabinoids bind to opioid receptors in the forebrain and may indirectly inhibit the vomiting center. THC is most useful in preventing the nausea and vomiting caused by certain anticancer agents, especially in younger patients. The drug is ineffective in cisplatin-induced vomiting. Oral absorption is variable, which could affect efficacy. Thus, incremental increases in dosage may be necessary. Drowsiness is the most common side effect, but orthostatic hypotension and dry mouth can also occur. Mood changes and distortions in visual and time senses may be unacceptable to some patients. Occasionally, dysphoria or hallucinations are encountered. THC may produce anxiety, tachycardia, depres-

sion, paranoia, and manic psychosis especially in older patients. THC is highly abusable and can produce both physical and psychologic dependence.

Diphenidol acts upon the aural vestibular apparatus. It is useful orally or parenterally in treating nausea and vomiting associated with malignancy, radiation sickness, anesthetics and antineoplastics, and is also effective in treating the vertigo of motion sickness and Meniere's disease. Diphenidol should be used only after safer agents have failed. Therapy should be closely supervised and discontinued if auditory or visual hallucinations, disorientation, or confusion occur. Drowsiness, dizziness, and dryness of the mouth may also occur. Diphenidol is eliminated almost entirely by the kidneys and is contraindicated in patients with severe renal impairment.

Trimethobenzamide is useful for preventing postanesthetic nausea and for treating the vomiting of pregnancy. The incidence of side effects is low, though drowsiness, diarrhea, extrapyramidal reactions, hypersensitivity reactions, and pain at the injection site or local irritation after rectal administration may occur.

---

282. NONNARCOTIC ANALGESICS; ANTIPYRETICS; NONSTEROIDAL ANTI-INFLAMMATORY DRUGS

MILD ANALGESICS

Analgesics for relief of mild to moderate pain include antipyretic/anti-inflammatory types (salicylates); para-aminophenol derivatives (acetaminophen); and anthranilic acid derivatives (mefenamic acid).

Aspirin (acetylsalicylic acid, ASA): Though salicylates are not identical, ASA can serve as a prototype for discussion of this group. Unlike narcotic analgesics, which act on the CNS, salicylates act, at least partially, at the peripheral or local level—the site of origin of the pain—and do not (in therapeutic dosage) alter consciousness or mood. ASA is often combined with a centrally acting analgesic. The exact mechanism of anti-inflammatory action of ASA is unknown. Its ability to decrease the synthesis of prostaglandins and lipoperoxides may explain its effects in rheumatoid arthritis. ASA also decreases fever, a usually desired but not always beneficial effect, perhaps by the same mechanism.

ASA 650 mg is an effective analgesic, equal to about 32 mg of codeine, 65 mg of propoxyphene, or 50 mg of oral pentazocine. Peak analgesic effects develop at about 45 min; duration of analgesia is generally 3 to 4 h. ASA is most useful in mild to moderate pain arising from injury or inflammation in structures such as the skin, teeth, or musculoskeletal system. ASA is rapidly absorbed from the gut and is hydrolyzed to free salicylate by nonspecific esterases shortly after entering the bloodstream. At higher doses, elimination of ASA follows zero-order kinetics; its metabolism is a capacity-limited process at higher doses; ie, there is a limit to the amount of drug that can be metabolized in any time period. Hence the elimination half-life and serum concentration of active drug may rise out of proportion to dose increases if the processes for metabolizing salicylate are saturated. Excretion of unchanged ASA may be promoted by alkalinization of the urine. This causes a larger percentage of the filtered drug to become ionized, and decreases its ability to diffuse passively from the glomerular filtrate across the tubular cells back into the blood.

ASA also has effects on uric acid secretion that are dose-dependent. Low doses compete with uric acid in the renal tubular organic acid secretory system and may

decrease urate excretion. However, larger doses compete for the more important, higher capacity renal tubular organic acid reabsorptive system, resulting in uricosuria and lower serum urate levels. In general, ASA should not be used by patients on uricosuric drugs. ASA is obsolete in the treatment of hyperuricemia or gout.

Dose-related and reversible **adverse effects** of aspirin include tinnitus and decreased hearing acuity, which may foretell more serious toxicity. Hyperventilation, resulting in respiratory alkalosis, may be followed by metabolic acidosis as a result of ASA overdose in children (see ACCIDENTS AND POISONINGS in Ch. 189). In adults, overdose usually results in respiratory alkalosis. Interference with the clotting mechanism occurs at doses lower than those causing acid-base disturbances: ASA decreases platelet aggregation by blocking the synthesis of thromboxane A_2 (TXA_2) and release of ADP, mediators of the second phase of platelet aggregation. This may be a serious problem in neonates or patients who have coagulation disorders, are taking anticoagulants, are undergoing surgery, or are receiving blood transfusions. Decreased platelet aggregation may be helpful in avoiding strokes and preventing recurrent myocardial infarctions. At higher doses, ASA interferes with prothrombin production or function, resulting in potentiation of the effects of oral anticoagulants. Aplastic anemia and thrombocytopenia are rare but serious adverse effects.

Direct GI irritation and subsequent GI blood loss can be caused by particles of ASA adhering to the mucosa, apparently a dose-related phenomenon. However, serious hemorrhage and peptic ulceration may occur at normally tolerated doses in susceptible patients. Various buffered preparations have been used in an attempt to decrease GI intolerance to ASA. Excessive buffer such as sodium bicarbonate present in several preparations of ASA including effervescent ones may lead to urinary and systemic alkalosis, with increased excretion of active drug. Delayed- or sustained-release formulations may cause less GI upset, but absorption may be variable. Various salts (aluminum, calcium, magnesium, choline, and sodium) and other salicylates have been used in efforts to decrease toxicity, prolong effect, or increase efficacy; none is as efficacious as ASA.

A small number of patients are hypersensitive to ASA and small doses may cause skin rashes and asthmatic-type anaphylactic reactions. The incidence is greater among those with asthma, hay fever, or nasal polyps. Salicylates other than ASA rarely cause these effects.

Some research points to a role for ASA in Reye's syndrome, a potentially fatal disease of unknown etiology occurring in the setting of influenza A or chickenpox (see under MISCELLANEOUS INFECTIONS in Ch. 191). Given effective alternatives, use of ASA to control fever in children with influenza or chickenpox should be avoided.

Diflunisal, a difluorophenyl derivative of salicylic acid, has analgesic and anti-inflammatory properties. It is useful for treatment of mild to moderate pain and rheumatoid and osteoarthritis. It is long-acting and usually a loading dose is given at the start of therapy. For mild to moderate pain, an initial dose of 1000 mg orally followed by 500 mg q 12 h is recommended for most patients.

Acetaminophen, a metabolic product of both phenacetin and acetanilid, is the major para-aminophenol derivative in common use today. It is an effective analgesic and antipyretic, but lacks major anti-inflammatory action and is a weak inhibitor of prostaglandin synthesis. The mechanism of its analgesic activity is unknown. In similar doses, it is therapeutically equivalent to aspirin in analgesic potency and duration of action; however, unlike aspirin it does not cause GI or bleeding disorders. There is no cross-sensitivity between aspirin and acetaminophen.

Acetaminophen is rapidly absorbed following oral administration. It is conjugated in the liver with glucuronide and sulfate; both the conjugates and some of the parent drug (< 10%) are then excreted in the urine. In overdose, acetaminophen can cause

hepatic necrosis through failure to inactivate a toxic metabolite. Administration of a sulfur containing amino acid such as acetylcysteine within 12 h of overdosing may decrease the extent and severity of this reaction (see Ch. 72 and also ACETAMINOPHEN POISONING in Ch. 189). Some patients (particularly those who are poorly nourished or alcoholics) on chronic acetaminophen therapy may also develop hepatic damage of a less dramatic type.

Acetaminophen (650 mg) is a useful drug for the relief of mild to moderate pain, especially in patients who are aspirin-sensitive, whose hemostatic system is impaired or under stress (eg, postpartum or after surgery), or who have gout. Acetaminophen is convenient for pediatric use because it can be formulated as a liquid. Acetaminophen provides a reasonable antipyretic in children with varicella or influenza. Following ingestion of large single doses, the acute toxicity of acetaminophen may be greater than that of aspirin, but it has fewer nuisance side effects. Combinations of centrally active agents (propoxyphene, codeine) and acetaminophen are effective.

Mefenamic acid, an anthranilic acid derivative, is a newer antipyretic, anti-inflammatory drug. Clinical evidence of its analgesic efficacy is limited. The initial dose is 500 mg, followed by 250 mg q 6 h as needed. Unwanted effects are generally mild and infrequent, but may include GI distress, diarrhea, dizziness, vertigo, skin rash, and, rarely, blood dyscrasias. Short courses of less than 1 wk are recommended to avoid serious adverse effects. If diarrhea or skin rash develop the drug should be discontinued immediately.

NONSTEROIDAL ANTI-INFLAMMATORY DRUGS (NSAIDs)

NSAIDs are a heterogeneous group of drugs (including ASA) that are useful in the symptomatic treatment of inflammation. Some appear to be most useful as analgesics. Most NSAIDs are organic acids that are rapidly absorbed and highly protein bound. Inhibition of synthesis of prostaglandins, also shown in vitro for some agents (eg, ASA, indomethacin), may be related to their clinical effects. NSAIDs are useful adjuncts in the treatment of rheumatoid arthritis, acute gout, ankylosing spondylitis, and osteoarthritis. Each "inflammatory disorder" may respond differently and only some aspects of inflammation (such as cellular infiltration) may respond to any given drug. Although the symptoms of a disease such as rheumatoid arthritis may be ameliorated by NSAIDs, tissue destruction may continue unabated. A single drug is often sufficient, but occasionally 2 agents that affect different aspects of inflammation may be more effective. NSAIDs work best in chronic conditions if given continuously rather than according to the presence of pain or other symptoms. Sudden cessation of therapy may result in a flare-up of disease activity.

NSAIDs may irritate the GI tract and predispose to peptic ulceration. All NSAIDs, to varying degrees, can cause sodium retention and edema in susceptible patients. NSAIDs have also been associated with renal disorders such as acute renal failure, proteinuria, the nephrotic syndrome, interstitial nephritis, and occasionally papillary necrosis.

Indomethacin, an indole derivative, also has analgesic, antipyretic, and anti-inflammatory actions, but because of its potential toxicity is not recommended as a simple analgesic. It is indicated primarily for rheumatoid arthritis and related diseases. Indomethacin is often helpful in the treatment of pain from bony metastases of cancer. (See also Ch. 108.)

Propionic acid derivatives: The newer NSAIDs such as ibuprofen, fenoprofen, ketoprofen, naproxen, and others are also useful as analgesics. Sodium naproxen, ibuprofen, and other agents of this class have been shown to be effective for dysmenorrhea.

NSAIDs are useful for mild to moderate pain from athletic injuries, skin, bone, and teeth disorders, postoperative pain, and rheumatoid and osteoarthritis. Propionic acid derivatives can help relieve pain in cancer patients as well, particularly the pain arising from bony metastasis. The availability of OTC ibuprofen has increased its use for nonarthritic pain, particularly dysmenorrhea.

Antiarthritic drugs, including salicylates, gold compounds, D-penicillamine, hydroxychloroquine, indomethacin, phenylbutazone, propionic acid derivatives, and several newer agents are also discussed in Ch. 108.

283. CORTICOTROPIN (ACTH) AND CORTICOSTEROIDS

While the adrenal corticosteroids are essential for life, they do not *initiate* cellular and enzymatic activity; they *permit* many biochemical reactions to proceed at optimal rates. Except as specific replacement therapy in adrenocortical insufficiency or for suppression of adrenal overactivity, clinical use of corticosteroids and their synthetic analogs depends on their anti-inflammatory, antiallergic, and lympholytic properties.

Endogenous ACTH and corticosteroids are not produced and do not function in isolation; they operate as an integral component of the hypothalamic-pituitary-adrenal system. This system is important in maintaining homeostasis under resting conditions and in response to many stimuli and stresses. The corticosteroids affect all organs and tissues. They aid in keeping the internal environment constant through their actions on the metabolism of water and electrolytes, carbohydrate, fat, and protein. The pituitary rapidly augments its release of ACTH into the circulation in response to environmental stress; the increased ACTH stimulates the adrenal cortex to secrete more hydrocortisone (cortisol). The mechanisms of interaction of the hypothalamic-pituitary-adrenal system and their clinical significance are detailed in Chs. 87, 88, and 91.

The best methods of assessing adrenocortical function, in addition to direct measurement of plasma ACTH, plasma corticosteroids, and urinary corticosteroids, are those which depend on the response of plasma or urinary corticosteroid levels to stimulation with ACTH or metyrapone, or suppression by exogenous corticosteroids. These are more specific and safer than the provocative tests. (For further discussion of tests, see Chs. 88 and 91.

CORTICOTROPIN (ACTH)

ACTH maintains the weight of the adrenal and stimulates its secretion of corticosteroid hormones. Excess ACTH, endogenous or administered, induces adrenal hypertrophy and provokes increased adrenocortical secretion of hydrocortisone. The increase in hydrocortisone and dehydroepiandrosterone **(DHEA)** production is reflected by sharp increases in urinary excretion of 17-hydroxycorticosteroids and 17-ketosteroids. The plasma hydrocortisone level rises in minutes in response to ACTH, which also causes some small and transient increases in adrenal aldosterone secretion.

ACTH given IV has a short plasma half-life. Repository, long-acting preparations such as ACTH in a gelatin vehicle or in combination with zinc are used for IM injection. Lyophilized preparations are partially inactivated in muscle. The therapeutic effects of ACTH are due to stimulation of hydrocortisone overproduction by the adrenal and can be achieved with corticosteroids, which are generally preferred to ACTH because they can be given orally. Some believe ACTH to be more effective in selected situations (eg, to avoid adrenal suppression, and, possibly, to lessen growth retardation

in children), but this has been questioned (see PRINCIPLES FOR USING CORTICOSTEROIDS, below).

THE CORTICOSTEROIDS

Chemistry and Classification

Over 50 steroids have been isolated from the adrenal cortex of animals and man, but few have biologic importance. They are classified according to their biologic activities as **glucocorticoids** (eg, hydrocortisone, cortisone, corticosterone), which affect mainly carbohydrate and protein metabolism and the immune system; **mineralocorticoids** (chiefly aldosterone, but also desoxycorticosterone), which regulate electrolyte and water metabolism; and **androgens** (eg, DHEA, androstenedione, testosterone, 11β-hydroxyandrostenedione), which are anabolic and cause masculinization.

The synthetic analogs of hydrocortisone (cortisol) possess no significant properties that hydrocortisone lacks; they differ chiefly in relative mineralocorticoid vs. anti-inflammatory potencies (see TABLE 283–1). The other chief difference is the long half-life of many of these synthetic analogs, which contributes significantly to their increased potency. **Desoxycorticosterone acetate,** which lacks the anti-inflammatory activity of hydrocortisone, is a potent mineralocorticoid that must be given parenterally. It has been supplanted in the treatment of Addison's disease by **fludrocortisone** (the most potent mineralocorticoid), which can be given orally.

Dehydrogenation at the 1 and 2 positions of the hydrocortisone and cortisone molecules yields **prednisolone** and **prednisone,** respectively, which possess more potent anti-inflammatory properties but have less sodium and water-retaining-effect. The addition of a 16α-hydroxyl, a 16α-methyl, and a 16β-methyl group to the 9α-fluoro substituent **(fludrocortisone)** forms **triamcinolone, dexamethasone,** and **betamethasone,** respectively, and reduces the sodium-retaining properties of the parent compound. All 3 compounds evoke little or no sodium retention in effective anti-inflammatory doses. Most synthetic corticosteroids disappear from the blood more slowly and are less firmly bound to serum protein than hydrocortisone.

TABLE 283–1. RELATIVE BIOLOGIC POTENCIES OF COMMONLY USED CORTICOSTEROIDS

Corticosteroid	*Relative Potency* (mEq)* Glucocorticoid (Anti-inflammatory)	Mineralocorticoid (Sodium-retaining)
Hydrocortisone (Cortisol)	1	1
Cortisone	0.8	0.8
Desoxycorticosterone	0	30–50
Fludrocortisone	10	125
Prednisone	4–5	0.8
Prednisolone	4–5	0.8
Methylprednisolone	5–6	0.5
Triamcinolone	4–5	Minimal
Paramethasone	10	Minimal
Fluprednisolone	10–15	Minimal
Dexamethasone	30	Minimal
Betamethasone	30	Minimal

* Hydrocortisone expressed as unity. Potencies vary considerably depending upon whether determination is at 4, 12, or 24 h following administration. The above rough approximations are taken chiefly from bioassays and do not necessarily apply to individual patients.

Absorption, Metabolism, and Excretion in Systemic Therapy

Hydrocortisone is readily and quickly absorbed from the gut, even in malabsorption syndromes or after total or partial gastrectomy. High corticosteroid blood levels are reached within 1 h and persist (though falling) for 6 to 8 h. Sustained action requires administration at 4- to 8-h intervals. The **oral route** is preferred for long-term therapy. Onset of action is rapid, but, for acute allergic emergencies (eg, status asthmaticus, angioedema), epinephrine acts faster.

The therapeutic effects of glucocorticoids are achieved most rapidly by the **IV route.** Hydrocortisone sodium succinate or hydrocortisone phosphate exemplify water-soluble preparations that can be dissolved in a small volume of sterile water and given as a rapid IV injection over a 2-min period. The ester hydrolyzes quickly in the blood, yielding free hydrocortisone; the level remains elevated for 4 h. An effect (eg, on blood pressure after adrenalectomy) may appear in minutes. These agents can also be given as a prolonged infusion in 5% dextrose or 0.9% sodium chloride solution (500 to 1000 mL over 4 to 12 h).

The **IM route** is probably the least satisfactory method of giving corticosteroids because absorption is slow and variable. However, the sustained action of IM hydrocortisone acetate makes it suitable for adrenal suppression when continuous adequate blood levels are essential. Hydrocortisone sodium succinate and similar esters can also be given IM, but are absorbed and metabolized more rapidly, thus requiring several injections daily for sustained effect.

Hydrocortisone enters all body tissues and compartments, including the CSF, and is eliminated from the body within 24 to 48 h. The major metabolic site is the liver, where the steroid undergoes degradation, yielding compounds readily excreted in the urine. Metabolism of hydrocortisone is delayed in patients with hepatic cirrhosis, hypothyroidism, and severe renal insufficiency.

Local or Topical Treatment

When the site of the disorder under treatment is accessible by local application, it may be preferable to give corticosteroids topically. Beclomethasone is often administered by inhalation as an aerosol or as microparticles in treating asthma; several esters are available as topical creams for treating dermatologic or ophthalmic inflammatory diseases, and various slowly-absorbed esters are administered intra-articularly for acute joint inflammation. Ulcerative colitis may respond to steroid enemas. All of these situations take advantage of the relatively high local concentration of steroids to produce a local effect while minimizing undesirable systemic effects. If steroids are given locally over long periods, however, absorption through the skin or mucous membranes may cause systemic effects like those described below.

Pharmacologic Actions and Undesirable Effects

Qualitatively, the pharmacologic actions of hydrocortisone and of the synthetic glucocorticoids are identical; quantitatively, they differ in their respective effects on various tissue and organ functions. See TABLE 283–1 for the relative biologic potencies of various corticosteroids.

Carbohydrate metabolism: Hydrocortisone repletes liver glycogen and raises blood glucose, largely through enhancement of gluconeogenesis from protein, and impedes peripheral utilization of glucose. While glucose intolerance occurs in many patients with spontaneous Cushing's syndrome, clinical diabetes mellitus is not common in corticosteroid-treated patients. **"Steroid diabetes"** is characterized by insulin resistance and, usually, the absence of ketosis and acidosis. When glucosuria occurs, latent or subclinical diabetes mellitus must be ruled out. A family history of diabetes mellitus demands extra vigilance when glucocorticoids are given.

Protein metabolism: Large doses of hydrocortisone invoke increased amino acid production from protein, negative nitrogen balance, and, after prolonged administration,

depletion of body protein, as in the severe muscle wasting and osteoporosis of both spontaneous and iatrogenic Cushing's syndrome.

Fat metabolism: Hydrocortisone is antiketogenic as a result of increased availability of carbohydrate. High doses cause redistribution of fat, with depletion in the extremities and increased deposition in the face and the cervicodorsal, interscapular, and abdominal regions.

Electrolyte and water metabolism: Mineralocorticoids and glucocorticoids produce Na and water retention. *Absence* of these hormones results in Addison's disease (see under ADRENAL HYPOFUNCTION in Ch. 91). Hydrocortisone acts with aldosterone to maintain electrolyte balance. Glucocorticoids (but not mineralocorticoids) also help maintain the capacity to excrete a water load. High dosages of any corticosteroid may produce Na and water retention with hypervolemia, edema, and, especially in elderly patients, congestive heart failure. Hypokalemic alkalosis occurs and can be treated with K salts.

Effects on the endocrine system: In addition to its diabetogenic effect, hydrocortisone causes adrenocortical atrophy by suppressing endogenous pituitary ACTH secretion. Such atrophy is accompanied by failure to secrete increased amounts of corticosteroid in response to an acute illness or other environmental stress; the ensuing adrenocortical insufficiency may be of clinical import (as in too hasty withdrawal) and occasionally is fatal.

Hydrocortisone may induce mild hirsutism in women. Disturbances in menstrual function are not likely to occur unless very high serum corticosteroid levels follow prolonged administration.

Effects on connective tissue: Glucocorticoids induce many chemical changes in ground substance and alter the response of connective tissue to injury. They inhibit inflammatory reactions, which explains their usefulness in suppressing manifestations of the collagen diseases but also accounts for their deleterious effect on wound healing. Since the anti-inflammatory actions are only suppressive, their withdrawal is generally followed by recrudescence of the disease. Suppression of the inflammatory reaction in patients receiving large doses may be so complete as to mask the clinical symptoms and signs of major diseases (eg, perforation of a peptic ulcer or spread of infection).

Effects on hypersensitivity reactions: The antiallergic action of hydrocortisone may be due to interference with the mechanism by which tissue injury results from an antigen-antibody reaction. Suppression of prostaglandin production may also be important.

Effects on cell-mediated immunity: All forms of delayed hypersensitivity are suppressed, including the tissue transplant rejection reaction. Glucocorticoids are therefore useful in controlling rejection of transplanted organs.

Effects on the musculoskeletal system: Hydrocortisone in physiologic quantities appears to be essential for muscular contraction. In large doses it evokes muscle weakness and atrophy due to inhibition of protein synthesis; K depletion may also play a role. Corticosteroids may induce myopathies characterized by loss of muscle substance and focal myositis.

Osteoporosis results from a decrease in the protein matrix of bone and an increased calcium removal. Hydrocortisone impedes growth in children, partially through its inhibition of protein synthesis. Daily doses of prednisone (or equivalent) of more than 4 mg/sq m of BSA retard skeletal maturation. Catch-up growth after treatment is stopped is slow and variable.

Effects on the hemopoietic system: Large doses of hydrocortisone induce peripheral lympholysis and slower lymphocyte production; polymorphonuclear leukocytes are relatively increased and may be markedly increased shortly after administration is

started. Leukemoid reactions rarely occur. Leukocytosis is uncommon in spontaneous Cushing's syndrome. The lympholytic property is exploited in the treatment of acute lymphoblastic leukemia, particularly in children.

Effects on the GI system: Gastric or duodenal ulcer may follow administration of hydrocortisone, especially in patients with RA. Corticosteroids combat the malabsorption of fat in sprue and in Whipple's disease through an unknown mechanism. Rarely, pancreatitis occurs during corticosteroid therapy.

Effects on the cardiovascular system: Hypervolemia, edema, and congestive heart failure occasionally follow administration of high doses of hydrocortisone. Hypertension occurs rarely.

Effects on the skin: Administration of excessive amounts of hydrocortisone is associated with thinning of the subcutaneous tissue and splitting of elastic fibers, with red or purple striae and ecchymoses. The acne and hirsutism of induced hypercorticism are due to androgenic breakdown products.

Effects on the CNS: Hydrocortisone increases brain excitability; seizures may result, especially in children and in those with established convulsive disorders. The abnormal EEG of Addison's disease usually becomes normal after a small dose of replacement hydrocortisone is taken.

Emotional disturbances including psychotic reactions with delusions and hallucinations may be seen in patients with Addison's disease or Cushing's syndrome. It cannot be predicted from the patient's underlying personality whether psychologic changes will occur in patients who receive large doses of glucocorticoids. Changes in affect vary from euphoria to depression. Agitation and insomnia are not uncommon. Pseudotumor cerebri is a rare untoward event. Serious psychiatric symptoms are directly, though roughly, correlated with higher dosage.

Corticosteroids, especially when applied topically to the eye, raise intraocular pressure. The increase is greater in patients with glaucoma.

PRINCIPLES FOR USING CORTICOSTEROIDS

Corticosteroids are used in physiologic replacement doses when normal adrenal function is absent, as in Addison's disease, or when overproduction of adrenal androgens occurs because of inadequate secretion of hydrocortisone, as in congenital adrenal hyperplasia (see Ch. 196). In these situations the dosage merely replaces normal secretion and is therefore kept low enough that it should not lead to toxic or side effects. Treatment should ordinarily be continued for the life of the patient. In supraphysiologic dosages, the pharmacologic properties of the corticosteroids also make them valuable in many other disorders (eg, RA, SLE, bronchial asthma, hypersensitivity diseases). Specific details of corticosteroid use in these conditions are discussed in their appropriate chapters. Topical corticosteroid preparations are discussed in Ch. 228. General principles of corticosteroid use are described here.

1. Possible benefits should be weighed against risks of undesirable effects.

2. Patients should be evaluated with regard to a history of (a) peptic ulcer; (b) emotional instability; (c) personal or family diabetes mellitus; or (d) tuberculosis. A chest x-ray and tuberculin skin test should be ordered routinely for all patients. If the latter is positive, isoniazid should be given concomitantly with corticosteroids.

3. The synthetic analogs are generally preferable to hydrocortisone or cortisone because of their lower sodium-retaining effects.

4. The lowest effective dose should be prescribed for the shortest possible time.

5. Committing a patient to long-term corticosteroid therapy should be considered only after other therapeutic measures have failed.

6. All dosages should be individualized. The effective dose varies with different diseases, with different phases of the same disease, and from patient to patient.

7. The dosage should be kept flexible, being raised or lowered according to the activity of the disease or the development of undesirable effects.

8. In stable treatment programs, use of the *alternate-day (intermittent) dosage schedule* should be considered; eg, prednisone 40 mg orally on alternate days instead of 20 mg/day. This regimen permits the hypothalamic-pituitary-adrenal axis to recover on alternate days from the suppressing effects of corticosteroid treatment. Longer-acting derivatives such as dexamethasone should not be used in alternate-day treatment, because their persistence prevents the advantages of alternate days without treatment. Usually, results are satisfactory with the alternate-day regimen and the undesirable effects are fewer and less severe.

9. If an acute infection, trauma, or surgery occurs during treatment, the dosage should be *increased* and given parenterally if necessary; eg, hydrocortisone sodium succinate 300 mg IV on the day of surgery, 200 mg on the 1st postoperative day, and 100 mg on the 2nd postoperative day, after which the previous prednisone doses are resumed. ACTH should not be used in these circumstances, since the adrenal response to ACTH is suppressed and the desired increases in endogenous hydrocortisone are not achieved.

10. Patients who have received cortisone 50 mg or more/day (or equivalent amounts of other corticosteroids) for periods of more than 1 to 2 mo should be considered to have some degree of pituitary-adrenal suppression for at least 1 yr after corticosteroid withdrawal.

11. Corticosteroids should be withdrawn gradually.

Contraindications

Active, healed, or questionably healed TB was once considered an absolute contraindication to corticosteroid use. However, corticosteroids, combined with antituberculous therapy, may be life-saving in overwhelming tuberculous infections and are essential in TB patients who develop adrenal insufficiency.

Ocular herpes simplex is an **absolute contraindication** to corticosteroid therapy. **Relative contraindications** are acute or chronic infections (especially chickenpox), pregnancy, diabetes mellitus, hypertension, peptic ulcer, osteoporosis, recent intestinal anastomoses, diverticulitis, psychotic tendencies, renal insufficiency, and diminished cardiac reserve or congestive heart failure other than that due to active rheumatic carditis. With any of these conditions, the advantages of corticosteroid therapy must be carefully weighed against the possibility of deleterious results.

Generally, corticosteroids should not be given if prophylactic immunization is imminent because of the possible interference with immune response. However, if the continued administration of corticosteroids is mandatory, as in adrenal insufficiency or SLE, concurrent immunization should be carried out as indicated.

No injection of these drugs should be made into an infected area.

Management During Long-Term Treatment

Precautions to be taken prior to corticosteroid therapy are outlined above. During treatment, close attention should be given to the appearance of undesirable effects: weight gain, edema, hypertension, signs of intercurrent infection, glucosuria, hyperglycemia, or psychiatric abnormalities. If back pain occurs, x-rays of the spine should be taken for possible osteoporosis or compression fractures. If pathologic fractures occur but the patient's condition requires continuation of corticosteroid therapy, additional Ca and protein are indicated with or without anabolic steroids. Abdominal pain or GI bleeding, major or minor, demands upper GI x-ray study to detect peptic ulcer. Peptic ulceration or severe mental disturbance requires stopping corticosteroids. With acute abdominal crisis (eg, perforated ulcer), increased corticosteroid dosage is needed during the acute phase or during surgery for its treatment; then the corticosteroid should be gradually withdrawn.

Dietary salt restriction is usually not needed at the outset, and need not be stringent with synthetic glucocorticoids. Body weight should be watched and, if edema develops, diuretics should be given or corticosteroid dosage reduced, or both. Hypokalemic alkalosis can be prevented or corrected with potassium chloride. Disturbances in carbohydrate metabolism may be controlled by dietary readjustment or by proper doses of insulin.

Infections occurring during therapy should be treated promptly with antibiotics, but not prophylactically. If the infecting organisms are not susceptible to antibiotics (as in candidiasis), corticosteroids should be discontinued gradually.

Withdrawal of ACTH and Corticosteroids

ACTH treatment produces adrenal hypertrophy, but suppresses secretion of endogenous ACTH. Cessation of ACTH therapy results in temporary relative adrenal insufficiency.

Administration of corticosteroids causes atrophy of the adrenal cortex and decreased production of endogenous hormones, and abrupt withdrawal produces a hypoadrenal state; therefore, drug dosage should be decreased gradually. Adrenal stimulation with exogenous ACTH is not helpful. Adrenal function is usually restored within a few weeks, but *relative adrenal insufficiency may occasionally persist for as long as 1 yr or more.* Clinically significant adrenal insufficiency is highly unlikely unless the steroid has been administered in a dosage of 50 mg/day of prednisone or equivalent for > 1 mo. It is also rare in patients who have received alternate-day treatment. Under these circumstances, discontinuation of steroid treatment is usually well tolerated even without special precautions, but the dangers of stress should not be ignored.

Patients with adrenal or pituitary suppression or both cannot tolerate stress (eg, surgery, trauma, infection). They must be prepared for surgery by increasing the amount of exogenous corticosteroid before, during, and after the stressful event. Stressed patients should be watched for fall in BP, weakness, circulatory collapse and shock, or other evidence of adrenal insufficiency. For emergency surgery, an IV solution of corticosteroid should be used until oral absorption is possible. After the stress has abated, dosage should be gradually decreased to previous maintenance levels. A small increase in corticosteroid dosage is advisable for minor surgery, slight injuries, or mild infections.

284. PROSTAGLANDINS, THROMBOXANES, AND LEUKOTRIENES

Prostaglandins **(PGs)** are a group of cyclic fatty acids that possess diverse and potent biologic activities affecting cell function in every organ system. Originally isolated as lipid-soluble extracts from sheep and human prostates, they are found in most mammalian tissues. The parent compound, prostanoic acid, contains a 20-carbon chain with a cyclopentane ring. Variations in the number and position of the double bonds and hydroxyl groups determine the physiologic activities of the different PGs. The important substitutions are on the cyclopentane ring.

PGA_1 primarily affects the cardiovascular-renal system, while PGE_1 has many other actions on the reproductive, gastrointestinal, respiratory, and immune systems. $PGF_{1\alpha}$ has diverse and potent physiologic effects on many organ systems but, unlike PGA_1 and PGE_1, does not lower BP. Although differences exist between PG_1s and PG_2s, in general they are physiologically similar. PG_2s are the most common naturally occurring PGs found in the body. PGD_2, PGI_2 (prostacyclin), thromboxane A_2, and the leukotrienes have been shown to be major end products of prostaglandin synthesis.

PGs are synthesized ubiquitously in the body from unsaturated fatty acid precursors with high rates of production by the seminal vesicles and renal medulla. These precur-

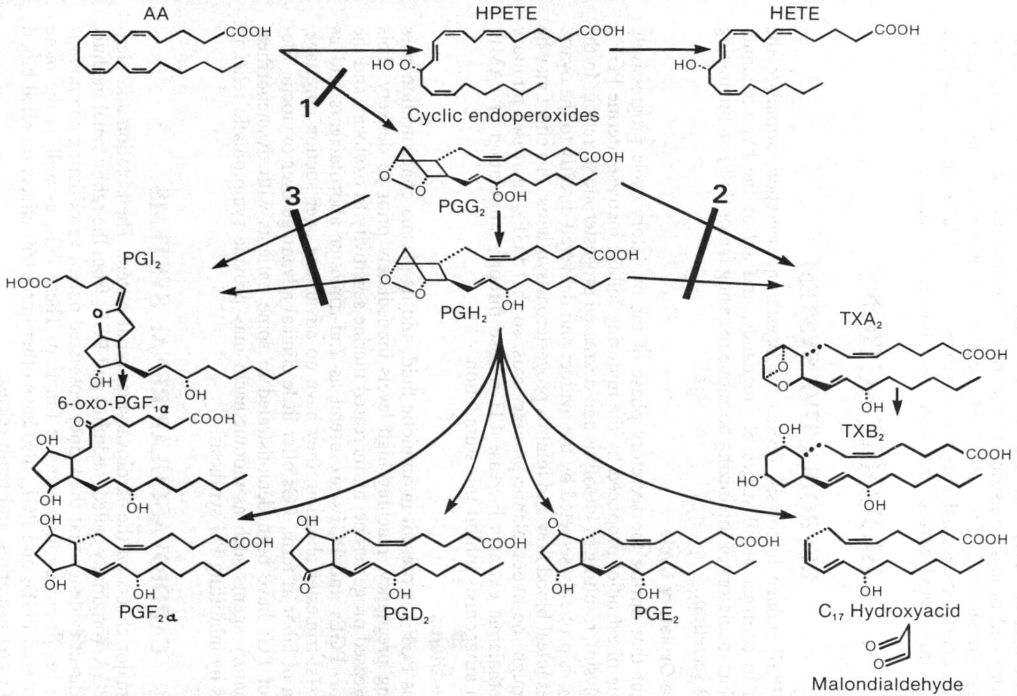

Fig. 284–1. Metabolic pathways of PG biosynthesis from arachidonic acid. The sites where cyclooxygenase inhibitors (aspirin-like drugs), thromboxane synthetase inhibitors (imidazole and 1-methyl imidazole) and prostacyclin synthetase inhibitors (15-hydroperoxyarachidonic acid and 13-hydroperoxylinoleic acid) act are indicated by the numerals 1, 2, and 3 respectively.

AA = arachidonic acid; HETE = 12-hydroxyarachidonic acid; HPETE = 12-hydroxyperoxyarachidonic acid; PGI_2 = prostacyclin; TXA_2 = thromboxane A_2; TXB_2 = thromboxane B_2

(From "Unstable metabolites of arachidonic acid and their role in haemostasis and thrombosis" by S. Moncada and J. R. Vane in *British Medical Bulletin* 34; 129–135, 1978. Published by Churchill Livingstone, Edinburgh. Used with permission.)

sors initially are converted to the cyclic endoperoxides PGG_2 and PGH_2 by PG cyclo-oxygenase, and then to various PGs and thromboxanes. An additional enzyme, lipoxygenase converts arachidonic acid to the intermediate 5-HPETE which in turn is converted to leukotrienes **(LTs)** A_4, B_4, C_4, D_4, and E_4 which possess marked proinflammatory and bronchoconstrictor properties. The structures and general synthetic pathways are shown in FIG. 284–1. PG synthesis is inhibited by aspirin, indomethacin, and other nonsteroidal anti-inflammatory agents. Metabolism takes place mostly in the lungs, renal cortex, and liver. Metabolites are excreted in the urine.

BIOLOGIC ACTIONS

REPRODUCTIVE SYSTEM

PGE and PGF induce luteolysis, decrease progesterone secretion, stimulate the gravid uterus to contract at all stages of pregnancy, and act at the hypothalamic-pituitary level as mediators of luteinizing hormone releasing factor **(LRF)** on luteinizing hormone **(LH)** secretion.

Effects on the Ovulatory Cycle

It is thought that during the secretory phase of the ovulatory cycle progressively larger amounts of estradiol produced by the maturing follicle increase uterine $PGF_{2\alpha}$ (uterine luteolysin), resulting in luteolysis and decreased progesterone secretion. In the human, $PGF_{2\alpha}$ is probably secreted by the oviduct and delivered directly to the ovary. $PGF_{2\alpha}$ reduces luteal blood flow and inhibits progesterone synthesis; this effect may be mediated through the hypothalamic-pituitary axis, so that $PGF_{2\alpha}$ increases pituitary cAMP. Hypothalamic extracts increase LH release through stimulation of cAMP; prostaglandin antagonists inhibit this stimulation.

Effects on the Uterus

Endogenous $PGF_{2\alpha}$ is present in amniotic fluid, and its plasma concentration rises steadily during pregnancy, reaching high levels immediately prior to delivery. This results in decreased progesterone, an increased uterine sensitivity to oxytocin, and the onset of labor. PGEs and PGFs are useful as 2nd-trimester abortifacients and as oxytocics. In 1st-trimester abortion, they have no advantage over suction curettage. For induction of labor at term, PGs offer little clinical advantage over oxytocin. Elevated levels of PGs have been demonstrated in some patients with dysmenorrhea. Anti-inflammatory agents such as indomethacin may provide symptomatic relief in these patients by inhibiting PG synthesis.

CARDIOVASCULAR-RENAL SYSTEMS

PGs have major effects on the cardiovascular-renal system. The isolation and identification of PGA_2 (originally called medullin) and PGE_2 from the rabbit renal medulla was the first direct evidence that the kidney possessed potent vasodilating compounds and, thus, an important *anti*hypertensive function. These PGs, as well as the more recently discovered PGD_2 and PGI_2, also have other important effects on renal blood flow, Na and water excretion, and renin release.

Renal Blood Flow and Sodium and Water Excretion

Administration of PGA, PGE, PGD, PGG, PGH, and PGI all increase renal blood flow and natriuresis. The natriuretic action of PGs may be due to nonspecific renovasodilation such as is observed with any renovasodilator (eg, acetylcholine, bradykinin, etc.). Similarly, the PG precursor arachidonic acid produces a rise in deep cortical and inner medullary flow accompanied by Na and water loss; these actions are inhibited by indomethacin. Loop diuretics (eg, ethacrynic acid and furosemide) also increase

renal blood flow, natriuresis, and urinary PGE excretion, suggesting that they act through PG release.

PGs probably do not directly maintain resting blood flow, but act to oppose renal vasoconstriction due to angiotensin, norepinephrine, sympathetic nervous stimulation, and renal artery occlusion by providing an offsetting vasodilatory action. This is important in diseases such as lupus nephritis, where renal blood flow becomes partially dependent on PG synthesis and release. Administration of indomethacin to such patients results in a marked deterioration of renal function. Thus, such compounds should be administered cautiously in patients with compromised renal blood flow, particularly those in renal failure.

Suppositions regarding the interaction of PGs with the renal handling of Na are controversial. Recent studies have shown a rise in plasma PGA and urinary PGE during volume depletion induced by low Na intake, diuretics, or hemodialysis. A major role of the renal PGs in volume depleted states such as low sodium diets or diuretic therapy is to counteract the antinatriuretic and prohypertensive effects of the renin-angiotensin-aldosterone axis. The rise in PGE_2 production in this instance is believed to be secondary to a direct stimulatory effect of angiotensin II on PG synthesis (see FIG. 284–2).

PGEs may attenuate vasopressin-stimulated adenyl cyclase and the accompanying increase in water movement. Aspirin, indomethacin, or meclofenamate can increase vasopressin-stimulated water reabsorption and maximal urinary osmolality. Thus PGE_2, which is normally secreted by the collecting duct cells, may be a physiologic antagonist of vasopressin acting at the site of vasopressin-induced water movement in the collecting duct cell.

Renin Release and Blood Pressure Regulation

Arachidonic acid, PGA_1, PGA_2, PGE_1, PGE_2, and PGI_2 all stimulate renin production. PG synthesis inhibition results in marked renin reduction and partial inhibition of the natriuretic and antihypertensive effects of loop diuretics, which suggests that

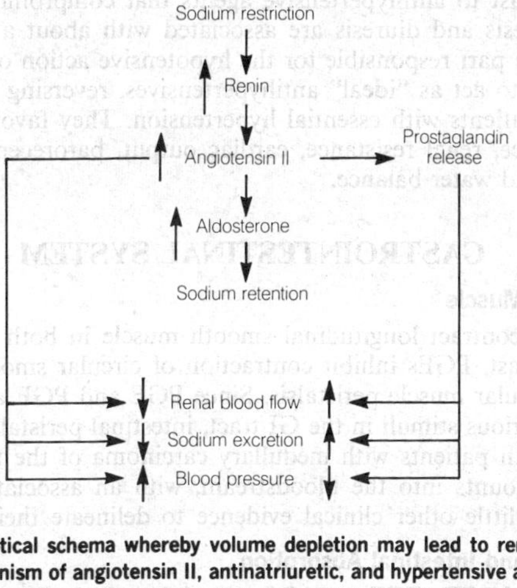

FIG. 284–2. Hypothetical schema whereby volume depletion may lead to renin-angiotensin release and physiological antagonism of angiotensin II, antinatriuretic, and hypertensive actions. (From "Prostaglandins and the renin-angiotensin axis" by J. B. Lee in *Clinical Nephrology* 14:159–163, 1980. Published by Dustri-Verlag, West Germany, Used with permission.)

volume depletion leads to a reduction in renal blood flow that triggers PG release leading to an increase in renin, angiotensin II, and aldosterone. Theoretically, volume depletion such as that resulting from a low Na intake or diuretic therapy should not lower BP as is clinically observed, since there is a marked activation of the renin-angiotensin-aldosterone axis under these conditions. Possibly the rise in plasma, renal, or local vascular PGs offsets the vasoconstricting effects of angiotensin II, thus lowering BP (see FIG. 284–2). The fact that indomethacin and aspirin increase BP in normotensives and hypertensives when plasma renin activity is markedly decreased supports this contention and suggests that inhibition of the vasodepressor PG system allows pressor mechanisms such as the renin-angiotensin system to act unopposed, even at lower plasma concentrations. Clinically, this has important connotations in **Bartter's syndrome** (see Ch. 155) where hyperreninemia, hyperaldosteronism, and hypokalemic alkalosis have been shown to be associated with increased plasma and urinary levels of PG, all of the above being temporarily reversed by PG synthesis inhibition with aspirin or indomethacin. However, it is now believed that this syndrome is not the result of a primary PG excess, but is the result of a defect in chloride transport in the thick ascending limb.

In summary, the evidence supports an antihypertensive function for renal and systemic PGs by antagonizing the vasopressor activity of the renin-angiotensin or the adrenergic nervous systems.

Effects in Hypertensive Humans

The first PG given to a hypertensive human was PGA_2. When given IV, the total calculated peripheral resistance fell as the result of direct peripheral arteriolar vasodilation and a fall in BP associated with a reflex baroreceptor-mediated increase in cardiac output. Subsequently, PGA_1 was shown to have the same mechanism of action as PGA_2. However, following infusion of PGA_1, the BP did not fall immediately; rather, there was an initial increase in renal blood flow and in Na, K, and water excretion. Later, when the BP fell to normotensive levels, there was a return to control levels in renal blood flow and in Na, K, and water excretion. Thus, normotension induced by PGAs is associated with normal renal blood flow and normal Na and water excretion, in contrast to antihypertensive agents that compromise renal blood flow. The initial natriuresis and diuresis are associated with about a 10% fall in plasma volume, which is in part responsible for the hypotensive action of PGA. Thus, PGA_1 and PGA_2 appear to act as "ideal" antihypertensives, reversing many of the known abnormalities in patients with essential hypertension. They favorably influence total peripheral resistance, renal resistance, cardiac output, baroreceptor activity, plasma volume, and Na and water balance.

GASTROINTESTINAL SYSTEM

Effect on Smooth Muscle

PGE and PGF contract longitudinal smooth muscle in both the small and large intestine. By contrast, PGEs inhibit contraction of circular smooth muscle, whereas PGFs increase circular muscle peristalsis. Since PGE and PGF are normally present and released by various stimuli in the GI tract, intestinal peristalsis may be mediated partially by PGs. In patients with medullary carcinoma of the thyroid, PGs are released in large amounts into the bloodstream, with an associated watery diarrhea. However, there is little other clinical evidence to delineate their role in peristalsis.

Gastric Secretion and Intestinal Absorption

Administration of PGE_1, PGE_2, and PGA_1 and their 16,16-dimethyl analogs inhibits gastric HCl secretion stimulated by histamine, pentagastrin, or food ingestion. In

addition, experimental ulcer production in animals (produced by pyloric ligation, stress, or steroids) is prevented by administration of PGEs and PGAs either orally, IV, or by inserting them into the jejunum. The hyperchlorhydric and ulcerogenic effects of aspirin and indomethacin are probably the result of inhibition of synthesis of anti-chlorhydric and antiulcerogenic PG.

Both PGE_1 and cholera toxin produce a rise in mucosal adenyl cyclase and cAMP that is capable of inhibiting intestinal Na and water transport. Diarrhea due to cholera toxin may be mediated by increased cAMP and inhibition of luminal Na and water transport resulting from increased intestinal PG release.

The most likely clinical GI use of PGEs and PGAs will be in the treatment of gastric hyperacidity and peptic ulceration. However, advantages over existing drugs and effectiveness in long-term therapy must be demonstrated.

RESPIRATORY SYSTEM

PGE_1 and PGE_2 relax human bronchiolar smooth muscle and increase pulmonary blood flow; $PGF_{2\alpha}$ and leukotrienes C and D contract bronchiolar smooth muscle and inhibit the bronchodilating effect of isoproterenol. This suggests that pulmonary synthesis and release of PGE may be clinically significant in increasing pulmonary blood flow in response to hypoxia. Furthermore, some bronchial asthma may be caused by a reduced PGE to PGF ratio, leading to bronchial vasoconstriction. PGE produces bronchial dilation by different mechanisms than isoproterenol, since PGE is devoid of β-adrenergic stimulation. Theoretically, PGEs could be very useful in the treatment of asthma, since they are metabolized by the lung and would not have the cardiovascular side effects associated with β-adrenergic stimulants.

Recent studies, however, appear to place the LTs rather than PGs as the most central agents in the etiologic genesis of bronchial asthma. They have been identified as the agents formerly known as slow-reacting substance and have 200 to 20,000 times the bronchoconstrictor activity as histamine. It is currently believed that an LT antagonist or synthesis inhibitor holds great promise in the treatment of bronchial asthma.

THE INFLAMMATORY RESPONSE

At high concentrations PGs are considered anti-inflammatory because they ameliorate experimental adjuvant arthritis in animals. However, at low concentrations, PGEs, PGD_2, and PGG_2 elicit all the typical signs of the inflammatory response. Furthermore, increased amounts of PGs are present in local areas of inflammation. PG synthetase activity is inhibited by nonsteroidal anti-inflammatory agents, and many of their actions, (as well as their side effects) have been attributed to this inhibition of PG synthesis.

PGs may play an important role during systemic, as well as local, inflammatory reactions. Pyrogen-induced fever, which has been associated with an increased $PGF_{2\alpha}$ content in the third ventricle, can be reduced by prior administration of a PG synthetase inhibitor such as indomethacin or aspirin. The analgesic effect of aspirin in headache may also be mediated by inhibition of PG synthesis, since PGE produces severe headaches in man.

In rheumatoid arthritis, large amounts of PGs and LTs in the synovium may contribute to inflammation and to periarticular bone demineralization from their Ca resorptive actions.

Recently, much attention has been given to the LTs as the major pathophysiologic mediators of the inflammatory response since they are much more potent than the PGs with regard to increasing vascular permeability, adhesion of leukocytes to the vessel wall, and edema production. Inhibitors of LT synthesis are currently being developed for possible clinical applications as anti-inflammatory agents.

IMMUNE RESPONSE

PGEs and PGAs, in contrast to the PGFs, have marked effects on the immune response. PGEs are capable of inhibiting antigen-induced histamine release from Ig-antibody-sensitized basophils and lung tissue; they are much more potent than catecholamines in this respect. Furthermore, catecholamine inhibition of histamine release can be blocked by propranolol, whereas no such inhibition occurs with PGE_1. Delayed hypersensitivity reactions are also inhibited. Lastly, phytohemagglutinin-induced lymphocyte transformation, as measured by protein DNA and RNA synthesis, is not only inhibited by cAMP but also by PGA and PGE, with a concomitant return of cell morphology toward normal.

In general, PGEs and PGAs inhibit both T and B cell activity, possibly in the former instance by inhibition of lymphokines. Since PGE is released by activated macrophages, a homeostatic feedback action of PGE inhibition of lymphocyte activation is believed to exist. However, it is premature to speculate on the clinical usefulness of PGs in various immune responses. The role of LTs in the immune response has been discussed under the RESPIRATORY SYSTEM above.

METABOLIC AND ENDOCRINE EFFECTS

Many of the actions of the PGEs and PGFs can be explained on the basis of their ability to stimulate or inhibit the production of cAMP, an intracellular hormonal mediator. Tropic hormones such as LH, TSH, and ACTH interact with cell membrane receptors, leading to increased PG synthetase activity and PG production. The increased levels of PG in turn stimulate the enzyme adenylate cyclase to convert ATP to cAMP where a biological action would be exerted. However, the same PG may accelerate production of cAMP within the target cell in one tissue and *inhibit* the activation of adenylate cyclase in another tissue. This puzzling and unexplained nonspecificity of PG interaction with cAMP does not occur with other hormone mediators. Specificity must relate to factors other than biochemical interactions between PGs and cAMP.

PGE_1 inhibits the lipolytic effects of ACTH, epinephrine, and glucagon, which act primarily by increasing adenylate cyclase activity and intracellular cAMP. In vitro, the antilipolytic effect of PGE_1 is associated with a decrease in cAMP, suggesting that it inhibits adenylate cyclase. Studies in humans, however, have shown both lipolytic and antilipolytic effects. The role of a deficiency in dietary essential fatty acids as a cause of hypertension, arthritis and other human disease states has received much attention in the lay press, but there is no scientific documentation to substantiate that such is the case, since most humans consume a diet containing large excesses of these compounds.

In carbohydrate metabolism, PGEs inhibit both basal and glucose-stimulated insulin release. Since PG synthesis inhibition with salicylates markedly improves the acute insulin response to glucose in diabetics, an excessive stimulation of pancreatic PG production has been postulated to be a contributing factor to impaired insulin release and carbohydrate intolerance in these patients. On the other hand, LTs have been shown to increase insulin secretion and an alternate current hypothesis is that carbohydrate intolerance in some patients with diabetes mellitus may result from an imbalance in the PG to LT ratio in the islet cell.

PGs stimulate thyroid, adrenal, and pituitary hormonogenesis. Thyroid hormone production is increased by PGE_1, apparently a TSH-like action with stimulation of adenylate cyclase and cAMP. In the adrenal gland, PGE_2 accelerates corticosterone and aldosterone production, the former in association with a rise in cAMP. PGs also act on the pituitary causing it to release growth hormone, prolactin, ACTH, and LH.

HEMATOLOGIC EFFECTS

PGE_1 is a potent inhibitor of platelet aggregation, while PGE_2 stimulates platelet aggregation. Both actions are mediated through cAMP, with PGE_1 causing a rise in cAMP and PGE_2 a fall in cAMP during the corresponding changes in platelet adherence. Although platelets normally contain PGE_2, which is released during clotting, the major compounds now believed to be involved in the clotting process are the recently discovered PGI_2 **(prostacyclin)** and thromboxane A_2 **(TXA_2)**. PGI_2 is synthesized ubiquitously in blood vessel walls from arachidonate derived either from the vessel wall or from the platelet. It is the most potent of all inhibitors of platelet aggregation and has vascular dilatory properties as well. Conversely, TXA_2, a potent platelet aggregator and vasoconstrictor, is synthesized primarily by the platelet.

Following endothelial damage, platelets adhere to the subendothelial connective tissue releasing catecholamines, serotonin, ADP, and TXA_2, which promote platelet aggregation through a decrease in platelet cAMP formation. TXA_2 is thought to be the main compound in this platelet aggregating process; it has a very short half-life and breaks down into the stable thromboxane B_2 (TXB_2). Conversely, once an interaction between the platelet and the vessel wall takes place, PGG_2 is converted to PGI_2 (prostacyclin), which tends to promote vasodilation and inhibition of TXA_2-induced platelet aggregation by stimulation of cAMP (FIG. 284–3). Whether or not physiologic or pathologic clot formation ensues appears to depend on the relative amount of PGI_2 versus TXA_2 production. The net effect appears to be on the anticlotting activity, since inhibition of TXA_2 synthesis occurs during the entire platelet lifetime and its effects on vascular PGI_2 synthesis is shorter lasting. This may be one of the main mechanisms involved in the beneficial effects of aspirin on thrombotic processes. The status of PGI_2 and TXA_2 in this process have important implications for the control of deep venous thrombosis, myocardial infarction, stroke and hypertension, and are receiving widespread attention.

CALCIUM AND BONE METABOLISM

PGE_1 and PGE_2, in contrast to the other PGs and thromboxanes, are potent stimulators of bone resorption in vitro, acting by increasing cAMP synergistically with parathyroid hormone. Excess PGE production has been attributed as a cause of bone resorption in periodontal inflammation, rheumatoid arthritis, and in the hypercalcemia of malignancy. Excess PGE has been demonstrated in hypercalcemic animals with experimental tumors. In such animals, indomethacin markedly reduces hypercalcemia caused by the tumor secreting PGE_2. In humans, the hypercalcemia of some solid tumors has been shown to be associated with low parathyroid hormone secretion and excessive plasma PGE, with both the high PGE levels and hypercalcemia being reversed by indomethacin. In contrast, hematologic tumors, hyperparathyroidism, and breast tumors are not associated with PG-induced hypercalcemia.

NERVOUS SYSTEM

Central

In animals, PGE_1 has sedative, tranquilizing, and anticonvulsant actions. Further, PGEs antagonize norepinephrine inhibition of Purkinje cell discharge, leading to the theory that PGs may function as CNS neuromodulators.

Peripheral

PGE_1, PGE_2, and PGI_2 reversibly inhibit norepinephrine in the peripheral nervous system with consequent inhibition of synaptic transmission. Presumably, a feedback mechanism exists whereby sympathetic stimulation leads to an increase in PGE_2 formation, thus reducing the amount of norepinephrine released.

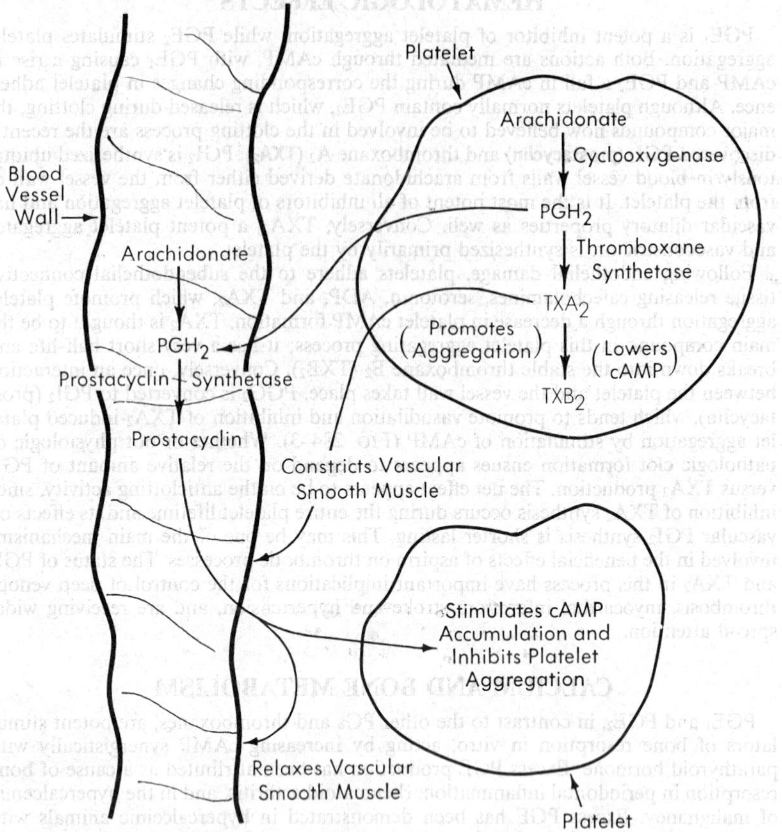

FIG. 284–3. Model of human platelet homeostais. (From "Modulation of human platelet function by prostacyclin and thromboxane A_2," pp. 83–88, by R. R. Gorman, in *Federation Proceedings* Vol. 38, No. 1, January 1979. Used with permission of the Federation of American Societies for Experimental Biology, and the author.)

OCULAR EFFECTS

In animals, PGE_1, PGE_2, and $PGF_{2\alpha}$ produce miosis; thus light-adapted miosis may be mediated in large part by local PG synthesis and release in the iris. This action is inhibited by norepinephrine. In rabbits, PGEs cause an increase in intraocular pressure, but this effect has not been duplicated in other animals. Nevertheless, PG antagonists may be found clinically useful in certain forms of wide-angle glaucoma. Currently, PG inhibition with indomethacin in patients undergoing corneal or lens transplant is being utilized as an effective method of reducing the degree and incidence of postoperative macular edema.

POTENTIAL THERAPEUTIC APPLICATIONS

TABLE 284–1 summarizes the current and potential therapeutic applications of the PGs. A major problem regarding the clinical use of PGs is finding an appropriate delivery system, particularly for the PGEs and PGFs. Since these compounds are metabolized during circulation through the lungs and appear to function as local hormones, their use would be limited if given orally or parenterally. However, PGA and PGI compounds, which are not degraded in the lungs, conceivably could be given as oral systemic antihypertensive agents.

In general, unique delivery systems that can provide local delivery are required for clinical use; eg, the intrauterine administration of PGE or PGF for abortion. Aerosol delivery of a PGE preparation may be feasible in bronchial asthma, and oral administration of PGA or PGE may have value for inhibition of HCl secretion.

To induce 2nd trimester abortion, PGE_2, $PGF_{2\alpha}$ and 15-methyl $PGF_{2\alpha}$ have been used since 1974 with an 80 to 90% success rate, but their superiority over saline infusion remains to be proven. The preferred routes are by intra- or extra-amniotic instillation in doses of 0.75 mg q 2 h ($PGF_{2\alpha}$), 0.25 mg q 2 h (PGE_2), and a single injection of 1 mg of 15-methyl $PGF_{2\alpha}$. The most common complications are GI with a high incidence of nausea and vomiting particularly with IV or IM administration. As of this writing, a definitive indication of prostaglandins for use in abortion has not been established.

PGE_1 is used in ductus arteriosus dependent cyanotic congenital heart disease (eg, interruption of the aortic arch proximal to ductus entry. To maintain patency of the ductus, an IV infusion rate of between 0.1 to 0.2 μg/kg/min has been utilized prior to and during surgical correction with considerable success. Conversely, in conditions where there is an abnormally prolonged patency of the ductus as a sole congenital abnormality, the use of indomethacin as adjuctive therapy to promote closure has received widespread attention (see PATENT DUCTUS ARTERIOSUS, in Ch. 187).

Aspirin, by virtue of its more prolonged inhibition of the platelet vasoconstrictor thromboxane than the arteriolar vasodilator PGI_2, is an effective agent in prolonging

TABLE 284–1. THERAPEUTIC APPLICATIONS OF THE PROSTAGLANDINS

Prostaglandins	*PG Synthesis Inhibition*
Current	
Midtrimester abortion	Rheumatoid arthritis
Peripheral vascular disease	Fever and headache
Hemodialysis	Bartter's syndrome
Induction of labor	Patent ductus arteriosus (closure)
Patent ductus arteriosus (maintenance)	
Potential	
Hypertension	Hypercalcemia of malignancy
Congestive heart failure	Periodontal inflammation
Infertility	Cholera and certain diarrheal states
Coronary and deep thrombosis	Burns
Peptic ulceration	Lupus erythematosus
Gastric hyperacidity	Glaucoma
Bronchial asthma (PGE)	Migraine headache
Nasal congestion	Bronchial asthma (leukotriene)

(Modified from "Prostaglandins, Thromboxanes and Leukotrienes" by J. B. Lee in Williams' *Textbook of Endocrinology*, ed. 7, edited by D. W. Foster and J. D. Wilson. Copyright 1985 by W. B. Saunders Company. Used with permission of W. B. Saunders Company and the author.)

the bleeding time in humans. It has been used in extensive clinical trials in low dosage (30 to 50 mg/day), alone or in combination with dipyridamole (a thromboxane synthetase inhibitor), to determine its effectiveness in prevention of deep venous thrombosis, coronary artery thrombosis, and cerebrovascular accidents. Although the results appear promising, much caution and many further trials await the establishment of this pharmaceutical regimen as effective in prevention of major cardiovascular thrombotic phenomena.

Nonsteroidal inflammatory agents have been used with considerable success in the treatment of the symptoms of dysmenorrhea, particularly abdominal cramps. The latter have been ascribed to elevated uterine pressure and ischemia that has been associated with elevated levels of $PGF_{2\alpha}$ in menstrual fluid. The abdominal discomfort may also result from enhanced PG-mediated intestinal tonic peristalsis. Although inhibition of PG synthesis by nonsteroidal anti-inflammatory agents may be of marked benefit in some cases of dysmenorrhea, others do not respond well.

---

285. ANTIHISTAMINES

Many antihistamines, in addition to blocking the effects of histamine, have other useful therapeutic effects. Pharmacologic differences among them are most apparent in their sedative, antiemetic, and other CNS effects, and in their anticholinergic, antiserotonin, and local anesthetic properties.

Histamine

Histamine is widely distributed in mammalian tissue. In man the highest concentrations are in skin, lungs, and GI mucosa. Histamine is present mainly in the intracellular granules of mast cells, but there is also an important extra-mast-cell pool in the gastric mucosa, with smaller amounts in the brain, heart, and other organs. The release of histamine from the mast-cell storage granules can be triggered by physical tissue disruption, various chemicals (including tissue irritants, surface active agents, and polymers), and most prominently by antigen-antibody interactions.

The specific homeostatic function of histamine remains unclear. Its actions in man are exerted primarily on the cardiovascular system, extravascular smooth muscle, and exocrine glands, and they appear to be mediated by 2 distinct histamine receptors, termed H_1 and H_2.

Histamine H_1 Receptor Effects

Cardiovascular system: Histamine is a potent arteriolar and capillary dilator that can cause extensive peripheral pooling of blood and hypotension. It also increases capillary permeability by distortion of the endothelial lining of the postcapillary venules, with widening of the gap between endothelial cells and exposure of basement membrane surfaces. This accelerates loss of plasma and plasma proteins from the vascular space and, combined with arteriolar and capillary dilation, can produce circulatory shock. Histamine also dilates cerebral vessels, which may be a factor in histamine headache.

The **"triple response"** is mediated by local *intracutaneous* histamine release, causing (1) local erythema from capillary dilation, (2) wheal due to local edema from increased capillary permeability, and (3) flare from a neuronal reflex mechanism producing a surrounding area of arteriolar vasodilation. **Other smooth muscle:** In man, histamine may cause severe bronchoconstriction in susceptible individuals. Histamine also stimulates GI motility. **Exocrine glands:** Histamine increases salivary and bronchial gland secretions. **Endocrine gland:** Stimulation of catecholamine release from adrenal chromaffin cells also appears to be H_1-receptor mediated. **Sensory nerve endings:** Local instillation of histamine may produce intense itching.

Histamine H_2 Receptor Effects

Cardiovascular system: Histamine increases heart rate, contractility, and coronary blood flow, and the H_2 receptor plays some role in the histamine vasodilator and depressor response. Administration of either a histamine H_1 or H_2 receptor blocker alone has little effect on histamine-induced vasodepression, but H_1 and H_2 receptor antagonists together can reverse the hypotension, suggesting that both types are involved in the vasodepressor response to histamine.

Exocrine glands: Histamine is a potent stimulator of gastric acid secretion. **Leukocytes:** H_2 receptor stimulation inhibits histamine release from sensitized basophils and mast cells (negative feedback system).

HISTAMINE H_1 RECEPTOR ANTAGONISTS

The conventional antihistamines, now termed histamine H_1 receptor antagonists, possess a substituted ethylamine side-chain (similar to that of histamine) linked to one or more cyclic groups. The similarity between the ethylamine moiety of histamine and the substituted ethylamine structure of the H_1 receptor antagonists suggests that this molecular configuration is important in receptor interactions. Histamine H_1 receptor antagonists appear to act by competitive inhibition; they do not significantly alter histamine production, or metabolism.

The H_1 blocker antihistamines are generally well absorbed from the GI tract following oral or rectal administration. Onset of action usually occurs within 15 to 30 min, with peak effects attained in 1 h; duration of action is generally 3 to 6 h, but some of these drugs act considerably longer.

Antihistaminic effects of H_1 receptor antagonists are noted only in the presence of increased histamine activity. They block the effects of histamine on GI tract smooth muscle, but in man the allergic reaction of the bronchial smooth muscle is not dependent primarily on histamine release and does not respond effectively to antihistamines. Histamine H_1 receptor antagonists effectively block histamine-induced increased capillary permeability and sensory nerve stimulation, thus inhibiting the wheal, flare, and pruritus responses. However, these agents are only partially effective in reversing histamine-induced vasodilation and hypotension.

Clinically useful effects other than histamine antagonism are discussed below.

Therapeutic Indications

Antihistamines are useful for treating the symptoms of allergies, including seasonal hay fever, allergic rhinitis, and conjunctivitis. They are mildly effective in perennial vasomotor rhinitis. Acute and chronic urticaria and certain allergic dermatoses respond well, and pruritus may be alleviated. They are also useful for treating minor transfusion incompatibility reactions and systemic reactions to IV x-ray contrast media. The H_1 blockers have no role, however, in the treatment of bronchial asthma or systemic anaphylaxis. They provide little benefit in the therapy of the common cold, but because of their anticholinergic effects (see below) they may control rhinorrhea.

TABLE 285–1 summarizes the dose, route, and frequency of administration of some commonly available histamine H_1 receptor antagonists. These agents are all effective H_1 receptor blockers; their pharmacologic differences are primarily in the type and intensity of their other effects.

Other Clinically Useful Effects

CNS depression is prominent with many H_1 receptor antagonists, and they have been used as sedatives and hypnotics. Most have some anticholinergic properties that may account centrally for modest antiparkinsonian activity and peripherally for symptomatic relief of rhinorrhea in URIs. Several of the H_1 blockers are potent local anes-

TABLE 285–1. DOSAGE, ADMINISTRATION, AND PREPARATIONS OF SOME HISTAMINE H_1 RECEPTOR ANTAGONISTS

Agent	*Usual Adult Dosage*	*Route of Administration*	*Frequency*	*Available Preparations*
I. Alkylamines				
Brompheniramine maleate	4–8 mg	Oral	tid or qid	4-mg tablets 2 mg/5 mL elixir 8- and 12-mg tablets (timed-release)
	5–20 mg	IM or IV	q 6–12 h	10 mg/mL
Chlorpheniramine maleate	2–4 mg	Oral	q 6–8 h	2-mg tablets 4-mg tablets 2 mg/5 mL syrup 8- and 12-mg tablets (timed-release)
	5–20 mg	IV, IM, or s.c.		10 mg/mL injection 100 mg/mL injection
Dexchlorpheniramine maleate	2 mg	Oral	tid or qid	2-mg tablets 2 mg/5 mL syrup 4- and 6-mg tablets (extended-release)
Triprolidine HCl	2.5 mg	Oral	bid or tid	2.5-mg tablets 1.25 mg/5 mL syrup
II. Ethanolamines				
Carbinoxamine maleate	4–8 mg	Oral	tid or qid	4-mg tablets 4 mg/5 mL elixir 8- and 12-mg tablets (timed-release)
Clemastine fumarate	2.68 mg	Oral	bid or tid	1.34 and 2.68 mg tablets
Dimenhydrinate	50–100 mg	Oral	q 4 h	50-mg tablets 12.5 mg/4 mL liquid
	100 mg	Rectal	bid	100-mg suppositories
	50 mg	IM or IV	q 4 h	50 mg/mL injection
Diphenhydramine HCl	25–50 mg	Oral	tid or qid	25-mg capsules 50-mg capsules 12.5 mg/mL syrup 12.5 mg/5 mL elixir
	10–50 mg	IV or deep IM	q 3–4 h	10 mg/mL injection 50 mg/mL injection
Diphenylpyraline HCl	2 mg	Oral	q 4 h	2-mg tablets 5-mg capsules (sustained-action)
Doxylamine succinate	12.5–25 mg	Oral	q 4–6 h	12.5- and 25-mg tablets 6.25 mg/5 mL syrup

(*Continued*)

thetics and are often applied to the skin in the form of creams and lotions to reduce itching. However, topical application of antihistamines incurs considerable risk of drug sensitization.

The alkylamines have relatively little sedative effect and are useful as H_1 antihista-

TABLE 285–1. DOSAGE, ADMINISTRATION, AND PREPARATIONS OF SOME HISTAMINE H_1 RECEPTOR ANTAGONISTS *(Cont'd)*

Agent	*Usual Adult Dosage*	*Route of Adminis-tration*	*Frequency*	*Available Preparations*
III. Ethylenediamines				
Tripelennamine citrate	25–50 mg	Oral	q 4–6 h	37.5 mg/5 mL elixir
Tripelennamine HCl	25–50 mg	Oral	q 4–6 h	25-mg tablets 50-mg tablets 50- and 100-mg tablets (timed-release)
IV. Piperazines				
Cyclizine HCl	50 mg	Oral	q 4–6 h	50-mg tablets
	50 mg	IM	q 4–6 h	50 mg/mL injection
Hydroxyzine HCl	25–100 mg	Oral	tid or qid	10-mg tablets 25-mg tablets 50-mg tablets 100-mg tablets 10 mg/5 mL syrup
	25–100 mg	IM	q 4–6 h	25 mg/mL injection 50 mg/mL injection
Meclizine HCl	25–50 mg	Oral	once daily	12.5-mg tablets 25-mg tablets
V. Phenothiazines				
Methdilazine HCl	8 mg	Oral	q 6–12 h	8-mg tablets 4-mg tablets (chewable) 4 mg/5 mL syrup
Promethazine HCl	12.5–25 mg	Oral	bid	12.5-mg tablets 25-mg tablets 50-mg tablets 6.25 mg/5 mL syrup 25 mg/5 mL syrup
	12.5–25 mg	Rectal	q 2 h prn q 6 h	12.5-mg suppositories 25-mg suppositories 50-mg suppositories
	12.5–25 mg	IV or IM IM only	q 6 h q 6 h	25 mg/mL injection 50 mg/mL injection
Trimeprazine tartrate	2.5 mg	Oral	qid	2.5-mg tablets 2.5-mg/5 mL syrup 5-mg capsules (timed-release)
VI. Other				
Azatadine maleate	1–2 mg	Oral	bid	1-mg tablets
Cyproheptadine HCl	4 mg not to exceed 0.5 mg/kg/day	Oral	tid or qid	4-mg tablets 2 mg/5 mL syrup
Terfenadine	60 mg	Oral	bid	60-mg tablets

mines for daytime use. Two new agents, astemizole (not currently available in the USA) and terfenadine, do not cause significant sedation. The ethanolamines are significant CNS depressants and are useful as sedatives and hypnotics, although they are less potent and dependable than the barbiturates and other central depressants. The

ethanolamines also have marked anticholinergic properties. The ethylenediamines produce less CNS depression but more GI side effects than the ethanolamines.

Diphenhydramine, an ethanolamine derivative, and dimenhydrinate, its chlorotheophyllinate salt, the phenothiazine congener promethazine, and the piperazines, cyclizine and meclizine, are all used to prevent or treat motion sickness and relieve the nausea and vertigo associated with labyrinthitis. Cyclizine, hydroxyzine, and meclizine have been implicated as teratogens in animals, and probably should not be given during pregnancy. The phenothiazine group of H_1 receptor antagonists, notably promethazine, are useful as sedatives and are effective in controlling the nausea associated with radiotherapy and certain antineoplastic drugs; for this latter use they are less effective than prochlorperazine and chlorpromazine.

Side Effects and Toxicity

Undesirable effects of the H_1 antihistamines include anorexia, nausea, vomiting, constipation, diarrhea, epigastric distress, decreased alertness, impaired ability to concentrate, muscular weakness, and drowsiness. Topical administration can produce dermatitis and urticaria. Blood dyscrasias, such as leukopenia, agranulocytosis, thrombocytopenia, and hemolytic anemia, occur relatively rarely. The manifestations of overdosage are dominated by anticholinergic effects, including dry mouth, palpitations, chest tightness, urinary retention, visual disturbances, convulsions, hallucinations, and, later, by respiratory depression, fever, hypotension, and mydriasis.

HISTAMINE H_2 RECEPTOR ANTAGONISTS

CIMETIDINE

In contrast to the H_1 receptor antagonists, which possess a side-chain similar to the ethylamine moiety of histamine, the H_2 receptor blocking agent, cimetidine, incorporates a longer and more complex side-chain but retains the imidazole ring structure of histamine.

Cimetidine is a competitive inhibitor of histamine at H_2 receptors. In the stomach it blocks gastric acid secretion stimulated by histamine, gastrin, parasympathetic activity, and food; it diminishes both basal and nocturnal gastric acid secretion. Pepsin secretion, gastric juice volume, and, to a lesser extent, intrinsic factor secretion are also reduced. In the gallbladder, H_2 blockers potentiate cholecystokinin-induced contraction. Cimetidine augments delayed hypersensitivity responses in the immune system.

Cimetidine is well absorbed from the GI tract after oral administration. Onset of action begins within 30 min after an oral dose, and peak effects are attained in 1 to 2 h. IV administration produces a more rapid onset of activity. Duration of action is generally 4 to 6 h with either route. Antacids may reduce the oral bioavailability of cimetidine; at least 1 h should elapse between administration of antacids and cimetidine. Cimetidine is largely eliminated unmetabolized from the body mainly by renal excretion, but several hepatic metabolites have been identified after oral doses. In renal failure the dosage should be reduced to prevent drug accumulation (see TABLE 285–2). Hemodialysis removes cimetidine, and patients on dialysis may need an extra dose at the end of the procedure.

Therapeutic Indications

The principal indication for cimetidine is treatment of peptic ulcer disease. Cimetidine 300 mg orally qid (with meals and at bedtime) relieves pain and promotes ulcer healing. Recent clinical studies indicate that 400 mg bid provides essentially equivalent pain relief and ulcer healing. Either regimen should be continued until the ulcer heals, and then be followed by maintenance therapy using 400 to 800 mg daily for 6 mo to 1 yr. Maintenance therapy can be given as a single 400-mg dose at bedtime. Cessation of therapy is often associated with recurrence of ulcers, and perforation of duodenal

TABLE 285–2. RECOMMENDED CIMETIDINE DOSAGE BASED ON RENAL FUNCTION

Creatinine Clearance	*Approximate Half-life*	*Recommended Dose Interval (300 mg dose)*
Normal	2 h	q 6 h
50–90 mL/min	2 1/2 h	q 6 h
20–35 mL/min	3 h	q 8 h
< 10 mL/min	4 h	q 12 h

ulcers has occurred when cimetidine was stopped abruptly. Patients should be cautioned that ulcers may recur weeks or months after discontinuing therapy.

Cimetidine has also been used to treat gastric ulcers, but clinical trials have given conflicting results and the role of cimetidine in gastric ulcer therapy is unclear.

Cimetidine is useful in the symptomatic treatment of patients with **Zollinger-Ellison syndrome** (see in ENDOCRINE TUMORS under CANCER OF THE PANCREAS in Ch. 55) but has no effect on tumor progression. Incapacitating pain, diarrhea, and peptic ulcers are often controlled with cimetidine, using oral doses of up to 2400 mg daily as long as needed; palliative surgery can often be avoided.

Prophylactic cimetidine administration reduces gastric mucosal damage and GI bleeding associated with aspirin use and decreases the risk of upper GI hemorrhage after renal transplantation. Cimetidine may be a useful adjunct to oral pancreatic enzyme replacement in patients with pancreatic insufficiency; it reduces acid-peptic degradation of the ingested enzymes.

Severe metabolic alkalosis may develop after prolonged nasogastric suction, especially in patients with gastric hypersecretion. Cimetidine decreases acid loss and allows correction of the metabolic alkalosis.

Side Effects and Toxicity

Cimetidine is generally well tolerated. A mild increase in serum creatinine and serum transaminases often occurs without apparent clinical significance. Diarrhea, rash, drug fever, and myalgias have been reported, and mental confusion with agitation and other neuropsychiatric disturbances may develop, especially in elderly patients with impaired renal function. Cimetidine increases plasma prolactin levels; gynecomastia and, rarely, galactorrhea may ensue. Depression of sperm count and impotence have been noted particularly with long-term high-dose cimetidine therapy. Other rare side effects include ileus in patients with extensive burns, sinus bradycardia, hypotension after rapid IV injection, and hyperglycemia. Reversible bone-marrow suppression with granulocytopenia, thrombocytopenia, and anemia has occurred. Potentiation of warfarin-type anticoagulants and theophylline may occur with concomitant administration of cimetidine, and the elimination of propranolol, morphine, lidocaine, and some benzodiazepines including diazepam, chlordiazepoxide, and flurazepam may be prolonged.

RANITIDINE

Unlike histamine and cimetidine, the H_2 receptor blocking agent, ranitidine, has a furan ring structure. It is a potent competitive inhibitor of histamine at H_2 receptors, and seems to be more specific than cimetidine, with less effect on androgen and hepatic receptors. Ranitidine blocks gastric acid secretion stimulated by histamine, gastrin, or food, and it diminishes both basal and nocturnal gastric acid secretion.

Ranitidine is rapidly absorbed from the GI tract, but about 30% is metabolized by

the liver during the first-pass effect; peak plasma levels are reached in 1 to 3 h. Gastric acid secretion is inhibited for 8 to 12 h, allowing bid dosage for most patients. Ranitidine is largely eliminated unchanged by the kidney. In renal failure (serum creatinine levels > 4 mg/dL) the dosage should be reduced to 75 mg bid.

Therapeutic Indications and Dosage

Ranitidine is indicated for treatment of peptic ulcer disease and gastric hypersecretory states. Doses of 150 mg orally bid inhibit gastric acid secretion by 70% over 24 h, and by 90% overnight in patients with duodenal ulcers. In clinical trials, 150 mg orally bid has been as effective in promoting ulcer healing as cimetidine, 1000 mg/day. Once the ulcer has healed, a single 150-mg dose at bedtime can prevent recurrence in most patients. Preliminary data suggest that ranitidine may also be useful in patients with benign gastric ulcers.

Ranitidine may also be effective for patients resistant to cimetidine, who develop unacceptable side effects from cimetidine, or who are taking other drugs that rely largely on hepatic clearance for their disposition. Patients with Zollinger-Ellison syndrome may respond to high oral doses of ranitidine (600 to 1200 mg/day).

Side Effects

Ranitidine is well tolerated and the side effects are mostly minor, but the drug has not been used as extensively as cimetidine. The most common adverse effects are headache, dizziness, malaise, nausea, constipation, and a rash that often resolves with continued use of the drug. Transient increases in serum transaminases have occurred. Ranitidine does not significantly prolong the hepatic clearance of propranolol, lidocaine, and morphine.

286. DIURETICS

Drugs that promote urine formation by increasing the GFR or by decreasing reabsorption in the renal tubules.

Diuretics are commonly used to prevent or eliminate edema; they improve function of vital organs and relieve symptomatic distress. Edema is always secondary to an underlying disorder and, except when due to obstruction of veins or lymphatics, represents an attempt by the body to restore its intravascular volume. Thus, its treatment should always be accompanied by other measures.

Diuretics are also used in nonedematous states such as hypertension, hypercalcemia, idiopathic hypercalciuria, and nephrogenic diabetes insipidus. This chapter emphasizes the pharmacology of diuretics and their clinical application; uses in specific disorders are discussed elsewhere in THE MANUAL.

General Guidelines

Since the success of a diuretic program is affected by the amount of Na in the diet, Na restriction usually accompanies use of a diuretic. In mild edema, such as may occur in chronic congestive heart failure, a "no-added salt" diet (about 2 to 4 gm [87 to 174 mEq] Na) will generally suffice; when Na retention is severe, a 1 gm (43 mEq) Na diet (the minimum most patients can manage at home) may be required. In the hospital, reduction of dietary Na to 500 mg (22 mEq) daily may occasionally be necessary in severe edema or poorly responsive patients.

Potent diuretics profoundly reduce ECF (and therefore intravascular) volume. Thus diuresis that is too rapid can produce **hypovolemia,** with orthostatic hypotension, tachycardia, azotemia, and impaired cardiac and CNS function.

Hypokalemia is probably the most common adverse effect of diuretics. Nearly all diuretics in effective doses, except those noted below to be K-sparing, inhibit Na and

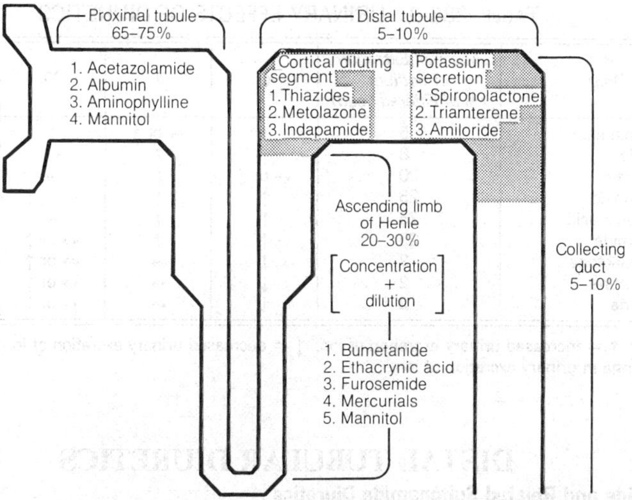

FIG. 286–1. Schematic diagram of a single nephron, indicating the normal ranges of sodium reabsorption (expressed as percent of filtered load) for each segment and the major site of action for various diuretics.

water reabsorption in the nephron at a point proximal to the site in the distal tubule where K is secreted. Thus they increase the load of Na and water delivered to the distal tubule where K secretion partly depends upon Na delivery. In some edematous patients, elevated aldosterone levels also augment K secretion. Serum K must be closely monitored when initiating diuresis, and supplemental K should be given to patients with low or low-normal values. Alternatively, a K-sparing diuretic may be used.

The combination of hypovolemia and hypokalemia frequently results in metabolic alkalosis. Since most potent diuretics produce urine in which Cl is the predominant anion with little or no HCO_3, the HCO_3 concentration in ECF is increased and that of Cl depressed. Hypokalemia also enhances renal HCO_3 reabsorption. The **hypokalemic-hypochloremic metabolic alkalosis** that results is not an indication that the diuretic should be discontinued, because the alkalosis and K deficit can be treated (or prevented) with potassium chloride. The more palatable K salts (eg, potassium bicarbonate, potassium citrate, potassium gluconate, or potassium acetate) deliver an alkali equivalent and thus will not correct the metabolic alkalosis. *Enteric-coated K preparations cause small-bowel ulcerations and should be avoided.*

Except in an emergency, therapy is begun with a single diuretic. Intermittent administration (once or twice/wk) is often sufficient to control fluid accumulation safely during the early stages of illness. As the disease state progresses, the dosage and frequency usually have to be increased. Since the principal sites of action within the nephron have been localized, appropriate drug combinations with additive effects can then be selected for patients who become refractory to a single-drug program.

In the following discussion, individual diuretics are classified by primary site of action within the nephron, as schematically diagrammed in FIG. 286–1. TABLE 286–1 summarizes the effect of the most important diuretics on urinary excretion of Na, K, Cl, HCO_3, and PO_4 ions.

TABLE 286–1. URINARY EFFECTS OF DIURETICS

Drug	*Maximal Excretion of Sodium (% of Filtered Load)*	K^+	Cl^-	HCO_3^-	PO_4^-
Acetazolamide	5	↑	↔ or ↑	↑	↑
Thiazides	8	↑	↑	↔	↔
Mercurials	20	↔ or ↓	↑	↔	↔
Bumetanide	25	↑	↑	↔ or ↑	↔ or ↑
Ethacrynic acid	25	↑	↑	↔	↔
Furosemide	25	↑	↑	↔ or ↑	↔ or ↑
Spironolactone	2	↓	↔	↔ or ↑	↔
Triamterene	2	↓	↔	↔ or ↑	↔
Amiloride	2	↓	↔	↔ or ↑	↔

Key: ↑ = increased urinary excretion of ion; ↓ = decreased urinary excretion of ion; ↔ = no change in urinary excretion of ion.

DISTAL TUBULAR DIURETICS

Thiazide and Related Sulfonamide Diuretics

The thiazides are sulfonamide derivatives and include bendroflumethiazide, benzthiazide, chlorothiazide, cyclothiazide, hydrochlorothiazide, hydroflumethiazide, methyclothiazide, polythiazide, and trichlormethiazide. They were the first potent oral diuretics. Certain general statements apply to all thiazides and related sulfonamides such as chlorthalidone, quinethazone, metolazone, and indapamide. The potency of thiazides varies widely between patients because of such factors as previous treatment and differing mechanisms of fluid retention. The thiazides all have a similar site of action, are equipotent when given in maximal doses, and, except for minor differences in onset and duration of action, are interchangeable.

These agents inhibit renal tubular reabsorption of Na, increasing urinary excretion of both Na and water. They also increase the urinary excretion of Cl and K ions. The thiazides probably have some action throughout the nephron, but their greatest effect appears to be in the distal tubule, at the cortical diluting site. Some carbonic anhydrase inhibitory activity occurs, but this effect is minimal at usual clinical doses; thiazides have little diuretic action in the proximal tubule.

Since the thiazides have a low incidence of side effects and are well tolerated orally, they are generally used before other diuretics. They are effective in edema associated with heart failure, renal and liver disease, pregnancy, the premenstrual syndrome, and edema caused by corticosteroids. Perhaps their most important use is in hypertension, either alone or in combination with other drugs. Thiazides decrease Ca excretion in hypercalciuric patients during chronic administration and also paradoxically reduce the polyuria of nephrogenic and central diabetes insipidus.

Thiazides are rapidly absorbed from the GI tract. The usual initial dose is 50 mg of hydrochlorothiazide orally once or twice daily. The maximum effective dose is 200 mg/day. Diuretic effects usually begin within 1 h. Peak action occurs at 3 to 6 h, and most of the drug is excreted during this interval. Thiazides differ mainly in duration of effect, which allows choice of a particular derivative. For example, trichlormethiazide may act for 24 h, and chlorthalidone for up to 72 h.

Hypovolemia and **hypokalemic metabolic alkalosis** are common with prolonged use of thiazides. Weakness, postural hypotension, and azotemia may result. Azotemia is a manifestation of decreased GFR, secondary to progressive ECF depletion, and is an indication for withholding all diuretics pending further evaluation. Serum K levels must be monitored; they may drop to 2 to 3 mEq/L, and occasionally ECG signs of K

deficiency appear. A suitable K preparation (eg, potassium chloride 40 to 80 mEq/day orally) should be given concurrently with the thiazide if dietary K intake is not adequate, especially during treatment of corticosteroid-induced edema, since steroids also increase K loss. K supplementation may not be needed if low doses, an intermittent dosage schedule, or combination therapy with spironolactone or triamterene is used. It is usually unnecessary when thiazides are used for the treatment of hypertension.

Hyperuricemia is a common side effect of the thiazides that is shared with furosemide, bumetanide, and ethacrynic acid (see below) and is due to impaired renal excretion of urate, but acute attacks of gout are rare. If thiazides must be used in the presence of severe hyperuricemia, allopurinol will nearly always reduce the serum level by blocking uric acid production.

An infrequent but worrisome side effect of the thiazides is the precipitation or worsening of **hyponatremia.** Since they block one of the Na reabsorptive sites responsible for urinary dilution, thiazides may interfere with water excretion. ECF depletion may induce the neurohypophysis to secrete antidiuretic hormone. Severe hyponatremia by these mechanisms is uncommon and can be corrected by discontinuing the drug or by water restriction.

Thiazides may also **impair glucose tolerance,** which is rarely of consequence in nondiabetic patients, but hyperglycemia in overt or prediabetic patients may be aggravated. This diabetogenic effect can occur with most diuretics.

Hypersensitivity phenomena are unusual, but include thrombocytopenic purpura, leukopenia, photosensitivity, and necrotizing vasculitis. **Other side effects** of thiazides include nausea, vomiting, and rashes. Serious toxicity resulting in exfoliative dermatitis, agranulocytosis, jaundice, acute pancreatitis, or interstitial nephritis is rare.

Metolazone, a nonthiazide sulfonamide diuretic, acts mainly at the cortical diluting segment, similar to the thiazides. The usual daily dose of 5 to 20 mg orally is rapidly absorbed from the GI tract. Natriuresis is comparable to that produced by the thiazides and begins about 1 h after ingestion, with a peak action at 2 h. However, because of enterohepatic recirculation of the drug, natriuretic effects persist for up to 24 h, allowing administration once a day. Another potential advantage of metolazone over thiazides is its effectiveness even with moderate degrees of renal insufficiency. In certain patients who appear refractory to "loop" diuretics, the addition of metolazone may produce a marked natriuresis.

Indapamide, the first of a new class of diuretics, the indolines, also acts at the cortical diluting segment. It is rapidly absorbed from the GI tract, and has a long half-life, allowing once daily dosage; 2.5 or 5 mg/day orally results in natriuresis equivalent to that of 50 to 100 mg of hydrochlorothiazide. Indapamide is extensively metabolized, with little intact drug excreted in the urine. Dosage is not modified in patients with moderate to severe renal failure, where the drug retains its antihypertensive action. However, indapamide's natriuretic potency diminishes, similar to the thiazides, with decreasing renal function.

POTASSIUM-SPARING DISTAL TUBULAR DIURETICS

Spironolactone competitively inhibits aldosterone at the distal tubule where Na is reabsorbed and reciprocal K and H ion secretion occurs. It does not affect electrolyte excretion in adrenalectomized animals, but in the presence of aldosterone, spironolactone can increase Na and HCO_3 excretion and decrease K excretion. Spironolactone may be absorbed poorly and promotes Na and water excretion slowly. Its immediate effect is much weaker than that of the "loop" diuretics, or the thiazides. Used alone, even in states of severe hyperaldosteronism, it is a relatively weak natriuretic agent, since Na reabsorption proximal to the distal tubule is enhanced. Nevertheless, it is

useful as an effective adjunct to K-losing diuretics, particularly when K depletion may cause cardiac arrhythmias (eg, in patients receiving digitalis).

Because of its different mode of action, spironolactone is useful in resistant cases to potentiate other agents and is most effective in edematous states associated with excessive aldosterone production, such as cirrhosis and the nephrotic syndrome. In congestive heart failure, results are less striking, possibly because hemodynamic factors are more important than hormonal factors in sustaining the edema.

The usual daily dose of spironolactone is 100 mg orally in divided doses, but as much as 400 mg/day may be required, particularly in patients with severe secondary hyperaldosteronism. The usual daily dose in children is 3.3 mg/kg body wt. Duration of action is 4 to 6 h. Spironolactone is usually well tolerated.

Hyperkalemia, the most significant adverse effect, is most likely to occur in uremic patients or those receiving supplemental K. **Metabolic acidosis** and hyperkalemia may occur, particularly in diabetics and patients with a decreased GFR. *Such patients should be treated with extreme caution. They should rarely be given spironolactone combined with potassium supplementation.* GI irritation has been reported. **Other side effects** are probably related to the drug's structural similarity to progesterone and include painful gynecomastia, hirsutism, and impotence. Spironolactone has been shown to be a tumorigen in chronic toxicity studies in rats; its use should be restricted to conditions in which the benefits justify the potential risks.

Triamterene and **amiloride** are mild natriuretics that decrease K excretion. They apparently act in the distal tubule and retard K loss during thiazide therapy. Their effect is similar to that of spironolactone, but they do not require aldosterone for their action, which can be demonstrated in patients with adrenal insufficiency. The combined effect of either of these drugs and spironolactone may be additive. They can be used interchangeably with spironolactone and may be preferred when the diagnosis of hyperaldosteronism is uncertain.

The usual oral dose of triamterene is 100 to 300 mg/day in divided dosage. It is readily absorbed from the GI tract. Action begins within 2 to 4 h and generally tapers off within 7 to 9 h. However, the maximum therapeutic effect may not appear for several days.

Amiloride is readily absorbed from the GI tract. Action begins within 2 h and lasts for about 24 h. The usual dose is 5 to 10 mg once daily.

Adverse reactions of triamterene and amiloride are uncommon and relatively mild but include nausea, vomiting, leg cramps, and light-headedness. BUN may be reversibly increased and they may at times cause mild H ion retention and **hyperchloremic acidosis.** As with spironolactone, **hyperkalemia** is the major danger, especially in azotemic patients. *Triamterene or amiloride can be dangerous when given concomitantly with K supplementation or in the presence of hyperkalemia.*

DIURETICS THAT ACT PRIMARILY IN THE LOOP OF HENLE

Furosemide, Ethacrynic Acid, and Bumetanide

Furosemide, ethacrynic acid, and bumetanide are the most potent diuretics currently in use (about 5 times as potent as the thiazides). At maximal effectiveness, they can cause as much as 25% of filtered Na to be excreted. All 3 induce K and H ion depletion, and all 3 interfere with urinary dilution and concentration. They are useful in patients refractory to other diuretics, particularly in chronic renal failure, the nephrotic syndrome, cirrhosis of the liver with ascites, and congestive heart failure. They are effective adjuncts in acute pulmonary edema and hypertensive crisis because IV administration produces a rapid diuresis and a transient reduction in peripheral vascular resistance. These drugs should be given initially in low doses with stepwise incre-

ments if necessary. Intermittent dosage regimens allow for correction of electrolyte derangements.

Furosemide, in usual doses, acts primarily in the ascending limb of the loop of Henle by inhibiting active Cl transport. It also has minor activity in the proximal tubule, possibly because it is a weak carbonic anhydrase inhibitor (like acetazolamide, it is a sulfonamide derivative). Normally, the proximal action is not important to natriuresis, but it may be responsible for significant increases in HCO_3 and PO_4 excretion. The urine resulting from a furosemide diuresis has a high Na and Cl content.

Furosemide is rapidly absorbed from the GI tract and is given orally in doses of 40 to 120 mg up to tid. Diuresis usually begins within 30 min, reaches a peak in 1 to 2 h, and is usually complete within 6 to 8 h. About ⅔ of the dose is excreted in the urine within 24 h; the remainder is excreted in the feces. In congestive heart failure refractory to thiazides, furosemide 40 mg orally once or twice daily is usually adequate. In acute pulmonary edema 20 to 40 mg should be given slowly IV over 1 to 2 min. Diuresis usually begins within 5 min, reaches a peak in 30 to 60 min, and ends within 3 to 4 h. This dose may be repeated once or twice until other measures to improve cardiac function have taken effect. In refractory edema, up to 240 to 320 mg/day may be needed, along with other diuretics such as thiazides, metolazone, or those that spare K. When large total IV or oral doses are needed, 1 or 2 daily doses are more effective than several smaller divided ones.

Aside from excessive diuresis and hypokalemia, toxicity is rare, but includes GI distress, skin rashes, thrombocytopenia, neutropenia, and paresthesias. Marked kaliuresis is also common, particularly in states of secondary hyperaldosteronism.

Ethacrynic acid is chemically dissimilar to furosemide, but its effects are remarkably similar, and the drugs can be used almost interchangeably. Most of the indications and precautions for furosemide apply. Ethacrynic acid is not a carbonic anhydrase inhibitor and therefore has limited action in the proximal tubule. It acts primarily in the ascending limb by inhibition of Cl transport, and is readily absorbed from the GI tract. It is given in doses of 25 to 100 mg (50 mg is equivalent to 40 mg of furosemide). Diuresis begins 1 to 2 h after oral and within 30 min of IV administration. The response usually lasts 6 to 8 h. Excretion is ⅔ renal and ⅓ hepatic.

Side effects of ethacrynic acid usually relate to excessive diuresis or kaliuresis. Less frequent side effects include gastric distress, vomiting, and diarrhea, particularly with long-term administration. GI bleeding has been reported. Large IV doses of ethacrynic acid, particularly in patients with renal insufficiency, can produce transient or permanent bilateral nerve deafness. This adverse effect is rare with furosemide.

Bumetanide is a new loop diuretic. Like furosemide, it is a sulfonamide derivative, with clinical effects virtually identical to furosemide. Bumetanide possesses some minimal proximal tubular activity as well, manifest clinically by phosphaturia. With respect to natriuretic activity, 1 mg bumetanide is equivalent to 40 mg furosemide. It is rapidly absorbed from the GI tract; diuretic activity peaks at 1 to 2 h and lasts 4 to 6 h. It is highly protein bound, reaching the tubular lumen by secretion. Its ototoxic potential appears less than that of ethacrynic acid and is probably similar to furosemide.

Mercurials

The organic mercurial diuretics are potent, must be given parenterally, and are contraindicated in the presence of renal disease; therefore, they are seldom used. Mersalyl (with theophylline) is the only organic mercurial diuretic available for clinical use in the USA.

However, mercurials are unique among the potent diuretics in being relatively nonkaliuretic. For any degree of natriuresis they cause less kaliuresis than ethacrynic acid or furosemide, and acute administration may produce no kaliuresis; hence, mercurials

are used occasionally in cirrhotic patients who have low K intake, or in patients with heart failure in whom acute K loss might precipitate digitalis toxicity.

DIURETICS ACTING IN THE PROXIMAL TUBULE

Carbonic Anhydrase Inhibitors

The enzyme carbonic anhydrase catalyzes the formation of carbonic acid and then of H^+ and HCO_3^- in the renal tubule; its inhibitors decrease the rate of carbonic acid formation and hence H^+ production. Renal tubular secretion of H^+ and reabsorption of HCO_3 and Na^+ are thereby inhibited. Urinary output is increased because of larger excretion of solutes. **Acetazolamide** is a potent inhibitor of carbonic anhydrase and also inhibits proximal NaCl reabsorption. Other carbonic anhydrase inhibitors include dichlorphenamide, methazolamide, and ethoxzolamide; they are primarily used in treating glaucoma and are not used as diuretics.

Although not usually useful alone, the carbonic anhydrase inhibitors may be combined with more distally acting diuretics, particularly in situations where proximal reabsorption is enhanced. The proximal inhibition produced by acetazolamide delivers more Na to distal sites where the second diuretic can act. Acetazolamide may be used to correct metabolic alkalosis, and it is helpful in glaucoma by decreasing the rate of aqueous humor secretion and reducing intraocular tension.

The usual dose of acetazolamide is 250 to 500 mg orally or IV daily or bid. This dosage may be used effectively on alternate days in some patients. Acetazolamide produces marked kaliuresis, because of increased delivery of Na to distal K secretory sites, and because distal K secretion is enhanced by alterations in intracellular pH produced by the drug. With repeated dosage hypokalemic metabolic acidosis occurs as a result of urinary excretion of potassium bicarbonate, but this effect is self-limiting, since acidosis prevents acetazolamide from producing its usual renal effects. Because of this loss of effectiveness after 2 or 3 days, carbonic anhydrase inhibitors should be given only when an interrupted dosage regimen is feasible. Serious toxicity is infrequent, although large doses may cause drowsiness and paresthesias. Hypersensitivity is rare, with occasional reports of skin rash, fever, and leukopenia.

Albumin Human, Concentrated

In nephrotic or cirrhotic patients with hypovolemia due to hypoalbuminemia, diuresis may sometimes be begun only by acutely expanding the intravascular volume. The osmotic effect of concentrated human serum albumin given IV expands the intravascular volume, thus increasing GFR and decreasing Na reabsorption in the proximal tubule. Albumin is most effective when used in conjunction with a diuretic acting in the loop of Henle. After pretreatment with a loop diuretic, 25 or 50 gm of albumin should be infused IV over 30 to 60 min. The dose may have to be repeated every 1 to 2 days, since the albumin is usually retained only transiently in the circulation. Albumin is expensive and should be used only for refractory edema that is life-threatening or that severely limits activity.

Osmotic Diuretics

Mannitol: Any nonreabsorbable solute in the proximal tubule or loop of Henle impairs Na and water reabsorption and thus increases the tubular fluid delivered to the distal nephron. As much as 5 to 10% of the filtered Na may be excreted during osmotic diuresis with IV mannitol. Mannitol is nontoxic, is not metabolized, and is excreted principally by glomerular filtration. Its most important natriuretic action occurs in the ascending limb of the loop of Henle. It is rarely used in the treatment of edema. Mannitol is specifically recommended for enhancing drug excretion (eg, salicylates and barbiturates) after poisoning, for reducing elevated CSF pressure, and for preventing oliguric renal failure during cardiopulmonary bypass operations.

Mannitol is given as 1 to 2 IV boluses of 12.5 gm administered in 15 to 30 min. To promote diuresis as an adjunct in drug intoxication, 100 to 200 gm may be given over 24 to 48 h. Serious adverse reactions are infrequent if that dose is not exceeded. *Extreme caution must be used in patients with cardiac disease because of the rapid expansion of vascular volume.* The patient must be constantly monitored for signs of circulatory decompensation. *Mannitol should not be used in patients with pulmonary vascular congestion.* Because osmotic diuretics cause more water than Na to be lost, prolonged use may result in water depletion and hypernatremia. Fluid and electrolyte balance should be monitored.

A special use of mannitol is in the reversal of acute oliguria and anuria secondary to hypovolemia and/or hypotension, in which it may prevent or modify the progression to acute renal failure. The mechanism of action is uncertain. If adequate ECF volume expansion does not restore urine flow, 25 gm of mannitol IV should be given cautiously. If urine flow is increased, up to 100 gm/24 h may be given in divided doses to maintain urine flow at approximately 100 ml/h. If the first 1 or 2 doses do not initiate diuresis within 2 h, no additional mannitol should be given since its primary route of excretion is renal.

ATRIAL NATRIURETIC FACTORS (ANF)

(Atrial Natriuretic Hormone; Atrionatriuretic Peptides; Atriopeptins)

A family of endogenous peptide diuretics have recently been discovered in "secretory" granules in cardiac atrial tissue. In a remarkably short time, the human peptide has been isolated, sequenced, synthesized, and its gene has been identified; sensitive radioimmunoassay procedures have been developed. It appears to be a relatively simple polypeptide with the chain length of the active portion between 25 and 28 amino acids. ANF appears to be released in response to atrial stretch and is an extremely potent natriuretic agent, rapidly producing a large natriuresis and diuresis. At the same time it is vasoactive, causing vasodilation and increased GFR. Some investigators believe ANF is part of a counter-regulatory system to the renin-angiotensin system.

Following administration of high physiologic or pharmacologic doses of ANF to animals and to a limited number of humans it has the following actions beginning 30 min after IV administration and lasting for about 45 min to 1 h: (1) There is rapid rise in urine flow and sodium excretion, exceeding baseline levels by several-fold and associated with a maximal fractional excretion of sodium of 6 to 8%. A rise in excretion of other ions occurs including chloride, calcium, and phosphorus. (2) In animals, GFR increases by 10 to 30%, whereas in humans the rise has been less consistently observed so far, but GFR does not decrease despite the natriuresis. (3) The peptide has potent vasodilator properties, exhibiting the capacity to overcome the vasoconstricting actions of certain catecholamines and especially angiotensin II. (4) ANF appears to have a direct action on the kidney to inhibit renin release and on the adrenal gland to inhibit aldosterone secretion (and possibly production).

Hence ANF is currently in a position to be classified as a major newly discovered hormone which might be playing a critical role in the regulation of ECF volume, sodium metabolism, and BP. Much more work remains to be done to clarify its ultimate biologic importance, its contribution to certain pathophysiologic conditions involving volume and BP disturbances, and its potential use in therapeutics as a diuretic and/or vasodilating agent.

287. RESPIRATORY DRUGS

NASAL DECONGESTANTS

Nasal decongestants provide symptomatic relief in many upper respiratory conditions, including allergic rhinitis, hay fever, acute coryza, and sinusitis.

Sympathomimetic Amines as Nasal Decongestants

The most important group of nasal decongestants are the sympathomimetic amines with α-adrenergic receptor stimulating action; they constrict the nasal mucosal blood vessels, lessening secretions and edema. Phenylephrine and the longer-acting congeners (imidazoline derivatives) are the most useful and are usually applied topically, although oral administration may be preferred if prolonged therapy is indicated.

Topical preparations are available as nasal drops, sprays, or inhalers containing the volatile bases of certain decongestants. Sprays and inhaled vapors reach a greater area of the mucous membrane. Adverse reactions, associated particularly with repeated application of nasal decongestants, include mucosal irritation, stinging or burning sensation, rebound congestion after the effect has worn off, allergic reactions, and **rhinitis medicamentosa,** *a chronic inflammation of the nasal mucosa caused by overuse of topical nasal decongestants*; it occurs when the drugs are used more frequently than q 3 h and for longer than 3 wk, and is treated by stopping the medication. Individual drugs in the group may have other adverse reactions. For example, systemic absorption of sympathomimetic amines may cause generalized vasoconstriction and tachycardia that may be undesirable in patients with hypertension, heart disease, hyperthyroidism, diabetes, and advanced arteriosclerosis. Other systemic adverse reactions may include nervousness, irritability, insomnia, headache, and dizziness. Systemic absorption of naphazoline and tetrahydrozoline can cause CNS depression and coma in children, especially infants. Sympathomimetic nasal decongestants are contraindicated in patients receiving a MAO inhibitor or a tricyclic antidepressant.

The common drugs in this group include the following: (1) Phenylephrine (0.125, 0.25, 0.5 and 1% solution), 2 to 3 drops or 2 to 4 sprays q 4 h. (2) Naphazoline (0.05% solution), 3 to 4 drops or 2 to 3 sprays tid or qid. CAUTION: *Avoid use in children; can cause CNS depression.* (3) Oxymetazoline (0.025 and 0.05% solution), 2 to 4 drops or 2 to 3 sprays bid. *Use with caution in children.* (4) Xylometazoline (0.05 and 0.1% solution), 2 to 3 drops or 1 to 2 sprays q 8 to 10 h. *Use with caution in children.* (5) Ephedrine (1 and 3% solution), 2 to 3 drops bid or tid and desoxyephedrine (inhaler). (6) Propylhexedrine (inhaler), two inhalations in each nostril as needed. (7) Other available topical decongestants, include epinephrine (0.1%), methylhexaneamine (inhaler), tetrahydrozoline (0.1%), and xylometazoline (0.05 and 0.1% solution).

Oral use: Sympathomimetic agents that are useful as oral decongestants include phenylpropanolamine (25 mg q 3 to 4 h), ephedrine (25 to 50 mg q 3 to 4 h), and pseudoephedrine (30 to 60 mg q 3 to 4 h). Phenylephrine (10 mg tid) is also a useful oral decongestant but it is available only in combination with other agents such as antihistamines. Systemic side effects due to sympathomimetic activity occur more frequently by this route, but rhinitis medicamentosa is avoided.

Other Nasal Decongestants

Other drugs are often used in combination with sympathomimetic amines, eg, antihistamines when an allergy such as acute allergic rhinitis is involved. They can be administered topically or orally. Intranasal topical corticosteroids (usually dexamethasone, beclomethasone, or flunisolide) exert a marked anti-inflammatory effect on the mucosa. They are useful alone or with nasal decongestants in the management of

allergic and inflammatory rhinitis and nasal polyps. Topical corticosteroids used alone may also be helpful in the treatment of rhinitis medicamentosa (see above). Corticosteroids for nasal use are usually available in the form of metered sprays. Usual dose range is 1 to 2 sprays in each nostril 2 to 4 times/day. Local reactions include burning sensation in the nose, sneezing, and rarely bloody nasal discharge or localized infections with *Candida*. Systemic absorption is low but may sometimes cause side effects (eg, adrenal suppression). Topical steroids should be used with caution or avoided entirely in patients with systemic bacterial, fungal, or viral infections, and those patients who have experienced recent nasal trauma or surgery.

COUGH REMEDIES

Cough is a protective reflex (FIG. 287–1) that can expel secretions, exudates, transudates, or extraneous materials from the respiratory tract (see also in COUGH in Ch. 31). When cough is productive, it should not be suppressed except in special circumstances (eg, when it is exhausting the patient or preventing rest and sleep). Useless cough should either be suppressed or made productive. Any symptomatic treatment of cough should be accompanied by measures aimed at diagnosis and treatment of the underlying cause.

Antitussives *inhibit or suppress coughing by acting on either the central or peripheral components of the cough reflex.*

Centrally Acting Antitussive Agents

These agents suppress the cough reflex by depressing the medullary cough center or associated higher centers. The most commonly used drugs in this group are codeine and dextromethorphan.

Codeine: Codeine has antitussive, analgesic, and slight sedative effects and is especially useful in relieving painful cough. It also exerts a drying action on the respiratory mucosa that may be useful (eg, in bronchorrhea) or deleterious (eg, when bronchial secretions are already viscous). The average adult dose is 10 to 20 mg orally q 4 to 6 h as required, but single doses as high as 60 mg may be necessary. The usual oral dose for children is 5 to 15 mg/day in divided doses. Codeine in these amounts has minimal

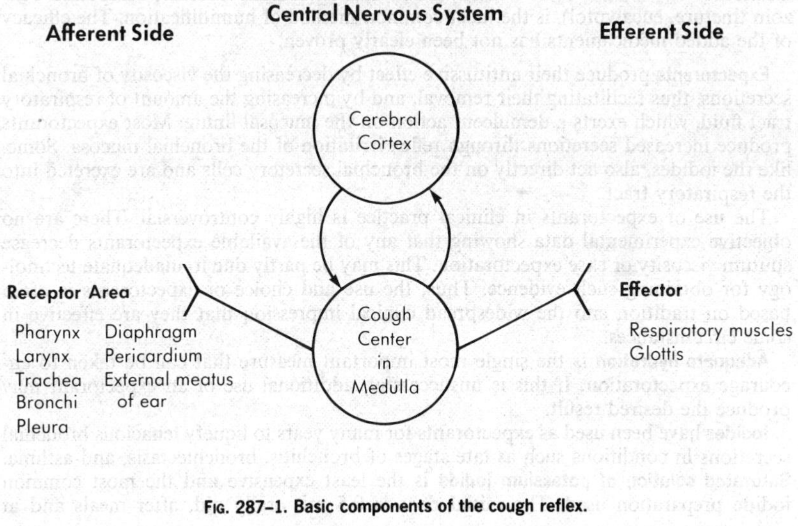

FIG. 287–1. Basic components of the cough reflex.

respiratory depressant effects. Nausea, vomiting, and constipation can occur, as well as tolerance and physical dependence, but abuse potential is low.

Dextromethorphan, a congener of the narcotic analgesic levorphanol, possesses no significant analgesic or sedative properties, does not depress respiration in usual doses, and is nonaddicting. No evidence of tolerance has been found during long-term use. The average dose for adults is 15 to 30 mg 1 to 4 times/day, given as a tablet or syrup; for children 1 mg/kg/day is given in divided doses. Extremely high doses may depress respiration.

Other agents in this group include benzonatate, chlophedianol, levopropoxyphene, and noscapine in the non-narcotic group; and hydrocodone, hydromorphone, methadone, and morphine in the narcotic group.

Peripherally Acting Antitussives

These may act on either the afferent or the efferent side of the cough reflex. On the afferent side, they may reduce the input of stimuli by acting as a mild analgesic or anesthetic on the respiratory mucosa, by modifying the output and viscosity of the respiratory tract fluid, or by relaxing the smooth muscle of the bronchi in the presence of bronchospasm. On the efferent side, they may render secretions more easily removable, increasing the efficiency of the cough mechanism. Peripherally acting agents are grouped as follows.

Demulcents are useful against cough arising above the larynx. They act by forming a protective coating over the irritated pharyngeal mucosa. They are usually given as syrups or lozenges and include acacia, licorice, glycerin, honey, and wild cherry syrups.

Local anesthetics such as benzocaine, cyclaine, and tetracaine are used to inhibit the cough reflex under special circumstances; eg, before bronchoscopy or bronchography. Benzonatate (100 mg orally tid), a congener of tetracaine, is a local anesthetic; its antitussive effect may be due to a combination of local anesthesia, depression of pulmonary stretch receptors, and nonspecific central depression.

Humidifying aerosols and steam inhalations exert an antitussive effect by demulcent action and by decreasing the viscosity of bronchial secretions. Inhalation of water as an aerosol or steam, with or without medicaments (sodium chloride, compound benzoin tincture, eucalyptol), is the most common method of humidification. The efficacy of the added medicaments has not been clearly proven.

Expectorants produce their antitussive effect by decreasing the viscosity of bronchial secretions, thus facilitating their removal, and by increasing the amount of respiratory tract fluid, which exerts a demulcent action on the mucosal lining. Most expectorants produce increased secretions through reflex irritation of the bronchial mucosa. Some, like the iodides, also act directly on the bronchial secretory cells and are excreted into the respiratory tract.

The use of expectorants in clinical practice is highly controversial. There are no objective experimental data showing that any of the available expectorants decrease sputum viscosity or ease expectoration. This may be partly due to inadequate technology for obtaining such evidence. Thus, the use and choice of expectorants is often based on tradition and the widespread clinical impression that they are effective in some circumstances.

Adequate hydration is the single most important measure that can be taken to encourage expectoration. If this is unsuccessful, additional use of an expectorant may produce the desired result.

Iodides have been used as expectorants for many years to liquefy tenacious bronchial secretions in conditions such as late stages of bronchitis, bronchiectasis, and asthma. **Saturated solution of potassium iodide** is the least expensive and the most common iodide preparation used. The initial dose is 0.5 mL orally qid, after meals and at

bedtime, and is increased gradually to 1 to 4 mL qid. It is usually given with milk to conceal its unpleasant taste. To be effective, iodides must be taken in doses approaching intolerance. Their usefulness is limited by low patient acceptance due to their unpleasant taste and also by the common occurrence of side effects in the form of acneiform skin eruptions, coryza, erythema of face and chest, and painful swelling of the salivary glands. The side effects are reversible and subside when the medication is stopped. **Iodinated glycerol** is better tolerated than potassium iodide solution but is probably less effective. The usual oral dose is 60 mg as tablets or elixir qid; *avoid in patients sensitive to iodide.*

Syrup of ipecac, 0.5 mL orally qid. (NOTE: This is much less than the emetic dose) can be used as an expectorant in patients sensitive to iodides. It is useful in relieving spasm of the larynx in children with croup and often clears up thick, tenacious mucus from the bronchi.

Guaifenesin (100 to 200 mg orally q 2 to 4 h) is the most commonly used expectorant in OTC cough remedies. It has no serious adverse effects, but there is no clear evidence for its efficacy.

Many of the other traditional expectorants, such as ammonium chloride, terpin hydrate, creosote, and squill, are found in numerous OTC cough remedies. Their efficacy is doubtful, particularly in the doses contained in most cough preparations.

Mucolytics: Chemical mucolytic agents, such as **acetylcysteine,** have free sulfhydryl groups that open mucoprotein disulfide bonds, reducing the viscosity of mucus. As a rule, their usefulness is restricted to a few special instances such as liquefying thick, tenacious, mucopurulent secretions in conditions like chronic bronchitis and cystic fibrosis. Acetylcysteine is given as a 10 to 20% solution by nebulization or instillation. In some cases, airway obstruction may be aggravated by these agents. If this occurs, use of the mucolytic may be preceded by inhalation of a nebulized sympathomimetic bronchodilator or use of a formulation containing acetylcysteine (10%) and isoproterenol (0.05%).

Proteolytic enzymes such as pancreatic dornase are useful only where grossly purulent sputum is a major problem. They seem to offer no advantage over chemical mucolytic agents. Local irritation of the buccal and pharyngeal mucosa and allergic reactions are common after repeated doses.

Antihistamines serve little or no use in the treatment of cough. Their drying action on the respiratory mucosa may be helpful in the early congestive phase of acute coryza, but may be deleterious especially to patients with a nonproductive cough resulting from retained viscous secretions.

Decongestants such as phenylephrine are *not* useful in relieving cough.

Bronchodilators such as ephedrine and theophylline may be useful if cough is complicated by bronchospasm. Atropine is *undesirable* because it thickens bronchial secretions.

Drug Combinations in the Treatment of Cough

Many prescription and nonprescription cough remedies are mixtures containing 2 or more drugs, usually in a syrup. Typically, they may include a centrally acting antitussive, an antihistamine, an expectorant, and a decongestant. Bronchodilators and antipyretics are also often present. These mixtures are aimed at treating the many symptoms of an acute URI. They should not be used for management of cough alone. Some combinations of antitussive drugs are rational (eg, a centrally acting antitussive such as dextromethorphan and a peripherally acting demulcent syrup for cough originating above the larynx). However, the components of some drug mixtures have opposing effects on respiratory tract secretions (eg, expectorants and antihistamines). Many combination cough remedies contain suboptimal or ineffective concentrations of potentially useful ingredients.

Choice of Drug Therapy in Cough

As a rule, when cough alone is a major problem, it is better to use full dosage of a single drug aimed at a specific component of the cough reflex. The following are some general principles and recommendations: (1) For simple suppression of useless cough, dextromethorphan is preferred, but codeine also is useful. The more potent narcotic antitussives should be reserved for patients in whom analgesic and sedative effects are required. (2) To increase bronchial secretion and liquefy viscous bronchial fluid, adequate hydration (water or steam inhalation) is used; saturated solution of potassium iodide or syrup of ipecac orally may be tried if hydration by itself is unsuccessful. (3) To relieve cough originating in the pharyngeal region, demulcent syrups or lozenges, combined if necessary with dextromethorphan, are used. (4) For bronchoconstriction complicating cough, bronchodilators, possibly combined with expectorants, are advised.

ASTHMA PREPARATIONS

(See Bronchial Asthma in Ch. 36)

288. SOME TRADE NAMES OF GENERIC (NONPROPRIETARY) DRUGS

Most prescription drugs placed on the market are given trade names (also called proprietary, brand, or specialty names) to distinguish them as being produced and marketed exclusively by a particular manufacturer. In the USA these names are usually registered as trademarks with the Patent Office and confer upon the registrant certain legal rights with respect to their use. A trade name may be registered as representing a product containing a single active ingredient (with or without additives) or one containing 2 or more active ingredients.

A drug marketed by several companies may have several trade names. Drugs manufactured in one country and marketed in many countries may have different trade names in each country.

Throughout this book we have used nonproprietary or "generic" names whenever possible. However, since trade names are found in many publications and are used extensively in clinical medicine, as a convenience to our readers, we have included a list of most of the drugs mentioned throughout The Manual, in alphabetic order, followed by many of their trade names (see Table 288-1 below).

With few exceptions, we have limited the trade names in this list to those marketed in the USA. This list is by no means all-inclusive and no effort has been made to list every trade name in current use for each drug. A few are investigational and may subsequently be released as approved new drugs. The inclusion of a drug in this list does not indicate approval or disapproval of its use in any category, neither does it imply efficacy nor safety of its action.

Finally, the reader must keep in mind that many drugs are marketed almost exclusively by their official nonproprietary name and that the inclusion of a trade name in this list does not indicate its endorsement by this book nor its preference as the product of choice.

Constant changes in information resulting from new research and clinical experience, reasonable differences in opinion among authorities, and the unique aspects of individual clinical situations require that the physician exercise his own best judgments in the choice and use of a drug. In particular, the physician is advised to check the

product information included in each package of drug that he plans to administer or prescribe, especially if the drug is one that is unfamiliar or is used only infrequently, or is one in which the effective therapeutic levels are close to the toxic levels.

TABLE 288–1. SOME TRADE NAMES OF COMMONLY USED GENERIC DRUGS

Generic Name	*Trade Name(s)*
Acebutolol	SECTRAL
Acetaminophen	DATRIL, TYLENOL
Acetazolamide	DIAMOX
Acetohexamide	DYMELOR
Acetophenazine	TINDAL
Acetylcysteine	MUCOMYST
ACTH	See Corticotropin
Acyclovir	ZOVIRAX
Allopurinol	ZYLOPRIM
Albuterol	PROVENTIL, VENTOLIN
Alprazolam	XANAX
Amantadine	SYMMETREL
Ambenonium	MYTELASE
Amikacin	AMIKIN
Aminocaproic acid	AMICAR
Aminophylline	AMINODUR, SOMOPHYLLIN
Amiodarone	CORDARONE
Amitriptyline	ELAVIL, ENDEP
Amoxicillin	LAROTID
Amoxicillin/clavulanate potassium	AUGMENTIN
Amphotericin B	FUNGIZONE
Ampicillin	AMCILL, OMNIPEN, POLYCILLIN, PRINCIPEN
Amrinone	INOCOR
Anisotropine	VALPIN
Anthralin	ANTHRA-DERM
Asparaginase	ELSPAR
Atenolol	TENORMIN
Auranofin	RIDAURA
Azathioprine	IMURAN
Baclofen	LIORESAL
Beclomethasone dipropionate	BECLOVENT, VANCERIL
Bendroflumethiazide	NATURETIN
Benzalkonium Cl	ZEPHIRAN
Benzene hexachloride, gamma	See Lidane
Benzonatate	TESSALON
Benzquinamide	EMETE-CON
Benzthiazide	AQUATAG, EXNA
Benztropine mesylate	COGENTIN
Benzylpenicilloyl-polylysine	PRE-PEN
Beta-Carotene	SOLATENE
Betamethasone	CELESTONE
Betamethasone benzoate	BENISONE
Betamethasone valerate	VALISONE
Bethanechol Cl	DUVOID, URECHOLINE
Bisacodyl	DULCOLAX
Bleomycin	BLENOXANE
Busulfan	MYLERAN
Bretylium	BRETYLOL
Bromocriptine	PARLODEL
Brompheniramine	DIMETANE
Bumetanide	BUMEX
Butaperazine	REPOISE
Butorphanol	STADOL
Calcifediol	CALDEROL
Calcitonin-salmon	CALCIMAR
Calcitriol	ROCALTROL
Calusterone	METHOSARB
Capreomycin	CAPASTAT
Captopril	CAPOTEN
Carbamazepine	TEGRETOL
Carbenicillin	GEOPEN, PYOPEN
Carbenicillin indanyl sodium	GEOCILLIN
Carbidopa-levodopa	SINEMET
Carbinoxamine	CLISTIN
Carboprost tromethamine	PROSTIN/15M
Carisoprodol	SOMA
Carmustine	BiCNU
Carphenazine	PROKETAZINE
Cefaclor	CECLOR
Cefadroxil	DURICEF
Cefamandole	MANDOL
Cefazolin	ANCEF, KEFZOL
Cefonicid	MONOCID
Cefoperazone	CEFOBID
Ceforanide	PRECEF
Cefotaxime	CLAFORAN
Cefotetan	CEFOTAN
Cefoxitin	MEFOXIN
Ceftazidime	FORTAZ; TAZIDIME
Ceftizoxime	CEFIZOX
Ceftriaxone	ROCEPHIN
Cefuroxime	ZINACEF
Cephalexin	KEFLEX
Cephalothin	KEFLIN
Cephapirin	CEFADYL

(*Continued*)

TABLE 288–1. SOME TRADE NAMES OF COMMONLY USED GENERIC DRUGS *(Cont'd)*

Generic Name	*Trade Name(s)*
Cephradine	ANSPOR, VELOSEF
Chenodiol	CHENIX
Chloral hydrate	NOCTEC, SOMNOS
Chlorazepate dipotassium	TRANXENE
Chlorazepate monopotassium	AZENE
Chlorambucil	LEUKERAN
Chloramphenicol	CHLOROMYCETIN
Chlordiazepoxide	LIBRIUM
Chlorhexidine	HIBICLENS, HIBITANE
Chlormezanone	TRANCOPAL
Chlorotrianisene	TACE
Chlorothiazide	DIURIL
Chlorphedianol	ULO
Chlorpheniramine	CHLOR-TRIMETON; TELDRIN
Chlorpromazine	THORAZINE
Chlorpropamide	DIABINESE
Chlorprothixene	TARACTAN
Chlorthalidone	HYGROTON
Cholestyramine	QUESTRAN
Cimetidine	TAGAMET
Cisplatin	PLATINOL
Clindamycin	CLEOCIN
Clofibrate	ATROMID-S
Clomiphene	CLOMID
Clonazepam	KLONOPIN
Clonidine	CATAPRES
Clotrimazole	LOTRIMIN, MYCELEX
Cloxacillin	TEGOPEN
Colestipol	COLESTID
Corticotropin (ACTH)	ACTHAR
Cortisol	CORTEF, HYDROCORTONE, SOLU-CORTEF
Cosyntropin	CORTROSYN
Co-Trimoxazole, see Trimethoprim-sulfamethoxazole	
Cromolyn sodium	INTAL, NASALCROM, OPTICROM
Cyclacillin	CYCLAPEN
Cyclandelate	CYCLOSPASMOL
Cyclizine	MAREZINE
Cyclobenzaprine	FLEXERIL
Cyclopentolate	CYCLOGYL
Cyclophosphamide	CYTOXAN
Cyclosporine	SANDIMMUNE
Cyproheptadine	PERIACTIN
Cytarabine	CYTOSAR-U
Dacarbazine	DTIC-DOME
Dactinomycin	COSMEGEN
Danazol	DANOCRINE

Generic Name	*Trade Name(s)*
Danthron	MODANE
Dantrolene	DANTRIUM
Dapsone	AVLOSULFON
Daunorubicin	CERUBIDINE
Deanol	DEANER
Deferoxamine	DESFERAL
Demeclocycline	DECLOMYCIN
Desipramine	NORPRAMIN, PERTOFRANE
Desmopressin	DDAVP
Dexamethasone	DECADRON, HEXADROL
Dexchlorpheniramine	POLARAMINE
Dextromethorphan	DELSYM, BENYLIN DM
Diazepam	VALIUM
Diazoxide, IV	HYPERSTAT
Diazoxide, Oral	PROGLYCEM
Dicloxacillin	DYNAPEN
Dicyclomine	BENTYL
Diethylpropion	TENUATE
Diflunisal	DOLOBID
Digitoxin	CRYSTODIGIN, PURODIGIN
Digoxin	LANOXIN
Dihydrotachysterol	HYTAKEROL
Diltiazem	CARDIZEM
Dimercaprol	BAL
Dinoprostone	PROSTIN E2
Diphenhydramine	BENADRYL
Diphenidol	VONTROL
Diphenoxylate with atropine	LOMOTIL
Dipivefrin	PROPINE
Dipyridamole	PERSANTINE
Disulfiram	ANTABUSE
Divalproex	DEPAKOTE
Dobutamine	DOBUTREX
Docusate sodium	COLACE
Dopamine	INTROPIN
Doxepin	ADAPIN, SINEQUAN
Doxorubicin	ADRIAMYCIN
Doxycycline	VIBRAMYCIN
Doxylamine	DECAPRYN
Dronabinol	MARINOL
Droperidol	INAPSINE
Echothiophate iodide	ECHODIDE; PHOSPHOLINE IODIDE
Edetate disodium (EDTA)	SODIUM VERSENATE
Edrophonium	TENSILON
Enalapril	VASOTEC
Ergocalciferol	CALCIFEROL, DRISDOL
Erythromycin	E-MYCIN, ERYTHROCIN, ILOSONE

(*Continued*)

TABLE 288–1. SOME TRADE NAMES OF COMMONLY USED GENERIC DRUGS *(Cont'd)*

Generic Name	*Trade Name(s)*	*Generic Name*	*Trade Name(s)*
Ethacrynic acid	EDECRIN	Indapamide	LOZOL
Ethambutol	MYAMBUTOL	Indomethacin	INDOCIN
Ethoheptazine	ZACTANE	Iodochlorhydroxyquin	VIOFORM
Ethosuximide	ZARONTIN	Iron dextran	IMFERON
Etidronate disodium	DIDRONEL	Isoetharine	BRONKOSOL
Factor IX complex (human)	KONYNE, PROPLEX	Isoflurophate	FLOROPRYL
Fenfluramine	PONDIMIN	Isoniazid	INH, NYDRAZID
Fenoprofen	NALFON	Isopropamide iodide	DARBID
Fentanyl	SUBLIMAZE	Isoproterenol	ISUPREL
Flecainide	TAMBOCOR	Isosorbide dinitrate	ISORDIL, SORBITRATE
Flucytosine	ANCOBON	Isotretinoin	ACCUTANE
Fludrocortisone	FLORINEF	Isoxsuprine	VASODILAN
Flumethasone pivalate	LOCORTEN	Kanamycin	KANTREX
Fluocinolone acetonide	FLUONID, SYNALAR	Ketoconazole	NIZORAL
Fluocinonide	LIDEX	Labetalol	NORMODYNE, TRANDATE
Fluoxymesterone	HALOTESTIN	Lactulose	CEPHULAC, CHRONULAC
Fluphenazine	PERMITIL, PROLIXIN	Levallorphan	LORFAN
Flurandrenolide	CORDRAN	Levarterenol bitartrate, see Norepinephrine bitartrate	
Flurazepam	DALMANE	Levodopa	DOPAR, LARODOPA
Furazolidone	FUROXONE	Levopropoxyphene	NOVRAD
Furosemide	LASIX	Levothyroxine (T_4)	SYNTHROID
Gemfibrozil	LOPID	Lidocaine	XYLOCAINE
Gentamicin	GARAMYCIN	Lincomycin	LINCOCIN
Glipizide	GLUCOTROL	Lindane	KWELL
Glutethimide	DORIDEN	Liothyronine (T_3)	CYTOMEL
Glyburide	DIABETA; MICRONASE	Liotrix	EUTHROID, THYROLAR
Gold sodium thiomalate	MYOCHRYSINE	Lithium carbonate	LITHANE, LITHONATE
Griseofulvin	GRIFULVIN, GRISACTIN, FULVICIN P/G, FULVICIN U/F	Lomustine	CeeNU
		Loperamide	IMODIUM
		Lorazepam	ATIVAN
Guaifenesin	HYTUSS, ROBITUSSIN	Loxapine	LOXITANE
Guanethidine	ISMELIN	Lypressin	DIAPID
Haloperidol	HALDOL	Mafenide	SULFAMYLON
Haloprogin	HALOTEX	Magaldrate	RIOPAN
Hydralazine	APRESOLINE	Maprotiline	LUDIOMIL
Hydrochlorothiazide	ESIDRIX, HydroDIURIL, ORETIC	Mazindol	SANOREX
		Mebendazole	VERMOX
Hydrocortisone	See Cortisol	Mecamylamine	INVERSINE
Hydromorphone	DILAUDID	Mechlorethamine	MUSTARGEN
Hydroquinone	ELDOPAQUE, ELDOQUIN	Meclizine	ANTIVERT, BONINE
Hydroxychloroquine	PLAQUENIL	Meclofenamate	MECLOMEN
Hydroxyprogesterone caproate	DELALUTIN	Medroxyprogesterone	PROVERA
		Mefenamic acid	PONSTEL
Hydroxyurea	HYDREA	Megestrol acetate	MEGACE
Hydroxyzine	ATARAX, VISTARIL	Melphalan	ALKERAN
Ibuprofen	MOTRIN, RUFEN, ADVIL	Menadiol	SYNKAYVITE
Idoxuridine	DENDRID, STOXIL	Menotropins	PERGONAL
Imipenem/cilastatin	PRIMAXIN	Meperidine	DEMEROL
Imipramine	PRESAMINE, TOFRANIL	Mephenytoin	MESANTOIN

(Continued)

TABLE 288–1. SOME TRADE NAMES OF COMMONLY USED GENERIC DRUGS *(Cont'd)*

Generic Name	*Trade Name(s)*
Mephobarbital	MEBARAL
Meprobamate	EQUANIL, MILTOWN
Mercaptopurine	PURINETHOL
Mesoridazine	SERENTIL
Metaproterenol	ALUPENT, METAPREL
Metaraminol	ARAMINE
Metaxalone	SKELAXIN
Methadone	DOLOPHINE
Methamphetamine	DESOXYN
Methandrostenolone	DIANABOL
Methaqualone	QUAALUDE, SOPOR
Methdilazine	TACARYL
Methanamine hippurate	HIPREX
Methenamine mandelate	MANDELAMINE
Methicillin	STAPHCILLIN
Methimazole	TAPAZOLE
Methocarbamol	ROBAXIN
Methohexital	BREVITAL
Methoxsalen	OXSORALEN
Methotrimeprazine	LEVOPROME
Methsuximide	CELONTIN
Methyldopa	ALDOMET
Methylphenidate	RITALIN
Methylprednisolone	MEDROL
Methyltestosterone	ORETON METHYL
Methyprylon	NOLUDAR
Methysergide	SANSERT
Metoclopramide	REGLAN
Metolazone	DIULO, ZAROXOLYN
Metoprolol	LOPRESSOR
Metronidazole	FLAGYL
Metyrapone	METOPIRONE
Mexiletine	MEXITIL
Miconazole	MICATIN, MONISTAT
Minocycline	MINOCIN
Minoxidil	LONITEN
Mithramycin	MITHRACIN
Mitomycin	MUTAMYCIN
Mitotane	LYSODREN
Molindone	LIDONE, MOBAN
Nadolol	CORGARD
Nafcillin	UNIPEN
Nalbuphine	NUBAIN
Nalidixic acid	NegGRAM
Naloxone	NARCAN
Naltrexone	TREXAN
Nandrolone	DURABOLIN
Naphazoline	PRIVINE
Naproxen	NAPROSYN
Neostigmine	PROSTIGMIN
Niclosamide	NICLOCIDE
Nifedipine	PROCARDIA

Generic Name	*Trade Name(s)*
Nitrofurantoin	FURADANTIN, IVADANTIN, MACRODANTIN
Nitrofurazone	FURACIN
Nitroprusside	NIPRIDE
Norepinephrine bitartrate	LEVOPHED
Nortriptyline	AVENTYL
Noscapine	TUSSCAPINE
Nylidrin	ARLIDIN
Nystatin	MYCOSTATIN, NILSTAT
Orphenadrine citrate	NORFLEX
Orphenadrine HCl	DISIPAL
Oxacillin	BACTOCILL, PROSTAPHLIN
Oxamniquine	VANSIL
Oxandrolone	ANAVAR
Oxazepam	SERAX
Oxolinic acid	UTIBID
Oxybutynin	DITROPAN
Oxymetazoline	AFRIN, DURATION
Oxymetholone	ADROYD, ANADROL
Oxytetracycline	TERRAMYCIN
Oxytocin	PITOCIN, SYNTOCINON
Pancreatin	ELZYME, VIOKASE
Pancrelipase	COTAZYM, ILOZYME
Pancuronium	PAVULON
Papaverine	CERESPAN, PAVABID
Paramethadione	PARADIONE
Paramethasone	HALDRONE
Pargyline	EUTONYL
Parmomycin	HUMATIN
Penicillamine	CUPRIMINE
Penicillin G benzathine	BICILLIN, PERMAPEN
Penicillin G potassium	PENTIDS
Pencillin G procaine	DURACILLIN A.S., DURACILLIN, CRYSTICILLIN A.S., WYCILLIN
Penicillin V	PEN·VEE, V-CILLIN
Penicilloyl-polylysine, see Benzylpenicilloyl-polylysine	
Pentaerythritol tetranitrate	PERITRATE
Pentamidine isethionate	PENTAM 300
Pentazocine	TALWIN
Pentobarbital	NEMBUTAL
Pentoxifylline	TRENTAL
Pentylenetetrazol	METRAZOL

(Continued)

TABLE 288–1. SOME TRADE NAMES OF COMMONLY USED GENERIC DRUGS *(Cont'd)*

Generic Name	*Trade Name(s)*	*Generic Name*	*Trade Name(s)*
Perphenazine	TRILAFON	Pyrvinium pamoate	POVAN
Phenacemide	PHENURONE	Quinacrine	ATABRINE
Phenazopyridine	PYRIDIUM	Quinethazone	HYDROMOX
Phenelzine	NARDIL	Quinidine	CARDIOQUIN, QUINAGLUTE, QUINIDEX, QUINORA
Phenmetrazine	PRELUDIN		
Phenobarbital	LUMINAL		
Phenoxybenzamine	DIBENZYLINE	Ranitidine	ZANTAC
Phensuximide	MILONTIN	Reserpine	RAU-SED, SERPASIL
Phentermine	IONAMIN	Ribavirin	VIRAZOLE
Phentolamine	REGITINE	Rifampin	RIFADIN, RIMACTANE
Phenylbutazone	AZOLID, BUTAZOLIDIN	Ritodrine	YUTOPAR
Phenylephrine	NEO-SYNEPHRINE	Secobarbital	SECONAL
Phenyl-propanolamine	DEXATRIM, PROPADRINE	Selenium sulfide	SELSUN
		Semustine	Methyl-CCNU
Phenytoin	DILANTIN	Silver sulfadiazine	SILVADENE
Physostigmine	ANTILIRIUM	Simethicone	MYLICON, SILAIN
Phytonadione	AquaMEPHYTON, MEPHYTON	Somatrem	PROTROPIN
		Spectinomycin	TROBICIN
Piperacetazine	QUIDE	Spironolactone	ALDACTONE
Piperacillin	PIPRACIL	Stanozolol	WINSTROL
Piperazine	ANTEPAR	Streptokinase	KABIKINASE, STREPTASE
Pipobroman	VERCYTE	Streptokinase-streptodornase	VARIDASE
Piroxicam	FELDENE		
Polythiazide	RENESE	Streptozocin	ZANOSAR
Pralidoxime	PROTOPAM	Sucralfate	CARAFATE
Prazepam	CENTRAX	Sulfacytine	RENOQUID
Praziquantel	BILTRICIDE	Sulfamethizole	THIOSULFIL
Prazosin	MINIPRESS	Sulfamethoxazole	GANTANOL
Prednisolone	DELTA-CORTEF, HYDELTRASOL	Sulfasalazine	AZULFIDINE
		Sulfinpyrazone	ANTURANE
Prednisone	DELTASONE, METICORTEN	Sulfisoxazole	GANTRISIN
		Sulfoxone	DIASONE
Primidone	MYSOLINE	Sulindac	CLINORIL
Probenecid	BENEMID	Tamoxifen	NOLVADEX
Probucol	LORELCO	Temazepam	RESTORIL
Procainamide	PRONESTYL, PROCAN SR	Terbutaline	BRETHINE, BRICANYL
Procaine	NOVOCAIN	Terfenadine	SELDANE
Procarbazine	MATULANE	Testolactone	TESLAC
Prochlorperazine	COMPAZINE	Testosterone	ORETON
Procyclidine	KEMADRIN	Testosterone cypionate	DEPO-TESTOSTERONE
Progesterone	PROGELAN		
Promazine	SPARINE	Testosterone enanthate	DELATESTRYL
Promethazine	PHENERGAN		
Propantheline	PRO-BANTHINE	Tetanus immune globulin (human)	HU-TET, HYPER-TET
Proparacaine	OPHTHETIC, OPHTHAINE		
Propiomazine	LARGON	Tetracycline	ACHROMYCIN V, TETRACYN, TETREX
Propoxyphene	DARVON, DOLENE		
Propranolol	INDERAL	Tetrahydrozoline	TYZINE
Propylhexedrine	BENZEDREX	Theophylline	ELIXOPHYLLIN, SUSTAIRE, THEO-DUR, THEOPHYL
Protriptyline	VIVACTIL		
Pseudoephedrine	SUDAFED		
Pyrantel pamoate	ANTIMINTH	Thiabendazole	MINTEZOL
Pyridostigmine	MESTINON	Thiethylperazine	TORECAN
Pyrimethamine	DARAPRIM	Thioridazine	MELLARIL

(Continued)

Table 288–1. SOME TRADE NAMES OF COMMONLY USED GENERIC DRUGS *(Cont'd)*

Generic Name	*Trade Name(s)*	*Generic Name*	*Trade Name(s)*
Thiothixene	NAVANE	Triflupromazine	VESPRIN
Thiphenamil	TROCINATE	Trihexyphenidyl	ARTANE, TREMIN
Thyroglobulin	PROLOID	Trimeprazine	TEMARIL
Thyrotropin	THYTROPAR	Trimethadione	TRIDIONE
Ticarcillin	TICAR	Trimethaphan	ARFONAD
Timolol maleate	BLOCADREN, TIMOPTIC	Trimethobenzamide	TIGAN
Tobramycin	NEBCIN	Trimethoprim	PROLOPRIM, TRIMPEX
Tocainide	TONOCARD	Trimethoprim-sulfamethoxazole	BACTRIM, SEPTRA, COMOXOL
Tolazamide	TOLINASE	Trimipramine	SURMONTIL
Tolazoline	PRISCOLINE	Tripelennamine	PBZ
Tolbutamide	ORINASE	Triprolidine	ACTIDIL
Tolmetin	TOLECTIN	Tromethamine	THAM
Tolnaftate	TINACTIN	Tropicamide	MYDRIACYL
Tranylcypromine	PARNATE	Tybamate	TYBATRAN
Trazodone	DESYREL	Urokinase	ABBOKINASE, BREOKINASE
Tretinoin	RETIN-A		
Triacetin	ENZACTIN	Valproic acid	DEPAKENE
Triamcinolone	ARISTOCORT, KENACORT, KENALOG	Vancomycin	VANCOCIN
Triamterene	DYRENIUM	Vasopressin	PITRESSIN
Triazolam	HALCION	Verapamil	CALAN; ISOPTIN
Trichlormethiazide	NAQUA	Vidarabine	VIRA-A
Triclofos	TRICLOS	Vinblastine	VELBAN
Trientine	CUPRID	Vincristine	ONCOVIN
Trifluridine	VIROPTIC	Warfarin	COUMADIN, PANWARFIN
Trifluoperazine	STELAZINE	Xylometazoline	OTRIVIN

§24. POISONING; VENOMOUS BITES AND STINGS

289. POISONING

(See also Ch. 189)

Some general principles for diagnosing and treating poisoning are discussed first. Highlights of symptoms and treatment for individual chemicals and drugs, or groups of substances follow alphabetically.

Poisoning due to bacterial or other toxins in food is discussed in Ch. 57. Venomous bites and stings are dealt with in Ch. 290. Alcoholism and drug dependence are discussed in Ch. 138. Drug reactions are discussed in Chs. 21, 237, and 277.

GENERAL PRINCIPLES OF TREATMENT

Diagnosis

Worldwide, > 9 million natural and synthetic chemicals have been identified; fortunately, fewer than 3000 cause more than 95% of accidental and deliberate poisonings. The identification of a poison and an accurate assessment of its potential toxicity are critical to a physician's successful management of poisoning. In their absence, one must rely on simple general supportive treatment unless a specific "toxidrome" (toxicologic symptom complex) is pinpointed. Increasingly, physicians are depending upon local or regional "Poison Centers" for technical information, particularly concerning ingredient data (toxic potentials) and consultations.

Poisoning should be considered in the differential diagnosis of any unexplained symptoms or signs, especially in children < 5 yr. Similarly, in the young adult, any disparity between expected history and clinical findings should suggest poisoning. Often the type and speed of onset of the total clinical picture will confirm or refute a suspicion of poisoning. Occasionally, the absence of a specific finding will be as important as its presence. Any pertinent history should be secured and the person and premises inspected for traces of drugs, ie, imprint identifications on solid medication forms, alcohol, etc, particularly for the unconscious patient.

> Ingredients, first aid measures, and antidotes often are printed on product containers, but may be inaccurate or out of date. Information about household and industrial chemicals can be obtained through poison centers in all parts of the USA and Europe. Consultation with the centers is encouraged. The nearest center is often listed under Emergency Numbers in the local telephone directory, or is available from the operator.

Immediate Care

1. Determine adequacy of cardiac and respiratory function and begin resuscitation if needed (see CARDIAC ARREST AND CARDIOPULMONARY RESUSCITATION in Ch. 27).

2. Determine quickly what has happened. Identify the substance ingested, its route of entry into the body, and its toxicity potential. *Save any containers and appropriate specimens of the product or of emetic returns.* Determine the need for medical care, recognizing that many substances (see TABLE 289–1) need no further treatment. At all times, recall that overtreatment per se may be a hazard.

3. Unless contraindicated, immediately dilute and remove the toxic substance from the body. A person who has ingested a toxic substance may also have spilled it on the skin and may be inhaling fumes as well.

Ingested poison: Emesis will usually remove more of the toxic substance than will gastric lavage. Immediately induce vomiting with ipecac syrup 15 to 30 mL (1 to 2

TABLE 289–1. SUBSTANCES GENERALLY NONTOXIC WHEN INGESTED*

Ball-point inks (amt. in 1 pen)	Lipstick
Barium sulfate	Magnesium silicate (antacid)
Bathtub toys (floating)	Matches
Blackboard chalk (calcium carbonate)	Methylcellulose
Candles (insect-repellent type may be toxic)	Modeling clay
Carbowax (polyethylene glycol)	Paraffin, chlorinated
Carboxymethylcellulose (dehydrating material packed with drugs, film, etc.)	Pencil lead (graphite)
	Pepper, black (except inhaled in mass)
Castor oil	Petrolatum
Cetyl alcohol	Polyethylene glycols
Crayons (children's: marked A.P., C.P., or C.S. 130–46)	Polyethylene glycol stearate
	Polysorbate (Tweens®)
Detergents, anionic and nonionic	Putty
Dichloral (herbicide)	Red oil (turkey-red oil, sulfated castor oil)
Dry cell battery	Silica (silicon dioxide)
Glycerol	Spermaceti
Glyceryl monostearate	Stearic acid
Graphite	Sweetening agents
Gums (acacia, agar, ghatti, etc.)	Talc
Hormones	Tallow
Kaolin	Thermometer fluid or mercury
Lanolin	Titanium oxide
Lauric acid	Triacetin (glyceryl triacetate)
Linoleic acid	Vitamins, multiple without iron
Linseed oil (not boiled)	

* Substances listed here may, however, be present in combination with phenol, petroleum distillate vehicles, or other toxic chemicals. Since manufactured products may be changed in their composition, this table is intended only as a guide, and prudence requires that a poison center be consulted for up-to-date information.

tbsp) for children and adults taken with water or soft drinks (orally: 15 mL/kg for infants; 1 qt [1 L] for adults); and keep the patient actively moving if possible. The dose of ipecac may be repeated in 15 min if necessary. If ipecac is not available, give soapy water, anionic or non-anionic detergent (handwashing liquid detergent) plus water, and induce vomiting by inserting a finger or blunt instrument into the patient's throat. Avoid being bitten. Place a child in the head-down position. Save a portion of the vomitus for analysis. (CAUTION: *Do not induce vomiting if the patient is comatose, is having convulsions [or is likely to], or has ingested petroleum distillates or corrosive substances. Emesis of petroleum distillates is hardly ever indicated unless some other compound has been dissolved in the distillates that requires evacuation [eg, parathion])*

When **gastric lavage** is carried out (*do not use lavage if the patient is convulsing or if the ingested substance is corrosive*), use the largest tube appropriate for the patient. For comatose or sedated patients > 2 yr of age, use a cuffed endotracheal tube to prevent aspiration. For those < 2, no cuff is needed on the endotracheal tube because of the snug fit. Have the patient in a head-low position. For adults, physiologic (0.9%) sodium chloride solution or tap water may be used; for children, 0.45% sodium chloride solution is recommended. Introduce lavage fluids in 20- to 30-mL aliquots and remove the stomach contents by siphon or syringe after each instillation. Continue the rinsing procedure until washings return free of toxin. After the return is clear, instill a specific antidote if one is available; otherwise instill a slurry of activated charcoal (see below).

The use of **cathartics** remains controversial; some evidence suggests that they may actually enhance absorption rather than promote excretion. If a cathartic is used, it is best limited to sodium sulfate 30 gm dissolved in 250 mL water, with proportionally reduced amounts for children.

When taken internally, **activated charcoal** with its molecular configuration and large surface area adsorbs significant amounts of many poisons, precluding their absorption from the gut. The earlier the charcoal is used, the more effective it is. From 5 to 10 times the amount of charcoal as that of the poison suspected of being ingested should be used. For children < 5 yr the usual dose is 25 gm; for older children and adults, 50 to 100 gm. Charcoal is administered as a slurry (20 to 200 gm in water), preferably by stomach tube; it should not be administered before or immediately after syrup of ipecac has been given.

Specific antidotes: While not numerous, specific antidotes are remarkably effective—eg, naloxone in opioid overdoses, atropine in organo-phosphate encounters, methylene blue for methemoglobinemia, N-acetylcysteine for acetaminophen. A poison center should be contacted to determine if new specific antidotes have been developed, particularly for new drugs.

Inhaled poison: The patient should be removed from the contaminated environment, his respiration supported, and other personnel protected from contamination.

Skin and eye contamination: Contaminated clothing (including shoes and socks) should be removed. The skin should be thoroughly washed and the eyes flushed with water (see also Chs. 215 and 254). Helpers should be protected from contamination.

CNS stimulation by the poison may require **sedation**. Usually, diazepam or a barbiturate is used. In pure amphetamine poisoning, chlorpromazine is the drug of choice. To terminate convulsions, diazepam (5 to 10 mg for adults; 0.1 to 0.2 mg/kg for children) is given slowly IV. Phenobarbital (100 to 200 mg for adults and 4 to 7 mg/kg for children) may be used IV or IM to either terminate or prevent the recurrence of a convulsion. Refractory seizures very rarely require general anesthesia; the above measures usually are satisfactory to control the hypoxic and cardiovascular consequences of convulsions.

Continuing Care

Symptomatic and supportive treatment depends on symptoms and signs and on anticipation of the clinical course, based upon identification of the poison. Continuation

of the appropriate measures already begun and attempts to enhance the excretion of poison already absorbed are basic considerations. Stimulants are unlikely to be effective and are generally *contraindicated.* **Severe CNS depression** requires support of the circulation and ventilation (see Ch. 34). Endotracheal intubation and, rarely, tracheostomy may be necessary. In suspected or known narcotic poisoning, naloxone should be used (see OPIOID ANALGESICS AND ANTAGONISTS in Ch. 281).

Cerebral edema is common in poisonings due to sedatives, carbon monoxide, lead, and other CNS depressants. A 20% mannitol solution (5 to 10 mL/kg) is given slowly IV over a 30- to 60-min period. Corticosteroids are also used (dexamethasone 1 mg/sq m of BSA q 6 h by IV drip). The use of intracranial monitoring with hyperventilation to alter the degree of cerebral edema enjoys widespread favor. The use of "barbiturate coma" in cerebral edema associated with hypoxic episodes has been advocated, but the practice must be considered experimental.

Renal failure may occur in poisoning, and dialysis may be required. Elimination of poisons sometimes can be hastened either by augmenting normal excretory pathways or by using artificial means such as dialysis, depending upon the nature of the poisoning, the availability of the facilities, and the condition of the patient. Flushing out the poison by simply increasing urine volume is rarely helpful. Alkalinization or acidification of the urine can occasionally be helpful (eg, in acute salicylate ingestions, giving 2 to 3 mEq/kg of sodium bicarbonate IV will augment excretion significantly). In general, weak acids are captured in alkalinized urine and weak bases in acidified urine.

Over the past decade, **hemo-** and **peritoneal dialysis** have been augmented by the development of **"lipid dialysis,"** aimed at removal of lipid-soluble substances from the blood, and **hemoperfusion,** to provide an even more rapid and efficient clearance of toxic substances from the blood. However, these technics are useless if the involved substance has a large "apparent volume of distribution"—ie, if it is stored in fatty tissue or extensively bound to tissue protein. In select circumstances these technics may be effective, but in many instances their yield is negligible. Thus, while digoxin is rapidly cleared from the blood via hemoperfusion, such a small amount (3 to 5%) of the total body digoxin is present in the blood that hemoperfusion is ineffective. Tricyclic antidepressants are also largely confined to other than the vascular compartment, and the use of hemoperfusion for overdoses is likewise not warranted. TABLE 289–2 lists some representative toxic substances that are dialyzable (see also Ch. 148).

TABLE 289–2. SOME DIALYZABLE TOXIC SUBSTANCES*

Alcohols	Chlorates	Methaqualone
Aminoglycoside antibiotics	Chlordiazepoxide	Methyprylon
Amphetamines	Chromic acid	Monoamine oxidase inhibitors
Aniline	Diphenhydramine	Paraldehyde
Barbiturates	Ethchlorvynol (lipid)	Penicillins
γ-Benzene hexachloride (lindane)	Ethinamate	Phenytoin (diphenylhydantoin)
Boric acid	Ethylene glycol	Potassium
Bromides and other halides	Glutethimide (lipid)	Salicylates
Calcium	Isoniazid	Sodium
Camphor	Lithium	Tetracycline
Cephaloridine	Meprobamate	Theophylline
Chloral hydrate	Metals (arsenic, copper, iron, lead, magnesium, strontium, zinc)	Thiocyanates
Chloramphenicol		

* It should be emphasized that only in unusual circumstances is dialysis or hemoperfusion actually clinically useful.

Chelating agents are useful in treating poisoning by many metals and other toxic substances. The most commonly used agents, the toxic substances that they effectively chelate, and the usual doses required are given in TABLE 289–3.

Prevention

Widespread, voluntary, and now mandatory use of child-resistant containers (safety caps) has produced a dramatic decline in aspirin poisoning. Labeling of household products and prescription items, use of drug imprints on solid medication forms, improved monitoring of toxic exposures within industry and throughout the environment, widespread public and professional education programs such as that built around the **Mr. Yuk Program®** or that of the American Association of Poison Control Centers, and intense community-wide efforts to make syrup of ipecac available in each home and to make each home aware of the nearest poison center's phone number are examples of successful and effective activities aimed at preventing poisoning.

TABLE 289–3. CHELATION THERAPY

Edetate calcium disodium (calcium disodium edathamil; $CaNa_2$-EDTA)

Toxic substances:

Cadmium	Lead	Tungsten
Chromium	Manganese	Uranium
Cobalt	Nickel	Vanadium
Copper*	Radium	Zinc
Copper salts	Selenium	Zinc salts

Dosage: Dilute to 3% (or less) for IV use
Give 25 to 35 mg/kg IV slowly (over 1 h) q 12 h for 5 to 7 days
Interrupt for 7 days, then repeat

Dimercaprol (BAL)

Toxic substances:

Antimony	Chromic acid*	Nickel
Arsenic	Chromium trioxide*	Tungsten
Bichromates*	Copper salts	Zinc salts
Bismuth	Gold	
Chromates*	Mercury	

Dosage: Use 10% BAL in oil; give IM only
1st day: 3 to 4 mg/kg q 4 h
2nd day: 2 mg/kg q 4 h
3rd day: 3 mg/kg q 6 h
Then 3 mg/kg q 12 h every 10 days until recovery

Penicillamine

Toxic substances:

Bichromates	Chromium trioxide	Mercury*
Cadmium	Cobalt	Nickel
Chromates	Copper salts	Zinc salts
Chromic acid	Lead	

Dosage: 15 to 20 mg/kg orally bid

NOTE: Neither iron nor thallium salts are chelated effectively by the above agents, but each has its own chelating agent (see Iron and Thallium salts in TABLE 289–4, below).

* Chelator of choice.

SPECIFIC POISONS

TABLE 289–4 lists the special toxicology for individual agents or groups of substances having related actions or similar treatment. However, the inclusion of a substance under a particular heading (eg, toluene under benzene) does not necessarily indicate that the toxicity is similar; it indicates that they are chemically related or that one substance may be found as an ingredient or impurity of another.

TABLE 289–4. SPECIFIC POISONS: SYMPTOMS AND TREATMENT

Poison	*Symptoms*	*Treatment*
Acetaminophen (see also ACETAMINOPHEN POISONING in Ch. 189)	Early: Often asymptomatic; mild nausea, vomiting, diaphoresis, pallor; beginning signs of hepatotoxicity; oliguria Later (at 24–48 h): Nausea & protracted vomiting, right upper quadrant pain, jaundice, coagulation defects, hypoglycemia, encephalopathy, hepatic failure; renal failure, myocardiopathy may occur	Emesis; gastric lavage. Monitor plasma drug levels for prognosis; if > 160–200 μg/mL at 4 h, hepatic necrosis may occur; if plasma level >300 μg/mL at 4 h, hepatic damage is almost certain. If given before 18 h, oral N-acetylcysteine (Mucomyst®) 140 mg/kg to start and 70 mg/kg q 4 h for 4 to 18 doses has been effective in preventing significant hepatotoxicity
Acetanilid Aniline (indelible) inks Aniline oils Chloroaniline Phenacetin (acetophenetidin)	Cyanosis due to formation of methemoglobin & sulfhemoglobin; dyspnea; weakness; vertigo; anginal pain; rashes & urticaria; vomiting; delirium; depression; respiratory & circulatory failure	(1) Inhalation: Give O_2; support respiration. Blood transfusion. For severe cyanosis, methylene blue 1–2 mg/kg IV (2) Skin: Remove clothing & wash area with copious soap & water; then as in (1) (3) Ingestion: Give ipecac emetic; if this fails, gastric lavage; then as in (1)
Acetic acid: see Acids and alkalis		
Acetone Nail polish remover Ketones Model airplane glues, cements	Inhalation: Bronchial irritation, pulmonary congestion & edema, decreased respirations, dyspnea, drunkenness, stupor, ketosis Ingestion: As above except direct pulmonary effect	Remove from source; evacuate stomach except for small amounts; support respirations; give O_2 & fluids; correct metabolic acidosis
Acetophenetidin: see Acetanilid		
Acetylene gas: see Carbon monoxide		
Acetylsalicylic acid: see ASPIRIN AND OTHER SALICYLATE POISONING in Ch. 189		
Acids & alkalis (see also specific acids & alkalis by name and INGESTION OF CAUSTICS in Ch. 189)		
Acids Acetic Hydrochloric Nitric Phosphoric Sulfuric (some drain or toilet bowl cleaners, some dishwasher detergents)	Corrosive burns from inhalation, skin contact, eye contact, & ingestion; local pain. In general, alkali is more damaging to the GI tract Drooling and striador are suggestive of damage	Skin or eye: Flush with water for 15 min Ingestion: Dilute with water or milk; *do not stimulate vomiting;* consider gastric lavage if large amounts of alkali granules have been consumed Hospitalize; give opiates for pain; treat shock if present; endoscopy is recommended; tracheostomy may be needed; for verified esophageal burns, give antibiotics and

TABLE 289–4. SPECIFIC POISONS: SYMPTOMS AND TREATMENT *(Cont'd)*

Poison	*Symptoms*	*Treatment*
Alkalis Ammonia water (ammonium hydroxide) Potassium hydroxide (potash) Sodium hydroxide (caustic soda, lye) Carbonates of the above Detergent powders Some drain or toilet bowl cleaners; some dishwasher detergents	NOTE: Even on the absence of mouth lesions, strong alkalies (pH > 10.5–11.0) can burn the esophagus; esophagoscopy is advised	dexamethasone 1 mg/sq m BSA q 6 h or equivalent for 2–3 wk
Airplane glues, cements (model-building): see Acetone, Benzene, Petroleum distillates		
Alcohol, ethyl (ethanol) Brandy, whiskey, & other liquors	Emotional lability, impaired coordination, flushing, nausea & vomiting, stupor to coma, respiratory depression	Emesis; gastric lavage; support respirations; IV glucose to prevent hypoglycemia; dialysis if blood levels > 300–350 mg/dL; generous fluid administration as serum alcohol increases serum osmolarity
Alcohol, isopropyl Rubbing alcohol	Dizziness, incoordination, stupor to coma, gastroenteritis, hypotension; *no* retinal injury	Emesis; gastric lavage; IV glucose; correct dehydration & electrolyte changes; dialysis
Alcohol, methyl (Methanol, wood alcohol) Paint solvent Varnish Antifreeze Solid canned fuel	Very toxic: 60–250 mL (2–8 oz) fatal in adults; 8–10 mL (2 tsp) in children. Latency period 12–18 h; headache, weakness, leg cramps, vertigo, convulsions, dimness of vision, decreased respiration	Combat acidosis with IV sodium bicarbonate; give 10% ethanol/5% dextrose solution IV; initially, a loading dose of 0.7 gm/kg of ethanol to impede methanol metabolism is infused over 1 h followed by 0.1 to 0.2 gm/kg hourly to maintain a blood ethanol level of 100 mg/mL; *hemodialysis*
Aldrin: see DDT		
Alkalis: see Acids & alkalis		
Aminophylline Caffeine Theophylline	Wakefulness, restlessness, anorexia, vomiting, dehydration, convulsions; with hypersensitivity, immediate vasomotor collapse may occur. Adults are more susceptible than children	If ingested use emetic; if by rectal suppository, use enema. Stop medication; obtain theophylline blood level; phenobarbital or diazapam for convulsions; give parenteral fluids; maintain blood pressure; if serum level > 50–100 mg/dL, consider dialysis
Amitriptyline: see Tricyclic antidepressants		

TABLE 289–4. SPECIFIC POISONS: SYMPTOMS AND TREATMENT *(Cont'd)*

Poison	*Symptoms*	*Treatment*
Ammonia gas	Irritation of eyes & respiratory tract; cough, choking; abdominal pain	Flush eyes with tap water for 15 min. *No gastric lavage or emetic.* If severe, positive pressure O_2 to prevent pulmonary edema; support respiration
Ammonia water: see Acids & alkalis		
Ammoniated mercury: see Mercury		
Ammonium carbonate: see Acids & alkalis		
Ammonium fluoride: see Fluorides		
Ammonium hydroxide: see Acids & alkalis		
Amobarbital: see Barbiturates		
Amphetamines Amphetamine sulfate, phosphate Dextroamphetamine Methamphetamine Phenmetrazine	Increased activity, exhilaration, talkativeness, insomnia, irritability, exaggerated reflexes, anorexia, dry mouth, arrhythmia, anginal chest pain, heart block, psychotic-like states and inability to concentrate or sit still	Emesis or lavage effective long after ingestion because of recycling via gastric mucosa Sedate with chlorpromazine 0.5–1 mg/kg IM or orally q 30 min as needed; reduce external stimuli; hypothermia; combat cerebral edema; peritoneal dialysis (NOTE: For amphetamine/barbiturate combination use 1/2 chlorpromazine dose)
Amyl nitrite: see Nitrites		
Aniline: see Acetanilid		
Ant poison: see DDT (chlordane); Thallium salts		
Antifreeze: see Alcohol, methyl; Ethylene glycol		
Antihistamines	Excitation or depression, drowsiness, nervousness, disorientation, hallucinations, tachycardia, arrhythmias, hyperpyrexia, delirium, convulsions	Ipecac emesis, gastric lavage; support respiration and blood pressure; control seizures with diazapam; physostigmine salicylate 0.5–2.0 mg IM or IV (slowly) if anticholinergic symptoms are obviously a problem
Antimony: see Arsenic & antimony		
Antineoplastic agents Methotrexate Mercaptopurine Vincristine	Effects on hematopoetic system; nausea; vomiting	Emesis > lavage; supportive care; "leucovorin rescue"
Arsenic & antimony Antimony compounds Stibophen Tartar emetic Arsenic Donovan's solution Fowler's solution Herbicides Paris green Pesticides	Throat constriction, dysphagia; burning GI pain, vomiting, diarrhea; dehydration; pulmonary edema; renal failure; liver failure	Emesis; gastric lavage, then a demulcent; chelation with penicillamine; BAL if patient cannot take oral medication; hydration; treat shock, pain; saline cathartic (sodium sulfate 15–30 gm in water)

TABLE 289–4. SPECIFIC POISONS: SYMPTOMS AND TREATMENT *(Cont'd)*

Poison	*Symptoms*	*Treatment*
Arsine gas	Acute hemolytic anemia	Transfusions; diuresis
Asphalt: see Petroleum distillates		
Aspirin: see ASPIRIN AND OTHER SALICYLATE POISONING in Ch. 189		
Atropine: see Belladonna		
Automobile exhaust: see Carbon monoxide		
Barbiturates Amobarbital Pentobarbital Phenobarbital Secobarbital	Headache, confusion, ptosis, excitement, delirium, loss of corneal reflex, respiratory failure, coma	Empty stomach up to 24 h after ingestion. If immediately after, use ipecac emetic; if sedated, use lavage with cuffed endotracheal tube. Consider saline cathartic (sodium sulfate 15–30 gm); good nursing care; support respirations, give O_2; correct any dehydration. Rarely hemodialysis or peritoneal lavage, especially for long-acting barbiturates
Barium compounds (soluble) Rodenticides Depilatories Fireworks Barium acetate carbonate chloride hydroxide nitrate sulfide	Vomiting, abdominal pain, diarrhea, tremors, convulsions, hypertension, cardiac arrest	To precipitate barium in stomach, give 60 gm sodium or magnesium sulfate orally. Then emesis or gastric lavage. 10% Sodium sulfate 10 ml slowly IV; repeat q 15 min until symptoms subside. Control convulsions with diazepam; atropine 0.5–1 mg for colic; sublingual nitroglycerin 1/100–1/50 for hypertension; O_2 for dyspnea & cyanosis; quinidine 100–300 mg to prevent ventricular fibrillation; correct hypokalemia
Belladonna Atropine Hyoscyamine Hyoscyamus Scopolamine (Hyoscine) Stramonium	Dry skin and mucous membranes; pupils dilated; flushing, hyperpyrexia; tachycardia, restlessness; coma; respiratory failure; convulsions	Emesis; support respiration; give fluids to augment excretion. May need to catheterize bladder. Physostigmine salicylate 0.5–2.0 mg IM or IV (slowly) may reverse peripheral and central effects
Benzene Benzol Hydrocarbons Toluene Toluol Xylene Model airplane glue	Dizziness, weakness, headache, euphoria, nausea, vomiting, ventricular arrhythmia, paralysis, convulsions; with chronic poisoning, aplastic anemia, leukemia	If sizeable ingestion (> 0.5–1 mL/kg), emesis or cautious gastric lavage. Give O_2; support respiration; monitor ECG—ventricular fibrillation can occur. Control seizures with diazepam. Blood transfusion for severe anemia. *Do not give epinephrine*
γ-Benzene hexachloride BHC Hexachlorocyclo-hexane Lindane	Irritability, CNS excitation, muscle spasms, atonia, clonic & tonic convulsions, respiratory failure, pulmonary edema	Emesis immediately after ingestion; gastric lavage; saline cathartic (sodium sulfate 15–30 gm). Diazepam for convulsions. Avoid all oils—they promote absorption. Charcoal hemoperfusion prn
Benzin, benzine: see Petroleum distillates		

TABLE 289–4. SPECIFIC POISONS: SYMPTOMS AND TREATMENT *(Cont'd)*

Poison	*Symptoms*	*Treatment*
Benzodiazapines Dalmane® Librium® Valium®	Sedation to coma, particularly if accompanied by alcohol	Emesis; lavage; supportive care
Benzol: see Benzene		
BHC: see γ-Benzene hexachloride		
Bichloride of mercury: see Mercury		
Bichromates: see Chromic acid		
Bishydroxycoumarin: see Warfarin		
Bismuth compounds	Poorly absorbed. Ulcerative stomatitis, anorexia, headache, rash, renal tubular damage	Ipecac emesis; gastric lavage; respiratory support; BAL (see TABLE 289–3, Chelation Therapy)
Bitter almond oil: see Cyanides		
Bitter almond oil, artificial: see Nitrobenzene		
Bleach, chlorine: see Hypochlorites		
Borates Boric acid	Nausea, vomiting, diarrhea, hemorrhagic gastroenteritis, weakness, lethargy, CNS depression, convulsion, "boiled lobster" skin rash, shock	Ipecac emesis; gastric lavage; remove from skin; prevent or treat electrolyte changes & shock; control convulsions. Dialysis for severe poisoning
Boric acid: see Borates		
Brandy: see Alcohol, ethyl		
Bromates: see Chlorates		
Bromides	Nausea, vomiting, rash (may be acneiform), slurred speech, ataxia, confusion, psychotic behavior, coma, paralysis	Ipecac emesis, gastric lavage for acute ingestion; stop use as medication; promote mild diuresis by hydration & sodium chloride IV; ethacrynic acid is specifically useful. Hemodialysis if severe
Bromine: see Chlorine		
Bulan: see DDT		
Cadmium Solder	Severe gastric cramps, vomiting, diarrhea; dry throat, cough, dyspnea; headache; shock, coma; brown urine, renal failure	Ipecac emesis; gastric lavage with milk or albumin; saline catharsis; respiratory support; hydration; IPPB for pulmonary edema. Give edetate calcium disodium (see TABLE 289–3, Chelation Therapy); *not BAL*
Caffeine: see Aminophylline		
Calomel: see Mercury		
Camphor Camphorated oils	Camphor odor on breath, headache; confusion, delirium, hallucinations, convulsions, coma	Ipecac emesis; gastric lavage. Prevent & treat convulsions with diazepam; support respiration. Lipid dialysis is being explored
Canned fuel, solid: see Alcohol, methyl		

TABLE 289–4. SPECIFIC POISONS: SYMPTOMS AND TREATMENT *(Cont'd)*

Poison	Symptoms	Treatment
Cantharides Spanish fly Cantharidin	Skin and mucous membranes irritated, vesicles; nausea, vomiting, bloody diarrhea; burning pain in back and urethra; respiratory depression; convulsions, coma; abortion, menorrhagia	Avoid all oils; ipecac emesis; support respiration; treat convulsions; maintain fluid balance
Cantharidin: see Cantharides		
Carbolic acid: see Phenols		
Carbon bisulfide: see Carbon disulfide		
Carbon dioxide	Dyspnea, weakness, tinnitus, palpitations	Respiratory support; O_2
Carbon disulfide Carbon bisulfide	Garlic-breath odor, irritability, weakness, manic depression, narcosis, delirium, mydriasis, blindness, parkinsonism, convulsions, coma, paralysis, respiratory failure	Wash skin; emesis; gastric lavage; O_2; diazepam sedation; support respiration & circulation
Carbon monoxide Acetylene gas Automobile exhaust Carbonyl iron Coal gas Furnace gas Illuminating gas Marsh gas	Toxicity varies with length of exposure, conc. inhaled, resp. & circ. rates. Symptoms vary with % carboxyhemoglobin in blood. Headache, vertigo, dyspnea, confusion, dilated pupils, convulsions, coma	100% O_2 by mask; respiratory support if needed; absolute bed rest (minimum 48 h); watch for cardiac problems & for nerve or brain injury (may appear up to 3 wk). *Do not use stimulants.* Hyperbaric O_2 is effective. See Ch. 267
Carbon tetrachloride Cleaning fluids (nonflammable)	Nausea, vomiting, abdominal pain, headache, confusion, visual disturbances, CNS depression, ventricular fibrillation, renal injury, hepatic injury	Wash from skin; emesis or gastric lavage; give O_2; support respiration; monitor renal & hepatic function & treat appropriately. *Avoid alcohol, epinephrine, ephedrine*
Carbonates (ammonium, potassium, sodium): see Acids & alkalis		
Caustic soda: see Acids & alkalis		
Chloral amide: see Chloral hydrate		
Chloral hydrate Chloral amide	Drowsiness, confusion, shock, coma; respiratory depression; renal injury, hepatic injury	Ipecac emesis; gastric lavage; saline enema if rectal instillation; respiratory support
Chlorates Bromates Nitrates Permanent wave neutralizers	Vomiting, nausea, diarrhea, cyanosis (methemoglobin), toxic nephritis, shock, convulsions, CNS depression, coma, jaundice	Ipecac emesis; gastric lavage; early renal or peritoneal dialysis; transfusion for severe cyanosis; *do not use methylene blue.* Treat shock; O_2
Chlordane: see DDT		
Chlorinated lime: see Chlorine		

TABLE 289–4. SPECIFIC POISONS: SYMPTOMS AND TREATMENT *(Cont'd)*

Poison	Symptoms	Treatment
Chlorine (see also Hypochlorites) Bromine Chlorinated lime Chlorine water Tear gas	Inhalation: Severe respiratory & ocular irritation, glottal spasm, cough, choking, vomiting; pulmonary edema; cyanosis Ingestion: Irritation, corrosion of mouth & GI tract, possible ulceration or perforation; abdominal pain, tachycardia, prostration, circulatory collapse	Inhalation: O_2; respiratory support; watch for & treat pulmonary edema Ingestion: Ipecac emesis; gastric lavage; treat shock
Chloroaniline: see Acetanilid		
Chloroform Ether Nitrous oxide Trichloromethane	Drowsiness, coma; with nitrous oxide, delirium	Inhalation: Respiratory, cardiac, and circulatory support Ingestion: Ipecac emesis; gastric lavage; observe for renal and hepatic damage
Chlorophenothane: see DDT		
Chlorothion: see Parathion		
Chlorpromazine: see Phenothiazine		
Chromates: see Chromic acid		
Chromic Acid Chromates Chromium trioxide Bichromates	Corrosive due to oxidation. Ulcer and perforated nasal septum; severe gastroenteritis; shock, vertigo, coma; nephritis	Milk or water to dilute; BAL (or penicillamine) for severe symptoms; fluids & electrolytes, with caution, to support renal function
Chromium: see TABLE 289–3, Chelation Therapy		
Chromium trioxide: see Chromic acid		
Cimitidine; ranitidine	Slight dryness and drowsiness; can alter metabolism of concomitant drugs	No specific antidotal treatment available: maintain a focus on metabolism of other drugs
Clonidine	Sedation; periodic apnea; hypotension	Emesis; lavage; supportive care; tolazoline IV and dopamine drip; naloxone 5 $\mu g/kg$ up to 2–20 mg, repeated as necessary
Coal gas: see Carbon monoxide		
Cobalt: see TABLE 289–3, Chelation Therapy		
Cobaltous chloride: see Nitrogen oxides		
Cocaine	Stimulation, then depression; nausea & vomiting; loss of self-control, anxiety, hallucinations; sweating; respiratory difficulty progressing to failure; cyanosis; circulatory failure; convulsions	Emetic early; gastric lavage; if needed, propranolol 10–15 mg orally or 0.1 mg IV, diazepam for excitation; O_2, respiratory & circulatory support
Codeine: see Narcotics		
Copper: see TABLE 289–3, Chelation Therapy		

TABLE 289–4. SPECIFIC POISONS: SYMPTOMS AND TREATMENT *(Cont'd)*

Poison	*Symptoms*	*Treatment*
Copper salts Zinc salts Cupric sulfate, acetate, subacetate Cuprous chloride, oxide	Emesis; burning sensation, metallic taste, diarrhea; pain; shock; jaundice; anuria; convulsions	Emesis; gastric lavage; penicillamine or BAL (see TABLE 289–3, Chelation Therapy); electrolyte & fluid balance; respiratory support; monitor GI tract; treat shock, control convulsions; monitor for hepatic & renal failure
Corrosive sublimate: see Mercury		
Creosote; cresols: see Phenols		
Cyanides Bitter almond oil Wild cherry syrup Hydrocyanic acid Nitroprusside Potassium cyanide Prussic acid Sodium cyanide	Tachycardia, headache, drowsiness, hypotension, coma, convulsions, death; plasma bright red; *very rapidly lethal* (1–15 min)	*Speed essential.* Remove from source of inhalation; immediate emesis or lavage, amyl nitrite inhalation, 0.2 mL (1 capsule) 30 sec of each min, 100% O_2, support respiration; 10 mL 3% sodium nitrite 2.5–5 mL/min IV (in child: 10 mg/kg) then 50 mL 25% sodium thiosulfate 2.5–5 mL/min IV; repeat the above if symptoms recur. Lilly kit
DDD: see DDT		
DDT(chlorophenothane) Chlorinated organic insecticides Aldrin Bulan Chlordane DDD Dieldrin Dilan Endrin Heptachlor Methoxychlor Prolan Toxaphene	Vomiting (early or delayed); paresthesias, malaise; coarse tremors, convulsions; pulmonary edema, ventricular fibrillation, respiratory failure	Emesis; gastric lavage if not convulsing; 15–30 gm sodium sulfate or charcoal left in stomach; diazepam or phenobarbital to prevent & control tremors & convulsions; avoid epinephrine & sudden stimuli; parenteral fluids; monitor for renal & hepatic failure
Deodorizers, household: see Naphthalene, Paradichlorobenzene		
Depilatories: see Barium compounds		
Detergent powders: see Acids & alkalis		
Dextroamphetamine: see Amphetamines		
Diazinon: see Parathion		
Dicumarol: see Warfarin		
Dieldrin: see DDT		
Diethylene glycol: see Ethylene glycol		
Digitalis, digitoxin, digoxin: see HEART FAILURE in Ch. 27		
Dilan: see DDT		

TABLE 289–4. SPECIFIC POISONS: SYMPTOMS AND TREATMENT *(Cont'd)*

Poison	*Symptoms*	*Treatment*
Dinitrobenzene: see Nitrobenzene		
Dinitro-*o*-cresol Herbicides Pesticides	Fatigue, thirst, flushing; nausea, vomiting, abdominal pain; hyperpyrexia, tachycardia, loss of consciousness; dyspnea, respiratory arrest. Absorbed through skin	Emesis; gastric lavage with 5% sodium bicarbonate; leave 0.5–1 L (1–2 pt) in stomach; saline catharsis; fluid therapy; O_2; anticipate renal & hepatic toxicity
Diphenoxylate with atropine	Lethargy, nystagmus, pinpoint pupils, tachycardia, coma, respiratory depression (NOTE: toxicity may be delayed up to 12 h)	Ipecac emesis, gastric lavage; activated charcoal; naloxone; admit all children to ICU for observation
Dipterex: see Parathion		
Dishwasher detergents: see Acids & alkalis		
Diuretics, mercurial: see Mercury		
Drain cleaners: see Acids & alkalis		
Endrin: see DDT		
Ergot derivatives	Thirst, diarrhea, vomiting, light-headedness, burning feet; convulsions, hypotension, coma, abortion; gangrene of feet; cataract	Ipecac emesis; gastric lavage; short-acting barbiturate for convulsions; amyl nitrite 0.3 mL by inhalation; papaverine 60 mg IV
Eserine: see Physostigmine		
Ethanol: see Alcohol, ethyl		
Ether: see Chloroform		
Ethyl alcohol: see Alcohol, ethyl		
Ethyl biscoumacetate: see Warfarin		
Ethylene glycol Diethylene glycol Permanent antifreeze	Eye contact iridocyclitis: Ingestion: Inebriation but no alcohol odor on breath; nausea, vomiting; carpopedal spasm, lumbar pain; oxalate crystalluria; oliguria progressing to anuria & acute renal failure; respiratory distress, convulsions, coma	Flush eyes Ingestion: Emesis; gastric lavage, support respiration, correct electrolyte imbalance; give ethanol (see Alcohol, methyl); hemodialysis
Explosives: see Barium compounds (fireworks); Nitrogen oxides		
Fava bean (favism): see NONBACTERIAL FOOD POISONING in Ch. 57		
Ferric salts: see Iron		
Ferrous gluconate, ferrous sulfate: see Iron		
Fireworks: see Barium compounds		

TABLE 289–4. SPECIFIC POISONS: SYMPTOMS AND TREATMENT *(Cont'd)*

Poison	*Symptoms*	*Treatment*
Fluorides Ammonium fluoride Hydrofluoric acid Rat poisons Roach poisons Sodium fluoride Soluble fluorides generally	Inhalation: Intense eye, nasal irritation; headache; dyspnea, sense of suffocation, glottal edema, pulmonary edema, bronchitis, pneumonia; mediastinal & subcut. emphysema from bleb rupture Skin & mucosa: Superficial or deep burns Ingestion: Salty or soapy taste; tremors, convulsions, CNS depression; shock; renal failure	Inhalation: O_2, respiratory support; prednisone for chemical pneumonitis (adults 30–80 mg/day in divided doses); manage pulmonary edema Skin: Copious flushing with cold water; debride white tissue; for late pain, inject 10% calcium gluconate locally & apply magnesium oxide paste Ingestion: Ipecac emesis; gastric lavage—leave aluminum hydroxide gel in stomach; IV glucose & saline; 10% calcium gluconate, 10 mL IV (1 mL/kg in child); monitor for cardiac irritability; treat shock & dehydration
Formaldehyde Formalin (NOTE: May contain methyl alcohol)	Inhalation: Irritation of eyes, nose, respiratory tract; laryngeal spasm & edema; dysphagia; bronchitis, pneumonia Skin: Irritation, coagulation necrosis; dermatitis, hypersensitivity Ingestion: Oral & gastric pain, nausea, vomiting, hematemesis, shock, hematuria, anuria, coma, respiratory failure	Inhalation: Flush eyes with saline; O_2; support respiration Skin: Wash copiously with soap & water Ingestion: Give water or milk to dilute; treat shock, correct acidosis with sodium bicarbonate; support respiration; observe for perforations
Fowler's solution: see Arsenic & antimony		
Fuel, canned: see Alcohol, methyl		
Fuel oil: see Petroleum distillates		
Furnace gas: see Carbon monoxide		
Gamma benzene hexachloride: see γ-Benzene hexachloride		
Gas Acetylene, automobile exhaust, coal, furnace, illuminating, marsh: see Carbon monoxide Ammonia: see Ammonia gas Tear: see Chlorine Nerve: see Parathion Sewer, volatile hydrides: see Hydrogen sulfide		
Gasoline: see Petroleum distillates		
Glues, model airplane: see Acetone, Benzene, Petroleum distillates		
Glutethimide	Drowsiness, areflexia, mydriasis, hypotension, respiratory depression, coma	Ipecac emesis; gastric lavage, activated charcoal; support respiration, maintain fluid & electrolyte balance; hemodialysis may help; treat shock
Gold salts: see TABLE 289–3, Chelation Therapy; see also RHEUMATOID ARTHRITIS in Ch. 108		
Guaiacol: see Phenols		
Halogenated hydrocarbons: see DDT		

TABLE 289–4. SPECIFIC POISONS: SYMPTOMS AND TREATMENT *(Cont'd)*

Poison	*Symptoms*	*Treatment*
Heptachlor: see DDT		
Herbicides: see Arsenic & antimony; Dinitro-*o*-cresol		
Heroin: see Narcotics		
HETP (hexaethyl tetraphosphate): see Parathion		
Hexachlorocyclohexane: see γ-Benzene hexachloride		
Hormones—single acute oral overdose—no toxicity		
Hydrides, volatile: see Hydrogen sulfide		
Hydrocarbons: see Benzene		
Hydrocarbons, halogenated: see DDT		
Hydrochloric acid: see Acids & alkalis		
Hydrocyanic acid: see Cyanides		
Hydrogen chloride, fluoride: see Nitrogen oxides		
Hydrogen sulfide Alkali sulfides Phosphine Sewer gas Volatile hydrides	"Gas eye" (subacute keratoconjunctivitis), lacrimation & burning; cough, dyspnea, pulmonary edema; caustic skin burns, erythema, pain; profuse salivation, nausea, vomiting, diarrhea; confusion, vertigo; sudden collapse & unconsciousness	Give O_2, support respiration; amyl nitrite & sodium nitrite as for cyanide (*no thiosulfate*)
Hyoscine, hyoscyamine, hyoscyamus: see Belladonna		
Hypochlorites Bleach, chlorine Javelle water	Usually mild pain & inflammation of oral & GI mucosa; cough, dyspnea, vomiting; skin vesicles	Usual 6% household preparations require little except milk dilution; treat shock; esophagoscope only if concentrated forms have been ingested
Illuminating gas: see Carbon monoxide		
Imipramine: see Tricylic antidepressants		
Indelible markers: see Acetanilid—usually no problem		
Ink, aniline: see Acetanilid—usually no problem		
Insecticides: see DDT, Paradichlorobenzene, Parathion, Pyrethrum		
Iodine	Burning pain in mouth & esophagus; mucous membranes stained brown; laryngeal edema; vomiting, abdominal pain, diarrhea; shock, nephritis, circulatory collapse	Give milk, starch, or flour orally; gastric lavage; fluid & electrolytes; treat shock; tracheostomy for laryngeal edema
Iodoform Triiodomethane	Dermatitis; vomiting; cerebral depression, excitation; coma; respiratory difficulty	Skin: Wash with sodium bicarbonate or alcohol Ingestion: Emetic or gastric lavage; respiratory support

TABLE 289–4. SPECIFIC POISONS: SYMPTOMS AND TREATMENT (Cont'd)

Poison	Symptoms	Treatment
Iron Ferric salts Ferrous salts Ferrous gluconate Ferrous sulfate Carbonyl iron: see Carbon monoxide Vitamins with iron	Vomiting; upper abdominal pain, pallor, cyanosis, diarrhea, drowsiness, shock; concern if >40–70 mg/kg of elemental iron ingested	Ipecac emesis, gastric lavage with sodium bicarbonate; if serum iron >400–500 mg/dL at 3–6 h, give deferoxamine 1 gm IV (max. rate of 15 mg/kg/h) or 1–2 gm IM q 3–12 h (urine turns red within 2 h; if no color change, no further dose is needed); for shock, give deferoxamine 1 gm IV (max. rate 15 mg/kg/h); exchange transfusion
Isoniazid	CNS stimulation, seizures, obtundation, and coma	Emesis; lavage; diazepam sedation; pyridoxine 200 mg slowly IV for seizures, with repeated doses as necessary; $NaHCO_3$ for acidosis
Isopropyl alcohol: see Alcohol, isopropyl		
Javelle water: see Hypochlorites		
Kerosene: see Petroleum distillates		
Ketones: see Acetone		
Lead Lead salts Some paints & painted surfaces Solder	Acute inhalation: Insomnia, headache, ataxia, mania, convulsions Acute ingestion: Thirst, burning abdominal pain, vomiting, diarrhea, CNS symptoms as above Lead encephalopathy: see LEAD POISONING in Ch. 189	See LEAD POISONING in Ch. 189
Lead, tetraethyl	Vapor inhalation, skin absorption, ingestion: CNS symptoms—insomnia, restlessness, ataxia, delusions, mania, convulsions	Supportive treatment; e.g., diazepam, chlorpromazine, fluid & electrolytes; eliminate the source
Lime, chlorinated: see Chlorine		
Lindane: see γ-Benzene hexachloride		
Liquor: see Alcohol, ethyl		
Lithium salts	Nausea, vomiting, diarrhea, tremors, drowsiness, renal failure, diabetes insipidus	Acute: emesis; diazepam—consider dialysis. Chronic: reduce dose; supportive therapy
Lye: see Acids & alkalis		
Lysergic acid diethylamide (LSD)	Confusion, hallucinations, hyperexcitability—coma. Flashbacks	Supportive therapy; diazepam; chlorpromazine (50–100 mg IM)
Malathion: see Parathion		
Manganese: see TABLE 289–3, Chelation Therapy		
Marsh gas: see Carbon monoxide		
Meperidine: see Narcotics		

TABLE 289–4. SPECIFIC POISONS: SYMPTOMS AND TREATMENT *(Cont'd)*

Poison	*Symptoms*	*Treatment*
Meprobamate: see Barbiturates		
Mercurial diuretics: see Mercury		
Mercuric chloride: see Mercury		
Mercury All mercury compounds Ammoniated mercury Bichloride of mercury Calomel Corrosive sublimate Diuretics Mercuric chloride Mercury vapor Merthiolate	Acute: Severe gastroenteritis, burning mouth pain, salivation, abdominal pain, vomiting; colitis, nephrosis, anuria, uremia. Skin burns from alkyl & phenyl mercurials Chronic: Gingivitis, mental disturbance; neurologic deficits Mercury vapor: severe pneumonitis	Gastric lavage, activated charcoal; give penicillamine (or BAL)—see TABLE 289–3, Chelation Therapy; maintain fluid & electrolyte balance; hemodialysis for renal failure, observe for GI perforation Skin: Scrub with soap & water Lungs: Supportive care
Merthiolate: see Mercury—usually no problem		
Metaldehyde	Nausea, vomiting, retching, abdominal pain, muscular rigidity, hyperventilation, convulsions, coma	Emesis, if not spontaneous; supportive therapy; diazepam
Metals	Symptoms vary with metals; see specific metals	See TABLE 289–3, Chelation Therapy
Methadone: see Narcotics		
Methamphetamine: see Amphetamines		
Methanol: see Alcohol, methyl		
Methoxychlor: see DDT		
Methyl alcohol: see Alcohol, methyl		
Methyl salicylate: see ASPIRIN AND OTHER SALICYLATE POISONING in Ch. 189		
Mineral spirits: see Petroleum distillates		
Model airplane glues, solvents: see Acetone, Benzene, Petroleum Distillates		
Morphine: see Narcotics		
Moth balls, crystals, repellent: see Paradichlorobenzene, Naphthalene		
Mushrooms, Poisonous: see NONBACTERIAL FOOD POISONING in Ch. 57		
Nail polish remover: see Acetone		
Naphtha: see Petroleum distillates		
Naphthalene (see also Paradichlorobenzene) Moth balls, crystals, repellent cakes Deodorizer cakes	Contact: Dermatitis, corneal ulceration Inhalation: Headache, confusion, vomiting, dyspnea Ingestion: Abdominal cramps, nausea, vomiting; headache, confusion; dysuria; intravascular hemolysis; convulsions. Hemolytic anemia in persons with G6PD deficiency	Contact: Remove clothing if formerly stored with naphthalene moth balls; flush skin and eyes Ingestion: Ipecac emesis, gastric lavage; blood transfusion for severe hemolysis; alkalize urine for hemoglobinuria; for severe hemolysis, blood transfusions as necessary; control convulsions

TABLE 289–4. SPECIFIC POISONS: SYMPTOMS AND TREATMENT *(Cont'd)*

Poison	*Symptoms*	*Treatment*
Naphthols: see Phenols		
Narcotics (see also Chs. 138 and 281) Alphaprodine Codeine Heroin Meperidine Methadone Morphine Opium Propoxyphene	Pinpoint pupils, drowsiness, shallow respirations, spasticity, respiratory failure	*Do not give emetics.* Gastric lavage, respiratory support. Naloxone 5 µg/kg IV to awaken & improve respiration; if patient does not respond, give 2–20 mg naloxone (dosage must be repeated as many as 10–20 times); fluids IV to support circulation
Neostigmine: see Physostigmine		
Nerve gas agents: see Parathion		
Nickel: see TABLE 289–3, Chelation Therapy		
Nicotine: see Tobacco		
Nitrates: see Chlorates		
Nitric acid: see Acids & alkalis		
Nitrites Amyl nitrite Butyl nitrite Nitroglycerin Potassium nitrite Sodium nitrite	Methemoglobinemia, cyanosis, anoxia; GI disturbance, vomiting; headache, dizziness, hypotension, respiratory failure, coma	Ipecac emesis, gastric lavage; O_2; for methemoglobinemia, 1% methylene blue 1–2 mg/kg slowly IV; when >40% methemoglobin, transfusion with whole blood
Nitrobenzene Artificial bitter almond oil Dinitrobenzene	Bitter almond odor (suggests cyanides); drowsiness, headache; vomiting; ataxia, nystagmus; brown urine; convulsive movements, delirium; cyanosis; coma, respiratory arrest	See Acetanilid
Nitrogen oxides (see also Chlorine; Hydrogen sulfide; Sulfur dioxide; and Ch. 42) (Air contaminants that form atmospheric oxidants. Liberated from missile fuels, explosives, agricultural wastes) Cobaltous chloride Fluorine Hydrogen chloride Hydrogen fluoride	Delayed onset of symptoms with nitrogen oxides unless heavy concentration; other irritant gases give warnings—local burning in eye, nasal, pharyngeal mucous membranes. Fatigue, cough, dyspnea, pulmonary edema; later, bronchitis, pneumonia	Absolute bed rest; pure O_2 as soon as symptoms develop; for excessive pulmonary foam: suction, postural drainage, tracheostomy; to prevent pulmonary fibrosis: prednisone 30–80 mg/day has been used
Nitroglycerin: see Nitrites		
Nitrous oxide: see Chloroform		
Oil of wintergreen: see ASPIRIN AND OTHER SALICYLATE POISONING in Ch. 189		
Oils Aniline: see Acetanilid Fuel, lubricating: see Petroleum distillates		
OMPA (octamethyl pyrophosphoramide): see Parathion		
Opiates: see Narcotics		

TABLE 289–4. SPECIFIC POISONS: SYMPTOMS AND TREATMENT *(Cont'd)*

Poison	*Symptoms*	*Treatment*
Oxalates: see Oxalic acid		
Oxalic acid Oxalates Ethylene glycol	Burning pain in throat, vomiting, intensive pain; hypotension, tetany, shock; glottal & renal damage; oxaluria	Give milk or calcium lactate; careful gastric lavage if at all; 10% calcium gluconate 10–20 mL IV; pain control, saline IV for shock; demulcents by mouth; watch for glottal edema & stricture
Paint solvents: see Mineral spirits (under Petroleum distillates) and Turpentine		
Paints: see Lead		
Paradichlorobenzene Insecticide Moth repellent Toilet bowl deodorant	Abdominal pain, nausea, vomiting, diarrhea, seizures, and tetany	Ipecac emesis, gastric lavage; fluid replacement; diazepam for seizure control
Paraldehyde	Paraldehyde odor on breath, incoherent, pupils contracted, respirations depressed, coma	Ingestion: Ipecac emesis, gastric lavage; support respiration, O_2
Paraquat	Immediate: GI pain and vomiting; within 24 h: respiratory failure	Emesis, fuller's earth plus Na_2SO_4; limit O_2; call poison center or manufacturer
Parathion Chlorothion Demeton Diazinon Dipterex (trichlorfon) HETP (hexaethyl tetraphosphate) Malathion Nerve gas agents OMPA (octamethyl pyrophosphor-amide) Systox TEPP (tetraethyl pyrophosphate)	Nausea, vomiting, abdominal cramping, excessive salivation; increased pulmonary secretion, headache, rhinorrhea, blurred vision, miosis; slurred speech, mental confusion; breathing difficulty, frothing at mouth, coma. Absorbed through skin	Remove clothing, flush & wash skin. Empty stomach; atropine: adults 2 mg, children 1–2 mg, IV or IM q 15–60 min, if no signs of atropine toxicity, repeat as needed; pralidoxime chloride (PAM): adults 1–2 gm, children 20–40 mg/kg, IV over 15–30 min, repeat in 1 h if needed; O_2; support respiration; correct dehydration. *Do not use morphine or aminophylline*
Paris green: see Arsenic & antimony		
Pentobarbital: see Barbiturates		
Permanent wave neutralizers (bromates): see Chlorates		
Pesticides: see Arsenic & antimony, Barium compounds, DDT, Dinitro-*o*-cresol, Fluorides, Paradichlorobenzene, Parathion, Phosphorus, Pyrethrum, Thallium salts, Warfarin		
Petroleum distillates (see also HYDROCARBON POISONING in Ch. 189) Asphalt Benzine (benzin) Fuel oil Gasoline Kerosene Lubricating oils Mineral spirits Model airplane glue Naphtha Petroleum ether Tar	Vapor inhalation: Euphoria; burning in chest; headache, nausea, weakness; CNS depression, confusion; dyspnea, tachypnea, rales Ingestion: Burning throat & stomach, vomiting, diarrhea; pneumonia, only if aspiration has occurred Aspiration: Early acute pulmonary changes	Since major problems are consequential to aspiration, as opposed to GI absorption, in most instances no gastric evacuation is warranted; gastric lavage only with rapid-onset depression from large amounts ingested; arterial blood gas levels to monitor care; supportive care for pulmonary edema; O_2, respiratory support

TABLE 289–4. SPECIFIC POISONS: SYMPTOMS AND TREATMENT *(Cont'd)*

Poison	*Symptoms*	*Treatment*
Petroleum ether: see Petroleum distillates		
Phenacetin: see Acetanilid		
Phencyclidine (PCP)	"Spaced-out," unconscious; hypertension	Quiet environment; prolonged gastric lavage; propranolol and diazepam
Phenmetrazine: see Amphetamines		
Phenobarbital: see Barbiturates		
Phenols Carbolic acid Creosote Cresols Guaiacol Naphthols	Corrosive. Mucous membrane burns; pallor, weakness, shock; convulsions in children; pulmonary edema; smoky urine; respiratory, cardiac, & circulatory failure	Remove clothing, wash external burns. Lavage with water, activated charcoal. *Do not use alcohol or mineral oil.* Demulcents; pain relief; O_2; support respiration; correct fluid balance; watch for esophageal stricture (rare)
Phenothiazine Chlorpromazine Prochlorperazine Promazine Trifluoperazine (etc.)	Extrapyramidal tract symptoms (ataxia, muscular & carpopedal spasms, torticollis), usually idiosyncratic; overdose results in dry mouth, drowsiness, coma, hypothermia, respiratory collapse. Leukopenia, jaundice, coagulation defect, skin rashes	Ipecac emesis, gastric lavage; diphenhydramine 2–3 mg/kg IV or IM for extrapyramidal symptoms; diazepam for convulsions; warm patient. Avoid levarterenol & epinephrine
Phenylpropanolamine	Nervousness, irritability, *hypertension* plus other sympathomimetic effects	Supportive therapy; diazepam; treat hypertension with phentolamine (Regitine® 5 mg) or nitroprussides
Phosphoric acid: see Acids & alkalis		
Phosphorus (Yellow or white) Rat poisons Roach powders (NOTE: Red phosphorus is unabsorbable & nontoxic)	3 Stages of symptoms: 1st—Garlicky taste; garlic odor on breath; local irritation, skin burns, throat burns; nausea, vomiting, diarrhea 2nd—Symptom-free 8 h to several days 3rd—Nausea, vomiting, diarrhea; liver enlargement, jaundice; hemorrhages; renal damage; convulsions, coma Toxicity enhanced by alcohol, fats, digestible oils	Protect patient & attendant from vomitus, gastric washing, feces. If phosphorus is imbedded in skin, keep patient's body submerged in water. Gastric lavage copiously—preferably with potassium permanganate (1:5000) or cupric sulfate (250 mg in 250 mL water); mineral oil 100 mL (to prevent absorption) & repeat in 2 h; combat shock; vit. K_1 IV; transfusion with fresh blood
Physostigmine Eserine Neostigmine (Prostigmin®) Pilocarpine Pilocarpus	Dizziness, weakness, vomiting, cramping pain; pupils dilated, then contracted	Atropine sulfate 0.6 to 1 mg s.c. or IV with repeat doses prn
Pilocarpine, pilocarpus: see Physostigmine		
Potash: see Acids & alkalis		
Potassium bichromate, Potassium chromate: see Chromic acid		
Potassium carbonate: see Acids & alkalis		

TABLE 289–4. SPECIFIC POISONS: SYMPTOMS AND TREATMENT *(Cont'd)*

Poison	*Symptoms*	*Treatment*
Potassium cyanide: see Cyanides		
Potassium hydroxide: see Acids & alkalis		
Potassium nitrate: see Chlorates		
Potassium nitrite: see Nitrites		
Potassium permanganate	Brown discoloration & burns of oral mucosa, glottal edema; hypotension; renal involvement	Gastric lavage, demulcents; maintain fluid balance
Prochlorperazine: see Phenothiazine		
Prolan: see DDT		
Promazine: see Phenothiazine		
Propoxyphene: see Narcotics		
Propranolol	Confusion and seizures	Emesis; lavage; supportive care; diazepam sedation
Prostigmin: see Physostigmine		
Prussic acid: see Cyanides		
Pyrethrin: see Pyrethrum		
Pyrethrum Pyrethrin	Allergic response (including anaphylactic reactions, skin sensitivity) in sensitive people. Otherwise low toxicity, unless vehicle is a petroleum distillate (see that entry)	For sizeable ingestion, emesis if patient is alert; otherwise, endotracheal tube & gastric lavage; wash skin well
Radium: see TABLE 289–3, Chelation Therapy		
Rat poison: see Barium compounds, Fluorides, Phosphorus, Thallium salts, Warfarin		
Resorcinol (resorcin)	Vomiting, dizziness, tinnitus; chills, tremor; delirium, convulsions, respiratory depression, coma	Emetic or gastric lavage; support respiration
Roach poison: see Fluorides, Phosphorus, Thallium salts		
Rodenticides (rat poison): see Barium compounds, Fluorides, Phosphorus, Thallium salts, Warfarin		
Rubbing alcohol: see Alcohol, isopropyl		
Salicylates: see ASPIRIN AND OTHER SALICYLATE POISONING in Ch. 189		
Salicylic acid: see ASPIRIN AND OTHER SALICYLATE POISONING in Ch. 189		
Scopolamine: see Belladonna		
Secobarbital: see Barbiturates		
Selenium: see TABLE 289–3, Chelation Therapy		
Sewer gas: see Hydrogen sulfide		
Silver salts Silver nitrate (NOTE: Chloride, bromide, iodide, & oxide salts are usually benign)	Stain on lips (white, then black); gastroenteritis, shock, vertigo, convulsions	Gastric lavage with saline soln; control pain; control convulsions with diazepam

TABLE 289–4. SPECIFIC POISONS: SYMPTOMS AND TREATMENT *(Cont'd)*

Poison	*Symptoms*	*Treatment*
Smog: see Sulfur dioxide		
Soda, caustic: see Acids & alkalis		
Sodium carbonate: see Acids & alkalis		
Sodium cyanide: see Cyanides		
Sodium fluoride: see Fluorides		
Sodium hydroxide: see Acids & alkalis		
Sodium nitrite: see Nitrites		
Sodium salicylate: see ASPIRIN AND OTHER SALICYLATE POISONING in Ch. 189		
Solder: see Cadmium; Lead		
Stibophen: see Arsenic & antimony		
Stramonium: see Belladonna		
Strychnine	Restlessness, hyperacuity of hearing, vision, etc.; convulsions from minor stimuli, complete muscle relaxation between convulsions; perspiration; respiratory arrest	Isolate & restrict stimulation to prevent convulsions. Activated charcoal orally; control convulsions with IV diazepam, curariform drugs; support respiration; acid diuresis with ammonium chloride or ascorbic acid; gastric lavage *after* convulsions controlled
Sulfur dioxide Smog	Respiratory tract irritation; sneezing, cough, dyspnea, pulmonary edema	Remove from contaminated area, give O_2; positive pressure breathing, respiratory support
Sulfuric acid: see Acids & alkalis		
Syrup of wild cherry: see Cyanides		
Systox: see Parathion		
Tar: see Petroleum distillates		
Tartar emetic: see Arsenic & antimony		
Tear gas: see Chlorine		
TEPP: see Parathion		
Tetraethyl lead: see Lead, tetraethyl		
Thallium salts Ant poison Rat poison Roach poison	Abdominal pain (colic), vomiting (may be bloody), diarrhea (may be bloody), stomatitis, excessive salivation; tremors, leg pains, paresthesias, polyneuritis, ocular & facial palsy; delirium, convulsions, respiratory failure; loss of hair approx. 3 wk after poisoning	Ipecac emesis, gastric lavage; activated charcoal; potassium chloride 5–25 gm/day orally; treat shock, control convulsions with diazepam; chelation (experimental) with sodium diethyldithiocarbamate 30 mg/kg/day orally or diphenylthiocarbazone 10 mg/kg orally; BAL, EDTA are of no use
Theophilline: see Aminophylline		
Thyroxine	Most are asymptomatic; rarely increasing irritability progressing to thyroid storm in 5–7 days	Emesis; observation at home; diazepam; consider antithyroid preparations and propranolol *only* if storm occurs

TABLE 289–4. SPECIFIC POISONS: SYMPTOMS AND TREATMENT *(Cont'd)*

Poison	*Symptoms*	*Treatment*
Tobacco Nicotine	Excitement, confusion, muscular twitching, weakness, abdominal cramps, clonic convulsions, depression, rapid respirations, palpitations, collapse, coma, CNS paralysis, respiratory failure	Ipecac emesis, gastric lavage; activated charcoal; support respiration, O_2; diazepam for convulsions; wash skin well if contaminated
Toilet bowl cleaners, deodorizers: see Acids & alkalis; Paradichlorobenzene		
Toluene, toluol: see Benzene		
Toxaphene: see DDT		
Trichlorfon: see Parathion		
Trichloromethane: see Chloroform		
Tricyclic antidepressants Amitriptyline Desipramine Doxepin Imipramine Nortriptyline Protriptyline	Anticholinergic effects (e.g., blurred vision, urinary hesitation); CNS effects (e.g., drowsiness, stupor, coma, ataxia, restlessness, agitation, hyperactive reflexes, muscle rigidity, and convulsions); CVS effects (tachycardia and other arrhythmias, bundle branch block, impaired conduction, congestive heart failure). Respiratory depression, hypotension, shock, vomiting, hyperpyrexia, mydriasis, and diaphoresis may also be present	Symptomatic and supportive; emesis, gastric lavage; monitor vital signs and ECG; maintain open airway and adequate fluid intake. Sodium bicarbonate as a rapid IV injection (0.5–2 mEq/L), repeat periodically to maintain blood pH >7.45, precludes development of arrhythmias. Diazapam controls most CNS problems; if symptoms persist, physostigmine salicylate (slowly IV) is reported to reverse both CNS and cardiac manifestations of overdosage—adults: 2 mg with repeat of 1–4 mg prn at 20- to 60-min intervals; children: 0.5 mg repeated prn at 5-min intervals to maximum 2 mg
Trifluoperazine: see Phenothiazine		
Triiodomethane: see Iodoform		
Tungsten: see TABLE 289–3, Chelation Therapy		
Turpentine Paint solvent Varnish	Turpentine odor; burning oral & abdominal pain, coughing, choking, respiratory failure; nephritis	Emesis (alert patient); if >1–4 oz, gastric lavage; support respiration, O_2; control pain; monitor renal function
Vanadium: see TABLE 289–3, Chelation Therapy		
Varnish: see Alcohol, methyl; Turpentine		
Verapamil; nifedipine; diltiazem	Nausea, vomiting, mental confusion, bradycardia, hypotension	Emesis; atropine has reversed bradycardia; avoid beta-agonists
Vitamins—single acute oral ingestion of isolated or multiple dose form—no toxicity		
Warfarin Bishydroxycoumarin Dicumarol Ethyl biscoumacetate Superwarfarins	Single ingestion not serious, multiple overdoses result in coagulopathy	For hemorrhagic manifestations, vitamin K_1 (see Ch. 81) till prothrombin time normal, transfusion with fresh blood if necessary

TABLE 289–4. SPECIFIC POISONS: SYMPTOMS AND TREATMENT (Cont'd)

Poison	Symptoms	Treatment
Wax, floor: see Carbon tetrachloride		
Whiskey: see Alcohol, ethyl		
Wild cherry syrup: see Cyanides		
Wintergreen oil: see ASPIRIN AND OTHER SALICYLATE POISONING in Ch. 189		
Wood alcohol: see Alcohol, methyl		
Xylene: see Benzene		
Zinc: see TABLE 289–3, Chelation Therapy		
Zinc salts: see Copper salts		

290. VENOMOUS BITES AND STINGS

POISONOUS SNAKES

In the USA, about 20 of the 120 species of snakes are venomous. These include mainly the **pit vipers** (Crotalidae), the **coral snakes** (Elapidae), and a few species of Colubridae. TABLE 290–1 lists some medically important snakes of the USA and their usual distribution.

Epidemiology

Although > 45,000 people/yr are bitten by snakes in the USA, < 8000 cases of snake venom poisoning are reported. Fewer than 15 fatalities/yr occur, mostly in children or the elderly, in untreated or undertreated cases, or in members of religious sects who handle venomous serpents. Rattlesnakes account for about 70% of venomous snake bites and for almost all the deaths. Most other venomous snake bites are by copperheads and, to a lesser extent, cottonmouths. Coral snakes inflict < 1% of all bites. Imported snakes found in zoos, schools, snake farms, and amateur and professional collections account for about 15 bites/yr.

Chemistry, Pharmacology, and Pathology

Snake venoms are complex mixtures, chiefly proteins, many having enzymatic activity. Although the enzymes contribute to the deleterious effects of the venom, some of the more important toxic components are smaller polypeptides, which are more toxic than the crude venom. Most venom components appear to have specific chemical and physiologic receptor sites.

Envenomation may be further complicated by the release of autopharmacologic substances (eg, histamine, serotonin) that can make diagnosis and treatment difficult. *Arbitrary grouping of snake venoms into categories such as "neurotoxins," "hemotoxins," "cardiotoxins" is pharmacologically superficial and can lead to grave errors in clinical judgment.* A so-called neurotoxic venom can produce marked cardiovascular changes or direct hematologic effects. The so-called hemotoxin venoms can also produce changes in the nervous system, or in vascular dynamics. A patient with snake venom poisoning must be considered as a victim of a complex poisoning.

Rattlesnake and many other viper venoms produce local tissue damage, blood cell changes, coagulation defects, blood vessel injury, changes in vascular resistance, and

TABLE 290–1. SOME MEDICALLY IMPORTANT

Snakes	Wash., Ore., Id.	Calif., Nev.	Ariz., New Mex.	Texas
PIT VIPERS (Crotalidae)				
Cottonmouths and Copperheads *(Agkistrodon)*				
Cottonmouths *(A. piscivorus)*				X
Copperheads *(A. contortrix)*				X
Rattlesnakes *(Crotalus)*				
Eastern diamondback *(C. adamanteus)*				
Western diamondback *(C. atrox)*		X	X	X
Sidewinder *(C. cerastes)*		X	Ariz.	
Timber *(C. horridus)*				X
Rock *(C. lepidus)*			X	X
Speckled *(C. mitchelli)*		X	Ariz.	
Black-tailed *(C. molossus)*			X	X
Twin-spotted *(C. pricei)*			Ariz.	
Red diamond *(C. ruber)*		Calif.		
Mojave *(C. scutulatus)*		X	X	X
Tiger *(C. tigris)*			Ariz.	
Western *(C. viridis)*				
Prairie *(C.v. viridis)*	Id.		X	X
Grand Canyon *(C.v. abyssus)*			Ariz.	
Southern Pacific *(C.v. helleri)*		Calif.		
Great Basin *(C.v. lutosus)*	Ore., Id.	X	Ariz.	
Northern Pacific *(C.v. oreganus)*	X	X		
Ridge-nosed *(C. willardi)*			Ariz.	
Massauga and Pigmy Rattlesnakes *(Sistrusus)*				
Massauga *(S. catenatus)*			X	X
Pigmy *(S. miliarius)*				X
CORAL SNAKES (Elapidae)				
Sonoran coral snake *(Micruroides euryxanthus)*			X	
Eastern coral snake *(Micrurus fulvius)*				X

Certain groups of adjoining states are treated here as units. The symbol X indicates that distribution of the species is widespread within the unit. Restriction of a species to a part of a unit is indicated appropriately.

neurologic defects. The Hct may fall rapidly, although hemoconcentration may occur during very early stages. Thrombocytopenia is common, and the coagulation profile is often abnormal. Pulmonary edema may be present in severe poisoning, and bleeding may occur in the lungs, peritoneum, kidneys, and heart. Renal failure may occur because of a critical deficit in glomerular filtration secondary to hypotension or because of the effects of hemolysis. Proteinuria, hemoglobinuria, or myoglobinuria are common in severe cases of some rattlesnake bites. Although cardiac dynamics may be disturbed, the early cardiovascular collapse seen in an occasional patient bitten by a rattlesnake is due chiefly to a sharp fall in circulating blood volume. This appears to be caused by a loss of blood plasma and protein through the vessel walls, and by blood pooling. Most North American crotalid venoms produce relatively minor changes in neuromuscular transmission, but Mojave rattlesnake venom may cause serious neurologic deficits.

SNAKES OF THE UNITED STATES

Mont., Mich., Wis., (W.) Minn., S. Dak., N. Dak., Neb., Iowa, Wyo., Utah, Colo.	*Kan., Okla., Ark., Mo.*	*Tenn., Ky., Ill., Ind., Ohio*	*N.C., S.C., Ga., Ala., Miss., La.*	*Fla.*	*Pa., N.J., Md., Del., Va., W. Va. N.Y., N. Eng.*
Neb., Iowa	X	Tenn., Ky., Ill.	X	X	Va.
Neb., Iowa	X	X	X	X	X
			X	X	
	Okla., Ark.				
Utah					
Minn., Wis., Neb., Iowa	X	X	X	X	X
Not Mich., Minn., Wis.	Kan., Okla.				
Utah					
Mich., Wis., Minn., Neb., Iowa, Colo.	Not Ark.	Ill., Ind., Ohio			N.Y., Pa.
	Not Kan.	Tenn.	X	X	
	Ark.			X	

(Adapted from *Snake Venom Poisoning* by F. E. Russell. Published 1983 by Scholium International. Used with permission.)

Most elapid venoms cause changes in neuromuscular transmission, in nerve conduction, and, to a much lesser extent, in the CNS. Some elapid venoms also cause local tissue damage and necrosis, blood changes, and severe renal complications.

Symptoms, Signs, and Diagnosis

Venomous snake bites are medical emergencies, requiring immediate attention and considerable judgment. Before any treatment is begun, it must be determined whether the snake was venomous and whether envenomation occurred, since a venomous snake may bite and *not* inject venom (no poisoning occurs in about 20 to 30% of pit viper bites and in about 50% of cobra and certain other elapid bites). When no envenomation occurs, or the bite is inflicted by a nonvenomous snake, it should be treated as a puncture wound.

Although the identity of the offending snakes can be suggested by the fang marks, *these should never be relied on for positive identification*. "Typical" fang-mark patterns

are based on the anatomy of the snake's jaw and laboratory studies and may not be seen under field conditions. Rattlesnakes may leave one or two fang marks, as well as other teeth marks; single fang punctures are very common and may also be seen with nonvenomous snake bites.

Numerical grading of rattlesnake bites is sometimes described in the literature, but it is more practical to describe cases as minor, moderate, or severe, depending on *all* the symptoms, signs, and laboratory findings, rather than on just 1 or 2 symptoms (eg, swelling and pain). Bites by the Mojave rattlesnake, for example, may cause only minimal edema, local tissue changes, and pain, and therefore be graded as 1, yet this snake's lethal index is the highest of the North American snakes. In the presence of minimal symptoms and signs, insufficient antivenin may be given and a poor, even fatal, outcome may ensue.

Pit viper envenomation: Symptoms and signs vary considerably, depending on the species of snake, the amount of venom injected, and other factors. If there is evidence of poisoning soon after a bite, the possible consequences must not be underestimated.

Bites by rattlesnakes, cottonmouths, and copperheads usually cause immediate swelling, edema, and pain. Contrary to popular opinion, severe pain is not a constant finding; it may be mild or absent. Usually, however, some pain immediately follows envenomation, and swelling and edema appear within 10 min—they are rarely delayed more than 15 to 20 min. By the time the patient arrives at the doctor's office, a diagnosis of crotalid bite with envenomation can usually be made (or envenomation excluded) on the basis of fang marks, swelling and edema, pain, and, in bites by some species, tingling or numbness periorally or in the fingers or toes, or a metallic or rubbery taste in the mouth, and other findings.

Untreated, the edema progresses rapidly and may involve the entire extremity within hours. There may be lymphangitis and enlarged, tender, regional lymph nodes. Skin temperature over the injured part and body temperature are usually elevated, although the patient may complain of chills. Weakness, a rapid and weak pulse, syncope, sweating, nausea, and vomiting may be present. BP often drops and shock may develop early. Respiratory distress may occur, particularly following bites by the Mojave rattlesnake; muscle fasciculations, spasms, and weakness are common, but true paralysis is rare. The patient may complain of headache, blurred vision, ptosis, and marked thirst.

Ecchymosis is common in moderate or severe rattlesnake poisoning and may begin to appear over the bite area within 3 to 6 h. It is severe following bites by the eastern and western diamondbacks and the prairie and Pacific rattlesnakes, less severe following copperhead and Mojave rattlesnake bites. The skin may appear tense and discolored; vesicles often appear in the area of the bite within 8 h, often becoming blood-filled. These changes are usually superficial, since North American rattlesnake bites tend to be limited to dermal and subcutaneous tissues. Necrosis is common around the bite area in untreated cases, and surrounding superficial blood vessels may be thrombosed. Most venom effects reach their peak by the 4th day.

There may be hemorrhage from the gums, hematemesis, melena, and hematuria. Bleeding and clotting times are prolonged, and platelet counts may fall sharply in moderate or severe envenomations. In most cases, a sharp rise in the packed cell volume is an early finding, although in severe cases hemolysis may cause a rapid fall in the Hct.

Coral snake envenomation: Pain and swelling are absent or minimal and often transitory. Paresthesia is often noted around the bite, and some weakness of the part may become evident within several hours. Muscular incoordination may develop, and the patient may complain of marked weakness and lethargy. There may be increased salivation, difficulties in swallowing and phonation, and visual disturbances. Respira-

tory distress and failure may ensue. In fatal cases, shock, leading to cardiovascular and respiratory failure, usually precedes death.

Laboratory Tests

In all but trivial cases, a CBC (including platelets), coagulation profile (PT, PTT, fibrinogen), blood typing, and urinalysis are essential. Other tests, such as ESR, serum electrolytes, BUN, creatinine, and RBC fragility tests, may be useful. An ECG is indicated in all severe cases.

Treatment

Pit viper: If the patient is within 30 to 40 min of a medical facility, he should be put at rest, reassured, kept warm, and transported there as quickly as possible. The injured part should be loosely immobilized in a functional position just below heart level, and all rings, watches, and constrictive clothing removed. If the patient is > 40 min from medical care, single incisions can be made through the fang marks (no longer than 1/4 in. and no deeper than 1/8 in.) within the first 5 min. Suction, using Sawyer's "extractor," applied directly over the incisions or even over the fang punctures is of value only during the first 30 to 60 min following the bite. The wound should be cleansed and covered with a sterile dressing.

If antivenin is needed, a skin test for horse serum sensitivity should be performed as described in the antivenin brochure. If the patient is mildly sensitive to horse serum and the poisoning is serious, diphenhydramine IV may be indicated before giving the antivenin. When a patient is 3+ or 4+ sensitive and life or limb are at stake, the patient should be placed in a critical or intensive care unit, carefully monitored, and antivenin given in the presence of a physician. The technic for this procedure has been described in the literature and consultation can be obtained by calling (602) 626-6016. A tourniquet, O_2, epinephrine, and other drugs and equipment for treating anaphylaxis should be available during antivenin therapy.

The amount of Antivenin (Crotalidae) Polyvalent to be given depends on many factors, the most important being the severity and progression of the symptoms and signs. In minimal rattlesnake poisoning, 50 to 80 mL (5 to 8 vials) of antivenin (reconstituted) will usually suffice; moderate cases may require 80 to 130 mL (8 to 13 vials); severe cases may need 150 mL (15 vials) or more. Water moccasin poisoning usually requires lesser doses, and in copperhead bites antivenin is usually required only for children and the elderly. Reconstituted antivenin should be diluted in sterile 0.9% saline or 5% dextrose and given by IV drip in most cases. If IM injection is necessary, it should be given in the buttocks. *Never inject antivenin into a toe or finger.* Measuring the circumference of the extremity at 3 points increasingly proximal to the bite and recording the measurements every 15 to 30 min provides one guide to antivenin dosage. If additional antivenin is needed, it is added to the IV drip and given over 3 to 4 h. Antivenin is probably of less value after 12 h; however, it can be effective, particularly for clotting defects, even after 24 h. IV fluids should be kept to a minimum, except when shock or hypovolemia is present.

Antitetanus therapy should always be given and a broad-spectrum antimicrobial administered in serious cases. Signs of hypovolemic shock, often with concomitant lysis of RBCs and platelet destruction, require fluid and blood component replacement; eg, plasma or albumin for hypovolemia and packed cells or whole blood for decreased RBC mass. Defects of hemostasis—ie, abnormal clotting or lysis of cells or clots, or a disturbance of platelet activity—require replacement with specific clotting factors, fresh frozen plasma, or platelets.

At the first sign of respiratory distress, O_2 should be given and mechanical support provided (see Ch. 34). Tracheal intubation or tracheostomy may be indicated, particularly if trismus, laryngeal spasm, or excessive salivation is present. Mild sedation with diazepam (which may reduce analgesic requirements) is indicated in all severe bites

when respiratory failure is not a problem. Aspirin or codeine may be used for pain and meperidine or morphine if the pain is severe. Cooling (10 to 15 C) reduces pain, but an extremity should never be iced for an extended period, as impairing circulation may lead to amputation.

Surgical debridement of blebs, bloody vesicles, or superficial necrosis, if present, should be carried out between the 3rd and 10th day, and may need to be done in stages. The injured part should be soaked in 1:20 Burow's solution tid for 15 min. O_2 bubbled through the solution at the same time may be of value.

Corticosteroids are of little or no value during the acute stages of poisoning and may be contraindicated, except in treating anaphylactic crisis; they are not a substitute for fluids and catecholamines in shock. Local infiltration of 0.5 mL of 0.05 M EDTA in isotonic saline around the bite area may reduce some of the local necrotizing effects of the venom if carried out within 20 min of the bite.

Follow-up care: Fasciotomy should be discouraged. It is usually unnecessary and reflects the use of insufficient or no antivenin during the first 12 h of the poisoning. Fasciotomy may be necessary, however, when there is clear evidence of severe vascular embarrassment as demonstrated by Wick measurements. Within several days of the injury, a complete evaluation should be made of joint motion, muscle strength, sensation, and girth measurements. To avoid contractures, immobilization is interrupted by frequent periods of gentle exercise, progressing from passive to active. Follow-up care also includes sterile whirlpool treatment, debridement as indicated, daily cleansing of the wound with 3% hydrogen peroxide followed by 15-min soaks in 1:20 Burow's solution, and twice weekly painting of the wound with an aqueous triple dye of brilliant green 1:400, gentian violet 1:400, and acriflavine 1:1000. A polymyxin-bacitracin-neomycin ointment can be applied at bedtime. Daily exposure to continuous flowing O_2 while the part is immobilized in a plastic bag may be of value. The lesion should be covered with a sterile dressing and a loose bandage when the patient is supine, and a reasonably firm bandage when the patient is ambulatory.

Coral snake: The general principles noted above for pit viper envenomation should also be considered in coral snake bites, but incision and suction and other such first aid measures are of little value. Three vials of antivenin (*Micrurus fulvius*) should be given when a diagnosis of coral snake envenomation has been established. If symptoms develop, 3 to 5 additional vials may be indicated. The physician should contact a poison control center, zoo, or Wyeth Laboratories for the nearest source of this antivenin. In severe cases, cardiopulmonary and intensive care may be indicated.

Imported species: The local zoo is the first place to call when dealing with a bite by an imported venomous snake. Most zoos maintain a list of consulting physicians as well as the *Antivenin Index* that lists the location and number of vials of antivenin available for imported species. Poison control centers in the major cities also maintain listings for antivenins. Federal regulations on the use of foreign-prepared antivenins indicate that it is prudent to contact a local public health officer before giving these antisera.

POISONOUS LIZARDS

Only 2 lizards, the Gila monster (*Heloderma suspectum*) found in Arizona and Sonora and adjacent areas, and the beaded lizard (*H. horridum*) of Mexico are known to be venomous. Their venom, somewhat similar to those of some snakes, contains hyaluronidase, phospholipase A, and one or more salivary kallikreins.

Symptoms and signs following poisoning include localized pain, swelling and edema, ecchymosis, lymphangitis, and lymphadenopathy. Systemic manifestations may develop in moderate or severe poisonings, including weakness, sweating, thirst, headache, and tinnitus. In severe cases, there may be cardiovascular collapse. The findings and

clinical course are generally similar to those of a mild to moderate case of western diamondback rattlesnake bite.

Treatment consists of supportive measures similar to those recommended above for pit viper envenomation. No specific antiserum is commercially available.

SPIDERS

With the exception of 2 small groups, all spiders are venomous. Fortunately, the fangs of most species are too short or fragile to penetrate the skin. Nevertheless, at least 60 species in the USA have been implicated in bites on humans. Species that are dangerous include the widow spiders, *Latrodectus mactans*, and related species; the brown or violin spider, *Loxosceles reclusa* (sometimes called the brown recluse), and related species; the jumping spiders, *Phidippus* species; the tarantulas, *Aphonopelma* and *Pamphobeteus* species; the trap-door spiders, *Bothriocyrtum* and *Ummidia* species; the so-called banana spiders, *Phoneutria* and *Cupiennius sallei*, *Lycosa* (wolf spider), and *Heteropoda*; the crab spider, *Misumenoides aleatorius*; the running spiders, *Liocranoides* and *Chiracanthium*; the orbweavers, *Neoscona vertebrata*, *Araneus* species, and *Argiope aurantia* (orange argiope); the running or gnaphosid spiders, *Drassodes*; the green lynx spider, *Peucetia viridans*; and the comb-footed or false black widow, *Steatoda grossa*. *Pamphobeteus*, *Cupiennius*, and *Phoneutria* are not native to the USA, but may be brought into the country on produce or other materials.

The incidence of spider bites in the USA is unknown. In Southern California, about 400/yr are reported to physicians. Fewer than 3 fatalities/yr occur in the USA, usually in children.

Chemistry and Pharmacology

Only a few spider venoms have been studied in any detail. Black widow venom consists chiefly of proteins, a few of which are enzymatic. The lethal fraction appears to be a peptide that markedly affects neuromuscular transmission. Brown or violin spider venom consists of at least 10 or 12 proteins. Its enzyme activity is greater than that of *Latrodectus* venom, but no fraction of *Loxosceles* venom has been isolated that produces the sequence of events that give rise to the unusual necrotic lesion characteristic of *Loxosceles* bites. Polymorphonuclear leukocyte infiltration plays a major role in the poisoning but the mechanism is not understood. Tarantula venom contains a number of proteins, of which at least one affects cardiovascular function; however, it is highly unlikely that the bite of one tarantula would produce a harmful cardiac effect in a human. Tarantulas native to the USA are not considered dangerous.

Symptoms and Signs

Widow spiders: A *Latrodectus* bite usually gives rise to a sharp pinprick-like pain, followed by a dull, sometimes numbing, pain in the affected extremity and by cramping pain and some muscular rigidity in the abdomen or the shoulders, back, and chest. Associated symptoms may include restlessness, anxiety, sweating, headache, dizziness, ptosis, eyelid edema, skin rash and pruritus, respiratory distress, nausea, vomiting, salivation, weakness, and increased skin temperature over the affected area. Blood and CSF pressures are usually elevated in the more severe cases.

Brown or violin spiders: A *Loxosceles* bite may cause little or no immediate pain, but some localized pain develops within an hour or so. The bite area becomes erythematous and ecchymotic. A bleb forms, often surrounded by either an irregular ecchymotic area or a more target-like lesion, as in the case of bites by the more western species. The lesion may present the appearance of a bull's eye; the central bleb becomes larger, fills with blood, ruptures, and leaves an ulcer over which a black eschar forms and eventually sloughs leaving a large tissue defect, which may include muscle. Pain can be severe and involve the entire injured area. Systemic symptoms and signs may develop,

including nausea and vomiting, malaise, hemolysis, thrombocytopenia, and kidney failure; death is a rare sequela.

Diagnosis

Far more common than spider bites are flea, bedbug, tick, mite, and biting fly bites; these are often mistaken for spider bites. Some arthropod bites may give rise to bullous lesions that rupture and ulcerate, resembling those produced by the violin and certain other spiders. Numerous reports of necrotic or gangrenous arachnidism attributed to *L. reclusa*, particularly in areas where this species is not found, are probably caused by spiders other than *Loxosceles* or more probably by other arthropods. Every attempt should be made to capture and identify the offending animal. Some cases of so-called brown recluse bites are misdiagnoses of epidermal necrolysis, erythema chronicum migrans, erythema nodosum, Lyell's syndrome, chronic herpes simplex, etc.

Treatment

Black widow spider: No first aid measures are of value. An ice cube may be placed over the bite to reduce pain. All patients < 16 or > 60 yr, or who have hypertensive heart disease, or have symptoms and signs of severe envenomation, should be hospitalized, and when symptomatic treatment is unsuccessful should be given 1 vial (6000 u.) of Antivenin *Latrodectus mactans* IV in 10 to 50 mL of 0.9% sodium chloride after the appropriate skin test. One vial is usually sufficient and is usually given over 3 to 15 min. Children may require respiratory assistance. Vital signs should be checked frequently during the first 12 h following the bite. In the elderly, acute hypertension can occur.

For muscle pain and spasms, 10 mL of 10% calcium gluconate may be given slowly IV. Several doses at 4-h intervals may be necessary. In adults, a relaxant, particularly methocarbamol or dantrolene sodium given IV, is often effective; diazepam 10 mg orally tid has had varying degrees of success. Meperidine 50 to 100 mg, or morphine 6 to 16 mg s.c. or IM q 6 h, may provide relief. Hot baths may afford relief in mild cases.

Brown or violin spider: A piece of ice can be placed over the bite area. Excision of the bite has been recommended in proven cases of envenomation seen within several hours of the bite, but is finding less favor today. In the past, persons bitten by this spider (or by an unidentified species) who developed a skin lesion within the first 12 h that increased in size during the next 12 h received a corticosteroid such as dexamethasone 4 mg IM q 6 h during the acute phase, then in decremental doses in accordance with standard practice. This protocol is still favored by many physicians. Presently, diaminodiphenylsulfone and acetyltrimethylcolchicinic acid are being evaluated. An antivenin has been prepared but is not yet commercially available.

Ulcerating lesions should be cleansed daily with 3% hydrogen peroxide; soaked in 1:20 Burow's solution tid for 15 min; painted 3 times/wk with the aqueous triple dye used for pit viper bites (see above); and debrided as needed. A polymyxin-bacitracin-neomycin ointment can be applied at bedtime. O_2 applied to the lesion several times a day through an improvised face mask or plastic bag may be of some value.

BEES, WASPS, HORNETS, ANTS

The venoms of these insects (order *Hymenoptera*) contain, among other components, peptides and nonenzymatic proteins (eg, apamin and melittin and/or kinins), enzymes (eg, phospholipase A and B, and hyaluronidase), and amines (eg, histamine and 5-hydroxytryptamine).

While it may take over 100 bees to inflict a lethal dose of venom in most adults, one sting can cause a fatal anaphylactic reaction in a hypersensitive person. There are 3 to 4 times more deaths in the USA from bee stings than from snakebites. In the few fatalities that have resulted from multiple bee stings, death has been attributed to acute cardiovascular collapse.

Treatment

The stings of many *Hymenoptera* may remain in the skin and should be removed by teasing or scraping rather than pulling. An ice cube placed over the sting will reduce pain; an antihistamine-analgesic–corticosteroid balm (Land/Sea Balm®) is often useful. Persons with known hypersensitivity to such stings should carry a kit containing an antihistamine and epinephrine when in endemic areas. Desensitization can be carried out using insect whole-body antigens or, preferably, whole-venom antigens. (See also Ch. 21, particularly ATOPIC DISEASES, ANAPHYLAXIS, and URTICARIA.)

OTHER BITING ARTHROPODS

Among the more common biting and sometimes bloodsucking arthropods in the USA are the ticks and mites; sand, horse, and deer flies; mosquitoes; fleas; lice; bedbugs; kissing bugs; and certain water bugs. The composition of the saliva of these arthropods varies considerably, and the lesions produced by the bites of these animals vary from a small papule to a large ulcer with swelling and acute pain. Dermatitis may also occur. Most serious bites are complicated by sensitivity reactions or infection. In hypersensitive persons, bites can be fatal.

Treatment

The offending arthropod should be quickly removed. For ticks and some of the bugs, this is best accomplished by direct application of a petroleum product or other irritant to the animal or by slowly withdrawing the arthropod while twisting it slowly with forceps. Care should be taken not to leave the capitulum in the wound, as it may induce chronic inflammation or migrate into deeper tissues and give rise to a granuloma. The bite should be cleansed and a corticosteroid lotion applied. Serious hypersensitivity reactions should be treated as described in Ch. 21, particularly ATOPIC DISEASES, ANAPHYLAXIS, and URTICARIA.

TICKS AND MITES

Ticks are vectors of many diseases. In addition to the reactions noted above under BITING ARTHROPODS, ticks are also involved in poisonings. In North America, some species of *Dermacentor* and *Amblyomma* cause **tick paralysis.** Symptoms and signs include anorexia, lethargy, muscle weakness, incoordination, nystagmus, and ascending flaccid paralysis. Bulbar or respiratory paralysis may develop. The bite of some *Ornithodorus* ticks ("pajaroello"), found in Mexico and southwestern USA, causes a local vesiculation, pustulation, rupture, ulceration, and eschar, with varying degrees of local swelling and pain. Similar reactions have been observed following the bites of other ticks.

Mite infestations are quite common and are responsible for **"chiggers"** (*intensely pruritic dermatitis caused by the mite larva, or chigger*), various forms of scabies, demodicidosis, and a number of other diseases. The bites produce varying degrees of local tissue reaction, with or without sensitization.

Treatment

Treatment of tick paralysis is symptomatic. O_2 and respiratory assistance may be needed. An antitoxin is presently under study. Pajaroello tick lesions should be cleansed, soaked in 1:20 Burow's solution, debrided, and painted with the aqueous triple dye used for pit viper bites (see above). Corticosteroids are of value in severe reactions. Infections are common during the ulcer stage, but rarely require more than local antiseptic measures.

Mite infestations may be treated as described under SCABIES in Ch. 233.

CENTIPEDES AND MILLIPEDES

Some of the larger centipedes of the genus *Scolopendra* can inflict a painful bite, with some localized swelling and erythema. Lymphangitis and lymphadenitis are common. Necrosis is rare and infection almost unknown. Symptoms and signs seldom persist for > 48 h. Millipedes do not bite, but when handled may secrete a toxin that can cause local skin irritation and, in severe cases, tissue changes. Some non-USA species can spray a highly irritating repugnant secretion that may cause severe conjunctival reactions.

Treatment

An ice cube will control the pain of most centipede bites. Toxic secretions of millipedes should be washed from the skin with copious amounts of soap and water; alcohol should not be used. A topical corticosteroid should be applied if a skin reaction develops. Eye injuries require immediate irrigation and the application of a corticosteroid-analgesic ointment.

SCORPIONS

All North American scorpions except *Centruroides exilicauda (sculpturatus)* are relatively harmless, their stings usually causing no more than some localized pain with minimal swelling, some lymphangitis with regional lymph gland swelling, and increased skin temperature and tenderness around the wound. Some localized tissue reaction may occur. *C. exilicauda (sculpturatus)* is found in Arizona, New Mexico, and the California side of the Colorado River. Its sting causes some immediate pain and sometimes numbness or tingling over the involved part. No swelling is present. Children become tense, restless, and display abnormal and random head, neck, and eye movements. In adults, tachycardia, hypertension, increased respirations, weakness, and motor disturbances may predominate. Respiratory difficulties may occur in both children and adults, often complicated by excessive salivation.

Treatment

The stings of most North American scorpions require no specific therapy. An ice cube over the wound area reduces pain. Hypertension can be controlled with diazoxide in doses of 5 mg/kg by slow IV push. For convulsions, diazepam is given IV 0.1 to 0.2 mg/kg up to 10 mg in adults and repeated q 15 min prn; in children the total dose is 10 mg. Muscle spasms usually respond to calcium gluconate, methocarbamol, or diazepam. Complete bed rest is indicated and no food for the first 8 to 12 h. Antivenin should be used in all severe cases. Information on its availability and use may be obtained from the Arizona Poison Control System at (606) 626-6016.

MARINE ANIMALS

Stingrays once caused about 750 stings/yr along North American coasts but the present incidence is unknown. The venom is contained in the one or more spines located on the dorsum of the animal's tail. Injuries usually occur when the unwary victim treads on the fish while wading in the ocean surf, bay, or slough. The pressure provokes the fish to thrust its tail upward and forward, driving the dorsal spine (or spines) into the victim's foot or leg. The integumentary sheath surrounding the spine is ruptured and the venom escapes into the victim's tissues, causing immediate severe pain. While often limited to the area of injury, the pain may spread rapidly, reaching its greatest intensity in < 90 min, and often persists (if untreated), though gradually diminishing, for 6 to 48 h. Syncope, weakness, nausea, and anxiety are common and may be due, in part, to peripheral vasodilation. Lymphangitis, vomiting, diarrhea, sweating, generalized cramps, inguinal or axillary pain, and respiratory distress have

been reported. The wound is usually jagged, bleeds freely, and is often contaminated with parts of the integumentary sheath. The edges of the wound are often discolored and some localized tissue destruction may occur. Generally, there is some swelling and edema. Wound infections are not common.

Molluscs include the cones, octopuses, and bivalves. *Conus californicus* is the only dangerous cone found in North American waters. Its sting produces localized pain, swelling, redness, and numbness. The bites of North American octopuses are rarely serious. Paralytic **shellfish poisoning,** caused by eating certain bivalves that have ingested toxic dinoflagellates, is discussed under NONBACTERIAL FOOD POISONING in Ch. 57.

Echinoderms contain several classes known to be venomous. Certain **sea urchins** have venom organs (globiferous pedicellariae) with calcareous jaws capable of penetrating human skin, but injuries from these are rare. Far more common are injuries by sea urchin spines, which can break off in the skin and give rise to local tissue reactions. If not removed they may migrate into deeper tissues, causing a granulomatous nodular lesion, or they may wedge against bone or nerve. Joint and muscle pains and dermatitis may also occur.

Coelenterates (Cnidaria) include the corals, sea anemones, jellyfishes, and hydroids (the Portuguese man-of-war is a colonial hydroid). Many possess a highly developed stinging unit (the nematocyst) that can penetrate the skin. These are particularly abundant on the animal's tentacles, and a single tentacle may fire thousands of nematocysts into the skin following contact. The lesions vary with the type of coelenterate involved. Generally, the initial lesions appear as small papular eruptions in one or several discontinuous lines, at times surrounded by an erythematous zone. The papules develop rapidly and the area becomes red and raised. Pain may be severe and itching is common. The papules may vesiculate and proceed to pustulation and desquamation. Systemic manifestations include weakness, nausea, headache, muscle pain and spasms, lacrimation and nasal discharge, increased perspiration, changes in pulse rate, and chest pain that increases on respiration.

Treatment

Stingrays and most other fish stings: Injuries to an extremity should be irrigated with the salt water at hand. An attempt should be made to remove the integumentary sheath if it can be seen in the wound. The extremity should then be submerged in water as hot as the patient can tolerate without injury, for 30 to 90 min. Sodium chloride or magnesium sulfate may be added to the hot water. The wound should again be examined for remnants of the sheath, debrided, and sutured if necessary. The appropriate antitetanus agent should be given and the injured extremity kept elevated for several days.

If the initial first aid measures are delayed, the wound may be anesthetized locally with procaine, although meperidine IM is the drug of choice for pain. The primary shock that sometimes immediately follows stingray injuries usually responds to simple supportive measures.

Molluscs: The treatment of *Conus* stings and octopus bites is largely empirical. Local measures appear to be of little value. Local injection of epinephrine, and subsequent use of neostigmine have been suggested. Severe *Conus* stings may require mechanical ventilation and measures to combat shock.

Echinoderms: Pedicellariae stings are treated by washing the area and applying an analgesic–corticosteroid cream (SeaBalm®). Sea urchin spines should be removed immediately. A bluish discoloration at the site of entry may help in locating the spine, which may sometimes be seen on x-ray. Vinegar dissolves most superficial spines, and soaking the wound in vinegar several times/day and covering the area with a wet

vinegar compress may be sufficient; surgery is seldom necessary. In time, the spine may migrate into deeper tissues. Removing these spines surgically may be tedious.

Coelenterates: Various remedies for coelenterate stings have been advocated. In some parts of the world, no treatment is advised except the local application of ammonia or vinegar. In the USA, the local application of meat tenderizers (eg, papain) has been popular. Sodium bicarbonate, boric acid, lemon or fig juice, alcohol, and many other agents have also been espoused, and it may be that merely changing the pH of the skin alleviates some of the localized pain. The following procedures are suggested: ocean water (not fresh water) is poured over the injured areas; the tentacles are removed, preferably with instruments or a gloved hand; the area is saturated with a slurry of baking soda for 10 min, or soaked in Burow's solution or vinegar for 30 min; flour or baking powder is poured over the wound area and scraped off with a sharp knife; the area is rinsed and a topical corticosteroid-antihistamine-analgesic (Sea-Balm®) applied.

More serious cases require additional therapeutic measures. O_2 or respiratory assistance may be required. Painful muscle spasms may be relieved with 10 mL of 10% calcium gluconate given IV. Meperidine is preferred for severe pain. IV fluids and epinephrine may be needed in the few cases where shock develops. An antivenin for the stings of certain Australian species of coelenterates is available.

INDEX

Page numbers followed by *f* indicate **FIGURE**; by *t*, **TABLE**

A

D

E

G

H

J

K

M

N

O

P

Q

R

S

U

V

W

X

Y

Z

The Fifteenth Edition of THE MERCK MANUAL is set in 9-point Times Roman, with sideheads and key words in News Gothic Bold. Figure legends and tables are in 7-point News Gothic. The original draft was produced on an AM Jacquard J100 word processor at the editorial office of THE MERCK MANUAL. The text was typeset by Donnelley/Rocappi Inc. of Cherry Hill, New Jersey, and the index was typeset by R. R. Donnelley & Sons Company, Chicago, Illinois. The book was printed on 19-pound Bible paper, by web offset, at National Publishing Company of Philadelphia, Pennsylvania.

NOTES

NOTES